Larry R. Kaiser M.D.
U of Penn Thoracic Surgery

THORACIC SURGERY

THORACIC SURGERY

Edited by

F. Griffith Pearson, M.D.
Professor
Division of Thoracic Surgery
Department of Surgery
University of Toronto Faculty of Medicine
Senior Surgeon
Division of Thoracic Surgery
The Toronto Hospital
Toronto, Ontario, Canada

Jean Deslauriers, M.D.
Professor
Department of Surgery
Laval University Faculty of Medicine
Head
Thoracic Surgery Division
Centre de Pneumologic
de L'Hôpital Laval
Ste-Foy, Quebec, Canada

Robert J. Ginsberg, M.D.
Professor
Department of Surgery
Cornell University Medical College
Chief
Division of Thoracic Surgery
and William G. Cahan Chair of Surgery
Memorial Sloan-Kettering
Cancer Center
New York, New York

Clement A. Hiebert, M.D.
Chairman Emeritus
Department of Surgery
Maine Medical Center
Portland, Maine

Martin F. McKneally, M.D., Ph.D.
Professor and Chairman
Division of Thoracic Surgery
Department of Surgery
University of Toronto Faculty of Medicine
Toronto, Ontario,
Canada

Harold C. Urschel, Jr., M.D.
Professor of Thoracic and Cardiovascular Surgery
University of Texa Southwestern Medical School
Dallas, Texas

Churchill Livingstone
New York, Edinburgh, London, Melbourne, Tokyo

Library of Congress Cataloging-in-Publication Data

Thoracic surgery / edited by F. Griffith Pearson ... [et al.].
    p. cm.
  Includes bibliographical references and index.
  ISBN 0-443-08798-9
  1. Chest—Surgery. I. Pearson, F. Griffith.
  [DNLM: 1. Thoracic Surgery. WF 980 T4865 1995]
  RD536.T458 1995
  617.5′4059—dc20
  DNLM/DLC
  for Library of Congress   94-42025
                                                       CIP

Distributed in the United Kingdom by Churchill Livingstone, Robert Stevenson House, 1–3 Baxter's Place, Leith Walk, Edinburgh EH1 3AF, and by associated companies, branches, and representatives throughout the world.

Accurate indications, adverse reactions, and dosage schedules for drugs are provided in this book, but it is possible that they may change. The reader is urged to review the package information data of the manufacturers of the medications mentioned.

The Publishers have made every effort to trace the copyright holders for borrowed material. If they have inadvertently overlooked any, they will be pleased to make the necessary arrangements at the first opportunity.

Acquisitions Editor: *Miranda Bromage*
Assistant Editor: *Ann Ruzycka*
Production Editor: *Katharine Leawanna O'Moore-Klopf*
Production Supervisor: *Laura Mosberg Cohen*
Cover Design: *Paul Moran*

Printed in the United States of America

First published in 1995   7   6   5   4   3   2   1

CONTRIBUTORS

John G. Armstrong, M.D.
Staff Member, Radiation Therapy Department, Memorial Hospital, New York, New York

Joseph E. Bavaria, M.D.
Assistant Professor, Division of Cardiothoracic Surgery, Department of Surgery, University of Pennsylvannia School of Medicine, Philadelphia, Pennsylvannia

Gilles Beauchamp, M.D.
Clinical Professor, Department of Surgery, Université de Montréal Faculty of Medicine; Head, Division of Thoracic Surgery, Department of Surgery, Hôpital Maisonneuve-Rosemont, Montreal, Quebec, Canada

Eugene Blackstone, M.D.
Professor, Division of Cardiothoracic Surgery, Department of Surgery, University of Alabama School of Medicine, University of Alabama at Birmingham, Birmingham, Alabama

H. G. Borst, M.D.
Professor, Division of Thoracic Surgery, University of Hannover, Hannover, Germany

Mario Brandolino, M.D.
Thoracic Surgeon, Montevideo, Uruguay

Carl E. Bredenberg, M.D.
Professor, Department of Surgery University of Vermont College of Medicine, Burlington, Vermont; Surgeon-in-Chief, Department of Surgery, Maine Medical Center, Portland, Maine

Michael Burt, M.D., Ph.D.
Associate Professor, Departments of Surgery and Biochemistry, Cornell University Medical College; Attending Surgeon, Division of Thoracic Surgery, Department of Surgery, Memorial Sloan-Kettering Cancer Center, New York, New York

Robert J. Caccavale, M.D.
Clinical Assistant Professor, Department of Surgery, University of Medicine and Dentistry of New Jersey Robert Wood Johnson Medical School; Senior Attending Surgeon, St. Peter's Medical Center and Robert Wood Johnson University Hospital, New Brunswick, New Jersey

José J. P. Camargo, M.D.
Professor, Department of Surgery, Fundação Faculdade Federal de Cincias Médicas de Porto Alegre; Head, Department of Thoracic Surgery, Pavilhão Pereira Filho Hospital, Santa Casa de Misericórdia de Porto Alegre, Porto Alegre, Brazil

Robert Cameron, M.D.
Chief, Section of General Thoracic Surgery, University of California, San Francisco, School of Medicine, San Francisco, California

Paulo Cardoso, M.D.
Associate Professor, Division of Thoracic Surgery, Department of Surgery, University of Porto Alegre; Surgeon, Division of Thoracic Surgery, Department of Surgery, University Hospital, Porto Alegre, Brazil

Guy Carrier, M.D.
Associate Professor, Department of Radiology, Laval University; Head, Department of Medical Imaging, Centre de Pneumologie de L'Hôpital Laval, Ste-Foy, Quebec, Canada

Andrea J. Cohen, M.D., C.M.
Instructor, Division of Pulmonary Sciences and Critical Care Medicine, Department of Medicine, National Jewish Center for Immunology and Respiratory Medicine and University of Colorado School of Medicine, Denver, Colorado

Joel D. Cooper, M.D.
Head, Section of General Thoracic Surgery, and Joseph C. Bancroft Professor, Department of Surgery, Washington University School of Medicine, St. Louis, Missouri; Surgeon, Division of Cardiothoracic Surgery, Department of Surgery, Barnes Hospital, St. Louis, Missouri

Denis A. Cortese, M.D.
Professor, Department of Medicine, Mayo Medical School, Rochester, Minnesota; Consultant, Thoracic Diseases and Internal Medicine, Jacksonville, Florida

R. J. Cusimano, M.D., M.Sc., B.Sc.
Assistant Professor, Department of Surgery, University of Toronto Faculty of Medicine; Staff Surgeon, Division of Cardiovascular Surgery, The Toronto Hospital, Toronto, Ontario, Canada

Pat O. Daily, M.D.
Director, Cardiac Surgery, Sharp Memorial Hospital, San Diego, California

Philippe G. Dartevelle, M.D.
Professor, Department of Thoracic and Cardiovascular Surgery, Paris-Sud University; Director, Department of Thoracic and Vascular Surgery and Heart-Lung Transplantation, Hôpital Marie-Lannelongue, Paris, France

Jacob Davtyan, M.D.
Chief Resident, Section of Cardiothoracic Surgery, Department of Surgery, Emory University School of Medicine, Atlanta, Georgia

Denis Desaulniers, M.D.
Clinical Professor, Department of Surgery, Laval University Faculty of Medicine; Surgeon, Division of Cardiac Surgery, Department of Surgery, Hôpital Laval, Ste-Foy, Quebec, Canada

Jean Deslauriers, M.D.
Professor, Department of Surgery, Laval University Faculty of Medicine; Head, Thoracic Surgery Division, Centre de Pneumologie de L'Hôpital Laval, Ste-Foy, Quebec, Canada

Marc Desmeules, M.D.
Professor and Chairman, Department of Medicine, Laval University Faculty of Medicine, Ste-Foy, Quebec, Canada

Carolyn M. Dresler, M.D.
Assistant Professor of Surgery, Division of Cardiothoracic Surgery, Section of General Thoracic Surgery, Washington University School of Medicine, St. Louis, Missouri

Ronald Feld, M.D.
Professor, Department of Medicine, University of Toronto Faculty of Medicine; Deputy Chief, Department of Medicine, Ontario Cancer Institute/Princess Margaret Hospital, Toronto, Ontario, Canada

Stanley C. Fell, M.D.
Professor, Department of Cardiothoracic Surgery, Albert Einstein College of Medicine of Yeshiva University; Director, Section of Thoracic Surgery, Department of Cardiothoracic Surgery, Montefiore Medical Center, Bronx, New York

Pasquale Ferraro, M.D.
Resident, Thoracic Surgery Division, Centre de Pneumologie de L'Hôpital Laval, Ste-Foy, Quebec, Canada

Robert M. Filler, M.D.
Professor, Division of General Surgery, Department of Surgery, University of Toronto Faculty of Medicine; Surgeon-in-Chief, Department of Surgery, Hospital for Sick Children, Toronto, Ontario, Canada

Eric D. Foster, M.D.
Clinical Professor, Department of Surgery, Albany Medical College, Albany, New York

David A. Fullerton, M.D.
Assistant Professor, Division of Cardiothoracic Surgery, Department of Surgery, University of Colorado School of Medicine; Chief, Department of Cardiothoracic Surgery, Denver Veterans Affairs Medical Center; Cardiothoracic Surgeon, Department of Surgery, The Children's Hospital, Denver, Colorado

Mitchell H. Gail, M.D., Ph.D.
Acting Chief, Biostatistics Branch, Division of Cancer Etiology, National Cancer Institute, National Institutes of Health, Bethesda, Maryland

Henning A. Gaissert, M.D.
Fellow, Division of Cardiothoracic Surgery, Department of Surgery, Washington University School of Medicine, St. Louis, Missouri

Robert J. Ginsberg, M.D.
Professor, Department of Surgery, Cornell University Medical College; Chief, Division of Thoracic Surgery, and William G. Cahan Chair of Surgery, Memorial Sloan-Kettering Cancer Center, New York, New York

Melvyn Goldberg, M.D.
Professor, Department of Surgery, Temple University School of Medicine; Chief, Thoracic Surgical Oncology, Fox Chase Cancer Center, Philadelphia, Pennsylvania

Andrew R. Golde, M.D.
Chief Resident, Department of Otolaryngology, University of Toronto Faculty of Medicine, Toronto, Ontario, Canada

Geoffrey M. Graeber, M.D.
Professor of Surgery, Section of Cardiovascular and Thoracic Surgery, and Director of Surgical Research, Department of Surgery, West Virginia University School of Medicine; Staff Cardiovascular and Thoracic Surgeon, Department of Surgery, Ruby Memorial and Monongalia General Hospitals, Morgantown, West Virginia

Jocelyn Grégoire, M.D.
Consultant, Division of Thoracic Surgery, Department of Surgery, Hôpital Sacre-Coeur, Montreal, Quebec, Canada

Hermes C. Grillo, M.D.
Professor, Division of General Thoracic Surgery, Department of Surgery, Harvard Medical School; Chief, Division of General Thoracic Surgery, Department of Surgery, Massachusetts General Hospital, Boston, Massachusetts

Ronald F. Grossman, M.D.
Associate Professor, Division of Respiratory Medicine, Department of Medicine, University of Toronto Faculty of Medicine; Head, Division of Respirology, Mount Sinai Hospital, Toronto, Ontario, Canada

Frederick L. Grover, M.D.
Head, Division of Cardiothoracic Surgery, and Professor, Department of Surgery, University of Colorado School of Medicine; Chief, Surgical Service, Denver Veteran's Administration Medical Center, Denver, Colorado

Carlos Alberto Guimarães, M.D.
Professor and Head, Division of Thoracic Surgery and Endoscopy, Department of Surgery, Institute of Phthisiology and Pneumology, Federal University of Rio de Janeiro, Rio de Janeiro, Brazil

Patrick J. Gullane, M.D.
Professor, Department of Otolaryngology, University of Toronto Faculty of Medicine; Director, Head and Neck Program, and Otolaryngologist-in-Chief, Department of Otolaryngology, The Toronto Hospital, Toronto, Ontario, Canada

Jeffrey A. Hagen, M.D.
Assistant Professor, Department of Surgery, University of Southern California School of Medicine; Staff Physician, Division of Cardiothoracic Surgery, Department of Surgery, Los Angeles County–University of Southern California Medical Center, Los Angeles, California

A. Haverich, M.D.
Director, Klinik fur Herz- und Gefasschirugie, Klinikum Der Christian-Albrechts, Universitat Zu Kiel, Kiel, Germany

W. Hardy Hendren III, M.D.
Robert E. Gross Professor of Surgery, Department of Surgery, Harvard Medical School; Chief, Department of Surgery, Children's Hospital, Boston, Massachusetts

Stephen J. Herman, M.D.
Associate Professor, Department of Radiology, University of Toronto Faculty of Medicine; Head, Division of Thoracic Imaging, Department of Radiology, The Toronto Hospital, Toronto, Ontario, Canada

Clement A. Hiebert, M.D.
Chairman Emeritus, Department of Surgery, Maine Medical Center, Portland, Maine

Richard V. Hodder, M.D.
Associate Professor, Department of Medicine, University of Ottawa Faculty of Medicine; Critical Care Specialist, Intensive Care Unit and Respirologist, Ottawa Civic Hospital, Ottawa, Ontario, Canada

E. Carmack Holmes, M.D.
Professor, Division of Oncology, Department of Surgery, University of California, Los Angeles, UCLA School of Medicine, Los Angeles, California

Alan R. Hopeman, M.D.
Professor Emeritus, Division of Cardiothoracic Surgery, Department of Surgery, University of Colorado School of Medicine; Consultant, Veterans Affairs Medical Center and Fitzsimons Army Hospital, Denver, Colorado

Jonathan C. Irish, M.D., M.Sc.
Assistant Professor, Department of Otolaryngology, University of Toronto Faculty of Medicine; Staff Otolaryngologist, Department of Otolaryngology and Head and Neck Program, and Staff Surgeon, Department of Surgical Oncology, Ontario Cancer Institute/Princess Margaret Hospital; Staff Otolaryngologist, The Toronto Hospital, Toronto, Ontario, Canada

Louis F. Jacques, M.D.
Clinical Instructor, Department of Surgery, Laval University Faculty of Medicine; Surgeon, Thoracic Surgery Division, Centre de Pneumologie de L'Hôpital Laval, Ste-Foy, Quebec, Canada

Robert H. Johnston, Jr., M.D.
Director, Department of Cardiothoracic and Vascular Surgery, Michael E. DeBakey Heart Institute of Wisconsin and Kenosha Hospital and Medical Center, Kenosha, Wisconsin

David R. Jones, M.D.
Chief Resident, Department of Surgery, West Virginia University School of Medicine; Chief Resident, Ruby Memorial, Morgantown, West Virginia; Chief Resident, Louis A. Johnson Veterans Affairs Medical Center, Clarksburg, West Virginia

William G. Jones II, M.D.
Attending Cardiothoracic Surgeon, Baylor University Medical Center and Methodist Medical Center, Dallas, Texas; Attending Cardiothoracic Surgeon, Medical Center of Mesquite, Mesquite, Texas

Larry R. Kaiser, M.D.
Associate Professor, Department of Surgery, University of Pennsylvania School of Medicine; Chief, General Thoracic Surgery, Division of Cardiothoracic Surgery, Department of Surgery, Hospital of the University of Pennsylvania, Philadelphia, Pennsylvania

Robert J. Keenan, M.D.
Assistant Professor, Section of Thoracic Surgery, Department of Surgery, University of Pittsburgh School of Medicine; Attending Surgeon, Division of Cardiothoracic Surgery, Department of Surgery, University of Pittsburgh Medical Center, Pittsburgh, Pennsylvania

M. Anne Keller, M.D.
Assistant Professor, Department of Radiology, University of Toronto Faculty of Medicine; Staff Neuroradiologist, Department of Radiology, The Toronto Hospital, Toronto, Ontario, Canada

Shafique Keshavjee, M.D., M.Sc.
Assistant Professor, Division of Thoracic Surgery, Department of Surgery, University of Toronto Faculty of Medicine; Staff Surgeon, Division of Thoracic Surgery, Department of Surgery, The Toronto Hospital; Staff Surgeon, Division of Cardiovascular Surgery, Hospital for Sick Children, Toronto, Ontario, Canada

Thomas J. Kirby, M.D.
Staff Surgeon and Director, Lung Transplantation, Department of Surgery, The Cleveland Clinic Foundation, Cleveland, Ohio

John Kirklin, M.D.
Professor, Division of Cardiothoracic Surgery, Department of Surgery, University of Alabama School of Medicine, University of Alabama at Birmingham, Birmingham, Alabama

Leslie J. Kohman, M.D.
Associate Professor, Division of Thoracic Surgery, Department of Surgery, State University of New York Health Science Center at Syracuse College of Medicine, Syracuse, New York

Rodney J. Landreneau, M.D.
Associate Professor of Surgery, Section of Thoracic Surgery, and Head, Department of Surgery, University of Pittsburgh School of Medicine; Attending Surgeon, Division of Cardiothoracic Surgery, Department of Surgery, University of Pittsburgh Medical Center, Pittsburgh, Pennsylvania

Michael P. La Quaglia, M.D.
Assistant Professor, Department of Surgery, Cornell University Medical College; Chief, Pediatric Surgical Service, Memorial Sloan-Kettering Cancer Center, New York, New York

Robert B. Lee, M.D.
Assistant Professor, Division of Cardiac and Thoracic Surgery, Department of Surgery, Emory University School of Medicine; Chief, Department of Cardiothoracic Surgery, Veterans Affairs Medical Center, Atlanta, Georgia

Ralph J. Lewis, M.D.
Clinical Professor, Department of Surgery, University of Medicine and Dentistry of New Jersey Robert Wood Johnson Medical School; Chief, Thoracic Surgery, St. Peter's Medical Center and Robert Wood Johnson University Hospital, New Brunswick, New Jersey

Paolo Macchiarini, M.D.
Staff Surgeon, Department of Thoracic and Vascular Surgery and Heart-Lung Transplantation, Hôpital Marie-Lannelongue, Paris, France

Michael Mack, M.D.
Clinical Assistant Professor, Division of Thoracic Surgery, Department of Surgery, University of Texas Southwestern Medical Center at Dallas Southwestern Medical School; Attending Surgeon, Section of Thoracic Surgery, Department of Surgery, Medical City Dallas, Dallas, Texas

Susan Mackinnon, M.D.
Professor, Division of Plastic Surgery, Department of Surgery, Washington University School of Medicine, St. Louis, Missouri

Michael Maddaus, M.D.
Assistant Professor, Division of Thoracic Surgery, Department of Surgery, University of Minnesota Medical School—Minneapolis, Minneapolis, Minnesota

Raphaël Maire, M.D.
Academic Staff , Department of Otorhinolaryngology, Head, and Neck Surgery, University of Lausanne Medical School, Lausanne, Switzerland

Richard A. Malthaner, M.D.
Chief Resident, Division of Thoracic Surgery, Department of Surgery, University of Toronto Faculty of Medicine, Toronto, Ontario, Canada

John C. Marshall, M.D.
Professor, Department of Surgery, University of Toronto Faculty of Medicine; Associate Surgical ICU Director and Staff Surgeon, The Toronto Hospital, Toronto, Ontario, Canada

Nael Martini, M.D.
Professor, Department of Surgery, Cornell University Medical College; Attending Thoracic Surgeon, Department of Surgery, Memorial Sloan-Kettering Cancer Center, New York, New York

Douglas J. Mathisen, M.D.
Associate Professor, Division of General Thoracic Surgery, Department of Surgery, Harvard Medical School; Associate Chief, Division of General Thoracic Surgery, Department of Surgery, Massachusetts General Hospital, Boston, Massachusetts

Kenneth L. Mattox, M.D.

Professor, Department of Surgery, Baylor College of Medicine; Chief of Staff and Chief of Surgery, Ben Taub General Hospital, Houston, Texas

Patricia M. McCormack, M.D.

Associate Professor, Department of Surgery, Cornell University Medical College; Attending Surgeon, Thoracic Service, Memorial Sloan-Kettering Cancer Center, New York, New York

Martin F. McKneally, M.D., Ph.D.

Professor and Chairman, Division of Thoracic Surgery, Department of Surgery, University of Toronto Faculty of Medicine, Toronto, Ontario, Canada

Reza John Mehran, M.D., C.M., M.Sc.

Assistant Professor, Department of Anatomy, Université de Montréal Faculty of Medicine, Montreal, Quebec, Canada; Resident, Thoracic Surgery Division, Centre de Pneumologie de L'Hôpital Laval, Ste-Foy, Quebec, Canada

Anthony B. Miller, M.D.

Professor and Chairman, Department of Preventive Medicine and Biostatistics, University of Toronto Faculty of Medicine, Toronto, Ontario, Canada

Joseph I. Miller, Jr., M.D.

Professor, Department of Cardiothoracic Surgery, Emory University School of Medicine; Surgeon, Department of Cardiothoracic Surgery, The Emory Clinic, Grady Memorial Hospital, Emory University Hospital, Veterans Affairs Medical Center, Egleston Hospital for Children at Emory, and Crawford W. Long Memorial Hospital, Atlanta, Georgia

Darroch W. O. Moores, M.D.

Clinical Associate Professor, Department of Surgery, Albany Medical College, Albany, New York

Albert Mudry, M.D.

Academic Staff, Department of Otorhinolaryngology, Head and Neck Surgery, University of Lausanne Medical School, Lausanne, Switzerland

David S. Mulder, M.D.

Professor, Department of Surgery, McGill University Faculty of Medicine; Surgeon-in-Chief, Department of Surgery, Montreal General Hospital, Montreal, Quebec, Canada

John Muscedere, M.D.

Staff Respirologist and Director, Intensive Care Unit, Hotel-Dieu Grace Hospital, Windsor, Ontario, Canada

Tsuguo Naruke, M.D., D.M.Sc.

Clinical Professor, Department of Surgery, University of Keio School of Medicine; Chief, Division of Thoracic Surgery, and Deputy Director and Chairman, Department of Surgery, National Cancer Center Hospital, Tokyo, Japan

Avery B. Nathens, M.D.

Resident, Department of Surgery, The Toronto Hospital, Toronto, Ontario, Canada

Bill Nelems, M.D.

Professor, Division of Cardiovascular and Thoracic Surgery, Department of Surgery, University of British Columbia Faculty of Medicine, Vancouver, British Columbia, Canada

Jorge Nin Vivo, M.D.

Thoracic Surgeon, Montevideo, Uruguay

Peter C. Pairolero, M.D.

Professor, Department of Surgery, Mayo Medical School; Chairman, Department of Surgery, Mayo Clinic and Mayo Foundation, Rochester, Minnesota

Philippe Pasche, M.D.

Academic Staff, Department of Otorhinolaryngology, Head, and Neck Surgery, University of Lausanne Medical School, Lausanne, Switzerland

Harvey I. Pass, M.D.

Senior Investigator, Clinical Oncology Program, Division of Cancer Treatment, and Head, Thoracic Oncology Section, Surgery Branch, National Cancer Institute, National Institutes of Health, Bethesda, Maryland

G. A. Patterson, M.D.

Professor, Division of Cardiothoracic Surgery, Department of Surgery, Washington University School of Medicine; Attending Surgeon, Barnes Hospital, St. Louis Children's Hospital, and The Jewish Hospital of St. Louis, St. Louis, Missouri

F. Griffith Pearson, M.D.

Professor, Division of Thoracic Surgery, Department of Surgery, University of Toronto Faculty of Medicine; Senior Surgeon, Division of Thoracic Surgery, The Toronto Hospital, Toronto, Ontario, Canada

Louis P. Perrault, M.D.

Resident, Thoracic Surgery Division, Centre de Pneumologie de L'Hôpital Laval, Ste-Foy, Quebec, Canada

Thomas L. Petty, M.D.

Professor, Department of Medicine, University of Colorado School of Medicine, Denver, Colorado; Professor, Department of Medicine, Rush Medical College of Rush University, Chicago, Illinois; Director, Academic and Research Affairs, Healthone Center for Health Sciences Education, Denver, Colorado

Steven Piantadosi, M.D., Ph.D.

Associate Professor, Department of Oncology, and Director of Biostatistics, Johns Hopkins Oncology Center, Johns Hopkins University School of Medicine; Associate Professor of Biostatistics and Epidemiology, Johns Hopkins School of Hygiene and Public Health, Baltimore, Maryland

Helen W. Pogrebniak, M.D.

Cancer Expert, Clinical Oncology Program, Division of Cancer Treatment, and Senior Staff Physician, Surgery Branch, National Cancer Institute, National Institutes of Health, Bethesda, Maryland

Marvin Pomerantz, M.D.

Professor, Department of Surgery, University of Colorado School of Medicine; Chief, General Thoracic Surgery Section, Division of Cardiothoracic Surgery, The University of Colorado Health Sciences Center; Chief, General Thoracic Surgery Section, Veterans Affairs Medical Center, Denver, Colorado

Celeste N. Powers, M.D., Ph.D.

Associate Professor, Departments of Pathology and Otolaryngology and Communication Sciences, State University of New York Health Science Center at Syracuse College of Medicine; Director of Cytopathology and Attending Pathologist, Department of Pathology, University Hospital, Syracuse, New York

A. C. Ralph-Edwards, M.D.

Fellow, Division of Thoracic Surgery, University of Toronto Faculty of Medicine, Toronto, Ontario, Canada

Salim Ratnani, M.D.

Clinical Fellow, Department of Cardiac Surgery, The Cleveland Clinic Foundation, Cleveland, Ohio

Thomas W. Rice, M.D.

Head, Section of General Thoracic Surgery, Department of Thoracic and Cardiovascular Surgery, The Cleveland Clinic Foundation, Cleveland, Ohio

M. Patricia Rivera, M.D.

Clinical Assistant Professor, Department of Medicine, University of North Carolina at Chapel Hill School of Medicine; Pulmonologist, Department of Medicine, University of North Carolina Hospitals, Chapel Hill, North Carolina

Jack A. Roth, M.D.

Professor and Chairman, Division of Surgery and Anesthesiology, Department of Thoracic and Cardiovascular Surgery, and Bud Johnson Chair and Professor of Tumor Biology, Department of Tumor Biology, University of Texas Medical School at Houston, Houston, Texas

Valerie W. Rusch, M.D.

Associate Professor, Department of Surgery, Cornell University Medical College; Attending Surgeon, Thoracic Service, Department of Surgery, Memorial Sloan-Kettering Cancer Center, New York, New York

Douglas E. Sanders, M.D.

Professor Emeritus, Department of Radiology, University of Toronto Faculty of Medicine; Staff Radiologist, Department of Radiology, The Toronto Hospital, Toronto, Ontario, Canada

Alan N. Sandler, M.B., Ch.B.

Associate Professor, Department of Anaesthesia, University of Toronto Faculty of Medicine; Anaesthetist-in-Chief, Department of Anaesthesia, The Toronto Hospital, Toronto, Ontario, Canada

J. Gordon Scannell, M.D.

Clinical Professor Emeritus, Department of Surgery, Harvard Medical School; Senior Surgeon, Massachusetts General Hospital, Boston, Massachusetts

Robert C. Shamberger, M.D.

Associate Professor, Department of Surgery, Harvard Medical School; Senior Associate, Department of Surgery, Children's Hospital, Boston, Massachusetts

Farid Shamji, M.D.

Assistant Professor, University of Ottawa Faculty of Medicine; Head, Division of Thoracic Surgery, Ottawa Civic Hospital, Ottawa, Ontario, Canada

Frances A. Shepherd, M.D.

Professor, Department of Medicine, University of Toronto Faculty of Medicine, Toronto, Ontario, Canada; Director of Medical Oncology, Division of Hematology and Oncology, Department of Medicine, The Toronto Hospital, Toronto, Ontario, Canada; Chairman, Lung Cancer Committee of the National Cancer Institute of Canada Clinical Trials Group, Kingston, Ontario, Canada

Thomas W. Shields, M.D., D.Sc. (Hon.)

Professor Emeritus, Department of Surgery, Northwestern University Medical School; Senior Staff Surgeon Emeritus, Department of Surgery, Northwestern Memorial Hospital, Chicago, Illinois

Glenn E. Sisler, M.D.

Clinical Associate Professor, Department of Surgery, University of Medicine and Dentistry of New Jersey Robert Wood Johnson Medical School; Senior Attending Surgeon, St. Peter's Medical Center and Robert Wood Johnson University Hospital, New Brunswick, New Jersey

Arthur S. Slutsky, M.D.

Professor, Division of Respirology, Department of Medicine, University of Toronto Faculty of Medicine; Staff Physician, Division of Respirology, Department of Medicine, Mount Sinai Hospital, Toronto, Ontario, Canada

Alma Smitheringale, M.B.

Assistant Professor, Department of Otolaryngology, University of Toronto Faculty of Medicine; Staff Surgeon, Department of Pediatric Otolaryngology, Hospital for Sick Children, Toronto, Ontario, Canada

Diane E. Stover, M.D.

Professor, Department of Medicine, Cornell University Medical College; Attending Physician and Head, Division of General Medicine, and Chief, Pulmonary Service, Department of Medicine, Memorial Sloan-Kettering Cancer Center, New York, New York

S. B. Sutcliffe, M.D.

Professor, Department of Radiation Oncology, University of Toronto Faculty of Medicine; Staff Physician, Department of Radiation Oncology, Ontario Cancer Institute/Princess Margaret Hospital, Toronto, Ontario, Canada

Thomas R. J. Todd, M.D.

Chairman, Division of Thoracic Surgery, and Professor, Department of Surgery, University of Toronto Faculty of Medicine; Head, Division of Thoracic Surgery, The Toronto Hospital, Toronto, Ontario, Canada

Ryosuke Tsuchiya, M.D.

Chief, Division of Thoracic Surgery, Department of Surgery, National Cancer Center Hospital, Tokyo, Japan

Harold C. Urschel, Jr., M.D.

Professor of Thoracic and Cardiovascular Surgery, University of Texas Southwestern Medical School, Dallas, Texas

Matthew J. Wall, Jr., M.D.

Assistant Professor, Department of Surgery, Baylor College of Medicine; Deputy Chief of Surgery, Ben Taub General Hospital, Houston, Texas

Paul F. Waters, M.D.

Professor of Surgery and Director, General Thoracic Surgery and Lung Transplantation, Division of Cardiothoracic Surgery, Department of Surgery, University of California, Los Angeles, UCLA School of Medicine, Los Angeles, California

Gordon L. Weisbrod, M.D.

Professor, Department of Radiology, University of Toronto Faculty of Medicine; Head, Division of Thoracic Imaging, Department of Radiology, The Toronto Hospital, Toronto, Ontario, Canada

Thomas H. Weisenburger, M.D.

Clinical Professor, Department of Radiation Oncology, University of California, Los Angeles, School of Medicine, Los Angeles, California; Director of Radiation Oncology, Cancer Foundation of Santa Barbara, Santa Barbara, California

Dov Weissberg, M.D.

Associate Professor, Department of Surgery, Tel Aviv University Sackler School of Medicine, Tel Aviv, Israel; Visiting Assistant Professor, Department of Surgery, Albert Einstein College of Medicine of Yeshiva University, New York; Chief, Department of Thoracic and General Surgery, E. Wolfson Medical Center, Holon, Israel

Earle W. Wilkins, Jr., M.D.

Clinical Professor Emeritus, Department of Surgery, Harvard Medical School; Senior Surgeon, Division of General Thoracic Surgery, Department of Surgery, Massachusetts General Hospital, Boston, Massachusetts

Ian J. Witterick, M.D.

Assistant Professor, Department of Otolaryngology, University of Toronto Faculty of Medicine; Staff Otolaryngologist, Department of Otolaryngology, Mount Sinai Hospital, Toronto, Ontario, Canada

Maureen Zakowski, M.D.

Assistant Professor, Department of Pathology, Cornell University Medical College; Assistant Attending Pathologist, Department of Pathology, Memorial Sloan-Kettering Cancer Center, New York, New York

Muhammad B. Zaman, M.D.

Professor, Department of Clinical Pathology, New York Medical College, Valhalla, New York; Attending Pathologist, Department of Pathology, Westchester County Medical Center, Valhalla, New York; Consulting Cytopathologist, Department of Pathology, Memorial Sloan-Kettering Cancer Center, New York, New York

Noe Zamel, M.D.

Professor, Division of Respirology, Department of Medicine, and Director, Trihospital Pulmonary Function Laboratories, University of Toronto Faculty of Medicine, Toronto, Ontario, Canada

FOREWORD

Unique.

As I sought to capture the character of this textbook with one word, I tried to imagine what accolades I might strive to merit were I the author of such a text. *Authoritative, comprehensive, informative,* and others came to mind. This text warrants them all, but I settled on *unique* as the one that best describes this important contribution to the field of general thoracic surgery.

In 1968, with the encouragement and support of Dr. Frederick Kergin, himself a distinguished thoracic surgeon, Dr. F. Griffith Pearson organized the General Thoracic Division at The Toronto General Hospital. Its structure was clearly influenced by Dr. Pearson's experience as a senior house officer in England under the tutelage of Mr. Ronald H. R. Belsey. The concentration of specialized resources in one service provided optimal care, which in turn attracted patients with interesting and challenging problems from far and wide. This "critical mass" of patients in turn stimulated an interest in thoracic surgical problems on the part of other related disciplines such as anesthesia, radiology, cytopathology, and chest physiotherapy, to name but a few. Perhaps most importantly, this division, and Dr. Pearson's enthusiasm for his specialty, kindled the interest of surgical trainees, who perceived general thoracic surgery as an exciting and distinguished career pathway. Indeed, Dr. Pearson has been referred to as the Pied Piper of general thoracic surgery, often to the chagrin of other surgical services, which witnessed some of their most prized trainees lured away by the magnetism of Dr. Pearson's personality, his love for general thoracic surgery, and his personal attention to trainees who vied to rotate on his service.

The specialty of general thoracic surgery is, in a certain sense, also unique among surgical disciplines. Our specialty has been fortunate in retaining for itself a major diagnostic as well as a therapeutic role. Whether to operate, when to operate, and what procedure to perform are as important to this specialty as the technical aspects of the numerous operative procedures. The general thoracic surgeon strives to embrace the disciplines of pulmonary medicine, gastroenterology, radiology, pathology, oncology, and intensive care. The multiplicity of conditions and diseases that afflict the thoracic organs, and the varying circumstances under which these conditions present, add challenge and variety. The permutations and combinations are almost limitless. It is for this reason that the most important attributes for practitioners of this specialty are judgment and experience.

It is exactly for this reason that the most senior members of the general thoracic surgical community are also the most esteemed, which brings me back to this textbook, *Thoracic Surgery,* and its companion, *Esophageal Surgery.* The books' very length speaks to both the variety and intricacy of our specialty. It is apparent that the goal of the editors was to impart both knowledge and wisdom. This alchemy, the infusion of knowledge with wisdom, is what in my opinion makes this text unique. Dr. Pearson assembled a "dream team" of coeditors and contributing authors. The editors, all senior, highly experienced thoracic surgeons, have had a long-standing close personal friendship with each other. Four of the five coeditors have either trained or practiced at one time in Toronto. The editors are characterized not only by their experience, but by their lifelong dedication to the education and training of general thoracic surgeons. The other contributing authors, many of whom trained in Toronto, were obviously selected for their specific expertise and ability. I have no doubt that all of the contributors undertook their assignments with particular energy and enthusiasm, engendered by admiration and affection for Dr. Pearson, and as an expression of gratitude for what he has contributed to our specialty and to our individual careers.

Each of the major sections of these textbooks was overseen by one of the senior editors, who added his own perspective and commentary. In addition, each chapter was modified or expanded by a process of simultaneous joint review by all six editors. By this process, the knowledge contained in both books was embellished with judgment and experience. Nowhere is this more apparent than in the companion to this book, *Esophageal Surgery.* Unlike many other areas in thoracic surgery, esophageal surgery is essentially reconstructive in nature. In addition to the usual yardsticks of morbidity and mortality, long-term functional outcome is the ultimate measure of success. The patient must live with the result for the rest of his or her life. *Esophageal Surgery* in particular clearly reflects the experience and expertise of the editors. Drs. Pearson and Clement A. Hiebert both trained at one time with Mr. Belsey at the Frenchay Hospital in Bristol, England, and both have subsequently had a career-long interest in the esophagus.

Mr. Belsey is undoubtedly proud of the accomplishments of his two pupils, though he often expresses a somewhat jaundiced view of textbooks. "Cooper," he would say, "when you personally observe, in your clinical practice, something that is at variance with what is written in a textbook, tear that page out of the book." I know Mr. Belsey would concur with me: this textbook is indeed unique. The reader will not have the occasion to tear out many of its pages.

Joel D. Cooper, M.D.
Head, Section of General Thoracic Surgery
and Joseph C. Bancroft Professor
Department of Surgery
Washington University School of Medicine
St. Louis, Missouri
Surgeon, Division of Cardiothoracic Surgery
Department of Surgery
Barnes Hospital
St. Louis, Missouri

PREFACE

Thoracic Surgery is published in an era of unprecedented expansion in medical knowledge, coupled with a revolution in worldwide communication skills and technology. It is difficult or impossible for a single editor to maintain a broad and perceptive awareness in all fields of thoracic surgery in the face of the sheer volume of important new information. Every effort was made to meet these challenges in the preparation of this book, and to create the ultimate reference book in thoracic surgery.

Each of the six medical editors was assigned responsibility for one or more sections in which the particular individual has internationally recognized expertise. The editors have known one another as friends and professional colleagues in the field of thoracic surgery for more than two decades, and share certain key spheres of activity and interest: All are operating surgeons with twenty or more years of experience and have been in charge of residency training programs. All have been examiners for the licensing boards for North American thoracic surgery. Most importantly, all are still actively involved in the practice of thoracic surgery. Authors were chosen because of their acknowledged expertise in their assigned topic.

The planning process developed as a concerted effort to create the best possible format for a book of value to the practicing thoracic surgeon, the residents in training, and for those physicians working in important collaborative specialities such as pulmonology and gastroenterology. Within the limits of practicality, every effort has been made to achieve uniformity of chapter presentation. The format includes a historical note with separately selected historical readings, followed by the usual sequences of anatomy, physiology or other relevant basic science, clinical presentation and diagnosis, management and results. Whenever available, long-term results are presented. A special feature includes commentary by the chapter author concerning areas of controversy and anticipated future change. The editors have also added commentary of their own for selected chapters. Technical chapters describe the common operations of thoracic surgery; clear illustrations and practical suggestions are included in order to provide a "manual for tomorrow morning's case," within a comprehensive text.

Throughout, there has been a strong and pervading influence from the University of Toronto Faculty of Medicine. Five of the six editors hold, or have held, academic positions in thoracic surgery in Toronto. The other, Harold C. Urschel, Jr., has had a close association with Toronto for many years and has tempered some of our parochial perspectives. Many chapter authors were trained at the University of Toronto Faculty of Medicine, or have had a close association with it.

Since the spheres of interest encompassed by general thoracic surgery vary in different countries, this text has been produced in two books. This book, *Thoracic Surgery*, encompasses surgery of the airways, lungs, chest wall, and mediastinum. The companion volume, *Esophageal Surgery*, is devoted to the esophagus, and will be of interest not only to thoracic surgeons, but to alimentary tract surgeons and gastroenterologists.

F. Griffith Pearson, M.D.
Jean Deslauriers, M.D.
Robert J. Ginsberg, M.D.
Clement A. Hiebert, M.D.
Martin F. McKneally, M.D., Ph.D.
Harold C. Urschel, Jr., M.D.

ACKNOWLEDGMENTS

I thank my secretaries, Jean Waters and Leah Wiscombe, for their invaluable assistance in the preparation of this text from beginning to end. I also acknowledge the enthusiasm and professionalism of the staff at Churchill Livingstone, particularly Kamely Dahir, Managing Editor; Katharine O'Moore-Klopf, Production Editor; and Avé McCracken, former Acquisitions Editor.

F. Griffith Pearson

I thank Debbie for her understanding, love, and encouragement. Thanks also to my to secretaries, Ann Julien and Claire Légaré, for their help with this project.

Jean Deslauriers

My thanks to Dorrel Granderson for holding it all together, and to my wife Charlotte and my children, Karyn, Jordan, and David and Haras, for their patience and understanding.

Robert J. Ginsberg

I thank the contributors and acknowledge special indebtedness to Miranda Bromage, International Surgery Editor; to Kamely Dahir, Managing Editor; and to Katharine O'Moore-Klopf, Production Editor, all of Churchill Livingstone. Avé McCracken, formerly Acquisitions Editor for the same publishing house, deserves credit for launching and guiding the original product. I must also thank my wife, May Cameron Hiebert (for many years head nurse of the Thoracic Surgical Unit at Toronto General Hospital) for her patience, understanding, and helpful criticism of my manuscripts.

Clement A. Hiebert

I thank Gregory McKneally for the cover design sketch and Deborah McKneally for managing the manuscripts and for her inspiration and advice.

Martin F. McKneally

I thank my loving wife Betsey and my wonderful children, Harold III, Brad, Locke, Amanda, and Susanna. I also thank Melanie and Mike Phillips, my invaluable office assistants.

Harold C. Urschel, Jr.

CONTENTS

III. Lung

V. Chest Wall and Sternum

VI. Diaphragm

VII. Mediastinum

1

GENERAL THORACIC SURGERY: ITS HISTORY AND DEVELOPMENT

Earle W. Wilkins, Jr.
Harold C. Urschel, Jr.

In his honored speaker's address to the American Association for Thoracic Surgery on the occasion of its fiftieth annual meeting, the scholarly Leo Eloesser (1970) referred to chest surgery as having "become a purposefully intended and scientifically directed art." That general thoracic surgery is indeed a science complemented by the skilled art of caring for the patient, few would disagree. That it has been purposefully intended may require appraisal and analysis, for which a historical review, seeking common threads of development, is quite admirably suited.

ORIGINS

There is no exact date or specific event that marks the birth of chest surgery. It did not arise de novo in a particular country or in one school of surgery. It appears that after the public demonstration of ether anesthesia by Warren in 1846 and the early understanding of sepsis following Semmelweiss' work in 1847, physicians in a number of countries began to explore the possible application of surgical techniques to the relief of diseases of the thorax. To ascribe priority is surely to pronounce error and invite rebuttal. A series of events and personalities is presented therefore, only to permit placement of the origins of general thoracic surgery in the context of time and to emphasize the multinational roots of its development.

Vincenz Czerny of Heidelberg, Germany, a former assistant of the early pioneer of surgery in Vienna, Theodor Billroth, performed one of the early resections for carcinoma of the cervical esophagus in 1877. M. H. Block of Danzig (now Gdansk, Poland) described his original experimental work in pulmonary resection in rabbits in 1881. Carlo Forlanini, professor of medicine in Pavia, introduced the concept of artificial pneumothorax for tuberculous cavities in 1882.

Édouard de Cérenville of Lausanne, although a professor of clinical medicine and internal pathology, described rib resections for collapsing the lung in 1885. W. I. Wheeler of Dublin described a successful resection of a pulsion diverticulum of the pharyngoesophageal junction in 1886. Ludwig Rehn of Frankfurt am Main in 1897 described the survival of a young man following suture of a stab wound of the right ventricle. Carl Beck of New York advocated visceral pleurectomy in the radical treatment of empyema in 1897. Finally, Hans Christian Jacobaeus of Stockholm introduced the thoracoscope for closed intrapleural pneumonolysis in 1911. Such were examples of the beginnings of thoracic surgery.

INTRAOPERATIVE CONTROL OF RESPIRATION

These pioneering ventures into chest surgery, as innovatively daring as they were, were doomed to limited success until control of respiration in the open chest was achieved. Johann von Mikulicz (1904) of Breslau (now Wroclaw, Poland) initiated research into the development of a differential pressure methodology for control of respiration during surgery. If there was a birth of modern chest surgery, this might be identified as its critical point in time. Eloesser (1965), in an editorial in the *Journal of Thoracic and Cardiovascular Surgery,* suggests that Mikulicz "stumbled on the very birth of modern chest surgery." He was recalling a 1904 scene in Breslau involving Mikulicz's pupil Ferdinand Sauerbruch: ". . . those fiery white-coats swarming out of the basement into the Silesian twilight heralded the beginnings of controlled respiration."

Sauerbruch developed the negative differential pressure chamber, a complicated system in which the patient and the operating team was closeted in a hermetically sealed space with only the patient's head outside at atmospheric pressure for administration of anesthesia and control of respiration. Meanwhile, Ludolf Brauer (1904) of Marburg, Germany was developing a positive-pressure method that enclosed only the patient's head, like a diver's helmet according to Borst (1985), for applying anesthesia and positive pressure. Samuel Robinson (1910) from the Massachusetts General Hospital in Boston, having worked with both Sauerbruch and Brauer, chose the latter's principle in constructing his own "box," a positive-pressure chamber in which the anesthetist was actually seated with the patient's head enclosed within the chamber.

All these cumbersome methods served as a prelude to the work of Samuel Meltzer and John Auer of New York (1909) with "continuous respiration without respiratory movements" by means of the intratracheal insufflation of a continuous stream of air and anesthetic vapor. This led ultimately to the intermittent, or phasic, application of positive-pressure respiration and its modern counterpart via the cuffed endotracheal tube. (It should be interjected here that Theodore Tuffier of Paris had reported in 1896 his actual development of an intratracheal tube with an inflatable cuff.)

Thus, the development of the methodology of intermittent positive-pressure inflation of the lungs, permitting all the phases of modern intrathoracic surgery, does seem "purposefully intended." It constituted what Eloesser called the first milestone in chest surgery.

THE BASIS OF PULMONARY RESECTION

With the ventilatory aspect of anesthesia for the open chest fully achieved, attention slowly turned toward both research and clinical application in pulmonary resection. Harold Brunn (1929) of San Francisco clearly stated the goal of lobectomy: "By this method the diseased lobe is removed at one stroke, the period of convalescence is diminished, and deformity does not result." The basic challenges in safe pulmonary resection were control of the hilar vessels and closure of the bronchial stump.

Lobectomy

Early efforts at lobectomy involved hilar mass ligature and two-stage resections. Frequently described as ghastly, the staged operation was considered essential because of the fear of bronchial stump blowout. Howard Lilienthal (1922) of New York reported 14 single lobectomies for bronchiectasis with 6 deaths (43 percent). In this series he used the presence of adhesions as a guide to staging the lower lobectomy. If the upper lobe were held in an expanded position, he proceeded with single-stage resection; if not, he induced adhesions with gauze abrading of the pleural surfaces and iodoform packing and continued to a two-stage operation. It is only fair to comment that this kind of suppurative lung disease with difficult adhesions and hypertrophy of the bronchial arterial system made early attempts at lobectomy the most hazardous and in large measure may have accounted in this preantibiotic era for the high mortality rate.

Despite this early experience of Lilienthal, Eloesser identifies the report of Brunn, including six lobectomies with a single death, as his second milestone in thoracic surgery, stating: "In 1918, Brunn did the first modern closed lobectomy, ligating the vessels, suturing the hilar stump of lung over the severed bronchus, and closing the chest." Brunn did employ a system of closed chest drainage to maintain expansion of residual lung. Wertheim hysterectomy clamps were used across the lung root pedicle, which was then ligated with double, heavy chromic catgut ties.

Apparently overlooked in these early lobectomies carried out with mass hilar ligature was the report of Morriston Davies (1913) of London. In 1912 he had performed a right lower lobectomy for carcinoma in which "the various structures at the pedicle of the lower lobe were ligated separately. . . . The proximal end of the bronchus was stitched over and covered with an adjacent portion of lung." Unfortunately, the patient developed an empyema and died on the eighth day but "at the autopsy, no evidence of leakage from the bronchus could be obtained." It may be assumed that the death of the patient discredited a technique reminiscent of the individual dissection technique developed by Edward Churchill of Boston (1931). In it Churchill carried out a successful lobectomy for a bronchial adenoma using individual dissection and ligation of vessels and continuous catgut suture of the bronchial stump with coverage by adjacent upper lobe parenchyma.

This work culminated in the classic report of Churchill and Ronald Belsey of Bristol, England (1939), working at that time in Churchill's department. In this report the individual dissection and ligature technique was extended to segmental pulmonary resection. The authors identified the lingula "for descriptive purposes . . . the homologue of the right middle lobe," emphasizing from bronchographic study its frequent (46 of 50 cases) involvement in bronchiectasis. The article concluded with a prophetic sentence: "It is suggested that the bronchopulmonary segment may replace the lobe as the surgical unit of the lung."

Richard Meade (1961) of Ann Arbor, Michigan, in *A History of Thoracic Surgery* insists that Edward Kent of Pittsburgh and Brian Blades of Washington, D.C. (1942) be credited with individual management of vessels and bronchus "for publicizing this technique" in their report on the surgical anatomy of pulmonary lobes.

Pneumonectomy

The concerns facing the pioneers in lobectomy were only magnified when it came to total removal of a lung, not only because of the risk of hemorrhage and the ever-present likelihood of bronchial fistula but also because of the fear of sudden occlusion of a main pulmonary artery. Would a ligature of the pulmonary artery simulate the clinical picture of a massive pulmonary embolus?

The prevention of hemorrhage was facilitated by the introduction by Norman Shenstone and Robert Janes of Toronto (1932) of their lung tourniquet. In this technique the lung root pedicle was encircled by a snare of heavy cord, which was then tightened, and the lung was cut away leaving a 2-cm cuff of tissue. In their words "obvious vessels were clamped and ligated and a running suture of chromic catgut was introduced across the pedicle." Evarts Graham of St. Louis and

J. J. Singer (1933) employed the tourniquet in their remarkable and successful one-stage pneumonectomy for carcinoma. Graham was apparently unaware of basic animal experiments, but his anxiety over occlusion of the pulmonary artery was relieved by preliminary tourniquet obliteration of arterial blood flow without apparent change in vital signs. Graham added a complementary thoracoplasty of the third to ninth ribs to reduce the size of the residual pleural space and to minimize the worrisome threat of mediastinal shift. The patient, a physician, survived 30 years until his death at age 78. Graham's pneumonectomy was Eloesser's third milestone in surgery, a courageous accomplishment and a turning point in history.

Edward Archibald of Montreal (1934) reported a successful dissection pneumonectomy performed just 3 months after Graham's feat. Ever after pneumonectomy would be carried out by individual ligation of pulmonary artery and veins. William Rienhoff (1933) of Baltimore provided the definitive technique for bronchial closure after pneumonectomy. His technique included "cutting the cartilages at various points, in order to do away with their spring-like action" and suturing "the bronchus with interrupted medium silk sutures." A classic paper by Rienhoff followed in 1942, the result of extensive experimentation with techniques of bronchial closure in dogs, including coverage of the stump with parietal pleura.

Here too, the techniques of hilar dissection and bronchial stump closure seem purposefully intended.

ESOPHAGECTOMY

Early efforts toward esophageal resection were confined to its cervical portion or to extrapleural approaches at the thoracic level. Billroth (1871) had demonstrated in dogs that resection and anastomosis of the cervical esophagus was feasible. His assistant in those animal experiments, Czerny (1877), carried out a partial cervical esophageal resection for carcinoma, as already noted. Meade (1961), the thoracic surgical historian, describes "the first successful intrathoracic resection and anastomosis of the esophagus" by Dobromysslow (1901). A 3- to 4-cm segment was resected, the ends united with two rows of silk sutures, and the anastomosis wrapped with a large posteriorly based skin flap. Although "complete union of the suture line" was demonstrated at 3 weeks, Meade reported that no further follow-up could be discovered. Wolfgang Denk (1913) of Vienna demonstrated in cadavers that the esophagus could be removed by blunt dissection through a subcostal transhiatal approach combined with a cervical dissection. Grey Turner (1933) reported a successful blunt esophagectomy followed by a second-stage completion of an antethoracic skin tube to connect the esophageal and gastric stomas.

The contemporary development of positive-pressure intratracheal anesthesia permitted the direct transthoracic approach to esophageal resection. The pioneering operation was that of Franz Torek (1913) of New York, who carried out a subtotal, left thoracic resection of the esophagus for a squamous carcinoma of the middle third. The 67-year-old woman survived 13 years, fed orally via a rubber tube that connected her cervical esophagostomy and gastrostomy. She refused any attempt at plastic, antethoracic skin tube reconstruction.

Restoration of alimentary continuity following esophagectomy now constituted the principal surgical challenge. Beck (1905) demonstrated in animal experiments the use of a tube of greater curvature than the stomach to replace the lower esophagus. César Roux (1907) of Lausanne developed the technique of esophagojejunoplasty for distal esophageal stricture. G. Kelling (1911) of Dresden devised a technique for use of the colon for esophageal replacement. In his initial case an isoperistaltic segment of transverse colon was brought up subcutaneously and its distal end was anastomosed to the stomach at the mid-sternal level in preparation for ultimate skin-tube connection to the cervical esophagostomy. Martin Kirschner (1920) of Leipzig originated the now standard use of a mobilized stomach to replace the esophagus by dividing the left gastric, left gastroepiploic, and short gastric arteries. He planned an antethoracic, subcutaneous placement of the stomach but never succeeded in using it in a patient with carcinoma.

In light of this burst of both animal experimentation and progressive attempts in humans, it is surprising that the final accomplishment of a successful esophagectomy with an intrathoracic esophagogastric anastomosis did not occur until 1937, when Samuel Marshall (1938) of Boston carried out an esophagogastrectomy with reestablishment of continuity by an end-to-side anastomosis. William Adams and Dallas Phemister (1938) of Chicago followed with a similar successful case, featuring for the first time a two-layer anastomosis using interrupted nonabsorbable sutures which in this case were linen. Churchill and Richard Sweet (1942) of Boston presented a classic report of 11 resections, emphasizing preservation of gastric blood supply and the meticulous suturing, with two-layer interrupted fine silk, of the anastomosis as the basis for avoiding anastomotic leakage and/or stricture formation.

Finally, Sweet (1945) and the British surgeon Ivor Lewis (1946) extended esophageal resection to any level of carcinoma within the esophagus, Sweet by the strictly left transthoracic double-rib resection approach and Lewis by the separate laparotomy and right thoracic incisions.

Mahoney and Sherman (1954) of Rochester, New York reintroduced use of the colon to replace the entire thoracic esophagus, utilizing isoperistaltic right colon placed in the anterior mediastinal position. Wilkins (1980) emphasized preference for use of left colon, always following preoperative angiographic mapping of mesenteric blood supply. The colon thus became the accepted alternative choice, after the stomach, for esophageal replacement.

Mark Orringer (1978) of Ann Arbor resurrected and perfected the technique of transhiatal-transcervical esophagectomy without thoracotomy. Once again in the esophagus, a purposefully intended art continued.

GLOBAL FACTORS

Tuberculosis: the White Plague

The late Norman Delarue (1989) of Toronto apparently coined the term *white plague* in noting that after the conquest of smallpox, tuberculosis remained a worldwide major public health threat. He recorded "little significant change . . . from Hippocratic times to the onset of the twentieth century." Indeed, Robert Koch had discovered the causative bacterial agent, the tubercle bacillus, only in 1882. That was the same year in which Forlanini reported his work with inducing artificial pneumothorax to treat cavitary pulmonary tuberculosis.

Thenceforth, the evolution of forms of therapy for tuberculosis was closely tied to the history of thoracic surgery, in fact defining early surgical techniques. Failure of pneumothorax to provide appropriate cavitary collapse led to the development of extrapleural thoracoplasty. As mentioned earlier, de Cérenville began this work in 1885 with resections of just a few ribs, usually the second and third. Brauer in 1909 related the number of ribs to be resected to the degree of collapse necessary to provide cavity closure. Paul Friedrich (1911) of Marburg described extensive thoracoplasty with removal of portions of ribs 2 through 10. The 3-month mortality, however, was 40 percent. Brauer then proposed certain modifications: operative staging of the rib resections, subperiosteal rib resection to permit better ultimate stability of the chest wall, and limiting the lengthy rib resections to those underlying the scapula. Max Wilms (1911) of Basel added removal of the transverse processes posteriorly and Noland Carter (1932) in the United States added removal the first rib. The final step in the evolution of extrapleural thoracoplasty was the addition of pulmonary extrafascial apicolysis described by Johann Holts (1933) and Carl Semb (1935) both of Oslo.

The operation of phrenicectomy, like use of pneumoperitoneum to elevate the diaphragm in an effort to promote collapse of lower lobe cavities, enjoyed a transient period of popularity in the 1920s. [*Editor's note:* Probably because it was easily performed.] It never proved effective in cavity closure and was largely abandoned, even before the modern antibiotic era.

The ingenuity of surgeons led to a rash of procedures to modify the standard operation that extrapleural thoracoplasty had become, primarily in an effort to avoid the major chest wall deformity caused by thoracoplasty. The underlying principles of all these were extra-parietal pleural dissection to free the lung from the chest wall and placement of substance in the extrapleural space to maintain pulmonary collapse. The variety of substances used included air (the original method), pedicled muscle, fat, and paraffin. A further modification was the subperiosteal stripping of ribs to provide an extraperiosteal space into which materials were introduced, providing a plombage. Popular substances included oil (oleothorax), polyethythene sheets, and Lucite balls. This trend toward plombage was terminated not so much by the onset of the antibiotic era as by the unacceptable rate of complications stemming from foreign body intolerance—tissue reaction, infection, and internal fistulae.

Pulmonary resection for tuberculous cavities dates back to Rudolf Krönlein (1882) of Zurich but was performed only sporadically and without signal success. Renewed interest followed the work of Churchill and R. Klopstock (1943), in which lobectomy was selectively carried out in cases not amenable to pneumothorax. However, in a consolidated report of these operations by Meade (1961), the "morbidity ranged from 37 to 70% and mortality rate was 6.2 to 33%."

The era of surgery for tuberculosis culminated, after the arrival of antituberculous agent therapy (streptomycin, para-amino-salicylic acid, and isoniazid) in segmental resection with Richard Overholt (Overholt, et al., 1950) of Boston and Max Chamberlain (Chamberlain and Klopstock, 1950) of New York as its principal advocates.

World War I

Two lessons learned from World War I were the management of open chest wounds and the treatment of empyema.

A long held physiologic concept that the mediastinum provided a rigid separation of the lungs was refuted by the deadly experience early in the war with open chest wounds. Meade quotes the 1917 directive from W. G. MacPherson for the Director General Medical Service, British Armies in France: "An open pneumothorax should be temporarily closed by suture at the earliest opportunity, either in the field ambulance or at the Casualty Clearing Station. If for any reason suturing is impossible, the wound should be packed, and strapped, so as to render it air tight." Only the modern technique of associated tube thoracostomy was missing from that order.

The other physiologic principle evolving from the war stemmed not from war wounding but from epidemic infection. Almost two-thirds of American army deaths were due to pneumonia and empyema complicating the 1918 influenza epidemic or tragically, to their treatment early on. Standard protocol had been open drainage of empyema as soon as diagnosed, but in these army cases the infecting organism was often the *Streptococcus*. Empyemas were being drained before the lung parenchyma had become adherent to the chest wall, and patients were dying from open pneumothorax. In their work with the Empyema Commission of the U.S. Army, Major E. A. Graham and Captain R. D. Bell (1918) concluded (once again to quote Meade): "the principles of treatment of acute empyema are (1) drainage, but with careful avoidance of open pneumothorax during the period of active pneumonia, (2) early sterilization and obliteration of the cavity, and (3) maintenance of the nutrition of the patient." It would take another 25 years and another world war before antibiotics, beginning with penicillin, could be added to the prescription of empyema therapy.

World War II

Whereas the lessons of the first World War I dealt with problems of pneumothorax, the principal advance in the handling of chest wounds in World War II involved the management of hemothorax. Contrary to civilian teaching at the time, war experience determined that clotted hemothorax was not uncommon. In spite of clotting, frequent aspiration was possible, or in some cases spontaneous resorption took place. Lt. Col. Paul Samson, Major Thomas Burford, Major Lyman Brewer (all later presidents of the American Association for Thoracic Surgery) and Major Benjamin Burbank (Samson, et al., 1946), in discussing the management of chest wounds in general, introduced the concept of early pulmonary decortication for organizing hemothorax. Their indications for operation included "patients in whom there is at least 50% compression of the lung . . . , those in whom aspiration has been unsuccessful and in whom there has been no appreciable pulmonary expansion at the end of 4 to 6 weeks following injury.'' Although appropriate credit must be given Carl Eggers (1923) of New York for his work with the radical treatment of empyema, it was this work beginning with Burford's 1943 innovative ''decortication in a case of uninfected organizing hemothorax five weeks after injury'' that culminated in the modern concept of total pulmonary decortication as expressed in the classic later report of Samson and Burford (1947).

The role of the thoracic center, in this case the Army Second Auxiliary Surgical Group's starting of the first Army Thoracic Surgical Center at Bizerte (Tunisia, North Africa), cannot be overstressed in studies on the wet lung syndrome and its treatment with intercostal block, tracheal suction, and repeated bronchoscopy. An abiding principle was that chest wounds in general do not require early thoracotomy.

EVOLUTION OF GENERAL THORACIC SURGERY

Eloesser's fourth milestone in chest surgery was the work of John Gibbon (1937, 1954) beginning in 1937 in the development of extracorporeal circulation, which Eloesser characterized as an ''idea and its elaboration . . . among the boldest and most successful feats of man's mind.'' This eventuated in opening the entire field of cardiac surgery, which in turn indirectly supported the distinct specialty of general thoracic surgery. The differences in its evolution in the United States and Canada are worthy of recounting.

United States

It is essential, in understanding the concept of general thoracic surgery as a specialty in its own right, to begin with the early interest in establishing thoracic surgical societies as a means of sharing ideas, techniques of surgery, and patient outcomes. These societies were all established within this century, the first being the New York Thoracic Surgical Society, founded in early 1917. Its prime mover was Willy Meyer, who immediately used this group as a focal point for discussing formation of a national thoracic society. That same year, at the American Medical Association meeting in New York, with the New York society as host to 23 physicians out of some 42 who had published on thoracic subjects, Meyer moved formation of the American Association for Thoracic Surgery (AATS). Its first meeting took place in Chicago in 1918 with Samuel Meltzer as president. There were 50 men in the founders' group, which was not limited to thoracic surgeons alone but included interested physicians ''*for* thoracic surgery.''

The proceedings of meetings were initially published in 1921 in the newly established *Archives of Surgery*. The *Journal of Thoracic Surgery* became the official organ of the Association in 1931; Graham was its first editor, a position he held untiil his death in 1957. In a move reflecting the exploding role of cardiac surgery and the burgeoning numbers of papers on cardiovascular surgery, its name was changed in 1959 to the *Journal of Thoracic and Cardiovascular Surgery*.

With a national society and a journal for the publication of its transactions now established, the next issue involved the need for a certifying mechanism and body. In 1937 the AATS appointed a seven-man committee chaired by Eggers to investigate the situation. Only John Alexander favored the establishment of a board of thoracic surgery. With only 18 surgeons in the country considering themselves to be thoracic surgeons, the committee advised the AATS that the time was not right for such a board. By 1946, however, particularly with the remarakble thoracic surgical developments during the war, the time was ripe. Another Eggers committee working with the American Board of Surgery (ABS), itself established only in 1937, reported favorably to the AATS this time. So, in 1948 the Board of Thoracic Surgery was created as an affiliate of the ABS. Reflecting the same pressures that beset the Journal, the Board ultimately (1971) became the independent American Board of Thoracic Surgery (ABTS). Although it retained the generic ''Thoracic'' in its title, the ABTS changed the wording of its certificate to specify accreditation in both thoracic and cardiovascular surgery.

The second national thoracic society was established in 1965, the Society of Thoracic Surgeons (STS). This organization permitted an unlimited membership of surgeons who strictly limited their practice to thoracic and cardiovascular surgery and who were accredited by the ABTS. It initiated and promoted its own journal, *The Annals of Thoracic Surgery*.

In his presidential address before the AATS entitled ''A Time for Assessment,'' Donald Paulson (1981) described three stages in the development of thoracic surgery—its establishment, expansion, and maturity. Much of the first two of these phases have been discussed earlier in this history. The first successful open heart operation by Gibbon (1953) was the catalyst in the phase of expansion. This took place primarily in the cardiac portion of the specialty, with the development of techniques for coronary bypass, valve replacement, correction of congenital defects, and excision of thoracic aneurysms. In the *maturity* phase, Paulson addressed an imbalance between programs for cardiac and what has come to be termed general thoracic surgery (GTS): ''The increase in volume of cardiac surgery has led to a serious imbalance in our educational programs, with subordination of general thoracic surgery to a secondary position in many thoracic surgical training centers.'' One of the several examples cited was the mean operative experience of ABTS candidates in the period 1971 to 1980, when only six to nine operations on the esophagus were encountered during an entire training career. This inadequate training experience resulted in either ill-equipped thoracic surgeons or non-board-certified surgeons performing these procedures.

In response to Paulson's recommendations, a Liaison Committee for Thoracic Surgery was established involving the Thoracic Surgery Directors Association, the ABTS, the Residency Review Committee, the STS, and the AATS. In a slowly increasing number of training centers, separate GTS programs with their own directors have been set up, collaborating with cardiac surgical programs to meet the ABTS requirements. A general thoracic surgeon finds that he must qualify and be certified in both fields to practice GTS.

Canada

The contrasting development of GTS in Canada was concisely described by Griffith Pearson (1990) in his presidential address to the AATS. He cited the combined specialty of thoracic and cardiovascular surgery prevalent in the United States, the United Kingdom, and Europe and then commented that "the evolution of training in thoracic surgery, in Toronto, however, was at variance with this pattern." A separate division of cardiovascular surgery had been created in 1958 with its own "dedicated residency." Thoracic surgery (now GTS) was continued within the two general surgical divisions until 1968, when a separate division of thoracic surgery was established. Pearson described the establishment of separate and autonomous divisions as "chance."

According to Pearson, "thoracic surgery was suffering the neglect of a 'poor relation' in departments of cardiovascular and thoracic surgery throughout the country." In 1976 the Royal College of Physicians and Surgeons of Canada, the one certifying body in Canada, established the Certificate of Special Competence in Thoracic Surgery, which "focused attention on training in thoracic surgery." The Toronto pattern thus had been recognized nationally, and the Certificate of Special Competence had helped enormously along the way in addressing the imbalance between cardiac surgery and GTS. In his expansive history of *Thoracic Surgery in Canada* the late Norman Delarue (1989) is quoted: "As a result, there is, at the present time, effective specialty coverage across the length and breadth of this huge country."

Canada, unlike the United States, has achieved a fifth milestone in thoracic surgery, recognition of the specialty of General Thoracic Surgery.

KEY REFERENCES

Borst HG: Hands across the ocean: German-American relations in thoracic surgery. J Thorac Cardiovasc Surg 90:477, 1985

This was the honored speaker's address before the 1985 annual meeting of the American Association for Thoracic Surgery. Borst, who is professor of surgery in Hannover, Germany and has experienced medical school and residency training in the United States, is uniquely qualified to trace the beginnings of thoracic surgery in Germany onward to the leadership role of the United States during the dark times in Europe.

Delarue NC: Thoracic Surgery in Canada. BC Decker, Toronto, 1989

In the words of the subtitle, this is a "a story of people, places, and events, the evolution of a specialty," told in a thoroughly authoritarian style by the late emeritus professor of surgery in the Faculty of Medicine, University of Toronto. It provides the details of the evolution of the specialty of general thoracic surgery in Canada and its credentialing with the Certificate of Special Competence in Thoracic Surgery.

Meade RH: A History of Thoracic Surgery. CC Thomas, Springfield, IL, 1961

This encyclopedic story of thoracic surgery from earliest times through 1960 is, in the words of Emile Holman in its preface, "less a history and more a textbook giving the development of surgical procedures, embellished by instructive details including results."

Naef AP: The Story of Thoracic Surgery: Milestones and Pioneers. Hogrefe & Huber, Bern, 1990

A Swiss surgeon's account of the evolution of both general thoracic and cardiovascular surgery, much of it from his own personal experience with the pioneers who created the milestones he has cited.

REFERENCES

Adams WE, Phemister DB: Carcinoma of the lower thoracic esophagus. Report of a successful resection and esophagogastrostomy. J Thorac Surg 7:621, 1938

Archibald EW: Unilateral pneumonectomy. Ann Surg 100:796, 1934

Beck C: Demonstrations of specimens illustrating a method of formation of a prethoracic esophagus. IMJ 7:463, 1905

Beck C: Discussion of Ferguson AH: Thoracoplasty in America and visceral pleurectomy, with report of a case. JAMA 28:58, 1897

Billroth CAT: Über die Resektion des Ösophagus. Arch Klin Chir 13;65, 1871

Block MH: Experimentelles zur Lungenresektion. Dtsch Med Wochenschr 7:634, 1881

Brauer L: Erfahrungen und Überlegungen zur Lungenkollapstherapie. Die ausgedehnte extrapleurale Thorakoplastik. Klin Tuberk 12:49, 1909

Brauer L: Die Ausschaltung der Pneumothoraxfolgen mit Hilfe des Überdruckverfahrens. Mitt Grenzgeb Med Chir 13:483, 1904

Brunn H: Surgical principles underlying one-stage lobectomy. Arch Surg 18:490, 1929

Cérenville ECB de: De l'intervention opératoire dans les maladies du poumon. Rev Med Suisse Rom 5:441, 1885

Carter BN: A technique for thoracoplasty. Surg Gynecol Obstet 57:353, 1933

Chamberlain JM, Klopstock R: Further experiences with segmental resection in pulmonary tuberculosis. J Thorac Cardiovasc Surg 20:843, 1950

Churchill ED, Belsey R: Segmental pneumonectomy in bronchiectasis; lingula segment of left upper lobe. Ann Surg 109:481, 1939

Churchill ED, Klopstock R: Lobectomy for pulmonary tuberculosis. Ann Surg 117:641, 1943

Churchill ED, Sweet RH: Transthoracic resection of tumors of the stomach and esophagus. Ann Surg 115:897, 1942

Czerny V: Neue Operationen. Zentralbl Chir 4:433, 1877

Davies HM: Recent advances in the surgery of the lung and pleura. Br J Surg 1:228, 1913

Denk W: Zur Radikaloperation des Ösophaguskarzinomas. Zentralbl Chir 40:1065, 1913

Dobromysslow VD: Ein Fall von transpleuraler Ösophagektomie ein Brustabschnitte. Zentralbl Chir 28:1, 1901

Eggers C: Radical treatment of chronic empyema. Ann Surg 77:327, 1923

Eloesser L: Milestones in chest surgery. J Thorac Cardiovasc Surg 60:157, 1970

Eloesser L: Birth of modern chest surgery and von Mikulicz's part in it. J Thorac Cardiovasc Surg 50:757, 1965

Forlanini C: A contribuzione della terrapie della tisi. Primo caso di tisi pulmonare curato col pneumotorace artificiale. Gaz Osped 68:537, 1882

Friedrich PL: Statisches und Prinzipielles zur Frage der Rippenresektion ausgedehnten oder beschränkten. Munch Med Wochenschr 58:2041, 1911

Gibbon JH Jr: The application of a mechanical heart and lung apparatus to cardiac surgery. Minn Med 37:171, 1954

Gibbon JH Jr: Artificial maintenance of circulation during experimental occlusion of pulmonary artery. Arch Surg 34:1105, 1937

Graham EA, Bell RD: Open pneumothorax: its relation to the treatment of acute empyema. Am J Med Sci 156:839, 1918

Graham EA, Singer JJ: Successful removal of an entire lung for carcinoma of the bronchus. JAMA 101:1371, 1933

Holst J: Local selective thoracoplasty in pulmonary tuberculosis. Norsk Mag Laegevidensk 94:361, 1933

Jacobaeus HC: Über Laparo und Thorakoscopie. Beitr Klin Tuberk 25:185, 1912

Kelling G: Ösophagoplastik mit Hilfe des Querkolon. Zentralbl Chir 38, 1209, 1911

Kent EM, Blades B: Surgical anatomy of the pulmonary lobes. J Thorac Surg 12:18, 1942

Kirschner MB: Eines neues Verfahren der Ösophagoplastik. Arch Klin Chir 114:606, 1920

Krönlein RV: Über Lungen-Chirurgie. Berl Klin Wochenschr 8:440, 1882

Lewis I: The surgical treatment of carcinoma of the oesophagus. With special reference to a new operation for growths of the middle third. Br J Surg 34:18, 1946

Lilienthal H: Pulmonary resection for bronchiectasis. Ann Surg 75:257, 1922

Mahoney EB, Sherman CD Jr: Total esophagoplasty using intrathoracic right colon. Surgery 35:937, 1954

Marshall SF: Carcinoma of the esophagus. Successful resection of lower end of esophagus with reestablishment of esophageal gastric continuity. Surg Clin North Am 18, 643, 1938

Meltzer SJ, Auer J: Continuous respiration without respiratory movements. J Exp Med 11:622, 1909

Mikulicz J von: Über Operationen in der Brusthöhle mit Hilfe der Sauerbruchschen Kammer. Cited in Eloesser L: Milestones in chest surgery. J Thorac Cardiovasc Surg 60:157, 1970

Naef AP: Hugh Morriston Davies: first dissection lobectomy in 1912. Ann Thorac Cardiovasc Surg 56:988, 1993

Orringer MB: Esophagectomy without thoracotomy. J Thorac Cardiovasc Surg 76:643, 1978

Overholt RH, Woods RM, Ramsay BH: Segmental pulmonary resection. Details of technique and results. J Thorac Cardiovasc Surg 19:207, 1950

Paulson DL: A time for assessment. J Thorac Cardiovasc Surg 82:163, 1981

Pearson FG: Adventures in surgery. J Thorac Cardiovasc Surg 100:639, 1990

Rehn L: Über penetrierende Herzwunden und Herznaht. Arch Klin Chir 55:315, 1897

Rienhoff WF Jr: Closure of bronchus following total pneumonectomy. Ann Surg 116:481, 1942

Rienhoff WF Jr: Pneumonectomy. A preliminary report on the operative technique in two successful cases. Johns Hopkins Med J 55:390, 1933

Robinson S: A positive pressure cabinet for thoracic surgery. Surg Gynecol Obstet 10:287, 1910.

Roux C: L'Esophago-jejuno-gastromie, nouvelle opération pour rétrécissement infranchissable de l'esophage. Semaine Med 27:37, 1907

Samson PC, Burford TH: Total pulmonary decortication. Its evolution and present concepts of indications and operative technique. J Thorac Cardiovasc Surg 16:127, 1947

Samson PC, Burford TH, Brewer LA, Burbank B: The management of war wounds of the chest in a base center. J Thorac Cardiovasc Surg 15:1, 1946

Sauerbruch JF: Über die physiologischen und physikalischen Grundlagen bei intrathorakalen Eingriffen in meiner pneumatischen Operationskammer. Arch Klin Chir 77:977, 1904

Semb C: Technique of plastic operation of apicolysis. Acta Chir Scand 76:84, 1935

Shenstone NS, Janes R: Experiences in pulmonary lobectomy. Can J Med 27:138, 1932

Sweet RH: Surgical management of carcinoma of the mid-thoracic esophagus. N Engl J Med 233:1, 1945

Torek F: The first successful case of resection of the thoracic portion of the esophagus for carcinoma. Surg Gynecol Obstet 16:614, 1913

Tuffier T: Régulation de la pression intrabronchique et de la narcose. Compt Rend Soc Biol 3:1086, 1896

Turner GG: Excision of thoracic oesophagus for carcinoma with construction of extra-thoracic gullet. Lancet 2:1315, 1933

Wheeler WI: Pharyngocele and dilatation of the pharynx, with existing diverticulum at lower part of pharynx lying posterior to the oesophagus. Dublin J Med Sci 82:349, 1886

Wilms M: Ein neue Methode zur Verengerung des Thorax bei Lungentuberkulose. Munch Med Wschr 50:777, 1911

Wilkins EW Jr: Long-segment colon substitution for the esophagus. Ann Surg 192:722, 1980

2

IMAGING

Stephen J. Herman

INTRODUCTION

The currently available methods of imaging the chest are indispensable tools in the investigation of patients with a thoracic problem. The importance of the chest radiograph in the workup of such patients cannot be overemphasized. Every patient with a suspicion of a potentially significant chest problem will have a chest x-ray. From an imaging point of view also, the importance of the chest x-ray cannot be overstated, since it is by far the most common imaging test performed. While the radiographic manifestations of hundreds of thoracic diseases have been described (Fraser et al., 1988), it is not the intention of this chapter to list these; instead, some principles of interpretation of the chest x-ray are discussed, with the goal of providing a basic understanding of the chest radiograph and giving a general approach to its interpretation. The correlation of pathologic patterns of pulmonary disease with their radiographic counterparts is emphasized. With this information, by knowing the pathology of a particular disease one can predict, in large part, what the radiographic manifestations will be.

Besides the chest x-ray, a number of other methods are available to image the chest. For each of these more advanced techniques, this chapter presents a brief discussion of the technique itself, followed by a discussion of its current uses. Knowledge of how the test is performed is necessary in that it provides a better understanding of what the test can be used for and what its limitations are. It must be kept in mind that while much of the information regarding the chest x-ray has changed little in recent years, most of the other techniques are still being improved and their uses are continually evolving; these sections of the chapter are therefore more heavily referenced. For each test, at least one recent in-depth review article of relevance is listed.

HISTORICAL NOTE

Within a few months of the discovery of x-rays by Wilhelm Roentgen in Germany on November 8, 1895, many investigators were realizing their extreme usefulness in diagnosing disease of the thorax (as well as other areas). Some of the injurious properties of the new rays, including skin burns and hair loss, were quickly recognized, but their oncogenic properties were not recognized until almost 10 years later.

Over the ensuing decades and continuing up to the present, many improvements were made in x-ray tube quality as well as in film and cassettes. Radiation-emitting materials began to be developed for diagnostic use, and newer isotopes and vehicles for injection, inhalation, and ingestion of these substances are still being produced. The technique of computed tomography (CT) was developed by Godfrey Hounsfield, for which he was awarded the Nobel Prize in 1979. In 1972 the first head CT scanner was installed in England; the first body scanner came into use in 1975. In 1946 the phenomenon of magnetic resonance was described, but it was not until 1980 that it was first used clinically (to demonstrate intracerebral pathology). Body imaging followed a few years later.

HISTORICAL READING

Eisenberg RL: Radiology: an Illustrated History. Mosby-Year Book, St. Louis, 1991

CHEST RADIOGRAPHY

Image Production

With a standard posteroanterior (PA) chest x-ray, the radiation passes through the patient from the back to the front, with the patient's chest lying in contact with the film cassette. Placing the patient in this position, as opposed to facing the x-ray source, minimizes the size of the heart and therefore the amount of lung it obscures, as it keeps the heart closer to the film, thus reducing magnification.

When the x-radiation passes through the patient's body, it is absorbed differently by different tissues. Tissues that adsorb little radiation (e.g., the lungs) allow most of this radiation to pass through the patient and expose the film. Since we are actually looking at a photographic negative, film regions that receive a large amount of radiation appear black. Tissues that absorb much radiation, for example bone, allow relatively little to reach the film, and these regions appear white. In practice, with plain chest radiography, we are able to distinguish four shades of gray representing the *four basic radiographic densities*. These include, from whitest to blackest, bone, water, fat, and gas. If the patient has any type of metal within the chest, for example a surgical prosthesis, this absorbs even more radiation than bone, and will appear even whiter. The patterns on the x-ray film thus created allow one to visualize the intrathoracic structures.

Technical Factors

Before beginning to interpret a chest x-ray, it is most important to determine if the study is technically adequate or not. Failing to do so may make one either under- or overstate disease. For example, on an underpenetrated film, in which it is difficult to see through the heart, even a large left lower lobe mass may be missed. Similarly, it is well known that a film obtained during a poor inspiration can mimic pulmonary edema (Fig. 2-1). Factors that must be checked include the patient's positioning, the depth of inspiration, and the degree of penetration of the radiograph.

Patient positioning must be proper in terms of both rotation and degree of lordosis. Rotation is easily checked by comparing the relationship of posterior structures (e.g., the spinous processes) with anterior structures (e.g., the medial ends of the clavicles). The spinous processes should project halfway between the clavicular heads. In terms of lordosis, the medial end of the clavicle anteriorly should project over the medial

end of (approximately) the fifth rib posteriorly. Deviations from either of these criteria may make it difficult to interpret the film properly.

Inspiration is best checked by comparing the height of the right hemidiaphragm with the anterior ribs. It is better to use the anterior than the posterior ribs because as can be seen on a lateral view, the top of the hemidiaphragm is much closer to the anterior than the posterior chest wall (Fig. 2-A). Changes in lordosis at the time of the PA film will cause a much bigger change in the relationship of the hemidiaphragm with the posterior ribs than in that with the anterior ribs, without any true change in the degree of inspiration. The dome of the right hemidiaphragm should project somewhere between the anterior fifth rib and the sixth interspace. If it is higher than this, the patient either has taken a poor inspiration or has some type of disease that is limiting the degree of inspiration. When the top of the hemidiaphragm is at or below the seventh rib, hyperinflation must be suspected.

A film is well penetrated if the disc spaces in the lower thoracic spine can be seen through the heart (Fig. 2-2B). If these cannot be seen, the film is underpenetrated and disease may be missed. At the same time, pulmonary vessels should be clearly visible within the lung parenchyma. A film is overpenetrated if the lungs appear black with poor visualization of these vessels.

Some miscellaneous information must be noted as well. For example, the patient's arms should be held high so as to not obscure the anterior mediastinum on the lateral view.

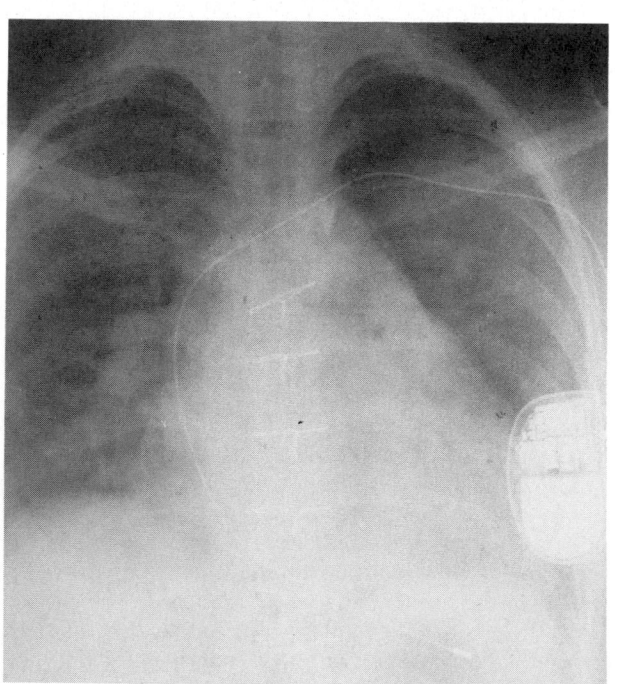

A

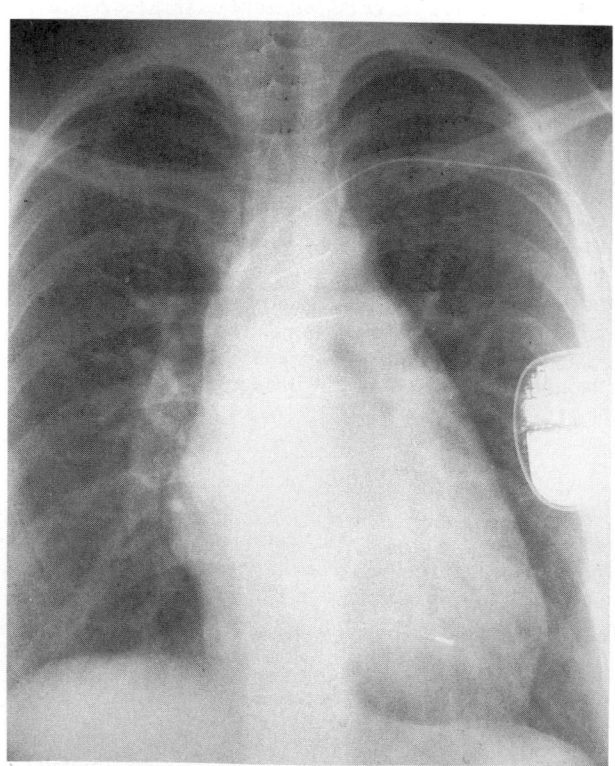

B

Figure 2-1. Poor inspiration mimicking pulmonary edema. **(A)** Film obtained during expiration reveals enlargement of the cardiac silhouette and bilateral perihilar haziness suggesting airspace disease, worse on the left. The appearance is highly suggestive of pulmonary edema. **(B)** Film obtained approximately 30 seconds later during a deep inspiration reveals complete clearing.

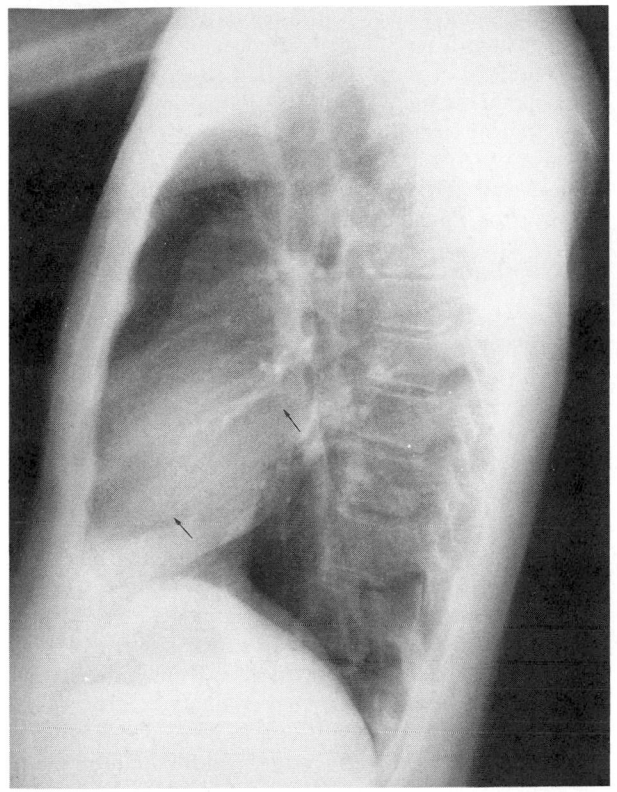

A

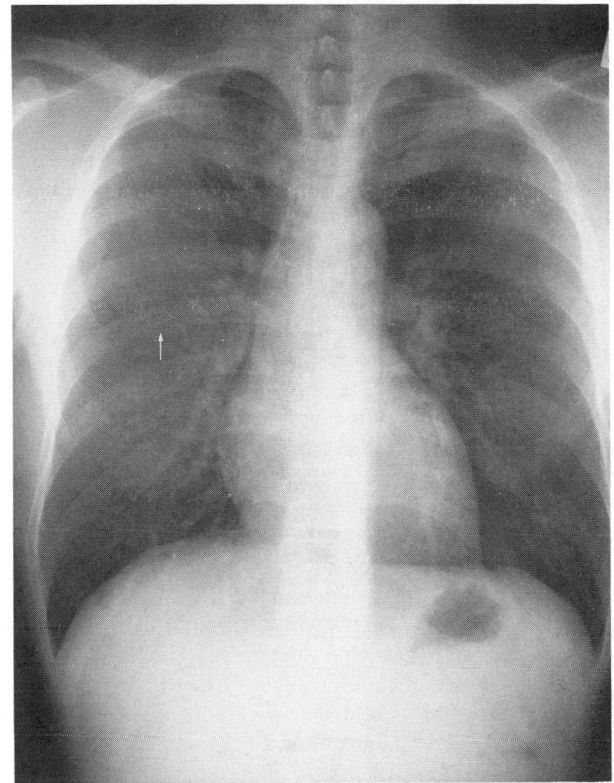

B

Figure 2-2. Normal chest radiograph. **(A)** Lateral view. **(B)** PA view. Note that (1) the spinous processes project midway between the clavicular heads; (2) the height of the right hemidiaphragm in the midclavicular line is at the level of the seventh rib; and (3) the vertebrae and disc spaces are clearly visible through the heart. The major fissures can be seen on the lateral view (*arrows*), and the minor fissure is well seen on the PA view (*arrow*). **(C)** Close-up view of mediastinum from PA film of another patient. This radiograph clearly reveals the medial margin of the azygoesophageal recess (*thick arrows*) as well as the anterior junction line (*small open arrow*). The former is the medial margin of the right lung anterior to the spine—note the positive Mach line (Fig. 2-12). The anterior junction line is formed where the two lungs meet in the retrosternal region. In addition, the interface between the left lung and the descending aorta (*medium thin arrows*) can be seen lateral to the left paraspinal line (*short thin arrows*), formed where the left lung contacts the mediastinum posterior to the descending aorta. The superior aspect of the posterior junction line (*long thin arrow*) is formed where posterosuperior aspects of both lungs come into contact in the retrotracheal region. The right paratracheal stripe (*large open arrow*) is visible because of air within the trachea and the adjacent right upper lobe.

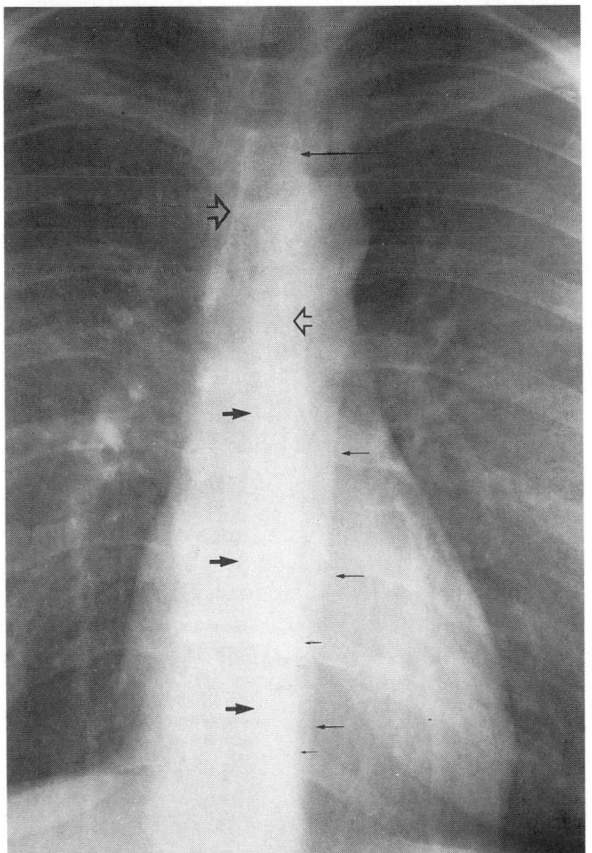

C

In addition, one should note if there is any material overlying the chest, such as a necklace (which may obscure disease) or hair braids (which may mimic disease). One has to remember that the x-ray beam is emitted from an x-ray tube and is absorbed by anything along its path toward the film. One usually thinks of intrathoracic structures only when looking at a chest radiograph, but keeping the above in mind will allow one to remember that a number of different extrathoracic objects can affect the appearance of the thorax.

Basic Principles

As stated above, on the plain chest x-ray there are four discernible radiographic densities: bone, water, fat, and gas. A structure is visible if its radiographic density is different than the density of adjacent tissue. For example, the heart is visible because its radiographic density (water) is different than that of surrounding lung tissue (air). The main right pulmonary artery, for example, is not visible because its water density is surrounded by the water density of the adjacent mediastinal structures.

This fact allows us to understand the so-called silhouette sign (Felson and Felson, 1950): A margin (or portion of a margin) of a structure that should be visualized but is not suggests the presence of disease. The right heart border should always be visible because there should always be water-density heart adjacent to air-density lung beside it. If the right heart border is not visible, this indicates that there is now water-density material in the lung adjacent to the part of the heart that forms the right heart border. The silhouette sign is extremely useful in detecting disease as well as in determining the location of the disease. For example, it is known that in most instances the portion of lung that is in contact with the right heart border is the right middle lobe. Therefore, loss of visualization of the right heart border implies disease in the right middle lobe (Fig. 2-3). A similar analysis allows detection of disease in many other parts of the chest. The silhouette sign is valid only if the film is adequately penetrated. If an inadequate amount of radiation has passed through the patient, it may not be possible to distinguish among the four radiographic densities, and one may diagnose the silhouette sign as being present when really it is not. In addition, in some individuals there will be anatomic reasons why a border that should be visible is not (e.g., the right heart border may not be visible in patients with pectus excavatum).

Approach to the Film

Besides remembering to check for technical adequacy before interpreting the film, one of the main differences between a trained and an untrained interpreter of chest radiographs is the way the film is analyzed. A trained observer will always remember to assess each and every structure that is present on the film, as opposed to merely honing in on the main abnormality while forgetting to search for other clues of disease. It is very natural to make this mistake, since the observer's eye is naturally directed to the main abnormality. In addition, a clinician who has seen the patient before looking at the radiograph has already formed an impression of what type of disease to suspect and will approach the film with this in mind, often forgetting to do a systematic search. Frequently, helpful clues to the patient's problem are found at sites distant from the main abnormality.

Therefore, it is most important to examine all structures present on the film. The order of examining these structures does not matter, but once a pattern is chosen, one should always try to use it. A suggested order is (1) written data, (2) chest wall, (3) abdomen, (4) diaphragm, (5) pleura, (6) heart, (7) mediastinum, (8) hila, and (9) lungs.

Written Data

One must always remember to check for the L (left) marker signifying the patient's left side. The PA film is always placed on the view box with the L marker to the observer's right, as if one is facing the patient, when interpreting the film. On the lateral projection, the L indicates that the patient's left side was placed against the cassette when the film was obtained, as is usually the case (again, so as to minimize the size of the heart). By convention, the lateral film is placed on the view box as if the observer is at the x-ray cassette looking back through the patient toward the x-ray source (i.e., the patient's back is placed to the observer's right, with the patient facing toward the observer's left).

On the PA view, if the L marker is inappropriate for the cardiac configuration, this may indicate dextrocardia; however, more commonly, a technical error is responsible.

One should always check the name written on the film to be certain that the correct patient is being assessed. Also, the date of the film must be noted to be certain that one is looking at the most current film and to determine if the timing of the film is adequate or if a more up-to-date study must be obtained.

Chest Wall

All bony structures must be assessed on both the PA and lateral views. Vertebral bodies should have an intact cortical rim around the entire perimeter of the body, which should be rectangular in shape on both views (Fig. 2-2). While loss of height of a vertebral body is most likely due to fracturing because of senile osteoporosis, in the right clinical setting metastatic disease could be the cause. Similarly, both pedicles should be visible on a well penetrated PA view throughout the thoracic spine. Again, an absent pedicle may indicate metastatic disease. On the lateral film the vertebral bodies should appear progressively blacker as one looks from superior to inferior. Any deviation from this suggests the presence of disease. Increased whiteness inferiorly may indicate lower lobe disease (consolidation or collapse, for example) or pleural fluid (see Fig. 18-5F).

Each rib should be checked individually in its entirety. In the upper ribs both superior and inferior margins are usually clearly visible (Fig. 2-2). In the mid- and lower chest, the lower rib margin often appears indistinct owing to the flange adjacent to the intercostal nerves and vessels. Rib expansion or focal loss of the cortical line may indicate a pathologic process, such as multiple myeloma or metastatic disease.

One should note the amount of soft tissue present in the chest wall since an abundant amount of fat may obscure underlying structures and may even simulate disease. For

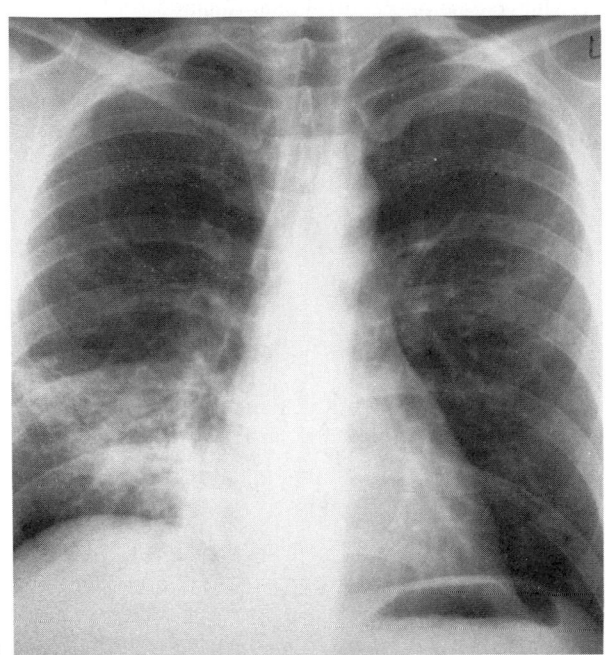

A

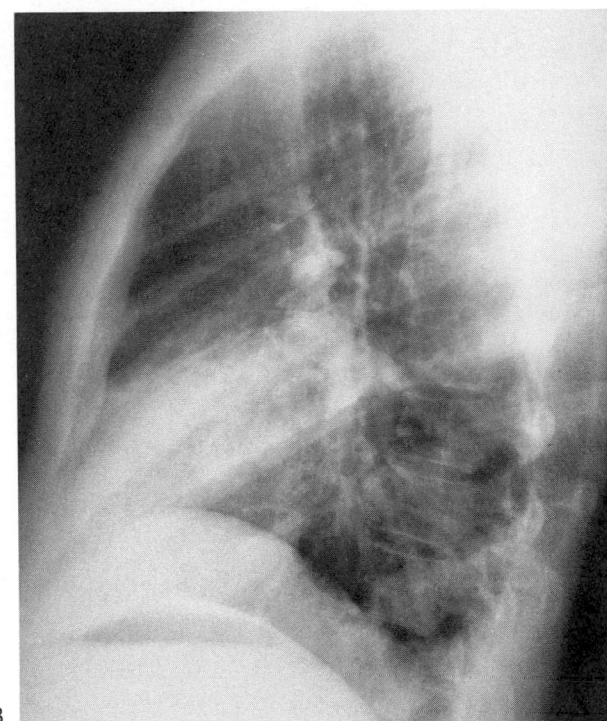

B

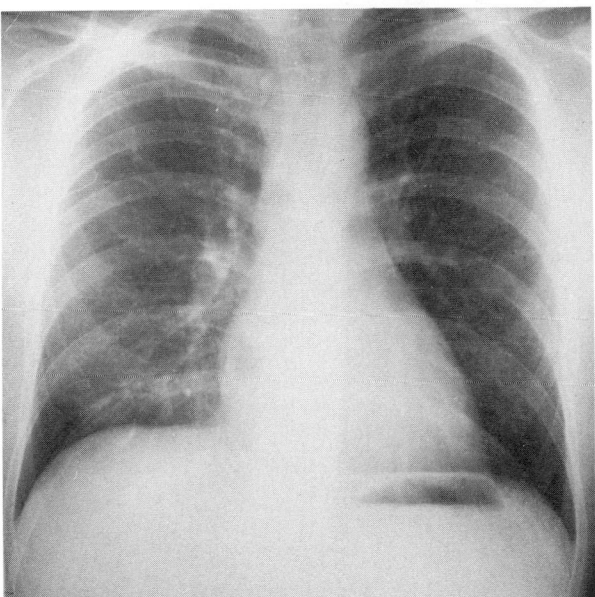

C

Figure 2-3. Silhouette sign. **(A)** PA radiograph reveals consolidation in the right lung base. The right heart border is not visible which indicates that this water-density process is located in lung adjacent to the right heart border; in most instances this is the right middle lobe. **(B)** The lateral view confirms the presence of consolidation in the right middle lobe. **(C)** PA radiograph obtained 3 weeks after Fig. A. The consolidation has cleared, and the right heart border is once again visible.

example, the hazy increase in density caused by overlying fat may simulate pneumonia or, on a supine view, pleural fluid. Similarly, one should note if there has been a mastectomy. While this may be known from the patient's clinical assessment, again the asymmetric soft tissue may mimic disease (Fig. 2-4).

Abdomen

On the chest radiograph, the amount of the abdomen that is visible is quite variable. One may be able to assess the size of the liver or spleen or to note distension of the stomach or loops of bowel. Also, one should also determine if free air is present under the diaphragm. Multiple tiny gas lucencies projecting beneath the diaphragm may indicate a subphrenic abscess, which may be the cause of intrathoracic abnormalities, such as basal atelectasis and/or pleural fluid.

Diaphragm

Usually each hemidiaphragm is smooth and on the PA film is somewhat horizontal medially with a gradual sloping laterally (Fig. 2-2). The point of maximal curvature is generally in the middle third of the hemidiaphragm. The point at which the

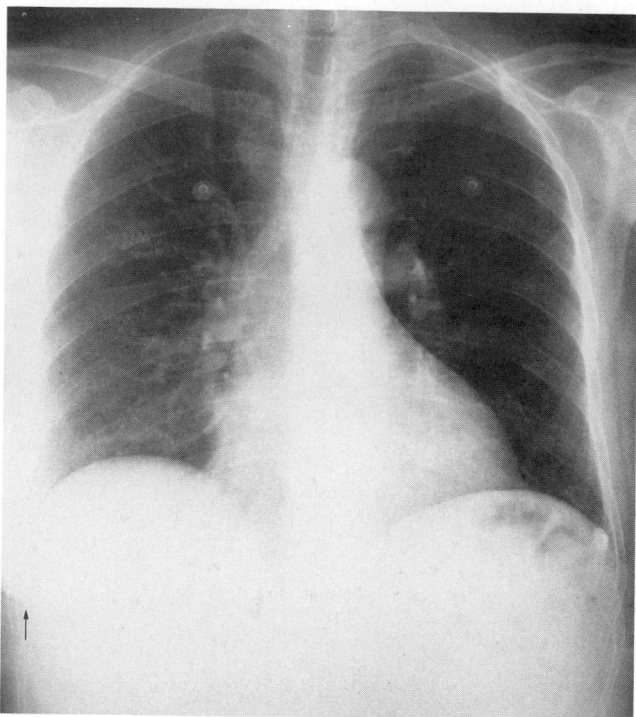

Figure 2-4. Mastectomy. The relative hyperlucency of the left hemithorax suggests the presence of left pulmonary parenchymal disease. However, the absent breast shadow and relative lack of soft tissues in the left axilla indicate that the hyperlucency is due to the reduced amount of overlying soft tissue. Note presence of right breast shadow (*arrow*).

diaphragm meets the chest wall laterally (on the PA film) and posteriorly (on the lateral film) forms a sharp acute angle, known as the *lateral* or *posterior costophrenic* angle, respectively (Fig. 2-5A). The diaphragm may normally have a slightly bumpy appearance known as *scalloping*. However, a very prominent bulge that forms acute angles with the rest of the hemidiaphragm suggests the presence of disease and warrants further investigation (Fig. 2-6).

The height of the right hemidiaphragm usually projects between the fifth rib and sixth interspace anteriorly (Lennon and Simon, 1965). The right hemidiaphragm is normally about 2 cm higher than the left. In Felson's series (1973c) the left hemidiaphragm was equal in height to or higher than the right in 9 percent of normal individuals, while in 2 percent the right hemidiaphragm was 3 cm or more higher than the left. Therefore, in the absence of any other pathology, minimal diaphragmatic displacement is probably due to normal variation.

Pleura

The costophrenic angles should be sharp and acute. If these angles are blunt, this usually indicates the presence of pleural fluid or thickening (Fig. 2-5B). One must study the entire perimeter of both lungs on both PA and lateral views, looking for any focal or diffuse areas of pleural thickening. While such areas may be benign (e.g., due to old fibrosis or pleural plaques), they may also represent malignancies such as metastatic disease or mesothelioma (Fig. 2-7).

The position of pleural fissures must be noted on each study since they may indicate the presence of lobar collapse. The major fissures are usually seen on the lateral view only and they run from about T4 in an anteroinferior direction to the junction of the anterior one-quarter and posterior three-quarters of the diaphragm (Fig. 2-2). The minor fissure is approximately horizontal or is gently curved (convex superiorly) on both views. On the PA view it contacts the chest wall laterally at about the level of the fifth rib (Felson, 1973d), and on the lateral view it contacts the anterior chest wall at about the midsternal level.

When pleural fluid forms, it generally first collects under the lung, in a so-called subpulmonic location. If a large amount of fluid remains in this location, this becomes evident on the PA film as a lateral shift of the most convex part of the hemidiaphragm from the middle third to the junction of the middle and lateral thirds (Fig. 2-8). The presence of a small or subpulmonic pleural effusion can be confirmed by obtaining a lateral decubitus view, with the suspicious side down. Free-flowing fluid will separate the lung from the chest wall; very small effusions (as small as 5 ml) can be detected by this technique (Moskowitz, et al., 1973). As the amount of fluid increases, one sees blunting of the posterior and lateral costophrenic angles. With further increases, water density is seen higher and higher within the hemithorax. If the effusion is large enough, there tends to be shifting of the mediastinum to the contralateral side. Lack of this shift indicates volume loss of the underlying ipsilateral lung. The combination of a large pleural effusion with lack of shift of the mediastinum suggests the presence of a bronchogenic carcinoma (causing airway obstruction and collapse) or of a mesothelioma.

A pneumothorax is manifested by the presence of a thin white line representing the visceral pleura, separated from the chest wall (Fig. 2-9A). This separation is usually seen in the lung apex because of the air rising to the top of the chest. However, it may be located anywhere in the thorax if the air is loculated. It is important that one diagnose a pneumothorax only when this thin white pleural line is seen. Paucity of vessels suggests but does not prove the presence of a pneumothorax. In addition, one must be careful to not confuse a skin fold with a pneumothorax. Skin folds can be problematic because they frequently parallel the chest wall (as does a partially collapsed lung in the presence of a pneumothorax) and have a sharp, well-defined peripheral margin (simulating the visceral pleura). However, a skin fold fades gradually medially, as opposed to the thin white line of the true visceral pleura (Fig. 2-9B).

On a supine view the appearance of a pneumothorax is quite different. In this position, pleural air rises to the most anterior aspect of the chest, which is at the base. The following are signs of a pneumothorax on a supine view (Ziter, et al., 1981; Gordon, 1980): basilar hyperlucency, visibility of the anterior costophrenic angle, a very deep lateral costophrenic angle (*deep sulcus sign*), a very sharp margin to the hemidiaphragm or heart, and visibility of a pericardial fat

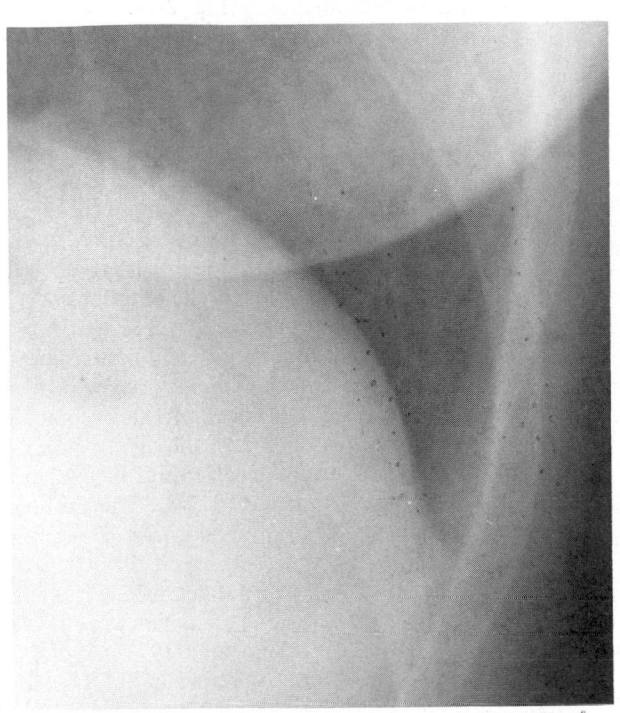

A

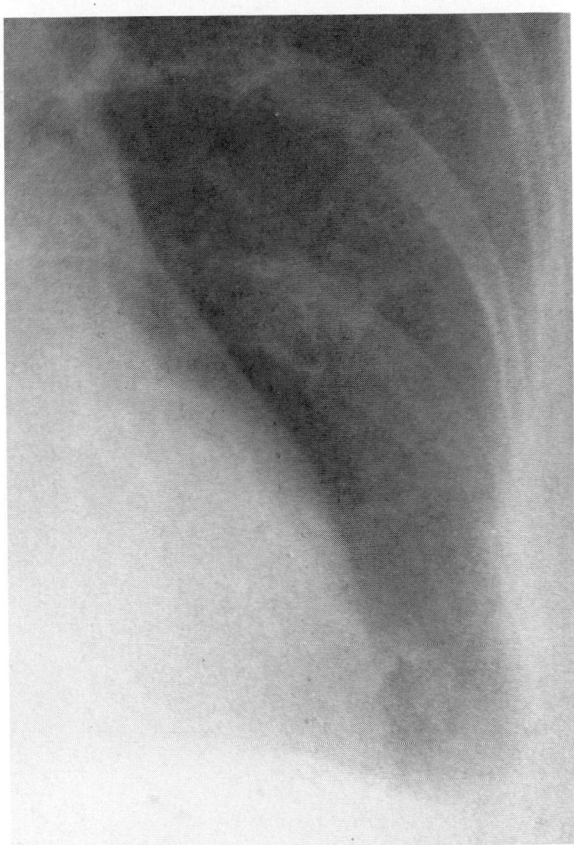

B

Figure 2-5. Sharp and blunted costophrenic angles. **(A)** Close-up of a normal left lateral costophrenic angle from PA chest radiograph. Note the sharp angle made by the diaphragm and chest wall and the fact that a lung is in direct contact with the chest wall. **(B)** Different patient with a small left pleural effusion. Note the blunting of the costophrenic angle.

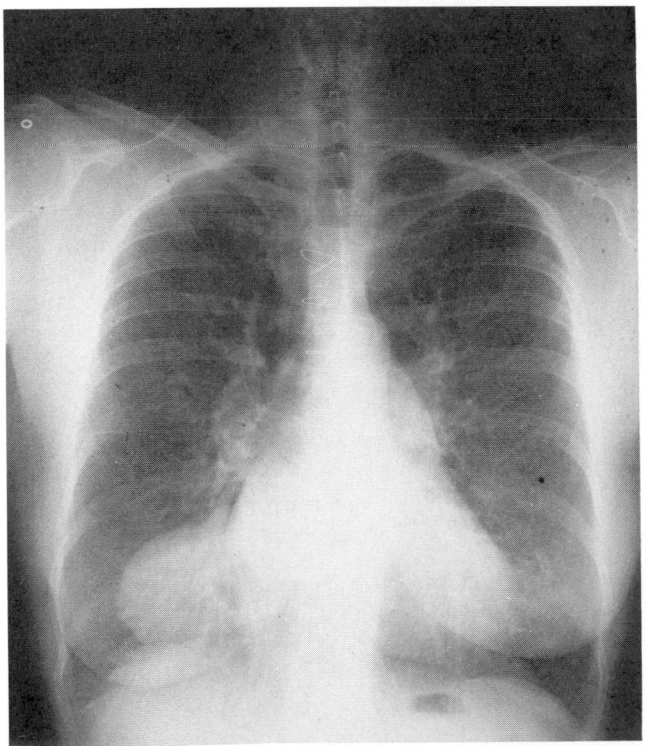

Figure 2-6. Cardiophrenic angle mass. A large mass lesion measuring approximately 7 cm in diameter is noted in the right cardiophrenic angle region. This degree of "lobulation" of the diaphragm is much more than normally seen and suggests a true mass (see Fig. 2-15A).

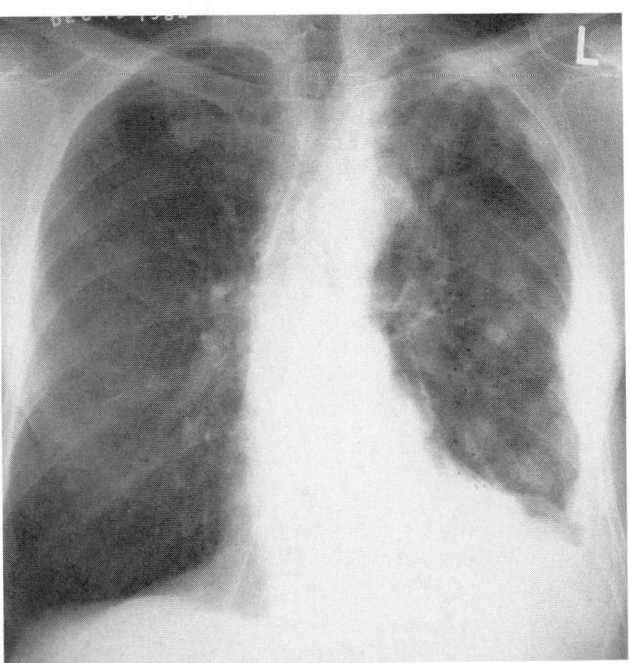

Figure 2-7. Mesothelioma. The PA chest radiograph of this 71-year-old man reveals marked nodular pleural thickening involving the left hemithorax circumferentially, as well as a significant decrease in the volume of the left lung.

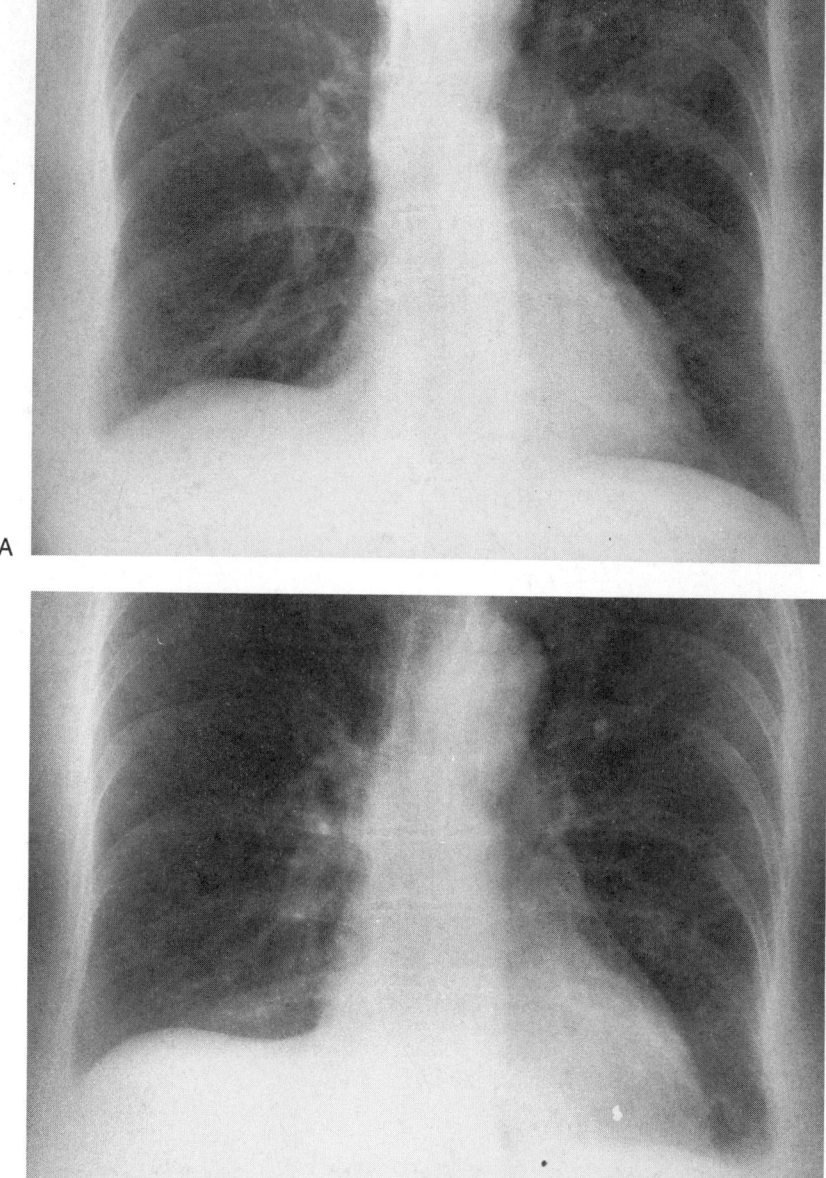

Figure 2-8.   Subpulmonic effusion. **(A)** Baseline PA chest radiograph. There is mild blunting of the right costophrenic angle. **(B)** The patient has developed bilateral pleural effusions, which on the right are mostly subpulmonic in location. Note the change in configuration of the hemidiaphragm, with apparent lateral shift of its most convex portion. In addition, there is increased blunting of both costophrenic angles.

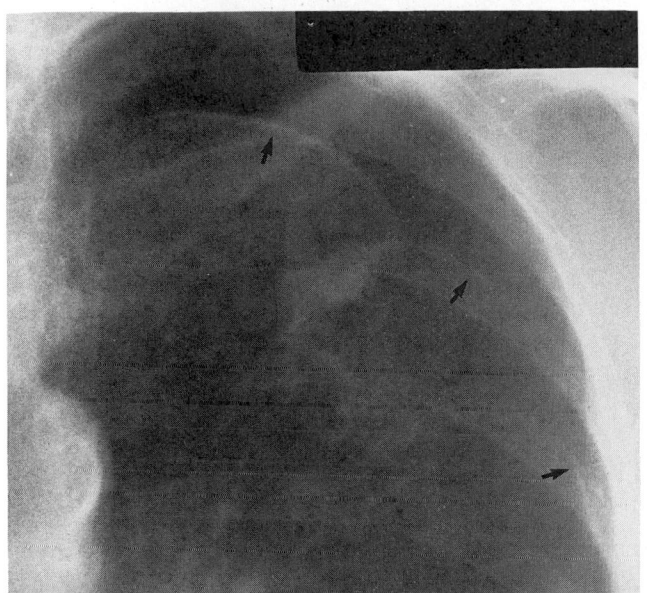

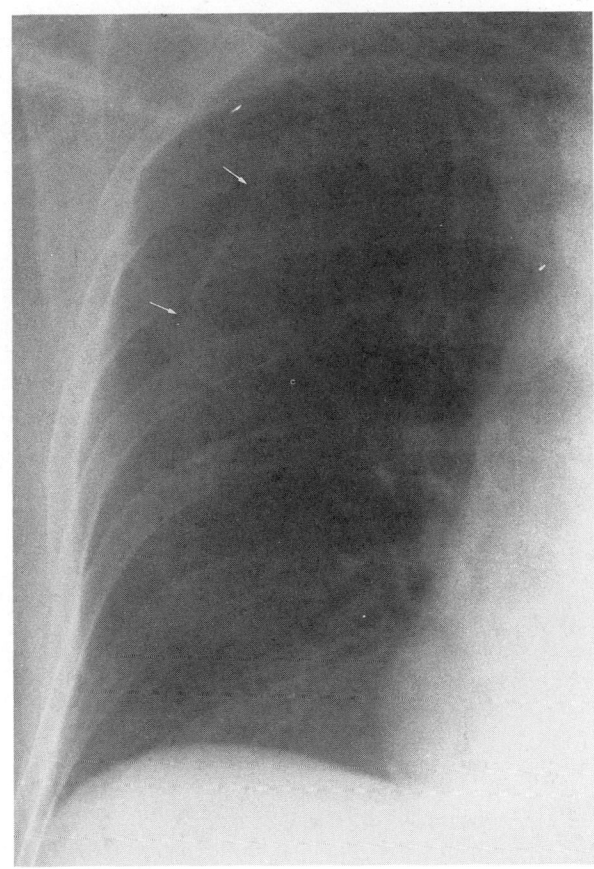

Figure 2-9. **(A)** Pneumothorax following a transthoracic needle biopsy of the left upper lobe nodule. Although the paucity of vessels in the periphery of the left upper lobe is suggestive of a pneumothorax, it can be diagnosed only because the visceral pleura (*arrows*), which is slightly thickened in this patient, is visible. **(B)** Upright portable chest radiograph obtained following insertion of right subclavian line. The line paralleling the chest wall in the right hemithorax (*arrows*) fades gradually medially, which indicates that it represents a skin fold rather than a pneumothorax.

pad (Fig. 2-10). If the pneumothorax is large enough, one may again see the thin white line of displaced visceral pleura. The presence of a pneumothorax can be confirmed by obtaining a lateral decubitus view with the suspicious side up. This allows the air to rise into the lateral pleural space separating the lung from the chest wall, thus allowing clear visibility of the visceral pleural line.

Heart

Details of the heart and vascular structures are beyond the scope of this chapter and are not discussed.

Mediastinum

The trachea is always well seen because it contains air and is surrounded by the water density of the mediastinum. It is a midline structure, but in middle-aged and older individuals, because of atherosclerosis, the aorta virtually always causes slight displacement of the lower trachea to the right. It is very important to specifically assess the trachea and main airways on every chest radiograph, looking for the presence

of intraluminal masses or thickening of the airway wall (Fig. 2-11). This is a frequently overlooked area and has been referred to as the "radiologist's blind spot."

Where various mediastinal structures contact adjacent lung, numerous lines and stripes are created. Familiarity with these increases one's ability to detect subtle mediastinal abnormalities. These interfaces are shown in Figure 2-2.

It is important that one be familiar with so-called Mach lines, since they may mimic disease. A water-density mediastinal structure, such as the aorta, which is convex into adjacent air-containing lung, is associated with a so-called negative Mach line (Fig. 2-12). What is meant by this is that the eye "sees" a thin, 1- to 2-mm wide, black line adjacent to the descending aorta. This line is a visual artifact and is not really present on the film (as can be proved by assessing the film with a densitometer). It is important to recognize this fact, since this black line may be confused with air, causing an erroneous diagnosis of pneumomediastinum. The corresponding positive Mach line is formed when air-density lung is convex into water-density mediastinum. In this case there is an apparent white line at the margin of the lung (e.g., at the left paraspinal region) (Fig. 2-12).

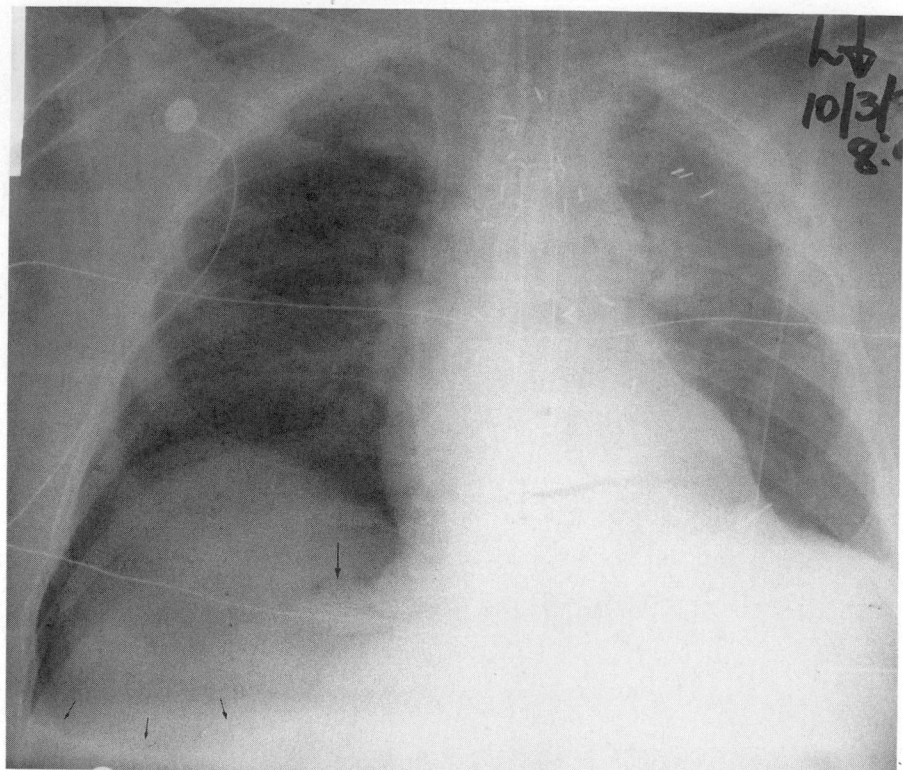

Figure 2-10. Basilar pneumothorax. On this supine chest radiograph, the right basilar pneumothorax is evidenced by the presence of the basilar hyperlucency, the visibility of the anterior costophrenic angle (*short arrows*), the deep sulcus sign (note how much more inferiorly the right costophrenic sulcus extends compared with the left), and the visibility of the right cardiophrenic fat pad (*long arrow*).

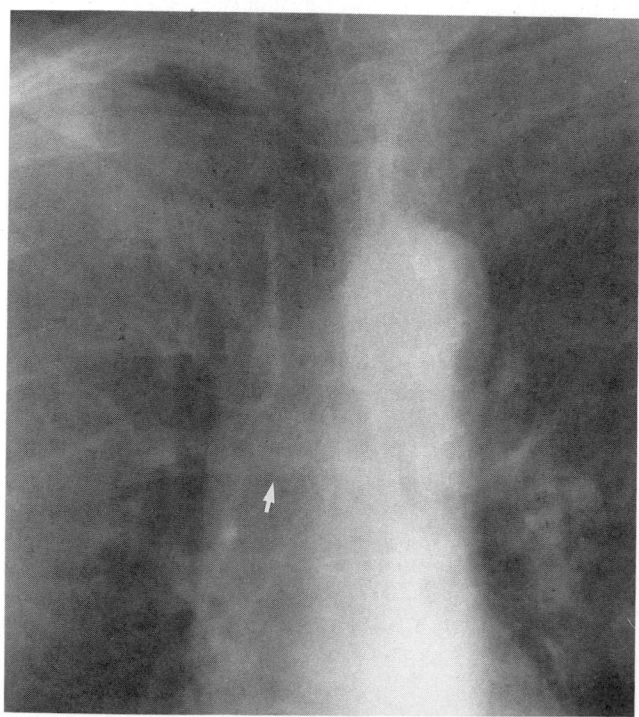

Figure 2-11. Close-up view of the central airways of a PA chest radiograph on this 65-year-old woman with a history of "asthma" for 2 years. Opacity in right mainstem bronchus (*arrow*) was shown at bronchoscopy to be a carcinoid tumor.

Pneumomediastinum presents as streaky linear gas densities along the fascial planes of the mediastinum, frequently adjacent to major mediastinal structures (Fig. 2-12C). Again, one must be certain that both sides of these gas densities are well marginated, differentiating them from the Mach line, which is well defined on one side only.

When abnormal mediastinal widening is present, it is important to determine in which compartment of the mediastinum the abnormality is located so as to narrow the differential diagnosis. The mediastinum is generally divided into anterior, middle, and posterior thirds on the lateral chest x-ray. Radiographically, the most commonly used system separates the anterior from the middle mediastinum by a line running down the front of the trachea and the back of the heart (Felson, 1973b). The middle mediastinum is separated from the posterior mediastinum by a line running parallel with and 1 cm posterior to the anterior margins of the vertebral bodies. Note that in this system the posterior mediastinum is not truly mediastinal at all by strict anatomic definition. However, masses defined as being posterior mediastinal by this system, such as neurogenic tumors, are considered to be mediastinal by most physicians.

One must consider lymphadenopathy, hematoma, abscess, and aortic aneurysm in all three mediastinal compartments. Other masses seen in the anterior mediastinum include thyroid or thymic lesions and germ cell tumors (Fig. 2-13A&B). Middle mediastinal masses also include esophageal lesions, hiatus hernias, and foregut cysts (Fig. 2-13C&D). Posterior mediastinal masses include neurogenic tumors (Fig. 2-13E&F).

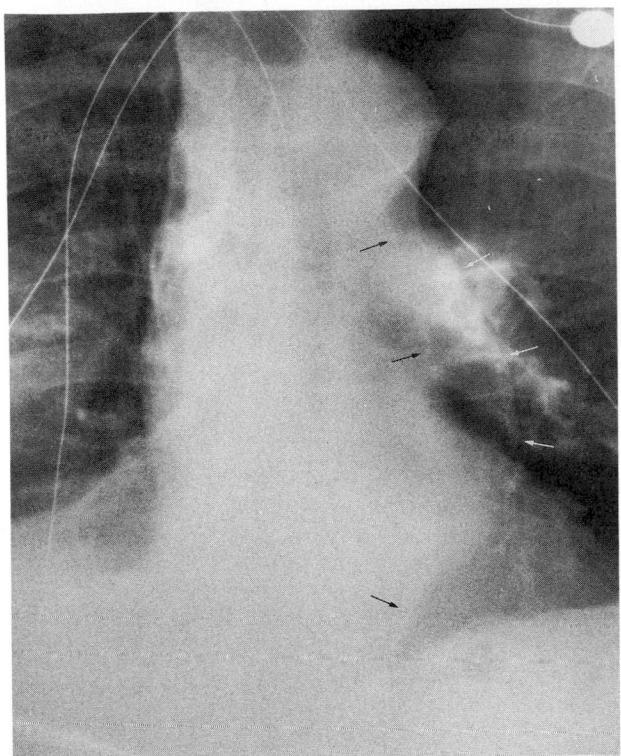

A

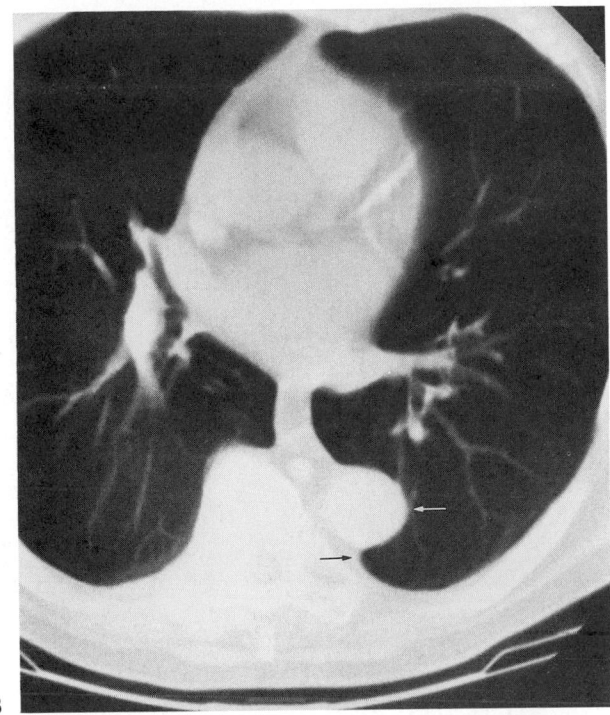

B

Figure 2-12.   Mach line. **(A)** In the left hemithorax medially, two convexities are seen. The more lateral one is marginated by a negative (black) Mach line (*white arrows*), indicating that this represents the descending aorta. The more medial convexity is marginated by a white (positive) Mach line (*black arrows*), indicating that this represents the left paraspinal line. **(B)** CT scan demonstrates the origin of these Mach lines. The water-density aorta protruding into the left lung (*white arrows*) causes the negative Mach line. Its margin is lateral to the most posterior aspect of the left lower lobe, which is convex into the mediastinal fat (*black arrows*) behind the aorta, producing the positive Mach line in Fig. A). **(C)** Spontaneous pneumomediastinum in a 20-year-old man. Note the linear lucency along the left superior cardiac margin (*large arrows*), which is bounded laterally by mediastinal pleura. These streaky linear lucencies can be seen extending superiorly within the mediastinum and into the lower neck (*small arrows*).

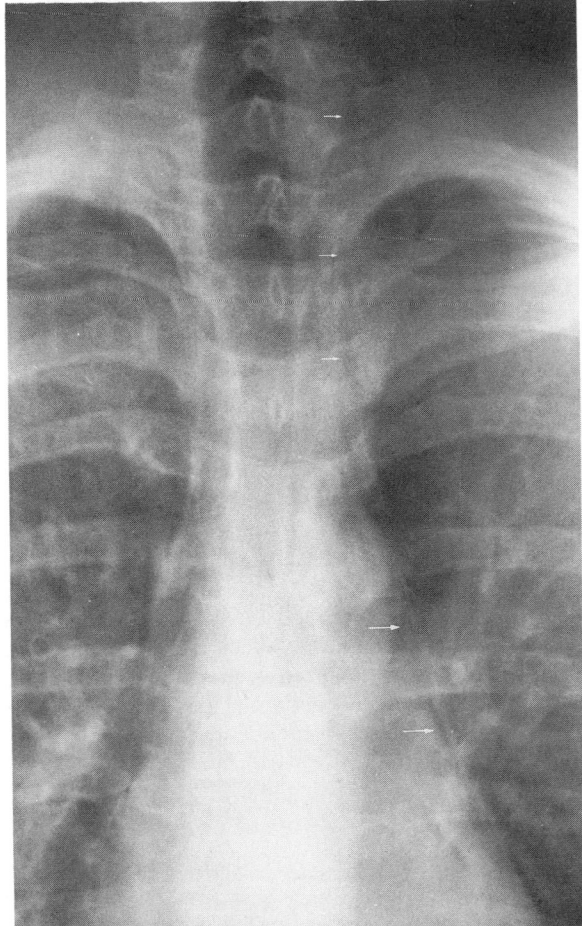

C

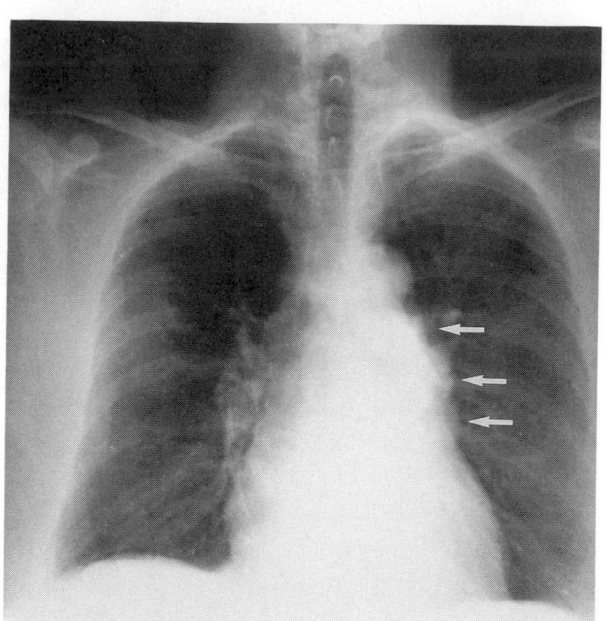

A

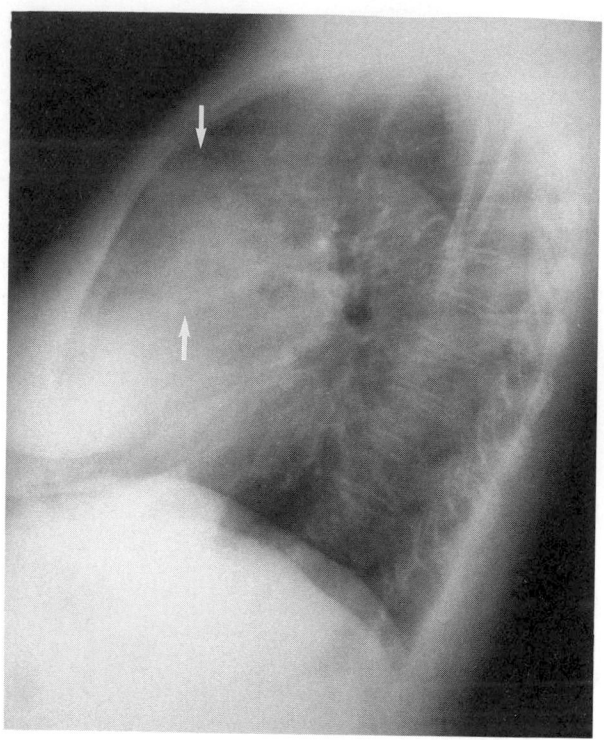

B

Figure 2-13. Mediastinal masses. **(A & B)** Anterior mediastinal mass—thymoma. A soft tissue opacity measuring approximately 7 cm in diameter is noted in the anterior mediastinum on the lateral view (*arrows*). Its lobulated contour is seen projecting to the left on the PA view (*arrows*). (*Figure continues.*)

Hila

The hila comprise the distal mainstem and lobar bronchi, as well as the central pulmonary arteries and veins. The left hilum is usually 1 to 2 cm superior to the right one (Felson, 1973a). Deviation from this pattern is usually due to lobar collapse or to lobectomy. The hila may be enlarged by large pulmonary arteries, which cause smooth hilar enlargement, by lymphadenopathy, which causes lobulated enlargement, or by a mass, which causes focal enlargement (Fig. 2-14).

Lungs

The radiographic appearance of the lungs is due to gas-filled alveoli, which appear black, and the pulmonary vessels, which appear white, coursing through the lungs. Bronchi are occasionally visible, if seen end-on near the hila, as very thin-walled, ring-like structures. Otherwise, bronchi do not contribute to the radiographic appearance of the lungs. Therefore, normal lungs are uniformly black except for the white vessels, which can be recognized as such because they taper and branch as they extend out from the hila peripherally. Any deviation from this appearance suggests the presence of disease.

PLAIN TOMOGRAPHY

The term *tomography* refers to visualization of a specific plane of tissue with the exclusion of all structures both above and below this plane. CT and magnetic resonance imaging

(MRI) are tomographic techniques, and these are discussed below. With plain tomography a specific plane is made visible by moving the x-ray tube and x-ray film in opposite directions during exposure of the film. By varying this motion, one can choose the level of the plane being brought into focus as well as its thickness. Since the advent of CT scanning, plain tomography is used much less frequently. In fact, it can probably be stated that when a tomogram is required, CT scanning, when available, is always the procedure of choice. However, there are instances in which plain tomography is very helpful, and in some radiology departments it is more readily available than CT scanning.

COMPUTED TOMOGRAPHY

Technical Considerations

CT differs from plain tomography in that the image is not made directly on radiographic film but rather is created by a computer. With CT, a moving x-ray tube emits radiation, which passes through the patient's body and interacts with radiographic detectors. The x-ray beam, which is highly collimated so that only a specific transverse plane of the patient's body is imaged, is directed from many different angles as the x-ray tube moves along a circular path around the patient. The information from each detector, which absorbs only a narrow portion of the emitted beam, is fed into a computer, which manipulates all this information and creates the CT image. On modern CT scanners, the CT image is composed

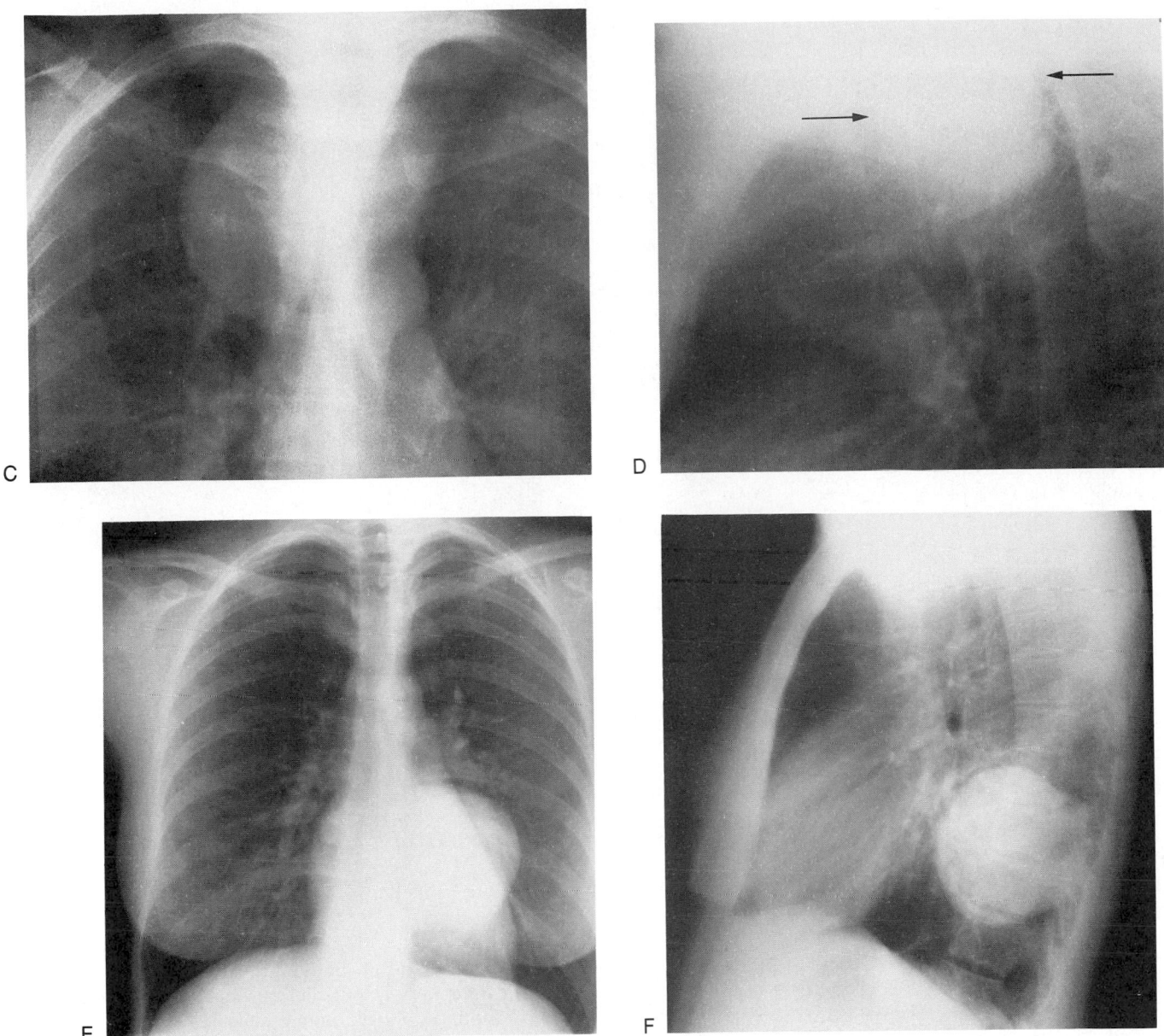

C

D

E

F

Figure 2-13 (*Continued*). **(C & D)** Middle mediastinal mass—goiter. On the PA view there is a large mass in the superior mediastinum, protruding bilaterally, more to the right. On the lateral view the mass is seen to lie in a retrotracheal location (*arrows*), placing it in the middle mediastinum. **(E & F)** Posterior mediastinal mass—schwannoma. There is a large mass lesion, with features of an extrapulmonary density (see Fig. 18-12), arising in the posterior mediastinum and protruding into the lung. Note that on the lateral view the mass appears to be arising from the costovertebral angle region.

of a 512 × 512 matrix, with each of the small squares, called pixels (for <u>pic</u>ture <u>el</u>ements), referring to a corresponding portion of the patient's body. A numerical value corresponding to the radiographic density is assigned to each of these pixels; by convention, these values vary between −1,000 Hounsfield units (HU) and +1,000 HU. These are set so that 0 HU corresponds to water, −1,000 HU to air, and +1,000 HU to bone. In this scheme fat measures about −100 HU and most normal soft tissues about 30 to 60 HU. The information thus obtained can be displayed on a television monitor

or radiographic film, and one can control the various shades of gray depicting the different radiographic densities.

CT images are usually viewed at two window settings, one bringing out mediastinal and chest wall structures and the other optimizing visualization of the lungs. Occasionally, views are selected that allow excellent visualization of bony structures (bone windows).

The main advantage of CT over plain radiography is the fact that one can resolve many more densities than the four basic radiographic densities; this is referred to as superior

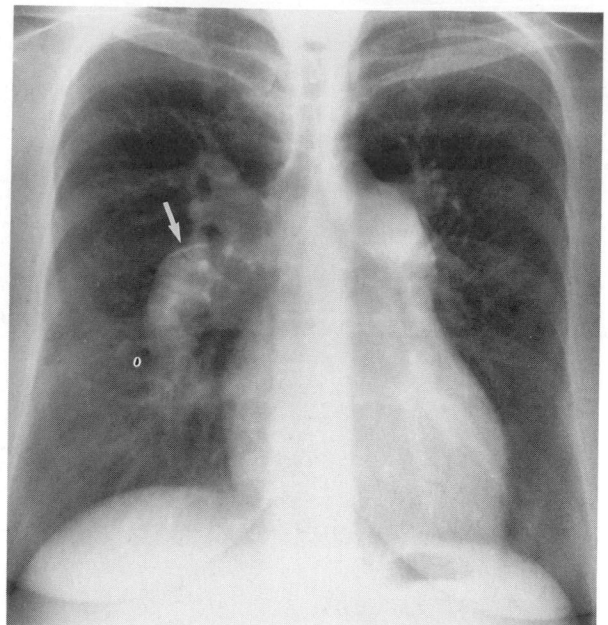
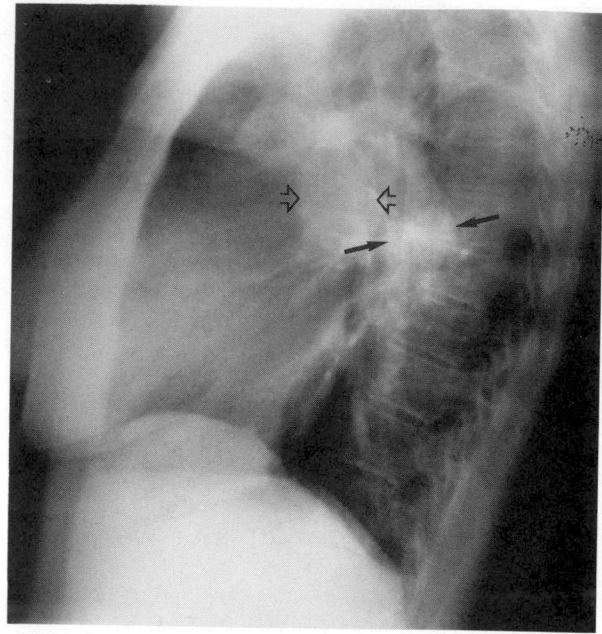

Figure 2-14. Hilar enlargement. **(A & B)** Pulmonary arterial enlargement in a 34-year-old woman with an atrial septal defect. Note the marked enlargement of both hila with a smooth configuration bilaterally. Calcium is noted in the right pulmonary artery on the PA view (*arrow*). Significant enlargement of both arteries is also well demonstrated on the lateral view (right pulmonary artery, *open arrows;* left pulmonary artery, *closed arrows*). (*Figure continues.*)

contrast resolution. Another advantage is the ability to image in the transverse plane. While spatial resolution was a problem with early machines, one can now visualize structures less than 1 mm in size. Disadvantages of CT scanning include its cost, the length of time required (about 30 minutes), the radiation dose (between 2 and 100 times more than a plain PA chest radiograph, depending on the CT technique), and the fact that intravenous contrast material is frequently needed to aid in visualization of vascular structures.

A standard CT study of the thorax consists of multiple 1-cm thick contiguous images from the lung apices to the lowest portions of the lungs. Depending on the clinical indication, intravenous contrast material may or may not be administered. It is important that the attending radiologist be provided with appropriate clinical information prior to the CT examination so that an informed decision regarding contrast (as well as other technical considerations) can be made. For example, in the workup of a patient with a solitary pulmonary nodule, it is very important that the study be done without contrast, while the investigation of a patient with suspected arteriovenous malformations must have contrast. In addition, there are instances in which the fine detail of the pulmonary parenchyma must be assessed. For example, the latter is necessary when working up patients with a solitary pulmonary nodule, a diffuse infiltrative lung disease, or bronchiectasis (see below). In these circumstances, so-called high-resolution CT (HRCT) is performed. With HRCT slices 1 to 1.5 mm thick are obtained. In addition, the images are created by using a high-detail type of reconstruction algorithm. With this technique, structures as small as 0.6 to 0.7 mm can be visualized. One can both detect disease that may otherwise be undetectable and accurately assess the type of disease

that is present, as well as its relationship to normal structures such as bronchi or interlobular septi.

Because of its superior contrast resolution, CT is extremely useful in determining if a mass lesion seen on the chest radiograph is solid, cystic, or fatty, features that obviously are of great benefit in determining the significance of the lesion as well as in narrowing the differential diagnosis (Fig. 2-15). For example, a cardiophrenic angle mass of uncertain etiology on plain radiography may be shown to definitely represent a foramen of Morgagni hernia, a pericardial cyst, or a solid mass such as a mesothelioma. In the mediastinum CT may provide other very helpful ancillary information. For example, if multiple enlarged lymph nodes in many mediastinal stations are seen in association with an anterior mediastinal mass, this suggests lymphoma rather than a thymoma. In addition, it may help determine if the mass is involving adjacent mediastinal structures (suspected by loss of the fat plane between the mass and these structures).

Uncommonly, there are instances in which plain tomography provides information less evident on CT. For example, in certain cases of round atelectasis, vessels curve into the mass from above downward; these are better visualized by anteroposterior (AP) or lateral plain tomography than by CT because of the restriction of the latter to the transverse plane.

MAGNETIC RESONANCE IMAGING

Although it has been shown to be very useful in many other areas, especially the central nervous system (CNS), MRI has limited practical use in the thorax (excluding cardiac and aortic indications, for which it is extremely useful). As with CT, images are created by manipulating raw data within a computer; however, with MRI ionizing radiation is not used

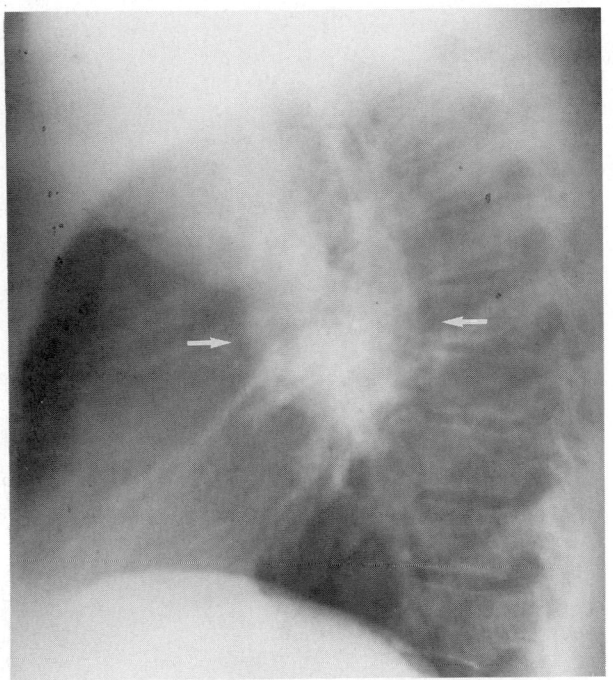

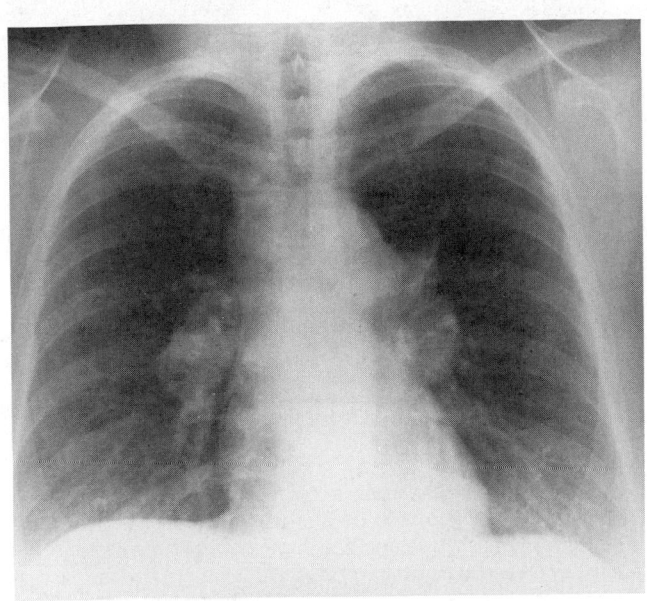

C

D

Figure 2-14 (*Continued*). **(C & D)** Lymphadenopathy. The hila are enlarged bilaterally in a lobulated fashion in this 29-year-old woman with sarcoidosis. The adenopathy is well seen on the lateral view as well (*arrows*). Enlarged nodes are also present in the right tracheobronchial angle region and AP window. **(E)** Hilar mass. Bronchogenic carcinoma involving the right hilum in a 29-year-old woman.

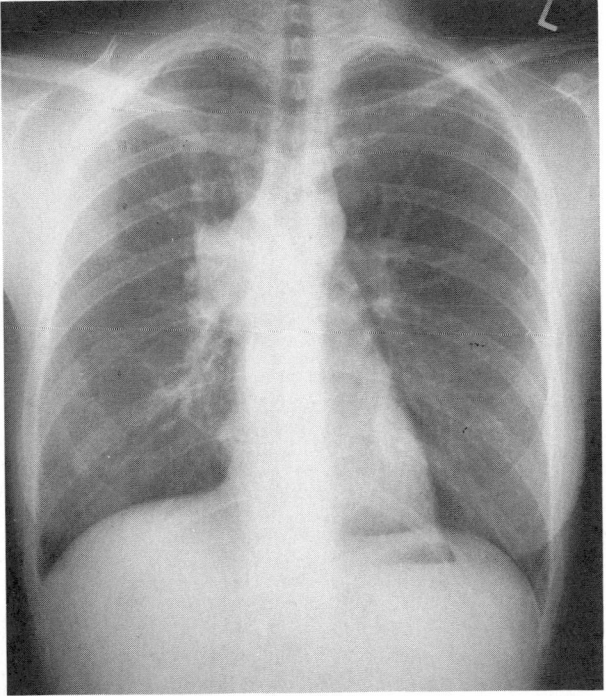

E

but instead one uses a very strong magnetic field and radio waves. Technical details are beyond the scope of this chapter, and the reader is referred to other sources (Newhouse and Wiener, 1991).

MRI is contraindicated in patients with pacemakers, ferromagnetic prosthetic cardiac valves (older Starr-Edwards valves only, all others are not magnetic), ferromagnetic intracranial aneurysm clips, or metallic fragments in the eye or spinal cord (Naidich, et al., 1991). In addition, a number of patients cannot tolerate the procedure because of claustrophobia.

Advantages of MRI over CT scanning include excellent visualization of vascular structures without the use of intravenous contrast material, avoidance of ionizing radiation, and the ability to image the patient in any plane desired, not just the transverse plane as with CT (Fig. 2-16). In addition, since MRI is based on physical properties different from those of CT, it may distinguish differences between two tissues that

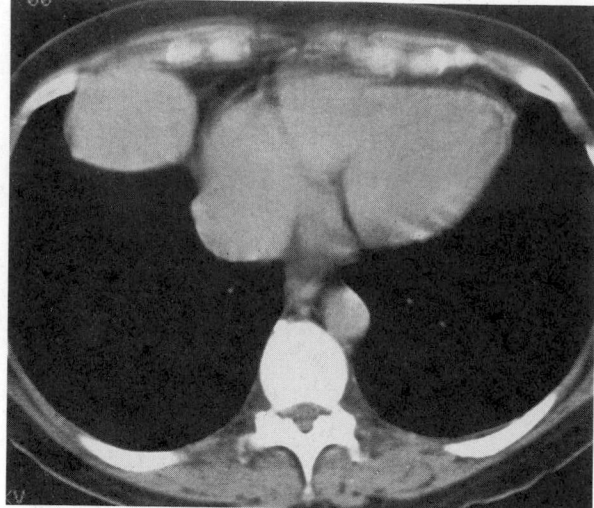

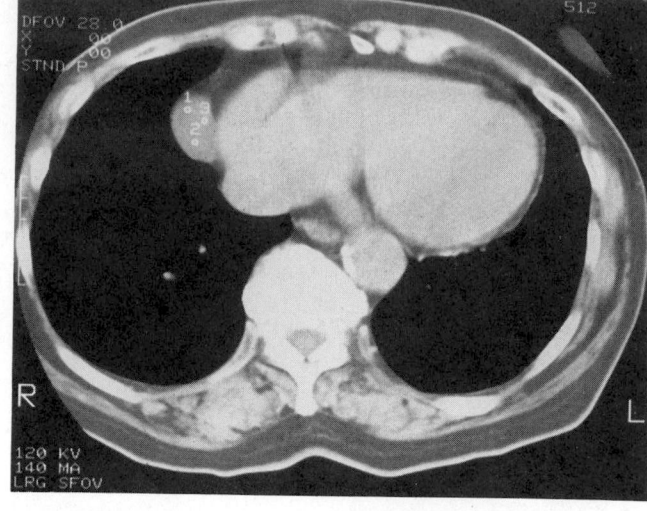

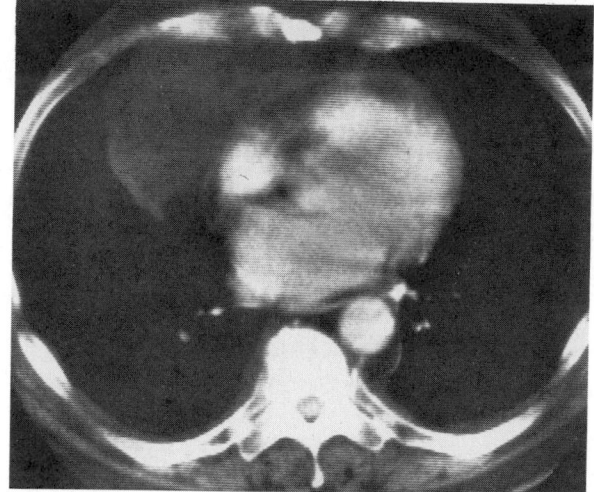

Figure 2-15.   Cardiophrenic angle masses. **(A)** CT scan on same patient shown in Figure 2-6. The right cardiophrenic angle mass is soft tissue in density (compare with paraspinal muscles) and was ultimately proved to be a benign mesothelioma. **(B)** Pericardial cyst. CT scan from a patient whose PA chest radiograph also showed a mass at the right cardiophrenic angle. In this case the CT scan shows that the mass is of water density (note that its density is lower than that of paraspinal muscles; its measured density was −1.7 HU). **(C)** Foramen of Morgagni hernia. Note the large "mass" in the region of the anterior right cardiophrenic angle, which has a density of fat. More inferiorly, colon was noted within these herniated abdominal contents.

CT cannot. In general, MRI is more expensive and less readily available than CT, and therefore its use should be confined to cases in which it provides information not obtainable with CT.

NUCLEAR IMAGING

Nuclear imaging studies differ fundamentally from conventional imaging in the way that images are produced. With conventional imaging, radiation is emitted by an external source, passes through the patient, and strikes a radiation detector (e.g. a film cassette or CT detector). With nuclear imaging, a radiation source is administered to the patient; the emitted radiation passes out from its sites of localization and strikes an external detector. A number of different radioisotopes are available, and each has certain advantages and disadvantages, a discussion of which is beyond the scope of this chapter. These radioisotopes are attached to one of a number of different vehicles, which can be delivered to the patient by one of a number of different methods; the choice of vehicle and delivery method determine the ultimate distri-

bution pattern of the radiation (see Fig. 18-31). Images can be created by so-called planar imaging or by single-photon emission CT (SPECT). In the former, a two-dimensional image is created by a stationary gamma camera located over a particular body part. With SPECT, three-dimensional information is obtained by having the gamma camera rotate around the patient while data are being collected; these data are then processed by a computer, and multiple tomographic images in one of many possible planes are created.

ANGIOGRAPHY

Pulmonary angiography involves placement of a catheter into the main pulmonary artery (frequently into the right or left pulmonary artery as well as into more peripheral branches) followed by injection of radiographic contrast material while rapid filming takes place. Images are obtained during both arterial and venous phases, providing visualization of pulmonary arteries and veins respectively.

Bronchial arteriography involves selective placement of a catheter into a bronchial artery followed by injection of con-

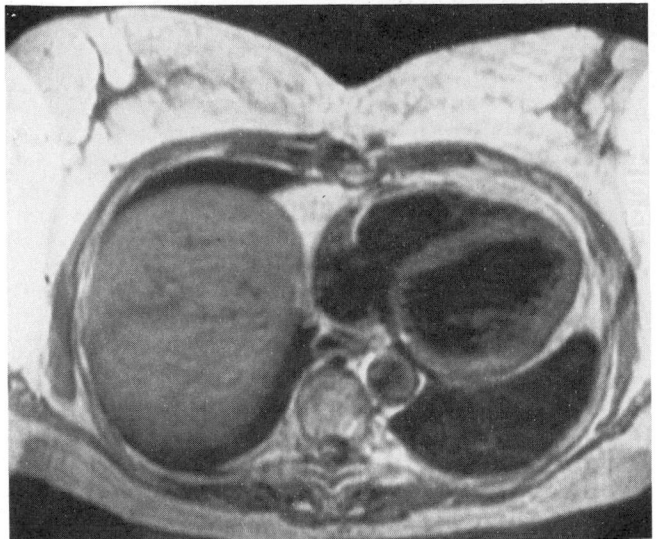

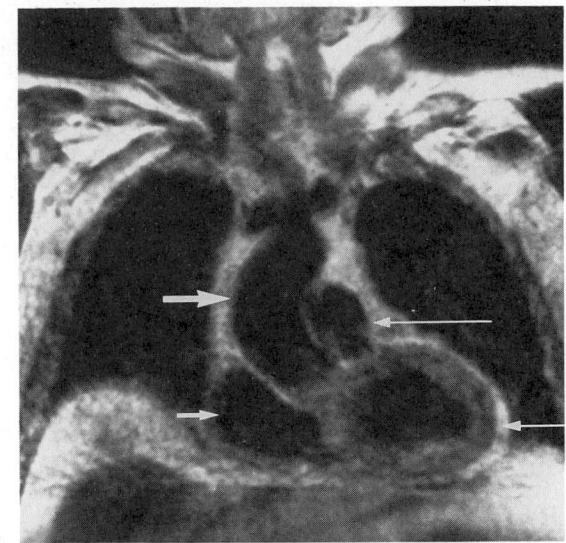

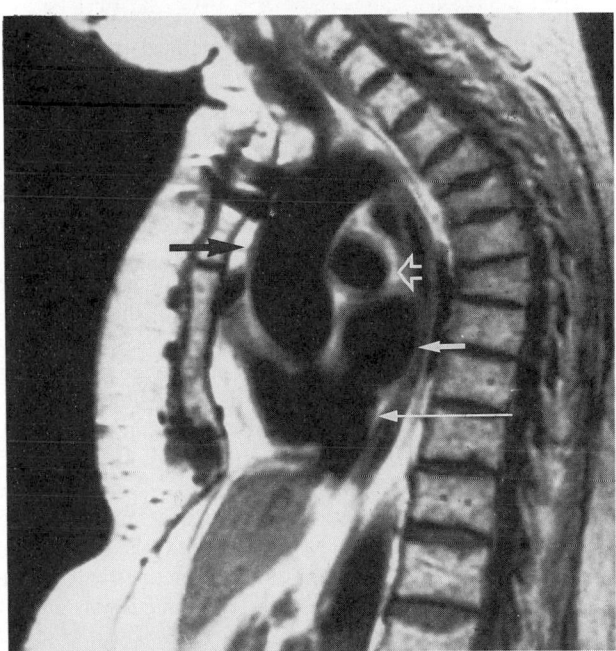

Figure 2-16. T₁-weighted MRI scans of the thorax. **(A)** Imaging in the transverse plane at the level of the heart. **(B)** Imaging in the coronal plane with visualization of the right atrium (*short wide arrows*), left ventricle (*short narrow arrows*), ascending aorta (*long wide arrow*), and main pulmonary artery (*long narrow arrow*). **(C)** Imaging in the sagittal plane with visualization of the left atrium (*short white arrow*), left ventricle (*long white arrow*), right pulmonary artery (*open arrow*), and ascending aorta (*black arrow*).

trast material (see Fig. 18-34). Similarly, aortography is performed by contrast injection after placement of a catheter into the aorta (see Fig. 18-35).

DIGITAL AND SCANNING EQUILIZATION RADIOGRAPHY

A standard (analog) chest radiograph differs from a digital one in that the latter is divided into a two-dimensional matrix of discrete sections while the former is a more continuous image. There are a number of technical problems with analog imaging, which can, at least theoretically, be overcome with digital imaging. Several excellent articles dealing with the potential advantages of digital imaging over conventional radiography, as well as much more detailed information than will be presented here, are available for the interested reader (Aberle, et al., 1990; Fraser, et al., 1989; Goodman, et al., 1988).

Briefly, a digital image is one that is divided up into discrete sections called pixels (for picture elements), each of which has an individual value. This value is determined by the amount of x-radiation passing through the overlying portion of the patient's chest. Current digital images are usually composed of a matrix containing 1024 × 1024 or 2048 × 2048 pixels. The image can be created by obtaining a single image of the whole chest at once and then dividing it up into discrete pixels by one of several methods or by creating the image one pixel at a time using a very focused x-ray beam. This digital information can be stored in a computer, can be manipulated to enhance certain features, and can be displayed on standard radiographic film or on a video display terminal. The image is fixed if recorded on film but can be further manipulated to enhance certain features if displayed on a video terminal. One main advantage of digital radiography is its so-called wide latitude, which means that even over- and underexposed images can be made interpretable, which decreases or even eliminates the need for repeat studies.

Another significant advantage of digital radiography is the fact that film is not necessary. This allows the image to be viewed in a remote location and by more than one person at the same time and eliminates the problem of unlocatable radiographs. However, the technology required to handle the huge amount of data, including the storage, transmission, and display of such information, is very expensive and still in need of improvement before it can be widely used (Gray, et al., 1984). The amount of information in a digital chest radiograph is enormous; for example, an optical disc capable of storing about 1 million typewritten pages (about 15 years' worth of a large newspaper) can hold only 166 standard radiographs (Gray, et al., 1984). In spite of this, some believe that the benefits of digital radiography are such that by the year 2020, all chest radiographs in large medical centers will be digital in type (Fraser, et al., 1989).

A related but nondigital newer form of chest imaging is so-called scanning equilization radiography (the first commercially available system is called AMBER [advanced multiple-beam equalization radiography] by its manufacturer, Optical Industries Oldelft, Delft, the Netherlands). With this technique a narrow, pencil-shaped beam of x-radiation passes sequentially over the patient's chest in a series of vertical bands, which move from left to right until the entire chest is imaged. As the beam is moving, the blackness of the image is constantly being monitored and the strength of the beam rapidly modified so as to maintain a constant degree of visualization of all intrathoracic structures. For example, when the beam first encounters the mediastinum, more radiation is absorbed, so that the detectors receive less; this then triggers the system to increase the strength of the beam so that more radiation reaches the film. By this method, the mediastinum and retrodiaphragmatic regions appear blacker than on a standard film, and visualization of overlying lung is consequently improved (Fig. 2-17).

This field of radiology is currently undergoing rapid change as newer technical developments are coming into use. At present, a number of the clinical aspects of digital radiography have been assessed, although it is difficult to compare many of the published studies owing to differences in experimental design (Aberle, et al.,1990). Generally, it may offer improved visualization of mediastinal and hilar detail (Templeton, et al., 1987) as well as hilar and mediastinal disease (Goodman, et al., 1986). However, in one study (Fajardo, et al., 1989), pneumothoraces were better detected by conventional imaging than by digital radiography, although for four of the eight readers, the two methods were equivalent. This latter finding points to the fact that evaluation of digital systems is not a straightforward task; some readers may be able to adapt to it more readily than others. In a more recent study, there was no significant difference between the two methods in the detection of bullous lung disease (Buckley, et al., 1991).

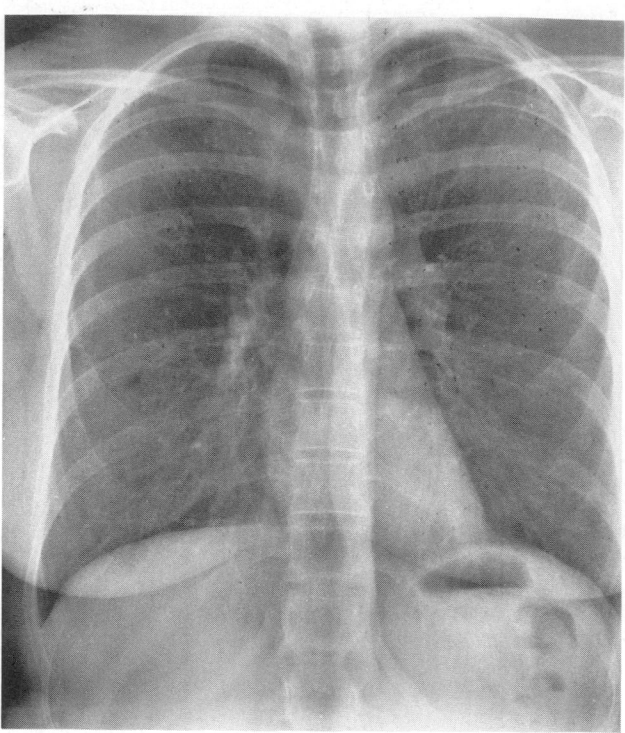

Figure 2-17. Scanning equalization radiograph. Note the clear visibility of both lungs in their entirety, including the retrocardiac and retrodiaphragmatic portions. (Courtesy of Dr. D. Plewes, Reichman Research Laboratory, University of Toronto.)

Pulmonary nodules were detected equally with both techniques in a study using a model of the thorax (Newell, et al,. 1988). Differing results were found in two other studies assessing the detection of pulmonary nodules: there was superior visualization with digital imaging in one (Cox, et al., 1990), whereas a second study revealed improved visualization with analog film (Aberle, et al., 1988). Similarly, in still another study, analog film was better than digital radiography in assessing both pneumothoraces and interstitial disease (Batra, et al., 1989). It is expected that as technology improves, digital radiography will become equivalent to, and in some instances better than, conventional imaging for all types of chest disease and will eventually replace it (Fraser, et al., 1989).

Definite improvement over standard radiography has been demonstrated with scanning equalization radiography in a number of studies for assessment of both normal structures (Wandtke, et al., 1985) and pathologic states (Wandtke and Plewes, 1985). Improved visualization of mediastinal, retrocardiac, and subdiaphragmatic regions has been demonstrated (Chotas, et al., 1991).

ACKNOWLEDGMENT

I wish to thank Rose Baldwin for her assistance with the preparation of this manuscript.

KEY REFERENCES

Fraser RG, Pare JAP, Pare PD et al.: Diagnosis of Diseases of the Chest, 3rd Ed. WB Saunders, Philadelphia, 1988–1991

This four-volume set is encyclopedic in scope and contains the answer to virtually any question that one could ask dealing with chest disease, whether it concerns etiology, epidemiology, pathology, clinical manifestations, or pulmonary function, in addition to imaging. Therapeutics are not covered. In addition to this information, it contains tables of differential diagnoses based on radiographic patterns, as well as over 20,000 references dealing with thoracic diseases.

Naidich DP, Zerhouni EA, Siegelman SS: Computed Tomography and Magnetic Resonance Imaging of the Thorax. 2nd Ed. Raven Press, New York, 1991, p. 21

This is a superb book, which thoroughly covers what its title suggests. It not only discusses the imaging findings in all important thoracic diseases, but it provides this information in a practical manner so that it is useful in day-to-day practice.

REFERENCES

Aberle DR, Batra P, Hayrapetian A et al.: Implementation of a dedicated digital projectional radiographic system in thoracic imaging. Radiology 169:354, 1988

Aberle DR, Hansell D, Huang HK: Current status of digital projectional radiolography of the chest. J Thorac Imaging 5:10, 1990

Batra P, Aberle DR, Brown K et al.: Computed radiography: a study of observer performance with a high-resolution dedicated chest unit. In Program of the Eighty-ninth Annual Meeting of the American Roentgen Ray Society, New Orleans. American Roentgen Ray Society, Pontiac, MI, 1989

Bergin CJ, Pauly JM, Macovski A: Lung parenchyma: projection reconstruction MR imaging. Radiology 179:777, 1991

Buckley KM, Schaefer CM, Greene R et al.: Detection of bullous lung disease: conventional radiography vs digital storage phosphor radiography. AJR 156:467, 1991

Chotas HG, Van Metter RL, Johnson GA, Ravin CE: Small object contrast in AMBER and conventional chest radiography. Radiology 180:853, 1991

Cox GG, Cook LT, McMillan JH et al.: Chest radiography: comparison of high-resolution digital displays with conventional and digital film. Radiology 176:771, 1990

Eisenberg RL: Radiology: an Illustrated History. Mosby-Year Book, St. Louis, 1991

Fajardo LL, Hillman BJ, Pond GD et al.: Detection of pneumothorax: comparison of digital and conventional chest imaging. AJR 152:475, 1989

Felson B: Chest Roentgenology. WB Saunders, Philadelphia, p. 105, 1973a

Felson B: Chest Roentgenology. WB Saunders, Philadelphia, p. 416, 1973b

Felson B: Chest Roentgenology. WB Saunders, Philadelphia, p. 498, 1973c

Felson B: Chest Roentgenology. WB Saunders, Philadelphia, p. 500, 1973d

Felson B, Felson H: Localization of intrathoracic lesions by means of the postero-anterior roentgenogram: the silhouette sign. Radiology 55:363, 1950

Fraser RG, Sanders C, Barnes GT et al.: Digital imaging of the chest. Radiology 171:297, 1989

Goodman LR, Foley WD, Wilson CR et al.: Digital and conventional chest images: observer performance with film digital radiography system. Radiology 158:27, 1986

Goodman LR, Wilson CR, Foley WD: Digital radiography of the chest: promises and problems. AJR 150:1241, 1988

Gordon R: The deep sulcus sign. Radiology 136:25, 1980

Gray JE, Karsell PR, Becker GP, Gehring DG: Total digital radiology: is it feasible? or desirable? AJR:1345, 1984

Lennon EA, Simon G: The height of the diaphragm in the chest radiograph of normal adults. Br J Radiol 38:937, 1965

Moskowitz H, Platt RT, Schachar R et al.: Roentgen visualization of minute pleural effusion: an experimental study to determine the minimum amount of pleural fluid visible on a radiograph. Radiology 109:33, 1973

Newell JD, Seeley G, Hagaman RM et al.: Computed radiographic evaluation of simulated pulmonary nodules: preliminary results. Invest Radiol 23:267, 1988

Newhouse JH, Wiener JI: Understanding MRI. Little, Brown, Boston, 1991

Templeton AW, Dwyer III SJ, Cox GG et al.: A digital radiology imaging system: description and clinical evaluation. AJR 149:847, 1987

Wandtke JC, Plewes DB: Improved chest disease detection with scanning equalization radiography. AJR 145:979, 1985

Wandtke JC, Plewes DP, Vogelstein E: Scanning equalization radiography of the chest: assessment of image quality. AJR 145:973, 1985

Ziter FM Jr, Westcott JL: Supine subpulmonary pneumothorax. AJR 137:699, 1981

3

PREOPERATIVE ASSESSMENT OF THE THORACIC SURGICAL PATIENT: A SURGEON'S VIEWPOINT

Robert J. Ginsberg

INTRODUCTION

The surgeon is trained to treat patients by invasive modalities. Despite the technical skills acquired, the surgeon first and foremost is a physician and must make use of the deductive skills acquired, not only to determine whether or not a therapeutic intervention is indicated or necessary but also to assess the suitability of the patient to undergo the surgical procedure. This initial assessment must not be delegated to other individuals.

In thoracic surgery, over two-thirds of postoperative complications are cardiopulmonary (Deslauriers, et al., 1989). In most cases cardiac complications tend to be minor (treatable arrhythmias), whereas pulmonary complications are more morbid and account for most deaths, usually due to respiratory failure.

In the field of general thoracic surgery, more often than not transthoracic or upper abdominal approaches are used. Because they inhibit postoperative respiratory mechanics, these interventions are associated with the highest postoperative cardiopulmonary morbidity rates. In most thorcic surgical practices the predominant illness treated is cancer-related. Our patients most frequently present between the sixth and eighth decades, each decade increasing the risk of postoperative morbidity and mortality (Ginsberg, et al., 1983, Deslauriers, et al., 1989). Associated cardiopulmonary disease is prevalent.

The necessity for a compulsive attitude toward preoperative evaluation cannot be emphasized enough. Technical misadventures do occur but rarely account for the problems seen following thoracic surgical procedures. The majority of postoperative complications and deaths are related to cardiopulmonary events, most of which can be identified and prevented prior to surgery. In addition, in pulmonary surgery, the surgeon must ensure that the anticipated resection will allow the patient a reasonable quality of life without chronic respiratory failure.

INITIAL PATIENT ENCOUNTER

The initial patient encounter is by far the most important step in preoperative assessment. Major predictors of postoperative complications include extent of resection, significant cardiopulmonary disease, age and other co-morbid conditions (e.g., diabetes, other systemic illnesses, immune-depressive diseases and drugs, obesity, recent weight loss) (Kohlman, et al., 1986, Wahi, et al., 1989). All these factors must be assessed. The Dripps–American Society of Anesthesiologists classification (Table 3-1) subdivides individuals into five risk categories, which have been correlated with both the morbidity and mortality of operative procedures.

The skills acquired in history taking, physical examination, and judicious use of laboratory investigation must be honed to perfection. It is a truism that over 75 percent of the first encounter with the patient should be devoted to accurate history taking. This initial step not only confirms the diagnosis and determines the indications and the necessity of the potential surgical intervention but also determines the suitability of the patient to undergo such a procedure, the extent of co-morbid disease, and the need for further testing. Accurate history taking can predict 95 percent of all diagnoses and can predict and hopefully thereby prevent most potential postoperative problems. A complete physical examination should never be ignored or delegated to a nonphysician. Use of these tools so painstakingly developed during the medical school apprenticeship in every patient encounter will serve the physician-surgeon well; failure to use them will lead to misdiagnoses, inappropriate treatment, and preventable disasters.

Table 3-1. Dripps–American Society of Anesthesiologists Risk Classification and Associated Estimated Mortality of General Anesthesia

Class	Description	% Mortality
1	Normal, healthy	0.08
2	Mild to moderate systemic disease	0.27
3	Severe systemic disease, limited activity	1.8
4	Incapacitating, life-threatening systemic disease	7.8
5	Moribund, 24-hour life expectancy without surgery	9.4

All premorbid conditions must be identified and optimized prior to surgical treatment. Although multivariant analyses have not consistently demonstrated the same adverse prognostic factors, those that seem to be most significant other than intrinsic cardiopulmonary disease include recent weight loss greater than 10 percent, age over 70 years, and in cancer surgery, the type and stage of the tumor.

Other factors that may predict a poor outcome from surgical intervention are difficult to classify. It has been my distinct impression that the patient's attitude toward the disease, the desire to have a favorable outcome, and confidence in the doctor are predictive of success. A prospective analysis of quality of life following lung cancer treatment, performed by the Lung Cancer Study Group (Ruckdeschel, et al., 1991), confirmed that the patient's attitude toward the disease was

---

Determinants of Postoperative Morbidity and Mortality[a]

Cardiac disease
Pulmonary disease
Tumor characteristics
    Stage
    Type
General medical conditions
    Diabetes
    Creatinine level
    Hemoglobin level
    Serum albumin level
    Immunosuppressed status
        Steroids
        Chemotherapy
        Other chronic illnesses
    Weight loss >10%
    Age >70
Anticipated surgery
Extent of resection
Additional procedures
Side of pulmonary resection (R > L)
Previous surgery

---

[a] Significant cardiopulmonary disease and tumor stage and extent of resection appear to be the most significant determinants.

---

the best predictor of long-term survival. Except in emergency life-threatening situations, patients should never be cajoled or forced into accepting surgery. In most cases this will lead to disastrous results. At times it is best to deny surgical intervention to the patient with a significant negative outlook, especially if other curative options (e.g., radiotherapy for cancer, medical therapy in reflux disease) are available.

PULMONARY ASSESSMENT

Pulmonary complications, especially retained secretions, atelectasis, pneumonia, and respiratory failure, are the most significant problems following thoracic surgical procedures (Deslauriers, et al., 1989; Ginsberg, et al., 1983). Most patients who are present or ex-smokers have underlying pulmonary problems, especially chronic obstructive lung disease and chronic bronchitis, and most have at least some compromise of pulmonary function.

History

Cardiopulmonary Reserve

A reasonable assessment of cardiopulmonary reserve can be determined by history taking alone. The dyspnea grade correlates well with pulmonary function testing.

Smoking

A smoking history is relevant. Patients who continue to smoke have a significantly increased risk of postoperative complications, and whenever possible surgery should be delayed until smoking has been stopped for a minimum of 1 to 2 weeks. The use of a transdermal nicotine patch has made preoperative smoking cessation an achievable goal.

Sputum Production

Daily sputum production, whenever present, should be quantified, and whenever possible, steps should be taken to decrease this production to minimal levels (cessation of smoking, antibiotics, postural drainage when indicated). If sputum production is present, preoperative sputum cultures may identify a chronic infection from a specific organism, which should be treated prior to surgical intervention.

Ability to Cough

The evaluation of the ability of patients to cough by using diaphragmatic and accessory respiratory muscles is an important but often ignored preoperative assessment of real value. Many patients do not know how to produce an effective cough but can be taught preoperatively, so that a more effective cough will be present in the postoperative period. I have found that this type of instruction together with the use of incentive spirometry improves postoperative pulmonary toilet.

Pulmonary Function Testing

Mountains of literature are available on the value of preoperative pulmonary function testing. The tests range from the

Table 3-2. Criteria of Pulmonary Function for Lung Resection

PFT	Normal	Pneumonectomy	Lobectomy	Wedge or Segment Resection	Inoperable
MVV	>80%	>55%	>40%	>35%	<35%
FEV$_1$	>2 L	>2 L	>1 L	>0.6 L	<0.6 L
FEV$_{25-75}$	>2 L	>1.6 L	>0.6 L	>0.6 L	<0.6 L
Stair climbing	>2 flights	2 flights	1 flight	<1 flight	

Abbreviations: PFT, pulmonary function test; MVV, maximal voluntary ventilation (% predicted); FEV$_1$, forced expiratory volume in 1 second, FEV$_{25-75}$, forced expiratory flow rate from 25 to 75%.

(Adapted from Miller JI: Thallium imaging in preoperative evaluation of the pulmonary resection candidate. Ann Thorac Surg 54:249, 1992, with permission.)

simplest medical assessment (history taking, physical examination, stair climbing, and the "match" test) to the most sophisticated exercise testing with calculation of maximal oxygen uptake (VO$_2$max) and invasive pulmomary artery pressure (PAP) measurements. All such testing has value (Tables 3-2 and 3-3). It has been well demonstrated that stair climbing of a fixed height, especially when combined with pulse oximetry, is probably the only cardiopulmonary test required in most patients who otherwise have normal function (Bolton et al., 1987; Olsen, ct al., 1991). However, for a variety of reasons, including medicolegal, preoperative spirometry, estimation of carbon monoxide diffusing capacity (DLCO), and determination of arterial blood gases should be carried out on all patients undergoing thoracic surgical procedures. These relatively simple tests are all that is necessary

Table 3-3. Predictors of Postoperative Mortality and Morbidity

Test	Predictive of Increased Morbidity	Prohibitive
Clinical		
Stair climbing	<3 flights (12 m height)	<1 flight
Match test	Failed	
Dyspnea grade	2–4	4
Pulmonary Mechanics		
MVV	<50 L/min	<35% predicted
FEV$_1$	<50% FVC	<0.6 L
FVC	<50% predicted	<1.0 L
FEV$_1$/FVC	<60% predicted	<50%
Gas Exchange		
DLCO	<50%	<30%
PO$_2$ & SaO$_2$	Desaturation on exercise	PO$_2$ <45 mmHg
PCO$_2$ & actual HCO$_3$ elevated		PCO$_2$ >50 mmHg
V̇/Q̇ Scanning Prediction		
FEV$_1$	<30% predicted	<0.8 L predicted
VC		<1 L predicted
Exercise Testing		
VO$_2$max	<20 ml/kg/min	<10 ml/kg/min
PVR		>190 dynes/s/cm^5

Abbreviations: MVV, maximal voluntary ventilation; FEV$_1$, forced expiratory volume in 1 second; FVC, forced vital capacity; DLCO, carbon monoxide diffusion capacity; V̇/Q̇, ventilation/perfusion; VC, vital capacity, VO$_2$max, maximal oxygen uptake; PVR, pulmonary vascular resistance.

(Data from multiple treatises.)

in most individuals. Abnormalities of these tests as outlined in Table 3-3 indicate a higher risk of developing postoperative complications. When resection of pulmonary tissue is anticipated, further pulmonary testing may be of value, including ventilation/perfusion scanning to predict postresection pulmonary capacity (Boysen, et al., 1977; Ali, et al., 1980) and function and exercise testing to determine oxygen saturation after exercise and VO$_2$max (Jones, 1975). The latter two tests assess general fitness as well as pulmonary function.

The forced expiratory volume in 1 second (FEV$_1$), which is used by many as the primary predictor of function and resectability, can be misleading in many patients, especially those who are of small stature or who have significant tracheomalacia. The latter patients will have an abnormally low FEV$_1$, and on physical examination, forced expiratory maneuvers will cause them to produce an audible large airway expiratory wheeze. This malacia can be confirmed by imaging maneuvers (tracheogram, dynamic computed tomography [CT] scan, or ultrasound) or by using fiberoptic bronchoscopy in an awake setting to assess airways collapse by forced expiratory maneuvers. Such patients frequently can tolerate pulmonary resection despite an unusually low FEV$_1$, especially if appropriate breathing instruction and preoperative control of excessive sputum can be accomplished. Other reasons for a falsely low FEV, include small body habitus or obstructed airways in diseased areas to be removed. The FEV$_1$/FVC ratio is a better predictor of postoperative complications, since it assesses the obstructive pulmonary component more accurately.

Blood Gas Assessment

Arterial blood gas analysis has become an essential preoperative assessment. On occasion, an unexpected extremely low preoperative oxygen pressure will indicate that further cardiopulmonary testing is required. Oxygen desaturation on exercise also indicates the need for further investigation. Patients with resting hypercarbia usually have cor pulmonale and can rarely tolerate a pneumonectomy but may be suitable candidates for lesser resections. In addition, patients who have an elevated bicarbonate as measured by serum electrolytes (not the bicarbonate calculated with blood gas analysis) must be investigated for possible carbon dioxide retention and cor pulmonale. Usually, abnormalities in blood gas analysis are associated with abnormalities seen on DLCO estimation, although the DLCO can vary enormously from laboratory to laboratory.

The risk of anesthesia and surgical intervention, especially when combined with pulmonary resection, cannot be exactly determined for any individual patient. Guidelines for prediction of high risks and contraindications to pulmonary resection have been suggested by many authors (Tables 3-2 and 3-3). Although most of these guidelines are relative, it appears that absolute contraindications to resection include a predicted postoperative FEV_1 of less than 0.8 L no matter the type of resection, a VO_2max of less than 10 ml/kg/min, and in the case of pneumonectomy, a resting elevated carbon dioxide pressure or cor pulmonale. However, even these criteria on occasion are not absolute, especially in dealing with small patients.

Despite all guidelines, the final preoperative pulmonary assessment of the patient depends on the experience of the assessor. There is no formula, no absolute criterion, and,in the case of curable lung cancer, in view of the alternative treatments, no absolute contraindication to surgical intervention. One must remember that these parameters predict morbidity, most of which is recoverable, and in the case of lung cancer treatment such recoverable morbidity may be acceptable. Moreover, I have been frequently pleasantly surprised at the improvement obtained by prolonged and intensive pulmonary rehabilitation and the smoothness of the postoperative course in patients initially deemed totally inoperable by standard functional assessments. An algorithm suggested by Miller (1992) is a valuable guideline, but even this cannot be considered absolute (Fig. 3-1).

Pulmonary Rehabilitation

Whenever possible, preoperative pulmonary assessment, especially in compromised individuals, should be performed at least 2 weeks prior to anticipated surgery. This allows enough time to correct deficiencies (by use of antibiotics, bronchodi-

lators when indicated, relief of airway obstructions to reduce infection, etc.) and improve function. In some individuals, prolonged preoperative intensive rehabilitation may significantly improve pulmonary function and thereby allow surgical intervention that otherwise would have been contraindicated. This should always be attempted before denying patients a curative surgical procedure. In some cases up to 2 months of preoperative therapy, including progressive pulmonary rehabilitation, may be required to optimally prepare the patient for surgery.

Preoperative bronchodilator therapy can be extremely useful in improving pulmonary function. If steroids are to be used, whenever possible the benefit of such therapy should be documented and as low a dose as possible should be employed in the perioperative period. Even in the minimally compromised individual, preoperative cardiopulmonary rehabilitation will have value. A program that we have found to be useful in our institution is outlined on the following page.

CARDIOVASCULAR ASSESSMENT

The risk of both morbidity and mortality from surgery increases exponentially in patients with significant cardiovascular disease. In the general population, the risk of a postoperative myocardial infarction following general anesthesia is 0.07 percent. However, this risk increases with a history of previous remote infarction, and is significant when a myocardial infarction has occurred within 3 months of the expected surgery (Arkins, et al., 1964, Steen, 1978). Similar risks have been identified for patients with angina, with an increasing risk for each class of the New York Heart Association Angina Classification (Table 3-4). Similarly, increasing postoperative morbidity and mortality correlate with the New York Heart Association functional class describing dyspnea associated with congestive heart failure. Cardiac predictors of increased

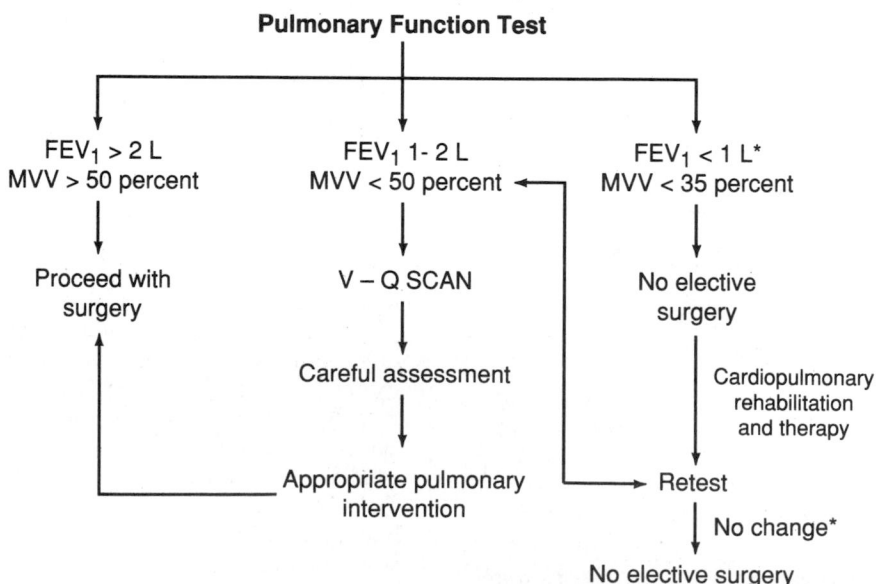

Figure 3-1. An algorithm suggesting the schema for evaluating pulmonary function. *The absolute numbers indicated are not absolute and depend on the individual. In selected cases FEV_1 may be as low as 0.6 L/min. (Adapted from Miller JI: Preoperative evaluation. Chest Surg Clin North Am 4:701, 1992, with permission.)

Preoperative Exercise Program[a]

This program includes strengthening and flexibility exercises to improve muscle conditioning before surgery.

Arm exercises—improve strength and flexibility

1. Sitting or standing position
2. Place arms out at shoulder level; arms are straight, parallel to floor
3. On breathing in: raise arms above head, touching both palms above head, hold for 2 seconds
4. On breathing out: lower arms slowly, exhale through pursed lips, stop when arms are parallel to floor

Leg exercises—improve strength

1. Sitting position
2. Lift leg off chair, tightening muscles on top of thigh, then extend leg straight, hold for 3 seconds
3. Bend knee and lower slowly, relax then repeat

Repeat 10 times; perform 10 times daily

Sniff and blow—improve strength of diaphragm

1. Sitting position
2. Sniff twice, hold breath for 2 to 3 seconds
3. Tighten stomach muscles and blow out slowly

Repeat 10 times; perform 10 times daily
Walk 1 mile twice daily, in less than 20 minutes
Climb 2 flights of stairs, quickly, 4 times daily
Use incentive spirometer for 10 minutes, 4 times daily

Mobilization—improve mobility and flexibility

1. Sitting position
2. Breathe in, raise arms above head, crossing wrists
3. Breathe out, pursed lip breathing
   Bend forward touching chest to top of thigh (if possible)
   Lowering arms to floor (try to touch fingers to floor)
4. Uncross arms
   Breathe in
   Raise upper body upright
   Stretch arms above head

Cough technique

1. Sitting position
2. Breathe in deeply 5 times, then
3. Hold breath for 2 seconds
4. Contract abdominal muscles (bearing down)
5. Cough, while maintaining contraction of abdominal muscles
6. Practice this 4 times daily

---

[a] Developed by my Thoracic Surgical Service and given to patients at their initial encounter. (Developed in association with D. Wilson R.N., R.T. and L. Wall, R.N.)

Table 3-4. The New York Heart Association Angina Classification

Class	Description
1	Angina with strenuous exercise
2	Angina with moderate exercise
3	Angina with 1 flight of stairs or 1 to 2 blocks
4	Angina with any activity

risk include hypertension, valvular heart disease, cardiac conduction abnormalities, and preoperative dysrhythmias.

For these reasons, an accurate cardiac history is of utmost importance in the preoperative assessment, including documentation of all cardiovascular medications used. A routine electrocardiogram is considered part of the physical examination, as important as auscultation of the heart, measurement of blood pressure, and examination for focal vascular lesions of the carotids, aorta and femoral vessels.

The overall estimation of cardiac risk has been documented by Goldman (1983), who used nine significant preoperative risk factors and assessed a point value by multivariant risk analysis (Table 3-5). It is likely that with modern postoperative care, the risks engendered are much less than originally predicted. Patients in class 3 or 4 according to this risk index require significant preoperative investigation and almost certainly benefit from intensive perioperative monitoring, including the use of intraoperative and postoperative pulmonary artery pressure monitoring. For pulmonary resectional

Table 3-5. Goldman Cardiac Risk Index (1983)[a]

Factors	Points
History	
Age >70	5
Myocardial infarction, <6 mo	10
Physical	
Congestive failure	11
Aortic stenosis	3
Electrocardiogram	
Rhythm abnormality	7
PVCs >5/min	7
General	
PO_2 <60 mmHg, PCO_2 >50 mmHg, HCO_3 <20 mg/L, ↑ creatinine Liver disease ↑ performance status	3
Type of operation	
Intraperitoneal or intrathoracic	3
Emergency	4
Total possible points	53

Class	Points	Severe Morbidity	Cardiac Death
1	0–5	0.7%	0.2%
2	6–12	5%	2%
3	13–25	11%	2%
4	>26	22%	56%

Abbreviation: PVCs, premature ventricular contractions.

[a] With more modern perioperative care, the risks for each class are probably less than those originally predicted.

surgery, Epstein et al. (1993) have correlated this type of risk index to VO_2max which is an estimate of total physical fitness, thus suggesting that VO_2max is as predictable as other indices already discussed.

Exercise Stress Testing

Much more difficult and germane is the need for preoperative identification of occult coronary artery disease in presumed healthy patients. With increasing frequency, exercise stress tests are being added to routine cardiac assessment for all preoperative thoracic surgical patients over age 45 or with other risk factors. Occult coronary artery disease can be revealed, which would indicate the need for more sophisticated testing.

Thallium Imaging

For those patients with a positive exercise stress test or a significant history of coronary artery or peripheral vascular disease, exercise thallium testing is indicated. In those patients with no coronary artery disease history, a normal exercise tolerance test, or a normal thallium test or fixed defect on thallium testing, the risk at surgery, especially in relation to postoperative major cardiac events, is minimal (Miller, 1992b; Lette, et al., 1989). The value of preoperative thallium imaging is its ability to identify reversible ischemia with viable myocardium that should be treated prior to thoracotomy. There have been several studies showing a high risk of perioperative cardiac events, including death, for those patients who have untreated reversible ischemic defect, in contradistinction to those patients who have fixed defects, in whom the risk of perioperative cardiac events is small (Lette, et al., 1990). Miller (1992b) has developed an algorithm for cardiovascular evaluation of patients older than 45 years of age (Fig. 3-2). On the basis of this algorithm, 275 of 2,340 patients were selected to undergo thallium imaging. Approximately 50 percent of these 275 patients had normal thallium imaging;

of those with abnormal imaging, 50 percent had fixed defects. Reversible ischemic changes were identified in approximately 25 percent of all patients undergoing imaging (1.5 percent of all patients) and were corrected prior to surgical exploration. The mortality was zero in this group of patients. However, some believe that documented ischemia on stress testing or a significant cardiac or vascular disease history warrants coronary angiography without the need for thallium testing (Jewell, 1985), pointing out the significant false negative rates of stress testing.

It appears that in future a more aggressive, proactive approach should be adopted for most patients who have an abnormal exercise tolerance test or history of coronary artery disease, despite a normal electrocardiogram. Whether or not all patients over the age of 60 should undergo routine thallium imaging despite a normal exercise tolerance test is yet to be determined.

CO-MORBID DISEASES

It is important to identify co-morbid diseases suffered by the patient (e.g., malnutrition, diabetes, peripheral vascular disease, other endocrinopathies), to ensure that these diseases have been optimally controlled and that no further preoperative intervention or treatment is required. Routine screening of significant electrolytes and blood chemicals will help to identify occult intercurrent disease. When necessary, appropriate consultations with specific specialists may be required for concurrent management of these illnesses. Whenever possible, all such co-morbid diseases should be stabilized and treated prior to surgical intervention.

CONCLUSIONS

The preoperative assessment of the thoracic surgical patient is of inestimable value in anticipating and preventing postoperative complications and lessening postoperative morbidity

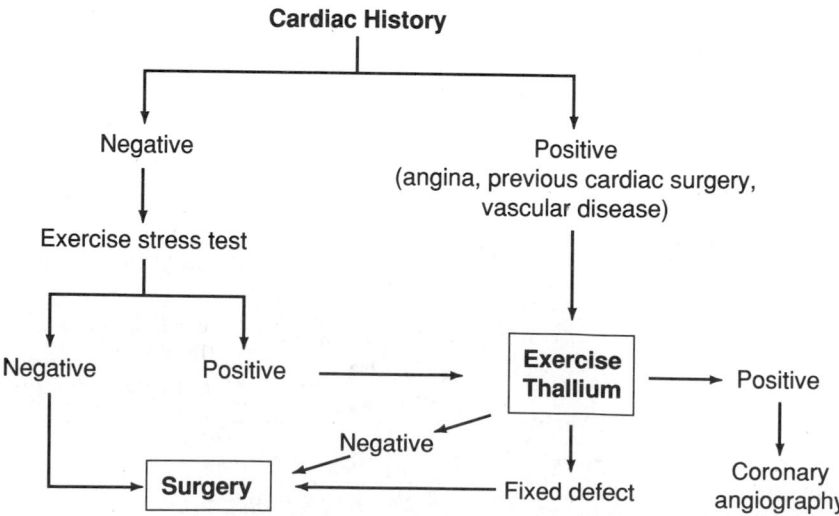

Figure 3-2. A suggested algorithm for investigating the cardiac status of all patients over the age of 45 or those with significant risk factors undergoing major thoracic surgery. (Adapted from Miller JI: Preoperative evaluation. Chest Surg Clin North Am 4:701, 1992, with permission.)

and mortality. The thoracic surgeon need not and should not abrogate the responsibility of this initial assessment, which requires a complete history and physical examination, judicious use of cardiopulmonary testing, and screening for other co-morbid diseases. Where indicated, pulmonary rehabilita-

tion, treatment of occult or manifest cardiac disease, and optimization of the treatment of other co-morbid disease will decrease the risks associated with major thoracic surgical interventions and hopefully lessen perioperative morbidity and mortality.

COMMENTS AND CONTROVERSIES

In this chapter, Dr. Ginsberg has shown the importance of careful preoperative assessment of the thoracic surgical patient. This assessment is important not only for identifying the patient at risk but also for preventing complications and predicting postoperative quality of life.

As outlined by Dr. Ginsberg, history taking is a most important step in preoperative assessment. It is worth noting, however, that the level of dyspnea does not always correlate with results of pulmonary function tests because patients often adjust their life style and level of activities according to their respiratory limitations. For this reason, all patients having thoracic operations should have screening pulmonary function studies. FEV at various time intervals are good predictors of operative risk, but it should be stressed that spirometric values are a function of age, sex, and height, so it is best to look at percentage of predicted value rather than absolute value. In addition, it has been shown that 6 to 12 months after resection, FEV_1 values often return to preoperative levels, especially if the patient has stopped smoking (which occurs in 80 to 85 percent of resected patients).

There is a large body of literature stressing the importance of predicted FEV_1 as measured by isotopic scanning methods. Depending on the author, the lower level of predicted FEV_1 acceptable for operability varies between 0.8 and 1.0 L. These figures are based on medical studies that have shown that once an emphysematous patient has reached an FEV_1 of 0.8 L or less, complications and/or death from respiratory failure are likely to occur. This situation may, however, be different than the one in which FEV_1 is brought down to similar levels by pulmonary resection and in which the re-

maining parenchyma is uninvolved with progressive emphysema.

Most emphysematous patients, even with advanced disease, are able to maintain relatively normal PO_2 at rest. It is therefore imperative to do a graded exercise tolerance test with $\dot{V}O_2max$ and blood gas measurements in patients felt to be high-risk candidates. An elevated PCO_2 at rest or during exercise or desaturation with exercise is indicative of poor reserve and high-risk surgery.

Preoperative rehabilitation is important in the prophylaxis of postoperative pulmonary complications in compromised individuals. In addition to the measures described by Dr. Ginsberg, preoperative teaching regarding respiratory maneuvers and the procedure to come are most important. This teaching, done by physiotherapists, nurses, and other specialized personnel, will improve postoperative cooperation and reduce the incidence of complications.

Two final points have to be made regarding preoperative evaluation: (1) with the advent of better techniques of anesthesia and surgery and of improved postoperative pain control, patients with compromised pulmonary function may be more suitable candidates for resection; and (2) among comorbid diseases, the clinician should always look for a previous history of thrombophlebitis or venous disease in the lower limbs because those patients should receive prophylactic lowdose heparin. The routine use of this prophylaxis remains controversial.

J.D.

KEY REFERENCES

Epstein SK, Faling JL, Daly B, Celli BR: Predicting complications after pulmonary resection: preoperative exercise testing vs a multifactorial cardiopulmonary risk index. Chest 104:694, 1993

This attempt to develop a cardiopulmonary risk index for patients undergoing pulmonary resection demonstrates the value of VO_2max as a single index, which correlates well with a multifactorial index.

Julio ER, Persson AV: Preoperative evaluation of high-risk patient. Surg Clin North Am 65:3, 1985

Another excellent review of preoperative assessment of the high-risk patient.

Miller JI: Preoperative evaluation. Chest Surg Clin North Am 4:701, 1992a

This outline of a surgeon's approach to preoperative pulmonary and cardiac evaluation of the thoracic surgical patient provides an excellent overview of current practice.

Olsen GN: The evolving role of exercise testing prior to lung resection. Chest 95:218, 1989

Dr. Olsen, a noted pulmonary physiologist interested in preoperative assessment, here discusses exercise testing including VO_2max assessment.

Tisi M: Preoperative evaluation of pulmonary function. Am Rev Respir Dis 119, 295, 1979

This excellent review of the early work in preoperative pulmonary function testing is very relevant despite its age.

REFERENCES

Ali KM, Mountain CF, Ewer MS et al.: Predicting loss of pulmonary function after pulmonary resection for bronchogenic carcinoma. Chest 77:337, 1980

Arkins R, Smesseart AA, Hicks RG: Mortality and morbidity in surgical patients with coronary artery disease. JAMA 190:485, 1964

Bolton JWR, Weiman DS, Haynes JL et al.: Stair climbing as an indicator of pulmonary function. Chest 82:783, 1987

Boysen PG, Block AJ, Olsen GN et al.: Prospective evaluation for pneumonectomy using the ^{99m}technetium quantitative perfusion lung scan. Chest 72:422, 1977

Deslauriers J, Ginsberg RJ, Dubois P et al.: Current operative morbidity associated with elective surgical resection for lung cancer. Can J Surg 32:335, 1989

Epstein TA, Tinker AH, Tarhan S: Myocardial re-infarction after anesthesia and surgery JAMA 339:2566, 1978

Ginsberg RJ, Hill LD, Eagan RT et al.: Modern 30 day operative mortality for surgical resections in lung cancer. J Thorac Cardiovasc Surg 86:654, 1983

Goldman L: Cardiac risks and complications of non-cardiac surgery. Ann Surg 198:780, 1983

Jones NL: Exercise testing in pulmonary evaluation: rational, methods in normal respiratory response exercise. N Engl J Med 393:541, 1975

Kohman LJ, Meyer JA, Ikins PM, Oates RP: Random versus predictable risks of mortality after thoractomy for lung cancer. J Thorac Cardiovasc Surg 91:551, 1986

Lette J, Waters D, Lapointe J: Usefulness of the severity and extent of reversible perfusion defects during thallium-dye dipyridamole imaging for cardiac risk assessment before non-cardiac surgery. Ann J Cardiol 64:276, 1989

Lette J, Waters D, Lasson DEJ: Postoperative myocardial infarction in cardiac death. Ann Surg 211:84, 1990

Miller JI: Thallium imaging in preoperative evaluation of the pulmonary resection candidate. Ann Thorac Surg 54:249, 1992b

Olsen GN, Bolton JWR, Weunab DS, Hornung CA: Stair climbing as an exercise test predict the postoperative complications of lung resection—2 years experience. Chest 99:587, 1991

Ruckdeschel J, Piantadori S (for the Lung Cancer Study Group): Quality of life assessment in lung surgery for bronchogenic carcinoma. J Theor Surg 6:201, 1991

Steen PA, Tinker JH, Tarhan S: Myocardial reinfarction after anesthesia and surgery. JAMA 220:1451, 1978

Wahi R, McMurtrey MJ, DeCaro LF et al.: Determinants of perioperative morbidity and mortality after pneumonectomy. Ann Thorac Surg 48:333, 1989

4

PHYSIOLOGY

John Muscedere
Noe Zamel
Arthur S. Slutsky

INTRODUCTION

The prominent role that the understanding of pulmonary physiology plays in the diagnosis and treatment of lung disease makes the lung unique. In no other organ system is function so closely related to relatively easily measured physiologic variables. The goal of this chapter is to provide an overview of this area, since comprehension of pulmonary physiology is essential for the provision of excellent care to the thoracic surgical patient.

The volume of literature devoted to pulmonary physiology is vast and is rapidly expanding. In this context, only important or classical articles are referenced in the present chapter. References are also provided to important review articles on selected topics so that information beyond the scope of this chapter may be readily accessible.

The structural basis of the observed physiology is discussed first, followed by discussions on the control of breathing, ventilation, and diffusion.

RESPIRATORY APPARATUS

Airways

The main purpose of the respiratory system is to deliver oxygen and remove carbon dioxide from the tissues. The anatomic arrangement required to carry out this task can be viewed of as consisting of two regions: the conducting airways and the alveolar region.

The conducting airways extend from the nasal passages to the terminal bronchioles, and in this region gas transport takes place largely by convection—the bulk transport of gas. Distal to the terminal bronchioles, the major gas transport mechanism is diffusion. The *anatomic dead space,* defined as the volume of the airways that serve only as conductive pathways for gas, is approximately 150 ml in a normal, upright subject (methods to measure this are discussed later in this chapter).

Starting from the trachea, successive branching of the bronchial tree occurs with subsequent narrowing of each individual bronchus. However, because of the increase in the number of airways, the total cross-sectional area increases with each division. As can be seen in Figure 4-1, the total cross-sectional area of the bronchi initially increases slightly and later starts to increase exponentially (West, 1985). Bronchial diameter reaches a minimum of about 0.5 to 0.7 mm at the level of the terminal bronchioles and remains constant despite subsequent division (Bastacky, et al., 1983; Horsfield and Cumming, 1968). It is postulated that the transition from bulk flow to diffusion occurs at this level, since the forward velocity of the inspired gas drops dramatically as the cross-sectional area rapidly increases. For this same reason, particulate matter is deposited in the terminal bronchioles. The average number of divisions, or generations, of airways from trachea to terminal bronchi is approximately 23 but there may be as few as 8 or as many as 25 divisions, as idealized in the schematic of Figure 4-2 (Horsfield and Cumming, 1968).

The primary gas exchange unit of the lung is the *acinus,* which is defined as the portion of the lung distal to the terminal bronchiole and comprises respiratory bronchioles, alveolar ducts, alveolar sacs, and alveoli (Fraser, et al., 1988). The acini are not completely isolated but are interconnected by small channels known as the *pores of Kohn.* Also, other poorly demarcated channels are present, which may serve the purpose of collateral ventilation (Raskin and Herman, 1975).

While the acinus is the primary gas exchange unit of the lung, it can be further broken down into many interrelated alveoli. The human lung had been thought to contain approximately 3×10^8 alveoli as determined in several studies (Horsfield and Cumming, 1968; Cumming, 1972). However, a more recent study found that the number of alveoli correlated with body length and ranged from about 2×10^8 to 6×10^8 (Angus and Thurlbeck, 1972). The total alveolar surface area has been found to range from 70 to 100 m^2 (Weibel, 1963; Thurlbeck, 1967).

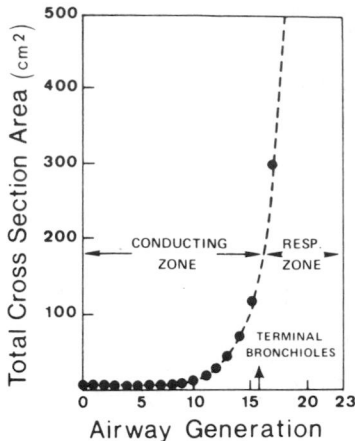

Figure 4-1. Cross-sectional area versus airway generation. Note that the total cross-sectional area increases exponentially as the number of airway generations increase. (From West JB: Respiratory Physiology—The Essentials. p. 7. 3rd Ed. Williams & Wilkins, Baltimore, 1985, with permission.)

Pulmonary Circulation

The pulmonary circulation is essential for the lungs to oxygenate and to eliminate CO_2. Although, the pulmonary circulation receives the entire cardiac output from the right ventricle, in comparison with the systemic circulation it is very compliant and pressures are quite low, with normal systolic pressures of about 25 mmHg, diastolic pressures of about 8 mmHg, and mean pressures of approximately 15 mmHg. It has several unique properties that make it ideally suited for

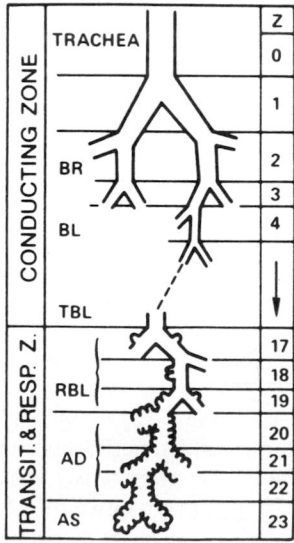

Figure 4.2. Diagram of human bronchial tree. Gas exchange cannot take place prior to division 17, and this volume constitutes the anatomic dead space. BR, bronchi; BL, bronchioli; TBL, terminal bronchioli; RBL, respiratory bronchioli; AD, alveolar ducts; AS, alveolar sacs: Z, number of airway generations. (From Weibel ER: Morphometry of the Human Lung. p. 111. Springer-Verlag, Berlin, 1963, with permission.)

the function of gas exchange. These are covered in this section, which explores its properties and how they relate to lung function as a whole.

As the pulmonary arteries enter the lungs from the hilum, they usually follow the divisions of the bronchi, branching with every bronchial division. However, the number of arterial branches is greater than the number of bronchial branches since the artery undergoes extra divisions, which serve the lung parenchyma. The number of extra branches increases with each additional bronchial branch (Elliot and Reid, 1965). These branches are not usually seen on pulmonary angiography since they tend to arise at very oblique angles, which tends to minimize blood flow under normal conditions.

Once the capillary level is reached, the capillary network becomes very extensive, and the total capillary cross-sectional area increases significantly at a rate analogous to the exponential increase in the area of the airways. The capillaries proceed to form a large plexus around each alveolus and do not become terminal vessels since they are all interconnected. The capillary network is so extensive that it can be thought of as a continuous sheet of blood enveloping the alveolus (Fung and Sobin, 1968). A red blood cell may pass several alveoli while in the capillary network. Because of this, the residence time of blood in the lung capillary is relatively long (~0.5 to 1.0 second), which under most conditions, at rest or exercise, is sufficient for the blood to become fully equilibrated with alveolar gas. The only situations in which the capillary transit time is thought to be a limiting factor in arterial oxygenation are heavy exercise in low oxygen atmospheres and abnormality of the alveolocapillary membrane, as pulmonary fibrosis (Staub, 1963).

Because the capillaries are arranged in extensive, multiple interconnected parallel networks, there is a large degree of reserve. A large number of capillaries can be occluded without an appreciable increase in pulmonary artery pressures. Also, the extensive endothelial surface of the pulmonary capillary network is very well suited for carrying out the metabolic functions of the lung.

Diffusion is facilitated by the fact that the air-blood barrier may be as thin as 0.5 μm and at its thinnest consists of only three layers (Weibel, 1963). These are the capillary endothelium, the fused basement membrane of the endothelial and epithelial layers, and the epithelium, which is composed of type I and II pneumocytes (Fig. 4-3) (Schneeberger, 1978). Because of the exceedingly thin air-blood barrier, the lung has several protective mechanisms to prevent alveolar flooding. First, the pulmonary capillary hydrostatic pressure is less than the oncotic pressure, and this tends to draw fluid into the vascular space (Landis and Pappenheimer, 1963). Also, interstitial pressure is subatmospheric (Meyer, et al., 1963), and surfactant reduces intra-alveolar surface tension (Prattle, 1965). These effects favor fluid migration from the air spaces to the interstitium. Once fluid arrives in the interstitium, there is efficient lymphatic drainage (Lauweryns, 1965). The final guard against alveolar flooding is the effective barrier of the air blood interface, with the main barrier to permeability residing in the epithelial layer (Schneeberger, 1978). Damage to the epithelial layer and the resultant increase in permeability account for the low-pressure pulmonary edema seen with the inhalation of noxious gases.

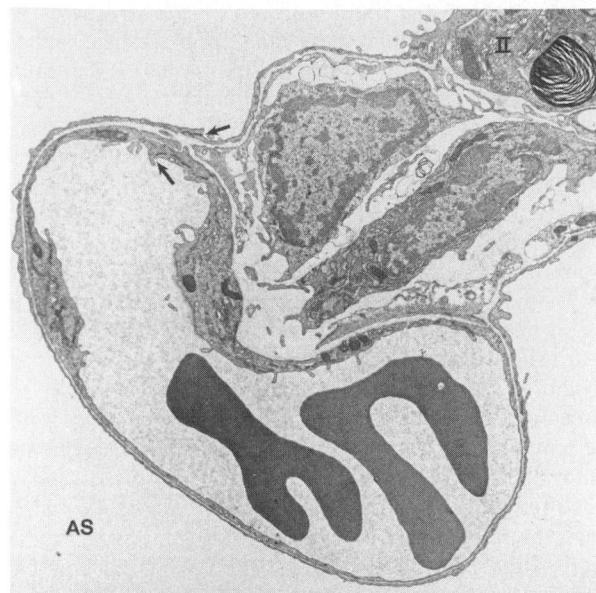

Figure 4-3. Alveolar capillary of rat lung. The alveolar space (AS) and intravascular compartment are closely approximated and are separated by the flattened epithelium of a type 1 pneumocyte, fused basement membrane, and nonfenestrated epithelium. (From Schneeberger, EE: Structural basis for some permeability properties of the air-blood barrier. FASEB J 37:2471, 1978, with permission.)

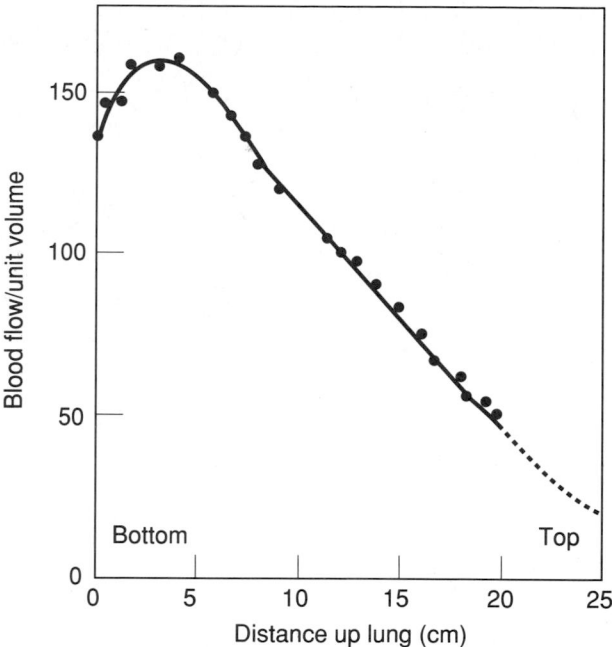

Figure 4-4. Perfusion versus blood flow per unit volume of lung in the upright position. The amount of blood flow per lung volume is increased in the bases and reduced in the apex. (Modified from Hughes JMB, Glazier JB, Maloney JE et al: Effect of lung volumes on the distribution of pulmonary blood flow. Respir Physiol 4:58, 1968, with permission.)

Since lung perfusion is accomplished with relatively low pulmonary artery pressures (mean, 15 mmHg) and because the lung is approximately 30 cm high in the upright position, the lung is uniquely affected by hydrostatic pressures. That is, perfusion pressure is the sum of the mean pulmonary artery pressure and hydrostatic pressure as measured from the right ventricle (West, et al., 1964). This results in large differences in pulmonary blood flow between dependent and nondependent regions of the lung (Fig. 4-4) (Ball, et al., 1962; West and Dollery, 1960; Hughes, et al., 1968). This gravitational effect can have a marked influence on oxygenation in the presence of markedly asymmetric lung injury. In such situations, oxygenation can be improved by simply placing the patient in a position such that the diseased lung receives a smaller fraction of the cardiac output (Norton and Conforti, 1985; Prokocimer, et al., 1983).

Much of the work on the influence of hydrostatic pressure on lung perfusion has been done by West and colleagues, who have divided the lung into three regions—zones I, II, and III—on the basis of perfusion pressure (Fig. 4-5) (Weibel, 1963; Elliot and Reid, 1965; West, et al., 1964; West, 1978). In zone I, which is found in the apex of the lung (in the upright posture), hydrostatic pressure is greater than perfusion pressure (Fig. 4-6) (Glazier, et al., 1969). As a result $P_A > Pa > Pv$, where P_A is atmospheric or alveolar pressure, Pa is pulmonary artery pressure, and Pv is the pulmonary venous pressure. Therefore, under normal conditions in the upright human, no flow occurs in the apex and ventilation occurs without perfusion.

In zone II conditions, $Pa > P_A > Pv$, and flow occurs only when P_A becomes subatmospheric, as during inspiration;

flow in this zone ceases during expiration. In zone III, $Pa > Pv > P_A$, and therefore, perfusion occurs throughout the respiratory cycle. This physiologic concept has a number of clinical implications. For example, estimation of capillary wedge pressure is based on the assumption that there is a

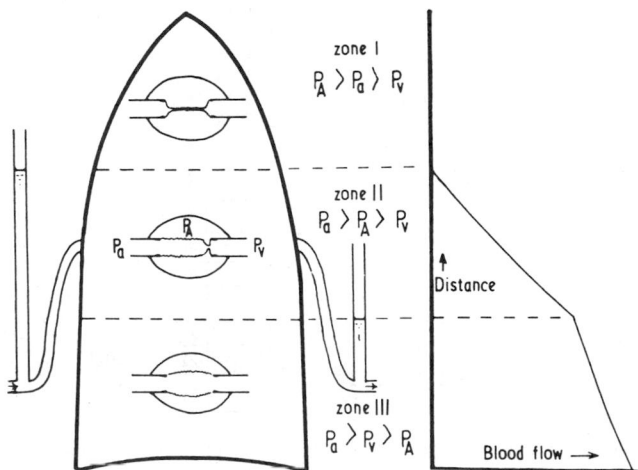

Figure 4-5. Three-zone model of lung perfusion. P_A, alveolar pressure; Pa, arterial pressure; Pv, venous pressure. (From West JB, Dollery CT, Naimark A: Distribution of blood flow in isolated lungs: relation to vascular and alveolar pressures. J Appl Physiol 19:713, 1964, with permission.)

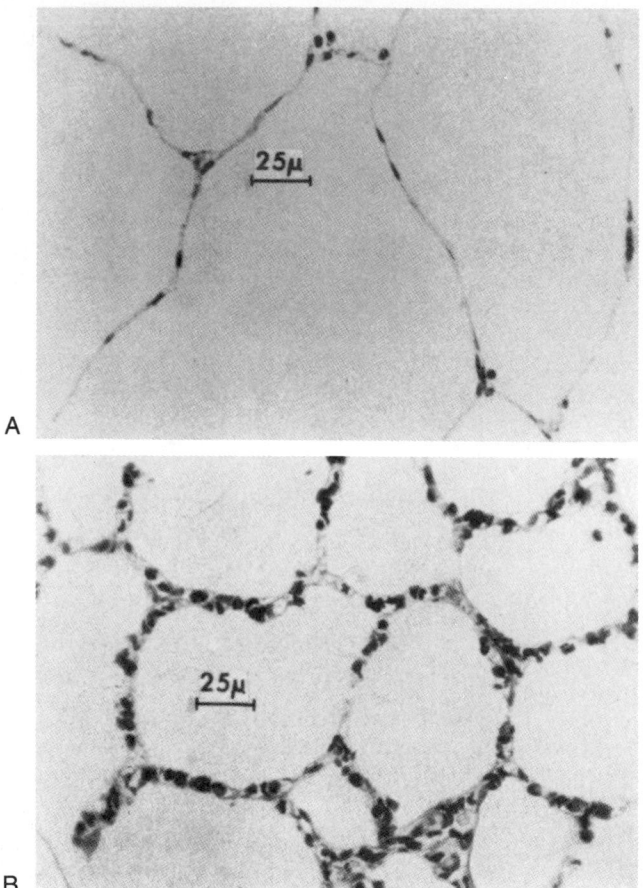

Figure 4-6. Rapidly frozen lung specimens taken from the apex **(A)** and basilar **(B)** regions of the lung. Note that the capillaries from the base (zone III conditions) are distended with blood, while capillaries in the apex (zone 1) are essentially empty of blood. (From Glazier JB, Hughes JMB, West JB: Measurement of capillary dimensions and blood volume in rapidly frozen lungs. J Appl Physiol 26:65, 1969, with permission.)

static column of blood between the site of measurement and the left atrium. If the pulmonary artery catheter is wedged in a part of the lung that is zone I, the pressure transducer will record alveolar pressure rather than left atrial pressure. For accurate readings, the catheter should be wedged in a part of the lung that is in zone III. This usually is the case, since the catheter is balloon-tipped and most of the pulmonary blood flow is to zone III; however, if the relationship among Pa, Pv, and PA changes (e.g., by addition of high positive end-expiratory pressure [PEEP]), the catheter tip may no longer be in zone III.

Respiratory Mechanics

The mechanical properties of the lung and chest wall are important determinants of function in health and disease. There can be measured and are important clues as to the presence of disease. In this section, the mechanics of respiratory function are delineated.

The lungs and the chest wall are elastic structures with inherent recoil and different mechanical properties, such that the function of the respiratory system in vivo is determined by the sum of individual characteristics (Fig. 4-7). These properties can be shown by plotting volume versus pressure, as in Figure 4-8, for each structure individually (Rahn, et al., 1946). In this diagram, the static pressure-volume curves of the lungs and relaxed chest wall are shown along with their sum, representing the pressure volume curve for the total respiratory system. The lung's resting volume, at which the transpulmonary pressure is zero, is near residual volume (RV), while the chest wall resting volume, at which the trans-chest wall pressure is zero, is near 80 percent of total lung capacity (TLC). As transpulmonary pressure increases with increasing lung volume, the trans–chest wall pressure is positive only over the top 20 percent of TLC and negative over the lower 80 percent.

The functional residual capacity (FRC) is the volume at which the inward recoil of the lungs balances the outward recoil of the chest wall (Fig. 4-8). As a consequence, any alteration in chest wall or lung compliance shifts the FRC. A practical example of this is the increase of FRC due to a loss of pulmonary elastic tissue as one ages. Also, FRC is reduced in the supine position, partly owing to the effect of gravity on outward chest recoil (Sykes, et al., 1976). If the FRC is below the volume at which the airways in the most dependent parts of the lung close, atelectasis in these regions may result.

Compliance

Compliance is defined as change in volume divided by change in pressure; therefore, compliance is the slope of the pressure-volume curve. It can be determined under static or dynamic conditions. Static compliance is measured under conditions such that there is zero flow and equilibration of the respiratory system is allowed to take place. A common way to make this measurement is to inflate the lungs with a known volume (via a ventilator or a large syringe), wait for equilibration to occur, and then measure the resulting airway pressure. When compliance is measured dynamically, factors related to distribution of the ventilation may have an influence, and as a result, dynamic compliance underestimates static compliance when there is uneven distribution of the ventilation. Lung compliance is directly related to lung volume and decreases with increasing volume (i.e., the lung behaves as if it were stiffer as one approaches TLC; the reverse is true with chest wall compliance, which decreases with decreasing volume.

Compliance is analogous to electrical conductance, and the compliance of two structures in series is added as follows:

$$\frac{1}{C_T} = \frac{1}{C_1} + \frac{1}{C_2}$$

where C_T is total compliance and C_1 and C_2 are the individual compliances. As an example, the compliance of chest wall and lungs is about 0.2 L/cmH$_2$O each, for a total respiratory system compliance of 0.1 L/cmH$_2$O (Grassino, et al., 1991).

Lung compliance is directly affected by diseases that affect the lung parenchyma. Diseases that lead to a loss of elastic

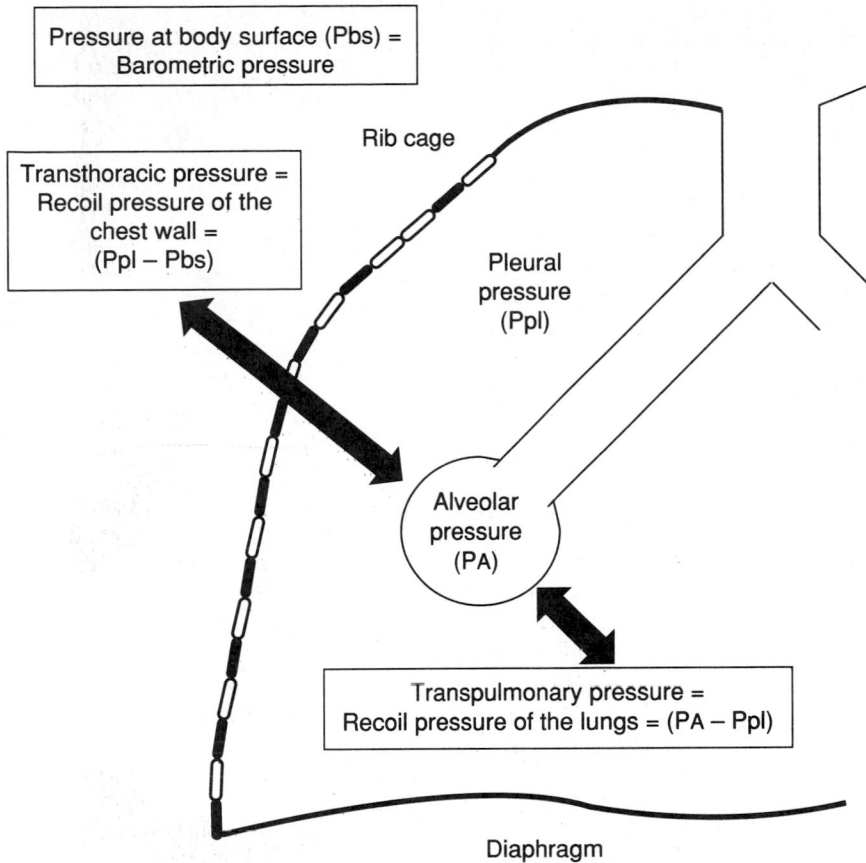

Figure 4-7. Schematic diagram illustrating the relationship between the lungs and chest wall.

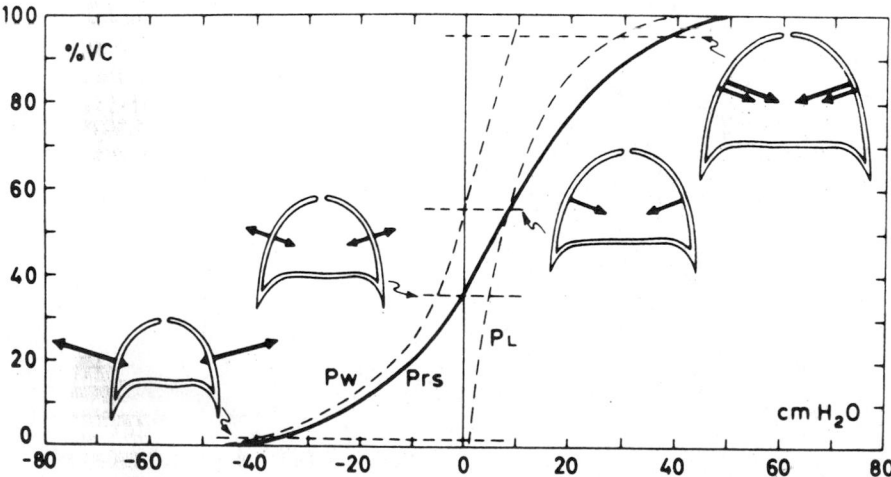

Figure 4-8. Pressure-volume curves of the lung (PL), chest wall (Pw) and total respiratory system (PRS). Size of large arrows indicates relative size of recoil forces. Functional residual capacity (FRC) is reached when outward chest recoil is equal to inward lung recoil. (From Sharp JT, Hammond MD: Pressure-volume relationships. p. 839. In Crystal RG, West JB (eds): The Lung: Scientific Foundations. Raven Press, New York, 1991, and from Knowles JH, Hong SK, Rahn H: Possible errors using an esophageal balloon in the determination of pressure-volume characteristics of lung and rib cage. J Appl Physiol 14:525, 1959, with permission.)

tissue and decreased recoil (e.g., emphysema), result in an increase in compliance, the opposite being true for diseases such as pulmonary fibrosis, as illustrated in Figure 4-9 (Zamel, 1989).

Pressure-Volume Curves

When pressure-volume curves are determined in isolated lungs by using air, the curves obtained depend on whether the measurements are made during inflation or deflation. This property is common to elastic tissues and is called *hysteresis*, which is defined as failure of a system to respond identically to the application versus the withdrawal of a force, in this case distending pressure (Landowne and Sacy, 1957). However, when the lungs are inflated with liquid, the inflation and deflation loops become virtually identical (i.e., the amount of hysteresis is reduced) as seen in Figure 4-10 (Bachofen, et al., 1970; Radford, 1957).

The characteristics of pressure-volume curves of excised lungs are dependent on the amount of lung recoil which is determined by the elasticity of lung parenchyma and the surface tension at the gas-liquid interface. Inflation with liquid abolishes the contribution of surface tension to lung recoil, so that the resultant pressure-volume curve is a reflection only of tissue forces and is shifted to the left.

When isolated lungs are deflated to transpulmonary pressures of zero, significant volume remains within the lung; in fact, even if the transpulmonary pressures become negative, little additional volume is removed. This effect is due to air trapping within alveoli from the closure of small airways and is relatively constant between air and liquid-filled lungs (Sharp and Hammond, 1991; West, 1985a). The retained volume is referred to as the *closing volume* and is approximately 15 percent of TLC; however, it increases with age and can be increased by some disease processes (Hoppin, et al.,

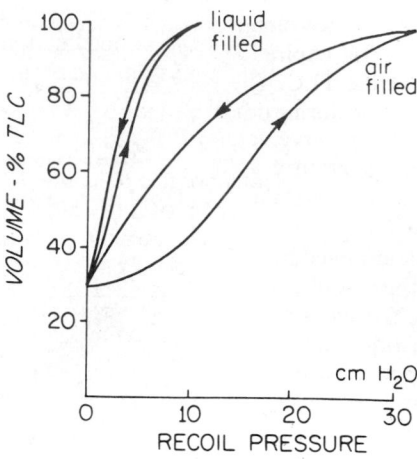

Figure 4-10. Static pressure-volume curve of the lung measured during inflation with saline and air. (From Culver BH: Mechanics of ventilation. p. 11. In Culver BH (ed): The Respiratory System. Syllabus for Human Biology. University of Washington Health Sciences Academic Services, Seattle, WA, 1990, with permission.)

1986). The in vitro closing volume is the volume at which all the airways are closed, while the in vivo closing volume is the lung volume at which the airway in the most dependent parts of the lungs start to close.

Pulmonary Functions Tests

Static Volumes

The volume of the lung can be divided into several compartments, the definitions of which are indicated in Figure 4-11. The TLC is the total amount of air within the lungs at maximal inspiration and is equal to the RV plus the vital capacity

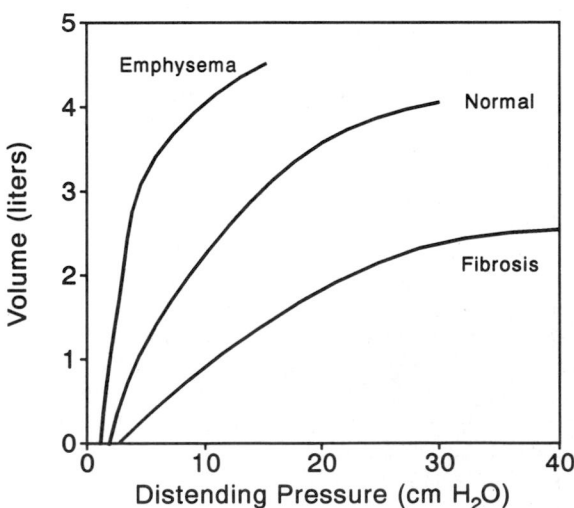

Figure 4-9. Static pressure-volume curves for patients with normal lungs, pulmonary fibrosis, and emphysema. Compliance represents the slope of the pressure-volume curve. (Adapted from Murray JF: The Normal Lung. p. 87. 2nd Ed. WB Saunders, Philadelphia, 1986, with permission.)

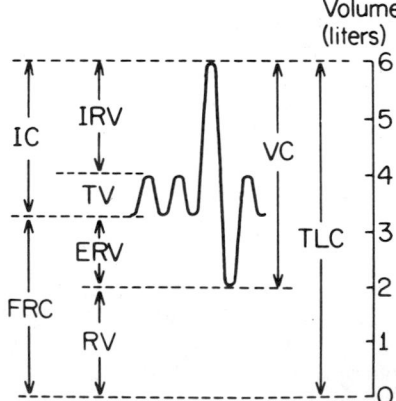

Figure 4-11. Divisions of lung volume. TLC, total lung capacity; FRC, functional residual capacity; VC, vital capacity; RV, residual volume; IC, inspiratory capacity; ERV, expiratory reserve volume; TV, tidal volume; IV, inspiratory reserve volume. (From Culver BH: Mechanics of ventilation. p. 11. In Culver BH (ed): The Respiratory System. Syllabus for Human Biology. University of Washington Health Sciences Academic Services, Seattle, WA, 1990, with permission.)

(VC). The VC is the volume obtained when a subject expires from TLC to full expiration and is approximately equal to 70 percent of the TLC. The volume present within the lung at end-expiration during tidal breathing is defined as the FRC. The inspiratory reserve volume is the volume between TLC and the end-inspiratory volume of normal tidal breathing, while the expiratory reserve volume is the volume between RV and FRC.

TLC is determined by a combination of inspiratory muscle strength, chest wall recoil, and lung recoil. A decrease in inspiratory muscle strength will decrease TLC, as will an increase in either lung or chest wall recoil. RV is determined by expiratory muscle strength, chest wall compliance, and the point at which airway closure takes place. In young persons the RV is greater than that at which airway closure takes place and is mainly dependent on muscle strength. However, with increasing age airway closure occurs at higher volumes and becomes relatively independent of expiratory muscle strength. As a result RV rises from approximately 25 percent of TLC at age 20 to 40 percent at age 70 (Freedman, 1990).

As seen previously, FRC is determined by the interplay between lung recoil and chest wall recoil. It may be reduced in states such as obesity and pregnancy and increased in patients with severe chronic obstructive pulmonary disease.

These volumes are measured by a combination of spirometry and more specialized tests. The volumes amenable to measurement with spirometry are the VC, tidal volume, and both the inspiratory and expiratory reserve volumes. FRC, TLC, and RV cannot be measured with spirometry, since the amount of RV cannot be measured unless specialized methods are used.

A common method for measuring static lung volumes is by helium dilution, as helium is relatively insoluble and is not taken up by the lungs. In this method a known concentration and volume of a helium-containing gas is inhaled and allowed to equilibrate with gas in the lung, and subsequently the helium concentration in the exhaled gas is measured. Based on the law of conservation of mass, the volume can be calculated as follows:

$$V_1 \times C_1 = V_2 \times C_2$$

where V_1 = volume of inhaled gas

C_1 = concentration of helium in the inspired gas

V_2 = unknown volume to be measured (volume of the lung)

C_2 = exhaled concentration of helium

The volume measured is a function of the lung volume at which the subject is asked to inhale the helium-containing gas. If inhalation commences at the end of a normal tidal volume, the lung volume measured is the FRC. If inhalation begins at end-expiration, the lung volume measured is TLC, and RV can be calculated by subtracting the VC from the TLC.

In practice there are two methods for measuring lung volume by helium dilution, the single breath hold technique, which is usually used to measure TLC, and the steady-state method, in which equilibrium is achieved over a few minutes (Meneely and Kaltrieder, 1949). FRC is usually measured by the steady-state method (Ogilvie, et al., 1957). A problem with these methods is that they only measure the volume of the air spaces in direct communication with the mouth and may seriously underestimate thoracic gas volume in disease states in which airway pathology or noncommunicating pockets of gas (as with bullous lung disease and pneumothoraces) are present.

Another method to measure FRC is to use a constant-volume body plethysmograph. This method meaures all compressible gas within the thorax by taking advantage of Boyle's law, which is applicable for constant temperature conditions.

$$PV = constant$$

The subject sits in an airtight chamber and pants against a closed mouthpiece. This produces pressure changes within the chamber, which are proportional to the thoracic gas volumes. Since the volume of the chamber is known and the pressure changes are measured, the FRC can then be calculated.

The advantage of constant-volume plethysmography is that it measures all gas within the thoracic cavity. However, if changes in abdominal pressure occur, this technique will measure intra-abdominal gas volume as well. Another source of artifact with this technique is the assumption that during a panting maneuver there is equilibration between alveolar and mouth pressure. This may not be the case in severe airways obstruction, where the lack of equilibration may lead to significant overestimation of TLC (Brown and Slutsky, 1984). Also, in patients with severe airways obstruction there may be large discrepancies between the two methods, since the airways obstruction may prevent full equilibration of the helium with all the air spaces. In normal individuals the two volumes should be nearly identical, and a volume greater than 500 ml is considered to be significant. In order to properly interpret lung volumes by plethysmography, a chest radiograph is required to exclude severe bullous disease or pneumothoraces.

Flow-Volume Curves

A large amount of information can be obtained with spirometry and examination of the relationship between maximal expiratory and inspiratory flow rates and lung volumes (Hyatt and Black, 1973; Macklem, 1975). Maximal expiratory and inspiratory flow rates are a function of lung volume, and plotting these on a graph produces a flow-volume curve (Fig. 4-12). In practice, the expiratory curve is constructed by having a subject inhale to TLC and then measuring the flows and changes in lung volume during a forced exhalation to RV. The inspiratory curve is constructed in a similar manner from the flow rates generated during maximal inspiration from RV to TLC. Typically, the expiratory curve is triangular, with the highest flows near TLC. The inspiratory curve is more symmetrical, with highest flows at mid-VC.

If markers of elapsed time are added during expiration, quantitative measurements of volume with respect to time can be derived. An example is the forced expiratory volume in 1 second (FEV_1). Other measurements, such as maximum flow at 50 percent and 25 percent VC ($Vmax_{50}$, $Vmax_{25}$,

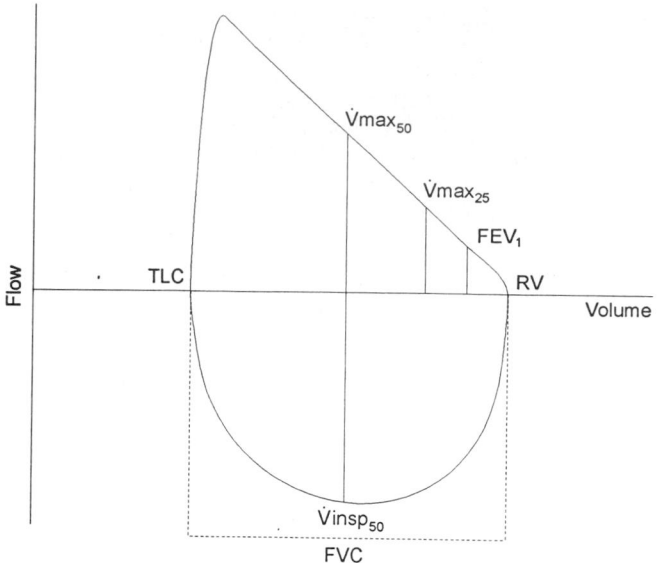

Figure 4-12.   Idealized diagram of maximal expiratory and inspiratory flow-volume curves. TLC, total lung capacity; RV, residual volume; FVC, forced vital capacity; $Vmax_{50}$, flow at 50 percent of vital capacity; $Vmax_{25}$, flow at 25 percent of vital capacity; $Vinsp_{50}$, inspiratory flow at 50 percent of vital capacity; FEV_1, forced expiratory flow in 1 second.

In restrictive lung disease, lung recoil is increased although total lung volume is reduced. Absolute flows are reduced because of the low lung volumes, but the airways are usually normal. When the flow measurements are standardized for lung volume, they are usually increased. An example is the reduction in FEV_1 seen in restrictive lung disease while the ratio of FEV_1 to forced vital capacity (FVC) (an indicator of lung volume) is increased (Gaensler, 1951). A normal FEV_1/FVC ratio is approximately 70 to 80 percent. In addition, the absolute values of $Vmax_{50}$ and $Vmax_{25}$ are reduced. However, when these are compared with lung volume, they are usually increased in the absence of airways disease ($Vmax_{50}$/VC is usually 1.0 L/S/L and $Vmax_{25}$/VC is 0.5 L/S/L in healthy subjects). This illustrates that it is difficult to evaluate flow measurements unless they are related to the lung volumes from which they are derived.

In obstructive lung disease, the FEV_1 is reduced, but lung volumes are increased and the FVC is much better preserved. Therefore, the FEV_1/FVC ratio is reduced. Although upper airways obstruction can mimic obstructive lung disease, both the inspiratory and expiratory limbs of the flow-volume loop are affected if the obstruction is fixed. This may help distinguish between the two disease processes. A useful measurement of inspiratory flow is the maximum inspiratory flow at 50 percent of VC. The FEV_1, and all other lung volumes vary directly with height and inversely with age and are greater in men than in women. Published tables for all lung volumes are available.

respectively) can also be derived (Fig. 4-12). $Vmax_{50}$ and $Vmax_{25}$ are reflective of small airways function and if reduced in comparison with lung volume, indicate small airways obstruction (Cosio, et al., 1978).

The shape of the flow-volume loop is dependent on the properties of the airways, lung recoil, and lung volume. For this reason it will be altered by disease states that affect any of these. The resultant curves can be divided into three categories, each having a clinical correlate; these are restrictive lung diseases, airways obstruction, and upper airways obstruction (Fig. 4-13).

If a flow-volume loop is obtained with minimal effort and then repeated with successively increasing effort until maximal effort is reached, an interesting phenomenon is observed. The peak flow is effort-dependent and increases with increasing effort, but 75 to 80 percent of the expiratory curve is effort-independent (Fig. 4-14). On this portion of the curve increasing effort will not increase flow. Several theoretical models have been proposed for this phenomenon, but the simplest is the equal pressure point model (Mead, et al., 1967). In this model the effort independence of flow is thought to result from the compression of intrathoracic airways. In-

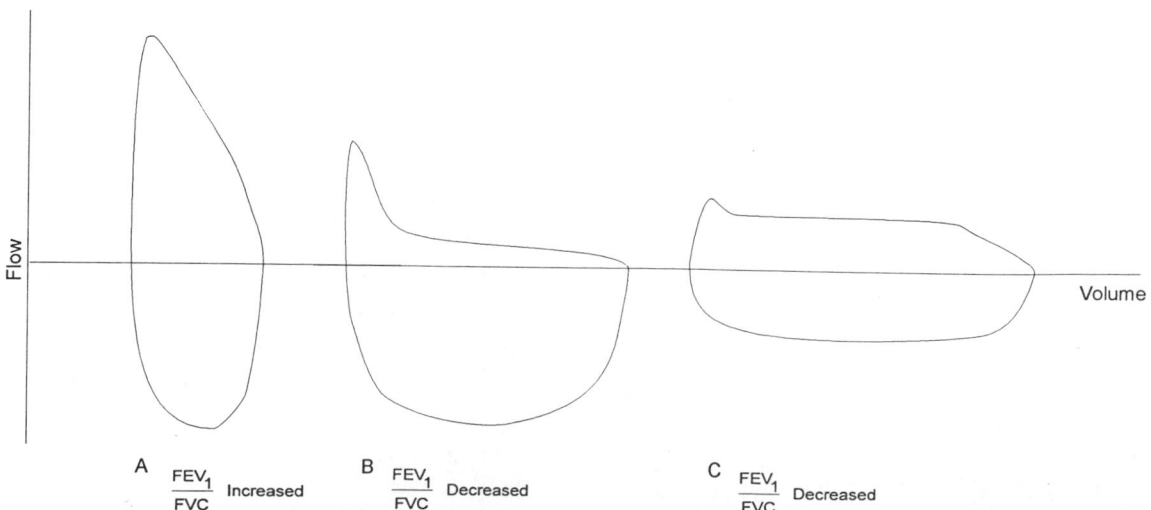

Figure 4-13.   Representative flow-volume curves of restrictive lung disease, obstructive lung disease, and upper airways obstruction. **(A)** Restrictive lung disease, **(B)** obstructive lung disease, and **(C)** upper airway obstruction.

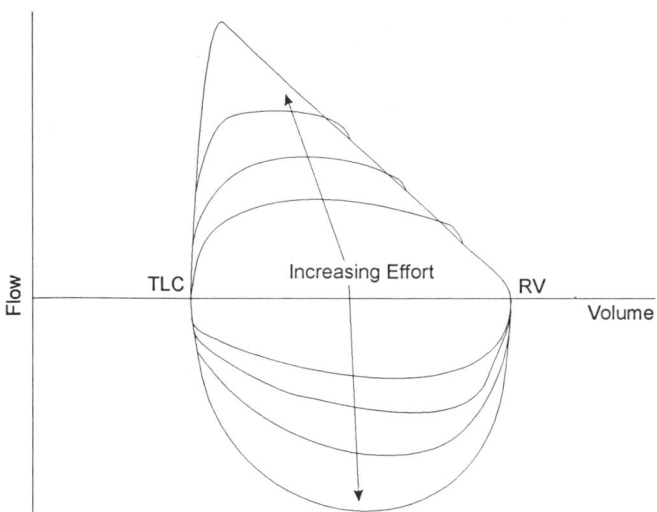

Figure 4-14. Effect of effort on the expiratory limb of a flow-volume curve. Note that at low lung volumes, increasing effort causes no increases in maximal flow.

creased effort results in the generation of increased positive pleural pressures, which are then transmitted to the intrathoracic airways, so that resistance to expiration increases in concert with driving pressure and flow remains constant.

Surfactant

Although von Neergaard in the 1920s was the first to suggest that surface tension played a role in lung expansion, it was not until the 1950s that surfactant was isolated and it was recognized that neonatal respiratory distress syndrome was due to surfactant deficiency (Floros, 1990). Since then surfactant has been shown to have multiple functions and to be crucial for normal lung function.

Surfactant is a heterogenous mixture consisting of 80 to 85 percent phospholipids, 5 to 10 percent protein, and 10 percent neutral lipids, with dipalmitoylphosphatidylcholine as the main surface-active agent (Hawgood, 1991; Morton, 1989). The protein components of surfactant are important for its function and are designated apoproteins A, B, and C. They appear to be essential for surfactant's secretion, regulation of turnover rate, and distribution into the alveolar liquid layer (Hawgood and Clements, 1990).

The main effect of surfactant is to reduce the surface tension at the interface between air and the alveoli, and in doing so it promotes lung stability. Intra-alveolar pressure can be estimated by Laplace's law.

$$p = \frac{2T}{r}$$

where p is the pressure, T is the tension, and r is the radius of curvature of the alveolus. From this equation it is evident that for a given surface tension, intra-alveolar pressure will rise as alveolar size falls, and smaller alveoli will tend to empty into larger alveoli, thereby initiating a cascade whereby the whole lung becomes unstable. Surfactant reduces surface tension, and when the surfactant film is com-

pressed as alveolar size falls, stability is enhanced (Schurch, et al., 1976).

Surfactant is important in alveolar fluid handling. Surface tension may be important in determining transvascular water flux, and there is experimental evidence that a reduction in surfactant activity or an increase in surface tension results in pulmonary edema (Nieman and Bredenberg, 1985; Albert et al., 1979). Surfactant also reduces the work of breathing by increasing pulmonary compliance (Bachofen, et al., 1979), functions as an antiadherence agent, and may have immunologic effects, such as increasing macrophage recruitment to the lungs (Dobbs, 1989).

Surfactant is synthesized by type II alveolar cells and stored in lamellar bodies (Fig. 4-15). Clearance is accomplished by several mechanisms, of which re-uptake by type II cells, degradation by alveolar macrophages and clearance up the mucociliary ladder are the most important (Wright, 1990). An example of a disease state arising from disordered surfactant metabolism is alveolar proteinosis, which is characterized by excess surfactant, although it is unclear if this results from increased production or decreased clearance.

CONTROL OF BREATHING

To meet the metabolic demands of the body, the process of respiration has to be tightly controlled so that delivery of oxygen, removal of carbon dioxide and maintenance of pH are ensured. This is accomplished by a central controller, a system of sensors, and a system to effect changes. For the respiratory system the central controller resides in the brain, with autonomic control residing in the brain stem and voluntary control in the cerebrum. The effector system consists of the lungs and the respiratory muscles. The system of sensors is complex and consists of chemoreceptors in the medulla as well as in the aortic and carotid bodies, which respond to changes in pH and in CO_2, and PO_2. Other receptors are the mechanoreceptors in the lungs and chest wall. In order to understand the coordination of breathing to meet metabolic demands, each component is discussed individually below.

Receptors

Peripheral Chemoreceptors

The peripheral chemoreceptors are situated within the aortic body and the carotid body, the carotid body being the more important of the two. They are extremely sensitive to changes in PO_2. Receptor activation and firing starts at a PO_2 of 500 mmHg, and its frequency increases as the PO_2 decreases, with a marked burst in activity as the PO_2 drops below 100 mmHg (Fig. 4-16) (Lahiri, et al., 1981).

These receptors are primarily responsible for the ventilatory response to hypoxia, and this response is enhanced in the presence of an elevated PCO_2. Overall, approximately 30 percent of the total ventilatory response to PCO_2 is mediated by the carotid bodies (Lugliani, et al., 1971). Clinically, this is important in disease states or procedures in which bilateral denervation or destruction of the carotid bodies occurs (e.g., bilateral carotid endarterectomies) in which the response to hypoxia is abolished and dangerous levels of hypoxemia may occur without compensatory ventilatory responses. There is also evidence that respiratory depression

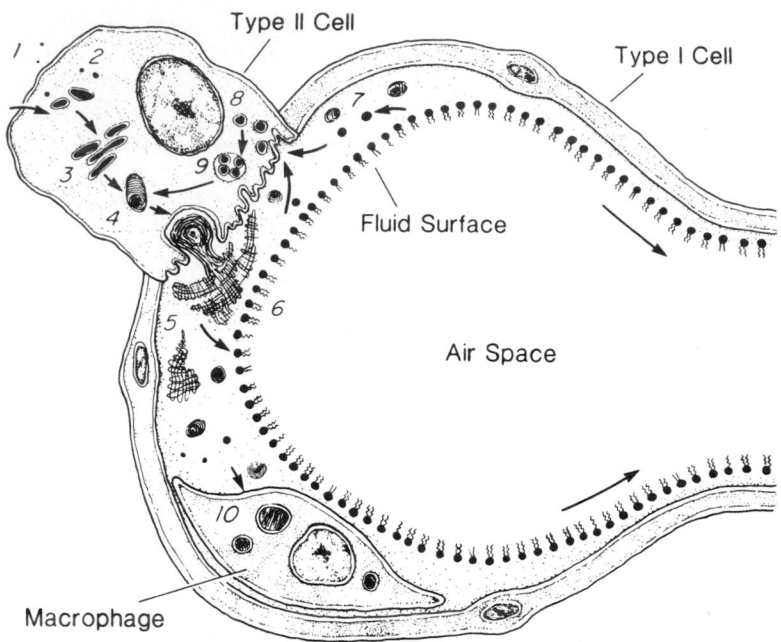

Type II Cell

Type I Cell

Fluid Surface

Air Space

Macrophage

Figure 4-15. Schematic diagram of the surfactant system. A single alveolus is shown, with the location and movement of surfactant components depicted. Surfactant components are synthesized from precursors (*1*) in the endoplasmic reticulum (*2*) and transported via the Golgi apparatus (*3*) into lamellar bodies (*4*), which are the intracellular storage granules for surfactant. After secretion into the liquid that lines the alveolus, the surfactant forms tubular myelin (*5*), which is thought to generate the surface monolayer (*6*), which lowers surface tension. Subsequently, surfactant components are taken back into type II cells, possibly in the form of small vesicles (*7*), apparently by a specific pathway involving endosomes (*8*) and multivesicular bodies (*9*) and culminating again in storage of surfactant in lamellar bodies. Some surfactant in the liquid layer is also taken up by alveolar macrophages (*10*). A single transit of the phospholipid components of surfactant through the alveolar lumen normally takes a few hours. The phospholipids in the lumen are taken back into the type II cell and used approximately 10 times before being degraded. (From Hawgood S, Clements JA: Pulmonary surfactant and its apoproteins. J Clin Invest 86:1, 1990, with permission.)

may occur in response to hypoxia without afferent input from the carotid bodies.

Stimulation of the carotid bodies also produces many other effects, including increased bronchomotor tone and increased catecholamine secretion, and during sleep it may cause arousal (Phillipson and Sullivan, 1978).

Central Chemoreceptors

The central chemoreceptors consists of a group of cells in the ventral-lateral surface of the medulla, approximately 200 to 500 μm below the surface. They respond to the hydrogen ion concentration of the extracellular fluid bathing the cells (i.e., the cerebrospinal fluid [CSF], with an increase in hydrogen ion concentration causing an increase in ventilation. Since bicarbonate and hydrogen ions do not cross the blood-brain barrier, in order for changes in CO_2 to effect a change in ventilation, CO_2 must diffuse across the blood-brain barrier and change the pH of the CSF. In order for full equilibration to take place, hours may be needed. Therefore the response to metabolic acidosis is less brisk than that to respiratory acidosis, since blood hydrogen ion concentration does not directly affect the central chemoreceptors and can only influence them by changing the concentration of bicarbonate in the serum and secondarily the plasma CO_2 levels.

Pulmonary Receptors

In the lung there are three major categories of receptors: pulmonary stretch receptors, irritant receptors, and J receptors. The pulmonary stretch receptors lie within airway smooth muscle and are activated by lung inflation. The primary effect of activation of these fibers, whose afferent impulses are carried within the vagus, is a slowing of inspiratory frequency due to an increase in expiratory time (Berger, et al., 1977a). Classically this is known as the Herring-Breuer reflex. However, this reflex seems to be much more important in some animals and does not seem to be activated for tidal volumes less than about 1 L in humans.

Receptors that respond to irritant stimuli are located between airway epithelial cells. They respond noxious gases, inhaled dust, smoke, cold air and histamine (Armstrong and Luck, 1974; Sampson and Vidruk, 1975). The afferent impulses are carried within the vagus, and receptor stimulation produces cough, bronchoconstriction and hyperpnea. These receptors may have a role in asthma, since contact with allergen produces histamine release with subsequent activation of the receptors.

Type J (juxtapulmonary-capillary) receptors are present within the walls of the pulmonary capillaries. They are believed to be activated by pulmonary congestion or by in-

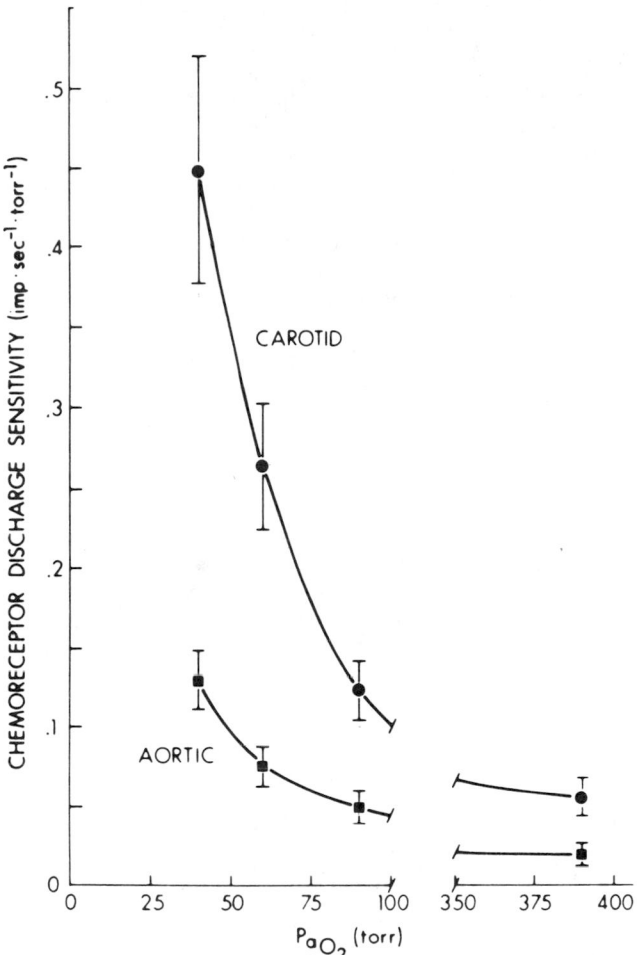

Figure 4-16. Response of aortic and carotid body receptors to hypoxia. (From Lahiri S, Mokasi A, Mulligan E, Nishino T: Comparison of aortic acid and chemoreceptor responses to hypercapnia and hypoxia. J Appl Physiol 51:55, 1981, with permission.)

creases in interstitial fluid volume (Paintal, 1973). The afferent impulses are conducted in nonmyelinated fibers in the vagus and result in rapid, shallow breathing. They are thought to play a role in the dyspnea associated with such disease states such as left ventricular failure and are not associated with normal respiration.

Other Receptors

Receptors are also located within the nasal passages, pharynx, and upper airways. These are sensitive to various chemical and mechanical stimuli and mediate reflexes such as sneezing, coughing, and laryngeal spasm. They are numerous and are beyond the scope of this review.

Central Control of Breathing

Respiration is governed by both voluntary and automatic controls, with the cerebral cortex respiratory for voluntary control and the brain stem responsible for automatic breathing. Brain stem control of breathing originates in neurons located within the pons and medulla, which are organized into separate groups called the respiratory centers. There are three separate areas named the pneumotaxic center, the apneustic center and the medullary center, which is divided into an expiratory center and a gasping center (Lumsden, 1923a,b; Berger et al., 1977b).

The pneumotaxic center is the most caudal of the three and is located in the upper pons. Stimulation of this area appears to inhibit inspiration and cause a swtich to expiration. The intensity of the stimulus needed decreases as inspiration progresses (Von Euler and Trippenbach, 1975). In this way, inspiratory volume is limited and respiratory rate is regulated.

The apneustic center lies in the lower pons, and it is so named because sectioning of the brain stem above this area results in prolonged inspiratory efforts with occasional expiratory gasps. This phenomenon, termed *apneustic breathing,* results from prolonged discharge of inspiratory neurons. Various inputs into this area can terminate inspiration by negative feedback.

The medullary center is located in the reticular formation of the medulla and consists of two centers, the dorsal respiratory group and the ventral respiratory group, with the dorsal group responsible for inspiration and the ventral group for expiration. These centers are capable of rhythmically driving the respiratory musculature in the absence of any other input, although the pattern of respiration is abnormal and gasping predominates. If these centers are destroyed, all automatic respiration ceases (Berger et al., 1977b). Respiratory rhythm generation is likely within the dorsal respiratory group.

Integration of Breathing Control

The respiratory system has a complex system of sensors and effectors (the lungs and respiratory muscles), with the central nervous system (CNS) coordinating the response to the stimuli received. Changes in PCO_2 or PO_2 are the main stimuli that elicit a response, and these are usually kept within narrow physiologic ranges. In this section they are considered separately in relation to the reactions that they elicit.

Carbon Dioxide

Carbon dioxide elimination is inversely related to alveolar ventilation, and if ventilation rises, PCO_2 falls until a new steady-state level is reached. At any given CO_2 production the relationship between PCO_2 and ventilation is a hyperbolic one (Fig. 4-17) (Berger et al., 1977c). For a normal subject, minute ventilation increases linearly with PCO_2. Fig. 4-18 plots the ventilatory response to changes in PCO_2, and as can be seen, the degree of response is altered by the subject's PO_2, greater degrees of hypoxia causing increased ventilation (Nielsen and Smith, 1951). The ventilatory response to hypercapnia is usually measured by the Read technique, in which the subject rebreathes from a small bag containing a mixture of CO_2 and oxygen (Read, 1967; Rebuck and Slutsky, 1981). The ventilatory response to CO_2 is quite variable among subjects, but in about 80 percent it is between 1 and 4 L/min/mmHg PCO_2, with women generally having a lower response than men. The ventilatory response to CO_2 diminishes with age, following the use of CNS depressants, and with increasing cardiovascular fitness.

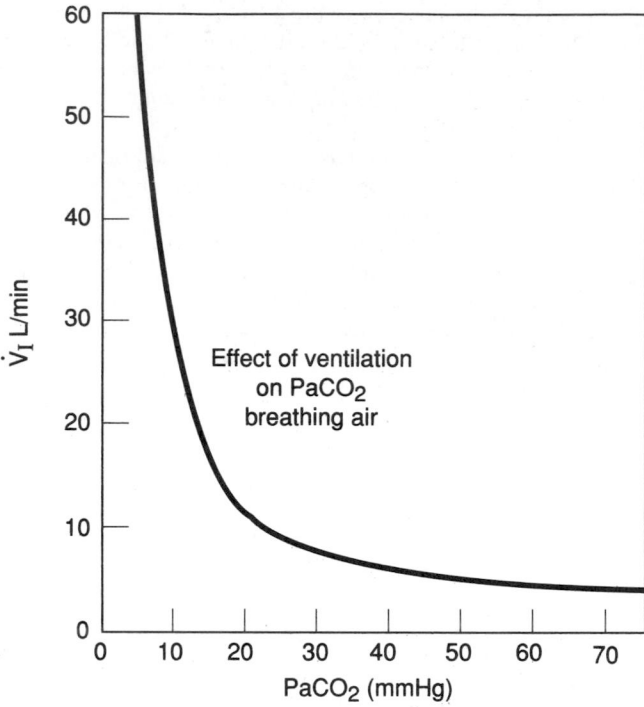

Figure 4-17. Effect of ventilation on $PaCO_2$.

The response to CO_2 is mainly central but there is a peripheral contribution. It is estimaed that peripheral chemoreceptors contribute 10 to 30 percent of the response to hypercapnia; however, the exact mechanism of this response is not fully known (Nielsen and Smith, 1951).

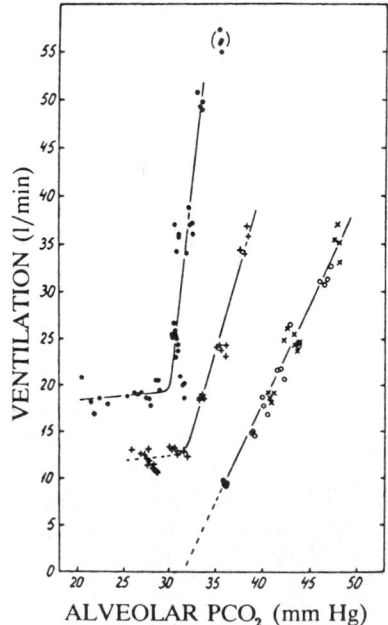

Figure 4-18. Ventilatory response to CO_2 at different $PaCO_2$ levels. The ventilatory response to CO_2 is enhanced by alveolar hypoxia. (From Nielsen M, Smith H: Studies on the regulation of respiration in acute hypoxia. Acta Physiol Scand 24:293, 1951, with permission.)

Oxygen

The response to hypoxia is mainly a peripheral phenomenon and originates in the carotid bodies, with minimal or no input from the aortic bodies, as manifested by the lack of hypoxic ventilatory drive in patients who have had bilateral carotid body resections (Nieman and Bredenberg, 1985). Ventilation increases as PO_2 and arterial hemoglobin saturation (SaO_2) fall; it is a hyperbolic function of PO_2 but a linear function of SaO_2 (Fig. 4-19) (Berger et al., 1977c). The response is variable, but about 80 percent of healthy subjects have a value between 0.6 and 2.8 L/min per 1 percent fall in SaO_2 (Rebuck and Woodley, 1975). This response is increased in the presence of elevated PCO_2 or decreased pH. The ventilatory response is blunted or reduced in chronic hypoxia (Sevringhaus, 1972).

Under normal circumstances hypoxic ventilatory drive plays a minimal role in the control of respiration. However, in the presence of a chronically elevated PCO_2, the ventilatory response to PCO_2 is reduced, partly because of the associated metabolic alkalosis in the CSF, which makes the pH of the CSF much less responsive to changes in PCO_2. In this situation hypoxic ventilatory drive assumes a prominent role, and administration of oxygen may severely depress respiration (West, 1985).

VENTILATION

Dead Space

Dead space is defined as the volume of the respiratory apparatus (including the upper airways) that is ventilated but in which gas exchange with the blood does not occur. This is arbitrarily divided into anatomic and physiologic dead space. Anatomic dead space is the volume of the conducting airways that are not specialized for gas exchange, including the nasal passages, pharynx, trachea, and airways up to the terminal bronchioles. In the normal human, the total volume of the anatomic dead space is approximately 150 ml. It also varies with inspiration, posture, and body size as the volume of the large airways changes. For normal, nonobese individuals in the seated position, the volume of dead space in milliliters approximaely equals body weight in pounds (West, 1985).

Abnormalities of perfusion and ventilation in regions of the lung specialized for gas exchange also produce dead space. This occurs when ventilation of gas exchange surfaces occurs in the absence of perfusion or when ventilation/perfusion mismatch occurs (i.e., when the amount of ventilation is out of proportion to the amount of perfusion). Physiologic dead space is the total amount of dead space present in the respiratory system, and as such it is the sum of anatomic dead space and dead space secondary to ventilation/perfusion ($\dot{V}/\dot{Q}$) mismatch. The total amount of dead space usually comprises about 25 to 35 percent of the normal tidal volume (expressed as the V_D/V_T ratio, where V_D is the volume of dead space and V_T is the tidal volume). During exercise, the tidal volume increases and V_D/V_T may fall as low as 10 to 15 percent.

The most common method of measuring anatomic dead space is Fowler's method (Fowler, 1952), in which the subject inhales a single breath of 100 percent oxygen and then ex-

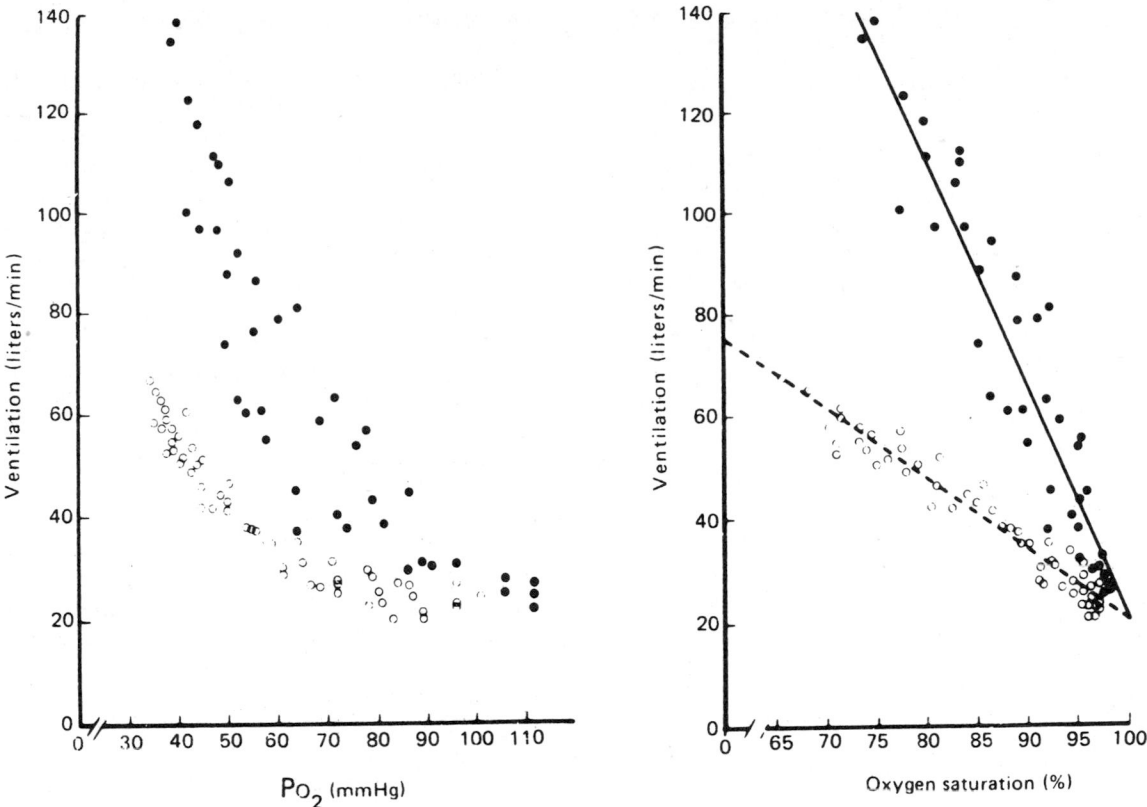

Figure 4-19. The ventilatory response to hypoxia in two subjects (open and closed circles). Illustrated are a hyperbolic response curve obtained by plotting PO_2 and a linear response curve obtained by plotting hemoglobin saturation against ventilation. (From Rebuck AS, Campbell EJM: A clinical method for assessing the ventilatory response to hypoxia. Am Rev Respir Dis 109:345, 1974, with permission.)

hales, and on expiration the nitrogen concentration is continuously measured at the mouth. The nitrogen concentration in the expired gas gradually rises as the 100 percent oxygen is washed out of the conducting airways by the alveolar gas and finally plateaus when only alveolar gas is being exhaled. If the slope of the plateau is zero, the volume of the anatomic dead space is taken as the volume halfway to the plateau point (Fig. 4-20).

Physiologic dead space can be measured by the Bohr method, which takes advantage of the fact that inspired air has virtually no CO_2 and that air ventilating perfused lung will equilibrate with the CO_2 within the blood. Thus

$$V_T \times F_{E}CO_2 = V_A \times F_{A}CO_2$$

where $F_{E}CO_2$ is the fractional concentration of CO_2 in the mixed expired gas and $F_{A}CO_2$ is the fractional concentration of CO_2 in the alveoli. Since $V_T = V_D + V_A$, where V_T is the tidal volume, V_D is the volume of dead space, and V_A is the volume of normally ventilated and perfused alveoli, rearrangement of the above equation produces

$$\frac{V_T}{V_D} = \frac{F_{A}CO_2 - F_{E}CO_2}{F_{A}CO_2}$$

Multiplication of the numerator and denominator of the right side by the atmospheric pressure minus the partial pres-

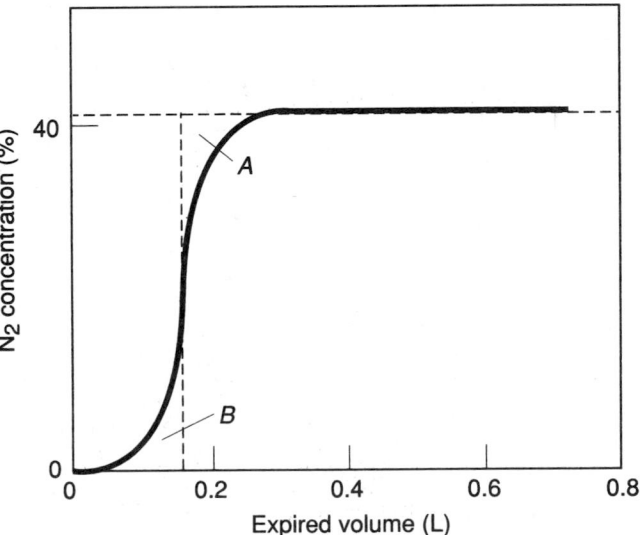

Figure 4-20. Fowler's method for determining anatomic dead space. (From Fowler WS: Intrapulmonary distribution of inspired gas. Physiol Rev 32:1, 1952, with permission.)

sure of water vapor converts the above equation to partial pressures

$$\frac{V_D}{V_T} = \frac{P_ACO_2 - P_ECO_2}{P_ACO_2}$$

where P_ACO_2 is the alveolar partial pressure of CO_2 and P_ECO_2 is the partial pressure of CO_2 in expired gas. P_ACO_2 is not easy to measure directly. Since P_ACO_2 is very close to arterial PCO_2, the value of P_ACO_2 is estimated by measuring $PaCO_2$. P_ECO_2 is measured by collecting an expired sample of gas.

Dynamic Aspects

In order for gas exchange to occur, O_2 must be delivered to the alveoli and CO_2 removed. This is accomplished by bulk transport to the small airways, where gas exchange by diffusion become predominant. In order for gas flow to occur, a pressure gradient must exist between the alveoli and the mouth. The relationship between the pressure gradient from the mouth to the alveoli and net flow is the resistance of the airways. The flow obtained from a given pressure gradient is dependent on whether gas flow is laminar or turbulent. This is determined largely by the Reynolds number (Re), which is given by the equation

$$Re = \frac{2rvd}{\eta}$$

where r is the radius, v is the velocity of the gas, d is the density, and η is the viscosity of the gas flowing in a cylinder. If the Reynolds number is greater than 2,000, flow is usually turbulent.

In the lung, flow is turbulent in the larger airways and becomes laminar in small peripheral airways. The flow is laminar at the level of the small airways partly because of their relatively small diameter individually but largely because the cross-sectional area of the lung increases markedly with distance into the lung and hence velocities are quite low. Thus the Reynolds number falls below the critical threshold of 2,000. Turbulent gas flow is proportional to gas density and to the square root of the driving pressure. It is this dependence on gas density which makes the use of gas mixtures such as helium and oxygen useful in some diseases in which there is upper airway obstruction (Curtis, et al., 1986; Ta-Shung, et al., 1976). A mixture of 80 percent helium and 20 percent oxygen has a density about one-third that of air, so that in situations in which the major pressure drop is related to turbulent flow, a decrease in density will decrease the pressure gradient necessary to generate a given flow rate (Houck, et al., 1990).

For laminar flow, flow is proportional to gas viscosity and directly proportional to the driving pressure. In a straight tube or airway, the flow profile is parabolic, with the velocity greatest in the center of the tube and zero at the wall. Laminar flow can be quantified by Poiseuille's law, which describes the relationship between flow and pressure:

$$\dot{V} = \frac{\pi r^4 \Delta P}{8\mu l}$$

where $\dot{V}$ is flow, r is the radius of the airway, ΔP is the driving pressure, μ is the gas viscosity, and l is the length of the airway.

Since airway resistance (Raw) is the relationship between a pressure gradient and the resultant flow, it is apparent from the above discussions that most of the resistance to flow occurs in the large airways, where flow is turbulent and the cumulative airway diameter is relatively small. Raw is also volume-dependent owing to the parenchymal recoil applied to the airway walls.

DIFFUSION

Diffusion is defined as the movement of a gas from an area of high partial pressure to an area of low partial pressure by the process of molecular mixing and not by bulk transfer. The rate of diffusion is determined by the pressure gradient that is driving the diffusion process, the cross-sectional area across which diffusion is taking place, and the properties of the gas in question and of the environment through which diffusion takes place.

Gas delivery by bulk transport is effective to the level of the respiratory bronchioles in the lung. At end inspiration, the fresh gas must distribute itself through the volume of the FRC. Therefore the mixing of residual alveolar gas and inspiratory gas is then dependent entirely on diffusion, augmented by cardiogenic oscillations (i.e., gas flow in the lung generated by the beating heart).

Once the inspiratory gas is delivered to the alveolar ducts, oxygen needs to reach the red cells in the alveolar capillaries. Oxygen must diffuse first into the alveolar spaces and then sequentially across the alveolocapillary membrane, the plasma in the capillaries, and the red cell membrane and finally must combine with hemoglobin within the red cells. The reverse process occurs with carbon dioxide (Fig. 4-21) (West, 1985).

The rate of diffusion of a gas in air is dependent on the molecular weight of the gas, while the diffusion of a gas in a liquid is dependent on the solubility of the gas in the liquid. Carbon dioxide is heavier than oxygen and diffuses through air at a slightly slower rate. However, because carbon dioxide is 20 times as soluble as oxygen, its rate of diffusion through the red cell, plasma, and alveolocapillary membrane is markedly faster than that of O_2.

The process of mixing within the alveolar spaces occurs very quickly and under normal conditions can be considered to be almost instantaneous; therefore, the rate determining step becomes the process of gas transfer from the alveoli to the red cell. Because of the greater ease with which carbon dioxide does this as compared with oxygen, pathologic states that impair diffusion affect oxygen transport to a much greater degree. For all intents and purposes, the reserve of carbon dioxide diffusion is so great that impairments of diffusion, unless extreme, can be considered not to have any effect on carbon dioxide elimination. The situation is much different, however, for oxygen which because of its relatively low diffusion reserve is very sensitive to pathologic process that impair diffusion.

Under normal circumstances, blood in the alveolar capillary becomes fully oxygenated in the first third of the time spent in the capillary (Fig. 4-22). In states of high cardiac

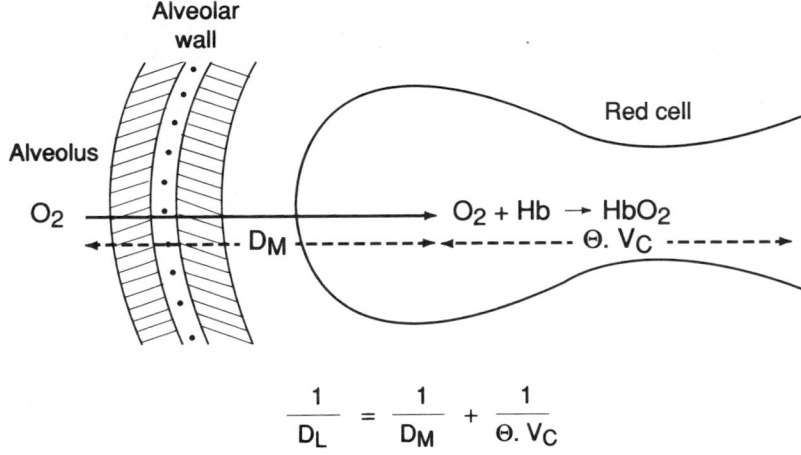

$$\frac{1}{D_L} = \frac{1}{D_M} + \frac{1}{\Theta \cdot V_C}$$

Figure 4-21. The components of diffusing capacity. (From West JB: Respiratory Physiology—The Essentials. p. 28. 3rd Ed. Williams & Wilkins, Baltimore, 1985, with permission.)

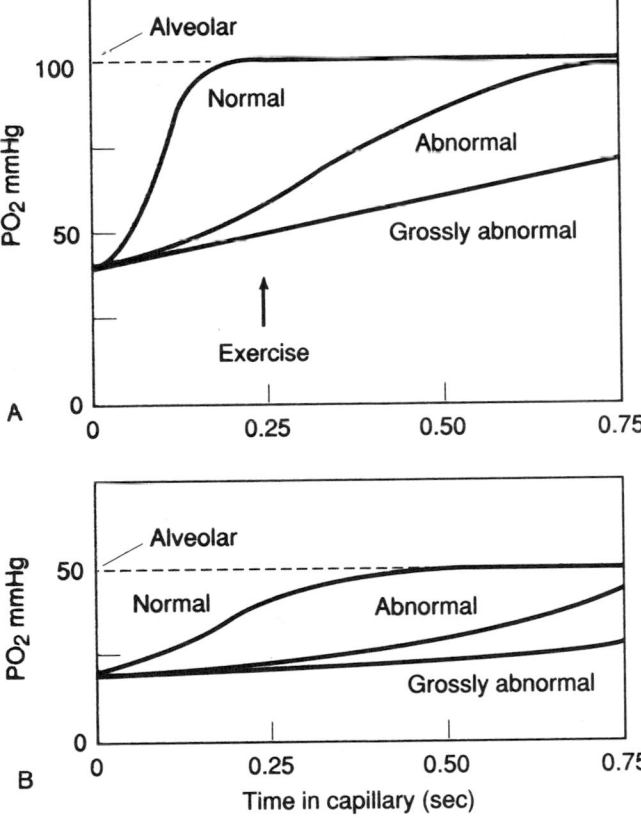

Figure 4-22. Alveolar capillary PO_2 versus the amount of time spent in the capillary by deoxygenated blood. **(A)** Graph is plotted with normal alveolar PO_2 levels, and **(B)** graph is plotted with an alveolar PO_2 of 50 mmHg. Both graphs are plotted with normal and abnormal alveolar membranes. Normal capillary transit time is approximately 0.75 second and may be reduced to as little as 0.25 second during exercise or other states of high cardiac output. End-capillary PO_2 is a function of transit time, alveolar membrane function, and alveolar PO_2. (From West JB: Respiratory Physiology—The Essentials. p. 28. 3rd Ed. Williams & Wilkins, Baltimore, 1985, with permission.)

output the capillary blood time is reduced, but the diffusion reserve is still adequate to ensure that the end-capillary blood is fully oxygenated. However, as the diffusion capability is reduced, the time required to fully oxygenate the blood during its course through the capillary becomes progressively longer and finally exceeds the capillary transit time, at which point end-capillary blood is not fully oxygenated and hypoxia results. In states of high cardiac output, in which the capillary transit time is reduced, hypoxia may be produced. This mechanism likely accounts for the hypoxia seen on exercise in patients with early interstitial lung disease who have normal blood gases at rest. It probably also accounts for a portion of the severe hypoxia seen in hyperdynamic septic patients with lung disease.

Diffusing Capacity

The measurement of diffusion efficiency is termed diffusing capacity. When the process of diffusion for O_2 is broken down into its individual components, three separate rate-limiting steps are found: the rate of passage of O_2 across the alveolocapillary membrane; the rate of combination of O_2 with hemoglobin in red blood cells; and the driving pressure for the diffusion, which is the difference in pressures between the PO_2 in the alveolus and the PO_2 in the red cell. In equation form, for the alveolocapillary membrane this becomes

$$D_M = \frac{V}{P_A - P_p} = \text{Conductance} = \frac{1}{\text{Resistance}}$$

$$\text{Resistance } (R_1) = \frac{1}{D_M}$$

where D_M is the diffusing capacity of the alveolocapillary membrane, V is the amount of diffusing gas, P_A is the partial pressure in the alveolus, and P_p is the partial pressure in plasma. Similarly, the rate at which a gas combines with the red cell (D_B) is proportional to the rate of the reaction and the capillary blood volume present.

$$D_B = \theta V_C = \text{conductance} = \frac{1}{R_2}$$

Therefore

$$\text{Resistance (R}_2) = \frac{1}{\theta V_C}$$

where θ is the rate of combination with hemoglobin and V_C is the volume of the capillary in contact with the blood. Similarly, the total diffusing capacity (D_L) is equal to the inverse of the total resistance to flow (R_L). However, the total resistance is obtained by adding R_1 and R_2. Therefore,

$$R_L = R_1 + R_2$$

which becomes

$$\frac{1}{D_L} = \frac{1}{D_M} + \frac{1}{\theta V_C}$$

Measurement of Diffusing Capacity

In practice, the diffusing capacity is measured by using carbon monoxide as the tracer gas. The advantage of using carbon monoxide as opposed to oxygen is that it has a very strong affinity for hemoglobin and under normal circumstances its partial pressure rises only slightly as it diffuses into the capillary. This is in contrast to oxygen, which has a moderate affinity for hemoglobin. The capillary partial pressure of oxygen starts to rise after about one-third of the blood capillary transit time, thereby reducing the pressure gradient for diffusion. As a result, the transfer of oxygen from the alveolar space to the red blood cell is initially diffusion-limited and later perfusion-limited. Also, carbon monoxide is readily measured and in low concentrations poses no hazard.

The single breath technique of measuring the diffusing capacity consists of the rapid inspiration from residual volume of a gas mixture of carbon monoxide (0.3 to 0.4 percent), helium, oxygen and nitrogen. The breath is held for 10 seconds, and a sample of alveolar gas is collected on expiration and analyzed for helium and carbon monoxide concentrations. The diffusing capacity D_LCO is defined as the volume of carbon monoxide transferred into the blood per minute per mmHg of carbon monoxide partial pressure.

Interpretation

The diffusing capacity can be either elevated or reduced depending on the disease process. The individual components of the equation for D_L provide useful clues as to the manner in which diseases affect the diffusing capacity.

D_M depends on the thickness and area of the alveolocapillary membrane, and diseases that affect either one tend to reduce the diffusing capacity. Examples of diseases that affect the area are emphysema and pneumonectomy, while those that affect the thickness are interstitial lung diseases and pulmonary edema.

Since θ remains relatively constant, V_C influences the diffusing capacity to a large extent. θV_C is reduced by anemia, pulmonary hypertension, pulmonary embolism, etc., diseases that reduce the amount of hemoglobin or cells in the capillary spaces. Diseases that increase the amount of blood or hemoglobin within the lung actually increase the measured diffusing capacity. Examples of this are polycythemia, early mitral stenosis, and left-right shunt. For this reason, in order to eliminate the effect of anemia or polycythemia, the diffusing capacity is usually reported after being corrected to a standard hemoglobin concentration. An interesting example of the extent of influence of intrathoracic hemoglobin is the elevation of diffusing capacity in pulmonary hemorrhage because of the free hemoglobin within the air spaces. In these situations, the diffusing capacity is a sensitive indicator of recurrent hemorrhage and may be used to follow up such diseases as Goodpasture syndrome.

MECHANISMS OF ALTERED GAS EXCHANGE

In order to gain a better understanding of pulmonary physiology, it is useful to look at the mechanisms of altered gas exchange. Within this context we will look at hypoxia and hypercarbia and the physiologic derangements that produce them. These are the problems that are frequently faced by clinicians, and an understanding of the physiology involved is crucial to dealing with them effectively.

Hypercapnia

The partial pressure of CO_2 in blood is inversely related to alveolar ventilation and directly related to CO_2 production. The relationship can be expressed as follows:

$$PaCO_2 = K \frac{\dot{V}CO_2}{\dot{V}_A}$$

where $PaCO_2$ is the partial pressure of arterial CO_2, $\dot{V}CO_2$ is CO_2 production, and $\dot{V}_A$ is alveolar ventilation. The constant K has a value of 0.863 mmHg (Weinberger, et al., 1989). Also, alveolar ventilation can be expressed in terms of tidal volume ($\dot{V}_T$) and dead space ($\dot{V}_D$):

$$\dot{V}_A = \dot{V}_T - \dot{V}_D$$

Therefore, the equation for $PaCO_2$ becomes

$$PaCO_2 = K \frac{\dot{V}CO_2}{\dot{V}_T - \dot{V}_D}$$

By looking at the individual terms in the equation, one can readily infer the causes of hypercapnia. CO_2 production is a function of the substrate metabolized for energy and is usually related to the amount of O_2 consumed. This is referred to as the respiratory quotient (RQ) and is expressed as

$$RQ = \frac{\dot{V}CO_2}{\dot{V}O_2}$$

where $\dot{V}O_2$ is the O_2 consumption. For carbohydrates RQ equals 1, for fat 0.7, and for protein 0.8, with an average of 0.8 for a typical diet. Excess CO_2 production does not usually cause hypercapnia in a normal individual since it can readily be compensated by increasing alveolar ventilation. However, in individuals who have underlying respiratory compromise, an increase in alveolar ventilation may not be possible and significant hypercapnia may result. Clinically, this may be significant in individuals who have respiratory failure secondary to severe chronic obstructive lung disease. In these patients high carbohydrate diets may significantly increase CO_2 production, with resultant hypercapnia. Although this is controversial, during the treatment of patients with severe ventilatory compromise, there may be a role for nutritional supplementation with high fat diets so that CO_2 production is minimized in the process of meeting caloric needs.

If CO_2 production is constant, $PaCO_2$ is inversely proportional to alveolar ventilation. In this case factors that reduces alveolar ventilation will cause hypercapnia. The causes of alveolar ventilation can be divided into three main groups: central hypoventilation ("lack of desire to breath"), neuromuscular disease (e.g., muscular dystrophy), and chest wall–lung disease.

From the equation for $PaCO_2$ in terms of $\dot{V}CO_2$, $\dot{V}_T$, and $\dot{V}_D$, it can also be deduced that as $\dot{V}_D$ increases in relation to $\dot{V}_T$, the denominator falls and $PaCO_2$ rises. In other words, the $\dot{V}_D/\dot{V}_T$ ratio is important in determining the amount of alveolar ventilation for a given respiratory rate and tidal volume. This may be an important mechanism of hypercapnia in patients with chronic obstructive lung disease who have areas of $\dot{V}/\dot{Q}$ mismatch (i.e., increased dead space) but who also tend to have relatively low tidal volumes because of this obstructive lung disease.

Hypoxia

The causes of arterial hypoxemia can be divided into two broad categories, depending on whether alveolar O_2 levels are normal or reduced.

Reduction of alveolar O_2, either focally or diffusely, is a relatively frequent cause of hypoxemia. Alveolar O_2 levels are the result of a balance between delivery of O_2 and its removal from the alveolus (Hlastala, 1991). Hypoxemia from low alveolar O_2 levels only occurs in situations where delivery of O_2 to the alveolus is reduced relative to the blood flow to that alveolus. This occurs throughout the lung at high altitudes, where the inspired PO_2 is low and although hyperventilation is usually present, total O_2 delivery to alveoli is reduced. It also occurs with hypoventilation, since the amount of air and consequently O_2 delivery is reduced. In this situation, if the fractional inspired concentration of O_2 is increased, it may compensate for the hypoventilation, and hypoxia may be circumvented.

Regional reduction of alveolar O_2 content occurs with $\dot{V}/\dot{Q}$ mismatch and shunt. In $\dot{V}/\dot{Q}$ mismatch, ventilation is inadequate to deliver sufficient amounts of O_2 to fully oxygenate the blood perfusing that alveolus, and shunt is present when there is no ventilation to a perfused alveolus. In $\dot{V}/\dot{Q}$ mismatch and shunt, arterial hypoxemia occurs when partially oxygenated blood mixes (in blood vessels downstream from alveolar capillaries) with fully oxygenated blood from regions with normal perfusion and ventilation. An example of hypoxia secondary to $\dot{V}/\dot{Q}$ mismatch occurs in obstructive airways disease, in which alveolar ventilation is not uniform and on a regional basis may be inadequate for the amount of perfusion present, while an example of shunt is provided by hypoxia secondary to lobar collapse, since continued perfusion may occur in the absence of ventilation.

Hypoxemia with normal alveolar O_2 levels occurs with abnormalities of diffusion and with very low mixed venous PO_2 ($P\bar{v}O_2$) levels. In these situations, equilibration of alveolar and capillary PO_2 does not occur during the transit time through the alveolar capillaries. In the normal situation, complete equilibration occurs in approximately one-third of the capillary transit time, and as a result there is a large degree of reserve present. Abnormalities of diffusion alone in the absence of $\dot{V}/\dot{Q}$ mismatch or shunt do not usually cause hypoxemia unless they are present with reduced pulmonary capillary transit times or they are associated with low $P\bar{v}O_2$ (Fraser, et al., 1988). An example in which hypoxia is secondary to impaired diffusion and reduced capillary transit time occurs during exercise in patients with pulmonary fibrosis.

A useful method of assessing gas exchange in the lung is to look at the alveolar-arterial PO_2 difference [$P(A\text{-}a)O_2$]. Under ideal circumstances, alveolar PO_2 (PAO_2) should be equal to arterial PO_2 (PaO_2). The PAO_2 is a function of the inspired O_2 concentration (PIO_2) and the subsequent uptake and replacement of O_2 by CO_2 in the alveolus. As previously stated, the amount of CO_2 exhaled from the lungs for a given O_2 uptake from the lungs is known as the respiratory quotient (RQ). Therefore

$$PAO_2 = PIO_2 - \frac{PaCO_2}{RQ}$$

$P(A\text{-}a)O_2$ then is

$$P(A\text{-}a)O_2 = PAO_2 - PaO_2$$

Combining these equations gives

$$P(A\text{-}a)O_2 = PIO_2 - \frac{PaCO_2}{RQ} - PaCO_2$$

In its full form the equation becomes

$$P(A\text{-}a)O_2 = (P_B - 47)\, FIO_2 - \frac{PaCO_2}{RQ} - PaO_2$$

where P_B is the barometric pressure, 47 mmHg is the partial pressure of water vapor in fully saturated air, and FIO_2 is the fraction of inspired oxygen. RQ is assumed to be approximately 0.8.

If $P(A\text{-}a)O_2$ is normal or less than 10, there unlikely to be any shunt or $\dot{V}/\dot{Q}$ mismatch. However, in the presence of $\dot{V}/\dot{Q}$ mismatch or shunt, the degree of elevation of $P(A\text{-}a)O_2$ does not correlate with the amount of shunt or $\dot{V}/\dot{Q}$ mismatch, since then it is also influenced by $P\bar{v}O_2$ and FIO_2. For example, in a patient with an elevated $P(A\text{-}a)O_2$, its calculated value will rise as the FIO_2 is increased, although the amount of lung disease remains constant.

The amount of shunt or venous admixture ratio is calculated from the following formula (for its full derivation see West (1985), p. 52):

$$\frac{\dot{Q}s}{\dot{Q}_T} = \frac{C\acute{c}O_2 - CaO_2}{C\acute{c}O_2 - C\bar{v}O_2}$$

where $\dot{Q}s/\dot{Q}_T$ is the shunt fraction, $C\acute{c}O_2$ is the O_2 content of end-capillary blood, CaO_2 is the O_2 content of arterial blood, and $C\bar{v}O_2$ is the O_2 content of mixed venous blood (Fig. 4-23).

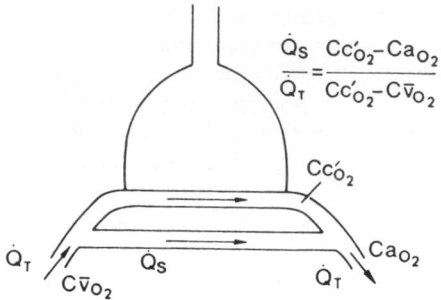

$$\frac{\dot{Q}_S}{\dot{Q}_T} = \frac{Cc'_{O_2} - Ca_{O_2}}{Cc'_{O_2} - C\bar{v}_{O_2}}$$

Figure 4-23. The influence of shunt on arterial PO_2.

The advantage of using this method to calculate shunt fraction is that it is independent of FIO_2. However, its main disadvantage is that it requires a sample of mixed venous blood, which normally requires insertion of a pulmonary artery catheter.

COMMENTS AND CONTROVERSIES

As important as it is for the surgeon to hone technical skills, the thoracic surgeon is obligated to assess a patient preoperatively with regard to pulmonary reserve and to manage difficult postoperative pulmonary problems. Without a basic understanding of pulmonary physiology and its application in preoperative assessment and the management of postoperative patients, one cannot practice modern thoracic surgery. The overview presented in this chapter provides the basis for such an understanding. However, a training thoracic surgeon is well advised to obtain and study a standard textbook of pulmonary physiology and its clinical applications. Similarly, every practicing thoracic surgeon should have spent time in a pulmonary function laboratory to obtain further understanding of the conduct of pulmonary function testing and its application in assessing patients.

Without this basic knowledge of physiology, advances made by thoracic surgeons in the fields of extracorporeal oxygen support and pulmonary transplantation could never have been made.

R.J.G.

KEY REFERENCES

Bates DV: Respiratory Function in Disease. 3rd ed., WB Saunders, Philadelphia, 1989

This very well referenced book summarizes key concepts relating to pulmonary function testing as well as clinical interpretation of these tests.

Crystal RG, West JB: The Lung. Vols. 1 and 2. Raven Press, New York, 1991

This comprehensive textbook deals with the scientific basis of respiratory medicine and biology. It covers topics ranging from basic molecular biology to mechanical ventilation.

Nunn JF: Applied Respiratory Physiology. 3rd Ed. Butterworths, London, 1987

This is an excellent comprehensive review of respiratory physiology, which covers the main concepts in depth.

Tisi GM: Preoperative evaluation of pulmonary function. Validity, indications, and benefits. Am Rev Respir Dis 119:293, 1979

This excellent summary of preoperative evaluation of pulmonary function, although relatively old, is a comprehensive review, and many of the concepts are still valid.

West JB: Respiratory Physiology—The Essentials, 4th Ed. Williams & Wilkins, Baltimore, 1989

This is an excellent short text that deals with the basics of respiratory physiology. It is much less comprehensive than Nunn's text.

Zibrak J, O'Donnell CR, Martin K: Indications for pulmonary function testing. Ann Intern Med 112:768, 1990

This article is the result of a consensus conference summarizing indications for pulmonary function testing.

REFERENCES

Albert RK, Lakshminarayan S, Hildebrandt WK, Butler J: Increased surface tension favours pulmonary edema formation in anesthetized dogs' lungs. J Clin Invest 63:1015, 1979

Angus GE, Thurlbeck WM: Number of alveoli in the human lung. J Appl Physiol 32:483, 1972

Armstrong DJ, Luck JC: A comparative study of irritant and type J receptors in the cat. Respir Physiol 21:47, 1974

Bachofen H, Hildebrandt J, Bachofen M: Pressure-volume curves of air and liquid filled excised lungs—surface tension in-situ. J Appl Physiol 29:422, 1970

Bachofen HP, Gehr P, Weibel ER: Alterations of mechanical properties and morphology in excised rabbit lungs rinsed with a detergent. J Appl Physiol 47:1002, 1979

Ball WC, Stewart PB, Newsham LGS, Bates DV: Regional pulmonary functions studied with xenon-133. J Clin Invest 41: 519, 1962

Bastacky, J., Hayes, TL, Schmidt, BV: Lung structure as revealed by microdissection. Am Rev Respir Dis 128:S7, 1983

Berger AJ, Mitchell RA, Severinghaus JW: Regulation of respiration (Part 1). N Engl J Med 297:92, 1977a

Berger AJ, Mitchell RA, Severinghaus JW: Regulation of respiration (Part 2). 297:139, 1977b

Berger AJ, Mitchell RA, Severinghaus JW: Regulation of breathing (Part 3). N Engl J Med 297:194, 1977c

Brown R, Slutsky AS: Frequency dependence of plethysmographic measurement of thoracic gas volume. J Appl Physiol 57:1865, 1984

Cosio M, Ghezzo H, Hogg JC: The relationship between structural changes in small airways and pulmonary function. N Engl J Med 298:1277, 1978

Cumming G: Airway morphology and its consequences. Bull Physiopathol Respir 8:527, 1972

Curtis JL, Mahlmeister M, Fink JB, et al.: Helium-oxygen gas therapy. Chest 90:455, 1986

Dobbs LG: Pulmonary surfactant. Annu Rev Med 40:431, 1989

Elliot FM, Reid L: Some new facts about the pulmonary artery and its branching pattern. Clin Radiol 16:193, 1965

Floros J: Sixty years of surfactant research. Am J Physiol 2:L238, 1990

Fowler WS: Intrapulmonary distribution of inspired gas. Physiol Rev 32:1, 1952

Fraser RG, Pare JAP, Pare PD, et al. (eds): Diagnosis of Diseases of the Chest. 3rd Ed. WB Saunders, Philadelphia, 1988, p. 29

Freedman S: Mechanics of ventilation. p. 114. In Brewes RAL, Gibbon GJ, Geddes DM (eds): Respiratory Medicine. Baillière Tindall, London, 1990

Fung YC, Sobin SS: Theory of sheet flow in lung alveoli. J Appl Physiol 26:472, 1968

Gaensler EA: Analysis of the ventilatory defect by timed vital capacity measurements. Am Rev Respir Dis 64:256, 1951

Glazier JB, Hughes JMB, West JB: Measurement of capillary dimensions and blood volume in rapidly frozen lungs. J Appl Physiol 26:65, 1969

Grassino AE, Roussos C, Macklem PT: Static properties of the chest wall. p. 855. In Crystal RG, West JB (eds): The Lung. Vol. 1. Scientific Foundations. Raven Press, New York, 1991

Hawgood S, Clements JA: Pulmonary surfactant and its apoproteins. J Clin Invest 86:1, 1990

Hawgood S: Surfactant: composition, structure and metabolism. p. 247. In Crystal RG, West JB (eds): The Lung. Vol. 1. Scientific Foundations. Raven Press, New York, 1991

Hlastala MP: Ventilation. p. 1209. In Crystal RG, West JB (eds): The Lung. Raven Press, New York, 1991

Hoppin FG, Stothert JC, Greaves IA, et al.: Lung recoil: elastic and rheological properties. p. 195. In Fishman AP, Macklem PT, Mead J, Greiger SR (eds): Vol. 3, The Respiratory System. Sec. 3. In Handbook of Physiology. American Physiological Society. Bethesda, 1986

Horsfeld K, Cumming G: Morphology of the bronchial tree in man. J Appl Physiol 24:373, 1968

Houck JR, Keamy MF, McDonough JM: Effect of helium concentration on experimental upper airway obstruction. Ann Otol Rhinol Laryngol 99:556, 1990

Hughes JMB, Glazier JB, Maloney JE, et al.: Effect of lung volumes on the distribution of pulmonary blood flow. Respir Physiol 4:58, 1968

Hyatt RE, Black LE: The flow-volume curve. Am Rev Respir Dis 107:191, 1973

Knowles JH, Hong SK, Rahn H: Possible errors using an esophageal balloon in the determination of pressure-volume characteristics of lung and rib cage. J Appl Physiol 14:525, 1959

Lahiri S, Mokasi A, Mulligan E, Nishino T: Comparison of aortic acid and chemoreceptor responses to hypercapnia and hypoxia. J Appl Physiol 51:55, 1981

Landis EM, Pappenheimer JR: Exchange of substances through capillary walls. p. 961. In Hamilton WE, Dao P (eds): Sec. 2. Circulation. Vol. 2. In Handbook of Physiology, American Physiological Society, Washington, 1963

Landowne M, Sacy WR: Glossary of terms. p. 197. In Remington JW (ed): Tissue Elasticity. American Physiological Society, Bethesda, 1957

Lauweryns J: The blood and lymphatic micro-circulation of the lung. Pathol Annu 6:365, 1965

Lugliani R, Whipp BJ, Seard C, Wasserman K: Effect of bilateral carotid-body resection on ventilatory control at rest and during exercise in man. N Engl J Med 285:1105, 1971

Lumsden T: Observations on the respiratory centres. J Physiol (Lond) 57:354, 1923

Lumsden T: Observations on the respiratory centres in the cat. J Physiol (Lond) 57:153, 1923

Macklem PT: New tests to assess lung function. N Engl J Med 293:339, 1975

Mead J, Turner JM, Macklem PT, et al.: Significance of the relationship between lung recoil and maximum expiratory effort. J Appl Physiol 22:95, 1967

Meneely GR, Kaltrieder NL: The volume of the lung determined by helium dilution. Description of the method and comparison with other procedures. J Clin Invest 28:129, 1949

Meyer BJ, Meyer A, Guyton AC: Interstitial fluid pressure versus negative pressure in the lung. Circ Res 22:263, 1968

Morton NS: Pulmonary surfactant: physiology, pharmacology and clinical uses. Br J Hosp Med 42:52, 1989

Nielsen M, Smith H: Studies on the regulation of respiration in acute hypoxia. Acta Physiol Scand 24:293, 1951

Nieman GF, Bredenberg CE: High surface tension pulmonary edema induced by detergent aerosol. J Appl Physiol 58:129, 1985

Norton LC, Conforti CG: The effects of body position on oxygenation. Heart Lung 14:45, 1985

Ogilvie CM, Forster RE, Blakemore WS, Morton JE: A standardised breath-holding technique for the clinical measurement of diffusing capacity. J Clin Invest 36:1, 1957

Paintal AS: Vagal sensory receptors and their reflex effects. Physiol Rev 53:159, 1973

Phillipson EA, Sullivan CE: Arousal: the forgotten response to respiratory stimuli (editorial). Am Rev Respir Dis 118:807, 1978

Prattle RE: Surface lining of lung alveoli. Physiol Rev 45:48, 1965

Prokocimer P, Garbino J, Wolff M, Regnier B: Influence of posture on gas exchange in artificially ventilated patients with focal lung disease. Intensive Care Med 9:69, 1983

Radford EP Jr: Recent studies of mechanical properties of mammalian lungs. p. 177. In: Remington JW (Ed): Tissue Elasticity. American Physiological Society, Bethesda, 1957

Radford EP: Static mechanical properties of mammalian lungs. p. 429. In Fenn WO, Rahn H (eds): Vol. 1. Respiration. In Handbook of Physiology. American Physiological Society, Bethesda, 1964

Rahn H, Otis AB, Chadwick LE, Fenn WO: The pressure-volume diagram of thorax and lung. Am J Physiol 146:161, 1946

Raskin PS, Herman P: Inter-acinar pathways in the human lung. Am Rev Respir Dis 111:489, 1975

Read DJC: A clinical method of assessing the ventilatory response to CO_2. Aust NZ J Med 16:20, 1967

Rebuck AS, Campbell EJM: A clinical method for assessing the ventilatory response to hypoxia. Am Rev Respir Dis 109:345, 1974

Rebuck AS, Woodley WE: Ventilatory effects of hypoxia and their dependence on PCO_2. J Appl Physiol 38:16, 1975

Rebuck AS, Slutsky AS: Measurement of the ventilatory response to hypercapnia and hypoxia. p. 745. Hornbein, TF (ed): Regulation of Breathing. Part II; Marcel Dekker, New York, 1981

Sampson SR, Vidruk EH: Properties of irritant receptors in canine lung. Respir Physiol 25:9, 1975

Schneeberger EE: Structural basis for some permeability properties of the air-blood barrier. FASEB J 37:2471, 1978

Schurch S, Goerke J, Clements JA: Direct determination of surface tension in the lung. Proc Natl Acad Sci USA 73:4698, 1976

Severinghaus JW: Hypoxic respiratory drive and its loss during chronic hypoxia. Clin Physiol 2:57, 1972

Sharp JT, Hammond MD: Pressure-volume relationships, p. 839. In Crystal RG, West JB (eds): The Lung; Scientific Foundations. Raven Press, New York, 1991

Staub NC: Alveolar-arterial oxygen tension gradient due to diffusion. J Appl Physiol 18:673, 1963

Sykes MK, McNicol MW, Campbell EJM: Respiratory Failure. 2nd Ed. Blackwell Scientific Publications, Oxford, 1976

Ta-Shung Lu, Ohmura A, Wong KC, Hodges MR: Helium-oxygen in treatment of upper airway obstruction. Anesthesiology 45:678, 1976

Thurlbeck WM: The internal surface of area on non-emphysematous lungs. Am Rev Respir Dis 95:765, 1967

Von Euler C, Trippenbach T: Cyclic excitability changes of the inspiratory 'off-switch' mechanism. Acta Physiol Scand 93:560, 1975

Weibel ER: Morphometry of the Human Lung. Springer-Verlag, Berlin, 1963

Weinberger SE, Schwartzstein RM, Weiss JW: Hypercapnia. N Engl J Med 321:1223, 1989

West JB: Regional differences in the lung. Chest 74:426, 1978

West JB: Ventilation. p. 17. In: Respiratory Physiology—The Essentials. 3rd Ed. Williams & Wilkins, Baltimore, 1985a

West JB: Mechanics of breathing. p. 88. In: Respiratory Physiology. The Essentials. 3rd Ed. Williams & Wilkins, Baltimore, 1985b

West JB; Control of ventilation. p. 124. In: Respiratory Physiology—The Essentials. 3rd Ed. Williams & Wilkins, Baltimore, 1985c

West JB, Dollery CT: Distribution of blood flow and ventilation-perfusion ratios on the lung measured with radioactive CO_2. J Appl Physiol 15:405, 1960

West JB, Dollery CT, Naimark A: Distribution of blood flow in isolated lungs: relation to vascular and alveolar pressures. J Appl Physiol 19:713, 1964

Wright JR: Clearance and recycling of pulmonary surfactant. Am J Physiol 259:L1, 1990

Zamel N: Normal lung mechanics. In Baum GL, Wolinsky E (eds): Textbook of Pulmonary Disease. Little, Brown, Boston, 1989

5

PULMONARY FUNCTION TESTING: A PRACTICAL APPROACH

Thomas L. Petty

The value of pulmonary function testing in health and disease is grossly underestimated. This chapter presents a practical approach to the assessment of lung mechanics and gas transfer, which is useful in diagnosis of pulmonary disease and responses to therapy, in preoperative assessment, and for estimation of the overall prognosis of surgical patients.

HISTORICAL NOTE

John Hutchinson, a surgeon, invented the spirometer and coined the term *vital capacity* (i.e., capacity for life). John Hutchinson was a very precise man. He was a violinist of some reputation. His exacting observations allowed him to learn that vital capacity was directly related to height and inversely related to the age of the patients he studied. In his landmark first paper (Huchinson, 1846), he cited measurements on 2,130 individuals, including deceased patients. John Hutchinson would inflate the body of a corpse immediately after death, using a bellows device equipped with a crude endotracheal tube and a valve system. He would then allow the corpse to "exhale" into his spirometer, which accurately measured exhaled volume. Thus he correctly concluded that elastic recoil of the lungs and thorax and open airways were essential for expiratory airflow. He believed that his device would be valuable for predictions of premature mortality by the insurance industry of London. Alas, the dogma of the era and the lack of vision of "experts" of the time prevented them from capitalizing on the brillance of John Hutchinson's predictions. In short, the spirometer was not accepted as a useful medical instrument until many years later. Even today many physicians and surgeons fail to take advantage of the immense value of simple pulmonary function tests in their daily practice.

Many years later in the landmark Framingham study, it was finally recognized that abnormalities in vital capacity were the best predictors of premature mortality, including deaths from all causes but especially from heart disease (Kannel et al., 1980). The reason that the vital capacity is such a powerful indicator of premature morbidity and mortality is because any compromise of ventilatory air space may result from an important heart or lung disease. A reduction in vital capacity may be a nonspecific indicator of poor health. Lung diseases can be classified as obstructive or restrictive, as described below. In addition, pulmonary congestion, cardiomegaly, space-preempting intrathoracic malignant or benign lesions, poor physical conditioning, neuromuscular disorders, and marked obesity can all affect the vital capacity. Thus, it is easy to understand how a simple measurement of expiratory airflow can be the true predictor of the capacity to live (i.e., the vital capacity).

Another surgeon, Gaensler (1951), developed the concept of the timed vital capacity, which ultimately became known as the forced expiratory volume as a function of time. Since Gaensler's original proposition that measurements of airflow were as important as air volume, clinicians have settled on the 1 second vital capacity, or forced expiratory volume in 1 second (FEV_1) as the standard. Similar conclusions could be drawn from the FEV in 0.75, 2, or 3 seconds, but there is no particular reason to do this. Thus, two key spirometric tests have become standard, the forced vital capacity (FVC) (volume test) and the FEV_1 (flow test). The ratio between the two is another important value, and normally this is greater than 70 percent. Thus, an FEV_1/FVC of 71 percent is considered the lower limit of normal (LLN).

HISTORICAL READINGS

Gaensler EA: Analysis of the ventilatory defect by timed vital capacity. Am Rev Respir Dis 69:256, 1951

Gilson JC, Hugh-Jones P: The measurement of total lung volume and breathing capacity. Clin Sci 7:185, 1949

Hutchinson J: On the capacity of the lungs and the respiratory function with a view of establishing a precise and easy method of detecting disease by the spirometer. Med Chir Trans (Lond) 29:137, 1846

Kannel WB, Lew EA, Hubert HB et al.: The value of measuring vital capacity for prognostic purposes. Trans Am Life Insurance Med Dir Am 64:66, 1980

Leiner GC, Abramowitz S, Small MJ et al.: Expiratory peak flow rate. Standard values for normal subjects. Use as a clinical test of ventilatory function. Am Rev Respir Dis 88:644, 1963

Ogilvie CM, Forster RE, Blakemore WS et al.: A standardized breath holding technique for the clinical measurement of the diffusing capacity of the lung for carbon monoxide. J Clin Invest 36:1, 1957

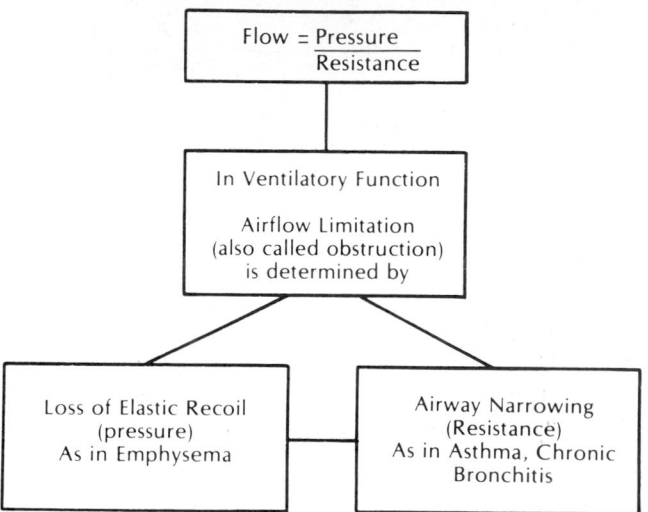

Figure 5-1. Origins of airflow. Airflow is a function of alveolar pressure and airways resistance. Expiratory pressure is caused by elastic recoil and muscular effort. Airways resistance is caused by anything that compromises the conducting air passages, such as mucus, bronchospasm, inflammation, mucosal edema, dynamic airways collapse, or combinations. (From Petty TL: Office spirometry. Semin Respir Med 4:184, 1983, with permission.)

ORIGINS OF AIRFLOW

Figure 5-1 schematically presents the origins of airflow from the complex respiratory system. After filling of the lungs by a forceful inspiratory effort, the fully inflated lungs and thorax empty, following another vigorous muscular effort during exhalation and by virtue of elastic recoil. Expiratory airflow is a result of the release of stored elastic energy and the fact that airways are normally open. Maximum emptying of the lungs is only possible with a forced expiration. The middle part of expiratory airflow is largely effort-independent and has been termed the forced expiratory flow between 25 and 75 percent of the total expiratory flow curve (FEF_{25-75}) or the maximum midexpiratory flow (MMEF). FEF_{25-75}, or MMEF, is not a more sensitive index of airflow; it is only more variable because it is affected by lung volume and thus elastic recoil. This measurement does not have any additional practical value as compared with FEV_1, FVC, and the percent of predicted (i.e., FEV_1/FVC), and accordingly both the measurement and term should be abandoned by clinicians. Contrary to previous dogma, it does not measure small airways function any more than the FEV_1 or the FEV_1/FVC ratio.

Not all the air in the lungs can be forcibly inhaled. The FVC is the amount of air that can be exhaled; the residual volume (RV) is the amount of air that cannot be exhaled. The RV and FVC together comprise the total lung capacity (TLC), as seen in Figure 5-2, which conceptualizes the elastic forces of lung and chest wall as equal but opposite forces at the resting level or functional residual capacity (FRC) (the heavily shaded area between vital capacity and RV).

Figure 5-3 graphically presents the radiographic features of normal lung emptying. The top of the lung and the diaphragm are outlined with wax pencil. On the left, one can see that the subject has filled his lungs by a forceful inspiratory muscular effort. The diaphragms have descended and the ribs have achieved a horizontal position at full inflation. As seen on the left, the man has now exhaled his FVC within

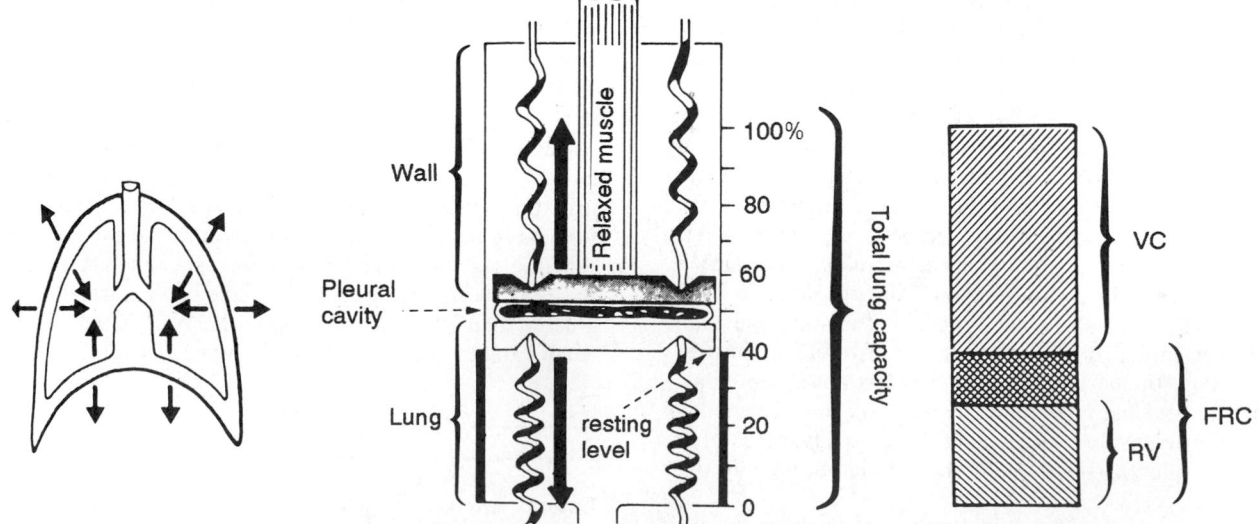

Figure 5-2. Balanced opposing elastic forces. Note that the elastic forces of the lung and chest wall are equal but pulling in opposite directions at the resting level or functional residual capacity. (From Cherniack RM: Mechanics of breathing. Semin Respir Med 4:171, 1983, with permission.)

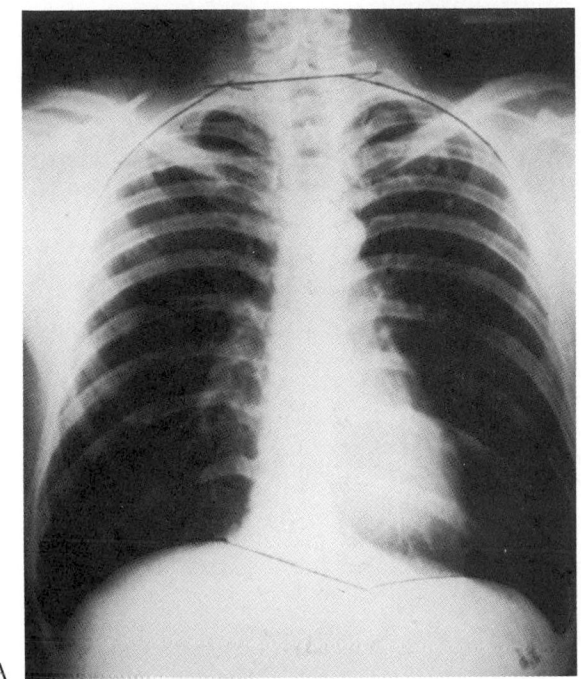

A

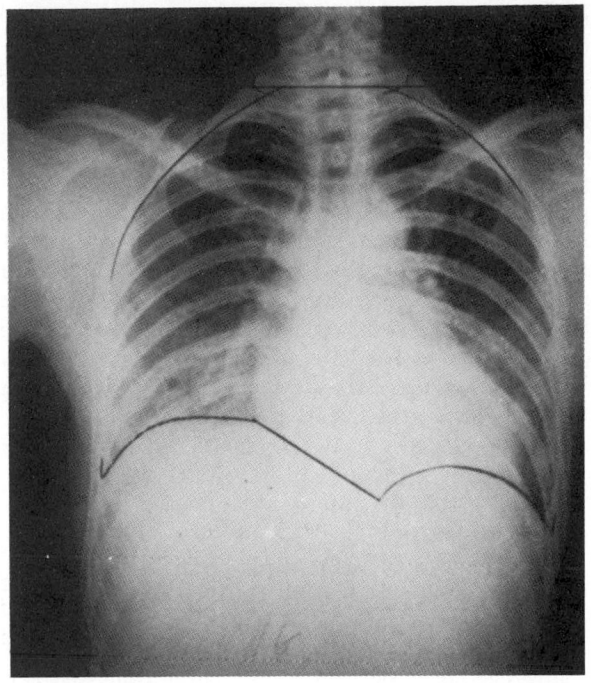

B

Figure 5-3.   Normal **(A)** inspiratory and **(B)** expiratory chest radiographs from a young, healthy 24-year-old male volunteer. Note that some air (i.e., the residual volume) remains at the top of the lung following a forced expiration. (From Petty TL: Office spirometry. Semin Respir Med 4:184, 1983, with permission.)

4 seconds; the FVC was 4.25 L, which is within the normal range. Thus, some air remains in the top of the lung, which constitutes the RV. This patient's TLC is 5.55 (4.25 FVC + 1.30), which is normal for his sex and height. That the RV is present in the top part of the lung is suggested by studies demonstrating that the upper lobes have less elastic recoil than the lower lobes (Silvers, et al., 1979).

In marked contrast are the inspiratory (left) and expiratory (right) films of a patient with advanced emphysema (Fig. 5-4). Notice the marked hyperinflation. There has been very little

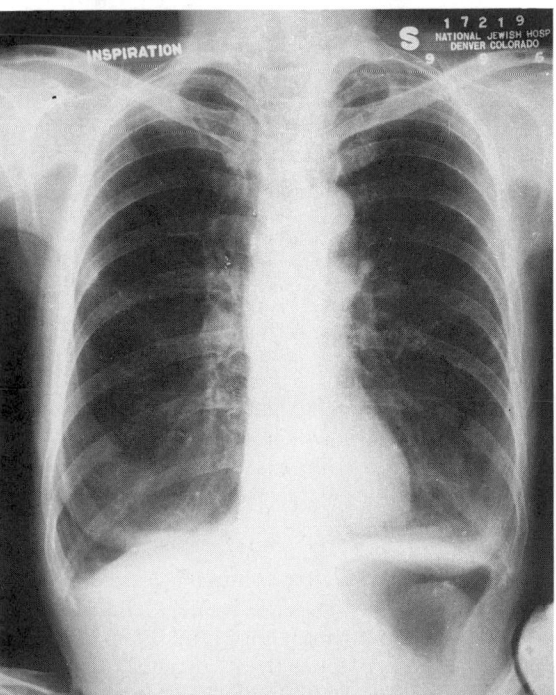

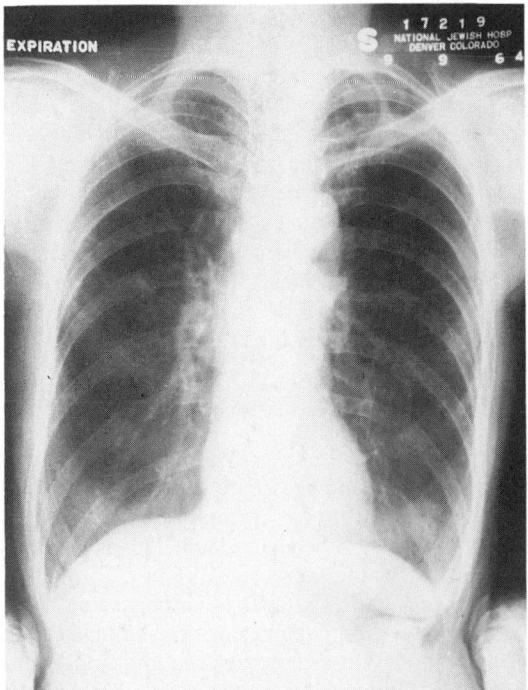

Figure 5-4.   Inspiratory-expiratory films of a patient with advanced emphysema. Notice that only a small amount of air has been exhaled; this proved to be 1.25 L. The residual volume (i.e., the air remaining in the lung) was 6.10 L. (From Petty TL: Office spirometry. Semin Respir Med 4:184, 1983, with permission.)

lung emptying between the inspiratory and expiratory maneuver. The FVC is 1.25 L, but a huge RV, 6.10 L, remains. Thus, the TLC is 1.25 plus 6.1, or 7.35 L, which is a markedly elevated total lung capacity (140 percent of normal).

Normal expiratory time is 6 seconds or less (Lal, et al., 1964). In obstructed breathing states, expiratory time is longer than 6 seconds. This can be easily observed by auscultation over the manubrium using a stopwatch or sweep second hand. A very short expiratory time (e.g., 1 to 2 seconds) strongly suggests increased elastic recoil from pulmonary fibrosis. Thus, the timing of the expiratory maneuver as well as the measures of volume and flow is important and is readily visualized by simple volume over time measurements in classic spirometry. These measurements can also be calculated from flow volume maneuvers, as illustrated below.

TESTING METHODS

Spirometry

John Hutchinson's "mysterious machine" was an inverted bell with a water seal. A reproduction of a slight modification of Hutchinson's spirometer is presented in Figure 5-5. Essentially this same technology was used in the Collins-type instruments which became the instruments of choice in many pulmonary function laboratories and are still used in some centers today. However, other technologies can accurately measure volume over time; flow transducers, one of which is shown in Figure 5-6, have become the most popular. Also, dry, direct-recording devices are commonly used, as shown in Figure 5-7.

Two methods of expressing the expiratory airflow curve are the volume over time curve, which I prefer, and the flow-volume curve, which is somewhat of a fad but also has value. The figures that follow show a comparison of flow-volume and time-volume curves in different situations.

Figure 5-8 presents both the flow-volume and time-volume expiratory airflow curves from a normal person. (The (LLN) is in parentheses.) Note the rapid emptying of the lung with FEV$_1$ 3.79 L as indicated by the arrow on both curves. Figures 5-9 to 5-12 present both the flow-volume and volume-time curves of patients with progressive degrees of obstructive ventilatory disorders. Figure 5-9 shows the pattern of mild airflow obstruction and reveals a concavity of the flow-volume curve. Note that the FVC is above the lower limit of normal but the FEV$_1$ (Gaensler, 1951) is below normal. This makes the FEV$_1$ 1 percent less than the normal 71 percent. Thus, there are actually two factors in the low FEV$_1$ percent—an increased denominator (volume) and a decreased numerator (flow). Studies in whole excised human lungs by my associates and me (Petty, et al., 1987) have shown that in the earliest stages of emphysema, TLC increases along with decreased elastic recoil. This is probably the best explanation for the increased FVC and low FEV$_1$/FVC ratio in the very earliest stages of emphysema.

Figure 5-10 shows the flow-volume and time-volume curves of a patient with moderate airflow obstruction, and Figure 5-11 presents the expiratory airflow curves of a patient with severe airflow obstruction. Finally, Figure 5-12 shows the expiratory flow curves of a patient with moderate airflow

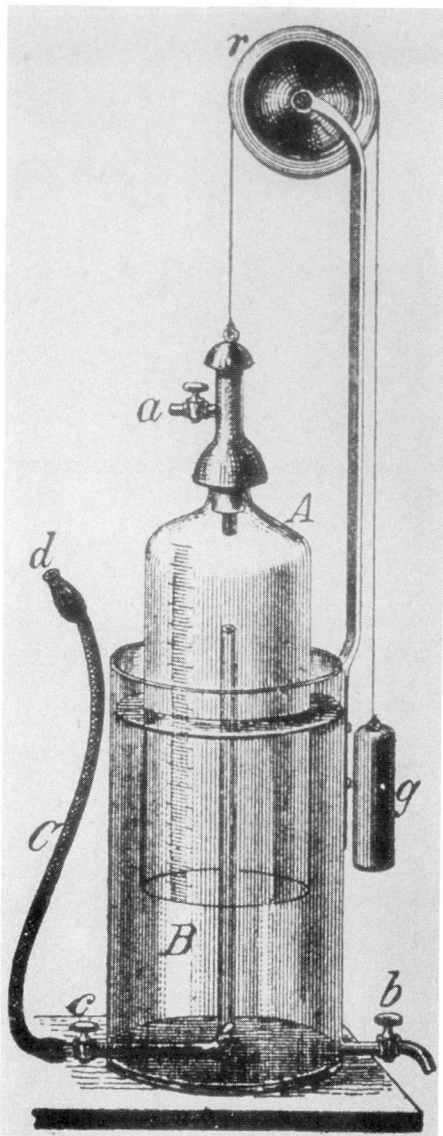

Figure 5-5. Reproduction of a slight modification of Hutchison's original water-sealed spirometer. This device is very similar to the Collins-type spirometers that are still in use and that were preferred the method in the past.

restriction. Note that in this case the expiratory time is shortened but peak flow is high, owing to excessive elastic recoil from pulmonary fibrosis.

Normal Values

Normal values are based upon age, sex, and height (Morris, et al., 1971). Younger, taller individuals have better air volume and flow than shorter, older individuals. Men have slightly higher values than women. For some reason certain ethnic groups, such as blacks, have slightly lower normal values (but most athletes would deny that this is true) (Rossiter and Weill, 1974).

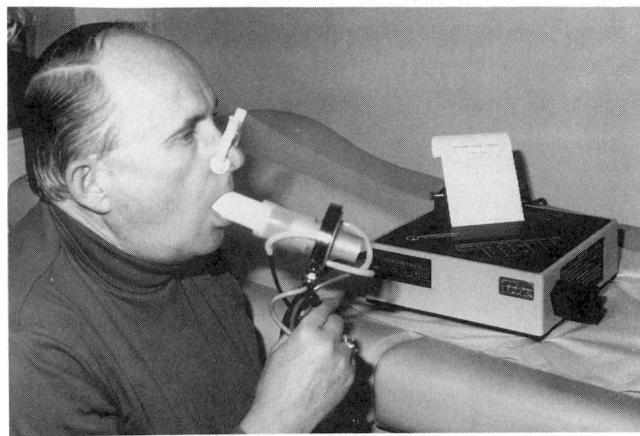

Figure 5-6. Flow transducer device, which accurately measures either flow-volume or volume-time curves. Volume is on the vertical and time on the horizontal axis. These devices are popular and convenient. They perform the calculations and give percentages of predicted normal values.

Figure 5-13 presents normal values for FVC, FEV_1 and the ratio between the two. A straight-edge to connect age and height helps to determine normal values. A range of ±20 percent is commonly taken as normal.

Below are listed the common disease states that are characterized by obstructive ventilatory defects, airflow disorders

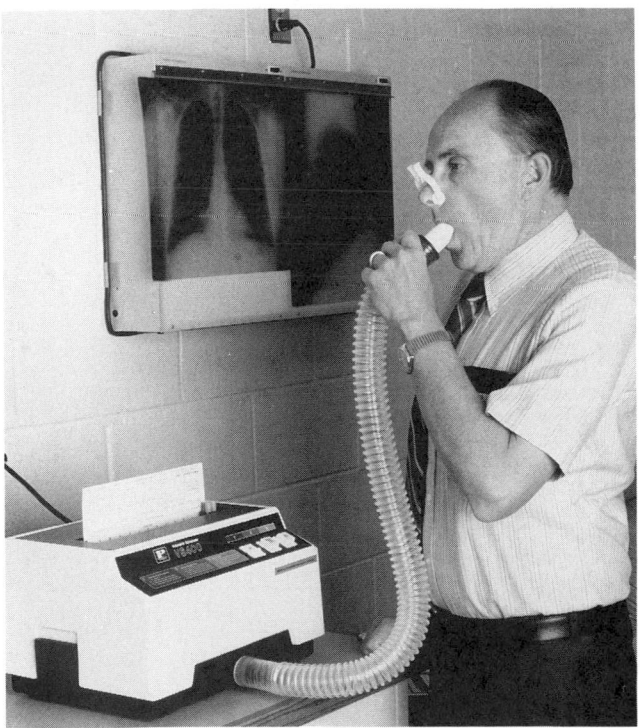

Figure 5-7. Example of a simple dry, direct-recording spirometer suitable for clinic or office use. Many of these spirometers are also used in modern pulmonary function laboratories because they possess accuracy equal to or greater than that of more complex spirometers, such as rolling-seal devices (which are not discussed in the text).

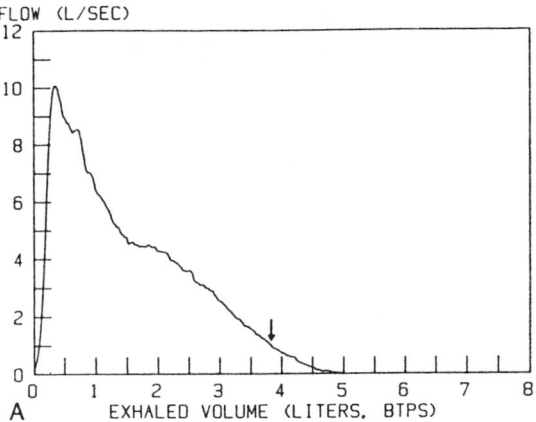

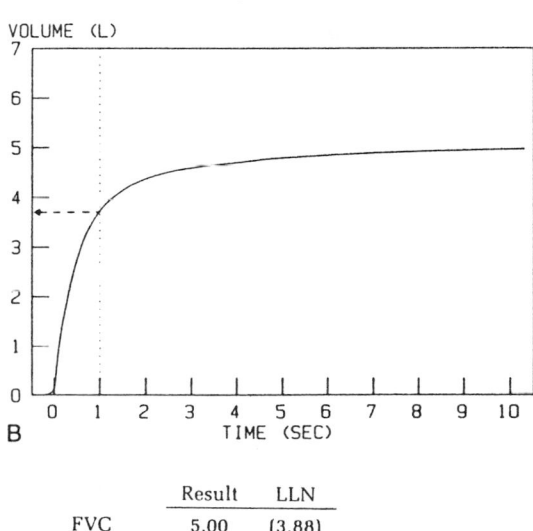

	Result	LLN
FVC	5.00	(3.88)
FEV_1	3.79	(3.12)
%FEV_1	76%	(71%)

Figure 5-8. Normal **(A)** flow-volume and **(B)** time-volume curves of a normal individual. LLN indicates lower limit of normal. Notice that the expiratory time can be visualized from the volume-time curve, but the peak flow can only be visualized from the flow-volume curve. Thus, both curves are useful. (From Enright PL, Hyatt PR: Office Spirometry—A Practical Guide to the Selection and Use of Spirometers. p. 34. Lea & Febiger, Philadelphia, 1987, with permission.)

Common Obstructive Ventilatory Disorders

Asthma

Asthmatic bronchitis

Chronic obstructive bronchitis

Chronic obstructive pulmonary disease (COPD) (This is a generic term, which lumps asthmatic bronchitis, chronic bronchitis, bronchitis, and emphysema. These states commonly overlap.)

Cystic fibrosis

Emphysema

Common Restrictive Ventilatory Disorders

Idiopathic fibrosing alveolitis

Interstitial pneumonitis and fibrosis associated with drug reactions (e.g., to bleomycin) or occupational exposures (e.g., asbestosis)

Fibrotic residue of disseminated granulomas (e.g., tuberculosis, histoplasmosis)

Sarcoidosis

Thoracic deformities

Congestive heart failure

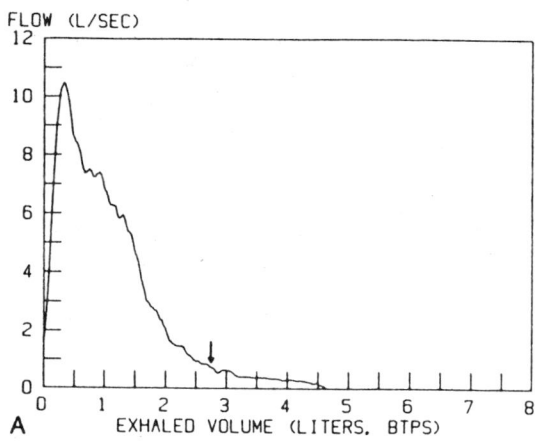

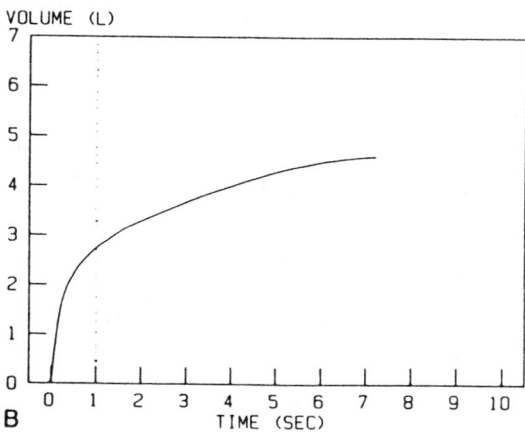

	Result	LLN
FVC	4.60	(3.88)
FEV₁	2.74	(3.12)
%FEV₁	59%	(71%)

Figure 5-9. **(A)** Flow-volume and **(B)** time-volume curves in a patient with a mild obstructive airflow disorder. (From Enright PL, Hyatt PR: Office Spirometry—A Practical Guide to the Selection and Use of Spirometers. p. 52. Lea & Febiger, Philadelphia, 1987, with permission.)

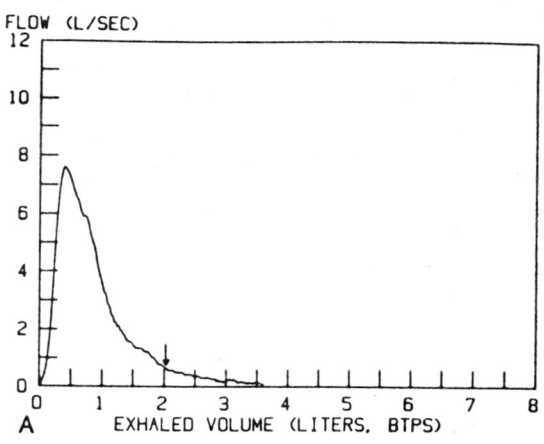

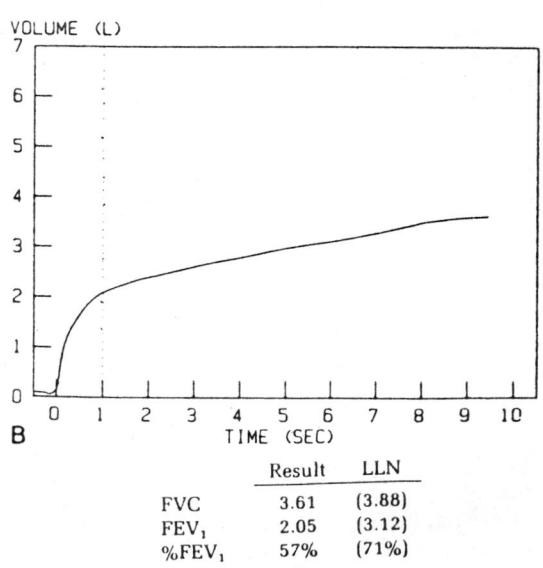

	Result	LLN
FVC	3.61	(3.88)
FEV₁	2.05	(3.12)
%FEV₁	57%	(71%)

Figure 5-10. **(A)** Flow-volume and **(B)** time-volume curves of a patient with moderate airflow obstruction. (From Enright PL, Hyatt PR: Office Spirometry—A Practical Guide to the Selection and Use of Spirometers. p. 46. Lea & Febiger, Philadelphia, 1987, with permission.)

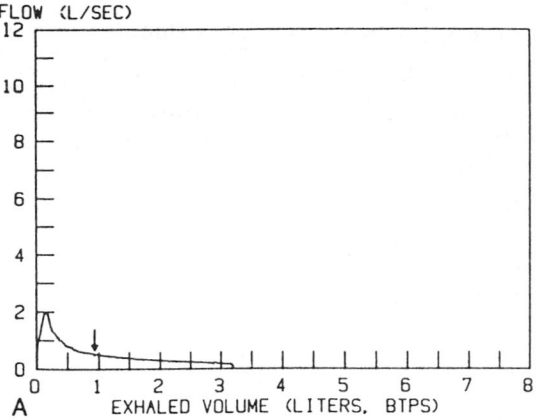

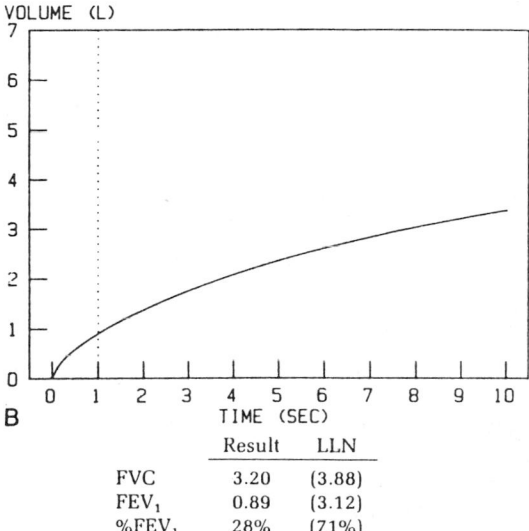

	Result	LLN
FVC	3.20	(3.88)
FEV$_1$	0.89	(3.12)
%FEV$_1$	28%	(71%)

Figure 5-11. **(A)** Flow-volume and **(B)** time-volume curves from a patient with advanced airflow obstruction from emphysema. (From Enright PL, Hyatt PR: Office Spirometry—A Practical Guide to the Selection and Use of Spirometers. p. 42. Lea & Febiger, Philadelphia, 1987, with permission.)

in less common disease states, and the common restrictive ventilatory disorders.

Alternatives to Spirometry

There really is no alternative to simple spirometry, but other methods can give insight into abnormalities of air flow and volume. Thus, the experienced clinician can easily estimate ventilatory function. The importance of the expiratory time has already been cited. In addition, use of a simple peak flowmeter gives a snapshot of flow. Peak flow does not measure the FEV$_1$, but it tracks FEV$_1$ accurately in a given individual. Normal values for peak flow have been established (Leiner, et al., 1963). Figure 5-14 shows a patient performing the peak flow maneuver.

Another simple device has been developed that also accurately estimates the FVC (Anders, et al., 1984). Use of this device is depicted in Figure 5-15. This *disposable* spirometer (named Spir-O-Meter) has been shown to be accurate to within 5 to 10 percent of a standard research spirometer. Both the peak flow and the Spir-O-Meter device could be easily used at the beside to obtain a simple estimate of ventilatory function in the preoperative patient if standard spirometry were not available.

A simple handheld microspirometer is shown in Figure 5-16. It gives values accurate to within 5 to 10 percent when compared with a standard flow transducer and a dry displacement spirometer.

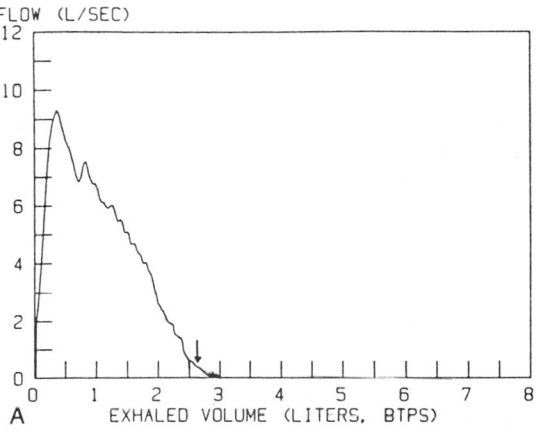

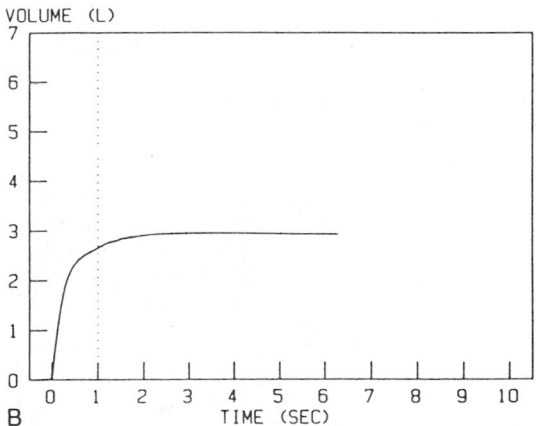

	Result	LLN
FVC	2.97	(3.88)
FEV$_1$	2.64	(3.12)
%FEV$_1$	89%	(71%)

Figure 5-12. **(A)** Flow-volume and **(B)** time-volume curves of a patient with a moderate restrictive ventilatory disorder. Notice that FEV$_1$ is nearly 90 percent of FVC; a restrictive disorder is often suggested when this ratio is high. However, normal individuals can often empty most of the lung in 1 second. (From Enright PL, Hyatt PR: Office Spirometry—A Practical Guide to the Selection and Use of Spirometers. p. 38. Lea & Febiger, Philadelphia, with permission.)

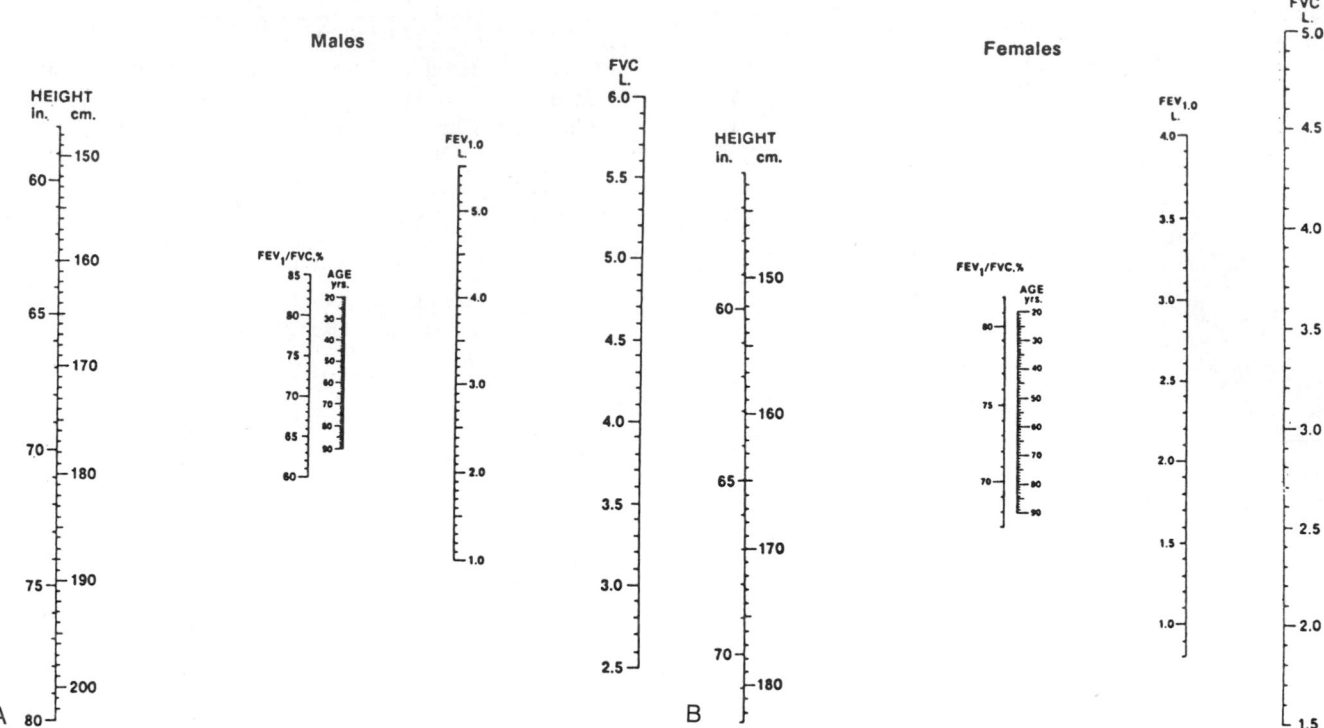

Figure 5-13. Nomogram to identify normal spirometry values for **(A)** men and **(B)** women. Place a straight edge to connect age and height to determine normal value. (Adapted from Morris JF, Koski A, Johnson LC: Spirometric standards for healthy nonsmoking adults. Am Rev Respir Dis 103:57, 1971, with permission.)

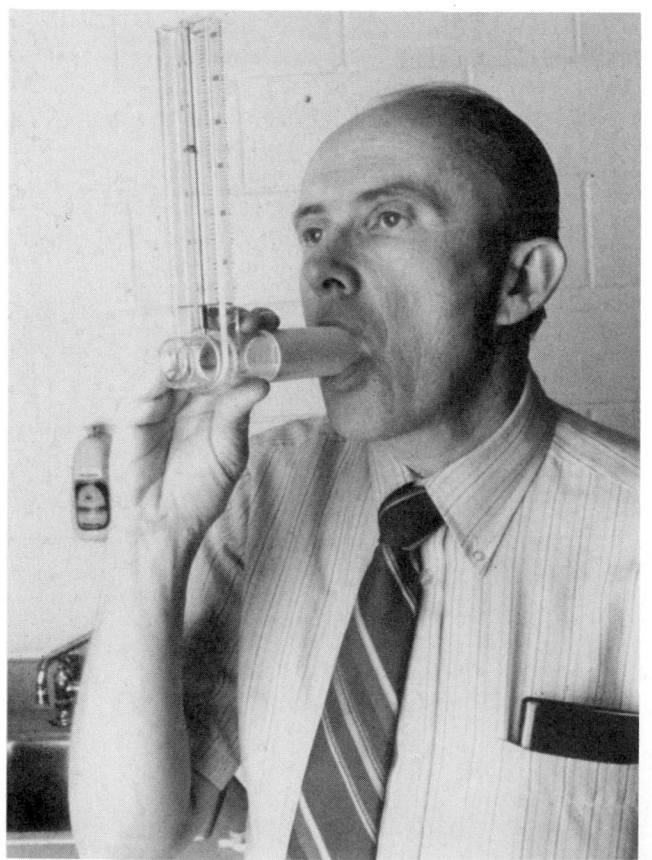

Figure 5-14. Popular peak flowmeter, which measures a snapshot of expiratory airflow. A peak flowmeter does not measure FEV_1 but tracks it in the individual. Conversion formulas exist.

Other Pulmonary Function Tests

Measurements or estimates of lung volumes have been briefly described above. These can be accurately estimated from chest x-rays. They can also be measured accurately by the application of Boyle's law through use of a "body box" (a volume body plethysmograph) (Mead, 1960) or by use of inert gases such as helium or nitrogen (Gilson and Hugh-Jones, 1949) to estimate the FRC, from which the RV can be derived following a forced expiration. The difference between FRC and RV is called the *expiratory reserve volume;* it is only measured in order to define the RV. TLC can be fairly accurately estimated from full inspiration posteroanterior and lateral chest x-rays. Subtracting the measured FVC from this estimate of TLC gives a fairly accurate estimate of the RV.

Gas Transfer Tests

There are basically two gas transfer tests. One, the diffusion test, measures the simple uptake of carbon monoxide. It measures the integrity of the air-blood interface (Ogilvie, et al., 1957). In emphysema, the diffusion test measurement is reduced owing to loss of alveolar walls; in fibrotic states, it is reduced by a barrier to gas transfer across the air-blood interface. Arterial blood gas determinations can also be used as indicators of gas transfer. The oxygen tension and carbon dioxide tension are also affected by ventilation.

Discussion of the role of arterial blood gases is beyond the scope of this chapter. Basically, oxygen tension, CO_2 tension,

Causes of Hypoxemia

Altitude

Hypoventilation

Shunt factors
    Ventilation/perfusion defect
    Diffusion defect
    Anatomic shunt

and the pH of arterial blood are measured. Oxygen saturation is a function of pH and oxygen tension. Factors that cause hypoxemia are listed below. A useful way of expressing PO_2 as a fraction of alveolar ventilation with shunt factors is presented in the following equation:

$$PO_2 \propto \frac{\text{alveolar ventilation}}{\text{shunt factors}}$$

Ventilation/Perfusion Scanning

Fairly accurate estimates of the contribution of each lung or lung region to global lung functions can be made from ventilation/perfusion lung scans. Details of the role of this increasingly popular form of lung imaging are beyond the scope of this chapter, except as commented on below.

CLINICAL APPLICATIONS OF PULMONARY FUNCTION TESTING

Internists primarily use pulmonary function testing for diagnostic purposes and to guide responses to therapy, such as improvements in airflow or volume with bronchodilators and, when indicated, with the use of corticosteroid drugs. Both internists and surgeons can also be guided in estimates of preoperative and postoperative risk by pulmonary function measurements. Various authors have published guidelines about the value of pulmonary function measurements to estimate risk of postoperative complications, but of course, no single estimate is absolute (Harmon and Lillington, 1979; Stein and Cassara, 1970; Stein, et al., 1962; Tisi, 1984). Identification of respiratory insufficiency before surgery can help to reduce postoperative complications by instituting smoking cessation and using bronchoactive drugs (e.g., bronchodilators and/or corticosteroids) if indicated (Harmon and Lillington, 1979; Stein and Cassara, 1970; Stein, et al., 1962; Tisi, 1984).

I firmly believe that any emergency surgery can be performed with relative safety in spite of severe degrees of respiratory impairment. However, it is important to know the degree of ventilatory impairment in order to predict the need for postoperative mechanical ventilation and the difficulties in weaning from mechanical ventilation. Nothing is more frustrating than to be consulted for a ventilator-dependent patient in the postoperative period when there are no mea-

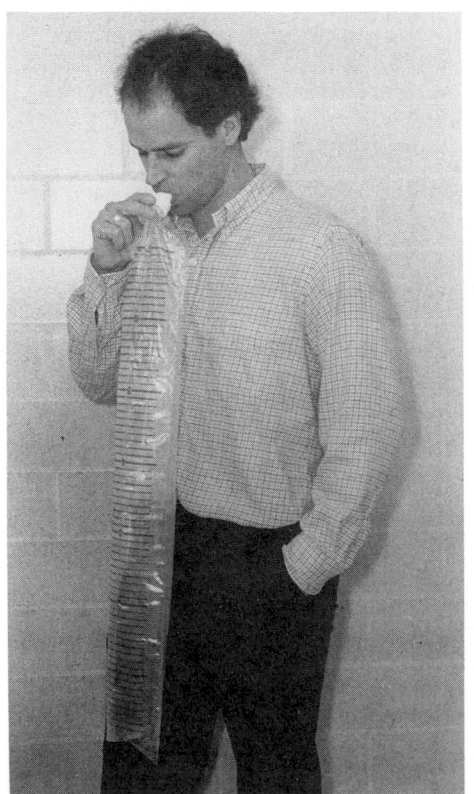

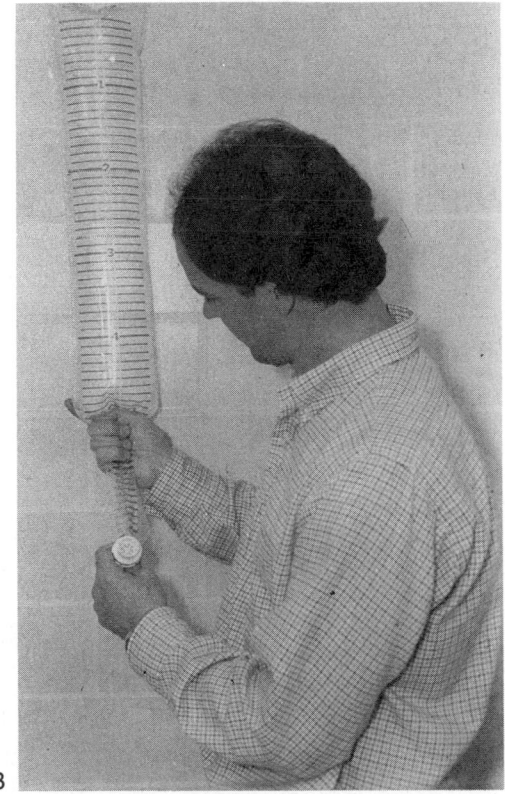

Figure 5-15. **(A)** A simple, disposable spirometer device, which measures FVC within 5 percent of the accuracy of a standard spirometer. **(B)** The method of estimating FVC in liters. Slight shrinkage of the volume occurs between the patient's body temperature and room air. This is known as ambient-temperature pressure and is approximately 8 percent less than under body temperature conditions.

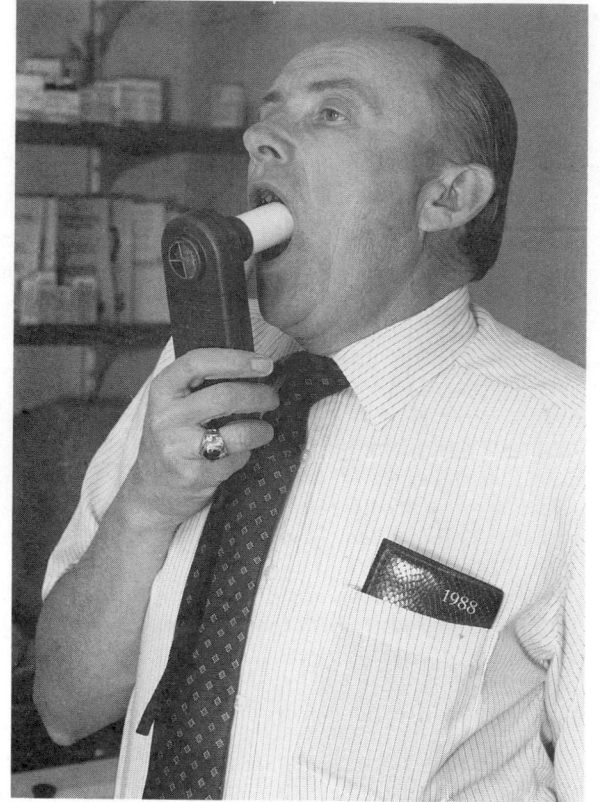

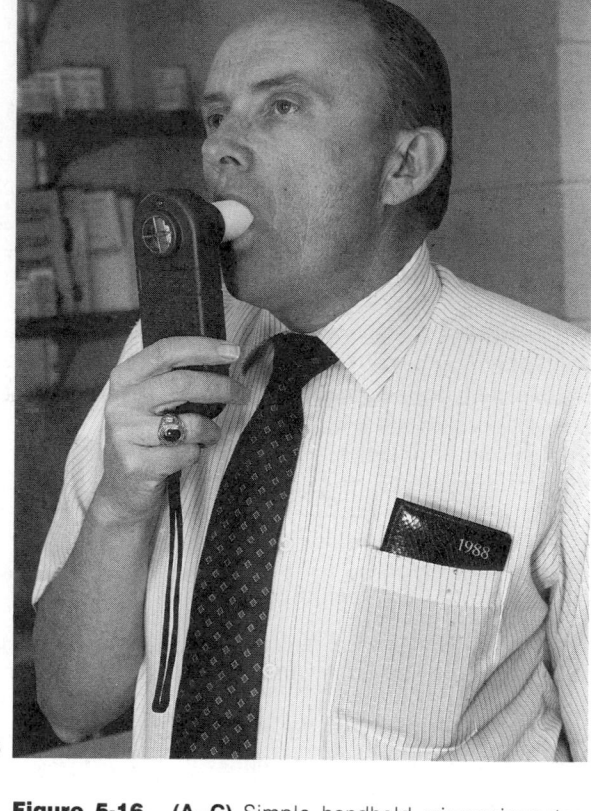

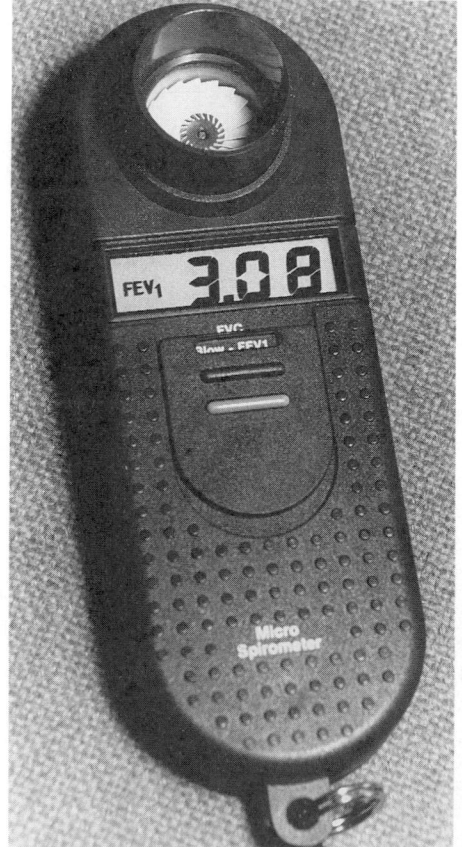

Figure 5-16. **(A–C)** Simple handheld microspirometer. This device has accuracy within 5 to 10 pecent of that of a standard spirometer. This is a very practical device for bedside, clinic, and office measurements of FVC and FEV_1. These devices are also used by some patients in the home, such as those who have received heart or lung transplants, in order to identify early stages of infection or rejection.

surements of pulmonary function prior to major thoracic surgery, including heart transplantation. Often every organ system of the body except the lungs has been measured prior to surgery. A recent study demonstrated that patients with respiratory impairment in the preoperative period had more postoperative complications and required longer stays in the intensive care unit than patients with normal pulmonary function. Patients requiring valve replacement have a much higher risk of pulmonary complications than patients undergoing other cardiac procedures (Bevelaqua, et al., 1990).

Pulmonary function measurements can also be used as crude but useful indicators of the functional success of resectional surgery for lung cancer and for benign lung disease. The amount of lung to be sacrificed is based upon knowledge of the contribution of each of the five lobes. Normally the right lung accounts for 55 percent of total lung function and the left lung for 45 percent. The right middle lobe and its counterpart, the lingula, on the left, can easily be resected with essentially no compromise in lung function. The large upper and lower lobes simply expand to fill the space previously occupied by these small lobes. Even an upper or lower lobectomy can be tolerated with fairly good postoperative pulmonary function if the remaining lobe or lobes can be expected to expand (i.e., in the absence of fibrosis, bronchial obstruction, etc.) Table 5-1 gives a crude estimate of the lower limits of lung function required with various degrees of lung resection. Of course, however, if a nonfunctional lung is resected as in cancer, these calculations would be modified. In some cases thoracic surgery results in actual restoration of lung function, as with draining of an empyema or decortica-

Table 5-1. Lower Limits of Lung Function Required for Various Degrees of Lung Resection[a]

Degree of Resection	Function Before Surgery	
	FEV_1 (L)	FVC (L)
Middle or lingular lobectomy	1.3	2.0
Upper or lower lobectomy	1.5	2.2
Left-sided pneumonectomy	1.8	2.8
Right-sided pneumonectomy	2.0	3.0

Abbreviations: FEV_1, forced expiratory volume in 1 second; FVC, forced vital capacity.

[a] For potential cure of cancer in 6-ft, 55-year-old man.

tion. A prospective study showed that fairly accurate estimates of postoperative lung function following resectional surgery can be obtained by estimating the relative contribution of each lung to overall lung function prior to pneumonectomy (Olsen, et al., 1974).

OTHER GLOBAL TESTS OF LUNG FUNCTION

For many years, experienced physicians and surgeons have asked patients about their ability to walk a flight or two of stairs. Many astute clinicians have actually taken corridor and stairwell walks with their patients while assessing respiratory rate, dyspnea, and use of respiratory muscles and feeling the pulse to note tachycardia. The anguished tachycardiac diaphoretic individual who cannot walk a half flight of stairs is a poor candidate for any form of surgery!

COMMENTS AND CONTROVERSIES

This chapter has presented a practical approach to pulmonary function testing and emphasized the importance of simple spirometry. Dry direct-recording devices measuring volume (FVC) and flow (FEV_1) are widely used. Only two values, namely the FEV_1 and FVC, and the ratio between the two are required. Estimates of expiratory time and simple measures of peak flow and FVC obtained with a disposable spirometer are reasonable alternatives to spirometry. A simple handheld spirometer may be of great practical value for bedside, clinic, or home measurements of FVC and FEV_1. Lung volume and diffusion tests do not often result in clinical decision making; these tests are primarily useful in categorizing disease states and for research purposes. As in all medicine and surgery, the values obtained by pulmonary function measurements must be put in the context of the patient, the patient's disease, the dynamics of the disease state, its trends, and the likelihood of improvement with surgical or medical intervention.

T.L.P.

KEY REFERENCES

Bevelaqua F, Garritan S, Haas F et al.: Complications after cardiac operations in patients with severe pulmonary impairment. Ann Thorac Surg 50:602, 1990

Although patients with severe lung impairment, as identified by abnormal pulmonary function, generally do well after cardiac operations, they have more postoperative pulmonary complications than patients with no impairment. Patients with restrictive ventilatory disorders have better outcomes than those with obstructive diseases. Preoperative pulmonary function tests (e.g., spirometry) can alert the surgeon to the possible risk of postoperative complica-

tions but alone do not exclude patients from necessary surgery. Patients with severe pulmonary impairment should be consideration for preoperative bronchodilator therapy to maximize pulmonary function prior to surgery. Although the history of pulmonary symptoms is important, it cannot replace spirometry to identify individuals at increased risk of cardiac surgery in the face of chronic obstructive pulmonary disease.

Harmon E, Lillington G: Pulmonary risk factors in surgery. Med Clin North Am 63:1289, 1979

Pulmonary complications following surgery are common and range from 6 to 60 percent. The most common complications are atelectasis, pneumonia, pulmonary embolism, and respiratory insufficiency in the immediate postoperative period. While all patients undergoing general anesthesia and surgery are at risk, those subjected to thoracic and upper abdominal surgery have the greatest chance of developing pulmonary complications.

Postoperative mortality from major surgery in patients over 60 years of age ranged from 10 to 33 percent, with most deaths due to respiratory and cardiac causes. Careful fluid management and early mobilization will help mitigate pulmonary complications.

The prediction of surgical risk in thoracic surgery is based on simple spirometric measurements. For example, the mortality following resection for bronchiogenic carcinoma is related to preoperative FEV_1 and age; 40 percent of patients with FEV_1 of less than 2 L and older than 60 years developed problems.

Kannel WB, Lew EA, Hubert HB et al.: The value of measuring vital capacity for prognostic purposes. Trans Am Life Insurance Med Directors Am 64:66, 1980

A simple test (i.e., the measurement of forced vital capacity, was the best predictor of mortality, including deaths from all causes, from the Framingham study. According, as John Hutchinson, a surgeon, stated, "the vital capacity" is clearly the capacity to live.

Lal S, Ferguson AD, Campbell EJM: Forced expiratory time. A simple test for airways obstruction. Br Med J 1:814, 1964

A simple measurement of expiratory time will help identify patients with airflow obstruction. Normal expiratory time is 6 seconds or less. If the total measured expiratory time is measured with a stopwatch or a sweep second hand while listening to a forced expiration over the manubrium and this time is significantly longer than 6 seconds, the patient likely has one of the diseases characterized by airflow obstruction.

Morris JF, Koski A, Johnson LC: Spirometric standards for healthy nonsmoking adults. Am Rev Respir Dis 103:57, 1971

These are important spirometric standards for nonsmoking healthy adults. Normal spirometric values are a function of age, sex, and height. Younger, taller men have higher FVC and FEV_1 than their older, shorter, female counterparts.

Stein M, Cassara EL: Preoperative pulmonary evaluation and therapy for surgical patients. JAMA 211:787, 1970

Simple pulmonary function tests using spirometry can help predict patients at poor risk. When patients were treated preoperatively and postoperatively with cessation of smoking, bronchodilator drugs, and inhaled bronchodilators, along with chest physical therapy techniques, a marked reduction in postoperative morbidity and mortality due to pulmonary complications, was observed. Identifying patients at poor risk, as strongly indicated by abnormal spirometric tests, and using aggressive therapy should reduce postoperative morbidity and mortality and allow discharge following a shorter hospital stay than without this identification or intervention.

REFERENCES

Anders NJ, Baidwan B, Petty TL: An evaluation of the vitometer, a simple device for measuring vital capacity. Respir Care 29:1144, 1984

Enright PL, Hyatt PR: Office Spirometry: A Practical Guide to the Selection and Use of Spirometers. Lea & Febiger, Philadelphia, 1987

Gaensler EA: Analysis of the ventilatory defect by timed vital capacity. Am Rev Respir Dis 69:256, 1951

Gilson JC, Hugh-Jones P: The measurement of total lung volume and breathing capacity. Clin Sci 7:185, 1949

Hutchison J: On the capacity of the lungs and on the respiratory function with a view of establishing a precise and early method of detecting disease by the spirometer. Med Chir Trans (Lond) 24:137, 1846

Leiner GC, Abramowitz S, Small MJ et al.: Expiratory peak flow rate. Standard values for normal subjects. Use as a clinical test of ventilatory function. Am Rev Respir Dis 88:644, 1963

Mead J: Volume displacement body plethysmograph for respiratory measurements in human subjects. J Appl Physiol 15:736, 1960

Ogilvie CM, Forster RE, Blakemore WS et al.: A standardized breath holding technique for the clinical measurement of the diffusing capacity of the lung for carbon monoxide. J Clin Invest 36:1, 1957

Olsen GN, Block AJ, Tobias JA: Prediction of postpneumonectomy pulmonary function using quantitative macroaggregate lung scanning. Chest 66:13, 1974

Petty TL, Silvers GW, Stanford RE: Mild emphysema is associated with reduced elastic recoil and increased lung size but not with air-flow limitation. Am Rev Respir Dis 136:867, 1987

Rossiter CE, Weill H: Ethnic differences in lung function: evidence for proportional differences. Int J Epidemiol 3:55, 1974

Silvers GW, Petty TL, Stanford RE et al.: The elastic properties of lobes of excised human lungs. Am Rev Respir Dis 120:207, 1979

Stein M, Koota GM, Simon M: Pulmonary evaluation of surgical patients. JAMA 181:765, 1962

Tisi GM: Evaluating pulmonary function before surgery. J Respir Dis 5:103, 1984

6

PERIOPERATIVE MANAGEMENT

Thomas R. J. Todd
A. C. Ralph-Edwards

INTRODUCTION

In the future thoracic surgical procedures will become more complex and will be undertaken upon an increasingly elderly population. Neoadjuvant treatment regimens for bronchogenic carcinoma ensure that pulmonary resections will be performed more frequently and that the procedures will be not only complex but also more challenging. The aging of the population has resulted in an increased number of older patients undergoing pulmonary and esophageal resection for malignant disease. In addition, the frequency of immunosuppressive disorders and the reappearance of mycobacterial infections will guarantee the presence of challenging cases of benign disease. These trends and the resulting increase in challenging surgery will demand careful preoperative assessment and rapid recognition and treatment of complications.

HISTORICAL NOTE

When thoracotomy first became feasible, the procedure was conducted without the benefit of readily available blood transfusions and critical care facilities. In addition, knowledge of fluid and electrolyte abnormalities and postoperative fluid shifts was poor. It would take the lessons learned from the Coconut Grove fire in Boston in 1947 and the experience gained from the Korean and Vietnamese conflicts before a thorough understanding of fluid requirements and the effect of resuscitation on pulmonary function was reached. More importantly, the advent of positive pressure ventilation was hastened by a polio epidemic, which largely led to the evolution of modern critical care units.

The technologic developments and the enhanced knowledge of cardiopulmonary physiologic interactions that were the result of this experience have greatly altered our ability to perform thoracic procedures on an increasingly complex patient population. As a result, perioperative management has become a much more involved and important aspect of surgical care.

HISTORICAL READINGS

Baily CC, Betts RH: Cardiac arrhythmias following pneumonectomy. N Engl J Med 229:356, 1943

Bettman RB, Tannenbaum WJ: Herniation of the heart through a pericardial incision. Ann Surg 128:1012, 1948

Cerney CI: The prophylaxis of cardiac arrhythmias complicating pulmonary surgery. J Thorac Surg 34:105, 1957

Claggett OT, Geraci JE: A procedure for the management of postpneumonectomy empyema. J Thorac Cardiovasc Surg 45:141, 1963

Eggers C: The treatment of bronchial fistulae. Ann Surg 72:345, 1920

Goldman L, Caldera DL, Nussbaum SR: Multifactorial index of cardiac risk in noncardiac surgical procedures. N Engl J Med 297:845, 1977

Shenstone NS: The use of intercostal muscle in the closure of bronchial fistulae. Ann Surg 104:560, 1936

GENERAL INCIDENCE

The overall perioperative mortality rate is 2.1 to 3.7 percent for pulmonary resection in most large series (Motta and Ratta, 1989; Deslauriers, et al., 1989; Ginsberg, et al., 1983; Nagasaki, et al., 1982; Wahi, et al., 1989). The 30-day postoperative mortality rate is 6.0 to 7.8 percent for pneumonectomy (right greater than left) and 2.0 to 2.9 percent for lobectomy. The overall major and minor complication rate of pulmonary resection is high (45.5 to 48 percent). Complications are noted in 36 to 75 percent of cases after pneumonectomy and in 41.4 to 50.0 percent of cases following lobectomy (Motta and Ratta, et al., 1989; Wahi, et al., 1989; Olsen, et al., 1991). DesLauriers, et al. (1989) report the incidence of major complications or death for lobectomy and pneumonectomy to be 10 percent. Extended lobectomy or pneumonectomy (on chest wall, tracheal, or pericardial block resection) carries significantly higher risks of death or major complication, at 20 and 17 percent, respectively. Over recent years the frequency of bronchial plastic procedures has increased nearly fourfold; 30-day postoperative mortality is 5.5 and 20.9 percent for sleeve lobectomy and sleeve pneumonectomy, respectively (Tedder, et al., 1992). Increased patient age has also been demonstrated to adversely affect outcome: patients under 60 years of age may be expected to have a perioperative mortality rate of 1.3 percent, those 60 to 69 years old, 4.1 percent, and those over 70 years old, 7 percent (Ginsberg, et al., 1983). The major causes of death after pulmonary resection include pneumonia and respiratory failure, bronchopleural fistula and empyema, myocardial infarction and pulmonary embolism (Ginsberg, et al., 1983).

In this chapter the principles of perioperative care and the recognition and treatment of selected complications are discussed. Preoperative preparation is discussed in the preceding chapters; only general comments follow here as they relate to the specific complications discussed.

PREOPERATIVE PREPARATION

More than two-thirds of the complications occurring in the postoperative period in general thoracic surgical patients are cardiopulmonary in nature. Postoperative respiratory failure, myocardial infarction, and pulmonary embolism may be reduced dramatically by careful patient selection, modification of operative intervention, and use of prophylactic heparin or antiembolic stockings. Strategies for preoperative cardiopulmonary assessment are outlined in Chapters 3 and 5. However, we would stress that careful and systematic evaluation of pulmonary function will lead to identification of a group of patients with poor pulmonary reserve who may benefit from a period of rehabilitation. Pulmonary rehabilitation should consist of graded and measurable supervised exercise over 3 to 4 weeks, accompanied by bronchodilator therapy and antibiotics when pathogenic organisms are identified in sputum.

Perioperative antibiotic prophylaxis has been demonstrated to reduce the incidence of wound infection from up to 18 percent to 1 to 5 percent (Krasnik, et al., 1991; Wertzel, et al., 1992; Ilves, et al., 1981). A single dose of antibiotic with adequate gram-positive and gram-negative coverage is suggested preoperatively and should be continued for no longer than 24 hours postoperatively. Cefuroxime, cefazolin, and penicillin G are all equally effective in reducing wound infections; however, the incidence of empyema and pneumonia is probably unaffected (Krasnik, et al., 1991; Wertzel, et al., 1992; Ilves, et al., 1981). A patient's nutritional status has also been found to correlate with postoperative morbidity. Deslauriers, et al. (1989) found an 11 percent increase in major morbidity and death among patients with a greater than 10 percent weight loss. When assessing patients for pulmonary resection, nutritional status should be considered and measures taken to supplement caloric intake if profound malnutrition is present. Perioperative use of total parental nutrition has been shown to benefit only severely malnourished surgical patients in the absence of specific indications for intravenous alimentation (Veterans Affairs Total Parenteral Nutrition Cooperative Study Group, 1991).

PROPHYLACTIC MEASURES IN THE POSTOPERATIVE PERIOD

Monitoring

In recent years significant improvements have been made in cardiorespiratory monitoring. Both cardiac and pulmonary complications after thoracotomy occur most frequently in the first 2 to 4 days, and this should correspond to the period of most intensive patient monitoring. The goals of monitoring include the provision of information regarding changes in a patient's cardiopulmonary status and the evaluation and appreciation of the results of therapeutic interventions. In order to provide this level of care, post-thoracotomy patients should be managed in a specialized unit. Ideally, frequent measurements of respiratory rate, heart rate, blood pressure, and arterial oxygen saturation are necessary. Oxygen saturation is readily measured noninvasively. Arterial blood gases should be drawn initially to provide information on postoperative ventilatory status via assessment of carbon dioxide partial pressure ($PaCO_2$). Transient elevations of $PaCO_2$ may occur secondary to excessive analgesia, failure to adequately reverse anesthesia, and the unmasking of previously unrecognized carbon dioxide retention, which may be seen in the postoperative period as a result of excessive oxygen administration. With carbon dioxide retention, oxygen supplementation should be guided by the saturation recordings from the pulse oximeter to achieve a saturation of no more than 90 percent. Newer intra-arterial electrodes that provide continuous oxygen partial pressure (PO_2) and PCO_2 measurements may in part resolve problems of sampling errors and delays in laboratory reporting. Preoperative knowledge of arterial oxygen and carbon dioxide content, combined with physical examination, is critical to direct oxygen therapy and analgesia.

Continuous cardiac rhythm monitoring should also be available, as cardiac arrhythmias are common after thoracotomy. Undiagnosed supraventricular tachycardia may lead to myocardial ischemia or congestive heart failure or may degenerate to a more malignant rhythm. If diagnosed early, the majority of arrhythmias are easily treated. Hypoxia, hypercarbia, anemia, electrolyte abnormalities and fluid overload are frequently associated inciting abnormalities.

More invasive monitoring is usually reserved for the ventilated patient in whom a widened alveolar-arterial oxygen gradient [$P(A-a)O_2$], hypotension, or both necessitate the availability of frequent arterial blood gas measurements, as well as assessments of cardiac output and oxygen transport. This requires insertion of a Swan-Ganz catheter in order to obtain cardiac output via thermal dilution, as well as measurements of left ventricular preload (via pulmonary arterial wedge pressure), pulmonary artery pressure, and mixed venous oxygen tension ($P\bar{v}O_2$).

These data permit the calculation of several other parameters, including oxygen transport and left ventricular stroke work. The former is particularly important in determining the optimal level of positive end-expiratory pressure (PEEP) in patients whose PEEP requirements exceed $10\,cmH_2O$. The optimal PEEP can also be obtained by repeated evaluations of static lung compliance, which is readily estimated by applying a clamp to the expiratory limb of the ventilator tubing at the end of inspiration. The peak airway pressure will fall to the degree determined by the relative contribution of airway resistance and pulmonary compliance to peak area pressure. In the absence of air flow, the plateau pressure obtained following application of the clamp to the expiratory tubing at end-inspiration must be solely due to pulmonary compliance. Some ventilators have an inspiratory hold and if so the application of the clamp is unnecessary.

Ventilatory Support

In some patients continued postoperative ventilation may be desirable as a prophylactic measure. Large-volume fluid resuscitation, hemodynamic instability, myocardial ischemia, prolonged anesthesia, and potential space problems may be more safely managed with a period of elective postoperative mechanical ventilation. This provides time to stabilize the patient and to appreciate the degree of pulmonary parenchymal damage. Short-term positive pressure ventilation in patients undergoing pulmonary decortication or major bullectomy may achieve more complete lung reexpansion, particularly if there is a reduction in pulmonary compliance. The latter is frequently the case for conditions that require decortication, and the procedure itself leads to excessive extravascular lung water, which will result in stiffer lungs.

Pain Control

Pain following thoracotomy can be severe and often results in an alteration in the pattern of breathing. The patient may generate low tidal volumes, maintaining adequate minute ventilation by an increase in rate. As a result, functional residual capacity will fall and airway closure with attendant atelectasis results. This is compounded by the suppression of cough, which in the presence of augmented secretions in the postoperative period further aggravates airway closure. The result is an impairment in oxygenation due to the consequent ventilation/perfusion mismatch.

As a result, it is imperative to control pain effectively and early following thoracotomy. There are several options. Narcotic administration has been a mainstay of therapy for decades. The mode of administration has markedly improved from the days of the intramuscular route. Hourly intravenous administration is satisfactory, and the advent of patient-controlled analgesia (PCA) has provided an even greater level of comfort. Adjuvant pain therapy with nonsteroidal compounds is often recommended, whether given orally or as a rectal suppository. In our experience, the latter provides significant improvement in pain control. Epidural administration of opiates takes advantage of the fact that there are specific opiate receptors on the dorsal columns of the spinal cord. A properly functioning epidural catheter permits excellent analgesia with narcotic doses that have few, if any, systemic effects and do not result in impairment of motor function. One must be alert to the possibility of respiratory depression, although this is less likely to occur if the epidural is placed in the lumbar region. In addition, an epidural catheter will usually require the insertion of a urinary catheter. Whether the epidural route offers any therapeutic advantage over PCA remains to be determined and must await randomized clinical trials. An important new area of research currently undergoing clinical trials is that of preemptive analgesia, which may increase patient comfort while possibly reducing analgesic requirements.

Oxygen Therapy

Oxygen should only be administered as needed. The availability of cutaneous saturation monitors allows one to titrate the amount required. Given the shape of the oxygen-hemoglobin dissociation curve (Fig. 6-1), the higher the saturation, the greater is the PaO_2 and hence the farther away is the patient from the steep portion of the curve. However, one must be mindful of the fact that oxygen administration can have deleterious effects. In a patient with chronic carbon dioxide retention, a hypoxic drive to breathing is required, and the elimination of hypoxemia can lead to respiratory depression and further carbon dioxide retention with respiratory acidosis. This emphasizes the need for preoperative blood gas determinations. The presence of an elevated $PaCO_2$ in the preoperative period will also be suggested by an abnormally elevated bicarbonate level on serum electrolyte determinations, on which basis the physician should suspect a compensated respiratory acidosis or a primary metabolic alkalosis (often secondary to chronic diuretic therapy). Other complications of excessive oxygen administration include alveolar damage and pulmonary fibrosis in either the ventilated patient (Fox et al., 1981; Sackner et al., 1976) or the patient who has received certain chemotherapeutic agents (Gilson and Sahn, 1985). In addition, excessive oxygen flow may predispose patients to infectious pulmonary complications by drying secretions, inhibiting mucus salivary clearance, and decreasing pulmonary macrophage function.

Intravenous Fluid

Patients undergoing thoracotomy for pulmonary resection should not receive excessive fluid, either in the operating room or postoperatively. Pulmonary surgery is not associated

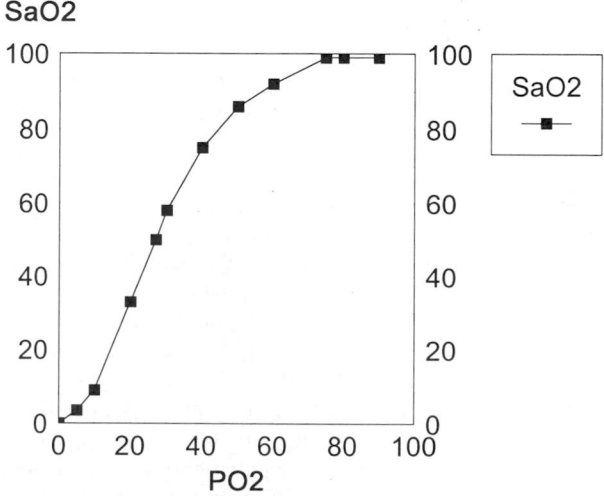

Figure 6-1. Oxygen-hemoglobin dissociation curve.

with large postoperative fluid shifts, and intraoperative lung manipulation and collapse not only may impair pulmonary lymphatic drainage in the early postoperative period but also may lead to the increased extravasation of fluid due to a disruption of the alveolar-capillary membrane. Excessive fluids given perioperatively may result in pulmonary edema, decreased alveolar gas permeability, and decreased pulmonary compliance, which will promote atelectasis and further hypoxia. It is important to remember that epidural analgesia may be associated with increased fluid administration because of induced hypotension. In patients undergoing resection for malignant disease, use of blood products has also been reported to decrease survival and increase the likelihood of recurrence through immunosuppression (Cade et al., 1983; Ziomek, et al., 1993). These observations are not, however, universal (Fox, et al., 1981).

MANAGEMENT OF COMPLICATIONS

Pulmonary Insufficiency

Respiratory failure is the major cause of perioperative mortality in patients undergoing pulmonary resection for lung cancer. Postoperative respiratory failure occurs in 0.2 to 2.6 percent of patients, and there is a 46 to 100 percent mortality from this complication (Deslauriers, et al., 1989; Nagasaki, et al., 1982). Pulmonary complications most frequently present in the first 2 to 4 days following surgery. As noted, preoperative pulmonary function testing is critical to minimize postoperative pulmonary complications and guide surgical decision making. Determination of the degree of pulmonary impairment and its reversibility will direct preoperative optimization and extent of resection and identify those patients at high risk for life-threatening pulmonary complications after resection (American College of Physicians, 1990). Antibiotics, bronchodilators, cessation of smoking, chest physiotherapy, postural drainage, and exercise may all be employed to enhance pulmonary function preoperatively. Spirometry, arterial blood gas analysis, split perfusion lung scanning, and exercise testing are suggested preoperative investigations in significantly impaired patients. Forced vital capacity in 1 second (FEV_1) is easily obtained and reproducible. Using this value, the expected postoperative FEV_1 can be determined by the formula

Postresection FEV_1
$$= \text{preoperative } FEV_1 - X \text{ (preoperative } FEV_1)$$

where X is the percent perfusion to the proposed area of resection. Regional pulmonary perfusion can be readily obtained preoperatively by quantitative perfusion lung scanning. A predicted postoperative FEV_1 less than 0.8 L/min in an adult of average size is associated with significantly increased perioperative morbidity and mortality (Nakahara, et al., 1988). Arterial blood gas analysis is also useful, identifying patients at high risk of respiratory complications postresection. Arterial hypercapnia ($PCO_2 > 45$ mmHg) is usually considered an indicator of significantly increased risk of respiratory failure and death following pulmonary resection. Arterial hypoxemia is also correlated with an increased risk of postoperative complications, although in some patients airway obstruction may cause intrapulmonary shunting, which will be eliminated with resection. In the patient with a mainstem bronchial obstruction, hypoxemia may be improved by pneumonectomy.

Because of their failure to either individually or collectively predict morbidity, all these apparent predictors must be assessed in the context of the individual patient. Indeed, we are more concerned with the presence of a preoperatively high PaO_2 (> 80 mmHg) in the presence of impaired pulmonary mechanics. As most patients presenting for pulmonary surgery are heavy smokers and have obstructive lung disease, various degrees of ventilation/perfusion mismatching are usually present. This is particularly the case if pulmonary function testing suggests a marginal FEV_1 or diffusing capacity. Under such circumstances a PaO_2 above 80 mmHg can only be achieved if the ventilation/perfusion mismatch has been either eliminated or maximized. In a patient with chronic bronchitis or emphysema, this can occur from destruction or obliteration of portions of the pulmonary capillary bed that have been poorly ventilated. As a result, a high PaO_2 may suggest the early development of pulmonary vascular hypertension. Under such circumstances, preoperative evaluation of pulmonary vascular pressure is advisable.

Chest physiotherapy has been demonstrated to be effective in preventing postoperative pulmonary complications and should be considered routine postoperative care for patients undergoing thoracotomy (Stiller and Munday, 1992). Patients identified preoperatively with lung diseases or excessive secretions or postoperatively with recurrent laryngeal nerve palsy, phrenic nerve palsy, diaphragmatic reimplantation, or chest wall resection are at higher risk and should receive more intensive evaluation and treatment. In patients with a history of excessive sputum production, prophylactic minitracheotomy may be advantageous to provide a route for frequent tracheal and bronchial suctioning without flexible bronchoscopy (Au, et al., 1989; Nelson, 1992). The development of recurrent laryngeal nerve palsy in the postoperative period may seriously impair the ability to cough and clear secretions. This is particularly a problem following pneumonectomy. When the diagnosis is suggested early, evaluation by laryngoscopy is warranted. If the paralyzed cord is abducted, augmentation should be considered. If one knows that the recurrent nerve has been divided, augmentation with Teflon is appropriate. However, if the paralysis is believed to be temporary, glycerol should be used, as it will be absorbed with time.

Arrhythmias

In 1943 the first recorded cases of cardiac arrhythmias occurring after pulmonary resection were simultaneously reported by Currens, et al. and Bailey and Betts. The occurrence of cardiac rhythm disturbances are likely related to the magnitude of the operative procedures performed. Cardiac arrhythmias (defined as atrial fibrillation, premature beats, atrial flutter, and ventricular arrhythmias) occurred in 3.1 to 14.3 percent of patients postlobectomy as compared with 19.4 to 40 percent for patients after pneumonectomy (Motta and Ratto, 1989; Wahi, et al., 1989; Cerney, 1957; Mowrey and Reynolds, 1964; Krowka, et al., 1987). The overall rate of postoperative arrhythmia in a large series was 3.2 to 20.8 percent (Deslauriers, et al., 1989; Nagasaki, et al., 1982; Cerney, 1957; Von Knorring, et al., 1992). In patients undergoing pneumonectomy, arrhythmias were associated with a significantly increased mortality. Of postoperative deaths in patients undergoing pneumonectomy, 81 percent were preceded by or associated with a tachyarrhythmia (Krowka, et al., 1987).

Atrial arrhythmias are the most common. Most arrhythmias (96 percent) occur within the first postoperative week, with a peak incidence at 48 hours (Mowry and Reynolds, 1964; Von Knorring, et al., 1992). Atrial fibrillation, atrial flutter, and atrial tachycardia account for the vast majority of postoperative arrhythmias encountered (42, 12.5, and 4.0 percent, respectively) (Ritchie, et al., 1992). The likelihood of arrhythmia increases with advancing age and previous cardiac history. Ventricular arrhythmias are rare. Prophylactic digitalization has been suggested for older patients (over 50 years) undergoing pulmonary resection. In several retrospective series, preoperative digitalization was shown to have a variable effect on the incidence of postoperative atrial arrhythmias and mortality (Juler, et al., 1969; Shields and Ujiki, 1968). In a prospective randomized series, prophylactic digitalization was found to increase the frequency and severity of postoperative arrhythmias (Ritchie, et al., 1992). Most authors do not advocate routine prophylactic digitalization. A prospective randomized trial using Flecainide after thoracic operations as prophylaxis for postoperative arrhythmia has demonstrated efficacy with no side effects (Borgeat, et al., 1989). These results await further testing in larger trials.

Much speculation exists regarding the etiology of postoperative arrhythmias. Most authors consider increased vagal tone, hypoxemia, and intraoperative fluid administration of more than 2 L to be the most important deciding factors. Intraoperative hypotension has also been found to significantly increase the risk of both arrhythmias and myocardial ischemia (Von Knorring, et al., 1992). Several series have failed to demonstrate any significant relation between preoperative pulmonary function, surgical indication, or TNM (tumor, node, metastasis) staging of lung cancer, and the subsequent development of a tachyarrhythmia. General investigations include serum electrolytes, cardiac enzymes, arterial blood gases, hemoglobin, and electrocardiography (ECG).

Therapy for atrial arrhythmias is dependent on correct diagnosis and careful assessment of the patient. Urgency and mode of therapy is dictated by the degree of hemodynamic impairment imposed by the new rhythm. Assessment for congestive heart failure should be made and supplemental oxygen given. Patients who are asymptomatic with a normal blood pressure and new-onset atrial fibrillation are easily treated with intravenous digoxin. Digoxin is the drug of choice in this situation, as it decreases ventricular response rate without impairment of myocardial contractility. The average-size adult should receive 0.5 mg IV, followed by two or three subsequent doses of 0.25 mg given every 6 hours or more rapidly if indicated. Subsequently, a maintenance dose of 0.25 mg PO is given daily; dosage may require adjustment based on renal function. Peak levels of digoxin occur approxi-

mately 90 to 120 minutes after intravenous administration; therefore, 1 or 2 hours may be required to obtain an effect. Digoxin levels have little correlation with effects, and adequacy of treatment is best judged by ventricular response rate. Additional doses of digoxin may be required in some cases to bring ventricular response rate below 120 beats/min.

Patients demonstrating evidence of circulatory compromise require more urgent therapy. If hypotension, dizziness, or angina is experienced, verapamil or propranolol may be used in addition to digoxin. Both verapamil (a calcium channel antagonist) and propranolol (a β-blocking agent) produce rapid slowing of ventricular response when administered intravenously. Both should be used in a monitored environment with dosage carefully titrated. Propranolol may be given in 1-mg aliquots every 5 to 8 minutes until the heart rate reaches 120 beats/min or less. Verapamil may be given as 2.5 mg IV as a slow push; the dose may be repeated every 10 to 15 minutes to a maximum of 15 mg. β-Blocking agents should not be used simultaneously with calcium channel blockers because of their possible synergistic negative inotropic and chronotropic effects, which could lead to hypotension or asystole in some patients.

Occasionally patients may experience extreme circulatory compromise with new-onset atrial fibrillation. Patients presenting with profound hypotension, severe angina, and obtundation require emergent treatment. Direct-current cardioversion is a fast and effective mode of treatment for patients in extremis. Following cardioversion, digoxin should be given to reduce the risk of recurrent atrial fibrillation and relative circulatory compromise. Patients who fail to convert to a normal sinus rhythm after the ventricular response rate has been controlled may be treated by chemical cardioversion with propranolol, sotalol, quinidine, or Pronestyl. Most patients, however, undergo spontaneous cardioversion after heart rate is controlled with digoxin. Patients with normal sinus rhythm prior to surgery who develop atrial tachyarrhythmias postoperatively are discharged home with digoxin for 6 weeks. This continuation of digoxin is arbitrary.

Postpneumonectomy Empyema

Empyema occurring after pneumonectomy presents as a suppurative contamination of the pneumonectomy space. The incidence of empyema occurring with or without a bronchial fistula has decreased in recent times and is now close to 1 percent (Eckersberger, et al., 1990). Empyema may occur early in the postoperative course or may develop years after the procedure. The majority of patients present within 12 weeks, with 77 percent having an associated bronchopleural fistula (Shamji, et al., 1983). Early empyema may be primary, due to bacterial contamination of the pleural fluid at the time of operation (most common), or secondary, due to contamination from infected residual lung (in the case of lobectomy or wedge resection) or to bronchopleural or esophagopleural fistula (Van Raemdonck, et al., 1990). Bronchopleural fistula in this setting is usually a complication of empyema. Empyema occurring months to years after resection is generally considered to arise from hematogenous seeding, but a late fistula should be ruled out.

Staphylococcus is the most frequently occurring pathogen. *Streptococcus* spp. and gram-negative and anaerobic organisms are also frequently cultured (Shamji, et al., 1983). Diagnosis is established by diagnostic thoracocentesis (Papadakis and Wall, 1990), and this procedure should be considered whenever patients are febrile, lethargic, and/or anorexic. Pleural fluid should be aspirated and sent for pH, protein, lactate dehydrogenase (LDH), and glucose determinations, cytology (if a late fistula), and aerobic and anaerobic cultures. Bronchoscopy and esophagography should be performed to rule out a bronchial or esophageal fistula when indicated. Delayed diagnoses may result in sepsis, bronchopleural fistula, pneumonia, or pericarditis.

Therapy consists of early drainage of the pleural space and administration of systemic antibiotics for 48 to 72 hours after drainage has been effected. Eventual obliteration of the space or closure of the draining sinus may be required. In approaching these difficult problems, the algorithm in Figure 6-2 is useful. Tube thoracostomy is essential initial treatment, and bronchoscopy should be performed to ensure that a bronchial fistula has not also developed. If the empyema occurs more than 3 weeks following thoracotomy, one can be assured that sufficient mediastinal fixation has occurred to allow creation of a thoracic window. If, however, the pulmonary resection was performed less than 3 weeks before the tube thoracostomy, a thoracic window should be delayed until the mediastinum has become stabilized. There is some controversy over the fate of the thoracic window. It can represent definitive treatment in high-risk patients with poor functional status. In our opinion, attempts at closure should be delayed

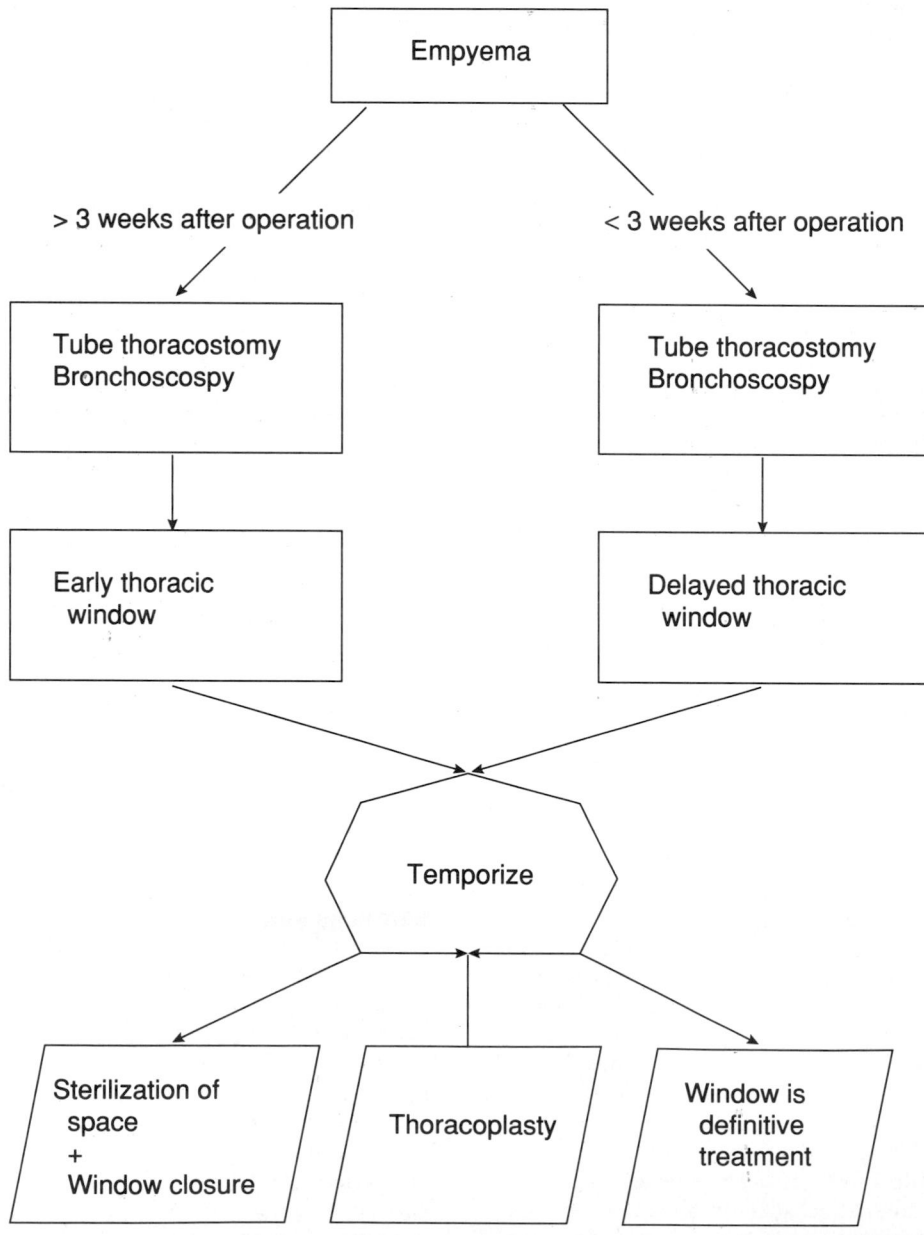

Figure 6-2.   Suggested algorithm for management of postpneumonectomy empyema.

for 12 to 24 months to ensure that the risk of recurrence of bronchogenic carcinoma is minimized and to allow the patient time to recover a normal nutritional status. Closure of the window following sterilization of the empyema cavity in the hospital has been reported with variable success (American College of Physicians, 1990; Shamji, et al., 1983; Pairoleiro, et al., 1991; Clagett and Geraci, 1963; Stafford and Clagett, 1972). Alternatively, thoracoplasty with or without muscle transposition represents a definitive approach to obliteration of the empyema space (Gregoire, et al., 1987).

Bronchopleural Fistulae

Bronchopleural fistulae with or without empyema has been identified as a major source of morbidity and mortality in patients undergoing pulmonary resections for malignancy (Deslauriers, et al., 1989; Ginsberg, et al., 1983; Nagasaki, et al., 1982). The incidence of postoperative fistula is approximately 1.6 to 6.2 percent (Motta and Ratto, 1989; Wahi, et al., 1989; Vester, et al., 1991; Asamura, et al., 1992). Wider resection, residual carcinoma in the bronchial stump, preoperative irradiation, and diabetes have been identified by multivariate analyses to be significant risk factors (Asamura, et al., 1992). Most bronchopleural fistulae occur following pneumonectomy (46 percent of cases), and approximately 75 percent are right-sided. Radical mediastinal lymphadenectomy also increases the risk of fistula formation because of bronchial

devascularization. In patients who have received preoperative radiation, the diagnosis of bronchopleural fistula is made significantly later than in patients who have not had radiotherapy (48 days average versus 18 days) (Vester, et al., 1991). Mortality from bronchopleural fistula may be as high as 71 percent (Asamura, et al., 1992). The diagnosis should be suspected if there is expectoration of copious amounts of infected material (when fistulae occur late) or serosanguineous fluid (early fistulae); this, however, is often not noted. The clinical scenario of a falling fluid level and a new contralateral infiltrate after pneumonectomy (Fig. 6-3) is virtually diagnostic and demands insertion of a chest tube into the space.

The initial therapy for a bronchial stump fistula involves immediate insertion of a chest drain and performance of bronchoscopy to verify the clinical suspicion. Prior to insertion of a thoracostomy tube, the patient should be nursed with the operative side dependent to reduce the incidence of contralateral soiling. Subsequent therapy depends on the time of occurrence of the fistula. Those fistulae that develop within the first week are usually secondary to technical difficulties and are unlikely to be associated with significant pleural infection. Following verification of bronchial stump dehiscence, thoracotomy is recommended in this situation. Reclosure of the bronchial stump is undertaken employing a buttress of pedicled intercostal muscle, pericardium, or omentum. The pleural space should be debrided and lavaged.

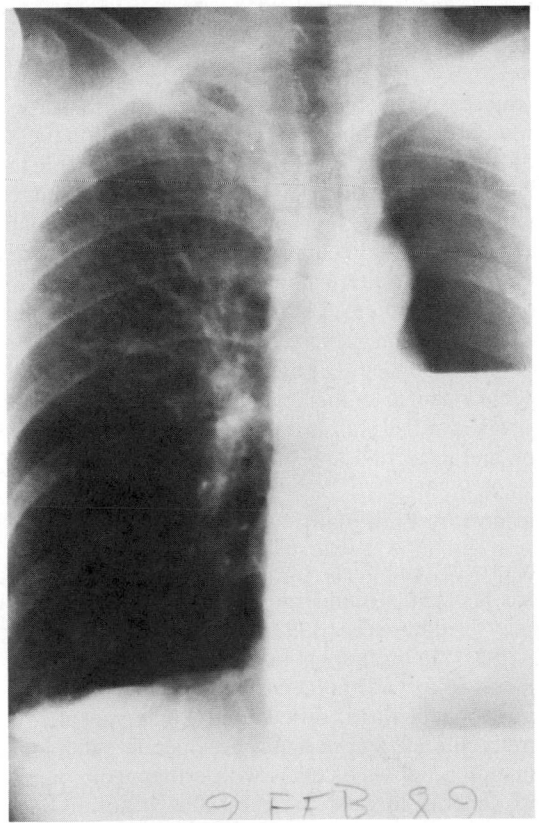
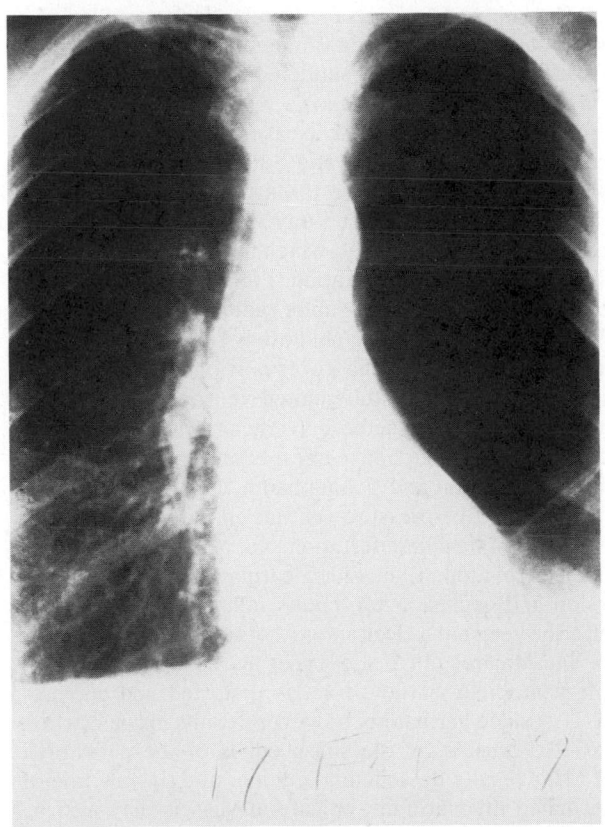

A   B

Figure 6-3. **(A)** Postpneumonectomy chest x-ray at discharge from hospital. **(B)** Follow-up chest x-ray demonstrating fallen fluid level.

The role of postoperative irrigation of the pleural space with or without antibiotic solutions—so-called balanced drainage—remains to be determined but empirically would seem to have merit.

Fistulae that occur beyond the tenth postoperative day are usually associated with an empyema. Under such circumstances reoperation is not recommended. Tube thoracostomy and antibiotic coverage for 5 to 7 days are appropriate. If there has been considerable soilage into the contralateral lung, mechanical ventilation may be required. If the fistula is large, high-frequency ventilation may be necessary (Panos, et al., 1986). If jet ventilation is unavailable, the fistula can be controlled with either a bronchus blocker or a balloon catheter or by insertion of an uncut endotracheal tube into the contralateral mainstem bronchus. For bronchopleural fistulae following lobectomy, tube thoracostomy may be all that is required. However, following pneumonectomy a thoracic window is a better option. The window is best created 2 to 3 weeks after the pneumonectomy to ensure that fixation of the mediastinum has occurred. Under these circumstances, closure of the fistula will occur in 30 percent of cases (Shamji, et al., 1983). Fistulae that fail to close can be managed by a thoracoplasty (Gregoire, et al., 1987) or by transsternal reamputation of the bronchial stump.

Cardiac Herniation

Cardiac herniation is an infrequently reported complication of intrapericardial pneumonectomy (right more common than left). This complication arises in the immediate postoperative period in patients with residual medium and large (>5 cm) pericardial defects. Onset is sudden and is marked by hypotension, tachycardia, and cyanosis, usually within 24 hours of operation. The mortality rate in cases recognized promptly approaches 50 percent (Groh and Sunder-Plassmann, 1987; Delranija, 1974). Diagnosis rests on clinical suspicion and critical appraisal of the chest x-ray. Right-sided herniation is unmistakable on chest x-ray, which frequently shows obvious right-sided cardiac subluxation (Fig. 6-4). Left-sided herniation demonstrates a more subtle radiographic change; often a left shift of the cardiac shadow is seen in conjunction with a rounded opacity in the lower portion of the left hemithorax, representing the strangulated ventricular mass.

Several predisposing factors have been described, including the application of suction to chest tubes, coughing, patient positioning (Bettman and Tannenbaum, 1948), tracheal suctioning, and positive-pressure ventilation. Hemodynamic alterations and clinical manifestations vary between right- and left-sided herniation. Right-sided cardiac herniation results in torsion and occlusion of venous inflow via the superior and inferior vena cava (Delraniya, 1974; Gates, et al., 1970; Takita and Majares, 1970; Levin, et al., 1971). In addition, the left ventricular outflow tract is distorted and compromised. Left-sided herniation, however, results in constriction of the left ventricle by the sharp edges of the pericardial defect. This results in ischemia, edema, and dysfunction of the herniated myocardium; epicardial vessels may also be lacerated, resulting in bleeding (Glass, et al., 1984; Papsin, et al., 1993). ECG changes may thus frequently accompany left-sided herniation (Yacoub, et al., 1968).

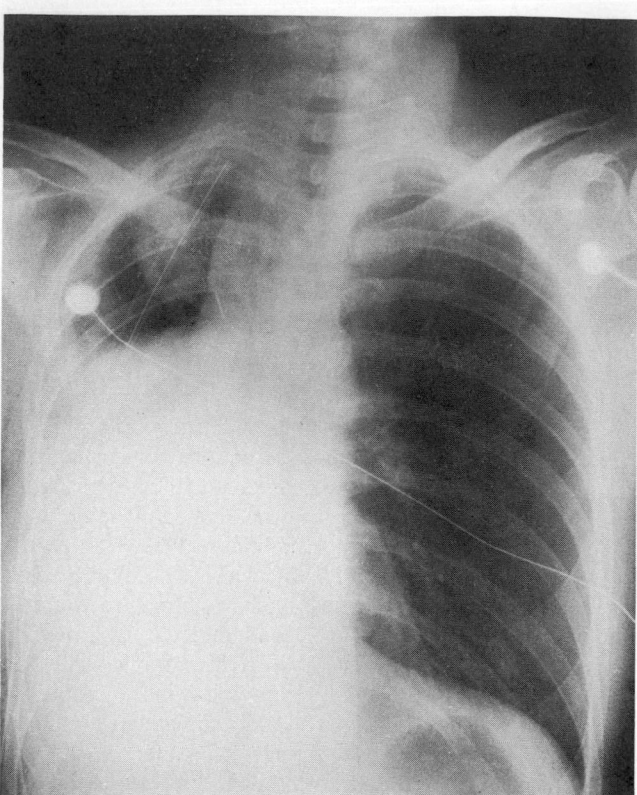

Figure 6-4. Chest x-ray after intrapericardial resection of lung tumor demonstrating right-sided cardiac herniation.

Successful management of cardiac herniation requires prompt diagnosis and operation. At operation the heart must be returned to its normal anatomic position within the pericardial sac, and the pericardial defect must be closed. Numerous methods of obliteration of the right-sided defect have been suggested, including approximation of the epicardium to the pericardium and patching the defect with pleura, fascia, or bovine pericardium. The use of Dacron to close pericardium defects has been associated with septic complications and is not recommended. On the left side, the pericardium may be widely opened to the diaphragm. With this maneuver the extreme cardiac shift is not eliminated, but cardiac strangulation and infarction are unlikely.

Pulmonary Embolism

Pulmonary embolism occurs in approximately 0.19 to 2.3 percent of patients undergoing pulmonary resection for malignancy (Tedder, et al., 1992; Asamura, et al., 1992; Rogiers, et al., 1991). In one series, postoperative pulmonary embolism accounted for 14.3 percent of early deaths in patients undergoing bronchoplastic procedures (Rogiers, et al., 1991). Most surgical literature concerning perioperative pulmonary embolism and prophylaxis deals with orthopaedic, neurosurgical, and general surgical patients. The reported incidence of symptomatic pulmonary embolism in thoracic surgical patients is low. Once pulmonary embolism is documented, however, the mortality is high (50 to 100 percent) (Tedder, et al., 1992; Asamura, et al., 1992; Waller, et al., 1993). This observation is likely related to poor cardiopulmonary reserve in this patient population.

Factors predisposing to venous thrombosis are stasis, hypercoagulability, and intimal damage. The majority of thoracic surgical patients have multiple risk factors, including advanced age, malignancy, and prolonged duration of general anesthesia (longer than 30 minutes). Some patients may have additional risk factors such as a previous history of deep venous thrombosis (DVT), a known hypercoagulable state, obesity, and heart disease. Thoracic surgical patients constitute a moderate risk group for perioperative thrombotic complications. Patients undergoing surgery without prophylaxis can be expected to have a 10 to 40 percent risk of calf vein thrombosis, a 2 to 10 percent incidence of proximal vein thrombosis, and a 0.1 to 0.7 percent risk of fatal pulmonary embolism (Papadakis and Wall, 1990). Preoperative patients should receive low-dose heparin administered subcutaneously, beginning 2 hours prior to surgery and continued every 8 to 12 hours, or should have antiembolic stockings applied. This regimen has been shown to decrease the incidence of DVT in thoracic surgical patients by approximately 50 percent (Jackaman, et al., 1978). Heparin prophylaxis is associated with an increased risk of bleeding and hematoma formation, but serious complications are minimal (Shirakusa, et al., 1990).

Diagnosis of DVT and pulmonary embolism is difficult. Physical examination is often misleading, swelling and tenderness are often subtle, and Homan's sign is not accurate. Pulmonary embolism is a complication of DVT; 90 percent of emboli originate in the deep veins of the lower extremities. Any patient suspected of having DVT should receive a duplex ultrasound scan or venogram. Pulmonary embolism can present in different forms, depending on the degree of obstruction to blood flow. Small emboli may produce minimal symptoms such as atrial arrhythmias, but if recurrent may lead to hypoxia and right-sided cardiac failure. Large emboli often present with significant hypoxemia and circulatory collapse. The most frequent patient symptoms include chest pain (89 percent), dyspnea (86 percent), apprehension (59 percent), and cough (51 percent). Dyspnea, cough, fever, and leg cramps are often the first symptoms reported by affected patients. Periodic chest pain and hemoptysis occur more frequently in patients with submassive emboli. Apprehension, syncope, increased pulmonic heart sound, gallop, and murmurs are more frequently present among patients with massive embolism.

Suspected pulmonary embolism mandates urgent investigation and treatment. Arterial blood gas measurements are nonspecific and should not be relied on for diagnosis (Hull, et al., 1986). Chest x-ray findings and ECG are useful in the initial investigation to confirm or rule out other important disorders with a presentation similar to that of pulmonary embolism and will be important in the evaluation of subsequent nuclear scans. Patients rarely have findings diagnostic of pulmonary embolism on routine chest x-ray or ECG.

Ventilation/perfusion scans remain the initial investigation of choice in the majority of patients; normal perfusion is associated with a very low incidence of angiographically documented emboli (Miller, 1990). A high-risk scan carries a reliable diagnostic accuracy (Lesser, et al., 1992) and should lead to the institution of systemic anticoagulation (Fig. 6-5). A moderate-risk scan presents uncertainty, and if the suspicion of pulmonary embolism is high, a pulmonary angiogram should be obtained. Ventilated patients and postoperative patients with other pulmonary complications frequently have multiple ventilation defects, rendering ventilation/perfusion scanning in this patient group less useful. Such patients should undergo perfusion scans to direct selective pulmonary angiography. Normally, pulmonary angiography is reserved for the patient with massive pulmonary embolism requiring surgical intervention, the patient with an indeterminant scan, or the patient in whom there is a contraindication to anticoagulation. Documented pulmonary embolism or DVT is treated with specific anticoagulation with heparin. Patients with low risk of anticoagulation-related complications should receive anticoagulants while confirmatory investigations are under way. In those patients who subsequently have a negative ventilation/perfusion scan or angiogram, the heparin therapy may be terminated. Those patients with documented embolism or thrombosis should be anticoagulated with heparin and then continued on oral anticoagulants for 3 to 6 months. Patients allergic to heparin can be anticoagulated with ancrod. Those with contraindications to systemic anticoagulation require surgical prophylaxis against recurrent embolism. Most commonly, a Greenfield filter can be placed radiographically in the inferior vena cava and positioned immediately below the renal veins (Forty, et al., 1990).

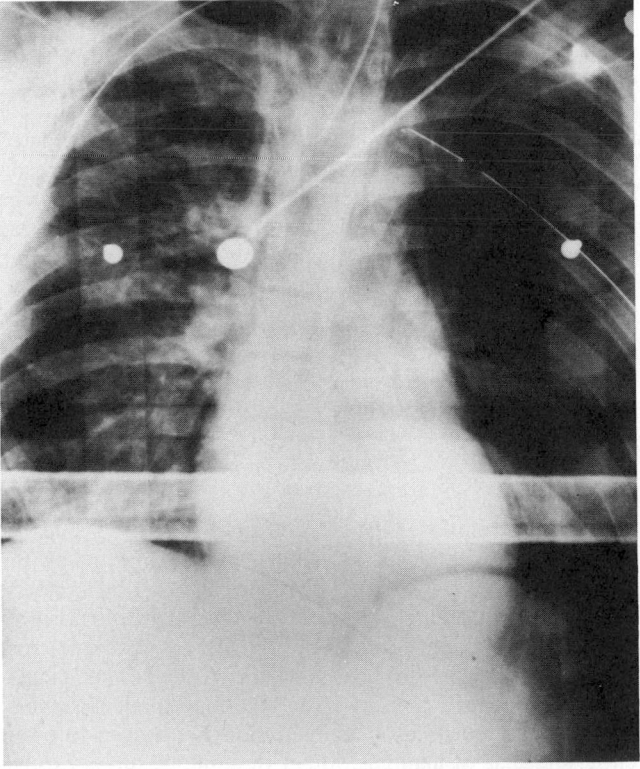

Figure 6-5. Chest x-ray of a postoperative patient demonstrating pneumomediastinum and pneumopericardium resulting from esophageal perforation.

Tumor Embolism

Massive systemic tumor embolism is a rare but potentially life-threatening complication of pulmonary resection for bronchogenic carcinoma. Embolism occurs most frequently during surgery or in the immediate postoperative period. In most cases the pulmonary vein is invaded by tumor, and embolization occurs either spontaneously or secondary to surgical manipulation. In 1967 Firor and Pearson reported the first successful removal of a massive tumor embolism situated at the aortic bifurcation. This patient did well after bilateral femoral Fogarty balloon embolectomy but 3 months later died of intracranial and systemic metastasis (Pairolero, et al., 1990). Subsequent case reports have stressed the importance of early pulmonary vein ligation prior to manipulation of the lung in order to prevent gross systemic tumor embolization (Van Raemdonck, et al., 1990; Arnold and Pairolero, 1990). Anticipation of the problem preoperatively will likely prevent most embolic phenomena.

Proximal tumors abutting the pulmonary veins or failure to visualize a pulmonary vein during a contrast computed tomography (CT) scan should lead to concern that the tumor is invading the lumen of the vessel or extending into the left atrium. If the problem is unsuspected preoperatively, it may first be recognized on palpation of the vein. Under this circumstance it is advisable to open the pericardium and apply an atrial clamp beyond the palpable abnormality. A two-dimensional echocardiogram or transesophageal echocardiogram will further elucidate the situation in such circumstances and alert the surgeon to the possibility of tumor embolism. The lower extremities have been the most frequent site of tumor emboli. Primary bronchogenic carcinoma has been diagnosed in a patient initially presenting with lower limb ischemia secondary to tumor embolism (Peters, 1989). It has been recently suggested that tumor embolism does not adversely affect prognosis and that outlook is best predicted by TNM staging (Shastri and Spaulding, 1989). Gradual respiratory decompensation secondary to subacute cor pulmonale from microscopic bronchogenic carcinoma embolization has also been well described (Postmus, et al., 1989). Massive tumor embolism can be diagnosed by careful physical examination and selective angiography when the latter is deemed necessary. Appropriate initial therapy involves systemic anticoagulation and urgent embolectomy. All extracted embolic material should be sent for pathologic examination.

Lobar Gangrene

Torsion of a remaining lobe following lobectomy or bilobectomy is a rare complication, occurring in approximately 0.2 percent of surgical patients (Rogiers, et al., 1991; Eggers, 1920). Without prompt diagnosis and treatment, torsion progresses to pulmonary infarction and finally fatal gangrene. The use of a double-lumen endotracheal tube has been implicated in inadvertent intraoperative lobar torsion (Eggers, 1920), but in most cases lobar torsion is believed to occur either because of manipulation at the time of surgery or because of the presence of a complete fissure between the middle lobe and either the upper or lower lobe. A complete oblique fissure, coupled with the narrow middle lobe hilum, make the right middle lobe the most frequently involved lobe (Pool and Garlock, 1929). Lobar torsion results in vascular and bronchial obstruction, predisposing the patient to ischemic lung injury. Patients often present with persistently high fever, hemoptysis, and bronchorrhea. Arterial blood gases may be deceptively normal, as the involved lobe may have no perfusion. Typically, serial chest radiographs demonstate increased volume and density of the involved pulmonary parenchyma. Prominent reticular markings may also be seen secondary to edema from venous obstruction (Wangensteen, 1935). Pleural effusion and abnormal location of bronchovascular markings are less specific associated findings (Eggers, 1920). Occasionally, a bronchial cutoff is also present. Differentiation from lobar opacification secondary to retained secretions may be difficult. Flexible bronchoscopy, CT scanning, and ventilation/perfusion scanning are adjuncts to diagnosis. Bronchoscopy shows no endobronchial lesion but rather a collapsed bronchus through which the scope may be passed. Removal of the bronchoscope results in prompt reclosure of the affected bronchus. Mucosal erythema and edema may also be evident.

When the diagnosis of lobar torsion is made, immediate operation is mandatory. Repeat thoracotomy is required to untwist the lobe and assess its viability. If diagnosis is early, the involved lobe may yet be viable and its fixation to the remaining lobe may be sufficient. If ischemic injury is advanced, lobectomy is indicated. Perioperative anesthesia management should include the use of a double-lumen tube. During detorsion, retained secretions or bleeding into the airway may occur; with isolation of the affected lung, soiling of the good lung may be prevented (Shenstone, 1936). Right middle lobe torsion may be prevented in suitable situations (complete fissure with a narrow bronchovascular pedicle) by suturing or stapling the middle lobe to adjacent lung (Pool and Garlock, 1929; Gray, 1938). During the conduct of intrathoracic procedures, care must be taken to avoid unrecognized lobar volvulus.

Esophageal Fistulae

A common cause of esophageal fistulae occurring postoperatively is an anastomotic leak from either an intrathoracic anastomosis or an esophagogastrostomy in the neck. Anastomotic leaks commonly present within the first 5 to 7 days. Those that are large or are secondary to major necrosis of the gastric tube may present earlier in more dramatic fashion. Although commonly presenting with symptoms and signs of sepsis, the intrathoracic anastomotic leak may declare itself with an increasing pleural effusion, supraventricular tachycardia, mediastinal air, and even pneumopericardium and cardiac tamponade (Fig. 6-6). Fistulae into the airway are not common but will usually heal spontaneously if adequate drainage is provided. Esophageal fistulae that occur in the neck usually heal quickly and are of little long-term consequence unless there has been substantial necrosis of the gastric transposition. The latter is suggested by the presence of a foul odor from the mouth and neck and is confirmed by gastroscopy.

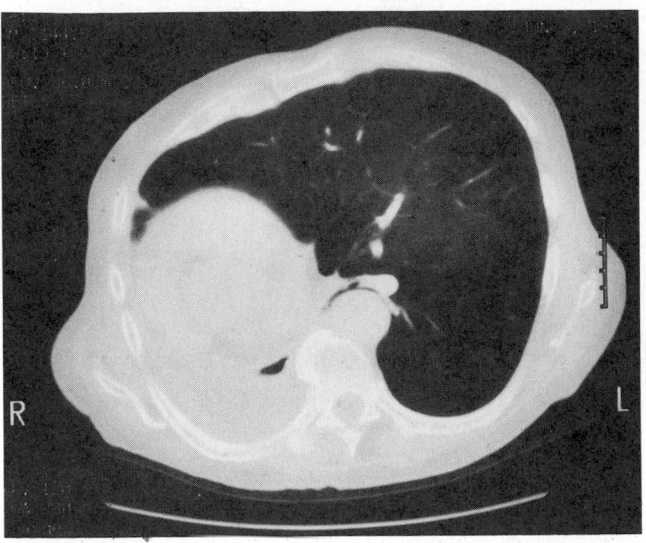

Figure 6-6. CT scan demonstrating extreme mediastinal shift and pulmonary hyperinflation occurring after pneumonectomy.

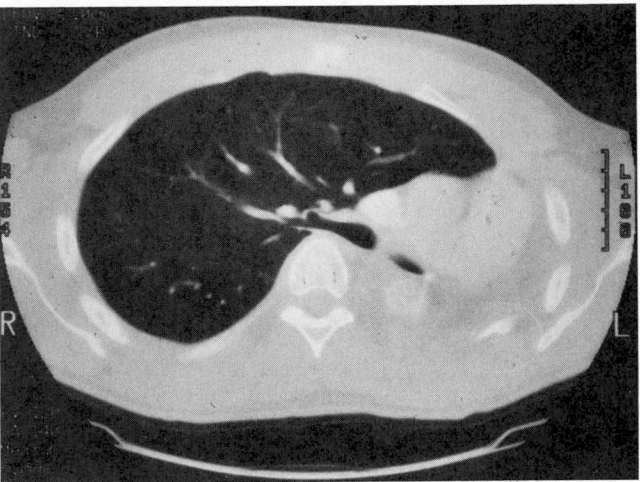

Figure 6-7. Obstruction of bronchus intermedius resulting from compression against the thoracic spine.

Pneumonia

Nosocomial pneumonia usually occurs between the third and seventh day postoperatively. The most common organisms are enteric gram-negative bacilli or those commonly seen colonizing the airways of patients with chronic obstructive lung disease (*Hemophilus influenzae* and *Pneumococcus*). The pathophysiology, diagnosis, and treatment are outlined in detail elsewhere in this book.

Postpneumonectomy Syndrome

Airway obstruction may occur following pneumonectomy accompanied by extreme mediastinal shift. This has most commonly been reported following pneumonectomy in children or adolescents. Although originally described following right pneumonectomy (Shepard et al., 1986), it has been observed after left pneumonectomy when there is a right aortic arch (Grillo, et al., 1992) or, in two of our cases, in the absence of associated congenital abnormalities. Following a right pneumonectomy, the mediastinum shifts to the right and the heart undergoes a counterclockwise rotation. The left main bronchus is compressed between the aortic arch and the left main pulmonary artery. The abnormality is best seen on CT scanning (Fig. 6-7) and confirmed with bronchoscopy. After a left pneumonectomy, the bronchus intermedius becomes compressed against the thoracic spine (Fig. 6-8) if there is extreme mediastinal shift and clockwise rotation of the heart. Diagnosis is made from a high degree of suspicion. The incidence of the condition is probably considerably greater than reported. It should be considered in any patient with dyspnea following pneumonectomy, particularly when there is significant mediastinal shift.

Surgical correction has involved several elaborate vascular procedures, such as division and bypass of the descending aortic arch. However, most successful corrections have involved mediastinal repositioning, either with autologous tissue (Grillo, et al., 1992) or expandable prostheses (Rasch, et al., 1990). In our experience, the latter has been straightforward and has resulted in reversal of the bronchial obstruction in all four cases attempted. The procedure involves reopening of the original thoracotomy with division of all adhesions between the parietal pleura and the mediastinal structures. The mediastinum can then be repositioned in the midline, correcting the rotation of the heart. On the right side the correction of the cardiac rotation is facilitated by division of the azygous vein. In our series of four cases, the pericardium was sutured to the anterior chest wall to maintain neutrality and an expandable tissue prosthesis was placed to ensure that no further mediastinal shift would occur. The correction of the airway obstruction is immediate, although bronchomalacia has been reported (Grillo, et al., 1992).

Myocardial Ischemia and Infarction

Preoperative assessment of cardiac risk is critical when evaluating potential patients prior to thoracic surgery. Perioperative cardiac complications can be reduced in patients identified as at high risk preoperatively by increased perioperative monitoring, performance of lesser procedures or medical optimization. Preoperative revascularization using either balloon angioplasty or coronary artery bypass grafting should be considered in appropriate patients with significant coronary artery disease.

Preoperative indicators of increased risk of perioperative cardiac morbidity (myocardial infarction, unstable angina, congestive heart failure, serious dysrhythmia, or cardiac death) include advanced age, history of previous myocardial infarction, congestive heart failure, poorly controlled hypertension, arrhythmias, severe valvular heart disease, angina, and previous coronary artery revascularization.

Age over 70 has been found by Goldman, et al. (1977) and Detsky, et al. (1986) to be an independent risk factor for perioperative cardiac events. Age alone may not be as im-

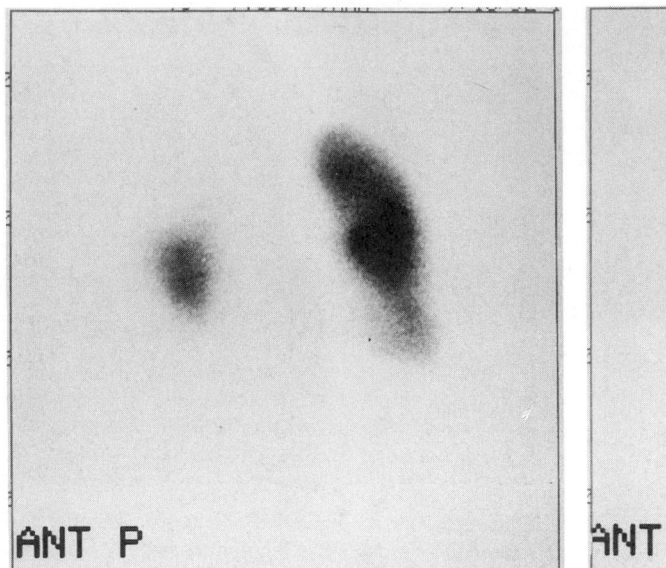 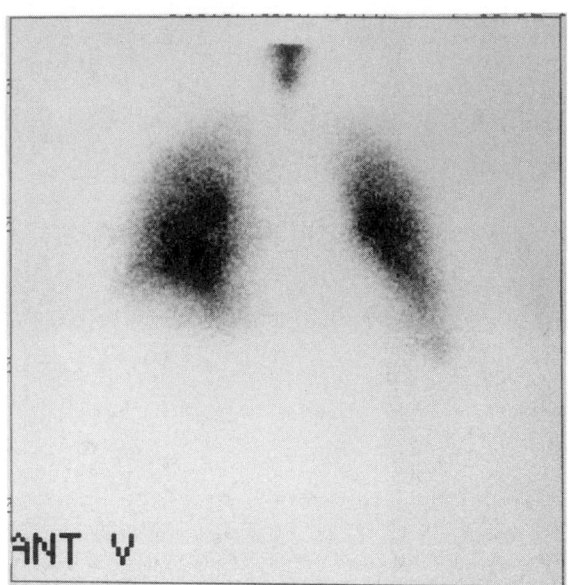

Figure 6-8. Ventilation/perfusion scan demonstrating mismatching over the right lung fields.

portant as the patient's overall physiologic status; however, the leading cause of death in elderly patients undergoing noncardiac surgery is cardiovascular disease.

Patients with a previous myocardial infarction are at greater risk of perioperative myocardial infarction and congestive heart failure as compared with those with no cardiac history. The time interval between surgery and the previous myocardial infarction significantly alters perioperative risk. Within 3 months of an infarction, surgery carries up to a 37 percent risk of perioperative cardiac morbidity. With time the risk diminishes, remaining constant at approximately 5 percent after 6 months (Dweyer, et al., 1984). Clinical or radiologic evidence of left ventricular failure is associated with a poor prognosis in patients with coronary artery disease. Patients with documented episodes of congestive heart failure may be expected to have a 5-year survival of less than 50 percent (Multicenter Postinfarction Research Group, 1983).

Hypertension is the most common cardiovascular disease in North America and a major risk factor for the development of atherosclerotic heart disease. Perioperative complications are frequent in hypertensive patients who develop either a 50 percent decrease in intraoperative blood pressure or a 33 percent or greater decrease for 10 minutes or more as compared with preoperative values (Goldman and Caldera, 1979). Untreated diastolic hypertension greater than 110 mmHg is also associated with increased frequency of intraoperative hypotension and perioperative myocardial ischemia and renal failure (Martin and Krammerer, 1983; Prys-Roberts, et al., 1971).

Arrhythmias are common and benign in normal individuals. In the presence of coronary artery disease or left ventricular dysfunction, however, dysrhythmias may pose considerable risk. In the setting of myocardial ischemia or electrolyte abnormalities, certain arrhythmias may precipitate ventricular fibrillation. Goldman et al. (1977) considered a rhythm other than sinus, premature atrial contractions, or more than five premature ventricular contractions per minute on preoperative ECG in patients with known atherosclerotic heart disease to be risk factors for perioperative cardiac morbidity.

Aortic stenosis is associated with left ventricular hypertrophy, subendocardial ischemia, and decreased coronary perfusion pressure. Patients with significant aortic stenosis have dramatically increased risk of perioperative cardiac morbidity.

In ambulatory patients with coronary artery disease, stable angina increases the risk of myocardial infarction and sudden death. The predictive value of stable angina in patients undergoing noncardiac surgery is less clear, however. In thoracic patients, activity level and anginal symptoms may be limited. Class III or IV angina is a significant predictor of cardiac morbidity.

Patients who have had previous coronary artery bypass surgery and have patent grafts are at low risk. In these patients the risk of surgery is equivalent to that in patients with no documented coronary artery disease for the corresponding age (Foster, et al., 1986). No similar data are available relating the risk of surgery in patients who have undergone angioplasty procedures.

Preoperatively, patients with multiple risk factors or symptomatic heart disease should be investigated (Table 6-1). Echocardiography is a noninvasive method or determining left ventricular function and regional wall motion and estimating pulmonary artery pressure. Persantine-thallium scanning reveals areas of myocardium with restricted perfusion. This test is a highly sensitive predictor of perioperative cardiac events with low specificity (Boucher, et al., 1985). In patients with curable pulmonary malignancy and a large reversible defect seen on persantine-thallium scan, coronary angiography should be pursued. These patients may be candidates for combined or staged revascularization and resection. In

Table 6-1. Preoperative Predictors of Perioperative Cardiac Events

Symptom	Two-Dimensional Echocardiogram	Persantine-Thallium Scan	Angiogram
Atrial arrhythmia	−	−	−
Ventricular arrhythmia	+	−	−
Stable angina	+	+	−
Congestive heart failure	+	−	−
Atypical chest pain	−	+	−
Unstable angina	+	−	+

patients with amenable significant single-vessel disease, angioplasty may be considered.

Patients undergoing thoracic surgical procedures are frequently at increased cardiac risk; many patients have significant underlying coronary artery disease. Thoracotomy-related supraventricular tachycardia, hypoxia, hypotension, fluid shifts, changes in pulmonary vascular resistance, and medications all may induce myocardial ischemia, which may progress to infarction. Principles of management are prevention and symptomatic care. Those patients who are identified preoperatively as being at increased risk and who are not candidates for revascularization procedures should have management plans carefully considered. Medical treatment or lesser surgical procedures may be appropriate. If these patients are to be treated surgically, preoperative anesthetic assessment should be sought, and patients should be managed postoperatively in an intensive care setting. Perioperative monitoring with a Swan-Ganz catheter allows more careful fluid management and hemodynamic optimization.

Episodes of myocardial ischemia should be treated promptly with nitrates, calcium channel blockers, β-blockade, and afterload reduction. Predisposing factors (i.e., hypotension, arrhythmia, tachycardia, hypoxia, and anemia) must be treated promptly. Patients with evidence of respiratory failure should be recognized early; those with refractory angina with any degree of respiratory insufficiency may benefit from early intubation and mechanical ventilation. If necessary, patients may be anticoagulated 24 to 48 hours after thoracotomy, and enteric-coated aspirin is indicated in all patients with myocardial ischemia or infarction.

KEY REFERENCES

Claggett OT, Geraci JE: A procedure for the management of postpneumonectomy empyema. J Thorac Cardiovasc Surg 45:141, 1963

A classic paper describing the difficulties managing postpneumonectomy empyema and the original description of the "Claggett drainage procedure."

Ilves R, Cooper JD, Todd TRJ, Pearson FG: Prospective, randomized, double-blind study using prophylactic cephalothin for major, elective, general thoracic operations. J Thorac Cardiovasc Surg 81:813, 1981

One of the earliest well-conducted studies demonstrating a significant reduction in the incidence of postoperative wound infections with the use of prophylactic antibiotics. No reduction in postoperative empyema or pneumonia was seen.

Ginsberg RJ, Hill LD, Eagan RT et al: Modern thirty-day operative mortality for surgical resections in lung cancer. J Thorac Cardiovasc Surg 86:654, 1983

Report from the lung cancer study group documenting mortality from pulmonary resection for lung cancer. Results from multiple institutions are reported, involving 2,200 resections performed over a 3-year period.

Deslauriers J, Ginsberg RJ, Dubois P et al: Current operative morbidity with elective surgical resection for lung cancer. Can J Surg 32:335, 1989

Experience at two teaching centers over a 6-year period is reported for 1,076 consecutive elective pulmonary resections. Frequency of complications and preoperative risk factors are described.

Tedder M, Anstadt MP, Tedder SD, Lowe JE: Current morbidity, mortality, and survival after bronchoplastic procedures for malignancy. Ann Thorac Surg 54:387, 1992

A report of 1,915 bronchoplastic procedures for carcinoma performed over a 12-year period. Morbidity, mortality, and survival statistics are presented.

REFERENCES

American College of Physicians: Preoperative pulmonary function testing. Ann Intern Med 112:793, 1990

Arnold PG, Pairolero PC: Intrathoracic muscle flaps. An account of their use in the management of 100 consecutive patients. Ann Surg 211:656, 1990

Asamura H, Naruke T, Tsuchiya R et al: Bronchopleural fistulas associated with lung cancer operations. Univariate and multivariate analysis of risk factors, management and outcome. J Thorac Cardiovasc Surg 104:1456, 1992

Au J, Walker WS, Inglis D, Cameron EW: Percutaneous cricothyroidostomy (minitracheostomy) for bronchial toilet: results of therapeutic and prophylactic use. Ann Thorac Surg 48:850. 1989

Bailey CC, Betts RH: Cardiac arrhythmias following pneumonectomy. N Engl J Med 229:356, 1943

Bettman RB, Tannenbaum WJ: Herniation of the heart through a pericardial incision. Ann Surg 128:1012, 1948

Borgeat A, Biollaz J, Bayer-Berger M et al: Prevention of arrhythmias by flecainide after noncardiac thoracic surgery. Ann Thorac Surg 48:232, 1989

Boucher CA, Brewster DC, Darling RC: Determination of cardiac risk by dipyridamole-thallium imaging before peripheral vascular disease. N Engl J Med 312:389, 1985

Cade JF, Clegg EA, Westlake GW: Prophylaxis of venous thrombosis after major thoracic surgery. Aust N Z J Surg 53:301, 1983

Cerney CI: The prophylaxis of cardiac arrhythmias complicating pulmonary surgery. J Thorac Surg 34:105, 1957

Clagett OT, Geraci JE: A procedure for the management of postpneumonectomy empyema. J Thorac Cardiovasc Surg 45:141, 1963

Currens JH, White PD, Churchill ED: Cardiac arrhythmias following thoracic surgery. N Engl J Med 229:360, 1943

Deiraniya AK: Cardiac herniation following intrapericardial pneumonectomy. Thorax 29:545, 1974

Deslauriers J, Ginsberg RJ, Dubois P et al: Current operative morbidity associated with elective surgical resection for lung cancer. Can J Surg 32:335, 1989

Detsky AS, Abrams HB, Mclaughlin JR: Predicting cardiac complications in patients undergoing noncardiac surgery. J Gen Intern Med 1:211, 1986

Dweyer EM, McMaster P, Greenberg H: Nonfatal cardiac events and recurrent infarction in the year after acute myocardial infarction. J Am Coll Cardiol 4:695, 1984

Eckersberger F, Moritz E, Klepetko W et al: Treatment of postpneumonectomy empyema. Thorac Cardiovasc Surg 38:352, 1990

Eggers C: The treatment of bronchial fistulae. Ann Surg 72:345, 1920

Forty J, Yeatman M, Wells FC: Empyema thoracis: a review of a 4½ year experience of cases requiring surgical treatment. Respir Med 84:147, 1990

Foster ED, Davis KB, Carpenter JA: Risk of noncardiac operation in patients with defined coronary artery disease: the coronary artery surgery study (CASS) registry experience. Ann Thorac Surg 41:42, 1986

Fox RB, Shasti DM, Harada N: A novel mechanism for pulmonary oxygen toxicity—phagocyte mediated lung injury. Chest 80 (suppl):35, 1981

Gates GF, Sette RS, Cope JA: Acute cardiac herniation with incarceration following pneumonectomy. Radiology 94:561, 1970

Gilson AJ, Sahn SA: Reactivation of bleomycin lung toxicity following oxygen administration. A second response to corticosteroids. Chest 88:304, 1985

Ginsberg RJ, Hill LD, Eagan RT et al: Modern thirty-day operative mortality for surgical resections in lung cancer. J Thorac Cardiovasc Surg 86:654, 1983

Glass JD, McQuillen EN, Hardin NJ: Iatrogenic cardiac herniation: post mortem case. J Trauma 24:632, 1984

Goldman L, Caldera DL: Risk of general anesthesia and elective operations in hypertensive patients. Anesthesiology 50:285, 1979

Goldman L, Caldera DL, Nussbaum SR: Multifactorial index of cardiac risk in noncardiac surgical procedures. N Engl J Med 297:845, 1977

Gray HK: The use of pedicle muscle grafts in facilitating obliteration of large, chronic, nontuberculous, pleural empyema cavities. Minn Med 21:608, 1938

Gregoire R, Deslauriers J, Beaulieu M, Piraux M: Thoracoplasty: its forgotten role in the management of nontuberculous postpneumonectomy empyema. Can J Surg 30:343, 1987

Grillo HC, Shepard JO, Mathisen DJ, Kanarek DJ: Postpneumonectomy syndrome: diagnosis, management, and results. Ann Thorac Surg. 54:638, 1992

Groh J, Sunder-Plassmann L: Heart dislocation following extensive lung resection with pericardial resection. Anaesthesist 36:184, 1987

Hull RD, Raskob GE, Hirsh J: The diagnosis of clinically suspected pulmonary embolism. Chest 89:417S, 1986

Ilves R, Cooper JD, Todd TRJ, Pearson FG: Prospective, randomized, double-blind study using prophylactic cephalothin for major, elective, general thoracic operations. J Thorac Cardiovasc Surg 81:813, 1981

Jackaman FR, Perry BJ, Siddons H: Deep vein thrombosis after thoracotomy. Thorax 33:761, 1978

Juler GL, Stemmer EA, Connolly JE: Complications of prophylactic digitalization in thoracic surgical patients. J Thorac Cardiovasc Surg 58:352, 1969

Krasnik M, Thiis J, Frimodt-Moller N: Antibiotic prophylaxis in non-cardiac thoracic surgery. A double-blind study of penicillin vs. cefuroxime. Scand J Thorac Cardiovasc Surg 25:73, 1991

Krowka MJ, Pairolero PC, Trastek VF et al: Cardiac dysrhythmia following pneumonectomy. Chest 91:490, 1987

Lesser BA, Leeper KV, Stein PD et al: The diagnosis of acute pulmonary embolism in patients with chronic obstructive pulmonary disease. Chest 102:17, 1992

Levin PD, Faber LP, Carleton RA: Cardiac herniation after pneumonectomy. J Thorac Cardiovasc Surg 61:104, 1971

Martin DE, Krammerer WS: Hypertensive surgical patient. Surg Clin North Am 63:1017, 1983

Miller JI: Empyema thoracis (editorial comment). Ann Thorac Surg 50:343, 1990

Motta G, Ratto GB: Complications of surgery in the treatment of lung cancer: their relationship with the extent of resection and preoperative respiratory function tests. Acta Chir Belg 89:161, 1989

Mowry FM, Reynolds EW: Cardiac rhythm disturbances complicating resectional surgery of the lung. Ann Intern Med 61:688, 1964

Multicenter Postinfarction Research Group: Risk stratification and survival after myocardial infarction. N Engl J Med 309:331, 1983

Nagasaki F, Flehinger BJ, Martini N: Complications of surgery in the treatment of carcinoma of the lung. Chest 82:25, 1982

Nakahara K, Ohno K, Hashimoto J: Prediction of postoperative respiratory failure in patients undergoing lung resection for lung cancer. Ann Thorac Surg 46:549, 1988

Nelson S: Minitracheostomy: the benefits for patient care. Br J Nurs 1:492, 1992

Olsen GN, Bolton JW, Weiman DS, Hornung CA: Stair climbing as an exercise test to predict the postoperative complications of lung resection. Two years' experience. Chest 99:587, 1991

Pairolero PC, Arnold PG, Trastek VF et al: Postpneumonectomy empyema. The role of intrathoracic muscle transposition. J Thorac Cardiovas Surg 99:958, 1990

Pairolero PC, Trastek VF, Allen MS: Empyema and bronchiopleural fistula. Ann Thorac Surg 51:157, 1991

Panos A, Demajo W, Todd TR: High frequency jet ventilation in the management of bronchopleural fistula (BPF). Chest 89 (suppl):521S, 1986

Papadakis MA, Wall SD: Failure to recognize late postpneumonectomy empyema. Role of diagnostic thoracentesis. West J Med 153:313, 1990

Papsin BC, Gorenstein LA, Goldberg M: Delayed myocardial laceration after intrapericardial pneumonectomy. Ann Thorac Surg 55:756, 1993

Peters RM: Empyema thoracis: historical perspective (see comments). Ann Thorac Surg 48:306, 1989

Pool EH, Garlock JH: A treatment of persistent bronchial fistula. An experimental and clinical study. Ann Surg 90:213, 1929

Postmus PE, Kerstjens JM, de Boer WJ et al.: Treatment of post pneumonectomy pleural empyema by open window thoracostomy. Eur Respir J 2:853, 1989

Prys-Roberts C, Meioche R, Foex P: Studies of anaesthesia in relation to hypertension: cardiovascular responses of treated and untreated patients. Br J Anaesth 43:122, 1971

Rasch DK, Grover FL, Schnapf BM et al: Right pneumonectomy syndrome in infancy treated with an expandable prosthesis. Ann Thorac Surg 50:127, 1990

Ritchie AJ, Danton M, Gibbons JR: Prophylactic digitalisation in pulmonary surgery. Thorax 47:41, 1992

Rogiers P, Van Miegham W, Engelaar D, Demedts M: Late-onset post-pneumonectomy empyema manifesting as tracheal stenosis with respiratory failure. Respir Med 85:333, 1991

Rogiers P, Verschakelen J, Knockaert D, Vanneste S: Occult tuberculous postpneumonectomy space empyema four years after lung resection. Postgrad Med J 67:672, 1991

Sackner MA, Landa J, Hirsh J: Pulmonary effects of oxygen breathing—a 6 hour study in normal men. Ann Intern Med 82:40, 1976

Shamji FM, Ginsberg RJ, Cooper JD et al: Open window thoracostomy in the management of postpneumonectomy empyema with or without bronchopleural fistula. J Thorac Cardiovasc Surg 86:818, 1983

Shastri KA, Spaulding MB: Late onset of post-pneumonectomy empyema. N Y J Med 89:582, 1989

Shenstone NS: The use of intercostal muscle in the closure of bronchial fistulae. Ann Surg 104:560, 1936

Shepard JO, Grillo HC, McLoud TC et al.: Right pneumonectomy syndrome: radiologic findings and CT correlation. Radiology 161:661, 1986

Shields TW, Ujiki GT: Digitalization for prevention of arrhythmias following pulmonary surgery. Surg Gynecol Obstet 126:743, 1968

Shirakusa T, Ueda H, Takata S et al: Use of pedicled omental flap in treatment of empyema. Ann Thorac Surg 50:420, 1990

Stafford EG, Clagett OT: Postpneumonectomy empyema: neomycin instillation and definitive closure. J Thorac Cardiovasc Surg 63:771, 1972

Stiller KR, Munday RM: Chest physiotherapy for the surgical patient. Br J Surg 79:745, 1992

Takita H, Majares WS: Herniation of the heart following intrapericardial pneumonectomy. Report of a case and review. J Thorac Cardiovasc Surg 59:443, 1970

Tedder M, Anstadt MP, Tedder SD, Lowe JE: Current morbidity, mortality, and survival after brochoplastic procedures for malignancy. Ann Thorac Surg 54:387, 1992

Van Raemdonck D, Kesteman J, Roekaerts F, Jadoul P: Treatment of postpneumonectomy empyema with or without bronchopleural fistula. Acta Chir Belg 90:50, 1990

Vester SR, Faber LP, Kittle CF et al: Bronchopleural fistula after stapled closure of bronchus. Ann Thorac Surg 52:1253, 1991

Veterans Affairs Total Parenteral Nutrition Cooperative Study Group: Perioperative total parenteral nutrition in surgical patients. N Engl J Med 325:525, 1991

Von Knorring J, Lepantalo M, Lindgren L, Lindfors O: Cardiac arrhythmias and myocardial ischemia after thoracotomy for lung cancer. Ann Thorac Surg 53:642, 1992

Wahi R, McMurtrey MJ, DeCaro LF et al: Determinants of perioperative morbidity and mortality after pneumonectomy. Ann Thorac Surg 48:33, 1989

Waller DA, Gebitekin C, Saunders MR, Walker DR: Noncardiogenic pulmonary edema complicating lung resection. Ann Thorac Surg 55:140, 1993

Wangensteen OH: The pedicled muscle flap in the closure of persistent bronchopleural fistula. With description of preservation and employment of the intercostal muscle bundles by a process of ribboning (for the avoidance of abdominal hernia) in the obliteration of large chronic empyema cavities. J Thorac Surg 5:27, 1935

Wertzel H, Swoboda L, Joos-Wurtemberger A et al: Perioperative antibiotic prophylaxis in general thoracic surgery. Thorac Cardiovasc Surg 40:326, 1992

Yacoub MH, Williams WG, Ahmad A: Strangulation of the heart following intrapericardial pneumonectomy. Thorax. 23:261, 1968

Ziomek S, Read RC, Tobler G et al: Thromboembolism in patients undergoing thoracotomy. Ann Thorac Surg 56:223, 1993

7

ANESTHESIA

Alan N. Sandler

INTRODUCTION

Anesthesia for noncardiac thoracic surgical procedures is continuing to evolve into a subspecialty in its own right as the number and complexity of thoracic surgical procedures increases (Rutkow 1986). To this end a number of specialized reference texts devoted to thoracic anesthesia are now available (Kaplan 1992, Marshall et al. 1987, Benumof 1987a). The increase in complexity of thoracic surgical procedures has often been associated with advances in anesthetic care, and this is highlighted by the success of lung transplantation (Demajo 1992) in recent years. This review summarizes some of the current aspects of anesthesia for thoracic surgery. The preoperative assessment, pathophysiology, pharmacology, and clinical considerations of thoracic surgical patients is presented first, followed by the physiology and implementation of one-lung ventilation. This is followed by sections on anesthesia for specialized thoracic surgical procedures and a section on postoperative care.

HISTORICAL NOTE

Anesthesia really only became a useful adjunct to surgery after 1846, when the use of general anesthesia with ether began and was followed by the use of chloroform and nitrous oxide. Although abdominal, gynecologic, urologic, orthopaedic, and ear, nose, and throat (ENT) procedures proliferated up until the 1880s, little thoracic surgery was performed. By the end of the 1930s, however, thoracotomy had become as safe as laparotomy and as widely practiced. Magill (1936) reported the anesthetic management of patients undergoing lobectomy in 1930 and again in 1936, when the number had increased to 128. Beecher (1940) also described anesthetic techniques for lobectomy and pneumonectomy, performed with surprisingly low hospital mortality. Tracheal intubation and control of the airway was a major refinement in the development of general anesthesia, especially for thoracotomy. Magill, as well as Rowbotham (1926), developed large-bore endotracheal tubes and also bronchial blockers. Carlens and Robertshaw later devised double-lumen tubes (DLTs) for selective endobronchial intubation, which were the forerunners of modern, disposable DLTs. Control of ventilation, which is critical for thoracic anesthesia, passed through stages of insufflation of gas at high flows to early positive-pressure ventilation to the complex mechanical ventilation used today. The introduction of potent, nonflammable inhalational anesthetics and muscle relaxants was also critical for thoracic surgery. The introduction of halothane by Raventos in the early 1950s eliminated the all too real risk of fire and explosion and allowed electrocautery to be used with impunity. Finally the rapid development of intensive monitoring of the respiratory and cardiovascular systems after the 1960s allowed quantum increases in anesthetic care of thoracotomy patients. The benefits of electrocardiographic (ECG) monitoring, intra-arterial pressure monitoring, flow-directed pulmonary artery catheters, and rapid analysis of arterial blood gases are essential for modern thoracic anesthesia. Continuous on-line noninvasive cardiac monitoring as well as continuous intra-arterial oxygen measurement are current developments that will make thoracic surgery safer and enable complex procedures such as lung transplantation to proliferate.

HISTORICAL READINGS

Beecher HK: Some controversial matters of anesthesia for thoracic surgery. J Thorac Surg 10:202, 1940
Magill IW: Anesthesia in thoracic surgery. Proc R Soc Med 29: 643, 1936
Rowbotham S: Intratracheal anesthesia. Lancet 2:583, 1926

PREOPERATIVE EVALUATION

History

The most relevant information for the anesthetist is related to the severity of attendant pulmonary and cardiovascular disease. Much of thoracic surgery is concerned with cancer resection, and this is reflected in the patient population (elderly, history of heavy cigarette smoking, recent weight loss). Symptoms arising from bronchopulmonary involvement include cough, sputum, chest pain, dyspnea, wheeze, and hemoptysis.

Dyspnea

Dyspnea is present when the patient's ventilatory requirements are greater than the physiologic ability to respond. Dyspnea is quantitated in relation to the level of physical activity at which it is present (e.g., walk on the level, climb stairs, etc.). Severe exertional dyspnea with marked impairment of physical activity implies decreased ventilatory reserve and a forced expiratory volume in 1 second (FEV_1) less than 1,500 ml, which may result in the need for postoperative ventilatory support.

Cough

The presence of cough and sputum may allow the diagnosis of chronic bronchitis (productive cough for 3 months of the year for 2 consecutive years). Cough is a very common symptom in chronic cigarette smokers and may be viewed as normal for them. Sputum should be cultured to determine whether preoperative antibiotic therapy is necesary. Hemoptysis may be indicative of bronchogenic carcinoma and occasionally can be present in massive quantities, making airway management extremely difficult. Wheezing may be related to bronchial obstruction.

Chest Pain

Chest pain may be present in up to 40 percent of patients with carcinoma of the lung. It is usually mild, constant, and related to the side of the tumor, in contrast to pleuritic pain, which is aggravated by breathing. In addition, other important causes of chest pain such as angina pectoris and gastric acid reflux must be differentiated.

Cigarette Smoking

Cigarette smoking is directly related to the incidence of chronic lung disease and carcinoma as well as to the occurrence of postoperative pulmonary complications such as atelectasis and arterial hypoxemia.

Tumor Growth

Symptoms may arise that are related to direct extension of tumor growth in the thorax or to metastatic invasion. These include pleural effusion, chest wall pain, esophageal obstruction, superior vena caval obstruction, brachial plexus invasion with arm pain or Horner syndrome, and recurrent laryngeal nerve invasion (hoarseness).

Endocrine Manifestations

Symptoms and syndromes related to endocrine function of thoracic tumors include Cushing syndrome, increased antidiuretic hormone (ADH) secretion, carcinoid syndrome, hypercalcemia, and hypocalcemia. Other syndromes include carcinomatous myopathies. Symptoms related to myasthenia gravis may also be associated with intrathoracic tumors (thymoma).

Physical Examination and Relevant Laboratory Investigations

Beside the routine general examination, particular attention should be paid to the respiratory and cardiovascular systems.

Respiratory System

Central cyanosis is usually secondary to arterial hypoxemia and indicates arterial saturation (SaO_2) of 80 percent or less (arterial oxygen tension [PaO_2] <50 mmHg) and greatly decreased pulmonary function. Clubbing of the fingertips may be seen in the presence of chronic lung disease, neoplasms, or right-to-left cardiac shunts. Tracheal placement should be midline. If displaced, problems with securing the airway or airway obstruction with anesthesia may occur. Abnormalities of respiratory pattern may reveal underlying disease. Paradoxical chest/abdominal movement, hyperinflation, asymmetrical chest expansion (phrenic nerve involvement), pleural effusion, and pneumothorax should be assessed. Breath sounds (crackles) may indicate fluid in the airways (sputum, edema) or obstruction/bronchospasm (wheezing). Faint or distant sounds indicate bullae or emphysema.

Chest X-Ray. Chronic obstructive pulmonary disease (COPD) produces hyperinflation and increased vascular markings, the latter also being present with chronic bronchitis. A retrosternal air space greater than 2 cm in diameter is present with hyperinflation. The location of the tumor should be assessed with posteroanterior (PA) and lateral views as well as by computed tomography (CT). Important specific anesthetic implications may be related to tracheal or carinal deviation or compression (due to airway management, ventilation), mediastinal mass (superior vena cava or pulmonary artery compression, ventilation), pleural effusions (decreased vital capacity [VC], functional residual capacity [FRC]), bullae (rupture, bronchopleural fistula, tension pneumothorax), and abscess with air fluid level or collapsed lobe (spillage, spread of infection).

Arterial Blood Gases. Severe COPD may present as chronic bronchitis with hypoventilation and carbon dioxide retention. These high-risk patients are in a state of chronic respiratory failure and are usually hypercarbic and hypoxemic (cyanotic) and have a reduced ventilatory response to carbon dioxide due to an increase in cerebrospinal fluid bicarbonate levels. A decreased hypoxic drive produces hypoventilation in this population when high concentrations of oxygen are given. Patients with primarily severe emphysematous disease present with dyspnea and essentially normal arterial blood gases (ABGs). An increase in minute ventilation maintains the normal arterial carbon dioxide tension ($PaCO_2$), resulting in an increase in the work of breathing and dyspnea.

Pulmonary Function Testing. Pulmonary function testing (PFT) is performed to assess those patients at risk of increased morbidity and mortality, the effect of bronchodilator therapy, the degree of lung resection possible and the need for postoperative ventilation. Anesthesia and surgery, primarily

Table 7-1. Minimal Pulmonary Function Test Criteria for Various Sized Pulmonary Resections

Test	Unit	Normal	Pneumonectomy	Lobectomy	Biopsy or Segmental
MBC	Liters/minute	>100	>70	40–70	40
MBC	Percentage predicted	100	>55	>40	>35
FEV_1	Liters	>2	>2	>1	>0.6
FEV_1	Percentage predicted	>100	>55	40–50	>50
FEV_{25-75}	Liters	2	>1.6	>0.6–1.6	>0.6

Abbreviations: MBC, maximum breathing capacity; FEV_1, forced expiratory volume in first second; FEV_{25-75}, forced expiratory volume from 25 to 75 percent of forced vital capacity.

(From Benumof JL, Alfery DD: Anesthesia for thoracic surgery. p. 1663. In Miller RD (ed): Anesthesia. 4th Ed. Churchill Livingstone, New York, 1994, with permission.)

abdominal and thoracic surgery, produce major decreases in lung volumes and alteration in respiratory patterns. Total lung capacity (TLC), VC, and FEV_1 are all markedly reduced even with control of postoperative pain (Shulman, et al., 1984; Tisi, 1979; Craig, 1981). Expiratory reserve volume (ERV) decreases by 25 percent after abdominal surgery and by 60 percent after thoracic surgery. Tidal volume (V_T) decreases by 20 to 30 percent, as does pulmonary compliance and FRC. These changes occur either immediately after surgery or in the early postoperative period and require from days to weeks to return to relatively normal levels. Spirometry can provide reasonable guidelines for the relative risk of patients presenting for various sized pulmonary resection (Table 7-1) and for pneumonectomy (Table 7-2). A VC at least three times the V_T is required for an effective cough (O'Donoghue, et al., 1976) and a VC less than 50 percent of predicted or less than 2 L is associated with increased risk (Gass and Olsen, 1986). FEV_1 testing provides an indication of airway obstruction. An FEV_1 of 0.8 L is an absolute contraindication to lung resection, and mortality increases as FEV_1 decreases from 2 L to less than 1 L (Lockwood 1973). The ratio of FEV_1 to forced vital capacity (FVC) is normal in restrictive disease but is decreased in obstructive disease as FEV_1 is reduced. Similarly, the ratio of residual volume (RV) to TLC if greater than 50 percent indicates increased risk (Mittman, 1961). With abnormal ABGs ($PaCO_2 > 45$ mmHg on room air), abnormal spirometry, and decreases in lung volumes, more sophisticated PFTs may be performed, especially if pneumonectomy is contemplated (Table 7-2). These include split-lung function tests (radioisotopic ventilation and perfusion scans) and temporary balloon occlusion of the major pulmonary artery on the operated side with or without exercise (Table 7-2).

Cardiovascular System

Pulmonary Vascular and Right Ventricular Function Testing. The presence of pulmonary hypertension caused by an increase in pulmonary vascular resistance (PVR) should be carefully assessed. Patients with COPD may have distension of the pulmonary capillary bed with reduced vascular compliance in relation to increases in cardiac output (CO) (Fig. 7-1). Signs of pulmonary hypertension include a split second heart sound, an increased pulmonary component of the second heart sound, and if severe, right atrial (RA) and right ventricular (RV) hypertrophy. The noninvasive diagnosis of pulmonary hypertension is summarized in Table 7-3. Factors that increase PVR include hypoxia (Abraham, et al., 1969), acidosis (Enson, et al., 1964), sepsis (Kinchi, et al., 1983), and the application of positive end-expiratory pressure (PEEP) (Hobelmann, et al., 1975; Canada and Benumof, 1982), which may contribute to RV failure. A rigid, restricted pulmonary vasculature may develop increased pulmonary hypertension after pneumonectomy, and this may contribute to postpneumonectomy pulmonary edema when it occurs (Zeldin, et al., 1984). Direct measurements of PVR have been made by mea-

Table 7-2. Preoperative Pulmonary Functions Tests (PFTs) and Operative Risk of Pneumonectomy

Testing Phase[a]	PFT[a]	Increased Operative Risk Result
1. Whole-lung tests	Arterial blood gas spirometry	Hypercapnia on room air $FEV_1 < 50\%$ of FVC $FEV_1 < 2L$ MBC < 50% predicted
	Lung volume	RV/TLC > 50%
2. Single-lung tests	Right-left (individual-lung) split-function tests	Predicted postoperative FEV_1 <0.85 L or >70% blood flow to diseased lung
3. Mimic postoperative condition	Temporary unilateral balloon occlusion of right or left pulmonary artery	Mean pulmonary artery pressure > 40 mmHg, $PaCO_2 > 60$ mmHg, or $PaO_2 < 45$ mmHg

Abbreviations: RV, residual volume; TLC, total lung capacity; MBC, maximum breathing capacity; FEV_1, forced expiratory volume in first second; FVC, forced vital capacity.

[a] The testing phases and PFT are listed in order of proper temporal performance and increasing invasiveness.

(From Benumof JL, Alfery DD: Anesthesia for thoracic surgery. p. 1663. In Miller RD (ed): Anesthesia. 4th Ed. Churchill Livingstone, New York, 1994, with permission.)

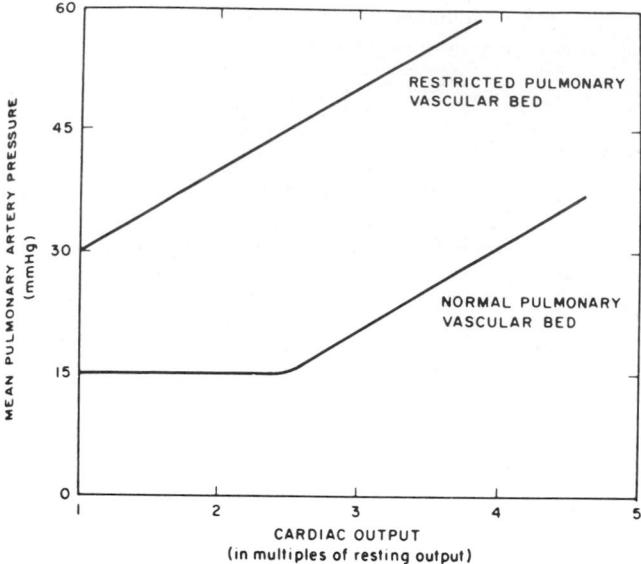

Figure 7-1. Mean pulmonary artery pressure (y axis) does not increase until cardiac output (x axis) has been increased to 2 to 2.5 times when the pulmonary vascular bed is normal, whereas mean pulmonary artery pressure increases linearly with cardiac output when the pulmonary vascular bed is restricted. (From Robin ED, Gaudio R: Cor pulmonale. Dis Mon [May]: 138, 1970, with permission.)

pulmonary vascular and RV function preoperatively that will provide indications as to the postoperative state after pneumonectomy (Olsen, et al., 1975; Tisi, 1979; Laros and Swierengo, 1967; Sloan, et al., 1955). If the mean pulmonary artery pressure increases above 40 mmHg, PaO_2 is less than 60 mmHg, or $PaCO_2$ is greater than 45 mmHg, pneumonectomy may not be tolerated without respiratory or RV failure postoperatively. Echocardiography (ECG) is also being increasingly used to assess the pulmonary vasculature and RV function.

Left Ventricular Function Testing. The main causes of left ventricular (LV) dysfunction in thoracic surgical patients are coronary artery disease, cardiac valvular disease, hypertension, and RV dysfunction (Zimmerman, et al., 1982; Kassis, 1977; Baum, et al., 1971; Kachel, 1978). The high incidence of smoking in this population is associated especially with an increased incidence of coronary artery disease. Further investigation of patients with ischemic heart disease requires exercise testing (ECG and thallium scanning), echocardiography, and if necessary, coronary angiography (Peters and Swain, 1982). In general, if coronary artery bypass grafting is necessary, this should be performed before pulmonary resection, although both procedures have been performed under the same anesthetic with limited resections (Piehler, et al., 1985; Dalton, et al., 1978).

suring pulmonary artery and pulmonary wedge pressures at different levels of CO (treadmill exercising). PVR measured in this fashion has provided a risk indicator for pneumonectomy (Fee, et al., 1978; Pecora and Hohenberger, 1979). PVR greater than 190 dyne/s/cm was found to be related to increased operative risk (Jones, 1980). If a pulmonary artery catheter is in place, additional PVR measurements can be made during temporary unilateral balloon occlusion at rest and during exercise. This will provide specific data about

Laboratory Investigations

Routine laboratory tests may disclose information pertinent to the thoracic surgical patient. Polycythemia may be associated with decreased hemoglobin saturation and leukocytosis with pulmonary infection. Gram stain of the sputum and culture and sensitivity tests allow bacterial diagnosis and antibiotic selection. Sputum cytology may assist in diagnosis of neoplasms. Metastatic spread may be indicated by abnormal liver and bone enzymes, blood urea nitrogen, creatinine, and urinalysis.

Table 7-3. Noninvasive Diagnosis of Pulmonary Hypertension, Increased Pulmonary Vascular Resistance, Right Atrial and Ventricular Hypertrophy, and Cor Pulmonale

Ausculatory Signs of ↑ PAP and ↑ PVR	Radiographic Signs of ↑ PAP and ↑ PVR	Electrocardiographic Signs of ↑ RA and ↑ RV	Additional Signs of CP
↑ Pulmonary component of second heart sound	Dilatation of main pulmonary artery	↑ RV Clockwise vector rotation	All those of ↑ PAP, ↑ PVR, ↑ RA, ↑ RV
Loss of normally present split in second heart sound	Fullness of apical pulmonary vessels	Right axis deviation	Pulmonary diastolic murmur
Presence of fourth heart sound	Counterclockwise cardiac rotation: globular shape on PA film (RV comprises left heart border, aortic knob)	↑ R and ↑ S wave V_2–V_6	Third heart sound
Appearance of high-pitched early systolic ejection click		Inverted T wave V_1–V_4	Prominent right sternal border pulsation plus retraction over left chest
		↑ RA	
		↓ ST segment V_2–V_6 ↑ P wave II and III; diphasic P wave V_1	Chronic dependent edema, large tender liver, ascites, distension neck veins (large A waves)

Abbreviations: ↑ PAP, pulmonary hypertension; ↑ PVR, increased pulmonary vascular resistance; ↑ RA, right atrial hypertrophy; ↑ RV, right ventricular hypertrophy; CP, cor pulmonale.

(From Benumof JL, Alfery DD: Anesthesia for thoracic surgery. p. 1663. In Miller RD (ed): Anesthesia. 4th Ed. Churchill Livingstone, New York, 1994, with permission.)

Preoperative Preparation

Preoperative preparation of thoracic surgical patients significantly decreases postoperative morbidity (atelectasis, pneumonia) (Stein, et al., 1962; Stein and Cassara, 1970; Gracey, et al., 1979; Palmer and Sellick, 1953; Veith and Rocco, 1959). Thoracic surgical patients are at risk of postoperative pulmonary complications because of preoperative, intraoperative, and postoperative factors. The high incidence of cigarette smoking and COPD increases the risk of postoperative pulmonary complications 6- to 20-fold (Morton and Camb, 1944; Stein, et al., 1962; Latimer, et al.,1971). Intraoperatively, atelectasis and edema in the dependent and nondependent lungs can contribute to postoperative morbidity. Postoperatively, pain control is an important factor, which if not adequately treated contributes to decreased ability to breathe deeply and produce an adequate cough, which in turn contributes to retained secretions, atelectasis and infections (Johnson, 1967; Ali, et al., 1974; Tarhan and Lundborg, 1973, Harmon and Lillington, 1979).

Preoperative preparation includes stopping smoking, dilating airways, and loosening and removing secretions in those patients with bronchospasm and increased secretions, as well as adequate education to improve patient participation in all aspects of perioperative care. Stopping smoking for several weeks to months prior to surgery produces an improvement in mucociliary transport and decreased airway reactivity and secretion production with consequent decrease in postoperative complications (Warner, et al., 1983; Pearce and Jones, 1984; Jones, 1985; Buist, et al., 1981). Stopping smoking for several days prior to surgery provides little of the benefits of a longer period but may decrease carboxyhemoglobin levels, reduce nicotine-induced tachycardia, and improve ciliary beating. Patients with a demonstrated reversible bronchospastic component should be treated with bronchodilating drugs. β_2-Sympathomimetic drugs such as albuterol, terbutaline, and metaproterenol are effective bronchodilating drugs when administered as inhaled aerosols. These drugs directly increase cyclic adenosine monophosphate (cAMP), which relaxes bronchial smooth muscle, in contrast to the methylxanthine drugs (theophylline, aminophylline), which inhibit the enzyme phophodiesterase, which breaks down cAMP. Methylxanthines added to β_2-sympathomimetics increase bronchial smooth muscle relaxation (Webb-Johnson, et al., 1977; Isles and Newth, 1983) and improve diaphragmatic contractility (Aubier, et al., 1981). Other agents may on occasion be useful, such as steroids (which decrease mucosal edema) and parasympatholytic agents (atropine improves bronchodilator therapy) (Marini, et al., 1981).

INTRAOPERATIVE PERIOD

Monitoring

Patients scheduled for thoracic surgery require all the standard monitoring devices currently recommended for major surgery plus a degree of invasive monitoring depending on the nature of the surgery and the severity of the pulmonary or associated diseases. Standard monitoring requirements include an ECG (leads II and/or V_5) to detect arrhythmias or ischemia, chest or esophageal stethoscopes to detect obstruction, secretions, or bronchospasm, and a temperature probe. Further standard noninvasive monitors include an automated oscillometric blood pressure monitor, capnography or a mass spectrometer to monitor end-tidal carbon dioxide ($EtCO_2$) and a pulse oximeter. End-tidal gas analysis allows breath-by-breath analysis of respiratory function and gas exchange (apnea, minute ventilaton, volatile anesthetic concentration), and as the carbon dioxide waveform/plateau corresponds roughly with airway resistance, airway mechanics (obstruction) can be estimated. Ventilation should be continuously monitored by observing the chest wall (lung movement when the chest is open).

Invasive Monitoring

Direct Arterial Catheterization. Peripheral arterial cannulation is an important feature in patients undergoing thoracic surgery. It allows for continuous beat-to-beat measurement of blood pressure as well as sampling for the determination of ABGs. The use of a 20-gauge Teflon catheter in the radial artery has decreased the risk of arterial cannulation to a very

---

Preoperative Respiratory Care Regimen

1. Stop smoking
2. Dilate airways
   a. β_2-Agonists
   b. Theophylline
   c. Steroids
   d. Cromolyn sodium
3. Loosen secretions
   a. Airway hydration (humidifier/nebulizer)
   b. Systemic hydration
   c. Mucolytic and expectorant drugs
   d. Antibiotics
4. Remove secretions
   a. Postural drainage
   b. Coughing
   c. Chest physiotherapy (percussion and vibration)
5. Increase education, motivation, and facilitation of postoperative care
   a. Psychological preparation
   b. Incentive spirometry
   c. Exposure to secretion removal maneuvers
   d. Exercise
   e. Weight loss/gain
   f. Stabilize other medical problems

(From Benumof JL, Alfery DD: Anesthesia for thoracic surgery. p. 1663. In Miller RD (ed): Anesthesia. 4th Ed. Churchill Livingstone, New York, 1994, with permission.)

low level. The risk is even lower if patency of the ulnar artery is assessed by a modified Allen test.

Continuous blood pressure readings are very useful during thoracic surgery, as major changes in blood pressure are common secondary to surgical manipulations or intravascular volume shifts. Rapid recognition of these changes allows time for diagnosis and rapid treatment (Nobak, 1983).

In addition, serial ABG determinations are essential during one-lung anesthesia, as arterial hypoxemia may be commonly seen owing to increased pulmonary shunting and inadequate hypoxic pulmonary vasoconstriction. Any changes in acid-base status as well as hyper- or hypoventilation can also be determined.

It is recommended that the radial artery catheter be placed in the right radial artery during anesthesia for mediastinoscopy, as this will allow monitoring of compression of the innominate artery by the mediastinoscope (Petty, 1979). Loss of the arterial blood pressure waveform indicates decreased blood flow to the brain through the innominate artery and allows repositioning of the mediastinoscope.

Central Venous Pressure Monitoring. Central venous pressure (CVP) is used as a measure of RA and RV pressures. The CVP reflects the patient's blood volume, venous tone, and RV performance. The CVP reflects right heart function and not left ventricular performance. It may be a useful monitor when large volume shifts or hypovolemia is expected. For monitoring of left heart function, a pulmonary artery catheter (PAC) is far more useful.

Pulmonary Artery Catheterization. Pulmonary artery catheterization allows measurements of left-sided filling pressures, measurement of CO by thermodilution, and calculation of derived hemodynamic and respiratory parameters (e.g., systemic vascular resistance and intrapulmonary shunt). Also, sophisticated versions of the PAC allow measurement of mixed venous oxygen saturation ($S\overline{v}O_2$) or RV ejection fraction as well as application of atrial or ventricular pacing.

Use of the PAC may be indicated during thoracic surgery during specific circumstances. PACs usually flow to and locate in the right lung (Benumof, 1977). However, data derived from the PAC may be misinterpreted, especially during one-lung ventilation owing to the effects of various factors on the functioning of the PAC; the factors include altered ventilatory modes, location of the PAC tip, ventricular compliance changes, and ventricular independence. It should be noted that in the lateral decubitus position, when the catheter is in the nondependent lung and the lung is collapsed, the measured CO and mixed venous oxygen pressure may be decreased as compared with the values available when the lung is inflated. Also, when the catheter is in the nondependent lung and PEEP is applied, pulmonary artery wedge pressure may not equal left atrial pressure. Finally, if the catheter is in the dependent lung, pulmonary artery wedge pressure is usually a good index of left atrial pressure even if PEEP is used (Benumof and Alfery, 1990).

More sophisticated PAC catheters are available such as the multipurpose PAC with five pacing electrodes, which can be used for atrial, ventricular, or atrioventricular (AV) sequential pacing in patients who require a PAC for hemody-

---

Relative Indications for Pulmonary Artery Catheterization in Thoracic Surgery

1. Patients with known cardiovascular disease, with or without heart failure
2. Surgery in which cross-clamping of the thoracic aorta is anticipated
3. Patients with respiratory failure
4. Patients with suspected or diagnosed pulmonary emboli
5. Patients who have undergone previous cardiac surgery
6. Pneumonectomy anticipated
7. Significant shifts of intravascular volume anticipated
8. Presence of sepsis
9. Patients who receive continuous infusions of inotropes or vasodilators
10. Patients with pulmonary hypertension or elevated pulmonary vascular resistance
11. Presence of cor pulmonale
12. Bleomycin-treated patients

(From Noback CR: Intraoperative monitoring. p. 231. In Kaplan JA (ed): Thoracic Anesthesia. 1st Ed. Churchill Livingstone, New York, 1983, with permission.)

---

namic monitoring. A further development in the area of PAC monitoring has been the addition of fiberoptic bundles for light transmission, allowing continuous measurement of $S\overline{v}O_2$.

Oxygenation

Adequate oxygenation of patients undergoing thoracotomy can be measured intermittently from arterial blood samples taken from an arterial catheter or continuously by using pulse oximetry, a transcutaneous oxygen sensor, or an indwelling intra-arterial "optode." The pulse oximeter is the most reliable and most widely used of these systems at present. Although subject to certain limitations (e.g., hypothermia, low CO, diathermy use) pulse oximeters are fairly accurate in estimating oxygenation over the range of 60 to 100 percent. Pulse oximetry does not eliminate the requirement for ABG analysis during thoracic surgery. The intra-arterial optode is a fiberoptic probe consisting of a single heparin-coated optical fiber, which passes easily through a 20-gauge cannula with a luminescent dye–coated tip. The mechanism of action is different from that of the pulse oximeter, as the amount of light emitted from the fiber when a flash lamp activates the luminescent dye is inversely proportional to the amount of oxygen. Improvements in accuracy are required at low PaO_2 (Barker, et al., 1987), but the device may be very useful as it allows simultaneous arterial pressure monitoring, arterial blood sampling, and direct oxygen measurements.

Ventilation

Modern anesthetic machines provide several measures for the assessment of ventilation parameters during controlled ventilation (i.e., circuit low- and high-pressure alarms, respiratory rate, V_T, minute volume, and inflation pressures). However, the final determinant of adequacy of ventilation is ABG analysis, $PaCO_2$ in particular. This may be estimated continuously and noninvasively with a capnometer or mass spectrometer used to sample expired gases. The $EtCO_2$ concentration represents alveolar carbon dioxide ($PACO_2$) which approximates $PaCO_2$. During one-lung ventilation the normal alveolar to arterial carbon arterial to dioxide gradient [$P(A - a)CO_2$] (4 to 6 mmHg) may be markedly altered and therefore capnographic measurements should be checked by ABG analysis.

PHYSIOLOGY OF THE LATERAL DECUBITUS POSITION

There are several potential physiologic situations affecting ventilation or perfusion of the lungs these thoracic surgical patients in the lateral decubitus position (LDP) may encounter. These are

1. Lateral position, awake, breathing spontaneously, chest closed
2. Lateral position, awake, breathing spontaneously, chest open
3. Lateral position, anesthetized, breathing spontaneously, chest closed
4. Lateral position, anesthetized, breathing spontaneously, chest open
5. Lateral position, anesthetized, paralyzed, chest open
6. One-lung ventilation, anesthetized, paralyzed, chest open

For an understanding of the changes in the ventilation and perfusion of the lungs in the lateral decubitus position, several of these situations need consideration.

Lateral Position, Awake, Breathing Spontaneously, Chest Closed

Gravity causes a vertical gradient affecting the distribution of blood flow in the lungs in LDP in a fashion similar to that in the upright position. As perfusion is gravity-dependent, the vertical hydrostatic gradient is smaller in the lateral than in the upright position (Fig. 7-2). Zone 1 in the upper region of the lung with low blood flow is thus smaller than in the upright position. However, blood flow to the dependent lung is still greater than to the nondependent lung (Fig. 7-2). Gravity also causes a vertical gradient in pleural pressure in the LDP, and thus ventilation is relatively increased in the dependent lung. In addition, in the LDP the dome of the lower diaphragm is pushed high into the chest by the abdominal contents and is thus able to contract more efficiently during spontaneous ventilation. Thus, ventilation and perfusion ($\dot{V}/\dot{Q}$) matching is good in this position and similar to that in the upright position (Fig. 7-3).

Lateral Position, Awake, Breathing Spontaneously, Chest Open

For a spontaneously breathing patient in the LDP with the chest open, two complications can arise. The first is mediastinal shift, which usually occurs during inspiration. The nega-

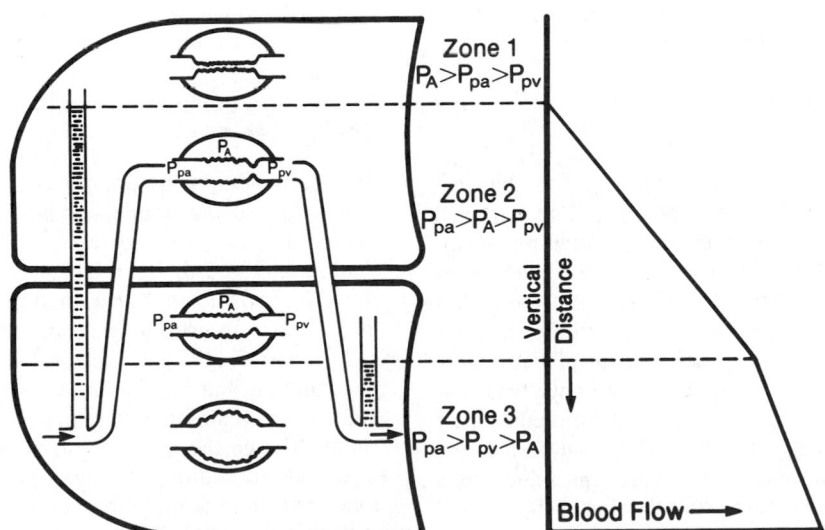

Figure 7-2. Schematic representation of the effects of gravity on the distribution of pulmonary blood flow in the lateral decubitus position. The vertical gradient in the lateral decubitus position is less than in the upright position; consequently, there is less zone 1 and more zone 2 and 3 blood flow in the lateral decubitus than in the upright position. Nevertheless, pulmonary blood flow increases with lung dependency and is greater in the dependent lung than in the nondependent lung. P_A, alveolar pressure; P_{pa}, pulmonary artery pressure; P_{pv}, pulmonary venous pressure. (From Benumof JL: Anesthesia for Thoracic Surgery. WB Saunders, Philadelphia, 1987, with permission.)

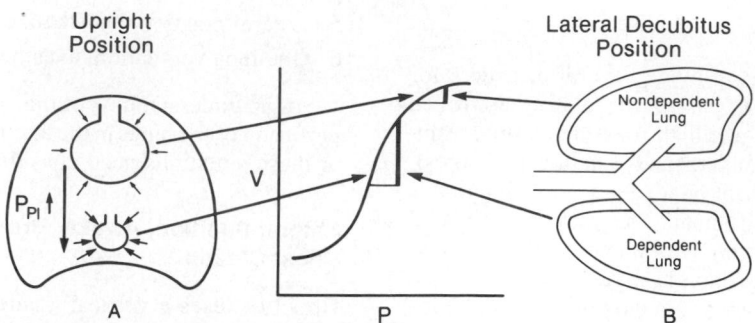

Figure 7-3. Awake, closed chest distribution of ventilation. **(A)** Pleural pressure (P_{pl}) in the awake upright patient is most positive in the dependent portion of the lung, and alveoli in this region are therefore most compressed and have the least volume. Pleural pressure is least positive (most negative) at the apex of the lung, and alveoli in this region are therefore less compressed and have the largest volume. When these regional differences in alveolar volume are translated over to a regional transpulmonary pressure–alveolar volume curve, the small dependent alveoli are on a steep (large-slope) portion of the curve, and the large nondependent alveoli are on a flat (small-slope) portion of the curve. In this diagram regional slope equals regional compliance. Thus, for a given and equal change in transpulmonary pressure, the dependent part of the lung receives a much larger share of the tidal volume than the nondependent part of the lung. **(B)** In the lateral decubitus position gravity also causes pleural pressure gradients and therefore similarly affects the distribution of ventilation. The dependent lung lies on a relatively steep portion and the nondependent lung on a relatively flat portion of the pressure–volume curve. Thus, in the lateral decubitus position the dependent lung receives the majority of the tidal ventilation. V, alveolar volume; P, transpulmonary pressure. (From Benumof JL: Anesthesia for Thoracic Surgery. WB Saunders, Philadelphia, 1987, with permission.)

tive pressure of the intact hemithorax relative to the positive pressure of the open hemithorax pushes the mediastinum vertically downward into the dependent hemithorax, which can create circulatory and reflex changes that result in decreased blood pressure and respiratory distress. Second, paradoxical breathing can occur. During inspiration the relatively negative pressure in the intact hemithorax as compared with atmospheric pressure in the open hemithorax can cause movement of air from the nondependent to the dependent lung. The opposite occurs during expiration. The movement of gas from one lung to the other in a reverse direction represents waste of ventilation and can compromise gas exchange.

Lateral Position, Anesthetized, Breathing Spontaneously, Chest Closed

With induction of general anesthesia most of the changes that occur affect the distribution of ventilation. The majority of the V_T passes to the nondependent lung, which results in a significant $\dot{V}/\dot{Q}$ mismatch. This is related to a reduction in FRC of both lungs with general anesthesia. However, the reduction of volume in the dependent lung is greater than in the nondependent lung owing to (1) cephalad displacement of the dependent diaphragm by the abdominal contents, which is increased by paralysis; and (2) pressure of the mediastinal structures on the dependent lung with or without poor positioning of the dependent side on the operating table, preventing the lung from expanding properly (Fig. 7-4).

Lateral Position, Anesthetized, Breathing Spontaneously, Chest Open

As in the chest-closed position, opening the chest has little impact on the distribution of perfusion. However, with an open chest the nondependent lung has increased compliance

and thus increased ventilation, which further increases the $\dot{V}/\dot{Q}$ mismatch seen when the chest is closed.

Lateral Position, Anesthetized, Paralyzed, Chest Open

During paralysis and positive-pressure ventilation, the diaphragm is displaced maximally over the nondependent lung, where there is least resistance by the abdominal contents. Conversely, the diaphragm is displaced minimally in the dependent portion, where the resistance to passive diaphragmatic movement by the abdominal contents is greatest (Froese and Bryan, 1974).

One-Lung Ventilation, Anesthetized, Paralyzed, Chest Open

During two-lung ventilation in the lateral position, the mean blood flow to the nondependent lung is assumed to be 40 percent of CO with 60 percent of CO directed to the dependent lung (Fig. 7-5). Normally, venous admixture (shunt) in the lateral position is 10 percent of CO and is equally divided as 5 percent to each lung. Thus, the average percentage of CO participating in gas exchange is 35 percent of the nondependent lung and 55 percent of the dependent lung. One-lung ventilation creates an obligatory right-to-left transpulmonary shunt through the nonventilated nondependent lung. Thus, in theory an additional 35 percent should be added to the total shunt during one-lung ventilation.

With normal hypoxic pulmonary vasoconstriction (HPV) (see below), blood flow to the nondependent hypoxic lung should be reduced by 50 percent. Thus blood flow to the nondependent lung should be 35/2 = 17.5 percent, all of which represents venous admixture (Marshall, 1981). Together with the obligatory 5 percent shunt in the dependent and nondependent lungs, total shunt during one-lung ventilation is thus

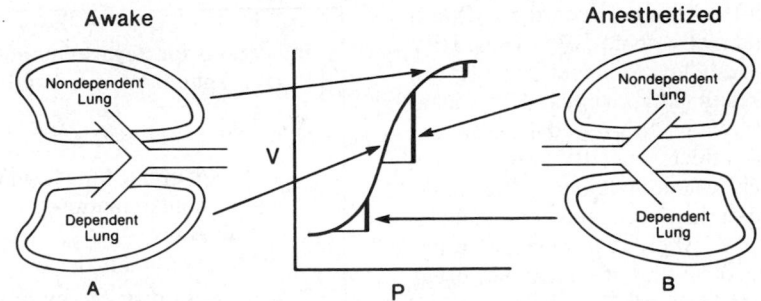

Figure 7-4. The distribution of ventilation in the patient in the lateral decubitus position when **(A)** awake, and **(B)** anesthetized. The induction of anesthesia has caused a loss of lung volume in both lungs, with the nondependent lung moving from a flat, noncompliant portion to a steep, compliant portion of the presusre-volume curve and the dependent lung moving from a steep, compliant part to a flat, noncompliant part of the pressure-volume curve. Thus, the anesthetized patient in a lateral decubitus position has more of the tidal ventilation in the nondependent lung (where there is the least perfusion) and less of the tidal ventilation in the dependent lung (where there is most perfusion). V, alveolar volume; P, transpulmonary pressure. (From Benumof JL: Anesthesia for Thoracic Surgery. WB Saunders, Philadelphia, 1987, with permission.)

$17.5 + 10 = 27.5$ percent of blood flow. With an FiO_2 of 1.0, this will result in a PaO_2 of approximately 150 mmHg. As 72.5 percent of the perfusion is directed to the dependent lung during one-lung ventilation, it is important to maximize gas exchange and match ventilation in the dependent lung. Because of reduced lung volume and reduced FRC, the dependent lung is no longer on the steep, compliant portion of the volume-pressure curve. Factors associated with the reduction of FRC include general anesthesia, paralysis, pressure of abdominal contents, compression by mediastinal structures, and poor positioning on the operating table. In addition, absorption actelectasis, accumulation of secretions, and the transudation of fluid into the dependent lung also impair the ability for gas exchange. All these factors create a low $\dot{V}/\dot{Q}$ ratio and a large alveolar to arterial oxygen gradient [$P(A - a)O_2$].

HYPOXIC PULMONARY VASOCONSTRICTION

HPV is a homeostatic mechanism whereby pulmonary blood flow is diverted away from hypoxic regions of the lung, and thus it optimizes the gas exchange function of the lung. First described by Von Euler and Liljestrand (1946) and characterized by others (Marshall, et al., 1981), HPV has been shown to cause a rise in perfusion (pulmonary arterial) pressure and flow diversion. The stimulus to HPV can be a function of both PaO_2 and mixed venous oxygen pressure ($P\bar{v}O_2$). When only small amounts of the lung are hypoxic, HPV has little effect on PaO_2, and similarly when most of the lung is hypoxic, there is no significant region of normoxic lung to which the hypoxic area can divert flow and thus HPV does not improve PaO_2. However during one-lung anesthesia when the amount of lung made hypoxic is between 30 and 70 per-

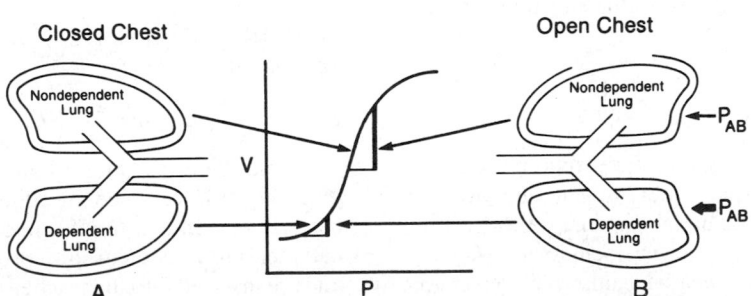

Figure 7-5. This schematic of a patient in the lateral decubitus position compares **(A)** the closed-chest anesthetized condition with **(B)** the open-chest anesthetized and paralyzed condition. Opening the chest increases nondependent lung compliance and reinforces or maintains the larger part of the tidal ventilation going to the nondependent lung. Paralysis also reinforces or maintains the larger part of tidal ventilation going to the nondependent lung because the pressure of the abdominal contents (P_{AB}) pressing against the upper diaphragm is minimal (*smaller arrow*), and it is therefore easier for positive pressure ventilation to displace this less resisting dome of the diaphragm. (V, alveolar volume; P, transpulmonary pressure. (From Eisenkraft JB, Neustein SM, Cohen E: Anesthesia for thoracic surgery. p. 905. In Barash PG, Cullen BF, Stoelting RK (eds): Clinical Anesthesia. 2nd Ed. JB Lippincott, Philadelphia, 1992, with permission.)

cent, there may be large differences between the PaO_2 expected with normal HPV and that with no HPV. Thus, HPV can raise PaO_2 from dangerously low to higher, safer levels, and inhibition of HPV may result in hypoxemia. All the inhalational and most of the intravenous drugs used in anesthesia have been studied for their effects on HPV. Most of the experiments have been performed in animals (Benumof, 1985). In animal experiments it has been shown that inhalational anesthetics inhibit HPV, whereas intravenous drugs do not; in humans the results of studies of inhalational drugs on HPV during one-lung anesthesia are not as clear-cut, although there are similarities to animal data. Other variables such as the effects of anesthetic agents on cardiac output may obscure the effects of inhalational anesthetics on HPV (Eisenkraft, 1990).

ONE-LUNG VENTILATION

It is currently unusual for thoracic procedures to be performed without one-lung ventilation being provided. However, there are several absolute and relative indications for separation of the lungs during thoracic procedures.

Absolute indications for one-lung ventilation include the need to prevent spillage of pus or blood from an infected or bleeding source to the opposite lung. Bilateral contamination can result in massive atelectasis, sepsis, or pneumonia, which can be life-threatening. Bronchopleural and bronchocutaneous fistulae represent low-resistance pathways for ventilation delivered by positive pressure and can prevent adequate alveolar ventilation. Giant cysts or unilateral bullae can rupture under positive-pressure ventilation. Finally, bronchopulmonary lavage requires effective separation of the lungs to avoid accidental spillage from the lavaged lung to the nondependent ventilated lung.

Although relative, the following indications for one-lung ventilation are most commonly used clinically for lung separation: lobectomies, especially upper lobectomy, pneumonectomy, and thorcic aortic aneurysm repair. Lower or middle lobectomy and esophageal resection are best performed with a quiescent lung field but are of lower priority. Thoracoscopy is greatly facilitated by collapse of the lung under examination.

Methods of Lung Separation

There are three techniques available for providing one-lung ventilation during anesthesia: double-lumen endotracheal tubes, bronchial blockers, and endobronchial tubes. Advantages of DLTs over bronchial blockers include (1) relatively ease of placement; (2) easy, repeated, and rapid conversion from two-lung ventilation to one-lung ventilation at any time during surgery; (3) suctioning of secretions, etc. from both lungs; and (4) provision of continuous positive airway pressure (CPAP) to the nonventilated lung. Bronchial blockers and endobronchial tubes do not allow ventilatory maneuvers to be used on the lung that is being operated on. Two relatively minor disadvantages of DLTs are (1) difficulty in passing suction catheters through the small lumen of the DLT, and (2) increased airway resistance of the narrower lumen

---

Indications for Separation of the Two Lungs (Double-Lumen Tube Intubation) and/or One-Lung Ventilation

Absolute

1. Isolation of one lung from the other to prevent spillage or contamination
   Infection
   Massive hemorrhage
2. Control of distribution of ventilation
   Bronchopleural fistula
   Bronchopleural cutaneous fistula
   Surgical opening of major conducting airway
   Giant unilateral lung cyst or bulla
   Tracheobronchial tree disruption
3. Unilateral bronchopulmonary lavage
   Pulmonary alveolar proteinosis

Relative

1. Surgical exposure: high priority
   Thoracic aortic aneurysm
   Pneumonectomy
   Upper lobectomy
2. Surgical exposure: low priority
   Middle and lower lobectomies and subsegmental resections
   Esophageal resection
   Thoracoscopy
   Procedures on the thoracic spine
3. Following removal of totally occluding chronic unilateral pulmonary emboli

---

(From Benumof JL, Alfery DD: Anesthesia for thoracic surgery. p. 1663. In Miller RD (ed): Anesthesia. 4th Ed. Churchill Livingstone, New York, 1994, with permission.)

---

of the DLT, which is easily overcome by positive-pressure ventilation.

Bronchial Blockers

Bronchial blockers with a lumen through them and a distal inflatable cuff have been used in the past but are not widely used at present. Arterial embolectomy catheters (Fogarty catheters) have been used to provide separation of the lungs and are inserted into the trachea before placement of a single-lumen endotracheal tube. A fiberoptic bronchoscope is then used to guide the catheter into either the right or left lung in position, so that when the balloon of the embolectomy catheter is inflated, the lung is obstructed (Ginsberg, 1981). The obstructed lung then collapses by absorption atelectasis.

A combination bronchial blocker/single-lumen endotracheal tube (the Univent tube) was introduced in 1982 by Fuji Systems Corp., Tokyo. This single-lumen endotracheal tube has a movable endobronchial blocker housed in a channel attached to the endotracheal tube wall. In a fashion similar to that used with the Fogarty catheter, the movable blocker is moved into the desired mainstem bronchus with the aid of a fiberoptic bronchoscope (Inoue, et al., 1982; Hultgren, et al., 1986).

Double-Lumen Endobronchial Tubes

These tubes are the most widely used means of achieving lung separation in one-lung ventilation at the present time. They consist of two catheters bonded together so that one lumen is long enough to reach a mainstem bronchus and the second lumen ends with an opening in the distal trachea. A proximal tracheal cuff and a distal endobronchial cuff located in the mainstem bronchus allow separation of the lungs when they are inflated. The endobronchial cuff of the right-sided tubes are slotted or designed to allow ventilation of the right upper lobe, as the right mainstem bronchus is too short to accommodate both the right-lumen tube and a right bronchial cuff.

Early designs of double-lumen endobronchial tubes included the Carlens tube, the White tube, and the Robertshaw tube (Wilson, 1992). Although still used today, most practitioners have discarded these red rubber tubes for modern designs. Modernday versions of the Robertshaw tube, made of clear polyvinyl disposable plastic are currently available from most manufacturers.

Double-lumen tubes have two curves (in planes approximately 90 degrees apart) that facilitate intubation and proper endobronchial placement. Disposable DLTs made of clear nontoxic tissue-implantable plastic are relatively easy to insert and have appropriate end-of-lumen and cuff arrangements that minimize lobar obstruction. The endobronchial cuff is colored blue, which is a very important recognition feature when using a fiberoptic bronchoscope. In addition, the ends of both lumina have black radiopaque lines that allow recognition when viewing a chest radiograph. The tubes have high-volume, low-pressure tracheal and endobronchial cuffs.

The slanted doughnut-shaped endobronchial cuff on the right-sided DLT allows the right upper lobe ventilation slot to ride off (away from) the right upper lobe orifice, which minimizes the chance of right upper lobe obstruction by the tube. The clear tubing allows continuous observation of the tidal movements of respiratory moisture as well as observation of secretions from each lung.

A left-sided double-lumen endotracheal tube is used for right thoracotomies requiring collapse of the right lung and ventilation of the left lung. A left- or right-sided tube may be used for left thoracotomies requiring collapse of the left lung and ventilation of the right lung (Fig. 7-6). There is considerable anatomic variation in the exact position of the right upper lobe orifice coming off the right main bronchus, and this makes it difficult to position the upper lobe ventilation slot of a right-sided DLT in exact opposition to the right upper lobe orifice. For this reason, the left-sided tube is preferable for most cases requiring one-lung ventilation. Removal of a left-sided DLT from the left mainstem bronchus and its use as a single-lumen tube allow clamping of the left mainstem bronchus if necessary during surgery.

Positioning of Double-Lumen Tubes

The DLT (after checking cuff inflation and lubricating) is passed with the distal curvature initially concave anteriorly (Fig. 7-7). After the tube tip passes the larynx, the stylet is removed and the tube is carefully rotated 90 degrees, so that the distal curve is now concave toward the appropriate side and the proximal curve is concave anteriorly to allow endobronchial intubation of the appropriate side (Fig. 7-7). The tube is then advanced until moderate resistance to further passage is encountered, indicating that the tube tip has been firmly seated in the mainstem bronchus, usually when 1 to 2 cm from the bifurcation of the two lumina is left outside

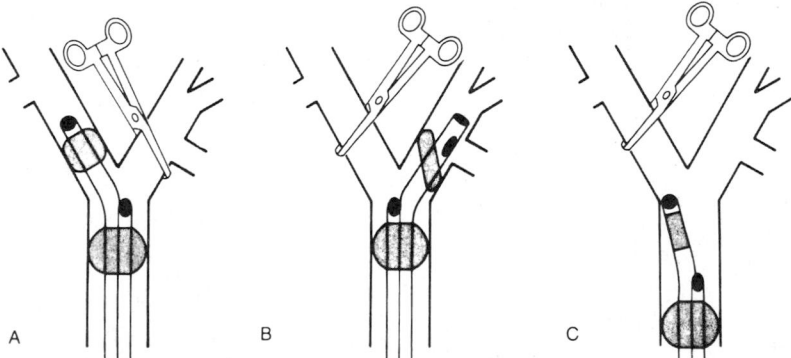

Figure 7-6. Use of the left-sided and right-sided double-lumen endotracheal tubes for left and right lung surgery (as indicated by the clamp). **(A)** When surgery is performed on the right lung, a left-sided double-lumen endotracheal tube should be used.**(B)** When surgery is performed on the left lung, a right-sided double-lumen endotracheal tube can be used. **(C)** However, because of uncertainty about the alignment of the right upper lobe ventilation slot to the right upper lobe orifice, a left-sided double-lumen endotracheal tube pulled back into the trachea should be used and the right lung ventilated through both lumina (use the double-lumen endotracheal tube as a single-lumen tube). (From Benumof JL: Anesthesia for Thoracic Surgery. WB Saunders, Philadelphia, 1987, with permission.)

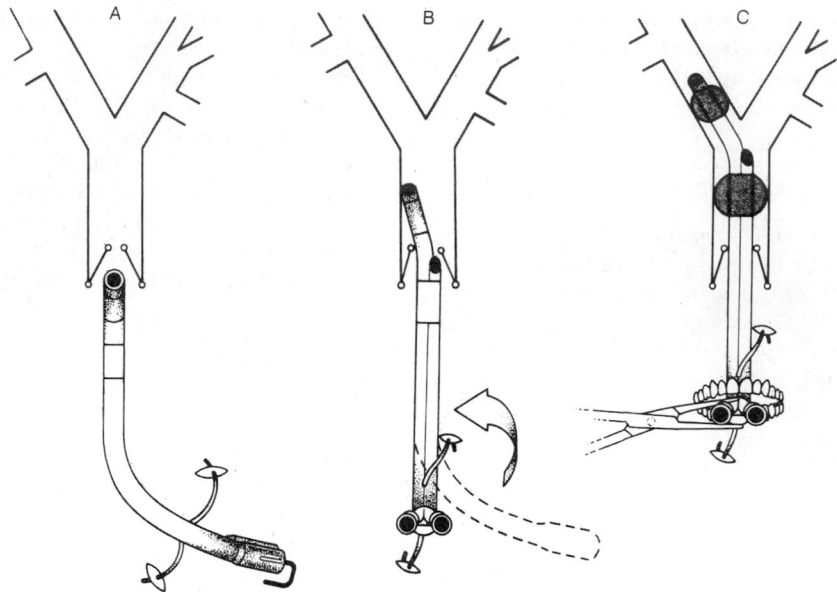

Figure 7-7. This schematic diagram depicts the passage of the left-sided double-lumen endotracheal tube in a supine patient. **(A)** The tube is held with the distal curvature concave anteriorly and the proximal curve concave to the right and in a plane parallel to the floor. The tube is then inserted through the vocal cords until the bronchial cuff passes the vocal cords. The stylet is then removed. **(B)** The tube is rotated 90 degrees counterclockwise so that the distal curvature is concave anteriorly and the proximal curvature is concave to the left and in a plane parallel to the floor. **(C)** The tube is inserted until either a mild resistance to further passage is encountered or the end of the common molding of the two lumina is at the teeth. Both cuffs are then inflated, and both lungs are ventilated. Finally, one side is clamped while the other side is ventilated and vice versa. (See text for further explanation.) (From Benumof JL: Anesthesia for Thoracic Surgery. WB Saunders, Philadelphia, 1987, with permission.)

the incisors. This depth of insertion for left DLTs has shown to be approximately 29 cm for patients of either sex, 170 cm tall. With each 10 cm increase in height there is an increase of 1 cm in the depth of insertion in the same direction (Brodsky, et al., 1991).

Once the DLT is judged to be in proper position, the cuffs are inflated, and proper endobronchial placement is then confirmed by a series of clamping, observation, and auscultation maneuvers. First, the tracheal cuff should be inflated and equal ventilation of both lungs established. If breath sounds are not equal, the tube is probably too far down and the tracheal lumen opening is in the mainstem bronchus or is lying at the carina. Withdrawal of the tube by 2 to 3 cm will restore equal breath sounds. The tracheal lumen is then clamped and the cap removed from the connector attached to the bronchial lumen. The bronchial cuff is then slowly inflated with 2 to 5 ml to prevent an air leak from the bronchial lumen around the bronchial cuff into the tracheal lumen. The clamp is then removed, and a check is made that both lungs are being ventilated with both cuffs inflated. This then shows that the bronchial cuff is not obstructing the contralateral hemithorax either totally or partially. The final step is to selectively clamp each side and watch for absence of movement and breath sounds on the contralateral side while the ventilated side should have clear breath sounds, chest movement that feels compliant, respiratory gas moisture with each tidal ventilation, and no air leak.

Sequence of Checks for Proper Placement of Double-Lumen Tubes

1. Insert tube to proper depth (moderate resistance)
   Bilateral chest elevation
   Inflate tracheal cuff
   Bilateral breath sounds
   Inflate bronchial cuff
2. Unilateral clamping
   Clamped side
      Loss of breath sounds
      No leak
      No respiratory moisture
   Unclamped side
      Normal breath sounds
      Normal feel to reservoir bag
      Exchange of respiratory moisture
      Elevation of ipsilateral chest wall with inspiration
3. Fiberoptic bronchoscopic examination

(From Hartman GS: Anesthesia for thoracic surgery. Anesth Analg, suppl. 74:93, 1992, with permission.)

Peak airway pressures during two-lung ventilation at 20 cmH$_2$O should not exceed 40 cmH$_2$O for the same tidal volume during one-lung ventilation. In situations in which absolute lung separation is needed, the use of an underwater seal can determine when bronchial and tracheal cuffs are correctly inflated. If the tracheal lumen is connected to an underwater seal system, gas will be seen to bubble up through the water when the bronchial cuff is not inflated and positive pressure is applied to the bronchial lumen of the DLT.

The most useful advance in checking the proper positioning of the DLT is the introduction of the pediatric fiberoptic bronchoscope to assess endoscopically where the tube is positioned. A guide to the size of pediatric bronchoscope required for different sizes of DLTs is given in Table 7-4. In one study 48 percent of tubes that were thought to be in the correct position by auscultation and physical examination were subsequently shown to be in an incorrect position when examined with fiberoptic bronchoscopy (Smith, et al., 1987).

Visualization through the DLT is usually first made through the tracheal lumen. The carina is visualized, and no bronchial cuff herniation should be seen. The upper surface of the blue endobronchial cuff should be just below the tracheal carina. The bronchoscope is then passed to the bronchial lumen, and the left upper lobe orifice should be identified. When a right-sided DLT is used, the carina should be visualized through the tracheal lumen, but more importantly, the orifice of the right upper lobe bronchus should be identified, which in some cases may be fairly difficult. The small size of the pediatric bronchoscope with its small suction channel is a disadvantage when copious secretions are present.

Problems Caused by Malpositioning of the Double-Lumen Tube

The principal problems occurring with the use of DLTs are associated with malposition of the tube. As the tube is inserted blindly, there are several possibilities for tube malposition.

First, the DLT may be accidently directed down the side opposite to the desired mainstem bronchus. This will result in collapse of the lung that is opposite to the side of the connector being clamped. In addition, inadequate separation, increased airway pressure, and instability of the DLT will occur. Several combinations of malpositions can occur, as illustrated in Figure 7-8.

1. If a left-sided DLT is inserted into the right mainstem bronchus, it will obstruct the ventilation of the right upper lobe.

2. The DLT may be passed too far down into either the right or left main bronchus. In this case breath sounds would be very diminished and not audible at all over the contralateral side. Withdrawing the DLT until the opening of the tracheal lumen is above the carina corrects the situation.

3. If the DLT is not inserted far enough so that the bronchial lumen opens above the carina, good breath sounds will be heard bilaterally when ventilating through the bronchial lumen but no breath sounds will be heard when the tracheal lumen is ventilated, as the inflated bronchial cuff obstructs gas flow through the tracheal lumen.

4. A right-sided DLT may occlude the right upper lobe orifice. The mean distance from the carina to the right upper lobe is approximately 2 to 2.3 cm for both men and women. Thus, there is little margin of error to allow positioning of the ventilatory slot in the side of the bronchial catheter when using right-sided DLTs over the opening of the right upper lobe.

5. The left upper lobe orifice may be obstructed by a left-sided DLT that is inserted too far down the left main bronchus. The mean distance between the left upper lobe orifice and the carina is between 5 and 5.5 cm for men and women (Benumof, et al., 1987b). The average distance between right and left lumen openings in a left-sided disposable DLT is approximately 7 cm, and therefore the left upper lobe can be obstructed while the tracheal lumen is still above the carina.

6. Finally, bronchial cuff herniation can occur and obstruct the bronchial lumen if excessive volume is used to inflate the cuff. The bronchial cuff has also been known to herniate over the tracheal carina if not inserted far enough down into the left main bronchus or if inserted too high up in the right main bronchus. Inflation and deflation of the bronchial cuffs should be observed directly using the fiberoptic bronchoscope at all times if possible.

Contraindications to Use of Double-Lumen Tubes

The use of a DLT to achieve lung separation is relatively contraindicated where there is a lesion in the airway itself or a difficult upper airway that results in poor laryngeal visual-

Table 7-4. Relationship of Fiberoptic Bronchoscope Size to Double-Lumen Endotracheal Tube Size

Fiberoptic Bronchoscope Size, Outside Diameter (mm)	Double-Lumen Tube Size (Fr)	Fit of Fiberoptic Bronchoscope Inside Double-Lumen Tube[a]
5.6	All sizes	Does not fit
4.9	41	Easy passage
	39	Moderately easy passage
	37	Tight fit, need lubricant, hard push
3.6–4.2	All sizes	Easy passage

[a] Lubricant recommended is a silicone-based fluid similar to that made by the American Cystoscope Co.

(From Benumof JL, Alfery DD: Anesthesia for thoracic surgery. p. 1663. In Miller RD (ed): Anesthesia. 4th Ed. Churchill Livingstone, New York, 1994, with permission.)

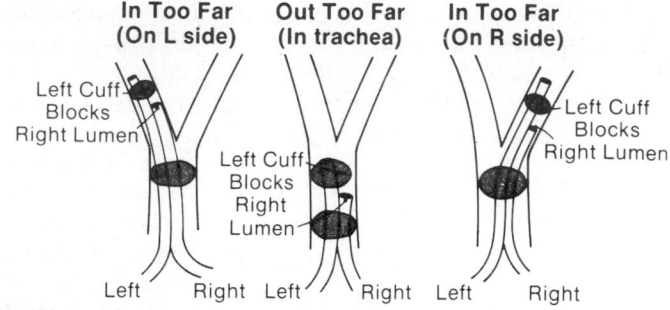

Procedure	Breath Sounds Heard		
Clamp Right Lumen Both Cuffs Inflated	Left	Left and Right	Right
Clamp Left Lumen Both Cuffs Inflated	None or Very ↓↓	None or Very ↓↓	None or Very ↓↓
Clamp Left Lumen Deflate Left Cuff	Left	Left and Right	Right

Figure 7-8. There are three major (involving a whole lung) malpositions of a left-sided double-lumen endotracheal tube. The tube can be in too far on the left (both lumina are in the left mainstem bronchus), out too far (both lumina are in the trachea), or down the right mainstem bronchus (at least the left lumen is in the right mainstem bronchus). In each of these three malpositions the left cuff, when fully inflated, can completely block the right lumen. Inflation and deflation of the left cuff while the left lumen is clamped create a breath sound differential diagnosis of tube malpositions. (See text for full explanation.) L, left; R, right: ↓, decreased. (From Benumof JL: Anesthesia for Thoracic Surgery. WB Saunders, Philadelphia, 1987, with permission.)

ization. Patients requiring rapid-sequence intubation do not constitute a contraindication to the use of DLTs as DLTs can usually be inserted as rapidly as single-lumen tubes.

Lung Separation with the Use of Bronchial Blockers and Single-Lumen Endotracheal Tubes

Lung separation can be effectively achieved with the use of a single lumen endotracheal tube and a fiberoptically placed bronchial blocker (Fig. 7-9). This is particularly useful in children, in whom DLTs may be too large to be used. The smallest DLT available is a left-sided 28 Fr tube, which can be used in patients from 10 to 14 years old and 30 to 45 kg. The bronchial blocker most often used for adults is a Fogarty occlusion (embolectomy) catheter with a 3-ml balloon (Ginsberg, 1981). The Fogarty catheter has a wire stylet so that it is possible to place a curvature at the distal tip. The Fogarty catheter is placed before intubating the larynx with an endotracheal tube and is passed down the trachea until some resistance is met with the curvature facing in the direction of the bronchus to be intubated. The trachea is then intubated with a single-lumen endotracheal tube, and a fiberoptic bronchoscope is passed down the single-lumen tube through a self-sealing diaphragm in the elbow connector, which allows continued positive-pressure ventilation around the fiberoptic bronchoscope. The end of the catheter is visualized below the tip of the single-lumen tube and directed into the desired mainstem bronchus. The wire stylet is then withdrawn and the balloon inflated until the bronchus is sealed. Lung collapse occurs via absorption atelectasis. Inflation and deflation of the lumen should always be conducted under direct visualization using the fiberoptic bronchoscope.

The Univent Tube (Fuji Systems Corp., Tokyo) is con-structed so that the bronchial blocker is housed in a small channel attached to the anterior wall of the endotracheal tube, which allows the blocker to be transmitted to the distal trachea by the endotracheal tube. Thus, the end of the blocker can be seen through a bronchoscope and manipulated into the desired mainstem bronchus in much the same way as the Fogarty catheter. The blocker attachment with an inflatable balloon at the end is different from the Fogarty catheter in that there is a small lumen through the blocker through which suction can be performed, although fairly minimally, and through which oxygen can be piped and CPAP can be provided as well (Inoue, et al., 1982; Kamaya and Krishna, 1985). In very small children (10 kg or less), bronchial blockage can also be performed by using a Fogarty embolectomy catheter with balloon capacity of 0.5 ml (Veil, 1969).

Although the technique of bronchial blockage can be learned relatively easily, it may occasionally take more time to perform than insertion of a DLT. In addition, the limited inability to suction and/or ventilate the lung distal to the blocker and the definite need for a fiberoptic bronchoscope are some of the disadvantages of bronchial blocker use as compared with DLTs. If absolute separation of the lungs is essential, as in severe infective or hemorrhagic situations, a bronchial blocker should not be used, as it is a relatively unstable system and may not guarantee absolute separation at all times.

Management of One-Lung Ventilation

The management of one-lung ventilation in a paralyzed patient in the LDP with an open chest involves manipulation of the inspired oxygen fraction (FiO_2), V_T, ventilatory rate, dependent-lung PEEP, and nondependent lung CPAP.

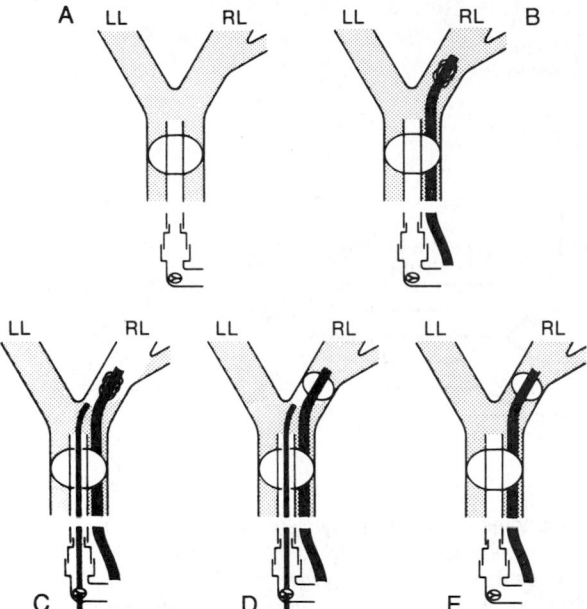

Figure 7-9. This figure shows how to separate the lungs with a single-lumen tube, fiberoptic bronchoscope, and right lung bronchial blocker. The sequence of events is as follows: **(A)** A single-lumen tube is inserted and the patient is ventilated. **(B)** A bronchial blocker is passed alongside the indwelling endotracheal tube. **(C)** A fiberoptic bronchoscope is passed through a self-sealing diaphragm in the elbow connector to the endotracheal tube and is used to place the bronchial blocker into the right main stem bronchus under direct vision. **(D)** The balloon on the bronchial blocker is also inflated under direct vision and is positioned just below the tracheal carina. **(E)** The fiberoptic bronchoscope is then removed (right lower diagram). During the insertion and use of the fiberoptic bronchoscope (Figs. C–E), the self-sealing diaphragm allows the patient to continue to be ventilated with positive-pressure ventilation (around the fiberoptic bronchoscope but within the lumina of the endotracheal tube). LL, left lung; RL, right lung. (From Benumof JL: Anesthesia for Thoracic Surgery. WB Saunders, Philadelphia, 1987, with permission.)

Inspired Oxygen Fraction

An FIO_2 of 1.0 is routinely used during one-lung ventilation and serves to protect against hypoxemia during the procedure. An FIO_2 of 1.0 has resulted in mean PaO_2 values between 150 and 210 mmHg during one-lung ventilation studies (Tarhan and Lundberg, 1971; Kerr, et al., 1974; Flacke, et al.,1976; Capan, et al., 1980). In addition, a high FIO_2 causes vasodilatation of the pulmonary vasculature in the dependent lung, which increases the capacity of this lung to accept blood flow redistribution due to nondependent lung HPV. Absorption atelectasis in the dependent lung (Dantzker, et al., 1975) can be minimized by the use of a high VT and PEEP.

Tidal Volume and Respiratory Rate

During one-lung ventilation, the dependent lung should be ventilated with a VT between 10 and 12 ml/kg. VTs between 8 and 15 ml/kg produce no significant effect on transpulmonary shunt or PaO_2 (Katz, et al., 1982). However, a VT less than 8 ml/kg can result in a decrease in FRC and increased atelec-

tasis in the dependent lung. A VT greater than 15 ml/kg may increase the pulmonary vascular resistance (PVR) of the dependent lung and divert blood flow into the nondependent lung. The respiratory rate should be adjusted to maintain a $PaCO_2$ of 35 to 40 mmHg. Elimination of carbon dioxide during one-lung ventilation is usually not a problem. Shunt during one-lung ventilation has little influence on $PaCO_2$ values as $P(A - a)CO_2$ is normally only 6 mmHg. In addition, carbon dioxide is 20 times as diffusible as oxygen. However, hyperventilation resulting in hypocapnia will increase the PVR of the dependent lung, inhibit nondependent lung HPV, increase shunt, and decrease PaO_2. One-lung ventilation also decreases the ratio of dead space (VD) to VT and enhances carbon dioxide elimination. Thus, at the commencement of one-lung ventilation, an FIO_2 of 1.0, a VT of 10 ml/kg, and a 10 to 20 percent increase in respiratory rate are used as the ventilation settings. If a problem with either ventilation or arterial oxygenation occurs, several maneuvers are available to improve the adverse effects.

Differential Management of One-Lung Ventilation

PEEP to the Dependent Lung. The beneficial effect of selective PEEP up to 10 cmH_2O to the dependent lung is due to an increased lung volume at end-expiration (FRC), which improves the $\dot{V}/\dot{Q}$ relationship in the dependent lung. The increase in FRC prevents airway and alveolar closure at end-expiration. However, results from several studies in which PEEP has been applied to the dependent lung with an FIO_2 of 1.0 have proved disappointing in that either a decrease or a slight increase in PaO_2 occurred (Capan, et al., 1980; Cohen, et al., 1988; Katz, et al., 1982; Tarhan and Lundberg, 1970). Thus, it is possible that when PEEP is applied to the dependent lung, the PaO_2 may increase, decrease, or not change at all. It is thought that PEEP induces an increase in lung volume that causes compression of the small interalveolar vessels and an increase in PVR. If this increase in resistance is limited to the dependent lung, blood flow is then diverted to the nondependent lung, increasing shunt and decreasing PaO_2.

CPAP to the Nondependent Lung. The most effective maneuver to increase PaO_2 during one-lung ventilation is application of CPAP to the nondependent lung (Capan, et al., 1980; Cohen, et al., 1988; Eisenkraft, et al., 1984; Merridew and Jones, 1985; Thiagarajah, et al., 1984; Hannenberg, et al., 1984; Brown and Davis, 1984). A CPAP level of 5 to 10 cmH_2O maintains patency of the nondependent alveoli and allows oxygen uptake to occur in the distended alveoli. The nondependent lung should be expanded slightly before CPAP is applied. The lower CPAP level of 5 to 10 cmH_2O does not inflate the lung and thus does not present a distended organ for surgery. However, application of higher levels of CPAP (15 cmH_2O) causes the lung to be overdistended and interferes with surgical exposure. CPAP can be applied to the nondependent lung by using several systems (Hannenberg, et al., 1984; Thiagarajah, et al., 1984; Lyons, 1984; Aalto-Setala, 1975; Brown and Davis, 1984). These systems feature an oxygen source, tubing to connect the oxygen source to the nonventilated lung, a pressure relief valve, and a pressure

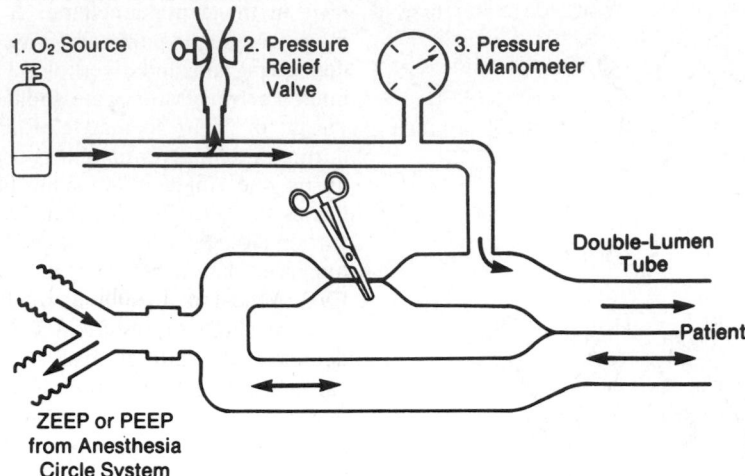

Figure 7-10. The three essential components of a nondependent lung continuous positive airway pressure (CPAP) system consist of (1) an oxygen source, (2) a pressure relief valve, and (3) a pressure manometer to measure the CPAP. The CPAP is created by the free flow of oxygen into the lung versus the restricted outflow of oxygen from the lung by the pressure relief valve. ZEEP, zero end-expiratory pressure. (From Benumof JL: Anesthesia for Thoracic Surgery. WB Saunders, Philadelphia, 1987, with permission.)

gauge. In addition, commercially prepared CPAP systems incorporating all these features are also available (Fig. 7-10).

Management of the Patient Receiving One-Lung Ventilation

The following outline is recommended for management of the patient receiving one-lung ventilation. With the patient in the lateral position, the position of the DLT should be rechecked. Two-lung ventilation should be maintained for as long as possible, and with institution of one-lung ventilation, an FiO_2 of 1.0 should be used. A V_T of 10 to 12 ml/kg at a rate adjusted to maintain $PaCO_2$ at 40 mmHg is recommended. Following initiation of one-lung ventilation, PaO_2 should be checked by measuring ABGs, as PaO_2 can continue to decrease for up to 45 minutes (Katz, et al., 1982). If hypoxemia occurs during one-lung ventilation, the position of the DLT should be rechecked with a fiberoptic bronchoscope. If a right-sided DLT is being used, the ventilation of the right upper lobe should be assessed and checked. With confirmation of correct tube position and continued hypoxemia, CPAP to the nondependent lung of 5 to 10 cm following a V_T that expands the lung should be instituted. If hypoxemia is not corrected with CPAP, PEEP can be applied to the dependent lung. The combination of CPAP with PEEP between 5 and 10 cmH$_2$O, respectively, can be applied in different combinations in search of optimal oxygenation. If PaO_2 remains low despite these maneuvers, intermittent two-lung ventilation should be reinstituted with the surgeon's cooperation so that surgery can be continued. In addition, if a pneumonectomy has been performed, ligation of the pulmonary artery through the surgical area will eliminate the shunt. The appearance of acute hypotension, cyanosis, or tachycardia should precipitate resumption of two-lung ventilation until the problems underlying these symptoms and signs have been resolved.

Overall One-Lung Ventilation Plan

1. Maintain two-lung ventilation until pleura is opened
2. Dependent lung
   $FiO^2 = 1.0$
   $TV = 10$ ml/kg
   $RR =$ so that $PaCO_2 = 40$ mmHg
   PEEP = 0–5 mmHg
3. If severe hypoxemia occurs
   a. Check position of double-lumen tube with fiberoptic bronchoscopy
   b. Check hemodynamic status
   c. Nondependent lung CPAP
   d. Dependent lung PEEP
   e. Intermittent two-lung ventilation
   f. Clamp pulmonary artery as soon as possible (for pneumonectomy)

Abbreviations: FiO_2, inspired oxygen fraction; TV, tidal volume; RR, respiratory rate; PEEP, positive end-expiratory pressure; CPAP, continuous positive airway pressure.

(From Benumof JL, Alfery DD: Anesthesia for thoracic surgery. p. 1663. In Miller RD (ed): Anesthesia. 4th Ed. Churchill Livingstone, New York, 1994, with permission.)

ANESTHESIA FOR THORACIC SURGERY

General Features

Thoracic surgical patients are more likely to have increased airway reactivity and bronchospasm owing to their high incidence of cigarette smoking and chronic bronchitis and/or

COPD. In addition, direct surgical manipulation of the airways and bronchial tree make bronchoconstriction more likely to occur. The potent inhalation anesthetics halothane, enflurane, and isoflurane all decrease the airways reactivity and bronchoconstriction, probably by a direct action on the airway musculature, and these agents are therefore the drugs of choice in patients with reactive airways. Synthetic opioids such as fentanyl, which do not affect bronchomotor tone, are preferable to other drugs such as morphine, which may increase bronchomotor tone by a central vagotonic effect and by releasing histamine.

For most patients, anesthesia is safely induced with a barbiturate, thiopental, thiamylal, or an alternative induction agent such as propofol. However, in patients with severe reactive airways, ketamine may be the drug of choice as it has a bronchodilator effect and has been successfully used in the treatment of asthma. Similarly, muscle relaxants of choice are those that do not release histamine or have vagotonic effects and/or have some sympathomimetic effect. Pancuronium and vecuronium probably represent the drugs of choice, whereas succinylcholine is useful to provide conditions for rapid intubation of the trachea and is not associated with an increase in airways reactivity. Intravenous lidocaine or

---

Instruments of Choice for Bronchoscopy

Rigid
  Foreign bodies
  Massive hemoptysis
  Vascular tumors
  Small children
  Endobronchial resections
Fiberoptic/Flexible
  Mechanical problems of neck
  Upper lobe and peripheral lesions
  Limited hemoptysis
  During mechanical ventilation
  Pneumonia, for selective cultures
  Positoning of double-lumen tubes
  Difficult intubation
  Checking position of endotracheal tube
  Bronchial blockade
Combination
  Positive cytology with negative chest x-ray

(Adapted from Landa JF: Indications for bronchoscopy. Chest 73(suppl):686, 1978, with permission.)

Indications for Bronchoscopy

Diagnostic
  Cough
  Hemoptysis
  Wheeze
  Atelectasis
  Unresolved pneumonia
  Diffuse lung disease
  Preoperative evaluation
  Rule out metastases
  Abnormal chest x-ray
  Assess local disease recurrence
  Recurrent laryngeal nerve palsy
  Diaphragm paralysis
  Acute inhalation injury
  Exclude tracheoesophageal fistula
  During mechanical ventilation
  Selective bronchoscopy
Therapeutic
  Foreign bodies
  Accumulated secretions
  Atelectasis
  Aspiration
  Lung abscess
  Repositioning of endotracheal tubes
  Placement of endobronchial tubes
  Laser surgery

(Adapted from Landa JF: Indications for bronchoscopy. Chest 73(suppl):686, 1978, with permission.)

---

nebulized lidocaine administered by the airways is also very useful to prevent reflex bronchospasm.

Finally, the rapidly metabolized agents such as propofol and alfentanil may be very useful for anesthesia involving short bronchoscopies where the patient needs to be awake soon after the procedure or for tracheal resections that may be much longer in duration, but again, in which the patient is required to be alert at the end of the procedure.

Anesthesia for Diagnostic Procedures

Bronchoscopy

Rigid translaryngeal bronchoscopy was first described around 1900 for removal of a foreign body from the right main bronchus under topical anesthesia. Indications for bronchoscopy and the instruments of choice for bronchoscopy are shown below.

The possibility of a more major procedure should always be anticipated, and thus bronchoscopy may lead to thoracotomy or sternotomy. Discussion and planning of the procedure with the surgeon is all-important. Monitoring equipment should include that described previously, depending upon the severity of the patient's condition and whether a thoracotomy may follow the bronchoscopy. Routine bronchoscopy often includes a rigid bronchoscopic examination of the tracheobronchial tree followed by intubation of the trachea with a single-lumen endotracheal tube, which will allow the use of a flexible fiberoptic bronchoscope to further examine the tracheobronchial tree. Bronchoscopic techniques can be carried out under local anesthesia with or without intubation of the trachea with a single-lumen endotracheal tube or under general anesthesia.

Local Anesthesia. Patients should first be pretreated with drying agents such as atropine or glycopyrrolate. The local anesthetics used most commonly are lidocaine and cocaine. The total dose of anesthetic used must always be held within the toxic total dose range. The oropharynx can be sprayed with the nebulizer, or the patient may gargle with viscous lidocaine. The superior laryngeal nerve can either be blocked with pledgets soaked in local anesthetic and held in the pyriform fossa or by an external approach. Tracheal anesthesia then can be achieved either by transtracheal injection of local anesthetic or by spraying the cords and trachea under direct vision with use of a laryngoscope or via the suction channel of the fiberoptic bronchoscope. If fiberoptic bronchoscopy is to be performed transnasally, the nasal mucosa is anesthetized with 4 percent cocaine and/or viscous lidocaine administered throughout the nares. Local anesthesia for bronchoscopy has the advantage that the patient is awake, cooperative, and breathing spontaneously.

General Anesthesia. General anesthesia is often combined with local anesthesia so that a decreased amount of general anesthetic is needed. A balanced technique using nitrous oxide–oxygen and incremental doses of intravenous drugs such as thiopental or propofol, plus the short-acting opioids such as alfentanil or fentanyl and a muscle relaxant such as succinylcholine, atracurium, or vecuronium, provides a satisfactory anesthetic mixture. Ventilation of the lungs is generally controlled.

Rigid Bronchoscopy. Modern rigid ventilating bronchoscopes are essentially hollow tubes with blunted beveled tips, which are available in various sizes and designs. In all of these a side arm is provided for connection to a ventilation source. Several techniques can be used to maintain ventilation and oxygenation during rigid bronchoscopy.

Apneic Oxygenation. Following preoxygenation and induction of general anesthesia and muscle paralysis, oxygen is insufflated at about 10 to 15 L/min via a small catheter placed above the carina. With adequate denitrogenation, this technique can provide adequate oxygenation for more than 30 minutes (Frumin, et al., 1959). However, the apneic period should not be allowed to extend beyond 5 minutes at a time, as the technique is limited by the buildup of carbon dioxide at the rate of 3 mmHg/min. Prolonged buildup of carbon dioxide will produce respiratory acidosis and cardiac dysrhythmias.

Apnea and Intermittent Ventilation. Oxygen and anesthesia gases are delivered to a closed-end bronchoscope fitted with an eyepiece via the anesthesia circuit. Ventilation is only possible when the eyepiece is in place, and this limits instrumentation by the surgeon. Intermittent ventilation of the lungs is achieved by using the reservoir bag. With a good bronchoscope fit, compliance is constantly monitored and V_T may be estimated. However, with prolonged bronchoscopies using this technique, hypoxemia and more particularly hypercarbia may result, leading to cardiac dysrhythmias.

Sanders Injection System. The Sanders injection system applies the venturi principle to provide ventilation of the lungs by attaching a jet ventilator to the bronchoscope. Oxygen from a high-pressure source (50 psi) is delivered by a pressure-reducing valve and toggle switch to an 18- or 16-gauge needle inside and parallel to the long axis of the bronchoscope. With a jet of oxygen entering the bronchoscope, air entrainment occurs, and the air-oxygen mixture resulting at the distal tip of the bronchoscope emerges at an adequate pressure to provide ventilation and oxygenation. As long as the proximal end of the bronchoscope is open, the system is strictly pressure-limited and the pressure will not rise because of obstruction at the distal end. The advantage of the Sanders system is that because continuous ventilation is possible, the duration of the bronchoscopy procedure is minimized although extended bronchoscopies are possible. The entrainment of air via the oxygen jet results in a variable FIO_2 at the distal end of the bronchoscope, and ventilation of the lungs may be inadequate if compliance is poor. $PaCO_2$ was lower and arterial pH higher with the Sanders injection technique than with intermittent ventilation, particularly after long procedures (Giesecke, et al., 1973).

High-Frequency Positive-Pressure Ventilation. High-frequency positive pressure ventilation (HFPPV) has been used with rigid bronchoscopy and compared with the Sanders injection technique. At HFPPV of up to 150 breaths/min, blood gases were identical with both techniques, but at frequencies of 500 breaths/min oxygenation deteriorated and carbon dioxide was not removed effectively. However, HFPPV has the advantage that the tracheobronchial wall remains immobile during ventilation (Vour'h, et al., 1983).

Fiberoptic Bronchoscopy. Modern fiberoptic bronchoscopes are invaluable instruments for airway management. Examination of the fifth order of bronchial branching is now possible, and the flexibility of the instrument has been applied in preoperative assessment of the airway, management of difficult tracheal intubations, endotracheal tube positioning and change, bronchial toilet, correct positioning of DLTs, bronchial blockade, and evaluation of the larynx and trachea (Sackner, 1975).

In all patients, insertion of the fiberoptic bronchoscope is associated with hypoxemia. The average decline in PaO_2 is 20 mmHg and lasts from 1 to 4 hours after the procedure. Thus, particularly if the PaO_2 is less than 70 mmHg on room air, bronchoscopy should be performed with administration of supplemental oxygen. In addition, during and after fiberoptic bronchoscopy, patients have developed increased airway obstruction. This included an increase in FRC and decreases in PaO_2, VC, FEV_1, and forced inspiratory flow (Matsushima, et al., 1984). These changes are thought to be secondary to mechanical activation of irritative reflexes in the airway and possibly also mucosal edema. Much of these changes may be avoided if atropine is administered either systemically or topically preoperatively.

Suctioning applied to the suction channel of the fiberoptic bronchoscope has the effect of causing decreases in FIO_2,

PaO_2, and FRC, leading to decreased PaO_2. The adult fiberoptic bronchoscope will pass through endotracheal tubes of 7.0 mm or greater internal diameter, and thus an endotracheal tube of the largest possible diameter should be used so that decreases in cross-sectional area available for ventilating the patient are kept to a minimum. Insertion of the bronchoscope also causes a significant PEEP effect, which occasionally may result in barotrauma in ventilated patients.

Neodymium-yttrium-aluminum-garnet (Nd-YAG) lasers have recently been used for the resection of obstructing tracheal and endobronchial lesions. The procedure is usually conducted under general anesthesia. The laser beam may be introduced into the bronchial tree through a fiberoptic bundle passed via the suction port of the fiberoptic bronchoscope or may be introduced via a rigid bronchoscope. During laser resection, FiO_2 should be kept to a minimum and titrated against oxygen saturation in order to make endotracheal fires less likely (Warner, et al., 1984). In addition, specially designed endotracheal tubes that are nonflammable have also been recommended for use (Eisenkraft and Neustein, 1992).

Complications of Bronchoscopy. Complications of rigid bronchoscopy include mechanical trauma to the teeth, hemorrhage, bronchospasm, loss of sponges, bronchial or tracheal perforation, subglottic edema, and barotrauma. In general, it is best to intubate the trachea with an endotracheal tube following rigid bronchoscopy under general anesthesia. This avoids increased airway irritability following rigid bronchoscopy, allows effective suctioning of the trachea and bronchi, and gives time for the patient to recover more gradually from a general anesthetic.

Mediastinoscopy

Mediastinoscopy was introduced as a means of assessing the spread of carcinoma of the bronchus. Mediastinoscopy allows examination of the lymphatic drainage of the bronchial tree, which drains first to the subcarinal and paratracheal areas and then to the sides of the trachea, the supraclavicular areas, and finally the thoracic duct. Mediastinoscopy provides tissue diagnosis and greater selectivity of patients for thoractomy. It has also been used to place electrodes for atrial-triggered pacing, and an adaptation of the technique allows removal of the thymus gland by the transcervical approach in patients with myasthenia gravis.

The mediastinoscope is passed via a transverse incision just above the suprasternal notch behind the innominate vessels and the aortic arch. In general, mediastinoscopy is performed under general anesthesia with use of an endotracheal tube and continuous ventilation. Muscle relaxation is important to prevent the patient from coughing, as this may produce venous engorgement in the chest or trauma by the mediastinoscope to surrounding structures.

Complications with mediastinoscopy include hemorrhage because of the proximity of major vessels and the vascularity of certain tumors. This may require treatment with tamponade or thoracotomy if hemostasis cannot be achieved. Other complications include pneumothorax, recurrent laryngeal nerve injury, and obstruction of the right radial pulse (Lee and Salvatore, 1976). The right radial pulse is obstructed by pressure on the innominate artery by the instrument. This may be of significance if there is a history of impaired cerebral circulation, particularly in the right carotid arterial system. Therefore, blood pressure should be monitored in the left arm, and the right radial pulse should be monitored continuously by pulse oximetry during mediastinoscopy.

Anesthesia for Mediastinal Masses

Patients with an anterior mediastinal mass present a special problem to the anesthetist. Such masses may cause superior vena cava (SVC) obstruction, which may or may not be obvious, and also may cause obstruction of major airways and cardiac compression, which may become apparent only upon induction of anesthesia (Neuman, et al., 1984).

A history of dyspnea in the supine position and examination of the CT/magnetic resonance imaging (MRI) scan to determine the extent of the tumor and its effect on surrounding structures are important preoperatively. If such obstruction occurs on induction of anesthesia, it may be relieved by the passage of a rigid bronchoscope or by changing the position of the patient. When a biopsy of the mass is required for diagnosis and the procedure cannot be performed under local anesthesia, an awake fiberoptic intubation, followed by general anesthesia with spontaneous ventilation, has been described for thoracotomy (Sibert, et al., 1987).

A flow chart has been described by Neuman et al. (1984) that is useful in the management of patients with anterior mediastinal masses (Fig. 7-11).

Thoracoscopy

Thoracoscopy allos direct visualization of the thoracic cavity and pleural space with an endoscope. It is useful for diagnostic and staging procedures as well as for some therapeutic maneuvers (laser treatment of spontaneous pneumothorax or malignant pleural tumors), chemical pleurodesis, and lung biopsy. The procedure can be performed under local, regional, or general anesthesia. Local anesthetic infiltration plus intercostal nerve blocks provide local and regional anesthesia and anesthetize the parietal pleura while the addition of an ipsilateral stellate ganglion block will supress the cough reflex. Introduction of the endoscope will produce a partial pneumothorax, which allows visualization of the pleural space. If the procedure is poorly tolerated, general anesthesia may be induced and the patient should be placed in the supine position and if possible intubated with a DLT. This will provide a quiescent lung field for proper examination of the pleural space and administration of any therapeutic procedures.

High-Frequency Ventilation

High-frequency ventilation (HFV) techniques have been used in certain circumstances for thoracic surgery (bronchopleural fistulae, empyema, giant cysts, and tracheal resection); a brief description is provided here. In contrast to conventional intermittent positive pressure ventilation (IPPV), HFV employs a smaller V_T and more rapid respiratory rates. Gas transport depends more on molecular diffusion, high-velocity flow, and coaxial gas flow than on convection and molecular diffusion as in IPPV. Two types of HFV have been used for thoracic surgery; HFPPV and high-frequency jet ventilation

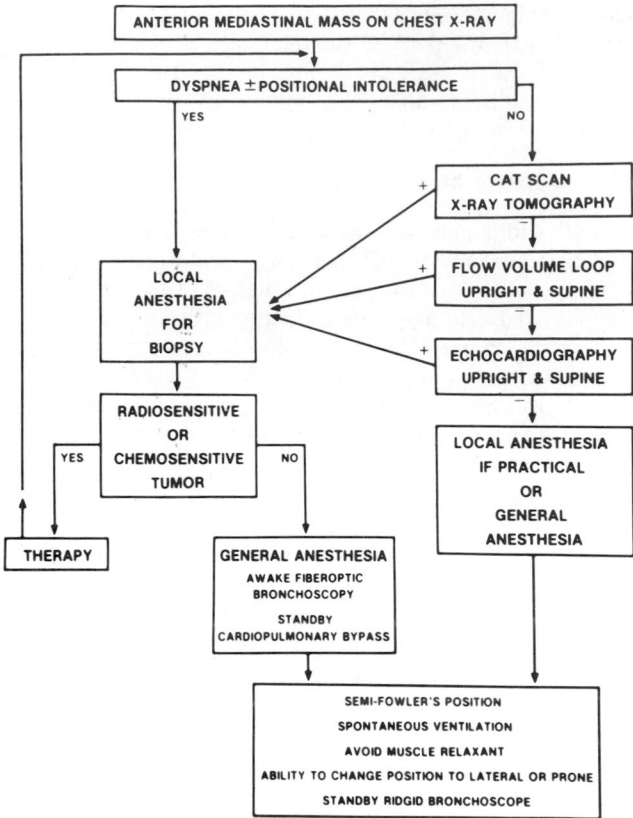

Figure 7-11. Flow chart describing the preoperative evaluation of the patient with an anterior mediastinal mass. +, positive finding; −, negative workup. (From Neuman G, Weingarten AE, Abramowitz RM et al.: The anesthetic management of the patient with an anterior mediastinal mass. Anesthesiology 60:144, 1984, with permission.)

(HFJV). HFPPV use small VT at rates of 60 to 120 breaths/min and the VT generated, which usually is similar to the dead space volume, represents all fresh gas flow. HFPPV may be delivered via an open or a closed system. An open system has the disadvantages of not using an endotracheal tube, so that the airway is subject to compromise and the gas outflow pathway is not mechanically established. Pulmonary aspiration is also possible. A closed system using an endotracheal tube provides better performance and is safer in that mechanical patency of the airway is provided and aspiration is prevented. In addition, PEEP can be provided with a closed system. HFJV use a pulse of fresh gas from a high-pressure (50 psi) source introduced into the endotracheal tube via a small catheter. Rates of 100 to 400 breaths/min are used. The fresh gas entrains gas in a fashion similar to that with the Sanders injector system. Although HFJV can be used as an open or closed system, the closed system allows the use of anesthetic gases and increased oxygen concentrations as well as PEEP if necessary. The potential advantages of HFV techniques relate to the small VT and low inspiratory pressures, which result in minimal movement of the lung and surrounding tissues, enhancing some surgical procedures. In addition, the lower pressures and VT produced by HFV result in a smaller leak via bronchopleural fistulae, and HFJV may

be useful in their repair. Another useful feature of HFV is that the rapid rate and small VT permit use of small catheters, so that ventilation of distal airways and lung tissue can be performed across divided airways. Thus, HFV has been used during sleeve resection, tracheal reconstruction, and surgery for tracheal stenosis, with the small catheters allowing surgery to be performed around them.

Bronchopleural Fistula and Empyema

A bronchopleural fistula is an abnormal communication between the bronchial tree and the pleural cavity. If there is additional communication to the surface of the chest, a bronchopleural-cutaneous fistula develops. A bronchopleural fistula occurs most commonly following pulmonary resection for carcinoma, but other causes include traumatic rupture of a bronchus or bulla, a penetrating chest wound, or spontaneous drainage into the bronchial tree of an empyema cavity or lung cyst. The incidence is higher following a pneumonectomy than following other types of lung resection.

Problems associated with bronchopleural fistula and empyema are related to positive-pressure ventilation, which may result in infectious contamination of healthy lung tissue, loss of air, decreased alveolar ventilation leading to carbon dioxide retention, and the development of a tension pneumothorax.

The anesthetic management of bronchopleural fistulae requires the isolation of the affected side to prevent contamination and permit adequate ventilation of the nonaffected side. Ideally, an awake intubation of the trachea using a DLT to separate the two lungs with the patient breathing spontaneously provides the best conditions. After satisfactory topical anesthesia of the airway down to the carina using techniques described previously and a fiberoptic bronchoscope, and with adequate sedation, the DLT is introduced so that the bronchial lumen is on the side opposite the bronchopleural fistula. If an empyema is present, there may be a considerable outpouring of pus from the tracheal lumen, which should be immediately suctioned with a large-bore suction catheter. The unaffected lung may then be ventilated, and adequacy of oxygenation and ventilation may be assessed by pulse oximetry or ABG analysis.

Alternatively, the DLT may be inserted under general anesthesia with the patient breathing spontaneously to avoid a tension pneumothorax. In patients who do not have an empyema, use of a single-lumen tube has been described and may be satisfactory if the bronchopleural fistula and air leak are small.

For large bronchopleural fistulae, HFJV may be the nonsurgical treatment of choice. However, Bishop et al. (1987) have demonstrated that HFJV may not always be superior to conventional ventilation in the conservative management of bronchopleural fistula; they concluded that HFJV should be used selectively in this application.

Lung Cysts and Bullae

Air-filled cysts of the lung can be bronchogenic, postinfective, infantile, or emphysematous. They may be associated with COPD. A bulla is a thin-walled space filled with air, which results from destruction of alveolar tissue. In general, bullae represent an area of end-stage emphysematous destruction of the lung. Indications for surgical bullectomy include incapacitating dyspnea, expanding bullae, repeated pneumothoraces due to rupture of bullae, and/or compression of a large area of normal lung. Most of these patients have severe COPD with carbon dioxide retention and little functional respiratory reserve.

Important anesthetic considerations include maintenance of a high FIO_2 and awareness that positive pressure ventilation may cause the cyst to expand and rupture, producing a tension pneumothorax. In addition, with highly compliant cysts most of the applied V_T may be wasted in this additional dead space. With the chest open, even more of the V_T may enter the bulla, which is no longer limited by the chest wall integrity.

For induction of anesthesia, arterial line monitoring and pulse oximetry are mandatory. A DLT should be inserted with the patient either awake or under general anesthesia but breathing spontaneously. Avoiding the use of positive pressure ventilation where possible helps to decrease the likelihood of increased dead space, rupture of bullae, or tension pneumothorax. Once the endotracheal tube is in place, each lung may be controlled separately, and adequate ventilation can be applied to the healthy lung if bilateral disease is not present. Positive pressure ventilation should be gentle, with small V_T, rapid respiratory rate, and airway pressures not to exceed 10 cmH_2O if at all possible. If positive pressure ventilation must be applied prior to opening the chest, the possibility of tension pneumothorax must be borne in mind. Treatment of a pneumothorax requires the rapid placement of a chest tube.

HFJV has been used in patients with large bullae undergoing coronary artery bypass grafting or bilateral bullectomy (Normandale, 1985; McCarthy, et al., 1987). In addition, a technique of sequential one-lung ventilation using a DLT has been described for the management of a bilateral bullectomy (Benumof, 1987c). Following bullectomy patients are left with a greater amount of functional lung tissue and the mechanics or respiration are improved. Patients commonly require postoperative ventilation and weaning for several days.

Anesthesia for Resection of the Trachea

Indications for resection of the trachea include congenital lesions (agenesis, stenosis), neoplasia, injuries (direct or indirect), infections, and postintubation injuries, usually due to endotracheal tubes or prolonged tracheostomies. The major problems associated with resection of the trachea are maintaining ventilation of the lungs while the airway is being operated on and maintaining the integrity of anastomoses postoperatively. The presence of lung disease that is of sufficient severity to require postoperative ventilatory support thus becomes a relative contraindication to tracheal resection and reconstruction.

All patients should have an arterial catheter placed in the left radial artery as the innominate artery, which supplies the right radial artery, crosses the trachea and may be compressed during surgery.

A variety of methods for providing ventilation during tra-

cheal resection have been described. These include (1) standard orotracheal intubation, (2) insertion of a tube into the open trachea distal to the area of resection, (3) HFJV through the stenotic area, (4) HFPPV, and (5) cardiopulmonary bypass. With mild stenosis, a small-bore tube may be pushed through and distal to an upper lesion so that resection can be performed around the tube. However, this may make completion of the tracheal anastomosis more difficult than otherwise. To overcome these problems, endotracheal or endobronchial tubes have been inserted into the open trachea distal to the site of the resection. Initially, a small endotracheal tube is passed distal to the obstruction, or a standard endotracheal tube is placed proximal to it if ventilation is possible through the stenotic segment. All further tracheoendobronchial intubations are performed with sheathed tubes passing to the airway, which is surgically opened distal to the lesion. These sterile sheathed tubes are then connected to breathing hoses, which are passed to the anesthetist and connected to the gas machine. After excision of the tracheal lesion and placement of the posterior tracheal sutures, the distal endotracheal tube is removed from the trachea and the original endotracheal tube is advanced past the anastomosis line and reconnected to the circuit, and the anastomosis completed.

With low tracheal or bronchial lesions, resection and reconstruction may be performed around an endobronchial tube or a DLT. The presence of large-bore tubes in the airway may make these resections more difficult, and the use of HFV may improve surgical access. HFPPV or HFJV has been used through small-diameter catheters placed across or through the stenotic lesion or transected airway(s), and ventilation to the distal airways and lungs has thus been maintained. Problems associated with these HFV techniques are that use of this open system may compromise egress of gas if the stenosis is tight. Also, the catheter may become occluded by blood or may become displaced, and distal aspiration of debris and blood may also occur. HFPPV to the left lung alone generally provides adequate oxygenation and ventilation.

Following tracheal resection or reconstructive surgery, patients are generally kept with their necks and heads flexed in order to reduce tension on the anastomotic suture lines. This may be maintained by using sutures between the chin and the anterior chest wall. It is desirable to have the trachea extubated as soon as possible so as to minimize tracheal trauma due to the endotracheal tube and cuff. For this reason, continuous infusion techniques with short-acting muscle relaxants (atracurium, vecuronium), plus rapidly metabolized intravenous anesthetic agents such as propofol and short-acting opioids such as alfentanil, are the current anesthetic agents of choice.

Anesthesia for Lung Transplantation

Single-lung, double-lung, and heart plus double-lung transplantations are being performed with increasing frequency in many parts of the world. Eligible recipients for lung transplantation are patients with end-stage progressive lung disease, which can be classified into four main groups: restrictive, obstructive, infective, and pulmonary vascular. Single-lung transplantation is indicated for patients not suffering from chronic infectious lung disease and has been performed for restrictive lung disease and pulmonary fibrosis. Double-lung transplantation is indicated for infectious disease, usually cystic fibrosis or bronchiectasis because of the risk of leaving an infected lung after single-lung transplantation. Heart-lung transplantation has been reserved for patients suffering from pulmonary hypertension and cor pulmonale. Selection criteria and preoperative evaluation are reviewed elsewhere in this book. Double-lung and heart-lung transplantation require standard cardiopulmonary bypass with a period of aortic cross-clamping and myocardial protection.

Single-lung transplantation is performed with extracorporeal bypass capabilities set up and available. Anesthetic technique includes insertion of arterial and intravenous catheters prior to surgery and insertion of a pulmonary artery catheter after induction. Insertion of a pulmonary artery catheter in a severely dyspneic patient while awake is difficult and hazardous (Demajo, 1992). Anesthesia consists of standard agents for thoracic anesthesia (see above)—that is, fentanyl, thiopental, and succinylcholine for tracheal intubation, pancuronium for muscle relaxation, isoflurane, and benzodiazepines for hypnosis. A left-sided DLT or blocker is absolutely necessary, as is a fiberoptic bronchoscope for repeated assessment of DLT or blocker position. Repeated ABG measurements are essential, as end-tidal carbon dioxide may be inaccurate owing to high dead space ventilation. An FiO_2 of 1.0 or an air-oxygen mixture as determined by ABG analysis is recommended. Recently double lung transplantation has been performed as a sequential procedure at the Toronto Hospital to avoid cardiopulmonary bypass, with only a limited requirement for bypass. In general, emphysematous patients do not usually require arteriovenous bypass, whereas approximately 30 percent of patients with pulmonary fibrosis required arteriovenous bypass (Demajo, 1992). The major anesthetic aspects in the management of lung transplantation are the level of right ventricular function and the effects on right ventricular competence of clamping the pulmonary artery. Preoperative data regarding oxygen requirements, exercise tolerance, and pulmonary artery pressures may assist in predicting the requirement for arteriovenous bypass. All patients are supported with positive pressure ventilation and appropriate intensive care postoperatively as the transplanted lung function is carefully observed. Epidural opioids are the agents of choice to control postoperative pain and assist early extubation.

THE POSTOPERATIVE PERIOD

Postoperative Complications

Complications related to thoracic surgery are summarized below. Complications related to the cardiovascular system include herniation of the heart after pneumonectomy and pericardial resection, major hemorrhage from the operative site, low CO syndrome, postoperative cardiac dysrhythmias, postoperative hypotension, myocardial ischemia and infarction, and occasionally pacing problems. Herniation of the heart through a pericardial defect after pneumonectomy causes twisting of the superior vena cava and inferior vena

---

Complications of Thoracic Surgery

I. Cardiovascular complications
1. Hypotension
2. Low-output syndrome
3. Dysrhythmias
4. Postoperative hypertension
5. Myocardial ischemia and infarction
6. Pacing problems

II. Pulmonary complications
1. Pulmonary emboli
2. Bronchopleural fistula
3. Empyema and mediastinitis
4. Pulmonary torsion
5. Tracheostomy problems
6. Diagnostic procedure complications
7. Chest wall complications
8. Pleural drainage
9. Pulmonary hemorrhage

III. Related complications
1. Monitoring equipment
2. Neurologic, central and peripheral

(From Eisenkraft JB, Neustein SM, Cohen E: Anesthesia for thoracic surgery. p. 905. In Barash PG, Cullen BF, Stoelting RK (eds): Clinical Anesthesia. 2nd Ed. JB Lippincott, Philadelphia, 1992, with permission.)

---

cava and results in pre–cardiac arrest conditions. The diagnosis of cardiac herniation almost always requires immediate reexploration.

Conservative measures that may improve cardiopulmonary function before and during transfer to the operating room after pneumonectomy include positioning the empty surgical side of the chest in a nondependent position, decreasing levels of pressure and volume in the ventilated lung if the patient is on a ventilator, removal of PEEP, discontinuing suction to the empty hemithorax if it is in place, and pharmacologic support of the circulation as required. Injection of 1 to 2 L of air into the surgical hemithorax may push the heart and mediastinum back into normal anatomic positions, but success of this latter technique has been variable (Benumof, 1987a; Kirsch, et al., 1975). Detection of postoperative hemorrhage is facilitated by drainage from a patent chest tube on the operated side. Significant hemorrhage is accompanied by hemodynamic signs of hypovolemia. Therapy requires replacement of blood volume and surgical exploration if necessary.

Right heart failure, low CO syndrome, and postoperative cardiac dysrhythmias are the most common and life-threatening of the cardiovascular complications. Advanced hemodynamic monitoring using pulmonary artery catheters may be necessary to make a differential diagnosis of low CO or acute right heart failure. Most patients at risk for developing right heart failure after pulmonary resection can be identified preoperatively, but right heart failure may also occur if new and active pulmonary vasoconstriction (caused by hypoxia, acidosis, vasoactive drugs, etc.) is placed on the right ventricle.

Therapy for right heart failure and low CO syndrome uses the same principles: control heart rate, optimize preload and the inotropic state of the right or left ventricle, and reduce pulmonary and/or systemic vascular resistance. Vasodilators are very effective at decreasing right ventricular afterload and improving right ventricular function, as this side of the heart is especially afterload-dependent (Prewitt and Ghignone, 1983). Combinations of inotropes and vasodilators, such as isoproterenol and nitroglycerin, or combined drugs such as amrinone, can be very useful in the treatment of right heart failure.

Postoperative cardiac dysrhythmias are common after thoracic surgery. Atrial fibrillation occurred in 20 percent of patients with malignant disease but in only 3 percent of patients with benign disease in one series (Beck-Nielsen, et al., 1973). However, the prophylactic use of digitalis in thoracic surgical patients is still a controversial issue, particularly in patients with signs of congestive heart failure. The use of digitalis does reduce the incidence of potentially fatal complications in older patients (Shields and Uyiki, 1968).

Respiratory complications include pulmonary emboli, bronchopleural fistulae, empyema and mediastinitis, pulmonary torsion, and acute respiratory insufficiency, as well as several others listed above. Acute respiratory insufficiency is probably the most common serious complication after pulmonary resection; it may occur with an incidence of 4 to 5 percent after bronchial carcinoma resections and may carry a mortality rate of up to 50 percent (Hirschler-Schulte, et al., 1985). Respiratory insufficiency is related to the development of atelectasis, which has been reported to occur in up to 100 percent of patients undergoing thoracotomy for pulmonary resection (Downs, 1983).

Atelectasis may occur intraoperatively and postoperatively because of the effects of surgical manipulation of the lung; transudation of fluid into the dependent lung during surgery; and the reduction of normal respiratory effort postoperatively due to pain, intrathoracic blood and fluid accumulation, and decreased compliance. A rapid, shallow, constant-V_T respiratory pattern produces small airway closure and obstruction, resulting in alveolar air resorption and terminal airway collapse.

Aggressive pain control associated with physiotherapy and "stir-up" regimens to produce vigorous coughing and clearance of secretions, plus the capacity to take long expansive breaths, is essential to prevent acute respiratory insufficiency

postoperatively. Standard physiotherapy techniques associated with incentive spirometry, plus use of effective analgesia, are the most widely used postoperative modalities to avoid and treat postoperative atelectasis and acute respiratory insufficiency.

Neural injuries can also occur after thoracic surgery and are both central and peripheral in location. Malpositioning of the patient on the table can result in peripheral nerve injury by either pressure or stretching (Seyfer, et al., 1985). The brachial plexus is especially vulnerable to trauma during thoracic surgery, and this should be protected against intraoperatively. Intrathoracic nerves can also be directly injured during the surgery by being either transected, crushed, stretched, or cauterized; this can occur with the intercostal nerves, the recurrent laryngeal nerve, or the phrenic nerve. Prevention is the therapy of choice for all of these intraoperative nerve injuries.

Management of Postoperative Mechanical Ventilation

In general, only a minority of patients undergoing thoracic surgery will require postoperative mechanical ventilation. These include patients with severe COPD who undergo extensive thoracic operations, as well as those who may have had extensive chest wall resection. Mechanical ventilation raises airway pressure and to a lesser extent intrapleural pressure, and therefore transpulmonary pressure increases. At the end of the procedure if postoperative ventilation is contemplated, the DLT should be replaced by a single-lumen tube.

Controlled mechanical ventilation is initiated with a tidal volume of 12 ml/kg, an intermittent mandatory ventilation (IMV) rate to maintain $PaCO_2$ at 40 mmHg (which usually requires an initial rate of 8 to 12 breaths/min), and an FIO_2 of 60 to 100 percent. IMV used in this way is a full-support ventilation modality allowing the patient to breathe spontaneously, but initially this spontaneous ventilation is not regarded as contributing to the minute ventilation. ABGs and chest radiographs are obtained shortly after institution of mechanical ventilation.

Reduction of FIO_2 to decrease oxygen toxicity (Winter and Smith, 1972; Lambertsen, 1965) is the first priority, and thus the FIO_2 is decreased to less than 0.5 to maintain an acceptable PaO_2 (Table 7-5). This is facilitated by performing a dose (PEEP)–response (PaO_2) titration. Thus, PEEP is progressively added in a range of 0 to 20 cmH_2O until the PaO_2 is relatively normal (about 60 mmHg) with an FIO_2 of less than 0.5. PEEP increments require 0.5 to 1 hour to complete and require repeated ABG measurements. Use of fiberoptic bron-

Table 7-5. Mechanical Ventilation and Weaning Plan

Temporal Goal Sequence to Be Followed	Goal		Method by Which Primarily Achieved
1. ↓ FIO_2	↓ FIO_2 < 0.5	PaO_2 > 60 mmHg	PEEP titration
2. ↓ PEEP	↓ FIO_2 < 0.5, ↓ PEEP < 10 cm H_2O	PaO_2 > 60 mmHg	Respiratory care regime
3. ↓ IMV rate	↓ FIO_2 < 0.5, ↓ PEEP < 10 cm H_2O, ↓ IMV < 1 breath/min	PaO_2 > 60 mmHg	Patient with adequate breathing power

Abbreviations: FIO_2, inspired oxygen fraction; PaO_2, arterial oxygen tension; PEEP, positive end-expiratory pressure; IMV, intermittent mandatory ventilation. (From Benumof JL, Alfery DD: Anesthesia for thoracic surgery. p. 1663. In Miller RD (ed): Anesthesia. 4th Ed. Churchill Livingstone, New York, 1994, with permission.)

choscopy to suction and lavage under direct vision areas of collapsed lung that are resistant to opening by PEEP obviates the need for very high levels of PEEP above 25 cmH₂O.

Patients who have a PEEP requirement greater than 10 cmH₂O to maintain a PaO_2 greater than 60 mmHg with an FIO_2 less than 0.5 are likely to have excessive work of breathing, and weaning the patient off the ventilator may fail owing to fatigue. Reduction of PEEP to less than 10 cmH₂O requires an intensive and aggressive respiratory care regimen, with use of coughing routines, tracheal suctioning, fiberoptic bronchoscopy, chest physiotherapy, humidification of inspired gases, and half-hourly to hourly turning of the patient. In addition, administration of antibiotics as required and bronchodilators, diuretics, and inotropic drugs may also be necessary.

There is a widespread consensus that this aggressive therapy of post-thoracotomy patients produces a clearing of atelectasis, eradication of infection, and a decrease in PEEP requirements (Petty, 1982; O'Donoghue, 1985). With achievement of an FIO_2 less than 0.5 and a PEEP level less than 10 cmH₂O with an acceptable PaO_2, the weaning process is accommodated by a progressive decrease in the IMV rate, allowing a gradual transition from 100 percent to zero ventilator dependence. The rate at which IMV can be reduced is proportional to VC and peak inspiratory flow rates. Thus, as the IMV is decreased, the patient is monitored for spontaneous respiratory rate, VC, peak inspiratory force, and $PaCO_2$.

Criteria for extubation include an FIO_2 less than 0.5, PEEP level less than 10 cmH₂O, VC greater than 15 ml/kg, peak inspiratory force more than −25 cmH₂O, IMV less than 1 breath/min, spontaneous respiratory rate less than 20 to 30/min, and $PaCO_2$ approximately 40 mmHg with a satisfactory PaO_2. There should be no other major organs systems in acute failure or instability, and the chest radiographic findings should be reasonably equivalent to preoperative appearances.

Management of Postoperative Pain

Pain after a posterolateral incision for thoracic lung resection is usually rated as "severe" and is generated from several sources following the procedure. These include soft tissue injury and inflammation, bone and joint trauma, and visceral damage (Conacher, 1990). Occasionally, a characteristic neuritic pain from damaged intercostal nerves is discernible. Pain is exacerbated by movement, especially obligatory ventilatory movements, and thus is associated with shallow breathing and the inability to cough. Many factors alter pulmonary function and hence gas exchange after thoracotomy. In general, a restrictive pattern of ventilation with decreased lung compliance is produced with reductions in timed forced expiratory volumes and peak flow rates of 75 percent in the first 24 to 48 hours postoperatively. In the few studies in which preoperative effort-elicited spirometry was compared with values after surgery, differences of 15 to 20 percent were achieved with effective analgesia (Shulman, et al., 1984). In addition effective analgesia is critical for allowing post-thoracotomy patients to take deep expansive breaths, cough

effectively to clear airways of secretions, and cooperate with physiotherapy in "stir-up" regimens.

Opioids

Opioids have been and continue to provide the mainstay of post-thoracotomy analgesia. Routes and techniques of administration include intravenous bolus, intravenous infusion, patient-controlled administration (PCA), epidural (bolus, PCA, continuous infusion, or in combination with local anesthetic), or intrathecal. Side effects of opioids are well known and dose-dependent and include pruritus, somnolence, urinary retention, and respiratory depression. The relative merits of different routes and methods of administratin of opioids have been the subject of much debate. The intravenous route is the most practical but may require constant nursing attention for repeated injections or adjustment of infusions. PCA devices have proved popular and effective in treating post-thoracotomy pain but may not provide as effective pain relief as neuraxially placed opioids. However, PCA sets the standard of analgesia for intravenous administration. Neuraxial placement of opioids has proved to be very effective for post-thoracotomy pain with only moderate increases in risk, particularly in severely compromised patients (Sandler, et al., 1986). As with intravenous administration, most of the opioids have been tried via neuraxial routes. Epidural catheter site placement does not seem to be important for lipid-insoluble opioids (morphine), and thus both lumbar and thoracic sites are equally effective. However with lipid-soluble opioids (fentanyl, sufentanil) catheter placement is critical, and there is evidence that lumbar catheter placement requires such high doses that systemic absorption produces blood concentrations equivalent to intravenous infusions (Sandler, et al., 1992). Combinations of epidural opioids and low-concentration local anesthetics have also produced excellent analgesic results while avoiding sympathetic blockade associated with epidural local anesthetics alone. There is some evidence that epidural opioids plus local anesthetics produce better analgesia and improve pulmonary function post-thoracotomy as compared with intramuscular or intravenous bolus opioid administration. It is more difficult to judge whether neuraxial opioids are superior to continuous intravenous infusions of opioids. Subarachnoid-placed opioids have also provided excellent prolonged analgesia (Gray, et al., 1986). Monitoring requirements for postoperative opioid analgesia requires repeated frequent nursing attention, although there is evidence that with proper dosage and administration intervals patients with epidural catheters can be monitored safely in a general ward bed after the early high dependency period.

Regional Techniques

Intercostal Nerve Block/Extradural Block. Because of their proximity, the intercostal nerves and the sympathetic chain may be blocked at the same time, usually by spread from the intercostal space to the paravertebral space. Intercostal blocks may be placed before surgery, during surgery under direct vision, or after surgery. Placement presurgery may result in improved analgesia and a reduced incidence of problems associated with deafferentiation. Strategically placed catheters allow continuous application of local anesthetic with prolonged analgesia. Catheters have been placed in intercostal spaces, in paravertebral spaces, and in the extradural space. There is often extensive spread of local anesthetic from the site of injection, with sensory block extending over several dermatomes. Although the analgesic effect of thoracic extradural block is similar to that of intercostal block, which may also provide bilateral analgesia (Matthews and Gorenden, 1989), extradural block tends to be associated with more sympathetic blockade and hypotension. Thoracic extradural blockade may be contraindicated after pneumonectomy because of the high incidence of hypotension, and these patients are more likely to be compromised by therapeutic measures such as volume loading and inotropic drugs.

Cryoanalgesia. Cryolesioning of intercostal nerves under direct vision near the angle of the ribs has been used to provide long-lasting analgesia (up to 3 months) while the nerve regenerates (Gough, et al., 1988). Not all investigators have found positive results with this technique, and there have been reports of association with deafferentiation symptoms and scar discomfort long after the operation.

Interpleural Analgesia. Interpleural analgesia is the percutaneous introduction of an epidural catheter into the thoracic cage between the parietal and the visceral pleura, usually placed at surgery at an interspace just below the level of the incision. Local anesthetic, usually bupivicaine (0.25 to 0.5

percent) with epinephrine is introduced through the catheter into the pleural space. Analgesia occurs as a result of diffusion of local anesthetic to the intercostal nerves and sympathetic chain and its direct action on pleural nerve endings. The results of several studies have varied from moderate to excellent analgesia to no analgesia (Ferrante, et al., 1991), and in some cases plasma concentration of bupivicaine reached near toxic levels. Further work on defining the exact role of interpleural analgesia post-thoracotomy is currently under way.

Multimodal Analgesia. Evidence is accumulating that combined use of local anesthesia blocks, nonsteroidal anti-inflammatory drugs, and opioids may provide excellent postoperative analgesia and improve pulmonary function. Excellent results have been reported when such triple-component analgesic regimens are used after abdominal surgery (Schulze, et al.,1988), and early results from my group's studies indicate that this may apply to postthoracotomy patients (Kavanagh, et al., 1992).

Preemptive Analgesic Therapy. Intense interest is also being directed to prevention of spinal cord plasticity and to controlling the "wind-up" phenomenon as related to postoperative pain. To this end application of opioids, local anesthetic blocks, and other analgesic modalities is being instituted and established *before* surgery to attempt to decrease the intensity and duration of postoperative pain (Katz, et al., 1992).

COMMENTS AND CONTROVERSIES

The chapter author is an experienced, practical anesthetist who has worked closely with general thoracic surgeons in Toronto for 15 years. Based on this experience, he has provided a comprehensive discussion of current anesthesia practice.

It is obvious from the information in this chapter that consultation and communication between surgeon and anesthetist is essential in the management of thoracic surgical patients. Both anesthetist and surgeon are frequently critically involved in a complementary fashion in perioperative care. The thoracic surgeon should find the information on specific conditions provided in this chapter useful in defining the nature of necessary preoperative assessment and the perioperative conduct of the surgery itself. Anesthesia issues must be addressed in advance of the surgical procedure.

F.G.P.

KEY REFERENCES

Benumof JL: Anesthesia for Thoracic Surgery. WB Saunders, Philadelphia, 1987

This single-author textbook provides an excellent review of all aspects of anesthesia for thoracic surgery in a very manageable size. The text is well written and easily understood, and the book is filled with numerous line drawings and diagrams, which complement the text extremely well. This book has definitely had a major impact on the anesthesia community in enhancing comprehension of the specific aspects of anesthesia for thoracic surgery.

Craig DB: Postoperative recovery of pulmonary function. Anesth Analg 60:46, 1981

A well written and comprehensive review of the time course and etiology of postoperative respiratory impairment, primarily after upper abdominal surgery. Important factors related to postoperative respiratory impairment include pain and impaired chest wall function. Inspiratory therapeutic maneuvers are much more effective than expiratory procedures.

Demajo WAP: Pulmonary transplantation. p. 555. In Kaplan JA (ed): Thoracic Anesthesia. 2nd Ed. Churchill Livingstone, New York, 1992

Authoritative review of anesthesia for pulmonary transplantation by the first anesthesia-surgical group to report consistent success with single and double lung transplantation. The review outlines the differing anesthesia requirements of patients with end-stage pulmonary disease of differing etiologies presenting for lung transplantation. Factors that influence the decision to proceed with full or partial cardiopulmonary bypass are also considered. Postoperative care in the intensive care unit is carefully detailed, as well as intraoperative data (hemodynamic, arterial blood gases, etc.) from this first group of long-term survivors of human lung transplantation.

Shulman M, Sandler AN, Bradley JW et al.: Postthoracotomy pain and pulmonary function following epidural and systemic morphine. Anesthesiology 61:569, 1984

One of the earliest carefully controlled trials comparing epidural with intravenous opioids for postthoracotomy pain relief. Epidural morphine was found to provide improved analgesia in the first 24 hours postoperatively. In addition, bedside pulmonary function tests (FVC, VC, peak expiratory flow rates) were improved by small but significant amounts in the epidural group as compared with the intravenous group in the first 24 hours postoperatively.

Slinger PD: Fiberoptic bronchoscopic positoning of double-lumen tubes. J Cardiothorac Anesth 3:486, 1989

An outstanding review of how to correctly position double-lumen tubes using the fiberoptic bronchoscope, which constitutes the recommended current standard of practice. The review includes a general discussion of the technique of intraoperative bronchoscopy. Color endoscopic photographs and line diagrams markedly enhance the thoroughness of this review.

REFERENCES

Aalto-Setala M, Heinonen J, Salorinne Y: Cardiorespiratory function during thoracic anesthesia: comparison of two-lung ventilation and one-lung ventilation with and without PEEP. Acta Anesthesiol Scand 19:287, 1975

Abraham AS, Cole RB, Green ID et al: Factors contributing to the reversible pulmonary hypertension of patients with acute respiratory failure: studies by serial observations during recovery. Circ Res 24:51, 1969

Ali J, Weisel RD, Layng AB et al: Consequences of postoperative alterations and respiratory mechanics. Am J Surg 128:376, 1974

Aubier M, De Troyer A, Sampson M et al.: Aminophylline improves diaphragmatic contractility. N Engl J Med 305:249, 1981

Barker SJ, Tremper KK, Heitzmann HA: Continuous fiberoptic arterial oxygen tension in dogs. Crit Care Med 15:403, 1987

Baum GI, Schwartz A, Llamas R et al: Left ventricular function in chronic obstructive lung disease. N Engl J Med 285:361, 1971

Beck-Nielsen J, Sorenson HR, Astroup P: Atrial fibrillation following thoracotomy for non cardiac disease; in particular, cancer of the lung. Acta Med Scand 193:425, 1973

Beecher HK: Some controversial matters of anesthesia for thoracic surgery. J Thorac Surg 10:202, 1940

Benumof JL, Partridge BL, Salvatierra C et al: Margin of safety in positioning modern double-lumen endotracheal tubes. Anesthesiology 67:729, 1987

Benumof JL: Sequential one-lung ventilation for bilateral bullectomy. Anestheisology 67:268, 1987

Benumof JL: One-lung ventilation and hypoxic pulmonary vasoconstriction: implications for anesthetic management. Anesth Analg 64:821, 1985

Benumof JL: Where do pulmonary artery catheters go: intrathoracic distribution. Anesthesiology 46:336, 1977

Benumof JL, Alfery DD: Anesthesia for thoracic surgery. p. 1517. In Miller RD (ed): Anesthesia, 3rd Ed. New York: Churchill Livingstone, 1990

Bishop MJ, Benson MS, Sato P et al: Comparison of high-frequency jet ventilation with conventional ventilation for bronchopleural fistula. Anesth Analg 66:833, 1987

Brodsky JB, Benumof JL, Ehrenwerth J: Depth of placement of left double-lumen endobronchial tubes. Anesth Analg 73:570, 1991

Brown DL, Davis RS: A simple device for oxygen insufflation with continuous positive airway pressure during one-lung ventilation. Anesthesiology 61:481, 1984

Buist AS, Sexton GV, Nagy JM et al: The effects of smoking cessation and modification of lung function. Am Rev Respir Dis 123:149, 1981

Canada E, Benumof JL: Pulmonary vascular resistance correlates in intact normal and abnormal lungs. Crit Care Med 10:719, 1982

Capan LM, Turndorf H, Patel K et al: Optimization of arterial oxygenation during one-lung anesthesia. Anesth Analg 59:847, 1980

Cohen E, Eisenkraft JB, Thys DM et al: Oxygenation and hemodynamic changes during one-lung ventilation. J Cardiothorac Anesth 2:34, 1988

Conacher ID: Pain relief after thoracotomy. Br Anaesth 65:806, 1990

Dalton ML Jr, Parker TM, Mistrot J et al: Concomitant coronary artery bypass and major noncardiac surgery. J Thorac Cardiovasc Surg 85:621, 1978

Dantzker DR, Wagner PD, West JB: Instability of lung units with low V/Q ratios during O_2 breathing. J Appl Physiol 38:886, 1975

Downs JB: Postoperative respiratory care. p. 635. In Kaplan JA (ed): Thoracic Anesthesia. 1st Ed. Churchill Livingstone, New York, 1983

Eisenkraft JB: Effects of anesthetics on the pulmonary circulation. Br J Anaesth 65:63, 1990

Eisenkraft JB, Neustein SM: Anesthetic management of therapeutic procedures of the lungs and airway. p. 419. In Kaplan JA (ed): Thoracic Anesthesia. 2nd Ed. Churchill Livingstone, New York, 1992

Eisenkraft JB, Neustein SM, Cohen E: Anesthesia for Thoracic Surgery. p. 905. In Barash PG, Cullen BF, Stoelting RK (eds): Clinical Anesthesia. 2nd Ed. JB Lippincott Philadelphia, 1992

Eisenkraft JB, Thys DM, Cohen E, Kaplan JA: Hemodynamic effects of CPAP and PEEP during one-lung anesthesia with isoflurane. Anesthesiology 61:A520, 1984

Enson Y, Guintini C, Lewis ML et al: The influence of hydrogen ion concentration and hypoxia on the pulmonary circulation. J Clin Invest 43:1146, 1964

Fee HJ, Holmes EC, Gewirltz HS et al: Role of pulmonary vascular resistance measurements in preoperative evaluation of candidates for pulmonary resection. J Thorac Cardiovasc Surg 75:519, 1978

Ferrante FM, Chan VWS, Arthur GR, Rocco AG: Interpleural analgesia after thoracotomy. Anesth Analg 72:105, 1991

Flacke JW, Thompson DS, Read RC: Influence of tidal volume and pulmonary artery occlusion on arterial oxygenation during endobronchial anesthesia. South Med J 69:619, 1976

Froese AB, Bryan CA: Effects of anesthesia and paralysis on diaphragmatic mechanics in man. Anesthesiology 41:242, 1974

Frumin MJ, Epstein R, Cohen G: Apneic oxygenation in man. Anesthesiology 20:789, 1959

Gass GD, Olsen GN: Clinical significance of pulmonary function tests. Preoperative pulmonary function testing to predict postoperative morbidity and mortality. Chest 89:127, 1986

Giesecke AH, Gerbershagen H, Dortman C et al: Comparison of the ventilating and injection bronchoscopes. Anesthesiology 38:298, 1973

Ginsberg RJ: New technique for one lung anesthesia using an endo-bronchial blocker. J Thorac Cardiovasc Surg 32:542, 1981

Gough JD, Williams AB, Vaughan RS et al: The control of post-thoracotomy pain. A comparative evaluation of thoracic epidural fentanyl infusions and cryoanalgesia. Anesthesia 43:780, 1988

Gracey DR, Divertie MB, Didier EP: Preoperative pulmonary prepa-ration of patients with chronic obstructive pulmonary disease. Chest 76:123, 1979

Gray JR, Fromme GA, Nauss LA et al: Intrathecal morphine for post-thoracotomy pain. Anesth Analg 65:873, 1986

Hannenberg AA, Satwicz PR, Pienes RS Jr, O'Brien JC: A device for applying CPAP to the non-ventilated upper lung during one lung ventilation. II. Anesthesiology 60:254, 1984

Harmon E, Lillington G: Pulmonary risk factors in surgery. Med Clin North Am 63:1289, 1979

Hartman GS: Anesthesia for thoracic surgery. Anesth Analg suppl. 74:93, 1992

Hirschler-Schulte CJW, Hylkema BS, Meyer RW: Mechanical venti-lation for acute postoperative respiratory failure after surgery for bronchial carcinoma. Thorax 40:387, 1985

Hobelmann CF Jr, Smith DE, Virgilio RW et al: Hemodynamic alterations with positive end-expiratory pressure: the contribution of the pulmonary vasculature. J Trauma 15:951, 1975

Hultgren BL, Krishna PR, Kamaya H: A new tube for one lung ventilation: experience with the Univent tube. Anesthesiology 65:3A, A481, 1986

Inoue H, Shohtsu A, Ogawa J et al: New device for one-lung anes-thesia: endotracheal tube with movable blocker. J Thorac Cardio-vasc Surg 83:940, 1982

Isles AF, Newth CJL: Combined beta agonists and methylxanthines in asthma. N Engl J Med 309:432, 1983

Johnson WC: Postoperative ventilatory performance. Dependence upon surgical incision. Am J Surg 41:615, 1967

Jones DP: Symposium on noncardiac thoracic surgery: diagnostic workup-up of chest disease. Surg Clin North Am 60:743, 1980

Jones RM: Smoking before surgery: the case for stopping smoking. Br Med J 290:1763, 1985

Kachel RG: Left ventricular function in chronic obstructive pulmo-nary disease. Chest 74:286, 1978

Kamaya H, Krishna PR: New endotracheal tube (Univent tube) for selective blockade of one lung. Anesthesiology 63:342, 1985

Kaplan JA (ed): Thoracic Anesthesia. 2nd Ed. Churchill Livingstone, New York, 1992

Kaplan JA (ed): Thoracic Anesthesia. 1st Ed. Churchill Livingstone, New York, 1983

Kassis E: Systemic hypertension, left ventricular hypertrophy and myocardial infarction in patients with chronic obstructive lung disease. Scand J Respir Dis 58:324, 1977

Katz J, Kavanagh BP, Sandler AN et al: Pre-emptive analgesia: clinical evidence of neuroplasticity contributing to post-operative pain. Anesthesiology 77:439, 1992

Katz JA, Larlane RC, Rairby HB et al: Pulmonary oxygen exchange during endobronchial anesthesia: effect of tidal volume and PEEP. Anesthesiology 56:164, 1982

Kavanagh B, Katz J, Sandler A et al: Is postoperative pain reduced by preoperative multimodal nociceptive blockade?: A randomized, double-blind, placebo controlled study. Can J Anesth 39:A76, 1992

Kerr JH, Crampton Smith A, Prys-Roberts C et al: Observations during endobronchial anesthesia II. Oxygenation. Br J Anaesth 46:84, 1974

Kinchi A, Ellrodt GA, Berman DS et al: Right ventricular perfor-mance in septic shock: radionuclide and hemodynamic observa-tions. Crit Care Med 11:229, 1983

Kirsch MM, Rotman H, Behrendt DM et al: Complications of pulmo-nary resection. Ann Thorac Surg 20:215, 1975

Lambertsen CJ: Effects of oxygen at high partial pressure. p. 1027.

In Fenn WO, Rahn E (eds).: Handbook of Physiology. Vol. 2. Williams & Wilkins, Baltimore, 1965

Laros CD, Swierengo J: Temporary unilateral pulmonary artery oc-clusion in the preoperative evaluation of patients with bronchial carcinoma. Respiration 24:269, 1967

Latimer G, Dickman M, Clinton DW et al: Ventilatory patterns and pulmonary complications after upper abdominal surgery deter-mined by preoperative and postoperative computerized spirometry and blood gas analysis. Am J Surg 122:622, 1971

Lee J, Salvatore A: Innominate artery compression simulating car-diac arrest during mediastinoscopy. A case report. Anesth Analg 55:748, 1976

Lockwood P: Lung function test results and the risk of post-thoracot-omy complications. Respiration 30:529, 1973

Lyons TE: A simplified method of CPAP delivery to the non-venti-lated lung during unilateral pulmonary ventilation. Anesthesiology 61:217, 1984

Magill IW: Anesthesia in thoracic surgery. J R Soc Med 29:643, 1936

Marini JJ, Lakshmimara Y, Kradyan WA: Atropine and terbutaline aerosols in chronic bronchitis. Chest 80:285, 1981

Marshall BE, Longnecker DE, Fairly HB: Anesthesia for Thoracic Procedures. Blackwell Scientific, Oxford, 1987

Marshall BE, Marshall C, Benumof JL et al: Hypoxic pulmonary vasoconstriction in dogs: effects of lung segment size and oxygen tension. J Appl Physiol 51:1543, 1981

Matsushima Y, Jones RL, King EG et al: Alterations in pulmonary mechanics and gas exchange during routine fiberoptic bronchos-copy. Chest 86:184, 1984

Matthews PJ, Govenden V: Comparison of continuous para-verte-bral and extradural infusions of bupivacaine for pain relief after thoracotomy. Br J Anaesth 62:204, 1989

McCarthy G, Coppel DL, Gibbons JR et al: High-frequency jet ventilation for bilateral bullectomy. Anesthesia 42:411, 1987

Merridew CG, Jones RDM: Nondependent lung CPAP (5 cm H_2O) with oxygen during ketamine, halothane, or isoflurane anesthesia and one-lung ventilation. Anesthesiology 63:A567, 1985

Mittman C: Assessment of operative risk in thoracic surgery. Am Rev Respir Dis 84:197, 1961

Morton HJV, Camb DA: Tobacco smoking and pulmonary complica-tions after operation. Lancet 1:368, 1944

Neuman G, Weingarten AE, Abramowitz RM et al: The anesthetic management of the patient with an anterior mediastinal mass. Anesthesiology 60:144, 1984

Nobak CR: Intraoperative monitoring. In Kaplan JA (ed): Thoracic Anesthesia. 1st Ed. Churchill Livingstone, New York, 1983

Normandale JP: Bullous cystic lung disease. Anesthesia 40:1182, 1985

O'Donoghue WJ: National survey of the usage of lung expansion modalities for the prevention and treatment of postoperative atel-ectasis following abdominal and thoracic surgery. Chest 87:76, 1985

O'Donoghue WJ, Baker JP, Bell GM et al: Respiratory failure in neuromuscular disease: management in respiratory intensive care unit. JAMA 235:733, 1976

Olsen GN, Block AJ, Swensen EW et al: Pulmonary function evalua-tion of the lung resection candidate: a prospective study. Am Rev Repsir Dis 111:379, 1975

Palmer KN, Sellick BA: The prevention of postoperative pulmonary atelectasis. Lancet 1:164, 1953

Pearce AC, Jones RM: Smoking and anesthesia: preoperative absti-nence and perioperative morbidity. Anesthesiology 61:576, 1984

Pecora DV, Hohenberger M: Effects of postpneumonectomy disten-sion on pulmonary compliance and vascular resistance. Am Surg 45:797, 1979

Peters RM, Swain JA: Management of the patient with emphysema, coronary artery disease and lung cancer. Am J Surg 143:701, 1982

Petty C: Right radial artery pressure during mediastinoscopy. Anesth Analg 58:428, 1979

Petty TL: Critical care for chronic air-flow limitation: emphysema, chronic bronchitis, and cystic fibrosis. Semin Respir Med 3:263, 1982

Piehler JM, Trastek VF, Pairolero PC et al: Concomitant cardiac and pulmonary operations. J Thorac Cardiovasc Surg 90:662, 1985

Prewitt R, Ghignone M: Treatment of right ventricular dysfunction in acute respiratory failure. Crit Care Med 5:346, 1983

Robin ED, Gaudio R: Cor pulmonale. Dis Mon (May): 138, 1970

Rowbotham S: Intratracheal anesthesia. Lancet 2:583, 1926

Rutkow IM: Thoracic and cardiovascular operations in the United States, 1979 to 1984. J Thorac Cardiovasc Surg 92:181, 1986

Sackner MA: State of the art—bronchofiberscopy. Am Rev Respir Dis 111:62, 1975

Sandler AN, Chovaz P, Whiting W: Respiratory depression following epidural morphine: a clinical study. Can J Anaesth 33:542, 1986

Sandler AN, Panos L, Stringer D et al.: A randomized, double-blind comparison of lumbar epidural and intravenous fentanyl infusions for post-thoracotomy pain relief: analgesic, pharmacokinetic and respiratory effects. Anesthesiology 77:626, 1992

Schulze S, Roikjaer O, Hasselstrom L et al.: Epidural bupivacaine and morphine plus systemic indomethacin eliminates pain but not systemic response and convalescence after cholecystectomy. Surgery 67:321, 1988

Seyfer AE, Grammer NY, Bogumill GP et al.: Upper extremity neuropathies after cardiac surgery. J Hand Surg 10:16, 1985

Shields TW, Uyiki GT: Digitalization for prevention of arrhythmias following pulmonary surgery. Surg Gynecol Obstet 126:743, 1968

Sibert K, Biondi JW, Hirsch NP: Spontaneous respiration during thoracotomy in a patient with a mediastinal mass. Anesth Analg 66:904, 1987

Sloan H, Morris JD, Figley M, Lee R: Temporary unilateral occlusion of the pulmonary artery in the preoperative evaluation of thoracic patients. J Thorac Surg 30:591, 1955

Smith G, Hirsch N, Ehrenwerth J: Sight and sound: can double-lumen endotracheal tubes be placed accurately without fiberoptic bronchoscopy? Br J Anaesth 58:1317, 1987

Stein M, Cassara EL: Preoperative pulmonary evaluation and therapy for surgical patients. JAMA 211:787, 1970

Stein M, Koota GM, Simon M et al.: Pulmonary evaluation of surgical patients. JAMA 181:765, 1962

Tarhan S, Lundborg RO: Carlens endobronchial catheter versus regular endobronchial tube during thoracic surgery: a comparison of blood gas tensions and pulmonary shunting. Can J Anaesth 18:594, 1961

Tarhan S, Lundborg RO: Effects of increased expiratory pressure on blood gas tensions and pulmonary shunting during thoracotomy with use of the Carlens catheters. Can J Anaesth 17:4, 1970

Tarhan S, Moffitt EA, Sessler AD et al.: Risk of anesthesia and surgery in patients with chronic bronchitis and chronic obstructive pulmonary disease. Surgery 74:720, 1973

Thiagarajah S, Job C, Rao A: A device for applying CPAP to the nonventilated upper lung during one lung ventilation. I. Anesthesiology 60:253, 1984

Tisi GN: Preoperative evaluation of pulmonary function: validity, indications, and benefits. Am Rev Respir Dis 119:293, 1979

Veil R: Selective bronchial blocking in a small child. Br J Anaesth 41:453, 1969

Veith FJ, Rocco AG: Evaluation of respiratory function in surgical patients: importance of preoperative preparation in the prediction of pulmonary complications. Surgery 45:905, 1959

Von Euler US, Liljestrand G: Observations on the pulmonary arterial blood pressure in the cat. Acta Physiol Scand 12:310, 1946

Vour'h G, Fishler M, Michon F et al.: Manual jet ventilation v high-frequency jet ventilation during laser resection of tracheo-bronchial stenosis. Br J Anaesth 55:973, 1983

Warner MA, Tinker JH, Divertie MB: Preoperative cessation of smoking and pulmonary complications in pulmonary dysfunction. Anesthesiology 59:A60, 1983

Warner ME, Warner M, Leonard P: Anesthesia for neodymium-YAG laser resection of major airway obstructing tumours. Anesthesiology 60:230, 1984

Webb-Johnson DC, Chir B, Andrews JL: Bronchodilator therapy. N Engl J Med 297:476, 1977

Wilson R: Endobronchial intubation. p. 371. In Kaplan JA (ed): Thoracic Anesthesia. 2nd Ed. Churchill Livingstone, New York, 1992

Winter PM, Smith G: The toxicity of oxygen. Anesthesiology 37:210, 1972

Zeldin RA, Normandin D, Landtwing D et al.: Postpneumonectomy pulmonary edema. J Thoracic Cardiovasc Surg 87:359, 1984

Zimmerman GA, Morris AH, Cegiz M: Cardiovascular alterations in the adult respiratory distress syndrome. Ann J Med 73:25, 1982

8

INCISIONS

Darroch W. O. Moores
Eric D. Foster
Martin F. McKneally

DEFINITION

The purpose of most surgical incisions is to provide optimal access to the underlying viscera requiring treatment. The ability to provide adequate exposure of the organs requiring operative attention is a fundamental skill learned early in surgical practice. Definitions of adequate exposure in a given procedure may vary, but it is undeniable that no surgeon feels at ease with unsatisfactory exposure of the operative field.

HISTORICAL NOTE

Incision of the thorax with therapeutic intent is recorded as early as the Hippocratic era (Adams, 1849). Hippocrates drained empyema by trephination through the rib to avoid injury to the intercostal artery. His skillful strategy of management of the wound was based on packing so that fluid and air could escape, but a semiocclusive dressing was laid over the packing to prevent open pneumothorax.

Larger incisions for drainage of empyema were facilitated by definition of the arterial anatomy of the interspace; Dulac (1874) recognized the subcostal position of the vascular bundle and described the safe passage still used by modern surgeons to enter the chest along the superior border of the rib. Rib resection and thoracoplasty to facilitate collapse of the tuberculous cavities represent the next major advance in thoracic incisions. These incisions were often performed under local anesthesia (Naef, 1990).

Deliberate entry into the pleural space was carefully avoided because of the fatal complication of open pneumothorax. Tuffier (1891) performed the first partial resection of a lung using an extrapleural approach, meticulously suturing the pleura to the lung to be certain that the free pleural space was not entered during surgery. The incisions of Monaldi for drainage of lung abscess depended on Tuffier's principle of maintaining pleural symphysis, as did the open drainage incisions introduced by Eloesser and others. Although positive pressure ventilation with endotracheal intubation had been described centuries before by Vesalius for open chest experi-

ments on pigs and redeveloped by Tuffier (1896), thoracic surgeons were distracted by the negative pressure chamber of Sauerbruch (1904) for several decades. Naef (1990) has pointed out how this ingenious approach actually retarded the progress of thoracic surgery. Solution of the problem of open pneumothorax allowed surgeons to open the chest more widely and apply their surgical skills to previously sacrosanct structures.

Ludwig Rehn performed the first repair of a cardiac laceration in 1896 and the first pericardiectomy in 1920 through a lateral thoracotomy. Posterolateral thoracotomies were performed for pulmonary resection as these techniques evolved under the leadership of Graham, Archibald, Nissen, and others. Garlock (1946) traced the history of the abdominothoracic incision and developed it for esophagectomy. Bilateral thoracotomy with transverse division of the sternum was used for a short time to gain access for heart surgery and was later abandoned in favor of the median sternotomy. Milton developed and applied the midline sternotomy in humans as early as 1897. Julian et al. (1957) popularized this approach for surgery on the heart. The median sternotomy has subsequently been widely employed for mediastinal and pulmonary surgery. It was the standard, and somewhat limiting, approach for double lung transplantation until Joel Cooper, at the suggestion of Hermes Grillo, resurrected the bilateral "clamshell" thoracotomy to facilitate dissection of the lungs for bilateral sequential lung transplantation in inflammatory lung disease.

HISTORICAL READINGS

Adams F: The Genuine Works of Hippocrates. London, 1849
Dulac: De la Blessure des Artères Intercostales dan les Plaies de Poitrine, et particulièrement dans la Paracentèse. Thesis, University of Paris, 1874; as quoted in Paget S: The Surgery of the Chest. p. 88. John Wright & Co, Bristol, England, 1896
Garlock JH: Combined abdominothoracic approach for carcinoma of cardia and lower esophagus. Surg Gynecol Obstet 83:737, 1946

Julian OC, Lopez-Belio M, Dye WS et al.: The median sternal incision in intracardiac surgery with extracorporeal circulation: a general evaluation of its use in heart surgery. Surgery 42:753, 1957

Milton H: Mediastinal surgery. Lancet 1:872, 1897

Naef AP: The Story of Thoracic Surgery; Milestones and Pioneers. Huber, Toronto, 1990

Sauerbruch F: Zur Pathologie des offenen Pneumothorax und die Grundlagen meines Verfahrens zu seiner Ausschaltung. Mitteil Grenzgeb Med Chir 13:399, 1904

Tuffier T: De la résection du sommet du poumon. Semin Med Paris 2:202, 1891

Tuffier T, Hallion: Regulation de la pression intrabronchique et de la narcose. Compt Rend Soc Biol 3:1086, 1896

SURFACE ANATOMY OF THE THORAX

The palpable landmarks on the chest wall serve as reference points locating the underlying viscera. A knowledge of these reference points allows precise placement of the incision and ideal exposure of the structures beneath it. These landmarks have taken on increased importance in the era of computed tomography (CT)-guided or video-assisted localization of lesions for excision through smaller and less disabling incisions.

Scapula and Bony Thorax

When the arms are at the sides, the root of the spine of the scapula lies opposite the spine of the third thoracic vertebra, and the inferior angle of the scapula lies over the seventh intercostal space. When the arm is moved forward, the inferior angle of the scapula rotates forward and upward to the fifth intercostal space. The spines of the vertebrae, particularly the prominent seventh cervical spine, can be palpated posteriorly. The sternal notch lies opposite the lower border of the second thoracic vertebra, the sternal angle of Louis lies opposite the lower border of the fourth thoracic vertebra, and the xiphisternal junction lies opposite the ninth thoracic vertebra. The first rib lies under the clavicle and is not easily palpated. The second rib is easily felt; its costal cartilage joins the sternum opposite the sternal angle.

Lungs and Pleura

With the shoulders depressed, the apex of the lung is 2 to 3 cm above the medial third of the clavicle. Figure 8-1 illustrates the lung and pleural boundaries in relation to the thoracic skeleton. The oblique fissure of the lung follows a line from the spine of the third thoracic vertebra (opposite the spine of the scapula) to the sixth costal cartilage, where it joins the sixth rib. The horizontal fissure of the right lung follows a line from the fourth costal cartilage back to the oblique fissure. During respiration the lungs move extensively; the markings shown in Figure 8-1 apply to a resting position. The surface markings of the pleura are congruent with those of the lung except where the pleura extends down in the costodiaphragmatic recess.

The hilum of the lung lies nearer to the posterior than to the anterior thoracic wall. On the back, its position is indicated by a line midway between the vertebral spines and the medial border of the scapula, extending from the level of the fourth to the sixth thoracic spine.

Mediastinal Structures

The apex beat of the heart is normally palpable at the fifth left intercostal space, 8 to 9 cm from the midline with the patient supine. In the upright position the apex drops down behind the sixth rib. In a healthy patient the apex moves to the left if the patient is rolled onto the left side but does not move when the patient is rolled onto the right side. Figure 8-2 illustrates the normal heart in relation to the thoracic skeleton. The position of these topographic sites of the cardiac outline and the valves varies with age and body build. In a slender, long thorax, they lie roughly one rib level higher than they do in a thorax that is broad.

The aorta ascends from the base of the heart to the right; it arches to the left and backward at the level of the fourth thoracic vertebra. The top of the arch of the aorta lies opposite the midpoint of the manubrium. The three great vessels of the arch of the aorta can be located by topographic points on the chest wall. The brachiocephalic artery arises in the midline from the top of the aortic arch and passes behind a point deep to the right sternoclavicular joint. The left common carotid artery passes behind a point deep to the left sternoclavicular joint. The left subclavian artery arises behind and slightly to the left of the left common carotid artery and ascends, maintaining this relationship.

The great veins in the mediastinum can be located by topographic points on the chest wall. The right brachiocephalic vein is formed at a point just below the right sternoclavicular joint. It descends along the right side of the brachiocephalic artery. The left brachiocephalic vein crosses in front of the roots of the left subclavian, left common carotid, and brachiocephalic arteries to form the superior vena cava behind the junction of the first right costal cartilage and the sternum.

GENERAL OPERATIVE CONSIDERATIONS IN THORACIC INCISIONS

The surgeon's responsibility for positioning the patient properly on the operating table should not be relinquished to assistants or to operating room personnel. Once properly positioned, the patient can be secured by using sandbags or kidney rests as well as long strips of wide adhesive tape attached to the table. We prefer the use of the "bean bag" (Olympic Vac-Pac, Olympic Medical, Seattle, WA) for positioning the patient. No skin preparation should begin until the proper position is secured.

Many different methods of skin preparation have proved satisfactory. Our preference is to paint the operative site over a wide area with alcohol. Following this an aqueous iodine solution is applied and the site covered with an adherent plastic drape. Sterile drapes are placed to allow for the placement of chest tubes, extension of the incision, identification of surface landmarks, or counting of ribs above or below the incision site. Accurate identification of the correct interspace for the planned operation is critically important for expeditious thoracic surgery.

Skin incisions are made with a scalpel. An electrocautery facilitates the division of the large muscles encountered in chest wall incisions. If the electrocautery current is used properly, it should not cause any more tissue necrosis than

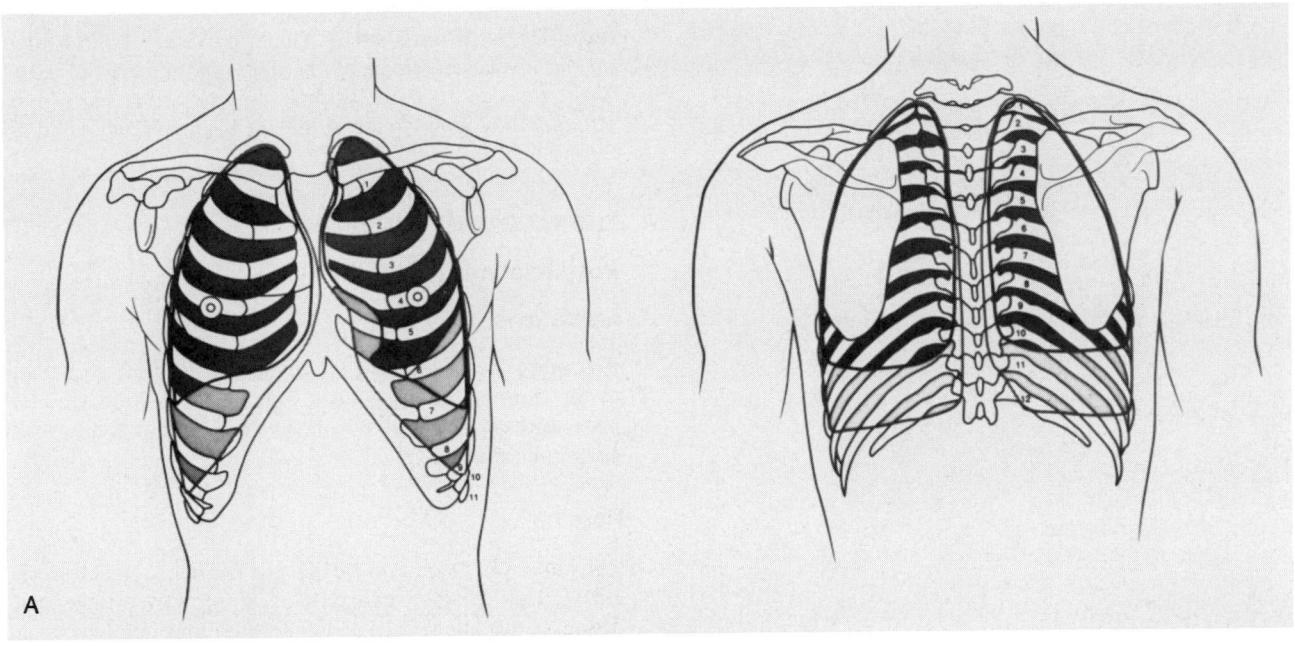

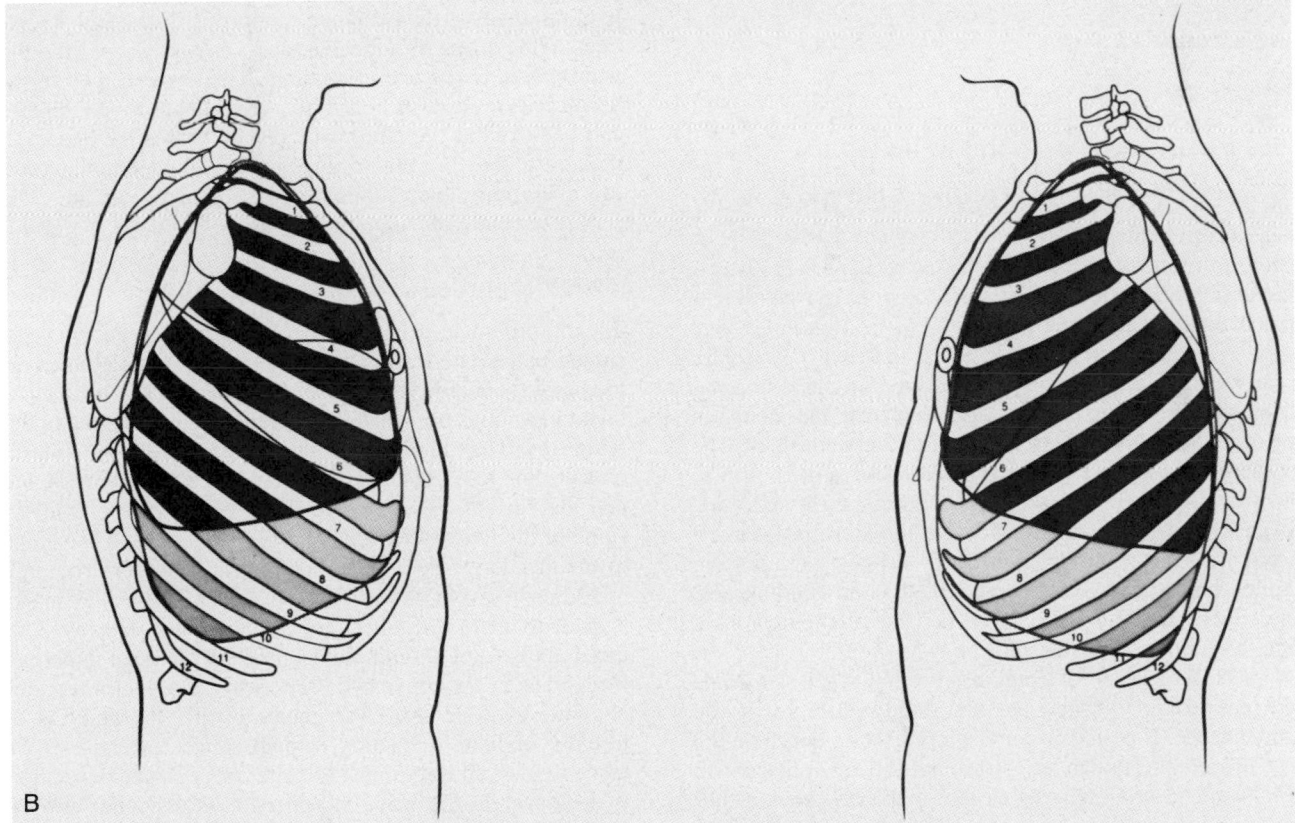

Figure 8-1. (A&B) Pulmonary and pleural boundaries.

would result if the muscle bulk were divided with a scalpel and each bleeding vessel ligated. Wide spreading of the ribs is responsible for a major component of post-thoracotomy pain (McKneally, 1992), and premature opening of the rib spreader before mobilization of the ribs may cause painful fractures.

In closing thoracic incisions, the point of entry for drainage tubes should not be placed too far posteriorly. Chest tubes posterior to the midaxillary line tend to kink and are uncomfortable for the recumbent patient. The course of the drainage tube through the chest wall should be oblique rather than a direct puncture. This oblique course permits closure of the

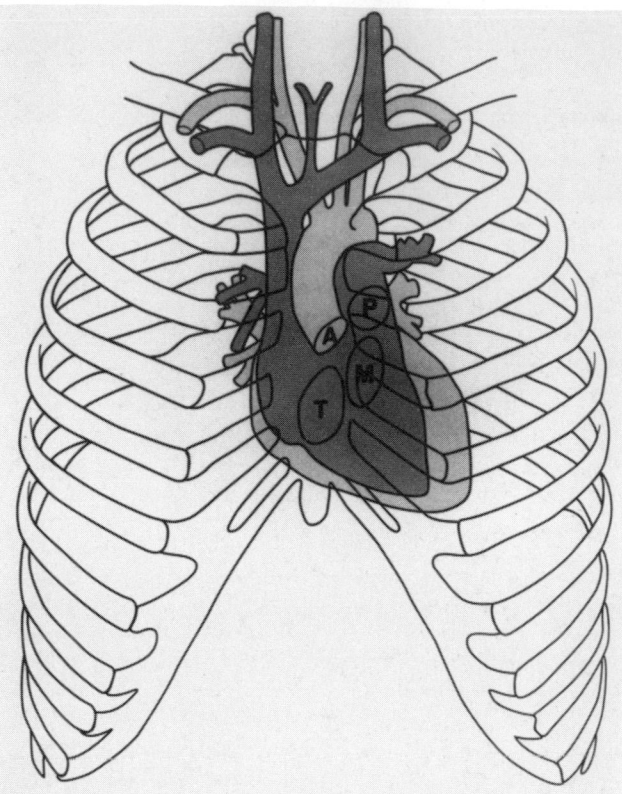

Figure 8-2. Surface anatomy of mediastinal structures. A, aortic valve; P, pulmonary valve; M, mitral valve; T, tricuspid valve.

chest tube tract when the catheter is removed. A tract is fashioned for the tube in the subcutaneous tissue over a distance equivalent to the width of one or two intercostal spaces. A location should be selected that will not require passing the tube through the pectoralis major, serratus anterior, or latissimus dorsi muscle. A chest tube site along the anterior axillary line avoids the bulk of these muscles. The tract should pass close to the superior border of the rib to avoid injury to the neurovascular bundle lying in the subcostal groove. The position of the tube within the chest can be secured with an absorbable suture (3–0 plain catgut) from the tip of the catheter to the parietal pleura and endothoracic fascia. Each chest tube should be secured at the skin level with a large nonabsorbable suture.

There is divergence of opinion among thoracic surgeons about reapproximating the ribs and divided muscles in the wound closure. If pericostal sutures are used to approximate ribs, we prefer to punch holes through the ribs adjacent to the incision and to pass the sutures through these holes rather than around the ribs (Boyd, et al., 1966).

Selection of the suture material to close muscle, fascial, subcutaneous, and skin layers remains a matter of the surgeon's preference. In a review on the selection of suture materials, Van Winkle and Hastings (1972) emphasize that the surgeon should make the choice with an understanding of the nature of the selected suture material and of the biologic forces involved in wound healing. The suture size should be sufficient in strength to hold the tissue securely. Our method of closure is to use continuous polyglycolic acid (PGA) su-

tures (Dexon, from Davis & Geck, or Vicryl, from Ethicon) on the fascial envelope of the deep and superficial aspects of the muscles. It is the fascial approximation that provides strength to wound closures; muscle tissue is friable and does not hold sutures well.

THORACOTOMY INCISIONS

Posterolateral Thoracotomy

Indications

A posterolateral incision is commonly used for exploration of the thoracic cavity and is suitable for a wide variety of procedures on the lung, esophagus, mediastinum, descending aorta, and diaphragm.

Position

The patient is placed on the side in the lateral position (Fig. 8-3A). The legs are separated by a pillow; the lower leg is flexed at the knee and hip, while the upper leg lies straight on the top of the pillow. The patient's position is secured with sandbags or the bean bag supporting the back and abdomen. Wide strips of adhesive tape are passed over the hips and secured to the operating table. The lower arm either can be placed on an arm board at a right angle to the table or can be flexed at the elbow and placed beside the head. The upper arm may be rotated forward and allowed to hang over the operating table, supported by adequate padding. This serves to rotate the scapula forward.

Incision

The inferior angle, spine, and vertebral border of the scapula should be palpated; the position of the vertebral spines and the nipple is noted. With these landmarks as guides, a curvilinear incision is prepared, following the course of the underlying ribs. The standard incision extends from the anterior axillary line to a point midway between the vertebral spines and the vertebral border of the scapula, at a level with the spine of the fourth thoracic vertebra (Fig. 8-3A). The length of the incision varies depending upon the surgery required.

The posterior half is similarly placed whether the incision is made in the fourth, fifth, or sixth interspace. However, the incision does not extend quite as high in the sixth interspace incision as in the other two. Anteriorly, the incision should continue to slope along the course of the rib, which is extremely oblique. Incisions through lower interspaces are made in their entirety along the interspace, since the scapula is no longer in the way. The incision is deepened through the subcutaneous tissue and superficial fascia until the fasciae overlying the serratus anterior, latissimus dorsi, and trapezius muscles are exposed (Fig. 8-3B). The latissimus dorsi and its fascial layers are divided; the trapezius muscle may be divided if wide exposure is required. The muscles and their fascial coverings are divided with the electrocautery. The serratus anterior muscle is usually elevated and retracted anteriorly. If necessary for exposure, the serratus anterior is divided as close as possible to its origins on the ribs (Fig. 8-3C). The surgeon's hand can be passed up beneath the scapula to palpate and count the ribs. The first rib can be palpated in this manner and identified by its horizontal border. The chest is generally entered through the fifth intercostal space or the bed of the fifth rib if it is resected (Fig. 8-3D). However, this incision may enter the chest anywhere from the third to the tenth rib. In dividing the rhomboid major and minor muscles, care should be taken to cut at least 3 to 4 cm medial to the vertebral border of the scapula so as to avoid the deep branch of the transverse cervical artery and the dorsal scapular nerve. It is not necessary to divide the thoracolumbar fascia or paravertebral muscles; the thoracolumbar fascia can be elevated by blunt dissection and retracted to expose the underlying rib posteriorly.

Entry into the pleural cavity through the deep layer of the thoracic wall may be made through an intercostal space or through the periosteal bed of a rib. Exposure of the selected entry site may be aided by retracting the scapula and its attached muscles with a Davidson scapula retractor. In the past, rib resection was considered a standard part of posterolateral thoracotomy incisions. At present most surgeons prefer not to resect a rib.

Entry into the pleural cavity through the selected intercostal space is made by using electrocautery to divide the intercostal muscles close to the upper border of the lower rib away from the neurovascular structures in the subcostal groove. With the lung retracted, the endothoracic fascia and parietal pleura are then opened the length of the incision with scissors or cautery. Exposure of the underlying thoracic contents is gained by retracting the wound margins with a rib spreader.

If a rib is resected, the periosteum is reflected superiorly and inferiorly with the periosteal elevator. Care is taken to avoid injury to the neurovascular bundle lying in the subcostal groove between the internal and innermost intercostal muscles. Separation of the periosteal bed posteriorly from the rib is aided by the use of Doyen raspatories (Fig. 8-3E). Separated from its periosteal bed, the rib is ready to be resected with Bethune rib shears (Fig. 8-3F). The cut ends may be shortened with a Sauerbruch rongeur.

Limited Thoracotomy (Muscle-Sparing Thoracotomy)

The majority of thoracic surgical procedures do not require the full standard posterolateral thoracotomy incisions. With increased technical competence and advances in anesthesia, particularly unilateral endobronchial ventilation, most procedures can be performed safely through a limited incision. The incision should be planned carefully to allow easy access to the operative site with division of as little muscle and rib as possible to obtain a safe working space. Limited thoracotomy incisions (1) cause less chest wall injury, (2) can be performed with less risk in patients with marginal pulmonary function, (3) provide adequate exposure for a wide range of intrathoracic procedures, and (4) heal with a cosmetically satisfactory scar.

Many satisfactory muscle-sparing incisions have been described (Becker and Munro, 1976; Mitchell, et al., 1976; Heitmiller and Mathisen, 1989; Kittle, 1988; Bethencourt and Holmes, 1988). Each technique has its advantages and disadvantages, and there is no one best incision. Any limited thora-

cotomy incision must be placed so that it can be safely extended if more exposure is required.

Axillary Thoracotomy

Publications advocating the use of the transaxillary incision indicate that it has been applied to nearly every mediastinal, chest wall, pulmonary, esophageal, and cardiovascular operation (Becker and Munro, 1976; Mitchell, et al., 1976; Baeza and Foster, 1976; Wada, et al., 1978; Massimiano, et al., 1988; Ginsberg, 1993).

Position

The arm on the operative side is abducted 90 degrees at the shoulder, flexed at the elbow, and supported on an arm stand (Fig. 8-4A&B). Care should be taken to secure the arm in a manner that allows some motion of the scapula and shoulder to facilitate operative exposure and avoid the possibility of injury during retraction.

Incision

The skin incision may be made in either a vertical or a horizontal direction, with the length dependent on the exposure needed for the planned procedure. Baeza and Foster (1976) and Ginsberg (1993) advocate a vertical incision beginning at the level of the third rib in the midaxillary line and extending in a caudal direction to approximately the eighth or ninth rib (Fig. 8-4A). Becker and Munro (1976) and Mitchell, et al. (1976) recommend horizontal incisions at the level of the third or fourth rib, extended to the level of the nipple anteriorly and to the tip of the scapula posteriorly if wide exposure is required (Fig. 8-4B). Both the vertical and the horizontal transaxillary thoracotomy incisions can be easily lengthened if necessary.

The incision is carried down through the subcutaneous fat and superficial fascia until the serratus anterior muscle is revealed. Tissue flaps can be developed with the plane of dissection between the superficial fascia and the fascia overlying the muscles of the middle layer of the chest wall until the pectoralis major muscle is exposed anteriorly and the latissimus dorsi muscle is exposed posteriorly (Fig. 8-4C). Skin flaps are not required, which eliminates postoperative seroma (Ginsberg, 1993). Care is required to protect the intercostobrachial and long thoracic nerves. The latissimus muscle is elevated and retracted posteriorly. The serratus is elevated from the chest wall, and by use of cautery it is detached from its rib insertions until the appropriate interspace to be opened is fully exposed (Fig. 8-4D). Occasionally, division of the lower fibers of the serratus anterior is required for complete exposure. The desired intercostal space is located, its muscle and fascial layers are divided, and the pleural cavity is entered. Exposure to attain an intercostal space incision is achieved by retracting the latissimus dorsi posteriorly and the pectoralis major and serratus anteriorly with a Richardson retractor. Usually, some pectoralis major muscle fibers originating from the fourth through the sixth intercostal cartilages must be divided to gain the full anterior intercostal space exposure. It is very rarely necessary to divide any of the latissimus dorsi muscle posteriorly. A second Tuffier rib

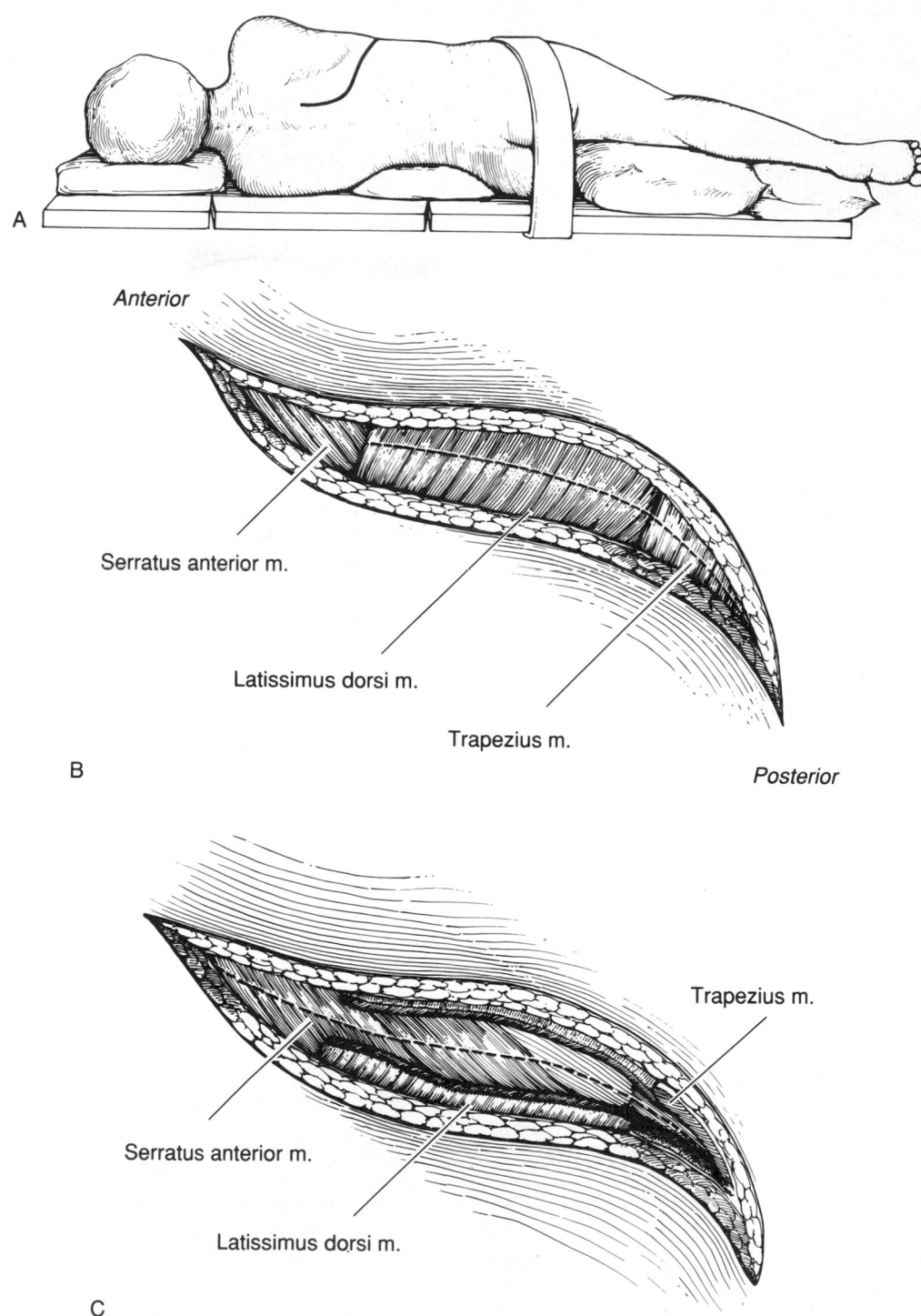

Figure 8-3. **(A–C)** Posterolateral thoracotomy incision (see text for explanation). (*Figure continues.*)

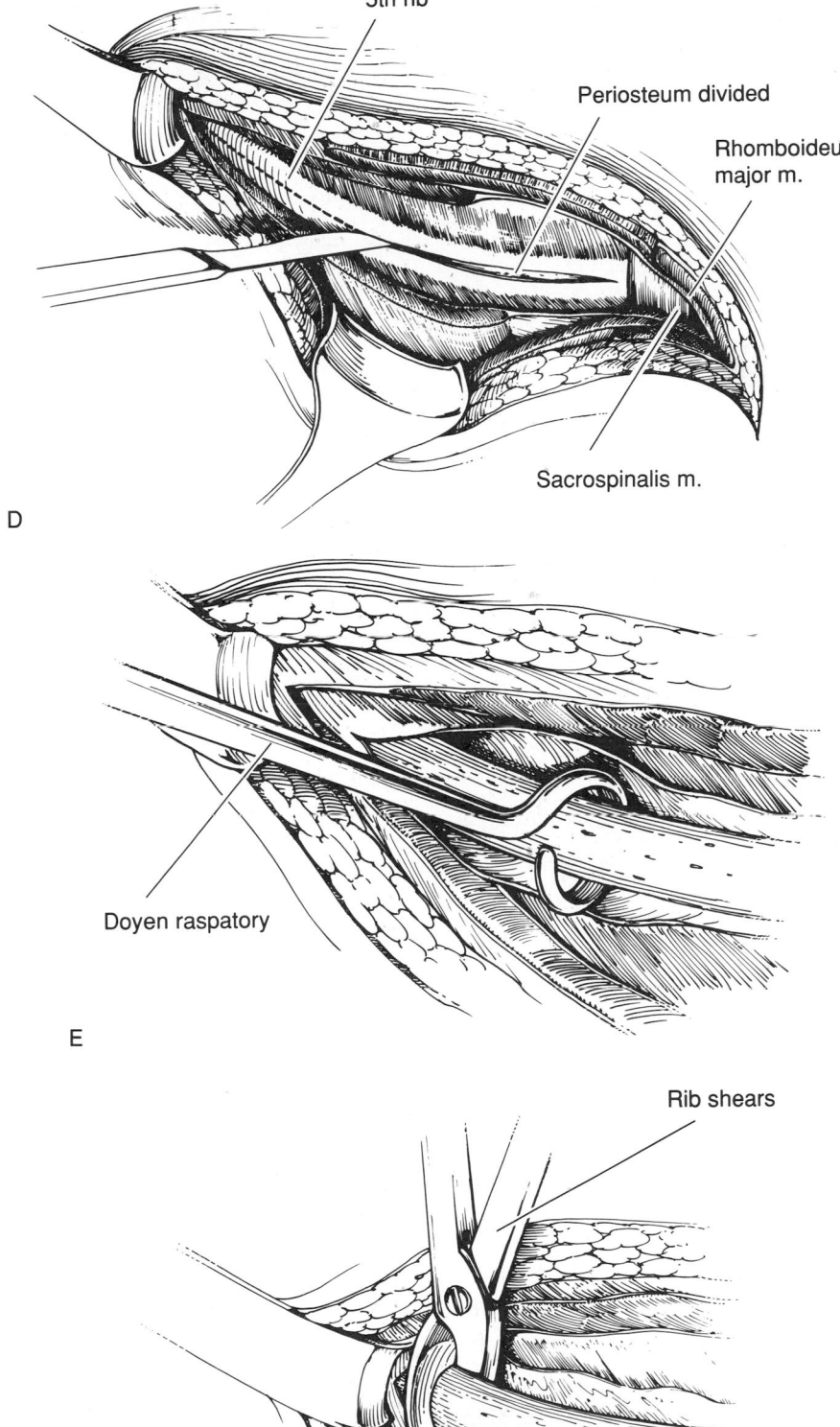

D

5th rib

Periosteum divided

Rhomboideus major m.

Sacrospinalis m.

E

Doyen raspatory

F

Rib shears

Figure 8-3 (*Continued*).   **(D–F).**

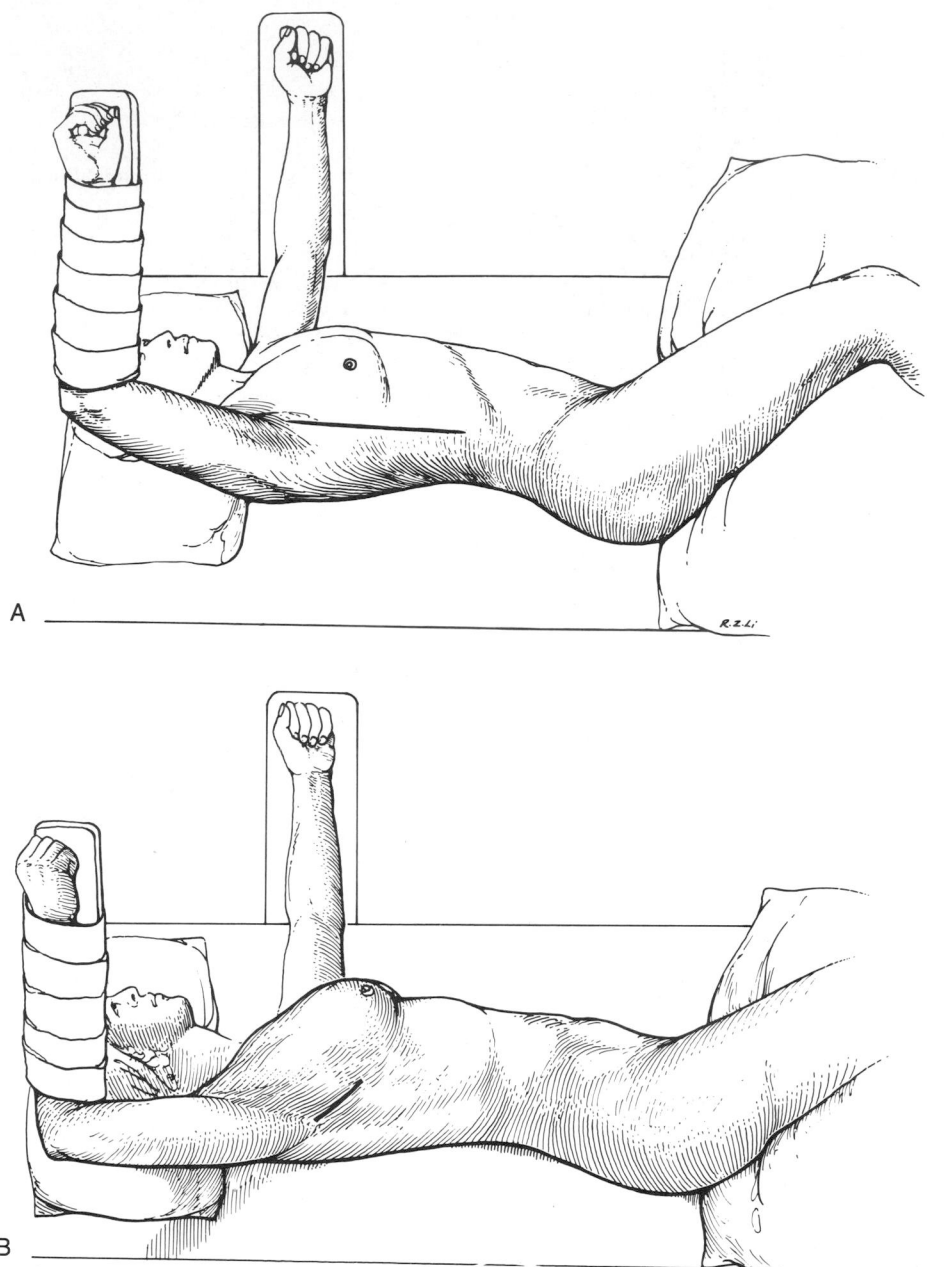

Figure 8-4. **(A&B)** Transaxillary thoracotomy incision (see text for explanation). (*Figure continues.*)

spreader or a Balfour abdominal retractor, placed at right angles to the intercostal retractor, retracts the muscles to improve intrathoracic exposure.

The intercostal space selected for entry into the pleural cavity depends on the planned intrathoracic procedure. The third intercostal space is best for operations on the sympathetic chain, apical lung lesions, and patent ductus arteriosus. The fourth intercostal space is used for wedge resection, upper lobectomy, pleurodesis, and biopsy or resection of a mediastinal lesion. The fifth intercostal space is employed

for lobectomy or pneumonectomy, while transthoracic hiatal hernia repair is performed through the sixth intercostal space.

Anterolateral Thoracotomy

Indications

An anterolateral thoracotomy can be used for a wide variety of thoracic procedures. The anterolateral incision may be used for resections of most segments of lung; however, expo-

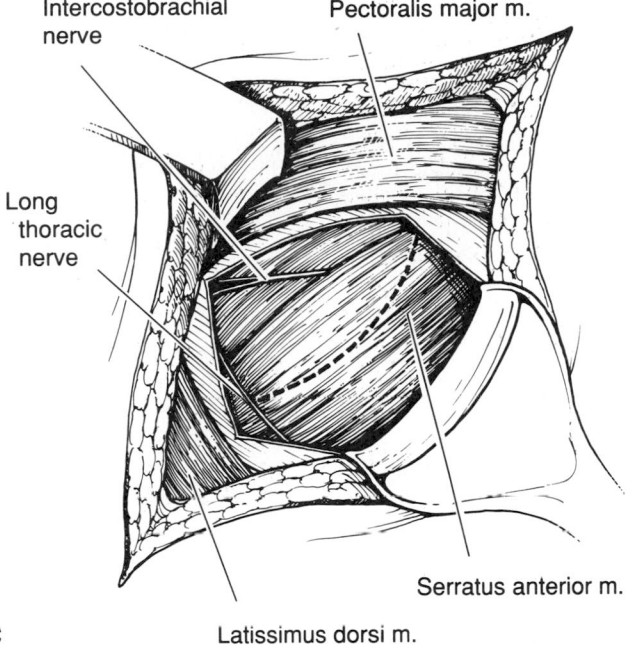

Intercostobrachial nerve

Pectoralis major m.

Long thoracic nerve

Serratus anterior m.

C

Latissimus dorsi m.

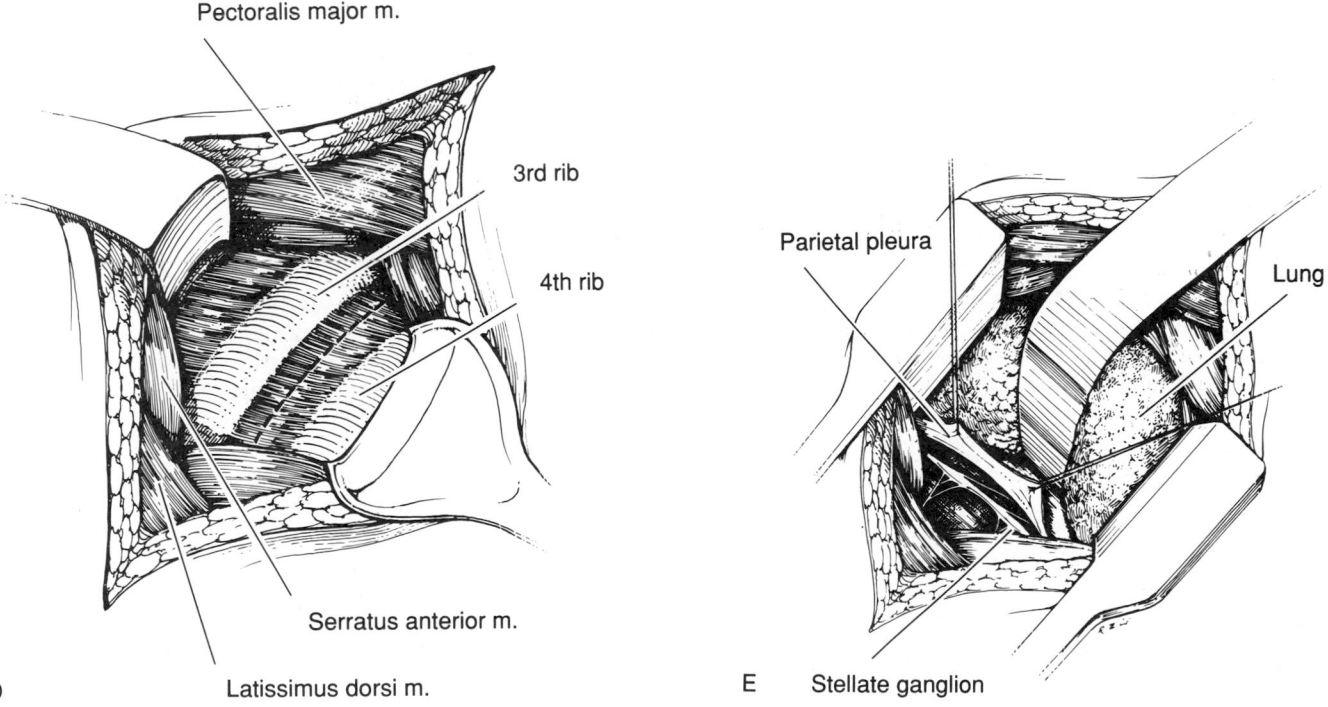

Pectoralis major m.

3rd rib

4th rib

Serratus anterior m.

D

Latissimus dorsi m.

Parietal pleura

Lung

E Stellate ganglion

Figure 8-4 (*Continued*). **(C–E).**

sure of the lower lobe may be difficult. This approach is particularly useful for right middle lobectomy. Total thoracic esophagectomy can readily be accomplished through a right anterior thoracotomy.

Position

The patient is placed in a supine position, and the operative side is elevated 20 to 45 degrees with use of a padded sandbag placed behind the buttocks and back (Fig. 8-5A). A wide strip of adhesive tape is passed across the hips to the edges of the operating table to secure the patient's position. The arm of the operative side should be flexed at the elbow, internally rotated at the shoulder, and placed behind the small of the back. This last maneuver reduces the necessity of dividing any fibers of the latissimus dorsi or serratus anterior muscle.

Incision

An anterolateral thoracotomy is performed through a curved submammary incision extending from the sternum anteriorly to the midaxillary line at the level of the fourth or fifth intercostal space (Fig. 8-5A). The skin incision is carried down through the subcutaneous tissue and superficial fascia until the superficial pectoral fascia overlying the pectoralis major muscle and the fascia over the serratus anterior muscle are exposed (Fig. 8-5B). The superficial pectoral fascia and the pectoralis major muscle are divided with electrocautery over the selected interspace. At the lateral end of the wound the pectoralis minor muscle is sectioned, and a portion of the serratus anterior muscle may have to be divided in the direction of its fibers to achieve exposure (Fig. 8-5C). In women it may be necessary to reflect the lower portion of the breast off the superficial pectoral fascia and pectoralis major muscle in order to reach the desired interspace level.

The intrathoracic fascia, endothoracic fascia, and parietal pleura are opened, and the pleural cavity is entered (Fig. 8-5D). The internal mammary vessels are ligated and divided at the anterior end of the wound as they pass behind the costal cartilages 1 cm lateral to the sternum. The wound margins are retracted with a rib spreader to provide exposure of the thoracic contents. Further exposure can be gained with this incision in several ways. Disarticulation of the chondrosternal joint at the anterior margin of the incision permits greater exposure anteriorly. Further exposure can be achieved by extending the incision across the midline and dividing the sternum horizontally. With the sternum divided and retracted, wide exposure of the mediastinum is achieved.

Dartevelle, et al. (1993) described an anterior transcervical-thoracic approach for radical resection of T4 Pancoast tumors that invade the cervical structures of the thoracic inlet. With this technique a large, L-shaped incision is made, with the vertical and horizontal arms following the anterior border of the sternocleidomastoid muscle and the inferior border of the internal half of the clavicle. The sternal attachments of the sternocleidomastoid muscle are divided, and the medial portion of the clavicle is resected to gain access.

Median Sternotomy

Indications

A median sternotomy is most commonly used in open heart surgery. This incision has long been used for exposure of the anterior mediastinum, particularly for anterior mediastinal tumors and thymectomy. Some tracheal tumors or stenoses require a median sternotomy incision to allow satisfactory operative exposure for resection. Bilateral pulmonary resections and combined cardiac and pulmonary operations are possible through this incision (Cooper, et al., 1978; Meng, et al., 1980; Takita, et al., 1977).

Position

The patient lies in a supine position on the operating table (Fig. 8-6A). The arms may be abducted and placed on arm boards, or they may be secured at the patient's sides. Movement of the head and neck should not be so restricted by the operative drapes or anesthesia equipment as to prevent extension or flexion; flexion of the neck may be of particular importance in tracheal resections.

Incision

The median sternotomy incision extends in the midline from the suprasternal notch to a point midway between the xiphoid and the umbilicus (Fig. 8-6A). This incision runs perpendicular to both Langer's lines and the crease lines, causing gaping of the wound edges and occasional hypertrophic scars. The skin incision is carried down through the subcutaneous tissue and superficial fascia to the superficial pectoral fascia overlying the sternal origins of the pectoralis major muscles and the linea alba. In the caudal portion of the wound the linea alba is divided, exposing the preperitoneal fat. Cephalad, the sternal origins of the two sternocleidomastoid muscles can be seen. The suprasternal space is a slitlike space between the two layers of the deep cervical fascia in the midline; it extends 2 to 3 cm above the suprasternal notch. Lying within the suprasternal space is the jugular arch, a vein of varying size that joins the two anterior jugular veins across the midline. To avoid troublesome bleeding, care should be taken to control the jugular arch at this stage of the median sternotomy incision.

With electrocautery the pectoral fascia and anterior periosteum of the sternum are divided in the midline. As the pectoral fascia and anterior periosteum of the sternum are divided, a nearly constant vein crossing the upper part of the xiphoid cartilage will be sectioned; this can result in a remarkable amount of bleeding at times.

The sternum is divided in the midline with a reciprocating electric saw, such as the Sarns sternal saw, a labor-saving device that allows rapid sectioning of the sternum (Fig. 8-6B). This saw has a footpad, which is placed behind the manubrium at the suprasternal notch. With the surgeon holding the saw in both hands and exerting upward traction to hold the footpad snugly against the posterior aspect of the sternum, the sternum is sectioned along the line made by the

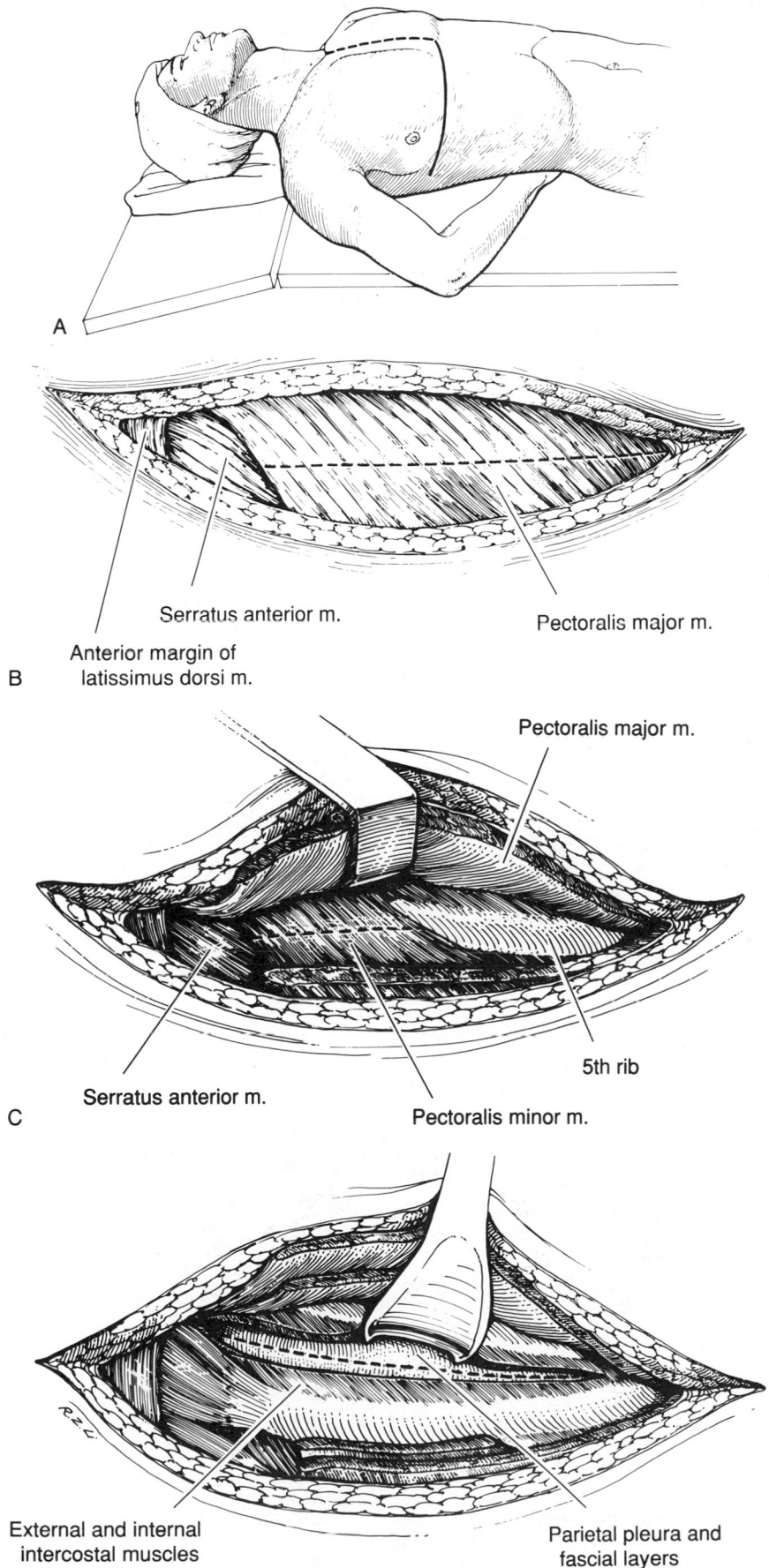

A

Serratus anterior m.

Pectoralis major m.

Anterior margin of
latissimus dorsi m.

B

Pectoralis major m.

5th rib

Serratus anterior m.

Pectoralis minor m.

C

External and internal
intercostal muscles

Parietal pleura and
fascial layers

D

Figure 8-5. (A–D) Anterolateral thoracotomy incision (see text for explanation).

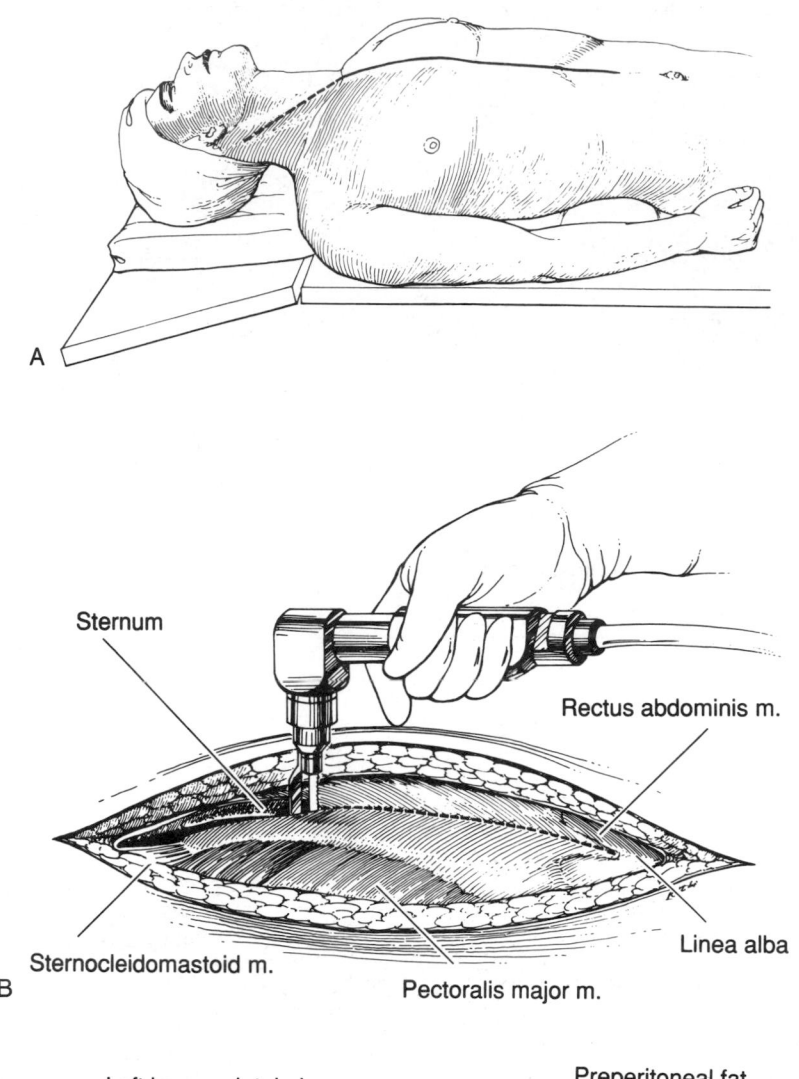

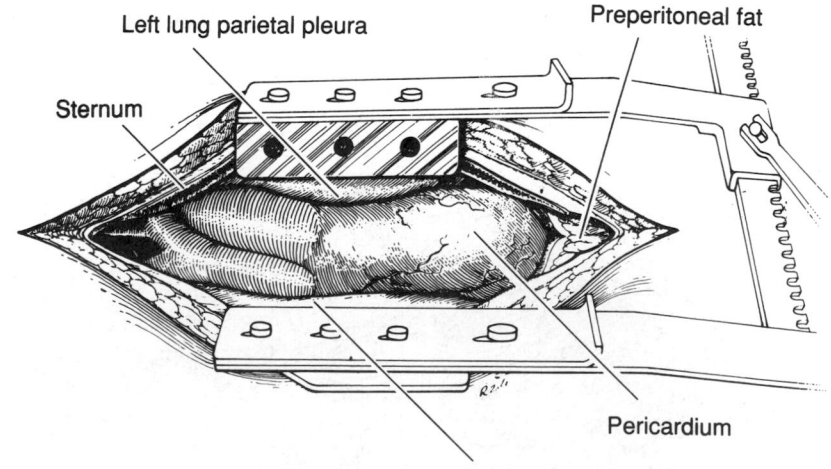

Figure 8-6. **(A–C)** Median sternotomy incision (see text for explanation).

electrocautery unit in dividing the anterior periosteum. In a patient who has had no previous mediastinal surgery and no lesion grossly distorting the mediastinal structures, the reciprocating elecric saw is a safe instrument to use in dividing the sternum provided that the footpad is kept firmly against the posterior aspect of the sternum. Positive pressure ventilation is discontinued during division of the sternum to reduce the risk of entering the pleural cavity. A pleural cavity, usually on the right side, may be opened occasionally with the electric saw. This is usually of little consequence other than requiring tube drainage at the conclusion of the operative procedure.

Alternative methods of dividing the sternum include use of either the Gigli saw or the Lebsche knife. To use the Gigli saw, a retrosternal tract is fashioned by blunt dissection, and the saw wire is passed down behind the sternum with a long-handled instrument. With the wire in place, the handles are attached, and the sternum is divided by applying a short back-and-forth motion to the saw wire. The Lebsche knife is a chisel with a footpad, or runner, similar to that on the sternal saw. The sternum is divided starting at the xiphoid end; the footpad is placed behind the sternum, and the back of the knife is struck with a mallet while upward traction is exerted on the knife handle. When the patient has had a prior sternotomy or a tumor lies immediately below the sternum, an oscillating sternal saw may be required to allow more gradual and precise control of the depth of the sternal incision.

After the sternum is divided, bone wax may be pressed into the marrow to seal the raw edges and prevent bleeding from this site. Both the anterior and posterior periosteal margins are searched for bleeding vessels; these are coagulated before the operation is continued. A number of sternal retractors are available to open the sternum widely to provide exposure of the underlying contents; it is best to use one with broad, shallow blades that will not cut into the sternum and damage it. Before the sternum can be widely retracted, it is often necessary to divide some of the anterior diaphragmatic fibers, to mobilize the brachiocephalic vein, or to open the pericardium (Fig. 8-6C).

Anterior Flap Incision

Indications

Excellent exposure of the upper mediastinum can be achieved by combining an anterolateral thoracotomy and an upper median sternotomy incision; procedures on the trachea, aortic arch, or its major branches can be performed by using this approach.

Position

The patient lies in a supine position with the arms secured at the sides, the neck extended slightly, and the head supported by a padded oval rest. Some surgeons prefer the patient's head to be rotated laterally away from the operative side.

Incision

The incision begins 4 to 6 cm above the suprasternal notch at the anterior border of the sternocleidomastoid muscle on the operative side; it runs down the anterior border of the sternocleidomastoid muscle to the manubrium and then follows the midline down the sternum before curving laterally over the second or third intercostal space to the anterior axillary line. In the cervical portion of the wound the incision is carried down through the platysma muscle until the deep cervical fascia investing the sternocleidomastoid muscle is revealed. Over the sternum and laterally over the intercostal space the skin incision is deepened until the superficial pectoral fascia is reached. The deep cervical fascia and the superficial pectoral fascia are opened. Care should be taken to control the anterior jugular vein running along the anterior border of the sternocleidomastoid muscle and the jugular arch lying in the suprasternal space. The pectoralis major muscle is divided by electrocautery. Entry through the deep layer of the thoracic wall is made next, as described for the anterolateral thoracotomy and median sternotomy incisions, and the pleural cavity is entered. The internal mammary vessels are isolated and tied with 2–0 silk. The anterior periosteum is incised over the manubrium and sternum down to the level of the intercostal space incision. The interclavicular ligament is divided with cautery, the sternum is sectioned with the sternal saw vertically in the midline from the suprasternal notch to the level of the intercostal incision, and the saw is then guided laterally out to the intercostal space.

This incision creates a large flap of tissue, which includes portions of the anterior chest wall, pectoral girdle, and cervical muscles. Acting as a hinge, this tissue flap can be retracted open to expose the upper mediastinal structures. A shorter version of the incision, which divides the sternum as described but does not include the lateral extension of the skin incision, provides good access to the superior mediastinum.

Transsternal Bilateral Thoracotomy (Clamshell Thoracotomy)

Indications

The transsternal bilateral thoracotomy incision was used as the standard approach to the pericardial contents in the early years of open heart surgery until it was replaced by the less traumatic median sternotomy. This incision is currently used for bilateral lung transplantation, resection of bilateral pulmonary metastases, pericardiectomy, or resection of a posterior ventricular aneurysm. It may also be a useful incision for trauma or for cardiac surgery in the patient with a tracheostomy (Marshall, et al., 1988).

Incision

With the patient supine with the arms abducted on arm boards, a transsternal bilateral thoracotomy is performed through a curvilinear bilateral submammary incision extending from the midaxillary lines across the anterior aspect of the chest at the level of the fourth intercostal space. The skin incision is carried down to the superficial pectoral fascia overlying the pectoralis major muscles, the sternum, and the fascia overlying the serratus anterior muscles at the lateral ends of the wound. These fascial layers are divided with the pectoralis major muscles. The portions of serratus anterior muscles that require division in this incision can be split in the direction of their fibers.

The deep layer of the thoracic wall is exposed at the level of the fourth intercostal space. The intercostal muscles and pleura are divided, with avoidance of injury to the lung. The internal mammary vessels are isolated at the anterior end of each intercostal space, tied with 2–0 silk, and sectioned.

The anterior periosteum of the sternum is divided horizontally with the electrocautery at the level of the fourth intercostal space. The Gigli saw wire is passed behind, and the sternum is divided with a Gigli or reciprocating saw. It is useful to offset the sternal tables by beveling the incision to allow a more stable closure. This can be accomplished by tipping the sternal saw to a 45-degree angle from the vertical plane. The sternal wires and the periosteal closure are thereby offset enough to prevent instability at the line of closure, an occasional annoying complication of simple transverse incision. As in the median sternotomy incision, the raw marrow edges of the divided sternum are sealed with bone wax, and any bleeding periosteal vessels are coagulated by electrocautery. The ribs are retracted bilaterally with rib spreaders.

Thoracoabdominal Incision

Indications

A thoracoabdominal incision converts the pleural and peritoneal cavities into a single space; this allows excellent exposure of the structures lying in the lower chest and upper abdomen. A right thoracoabdominal incision is useful in reconstructive procedures on the biliary tract, excision of the right lobe of the liver, portacaval shunt operations, and excision of bulky tumors of the right adrenal gland or kidney. Left thoracoabdominal incisions facilitate resection of the lower esophagus, total gastrectomy, removal of a large spleen, splenorenal vein shunt, and exposure of large adrenal, renal, or other retroperitoneal tumors. The thoracoabdominal incision provides excellent exposure for aortic surgery (Williams, et al., 1980; Corson, et al., 1987).

Incision

Thoracoabdominal incisions commonly overlie the fifth, sixth, seventh, or eighth intercostal space and run from the posterior axillary line across the costal arch toward the midline. The choice of interspace depends on the intrathoracic surgical mission. The skin incision is deepened through the subcutaneous tissue and superficial fascia until the fasciae overlying the latissimus dorsi, serratus anterior, and external oblique muscles are revealed. Anteriorly, the aponeurosis of the external oblique muscle and the anterior rectus sheath are exposed and divided. At the posterior end of the incision, a portion of the latissimus dorsi and serratus anterior muscles is divided if necessary. The external oblique is divided in the direction of its fibers.

The internal oblique muscle and the posterior rectus sheath are exposed and divided. The intercostal space for entry into the chest is selected, and the intercostal structures are divided as in a posterolateral thoracotomy incision. Care must be taken to avoid injuring the lung as the pleural cavity is entered. In the anterior portion of the wound the interal oblique muscle is divided at right angles to the direction of its fibers, exposing the underlying transversus abdominis muscle.

The costal margin is sectioned in the line of the incision. A 2- to 3-cm section of the costal arch should be resected to prevent a "clicking" sensation caused by overriding of the costal arch ends in the postoperative wound. The transversus abdominis muscle, posterior rectus sheath, and peritoneum are divided as the abdominal cavity is entered. A rib spreader is used to retract the margins of the chest portion of the wound; this reveals the diaphragm, which is divided circumferentially approximately 1 in. from the chest wall. Circumferential division of the diaphragm allows excellent exposure and preserves phrenic function. A self-retaining Balfour retractor can then be used to retract the abdominal wound margins to expose the desired operative site.

Drainage of the Pericardium

Pericardial drainage is indicated in patients with pericardial effusions causing tamponade and in those with purulent pericarditis. It may be performed through the subxiphoid approach, through the left anterolateral approach, or thorascopically.

Subxiphoid Approach

The subxiphoid route provides expeditious and safe access to the pericardium (Prager, et al., 1982; Larrieu, et al., 1986; Hankins, et al., 1980). Drainage through this incision can usually be performed under local anesthesia. If necessary, this incision can be extended into a standard median sternotomy.

Indications

Subxiphoid thoracotomy provides limited access to the anterior mediastinum and heart within the pericardial cavity for diagnostic and therapeutic procedures. The primary indications for this incision are (1) creation of a pericardial window for relief of pericardial tamponade produced by malignant tumors, infective pericarditis, or renal failure; (2) diagnostic pericardial biopsy and or defibrillators; (3) insertion of permanent epicardial pacemaker leads (Arom, et al., 1977; Santos and Frater, 1977; Stewart, 1974). It is our procedure of choice for initial drainage of the pericardium.

Incision

With the patient supine, a 10-cm vertical midline skin incision centered over the xiphoid process is fashioned, extending from the caudal end of the sternum toward the umbilicus (Fig. 8-7). The subcutaneous fat and superficial fascia are divided to expose the caudal end of the sternum, the xiphoid process, and the linea alba at the caudal end of the wound. The linea alba is divided, and the tip of the xiphoid process is grasped with a Kocher clamp. While retracting the process

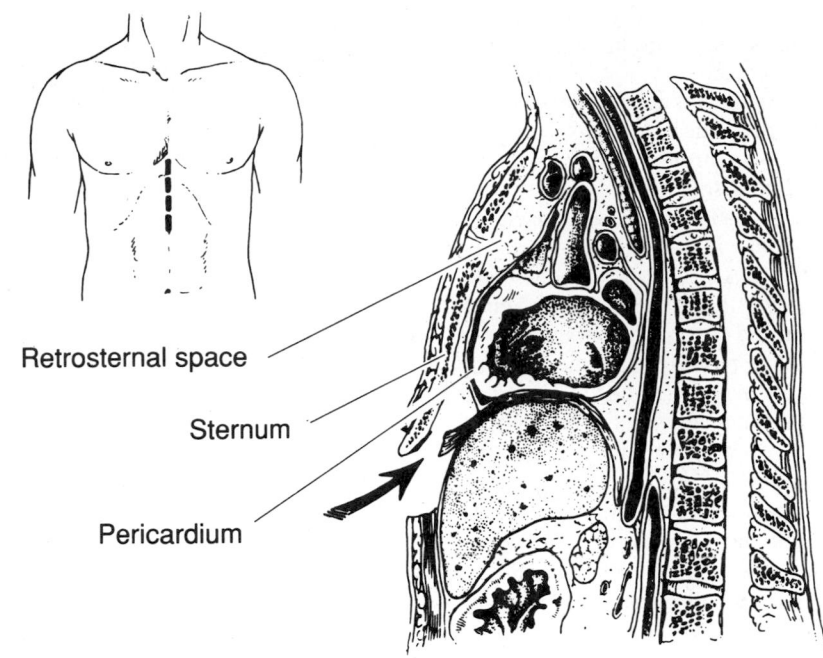

Figure 8-7. Skin incision for subxiphoid thoracotomy. Access to pericardium and retrosternal space.

upward, a plane of dissection is developed along the posterior perichondrium, freeing it from the preperitoneal fat. The xiphoid may be removed or divided. The communicating vein between the two internal mammary veins lies across the anterior aspect of the xiphoid process and should be controlled. Two narrow, right-angled retractors (Army-Navy) are placed beneath the rectus abdominis muscle attachments to the sternum, allowing the assistant to lift the sternum upward. A plane of dissection is continued along the posterior periosteum of the sternum. The diaphragmatic attachments to the sternum are cut with the electrocautery, exposing the pericardium and anterior mediastinum (Fig. 8-7).

Anterolateral Approach for Pericardial Drainage

With the patient positioned as described above for an anterolateral thoracotomy incision, the pericardium is approached through a left anterolateral thoracotomy incision in the fourth or fifth intercostal space. Drains are placed in the pericardial sac and pleural cavity. Care must be taken not to leave cartilage denuded of its perichondrium or bone denuded of its periosteum if purulent material is being drained, as necrosis and sequestration may result.

Thoracoscopy

Video-assisted thoracoscopy has become a popular method for pericardial drainage. The pericardium can be examined and opened widely with use of this technique, and pericardial window drainage or extensive pericardiectomy can be performed. Despite the recent interest in this technique, transxiphoid pericardial drainage remains our method of choice, as this procedure can be performed rapidly with local or general anesthesia and is no more painful than the thoraco-

scopic approach. Single-lung anesthesia is not required for the collapse of the lung.

INCISIONS FOR UPPER DORSAL SYMPATHECTOMY

Anterior Approach

Indications

The anterior approach was the first route advocated for reaching the upper thoracic sympathetic ganglia and exploring the neurovascular structures in the costoclavicular space. Through this incision a scalenotomy and resection of a cervical or first thoracic rib can be performed with decompression of the subclavian artery and brachial plexus in the costoclavicular space. The advantages of the anterior approach incision have been reviewed by Nanson (1957). However, it is a confining incision, and vital structures leading to the arm and diaphragm are in some jeopardy. An excess of stellate ganglion is often removed through this incision, which produces Horner syndrome.

Position

The patient is placed supine with the head elevated slightly and rotated away from the operative side. The arm on the operative side is secured to the operating table on an armboard so that the shoulder is held down firmly against the table.

Incision

The incision for the anterior approach is placed parallel to and 1 cm above the clavicle. The medial end of the incision is just cephalad to the clavicular head; the lateral extent of the incision depends on the anticipated procedure. If a scalenotomy and upper dorsal sympathectomy are planned, an 8-cm incision above the medial end of the clavicle is sufficient. If a rib resection is undertaken, the skin incision should extend nearly the length of the clavicle.

The skin incision is carried down through the subcutaneous tissue, superficial fascia, and platysma muscle. The superficial layer of the deep cervical fascia is incised, and the clavicular head of the sternocleidomastoid muscle is divided. The external jugular vein and fat pad lying superficial to the scalenus anterior muscle are exposed; the external jugular vein is tied and divided. At the lateral end of the incision, the inferior belly of the omohyoid muscle is retracted laterally. For rib resection the omohyoid muscle may be divided. The prescalene fat pad is dissected off the scalenus anterior muscle to reveal the phrenic nerve, which is carefully preserved. Retraction at the medial end of the incision reveals the medial edge of the scalenus anterior muscle and the internal jugular vein. For scalenotomy the phrenic nerve is retracted gently off the anterior aspect of the scalenus anterior muscle.

To perform an upper dorsal sympathectomy following the scalenotomy, the subclavian artery is retracted downward and Sibson's fascia in the base of the wound is incised to permit entry into the extrapleural space. Adequate retraction of the subclavian artery may require that the thyrocervical trunk be tied and divided. With blunt dissection, the parietal pleura is stripped down posteriorly off the vertebral bodies and posterior thoracic wall to the neck of the third rib. The sympathetic chain overlies the necks of the ribs.

Axillary Approach

Indications

The axillary approach, as popularized by Atkins (1954), can be used for either upper dorsal sympathectomy or first rib resection. The advantages of the axillary approach for sympathectomy include (1) the simplicity of the incision, in that no large muscle of the middle layer of the thoracic wall must be divided; (2) the accuracy of sympathectomy afforded by the excellent exposure of the sympathetic chain; (3) the ease with which bleeding from intercostal vessels at the dissection site can be controlled; and (4) the fact that the axillary incision when healed is hidden by the arm.

Position

After induction of general anesthesia, the patient is placed and secured in a lateral position, as described for a posterolateral thoracotomy (Fig. 8-3A). The arm on the operative side is abducted 90 degrees at the shoulder, flexed at the elbow, and supported on an arm stand (Fig. 8-4A or B).

Incision

The skin incision is made in the line of the second intercostal space; it extends posteriorly to the edge of the latissimus dorsi and anteriorly to the pectoralis major muscle (Fig. 8-4B). Rarely, some fibers of the pectoralis major and latissimus dorsi muscles will have to be divided to achieve adequate exposure. The incision is carried down through the subcutaneous tissue and superficial fascia until the serratus anterior muscle is exposed overlying the third intercostal space. The long thoracic nerve is exposed as it lies on the serratus anterior muscle at the posterior end of the incision; this nerve must be preserved to avoid a winged scapula deformity postoperatively. The intercostobrachial nerve can be seen emerging from the second intercostal space (Fig. 8-4C).

To enter the pleural cavity for an upper dorsal sympathectomy or pulmonary resection through this incision, the serratus anterior muscle overlying the third intercostal space is split in the direction of its fibers. The intercostal structures are divided, and the pleural cavity is entered (Fig. 8-4D). A small rib spreader is placed to retract the ribs. The lung is retracted, and the sympathetic chain is exposed as it lies against the necks of the ribs. The parietal pleura overlying the sympathetic chain is opened, and the sympathectomy is performed (Fig. 8-4E).

Thoracoscopic Upper Dorsal Sympathectomy

Video-assisted thoracoscopic surgery has generally replaced the open operative approach for upper dorsal sympathectomy. With video surgery the sympathetic chain can readily be exposed and resected or ablated with laser (Massad, et al., 1991).

The technique of incision for mediastinoscopy, anterior mediastinotomy, pleural drainage, tracheotomy, and treatment of thoracic outlet syndrome are described in the chapters discussing their application.

REFERENCES

Adams F: The Genuine Works of Hippocrates. London, 1849

Arom KV, Richardson JD, Webb G et al.: Subxiphoid pericardial window in patients with suspected traumatic pericardial tamponade. Ann Thorac Surg 23:545, 1977

Atkins TIJB: Sympathectomy by the axillary approach. Lancet 1:538, 1954

Baeza OR, Foster ED: Vertical axillary thoracotomy: a functional and cosmetically appealing incision. Ann Thorac Surg 22:287, 1976

Becker RM, Munro DD: Transaxillary minithoracotomy: the optimal approach for certain pulmonary and mediastinal lesions. Ann Thorac Surg 22:254, 1976

Bethencourt DM, Holmes EC: Muscle-sparing posterolateral thoracotomy. Ann Thorac Surg 45:337, 1988

Boyd AD, Gonzalez LL, Altemeier WA: Disruption of chest wall closure following thoracotomy. J Thorac Cardiovasc Surg 52:47, 1966

Cooper JD, Nelems JB, Pearson FG: Extended indications for median sternotomy in patients requiring pulmonary resection. Ann Thorac Surg 26:413, 1978

Corson JD, Leather RP, Shah DM et al.: Extraperitoneal aortic bypass with exclusion of the intact infra-renal aortic aneurysm: the in-situ management of aortic aneurysms. J Cardiovasc Surg 28:274, 1987

Dartevelle FG, Chapelier AR, Macchiarini P et al.: Anterior transcervical-thoracic approach for radical resection of lung tumors invading the thoracic inlet. J Thorac Cardiovasc Surg 105:1025, 1993

Dulac: De la Blessure des Artères Intercostales dans les Plaies de Poitrine, et particulièrement dans la Paracentèse. Thesis, Univ. Paris, 1874; quoted in Paget S: The Surgery of the Chest. p. 88. John Wright & Co., Bristol, England, 1896

Garlock JH: Combined abdominothoracic approach for carcinoma of cardia and lower esophagus. Surg Gynecol Obstet 83:737, 1946

Ginsberg RJ: Alternative (muscle-sparing) incisions in thoracic surgery. The First International Symposium of Thoracoscopic Surgery. Ann Thorac Surg 56:752, 1993

Hankins JR, Satterfield JR, Aisner J et al: Pericardial window for malignant pericardial effusion. Ann Thorac Surg 30:465, 1980

Heitmiller RF, Mathisen DJ: The French incision. p. 268. In Grillo HC, Austen WG, Wilkins EW Jr et al (eds): Current Therapy in Cardiothoracic Surgery. BC Decker, Toronto, 1989

Julian OC, Lopez-Belio M, Dye WS et al: The median sternal incision in intracardiac surgery with extracorporeal circulation: a general evaluation of its use in heart surgery. Surgery 42:753, 1957

Kittle CF: Which way in? The thoracotomy incision. Ann Thorac Surg 45:234, 1988

Larrieu AJ, Ghosh SC, Ablaza SG et al: Favorable results with the subxiphoid pericardial window technique, letter. J Thorac Cardiovasc Surg 91:639, 1986

Marshall WG Jr, Meng RL, Ehrenhaft JL: Coronary artery bypass grafting in patients with a tracheostomy: use of a bilateral thoracotomy incision. Ann Thorac Surg 46:465, 1988

Massad M, LoCicero J, Matano J et al: Endoscopic thoracic sympathectomy: evaluation of pulsatile laser, non-pulsatile laser, and radiofrequency-generated thermocoagulation. Lasers Surg Med 11:18, 1991

Massimiano P, Ponn RB, Toole AL: Transaxillary thoracotomy revisited. Ann Thorac Surg 45:559, 1988

McKneally MF: Lobectomy without a rib spreader, editorial. Ann Thorac Surg 54:2, 1992

Meng RL, Jensik RJ, Kittle CF et al: Median sternotomy for synchronous bilateral pulmonary operations. J Thorac Cardiovasc Surg 80:1, 1980

Milton H: Mediastinal surgery. Lancet 1, 872, 1897

Mitchell R, Angell W, Wuerflein R et al: Simplified lateral chest incision for most thoracotomies other than sternotomy. Ann Thorac Surg 22:284, 1976

Naef AP: The Story of Thoracic Surgery: Milestones and Pioneers. Huber, Toronto, 1990

Nanson EM: The anterior approach to upper dorsal sympathectomy. Surg Gynecol Obstet 104:118, 1957

Prager RL, Wilson CH, Bender HW Jr: The subxiphoid approach to pericardial disease. Ann Thorac Surg 34:6, 1982

Santos GH, Frater RWM: The subxiphoid approach in the treatment of pericardial effusion. Ann Thorac Surg 23:467, 1977

Sauerbruch F: Zur Pathologie des offenen Pneumothorax und die Grundlagen meines Verfahrens zu seiner Ausschaltung. Mitteil Grenzgeb Med Chir 13:399, 1904

Stewart S: Placement of the sutureless epicardial pacemaker lead by the subxiphoid approach. Ann Thorac Surg 18:308, 1974

Takita H, Merrin C, Didolkar MS et al: The surgical management of multiple lung metastases. Ann Thorac Surg 24:359, 1977

Van Winkle W Jr, Hastings JC: Considerations in the choice of suture materials for various tissues. Surg Gynecol Obstet 135:113, 1972

Wada J, Ajika H, Kitano I: Left axillary incision (minithoracotomy) for PDA division. Ann Thorac Surg 26:189, 1978

Tuffier T: De la resection du sommet du poumon. Semin Med Paris 2:202, 1891

Tuffier T, Hallion: Régulation de la pression intrabronchique et de la narcose. Compt Rend Soc Biol 3:1086, 1896

Williams GM, Ricotta J, Zinner M et al: The extended retroperitoneal approach for treatment of extensive atherosclerosis of the aorta and renal vessels. Surgery 88:846, 1980

9

VIDEO-ASSISTED THORACIC SURGERY

Robert J. Keenan
Rodney J. Landreneau
Martin F. McKneally

INTRODUCTION

Improvements in video technology and endoscopic surgical equipment have fostered a resurgence of interest in thoracoscopy. These advances have allowed thoracic surgeons to move beyond use of the thoracoscope for simple pleural biopsy or management of pleural effusions to more complex video-assisted thoracic surgery (VATS) as therapy for diseases classically managed by open thoracotomy. Through ports and small but not rib-spreading incisions, pulmonary, mediastinal, and esophageal resections have been carried out with excellent visualization and without the need for large, disabling incisions. The general surgical and gynecologic literature suggests that postoperative pain and disability may be reduced by using video technology. This chapter discusses the basic operative setting and the positioning of endoscopic instruments and video equipment for various VATS procedures.

HISTORICAL NOTE

H. C. Jacobaeus, professor of medicine at the University of Stockholm, is generally credited with the first thoracoscopy using a rigid cystoscope introduced into the thoracic cavity through a small incision. His first description in the English literature (Jacobaeus, 1922) detailed an experience with lysis of pleural adhesions, drainage of empyemas, and biopsy of pleural tumors dating back to 1910. Thoracoscopy offered an exciting viewpoint into the pleural space without the need for a major surgical incision.

Widespread adoption of thoracoscopy in the United States was discouraged by leading thoracic surgeons of the time such as J. Alexander (1937), who admonished internists against performing the procedure after a patient died from uncontrolled pulmonary arterial hemorrhage. In Europe thoracoscopy continued to be performed for diagnosis of pleural tumors and effusions and for treatment of spontaneous pneumothorax. Its widest application was in the treatment of tuberculosis by collapse therapy. Interest in this procedure dwindled markedly with the advent of successful antituberculous therapy. By the early 1970s there was a resurgence of interest in thoracoscopy for malignant pleural and mediastinal disease and for the diagnosis and treatment of pleural effusions and empyemas. This interest led to the organization of an international symposium on thoracoscopy (Boutin, et al., 1981). Use of the mediastinoscope by Deslauriers, et al., (1976) and fiberoptic or rigid endoscopes by Lewis, et al., (1976) prompted a renewed interest in thoracoscopy by thoracic surgeons in North America. The application of video technology and improvements in endoscopic instrumentation in the 1980s led to widespread adoption of video endoscopy in the fields of gynecology and orthopedics. The development of laparoscopic cholecystectomy and its rapid diffusion into practice spurred the development of present-day VATS procedures.

HISTORICAL READINGS

Alexander J: The Collapse Therapy of Pulmonary Tuberculosis. p. 313. Charles C Thomas, Springfield, IL, 1937

Boutin C, Viallat JR, Cargnino P, Farisse P: Indications actuelles de la thoracoscopie. Etude préliminaire. Rev Franc Mal Respir 9:309, 1981

Deslauriers J, Beaulieu M, Dufour C et al: Mediastinopleuroscopy: A new approach to the diagnosis of intrathoracic diseases. Ann Thorac Surg 22:265, 1976

Jacobaeus HC: The practical importance of thoracoscopy in surgery of the chest. Surg Gynecol Obstet 34:289, 1922

Lewis RJ, Kunderman PJ, Sisler GE: Direct diagnostic thoracoscopy. Ann Thorac Surg 21:536, 1976

BASIC OPERATIVE SETTING AND GENERAL PRINCIPLES OF MANAGEMENT

VATS must be performed in an appropriate operating room environment that will allow the thoracic surgeon to convert to an open thoracotomy immediately should complications arise or difficulty in performing the procedure develop. The operating team must be familiar with standard thoracic surgical procedures before attempting VATS. Anesthesia personnel should be experienced in open thoracic procedures and well versed in the principles of single-lung ventilation as discussed by Benumof (1983). Since many VATS procedures can be accomplished in under 1 hour, short-acting intravenous drugs may be used to augment inhalational anesthetics. Immediately following confirmation of proper placement of the double-lumen endotracheal tube, the operative side should be isolated and opened to the outside atmosphere to initiate collapse of the lung. This maneuver avoids unnecessary delay in waiting for complete deflation.

The patient is positioned in a full lateral position with the thorax surgically prepared for conversion to an open thoracotomy if necessary. The table and viewing monitor(s) should be positioned to place the surgeons, patient, and video screen in a straight line for best orientation of instruments and pathology within the chest (Fig. 9-1). This positioning may require that anesthesia personnel be displaced from their usual position at the head of the table. Several general principles have been developed that simplify and expedite the VATS procedure.

Orientation

It is critically important to orient the surgeon, endoscopic instruments, camera, lung pathology, and video monitor during VATS procedures. The surgeon, camera, and instruments should all be looking in the same direction toward the pathol-

---

Basic Operative Setting and Instruments

General anesthesia in the operating room
(Double-lumen endotracheal tube preferred)
Open thoracotomy instrument tray available
    A reduced but adequate set should be open on the back table
Zero-degree thoracoscope
    A 10-mm operative scope is preferred with a 5-mm operative channel
High-resolution video monitor
    Two monitors preferably positioned on opposite sides of operating table for surgeon and assisting team. If one monitor is used, it is usually placed at the head of the table.
Two to five ports of intercostal operative access
Videoscopic instruments
    Endoscopic graspers, scissors, coagulator, and selected standard surgical instruments
Endoscopic staplers and clip appliers
Adequate suction and smoke evacuation system

---

ogy. The video monitor is placed so that the surgeon, camera, pathology, and screen are all aligned in a straight line (Fig. 9-2). This will avoid awkward handling of instruments due to the "mirror imaging" that results when the instruments are pointed toward the camera.

Initiating the Procedure

The VATS procedure is begun by choosing an appropriate intercostal space for insertion of the video thoracoscope to explore the hemithorax. The initial access site must be planned to visualize the lesion from an adequate distance for instrument manipulation. Posterior lesions are approached through a slightly anterior intercostal space access site; anterior lesions are approached through posterior axillary intercostal space sites. Careful review of the preoperative chest x-ray and computed tomography (CT) scans help to identify the three-dimensional location of the lesion within the hemithorax in order to decide which intercostal spaces are appropriate to place viewing and operating ports. The operating table should be tilted to allow gravity to assist displacement and retraction of the lung. The sixth or seventh intercostal space in the mid to posterior axillary line usually provides an unobstructed panoramic view of the entire hemithorax. Sharp dissection and direct digital exploration is used to rule out local pleural adhesions that can impede the introduction of the thoracoscope and potentially result in pulmonary injury (Fig. 9-3). Flimsy local adhesions can often be digitally separated. The presence of more extensive pleural symphysis may require repositioning the port to a different site. If extensive pleural fusion is found, thoracoscopy is abandoned and the procedure converted to an open thoracotomy.

Ports

A trocar port rather than an unprotected small incision should be used at the camera site to reduce lens smudging as the thoracoscope is introduced into the chest. Exploratory thoracoscopy is then performed. The relatively inferior and posterior initial intercostal placement of the thoracoscope assists in maintaining intrathoracic orientation as the mediastinum, lung surface, major pulmonary fissures, and apex of the thorax are viewed. The enhanced visibility of the entire thoracic cavity obtained by the video telescope is generally superior to the limited view obtained through an axillary, inframammary, or lateral thoracotomy (Daly, et al., 1991). When the initial thoracoscopic exploration of the pleural cavity is concluded, intercostal access for VATS instrumentation is developed under direct thoracoscopic vision. It is sometimes useful to insert a 20-gauge spinal needle at the proposed site of additional ports to visualize its intrathoracic position and ensure that the location is appropriate. In general, 10-mm ports should be inserted to give maximum flexibility for using the port for larger instruments or the camera.

Intercostal access sites should be positioned at a comfortable working distance from the pathology. The camera port must give sufficient visibility to see all instruments as they are being introduced into the chest and maneuvered into position. Stapling devices require insertion to a minimum depth of 30 to 60 mm before they can be opened. This is difficult if the access port is close to the lesion. A 10-mm

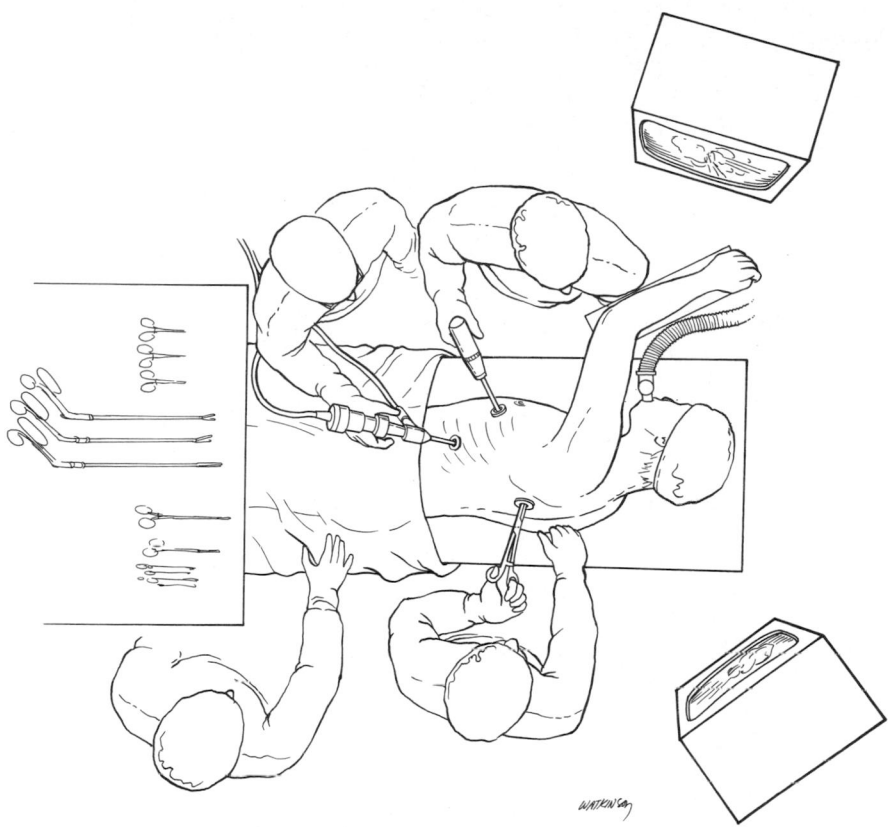

Figure 9-1. Orientation of patient and video equipment using two monitors. The operating team aligns itself depending on the intrathoracic location of the pathology. Alternatively, a single monitor, placed at the head of the bed, can be used. In this case, the anesthetic team takes a position to one side of the patient.

thoracoscope with a 5-mm operative channel is available, which provides the opportunity for "single stick" diagnostic thoracoscopy and may allow VATS procedures to be performed with one less intercostal access site.

Camera and Telescope

The camera operator, who may be the primary surgeon or an assistant, coordinates the manipulation of instruments used by all other surgeons and assistants. The use of anti-fogging agents, irrigation, and periodic warming of the thoracoscope shaft with hot saline solution are necessary to reduce fogging of the lens by condensation due to differences between the temperature within the thorax and the ambient temperature in the operating room.

The thoracoscope should periodically be retracted from a close-up, magnified image of the intrathoracic "target" to obtain a panoramic view of the operative field and to confirm a proper position of all intrathoracic instruments. This scanning maneuver is also used whenever an additional instrument is introduced into the thorax. The enhanced visualization of the target pathology is then regained once instrument alignment is achieved. It is best for the surgical team to position only one instrument at a time to avoid operative chaos.

Instruments

Most VATS procedures are performed with a variety of reusable instruments, including some taken straight from the open thoracotomy tray, such as standard operating scissors, ring forceps, and right angle clamps. There are some disposable endoscopic instruments, such as the endoscopic stapling devices and multiload endoscopic clip appliers, that are not available in reusable form. We prefer disposable endoscopic scissors for sharp dissection because of rapid dulling of presently available reusable endoscopic scissors. The present medical economic environment dictates judicious use of disposable instruments by active thoracoscopy programs.

Specimen Removal

A potential problem encountered with VATS procedures involves the removal of infected or malignant tissues from the thoracic cavity. These specimens should always be extracted by placing them in a sterile glove or a commercially available plastic-sleeved device introduced through one of the intercostal access sites. For larger specimens we have simply expanded one of the intercostal access incisions to 3 to 4 cm without spreading the ribs to allow extraction of the specimen.

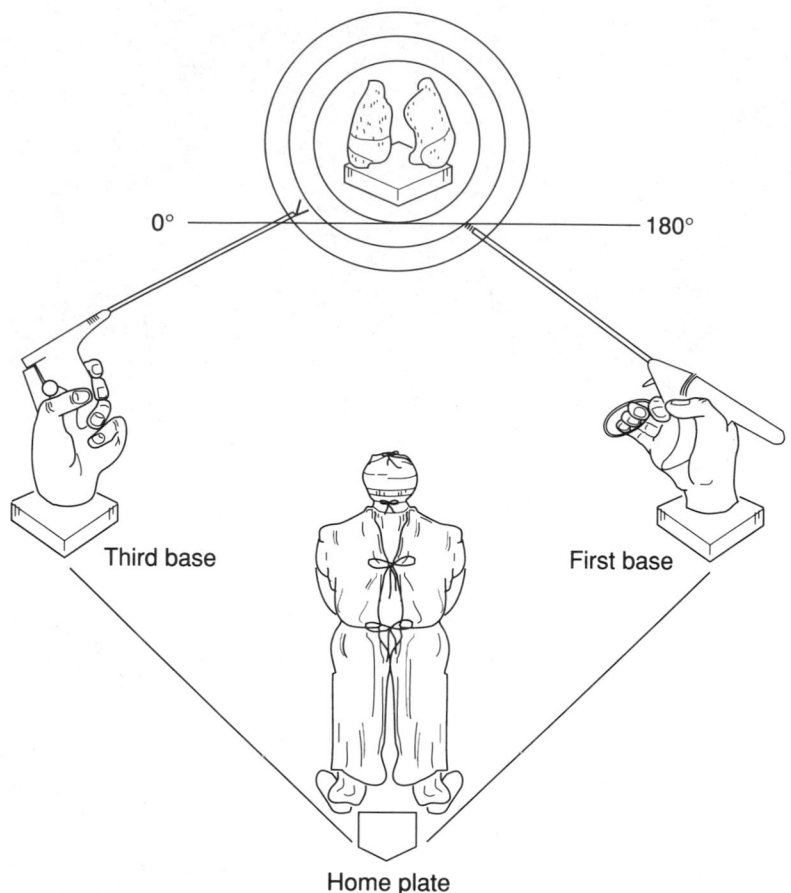

Figure 9-2. "Baseball diamond" concept for triangulation of the instruments and thoracoscope for stratgic visibility and manipulation of the target pathology. (From Landreneau RJ: Video-assisted surgery: basic technical concepts and intercostal approach strategies. Ann Thorac Surg 54:800, 1992, with permission.)

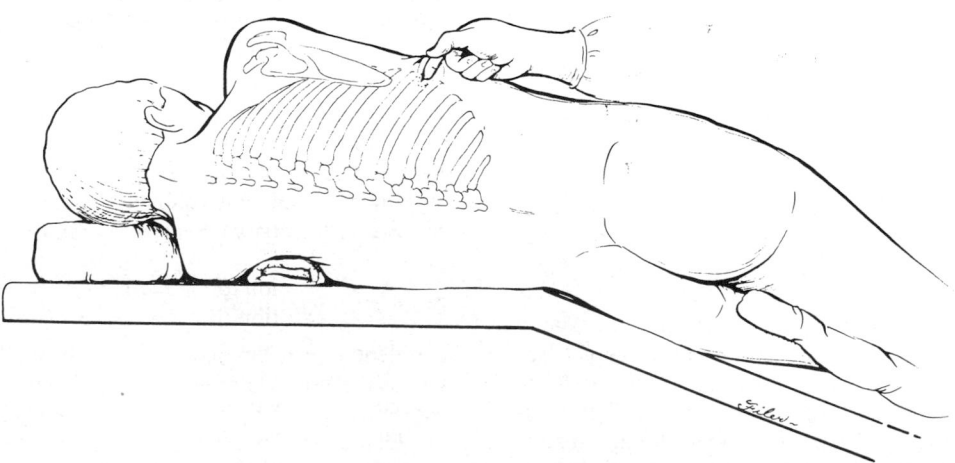

Figure 9-3. Patient in the right lateral decubitus position with digital exploration of the proposed initial trocar site to ensure that a free pleural space is present. (From Landreneau RJ: Video-assisted surgery: basic technical concepts and intercostal approach strategies. Ann Thorac Surg 54:800, 1992, with permission.)

Closure

Incisions should be inspected from within the chest for bleeding. They should be closed with care, with use of absorbable subcutaneous and subcuticular sutures.

SPECIFIC VATS APPLICATIONS

VATS Wedge Resections of the Lung

VATS wedge resection is well suited for the evaluation of diffuse infiltrative lung disease, yielding pulmonary tissue equivalent to that achieved through limited thoracotomy (Mack, et al., 1992; Landreneau, et al., 1992a). A standard intercostal access strategy is best for biopsy of diffuse infiltrative disease (Ferson, et al., 1993).

An initial camera site at the sixth or seventh intercostal space in the mid- to posterior axillary line offers excellent visualization of the hemithorax and pulmonary parenchyma. After exploration a second access site is chosen, usually in the fifth intercostal space along the anterior axillary line. These two sites align the instruments along the interlobar fissures, facilitating exposure and manipulation of most areas of the lung and application of the endoscopic stapler along a variety of parenchymal edges. The endoscopic stapler should be introduced through a trocar port to keep the jaws clean and avoid entanglement in subcutaneous tissues. The port should be located at a sufficient distance from the target lesion that the jaw mechanism of the stapler can be fully opened and freely maneuvered.

An operating thoracoscope frequently allows wedge resection to be accomplished with only two sites of intercostal space access. An endoscopic forceps, 5 mm in diameter, is introduced through the operative channel of the thoracoscope to grasp an appropriate site along the edge of the lung. The endoscopic stapler is then introduced through the second intercostal space site and positioned to begin the V wedge resection. The positions of the thoracoscope with forceps and stapler are then reversed to complete the V wedge resection. Alternatively, a third intercostal space access site through the posterior seventh to ninth intercostal space can be made to position the thoracoscope and directly view the endoscopic stapler and grasping forceps to confirm proper positioning.

A more flexible approach must be used for VATS resection of the indeterminate pulmonary nodule (Fig. 9-4). Careful examination of the preoperative CT scan of the chest is important prior to deciding on trocar port placement for VATS pulmonary nodular resection (Landreneau, et al., 1991; Daly, et al., 1991). Lesions deep within the substance of the parenchyma or on convex surfaces of the lung can be difficult to resect by using staplers alone. In these circumstances, excision using the neodymium-yttrium aluminum garnet (Nd:YAG) laser spares unnecessary resection of surrounding normal tissue (Keenan, et al., 1993). The laser fiber is introduced through one of the trocar ports or through the operating channel of the thoracoscope, with a smoke evacuator system inserted through another site.

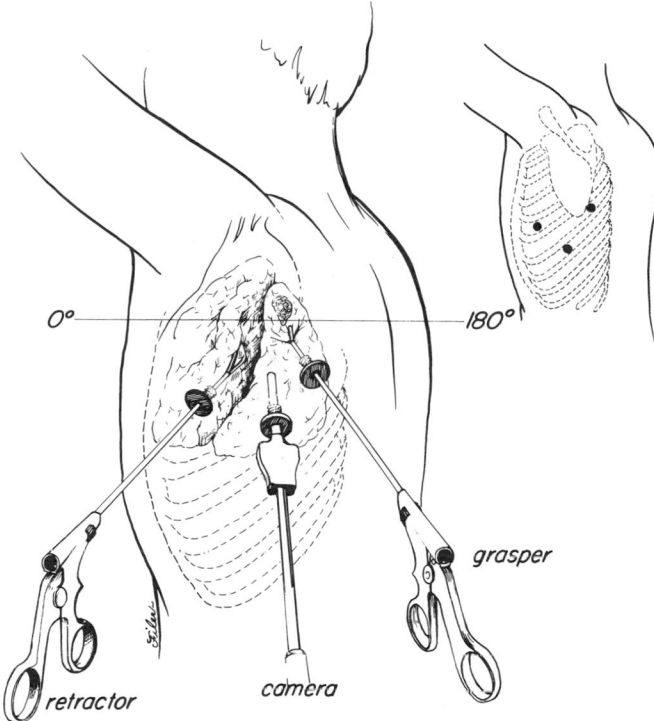

Figure 9-4. Typical positioning of the thoracoscopic instruments and thoracoscopic camera for an approach to a lesion in the superior segment of the left lower lobe of the lung. (From Landreneau RJ: Video-assisted surgery: basic technical concepts and intercostal approach strategies. Ann Thorac Surg 54:800, 1992, with permission.)

Bullectomy

Proper placement of instruments and the thoracoscope is critical for accurate VATS exploration and stapled resection of apical bullous disease (Hazelrigg, et al. 1993). The thoracoscopic camera is positioned through the sixth intercostal space along the midaxillary line (Fig. 9-5). Operating instruments are best introduced through trocar sites along the posterolateral fourth or fifth intercostal space in the area of the auscultatory triangle and at the lateral border of the pectoralis muscle in the fourth intercostal space. This instrument and camera positioning allows easy resection of bullous disease at the apex of the upper lobe and/or superior segment of the lower lobe. A mechanical pleurodesis or apical pleurectomy can be performed with use of these intercostal space access sites.

VATS resection for more diffuse bullous disease is gaining increased attention. Bullectomy has been reported by Wakabayashi (1993) using carbon dioxide and Nd:YAG lasers and by Lewis et al. (1993) using staplers and argon beam coagulation. Two or three trocar port sites located in the seventh intercostal space along the mid- to posterior axillary line and in the fifth intercostal space anteriorly provides exposure of most large bullae. Late development of bronchopleural fistula and poor definition of indications continue to be problems in this application of VATS.

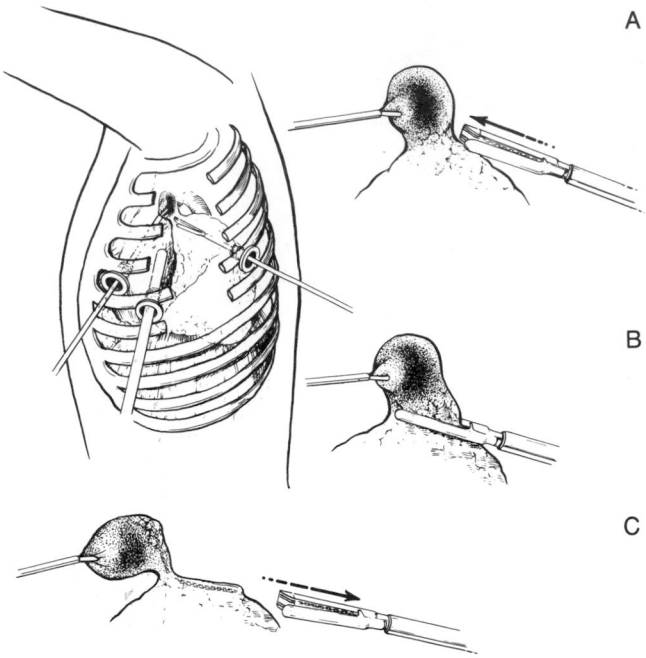

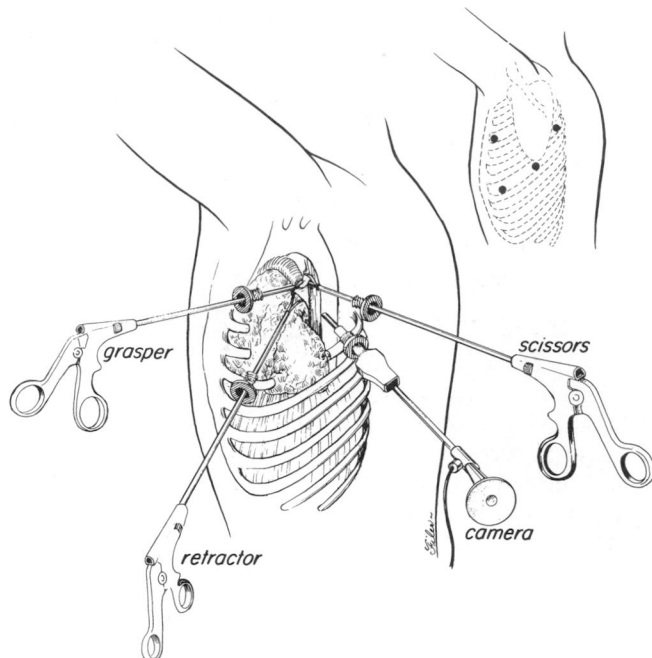

Figure 9-5. Thoracoscopic approach to left upper lobe apical bullous disease. **(A)** The bulla is identified and retracted with a grasper to facilitate placement of the endoscopic stapler. **(B)** The stapler is placed across the bulla to encompass a small amount of normal tissue. **(C)** Additional applications of the stapler may be required to complete the resection of the bulla. (From Landreneau RJ: Video-assisted surgery: basic technical concepts and intercostal approach strategies. Ann Thorac Surg 54:800, 1992, with permission.)

Figure 9-6. Thoracoscopic approach to the aorticopulmonary window or alternatively the subazygous and subcarinal lymph node group on the right. (From Landreneau RJ: Video-assisted surgery: basic technical concepts and intercostal approach strategies. Ann Thorac Surg 54:800, 1992, with permission.)

Lobectomy

VATS lobectomy is not recommended for the occasional or inexperienced thoracoscopic surgeon. Objective analyses of the morbidity, cost, and therapeutic effectiveness of VATS lobectomy versus open lobar resection will be required before the VATS approach can be considered a reasonable treatment option for most patients. Thoracoscopic ports are placed in the sixth or seventh intercostal space in the anterior to midaxillary line and in the auscultatory triangle for camera position and operating instruments. The anterior port is used later as a chest tube site. A small fourth or fifth intercostal space thoracotomy incision 6 to 10 cm in length is used without spreading the ribs to introduce standard instruments during the course of the dissection and to extract the resected lobe.

Mediastinal Nodes

VATS may be used as an adjunct to cervical mediastinoscopy for the staging of lower mediastinal lymph nodes and as an alternative to the Chamberlain anterior mediastinotomy to assess the aorticopulmonary window and subazygous lymph node regions (Fig. 9-6). Many surgeons use VATS routinely to assess these latter nodal stations in order to avoid the discomfort associated with resection of the costal cartilage

and the limited exposure that is gained when the mediastinoscope is inserted through the intercostal space.

The thoracoscope is introduced through the fifth or sixth intercostal space along the posterior axillary line. Second and third intercostal space access sites are created through the fifth intercostal space in the auscultatory triangle and along the anterior axillary line at the fourth intercostal space for dissecting instruments and the endoscopic clip applier. A seventh intercostal space access site, usually in the midaxillary line, is used to introduce a lung-retracting instrument and improve visibility to these nodal regions. The VATS approach offers consistently good access to these sometimes difficult nodal stations.

As an alternative, the video telescope can be placed in the second intercostal space incision used for anterior mediastinotomy, thus expanding visibility and allowing palpation and dissection through the same incision with standard instruments. The pleural space should be entered and a port in the fourth or fifth intercostal space used for retraction of the lung. This procedure is carried out in combination with mediastinoscopy when appropriate, with the patient in the supine position.

Mediastinal Masses

VATS techniques are easily adaptable for biopsy and occasionally for resection of some mediastinal masses (Lewis, et al., 1992; Landreneau, et al., 1992b; Landreneau, 1992c). The patient is positioned in the lateral thoracotomy position with the camera port located posteriorly for anterior masses and anteriorly for posterior lesions. The thoracoscope is best introduced through a fifth intercostal space site. For anterior masses, additional ports are placed in the second or third intercostal space in the midaxillary line and in the fifth or sixth intercostal space in the anterior axillary line. A fourth site of instrument access is often established through the seventh intercostal space in the mid- to anterior axillary line for the alternate positioning of scissors and graspers or to provide retraction of the lung during the course of the dissection.

For posterior neurogenic tumors located in the superior costovertebral recess, the thoracoscope is introduced through the fifth intercostal space at the midaxillary line, and additional ports for operating instruments are placed through the mid- to anterior axillary line at the third to fourth intercostal space. The table should be tilted in a face-down and foot-down direction for gravity displacement. Lung retraction is best achieved through a port located in the fourth or sixth intercostal space in the anterior axillary line.

Pericardium

Pericardiectomy is discussed in more detail in Chapter 56. The emergent treatment of pericardial tamponade should be carried out expeditiously by catheter pericardiocentesis or subxiphoid pericardial resection to avoid unnecessary delays for double-lumen endotracheal intubation and patient positioning.

VATS pericardiectomy is used instead of the subxiphoid pericardial window technique for elective decompression in patients requiring diagnosis and management of associated pleural or lung pathology. The thoracoscope and instrument placement is planned to approach the pericardium from slightly posterior and lateral fifth, seventh, and ninth intercostal space positions (Fig. 9-7). A posterolateral approach well away from the expanded pericardium is essential to give visibility of the entire operative field and maneuverability of the endoscopic instruments. The surgical team should have sterile external defibrillation equipment on the operative field to electrically convert the patient's rhythm if manipulation should cause ventricular tachycardia or fibrillation.

Esophagus

The VATS approach to the distal esophagus for transthoracic truncal vagotomy or esophagomyotomy for the management of achalasia usually requires positioning of the thoracoscope through the seventh intercostal space in the mid- to posterior axillary line (Fig. 9-8). The thoracoscope is directed toward the esophageal hiatus, and accessory intercostal space access

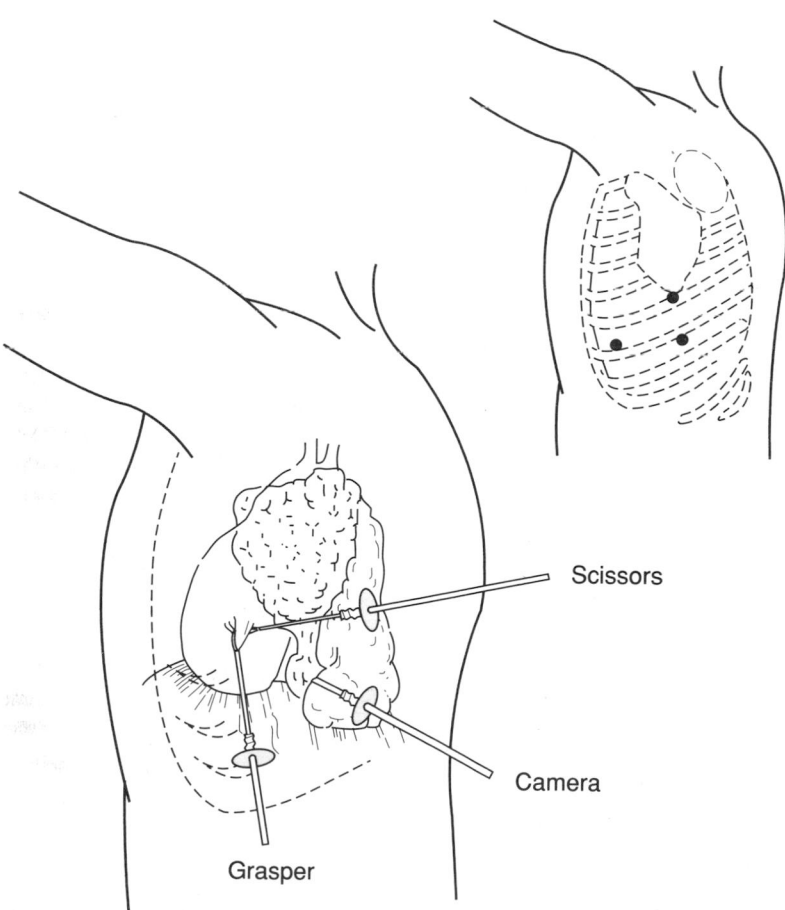

Figure 9-7.   Left-sided thoracoscopic approach for pericardiectomy. (From Landreneau RJ: Video-assisted surgery: basic technical concepts and intercostal approach strategies. Ann Thorac Surg 54:800, 1992, with permission.)

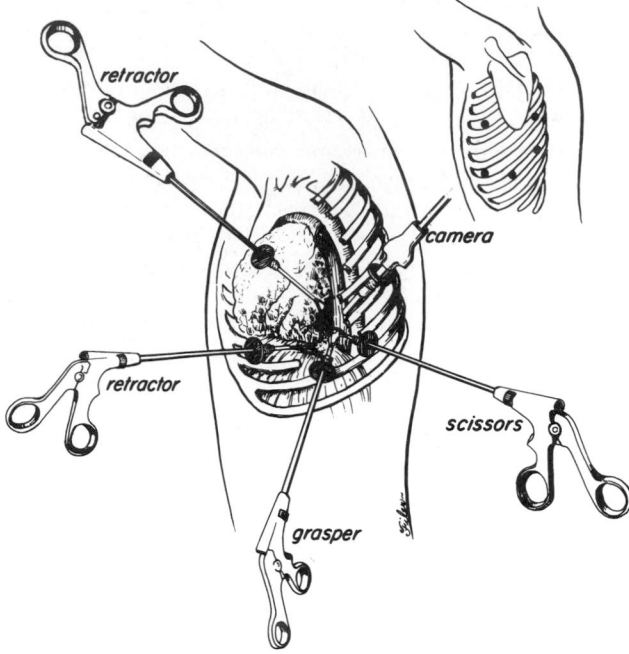

Figure 9-8. Right thoracoscopic approach to the distal esophagus for esophagomyotomy. (From Landreneau RJ: Video-assisted surgery: basic technical concepts and intercostal approach strategies. Ann Thorac Surg 54:800, 1992, with permission.)

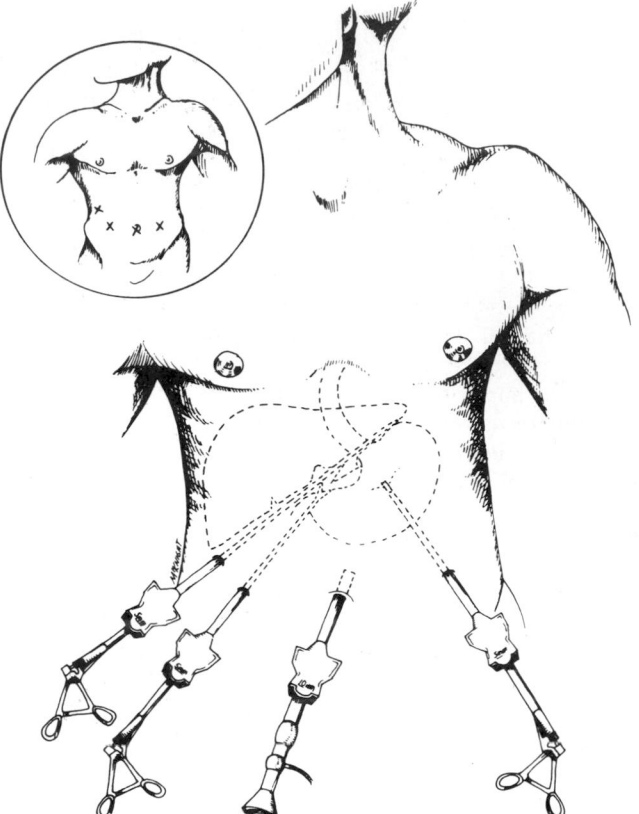

Figure 9-9. Positioning of the patient and placement of ports for laparoscopic fundoplication. (From Landreneau RJ: Video-assisted surgery: basic technical concepts and intercostal approach strategies. Ann Thorac Surg 54:800, 1992, with permission.)

sites are established at the fourth intercostal space in the anterior axillary line for retraction of the lung, the seventh intercostal space in the anterior axillary line for diaphragmatic retraction, and the sixth and eighth intercostal spaces along the posterior axillary line for grasping forceps and endoscopic scissors. A 40 to 48 Fr Maloney esophageal bougie is introduced into the esophagus through the mouth to assist in identifying the esophagus and the plane of submucosal dissection. A flexible esophagogastroscope may be used to stent the esophagus and transilluminate and insufflate the lumen of the esophagus to ensure mucosal integrity during the course of the dissection. It is extremely helpful to position the television monitor(s) toward the foot of the operating table to give the operators in-line orientation during the procedure and prevent reversal of the image.

Laparoscopic fundoplication is now being performed with increasing frequency in Europe (Weerts, et al., 1993) and North America (McKernan, et al., 1992). Access is achieved through multiple abdominal ports and requires that surgical personnel be familiar with the use of carbon dioxide insufflation and laparoscopic techniques. Insufflation is achieved by inserting an initial 10-mm port, to be used for the camera, in the midline 3 to 4 cm above the umbilicus. Three or four additional ports are placed across the abdomen (Fig. 9-9). The lateral 10-mm ports are used for retraction, while the medial 5-mm ports are for operating instruments. The most popular procedure is the Nissen fundoplication, although other repairs have been reported.

In addition to the usually recognized complications of laparoscopic surgery, several deaths have been reported from bilateral tension pneumothoraces after mediastinal mobilization of the esophagus. Patients are usually placed in the lithotomy position for these procedures, which requires special emphasis on prophylaxis against pulmonary emboli.

COMMENTS AND CONTROVERSIES

The initial unbridled enthusiasm for video-assisted thoracic procedures has been replaced by critical evaluation of its role in comparison with traditional open techniques. A reduction in the incidence and severity of post-thoracotomy discomfort was initially expected to be a major advantage of VATS. Recent trials suggest that while early requirement for narcotics is reduced following VATS operations, the incidence of long-term (>12 months) pain is unchanged when compared with muscle-sparing thoracotomy (Landreneau, et al., 1994a; Landreneau, et al., 1994b). Intercostal neuritis or neuroma formation, secondary to spreading of the ribs during open procedures, may also develop from traction injury when screw-in trocar ports are used or from excessive levering against the ribs during movement of thoracoscopic instruments.

Intraoperative hypotension may develop from excessive carbon dioxide insufflation, causing mediastinal shift and reduction in venous return to the heart (Jones, et al., 1993). Insufflation is rarely required to obtain lung deflation during thoracic procedures except in patients with significant obstructive disease. In general, isolation of the ipsilateral lung as soon as proper position of the double-lumen tube is confirmed and suctioning through the tube are adequate in most cases. If required, carbon dioxide should be insufflated at the minimum pressure and rate necessary, generally less than 10 mmHg and 1.5 L/min.

All trocar sites must be inspected from within the hemithorax for bleeding, as laceration of the intercostal vessels can occur during insertion of the trocar, which may then result in tamponade. The injury may not be recognizable until after the port is removed.

The thoracic surgical community has attempted to avoid the uncontrolled proliferation of video-assisted procedures by establishing credentialing through courses approved by the Joint Committee of the American Association for Thoracic Surgery and the Society of Thoracic Surgeons (McKneally, 1993), by sponsorship of peer review through the VATS registry, and by critical evaluation through the VATS study group. Credible conclusions about the efficacy of this technology in basic thoracic procedures such as lung biopsy, apical bullectomy, and pleurodesis will be derived from these sources. More complex or controversial procedures, such as lobectomy and esophagectomy, can be developed and studied scientifically through group efforts such as these before diffusion into community practice.

VATS may offer the potential benefit of reduced morbidity for patients with a number of thoracic surgical problems. This advantage will be diminished if extended operating time and imprecise handling of the intrathoracic tissues result from poorly planned surgical approaches to the target pathology. The VATS learning curve can be steep, slow, and discouraging if repeated difficulties with endoscopic instruments and camera positioning limit the dexterity of the thoracic surgical team. This chapter has outlined the basic approaches to VATS with the hope that some of these early difficulties can be minimized.

M.F.M.

KEY REFERENCES

Boutin C, Viallat JR, Aelony Y: Practical Thoracoscopy. Springer-Verlag, Berlin 1991

These authors represent the predominant European influence of pulmonologists on the field of diagnostic thoracoscopy. Concentrating on pleural disease, the chapters are devoted to the practical aspects of the procedures.

Brandt H, Loddenkemper R, Mai J: Atlas of Diagnostic Thoracoscopy. Thieme, New York, 1985

The authors were instrumental in the organization of the first international symposium on thoracoscopy, held in Marseilles in 1980. The text offers practical guidelines supplemented with case reports to illustrate the techniques of diagnostic thoracoscopy.

Kaiser LR, Daniel TM: Thoracoscopic Surgery. Little, Brown, Boston, 1993

The editors have assembled a list of North American thoracic surgeons who represent the most enthusiastic proponents of video-assisted thoracic surgery. The emphasis is less on diagnostic techniques and more on therapeutic surgical procedures.

Krasna MJ, Mack MJ: Atlas of Thoracoscopic Surgery. Quality Medical Publishing, St. Louis, 1994

This practical text offers a minimum of literature review and a maximum of practical description of operative techniques. The approaches reflect the experience of the editors, but all chapters are accompanied by an invited commentary by surgeons recognized for their expertise, who offer alternative views.

Lewis RJ: Video-assisted thoracic surgery. Chest Surg Clin North Am 3(2): 1993

This issue presents up-to-date information, with complete references, covering the breadth of video-assisted thoracic surgery. The contributors are recognized experts in the field.

REFERENCES

Alexander J: The Collapse Therapy of Pulmonary Tuberculosis. p. 313. Charles C Thomas, Springfield, IL, 1937

Benumof JL: Physiology of the open chest and one-lung ventilation. p. 287. In Kaplan JA (ed): Thoracic Anesthesia. Churchill Livingstone, New York, 1983

Boutin C, Viallat JR, Cargnino P, Farisse P: Indications actuelles de la thoracoscopie. Etude préliminaire. Rev Franc Mal Respir 9:309, 1981

Daly BDT, Faling LJ, Diehl JT et al: Computed tomography-guided minithoracotomy for the resection of small peripheral pulmonary nodules. Ann Thorac Surg 51:465, 1991

Deslauriers J, Beaulieu M, Dufour C et al: Mediastinopleuroscopy: a new approach to the diagnosis of intrathoracic diseases. Ann Thorac Surg 22:265, 1976

Ferson PF, Landreneau RJ, Dowling RD et al: Thoracoscopic vs. "open" lung biopsy for the diagnosis of infiltrate lung disease. J Thorac Cardiovasc Surg 106:194, 1993

Hazelrigg SR, Landreneau RJ, Mack MJ et al: Thoracoscopic stapled resection for spontaneous pneumothorax. J Thorac Cardiovasc Surg 105:389, 1993

Jacobaeus HC: The practical importance of thoracoscopy in surgery of the chest. Surg Gynecol Obstet 34:289, 1922

Jones DR, Graeber GM, Tanguilig GC et al: Effects of insufflation on hemodynamics during thoracoscopy. Ann Thorac Surg 55:1379, 1993

Keenan RJ, Landreneau RJ, Hazelrigg SR, Ferson PF: Video-assisted thoracic surgical resection using the Nd:YAG laser. J Thorac Cardiovasc Surg 1994 (in press)

Landreneau RJ, Dowling RD, Castillo R, Ferson PF: Thoracoscopic resection of an anterior mediastinal tumor. Ann Thorac Surg 54:142, 1992b

Landreneau RJ, Dowling RD, Ferson PF: Thoracoscopic resection of a posterior mediastinal mass. Chest 102:1288, 1992c

Landreneau RJ, Hazelrigg SR, Ferson PF et al: Thoracoscopic resection of 85 pulmonary lesions. Ann Thorac Surg 54:415, 1992a

Landreneau RJ, Hazelrigg SR, Mack MJ et al: Postoperative pain-related morbidity: video-assisted thoracic surgery vs thoracotomy. Ann Thorac Surg 56:1285, 1993

Landreneau RJ, Herlan DB, Johnson JA et al: Thoracoscopic Nd:YAG laser assisted pulmonary resection. Ann Thorac Surg 52:1176, 1991

Landreneau RJ, Mack MJ, Hazelrigg SR et al: Prevalence of chronic pain following pulmonary resection by thoracotomy or video-assisted thoracic surgery. J Thorac Cardiovasc Surg 107:1079, 1994

Lewis RJ, Caccavale RJ, Sisler GE: VATS-argon beam coagulator treatment of diffuse end-stage bilateral bullous disease of the lung. Ann Thorac Surg 55:1394, 1993

Lewis RJ, Caccavale RJ, Sisler GE: Imaged thorascopic surgery: a new thoracic technique for resection of mediastinal cysts. Ann Thorac Surg 53:38, 1992

Lewis RJ, Kunderman PJ, Sisler GE: Direct diagnostic thoracoscopy. Ann Thorac Surg 21:536, 1976

Mack MJ, Aronoff R, Acuff T et al: The present role of thoracoscopy in the diagnosis and treatment of diseases of the chest. Ann Thorac Surg 54:403, 1992

McKernan JB, Wolfe BM, MacFadyen BV Jr: Laparoscopic repair of duodenal ulcer and gastroesophageal reflux. Surg Clin North Am 72:1153, 1992

McKneally MF: Credentialling and privileging. In Kaiser LR, Daniel TM (eds): Thoracoscopic Surgery. Little, Brown, Boston, 1993

Wakabayashi A: Thoracoscopic technique for management of giant bullous lung disease. Ann Thorac Surg 56:708, 1993

Weerts JM, Dallemagne B, Hamoir E et al: Laparoscopic Nissen fundoplication: detailed analysis of 132 patients. Surg Laparosc Endosc 3:359, 1993

10

ANATOMY AND PHYSIOLOGY

Larynx

Jonathan C. Irish
Patrick J. Gullane

PHYSIOLOGY

The larynx plays an important role in the swallowing mechanism. The first two phases of swallowing, the oral and oral preparatory phases, are voluntary, while the third and fourth phases, the pharyngeal and esophageal phases, are involuntary (Mandelstam and Lieber, 1970). During the involuntary phase of swallowing, coordinated activity between the swallowing center, mediated in the reticular formation of the brain stem, and the adjacent respiratory center is critical for respiration to cease during the initiation of the swallow (Miller, 1972). In addition to the brief cessation of respiration and the coordinated neuromuscular activity of the pharyngoesophageal complex for propulsion of the food bolus, airway protection during the swallow is also performed by the sphincteric actions of the larynx. These sphincters include the epiglottis, the false vocal folds, and the true vocal folds (Ardran and Kemp, 1967).

During the normal swallow the larynx is elevated and moves anteriorly under the base of the tongue, allowing the passive closure of the epiglottis over the laryngeal aperture (Fink and Demarest, 1978). Anterior movement of the larynx away from the esophagus also "stretches" the cricopharyngeus muscle, allowing the food bolus to pass through the upper esophageal sphincter.

Speech production is an obvious function of the larynx. The current theory of speech production, the myoelastic theory, suggests that the larynx is pivotal (Van Len Berg, 1958). This theory recognizes that the larynx is a pliable, elastic, muscular organ, with the ability to generate closure with vocal cord adduction and the ability to finely tune speech by alteration of the mass and tension of the vocal folds. The ability to generate glottic closure enables subglottic pressure to build up until it is greater than the glottic closing pressure, allowing escape of air. This periodic opening and closing of the glottis, causes compression and rarefaction of air, re-

sulting in the physical phenomenon of sound. The frequency of vocal cord opening corresponds to the frequency of the sound produced. Fine tuning of the sound is secondary to finer alterations in the intrinsic muscles of the larynx allowing variation of vocal fold mass (greater mass, lower frequency) and vocal fold tension (increased tension, higher frequency). Vocal cord pathology such as a polyp results in a "raspy" voice often lower in frequency (secondary to increased mass) and diplophonic in quality.

Effort-induced approximation of the false and true vocal folds is critical for producing the "tussive squeeze" and "becchic blast" so necessary for normal cough production (Adrian, et al., 1953). This function also allows performance of Valsalva maneuvers, which are essential for lifting heavy objects and for normal defecation. Failure to generate effort-induced approximation of the glottis, as in recurrent laryngeal nerve paralysis, can result in aspiration, with the situation further aggravated by the inability of the patient to produce an effective cough, often resulting in pneumonia. Teflon augmentation of the paralyzed cord can restore this ability.

EMBRYOLOGY

At approximately the 26th day of embryonic development, the endodermally lined rudiment of the respiratory tree develops as the median laryngotracheal groove (Fig. 10-1A). This groove develops in the caudal end of the ventral wall of the pharynx, and over the course of the fourth week of development it deepens and elongates to form a diverticulum. The edges of the tube fuse, forming a septum, and thus provide a functional and anatomic separation of the pharyngoesophageal complex from the laryngotracheal complex. The fusion commences caudally and extends cranially and excluding the slitlike opening into the pharynx. Failure of fusion during this period of embryonic development may result in a posterior laryngeal cleft, while failure of caudal septal fusion is the

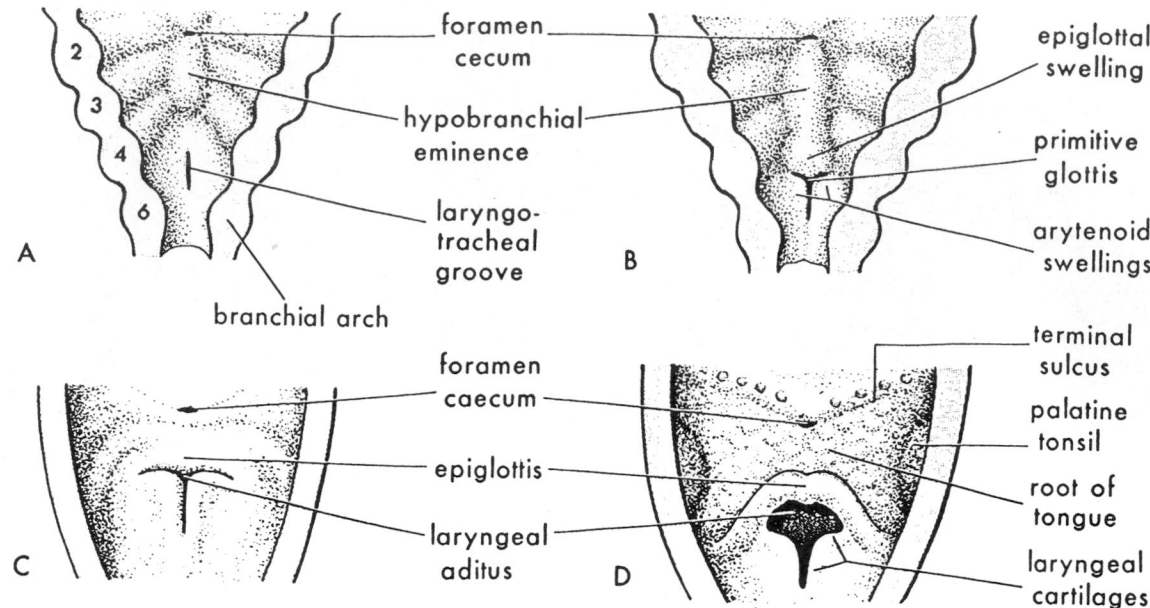

Figure 10-1. Successive stages of development of the larynx at **(A)** 4 weeks, **(B)** 5 weeks, **(C)** 6 weeks, and **(D)** 10 weeks. (From Moore K: The Developing Human: Clinically Oriented Embryology. p. 188. 2nd Ed. WB Saunders, Philadelphia, 1977, with permission.)

presumed etiologic basis of a congenital tracheoesophageal fistula. The endodermally lined tube gives rise to the mucosal epithelium and glandular elements of the larynx, trachea, and bronchi, while the splanchic mesenchyme, into which the diverticulum grows, gives rise to the supporting connective tissue, cartilage, nonstriated muscle, and vasculature of the laryngotracheal complex.

The primitive larynx in the fourth week of development is bounded cranially by the hypobranchial eminence (formed by the third and fourth arch), and bounded laterally by the folds of the sixth branchial arch. By the sixth week of embryonic development, mesenchymal proliferation occurs on both sides of the laryngotracheal groove, forming the arytenoid swellings (Fig. 10-1B). With this proliferation the laryngeal aperture changes from a vertical slit or cleft shape to a T shape. During the second month of prenatal development the arytenoid swelling differentiates into the arytenoid and corniculate cartilages as derivatives of the sixth branchial arch. At this time the aryepiglottic folds develop, joining the arytenoids to the epiglottis, which has developed from the hypobranchial eminence (Fig. 10-1C). During this time the laryngotracheal lumen is obstructed by an epithelial plug and by mucosa-mucosa adherence, which during the third month of prenatal life undergoes recanalization. Failure of recanalization has been proposed as an etiology of congenital glottic and subglottic stenosis.

The thyroid cartilage develops from the fourth branchial arch with the fusion of two lateral plates, each with two chondrification centers. The cricoid cartilage and tracheal cartilages develop during the sixth week of embryologic development from the sixth branchial arch.

The development of each branchial arch is accompanied by that of an accompanying arch nerve and artery. The artery from the third arch ultimately forms the proximal part of the common carotid artery and the internal carotid artery. The superior laryngeal nerve and subclavian artery are the nerve and artery of the fourth arch, while the recurrent laryngeal nerve and ligamentum arteriosum are the neurovascular structures of the sixth branchial arch.

DESCRIPTIVE ANATOMY

The larynx in men is opposite the third to sixth cervical vertebrae while in women and children it lies in a more cranial position. Although there is little difference in the size of the laryngeal aperture between boys and girls before puberty, after puberty the anteroposterior diameter of the larynx increases dramatically in boys to 36 mm as compared with 26 mm in girls.

Laryngeal Cartilages

The rigid framework of the larynx is provided by nine cartilages. (Fig. 10-2) The thyroid, cricoid, and epiglottic cartilages are unpaired, while the arytenoid, corniculate, and cuneiform cartilages are paired.

Thyroid Cartilage

The longest and largest of the laryngeal cartilages is the thyroid cartilage consisting of two laminae fusing in the midline with a 90-degree angle in men and a 120-degree angle in women. From the posterior border of the thyroid cartilage two slender processes extend superiorly and inferiorly, forming the superior and inferior cornua, respectively. A facet on the medial surface of the inferior cornu marks the cricothyroid joint and allows the thyroid cartilage to tilt or glide anteriorly or posteriorly on the cricoid cartilage. The superior border of the thyroid cartilage is attached to the hyoid bone

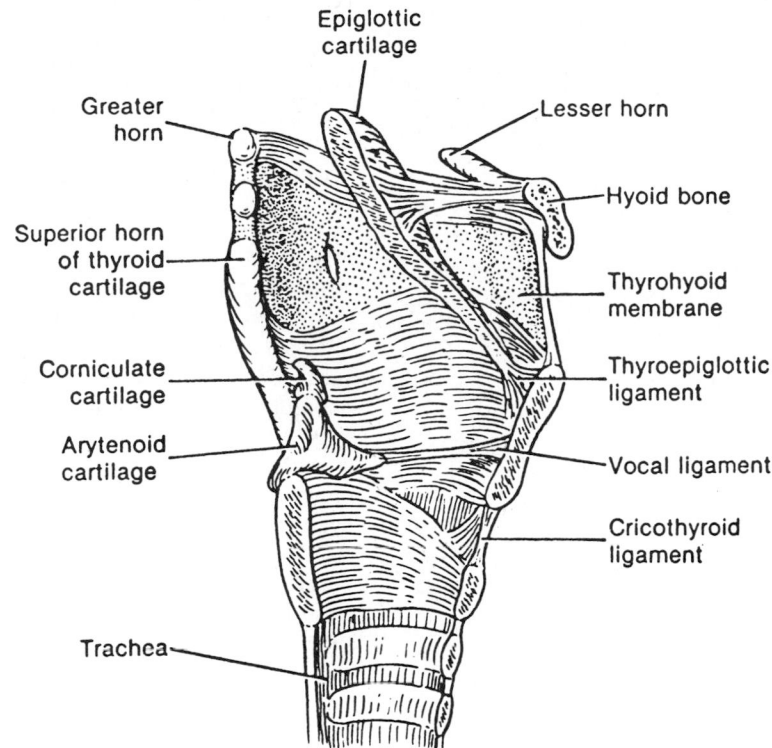

Figure 10-2. The laryngeal bones and cartilages in saggital section. (From Graney DO: Larynx/hyperpharynx anatomy. p. 1729. In Cummings C et al. (eds): Otolaryngology—Head and Neck Surgery. 1st Ed. CV Mosby, St. Louis, 1986, with permission.)

by the thyrohyoid membrane, while the inferior attachment to the cricoid is provided by the cricothyroid membrane, which attaches to the inner aspect of the medial portion of the inferior border of the thyroid cartilage. The external surface of the thyroid laminae is marked by an oblique line curving downward and forward from the superior cornu. This line marks the attachment for the inferior constrictor muscle of the pharynx and for the sternothyroid and thyrohyoid muscles.

Cricoid Cartilage

The signet ring–shaped cricoid cartilage is the only complete cartilaginous ring in the air passage. The posterior lamina is deep and thick, while the anterior arch is narrow. The cricoid is attached to the first tracheal ring by the cricothyroid ligament. At the junction of the lamina and arch is a facet that articulates with the inferior cornu of the thyroid. The other important joints of the cricoid are the paired cricoarytenoid joints, which are synovial joints that allow rotation and glide of the arytenoids on the sloping shoulders of the cricoid lamina. As with any synovial joint, arthritic processes such as rheumatoid arthritis may cause inflammation and ultimately ankylosis of the cricoarytenoid joint.

Arytenoid Cartilages

The paired arytenoid cartilages are shaped like irregular three-sided pyramids. The three points of the pyramid are the superiorly projecting apex, the anteriorly projecting vocal

process attaching to the vocal ligament, and the laterally projecting muscular process to which the lateral and posterior cricoarytenoid muscles attach. The base of the arytenoid is concave, providing an articulating relationship with the gently sloping shoulders of the cricoid lamina.

Corniculate and Cuneiform Cartilages

The corniculate cartilages are conical nodules of elastic fibrocartilage attached to the apices of the arytenoid cartilages. The cuneiform cartilages are elongated pieces of fibrocartilage lying in the aryepiglottic folds. The function of these small cartilages is not clear, but they may provide increased structure and prevent collapse of the aryepiglottic folds into the laryngeal inlet.

Epiglottis

The epiglottis is a thin sheet of elastic fibrocartilage shaped like a leaf. In neonates and infants the epiglottis is omega-shaped, forming a long, floppy, deeply grooved structure, while in adults it has a gradually curving semielliptical shape. The epiglottis is attached to the thyroid cartilage anteriorly by the thyroepiglottic ligament. The epiglottis forms the anterior wall of the laryngeal inlet, and laterally its margins are continuous with the aryepiglottic folds forming the lateral walls of the inlet. Anteriorly the epiglottis is attached to the hyoid bone by the hyoepiglottic ligament, thereby dividing the epiglottis into an infrahyoid and a suprahyoid segment. The mucous membrane covering the epiglottis is continuous with that of the posterior tongue. Three folds of mucous membrane are reflected onto the pharyngeal part of the tongue and onto the lateral walls of the pharynx, forming a median glossoepiglottic fold and two lateral glossoepiglottic folds. Between each of the lateral folds and the median fold are depressions called the epiglottic valleculae.

While the corniculate, cuneiform, and arytenoid apices are composed of elastic fibrocartilage with little tendency to calcify, the thyroid, cricoid, and the greatest part of the arytenoid cartilages are composed of hyaline cartilage and can begin calcification in early adulthood, which can mimic the appearance of a foreign body on lateral soft tissue x-rays.

Ligaments

The extrinsic ligaments of the larynx, including the thyrohyoid ligament, the cricotracheal ligament, and the hyoepiglottic ligament have been previously discussed. The intrinsic ligaments are divided into two major groups by the laryngeal vestibule. Superior to the vestibule is the quadrangular membrane, the free inferior margins of which constitute the ventricular ligament, which when covered by mucous membrane forms the false cords or vestibular folds.

The second network of ligaments is positioned inferior to the laryngeal ventricle and consists of the vocal ligament and conus elasticus. The vocal ligament runs anteriorly from the junction of the laminae of the thyroid cartilage to its posterior attachment with the vocal processes of the arytenoid. The vocal ligament forms the superior free edge of the conus elasticus. The conus spreads like a draped tent from the vocal ligament to its attachment to the cricoid cartilage. The vocal ligament forms the fibrous core of the true vocal cord. The ligament and fibrous layers of the larynx can play critical roles as barriers in the prevention of tumor spread. Breach of tumor across these anatomic barriers into the paraglottic and pre-epiglottic spaces portends poor patient outcome and survival.

Interior of the Larynx

The cavity of the larynx extends from the pharynx at the laryngeal inlet to the trachea beginning at the lower border of the cricoid cartilage. The larynx is divided into three parts by the vestibular and vocal folds. Above the vestibular folds the cavity of the larynx is called the vestibule. Between the vestibular and vocal folds lies the ventricle, which arises through a narrow horizontal slit laterally. Extending superiorly from the anterior part of the ventricle is a pouchlike structure, which ascends between the ventricular folds and the inner surface of the thyroid cartilage (Fig. 10-3).

The high density of mucous glands in the ventricle and saccule has led to the belief that they play a particularly important role in lubrication of the larynx and therefore are important in voice production. The ventricle is separated from the subglottis by the vocal folds, which are two folds of mucous membrane closely adherent to the underlying vocal ligaments, consisting of the free upper thickened margins of the conus elasticus. Lateral to the vocal ligament lies the vocalis muscle, which by contraction and stretching plays an integral role in the determination of voice quality. The subglottic space extends from the vocal folds to the lower border of the cricoid cartilage, where the trachea begins.

Laryngeal Musculature

The muscles of the larynx are divided into intrinsic and extrinsic groups.

Extrinsic Musculature

The extrinsic muscles move the larynx as a whole and originate outside the larynx. These muscles are further subdivided into depressors of the larynx (omohyoid, sternohyoid, and sternothyroid) and elevators of the larynx (stylohyoid, digastric, mylohyoid, geniohyoid, stylopharyngeus, and an thyrohyoid). Except for the thyrohyoid muscle, which elevates the

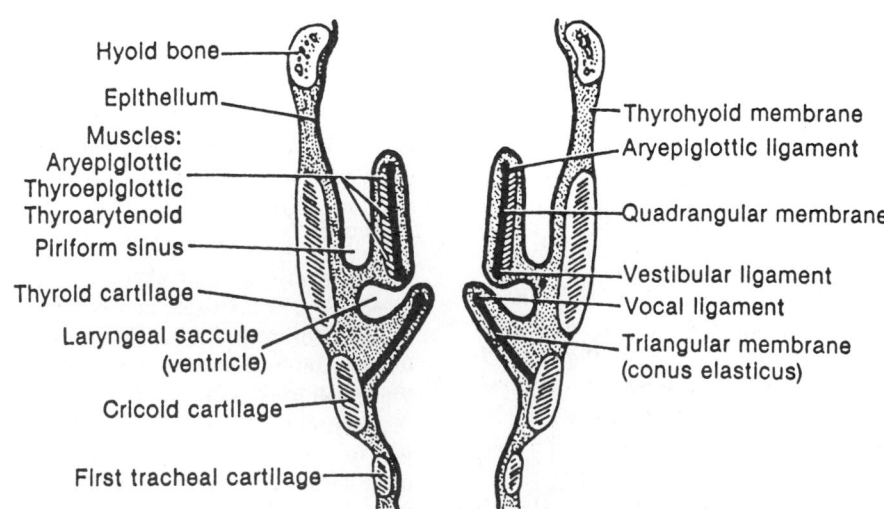

Hyoid bone
Epithelium
Muscles:
Aryepiglottic
Thyroepiglottic
Thyroarytenoid
Piriform sinus
Thyroid cartilage
Laryngeal saccule (ventricle)
Cricoid cartilage
First tracheal cartilage

Thyrohyoid membrane
Aryepiglottic ligament
Quadrangular membrane
Vestibular ligament
Vocal ligament
Triangular membrane (conus elasticus)

Figure 10-3. Schematic drawing of a coronal section of the larynx demonstrating the supporting ligaments and membranes. (From Graney DO: Larynx/hyperpharynx anatomy. p. 1729. In Cummings C et al. (eds): Otolaryngology—Head and Neck Surgery, 1st Ed. CV Mosby, St. Louis, 1986, with permission.)

larynx but draws the hyoid and thyroid cartilages together, all the elevators elevate both the hyoid and the larynx as a unit.

Intrinsic Musculature

The intrinsic muscles (Fig. 10-4) are concerned with movements of the laryngeal parts and have both their origin and insertion within the larynx. The prime function of these muscles is to make alterations in vocal cord length and tension and to change the size and shape of the rima glottis. The intrinsic muscles of the larynx are best subdivided into three groups.

The first group of muscles consists of those that open and close the glottis. The posterior cricoarytenoid muscles are the primary abductors of the vocal cords, while the lateral cricoarytenoid muscles are the primary adductors of the vocal cords. The interarytenoid muscles comprise the transverse and the oblique arytenoid muscle, both of which act as adductors of the vocal cords by approximation of the arytenoids. Some of the fibers of the oblique arytenoid muscle continue as the aryepiglottic muscle, which ensures that the epiglottis is drawn inferiorly simultaneously with vocal cord adduction. This action of laryngeal inlet closure plays an important role in the normal swallow.

The second group of intrinsic laryngeal muscles comprises those that control the tension of the vocal ligaments. The main tensor of the vocal folds is the cricothyroid muscle. This muscle arises on the cricoid cartilage and inserts into the anterior aspect of the inferior margins of the thyroid cartilage. Therefore, contraction of this muscle tilts the thyroid cartilage anteriorly on the cricoid, increasing the distance between the thyroid and arytenoid cartilages and thereby elongating the vocal ligaments and increasing vocal pitch. The main relaxors of the vocal folds are the thyroarytenoid muscles, which arise from the posterior surface of the thyroid cartilage and insert on the anterolateral surfaces of the arytenoid cartilages. The vocalis muscle is part of the thyroarytenoid muscle.

The final group of intrinsic muscles are those whose primary function is to alter the shape of the laryngeal inlet. The thyroepiglottic muscle is formed from the superior fibers of the thyroarytenoid muscles and functions to widen the laryngeal inlet. The aryepiglottic muscle is formed from fibers of the oblique arytenoid muscles and closes the inlet.

Blood Supply

The blood supply of the larynx is derived from the superior thyroid artery through its superior laryngeal and cricothyroid branches and from the inferior thyroid artery through its inferior laryngeal branch (Fig. 10-5).

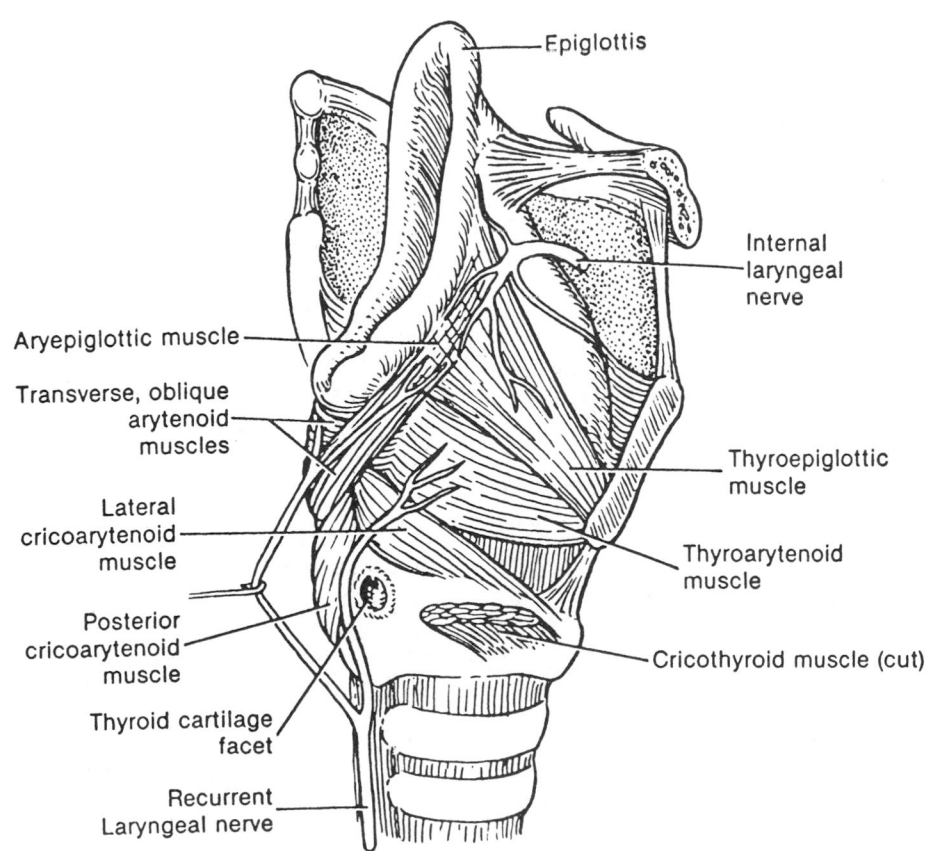

Figure 10-4.   Lateral view of laryngeal muscles and nerves. (From Graney DO: Larynx/hyperpharynx anatomy. p. 1729. In Cummings C et al. (ed): Otolaryngology—Head and Neck Surgery. 1st Ed. CV Mosby, St. Louis, 1986, with permission.)

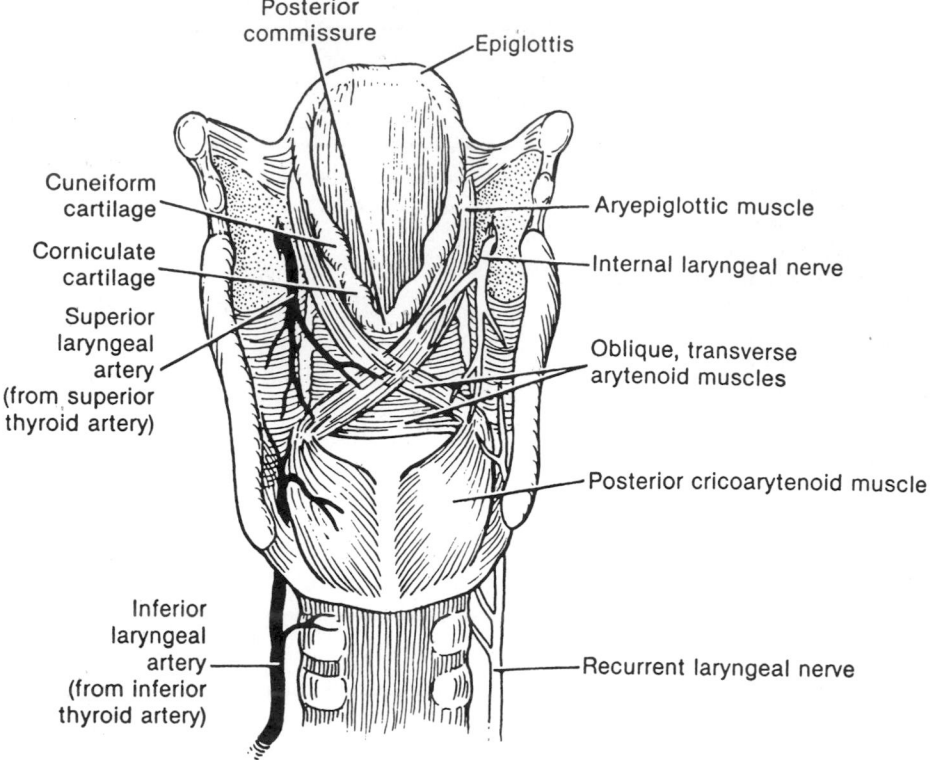

Figure 10-5. Posterior view of the larynx demonstrating intrinsic muscles, nerves, and vascular supply. (From Graney DO: Larynx/hyperpharynx anatomy. p. 1729. In Cummings C et al. (eds): Otolaryngology—Head and Neck Surgery. 1st Ed. CV Mosby, St. Louis, 1986, with permission.)

The superior thyroid artery which arises from the external carotid artery and passes deep to the thyrohyoid muscle, piercing the thyrohyoid membrane with the internal branch of the superior laryngeal nerve, supplies the internal surface or the larynx. The inferior thyroid artery arises from the thyrocervical trunk of the first part of the subclavian artery and gives rise to the inferior laryngeal branch at the level of the lower border of the thyroid gland. The artery, which enters the larynx and runs along with the recurrent laryngeal nerve beneath the lower border of the inferior constrictor, supplies the inferior internal larynx.

The veins leaving the larynx accompany the arteries, with the superior vessels entering the internal jugular vein by way of the superior thyroid vein and the inferior veins draining into the brachiocephalic vein through the inferior thyroid vein. Additional venous drainage is through the middle thyroid vein into the internal jugular vein.

Lymphatics

Lymphatic drainage of the larynx occurs by way of two main pedicles. Superior to the vocal folds the lymphatic circulation accompanies the superior laryngeal artery through the thyrohyoid membrane. The superior pedicle ultimately drains into the superior deep cervical lymph nodes. Inferior to the vocal folds the lymphatics drain to the inferior deep cervical lymph nodes via the prelaryngeal, pretracheal, and paratracheal lymph nodes.

Innervation

The innervation of the larynx is provided by the vagus nerve by way of the superior and recurrent laryngeal branches (Fig. 10-5). The motor innervation arises within the nucleus ambiguus while the parasympathetic supply arises from the dorsal motor nucleus of the vagus (Yoshida, et al., 1982).

The superior laryngeal nerve divides within the carotid sheath into two terminal branches, the internal laryngeal nerve (sensory and autonomic) and the external laryngeal nerve (motor). The internal laryngeal nerve pierces the thyrohyoid membrane with the superior laryngeal artery, supplying sensation (including stretch receptor and proprioceptive information) to the larynx superior to the vocal folds. The external laryngeal nerve accompanies the superior thyroid artery descending posterior to the sternothyroid muscle, supplying motor innervation to the cricothyroid muscle.

The recurrent laryngeal nerve on the right loops under the right subclavian artery and ascends in the tracheoesophageal groove. On the left the nerve passes under the aortic arch and ligamentum arteriosum to reach the tracheoesophageal groove. On both sides the nerve accompanies the laryngeal branch of the inferior thyroid artery and passes deep to the inferior constrictor muscle behind the cricothyroid joint. The motor supply innervates all the intrinsic laryngeal musculature except the cricothyroid muscle, while the sensory branch supplies the laryngeal mucosa inferior to the vocal folds.

The extrinsic muscles of the larynx receive their motor innervation from the ansa cervicalis derived from cervical roots C1, C2, and C3.

KEY REFERENCES

Basmajian, JB: Grant's Method of Anatomy. 10th Ed. Williams & Wilkins, Baltimore, 1980

A traditional text, but remains highly regarded as concise, with simple, easily reproducible line drawings.

Fink BR, Demarest RI: Laryngeal Biomechanics. Cambridge University Press, Cambridge, MA, 1978

Good, detailed review of the physiologic detail of laryngeal function.

Hollinshead WH: Anatomy for Surgeons: the Head and Neck. 2nd Ed. Harper & Row, Hagerstown, MD, 1968

Clinically applied anatomy of the head and neck, with excellent accompanying text.

Moore KL: The Developing Human: Clinically Oriented Embryology. p. 188. 3rd Ed. WB Saunders, Philadelphia, 1982

Development of the larynx, esophagus, and related structures of the upper aerodigestive tract are fully described and illustrated with clinical relevance.

REFERENCES

Adrian GM, Kemp FH, Manen L: Closure of the larynx. Br J Radiol 26:497, 1953

Ardran J, Kemp F: The mechanism of the larynx. II. The epiglottis and closure of the larynx. Br J Radiol 40:372, 1967

Graney DO: Larynx/hypopharynx anatomy. p. 1729. In Cummings C et al (eds): Otolaryngology—Head and Neck Surgery. 1st Ed. CV Mosby, St. Louis, 1986

Mandelstam P, Lieber A: Cineradiographic evaluation of the esophagus in normal adults. Gastroenterology 58:32, 1970

Miller A: Characteristics of the swallowing reflex, induced by peripheral nerve and brain stem stimulation. Exp Neurol 34:210, 1972

Van den Berg J: Myoelastic-aerodynamic theory of voice production. J Speech Hear Res 1:227, 1958

Yoshida Y, Miyazaki T, Hirano M et al: Arrangement of motoneurons innervating the intrinsic laryngeal muscles of cats as demonstrated by horseradish peroxidase. Acta Otolaryngol (Stockh) 94:329, 1982

Upper Airway

R. J. Cusimano
F. Griffith Pearson

EMBRYOLOGY

Trachea

The development of the respiratory system begins at 4 weeks of gestation with the development of an endodermal bud growing into the splanchnic mesenchyme. The endodermal components become the epithelium and glands, while the mesenchyme becomes cartilage, connective tissue, and muscular components (Moore, 1977; Salassa, et al., 1977). Growth occurs in both length and circumference. Longitudinal growth occurs first by the laying down of new cellular elements followed by a lengthening of the cartilage, intervening connective tissue, and muscle. Circumferential growth of the trachea is uniform, unlike the growth and lengthening of bones, which grow at each end. Burrington (1978) found, in examinations of both animal and human material, that increases in the circumference of the trachea occur by the simultaneous process of uniform growth of the convex side of the trachea and remodeling by resorption along the concave surface. In this manner, the whole cartilage grows as a unit. Interestingly, while the growth at each segment is uniform, the different levels grow to different extents so that the trachea is funnel-shaped, being larger at the larynx than at the carina (Wailoo and Emery, 1982). This funnel shape is especially evident in the antenatal period and in the youngest babies and children. Because of the uniform, almost radial growth along the surface of each tracheal ring, incisions made in a vertical direction can be expected to have little influence on the final cross-sectional area of a growing trachea.

Tracheal Glands

Tracheal glands develop from the endodermal layer of the developing embryo, development generally occuring after that of the cartilage, between 10 and 25 weeks' gestation. Thereafter, there is no further increase in the number of new glands (Reid, 1976). Glandular development after this stage occurs by an increase in the acinar components, thus increasing the mass but not the number of glands. After birth the density of glands gradually decreases. Thus, while there are 7.3 glands per square millimeter at birth, by 8 years of age the density has decreased to 2.3. The adult trachea generally contains less than one gland per square millimeter (Tos 1970).

Cilia

The cilia of the trachea develop within the first half of gestation, and by 24 weeks their development is complete (Galliard, et al., 1989). There is constant differentiation from columnar undifferentiated epithelium through primitive ciliated cells to the final form.

Blood Supply

During prenatal life the blood supply of the trachea is segmental. Thus, multiple pairs of arteries arise in segmental fashion from the aorta to supply both trachea and esophagus. With time, the segmental distribution disappears, and branches that originate from the thyroid artery and aorta (via bronchial vessels) become the major sources of blood supply (Reid, 1976).

ANATOMY

Trachea

Length

The trachea is a cartilaginous and membranous tube, which connects the larynx with the bronchi. It is continuous with the larynx at the level of the cricoid cartilage. The upper trachea is normally found at the level of the sixth or seventh cervical vertebra, and the lower end lies at the fourth or fifth thoracic vertebra. On full inspiration, the distal end of the trachea may descend to the level of the sixth vertebra. In the adult resting state, the total length of the trachea is 10 to 11 cm, with approximately 5 cm lying superior to the suprasternal notch.

The noncartilaginous portions of the trachea between rings is elastic and allows lengthening or shortening of the trachea during respiration (or neck flexion or extension). Thoracic surgeons use this knowledge in the management of tracheal resections. It is desirable to minimize anastomotic tension by maintaining neck flexion after segmental tracheal resections. Surgeons commonly suture the chin to the skin of the manubrium in order to prevent neck extension during the first postoperative week.

Projected anteriorly, the tracheal bifurcation, or carina lies at the level of the manubriosternal junction, or the second inner end of the costal cartilage. In children, the carina lies at the level of the third costal cartilage (Nagaishi, 1972; Williams

and Warwick, 1981). While the trachea runs in the median plane, the carina is usually slightly to the right of the midline.

Shape

The cross-sectional shape of the trachea is determined by the horseshoe-shaped cartilage anteriorly and the membranous portion posteriorly. The most common cross-sectional configuration of the trachea is elliptical (larger transverse than anteroposterior diameter, 33 percent of cases). A C shape (equal transverse and anteroposterior diameters) is found in 26 percent of cases, and the U-shaped trachea accounts for 21 percent. A triangular cross-sectional shape occurs in less than 10 percent of the population, and a circular variant accounts for less than 1 percent of cases (Meta and Myat, 1984). Asymmetric shapes are found, and males and females differ not only in the size of their tracheas but also in the most common shape. Meta and Myat reported that the U-shaped trachea was the most common variant in adult men, and an elliptical shape was most common in adult women. Tracheal shape also changes as the individual grows and during the different phases of a respiratory cycle (Kawakami, et al., 1991).

While the adult trachea has an almost constant dimension for its entire length, the same cannot be said for the pediatric trachea. Wailoo and Emery (1982) studied humans from 28 weeks of gestation to 4 years of age and found that the trachea was a funnel-shaped structure, being larger at the larynx than at the carina. This was most pronounced in the prenatal and neonatal stages. With growth, the difference in size between larynx and carina decreased until it was negligible, creating a cylindrical rather than a funnel-shaped trachea. While there is generally no difference between the dimensions in young children, after the age of 14 the size of the female trachea tends to remain constant while the male trachea continues to enlarge (but not lengthen), even after somatic growth ceases (Griscom and Wohl, 1986).

Tracheal Rings

There are between 16 and 20 horseshoe-shaped tracheal rings, composed of hyaline cartilage. While there is variation in size and shape, the average ring in an adult is approximately 4 mm wide and 1 mm thick. Some rings are fused over variable circumferential distances, and there is a great variability among individuals in this respect. Although the cartilaginous rings are resilient and compliant in childhood and early adulthood, they tend to calcify with age. Calcification may occur earlier when certain lung diseases are present, and it is thought to occur through the chelation of calcium by the acid glycoprotein of the cartilage (Reid, 1976). Each cartilage is enveloped by perichondrium, which is continuous with a sheet of dense connective tissue made up primarily of collagen with some elastin. The collagen and elastin are diagonally apposed, allowing both for changes in diameter of the airway and for some elastic recoil when the distending stress is removed. The connective tissue is continuous with the posterior or membranous trachea. This gradual calcification and resultant loss of compliance with age has clinical implications: blunt trauma may be better tolerated by the young patient, because of higher compliance as compared with the elderly. During tracheal resections, mobilization of a compliant trachea may allow a greater extent of resection without undue anastomotic tension than is possible in the elderly patient with a rigid, calcified upper airway.

Membranous Trachea

The membranous trachea consists of an enveloping fibrous sheath, smooth muscle, epithelium, and glands. The smooth muscle component consists mostly of transverse fibers with some vertical elements external to the transverse layer. The cartilaginous part of the trachea also contains small amounts of muscle (Håkansson et al., 1976). It is the soft, distensible membranous trachea that allows for most of the moment to moment change in size of the tracheal lumen.

Glands

The luminal surface of the trachea consists of pseudostratified columnar cells, some goblet cells, and many glandular openings. The glands are situated in the membranous trachea and in the intercartilaginous components of the cartilaginous trachea. They are layered in the submucosa, with ducts extending through the mucosa and opening into the lumen. Glands are distributed in three layers: the first layer lies immediately below the mucosa; deep to this lies the transverse muscle layer, which contains the greatest concentration of glands; and a third deep layer lies on the fibrous sheath with a flattened, platelike distribution. External to the fibrous sheath and perichondrium of the trachea there is an envelope of fascia, which blends with the surrounding muscle. External to the enveloping fascia there is no glandular tissue.

Blood Supply

Macroscopic. The blood supplies of the trachea and esophagus are similar and closely linked. While that of the trachea is segmental prenatally, there are primarily two sources after birth. The cervical trachea receives its' arterial blood supply from the inferior thyroid artery and its' branches. There is a rich anastomotic connection between the ascending branches of the bronchial vessels and the descending branches of the inferior thyroid vessels. As their name implies, the bronchial vessels also supply the bronchi themselves. Figure 10-6 demonstrates the rich anastamotic network of the trachea and the major origins from the inferior thyroid and bronchial vessels.

Miura and Grillo (1966) studied the blood supply of the cervical trachea and found that the inferior thyroid artery gives rise to branches that not only serve the esophagus but also the trachea. They found that a variable number of vessels pass to the trachea on the way to the thyroid gland. Typically there are three parathyroid branches with one of the three dominant, most commonly the inferior one. Occasionally, a vessel arises directly from the subclavian artery, usually on the right side. When this occurs, two rather than three prethyroid branches of the inferior thyroid artery are present. These branches, regardless of origin, anastomose with the bronchial vessels and also provide blood supply to the esophagus (Fig. 10-7). The superior thyroid artery has anastomotic connec-

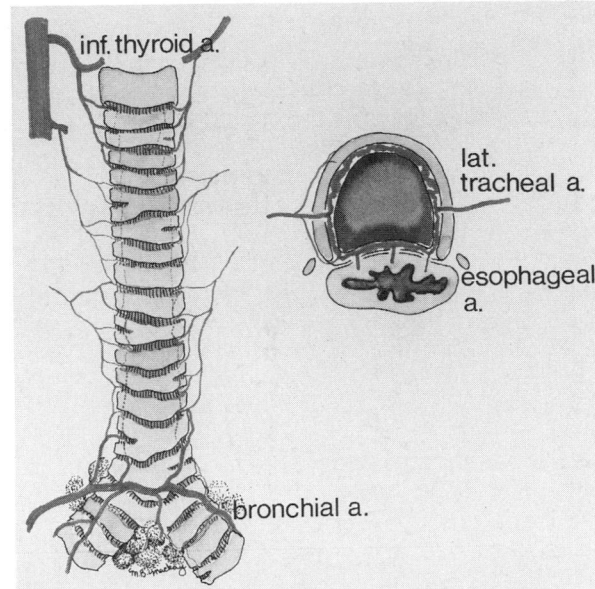

Figure 10-6. The important components of the tracheal circulation. Substantial contributions are provided by the inferior thyroid vessels above and the bronchial vessels below. These vessels anastomose with one another and, along with additional contributions from the aorta and other great vessels, form a lateral arcade, which then supplies the rich submucosal plexus through vessels passing between the cartilages anterior to the tracheal esophageal grooves. These lateral tracheal vessels supply the trachea in segmental fashion.

tions with the inferior thyroid artery and thus supplies the trachea (and esophagus) only indirectly.

From the work of Cauldwell et al. (1948) and Salassa et al. (1977), it is known that the bronchial vessels are also a major source of blood to the trachea. While there may be some variation in the origin and number of bronchial vessels, both between species (McLaughlin, 1983) and between individuals, the most common arrangement (40 percent of cases) is to have two left and one right bronchial vessel originating directly from the aorta. Approximately 50 percent of such bronchial arteries arise at the level of the sixth thoracic vertebra, while a smaller number (35 percent) arise at the level of the fifth vertebra. Occasionally there is only one left bronchial vessel (20 percent of cases), and occasionally there are two right vessels (20 percent). Two-thirds of all right lungs are supplied by a single bronchial vessel while only one-third of all left lungs are singly supplied (Cauldwell, et al., 1948).

The trachea is also supplied by branches that originate from the subclavian artery, internal mammary artery, and/or brachiocephalic (innominate) artery (Fig. 10-8). While the bronchial vessels usually arise from the aorta (the right from the lateral or posterolateral part and the left from the anterior surface or the convex surface of the aortic arch), they can and frequently do originate from a common trunk with an intercostal artery. This is found more commonly on the right side. More recently, Schreinemakers, et al. (1990) and Couraud, et al. (1992) studied the tracheal and bronchial vasculature in humans in order to better evaluate the role of the bronchial circulation in human lung transplantation. Their

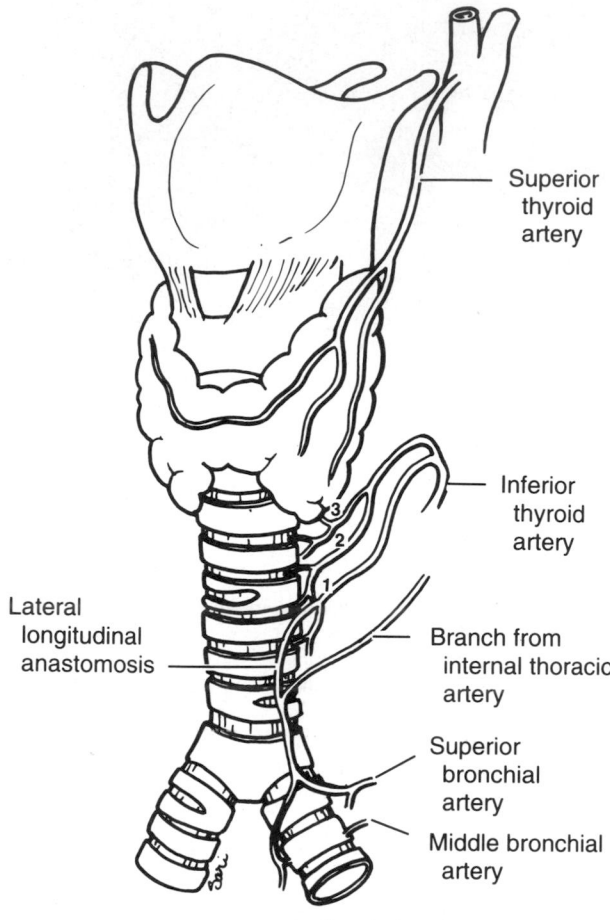

Left anterior view

Figure 10-7. Left anterior view of the blood supply of the trachea. A most important supply to the cervical trachea arises from the three branches of the inferior thyroid artery, one of which is usually dominant. There is an occasional branch derived from the subclavian artery. The superior thyroid artery only provides contributions through its anastomoses with the inferior thyroid artery. (From Salassa JR, Pearson BW, Payne WS: Gross and microscopical blood supply of the trachea. Ann Thorac Surg 24:100, 1977, with permission.)

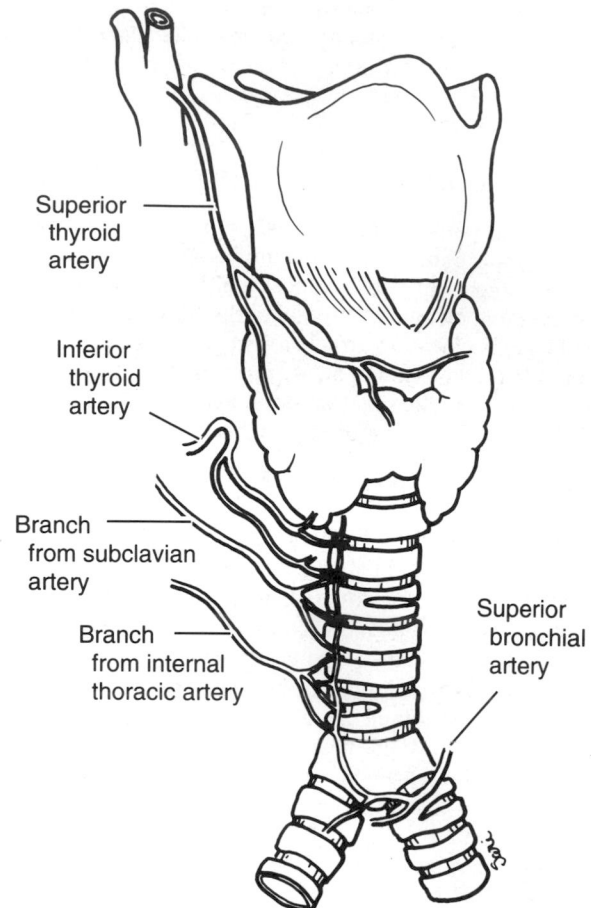

Figure 10-8. Right anterior view of the tracheal blood supply, demonstrating alternate mechanisms of supply. In this diagram arterial branches arise from the innominate artery, a supreme intercostal artery, and the internal thoracic or vertebral artery. Such vessels usually anastomose with the lateral longitudinal arcade which is supplied inferiorly through the bronchial circulation originating directly from the aorta or from intercostal vessels. The first intercostal artery on the right side is commonly the most important contributor to the tracheal circulation. (From Salassa JR, Pearson BW, Payne WS: Gross and microscopical blood supply of the trachea. Ann Thorac Surg 24:100, 1977, with permission.)

findings confirmed the observations of Cauldwell, et al. and Salassa, et al. They also documented the importance of the right first intercostal artery, noting that many bronchial trunks arise from the *right* but not the left first intercostal artery. Cauldwell, et al. (1948) found that 90 percent of the intercostobronchial arteries arose from the right first intercostal artery and only 6 percent arose from the left (Fig. 10-9). The esophagus is supplied by twigs from these vessels as they supply the trachea. A knowledge of the anatomy of the bronchial arteries has allowed some surgeons to incorporate a bronchial artery anastomosis into the lung transplant operation. There appears to be early improvement in the mucosal circulation of the donor airway and theoretical benefits for tracheal healing (Laks, et al., 1991; Couraud, et al., 1992; Daly, et al., 1993).

Microcirculation. Once the arteries reach the tracheoesophageal groove, they divide into primary tracheal and primary esophageal branches. Tracheal vessels enter the trachea in its' lateral wall 0.7 to 1.5 cm anterior to the tracheoesophageal groove. After entering the trachea, lateral longitudinal and transverse intercartilaginous arteries are formed that connect the superior to the inferior vessels and supply blood in a circumferential manner to the trachea (Fig. 10-10). The lateral longitudinal arteries may be large—up to 1 to 2 mm in diameter—and form an important anastomotic connection for the entire trachea. In order to safely preserve blood supply, mobilization of long segments of trachea, especially along the posterolateral aspects, should be minimized during tracheal surgery. Bleeding from these vessels can be brisk and alarming in the case of accidental laceration, as may occasion-

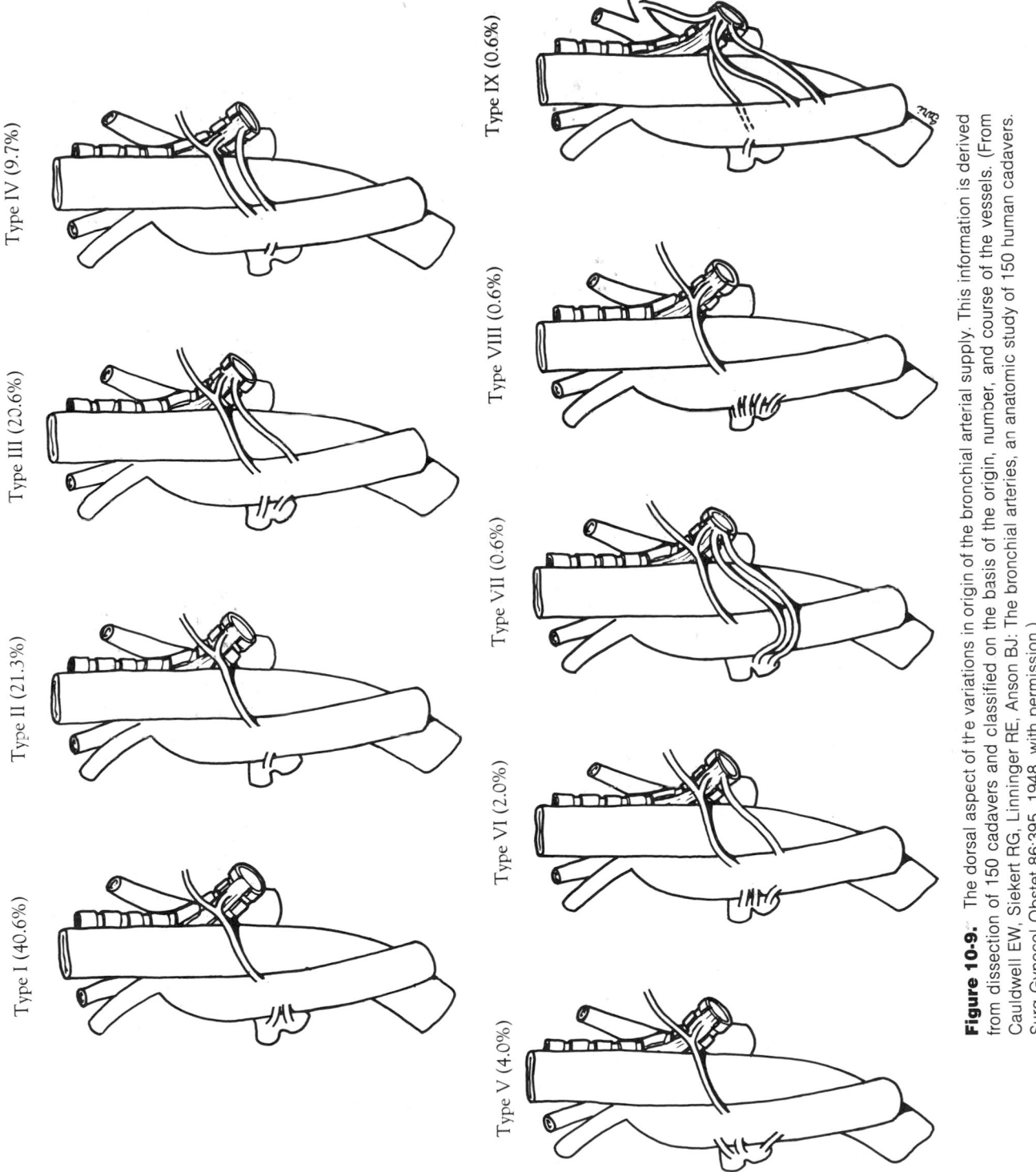

Type IV (9.7%) Type III (20.6%) Type II (21.3%) Type I (40.6%)

Type IX (0.6%) Type VIII (0.6%) Type VII (0.6%) Type VI (2.0%) Type V (4.0%)

Figure 10-9. The dorsal aspect of the variations in origin of the bronchial arterial supply. This information is derived from dissection of 150 cadavers and classified on the basis of the origin, number, and course of the vessels. (From Cauldwell EW, Siekert RG, Linninger RE, Anson BJ: The bronchial arteries, an anatomic study of 150 human cadavers. Surg Gynecol Obstet 86:395, 1948, with permission.)

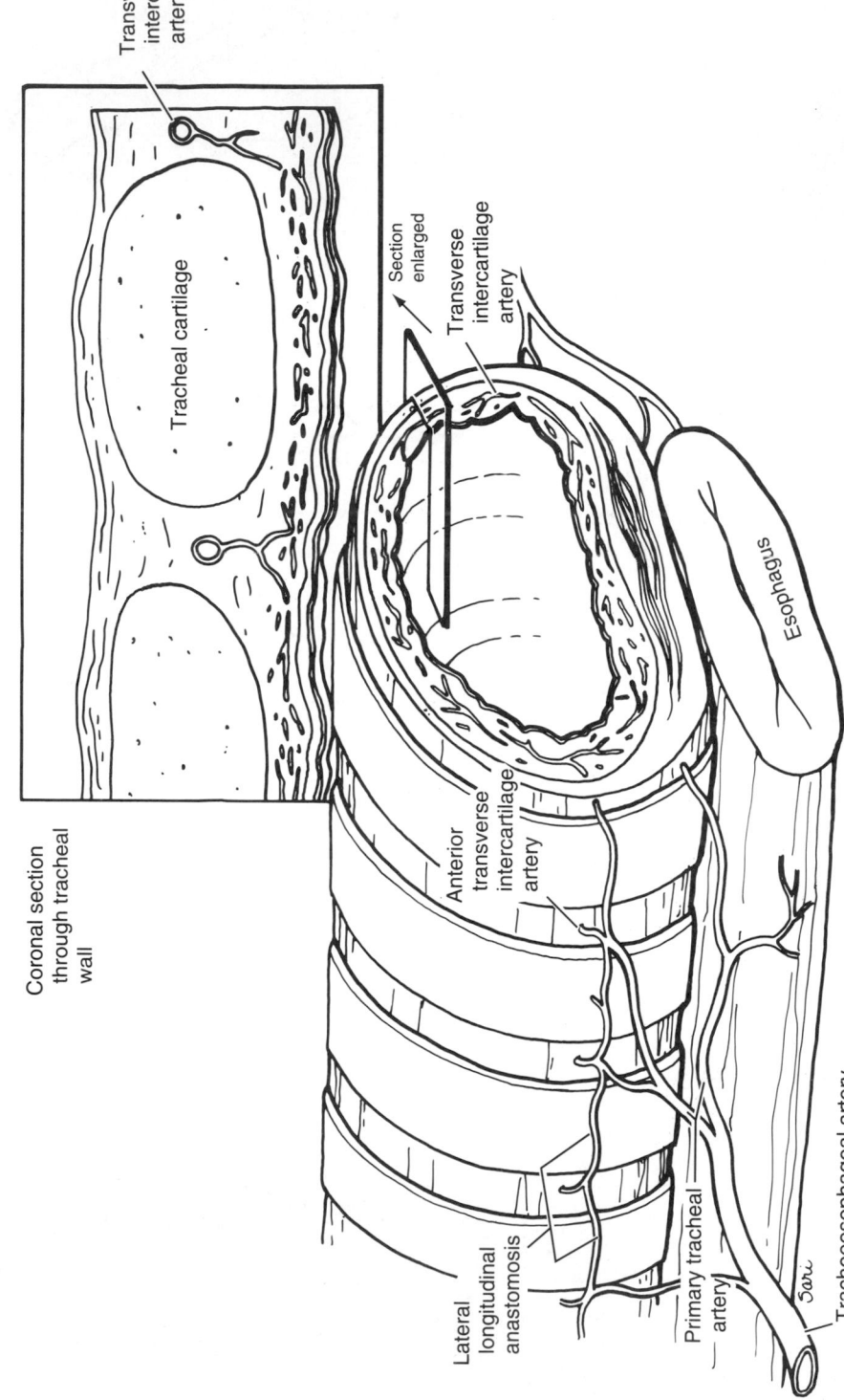

Coronal section
through tracheal
wall

Transverse
intercartilage
artery

Tracheal cartilage

Section
enlarged

Transverse
intercartilage
artery

Esophagus

Anterior
transverse
intercartilage
artery

Lateral
longitudinal
anastomosis

Primary tracheal
artery

Tracheoesophageal artery

Figure 10-10. Microcirculation of the trachea and esophagus. There is a rich submucosal plexus but no similar plexus of vessels on the external surface. Tracheal cartilage is nourished entirely from the submucosal circulation. (From Salassa JR, Pearson BW, Payne WS: Gross and microscopical blood supply of the trachea. Ann Thorac Surg 24:100, 1977, with permission.)

ally occur during lymph node biopsy in the paratracheal or subcarinal space.

Throughout the length of the trachea is an extensive submucosal plexus, fed by transverse intercartilaginous arteries, each of which penetrates the soft tissue space between the cartilaginous rings and runs anteriorly. As they reach the midline, they dive more deeply and terminate in the submucosal plexus. Conversely, there is *no* blood supply external to the cartilages. Thus, the cartilages receive their nutrient supply from the submucosal arterial plexus. It is therefore understandable that the tracheal rings may be damaged by ischemic injury due to overinflation of endotracheal tube cuffs.

The membranous trachea is not supplied by the transverse intercartilaginous arteries. While small twigs from these vessels pass posteriorly, they tend to stop at the cartilage-membrane junction. The membranous portion is supplied by secondary tracheal twigs, which arise from primary esophageal branches of the tracheoesophageal arteries. These secondary tracheal twigs enter the membranous portion of the trachea and feed the submucosal plexus of the posterior wall of the trachea. These secondary arteries are well developed and form longitudinal arcades that span several segments.

Carina

The most inferior portion of the trachea, the bifurcation, is called the carina. It normally lies slightly to the right of the midline and is at the level of the fourth or fifth vertebra posteriorly and the sternomanubrial junction anteriorly. In normal individuals the left mainstem bronchus lies under the aortic arch, and for this reason, the carina, proximal left mainstem bronchus, and distal trachea are difficult to access through a left thoracotomy. Exposure is excellent through a high (fourth interspace) right thoracotomy. The angle between the two mainstem bronchi varies among individuals and is generally greater in children than in adults (Kubota, et al., 1986). The configuration of the cartilages at the carina is quite variable. Occasionally a tracheal ring arising from the right or left mainstem bronchus extends under the crotch of the carina. Most often however, there is a symmetric contribution from each side, with or without fusion at the carinal bifurcation (Vanpeperstraete, 1973). The blood supply at the carina is very robust and comes primarily from bronchial vessels, which branch to supply both the trachea and the bronchi. There is an abundance of lymph nodes in the crotch of the carina, which drain each side of the tracheobronchial tree and the lungs.

PHYSIOLOGY

There are three aspects of tracheal physiology that warrant discussion: changes in airway size, ciliary clearance, and humidification of tracheobronchial secretions.

Airway Size

Alterations in tracheal diameter and length occur with each respiration. During inspiration both the length and diameter increase in size, which facilitates airflow. The airway resistance is decreased (it is inversely related to the fourth power of the radius), as is the muscular work to move air. It is this capacity to change radius that accounts for different lung volumes in individuals with similar tracheal areas. Tracheal area is related more to sex (males having larger tracheas than females despite equivalent total lung capacities) than it is to lung volume (Martin, et al., 1987). The length of the trachea can increase by one vertebral size on full inspiration, which allows for the descent of the diaphragm during inspiration.

Ciliary Action

The epithelium of the trachea consists of pseudostratified ciliated columnar epithelium with interspersed goblet cells. Ciliary action gently wafts debris proximally from more distal airways, and the mucoid material is then either expectorated or swallowed. This occurs by a rhythmic contraction of the cilia at a rate of 160 to 1,500 times per minute and moves debris at a rate of about 16 mm/min (Paparella and Shumrick, 1980). Hypoxia as well as hyperoxia can decrease the beat frequency of these cilia. While it is said that cigarette smoking also decreases the frequency and thus the clearance, some find this not to be the case (Konietzko, et al., 1981). The average beat frequency is similar regardless of the primary disease process (Konietzko, et al., 1981). A rise in temperature causes an increase in beat frequency. The metabolic rate of the tracheal mucosa is quite high owing to the ciliary and glandular function. In fact, the oxygen consumption of the tracheal mucosa exceeds that of both the liver and the beating heart (Widdicombe, 1993).

Tracheobronchial Secretions

Tracheobronchial secretions consist of the output of the mucous glands under vagal and parasympathetic drug stimulation and of the goblet cells under the influence of local irritants. The sympathetic nervous system plays no known role in the production of these secretions. The total volume of the secretions is difficult to measure but under normal circumstances varies from 10 to 100 ml/day. The mucous layer forms a coat on the surface of the airway, which not only moistens the inspired air, but also may limit evaporation from the trachea and bronchi. This mucous coat, which is about 5 μm in thickness, also carries foreign debris out of the airway. These secretions contain immunoglobulins, lysozymes, and other bacteriostatic and bacteriocidal components; they are 95 percent composed of water, with carbohydrates, proteins, and lipids making up most of the remaining 5 percent (Yeager, 1971). Output from the goblet cells is strongly stimulated by local irritants.

KEY REFERENCES

Cauldwell EW, Siekert RG, Linninger RE, Anson BJ: The bronchial arteries, an anatomic study of 150 human cadavers. Surg Gynecol Obst 86:395, 1948

The most comprehensive study of the tracheal and bronchial circulations. All subsequent studies have confirmed the findings in this report.

Salassa JR, Pearson BW, Payne WS: Gross and microscopical blood supply of the trachea. Ann Thorac Surg 24:100, 1977

A study of the tracheal blood supply that is pertinent to surgery of the trachea, particularly circumferential resection and reconstruction by primary anastomosis. The report was written by an anatomist and two Mayo Clinic surgeons.

REFERENCES

Burrington JD: Tracheal growth and healing, J Thorac Cardiovasc Surg 76:453, 1978

Couraud L, Baudet E, Martigne C, et al.: Bronchial revascularization in double lung transplantation: a series of 8 patients. Ann Thorac Surg 53:88, 1992

Daly RC, Tadjkarimi S, Khaghani A, et al.: Successful double-lung transplantation with direct bronchial artery revascularization. Ann Thorac Surg 56:885, 1993

Galliard DA, Lallement AV, Petit AF, Puchelle ES: In vivo ciliogenesis in human fetal tracheal epithelium. Am J Anat 185:415, 1989

Griscom NT, Wohl ME: Dimensions of the growing trachea related to age and gender. AJR 146:233, 1986

Håkansson CH, Mercke U, Sonesson B, Toremalm NG: Functional anatomy of the musculature of the trachea. Acta Morphol Neerl Scand 14:291, 1976

Kawakami Y, Nishimura M, Kusaka H: Tracheal dimensions at full inflation and deflation in adolescent twins. J Appl Physiol 70:1781, 1991

Konietzko N, Nakhosteen JA, Mizera W et al.: Ciliary beat frequency of biopsy samples taken from normal persons and patients with various lung diseases. Chest 80(suppl):855, 1981

Kubota Y, Toyoda Y, Nagata N, et al.: Tracheo-bronchial angles in infants and children. Anesthesiology 64:374, 1986

Laks H, Louie HW, Haas GS, et al.: New technique of vascularization of the trachea and bronchus for lung transplantation. J Heart Lung Transplant 10:280, 1991

Martin R, Castile RG, Fredberg JJ, et al.: Airway size is related to sex but not lung size in normal adults. J Appl Physiol 63:2042, 1987

McLaughlin RF: Bronchial artery distribution in various mammals and in humans. Am Rev Respir Dis 128(2):S57, 1983

Meta S, Myat HM: The cross-sectional shape and circumference of the human trachea. Ann R Coll Surg Engl 66:3568, 1984

Miura T, Grillo JC: The contribution of the inferior thyroid artery to the blood supply of the human trachea. Surg Gynecol Obstet 123:99, 1966

Moore K: The Developing Human. 2nd Ed WB Saunders, Philadelphia, 1977

Nagaishi C: Functional Anatomy and Histology of the Lung. University Park Press, Baltimore, 1972

Paparella MM, Shumrick DA: Otolaryngology. 2nd Ed. WB Saunders, Philadelphia, 1980

Reid L: Visceral cartilage. J Anat 122:349, 1976

Schreinemakers HHJ, Weder W, Miyoshi S, et al.: Direct revascularization of bronchial arteries for lung transplantation: an anatomical study. Ann Thorac Surg 49:44, 1990

Tos M: Anatomy of the tracheal mucous glands in man. Arch Otolaryngol Head Neck Surg 92:132, 1970

Vanpeperstraete F: The cartilaginous skeleton of the bronchial tree. Adv Anat Embryol Cell Biol 48:1, 1973

Wailoo MP, Emery JL: Normal growth and development of the trachea. Thorax 37:584, 1982

Widdicombe J: New perspectives on basic mechanisms in lung disease 4: Why are the airways so vascular? Throax 48:290, 1993

Williams PL, Warwick R: Gray's Anatomy. 33rd Ed. Churchill Livingstone, Edinburgh, 1981

Yeager H: Tracheobronchial secretions. Am J Med 50:493, 1971

11

IMAGING

Plain Radiography, Tomography, and Contrast Radiography

Douglas E. Sanders

PLAIN RADIOGRAPHY

Plain chest radiography in two or more views will not define the central airways adequately because of the complex anatomy of the superior mediastinum. Superimposition of overlying vessels often prevents the demonstration of these structures throughout their entire course. On occasion, however, excellent demonstration of significant abnormalities can be recognized in standard plain films. Anomalies, masses, displacements, and compromise of the trachea and carina can be clearly identified; therefore, careful inspection of these structures in plain films is required prior to further radiographic or direct examination (Figs. 11-1 and 11-2).

TOMOGRAPHY

Tomography can be carried out in frontal, lateral, or oblique views and will provide sharp detail of morphology without superimposition of adjacent structures. It has been used with xeroradiography with some success although owing to relatively high patient doses this method of study of the central airways has fallen into disfavor (Harle, et al., 1975) (Fig. 11-3). Tomograms will aid in identification of calcification in masses, cartilage, aneurysms, lymph nodes, etc. It is easily performed, fast, and ideal for the evaluation of patients with respiratory difficulty, and it is useful for the follow-up of patients with obstructive lesions or those operated patients who cannot tolerate prolonged investigative workup. It is the procedure of choice for periodic follow-up and is not associated with any preparation or risk (Figs. 11-4 and 11-5). When narrowing of the major airways is suspected from historical data, physical examination, or plain films, tomography will frequently provide helpful information, and on the basis of the findings, subsequent studies can be selected if required (George, et al., 1990; Standertskjöld-Nordenstam, et al., 1981; Gamsu and Webb, 1983).

CONTRAST RADIOGRAPHY

The rapid motion of the trachea during cough requires special attention, since static imaging procedures (oblique view xerography, plain film tomography, computed tomography [CT], and magnetic resonance imaging [MRI]) may not indicate the stability of the central airways during peak air flow. High-resolution computed tomography (HRCT) is the method of choice for evaluating morphology of the peripheral airways. In conjunction with endoscopy, it provides highly reliable data. It is carried out during quiet breathing or suspended respiration.

Dynamics of the central airways can be assessed by cinefluorography or video fluorography with rapid frame speeds (30/s), stop framing, and slow motion. These methods are used to evaluate rapid motion in other areas such as cardiac valve prostheses, swallowing, etc. (Feinberg and Ekberg, 1991; Ott, et al., 1989). In order to demonstrate the trachea during cough and other breathing maneuvers, a contrast tracheogram is obtained prior to filming.

Indirect cine or video fluoroscopy of the trachea has been used by coating the esophagus with thick barium sulfate and recording the motion of the esophagus against the posterior tracheal wall during coughing. This does not provide mucosal detail or circumferential demonstration of the trachea, so opacification of the airway is preferred but is reserved for selected patients who may be candidates for surgical reconstruction (Pearson, et al., 1968; Pearson, et al., 1968a; Pearson and Andrews, 1971; Pearson, et al., 1984; James, et al., 1970).

Conduct of Contrast Videotracheogram

Patients have usually had repeated direct endoscopic procedures, so premedication is not used routinely. When required, mild sedation similar to that used for endoscopy is given.

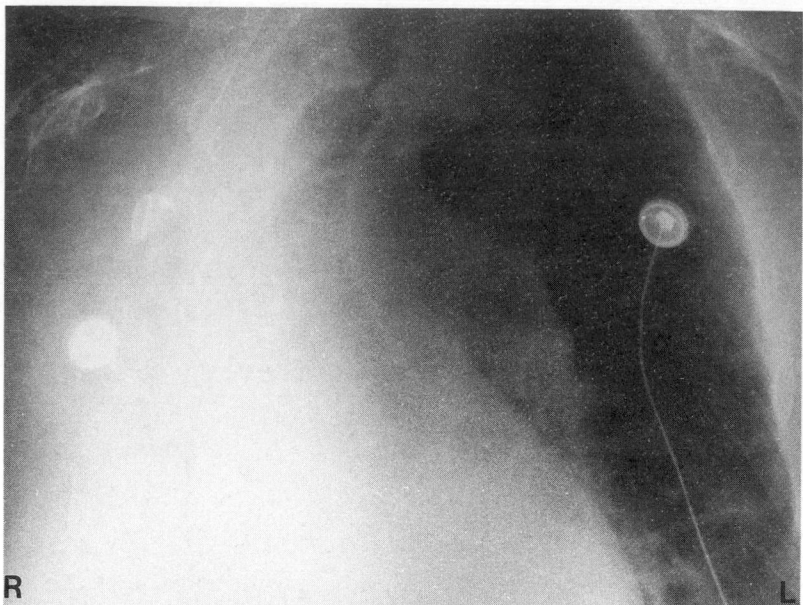

Figure 11-1. Anteroposterior (AP) bedside film demonstrates tracheal stenosis following a previous tracheotomy. This was not a fixed narrowing, and the bronchoscope could be passed through it without difficulty.

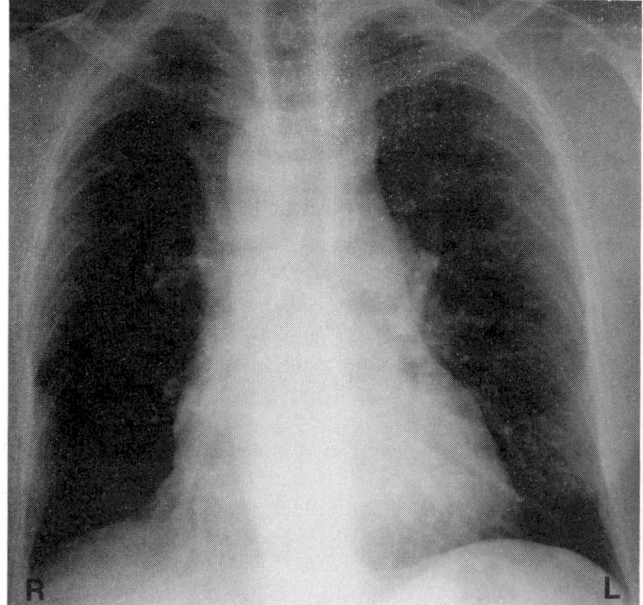

Figure 11-2. Tracheal bronchus. The bronchus to the right upper lobe arises 3 cm proximal to the carina. Multiple anomalies frequently associated include those of the cardiovascular system as in this patient, who has an atrial septal defect and a right-sided aorta.

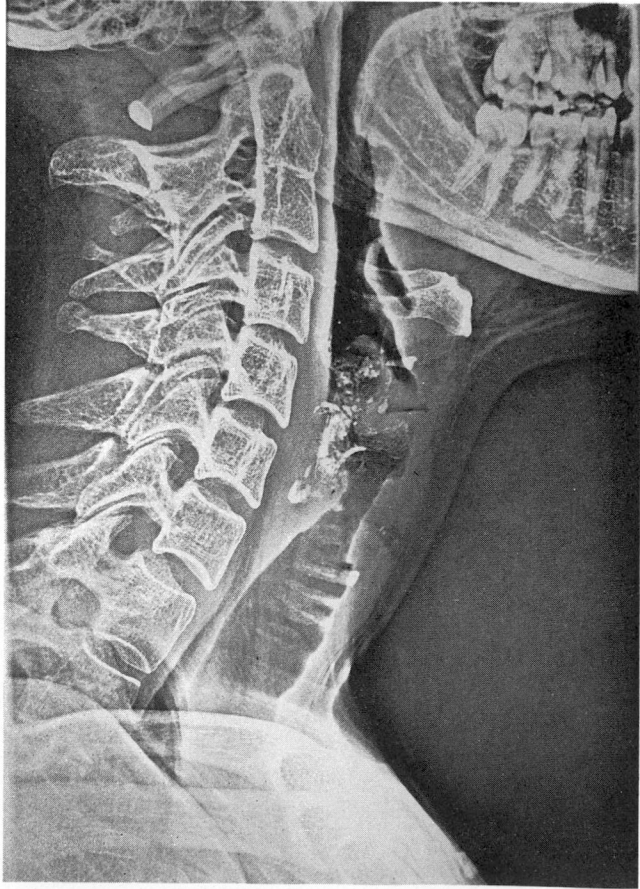

Figure 11-3. Lateral xeroradiography demonstrates tight sub-glottic stenosis following direct trauma in motor vehicle accident.

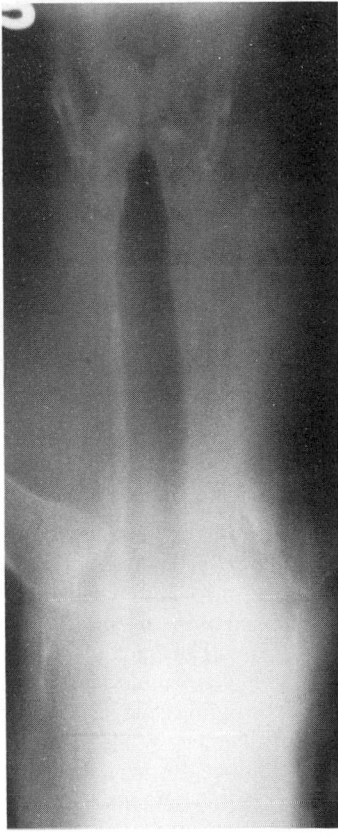

Figure 11-4. Anteroposterior (AP) tomogram. Tracheal airway (normal) well demonstrated in the neck. Note calcification in thyroid and arytenoid cartilages.

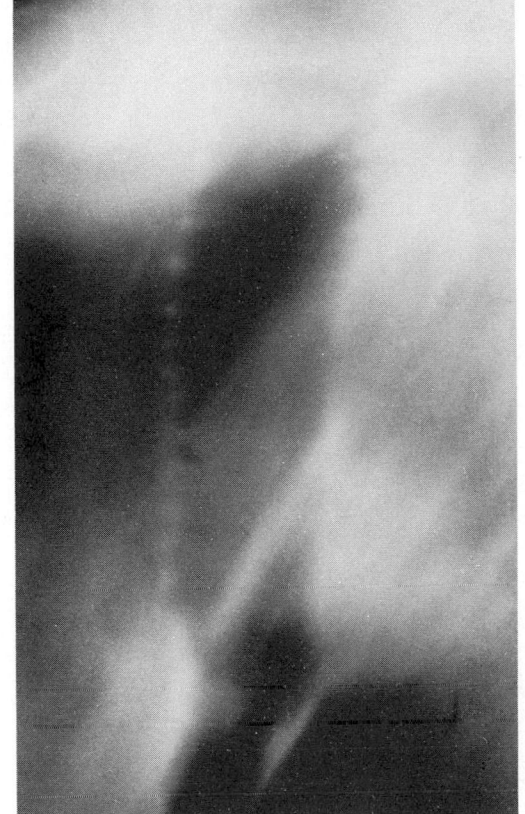

Figure 11-5. Lateral tomogram (normal) of intrathoracic trachea.

Differential Diagnosis of Tracheal Narrowing

Congenital
  Atresia
  Elliptical cricoid cartilage
  Chondrodysplasia
Acquired
  Traumatic
    Direct injury
    Postintubation
    Inhalation injury, toxic fumes, etc.
  Inflammatory
    Infection
      Bacterial
      Mycobacterial
      Fungal
    Noninfectious
      Granuloma
      Sarcoid
      Wegener's granuloma
Autoimmune
  Relapsing polychondritis
Degenerative
  Tracheopathia osteoplastica (polypoid or sessile)

(Continues)

Neoplastic
  Benign
    Chondroma
    Papilloma
    Hemangioma
    Granular cell myoblastoma
  Malignant
    Carcinoid tumor
    Adenoid cystic carcinoma
    Carcinoma
    Lymphoma
    Plasmacytoma
    Sarcoma
Pseudo
  Obstruction
  Saber sheath trachea
Idiopathic
  Amyloid disease
  Extrinsic compression
    Primary neoplasm
    Metastasis
    Mediastinal fibrosis
    Postradiation fibrosis
    Aneurysm

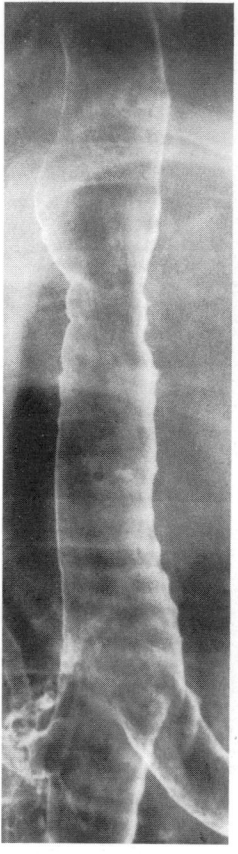

Figure 11-6. Contrast tracheogram, oblique projection shows characteristics of COPD. Occasional dilated mucous gland ducts and posterior bulge at sternal notch.

Those patients with allergies or a history of hypersensitivity to topical anesthetic agents or contrast agents are not examined by this method. Anesthesia is carried out with lidocaine spray. A gently curved preshaped Metras catheter is lubricated with lidocaine gel and passed through the nose into the proximal trachea with use of a laryngeal mirror or fluoroscopic guidance with the patient in the sitting position. When the catheter is secure, the patient is placed in the semiupright position on the fluoroscopy table. Contrast is fractionally injected and the video sequence performed with Valsalva and Mueller maneuvers and coughing. Recording is done while the patient is rotated into both oblique and lateral views. The catheter is then withdrawn and the filming sequence repeated. Remote control is preferred. Conventional static films and 105-mm spot films are obtained simultaneously with the video record.

The various commercially available contrast agents have been used. All have potential limitations and are used in small amounts (usually 4 to 8 ml). Care must be taken to mix the contrast material thoroughly at room temperature. The vial is opened just prior to use. The injection must be made slowly and cautiously, and oxygen should be available. Peripheral filling is prevented by avoiding deep inspiration prior to cough while the contrast is injected. While Hytrast (Therapex) is preferred, it is not universally available, and other water-soluble agents such as oily Dionosil (Glaxo) can be used (Erickson, et al., 1979; Strecker, et al., 1979; Friedell, et al., 1962; Light and Oster, 1964; Grainger, et al., 1970; Nelson, et al., 1959).

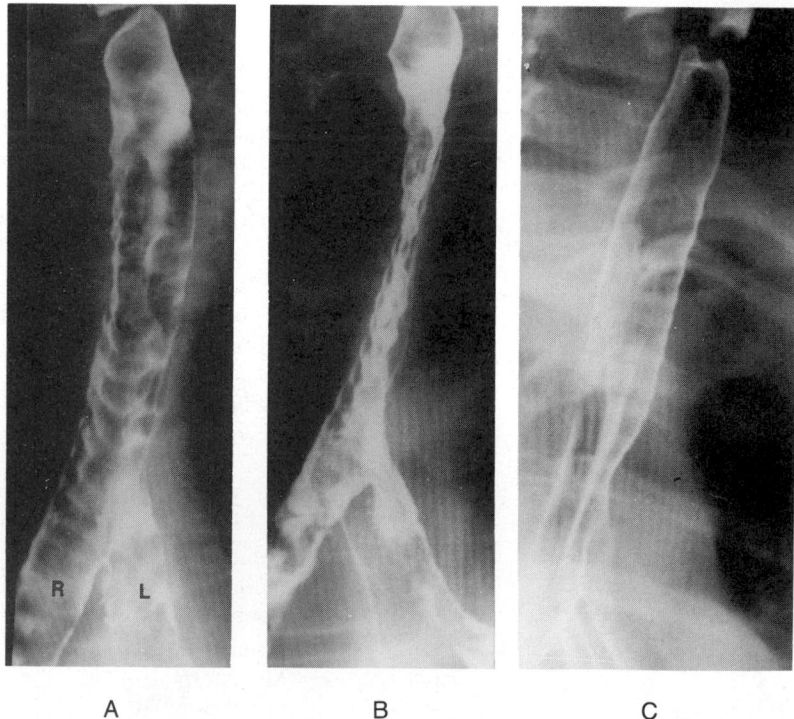

A   B   C

Figure 11-7. **(A)** Full inspiration. Anteroposterior (AP) tracheogram of patient with diffuse COPD. Note coarse striation and filling defects due to thickened mucosal folds and retained secretions. **(B)** Cough. AP tracheogram during peak cough (spot film) of same patient. Note marked, slightly asymmetric narrowing of airway ("twisted rope" appearance). Short segmental narrowing in left main bronchus. **(C)** Full inspiration. Oblique tracheogram normal.

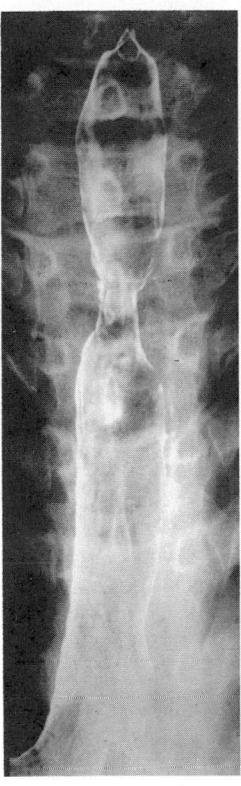

Figure 11-8. Anteroposterior (AP) tracheogram. Rigid post-tracheostomy stenosis with normal intrathoracic trachea.

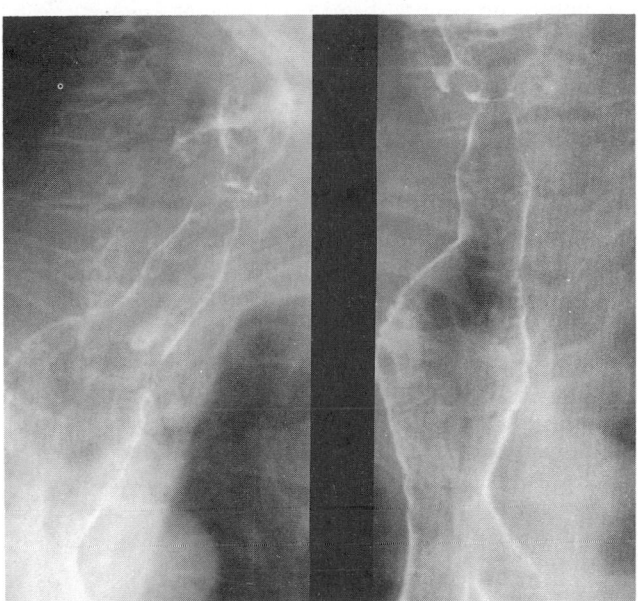

Figure 11-9. Fixed right lateral dilatation of trachea following right upper lobectomy in a patient with tracheomalacia and ineffectual clearing of secretions.

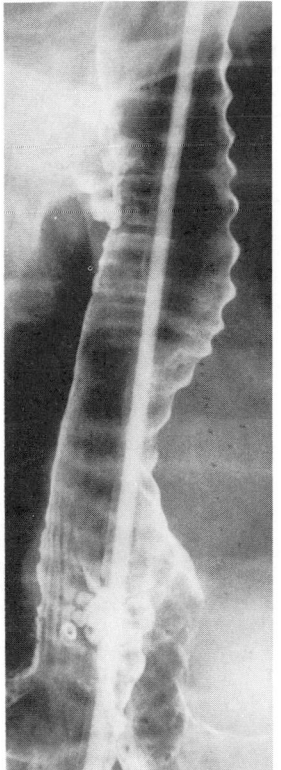

Figure 11-10. Oblique tracheogram demonstrates large diverticula on right posterolateral wall. Intratracheal catheter in place.

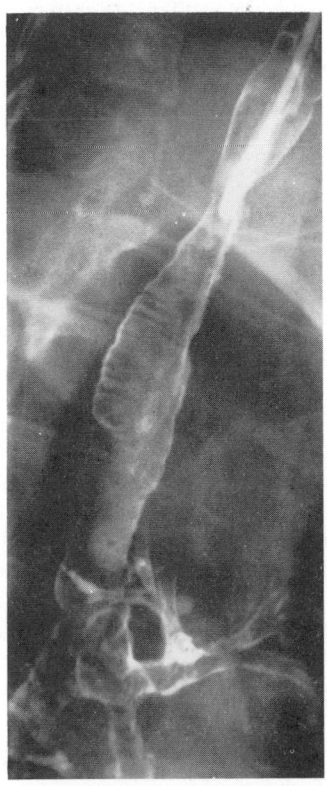

Figure 11-11. Spot film during injection of contrast. Note tracheal stenosis at level of catheter.

Analysis of Videotracheogram

The purpose is to assess airway motion during deep breathing and cough. Normal upper limits of measurement of the trachea in men is considered to be 25 mm in the coronal and 27 mm in the sagittal diameter at a point 2 cm above the aortic arch in chest radiographs (Breatnach, et al., 1984). It should be noted that a short narrow segment, or web, in the trachea may not be demonstrated by CT owing to volume averaging (Gamsu and Webb, 1983). This type of lesion is readily detected by the contrast tracheogram.

Abnormal findings during cough include segmental collapse, kinking or buckling, retention of secretions, filling of dilated mucous glands and ducts, fistulae, and paradoxical movement of membranous tracheal wall. One of the main purposes of the dynamic study is to assess the stability of the airway distal to a stenotic lesion. Localized tracheomalacia may be very obvious, but an unstable distal segment may significantly compromise the results of resection of a stenotic lesion and may be more difficult to identify.

The main considerations are the degree of narrowing and the length of the affected segment. The airway may be rigid in patients with long-standing stenoses and chronic infection. The motion of the entire airway is evaluated. Videotracheogram findings regarding distal airways and pulmonary function are evaluated together with the clinical findings. HRCT and pulmonary function tests provide this information. Bronchography is avoided since these studies have now been replaced by thin-section CT.

Normal motion during cough is characterized by rapid reduction in caliber and forward uniform herniation of the posterior wall, followed by sudden return to resting dimensions. The degree of caliber change appears to be less important than the uniformity. The sequence is rapid, occurring in about 40 ms (Fraser, et al., 1988). There is simultaneous upward movement and shortening. Abnormal dynamics are characterized by cough that is ineffectual in clearing the airways of mucus and contrast material, by paradoxical motion of the posterior membranous wall, and by kinking. A high intraluminal pressure is required for an effective cough. Accentuated generalized tracheal collapse during cough is characteristic of advanced chronic obstructive pulmonary disease (COPD) (Sabel, et al., 1968) (Figs. 11-6 and 11-7). Static and dynamic caliber changes in the trachea cannot be evaluated in isolation, and each patient must be investigated thoroughly, with emphasis on causative factors, endoscopic findings, and functional impairment in addition to the appropriate imaging studies (Figs. 11-8 to 11-12). Aftercare is important following use of intrabronchial contrast agents. Avoiding ingestion of food or fluids and avoiding sedation is advised, and vigorous cough to clear secretions is encouraged.

So-called saber-sheath tracheal deformity (i.e., increase in sagittal diameter and decrease in coronal diameter), which is not uncommon, has been defined to consist of a decrease of two-thirds or more of the coronal measurement as compared with the sagittal (Greene, 1978). It is confined to the intrathoracic segment of the trachea and may have segmental accentuation. It results from COPD, is rarely seen in females, and is uncommon in males under the age of 50 (Greene, 1978, Rubinstein, et al., 1978).

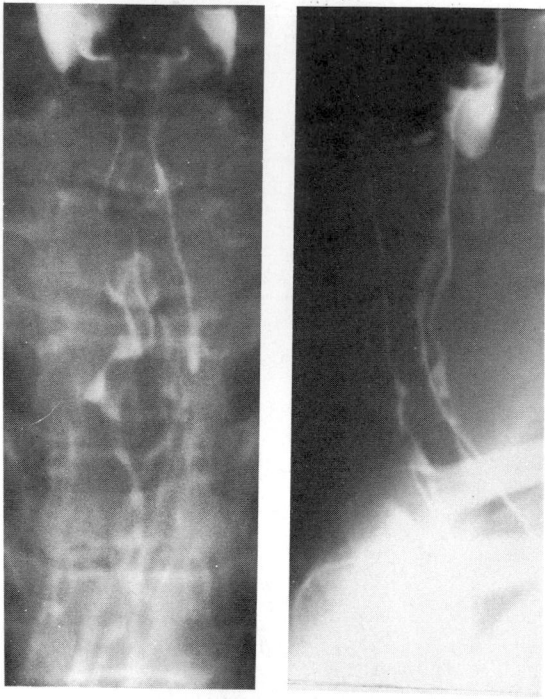

Figure 11-12. Anteroposterior (AP) and lateral tracheograms demonstrate long, smooth intramural filling defect due to adenoid cystic carcinoma in 26-year-old patient.

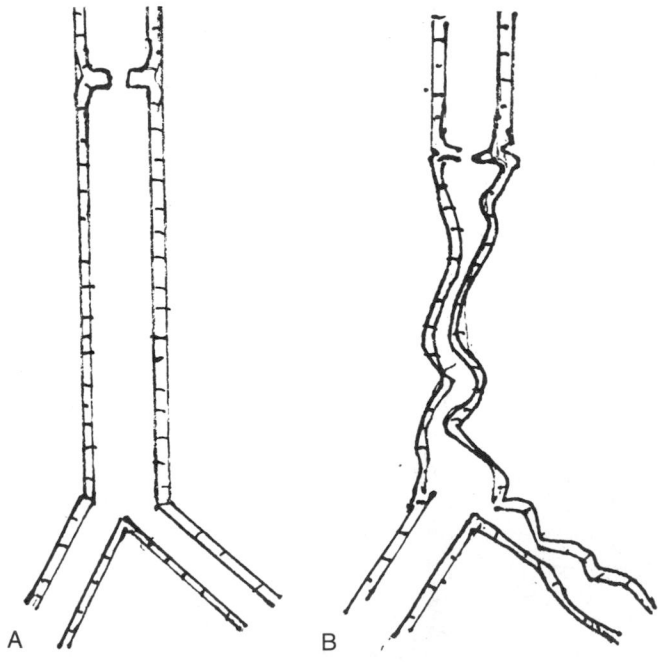

Figure 11-13. **(A)** Schematic drawing of post-tracheotomy stenosis. **(B)** During peak cough, marked shortening, asymmetric narrowing, and instability of airway are found. Such findings may be associated with retention of secretions, granulomatous changes in the trachea, and more distal infections.

Minor bronchographic features of chronic bronchitis have been described in normal patients, so these changes must be interpreted with caution (Gamsu, et al., 1981). Relapsing polychrondritis can be recognized by its extrathoracic manifestations and general as well as local involvement (Mendelson, et al., 1985; Johnson, et al., 1973; Horns and O'Laughlin, 1962; Killman, 1978; Casselman, et al., 1988; Davis, et al., 1989). There is gross collapse and progressive narrowing, which is eventually complicated by infection. Involvement of the cartilaginous structures of the ear, nose, larynx, trachea, bronchi, peripheral joints, and costochondral junctions is characteristic of this disease. Saddle-nose deformity, history of repeated and progressive lower respiratory tract infection, and biopsy findings are required to establish this diagnosis.

Infections, granulomas, amyloid disease, and neoplasms will also require appropriate bacteriologic and/or tissue diagnosis.

In each patient the etiology of a segmental stenosis should be established prior to dynamic studies (Fig. 11-12). Those with benign segmental lesions may then be evaluated by the contrast videotracheogram to aid in selection of suitable candidates for surgical resection. Diffuse instability of the intrathoracic trachea and main bronchi during coughing is secondary to chronic obstructive disease in small distal airways and secondary tracheomalacia (Fig. 11-13). This and/or the presence of other intrinsic central airway lesions can be demonstrated by rapid-motion study during cough and other breathing maneuvers.

REFERENCES

Breatnach E, Abbott GC, Fraser RG: Dimensions of the normal human trachea. AJR 141:903, 1984

Casselman JW, Lemahieu P, Peene P, Stoffels G: Polychondritis affecting the laryngeal cartilages: CT findings. AJR 150:355, 1988

Christiforidis AJ, Nelson SW, Tomashefski JF: Effects of bronchography on pulmonary function. Am Rev Respir Dis 85:127, 1962

Davis SD, Berkman YM, King T: Peripheral bronchial involvement in relapsing polychondritis demonstration by thin-section CT. AJR 153:953, 1989

Erickson LM, Shaw D, Macdonald FR: Prolonged barium retention in the lung following bronchography. Radiology 39:635, 1979

Feinberg MJ, Ekberg O: Videofluoroscopy in elderly patients with aspiration. AJR 156:293, 1991

Fraser RF, Paré JAP, Paré PD et al.: Diagnosis of Diseases of the Chest. 3rd Ed. WB Saunders, Philadelphia, 1988

Friedell GH, Kaufman SA, LaForet EG, Strieder JW: Granulomatous lung reaction following repeat bronchography with propyliodone. AJR 87:847, 1962

Gamsu G, Forbes AR, Overfors C: Bronchographic features of chronic bronchitis in normal men. AJR 36:317, 1981

Gamsu G, Webb R: CT of the trachea and main stem bronchi. Semin Roentgenol 18:51, 1983

George PJM, Pearson MC, Edwards D: Bronchography in the assessment of patients with lung collapse for endoscopic laser treatment. Thorax 45:503, 1990

Grainger RG, Castellino RA, Lewin K, Steiner RN: Hytrast: experimental bronchography comparing two different formulations. Clin Radiol 21:390, 1970

Greene R: Sabre sheath trachea: Relation to chronic obstructive pulmonary disease. AJR 130:44, 1978

Harle TS, Hevezi JM, Rogers LF et al.: Xerotomography of the tracheobronchial tree. AJR 124:353, 1975

Horns JW, O'Loughlin BJ: Tracheal collapse in polychondritis. AJR 87:844, 1962

James AE, MacMillan AS, Eaton SB, Grillo HC: Roentgenology of tracheal stenosis resulting from cuffed tracheostomy tubes. AJR 109:455, 1970

Johnson TH, Mital N, Rodnan GP, Wilson RJ: Relapsing polychondritis. Radiology 106:313, 1973

Killman WJ: Narrowing of the airway in relapsing polychondritis. Radiology 126:373, 1978

Light JP, Oster WP: A study of clinical and pathological reaction to the bronchographic agent Hytrast. AJR 92:615, 1964

Mendelson DS, Som PM, Crane R et al.: Relapsing polychondritis studied by CT. Radiology 157:489, 1985

Nelson SW, Christiforidis A, Pratt PC: Barium sulphate and bismuth subcarbonate suspensions in bronchographic contrast media. Radiology 72:829, 1959

Ott J, Chen YM, Hewson EG et al.: Esophageal motility: assessment with synchronous video tape fluoroscopy and manometry. Radiology 173:419, 1989

Pearson FG, Goldberg M, da Silva AJ: Tracheal stenosis complicating tracheostomy with cuffed tubes. Arch Surg 97:380, 1968

Pearson FG, Henderson RD, Gross AE et al.: The reconstruction of circumferential tracheal defects with a porous prosthesis. J Thorac Cardiovasc Surg 55:605, 1968b

Pearson FG, Andrews MJ: Detection and management of tracheal stenosis following cuffed tube tracheostomy. Ann Thorac Surg 12:359, 1971

Pearson FG, Todd TRJ, Cooper JD: Experience with primary neoplasms of the trachea and carina. J Thorac Cardiovasc Surg 88:511, 1984

Rubinstein J, Weisbrod G, Steinhardt M: Atypical appearances of "saber-sheath" trachea. Radiology 127:41, 1978

Sabal IA, Sanders DE, Suero, JT, Woolf CR: The relationship between tracheobronchial collapse and pulmonary function in COPD. Chest 53:407, 1968

Standertskjöld-Nordenstam CG, Halttunen PA, Meurala HG: Cinetracheobronchography and surgical correction of central airway collapse in an asthmatic patient. Eur J Radiol 1:20, 1981

Strecker EP, Kraemer C, Reinbold WD, Speck U: Inhalation bronchography using powdered calcium/ioglycamic acid. Radiology 130:303, 1979

Computed Tomography and Magnetic Resonance Imaging

M. Anne Keller
Stephen J. Herman
Gordon L. Weisbrod

HISTORICAL NOTE

Imaging of the larynx and trachea was, until the 1980s, restricted solely to radiography. Plain radiography, xeroradiography, and tomography have been the only useful imaging tools at our disposal. However, only the effect on the airway by adjacent soft tissue or bone is identified by these methods, and no intrinsic information about the soft tissues is obtained. Hence, the utility of radiography depended on lesions causing airway narrowing, filling defects within the air column, or irregularity of the airway walls. The magnitude of the lesion could in no way be accurately predicted. The introduction in the mid-1970s of computed tomography (CT) with a body-sized gantry and, more recently, magnetic resonance imaging (MRI) has provided enormous benefits in the evaluation of the airways by allowing soft tissue to be visualized.

HISTORICAL READING

Eisenberg RL: Radiology: An Illustrated History. Mosby-Year Book, St. Louis, 1991

IMAGING TECHNIQUES

Some CT features of neoplastic diseases of the airways are described in another chapter. Generally speaking, CT and MRI are quite accurate in the detection of airway lesions but are unreliable in determining if the lesion is mucosal or submucosal in origin (Naidich, et al., 1990). The mucosa is identified only by its proximity to air and is better visualized endoscopically. However, the endoscopist can not appreciate alteration of planes deep to the mucosa. In particular, laryngeal tumor spread along fat planes in the pre-epiglottic space, across the anterior commissure, and into the paraglottic fat stripe of the vocal cord is well visualized by axial CT or MRI. Involvement of cartilages cannot be easily detected clinically, but axial imaging does quite reliably demonstrate erosion of these structures. Imaging in the axial plane provides excellent assessment of airway caliber.

Airway tumor can appear as an intraluminal soft tissue mass, thickening of the airway wall, extraluminal mass, or any combination of these. In addition to assessing the primary tumor (Li, et al., 1990), CT is particularly helpful in detecting enlarged neck and mediastinal nodes. Small positive nodes, however, can still be missed in either location. The patient with tumor recurrence can also be well evaluated by CT (Naidich, et al., 1982).

The larynx and trachea are evaluated by CT with 5-mm thick contiguous scans from the skull base to the carina following a bolus and infusion of intravenous radiographic contrast agent. Additional 1.0- to 1.5-mm contiguous scans through the laryngeal cartilages using a bone algorithm are necessary to appreciate erosion. Intravenous radiographic contrast is necessary to differentiate lymph nodes from adjacent vascular structures. Unfortunately, enhanced CT often does not reliably provide differentiation between edema and tumor within the airway. MRI suffers from the same inability to separate malignant tissue from edema. MRI does not offer a major advantage over CT in the larynx, but in the trachea it is better able to assess the effect of extra- or intraluminal masses on the adjacent tracheal rings. MRI scans are performed by using a neck surface coil, and both T_1- and T_2-weighted images in the axial plane are obtained. Occasionally, sagittal and coronal images will be beneficial, particularly when assessing small lesions, which may be volume-averaged and therefore missed on axial scans. The use of intravenous paramagnetic contrast agents such as gadolinium diethylenetriamine penta-acetic acid has not yet been fully evaluated.

INTRINSIC AIRWAY LESIONS

Inflammatory Lesions

Acute and chronic inflammatory lesions involving the larynx and trachea present either as diffuse or focal masses. All may present a diagnostic challenge by mimicking malignant tumors. The role of imaging is not to primarily make the diagnosis but to provide the clinician with essential data necessary for planning therapy. The site of origin of pathology, the extent of the pathologic process, and its effect on adjacent intra- or extralaryngeal structures constitute essential pretreatment information. In nearly all cases endoscopic biopsy provides the definitive diagnosis.

Focal inflammatory masses are more common in the larynx than the trachea (Fig. 11-14). Mucus retention cysts can arise in mucus-secreting glands anywhere along the respiratory mucosa, sparing only the free edge of the vocal cords (Fig. 11-15). They are well-defined masses with a relatively sharply marginated thin capsule and central homogeneous low density on CT and high signal on T_2-weighted MRI. An obstructed laryngocele has a similar appearance. Differentiation can be aided by following the origin of a laryngocele to the laryngeal ventricle (Fig. 11-16). Extralaryngeal extension through the thyrohyoid membrane is also characteristic of the external or mixed internal-external laryngocele. While laryngoceles are benign, they can be associated with laryngeal malignancy. The presence of adjacent tumor may obstruct the ventricle, producing a secondary laryngocele (Som and Bergeron, 1991).

A thyroglossal duct cyst can arise anywhere along the embryologic course of the thyroglossal duct, from the foramen cecum at the base of the tongue to the normal position of the thyroid gland overlying the upper trachea (Fig. 11-17). Secretory lining epithelium in the face of an obstructed duct may produce fluid accumulation, which may on occasion become acutely infected. The cystic collection is in or around the hyoid bone (15 percent), suprahyoid (20 percent), or infrahyoid (65 percent) (Batsakis, 1979). A noninfected cyst is of homogeneous low density, has a thin peripheral margin (or capsule), and may be multiseptated. When infected, the internal fluid attains a higher density, and the capsule becomes thickened and irregular, particularly at the external border, reflecting the acute inflammatory reaction, which extends within and beyond the margins of the cyst. Carcinoma of thyroid origin occurs within a thyroglossal duct cyst in less than 1 percent of patients (Som and Bergeron, 1991).

Acute diffuse inflammatory lesions of the laryngotracheobronchial tree usually are caused by bacterial or viral infections (Choplin, et al., 1983; Rosai, 1981). Laryngotracheobronchitis is thought to be due to bacterial infection superimposed on viral infection. In adults, *Haemophilus* is the commonest cause of epiglottitis. Other frequent pathogens are *Staphylococcus aureus, Klebsiella, Pneumococcus,* influenza and parainfluenza viruses, and enteroviruses. There are no specific imaging characteristics for these infectious processes (Fig. 11-18). Increased soft tissue is seen in all or parts of the laryngotracheal mucosa/submucosa in a diffuse rather than focal pattern. The epiglottis may be enlarged with edematous change affecting one or both aryepiglottic folds,

the vocal cords, and the subglottic trachea, where the involvement often becomes more circumferential. Irregular soft tissue densities along the mucosal surface, representing the bacterial pseudomembrane, may be seen.

The incidence of tuberculosis affecting the major airways has decreased paralleling the overall decrease in tuberculosis. Laryngeal and tracheal involvement now are rare (Choplin, et al., 1983; Rosai, 1981). The most common manifestation is mucosal ulceration, usually on the distal posterior tracheal wall. Occasionally, extensive granulation tissue associated with these ulcerations results in tracheal stenosis. The vocal cords are usually involved first if the larynx is affected. Endoscopy reveals ulcerated lesions amenable to biopsy on the posterior tracheal wall. Diagnosis depends on acid-fast bacilli being demonstrated on biopsy or culture.

Chronic inflammatory processes can also mimic neoplasms. Active rheumatoid arthritis can involve the cricoarytenoid and cricothyroid joints, the only synovial joints in the larynx. The surrounding localized granulation tissue mass causes erosion of the joint space and cartilages and airway obstruction (Fig. 11-19). Multiple deep biopsies and an appropriate clinical history are necessary to differentiate this lesion from carcinoma.

Primary laryngeal sarcoidosis is rare, but laryngeal involvement in systemic sarcoidosis occurs in 1 to 3 percent of patients (Choplin, et al., 1983). Usually the supraglottic larynx is involved, but the disease can extend into the subglottic region and less frequently into the distal trachea (Brandstetter, et al., 1981). Biopsy is necessary for diagnosis, as no specific imaging pattern is seen. Similarly, Wegner's granulomatosis (Choplin, et al., 1983) can infrequently produce subglottic laryngeal and upper tracheal airway narrowing (Fig. 11-20). Biopsy is necessary for diagnosis but can usually be more easily obtained from other, more frequently involved sites, such as lung or upper airways.

Relapsing polychondritis (Choplin, et al., 1983; Crockford and Kerr, 1988; Takasugi and Godwin, 1991) involves the larynx and trachea in 50 percent of affected patients. A characteristic clinical picture includes recurrent inflammatory symptoms involving nasal, ear, laryngeal, and tracheal cartilages. Systemic involvement with nonerosive polyarthritis, ocular inflammation, vestibulocochlear abnormality, and arteritis can coexist. The disease is thought to be related to abnormal acid mucopolysaccharide metabolism with a possible relationship to autoimmune vasculitis (Im, et al., 1988). Inflammatory reaction involving the cartilages produces softening, resulting in partial collapse of the laryngeal and tracheal airways (Horns and O'Loughlin, 1962; Killman, 1978; Mendelson, et al., 1985). The healing phase of fibrous tissue replacement results in further narrowing of the collapsed airway, with wall thickening and dense calcification of the destroyed cartilage remnants (Im, et al., 1988) (Fig. 11-21). This process usually does not remain confined to the larynx (Casselman, et al., 1988) and subglottic region, but involves the entire trachea and the mainstem bronchi. The radiologic appearance is diagnostic in a clinical setting of recurrent airway obstruction and pneumonia.

The most common noninfectious inflammatory lesion seen in the larynx and subglottic trachea is granulation tissue secondary to injury (Wiot, 1983). Intubation injuries (Fig.

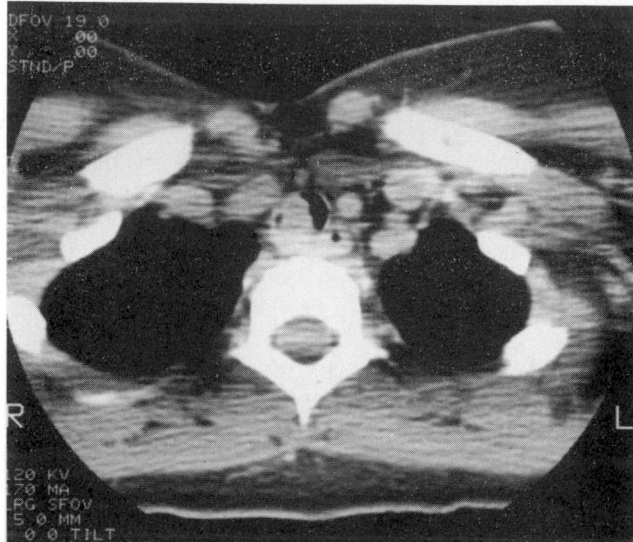

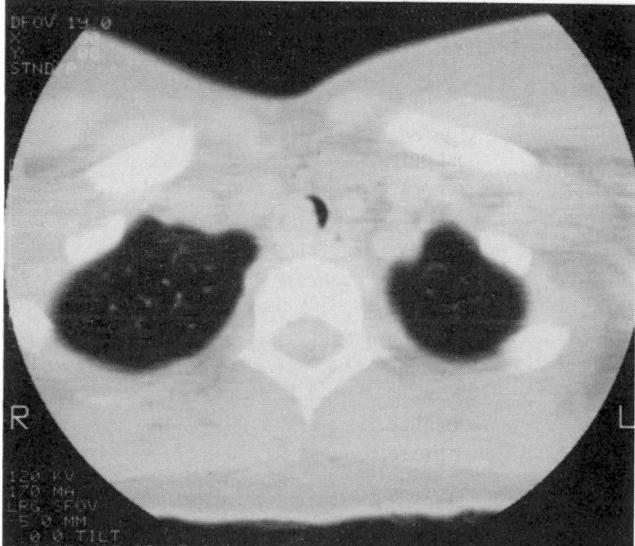

Figure 11-14. Tracheal granuloma in a 25-year-old woman with shortness of breath on exertion for 4 months and one episode of hemoptysis. CT scan of the trachea shows a mass obstructing the right half of the tracheal lumen without extratracheal extension. Bronchoscopy showed a polypoid vascular lesion arising 7 cm below the vocal cords from the right posterolateral wall of the trachea and obstructing 80 percent of the lumen. Tracheal resection revealed a broad-based polypoid mass composed primarily of plasma cells but also lymphocytes and histiocytes. Pathologic diagnosis was plasma cell granuloma of the trachea.

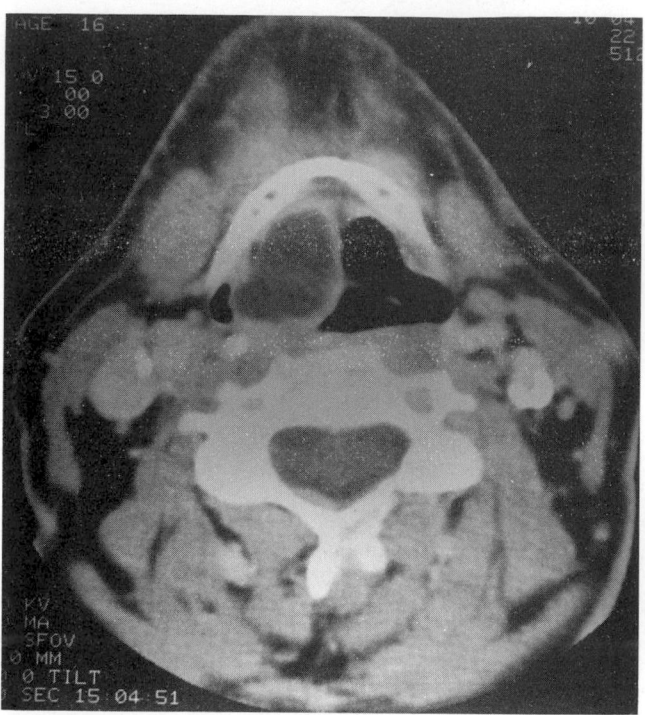

Figure 11-15. Mucus retention cyst. Note the well-encapsulated low-density mass arising in the pre-epiglottic space and compressing the epiglottis. Only the anatomic location well above the laryngeal ventricle differentiates the lesion from an obstructed internal laryngocele.

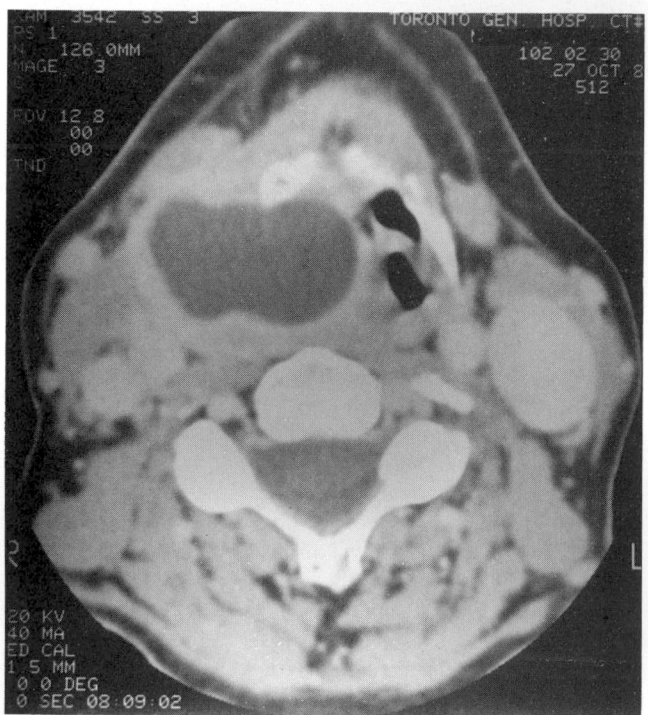

Figure 11-16. Obstructed laryngocele. Note the similarities to the mucous retention cyst (Fig. 11-15). This mass could be seen down to its origin from the laryngeal ventricle. The mixed intra- and extralaryngeal components are diagnostic for laryngocele.

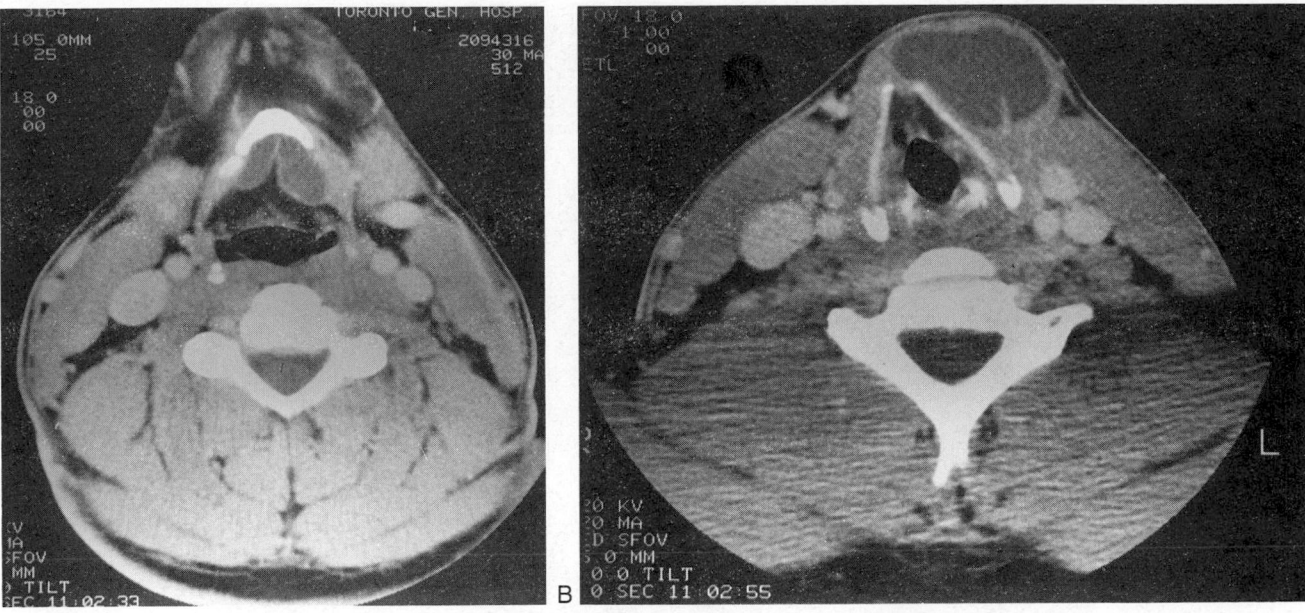

Figure 11-17. Thyroglossal duct cyst. **(A)** A cystic encapsulated mass in the midline is deep to the hyoid bone. **(B)** It becomes superficial to the thyroid cartilage in its inferior extension along the tract of the thyroglossal duct.

11-22), in spite of soft-cuffed endotracheal tubes, are still seen more commonly than inhalation of toxic gases (smoke, industrial exposure). Although the supraglottic larynx and vocal cords may be affected, the predominant airway obstruction postintubation is in the subglottic larynx. The pattern of soft tissue thickening is extremely variable and can involve all walls of the trachea. Chronic inflammatory changes often involve tracheal cartilages to eventually produce tracheomalacia. The functional airway caliber, the position and extent of intraluminal soft tissue, and tracheal ring involvement can be accurately assessed by axial imaging. Thin, contiguous axial sections (1.0 to 1.5 mm) are required to accurately define the segment of the tracheal involvement. In the evaluation of the post-traumatic larynx and trachea, intravenous radiographic contrast agent is not necessary to assess mucosal thickening. Although sagittal and coronal views provide excellent pictures, axial images are the most useful and the most accurate for measuring the extent of the mucosal and tracheal cartilage change.

Tumors of the Larynx and Trachea

Benign tumors of the larynx and upper trachea do not present major diagnostic problems. First visualized by endoscopy, polyps and papillomas often do not require further imaging and can be biopsied and/or removed by the endoscopist. Malignant tumors, however, require either CT or MRI to assess the full extent of the lesion. Although invasive malignant tumor can not usually be accurately marginated from tumor edema, the full extent of the pathologic process can be well mapped. Of particular importance is the ability to appreciate laryngeal cartilage erosion and submucosal spread of tumor across the anterior commissure, into the pre-epiglottic space, and into the subglottic region.

Squamous cell carcinoma (SCC) accounts for 99 percent (Rosai, 1981) of all malignant laryngeal tumors (Thedinger, et al., 1991), subdivided by anatomic location into the supraglottic, glottic, transglottic, and subglottic larynx (Batsakis, 1979). For the most part, the tough cartilaginous and membranous laryngeal framework encourages superior and inferior extension rather than lateral spread into the neck. Since lymphatic spread is relatively common, the entire neck must be scanned with particular attention to the internal jugular lymph node chains. Pretracheal lymph nodes can occasionally be seen on CT and are always pathologic when identified.

Glottic SCC most often occurs in the anterior third of the glottis and tends to spread across the anterior commissure to the opposite vocal cord. The paucity of lymphatics at this level accounts for the relatively localized form of the disease. Supraglottic SCC involves the false cord, the ventricle, and the laryngeal surface of the epiglottis. Tumor commonly extends to the pre-epiglottic space (Fig. 11-23). Lymph node metastases are more common than from glottic SCC. Transglottic carcinoma crosses the laryngeal ventricle and may extend into the subglottis by as much as 1 cm (Fig. 11-24). It has the highest incidence of lymph node metastases. Subglottic SCC either originates on the cord and extends into the subglottis by more than 1 cm or originates solely in the subglottic region. The latter is very uncommon. Subglottic cancers tend to invade the upper tracheal wall and the thyroid gland. The incidence of lymph node metastases is relatively high.

Chondrosarcoma (Felson, 1983; Nicalai, et al., 1990; Rosai, 1981) usually arises from the posterior cricoid cartilage and presents with an exophytic calcium-containing mass in the subglottis. The lesion tends to be destructive of the adjacent cartilages, extending outside the larynx and trachea (Fig. 11-25). Because the lesion is submucosal, small tumors can

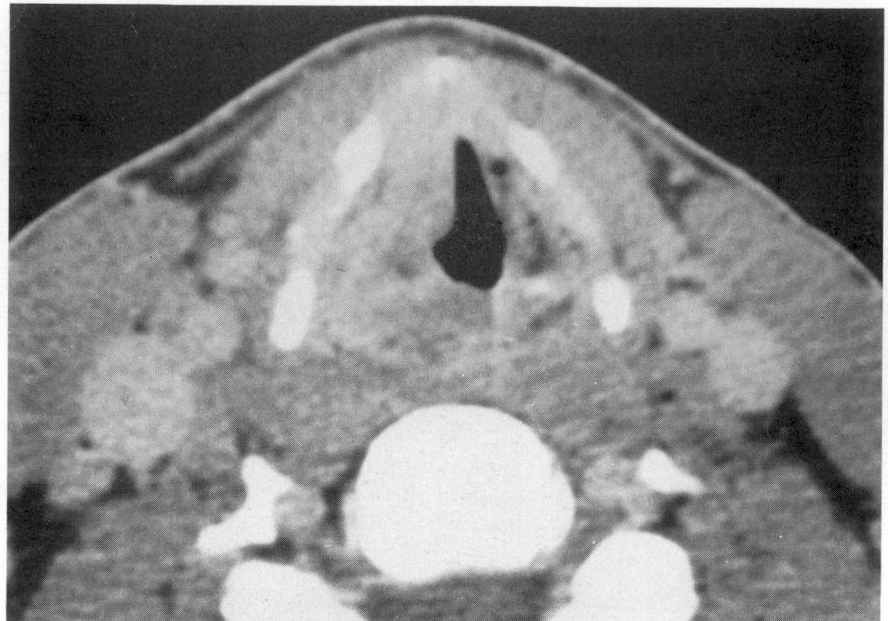

Figure 11-18.   Viral laryngotracheitis. A 27-year-old man presented with a 3-day history of progressive respiratory distress. Endoscopy and CT showed minimal epiglottic swelling and diffuse unilateral increase in soft tissue throughout the right side of the supraglottic and glottic larynx, with obliteration of the paraglottic fat stripe. Biopsy was compatible with inflammation. Electron microscopy confirmed herpes simplex.

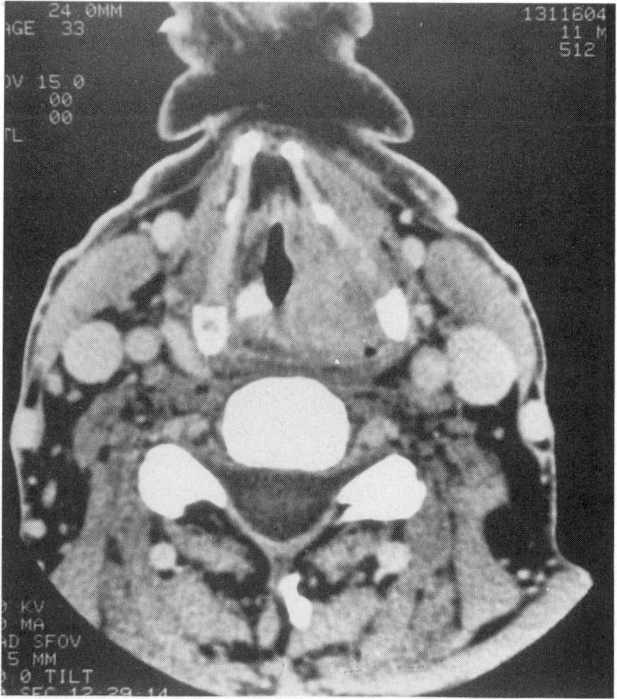

Figure 11-19.   Active rheumatoid arthritis. A soft tissue mass surrounds and destroys the left arytenoid cartilage. The left paraglottic fat stripe has also been obliterated. These findings are indistinguishable from malignancy. The patient had a 40-year history of rheumatoid arthritis, and multiple biopsies revealed only inflammatory tissue. The mass regressed over the course of several months following oral steroids.

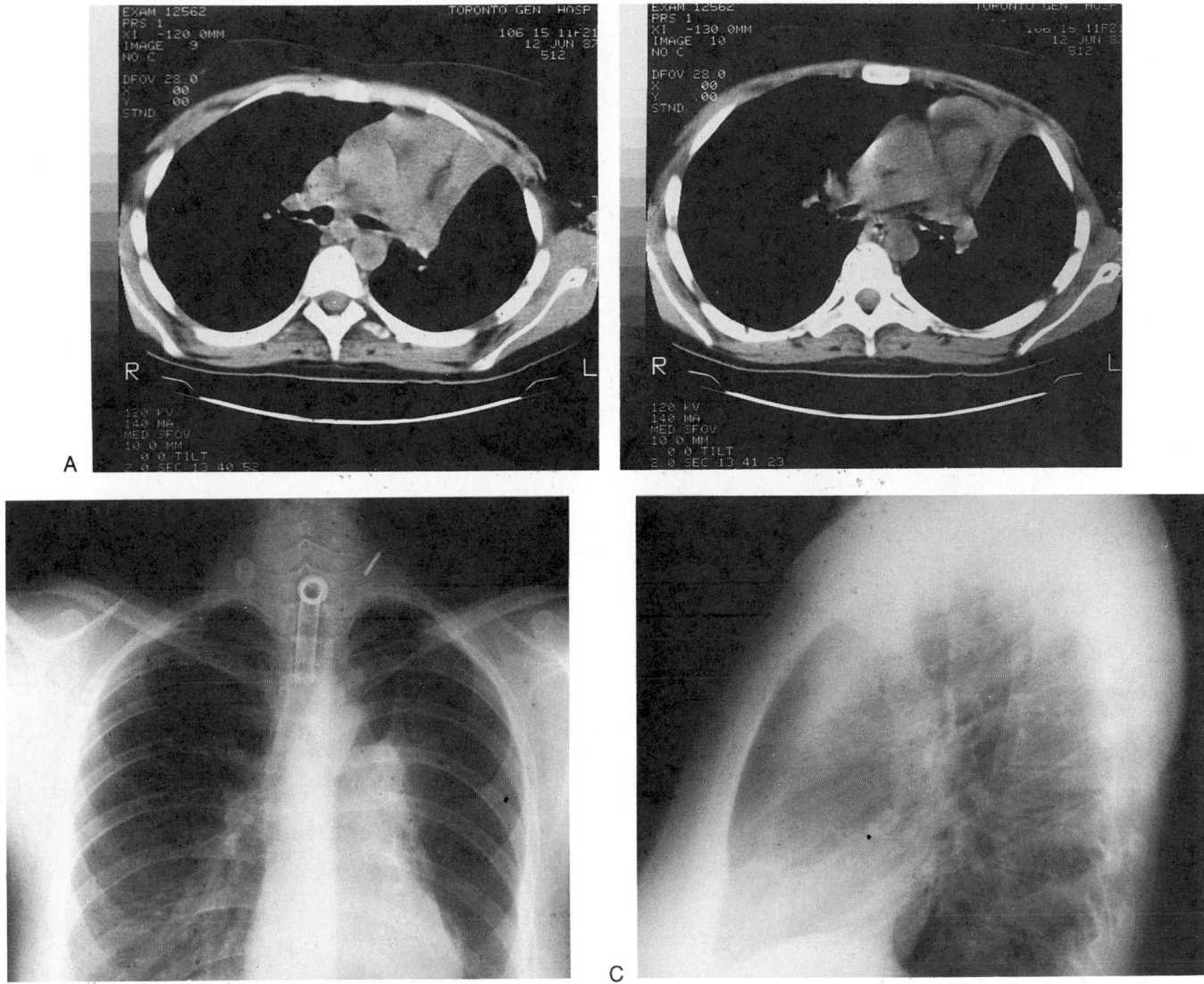

Figure 11-20.   Wegener's granulomatosis. **(A)** This 20-year-old woman had a history of Wegener's granulomatosis and a history of subglottic stenosis treated by tracheostomy. CT scans show narrowing and irregularity of the right and left main bronchi. Note the atelectasis in the left upper lobe. Bronchoscopy showed a stricture of the right upper lobe bronchus and bronchus intermedius and a tight stricture of the left main bronchus and the left lower lobe orifice. Biopsy showed nonspecific granuloma. Treated with chemotherapy. **(B)** Posteroanterior and **(C)** lateral chest radiographs show tracheostomy tube in place. Stenosis of the main bronchi poorly seen. Note total atelectasis of the left upper lobe.

be easily overlooked by the endoscopist. A chondrosarcoma may be difficult to differentiate from a chondroma without a biopsy. Chondromas may infrequently undergo sarcomatous change.

Lymphoma (Felson 1983; Wiggins, et al., 1988), either primary or secondary, in the laryngotracheal tree is uncommon, accounting for 2.8 percent of all malignancies in this area and for 1.8 percent of all lymphomas (Hesson, et al., 1988). There are no characteristic radiologic features, although an extensive homogeneous mass of low CT attenuation numbers may be suggestive (Fig. 11-26). Disproportionate extensive lymphadenopathy may also be suggestive, but biopsy is necessary for diagnosis.

About 0.5 percent of bronchogenic carcinomas arise in the trachea. Most of these are squamous cell in type, which makes this the most common tumor affecting the trachea (Houston, et al., 1969; Li, et al., 1990; Shapshay, et al., 1988). Adenoid cystic carcinoma is second in incidence. This tumor almost always arises within the upper trachea or mainstem bronchi. It tends to grow into the airway lumen in a polypoid fashion, although occasionally it may have a more circumferential growth pattern. Not uncommonly, there is submucosal extension of the tumor along the airway wall, often for a considerable distance. Axial imaging, particularly MRI, is useful to determine if there is extension through the tracheal cartilage into the adjacent thyroid gland and

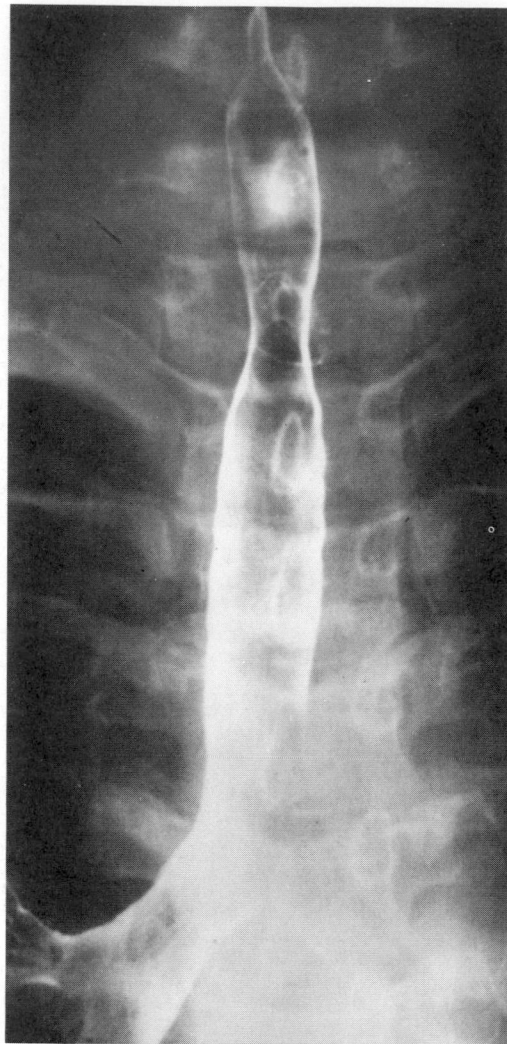

Figure 11-21. Relapsing polychondritis. Tracheo-gram shows stenosis of the lumen of the upper trachea in the coronal plane.

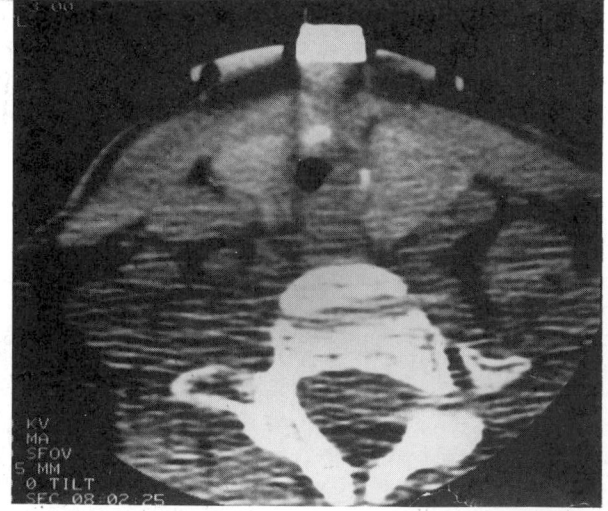
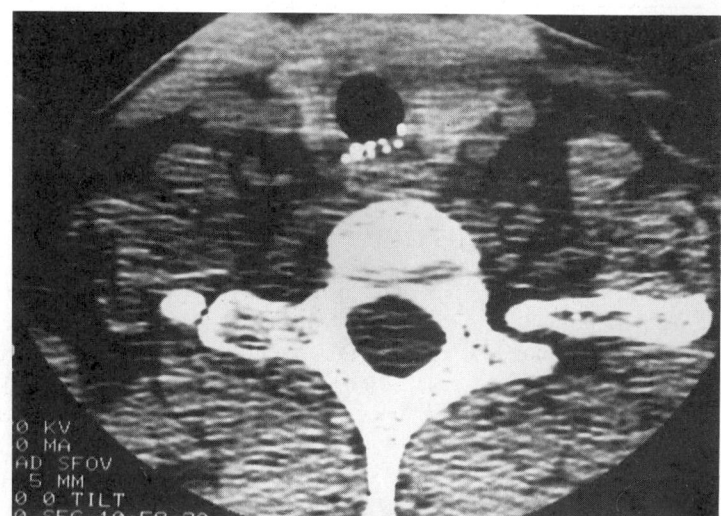

Figure 11-22. Postintubation subglottic stenosis. **(A)** Extensive asymmetric circumferential granulation tissue in the subglottic region has markedly narrowed the airway in this patient, who had prolonged intubation several months earlier. **(B)** The length of scarred trachea was resected with an end-to-end anastomosis as evidenced by tiny surgical wires along the posterior wall. The residual airway is of normal caliber, without intraluminal tissue.

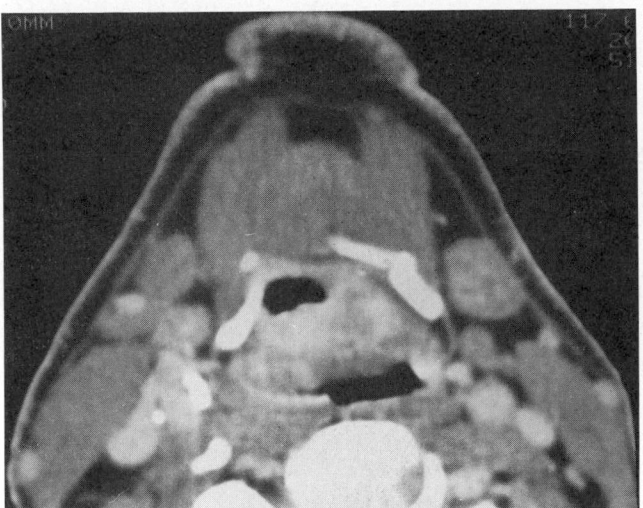

Figure 11-23. Supraglottic squamous cell carcinoma. A large, slightly inhomogeneous mass occupies the supraglottic larynx and infiltrates the pre-epiglottic fat, extending to the posterior aspect of the hyoid bone.

esophagus (Figs. 11-27 and 11-28). In one study of patients with adenoid cystic carcinoma (Spizarny, et al., 1986), CT consistently underestimated the extent of tumor growth along the trachea and the presence of mediastinal nodal metastases. However, it was accurate in the assessment of the extraluminal component of the tumor. Therefore, CT is helpful but imperfect in the determination of operability, including assessment of nodal and distant metastatic disease, involvement of adjacent structures, and the longitudinal extent of the tumor.

Approximately 75 percent of carcinoid tumors arise centrally within a lobar, segmental, or subsegmental bronchus. They may occur in the trachea, although this is rare (Briselli, et al., 1978). These tumors may primarily grow intraluminally, although many have a larger extrabronchial than intrabronchial component, which leads to their designation as "iceberg" tumors. This fact makes CT scanning important in the work-up of these tumors, since bronchoscopy can evaluate only the endobronchial component. Carcinoid tumors (Fig. 11-29) frequently exhibit calcification on CT; this was noted in three of five central tumors in one study (Magid, et al., 1989). The calcium can be either within necrotic cartilage or in bone within the tumor. This calcification has caused this tumor to be confused with broncholithiasis (Shin, et al., 1989). Calcification has also been reported in a tracheal chondroma (Swain and Coblentz, 1988). In addition, carcinoid tumors may, but do not always, enhance following administration of intravenous contrast material (Aronchick, et al., 1986), a finding consistent with their very vascular nature. Generally they are not associated with hilar or mediastinal lymphadenopathy. If adenopathy is seen on CT, one must be suspicious that the tumor is actually an atypical carcinoid tumor (well-differentiated neuroendocrine carcinoma, Kulchitsky cell tumor II). However, adenopathy has been reported in association with a typical carcinoid (Webb, et al., 1983); in this case it was caused by recurrent pneumonia due to bronchial obstruction. These nodes may be mistaken for a large extrabronchial component of the tumor.

Mucoepidermoid carcinoma occurs in main or lobar bronchi, being quite rare in the trachea itself. This tumor tends to grow within the airway lumen, generally without a large extrabronchial component.

Metastatic disease to the airway wall is generally an incidental finding at autopsy. However, there are cases in which

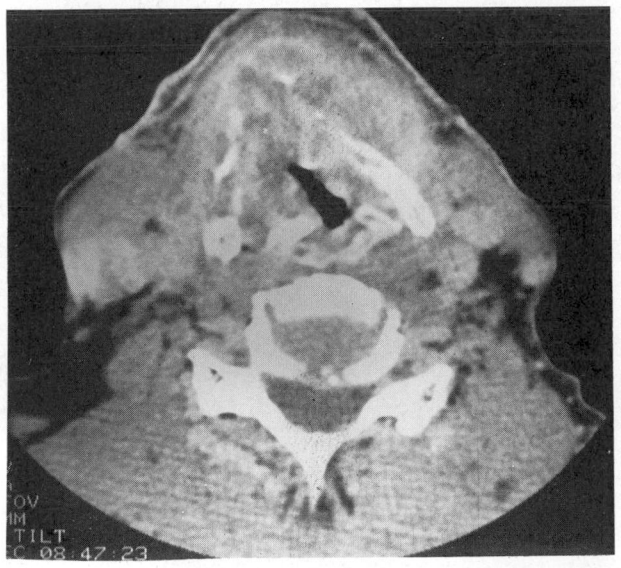

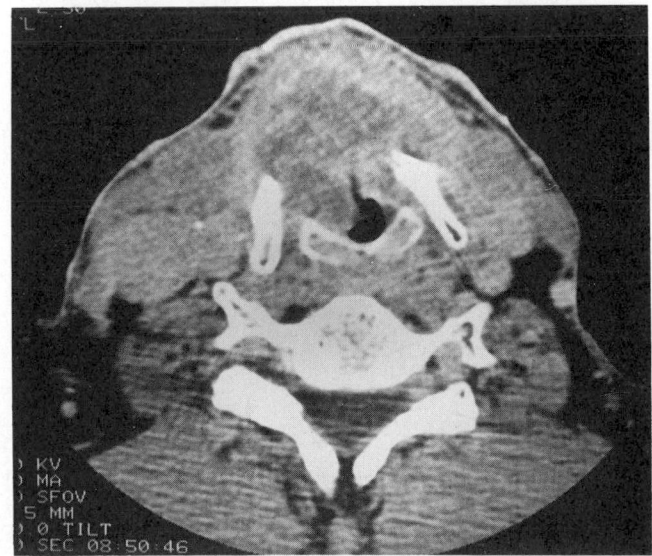

Figure 11-24. Transglottic squamous cell carcinoma. Massive tumor bulk is present, predominantly extralaryngeal, with destruction of the thyroid cartilage anteriorly and on the right. Tumor crosses the anterior commissure onto the left vocal cord. Note the infiltration of the thyroid strap muscles bilaterally, an unusual manifestation of squamous cell carcinoma.

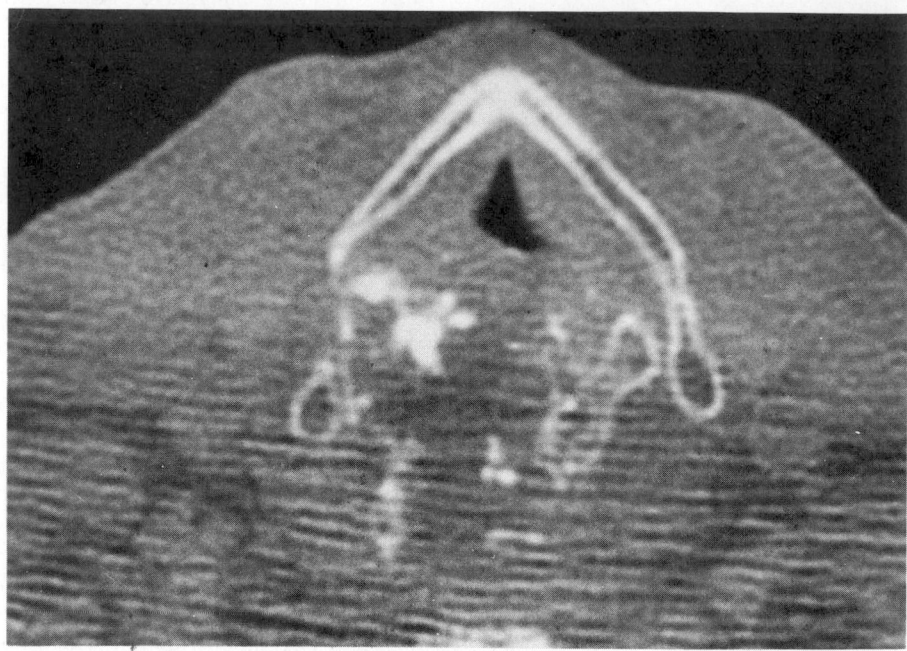

Figure 11-25.   Chondrosarcoma. A destructive bone-forming mass arising from laryngeal cartilage is diagnostic of chondrosarcoma. Extensive soft tissue tumor contributes to airway obstruction.

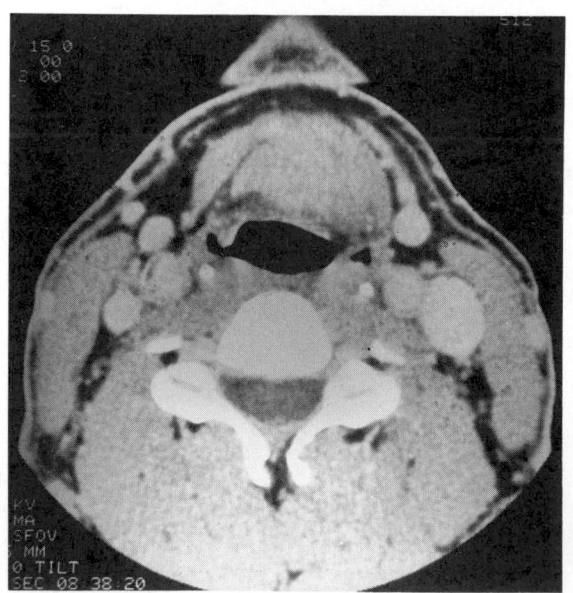
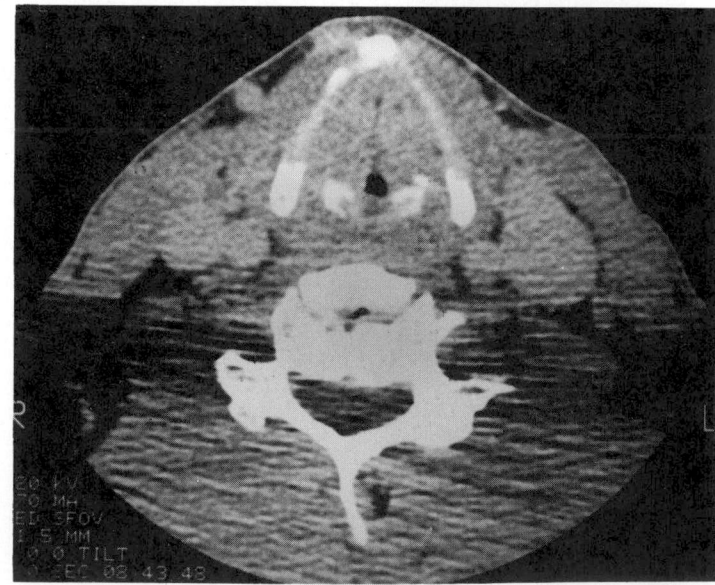

Figure 11-26.   Lymphoma. **(A)** Lymphoma is frequently homogenous and isodense with muscle. The margins are ill-defined and tumor infiltrates the pre-epiglottic space. **(B)** At the level of the glottis, both vocal cords are involved, with obliteration of the fat in the paraglottic regions bilaterally and the anterior commissure.

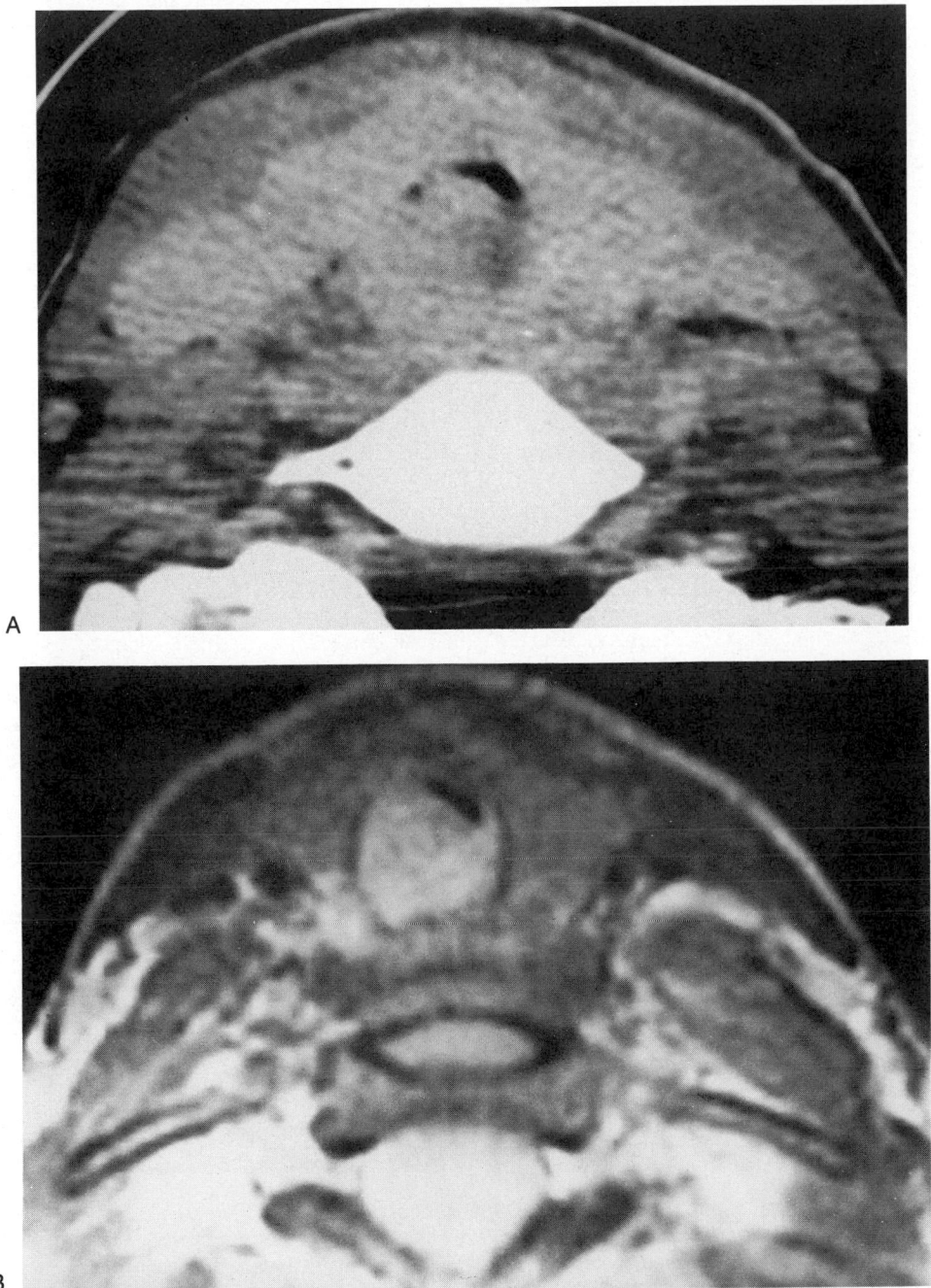

Figure 11-27. Adenoid cystic carcinoma. **(A)** The CT scan does not allow differentiation between the intraluminal tracheal mass and the thyroid gland. The tracheal cartilage cannot be identified. **(B)** T_2-weighted MRI scan clearly indicates that the intraluminal tracheal tumor does not breach the tracheal rings.

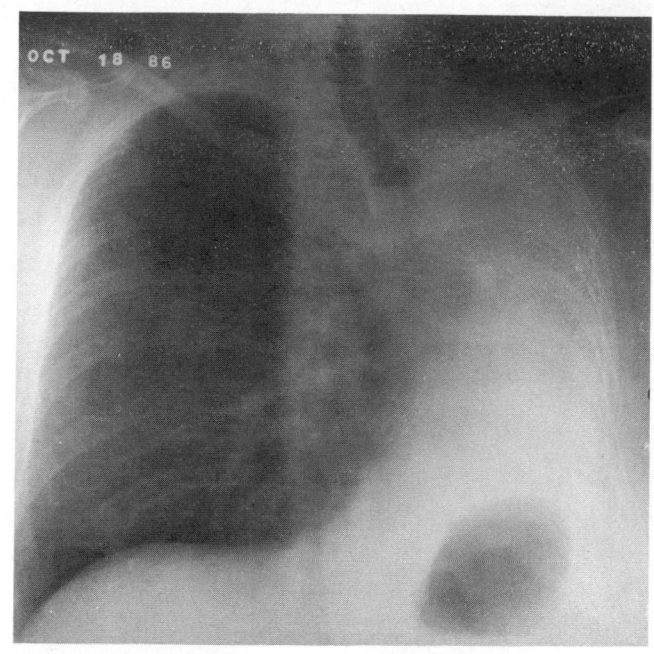

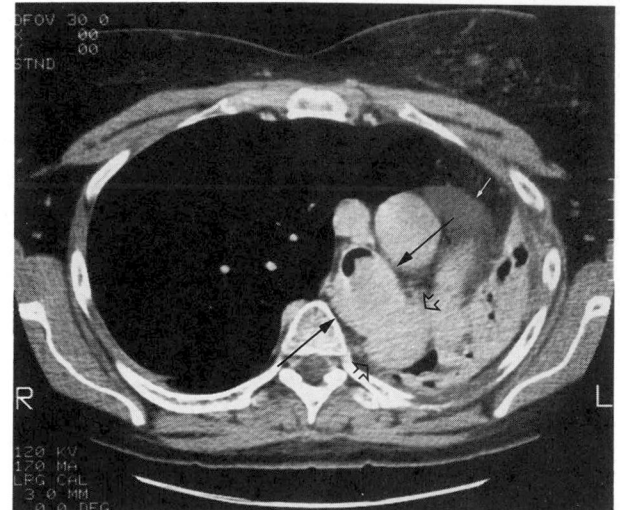

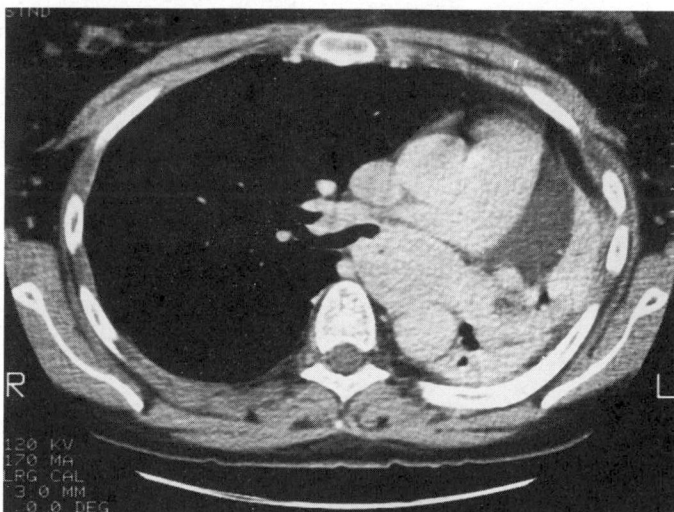

Figure 11-28. Adenoid cystic carcinoma. **(A)** Posteroanterior chest radiograph. There is complete collapse of the left lung with marked shift of the mediastinum to the left, along with elevation of the left hemidiaphragm. **(B)** CT image from lower tracheal region. There is marked obliteration of the tracheal lumen by a large soft tissue mass (*black arrows*). Note the very large extrabronchial component. (*Descending aorta marked by open arrows.*) Note as well the pericardial effusion (*white arrow*). **(C)** CT scan just inferior to carina. There is complete obstruction of the left mainstem bronchus by the large tumor mass. Again note the very large extrabronchial component. There is complete collapse of the left lung.

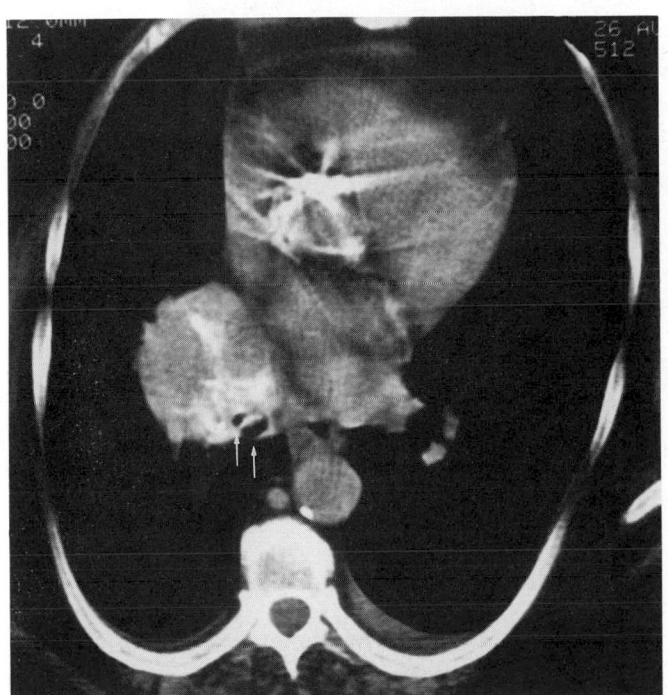
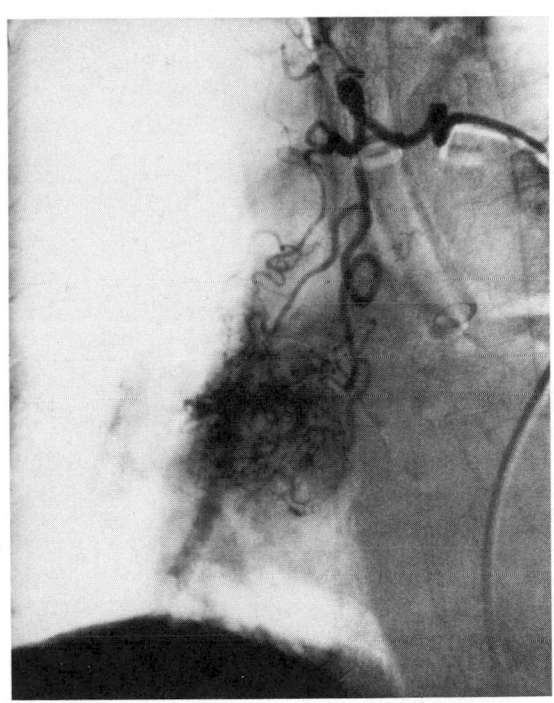

Figure 11-29. Carcinoid tumor. **(A)** CT scan. There is a soft tissue mass, measuring approximately 5 cm in diameter, causing marked narrowing of the right middle and lower lobe bronchi (*arrows*). Large portions of the mass contain calcium. **(B)** Bronchial arteriogram. Note the marked vascularity of the tumor.

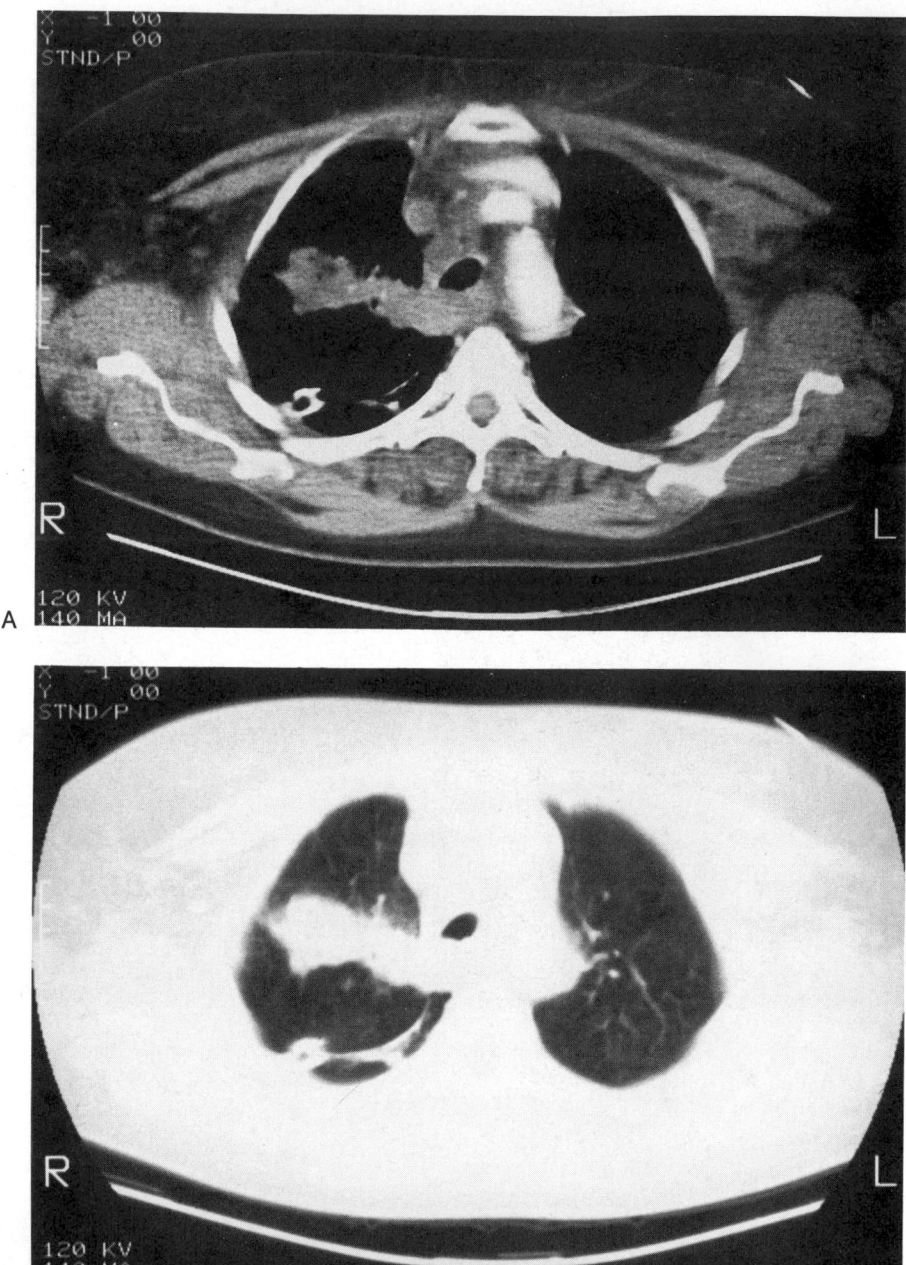

Figure 11-30. Metastatic disease from carcinoma of the breast. **(A)** Mediastinal windows. **(B)** Lung windows. A large amount of soft tissue is seen surrounding the trachea, causing distortion of the lumen. The tumor mass extends into the right upper lobe. Much of the more peripheral density represents postobstructive change, as more inferiorly (not shown) there was some obstruction of the right upper lobe bronchus.

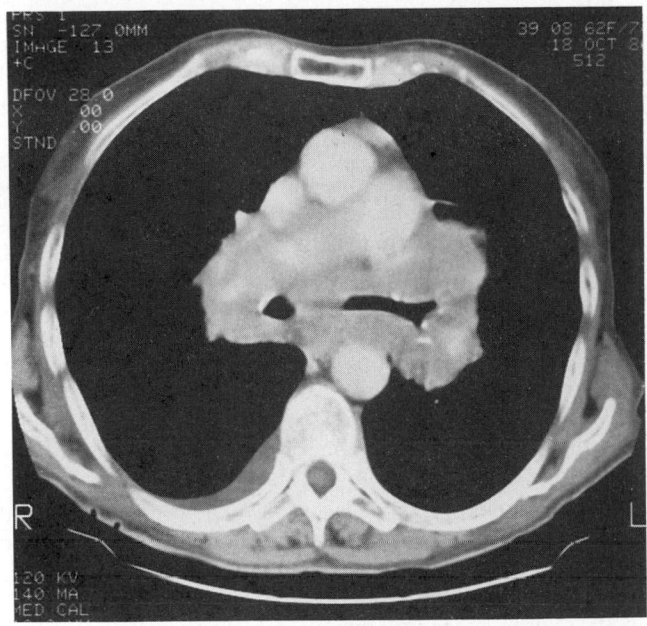
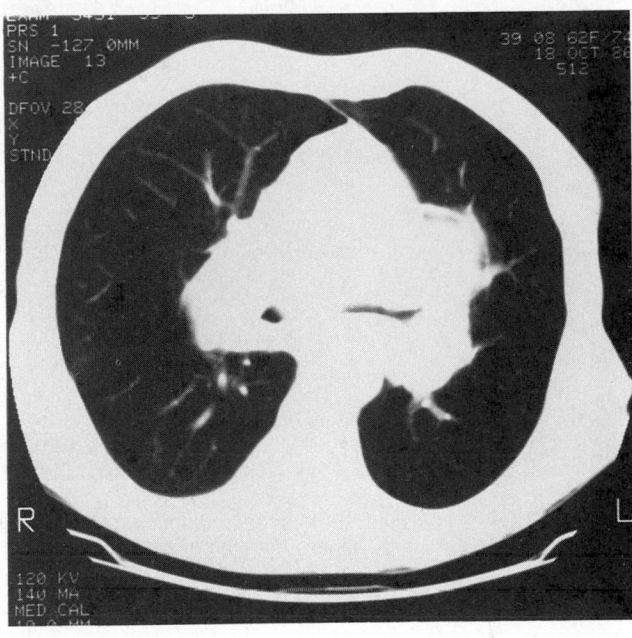

Figure 11-31. Non-Hodgkin's lymphoma. **(A)** Mediastinal windows. **(B)** Lung windows. The lung windows reveal marked narrowing of the bronchus intermedius as well as the left mainstem bronchus and origins of the left upper and lower lobe bronchi. On the mediastinal windows, the airways are seen to be completely surrounded by homogeneous soft tissue, which is infiltrating the mediastinum extensively, with involvement of both hila. In addition, there is a small right pleural effusion.

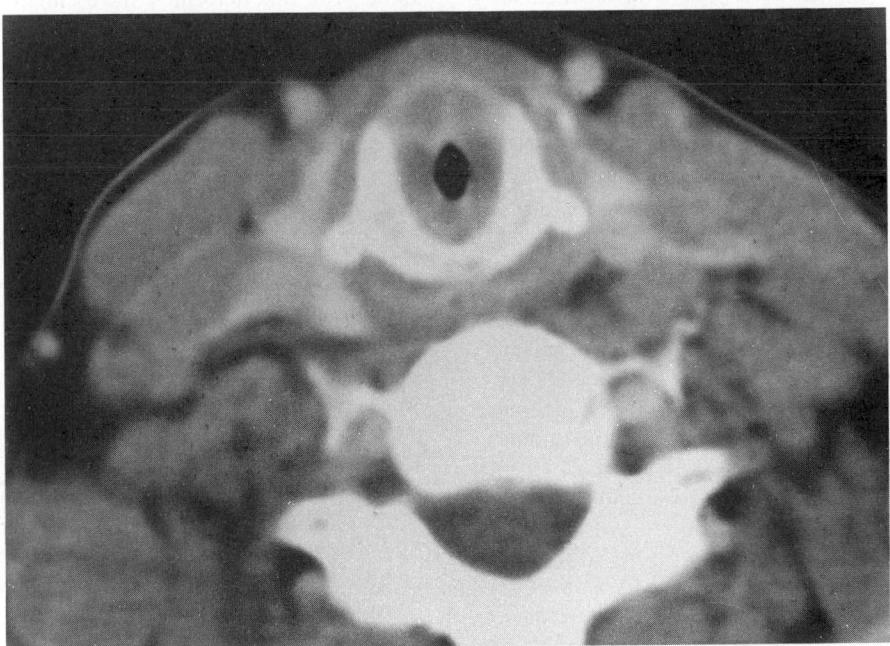

Figure 11-32. Leukemia. CT shows an inhomogeneous circumferential mass in the subglottic larynx. The appearance is nonspecific and requires biopsy for diagnosis.

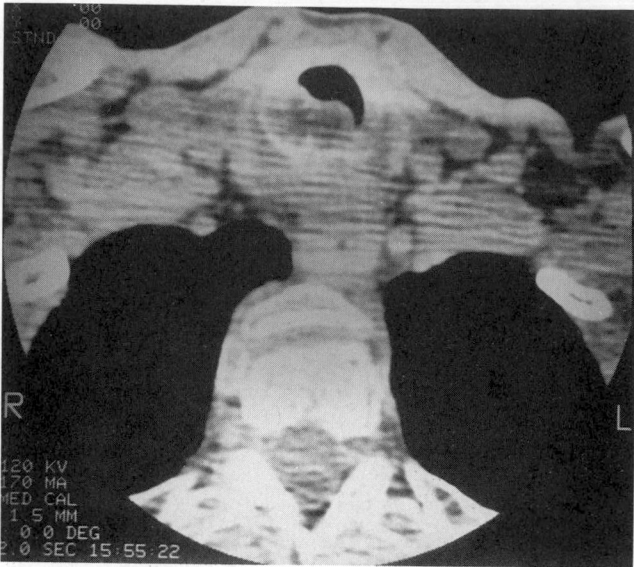

Figure 11-33. Amyloid. Asymmetric circumferential soft tissue is present in the tracheal lumen. Note the marked involvement of the posterior wall.

intraluminal growth may cause symptoms due to bronchial obstruction. Metastatic disease (Fig. 11-30) and lymphoma (Fig. 11-31) cause airway abnormalities that are typical of this group, namely nonspecific thickening of the bronchial wall and/or an endo- or extrabronchial mass, as well as enlargement of mediastinal nodes. Biopsy is necessary for diagnosis. The primary tumors most likely to metastasize to airway wall are breast, kidney, melanoma, and colorectal (Felson, 1983). Occasionally Hodgkin's disease can extend from peribronchial lymphatics and interstitial tissues into the bronchial mucosa, leading to bronchial obstruction (Stolberg, et al., 1964; Seward and Safdar, 1972). Airway involvement with multiple myeloma is uncommon, although both upper and lower airways can be affected (Kintzer, et al., 1978). Endobronchial plasmacytoma has been reported as well (Tenholder, et al., 1982).

Rarely, the airway can be involved by benign or malignant smooth muscle tumors (Allen, et al., 1972; Guccion and Rosen, 1972; Thedinger, et al., 1991), vascular tumors such as hemangiopericytoma (Gavilan, et al., 1987), Kaposi's sarcoma, chondromas (Swain and Coblentz, 1988), lipomas (Schraufnagel, et al., 1979; Chen, et al., 1990), fibrosarcomas (Guccion and Rosen, 1972), glomus tumor (Kim, et al., 1989), neurilemmoma (Felson, 1983), rhabdomyosarcoma, and leukemic deposits (Fig. 11-32).

Miscellaneous Conditions

Amyloidosis (Simpson, et al., 1984; Takasugi and Godwin, 1991), is a tumorlike condition characterized by extracellular deposition of amyloid in tissue. In the systemic form of the disease, 90 percent of patients have amyloid deposits in the head and neck, upper digestive tract, and the lower respiratory tract. The localized form, much rarer, is characterized by amyloid deposits in the eye, major and minor salivary glands, submucosa of the nose, paranasal sinuses, nasopharynx, oral cavity, pharynx, larynx, tracheobronchial tree, and lung. Radiographically, amyloid may cause diffuse narrowing of the tracheal air column or may cause nodular protrusions into the tracheal lumen, which may calcify or ossify (Fig. 11-33). In the trachea, the posterior wall is involved, which allows for differentiation from tracheobronchopathia osteochondroplastica, which spares the posterior wall.

Tracheobronchopathia osteochondroplastica (Takasugi and Godwin, 1991; Neinhuis, et al., 1990) is an idiopathic disease, usually seen in men over 50, in which multiple 1- to 3-mm osseous and cartilaginous submucosal nodules project intraluminally from the anterior and lateral walls of the trachea. The disease is rare in the larynx alone. Radiographically, multiple nodules, with or without calcification, project into the lumen over a long segment of trachea (Fig. 11-34). Extension into the mainstem bronchi also occurs. Obstructive hyperinflation, atelectasis, and recurrent pneumonia may develop as secondary manifestations of the tracheobronchial involvement.

"Saber sheath" trachea is a tracheal deformity associated with chronic obstructive pulmonary disease and is found almost exclusively in men (Greene, 1978). The trachea is flattened from side to side so that the coronal diameter is equal to or less than two-thirds of the sagittal when measured 1 cm above the top of the aortic arch. Since the deformity affects only the intrathoracic trachea, there is abrupt widening above the thoracic inlet. The trachea usually has a smooth inner margin, but a nodular appearance has been described (Rubenstein, et al., 1978). Calcification of the tracheal cartilages is frequently present. Although over 95 percent of patients with this deformity have clinical evidence of chronic obstructive pulmonary disease, only 55 percent have radiographic evidence of it (Greene, 1978). The pathogenesis of the deformity is unknown.

Idiopathic fibrosis may also result in areas of narrowing in the subglottic region, distal trachea, and mainstem bronchi.

Tracheal Widening

Diffuse tracheal widening is much less common than tracheal narrowing. Tracheobronchomegaly (Mounier-Kuhn syndrome) primarily affects men in the fourth and fifth decades. The etiology is unknown. The cartilaginous rings dilate and the intercartilaginous portions of the tracheal wall bulge outward, forming broad diverticulum-like protrusions. The trachea is involved from the subglottic region to the carina. Bronchiectasis involving the first- to fourth-order branchings is present in many patients (Dunne and Reiner, 1988; Shin, et al., 1988; Rindsberg, et al., 1987). Dilatation of the tracheal lumen can also occur in patients with tracheomalacia, chronic obstructive airways disease, and diffuse pulmonary fibrosis (Woodring, et al., 1989).

EXTRINSIC AIRWAY LESIONS

The subglottic larynx and trachea are occasionally invaded by malignancies arising from the adjacent tissues. This occurs most commonly in thyroid carcinoma, where the tumor erodes through the thyroid cartilage and extends within the

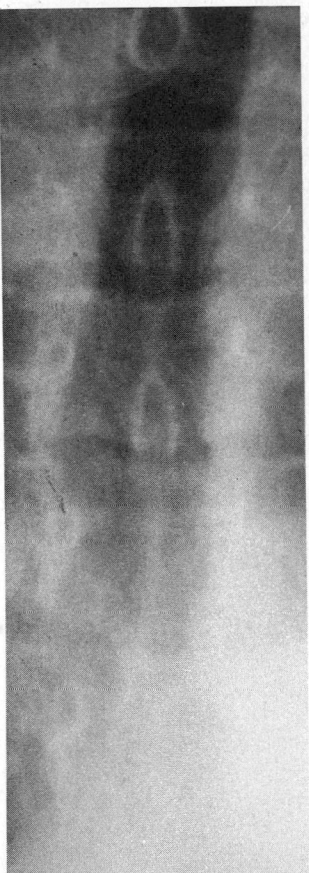

A

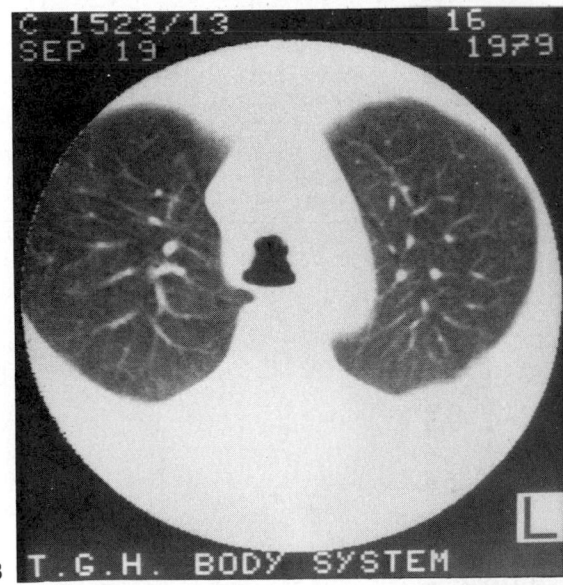

B

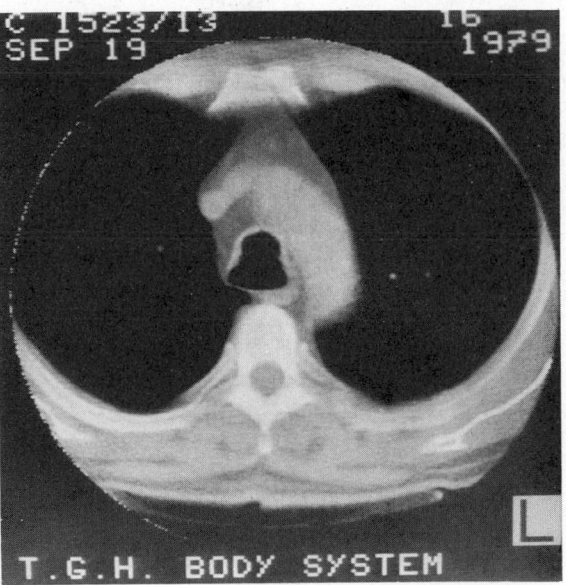

Figure 11-34. Tracheobronchopathia osteochondroplastica in a 57-year-old man. **(A)** Coned view of trachea from a posteroanterior chest radiograph shows irregularity in contour of the right and left lateral walls of the trachea. **(B)** CT scans show irregular nodularity of the right and left lateral walls of the trachea.

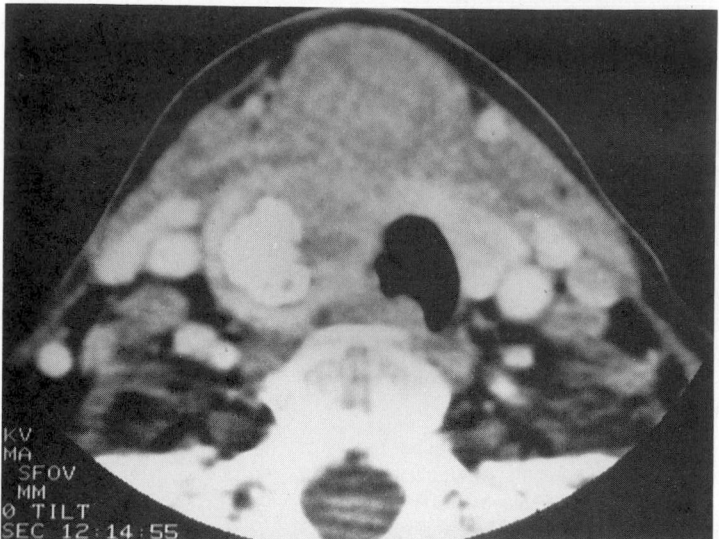

Figure 11-35. Thyroid carcinoma. A large mass with a focal calcified nodule involves the right lobe of the thyroid. Nodular irregularity of the right lateral wall of the trachea indicates invasion of the tracheal wall by malignancy. The lateral margin of the thyroid tumor does not exhibit extracapsular invasion, as the neurovascular bundle is sharply defined by the fat separating the carotid artery from the capsule of the thyroid.

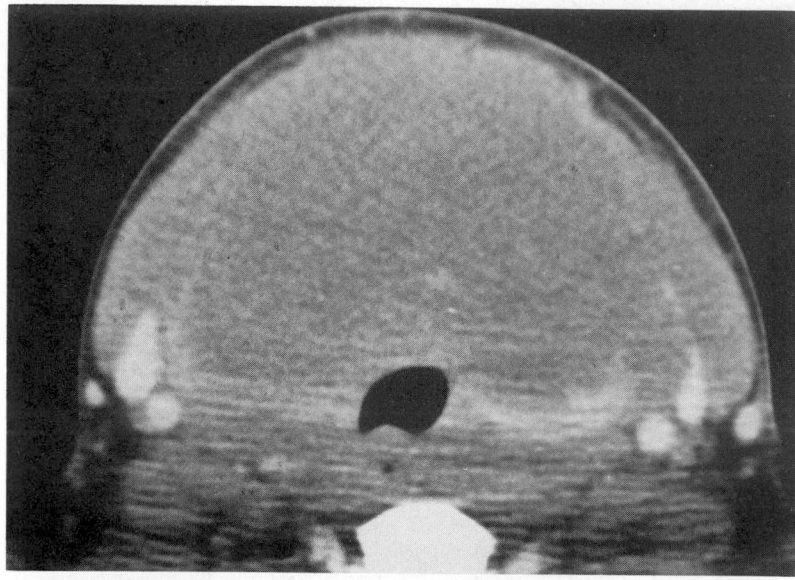

A

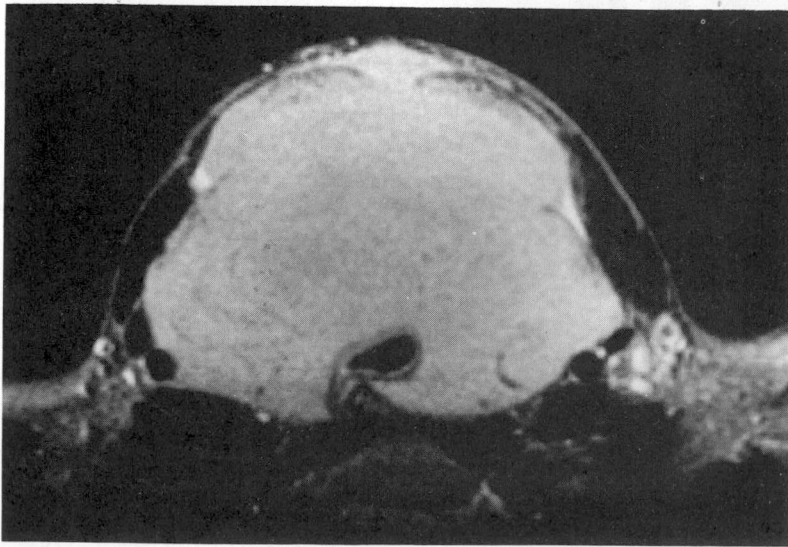

B

Figure 11-36. Thyroid lymphoma. **(A)** CT demonstrates a low-density homogenous mass in the thyroid gland. Tracheal compression is obvious, but tracheal cartilage involvement can not be defined, as the cartilage is indistinct from tumor. **(B)** The T_2-weighted MRI scan clearly demarcates cartilage from tumor. Although the cartilage is flattened and compressed, it is intact.

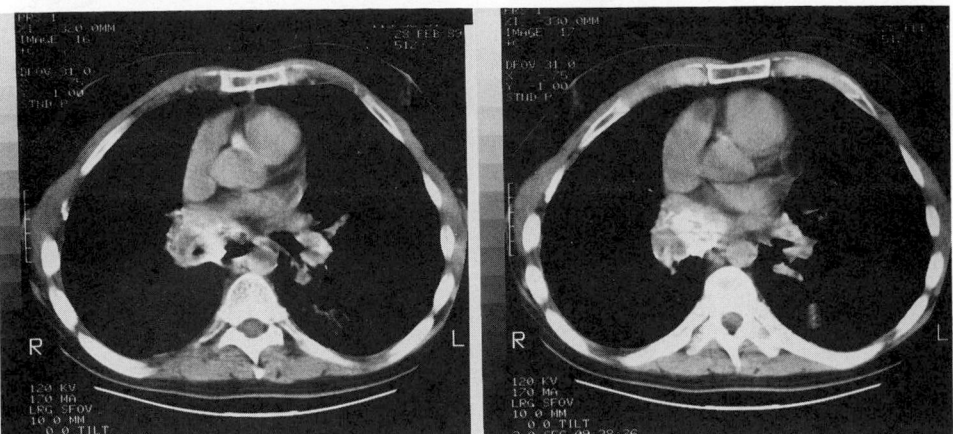

Figure 11-37. Fibrosing mediastinitis in a 43-year-old man with a 20-year history of fibrosing mediastinitis believed to be secondary to histoplasmosis. CT scan of the chest shows a mass in the right hilum containing dense calcification consistent with calcific adenitis. There is marked narrowing and eventual occlusion of the bronchus intermedius. Bronchoscopy revealed complete obstruction of the right lower lobe bronchus and almost complete obstruction of the right middle lobe bronchus. The patient died shortly after a left lung transplant. Autopsy revealed fibrosing mediastinitis and hilar lymphadenitis resulting in obstruction of the right pulmonary artery and bronchial tree.

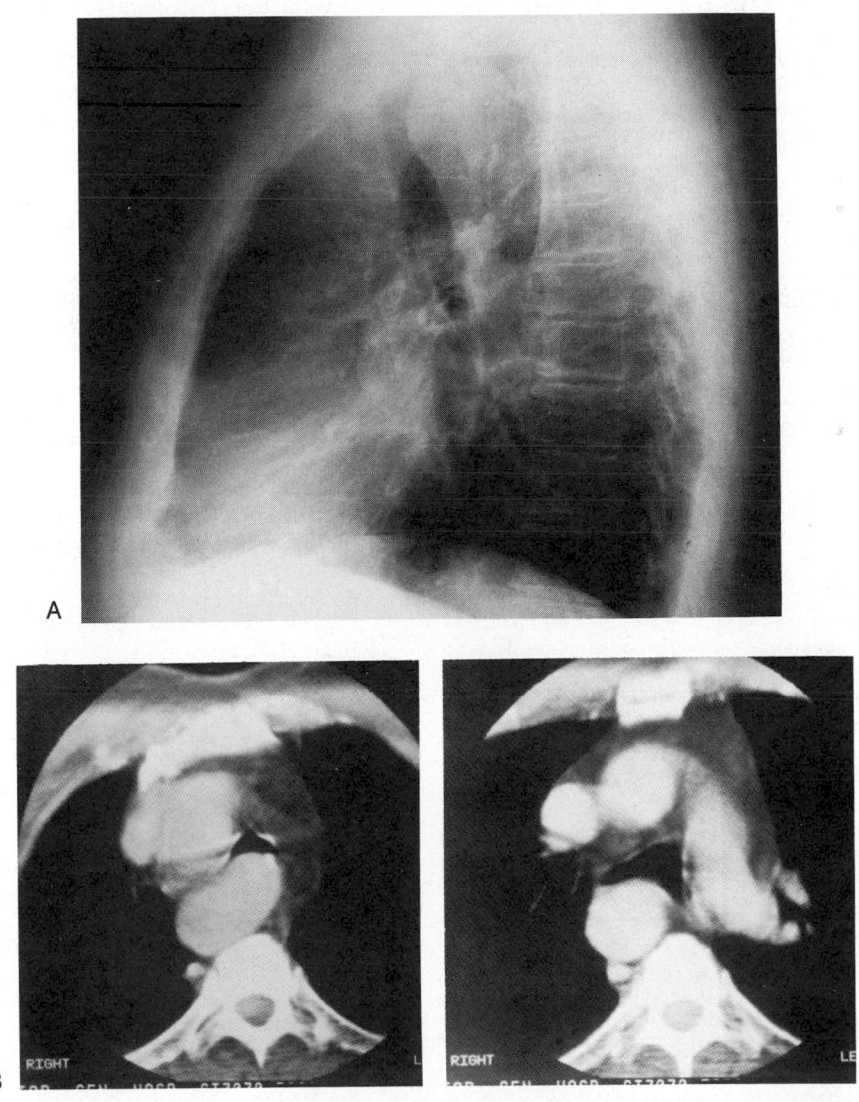

Figure 11-38. Righrt aortic arch in a 52-year-old man with a mediastinal mass. **(A)** Lateral chest radiograph shows a mass indenting the tracheal air column on its posterior aspect. **(B)** Contrast-enhanced CT scan shows a right aortic arch. The posterior portion of the aortic arch and the dilated origin of the anomalous left subclavian artery press upon the posterior distal trachea with moderate narrowing of the lumen.

trachea, producing some element of airway obstruction and deviation (Fig. 11-35). Similarly, carcinoma of the esophagus can invade the tracheal lumen. MRI is particularly helpful in differentiating extrinsic compression of the trachea from frank tumor invasion of the cartilage of the anterior and lateral walls (Fig. 11-36) or invasion through the posterior wall from the esophagus.

Fibrosing mediastinitis, either idiopathic or resulting from histoplasmosis, may result in narrowing of the tracheobronchial tree in about 30 to 50 percent of patients. The CT manifestations include mediastinal or hilar mass, calcification of the central mass or associated lymph nodes, tracheobronchial narrowing, and pulmonary infiltrates (Weinstein, et al., 1983). MRI is useful in assessing vascular patency, precluding the need for intravenous contrast material (Rholl, et al., 1985). The fibrosis typically involves the distal trachea and one or both mainstem bronchi (Fig. 11-37). The narrowing is of variable length and usually has a smooth margin. Calcification within mediastinal lymph nodes is a clue to the correct diagnosis (Farmer, et al., 1984).

Vascular lesions such as aortic aneurysm, congenital aortic anomalies (double aortic arch, right aortic arch), and anomalous left pulmonary artery can cause a mediastinal mass with tracheal narrowing on plain films. A good clue to the presence of a right aortic arch is indentation of the posterior wall of the trachea (Fig. 11-38). CT and MRI are diagnostic (Gomes, et al., 1987; Kersting-Sommerhoff, et al., 1987).

REFERENCES

Allen HA, Angell F, Hankins J, Whitley NO: Leiomyoma of the trachea. AJR 141:683, 1972

Aronchick JM, Wexler JA, Christen B et al.: Computed tomography of bronchial carcinoid. J Comput Assist Tomogr 10:71, 1986

Batsakis JG: Tumors of the Head and Neck. Clinical and Pathological Considerations. 2nd Ed. Williams & Wilkins, Baltimore, 1979

Brandstetter RD, Messina MS, Sprince NL: Tracheal stenosis due to sarcoidosis. Chest 86:56, 1981

Briselli M, Mark GJ, Grillo HC: Tracheal carcinoids. Cancer 42:2870, 1978

Casselman JW, Lemahieu P, Peene P, Stoffels G: Polychondritis affecting the laryngeal cartilages: CT findings. AJR 150:355, 1988

Chen TF, Braidley PC, Shneerson JM, Wells FC: Obstructing tracheal lipoma: management of a rare tumor. Ann Thorac Surg 49:137, 1990

Choplin RH, Wehunt WD, Theros EG: Diffuse lesions of the trachea. Semin Roentgenol 18:38, 1983

Crockford MP, Kerr IH: Relapsing polychondritis. Clin Radiol 39:386, 1988

Dunne MG, Reiner B: CT features of tracheobronchomegaly. J Comput Assist Tomogr 12:388, 1988

Eisenberg RL: Radiology: An Illustrated History. Mosby-Year Book, St. Louis, 1991

Farmer DW, Moore E, Amparo E et al.: Calcific fibrosing mediastinitis: demonstration of pulmonary vascular obstruction by magnetic resonance imaging. AJR 143:1189, 1984

Felson B: Neoplasms of the trachea and main stem bronchi. Semin Roentgenol 18:23, 1983

Gavilan J, Rodriguez-Peralto JL, Tomas MD et al.: Hemangiopericytoma of the trachea. J Laryngol Otol 101:738, 1987

Gomes AS, Lois JF, George B et al.: Congenital abnormalities of the aortic arch: MR imaging. Radiology 165:691, 1987

Greene R: ''Saber-sheath'' trachea: relation to chronic obstructive pulmonary disease. AJR 130:441, 1978

Guccion JG, Rosen SH: Bronchopulmonary leiomyosarcoma and fibrosarcoma. A study of 32 cases and review of the literature. Cancer 30:836, 1972

Hesson H, Houck J, Harvey H: Airway obstruction due to lymphoma of the larynx and trachea. Laryngoscope 18:176, 1988

Horns JW, O'Loughlin BJ: Tracheal collapse in polychondritis. AJR 87:844, 1962

Houston HE, Payne WS, Harison EG Jr, Olsen AM: Primary cancers of the trachea. Arch Surg 99:132, 1969

Im JG, Chung JW, Han SK: CT manifestations of tracheobronchial involvement in relapsing polychondritis. J Comput Assist Tomogr 12:792, 1988

Kersting-Sommerhoff BA, Sechtem UP, Fisher MR, Higgins CB: MR imaging of congenital anomalies of the aortic arch. AJR 159:9, 1987

Killman WJ: Narrowing of the airway in relapsing polychondritis. Radiology 126:373, 1978

Kim YI, Kim JH, Suh JS et al.: Glomus tumor of the trachea. Report of a case with ultrastructural observation. Cancer 64:881, 1989

Kintzer JS, Rosenow EC, Kyle RA: Thoracic and pulmonary abnormalities in multiple myeloma. Arch Intern Med 138:727, 1978

Li W, Ellerbroek NA, Libshitz HI: Primary malignant tumors of the trachea: a radiologic and clinical study. Cancer 66:894, 1990

Magid D, Siegelman SS, Eggleston JC et al.: Pulmonary carcinoid tumors: CT assessment. J Comput Assist Tomogr 13:244, 1989

Mendelson DS, Som PM, Crane R et al.: Relapsing polychondritis studied by computed tomography. Radiology 157:489, 1985

Naidich DP, Funt S, Ettenger NA, Arranda C: Hemoptysis: CT-bronchoscopic correlations in 58 cases. Radiology 177:357, 1990

Naidich DP, McCauley DI, Siegelman SS: Computed tomography of bronchial adenomas. J Comput Assist Tomogr 6:725, 1982

Nicalai P, Sasaki CT, Ferlito A, Kirchner JA: Laryngeal chondrosarcoma: incidence, pathology, biological behavior, and treatment. Ann Otol Rhinol Laryngol 99:515, 1990

Neinhuis DM, Prakash UB, Edell ES: Tracheobronchopathia osteochondroplastica. Ann Otol Rhinol Laryngol 99:689, 1990

Rholl KS, Levitt RG, Glazer HS: Magnetic resonance imaging of fibrosing mediastinitis. AJR 145:255, 1985

Rindsberg S, Friedman AC, Fiel SB, Radecki PD: MRI of tracheobronchomegaly. J Can Assoc Radiol 38:126, 1987

Rosai J: Ackerman's Surgical Pathology. p. 213. Vol. 1. 6th Ed. CV Mosby, St. Louis, 1981

Rubenstein J, Weisbrod GL, Steinhardt MI: Atypical appearances of ''saber-sheath'' trachea. Radiology 127:41, 1978

Seward CW, Safdar SH: Endobronchial Hodgkin's disease presenting as a primary pulmonary lesion. Chest 62:649, 1972

Shapshay SM, Ruah CB, Bohigian RK, Beamis JF Jr: Obstructing tumors of the subglottic larynx and cervical trachea: airway management and treatment. Ann Otol Rhinol Laryngol 97:487, 1988

Shin MS, Berland LL, Myers JL et al.: CT demonstration of an ossifying bronchial carcinoid simulating broncholithiasis. AJR 153:51, 1989

Shin MS, Jackson RM, Ho K-J: Tracheobronchomegaly (Mounier-Kuhn syndrome): CT diagnosis. AJR 150:777, 1988

Simpson GT II, Skinner M, Strong MS, Cohen AS: Localized amyloidosis of the head and neck and upper aerodigestive and lower respiratory tracts. Ann Otol Rhinol Laryngol 93:374, 1984

Som PM, Bergeron RT: Head and Neck Imaging. 2nd Ed. Mosby-Year Book, St. Louis, 1991

Spizarny DL, Shepard JO, McLoud TC et al.: CT of adenoid cystic carcinoma of the trachea. AJR 146:1129, 1986

Stolberg HO, Patt NL, MacEwen KF et al.: Hodgkin's disease of the lung. Roentgenologic-pathologic correlation. AJR 92:96, 1964

Swain ME, Coblentz CL: Tracheal chondroma: CT appearance. J Comput Assist Tomogr 12:1085, 1988

Takasugi JE, Godwin JD: The airway. Semin Roentgenol 26:175, 1991

Tenholder MF, Scialla SJ, Weisbaum G: Endobronchial metastatic plasmacytoma. Cancer 49:1465, 1982

Thedinger BA, Cheney ML, Montgomery WW, Goodman M: Leiomyosarcoma of the trachea. Case report. Ann Otol Rhinol Laryngol 100:337, 1991

Webb WR, Gamsu G, Birnberg FA: CT appearance of bronchial carcinoid with recurrent pneumonia and hyperplastic hilar lymphadenopathy. J Comput Assist Tomogr 7:707, 1983

Weinstein JB, Aronberg DJ, Sagel SS: CT of fibrosing mediastinitis: findings and their utility. AJR 141:247, 1983

Wiggins J, Sheffield E, Green M: Primary B cell malignant lymphoma of the trachea. Thorax 43:497, 1988

Wiot JG: Tracheobronchial trauma. Semin Roentgenol 18:15, 1983

Woodring JH, Barrett PA, Rehm SR, Nurenberg P: Acquired tracheomegaly in adults as a complication of diffuse pulmonary fibrosis. AJR 152:743, 1989

12

ENDOSCOPY

Laryngoscopy

Ian J. Witterick
Patrick J. Gullane

Laryngoscopy is an important part in the examination of the upper aerodigestive tract to (1) identify benign and malignant disease, (2) evaluate vocal cord mobility, and (3) assess laryngeal trauma and stenosis. Direct laryngoscopy implies that the larynx is seen in a direct line from the examiner's eye to the area of interest. It usually requires a hollow metal scope to be placed through the mouth to the area of interest. Indirect laryngoscopy uses various devices, including mirrors and fiberoptic scopes (flexible or rigid), to direct an image of the larynx and pharynx to the examiner's eye.

INDIRECT LARYNGOSCOPY

Indications

Indirect laryngoscopy is a routine part of the examination of the head and neck. It is particularly important in patients with a history of smoking and alcohol abuse because of the known risk of upper aerodigestive tract malignancies associated with these habits. It is advisable to perform indirect laryngoscopy in any patient who complains of dysphagia, odynophagia, or hoarseness for greater than 2 to 3 weeks. It can also be used with appropriate instrumentation to sample lesions in the larynx, remove foreign bodies, and augment the vocal cords with temporary (Gelfoam, glycerin) or permanent (Teflon) materials.

When indirect laryngoscopy is properly performed in a cooperative patient, a good view of the base of tongue, vallecula, supraglottic and glottic larynx, and posterior pharyngeal wall can be obtained. It may be difficult to assess the pyriform sinuses, laryngeal surface of the epiglottis, and subglottic larynx fully. The postcricoid area cannot usually be fully visualized.

The one contraindication to indirect laryngoscopy is a suspected case of supraglottitis or epiglottitis in a child. Traction on the tongue and insertion of a laryngeal mirror may precipitate an acute airway obstruction. If the diagnosis is in question, it may be possible to examine these patients with a flexible fiberoptic scope inserted transnasally. Alternatively, the patient can be taken to the operating room for inhalational induction, direct laryngoscopy, and intubation.

Instruments

The larynx may be examined indirectly with a mirror or flexible or rigid fiberoptic scopes. The mirror has stood the test of time and is adequate for the examination of most patients. Good illumination is required. Either a head mirror and appropriate light source or a head light with its own built-in light source is used. Flexible and rigid fiberoptic scopes have revolutionized the examination of the larynx and pharynx. The flexible scope in particular is superior in patients who are difficult to examine with a mirror or rigid scope because of gagging or an overhanging epiglottis. The flexible scope usually does not trigger the pharyngeal gag reflex and can be manipulated posterior to the epiglottis.

Rigid scopes come in a variety of designs, but basically they are like a 90-degree periscope (Fig. 12-1). The light is conducted along fiberoptic cables out the end of the instrument and directed at the target. Some scopes have built-in zoom lenses to magnify the larynx and give an excellent view of vocal cord pathologic conditions. Rigid scopes may be ineffective in patients with a prominent gag reflex or in those in whom the epiglottis is displaced posteriorly.

Flexible laryngoscopes are similar to bronchoscopes except they are shorter, have a smaller diameter, and usually do not come equipped with suction (Fig. 12-2). A lever mechanism manipulates the end forward or backward but not from side to side. Therefore, orientation of the end of the scope is important before insertion. Transnasal insertion usually does not trigger the pharyngeal gag reflex. Flexible bronchoscopes can be substituted, but the diameter of some may

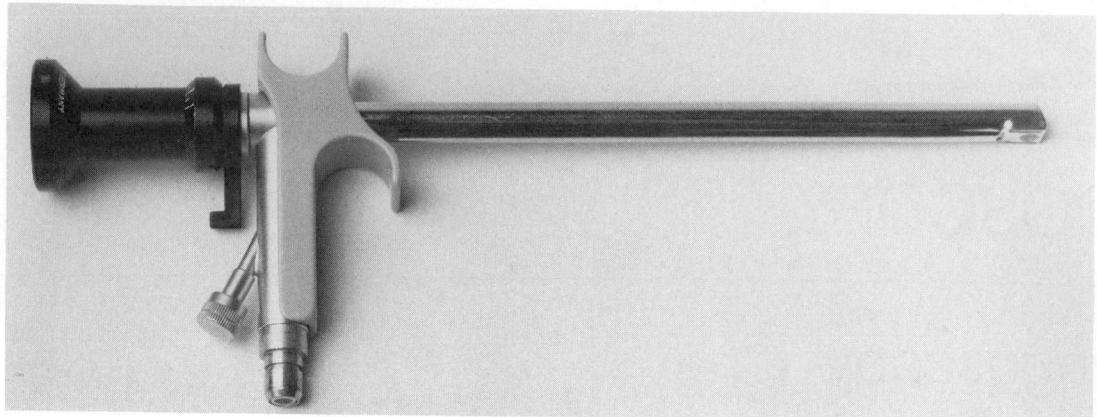

Figure 12-1. Rigid fiberoptic scope for examination of the pharynx and larynx.

be too large to fit comfortably through the nose. Pediatric bronchoscopes are of similar caliber but more difficult to manipulate because of the added length. They do not give as wide or as bright a view as a flexible laryngoscope does.

Another advantage of the fiberoptic systems is the ability to connect them to camera and video devices. High-quality still and motion pictures can be produced for documentation, discussion with colleagues, or teaching. A strobe light can be connected to slow laryngeal vocal cord vibrations perceptively and allow an assessment of subtle laryngeal pathologic conditions (Sodersten and Lindestad, 1992).

Anesthesia

Most patients can be examined without anesthesia. If the patient has a prominent gag reflex, the anterior tonsillar pillars, base of the tongue, and posterior oropharyngeal wall can be sprayed with a topical anesthetic (e.g., 10 percent lidocaine spray). Having the patient gargle with a topical

anesthetic (e.g., 2 to 5 percent lidocaine) is also effective. Rarely is a superior laryngeal nerve block required (subcutaneous infiltration of a local anesthetic 1 cm anterior to the superior thyroid cornu and 1 cm superior to the thyroid ala). When a flexible laryngoscope is passed transnasally, the procedure is much more comfortable for the patient when topical nasal anesthesia is used. Topical cocaine (4 to 5 percent) is particularly effective because it decongests and anesthetizes at the same time. Attention to the maximum dose of the anesthetic per kilogram of weight must be observed, particularly in children.

Technique

Mirror

Laryngeal mirrors are readily available and inexpensive, but they require some practice to use them effectively. The examiner and patient are seated comfortably at eye level (Fig. 12-3). A head mirror or head light is used to focus light at

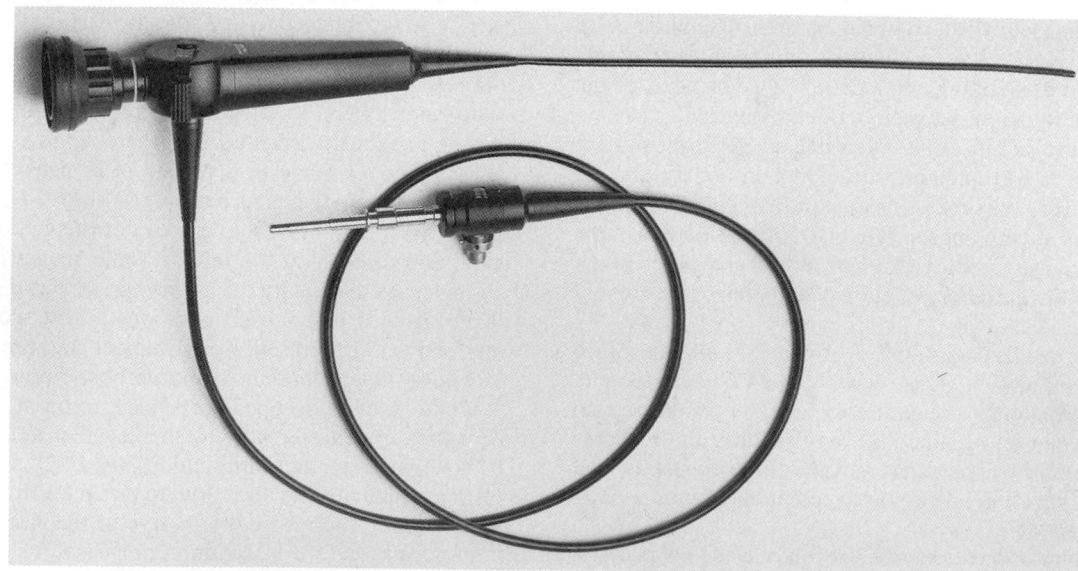

Figure 12-2. Flexible fiberoptic scope for examination of the pharynx and larynx.

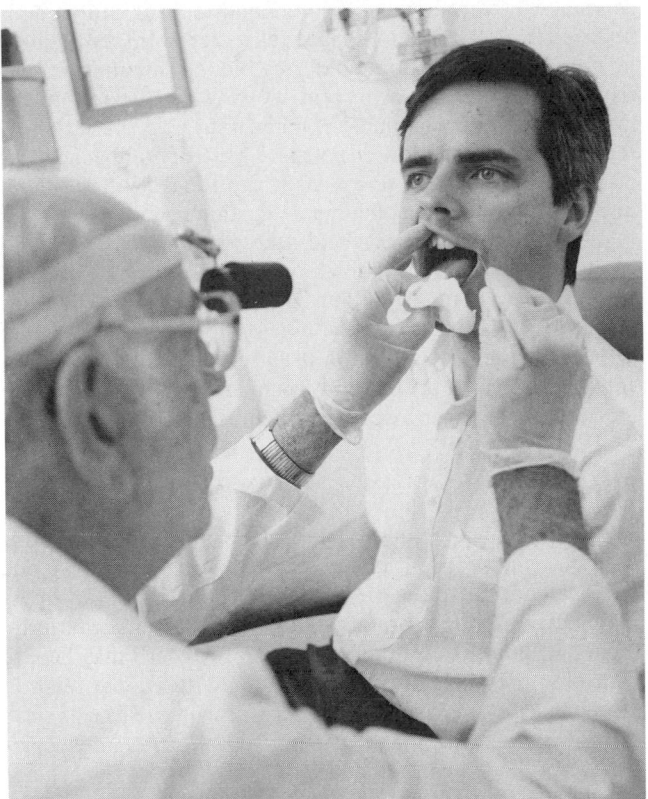

Figure 12-3. Indirect mirror laryngoscopy. Note the examiner's left hand retracting the tongue with a folded gauze while the right hand positions the mirror.

the soft palate and posterior pharyngeal wall. The mirror is warmed with hot water, heated beads, or a flame to prevent the patient's respirations from fogging the mirror during the examination. The temperature should be tested on the examiner's hand before the instrument is inserted to avoid burning the patient. Alternatively defogging solution may be used. If the examiner is right-handed, the left hand is used to hold the tongue protruded with a folded gauze. If the examiner needs one hand free, patients can hold their own tongue. The right hand directs the mirror toward the posterior oropharyngeal wall and angles it so a view of the base of tongue, vallecula, pharynx, and larynx is obtained. It is helpful to have the patient pant, and it is often necessary to touch and elevate the soft palate to gain an adequate view. The patient attempts to vocalize "eee" so that vocal cord mobility may be assessed. The larynx and pharynx should be examined in a systematic fashion, which may require several trials.

It is important to remember that, with a mirror, the anterior and posterior relationships of the larynx are reversed but right and left remain the same when the examiner looks at the reflected image. An easy way to understand this is to draw two labeled vocal cords on a piece of paper and position them so the anterior commissure is pointed at the examiner (i.e., the patient is facing the examiner). When a mirror is held over the drawing, as if the patient were being examined, it will be noted how the right and left cords remain on the same side but the anterior and posterior dimensions are re-

versed. This reversal makes instrumentation of the larynx with a mirror confusing. An advantage of both the rigid and flexible telescopes is that there is no reversal and a true image of the larynx is obtained.

Rigid Telescope

Examination with the rigid scope is similar to that with the mirror. The tongue is held protruded with one hand while the telescope is inserted through the mouth toward the posterior oropharyngeal wall. It often touches the wall. The telescope can be rotated to view the entire larynx and pharynx while the patient pants or attempts to vocalize "eee." If the telescope is equipped with a zoom lens, particular areas can be examined with magnification.

Flexible Telescope

The patient is asked if one nasal passage is more patent, or preferably patency is assessed by anterior rhinoscopy. After topical anesthesia is administered, the scope is directed along the floor of the nose adjacent to the inferior turbinate or between the inferior and middle turbinates. In the nasopharynx the scope is directed posterior to the soft palate, and a panoramic view of the base of tongue, larynx, and pharynx is obtained. The scope is then directed toward areas of interest for a closer examination in a systematic fashion. The subglottis and trachea can be examined through the vocal cords. The access to difficult-to-examine areas is superb, although the illumination and clarity may not always be as good as those with a mirror or rigid scope (Fig. 12-4).

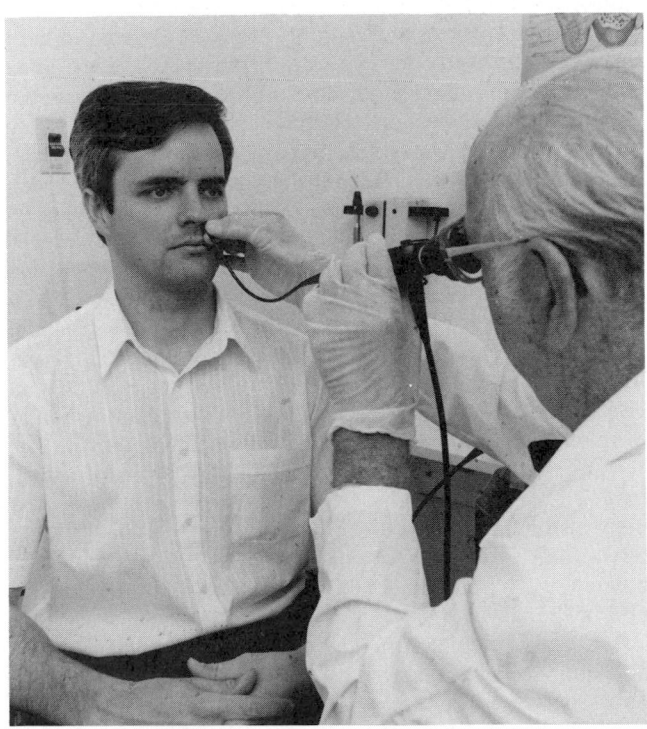

Figure 12-4. Flexible laryngoscopy.

DIRECT LARYNGOSCOPY

Indications

Direct laryngoscopy is the preferred technique for the detailed evaluation of laryngeal growths, stenosis, and trauma (Benjamin, 1990; Kleinsasser, 1991; Benjamin, 1993). The extent of any disease process can be precisely mapped out, and appropriate biopsy specimens can be taken. Areas that are difficult to examine by indirect laryngoscopy can be evaluated (e.g., laryngeal ventricles, postcricoid area, and pyriform sinuses). The vocal cords and arytenoids may be palpated to ascertain whether vocal cord immobility is due to paralysis or ankylosis. Vocal cord augmentation with a direct laryngoscope is preferred by many surgeons. Laryngeal laser surgery is usually performed with direct laryngoscopy.

Contraindications and Precautions

It is inappropriate to administer general anesthesia when the patient has a laryngeal obstruction (e.g., neoplasm, foreign body, or edema). When the pharyngeal tone is lost, a marginal airway may advance to total obstruction. There are several options in this situation, including awake intubation [often with the aid of a flexible bronchoscope (Roberts, 1991)] and tracheotomy under local anesthesia. Unfavorable patient anatomy may create impossible or dangerous situations for direct laryngoscopy. Examples include ankylosing spondylitis, rheumatoid arthritis, and cervical spine fractures or dislocation. Other anatomic features that may make laryngoscopy difficult include a small mandible, trismus, long central incisors, a short thick neck, or inability to extend the neck.

Preoperative Preparation

The patient is placed in the supine position on a head support that raises the head approximately 10 cm above the operating room table. This flexes the neck on the chest and places the patient in the Boyce or "sniffing" position, which is the optimal endoscopic position for visualization of the larynx. Secretions can be minimized if the patient is given a drying agent preoperatively, such as atropine or glycopyrrolate.

Anesthesia

Direct laryngoscopy can be performed under local or general anesthesia. General anesthesia is preferred for patient comfort and muscular relaxation. Local anesthesia is used in circumstances in which vocal cord mobility or assessment of the voice is important (e.g., Teflon augmentation).

Ventilation is carried out by a jet Venturi or endotracheal tube. The advantage of the jet Venturi tube is an unobstructed view of the larynx. An endotracheal tube provides a stable airway and prevents aspiration of blood and debris. Unfortunately the tube may obstruct visualization and instrumentation of the larynx.

The Venturi tubing commonly has a large-bore plastic cannula attached to its end that can be placed in the main lumen or a separate port of the laryngoscope. The patient is ventilated in short bursts to allow sufficient time for expiration (Bourgain, et al., 1990). Restrictive lung disease or obesity can make jet ventilation difficult. Endotracheal intubtaion is required if jet ventilation is inadequate. Jet ventilation should be temporarily discontinued during biopsy sampling and removal of specimens to prevent blowing the tissue into the lungs. In addition, care must be taken if the jet is placed below the vocal cords or another potential obstruction because air may not be able to escape from the lungs with resultant pneumothorax and/or pneumomediastinum.

A small cuffed endotracheal tube (number 24 to 28) and positive pressure ventilation can provide adequate gas exchange for as long as 1 hour. In most cases the tube lies posterior to the laryngoscope unless the posterior larynx is to be examined. The tube is usually taped or held by the anesthesiologist at the left oral commissure to remove it from the path of the laryngoscope through the right oropharynx.

Protection of the Teeth

The patient's upper dentition is at risk for damage during direct laryngoscopy. It is important to note dental work and loose teeth prior to the procedure and point these out to the patient. Gauze or a prefabricated plastic dental guard are most useful to prevent dental abrasion. A guard may help to distribute pressure, but it does not allow the upper teeth to be used as a fulcrum during exposure of the larynx in a difficult patient. In patients who require frequent endoscopies or those with precarious dentition, a customized acrylic or plastic plate of the upper dentition is useful to reduce dental trauma. It is much easier to position the scope in patients who do not have teeth or who have large gaps in their upper teeth.

Instruments

There are many laryngoscopes that can be used to carry out direct laryngoscopy. To examine the entire larynx and pharynx in detail, an anterior commissure scope is excellent because it can reach most sites (Figs. 12-5 and 12-6). Unfortunately the overall panoramic view is lost, and different sites must be sequentially examined. For delicate laryngeal surgery, it is preferable to select the widest scope that can be inserted to expose the anterior commissure. A variety of shapes and sizes of laryngoscopes is required to meet the needs of the entire spectrum of patients (Fig. 12-6). Laryngoscopes have ports for one or two fiberoptic light carriers, and some have extra ports for jet ventilation and smoke evacuation.

The laryngoscope may be held by one hand, but it is often preferable to suspend it and free up both hands. Two commonly used suspension devices are the Lewy and Boston suspension systems. The Lewy system is light, is easily attached and detached, and provides excellent stabilization of the laryngoscope within the larynx (Fig. 12-7). Unfortunately when exposure of the larynx is difficult, the Lewy system may exert unacceptable pressure on the maxillary dentition. In these patients the Boston system is favored because it allows proper positioning of the head and neck and minimizes pressure on the maxillary teeth (Fig. 12-8). This system takes longer to set up and position accurately.

Magnification of laryngeal structures can be accomplished with an operating microscope (Fig. 12-9). The axis of the

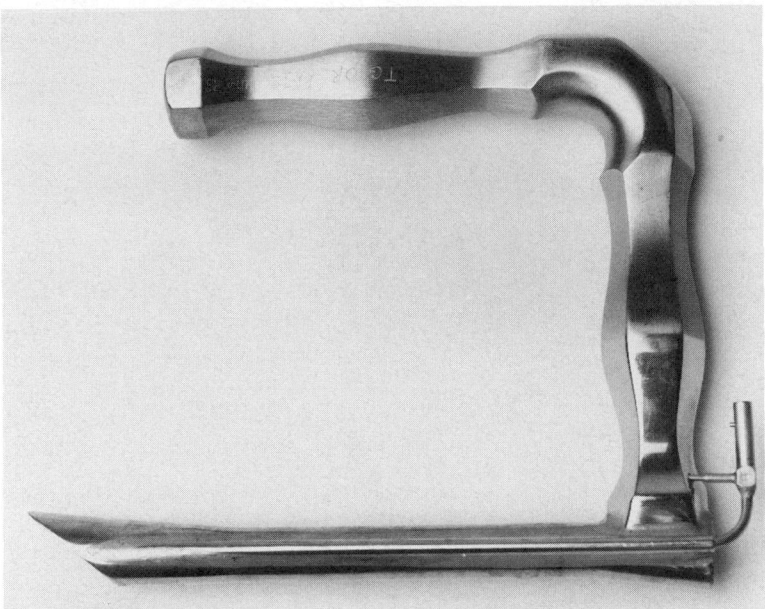

Figure 12-5. Anterior commissure scope.

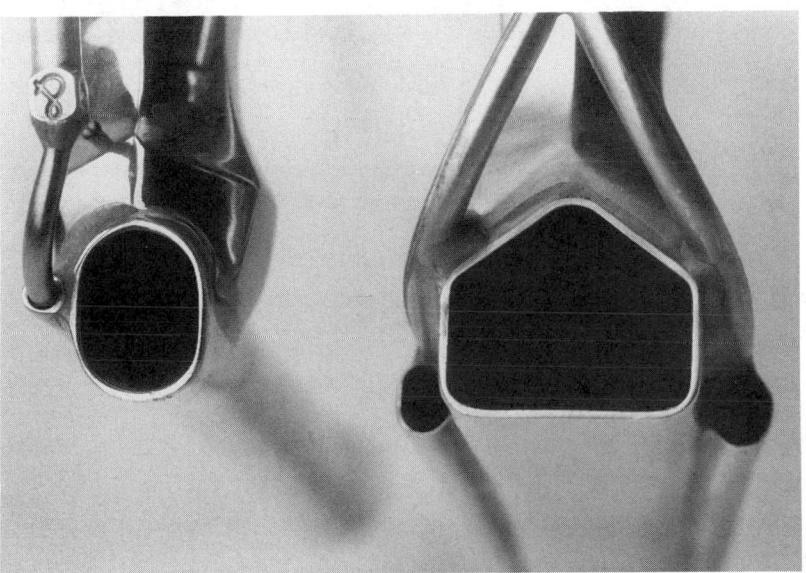

Figure 12-6. Two examples to illustrate the different luminal sizes of direct laryngoscopes: anterior commissure scope (*left*) and Dedo scope (*right*).

microscope is aligned with the axis of the scope. A 400-mm objective lens has a focal length long enough to allow instrumentation of the larynx without the instrument hitting the microscope. It is usually not possible to get binocular vision through narrow scopes, and hence there is a need for the widest scope possible that will expose the area of interest. For microlaryngeal surgery it is advantageous to have a support (e.g., Mayo stand) at the head of the table to brace and rest the elbows. In addition, rigid fiberoptic telescopes can be inserted through the suspended laryngoscope to magnify

and examine the larynx in detail. These telescopes are available in various angles of view from 0 to 90 degrees.

Technique

The airway must be stable, and the patient must be relaxed. This is best provided through close collaboration between surgeon and anesthesiologist. It is again stressed that general anesthesia should not be administered if there is concern in regard to the patency of the airway. In most cases induction

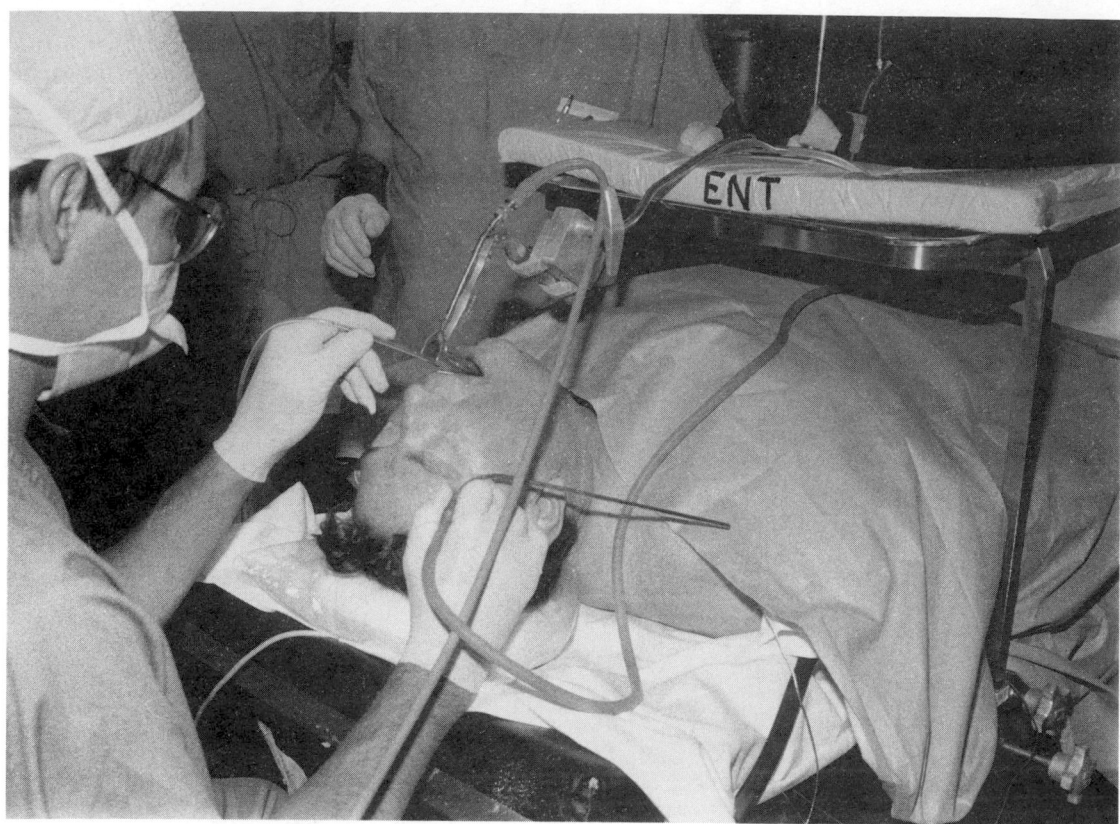

Figure 12-7. Lewy suspension system with jet Venturi. This system is placed on a Mayo stand over the patient's upper chest and attached to the laryngoscope.

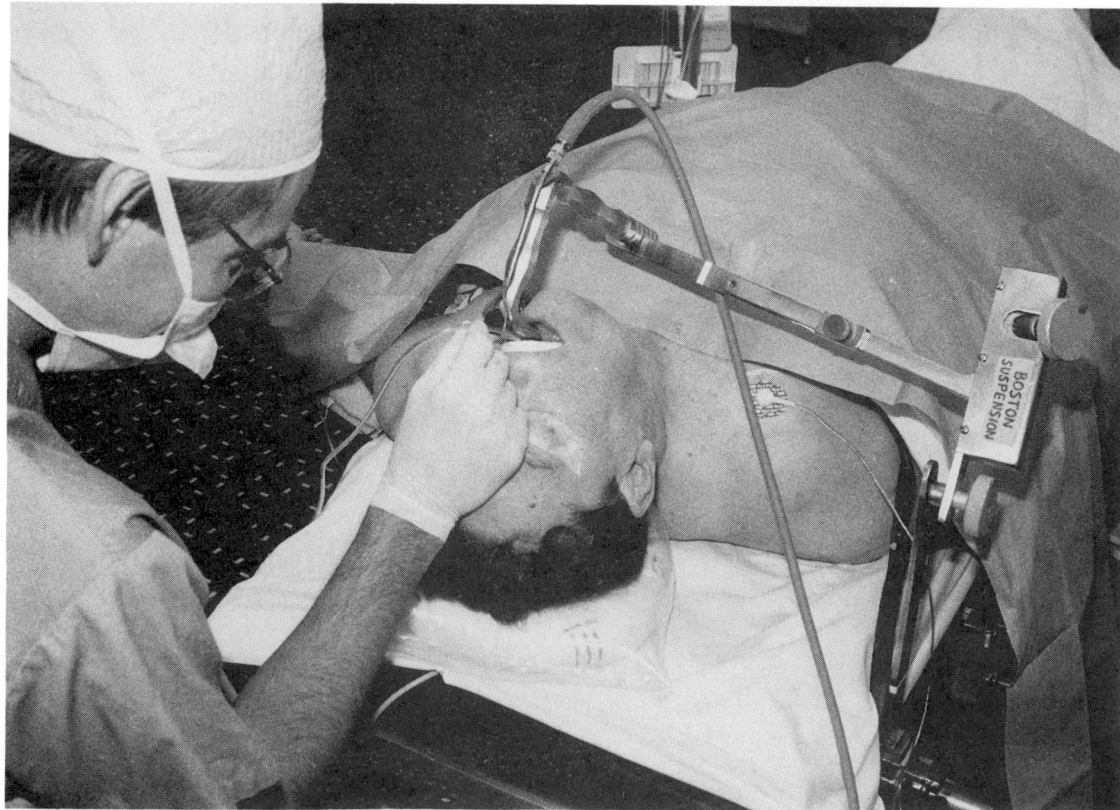

Figure 12-8. Boston suspension system. The teeth are not used as a fulcrum with this system to avoid excessive pressure on the maxillary dentition.

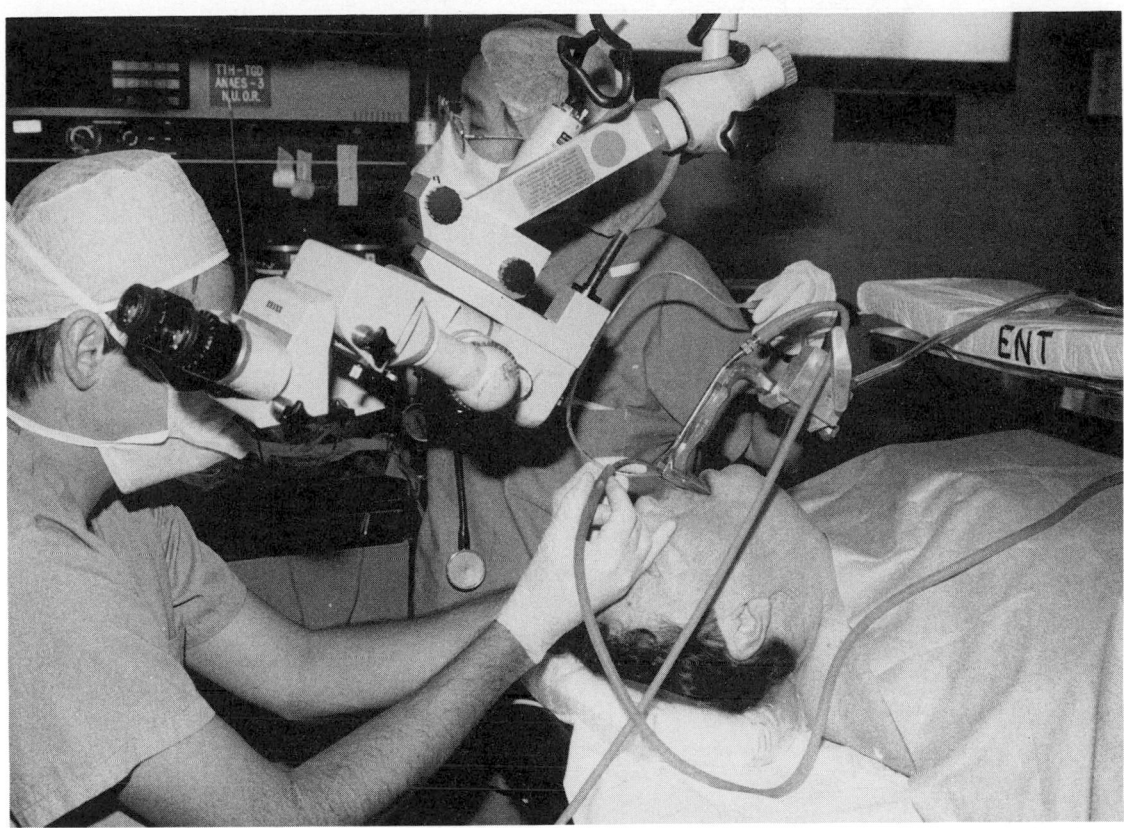

Figure 12-9. Direct microlaryngoscopy.

is carried out with an intravenous agent after preoxygenation. The patient is paralyzed (e.g., succinylcholine), and maintenance of anesthesia is commonly carried out with nitrous oxide, oxygen, and halothane or enflurance. Newer intravenous anesthetics also work well (e.g., propofol). The eyes are taped shut to prevent corneal abrasion, and the teeth or gingiva are protected. Ventilation is achieved by intubation or jet Venturi, as discussed above. The surgeon sits at the head of the table and introduces the laryngoscope through the patient's mouth to the epiglottis. It is important not to crush the lips or tongue during manipulation of the laryngoscope. The tip of the scope is passed under the epiglottis, which is displaced anteriorly. The scope is advanced to the laryngeal inlet as far as necessary to expose the internal surface of the larynx. The scope can be suspended at this point or held in the hand to examine various parts of the larynx systematically, including the true and false vocal

cords, anterior and posterior commissures, ventricles, subglottis, epiglottis, pyriform sinuses, vallecula, and postcricoid area. It is often necessary to push on the thyroid or cricoid cartilage externally to bring structures into view through the scope. Fine dissecting instruments are required for microsurgery of the larynx.

Local anesthesia, such as lidocaine or cocaine, is commonly applied topically to the larynx at the conclusion of laryngoscopy to prevent postoperative laryngospasm. Most patients have minimal pain and can tolerate their regular diets when they are fully recovered from the anesthesia. The patient's voice is often hoarse, depending on the nature of the procedure. They should be encouraged to talk softly for short periods only and avoid whispering, shouting, or long conversations, which put excessive strain on the vocal apparatus.

KEY REFERENCES

Benjamin B: Diagnostic Laryngology: Adults and Children. p. 1. WB Saunders, Philadelphia, 1990

This atlas of laryngology will assist the reader in the differential diagnosis and correct interpretation of various laryngeal abnormalities in both adults and children.

Kleinsasser O: Microlaryngoscopy and Endolaryngeal Microsurgery: Techniques and Typical Findings. 3rd Ed. p. 1. Mosby Year Book, St. Louis, 1991

This is a beautifully illustrated book of typical findings seen with direct laryngoscopy. It will give the reader an appreciation of the variety of laryngeal pathologic conditions examined under the operating microscope.

REFERENCES

Benjamin B: Prolonged intubation injuries of the larynx: endoscopic diagnosis, classification, and treatment. Ann Otol Rhinol Laryngol 160 (suppl):1, 1993

Bourgain JL, McGee K, Cosset MF et al: Carbon dioxide monitoring during high frequency jet ventilation for direct laryngoscopy. Br J Anaesth 64:327, 1990

Roberts JT: Preparing to use the flexible fiber-optic laryngoscope. J Clin Anesth 3:64, 1991

Sodersten M, Lindestad PA: A comparison of vocal fold closure in rigid telescopic and flexible fiberoptic laryngostroboscopy. Acta Otolaryngol (Stockh) 112:144, 1992

Rigid Bronchoscopy

Shafique Keshavjee
Robert J. Ginsberg

HISTORICAL NOTE

Bronchoscopy is an invaluable tool for the management of thoracic disease. In addition to being an essential diagnostic modality, it provides direct therapeutic benefits in many situations. Until 1970 the only access to the tracheobronchial tree was the rigid bronchoscope, initially designed by Chevalier Jackson (Boyd, 1994; Jackson and Jackson, 1950). Although this provided a limited view, the operator could usually visualize the pulmonary segmental orifices of most lobes. The rigidity of the instruments limited our ability to obtain biopsy specimens to the major bronchi. The development of rigid telescopes with high-quality optics enhanced our ability to examine the subsegmental bronchi and lesions of the central airway in detail.

The introduction of flexible fiberoptic bronchoscopic equipment has enhanced our ability to view the distal segmental bronchi and has simplified the procedure considerably. Both techniques of bronchoscopy—rigid and flexible—have evolved to define their own diagnostic and therapeutic indications. Each system has its strengths and limitations, and the thoracic surgeon should be competent in the use of both modalities to manage the spectrum of thoracic disease that may be confronted. Flexible bronchoscopy is dealt with in detail in the next part of this chapter by Cortese.

HISTORICAL READINGS

Boyd AD: Chevalier Jackson: the father of American bronchoesophagoscopy. Ann Thorac Surg 57:502, 1994

Jackson C, Jackson CL: Bronchoesophagology. WB Saunders, Philadelphia, 1950

INDICATIONS FOR RIGID BRONCHOSCOPY

Hemoptysis

Although many common respiratory symptoms can be investigated by fiberoptic bronchoscopy, one specific indication for rigid equipment is massive hemoptysis (Wedzicha and Pearson, 1990). A rigid endoscope provides the operator with immediate control of the airway. In addition, it permits the use of large-bore suction equipment to keep the airway clear of blood and clots. Although occlusive balloon catheters or packing (to tamponade bleeding) may be placed in certain circumstances with flexible fiberoptic equipment, they can be positioned with greater control and accuracy under direct vision with the rigid scope, especially when there is significant bleeding that requires efficient suctioning.

Indications for Rigid Bronchoscopy

Massive hemoptysis

Airway obstruction: diagnostic and therapeutic
    Foreign body
        Tumor: endobronchial, extrinsic compression
        Benign stricture

Laser therapy

Endobronchial stenting

Tracheobronchial toilet

Pediatric bronchoscopy

Miscellaneous

Airway Obstruction

In conditions that cause the obstruction of the airway (larynx, trachea, or main bronchi), the use of the rigid bronchoscope is the safest modality to obtain a diagnosis because it enables secure control of the airway should a problem arise. In many instances it is both diagnostic and therapeutic.

Foreign Bodies

The need for a rigid bronchoscope for the extraction of foreign bodies is self-evident. In fact this was the initial indication for which Jackson developed the instrument (Boyd, 1994). With the varied forceps available and the operator working through the scope, a foreign body can be manipulated and extracted directly (Weissberg and Schwartz, 1987; Holinder, 1978).

Malignant Disease

In cases of malignant obstruction, the first priority is the establishment of a safe airway. This is readily achieved with a rigid bronchoscope. Endobronchial tumors may be debrided directly with biopsy forceps, electrocautery, or a laser to establish an improved airway. Such debridement is often impossible with flexible equipment (Hetzel and Smith, 1991). Such cases should be handled in an operating room where problems with airway control can be readily dealt with if necessary. In cases of obstruction caused by endobronchial pathologic conditions or extrinsic compression, it is safer to keep the patient breathing spontaneously until a secure airway is established.

Once an airway is established, the obstructing lesion can be dilated as the first step. Dilatation may be carried out by the surgeon first passing the smallest scope that will fit through the stricture and then using sequentially larger scopes for dilatation in a stepwise fashion. Gum-tipped Jackson bougies inserted under direct vision through the bronchoscope can be used in selected cases of tumor obstruction to define the lumen prior to the use of the laser (see below).

Benign Stricture

Rigid bronchoscopy is often the first step in the management of a benign stricture. Tracheal or mainstem bronchial stenoses are often readily dilated with sequential passage of bronchoscopes of increasing diameter. Narrow, tight strictures that will not easily admit the tip of a scope may be initially dilated with gum-tipped Jackson bougies that are passed under direct vision through the bronchoscope. Rigid equipment allows an accurate assessment of the location, caliber, length, and rigidity of the stricture and the status of the distal airway. This detailed examination is essential in the preoperative assessment and planning for airway resection (see Ch. 16).

Laser Therapy

Laser therapy of the airway is dealt with in detail in the part of this chapter by Goldberg, et al. It is apparent that the use of rigid equipment extends the surgeon's ability to remove a tumor more rapidly and use laser coagulation. The CO_2 laser, which cannot be used with a fiberoptic system, mandates the use of rigid equipment. Once again in cases of airway obstruction, the rigid bronchoscope enables the surgeon to obtain immediate control of the airway safely. The tumor can then be managed by dilatation or debridment prior to the application of the laser. In many such cases, the laser may not be required because gross tumor can be adequately debrided with the biopsy forceps and bleeding can be controlled with epinephrine solution or electrocautery.

Endobronchial Stents

The placement of endobronchial stents frequently requires the use of the rigid bronchoscope (Cooper, et al., 1989). Stents are used both in the palliation of obstructing tumors and to stent the airway for benign stenoses. The indications and techniques for stent placement are described in detail in the part of this chapter by Gaissert and Patterson.

Tracheobronchial Toilet

In rare instances the tracheobronchial toilet of thick secretions cannot be managed adequately with a fiberoptic bronchoscope. Rigid equipment allows the use of larger-bore suction equipment and facilitates the removal of such viscid secretions.

Pediatric Bronchoscopy

In children with tiny airways, rigid bronchoscopy is the only option available to inspect the airway because tiny endotracheal tubes will not permit the passage of flexible equipment.

Miscellaneous

Proponents of rigid endoscopy maintain that the assessment of airway invasion by surrounding or extrinsic tumors (e.g., esophageal carcinoma) can be done better with a rigid instrument than with flexible bronchoscopy. The rigidity of the airway is best "felt" with a rigid scope, and the larger biopsy specimens obtained will be more accurate in the assessment of microscopic submucosal invasion.

METHODS OF ANESTHESIA AND VENTILATION

General Anesthesia

When bronchoscopy is performed under general anesthesia, the patient is supine, usually on an operating table. Intravenous or inhalation general anesthesia, or a combination of both, can be used. The induction is rapid if intravenous agents are used, but it can take 10 to 20 minutes if one "breathes down" the patient with inhalational agents. Once suitable induction has occurred and a muscle relaxant has been administered, the lower jaw should be loose and mobile. This indicates a suitable depth of anesthesia and muscle relaxation for the procedure. The patient should be fully monitored xygen saturation, blood pressure, and electrocardiography) throughout the procedure. Further details on the anesthetic management for rigid bronchoscopy are found in Chapter 7.

Techniques of Ventilation

For rigid bronchoscopic examination, four techniques of ventilation are available as follows: intermittent insufflation, continuous insufflation, Venturi (jet) ventilation, and spontaneous inhalation ventilation.

Intermittent Insufflation

This classic technique of ventilation through the bronchoscope involves intermittent ventilation through either a side port or through the proximal end of the bronchoscope to ventilate, oxygenate, and maintain anesthesia. This is simply carried out by the examiner inserting an endotracheal tube, attached to the ventilating system, to either the side port or the open end of the bronchoscope. Endoscopists may have to occlude the upper airway with packing or occlude the nose and mouth with their hands if there is a large air leak. This technique is cumbersome and does not allow for continuous viewing through the scope.

Continuous Insufflation

The end of the bronchoscope is fitted with a lens, and a side port is used to ventilate the patient continually while the endoscopist proceeds with the bronchoscopy. This has the advantages of allowing uninterrupted bronchoscopy and using inhalational agents throughout the procedure, thus minimizing the need for intravenous anesthesia. However, it has the disadvantages of fogging the lens and not permitting suctioning the biopsy sampling in an expeditious fashion because the lens must be removed for these maneuvers. However, this technique is a simple and reliable compromise that provides relatively continuous viewing and continuous ventilation. The middle bronchoscope in Figure 12-10 is shown fitted with the viewing lens. With the use of rigid telescopes, this ventilation technique provides excellent conditions for continuous, detailed viewing. The lower bronchoscope in Figure 12-10 is shown with the ventilation tubing attached and a Hopkins telescope in place.

Jet Ventilation

The most common form of ventilation used during rigid bronchoscopy is the Venturi technique (Fig. 12-11). This is based on the principle of air entrainment. With a side port or the open proximal end of the scope, a high-pressure (25 to 30 psi) jet of oxygen (delivered at 10 to 20 breaths per minute through an 18-gauge catheter) entrains surrounding ambient air, thereby ventilating the patient throughout the procedure. The modified Sanders ventilating system (Fig. 12-11) and a

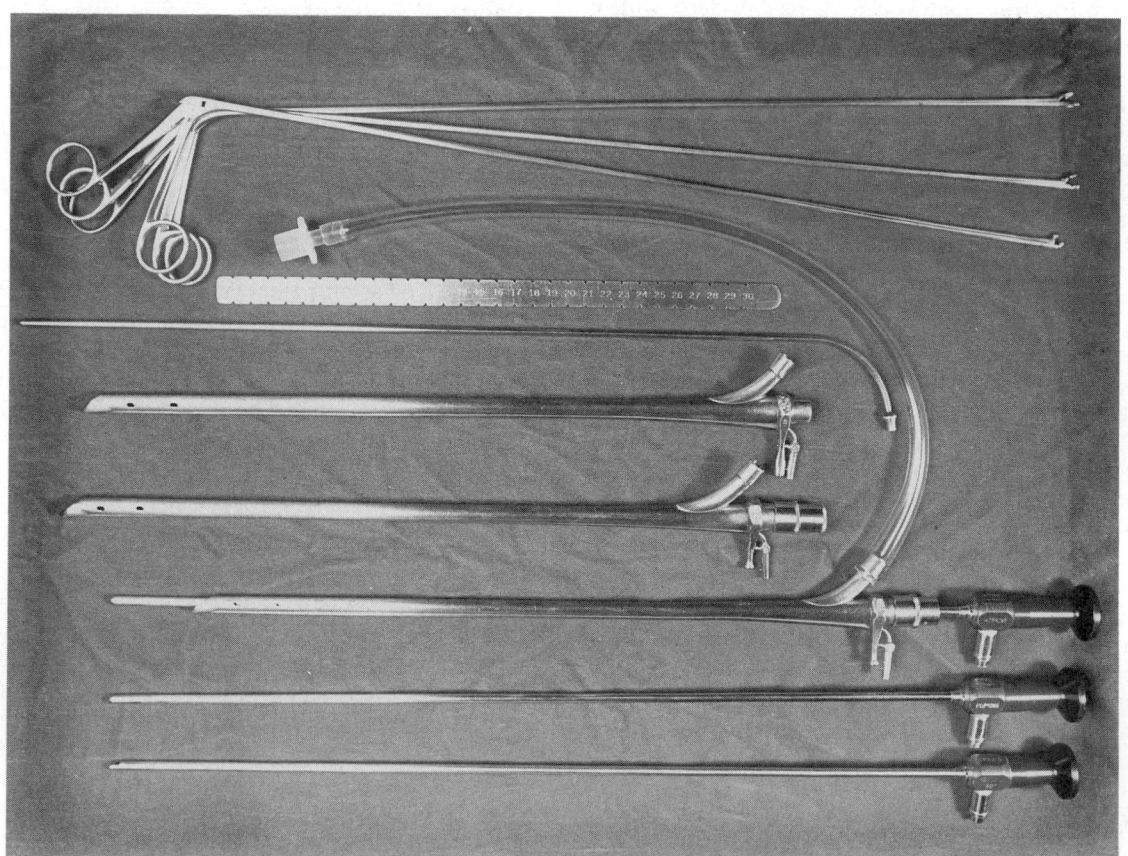

Figure 12-10. Basic equipment for rigid bronchoscopy. From top to bottom, biopsy forceps, ruler, rigid suction cannula, rigid bronchoscopes of varying sizes, and rigid Hopkins telescopes. The middle bronchoscope is shown with the viewing lens fitted. The lower bronchoscope is illustrated with the ventilation tubing attached to the side port and a 0-degree telescope inserted as it would be during use. The light source and fiberoptic cable are not shown.

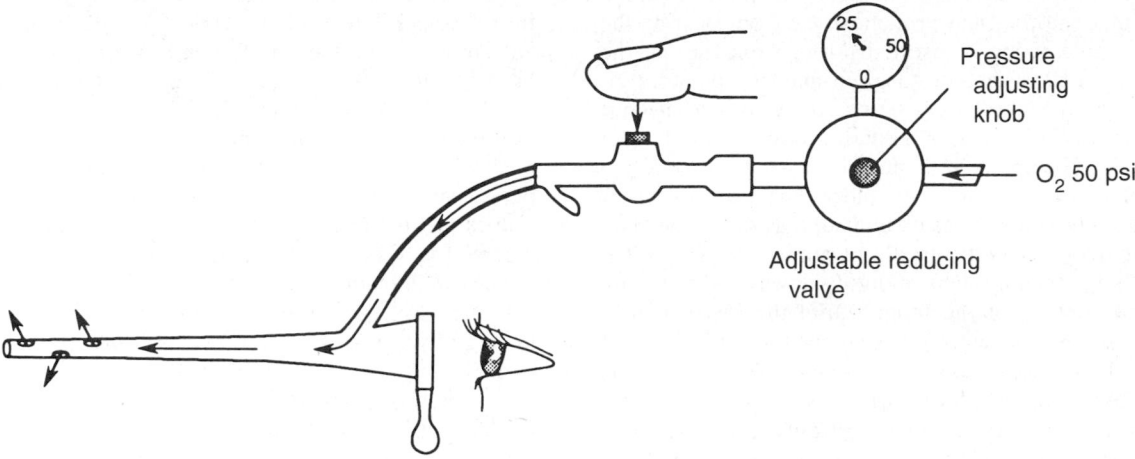

Figure 12-11. A schematic illustrating the modified Sanders jet ventilation technique for ventilation through a rigid bronchoscope. The wall oxygen supply at 50 psi is connected to a reducing valve that allows the pressure to be adjusted from 0 to 50 psi. The side port of the bronchoscope is used as the Venturi injector site, and the open end can be used for continuous viewing by the endoscopist. (From Ehrenwerth J, Brull S: Anesthesia for thoracic diagnostic procedures. p. 331. In Kaplan JA (ed): Anesthesia. 2nd Ed. Churchill Livingstone, New York, 1991, with permission.)

reducing valve are required (Sanders, 1987; Ehrenwerth and Brill, 1991). With this technique it is essential that the surgeon wear eye protection because droplets of secretions or blood can be drawn out of the open end of the bronchoscope. Anesthesia is maintained with intravenous agents and/or muscle relaxants.

Spontaneous Inhalation Ventilation

The technique of spontaneous inhalation ventilation demands a nonapneic patient. Inhalational agents are administered through the side port, and the anesthesia is kept light enough to maintain spontaneous respiration. The major disadvantages are lack of relaxation and exposure of the operator to the anesthetic gases. This technique is useful for the reduction of a patient with an obstructive lesion of the airway when the surgeon anticipates that airway control is precarious. With this technique it is not catastrophic if an airway is not obtained immediately because patients continue to breathe on their own.

Local Anesthesia

Rigid bronchoscopy can be carried out under local anesthesia. However, in most cases general anesthesia is the usual and preferred technique. The technique of local anesthesia is similar to that used with flexible bronchoscopy (see the part of this chapter by Cortese) and includes adequate topical anesthesia of the mouth, pharynx, and vocal cords and intravenous sedation as required. The use of atropine to decrease secretions and inhibit vagal reflexes is helpful. The authors' technique is as follows: administration of a local spray anesthetic to the pharynx and larynx, a transcricoid injection of 2 ml of 1 percent lidocaine, and premedication with an intravenous narcotic analgesic (e.g., morphine 2 to 5 mg IV). Intravenous sedation with diazepam or midazolam is then titrated to the patient's needs. The need for an adequately

sedated and reasonably comfortable patient cannot be overemphasized because intubation of the airway under local anesthesia requires the patient's cooperation. This can be enhanced with moderate sedation and effective local anesthesia, as described above. The procedure may be performed with the patient in a chair (preferably a dental chair) or supine on an operating table. If necessary in an emergency, intubation can be carried out on a stretcher or hospital bed. The technique for intubation under local anesthesia is identical to that for general anesthesia (described below).

TECHNIQUE OF RIGID BRONCHOSCOPY

Prior to the induction of anesthesia, the equipment and light source should be checked for proper function. The basic setup includes at least two sizes of bronchoscopes, appropriate suctioning cannulas, a variety of biopsy forceps, and a variety of telescopes (see Figure 12-10 and Equipment, below).

Care must be taken to protect the patient's eyes, usually with padding and adhesive tape. At all times the operator must protect the lips and teeth or gums of the patient from injury. A commercial rubber tooth guard is available, but a saline-soaked gauze sponge is adequate. The largest bronchoscope sufficient for the needs of the operator should be chosen. In most instances an 8- or 9-mm (outer diameter) scope is used for men, and a 7- or 8-mm scope is used for women (Fig. 12-11). Larger-diameter scopes may damage the larynx and may preclude intubation of the smaller distal bronchi. Much smaller equipment is required for infants and children; the selection of the size depends on the size of the child; scopes as small as 2.5 to 3 mm are required for patients who weigh less than 10 kg.

Placement of the patient's head on a pillow and then extension of the patient's neck so that the chin points vertically (the "sniffing" or "intubating" position) facilitates the introduction of the bronchoscope. With the examiner's thumb always protecting the rigid bronchoscope from injuring the upper teeth, the scope is inserted through one side of the mouth (usually the right side for right-handed operators) or in the midline in edentulous patients. Under direct vision it is advanced to the posterior median groove of the tongue (Fig. 12-12A). The upper teeth must never serve as a fulcrum to lever the bronchoscope into place; the operator's left thumb should bear this pressure and support the scope at all times. The scope is first introduced almost vertically; the proximal end is then brought smoothly downward as the tip follows the contour of the tongue until the instrument is almost horizontal. By gently elevating the tongue and slowly advancing the scope, the operator can identify the epiglottis (Fig. 12-12A). If the epiglottis is not seen (usually because of the instrument was advanced too rapidly past it), the scope should be partially withdrawn, and the maneuver should be repeated. The tip of the bronchoscope is insinuated a short distance beyond and posterior to the epiglottis, just far enough to raise it without having it slip off the end of the instrument (Fig. 12-12B). Once the epiglottis is lifted anteriorly with the tip of the bronchoscope, the posterior part of the laryngeal inlet, the arytenoids, and the vocal cords are identified (Fig. 12-12B). Occasionally external pressure on the larynx by an assistant, to displace it posteriorly, might be required to visualize the cords. In difficult cases the glottis can be displayed with a laryngoscope held in the left hand, and the bronchoscope is then inserted with the right hand.

Once the glottis is visualized, the bronchoscope is advanced toward the cords (Fig. 12-12C). As the cords are approached, the scope is turned 90 degrees to align the vertical orifice of the glottic chink with the tip of the scope (Fig. 12-12D). The scope is then gently advanced through the larynx into the upper airway. With a gentle twisting motion, the scope is rotated back to the original orientation. No force must be used at this stage. When the examiner advances the scope gently, injuries will not occur. If significant resistance is met, a smaller-sized bronchoscope should be used. Also the surgeon should ensure that the lips or pharyngeal tissues are not being inadvertently compressed and injured by the advancing scope.

After intubation the patient's head is extended; care is taken to prevent injury to cervical spine. The operator is advised to use a mobile stool to sit on and to raise the operating table to a comfortable position before beginning the examination. The scope is then slowly advanced, and the glottis, trachea, and carina are examined. To inspect the left or right side, the patient's head is turned in the opposite direction so that a ''straight line'' is developed between the oropharynx, trachea, and the mainstem bronchus to be examined.

To examine the left side, the bronchoscope is placed in the right corner of the mouth, and the patient's head is turned to the right. The scope is gently advanced down the left main bronchus. The lingular and lower lobe bronchi are easily seen. To visualize the segmental and subsegmental bronchi clearly, a telescope (Fig. 12-10) should be used. A lateral or oblique viewing telescope is required to see the left upper lobe bronchus. The presence of an aortic arch aneurysm is a contraindication to the passing of a rigid instrument down the left mainstem bronchus.

To examine the right bronchial tree, the patient's head is turned to the left, and the bronchoscope is moved to the left corner of the mouth. The right main bronchus and the bronchus intermedius are easily examined. The lower lobe is relatively easily visualized. To examine the middle lobe orifice, the patient's head may have to be extended further to allow the operator an adequate angle to view the anteriorly placed middle lobe orifice. Oblique or lateral viewing telescopes facilitate this task. The lateral viewing telescope is essential to visualize the right upper lobe bronchus and its segmental divisions.

Removal of the rigid bronchoscope should be performed as carefully as its insertion. The opportunity should be taken to examine the entire airway carefully on the way out. This is especially important for the proximal trachea and the subglottic, glottic, and supraglottic areas that may not have been visualized in detail on the way in. Furthermore if the patient is starting to ''lighten'' from the anesthetic, this will provide an opportunity to assess the function of the vocal cords.

EQUIPMENT

The performance of rigid bronchoscopy requires several essential pieces of equipment (Fig. 12-10). Additional components or modifications are available for specialized procedures or are based on operator preference. The basic components will be discussed under the categories of bronchoscopes and light sources, suction devices, forceps, and enhanced visualization.

Bronchoscopes

There are a variety of rigid bronchoscopes available; all are variations of the original design by Jackson (Jackson and Jackson, 1950; Boyd, 1994). Several standard rigid bronchoscopes are illustrated in Figure 12-10. The most commonly used sizes in adult practice are in the range of 6 to 9 mm in external diameter and 40 cm in length. For pediatric use a range of smaller (3 to 6 mm) and shorter scopes are available. A cold halogen light source is connected by a fiberoptic cable to the bronchoscope. The light is transmitted down a fiberoptic fibre bundle along the side wall of the tube such that the light is emitted from a point just inside the distal tip of the scope.

Suction Devices

One of the major advantages of rigid bronchoscopy is the ability to suction out the airway effectively, especially in cases of massive hemoptysis. An effective (operating room-type) suction source is required. The rigid suction cannula (Fig. 12-10) must be long enough to protrude from the distal end of the scope that is being used. An insulated suction tube is useful for the application of electrocautery to deal with bleeding after tumor debridement or biopsy.

Forceps

A wide variety of forceps are available for use in varying circumstances. Some of these are illustrated in Figure 12-10. Tissue biopsy forceps come in several sizes. The large biopsy

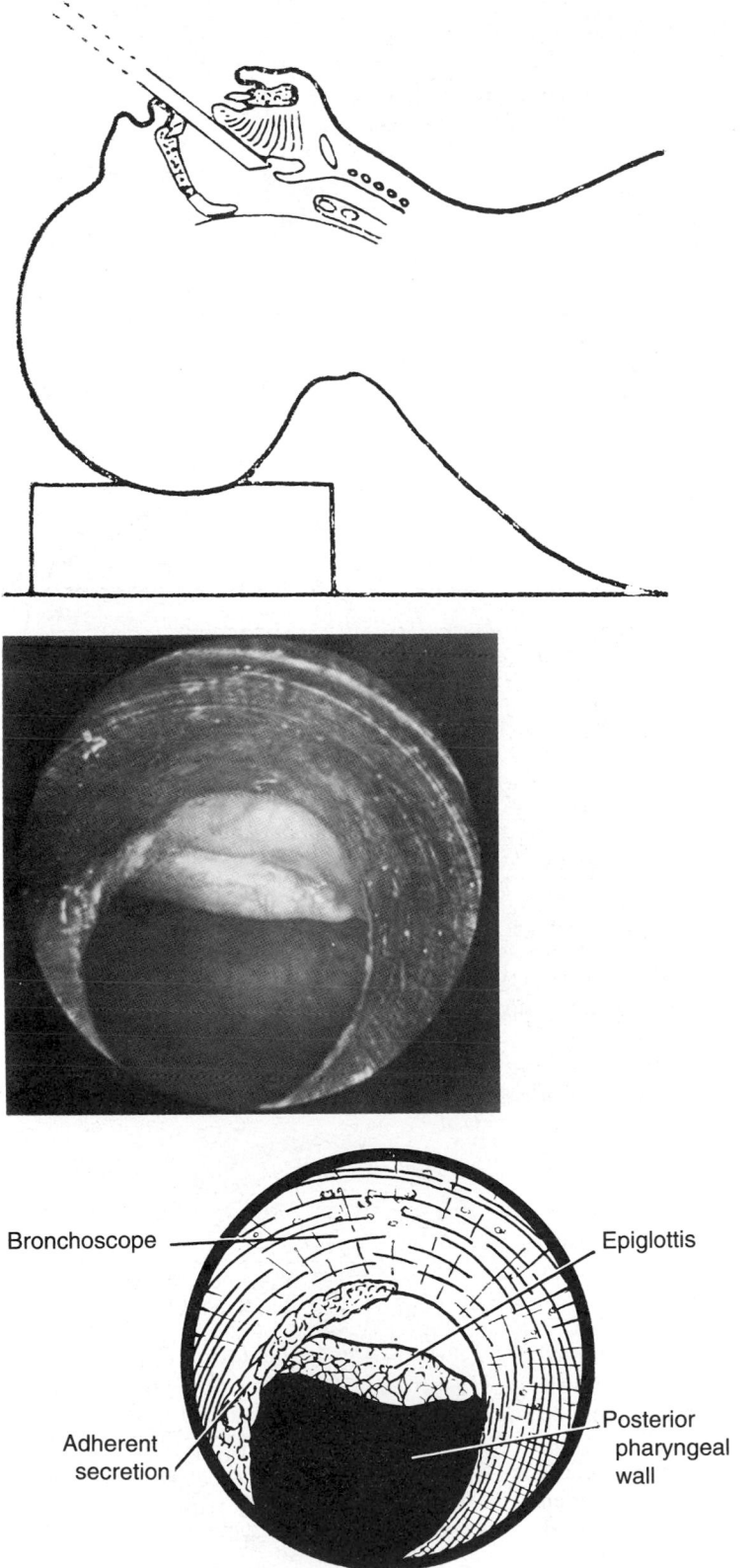

A

Figure 12-12 **(A)** Visualization of the epiglottis. The tip of the bronchoscope has followed the contour of the tongue toward its root, and the epiglottis has been located and centered in the field of vision. (*Figure continues.*)

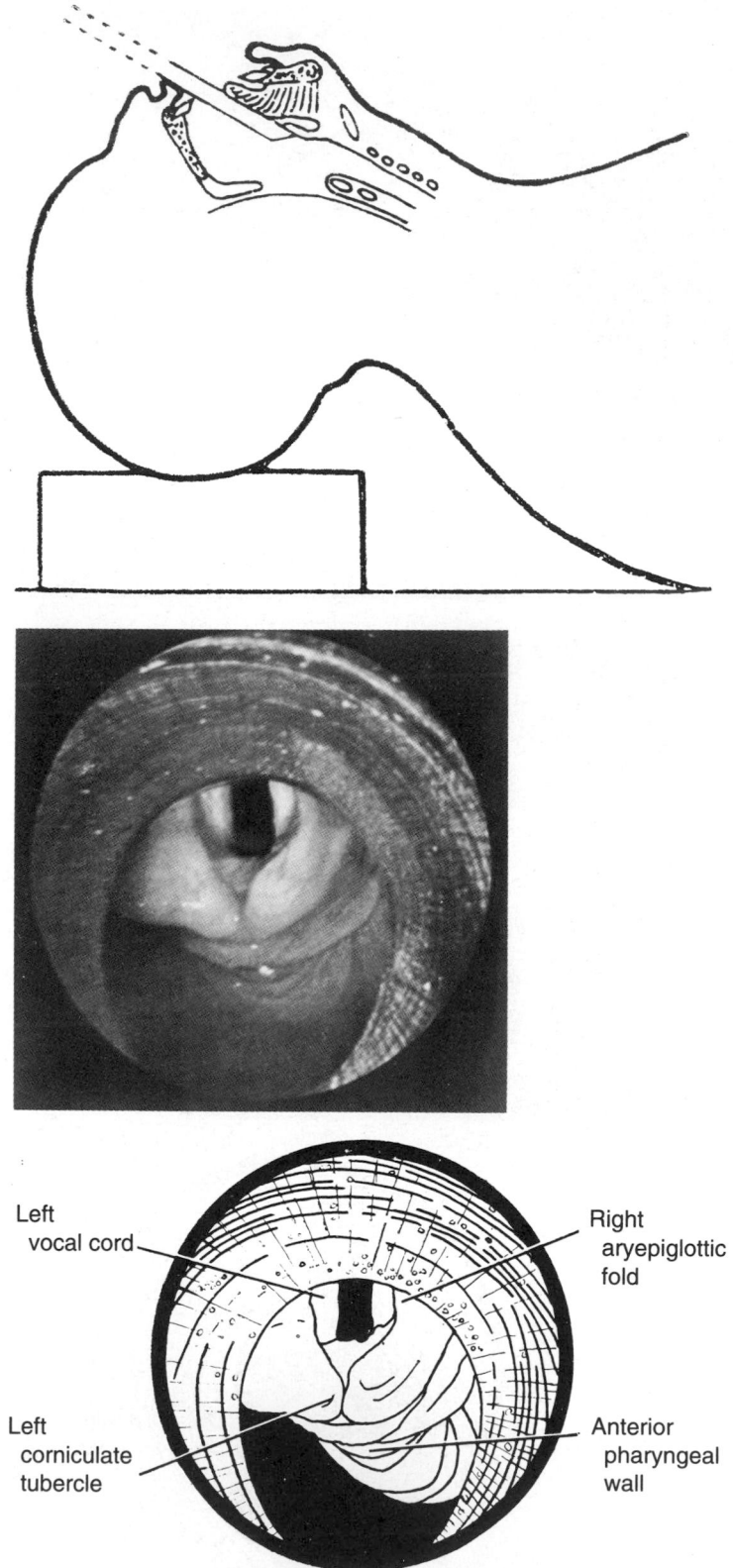

B

Figure 12-12 (*Continued*).   **(B)** The epiglottis is elevated with the tip of the scope and the scope is advanced just beyond to demonstrate the glottis. The posterior larynx and vocal cords are clearly visualized. (*Figure continues.*)

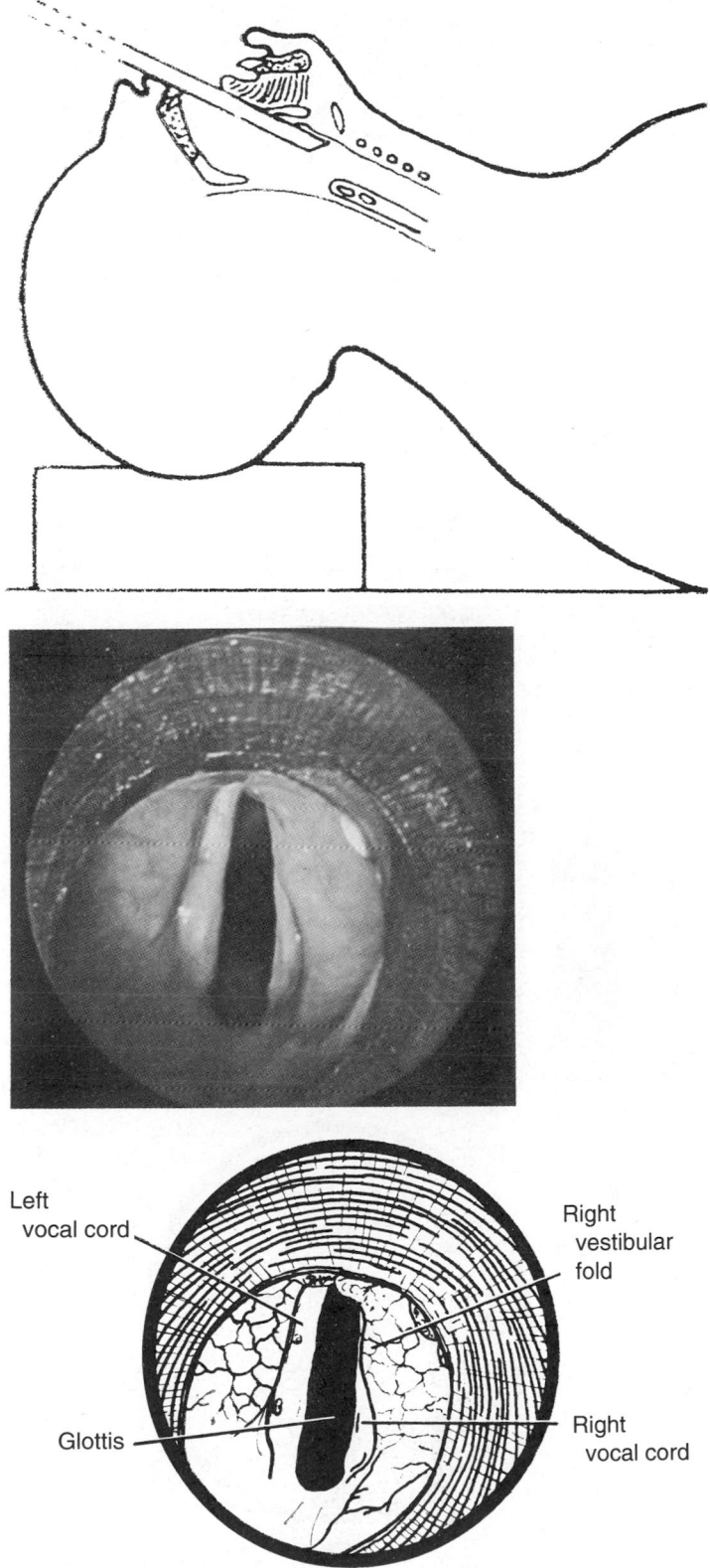

C

Figure 12-12 (*Continued*). **(C)** The bronchoscope is advanced a little further, and its axis is carefully aligned with that of the glottis and trachea. (*Figure continues.*)

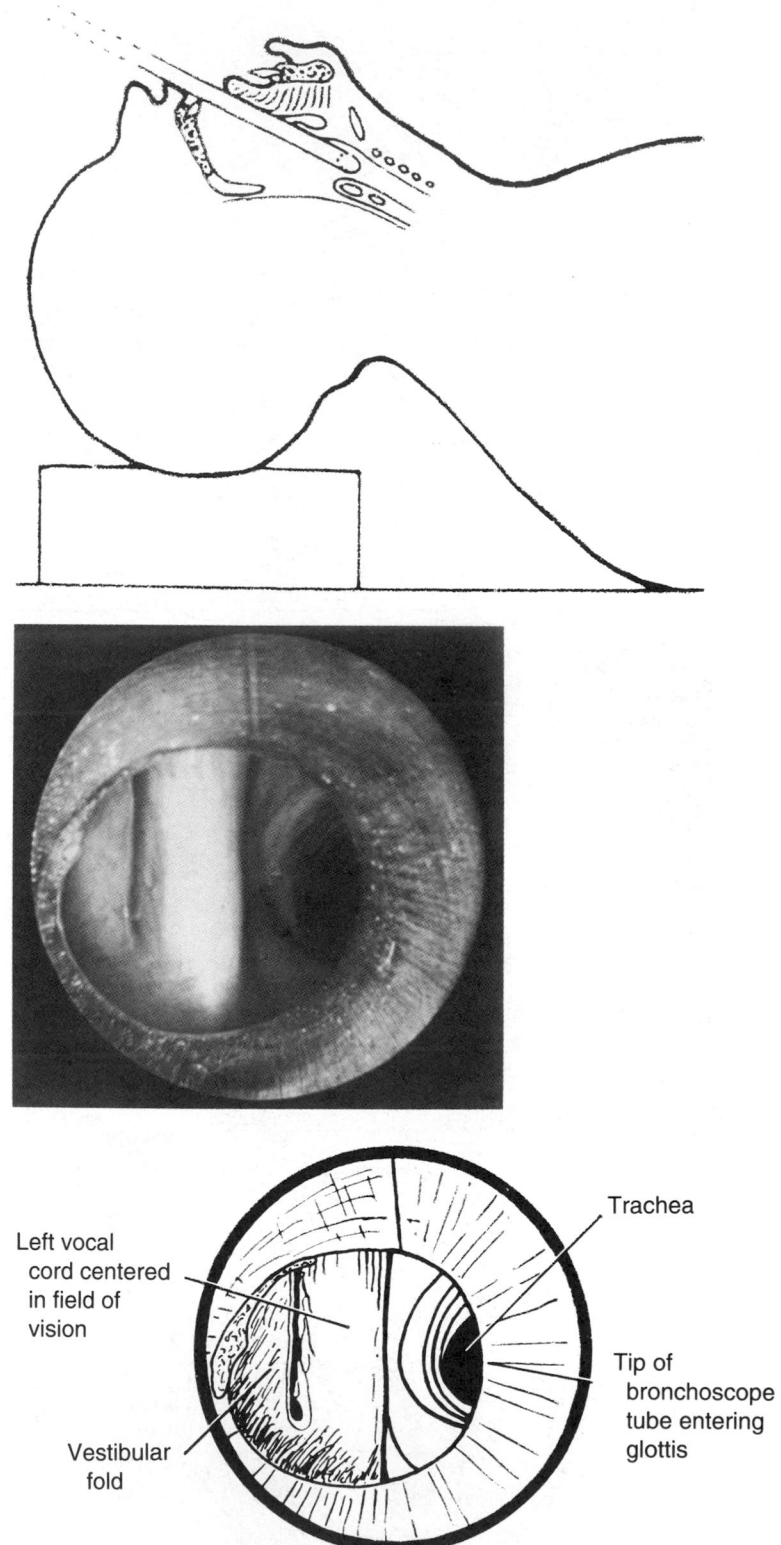

D

Figure 12-12 (*Continued*).   **(D)** The bronchoscope is turned 90 degrees and gently advanced between the cords into the trachea. The tracheal cartilages are seen in the distance. Once the bronchoscope is in the trachea, it is rotated back to its original orientation for comfortable manipulation, and the pillow behind the patient's head is removed. (From Stradling P: Diagnostic Bronchoscopy—an Introduction. 2nd Ed. Williams & Wilkins, Baltimore, 1973, with permission.)

forceps allow for deeper biopsy specimens to be sampled than are generally obtainable with the flexible bronchoscope, but caution must be used to avoid hemorrhage. Aggressive, deep biopsy sampling can remove the full thickness of airway cartilage and lead to troublesome bronchial arterial bleeding. The larger forceps can be used to debride an obstructing tumor or to extract a clot from the airway. A number of forceps are also available that can be used to manipulate, grasp, and extract foreign bodies in the airway. These are stronger than biopsy forceps and more suitably designed for grasping and removing objects.

Enhanced Visualization: Telescopes and Video Display

Rigid Hopkins rod-type telescopes have been developed to examine distal segmental orifices and improve the image (Hopkins, 1976). These solid rod telescopes produce the best image available, far superior to that seen with fiberoptic equipment. Zero (forward), 30-, 60-, and 90-degree telescopes are available (Fig. 12-10). Some telescopes are also equipped with malleable forceps so that biopsy specimens can be taken when this equipment is used. However, in most instances the need to examine segmental and subsegmental orifices is best handled by the insertion of the fiberoptic bronchoscope through the rigid scope to examine the distal structures. Specimens can be taken in the usual fashion with fiberoptic equipment. For this examination, a 7- or 8-mm bronchoscope is necessary to allow passage of the fiberoptic scope, although flexible pediatric bronchoscopes are available for use through smaller tubes.

It can be difficult to teach the fine points of rigid bronchoscopy because of the nature of the examination (Stradling, 1973). However, connectors are now available that fit on the end of the telescope and allow the display of the image on a video monitor. This is of obvious value in the teaching environment and to obtain permanent records of the surgeon's observations.

LIMITATIONS AND COMPLICATIONS

There are many potential complications of rigid bronchoscopy, but most can be avoided with careful technique. The major disadvantages of rigid endoscopy include the limitation of view necessitated by the rigid equipment and the need for general anesthesia during this procedure. Because of the rigid nature of the equipment, injury to the upper aerodigestive tract is also a potential complication. The unique complications of rigid endoscopy are injuries to the mouth, pharynx, and upper airway as a result of poor application of the technique. Injuries to the lips, gums, and incisor teeth are avoided with care in the insertion and manipulation of the instrument.

Lacerations of the peripharyngeal tissues and injuries to the glottis (e.g., dislocation of the arytenoids) are rare but can occur with forceful manipulation of the scope. A traumatic bronchoscopic examination can result in laryngeal edema, especially in children when the bronchoscope is larger than the laryngeal orifice. Rigid bornchoscopy may be difficult or impossible in patients with certain physical disabilities (e.g., tempromandibular joint fixation or cervical spondylosis) because of the restriction of the opening of the mouth or of the extension of the neck.

Major hemorrhage may occur only when excessive or ill-advised biopsy specimens are taken. The examiner must always remember that the biopsy forceps are large, that bronchial vessels lie in the submucosa, and that certain tumors (e.g., carcinoid) can be highly vascular. If sudden hemorrhage does occur, the main bronchus on the side of bleeding should be intubated with the bronchoscope to diminish spillage into the contralateral lung. Working through the bronchoscope lumen, the surgeon can deal directly with the bleeding site. The topical application of epinephrine solutions (0.2 mg of epinephrine in 500 ml of Ringer's lactate) for vasoconstriction is helpful in some instances. Ventilation of the contralateral lung is maintained through the side ports of the bronchoscope (Fig. 12-10), which by design will always be in the tracheal lumen. Cauterization, tamponade with epinephrine-soaked gauze, or selective balloon catheterization can be performed through the bronchoscope.

The major anesthetic complication that is seen occurs with the misuse of the Venturi technique. High-pressure jets can produce surgical emphysema, especially if the airway is injured during the procedure. This is extremely rare and is totally avoidable. On occasion rupture of peripheral pulmonary blebs or bullae can result in a pneumothorax. This complication can occur with any positive pressure ventilation technique.

SUMMARY

The rigid bronchoscope remains an extremely valuable tool for the diagnosis and management of many thoracic conditions. In certain instances of upper airway obstruction, it may in fact be the only modality that can save a patient's life. It has specific advantages but requires expertise to avoid unnecessary complications. Flexible and rigid bronchoscopy are complementary, rather than mutually exclusive, tools to be used in the diagnosis and therapy of thoracic disease. Although there is some overlap of indications, each modality has its unique indications and limitations, and the thoracic surgeon should be experienced with both techniques to diagnose and treat the spectrum of thoracic disease that may be encountered effectively.

REFERENCES

Boyd AD: Chevalier Jackson: the father of American bronchoesophagoscopy. Ann Thorac Surg 57:502, 1994

Cooper JD, Pearson FG, Patterson GA et al: Use of silicone stents in the management of airway problems. Ann Thorac Surg 47:371, 1989

Ehrenwerth J, Brull S: Anesthesia for thoracic diagnostic procedures. In Kaplan JA (ed): Thoracic Anesthesia. 2nd Ed. Churchill Livingstone, New York, 1991

Hetzel MR, Smith STT: Endoscopic palliation of tracheobronchial malignancies. Thorax 46:225, 1991

Holinder LD: Use of the open tube bronchoscope in the extraction of foreign bodies. Chest 73:721, 1978

Hopkins HH: Optical principles of the endoscope. p. 3. In Berci G (ed): Endoscopy. Appleton-Century-Crofts, New York, 1976

Jackson C, Jackson CL: Bronchoesophagology. WB Saunders, Philadelphia, 1950

Sanders RD: Two ventilating attachments for bronchoscopy. Del Med J 39:170, 1967

Stradling P: Diagnostic Bronchoscopy—an Introduction. 2nd Ed. Williams and Wilkins, Baltimore, 1973

Wedzicha JA, Pearson NC: Management of massive hemoptysis. Respir Med 84:9, 1990

Weissberg D, Schwartz I: Foreign bodies in the tracheobronchial tree. Chest 91:730, 1987

Flexible Bronchoscopy

Denis A. Cortese

INTRODUCTION

The flexible bronchofiberscope was a unique diagnostic tool when first introduced in 1968 by Ikeda, et al. (1968, 1971). Since then it has become the standard in medical practice. It is a useful tool in patient care and medical research because it significantly extends the utility of bronchoscopy compared with that of the rigid bronchoscope for endoscopists. However, the rigid bronchoscope continues to play an important role in the management of hemorrhage, removal of foreign bodies, control of the airway in cases of bronchial and tracheal strictures, placement of Silastic stents, and laser therapy.

The flexible bronchoscope has replaced the rigid instrument for almost all routine diagnostic procedures and is used in situations in which previously there was no other instrument available. It is easy to use and is highly portable. A wide range of medical specialists use the flexible bronchoscope in their practice, including anesthesiologists, critical care specialists, otorhinolaryngologists, pulmonologists, and thoracic surgeons. Bronchoscopy has moved from the operating suite into procedure rooms, outpatient settings away from the hospital, and intensive care units. The diagnostic role of the flexible bronchoscope has expanded because of its usefulness in obtaining lung biopsy specimens, needle aspirates, bronchoalveolar lavage specimens, and protected catheter brushings with low risk to patients. Flexible bronchofibroscopy has therapeutic utility for the removal of secretions and obstructions. It assists in dilatation, laser therapy, and brachytherapy. The ability to collect bronchoalveolar lavage specimens also provides a role for the flexible bronchoscope in research.

This chapter describes the equipment, procedures, indications (both diagnostic and therapeutic), and complications in the field of flexible bronchofibroscopy.

HISTORICAL NOTE

Inspection of the airway was probably first accomplished with polished metal mirrors, but there is no historical record of such use. In 1743 Leuret developed a speculum through which he removed polyps from the nose and throat of patients (Tyson, 1957). In 1807 the interior of various canals of the human body were illuminated with small metal tubes developed by Bozini (Jackson, 1928). Endoscopic examination of the larynx was first conceived in 1828 when Green noted that the larynx could tolerate the presence of a foreign body (Donaldson, 1891). With topical applications of silver nitrate solution, Green became proficient in catheterizing the larynx and bronchi. In 1885 O'Dwyer perfected an intubation tube that he used to dilate strictures of the upper airway caused by diphtheria (Birkett, 1923). In 1895 Kirstein examined the interior of a patient's larynx directly using O'Dwyer's tube. He was also able to intubate the upper trachea (von Eiken, 1904). In 1987 Gustav Killian, the father of bronchoscopy, investigated the lower trachea and mainstem bronchi using a Kirstein laryngoscope (von Eiken, 1904). The following year he reported the removal of three foreign bodies from the tracheobronchial tree. The first rigid bronchoscopy done in the United States was by Coolidge. Using an open urethroscope, a head mirror, and reflected sunlight, he removed a hard rubber tracheotomy cannula from the right mainstem bronchus of a 22-year-old man (Jackson, 1928). In 1899 Chevalier Jackson modified an esophagoscope and began his extraordinary career in the use of rigid bronchoscopy. Some of Jackson's students included Louis Clerf, Jo Ono, Gabriel Tucker, Sr., Edwin Broyles, and his son, C. L. Jackson. Under Jackson's supervision, the bronchoscope was developed and included a small light at the distal end. An instrument with an auxiliary tube for lighting the distal airway was developed as was a tube for drainage. By 1912 the bronchoscope had become an accepted instrument for inspection of the trachea and mainstem bronchi. Its use was limited almost exclusively to the removal of foreign bodies. Broyles developed the optical telescope with forward and angled viewing, which permitted inspection of the upper and lower lobes of each lung. During the midportion of the twentieth century, the bronchoscope evolved for therapy of disorders of the trachea and mainstem bronchi and tuberculosis and for diagnosis of lung cancer. Andersen and Fontana described the use of the rigid bronchoscope to obtain transbronchoscopic lung biopsy specimens in patients with diffuse lung disease (Anderson, et al., 1965; Andersen and Fontana, 1972).

In the late 1800s, the optical properties of glass fibers were discovered. In 1930 Lamb advocated the application of glass fibers in a flexible gastroscope. Progress was not made in this field until the 1950s when van Heel and O'Brien developed the process of cladding glass fibers so that they could carry light (van Heel, 1954). Hopkins and Kapan arranged these fibers in a fashion that has evolved into the current fiberscopes (Ikeda, et al., 1968). Shigeta Ikeda performed the pioneering work in the 1960s that led to the introduction of the first flexible fiberoptic bronchoscope.

HISTORICAL READINGS

Andersen HA, Fontana RS: Transbronchoscopic lung biopsy for diffuse pulmonary diseases: technique and results in 450 cases. Chest 62:125, 1972

Andersen HA, Fontana RS, Harrison EG Jr: Transbronchoscopic lung biopsies in diffuse pulmonary disease. Dis Chest 48:187, 1965

Birkett HS: Transatlantic development of rhinolaryngology. Laryngoscope March, 1923

Donaldson F: The laryngology of Trousseau and Horace Green. An historical review. Proc Am Laryngol Assoc 10, 1891

Jackson C: Bronchoscopy: past, present, and future. N Engl J Med 199:758, 1928

Tyson EB: Development of the bronchoscope. N J Med 54:26, 1957

van Heel ACS: A new method of transporting optical images without aberrations. Nature 173:39, 1954

von Eiken C: The clinical application of the method of direct examination of the respiratory passes and the upper alimentary tract. Arch Laryngol Rhinol Nov: 15, 1904

EQUIPMENT

A wide range of flexible bronchofiberscopes is available today. The bronchoscopes vary with respect to external diameter, the size of the internal working channel, the presence of additional working channels, and the degree of flexion at the distal tip (Figs. 12-13 and 12-14). Also, there are video endoscopes available for bronchoscopic work. All of the flex-

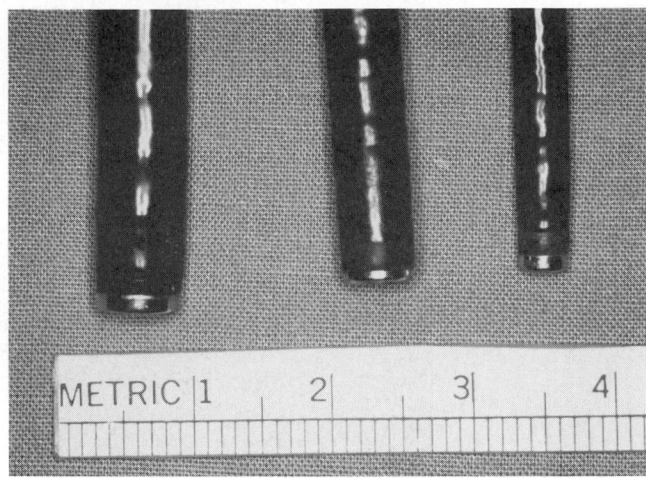

Figure 12-13. Distal ends of three Olympus bronchoscopes demonstrate the differences in external diameters. From left to right, 1T20, P20D (standard scope), and 3C10 (pediatric scope).

ible bronchoscopes are high quality and perform well in the hands of an experienced bronchoscopist. The proper selection of equipment is important to ensure a safe and effective procedure. Therefore the endoscopist should give careful consideration to the goals of the procedure as the bronchoscope is selected. Equipment that could be placed on a portable cart and moved to wherever the bronchoscopy is to be performed is listed below. The bronchoscopes should be stored in the vertical position so they hang straight and are protected from injury. They may be stored on the cart or in some other convenient location in the bronchoscopy suite. Individual bronchoscopes can be placed in trays and stored for use, but they should be coiled with care to prevent damage to the fiber bundles. Suction apparatus, supplemental oxygen, and a cardiac monitor should be available for the procedure.

PATIENT EVALUATION

The patient's history should be carefully reviewed for possible contraindications to the procedure. Most contraindications are relative contraindications. If the benefit of bronchoscopy outweighs the risk, then the procedure should be performed by an experienced bronchoscopist. Bronchoscopy, particularly when suction is applied in the tracheobronchial tree, is a frequent cause of a decrease in arterial oxygen tension and hemoglobin saturation both during and after the procedure. Supplemental oxygen should be provided throughout the procedure, and a finger-pulse oximeter should be used (Brutinel, et al., 1983; Hendy, et al., 1984; Matsushima, et al., 1984; Lennon, et al., 1987; Breuer, et al., 1989; Macgillivray and Zulu, 1989). If the patient already has hypoxemia and is receiving oxygen supplementation or mechanical ventilation, the bronchoscopy may worsen the hypoxemia and could be a serious risk to the patient.

Acute hypercapnia with acidosis is a major concern because bronchoscopy will increase airway resistance and the work of breathing. Mechanical ventilation might be required

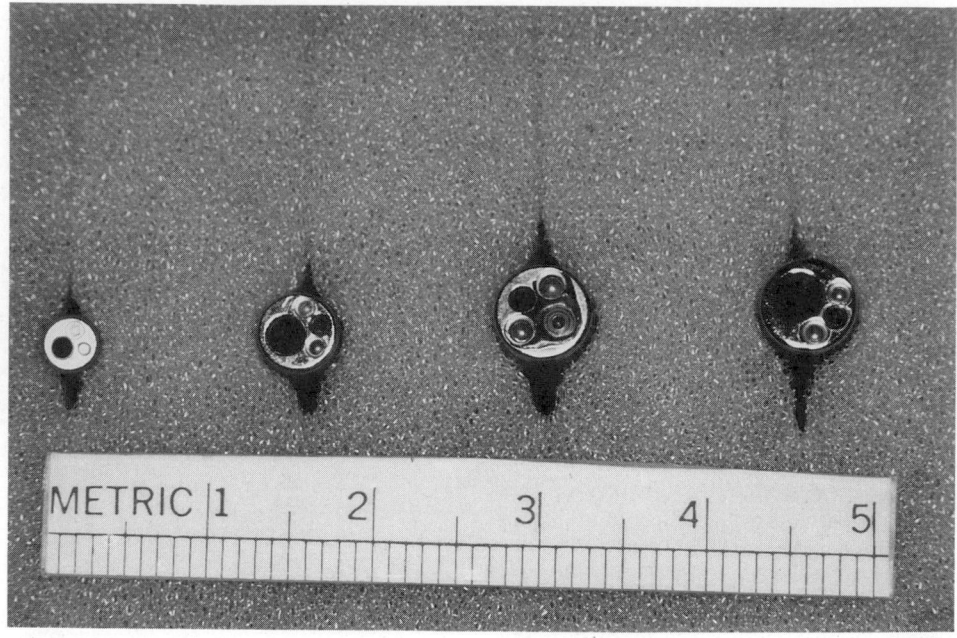

Figure 12-14. Distal tips of four Olympus bronchoscopes demonstrate various sizes of scopes, diameters of the working channels, and imaging bundles. From left to right, 3C10 (pediatric scope), P20D (standard), 6C20 (photographic), and IT20 (large channel).

Bronchoscopy Equipment

Assortment of endotracheal tubes

Benzocaine 20 percent oral spray

Biopsy forceps

Bronchoalveolar lavage kit

Bronchoscopes
    Adult scope (5.0-mm outside diameter)
    Adult lavage scope (6.0-mm outside diameter)
    Pediatric scope (3.5-mm outside diameter)

Bronchoscopic needles

Cardiac monitor

Cytology brushes

Direct laryngoscopes

Head lamp

Laryngeal mirror

Lidocaine

Light source

Oxygen source

Protected catheter brush

Pulse oximeter

Specimen containers

Suction tubing and connectors

Swivel adapters with rubber diaphragms

Syringes (non-Luer-lock)

Wall suction adapters

---

either before or after the procedure, depending on the patient's response to sedation. A patient with stable, compensated respiratory acidosis can undergo bronchoscopy if there is careful attention to the use of premedication, sedation during the procedure, and awareness about the possibility of respiratory depression related to oxygen supplementation.

Cardiac instability should be treated and controlled before elective bronchoscopy. Of course if the cardiac instability is related to a condition that can be corrected by bronchoscopy, then the benefits of the procedure are likely to outweigh the risks.

Asthma can be triggered and worsened by bronchoscopy because bronchial edema and bronchospasm can result from the procedure. If the asthma is adequately treated and controlled, asthmatic patients can be examined safely.

Coagulopathy, platelet dysfunction, and prolonged bleeding associated with uremia are contraindications only to the

---

Relative Contraindications to Bronchoscopy

Hypoxemia

Hypercapnia

Cardiovascular instability
    Hypotension
    Uncontrolled angina
    Myocardial infarction
    Malignant arrhythmias

Asthma

Patient unable to cooperate with the procedure

performance of brushings, needle aspirations, and biopsies. Special consideration in planning the procedure is required when the prothrombin time is 1 second longer than the control time, when the platelet count is less than $50 \times 10^9/L$, and when the bleeding time is prolonged. Patients can undergo bronchoscopy even when fully treated with anticoagulants as long as care is taken not to irritate the mucosa. Bronchoalveolar lavage can be performed in patients with low platelet counts and is routinely used in immunocompromised patients with hematologic disorderws who often have coagulopathies. Uremia increases the risk of bleeding owing to platelet dysfunction, which may be a significant problem when brushings, needle aspirations, or biopsies are planned.

The patient who is unable to cooperate completely with the procedure may need bronchoscopy under heavy sedation or general anesthesia. Of course this should be done in an operating room, an outpatient surgical area, or an intensive care unit with the assistance of an anesthesiologist.

Bronchoscopists perform elective procedures while the patient is seated or lying supine. The bronchoscope may be inserted through an anesthetized naris without an endotracheal tube. Lidocaine (2 percent) is administered through the suction channel of the bronchoscope to anesthetize the hypopharynx, the larynx, the vocal cords, and the tracheobronchial tree in a progressive fashion as the bronchoscope is advanced. Other alternatives include the use of an endotracheal tube, which could be placed through the naris or through the anesthetized mouth. The bronchoscope also can be passed through the mouth without an endotracheal tube. The use of an endotracheal tube during the procedure facili-

tates the administration of supplemental oxygen; ventilatory support, if it should be needed during the procedure; removal of tenacious secretions; and repeated passage of the bronchoscope when diagnostic and therapeutic procedures are performed. A swivel adapter attached to the endotracheal tube allows assisted ventilation during the procedure. To examine the patient through the mouth, topical anesthesia can be administered to the mouth, tongue, and back of the throat with an oral spray, such as 20 percent benzocaine followed by the application of 2 percent lidocaine into the hypopharynx and larynx. Other anesthetic techniques include the use of 4 percent lidocaine (5 ml) delivered by a nebulizer, superior laryngeal nerve block, and direct instillation of 2 percent lidocaine (2 ml) through the cricothyroid membrane into the trachea with a syringe and a small-gauge needle.

PROCEDURES

There are several categories of specimens obtained at bronchoscopy; these include material for microbiologic, histologic, and cytologic examinations. The handling of specimens depends on the requirements of the microbiology and pathology departments in each institution.

If secretions are to be collected for culture, suction should not be attached to the bronchoscope until it has been advanced into the trachea. This prevents the aspiration of saliva and pharyngeal contents through the working channel and into the specimen bottle.

Several biopsy forceps are available for both endoscopic biopsy and transbronchoscopic lung biopsy (Fig. 12-15). The

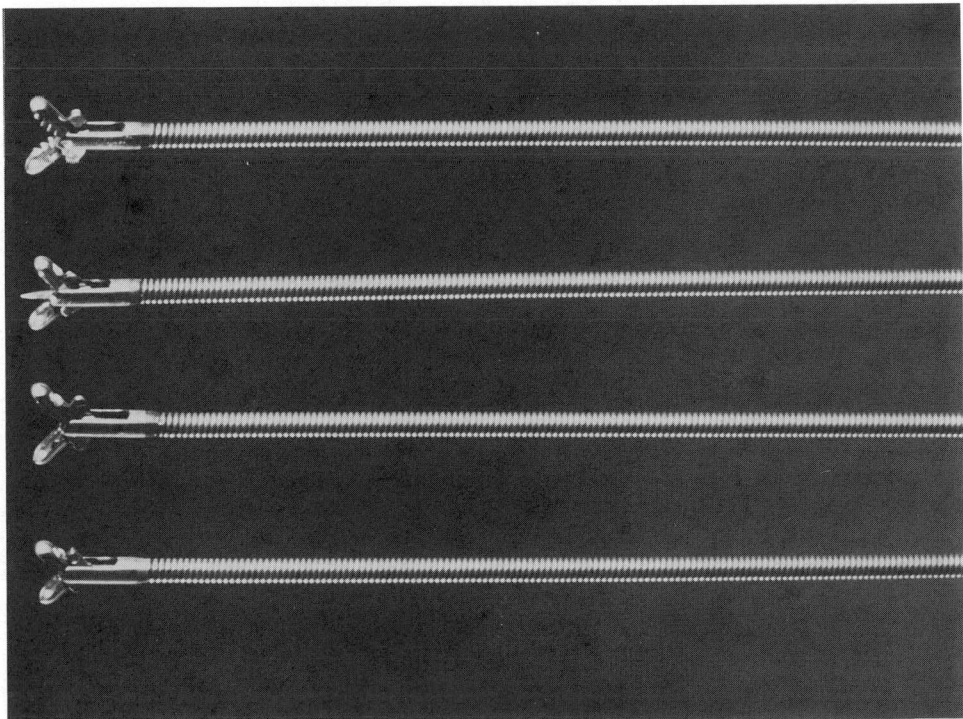

Figure 12-15. Four biopsy forceps. From top to bottom, alligator forceps, needle-nose forceps, large cups, and standard cups.

forceps cups are hinged and have a cutting edge or a serrated edge (alligator forceps). Some forceps have a small, needle-like projection in the center to help maintain the position of the forceps as the cups are closed and the biopsy specimen is obtained. Some forceps have fenestrated cups, reportedly to reduce the crush artifact. After the sample is obtained, the forceps can be removed through the working channel, or the entire bronchoscope with the forceps can be withdrawn from the endotracheal tube. The sample is placed either on a glass slide in a drop of isotonic saline for frozen sections or into formaldehyde solution for microscopic examination.

To obtain cytologic specimens, brushes are available that are 2 to 7 mm in diameter. Some brushes are available in a protective outer plastic sheath (Fig. 12-16). The sheath with the brush in place or a nonsheathed bronchial brush is inserted through the suction channel, and brushings are performed. At this point the brush can be pulled back through the suction channel, or the entire bronchoscope can be removed with the brush still protruding from the distal end of the suction channel. This latter procedure seems to produce a larger specimen. The material on the brush should be smeared on a series of slides that are placed in the fixative. In most cases the brush is clipped off and also placed in the fixative.

A double-sheath protected catheter brush is available to obtain sterile specimens for bacterial cultures from the tracheobronchial tree. There are several commercially available; instructions are included in their packaging. In general this procedure should be performed before any suction is applied to the suction channel. Consequently if the protected catheter brush is to be used, this procedure should be performed immediately after intubation and before the airway

is inspected. It is important that the tip of this catheter be treated in a sterile fashion. The protected catheter is advanced into the area to be brushed. The inner catheter is then advanced out through the outer catheter sheath. As this is done, a glycerol plug is ejected from the outer catheter sheath and will be absorbed subsequently by the airway. The brush is then advanced out of the inner catheter sheath to collect the specimen. At this point the brush is withdrawn into the inner catheter sheath, and the whole protected catheter is removed from the channel of the bronchoscope. The inner catheter sheath is wiped with alcohol, and its distal tip is cut off with a sterile scissors. The brush is then advanced out of the inner catheter sheath again and clipped into a small vial that contains isotonic saline (1 ml). The vial is sealed tightly and transported to the microbiology laboratory where quantitative cultures for aerobic and anaerobic bacteria are performed.

Bronchoalveolar lavage is a procedure that also should be performed before any secretions are aspirated through the suction channel. If both bronchoalveolar lavage and a protected catheter brushing are planned, the brushing should be completed first. For bronchoalveolar lavage the wall suction should be set at a low level, approximately 80 mmHg. The bronchoscope should be advanced until it is wedged into the segmental bronchus. Suction tubing with a three-way stopcock between the scope and the collecting jar is then attached. Usually the contents of five syringes—each filled with 20 ml of isotonic saline and 10 ml of air—are injected sequentially. After the contents of a syringe have been injected slowly, the three-way stopcock is turned to the suction position. Suction is applied until the return of isotonic saline stops. The procedure is repeated with all five syringes. A

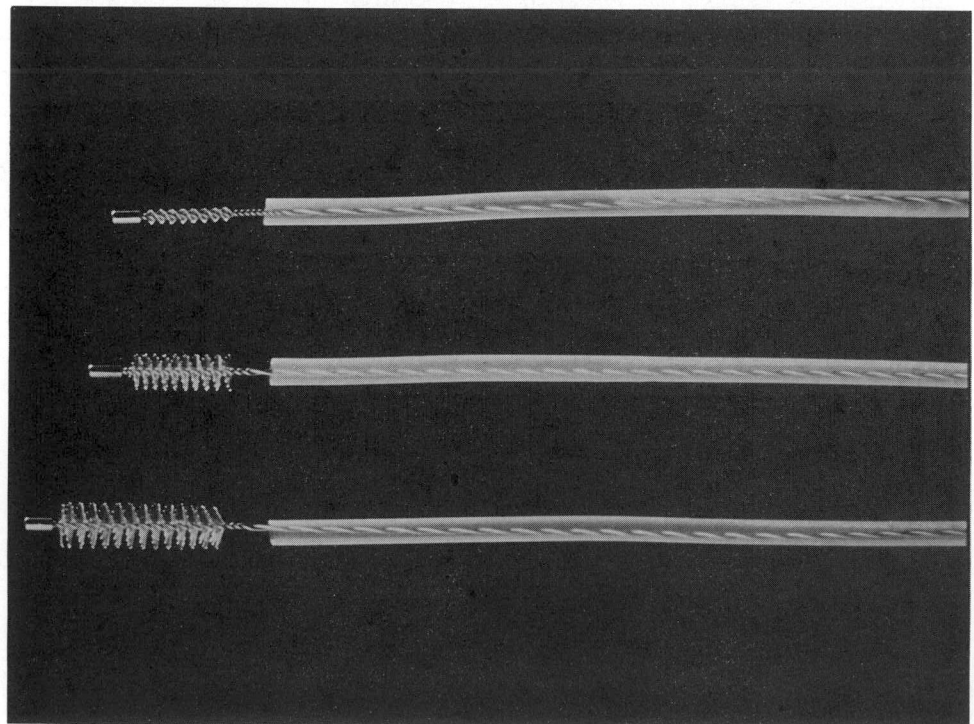

Figure 12-16. Bronchial brushes in protective plastic catheter sheath. From top to bottom, 2-, 5-, and 7-mm brushes.

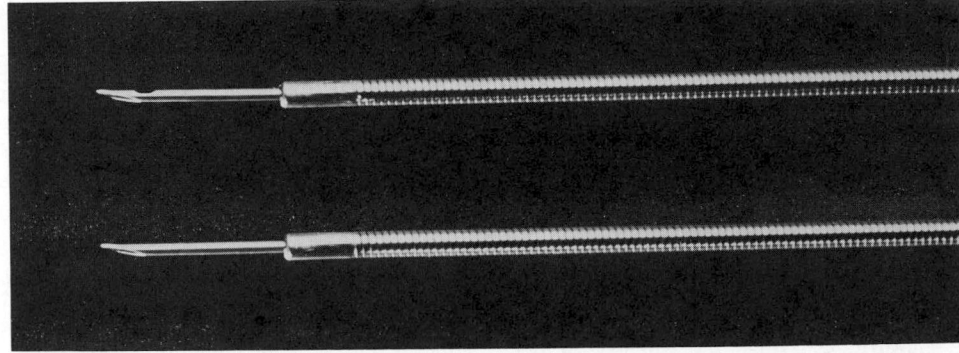

Figure 12-17. Needle catheters for transbronchial needle aspiration: 18 (above) and 21 gauge (below).

successful lavage results in the retrieval of approximately 40 to 50 percent of the injected volume. The aspirated material can be sent for a special cell analysis, cytologic examination, and complete cultures.

Transbronchial and transtracheal needle aspirations are performed with needle catheters, which come in various sizes (usually 18 to 21 gauge) and styles (Fig. 12-17). The needle catheters are inserted through the suction channel of the bronchoscope. Most needles are prepared either by withdrawal of a stylet or extension and locking of a needle into place. The bronchoscopist punctures the tracheal or bronchial wall. At this time suction is created with a syringe attached to the end of the needle catheter. The syringe should contain a small amount of isotonic saline to help flush the specimen when the procedure is completed. Once the needle is through the bronchial or tracheal wall, it is agitated slightly to help facilitate collection of the specimen. Then it is withdrawn through the suction channel of the bronchoscope. An assistant flushes the catheter and needle with the saline in the syringe. Some of the aspirate can be placed on a slide and submitted in fixative for cytologic study. The excess aspirate fluid is submitted in a jar as a cytologic specimen. If an 18-gauge needle is used, a core of tissue is sometimes obtained and can be flushed into a fixative jar for histologic examination. Usually multiple aspirations or biopsy samples can be performed with little risk to the patient.

DIAGNOSTIC INDICATIONS

The most common indication is an abnormal chest radiograph, but other imaging studies may also provide an indication (tomogram, computed tomographic [CT] scan, or magnetic resonance imaging scan). Lesions that justify bronchoscopy include a mass; a pulmonary nodule; a recurring pulmonary infiltrate; an unresolving pulmonary infiltrate; persistent atelectasis; collapse of a segment, a lobe, or a lung; a mediastinal or hilar mass; a persistent pleural effusion; and an abnormal air shadow of the trachea or bronchi.

Bronchoscopy may be required to help diagnose diffuse parenchymal lung disease when the differential diagnosis includes neoplastic, infectious, or certain interstitial lung diseases. In the immunocompromised patient, bronchoalveolar lavage, protected catheter brushing, and transbronchoscopic

lung biopsies are frequently required. In this situation the bronchoscope has been highly efficacious to establish infectious causes of new pulmonary infiltrates (Martin, et al., 1987; Frankel, et al., 1988; Pattishall, et al., 1988; Luce and Clement, 1989; Xaubet, et al., 1989). Bronchoalveolar lavage is used routinely to diagnose bacterial (e.g., Legionella), fungal, protozoan (e.g., Pneumocystis), and viral infections in the immunocompromised host. The yield from this procedure is high and has reduced the need for open-lung biopsy in these patients.

Acute inhalation injury from toxic gases or smoke can be a life-threatening situation. Bronchoscopy of the upper and lower airways is helpful to define the extent of damage and plan therapy. The larynx can be examined carefully to rule out the immediate concern of laryngeal edema. An experienced bronchoscopist can then decide whether to proceed with elective intubation, depending on the appearance of the larynx. Knowledge of the extent of mucosal damage can help

---

Diagnostic Indications for Bronchoscopy

Abnormal radiographic findings

Acute inhalation injury

Bronchiectasis

Broncholithiasis

Bronchopleural fistulae

Cough

Diaphragmatic paralysis

Esophageal lesions

Foreign body

Hemoptysis

Intubation damage

Lung abscess

Sputum cytologic findings that indicate cancer

Stridor or localized wheezing

Thoracic trauma

Vocal cord paralysis

determine whether early therapy with steroids and antibiotics is indicated (Robinson and Miller, 1986; Bingham, et al., 1987; Schneider, et al., 1988).

After a difficult intubation, prolonged oral intubation, or nasotracheal intubation, the bronchoscope is an excellent tool to assess the possibility of tracheal damage. Hemoptysis from an endotracheal tube should be assessed with bronchoscopy. Flexible bronchoscopy also helps rule out a tracheal stricture in patients who present with shortness of breath, stridor, or wheezing after prolonged intubation. Bronchoscopy can be used to check the placement of an endotracheal tube and to clear mucus, blood, or a foreign body that might be obstructing the endotracheal tube, the trachea, or the mainstem bronchus. A patient who is undergoing mechanical ventilation and in whom high peak pressures develop or in whom the suction catheter can only be passed with difficulty should also have the airway examined (Messeter and Pettersson, 1980; Edens and Sia, 1981; Rogers and Benumof, 1983).

Bronchiectasis, particularly when it is localized, should lead to endoscopy to rule out a localized endobronchial cause, such as a foreign body or another obstructing process.

The flexible bronchoscope can be used in an attempt to localize the segmental or subsegmental bronchus that is feeding a bronchopleural fistula, particularly after a lung resection when inspection of the suture line is important.

Broncholithiasis, which may present with hemoptysis, lithoptysis, or bronchial obstruction, can be diagnosed with a flexible bronchoscope. Occasionally the broncholith can be retrieved as a foreign body if it is free in the airway. More commonly the broncholith is firmly embedded and should not be removed because of the danger of massive hemoptysis (Rees, 1985; Lan, et al., 1989).

Diaphragmatic paralysis, particularly unilateral, can be idiopathic, iatrogenic from a previous surgical procedure, or caused by a neoplasm of the airway with mediastinal involvement. The advent of CT scanning has made bronchoscopy less common in this situation because the likelihood is small that a visible endobronchial lesion could be causing phrenic nerve paralysis when the CT scan results of the chest are negative.

The flexible bronchoscope is excellent to diagnose the presence of a foreign body in the major airways. Occasionally the foreign body can be removed with the flexible bronchoscope, as reported by Lan, et al. (1989). The rigid bronchoscope, however, is the instrument of choice for the removal of a foreign body because it simultaneously facilitates ventilation and the safe delivery of a foreign body through the subglottic area and the larynx (Wood and Gauderer, 1984; McGuirt, et al., 1988; Mantor, et al., 1989).

Bronchoscopy is indicated in patients with hemoptysis. The most common cause of hemoptysis is benign bronchitis, but it is also common in bronchiectasis and broncholithiasis and in the presence of a foreign body, endobronchial tumor, or bronchogenic carcinoma. Bronchoscopy is indicated in patients with increased risk factors for cancer or those in whom the clinical situation suggests a diagnosis that involves the tracheobronchial tree (Poe, et al., 1988; Johnston and Reisz, 1989; Lederle, et al., 1989).

A persistent lung abscess may be the result of an endobronchial obstruction, such as a foreign body, tumor, or extrinsic compression. Occasionally flexible bronchoscopy can help establish drainage from the affected area of the lung (Sosenko and Glassroth, 1985; Schmitt, et al., 1988). Major blunt thoracic trauma can result in lung contusions or a mechanical disruption of the tracheobronchial tree, which ranges from small tears to complete transsection of the trachea or a major bronchus. A patient who presents with pneumothorax, pneumomediastinum, or subcutaneous emphysema after blunt trauma should undergo flexible bronchoscopy (Hara and Prakash, 1989).

Bronchoscopy is indicated in patients when the cytologic examination of their sputum reveals cancer cells. In those cases with radiographically occult lung cancer, an ear, nose, and throat examination followed by bronchoscopy is indicated to search for the origin of the cancer cells from the upper airway and the tracheobronchial tree. Occasionally the initial bronchoscopy is nondiagnostic. In this situation another bronchoscopy performed under general anesthesia with a thorough inspection, selective brushings from all the lobar and segmental segments, and multiple biopsy specimens is indicated. Malignancy should be considered localized if the cancer is bronchoscopically visible or a diagnostic biopsy is obtained. If the results of brush cytologic analysis are only diagnostic of cancer, the lesion may be considered localized if the brushings were obtained from the same segment at two separate bronchoscopic procedures several weeks apart. Occasionally the cancer eludes localization despite these studies. Careful observation is advised, with repeat radiographs and bronchoscopic studies in 4 to 6 months. Localization with hematoporphyrin-derivative fluorescence bronchoscopy is another technique that can be used but requires special instrumentation and an experimental drug (Edell and Cortese, 1989).

Paralysis of a vocal cord may be due to recurrent laryngeal nerve damage and raises the possibility of a lesion along the distribution of the recurrent laryngeal nerve. A CT scan of the chest is indicated. If the results are abnormal, bronchoscopy should be performed to look for an endobronchial lesion that has a high probability of being a malignant process. If a mediastinal mass is present, a transbronchial or transtracheal needle aspiration may be helpful (Shure, 1989).

Stridor or localized wheezing may be due to a dynamic abnormality or a structural narrowing of the upper airway and trachea, such as a vocal cord paralysis, laryngeal abnormality, benign and malignant tumors, extrinsic compression of the tracheobronchial tree, tracheal strictures caused by a mucosal process, or tracheomalacia (Filston, et al., 1987; Zalzal, 1989).

Unexplained chronic cough requires bronchoscopy once the common causes, such as respiratory infection, chronic obstructive pulmonary disease, and asthma, have been ruled out or treated. An occult endobronchial lesion, such as malignancy, carcinoid tumor, broncholithiasis, or a foreign body, may be the cause of the cough. Poe, et al. (1982) suggested that if no cause for cough is found and no significant improvement occurs after all treatable causes have been evaluated, bronchoscopy should be performed within 2 to 3 months of the initiation of the evaluation.

Carcinoma of the upper or midportion of the esophagus may invade the tracheobronchial tree. This has significant implications for the thoracic surgeon, and bronchoscopic examination of the trachea and main bronchi is indicated in this situation (Weaver, et al., 1979; Choi, et al., 1984; Leipzig, et al., 1985).

THERAPEUTIC INDICATIONS

The flexible bronchoscope facilitates the placement of an oral or nasal endotracheal tube, particularly in patients who have limited neck motion or abnormal upper airway anatomy and in those who must be awake during intubation (Messeter and Pettersson, 1980; Rogers and Benumof, 1983).

The therapeutic use of the bronchoscope to remove retained secretions is indicated in patients who have new atelectasis that does not respond to chest physical therapy, deep suctioning, and intensive respiratory management within 12 to 24 hours. These guidelines are normally followed for patients whose conditions are stable and who have an adequate arterial oxygen level. Of course for patients who become hypoxemic and whose conditions are unstable, immediate bronchoscopy should be performed and may be life saving (Marini, et al., 1979; Jaworski, et al., 1988).

The use of the flexible bronchoscope for the management of foreign bodies has been mentioned. It is the opinion of many that the flexible bronchoscope is useful to identify the presence of a foreign body, but the rigid bronchoscope is the preferred tool for the removal of foreign bodies. The rigid bronchoscope facilitates safe and rapid removal of the foreign body and provides an excellent airway for ventilation.

Flexible bronchoscopy can be useful to manage hemoptysis, depending on the site and degree of the hemorrhage. The flexible bronchoscope can be used to localize the site of bleeding, remove blood and clots from the airway, and facilitate the placement of a single-lumen endotracheal tube or a double-lumen tube to isolate the two bronchial trees or of small balloon catheters to help tamponade the bronchus from which the bleeding is identified (McCollun, et al., 1975; Porter, et al., 1983; Conlan, 1985; Imgrund, et al., 1985; Rees,

---

Therapeutic Indications for Bronchoscopy

Endotracheal intubation

Retained secretions or mucus plugs

Foreign body aspiration

Management of hemoptysis

Bronchopleural fistulae

Lung abscess

Bronchial strictures
    Dilatation (rigid bronchoscopy)
    Placement of stents (rigid bronchoscopy)
    Laser therapy (rigid and flexible bronchoscopy)

Endobronchial malignant obstruction
    Dilatation (rigid bronchoscopy)
    Placement of stents (rigid bronchoscopy)
    Laser therapy (rigid and flexible bronchoscopy)

Brachytherapy

1985; Shivaram, et al., 1987; Lederle, et al., 1989). However, in the case of massive hemoptysis, the flexible instrument is not adequate. The rigid bronchoscope should be used. It provides an excellent airway, allows the use of one or more large suction catheters, and facilitates the placement of umbilical tape soaked with epinephrine to pack the bleeding bronchus. A combination of the rigid bronchoscope and the flexible bronchoscope can be used to help control bleeding from the upper lobes when necessary.

In the therapy of bronchial strictures, the flexible bronchoscope has a role limited to defining the anatomy and location of the stricture and helping to determine whether surgical resection or bronchoscopic therapy would be possible. The flexible bronchoscope facilitates the use of the neodymium:yttrium-aluminum-garnet Nd:YAG laser by directing the laser fiber into locations that are difficult to reach with the rigid bronchoscope. However, in the usual situation, the management of strictures is best and most safely performed by the use of a rigid bronchoscope to accomplish dilatation and laser resection with a Nd:YAG or CO_2 laser to allow the placement of Silastic bronchial stents (Dumon, 1982, 1990; Shapshay, et al., 1987; Cavaliere, et al., 1988; Cooper, et al., 1989; Tsang and Goldstraw, 1989).

Similarly the endoscopic management of endobronchial malignant obstruction is safely and effectively treated with the rigid open-tube bronchoscope (Dumon, 1982; McDougall and Cortese, 1983; Brutinel, et al., 1987; Cavaliere, et al., 1988; Diaz-Jiménez, et al., 1990). These techniques can help palliate respiratory symptoms and prolong life. Frequently the use of laser therapy with either the CO_2 or the Nd:YAG laser has been helpful. Silastic stents can also be placed to maintain the airway in these situations (Cooper, et al., 1989; Dumon, 1990; Tsang and Goldstraw, 1989). Photodynamic therapy has been used with success by some clinicians to treat malignant airway-obstructing lesions (Balchum and Doiron, 1985; Lam, et al., 1986; McCaughan, et al., 1988; LoCicero, et al., 1990). This can be performed with the flexible bronchoscope but requires repeat bronchoscopy to clean the airway and remove necrotic tumor several days after photodynamic therapy (PDT). Laser therapy, using the rigid bronchoscope, facilitates the complete removal of an obstructing tumor in one therapeutic session and is therefore the preferred tool of other clinicians to remove cancers that significantly obstruct a major airway.

Bronchoscopic PDT with the flexible bronchoscope has been used to treat early-stage squamous cell carcinoma of the lung. In the situation of an in situ and minimally invasive squamous cell carcinoma, PDT has been reported to produce a complete response (complete disappearance of tumor) in 60 to 80 percent of patients (Hayata, et al., 1984; Edell and Cortese, 1987).

If PDT is used in nonsuperficial early-stage lung cancer, it should be combined with other therapeutic modalities. The current indications for PDT include a superficial cancer that is less than 3 cm^2 in surface area and entirely within the reach of the flexible bronchoscope, radiographically occult cancer, and a patient who is not a candidate for surgical resection.

Endobronchial brachytherapy can be performed with small plastic catheters placed through the working channel of the flexible bronchoscope. These catheters can be loaded subsequently with [197]Ir beads to provide local radiotherapy to endo-bronchial cancers (Schray, et al., 1988).

COMPLICATIONS

Pereira, et al. (1978) summarized the complications of flexible fiberoptic bronchoscopy. The overall mortality should be less than 0.1 percent. The reported incidence of other complications ranges widely, depending on the procedure, but all complications should be less than 8.1 percent. The complications include vasovagal reaction, 2.4 percent; fever, 1.2 percent; cardiac arrhythmia, 0.9 percent; pneumothorax, 0.7 percent; nausea and vomiting, 0.2 percent; respiratory arrest, 0.1 percent; and aphonia, 0.1 percent.

KEY REFERENCES

Cavaliere S, Foccoli P, Farina PL: Nd:YAG laser bronchoscopy: a five-year experience with 1,396 applications in 1,000 patients. Chest 94:15, 1988.

This is an excellent treatise on the spectrum of disease that is treatable with YAG laser photoresection. The complication rate was exceedingly low, and the rigid bronchoscope was the instrument of choice because it was safer and faster to use.

Dumon JF: A dedicated tracheobronchial stent. Chest 97:328, 1990.

This is a description of a significantly improved Silastic tracheobronchial stent for use in the management of patients with benign and malignant airway compromise. The advantages of the rigid bronchoscope over the flexible bronchoscope for interventional bronchoscopy were emphasized.

Dumon JF: Treatment of tracheobronchial lesions by laser photoresection. Chest 81:278, 1982

This is a description of the use of Nd:YAG laser photoresection of malignant airway obstruction using both rigid and flexible bronchoscopes. The distinct advantage of the rigid bronchoscope in this setting was emphasized.

Edell ES, Cortese DA: Bronchoscopic localization and treatment of occult lung cancer. Chest 96:919, 1989

This is a summary of the usefulness of flexible fiberoptic bronchoscopy in the localization and therapy of radiographically occult superficial squamous cell carcinoma of the lung.

Hayata Y, Kato H, Konaka C et al: Photoradiation therapy with hematoporphyrin derivative in early and stage I lung cancer. Chest 86:169, 1984

This is an excellent review of the usefulness of photodynamic laser therapy applied with the flexible fiberoptic bronchoscope for the therapy of early and stage I lung cancer.

Ikeda S, Yanain N, Ishikawa S: Flexible bronchofiberscope. Keio J Med 17:1, 1968

This is the first description of the use of a flexible fiberoptic bronchoscope in the tracheobronchial tree. This pioneering article laid the groundwork for the future of flexible fiberoptic bronchoscopy.

Pereira W Jr, Covenat DM, Snider GL: A prospective cooperative study of complications following flexible fiberoptic bronchoscopy. Chest 73:813, 1978

This large study demonstrates the usefulness and safety of the flexible fiberoptic bronchoscope.

Schray MF, McDougall JC, Martinez A et al: Management of malignant airway compromise with laser and low-dose rate brachytherapy: the Mayo Clinic experience. Chest 93:264, 1988

This is a summary of the experience of endobronchial radiotherapy facilitated by the use of flexible fiberoptic bronchoscopy.

Shure D: Transbronchial biopsy and needle aspiration. Chest 95:1130, 1989

This is an excellent review of the utility of the transbronchoscopic lung biopsy using the flexible fiberoptic bronchoscope and the safe use of the transbronchial needle aspiration for diagnosis and staging of malignant disease.

REFERENCES

Andersen HA, Fontana RS: Transbronchoscopic lung biopsy for diffuse pulmonary diseases: technique and results in 450 cases. Chest 62:125, 1972

Andersen HA, Fontana RS, Harrison EG Jr: Transbronchoscopic lung biopsies in diffuse pulmonary disease. Dis Chest 48:187, 1965

Balchum OJ, Doiron DR: Photoradiation therapy of endobronchial lung cancer: large obstructing tumors, nonobstructing tumors, and early-stage bronchial cancer lesions. Clin Chest Med 6:255, 1985

Bingham HG, Gallagher TJ, Powell MD: Early bronchoscopy as a predictor of ventilatory support for burned patients. J Trauma 27:1286, 1987

Birkett HS: Transatlantic development of rhinolaryngology. Laryngoscope March, 1923

Breuer H-WM, Charchut St, Worth H: Effects of diagnostic procedures during fiberoptic bronchoscopy on heart rate, blood pressure, and blood gases. Klin Wochenschr 67:524, 1989

Brutinel WM, Cortese DA, McDougall JC et al: A two-year experience with the neodymium-YAG laser in endobronchial obstruction. Chest 91:159, 1987

Brutinel WM, McDougall JC, Cortese DA: Bronchoscopic therapy with neodymium-yttrium-aluminum-garnet laser during intravenous anesthesia: effect on arterial blood gas levels, pH, hemoglobin saturation, and production of abnormal hemoglobin. Chest 84:518, 1983

Choi TK, Siu KF, Lam KH, Wong J: Bronchoscopy and carcinoma of the esohpagus [parts I and II]. Findings of bronchoscopy in carcinoma of the esophagus; carcinoma of the esophagus with tracheobronchial involvement. Am J Surg 147:757, 1984

Conlan AA: Massive hemoptysis—diagnostic and therapeutic implications. Surg Annu 17:337, 1985

Cooper JD, Pearson FG, Paterson GA et al: Use of silicone stents in the management of airway problems. Ann Thorac Surg 47:371, 1989

Diaz-Jiménez JP, Canela-Cardona M, Maestre-Alcacer J: Nd:YAG laser photoresection of low-grade malignant tumors of the tracheo-bronchial tree. Chest 97:920, 1990

Donaldson F: The laryngology of Trousseau and Horace Green. An historical review. Proc Am Laryngol Assoc 10, 1891

Edell ES, Cortese DA: Bronchoscopic phototherapy with hemato-porphyrin derivative for treatment of localized bronchogenic carci-noma: a 5-year experience. Mayo Clin Proc 62:8, 1987

Edens ET, Sia RL: Flexible fiberoptic endoscopy in difficult intub-ations. Ann Otol Rhinol Laryngol 90:307, 1981

Filston HC, Ferguson TB Jr, Oldham HN: Airway obstruction by vascular anomalies: importance of telescopic bronchoscopy. Ann Surg 205:541, 1987

Frankel LR, Smith DW, Lewiston NJ: Bronchoalveolar lavage for diagnosis of pneumonia in the immunocompromised child. Pedia-trics 81:785, 1988

Hara KS, Prakash UBS: Fiberoptic bronchoscopy in the evaluation of acute chest and upper airway trauma. Chest 96:627, 1989

Hendy MS, Bateman JRM, Stableforth DE: The influence of trans-bronchial lung biopsy and bronchoalveolar lavage on arterial blood gas changes occurring in patients with diffuse interstitial lung dis-ease. Br J Dis Chest 78:363, 1984

Ikeda S, Tsuboi E, Ono R, Ishikawa S: Flexible bronchofiberscope. Jpn J Clin Oncol 1:55, 1971

Imgrund SP, Goldberg SK, Walkenstein MD et al: Clinical diagnosis of massive hemoptysis using the fiberoptic bronchoscope. Crit Care Med 13:438, 1985

Jackson C. Bronchoscopy: past, present, and future. N Engl J Med 199:758, 1928

Jaworski A, Goldberg SK, Walkenstein MD et al: Utility of immedi-ate postlobectomy fiberoptic bronchoscopy in preventing atelecta-sis. Chest 94:38, 1988

Johnston H, Reisz G: Changing spectrum of hemoptysis: underlying causes in 148 patients undergoing diagnostic flexible fiberoptic bronchoscopy. Arch Intern Med 149:1666, 1989

Lam S, Müller NL, Miller RR et al: Predicting the response of obstructive endobronchial tumors to photodynamic therapy. Can-cer 58:2298, 1986

Lan R-S, Lee C-H, Chian Y-C, Wang W-J: Use of fiberoptic bron-choscopy to retrieve bronchial foreign bodies in adults. Am Rev Respir Dis 140:1734, 1989

Lederle FA, Nichol KL, Parenti CM: Bronchoscopy to evaluate hemoptysis in older men with nonsuspicious chest roentgeno-grams. Chest 95:1043, 1989

Leipzig B, Zellmer JE, Klug D: the Panendoscopy Study Group: The role of endoscopy in evaluating patients with head and neck cancer: a multi-institutional prospective study. Arch Otorhinolar-yngol Head Neck Surg 111:589, 1985

Lennon RL, Hosking MP, Warner MA et al: Monitoring and analysis of oxygenation and ventilation during rigid bronchoscopic neo-dymium-YAG laser resection of airway tumors. Mayo Clin Proc 62:584, 1987

LoCicero J III, Metzdorff M, Almgren C: Photodynamic therapy in the palliation of late stage obstructing non-small cell lung cancer. Chest 98:97, 1990

Luce JM, Clement MJ: Pulmonary diagnostic evaluation in patients suspected of having an HIV-related disease. Semin Respir Infect 4:93, 1989

Macgillivray RG, Zulu S: Oxygen saturation after bronchography under general anaesthesia. S Afr Med J 76:151, 1989

Mantor PC, Tuggle DW, Tuneel WP: An appropriate negative bron-choscopy rate in suspected foreign body aspiration. Am J Surg 158:622, 1989

Marini JJ, Pierson DJ, Hudson LD: Acute lobar atelectasis: a pro-spective comparison of fiberoptic bronchoscopy and respiratory therapy. Am Rev Respir Dis 119:971, 1979

Martin WJ II, Smith TF, Sanderson DR et al: Role of bronchoalveolar lavage in the assessment of opportunistic pulmonary infections: utility and complications. Mayo Clin Proc 62:549, 1987

Matsushima Y, Jones RL, King EG et al: Alterations in pulmonary mechanics and gas exchange during routine fiberoptic bronchos-copy. Chest 86:184, 1984

McCaughan JS Jr, Hawley PC, Bethel BH, Walker J: Photodynamic therapy of endobronchial malignancies. Cancer 62:691, 1988

McCollun WB, Mattox KL, Guinn GA, Beall AC Jr: Immediate operative treatment for massive hemoptysis. Chest 67:152, 1975

McDougall JC, Cortese DA: Neodymium-YAG laser therapy of ma-lignant airway obstruction: a preliminary report. Mayo Clin Proc 58:35, 1983

McGuirt WF, Holmes KD, Feehs R, Browne JD: Tracheobronchial foreign bodies. Laryngoscope 98:615, 1988

Messeter KH, Pettersson KI: Endotracheal intubation with the fibre-optic bronchoscope. Anaesthesia 35:294, 1980

Pattishall EN, Noyes BE, Orenstein DM: Use of bronchoalveolar lavage in immunocompromised children with pneumonia. Pediatr Pulmonol 5:1, 1988

Poe RH, Israel RH, Marin MG et al: Utility of fiberoptic bronchos-copy in patients with hemoptysis and a nonlocalizing chest roent-genogram. Chest 93:70, 1988

Poe RH, Israel RH, Utell MJ, Hall WJ: Chronic cough: bronchos-copy or pulmonary function testing? Am Rev Respir Dis 126:160, 1982

Porter DK, Van Every MJ, Anthracite RF, Mack JW Jr: Massive hemoptysis in cystic fibrosis. Arch Intern Med 143:287, 1983

Rees JR: Massive hemoptysis associated with foreign body removal. Chest 88:475, 1985

Robinson L, Miller RH: Smoke inhalation injuries. Am J Otolaryngol 7:375, 1986

Rogers SN, Benumof JL: New and easy techniques for fiberoptic endoscopy-aided tracheal intubation. Anesthesiology 59:569, 1983

Schmitt GS, Ohar JM, Kanter KR, Naunheim KS: Indwelling trans-bronchial catheter drainage of pulmonary abscess. Ann Thorac Surg 45:43, 1988

Schneider W, Berger A, Mailänder P, Tempka A: Diagnostic and therapeutic possibilities for fiberoptic bronchoscopy in inhalation injury. Burns 14:53, 1988

Shapshay SM, Beamis JF Jr, Hybels RL, Bohigian RK: Endoscopic treatment of subglottic and tracheal stenosis by radial laser incision and dilation. Ann Otol Rhinol Laryngol 96:661, 1987

Shivaram U, Finch P, Nowak P: Plastic endobronchial tubes in the management of life-threatening hemoptysis. Chest 92:1108, 1987

Sosenko A, Glassroth J: Fiberoptic bronchoscopy in the evaluation of lung abscesses. Chest 87:489, 1985

Tsang V, Goldstraw P: Endobronchial stenting for anastomotic ste-nosis after sleeve resection. Ann Thorac Surg 48:568, 1989

Tyson EB: Development of the bronchoscope. N J Med 54:26, 1957

van Heel ACS: A new method of transporting optical images without aberrations. Nature 173:39, 1954

von Eiken C: The clinical application of the method of direct exami-nation of the respiratory passes and the upper alimentary tract. Arch Laryngol Rhinol Nov: 15, 1904

Weaver A, Fleming SM, Knechtges TC, Smith D: Triple endoscopy: a neglected essential in head and neck cancer. Surgery 86:493, 1979

Wood RE, Gauderer MWL: Flexible fiberoptic bronchoscopy in the management of tracheobronchial foreign bodies in children: the value of a combined approach with open tube bronchoscopy. J Pediatr Surg 19:693, 1984

Xaubet A, Torres A, Marco F et al: Pulmonary infiltrates in immuno-compromised patients: diagnostic value of telescoping plugged catheter and bronchoalveolar lavage. Chest 95:130, 1989

Zalzal GH: Stridor and airway compromise. Pediatr Clin North Am 36:1389, 1989

Endoscopic Laser Therapy for Bronchogenic Carcinoma

Melvyn Goldberg   Albert Mudry
Philippe Pasche   Raphaël Maire

HISTORICAL NOTE

Although the principles of light amplified stimulated emission of electromagnetic radiation have been known since the beginning of the century (Einstein, 1917), the first laser (a ruby laser) was not developed until 1960. Since the mid 1960s, ruby lasers in ophthalmology have pioneered the use of lasers in medicine. Subsequently, new sources for emitting in ultraviolet, visible, and infrared light appeared: excimer laser, krypton laser, argon laser, KTP laser, dye laser, neodymium: yttrium aluminum garrett (Nd:YAG) laser, erbium and holmium laser, and carbon dioxide (CO_2) laser.

The first applications of laser technology for use in bronchology date from 1970; Strong and Jako (1972) used the CO_2 laser for removing benign tumors, specifically tracheobronchial papillomas. In 1976, Laforet, et al. reported the first application of this laser for treating malignant obstructive lesions of the trachea and the bronchi. Later on, the indications for employing the CO_2 laser were expanded to include benign tracheal stenoses. At the end of the 1970s, the Nd:YAG laser was introduced in France by Toty, et al. (1979) and Dumon, et al. (1982) and in Japan by Oho, et al. (1983) for palliative therapy of tracheobronchial tumors. In the United States, these techniques were developed by Shapshay (1983) and Brutinel, et al. (1987) in the beginning of the 1980s. Due to its physical properties, the Nd:YAG laser remains the current laser of choice for the removal of obstructive tumors in the tracheobronchial tree. A second laser application in bronchoesophagology is represented by photodynamic therapy with the goal of curing superficial cancers (in situ and microinvasive carcinomas). Palliative photodynamic therapy for inoperable bronchial cancers has not been indicated, due to potential complications (hemorrhages and fistulae) and the risk of cutaneous photosensitization to the sun (Smith, et al., 1993).

HISTORICAL READINGS

Brutinel WM, Cortese DA, McDougall JC et al: A two year experience with neodynium-YAG laser in endobronchial obstruction. Chest 91:159, 1987

Dumon JF, Reboud E, Garbe L, et al: Treatment of tracheobronchial lesions by laser photoresection. Chest 81:278, 1982

Laforet EG, Berger RL, Vaughn CW: Carcinoma obstructing the trachea: treatment by laser resection. N Engl J Med 214:941, 1976

Oho K, Ogawa I, Amemiya R et al: Indication for endoscopic Nd:YAG laser surgery in the trachea and bronchus. Endoscopy 15:302, 1983

Shapshay S: Endoscopic treatment of subglottic and tracheal stenosis by radial laser incision and dilatation. Ann Otol Rhinol Laryngol 99:661, 1987

Smith SGT, Bedwell J, MacRobert AJ et al: Experimental studies to assess the potential of photodynamic therapy for the treatment of bronchial carcinomas. Thorax 48:474, 1993

Strong MS, Jako JG: Laser surgery in the larynx: early clinical experience with continuous CO_2 laser and soft fisme. Ann Otol Rhinol Laryngol 81:791, 1972

Toty L, Personne C, Hertzog P et al: Utilisation d'un faisceau laser (YAG) à conducteur souple, pour le traitement endoscopique de certaines lésions trachéobronchiques. Rev Fr Mal Respir 7:57, 1979

PROPERTIES OF LASERS

Each laser possesses particular properties (Table 12-1) based on its wavelength. Nevertheless, even though they may possess very different configurations, all lasers are composed of 3 fundamental elements:

1. An active substance (lasing medium), either atoms or molecules, which are excited by an energy source and emit photons of a concisely defined wavelength. The choice of

Table 12-1. Characteristics of Lasers in Clinical Use

Variable	CO_2	Nd:YAG	Argon	Argon-Tunable Dye
Wavelength (nm)	10,600	1,060	500	630
Power (W)	40	100	5–20	2
Transmission system	Mirrors	Fiberoptic	Fiberoptic	Fiberoptic
Absorption in tissues	High	Low	Selective	Selective for photodynamic therapy
Coagulation effect	Low	High	Medium	None
Cutting effect	High	Low	Low	None
Penetration	1 mm	10–15 mm	5 mm	8–10 mm

medium (e.g., gas, crystal, or dye) defines the wavelength of the laser and thus its properties.

2. The energy source that excites the active substance; this is the pumping source.

3. The optical resonator is formed by two mirrors separated by a cylindrical cavity in which the active substance is found.

We differentiate the following lasers: crystal solids lasers (ruby, 696 nm; Nd:YAG, 1,064 nm), gas lasers (He Ne, 632.8 nm; CO_2, 10,600 nm; argon, 488 and 514 nm; krypton, 407 nm), dye lasers (variable wavelength depending on the dye), and semiconductor lasers.

Effects on Tissue

The effects of laser beams on tissue is primarily dependent on the type of laser used (wavelength of the laser) and the type of tissue under consideration (optical properties of biologic tissues).

When a laser comes in contact with a tissue, four phenomena, of varying degrees, can be produced:

1. *Reflection:* partially seen on the surface of biologic tissues

2. *Transmission:* total or partial (e.g., the total transmission of the argon laser through water and glass, through the cornea and the vitreous body of the eye, and through the urinary bladder filled with fluid, just to name a few examples. The same is true to a lesser degree for the Nd:YAG laser.)

3. *Absorption:* Based on the wavelength and the biologic tissue composition, a laser beam may be absorbed to a greater or lesser degree (e.g., strong absorption of the CO_2 laser by water, strong absorption of the argon and the KTP lasers by hemoglobin and melanin pigments.

4. *Diffusion with tissue contact:* coherence and collimation properties of the laser beams are partially lost in relation to the wavelength and the type of tissue considered. The energy concentration is lost due to its diffusion in the tissue (e.g., strong diffusion of the Nd:YAG laser in biologic tissues).

Thermal Effect

In prevailing use, it is the thermal effect of the laser beam that is exploited. Laser energy, absorbed by the tissue, is converted into heat. According to the temperature reached, various tissue effects are observed: coagulation (blanching of the lesion), protein denaturation (gray coloring of the lesion), carbonization (black coloring of the lesion) and vaporization (tissue volatilization) (Fig. 12-18).

While the effects achieved on the tissue are, to a large part, dependent on the types of laser and tissue, two other important parameters enable one to control the laser effects on the tissue: (1) power density and (2) time of tissue exposure to the action of the laser beam. The power density decreases by the square of the diameter at the point of focalization.

Photochemical Effect

In general, a pump laser (argon, KTP [potassium-titanyl-phosphate], Nd:YAG) is required to excite the dye, the wavelength of which depends upon its type. Dye lasers are basically used in bronchology for photodynamic therapy for early cancers (in situ carcinoma and microinvasive carcinoma), which do not infiltrate the cartilage or cause lymphnode metastases (Monnier, et al., 1991). The effect is not thermal but photochemical. The principle is such that a photosensitizer, usually from the porphyrin group, is injected intravenously several hours or days before therapeutic endoscopy. Its preferential accumulation in cancer cells leads to the tumoral destruction by a photochemical effect due to a weak irradiation (0.1 W) by a dye laser the wavelength of which is selected according to the peak absorption of the photosensitizer and the desired tissue penetration. The majority of the porphyrins have strong fluorescent properties, and these same substances can therefore be used equally well for the photodetection of early cancers still invisible by traditional endoscopic methods (photodiagnostic imaging).

THERMAL LASERS

Carbon Dioxide Lasers

The carbon dioxide (CO_2) laser is a gas laser emitting light with a wavelength of 10,600 nm. The spot size varies in diameter from 0.16 to 2 mm, as a function of the focal distance and the transmission systems (microspot, guide). The beam is strongly absorbed by water and by all biologic tissues whose composition is 90 percent water. Absorption is totally independent on the presence of hemoglobin or melanin. All the beam's energy contributes to the destruction-coagulation of a certain tissue volume element almost without heat dispersion by conduction. These properties make it a precise scalpel that ensures hemostasis of all vessels with a caliber less than 0.5 mm. Thus, the tissue neighboring a zone excised by a

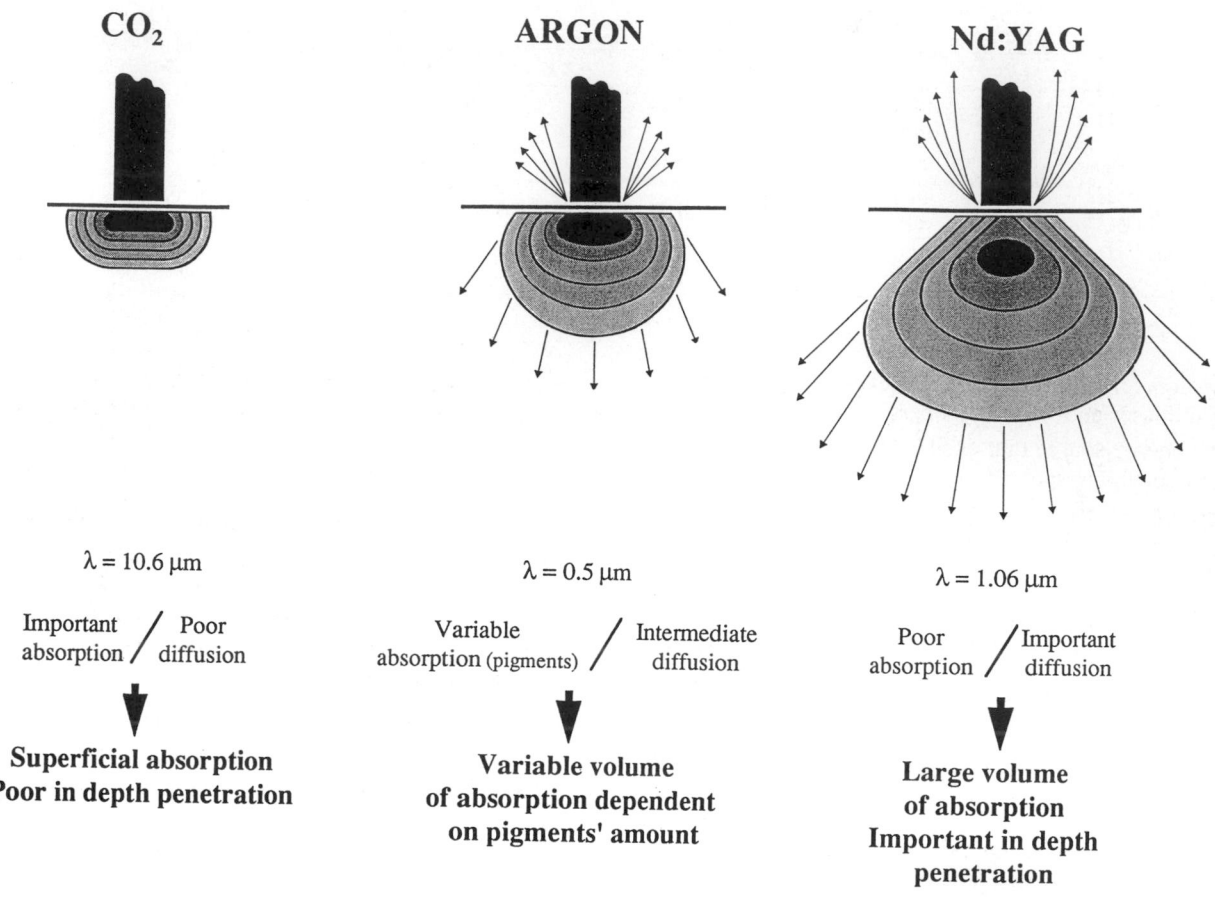

Figure 12-18. Comparison of the effects on tissue with carbon dioxide, argon and Nd:YAG lasers.

CO_2 laser remains intact. This causes a weak inflammatory reaction and a diminution of fibrous scarring reactions. A major inconvenience lies in the fact that the beam is transmittable only in a straight line, necessitating the use of articulating arms and mirrors as intermediaries. The improvement of adding hand-regulated accessories to the rigid bronchoscope has facilitated its use in the trachea and in the mainstem bronchi, but its capabilities are practically excluded at the level of the distal airway routes (lobar and segmental bronchi), despite the development of semiflexible guides that can convey the beam through the biopsy channel of the fibroscope. Nevertheless, these guides do not allow as comparable an angulation as those of a true fiberoptic used with Nd:YAG, argon, and KTP lasers. The CO_2 laser represents the ideal laser for therapy for certain benign pathologies of the tracheobronchial tree, and is especially helpful in the vaporization of thin fibrous strictures of the airway.

Methodology

Because a rigid bronchoscope must be used, patients receive a general anesthetic. The method of ventilation may vary from spontaneous, to controlled, to jet ventilation with a Sanders injector at conventional frequencies, to jet ventilation with appropriate equipment at high frequencies. With jet ventilation, total intravenous anesthesia is necessary. The patient's eyes are protected with moist gauze, all personnel in the operating theater must wear protective goggles, and

the addition of ear oximetry to continuously monitor serum oxygen saturation is essential.

Once adequate ventilation has been established, the laser port is connected to the ventilating bronchoscope by means of a coupler (Fig. 12-19) and the laser beam can be fired directly down the bronchoscope into the area of pathology. The oxygen environment at the focal point must be below 40 percent in order to minimize intraoperative combustion and fire.

Advantages and Disadvantages

The CO_2 laser is a precise cutting instrument, and it affords hemostasis only to the microcirculation. There is little perioperative edema next to the focal point of the beam, and excellent healing ability exists in the adjacent tissue. The advantage to the surgeon of using the rigid ventilating system is that it allows the use of a large-bore suction catheter to remove secretions, blood, and the products of coagulation. It also permits physical debridement of the tumor mass by literally coring out the tumor with the end of the rigid bronchoscope. Excellent airway control is available if hemorrhage occurs, and the bronchoscope can be used to tamponade the bleeding surface of a tumor by lateral compression.

Unfortunately, there is poor hemostasis with CO_2 laser therapy in vessels greater than 0.5 mm. The CO_2 laser requires a cumbersome delivery system of articulated arms because its light cannot at present be transmitted through

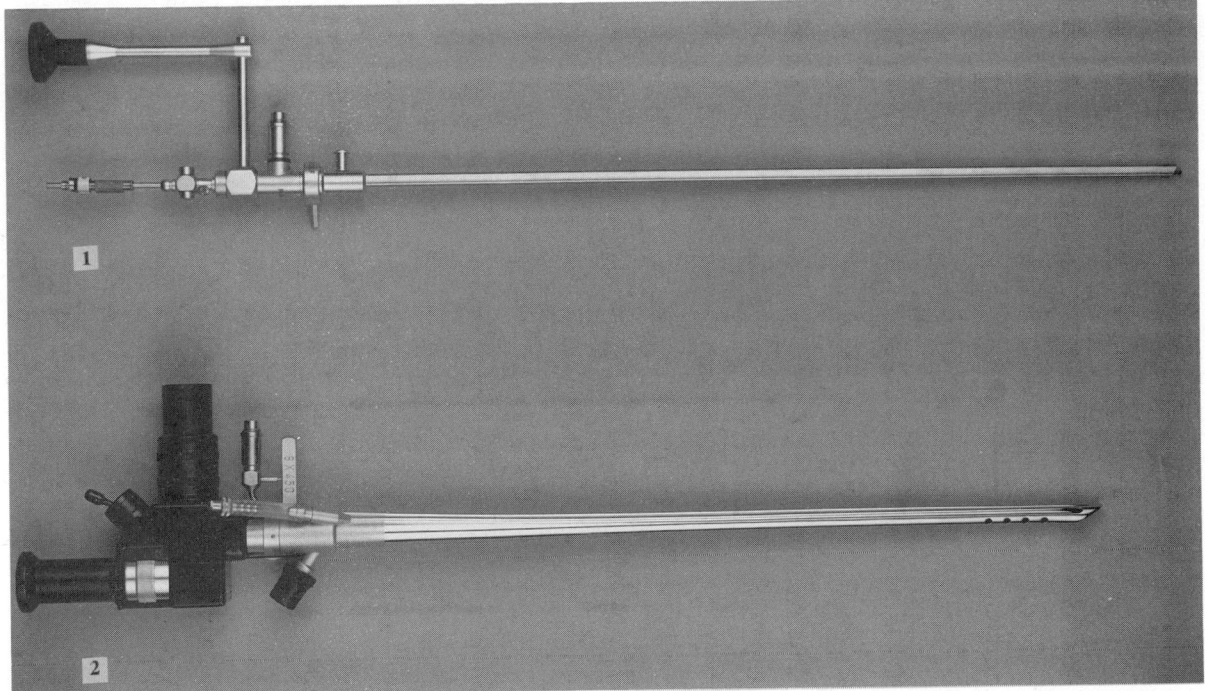

Figure 12-19.   Bronchoscopes for CO_2 laser: (1) Exelite guide (Coherent), adapted on a bronchoscope whose optical element is mounted in a bayonet shape; (2) bronchoscope with CO_2 laser coupler (Storz).

fiberoptic bundles but must be reflected in transit off prisms in the articulations. The special tips that are used with the Nd:YAG laser are not available (e.g., thermal, divergent, convergent, and contact tips). A general anesthetic with rigid endoscopy is required, and because of the mechanics of delivery, only tracheal and proximal bronchial lesions are accessible.

The use of the CO_2 laser is contraindicated in patients with obstruction due to loss of cartilaginous support or to extrinsic compression of the tracheobronchial tree. It should not be used to open obstructed lobar or more distal orifices. With the advent of the Nd:YAG laser for similar lesions, most laser therapists have abandoned the CO_2 laser, using it solely for therapy for localized benign lesions of the upper airway and for benign short circumferential strictures of the trachea. Ablation of tumor mass in major airways is much more effectively and safely performed with the more recently developed Nd:YAG laser.

Nd:YAG Lasers

The Nd:YAG is a crystal solid laser emitting at 1064 nm, with a minimum diameter spot size of 0.6 mm. In contrast to the CO_2 laser, the Nd:YAG laser is poorly absorbed by water. A large part of its energy is diffused by conduction in the tissue; thus, an increased power is necessary to achieve a vaporization effect. With respect to the mucous membranes, underlying tissue injury is approximately 600 times more prominent than with the CO_2 laser and reaches a depth of several millimeters. With this laser, edema and a more marked inflammatory reaction is seen than with the CO_2 laser. The Nd:YAG laser thus lends itself less well to precise tissue

resection than does the CO_2 laser, but its coagulation and vaporization effects are excellent. Its beam is transmitted by a Teflon-coated flexible quartz fiber with a diameter from 1.8 to 2.2 mm, which can easily be introduced into a rigid or flexible endoscope and oriented in any angle.

Due to its effects of coagulation and capability of vaporizing large amounts of tissue, the use of the Nd:YAG laser is indicated in bronchology to remove tumoral obstructions, but is less valuable in treating benign strictures.

Methodology

The preoperative assessment involves a history, physical examination, recent chest x-ray, and routine blood tests, including arterial blood gases. On occasion a ventilation/ perfusion scan is helpful in identifying an occluded pulmonary artery to the involved lung that might preclude an attempt to open the airway. The need for absolute cooperation between the surgeon and the anesthetist cannot be overstated. For both, the airway is a shared facility, and discussion is essential before the procedure commences and throughout its course. If the patient has not had bronchoscopy in our facility previously, either bronchoscopy is done initially under local anesthesia or the patient is given general anesthesia and bronchoscopy is done through the endotracheal tube with a fiberoptic bronchoscope. After the tumor has been assessed by this means and if a decision has been made to perform laser therapy, the patient is extubated and reintubated with a rigid ventilating bronchoscope. Although a variety of specific laser bronchoscopes has been developed (Fig. 12-20), we routinely use a more standard ventilating bronchoscope and jet ventilate with a Sanders injector at conventional

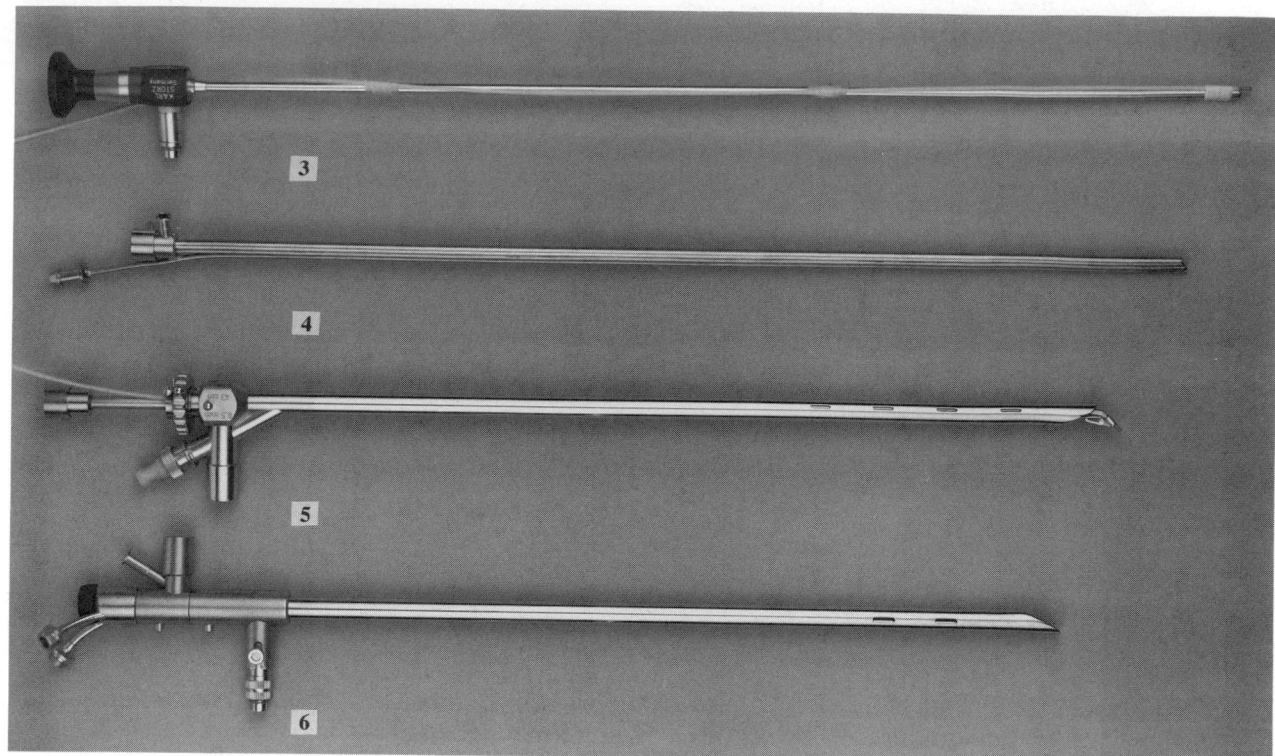

Figure 12-20. Bronchoscopes for Nd:YAG laser: (3) the laser fiber is attached with adhesive strips directly to the optic; (4) in order to easily retract the laser fiber, we have added an external canal to the intermediary guide of the bronchoscope allowing the passage of the fiber; (5) the diagnostic bronchoscope of Storz as a single canal that can be adjusted to 45 degrees from the access of the bronchoscope; (6) bronchoscope by Shapshay (Storz) with three channels (laser fiber, aspiration of secretion, aspiration of smoke).

frequencies. The FiO_2 should be less than 0.4 to prevent combustion and/or fire. The tumor is then assessed through the rigid bronchoscope. Any large, bulky portions are dislodged by manipulation of the tip of the bronchoscope into the tumor mass, and large fragments are removed with large biopsy forceps and a large-bore suction catheter. Hemorrhage from the bed of the tumor is only mild to moderate. Indeed, most of the tumor bulk can be removed by this simple method of debridement (Fig. 12-21). By attaching a ventilator to the side port of the bronchoscope and occluding its open end, the anesthesia system can be converted to a conventional closed ventilation system (Figure 12-22). A flexible bronchoscope can then be passed through a grommet occluding the open end of the bronchoscope, and a laser fiber can be passed through the channel of the fiberoptic bronchoscope and positioned under the direct vision of the operator in the area to be treated (Figure 12-23). This allows for excellent manipulation of the fiber tip with the flexible bronchoscope and endoscopic visualization of the fiber tip, tumor mass, and therapy. A vinyl suction catheter with its tip at the end of the rigid bronchoscope can be attached to its outer length with tape before the procedure commences. This allows for aspiration of smoke in the area during therapy. The power output is between 45 and 55 W in 0.5-second pulses. Various tips can be applied to the end of the laser fiber to vary the effect on the tissue. With the fiber tips that have lenses applied

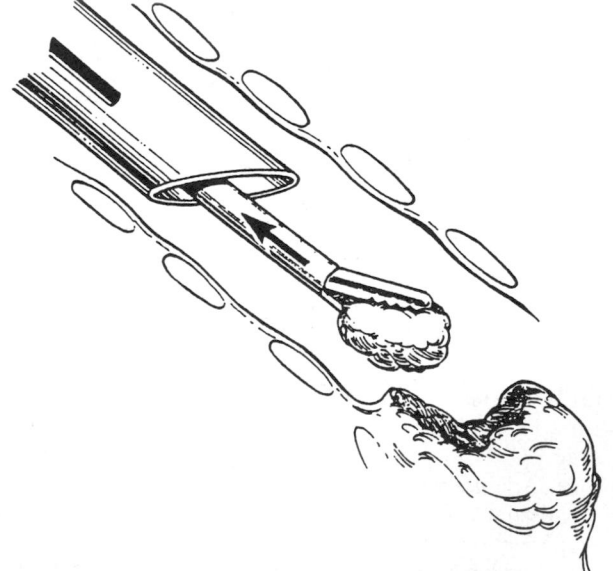

Figure 12-21. Most of the tumor bulk can be removed by physical debridement using large biopsy forceps through the ventilating bronchoscope. Bleeding is usually minimal and can be controlled with locally epinephrine (1 : 200,000).

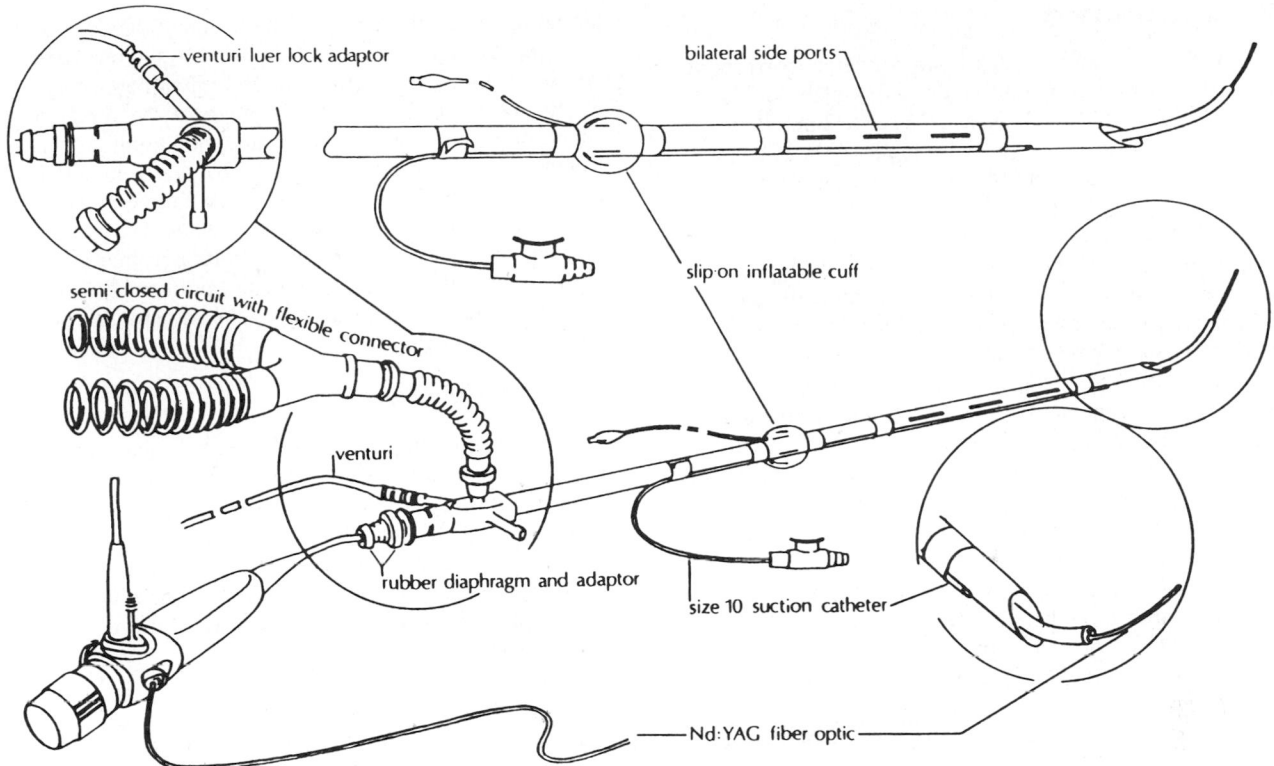

Figure 12-22. A technique illustrated by Perera (1987) demonstrating the bronchoscopy/anesthesia technique for laser resection of airway lesions (see text). (From Perera ER, Mallon JS: General anesthetic management for laser resection of central airway lesions in 85 procedures. Can J Anaesth 34:383, 1987, with permission.)

to them, the closer the lens is to the tissue, the more vaporization takes place; moved slightly away from the tissue, the laser produces more coagulation for hemostasis.

If, during the laser therapy, there is need for suctioning of secretions, purulent material, or blood or the removal of large portions of necrotic debris, the flexible bronchoscope can be

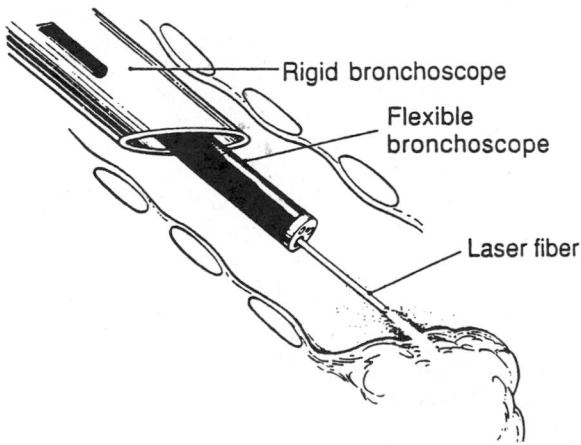

Figure 12-23. Laser therapy is performed by direct observation of the laser fiber through the fiberoptic bronchoscope, which is passed initially through the rigid endoscope. If suctioning is required during therapy, the flexible bronchoscope can be removed and ventilation converted to a jet system, and debridement can occur simply through the rigid bronchoscope.

removed, the ventilation converted to a jet system, and the large-bore suction catheter and the biopsy forceps inserted directly into the open end of the bronchoscope. This particular technique allows for simple and rapid conversion from one delivery system to the other when required.

The initial procedure may be life-saving in patients who have airway compromise. Therefore, just opening the airway to relieve the initial distress may suffice, with the return of the patient to the operating room for repeated laser therapy at a future date. Repetitive therapy sessions are often necessary to obtain optimal airway patencies. All of our patients are monitored conventionally as well as with ear oximetry. A solution of epinephrine (1 : 200,000) is occasionally injected into the bronchoscope to arrest bleeding from the raw tumor bed. This technique is quite effective and has not yet interfered with patient stability.

The patient can either be extubated in the operating room or reintubated with an endotracheal tube after the rigid bronchoscope has been removed and then extubated in the recovery room.

Advantages

The Nd:YAG laser has characteristics that produce excellent vaporization, excellent coagulative necrosis, and deeper penetration than the CO_2 laser. Safe and effective ablation can be performed much more quickly with this laser, and the procedure may be done either through a flexible bronchoscope as described or through a rigid bronchoscope exclusively, as described by Dumon (1987).

KTP and Argon Lasers

The KTP (532 nm, spot size 0.15 mm diameter) corresponds to a Nd:YAG Laser coupled to a crystal, which doubles the wavelength of the Nd:YAG from 1,064 to 532 nm. The laser can be used either in the Nd:YAG mode or in the KTP mode.

The argon laser (488 and 514 nm, spot size 0.15 mm diameter) has a wavelength close to the KTP laser, and based on this, also similar effects on tissue. Nevertheless, the absorption peak in hemoglobin is somewhat lower than that of the KTP laser. Its tissue penetration depth is difficult to predict and is extremely dependent on the degree of tissue vascularization and tissue pigmentation. The use of these two lasers requires a perfect knowledge of the tissue interactions themselves with each organ and with each lesion. For the mucous membranes, tissue damage is approximately 10 times greater than that of the CO_2 laser (i.e., approximately 1 to 2 mm). The laser beam of argon and KTP is transmitted through a flexible fiber. With lower strength, it has a coagulating effect, and with higher strengths, it has a vaporization effect.

The KTP laser is not widely used in bronchology due to the physical properties listed here and to its purchase cost comparable to that of a CO_2 and a Nd:YAG laser together. In comparison to the CO_2 laser, the KTP laser has the advantage of being used with a bronchofibroscope. In bronchology, the argon laser is especially used in photochemotherapy at 514 nm or as a pump laser on a dye-emitting laser in the red (630 nm; see page 220).

Complications of Thermal Laser Therapy

Hypoxemia

Hypoxemia can occur both intraoperatively and postoperatively. During the operative procedure it is essential to obtain airway control immediately after anesthesia is given. This is initially accomplished by forcibly dilating the airway and inserting the rigid bronchoscope through either the tracheal or the mainstem bronchial obstruction. At that time secretions that have accumulated beyond the obstruction can be aspirated, as can the necrotic debris that has been dislodged during the manipulation. During the procedure both the right and left lungs should be irrigated with saline and aspirated occasionally to keep them maximally patent. Hypoxemia is identified either by analysis of arterial blood gases or by oximetry. Laser therapy may have to be discontinued until the abnormality is corrected; correction is usually accomplished by jet ventilation with higher concentrations of oxygen or by changing to a closed ventilation system. Postoperatively, in the recovery room, pooling of secretions and blood may compromise the airway. Patients who experience this may benefit from flexible bronchoscopy with or without 1 to 2 hours of assisted ventilation. On occasion, the patency of the main airway is improved by the laser therapy, but the patient remains hypoxemic following therapy, owing to a nonfunctioning nonperfused ventilated lung.

Hemorrhage

This complication rarely occurs during or immediately after laser therapy. During therapy, hemorrhage is controlled by tamponading the tumor bed with the end of the rigid bronchoscope or directly by laser coagulation. A mild ooze can easily be controlled by the instillation of 5 ml epinephrine solution (1 : 200,000) directly down the lumen of the rigid bronchoscope onto the tumor. The pulmonary vasculature is more closely related to the lobar bronchi than to the major airways, and the wall of the airway is much thinner distally. The chance of producing fistulization between the pulmonary artery and the airway is much higher with peripheral therapies. Familiarity with the anatomy of the pulmonary vasculature and its relationship to the airway is essential for any practicing laser endoscopist.

Perforation and Fistulae

This is a rare complication and is usually due to aggressive therapy in the posterior carina or at the origin of the left mainstem bronchus, with penetration and perforation into the underlying esophagus. When isolated lesions are identified bronchoscopically in these particular locations, esophagoscopy must be performed to rule out a primary malignancy in the esophagus with anterior penetration into the back wall of the airway.

Fire

Fire in the area of laser therapy can always be avoided with proper care. The area of therapy should always be visible to the operator, and nothing, such as a suction catheter or normal tissues, should inadvertently be fired upon. The tip of the laser fiber should be at least 5 mm beyond the end of the flexible bronchoscope. If it is retracted into the bronchoscope, then the tip of the bronchoscope will be severely damaged. The FIO_2 during therapy should always be less than 0.4.

Pneumothorax

Pneumothorax is a rare complication of barotrauma associated with both jet and conventional positive-pressure ventilation. It does happen on occasion, and once recognized it should be treated simply by chest tube drainage.

Endobronchial Spill

Occasionally when an obstructing malignancy has been removed, the airway and lung beyond contain purulent material due to obstruction and accumulation or to acute endobronchial drainage of a parenchymal abscess cavity. Care must be taken to avoid spillage to the contralateral lung, both during the operation and immediately postoperatively.

Clinical Applications of the Thermal Laser in Airway Obstruction

Palliative Endoscopic Therapy for Tracheobronchial Cancer

Indications. It is important to choose those patients capable of being helped by laser obstruction removal in order to eliminate unnecessary surgical risks. One must ensure that the patient can indeed realize a genuine benefit from the intervention. The primary indication is the amelioration of respiratory obstruction. The draining of an obstructive pneumonia and hemostasis of a hemorrhaging tumor are rarer indications. Our eligibility criteria, taking into account only the use of the rigid endoscope under general anesthesia, include the following:

1. The tumor should basically be exophytic if therapy is to be laser alone (Fig. 12-24). However, since the appearance of the autoexpandable prostheses (Dumon, et al., 1994; Mudry and Monnier, 1994), this condition is less strict. If mixed compression is present, a lumen is created by the laser which is large enough to allow the introduction of

the expandable prosthesis, which, upon unfolding, acts on the extrinsic compression to restore a sufficient lumen (Fig. 12-25).

2. If possible, a lumen should always be present in order to reduce the risk of creating a perforation of the bronchus or of the large vessels. With inoperable cases, preventive vaporization of the tumor is recommended before it completely obstructs the lumen, even if it is producing no symptoms, or if these symptoms are minor (Dierkesmann, 1990).

3. In the bronchi, the length of the tumor should not exceed 4 cm (Edell and Shapsay, 1994).

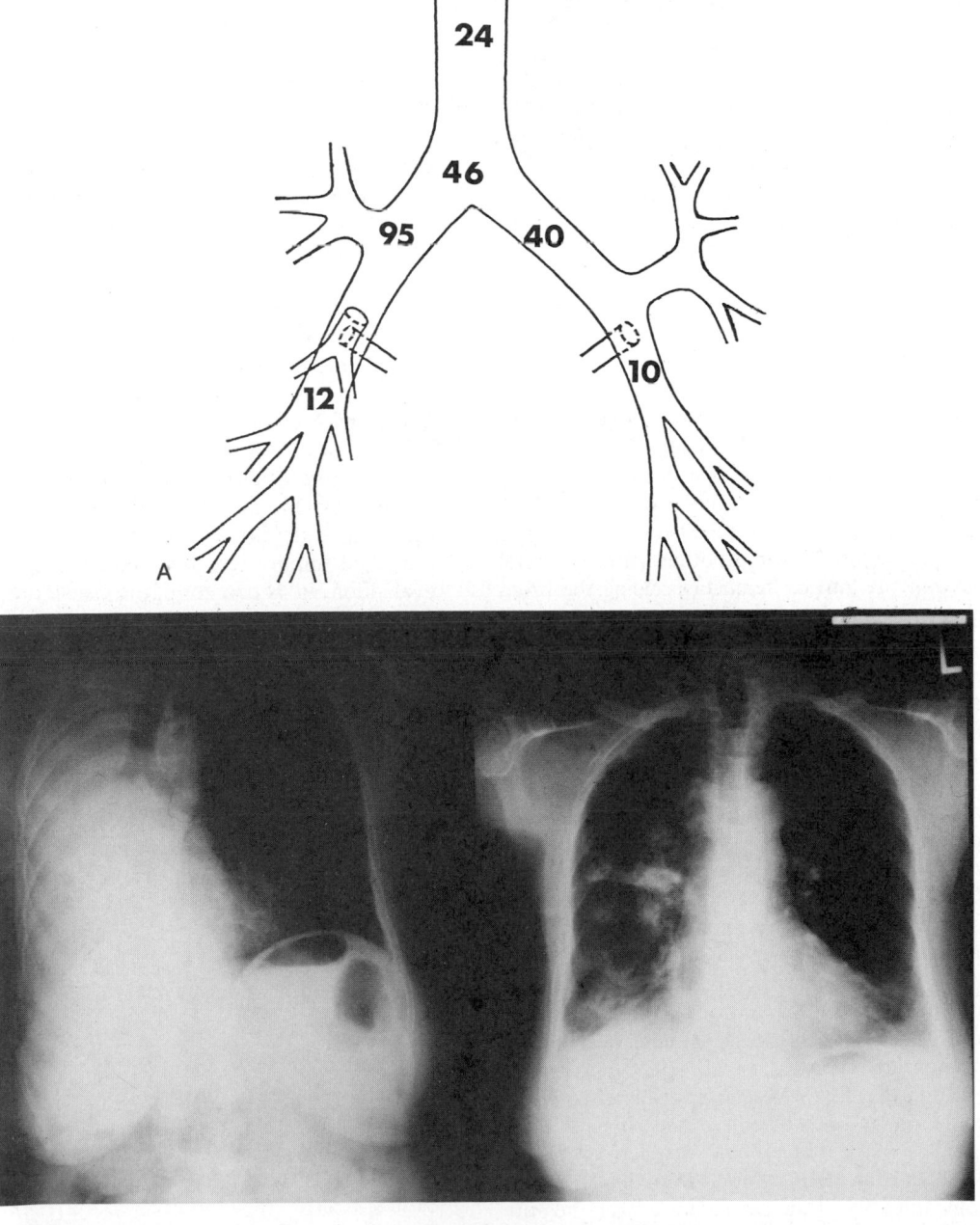

Figure 12-24. **(A)** Sites of airway obstruction at first therapeutic session (227 patients). **(B)** Radiographs of the chest demonstrating aeration of the right lung both before and after laser ablation to a tumor obstructing the right main bronchus.

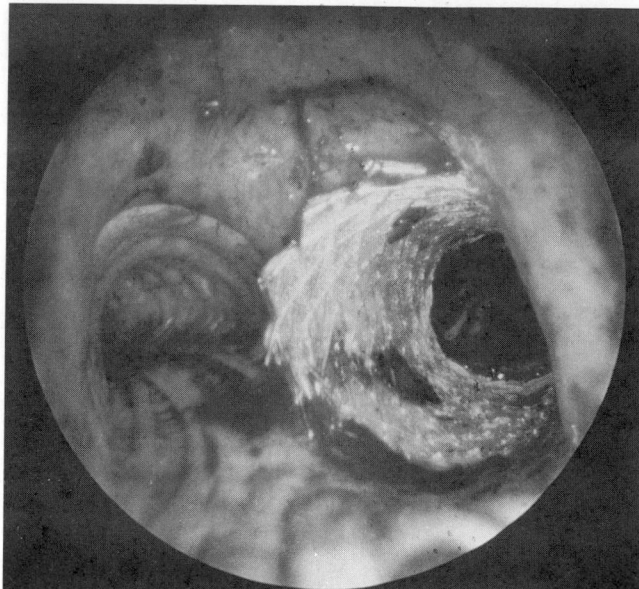

Figure 12-25. Covered Wallstent in place in the right main bronchus after removal of obstruction with Nd:YAG laser for an adenocarcinoma of the right main bronchus with extension on the lateral wall of the trachea.

4. Since the therapeutic effect increases the more proximal the obstruction, the best indications for therapy are obstructions of the trachea and mainstem bronchi. In the periphery (lobar and segmental bronchi), the proportion of the tumoral obstruction by extrinsic components increases the same as the risk of vascular perforation; the relationship between the risks and the benefits of therapy thus becomes less favorable. On the other hand, a tumoral coagulation with the aim of hemostasis using the bronchofibroscope introduced in the rigid bronchoscope could be indicated.

5. The pulmonary parenchyma beyond the obstruction must still be functional. An atelectic lobe of more than 1 week's duration has little chance of reexpanding after the reopening of the obstructed bronchus.

Results. Dumon, et al. (1982), using a specially constructed rigid bronchoscope for laser endoscopy, performed 1,500 procedures in 817 patients. The immediate results in main airway disease, including the trachea and right and left mainstem bronchi, were excellent in 75 percent, fair in 15 percent, and poor in 10 percent. As therapy became more distal, the efficacy of the procedure was directly reduced. Dumon's group also performed laser endoscopy on 122 benign lesions, achieving good results in 90 of these patients over 1 year after the initial therapy. Hayata, et al. (1989) and Unger (1985) demonstrated that Nd:YAG therapy was effective in improving ventilation by both objective and subjective assessment in 78 and 77 percent of patients, respectively. Therapy was most effective in patients who had proximal tracheobronchial lesions, integrity of the cartilaginous wall, healthy parenchyma distal to the lesion, benign lesions, and those with partial obstructions.

Miller (1989) has compared CO_2 to Nd:YAG laser endoscopy for obstructing lesion in 89 patients with 102 procedures performed. This study demonstrated good to excellent results in 81 percent of those treated by CO_2 laser and 91.5 percent in those treated by Nd:YAG laser. The Nd:YAG therapy was easier to use, involved a shorter anesthesia time and a shorter operating room time, and was less expensive overall.

Hetzel, et al. (1985), in treating 100 tracheobronchial tumors, identified a much better response in the more proximally and centrally located pathologies. His indications for laser therapy include partial obstruction in 70 percent, complete lobar or lung atelectasis in 35 percent, and hemoptysis in 60 percent.

Brutinel, et al. (1987) and Cavalière, et al. (1988) reported the restoration of the tracheobronchial lumen in 83 and 92 percent of cases, respectively. An amelioration of pulmonary function is seen in a similar percentage (Mohsenifar, et al., 1988; George, et al., 1990), and increases the more proximal the lesion. For the majority of patients, the quality of life is considerably improved and death by asphyxiation is avoided. There is no way of determining if the survival of patients is prolonged due to the impossibility of carrying out randomized studies in patients with severe dyspnea. We believe there is an increase in the survival of patients treated by laser and radiotherapy compared to those treated solely with radiotherapy (Ross, et al., 1990). The association of laser therapy with radiochemotherapy seems to significantly prolong symptom remission and survival (Jain, et al., 1985; Joyner, et al., 1985; Maire and Monnier, 1989).

From May 1983 to January 1994 at Hospitalier Universitaire Vaudois (Lausanne, Switzerland), 272 patients (211 men and 61 women, ranging from 25 to 95 years old; average age, 64 years) who suffered from an untreatable tracheal or bronchial tumor were referred for palliative laser therapy evaluation. In 44 percent of the cases, the localization of the cancer, the advanced stage, or the poor condition of the patient did not permit the contemplation of curative therapy. The other 56 percent of the patients presented with tumor progression after surgical therapy or radiotherapy. All the patients complained of severe dyspnea (stage 3 or 4, the Medical Research Council's Grading System of Dyspnea, 1966) or suffered from hemoptysis. Based on the above-mentioned selection criteria, we treated 227 patients (83.5 percent). The site and histologic type of the tumor are summarized in Fig. 12-24A and Table 12-2. We performed 333

Table 12-2. Histology of Malignant Primary and Metastatic Lesions (May 1983–January 1994)

Lesion Type	No.	
Squamous cell carcinoma	158	}78%
Anaplastic carcinoma	20	
Adenocarcinoma	13	
Adenoid cystic carcinoma	4	
Carcinoid	2	
Carcinosarcoma	1	
Metastasis or local infiltration (esophagus, thyroid, breast, bone, kidney, colon)	29	

Table 12-3. Nd:YAG Laser Therapy for Endobronchial Lesions: Immediate Results

Patients (n = 227)	Site of Tumor	No. (%) of Satisfactory Results (Restoration of at Least 40% of Normal Lumen)
24	Trachea	24/24 (100)
46	Carina	42/46 (91)
135	Main bronchi and right intermedius bronchus	104/135 (77)
22	Lobar bronchi (upper lobe excluded)	10/22 (45)

operations, 26 percent of the patients having 2 to 8 laser treatments. In 33 cases over the past 3 years, we have combined laser removal of the obstruction with endoprostheses placement (Dumon, Hood, and Wallstent types). We consider reopening satisfactory if a restitution of at least 40 percent of the bronchial lumen is obtained, the value estimated sufficient for the reestablishment of a normal airflow. A restitution of the lumen less than this is considered to be a therapy failure. Therapeutic success is established if the patient indicates a significant lessening of dyspnea (improvement of at least one stage) or the disappearance of hemoptysis. Table 12-3 shows that the success of therapy increases when the obstruction is proximal. Symptom improvement is correlated with endoscopic results if the ventilation/perfusion function of the lung is normal. The average duration of symptom amelioration is 6 weeks after a single laser treatment. Survival after 3 months does not surpass 50 percent, reflecting the advanced stage of the disease. The complication rate is 8.4 percent and the mortality rate, 2.1 percent. These complications are detailed in Table 12-4. With cases of severe hemorrhage, perioperative hemostasis was always capable of being carried out and blood loss never exceeded 300 ml. Pneumothoraces were conservatively treated with success. Seven patients died in the first 36 hours after surgery; the cause of death was complications from anesthesia in 4 cases, and in 3 cases, respiratory distress due to an extensive necrosis and a collapse of the terminal bronchi. Late complications were a progressive collapse of the cartilage in 11 cases. The therapy here depends on an endoprosthesis.

Table 12-4. Nd:YAG Laser Therapy: Complications of 333 Palliative Laser Resections of Endobronchial Tumors

Complications	No. (%)	Death
Immediate		
Perioperative hemorrhage (≥200 ml)	17 (5)	0
Pneumothorax	3 (0.9)	0
Bronchial collapse with acute respiratory distress syndrome	3 (0.9)	3
Cardiogenic shock	5 (1.5)	4
Late		
Cartilaginous subsidence	11 (3)	0

Therapy for Tracheobronchial Cicatricial Stenoses

The handling of these stenoses remains a difficult therapeutic problem. They are most often associated with a lesion of the larynx and are frequently localized to the subglottic and superior tracheal regions (sequelae of intubation, tracheotomy, or trauma). The pretherapeutic endoscopic assessment must be carried out in a rigorous manner. It comprises a functional examination of the vocal cords and a laryngotracheoscopy ranging at least from the epiglottis to the carina. This examination should provide the following information: (1) mobility of the vocal cords, (2) exact location of the lesion (distance in centimeters and the number of rings between the level of the glottis and the superior pole of the stenosis on one side; the distance between the inferior pole of the stenosis and the carina on the other); and (3) the length and the diameter of the lesion (Mudry and Monnier, 1994). Based on the type of stenosis encountered, various therapeutic surgical or endoscopic modalities exist. Thanks to the development of the therapeutic bronchoscopy with the CO_2 laser, certain endoscopic therapies have become possible. In all cases of cicatricial stenosis, the risk of aggravating the initial situation exists; it is thus necessary to rigorously respect the indications and to know when to propose surgical resection before "attempting" laser therapy as a first step. Unfortunately, the latter view is often promoted by our pulmonology colleagues; it must be severely fought. There are either primary or secondary indications for endoscopic laser therapy (Simpson, et al., 1982; Mudry and Monnier, 1994).

Indications. Indications include the following:

1. A thin, scarred diaphragm less than 1 cm in length without cartilaginous collapse or localized malacia. Preferentially chosen should be a microspot CO_2 laser set on discontinuous mode to avoid heat diffusion in the tissue. A circular vaporization is possible, but we prefer to carry out radial incisions on the stenosis to maintain intact mucosal bridges, which also affords a better reepithelialization, based on the technique proposed by Shapsay (1987).

2. Bridle scar without changes in the cartilaginous structure. Here there is also an indication for the CO_2 laser. The bridle scar may be completely vaporized on the provision that they are not circular. Everything possible must be done to avoid vaporization of the perichondrium and cartilage, as this may lead to serious deformations of the framework, which could make further therapy necessary.

3. Failures of previous surgical therapy that exclude further intervention. With this type of indication, it is most difficult to give guidelines concerning the techniques to be used. The most conservative therapy is indicated in order to avoid further aggravating the situation. In the face of such restricting situations, sometimes one must refrain from making any endoscopic therapy attempt and rely on endoluminal stenting.

4. Postoperative inflammatory granulations at the level of an anastomosis, at the level of a suprastomal spur, or at the level of the tip of the canula. The CO_2 laser remains the best laser for vaporization of granulations.

5. Laryngotracheal papillomatosis is a rather frequent indication. We have carried out more than 100 instances of therapy for this type of pathology. Therapy at the tracheobronchial level is most often accompanied by therapy at the larynx level, where the pathology is most frequently seen. The CO_2 laser is the one most often used for vaporization of papillomas, even though it is well known that the risk of recurrence is relatively high. Among the other indications, we include benign tumors that are not surgically resectionable, tracheobronchial amyloidosis, and Wegener's granulomatosis.

Contraindications. Contraindications include destruction of cartilaginous framework, tracheomalacia, stenosis longer than 1 cm, and total stenosis. If the indications and contraindications for endoscopic therapy (above) are ignored, irreversible damage may ensue from repeated laser therapy. As stenoses are frequently associated with laryngeal disease, it is most imperative to have the opinion of an ear, nose, and throat specialist. For the past few years, it has been the trend of certain practitioners to combine laser therapy with an endotracheal stent placement. The long-term consequences of these current prostheses in use are not yet known. Perhaps when a resorbable prosthesis makes its debut, this difficult therapeutic problem will be resolved. Those stenoses that can be treated surgically should be treated surgically. One should not forget that it is often the first therapeutic manipulation that determines the final outcome; thus, one must choose well this initial therapy.

Between 1973 and 1993, we treated 45 cases of tracheal stenoses; 25 were successfully treated with tracheal resection. Nineteen required endoscopic therapy and 6 of these should have first been subjected to surgical therapy, which unfortunately was not possible for various reasons. The postoperative endoluminal size after endoscopic therapy in these selected cases was, on average, 80 percent, and 79 percent of the patients no longer presented with dyspnea or dyspnea on intense exertion (Lang, 1994).

Conclusion

The role of interventional bronchoscopy has expanded with the advent of lasers. Our experience has shown that the use of the rigid endoscope can effectively treat lesions, and when both safety measures and indications are respected, low mortality and morbidity rates are observed. For inoperable tumors, tracheal or bronchial prostheses are becoming a very useful adjunct to laser removal of obstructions. Nevertheless, progress remains to be made in the development of new prostheses which are better tolerated, and an instrumentation which more easily permits their insertion and retraction. Endoscopic treatment of benign stenoses should be reserved for certain cases. In numerous situations, surgery remains the treatment of choice. As we do not yet know the long-term outcomes of prostheses, these should only be used as the last choice in cases of benign pathology, when no other treatment can be proposed. In this context, the resorbable prosthesis could be a solution for the future (see the section by Gaissert and Patterson).

PHOTOCHEMICAL LASER THERAPY

Argon Tunable Dye Laser and Photodynamic Therapy

In the argon tunable pump laser system, the argon laser produces a high-intensity beam that is focused on a dye that is continuously circulating in front of it. This energizes the dye and produces a laser beam. By changing the type of dye, different desired wavelengths can be obtained. Currently the major clinical use of this laser is a photochemical effect in conjunction with the selective PDT of malignant tumors of the airway following the intravenous injection of a photosensitizer, hematoporphyrin derivative (HpD). Lipson, et al. (1961) at the Mayo Clinic found that HpD, prepared by acetic and sulfuric acid treatments of hematoporphyrin, had good tumor-localizing properties in a variety of cancers. Dougherty, et al. (1978) at the Roswell Park Memorial Institute pioneered the first clinical study, and Hayata, et al. (1982) were the first to apply HpD PDT to therapy for lung malignancies.

After the intravenous injection, the HpD is distributed to all cells of the body. It then rapidly moves out of the normal cells but remains for a much longer time in the neoplastic cells. After a few days, there is a differential concentration of the sensitizer between the tumor cells and the normal ones. When the tumor is exposed to red light (630 nm), the HpD absorbs the light, which initiates a photochemical reaction within the cell that gives off singlet oxygen. This causes cell destruction by the oxidation of cellular biologic components. The cell membrane and mitochondrial function and integrity are impaired, and slow cell death occurs within 24 hours. Because there is less photosensitizer in normal tissue, a much less severe reaction, if any, occurs there. No immediate visible effects are seen (i.e., no edema, coagulation, char, or smoke). The reaction is primarily photochemical and not thermal, although hyperthermia may promote the cytotoxic reaction. The patient can be treated again within the first week of injection and at any time in the future in the event of a recurrence.

Methodology

Currently HpD or its more efficient derivative, dihematoporphyrin ester, is manufactured in only a few facilities in the United States and Canada. Therefore, its use in PDT is somewhat restricted. It is supplied in a sterile dehydrated form that is reconstituted on site into an injectable solution or in a frozen solution, which requires thawing before injection. The dosage is 2.0 to 4.0 mg/kg of body weight injected through an open intravenous line of 0.5 N saline over 5 to 10 minutes at 48 hours prior to PDT. Red light (630 nm) from the continuous argon-pumped tunable dye laser is delivered by simple single-step index quartz fibers inserted into the channel of a flexible fiberoptic bronchoscope. Surface illumination of the endobronchial tumors is performed directly by the red light that exits from the end of a flat cutoff fiber tip to cover the given tumor area and/or by the endoscopist sweeping the light over the desired area to be treated. Insertion illumination is performed by inserting the fiber directly into the tumor mass. In both types of illumination, either a flat cutoff fiber tip or a cylindric end, which yields a 360-

degree radius of light with isotropic distribution over a given length, may be used.

The diffusion of light throughout the tumor must be adequate (bright) throughout the entire period of illumination and should be inspected and reapplied whenever necessary. Dosimetry is based on the tumor's size, configuration, and location; the type of illumination (fiber tip variation); and the laser output (in watts). The average period of light exposure is 15 to 20 minutes.

PDT can be performed under local or general anesthesia. The fiber is positioned by direct observation through the fiberoptic bronchoscope. One hundred percent oxygen can be used if necessary, because the reaction is nonthermal. Forty-eight to 72 hours postoperatively, patients are examined bronchoscopically, and necrotic and exudative debris is removed by suction and biopsy forceps. If necessary a repeat PDT can be performed up to 1 week after the initial injection of HpD.

The only side effect reported with HpD is photosensitivity (sunburn) to sunlight for up to 4 weeks after injection. This need not be a major problem if proper precautions are taken by the patient (i.e., remain out of direct sunlight, wear sunglasses, and keep the skin covered with clothing). The incidence of notable reactions is less than 5 percent.

Complications

Complications are minimal now that post-PDT bronchoscopy is used for debridement. Initially, retained secretions mixed with necrotic tumor produced major post-therapy airway compromise, which necessitated intensive care unit management with intubation and assisted ventilation. At present, the only major acute problems after this therapy are delayed hemorrhage, which is rare, and hypoxemia, which can usually be managed by toilet bronchoscopy.

Results

Lam, et al. (1986), in evaluating 24 patients treated with PDT for tracheobronchial malignancy, found that CT and radionuclide quantitative ventilation/perfusion lung scans were useful in addition to bronchoscopic examination in determining the response of patients with obstructive endobronchial tumors to photodynamic therapy. PDT was found to be most effective when the tumor was bronchoscopically polypoid in appearance, with little or no submucosal invasion or peribronchial extensions seen on CT scan. With increasing submucosal and/or peribronchial extension, the immediate response to therapy was poor. Patients who had 50 percent or more airway obstruction due to mucosal tumor had no evidence of local tumor recurrence for a median interval of 22 weeks after therapy. In patients with predominate submucosal and/or peribronchial tumor, the duration of response was 7 weeks.

Hayata, et al. (1989), in treating 127 patients during 151 therapeutic courses, identified a complete response in 27 percent, a significant response (greater than 60 percent reduction) in 56 percent, a partial response (20 to 59 percent reduction) in 18.5 percent, and no response (less than 20 percent reduction) in 0 percent. Thirteen early lesions were treated initially with PDT and then followed by surgery. In 4 instances complete pathologic responses (31 percent) were found at the time of resection. Of these, 12 of 13 patients were alive and free of disease 3 to 61 months postoperatively.

Cortese (1987) reported the results of PDT in patients with small tumors less than 3 cm.³ In 10 such tumors, a complete response was identified after PDT, and the patients were followed from 3 to 38 months post-therapy. Seven of these patients were alive and free of disease at follow-up. One at death due to other causes; there was no local recurrence in this patient. All these patients had lesions less than 3 cm³ and had negative pretherapy chest radiographic findings. Contrasted with these results were those in 20 patients with larger tumors who had less than complete pathologic responses to PDT and were followed 6 days to 46 months post-therapy. Of these 11 were alive at follow-up; most had local recurrences identified by bronchoscopy. These represented larger tumors that were visible on the chest radiograph in 12 of 20 instances.

Discussion

The indications for therapy are similar to those for patients treated by Nd:YAG laser therapy. They include obstructive lesions of the trachea, carina, and mainstem bronchi in patients with major life-threatening symptoms caused by progressive occlusion that may have been previously treated with conventional therapies. The favorable response to therapy approximates 80 to 85 percent—much the same as with the other, more conventional laser therapies.

The recent introduction of the Nd:YAG laser, which can provide dramatic and rapid palliation by debulking large endobronchial tumors, has limited the role of PDT in the palliation of major tracheobronchial malignancies. However, PDT can offer an alternative to other forms of therapy in carefully selected patients with in situ or early invasive squamous cell carcinoma of the bronchus and in patients who have diffuse endothelial malignant changes primarily postoperatively and who have been rejected for or have not responded to conventional radiotherapy and chemotherapy.

SUMMARY

The use of laser therapy for endobronchial lesions has met with general enthusiasm. From published series it is difficult to determine specific indications for its use, based on patients' complaints, locations of the tumor, and any concomitant therapies. Most reports do not provide sufficient information to permit adequate comparisons in regard to improvement in symptoms and long-term efficacy. Exophytic lesions of the trachea and mainstem bronchi are most amenable to therapy by laser, and the improvement in symptoms correlates best with the improved patency of large airways. In most patients, the major portion of the endobronchial debulking procedure can be performed quickly and safely by physically coring out the exophytic tumor mass with the rigid end of the bronchoscope. A large biopsy forceps can help accomplish this with very little bleeding. The laser can then remove any remaining tumor and produce hemostasis by coagulation of the tumor bed.

The major purpose of laser therapy is to lessen or completely relieve the symptoms of airway obstruction. Laser therapy to obstructed lobar or segmental bronchi rarely reduces symptoms unless they are associated with postobstructive pneumonia. When the obstruction is long-standing, laser ablation may not establish airway patency. Hemoptysis from exophytic lesions can usually be well controlled. Therapy for lesions that produce extrinsic compression of the trachea or bronchi is of little value.

At present, laser therapy is one of several therapies available for neoplastic endotracheal or endobronchial obstruction. Other local therapies include external beam irradiation, cryotherapy, electrocoagulative therapy, and intraluminal brachytherapy with the insertion of afterloading catheters.

Most of these modalities are available in large oncologic centers, and it will take the better part of the next decade to identify specific indications for each of these therapies individually and in combination.

Currently, Nd:YAG therapy plays an established role in palliative therapy for obstructive endobronchial disease. The response rates to therapy with the relief of obstruction are in the range of 80 to 85 percent. Nd:YAG therapy is easy, quick, and (with proper caution) safe. In most cases, it must be repeated on one or several occasions. PDT is now being critically evaluated for therapy for similar lesions.

COMMENTS AND CONTROVERSIES

Other than the use of the argon laser with hematoporphyrin derivatives, laser endoscopy is usually a palliative technique using yet another form of thermal destruction. Other methods to relieve airway obstructions include the simple coring-out technique best described by Mathisen, endoscopic electrocautery, and endoscopic cryotherapy. All of these techniques form the armamentarium that may be of value in opening airways.

The authors do not discuss post-laser management in detail. In many instances, where the patient has not been exposed to radiotherapy, following such laser palliation, the patient should be referred for palliative radiotherapy to delay onset of further obstruction and avoid repeated laser treatments. Similarly, in those patients who have received all palliative modalities or present with extrinsic compressing lesions, intraluminal stents of the silicone or expandable wire

mesh variety can be employed to avoid repeated hospitalizations for airway obstruction (see the following section of this chapter).

This laser technology is valuable. I personally prefer the CO_2 laser for large airway obstructions. With increased wattage, the rapidity of destruction can be almost equivalent to that seen with the Nd:YAG system. The big advantage of the CO_2 laser is you can coagulate only what you see. With the Nd:YAG system, tissue destruction occurs for at least 4 or 5 mm beyond the tumor into the wall of the airway. This can lead to late hemorrhage and exsanguination. This is especially dangerous if lobar bronchi are treated where the pulmonary arteries lie extremely close to the bifurcation of the lobar airways.

R.J.G.

REFERENCES

Brutinel WM, Cortese DA, McDougall JC et al: A two year experience with neodymium-YAG laser in endobronchial obstruction. Chest 91:159, 1987

Cavalière S, Foccoli P, Farina PL: Nd:YAG laser bronchoscopy. A five-year experience with 1396 applications in 1000 patients. Chest 94:15, 1988

Cortese DA: Bronchoscopic phototherapy with hematoporphyrin derivative and argon dye laser. In: Endoscopic Laser Surgery Handbook. Marcel Dekker, New York, 1987

Dierkesmann R: Indication and results of endobronchial laser therapy. Lung (suppl):1095, 1990

Dougherty TJ, Kaufman JE, Goldfarb A et al: Photoradiation therapy for the treatment of malignant tumors. Cancer Res 38:2628, 1978

Dumon JF, Meric B, Dumon MC: Tracheobronchial stent. The 8th world congress for bronchology and bronchoesophagology, abstracted Munich, 1994

Dumon JF: Applications of the neodymium:yttrium-aluminum-garnet laser in bronchology. p. 206. In: Endoscopic Surgery Handbook. Marcel Dekker, New York, 1987

Dumon JF, Rebund E, Garbe L et al: Treatment of tracheobronchial lesions by laser photoresection. Chest 81:278, 1982

Edell E, Shapsay S: Laser bronchoscopy. In Prakush U (ed): Bronchoscopy. Raven Press, New York, 1994

Einstein A: On the quantum theory of radiation. Physikal Z 18:121, 1917

George PJM, Clarke G, Tolfree S et al: Changes in regional ventilation and perfusion of the lung after endoscopic laser treatment. Thorax 45:248, 253, 1990

Hayata Y, Oho K, Kato H: Laser treatment of tracheobronchial lesions. In: Thoracic Surgery: Frontiers and Uncommon Neoplasms. CV Mosby, St. Louis, 1989

Hetzel MR, Nixon C, Edmondstone WM et al: Laser therapy in 100 tracheobronchial tumors. Thorax 40:341, 1985

Jain PR, Dedhia HV, Lapp NL et al: Nd:YAG laser followed by radiation for treatment of malignant airway lesions. Lasers Surg Med 5:47, 1985

Joyner LR, Maran AG, Sarama R et al: Neodymium-YAG laser treatment of intrabronchial lesions. Chest 87:418, 1985

Laforet EG, Berger RL, Vaughn CW: Carcinoma obstructing the trachea: treatment by laser resection. N Engl J Med 214:941, 1976

Lam S, Muller NL, Miller RR et al: Predicting the response of obstructive endobronchial tumors to photodynamic therapy. Cancer 58:2298, 1986

Lipson RL, Baldes EJ, Olsen AM: The use of a derivative of hematoporphyrin in tumor detection. J Natl Cancer Inst 26:1, 1961

Maire R, Monnier PH: Le laser-YAG dans le traitement endoscopique palliatif du cancer trachéo-bronchique: indications, modalités et résultats. ORL, Aktuelle Probleme der Otorhinolaryngologie 12:146, 1989

Miller JI: Comparison of Nd:YAG and CO_2 laser bronchoscopy in the management of tracheobronchial lesions. In: Thoracic Surgery: Frontiers and Uncommon Neoplasms. CV Mosby, St. Louis, 1989

Mohsenifar Z, Jasper AC, Koerner SK: Physiologic assessment of lung function in patients undergoing laser photoresection of tracheobronchial tumors. Chest 93:65, 1988

Monnier PH, Fontolliet CH, Wagnières G et al: The possibilities and limitations of the endoscopic and photodynamic treatments of early squamous cell cancer of the upper aero-digestive tract, bronchi and oesophagus. Acta endoscopica 21:641, 1991

Mudry A, Monnier PH: Les sténoses cicatricielles glotto-sous-glottiques: place du traitement endoscopique. ORL Aktuelle Probleme der Otorhinolaryngologie 17:137, 1994

Oho K, Ogawa I, Amemiya R et al: Indication for endoscopic Nd:YAG laser surgery in the trachea and bronchus. Endoscopy 15:302, 1983

Ross D, Mohsenifar Z, Koerner SK: Survival characteristics after Neodymium:YAG laser photoresection in advanced stage lung cancer. Chest 98:581, 1990

Shapshay S: Endoscopic treatment of subglottic and tracheal stenosis by radial laser incision and dilatation. Ann Otol Rhinol Laryngol 96:661, 1987

Simpson GT, Strong MS, Healy GB et al: Predictive factors of success or failure in the endoscopic management of laryngeal and tracheal stenosis. Ann Otol Rhinol Laryngol 91:384, 1982

Smith SGT, Bedwell J, MacRobert AJ et al: Experimental studies to assess the potential of photodynamic therapy for the treatment of bronchial carcinomas. Thorax 48:474, 1993

Strong MS, Jako JG: Laser surgery in the larynx: early clinical experience with continuous CO_2 laser and soft tissues. Ann Otol Rhinol Laryngol 81:791, 1972

Toty L, Personne C, Hertzog P et al: Utilisation d'un faisceau laser (YAG) à conducteur souple, pour le traitement endoscopique de certaines lésions trachéobronchiques. Rev Fr Mal Respir 7:57, 1979

Unger M: Neodymium:YAG laser therapy for malignant and benign endobronchial lesion. Clin Chest Med 6:277, 1985

Tracheobronchial Stents

Henning A. Gaissert
G. A. Patterson

The purpose of tracheobronchial stents is to maintain airway patency through strictures not amenable to resection and reconstruction. In contrast to tracheostomy tubes, these stents permit translaryngeal air flow and thereby provide for a humidified airway and preservation of the voice. Stents have been used successfully in a variety of benign and malignant airway strictures. They are placed under bronchoscopic control and may reside in the airway lumen for extended periods. Most experience has been gained with tubes made of silicone rubber. Wire mesh tubes have been introduced in recent years; however, long-term experience with their use is limited.

HISTORICAL NOTE

The concept of stenting to treat airways disease probably originated toward the end of the last century, although tracheostomy tubes have been known for much longer. Trendelenburg (1872) of Berlin reported the use of a metal coil spring covered with rubber tubing to stent a stenosis of the cervical trachea temporarily in a young woman. The T-shaped tracheotomy tube depicted in Figure 12-26 was described in a brief case report by the surgeon Bond (1891) in 1891. This metal cannula was made for a tracheal stricture caused by a suicidal knife wound. It consisted of two halves that were separately introduced into the trachea and held together by a metal collar fixed with a screw over an external sidearm. The sidearm was closed to allow the patient to breathe and talk naturally.

Montgomery (1965) used a similar device made of rigid acrylic in 1964 and later modified this tube with flexible silicone rubber. Subsequent reports emphasized the safety and success of T tubes in the therapy of subglottic stenosis (Montgomery, 1968), in the palliation of malignant strictures, as a temporizing therapy prior to definitive tracheal resection, and for salvage of the airway after failed reconstruction (Cooper, et al., 1981). Tracheobronchial Y stents and straight endobronchial stents have been developed more recently as permanent palliative devices. Such stents have been invaluable in the management of airway complications after lung transplantation.

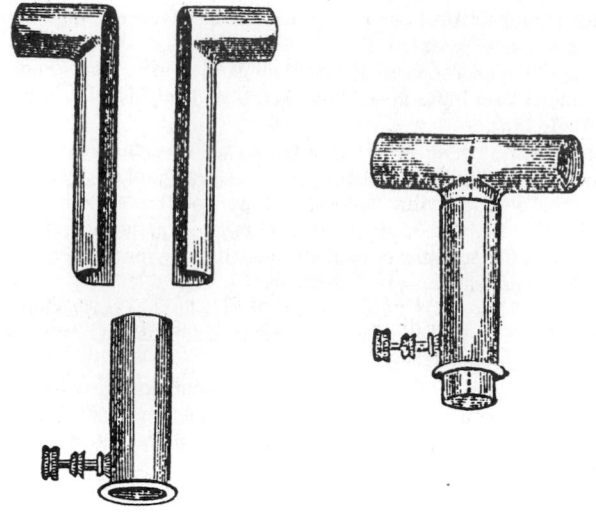

Figure 12-26. Bond's tracheal T tube. (From Bond CJ: Note on the treatment of tracheal stenosis by a new T-shaped tracheotomy tube. Lancet 1:539, 1891, with permission.)

The purpose of the original Montgomery tube was the definitive therapy of strictures in the cervical trachea. It has been repeatedly demonstrated that the inert Silastic material allows airway epithelium to resurface a granulating stricture. However, current experience suggests that most tracheal strictures will not respond to transient stenting alone and require additional reconstructive procedures because of the concurrent loss of stabilizing cartilage.

HISTORICAL READINGS

Bond CJ: Note on the treatment of tracheal stenosis by a new T-shaped tracheotomy tube. Lancet 1:539, 1891

Montgomery WW: T-tube tracheal stent. Arch Otolaryngol Head Neck Surg 82:320, 1965

Trendelenburg F: Beitraege zu den Operationen an den Luftwegen. Langenbecks Arch Chir 13:335, 1872

INDICATIONS

Airway stents are used for benign and malignant strictures that require repeated dilatation and are unsuitable for surgical reconstruction. The general condition of the patient may preclude safe resection because of the presence of prohibitive perioperative risk factors, the likelihood of postoperative ventilator dependence, or the use of high-dose steroid medication. The stricture may have anatomic characteristics that indicate the need for stenting, such as extensive length or poor quality of the remaining airway. The presence of active tracheobronchial inflammation may call for a delay of reconstructive procedures to allow an accurate estimation of the true length of the involved airway at a later date.

Tracheal lesions most commonly in need of stenting are produced by the effects of long-term mechanical ventilatory support. Strictures at the site of the endotracheal tube cuff, a previous tracheostomy site, or in the subglottic space may require stenting prior or subsequent to resection. Such postintubation strictures and inflammatory strictures that occur as a result of burn injury were among the most common indications for T-tube insertion in the Massachusetts General Hospital experience (Table 12-5). The palliation of malignant obstruction by either an intrinsic endoluminal tumor or an extrinsic tumor compression is a further important indication.

Isolated bronchial stenosis that is not amenable to surgical resection or dilatation is rare. The emergence of lung transplantation as an accepted therapy for end-stage lung disease has been accompanied by complications at the airway anastomosis. The incidence of such complications is high after en bloc double-lung transplantations that use a single tracheal anastomosis without bronchial revascularization. The incidence of airway complications has been reduced dramatically by improved allograft preservation, superior immunosuppression, and the introduction of bilateral bronchial anastomoses (Patterson, et al., 1990). However, ischemia at the bronchial suture line remains an important cause of delayed anastomotic healing in approximately 19 percent of patients and results in stricture development in 6 percent of patients (Cooper, et al., 1994).

STENT TYPES

An airway stent should not interfere with usual daily activities and be easily placed and replaced in the event of dislodgement. The properties expected from an airway stent are restoration of a sufficient luminal diameter, undisturbed passage of air through the larynx to provide for humidification of inspired air and phonation, minimal interference with clearance of secretions, a simple cleaning procedure (if at all necessary), and uncomplicated removal once it becomes obstructed or is no longer needed.

Table 12-5. Diagnosis in 140 Patients Undergoing T-Tube Placement at the Massachusetts General Hospital

Diagnosis	No. Patients
Postintubation stenosis	86
Burn	13
Malignant airway tumor	12
Radiation stenosis	4
Relapsing polychondritis	4
Tracheomalacia	4
Vascular malformation	3
Sarcoidosis	2
Trauma	2
Necrotizing tracheitis	2
Mucopolysaccharidosis	2
Postpneumonectomy syndrome	2
Tracheobronchomegaly (Mounier-Kuhn)	1
Tuberculosis	1
Idiopathic stenosis	1
Tracheopathia osteoplastica	1

(From Gaissert HA, Grillo HC, Mathisen DJ, Wain JC: Temporary and permanent restoration of airway continuity with the tracheal T-tube. J Thorac Cardiovasc Surg 107:600, 1994, with permission.)

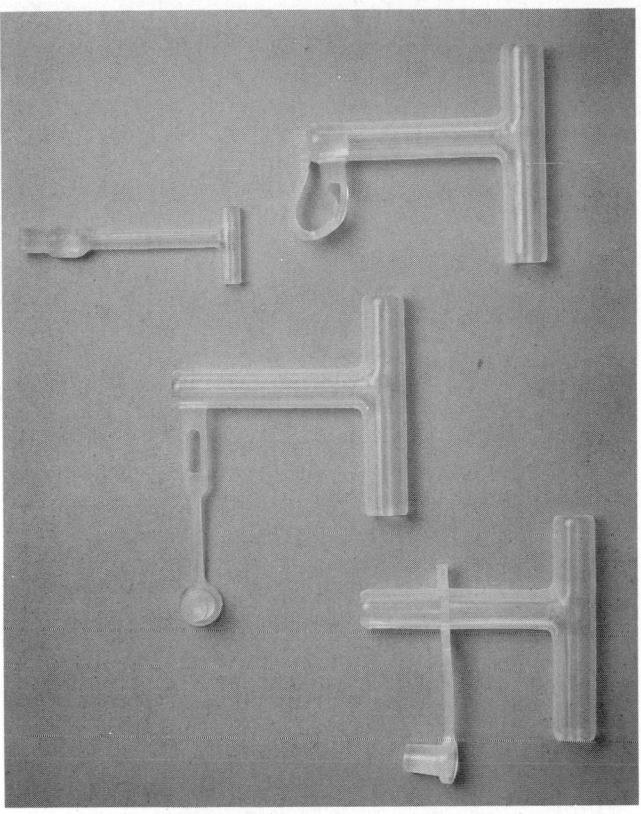

Figure 12-27.   Silicone tracheal T-tube. (Courtesy of Hood Laboratories, Pembroke, MA.)

Tracheal T Tube

The largest clinical experience in the therapy of tracheal strictures has been gained with the silicone T tube. These tubes are generally well tolerated and reliable. Once they are inserted, they function for long periods, in some patients for many years, without causing further damage to the tracheal wall.

The T tube is a hollow cylinder made of medical-grade silicone rubber, in continuity with a sidearm that is closed with a plug (Fig. 12-27). The tube is produced in sizes from 4.5 to 16 mm outer diameter (Hood Laboratories, Pembroke, MA). Sizes 4.5 to 9 are generally used for infants and children, 10 to 14 for women, and 12 to 16 for men. The upper and lower limbs of the tube are manufactured in various lengths and can be custom-made to meet individual specifications. Further modifications of the T tube, with and without the sidearm, are used to stent unilateral main bronchial strictures.

TY Tube

The therapy of benign and malignant strictures with diffuse involvement of the trachea and main bronchi or local obstruction at the carina is challenging. Westaby, et al. (1982) described a modified T tube by the addition of a Y-shaped extension for intubation of both main bronchi. TY tubes contain a bifurcated extension to fit into carina and both main bronchial lumina (Fig. 12-28). Accurate placement of this tube is particularly important to achieve a correct fit for the two angulations at the stoma and the carina. TY tubes are therefore usually custom-made for an individual patient. Be-

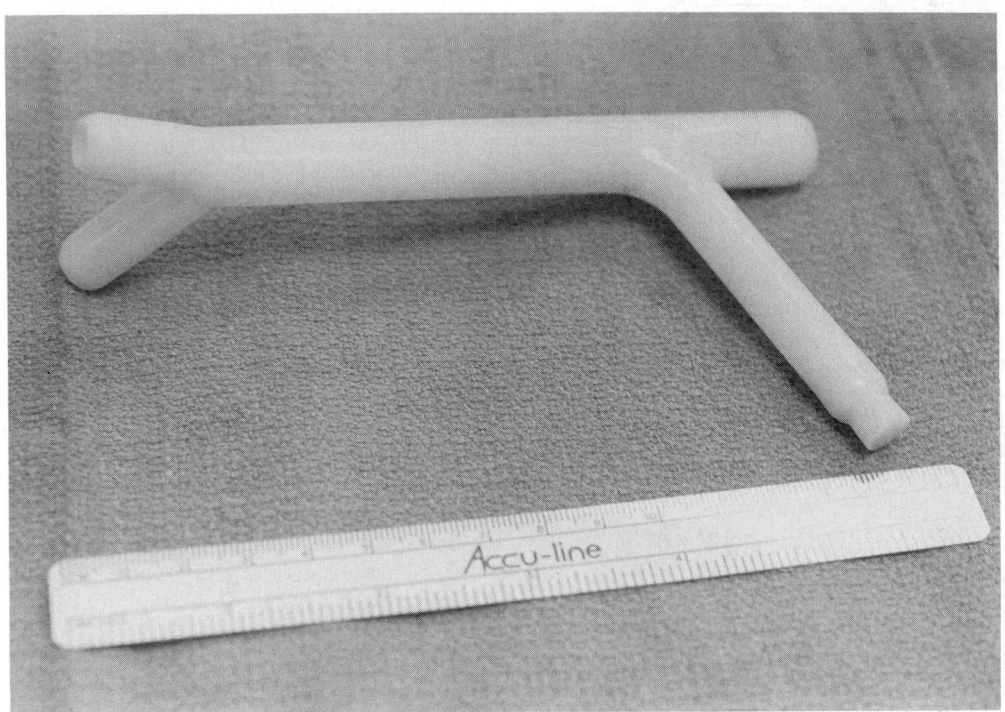

Figure 12-28.   TY tube.

cause of their length and two points of fixation, these tubes may cause granulations in the area where the edge of the tube is in contact with the wall of the smaller-caliber main bronchus. However, successful long-term intubation has been performed in many children and adults.

Y Stent

The bifurcated Y tubes have been particularly useful in patients without tracheal stomas who have tracheal or proximal main bronchial strictures. Tracheal, carinal, or proximal bronchial compression by a tumor can be effectively palliated by such stents. Various left main bronchial limb lengths are available (Fig. 12-29).

Bronchial Stent

Straight silicone endobronchial stents are available with outer diameters from 6 to 10 mm or as customized tubes (Hood Laboratories, Pembroke, MA) (Fig. 12-30). These tubes are flanged on both ends to prevent dislodgement and have remained in place in patients for extended periods. The selection of a correct stent size and length is critically important. The tube must be long enough to enable its flanges to anchor the tube within the stricture, short enough to avoid compromise of a lobar bronchus distally or the trachea proximally, and of satisfactory diameter to maintain the caliber of the airway. In our early experience, we fashioned bronchial stents from the side arm of a T tube. This is still used on

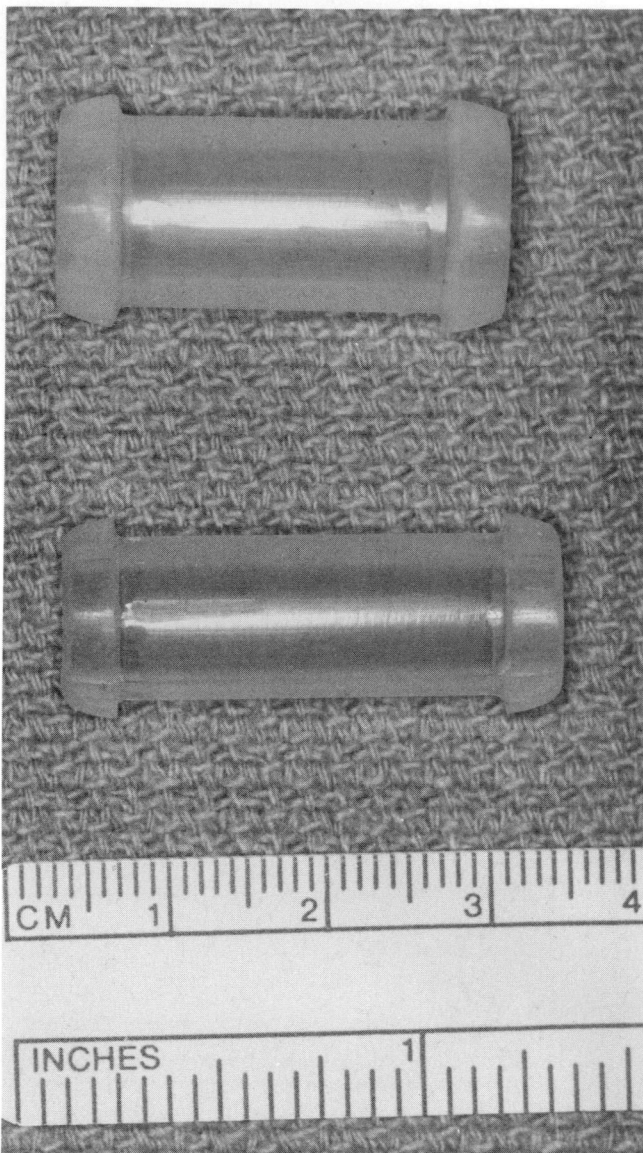

Figure 12-30. Bronchial stent with flange.

...ccasion to create an elliptic distal flange that will seat nicely at the point of bronchial bifurcation.

Dumon (1990) introduced a Silastic stent for use specifically in the trachea and bronchus (Fig. 12-31). Four rows of studs oriented at 90-degree angles on the external surface are intended to prevent dislodgement (Bryan, Woburn, MA). He reported on 118 stents placed in 66 patients, of whom 38 had malignant disease. Eleven patients had more than one stent placed simultaneously. Cannular migration occurred in 12 instances. Relief of obstructive symptoms was achieved in all but two patients. The overall tolerance appears to be similar to that of other silicone tubes.

Wire Stent

Wire stents of the Gianturco or Wallstent type have been introduced to palliate strictures of the biliary tree, but they

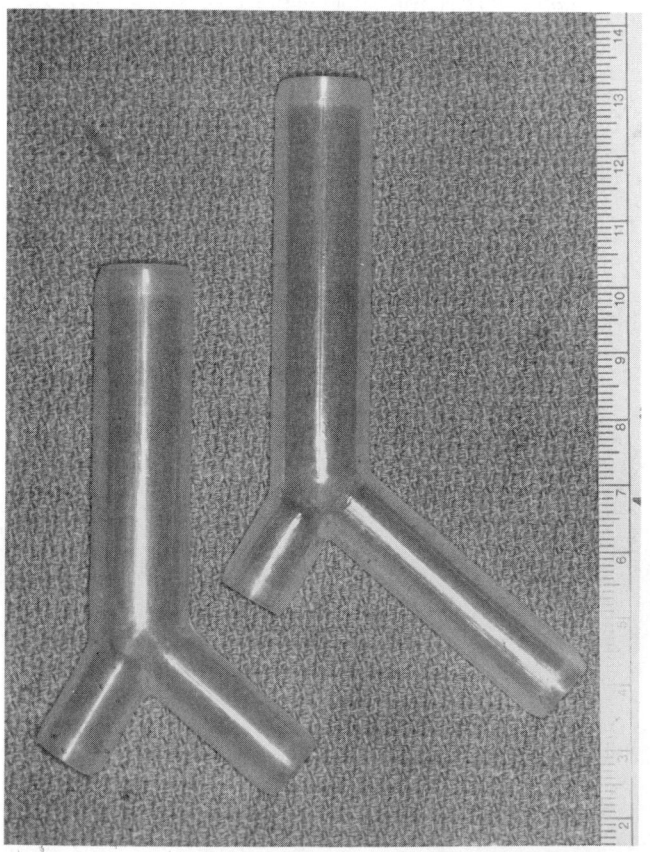

Figure 12-29. Y stent.

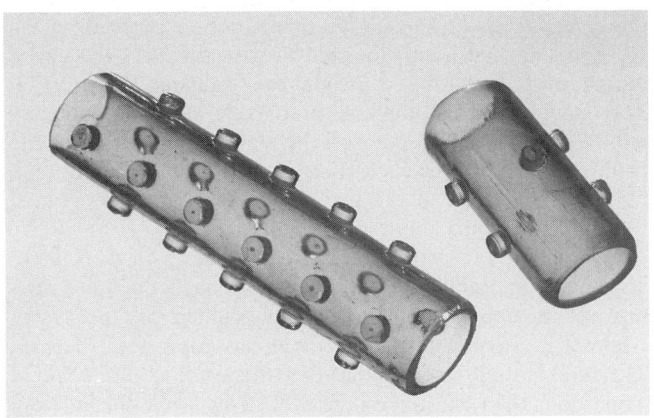

Figure 12-31. Dumon studded endobronchial stent. (Courtesy of Bryan Corp., Woburn, MA.)

were more recently applied in the therapy of airways disease. The Gianturco stent (Cook Co., Bloomington, IN) is a stainless steel wire shaped in a cylindric zig-zag formation of 5 to 10 turns (Fig. 12-32). These stents are discharged from a cartridge. The Wallstent (Schneider Co., Minneapolis, MN) consists of woven filaments of alloy steel released from an introducer catheter. Currently neither model is approved for use in the airway in the United States or Canada. Their presumed advantage is a thinner wall, which consists of a large-pore mesh and thus takes up less of the airway diameter and allows the tube to ride across while aeration is provided to a lobar or segmental bronchial orifice. After insertion the wire tube expands to a predetermined diameter, and overgrowth of epithelium embeds the wire. Although this process is desirable to facilitate natural mucociliary clearance, the

wire is difficult if not impossible to remove at this point. These stents have a particular attraction when the airway mucosa is intact, as in tracheobronchial malacia or extrinsic compression by a tumor.

In inflammatory strictures with active granulation tissue, the stricture often recurs inside the lumen of the wire mesh. In an effort to avoid this problem, Cooper designed a modification of the Gianturco stent (Fig. 12-32). A thin film of plastic is secured to the outer wall of the expanded wire stent. These stents can be collapsed into a small-caliber rigid bronchoscope released into place under direct vision. We were encouraged by the preliminary results in a small number of patients. Because most wire stents have been inserted for only brief periods to palliate malignant obstruction, limited information is available in regard to the long-term outcome and complications.

INSERTION TECHNIQUE

All patients under consideration for the placement of a tracheobronchial stent undergo a complete examination of their airway. Endoscopic evaluation of the airway must be performed in an anesthetized, spontaneously breathing patient. Muscular paralysis, while advantageous for vigorous dilatation and stent placement, must not be instituted until a detailed examination is completed and the surgeon is certain an airway can be subsequently maintained. Optimal assessment of the lower airway anatomy is obtained with flexible bronchoscopy. Assessment of fixation, precise measurements, and satisfactory dilatation is best achieved by rigid bronchoscopic equipment. The patency and function of the larynx should be ascertained with a laryngoscopic examination, particularly if the stent replaces a tracheostomy. The condition of the vocal cords, the size of the subglottic space,

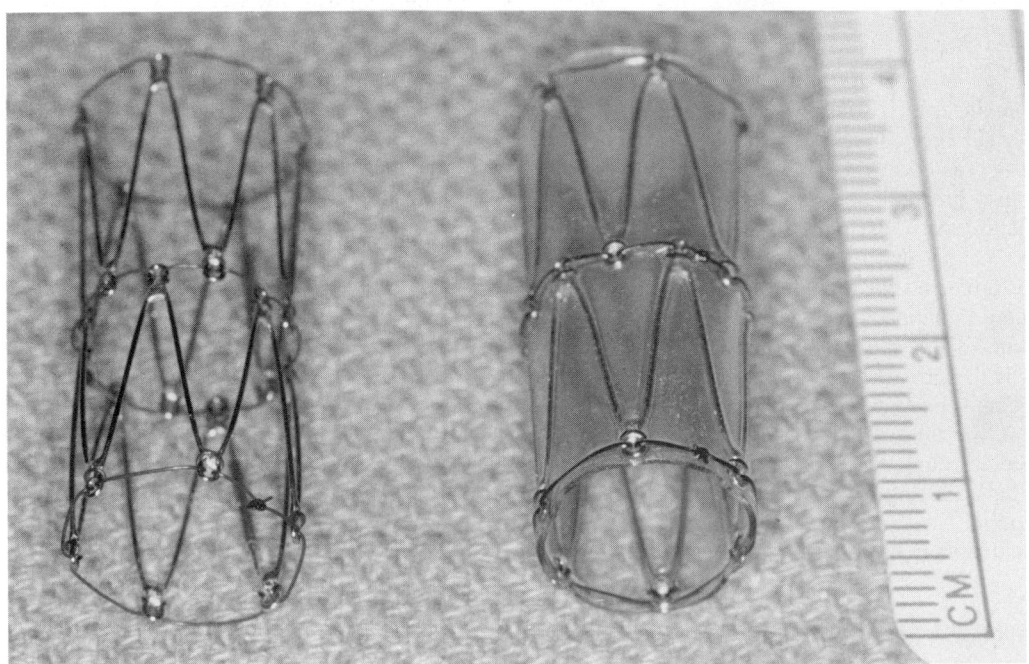

Figure 12-32. Gianturco wire stent. Original stent on the left; modified, Craton-covered version on the right.

and the proximity of the stricture to the larynx should be visualized. The distance from the vocal cords to the carina and tracheal stoma and from the upper and lower extent of the stricture to these reference points is recorded. The required stent dimensions and the need for a custom-designed tube are determined.

Dilatation

Rigid endoscopy should be used exclusively for dilatation of airway strictures. The Holinger bronchoscope is suitable to dilate tracheal and bronchial strictures with a preserved, recognizable lumen. This endoscope has a round lip, which for this purpose, is insinuated into the stricture and advanced in a corkscrew motion. The dilatation is started with a small pediatric-size instrument and continued with larger sizes. A particularly tight stricture can be initially stretched with peripheral vascular angioplasty catheters of various sizes inflated under direct bronchoscopic vision. Gum-tipped Jackson esophageal dilators are used when there is uncertainty about the course of the lumen. They are also helpful in the dilatation of laryngeal and subglottic strictures. Hegar dilators are well suited for tracheal dilatation through a stoma. Dilatation to a diameter at least as big as the external diameter of the intended stent is advisable.

Ventilation

Jet ventilation with Venturi ventilation is used through the rigid bronchoscope for most routine dilatations and stent placements. Intraoperative ventilation through a T tube is provided by the operator fitting the sidearm with a suitable 15-mm endotracheal tube adapter and ventilating with high tidal volumes to compensate for the escape of gases through the upper limb. Alternatively intermittent ventilation through the stoma can be used.

T-Tube Insertion

T tubes may be inserted through the tracheal stoma or, mounted on a rigid bronchoscope, through the mouth. A tracheal stoma is created at the time of T-tube insertion, if it is not previously present. Standard insertion through the stoma is satisfactory for most patients; the latter technique provides control of the airway during the entire procedure and is therefore preferred for unstable patients with critical stenosis or limited pulmonary reserve.

Correct seating of the stent in the airway is critical for success. In particular pressure of the edge of the tube on the mucosal surface must be avoided to prevent granulation. For the same reason, the tube should terminate well below the cords or be placed through the true vocal cords. The cannula is trimmed in the operating room with a scalpel blade, and the edges are rounded with sterilized sandpaper. To achieve a perfect fit, the tube may have to be reinserted and trimmed several times.

Insertion Through the Stoma

For standard insertion of a T tube, the lower limb of the tube is introduced into the tracheal stoma and advanced toward the carina (Fig. 12-33A). The upper limb is grasped with a Kelly clamp and gently pushed downward until the entire length of the T tube is inside the tracheal lumen (Fig. 12-33B&C). At this point the first Kelly clamp is detached while a second clamp pulls on the sidearm to straighten the cannula inside the trachea (Fig. 12-33D). This maneuver is difficult to perform if the tip of the tube has to be guided through a stricture above the stoma.

For modified insertion through the stoma with a bronchoscope, a long umbilical tape is passed both through the sidearm and the upper limb of a T tube and guided into the stoma, where it is grasped with a rigid bronchoscope (Fig. 12-34A). The tube is then inserted into the trachea (Fig. 12-34B&C). Traction is then exerted on the oral string while the sidearm tape is kept steady (Fig. 12-34D).

Peroral Insertion

To place a T tube through the mouth, a well-lubricated endotracheal tube is passed over a rigid bronchoscope. The silicone cannula is mounted on the tip of the bronchoscope, and the entire assembly is advanced into the airway. When the stent is in the proposed position, it is pushed off with the endotracheal tube while the bronchoscope is withdrawn. A heavy-gauge suture fixed to the sidearm and previously passed by mouth through the stoma is then grasped to guide the sidearm properly through the stoma. The position of the tube is inspected with a fiberoptic bronchoscope.

An alternative peroral method was described by Cooper, et al. (1989). A Pilling bronchoscope is fitted with a balloon. When this is inflated, it will firmly hold a T tube in place for insertion (Fig. 12-35). The advantage of this technique is that direct vision of the airway and ventilation is maintained throughout the placement.

Stenting Glottic Airway

In strictures that extend to the vocal cords, in the presence of active mucosal inflammation that involves the glottic or subglottic larynx or in the immediate postoperative period after a high subglottic anastomosis, the laryngeal airway is often obstructed. The placement of the upper end of a T tube immediately below the cords results in granulations beneath the cords and increased obstruction. In this circumstance the tube is positioned above the true vocal cords to terminate below the false cords, as proposed by Cooper, et al. (1981). Aspiration is prevented by an approximation of the false cords and epiglottic closure, and any contact with the undersurface of the epiglottis must be prevented. Patients are able to talk with a whispered voice, which usually improves over time. A supraglottic tube may remain in place for periods of months to more than 1 year, without deterioration of vocal cord function. This use of the T tube has particular application in the therapy of inflammatory strictures related to inhalation injury (Gaissert, et al., 1993).

TY-Tube Insertion

Insertion of the TY tube is accomplished through the tracheal stoma with two ureteral catheters or small-caliber gum-tipped bougies in both mainstem bronchi as guides. The cannula is

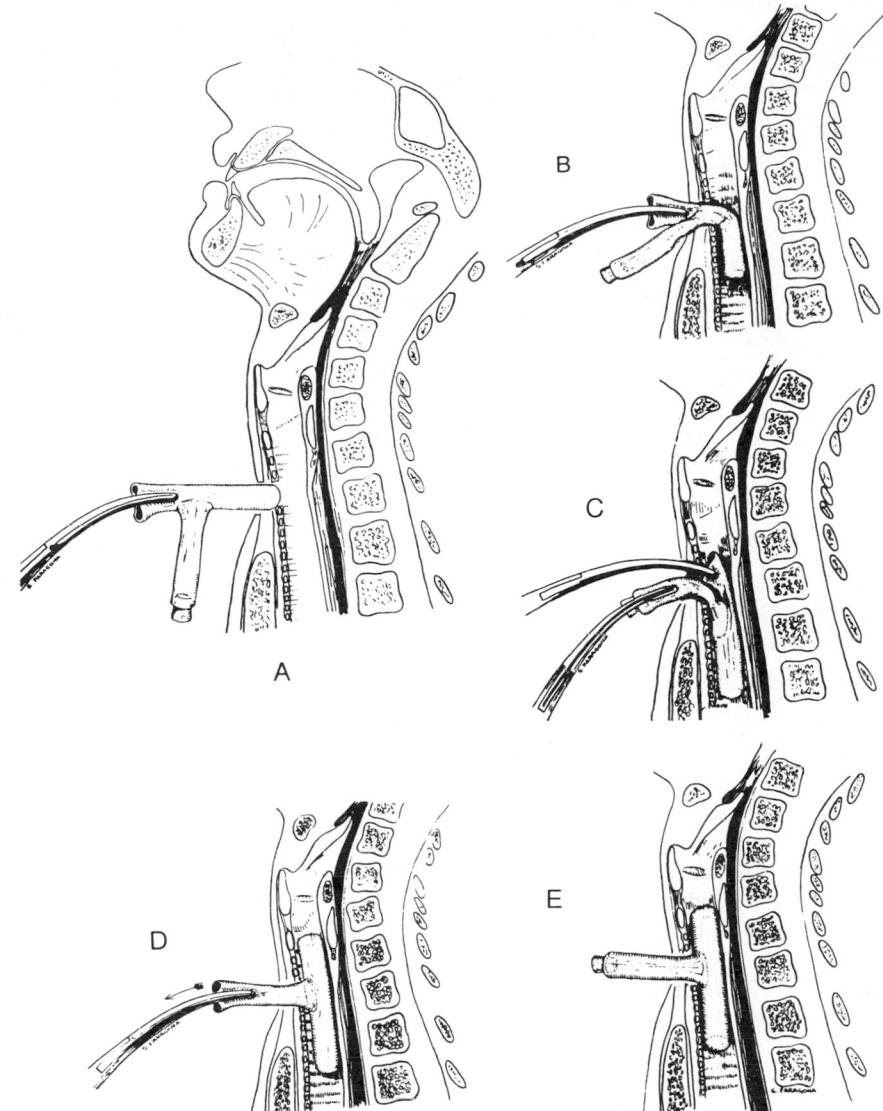

Figure 12-33. **(A–E)** T-tube insertion through the stoma. See explanation in the text. (From Landa L: The tracheal T tube: in tracheal surgery. p. 124. In Grillo HC, Eschapasse H (eds): International Trends in General Thoracic Surgery. Vol. 2. WB Saunders, Philadelphia, 1987, with permission.)

then advanced over the catheters toward the carina, and its upper limb is inserted into the cervical trachea with the standard or modified technique. Proper seating of the tube is ascertained with a flexible bronchoscope.

Y-Stent Insertion

In patients without tracheal stomas, Y tubes are placed as shown in Figure 12-36. The right limb is inverted into the tracheal limb. A rigid bronchoscope, premounted with an 8.5- or 9-mm endotracheal tube, is advanced through the left limb of the Y tube. The bronchoscope is passed to the desired location in the left main bronchus and then withdrawn; the stent is left in place. Through the rigid scope, now in the tracheal portion of the stent, a biopsy forceps is used to place the invaginated right limb out into the right main bronchus.

The above described technique for the insertion of TY tubes with catheters or bougies as guides may also be used but is more tedious.

Bronchial Stent Insertion

In our experience the Hood stent was used for bronchial stent insertion. The technique is similar to that described for Y tubes. This method is straightforward for proximal right main bronchial strictures and satisfactory for proximal left main bronchial strictures. However, positioning of stents is difficult in small-caliber distal left main bronchial strictures. In lowering a 5-mm or smaller bronchoscope to pass into the distal bronchus, the surgeon's vision is obstructed by the bend in the instrument. In this circumstance the stent should be mounted on a rigid 0-degree telescope.

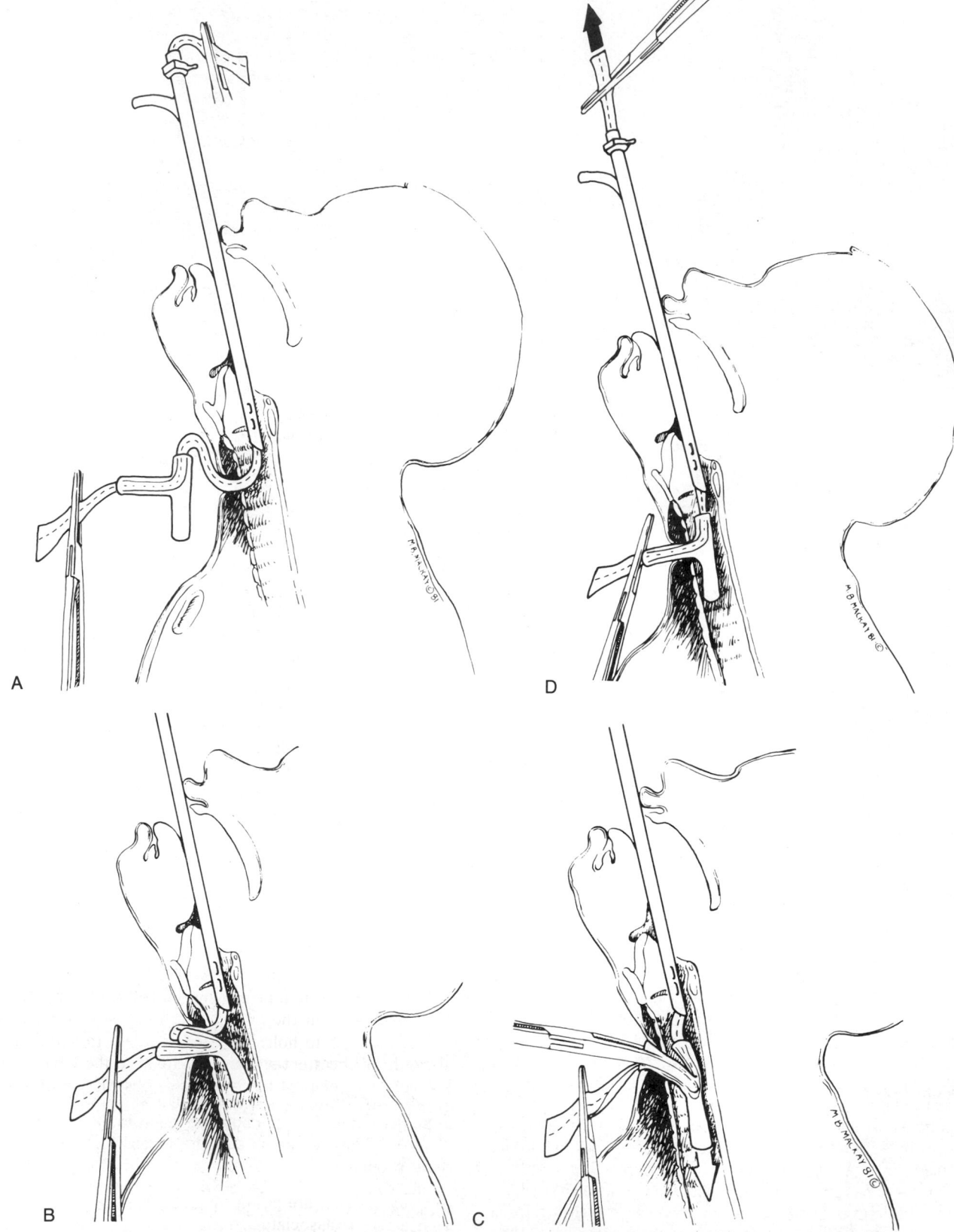

Figure 12-34.   **(A–D)** Modified T-tube insertion into the stoma using umbilical tape. See explanation in the text. (From Cooper JD, Todd TRJ, Ilves R, Pearson FG: Use of the silicone tracheal T-tube for the management of complex tracheal injuries. J Thorac Cardiovasc Surg 82:559, 1981, with permission.)

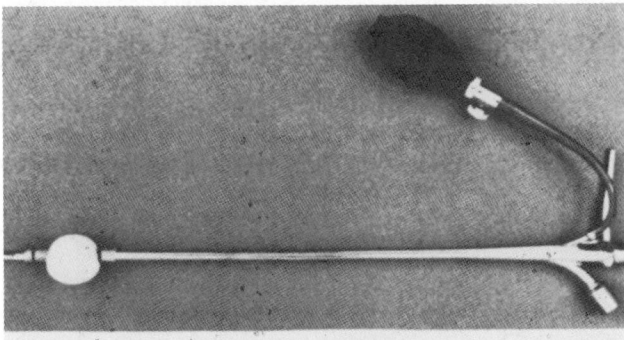

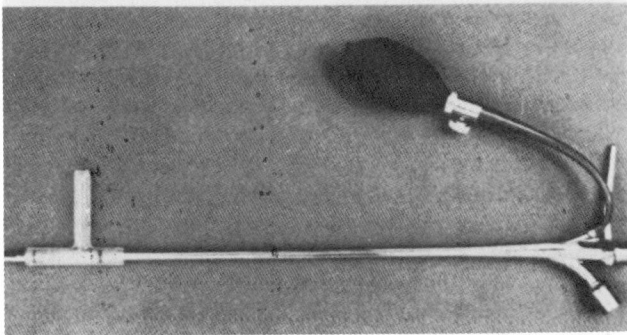

Figure 12-35. Pilling bronchoscope adapted for peroral insertion of tracheal T tube. The inflatable balloon at the tip of the bronchoscope secures the T tube during insertion. A heavy silk tie is passed through the stoma and attached to the sidearm. After translaryngeal insertion of the bronchoscope, the balloon is released, and traction on the silk tie guides the horizontal limb through the stoma. (From Cooper JD, Pearson FG, Patterson GA et al: Use of silicone stents in the management of airway problems. Ann Thorac Surg 47:371, 1989, with permission.)

T Tube in Children

T-tube placement in children is more difficult than in adults. Of 21 patients younger than the age of 20 years reported in one study, T tubes were tolerated in all 11 patients older than 10 years but failed in one-half of the children younger than 10 years (Gaissert, et al., 1994). Most failures were due to obstruction at the subglottic end of the tube. Although the success rate is lower than in adults, T-tube stenting is an important part of the management of airways disease because it allows the postponement of reconstruction until the airway has completed its growth and the chances for success are greatest.

Postoperative Care

After T-tube insertion, the sidearm is plugged when the patient has recovered from anesthesia. Transient laryngeal edema may cause temporary obstruction of the airway, which usually improves within the first 2 days. If occlusion of the sidearm is not tolerated, the sidearm is left open. Adjustments in the length or position of the tube in the operating room may be necessary. A short course of parenteral steroids may on occasion improve the local swelling.

In the first postoperative week, constant humidification of inspired air is important to keep secretions moist and prevent crusting. This is particularly important for T tubes with open sidearms and small-caliber bronchial stents. Humidity is administered with a tracheostomy mask while the sidearm is unplugged and with a face mask when it is closed. For T tubes, sterile saline solution is instilled three times daily, and the T tube is suctioned through the sidearm. After the first week, humidification is discontinued. Daily inhalations with N-acetylcysteine are continued for bronchial stents and in some patients with T tubes. The patient is taught to clean and suction the T tube independently before discharge from the hospital.

Pitfalls

T Tube

A T tube fails for three reasons: anatomic obstruction, dried secretions, or aspiration. Anatomic obstruction occurs when the tube is wedged against the wall of the airway or when contact with the sidewall causes granulation. Most commonly the point of obstruction is in the subglottic space or, in TY tubes, in the bronchus. The tip of the T tube must be tailored to avoid contact with the conus elasticus or the vocal cords during normal laryngeal excursion or cough. If the subglottic space is markedly narrowed, the T tube may have to be placed above the vocal cords. Dried secretions may occlude the lumen. This occurs when the sidearm is left open for extended periods without humidification or when the patient does not clean the tube. Aspiration may ensue when the T tube interferes with epiglottic descent and glottic closure during swallowing. However, prior episodes of aspiration, masked by a tracheostomy, may only become apparent after T-tube insertion. These problems typically occur immediately or within the first 2 months after tube placement. Often they can be corrected, and T-tube stenting should therefore not be prematurely abandoned without a further effort at placement. When the T tube is used liberally in an effort to restore translaryngeal air flow and the patient's voice, insertion may not be tolerated in as many as 20 percent of patients (Gaissert, et al., 1994).

Bronchial Stents

Because bronchial stents are not anchored to the airway like T tubes, they are prone to movement. Overdilatation of a stricture prior to stent placement or the use of a small, loose stent may prevent the tight fit at the waist of the stenosis that is required to hold the stent in place. In addition, the distal tip of the stent sits just proximal to the lobar carina. Inaccurate placement leads easily to obstruction of a lobar orifice. The stent may be placed too distally if two segmental orifices are mistaken for the lobar carina.

Wire Stent

Gianturco stents are poorly tolerated in inflammatory strictures and were associated with a high rate of migration or wire rupture in a recent study (Rousseau, et al., 1993). Erosion of adjacent pulmonary vascular structures with fatal hemorrhage has been reported (Nashef, et al., 1992).

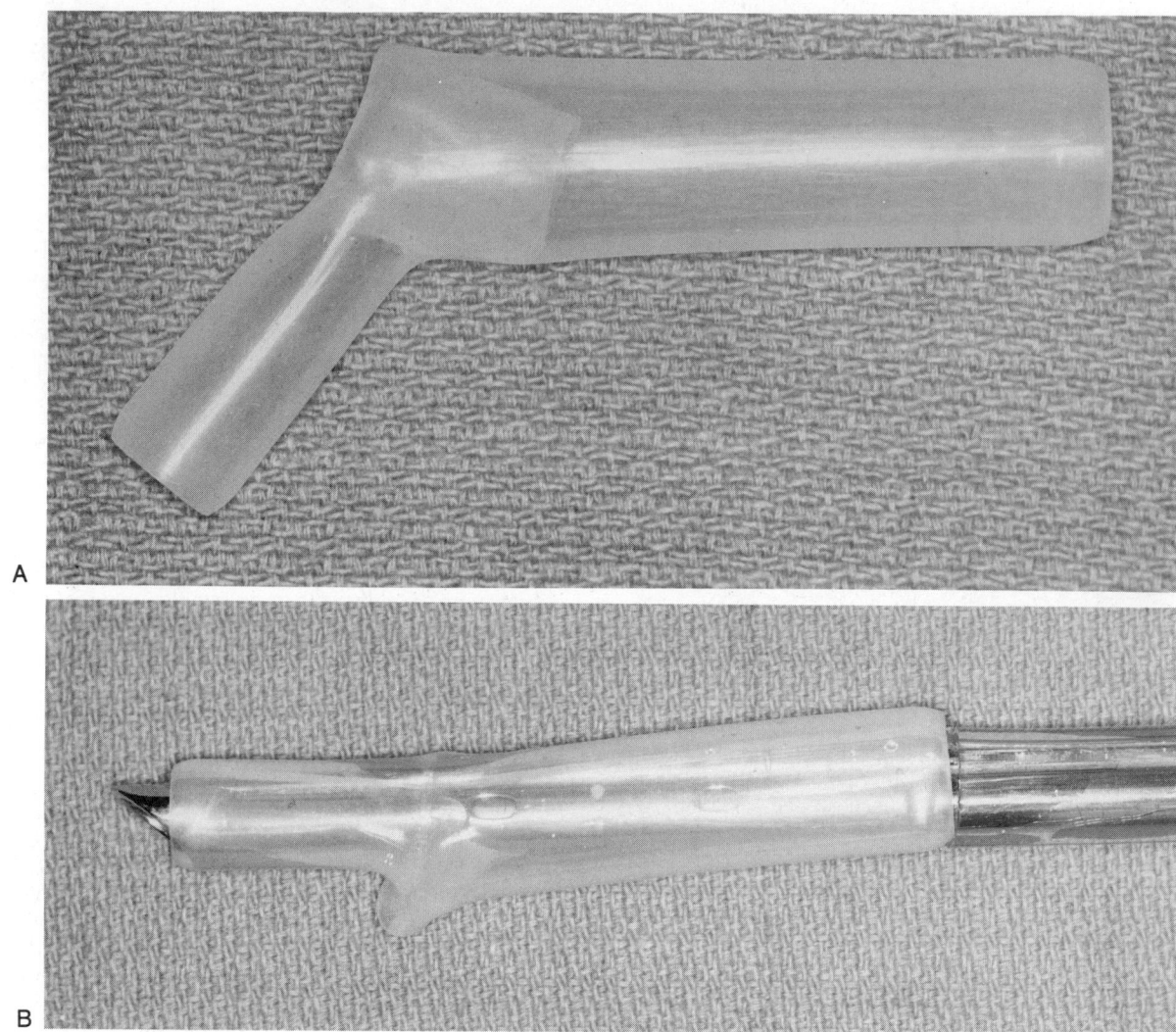

Figure 12-36. Insertion of bronchial stent. **(A)** Y stent with inverted right bronchial arm. **(B)** Bronchial stent and endotracheal tube, used as a pusher, both fitted over bronchoscope.

RESULTS

The reports by Cooper, et al. (1981, 1989) and Gaissert, et al. (1994) document the wide spectrum of airway problems approached with the T tube in a large number of patients with long follow-up periods. Table 12-6 shows the duration of

Table 12-6. Duration of T-Tube Intubation in 112 Patients

Duration of Intubation	No. Patients
Less than 1 month	5
1–3 months	12
3–12 months	46
1–5 years	37
Longer than 5 years	12

(From Gaissert HA, Grillo HC, Mathisen DJ, Wain JC: Temporary and permanent restoration of airway continuity with the tracheal T-tube. J Thorac Cardiovasc Surg 107:600, 1994, with permission.)

intubation in 112 patients after successful T-tube placement. Patients accept the T tube despite the presence of an unattractive silicone sidearm in the neck. This sidearm may even be shortened and buried under the skin, as described by Keszler (1987). Complications that necessitate stent removal occur typically within the first 2 months. Once a silicone tube remains beyond this period, long-term stenting will in all likelihood be well tolerated.

Patients typically feel immediate relief of airway obstruction after stent insertion. Gelb, et al. (1992) documented significant improvement of forced expiratory volume in 1 second and maximum expiratory flow rates in 15 patients with tracheal Y and bronchial stents. Post-transplant strictures may stabilize after prolonged intubation. Indeed in our experience, most stents are only temporarily required. The anastomotic site should therefore be inspected 6 to 12 months after insertion to determine whether bronchial patency can be maintained without the stent.

COMMENTS AND CONTROVERSIES

Surgical reconstruction is the primary and preferred therapy of a tracheal or bronchial stricture because resection removes the obstruction, is followed by excellent long-term results, and rids the patient from the nuisance of tubes. Under certain circumstances an operation is not advised, and a tracheobronchial stent may offer excellent palliation. We prefer silicone cannulas, such as the T tube or bronchial stent, because they are nonreactive, well tolerated, and easily removable.

Although some features of the wire mesh stent appear to offer important advantages, such as a thinner wall and the nonocclusive mesh, the incorporation of wire stents into the airway may be irreversible and is associated with problems. We therefore do not expect widespread use of the Gianturco stent or the Wallstent until these problems are resolved.

H.A.G.
G.A.P.

KEY REFERENCES

Cooper JD, Pearson FG, Patterson GA et al: Use of silicone stents in the management of airway problems. Ann Thorac Surg 47:371, 1989

This is a detailed description of the indications for tracheobronchial stents and the techniques of their placement.

Gaissert HA, Grillo HC, Mathisen DJ, Wain JC: Temporary and permanent restoration of airway continuity with the tracheal T-tube. J Thorac Cardiovasc Surg 107:600, 1994

This is a summary of the extensive Massachusetts General Hospital experience with the tracheal T tube.

Montgomery WW: Manual care of the Montgomery silicone tracheal T-tube. Ann Otol Rhinol Laryngol 73(suppl):1, 1980

This is a concise guide for inpatient and outpatient care of the tracheal T tube written by its inventor.

REFERENCES

Bond CJ: Note on the treatment of tracheal stenosis by a new T-shaped tracheotomy tube. Lancet 1:539, 1891

Cooper JD, Patterson GA, Trulock EP: Results of single and bilateral lung transplantation in 131 consecutive recipients. J Thorac Cardiovasc Surg 107:460, 1994

Cooper JD, Todd TRJ, Ilves R, Pearson FG: Use of the silicone tracheal T-tube for the management of complex tracheal injuries. J Thorac Cardiovasc Surg 82:559, 1981

Dumon JF: A dedicated tracheobronchial stent. Chest 97:328, 1990

Gaissert HA, Lofgren RH, Grillo HC: Upper airway compromise after inhalation injury: complex strictures of larynx and trachea and their management. Ann Surg 218:672, 1993

Gelb AF, Zamel N, Colchen A et al: Physiologic studies of tracheobronchial stents in airway obstruction. Am Rev Respir Dis 146:1088, 1992

Keszler P: The tracheal T-tube: for indwelling intubation as an alternative management method. p. 133. In Grillo HC, Eschapasse H (eds): International Trends in General Thoracic Surgery. Vol. 2. WB Saunders, Philadelphia, 1987

Landa L: The tracheal T tube: in tracheal surgery. p. 124. In Grillo HC, Eschapasse H (eds): International Trends in General Thoracic Surgery. Vol. 2. WB Saunders, Philadelphia, 1987

Montgomery WW: The surgical management of supraglottic and subglottic stenosis. Ann Otol 77:534, 1968

Montgomery WW: T-tube tracheal stent. Arch Otolaryngol Head Neck Surg 82:320, 1965

Nashef SAM, Dromer C, Velly JF et al: Expanding wire stents in benign tracheobronchial disease: indications and complications. Ann Thorac Surg 54:937, 1992

Patterson GA, Todd TR, Cooper JD et al: Airway complications after double lung transplantation. J Thorac Cardiovasc Surg 99:14, 1990

Rousseau H, Dahan M, Lauque D et al: Self-expandable prostheses in the tracheobronchial tree. Radiology 188:199, 1993

Trendelenburg F: Beitraege zu den Operationen an den Luftwegen. Langenbecks Arch Chir 13:335, 1872

Wallace MJ, Charnsangavej C, Ogawa K et al: Tracheobronchial tree: expandable metallic stents used in experimental and clinical applications. Radiology 158:309, 1986

Westaby S, Jackson JW, Pearson FG: A bifurcated silicone rubber stent for relief of tracheobronchial obstruction. J Thorac Cardiovasc Surg 83:414, 1982

13

BENIGN CONDITIONS

Congenital Anomalies

Robert M. Filler

DEFINITION

The two most common congenital anomalies of the trachea are tracheomalacia and tracheal stenosis. *Tracheomalacia* is decreased rigidity of the trachea due to a structural abnormality of its wall. In childhood, this arises from faulty development of the trachea, whereas in adults, it is usually secondary to obstructive lung disease. This anomaly is most commonly present in children born with esophageal atresia and tracheal esophageal fistula, but it is also associated with lesions that apply external pressure to the trachea, such as a double aortic arch or a paratracheal tumor (Baxter, et al., 1963). Tracheomalacia may also occur as an isolated event. Congenital *tracheal stenosis,* which may involve all or a portion of the length of the trachea, is almost always secondary to a developmental defect in which the pars membranacea of the trachea is deficient and the wall consists of complete or almost complete cartilaginous rings.

In the following discussion of the clinical syndromes associated with these abnormalities, there will be a special focus on diagnosis and management.

TRACHEOMALACIA

HISTORICAL NOTE

In 1948 Gross and NeuHauser described a condition in which the trachea was compressed by "an anomalous innominate artery," for which suspension of the innominate artery gave relief. In the subsequent years the existence of the so-called innominate artery syndrome was questioned by many because anatomic dissections and angiographic findings failed to corroborate the presence of an anomalous innominate artery. In 1969 Mustard, et al. reported 285 cases of symptomatic tracheal compression by the innominate artery, 39 of which were treated surgically. These authors believed that

tracheal compression was due to mediastinal crowding and that suspension of the innominate artery provided more space in the mediastinum. Many of the children in the series of Mustard et al. had been born with esophageal atresia. Subsequent reports suggest that the innominate artery syndrome is identical to what we now call a tracheomalacia. In 1969 Benjamin, et al. demonstrated that an abnormally soft trachea (tracheomalacia) rather than aortic root anomalies was responsible for tracheal obstruction, at least in those children who also had been born with esophageal atresia. In 1976 Filler, et al. described life-threatening anoxic spells caused by tracheomalacia after repair of esophageal atresia and indicated that displacement of the aorta anteriorly to the undersurface of the trachea (aortopexy) could be curative. Further experience in a variety of pediatric centers has now indicated that aortopexy will alleviate the symptoms associated with severe tracheomalacia, and a definite anatomic abnormality has been identified (Delorimier, et al., 1990; Heimansohn, et al., 1991; Kiely, et al., 1987; Schwartz and Filler, 1980; Wailoo and Emery, 1979.

HISTORICAL READINGS

Benjamin B, Cohen D, Glasson M: Tracheomalacia in association with congenital tracheoesophageal fistula. Surgery 79:504, 1969

DeLorimier A, Harrison M, Hardy K et al.: Tracheobronchial obstructions in infants and children. Ann Surg 212:277, 1990

Filler RM, Rossello PJ, Lebowitz RL: Life-threatening anoxic spells caused by tracheal compression after repair of esophageal atresia: correction by surgery. J Pediatr Surg 11:739, 1976

Gross RE, Neuhauser EB: Compression of the trachea by an anomalous innominate artery. An operation for its relief. Am J Dis Child 75:570, 1948

Heimansohn D, Kesler K, Turrentine M: Anterior pericardial tracheoplasty for congenital tracheal stenosis. J Thorac Cardiovasc Surg 102:710, 1991

Kiely EM, Spitz L, Brereton R: Management of tracheomalacia by aortopexy. Pediatr Surg Int 2:13, 1987

Mustard WT, Bayliss CE, Fearon B et al.: Tracheal compression by the innominate artery in children. Ann Thorac Surg 8:312, 1969

Schwartz MZ, Filler RM: Tracheal compression as a cause of apnea following repair of tracheoesophageal fistula: treatment by aortopexy. J Pediatr Surg 15:842, 1980

Wailoo MP, Emery JL: The trachea in children with tracheoesophageal fistula. Histopathology 3:329, 1979

BASIC SCIENCE

The size of the tracheal lumen depends on the rigidity of its wall and the difference between the intraluminal and extraluminal forces that act upon it. Because of these relationships the lumen of the normal, somewhat flexible intrathoracic trachea increases during inspiration and decreases during expiration in response to a decrease and then an increase in intrathoracic pressure. In the patient with an abnormally soft trachea, the changes in tracheal caliber caused by ventilation are magnified, so that in the most severe cases complete collapse of the trachea may occur, even during unlabored expiration. When higher intrathoracic pressures are generated, as during a cough or in clinical situations in which lung compliance is reduced, obstruction to the outflow of air is even greater. Since inspiratory efforts cause the trachea to enlarge, obstruction to air inflow does not occur in tracheomalacia. Tracheomalacia in the cervical trachea rarely produces airway obstruction during quiet or forceful respiration because the pressures inside and outside the cervical trachea are equal (i.e., atmospheric) when the glottis is open. The dynamics of airway collapse have been discussed in detail by Wittenborg, et al. (1969).

In addition to changes in airway size that occur in response to variations in intrathoracic pressure, changes can occur from compression of an abnormally soft trachea by adjacent intrathoracic structures, especially the esophagus posteriorly and the ascending aorta and aortic arch and its branches anteriorly. The size and position of the aorta are relatively constant, but esophageal diameter is increased by swallowing, gastroesophageal reflux, and the presence of obstructive lesions of the lower esophagus. As a result, patients with tracheomalacia often have their most severe symptoms during or shortly after eating, when the esophagus is most distended.

A variety of structural abnormalities can produce tracheomalacia; however, the most common type encountered in childhood is found in children also born with esophageal atresia. The structural defect was first described by Wailoo and Emery (1979), who studied an unselected sequential series of tracheas obtained from 53 deceased infants and children born with esophageal atresia and tracheoesophageal fistula (TEF). Their evaluations showed that in 75 percent of these cases there was a segment of trachea in which cartilaginous rings were fragmented and/or had an elliptical rather than a C shape. The membranous portion of this segment of the trachea was extremely wide and floppy, so that even minor forces acting on the trachea would cause apposition of its anterior and posterior walls. These pathologic findings correspond precisely to those seen at bronchoscopy in children with symptomatic tracheomalacia (Fig. 13-1).

Several causes have been postulated for the association between tracheomalacia and esophageal atresia. Since the trachea and esophagus are derived from the foregut, a faulty division of the foregut, which is the presumed cause of esoph-

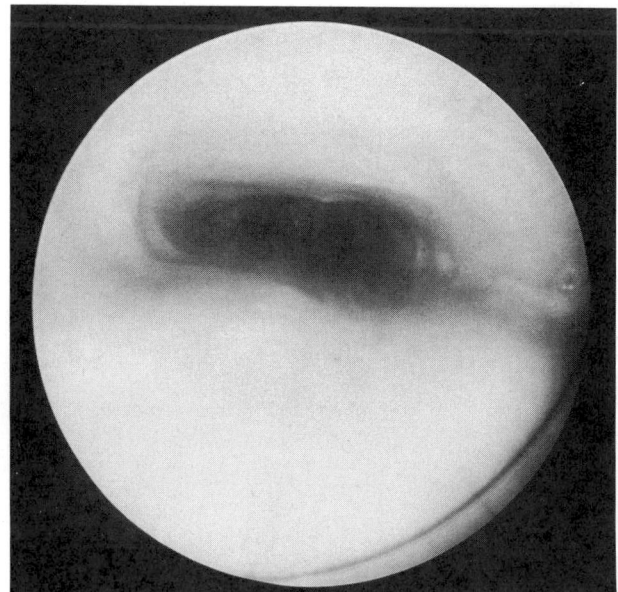 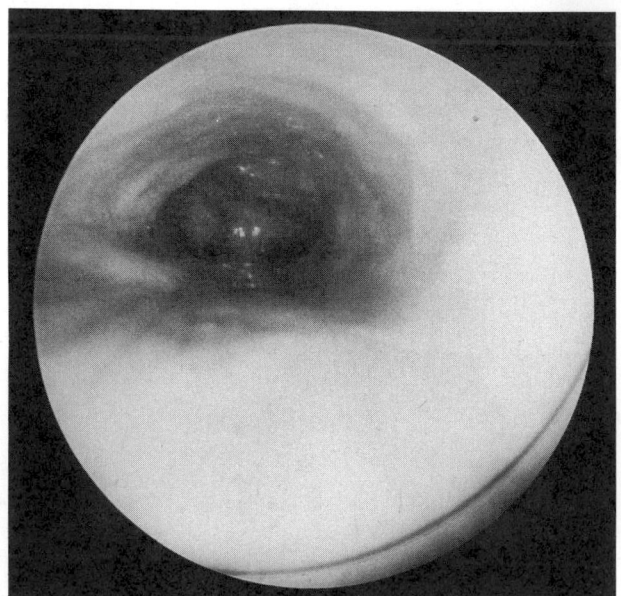

A   B

Figure 13-1. Endoscopic view of trachea above carina in spontaneously breathing 3-month-old child with tracheomalacia. **(A)** Before aortopexy. Note elliptical narrowed lumen and bulging of elongated membranous trachea posteriorly. **(B)** After aortopexy. The incomplete cartilaginous rings can be appreciated in the anterior wall of the trachea, whose lumen is now wider during all phases of respiration and during coughing.

ageal atresia, can be expected also to affect the adjacent trachea. Evidence to support this possibility can be found in Wailoo and Emery's (1979) studies, in which esophageal muscle was often present in the membranous trachea at the site of the other tracheal abnormalities. This finding suggests that when the foregut divides, the esophagus receives too little (atresia) and the trachea receives too much (tracheomalacia). Davies and Cywes (1978) surmised that the dilated esophagus above the site of atresia may compress the fetal trachea and prevent its normal development. They also suggested that abnormal tracheal development could be due to the loss of intratracheal pressure in the fetus through a TEF, since the fluid that normally fills the embryonic airway may provide the mechanism of internal support for the growing trachea.

Tracheomalacia sometimes becomes apparent only after surgery for lesions that mechanically compress the trachea, such as a vascular ring or a tumor. While it is possible that trauma during surgery contributes to postoperative tracheomalacia, it is more likely that long-term compression of the trachea is responsible for abnormal tracheal development. Other developmental defects of cartilage and complete absence of tracheal cartilage are much less common causes of tracheomalacia (Cox and Shaw, 1965; Johner and Szanto, 1970).

DIAGNOSIS

Clinical Features

The symptoms of tracheomalacia are due to airway obstruction during expiration. Most children have a typical barking cough, which is probably due to vibration of the opposing anterior and posterior tracheal walls (Benjamin, et al., 1969). Recurrent pneumonia is common in these patients, presumably because airway collapse during coughing prevents effective clearance of airway secretions. In some children airway obstruction during normal ventilation is so severe that airway intubation is necessary and in others the diagnosis of tracheomalacia is not really appreciated until the airway cannot be extubated after a surgical procedure such as repair of esophageal atresia or a vascular ring. The most serious symptom and the one that is the most frequent reason for surgery is a life-threatening "dying spell." Spells, which often do not appear until 2 or 3 months of age, are characterized by cyanosis that rapidly progresses to apnea, bradycardia, and if uninterrupted, even cardiac arrest. Characteristically, spells occur during feeding or within 5 to 10 minutes of a meal. Benjamin, et al. (1969) and Mustard, et al. (1969) suggested that the spells are due to a vagal reflex that arises from the tracheal wall when the trachea collapses.

Our experience, however, suggests another mechanism. Transcutaneous oxygen pressure (tcPO$_2$) monitoring during feedings in a small group of infants with spells associated with tracheomalacia showed a progressive fall in tcPO$_2$ during uninterrupted bottle feeding, with bradycardia developing as tcPO$_2$ fell; tcPO$_2$ and heart rate returned to normal as soon as the feeding was interrupted. We theorize that the spell is secondary to progressive hypoxia, which occurs because the lumen of the malacic trachea is compressed by an esophagus filled with milk. Since esophageal dilatation is extremely common in children after repair of esophageal atresia because of poor esophageal peristalsis, esophageal stricture, and/or gastroesophageal reflux, it is not surprising that spells are extremely common in this subset of tracheomalacia patients. Since similar-type spells can be due to cardiac or neurologic causes, complete evaluation of the child's neurologic and cardiac status is also necessary in these cases.

Natural History

Symptoms due to tracheomalacia tend to improve with time, presumably because the trachea becomes more rigid with growth. In patients with the most severe symptoms, such as dying spells, one cannot delay treatment to see how much improvement occurs with time. However, for those with mild or even intermediate symptoms, such as recurrent pneumonia, a wait-and-see attitude is sometimes justified.

Differential Diagnosis

Symptoms of tracheomalacia can be caused by a variety of conditions. However, in the setting in which they occur the primary diagnosis that must also be considered are gastroesophageal reflux, esophageal stricture, recurrent tracheoesophageal fistula, and neurologic and cardiac conditions that could cause anoxic syncopal attacks.

Investigative Techniques

The diagnosis of tracheomalacia should be suspected on the basis of a clinical history of apneic spells, recurrent pneumonia, or inability to extubate the airway because of expiratory obstruction, especially in children with a history of esophageal atresia, vascular ring, or a previous mass around the trachea. Investigations to confirm the diagnosis are relatively straightforward. A narrowing of the air-filled trachea can be noted on the lateral view of a plain chest x-ray in almost all children with tracheomalacia whose airway is not intubated. A better evaluation of tracheal dynamics is obtained radiographically with the image intensifier by continuous visualization of the trachea during several respiratory cycles. At the same time, the esophagus should be filled with radiocontrast material so that the relationship between esophageal size and tracheal diameter can be appreciated. The radiocontrast study is also needed to determine if gastroesophageal reflux, esophageal stricture, recurrent tracheoesophageal fistula, and/or poor esophageal motility is present. Typical radiographic findings in tracheomalacia are shown in Figure 13-2.

Bronchoscopy provides a definitive diagnosis in these cases (Fig. 13-1). General anesthesia is usually necessary for bronchoscopy, but the child must be breathing spontaneously and not paralyzed for proper evaluation of the trachea. In the symptomatic case, the tracheal lumen has an elliptical shape. Anterior vascular pulsations are usually evident, and the membranous portion of the trachea is usually enlarged and bulging into the lumen, more on the left than on the right. The cartilaginous tracheal rings may appear to be discontinuous. Anterior and posterior collapse of the lumen occurs during expiration, and in severe cases complete airway occlu-

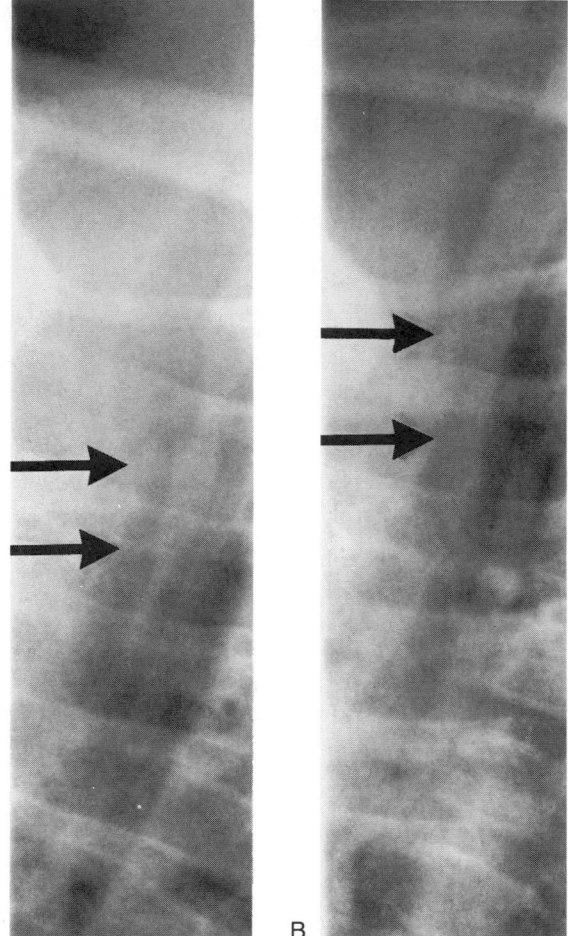

A   B

Figure 13-2. Lateral chest films in 2-month-old child with tracheomalacia. Note tracheal air shadow. **(A)** During inspiration a slight indentation related to the aorta is seen on the anterior wall of the trachea (*between arrows*). **(B)** During expiration the tracheal air shadow disappears in this same region (*between arrows*) as the trachea collapses.

sion is noted when a cough is stimulated. Because of the need for general anesthesia, bronchoscopy is usually the last test to be performed in suspected cases of tracheomalacia. In general, one should be prepared to proceed with definitive surgery at the time of bronchoscopy if the diagnosis of severe tracheomalacia is confirmed.

MANAGEMENT

Principles

Many children with minor degrees of airway collapse do not require specific therapy. The abnormally soft trachea tends to become more rigid with continued growth and development, and symptoms can be expected to improve in the first 1 or 2 years of life.

Symptoms that are life-threatening or are likely to represent a significant health hazard require surgical intervention. The major indications for surgery are noted in Table 13-1. We believe that a single dying spell due to tracheomalacia is

Table 13-1. Primary Indication for Surgery in 46 Cases of Tracheomalacia (1978–1991)

Indication	No.
Dying spells	33
Airway intubation needed	
Nasotracheal	5
Tracheostomy	4
Recurrent pneumonia	4
Total	46

an indication for surgery. Likewise, there appears to be little justification for delaying surgical correction for the child who requires a tracheostomy or an endotracheal tube to keep the airway patent. Sometimes it is difficult to decide how many episodes of pneumonia are acceptable before advising surgery. Certainly more than three documented episodes in a year would seem excessive, especially if a severe anatomic abnormality is seen at bronchoscopy.

Surgical Therapy

Tracheomalacia can be treated by several surgical techniques. A tracheostomy will provide an internal tracheal splint and has been used by some in the hope that improvement would accompany growth (Shapiro and Martin, 1981). Wiseman, et al. (1985) successfully treated tracheomalacia and bronchomalacia with airway intubation and continuous positive airway pressure (CPAP) for 14 weeks. This duration of CPAP is probably not sufficient for most infants with airway collapse, since significant spontaneous improvement in tracheomalacia is unlikely before 1 or 2 years of age. Johnston, et al. (1980) used a free rib graft as a splint for the trachea in two children in whom a tracheostomy tube failed to stabilize the malacic segment. Our experience indicates that aortic suspension is an effective and safe method of therapy for most tracheomalacia patients. In a small number of cases the abnormal airway segment is so long that aortopexy is not sufficient and application of an airway splint is necessary.

Aortopexy

Our original decision to use aortopexy (Fig. 13-3) for tracheomalacia was based on the favorable reports of Gross and Neuhauser (1948) and Mustard, et al. (1969) in treating what they called the innominate artery compression syndrome. Many of their patients undoubtedly had what we are now calling tracheomalacia. The rationale for the procedure assumes that the trachea will be pulled anteriorly when the aorta is suspended from the sternum if the connective tissue between the two is not disturbed. This translocation will change the configuration of the cross-section of the malacic trachea from an ellipse to a circle and prevent apposition of its anterior and posterior walls. In addition, anterior displacement of the trachea will minimize airway compression by the esophagus.

Anesthesia for aortopexy is planned to permit intraoperative endoscopic examination of the affected portion of the airway and immediate assessment of the adequacy of repair.

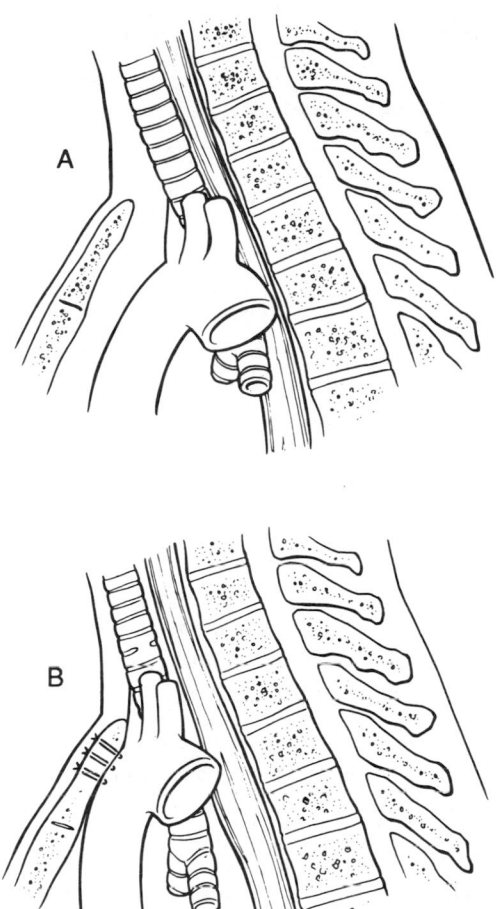

Figure 13-3. Mediastinal anatomy in tracheomalacia and effect of aortopexy. **(A)** Sagittal view of chest showing the relationships between aorta, trachea, and esophagus. The malacic trachea can be compressed by the adjacent aorta, but when the esophagus is empty or the child is not coughing, there is usually no appreciable airway obstruction. However, when the esophagus dilates (during swallowing or reflux), the trachea collapses between it and the aorta. Respiratory symptoms and apneic spells occur at this time. **(B)** The operative procedure pulls the aorta anteriorly and displaces the anterior wall of the trachea as well. The filled esophagus no longer causes critical airway narrowing.

For this purpose, anesthetic gases are delivered through a ventilating bronchoscope with a telescope attachment. Although the telescope takes up a portion of the lumen of the bronchoscope and resistance to airflow is increased, the anesthetist can still maintain satisfactory ventilation.

A left anterior thoracotomy through the third interspace is used to gain access to the anterior mediastinum for aortopexy. The left lobe of the thymus is excised to expose the aorta and its first branches and to create a space to translocate these vessels. The tissue plane between the aorta and trachea is not dissected, since it is this attachment that pulls the trachea forward when the aorta is suspended from the sternum. Three or four 3–0 nonabsorbable vascular sutures are placed into the adventitia and a portion of the media at three locations, namely, the ascending aorta, the origin of the right

innominate artery, and the aortic arch just beyond the origin of the innominate artery. A subcutaneous pocket is created anterior to the upper sternum, and both ends of the vascular sutures are passed through the entire thickness of the sternum into this pocket. The sutures are pulled up simultaneously, and they are tied sequentially after bronchoscopic observation indicates a satisfactory improvement in the tracheal configuration. If the correction is not satisfactory, one or two additional sutures may be of help; otherwise, a splinting procedure will be necessary.

In patients with a tracheostomy tube in place prior to surgery, we have removed it and replaced it with a nasotracheal tube 1 week before aortopexy. This allows the stoma to close, which minimizes the possibility of bacterial contamination of the wound at the time of aortopexy. This step is especially important if a prosthetic splint is implanted.

Splinting Operation

Collapsing airways have been stabilized with a variety of external splints. Herzog, et al. (1968) described the use of a free autologous rib graft to stent the adult trachea. Johnston, et al. (1980) applied the same technique in two children, but long-term results have not been published. Rainier, et al. (1968) first used prosthetic splinting in 23 adults with tracheomalacia due to severe chronic obstructive lung disease. In their cases, the widened membranous trachea was plicated and covered with a Dacron-reinforced Silastic prosthesis.

Since 1978 we have implanted a Silastic-reinforced Marlex mesh device in five children with tracheomalacia. The device has not adversely affected tracheal growth in animals or in long-term clinical follow-up of these and other children (Filler, et al., 1982; Murphy, et al., 1983).

The indication for application of an airway splint in tracheomalacia is long-segment tracheal collapse or collapse that is not corrected by aortopexy. In three of the patients splinted, aortopexy was planned to be the primary corrective procedure. However, when bronchoscopy at the completion of the procedure indicated that aortic suspension had failed to prevent tracheal collapse, the splinting procedure was undertaken under the same anesthetic. The average length of splint applied was 4.5 cm (range 3 to 6 cm), which is about 1.5 cm longer than the length of tracheomalacia usually cured by aortopexy alone (Murphy, 1983).

The exact operative technique and selection of the size and shape of prosthetic splint are determined by the site and extent of airway collapse. We have a set of splints of different size and shape, which can be cut and modified as needed. The involved trachea can be approached either by median sternotomy or by right posterior lateral thoracotomy. The splint, which is sized to encircle 75 percent of the circumference of the trachea, is sewn to the airway with interrupted 3–0 Dexon sutures. Application of the splint to the entire circumference of the trachea should be avoided, since this will limit growth and produce tracheal stenosis in a growing trachea. As fibrous tissue grows into the interstices of the Marlex mesh, the prosthesis becomes permanently fixed to the tissues. The flexible Silastic attached to the mesh is sufficiently soft and thin that erosion into the esophagus or a major artery is very unlikely.

Table 13-2. Clinical Data in Group 1 Children in Whom Tracheomalacia Was Associated with Esophageal Atresia and Tracheoesophageal Fistula

Primary Indication for Surgery	No. Patients	Operation			Result	
		Aortopexy	Aortopexy + Splint	Splint	Success	Failure
Dying spells	24	23	1		23	1[c]
Airway intubation needed						
Nasotracheal	5	5[a]			5	0
Tracheostomy	3	2	1		1	2
Recurrent pneumonia	3	2[b]		1	2	1
Total	35	32	2	1	31	4

[a] Membranous trachea plicated in one.

[b] Periosteal graft placed around trachea in one.

[c] Dead of undetermined cause.

Perioperative Care

Management of the child after surgery is relatively simple. The airway is extubated immediately in most patients. Antibiotics are not used, and analgesics are needed for 1 to 3 days postoperatively. Physiotherapy to ensure adequate coughing and ventilation is necessary, but endotracheal suctioning is almost never needed.

Results

Aortopexy

For analysis of my group's care material from 1978 to 1991, patients were divided into two groups according to whether or not tracheomalacia was associated with esophageal atresia. In Tables 13-2 and 13-3, comparisons are made between the major indication for surgery, the operation performed, and the long-term result. Additional details have been recently published (Filler, et al., 1992).

Aortopexy has been well tolerated, and operative complications in our hands and those of others have been minimal. Evaluation of the aortic suspension by postoperative echocardiogram in a limited number of patients indicates that the aorta remains attached to the sternum for at least a year following surgery. Although this is theoretically a problem, there have been no reports of long-term vascular complications from aortopexy.

Treatment of tracheomalacia by aortopexy has been the subject of several reports by other authors, and their results are similar to our own. Kiely, et al. (1987) reported on 25 aortopexies in 22 children with associated esophageal anomalies, mostly esophageal atresia and tracheoesophageal fistulas. Excellent results were obtained in 17 children, with only one long-term failure. Of interest is that symptoms worsened after aortopexy in two of children, both of whom had recurrent tracheoesophageal fistula and severe gastroesophageal reflux. Division of the fistula and fundoplication in each case proved to be curative.

In our series, of the 41 patients who had only aortopexy, symptoms were relieved in 37. Of the nine children who required surgery for inability to extubate the airway, only one still had a tracheostomy in place 2 years later, although immediate extubation was not possible in two others. The only death in the series was that of a child who had a vascular ring that was unrecognized at the time of aortopexy. This child's dying spells recurred in the week following aortopexy, and they ceased permanently after division of the ring. One month later, however, the child died unexpectedly and suddenly at home. Autopsy failed to reveal the cause of death.

Three children had a splint applied when intraoperative bronchoscopy indicated that tracheomalacia persisted after aortopexy. These children are all well.

Splinting

Relatively few children have been treated for tracheomalacia by splinting, so that one must still be cautious in evaluating the results. Tracheal collapse was eliminated in all five cases in which the trachea was splinted. My associates and I have reported the result of the splinting operation in five children who have been followed for more than 4 years (Vinograd, et al., 1987). They were evaluated clinically and by bronchoscopy, computed tomography (CT) scan, and pulmonary function tests, and all were found to be leading normal lives. The only complication occurred in a child who developed a serous effusion around the splint, which compressed the treachea 2 years after implantation. Removal of the splint was necessary, but the rigidity of the trachea at that time prevented airway collapse. There was no adverse effect on tracheal growth in any case.

Table 13-3. Clinical Data in Group II Children in Whom Tracheomalacia Was an Isolated Finding

Primary Indication for Surgery	No. Patients	Operation			Result	
		Aortopexy	Aortopexy + Splint	Splint	Success	Failure
Dying spells	9	8		1	9	
Airway intubation needed (Tracheostomy)	1		1		1	
Recurrent pneumonia	1	1				1
Total	11	9	1	1	10	1

COMMENTS AND CONTROVERSIES

One of the frequent clinical decisions to be faced is how to deal with the severely symptomatic child who is found to have both tracheomalacia and gastroesophageal reflux. This complex of abnormalities occurs frequently in the group of children born with esophageal atresia. The reflux of gastric contents into the esophagus may actually cause tracheal collapse if a dilated esophagus filled in retrograde fashion impinges on a flaccid trachea. In our series, 14 of the 35 children who had esophageal atresia were diagnosed as having reflux before surgery for tracheomalacia. Five of these had undergone an antireflux procedure elsewhere because of the belief that gastroesophageal reflux was responsible for the life-threatening respiratory symptoms, and three others required a fundoplication after aortopexy. Four additional children who developed gastroesophageal reflux after aortopexy also needed fundoplication, although not for respiratory symptoms.

In those children who are found to have gastresophageal reflux during evaluation for tracheomalacia or vice versa, if the major symptom is a dying spell or recurrent pneumonia and if radiography and bronchoscopy show complete or near-complete closure of the trachea on swallowing and coughing, we and others (Kiely, et al., 1987) would elect to proceed with aortopexy rather than fundoplication as the initial step in surgical management.

For aortopexy, the aorta can be approached through a left or right anterior thoracotomy or a sternal split. We have found the left-sided approach to be the easiest, although this is not always possible because of a previous surgical procedure. With sternotomy the effect of the aortic suspension cannot be determined until the sternum is closed; if the desired change in tracheal shape is not achieved, the sternum must be reopened. In contrast, closure of an anterior thoracotomy does not change the spatial relationships of the structures affected by aortopexy.

To reduce the possibility of aortic tear from the deep sutures that we use to suspend the aorta, some surgeons prefer to attach a patch of synthetic material to the adventitia of the aorta with many superficial sutures and then to sew the synthetic fabric to the undersurface of the sternum. Since we have had no complication from sutures placed through a partial thickness of the aortic wall, this additional step seems unnecessary. The bleeding that sometimes occurs when the aortic suture is placed indicates that the lumen has been entered. If this occurs, the suture is removed and gentle pressure is applied to the needle hole. When bleeding stops, a new suture can be placed.

R.M.F.

TRACHEAL STENOSIS

HISTORICAL NOTE

Wolman (1941) reported 11 cases of congenital tracheal stenosis, including one of his own, that had been documented since 1832. One child with dyspnea for the first 7 years of life improved after tracheostomy, but all others died. Benjamin, et al. (1981) reviewed 21 cases of congenital tracheal stenosis seen in Sydney, Australia, between 1971 and 1980. Despite nine deaths in that series, the authors emphasized that 12 of the 21 patients survived after mostly conservative treatment (excepting one pneumonectomy and one tracheopexy), and they concluded "there appears to be little place for surgical resection of the stenosis. . . ." Case reports of successful segmental resection of tracheal stenosis in babies started to appear in the 1980s (Harrison, et al., 1980; Mansfield, 1980; Mattingly, et al., 1981; Weber, et al., 1982; Nakayama, et al., 1982; Minato, et al., 1986; Healy, et al., 1988). Aggressive surgical treatment of symptomatic lesions is now the accepted standard, although methods of tracheoplasty have varied at different surgical centers.

HISTORICAL READINGS

Benjamin B, Pitkin J, Cohen D: Congenital tracheal stenosis. Ann Otol Rhinol Laryngol 90:364, 1981

Harrison MR, Heldt GP, Brasch RC et al: Resection of distal tracheal stenosis in a baby with agenesis of the lung. J Pediatr Surg 15:938, 1980

Healy GB, Schuster SR, Jonas RA et al: Correction of segmental tracheal stenosis in children. Ann Otol Rhinol Laryngol 97:444, 1988

Mansfield PB: Tracheal resection in infancy. J Pediatr Surg 15:79, 1980

Mattingly WT Jr, Belin RP, Todd EP: Surgical repair of congenital tracheal stenosis in an infant. J Thorac Cardiovasc Surg 81:738, 1981

Minato N, Itoh K, Ohkawa Y et al: Surgical treatment of congenital distal tracheal stenosis involving the carina. Ann Thorac Surg 42:326, 1986

Nakayama DK, Harrison MR, de Lorimier AA et al: Reconstructive surgery for obstructing lesions of the intrathoracic trachea in infants and small children. J Pediatr Surg 17:854, 1982

Weber TR, Eigen H, Scott PH et al: Resection of congenital tracheal stenosis involving the carina. J Thorac Cardiovasc Surg 84:200, 1982

Wolman IJ: Congenital stenosis of the trachea. Am J Dis Child 61:1263, 1941

BASIC SCIENCE

With rare exception, congenital tracheal stenosis is caused by absence of all or most of the membranous portion of the affected tracheal segment. From their review of the literature, Cantrell and Guild (1964) described three basic anatomic patterns: generalized tracheal hypoplasia, funnel-like stenosis, and segmental stenosis. These stenoses are often associated with other anomalies of the tracheobronchial tree, the most common of which are pulmonary artery sling; aberrant right middle and lower lobe bronchi arising from the left mainstem bronchus; and unilateral pulmonary agenesis or hypoplasia (Fig. 13-4).

The so-called pulmonary artery sling represents an aberrant left pulmonary artery, which arises from the right pulmonary artery and passes behind the trachea to the left lung (Fig. 13-5). In children with congenital tracheal stenosis, a

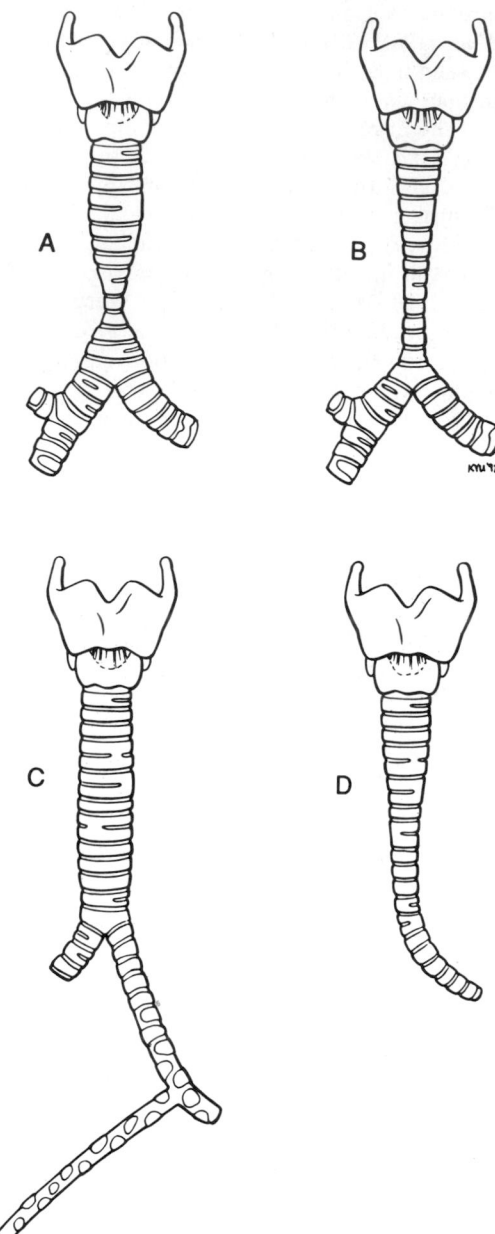

Figure 13-4. Types of congenital tracheal stenosis commonly encountered. **(A)** Short segment. **(B)** Long, funnel-like narrowing. The carina and upper bronchi can be involved. **(C)** Abnormal branching of bronchi. In this example the two lower lobes on the right are supplied by a bronchus originating on the left. Major stenosis in this type usually begins at the carina and extends distally often on both right and left sides. **(D)** Tracheal stenosis is associated with pulmonary agenesis on the right.

pulmonary artery sling coexists in about 50 percent of the cases. Similarly, among children in whom a sling is identified, about 50% also have congenital tracheal stenosis. The severity and type of tracheal stenosis is independent of the presence of the vascular sling. Berdon, et al. (1984) coined the

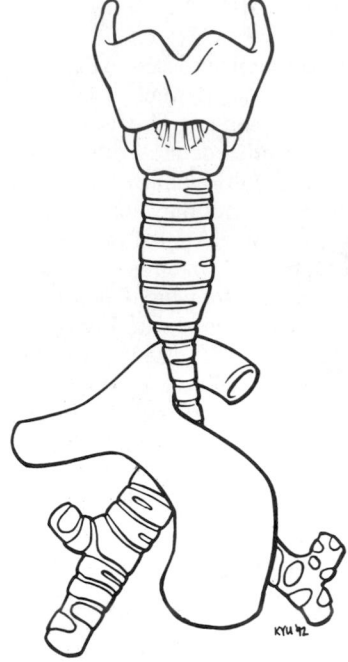

Figure 13-5. Tracheal stenosis is associated with aberrant left pulmonary artery (sling) in 50 percent of cases. Repair of sling will not correct the intrinsic tracheal problem.

term *ring-sling syndrome* for those cases in which a pulmonary artery sling coexists with complete cartilaginous O tracheal rings. The surgeon must be aware of this association, for in these cases repair of the vascular anomaly alone will not eliminate intrinsic airway obstruction.

DIAGNOSIS

Clinical Features

Clinical features associated with congenital tracheal stenosis are listed in Table 13-4 (Loeff, et al., 1988b). Most commonly, children present in the first few months of life because of stridor and/or pneumonia.

Natural History

The length and degree of narrowing varies significantly between cases. Children without life-threatening symptoms may grow and develop normally although a degree of airway obstruction and stridor may be obvious during exercise, when ventilation increases. It appears that at least in some cases the airway diameter can increase with growth even in the absence of a membranous trachea (Benjamin, et al., 1981). However, in children with severe stridor due to tracheal stenosis, death can be expected in hours or days.

Table 13-4. Clinical Features in 22 Cases of Congenital Tracheal Stenosis

Characteristics	No. of Patients
Total number of patients	22
Boys	13
Girls	9
Age of onset of symptoms	
0–3 months	18
4–12 months	4
Presenting symptoms	
Stridor	18
Recurrent pneumonia	10
Cyanosis	7
Wheezing	2
Respiratory arrest	2
Associated anomalies	
Vascular ring or sling	11
Hypoplastic aortic arch	2
Other aberrant vessels	4
Osteocartilaginous	9
Cardiac	8
Gastrointestinal	4
Renal	3
TEF = EA, H-type TEF	2

Abbreviations: TEF, tracheoesophageal fistula; EA, esophageal atresia.

(Data from Loeff DS, Filler RM, Vinograd I et al.: Congenital tracheal stenosis: a review of 22 patients from 1965 to 1987. J Pediatr Surg 23:744, 1988b)

Differential Diagnosis

In young infants who present with stridor due to airway obstruction, the differential diagnosis includes congenital tracheal stenosis; complete vascular ring, including double aortic arch; subglottic hemangioma; and more rarely, unusual pharyngeal and paratracheal tumors, cysts, and infections.

Investigative Techniques

High-contrast radiographs plus fluoroscopy in two projections will give fairly accurate information about an infant's airway. However, additional information is usually necessary to make an accurate anatomic diagnosis and plan appropriate therapy. Barium swallow is useful in children with airway obstruction to see if a vascular ring or pulmonary artery sling is present. In addition, paratracheal or esophageal masses can be identified by the impression that they make on the esophageal lumen.

Tracheobronchography

Until recently we relied primarily on tracheobronchography for the most accurate evaluation of children with congenital tracheal stenosis. When performed properly, this technique will clearly outline the degree and extent of narrowing and delineate anomalies of airway branching. It will allow the surgeon to decide whether or not surgery will help and what procedure might be best suited for the specific anatomic abnormality.

The major problem with tracheobronchography is that the injection of contrast material into a severely narrowed airway may convert a partial obstruction into a complete one, either by plugging the narrowed lumen with contrast agent or by inciting an inflammatory reaction within its wall. If tracheobronchography is attempted, fluoroscopic control is essential. Minimal quantities of contrast material should be used, and contrast must be carefully aspirated after the study. An operating room must be ready to accept the infant for urgent surgical repair should condition deteriorate. Because other diagnostic procedures have largely replaced tracheobronchography, radiocontrast agents designed specifically for airway use are no longer being manufactured. As a result, alternate radiocontrast agents have been used, but these have not yet been approved for young infants. In fact, our limited use of intravenous contrast media for bronchography suggests that these agents do indeed carry a greater risk of airway and lung inflammation than the bronchography media formerly used.

Computed Tomography

CT scanning with three-dimensional reconstruction is now our procedure of choice to evaluate the airway in cases of congenital tracheal stenosis. This technique can detect a pulmonary artery sling, abnormal tracheobronchial branching, aortic arch anomalies, and most of the rarer causes of tracheal obstruction. The display of the length and degree of airway narrowing is appropriate for surgical decision making. An example is shown in Figure 13-6.

Magnetic Resonance Imaging

We have had no significant experience with magnetic resonance imaging (MRI) in these cases. Because many infants with severe congenital tracheal stenosis have a precarious airway, and/or require ventilatory support, MRI with the current techniques used in most centers may be hazardous.

Bronchoscopy

Bronchoscopy is useful to resolve any doubt concerning the diagnosis of congenital tracheal stenosis and to confirm the site and degree of stenosis at the upper end of the narrowed trachea. However, when tracheal obstruction is severe, even the smallest bronchoscope will not pass into the narrowed segment, so that the total length of stenosis and the presence of abnormal airway branching cannot be evaluated endoscopically. If bronchoscopy is attempted, the surgeon must be prepared to proceed immediately with surgical repair, since trauma to the narrowed tracheal wall may precipitate total airway obstruction.

Cardiac Evaluation

Cardiac catheterization is not necessary to determine whether a pulmonary artery sling is present if a CT scan with injection of radiocontrast material scan has been obtained. However, in those children with associated heart defects, complete cardiac evaluation, including echocardiogram and heart catheterization, may be indicated.

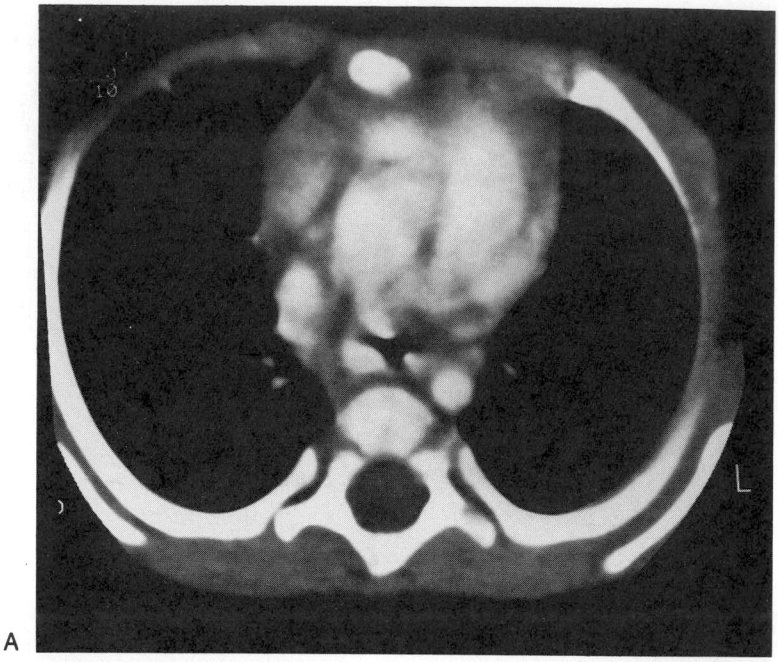

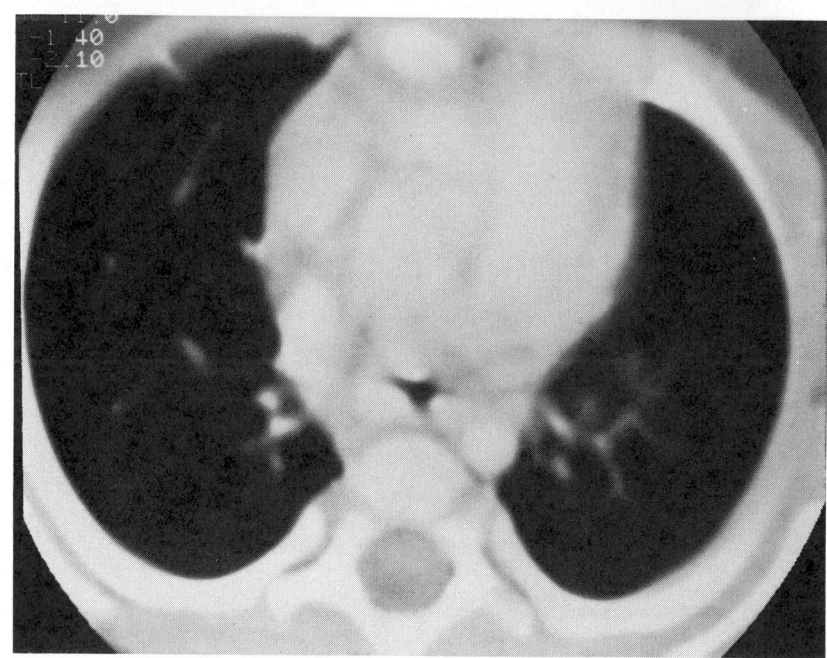

Figure 13-6. CT scan in 7-month-old child with tracheal stenosis involving 2.5 cm of distal trachea but not carina. Stenosis associated with aberrant left pulmonary artery (sling). **(A)** Mediastinal window is cut just above carina. The contrast-filled aberrant pulmonary artery can be seen behind the tracheal air shadow. **(B)** Tracheal window gives a more accurate measurement of the size of the tracheal lumen, which in this case measures 2.5 mm.

MANAGEMENT

Principles

The obvious goal of surgery is to eliminate airway narrowing without compromising future growth of the tracheobronchial tree. In the small infant and child procedures to accomplish this end are not without significant risks, and sophisticated surgical judgment is required to reach a satisfactory conclu-

sion. The decision to proceed with operative correction depends on the magnitude of ventilatory embarrassment and on the surgeon's experience in the use of available corrective procedures, knowledge of what such an operation can be expected to achieve, and complete understanding of the mortality and morbidity associated with the corrective operation. For example, we would usually advise surgery for the child with moderate respiratory obstruction with a short stenotic segment manageable by resection. However, in the child with identical symptoms due to long-segment stenosis, a nonoperative approach might be chosen initially since the risk and morbidity of tracheoplasty is so much greater. Postponement to a later date when the child is larger might improve outcome. Help in making this decision can be obtained by measuring the diameter of the airway lumen on a CT scan with proper window and comparing it with predicted normals (Griscom and Wohl, 1986). Loeff, et al. (1988b) published a graph showing the relationship between airway diameter and body length in normal infants and children. By comparison, in 13 patients who died with severe tracheal stenosis, the airway was consistently 50 percent of normal. In the small infant this translates to a tracheal diameter of 2 to 2.5 mm. These data suggest that if the airway diameter is significantly greater than 50 percent of normal, imminent death is unlikely and the decision for repair can be safely deferred.

Operative Technique

Operations to correct tracheal stenosis fall into three categories: dilatation, resection and anastomosis, and tracheoplasty.

Balloon Dilatation

Although there has been little clinical experience to date, a few reports suggest that balloon dilatation may have a place in the treatment of congenital tracheal stenosis (Bagwell, et al., 1991; Messineo, et al., 1992b). We have used balloon dilatation on many occasions to treat tracheal strictures that develop after tracheal resection, tracheoplasty, and tracheal intubation injuries. Equipment developed for balloon angioplasty is well suited for the small trachea. Radiographic control is useful to ensure that the balloon is in proper position and that the airway is not overdistended to the point of rupture. Dilatation as a primary treatment for congenital stenosis awaits further experience. Certainly in the neonate or premature infant it may be the only procedure that can be performed.

Resection and Anastomosis

Segmental resection of stenotic lesions less than five rings in length with end-to-end anastomosis is accepted by most tracheal surgeons as the treatment of choice. My group and others (DeLorimier, et al., 1990; Grillo and Zannini, 1984) have had success with resection of 50 percent of the tracheal length (up to nine rings). The techniques of resection enunciated by Grillo and Mathisen (1988) have been adopted by most surgeons performing these operations. The trachea can be exposed anteriorly through the neck, by sternotomy, or through a right posterior lateral thoracotomy. The anterior or posterior surface of the trachea can be exposed along its entire length, but care should be taken to preserve the lateral tracheal blood supply. Initial circumferential tracheal dissection should be limited to 1 to 2 cm above and below the narrowed area in order to preserve the tracheal blood supply. Any posterolateral dissection must be on the tracheal wall to avoid recurrent nerve injury. Both ends of the stenosis should be resected to normal-diameter trachea.

For tracheal anastomosis, four to five sutures are placed in the posterior trachea with knots on the outside and are not tied until all are in place. Ventilation is maintained through a separate anesthesia circuit connected to the distal trachea. After the posterior sutures are tied, a translaryngeal endotracheal tube is advanced across the anastomosis, and the anterior row of sutures is placed. When the distal stenosis extends to the carina, it is easier to perform the operation with cardiopulmonary bypass rather than to have ventilation tubes providing a precarious airway in the operative field. Absorbable suture material should be used to minimize formation of intraluminal granulation tissue after surgery. Polyglycolic acid, polydioxanone, and polyglactin all seem adequate (Friedman, et al., 1990). Traction sutures placed in the midlateral trachea on either side of and at least 1 cm proximal and distal to the anastomosis may be tied together after completion of the anastomosis to relieve tension on the suture line. Head-restraining sutures between the chin and the chest wall or a prosthetic brace to keep the neck flexed postoperatively can be helpful to reduce anastomotic tension when long segments of trachea are removed. My colleagues and I have had no experience with laryngeal release procedures (Dedo and Fishman, 1969; Montgomery, 1974) for severe length problems.

Tracheoplasty

Tracheoplasty is reserved for long-segment tracheal stenosis, which cannot be treated by resection and end-to-end anastomosis. The basic technique, which is similar in all tracheoplasties described, is illustrated in Figure 13-7.

The stenotic section of the trachea is incised in the anterior midline (or posterior midline if a posterior lateral approach is used) to one ring beyond the narrowing, which often means extension into the upper end of a bronchus. An interposition graft is then sutured to the edges of the open trachea to enlarge the lumen. A variety of grafts have been employed, including tantalum (Loeff, et al., 1988a), esophagus (Ein, et al., 1982), dura (Lobe, et al., 1987), cartilage (Kimura, et al., 1982; Lobe, et al., 1987; Campbell and Lilly, 1986), pericardium (Idriss, et al., 1984; Heimansohn, et al., 1991), and periosteum (Cohen, et al., 1986).

In the literature pericardium and costal cartilage have been used most frequently. We have had experience with all types of grafts, and unfortunately none have been ideal. The pericardial graft is taken from the anterior pericardium, and its size is designed to enlarge the trachea 1.5-fold. It is sewn to the edge of the trachea with a continuous stitch of absorbable 5–0 or 6–0 sutures. The pericardial patch should be sutured to the undersurface of the aorta and mediastinal structures to prevent collapse until the graft become stiff, presumably by fibrosis. In addition, after surgery the trachea is kept intubated with a nasotracheal tube for 10 to 14 days. Heimansohn, et al. (1991) recommend that children be kept pharmacologically paralyzed and sedated until the pericardium adheres to mediastinal structures.

When cartilage is inserted as a graft, its rigidity precludes the need to fix it to other mediastinal structures. Also, intubation and paralysis beyond 1 or 2 days after surgery are often not necessary. However later complications may require pro-

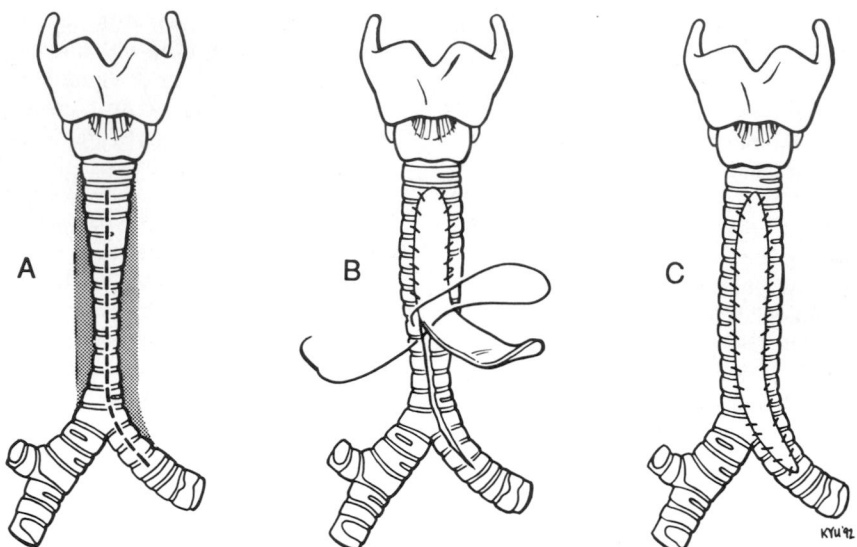

Figure 13-7.   General technique of tracheoplasty. **(A)** The stenotic segment of trachea is opened longitudinally to an airway of normal diameter superiorly and inferiorly. **(B)** Tissue selected for grafting is sutured to the defect with running or interrupted sutures of absorbable material. **(C)** Completed tracheoplasty.

longed endotracheal intubation. We have found that sufficient length of cartilage can be obtained from the costal margin by subperichondrial resection. The thickness of the cartilage can be reduced by scraping it with a scalpel, leaving the side facing the lumen slightly concave. Continuous or interrupted sutures of 5–0 to 6–0 absorbable material pass easily through the cartilage of the young child so that implantation is not a problem. The goal is to use a piece of cartilage that will give maximum luminal size.

Periosteum for a tracheal graft is obtained by making a longitudinal incision over the anterior aspect of the tibia. A graft that starts below the tibial tubercle and extends to just above the ankle is adequate to cover the longest tracheal defects. A graft 7 to 10 mm wide can be obtained. Tibial periosteum in the infant is quite thick and has a leathery quality, which makes for easy handling and suturing. The outermost surface of periosteum should face the lumen. The graft is best obtained prior to thoracotomy and cardiopulmonary bypass if that is to be used, so that it is available when needed and at a time when the child is not heparinized. Hemostasis should be complete by the time heparin is given for cardiopulmonary bypass. Animal and clinical experience with free grafts of periosteum show that bone will grow from the graft, which becomes rigid within 2 weeks (Cohen, et al., 1986).

When the esophagus is used to cover the tracheal defect, the trachea is opened in the posterior midline. The intact anterior wall of the esophagus is sutured to the edges of the defect to eliminate air leak (Ein, et al., 1982).

In 1989 Tsang and colleagues described a slide tracheoplasty for tracheal stenosis, which obviates the need for a graft. This tracheoplasty was used in two children, ages 10 months and 3 months. Each had a funnel-type stenosis of the trachea not involving the carina. The trachea was divided at the midpoint of the stenosis. Both segments of the trachea

were opened longitudinally and spatulated, the upper segment posteriorly and the lower segment anteriorly. The open segments were slid on top of one another and sutured in place. This tracheoplasty shortens the trachea and uses living tracheal tissue for coverage. One child was well 12 months later.

A critical issue in tracheoplasty is the maintenance of ventilation during the operation. We believe, as do others (Idriss, et al., 1984; Heimansohn, et al., 1991), that cardiopulmonary bypass is the most reliable and safest method to ensure adequate oxygenation and still allow excellent exposure of the entire trachea and upper bronchi. Through a sternotomy incision we have used right atrial and aortic cannulas for bypass. The catheters can be fixed in place and kept out of the surgeon's way even in the smallest infant. We have not found a need to use the femoral artery for arterial inflow. Cardiopulmonary bypass also allows easy rerouting of an aberrant left pulmonary artery and the repair of other cardiac defects that may be present (Yamaguchi, et al., 1990). With the trachea open during bypass, it is helpful to place balloon catheters through an endotracheal tube into each bronchus to prevent accumulation of blood in the lower airways. Excessive bleeding at the cut edges of the trachea due to heparinization has not been troublesome during or after bypass.

Formerly we used fibrin glue at the junction of the graft and trachea to minimize the possibility of an air leak at the completion of tracheoplasty. However, in several children who needed a second operation, we believed that excessive fibrous tissue at the graft site might have been due in part to use of the fibrin. Since small air leaks around the graft close spontaneously in a few minutes when airway pressures are not excessive, fibrin glue does not seem to be needed.

The adequacy of tracheoplasty can be judged by the pressures required for lung expansion and the rapidity of lung collapse during expiration. When the extracorporeal circuit is turned off, arterial and venous bypass cannulas should be left in place until one is certain that adequate ventilation can be achieved through an endotracheal tube with reasonable airway pressures.

Airway stenting is important after tracheoplasty, not only to ensure adequate ventilation and airway toilet following surgery but also to provide temporary ridigity to an airway that might collapse following tracheoplasty, especially when a nonrigid tissue such as pericardium is used to cover the tracheal defect. Standard endotracheal tubes suffice in most cases, but when the bronchi must be stented, this presents an enormous problem in the small child. We have tried to intubate one bronchus and leave an opening at the carina for ventilation of the other, but this has invariably failed. Similarly, the development of Y-shaped stents for small children has been unsuccessful because the small lumen of these stents plugs frequently and the distal ends cannot be prevented from occluding upper lobe bronchi. We believe that this contributes to the poor long-term results of tracheoplasty in infants and children with stenosis extending well into one or both bronchi.

Postoperative Care

The major problem following tracheoplasty is maintenance of a patent airway. In the first 2 weeks after surgery airway secretions seem to be the main problem. Usually these can be handled easily with suctioning, especially when an endotracheal tube has been left in place. Suction catheters must be used with care, for the delicate, narrow airway of the infant can be traumatized easily by these catheters, especially since the distal end of the tracheoplasty is usually beyond the end of the endotracheal tube.

In the next several weeks to months after surgery three more difficult to treat problems causing airway obstruction may arise; these are formation of granulation tissue, airway collapse, and airway stricture.

Despite all precautions to minimize formation of granulation tissue, such as the use of low-reactive absorbable suture material and the avoidance of airway trauma by suction catheters, the healing of the tracheal repair is often associated with the formation of granulation tissue at suture lines and on the surface of grafts. Even a ring of granulation tissue 1 to 2 mm thick in the lumen of a small infant's airway can result in significant obstruction, in contrast to a ring of equal thickness in an adult. Its presence is signaled by airway obstruction, usually in the region of the carina and bronchial orifices. The granulations can be identified by bronchoscopy and can be removed by suction and/or foreign body forceps. Rarely, excision with a laser can be helpful. Because the trauma of removal (by whatever method) often begets more granulations, this complication can be extremely troublesome. The need for repeated endoscopic procedures is to be expected. Granulation tissue formation ceases only when the grafted tissues and/or sutures are completely epithelialized. Since any manipulation of a healing tracheoplasty tends to produce granulation tissue, we remove such tissues only when they cause significant airway obstruction and not prophylactically.

Intrathoracic airway collapse causing airway obstruction tends to occur at a grafted area of the trachea when the graft has little or no rigidity. Pericardium is a flexible tissue, which allows airway collapse at least until it becomes more rigid by ingrowth of fibrous tissue. Therefore when pericardium is used, the graft should be sutured to other mediastinal structures, and the grafted area should be stented with an endotracheal tube for approximately 2 weeks (Heimansohn, et al., 1991). Since there are no satisfactory stents for small bronchi, complete stenting of the repair site may not be possible when the graft extends into one or both bronchi. Providing high end-expiratory pressures with a ventilator may help keep the airway open until the graft becomes rigid. Using the wall of the esophagus for tracheoplasty can also be associated with significant tracheal collapse. The muscular esophageal wall ordinarily does not become rigid after surgery, and long-term airway intubation can be anticipated postoperatively with this type of repair. Free periosteal grafts tend to become rigid in 1 to 2 weeks, at which time calcium can be seen radiographically (Cohen, et al., 1986).

In our experience, stricture at the tracheoplasty site as a complication of the tracheoplasty procedure occurs commonly regardless of the tissue used for grafting. Usually the stricture develops in the distal trachea and carina just beyond the tip of the endotracheal tube stent. This complication is often blamed on faulty blood supply and/or a lack of stenting. It seems likely that trauma from suction catheters is also at least a part of the problem. Our first approach to treating the stricture has been balloon dilatation. By using balloons designed for angioplasty, satisfactory dilatation can be achieved, at least temporarily. The need for repeat dilatation is the rule. With epithelialization of the graft, the intervals between dilatations increases; however, dilatations over many weeks are usually necessary. As noted in Table 13-5, we have also resorted to surgical resection of the stricture with end-to-end anastomosis or regrafting using cardiopulmonary bypass. Despite many frustrations and long hospitalizations, some infants can be salvaged after apparent initial failure.

In 1988 my colleagues and I reported the use of a coiled stainless steel stent, which could be inserted endoscopically, to treat recurrent tracheoplasty strictures (Loeff, et al., 1988a). This type splint was not successful over the long term because granulation tissue formed through and over the coils and obstructed the airway. More recently we and others (Domschke, et al., 1990; Dumon, 1990) have treated strictures by inserting expandable metal stents and silicone stents into the trachea through a bronchoscope with radiographic control. Since the stents we use have been developed and marketed to supplement percutaneous balloon angioplasty, special approval should be obtained for their use in the trachea in these desperate situations. Although granulation tissue still tends to be a problem with this type of splint, it has been less exuberant than with the coils, and we have been able to cope with the problem by repeated bronchoscopic removal. We have followed two children with airway stents of this type (Table 13-5 and Fig. 13-8), one of whom, with two stents in place, went home and has been ventilating normally. The other was still hospitalized 4 months after placement of three stents and still required weekly bronchoscopy for removal of granulation tissue although his airway was not intubated.

Table 13-5. Clinical Data for Five Recent Cases of Long-segment Congenital Tracheal Stenosis

Patient (Age 3–6 mo)	Months in Hospital	Stenosis			Plasty (Graft)	Left Hospital	Current Status
		L (cm)	W (mm)	Br (+, −)			
1	3	5	2	−	PO		
					R	No	Died (OR)
2	4	5	2	+	PO & S		
					PC & S	Yes	Died, 1 yr (home)
3	7	3	2	+	PC		
					R		
					R	Yes	Died, 8 mo (home)
4	6	5	2.5	+	CA & S	Yes	Alive (home)
5	6+	6	2	+	PC		
					CA & S	No	Alive (hospital)

Abbreviations: PO, periosteum; PC, pericardium; CA, cartilage; S, metallic stent; L, length of stenosis; W, width of stenosis; BR, bronchial involvement; OR, operating room.

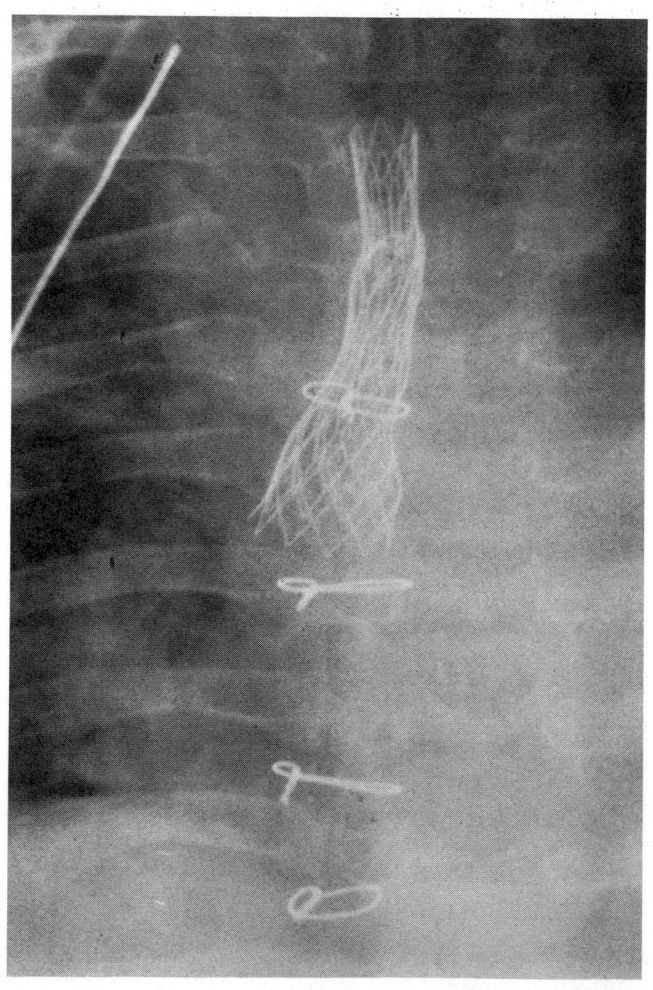

Figure 13-8. Chest x-ray in 7-month-old infant who had tracheoplasty using cartilage (case 4, Table 13-5). Because of recurrent stricture at lower end of the repair, two expandable metallic stents were inserted bronchoscopically. This child was at home 6 months later.

Results

Since congenital tracheal stenosis is relatively rare, the number of cases in the largest series ranges from 5 to 13 (Lobe, et al., 1987; Loeff, et al., 1988b; Tsugawa, et al., 1988; Idriss, et al., 1984; DeLorimier, et al., 1990; Heimansohn, et al., 1991; Grillo and Zannini, 1984). The children treated in these reports had varying lengths of tracheal stenosis, and the degree of narrowing in each case was not similar. In addition, follow-up was often inadequate for judging the long-term results, which is especially important since laboratory and clinical experience suggest that tracheoplasty may reduce subsequent tracheal growth (Dykes, et al., 1990). Because of the small numbers and these other variables, one cannot draw clear-cut conclusions as to the best method of repair. Nevertheless, some generalizations seem warranted. When resection of the narrowed segment and end-to-end anastomosis are possible, survival is the rule by methods currently available in most centers. No current method will correct all the variants of congenital tracheal stenosis. When severe stenosis extends into one or both bronchi, the results from all types of tracheoplasty are poor.

Most tracheoplasty experience has been with cartilage and pericardial grafts. Given the limitations in evaluating surgical results, encouraging results have been reported, especially with pericardium. In the series of Heimansohn, et al. (1991), seven of eight patients survived, and Idriss, et al. (1984) had five of five survivors. In 10 of these 12 survivors grafted with pericardium, the airway was eventually extubated.

As an example of the trials and tribulations that one can encounter in treating long-segment tracheal stenosis, I have noted the status and outcome of the last five children with extensive stenosis whom we have treated (Table 13-5). All except one had involvement of the proximal bronchi on one or both sides. Pericardium, cartilage, and periosteum were all used as grafts. The selection of a graft at any particular time was based on the current reports in the literature and/or on the results of trials in our animal laboratory. All five children survived initial surgery and the immediate postoperative period. One child died during surgery for resection of a tracheoplasty stricture (case 1). Two children had a second tracheoplasty 4 and 6 weeks after failure of the initial procedure (cases 2 and 5). A tracheoplasty stricture with reanastomosis was resected successfully on two occasions in case 3.

Metallic splints were used for persistent tracheal stricture in cases 2, 4, and 5 and are currently in place in patients 4 and 5. Innumerable bronchoscopic procedures were performed in all patients for removal of granulation tissue, dilatation of strictures, and/or insertion of an airway splint. Three of these children could be sent home but two subsequently died, primarily because of an abnormal airway. Patient 4 is home and so far is well, and patient 5 still requires weekly removal of tracheal granulation tissue and dilatation but remains extubated.

COMMENTS AND CONTROVERSIES

My group's experience and that of others indicates that there is still much to be accomplished in treating congenital tracheal stenosis.

As noted throughout this entire section on congenital tracheal stenosis, the primary issues involved in its treatment include indications for surgery; type of operation to be selected; graft selection when tracheoplasty is performed; the value of dilatation as primary treatment; and the exclusive use of cardiopulmonary bypass for extensive tracheoplasties. Except perhaps for the last issue, defensible recommendations await further laboratory and clinical experience.

Our recent limited experience with intraluminal splints suggests that this is one area for further fruitful exploration. Questions still to be answered include long-term effects of splints on tracheal growth; the necessity for removal at a later date; ideal prosthetic material; ideal size and shape of splint; and the value of implanting splints at the time of initial tracheoplasty.

Replacement of narrowed segments of trachea and bronchi with allografts of appropriate size is currently being explored in our laboratory. Using a pig model we have replaced airway segments with free nonvascularized fresh and cryopreserved tracheal allografts and cryopreserved cartilage. Transplanted cartilage tends to be replaced with fibrous tissue, and its growth is less than that of the normal adjacent trachea. However, the luminal surface of the grafts becomes epithelialized. In addition, the ability to use cryopreserved tissue would allow us to store tracheas and cartilage for later use (Messineo 1992a).

R.M.F.

KEY REFERENCES

Filler RM, Messineo A, Vinograd I: Severe tracheomalacia associated with esophageal atresia: results of surgical treatment. J Pediatr Surg 27:1136, 1992

This study reviews a 15-year experience with the surgical treatment of tracheomalacia in 32 children. Indications for surgery, types of operative procedures, and their techniques are reviewed.

Heimansohn DA, Kesler KA, Turrentine MW et al.: Anterior pericardial tracheoplasty for congenital tracheal stenosis. J Thorac Cardiovasc Surg 102:710, 1991

This paper clearly outlines the technique of tracheoplasty using a pericardial patch. The authors indicate the value of cardiopulmonary bypass for the procedure and outline the details of postoperative care, including paralysis and ventilation. The surgical approach used in this paper can be applied equally well to tracheoplasties when tissue other than pericardium is used. These authors report their experience with eight cases with very good results.

Tsang V, Williams AM, Goldstraw P: Sequential Silastic and expandable metal stenting for tracheobronchial strictures. Ann Thorac Surg 53:856, 1992

The use is reported of metal expandable stents, which were inserted into the tracheal lumen via the bronchoscope to treat benign and malignant tracheal and bronchial strictures in five adults. The basic technique described should also be considered when indicated for infants and children on the basis of our early limited experience.

Tsugawa C, Kimura K, Muraji T et al.: Congenital stenosis involving a long segment of the trachea: further experience in reconstructive surgery. J Pediatr Surg 23:471, 1988

The authors describe their technique of tracheoplasty with costal cartilage, performed in five children with use of jet ventilation. Four of the children are doing well.

REFERENCES

Bagwell C, Talbert J, Tepas J: Balloon dilatation of long-segment tracheal stenosis. J Pediatr Surg 26:153, 1991

Baxter JD, Dunbar JS: Tracheomalacia. Ann Otol Rhinol Larnygol 72:1013, 1963

Benjamin B, Cohen D, Glasson M: Tracheomalacia in association with congenital tracheoesophageal fistula. Surgery 79:504, 1969

Benjamin B, Pitkin J, Cohen D: Congenital tracheal stenosis. Ann Otol Rhinol Laryngol 90:364, 1981

Berdon WE, Baker DH, Wung JT et al.: Complete cartilage-ring tracheal stenosis associated with anomalous left pulmonary artery: the ring-sling complex. Radiology 152:57, 1984

Blair GK, Filler RM, Cohen R: Treatment of tracheomalacia: 8 years' experience. J Pediatr Surg 21:781, 1986

Campbell AH, Young IF: Tracheobronchial collapse, a variant of obstructive respiratory disease. Br J Dis Chest 57:174, 1963

Campbell DN, Lilly JR: Surgery for total congenital tracheal stenosis. J Pediatr Surg 21:934, 1986

Cantrell JR, Guild HG: Congenital stenosis of the trachea. Am J Surg 108:297, 1964

Cogbill TH, Moore FA, Accurso FJ et al.: Primary tracheomalacia. Ann Thorac Surg 35:538, 1983

Cohen RC, Filler RM, Konuma K et al.: A new model of tracheal stenosis and its repair using free periosteal grafts. J Thorac Cardiovasc Surg 92:296, 1986

Cox WL Jr, Shaw RR: Congenital chondromalacia of the trachea. J Thorac Cardiovasc Surg 49:1033, 1965

Davies MR, Cywes S: The flaccid trachea and tracheoesophageal congenital anomalies. J Pediatr Surg 13:363, 1978

Dedo HH, Fishman NH: Laryngeal release and sleeve resection for tracheal stenosis. Ann Otol Rhinol Laryngol 78:285, 1969

DeLorimier A, Harrison M, Hardy K et al.: Tracheobronchial obstructions in infants and children. Ann Surg 212:277, 1990

Domschke W, Foers EC, Matek W et al.: Self-expanding mesh stent for esophageal cancer stenosis. Endoscopy 22:134, 1990

Dumon J: A dedicated tracheobronchial stent. Chest 97:328, 1990

Dykes EH, Bahoric A, Smith C et al.: Reduced tracheal growth after reconstruction with pericardium. J Pediatr Surg 25:25, 1990

Ein SH, Friedberg J, Williams WG et al.: Tracheoplasty: a new operation for complete congenital tracheal stenosis. J Pediatr Surg 17:872, 1982

Fallis J, Filler RM, Lemoine G: Pediatric Thoracic Surgery. Elsevier Science, New York, 1991

Filler RM, Buck JR, Bahoric A et al.: Treatment of segmental tracheomalacia and bronchomalacia by implantation of an airway splint. J Pediatr Surg 17:597, 1982

Filler RM, Rossello PJ, Lebowitz RL: Life-threatening anoxic spells caused by tracheal compression after repair of esophageal atresia: correction by surgery. J Pediatr Surg 11:739, 1976

Friedman E, Perez-Atayde A, Silvera M et al.: Growth of tracheal anastomoses in lambs. J Thorac Cardiovasc Surg 100:188, 1990

Grillo HC, Mathisen DJ: Surgical management of tracheal strictures. Surg Clin North Am 68:511, 1988

Grillo HC, Zannini P: Management of obstructive tracheal disease in children. J Pediatr Surg 19:414, 1984

Griscom NT, Wohl ME: Dimensions of the growing trachea related to age and gender. AJR 146:233, 1986

Gross RE, Neuhauser EB: Compression of the trachea by an anomalous innominate artery. An operation for its relief. Am J Dis Child 75:570, 1948

Harrison MR, Heldt GP, Brasch RC et al.: Resection of distal tracheal stenosis in a baby with agenesis of the lung. J Pediatr Surg 15:938, 1980

Healy GB, Schuster SR, Jonas RA et al.: Correction of segmental tracheal stenosis in children. Ann Otol Rhinol Laryngol 97:444, 1988

Heimansohn D, Kesler K, Turrentine M: Anterior pericardial tracheoplasty for congenital tracheal stenosis. J Thorac Cardiovasc Surg 102:710, 1991

Herzog H, Keller R, Maurer W et al.: Distribution of bronchial resistance in obstructive pulmonary diseases and in dogs with artificially induced tracheal collapse. Respiration 25:381, 1968

Idriss F, DeLeon SY, Ilbawi MN et al.: Tracheoplasty with pericardial patch for extensive tracheal stenosis in infants and children. J Thorac Cardiovasc Surg 88:527, 1984

Johner CH, Szanto PA: Polychondritis in a newborn presenting as tracheomalacia. Ann Otol Rhinol Laryngol 79:1114, 1970

Johnston MR, Loeber N, Hillyer P et al.: External stent for repair of secondary tracheomalacia. Ann Thorac Surg 30:291, 1980

Kiely EM, Spitz L, Brereton R: Management of tracheomalacia by aortopexy. Pediatr Surg Int 2:13, 1987

Kimura K, Mukohara M, Tsugawa C et al.: Tracheoplasty for congenital stenosis of the entire trachea. J Pediatr Surg 17:869, 1982

Lobe TE, Hayden K, Nicolas D: Successful management of congenital tracheal stenosis in infancy. J Pediatr Surg 22:1137, 1987

Loeff DS, Filler RM, Gorestein A et al.: A new intratracheal stent for tracheobronchial reconstruction. J Pediatr Surg 23:1173, 1988a

Loeff DS, Filler RM, Vinograd I et al.: Congenital tracheal stenosis: review of 22 patients from 1965 to 1987. J Pediatr Surg 23:744, 1988b

Mansfield PB: Tracheal resection in infancy. J Pediatr Surg 15:79, 1980

Mattingly WT Jr, Belin RP, Todd EP: Surgical repair of congenital tracheal stenosis in an infant. J Thorac Cardiovasc Surg 81:738, 1981

Messineo A, Filler RM, Bahoric A et al.: Repair of long tracheal defects with cryopreserved cartilaginous allografts. J Pediatr Surg 27:1131, 1992a

Messineo A, Forte V, Joseph T et al.: The balloon posterior tracheal split: a technique for managing tracheal stenosis in the premature infant. J Pediatr Surg 27:1142, 1992b

Minato N, Itoh K, Ohkawa Y et al.: Surgical treatment of congenital distal tracheal stenosis involving the carina. Ann Thorac Surg 42:326, 1986

Montgomery WW: Suprahyoid release for tracheal stenosis. Arch Otolaryngol Head Neck Surg 99:225, 1974

Murphy P, Filler RM, Muraji T et al.: Effect of prosthetic airway splint on the growing trachea. J Pediatr Surg 18:872, 1983

Mustard WT, Bayliss CE, Fearon B et al.: Tracheal compression by the innominate artery in children. Ann Thorac Surg 8:312, 1969

Nakayama DK, Harrison MR, de Lorimier AA et al.: Reconstructive surgery for obstructing lesions of the intrathoracic trachea in infants and small children. J Pediatr Surg 17:854, 1982

Rainier WG, Newby JP, Kelble DL: Long-term results of tracheal support surgery for emphysema. Chest 53:765, 1968

Schwartz MZ, Filler RM: Tracheal compression as a cause of apnea following repair of tracheoesophageal fistula: treatment by aortopexy. J Pediatr Surg 15:842, 1980

Shapiro RS, Martin WM: Long custom-made plastic tracheostomy tube in severe tracheomalacia. Laryngoscope 91:355, 1981

Tsang V, Murday A, Gillbe C et al.: Slide tracheoplasty for congenital funnel-shaped tracheal stenosis. Ann Thorac Surg 48:632, 1989

Vinograd I, Filler RM, Bahoric A: Long-term functional results of prosthetic airway splinting in tracheomalacia and bronchomalacia. J Pediatr Surg 22:38, 1987

Vinograd I, Filler RM, England SJ et al.: Tracheomalacia: an experimental animal model for a new surgical approach. J Surg Res 42:597, 1987

Wailoo MP, Emery JL: The trachea in children with tracheoesophageal fistula. Histopathology 3:329, 1979

Weber TR, Eigen H, Scott PH et al.: Resection of congenital tracheal stenosis involving the carina. J Thorac Cardiovasc Surg 84:200, 1982

Wiseman NE, Duncan PG, Cameron CB: Management of tracheobronchomalacia with continuous positive airway pressure. J Pediatr Surg 20:489, 1985

Wittenborg MM, Gyepes MT, Crocker D: Tracheal dynamics in infants with respiratory distress, stridor and collapsing trachea. Radiology 88:653, 1969

Wolman IJ: Congenital stenosis of the trachea. Am J Dis Child 61:1263, 1941

Yamaguchi M, Yoshihiro O, Hosokawa Y et al.: Concomitant repair of congenital tracheal stenosis and complex cardiac anomaly in small children. J Thorac Cardiovasc Surg 100:181, 1990

Postintubation Injury

Michael Maddaus
F. Griffith Pearson

STENOSIS

DEFINITION

Postintubation injury is the most common cause of benign, stenotic lesions of the upper airway. Such injury may be produced by either translaryngeal intubation or tracheostomy.

Following tracheostomy, stenotic lesions may be the result of injury at the level of the tracheostoma or at the level of the inflatable cuff. Full-thickness erosion of the tracheal wall occasionally results in tracheoinnominate artery fistula (TIF) or tracheoesophageal fistula (TEF).

Translaryngeal intubation may result in damage to the glottis, the subglottic segment, or the trachea itself and usually follows periods of more prolonged intubation in which a translaryngeal cuffed tube has been used in an intensive care setting for the support of ventilation. The laryngeal injury most commonly occurs in the posterior interarytenoid area and restricts abduction of the vocal cords. Significant subglottic lesions usually result in circumferential stenosis.

HISTORICAL NOTE

Postintubation injury is a rare complication of tracheostomy with an uncuffed tube and only became a significant problem with the advent of mechanical ventilatory support using cuffed endotracheal tubes. Although Trendelenburg reported on the use of a cuffed tracheostomy tube in 1871, the use of cuffed tubes did not become widespread until the introduction of mechanical ventilators and cuffed tracheostomy tubes during the 1952 epidemic of poliomyelitis in Europe (Lassen, 1956). During the early 1960s postintubation tracheal stenosis was increasingly recognized as a frequent and life-threatening complication of assisted ventilation with cuffed tubes. A prospective study, initiated in 1967, and identified a 17.5 percent incidence of functionally significant tracheal stenosis in 153 patients surviving management by mechanical ventilation and cuffed tracheostomy tubes (Pearson, et al., 1968; Andrews and Pearson, 1971). Most of the postintubation strictures occurred either at the stoma or under the inflatable cuff, and the most severe lesions were seen at the cuff level.

Subsequent investigation focused on the mechanisms of injury, and it soon became apparent that the greatest damage resulted from pressure ischemia under the small-volume, noncompliant inflatable cuffs that were in use during those early years. In 1969 Cooper and Grillo showed that mucosal ulceration with exposure of underlying cartilage occurred within as little as 48 hours of cuff inflation. Inflation pressures of up to 100 mmHg were necessary to obtain an airtight seal with these low-volume cuffs (Webb, et al., 1973). Such high pressures deformed the wall of the trachea until the tracheal contour matched that of the balloon.

Having identified the pathophysiology of these injuries, Grillo, et al. (1971) developed a large-volume low-pressure cuff, which was a prototype for the cuff design in current use on tracheostomy and endotracheal tubes. These cuffs are large-volume and "floppy," with a resting diameter of approximately 3 cm. Inflation with as little as 2 to 6 ml of air usually fills the trachea, allows the cuff to conform to the normal tracheal shape, and provides an airtight seal with inflation pressures that are in the same range as the peak airway pressures generated during mechanical ventilation.

These early experiences were recorded during a time when translaryngeal intubation was maintained for relatively brief periods before proceeding to tracheostomy. During the 1970s translaryngeal intubation was rarely maintained beyond 48 to 72 hours. Since then, however, there has been an ongoing trend to maintain patients with longer and longer periods of nasotracheal or orotracheal intubation. Although the incidence of post-tracheostomy stenosis is now markedly reduced, the application of longer periods of translaryngeal intubation (often continued for 2 or 3 weeks), has resulted in an increased incidence of postintubation stenosis at the level of the glottis and subglottic segment.

HISTORICAL READINGS

Andrews MJ, Pearson FG: The incidence and pathogenesis of tracheal injury following cuffed tube tracheostomy with assisted ventilation: an analysis of a two year prospective study. Ann Surg 173:249, 1971

Cooper JD, Grillo HC: Experimental production and prevention of injury due to cuffed tracheal tubes. Surg Gynecol Obstet 129:1235, 1969

Grillo HC, Cooper JD, Geffin B et al.: A low pressure cuff for tracheostomy tubes to minimize tracheal injury—a comparative clinical trial. J Thorac Cardiovasc Surg 62:898, 1971

Lassen HCA: Management of Life-Threatening Poliomyelitis. E & S Livingstone, London, 1956

Pearson FG, Goldberg, DaSilva: A prospective study of tracheal injury complicating tracheostomy with a cuffed tube. Ann Otol Rhinol Laryngol 77:867, 1968

Trendelenburg F: Beitrage zu den Operationen an den Luftwegen. Arch Klin Chir 12:112, 1871

Webb WR, Ozdenin IA, Ikins PM et al.: Surgical management of tracheal stenosis. Ann Surg 179:819, 1973

BASIC SCIENCE

Anatomy

The trachea extends from the inferior cricoid margin to the carina, averages between 10 and 13 cm in length, and contains between 18 and 22 cartilaginous rings (approximately two rings per centimeter of length). The average internal diameter of the trachea is 2.3 cm. The tracheal blood supply arises above from the inferior thyroid arteries and from the bronchial circulation below. Anastomosing branches of these vessels enter the trachea at its posterolateral margin and are segmental in their distribution. In view of this segmental distribution, the tracheal circulation may be impaired if circumferential mobilization is extended beyond 1 to 2 cm (Fig. 13-9).

The anatomy and relationships of the recurrent laryngeal nerves at the level of the larynx and upper airway are illustrated in Figure 13-10. A knowledge of this anatomy is essential during any circumferential resection of the trachea or

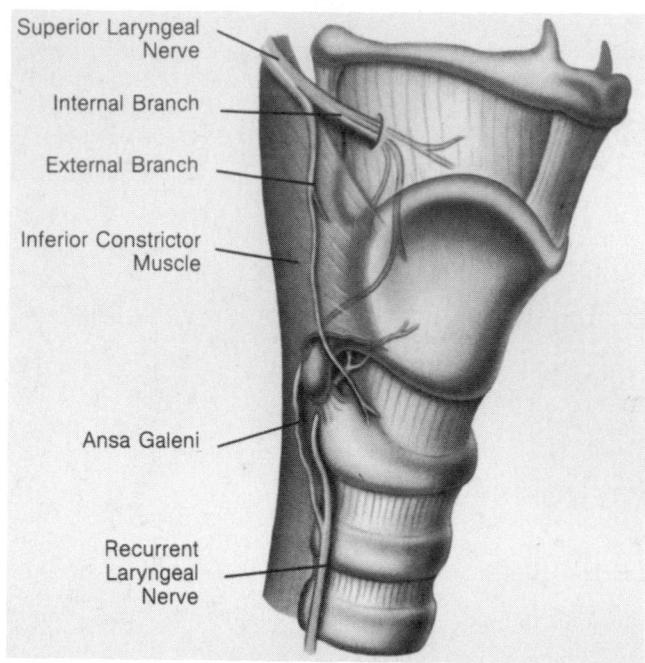

Figure 13-10. Diagram illustrating the course and anatomic relations of the recurrent laryngeal nerves in the upper trachea and cricoid levels.

adjacent cricoid cartilage. These nerves ascend in the tracheoesophageal groove and pass deep to the inferior border of the cricothyroid muscle and posterior to the cricothyroid articulations. It is only above this level that the nerves enter the laryngeal musculature. Thus, it is possible to preserve the recurrent nerves when operating in the region of the posterior cricoid cartilage as long as the posterior perichondrium or a thin shell of posterior cricoid plate is maintained intact.

The anatomy of the larynx and upper airway is described in detail in Chapter 10. To provide a clear understanding of postintubation injury at the level of the larynx and subglottis, however, some details of anatomy warrant emphasis. The

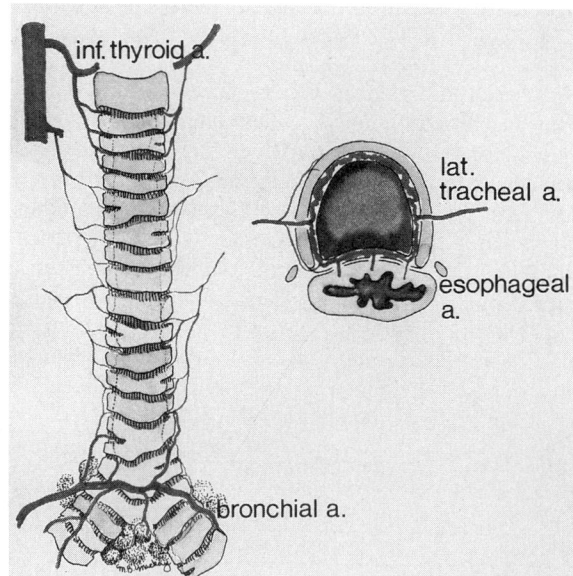

Figure 13-9. Diagram illustrating the important features of the tracheal circulation. The most robust contributions to the circulation arise from the inferior thyroid arteries above and the bronchial arteries below. These vessels anastomose in an arcade lying along the posterolateral margins of the trachea, and feed the submucosal plexus by intercartilaginous branches, which are segmental in distribution.

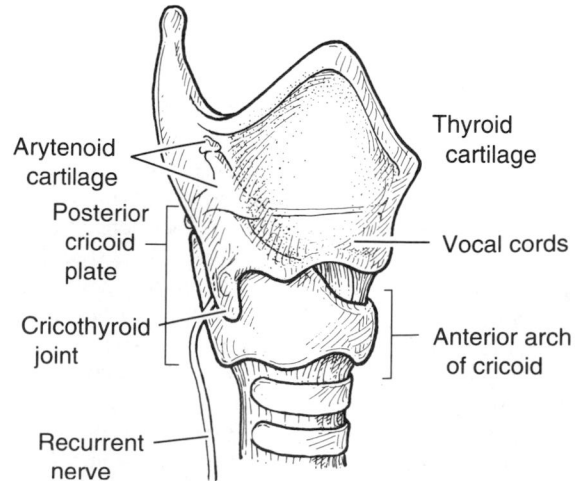

Figure 13-11. Diagram illustrating the thyroid, cricoid, and arytenoid cartilages and their interrelationships.

larynx has three key cartilaginous components that provide skeletal support for the airway and vocal function, namely, the thyroid cartilage, the cricoid cartilage, and the paired arytenoid cartilages. The thyroid cartilage is the outer protective cover for the entire larynx and articulates inferiorly with the cricoid cartilage at the cricothyroid joints (Fig. 13-11). The cricoid cartilage is the first full ring of the upper airway and has an anterior arch approximately similar in height to a normal tracheal ring, which expands into a broadly based posterior plate or rostrum. Both the inner and outer aspects of the cricoid cartilage are covered with a stout perichondrial layer, which may be an important feature during segmental resection and primary reconstruction in the subglottic level. The paired arytenoid cartilages rest on the superior surface of the posterior cricoid plate and articulate with the cricoid cartilage at the cricoarytenoid joints. The vocal ligaments, or cords, arise behind from the vocal processes of the arytenoid cartilages and attach anteriorly to the thyroid cartilage (Fig. 13-11).

The action of vocal muscles on the arytenoid cartilages produces changes in both the position and tension of the vocal cords. These changes are responsible for important aspects in the normal range of vocal function and require full mobility in the cricoarytenoid articulations. The subglottic larynx begins immediately below the vocal folds and extends to the inferior margin of the cricoid cartilage and the interface with the first tracheal ring. The subglottic space is the narrowest part of the upper airway aside from the larynx. The subglottis has an internal diameter between 1.5 and 2 cm and is surrounded throughout by the cricoid cartilage, which provides a rigid structural support for both the subglottic and laryngeal apertures.

Pathophysiology

The mechanisms by which translaryngeal intubation or tracheostomy produce airway injury are diverse: the injury may be due to the inflated cuff, the rigid walls of the endotracheal tube, or the site of creation of a tracheostomy or cricothyroidotomy.

Cuff Level Injury

Injury of various degrees under the inflatable cuff continues to be the most frequent complication following either endotracheal intubation or tracheostomy. These injuries continue to occur despite the widespread use of high-volume, low-pressure floppy cuffs. Normal capillary perfusion pressure is no more than 20 to 30 mmHg, and hyperinflation of the cuff may lead to circumferential mucosal ischemia and ulceration. Schmidt, et al. (1979) demonstrated the occurrence of mucosal injury within as little as 4 hours after overinflation of a floppy cuff. When mucosal ulceration occurs, the underlying tracheal cartilage is exposed and may subsequently become devitalized and disappear. Following extubation, the ulcerated area usually heals with the formation of a firm fibrous scar, which results in varying degrees of stenosis (Fig. 13-12). Circumferential injury and cicatrix produce the most extreme degrees of obstruction. On occasion, relatively little collagen may be laid down in an area of destruction, which results in a malacic segment.

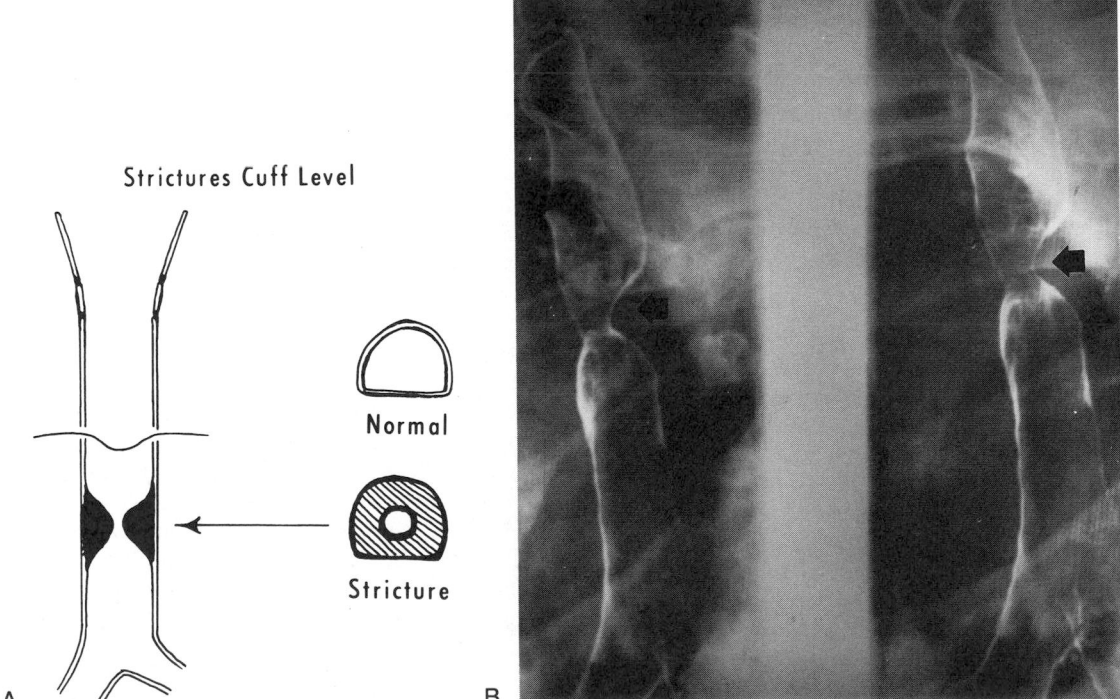

Figure 13-12. **(A)** Diagrammatic illustration of a typical concentric, fibrous stricture due to injury under the inflatable cuff. These lesions are usually short (no more than 2 to 3 cm in extent). **(B)** Contrast tracheogram illustrating a relatively tight cuff stricture (*black arrows*).

To minimize cuff-related injury, cuff pressure should be maintained below 20 mmHg whenever possible. Alternatively, the cuff may be inflated to a level that provides an airtight system and then repeatedly checked to ensure that minimal inflation is maintained. In some cases involving unduly high peak airway pressures, maintaining a small leak around the cuff may be desirable in order to avoid hyperinflation injury.

Stomal Injury

Stomal stenosis was clearly identified as a complication of cuffed tracheostomy tubes in a prospective study by Pearson and associates (1968; Pearson and Andrew 1971). In this early study, functionally significant stomal stenosis occurred in 12 percent of patients surviving mechanical ventilation with a cuffed tracheostomy tube. It was apparent that the incidence of stomal stenosis increased significantly with the use of larger-diameter tracheostomy tubes. The smallest tube that is satisfactory for ventilation and tracheal toilet is recommended for either translaryngeal intubation or tracheostomy. The factors promoting stenosis include pressure and leverage on the stomal margins, due to fixation of the ventilator attachments, and pooling of infected secretions above the inflated tracheostomy cuff. Following extubation, the stomal margins fall together, and there is some degree of anterolateral scarring with loss of luminal diameter in every patient (Fig. 13-13A). In functionally significant lesions, the defect is usually triangular in shape with preservation of the posterior membranous airway (Fig. 13-13B and C).

On occasion, airway obstruction may be due to soft inflammatory granulations, which develop at the margins of the stoma or adjacent to areas of ulceration under the inflatable cuff. These may result in airway obstruction following decannulation and are usually easily managed by endoscopic removal. To prevent stomal stenosis, the tracheostomy tube should be introduced at the level of the second or third ring with removal of the least amount of cartilage that permits introduction of the tube. The smallest tracheostomy tube providing a satisfactory airway is recommended. Ventilator connections that result in leverage and pressure at the stomal margins, with tubing supports and swivel connectors, will reduce lateral pressure at the stoma.

Glottic and Subglottic Injury

Following translaryngeal intubation, the most common site of injury is the larynx or subglottis. This is the narrowest part of the upper airway, and the subglottic segment is circumferentially encased with unyielding cricoid cartilage. At the level of the glottis and vocal cords, endolaryngeal tubes most commonly damage the posterior structures, with ulceration of the interarytenoid mucosa. This may be followed by the development of a fibrous posterior glottic stenosis. The most severe of these posterior injuries may involve one or both cricoarytenoid joints. The usual result is limitation of abduction of one or both vocal cords.

Subglottic stenosis is more commonly results from circumferential injury resulting in a concentric stricture than from an isolated posterior injury. Occasionally, anterior commissure stenosis is produced at the glottic level.

It is very likely that some degree of mucosal injury occurs in a majority of patients undergoing translaryngeal intubation for more than a few days. In most, recovery may leave the patient with reasonably normal function. There is only one report of a prospective study (Whited, 1984) that demonstrated a relationship between the incidence of posterior commissure stenosis and the length of time the patient was intubated: such a stenosis was identified in 12 percent of patients intubated for longer than 11 days. Colice, et al. (1989) and Kastanos, et al. (1983) reported a high incidence of acute injury (mucosal ulceration) but did not register a clear correlation between the length of intubation and the degree of significant permanent injury.

Subglottic injury may occur when the tracheostomy is incorrectly placed through the first tracheal or anterior cricoid ring. It may also occur following cricothyroidotomy. In each of these circumstances the anterior cricoid arch may be lost, with more or less damage occurring on the posterior cricoid plate.

Clinical Presentation

Symptoms usually appear within 1 to 6 weeks after extubation. This delay in onset is due to the ongoing development and maturation of scar tissue at the site of airway damage. Both Andrews and Pearson (1971) and Couraud and Hafez (1987) noted that 80 percent of patients develop symptoms within 3 months of extubation. Less commonly, symptoms may be evident immediately after extubation, and very rarely they may be delayed for up to several years (Couraud and Hafez, 1987).

Dyspnea on exertion is the primary symptom in all patients with clinically significant obstruction. Depending on the degree of stenosis, dyspnea ranges from a mild limitation of breathing during heavy exertion to marked shortness of breath with minimal activity such as speaking. In most patients narrowing of the lumen to less than 50 percent of normal cross-sectional area results in dyspnea only with significant exertion. Narrowing of the lumen to less than 25 percent of normal cross-sectional area will usually produce dyspnea and stridor at rest; such patients may be at risk of asphyxia from inability to clear secretions.

Stridor is classically accentuated during inspiration. However, if the obstructive lesion is in the mediastinal trachea (where intrathoracic pressure increases with exhalation against an obstruction) or if there is associated tracheomalacia, the stridor may be predominantly expiratory. Frequent but often overlooked symptoms of severe airway narrowing are a characteristic brassy cough and difficulty in raising secretions.

Not infrequently, these symptoms lead to a misdiagnosis of asthma or bronchitis. Understandably, symptoms are often attributed to manifestations of the original respiratory illness that led to the need for assisted ventilation, and the correct diagnosis is frequently delayed.

Symptom severity usually correlates with the degree of stenosis. If the lumen is greater than 5 mm (in adults), symptoms may be subtle and diagnosis difficult. Such patients may accept a modest restriction of exercise tolerance without seeking help. In patients whose pulmonary function is already

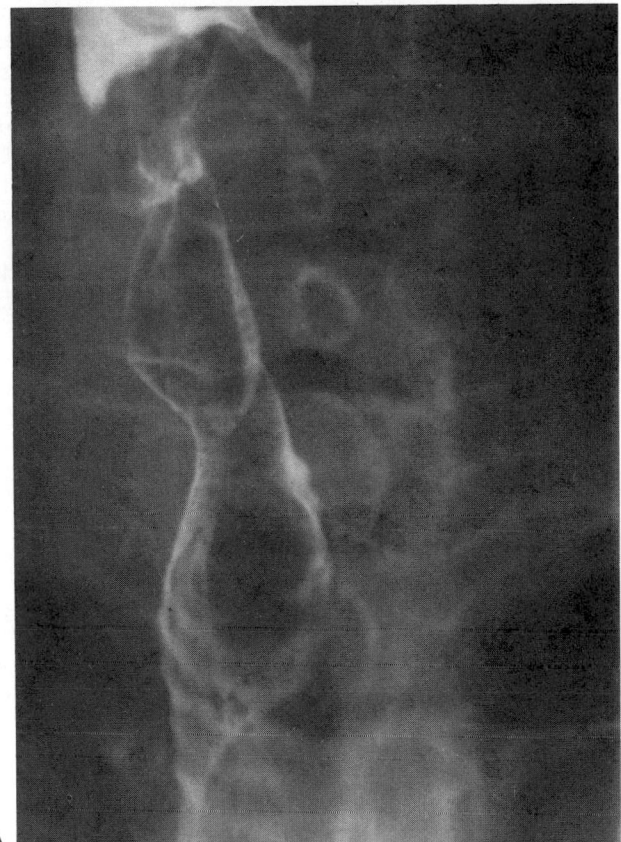

A

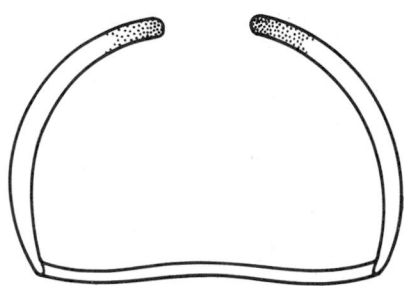

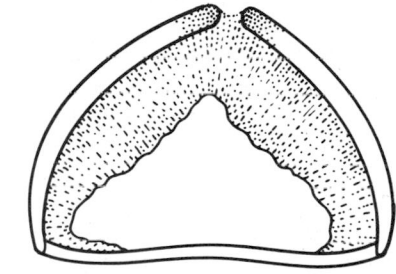

B

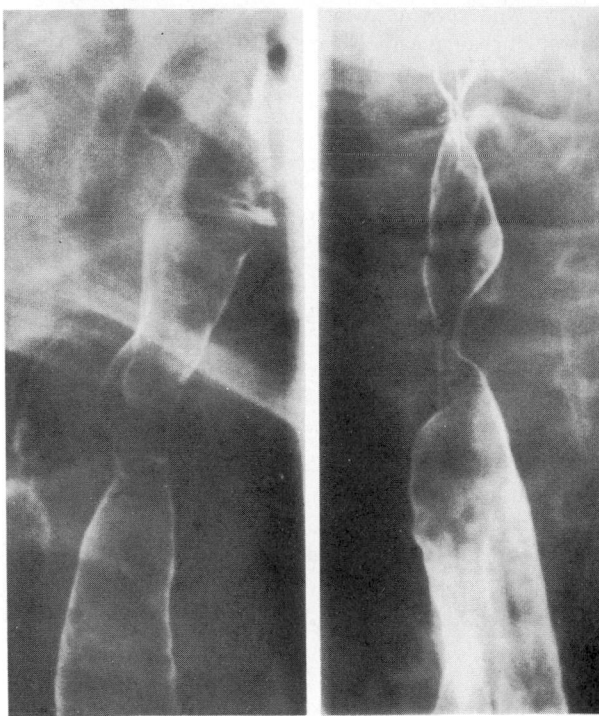

C

Figure 13-13. **(A)** Contrast tracheogram showing the typical anterolateral defect at the stomal level following tracheostomy. This relatively mild lesion was asymptomatic. **(B)** Diagramatic illustration of the mechanism of stomal stenosis. A variable segment of cartilage is lost anteriorly (*top*), and with healing the remaining margins fall together with formation of scar in the anterolateral parts of the trachea. The membranous trachea is relatively preserved, and a triangular-shaped stenosis results (*bottom*). **(C)** Severe stomal stenosis illustrated in a contrast tracheogram.

impaired (e.g., by chronic obstructive pulmonary disease), a lesser reduction in airway diameter may result in more severe symptoms. Stridor is present only when the diameter of the airway is reduced to 4 or 5 mm and may be noticeable only with exertion or during forcible inspiration and exhalation.

Changes in vocal function occur with lesions involving the glottis. Patients suffering from postintubation laryngeal injury and stenosis have variable degrees of hoarseness and loss of vocal power. Rarely, recurrent nerve injury occurs as a complication of tracheostomy and may be the cause of hoarseness.

Investigative Techniques

Radiology

Radiologic evaluation begins with a plain posteroanterior and lateral chest x-ray. This will provide information about the status of the lungs, and on occasion a narrowing in the airway may be apparent and obvious. Laryngeal and subglottic stenosis are never easily defined in the plain chest x-ray. Stomal stenosis in the cervical airway is sometimes evident in the plain film at a level above the manubrium, but the mediastinal airway is rarely accurately defined. Tomograms of the larynx, trachea, and main bronchi are useful and provide reasonably precise information about the location, length, and extent of the stenosis. Anteroposterior and lateral tomography provides three-dimensional information and is still easier for many practitioners to interpret than the images produced from the CT scan. CT does provide accurate information and will allow an evaluation of location, length, and extent of narrowing. In addition, the CT scan provides information about the tracheal wall and adjacent soft tissues, which is not available from tomography or plain chest films. The CT scan may be particularly useful in evaluating lesions involving both the larynx and the subglottis, for which fine intervals (1.5-cm cuts) are recommended. A more detailed evaluation of upper airway and laryngeal radiology is provided in Chapter 11.

Bronchoscopy

Bronchoscopy is a mainstay of evaluation. Much can be learned from flexible endoscopy under topical anesthesia. With the patient breathing spontaneously and able to vocalize, assessment can be made of vocal cord function and the more distal airway dynamics during inspiration, expiration, forced expiration, and coughing. Segments of tracheomalacia may only be evident at such an examination. It is important to note, however, that the operator has no control over a critically obstructed airway when using a flexible bronchoscope. It cannot be used to maintain the airway, as can a rigid bronchoscope, nor is the suction satisfactory in the face of abundant or tenacious secretions lying distal to a point of obstruction.

Rigid bronchoscopy conducted in an operating room and preferably under general anesthesia is desirable at some point in the evaluation of all patients with functionally significant stenosis. With the patient awake, vocal cord function and areas of malacia may be assessed with the rigid bronchoscope

as well. At rigid bronchoscopy it is possible to identify the exact anatomic location and diameter of the stenosis, to determine its position relative to the larynx above and the carina below, and to assess the rigidity of the stenosed segment. During either rigid or flexible bronchoscopy, it is important to evaluate the status of the mucosa adjacent the proximal and distal margins of the damaged segment. Most importantly, a tight and disabling stricture may be dilated at the time of rigid bronchoscopy: dilatation may be initiated by passing gum-tipped bougies through the bronchoscope, after which progressively larger diameter bronchoscopes are passed fully through the stenosis until a safe and adequate airway has been obtained. This allows safe and satisfactory relief of obstruction in almost all patients for a period usually measured in days or weeks and permits a more leisurely approach to the planning of subsequent management.

MANAGEMENT

Emergency Management

On occasion, patients with severe stenosis and disabling, life-threatening obstruction require emergency intervention. Therapy is initiated with humidified oxygen or a mixture of helium and oxygen, and the institution of measures that may reduce the inflammatory or edematous component of the obstruction. These include nebulized racemic epinephrine inhalation, intravenous steroid (Solu-Medrol 500 mg as a bolus), or steroid-containing inhalants such as Beclovent. These initiatives can be undertaken while preparing for emergency bronchoscopy in the operating room. Rigid bronchoscopy, with general anesthesia available, is preferable. The techniques of anesthesia are described in detail in Chapter 7. In patients with postintubation strictures, it is almost always possible to obtain control of the airway by using a rigid bronchoscope. Indeed, Couraud and Hafez (1987) report that they have never found it necessary to perform an emergency tracheostomy in these patients. If possible, every effort should be made to avoid tracheostomy since this will only complicate the pathology and may make subsequent surgery more difficult. In that rare instance when tracheostomy is deemed unavoidable, the tube should be introduced through an area of damaged trachea so that the extent of any subsequent resection is not increased. There is no role for emergency resection in these patients.

Elective Management

The options in elective management for patients with subglottic or tracheal stenosis include interval dilatation, laser resection, internal stents, staged plastic reconstructions, circumferential resection and primary anastomosis, or permanent tracheostomy.

Dilatation

Dilatation is useful to establish a safe airway at the onset of treatment. Further interval dilatation may be useful in maintaining the airway while acute inflammatory features of the original injury resolve and mature. With the exception of very short strictures (<0.5 cm in length), dilatation alone is rarely if ever successful in restoring an adequate airway.

Laser Resection

Laser resection has been popularized in recent years for the management of many lesions of the airway. For benign strictures, however, the benefit of the laser is almost always temporary. Only very short strictures are amenable to definitive management by laser resection. These are usually web-like lesions in which a four-quadrant laser incision may be successful (Fig. 13-14). In the subglottic region laser resection is generally contraindicated because of the potential for damaging the underlying cricoid cartilage.

Internal Stents

Although there are a variety of stents, a silicone T tube is most commonly used in the trachea. A stent is useful (1) as a temporary measure to avoid the need for repeated dilatations while waiting for inflammation to subside or for the general condition of the patient to improve prior to definitive surgical resection and (2) as an alternative to permanent tracheostomy in patients who are not candidates for resection and primary anastomosis. A Silastic T tube has the distinct advantage over open tracheostomy of maintaining both adequate humidification of the airway and normal speech. In cases of subglottic stenosis, the proximal arm of the T tube must be positioned with the open end lying just above the level of the vocal cords. In this position the tube is remarkably well tolerated. "Hypopharyngeal voice" is sufficient for reasonable communi-

nication. The problem of aspiration is common but usually resolves completely within a few days or weeks, except in some elderly patients or in the presence of additional pathology.

Staged Plastic Reconstruction

Staged plastic reconstruction has been popularized by otolaryngologists and is most widely used in the management of subglottic strictures. Most procedures involve vertical division of the anterior and posterior walls of the subglottic space (cricoid cartilage) and placement of some type of autogenous tissue graft between the divided ends of the cartilage. This is designed to achieve permanent enlargement of the subglottic airway. Grafts have been obtained from many sources and include free segments of bone or cartilage or composite pedicled grafts. As recently as 1991, McCaffrey reported results with costal cartilage grafts placed in anterior vertical incisions in the thyroid and cricoid cartilages. Of 21 patients with isolated subglottic stenosis, McCaffrey reported 16 (76 percent) with a satisfactory postoperative airway, while the other 5 (24 percent) could not be extubated.

Segmental Resection and Primary Anastomosis

The majority of functionally significant postintubation strictures are best managed by segmental resection and reconstruction with primary anastomosis. Most postintubation injuries involve relatively short segments (1 to 4 cm) and are reliably managed by circumferential resection and end-to-end anastomosis without resorting to special techniques of airway mobilization at the upper and lower ends of the trachea. On occasion, longer segments are damaged, and it is usually possible to resect approximately half the length of the adult trachea with the addition of supraglottic and infracarinal mobilization techniques.

Details of operative technique, including indications, perioperative management, complications, and results, are provided in Chapter 16.

Several principles for successful reconstruction by primary anastomosis warrant emphasis:

1. Accurate preoperative identification of the precise level and length of the lesion to be excised is essential, particularly in the case of benign strictures, and determines the anticipated operative exposure and mobilizing procedures. This information is most accurately obtained from the preoperative tomograms and CT scans, combined with the findings at bronchoscopy.

2. The tracheal margins at the level of the anastomosis should be as healthy as possible. When appropriate, acute mucosal inflammation should be allowed to subside before undertaking resection, and the excision should include all significantly diseased tissue. Both preoperative and postoperative tracheostomy should be avoided if possible, since an open tracheostomy inevitably results in some degree of chronic inflammatory change.

3. It is essential to preserve the tracheal circulation and avoid undue tension at the anastomosis. These are surgical platitudes, but nevertheless are of critical concern in obtaining a healthy, healing suture line. With the mobilization re-

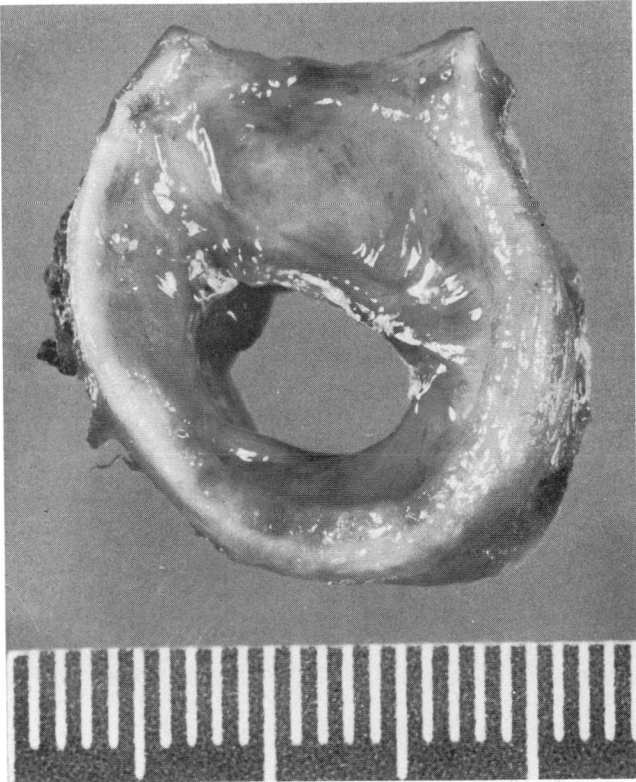

Figure 13-14. Photograph of a resected short postintubation stricture at the cuff level. This stricture, less than 5 mm in length, was resected in 1969 prior to the availability of an endobronchial laser and would be suitable for laser management today.

quired for resection, it is important to preserve the segmental blood supply which enters the trachea through a series of small, posterolateral branches. Once the lesion has been resected, the remaining tracheal ends should not be mobilized circumferentially for more than about 1 cm.

Grillo (1979) has clearly defined the contraindications to resection as (1) a continued need for, or high likelihood of future, ventilatory support; (2) medical unfitness to withstand operation (rarely a contraindication in patients requiring resection that is manageable through a cervical incision); (3) tracheal lesions requiring resection of lengths that cannot be technically reconstructed by primary anastomosis; and (4) anticipated requirement for future tracheostomy and management of certain neurologic diseases in which the patient is unable to avoid disabling aspiration. In addition, resection is relatively contraindicated in patients receiving high-dose steroids at the time of surgery or those who have previously undergone radical local irradiation in the field of resection (Grillo, 1979).

Results

In general, the results of resection and reconstruction by primary anastomosis for benign stenosis are excellent. We reported results in 34 patients with benign postintubation strictures (Andrews and Pearson, 1973). There were 30 good to excellent results, 3 unsatisfactory results, and 1 operative death. In this early series, seven patients developed restenosis, requiring reoperation and resection, and five of the seven ultimately obtained a good result. Grillo (1979) reported the results of resection and primary anastomosis in 208 patients with postintubation strictures. Of these lesions, 185 were produced by cuffed tracheostomy tubes. Between 2 and 7 cm of trachea was resected, with overall good results were obtained in 168 patients, satisfactory results in 21, and failure in only 9 (4 percent). These early reports by Pearson (1973) and Grillo (1979) provide results in patients with postintubation strictures involving the trachea in which only an occasional lesion extended above the lower border of the cricoid cartilage.

The results of resection in patients with subglottic stenosis have been reported separately. A technique of partial cricoid resection, preservation of recurrent nerves, and primary thyrotracheal anastomosis (Pearson, 1975) was used in 38 patients with isolated, benign subglottic stenosis (Maddaus, et al., 1992). There was no operative mortality, and all 38 patients were decannulated. Restenosis occurred in two cases, of which one was successfully managed by re-resection and the other by dilatation and laser ablation of anastomotic granulation tissue. Ultimately, therefore, all 38 patients achieved a satisfactory result. In this same publication (Maddaus, et al., 1992) we reported results in 16 patients with combined laryngeal and subglottic lesions, who were managed in collaboration with otolaryngology, by a synchronous subglottic resection combined with laryngeal reconstruction. Of the 16 patients so managed, 15 were decannulated and maintained a satisfactory glottic and subglottic airway.

Grillo, et al. (1992) have reported on 80 patients with subglottic stenosis managed by segmental resection and primary thyrotracheal anastomosis according to Grillo's own modified

technique for subglottic resection and reconstruction. Of these patients 50 had postintubation injuries, and in this group there was one operative mortality. All 49 survivors were improved, and a majority had good to excellent results, with none requiring long-term tracheostomy.

Couraud, et al. (1988) have reported experience with a large number of postintubation injuries involving either subglottal injury alone or subglottal concomitant laryngeal injury. Good to excellent results were obtained in 95 percent of cases, and all patients were extubated.

TRACHEOINNOMINATE ARTERY FISTULA

DEFINITION

TIF is a rare but frequently lethal complication of intubation or tracheostomy resulting from full-thickness erosion of the anterior wall of the mediastinal trachea. Nelems reviewed the literature in 1988. Of 175 reported cases, only 24 patients survived, a mortality rate of 86 percent.

HISTORICAL NOTE

The first report of massive hemorrhage due to a TIF following tracheostomy was by Korte in 1897. The patient, a 5-year-old girl with diphtheria, died of exsanguinating hemorrhage. In 1924 Schlaepfer reviewed the literature and summarized the findings in 115 patients with TIF, noting an incidence of 0.5 to 4.5 percent following tracheostomy. Couraud, et al. (1966) reported detailed pathologic observations in six clinical cases. Four of the fistulae were due to circumferential tracheal erosion by the cuff, extending through the anterior wall into the innominate artery. The anterior wall of the trachea was adherent to the artery, and hemorrhage occurred directly into the airway through a fistula measuring between 0.5 and 3.0 mm in diameter. In two cases erosion occurred at the inferior border of the tracheal stoma owing to pressure necrosis of the arterial wall against the undersurface of the tracheostomy tube. Two of the six patients had a premonitory hemorrhage of bright red blood, which occurred at 8 and 124 days, respectively, following creation of the tracheostomy.

HISTORICAL READINGS

Couraud L, Favarel-Garrigues JC, Chevais G et al.: Cataclysmic creation of the tracheal hemorrhage following tracheostomy. Anatomical etiological and therapeutical consideration. Ann Chir Thorac Cardiovasc 5:772, 1966

Korte W: Über einige seltenere nach Krankheiten nach der Tracheotomie wegen Diphtheritis. Arch Klin Chir 24:238, 1897

Schlaepfer K: Fatal hemorrhage following tracheotomy for laryngeal diphtheria. JAMA 82:1581, 1924

BASIC SCIENCE

Figure 13-15 illustrates the mechanisms of postintubation TIF. The most common cause is the result of erosion following a low placement of the tracheal stoma, allowing the can-

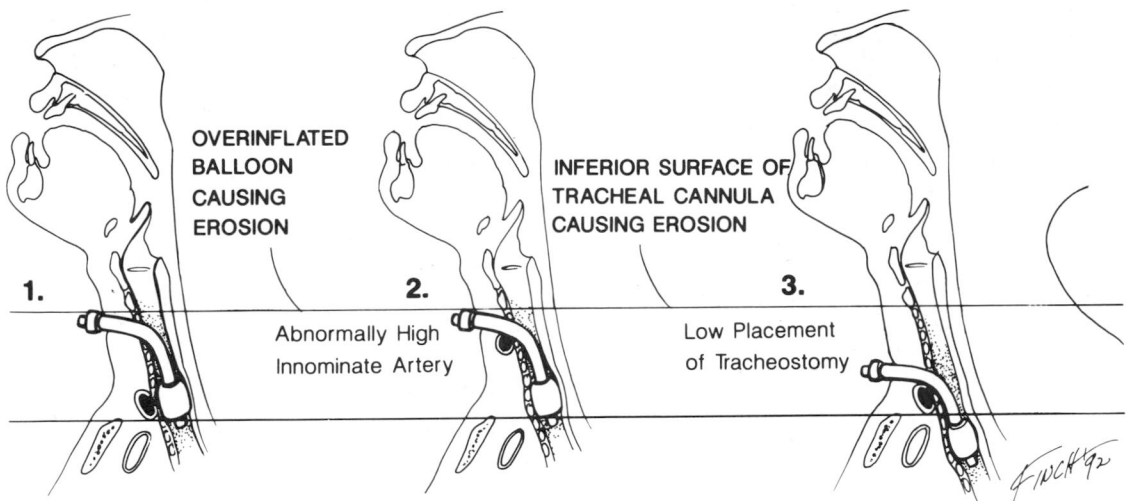

Figure 13-15. Diagram illustrating the mechanisms of TIF. The fistula may occur from erosion of the anterior wall under the inflatable cuff or at the level of the stoma owing to pressure from the tracheostomy tube itself. This latter mechanism occurs when the innominate artery courses above the manubrium in the neck or when the tracheal stoma is created at too low a level.

nula to abut and erode the innominate artery. This mechanism of fistula formation is preventable by placing the stoma at the level of the second or third tracheal ring. The innominate artery normally lies at the level of the fifth or sixth tracheal ring behind the manubrium. In children and young adults, however, it may lie in the neck above the sternal notch. In such patients mobilization of the arterial wall adjacent to the stoma should be avoided and the stoma placed so as to avoid possible contact and erosion.

Another etiology is tracheal wall necrosis due to cuff hyperinflation, resulting in erosion of the anterior tracheal wall into the innominate artery. Also, normally placed tracheostomy may occasionally erode the adjacent distal tracheal cartilage and ultimately abut the innominate artery, with subsequent fistula formation.

TIF can complicate tracheal resection, extended laryngectomy, and prosthetic tracheal reconstruction. Arterial fistula following tracheal resection has been reported by Grillo (1979) in 0.5 percent and by Deslauriers, et al. (1975) in 3.0 percent of tracheal reconstructions with end-to-end anastomosis. These fistulae result from erosion against the contiguous tracheal anastomosis and the associated suture material. Grillo (1979) recommends protecting any tracheal anastomosis that lies near the innominate artery, for which he uses local tissue such as surrounding fat, thymus, or strap muscle.

Nelems (1987) described fistula formation after extended laryngectomy in two patients who required extensive tracheal resection for distal tracheal spread of a laryngeal tumor. Following dehiscence of the cutaneous tracheostomy stoma due to undue tension, the innominate artery was exposed and eroded by the laryngectomy tube.

DIAGNOSIS

TIF presents with massive bleeding. Jones, et al. (1976) noted that 72 percent of such patients bled within 21 days of establishing the tracheostomy. Premonitory hemorrhage, often sig-

nificant but not life-threatening, may precede massive bleeding. Premonitory bleeding can manifest around the tracheostomy tube (attributed to the tracheostomy wound), through the tracheostomy tube (attributed to tracheal suctioning or tracheitis), or through the mouth or nose (often ignored). It is critical to recognize that bleeding from any of the above sites may represent a TIF.

MANAGEMENT

In all patients with a tracheostomy and possible premonitory bleeding, flexible bronchoscopy is performed to define the etiology. If the findings suggest arterial injury, the neck incision is reopened and the wound explored in the operating room. Prior to exploration of the wound, an endotracheal tube is placed with the tip above the tracheostomy. With the airway thus controlled, the tracheostomy tube is partially withdrawn and the wound opened laterally as far as necessary to fully assess the tracheostomy site. If no fistula is found, the wound is closed and the tracheostomy tube replaced. If a fistula is found, it is managed by resection of the damaged arterial segment, with subsequent closure of the divided ends.

In patients with massive bleeding, which is the usual scenario, management involves three simultaneous priorities, namely, control of the airway, control of bleeding, and resuscitation. Initially, the tracheostomy balloon is hyperinflated in an effort to compress the artery anteriorly (Fig. 13-16). If this is successful, an assistant is assigned to hold the tracheostomy tube securely in position. Simultaneously, an endotracheal tube is passed with the tip placed just above the tracheostomy site to ensure control of the airway. If balloon hyperinflation is unsuccessful, the tracheostomy wound is widely opened and the innominate artery is compressed anteriorly against the manubrium with a finger (Fig. 13-16). A rigid bronchoscope can be used to compress the hyperinflated tracheostomy balloon against the innominate artery and the sternum with control of the bleeding (Cooper, 1987) (Fig.

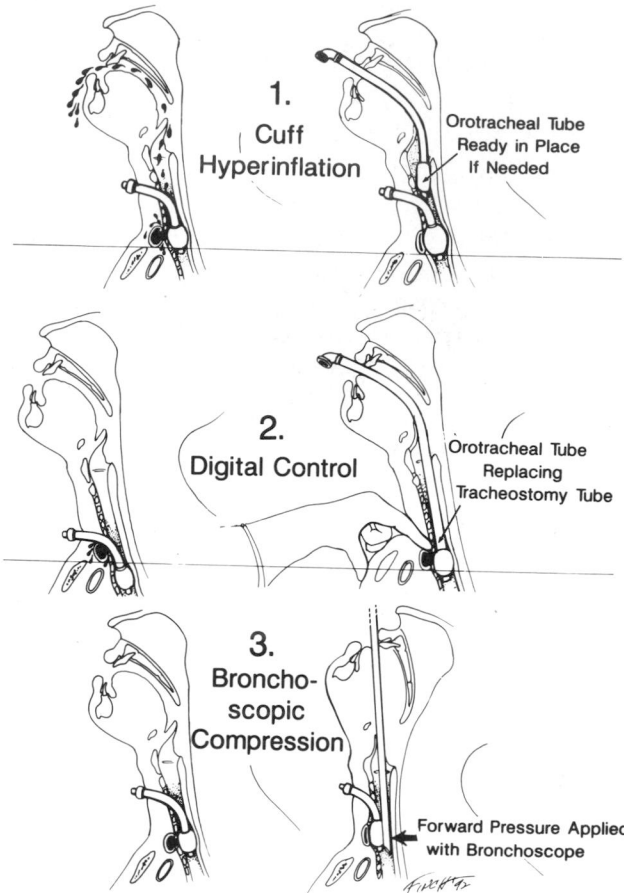

Figure 13-16. Diagram illustrating the steps in the emergency management of TIF.

13-16). One can then clear blood from the distal tracheobronchial tree and ventilate the patient. Jet ventilation may be preferable in this situation, if available.

With the airway secure and bleeding controlled, the patient is cross-matched, sedated as necessary, and if not already there, transported to the operating room. Under general anesthesia, the entire neck and chest are prepared and draped. The incision for repair of the fistula is an extension of the tracheotomy incision and a partial upper sternotomy with extension into the right third or fourth intercostal space (Cooper, 1987; Nelems, 1987). Full sternotomy adds a higher risk of infection from the contaminated tracheostomy site. After clearing the thymus and retracting the innominate vein, proximal and distal control of the innominate artery is obtained. The artery is dissected free from the trachea and the fistula resected. It may be necessary to resect the innominate artery at its point of origin from the aorta, and the suture line may be flush with the aortic wall. Repair of the arterial wall is contraindicated. Jones, et al. (1976) reported only an 18 percent survival in cases managed by repair. Deslauriers, et al. (1975) noted that repair almost inevitably fails even when bolstered with autogenous tissue.

The controversy about vascular reconstruction is still unresolved, although anecdotal reports strongly suggest that bypass to the right carotid system is unnecessary. Most authors therefore advise resection of the innominate artery without vascular bypass.

If the field is grossly infected, the tracheal defect may be packed open to await secondary closure with granulation tissue. It may be closed primarily and covered with soft tissue if the operative field is clean. The airway is managed by translaryngeal intubation with positioning of the balloon cuff below the tracheal wall defect.

TRACHEOESOPHAGEAL FISTULA

DEFINITION

TEF results from the destruction of the posterior membranous trachea, which occurs predominantly after prolonged mechanical ventilation and nasogastric intubation.

HISTORICAL NOTE

Prior to 1960 the most common etiology of benign TEF was granulomatous mediastinal infection or trauma. In 1967 Flege reported on TEF due to injury caused by cuffed endotracheal tubes. By 1973 Thomas (1973) had collected 46 cases of benign postintubation TEF and documented cuffed tube intubation as the leading cause. A variety of methods have been used in the management of these fistulae. Early attempts at direct repair of the fistula were made by Braithwaite (1961), Flege (1967), and Thomas (1973) with some success. In 1976 Grillo, et al. noted that these fistulae were frequently associated with a damaged and stenosed tracheal segment at the same level as the fistula. They described a single-stage technique for simultaneous closure of the esophageal defect, circumferential tracheal resection, and primary tracheal anastomosis, performed through an anterior cervical approach.

HISTORICAL READINGS

Braithwaite FC: Closure of a tracheo-esophageal fistula. Br J Plast Surg 14:138, 1961

Flege JB Jr: Tracheoesophageal fistula caused by cuffed tracheostomy tube. Ann Surg 166:153, 1967

Grillo HC, Moncure AC, McEnany MT: Repair of inflammatory tracheoesophageal fistula. Ann Thorac Surg 22:112, 1976

DIAGNOSIS

TEFs occur predominantly in patients who have required prolonged mechanical ventilation combined with nasogastric intubation. Cuff inflation compresses the membranous trachea and anterior esophageal wall against the nasogastric tube, leading to full-thickness necrosis and fistula formation. In most cases there is a concurrent circumferential injury to the tracheal wall at cuff level.

A TEF may be heralded by a marked increase in tracheal secretions with the characteristics of saliva. Patients receiving oral nutrition may cough during swallowing, with liquids or particulate food appearing in the tracheal aspirate. Patients with reflux may have repeated aspiration of gastric juice through the fistula and into the tracheobronchial tree. Gross gastric distension due to "ventilation" of the esophagus and stomach through the fistula occurs if the cuff is positioned above the fistula.

Confirmation of the suspected diagnosis is usually simple. TEFs are usually sizable and easy to identify directly through the stoma, after removing the tracheostomy tube. Alternatively, the tracheostomy tube can be pulled back and a flexible bronchoscope inserted through the tracheostomy to visualize the defect. Esophagoscopy, with the tracheostomy cuff inflated, allows visualization of the fistula, which is typically located on the anterior wall of the esophagus 1 to 2 cm below the stoma. Contrast studies are usually unnecessary. The large size of the fistula allows direct visualization in nearly all cases.

MANAGEMENT

Mathisen (1991) has eloquently reported an extensive experience with nonmalignant TEF. The initial dilemma is whether or not the fistula should be repaired while the patient still requires assisted ventilation. The few reported attempts to achieve closure in this circumstance have been failures. With a documented TEF in a patient who still requires ventilation, Mathisen (1991) recommends the following steps: (1) Remove the nasogastric tube. (2) Ensure that the tracheostomy has a low-pressure cuff that is not overinflated and attempt to place the cuff below the fistula; if absolutely necessary the cuff can be kept at the level of the fistula. (3) Establish a gastrostomy (to prevent gastroesophageal reflux) and a feeding jejunostomy.

Salivary secretions are usually easily managed by frequent suctioning. In the rare patient who appears disabled because of aspiration of salivary secretions, a tube pharyngostomy or cervical esophagostomy may be necessary. The patient is weaned as tolerated from ventilator support. Esophageal diversion is only used when disabling and life-threatening aspiration continues despite the above measures or in cases of supracarinal fistula that cannot be controlled with the cuffed tube.

Once the patient is weaned from the ventilator, a single-stage repair is performed. Since many fistulae are accompanied by simultaneous circumferential tracheal injury, repair often requires a segmental tracheal resection and reanastomosis, along with repair of the esophageal defect.

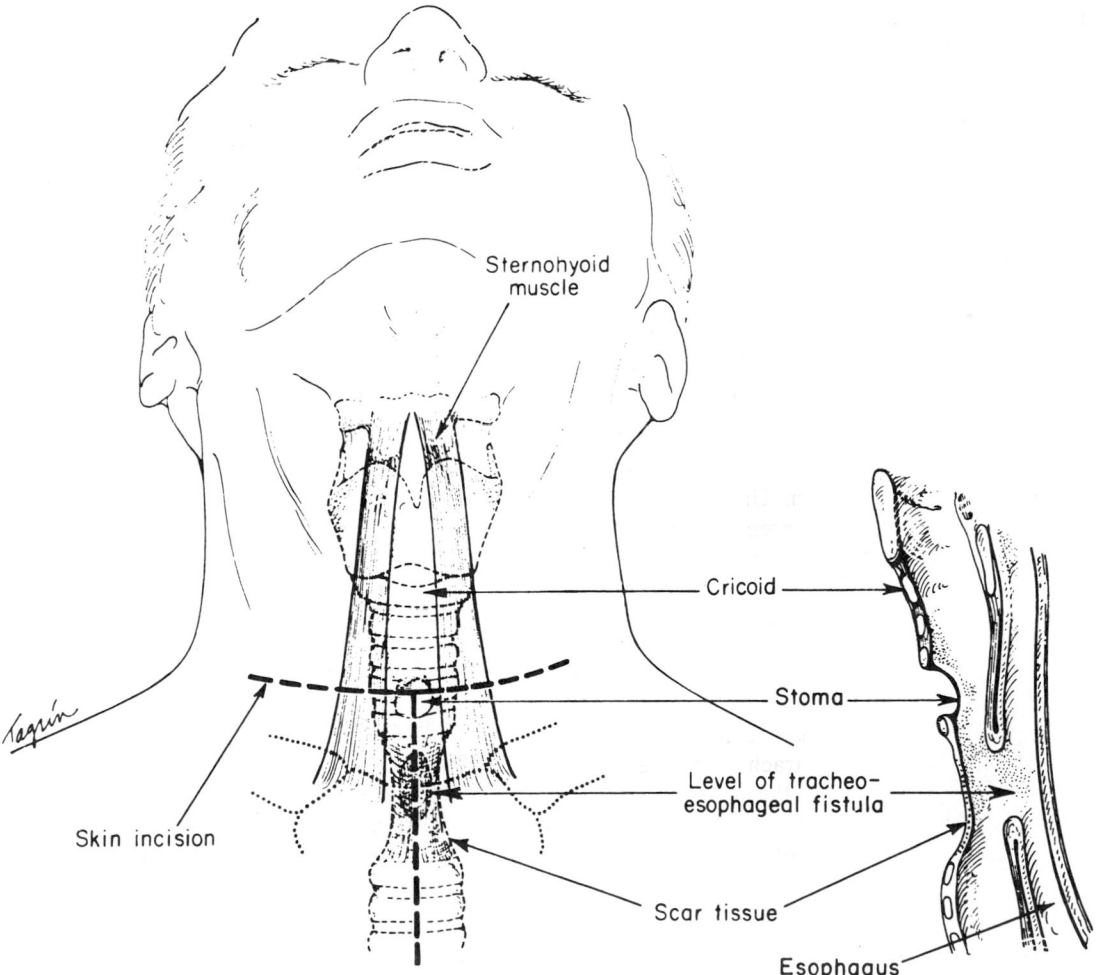

Figure 13-17. Diagram illustrating the position of a cervical incision centered over the tracheostomy stoma, with a vertical extension for partial upper sternotomy, in the management of postintubation TEF.

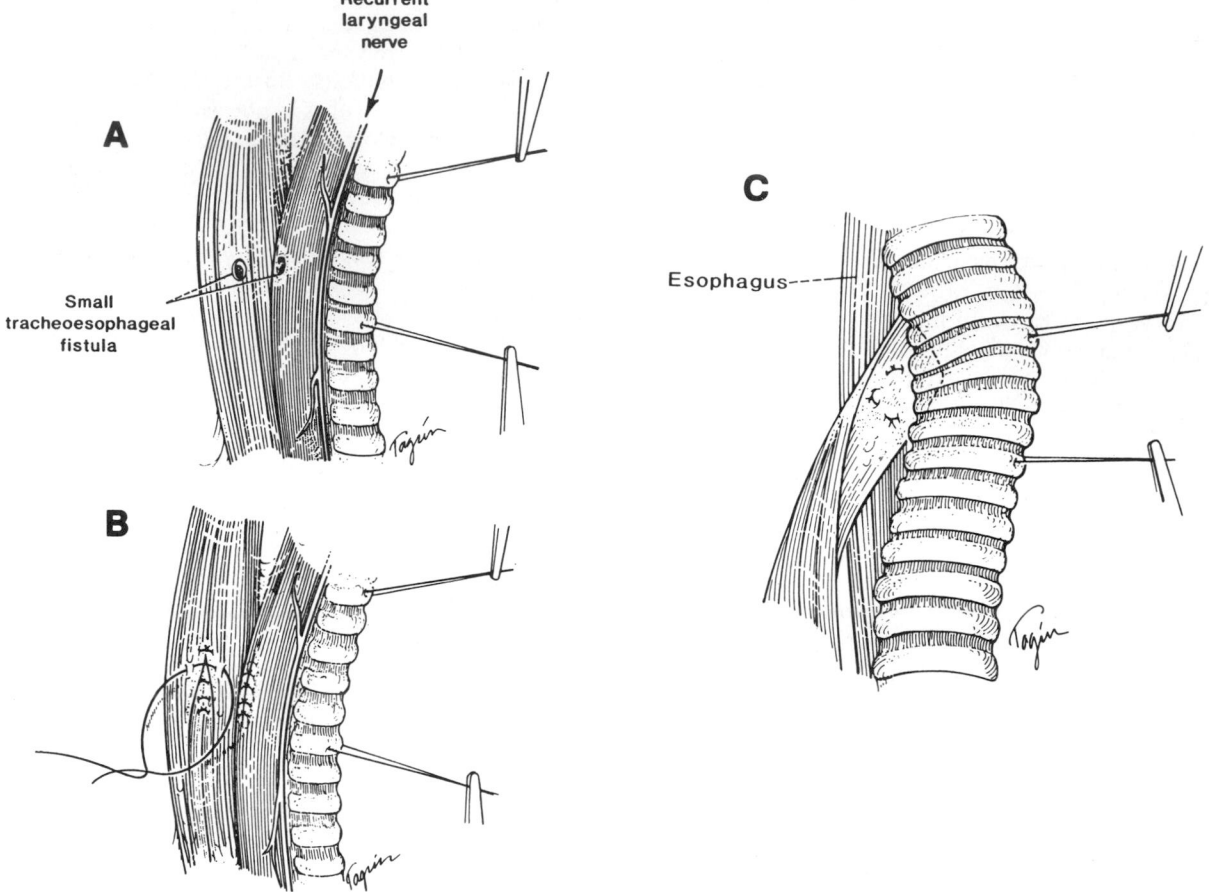

Figure 13-18. Diagrammatic illustration of repair for **(A)** a small TEF without significant tracheal injury. **(B)** The fistula is closed on both tracheal and esophageal sides, and **(C)** a pedicle flap of strap muscle is interposed between esophagus and trachea at the level of the suture lines.

Figure 13-17 illustrates placement of a collar incision over the tracheostomy stoma. Since many of these fistulae are at a level below the manubrium, partial upper sternotomy may be necessary.

With small fistulae and lesser degrees of tracheal damage, repair consists of identification and division of the fistula, closure of the tracheal defect with interrupted 4–0 Vicryl sutures, and a two-layer closure of the esophageal defect. A pedicle of strap muscle is interposed between the esophageal and tracheal suture line to prevent recurrence (Fig. 13-18).

In patients with extensive or circumferential tracheal damage, the fistula is identified and divided, the damaged trachea is resected, and a primary tracheal anastomosis is performed. The esophageal defect is closed in two layers (Fig. 13-19), and strap muscle is interposed between the two suture lines. If a tracheostomy is required for postoperative airway man-

agement, it is preferably placed at least two tracheal rings below the tracheal anastomosis if possible.

Mathisen (1991) reported on 38 patients with nonmalignant TEF in whom 41 operations were performed. In 9 patients with smaller fistulae and normal tracheas, the procedure was simple division and closure of the fistula, while the other 29 patients were managed by tracheal resection and esophageal repair. There were three recurrent fistulae, of which two were managed by re-resection and the other healed spontaneously with simple drainage. Of the 34 surviving patients, 33 were capable of normal oral intake. Five patients required esophageal dilatation owing to narrowing at the level of the repair of the esophageal fistula. Thus, in the majority of patients, a single-stage repair can be performed with a low rate of recurrence and with a good prospect of restoring normal oral alimentation.

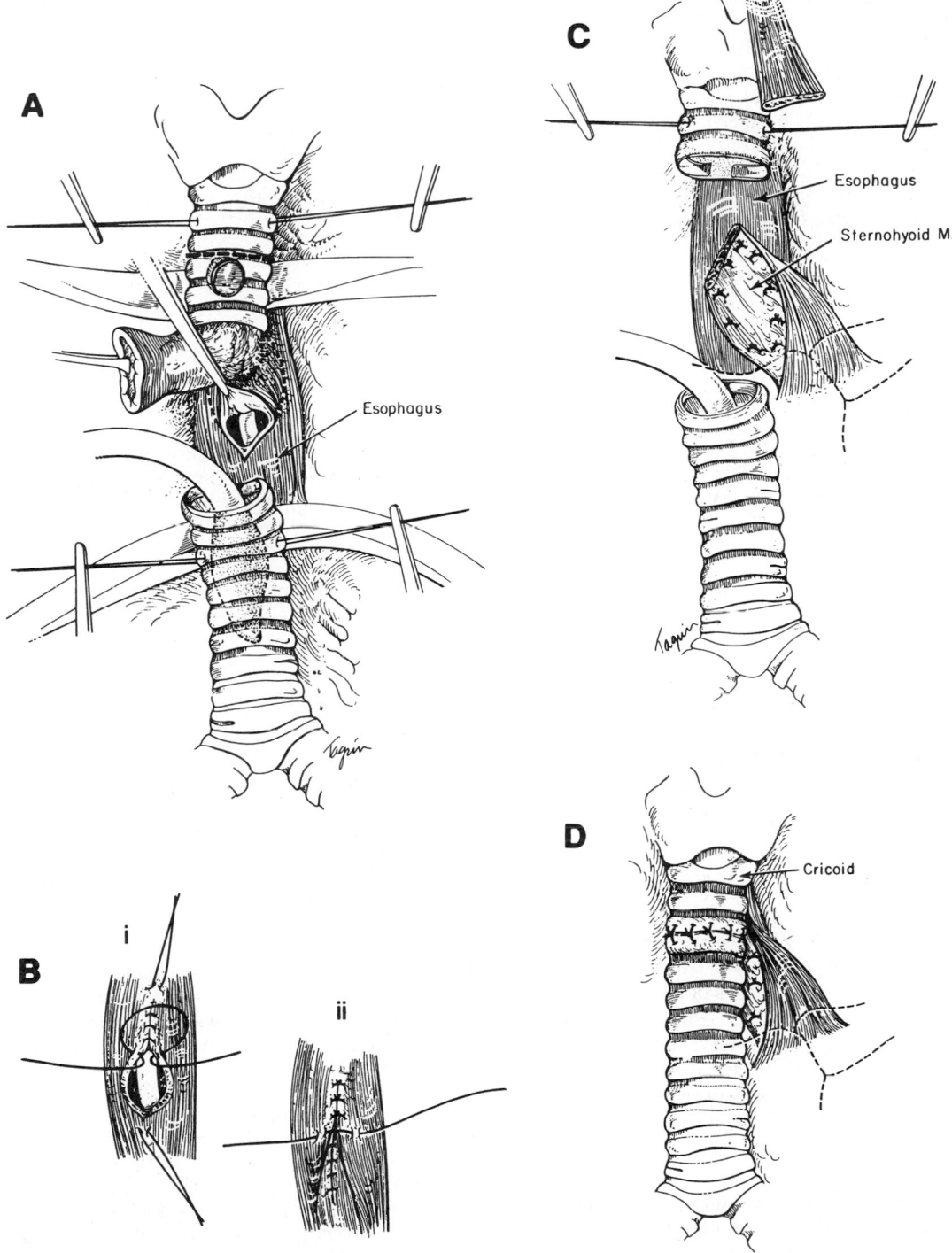

Figure 13-19. Illustration of steps for closure in a TEF in which there is extensive tracheal damage requiring a concomitant tracheal resection. **(A)** The fistula is divided and the trachea transected below the level of the tracheal injury. **(B)** The tracheal side of the fistula is closed with a single layer of interrupted absorbable suture, and the esophageal side of the defect is closed in two layers. **(C)** The damaged tracheal segment is removed, usually with inclusion of the tracheostomy stoma, and a pedicled flap of sternohyoid muscle is sutured in place over the esophageal closure. **(D)** The tracheal anastomosis is then completed.

KEY REFERENCES

Cooper JD: Complications of tracheostomy: pathogenesis, treatment, and prevention. In International Trends in General Thoracic Surgery. Vol 2. WB Saunders, Philadelphia, 1987

A comprehensive review of postintubation injury due to tracheostomy, which provides a clear exposition of pathogenesis and recognition and important statements about prevention of injury in the current era.

Couraud L, Hafez A: Acquired and non-neoplastic subglottic stenoses. In In International Trends in General Thoracic Surgery. Vol. 2. WB Saunders, Philadelphia, 1987

A comprehensive report of a large and carefully documented experience with laryngotracheal injury. The report, which catalogs

Couraud's experience beginning in the early 1960s, parallels the evolution in management of subglottic stenosis from simple dilatation through staged plastic reconstruction and the ultimate evolution of techniques for circumferential resection and primary anastomosis.

Mathisen DJ, Grillo HC, Wain JC et al.: Management of acquired nonmalignant tracheoesophageal fistula. Ann Thorac Surg 52:759, 1991

A detailed review of the largest reported experience with postintubation tracheoesophageal fistula in the world. Pathogenesis, diagnosis, and details of management are provided, and the importance of identifying significant associated tracheal injury is documented and emphasized.

REFERENCES

Andrews MJ, Pearson FG: An analysis of 59 cases of tracheal stenosis following tracheostomy with cuffed tube and assisted ventilation, with special reference to diagnosis and treatment. Br J Surg 60:208, 1973

Andrews MJ, Pearson FG: The incidence and pathogenesis of tracheal injury following cuffed tube tracheostomy with assisted ventilation: an analysis of a two year prospective study. Ann Surg 173:249, 1971

Braithwaite FC: Closure of a tracheo-esophageal fistula. Br J Plast Surg 14:138, 1961

Colice GL, Stukel TA, Dain B: Laryngeal complications of prolonged intubation. Chest 96:877, 1989

Cooper JD, Grillo HC: The evolution of tracheal injury due to ventilatory assistance through cuffed tubes—a pathologic study. Ann Surg 169:334, 1969a

Cooper JD, Grillo HC: Experimental production and prevention of injury due to cuffed tracheal tube. Surg Gynecol Obstet 129:1235, 1969b

Couraud L, Brichon PY, Velly JF: The surgical treatment of inflammatory and fibrous laryngotracheal stenosis. Eur J Cardiothorac Surg 2:410, 1988

Couraud L, Favarel-Garrigues JC, Chevais G et al.: Cataclysmic creation of the tracheal hemorrhage following tracheostomy. Anatomical etiological and therapeutic consideration. Ann Chir Thorac Cardiovasc 5:772, 1966

Deslauriers J, Ginsberg RJ, Nelems JM, Pearson FG: Innominate artery rupture. A major complication of tracheal surgery. Ann Thorac Surg 20:671, 1975

Donnelly WH: Histopathology of endotracheal intubation: an autopsy study of 99 cases. Arch Pathol Lab Med 88:511, 1969

Flege JB Jr: Tracheoesophageal fistula caused by cuffed tracheostomy tube. Ann Surg 166:153, 1967

Gerwat J, Bryce DP: The management of subglottic laryngeal stenosis by resection and direct anastomosis. Laryngoscope 84:940, 1974

Grillo HC: Surgical treatment of post-intubation tracheal injuries. J Thorac Cardiovasc Surg 78:860, 1979

Grillo HC, Cooper JD, Geffin B et al.: A low pressure cuff for tracheostomy tubes to minimize tracheal injury—a comparative clinical trial. J Thorac Cardiovasc Surg 62:898, 1971

Grillo HC, Mathisen DJ, Wain JC: Laryngotracheal resection and reconstruction for subglottic stenosis. Ann Thorac Surg 53:54, 1992

Grillo HC, Moncure AC, McEnany MT: Repair of inflammatory tracheoesophageal fistula. Ann Thorac Surg 22:112, 1976

Grillo HC, Zannini P, Michelassi F: Complication of tracheal reconstruction. J Thorac Cardiovasc Surg 91:322, 1986

Jones JW, Reynolds M, Hewitt RL et al.: Tracheoinnominate artery erosion: successful surgical management of a devastating complication. Ann Surg 184:194, 1976

Kastanos N, Epoa Miro R, Marin Perez A et al.: Laryngotracheal injury due to endotracheal intubation: incidence, evolution, and predisposing factors. A prospective long-term study. Crit Care Med 11:362, 1983

Korte W: Über einige seltenere nach Krankheiten nach der Tracheotomie wegen Diphtheritis. Arch Klin Chir 24:238, 1897

Lassen HCA: Management of Life-Threatening Poliomyelitis. E & S Livingstone, London, 1956

Maddaus MA, Toth JL, Gullane PJ, Pearson FG: Subglottic tracheal resection and synchronous laryngeal reconstruction. J Thorac Cardiovasc Surg 104:1443, 1992

McCaffrey TV: Management of subglottic stenosis in the adult. Ann Otol Rhinol Laryngol 100:90, 1991

Montgomery WW: Suprahyoid release for tracheal anastomosis. Arch Otolaryngol Head Neck Surg 99:255, 1974

Mulliken JB, Grillo HC: The limits of tracheal resection with primary anastomosis. J Thorac Cardiovasc Surg 55:418, 1968

Nelems B: Tracheoarterial fistula. p. 69. In In International Trends in General Thoracic Surgery. Vol. 2, WB Saunders, Philadelphia, 1987

Ogura JH, Powers WE: Functional restitution of traumatic stenosis of the larynx and pharynx. Laryngoscope 74:1081, 1964

Pearson FG: Primary tracheal anastomosis after resection of the cricoid cartilage with preservation of recurrent laryngeal nerves. J Thorac Cardiovasc Surg 70:806, 1975

Pearson FG, Goldberg, DaSilva: A prospective study of tracheal injury complicating tracheostomy with a cuffed tube. Ann Otol Rhinol Laryngol 77:867, 882, 1968

Pearson FG, Andrew MJ: Detection and management of tracheal stenosis following cuffed tube tracheostomy. Ann Thorac Surg 12:359, 1971

Pearson FG, Brito-Filomen L, Cooper JD: Experience with partial cricoid resection and thyrotracheal anastomosis. Ann Otol Rhinol Laryngol 95:582, 1986

Schlaepfer K: Fatal hemorrhage following tracheotomy for laryngeal diphtheria. JAMA 82:1581, 1924

Schmidt WA, Schaap RN, Mortensen JD: Immediate mucosal effects of short-term, soft-cuff, endotracheal intubation. Arch Pathol Lab Med 103:516, 1979

Streitz JM, Shapshay SM: Airway injury after tracheostomy and endotracheal intubation. Surg Clin North Am 71:1211, 1991

Thomas AN: Management of tracheo-esophageal fistula caused by cuffed tracheal tubes. Am J Surg 124:181, 1972

Trendelenburg F: Beitrage zu den Operationen an den Luftwegen. Arch Klin Chir 12:112, 1871

Tucker HM: The Larynx. Thieme, New York, 1987

Webb WR, Ozdenin IA, Ikins PM et al.: Surgical management of tracheal stenosis. Ann Surg 179:819, 1973

Whited RE: A prospective study of laryngo-tracheal sequelae in long-term intubation. Laryngoscope 94:367, 1984

Idiopathic Stenosis

Hermes C. Grillo

DEFINITION

A lower laryngeal and upper tracheal circumferential fibrous stenosis that is of idiopathic origin is occasionally seen. While such patients are characterized principally by the fact that they have no known cause for the stenosis, the lesions also share typical features of location, configuration, clinical evolution, and specific pathology.

HISTORICAL NOTE

Brandenburg (1972) described three cases of idiopathic subglottic stenosis seen over 10 years, two of which were complicated by retro-orbital pseudotumor. Several other case reports have appeared (Mikaelian, 1974; Jazbi, et al., 1977; Havas, et al., 1984). Grillo (1982), Grillo, et al., (1992), and Maddaus, et al. (1992) noted a number of these patients in reports on single-stage laryngotracheal resection and reconstruction. In 1993, Grillo, et al. reported 49 patients with this entity, provided a detailed picture of the pathology, and described the natural history, surgical management, and results of treatment.

HISTORICAL READINGS

Brandenburg JH: Idiopathic subglottic stenosis. Trans Am Acad Ophthalmol Otolaryngol 76:1402, 1972

Grillo HC: Primary reconstruction of airway after resection of subglottic laryngeal and upper tracheal stenosis. Ann Thorac Surg 33:3, 1982

Grillo HC, Mathisen DJ, Wain JC: Laryngotracheal resection and reconstruction for subglottic stenosis. Ann Thorac Surg 53:54, 1992

Havas T, Dodd M, Weldon B et al.: A case report of subglottic stenosis. Aust N Z J Surg 54:291, 1984

Jazbi B, Goodwin C, Tackett D, Faulkner S: Idiopathic subglottic stenosis. Ann Otol Rhinol Laryngol 86:644, 1977

Maddaus MA, Toth JLR, Gullane PJ, Pearson FG: Subglottic tracheal resection and synchronous laryngeal reconstruction. J Thorac Cardiovasc Surg 104:144, 1992

Mikaelian DO: Idiopathic subglottic stenosis in an adult. J Laryngol Otol 88:467, 1974

BASIC SCIENCE

The lesion presents as circumferential fibrotic stenosis, which begins at varying distances from the vocal cords, usually in the subglottic larynx but occasionally in the upper trachea only, and extends into the upper trachea. The tissue is dense and fibrous, although mucosal bleeding occurs easily on instrumentation. In a few patients more florid granulation tissue or even ulceration is present, but this is unusual. While the proximal end of the stricture begins subtly somewhere below the vocal cords, its inferior border in the trachea is usually quite sharp. The usual length of stenosis measures between 2 and 3 cm with a range of 1.5 to 5 cm. Trachea distal to the lesion is normal. The effective lumen may be as narrow as 2 mm but more frequently ranges from 5 to 7 mm.

Dense, white, fibrous tissue replaces the lamina propria of the trachea. No calcification or ossification is encountered. Fibrosis is of the keloidal type, with thick bundles of eosinophilic collagen separated by sparse fibroblasts (Fig. 13-20). Some patients have areas of spindle cell proliferation with regimentation of nuclei, but such cellular regions represent a minority of the affected area. Mucous glands may be entrapped by fibrosis and become dilated. Lymphocytes are

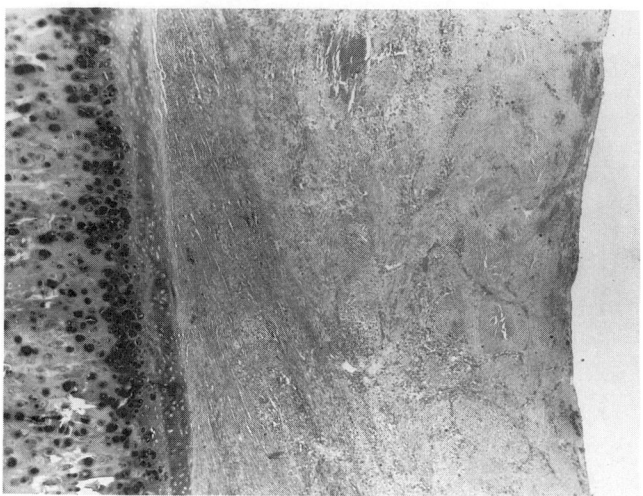

Figure 13-20. Histopathology of idiopathic tracheal stenosis. Dense fibrosis of the keloidal type replaces the lamina propria of the mucosa. Epithelium (*right*) has squamous metaplasia. Inner perichondrium (*left*) is normal (× 30). (From Grillo HC, Mark EJ, Mathisen DJ, Wain JC: Idiopathic laryngotracheal stenosis and its management. Ann Thorac Surg 56:80, 1993, with permission.)

modest in number and sometimes are almost lacking. Small numbers of histiocytes associated with lymphocytes are embedded in the cellular fibrosis.

The surface epithelium usually shows squamous metaplasia (Fig. 13-20), sometimes with granulation tissue noted. Cartilaginous rings remain intact or in some cases show slight loss of basophilic chondroitin sulfate from chondrocytes along the inner perichondrium. Little, if any destruction of cartilage is seen, and no pus, eosinophiles, plasma cells, polychondritis, granulomas, vasculitis, granulomatosis of the Wegener type, amyloid, organisms, or foreign particles are seen. Cultures for bacteria, mycobacteria, and fungi have been repeatedly negative. Antineutrophil cytoplasmic antibody (ANCA) tests have been negative in all but one patient with poorly defined periarteritis.

DIAGNOSIS

Clinical Features

Of 49 patients seen by Grillo, et al. (1993), 46 were women ranging in age from 18 years to the 70s, with most in their 30s to 60s. Symptoms were initially dyspnea on effort, progressing to dyspnea at rest, noisy breathing, wheezing, or stridor. The duration of symptoms before evaluation varied from 4 months to 15 years, with the majority of patients reporting symptoms of 1 to 3 years duration. None had been intubated for ventilation. A few had had brief anesthesias, with or without intubation, probably unrelated to their pathology. None had had bacterial tracheitis, tuberculosis, histoplasmosis, diphtheria, scleroma, or other specific tracheal infections. None had suffered external trauma to the trachea, inhalation burns, or irradiation. The age of onset, relative brevity of symptom duration, and pathologic findings ruled out congenital lesions. Sarcoid, relapsing polychondritis, Wegener's granulomatosis, and amyloid disease were not present. Two patients had vague arthralgia, and in one polyarteritis was suspected. The remaining 46 had no systemic symptoms or illnesses previously, concurrently, or subsequently.

Natural History

Most patients had had symptoms for 1 to 3 years prior to their clinical recognition, but in others the symptoms could be traced back for as long as 15 years. Initially, and continuing in many cases, the therapy was dilatation. Stenosis then recurred with its original or even greater tightness over varying periods, sometimes weeks and sometimes years. Lesions have never regressed spontaneously over long periods of follow-up. In only 2 of the 49 patients was there evidence of extension of stenosis into more distal areas of the trachea following initial resection. As noted, no signs of disease elsewhere or of systemic illness appeared. No association with gastroesophageal reflux was found.

Differential Diagnosis

Idiopathic stenosis is a diagnosis made initially by its typical clinical characteristics and by exclusion of any other etiology. These conditions have been noted in previous paragraphs. The pathology of a resected specimen is quite typical and rules out the diagnoses of polychondritis, Wegener's granulomatosis, and other entities.

Investigative Techniques

Simple radiologic techniques (Momose and MacMillan, 1978) demonstrate the location and extent of the lesion very well (Fig. 13-21). These may be supplemented with tomograms. Crisp, linear images such as these are generally of more use than CT scans, which provide cross-sectional images. Linear pictures show where the lesion begins and ends and its severity, as well as the amount of subglottic space remaining for reconstruction. Flow-volume loops demonstrate extrathoracic fixed obstruction as might be expected (Fig. 13-22). Direct endoscopy usually demonstrates normal vocal cord function with subglottic stenosis, as described (Fig. 13-23). The proximity and severity of the process in relation to the undersurface of the vocal cords are of greatest importance in determining the ease with which surgical correction may be done with a reasonable chance of success.

MANAGEMENT

Principles

Because of the unknown nature of the disease process and uncertainty about its future progression, patients were approached conservatively. Therapy consisted of dilatation at intervals, as necessary for relief of severe symptoms. The period of relief obtained varied greatly. Surgical resection and reconstruction have been increasingly performed, as favorable results were obtained. When the disease involves the larynx, as is often the case, techniques are used that provide correction in a single stage.

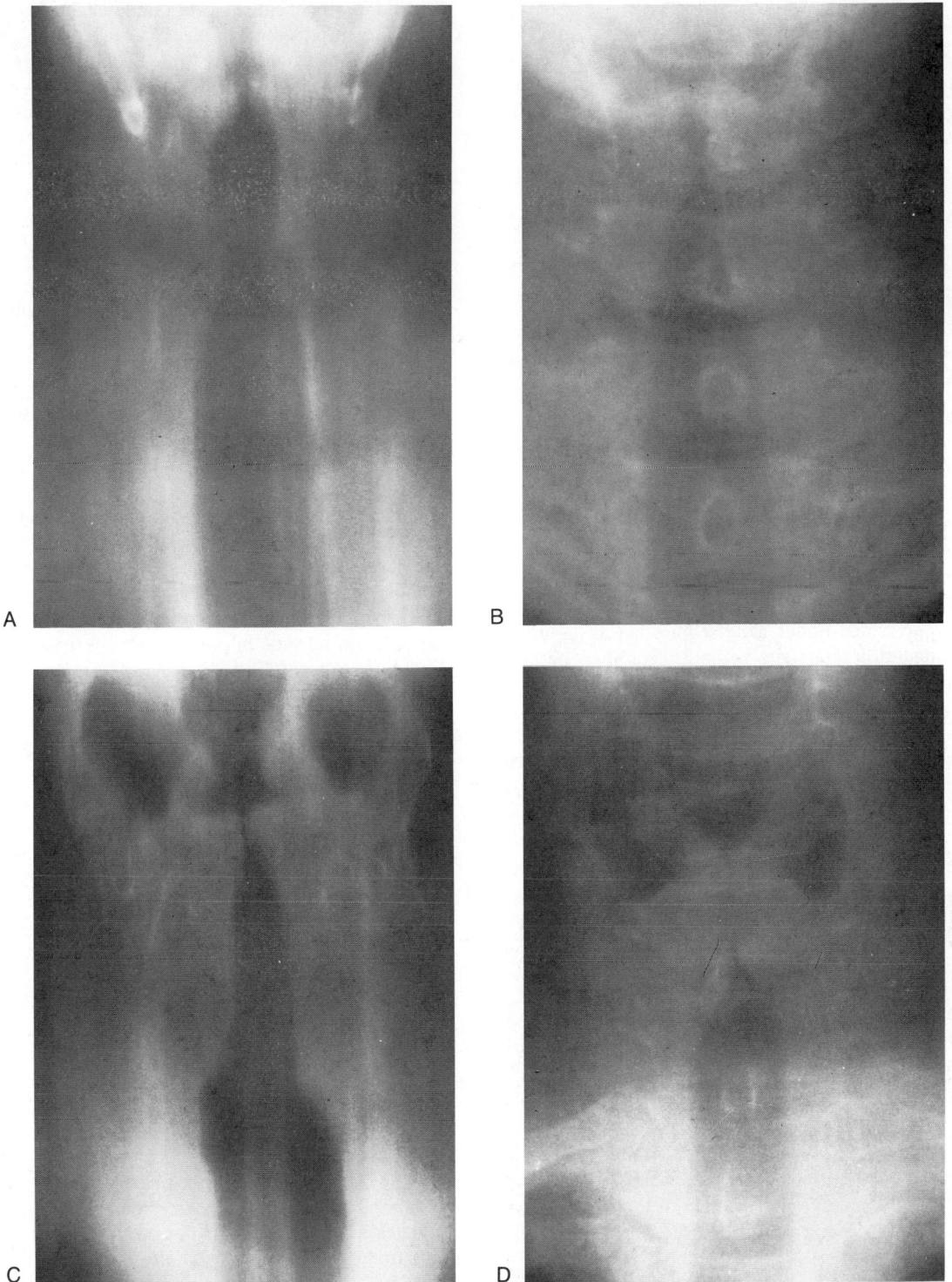

Figure 13-21.   Radiographs of larynx and upper trachea in idiopathic laryngotracheal stenosis. **(A)** Tomographic cut showing false and true vocal cords and a narrowed but still quite adequate immediate subglottic space, with maximal narrowing in the lower subglottic larynx and uppermost trachea. The distal trachea is normal in diameter. **(B)** Postoperative radiograph using a copper filter for clarity. A nearly normal subglottic configuration has been attained. **(C)** The subglottic narrowing here is more severe and commences immediately below the vocal cords. **(D)** Postoperative view. (From Grillo HC, Mark EJ, Mathisen DJ, Wain JC: Idiopathic laryngotracheal stenosis and its management. Ann Thorac Surg 56:80, 1993, with permission.)

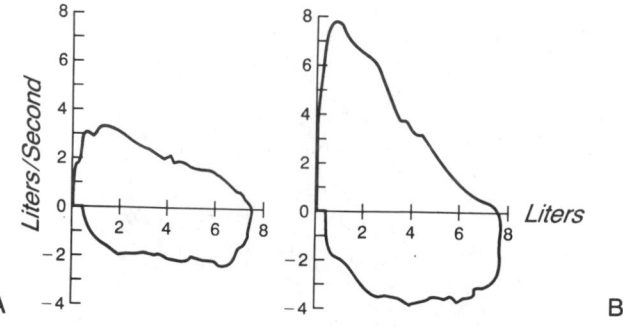

Figure 13-22. **(A)** Preoperative and **(B)** postoperative flow-volume loops in idiopathic stenosis. Measurements were made at a 3-year interval. Forced expiratory volume in 1 second rose from 2.7 to 3 L, and peak expiratory flow rate from 4 to 7.7 L/s. Operation corrected the marked reduction in inspiratory flow. (From Grillo HC, Mark EJ, Mathisen DJ, Wain JC: Idiopathic laryngotracheal stenosis and its management. Ann Thorac Surg 56:80, 1993, with permission.)

Operative Technique

Dilatation

Dilatation is performed under general anesthesia, administered by an inhalation technique without respiratory paralysis. The subglottic larynx is visualized with use of a rigid ventilating bronchoscope, through which small Jackson bougies are introduced to initiate dilatation. When lumen of adequate size is achieved, Jackson-type rigid bronchoscopes are passed serially, appropriate sizes from the range of 3.5-, 4-, 5-, and 6-mm laryngoscopes being selected. If dilatation is to be therapeutic, adult-sized rigid bronchoscopes may also

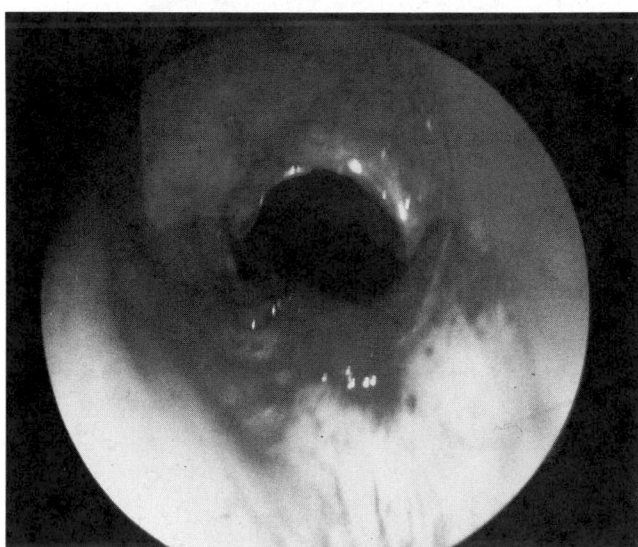

Figure 13-23. Bronchoscopic view of typical subglottic stenosis. Lesions are concentric, although sometimes eccentric. Mucosal vascularity but no granulation tissue is present. (From Grillo HC, Mark EJ, Mathisen DJ, Wain JC: Idiopathic laryngotracheal stenosis and its management. Ann Thorac Surg 56:80, 1993, with permission.)

be used to obtain satisfactory diameter, but these should not be so large that severe damage is caused. I prefer not to use a laser in these maneuvers for fear of creating more damage, which may interfere with future surgical repair. A tracheotomy is never performed, since this would complicate surgical repair. However, if a tracheostomy is already in place, anesthesia is delivered through the tracheostomy tube and the dilatation becomes a simpler process.

Surgical Correction

When idiopathic stenosis involves only the upper trachea or extends only to the lower margin of cricoid cartilage, standard segmental circumferential resection is performed with end-to-end anastomosis. This usually requires anastomosis of the trachea to the inferior margin of the cricoid cartilage. However, when stenosis involves the subglottic larynx, as is most often the case, resection must be modified to preserve the posterior skeleton of the larynx with the entry point of the two recurrent laryngeal nerves (Grillo, 1982; Grillo, et al., 1992). In these cases the anteroinferior portion of the larynx below the glottic commissure is resected, including the anterior portion of the circumferential stenosis. An arcuate line of incision transects the midpoint of the lateral laminae of the cricoid cartilage and sweeps up in a curve that goes beneath the inferior margin of the thyroid cartilage in the midline anteriorly (Fig. 13-24A). The posterior portion of circumferential stenosis which remains is resected from the anterior surface of the posterior cricoid plate, baring the cartilage. The proximal line of resection may be almost at the arytenoid cartilages. The distal normal trachea is beveled for use in the reconstruction (Fig. 13-24B). The first good cartilage below the stricture is salvaged and is cut backward in a sloping line toward its posterior ends on either side, so that a "prow" is created of this single cartilage. This slides into the similarly shaped defect in the inferior part of the anterior laryngeal wall. Posteriorly, a broad-based flap of membranous wall is fashioned, which serves to resurface the bared posterior cricoid plate.

Lateral traction sutures (2–0 Vicryl) are placed in lateral midpoints of the trachea on either side below the line of anastomosis and proximally in the lateral laryngeal wall at the junction of the thyroid cartilage and remaining cricoid plates. Anastomosis is commenced with 4–0 Vicryl sutures, which are placed from the posterior mucosa of the larynx to the membranous wall flap, with knots inverted from the lumen (Fig. 13-24C). The sutures are placed but not tied. Four nonabsorbable sutures (4–0 Tevdek) are placed in a line across the back of the base of this flap to the inferior margin of the posterior cricoid plate to fix the flap against the cartilage (Fig. 13-24D). These are clipped to the drapes, two on each side.

Sutures lateral to the midline traction sutures on either side are placed through the cartilage of the larynx and the trachea, along with one or two sutures anterior to the location of the traction sutures. The traction sutures are then approximated, with cervical flexion, to relieve tension on the anastomosis. The sutures are tied in the following order: (1) posterior Tevdek approximating sutures; (2) posterior mucosal flap sutures; (3) anastomotic sutures posterior to the lateral

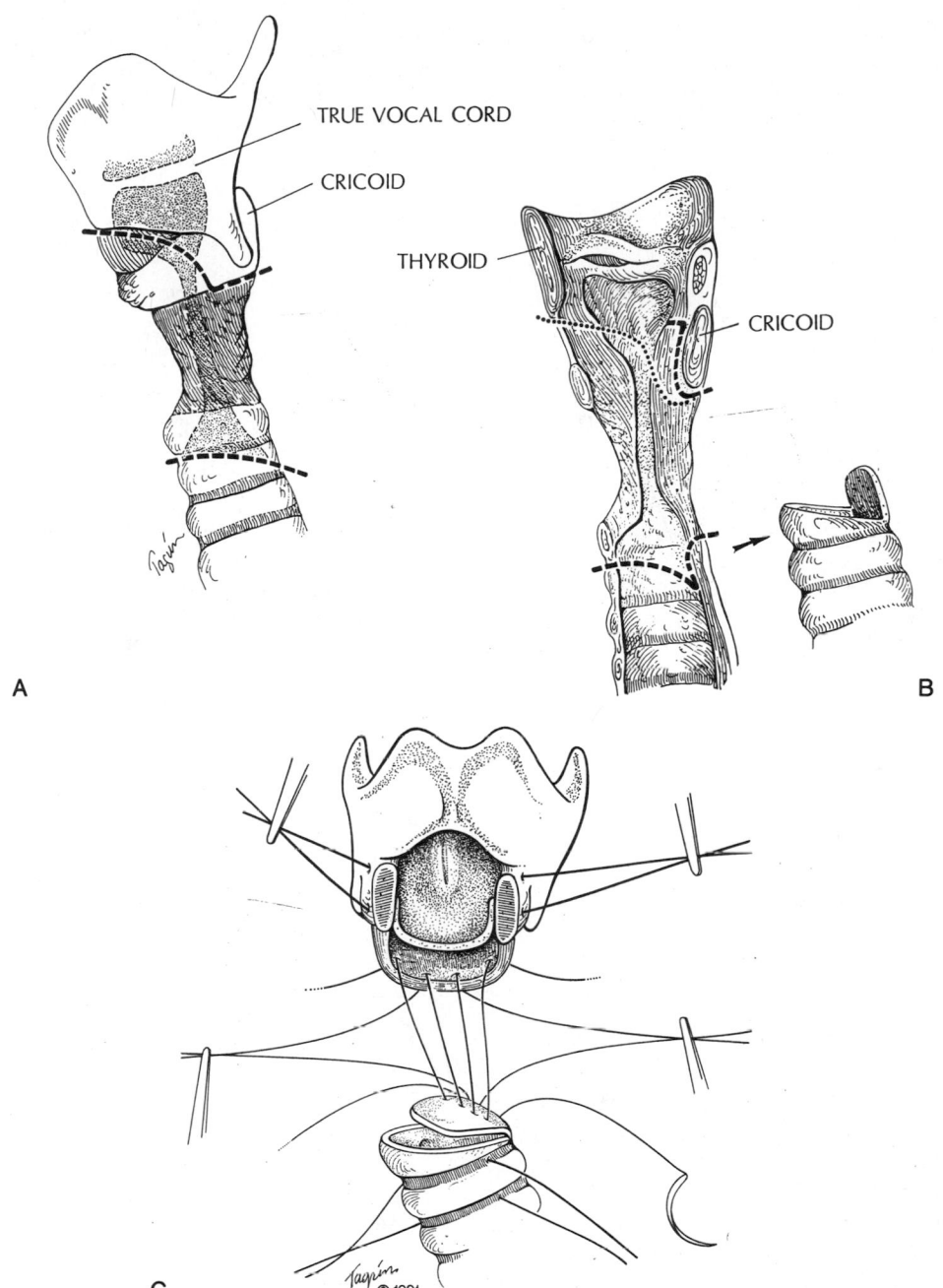

Figure 13-24. Technique of laryngotracheal resection and reconstruction. **(A)** External lines of division of the larynx and trachea are indicated by dashed lines. The anterior cricoid arch is removed. **(B)** When the subglottic intralaryngeal stenosis is circumferential, scar is removed from the front of the posterior cricoid lamina, baring the cartilage, as shown. The residual posterior cricoid lamina protects the recurrent laryngeal nerves. Distally, the trachea is beveled over the length of one cartilage, as shown, to fit the anterolateral subglottic defect that has been created. A broad-based flap of membranous tracheal wall is fashioned to resurface the bared cricoid plate. **(C)** The posterior flap is fixed to the lower margin of the cricoid plate with four extraluminal sutures (4–0 Tevdek). The lateral traction sutures (2–0 Vicryl) are also shown in the larynx proximally and in the trachea distally. (*Figure continues.*)

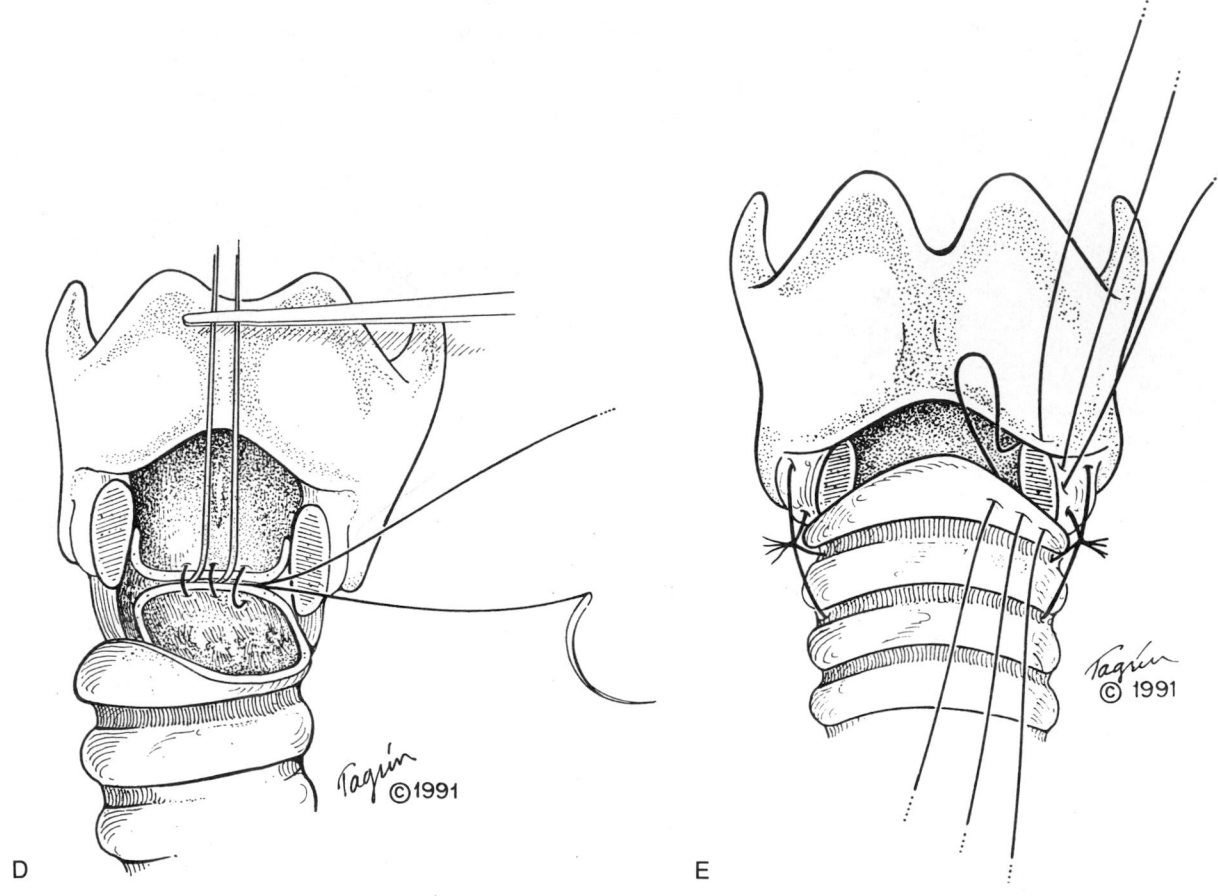

D

E

Figure 13-24. *(Continued.)* **(D)** Posterior mucosal anastomotic sutures (4–0 Vicryl) are placed with knots to lie behind the mucosa. Traction sutures are omitted in this diagram for simplicity. **(E)** After placement of all the posterior and posterolateral anastomotic sutures as far anteriorly as the lateral stay sutures, the patient's neck is flexed, and the stay sutures, external fixing Tevdek sutures, and posterior mucosal sutures are tied, in that order. The anterior and anterolateral anastomotic sutures are then placed and finally tied serially. (Figs. A and B from Grillo HC: Primary reconstruction of airway after resection of subglottic laryngeal and upper tracheal stenosis. Ann Thorac Surg 33:3, 1982, with permission. Figs. C–E from Grillo HC, Mathisen DJ, Wain JC: Laryngotracheal resection and reconstruction for subglottic stenosis. Ann Thorac Surg 53:54, 1992, with permission.)

traction sutures. The remaining anterior anastomotic sutures are then placed, and the anastomosis is completed (Fig. 13-24E). The anterior flap of cartilage from the trachea that is used to fill in the defect in the larynx is fashioned from a single ring in order to avoid floppiness.

Of the 35 patients who underwent single-stage resection and reconstruction, 32 achieved good or excellent results in terms of respiration and voice. Two needed annual dilata-cartilage. The other 29 patients with involvement of the subglottic larynx in varying degrees of severity were managed by laryngotracheal resection as described. In 7 of the 29, a posterior flap was not necessary because of the location of the posterior portion of the stenosis, which could be removed by simple resection. In the others a flap was necessary to resurface the posterior plate of the cricoid cartilage. Concomitant temporary tracheostomies for 2 to 4 weeks were necessary in 3 of 22 undergoing laryngotracheal resection and reconstruction. In only one was suprahyoid laryngeal release

necessary. The approach for all was through a cervical incision.

Perioperative Care

In all laryngotracheal anastomoses in which a normal subglottic airway is not present even at the final point of anastomosis, patients must be observed closely following surgery for signs of airway obstruction. If progressive glottic or subglottic edema occurs postoperatively, the patient should be intubated promptly with a small-bore, uncuffed, endotracheal tube. After several days a trial of tube removal is made. If the airway is inadequate, a small tracheostomy tube is inserted very carefully in the now sealed tissue planes at a preselected point inferior to the anastomotic line. The anastomosis itself is protected at the original operation with thyroid isthmus or other tissue, and if the innominate artery is close to the area of potential tracheostomy, a strap muscle is sutured down to the trachea over the innominate artery to protect it. Using this technique we have had no difficulties involving arterial injury in these resections or others of this type. In the series of 35 patients who underwent operation for idiopathic stenosis, no late intubations or tracheostomies were necessary.

Results

Of the 49 patients seen with this diagnosis (Grillo, et al., 1993), 35 underwent surgical resection. The reasons for nonresectional therapy in 9 of the other 14 patients were severe stenosis close to the vocal cords, which prohibited reconstruction, in four patients; an excessive length of involvement, prohibiting anastomosis, in one; ease of conservative management in three; demonstrated mucosal ulcerations in one. The other five patients were seen in consultation but underwent therapy elsewhere.

Of the 35 patients who underwent single-stage resection and reconstruction, 32 achieved good or excellent results in terms of respiration and voice. Two needed annual dilatations, and in one, failure demanded permanent tracheostomy. Of 26 patients followed for 1 to 15 years, 10 attained excellent results with respect to both airway and voice, and 22 had good results. A patient with a good result was considered to be one who is left with a slight change in vocal characteristics such as weakness in ability to project the voice or inability to sing as well as preoperatively. Minimal dyspnea on major exertion was also so categorized. Two patients had fair results, meaning either vocal hoarseness or an intermittently weak voice and low exercise tolerance due to limited airway diameter, which limited activity. Failure occurred in one patient operated upon elsewhere previously. Patients with good or excellent results have not required further dilatations or other therapy of any type.

KEY REFERENCE

Grillo IIC, Mark EJ, Mathisen DJ, Wain JC: Idiopathic laryngotracheal stenosis and its management. Ann Thorac Surg 56:80, 1993

Clinical characteristics, diagnosis, pathology, management, and results in idiopathic laryngotracheal stenosis are described as studied in 49 patients, 35 of whom were treated surgically. This appears to be the first definitive study of this topic.

REFERENCES

Brandenburg JH: Idiopathic subglottic stenosis. Trans Am Acad Ophthalmol Otolaryngol 76:1402, 1972

Grillo HC: Primary reconstruction of airway after resection of subglottic laryngeal and upper tracheal stenosis. Ann Thorac Surg 33:3, 1982

Grillo HC, Mathisen DJ, Wain JC: Laryngotracheal resection and reconstruction for subglottic stenosis. Ann Thorac Surg 53:54, 1992

Havas T, Dodd M, Weldon B et al.: A case report of subglottic stenosis. Aust N Z J Surg 54:291, 1984

Jazbi B, Goodwin C, Tackett D, Faulkner S: Idiopathic subglottic stenosis. Ann Otol Rhinol Laryngol 86:644, 1979

Maddaus MA, Toth JLR, Gullane PJ, Pearson FG: Subglottic tracheal resection and synchronous laryngeal reconstruction. J Thorac Cardiovasc Surg 104:1443, 1992

Mikaelian DO: Idiopathic subglottic stenosis in an adult. J Laryngol Otol 88:467, 1974

Momose K, MacMillan AS Jr: Roentgenologic investigations of the larynx and trachea. Radiol Clin North Am 16:321, 1978

Tracheomalacia

Michael Maddaus
F. Griffith Pearson

DEFINITION

In normal individuals, the trachea and main bronchi are pliant, elastic structures, which undergo significant changes in length during extension of the neck and with each inspiration. Shortening occurs during neck flexion, expiration, and coughing. A concomitant and relatively diffuse change in the diameter of the tracheal lumen occurs during the phases of respiration. During forced expiration or coughing, the tracheal cartilages are compressed, with reduction of the diameter between the lateral walls of the cartilaginous rings. In addition, there is usually some forward displacement, or "herniation" of the posterior, membranous wall. The condition of *tracheomalacia* is defined as a pathologic exaggeration of these changes and may result in functionally significant interference with air flow and impaired clearance of tracheobronchial secretions. On occasion, extreme degrees of malacic collapse may result in cough syncope.

HISTORICAL NOTE

In 1954 Herzog and Nissen of Switzerland were the first to describe a syndrome of "expiratory stenosis of the trachea and main stem bronchi," which is now identified as tracheomalacia secondary to emphysema. They defined the condition as "an alteration of the elastic fibers of unknown etiology, always associated with chronic inflammation" and found primarily in "men over the age of 50 with chronic bronchitis." Herzog and Nissen (1954) described the first clinical attempts at surgical treatment of this condition by stabilizing the membranous trachea with thin bone grafts. Rainer, et al. in 1963 and 1965 reported their clinical experience with their own technique of stabilization of the membranous trachea. In the region of the malacic segment, a thin plate of silicone rubber covered with Marlex mesh was sutured over the plicated membranous trachea and fixed to the free margins of the tracheal cartilages. Both subjective and objective improvement was noted in some patients.

HISTORICAL READINGS

Herzog H, Nissen R: Erschlaffung und expiratorische Invagination des membranosen Teils der intrachorakalen Luftrohre und der Hauptbronchien als Ursache der asphyktischen Anfalle beim Asthma bronchiale und bei der chronischen asthmoiden Bronchitis des Lungenemphysems. Schweiz Med Wochenschr 84:217, 1954

Rainer WG, Hutchinson D, Newby JP et al.: Major airway collapsibility in the pathogenesis of obstructive emphysema. J Thorac Cardiovasc Surg 46:559, 1963

Rainer WG, Feilder EM, Kelble L: Surgical technic of major airway support for pulmonary emphysema. Am J Surg 110:788, 1965

ETIOLOGY

Congenital

Congenital anomalies include (1) rare, segmental cartilaginous defects (more commonly of the main bronchi); (2) congenital vascular rings and anomalous innominate artery (discussed in the first part of this chapter); and (3) the syndrome of tracheobronchomegaly (also known as tracheal diverticulosis and the Meunier-Kuhn syndrome).

The Meunier-Kuhn syndrome is a diffuse dilatation of the tracheobronchial tree, which may involve the airway from the larynx to the subsegmental bronchi (Meunier-Kuhn, 1932; Johnson and Green, 1965). In 1973 Bateson and Woo-Ming reviewed 55 reported cases and noted the following: the syndrome occurs primarily in males and usually presents with bouts of cough, purulent sputum, or pneumonia during the third and fourth decades; chest x-ray is often diagnostic and reveals a striking enlargement of the trachea and bronchi; bronchoscopy reveals redundant semicircular folds of mucous membrane with the formation of saccular pouches (hence the name tracheal diverticulosis).

The etiology of the Meunier-Kuhn syndrome is unknown; however, a decrease in the number of airway elastic fibers has been reported, and association with the Ehlers-Danlos syndrome and other connective tissue disorders has been observed (Aaby and Blake, 1966; Ayres, et al., 1981). The trachea and bronchi are abnormally compliant owing to atrophic changes in the cartilage and collapse easily with coughing or forced expiration (Katz, et al., 1962; Al-Mallah and Quantock, 1968). Fluoroscopy demonstrates a striking airway dilatation during inspiration, collapse on forced expiration or cough, and pooling of secretions in the trachea and main bronchi (Johnson and Green, 1965).

Acquired

Post-traumatic

Segmental areas of tracheomalacia may occur following any injury that results in loss of cartilage. The most common cause is postintubation injury at the stomal or cuff sites. Postintubation tracheomalacia is more frequently observed in the early phase of injury in association with acute inflammation. In most patients the "softening" disappears as the scar matures and inflammation subsides. Although most postintubation injuries heal by dense scar formation and stenosis, in some cases (most notably with administration of high-dose steriods) scar formation is minimal, and malacia rather than fibrous stenosis occurs.

Emphysema and Chronic Bronchitis

Most patients with advanced emphysema and chronic bronchitis have some degree of malacia affecting part or all of the trachea and main bronchi. The etiology appears related to a decrease in the amount of cartilage (Thurlbeck, et al., 1974; Maiscl, et al., 1968). On occasion the degree of malacia results in functional air flow impairment and inability to raise secretions across the malacic segment. In such patients there is a pathologic exaggeration of the changes in airway diameter that normally occur with changes in intrathoracic pressure.

Saber sheath trachea is characterized by the presence of marked coronal narrowing of the trachea to less than two-thirds the sagittal diameter. The coronal narrowing, usually easily identified on a posteroanterior chest x-ray, involves only the intrathoracic trachea and ends abruptly above the level of the thoracic inlet. The cause is unknown. Because this narrowing is invariably associated with significant chronic obstructive pulmonary disease, it has been proposed that the deformity may be due to chronic compression by the overinflated lungs. Saber sheath narrowing appears to be a fixed abnormality with no tendency to malacia and collapse; this may be the result of extensive tracheal calcification, which is seen in the majority of cases (Greene and Lechner, 1975).

Chronic External Compression

Chronic external compression most commonly involves compression of the upper mediastinal trachea by a benign mediastinal goiter. On occasion other mediastinal lesions contiguous with the trachea (teratoma, thymoma, bronchogenic cyst, etc.) may induce an area of segmental tracheomalacia. Segmental malacia of a main bronchus may occur following pneumonectomy when the carinal airway is markedly displaced and a main bronchus is compressed by the underlying thoracic spine.

Relapsing Polychondritis

Relapsing polychondritis is a systemic disease affecting cartilage in multiple areas of the body, including the ear, nose, larynx, and tracheobronchial tree. It is an autoimmune connective tissue disease, thought to be secondary to production of autoantibodies to cartilage (Ebringer, et al., 1981; Foidart, et al., 1978). Occasionally it is associated with other systemic connective tissue disorders such as systemic lupus erythematosus. Pathologically (as is most often demonstrated by nasal biopsy) a tracheal chondritis is initially seen and characterized by an infiltration of lymphocytes and plasma cells; with time, the destroyed cartilage is replaced by fibrous tissue. Although it is a diffuse disease, there may be variable and segmental involvement of the airway. Dolan, et al. (1966) noted that the involved segments may demonstrate either a fixed obstruction or a variable malacic obstruction. Relapsing polychondritis usually occurs in the third or fourth decade and with equal incidence in males and females. Involvement of the tracheobronchial tree, as noted by McAdam, et al. (1976), is present in over 50 percent of patients and when severe can lead to disabling airway symptoms. Respiratory involvement is the leading cause of death in this disease (Hughes, et al., 1972).

DIAGNOSIS

Symptoms are related to collapse of the airway and occur with increases in intrathoracic pressure; they include expiratory wheezing and/or stridor, particularly with exertion, a barking cough, and an inability to clear secretions. Physical examination may reveal an audible wheeze or stridor with forced expiration. Auscultation over the suprasternal notch during forced expiration or cough may disclose a sharp, loud "knock" early in expiration. Postintubation malacia in the cervical trachea may be palpable on physical examination.

Investigative Techniques

Pulmonary Function Studies

Pulmonary function studies show a "break" in the expiratory phase of the spirogram, which has been described and discussed in detail by Gandevia (1963) and by Campbell and Gaulks (1965). The break in the expiratory curve to a flat plateau is assumed to represent the moment of large airway collapse after dead space air has been exhaled. It is at this point in the cycle that a sharp knock may be heard with a stethoscope placed over the upper sternum.

Imaging

Static Imaging. Plain posteroanterior and lateral chest x-rays, tracheal tomograms, and CT scans may show no abnormality, since these studies provide only static images of the airways. However, some changes are seen in specific types of tracheomalacia. In the Meunier-Kuhn syndrome the diagnosis is immediately manifest on the plain chest x-ray by an overall increase in the caliber of the trachea and bronchi and a unique corrugated diverticular appearance of the airways. With saber sheath trachea, the coronal diameter of the trachea is markedly reduced on the posteroanterior chest x-ray while the sagittal diameter, seen in the lateral film, is increased (normally the two diameters are roughly equal). Any mediastinal mass compressing the trachea, such as a benign goiter may be evident in the plain chest films.

Cine Studies. If the diagnosis is not apparent on static images, cine studies of the trachea and main bronchi, with or without contrast medium, will provide a dynamic display of the airways and critical diagnostic information. Such studies demonstrate the presence of airway collapse and the anatomic levels involved. The lateral projection is an essential component of this examination, particularly in patients with malacia due to emphysema and bronchitis (Fig. 13-25).

Bronchoscopy. Bronchoscopy is an important diagnostic modality and may be performed with either rigid or flexible instruments. It should be done under local anesthesia, allowing observation of the airway during spontaneous respiration, deep breathing, forced expiration, and cough. Abnormal collapse of the airway is typically identified during expiration, especially forced expiration and cough. In cases of malacia associated with emphysema, the membranous trachea is widened, and redundant and may lack the normal longitudinal folds. During expiration, pronounced anterior displacement of the redundant membranous trachea occurs, resulting in a semilunar "new moon" configuration of the airway lumen. In some cases the airway closes completely at certain points in the cycle as the redundant membranous trachea becomes apposed to the inner surface of the cartilaginous rings. These changes may be diffuse or segmental in distribution and commonly involve the origins of the main bronchi.

The dynamic changes seen on cineradiography or at bronchoscopy may be dramatically demonstrated at the time of surgery. If the malacia is due to emphysema, gross widening of the posterior tracheal wall is evident, and abnormal softening of the cartilages is readily palpable. With the patient breathing spontaneously, expiration will produce invagination of the membranous wall in that part of the malacic airway beyond the endotracheal tube. Stimulation of cough

by carinal irritation will produce abrupt collapse and forward herniation of the posterior wall, even in the open thorax.

MANAGEMENT

Postintubation Tracheomalacia

Postintubation tracheomalacia results in defects that are usually short and similar in length to the more common postintubation fibrous strictures. Some degree of malacia is often observed during the early phase of postintubation injury in association with acute inflammation. In the majority of patients, this softening disappears as the inflammation subsides and the scar matures. High-dose steroids undoubtedly interfere with the formation of normal scar and predispose to malacia rather than cicatricial stenosis.

At bronchoscopy, malacic segments are easily "dilated," since the luminal circumference is often normal. A rigid bronchoscope is easily advanced through the collapsed segment. Obviously, such dilatation is of no therapeutic benefit. Disabling postintubation malacia is usually best managed by segmental resection and primary anastomosis. Otolaryngologists have reported successful alternative techniques, such as ceramic ring reinforcement of the malacic segment (Amedee, et al., 1992). In our opinion such techniques are unwarranted in view of the need to implant foreign material and the demonstrated safety and effectiveness of resection and primary repair. In those rare instances in which operation is deemed impossible, internal stenting with a Montgomery silicone rubber T tube may provide a safe and satisfactory airway.

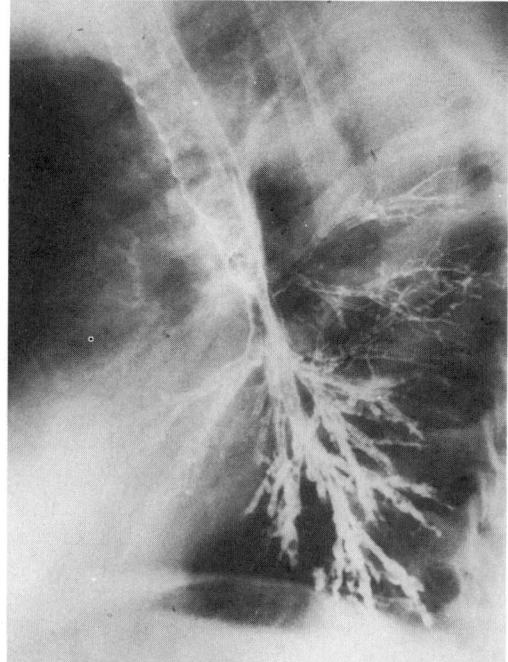
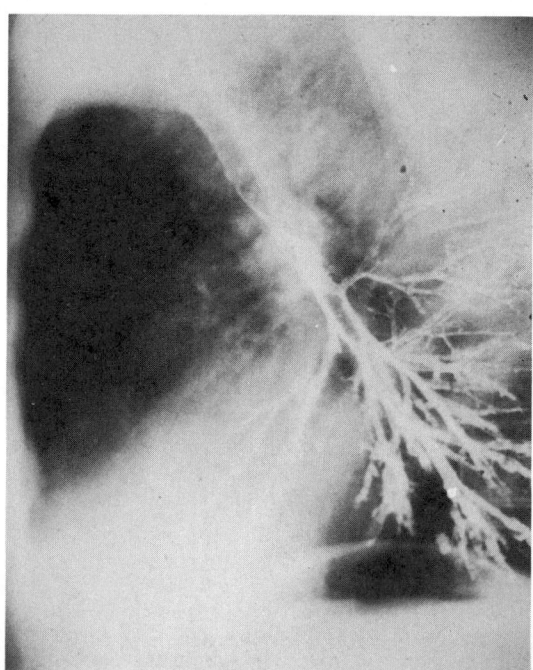

A   B

Figure 13-25.   Contrast tracheogram illustrating pronounced narrowing of the trachea during cough in a patient with chronic bronchitis and emphysema.

Emphysema and Chronic Bronchitis

A number of surgical techniques have been described to provide external support of the trachea and main bronchi in selected patients with functionally disabling malacia secondary to emphysema and chronic bronchitis.

Herzog and Nissen (1954) were the first to describe a technique of external support using either autologous or homologous arches or rings of bone. Rainer, et al. (1965) reported on 12 patients in whom a "slab" of specially prepared silicone and Marlex was secured to the membranous wall of the trachea, with "reefing" of the redundant membranous component. In some patients with significant cartilaginous malacia, polypropylene rings were added anterolaterally. Exposure was obtained in all cases through a right posterolateral thoracotomy through the bed of the fifth rib. Four late deaths (3 to 11 months postsurgery) occurred, of which three were due to unrelated disease and one was due to erosion of the prosthesis into the airway, resulting in a fatal distal pneumonia. Of the eight longer-term survivors, four were significantly improved clinically, and in each case there was quantitative documentation of improvement in pulmonary function tests. In a later publication Rainer (1968) reported experience in

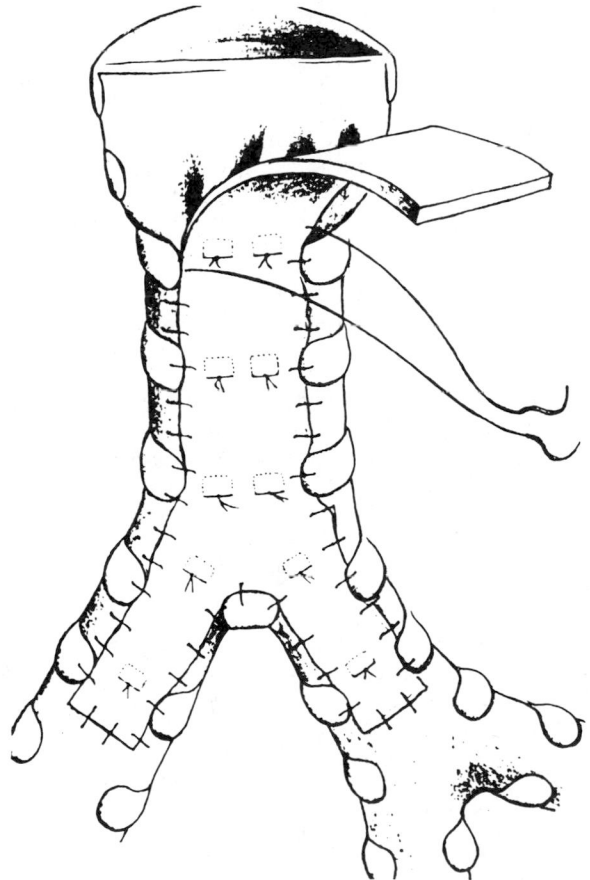

Figure 13-26. Diagram illustrating Urschel's modification of Rainer's technique of tracheal stabilization using a silicone and Marlex plate to "reef" and stabilize the membranous part of the trachea and main bronchi.

19 patients, in 3 of whom fatal complications of esophageal and aortic erosion by the prosthesis occurred.

Urschel (personal communication) has collected experience with approximately 40 patients, in all but 2 of whom the malacia was secondary to emphysema and bronchitis. (One of the two had a congenital Meunier-Kuhn syndrome and the other a "giant trachea" of no known etiology in the emphysema group.) Urschel used a modification of the posterior Marlex support developed by Rainer (Fig. 13-26). Urschel's experience has yet to be critically assessed with long-term evaluation. Severe and fatal complications due to erosion of the airway or adjacent organs and infection were observed. There were, however, some excellent immediate and long-term results.

An alternative technique described by Hanawa, et al. (1990) involved stabilization of the membranous wall using Marlex mesh with lyophilized human dura. The support is secured by bonding with fibrin glue. Hanawa, et al. used this technique in one patient with emphysematous tracheomalacia; the patient's cough syncope and airway collapse disappeared completely after surgery.

Dunn, et al. (1990), in a recent case report, emphasized an important feature of the pathology of tracheomalacia secondary to emphysema. On preoperative cine studies and bronchoscopy, their patient had evidence of collapse of a segment of trachea above the aortic arch and underwent thoracotomy for the intended purpose of resection with primary anastomosis. However, at surgery the defect in cartilaginous support was found to extend from the thoracic inlet to the carina and major bronchi. The authors noted the reason for the discrepancy in the preoperative assessment and the operative findings: Collapse will occur predominantly at the weakest site of the tracheal wall, and repair of the "weakest link" may lead to subsequent collapse of the adjacent segment.

Chronic Compression

It is not possible to evaluate the extent of malacia in a patient with tracheal compression due to a mediastinal goiter before the enlarged gland has been resected and the pressure relieved. In most of these cases the compressed segment of trachea is abnormally soft but presents no airway problem following extubation. Most cases are manageable without a period of postoperative airway support. If, however, breathing and coughing are critically impaired following extubation, an indwelling T tube offers an immediate solution and can almost always be removed within a few weeks or months. A T tube is unquestionably superior to a conventional open tracheostomy. Other reported options include application of a Marlex mesh wrap (Meurala, et al., 1982) or artificial rings of Gortex and stainless steel wire (Geelhoed, 1988) to provide external support. Depending on the length of the involved segment, resection with primary anastomosis may be used.

In cases of relapsing polychondritis, with either diffuse or segmental malacic segments, some type of internal stent (T tube, T-Y tube, or Y tube) may provide good palliation.

COMMENTS AND CONTROVERSIES

In summary, there is a scarcity of experience with surgical treatment of the type of diffuse malacic change discussed above. There are undoubtedly patients who would benefit from the available management techniques, but the indications for selection have yet to be clearly defined. More sophisticated tests of airway dynamics may be necessary to better delineate the future indications for surgery. There may well be a place for internal stenting with silicone rubber tubes (T tubes, T-Y tubes, or Y tubes) as an alternative to external surgical stenting in selected cases.

M.M.
F.G.P.

KEY REFERENCES

Rainer WG, Hutchinson D, Newby JP et al.: Major airway collapsibility in the pathogenesis of obstructive emphysema. J Thorac Cardiovasc Surg 46:559, 1963

This report clearly defines the pathophysiology of the commonest form of tracheomalacia, which is secondary to obstructive emphysema.

Rainer WG, Newby JP, Kelble DL: Long term results of tracheal support surgery for emphysema. Chest 53:765, 1968

This is the first paper reporting longer-term follow-up in patients with tracheomalacia secondary to emphysema, managed by surgical stabilization of the redundant membranous trachea. The authors also define details of surgical technique, which might still be applied today.

REFERENCES

Aaby GV, Blake HA: Tracheobronchomegaly. Ann Thorac Surg 2:64, 1966

Al-Mallah Z, Quantock OP: Tracheobronchomegaly. Thorax 23:230, 1968

Amedee RG, Mann WJ, Lyons GD: Tracheomalacia repair using ceramic rings. Otolaryngol Head Neck Surg 106:270, 1992

Ayres J, Rees J, Cochrane GM et al.: Hemoptysis and non-organic upper airways obstruction in a patient with previously undiagnosed Ehlers-Danlos syndrome. Br J Dis Chest 75:309, 1981

Bateson EM, Woom-Ming M: Tracheobronchomegaly. Clin Radiol 24:354, 1973

Campbell AH, Gaulks LW: Expiratory air-flow pattern in tracheobronchial collapse in emphysema. Am Rev Respir Dis 92:781, 1965

Dolan DL, Lemmon GB, Teitelbaum SL: Relapsing polychondritis. Analytical literature review and studies on pathogenesis. Am J Med 41:285, 1966

Dunn WF, Hubmayr RD, Pairolero PC et al.: The assessment of major airway function in a ventilator-dependent patient with tracheomalacia. Chest 97:939, 1990

Ebringer R, Rook G, Swana GT et al.: Autoantibodies to cartilage and type II collagen in relapsing polychondritis and other rheumatic diseases. Ann Rheum Dis 40:473, 1981

Foidart JM, Abe S, Martin GR et al.: Antibodies to type II collagen in relapsing polychondritis. N Engl J Med 299:1203, 1978

Gandevia B: The spirogram of gross expiratory tracheobronchial collapse in emphysema. Q J Med 32:23, 1963

Geelhoed GW: Tracheomalacia from compressing goiter: management after thyroidectomy. Surgery 104:1100, 1988

Greene R, Lechner GL: "Saber-sheath trachea": a clinical and functional study of marked coronal narrowing of the intrathoracic trachea. Radiology 115:265, 1975

Hanawa T, Ikeda S, Funatsu T et al.: Development of a new surgical procedure for repairing tracheobronchomalacia. J Thorac Cardiovasc Surg 100:587, 1990

Herzog H, Nissen R: Erschlaffung und expiratorische Invagination des membranosen Teils der intrachorakalen Luftrohre und der Hauptbronchien als Ursache der asphyktischen Anfalle beim Asthma bronchiale und bei der chronischen asthmoiden Bronchitis des Lungenemphysems. Schweiz Med Wochenschr 84:217, 1954

Hughes RAC, Berry CL, Seifert M et al.: Relapsing polychondritis: three cases with a clinico-pathological study and literature review. Q J Med 41:363, 1972

Johnson RF, Green RA: Tracheobronchiomegaly. Report of five cases and demonstration of a familial occurrence. Am Rev Respir Dis 91:35, 1965

Katz I, LeVine M, Herman P: Tracheobronchomegaly. The Mounier-Kuhn syndrome. AJR 88:1084, 1962

Maisel JC, Silvers GW, Mitchell RS et al.: Bronchial atrophy and dynamic expiratory collapse. Am Rev Respir Dis 98:988, 1968

McAdam LP, O'Hanlan A, Bluestone R et al.: Relapsing polychondritis: prospective study of 23 patients and a review of the literature. Medicine (Baltimore) 55:193, 1976

Meurala H, Halttunen P, Standertskjold-Nordenstam C-G, Keskitalo E: Surgical support of collapsing intrathoracic tracheomalacia after thyroidectomy. Acta Chir Scand 148:127, 1982

Meunier-Kuhn P: Dilatation de la trachée: Constatations radiographiques et bronchoscopiques. [Tracheal dilatation: roentgenographic and bronchographic findings.] Lyon Med 150:106, 1932

Rainer WG, Feilder EM, Kelble L: Surgical technic of major airway support for pulmonary emphysema. Am J Surg 110:788, 1965

Rainer WG, Hutchinson D, Newby JP et al.: Major airway collapsibility in the pathogenesis of obstructive emphysema. J Thorac Cardiovasc Surg 46:559, 1963

Thurlbeck WM, Pun R, Toth J et al.: Bronchial cartilage in chronic obstructive lung disease. Am Rev Respir Dis 109:73, 1974

14

RECURRENT LARYNGEAL NERVE PALSY

Clement A. Hiebert

DEFINITION

Like other functions of the healthy body that get taken for granted, that precious instrument, the human voice, gains the doctor's attention only when it breaks down. The laryngeal nerves cross the domain of the thoracic surgeon in the mediastinal corridor and neck close by those stouter conduits for air, blood, and food with which the surgeon regularly deals. In comparison with the trachea, great vessels, and esophagus, the recurrent nerves are inconspicuous and flimsy. They tend to quit if compressed by an aneurysm, invaded by cancer, or straddled by a nerve sheath tumor. Trauma—blunt or sharp—will do it. It is an uncomfortable fact that most laryngeal nerve trauma is iatrogenic (Table 14-1). (Montgomery, 1989). The purpose of this chapter is to review the anatomy of the recurrent laryngeal nerves and to call attention to the consequences of their being disabled.

HISTORICAL NOTE

Although Hippocrates recognized hoarseness and dysphagia, it remained for Marinos, an anatomist in 100 A.D., to identify the inferior nerves to the larynx and for the second-century surgeon Galen to prove their function. Major (1954) reports how Galen returned to Pergamon after eleven years of anatomic study in Alexandria and shortly thereafter was appointed surgeon at the gladiatorial ampitheater, a natural arena for studying cross-sectional anatomy of the neck. It was, after all, an era when the dissection of human cadavers was reckoned an unholy act. Among Galen's conclusions was that transection of the nerves to the larynx abolishes the normal voice. In tracing the parent nerve (i.e., the vagus) to the brain he disproved the intuitively agreeable but archaic dogma that speech emanates from the heart. On a prosaic but more scientific note, he demonstrated that division of the laryngeal nerves in a laboratory pig destroyed the animal's ability to squeal.

Except for observations on wounds produced by swords and spears, surgeons had little opportunity to study cadavers until the renaissance ushered in an enlightened attitude toward dissection of the human body. All the same, the 1,700 years between Galen and the nineteenth century produced little useful information until operations on the thyroid gland and cervical esophagus reintroduced the surgeon to the subject of transected nerves to the larynx.

In 1883 Hooper first observed the complementary role of the external branch of the superior laryngeal nerve in raising the pitch of a singer's voice. Half a century later (in 1931), Terracol confirmed the cricothyroid muscle as an essential cord adductor. The earliest observation of a nonrecurrent laryngeal nerve was made in a cadaver by Stedman (1823), but it was Pemberton and Beaver (1932) who recognized the implications of this anomaly for surgeons operating in the area of the neck or thoracic inlet.

HISTORICAL READINGS

Major RH: A History of Medicine. pp. 191, 220. Vol. 1. 1st Ed. Charles C Thomas, Springfield, IL, 1954

Pemberton J, Beaver MG: Anomaly of the right recurrent laryngeal nerve. Surg Gynecol Obstet 54:594, 1932

Stedman GW: A singular distribution of some of the nerves and arteries of the neck and the top of the thorax. Edinb Med Surg J 19:564, 1823 (cited by Henry JF, Audifrett J, Denizot A, Plan M: The nonrecurrent inferior laryngeal nerve: review of 33 cases, including two on the left side. Surgery 104:6, 1988)

BASIC SCIENCE

Laryngeal Function

The threefold function of the laryngeal muscles is to open the cords for breathing, approximate them for phonation, and close them tightly for swallowing. Four abductors and one adductor are innervated by the ipsilateral recurrent nerve. (Adductor force is further enhanced by the cricothyroid muscle, an important muscle with separate innervation.)

Phonation and swallowing are reciprocal functions. Both require the cords to be adducted, but to swallow and speak

Table 14-1. Incidence of the Causes of Vocal Cord Paralysis in Various Series Reported[a]

	Hagan (100 cases)	Maisel and Ogura (181 cases)	Titche (134 cases)	Parnell and Brandenburg (100 cases)	Average
Neoplastic	23	20	38	35	29
Trauma	9	23	11	12	14
Surgery	35	23	11	28	24
CNS disease	13	8	16	7	11
Inflammatory	10	6	20	6	10.5
Toxic	5	—	—	2	1.5
Idiopathic	5	20	4	10	10

[a] Figures given are percentages.

(From Montgomery WW: Laryngeal paralysis. p. 607. In: Surgery of the Upper Respiratory System. Vol. 2. 2nd Ed. Lea & Febiger, Malvern, PA, 1989, with permission.)

at the same time is impossible. Abduction is useful only for taking a breath and is normally abruptly canceled with the onset of a swallow. Trouble looms when it cannot be, as is the case when nerve damage maroons a cord off center.

Rice (1982) states the assumed position of a paralyzed cord to be the resultant of forces generated by (1) the cricothyroideus muscle, which is innervated by the superior laryngeal nerve, and (2) the interarytenoid adductor, which has bilateral innervation. The airway may be adequate as long as the opposing cord can abduct during inspiration, provided that the patient's pulmonary reserve is unimpaired.

Recurrent Laryngeal Nerve Anatomy

The recurrent laryngeal nerves arise from the vagi (Fig. 14-1). On the left side, the nerve originates at the ligmentum arteriosum, behind which it loops before ascending in the tracheoesophageal groove to the neck. It courses posterior to the left thyroid lobe, either in front of or, more commonly, behind the inferior thyroid artery, and enters the larynx at the point of articulation between the thyroid and cricothyroid cartilages; this prominence at the inferior and posterior pole of the thyroid cartilage is easily palpated. On the right side, the recurrent nerve loops posteromedially around the first portion of the subclavian artery and crosses obliquely to the tracheoesophageal groove and thence to the larynx. The asymmetric origin of the recurrent nerves is of interest to thoracic surgeons, who generally favor the left thoracic inlet as the avenue for transposing stomach or colon to the neck—the nerve is less in the way.

Before the recurrent nerve enters the larynx, it sprouts fine branches to the upper trachea, esophagus, and cricopharyngeus muscle, branches that are visible during operations on the upper esophageal sphincter, especially if one wears 2X or 3X optical loupes. Upon entering the larynx, each nerve divides into abductor and adductor limbs plus a small posterolateral sensory twig known as Galen's loop, which anastomases with the internal branch of the superior laryngeal nerve (Crumley, 1990) (Fig. 14-2).

The Nonrecurrent Nerve

Of special anatomic concern to surgeons is the nonrecurrent laryngeal nerve, an uncommon but important anomaly associated with a retroesophageal right subclavian artery. In this circumstance the artery, which is normally a branch of the innominate artery, arises distal to the left subclavian, leaving no vessel around which the developing recurrent nerve can hook (Fig. 14.3). An unexpected encounter with a retro-

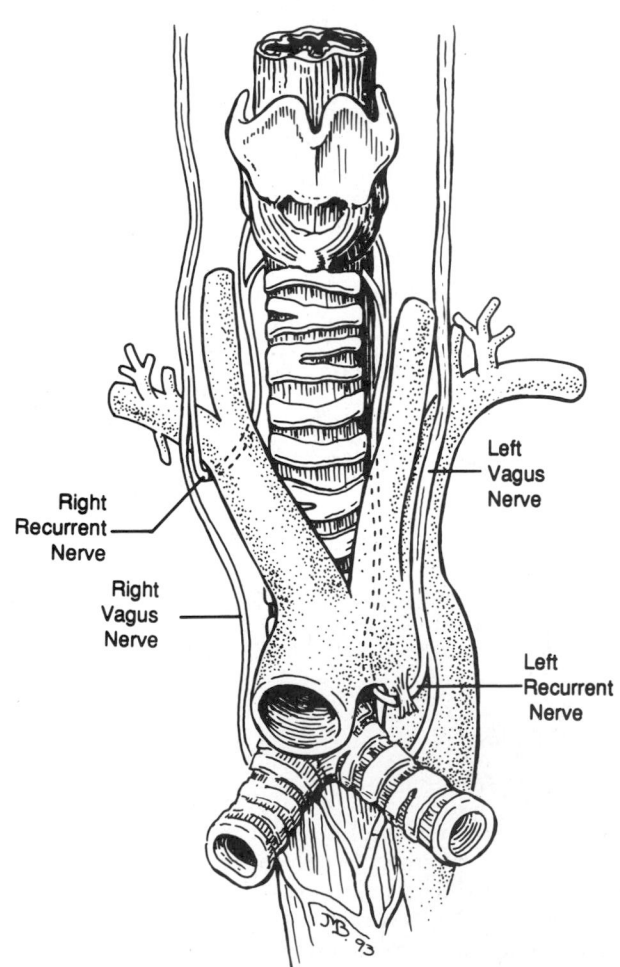

Right Recurrent Nerve

Right Vagus Nerve

Left Vagus Nerve

Left Recurrent Nerve

Figure 14-1. Anatomy of the left and right recurrent laryngeal nerves.

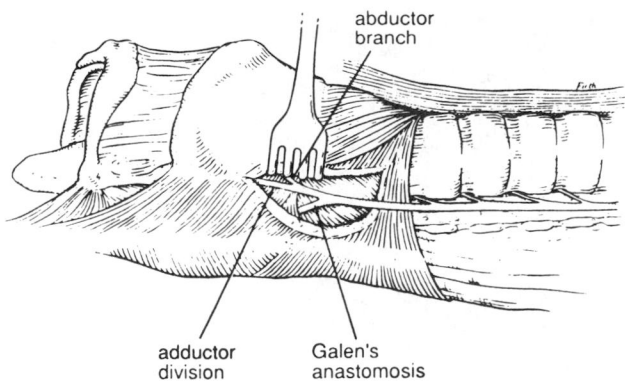

Figure 14-2. Dissection of the terminal portion of the right recurrent nerve. Branches to the trachea but not to the esophagus are shown. (From Crumley RL: Repair of the recurrent laryngeal nerve. Otolaryngol Clin North Am 23:553, 1990, with permission.)

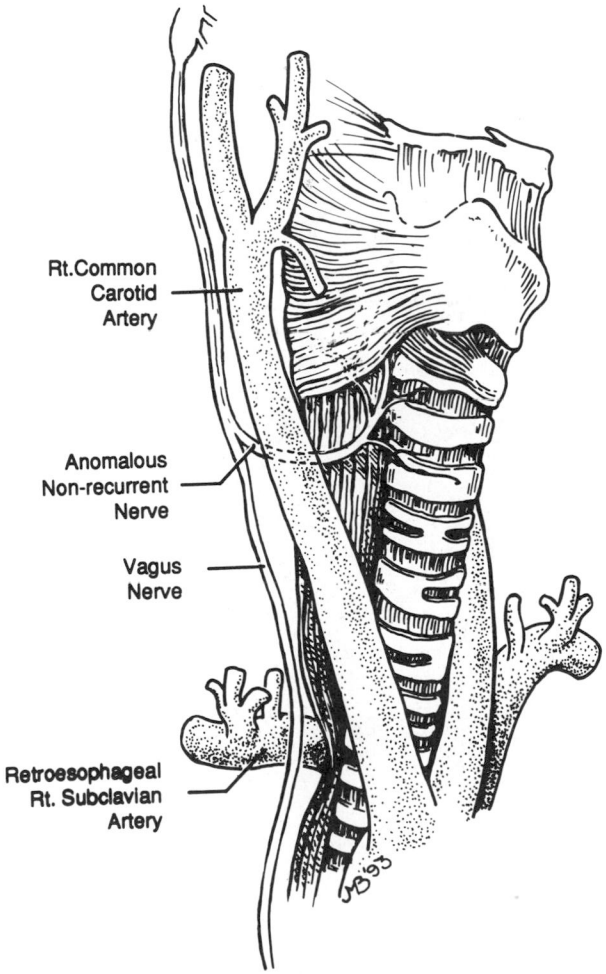

Figure 14-3. Anatomy of the nonrecurrent nerve. Note the compression of the retroesophageal right subclavian artery.

esophageal subclavian artery during esophagectomy is less than ideal. The investigation of dysphagia lusoria, with contrast studies of the esophagus and aortic arch, makes the diagnosis. In a review of 6,307 operations on the thyroid or parathyroid glands, Henry (1988) found 33 instances of nonrecurrent inferior laryngeal nerves, 31 of which were on the right side. The remaining two patients, with a left nonrecurrent nerve, both had situs inversus and a right-sided arch.

Nerve Injury and Regeneration

The ultimate anatomic unit of nerve is the nerve fiber or axon, a microscopic filament connecting the nerve cell in the brain stem on the one hand to the motor endplates or specialized sensory receptors of the larynx, upper esophagus, and trachea on the other. As compared with the parent cell, each axon is rather long. Ducker (1980) has suggested that if the tiny cell body tucked away in the central nervous system (CNS) were the height of an average man, its axon would have a diameter of about 1 in. and would extend over 2 miles!

Undulating bundles of axons lie within a connective tissue sleeve called the perineurium; a myriad of these fascicles in turn are sheathed in another diaphanous sleeve, known to the neuroanatomist as the external epineurium and to the surgeon, peering through $3\times$ optical loupes, as the nerve sheath.

Axons are embraced by splayed out Schwann cells. Perhaps one-quarter of the axons are coated with a waxy insulation called myelin. When a nerve is injured, the Schwann cells proliferate and phagocytose the detritus of degenerating axons and myelin sheaths, a process known as Wallerian degeneration, described by Waller in 1850 (MacKinnon and Dellon, 1988). But even as degeneration proceeds, regeneration begins. MacKinnon (1992) describes degrees of nerve damage that relate the histologic events to the potential for recovery (Fig. 14-4).

When a nerve is injured, the cell itself senses the situation, for within a few hours it swells and the nucleus drifts over to the periphery of the cytoplasm. Intracellular substances associated with neurotransmission decrease, and RNA and other protein components required for regeneration of the axon increase (MacKinnon and Dellon, 1988). Propelled by trophic factors and guided by the potential tubes formed by Schwann cell bodies, proximal axonal sprouts either cross the site of injury and enter the distal endoneurial tubes or else become snarled in trying to do so (Fig. 14-5). The latter circumstance is likely to obtain when the distance between the ends of the divided nerve allows axons to lose their way. A similar tangle can result when the repair is excessively delayed and the distal endoneurial tubes collapse and fibrose.

DIAGNOSIS

Clinical Features of Recurrent Nerve Injury

The most conspicuous evidence of unilateral nerve failure is change in the pitch, force, and timber of phonation, but the spectrum of symptoms varies from near normal speech to hoarseness, breathlessness, choking, and aspiration. Montgomery (1989) notes three variables: (1) unilaterality or bilat-

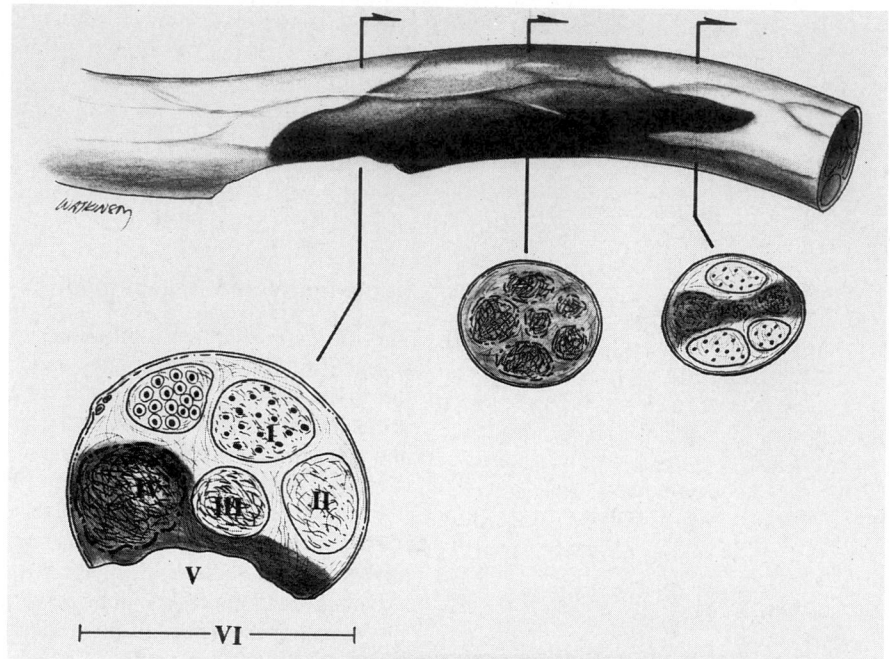

Figure 14-4. Mackinnon's sixth degree injury, a situation where fibers and fascicles are variably injured. The likelihood of spontaneous recovery is certain with first- and second-degree injuries and nil for fourth- and fifth-degree injuries.

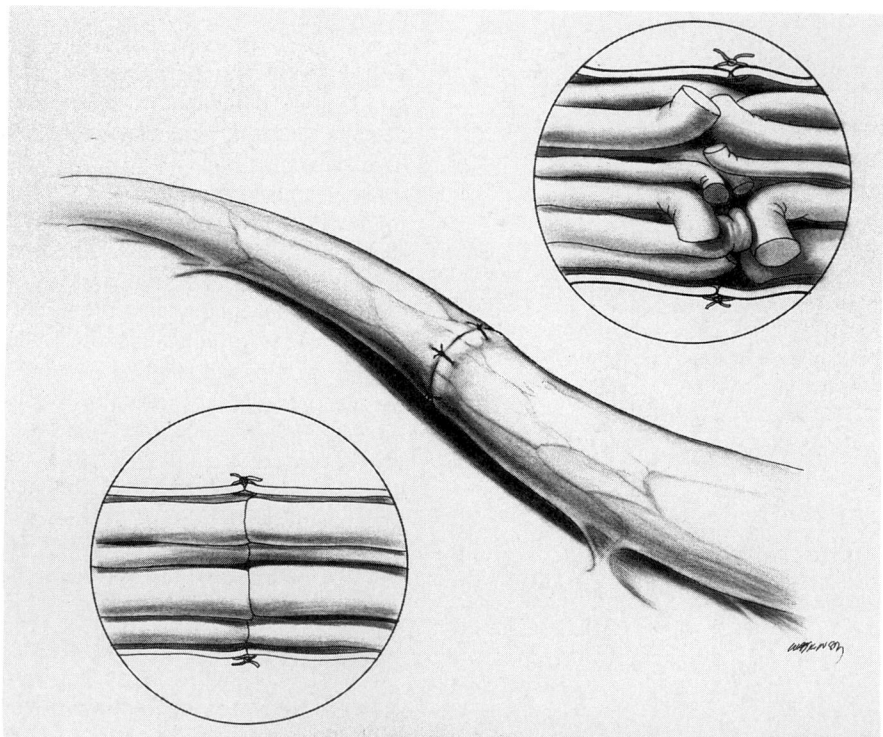

Figure 14-5. Repaired laryngeal nerve. The surgeon's expectation (*lower left*) is contrasted with the all too frequent result (*upper right*). Accurate orientation is elusive, and such axons as successfully cross the gap may still reach a motor end-plate with discordant function. (From Mackinnon SE: In Cohen ML (ed): Mastery of Surgery—Plastic Surgery. Little, Brown, Boston, 1992, with permission.)

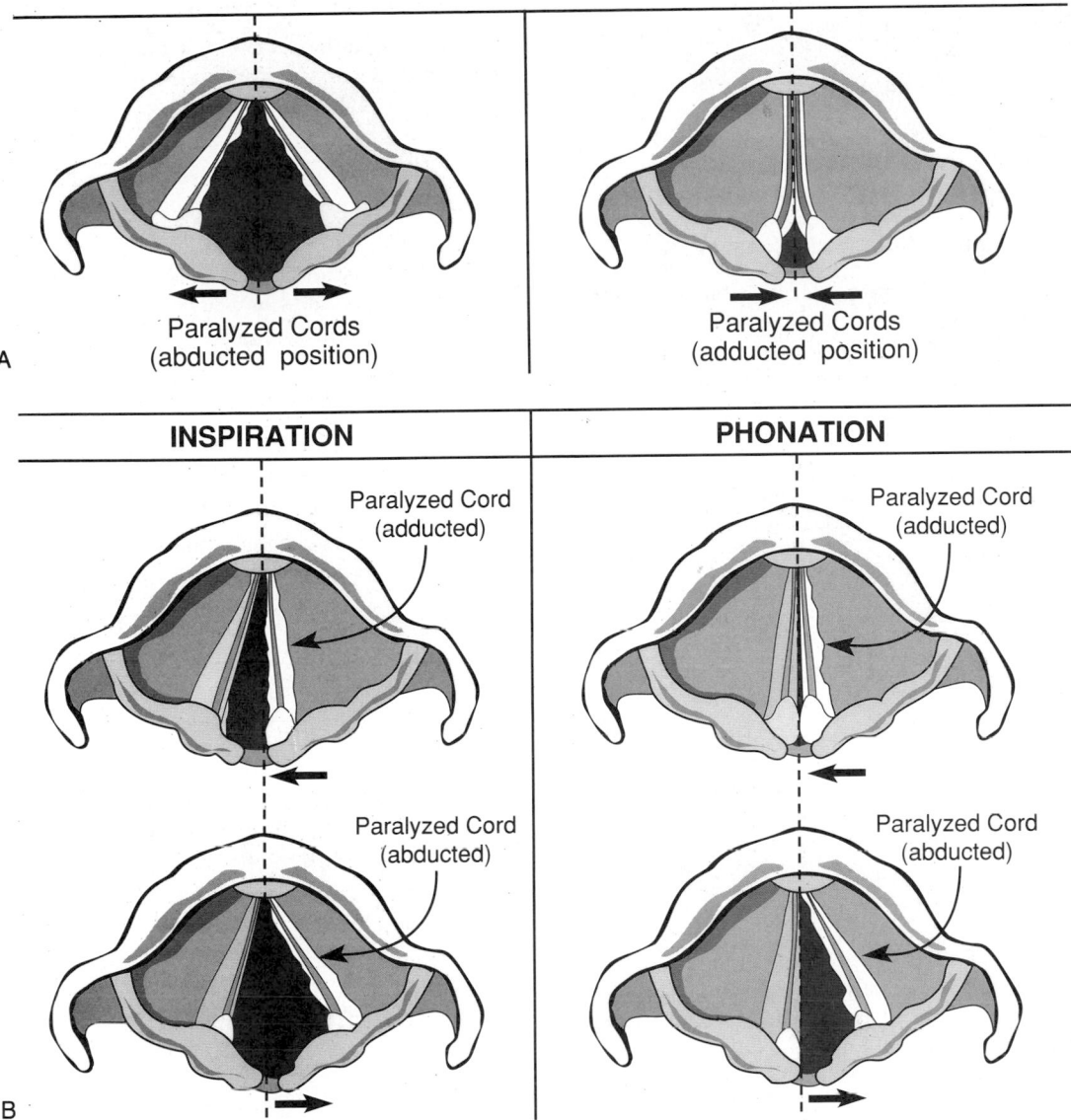

INSPIRATION   **PHONATION**

Paralyzed Cords
(abducted position)

Paralyzed Cords
(adducted position)

A

Paralyzed Cord
(adducted)

Paralyzed Cord
(adducted)

Paralyzed Cord
(abducted)

Paralyzed Cord
(abducted)

B

Figure 14-6. **(A)** Bilateral paralysis. Contrasting clinical pictures depending on whether the paralysed cords are in the abducted or adducted position. Abducted cords leaves the airway defenseless and the patient voiceless. Adducted cords may obstruct to the point of asphyxiation. **(B)** The clinical description of unilateral paralysis requires (1) naming the side and (2) stating the cord's position (e.g., "The left cord is paralyzed in the abducted position.")

erality of recurrent nerve failure, (2) position of the cords, and (3) compensatory movement of the functioning cord (Fig. 14-6).

Bilateral Recurrent Laryngeal Nerve Paralysis with Cords Adducted

Bilateral recurrent laryngeal nerve paralysis with the cords adducted places the patient in constant danger of obstruction and almost always requires a permanent tracheostomy. With-

out such a vent the patient must endure inspiratory stridor and the specter of sudden unheralded asphyxiation.

Bilateral Paralysis with Cords Abducted

Bilateral paralysis with the cords abducted leaves the patient without a voice. Coughing is ineffective. Aspiration of saliva and food is severe, and tracheostomy with a cuffed tube may be required as a temporizing measure. Over the long term, Montgomery (1989) suggests either laryngectomy and end tracheostomy or Habal and Murray's operation (1972) of sealing the larynx permanently with a flap of epiglottis.

Unilateral Paralysis with Cord Adducted

Unilateral paralysis with the cord in the position of adduction impairs pitch in singing, but the speaking voice and airway may be close to normal otherwise. No treatment is required.

Unilateral Paralysis with Cord Abducted

Unilateral paralysis of the recurrent laryngeal nerve and the cord in the position of abduction results in breathy hoarseness or aphonia, depending on the degree of abduction. The patient is unable to cough or laugh. Aspiration, especially of liquids, is the rule. Over time, the normal cord may swing across the midline and partially close the chink, but given no improvement within 6 months to 1 year, either injection of the immobile cord or a phonoplastic operation may be performed to enhance cord approximation (see Management).

There is a human side to the loss of recurrent nerve function that is not conveyed by anatomic descriptions. Explanation is less awkward for the surgeon when nerves succumb to natural events, such as invasion by a tumor; then we tell the patient, "You have a paralyzed vocal cord." When the nerve has been cut with the scalpel or Bovie a less painful euphemism emerges—"hoarseness," we say. The patient could tell us more if we took the time to ask: Aspiration results when reflexes that shunt air to the trachea and food to the pharynx falter. With time the patient learns to swallow without aspirating by pressing the chin against the chest. Coughing is ineffectual, as are efforts to clear the throat. A Valsalva maneuver is impossible. Singing, laughing, and raising the voice, let alone shouting, are out of the question. Hoarseness is a joke to all but the afflicted, and strangers react as if encountering someone with a contagious disease. Time may also add force and timber to the voice as the working cord stretches across the midline, but in the stretching it appears to fatigue more easily, and toward evening the voice weakens.

Causes of Recurrent Nerve Paralysis

Among the causes of recurrent laryngeal nerve paralysis are cancer of the lung, primary or metastatic malignancy of mediastinal nodes, and carcinoma of the trachea, thyroid, or esophagus. Dayal (1981) states that the left nerve is twice as frequently involved as with the right, a not surprising fact given its longer course and close proximity to the lung, pleura, trachea, and esophagus. Less commonly, an aortic aneurysm or dilated left atrium will put the left nerve on stretch. Other natural causes of nerve dysfunction include neuritis due to lead poisoning and alcoholism. One-third of all cases of vocal cord paralysis have no demonstrable cause (Dayal, 1981).

Surgical Damage

Surgical damage to the recurrent laryngeal nerves is said to occur in 0.5 to 37 percent of operations on the neck and upper chest. Injury is unavoidable at times, especially if one is operating for cancer with wide margins indicated. An in-

---

> **Some Operations That Are Inherently Risky for the Recurrent Laryngeal Nerves**
>
> Correction of Zenker's diverticulum
> Resection of the cervical esophagus
> Parathyroid exploration
> Thyroidectomy
> Carotid endarterectomy
>   (Vagus may be clamped with artery)
> Radical neck dissection
> Mediastinoscopy
> Tracheal resection
> Correction of persistent ductus arteriosus
> Left pheumonectomy, left upper lobectomy
> Left hilar dissections
> Resection of mediastinal tumor
> Operations on the aortic arch or isthmus
> Transhiatal esophagectomy
> Resection carotid body tumor
> Nerve sheath tumors

complete list of operations that are inherently risky for the recurrent laryngeal nerves is presented above. The pivotal points in a few of these operations bear reviewing.

Transhiatal esophagectomy. Transhiatal esophagectomy inevitably exposes the left recurrent nerve to the risk of neuropraxis from traction or even avulsion during stripping in the region of the aorta. This is the least accessible point, where hopeful fingertips strain to stroke away the final tethers. Orringer and Orringer (1983) recommend keeping the index and third fingers of each hand closely applied to the anterior and posterior aspects of the esophagus (see Ch. 43 in *Esophageal Surgery,* a companion book to this one), advice that is not easy to follow when the operation is for stage III middle-third carcinoma.

A second area of vulnerability is in the neck, where the nerve lies parallel to the trachea and in front of and to the left of the esophagus. Medial retraction of the trachea with a self-retaining retractor can cause pressure damage to the nerve and ostensibly did so in 37 percent of Orringer and Orringer's (1983) first series of patients undergoing transhiatal esophagectomy. The Orringers now eschew the use of a self-retaining retractor. My recommendation is to expose and identify the nerve and to position the retractor(s) with the nerve in view.

The right recurrent nerve is most vulnerable during encirclement of the cervical esophagus with a rubber drain or tube such as is routinely used for traction. The far side of the esophagus is not visible, and if the right-angled clamp or Semb dissector drifts from the outer esophageal muscle layer it can capture the contralateral laryngeal nerve. A 46 Fr bougie can be passed through the mouth and to help define the far unseen edge of the esophagus.

Tracheal Resections. Operations about the cervical trachea inevitably carry a risk for disrupting the recurrent laryngeal nerves. Pearson (personal communication, 1984) and Grillo (1983) both agree that the safest approach when operating for benign disease is to keep the dissection very close to the trachea. All the same, there is a risk of current spreading from the Bovie tip to the unseen nerves, a risk thought to be minimized by using a bipolar electrode and reducing the current to the lowest hemostatically useful level.

Visualization of the recurrent nerves makes more sense when contemplating wider resections for malignant tracheal tumors or in operations for tumors of the thyroid gland or esophagus that have invaded the trachea. When paresis of a single vocal cord already exists, it is in the patient's interest to identify and preserve the contralateral recurrent nerve. Even the nerve on the paralyzed side should be protected until it is clear that the tumor is otherwise irresectable, in a single instance (my own case) of advanced upper-third esophageal cancer radiation and chemotherapy successfully reversed a recurrent nerve palsy, albeit for only a few months.

In contrast to operations on the larynx or cervical trachea, when the patient is forewarned of the possibility of laryngeal dysfunction, awakening to the reality of permanent hoarseness following other procedures, especially those anatomically remote from the larynx, can be troublesome for the doctor to explain and for the patient to endure. Better that the surgeon take the time to warn of the possibility before embarking on any lung resection on the left that could eventuate in a pneumonectomy. A subaortic lymphadenectomy, whether for staging or for cure, merits a similar preoperative discussion, as do operations that expose the proximal portion of the right subclavian artery; the same applies to right apical pleurectomy, resection of a Pancoast tumor, mediastinoscopy, and any operation for malignancy in the mid-mediastinum. Any search for parathyroid glands, especially aberrant ones, puts the nerves at risk. The special circumstance a right-sided parathyroid tumor that presents as a thoracic shadow and is more safely approached through the neck deserves emphasis (see Ch. 58).

MANAGEMENT

The bruised but intact recurrent laryngeal nerve possesses remarkable regenerative potential. Trauma from an inadvertent ligature, excessive retraction, partial clamping, or minimal cauterization can eventuate in complete or nearly complete restoration of function. (I personally experienced just such recovery 4 months after I underwent a partial thyroidectomy associated with a complete right cord paresis).

Recognizing the actual severance of the nerve, say, in the course of removing a substernal goiter, poses a dilemma for the thoracic surgeon. The issue of immediate repair is clouded by pessimistic reports of imperfect results, presumed to be secondary to proximal adductor fibers reaching distal abductor axons and vice versa. The practical consideration is that vocal cords that close on inspiration and separate on phonation are less than ideal. Reports of satisfactory return to normal function following primary repair notwithstanding, recurrent laryngeal nerve repair remains controversial (Sa-

toh, 1973; Ezaki, et al., 1982; Montgomery, 1989; Crumley, 1990).

Mackinnon (1994) recommends an epineurial repair for a clean transection and a short nerve graft for actual nerve loss. A cervical sensory nerve can ordinarily be found and would be appropriate for an injury in the neck. When a nerve palsy with functional loss has become established, either a cord injection or Crumley's neurotization could be performed.

Based on the results of two patients with schwannoma, Crumley (1990) recommends dividing the ansa hypoglossal nerve and suturing its proximal end to the distal stump of the recurrent laryngeal nerve. Normal tension and bulk of all intrinsic ipsilateral laryngeal muscles plus a normal voice are said to have returned in 3 months. In this operation the proximal end of the ansa hypoglossi branch to the sternothyroid muscle is sutured to the distal stump of the recurrent nerve by using three to four sutures of 10–0 nylon.

Isshiki et al. (1974) described tightening the paralyzed cord through placement of a silicone block through a window in the thyroid cartilage. Local anesthesia is proposed to facilitate fine tuning of the voice. The principal drawback to thyroplasty appears to be the potential for further complications within the larynx itself (Crumley, 1990).

Teflon injection has been widely used for the "permanent" treatment of patients with unilateral cord paralysis since its introduction by Arnold (1962). A number of complications and drawbacks have caused concern, including granuloma, migration of the injected mass, inability to remove the paste, and troublesome problems relating to injecting too much or too little of the material.

PREVENTION

The best remedy for recurrent nerve injury is prevention. On the basis of personal experience of deliberately exposing over 600 recurrent laryngeal nerves in the neck and mediastinum without a single instance of inadvertently caused permanent paralysis, I offer the following:

1. It is better to learn the anatomic course of the recurrent nerve in the dissecting room than in the operating room.
2. Use 2 to 3 optical loupes and a headlamp.
3. Sit down on a stool and work in unhurried fashion.
4. Be wary of grasping with forceps or clamping with hemostats any filamentous structure until the recurrent laryngeal nerve has been positively identified. (There are a few exceptions to this rule, notably tracheal surgery and mediastinoscopy.)
5. Even after the nerve has been identified, remember that its somewhat slack and meandering course may catch the inattentive operator unaware.
6. Be gentle with retraction and careful with the electrocautery.
7. Alert the patient beforehand that the conditions for which the thoracic surgeon usually operates, if uncorrected, also place the respiratory, swallowing, and speech functions at risk.

KEY REFERENCES

Crumley RL: Repair of the recurrent laryngeal nerve. Otolaryngol Clin North Am 23:553, 1990

An excellent overview for those who prefer a concise, readable summary of the state of the art.

Mackinnon SE, Dellon AL: Surgery of the Peripheral Nerve. Thieme, New York, 1988

A thorough, scholarly, and beautifully illustrated examination of nerve injury and repair.

Montgomery WW: Laryngeal paralysis, p. 607. In: Surgery of the Upper Respiratory System. Vol. 2, 2nd Ed. Lea & Febiger, Malvern, PA, 1989

An excellent overview covering all aspects of laryngeal paralysis.

Rice DH: Laryngeal reinnervation. Laryngoscope 92:1049, 1982

A useful review of the multitude of procedures attempted to improve the lot of patients with vocal cord paralysis, with discussion and suggestions for further research.

REFERENCES

Arnold GE: Vocal rehabilitation of paralytic dysphonia. Arch Otolaryngol Head Neck Surg 76:358, 1962

Dayal DS: Clinical Otolaryngology. JB Lippincott, 1981

Ducker TB: Pathophysiology of peripheral nerve trauma. p. 476. In Omer GE, Spinner M (eds): Management of Peripheral Nerve Problems. WB Saunders, Philadelphia, 1980

Ezaki H, Ushio H, Harada Y et al: Recurrent laryngeal nerve anastomosis following thyroid surgery. World J Surg 6:342, 1982

Grillo HC: Congenital lesions, neoplasms, and injuries of the trachea. In Sabiston DC, Spencer FC (eds): Gibbon's Surgery of the Chest. Vol. 1. 4th Ed., WB Saunders, Philadelphia, 1983

Habal MB, Murray JE: Surgical treatment of life-endangering chronic aspiration pneumonia. Use of an epiglottic flap to the arytenoids. Plast Reconstr Surg 49:305, 1972

Henry JF: Nonrecurring recurrent laryngeal nerve. Surgery 104:977, 1988

Isshiki N, Morita H, Okamura H et al: Thyroplasty as a new phonosurgical technique. Acta Otolaryngol (Stockh) 78:451, 1974

Major RH: A History of Medicine. Vol. 1. 1st Ed. Charles C Thomas, Springfield, IL, 1954, pp. 191, 220

Mackinnon SE: Upper extremity nerve injuries: primary repair and reconstruction. In Cohen ML (ed): Mastery of Surgery—Plastic Surgery. Little, Brown, Boston, 1992

Mackinnon SE, Dellon AL: Surgery of the Peripheral Nerve. p. 35. Thieme, New York, 1988

Montgomery WW: Laryngeal paralysis. p. 607. In: Surgery of the Upper Respiratory System. Vol. 2. 2nd. Ed. Lea and Febiger, Malvern, PA, 1989

Orringer MB, Orringer JS: Esophagectomy without thoracotomy: a dangerous operation? J Thorac Cardiovasc Surg 85:72, 1983

Pemberton J, Beaver MG: Anomaly of the right recurrent laryngeal nerve. Surg Gynecol Obstet 54:594, 1932

Satoh I, Harvey JE, Ogura JH: Impairment of function of the intrinsic laryngeal muscles after regeneration of the recurrent laryngeal nerve. Laryngoscope 88:1268, 1978

Stedman GW: A singular distribution of some of the nerves and arteries of the neck and the top of the thorax. Edinb Med Surg J 19:564, 1823 (as cited by Henry JF, Audifrett J, Denizot A, Plan M: The nonrecurrent inferior laryngeal nerve: review of 33 cases, including two on the left side. Surgery 104:6, 1988)

Waller AV: Experiments on the glossopharyngeal and hypoglossal nerves of the frog and observations produced thereby in the structure of their primitive fibers. Phil Trans R Soc Land 140:423, 1850

15

UPPER AIRWAY TUMORS

Primary Tumors

F. Griffith Pearson
Paulo Cardoso
Shafique Keshavjee

Primary tumors of the trachea are much less common than neoplasms of either the lung or larynx. A majority of primary tumors in adults are malignant, whereas in children most are benign. In general, the incidence is equally distributed between the sexes and is highest between the third and fifth decades. In adults primary malignant neoplasms of the trachea represent 2 percent of upper airway tumors (Barak, 1984). Aside from anecdotal case reports, only a few centers throughout the world have reported any significant experience with the surgical management of primary tracheal tumors.

This chapter does not discuss laryngeal neoplasms. Tumors involving the main carina are considered in Chapters 16 to 27, and secondary neoplasms of the upper airway are dealt with later in this chapter.

HISTORICAL NOTE

Prior to the 1960s tracheal resection was limited by the assumption that no more than three or four tracheal rings (up to 3 cm) could be resected circumferentially and reconstructed by primary anastomosis (Barclay, et al., 1957). During these early years there were numerous reports of experimental and clinical efforts to replace segments of the resected trachea with a variety of prosthetic materials, both solid and porous. Belsey (1950) was the first to report reconstruction of the human trachea using fascia lata reinforced with stainless wire. Beall, et al. (1963) reported on experimental and clinical experience with a porous prosthesis of heavy Marlex mesh, and our group subsequently reported our preliminary clinical experience with this same prosthesis (Pearson, et al., 1968). Neville, et al. (1972) introduced a solid silicone prosthesis for both tracheal and carinal replacement, and Neville updated this initial report in 1987.

Between 1960 and 1970, significant technical advances re-

sulted from increased experience with postintubation tracheal injury secondary to cuffed tubes and mechanical ventilation. Techniques of mobilization were developed (Grillo, et al., 1964) that made it possible to resect up to half the length of the adult trachea and achieve reconstruction by primary end-to-end anastomosis. Furthermore, techniques were developed for circumferential resection and primary reconstruction at both the subglottic (Pearson, et al., 1975) and carinal (Grillo, 1982) levels.

HISTORICAL READINGS

Barclay RS, McSwan N, Welsh TM: Tracheal reconstruction without the use of grafts. Thorax 12:177, 1957

Beall AC Jr, Harrington OB, Greenberg SD et al.: Circumferential replacement of thoracic trachea with Marlex mesh. JAMA 183:1082, 1963

Belsey R: Resection and reconstruction of the intrathoracic trachea. Br J Surg 38:200, 1950

Neville WE, Hamouda F, Andersen J, Dwan FM: Replacement of the intrathoracic trachea and both stem bronchi with a molded Silastic prosthesis. J Thorac Cardiovasc Surg 63:569, 1972

Pearson FG, Henderson RD, Gross AE et al.: The reconstruction of circumferential tracheal defects with a porous prosthesis: an experimental and clinical study using heavy Marlex mesh. J Thorac Cardiovasc Surg 55:605, 1968

BASIC SCIENCE: PATHOLOGY

Benign Tracheal Neoplasms

Benign tumors of the trachea may arise from any component of the tracheal wall and account for 90 percent of primary neoplasms in children. Conversely, less than 10 percent of primary neoplasms in the adult trachea are benign.

Papillomas are the most common neoplasms in the pediatric population and are usually multifocal, with diffuse involvement of the larynx, trachea, and bronchial tree. Juvenile papillomatosis almost always regresses following puberty. The origin of this condition remains obscure; both viral and endocrine disorders have been considered as causative factors, and improvement has been reported in patients given interferon therapy (Goepfert, et al., 1982). Therapy of symptomatic lesions is primarily surgical, using various modalities of endoscopic ablation.

Another ostensibly benign tumor of epithelial origin is the neuroendocrine carcinoid neoplasm (Briselli, et al., 1978; Perelman and Koroleva, 1987). Although carcinoids are listed in this benign category, these tumors are undoubtedly of low-grade malignancy, with histologic evidence of direct local invasion of contiguous structures.

Tumors of mesenchymal origin include chondroma, neurilemmoma, schwannoma, fibroma, and lipoma. Of these, chondroma is the most frequent and is commonly located in the upper trachea at the cricoid level (Neis, et al., 1989). It is often difficult or impossible for the pathologist to distinguish between a benign chondroma and a low-grade chondrosarcoma on the basis of histology. Rarer mesenchymal tumors include leiomyoma, hemangioma and benign epithelial polyp (Grillo, 1978; Xu, et al., 1987; and Perelman and Koroleva, 1987).

Malignant Tracheal Neoplasms

Once more, we emphasize that more than 90 percent of primary tumors of the trachea and carina in the adult population are malignant. By far the most common of these malignant neoplasms are squamous cell carcinomas and adenoid cystic tumors. Five major publications have reported experience with surgical resection of primary tumors of the trachea and carina between 1969 and 1990 (Table 15-1). It is apparent from a summary of these reported data that 153 (38 percent) of 397 resections were performed for adenoid cystic carcinoma and 88 (22 percent) for squamous cell carcinoma. The pathology and clinical features of these two tumor types is described below in some detail.

Adenoid Cystic Carcinoma

Adenoid cystic carcinoma, first described by Billroth in 1859, for many years was called "cylindroma" and considered to be a slowly growing benign adenoma. The gross appearance of the tumor may suggest benignity, since the overlying tracheal mucosa is frequently intact (Fig. 15-1) and the progression of these tumors is often exceedingly slow. It is apparent, however, that these are malignant neoplasms with universal evidence of local invasion on histologic examination. Indeed, this tumor is nearly always found to extend beyond the visible and palpable confines of the gross lesion at the time of surgery. Invisible, microscopic spread occurs both circumferentially and longitudinally in the tracheal wall, particularly in the submucosal plane and on the external surface of the trachea in the perineural lymphatic spaces. The gross and microscopic features of this tumor are illustrated in Figures 15-1 to 15-4. It is evident from this information that frozen section evaluation of resection margins is of critical importance at the time of resection if a complete and potentially curative operation is the objective.

Metastases to regional lymph nodes are reported in approximately 10 percent of patients. Hematogenous metastasis occur most commonly in the lungs, but there is occasional spread to brain and bone (Pearson, et al., 1974). The natural history of this tumor, even in untreated cases, is often that of a slow and insidious progression. Local recurrences have been observed by one of us (F.G.P.) more than 25 years following a presumably complete resection (Figs. 15-5 to 15-9). Pulmonary metastases are frequently asymptomatic when first identified in plain chest films and may remain so for long periods (years) in some patients (Pearson, et al., 1974).

Adenoid cystic carcinoma occurs with equal frequency in men and women and in all age groups from the teens through the nineties. There is no relationship to cigarette smoking.

Table 15-1. Primary Tumors of the Trachea and Carina: Reported Series of Resected Cases

Author (Year)	Total Cases Resected	Adenoid Cystic Carcinoma	Squamous Cell Carcinoma
Houston, et al. (1969)	11	6	2
Echapasse (1974)	75	19	27
Pearson, et al. (1984)	44	28	9
Perelman and Koroleva (1987)	135	56	20
Grillo and Mathisen (1990)	132	50	41
Total	397	153	88

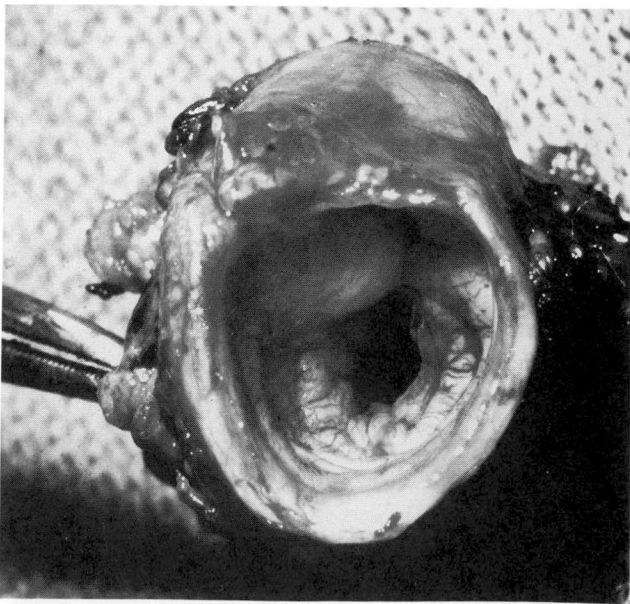

Figure 15-1. Photograph illustrating the gross appearance of a freshly resected specimen of adenoid cystic carcinoma, such as might be seen at bronchoscopy. The overlying mucosa is intact, and the gross margins of the tumor appear circumscribed.

Figure 15-2. A whole mount histologic section of a resected specimen of adenoid cystic carcinoma. The tumor extends through the full thickness of the tracheal wall, and there is as much gross tumor lying outside the lumen as within. TU, tumor; TR, tracheal cartilage; LN, lymph node.

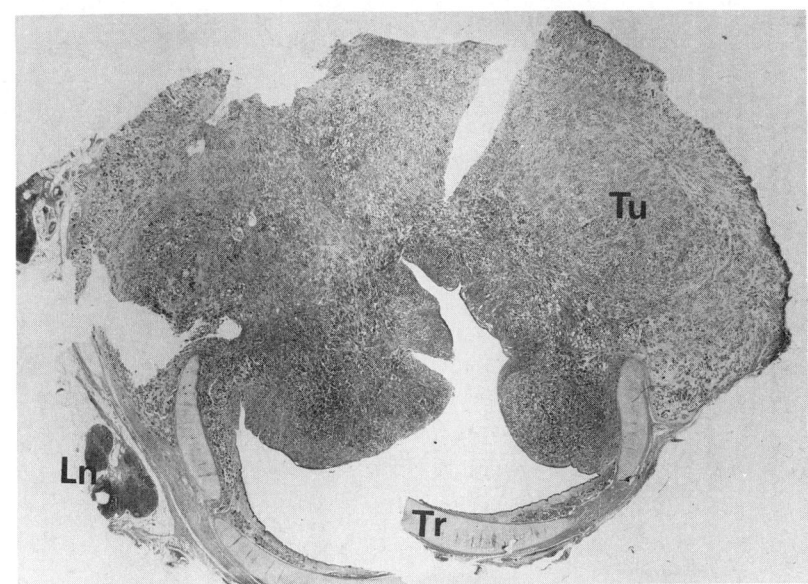

Figure 15-3. Photomicrograph illustrating the extensive submucosal spread of adenoid cystic carcinoma. The spread occurs both longitudinally and circumferentially and is neither visible nor palpable to the operating surgeon. The overlying mucosa is intact. Only intraoperative frozen section assessment will identify such involvement. TR, tracheal cartilage.

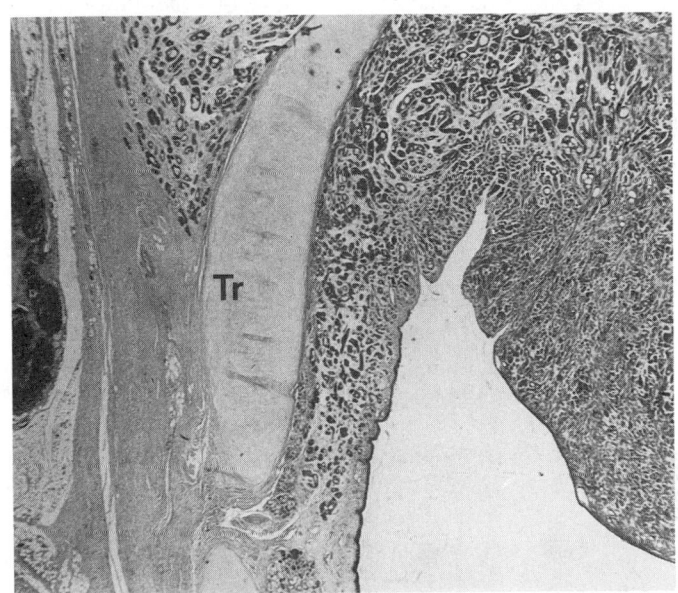

Figure 15-4. Photomicrograph illustrating adenoid cystic carcinoma, spreading longitudinally on the outer surface of the trachea, in the perineural lymphatics. This type of microscopic spread is invisible and produces no gross abnormality in the appearance of the external tracheal wall.

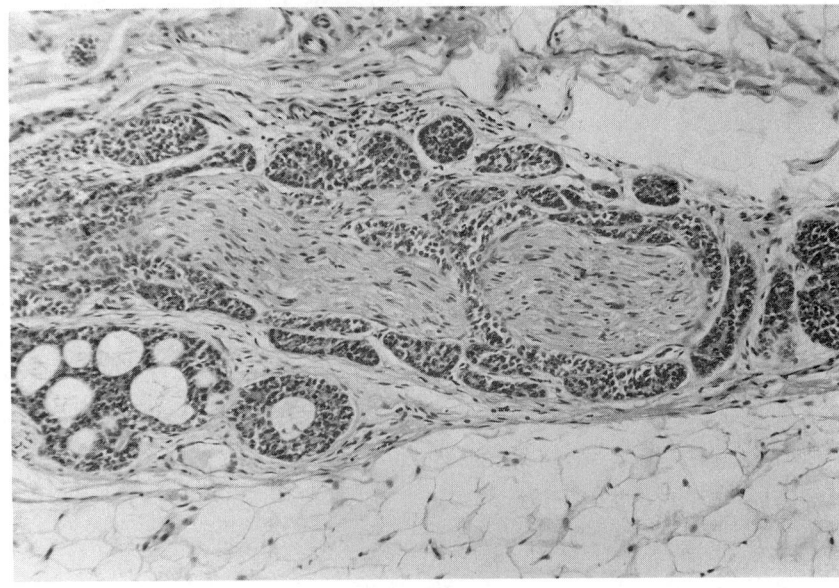

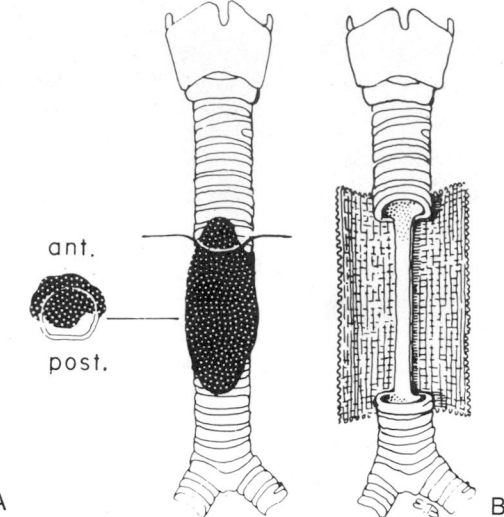

Figure 15-5. **(A)** Diagram illustrating a tumor in the upper medi-astinal trachea in a 15-year-old girl. This patient had a 2-year history of a condition diagnosed as "asthma and chronic bronchitis." The tumor was an adenoid cystic carcinoma. **(B)** This tumor was re-sected in 1963 in the first case in which the author (F.G.P.) used a cylinder of heavy-duty Marlex mesh for replacement. A 6.5-cm segment was resected, and a strip of membranous trachea was preserved as a potential source for early epithelialization of the internal surface of the prosthesis.

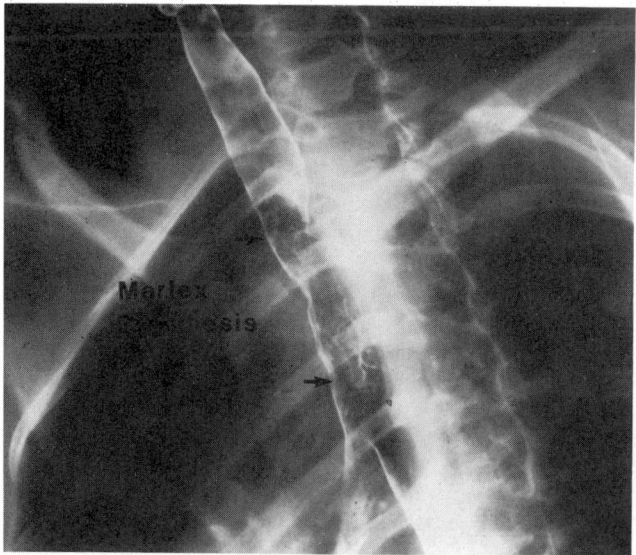

Figure 15-6. A contrast tracheogram from the same patient shown in Figure 15-5. This tracheogram was taken 4 years after prosthetic replacement, and the patient maintained had an excellent airway until that time. During the following year she developed slowly progressive narrowing at the upper end of the prosthesis, with associated dyspnea. Arrows indicate ends of Marlex prosthesis.

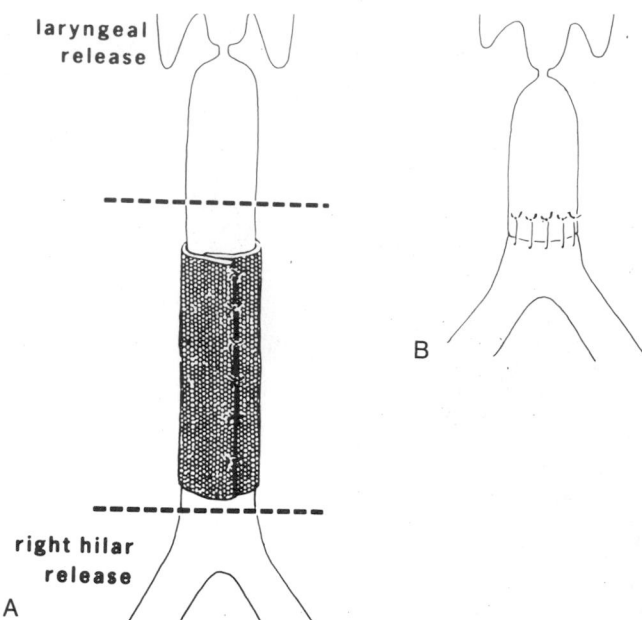

Figure 15-7. The same patient shown in Figures 15-5 and 15-6. The diagram illustrates the operative procedure performed in 1968, 5 years after the initial prosthetic replacement. The entire prosthesis was resected. **(A)** By using a suprathyroid release proce-dure above and a right intrapericardial release below, it was possi-ble to achieve **(B)** a successful primary anastomosis.

Squamous Cell Carcinoma

Squamous cell carcinoma occurs predominantly in men (3 : 1 male/female ratio), and has an age distribution similar to that of squamous cell carcinoma of the lung. All the squamous cell tumors in Grillo and Mathisen's (1990) series were associated with cigarette smoking.

The gross appearance of these tumors is like that of squa-mous cancer of the bronchus in any other location. They are almost always ulcerated lesions, and hemoptysis is a common presenting symptom. Unfortunately, the incidence of re-gional lymph node metastasis is high, and the tumor is fre-quently locally advanced and unresectable at the time of presentation. Hematogenous spread is similar to that of bron-chogenic carcinoma.

Other Primary Malignancies

The remaining primary malignancies are rare and include chondrosarcoma, leiomyosarcoma, carcinosarcoma, and spindle cell sarcoma. Mucoepidermoid carcinoma and mixed adenosquamous tumors may also arise from the tracheal or carinal epithelium. Monocytic leukemia and plasmacytoma have been reported (Hadju, et al., 1970; Grillo, 1978; Kairalla, et al., 1988; Neis, et al., 1989).

DIAGNOSIS AND CLINICAL FEATURES

Signs and Symptoms

The clinical presentation of tracheal tumors may be due to upper airway obstruction (dyspnea, wheezing, and stridor), mucosal irritation and ulceration (cough and hemoptysis),

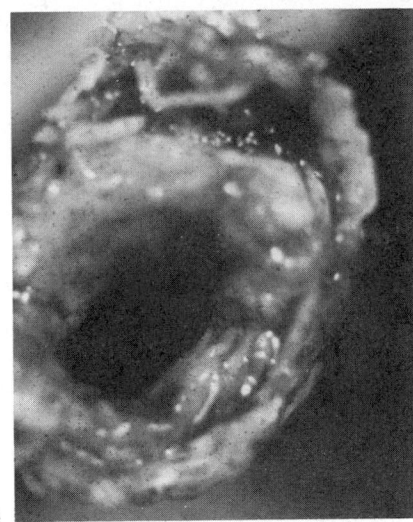 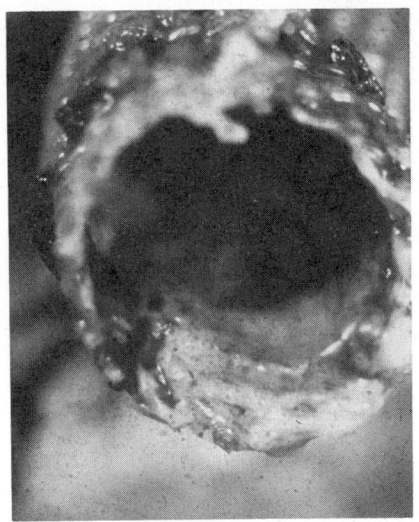

Figure 15-8. Photograph of same patient as in Figures 15-5 to 15-7, showing the gross appearance of the resected prosthesis. **(A)** There was concentric stenosis due to fibrosis and granulations at the upper end. **(B)** The lower end was epithelialized and widely patent.

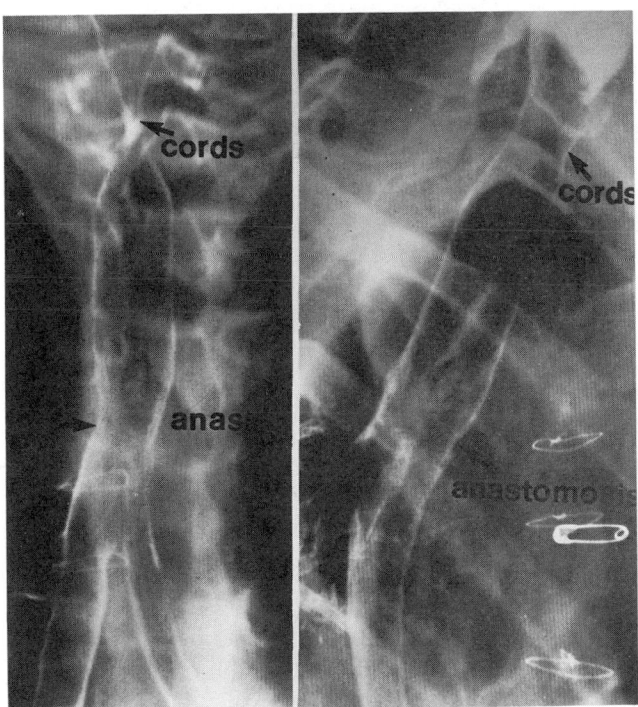

Figure 15-9. A contrast tracheogram in the same patient as in Figures 15-5 to 15-8, obtained 1 year following resection and primary reconstruction. A widely patent airway was obtained, and the degree of tracheal shortening is apparent. This patient survived for an additional 24 years before succumbing to airway obstruction from a *local recurrence* in the distal remaining trachea. This recurrence did not become clinically evident until 1989, 26 years following the first operation with prosthetic reconstruction. Cords, upper arrows; anastomosis, lower arrows.

direct invasion and involvement of contiguous structures (recurrent nerve palsy, dysphagia) or may be the result of distant metastasis. Upper airway obstruction is characterized by dyspnea, stridor, wheezing, and cough. These are common symptoms of respiratory dysfunction, and many patients with tracheal tumors are treated for "asthma" or "chronic bronchitis" for long periods prior to correct diagnosis. Furthermore, many of these tumors do grow very slowly (benign tumors, adenoid cystic carcinoma, carcinoid tumors, mucoepidermoid carcinoma), and symptoms of obstruction may continue for months or even years without development of life-threatening airway impairment.

It is understandable that the correct diagnosis of primary tracheal tumor is so frequently delayed, since these neoplasms are so uncommon that they are rarely if ever encountered by most physicians. When symptoms of cough, wheezing, and dyspnea are investigated with plain chest films, there may be no apparent abnormality in the mediastinum or tracheal air column. If abnormalities do exist in the plain chest film, they are often subtle and easily overlooked.

Radiology

Plain chest films, anteroposterior and lateral tomograms, and contrast tracheograms are all valuable modalities for imaging tracheal tumors. Computed tomography (CT), however, provides the most informative evaluation, with delineation of both intraluminal and extraluminal extent of tumor and relatively accurate evaluation of the relationship of tumor to adjacent structures. CT is recommended in all cases for staging and for directing management (Morency, et al., 1989). A contrast esophagogram will identify esophageal involvement and may be obtained as part of the CT scan.

The role of magnetic resonance imaging (MRI) is still under review. A major advantage of MRI is the creation of sagittal and coronal images, which better demonstrate the luminal dimensions and the extent of extramural disease (Naidich,

1990). This same detail can be reconstructed from fine-interval CT scans, and at present there is no clear advantage of MRI over CT imaging.

Pulmonary Function Studies

Pulmonary function tests may alert the physician to the possibility of upper airways obstruction and a correct diagnosis. An obstructive pattern combined with a lack of response to bronchodilator medication may suggest a fixed upper airway obstruction. Flow-volume loops may clearly indicate upper airway obstruction, with plateauing of the inspiratory or expiratory phase depending on the location of the tumor in relation to the mediastinum. In most cases both limbs of the flow-volume loop are flattened (Fig. 15-10). The problem of interpreting false negative results has been addressed by Gelb, et al. (1988). Fredberg, et al. (1980) have described a technique for measuring upper airway diameters by acoustic reflection directly at the patient's mouth; these "tracheal echograms" provide relatively accurate quantitative measurements of airway diameters and the precise level of obstruction relative to the vocal cords. This technique also identifies areas of lesser obstruction that would not be picked up in the flow-volume curves.

Endoscopy

Bronchoscopy is essential in all cases and provides the simplest and most reliable approach for biopsy and tissue diagnosis. The extent of intraluminal involvement is ascertained, and precise measurements define the margins of the tumor and the relationship to carina, cricoid, and vocal cords. This information is essential for planning the operative approach and the details of surgical resection. Biopsies taken at and beyond the margins of visible tumor may detect microscopic extension of disease and further facilitate judgment concerning the necessary extent of resection.

In patients with significant upper airways obstruction or massive hemoptysis, the flexible bronchoscope is ineffective. These are potentially life-threatening conditions and require

rigid bronchoscopy to provide adequate control of the airway. In most cases the bronchoscope can be advanced beyond the tumor and provide access for ventilation. The tracheal lumen may be enlarged by endoscopic removal of tumor using biopsy forceps, coagulation, or laser resection. Whenever possible, tracheotomy is to be avoided, since it may complicate any subsequent resection.

MANAGEMENT

We again emphasize that most primary tracheal tumors are malignant, are usually locally advanced at the time of symptomatic presentation and diagnosis, and are frequently at a stage that precludes a complete resection. Both curative and palliative approaches are presented below.

Tracheal Resection and Primary Reconstruction

With few exceptions, surgical excision is the best therapy for those neoplasms that can be completely resected with restoration of continuity by primary reconstruction. It is assumed that all malignant tumors extend through and beyond the trachea wall, which makes endoscopic resection (including laser resection) inevitably incomplete, and therefore inadequate, in otherwise operable patients.

A cervical collar incision provides adequate access for most tumors confined to the cervical and upper mediastinal trachea. The mediastinal trachea is well exposed throughout its length via a median sternotomy, although a right posterolateral thoracotomy may provide preferable exposure for selected tumors that involve the distal trachea and require a concomitant carinal resection (Pearson, et al., 1984; Grillo and Mathisen, 1990). The technique of resection for a tumor in the mediastinal trachea is illustrated in Figures 15-11 to 15-14. An extended resection is necessary for the management of many of these tracheal neoplasms. With few exceptions, it is usually possible to remove approximately half the length of the adult trachea and achieve reconstruction by primary anastomosis. Such extended resections require mobilization of the anterior and lateral aspects of the trachea from top to bottom and may necessitate the addition of release procedures at the upper and lower ends of the trachea. The operative details describing these procedures are provided in Chapter 16. An illustrative case of a patient requiring extended resection for adenoid cystic carcinoma is depicted in Figures 15-15 through 15-17.

A difficult problem for the surgeon in many of these operations relates to the extent of resection that is undertaken. Until the airway has been divided and the information provided by frozen section assessment of the resection margins is available, it is impossible to judge the extent of resection required to remove all identifiable tumor. It may be necessary to accept microscopic disease at one or both margins rather than to further extend the resection beyond the limits judged to be safe. This decision must be made at a time when the airway has already been divided, the tumor resected, and there is no option other than reconstruction. Microscopic tumor at the resection margin does not appear to impair healing, and long-term survival may still be possible, particu-

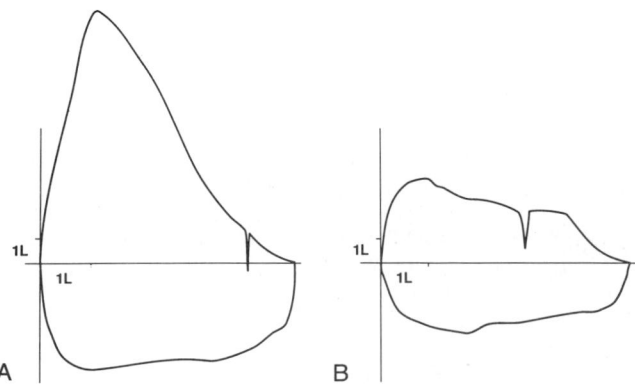

Figure 15-10. A flow-volume loop illustrating the typical flattening of both inspiratory and expiratory curves associated with a fixed obstruction in the trachea due to neoplasm. **(A)** Normal. **(B)** Tracheal obstruction.

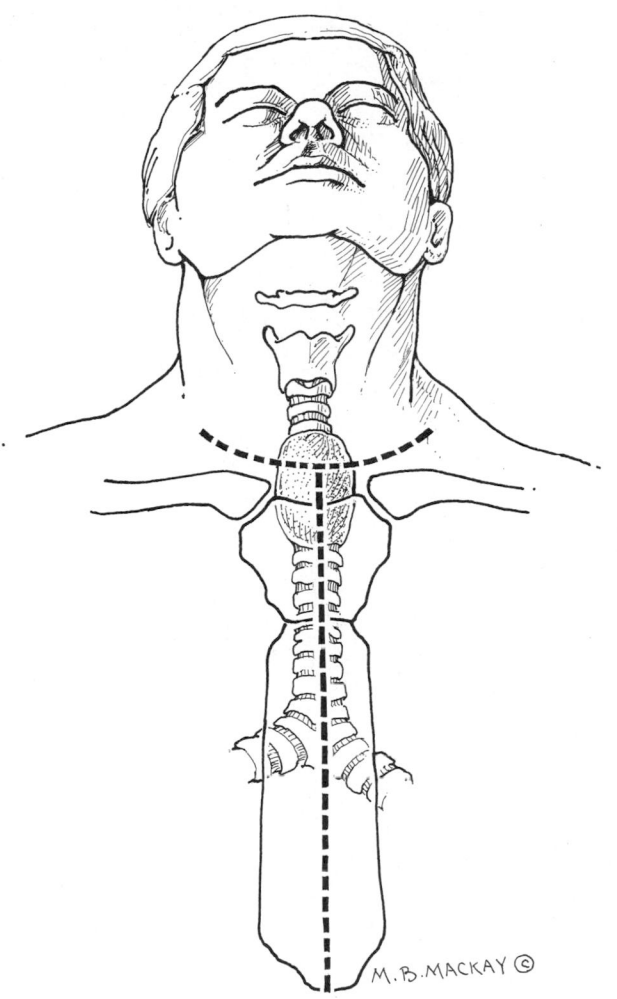

Figure 15-11. Diagram illustrating the incision most comonly used for tracheal tumors that extend to the mediastinal trachea: a generous collar incision and a full median sternotomy.

larly in patients with adenoid cystic tumors (Pearson, et al., 1984; Grillo and Mathisen, 1990).

There are technical problems that complicate resection at the upper and lower ends of the trachea. The various approaches to carinal resection are well described by Grillo (1982) and Grillo and Mathisen (1990). In selected cases neoplasms involving the subglottic airway may be managed by circumferential resection of the distal cricoid with preservation of the larynx and vocal function (Pearson, et al., 1986).

Results of Resection and Primary Reconstruction

Complications

Operative mortality reported in the four major publications dealing with resection and primary anastomosis for primary tracheal tumors is summarized in Table 15-2. The mortality reported in these four publications varies between 5 and 17 percent. Lethal complications included anastomotic dehiscence, pneumonia and respiratory failure, pulmonary embolism, and tracheal innominate artery fistula. Nonlethal complications included pneumonia, recurrent nerve palsy

Table 15-2. Primary Tracheal Tumors: Resection and Primary Anastomosis Operative Mortality

Author (Year)	No. Cases Resected	Operative Mortality No.	Operative Mortality %
Echapasse (1974)	75	13	17
Pearson, et al. (1984)	33	2	6
Perelman and Koroleva (1987)	75	11	15
Grillo and Mathisen (1990)	132	7	5

(usually transient), aspiration with deglutition following superior release procedures, and late stenosis at the anastomosis. These late strictures were the result of either dehiscence or ischemia at the anastomotic margins. Successful management included dilatation (Pearson, et al., 1984) and reoperation (Grillo and Mathisen, 1990).

Survival

Long-term survival is excellent in patients with adenoid cystic carcinoma. Perelman and Koroleva (1987), reporting on 56 patients with adenoid cystic tumors, recorded a 5-year survival of 66 percent and a 10-year survival of 56 percent. Grillo and Mathisen (1990), reporting on 41 patients with adenoid cystic tumors, recorded a 5-year survival of 75 percent. Echapasse (1974) reported 5 of 19 patients with adenoid cystic carcinoma (26 percent) alive and free of recurrence after 3 to 9 years. Pearson, et al. (1984) reported survival data on 21 patients with adenoid cystic carcinoma managed by resection. Of the 12 patients who underwent a complete resection, 9 were living 1 to 20 years after operation. At present, it is known that all nine (75 percent) survived beyond 5 years. The other 3 of the 12 patients died of unrelated disease, no patient succumbing to local recurrence. Of the other 9 of the 21 patients who had incomplete resections, 7 of the 9 died with recurrent disease between 2 and 9 years after operation. Among these 7 patients, 5 deaths were due to local recurrence, 1 to cerebral metastasis, and 1 to diffuse pulmonary metastasis. It is important to note that all the patients with adenoid cystic tumors reported by Grillo and Mathisen (1990) and by Pearson, et al. (1984) received adjuvant radiotherapy.

Survival following resection for squamous cell carcinoma is less favorable, and the reported experience is smaller. Perelman and Koroleva (1987) reported a 15 percent 5-year survival in 20 patients. Grillo and Mathisen (1990) reported 14 of 41 patients alive and free of disease between 3 and 15 years after resection. If it is assumed that these probably represent ultimate 5-year survivors, the projected survival rate is as high as 35 percent. Pearson, et al. (1984) reported four of nine patients living and clinically free of disease at 6, 16, 21, and 56 months after operation. Two patients died at 6 and 46 months, respectively, with recurrent cancer.

Miscellaneous Reports

A number of publications, reporting on small numbers of patients managed by resection, identify both modifications in management and the results of resection for unusual primary tracheal tumors.

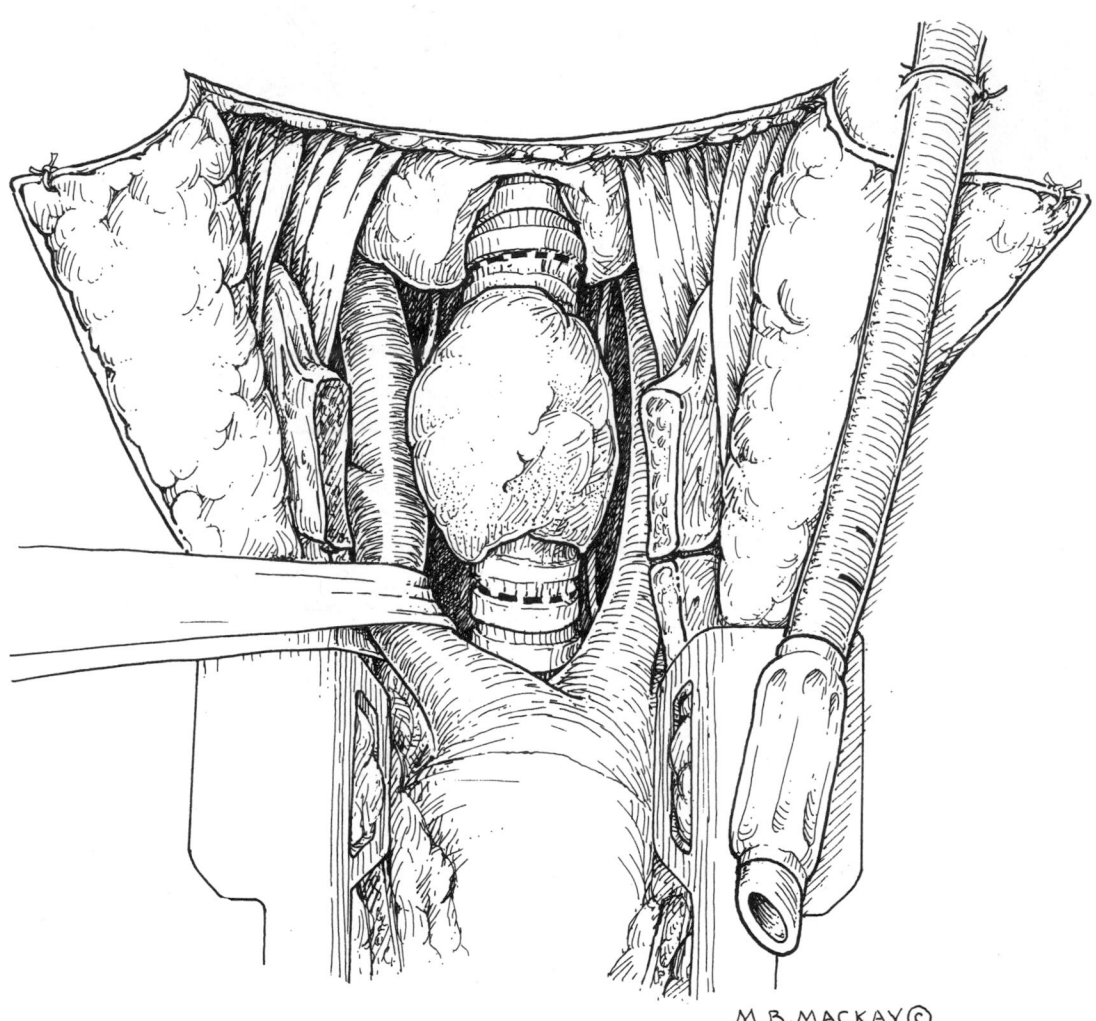

Figure 15-12. The intraoperative appearance following retraction of the sternal margins, reflection of the strap muscles above, and exposure of the trachea from the thyroid isthmus above to the top of the aortic arch below. In this patient the resection can be achieved with this exposure. The proposed resection margins are illustrated with dotted lines. For more distal resections, it may be necessary to open the pericardium vertically front and back, with lateral retraction of the ascending aorta to the patient's left, and the superior vena cava to the patient's right. This will expose the entire mediastinal trachea, the carina, and the origin of both main bronchi.

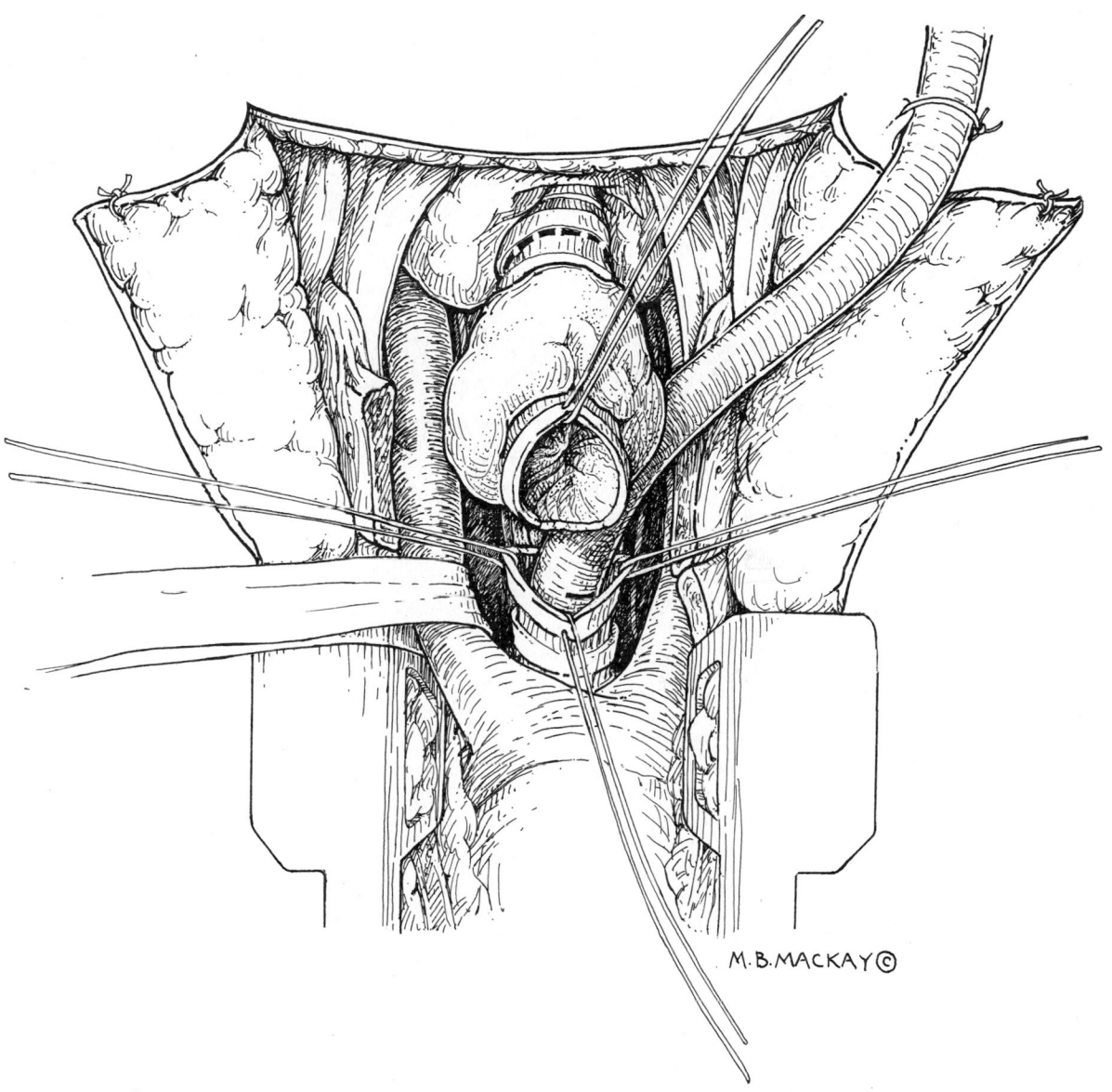

Figure 15-13. The airway has been divided 1 cm beyond the gross distal margin of the tumor. Three stay sutures are used to stabilize the distal tracheal stump, which has been intubated with an armored endotracheal tube for ventilation. At this point a circumferential ring is taken from the distal trachea and submitted to pathology for frozen section assessment.

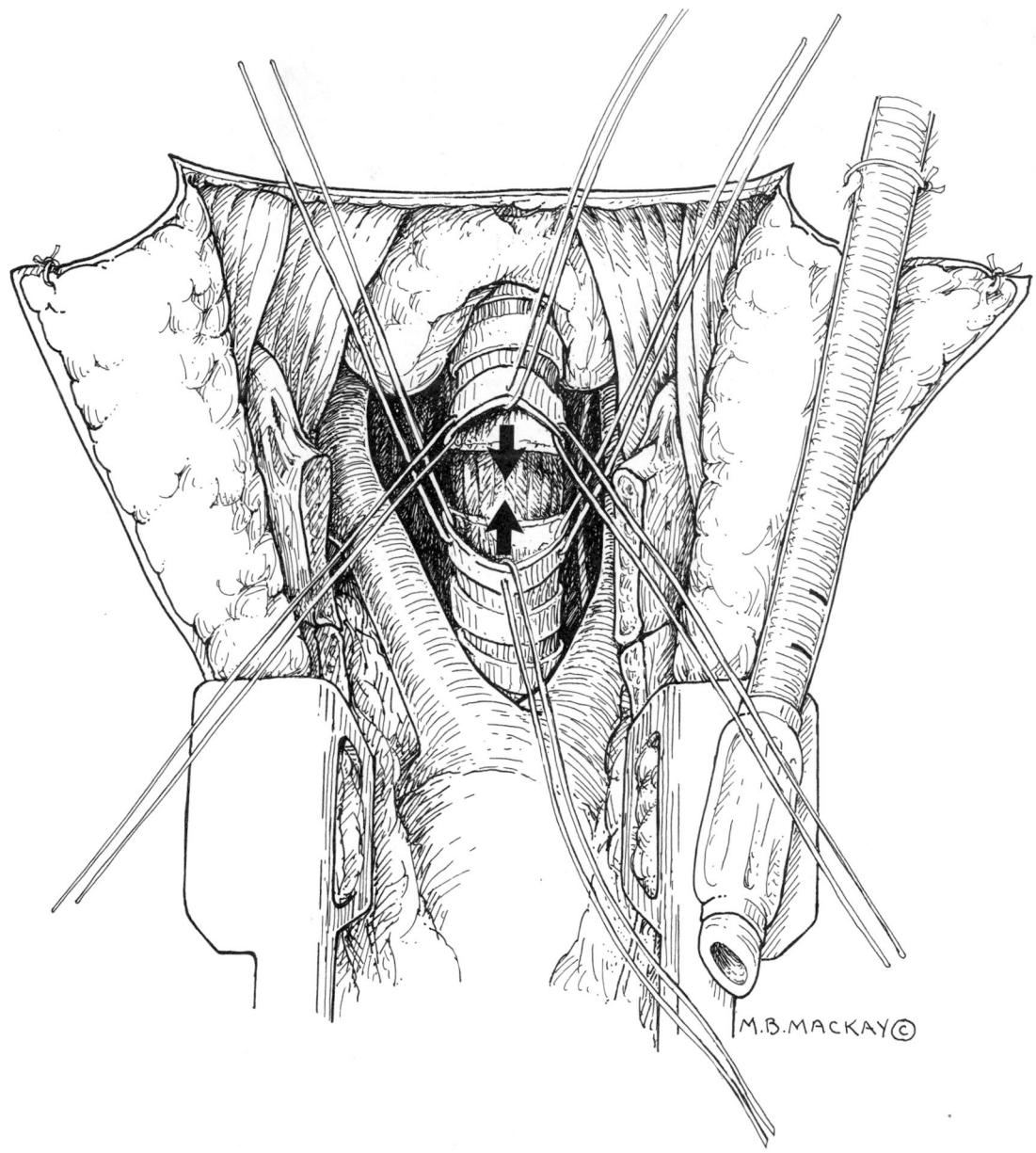

Figure 15-14.   The tumor has been resected, the divided tracheal ends evaluated by frozen section assessment, and each end stabilized with three stay sutures in preparation for primary anastomosis. Details of anastomotic technique will be found in Chapter 16.

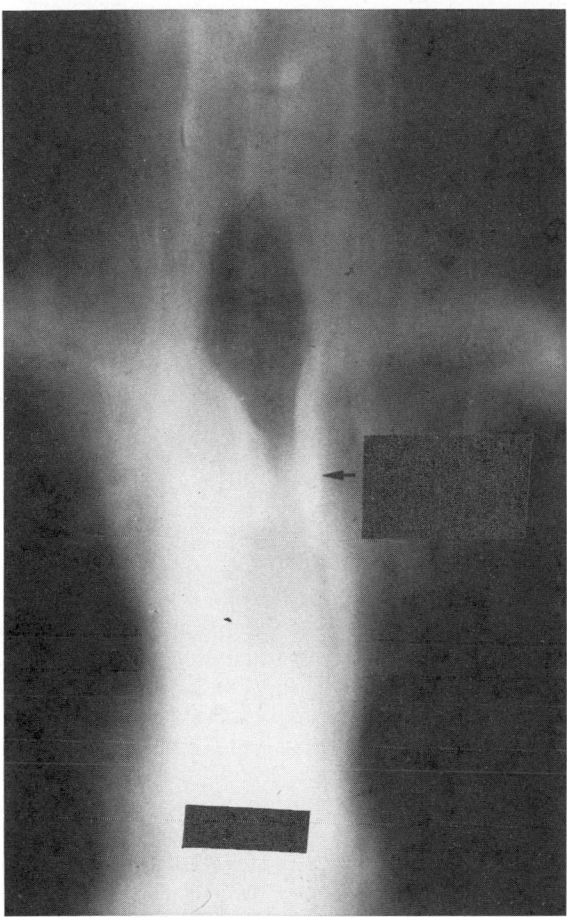

Figure 15-15. Contrast tracheogram illustrating a large, lobulated filling defect in the mediastinal trachea. This was due to an adenoid cystic carcinoma in a 58-year-old patient with a 1-year history of slowly progressing wheezing and dyspnea.

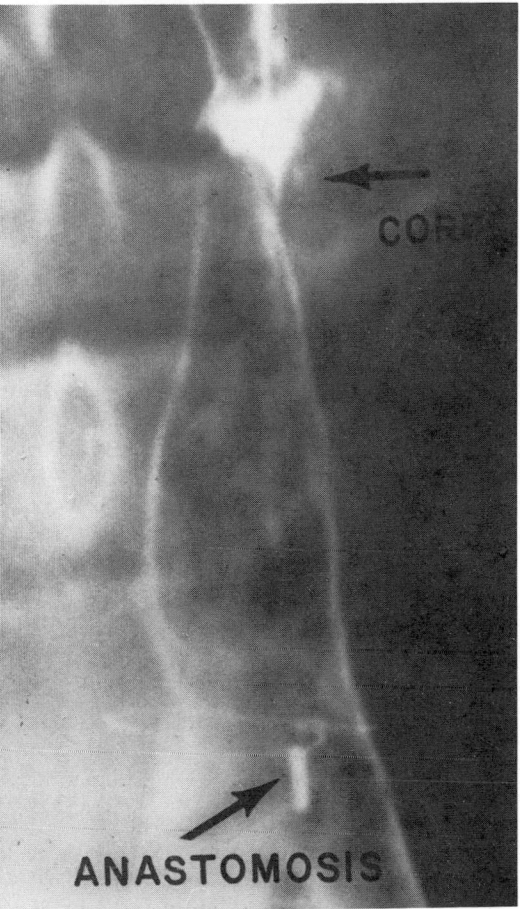

Figure 15-17. A contrast tracheogram in the same patient shown in Figures 15-15 and 15-16, obtained 1 year after resection. There is a widely patent airway, and a marked degree of tracheal shortening is evident.

Figure 15-16. The gross appearance of the freshly resected specimen. In this longitudinal cross-section of the airway, it is evident that 10 tracheal rings have been removed. Including separately submitted resection margins, this represented removal of more than half of the trachea, a length of 8.0 cm. A diffusely infiltrating adenoid cystic tumor is seen invading the full circumference of the resected segment.

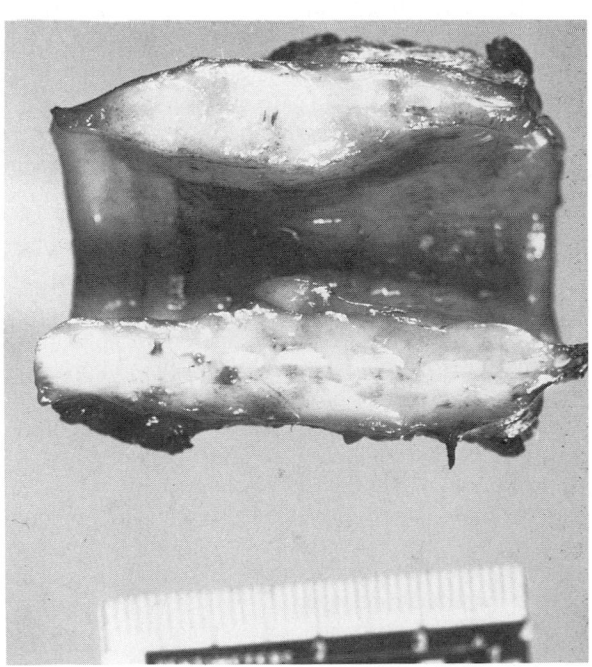

Heitmiller, et al. (1989) reported experience with resection for mucoepidermoid tumors of the tracheobronchial tree. There were 3 patients with primary tracheal tumors seen during a 41-year period at the Massachusetts General Hospital. These authors confirmed previous observations that mucoepidermoid carcinoma presents with differing grades of malignancy. All patients who underwent complete resection for well differentiated, low-grade tumors were long-term survivors. Patients with the highest grades of malignancy all died within 2 years of resection.

Daniel, et al. (1980) reported on a single case of granular cell myoblastoma of the trachea managed by resection; this was part of a literature review identifying management and outcome in 44 patients with this type of tumor. There were no instances of tumor recurrence in patients managed by surgical resection. In cases managed by bronchoscopic removal, however, the recurrence rate was 54 percent. Their obvious recommendation was that surgical resection is the treatment of choice.

Maeda, et al. (1981) reported on a patient with primary malignant lymphoma of the trachea, which was managed by segmental resection and primary anastomosis. No adjuvant therapy was given, and the patient remained well and free of tumor more than 5 years following operation.

Shankar, et al. (1990) reported on four patients in whom the primary tracheal malignancy was initially managed by resection using the neodymium-yttrium-aluminum-garnet (Nd-YAG) laser to open an obstructed airway. In these cases 2 months elapsed before elective tracheal resection was performed, presumably in order to avoid impaired healing, which might be secondary to thermal damage created by the laser. There were no anastomotic complications in these four patients, and good long-term results were reported.

Terz, et al. (1980) reported an unusual experience with 21 patients managed by tracheal resection and reconstruction of the airway with mediastinal tracheostomy. The tracheostomy tube was brought out through a bipedicled flap of soft tissue and skin. A mediastinal lymphadenectomy was performed in all 21 patients, and simultaneous neck dissections were done in 9. Of the 21 patients, 8 (38 percent) died during their hospital stay as a result of rupture of a major vessel, mediastinitis, or pulmonary insufficiency. Three patients (14 percent) were long-term survivors. The authors concluded their report with a statement of caution about the application of this approach.

Resection and Prosthetic Replacement

Belsey in 1950 was the first to describe prosthetic replacement of a circumferential tracheal defect in a patient. He fashioned a tubular prosthesis from autogenous fascia lata reinforced with a coil of stainless steel wire. During the next decade there were anecdotal reports of clinical reconstructions using a variety of solid tubes, which included such substances as glass, stainless steel, and tantalum. Both solid and porous materials were used. A porous substance used for tracheal replacement has the presumed advantage of becoming infiltrated with host granulation tissue, which may penetrate to the endoluminal surface and create a base for subsequent epithelization. Bucher (1951) was the first to report on the use of a porous stainless steel wire mesh prosthesis. In 1960 Usher reported laboratory studies with a porous prosthesis of "heavy-duty" Marlex mesh, and in 1963 Beall, et al. reported its application in two patients.

Pearson and colleagues initiated laboratory studies with the same Marlex prosthesis in 1962 and reported results along with a preliminary report of replacement in two patients (Pearson, et al., 1968). They subsequently reported experience in seven patients with a cylinder of heavy Marlex mesh for replacement of extensive circumferential defects (Pearson, et al., 1984). In three of the seven an excellent functional airway was obtained and functioned well for 2, 5, and 7.5 years, respectively. (One of these patients is shown in Figures 15-5 to 15-9.) There were, however, four deaths, all related to the replacement: dehiscence at the distal end caused one of these, and fatal hemorrhage from tracheoinnominate artery fistula caused the other three. These vascular fistulae all occurred within 3 weeks of operation.

The seventh patient in this series was operated on in 1972 for recurrent adenoid cystic carcinoma following a prior extended resection. At the second operation, the surgery required esophageal replacement, laryngectomy, and removal of the entire trachea to the level of the carina (Fig. 15-18). The airway was reconstructed with a cylinder of heavy Marlex mesh, which was anastomosed distally at the carina and sutured to the skin above as a terminal stoma in the suprasternal notch. The innominate artery was deliberately resected in this patient to avoid tracheo-innominate artery fistula. The patient, a 65-year-old man, lived for 7½ years with a satisfactory airway and subsequently died of unrelated disease at age 72.

Neville was the first to report on the clinical use of a solid silicone rubber tube for tracheal replacement (Neville, 1968). Neville and colleagues subsequently accumulated a significant experience and reported on 51 patients managed by reconstruction with a tube of solid, silicone rubber (Neville, et al., 1972). A straight prosthesis was used for tracheal replacement in 37 patients (29 with postintubation strictures and 8 with neoplasms), and a bifurcation stent was used for carinal replacement in 14 patients, all with neoplastic disease. A Dacron-reinforced sewing ring was devised at each end of the prosthesis to secure better fixation at the proximal and distal margins. Cardiopulmonary bypass was recommended and was used in a majority of these cases.

It was observed that the silicone replacement was never intimately incorporated into the host tissues but remained in an encapsulated pocket of connective tissue, similar to the envelope that surrounds a silicone breast implant. Granulation tissue developed unpredictably at the interface between the native trachea or bronchus and the prosthesis. The inner surface never became epithelialized. Complications included obstruction due to granulation tissue, dehiscence requiring reoperation, erosion of the innominate artery, and retention of secretions. It is impossible to precisely quantitate the incidence of complications in this report. It is also clear that a majority of the 29 patients with postintubation strictures could have been managed by circumferential resection and primary anastomosis; it is exceptional for postintubation in-

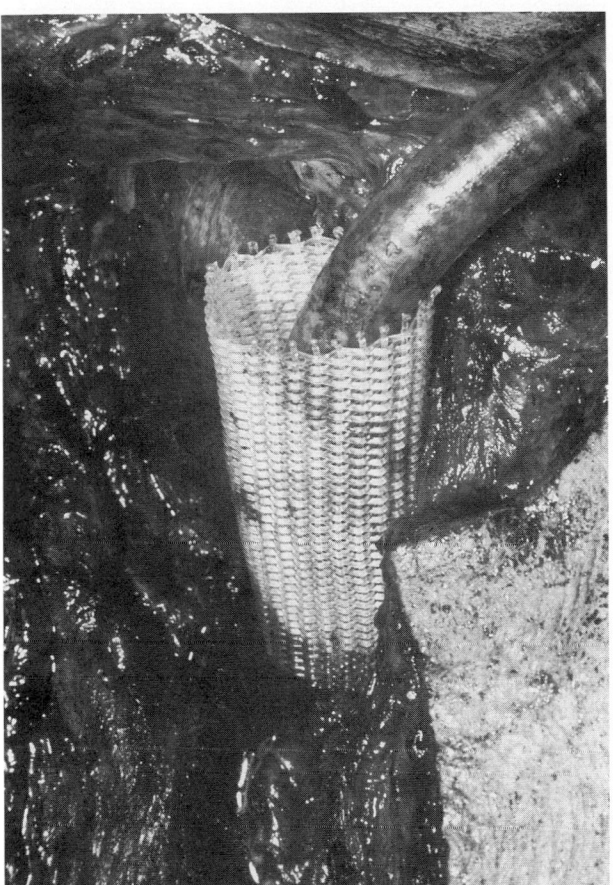

Figure 15-18. Intraoperative photograph illustrating replacement of the entire remaining upper airway with a cylindrical prosthesis of heavy Marlex mesh. At operation, the larynx and entire trachea were removed through a cervical incision, median sternotomy, and laparotomy, and the mediastinal trachea was replaced with the Marlex prosthesis. The distal end has been sutured to the main carina and the upper end intubated for intraoperative ventilation. The upper end was brought out as a terminal stoma through the skin of the suprasternal notch. The overlying innominate artery was resected, and the involved thoracic esophagus was replaced with stomach.

juries to involve an extent of airway that precludes primary reconstruction. Neville and associates are the only surgeons to have recommended widespread application of cardiopulmonary bypass for tracheal replacement surgery.

Subsequent to the report of Neville et al. (1972), Toomes, et al. (1985) published experience with nine patients who were operated on between 1979 and 1984 with use of the Neville prosthesis. Eight of these nine patients were operated on for locally advanced malignancy and the remaining patient had relapsing polychondritis. Resection and reconstruction required the use of a straight Neville prosthesis in five cases and a bifurcation prosthesis in four. Circumferential segments between 6 and 9 cm in length were resected, and resections of this extent may indeed require prosthetic replacement. None of the nine patients required cardiopulmonary bypass for the procedure. Five of these patients died of complications

of the prosthesis and operation: two of cardiorespiratory insufficiency, two of tracheoinnominate artery erosion (15 days and 10 months postsurgery, respectively), and one of dehiscence. Toomes, et al. concluded that the morbidity and mortality with this method of tracheal replacement were unacceptable.

We emphasize that the need for prosthetic reconstruction of the airway appears very limited at present. With use of currently available techniques, the majority of resectable lesions can be reconstructed by primary anastomosis with autologous tissues. In those rare cases in which prosthetic replacement is considered, one of us (F.G.P.) would recommend using a porous material and would select heavy-duty Marlex mesh as the best available. The prosthesis should be enveloped with a pedicle graft of omentum. Since soft tissue interposition does not provide dependable protection to the innominate artery, resection of the overlying segment of the innominate artery at the time of operation is recommended. If a prosthesis is used, the shortest possible length of cylinder should be employed. If, for example, 80 percent of the trachea is resected, it is not necessary to use a prosthesis representing the full length of the missing segment. By employing known techniques of mobilization, the ends of the airway can be approximated, and a prosthesis that may be less than half the length of the normal airway can be inserted without anastomotic tension. The shorter the prosthesis, the less formidable the problem of obtaining endoluminal epithelial cover and avoiding late stenosis.

Endoscopic Clearance

Endoscopic procedures are obviously for palliation only. As with any form of upper airways obstruction, it may be possible to secure an improved and safer airway by using a rigid bronchoscope and removing the endoluminal neoplasm with biopsy forceps, suction, and/or electrocoagulation. Laser resection has become increasingly popular since the mid-1980s, and is often combined with other bronchoscopic techniques. Techniques of laser bronchoscopy are described in Chapter 12.

Internal Stents

Some form of internal stent may be used to secure a patent airway in patients with otherwise unmanageable neoplasms. Such therapy is obviously palliative. The options include silicone tubes of various configuration (T, Y, and TY tubes) and internal metal mesh supports such as the Gianturco and Wall stents. A detailed description of the indications and techniques for the employment of tracheobronchial stents is provided in Chapter 12, in which it is concluded that tracheobronchial stents offer excellent palliation, the preference being for silicone cannulas, since they are nonreactive, well tolerated, and easily removed. Although some features of the wire stents appear advantageous (no external limb, wider diameters), incorporation of these stents into the airway may be difficult to reverse and is contraindicated in patients with neoplasms, since the tumor may grow through the interstices of the mesh.

COMMENTS AND CONTROVERSIES

Most primary neoplasms of the trachea are malignant, and adenoid cystic carcinoma and squamous cell carcinoma are by far the most common histologic types.

Using currently available techniques of mobilization and "release," the surgeon can safely resect long circumferential segments and achieve primary reconstruction without the need for a prosthesis in the majority of operable patients. As experience with carinal resection improves, the innovations in techniques of reconstruction have advanced the capability to manage tumors at this level. Cervical collar incision, with a full median sternotomy, is our incision of choice in most patients requiring a concomitant carinal resection for a primary tracheal tumor.

Worthwhile survival can be obtained in patients with adenoid cystic carcinoma, squamous cell carcinoma, and the rarer sarcomas of the trachea as long as a complete and potentially curative resection is done. In the majority of patients with adenoid cystic tumors, even an incomplete resection may be compatible with long periods of symptom-free palliation. Most adenoid cystic carcinomas are radiosensitive, and adjuvant radiation is recommended in all resectable tumors of this cell type. Radical radiation therapy is the treatment of choice in patients with unresectable adenoid cystic carcinoma and often results in dramatic regression of the tumor and palliation, which may endure for years. Pulmonary metastasis occur in about one-third of patients with adenoid cystic carcinoma. When first seen, the metastases are often asymptomatic, progress slowly, and may remain symptom-free for many years. In selected patients, therefore, the presence of asymptomatic, synchronous pulmonary metastases is not necessarily a contraindication to resection of an obstructing primary adenoid cystic carcinoma.

Safe and reliable methods of prosthetic replacement remain elusive. The experience of one of us (F.G.P.) with heavy-duty Marlex mesh was unsatisfactory owing to an unacceptable operative mortality. The relatively favorable clinical experience reported by Neville and associates with a solid, silicone rubber prosthesis has not been reproduced by others. We emphasize again that the need for prosthetic reconstruction is very limited. By using currently available techniques, the majority of resectable lesions can be reconstructed by primary anastomosis with autologous tissue.

Although there is some experimental work evaluating homotransplantation of the larynx and trachea, no clinical success has been reported up to now.

F.G.P.
P.C.
S.K.

KEY REFERENCES

Grillo HC, Mathisen DJ: Primary tracheal tumors: treatment and results. Ann Thorac Surg 49:69, 1990

This is a detailed review and analysis of the largest reported series of primary tracheal tumors, in which 132 cases were managed by resection, with an operative mortality of 5 percent.

Pearson FG, Todd TRJ, Cooper JD: Experience with primary neo-plasms of the trachea and carina. J Thorac Cardiovasc Surg 88:511, 1984

This report includes an analysis of the unique pathology and natural history of 28 patients with adenoid cystic carcinoma. A description of the transpericardial approach to the mediastinal trachea and carina is provided.

REFERENCES

Barak E: Malignant tumors of the trachea. Ann R Coll Surg Engl 66:27, 1984

Barclay RS, McSwan N, Welsh TM: Tracheal reconstruction without the use of grafts. Thorax 12:177, 1957

Beall AC Jr, Harrington OB, Greenberg SD et al.: Circumferential replacement of thoracic trachea with Marlex mesh. JAMA 183:1082, 1963

Belsey R: Resection and reconstruction of the intrathoracic trachea. Br J Surg 38:200, 1950

Briselli M, Mark EJ, Grillo HC: Tracheal carcinoids. Cancer 42:2870, 1978

Bucher RM, Burnett WE, Rosemond GP: Experimental reconstruction of tracheal and bronchial defects with stainless steel wire mesh. J Thoracic Surg 21:572, 1951

Daniel TM, Smith RH, Faunce HF, Sylves VM: Transbronchoscopic versus surgical resection of tracheobronchial granular cell myoblastomas. Suggested approach based on follow up of all treated cases. J Thorac Cardiovasc Surg 80:898, 1980

Echapasse H: Les tumeurs trachéales primitives. Traitement chirurgical. Rev Fr Mal Respir 2:425, 1974

Fredberg JJ, Wohl MEB, Glass GM, Dorkin HL: Airway area by acoustic reflections measured at the mouth. J Appl Physiol 48:749, 1980

Gelb AF, Tashkin DP, Epstein JD et al.: Diagnosis and Nd-YAG laser treatment of unsuspected malignant tracheal obstruction. Chest 94:767, 1988

Goepfert H, Sessions RB, Gutterman JV et al.: Leukocyte interferon in patients with juvenile laryngeal papillomatosis. Ann Otol Rhinol Laryngol 91:431, 1982

Grillo HC: The trachea. p. 668. In Shields TW (ed): General Thoracic Surgery. Lea & Febiger, Philadelphia, 1989

Grillo HC: Carinal reconstruction. Ann Thorac Surg 34:356, 1982

Grillo HC: Tracheal tumors: surgical management. Ann Thorac Surg 26:112, 1978

Grillo HC, Dignan EF, Miura T: Extensive resection and reconstruction of mediastinal trachea without prosthesis or graft: an anatomical study in man. J Thorac Cardiovasc Surg 48:741, 1964

Hadju SI, Huvos AG, Goodner JT et al.: Carcinoma of the trachea: clinicopathologic study of 41 cases. Cancer 25:1448, 1970

Heitmiller RF, Mathieson DJ, Ferry JA et al.: Mucoepidermoid lung tumors. Ann Thorac Surg 47:394, 1989

Houston HE, Payne WS, Harrison EG Jr, Olsen, AM: Primary cancers of the trachea. Arch Surg 99(2):132, 1969

Kairalla RA, Carvalho CRR, Parada AA et al.: Solitary plasmacytoma of the trachea by loop resection and laser therapy. Thorax 43:1011, 1988

Maeda M, Kotake Y, Monden Y et al.: Primary malignant lymphoma of the trachea. Report of a case successfully treated by primary end-to-end anastomosis after circumferential resection of the trachea. J Thorac Cardiovasc Surg 81:835, 1981

Morency G, Chalaoui J, Samson L, Sylvestre J: Malignant neoplasms of the trachea. J Can Assoc Radiol 40:198, 1989

Naidich DP: CT/MR correlation in the evaluation of tracheobronchial neoplasia. Radiol Clin North Am 28:555, 1990

Neis PR, McMahon MF, Norris CW: Cartilaginous tumors of the trachea and larynx. Ann Otol Laryngol 98:31, 1989

Neville WE: Prosthetic replacement of the trachea. p. 138. In Grillo HC, EH (eds): International Trends in General Thoracic Surgery. Vol. 2. WB Saunders, Philadelphia, 1987

Neville WE: Reconstruction of the trachea and both stem bronchi with Neville prosthesis. Int Surg 67:229, 1982

Neville WE, Hamouda F, Andersen J, Dwan FM: Replacement of the intrathoracic trachea and both stem bronchi with a molded Silastic prosthesis. J Thorac Cardiovasc Surg 63:569, 1972

Pearson FG, Brito Flomeno LT, Cooper JD: Experience with partial cricoid resection and thyrotracheal anastomosis. Ann Otol Rhinol Laryngol 95:582, 1986

Pearson FG, Cooper JD, Nelems JM, Van Nostrand AWP: Primary tracheal anastomosis safer resection of the cricoid cartilage with preservation of recurrent laryngeal nerves. J Thorac Cardiovasc Surg 70:806, 1975

Pearson FG, Henderson RD, Gross E et al.: The reconstruction of circumferential tracheal defects with a porous prosthesis: an experimental and clinical study using heavy Marlex mesh. J Thorac Cardiovasc Surg 55:605, 1968

Pearson FG, Thompson DW, Weissberg D et al.: Adenoid cystic carcinoma of the trachea. Ann Thorac Surg 18:16, 1974

Perelman MI, Koroleva NS: Primary tumors of the trachea. p. 91. In Grillo HC EH, (eds) International Trends in General Thoracic Surgery. Vol. 2. WB Saunders, Philadelphia, 1987

Shankar S, George PJ, Hetzel MR, Goldstraw P: Elective resection of tumors of the trachea and main carina after endoscopic laser therapy. Thorax 45:493, 1990

Terz JJ, Wagman LD, King RE et al.: Results of extended resection of tumors involving the cervical part of the trachea. Surg Gynecol Obstet 151:491, 1980

Toomes H, Mickisch G, Bogt-Moykopf I: Experiences with prosthetic reconstruction of the trachea and bifurcation. Thorax 40:32, 1985

Usher FC, Ochsner JL: Marlex mesh: a new polyethylene mesh for replacing tissue defects. Surg Forum 10:319, 1960

Xu L-T, Sun Z-F, Li Z-J et al.: Clinical and pathological characteristics in patients with tracheobronchial tumor. Report of 50 patients. Ann Thorac Surg 43:276, 1987

Secondary Tumors

Hermes C. Grillo
Douglas J. Mathisen

DEFINITION

Secondary tumors most often involve the trachea or carina by direct invasion from the adjacent organ of origin—larynx, thyroid, lung or esophagus. The two categories of secondary tumors involving trachea and carina that are most appropriately treated surgically are carcinoma of the thyroid and bronchogenic carcinoma.

This chapter section is divided into three parts: (1) thyroid cancer invading the airway; (2) bronchogenic carcinoma involving the carina; and (3) other secondary tumors involving the airway.

THYROID CANCER

HISTORICAL NOTE

Resection of the larynx and upper trachea was early performed for both well and poorly differentiated invasive carcinoma of the thyroid (Frazell and Foote, 1958; Hendrick, 1963), sometimes with surprisingly long-term palliation or apparent cure. Patients are few in number who have well-differentiated carcinoma involving the trachea or adjacent larynx in limited enough fashion to be resectable with the involved airway and yet permit primary reconstruction. The techniques of airway reconstruction that have evolved in the last 30 years have been applied only slowly to these cases. Ishihara and associates (1978) reported on 11 such patients. In the Western Hemisphere, Grillo reported an initial case in 1965 and with Zannini (1986) described 19 patients who underwent resection for papillary or mixed papillary and follicular carcinoma of the thyroid and 3 who underwent this surgery for undifferentiated carcinoma. In 16, primary reconstruction was performed, and for the other 6 therapy was en bloc cervicomediastinal resection with end tracheostomy. Of the 16 having airway reconstruction, 15 had good surgical results with speech preservation. Eight patients were alive without disease at up to 9 years, and only two developed airway recurrence. By 1991 Ishihara had performed 60 resections for thyroid cancer invading the airway. Maeda, et al. (1989) recorded 151 patients in Japan with tracheoplasty for thyroid cancer (26.7 percent of all tracheoplasties in Japan). Grillo, et al. (1992) described 34 patients at Massachusetts General Hospital who underwent resection for thyroid cancer invading the airway out of 52 who presented with such involvement.

HISTORICAL READINGS

Grillo HC, Zannini P: Resectional management of airway invasion by thyroid carcinoma. Ann Thorac Surg 42:287, 1986
Ishihara T, Kikuchi K, Ikeda T et al.: Resection of thyroid carcinoma infiltrating the trachea. Thorax 33:378, 1978

BASIC SCIENCE

Well-differentiated thyroid carcinoma usually runs an indolent course, frequently with long-term survival (Beahrs, et al., 1981). Airway invasion, however, is directly responsible for many late deaths due to thyroid cancer and is a source of profound morbidity due to airway hemorrhage and suffocation (Silliphant, et al., 1964). Thyroid cancer that invades the airway early usually does so by direct involvement of the airway closest to the tumor; it occurs in 1 to 6.5 percent of patients (Lawson, et al., 1977). Tsumori, et al. (1985) reported that 50 percent of papillary and follicular carcinomas that invaded the airway showed poor differentiation, as compared with 11.4 percent of noninvasive thyroid cancers of the same histology. Invasion also tends to be seen in older patients, in whom papillary and follicular thyroid cancer are more aggressive, although the spectrum is broad. Nomori, et al. (1990) found that the nuclear area of tumor cells was significantly greater in cases with tracheal invasion than in those without. Both Tsumori, et al. and Nomori, et al. noted that the tumors had sometimes become less well differentiated than originally.

The prognosis of thyroid cancers invading the airway appears to correlate with the site and depth of invasion (Tsumori, et al., 1987). Shin, Mark, Suen, and Grillo (1993) classified papillary thyroid cancer invading the trachea as follows: stage 0, tumor confined to the thyroid gland; stage I, extension through the capsule to abut perichondrium but without cartilaginous erosion or intercartilaginous invasion; stage II,

destruction of cartilage or intercartilaginous invasion; stage III, extension into lamina propria of tracheal mucosa; stage IV, extension through tracheal mucosa. Clinical results correlated well with these stages, in general confirming the observations of Tsumori et al. (1987).

Because of the location of the thyroid gland, the subglottic larynx may also be invaded. The corresponding recurrent laryngeal nerve is often paralyzed, paretic, or encircled by tumor. Adjacent esophagus or cricopharyngeus may be involved. The tumor may penetrate into any depth of the airway. Recurrent tumors are too often permitted to grow to large sizes even though they frequently respond little to radioactive iodine therapy (RaI) or external radiotherapy. Poorly differentiated tumors in their initial presentation may involve the larynx to such a degree that its salvage is not possible. Invasion may include the pharynx and esophagus as well.

DIAGNOSIS

The patient with differentiated thyroid carcinoma involving the airway may present with classical signs of airway involvement, mainly hemoptysis and sometimes dyspnea on exertion or wheezing. More often airway involvement is not symptomatic, since the tumor has not yet penetrated the mucous membrane or projected any distance into the lumen. A firm mass that is not freely movable over the airway may be palpable. All too often tracheal and laryngeal involvement are detected only at thyroidectomy. Under these circumstances the thyroid surgeon, often unskilled in techniques of airway resection and reconstruction, will "shave off" the tumor from the airway wall.

In addition to the usual diagnostic approach to thyroid cancer (thyroid function studies, thyroid scan, and needle biopsy) flexible bronchoscopy is advisable in *every* patient. CT scanning should include the chest to search for pulmonary metastases. MRI is also useful in defining these lesions. The neck should be imaged by means of thin-section CT scans, which are most likely to identify involvement of the tracheal wall or intrusion into the lumen. Linear radiographic studies of the trachea, including filtered views and crisp tomography, are of great use in determining the extent of gross involvement of the larynx and trachea and also the relative proportion of uninvolved airway, which is important to the surgeon considering resection and reconstruction (Fig. 15-19). Fluoroscopy of the larynx adds information about function of the vocal cords to that obtained by direct laryngoscopy. A barium swallow may define the bulk of the tumor and detect involvement of the proximal esophagus.

In some cases considered for cervical exenteration, arch angiography may detect involvement of mediastinal vessels and may be useful to study cerebral blood supply in the event that mediastinal tracheotomy should become necessary and require prophylactic division of the brachiocephalic artery. Bone scan is performed to search for skeletal metastases.

MANAGEMENT

Principles

The purposes of resection of thyroid cancer invading the airway are (1) to attempt to achieve cure by accomplishing complete resection of the tumor; (2) to provide prolonged

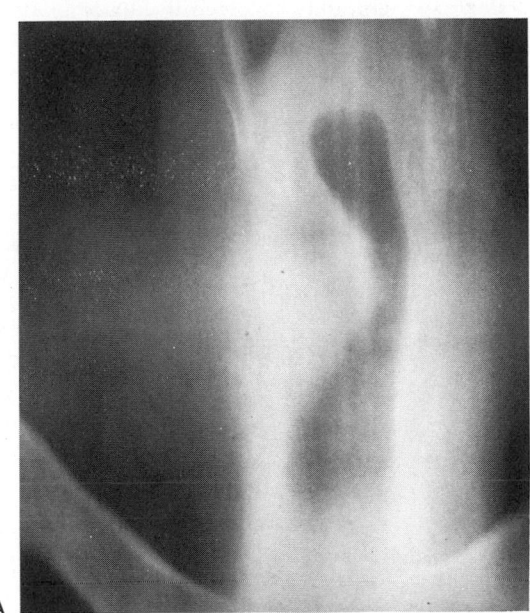
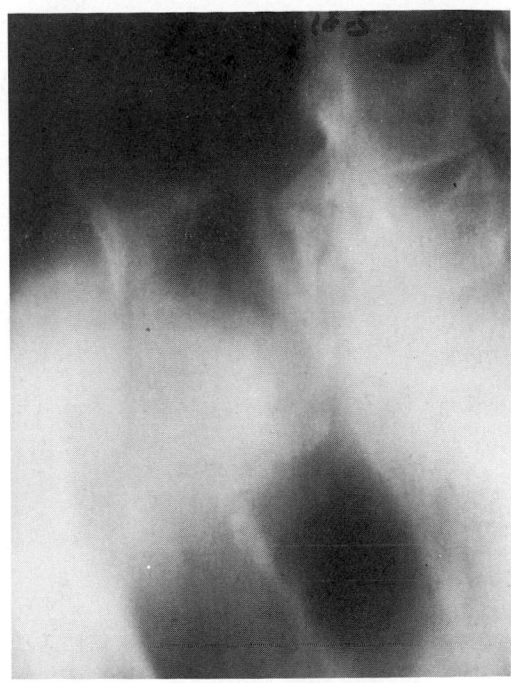

Figure 15-19. Tomograms of mixed papillary and follicular carcinoma invading the subglottic larynx and upper trachea. **(A)** Anterior view: tumor is seen protruding on the right invading the subglottic larynx just below the conus elasticus. The alae of the thyroid cartilage may be seen just above the tumor mass on the right. **(B)** Lateral view: the calcified thyroid cartilage is seen just above the mass. (From Grillo HC, Zannini P: Resectional management of airway invasion by thyroid carcinoma. Ann Thorac Surg 42:287, 1986, with permission.)

palliation by relief or prevention of airway obstruction in patients with slowly progressive neoplasms; and (3) to prevent death by asphyxiation or hemorrhage. Resection and reconstruction of involved airway as part of the complete local excision of thyroid cancer, particularly as an initial procedure, accomplishes the primary goals of conventional thyroid cancer surgery. It does not represent a radical extension of surgery for thyroid cancer. Where resection and reconstruction of the airway can effect complete removal of the disease, it is illogical simply to shave off a cancer, leaving the local tumor to recur in the airway. This is done all too frequently, however, because a surgeon performing thyroidectomy may not be competent to perform airway surgery. Hence, it is important to attempt to diagnose such involvement in advance of surgical exploration in order to refer the patient for the needed care. The alternative is to refer a patient immediately after discovery of such involvement in the operating theater for resection of the airway.

Follow-up results suggest strongly that patients in whom either of these alternatives has been followed are the two groups in whom the best long-term results and even cure may be expected (Grillo, et al., 1992). Late removal of recurrent tumor obstructing the airway, occurring sometimes years after the initial tumor has been shaved off the trachea, is effective palliation but not often curative. Remote metastases have often occurred by this time. The finding of pulmonary metastases from slowly progressive differentiated carcinoma of the thyroid is not an absolute contraindication to therapy of the airway disease, however. Almost uniformly, localized involvement of the airway by carcinoma of the thyroid in-

volves only one recurrent laryngeal nerve. Thus, a still functional larynx will be preserved by conserving the nerve on the opposite side.

Radical techniques of cervical or cervicomediastinal exenteration, on the other hand, should be applied very selectively. Such radical technique appears justifiable when the tumor is localized but involves larynx too extensively for salvage, and sometimes pharynx and esophagus as well. This occurs more commonly with aggressive, poorly differentiated carcinoma. A second situation justifying radical technique is massive recurrence of differentiated carcinoma, often over years and usually after unsuccessful treatment with RaI and external radiotherapy. Such patients may be wretched, with poorly functioning tracheostomies accompanied by local bleeding, loss of voice, and inability to swallow food or even saliva. Cervical pain further aggravates their condition. In such patients radical excision may offer palliation even if pulmonary metastases are present.

Operative Technique

Resection and Reconstruction

Careful endoscopic examination uses a rigid instrument with a Storz-Hopkins magnifying telescope rather than a flexible bronchoscope, in order to obtain precise information about the gross extent of involvement proximally and distally. Measurements are made of the extent of grossly uninvolved trachea that will be available for reconstruction. The same general guiding principles of extent of resection that apply in surgery for primary tracheal tumors (Grillo and Mathisen,

1990) also apply here. Since resection will often extend proximally to include a portion of the subglottic larynx on one side, the distal trachea will have to be divided in an irregular, bayonet-like pattern in order to slide the two ends of the airway together for reconstruction (Grillo and Zannini, 1986). This requires a longer resection than simply the distance from the inferior border of the cricoid cartilage to a point just distal to the tumor. This length must be considered in planning the reconstruction.

Approach is almost uniformly through a low collar incision, elevating flaps well up onto the larynx as necessary and extending to the sternal notch below. If the tumor is recurrent or invasive, strap muscles or residual tissue overlying the tumor are excised en bloc. The limits of tumor are defined by dissection before irrevocable steps are taken. This includes superior and inferior definition of the extent of tumor, lateral definition of the carotid arteries and internal jugular veins, and later in the dissection the extent, if any, of involvement of the upper esophagus and cricopharyngeus. Since such involvement is proximal, at the level where the thyroid gland is most closely adjacent to the trachea, upper sternal division has not been required.

There are three principal patterns by which the trachea has been resected for invasive differentiated thyroid carcinoma (Grillo and Zannini, 1986) (Fig. 15-20). The first consists of sleeve resection, performed when the trachea alone is involved. The superior margin is usually at the inferior border of the cricoid cartilage. In a second situation, in which the tumor involves the cricoid on one side, the line of proximal division may be beveled to transect the larynx above the

point of involvement, including part of the cricoid cartilage on one side. Since the recurrent laryngeal nerve on that side is almost uniformly involved by tumor in such a case, no additional avoidable functional loss is incurred by deliberate division of the paralyzed nerve as it enters the larynx posteriorly on that side.

More complicated is the third situation, in which the tumor creeps up higher into the larynx on one side, so that a straight beveled line of resection is not feasible (Fig. 15-21). In such a case we prefer to commence division beneath the cricoid cartilage on the uninvolved side and angle the incision upward anteriorly, staying away from the gross border of the tumor; we then curve the incision to divide the larynx beneath the paralyzed vocal cord, carrying it down in a curve to leave a margin of uninvolved tissue around tumor, and finally dropping vertically or obliquely in the posterior part of the laryngeal wall. Each resection is necessarily individualized (Fig. 15-22). Frozen sections are obtained at the points nearest the tumor, preferably sampled from tissue that remains in the patient rather than from the resected specimen. This is definitive for the surgeon and pathologist, eliminating any question about location of cancer cells. If tumor is still present, the surgeon may take additional tissue, remembering, however, that reconstruction is the goal. The trachea distal to the tumor is trimmed to fit the irregular lateral defect that has been created in the larynx.

Microscopically positive margins may have to be accepted occasionally if this is necessary to salvage a functional larynx. With well-differentiated carcinoma, often characterized by slow clinical progression, this seems preferable to laryngec-

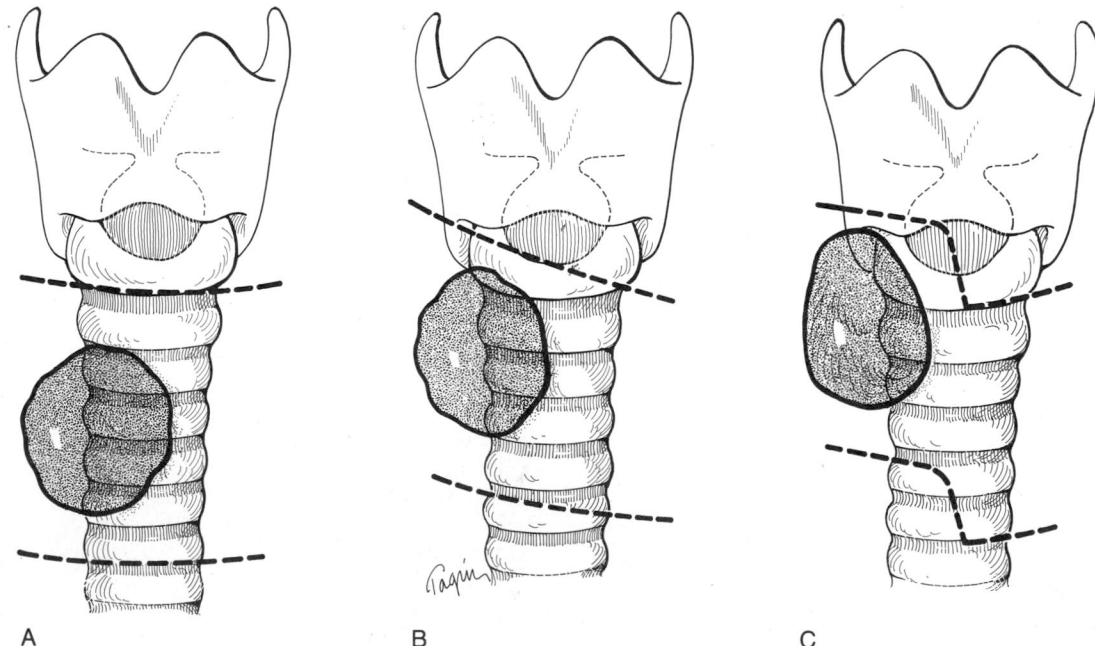

A   B   C

Figure 15-20. Types of resection of upper airway for thyroid carcinoma. **(A)** Sleeve resection of trachea. **(B)** A portion of the lower cricoid is beveled to remove an additional margin above the tumor. The recurrent laryngeal nerve may or may not be involved in such a case. **(C)** Tailored line of resection to obtain a margin around the tumor with deeper and more proximal invasion of the cricoid cartilage. The recurrent laryngeal nerve in such a case is almost uniformly paralyzed prior to resection. (From Grillo HC, Zannini P: Resectional management of airway invasion by thyroid carcinoma. Ann Thorac Surg 42:287, 1986, with permission.)

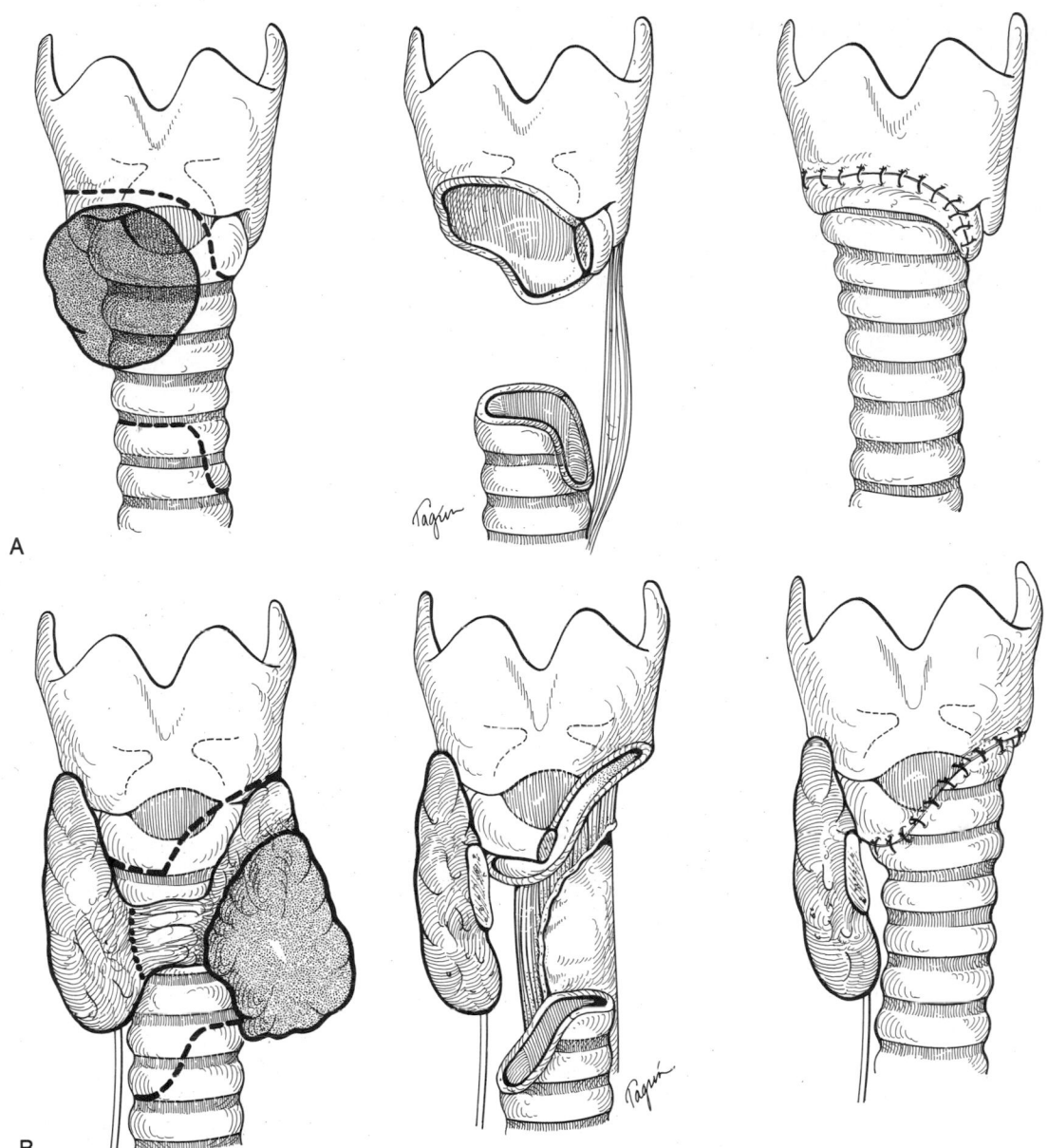

Figure 15-21. Examples of complex resections. **(A)** Resection of mixed papillary and follicular carcinoma for recurrence 2 years after total thyroidectomy. The left recurrent laryngeal nerve was preserved anatomically and functionally. **(B)** Mixed papillary and follicular carcinoma, not previously treated, managed by resection of part of the larynx, trachea, and anterolateral muscular wall of the esophagus. (From Grillo HC, Zannini P: Resectional management of airway invasion by thyroid carcinoma. Ann Thorac Surg 42:287, 1986, with permission.)

tomy. External radiation is administered after healing, provided that prohibitive doses have not been given in the past. It appears likely that laryngectomy could be performed later should tumor recur locally in the larynx. Thus far, this has not occurred.

Reconstruction is accomplished with 4–0 Vicryl sutures, all sutures being placed prior to tying any of them (Grillo, 1988). Lateral traction sutures are employed to take tension off the anastomosis while it is being accomplished. Ventilation is managed across the operative field in the usual manner in methodical and unhurried fashion. With very extensive resection suprahyoid laryngeal release (Montgomery, 1974)

may be employed, although this has rarely been necessary in these cases. Even with the known occurrence of microscopic foci of papillary carcinoma elsewhere in an involved gland, we have not considered it necessary to remove the opposite lobe of thyroid in all cases; a second clinically significant cancer on the opposite side is rare. This conservative approach further ensures that damage will not be done to the opposite and uninvolved recurrent laryngeal nerve. Total thyroidectomy is performed if indicated.

If reconstruction is particularly high or if the laryngeal airway seems to be tenuous because of edema, protective tracheostomy is advised. The anastomosis is covered with

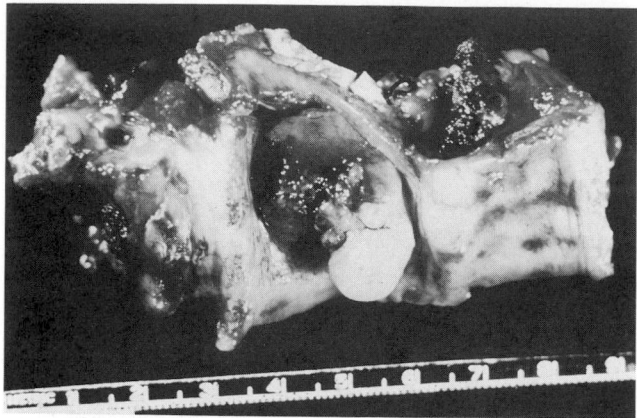

Figure 15-22. Follicular carcinoma recurrent 4 years after total thyroidectomy, which in turn was preceded by right hemithyroidectomy 2 years earlier. The proximal resection line includes a beveled portion of the cricoid cartilage. The right recurrent laryngeal nerve was paralyzed preoperatively. The patient died almost 7 years following this resection from mediastinal metastases. (From Grillo HC: Congenital lesions, neoplasms and injuries of the trachea. p. 335. In Sabiston DC Jr, Spencer FC (eds): Gibbon's Surgery of the Chest. 5th Ed. WB Saunders, Philadelphia, 1983

available adjacent tissue (muscle). The brachiocephalic artery is protected by suturing strap muscle or other available tissue over the artery against the trachea in order to prevent potential erosion of the artery by a low-placed tracheostomy tube (in a shortened trachea). A small tracheostomy tube is inserted in the resulting triangular space 1.5 to 2 cm distal to the anastomosis.

If it is uncertain whether the airway might be edematous postoperatively or if there is concern about the short distance available for placement of a tracheostomy tube adjacent to the anastomosis, the anastomosis and brachiocephalic artery are walled off as described, and a single silk marking suture is placed on the tracheal wall at the point where a tracheostomy may later be placed (Grillo, 1982b). The patient is awakened and the airway examined with a flexible bronchoscope. If there is any question about adequacy of the glottis because of edema, an uncuffed small-bore nasotracheal tube is placed. After 5 days, this is removed in the operating room and the airway again examined. If it is adequate, the patient is observed closely for another period of days. If it does not appear adequate, tracheotomy is performed in the premarked spot without interfering with the now sealed suture lines. The tracheostomy is removed when glottic edema subsides. Decadron, as well as racemic epinephrine, is administered perioperatively and immediately postoperatively in most patients.

When the outer esophageal wall is involved, we have removed the full thickness of the muscularis, leaving an intact mucosa. In other patients we have removed the full thickness of the esophageal wall, closing the esophagus in linear fashion with two layers of interrupted 4–0 silk sutures in the manner described by Sweet (1950). A thus narrowed esophagus remains an adequate conduit for saliva and for initial liquid feedings. It usually dilates spontaneously later without the need even for mechanical dilatation, which may, however, occasionally be needed. A pedicled strap muscle or other tissue is placed between an esophageal suture line and the airway anastomosis to prevent fistulization.

The surgery is precise and demanding, but functional results are excellent. The patient will initially have a hoarse voice if one recurrent laryngeal nerve has been sacrificed. Often this is largely self-corrected over 6 to 12 months. If at the end of that time the voice remains inadequate, the vocal cord may be stiffened by a variety of procedures such as Teflon injection. Since so many patients improve spontaneously, such procedures are deferred for 1 year. The airway is usually wholly satisfactory.

Cervical Exenteration

There is limited application for the drastic approach of cervical exenteration to airway involvement by thyroid cancer. However, exenteration can be a remarkably effective palliative measure for a patient who is facing strangulation by tumor, usually recurrent, or less commonly, for the patient who is faced with a primary carcinoma of rapid local growth that is still resectable (Fig. 15-23). Rarely, resection may be curative.

If the pharynx and esophagus are also involved, our technique of resection consists of blocking out all tissue from above the hyoid bone, including the lower pharynx, and from carotid sheath to carotid sheath laterally to the upper mediastinum below (Grillo and Mathisen, 1990). The vertebral spine forms the floor of the dissection. A long horizontal incision along the top of the clavicles is used. If tumor extends low on the trachea, a mediastinal tracheotomy is performed, with removal of the heads of the clavicles and the first two costal cartilages and division of the sternum at the level of the second interspace. The feasibility of resection is determined initially by dividing the sternum horizontally through the second interspace and vertically through the manubrium. If resection is safely possible, the bony plaque is removed.

The trachea is divided well below the tumor but is not mobilized except on its anterior surface, with careful preservation of the lateral blood supply. A second inferior horizontal incision beneath the mammary crease allows a bipedicled cutaneous flap to fall into the mediastinum for stomal anastomosis without tension. The inferior deficit in skin is closed with a skin graft (Fig. 15-24). In the case of a very low mediastinal tracheostomy (within 2 to 3 cm of the carina)—rarely necessary for thyroid cancer, even for recurrent disease—the brachiocephalic artery may be electively divided after first occluding it and checking the electroencephalographic monitors, which are placed in all such cases. Esophageal continuity is established with stomach or left colon.

The omentum is also advanced substernally in such cases, particularly if the patient has received heavy irradiation, as many have. The omentum covers major mediastinal vessels, buttresses the neoesophageal anastomosis, and surrounds the trachea just beneath its anastomosis to the skin (Mathisen, et al., 1988). Postoperative separation of the anastomosis in the vicinity of the innominate artery, due to irradiation or tension, thus will not necessarily produce a disastrous vascular fistula. Cervicomediastinal exenteration is a lengthy and

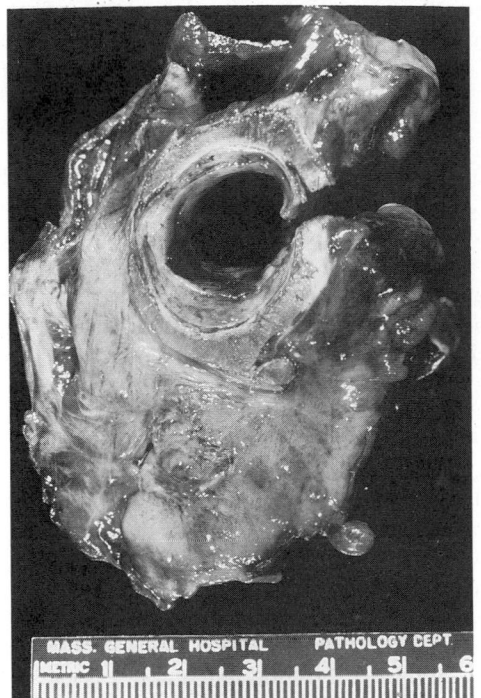
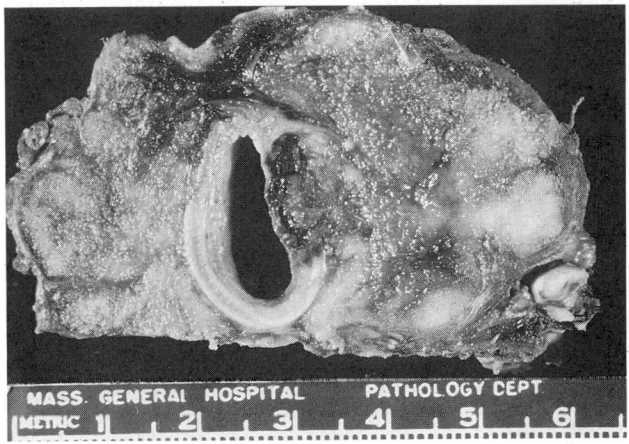

Figure 15-23. **(A)** Squamous cell carcinoma of the thyroid, which required resection of larynx, trachea, and esophagus. **(B)** Papillary carcinoma, which required tracheal resection, neck dissection, and removal of the anterolateral wall of the esophagus. (From Grillo HC, Zannini P: Resectional management of airway invasion by thyroid carcinoma. Ann Thorac Surg 42:287, 1986, with permission.)

complex procedure that demands rigorous indications and considerable experience.

Early Results

Of 52 patients with thyroid cancer invading the airway seen between 1964 and 1991, resection was not performed in 18, because of either distant disease, extensive local disease, or the desire to preserve laryngeal function where only an operation including laryngectomy would have been adequate (Grillo, et al., 1992). The other 34 patients underwent resectional therapy; 27 of these had reconstruction of the airway and 7 had exenteration with end tracheostomies. The distribution was even between males and females, and their ages ranged from 17 to 79 years, with a mean of 61. Among the patients who had the reconstructive procedure, there were 16 with papillary carcinoma, 5 with follicular carcinoma, 4 with carcinomas of mixed histology, and 2 with poorly differentiated carcinomas. The cancers of those undergoing resection without reconstruction comprised 3 of papillary, 1 of follicular, and 3 of more aggressive histology. Of those who had reconstruction, 15 had unilateral recurrent laryngeal nerve paralysis, but 11 of these had had prior surgery. Only 9 of the 27 patients undergoing reconstruction had had no prior therapy, and 1 had had ^{131}I radiotherapy only. The other 17 had undergone resection, including hemithyroidectomy and subtotal thyroidectomy. Neck dissections had been performed in some. Five of the patients were referred immediately after the surgeon identified tracheal invasion, but 13 others were referred at the time of recurrence, the original

tumor having been shaved off the trachea. The interval between initial surgical treatment and airway resection ranged from 1 to 47 years. A number had undergone ^{131}I therapy, chemotherapy, and external irradiation. Some had tracheostomies. Only 3 of those undergoing exenteration had had no prior therapy, while the other 4 had had thyroidectomy, ^{131}I therapy, and external irradiation.

Ten patients underwent tracheal sleeve resection; 6 had partial oblique resection of the cricoid cartilage with a laryngotracheal anastomosis; and 10 underwent complex resections with individually designed lines of resection through the larynx to accomplish maximal tumor removal but preservation of laryngeal function. In 3 patients a complementary tracheotomy was performed because the immediate adequacy of the airway at the conclusion of the surgery was in question. Laryngeal release was not required. Of the 27, 15 showed lymph node metastases, and in 13 positive resection margins were accepted in order to salvage the larynx. Eight patients received radioactive iodine therapy and 7 received external radiation.

Two deaths occurred in this group of 27 patients. The first was the result of failure of anastomotic healing in a patient who had undergone 7,800 cGy of irradiation 6 years prior to reconstruction, following incomplete resection of cancer. This resection was attempted prior to the time when omental augmentation was used for irradiated airways. A second patient died from respiratory arrest due to airway obstruction; a temporary tracheostomy would have obviated this occurrence. One patient suffered right vocal cord paralysis not present preoperatively and not the result of elective resection

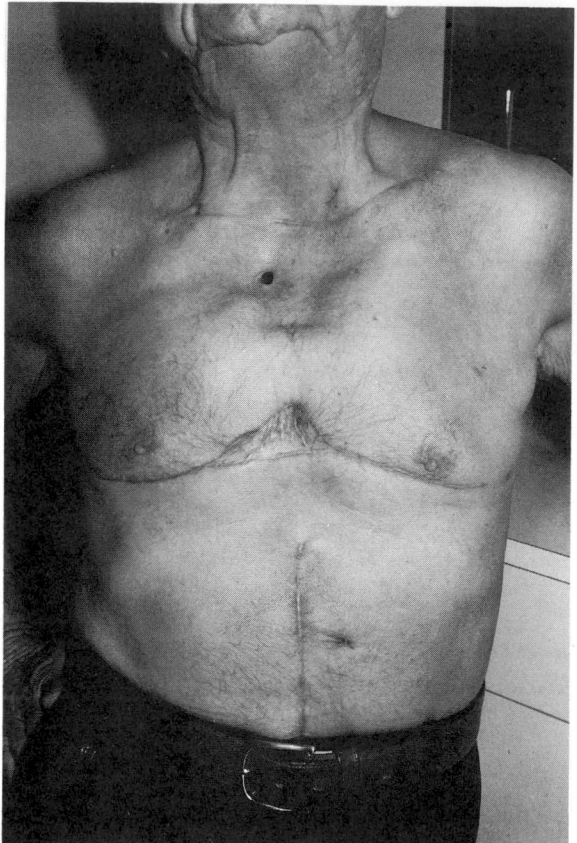

Figure 15-24. Postoperative status of patient whose specimen is shown in Figure 15-23A. The mediastinal tracheostomy may be seen in a depressed portion of the chest wall, where the upper part of sternum, the heads of the clavicles, and the first two cartilages have been removed. A skin graft covers the relaxing incision, which permitted the flap to drop into the mediastinum.

of a recurrent laryngeal nerve. Mild dysphagia in 3 patients resolved, 1 patient requiring dilatation.

Late Results

In the reconstruction group, 11 of the 25 survivors of surgery died of cancer from 3 months to 10 years and 3 months following reconstruction (Fig. 15-25). Two patients with undifferentiated thyroid cancer died from distant metastases within 6 months of resection. Cancer of the airway recurred in only 2 patients in the group, which indicates the accomplishment of one of the primary goals of surgery, obviation of death by airway obstruction. The average duration of survival among these 11 patients was 3 years and 7 months. The usual cause of death was metastatic disease in the mediastinum, lungs, or brain. One patient died of leukemia, which was possibly related to earlier ^{131}I therapy. Of the 13 surviving patients, 12 were without evidence of cancer at the time of follow-up (1 month to 14½ years following airway surgery); the other one had pulmonary metastases. The average survival of the 13 patients was 5 years and 9 months at the time of follow-up. In 2, local nodal recurrences had been excised at varying intervals following the initial airway resection.

Of the 13 surviving patients, 9 had undergone airway resection as part of the initial surgical treatment or had been referred immediately after a surgeon found evidence of tracheal invasion at thyroidectomy (Fig. 15-25). Of 17 patients eligible for 5-year follow-up, 10 were alive at 5 years and 9 at 10 years. Of 11 survivors with positive microscopic margins, 3 were alive without evidence of disease up to 6 years after resection. Six of the others died of thyroid cancer, 1 died of leukemia, and 1 was alive with pulmonary metastases. The 6 who died of thyroid cancer lived from 3 months to over 10 years following resection.

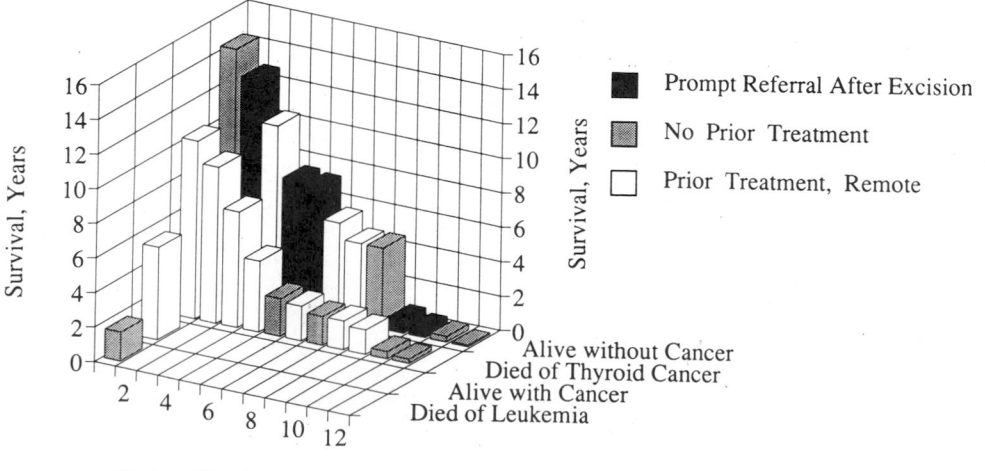

Figure 15-25. Performance of 25 survivors in the reconstructed group. Long-term palliation achieved in some patients who died of thyroid cancer is to be noted. Also striking is the number of patients alive without cancer who had undergone resection either primarily or following prompt referral upon discovery of airway invasion. (From Grillo HC, Suen HC, Mathisen DJ, Wain JC: Resectional management of thyroid carcinoma invading the airway. Ann Thorac Surg 54:3, 1992, with permission.)

It is also worth noting that 7 patients had evidence of pulmonary metastases at the time of airway resection performed to achieve palliation. The metastases were known to be slowly enlarging. While 2 of these died within 1 year of the airway procedure (with undifferentiated carcinoma), the average survival for the whole group was 4.2 years and the patient surviving the longest was still alive over 10½ years following surgery.

In the nonreconstruction group who underwent radical resection, 1 patient with sarcoma died of metastases 2 years and 7 months following resection, 1 with squamous carcinoma died 7 years and 4 months after resection, 3 died of other diseases without evidence of recurrence, and 1 remains alive 3 years later but now has asymptomatic pulmonary metastases.

COMMENTS AND CONTROVERSIES

Although differentiated carcinoma that invades the airway appears often to be more aggressive in character, many tumors run an indolent course, with potential for long-term survival. Complete resection of the local disease including involved airway appears to be the best therapy, providing potential for cure when it is done as part of the initial therapy and for prolonged palliation when it is done for late recurrent disease. External irradiation, radioactive iodine, and chemotherapy have often not proved to be effective agents for management of such residual disease. Various techniques of coring out the airway, either mechanically or by laser, provide temporary palliation but should otherwise be applied only when resection is not possible. Even when cure is not achieved, prolonged palliation is often obtained by resection, and devastating airway complications are avoided.

For these reasons bronchoscopy and careful CT examination should be part of preoperative investigation of all patients with thyroid carcinoma. Either the preoperative discovery of invasion or its finding at thyroidectomy should dictate prompt referral to a center where appropriate airway reconstruction can be performed. Every effort should be made to save the larynx. In a highly selected group of patients, radical resection, including laryngectomy in patients with no hope of laryngeal salvage, is indicated. Even the presence of slowly growing pulmonary metastases is not a contraindication for resection, since this is compatible with prolonged survival.

H.C.G.
D.J.M.

BRONCHOGENIC CARCINOMA

HISTORICAL NOTE

Techniques of carinal resection and reconstruction (Grillo, 1982a) have been applied infrequently for bronchogenic carcinoma. Mathey, et al. (1966) and Jensik, et al. (1972) were among the earliest to practice sleeve pneumonectomy for bronchogenic carcinoma. Indeed, classification of bronchogenic cancer invading the carina into stage IV was dictated largely by the rarity of technical expertise for such resections. Even main bronchial invasion has been classified as stage IIIB. Since the late 1970s carinal resection for bronchogenic carcinoma has been reported in North America by Deslauriers, et al. (1978), Jensik, et al. (1982), and Mathisen and Grillo (1991); in Europe by Dartevelle, et al. (1988) and Perelman and Koroleva (1980); and in Japan by Ishihara, et al. (1977) and Naruke (1982), among others. Excessive mortality has attended extension of surgery to this group of patients. Mathisen and Grillo (1991) called attention to the alarming occurrence of acute postoperative adult respiratory distress syndrome (ARDS) in these patients.

HISTORICAL READINGS

Jensik RJ, Faber P, Milloy FJ, Goldin MD: Tracheal sleeve pneumonectomy for advanced carcinoma of the lung. Surg Gynecol Obstet 134:231, 1972
Mathey J, Binct JP, Galcy JJ et al: Tracheal and tracheobronchial resection. J Thorac Cardiovasc Surg 51:1, 1966

BASIC SCIENCE

When bronchogenic carcinoma invades the trachea directly from parenchymal contiguity, the disease is usually so extensive that segmental resection of the trachea is precluded. On the other hand, when bronchogenic carcinoma is centered in the proximal main bronchus or involves the carina, it should be considered for resection. The disease must be localized enough so that resection of the involved carina will not result in reconstruction under tension. The generally safe limit of such resection in right carinal pneumonectomy is approximately 4 cm between the distal end of the trachea and the left main bronchus. With carinal resection alone, which preserves the right lung, resection may be somewhat more extensive because of greater possibility for mobilization of the right lung unhindered by the aortic arch. This applies also to the rare left carinal pneumonectomy for bronchogenic carcinoma.

Considerations regarding lymph node involvement are the same as for any other resection of carcinoma of the lung. N3 disease is out of bounds, and N2 disease would be resected only as part of a protocol approach with adjunctive therapy. Because of the extensiveness of the operation and the still high mortality, it is important to search exhaustively for remote metastases prior to performing resection.

Carcinoma involving the right upper lobe at its origin may easily extend up the short length of right main bronchus to involve the carina. On the left side the bronchus is considerably longer, and carcinoma of the left upper lobe, which is less common than that of the right upper lobe, is not likely to extend to the carina. In all series the number of right carinal pneumonectomies for bronchogenic carcinoma is far greater than the rare left-sided resection.

Of 37 patients undergoing carinal resection for broncho-genic carcinoma, 26 had squamous carcinoma, 9 adenocarci-noma, 1 large cell carcinoma, and 1 adenosquamous carci-noma (Mathisen and Grillo, 1991).

Particularly in right carinal pneumonectomy, significant interruption of tracheobronchial lymphatics necessarily oc-curs even when no effort is made to perform radical lymphad-enectomy of the subcarinal, precarinal, and right paratracheal lymph nodes.

DIAGNOSIS

Involvement of the carina by bronchogenic carcinoma must be assessed with great care by conventional imaging, which includes CT scanning of the chest and upper abdomen. Crisp carinal tomograms are useful to demonstrate the gross extent of the lesion both within and without the lumen of the trachea and equally important, to make clear the relative proportion of airway that may be uninvolved by tumor (Fig. 15-26). This is confirmed intraluminally by bronchoscopy. Even when flexible bronchoscopy has been performed for preliminary assessment, we prefer to carry out rigid bronchoscopy with Storz-Hopkins magnifying telescopes under general anesthe-sia for precise definition at the time of resection. The lengths of airway that are and are not involved are determined by difference with a rigid bronchoscope, the level of carina, proximal extent of gross tumor, and the inferior border of the cricoid cartilage being noted successively. Particular at-tention is paid to extent of involvement of the opposite main bronchus. Extension of tumor down the opposite main bron-chus for any distance, particularly down the left side when the tumor is predominantly on the right, may severely com-promise or make impossible the approximation of the airway without tension. Mediastinoscopy is important for assess-ment of lymph node involvement to supplement information from the CT scan. Mediastinoscopy is preferably performed concurrently with the planned resection so that tissue planes and definition between scar and tumor will not be obscured.

All patients who are being considered for carinal resection in connection with bronchogenic carcinoma must be evalu-ated by pulmonary function studies and quantitative ventila-tion/perfusion scans to determine what pulmonary function will be present postoperatively. In a few patients in whom pneumonectomy would not have been tolerated and whose tumor was localized, it was possible to perform carinal resec-tion and right upper lobectomy with reimplantation of the middle and lower lobes or the lower lobe. Exploration was necessary before final decision could be made about resect-ability.

MANAGEMENT

Principles

The patient must have disease that is not so extensive locally that the resulting resection will run a high risk of technical failure due to tension at the anastomosis. Lymph node involvement must be carefully analyzed and an appropriate decision must be made according to the surgeon's policy for the management of involved mediastinal lymph nodes. Distant metastases must be ruled out. The patient's functional limitations for resection must be defined. It must be made clear to the patient that the risk of carinal resection is pres-ently greater than that of total pneumonectomy.

Operative technique is discussed in Chapter 16.

Early Results

Among 37 patients (age range, 29 to 70; mean, 53 years) some had had prior pneumonectomy, others, thoracotomy and bi-opsy. Mediastinoscopy was negative in all but 3, who were entered into a protocol for therapy of N2 disease with neoad-

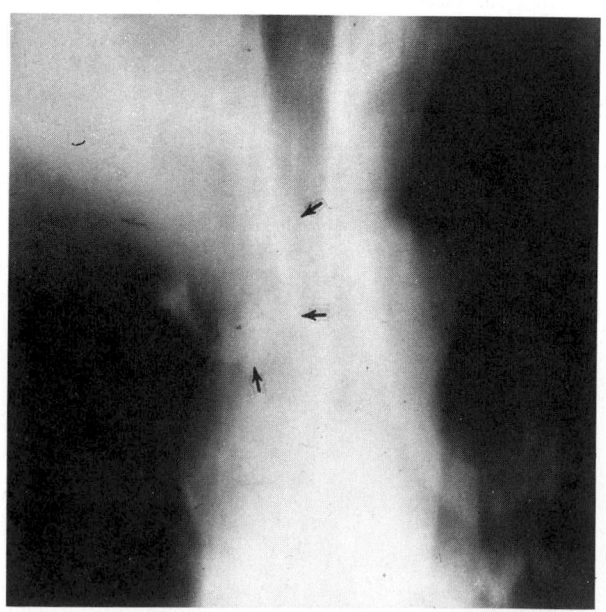
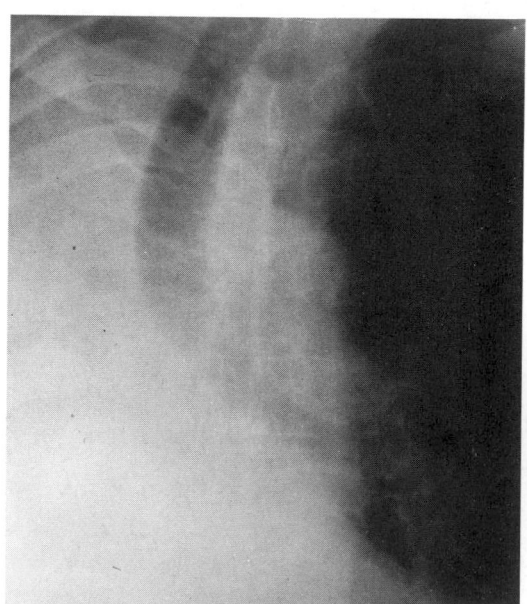

Figure 15-26. (A) Preoperative tomogram demonstrating a large cell carcinoma invading the carina and lower trachea. (B) Postoperative image. The patient achieved a 5-year survival.

juvant chemotherapy and radiotherapy. Right carinal pneumonectomy was performed in 21 patients, lymph node dissection in 7, partial lateral resection of superior vena cava in 3, and partial resection of muscular wall of the esophagus in 1. Seven patients underwent carinal resection with preservation of all pulmonary parenchyma, and 7 underwent right upper lobectomy and carinal resection with salvage and reimplantation of middle and lower lobes. In 2 patients with recurrent bronchial stump cancer, 1 on the right and 1 on the left, resection of the involved airway was performed through the right chest. Since both had received 4,400 cGy of radiation 3 years previously, the anastomoses were wrapped with omentum.

In 17 patients, there were no complications. Many in this population with a history of smoking required frequent postoperative chest physiotherapy and flexible bronchoscopy to clear secretions. Six developed atelectasis, 5 developed pneumonia, and 9 had postoperative atrial fibrillation. The ominous complication of pulmonary infiltration and respiratory failure occurred in 3 (8 percent), and all died despite vigorous therapy. Bacteriologic findings were unimpressive. Seven patients developed anastomotic problems, which in 2 consisted of stenosis of the right main bronchial anastomosis with the side of the trachea and in 1 involved the bronchus intermedius. Two stenoses were repaired successfully surgically and others were managed conservatively by dilatation or laser therapy. Three patients died ultimately of anastomotic complications, principally separation: In 1 of them much more than 4 cm of trachea had been resected after prior resection 9 years earlier; 1 required prolonged mechanical ventilation, and separation followed; and the third died during endoscopic manipulation of an occluded reimplanted right lower lobe bronchus. Three patients had left vocal cord dysfunction, presumably due to injury to the left recurrent nerve; in 2 the problem resolved spontaneously, but 1 required vocal cord injection with Teflon. Early postoperative mortality was 8 percent, but delayed mortality was nearly 11 percent. The late deaths were due to anastomotic complications related to either tension or ischemia. Overall mortality rate was therefore 18.9 percent.

Mortality rates of 29 and 27 percent were reported, respectively, by Jensik and colleagues (1982) and by Deslauriers and colleagues (1985). The series of Dartevelle et al. (1988) showed mortality reduced to 11 percent. A significant number of early postoperative deaths following right carinal pneumonectomy are due to a particularly aggressive and rapidly moving ARDS-like syndrome. The operation may go smoothly, after which the patient may be extubated early and appear to be in fine condition for 24 hours. At 36 to 48 hours a diffuse infiltrate appears in the remaining lung (Fig. 15-27). This progresses relentlessly to complete "whiteout" of the lung and ultimately to death. At postmortem the lung is wet and heavy, and nonspecific bacteria, if any, are cultured. A postmortem diagnosis of bronchopneumonia does not appear to be supported. This syndrome also follows conventional right pneumonectomy, but rarely. Peters and associates (1987) describe this sequence as postpneumonectomy pulmonary edema, attributing it most likely to perioperative intravenous fluid overload. In reviewing our case data, we have not found a correlation between the amount of perioperative fluid administered and occurrence of this dreaded complication. Nonetheless, we manage these patients with minimum fluid administration. It is possible that interference with pulmonary lymphatics impairs the ability of the remaining lung to clear interstitial fluid. This remains conjectural. Once the syndrome appears, the patient is unlikely to survive despite all measures, including fluid restriction, diuresis, ventilatory support, and adjunctive medications.

Late Results

Our series produced 5 absolute 5-year survivors (5 to 10 years), 9 patients alive between 1½ and 3½ years without evidence of disease, and 2 dead of other causes at 2½ years.

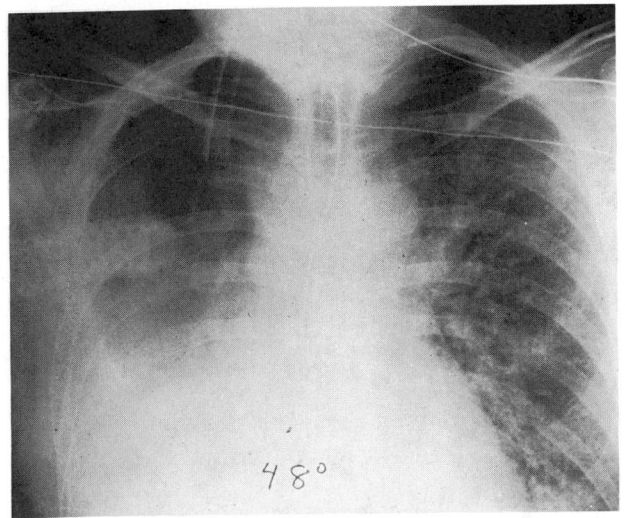
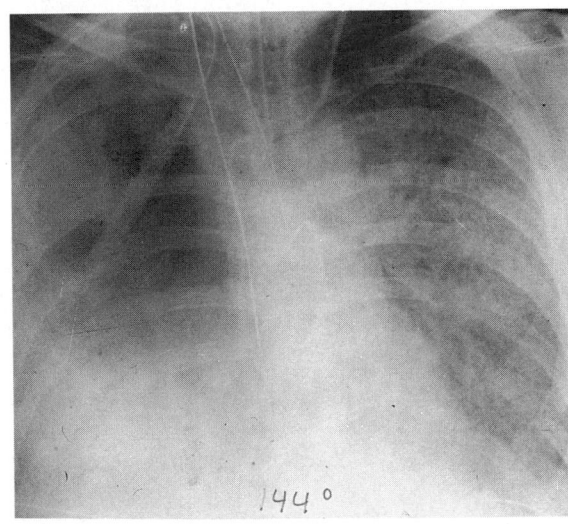

Figure 15-27. Postpneumonectomy pulmonary edema. Following an uneventful right carinal pneumonectomy, this patient developed a "ground glass" infiltrate in his left lung at approximately 36 hours. **(A)** Pulmonary infiltrate at 48 hours. **(B)** Progression of ARDS at 6 days. Death followed despite maximum therapy.

Five patients were alive without disease less than 1 year after surgery. Eight patients died of recurrent disease between 1 and 3½ years after operation. Actuarial survival is 19 percent. This compares with a 5-year actuarial survival of 15 percent in the series of Jensik, et al. (1982) and 23 percent in the series of both Deslaurier, et al. (1985) and Dartevelle, et al. (1988). The patients of Jensik, et al. (1982) were not staged with respect to mediastinal lymph node metastases.

COMMENTS AND CONTROVERSIES

With the development of carinal surgery, carinal pneumonectomy or carinal resection with various types of reconstruction has become feasible with growing safety. The techniques are applicable to bronchogenic carcinoma that involves the carina and that would otherwise be potentially curable. Involvement of the main bronchus or carina therefore should not by itself exclude surgical consideration even if currently classified in stage IIIB or IV. Such patients must be very carefully appraised for extent of local and distant disease and for anatomic feasibility of safe resection. With careful attention to selection of patients, surgical technique, and perioperative management, complications from the surgery itself will decrease steadily. The ominous exception is postpneumonectomy pulmonary edema or ARDS. Its cause remains uncertain, as do, therefore, methods for prevention and treatment. A 5-year survival rate between 20 and 25 percent may be anticipated if patients with N2 disease are excluded. The N0 patients should probably be reclassified into stage IIIA.

H.C.G.
D.J.M.

OTHER TUMORS

Recurrence of squamous carcinoma of the larynx at the tracheal stoma after laryngectomy has been approached by radical resection (Sisson, et al., 1962). This has usually followed either postoperative irradiation that failed to prevent recurrence or failed radiation therapy for recurrence. Such resection frequently requires radical excision, including adjacent cervical tissues and esophagus. Reconstruction is performed much as described for cervical exenteration for extensive thyroid carcinoma. Because of cutaneous involvement by recurrent tumor and irradiation, it is frequently necessary to rotate unirradiated myocutaneous flaps to cover the lower neck and upper mediastinum and to establish a low mediastinal tracheostomy.

All too often, however, cancer recurs soon after resection (Krespi, et al., 1985). Lymphatics are probably permeated with cancer paratracheally for some distance distally. Justification for such extensive surgery is therefore questionable.

Cervicomediastinal exenteration has also been performed for other secondary tumors invading the trachea, including postcricoidal squamous carcinoma of the esophagus that involves the larynx and upper trachea, so that laryngeal salvage is impossible (see Ch. 16). Adenoid cystic carcinoma may also invade the larynx in an unsalvageable manner, as well as the upper portion of the trachea and less often the wall of the esophagus.

Generally, resection of the trachea for direct involvement by esophageal carcinoma other than postcricoidal is not advised. The extent of involvement is usually so great that curative resection is unlikely. Tracheoesophageal fistula due to esophageal carcinoma is an extreme example. In a rare patient following preoperative neoadjuvant therapy, if the only point of apparent nonresectability is a short segment of trachea, it has seemed worthwhile to resect this segment and perform direct tracheotracheal anastomosis. One must be particularly cautious in such cases because the blood supply of the trachea may well be damaged by the extensive dissection performed for removal of the esophagus. Through a large part of the body of the trachea, segmental arteries provide an anterior branch to the trachea and a posterior one to the esophagus. If combined resection is performed, advancement of the omentum is advisable. This is brought up with the stomach, which is used to reconstruct the esophagus. Extension of radical esophageal resection to include tracheal segmental resection in any programmatic way is not advised.

KEY REFERENCES

Dartevelle PG, Khalife J, Chepelier A et al.: Tracheal sleeve pneumonectomy for bronchogenic carcinoma: report of 55 cases. Ann Thorac Surg 46:68, 1988

In 55 tracheal sleeve pneumonectomy patients, mortality was 10.9 percent, the lowest recorded. Actuarial survival was 23 percent at 5 years and correlated with node involvement.

Deslauriers J: Involvement of the main carina. p. 139. In Delarue NC, Eschapasse H (eds): Lung Cancer. International Trends in General Thoracic Surgery. Vol. 1. WB Saunders, Philadelphia, 1985

In 27 patients a 23 percent 5-year survival was obtained, but operative mortality was 27 percent. The authors identify the cause of death as infection but describe what may well be "postpneumonectomy pulmonary edema" (ARDS).

Grillo HC, Suen HC, Mathisen DJ, Wain JC: Resectional management of thyroid carcinoma invading the airway. Ann Thorac Surg 54:3, 1992

The principles of application of airway resection for invading thyroid carcinoma are stated on the basis of 34 resections including 27 with reconstruction. Results and long-term follow-up are detailed.

Ishihara T, Kobayashi K, Kikuchi K et al.: Surgical treatment of advanced thyroid carcinoma invading the trachea. J Thorac Cardiovasc Surg 102:717, 1991

In 60 patients thyroid cancer invading the trachea was removed, resulting in 5- and 10-year survival rates for complete resection of 78 percent and for incomplete resection of 44 and 24 percent, respectively.

Jensik RJ, Faber JP, Kittle CF et al.: Survival in patients undergoing tracheal sleeve pneumonectomy for bronchogenic carcinoma. J Thorac Cardiovasc Surg 84:489, 1982

This is the first large series of such patients, listing 34, with a 15 percent 5-year survival but 29 percent mortality. The high mortality clearly differentiated the magnitude of the procedure from standard pneumonectomy.

Mathisen DJ, Grillo HC: Carinal resection for bronchogenic carcinoma. J Thorac Cardiovasc Surg 102:16, 1991

Of the 37 patients in this series, 8 percent suffered early death, principally due to respiratory distress syndrome of a characteristic type. Late operative deaths were due to anastomotic complications. Actuarial 5-year survival was 19 percent.

REFERENCES

Abbruzzini P: Trattamento chirurgico delle fistole del broncho principale consecutive a pneumonectomia per tubercolosi. Chir Torac 14:165, 1961

Beahrs OH, Kiernan PD, Hubert JP Jr: Cancer of the Head and Neck. Churchill Livingstone, New York, 1981

Deslauriers J, Beaulieu M, Benazera A, McClish A: Sleeve pneumonectomy for bronchogenic carcinoma. Ann Thorac Surg 28:465, 1978

Frazell EL, Foote FW Jr: Papillary cancer of the thyroid: a review of 25 years of experience. Cancer 11:895, 1958

Grillo HC: Atlas of General Thoracic Surgery. WB Saunders, Philadelphia, 1988

Grillo HC: Congenital lesions, neoplasms and injuries of the trachea. p. 335. In Sabiston DC, Jr, Spencer FC (eds): Gibbon's Surgery of the Chest. 5th Ed. WB Saunders, Philadelphia, 1983

Grillo HC: Carinal resection. Ann Thorac Surg 34:356, 1982a

Grillo HC: Primary reconstruction of airway after resection of subglottic and upper tracheal stenosis. Ann Thorac Surg 33:3, 1982b

Grillo HC: Circumferential resection and reconstruction of mediastinal and cervical trachea. Ann Surg 162:374, 1965

Grillo HC, Mathisen DJ: Cervical exenteration. Ann Thorac Surg 49:401, 1990a

Grillo HC, Mathisen DJ: Primary tracheal tumors: treatment and results. Ann Thorac Surg 49:69, 1990b

Grillo HC, Zannini P: Resectional management of airway invasion by thyroid carcinoma. Ann Thorac Surg 42:287, 1986

Hendrick JW: An extended operation for thyroid carcinoma. Surg Gynecol Obstet 116:183, 1963

Ishihara T, Ikeda T, Inoue H, Fukai S: Resection of cancer of the lung and carina. J Thorac Cardiovasc Surg 73:936, 1977

Ishihara T, Kikuchi K, Ikeda T et al.: Resection of thyroid carcinoma infiltrating the trachea. Thorax 33:378, 1978

Jensik RJ, Faber P, Milloy FJ, Goldin MD: Tracheal sleeve pneumonectomy for advanced carcinoma of the lung. Surg Gynecol Obstet 134:231, 1972

Krespi YP, Wurster CF, Sisson GA: Immediate reconstruction after total laryngopharyngoesophagectomy and mediastinal dissection. Laryngoscope 95:156, 1985

Lawson W, Som MP, Biller HF: Papillary carcinoma of the thyroid invading the upper air passages. Ann Otol Rhinol Laryngol 86:751, 1977

Maeda M, Nakamoto K, Ohta M et al.: Statistical survey of tracheobronchoplasty in Japan. J Thorac Cardiovasc Surg 97:402, 1989

Mathey J, Binet JP, Galey JJ et al.: Tracheal and tracheobronchial resection. J Thorac Cardiovasc Surg 51:1, 1966

Mathisen DJ, Grillo HC, Vlahakes GJ, Daggett WM: The omentum in the management of complicated cardiothoracic problems. J Thorac Cardiovasc Surg 95:677, 1988

Montgomery WW: Suprahyoid release for tracheal stenosis. Arch Otolaryngol Head Neck Surg 99:255, 1974

Naruke T, Yoneyama T, Ogata T et al.: Bronchoplastic procedures for lung carcinoma. J Thorac Cardiovasc Surg 84:489, 1982

Nomori H, Kobayaski K, Ishihara T et al.: Thyroid carcinoma infiltrating the trachea: clinical histologic, and morphometric analyses. J Surg Oncol 44:78, 1990

Perelman MI, Koroleva NS: Primary tumors of the trachea. p. 91. In Grillo HC, Eschaparre H (eds): Major Challenges. In International Trends in General Thoracic Surgery. Vol. 2. WB Saunders, Philadelphia, 1987

Perelman MI, Koroleva NS: Surgery of the trachea. World J Surg 4:583, 1980

Peters RM: Postpneumonectomy pulmonary edema. p. 460. In Grillo HC, Eschaparre (eds): Major Challenges. In International Trends in General Thoracic Surgery. Vol. 2. WB Saunders, Philadelphia, 1987

Shin DH, Mark EJ, Suen HC, Grillo HC: Pathological staging of papillary carcinoma of the thyroid with airway invasion based upon the anatomic manner of extension to the trachea. Hum Pathol 24:866, 1993

Silliphant WM, Klinck GH, Levitin MS: Thyroid carcinoma and death: a clinicopathological study of 193 autopsies. Cancer 17:513, 1964

Sisson GA, Straehley CJ Jr, Johnson NE: Mediastinal dissection for recurrent cancer after laryngectomy. Laryngoscope 72:1064, 1962

Sweet RH: Thoracic Surgery. WB Saunders, Philadelphia, 1950

Tsuchiya R, Goya T, Naruke T, Suemasu K: Resection of tracheal carina for lung cancer. J Thorac Cardiovasc Surg 99:779, 1990

Tsumori T, Nakao K, Miyata M et al.: Clinicopathologic study on the mode and degree of invasion of the trachea by thyroid carcinoma. Nippon Geka Gakkai Zasshi 88:600, 1987

Tsumori T, Nakao K, Miyata M et al.: Clinicopathologic study of thyroid carcinoma infiltrating the trachea. Cancer 56:2843, 1985

16

SURGICAL TECHNIQUES

Tracheotomy

Andrew R. Golde
Jonathan C. Irish
Patrick J. Gullane

Currently, four methods of obtaining a surgical airway are recognized: (1) tracheotomy, (2) percutaneous tracheotomy, (3) cricothyroidotomy, and (4) minitracheotomy.

HISTORICAL NOTE

The oldest known reference identifying a procedure akin to a tracheotomy is found in a sacred Hindu book, the *Rigveda,* from the second millennium B.C. (Goodall, 1934). Mention of the procedure is also found in the writings of Galen and Aretaeus in the second century A.D. However, lack of both anatomic knowledge and surgical experience produced uniformly poor results, resulting in tracheotomy being labeled "the scandal of surgery" (Goodall, 1934).

The first successful tracheotomy was recorded in 1546 by an Italian physician, Antonio Musa Brasavola, who operated upon a patient suffering from "an abscess in the windpipe" (Frost, 1976). By the year 1825, as cited by Goodall (1934), roughly 30 tracheotomies had been documented in the medical literature. The indications varied from removal of gold coins and blood clots from the upper airway to an unsuccessful attempt at cheating the hangman's noose with a surreptitious secondary airway.

By the mid 1800s Trousseau (1833) reported the procedure as having saved the lives of one-quarter of approximately 200 children dying with diphtheria. Despite technical refinements, widespread acceptance of the procedure did not come until the 1920s, when the work of Chevalier Jackson clearly delineated the indications for tracheotomy and standardized the technique for performing the procedure (Jackson and Jackson, 1937). Jackson (1923) strongly condemned other methods of airway control, particularly cricothyroidotomy, which he considered to be associated with an unacceptable incidence of laryngeal and subglottic stenosis.

HISTORICAL READINGS

Frost EA: Tracing the tracheotomy. Ann Otol Rhinol Laryngol, 85:618, 1976

Goodall EW: The story of tracheotomy. Br J Child Dis 31:167, 253, 1934

Jackson C: High tracheotomy and other errors—the chief causes of chronic laryngeal stenosis. Surg Gynecol Obstet 32:392, 1923

Jackson C, Jackson CL: The Larynx and Its Diseases. WB Saunders, Philadelphia, 1937

Trousseau A: J Commun Med Chir Paris:541, 1833

TRACHEOTOMY

In no era has the operation dubbed *tracheotomy* been called by the same name. Laryngotomy and bronchotomy were used interchangeably up to the eighteenth century, as are tracheotomy and tracheostomy today. In practical terms, *tracheotomy* is the operation of "opening the trachea" (Jackson, 1923), derived from the Greek words *trachea arteria* (rough artery) and *tome* (cut); *tracheostomy,* however, has an ending derived from the Greek word *stoma* (opening or mouth). Unless the procedure is performed with the intent of placing a permanent opening, the more correct term would be tracheotomy (Eavey, 1985).

Indications

Four main goals are achieved when the trachea is intubated, regardless of the route employed (oral, nasal, laryngeal, or tracheal). Tracheotomy may be employed for any of the four, alone or in *either* combination: (1) to treat upper airway obstruction; (2) to protect the airways from aspiration and provide access to improve tracheobronchial toilet; (3) to provide respiratory support with mechanical ventilation; and

(4) to eliminate ventilatory dead space and treat obstructive sleep apnea.

Upper Airway Obstruction

Traditionally, the primary role of tracheotomy has been to relieve upper airway obstruction. Etiologies of airway obstruction that may necessitate tracheotomy include laryngeal and tracheal injuries that preclude routine methods of intubation; severe maxillofacial trauma; foreign bodies in the upper airway; bilateral vocal cord paralysis; congenital anomalies of the upper airway; tumors of the upper aerodigestive tract; and inflammatory swellings of the oral cavity, pharynx, larynx, and trachea (as a result of surgery in the head and neck or from infection).

With the advent of flexible fiberoptic laryngoscopes and bronchoscopes, some of the more traditional applications for tracheotomy have changed. For example, there has been a trend toward using oral or nasal intubation in the treatment of acute epiglottitis (Baxter and Dunn, 1988). Other circumstances that previously warranted tracheotomy, such as cervical spine disorders and injuries that prevent neck movement, may now be intubated by using a flexible fiberoptic endoscope (Wenig, 1991).

In the setting of acute airway obstruction, tracheotomy should not be considered the procedure of last resort. Instead, it should be performed quickly, and when possible, in a controlled setting. Needless to say, it is usually not the first step in airway management. Clinical judgment warrants a logical and safe approach using a variety of techniques to secure a safe airway.

Endotracheal intubation has become the procedure of choice in the emergency situation, and effective ventilation, bronchial toilet, airway control, and general anesthesia can be achieved with this method. This has obviated the precipitous emergency tracheotomy on a struggling patient in the corridor with improper lighting or instrumentation, resulting in an unacceptably high mortality rate. Patients subsequently requiring long-term ventilatory support may be considered for elective tracheotomy within 7 to 10 days postintubation. Therefore, there are very few and specific indications for an emergency tracheotomy without the benefit of previous endotracheal intubation. The only indication for emergency tracheotomy occurs when airway control cannot be secured by endotracheal intubation or cricothyroidotomy. This is usually in the setting of trauma to the larynx or hypopharynx or a deforming injury to the mandible or maxillofacial areas (Mulder and Marelli, 1992; Hardy, 1973; Orringer, 1980).

Tracheobronchial Toilet

Tracheotomy may be necessary to maintain adequate pulmonary toilet in patients who have pneumonia, bronchiectasis, or chronic aspiration secondary to either a neurologic or a structural disorder affecting laryngeal function.

Respiratory Support

Patients receiving prolonged ventilatory support are exposed to a variety of delayed complications from endotracheal intubation. These include mucosal lesions, posterior glottic and subglottic stenosis, tracheal stenosis, and cricoid abscess.

In a prospective study, Santos and associates (1989) showed that after a mean of 10 days intubation, 94 percent of patients had laryngeal erythema and 67 percent had vocal cord ulceration. In the majority of patients, both the erythema and ulceration resolved within 8 weeks following extubation. The presence of a nasogastric tube and the use of a larger endotracheal tube appear to increase the risk of laryngeal injury.

The true frequency of laryngeal stenosis and its relation to the duration of intubation remains unknown (Bishop, et al., 1984). A review of the literature suggests an incidence of less than 5 percent of long-term laryngeal dysfunction (Bishop, et al., 1984). The study by Whited in 1983 showed no evidence of postintubation stenosis in 50 patients intubated for less than 5 days and a 5 percent incidence of stenosis in 100 patients intubated for between 6 and 10 days; Whited noted, however, that 14 percent of 50 patients intubated for more than 10 days developed either glottic, subglottic, or tracheal stenosis. No consensus exists, however, regarding the specific time when conversion from endotracheal intubation to a tracheostomy tube should occur. A flexible, prospective, and anticipatory approach that emphasizes individualization of care is recommended. Endotracheal tubes are maintained if extubation appears probable within 7 to 10 days from the onset of respiratory failure. After 7 days of mechanical ventilation, if extubation seems unlikely in the next 5 to 7 days, tracheotomy should be considered. In patients who are likely to require airway support beyond 21 days, early tracheotomy should be performed to enhance patient care and comfort. Consideration of tracheotomy should not be postponed until patients have completed an arbitrary 14 to 21 days of translaryngeal intubation (Heffner, 1991).

Elimination of Dead Space

Gas exchange occurs in the alveoli and bronchioles. The larger bronchi and upper aerodigestive tract do not participate in diffusion of gases and thus are termed the *anatomic dead space*. Tracheotomy in some cases will eliminate a substantial portion of the anatomic dead space and thus improve the efficiency of ventilation.

Sleep Apnea

Persons suffering from obstructive sleep apnea represent a special group of patients requiring a tracheotomy. These patients have a normal airway while awake; however, collapse of the pharyngeal muscles occurs during sleep, and airway obstruction ensues. These patients can maintain normal oxygen saturation levels with a patent tracheostomy during sleep. The tracheostomy tube may be "corked" during waking hours to enable the patient to phonate normally. Only those apneic patients with severe ventilatory compromise who fail more conservative treatment are selected for this procedure.

Technique

Elective conventional tracheotomy is ideally undertaken in the operating room with adequate lighting, instrumentation, and assistance. However, bedside tracheotomy is sometimes performed in an intensive care unit (ICU) setting. Movement of these patients out of the ICU to an operating room entails logistic problems and risk of complications. Concerns have been expressed regarding the possibility of an increased complication rate when bedside tracheotomy is performed. Stevens and Howard (1988) found no increased incidence of complications or infection attributable to that setting. However, an operating room environment must then be provided in the ICU, with adequate sterile fields, instrumentation, lighting, and suction.

Tracheotomy may be performed under either local or general anesthesia. The patient is placed in a supine position with the neck hyperextended. Reassurance from both the surgeon and the anesthetist, in addition to adequate sedation and oxygenation, help in maintaining an orderly environment.

Following proper patient positioning, the skin of the anterior neck and chest is prepared and draped for surgery. The patient's face is best left exposed when awake. Xylocaine with 1 : 100,000 epinephrine is infiltrated locally. A horizontal incision, preferably in a skin crease, one fingerbreadth below the cricoid cartilage is used. In an emergent situation a vertical incision can be employed. The incision is carried through skin and subcutaneous tissue until the strap muscles are encountered. The strap muscles are separated at the midline and retracted laterally. The dissection proceeds bluntly in the midline until the thyroid isthmus is encountered. Several options exist to manage the thyroid isthmus. We prefer to reflect it superiorly or inferiorly without division if possible. On occasion, an enlarged thyroid isthmus must be divided for access to the trachea. This is carried out between two Kelly clamps, and the ends are oversewn with 4–0 chromic catgut.

The trachea is then stabilized and retracted cephalad with a cricoid hook. A horizontal, intercartilaginous incision is made, and the trachea is entered between the third and fourth tracheal rings. We do not routinely excise any of the tracheal wall or develop a tracheal flap. In obese patients or in those with short necks, two stay sutures of 2–0 silk may be placed in the cartilaginous rings on either side of the horizontal opening. This facilitates changing the tracheostomy tube until the stoma has matured. A tracheostomy tube of appropriate size is chosen and is inserted into the trachea with the aid of the tracheostomy tube obturator. The position of the tube is confirmed, an inner cannula is inserted (depending on the style of tube), and ventilation is then continued through the tracheostomy tube. We routinely suture a fresh tracheostomy tube to the skin with 2–0 silk sutures to help eliminate the risk of tube displacement in the early postoperative period. Tracheotomy ties may also be placed around the neck while the patient's head is held in the flexed position. A postoperative chest x-ray is recommended to exclude early complications of malposition or pneumothorax.

Complications

Following the work of Chevalier Jackson, the operative mortality rate from tracheotomy was reduced from 25 to 1 percent by the late 1920s. This figure compares well with those of more recent publications reporting 0 to 5 percent mortality rates according to circumstances and population (Stock, et al., 1986).

Since the early 1970s the reported incidence of complications associated with tracheotomy has been reduced significantly. In part, this reduction is related to the development of an improved, controlled intraoperative environment, selection of the most appropriate tube and cuff, and improved postoperative care. Complications can be divided into those occurring in the intraoperative, immediate postoperative, and late postoperative periods.

Intraoperative

Hemorrhage. Major hemorrhage during the procedure is rare, unless an unusually high innominate artery is inadvertently cauterized or otherwise injured. Minor bleeding from the anterior jugular veins or thyroid isthmus is easily controlled locally with ligatures and cauterization.

Cardiorespiratory Arrest. Cardiorespiratory arrest, a potentially fatal event, may arise from vagal reflexes, failure to obtain an airway, tension pneumothorax, postobstructive (negative-pressure) pulmonary edema, oxygen administration to a patient with chronic carbon dioxide retention, or malplacement of the tube into the soft tissues or mainstem bronchus. Patients who have a known history of carbon dioxide retention should be monitored and ventilated in the immediate postoperative period.

Pneumothorax and Pneumomediastinum. Pneumothorax and pneumomediastinum may occur secondary to direct damage to the pleura, dissection of air through soft tissue planes, or rupture of a bleb. The reported incidence of pneumothorax after tracheotomy in adults is 0 to 4 percent (Goldstein, et al., 1987). It is more common in children because the dome of the pleura often extends above the clavicles. Peritracheal dissection should be kept to a minimum, and the tracheostomy tube should be inserted under direct vision. A postoperative chest film is mandatory.

Immediate Postoperative

Hemorrhage. Minor local oozing can be controlled by packing and ensuring that the cuff on the tracheostomy tube is inflated. Major bleeding not controlled by local measures will require reoperation, under a controlled setting with good exposure and lighting, to isolate and ligate the offending vessel.

Wound Infection. A tracheotomy is considered a clean-contaminated wound. It is rapidly colonized by hospital flora, usually *Pseudomonas* and *Escherichia coli*. Prophylactic antibiotics are usually not warranted, as the wound is left open to facilitate drainage. True infection is rare and requires only local therapy. Antibiotic coverage is needed only if surrounding cellulitis develops (Myers and Carrau, 1991).

Subcutaneous Emphysema. In the early postoperative period, subcutaneous emphysema is caused by positive-pressure ventilation or coughing against a tightly sutured or packed wound. It can be prevented by not suturing the wound around the tube or by packing the wound closed. The emphysema will resolve spontaneously within a few days. A chest radiograph should be obtained to rule out a pneumothorax.

Tube Obstruction.   The tube can be obstructed by inspissated mucus, blood clot, displacement into surrounding soft tissues, or abutment of the tube's open tip against the tracheal wall. Failure to reestablish adequate ventilation by sectioning through the tube requires immediate replacement of the inner cannula or the entire tube (Myers and Carrau, 1991).

Tube Displacement.   Early displacement or attempted replacement of the tube can create an airway emergency. The multiple layers of subcutaneous fascia, strap muscles, and pretracheal fascia slide over each other, obliterating the fresh tract. *Orotracheal intubation should be performed when the tract cannot be reestablished immediately.* This early complication can be prevented by suturing the breastplate of the tracheostomy tube to the skin: two stay sutures in the tracheal wall on either side of the stoma can be left in place to provide quick access in the event of displacement in the early postoperative period. Fusion of the multiple layers of fascia occurs at 5 to 7 days, making tracheostomy tube replacement safe.

Swallowing Problems.   The major swallowing disorder associated with tracheotomy is aspiration. Both mechanical and neurophysiologic factors in the tracheotomized patient contribute to an abnormal swallow. Mechanical factors include (1) decreased laryngeal elevation and (2) esophageal compression and obstruction from the tracheostomy tube cuff, resulting in overflow of esophageal contents into the airway. Neurophysiologic factors include (1) desensitization of the larynx, with loss of protective reflexes, and (2) uncoordinated laryngeal closure due to chronic upper airway bypass. Postoperative nursing care is of the utmost importance in minimizing aspiration (Nash, 1988).

Late

Trachea–Innominate Artery Fistula.   Trachea–innominate artery fistula is a rare but life-threatening complication, occurring in less than 1 percent of tracheotomies (Jones, et al., 1976). Most fistulae appear to result from direct pressure of the cannula against the innominate artery. This problem results from the creation of the tracheostoma lower than the fifth cartilaginous ring, with downward migration of the stoma, or from an aberrant, high-riding innominate artery. A ''sentinel bleed'' of bright, red blood may herald this particular complication. Temporary occlusion of the arterial injury may be attempted by a combination of digital pressure within the stoma and overinflation of the tracheostomy tube cuff. At times orotracheal intubation is necessary to provide room for finger pressure in the stoma. Emergency median sternotomy and arterial repair are required as definitive management. The prognosis of survival after developing a fistula is poor. There were only 24 survivors among 175 patients who suffered such fistulae, as reported in a review of the world literature (Nelems, 1987).

A sentinal bleed suggesting a trachea–innominate artery fistula is a brief, dramatic, bright red bleeding episode, which stops promptly. A small crack in the innominate artery opens and closes because of changes in position of the tracheostomy tube or the vessel. It may be difficult to detect this crack even at postmortem examination. It is not practical to try to identify such a lesion by bronchoscopy, although endoscopy can provide evidence of other sources of bleeding if the diagnosis is less clear. Occlusion of the arterial side of the trachea–innominate artery fistula can be accomplished by placing a gloved finger on the fracture line just anterior to the tracheostomy tube.

The bleeding is more easily and better controlled when the tracheostomy tube is replaced with a standard endotracheal tube brought out through the tracheal stoma. Some authors have recommended using two tubes so that the balloon of one can be used as a replacement for the finger and the second endotracheal tube can be passed either through the mouth or through the tracheostomy. Inflation of the second cuff below the occluding cuff secures the airway while the first cuff controls the bleeding. Stabilization of this double intubation of the stoma should be maintained by the surgeon's hand during immediate transfer to the operating room for sternotomy with the tamponading and ventilating tubes in place. Bleeding is not controllable until the proximal and distal inflow to the fistula via the subclavian, carotid, and innominate arteries has been secured. Suture ligation of the injured artery, with or without extra-anatomic bypass, is required to separate the bleeding site from the trachea. Ligation without extra-anatomic bypass is associated with cerebral infarction, particularly in older patients, in whom occlusion of the contralateral, carotid, or vertebral arteries may be present. Closure packing or repair of the trachea may be necessary. If possible, the tracheostomy tube should be removed and the patient intubated orotracheally.

Tracheal Stenosis.   Stenosis may occur at the stoma, the cuff site, or the tip of the tracheostomy tube. Since the development of soft, compliant, high-volume cuffs, the incidence of tracheal complications has greatly diminished. Cooper and Grillo (1969) showed that tracheal damage following prolonged use of a tracheostomy tube was largely due to ischemia of the tracheal mucosa, which resulted from high pressure within a stiff, noncompliant cuff. Subsequent colonization of mucosal ulcers by bacteria contributes to destruction of the cartilaginous rings, resulting in circumferential fibrous scarring. The recommended intracuff pressure should not exceed 25 cmH_2O, and, if monitored regularly, this should reduce the incidence of tracheal stenosis significantly.

Granuloma Formation.   Granuloma formation is not an uncommon complication in the late postoperative period. These lesions should be excised or removed with forceps and the base cauterized.

Tracheoesophageal Fistula.   Tracheoesophageal fistula occurs in less than 1 percent of patients undergoing tracheotomy (Stauffer, et al., 1981). It results either from inadvertent injury to the posterior tracheal wall at the time of surgery or secondarily from local irritation of the tracheostomy tube. Increased tracheal secretions or an air-filled upper digestive tract during mechanical ventilation should alert one to this complication. Initially, bypass with a nasogastric tube is imperative. Multiple surgical techniques are available for definitive closure, including direct suture closure of the defect, closure with muscle flaps, staged tracheal closure with a defunctionalized esophagus, and staged esophageal diversion (Thomas, 1972; Utley, et al., 1978).

Tracheocutaneous Fistula.   Persistent tracheocutaneous fistula occurs more frequently in patients who have had tracheostomy tubes in place for a lengthy period. In these cases the epithelium grows inward, maintaining a tract that communicates with the tracheal mucosa. Excision of this epithelial tract, while leaving a surface to granulate primarily, results in closure of a great majority of these fistulae. Alternatively, skin flaps may be elevated locally, with one layer of advancement flaps providing internal lining and the second layer of advancement flaps providing external cover.

PERCUTANEOUS TRACHEOTOMY

The percutaneous tracheotomy technique was described by Toye and Weinstein, first in 1969 and again in 1986. Commercial kits have become available since 1985 (Shiley Inc.; Cook Inc.) (Fig. 16-1). The technique is adapted from percutaneous nephrosotomy tube insertion (Ciaglia, et al., 1985). The advantages of the percutaneous method are that it is quick, efficient, and relatively inexpensive as compared with conventional tracheotomy performed in an operating room. Initial enthusiasm for this technique as a widespread tool for all physicians has been tempered by numerous reports of significant complications (Wavey, et al., 1992).

Indications

Percutaneous tracheotomy by dilatation is an approach to be used only under elective conditions. The indications are essentially the same as for conventional elective tracheotomy. The relative contraindications to percutaneous tracheotomy include young age (less than 16 years), inability to palpate a normal laryngeal cartilage and cricoid ring, an enlarged thyroid gland, calcified tracheal rings, and bleeding dyscrasias. An absolute contraindication is the need for an emergency airway (Anderson and Bartlett, 1991).

Technique

The technique is best learned by observation of and assistance to an experienced operator. The surgeon must be experienced in conventional operative tracheotomy should this become necessary owing to failure of the percutaneous approach.

Positioning of the patient, preparation of the skin, and draping are similar to those for a conventional tracheotomy. Percutaneous introducer sets, as supplied by Cook Inc. (Bloomington, IN), contain all the equipment to gain access to the trachea and dilate the stoma to the desired size. A tracheotomy tray and intubation equipment should be readily available. Three people are required to safely perform the procedure: the surgeon placing the tracheostomy, a surgical assistant, and an anesthetist. At our institution a long, jet ventilation–style catheter (endotracheal tube ventilation catheter) is introduced into the endotracheal tube to act as a guide for rapid reintubation should this become necessary (Fig. 16-2).

Sedation or light anesthesia is generally required. The skin overlying the second and third tracheal rings is infiltrated with xylocaine and 1 : 100,000 epinephrine. A 1-cm long vertical skin incision, extending from the inferior edge of the cricoid cartilage, is made. The endotracheal tube is withdrawn, so that the tip is below the vocal cords. The catheter-introducer needle is advanced through the anterior tracheal wall, at an angle of 45 degrees directed caudally, until air is freely aspirated from the tracheal lumen. The J-tip wire and guiding catheter assembly is then used to introduce sequentially larger-diameter (12 to 36 Fr) dilators until the desired size of opening is achieved (Fig. 16-3). The tracheostomy tube is then placed over an appropriate-sized dilator and advanced into the trachea over the guidewire assembly. The

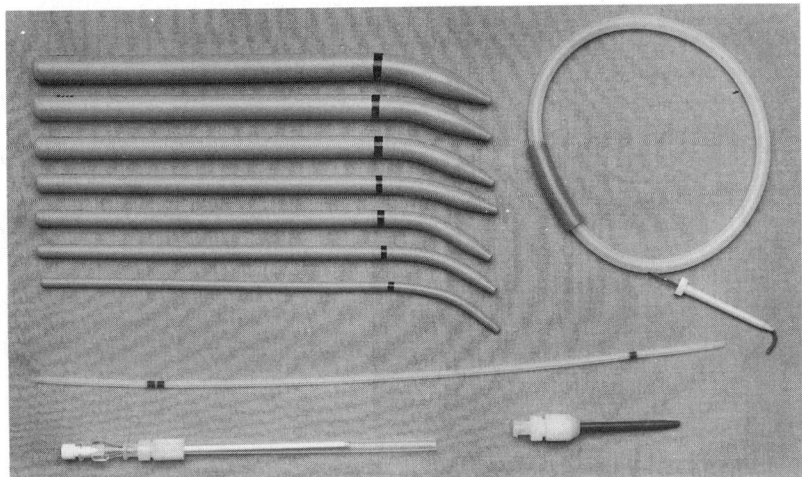

Figure 16-1.   Percutaneous tracheotomy kit as available from Cook Inc. Needle puncture of the anterior tracheal wall is followed by J-wire cannulation with Teflon oversheath. Sequential dilatation of the tracheotomy site with plastic dilators over the J wire is performed, allowing placement of a tracheostomy tube.

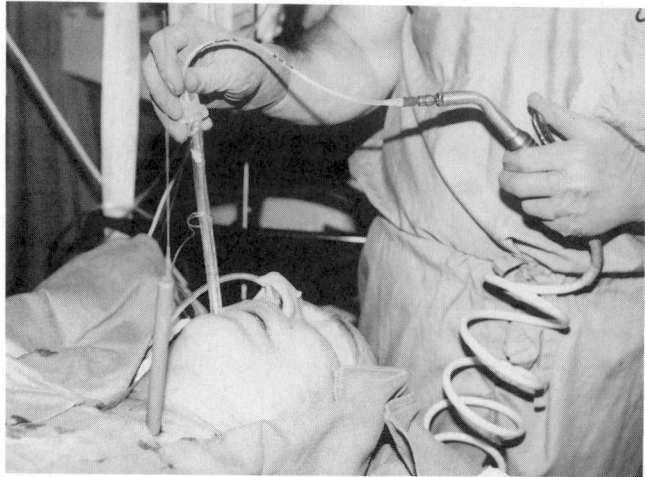

Figure 16-2. Intraoperative photograph demonstrating percutaneous tracheotomy technique with tracheal dilator in place. The patient is being ventilated through an endotracheal ventilation catheter through the mouth.

dilator assembly is removed, and the tracheostomy tube is sutured to the skin. Postoperative care is similar to that for a conventional tracheotomy.

Complications

As with any new technique, few well controlled prospective studies of the potential advantages, limitations, and possible complications of percutaneous tracheotomy have been completed. At our institution a randomized, controlled trial comparing percutaneous with conventional tracheotomy is currently underway.

Reports in the literature regarding the safety of percutaneous tracheotomy have been mixed. Several authors have

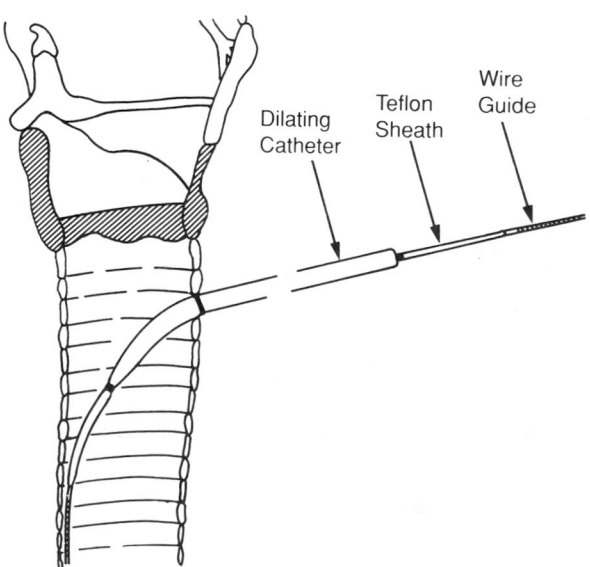

Figure 16-3. Dilators, guidewire, and introducer used in percutaneous tracheotomy.

reported success with this technique (Hazard, et al., 1988; Ciaglia, et al., 1985; Schachner, et al., 1989). Our own initial experiences have mirrored those of some other authors, who described intraoperative complications of false passage, pneumothorax, and death (Wavey, et al., 1992). With over 100 percutaneous tracheotomies performed among our university's teaching hospitals to date, the complication rates approach those of conventional tracheotomy.

EMERGENCY CRICOTHYROIDOTOMY

There is little discussion today over the value of emergency cricothyroidotomy for rapid airway access. It is recommended for immediate airway control in patients with severe facial trauma or upper airway obstruction and in those for whom endotracheal intubation or other methods of airway access are contraindicated or not possible (Walls, 1988). The procedure carries with it a complication rate roughly five times that of its elective counterpart, but it may be lifesaving in skilled hands (Esses and Jafek, 1987). In unskilled hands it may be less helpful and can be replaced by needle (14-gauge) cricothyroidotomy with high-pressure jet or bag ventilation if available (Roven and Clapham, 1983). Special cricothyroidotomy kits (Cook Inc.) are available for use in the emergency room or in the field (Fig. 16-4). Any emergency cricothyroidotomy should be converted to a formal tracheotomy as soon as possible.

Technique

The patient should be placed supine with the neck in a neutral position. After surgical preparation and the infiltration of local anaesthesia, the thyroid cartilage is stabilized while a skin incision is made horizontally over the lower half of the cricothyroid membrane. The membrane itself should be carefully incised. The scalpel handle is inserted into the incision and rotated 90 degrees to open the airway. (A tracheal spreader may be used in place of the scalpel handle.) An appropriate-size cuffed endotracheal tube or cuffed tracheostomy tube is inserted through the cricothyroid membrane incision and directed distally into the trachea. The cuff is

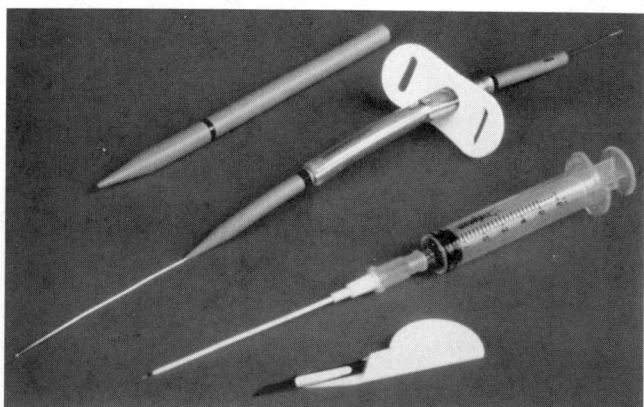

Figure 16-4. Percutaneous cricothyroidotomy kit as marketed by Cook Inc. The airway is introduced over a single dilator, which in turn is introduced over a guidewire.

then inflated and the patient ventilated. The tube is secured in position by the safest means available at the time (American College of Surgeons, 1985).

ELECTIVE CRICOTHYROIDOTOMY

Controversy regarding cricothyroidotomy has to do with its use as an elective procedure for long-term airway management. As a result of Chevalier Jackson's 1921 paper entitled "High tracheotomy and other errors—the chief causes of chronic laryngeal stenosis," cricothyroidotomy was eschewed as a method of long-term airway management for the next 50 years. As a method for elective long-term airway management it was reintroduced to the medical community by Brantigan and Grow in 1976. They reported on 655 patients who underwent elective cricothyroidotomy over a 10-year period, both for airway control during cardiac surgery and later for patients requiring long-term airway management. Complications occurred in only 6.1 percent of patients and consisted of bleeding, airway obstruction, and voice changes. There were no cases of chronic subglottic stenosis requiring resection.

The study of Brantigan and Grow had significant limitations. Most of their candidates would today be managed intraoperatively by endotracheal intubation instead of cricothyroidotomy. Moreover, the average duration of cannulation was only 7 days. Finally, follow-up on the patients was poor (completed in only 43 percent of patients), with no laryngoscopic or bronchoscopic information provided. In addition, little attention was paid to voice. It was this study, however, that spurred other clinical and experimental trials.

The suspicion that long-term endotracheal intubation was a risk factor for development of subglottic stenosis following cricothyroidotomy was confirmed by several prospective studies (Weymuller and Cummings, 1982; Sise, et al., 1984). The frequency of associated voice dysfunction was also brought to light (Weymuller and Cummings, 1982; Jakobsson, et al., 1984; Gleeson, et al., 1984). By collating all available studies looking at the complication rates from elective cricothyroidotomy, Berkey and associates (1991) were able to extrapolate the following statistics: (1) the rate of subglottic stenosis averaged approximately 4 percent; (2) voice dysfunction occurred in an average of 15 percent of patients; (3) the complication rate for this procedure averaged 25 percent.

We believe it would be a rare situation in which a more appropriate method would not be available for long-term airway management, and we would not advise the use of elective cricothyroidotomy (Burkey, et al., 1991).

MINITRACHEOTOMY

Since the early 1980s numerous methods of percutaneous transtracheal ventilation have been described in the literature. They all have in common the idea of cannulating the trachea either through the cricothyroid membrane or directly between its cartilaginous rings. Oxygen and anesthetic gases can be delivered at various rates, including maximal flow provided by high-frequency jet ventilation. The simplest form of this technique is needle cricothyroidotomy, whereby a 14-gauge intravenous catheter is plunged through the cricothyroid membrane. In an emergency, adequate gas exchange can be established temporarily at high flow rates (10 L/min) from a wall-mounted oxygen unit. Conversion to a more definitive method of airway control (e.g., by endotracheal intubation or tracheotomy) is subsequently carried out as soon as possible.

For the purpose of ventilating a patient during general anesthesia, numerous methods of elective needle cricothyroidotomy have been developed (Boyce and Peters, 1989; Monnier, et al., 1988). They are available in a variety of kit formats. The major indications for the use of such catheters include (1) emergency situations, until the patient can be better ventilated by other means; (2) elective microlaryngeal surgery in which maximum endoscopic exposure is required; and (3) prophylactic, temporary transtracheal ventilation while a difficult intubation is attempted.

The technique of minitracheotomy was first described by Matthews and Hopkinson in 1984. It varies from other percutaneous needle ventilation procedures in that it was intended for use in a more prolonged fashion.

Technique

The procedure begins with the injection of local anesthetic with 1:100,000 epinephrine into the skin overlying the cricothyroid membrane. A 1-cm stab incision, referred to as a *coniotomy,* is made in the cricothyroid membrane. A 4-mm inner diameter cannula is then passed through this opening into the trachea. The cannula has a flange attached to it for the purpose of securing ties around the neck (Minitrach II set) (Hutchinson and Hopkinson, 1989).

This technique is effective in the management of postoperative sputum retention and atelectasis. However, in a prospective evaluation by Campbell and associates (1988), it fell short of providing an adequate portal for longer-term mechanical ventilation. It is therefore not recommended as a safe alternative to conventional tracheotomy for providing a reliable airway.

KEY REFERENCES

Cole RR, Aguilar EA: Cricothyroidotomy versus tracheotomy otolaryngologist's perspective. Laryngoscope 98:131, 1988

   The authors review the literature on elective cricothyroidotomy and its complications. Their recommendations regarding indications for cricothyroidotomy and currently accepted standards of practice are presented.

Tracheotomy. Clin Chest Med 12(3) 1991

   Contributions from several disciplines, including otolaryngology and cardiothoracic surgery, offer an excellent overview on the subject of surgical airway management. The entire volume is worth reading.

Wang MB, Berke GS, Ward PM et al.: Experience with percutaneous tracheotomy. Laryngoscope 102:157, 1992

The serious complications resulting from percutaneous tracheot-

omy are well represented in this small series. Subsequent improvements in both technique and instrumentation have led to much improved outcomes for this procedure, at least in our hands.

REFERENCES

American College of Surgeons: Advanced Trauma Life Support Course—Student Manual. 1985, p. 42

Anderson HL, Bartlett RH: Elective tracheotomy for mechanical ventilation by the percutaneous technique. Clin Chest Med 12:555, 1991

Baxter FJ, Dunn GL: Acute epiglottitis in adults. Can J Anaesth 35:428, 1988

Bishop MJ, Weymuller EA, Fink BR: Laryngeal effects of prolonged endotracheal intubation. Anesth Analg 63:335, 1984

Boyce JR, Peters G: Vessel dilator cricothyrotomy for transtracheal jet ventilation. Can J Anesth 36:350, 1989

Brantigan CO, Grow JB: Cricothyroidotomy: elective use in respiratory problems requiring tracheotomy. J Thorac Cardiovasc Surg 71:72, 1976

Burkey B, Esclamado R, Morganroth M: The role of cricothyroidotomy in airway management. Clin Chest Med 12:561, 1991

Campbell JB, Watson MG, Povey L et al.: Minitracheotomy and laryngeal function. J Laryngol Otol 102:49, 1988

Ciaglia P, Firshing R et al.: Elective percutaneous dilational tracheostomy. Chest 87:715, 1985

Cooper JD, Grillo HC: Experimental production and prevention of injury due to cuffed tracheal tubes. Surg Gynecol Obstet 129:1235, 1969

Eavey RD: The Evolution of Tracheotomy-Tracheotomy. Churchill Livingstone, New York, 1985

Esses BA, Jafek BW: Cricothyroidotomy: a decade of experience in Denver. Ann Otol Rhinol Laryngol 96:519, 1987

Frost EA: Tracing the tracheotomy. Ann Otol Rhinol Laryngol 85:618, 1976

Gleeson MJ, Pearson RC, Armistead S et al.: Voice changes following cricothyroidotomy. J Laryngol Otol 98:1015, 1984

Goldstein SI, Breda SD, Schneider KL: Surgical complications of bedside tracheotomy in an otolaryngologic residency program. Laryngoscope 97:1407, 1987

Goodall EW: The story of tracheotomy. Br J Child Dis 31:167, 253, 1934

Hardy KL: Tracheostomy: indications, technics and tubes. A reappraisal. Am J Surg 126:300, 1973

Hazard PB, Garrett HE et al.: Bedside percutaneous tracheostomy. Ann Thorac Surg 46:63, 1988

Heffner JE: Timing of tracheotomy in ventilator-dependent patients. Clin Chest Med 12:611, 1991

Hutchinson J, Hopkinson RB: How to insert a Minitrach. Br J Hosp Med 42:2, 112, 1989

Jackson C: High tracheotomy and other errors—the chief causes of chronic laryngeal stenosis. Surg Gynecol Obstet 32:392, 1923

Jackson C, Jackson CL: The Larynx and Its Diseases. WB Saunders, Philadelphia, 1937

Jakobsson J, Andersson G, Wiklund PE: Experience with elective coniotomy. Acta Chir Scand Suppl 520:101, 1984

Jones JW, Reynolds M et al.: Tracheoinnominate artery erosion. Ann Surg 184:194, 1976

Matthews HR, Hopkinson RB: Treatment of sputum retention by minitracheotomy. Br J Surg 71:147, 1984

Monnier P, Ravussin P et al.: Percutaneous transtracheal ventilation for laser endoscopic treatment of laryngeal and subglottic lesions. Clin Otolaryngol 13:209, 1988

Mulder DS, Marelli D: Evolution of airway control in the management of injured patients. J Trauma 33:856, 1992

Myers EN, Carrau RL: Early complications of tracheotomy. Clin Chest Med 12(3):1991

Nash M: Swallowing problems in the tracheotomized patient. Otolaryngol Clin North Am 21:701, 1988

Nelems B: Tracheoarterial fistula. p. 69. In Grillo HC, Eschepasse H (eds): Major Challenges. In International Trends in General Thoracic Surgery. Vol. 2. WB Saunders, Philadelphia, 1987

Orringer MB: Endotracheal intubation and tracheostomy: indications, techniques, and complications. Surg Clin North Am 60:1447, 1980

Roven AN, Clapham MCC: Cricothyroidotomy. Ear Nose Throat J 62:489, 1983

Santos PM, Afrassiabi A, Weymuller EA et al.: Prospective studies evaluating the standard endotracheal tube and a prototype endotracheal tube. Ann Otol Rhinol Laryngol 95:935, 1989

Schachner A, Ovil Y et al.: Percutaneous tracheostomy—A new method. Crit Care Med 17:1052, 1989

Sise MJ, Shackford SR et al.: Cricothyroidotomy for long-term tracheal access. Ann Surg 200:13, 1984

Stauffer JL, Olson DE et al.: Complications and consequences of endotracheal intubation and tracheostomy. Am J Med 70:65, 1981

Stevens DJ, Howard DJ: Tracheotomy service for ICU patients. Ann R Coll Surg Engl 70:241, 1988

Stock MC, Woodward CG, Shapiro BA et al.: Perioperative complications of the elective tracheotomy in critically ill patients. Crit Care Med 14:861, 1986

Thomas AN: Management of tracheoesophageal fistula caused by cuffed tracheal tubes. Am J Surg 124:181, 1972

Toye FJ, Weinstein JD: Clinical experience with percutaneous tracheostomy and cricothyroidotomy in 100 patients. J Trauma 26:1034, 1986

Toye FJ, Weinstein JD: A percutaneous tracheostomy device. Surgery 65:384, 1969

Trousseau A: J Commun Med-Chir Paris: 541, 1833

Utley JR, Dillon ML et al.: Giant tracheoesophageal fistula. J Thorac Cardiovasc Surg 75:373, 1978

Walls RM: Cricothyroidotomy. Emerg Med Clin North Am 6:7725, 1988

Wavey MD, Berka GS et al.: Early experience with percutaneous tracheotomy. Laryngoscope 102:157, 1992

Wenig BL: Indications for and techniques of tracheotomy. Clin Chest Med 12(3): 1991

Weymuller EA, Cummings CW: Cricothyroidotomy: the impact of antecedent endotracheal intubation. Ann Otol Rhinol Laryngol 91:437, 1982

Whited RE: Posterior commissure stenosis post long-term intubation. Laryngoscope 93:1314, 1983

Subglottic Resection

Michael Maddaus
F. Griffith Pearson

DEFINITION

The subglottic airway extends from the inferior margin of the vocal cords above to the lower border of the cricoid cartilage below. Resection of the subglottic airway is complicated by the following factors:

1. It is in close proximity to the vocal cords.
2. Complete transsection of the subglottic airway at any level above the cricothyroid joints will divide the recurrent laryngeal nerves.
3. The posterior rim of the upper border of the cricoid cartilage supports the arytenoid cartilages, which play a critical role in vocal function.

The technique of subglottic resection, which is described in detail below, allows transverse division of the airway up to the level of the inferior border of the vocal cords *without* transsection of intact recurrent laryngeal nerves. At the level of the inferior border of the posterior cricoid plate, the recurrent nerves pass behind the cricoid cartilage. On each side the nerve passes behind the cricothyroid articulation and continues a vertical ascent to the superior border of the cricoid cartilage, at which point it passes forward to supply the glottic muscles. As long as the tissues lying behind the cricoid cartilage are undisturbed, both recurrent laryngeal nerves can be predictably preserved.

HISTORICAL NOTE

Ogura and Powers (1964) were the first to describe a segmental resection of the cricoid cartilage with primary thyrotracheal anastomosis. They reported on seven patients with subglottic obstruction secondary to blunt trauma. In all these patients, however, the recurrent laryngeal nerves were avulsed and paralyzed on both sides as a result of the original trauma. In 1974 Gerwat and Bryce described a technique of partial cricoid resection using an oblique line of transsection of the subglottic airway (Fig. 16-5), which removed the anterior cricoid arch but preserved the posterior cricoid cartilage and recurrent nerves above the level of the cricothyroid joints. With this technique, however, the level of resection of the posterior subglottic airway was limited.

In 1975 Pearson, et al. described a technique of *transverse* resection of the subglottic airway at any level below the vocal cords but with preservation of intact recurrent laryngeal nerves. This was accomplished by maintaining a posterior shell of cricoid cartilage. A primary thyrotracheal anastomosis was performed within 1 cm or less of the inferior margin of the vocal cords. This is the technique that we describe in detail in the section, Operative Technique.

HISTORICAL READINGS

Gerwat J, Bryce DP: The management of subglottic laryngeal stenosis by resection and direct anastomosis. Laryngoscope 84:940, 1974

Ogura JH, Powers WE: Functional restitution of traumatic stenosis of the larynx and pharynx. Laryngoscope 74:1081, 1964

Pearson FG, Cooper JD, Nelems JM et al.: Primary tracheal anastomosis after resection of the cricoid cartilage with preservation of recurrent laryngeal nerves. J Thorac Cardiovasc Surg 70:806, 1975

ANATOMY

A clear knowledge of the anatomy of the region is essential to an understanding of this operative technique. The anatomy of the larynx and upper airway is described in detail in Chapter 10. Some features warrant emphasis (Fig. 16-6). The cricoid cartilage is the first full ring of the upper airway, has an anterior arch similar in height to a normal tracheal ring, and expands into a broad posterior plate or rostrum. Both the inner and outer aspects of the cricoid cartilage are covered with a stout perichondrial layer, which may be freed from the underlying cartilage during certain stages of the operation. Paired arytenoid cartilages rest on the superior border of the posterior cricoid plate and articulate at the cricoarytenoid joints. The vocal cords are attached posteriorly to the vocal processes of the arytenoid cartilages and attach anteriorly to the thyroid cartilage. The subglottic larynx begins immediately below the vocal folds and extends to the inferior margin of the cricoid cartilage. The subglottic space is the narrowest part of the upper airway aside from the larynx. The subglottis has an internal diameter between 1.5 and 2 cm in the adult and is completely surrounded by the cricoid cartilage.

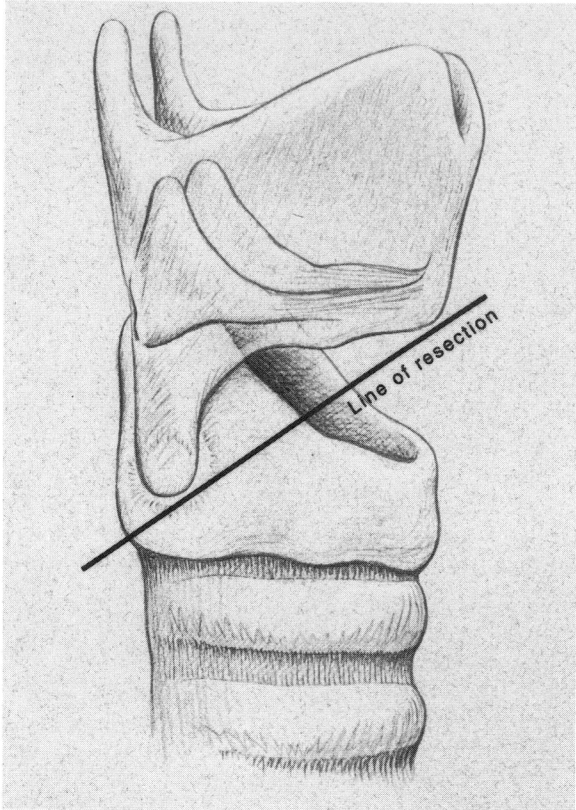

Figure 16-5. Diagram illustrating lateral view of the larynx and upper airway. The line of resection begins at the inferior border of the thyroid cartilage anteriorly and passes below the cricothyroid joint behind. This line of resection allows preservation of the recurrent laryngeal nerves and was the technique of partial cricoid resection described by Gerwat and Bryce (1974).

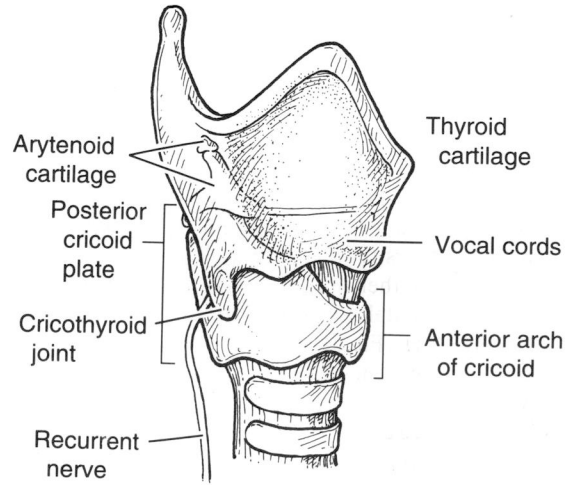

Figure 16-6. Diagrammatic illustration, lateral view, showing the pertinent anatomy of the larynx and the subglottic and upper tracheal airways.

ANESTHETIC TECHNIQUE

When necessary, the stenosis is dilated prior to operation. With the patient asleep, gum-tipped esophageal bougies are directed through a conventional intubating laryngoscope. This is the least traumatic technique for dilatation of the subglottic region. Following passage of a 34 Fr gum-tipped bougie, the anesthetist should easily pass a no. 6 or 6.5 endotracheal tube. If the intubation is difficult owing to a tight stenosis, an uncuffed tube may be preferable, since an air seal will be secured at the level of the stricture. A rigid bronchoscope can be used as the dilating instrument, but this procedure is more traumatic than use of the tapered bougies.

Once the distal airway is divided, an armored endotracheal tube is introduced through the distal trachea, and the proximal end of the tube is passed under the drapes at the side of the cheek to the anesthetist (Fig. 16-7A).

INDICATIONS

Postintubation injury remains the most common cause of subglottic stenosis that is amenable to resection and primary reconstruction (Fig. 16-8). The injury follows translaryngeal intubation, with or without a subsequent tracheotomy. A high tracheotomy or cricothyroidotomy may result in injury within the cricoid ring, even in the absence of prior translaryngeal intubation. Other causes of benign stenosis are blunt trauma with cricotracheal disruption, idiopathic subglottic stenosis, inhalation injury due to thermal or chemical burns, and rare miscellaneous conditions such as primary amyloidosis. On occasion, neoplasms of the upper airway may be amenable to subglottic resection with sparing of the larynx and voice. To date we have used this approach in 11 patients, including 3 with adenoid cystic carcinoma, 2 with squamous cell carcinoma, 2 with mucoepidermoid carcinoma, 2 with neurofibroma, and 2 with thyroid carcinoma. It should be emphasized, however, that a majority of primary malignancies involving the subglottic airway will be best managed by a resection that includes a laryngectomy.

Monnier and Savary (1993) were the first to demonstrate the successful application of this operation in infants and children suffering from obstruction due to postintubation stenosis or congenital subglottic stenosis. They have shown that such resections do not interfere with the normal growth and development of the larynx and subglottis in long-term follow-up. Of their 15 pediatric patients, 4 were less than 1 year of age at the time of operation, and 14 of the 15 were successfully extubated, with follow-up of 1 to 15 years.

MANAGEMENT

Operative Technique

Subglottic Resection

The neck is fully extended, with some type of bolster placed behind the scapulae. Exposure is obtained with a generous collar incision, which is located at a level that will best expose the pathology in the upper airway. Subplatysmal skin flaps are developed to provide exposure from the thyroid notch above to the suprasternal notch below. The strap muscles

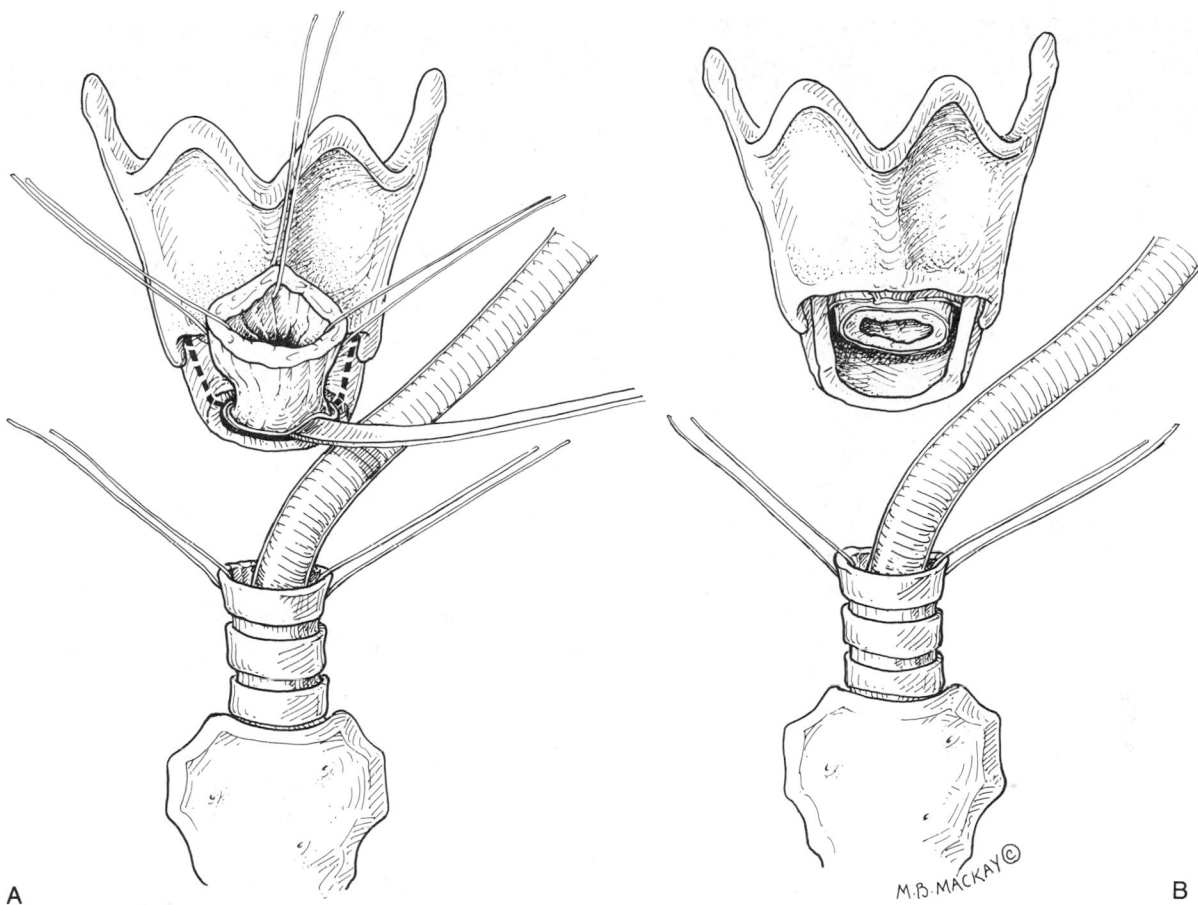

A   M.B. MACKAY©   B

Figure 16-7. **(A)** The airway has been divided just beyond the stenotic lesion and the distal trachea intubated with the armored endotracheal tube. Stay sutures have been placed in the divided tracheal ends. The anterior and lateral components of the cricoid cartilage have been removed, and it is now possible to develop the subperichondrial plane in front of the posterior cricoid plate. This is usually done with a small orthopedic elevator. This avascular plane can be developed posteriorly and laterally to a level just below the arytenoid cartilages and vocal folds. **(B)** The soft tissue airway is now divided above the lesion, through an area of healthy mucosa in the subglottic region. This line of division may lie within a few millimeters of the inferior margins of the vocal cords. A posterior shell of the remaining cricoid cartilage is exposed and protects the posteriorly situated recurrent nerves.

are reflected from the midline to expose the anterior aspect of the thyroid and cricoid cartilages and the adjacent cervical trachea (Fig. 16-9). In these cases the pathology lies within the cricoid ring and commonly extends to the adjacent cervical trachea. The lines of resection for this isolated subglottic lesion are illustrated in Figure 16-10.

The upper trachea in the region of the diseased segment is freed circumferentially to the level of the inferior border of the cricoid ring. Dissection is maintained immediately against the outer surface of the airway, which protects the recurrent laryngeal nerves posterolaterally. In patients with benign lesions, no attempt is made to identify the recurrent nerves, which are frequently obscured by peritracheal scar. When operating for neoplasm, however, it may be necessary to identify one or the other recurrent laryngeal nerve in order to determine the extent of neoplastic involvement.

Once the inferior border of the cricoid cartilage has been identified, the exposed perichondrium is incised with a scalpel or by cautery. In most patients it is possible to free the

perichondrium from the underlying cartilage by using a small orthopedic elevator (Fig. 16-11). The entire circumference of the inferior border of the cricoid cartilage is exposed under the perichondrium, and the entire anterolateral ring of the cricoid cartilage is then freed from its perichondrial cover (Fig. 16-12). The exposed anterior and lateral aspects of the cricoid arch are then removed, usually in piecemeal fashion with small rongeurs (Fig. 16-13).

The trachea is then transected at the distal end of the lesion, and the distal airway is intubated with an armored endotracheal tube (Fig. 16-7A). Stay sutures are placed in the divided tracheal ends, above and below. It is now possible to develop the subperichondrial plane in front of the posterior cricoid plate. Once again, by using an orthopedic elevator this avascular plane can be freed almost to the inferior margins of the cricoarytenoid joints (Fig. 16-7A). The airway is then divided above the stenosis, through healthy mucosa in the subglottic region (Fig. 16-7B). This line of division may lie within a few millimeters of the inferior margins of the vocal

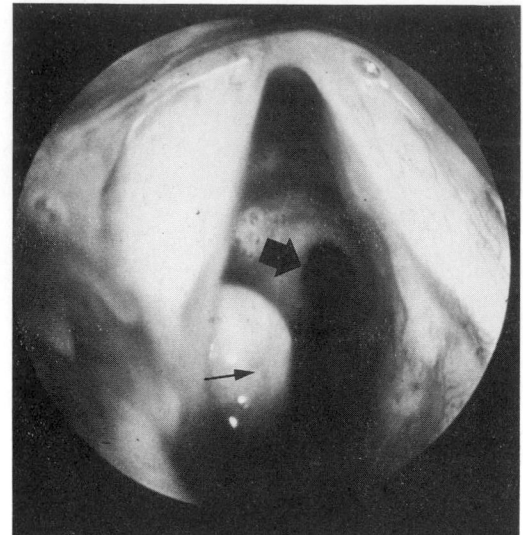

A

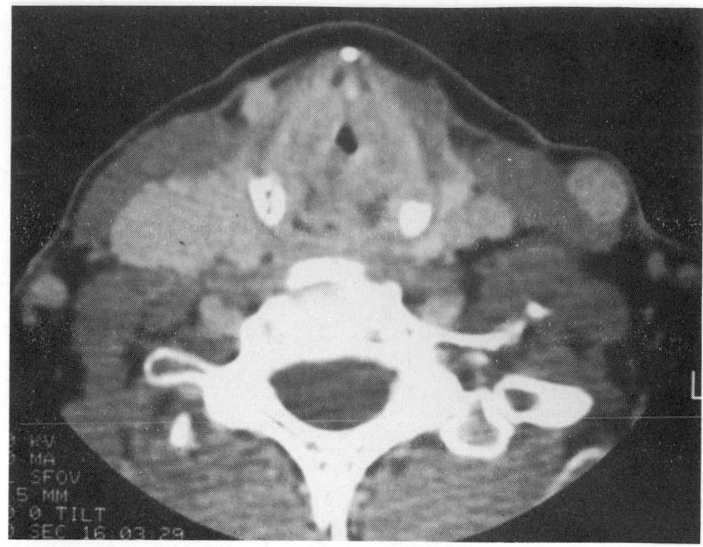

B

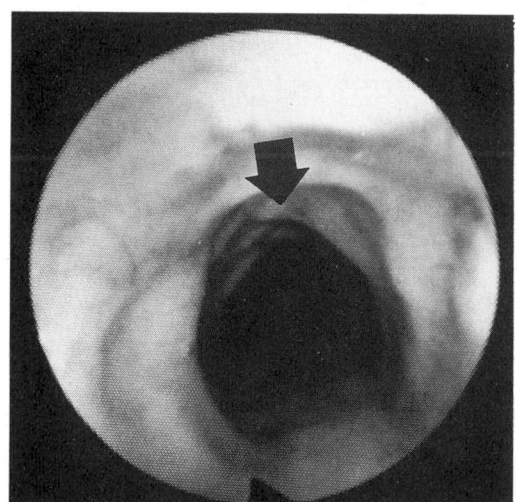

C

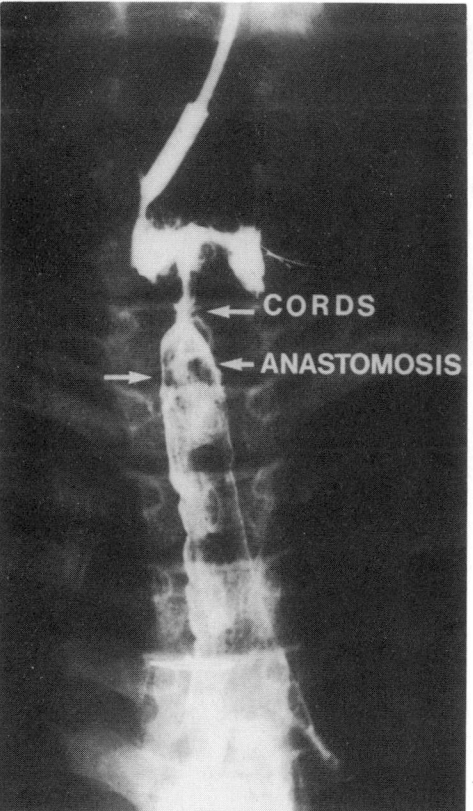

D

Figure 16-8. **(A)** Postintubation injury. There is a polypoid granulation projecting from the posterior third of the left vocal cord (*small arrow*). In the subglottic area, a concentric stenosis is just visible (*large arrow*). **(B)** CT scan (1.5-mm-interval cut) at the subglottic level showing a severe stenosis with marked circumferential submucosal thickening (scar). (Same patient as in Fig. A.) **(C)** Photograph obtained 1 year after subglottic resection and reconstruction by primary thyrotracheal anastomosis. The subglottic airway is healthy throughout, with a complete mucosal covering, and normal airway diameters. The thin line of scar that identifies the anastomosis is almost invisible (*arrow*). (Same patient as in Figs. A and B). **(D)** Contrast tracheogram obtained 1 year after operation in the same patient. The anastomosis is widely patent, and lies within 1 cm of the inferior aspect of the vocal cords.

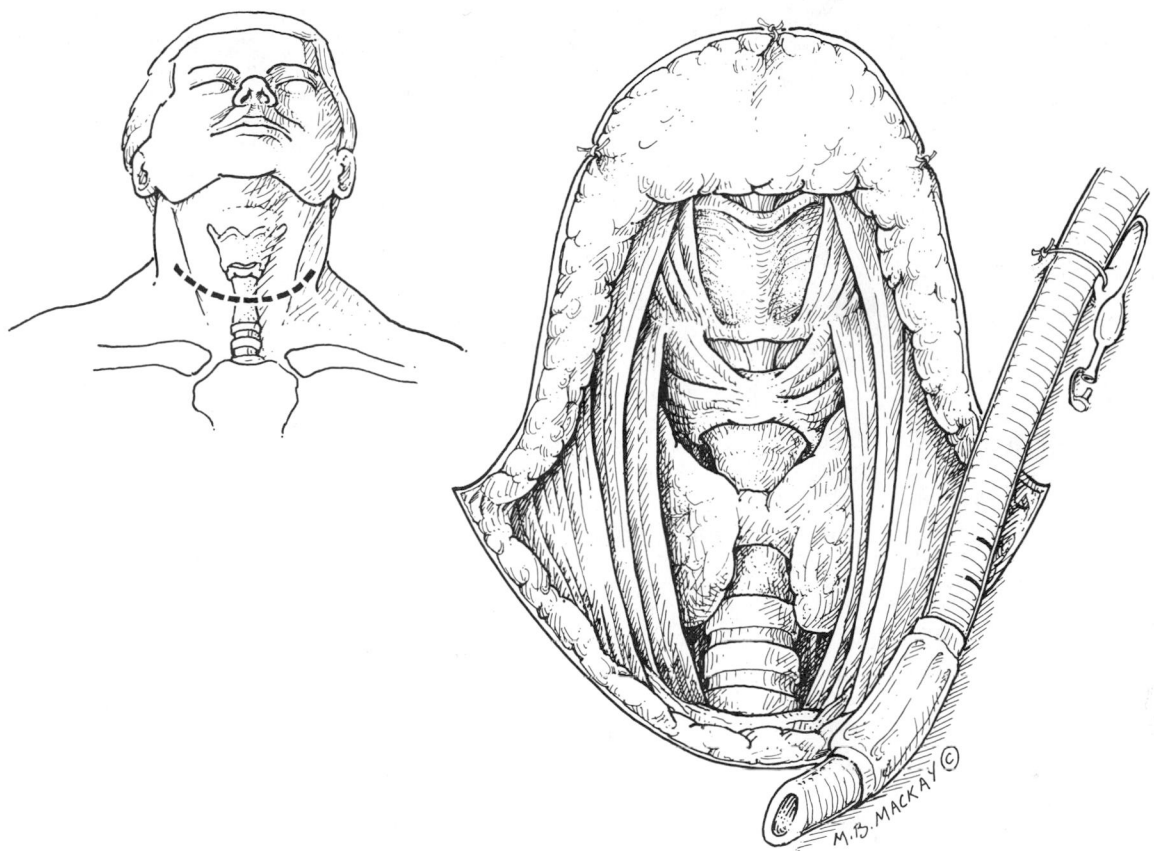

Figure 16-9. Diagram illustrating the location of a generous collar incision (*upper left inset*) and the subsequent exposure of the upper airway following retraction of upper and lower skin flaps developed in the subplastimal plane. The airway is exposed from the level of the thyroid notch above to the suprasternal notch below. The strap muscles have been reflected from the midline, and the anterior aspects of the thyroid, cricoid and upper tracheal cartilages have been exposed.

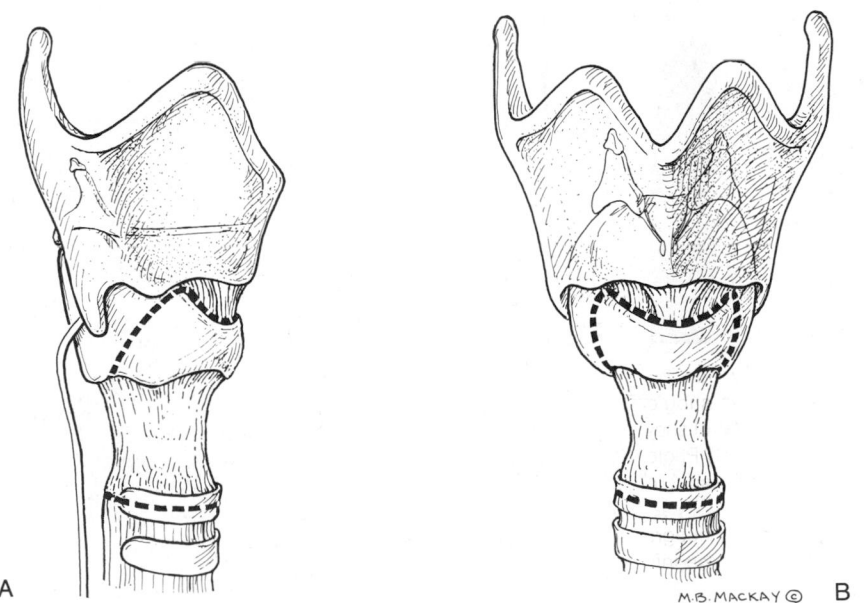

Figure 16-10. **(A)** Lateral and **(B)** anteroposterior (AP) projections showing the resection margins for a benign postintubation stenosis, which involves the subglottic airway, within the cricoid ring, as well as the proximal cervical trachea.

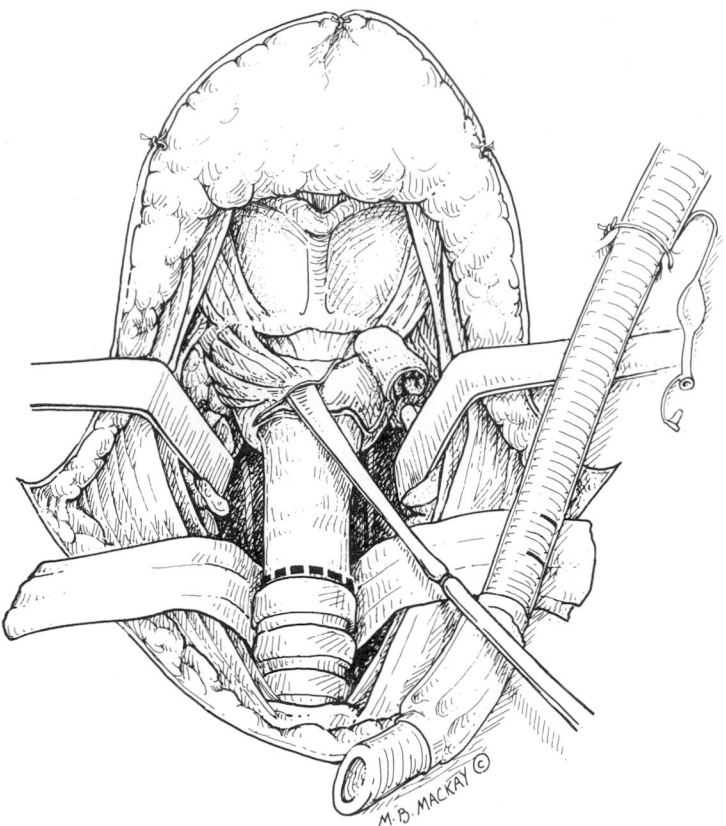

Figure 16-11. Diagram illustrating technique of subperichondrial exposure of the anterior and lateral aspects of the cricoid cartilage. The perichondrium has been incised along the inferior border of the arch and is being freed from the underlying cartilage by means of a small orthopedic elevator. The damaged and stenotic lesion extends for several centimeters below the cricoid and has been mobilized circumferentially. The distal airway will be divided at the level of the dotted line, and an armored orotracheal tube has been secured along the left side of the neck for intubation of the distal airway following transsection.

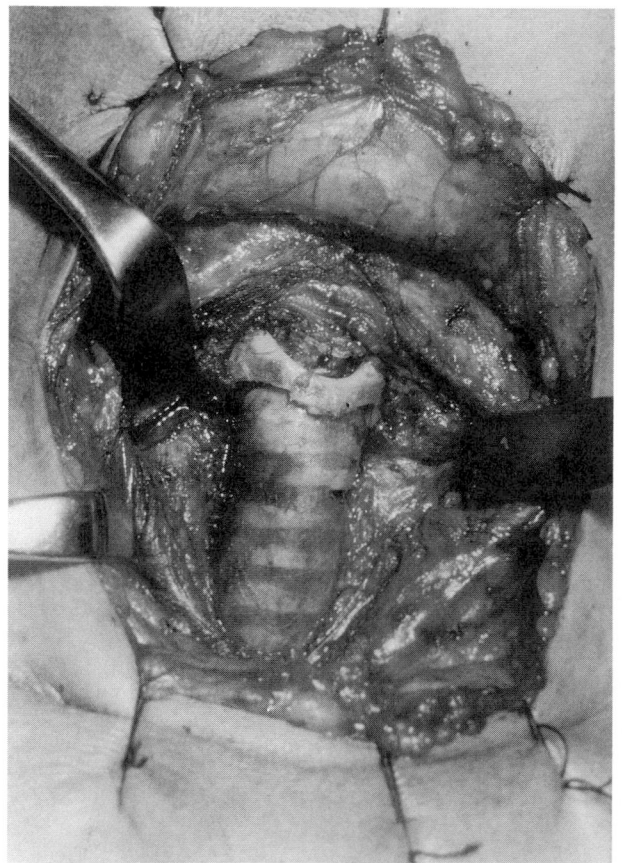

A

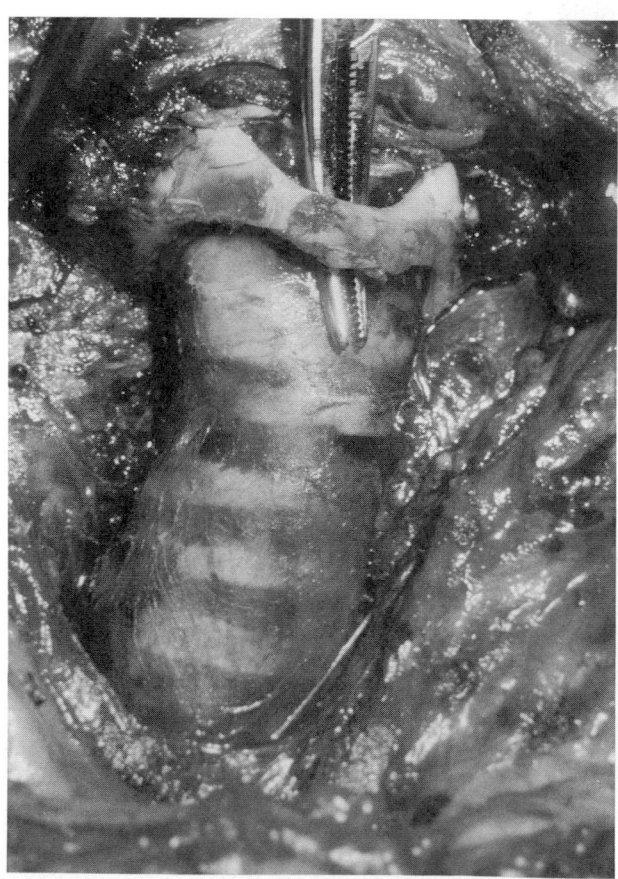

B

Figure 16-12. **(A)** Operative photograph illustrating the anterior cricoid cartilage after it has been freed completely of its perichondrial cover. **(B)** The tip of a hemostat has been passed behind the anterior cricoid arch, demonstrating the circumferential mobilization.

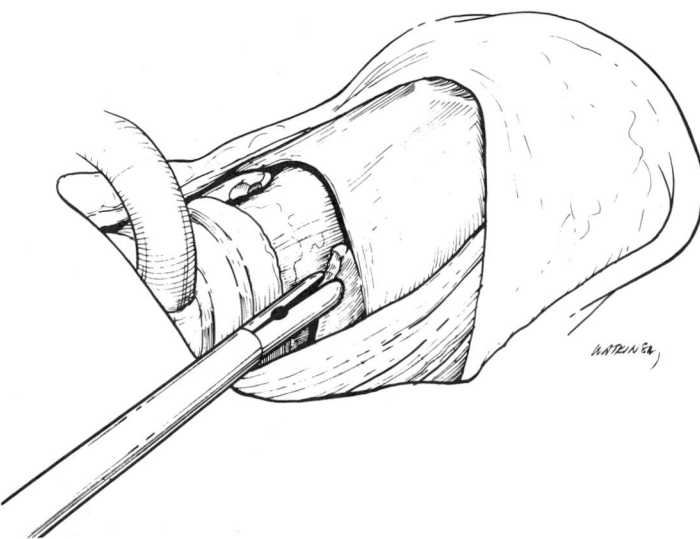

Figure 16-13. Diagram illustrating removal of the exposed anterior and lateral aspects of the cricoid arch using a small rongeurs.

cords. The posterior shell of the remaining cricoid cartilage is exposed and protects the posteriorly situated recurrent laryngeal nerves.

If the external, posterior aspect of the cricoid plate is freed subperichondrially, the posterior cartilage may also be removed up to the level of the proposed anastomosis. This may be necessary in patients with a damaged or chronically infected posterior cricoid cartilage. The remaining subglottic airway now consists of a stout tube of perichondrium with underlying mucosa and submucosa. There will inevitably be a discrepancy in luminal diameter between the subglottic airway (smaller) and the cut end of the distal trachea. It is usually desirable to plicate the membranous component of the distal trachea in order to accommodate these differences in diameter (Fig. 16-14A).

An end-to-end thyrotracheal anastomosis is performed with use of interrupted sutures (Fig. 16-14B). Our preference is to use 35-gauge stainless steel wire on the posterior wall with knots tied on the inside. The lateral and anterior part of the anastomosis is completed with interrupted sutures of 3–0 or 4–0 Vicryl, with knots tied on the outside.

Subglottic Resection and Synchronous Laryngeal Reconstruction

Synchronous laryngotracheal injury is commonly seen following prolonged translaryngeal intubation (Maddaus, et al., 1993). The most common glottic injury is a posterior interarytenoid stenosis, which restricts abduction of the vocal cords. These combined injuries are best managed collaboratively with the otolaryngologist. A review of our group's experience with postintubation glottic injury was recently reported by Gullane, et al. (1994).

The lines of incision and transection for a synchronous combined procedure are illustrated in Figure 16-15. The technique of mobilization of the cervical trachea and cricoid is similar to that used for resection of isolated subglottic stenosis (Fig 16-16). In these cases, however, the thyroid cartilage

is divided in the midline anteriorly (Fig. 16-17A). When the margins of the laryngofissure are retracted laterally, the vocal cords and upper subglottic region are exposed (in Figure 16-17B the subglottic pathology is resected, but the interarytenoid scar remains—see dotted line).

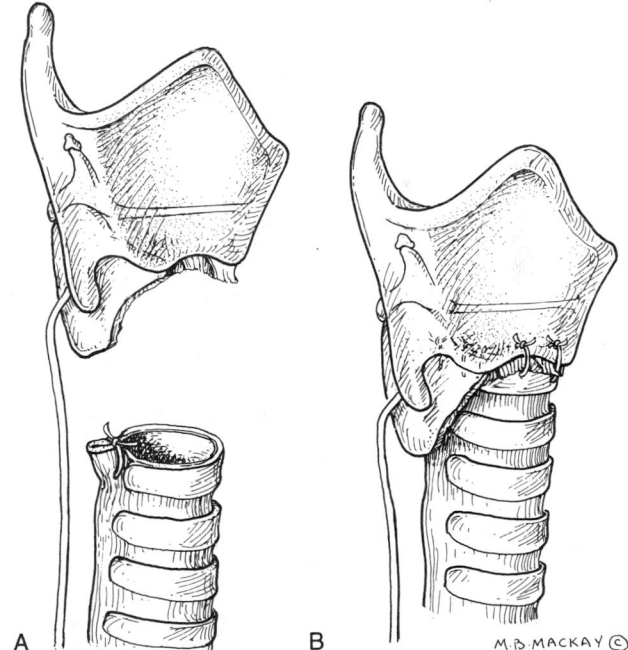

Figure 16-14. **(A)** Diagram illustrating the technique of plication of the membranous trachea in order to match the luminal diameters of the tracheal and subglottic airways at the level of anastomosis. This also restores a complete cartilaginous ring in the subglottic larynx. **(B)** Diagram illustrating an end-to-end thyrotracheal anastomosis. This anastomosis is begun posteriorly using interrupted sutures of fine-gauge (35 Fr) stainless steel wire, with the knots tied inside. The lateral and anterior margins of the anastomosis are then closed by interrupted sutures of 3–0 or 4–0 Vicryl with the knots tied on the outside.

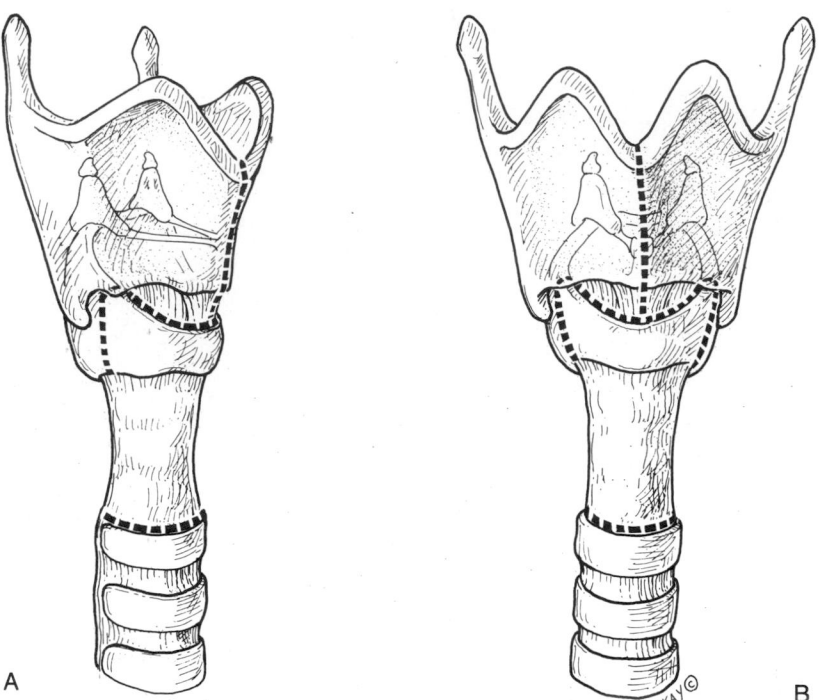

Figure 16-15. **(A)** Lateral and **(B)** AP diagrams illustrating the lines of incision and transsection for subglottic resection and synchronous laryngeal reconstruction. In this operation a laryngofissure is made by using a vertical incision in the midline of the thyroid cartilage anteriorly.

A

B

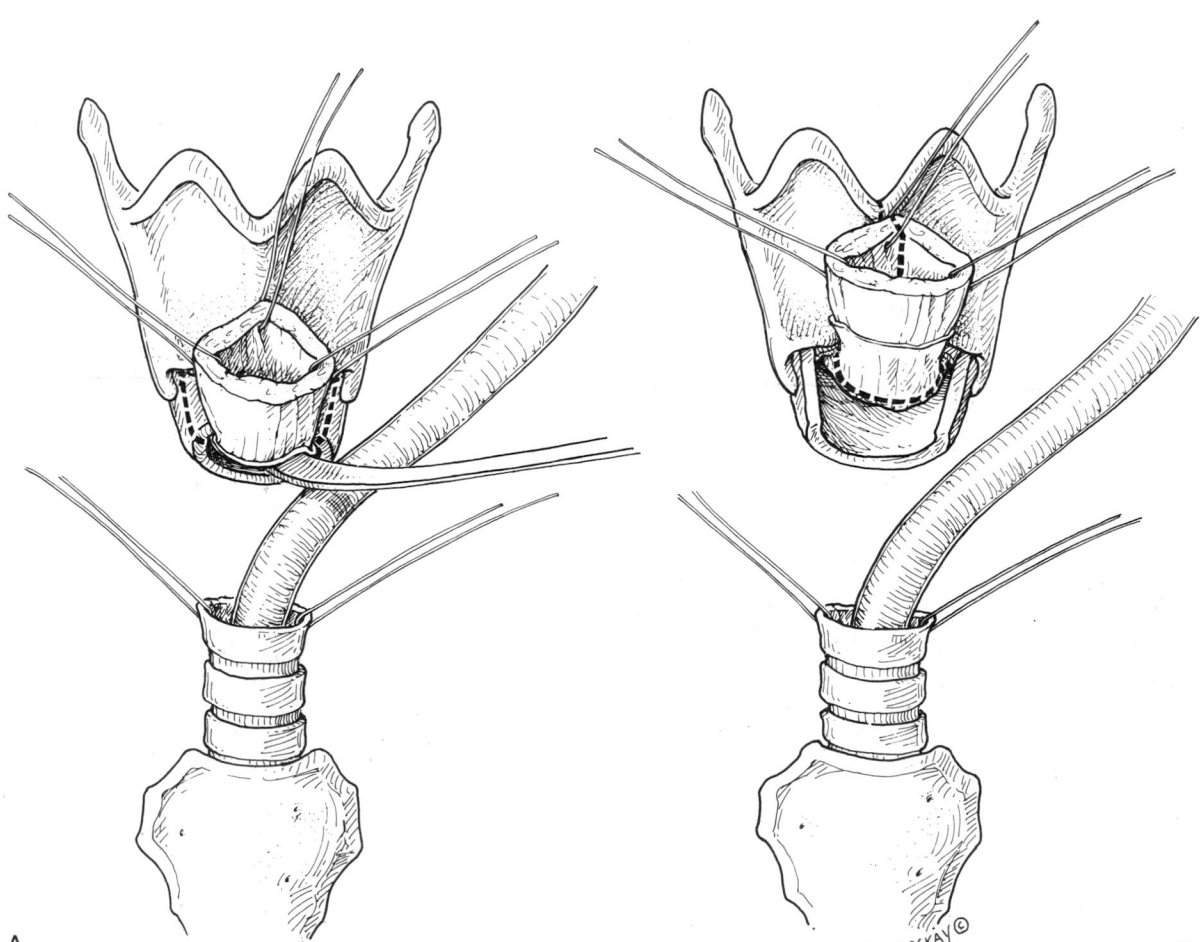

A

B

Figure 16-16. **(A)** Diagram illustrating mobilization and resection of the subglottic defect. The cricoid arch has been freed subperichondrially and resected, and the trachea has been divided below the lesion and intubated for ventilation. The avascular, subperichondrial plane in front of the posterior cricoid plate is being developed with a small orthopaedic elevator. **(B)** The stenotic lesion in the subglottic airway has been freed posteriorly to a level above the pathology.

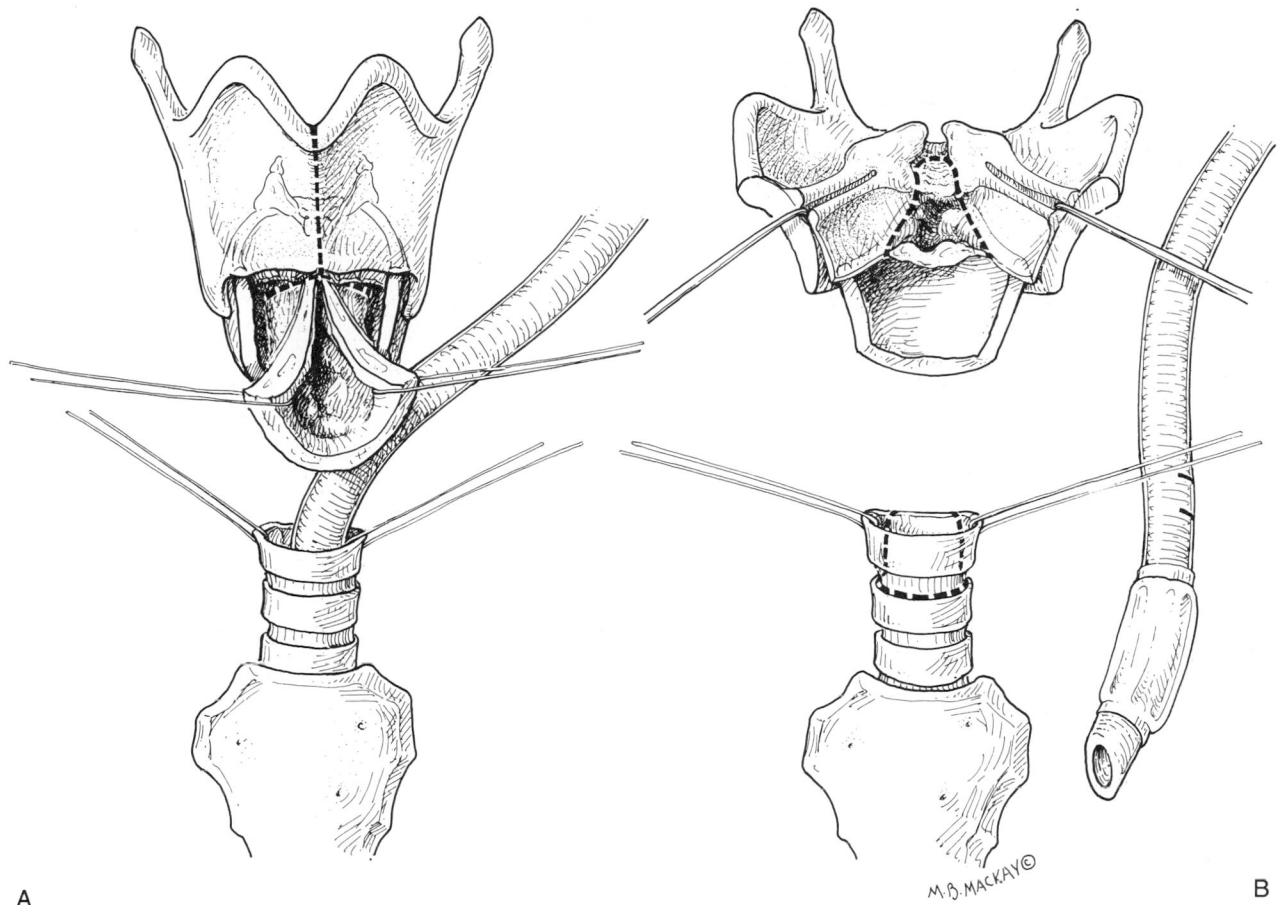

A

B

M.B. MACKAY©

Figure 16-17. **(A)** Diagram illustrating the diseased and stenotic airway, which has been opened anteriorly in the midline to the level of the thyroid cartilage. The subglottic airway will be transsected above the pathology (*transverse dotted line*) and the larynx exposed by a laryngofissure. **(B)** The laryngofissure has been completed and the diseased subglottic segment resected. The margins of the thyroid cartilage are separated with small retracting hooks, which are positioned at the anterior ends of the vocal cords in the diagram. Following resection of the subglottic stenosis, a broad plate of inferior cricoid cartilage is exposed. There is still a dense interarytenoid scar, which will be excised within the margins of the upper dotted line. A posterior pedicled flap of membranous trachea will be fashioned from the distal cut margin of the airway (*lower dotted line*) and will be used to resurface the interarytenoid defect.

When the interarytenoid scar is excised, a posterior mucosal defect is created, which extends to the upper margins of interarytenoid mucosa (Fig. 16-18A). This defect will be resurfaced by using a pedicled flap of membranous trachea fashioned from the distal tracheal margins (Fig. 16-18B). To create this vascularized pedicle of membranous trachea, it is necessary to resect one or two of the anterolateral cartilaginous rings. The mucosal flap is then secured with interrupted sutures of fine-gauge stainless steel wire, as illustrated in Figure 16-18. Figures 16-19 to 16-23 are operative photographs illustrating laryngofissure, excision of interarytenoid scar, and preparation of a pedicled flap of posterio membranous distal trachea, which will be used to resurface the posterior glottic defect. The remainder of the thyrotracheal anastomosis is completed with interrupted 3–0 or 4–0 Vicryl sutures. The laryngofissure is closed anteriorly with interrupted 3–0 or 4–0 Vicryl sutures (Fig. 16-24). When the subglottic anastomosis lies within a few millimeters of the vocal cords, there is an unpredictable risk of postoperative glottic edema. This problem is managed by placement of a small distal tracheostomy tube or placement of a silicone Montgomery T tube, with the upper limb of the T tube lying 0.5 to 1 cm above the vocal cords, as illustrated in Figure 16-24. Depending on the status of the airway at the margins of this high anastomosis, the T tube may be left in position for intervals varying from a few weeks to 3 or more months.

The incision is closed as described previously. A stout suture of 5–0 Tevdek secures the skin of the chin to the skin of the chest to maintain neck flexion during the first postoperative week.

Postoperative Management

If a Montgomery T tube is placed, the cervical arm should be closed or corked, so that breathing occurs through the nose and mouth and the normal mechanisms for humidification of

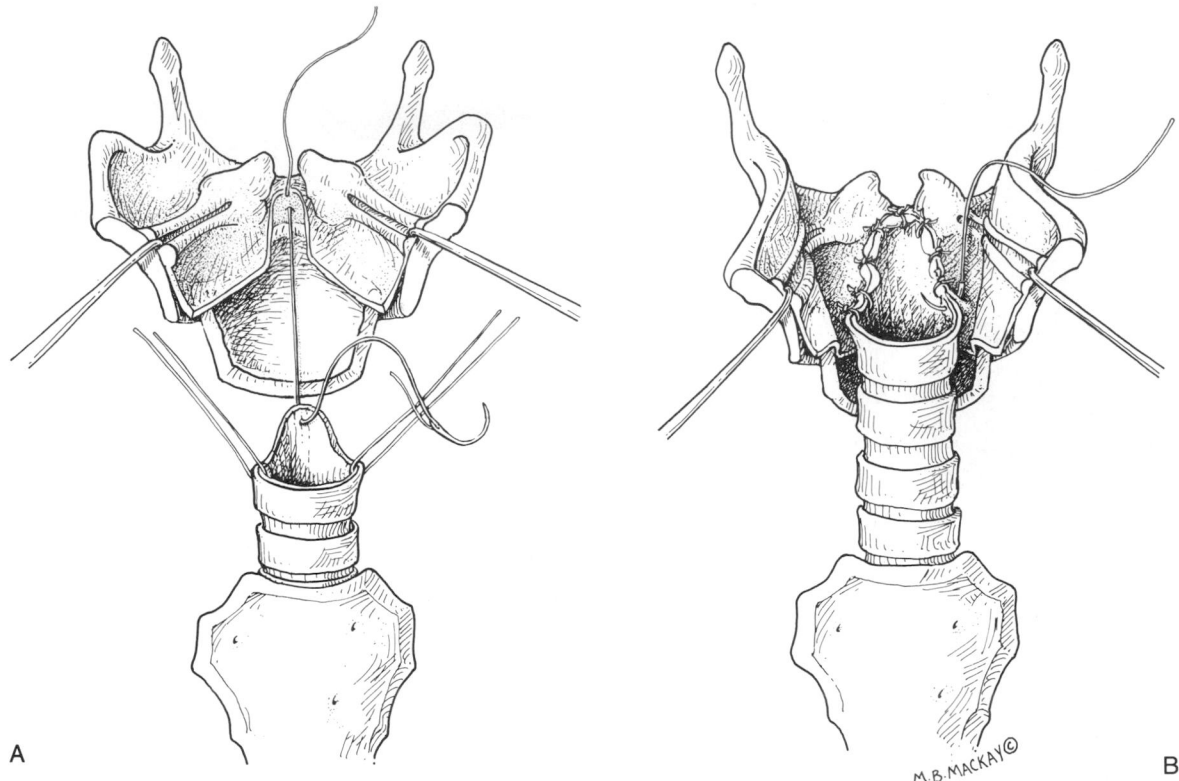

A   B

Figure 16-18. **(A)** The posterior mucosal flap has been developed at the distal resection margin, and the first of a series of interrupted sutures is placed in order to secure the flap in the interarytenoid defect. **(B)** The completed closure of the posterior defect is illustrated. We prefer fine-gauge stainless steel wire for this part of the anastomosis, with the knots tied on the inside.

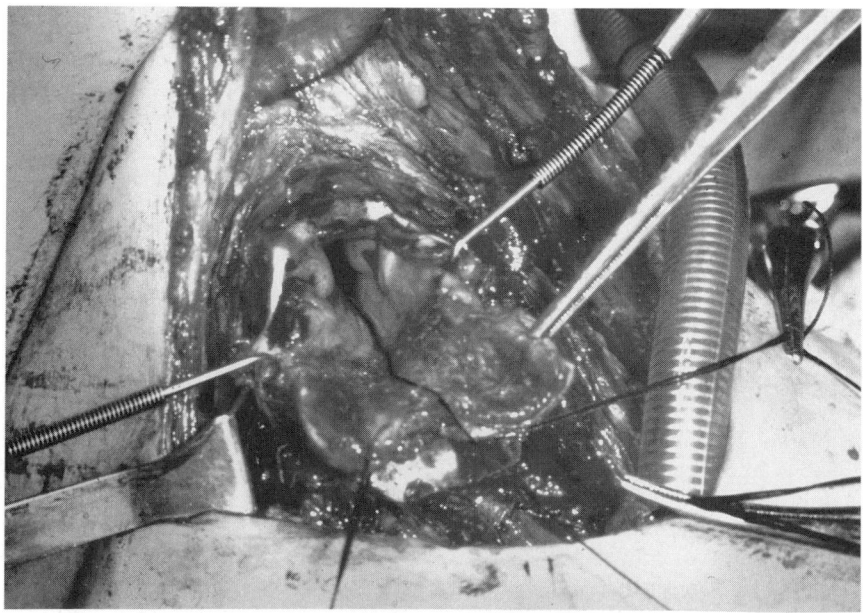

Figure 16-19. Operative photograph showing the larynx and subglottic areas following resection of the anterior cricoid arch and laryngofissure. Fine hook retractors are being used to spread the anterior margins of the thyroid cartilage. In the photograph, the vocal cords lie about 5 mm superior to the position of the hook retractors. The ulcerated, thickened, and stenosed subglottic segment begins immediately below these small retractors and extends posteriorly into the interarytenoid mucosa.

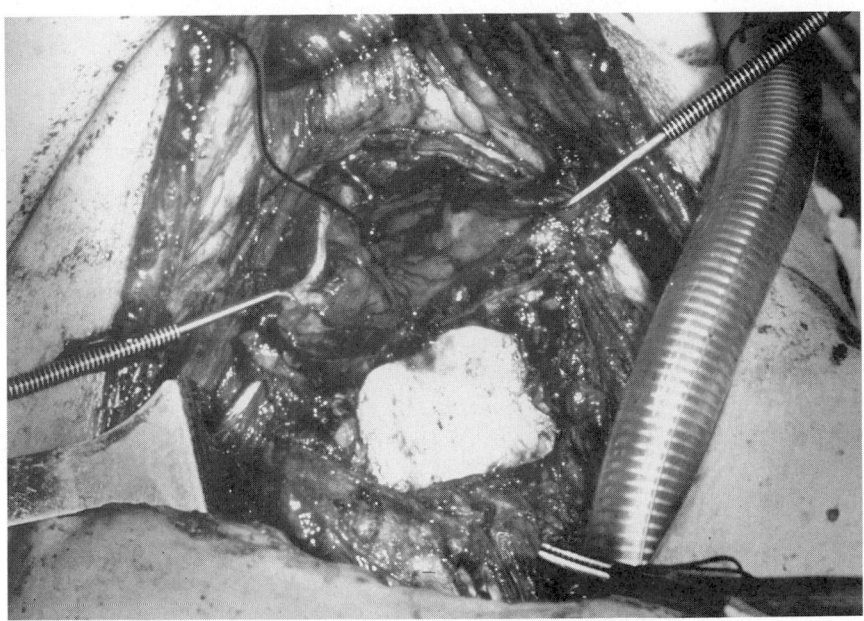

Figure 16-20. Photograph of the same patient shown in Figure 16-18, following resection of the stenosed subglottic segment and interarytenoid scar. A broad plate of posterior cricoid cartilage is exposed below. The fine hook retractors lie just below the inferior margin of the vocal folds.

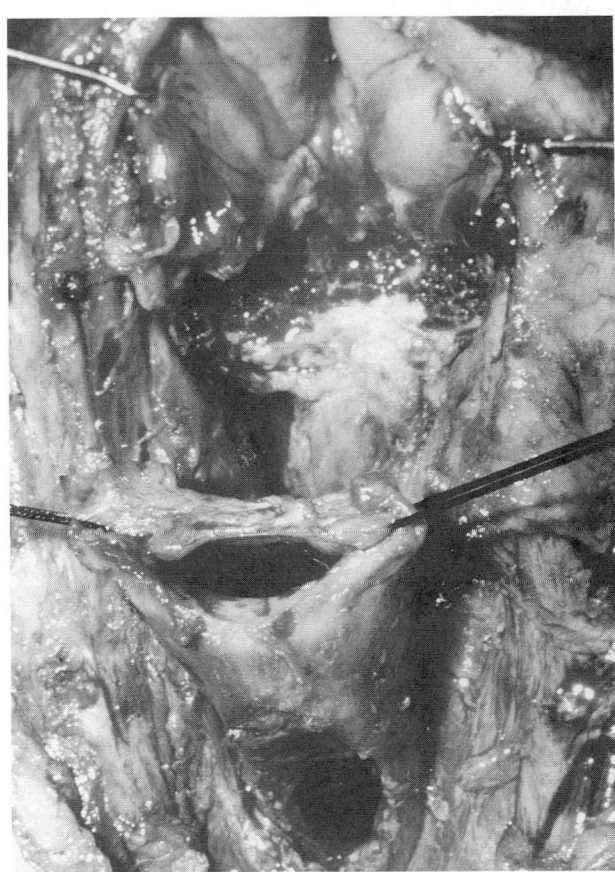

Figure 16-21. The distal airway has been stabilized with two posterolateral stay sutures. At the bottom of the photograph the stoma of a prior tracheostomy is seen. The uppermost cartilaginous rings of the distal airway will be resected in order to develop a vascularized posterior mucosal flap.

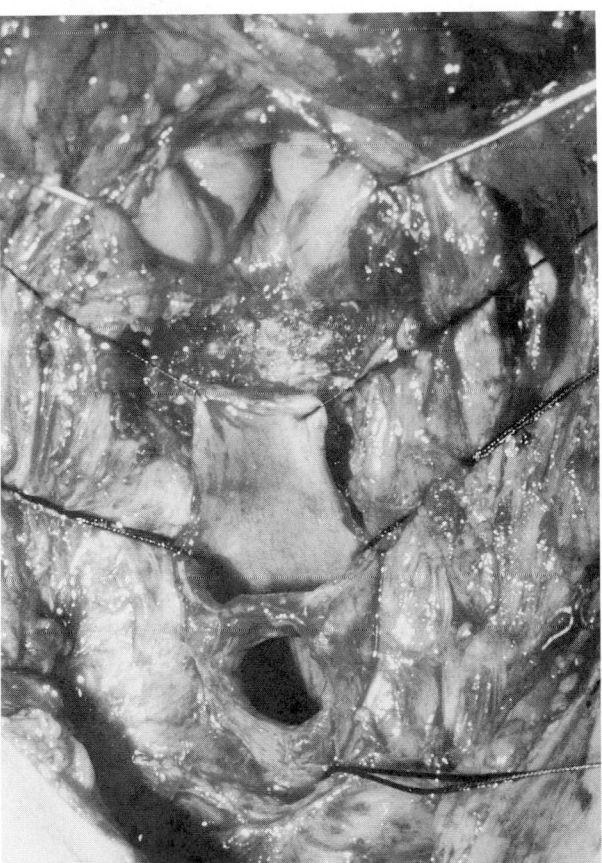

Figure 16-22. The anterolateral margins of the distal airway have been trimmed back, with preservation of a pedicle of posterior membranous trachea. The pedicled flap has been stabilized with two fine stay sutures. The old tracheostomy stoma now lies within a few millimeters of the tracheal margin. Just above the mucosal flap a bare area of cricoid is seen, and above this the mucosal surface of the airway lies immediately below the vocal cords.

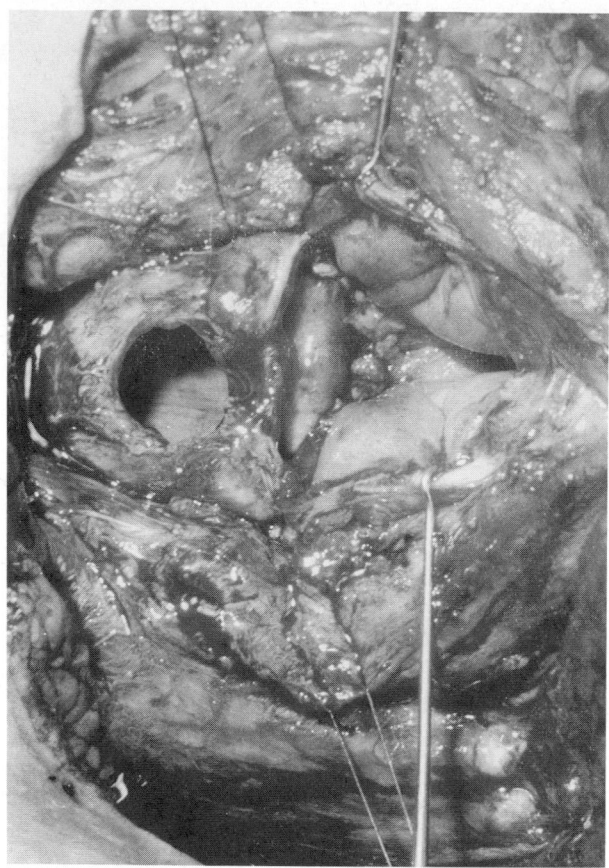

Figure 16-23. The distal airway has been elevated in preparation for the anastomosis. The posterior flap is now lying just below the mucosal defect between the arytenoid cartilages. This pedicle will be secured in place with interrupted sutures of fine gauge (35 Fr) stainless steel wire with the knots tied inside.

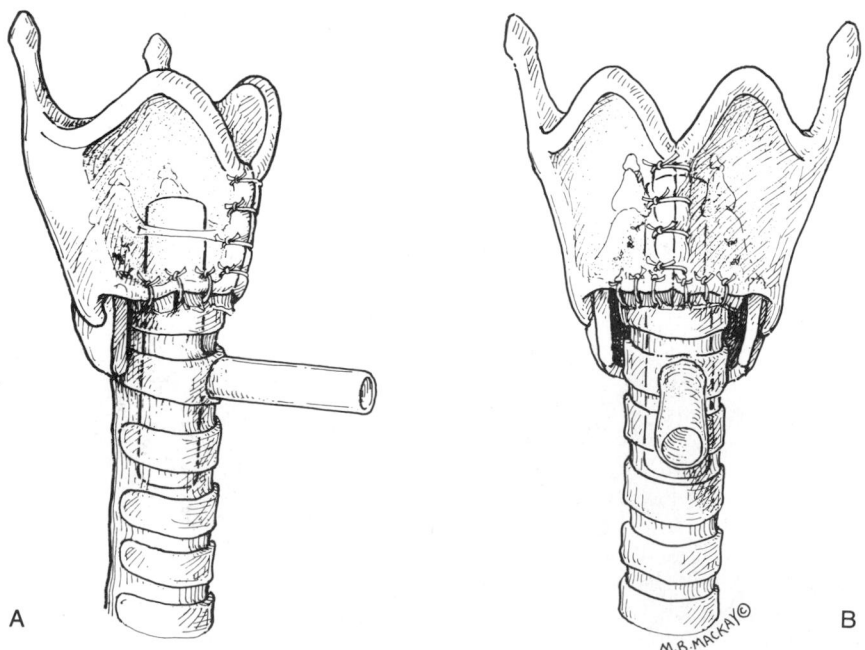

A   B

Figure 16-24. (A) Lateral and (B) AP diagrams illustrating the completed thyrotracheal anastomosis and closure of the laryngofissure. A silicone T tube has been placed with the proximal limb lying 0.5 cm above the vocal cords.

the airway are preserved. If a small distal tracheostomy is placed, this too may be corked if the patient can breath adequately around it. If not, it is important to provide adequate humidification with a tracheostomy mask during the early postoperative period.

The chin suture is removed at the end of 1 week. It is recommended that the anastomosis be examined by flexible bronchoscopy at that time. If the margins are well vascu-larized and healing cleanly, it is almost certain that a satisfactory result will be obtained, and it is safe to discharge the patient.

The complications and results of subglottic and laryngotracheal resection are reported in publications by Pearson et al. (1975, 1986), Maddaus, et al. (1992), Couraud and Hafez (1987), Grillo (1982), Grillo, et al. (1992) and Monnier and Savary (1993). These reports are summarized in Chapter 13.

KEY REFERENCES

Monnier P, Savary M: Partial cricoid resection with primary tracheal anastomosis for subglottic stenosis in infants and children. Laryngoscope 103:1273, 1993

These authors are the first in the world to report a successful experience with subglottic resection in infants and children. The indications for operation and the details of technique in this age group are clearly outlined.

Pearson FG, Cooper JD, Nelems JM et al.: Primary tracheal anastomosis after resection of the cricoid cartilage with preservation of recurrent laryngeal nerves. J Thorac Cardiovasc Surg 70:806, 1975

The operative technique of partial cricoid resection, preservation of recurrent laryngeal nerves, and primary thyrotracheal anastomosis is described in detail in this original report. The description includes anatomic diagrams, intraoperative photographs, and photographs of cadaver dissections illustrating pertinent details of anatomy in this region.

REFERENCES

Couraud L, Hafez A: Acquired and non-neoplastic subglottic stenoses. In Grillo HC, Eschapasse H (eds): Major Challenges. In International Trends in General Thoracic Surgery. Vol. 2. WB Saunders, Philadelphia, 1987

Gerwat J, Bryce DP: The management of subglottic laryngeal stenosis by resection and direct anastomosis. Laryngoscope 84:940, 1974

Grillo HC, Mathisen DJ, Wain JC: Laryngotracheal resection and reconstruction for subglottic stenosis. Ann Thorac Surg 53:54, 1992

Grillo HC: Primary reconstruction of airway after resection of subglottic and upper tracheal stenosis. Ann Thorac Surg 33:3, 1982

Gullane PJ, Pearson FG, Maddaus MA: Laryngotracheal stenosis. Outcome analysis 73 Cases. Laryngoscope (in press)

Maddaus MA, Toth JL, Gullane PJ, Pearson FG: Subglottic tracheal resection and synchronous laryngeal reconstruction. J Thorac Cardiovasc Surg 104:1443, 1992

Ogura JH, Powers WE: Functional restitution of traumatic stenosis of the larynx and pharynx. Laryngoscope 74:1081, 1964

Pearson FG, Brito-Filomen L, Cooper JD: Experience with partial cricoid resection and thyrotracheal anastomosis. Ann Otol Rhinol Laryngol 95:582, 1986

Tracheal Resection

Shafique Keshavjee
F. Griffith Pearson

HISTORICAL NOTE

Prior to 1960 reports of segmental tracheal resection and reconstruction by primary anastomosis were rare and anecdotal. At most, it was assumed that no more than two or three tracheal rings (3 cm) could be resected and restored by primary anastomoses. With the advent of mechanical ventilation and the increasing use of cuffed endotracheal tubes, a spate of postintubation tracheal injuries were reported in North America and Europe. The management of these injuries provided a major stimulus to the development of new techniques of resection and reconstruction. Grillo (1970) described techniques of mobilization of the anterolateral aspects of the trachea and elevation of the main carina by an intrapericardial release of the right pulmonary hilum and also highlighted the importance of neck flexion in minimizing tension on a primary anastomosis. By using these maneuvers it became possible to resect 4- to 5-cm long segments of the adult trachea and obtain predictable healing by primary anastomosis.

The addition of the superior laryngeal release operation (Dedo and Fishman, 1969) and the technique of suprahyoid release (Montgomery, 1974) increased the capability of extended tracheal resection and primary reconstruction. By using these superior release procedures, it is usually possible to remove about half the length of the adult trachea and reconstitute the airway by end-to-end anastomosis. During the same decade techniques were developed for resection of the carina below and the subglottic airway within the cricoid ring. The techniques of subglottic and carinal resection are detailed in separate parts of this chapter, by Maddaus and Pearson and by Mathisen and Grillo, respectively.

HISTORICAL READINGS

Dedo HH, Fishman NH: Laryngeal release and sleeve resection for tracheal stenosis. Ann Otol Rhinol Laryngol 78:285, 1969

Grillo HC: Surgery of the trachea. In Ravitch MM (ed): Current Problems in Surgery. Year Book Medical Publishers, Chicago, 1970

Montgomery WW: Suprahyoid release for tracheal stenosis. Arch Otolaryngol 99:255, 1974

INDICATIONS

Among the indications for tracheal resection and reconstruction are postintubation strictures (including upper airways burns), idiopathic stenosis, benign and malignant neoplasms, some congenital anomalies, and rare conditions such as selected cases of tracheomalacia. The incidence, pathogenesis, and principles of management of these conditions are discussed in Chapters 13 and 15. At present, postintubation stricture is the commonest indication for resection. These lesions are frequently no more than a few centimeters in length and rarely require special mobilization techniques for management. In contrast, a majority of tracheal neoplasms are malignant and locally extensive at the time of symptomatic presentation, and they frequently require extended resection using many or all of the available maneuvers to achieve a satisfactory primary reconstruction.

MANAGEMENT

Preoperative Assessment

Preoperative assessment includes history and physical examination, a combination of imaging modalities, and bronchoscopy. From the information obtained by imaging and endoscopy, it is possible to obtain a precise evaluation of the nature, location, and extent of the lesion prior to resection. This information determines the operative exposure and mobilizing procedures that are anticipated. Details of preoperative evaluation are provided in the section on postintubation injury by Maddaus and Pearson in Chapter 13.

Risk Factors

It is important to identify several important risk factors: (1) the presence of ongoing inflammation or infection, (2) diabetes, (3) previous radiation in the operative field, (4) therapy with high-dose steroids, and (5) age.

Particularly in patients with postintubation injury, it is desirable to delay resection and reconstruction until active inflammatory changes beyond the margins of the stricture subside. Early in the evolution of such injury these changes are common, and time is required simply to allow the process to mature and the adjacent inflammatory changes to settle. On occasion, the resolution of inflammation is expedited by removing an indwelling tracheostomy tube and maintaining the airway by interval dilatation if necessary. Alternatively, in selected cases the tracheostomy tube may be replaced with a T tube, which provides a well humidified and closed airway and is less irritating to the tracheal mucosa than an open tracheostomy tube (Pearson, 1983; Montgomery, 1968; Cooper, et al., 1989).

Radical radiotherapy (dosage of 400 cGy or greater) creates a significant risk to airway healing (Mathisen, et al., 1988; Tsubota, et al., 1975). Unless some form of additional protection is provided, the anastomosis frequently fails in an irradiated field, with dehiscence, progressive necrosis, and further destruction of the remaining airway. For some time Grillo refrained from operating on these patients because of the anticipated high morbidity and mortality. He was the first to recommend use of a vascularized pedicle to support healing at the anastomosis and with Mathisen (1988) reported on a group of successful cases managed with the addition of an omental pedicle. The effects of irradiation on tracheal healing were documented in an animal study by Tsubota, et al. (1975).

Diabetics have a known propensity for impaired healing and a reduced tolerance to contamination and infection. Needless to say, all airway surgery is relatively contaminated with oropharyngeal pathogens. Similarly, administration of steroids (especially in high dosage) appears to impede healing and increase the risk of infection. Whenever possible, patients should be weaned from steroid medication preoperatively. In diabetics or patients requiring perioperative high-dose steroids, it may be desirable to support the anastomosis with some form of vascularized pedicle, such as omentum, muscle flap, pericardium, or thymus.

Age is a variable risk factor owing to loss of elasticity in older patients, which may limit the extent of segmental resection that is possible.

Anesthesia

The management of anesthesia for tracheal resection is challenging and requires close cooperation between the anesthesiologist and the surgical team. The induction must be carefully planned, and the surgeon should be present and available to secure the airway with a rigid bronchoscope whenever necessary. A rigid bronchoscope can be used to dilate a stenotic airway when necessary to accommodate the appropriate-size endotracheal tube.

A detailed description of the anesthetic techniques for tracheal resection is provided by Sandler in Chapter 7. Some important steps in management are repeated here for emphasis: the airway is usually transected on the distal side of the lesion and the distal trachea intubated with a cuffed, armored, endotracheal tube. In all operations done through a cervical incision, the proximal end of the armored tube can be passed under the surgical drape alongside the upper neck and jaw, directly to the anesthetic connections at the patient's head. When the operative field requires either a sternotomy or a thoracotomy, it will be necessary to use a set of sterile anesthetic connections extending from the armored tube across the operative field and under the drapes to the anesthetist. The armored tube is intermittently withdrawn and reinserted during the conduct of the tracheal anastomosis.

Jet ventilation offers an alternative technique and has the advantage of permitting continuous operation without intermittent withdrawal and reinsertion of the endotracheal tube. Familiarity with the technique of jet ventilation is essential in order to avoid forceful insufflation, barotrauma, or air embolism. Jet ventilation is preferred in those circumstances in which one is obligated to ventilate an airway that cannot be easily or reliably intubated, such as the bronchus intermedius or distal left main bronchus. Oxygen saturation and carbon dioxide tension should be recorded throughout the procedure.

In most cases it is desirable to have the patient resume spontaneous respiration and awaken as quickly as possible following termination of surgery. The sooner the orotracheal tube is removed, the better, since the cuffed tube may impair circulation at the anastomosis as long as it remains inflated in the upper airway.

Operative Technique

The patient is placed in the supine position. An inflatable bag is positioned transversely beneath the scapulae so that reversible hyperextension of the neck is easily obtained. A generous collar incision usually provides ample exposure (Fig. 16-25) for lesions involving the upper one-half to two-thirds of the trachea. Occasionally, extension to a sternotomy may be required. Lesions in the distal one-third of the trachea

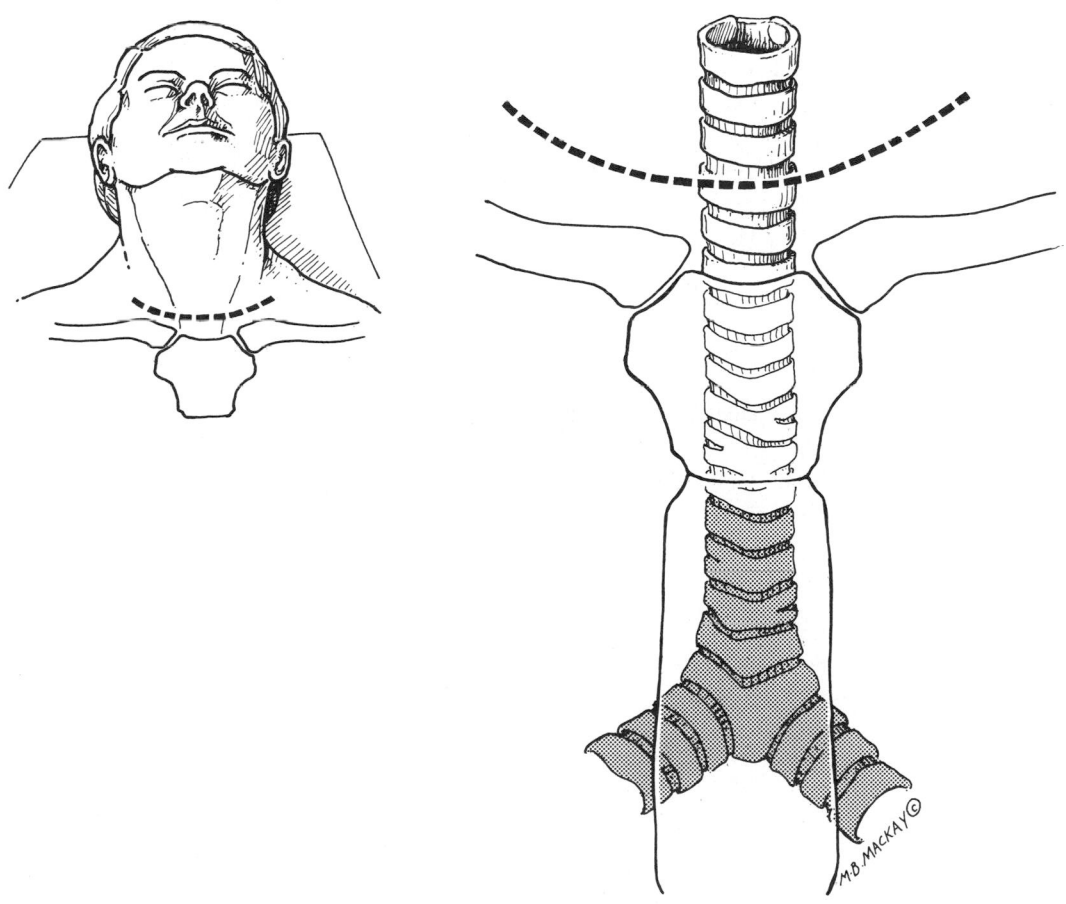

Figure 16-25. Diagram illustrating the position of a generous collar incision. In most patients this incision permits exposure of the larynx and upper cervical trachea and the proximal one-half to two-thirds of the mediastinal trachea (*unshaded area*). Exposure of the distal mediastinal trachea and carina (*shaded area*) requires either a right posterolateral thoracotomy (fourth intercostal space) or a median sternotomy.

are commonly approached with a right posterolateral thoracotomy through the fourth intercostal space.

An alternate approach to the mediastinal trachea is through a full median sternotomy. This exposure has several distinct advantages over a right posterolateral thoracotomy in selected cases. A median sternotomy should be selected in situations (usually involving neoplasms) in which there is the possibility of extension to a carinal or more distal resection. This is particularly useful in cases of malignancy involving the carina, in which the extent of involvement of the left main bronchus cannot be assessed with certainty preoperatively. In some cases extensive involvement of the left main bronchus precludes anastomosis, necessitating a left pneumonectomy, which is possible through a median sternotomy. To obtain exposure of the distal trachea, carina, and both main bronchi through a median sternotomy, it is necessary to divide the pericardium both anteriorly and posteriorly, using vertical incisions extending from the innominate artery above to the right main pulmonary artery below. The ascending aorta and superior vena cava are freed intrapericardially and then retracted laterally. Once the posterior pericardium is divided, the carina and main bronchi are clearly displayed and accessible. Through this midline exposure, bilateral intrapericardial releases can be performed, and a cervical incision may be added if a suprathyroid or suprahyoid laryngeal release is required. Thus exposure from the hyoid bone to the carina can be obtained through a median sternotomy combined with a cervical incision.

The technique for circumferential resection of short tracheal segments is relatively straightforward. Several important principles should again be emphasized:

1. Accurate preoperative identification of the precise level and length of the lesion to be resected is necessary.
2. Resection should be performed through healthy trachea. Reconstruction with inflamed tissue will prejudice the success of a primary anastomosis.
3. The airway should not be circumferentially mobilized for more than 1 cm beyond the resection margin in order to preserve its circulation. The anterior and anterolateral aspects of the trachea from the cricoid to the carina can be mobilized without compromising the circulation that enters posterolaterally. This mobilization often improves the mobility of the distal trachea and decreases tension on the anastomosis. The membranous trachea can be mobilized posteriorly in the midline in circumstances in which there is a desperate need for additional length. This maneuver is rarely necessary, and it is usually not performed since it will diminish some blood supply provided by esophageal collaterals.
4. Tension at the anastomosis should be avoided.

Resection of the Trachea

The airway between the hyoid bone above and the junction between the middle and lower thirds of the mediastinal trachea is usually accessible through a generous collar incision (Fig. 16-25). Resection within these boundaries rarely requires a median sternotomy except in patients with a very

short neck, those with a dorsal kyphosis, or some older patients with a rigid, inelastic trachea.

Skin flaps are elevated in the plane deep to platysma and are developed to expose the airway from the inferior border of the thyroid cartilage to the suprasternal notch. The strap muscles are separated in the midline to expose the anterior tracheal wall (Fig. 16-26). The thyroid isthmus is divided between suture ligatures if necessary for exposure. With the neck in full extension, the upper mediastinal trachea is elevated into the operative field and the area to be resected is identified. In the case of benign stricture, the tracheal wall is often deformed, may be enveloped by fibrous tissue, and can be densely adherent to adjacent structures (Fig. 16-26). Occasionally, the area to be resected is not readily apparent, and the external aspect of the trachea looks normal. In such cases the location of the lesion can be determined from the measurements obtained at preoperative (or intraoperative) bronchoscopy. These predetermined distances can be confirmed by using a sterile ruler intraoperatively, with the lower border of thyroid cartilage, cricoid cartilage, or main carina as an identifiable external landmark. If there is still doubt about the location of the lesional margins, their position can be confirmed with flexible bronchoscopy: the combination of the site of the bronchoscope light seen in the operative field and a transtracheally positioned needle viewed through the bronchoscope will accurately localize the position for the initial incision in the airway.

In benign disease the strictured segment is mobilized circumferentially by sharp dissection, which is maintained as close to the tracheal wall as possible, particularly at the tracheoesophageal angles in which the recurrent laryngeal nerves run. No effort is made to identify the nerves in these cases. In resection for malignant disease, however, the recurrent nerves should be clearly defined above and below the tumor. A decision can then be made as to whether the nerve has to be sacrificed to achieve complete resection. Circumferential mobilization should not extend more than 1 cm above and below the segment to be resected (Fig. 16-27).

The airway is divided transversely through healthy trachea immediately below the segment to be resected. This incision is placed conservatively, with the surgeon choosing to divide the trachea through abnormal tissue if in doubt, since a more distal resection is always possible. Following incision of the cartilaginous wall anteriorly and laterally, 2–0 Vicryl stay sutures are placed in the midline anteriorly and also on each side at the junction between the cartilaginous and membranous trachea, approximately one ring away from the divided edge (Fig. 16-28A). Traction on these sutures will accurately display the normal shapes and diameters of the tracheal lumen and membranous tracheal wall, which otherwise may be deformed and contracted. These stay sutures also prevent retraction of the distal tracheal stump into the mediastinum once the trachea is completely transected.

Following division of the trachea, the oral endotracheal tube is pulled back into the proximal airway, and the distal trachea is intubated with a flexible, cuffed, armored endotracheal tube (Fig. 12-28B). The trachea is then divided above the lesion through healthy airway, and similar stay sutures are placed to display the upper tracheal margin. In the case

Figure 16-26. Subplatysmal skin flaps have been developed to allow exposure of the airway from the suprasternal notch below to the thyroid notch above. The soft tissues are divided vertically in the midline from the thyroid cartilage to the suprasternal notch, with lateral mobilization and retraction of the strap muscles. This exposes the anterior wall of the larynx and trachea with the overlying thyroid isthmus in the region of the cricoid cartilage. A short area of circumferential scarring is depicted in the airway just above the suprasternal notch. Exposure of this segment has been facilitated by hyperextension of the neck and a bolster between the shoulders. An endotracheal tube has been positioned on the left side of the neck prior to division of the airway at the lower border of the stricture.

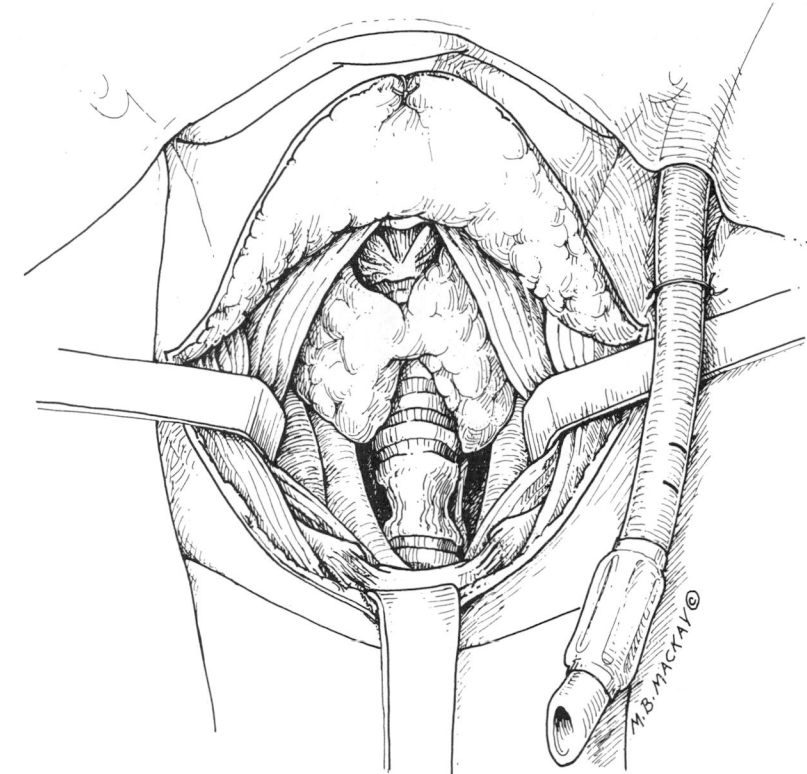

Figure 16-27. In this diagrammatic representation of a benign, postintubation stricture, the lesion has been mobilized circumferentially by maintaining sharp dissection immediately against the tracheal wall. The normal trachea on each side of the lesion is mobilized circumferentially for no more than 1 cm in order to preserve a good circulation at the subsequent tracheal margins (*dotted line*).

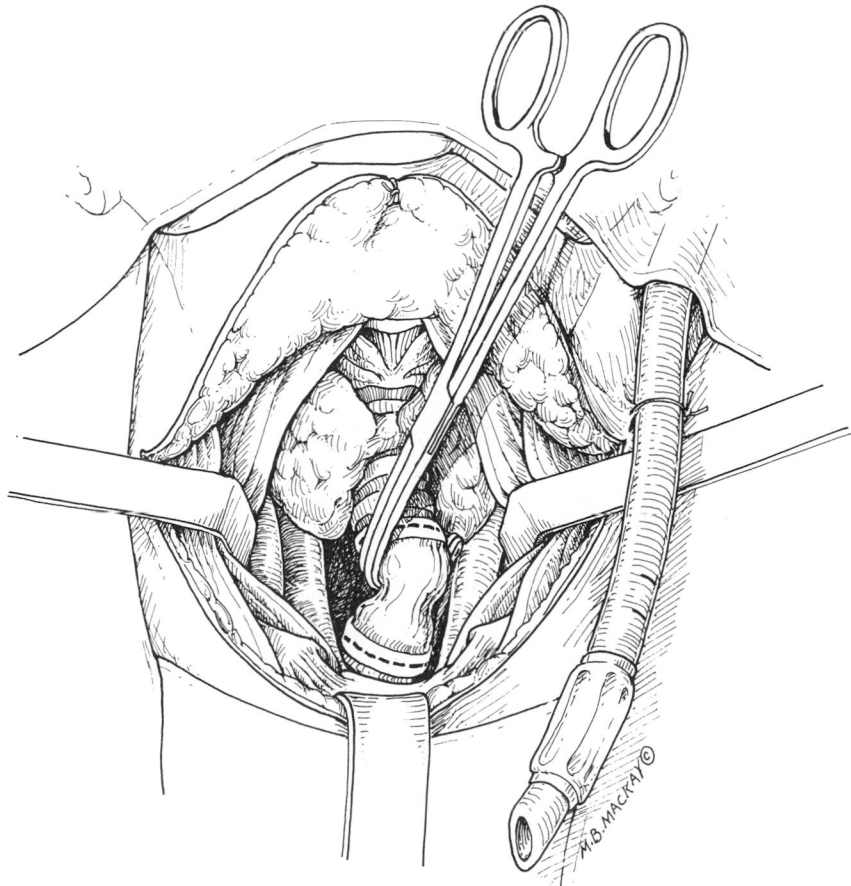

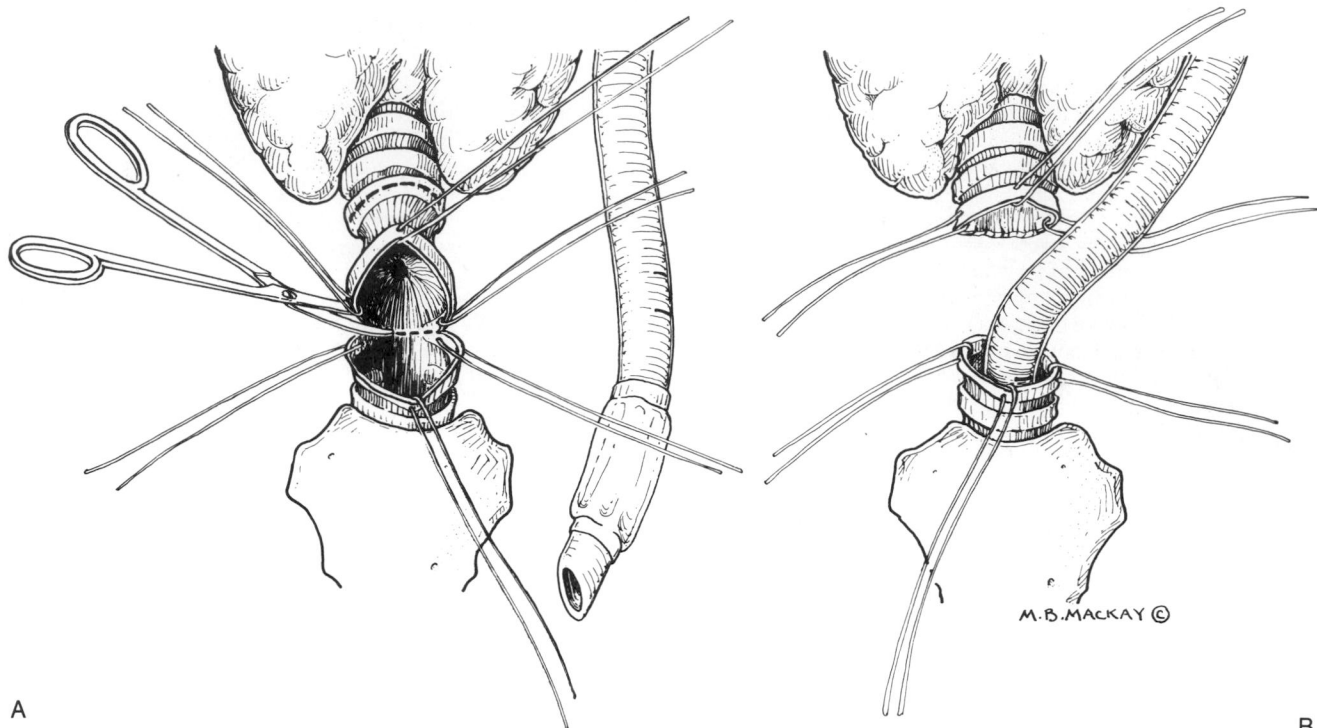

A

B

Figure 16-28. **(A)** The airway is divided distally just beyond the stricture. Stay sutures have been placed in the midline anteriorly and posterolaterally at the junction between tracheal cartilage and membranous trachea. **(B)** With the airway completely divided, the distal end is intubated with an armored tube, which has been secured laterally to the skin of the neck and passed alongside the jaw and under the drapes to the anesthetic connections at the head of the operating table.

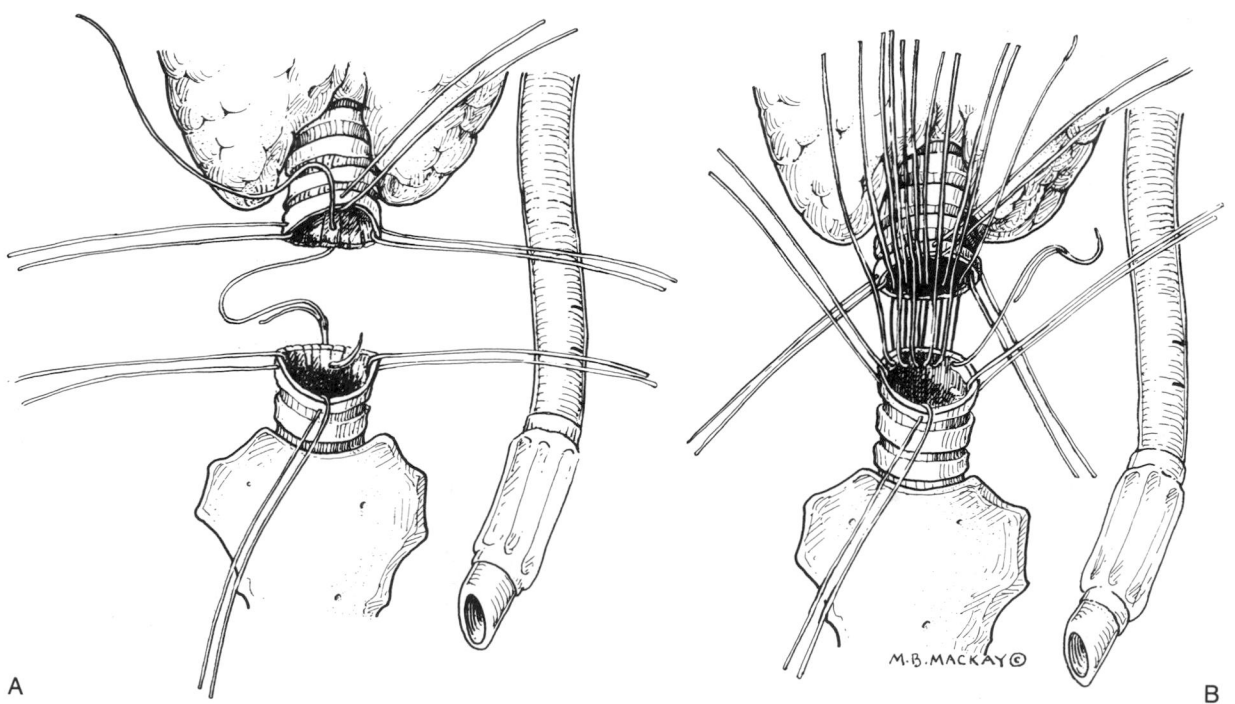

A

B

Figure 16-29. **(A)** The stricture has been resected, stay sutures placed in the proximal tracheal margin, and the posterior layer of anastomotic sutures begun. Reasonably deep 3- to 4-mm bites are taken in the tracheal wall on each side. **(B)** Interrupted sutures are placed across the entire posterior wall of the anastomosis without being tied. An absorbable suture such as 3–0 or 4–0 Vicryl may be used for this part of the anastomosis. We prefer fine (35-gauge) stainless steel wire for this part of the anastomosis with the knots tied on the inside.

of malignant disease, frozen section evaluation of the tracheal margins is an essential requirement.

Prior to performance of the anastomosis, the inflatable bag beneath the scapulae is deflated and the neck is flexed to shorten the distance between the tracheal ends. The anastomosis is begun by placing a row of interrupted sutures in the posterior membranous trachea (Fig. 16-29A). These sutures are placed at 2- to 3-mm intervals, taking approximately a 3-mm bite of trachea on each side of the tracheal margin. The endotracheal tube is intermittently removed and replaced, as required, in order to place the sutures. The entire posterior row is placed before any sutures are tied (Fig. 16-29B). Our preference is to use fine (35-gauge) stainless steel wire with knots tied on the inside. This technique permits precise approximation of the posterior tracheal wall under direct vision. By means of appropriate traction on the stay sutures, all tension is removed from the tracheal ends while the posterior sutures are being tied. Once the sutures in the membranous trachea have been tied, the distal airway is extubated, and the original orotracheal tube is carefully advanced across the anastomosis into the distal airway. The anastomosis is then completed by using similarly placed, interrupted sutures of 4-0 Vicryl in the anterolateral cartilaginous wall, with the knots tied on the outside (Fig. 16-30).

In an alternative technique, practiced by Grillo (1970), the anastomosis is performed by using interrupted 4-0 Vicryl sutures only. All sutures are placed without tying, starting in the middle of the membranous trachea and progressing around each side to the front. The tracheal ends are then approximated, and the stay sutures of 2-0 Vicryl are tied to ablate tension when the 4-0 Vicryl sutures are tied. The 4-0 Vicryl sutures are tied sequentially, with knots on the outside, beginning in the midline anteriorly and working around the back on both sides.

Tension on the completed anastomosis should be minimal, and secure apposition should be possible with use of relatively fine suture material. Unfortunately, there is no practical method to quantitate tension at the anastomosis, and this evaluation must be learned through experience.

After completion of the anastomosis, its integrity can be checked by manual ventilation of the patient to 20 to 30 cmH_2O with the cuff deflated. The thyroid gland and/or strap muscles are approximated in the midline to buttress the anastomosis. A drain is placed alongside the trachea and brought out through a separate stab wound.

It is essential to maintain neck flexion during the postoperative period. This is simply and effectively achieved by securing a stout suture between the skin of the chin and the skin of the anterior chest (Fig. 16-31). This suture is left in place for 7 days to protect the tracheal anastomosis. It is surprisingly well tolerated by the patient.

It is desirable to extubate the patient in the operating room. If patency of the airway is equivocal—a situation usually due to acute edema—a distal (nos. 4 or 5) uncuffed tracheostomy tube is placed prior to closure. Alternatively, if the airway obstruction is minor or expected to be short-lived, translaryngeal intubation with a small uncuffed tube may suffice. In those cases in which there is concern about the viability of the anastomosis, a silicone Montgomery T tube can be used to stent the anastomosis. This not only protects and maintains continuity of the airway but may prevent or diminish stricture development during the healing phase.

Mobilization and Release Procedures

If attempts to approximate the ends of the divided airway suggest that undue tension would result, there are several mobilization and release procedures that can be used to re-

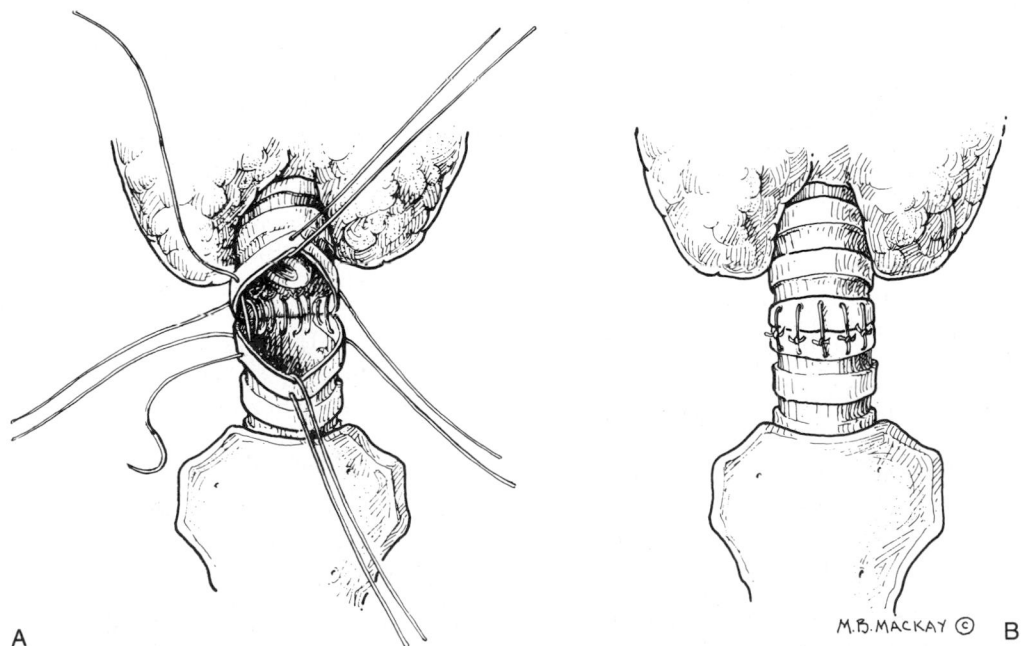

Figure 16-30. **(A)** Sutures on the posterior wall have been tied. At this point the orotracheal tube (lying just proximal to the anastomosis) is advanced across the anastomosis into the distal trachea, and **(B)** the anastomosis is completed.

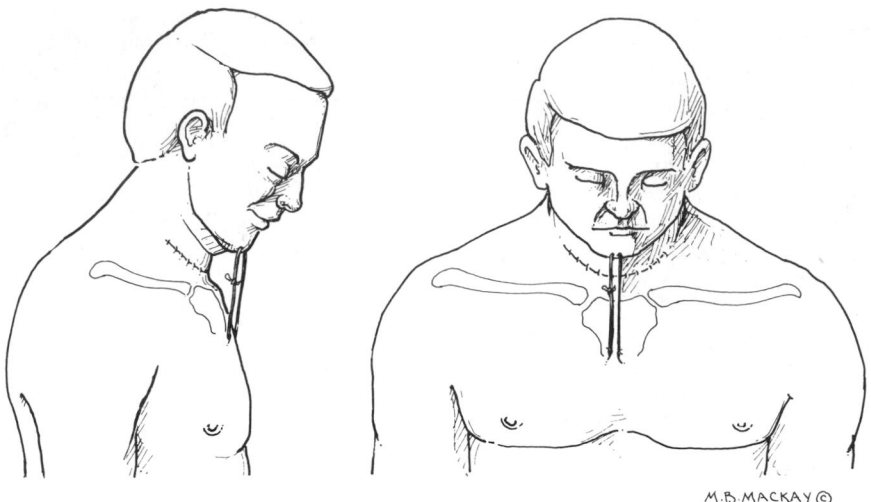

Figure 16-31. At the end of the operation and before the patient is awake, a stout suture (#5 Tevdek) is secured as shown in the diagrams, between the skin of the point of the chin and the midline of the chest over the manubrium. This maintains neck flexion for the first postoperative week.

solve the problem. These include neck flexion, which has its maximal effect in the cervical trachea but still reduces some tension in resections involving the lower trachea. Digital dissection of the trachea along the anterior, pretracheal "mediastinoscopy plane" is a useful technique which will provide additional mobility. The suprahyoid and suprathryoid laryngeal release procedures and the intrapericardial hilar releases are mobilization techniques that reduce anastomotic tension by elevation of the carina.

Suprathyroid Laryngeal Release

The suprathryoid laryngeal release operation, described by Dedo and Fishman in 1969, permits resection of an additional 2 to 3 cm of trachea by "dropping" the larynx and reducing tension at the anastomosis. To perform this procedure, the upper skin flap of the cervical incision is extended to the level of the hyoid bone. The sternohyoid strap muscles are retracted laterally, and the thyrohyoid muscles on each side are freed and divided transversely (Fig. 16-32, *dotted lines*). This exposes the thyrohyoid membrane and a centrally placed thyrohyoid ligament. The membrane and ligament are divided anteriorly and laterally between the superior cornua of the thyroid cartilage (Fig. 16-33A). The tips of the superior cornua are amputated (Fig. 16-33B), with care taken to avoid injury to the superior laryngeal nerves and their accompanying vessels, which are usually readily identified on each side.

After division of the thyrohyoid membrane and ligament, the submucosa of the anterior pharyngeal wall is exposed. It is easily recognized by the rich submucosal plexus of vessels that it possesses. Thus, all the anterior and lateral soft tissue attachments lying between the inferior border of the hyoid bone and the superior border of the thyroid cartilage except for the underlying mucous membrane, have been divided. It is now possible to drop the larynx at least 2 to 3 cm inferior to its original position (Fig. 16-33B). This opera-

tion may be complicated by transient postoperative supraglottic edema and is frequently associated with uncoordinated swallowing and with aspiration. Although these problems are usually transient, troublesome or disabling aspiration may be more prolonged and pronounced in elderly patients.

Suprahyoid Laryngeal Release

The suprahyoid release, originated by Montgomery in 1968, results in a laryngeal drop of similar magnitude to that achieved with the suprathyroid release. It has the reported advantage, however, of causing a diminished incidence and severity of incoordinate swallowing.

To perform this procedure, the upper skin flap is extended to the suprahyoid region. Alternatively, this operation may be performed through a separate transverse incision, which is centered over the hyoid bone. The muscular attachments (mylohyoid, geniohyoid, and genioglossus muscles) on the central two-thirds of the superior aspect of the hyoid bone are completely transected to expose the preepiglottic space (Fig. 16-34A). The lesser cornua of the hyoid bone are transected, and the body of the hyoid bone is then divided just anterior to the tendinous attachments of the digastric muscles on each side. This separates the body of the hyoid from the greater horns and allows the larynx to drop for 2 to 3 cm (Fig. 16-34B).

Intrapericardial Pulmonary Hilar Release

A right hilar release (Fig. 16-35) allows elevation of the carina or distal trachea for approximately 2 cm. To begin, the inferior pulmonary ligament is divided. Intrapericardial mobilization of the right pulmonary hilus is then accomplished by circumferential division of the pericardium and its reflections a few millimeters beyond the pericardial reflection on the superior and inferior pulmonary veins and the right pulmonary artery. The pericardium is divided close to the hilar

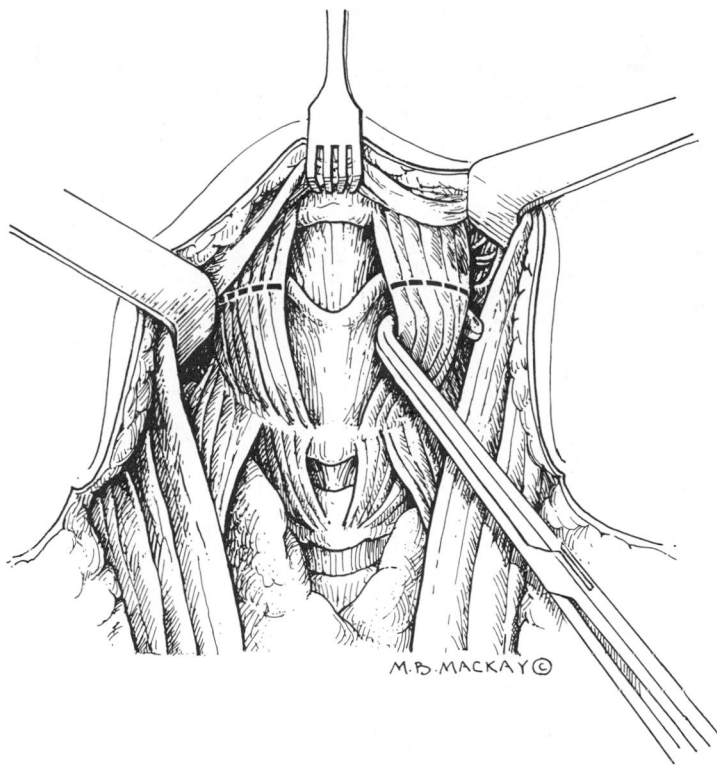

Figure 16-32. Diagram illustrating the suprathyroid laryngeal release: the sternohyoid strap muscles have been retracted laterally, the thyrohyoid muscles on each side have been freed circumferentially, and the dotted line identifies the point of division of the thyrohyoid muscles.

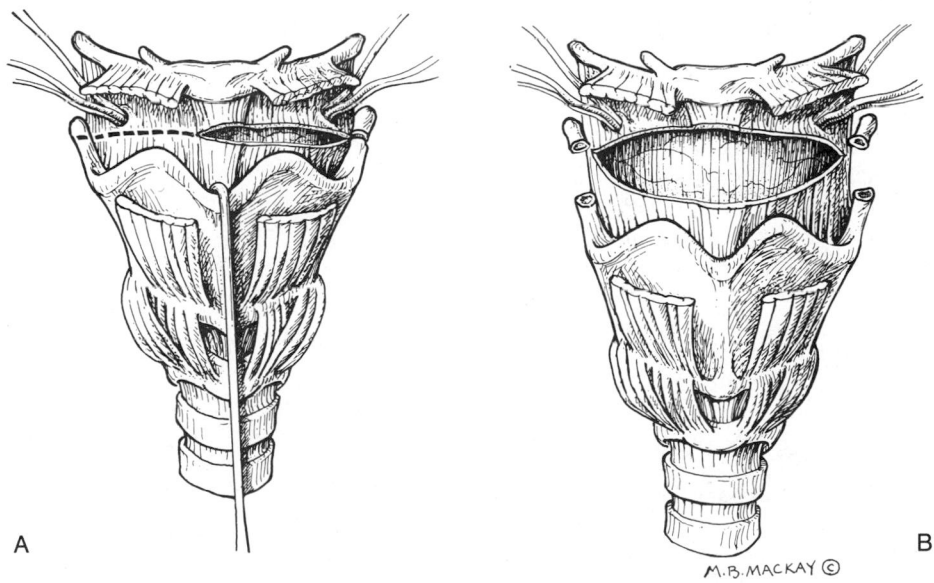

Figure 16-33. **(A)** Following division of the thyrohyoid muscles, the thyrohyoid membrane and a centrally placed thyrohyoid ligament are displayed. **(B)** The thyrohyoid membrane and ligament are divided anteriorly and laterally between the superior cornua of the thyroid cartilage. The tips of the superior cornua are amputated, with care taken to avoid injury to the superior laryngeal nerves and vessels. It is now possible to "drop" the larynx at least 2 to 3 cm inferior to its original position.

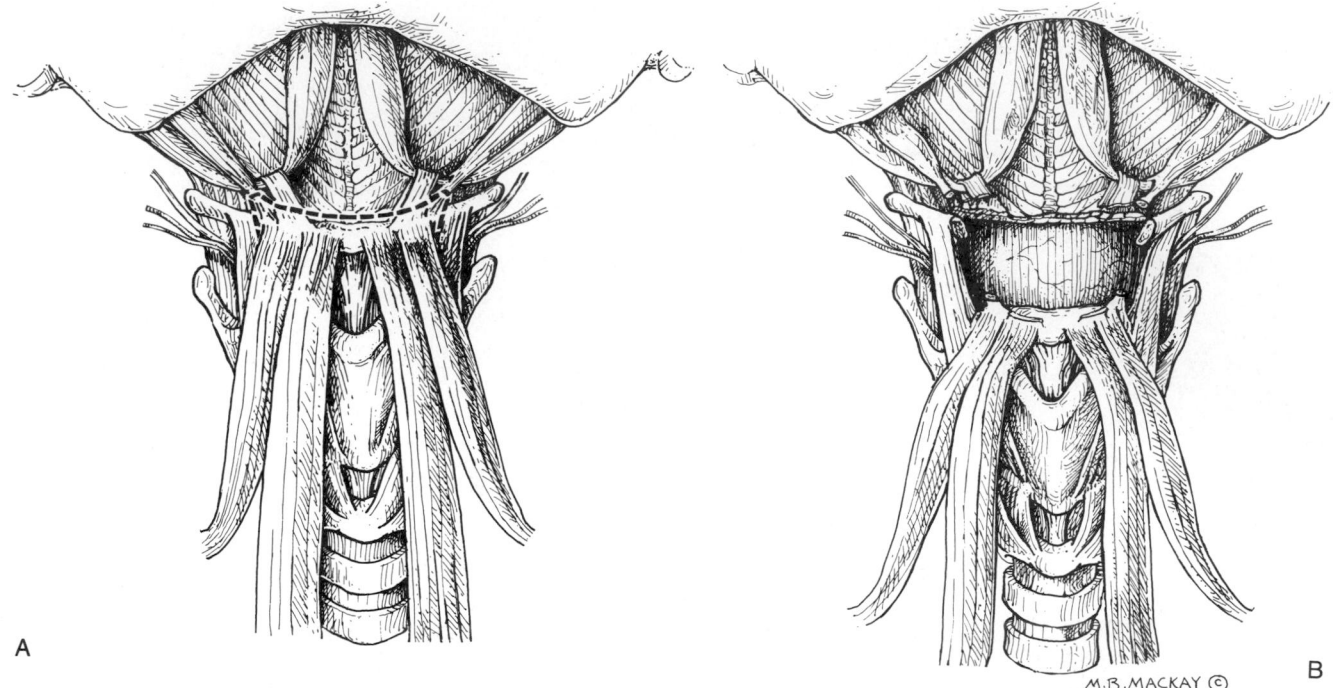

A

B

M.B. MACKAY ©

Figure 16-34. **(A)** Diagram illustrating the suprahyoid laryngeal release: Muscular attachments on the central two-thirds of the upper margin of the hyoid bone are transected *(dotted line)* to expose the pre-epiglottic space. The lesser cornua of the hyoid bone are amputated, and the body of the hyoid bone is divided just anterior to the tendinous attachments of the digastric muscles on each side. **(B)** This procedure separates the body of the hyoid from the greater horns and allows the larynx to "drop" 2 to 3 cm.

reflection, and the right pulmonary artery is freed to its origin. In freeing the origin of the right main bronchus, care is taken to preserve the bronchial arterial circulation. In order to complete the release on the right side, the intrapericardial septum, which joins the lateral aspect of the atrium and inferior vena cava to the pericardium, is divided from the level of the inferior pulmonary vein to the diaphragm. There is no such septum on the left side.

A hilar release on the left side does not yield as much additional length as is obtained on the right. On the left side the aortic arch restricts upward movement of the left main bronchus. The mobilization procedure is similar to that described for the right side, except that there is no intrapericardial septum to divide, and the ductus arteriosus must be divided to allow the hilum to shift upwards. The left main bronchus is freed, but care is taken to preserve its systemic, bronchial blood supply.

Complications

The potential early and late complications of tracheal resection are listed below.

Mild to moderate airway obstruction can be treated with heliox (80 percent helium, 20 percent oxygen), racemic epinephrine inhalational therapy, and bolus administration of steroid (500 mg Solumedrol) as necessary. One or two such doses of steroid do not appear to significantly impair tracheal healing. Severe airway obstruction should be anticipated and treated intraoperatively with a distal tracheotomy under care-

fully controlled conditions, preferably with use of a flexible bronchoscope.

Minor air leaks at suture holes usually seal spontaneously and promptly. Larger leaks, if noticed at surgery, should be closed, usually by buttressing the leak site with vascularized tissue. If postoperative subcutaneous emphysema develops, the incision may have to be partially opened to achieve decompression. Pneumothorax is another potential postopera-

---

Potential Complications of Tracheal Resection

Early
    Airway obstruction—edema
    Air leak, subcutaneous emphysema
    Recurrent laryngeal nerve injury—transient, permanent
    Aspiration, dyscoordinate swallowing
    Anastomotic dehiscence
    Bleeding
    Infection, abscess
Late
    Restenosis, failure of healing
    Suture-line granuloma
    Tracheoesophageal fistula
    Trachea–innominate artery fistula

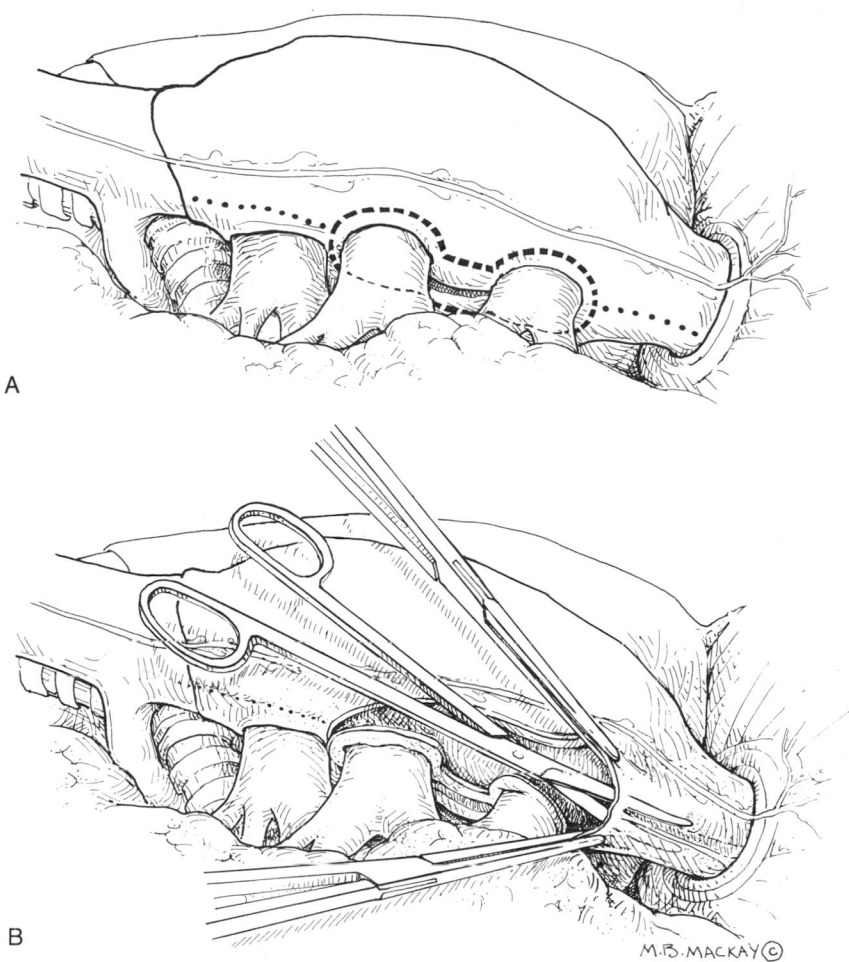

A

B

M.B. MACKAY©

Figure 16-35. **(A)** Diagram illustrating the technique of right hilar pulmonary release. The dotted lines indicate the line of incision of the pericardium, a few millimeters outside the pericardial reflections on the pulmonary veins. The upper dotted line indicates the extension of the incision anterior to the right main pulmonary artery and bronchus, which gives exposure for circumferential mobilization of these two structures, which lie outside the free pericardial space. The lower dotted line indicates the location of the fibrous pericardial septum, which lies between the pericardium and the inferior vena cav, and separates the pericardial space on the right side into anterior and posterior compartments. **(B)** The pericardium has been opened circumferentially around the pulmonary veins. The fibrous septum between the pericardium and the inferior vena cava is being divided from the lower border of the inferior pulmonary vein to the diaphragm. This allows the right side of the heart (right and left atria), pulmonary artery, and the right main bronchus and carina to be elevated in a cephalad direction by several centimeters.

tive complication and should be ruled out by an early postoperative chest x-ray.

Permanent *inadvertent* injury to the recurrent laryngeal nerve is not common if the operative principles described above are followed. Transient dysfunction may be seen, however, and is presumably the result of reversible injury due to traction or mobilization.

Patients are started on clear fluids on the first postoperative day and are usually quickly advanced to a full diet. Following a laryngeal release procedure, however, patients may experience considerable difficulty with swallowing and aspiration.

Incoordinate swallowing and aspiration are usually most troublesome with liquids and less of a problem with solid food. In most patients the disability is transient and short-lived and results in a minor delay of a full recovery. Longer-

term and disabling problems with aspiration are more often seen in the elderly patient or in cases in which laryngeal mobility is impaired by prior neck surgery or cervical irradiation.

A bronchoscopic examination should be performed postoperatively to evaluate healing of the anastomosis in all patients. This is usually done prior to discharge from the hospital about 1 week after surgery, or sooner if there is concern about the integrity of the anastomosis. If a dehiscence involving more than one-third of the circumference of the airway is encountered, a Montgomery T-tube stent should be placed. Smaller areas of separation usually heal without stricture formation but warrant follow-up with repeated bronchoscopic examination. Bleeding is an uncommon complication of tracheal surgery.

Infections occur infrequently in view of considering the contamination that accompanies all tracheal surgery. Prophylactic antibiotics are given immediately before surgery, and one or two doses are given postoperatively. The course of antibiotics may be extended in patients with residual sepsis or risk factors such as diabetes or steroid therapy. If the patient does develop a wound infection or is suspected of having a deep infection, the wound should be widely opened to provide immediate drainage. An undrained abscess may abut and necrose the tracheal anastomosis and drain internally.

Re-stenosis is a delayed complication, which is usually manifest within 4 to 6 weeks of surgery. Therapy consists of dilatation (repeated if necessary) and re-resection in selected cases. Where re-resection is not possible, insertion of a permanent stent may be the only option. Suture line granulomas are uncommon with the use of absorbable suture or stainless steel suture. If they do occur, the granulomatous tissue can be removed through the rigid bronchoscope with biopsy forceps. Granulation tissue can also be treated with a silver nitrate stick or a judiciously applied laser.

Another potential late complication is fistulization between the tracheal anastomosis and the esophagus or the innominate artery. The management of these conditions is discussed elsewhere in this chapter. These complications can be avoided in most cases. During dissection of the trachea, the innominate artery should not be unduly mobilized of denuded. If the artery lies near the completed anastomosis, it can be protected with a muscular or omental pedicle. Similarly, if an esophageal repair is part of the tracheal operation, a buttress of vascularized tissue (usually strap muscle) should be interposed between the esophagus and trachea at the level of anastomosis or repair.

KEY REFERENCES

Grillo HC: Surgery of the trachea. In Ravitch MM (ed): Current Problems in Surgery. Year Book Medical Publishers, Chicago, 1970

A comprehensive review of the advances in surgical techniques for tracheal resection that occurred prior to 1970. The basic principles pertaining to segmental resection were established and have changed little since this publication.

Pearson FG: Advances in Tracheal Surgery. Year Book Medical Publishers, Chicago, 1983

A review of advances in tracheal surgery following Grillo's landmark publication in 1970. Among these advances are improved techniques for segmental resection, including the carina below and the subglottis above, and the use of median sternotomy for selected cases of segmental resection.

REFERENCES

Cooper JD, Pearson FG, Patterson GA et al.: Use of silicone stents in the management of airway problems. Ann Thorac Surg 47:371, 1989

Dedo HH, Fishman NH: Laryngeal release and sleeve resection for tracheal stenosis. Ann Otol Rhinol Laryngol 78:285, 1969

Mathisen DJ, Grillo HC, Vlahakes GJ, Daggett WM: The omentum in the management of complicated cardiothoracic problems. J Thorac Cardiovasc Surg 95:677, 1988

Montgomery WW: The surgical management of supraglottic and subglottic stenosis. Ann Otol Rhinol Laryngol 77:534, 1968

Tsubota N, Simpson WJ, Van Nostrand AWP, Pearson FG: The effects of pre-operative irradiation on primary tracheal anastomosis. Ann Thorac Surg 20:152, 1975

Carinal Resection

Douglas J. Mathisen
Hermes C. Grillo

The intrathoracic portion of the trachea is the last unpaired organ of the body to fall to the surgeon, and the successful solution of the problem of its reconstruction may mark the end of the "expansionist" epoch in the development of surgery.

—Ronald H. R. Belsey
Bristol, England
1946

In 1946, Belsey could not have predicted the challenges of organ transplantation to the thoracic surgeon, but his admonition regarding resection and reconstruction of the intrathoracic trachea remains true even today. Techniques for resection and reconstruction of the trachea and carina are available, but many hurdles remain before they are widely accepted and practiced. Unique perioperative complications, high operative mortality rates, technical challenges, and evolution of the understanding of the limits of resection are but a few of the hurdles remaining. Until these hurdles are cleared, experience with carinal resection remains limited to a small number of institutions around the world.

Successful resection and reconstruction of the carina initially faced four major challenges: preoperative evaluation of the extent of disease, technique of surgery, anesthetic management, and postoperative care. The techniques for reconstruction and anesthesia have been established but need continued refinement to improve current results. Postoperative care needs further refinement to reduce the complications and improve the operative mortality rates, thereby improving the chances for long-term survival.

HISTORICAL NOTE

Early surgical efforts involved lateral or wedge resections of the airway. Prosthetic materials were used because of the uncertainty of airway healing and concern about the extent of resection of the airway that would allow safe reconstruction. Belsey's initial report (1946) of intrathoracic tracheal resection described reconstruction with prosthetic material after lateral resection of the distal airway, including the carina, in one patient. Juvenelle and Citret in 1951 were among the earliest to report experimental results of carinal resection in dogs. The first report of complicated carinal resection and reconstruction in humans was in 1957 by Barclay, et al. They reported successful resection of the carina for a cylindroma, with end-to-end reconstruction between the trachea and right mainstem bronchus and implantation of the left mainstem bronchus into the side of the bronchus intermedius. Grillo, et al. in 1963 and Grillo in 1982 described carinal resection and reconstruction. Grillo presented a comprehensive approach to carinal reconstruction based on experience with 36 cases. Other significant reports of carinal resection and reconstruction included those by Mathey, et al. (1966), Eschapasse (1974), and Perelman (1976). Jensik, et al. (1972) reported 17 patients undergoing tracheal sleeve pneumonectomy for lung cancer. Current results, mostly for lung cancer, report operative mortality ranging from 10.9 to 29 percent (Darteville and Chapelier, 1988; Deslauriers, 1985; Jensik, et al., 1982; Mathisen and Grillo, 1991; Perelman and Koroleva, 1980; Tsuchiya, et al., 1990).

HISTORICAL READINGS

Barclay RS, McSwan N, Welsh TM: Tracheal resection without the use of grafts. Thorax 12:177, 1957

Belsey R: Resection and reconstruction of the intrathoracic trachea. Br J Surg 38:200, 1946

Dartevelle PG, Chapelier A: Tracheal sleeve pneumonectomy for bronchogenic carcinoma: a report of 55 cases. Ann Thorac surg 46:68, 1988

Deslauriers J: Involvement of the main carina. p. 139. In Delarue NC, Eschapasse H (eds): International Trends in General Thoracic Surgery. Vol. 1. WB Saunders, Philadelphia, 1985

Eschapasse H: Les tumeurs tracheales primitives. Traitement chirurgical. Rev Fr Mal Respir 2:425, 1974

Grillo HC: Carinal resection. Ann Thorac Surg 34:356, 1982

Grillo HC, Bendixen HH, Gephart T: Resection of the carina and lower trachea. Ann Surg 158:889, 1963

Jensik RJ, Faber JP, Kittle CF et al.: Survival in patients undergoing tracheal sleeve pneumonectomy for bronchogenic carcinoma. J Thorac Cardiovasc Surg 84:489, 1982

Jensik RJ, Faber LP, Milloy FJ, Goldin MD: Tracheal sleeve pneumonectomy for advanced carcinoma of the lung. Surg Gynecol Obstet 134:232, 1972

Juvenelle A, Citret C: Transplantation de la bronche souche et résection de la bifurcation trachéale. J Chir (Paris) 67:666, 1951

Mathey J, Binet JP, Galey JJ et al.: Tracheal tracheobronchial resection. J Thorac Cardiovasc Surg 51:1, 1966

Mathisen DJ, Grillo HC: Carinal resection for bronchogenic carcinoma. J Thorac Cardiovasc Surg 102:16, 1991

Mathisen DJ, Grillo HC: Endoscopic relief of malignant airway obstruction. Ann Thorac Surg 48:469, 1989

Mathisen DJ, Grillo HC, Vlahakes GJ, Daggett WM: The omentum in the management of complicated cardiothoracic problems. J Thorac Cardiovasc Surg 95:677, 1988

Perelman MI: Surgery of the Trachea. Moscow Mir, Moscow, 1976

Perelman M, Koroleva N: Surgery of the trachea. World J Surg 4:583, 1980

Tsuchiya R, Goya T, Naruke T, Suemasu K: Resection of tracheal carina for lung cancer. J Thorac Cardiovasc Surg 99:941, 1990

Preoperative Evaluation

The risks of surgery demand careful preoperative assessment of each patient. Computed tomography (CT), magnetic resonance imaging (MRI), and plain linear tomography are all helpful in assessing the extent of disease and involvement of the airway. Conventional tomography has been particularly helpful in determining the extent of airway involvement and defining the carina radiologically regardless of the etiology of the problem. All patients with lung cancer should undergo routine radiologic evaluation for metastatic disease.

Patients should be carefully screened from a general medical point of view, and each patient should be particularly screened for coronary disease. Stress thallium studies and echocardiography are used when indicated. Most importantly, all patients should be evaluated to be certain they will have adequate pulmonary function to tolerate such operations and such pulmonary resection as may be indicated. Smoking must stop and medical regimens must be optimized for underlying chronic obstructive lung disease. Chronic bronchitis should be treated with antibiotics and steroids; steroids should be discontinued prior to the time of surgery, however. Arterial blood gases, spirometry, and quantitative ventilation/perfusion scans have become routine. Diffusion capacity, maximum oxygen uptake, and exercise testing are also useful in assessing high-risk patients. Predicted postoperative forced expiratory volume in 1 second should be at least 800 ml/s, but this figure is only a guideline in the context of the patient's size and general medical condition.

Preoperative irradiation for lung cancer is advocated by some authors but is probably associated with a higher incidence of complications (Jensik, et al., 1982). Preoperative irradiation should not exceed 4,000 cGy and is generally given over a period of 3 to 4 weeks. An additional interval of 3 to 4 weeks is allowed for the acute inflammatory effects of irradiation to subside. Irradiation in excess of 5,000 cGy given 1 year or more prior to planned resection should be viewed as a relative contraindication. If circumstances dictate carinal resection, omentum should be wrapped around the anastomosis to aid healing and buttress the anastomosis (Mathisen, et al., 1988). Chronic steroid dependency also precludes safe carinal resection.

Anesthesia

Anesthetic management is an important consideration in patients undergoing carinal resection. If an obstructing tumor exists, an adequate airway must be provided to allow safe conduct of anesthesia. This can be accomplished at the time of planned resection by rigid bronchoscopes and biopsy forceps or by laser (Mathisen and Grillo, 1989; Shapshay, et al. 1985). The risk of bleeding is minimal with either technique. If postobstructive pneumonia is present, it may be desirable to relieve the obstruction and treat the pneumonia prior to proceeding to carinal resection. In the face of severe obstruction, preliminary "coring out" of the airway may provide time for any necessary study, medical therapy, or weaning from steroids.

The anesthetic technique of choice in our institution has been a deep Ethrane anesthesia that avoids long-acting muscle relaxants and narcotics (Wilson, 1988). This technique allows spontaneous ventilation by the patient, which is especially important in difficult airway situations and facilitates extubation at the end of the procedure.

The choice of endotracheal tube is also important. Double-lumen tubes are generally not useful for carinal resection. Abbott (1950) initially recommended the use of a long tube advanced through the divided end of the trachea into the remaining mainstem bronchus. Grillo, et al. (1963) advocated intubation of the left mainstem bronchus across the operative field, with sterile tubing passed off to the anesthesiologist. El-Baz and colleagues (1981) later advocated high-frequency ventilation, which has become the preferred method of airway management for some. Our preferred method of airway management is with an extralong oral endotracheal tube initially. This can be directed into the opposite bronchus if collapse of the operated lung is desired, or a bronchial blocker can be used. Once the carina has been resected, the opposite bronchus (usually the left mainstem) is intubated with a sterile, flexible Tovell tube. Sterile connecting tubing is passed to the anesthesiologist. The tube can be removed for brief periods to allow precise placement of sutures. When the anastomosis is ready to be approximated, the original long oral endotracheal tube is advanced from above across the anastomosis into the mainstem bronchus. Previously placed stay and anastomotic sutures are then tied. Special circumstances occasionally arise that require bifid catheters for selective high-frequency ventilation of upper and lower lobes or, rarely, two separate anesthesia machines and small Tovell tubes to accomplish the same effect. Cardiopulmonary bypass is almost never required for carinal resection. In the extraordinarily complex situation in which bypass might seem useful, the risk of parenchymal hemorrhage negates its use.

Any surgical team performing carinal resection must be equipped and familiar with all the techniques of airway management to ensure safe conduct of the operation. Complete control of ventilation and oxygenation must be maintained continuously.

Operative Technique

Bronchoscopy

Careful bronchoscopic evaluation to determine the extent of involvement and the adequacy of the remaining airway is invaluable. The distal trachea, carina, and mainstem bronchi should be carefully inspected for signs of involvement. We find that more precise assessment is possible with rigid ventilating bronchoscopes and Storz-Hopkins telescopes than with flexible fiberoptic instruments. It is always difficult to know the maximum amount of airway that can be removed to allow safe, tension-free anastomosis, and this varies from patient to patient. For the most common carinal resection, namely right carinal pneumonectomy, the length of distal trachea, carina, and left mainstem bronchus resection should not exceed 4 cm in most patients. Length in excess of 4 cm will produce excessive anastomotic tension and predisposes to separation or stenosis. This does not apply to anastomosis of right main bronchus to trachea.

Mediastinoscopy

All patients with lung cancer should undergo mediastinoscopy to evaluate mediastinal nodes and degree of extraluminal tumor involvement. The presence of positive mediastinal nodes should preclude resection in most patients with primary carinal tumors since these are first-level nodes for such tumors in lung cancer cases. The management of N_2 nodes should follow the surgeon's protocol for such a stage. It is preferable to perform mediastinoscopy at the time of planned resection in order to avoid fibrosis, which would limit mobility of the airway and avoid intraoperative confusion between scar and tumor. Dissection of the pretracheal plane increases mobility of the airway in patients without lung cancer as well, although the plane is easily dissected intrathoracically. Blunt dissection of the carina at mediastinoscopy may facilitate dissection of this area at the time of thoracotomy and may be useful in separating the left recurrent nerve from the left lateral wall of the trachea.

Incisions

The most common incision to gain access to the carina for carinal resection or right carinal pneumonectomy or to the stump of either mainstem bronchus and the carina is a right posterolateral thoracotomy. Median sternotomy is adequate for limited carinal resection; this is carried out transpericardially between the superior vena cava and the ascending aorta laterally and the innominate vein and the pulmonary artery superiorly and inferiorly. These structures need to be fully mobilized to give adequate exposure. The pericardium is opened anteriorly and posteriorly.

Left carinal pneumonectomy poses difficult exposure problems. Limited resection of the carina can be done through a left thoracotomy but requires mobilization of the aorta to gain access to the carina. Tapes can then be passed around the distal trachea and right mainstem bronchus to facilitate exposure (Newton, et al., 1991) (Fig. 16-36). Cervical flexion to devolve the lower trachea is essential to the exposure. More extensive involvement of the carina, distal trachea, or right mainstem bronchus precludes this approach. Bilateral, submammary, transsternal (clamshell) thoracotomy has been the most useful approach under these conditions. Access is adequate but is to be used only for the fittest of patients. Median sternotomy also has a limited role in very limited lesions involving the left mainstem and carina. Left hilar mobilization, if required, is difficult or impossible in many patients through sternotomy, since excessive traction on the heart is required.

Release Maneuvers

One of the most important reasons for technical failure following carinal resection is excessive anastomotic tension. Surgeons performing carinal resection should be very familiar with the available maneuvers to reduce anastomotic tension. The simplest maneuver, as with tracheal resection, is flexion of the neck. This allows development in the trachea into the mediastinum and should be done in all cases just prior to approximation of the airway. Mobilization of the anterior pretracheal plane, avoiding injury to the lateral blood supply to the trachea, increases the mobility of the airway and should be done in all patients, often by mediastinoscopy. Dissection of the left mainstem bronchus in a similar fashion, avoiding its lateral blood supply, will slightly increase the mobility of the distal airway as well. A stitch between the chin and chest placed at the completion of the operation holds the patient's head in flexion, avoiding excessive tension in the early postoperative period. The stitch is cut on the seventh postoperative day. Laryngeal release for carinal reconstruction has

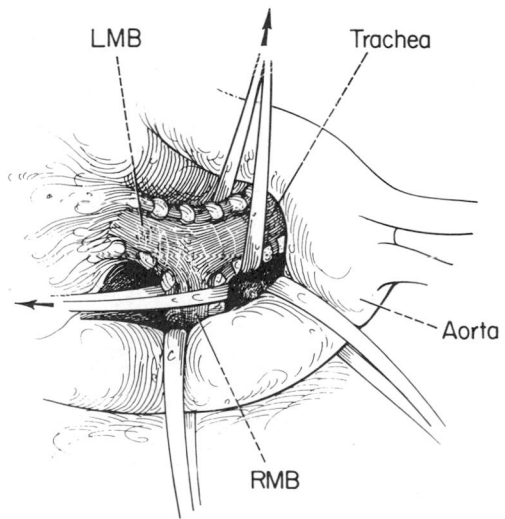

Figure 16-36. Exposure for left carinal resection through left thoracotomy. The aortic arch is mobilized and retracted. Tapes are passed around the distal trachea and right main bronchus (RMB) and retracted to bring the carina into the operative field.

not been helpful in gaining additional length and has been abandoned in most cases.

For carinal resection involving anastomosis of the trachea to right mainstem bronchus, division of the inferior pulmonary ligament and mobilization of the right hilum are important. A U-shaped incision in the pericardium below the inferior pulmonary vein will allow the hilar structures and bronchus to advance (Fig. 16-37). Additional length may be obtained by completely incising the pericardium around the hilar vessels. It is best to preserve a posteriorly based pedicle of tissue that includes bronchial vessels and lymphatics whenever complete incision of the pericardium is performed.

Special mention should be made of those resections involving only the carina. Attempting to ''recreate'' a carina by joining the left and right mainstem bronchi will not allow much, if any, cephalad advancement of the neocarina, since in this case length can be obtained largely by devolvement of the trachea from above. The left main bronchus remains tethered by the aortic arch.

Surgical Technique

Because of the narrow margin between success and failure, precise surgical technique is required. Careful, gentle handling of the tissues is crucial; every attempt should be made to avoid trauma to the bronchial mucosa. Sharp, single, clean transection lines are imperative. The blood supply to the trachea is predominantly segmental, and every effort should be made to avoid interruption. Lateral dissection proximal and distal to the proposed lines of transection should be limited to 1 to 2 cm. Size discrepancy usually exists between the proximal and distal ends of the airway, and no attempt should be made to alter either end; narrowing the proximal end or creating a V in the distal end, is unnecessary. All airway anastomoses should be covered by local vascularized tissues. This may add to the blood supply but, most impor-

tantly, separates these suture lines from nearby vascular structures and suture lines. Pleural flaps, pericardial fat pads, pedicled intercostal muscle flaps, and even omentum can be used. The principles apply to all the reconstructive procedures discussed below.

The goal of surgery should be a tension-free anastomosis with clear surgical margins. Because of the limits of safe resection, a balance must be struck between the desire for clear margins and the ability to safely reconstruct the airway. Clear margins are most desirable for invasive carcinoma. Failure to achieve clear margins, even with postoperative radiotherapy, will invariably lead to recurrence in squamous carcinoma, but this does not appear to be equally true for adenoid cystic carcinoma, in which microscopically positive margins seem to be successfully managed with postoperative radiotherapy.

Modes of Reconstruction

A variety of techniques for reconstruction of the carina have been proposed and used (Fig. 16-38). In practice, the applicability of each technique is determined by the required extent of resection of various parts of the carina. The first reconstructive technique described below applies when no pulmonary tissue is resected, and the other techniques are used after varying amounts of pulmonary resection have been performed.

The simplest technique would appear to be the approximation of the medial walls of the right and left main bronchi to one another to fashion a new carina with the trachea. This technique is applicable only in cases of very small tumors, requiring limited resection of the trachea and bronchi (Fig. 16-39). Suturing the two bronchi together restricts the mobilization of the newly created carina. The left main bronchus has very little mobility, even if its anterior surface has been bluntly dissected; it is held in position by the aortic arch.

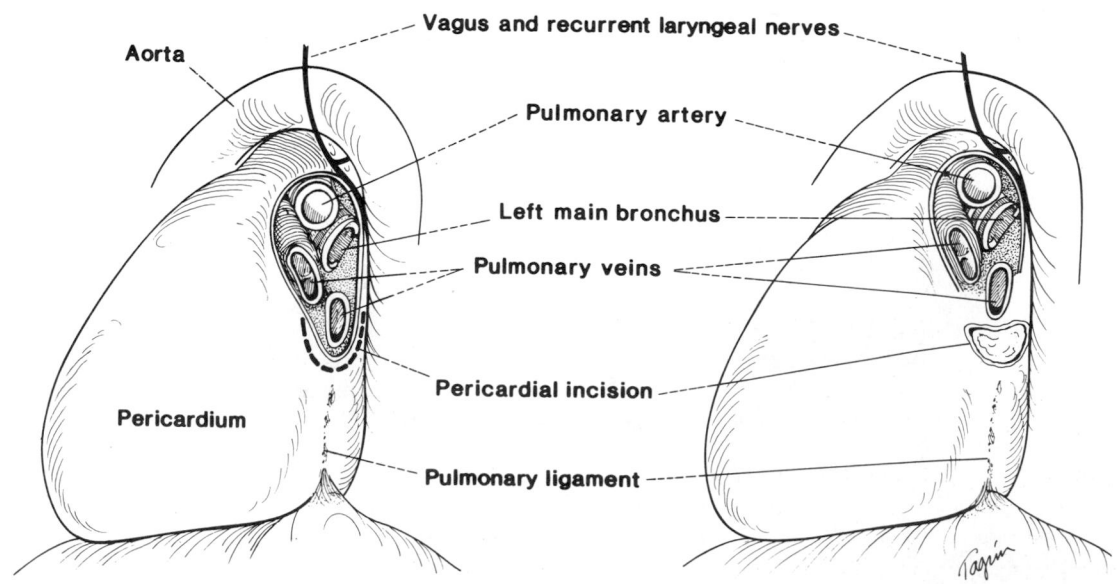

Figure 16-37. The left-sided intrapericardial hilar release technique showing the U-shaped pericardial incision, which allows 1 to 2 cm of upward hilar mobility to facilitate the creation of a tension-free anastomosis.

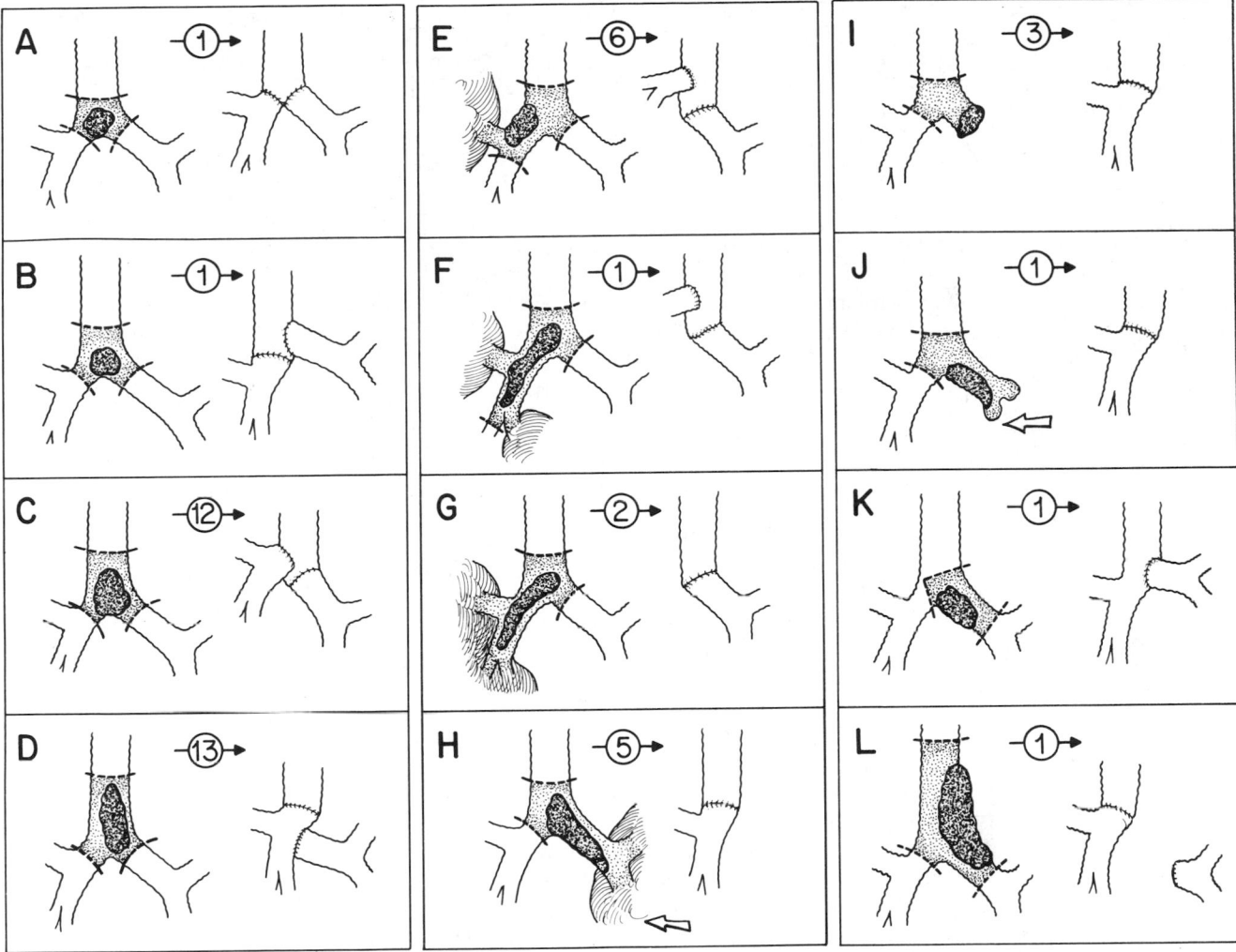

Figure 16-38.   Modes of carinal resection and reconstruction that have been used for tracheal and carinal tumors. Circled number is number of patients. Open arrow indicate side of approach when not conventionally right-sided. **(A)** Limited resection permits carinal restitution; **(B)** technique used in initial carinal resection; technique in Fig. A would now be used. **(C)** More extensive resection; **(D)** greater length of trachea (technique of Barclay and co-workers [1957]); **(E)** involvement of right main bronchus and right upper lobe bronchus, requiring right upper lobectomy. **(F)** middle lobe also removed; right lower lobe bronchus may be anastomosed to left main bronchus. **(G)** Right carinal pneumonectomy; **(H)** left carinal pneumonectomy. **(I)** Resection of carina after previous left pneumonectomy. **(J)** Resection of carina with extra long stump; **(K)** wedge removal of left main bronchus from the right. **(L)** Tracheocarinal resection with long segment of left main bronchus, and exclusion of remaining left lung from the right; left pneumonectomy also through bilateral thoracotomy.

Closure of the gap must therefore be accomplished by bringing the trachea down to the new carina.

When the tumor is more extensive, requiring a larger portion of trachea to be resected, end-to-end plus end-to-side tracheobronchial anastomosis is the method of choice (Fig. 16-40). The possibility of approximation after resection is determined, with the patient's neck flexed, by drawing together lateral traction sutures that have been placed in the trachea and bronchi. In some cases it is easier to approximate the trachea to the left than to the right main bronchus. The tube across the operative field may be intermittently removed, if necessary, during placement of the sutures. It is preferable to place all the anastomotic sutures prior to drawing the lateral traction sutures together and then to tie each

of the anastomotic sutures in sequence. In this anastomosis most of the length is gained by bringing the proximal trachea down to the end of the left main bronchus. After completion of this anastomosis, the endotracheal tube is passed into the left main bronchus and the right main bronchus is elevated and anastomosed to the side of the trachea. The opening is ovoid and is placed in the cartilaginous wall to provide more rigidity. Rarely, it is easier to anastomose the trachea to the right main bronchus and to implant the left main bronchus into the left lateral wall of the trachea. Access for this anastomosis is not as easy.

When a greater length of trachea must be removed, the distance between the relatively immobile left main bronchus and the stump of the trachea is too great to be spanned by

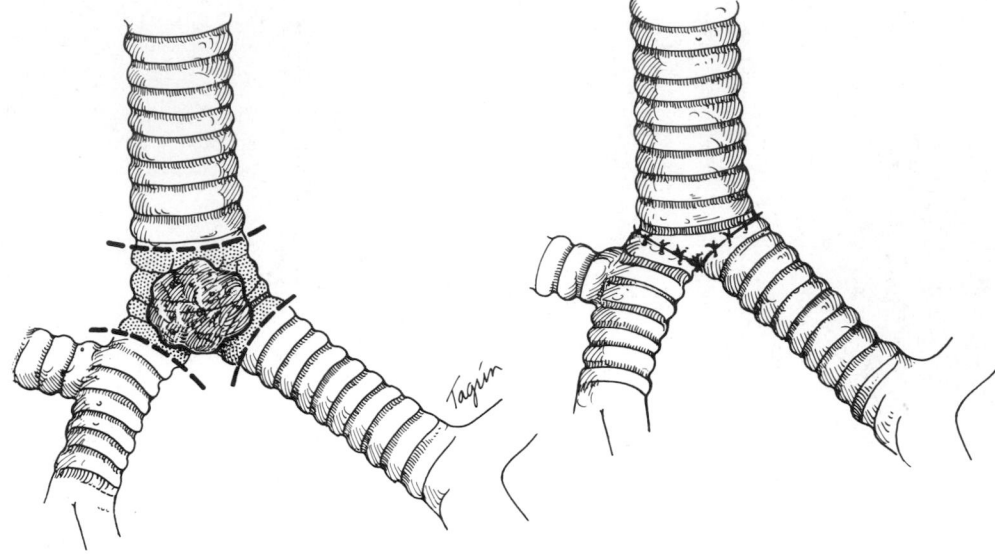

Figure 16-39. Resection with restitution of newly created carina. This technique is applicable only for small, centrally placed tumors.

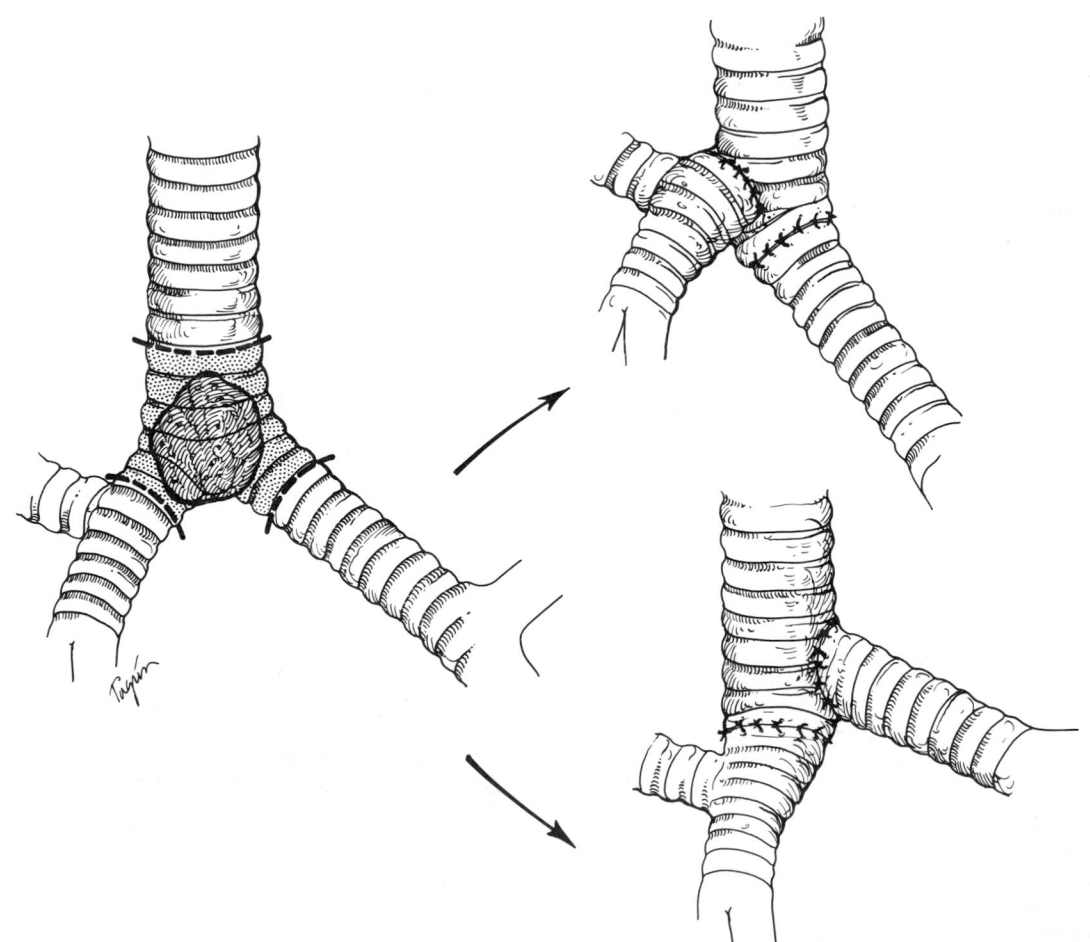

Figure 16-40. Carinal reconstruction after resection, with the trachea anastomosed end-to-end to either the left or the right main bronchus and the other bronchus placed into the lateral wall of the trachea above the first anastomosis. The diagram at upper right shows the more commonly used technique.

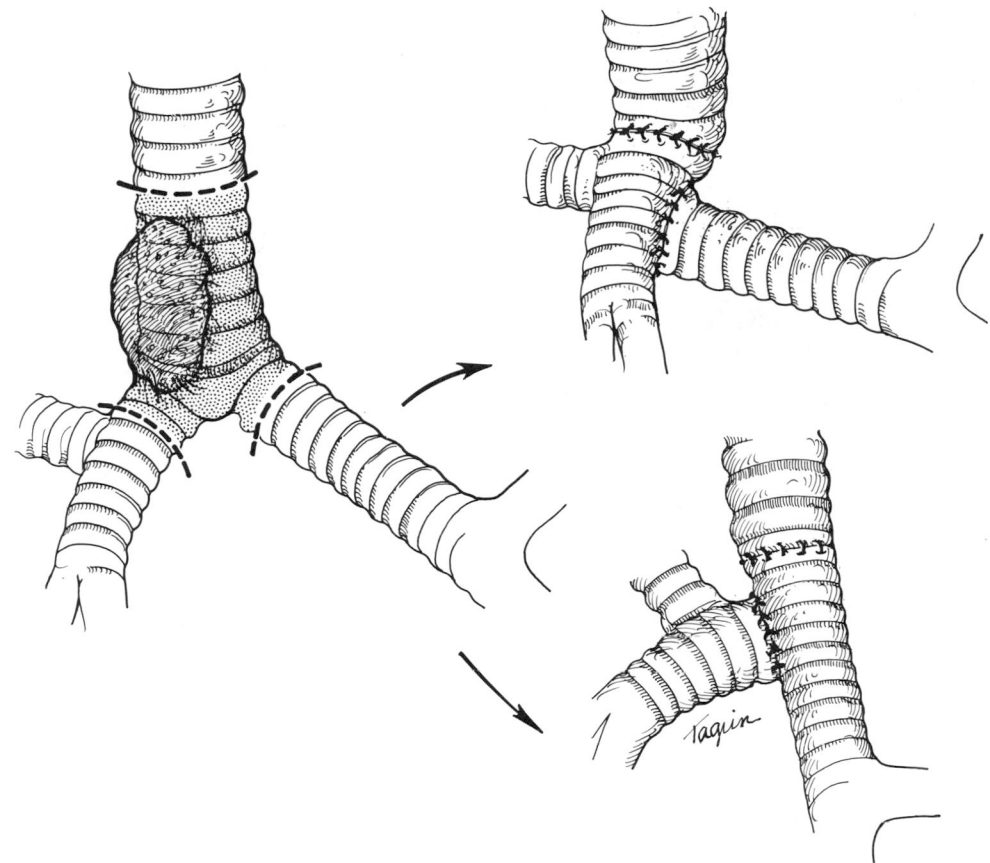

Figure 16-41. More extensive tracheal resection, with advancement of the right main bronchus to the end of the trachea and implantation of the left main bronchus into the bronchus intermedius (*upper right*). The reverse procedure (*lower right*) is rarely applicable, since the left main bronchus is quite fixed.

bringing the trachea down. Under these circumstances the right lung is mobilized, the right main bronchus is brought up for direct end-to-end anastomosis to the trachea, and the left main bronchus is implanted across the mediastinum into the side of the bronchus intermedius (Fig. 16-41). A "reverse" procedure can be done but is rarely required (Fig. 16-41).

If the lesion involves the carina and the right main bronchus to the right upper lobe bronchus, the problem is more complex. The lower trachea and carina, plus the right main bronchus and upper lobe, are resected. The bronchus intermedius is transected below the takeoff of the upper lobe bronchus; the trachea and left main bronchus are anastomosed; and after mobilization of the right hilum intrapericardially, the bronchus intermedius is elevated and implanted in the lateral wall of the trachea, about 1 cm above the previously described anastomosis (Fig. 16-42). This may lead to excessive anastomotic tension, dictating implantation of the bronchus intermedius into the left main bronchus, or to sacrifice of the residual right lung if feasible.

The most common resection of the carina involves the entire right lung and carina (Fig. 16-43) because of the frequency of bronchogenic carcinoma relative to other primary carinal neoplasms. Anastomosis is between the distal trachea and left mainstem bronchus. The procedure is performed for tumors of the right lung involving the carina that require pneumonectomy. The hilar structures are carefully dissected as for right pneumonectomy. The azygous vein is divided, and the distal trachea and left mainstem bronchus are encircled with tape.

Once it has been determined that resection is feasible, vascular structures are divided as for right pneumonectomy. Sterile tubing is passed from the operative field to the anesthesiologist to allow ventilation of the left lung across the operative field. Two midlateral traction sutures are placed proximally on the trachea and distally on the left mainstem bronchus. These sutures are 2–0 Vicryl and are placed full thickness and vertically 4 mm from the point of transection. The airway is then divided and the oral endotracheal tube pulled out of the way into the proximal trachea. The left mainstem bronchus is intubated with a sterile Tovell tube. Frozen section specimens are taken from the proximal and distal margins. With cervical flexion, the traction sutures are used to approximate the two ends tentatively to ensure that the airway can be reconstructed. A balance must be struck between extent of resection for margin and the ability to reconstruct the airway. The pretracheal plane should have been dissected at mediastinoscopy, but if not, it can be done

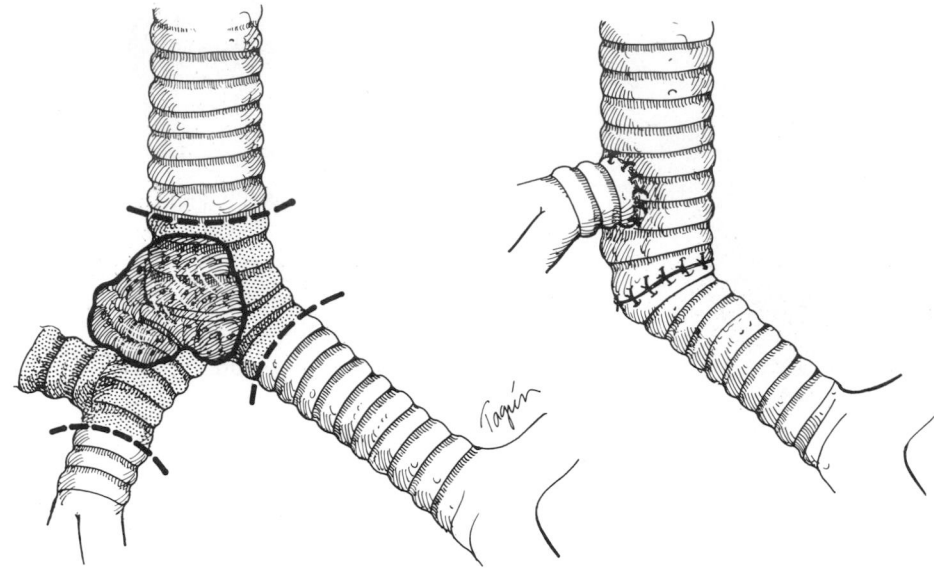

Figure 16-42. Carina resection with right upper lobectomy. With mobilization, the bronchus intermedius is advanced to the side of the trachea and implanted above the anastomosis of the trachea and the left main bronchus.

at this time. To improve mobility, the left mainstem can be dissected anteriorly, avoiding the lateral blood supply.

Once clear frozen section margins have been confirmed, individual anastomotic sutures of 4–0 Vicryl are placed. The sutures are placed so the knots are on the outside 3 to 4 mm from the cut edge of the airway. The first suture is placed in the 6 o'clock position of airway as seen from the operative field. Individual sutures for the anastomosis are completed, the operating table is leveled, the patient's head is maximally flexed, the original oral tube is advanced carefully from above, and the traction sutures are drawn together and tied. The individual sutures are tied in the reverse order of that in which they were placed, so that the last suture to be tied is the first stitch in the 6 o'clock position.

Occasionally the oral endotracheal tube will push against the left mainstem distracting it and preventing approximation with the trachea. If this occurs, the tube is withdrawn and a high-frequency ventilation catheter is passed through the oral endotracheal tube across the anastomosis and into the left mainstem bronchus. High-frequency ventilation is terminated when the anastomosis is completed. The anastomosis is inspected through the oral endotracheal tube with a flexible bronchoscope. The anastomosis is checked to be certain it is airtight by flooding the operative field with saline and sustaining a breath at 30 or 40 cmH$_2$O. A superiorly based pericardial fat pad or a pleural flap is elevated and passed circumferentially around the anastomosis and secured to the airway with fine interrupted sutures. The pleural space is irrigated

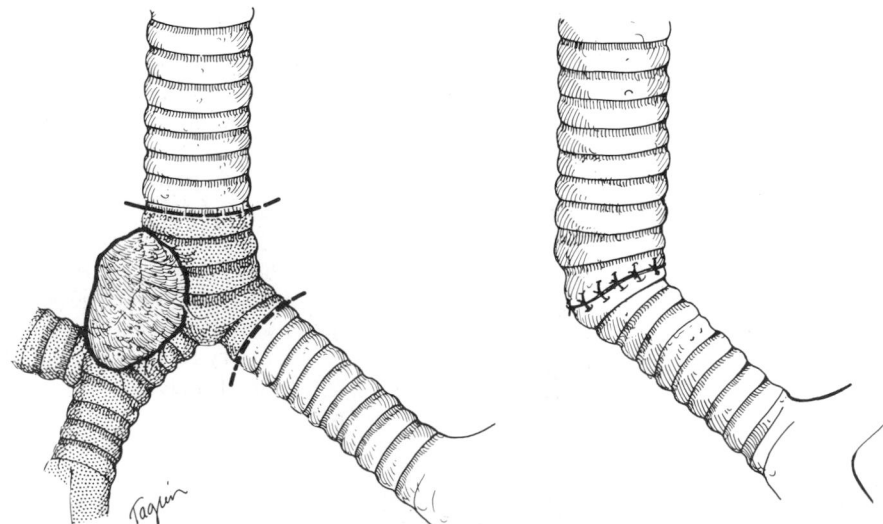

Figure 16-43. Lung cancer involving carina. In this situation the right lung is involved. The right lung and carina are resected and the trachea is anastomosed to the left main bronchus.

copiously, and a chest tube is placed to be managed as for a pneumonectomy.

When tumor involves the lower trachea and a large part of the left main bronchus, the problem becomes very difficult. When the left main bronchus is divided close to the bifurcation into the upper and lower lobes from beneath the aorta and the trachea cannot be brought down to that point, there is currently no way to advance the residual left main bronchus to a resected trachea. Perelman and Koroleva (1980) have managed this problem by stapling the left main bronchus distal to the tumor and reanastomosing the trachea to the right main bronchus. In 10 patients they noted no difficulty with shunting or infection in the left lung; however, massive vascular shunting through the nonaerated left lung may occur, requiring left pneumonectomy. These authors now recommend ligation of the left pulmonary artery also. Bilateral anterolateral thoracotomy can be performed for tracheal resection, left pneumonectomy, and anastomosis of the trachea to the right main bronchus. Such procedures produce major physiologic stresses.

In patients with involvement of most of the left main bronchus and very limited involvement of the carina, pneumonectomy and carinal resection can be performed from the left hemithorax. With flexion of the neck and with tapes placed around the lower trachea and the right main bronchus, it is possible to draw the airway up beneath the aortic arch and to place appropriate traction sutures, excise the carina, and anastomose the trachea to the right main bronchus. Exposure is difficult, and fortunately this approach is rarely required. Bilateral submammary transsternal thoracotomy, another approach giving better access, is suitable only for the fittest of patients. Prolonged mechanical ventilation can be anticipated.

Tumor recurrence in the stump following left pneumonectomy may require resection of the carina (Fig. 16-44). Resection is performed through the right chest while maintaining ventilation in the right lung but working with the lung gently retracted and incompletely collapsed. High-frequency ventilation may be of value, and a great deal of understanding, patience, and cooperation must exist between surgeon and anesthesiologist. Recurrence in the stump following right pneumonectomy can be approached through the right chest. Dissection is difficult and mobility reduced because of the associated fibrosis, but the procedure is applicable for selected patients.

Staged resections of the carina have been abandoned because of the excessive mortality and morbidity associated with these procedures. There is presently no uniformly dependable prosthesis for tracheal or carinal replacement.

Postoperative Care

Postoperative care begins in the operating room. The anesthesiologist must be constantly vigilant to clear secretions and blood from the airway in an aseptic manner. Fluids must be minimized to avoid fluid overload and subsequent pulmonary edema. It is always best to perform bronchoscopy at the completion of the procedure to remove any retained secretions and inspect the anastomosis.

Early postoperative management requires great attention to detail and dedication on the part of all involved. Adequate pain control is paramount and has been greatly facilitated by epidural analgesia, patient-controlled analgesia, and intercostal nerve blocks. Vigorous chest physiotherapy should be instituted early and often. Nasotracheal suction or direct aspiration with a flexible bronchoscope should be performed whenever needed. Minitracheotomy through the cricothyroid membrane with a small (4 Fr) cannula has greatly aided pulmonary toilet in some patients (Wain, et al., 1990). Sputum cultures should be monitored daily and antibiotics adjusted accordingly.

Fluid and electrolyte management are crucial in the early postoperative period. A problem resembling the adult respiratory distress syndrome (ARDS) is the leading cause of early mortality in some series, and fluid overload is almost certainly a contributing factor in some patients (Mathisen and Grillo, 1991). Early presentation has been with hypoxia, tachypnea, and a "ground glass" appearance on radiography of the remaining lung. It usually presents 36 to 72 hours postoperatively. Measures to treat it include intubation, diuresis, fluid restriction, broad-spectrum antibiotics, and frequent suctioning. It is often fatal despite all these measures.

Atrial arrhythmias are common, just as in patients undergoing conventional pneumonectomy. Digoxin and calcium channel blockers are indicated. β-Blockers should be used with caution in this group of patients because of the limitations of pulmonary reserve.

Patients should undergo bronchoscopy at about 1 week postoperatively to check the adequacy of healing. Any sign of early ischemia or necrosis must be followed *very* closely. Bronchopleural fistula must be treated with drainage and antibiotic coverage. If dehiscence and anastomotic separation occur, internal stenting is necessary with a long, custom-made Silastic T tube or a tracheostomy tube. Initial management may require a carefully placed long endotracheal tube.

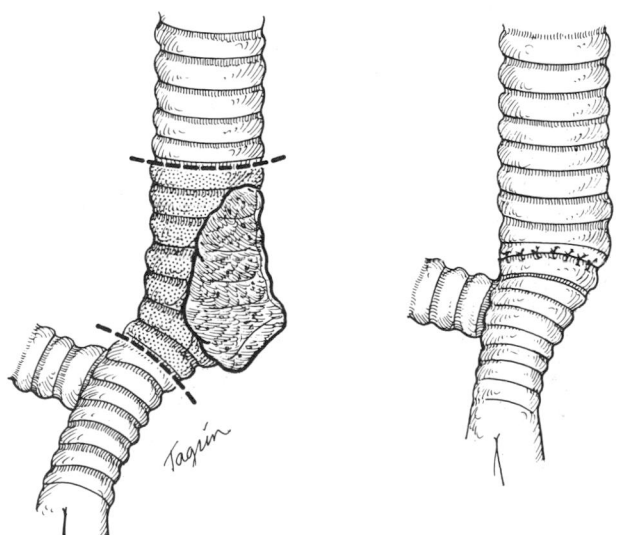

Figure 16-44. Carinal resection after prior pneumonectomy. Except for one patient who had an abnormally long residual left main bronchial stump, these procedures were carried out through the right hemithorax.

It may be necessary in these extreme situations to buttress the anastomosis with pedicled intercostal muscle or omentum. Delayed stenosis should be managed with dilatations or stenting. Re-resection is possible in a limited number of patients, but a sufficient period should elapse to allow resolution of inflammation and fibrosis. Anastomotic complications represent the leading cause of delayed mortality in most series.

The challenge for carinal resection is to reduce the operative mortality to under 10 percent. A better understanding of the early postoperative ARDS problem is essential to reduce early mortality. A better understanding of the limits of safe resection will reduce the late mortality from technical complications. With proper patient selection, attention to technical detail, and dedicated postoperative care, carinal resection can be performed relatively safely and remains an important surgical option in a narrow spectrum of cases. The rarity of such cases makes if difficult for many surgical teams to acquire the requisite skills and experience.

KEY REFERENCES

Dartevelle PG, Chapelier A: Tracheal sleeve pneumonectomy for bronchogenic carcinoma: a report of 55 cases. Ann Thorac Surg 46:68, 1988

This is a report of the largest series available on sleeve pneumonectomy for bronchogenic carcinoma. The results are excellent, with the lowest operative mortality reported to date, 10.9 percent.

Grillo HC: Carinal resection. Ann Thorac Surg 34:356, 373, 1982

This report describes a variety of techniques suitable for carinal resection. A great deal of detailed information on the different techniques is provided. Many etiologies other than lung cancer that require carinal resection and reconstruction are also included.

Jensik RJ, Faber LP, Milloy FJ, Goldin MD: Tracheal sleeve pneumonectomy for advanced carcinoma of the lung. Surg Gynecol Obstet 134:232, 1972

This is a report of the first series of any significant number of patients undergoing sleeve pneumonectomy for carcinoma of the lung. The authors describe in detail their results, their techniques, complications, mortality, and long-term results.

Mathisen DJ, Grillo HC: Carinal resection for bronchogenic carcinoma. J Thorac Cardiovasc Surg 102:16, 1991

This contemporary report of the authors' experience with carinal resection for bronchogenic carcinoma includes techniques other than sleeve pneumonectomy. This represents one of the few series to include procedures of re-creation of the carina and carinal resection plus right upper lobectomy for cancer.

Wilson RS: Tracheal resection. p. 415. In Marshall BE, Longnecker DE, Fairley HB (eds): Anesthesia for Thoracic Procedures. Blackwell Scientific, Boston; 1988

This is an excellent reference on anesthetic techniques for thoracic procedures in general and carinal resections in particular. A variety of different techniques are described, all of which should be well known to those working in the area of carinal resection and reconstruction.

REFERENCES

Abbott OA: Experiences with the surgical resection of the human carina, tracheal wall, and contralateral bronchial wall in cases of right toal pneumonectomy. J Thorac Cardiovasc Surg 19:906, 1950

Barclay RS, McSwan N, Welsh TM: Tracheal resection without the use of grafts. Thorax 12:177, 1957

Belsey R: Resection and reconstruction of the intrathoracic trachea. Br J Surg 38:200, 1946

Deslauriers J: Involvement of the main carina. p. 139. In Delarue NC, Eschapasse H (eds): International Trends in General Thoracic Surgery. Vol 1. WB Saunders, Philadelphia, 1985

El-Baz J, Jensik R, Faber LP, Faro RS: One-lung high-frequency ventilation of tracheoplasty and bronchoplasty: a new technique. Ann Thorac Surg 34:564, 1982

Eschapasse H: Les tumeurs tracheales primitives. Traitement chirurgical. Rev Fr Mal Respir 2:425, 1974

Grillo HC, Bendixen HH, Gephart T: Resection of the carina and lower trachea. Ann Surg 158:889, 1963

Jensik RJ, Faber JP, Kittle CF et al.: Survival in patients undergoing tracheal sleeve pneumonectomy for bronchogenic carcinoma. J Thorac Cardiovasc Surg 84:489, 1982

Juvenelle A, Citret C: Transplantation de la bronche souche et résection de la bifurcation tracheale. J Chir (Paris) 67:666, 1951

Mathey J, Binet JP, Galey JJ et al.: Tracheal tracheobronchial resection. J Thorac Cardiovasc Surg 51:1, 1966

Mathisen DJ, Grillo HC: Endoscopic relief of malignant airway obstruction. Ann Thorac Surg 48:469, 1989

Mathisen DJ, Grillo HC, Vlahakes GJ, Daggett WM: The omentum in the management of complicated cardiothoracic problems. J Thorac Cardiovasc Surg 95:677, 1988

Newton JR Jr, Grillo HC, Mathisen DJ: Main bronchial sleeve resection with pulmonary conservation. Ann Thorac Surg

Perelman MI: Surgery of the trachea. Mir (Moscow) 1976

Perelman M, Koroleva N: Surgery of the trachea. World J Surg 4:583, 1980

Shapshay SM, Dumon JF, Beamis JF: Endoscopic treatment of tracheobronchial malignancy: experience with the Nd-YAG and CO_2 lasers in 506 operations. Otolaryngol Head Neck Surg 93:205, 1985

Tsuchiya R, Goya T, Naruke T, Suemasu K: Resection of tracheal carina for lung cancer. J Thorac Cardiovasc Surg 99:941, 1990

Wain JC, Wilson DJ, Mathisen DJ: Clinical experience with minitracheostomy. Ann Thorac Surg 49:881, 1990

17

ANATOMY

Thomas W. Rice

HISTORICAL NOTE

Graham and Singer (1933) reported the first successful pneumonectomy for therapy for bronchogenic carcinoma. The left pneumonectomy was performed by mass ligation of the pulmonary hilum. Although not the first pulmonary resection, this landmark procedure marked the beginning of modern thoracic surgery. However, mass ligation soon became a historical curiosity, and careful identification and precise control of the individual structures of the pulmonary hilum, lobes, and segments swiftly became the norm. Recognition and preservation of the pulmonary arterial supply, pulmonary venous drainage, and bronchial anatomy permit conservation of the parenchyma, and this is the cornerstone of pulmonary surgery.

HISTORICAL READING

Graham EA, Singer JJ: Successful removal of an entire lung for carcinoma of the bronchus. JAMA 101:1371, 1933

BRONCHOPULMONARY SEGMENT

The anatomic and surgical unit of the lung is the bronchopulmonary segment. A review of pulmonary embryology is helpful in understanding this pulmonary element and the congenital abnormalities of the lung bud (i.e., congenital lobar emphysema, cystic adenomatoid malformation, pulmonary sequestration, and bronchogenic cyst). The lung develops from a foregut bud with continual branching of the principal structures. The lung bud is first seen in the embryo at 3 weeks. In the 4th week, the branching begins with the growth of the right and left main bronchi. Further development is asymmetric, and absorption of the left eparterial bud principally accounts for this. Rapid growth of the airway by terminal branching ensues. By the 17th week, 70 percent of the airway has been formed. The alveoli appear between 20 and 24 weeks in utero.

The pulmonary vascular plexus and venous drainage originates from the splanchnic plexus, which is carried with the developing lung buds. The pulmonary arteries arise from the sixth aortic arch as bilateral buds. These grow into the lung and connect with the developing pulmonary plexus. On the right, absorption of the dorsal sixth aortic arch bud allows for the potential separation of the pulmonary vasculature from the systemic. On the left, persistence and growth of the dorsal bud and its connection to the ventral bud forms the fetal and neonatal communication between the pulmonary and systemic vascular circuits, the ductus arteriosus.

The repetitive branching of the airway and vasculature allows the evolution of independent lung units. Bronchopulmonary segments are subdivisions of the lung that function as individual units because they possess their own bronchus, pulmonary arterial supply, and venous drainage. Each segment may be individually removed without disturbing the function of adjacent segments if the bronchovascular anatomy is appreciated and precisely controlled. The bronchial anatomy of the segment is most constant. The pulmonary artery accompanies the bronchus but with a more variable pattern. The pulmonary veins do not accompany the artery and bronchus in the center of the bronchopulmonary segment but run in the intersegmental planes. Pulmonary veins drain adjacent segments and mark the boundaries of this anatomic unit (Fig. 17-1). Ramsey (1949) emphasized the importance of the venous drainage pattern of the bronchopulmonary segments. Appreciation of the venous drainage is crucial in the identification of the segment and the successful completion of a segmental or lobar resection.

The right lung, which is the larger of the two lungs, has three lobes: the upper, middle, and lower. The right major fissure runs obliquely along the lateral surface of the lung from a superior and posterior position to an inferior and anterior position. The major fissure separates the lower lobe from the upper and middle lobes. The minor fissure, which is less well developed, runs horizontally to separate the upper lobe from the middle lobe. The right lung is composed of 10 segments (Fig. 17-2). The upper lobe has three segments: apical, posterior, and anterior. The middle lobe has two seg-

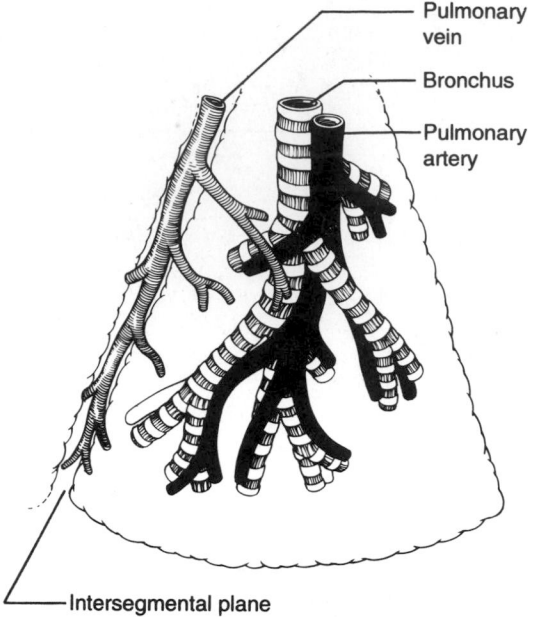

Figure 17-1. The bronchopulmonary segment.

ments: lateral and medial. The lower lobe has five segments: superior, medial basal, anterior basal, lateral basal, and posterior basal.

The left lung has two lobes: upper and lower. The lingula, which is the anatomic equivalent of the middle lobe, is part of the left upper lobe. The left major fissure runs obliquely along the lateral surface of the lung from a superior and posterior position to an inferior and anterior position. The major fissure separates the upper lobe from the lower lobe. The left lung is composed of eight segments (Fig. 17-2). The upper lobe has four segments: apical posterior, anterior, superior (lingular), and inferior (lingular). The lower lobe has four segments: superior, anteromedial basal, lateral basal, and posterior basal. There are fewer segments in the left lung because of sharing of the segmental bronchi by subsegmental bronchopulmonary units, which in the right lung, are segments. The apical and posterior segments of the right upper lobe are one segment in the left upper lobe where these two subsegments share a common segmental bronchus (apical posterior). Similarly the anterior basal and medial basal subsegments of the left lower lobe share the common anteromedial basal segmental bronchus. This variation is of greatest interest at bronchoscopy. At surgery these subsegments can

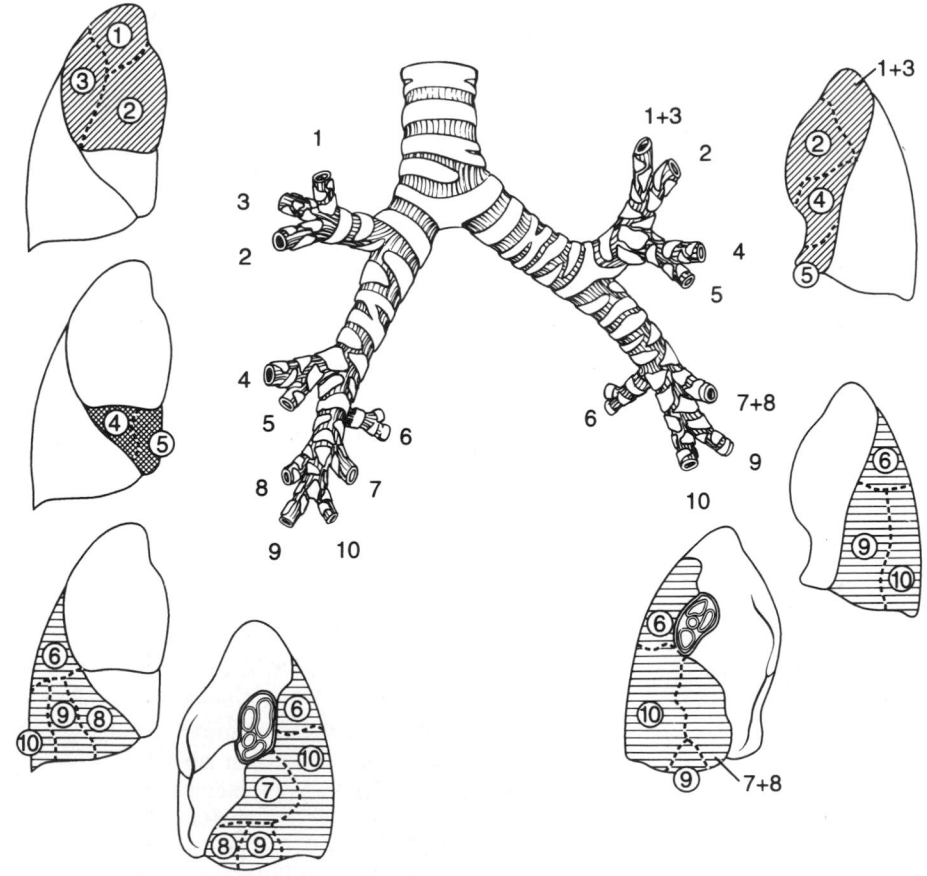

Figure 17-2. The lobes and segments of the lung. Right upper lobe segments: 1. apical, 2. anterior, 3. posterior; right middle lobe segments: 4. lateral, 5. medial; right lower lobe segments: 6. superior, 7. medial basal, 8. anterior basal, 9. lateral basal, 10. posterior basal; left upper lobe segments: 1 and 3. apical posterior, 2. anterior, 4. superior (lingular), 5. inferior (lingular); left lower lobe segments: 6. superior, 7 and 8. anteromedial basal, 9. lateral basal, and 10. posterior basal.

be dissected; this may be useful in surgery of the left upper lobe but is generally not advantageous in the left lower lobe.

Anomalies of lobation are usually the result of too few or too many fissures. Absences or incomplete development of the major or minor fissures cause fusion of adjacent lobes. Accessory fissures correspond to the planes of division between bronchopulmonary segments and account for many of the previously reported accessory lobes. The cardiac lobe is the medial basal segment of the lower lobe, demarcated by an intersegmental fissure. Similarly the superior segment of the lower lobe and the lingula can be separated by an accessory fissure. Accessory lobes are seen in two instances. If no bronchial communication exists, these accessory lungs are really extralobar sequestrations. Rarely an accessory lobe has a bronchial connection; this is seen in the tracheal lobe. This lobe is the apical segment of the right upper lobe with a tracheal origin of the segmental bronchus. Agenesis or aplasia of the lung results from maldevelopment of the lung bud.

INTRAPERICARDIAL ANATOMY

The control of the pulmonary vessels within the pericardium was first advocated by Allison (1946) and further refined by Healey and Gibbon (1950). The ability to control the pulmonary vasculature within the pericardium is crucial for the resection of central tumors and tumors with hilar invasion and for the management of distal vascular problems in which proximal control is required. The serous pericardium reflects onto the pulmonary vessels, as they originate within or enter the fibrous pericardial sac, and must be divided to mobilize these vessels. The lack of complete pericardial investage sometimes obscures the vessel and may make identification and mobilization difficult.

The pulmonary trunk arises from the infundibulum of the right ventricle, and at its origin overlies the aorta. It then passes to the left, rising superiorly and posteriorly for approximately 4 to 6 cm. It is contained in the serous pericardium with the aorta. In this position, it lies between the right and left atria. Below the aortic arch, it bifurcates into the right and left main pulmonary arteries.

The right main pulmonary artery (Fig. 17-3) arises from the main pulmonary artery to pass transversely posterior to the aorta and superior vena cava. More than three-quarters of its length is within the pericardial sac. Behind the aorta and superior vena cava, it constitutes the superior border of the transverse sinus. It is covered by serous pericardium for more than three-quarters of its circumference. Its posterior surface is directly applied to the fibrous pericardium and is not covered by serous pericardium. The pulmonary artery may be safely controlled in this location by retracting the aorta medially and superior vena cava laterally. After the right pulmonary artery is mobilized, it may be retracted, and division of the posterior fibrous pericardium provides transpericardial access to the trachea and main bronchi. As the right pulmonary artery passes from behind the vena cava, it exits the pericardial sac. In this position, it forms the superior border of the postcaval recess of Allison. The medial border is the superior vena cava; the inferior border, the superior pulmonary vein; and the lateral border, the pericar-

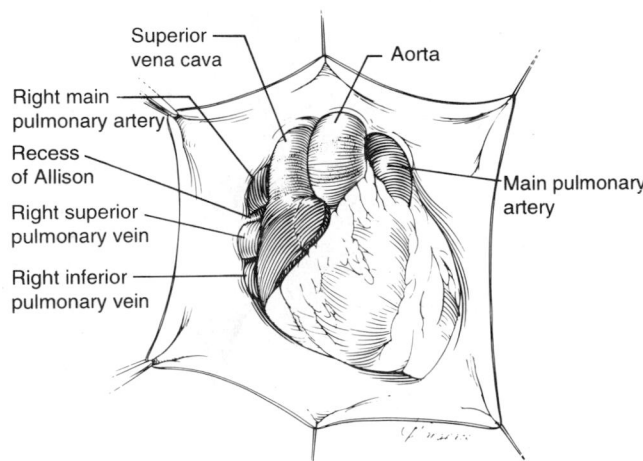

Figure 17-3. The right intrapericardial anatomy.

dial sac. In approximately 5 percent of patients, there is no postcaval recess. The right pulmonary artery exits the pericardial sac when it is still in the retrocaval position.

The right superior pulmonary vein enters the pericardium and is covered by serous pericardium for more than two-thirds of its circumference. It immediately drains into the left atrium. The right inferior pulmonary vein is covered by serous pericardium over only one-third of its circumference, and total lack of this covering in one-half of patients makes it appear that the right inferior pulmonary vein has no intrapericardial component. Mobilization of the inferior pulmonary vein's short stubby pericardial attachments and division of the frenulum of pericardium that runs to the inferior vena cava provide additional mobility of the hilum. This maneuver is sometimes required during intrathoracic tracheobronchial resections for the relief of tension at the airway anastomosis. The vein then drains into the left atrium. On the right, a common pulmonary vein is found in approximately 3 percent of patients. The junction between the right and left atria lies just anterior to the termination of the right pulmonary veins. Added pulmonary venous length may be obtained by dissection within (developing) the intra-atrial groove.

The left pulmonary artery (Fig. 17-4) arises from the main pulmonary artery and passes inferiorly and posteriorly before exiting the pericardium from under the aortic arch. As it leaves the pericardial sac, 50 percent of its circumference is covered by serous pericardium, and this must be divided to control the pulmonary artery at this point. The left pulmonary recess is bordered by the left main pulmonary artery superiorly, the left superior pulmonary vein inferiorly, and the fibrous pericardium laterally. The medial border is the fold of Marshall, which contains the remnant of the left superior vena cava. This is patent in less than 1 percent of patients and may be divided to provide improved intrapericardial access to the left main pulmonary artery and left superior pulmonary vein.

The left superior pulmonary vein enters the pericardium to be covered by serous pericardium on two-thirds of its circumference. Immediately below and inferior to this, is the left inferior pulmonary vein. It is the most distinct and free of

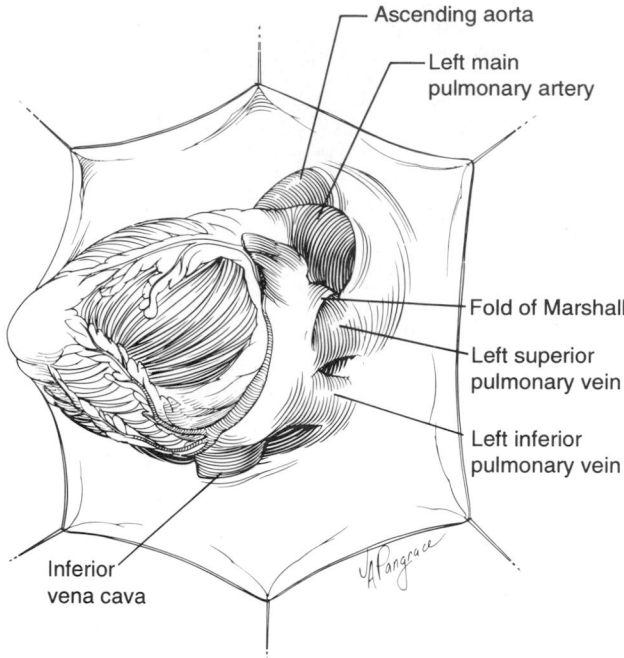

Figure 17-4. The left intrapericardial anatomy.

all the pulmonary vessels with 90 percent of its circumference covered by serous pericardium. Unlike the pulmonary veins on the right, approximately 25 percent of patients have a common left pulmonary vein within the pericardium.

Anomalies of the pulmonary arteries and pulmonary veins may be classified as abnormalities of number or of site of origin or termination. Aberrations of the main pulmonary artery are typically accompanied by anomalies of the heart and great vessels. Main pulmonary artery anomalies are uncommon and consist of agenesis, hypoplasia, or abnormal origin, causing vascular rings that result in airway and esophageal compression. There may be accessory pulmonary arteries arising from the aorta or its branches. This is usually seen in pulmonary sequestrations or pulmonary atresia with ventricular septal defect but may occur without associated disease. Anomalies of pulmonary veins are more common. An abnormal number of veins is seen most frequently as a common left pulmonary vein or separate veins that drain the upper, middle, and lower lobes on the right. Anomalous pulmonary venous drainage can be partial or complete. The veins typically drain into the superior vena cava, right atrium, coronary sinus, inferior vena cava, persistent left vena cava, or systemic veins.

HILUM

The principal structures passing to and from the lung at the mediastinal border are the bronchus, pulmonary artery, and superior and inferior pulmonary veins. These constitute the pulmonary hilum. The lung is fixed centrally by the hilum and the inferior pulmonary ligament. The inferior pulmonary ligament is the reflection of the inferior mediastinal parietal pleura onto the lung, where it envelops the inferior pulmonary vein. On both sides, the hilum is subtended by a vascular

arch; on the right, by the azygous vein; and on the left, by the aortic arch. The hilum is bordered by nerves and systemic vessels: the phrenic nerve and its vascular bundle anteriorly and the vagus nerve and bronchial vessels posteriorly.

The right main bronchus is the most superior and posterior of the right hilar structures and passes into the hilum after exiting the mediastinum below the azygous vein (Fig. 17-5). The right pulmonary artery leaves the pericardium to rise above the superior vena cava and enters the hilum. In the right hilum, the right pulmonary artery lies inferiorly and anteriorly to the bronchus, partially obscuring the bronchus. The truncus anterior, the first branch of the right pulmonary artery, originates from the pulmonary artery before it enters the lung. The superior pulmonary vein passes from the pulmonary parenchyma to lie anteriorly to the pulmonary artery and slightly inferiorly to the truncus anterior branch of the right pulmonary artery. Here it overlaps and obscures the intraparenchymal continuation of the pulmonary artery, the pars intralobares. The superior pulmonary vein receives four component branches. Three drain the upper lobe, and three are superficial. The most superior is the apical anterior vein and, just below this, is the inferior vein, which drains the inferior surface of the anterior segment. Entering the vein deep from the pulmonary parenchyma and from its posterior aspect is the posterior vein, which principally drains the posterior segment of the right upper lobe. The most inferior venous tributary is the middle lobe vein. The inferior pulmonary vein lies posteriorly and inferiorly to the superior pulmonary vein. It is composed of two tributaries: the superior and common basal branches. Lying anteriorly to the hilum on the superior vena cava and pericardium is the right phrenic nerve.

The posterior right hilum (Fig. 17-6) is bordered superiorly by the azygous vein. The short membranous portion of the right main bronchus passes from under the arch of the azygous vein to terminate as the right upper lobe bronchus and the bronchus intermedius. Lying inferiorly and posteriorly to the bronchus intermedius is the inferior pulmonary vein.

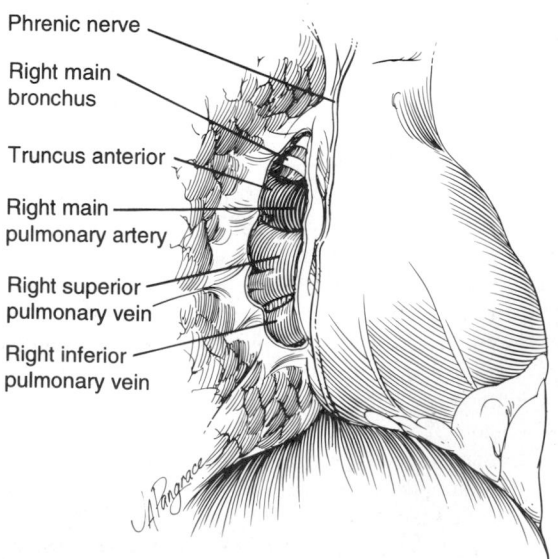

Figure 17-5. The right hilar anatomy, anterior view.

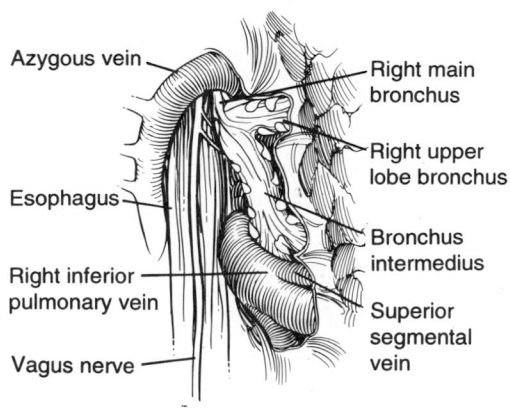

Figure 17-6. The right hilar anatomy, posterior view.

The superior branch of the inferior pulmonary vein, which drains the superior segment of the right lower lobe, is best identified posteriorly. The esophagus and right vagus nerve lie immediately posterior to the right hilum. Lying behind these structures is the azygous vein, which arches over the right main bronchus just above the origin of the right upper lobe. The most constant position of the thoracic duct in the thoracic cavity is inferior to the right hilum (Fig. 17-7). Here, in its supradiaphragmatic location, it can be found between the azygous vein and aorta, bordered anteriorly by the esophagus and posteriorly by the vertebral column.

The left main bronchus is 4 to 6 cm long and passes under the aortic arch to lie posteriorly in the hilum. Unlike the right, where the bronchus remains the most posterior structure, on entering the lung on the left, the left main bronchus is sandwiched between the superior pulmonary vein anteriorly, the pulmonary artery superiorly and posteriorly, and the inferior pulmonary vein inferiorly.

The left pulmonary artery (Fig. 17-8) is the most anterior superior structure in the left pulmonary hilum. The ligamentum arteriosum is found as the pulmonary artery exits from the pericardium. This is the remnant of the ductus arteriosus, which connects the aortic arch to the left pulmonary artery in utero. At this point, the left recurrent laryngeal nerve loops around the aorta at the lateral margin of the ligamentum arteriosum (Fig. 17-9). The pulmonary artery leaves the pericardium and passes over the left main bronchus. The first branch of the artery, the truncus anterior, which supplies the anterior segment of the left upper lobe,

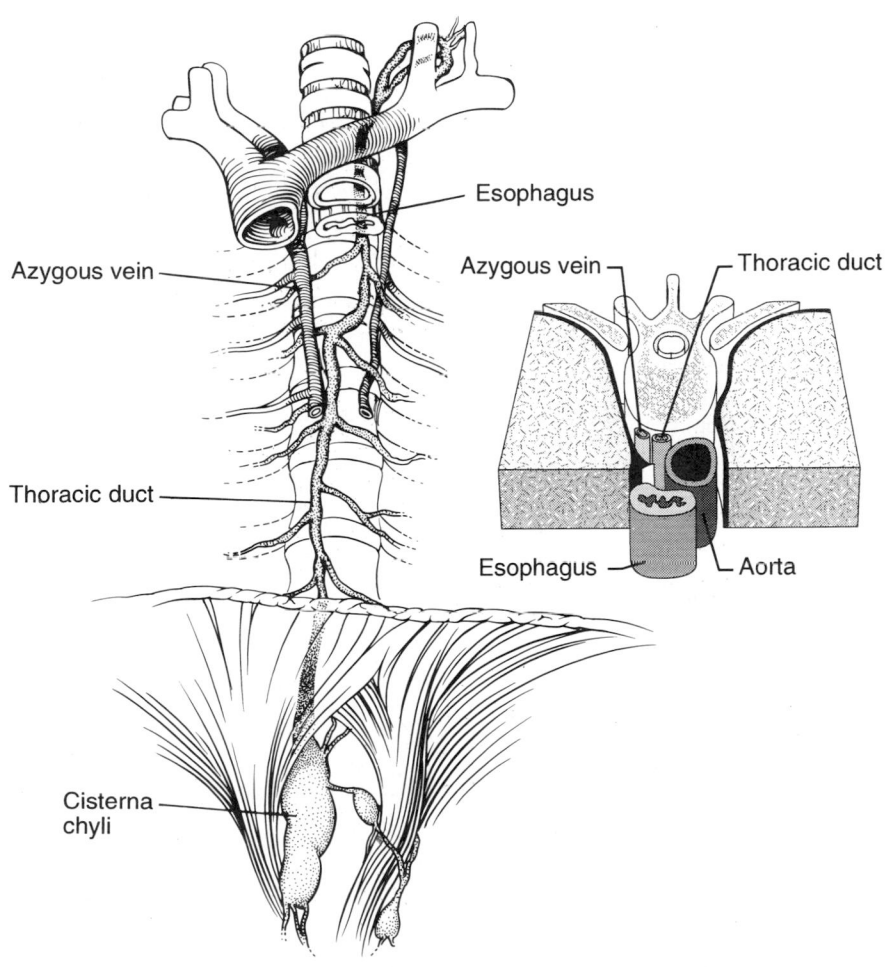

Figure 17-7. The course and relationship of the thoracic duct.

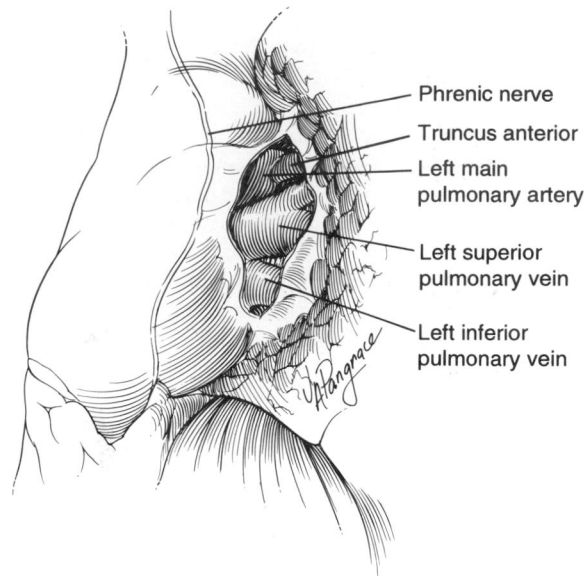

Figure 17-8. The left hilar anatomy, anterior view.

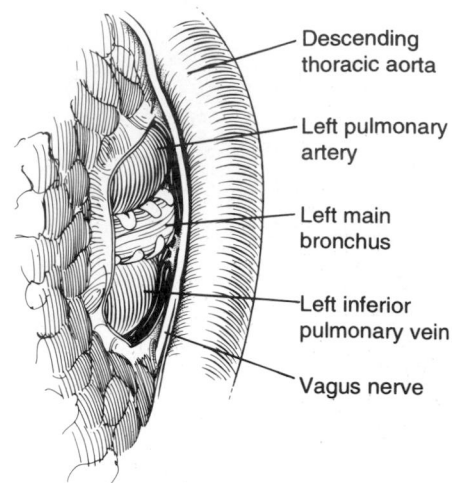

Figure 17-10. The left hilar anatomy, posterior view.

originates before the pulmonary artery passes around the left upper lobe bronchus to enter the left lung posteriorly. The superior pulmonary vein lies anteriorly and inferiorly to the pulmonary artery and is composed of three draining veins: apical posterior, anterior, and lingular. The inferior pulmonary vein lies inferiorly and posteriorly to the superior pulmonary vein and is found at the apex of the pulmonary ligament.

The posterior left hilum (Fig. 17-10) consists of the pulmonary artery superiorly, the left main bronchus, and the inferior pulmonary vein inferiorly. The esophagus and left vagus

nerve lie immediately posterior to the left pulmonary hilum. Behind these structures lies the descending thoracic aorta.

RIGHT UPPER LOBE

The right upper lobe bronchus arises from the lateral wall of the right main bronchus immediately after the origin of the right main bronchus from the trachea. The bronchus passes at right angles to the right main bronchus and bronchus intermedius to enter the right upper lobe. The anomalies of the right upper lobe bronchus have been outlined by le Roux (1962). The origin of the right upper lobe bronchus is anomalous in 3 percent of patients. The most common bronchial anomaly of the right upper lobe is the origin of the apical segmental bronchus from the trachea or right main bronchus, which is reported in 1.4 percent of patients. Absence of a true right upper lobe bronchus with immediate division into the segmental bronchi is seen in 1.1 percent of patients. The entire right upper lobe bronchus may originate from the trachea in 0.5 percent of patients.

The pulmonary arterial supply of the right upper lobe arises from two main branches: the truncus anterior, which originates in the hilum, and the ascending branches, which originate within the pulmonary parenchyma. The variations of the pulmonary artery anatomy of the right upper lobe are well outlined by Milloy, et al. (1963). The truncus anterior is the first and largest branch of the right pulmonary artery. It usually bifurcates after traveling for about 1 cm. In 3.6 percent of patients, there is a split anterior trunk in which two small branches arise separately from the main pulmonary artery. Rarely it may have three branches. The truncus anterior is found in all patients. In 10 percent of patients, the truncus anterior is the only arterial supply of the right upper lobe.

The ascending branches of the right upper lobe originate from the pulmonary artery after it enters the pulmonary parenchyma. These branches ascend to enter the inferior surface of the right upper lobe. In 90 percent of patients, there is an ascending arterial contribution. In 60 percent of patients, there is one branch; in 29 percent, two branches; and in 1

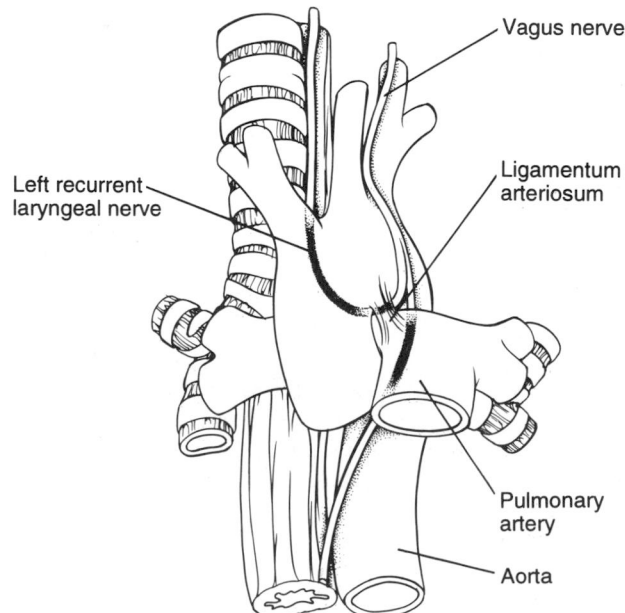

Figure 17-9. The course and relationship of the left vagus and left recurrent laryngeal nerves.

percent, three ascending branches. The ascending artery may be a posterior ascending branch that supplies the posterior segment of the right upper lobe. This is the most common ascending artery and is seen in 88 percent of patients with ascending arteries. This artery arises from the lateral and posterior aspect of the pulmonary artery, opposite the middle lobe branch, and it lies anteriorly to the junction of the inferior margin of the upper lobe bronchus and the bronchus intermedius. In 12 percent of patients, this artery originates from a common trunk with the superior segmental artery. The anterior ascending artery is seen in 25 percent of patients and supplies a portion of the anterior segment of the right upper lobe. It arises from the lateral aspect of the pulmonary artery opposite the middle lobe branch. Ninety-nine percent of these arterial branches are single, and only 1 percent arise from a common trunk with the middle lobe artery.

The superior pulmonary vein drains both the upper and middle lobes. It is crucial during a right upper lobectomy to identify and preserve the middle lobe vein. The venous drainage of the upper lobe is variable but usually consists of three venous tributaries: the apical anterior, the inferior, and the posterior veins.

The azygous lobe is the major anomaly in the segmentation of the right upper lobe, and it is seen in less than 1 percent of patients. It is not a supernumerary lobe but a segregated portion of the right upper lobe. As such it does not have an individual or anomalous bronchovascular supply. The azygous lobe is associated with an azygous vein, which has a long dangling mesentery, and this accessory lobe is formed medially to the pleural septation of the azygous vein.

RIGHT MIDDLE LOBE

The bronchus intermedius is the continuing right bronchus after the origin of the right upper lobe. It is approximately 2 to 4 cm long and terminates at the origin of the middle and lower lobe bronchi. The middle lobe bronchus is on average 1.8 cm long. Generally the bronchus bifurcates to form the two segmental bronchi; rarely in 3 percent of patients, a trifurcate bronchus is seen (Boyden and Hamre, 1951).

An analysis of 225 specimens by Wragg, et al. (1968) demonstrated that the pulmonary arterial supply of the middle lobe is from one artery in 46.5 percent of patients. It usually arises as the first branch of the pars intralobares after the origin of the truncus anterior. It originates from the anterior and medial surface of the pulmonary artery at the level of the ascending branch of the upper lobe. More commonly in 51.5 percent of patients, the middle lobe is supplied by two arteries. This second artery arises, in 48.5 percent of patients, from the pulmonary artery at the level of and opposite to the branch to the superior segment of the right lower lobe. This second branch arises from the ascending branch of the right upper lobe in 0.5 percent of patients and from a common trunk with a basal segmental artery, in 2.5 percent of patients. Rarely in 2 percent of patients, there are three branches that supply the middle lobe.

The middle lobe vein joins the upper lobe vein to form the superior pulmonary vein. Lindskrog, et al. (1949) demonstrated that, in the majority of patients (64 percent), the two segmental veins joined to form the middle lobe vein. In 36 percent of patients, the two segmental veins terminated separately at the superior pulmonary vein.

RIGHT LOWER LOBE

The segmental bronchi of the right lower lobe arise with the middle lobe bronchus at the termination of the bronchus intermedius. The superior segmental bronchus originates from the posterior and lateral aspect of the bronchus intermedius, usually opposite or slightly above the middle lobe bronchus. In 6 percent of patients, the superior segmental bronchus arises as two separate orifices 6 to 10 mm apart (Ferry and Boyden, 1951). Below this are the four basal segmental bronchi of the right lower lobe. Usually the medial basal segmental bronchus is the most proximal basal branch. The anterior basal bronchus is next, and then a common stem for the lateral basal and posterior basal bronchi is usually seen. The middle lobe bronchus must be protected during right lower lobectomy. The abrupt termination of the bronchus intermedius into the middle lobe bronchus and superior and basal segmental bronchi makes compromise of the middle bronchial lobe bronchus a distinct possibility if the lower lobe segmental bronchi are taken en masse. Identification of all three bronchi and separate control of the superior segmental and basal segmental bronchi minimizes this complication.

Wragg, et al. (1968) provides the largest modern description of the arterial supply of the right lower lobe. In 78 percent of patients, the superior segment of the right lower lobe is supplied by a single arterial branch. Two branches to the superior segment are seen in 21 percent of patients. Rarely in less than 1 percent of patients, three branches to this segment are found. Branches to the segment may be displaced in their origin or arise as common trunks, either from the ascending branch of the upper lobe or from the basal segmental arteries of the lower lobe. Twelve to 14 percent of arterial branches to the superior segment may arise from a common branch with the ascending branch of the upper lobe. In 6 percent of patients, the superior segmental artery may arise from a basal segmental artery. The basal segmental arterial supply is variable, but generally this artery, which lies posterolateral to the bronchus, sends branches to the anterior basal and medial basal segments. Then the pulmonary artery terminates by division into the lateral basal and posterior basal segmental arteries.

The inferior pulmonary vein is usually composed of two segmental tributaries: the superior and the common basal veins. Generally the common basal vein is composed of two major veins, the superior basal vein (which drains the medial basal, anterior basal, and lateral basal segments) and the inferior basal vein (which usually drains the lateral basal and posterior basal segments). In one-third of patients, there may be three and four branches of the common basal vein. Rarely venous drainage is received from the posterior segment of the right upper lobe or from the middle lobe.

LEFT UPPER LOBE

The left main bronchus, which is 4 to 6 cm long, passes at an oblique angle under the aortic arch and bifurcates to form the upper and lower lobe bronchi. The upper lobe bronchus, which originates much lower than does the right upper lobe bronchus, bifurcates immediately, forming the lingular orifice and the common bronchus to the anterior and apical posterior segments.

The pulmonary arterial supply of the left upper lobe is the most variable of all lobes. In an analysis of 300 specimens, Milloy, et al. (1968) provided the most complete description of the left upper lobe arterial supply. The number of branches varies from one to eight. In 46 percent of patients, three branches supply the left upper lobe, and in 36 percent, four branches are found. The arterial branches arise as two groups: the truncus anterior and the posterior arterial branches, which originate in the fissure along the inner curve of the pulmonary artery.

The truncus anterior is large, short, and partially hidden by the superior pulmonary vein. It is the origin of a hidden deep branch to the anterior or lingular segments in one-quarter of patients, and frequently it is invaded by large left upper lobe tumors. All these factors make mobilization of the truncus anterior hazardous. In less than 1 percent of patients, it is the only arterial supply of the left upper lobe. In approximately 70 percent of patients, there are two branches of the anterior trunk and, in near-equal proportions, one or three branches. In the majority of patients, the apical posterior and anterior segments are supplied by this branch (62.3 percent). In 8 percent the anterior and lingular segments are supplied by this branch. In 15.6 percent of patients, three branches of this artery supply all segments of the left upper lobe. In 13.9 percent of patients, only one branch is seen, supplying variably the apical posterior or anterior segments.

The remaining blood supply of the left upper lobe comes from the posterior segmental arteries. These arise along the inner curve of the pulmonary artery, in the fissure, as it wraps around the left upper lobe bronchus. These vessels pass into the posterior aspect of the left upper lobe. There may be zero to five posterior artery branches. In 65 percent of patients, no common trunks are seen. However, in 35 percent of patients, common trunks of these posterior branches are found. In 5 percent of patients, there is only one posterior branch to the left upper lobe; in 46 percent, two; in 36 percent, three; in 12 percent, four; and in 1 percent, five posterior branches. The segmental arterial supply to the left upper lobe is variable, with anterior and lingular segments receiving one to three branches. The apical posterior segment may receive as many as four separate branches.

The venous drainage of the left upper lobe is similarly divergent. The superior pulmonary vein may receive two major branches, three major branches, or a number of radiating veins. Generally it is the terminus of the anterior, apical posterior, and lingular veins. However these veins may have multiple branches. Because the vein lies anterior to the pulmonary artery, all except its deep branches may be appreciated in the anterior dissection of the hilum.

LEFT LOWER LOBE

The lower lobe bronchus arises with the upper lobe bronchus at the termination of the left main bronchus. The first segmental branch, the superior segmental bronchus, originates poste-

riorly and laterally. In less than 1 percent of patients, it has a bifurcate origin. Approximately 1 to 2 cm beyond this, the common basal trunk is found. In 80 percent of patients, it immediately bifurcates; in the remainder, it branches into the three segmental bronchi (Pitel and Boyden, 1953).

The arterial supply of the left lower lobe is derived solely from arteries arising in the fissure. The superior segment of the lower lobe is supplied by a single artery in 72 percent of patients (Wragg, et al., 1968). In 26 percent two superior segmental arteries are found. In 2 percent of patients, three arteries supply the superior segment. These arteries usually arise directly from the pulmonary artery; however in less than 3 percent of patients, one may originate from a common trunk with a posterior artery of the left upper lobe. In as many as 12 percent of patients, a common trunk with a basal segmental artery is found. The frequency of a shared trunk with a basal segmental artery is similar for the superior segments of both the right and left lower lobes. A common trunk with an upper lobe artery is seen more commonly on the right.

The basal segmental artery is the termination of the left pulmonary artery after the origin of the superior segmental and lingular branches. In approximately 50 percent of patients, the artery bifurcates to supply the anteromedial segment and the combination of the posterior and lateral segments. In the remaining patients, the branching is variable and ranges from two to four segmental branches.

The venous drainage of the left lower lobe is similar to that of the right lower lobe. The inferior pulmonary vein receives two major branches: the superior segmental and the common basal veins.

FISSURES

The relationships of the bronchovascular structures of the lobes and segments is best appreciated by describing their relationship during control of the fissures.

Right Major Fissure

The pulmonary artery may be palpated at the confluence of the major and minor fissures (Fig. 17-11). Dissection of the pulmonary parenchyma permits the pulmonary artery to be identified in its interlobar position. The posterior branch of the superior pulmonary vein commonly runs in this interlobar plane and may overlay and obscure the pulmonary artery. In addition, an interlobar lymph node, commonly referred to as the sump node, is found overlying the pulmonary artery. After identification of the pars intralobares, the branches of the pulmonary artery in this area may be mobilized. They are identified as follows: anteriorly, the superior branch of the middle lobe; posteriorly and superiorly, the posterior ascending branch of the right upper lobe; posteriorly and inferiorly, the superior segmental arterial branch of the right lower lobe; and inferiorly, the bifurcating termination of the pulmonary artery supplying the basal segments. Dissection in the notch between the posterior ascending and superior segmental arterial branches allows the identification of a posterior interlobar lymph node (number 11, Fig. 17-11A).

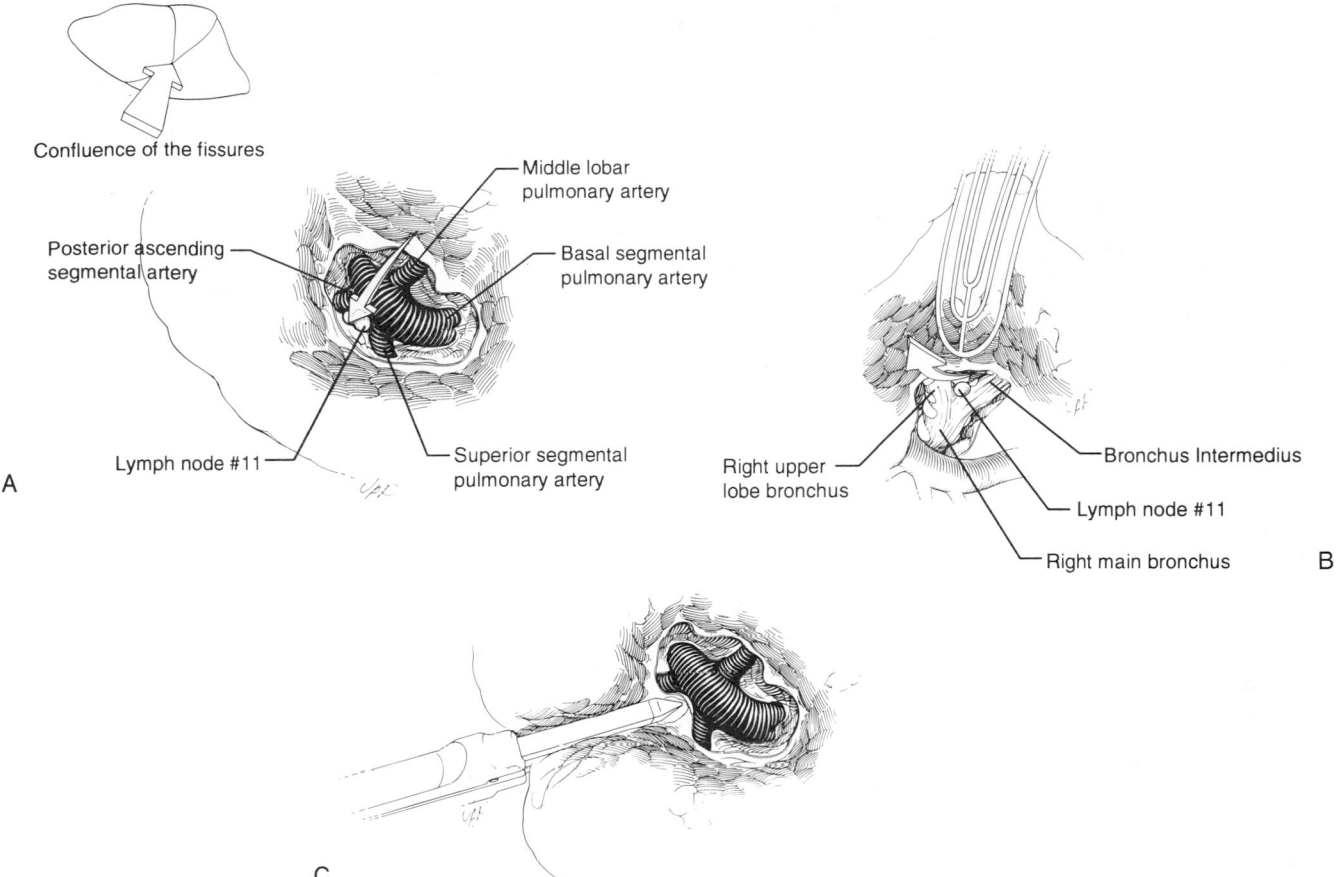

Confluence of the fissures

Posterior ascending segmental artery

Middle lobar pulmonary artery

Basal segmental pulmonary artery

Lymph node #11

Superior segmental pulmonary artery

A

Right upper lobe bronchus

Bronchus Intermedius

Lymph node #11

Right main bronchus

B

C

Figure 17-11. The posterior, superior dissection of the right major fissure. **(A)** Dissection at the confluence of the fissures allows identification of the pars intralobares of the pulmonary artery and its major branches. The dissection is carried out between the posterior ascending segmental artery and the superior segmental artery. **(B)** The posterior hilar dissection is carried out between the inferior margin of the right upper lobe bronchus and the bronchus intermedius. **(C)** The posterior superior portion of the right major fissure is completed by connecting the dissections of both the pulmonary artery (Fig. A) and the bronchus (Fig. B).

Next the hilum is approached posteriorly, and the angle between the inferior margin of the right upper lobe bronchus and the bronchus intermedius is dissected (Fig. 17-11B). In this notch between the bronchi, the posterior aspect of the posterior interlobar lymph node is seen. The posterior superior portion of the major fissure may be controlled if the posterior interlobar lymph node is mobilized and the posterior dissection about the bronchi is then connected to the posterior and lateral pulmonary arterial dissection in the fissure (Fig. 17-11C).

Return to the confluence of the fissures allows control of the anterior inferior portion of the right major fissure (Fig. 17-12A). Dissection in the notch between the inferior pulmonary artery branch of the middle lobe and the adjacent basal segmental artery reveals the bronchi deep to these arteries. An anterior interlobar lymph node (number 11) is found lying in the notch between the middle lobe and basal segmental bronchi.

Next the hilum is approached anteriorly, and the space between the superior and inferior pulmonary veins is cleared (Fig. 17-12B). Dissection in this notch allows the identification of the middle lobe and basal segmental bronchi and the anterior surface of the previously identified anterior interlobar lymph node. The anterior inferior portion of the major fissure may be controlled if the anterior interlobar lymph node is mobilized and the anterior dissection about the pulmonary veins is connected to the anterior and lateral pulmonary arterial dissection in the fissure (Fig. 17-12C).

Right Minor Fissure (Horizontal Fissure)

The horizontal fissure is usually incomplete (poorly developed). Generally it is the last structure controlled in a middle or upper lobectomy. However, management of this fissure may be necessary as an early step in these surgical procedures. Again the control of this fissure commences with a dissection at the confluence of the fissures. The pars intralobares of the pulmonary artery is identified in the fissure. The superior arterial branch of the middle lobe is identified anteriorly. In approximately one-quarter of patients, the ante-

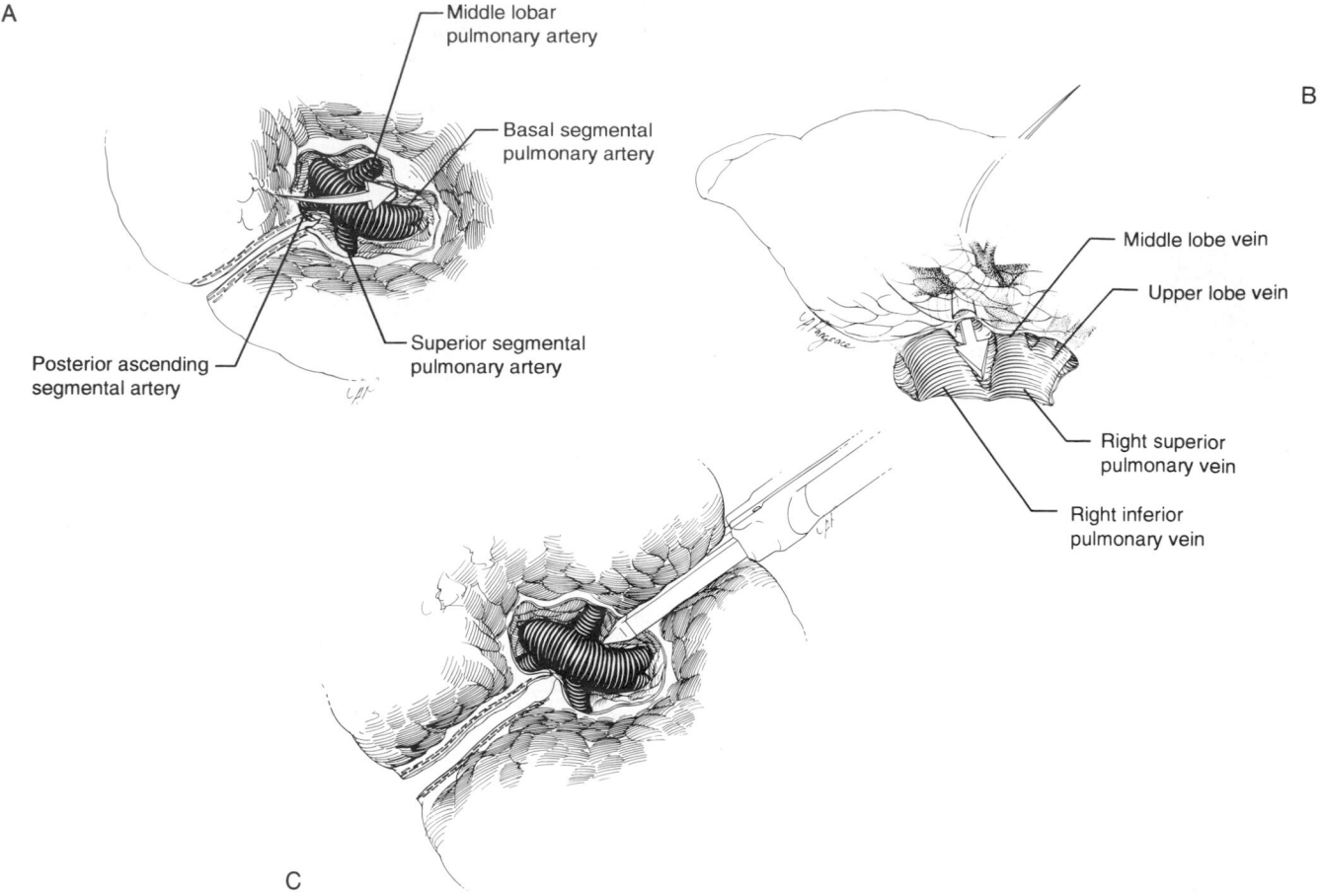

A

B

C

Figure 17-12.   The anterior inferior dissection of the right major fissure. **(A)** Dissection at the confluence of the fissures allows identification of the pars intralobares and its branches in the fissure. The dissection is carried out between the inferior middle lobe artery and the basal segmental artery. **(B)** The anterior hilar dissection is carried out between the superior and inferior pulmonary veins. **(C)** The anterior inferior portion of the right major fissure is completed by connecting the dissection of both the pulmonary artery (Fig. A) and the pulmonary veins (Fig. B).

rior ascending branch of the right upper lobe is found at this level, lying opposite the highest middle lobe branch (Fig. 17-13A).

Next the hilum is approached anteriorly, and the space between the middle lobe vein and the inferior segment vein of the upper lobe is dissected (Fig. 17-13B). Care must be taken during dissection not to damage the posterior vein branch, which joins the upper lobe vein from deep within the pulmonary parenchyma. The minor fissure may be controlled if the anterior dissection about the superior pulmonary vein is connected to the lateral pulmonary arterial dissection in the fissure (Fig. 17-13C).

Left Major Fissure

The pulmonary artery may be palpated in the midportion of the major fissure (Fig. 17-14). Dissection of the pulmonary parenchyma permits the pulmonary artery to be identified in its interlobar position. An interlobar lymph node (number 11), the left sump node, is found overlying the pulmonary artery. The branches of the pulmonary artery may now be

mobilized: anteriorly, the posterior branches of the upper lobe supplying the apical posterior and lingular segments; posteriorly, the superior segmental artery; and inferiorly, the basal segmental arteries (Fig. 17-14A).

Next the hilum is approached posteriorly, and the main pulmonary artery is mobilized as it enters the pulmonary parenchyma (Fig. 17-14B). Dissection allows the posterior surface of the superior segmental artery to be defined. The posterior superior portion of the major fissure may be controlled if the posterior dissection of the pulmonary artery at the hilum is connected in the plane of the pulmonary artery to the lateral pulmonary arterial dissection in the fissure (Fig. 17-14C). Care is taken to dissect in the plane above the pulmonary arterial adventitia and between the posterior branches to the upper lobe and the superior segmental branch to the lower lobe.

Return to the fissure allows control of the anterior inferior portion of the left major fissure. Dissection in the notch between the lingular segmental artery branch and the adjacent basal segmental artery reveals the bronchi deep to these arteries. An anterior interlobar lymph node (number 11) is

A

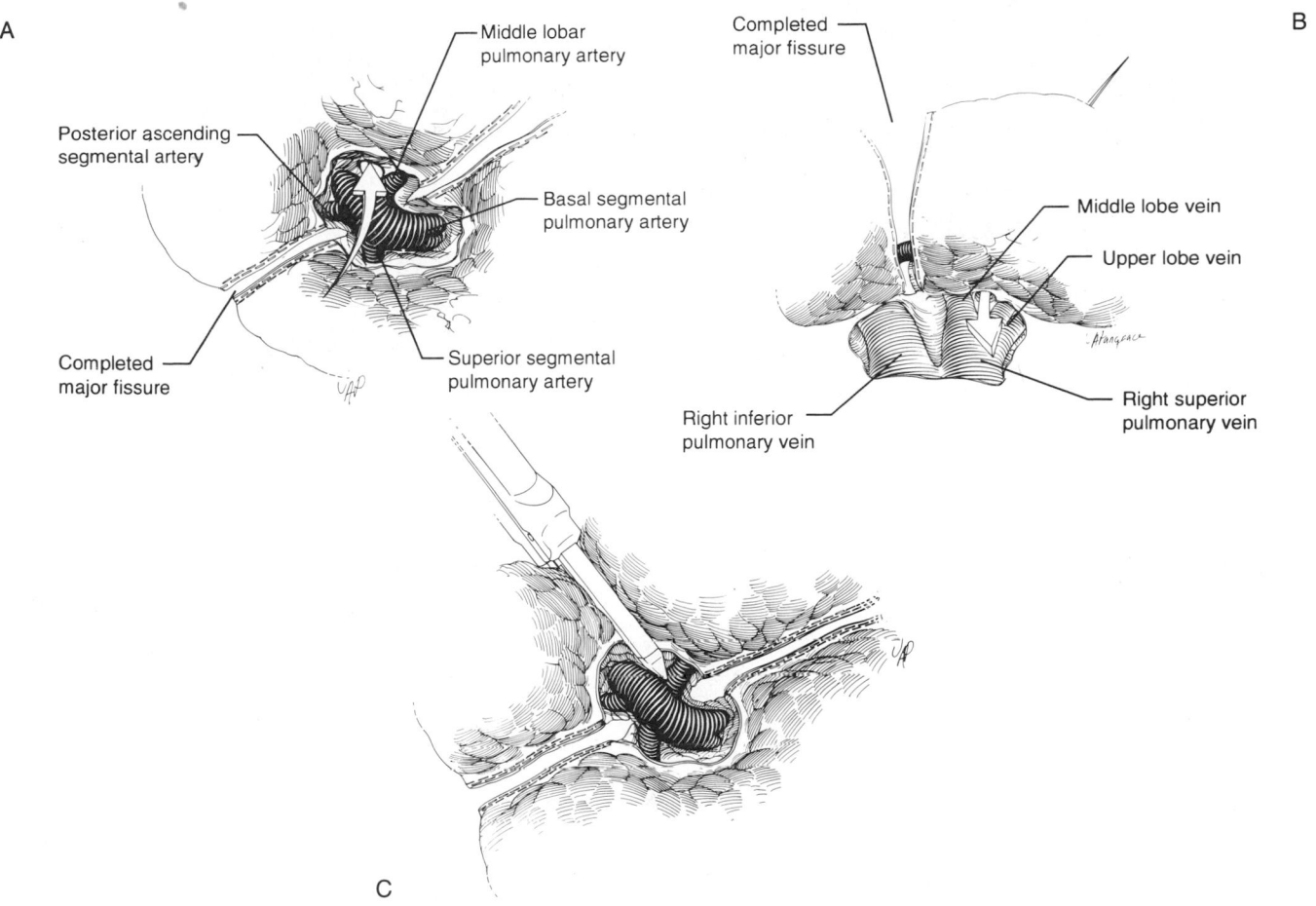

Posterior ascending
segmental artery

Middle lobar
pulmonary artery

Basal segmental
pulmonary artery

Completed
major fissure

Superior segmental
pulmonary artery

B

Completed
major fissure

Middle lobe vein

Upper lobe vein

Right inferior
pulmonary vein

Right superior
pulmonary vein

C

Figure 17-13.   The dissection of the minor (horizontal) fissure. **(A)** Dissection at the confluence of the fissures allows identification of the pars intralobares and the branches to the middle lobe. **(B)** The anterior hilar dissection carried out between the middle lobe vein and the inferior segmental vein of the upper lobe. **(C)** The minor fissure is completed by connecting the dissections of both the pulmonary artery (Fig. A) and the pulmonary veins (Fig. B).

found lying in the notch between the lingular and basal segmental bronchi (Fig. 17-15A).

Next the hilum is approached anteriorly, and the space between the superior and inferior pulmonary veins is cleared (Fig. 17-15B). Dissection in this notch allows identification of the lingular and basal segmental bronchi and the anterior surface of the previously identified anterior interlobar lymph node. The anterior inferior portion of the major fissure may be controlled if the anterior interlobar lymph node is mobilized and the anterior dissection about the pulmonary veins is connected to the anterior and lateral pulmonary arterial dissection in the fissure (Fig. 17-15C).

PULMONARY LYMPHATICS

Naruke, et al. (1978) were the first to propose a mapping system for the regional lymph nodes of the lung. This refined map is now a mainstay in the staging of primary bronchogenic carcinomas (Fig. 17-16). The regional lymph nodes of the lung are arranged into 1 of 14 lymph node stations. Lymph nodes 1 through 9 are mediastinal lymph nodes. Metastases

to mediastinal lymph nodes represent stage N2 or N3 disease (in the tumor-node-metastasis staging system), depending on whether the metastases are ipsilateral or contralateral. Hilar lymph nodes are designated as station 10. Lymph nodes 11 through 14 are intrapulmonary lymph nodes. Metastases to lymph nodes 10 through 14 are termed stage N1 disease. If no lymph node metastases are found, the regional lymph node status is stage N0. Supraclavicular lymph nodes are not included in this map, but metastases to regional lymph nodes on either side of the neck are classified as stage N3 disease.

The highest mediastinal node is a pretracheal node, sometimes called the delphian lymph node. It is frequently involved with thyroid carcinoma but infrequently is a site of metastasis in primary lung cancer. It is encountered at the beginning of mediastinoscopy during the identification of the pretracheal plane. Lymph nodes 2, 3, 4, and 7 are found about the trachea and are easily assessed at mediastinoscopy. These are the right and left paratracheal (2R and 2L), the right and left tracheobronchial angle (4R and 4L), pretracheal (subinnominate, 3), and subcarinal (7) lymph nodes. These

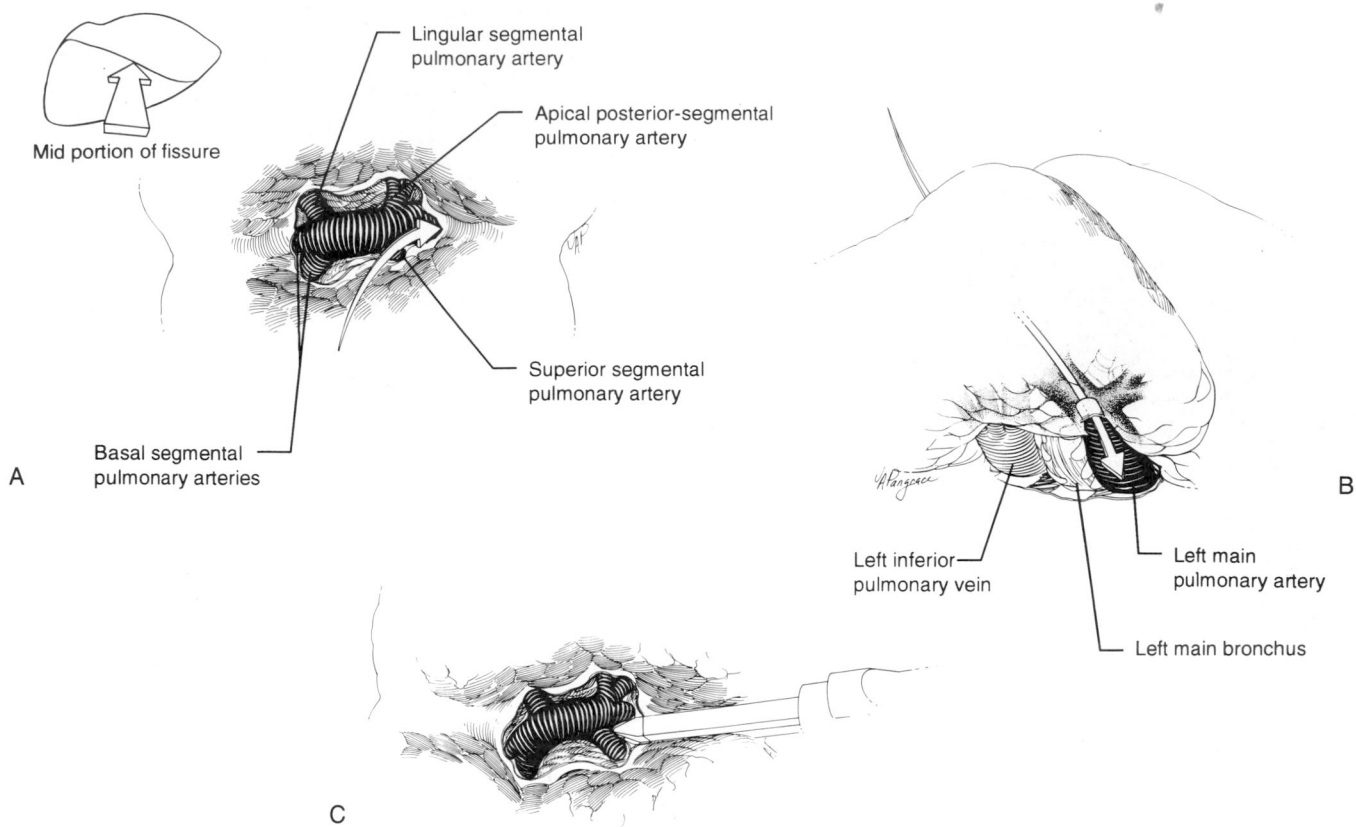

Figure 17-14. The posterior superior dissection of the left major fissure. **(A)** Dissection in the midportion of the left major fissure allows the pulmonary artery to be identified in its interlobar position. Dissection allows the branches of the pulmonary artery to be identified. **(B)** The posterior hilar dissection of the pulmonary artery allows identification of the branches to the upper and lower lobes. **(C)** The posterior superior portion of the left major fissure is developed by connecting the pulmonary arterial dissection in the fissure (Fig. A) to the posterior hilar arterial dissection (Fig. B).

nodes may also be identified at thoracotomy, but sampling of 2L and 4L may be difficult because they are obscured by the aortic arch.

Not obtainable by standard cervical mediastinoscopy are lymph nodes in the subaortic window (5) and para-aortic area (6). These may be obtained by extended cervical mediastinoscopy (Ginsberg, et al., 1987), anterior mediastinotomy (Chamberlain procedure), thoracoscopy, or thoracotomy. The paraesophageal (8) and inferior pulmonary ligament (9) lymph nodes can be sampled by thoracoscopy or dissected at thoracotomy. Hilar lymph nodes (10) may be obtained by mediastinotomy, thoracoscopy, or thoracotomy.

Interlobar lymph nodes (11) are found in the fissures, surrounding the pulmonary arteries or bronchi. Lobar (12), segmental (13), and subsegmental (14) lymph nodes can only be reliably sampled at thoracotomy.

The classic drainage pathway of the pulmonary lymphatics is from subpleural lymphatic vessel along lymphatic channels associated with the pulmonary veins to reach larger channels that run with the arteries and bronchi. These deeper lymphatic channels drain into segmental, lobar, interlobar, hilar, and mediastinal nodes. Riquet, et al. (1989) demonstrated segmental drainage of subpleural lymphatic in 90.5 percent of patients. In 9.5 percent of patients, the drainage is interseg-

mental. In 77.8 percent of right-sided studies, intrapulmonary drainage was demonstrated; however, 22.2 percent had direct drainage to mediastinal lymph nodes, bypassing the classic drainage pattern. On the left, this was slightly more common, with 25 percent of studies showing direct mediastinal drainage, circumventing the classic intrapulmonary pathway.

The drainage of the parenchymal lymphatic channels to mediastinal lymph nodes is generally ipsilateral and directed toward the trachea. Anomalies of drainage are more likely to be found on the left. The left lower lobe lymphatic vessels may drain through the subcarinal lymphatic channels to the right-sided mediastinal nodes in up to one-third of all patients. However, it appears that drainage is predominantly left sided. Baker, et al. (1967) demonstrated, in live human subjects, drainage of left lower lobe lymphatic channels to left scalene nodes in eight of nine patients, but to right-sided scalene nodes, in only three of nine. The left upper lobe has a dual drainage, with lymph flowing from lobar, interlobar, and hilar nodes to subcarinal, left tracheobronchial, and paratracheal lymph nodes. The alternate pathway is to the subaortic, periaortic, and anterior mediastinal nodes. In patients with left upper lobe tumors and stage N2 disease, one-third have metastases confined to the classic pathway, one-third have me-

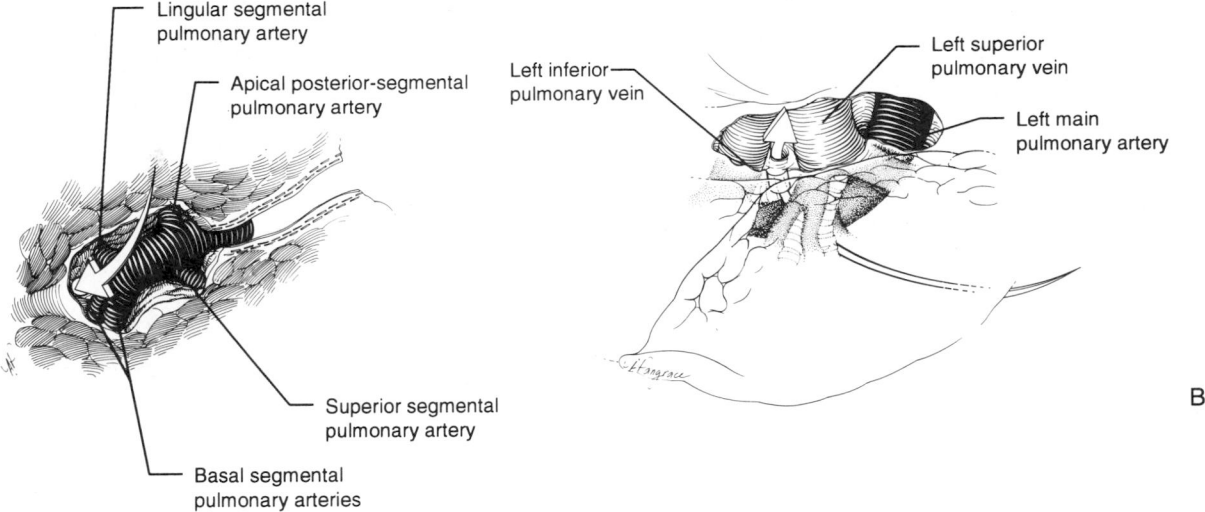

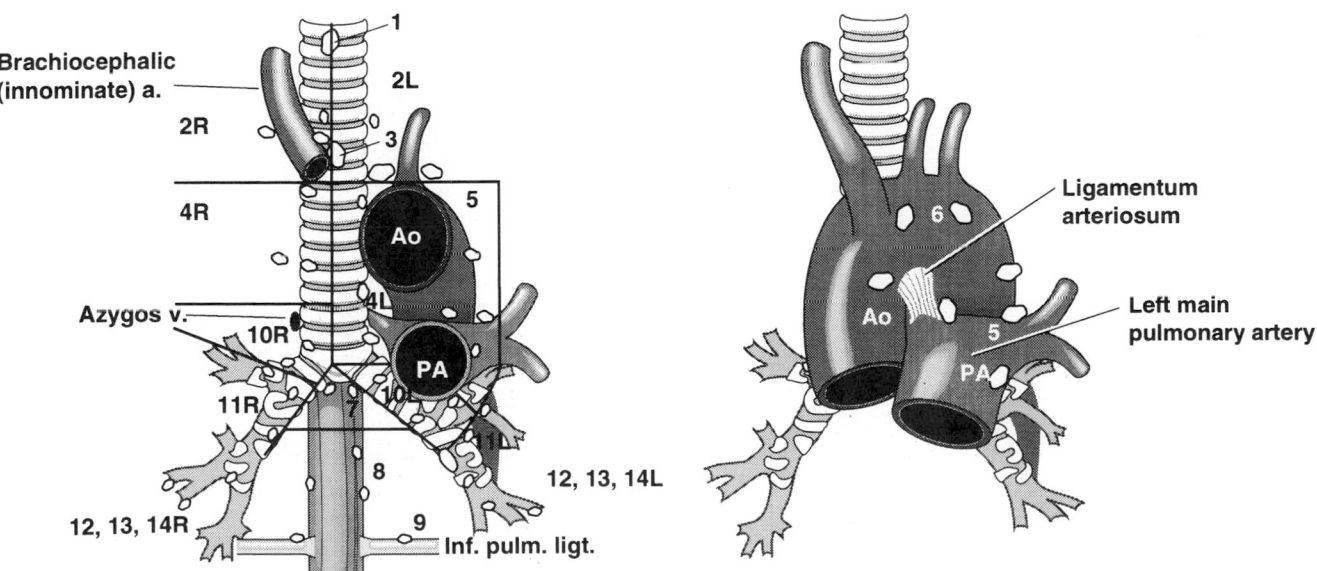

Figure 17-15.   The anterior inferior dissection of the left major fissure. **(A)** Dissection at the midportion of the major fissure allows identification of the pulmonary artery and its branches. The dissection is carried out between the lingular pulmonary artery and the basal segmental pulmonary artery. **(B)** The anterior hilar dissection is carried out between the superior and inferior pulmonary veins. **(C)** The anterior inferior portion of the left major fissure may be developed by connecting the dissection about the pulmonary arteries (Fig. A) with dissection about the veins (Fig. B).

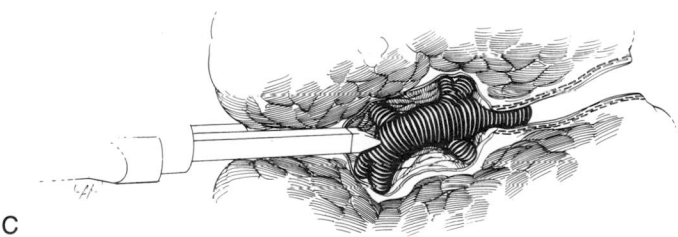

Figure 17-16.   Regional lymph nodes: 1. highest mediastinal, 2R. right paratracheal, 2L. left paratracheal, 3. pretracheal (subinnominate), 4R, right tracheobronchial; 4L. left tracheobronchial, 5. aortopulmonary, 6. para-aortic, 7. subcarinal, 8. paraesophageal, 9. pulmonary ligament, 10R. right hilar, 10L. left hilar, 11. interlobar, 12. lobar, 13. segmental, and 14. subsegmental. a., artery; Ao, aorta; Inf. pulm. ligt., inferior pulmonary ligament; PA, pulmonary artery; v., vein.

tastases confined to the alternate pathway by the subaortic window, and one-third have metastases to both chains.

In patients with bronchogenic carcinoma and positive mediastinoscopy, Funatsu, et al. (1992) found the greatest incidence of contralateral mediastinal metastases in left lung and lower lobe tumors. Spread to contralateral mediastinal nodes (stage N3 disease) was found in 50 percent of left lower lobe tumors and 35 percent of left upper lobe tumors. For right lung tumors with positive mediastinoscopy, 42 percent of right lower lobe tumors, 18 percent of right upper lobe tumors, and none of the middle lobe tumors had metastases to contralateral mediastinal nodes.

BRONCHIAL CIRCULATION

The majority of bronchial arteries arise from the anterolateral aspect of the aorta or its branches within 2 to 3 cm of the origin of the left subclavian artery (Fig. 17-17). About 20 percent of origins are either higher or lower. Usually the arteries to the right and left lungs arise separately; however, common trunks may be found in 25 percent of patients. Origin from the intercostal arteries is uncommon on the left but frequent on the right. Liebow (1965) and Cauldwell, et al. (1948), in two large autopsy series, found an intercostal origin for a right bronchial artery in 43 to 89 percent of specimens. There are two arteries to each lung in 20 to 30 percent of patients. The most frequent distribution of the bronchial arteries is three bronchial arteries, with dual supply to the left being more common. There are two left and one right arteries in 20 to 40 percent of patients, and two right and one left arteries in 10 to 16 pecent of patients. There may be one artery to each lung in 10 to 21 percent of patients.

Before reaching the airway, the bronchial arteries give off esophageal branches. These, along with direct branches from the aorta, account for a significant portion of the midthoracic esophageal blood supply. The arteries then pass posteriorly to the airway to lie on the membranous portion of the mainstem bronchi. They divide to supply lobar and segmental branches. There is a rich anastomosis with the pulmonary artery, and these anastomoses are important for the initial blood supply of the airway after bronchoplastic resections and pulmonary transplantation.

The majority of venous drainage from the bronchial arteries passes into the pulmonary venous system. However, Marchand, et al. (1950) pointed out that there is a second group of veins that form a venous network about the first two or three divisions of the bronchi that drain a small portion of bronchial arterial blood main into the azygous system on the right or the hemiazygous on the left.

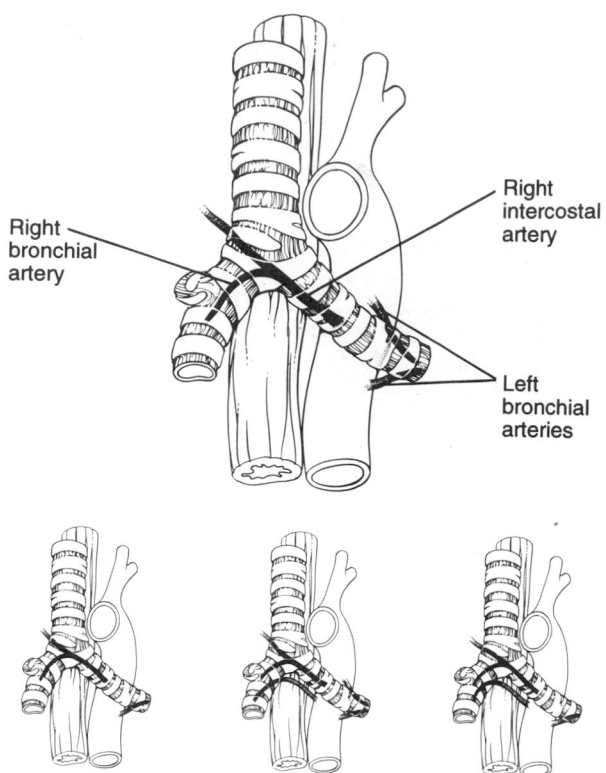

Figure 17-17. The bronchial arterial anatomy is variable. The most frequent bronchial aterial supply is one right artery arising from an intercostal artery and two left arteries with separate aortic origins. The inset (*bottom*) demonstrates the next three most common bronchial arterial arrangements.

PULMONARY NERVES

The vagus nerves and the sympathetic plexus send branches to the lungs. In the hilum they form a poorly developed anterior plexus about the main pulmonary arteries and a well-developed posterior plexus about the bronchi. The nerves then pass into the pulmonary parenchyma where they divide into the periarterial plexus or the peribronchial plexus. The periarterial plexus contains only nonmyelinated fibers; both myelinated and nonmyelinated fibers are found about the bronchus. Bronchoplastic procedures, lung transplantation, and sometimes hilar dissections result in denervation of the lung. The loss of neural control of the bronchial glands and the smooth muscle of the bronchi and arteries is of minimal clinical importance. Loss of the cough reflex as a result of this denervation can be critical.

COMMENTS AND CONTROVERSIES

The importance of a detailed knowledge of the physical anatomy of the thorax cannot be underestimated in the training and practice of a general thoracic surgeon. Intimate knowledge of the anatomy of the fissures, the recesses of the pericardium, and the relationships of the lobes and vascular structures of the mediastinum allows the thoracic surgeon complete command in the operating room, despite the intricacies of the surgery.

After obtaining this knowledge, before embarking on an unusual or new surgical procedure, it has always been our practice to reinforce this knowledge by time in the postmortem room, dissecting the area of concern on cadavers before embarking on a new adventure.

Dr. Rice's chapter provides a basis for knowledge of the surgical anatomy and the practical applications in performing pulmonary resections and reconstructions.

R.J.G.

KEY REFERENCES

Milloy FJ, Wragg LE, Anson BJ: The pulmonary arterial supply to the right upper lobe of the lung based upon a study of 300 laboratory and surgical specimens. Surg Gynecol Obstet 116:34,1963

A large modern study using current terminology describes the variations in the pulmonary arterial supply of the right upper lobe. It is the first in a series of three articles detailing the lobar pulmonary artery supply.

Milloy FJ, Wragg LE, Anson BJ: The pulmonary artery supply to the upper lobe of the left lung. Surg Gynecol Obstet 126:811, 1968

The second in the series, this article outlines the variations in the pulmonary arterial supply of the left upper lobe.

Wragg LE, Milloy FJ, Anson BJ: Surgical aspects of the pulmonary artery supply to the middle lobe and lower lobes of the lungs. Surg Gynecol Obstet 127:531, 1968

The last of this series, this large modern study describes the variations in pulmonary arterial supply of the middle and lower lobes.

REFERENCES

Allison PR: Intrapericardial approach to the lung root in the treatment of bronchial carcinoma by dissection pneumonectomy. J Thorac Cardiovasc Surg 15:99, 1946

Baker NK, Hill N, Ewy GH, Marable S: Pulmonary lymphatic drainage. J Thorac Cardiovasc Surg 54:695, 1967

Boyden EA, Hamre CJ: An analysis of variations in the bronchovascular patterns of the middle lobe in fifty dissected and twenty injected lungs. J Thorac Cardiovasc Surg 21:172, 1951

Cauldwell EW, Siekert RG, Lininger RE, Anson BJ: The bronchial arteries: an anatomic study of 150 human cadavers. Surg Gynecol Obstet 86:395, 1948

Ferry RM Jr, Boyden EA: Variations in the bronchovascular patterns of the right lower lobe of fifty lungs. J Thorac Cardiovasc Surg 22:188, 1951

Funatsu T, Yoshito M, Hatakenaka R et al.: The role of mediastinoscopic biopsy in preoperative assessment of lung cancer. J Thorac Cardiovasc Surg 104:1688, 1992

Ginsberg RJ, Rice TW, Goldberg M et al.: Extended cervical mediastinoscopy. A single staging procedure for bronchogenic carcinoma of the left upper lobe. J Thorac Cardiovasc Surg 94:673, 1987

Graham EA, Singer JJ: Successful removal of an entire lung for carcinoma of the bronchus. JAMA 101:1371, 1933

Healey JE Jr, Gibbon JM: Intrapericardial anatomy in relation to pneumonectomy for pulmonary carcinoma. J Thorac Cardiovasc Surg 19:864, 1950

le Roux BT: Anatomical abnormalities of the right upper bronchus. J Thorac Cardiovasc Surg 44:225, 1962

Liebow AA: Patterns of origin and distribution of the major bronchial arteries in man. Am J Anat 117:19, 1965

Lindskrog GE, Liebow AA, Hales MR: Bilobectomy—surgical and anatomic considerations in resection of right middle and lower lobes through the intermediate bronchus. J Thorac Cardiovasc Surg 18:616, 1949

Marchand P, Gilroy JC, Wilson VH: An anatomical study of the bronchial vascular system and its variations in disease. Thorax 5:207, 1950

Naruke T, Suemasu K, Ishikawa S: Lymph node mapping and curability at various levels of metastasis in resected lung cancer. J Thorac Cardiovasc Surg 76:832, 1978

Pitel M, Boyden EA: Variations in the bronchovascular patterns of the left lower lobe of fifty lungs. J Thorac Cardiovasc Surg 26:633, 1953

Ramsey BH: The anatomic guide to the intersegmental plane. Surgery 25:533, 1949

Riquet M, Hidden G, Debesse B: Direct lymphatic drainage of lung segments to the mediastinal nodes. J Thorac Cardiovasc Surg 97:623, 1989

18

IMAGING

Stephen J. Herman

HISTORICAL NOTE

Shortly after the discovery of x-rays in November 1895, their use as an aide to recognizing thoracic disease became quickly apparent (Eisenberg, 1991). As early as May 1896, descriptions of both film and fluoroscopic findings in diseases of the lungs and heart were published. It soon was evident that chest radiography could detect some diseases much earlier than was ever possible before; for example, in 1897 it was noted by Dr. Williams of Boston that pulmonary tuberculosis was detectable earlier by chest radiography than by any other method. The diagnosis of bronchogenic carcinoma was similarly improved.

The development of computed tomography (CT) in the 1970s greatly improved the detection of diseases of both the lungs and the mediastinum. In addition it led to a much better understanding of many of the poorly understood patterns of disease as seen on the plain chest radiograph. High-resolution CT improved our ability to image lung disease by another order of magnitude.

Magnetic resonance imaging (MRI), developed in the 1980s, has been of great use in the diagnosis of cardiovascular disorders. Its utility in assessing other thoracic regions is less significant but newer techniques that allow better visualization of lung parenchyma may make this test more important for pulmonary problems in the near future.

HISTORICAL READING

Eisenberg RL: Radiology: An Illustrated History. Mosby-Year Book, St. Louis, 1991

CHEST RADIOGRAPHY

Air Space Versus Interstitial Disease

Pulmonary parenchymal diseases can be subdivided radiologically and pathologically into air space and interstitial categories (Fig. 18-1). With air space disease, the pathologic process is the result of increased amounts of water-dense material located predominantly within alveolar air spaces. Interstitial disease is manifested by increased water-dense material located predominantly within the pulmonary interstitial tissues, which include the alveolar walls, interlobular septa, subpleural spaces, and bronchovascular bundles (Heitzman, 1984).

Air space disease is manifested radiologically by the appearance of small (5 to 10 mm in diameter) fluffy ill-defined nodular densities that tend to coalesce when adjacent to each other (Fig. 18-2). Each of these individual opacities is known as an "acinar shadow." Although there is no universal agreement, it is believed that these opacities represent a single pulmonary acinus filled with a water-dense material (Ziskind, et al., 1963). In many air space diseases, the bronchi in the affected lung remain air filled and can therefore be seen as tapering, branching lucent structures within the diseased area (Fleischner, 1948). These lucencies are known as "air bronchograms" (Felson, 1973), a highly indicative (but not absolute because rarely they can be seen with interstitial disease) finding that air space disease is involved. The individual acinar shadows coalesce to from larger and larger areas of opacification, which are somewhat ill defined and irregular in outline. Depending on the cause, these areas of opacification are either distributed in a patchy distribution in the lungs or more focally in one region. With some causes, for example pneumococcal pneumonia, there may be rapid spread of the disease centrifugally with time. Such spread is usually limited by a pleural surface (i.e., the process appears to stop at a pleural fissure).

Interstitial diseases manifest radiologically in a nodular, reticular, or reticulonodular pattern, the last one being a combination of the first two. Interstitial nodules are tiny (2 to 3 mm in diameter) multiple discrete round densities that are usually easily distinguished from air space nodules in that they are smaller and remain discrete where they appear to be adjacent to one another (Fig. 18-3). There is the feeling that these can be plucked out with tweezers. Reticular densities are a network of lines that are thin (1 to 2 mm in width) and well defined. This network can be either fine (in which case the black spaces between the linear densities are small and the linear densities themselves are thin) or coarse (in which case the black spaces are larger, up to 1 cm or so in

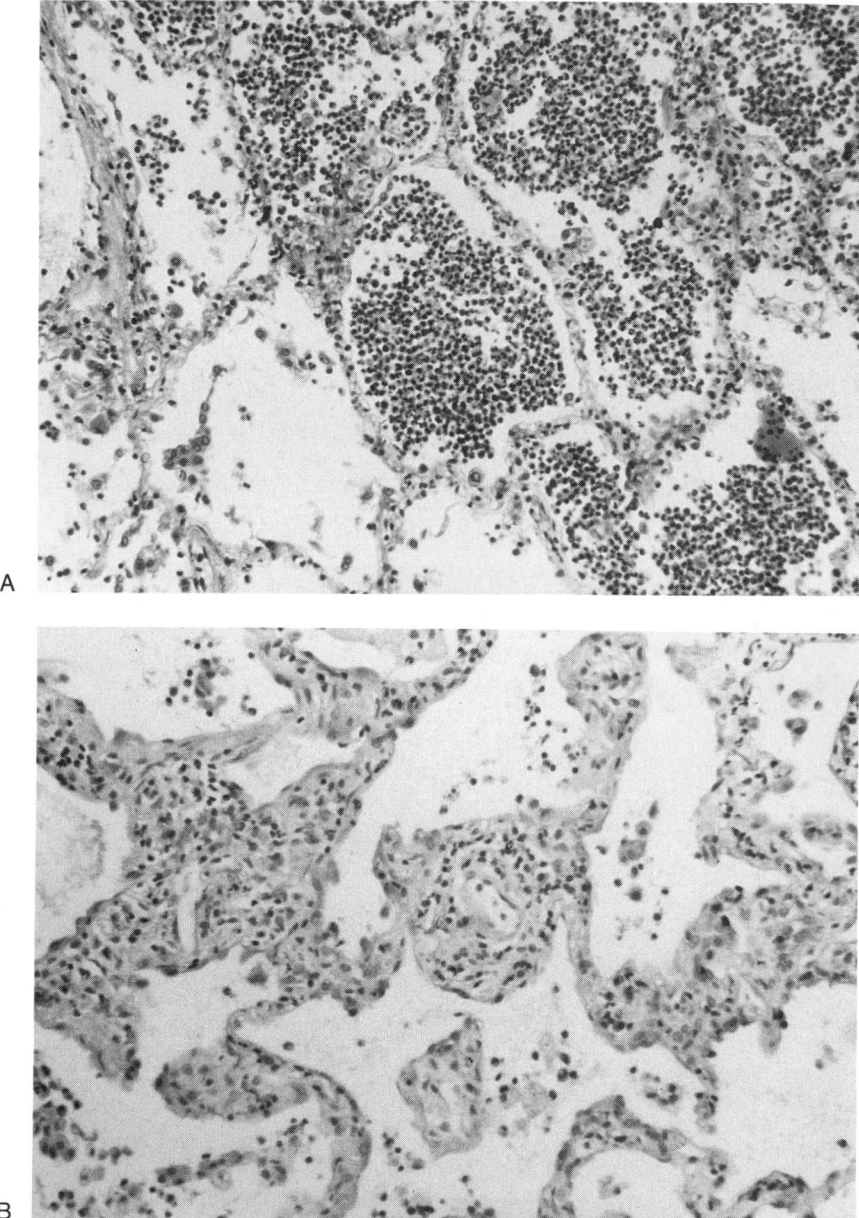

Figure 18-1. Microscopic pathologic specimens. **(A)** Air space disease. In this patient with bronchopneumonia, innumerable polymorphonuclear cells fill the air spaces; the alveolar walls are intact. **(B)** Interstitial disease. In this patient with fibrosing alveolitis, the air spaces are relatively free of disease; there is marked thickening of the pulmonary interstitium.

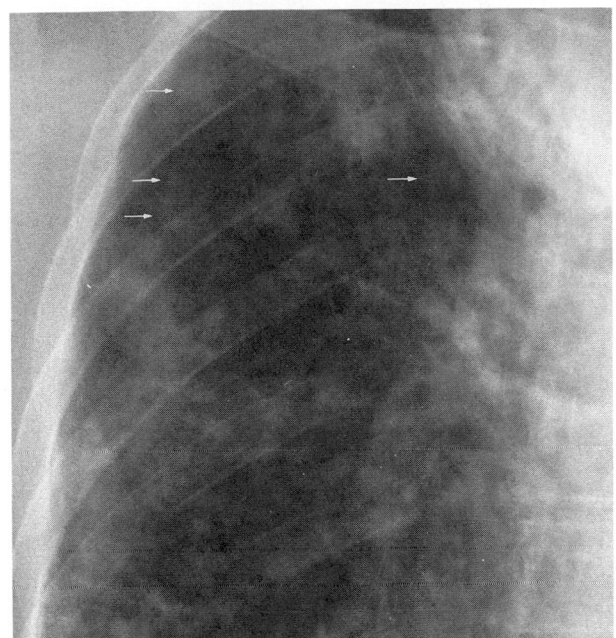

A

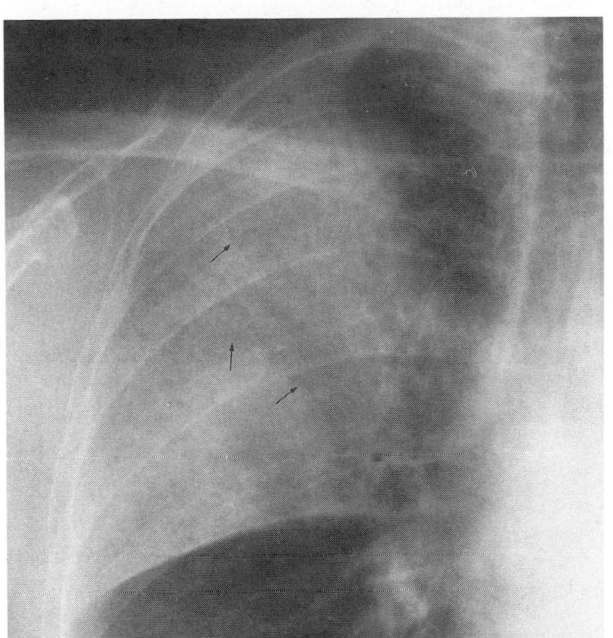

B

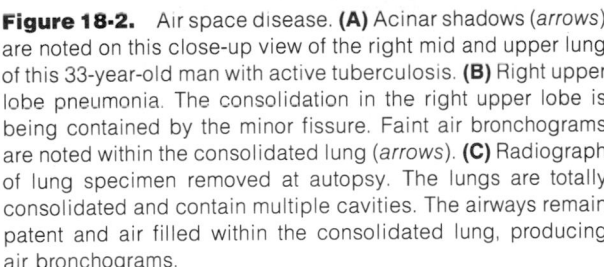

Figure 18-2. Air space disease. **(A)** Acinar shadows (*arrows*) are noted on this close-up view of the right mid and upper lung of this 33-year-old man with active tuberculosis. **(B)** Right upper lobe pneumonia. The consolidation in the right upper lobe is being contained by the minor fissure. Faint air bronchograms are noted within the consolidated lung (*arrows*). **(C)** Radiograph of lung specimen removed at autopsy. The lungs are totally consolidated and contain multiple cavities. The airways remain patent and air filled within the consolidated lung, producing air bronchograms.

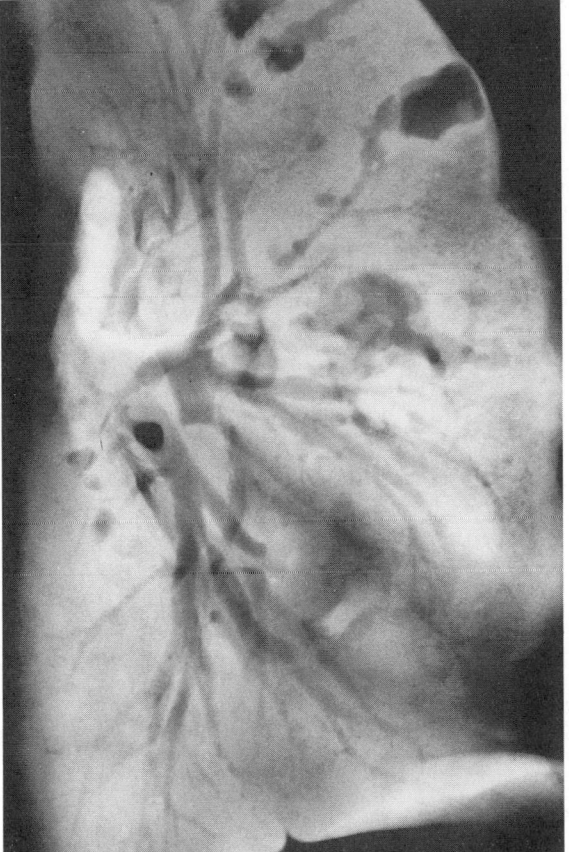

C

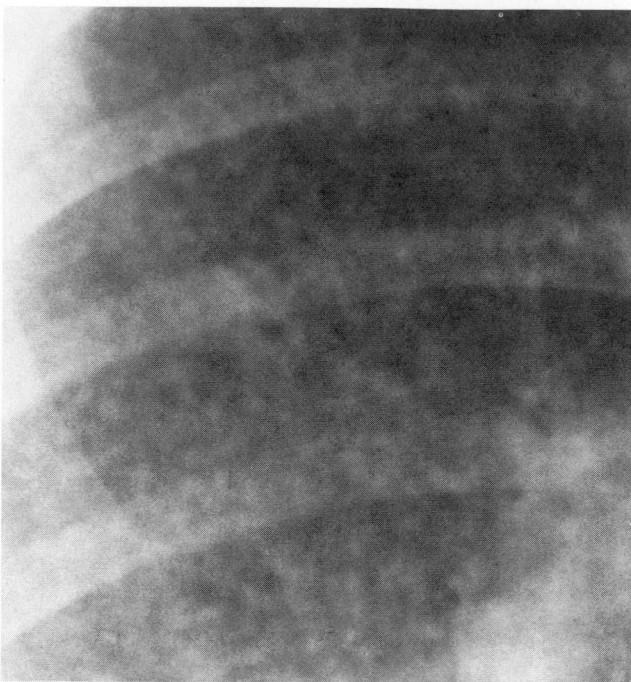

Figure 18-3. Interstitial nodules. Close-up view of PA chest radiograph of a 16-year-old girl with sarcoidosis. Note the innumerable well-defined nodular densities each measuring 1 to 2 mm in diameter.

diameter, with thicker white linear margins) (Fig. 18-4). When the interstitial process involves an interlobular septum, the so-called Kerley B lines appear. These appear as thin (about 0.5 to 1 mm thick) linear densities about 1 cm in length, which meet the pleural surface at right angles. Although they are often considered to indicate pulmonary edema (which *is* a common a cause of their occurrence), they can be caused by any condition in which a water-dense process accumulates in the interlobular septi (e.g., lymphangitic carcinoma). Disease in the interstitium that accompanies bronchovascular bundles causes these structures to be somewhat prominent and more poorly defined.

Lobar Collapse

Lobar collapse is extremely important to recognize because it may be missed clinically and may be the result of significant potentially treatable diseases, such as bronchogenic carcinoma or possibly an aspirated foreign body. Lobar collapse can be recognized by direct and indirect signs (Fraser, et al., 1988; Fig. 18-5). The main direct sign of lobar collapse is displacement of a pleural fissure because this represents the margin of a lobe itself; if this moves, this indicates that one of the lobes has lost volume. With this loss of volume, a number of compensatory mechanisms come into play, and these form the so-called indirect signs. These include elevation of the ipsilateral hemidiaphragm (most prominent when a lower lobe is collapsed), hilar displacement, mediastinal shift, and compensatory hyperinflation. The part of the mediastinum that shifts is usually that which is closest to the collapsed lobe. For example, with upper lobe collapse, tracheal shift is the main finding; with lower lobe collapse, there is a shift of the heart. Compensatory hyperinflation is noted in the lung closest to the collapsed lobe. For example, with left lower lobe collapse, the left upper lobe appears relatively hyperlucent compared with the right lung. This is because it has expanded into the space formally occupied by the left lower lobe and its vessels and parenchyma are now more spread out than they were previously. A collapsed lobe is generally of increased density because of the relative lack of air within it. Occasionally the ribs adjacent to the collapsed lobe are more crowded than are the corresponding ribs on the contralateral side, although this is a poor sign of collapse.

Patterns of collapse of each of the five pulmonary lobes and combinations of lobes have been described in detail elsewhere (Robbins and Hale, 1945a to 1945f; Robbins et al., 1945; Proto and Thomas, 1980; Fraser, et al., 1988). Examples of these are shown in the accompanying figures (Fig. 18-5).

The causes of atelectasis have been divided into four main types: resorptive (obstructive), passive (relaxation), adhesive, and cicatrization (Fraser, et al., 1988). Resorptive or obstructive atelectasis occurs when the normal communication between the trachea and alveoli is lost; this form is discussed below. Passive or relaxation atelectasis occurs when a space-occupying lesion, most often a pneumothorax or pleural effusion, "compresses" adjacent lung (in fact, the lung is not truly compressed by these processes but rather allowed to return to its resting size by the local loss of "negative" pleural pressure). Adhesive atelectasis refers to situations in which increased surface tension in the alveoli, probably caused by loss of surfactant, causes the alveoli to collapse (e.g., acute radiation-induced pneumonitis). Cicatrization atelectasis occurs secondary to pulmonary fibrosis, which may be local or general.

It is most important to distinguish resorptive atelectasis from the other three forms because the bronchial obstruction must be recognized and treated. Generally this is not a problem because obstructive atelectasis is the only form that tends to involve an entire lobe or segment of lung. Rarely some cicatrizing diseases, such as tuberculosis, can involve an entire lobe and leave it scarred and atelectatic, but this is not difficult to distinguish from an obstructive collapse (Fig. 18-6). In addition, the other three forms should contain air bronchograms by their nature. In contrast, all air distal to an obstructing airway lesion is absorbed, and therefore, usually air bronchograms are not seen with resorptive atelectasis. However air bronchograms by themselves should not be used to determine if the cause of a lobar collapse is caused by airway obstruction (Woodring, 1988). Two other radiographic signs, central bronchial narrowing or cutoff and the so-called Golden S sign, are accurate in determining if the atelectasis is the result of an obstructing tumor or not (Woodring, 1988). The latter refers to the presence of a central convexity at the hilum, the convexity being the margin of the central tumor itself (Golden, 1925; Fig. 18-5A).

A somewhat unique form of parenchymal collapse, known as round atelectasis, has some well-described characteristic features (Schneider, et al., 1980). It appears as a pleural-based well-defined round or oval opacity, usually occurring in the lung base posteriorly with adjacent pleural thickening

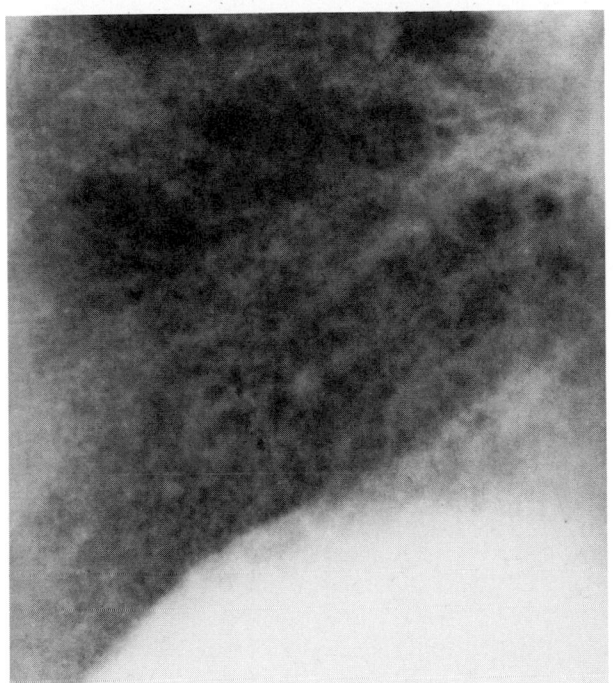

A

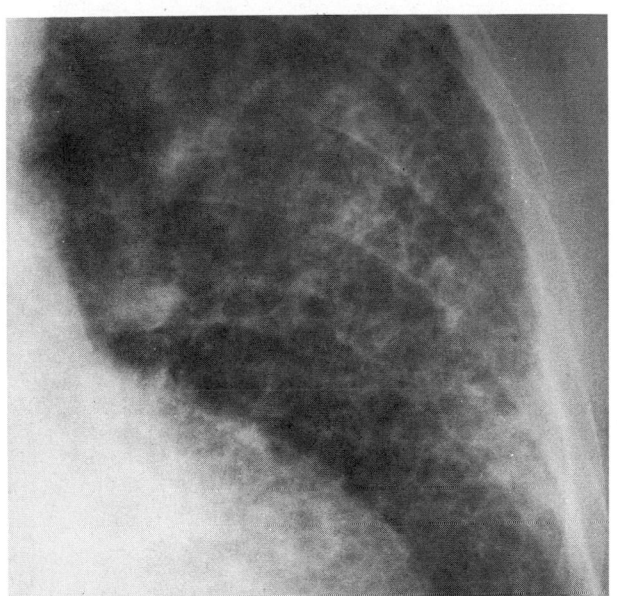

B

Figure 18-4. Reticular interstitial disease. **(A)** Fine reticular disease. Close-up view of right lung base of 59-year-old woman with fibrosing alveolitis. **(B)** Close-up view of left midlung reveals a course reticular pattern in this 62-year-old man with farmer's lung. **(C)** Close-up view of PA chest radiograph of a patient with pulmonary edema. Kerley B lines (*arrows*) are short straight thin lines running perpendicular to and abutting the pleural surface.

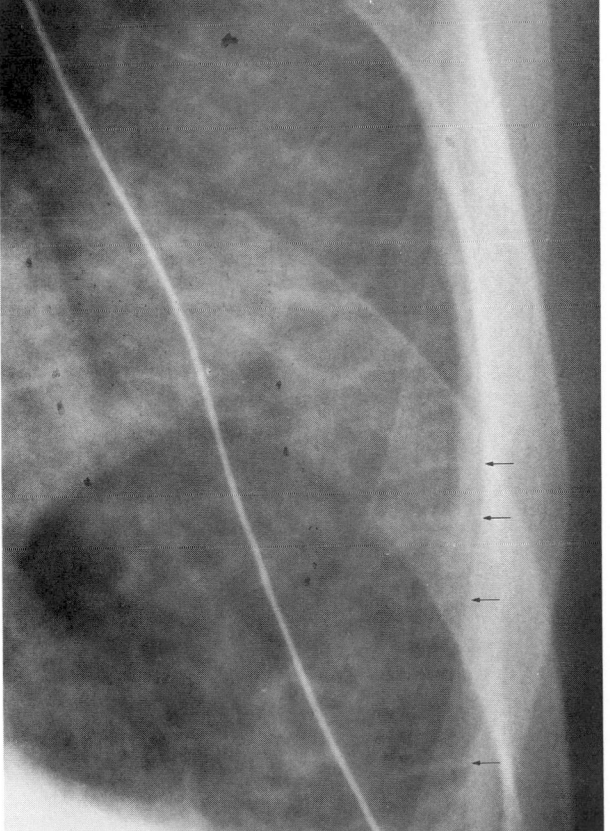

C

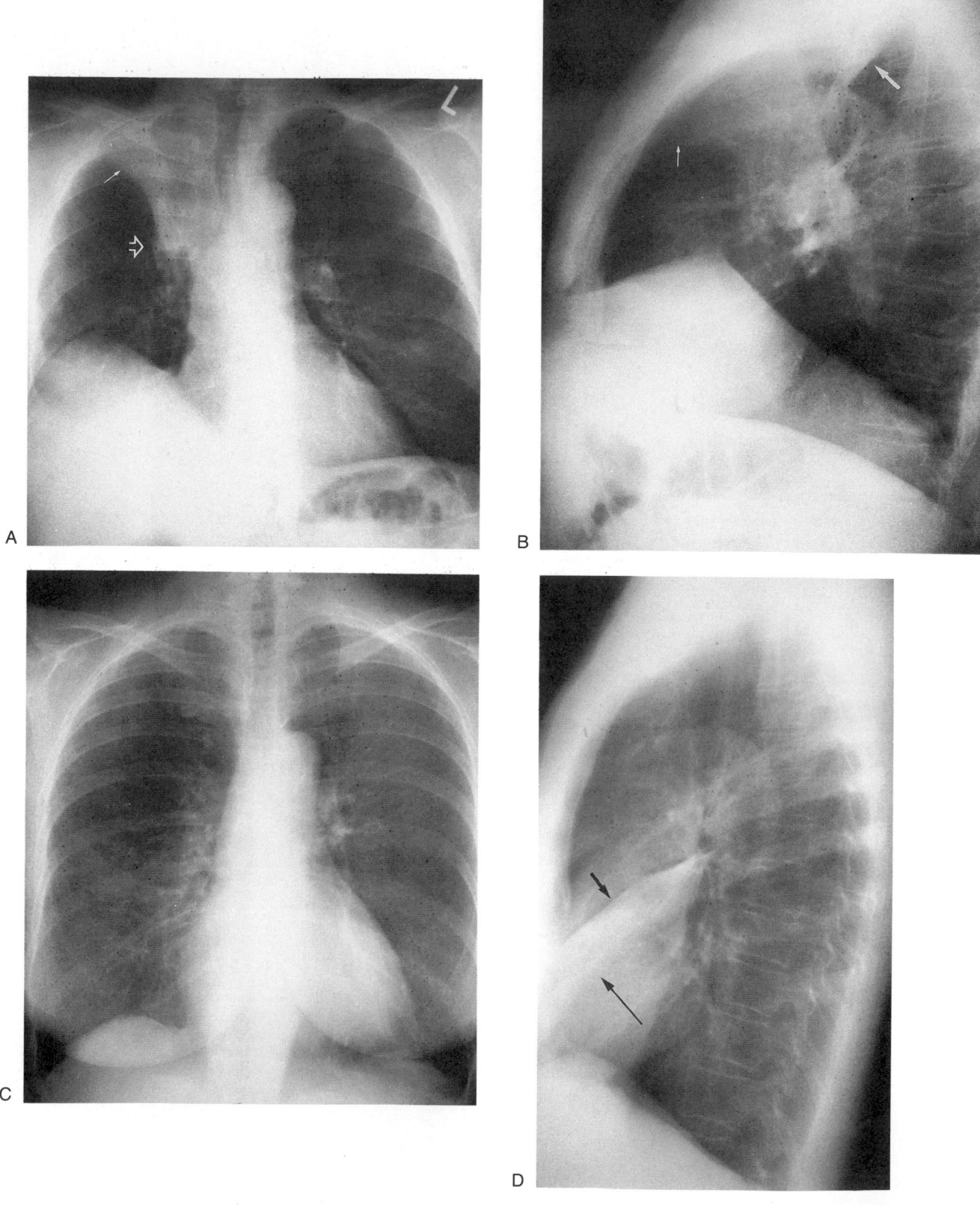

Figure 18-5. **(A and B)** Right upper lobe collapse. The minor fissure is displaced superiorly on the posteroanterior and lateral views (*small arrows*); the superior aspect of the major fissure is displaced anteriorly on the lateral view (*large arrows*). There is elevation of the right hilum and right hemidiaphragm and displacement of the trachea to the right. Note the presence of a central convexity in the region of the hilum (*open arrows*), the Golden S sign. **(C and D)** Right middle lobe collapse. On the PA view, there is loss of visualization of the right heart border (silhouette sign), with a slight increase in the density of the right base medially. On the lateral view, there is displacement of the minor fissure inferiorly (*short arrow*) and the inferior aspect of the major fissure anterosuperiorly (*long arrow*). Because of the relatively small size of the middle lobe, indirect compensatory signs are not present. (*Figure continues.*)

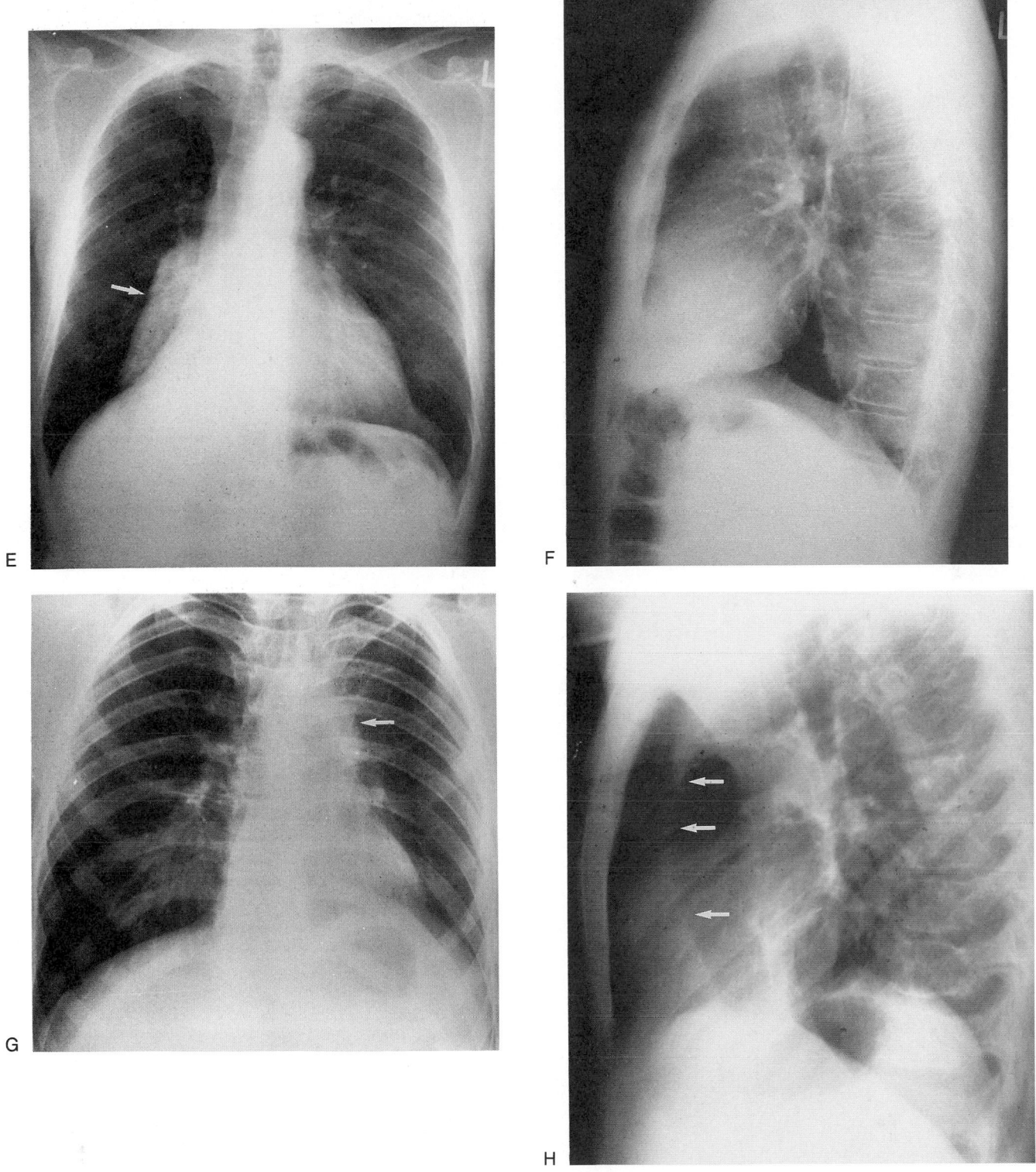

E

F

G

H

Figure 18-5 (*Continued*). **(E and F)** Right lower lobe collapse. The major fissure is displaced inferomedially (*arrow*). Indirect signs include relative hyperlucency of the right lung, especially the right middle lobe (compare with corresponding locations on the left), inferior displacement of the right hilum, shift of trachea to the right, and slight elevation of the right hemidiaphragm, especially medially. On the lateral view, note that the density of the thoracic spine decreases from the upper to the midthoracic spine but then increases inferiorly because of the overlying airless lobe. **(G and H)** Left upper lobe collapse. On the lateral view, there is displacement of the left major fissure anteriorly with increased density of the collapsed lobe anterior to it. On the posteroanterior view, there is elevation of the left hemidiaphragm, elevation of the left hilum (*arrow*), shift of the trachea and the heart to the left, and a generalized increase in the density of the left hemithorax. (*Figure continues*.)

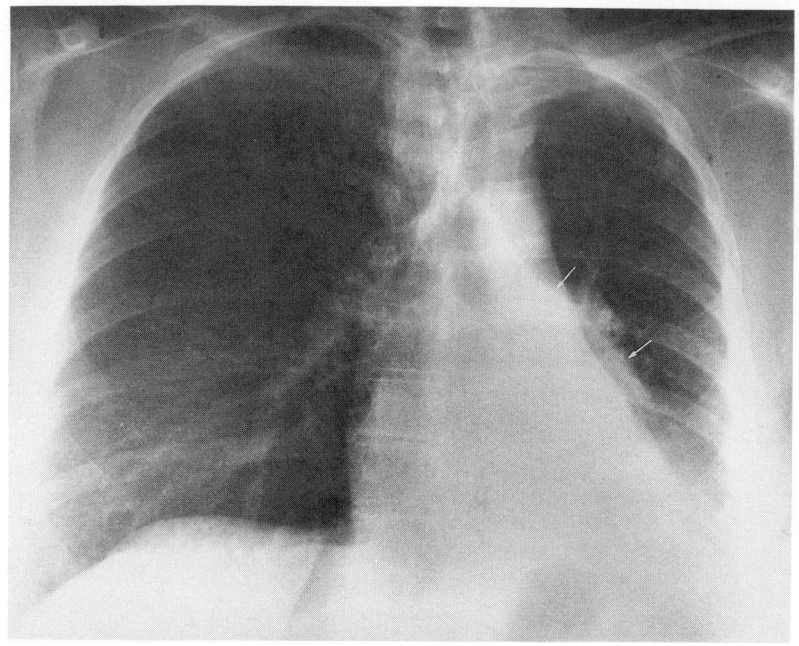

I

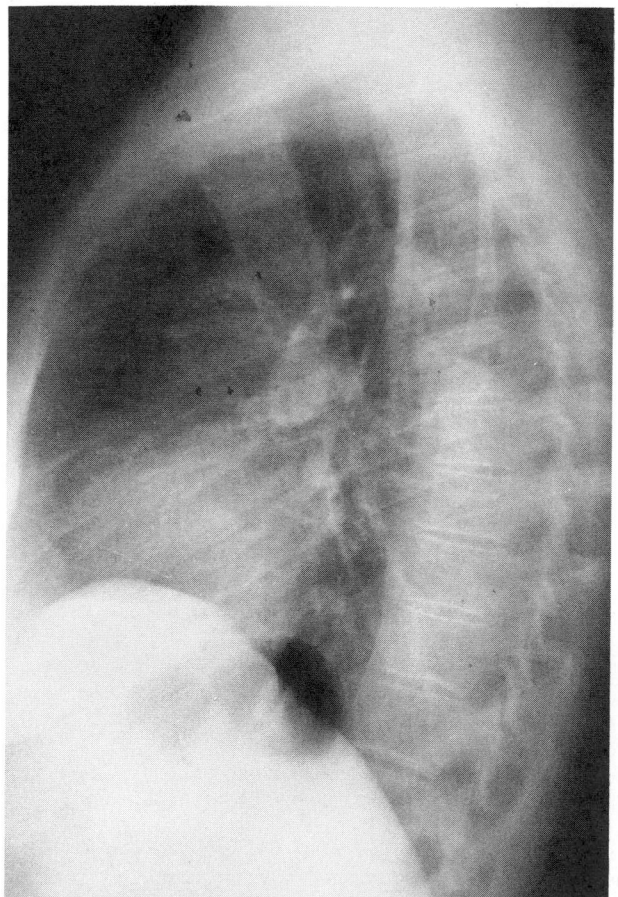

J

Figure 18-5 (*Continued*). **(I and J)** Left lower lobe collapse. The inferomedially displaced left major fissure is seen (*arrows*) just lateral to the left cardiac margin. In addition there is increased density within the lobe, shift of the heart and trachea to the left, inferior displacement of the left hilum, and elevation of the left hemidiaphragm. On the lateral views, note the increase in the density of the lower thoracic spine compared with the upper spine. Note also the loss of visualization of the left hemidiaphragm as a result of the now airless left lower lobe.

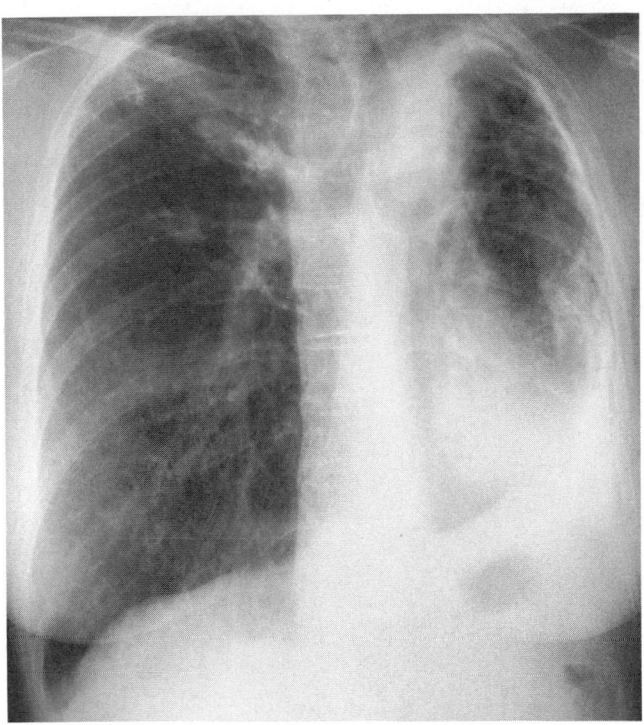

Figure 18-6. This elderly woman with known tuberculosis from many years earlier has significant bilateral upper lobe atelectasis, especially on the left. The type of atelectasis demonstrated in this patient does not make the clinician suspicious of an endobronchial tumor.

and curving pulmonary vessels sweeping into it (Fig. 18-7). These features may be better seen on CT (see section, Computed Tomography). A mass exhibiting these characteristic features needs no further workup.

Pulmonary Nodules and Masses

When a pulmonary nodule or mass is seen, the main consideration is whether the lesion is benign or malignant. A number of signs suggest one or the other. One that suggests malignancy is the presence of poorly defined margins, especially if there is spiculation forming so-called corona radiata (Fig. 18-8). The latter refer to short linear opacities extending from the margin of the mass into the adjacent lung. Although formerly believed to be definitely an indication of malignancy (and known as corona maligna), they are now known to be seen also in some benign diseases. However, they are definitely highly suggestive of malignancy. Malignant nodules tend to be lobulated in contour and generally do not contain calcium. The rare malignant nodule that does contain calcium is usually larger than 2 cm, and when present, the calcium is most often eccentrically located. If old films are available, any increase in the size of the mass makes the clinician suspicious of the presence of a malignancy (see below). In addition, malignancy should be suspected when there are associated signs, such as lymphadenopathy, bone destruction, or pleural effusion. Cavitation, per se of the mass does not help in making the distinction; however, the thickness

of its wall does (Woodring, et al., 1980; Woodring and Fried, 1983). If the maximum wall thickness is 4 mm or less, the mass is most likely benign. If the thickness is greater than 1.5 cm, the mass is likely to be malignant; otherwise the mass must be considered indeterminate.

Signs that the nodule or mass is benign include well-defined margins and a smooth contour, although both features are also seen with metastases. However, the most important signs that a nodule is benign include calcification and growth rate. There are certain patterns of calcification that are virtually pathognomonic of benign disease (Fig. 18-9). If the nodule contains a central nidus of calcification, diffuse calcification, or lamellated (ringlike) calcification, then granulomatous disease is almost certain. So-called popcorn calcification (i.e., lumps of calcium seen throughout the mass) indicates that the mass is probably a benign hamartoma. If old films are available, the clinician can estimate the growth rate of the nodule. By measuring its diameter on both studies and calculating its volume, the doubling time of the nodule can be determined. If the doubling time is 7 days or less, or 465 days or greater, then benign disease is almost certain (Nathan, et al., 1962).

Pragmatically, a nodule that either (1) exhibits a benign calcific pattern or (2) exhibits no growth over a 2-year period may be considered benign; otherwise, it must be considered suspicious for malignancy. Having said this, it must be noted that occasionally some tumors, especially bronchoalveolar cell carcinoma, exhibit no growth over 2 years. This possibility must always be kept in mind.

Line Shadows

Linear densities are a common finding in the lungs and can be the result of a number of different causes, the most common on which are scarring, subsegmental (discoid or plate) atelectasis, and Kerley B lines (described above, Fig. 18-10). Any parenchymal process that heals with the development of scar tissue can leave behind permanent thin linear opacities that can run in any direction and remain visible for the rest of the patient's life. Subsegmental atelectasis appears as a linear density up to about 1 cm in diameter and many centimeters in length, which abuts a pleural surface. Its pathogenesis is poorly understood (Westcott and Cole, 1985).

Other causes of line shadows include mucoid impaction (dilated mucus-filled bronchi caused by bronchial obstruction or thick inspissated mucus), bronchial wall thickening (which can cause the appearance of parallel lines, so-called tram tracks, or thickening of the circular shadow of a bronchus seen end on), and the walls of bullae. Of course, an extrathoracic cause, such as a skin fold, clothing, or a bed sheet, must always be kept in mind.

Increased Radiolucency

There are many causes of increased radiolucency of the lungs, and these can be categorized into four main groups: artifactual, extrapulmonary, decreased perfusion, and increased aeration. Artifactual lucency occurs when the film is obtained with the patient is rotated to one side, with the side to which the patient is rotated being more radiolucent. A relative lack

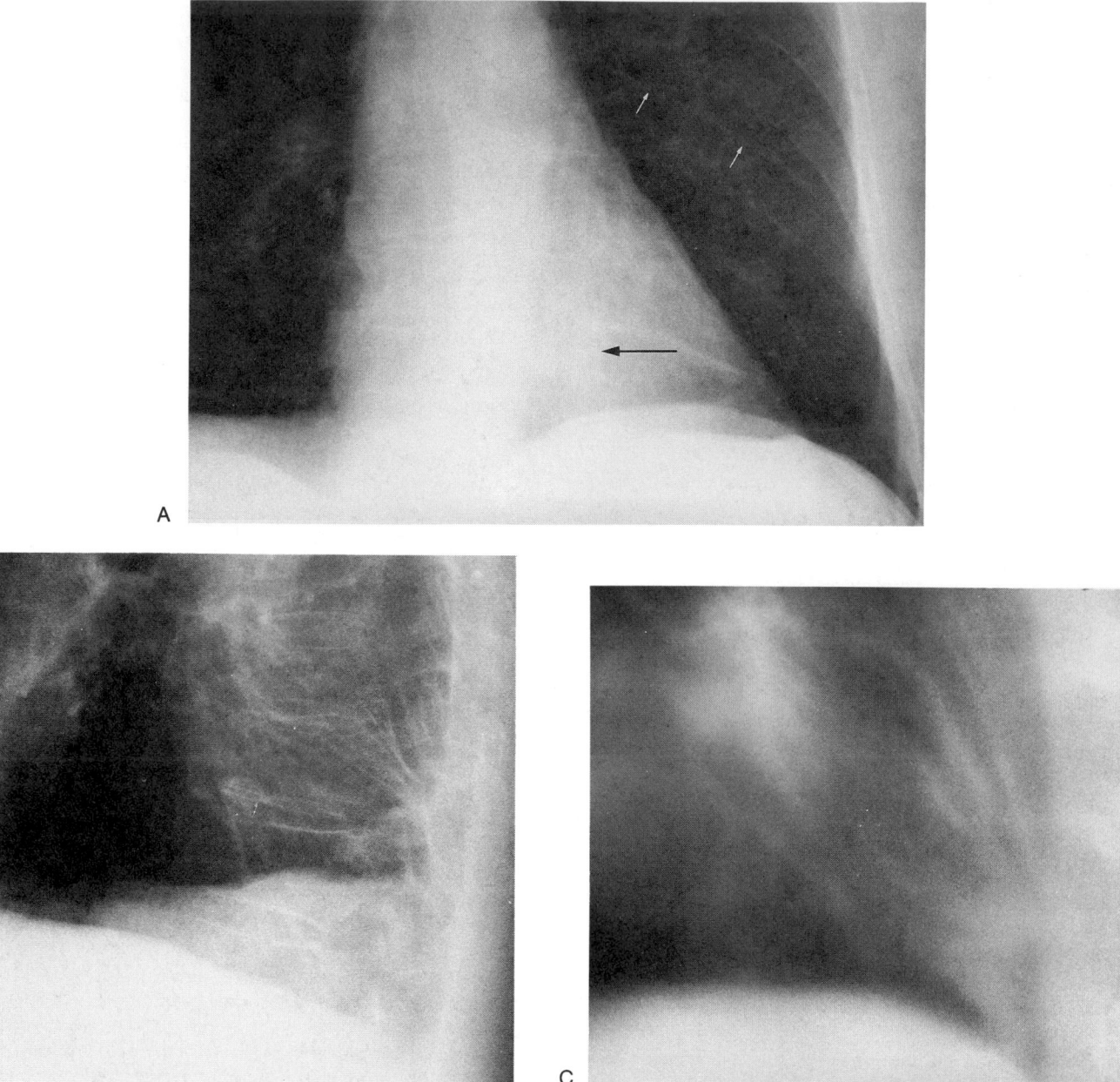

Figure 18-7. Round atelectasis. **(A)** Close-up view of PA chest radiograph reveals a nodular density measuring 2 cm in diameter in the left lower lobe (*black arrow*). Note the mild left lower lobe volume loss, as evidenced by the slightly inferiorly displaced left major fissure (*white arrows*). **(B)** On the lateral view, linear densities are seen extending posteriorly toward the thickened pleura. **(C)** Plain lateral tomogram. This study clearly reveals curving vessels sweeping into the nodular density in the left lower lobe. There is adjacent pleural thickening (note that the lung is separated from the posterior rib by a water-dense band).

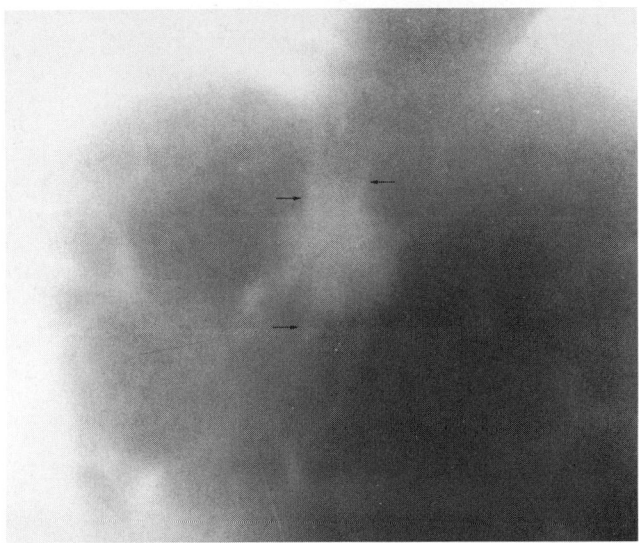

Figure 18-8. Bronchogenic carcinoma in a 60-year-old man. This somewhat ill-defined nodule has prominent spiculated margins. Specifically there are linear opacities extending from the surface of the nodule into the adjacent lung, so-called corona radiata (*arrows*).

of overlying soft tissues (e.g., mastectomy) causes ipsilateral lucency. One of many possible causes of decreased perfusion (e.g., pulmonary embolism, arterial obstruction by tumor, or congenital pulmonary arterial agenesis) causes focal lucency. Relative hyperinflation of a portion of the lung is a significant cause that must be recognized because it can be the result of bronchial obstruction; however, compensatory hyperinflation (e.g., atelectasis or resection of another lobe) and the presence of emphysema or a bulla are more common causes. A film obtained during expiration can often be helpful in assessing hyperlucent lung; if it is the result of a bronchial obstruction, the hyperlucency is accentuated on the expiratory film (Fig. 18-11).

Pulmonary Versus Extrapulmonary Disease

When an opacity is seen in the periphery of the lung, the clinician must determine if it is a pulmonary lesion extending to the pleura or if it actually represents an extrapulmonary lesion that is bulging into the lung. It is not always possible to be certain which of these is the correct situation; however, a number of signs can be helpful (Fig. 18-12). If the opacity forms acute angles with the chest wall, then most likely it is of pulmonary origin. If the angles are obtuse, then it more often represents an extrapulmonary lesion. Extrapulmonary lesions tend to be uniform in density (although so may be pulmonary lesions); however, if an air bronchogram is seen within the lesion, then it is definitely pulmonary in origin. A pulmonary lesion may have well- or ill-defined margins, but an extrapulmonary lesion has extremely well-defined margins (as a result of the overlying visceral pleura), and these margins are convex toward the lung.

PLAIN TOMOGRAPHY

When investigating a pulmonary nodule seen by chest radiography, CT scanning is definitely better than plain tomography in detecting calcification. However, there are many instances in which a vague opacity is seen on the plain radiograph and the clinician may or may not be certain if it represents a pulmonary nodule or not. In these instances plain tomography can be very helpful (Huston and Muhm, 1987). For example it may reveal that the suspicious opacity lies in an overlying rib (e.g., a bone island) or just represents a linear scar. Even if it does turn out to represent a pulmonary nodule, plain tomography may still show calcium within it. Frequently, however, patients still need to undergo CT.

Occasionally if the clinician is suspicious of a lesion within one of the large airways on the plain chest radiograph, plain tomography is helpful in visualizing these airways. However, an overpenetrated plain film often also suffices.

COMPUTED TOMOGRAPHY

Solitary Pulmonary Nodule

The main advantage of CT over the chest radiography and plain tomography in the assessment of the solitary pulmonary nodule is its ability to detect small amounts of calcium, which may otherwise be undetectable.

During a single breath-hold maneuver, multiple thin (1.5 to 3 mm) contiguous sections are obtained through the nodule. By this method an accurate picture of the internal characteristics of the nodule can be obtained without any effects of partial volume averaging. That is, because the thickness of tissue being imaged is such that no lung is included with the nodule, the CT numbers obtained are not affected by the air in the adjacent lung. The CT density thus obtained reflects relatively accurately the nature of the lesion in terms of the amount of radiation absorbed. An idea of the amount and distribution of calcium (and fat) in the nodule is therefore determined. The resultant image is viewed in both the standard fashion and as a matrix of numbers (Fig. 18-13). Generally densities of 200 HU or greater are said to reflect calcium; numbers in the −40 to −120 HU range indicate fat.

If no calcium or fat is seen within the nodule, then it is considered suspicious for malignancy. If fat is seen within the nodule, then it most likely represents a hamartoma (Fig. 18-14). If calcium is seen in the nodule, then the pattern of calcification is examined. As with plain film techniques, benign patterns include central, diffuse, or laminated calcification (Fig. 18-13). If one of these patterns is seen, then the nodule is considered benign, most likely caused by previous granulomatous disease or possibly a hamartoma. If calcium is seen in an eccentric location, then the lesion is probably benign; however, nodules such as this are usually investigated further because these may represent a tumor that has engulfed adjacent granulomatous disease.

The technique of CT densitometry was first introduced in 1980 by Siegelman, et al. (1980). Although not initially accepted as clinically valuable by all investigators (Godwin, et al., 1982), it is now considered extremely useful (Webb, 1990; Zerhouni, et al., 1986; Proto, et al., 1985), pending a number

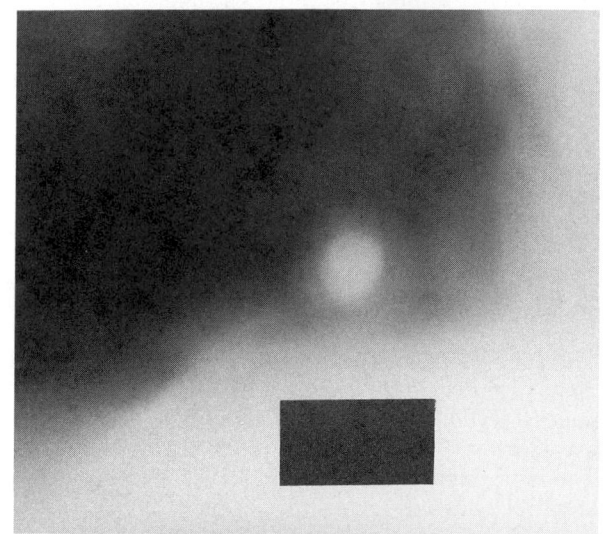

A

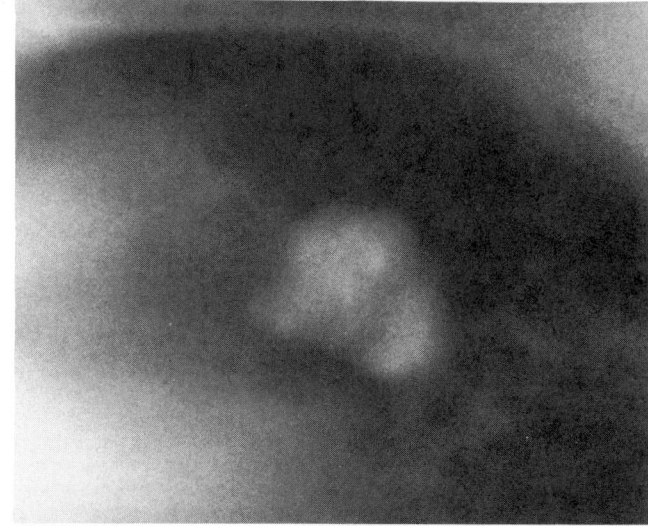

B

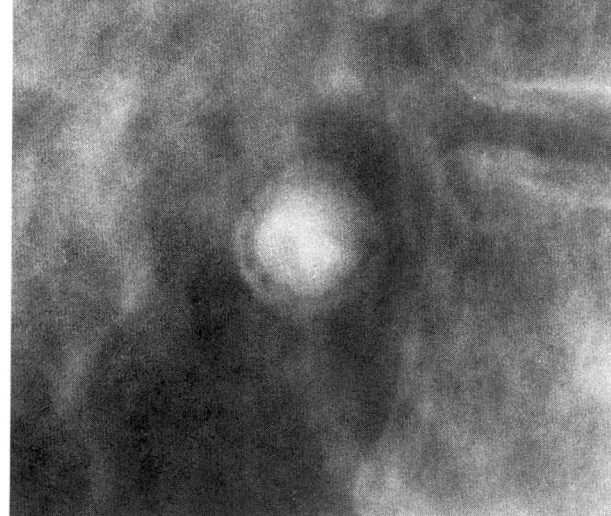

C

Figure 18-9. Patterns of calcification in benign nodules. **(A)** Close-up view of a tomogram of a smooth well-defined nodule with dense central calcification. **(B)** Popcorn calcification in a presumed pulmonary hamartoma. **(C)** Close-up view of a nodule containing a large central nidus of calcification and peripheral lamellated calcification.

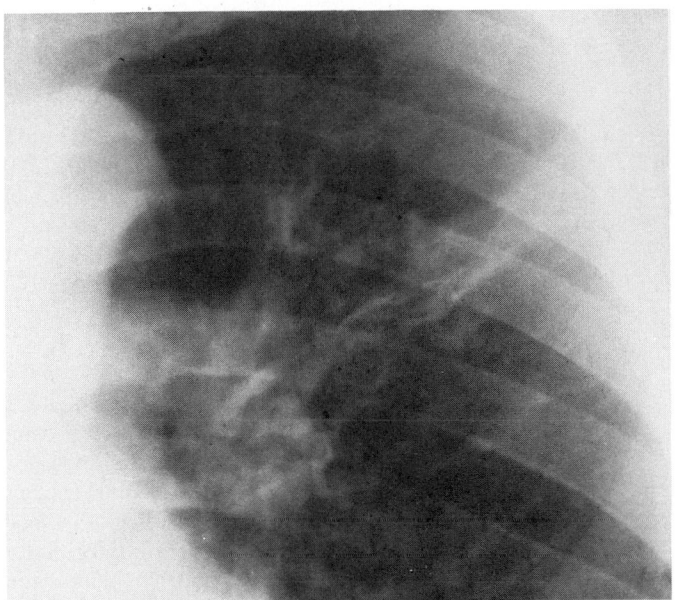
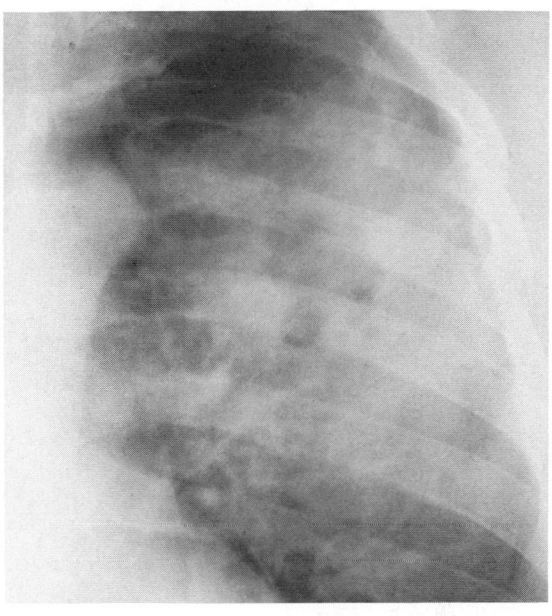

Figure 18-10. **(A)** The linear densities in the left perihilar region are typical of both pulmonary fibrosis and subsegmental atelectasis. **(B)** One year earlier, this patient had a necrotizing pneumonia in this region and was left with permanent linear scarring.

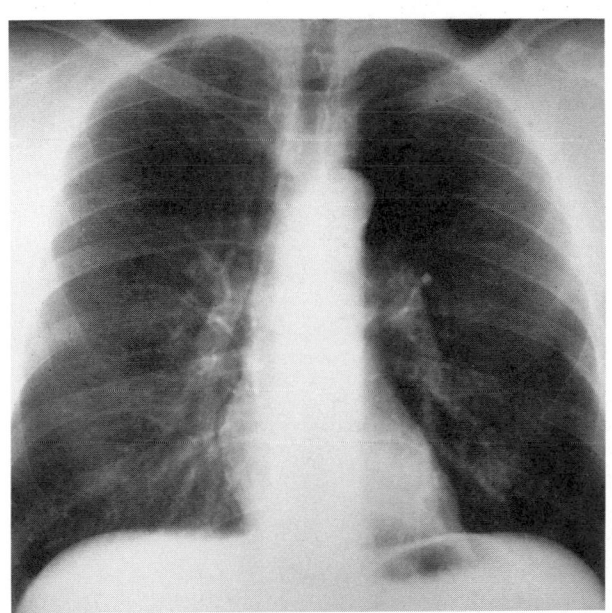
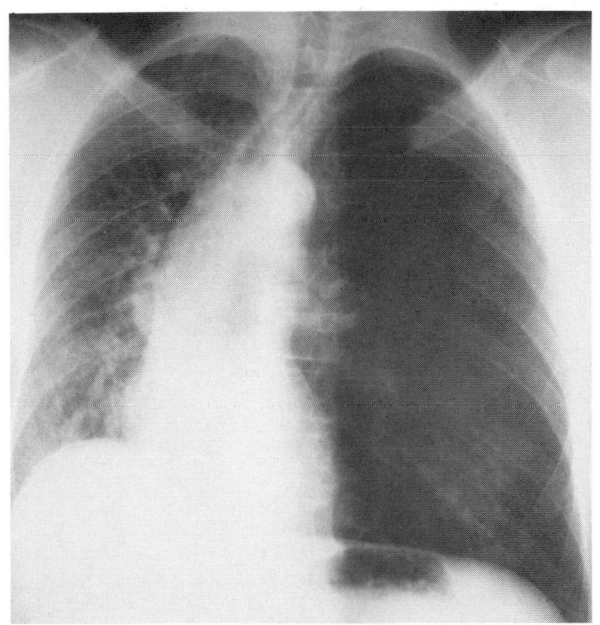

Figure 18-11. **(A)** Inspiration PA chest radiograph reveals mild hyperlucency of the left hemithorax. **(B)** Expiration view reveals marked hyperlucency of the left lung with significant shift of the mediastinum to the right. These findings suggest bronchial obstruction. At bronchoscopy, this 49-year-old man was found to have a bronchogenic carcinoma completely occluding the left mainstem bronchus.

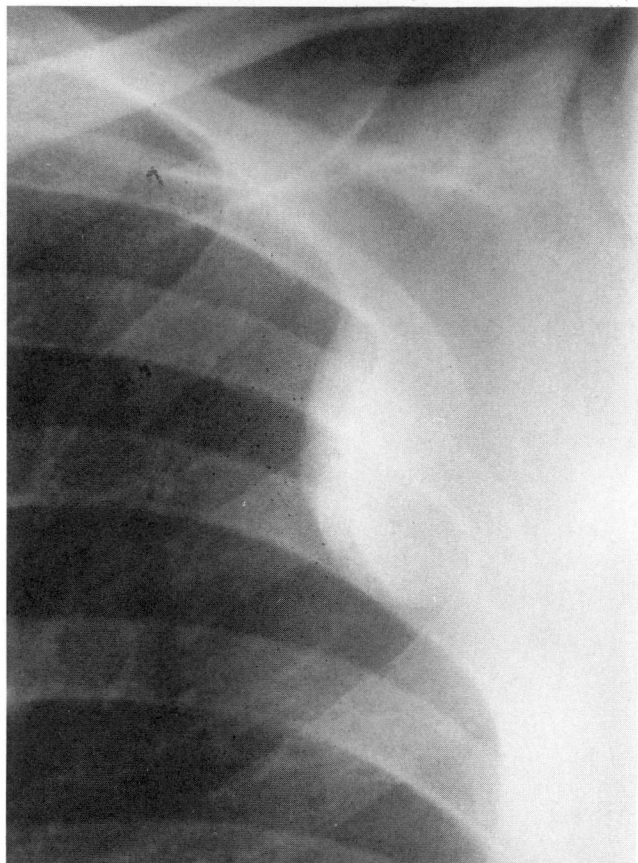

Figure 18-12. Intercostal lipoma. Note the typical characteristics of this extrapulmonary lesion, which is protruding into the thorax. It is well defined and makes obtuse angles where it contacts the chest wall. In addition it is homogeneous in density and convex toward the lung.

of caveats. Since the initial article, a number of controversies regarding the technique have arisen. At that time it was believed that there was an exact relationship between the attenuating characteristics of the nodule and the subsequently obtained CT numbers. However, this was found not to be such a simple relationship (Zerhouni, et al., 1982). A number of variables were found that affected the CT numbers, including the location and size of the nodule, the amount of patient body fat, the reconstruction algorithm used to generate the CT image, and the CT scanner itself. For example, a nodule located adjacent to the spine may have different CT numbers than does a similar nodule located in the midlung. Since 1980, some improvements have been made in CT scanners, which have reduced the effects of some of these variables (de Geer, et al., 1986; Im, et al., 1988).

In an attempt to remove these effects completely, a reference phantom (a model that simulates the patient's thorax) was created (Zerhouni, et al., 1983). A plastic cylinder of the same size as the patient's nodule is attached to this model in the same location as the true nodule and a ring corresponding to the amount of the patient's body fat is placed around it. The technique involves first scanning the patient's thorax at the level of the pulmonary nodule, using thin sections. Immediately after this, the appropriately configured reference phantom is scanned. The simulated nodules are constructed of a material with a density of 185 to 264 HU (Swensen, et al., 1991; Khouri, et al., 1987). After both images have been obtained, they are placed one above the other on the CT television monitor. The window level is manipulated so that both the true nodule and simulated nodule begin to disappear. If the true nodule disappears before the simulated nodule, then its density is lower than that of the simulated nodule (and it therefore does not contain calcium). Therefore, the clinician must be suspicious that it may represent a tumor. However if the simulated nodule disappears first, then the

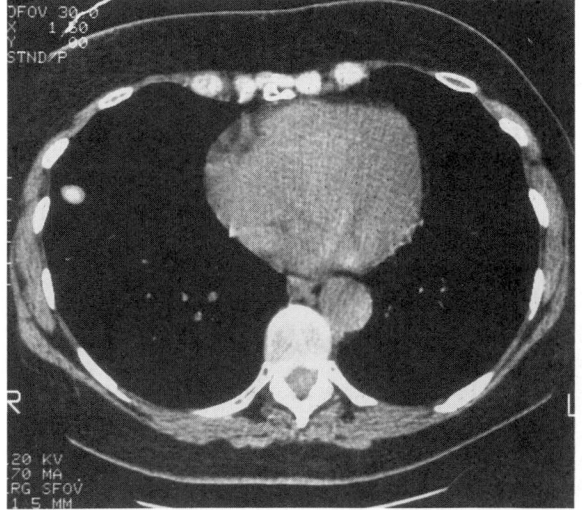

Figure 18-13. **(A)** Old granulomatous disease. Thin-section CT scan through the lower lung reveals a nodule in the right lower lobe, measuring 1 cm in diameter and containing a dense calcified central nidus. **(B)** Computer readout of the density (in Hounsfield units) of each of the pixels in the central part of this nodule. Note that many of these pixels have values greater than 200, indicating calcification.

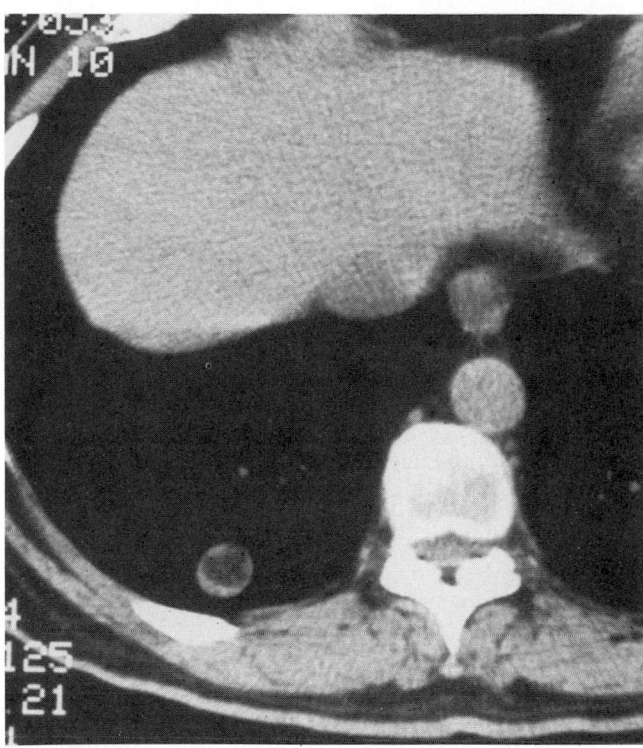

Figure 18-14. Pulmonary hamartoma. Thin-section CT scan thought to be a nodule in the right lower lobe, which is composed almost entirely of fat.

nodule in question has a higher density than does the simulated one and can be considered benign. Although CT densitometry was shown to be a useful test in the workup of patients with pulmonary nodules, there is some controversy as to the exact role that the phantom plays. Some think that it is useful (Zerhouni, et al., 1986; Khan, et al., 1991); others believe it is not necessary (Webb, 1990).

There are some aspects of CT densitometry that complicate its use. It is important to keep in mind that some pulmonary malignancies may contain calcium pathologically and radiographically (Mahoney, et al., 1990); therefore, all nodules diagnosed as benign by CT must still be followed by plain radiography to be certain that they do not enlarge (Siegelman, et al., 1986a). Most tumors that appear calcified are greater than 2.0 cm in diameter; in general therefore it is most useful for nodules less than this size (Siegelman, et al., 1986a). Similarly the margins of the nodules must be studied carefully. If the margins are smooth and the nodule is not lobulated, then the finding of calcium in a benign pattern can make the clinician confident of the benign diagnosis. However if the margins of the nodule are irregular, then again the clinician must be suspicious of its malignant potential no matter what the CT numbers reveal (Siegelman, et al., 1986a). The misdiagnosis rate (i.e., carcinomas called benign on the basis of CT, using the reference phantom) ranged from 0 to 9 percent (Zerhouni, et al., 1986; Swensen, et al., 1991; Huston, et al., 1989; Jones, et al., 1989; Ward, et al., 1989). Therefore, although the vast majority of CT-negative nodules are truly benign, proper follow-up of these patients is critical.

Other Focal Lesions

CT is useful in determining if a suspicious nodule seen on the plain radiograph lies within the lung or not (Fig. 18-15). For example, lesions, such as bone islands, costochondral junctions, tortuous mediastinal vessels, and focal areas of pleural thickening, can all be clearly distinguished from true pulmonary nodules by CT.

Pulmonary hamartomas can often be diagnosed as such by CT densitometry by finding a well-defined nodule containing fat (-40 to -120 HU) with or without calcium. In one large study of 47 patients with this lesion (Siegelman, et al., 1986b), fat without calcium was found in 18, fat with calcium in 10, and calcium alone in 2.

CT demonstrates vessels and bronchi coursing into a region of round atelectasis, thereby proving the true nature of what might otherwise be considered a nonspecific pulmonary mass by chest radiography. In certain instances, these curving vessels, which form the so-called comet tail sign, are sometimes more readily appreciated on plain tomography. Other CT features of round atelectasis include its peripheral mass-like nature, adjacent pleural thickening, an ill-defined margin medially where it contacts the incoming vessels, and the frequent presence of air bronchograms within it (Doyle, et al., 1984; McHugh, et al., 1989).

CT is useful in demonstrating arteriovenous malformations as the cause of a pulmonary nodule (Fig. 18-16). The feeding vessels are usually clearly visualized. In addition, by performing dynamic scanning (multiple images at 2-second intervals at the same level during the injection of a bolus of intravenous contrast material), the clinician can demonstrate that free-flowing blood is present within the lesion in question. However, a number of other lesions may also rapidly take up contrast material. These include bronchogenic carcinoma (Halbsguth, et al., 1983), peripheral carcinoid tumor (Davis, et al., 1990), and metastatic disease (Cirimelli, et al., 1988).

Bronchogenic Carcinoma

The role of CT in the initial workup of patients with bronchogenic carcinoma is controversial. It has been used in assessing all of the tumor (T), node (N), and metastasis (M) aspects of the disease, but the following discussion is limited to only the N and T factors.

The CT technique that is most often used includes 1-cm thick contiguous images from the thoracic apex into the upper abdomen, including the liver and adrenal glands. Intravenous contrast material aids in detecting hepatic lesions and in assessing hila and the mediastinum in problematic situations. Additional 3-mm thick images through the anteroposterior AP window and subcarinal regions are also helpful. The nodes may be round or oblong on the CT transverse images, and some interpreters measure the long axis of the nodes. Others measure the short axis. There is no definite consensus as to which is superior. Nodes tend to be oblong in the superoinferior direction, but this is difficult to assess on CT scanning. For example if a lymph node in the right paratracheal region is seen on two contiguous images, the clinician cannot be certain if this actually represents one oblong node or two separate nodes lying one above the other. Therefore, lymph

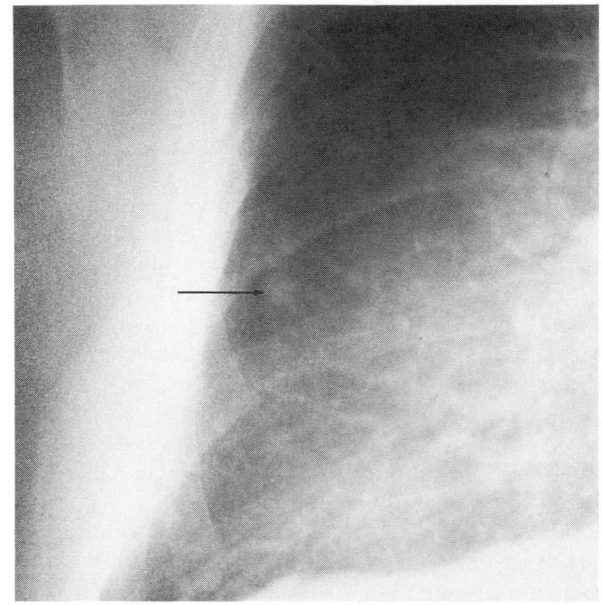

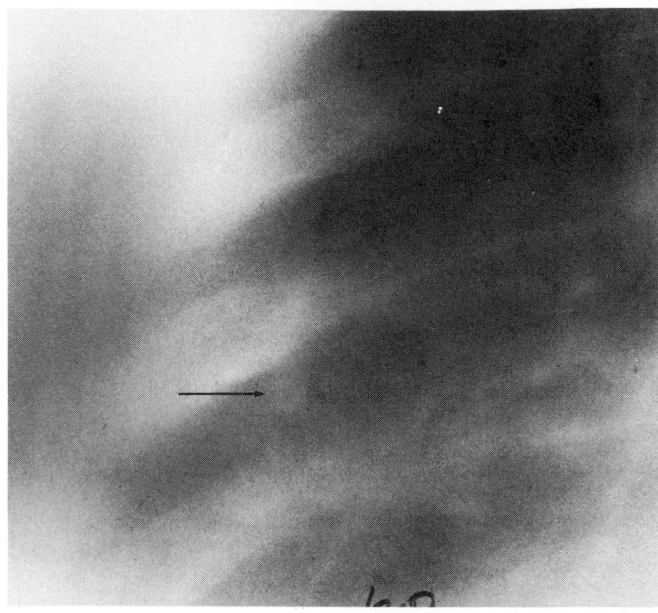

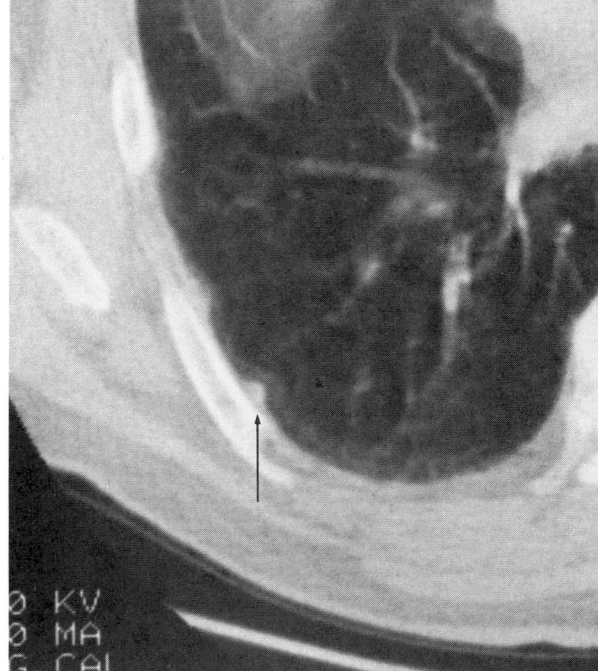

Figure 18-15. "Pulmonary" nodule. **(A)** Close-up view of PA chest radiograph reveals a nodular density (*arrow*), measuring 8 mm in diameter and projecting over the lateral aspect of the right midchest. **(B)** Plain tomogram. This study confirms the presence of this nodule but cannot determine its exact location. Because the nodule is in focus with the adjacent rib, we can state that the nodule lies in a peripheral location. **(C)** CT scan. This study reveals that the nodular density represents a focal area of pleural thickening rather than a true (*arrow*) pulmonary nodule.

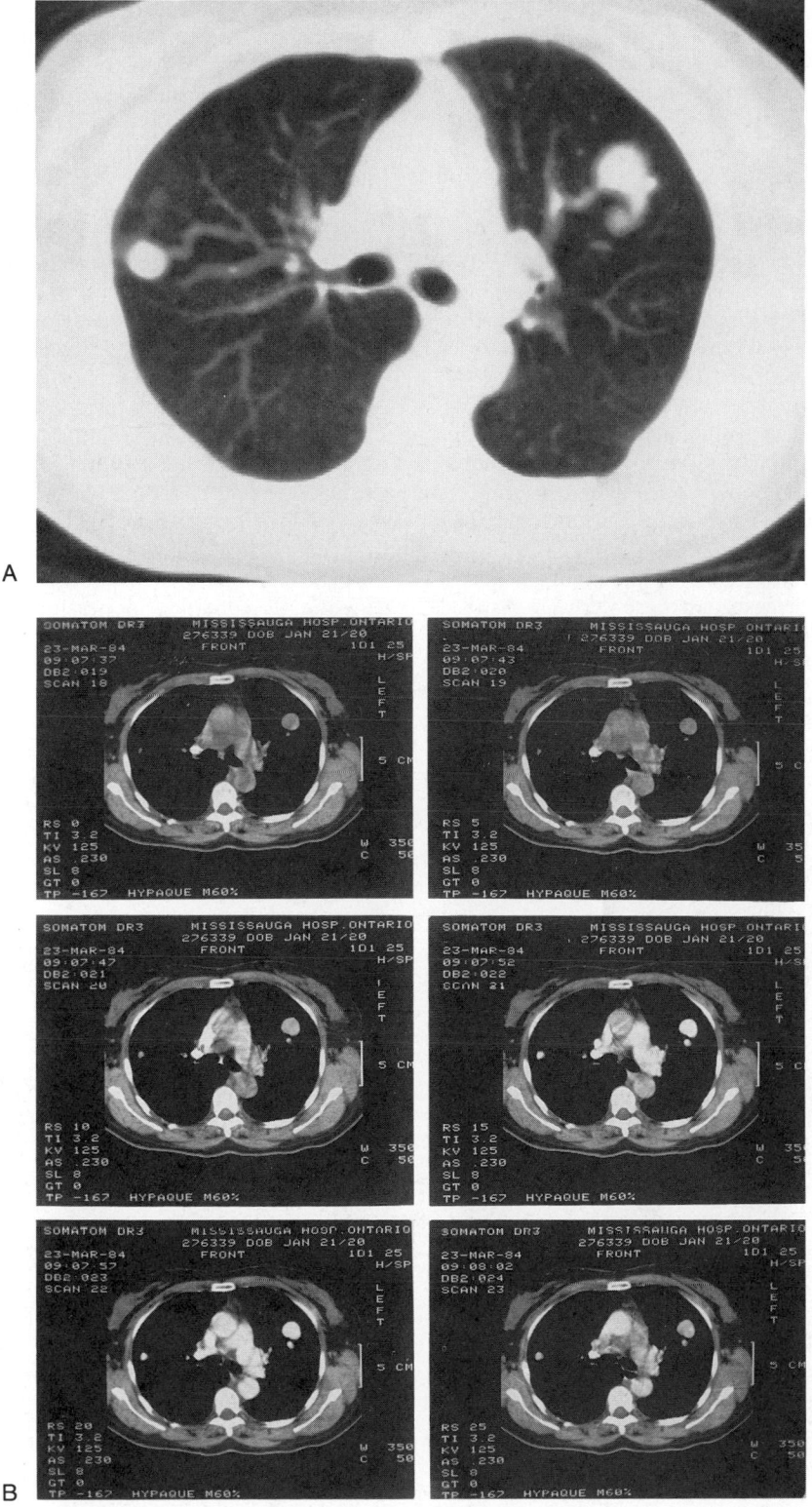

Figure 18-16. A 64-year-old woman with known Rendu-Osler-Weber disease. **(A)** CT scan. Bilateral upper lobe pulmonary nodules are noted, along with dilated feeding vessels. **(B)** Six images from a dynamic scan through the same level. The pulmonary nodules pick up contrast as soon as it is seen in the left pulmonary artery (third image). Maximum opacification is present on the fourth image, and by the sixth image, the density of the nodules has returned almost to baseline.

node size as measured by CT may not be equal to the size measured pathologically. In addition, there are some specific pitfalls that are well known in the assessment of mediastinal nodes. For example, the clinician must be careful not to interpret the top of the left pulmonary artery as an AP window node. Similarly the transverse sinus of the pericardium, located just posterior to the ascending aorta and just above the right pulmonary artery, must not be mistaken for a lymph node.

N Factor

A number of studies were performed on normal patients to determine the upper limits of normal for each of the American Thoracic Society nodal stations (Genereux, et al., 1984; Glazer, et al., 1985b, Quint, et al., 1986; Kiyono, et al., 1988). The largest nodes are generally found in the right tracheobronchial angle region (station 10R) and in the subcarinal region (7). In practice, the upper limit of normal is considered to be 1.0 cm; this size is used whether the long or short axis is measured.

A large number of studies looked at the ability of CT to detect mediastinal nodal disease, and these were summarized in numerous reviews (Webb, 1987; Libshitz, 1990; Aronchick, 1990). Using 1 cm as the criterion for abnormality, from these studies a range of sensitivities of 29 to 95 percent is found with a range of specificities from 46 to 94 percent (Libshitz, 1990). Obviously clinicians can pick whatever values they choose. The published studies differ greatly in a number of details, including the prevalence of granulomatous disease, prevalence of metastatic disease, relative proportion of each T stage, prospective versus retrospective, CT tech-

nique, and very importantly, the extent of nodal dissection (Freedman, 1992). Those studies in which complete nodal dissection is the therapy of choice noted relatively lower sensitivities (Freedman, 1992; McLoud, et al., 1992; Webb, et al., 1991), as would be expected. If a normal-sized node is not resected (e.g., as might occur if it is not palpable during thoracotomy), then the result is called a true negative by CT; however, this would be a false negative if this node were found to contain a tumor if a complete nodal dissection had been performed.

In clinical practice, two specific questions arise in the individual patient. These are (1) what is the clinical significance of having one or more nodes greater than 1 cm in diameter, and (2) what is the clinical significance if all nodes are less than 1 cm in size?

Nodes between 1 and 2 cm in diameter have a 25 to 30 percent chance of harboring a tumor; nodes greater than 2 cm in diameter have a 70 to 75 percent chance of harboring a tumor (Libshitz, 1990) (Fig. 18-17). Therefore, even patients with nodes larger than 2 cm in diameter have a 25 to 30 percent chance of having no tumor within these lymph nodes. Thus, nodal enlargement alone on CT scanning does not make a patient's condition inoperable; biopsy proof is required.

In patients with no enlarged lymph nodes, the chance of the patient who actually has mediastinal involvement is generally in the 3 to 16 percent range (Whittlesey, 1988; Gross, et al., 1988; McKenna, et al, 1985b) (Fig. 18-18). Some interpret these figures as meaning the patient can undergo thoracotomy directly (Whittlesey, 1988); others believe that mediastinoscopy is still necessary (Patterson, et al., 1987). At the present time, the issue must be individualized to the particular institution, and there must be good communication between the

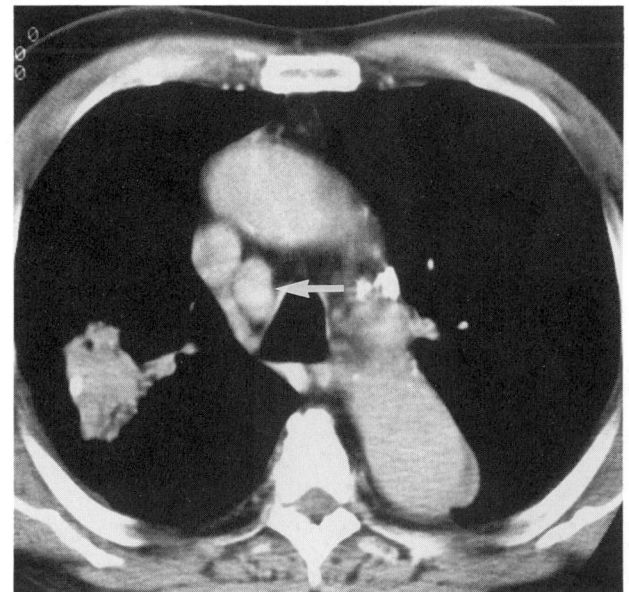
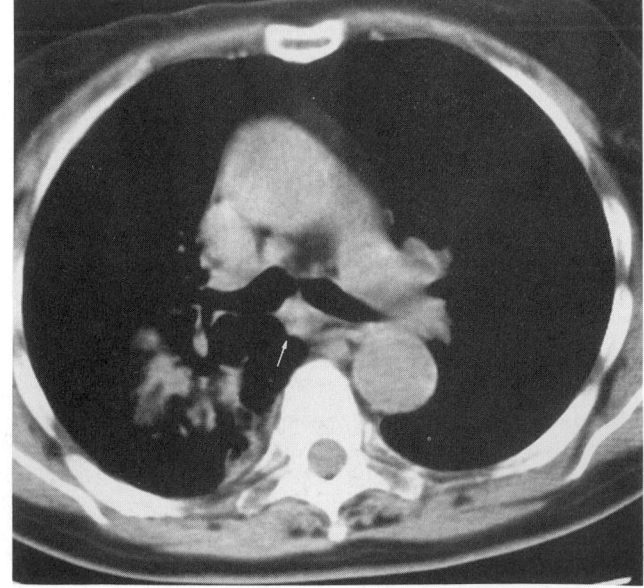

Figure 18-17. **(A)** CT scan in this 74-year-old man reveals a right upper lobe bronchogenic carcinoma with an enlarged lymph node in the right tracheal bronchial angle region (*arrow*). Pathologic examination revealed malignant cells in this node, which had been removed at mediastinoscopy. **(B)** In this 70-year-old woman with a right upper lobe bronchogenic carcinoma, an enlarged node measuring 1.7 × 1.3 cm in size is seen in the posterior subcarinal region (*arrow*). This node was found to be free of tumor at thoracotomy.

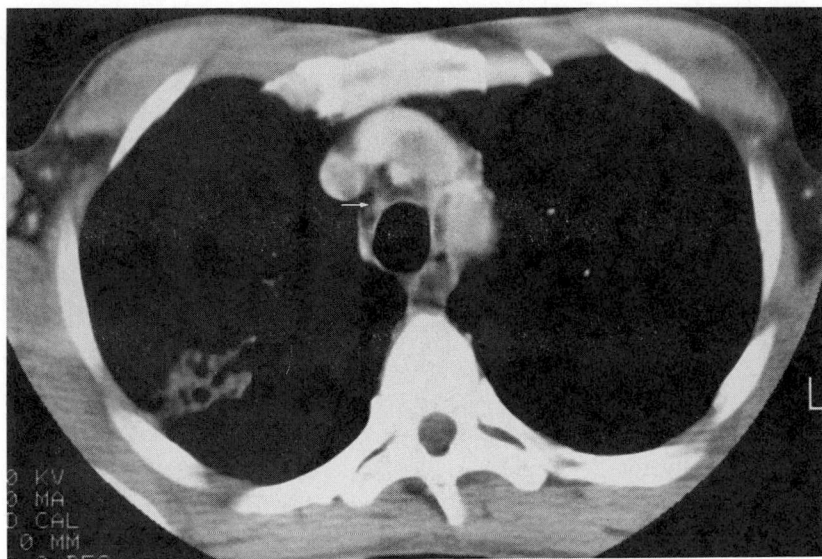

Figure 18-18. CT scan of high paratracheal region in this 53-year-old man with a right upper lobe bronchogenic carcinoma. A tiny 2R node, measuring about 2 mm in diameter (*arrow*), was found to contain tumor at mediastinoscopy.

surgeon and radiologist as to what is thought to be significant and what is not.

The finding of normal-sized mediastinal nodes by CT does not mean that the patient does not require a search for metastatic disease. In fact such patients have a 25 percent chance of having stage M1 disease (Sider, et al., 1988).

A number of questions still remain in this field of study. For example, there is some evidence that CT scanning accuracy can be improved by using different nodal sizes in different stations. As stated earlier, superior mediastinal nodes are normally smaller than are pericarinal nodes. Average normal 2R nodes measure 3 mm in diameter; average normal 10R nodes measure 7 mm. If the clinician assumes that the presence of tumor enlarges the lymph node diameter by 5 mm, then a 2R node becomes 8 mm in size and will still be called normal, using 1 cm as the cutoff. A 10R node becomes 12 mm in size and is considered positive. From this analysis, we might predict that the sensitivity for the 2R nodal station would be low but the specificity would be high. This is exactly what was found. For example, in one study (Staples, et al., 1988) the sensitivity in the 2R region was found to be 0.22; the specificity was 0.98. This is in contrast to the observed 10R sensitivity and specificity of 0.63 and 0.73, respectively.

Similarly cell type may play a role in affecting the CT accuracy. False-negative nodal disease appears more likely with adenocarcinoma than with squamous cell carcinoma (Staples, et al., 1988). In addition, the location of the primary tumor is believed by some to be a factor, although this is also controversial. Although some demonstrated that the sensitivity of CT scanning is higher for central rather than for peripheral tumors (Staples, et al., 1988), the opposite was found to be the case in a recent metanalysis study (Dales, et al., 1990).

In summary it appears that the use of CT scanning versus mediastinoscopy in working up patients with mediastinal

nodal disease varies from institution to institution and it is important that the radiologist and surgeon discuss each case individually to fit the practice for that institution best. Although it is invasive and requires a general anesthetic, mediastinoscopy has a better sensitivity and specificity than does CT scanning. In addition, it must be stressed that the clinician must prove the presence of metastatic disease in enlarged nodes and not deem the patient's condition inoperable by CT alone.

T Factor

Although a large number of studies have looked at mediastinal nodal disease, fewer have examined chest wall and mediastinal invasion by the primary tumor. The surgeon may want to know if the chest wall is involved prior to thoracotomy because of the increased morbidity and mortality rates associated with chest wall resection (Patterson, et al., 1982) compared with the general situation (Ginsberg, et al., 1983). In addition, it affects the surgical approach because the surgeon does not want to make the thoracotomy incision at the level of chest wall invasion. The prognosis for a patient with stage N1 or N2 disease and chest wall involvement also is poor (Patterson, et al., 1982; Piehler, et al., 1982).

Generally speaking, CT performs poorly in the assessment of chest wall involvement in most cases (Pennes, et al., 1985; Glazer, et al., 1985a). Many different CT signs were looked at, including the length of contact of the tumor with the chest wall, the angles that were made at the point of contact, and the presence of asymmetry of the chest wall soft tissues adjacent to the tumor. None of these signs was reliable. Highly predictive signs of chest wall invasion are definite rib destruction and the presence of a large soft tissue mass in the adjacent chest wall (Pennes, et al., 1985; Glazer, et al., 1985a; Fig. 18-19). If there is no evidence of pleural thick-

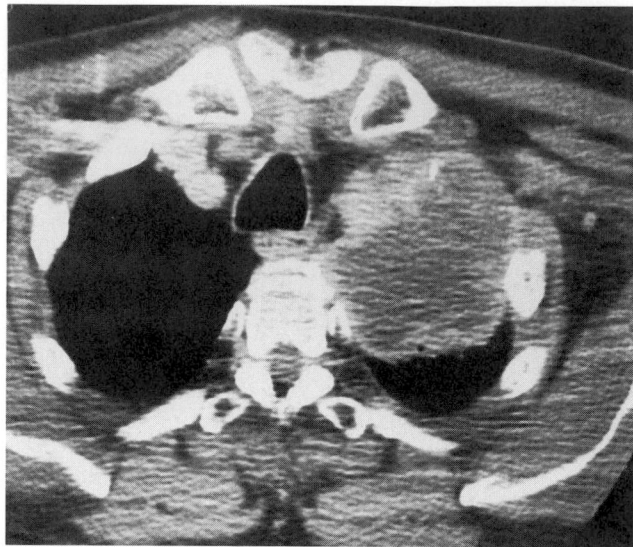

Figure 18-19. CT scan in this 78-year-old man with a left upper lobe bronchogenic carcinoma reveals that the tumor is extending directly into the chest wall, almost completely destroying the left first rib.

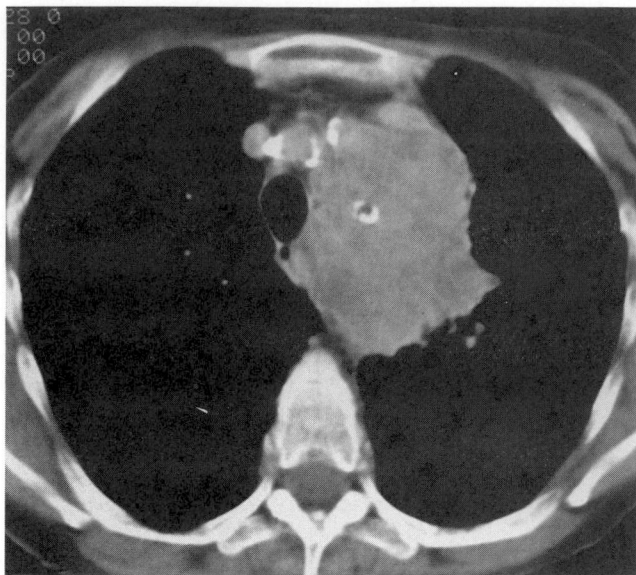

Figure 18-20. This left upper lobe carcinoma has extended directly into the mediastinum where it can be seen to be surrounding the calcified left subclavian artery completely.

ening, then the chest wall is not involved (Pennes, et al., 1985; Glazer, et al., 1985a). MRI is better than CT scanning in assessing chest wall involvement.

However, this does not mean that CT plays no role. For example, it may demonstrate clearly that a mass that appears to be contiguous with the chest wall on the plain chest radiograph is actually separate from it on the CT scan.

Similar to chest wall involvement, CT assessment of mediastinal invasion is poor (Webb, et al., 1991; Scott, et al., 1988; Glazer, et al., 1989b). Most investigators used the findings of gross interdigitation of the tumor with mediastinal fat or encasement of mediastinal structures as indicative of mediastinal invasion (Fig. 18-20). However even these signs were shown to lack sensitivity and to be poor predictors of mediastinal invasion (Herman, et al., 1991b). A number of other criteria were also studied in this regard, including the angle that the tumor makes with the mediastinum, the length of contact, whether vessels are indented by the tumor, whether there is bronchial wall thickening, the presence or absence of a fat plane between the mass and mediastinal structures, and the degree of contact with the aorta. Using these criteria, sensitivity was found to range from 53 to 84 percent and specificity, from 57 to 94 percent (Webb, et al., 1991; Baron, et al., 1982; Rendina, et al., 1987; Martini, et al., 1985; Kameda, et al., 1988; Wursten and Vock, 1987). Of importance is the fact that the positive predictive value is in the 64 to 84 percent range (Baron, et al., 1982; Wursten and Vock, 1987), and therefore the clinician must not assume that a tumor is inoperable by CT criteria alone.

Conclusions

Therefore, although CT scanning provides excellent visualization of the mediastinum, it appears that it is not accurate enough to allow the clinician to deem a patient's condition inoperable by CT criteria alone. This applies to both the presence of nodal involvement and mediastinal invasion. Other means of detecting involvement with certainty must be used. That is, enlarged lymph nodes required histologic proof of metastatic involvement. Similar proof of direct mediastinal invasion may be necessary, although not uncommonly, certain clinical features are sufficient. For example, tumor surrounding the superior vena cava in the presence of clinical superior vena caval syndrome or a tumor in the AP window in the presence of a left vocal cord paralysis are good evidence of direct mediastinal invasion.

Some other uses of CT in patients with bronchogenic carcinoma include its use as a guide to the radiotherapist, its ability to detect recurrent disease in patients who have had a pneumonectomy (Peters, et al., 1983; Glazer, et al., 1984a), and its ability to distinguish recurrent tumor from radiation fibrosis (Bourgouin, et al., 1987).

Central Airways Disease

Bronchoscopy is superior to CT scanning in determining if an airway lesion is endobronchial, submucosal, or extrabronchial in location (Naidich, et al., 1990). Although an unequivocal filling defect within an airway is highly suggestive of endobronchial disease, the CT finding of narrowing cannot be definitive in distinguishing among these three (Fig. 18-21). However, CT scanning is much better for detecting the extent of extrabronchial disease than is bronchoscopy and can therefore be useful in guiding the bronchoscopist to the site of a transbronchial needle biopsy (Fig. 18-22). In addition by demonstrating the extent of peribronchial tumor, CT scanning was shown to be useful in predicting which patients will benefit from photodynamic therapy (Zwirewich, et al., 1988).

A number of studies have been performed that compared CT and fiberoptic bronchoscopy in the detection of abnormal-

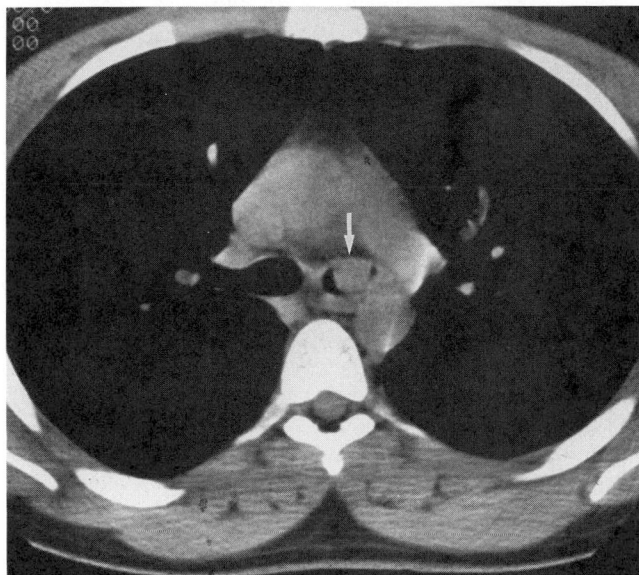

Figure 18-21. CT scan of a 20-year-old man with a mucoepidermoid tumor in the left mainstem bronchus (*arrow*). The presence of soft tissue within an airway, as exemplified by this case, is highly suggestive of endobronchial tumor.

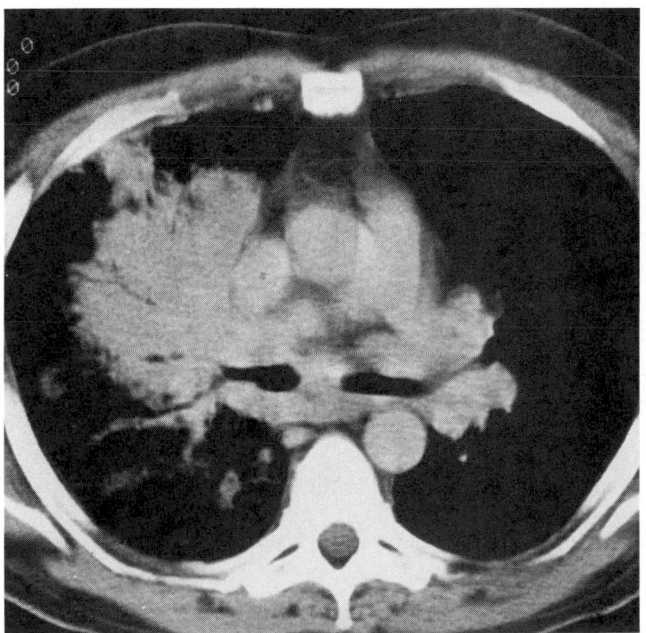

Figure 18-22. Bronchoscopy in this 51-year-old man with bronchogenic carcinoma revealed a splayed carina and occlusion of one segmental branch of the right upper lobe by extrinsic compression. The right upper lobe bronchus itself is normal. The CT scan in this patient reveals extensive tumor surrounding the right upper lobe airways and the right mainstem bronchus itself.

ities of the central airways. In one large study (Naidich, et al., 1987) using 1.5- and 10-mm thick sections and bronchoscopy as the procedure of choice, CT had a sensitivity of 90 percent and a specificity of 92 percent; all malignant lesions were accurately visualized. In another study Mayr, et al., 1989), the use of contiguous 4-mm-thick sections was found to yield a sensitivity and specificity of 100 percent.

If a specific airway is closely associated with a pulmonary mass, forming the so-called positive bronchus sign, it has been shown that a transbronchial biopsy is more likely to have a positive yield (Naidich, et al., 1988). In this study, the yield from transbronchial biopsy was 60 percent in patients with this sign but only 30 percent in those without it. In a more recent study of 33 patients with proved bronchogenic carcinoma (Gaeta, et al., 1991), transbronchial biopsy and brushing revealed tumor in 13 of 22 (59 percent) patients with the sign but only 2 of 11 (18 percent) without it. If the sign was present in a fourth-order bronchus, then there was a 90 percent success rate at bronchoscopy, compared with a 33 percent success rate when the sign was present in fifth-through seventh-order bronchi.

CT has been shown to be very useful in evaluating patients with hemoptysis (Naidich, et al., 1990). In this study of 58 patients investigated by plain radiography, CT, and fiberoptic bronchoscopy, airway abnormalities were detected at CT in 28 patients (48 percent). Eighteen of these patients had central airway problems (including all such lesions detected by bronchoscopy), and 10 had bronchiectasis. All 24 patients ultimately proved to have malignant disease had abnormal CT scan results (17 had a central airway abnormality, and 21 had a mass lesion).

Lobar Collapse

CT was shown to be useful in working up patients with lobar collapse (Naidich, et al., 1983a; Naidich, et al., 1983b). It may demonstrate evidence of a central bronchial abnormality or hilar mass that is causing a bronchial obstruction when no such mass is evident on the plain radiograph (Woodring, 1988). Occasionally a small hilar mass can be simulated by lobar vessels, and if this is considered a possibility, images through this region must be obtained following a bolus of intravenous contrast material.

A characteristic finding of central bronchial obstruction on CT, which cannot be seen by plain tomography or chest radiography, is the presence of so-called mucus bronchograms (Woodring, 1988) (Fig. 18-23). In this situation dilated bronchi filled with low-density material can be seen within the collapsed lobe. This finding suggests a central obstructing lesion (Glazer, et al., 1989a). Similarly, the absence of air bronchograms on CT suggests, but not definitely, the presence of obstruction; in one study (Woodring, 1988) it was associated with obstruction 89 percent of the time. In 34 percent of those *with* air bronchograms, a central obstruction was present (Woodring, 1988).

Bronchiectasis

In the early years of CT scanning, some controversy existed regarding the accuracy of CT in the diagnosis of bronchiectasis. On a segment-by-segment basis, the sensitivity of CT

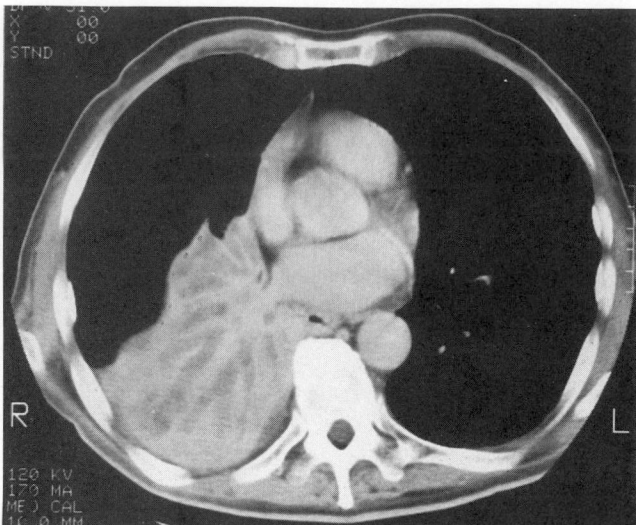

Figure 18-23.   This 74-year-old man had a bronchogenic carcinoma causing complete obstruction of the bronchus intermedius and complete collapse of the right middle and lower lobes. The CT scan reveals dilated bronchi filled with relatively low-density bronchial secretions (mucus bronchograms).

accurately assessed, and CT is now considered to be the procedure of choice for this condition (Muller, 1991).

Bronchiectasis is diagnosed with high-resolution CT when abnormally dilated thick-walled airways are seen (Fig. 18-24). Normally bronchi are visualized only in the inner and middle thirds of the lung with high-resolution CT. With bronchiectasis, because of the dilation of the airways and thickening of their walls, bronchi can be seen more peripherally. A length of an abnormal bronchus will be seen if it is running in the transverse plane. When oblique or vertical, the abnormal bronchus appears to be oval or round in configuration, respectively. Because bronchi are accompanied by branches of the pulmonary artery, a signet ring appearance is frequently seen when these abnormal airways are seen in cross-section. Varicose bronchiectasis can be recognized by the beaded appearance of the bronchial wall. With cystic bronchiectasis there are multiple large air-containing spaces, with water-dense walls, which may contain air-fluid levels. The cysts frequently are arranged linearly, which can be noted either directly on a single transverse image or more indirectly by analyzing contiguous images.

The accuracy of CT in the diagnosis of bronchiectasis, using bronchography as the procedure of choice, has been assessed in a number of studies (Grenier, et al., 1986; Joharjy, et al., 1987; Munro, et al., 1990) (Fig. 18-25). In one (Grenier, et al., 1986), 44 lungs in 36 patients were assessed by using 1.5-mm thick sections every 10 mm throughout the thorax. The sensitivity was found to be 96 percent and the specificity, 93 percent. CT underestimated the extent of the disease in one patient; however, it detected bronchiectasis in one instance where it was not diagnosed by bronchography because of incomplete filling of mucus-filled airways by the broncho-

compared with that of bronchography was found to be low, in the 63 to 66 percent range (Silverman and Godwin, 1987; Cooke, et al., 1987). Cystic bronchiectasis was clearly seen, but varicose and cylindrical bronchiectases were more difficult to detect (Muller, et al., 1984). However, with the advent of high-resolution CT, even cylindrical bronchiectasis is now

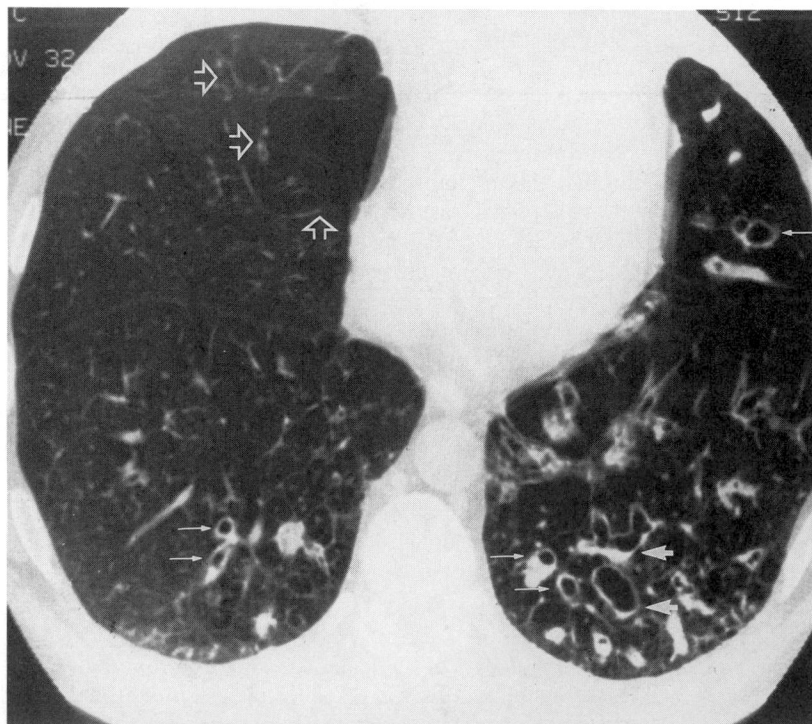

Figure 18-24.   Bronchiectasis. This high-resolution CT image reveals moderately severe cystic bronchiectasis in the left lower lobe, with small amounts of fluid present in some of the cysts (*short solid arrows*). Cylindrical bronchiectasis is seen in both lower lobes and in the lingula (*long narrow arrows*). Note also the emphysema in the right middle lobe (*open arrows*).

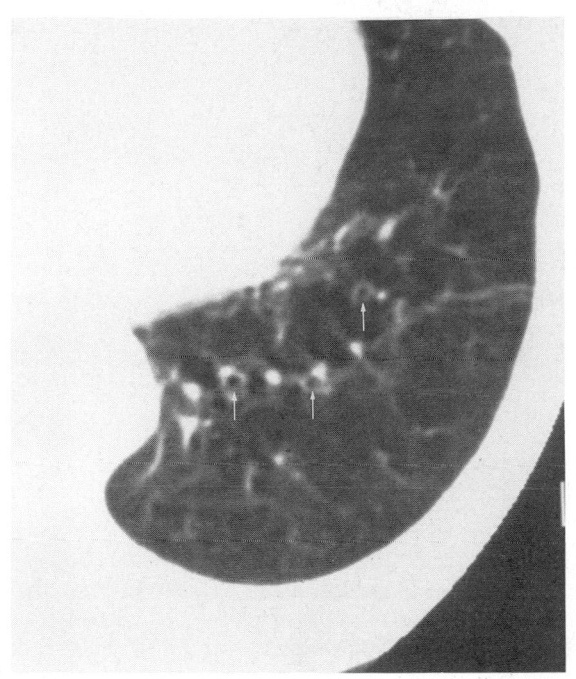

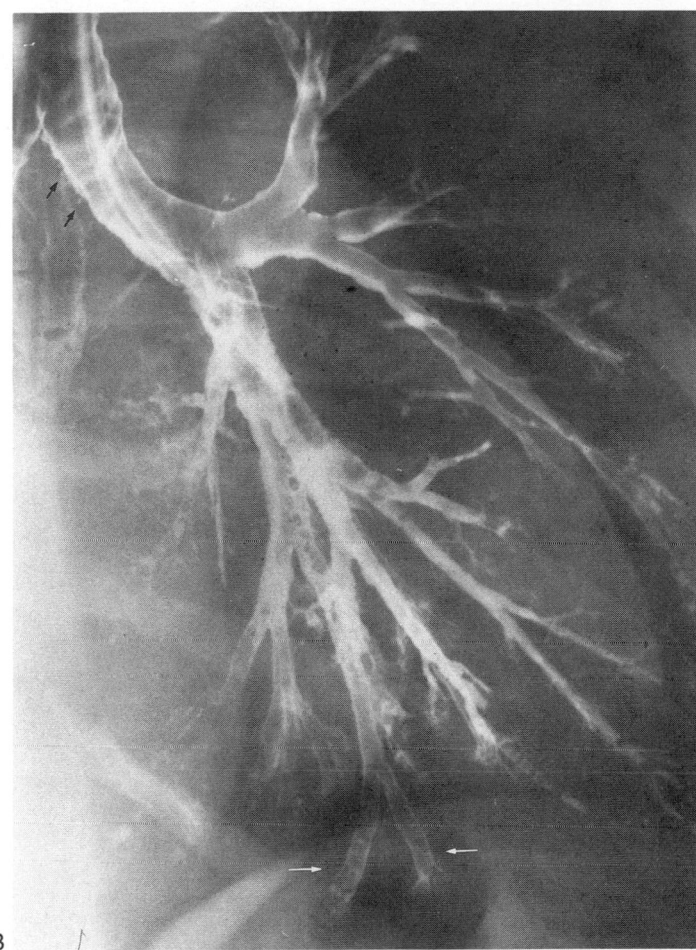

Figure 18-25. Bronchiectasis. **(A)** Close-up view of high-resolution CT scan of the left lower lobe. Note that the bronchi (*arrows*) are larger than their accompanying pulmonary artery, indicating mild cylindrical bronchiectases. **(B)** A left bronchogram reveals mild cylindrical bronchiectasis in the left lower lobe, as evidenced by the lack of tapering of multiple airways (*white arrows*). In addition, note the bronchographic contrast filling the necks of dilated bronchial glands along the inferior aspect of the left mainstem bronchus (*black arrows*).

graphic contrast. In a second study (Joharjy, et al., 1987), in which 4-mm-thick sections at 5-mm intervals were used, the sensitivity of CT was found to be 97 percent. Somewhat poorer results were noted in a third study comparing 3-mm-thick images with bronchography in 27 patients (Munro, et al., 1990); a sensitivity of 84 percent and specificity of 82 percent were found.

High-resolution CT is therefore very useful in the workup of patients with suspected bronchiectasis. It may clearly demonstrate disease in multiple locations, obviating surgery in most instances. High-resolution CT does not demonstrate the necks of dilated mucus glands, which can be seen during bronchography (Fig. 18-25). If the presence of such a finding in a lobe other than the one under consideration for resection would make a surgeon decide that resection is contraindicated, then bronchography may still be indicated in some patients. Because of the differing findings in these studies, it is still controversial if high-resolution CT can exclude bronchiectasis with enough certainty in patients being considered for surgery.

Diffuse Lung Disease

In recent years a huge amount of literature has been devoted to the assessment of diffuse lung disease by CT scanning. A number of excellent reviews (Muller, 1991; Genereux, 1989; Muller, et al., 1990a; Muller, et al., 1990b; Klein and Gamsu, 1989) and an entire book are available for the interested reader (Webb, et al., 1992). In this section a few highlights are summarized.

Both standard CT scanning and high-resolution CT (especially) have been shown to be very useful in working up patients with diffuse lung disease (Fig. 18-26). These techniques are able to reveal definite abnormalities in cases in which the chest radiograph is normal; this has been reported for a number of conditions, including fibrosing alveolitis (Strickland and Strickland, 1988), sarcoidosis (Brauner, et al., 1989), asbestosis (Aberle, et al., 1988), and lymphangitic carcinomatosis (Stein, et al., 1987). High-resolution CT should therefore be performed in patients with clinical or pulmonary function evidence of diffuse lung disease and a

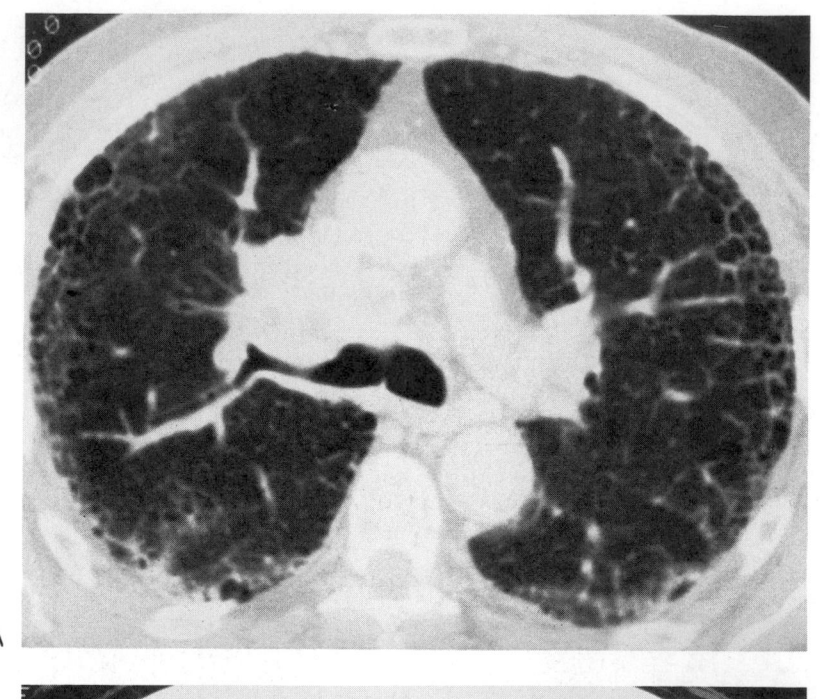

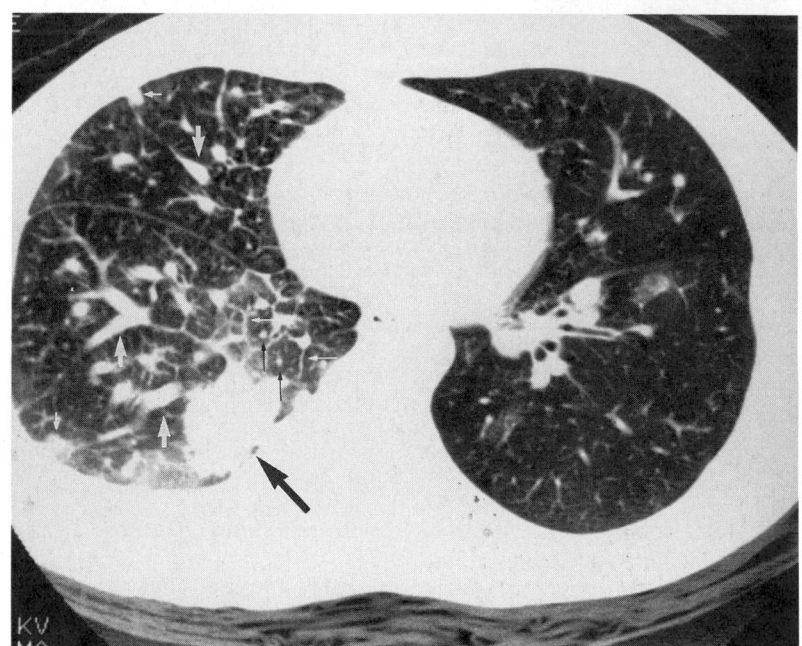

Figure 18-26 **(A)** Fibrosing alveolitis. This high-resolution CT scan reveals reticular interstitial disease, with cyst formation, in a characteristic peripheral distribution. The patient also has a right upper lobe bronchogenic carcinoma, which extends into the mediastinum. **(B)** Lymphangitic carcinomatosis. High-resolution CT scan from a 36-year-old man with a right lower lobe adenocarcinoma (*large black arrow*). In the right base, there are prominent bronchovascular bundles (*wide white arrows*), nodules (*short white arrows*), and polygonal shadows with irregular walls (*long white arrows*) and a central dot (*small black arrows*).

normal chest radiograph. Even when a definite diagnosis cannot be made by CT, it may still be helpful by suggesting both the most appropriate type of biopsy that should be performed and the optimal location for the biopsy.

Besides the ability to detect disease in the presence of a normal chest radiograph, CT (and high-resolution CT) scan-

ning have been shown to allow the clinician to be much more specific in diagnosing the patient's disease (Mathieson, et al., 1989; Grenier, et al., 1991). In addition, this diagnosis can be made with much more confidence (Mathieson, et al., 1989; Grenier, et al., 1991). Even if a specific diagnosis cannot be made, the techniques have been shown to be excellent for determining whether the patient needs a transbronchial or open lung biopsy (Mathieson, et al., 1989). The former is suggested when there is evidence of peribronchial disease, as is the case with diseases such as sarcoidosis or lymphangitic carcinoma. When the lung disease is seen to be more peripheral within the parenchyma, then an open lung biopsy is more likely necessary. CT has also been shown to be useful in directing the surgeon to the optimal site for the open lung biopsy (Fig. 18-27). Not only can abnormal areas be clearly seen, but regions suggesting the presence of active disease can also be detected. This was shown in patients with fibrosing alveolitis (Muller, et al., 1987) in whom ''ground glass'' densities, as opposed to more reticular densities, have been shown to be associated more likely with active disease, as opposed to residual fibrosis. If a biopsy is obtained from the region of fibrosis, then it might be impossible to determine the cause of the original process. However, if a biopsy can be obtained from the more active areas, then characteristic pathologic lesions are frequently seen that allow a more specific diagnosis to be made (Miller, et al., 1987).

Metastatic Disease

CT is currently the procedure of choice for the detection of pulmonary metastatic disease in patients with a known extrathoracic primary tumor (Davis, 1991). CT has been shown to be much more sensitive than both plain radiography and full lung tomography in this regard (Vanel, et al., 1984; Heaston, et al., 1983) because it detects both smaller and more nodules than either of these techniques (Fig. 18-28). However still more nodules are found by thoracotomy (Schaner, et al., 1978). Unfortunately not all of the nodules that are detected turn out to be metastases but are instead

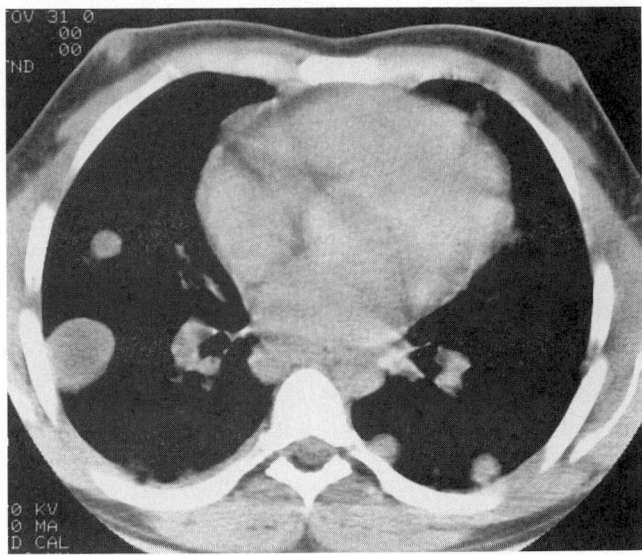

Figure 18-28.   CT scan of 22-year-old man with metastatic choriocarcinoma of the testis. There are multiple pulmonary nodules of varying size bilaterally. Note the gynecomastia; this patient's β-human chorionic gonadotropin level was greater than 300,000 units.

the result of other conditions, such as old granulomatous disease, intrapulmonary lymph nodes, or areas of fibrosis (Peuchot and Libshitz, 1987). The false-positive rate depends on a number of factors, including the site of the primary tumor, the patient's age, and whether prior therapy was given. For example sarcomas are more likely to metastasize to the lungs than are carcinomas; therefore pulmonary nod-

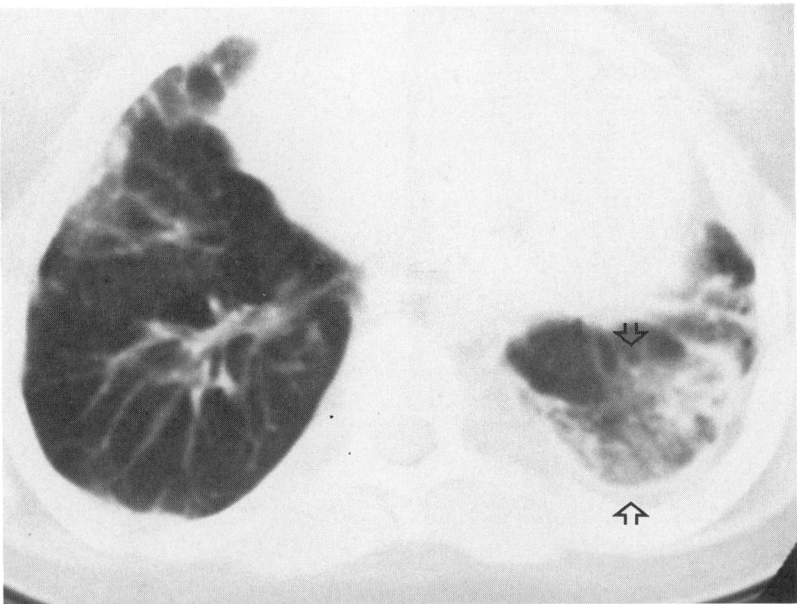

Figure 18-27.   The presence of the air space disease in the left lower lobe (between arrows) suggests active disease in this patient with biopsy-proved fibrosing alveolitis. Areas such as this are more likely to yield active disease than are more peripheral areas of reticular disease, which generally represent scarring (as shown in Fig. 18-26A).

ules in a patient with the former are more likely to be metastases than those in a patient with a carcinoma (Peuchot and Libshitz, 1987). Similarly younger patients are less likely to have previous granulomatous disease; their nodules are therefore more likely to be caused by metastatic disease (Putnam, et al., 1984; Wellner and Putnam, 1986). A patient being investigated after having been treated may have so-called sterile metastases, residual areas of scar tissue where viable tumor had originally been; these can be confused with true metastases on CT (Hidalgo, et al., 1983).

In a study comparing the features of metastases and benign nodules (Gross, et al., 1985), the former were found to be more numerous, larger, and more rounded. The presence of calcium was associated with benign disease. Other features that suggest that a nodule is a metastasis are the presence of a feeding vessel into the center of the nodule (Milne and Zarhouni, 1987), beaded adjacent interlobular septi (Ren, et al., 1989), and possibly a zone of hyperlucency distal to the nodule (Naidich, et al., 1991).

In practice it can be difficult to be certain whether the multiple pulmonary nodules demonstrated by CT in a patient with a known primary tumor represent metastases or not, and the probability is subjectively assigned based on the above factors. If large enough, one of these nodules can be sampled by transthoracic needle lung biopsy (see the section, Transthoracic Needle Biopsy). However, they are often too small for this to be possible. In these instances, a clinical decision must be made to either obtain tissue by open lung biopsy or repeat the CT in 1 to 2 months' time, assuming that metastases are likely to enlarge.

Lung Abscess Versus Empyema

It is important to be able to distinguish between a lung abscess and empyema because patient management differs, depending on which condition is present. Generally lung abscesses tend to be spherical, with thick irregular lobulated walls, and they cause little compression of the adjacent lung. Empyemas tend to be oblong, have smooth thin walls, and may cause compression of adjacent lung.

Although they frequently can be differentiated on the chest radiograph, CT has been shown to be excellent at distinguishing between them (Fig. 18-29). Lung abscesses have thick irregular walls; the walls of empyemas tend to be uniformly thin and smooth (Stark, et al., 1983; Baber, et al., 1980; Pugatch, et al., 1978). These latter walls, which are better assessed if the study is performed after the injection of contrast, represent the separated visceral and parietal pleura. Their visibility forms the so-called split pleura sign, an excellent sign of an empyema (Stark, et al., 1983). Compression of the adjacent lung is much more commonly seen with empyema, as would be expected. If the entire lesion is considered

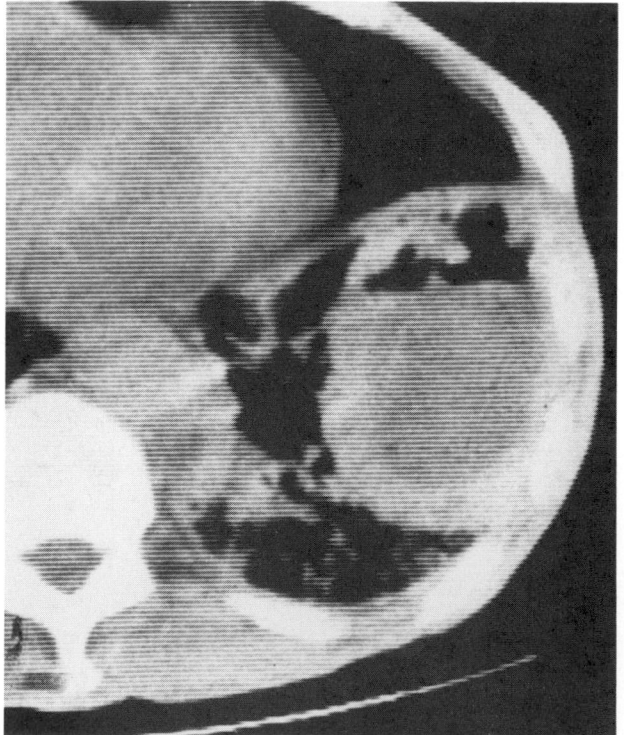
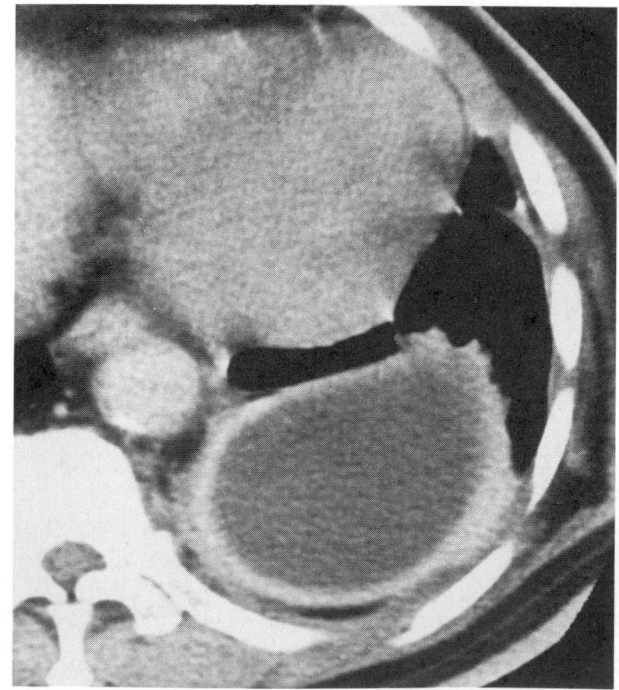

A   B

Figure 18-29. **(A)** Close-up view of CT scan of a patient with a left lower lobe abscess. The walls of this abscess are thick and irregular. The mass is spherical in shape (confirmed by synthesis of multiple adjacent images, not shown). The abscess makes acute angles with the chest wall. Lung windows (not shown) did not show adjacent atelectases. **(B)** Empyema. The walls of this left lower lobe lesion are thin and smooth. Its shape is only slightly oblong on this view, but examination on multiple other images reveals that it was oblong in a craniocaudad direction. Although it is making acute angles with the chest wall, the other features are highly indicative of empyema.

three dimensionally, then lung abscesses tend to be spherical. Empyemas are oblong, either in an AP, lateral, or craniocaudad direction. Another helpful but less definite feature is the fact that lung abscesses tend to form acute angles with the chest wall or mediastinum; empyemas tend to form obtuse angles.

MAGNETIC RESONANCE IMAGING

At the present time, MRI has very limited use in investigating pulmonary parenchymal problems. This is because of the inherent magnetic properties of the lung itself and problems of cardiac and respiratory motion. However, newer MRI techniques are currently under development, and the situation is beginning to change (Bergin, et al., 1991). It is anticipated that in the near future some of the current physical problems will be surmounted by newer MRI techniques that will lead to applications in both focal and diffuse lung disease (Webb and Sostman, 1992).

There are a number of aspects of bronchogenic carcinoma in which MRI plays a definite role. It has been shown to be better than CT in diagnosing chest wall invasion by the tumor (Musset, et al., 1986; Haggar, et al., 1987) and is especially useful in patients with Pancoast tumors (Heelan, et al., 1989) (Fig. 18-30). The ability to image in coronal and sagittal planes is very advantageous in this region, allowing MRI to accurately assess the brachial plexus, subclavian artery, and vertebral bodies. In addition, MRI may be better than CT in the diagnosis of mediastinal invasion by the primary tumor (Webb, et al., 1991; Kameda, et al., 1988).

However it is no different than CT scanning in detecting mediastinal nodal involvement with bronchogenic carcinoma (Webb, et al., 1991; Musset, et al., 1986; Poon, et al., 1987; Webb, et al., 1985). It was originally hoped that MRI would

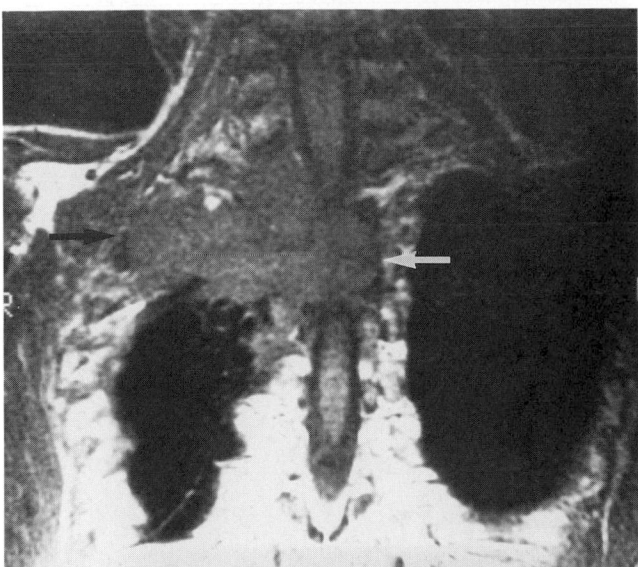

Figure 18-30. T1-weighted image in the coronal plane of a 66-year-old man with a right upper lobe Pancoast tumor. Note extension of this tumor into the chest wall (*black arrow*) and spinal canal (*white arrows*).

be able to detect certain tissue characteristics of nodes that were enlarged by a tumor as opposed to those enlarged by inflammation. However, this has been shown not to be the case, even if the nodes are examined in vitro (Glazer, et al., 1988). In practice therefore, MRI uses size criteria as does CT. In this regard, CT scanning is probably better than MRI because of its increased spatial resolution; what appears as one large node on MRI may actually turn out to be multiple smaller nodes on CT scanning. Similarly because MRI cannot detect calcification, it may misrepresent calcified nodes as malignant when CT would have correctly identified them as benign. However, because of its ability to image in the coronal plane, MRI may be better than CT in depicting certain nodal groups, specifically those in the AP window and subcarinal regions.

MRI has been shown to be accurate in distinguishing obstructive from nonobstructive atelectasis by differenes in the signal pattern of the collapsed lung (Herold, et al., 1991). In patients with lobar collapse caused by bronchogenic carcinoma, MRI can often distinguish the central tumor mass from the more peripheral atelectasis (Kameda, et al., 1988; Tobler, et al., 1987; Shioya, et al., 1988). However in some instances, CT is able to do this at least as well if a bolus of contrast material is administered (Tobler, et al., 1987).

A common problem in patients being followed for treated malignancies is whether a residual opacity represents recurrent tumor or postirradiation fibrosis. Although MRI has been shown to be useful in this regard (Glazer, et al., 1984b), it is not perfect. For example, it can be difficult to differentiate tumor from an inflammatory response, a common sequela following irradiation (Glazer, et al., 1985c; Lee and Glazer, 1990).

Early work in the use of MRI in patients with pulmonary vascular disease shows much promise, particularly in patients with pulmonary arterial hypertension (Gefter, et al., 1990). In addition, MRI can detect pulmonary thromboemboli within the central pulmonary arteries, although it is less accurate for peripheral emboli (Posteraro, et al., 1989; Shah, et al., 1989).

The interested reader is invited to refer to reviews on the uses of MRI in the assessment of mediastinal diseases, a discussion beyond the scope of this chapter (Gamsu and Sostman, 1989; Swensen, et al., 1989). It has been shown to be useful in cardiac, paracardiac, and aortic disease and in the workup of patients with posterior mediastinal masses and residual masses following treatment of lymphoma.

NUCLEAR IMAGING

V̇/Q̇ Scanning

A perfusion lung scan, as its name implies, produces an image of the distribution of pulmonary blood flow throughout both lungs (Fig. 18-31). While in the supine position (to minimize the effects of gravity), the patient is given an intravenous injection of macroaggregated albumin, which has been radiolabelled with technetium (^{99m}Tc). This material is composed of particles of such a size (5 to 100 μm) that they become trapped in the pulmonary capillaries. The amount given (1 to 4 $\times$ 10^5 particles) is such that less than 1 in 1,000 capillaries,

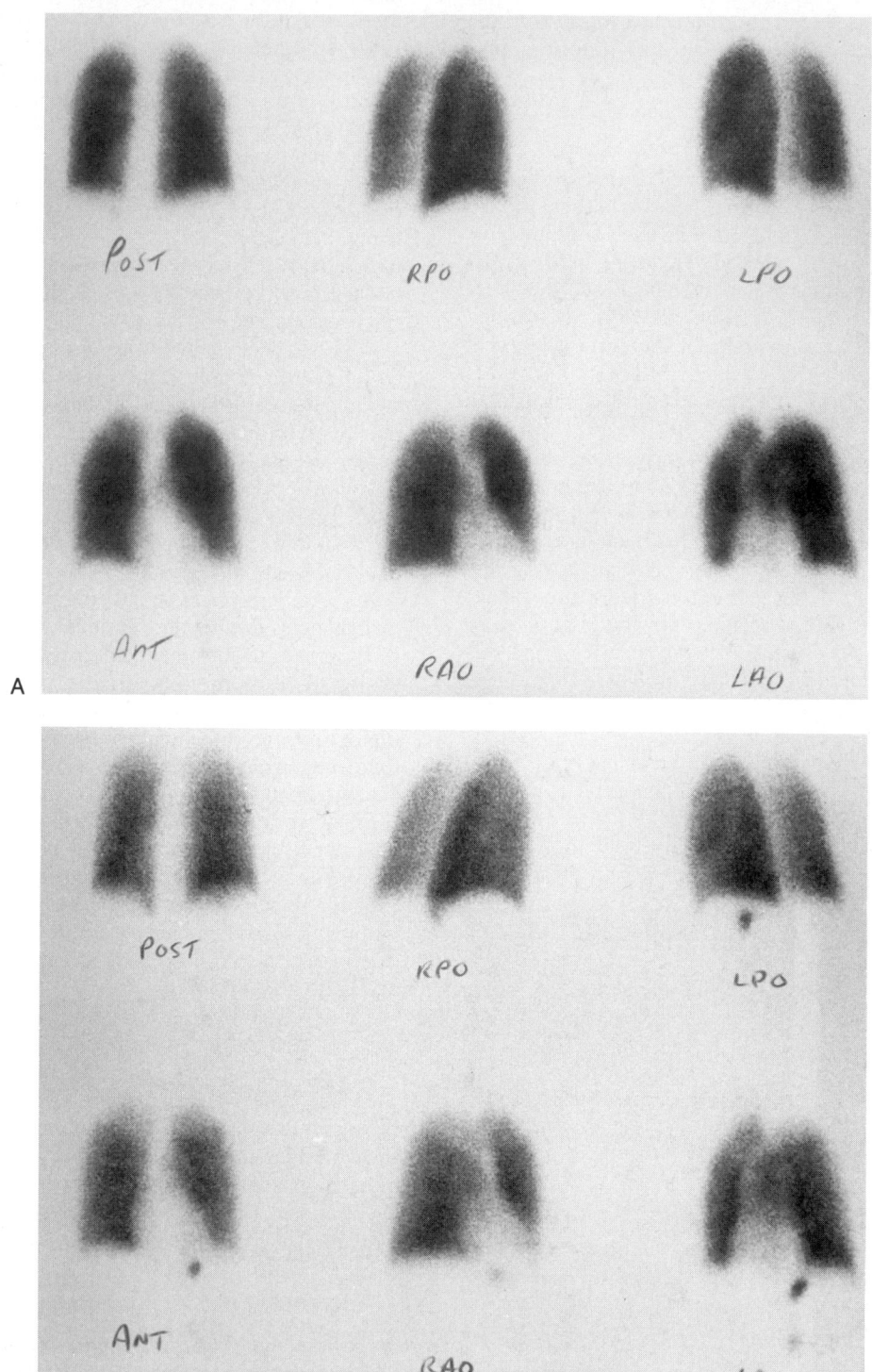

Figure 18-31. Normal V̇/Q̇ scan. **(A)** Perfusion scan. **(B)** Ventilation scan. There is homogeneous distribution of radioactivity throughout the lungs on both studies. (Courtesy of Dr. K. Yip, The Toronto Hospital, Toronto, Canada.)

in normal lungs, become obstructed (Metter and Guiberteau, 1991). A gamma camera is placed over the patient's chest, and an image reflecting pulmonary blood flow is obtained from six to eight directions.

A ventilation scan is used in a corresponding manner to obtain images reflecting the distribution of air flow to the lungs (Fig. 18-31). A number of different radioactive gases are available for this purpose. Some, such as ^{133}Xe, are inhaled with the patient in the sitting position while a gamma camera records the distribution of the radioactivity. Multiple images are obtained during the washin, equilibrium, and washout phases of the test. Areas of abnormal ventilation, including air trapping, are therefore recorded. A different technique involves the use of radioactive aerosols, the most common one being nebulized ^{99m}Tc-DTPA (diethyltriamine-pentaacetic acid). This mixture is inhaled, and the gas is deposited in the lungs again in a distribution reflecting alveolar ventilation. The advantage of this technique is that multiple images can be obtained from different directions, and these are chosen to correspond to those obtained during the perfusion scan. In this way pairs of images reflecting both ventilation and perfusion are obtained in multiple directions, allowing accurate comparison of these two aspects of pulmonary function in each lung region.

Two large prospective trials (The PIOPED Investigators, 1990; Hull, et al., 1985) helped to define the role of $\dot{V}/\dot{Q}$ scanning in the workup of patients with suspected pulmonary embolism (Fig. 18-32). A discussion of this topic is a chapter unto itself, and only a summary is presented here. Most investigators believe that a normal perfusion scan rules out pulmonary embolism with enough certainty that no further consideration need be given to this diagnosis and another cause for the patient's problems must be sought. In general a high-probability $\dot{V}/\dot{Q}$ pattern is specific enough that therapy may be given without further testing. However, if there is a contraindication to anticoagulation, then pulmonary angiography should be performed to increase the certainty of the diagnosis. In addition, because emboli may take years to resolve, a high-probability scan may reflect old embolic disease. In the PIOPED study (The PIOPED Investigators, 1990), the positive predictive value of a high probability scan was 91 percent in those without a history of prior pulmonary emboli, but it fell to 74 percent in those with a prior history.

The clinical situation of a low- or intermediate-probability scan is much more controversial (Juni and Alavi, 1991). In this circumstance, the clinician must always keep in mind that pulmonary emboli result, almost always, from deep venous thrombosis in the leg or pelvic veins. Therefore, attention must be paid to this primary disease. The finding of venous thrombosis necessitates anticoagulation. Patients with a low- or intermediate-probability scan and no evidence of venous thrombosis may be safely followed (closely) without anticoagulation (Hull, et al., 1989).

Gallium Scanning

Both inflammatory and neoplastic tissues take up and concentrate ^{67}Ga citrate. It can therefore be used to locate abscesses and assess diffuse inflammatory conditions in the lungs; in addition it has been used in the staging of patients with bronchogenic carcinoma and lymphoma. One disadvantage of ^{67}Ga is that imaging cannot take place until about 48 hours following its administration.

This radiopharmaceutical is useful in detecting otherwise hidden abscesses, although if a specific site is suspected of harboring an abscess by clinical criteria, it is better to perform CT or ultrasound of the region rather than ^{67}Ga imaging. A number of conditions are associated with diffuse pulmonary uptake of ^{67}Ga. These include pneumonia from *Pneumocystis carinii,* active sarcoidosis, active idiopathic pulmonary fibrosis, miliary tuberculosis, bleomycin toxicity, acute radiation pneumonitis, and lymphangitic carcinoma (Metter and Guiberteau, 1991).

In addition, ^{67}Ga imaging has been investigated by numerous groups in regard to its ability to stage bronchogenic carcinoma (Alazraki, et al., 1978; Fosburg, et al., 1979; Freedman, et al., 1984; McKenna, et al., 1985a). In 4 to 32 percent of cases, the primary tumor itself does not take up the radionuclide. In these cases, it is impossible to make a statement about mediastinal nodal status. Even when the tumor does take up ^{67}Ga, the reported sensitivities of detecting mediastinal nodal involvement range from 23 to 100 percent and specificities, from 55 to 86 percent. Because CT is at least as accurate as ^{67}Ga scanning and the result is known immediately, ^{67}Ga is not used by many physicians to stage bronchogenic carcinoma at the present time.

Recently ^{67}Ga single-photon emission CT has been shown to improve significantly both the sensitivity and specificity over ^{67}Ga planar imaging in the staging of patients with lymphoma (Tumeh, et al., 1987; Front, et al., 1990). In addition, ^{67}Ga scanning appears to be better than CT for predicting the outcome of these patients (Front, et al., 1992). Following treatment of lymphoma, patients are commonly left with a so-called residual mass on CT. It is impossible to know whether such a mass represents residual tumor requiring further treatment or is just scar tissue requiring observation only. ^{67}Ga scanning (Front, et al., 1990) and MRI (described earlier) were shown to be useful in determining whether such a residual mass represents a residual tumor.

ANGIOGRAPHY

Pulmonary Angiography

At the present time, the main indication by far for pulmonary angiography is in the diagnosis of pulmonary embolism (Fig. 18-33). Other indications include the investigation of congenital lesions (e.g., pulmonary arteriovenous malformations), acquired vascular abnormalities (e.g., pulmonary arterial and/or venous obstruction from mediastinitis), involvement of central vessels by bronchogenic carcinoma (rarely used for this reason since the advent of CT), and again rarely, the investigation of hemoptysis.

Pulmonary angiography is currently the procedure of choice in the diagnosis of pulmonary embolism. It is believed to be underused in this regard, probably because of the impression that it is an invasive expensive test associated with significant complications (Goodman, 1984; Newman, 1989). In fact the morbidity and mortality rates of the procedure are quite low, with reported mortality rates being about 0.1 to 0.2 percent (Goodman, 1984; Mills, et al., 1980; Perlmutt,

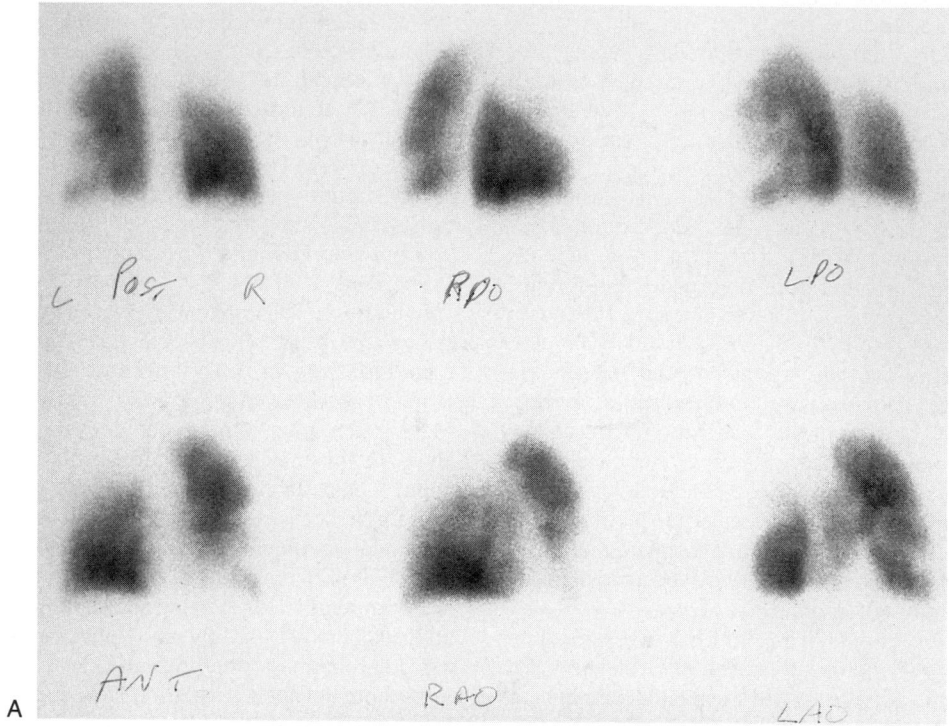

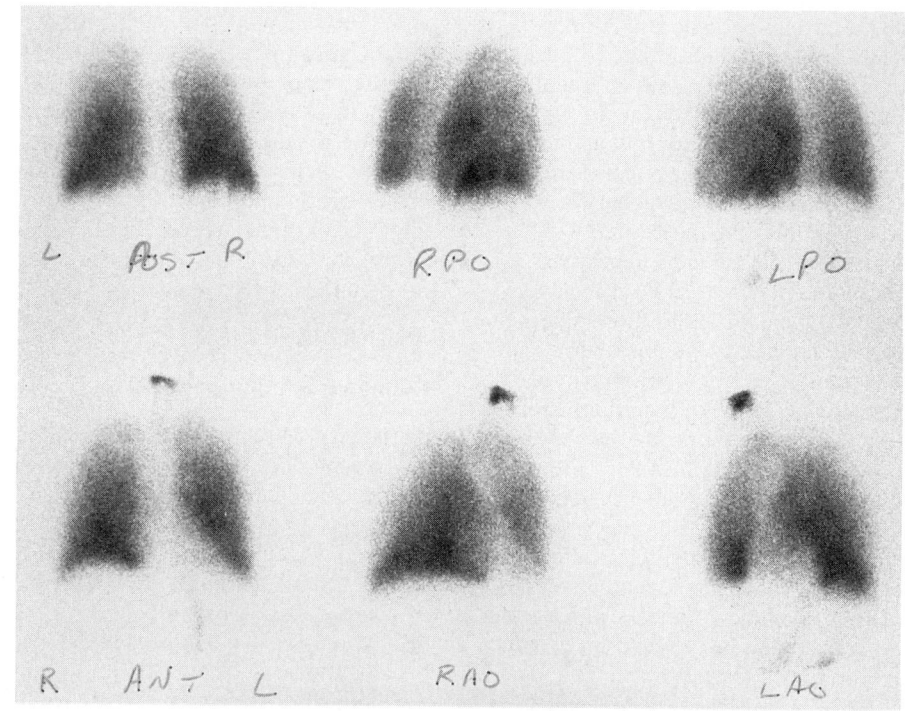

Figure 18-32. V̇/Q̇ scan of pulmonary emboli. **(A)** Perfusion scan. **(B)** Ventilation scan. There is no flow to the entire right upper lobe, the anteromedial basal segment of the left lower lobe, or the lingula. Ventilation to these regions, and to the rest of both lungs, is normal. These multiple large areas of V̇/Q̇ mismatch are highly predictive of pulmonary emboli. (Courtesy of Dr. K. Yip, The Toronto Hospital, Toronto, Canada.)

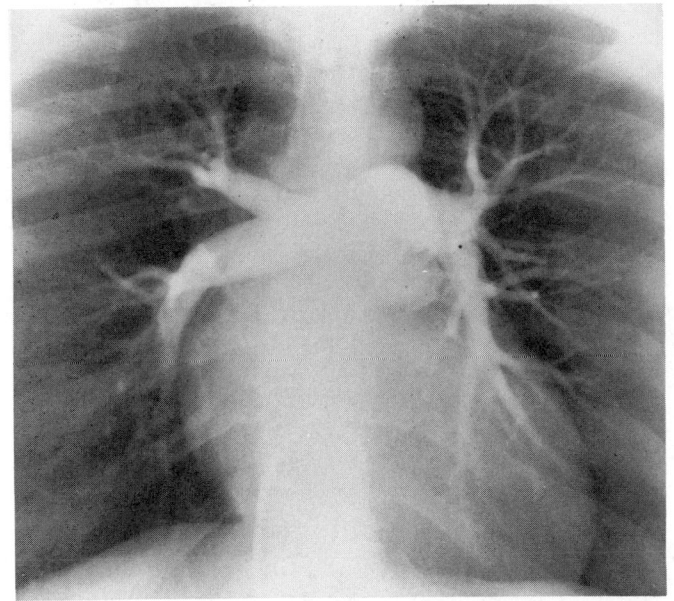

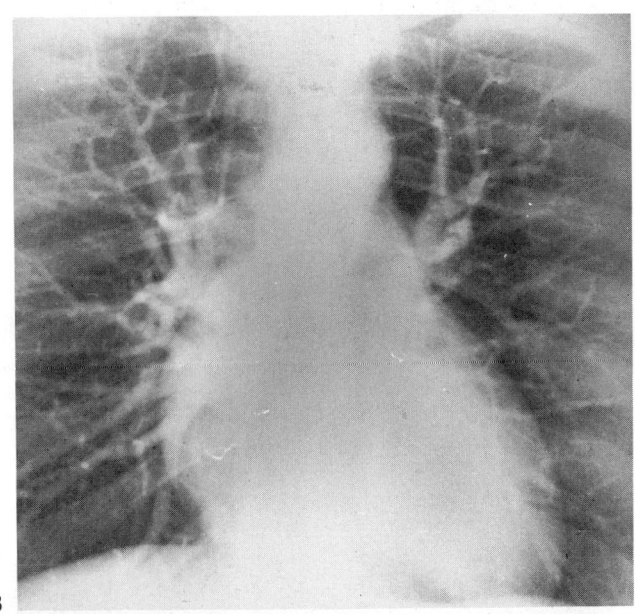

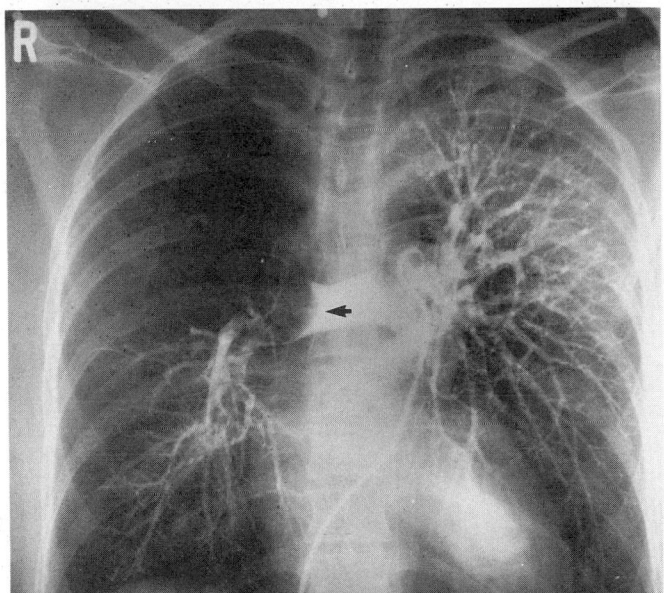

Figure 18-33. Pulmonary arteriogram. **(A)** Normal arterial phase. Contrast has been injected through a catheter with its tip just into the left main pulmonary artery. **(B)** Normal venous phase. **(C)** Pulmonary embolism. A large filling defect (*arrows*), representing a large obstructing pulmonary embolism, is seen in the distal right main pulmonary artery. Note the paucity of flow to the right upper lung (compare with the left side).

et al., 1987) and morbidity of significance rates of about 1.5 to 3 percent (Goodman, 1984; Mills, et al., 1980). The major cause of mortality is acute right heart failure, which is generally limited to patients with severe pulmonary arterial hypertension and elevated right ventricular end-diastolic pressures of 20 mmHg or more (Mills, et al., 1980; Perlmutt, et al., 1987). This problem can be minimized by using small amounts of contrast in these patients and delivering it slowly by hand injection. The causes of significant morbidity include cardiac perforation and endocardial or myocardial injury, cardiac arrest, and significant arrhythmias (Mills, et al., 1980), although cardiac perforation is no longer a problem now that pigtail catheters are used. In addition because contrast material is administered, the possibility of a hypersensitivity reaction must also be kept in mind.

Although angiography is considered the procedure of choice for the diagnosis of pulmonary embolism, it is not a perfect test. The exact sensitivity is unknown, but it is certainly not 100 percent. In part this is caused by interobserver interpretation differences (The PIOPED Investigators, 1990) and in part by the occasional finding of emboli at autopsy following a negative angiogram (Cheely, et al., 1981). However, for practical purposes, a negative study, when properly performed, essentially rules out clinically significant pulmonary emboli (Cheely, et al., 1981; Novelline, et al., 1978). The specificity is believed to be high (i.e., if an abrupt arterial cutoff or a definite filling defect is seen, the clinician can be virtually sure that a pulmonary embolism is present) (Goodman, 1984).

In regard to the timing of pulmonary angiography in patients with possible pulmonary embolism, statements suggesting that it must be performed within 48 hours of the suspected episode are unfounded. In fact available data suggest that emboli should remain present and detectable for 1 week after embolization occurs (Dalen, et al., 1969).

Bronchial Arteriography

Bronchial arteriography is frequently performed for the diagnosis of severe hemoptysis (Johnsrude, et al., 1987; Remy-Jardin and Remy, 1991). The procedure involves selective

placement of a catheter into a bronchial artery followed by the injection of contrast material (Fig. 18-34).

When performing bronchial arteriography, it must be kept in mind that an intercostal, or some other nonbronchial, arterial source may be contributing to the hemoptysis, especially when the patient has associated pleural inflammatory disease. If the bleeding is found to be the result of a bronchial arterial cause, then it can often be controlled by therapeutic embolization, using one of a number of different materials, including

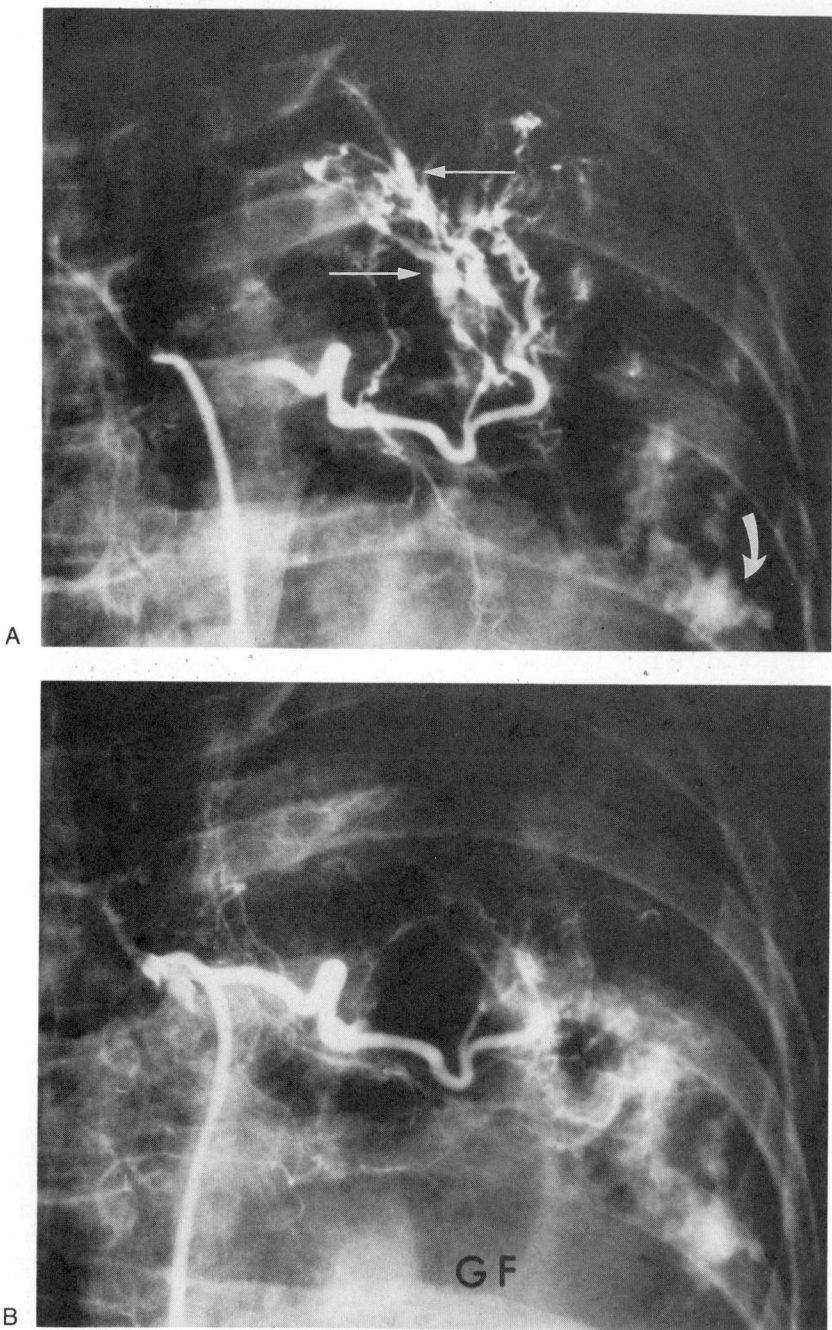

Figure 18-34. (A) Bronchial arteriogram in a patient with previous tuberculosis and recurrent hemoptysis. Arteriography reveals multiple dilated abnormal vessels (*straight arrows*). (B) Following the injection of absorbable gelatin sponge, there is no flow to these abnormal vessels. The calcific density (curved arrow in A) is related to the previous tuberculous infection. (Courtesy of Dr. K. Sniderman, The Toronto Hospital, Toronto, Canada.)

polyvinyl alcohol (Ivalon) microparticles or absorbable gelatin sponge (Gelfoam) (Fig. 18-34B). The main problem that must be avoided is inadvertent obstruction of the anterior spinal artery, which may lead to transverse myelitis.

Aortography

Although aortography has many uses in the investigation of various pathologic processes involving the aorta, the main indication in the context of this chapter is for the diagnosis of bronchopulmonary sequestration (Fig. 18-35). In this in-

stance, a catheter is first placed within the lower thoracic aorta, and contrast is injected. The finding of an anomalous vessel (or vessels) feeding an abnormal portion of the lung is diagnostic of sequestration. The clinician must not confuse this anomalous vessel with a hypertrophied inferior phrenic or intercostal artery, which may be feeding a noncongenital chronic inflammatory pulmonary process. In addition, it must be kept in mind that the finding of an anomalous vessel alone is not diagnostic of sequestration; systemic supply to a normal portion of lung is a well-described phenomenon.

The aortic injection may be followed by selective catheter-

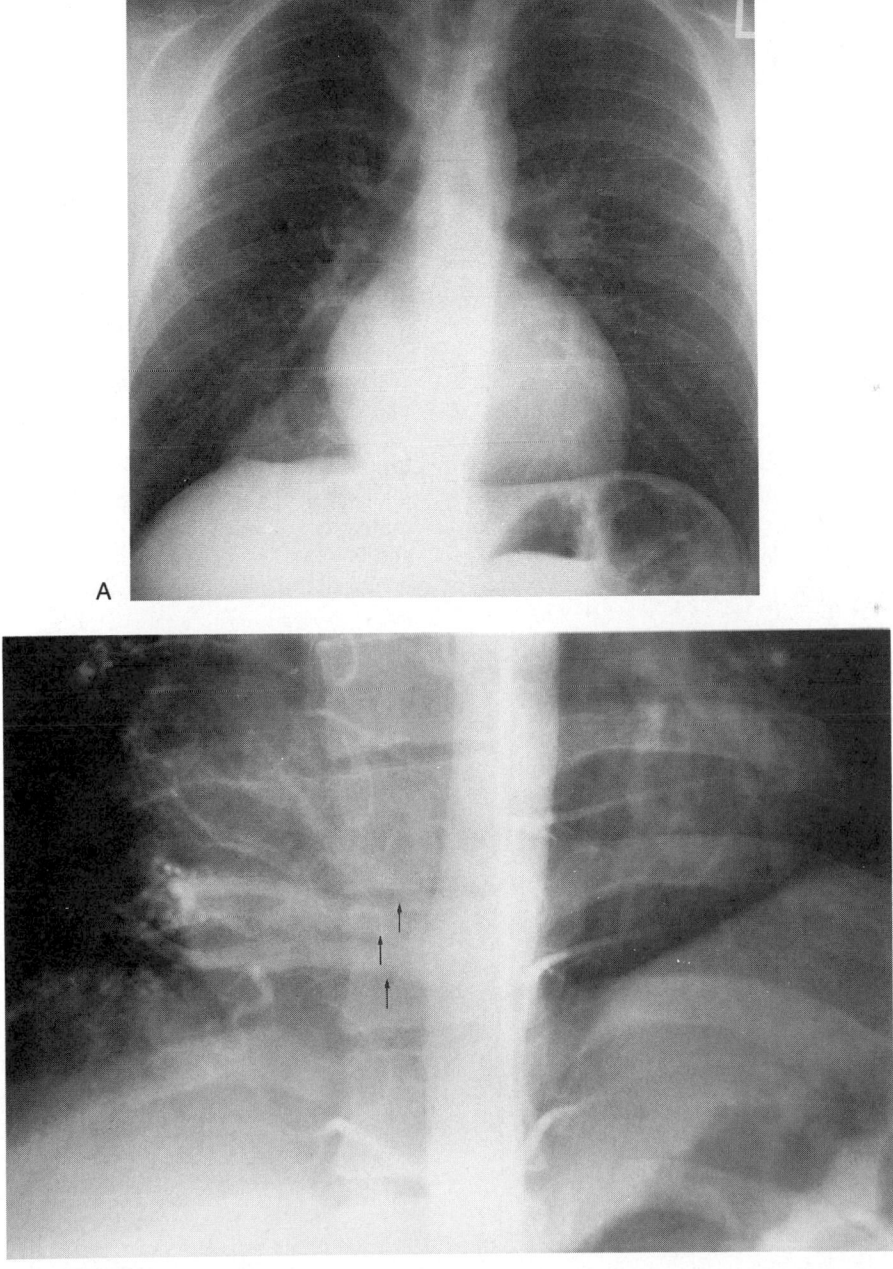

Figure 18-35. Bronchopulmonary sequestration. **(A)** PA chest radiograph. This 27-year-old man had a history of recurrent fever, chills, and dry cough. The radiograph reveals an ill-defined mass in the medial aspect of the right lower lobe. **(B)** Aortogram reveals three anomalous vessels (*arrows*) feeding this bronchopulmonary sequestration.

ization of the anomalous vessel. In this way, both the number of anomalous vessels (by the aortogram) and their venous drainage (by the selective studies) can be determined. Intralobar sequestrations generally have pulmonary venous drainage; extralobar ones usually have systemic drainage, most often into the inferior vena cava or hepatic veins.

BRONCHOGRAPHY

During the past decade, the indications for bronchography have diminished to the point where this procedure is now rarely performed in most imaging departments. The procedure consists of the application of topical anesthesia into the oro- and hypopharynx, larynx, and the airways to be examined, followed by the instillation of contrast material by a directable rubber catheter into the appropriate bronchi. Exquisite visualization of these airways is generally achieved (Figs. 18-25B and 18-36). Although somewhat unpleasant for the patient, most are able to cooperate adequately and tolerate the procedure well. The majority of the instilled contrast is expectorated during the first 15 minutes following the procedure and almost all of it, by 24 hours. In our experience, the test causes few side effects, the main one being mild chemical pneumonitis, which may occur if too much contrast flows too peripherally within one region of the lung. However, it can cause allergic reactions, pulmonary collapse, and a foreign-body reaction (Light and Oster, 1966; Fraser, et al., 1988).

The main indication for the procedure has been the investigation of patients with suspected or known bronchiectasis. It now appears this disease can be assessed as accurately by high-resolution CT, which is completely noninvasive. At the present time, therefore, there is no definite indication for bronchography.

TRANSTHORACIC NEEDLE BIOPSY

Although transthoracic needle lung biopsy was first performed more than 100 years ago, the technique did not achieve widespread popularity until the 1960s, when Nordenstrom (1966) introduced thin needles (18 to 20 gauge) along with biplanar fluoroscopic guidance and improved cytologic methods (Fig. 18-37). Although cytologic examination continues to be the principle pathologic method of assessment, newer needles may now acquire tissue fragments large enough for histologic examination (Westcott, 1980). In addition, although fluoroscopic guidance is used in most instances, CT guidance allows the clinician to assess more difficult pulmonary lesions (vanSonnenberg, et al., 1988). Also, it is now possible to obtain diagnostic material from hilar, mediastinal, and pleural lesions by using either fluoroscopic, CT, or even ultrasound guidance (Weisbrod, 1987; Westcott, 1987; Wernecke, et al., 1989).

Transthoracic needle biopsy is indicated for the diagnosis of many intrathoracic pathologic processes, including pulmonary nodules and masses; pleural, rib, hilar, or mediastinal masses; or undiagnosed pulmonary infiltrates, especially when neoplasia or infection are considered possible (Weisbrod, 1990; Westcott, 1988; Perlmutt, et al., 1989).

Some have questioned the value of transthoracic needle biopsy on the grounds that the patient will need to undergo thoractomy whether malignancy is found or not. However, many surgeons use transthoracic needle biopsy in such cases for a number of reasons. Knowing that a patient has definite bronchogenic carcinoma prior to thoracotomy allows better planning of operating room time, reduces the need for intraoperative quick sections of the nodule, and allows the patient and family to be better informed of what to expect from the operation. In addition, transthoracic needle biopsy can make

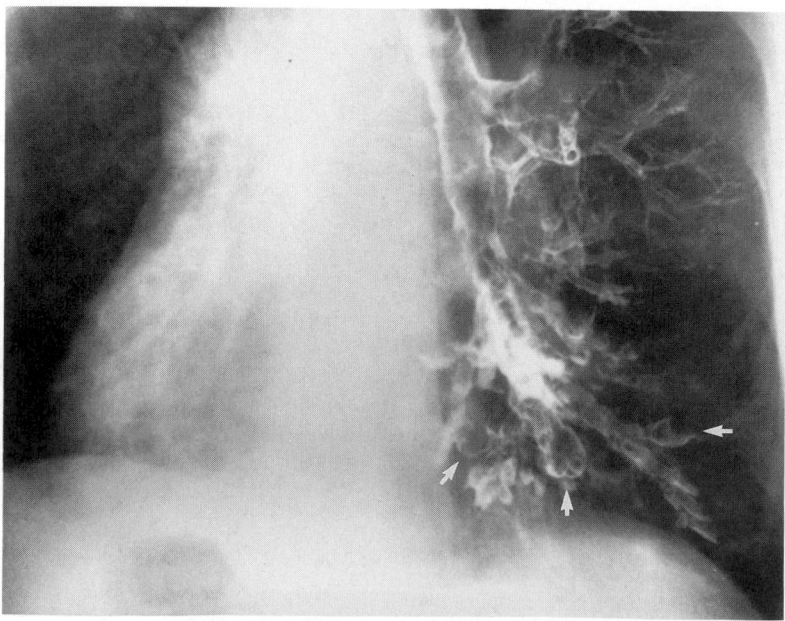

Figure 18-36. Left bronchogram reveals cystic bronchiectasis (*arrows*) in the left lower lobe of this 51-year-old man with Kartagener's syndrome.

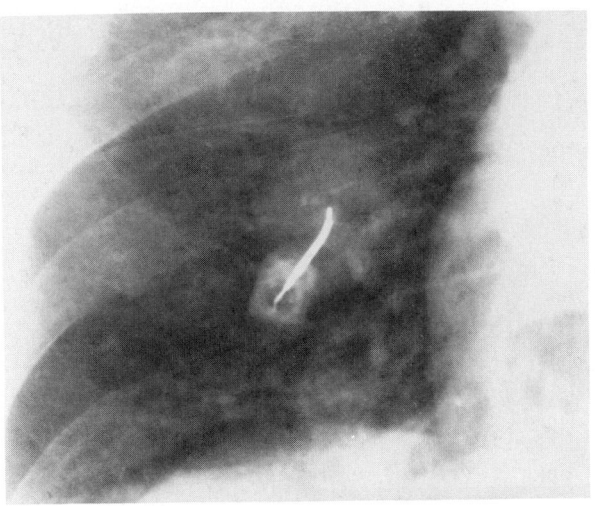 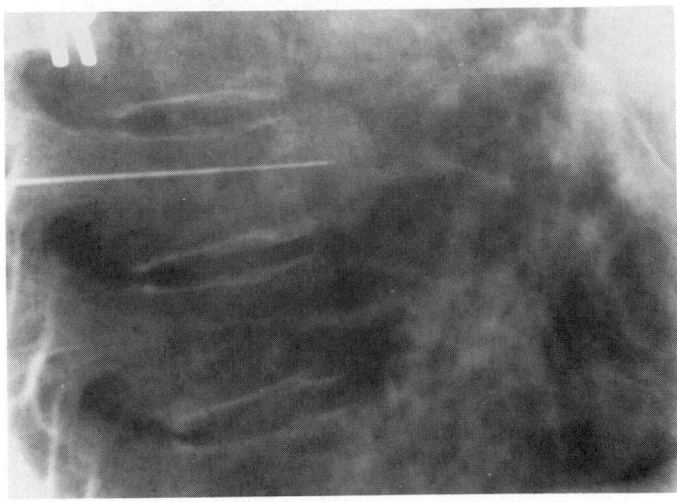

Figure 18-37. Transthoracic needle biopsy. **(A)** Frontal and **(B)** lateral views reveal the tip of the needle within the central portion of the pulmonary nodule, an optimal position for sampling a lesion such as this.

a definite benign diagnosis on occasion or may find small cell carcinoma (which can be reliably diagnosed), both of which may obviate thoracotomy. Furthermore, it has been shown that transthoracic needle biopsy can shorten both the time from admission to diagnosis and the length of hospital stay and reduce the number of thoracotomies and hospitalization costs (Gobien, et al., 1983).

Transthoracic needle biopsy can be safely performed on outpatients (Stevens and Jackman, 1984). In these instances, it is prudent to restrict the procedure to those 70 years of age or younger who do not have significant cardiopulmonary compromise. In addition to the usual follow-up procedures, these patients must be accompanied by a responsible adult for the next 24 hours and remain near a medical facility during this period.

Absolute contraindications to the procedure include patients with uncorrected bleeding disorders, uncooperative patients, including those with intractable coughing, and patients with suspected hydatid cysts. Relative contraindications include severe emphysema and significant pulmonary arterial hypertension.

Patients undergoing transthoracic needle biopsy do not require premedication. After obtaining informed consent, the patient is placed on the fluoroscopic table, and the opacity to be sampled is localized. The skin is washed with antiseptic solution, and a local anesthetic is instilled, with particular attention to the skin and subpleural regions. An attempt is made to avoid pleural transgression with the local anesthetic needle. The biopsy needle is then slowly advanced into the lesion, using frequent fluoroscopic assessment of its course. We currently use a coaxial needle (Greene Needle Biopsy Set, Cook Catheter Corp., Bloomington, IN), that is, an outer 19-gauge needle is placed close to the lesion, and a 22-gauge needle is passed into it. This allows the on-site cytopathologic technician to check for specimen adequacy before the outer needle is withdrawn. Multiple passes can therefore be made with a single pleural transgression.

Following the procedure, patients are closely watched for

the development of a pneumothorax by performing vital signs every 15 minutes for 1 hour and then every 30 minutes until the first chest radiograph. This is obtained routinely at 4 hours with inpatients and at 2 hours with outpatients. In a series of 2,421 transthoracic needle biopsies at our institution, pneumothorax occurred in 34.1 percent, and chest tubes were required in 7.8 percent of the biopsies (Weisbrod, 1990). If a chest tube is required, it generally becomes apparent within the first hour following the procedure, often within the first few minutes (Perlmutt, et al., 1986).

Hemoptysis occasionally occurs following the procedure, also almost always within the first few minutes, and is usually self-limited. However, fatalities caused by massive hemorrhage were reported (Berquist, et al., 1980); in these cases, bronchial blockers must be placed immediately. Other less common complications include air embolism (Tolly, et al., 1988) and hemopericardium (Kucharczyk, et al., 1982). The theoretical possibility of spread of the tumor along the needle track is extremely unlikely with the use of small-gauge needles; it is limited to case reports (Muller, et al., 1986).

The sensitivity of transthoracic needle biopsy in diagnosing malignancy has been reported to range from 64 to 97 percent (Weisbrod, 1990). The correlation between the cytologic and final histologic diagnosis of cell type has been good. For example, in the series from our hospital, 80 percent of the transthoracic needle biopsies diagnosed as squamous cell carcinoma turned out to have this cell type on tissue section (Weisbrod, 1990). Similar results were found with both adenocarcinoma and small cell carcinoma. The positive predictive value for small cell carcinoma rose to 93.9 percent if those cases that were called ''suggestive of'' (as opposed to ''diagnostic of'' or ''definite'') small cell carcinomas were excluded (Weisbrod, 1990).

Transthoracic needle biopsy has been shown to be of significant value in the diagnosis of pulmonary infections, with clinically useful information being found in 81 percent of those with suspected infection and with a specific organism being found in 76 percent of those in whom infection was ultimately diagnosed (Conces, et al., 1989). However, because fiberoptic bronchoscopy has a very high diagnostic yield and a lower chance of causing pneumothorax, transthoracic needle biopsy should probably be used only in those patients in whom bronchoscopic results are negative.

Besides infection, other specific benign diagnoses that can be identified include hamartoma and pulmonary infarction (Westcott, 1988). When a proved benign condition is ultimately shown to be present, transthoracic needle biopsy makes a specific diagnosis in 11.7 to 68 percent of instances (Perlmutt, et al., 1989). In the absence of a specific benign diagnosis, the procedure should be repeated at least once. The reliability of a nonmalignant result depends to a large degree on the radiologist performing the biopsy and the cytopathologist interpreting the specimen. In our institution, there were only 5 instances of more than 1,000 malignancies in which surgery was delayed because of a false-negative transthoracic needle biopsy result. However, if the clinician still suspects malignancy after a negative biopsy result (e.g., lesion is new or enlarging or has spiculated margins), then an open biopsy should be performed. If the clinician is less suspicious, then regular follow-up chest radiographs must still be performed to be certain that the lesion is stable or becoming smaller. In one study (Calhoun, et al., 1986) of 116 patients with nonmalignant nonspecific benign diagnoses after transthoracic needle biopsy, 33 percent were subsequently found to have a malignant process.

In addition to pulmonary lesions, transthoracic needle biopsy has been shown to be useful in the diagnosis of hilar and mediastinal masses (Weisbrod, et al., 1984; Westcott, 1981). It is safe in these regions, with pneumothorax and chest tube insertion rates of 19.2 and 4.8 percent, respectively (Weisbrod, 1987). Because the pleura is frequently not transgressed in many of these instances, these rates are actually lower than those found with pulmonary biopsies. When these biopsies are interpreted cytologically, immunohistochemical analysis is of the utmost importance, especially in distinguishing lymphoma from thymoma (Herman, et al., 1991a). Although the accuracy is high in the diagnosis of metastatic disease and germ cell tumors, it is lower with thymoma, lymphoma, and neurogenic tumors (Weisbrod, 1987; Herman, et al., 1991a).

ACKNOWLEDGMENT

I wish to thank Rose Baldwin for her assistance with the preparation of this manuscript.

COMMENTS AND CONTROVERSIES

Because of the importance of imaging in the practice of thoracic surgery, this expanded chapter has been provided. As editors, it is our belief that thoracic surgeons must be as accomplished as radiologists in interpreting chest radiographs and CT and MRI scans. The importance of a continuing dialogue between surgeons and radiologists cannot be overemphasized. This is best accomplished by personal review of the radiographic films with the radiologist rather than by depending on reading their reports. The value of the thoracic surgeon attending weekly pathologic-radiologic conferences to maintain these skills cannot be overemphasized.

There is no doubt that the field of imaging has accelerated faster than any other clinically applied area of medicine. In the future, we can look forward to further advances in imaging spectroscopy, computerized three-dimensional imaging, further refinements in invasive imaging, and computerized transmission of imaging materials.

This chapter, written by a radiologist specializing in the field of thoracic imaging, provides a basis for understanding the expanding field of pulmonary imaging. However, the thoracic surgical trainee or practitioner is well advised to read thoroughly the four textbooks identified by the author in the annotated references. Unfortunately, not all thoracic surgeons have the advantage of an expert chest radiographer in their own institutions. Therefore, the surgeon must be as well versed in the imaging of the thorax as are general radiologists.

R.J.G.

KEY REFERENCES

Felson B: Chest Roentgenology. WB Saunders, Philadelphia, 1973

This book is a classic and is mandatory reading for any serious student of chest radiology. Although lacking in some up-to-date details of specific thoracic diseases, it contains a wealth of information regarding plain film image interpretation, both of the lung and nonpulmonary thoracic structures.

Fraser RG, Pare JAP, Pare PD et al: Diagnosis of Diseases of the Chest. 3rd Ed. Vols. 1–4. WB Saunders, Philadelphia, 1988–1991

This four-volume set is encyclopedic in scope and contains the answer to virtually any question that could be asked dealing with chest disease, whether it be regarding the cause, epidemiology, pathologic conditions, clinical manifestations, or pulmonary function, in addition to imaging. Therapeutics are not covered. In addition to this information, it contains tables of differential diagnoses based on radiographic patterns and more than 20,000 references dealing with thoracic diseases.

Heitzman ER: The Lung: Radiologic-Pathologic Correlations. 2nd Ed. CV Mosby, St. Louis, 1984

This book provides an explanation of all major radiographic signs of disease by demonstrating their genesis based on pathologic correlations, both gross and microscopic. By reading the book, the clinician gains a thorough understanding of the pathologic and radiologic signs of pulmonary diseases; it is mandatory reading for radiology residents.

Naidich DP, Zerhouni EA, Siegelman SS: Computed Tomography and Magnetic Resonance Imaging of the Thorax. 2nd Ed. Raven Press, New York, 1991.

This is a superb book that thoroughly covers what its title suggests. Aside from a discussion of the imaging findings in all important thoracic diseases, it provides this information in a practical manner so that it is useful in day-to-day practice.

REFERENCES

Aberle DR, Gamsu G, Ray CS, Feuerstein IM: Asbestos-related pleural and parenchymal fibrosis: detection with high-resolution CT. Radiology 166:729, 1988

Alazraki NP, Ramsdell JW, Taylor A et al.: Reliability of gallium scan chest radiography compared to mediastinoscopy for evaluating mediastinal spread in lung cancer. Am Rev Respir Dis 117:415, 1978

Aronchick JM: CT of mediastinal lymph nodes in patients with non-small cell lung carcinoma. Radiol Clin North Am 28:573, 1990

Baber CE, Hedlung LW, Oddson TA, Putman CE: Differentiating empyemas and peripheral pulmonary abscesses. Radiology 135:755, 1980

Baron RL, Levitt RG, Sagel SS: Computed tomography in the preoperative evaluation of bronchogenic carcinoma. Radiology 145:727, 1982

Bergin CJ, Pauly JM, Macovski A: Lung parenchyma: projection reconstruction MR imaging. Radiology 179:777, 1991

Berquist TH, Bailey PB, Cortese DA, Miller WE: Transthoracic needle biopsy accuracy and complications in relation to location and type of lesion. Mayo Clin Proc 55:475, 1980

Bourgouin P, Cousineau G, Lemire P et al.: Differentiation of radiation-induced fibrosis from recurrent pulmonary neoplasm by CT. J Can Assoc Radiol 38:23, 1987

Brauner MW, Grenier P, Mompoint D et al.: Pulmonary sarcoidosis: evaluation with high-resolution CT. Radiology 172:467, 1989

Calhoun P, Feldman PS, Armstrong P et al.: The clinical outcome of needle aspirations of the lung when cancer is not diagnosed. Ann Thorac Surg 41:592, 1986

Cheely R, McCartney WH, Perry JR et al.: The role of noninvasive tests versus pulmonary angiography in the diagnosis of pulmonary embolism. Am J Med 70:17, 1981

Cirimelli KM, Colletti PM, Beck S: Metastatic choriocarcinoma simulating an arteriovenous malformation on chest radiography and dynamic CT. J Comput Assist Tomogr 12:317, 1988

Conces DJ Jr, Clark SA, Tarver RD, Schwenk GR: Transthoracic aspiration needle biopsy: small value in the diagnosis of pulmonary infections. AJR 152:31, 1989

Cooke JC, Currie DC, Morgan AD et al.: Role of computed tomography in diagnosis of bronchiectasis. Thorax 42:272, 1987

Dalen JE, Banas JS Jr, Brooks HL et al.: Resolution rate of acute pulmonary embolism in man. N Engl J Med 280:1194, 1969

Dales RE, Stark RM, Raman S: Computed tomography to stage lung cancer. Approaching a controversy using meta-analysis. Am Rev Respir Dis 141:1096, 1990

Davis SD: CT evaluation for pulmonary metastases in patients with extrathoracic malignancy. Radiology 180:1, 1991

Davis SD, Zirn JR, Govoni AF, Yankelevitz DF: Peripheral carcinoid tumor of the lung: CT diagnosis. AJR 155:1185, 1990

de Geer G, Gamsu G, Cann C, Webb WR: Evaluation of a chest phantom for CT nodule densitometry. AJR 147:21, 1986

Doyle TC, Lawler GA: CT features of rounded atelectasis of the lung. AJR 143:225, 1984

Eisenberg RL: Radiology: An Illustrated History. Mosby-Year Book, St. Louis, 1991

Felson B: Chest Roentgenology. WB Saunders, Philadelphia, 1973

Fleischner FG: The visible bronchial tree: a roentgen sign in pneumonic and other pulmonary consolidations. Radiology 50:184, 1948

Fosburg RG, Hopkins GB, Kan MK: Evaluation of the mediastinum by gallium-67 scintigraphy in lung cancer. J Thorac Cardiovasc Surg 77:76, 1979

Fraser RG, Pare JAP, Pare PD et al.: Diagnosis of Diseases of the Chest. 3rd Ed. Vol. 1. WB Saunders, Philadelphia, 1988

Freedman P: Editorial. Radiology 182:307, 1992

Freedman PJ, Feigin DS, Liston SE et al.: Sensitivity of chest radiography, computed tomography, and gallium scanning to metastasis of lung carcinoma. Cancer 54:1300, 1984

Front D, Ben-Haim S, Isreal O et al.: Lymphoma: predictive value of Ga-67 scintigraphy after treatment. Radiology 182:359, 1992

Front D, Israel O, Epelbaum R et al.: Ga-67 SPECT before and after treatment of lymphoma. Radiology 175:515, 1990

Gaeta M, Pandolfo I, Volta S: Bronchus sign on CT in peripheral carcinoma of the lung: value in predicting results of transbronchial biopsy. AJR 157:1181, 1991

Gamsu G, Sostman D: Magnetic resonance imaging of the thorax. Am Rev Respir Dis 139:254, 1989

Gefter WB, Hatabu H, Dinsmore BJ et al.: Pulmonary vascular cine MR imaging: a noninvasive approach to dynamic imaging of the pulmonary circulation. Radiology 176:761, 1990

Genereux GP: The Fleischner Lecture: computed tomography of diffuse pulmonary disease. J Thorac Imaging 4:50, 1989

Genereux GP, Howie JL: Normal mediastinal lymph node size and number: CT and anatomic study. AJR 142:1095, 1984

Ginsberg RJ, Hill LD, Eagan RT et al.: Modern 30 day operative mortality for surgical resections in lung cancer. J Thorac Cardiovasc Surg 86:654, 1983

Glazer HS, Anderson DJ, Sagel SS: Bronchial impaction in lobar collapse: CT demonstration and pathologic correlation. AJR 153:485, 1989a

Glazer HS, Aronberg DJ, Sagel SS, Emami B: Utility of CT in detecting postpneumonectomy carcinoma recurrence. AJR 142:487, 1984a

Glazer HS, Duncan-Meyer J, Aronberg DJ et al.: Pleural and chest wall invasion in bronchogenic carcinoma: CT evaluation. Radiology 157:191, 1985a

Glazer GM, Gross BH, Quint LE et al.: Normal mediastinal lymph nodes: number and size according to American Thoracic Society mapping. AJR 144:261, 1985b

Glazer HS, Kaiser LR, Anderson DJ et al.: Indeterminate mediastinal invasion in bronchogenic carcinoma: CT evaluation. Radiology 173:37, 1989b

Glazer HS, Lee JK, Levitt RG et al.: Radiation fibrosis: differentiation from recurrent tumor by MR imaging. Radiology 156:721, 1985c

Glazer HS, Levitt RG, Lee JKT et al.: Differentiation of radiation fibrosis from recurrent pulmonary neoplasm by magnetic resonance imaging. AJR 143:729, 1984b

Glazer GM, Orringer MB, Chenevert TL et al.: Mediastinal lymph nodes: relaxation time/pathologic correlation and implications in staging of lung cancer with MR imaging. Radiology 168:429, 1988

Gobien RP, Bouchard EA, Gobien BS et al.: Thin needle aspiration biopsy of thoracic lesions: impact on hospital charges and patterns of patient care. Radiology 148:65, 1983

Godwin JD, Speckman JM, Fram EK et al.: Distinguishing benign from malignant pulmonary nodules by computed tomography. Radiology 144:349, 1982

Golden R: The effect of bronchostenosis upon the roentgen-ray shadows in carcinoma of the bronchus. AJR 13:21, 1925

Goodman PC: Pulmonary angiography. Clin Chest Med 5:465, 1984

Grenier P, Maurice F, Musset D et al.: Bronchiectasis: assessment by thin-section CT. Radiology 161:95, 1986

Grenier P, Valeyre D, Cluzel P et al.: Chronic diffuse interstitial lung disease: diagnostic value of chest radiography and high-resolution CT. Radiology 179:123, 1991

Gross BH, Glazer GM, Bookstein FL: Multiple pulmonary nodules detected by computed tomography: diagnostic implications. J Comput Assist Tomogr 9:880, 1985

Gross BH, Glazer GM, Orringer MB et al.: Bronchogenic carcinoma metastatic to normal-sized lymph nodes: frequency and significance. Radiology 166:71, 1988

Haggar AM, Pearlberg JL, Froelich JW et al.: Chest-wall invasion by carcinoma of the lung: detection by MR imaging. AJR 148:1075, 1987

Halbsguth A, Schulze W, Ungeheur E, Hoer PW: Pitfall in the CT diagnosis of pulmonary arteriovenous malformation. J Comput Assist Tomogr 7:710, 1983

Heaston DK, Putman CE, Rodan BA et al.: Solitary pulmonary metastases in high-risk melanoma patients: a prospective comparison of conventional and computed tomography. AJR 141:169, 1983

Heelan RT, Demas BE, Caravelli JF et al.: Superior sulcus tumors: CT and MR imaging. Radiology 170:637, 1989

Herman SJ, Holub RV, Weisbrod GL, Chamberlain DW: Anterior mediastinal masses: utility of transthoracic needle biopsy. Radiology 180:167, 1991a

Herman SJ, Winton T, Weisbrod GL et al.: Mediastinal invasion by bronchogenic carcinoma: CT signs. Radiology 190:841, 1994

Herold CJ, Kuhlman JE, Zerhouni EA: Pulmonary atelectasis: signal patterns with MR imaging. Radiology 178:715, 1991

Hidalgo H, Korobkin M, Kinney TR et al.: The problem of benign pulmonary nodules in children receiving cytotoxic chemotherapy. AJR 140:21, 1983

Hull RD, Hirsh J, Carter CJ et al.: Diagnostic value of ventilation-perfusion lung scanning in patients with suspected pulmonary embolism. Chest 88:819, 1985

Hull RD, Raskob GE, Coates G et al.: A new noninvasive management strategy for patients with suspected pulmonary embolism. Arch Intern Med 149:2549, 1989

Huston J III, Muhm JR: Solitary pulmonary opacities: plain tomography. Radiology 163:481, 1987

Huston J III, Muhm JR: Solitary pulmonary nodules: evaluation with a CT reference phantom. Radiology 170:653, 1989

Im JG, Gamsu G, Gordon D et al.: CT densitometry of pulmonary nodules in a frozen human thorax. AJR 150:61, 1988

Joharjy IA, Bashi SA, Adbullah AK: Value of medium-thickness CT in the diagnosis of bronchiectasis. AJR 149:1133, 1987

Johnsrude IS, Jackson DC, Dunnick NR: A Practical Approach to Angiography, 2nd Ed. Little, Brown, Boston, 1987

Jones FA, Wiedemann HP, O'Donovan PB, Stoller JK: Computerized tomographic densitometry of the solitary pulmonary nodule using a nodule phantom. Chest 96:779, 1989

Juni JE, Alavi A: Lung scanning in the diagnosis of pulmonary embolism: the emperor redressed. Semin Nucl Med 21:281, 1991

Kameda K, Adachi S, Kono M: Detection of T-factor in lung cancer using magnetic resonance imaging and computed tomography. J Thorac Imaging 3:73, 1988

Khan A, Herman PG, Vorwerk P et al.: Solitary pulmonary nodules: comparison of classification with standard, thin-section, and reference phantom CT. Radiology 179:477, 1991

Khouri NF, Meziane MA, Zerhouni EA et al.: The solitary pulmonary nodule: assessment, diagnosis, management. Chest 91:128, 1987

Kiyono K, Sone S, Sakai F et al.: The number and size of normal mediastinal lymph nodes: a postmortem study. AJR 150:771, 1988

Klein J, Gamsu G: High resolution computed tomography of diffuse lung disease. Invest Radiol 24:805, 1989

Kucharczyk W, Weisbrod GL, Cooper JD et al.: Cardiac tamponade as a complication of thin needle aspiration lung biopsy. Chest 82:120, 1982

Lee JKT, Glazer HS: Controversy in the MR imaging appearance of fibrosis. Radiology 177:21, 1990

Libshitz HI: Computed tomography in bronchogenic carcinoma. Semin Roentgenol 25:64, 1990

Light JP, Oster WF: Clinical and pathological reactions to the bronchographic agent Dionosil aqueous. AJR 98:468, 1966

Mahoney MC, Shipley RT, Corcoran HL, Dickson BA: CT demonstration of calcification in carcinoma of the lung. AJR 154:255, 1990

Martini N, Heelan R, Westcott J et al.: Comparative merits of conventional, computed tomographic, and magnetic resonance imaging in assessing mediastinal involvement in surgically confirmed lung carcinoma. J Thorac Cardiovasc Surg 90:639, 1985

Mathieson JR, Mayo JR, Staples CA, Muller NL: Chronic diffuse infiltrative lung disease: comparison of diagnostic accuracy of CT and chest radiography. Radiology 171:111, 1989

Mayr B, Ingrisch H, Haussinger K et al.: Tumors of the bronchi: role of evaluation with CT. Radiology 172:647, 1989

McHugh K, Blaquiere RM: CT features of rounded atelectasis. AJR 153:257, 1989

McKenna RJ Jr, Haynie TP, Libshitz HI et al.: Critical evaluation of the gallium-67 scan for surgical patients with lung cancer. Chest 87:428, 1985a

McKenna RJ Jr, Libshitz HI, Mountain CT: Roentgenographic evaluation of mediastinal nodes for preoperative assessment in lung cancer. Chest 88:206, 1985b

McLoud TC, Bourgouin PM, Greenberg RW et al.: Bronchogenic carcinoma: analysis of staging in the mediastinum with CT by correlative lymph node mapping and sampling. Radiology 182:319, 1992

Metter FA, Guiberteau MJ: Essentials of Nuclear Medicine Imaging. 3rd Ed. WB Saunders, Philadelphia, 1991

Miller RR, Nelems B, Muller NL et al.: Lingular and right middle lobe biopsy in the assessment of diffuse lung disease. Ann Thorac Surg 44:269, 1987

Mills SR, Jackson DC, Older RA et al.: The incidence, etiologies, and avoidance of complications of pulmonary angiography in a large series. Radiology 136:295, 1980

Milne ENC, Zerhouni EA: Blood supply of pulmonary metastases. J Thorac Imaging 2:15, 1987

Muller NL: Clinical value of high-resolution CT in chronic diffuse lung disease. AJR 157:1163, 1991

Muller NL, Bergin CJ, Miller RR, Ostrow DN: Seeding of malignant cells into the needle track after lung and pleural biopsy. J Can Assoc Radiol 37:192, 1986

Muller NL, Bergin CJ, Ostrow DN, Nichols DM: Role of computed tomography in the recognition of bronchiectasis. AJR 143:971, 1984

Muller NL, Miller RR: Computed tomography of chronic diffuse infiltrative lung disease. Part 1. Am Rev Respir Dis 142:1206, 1990a

Muller NL, Miller RR: Computed tomography of chronic diffuse infiltrative lung disease. Part 2. Am Rev Respir Dis 142:1440, 1990b

Muller NL, Staples CA, Miller RR et al.: Disease activity in idiopathic pulmonary fibrosis: CT and pathologic correlation. Radiology 165:731, 1987

Munro NC, Cooke JC, Currie DC et al.: Comparison of thin section computed tomography with bronchography for identifying bronchiectatic segments in patients with chronic sputum production. Thorax 45:135, 1990

Musset D, Grenier P, Carette MF et al.: Primary lung cancer staging: prospective comparative study of MR imaging with CT. Radiology 160:607, 1986

Naidich DP, Funt S, Ettenger NA, Arranda C: Hemoptysis: CT-bronchoscopic correlations in 58 cases. Radiology 177:357, 1990

Naidich DP, Lee JJ, Garay SM et al.: Comparison of CT and fiberoptic bronchoscopy in the evaluation of bronchial disease. AJR 148:1, 1987

Naidich DP, McCauley DI, Khouri NF et al.: Computed tomography of lobar collapse: 1 Endobronchial obstruction. J Comput Assist Tomogr 7:745, 1983a

Naidich DP, McCauley DI, Khouri NF et al.: Computed tomography of lobar collapse: 2. Collapse in the absence of endobronchial obstruction. J Comput Assist Tomogr 7:758, 1983b

Naidich DP, Sussman R, Kutcher WL et al.: Solitary pulmonary nodules: CT-bronchoscopic correlation. Chest 93:595, 1988

Naidich DP, Zerhouni EA, Siegelman SS: Computed tomography and magnetic resonance imaging of the thorax. 2nd Ed. Raven Press, New York, 1991

Nathan MH, Collins VP, Adams RA: Differentiation of benign and malignant pulmonary nodules by growth rate. Radiology 79:221, 1962

Newman GE: Pulmonary angiography in pulmonary embolic disease. J Thorac Imaging 4:28, 1989

Nordenstrom B: New technique for transthoracic biopsy of lung changes. Br J Radiol 38:550, 1965

Novelline RA, Baltarowich OH, Athanasoulis CA et al.: The clinical course of patients with suspected pulmonary embolism and a negative pulmonary arteriogram. Radiology 126:561, 1978

Patterson GA, Ginsberg RJ, Poon PY et al.: A prospective evaluation of magnetic resonance imaging, computed tomography, and mediastinoscopy in the preoperative assessment of mediastinal node status in bronchogenic carcinoma. J Thorac Cardiovasc Surg 94:679, 1987

Patterson GA, Ilves R, Ginsberg RJ et al.: The value of adjuvant radiotherapy in pulmonary and chest wall resection for bronchogenic carcinoma. Ann Thorac Surg 34:692, 1982

Pennes DR, Glazer GM, Wimbish KJ et al.: Chest wall invasion by lung cancer: limitations of CT evaluation. AJR 144:507, 1985

Perlmutt LM, Braun SD, Newman GE et al.: Pulmonary arteriography in the high-risk patient. Radiology 162:187, 1987

Perlmutt LM, Braun SD, Newman GE et al.: Timing of chest film follow-up after transthoracic needle aspiration. AJR 146:1049, 1986

Perlmutt LM, Johnston WW, Dunnick NR: Percutaneous transthoracic needle aspiration: a review. AJR 152:451, 1989

Peters JC, Desai KK: CT demonstration of postpneumonectomy tumor recurrence. AJR 141:259, 1983

Peuchot M, Libshitz HI: Pulmonary metastatic disease: radiologic-surgical correlation. Radiology 164:719, 1987

Piehler JM, Pairolero PC, Weiland LH et al.: Bronchogenic carcinoma with chest wall invasion: factors affecting survival following en bloc resection. Ann Thorac Surg 34:684, 1982

Poon PY, Bronskill MJ, Henkelman RM et al.: Mediastinal lymph node metastases from bronchogenic carcinoma: detection with MR imaging and CT. Radiology 162:651, 1987

Posteraro RH, Sostman HD, Spritzer CE, Herfkens RJ: Cine-gradient-refocused MR imaging of central pulmonary emboli. AJR 152:465, 1989

Proto AV, Thomas SR: Body computed tomography. Pulmonary nodules studied by computed tomography. Radiology 156:149, 1985

Proto AV, Tocino I: Radiographic manifestations of lobar collapse. Semin Roentgen 15:117, 1980

Pugatch RD, Faling LJ, Robbins AH, Snider GL: Differentiation of pleural and pulmonary lesions using computed tomography. J Comput Assist Tomogr 2:601, 1978

Putnam JB, Roth JA, Wesley MN et al.: Analysis of prognostic factors in patients undergoing resection of pulmonary metastases from soft tissue sarcomas. J Thorac Cardiovasc Surg 87:260, 1984

Quint LE, Glazer GM, Orringer MB et al.: Mediastinal lymph node detection and sizing at CT and autopsy. AJR 147:469, 1986

Remy-Jardin M, Remy J: Embolization for the treatment of hemoptysis. p. 194. In: Current Practice of Interventional Radiology. BC Decker, Philadelphia, 1991

Ren H, Kuhlman JE, Hruban RH et al.: Computed tomography of inflation-fixed lungs: the beaded septum sign of pulmonary metastasis. J Comput Assist Tomogr 13:411, 1989

Rendina EA, Bognolo DA, Mineo TC et al.: Computed tomography for the evaluation of intrathoracic invasion by lung cancer. J Thorac Cardiovasc Surg 94:57, 1987

Robbins LL, Hale CH: The roentgen appearance of lobar and segmental collapse of the lung: preliminary report. Radiology 44:107, 1945a

Robbins LL, Hale CH: The roentgen appearance of lobar and segmental collapse of the lung. II. The normal chest as it pertains to collapse. Radiology 44:543, 1945b

Robbins LL, Hale CH: The roentgen appearance of lobar and segmental collapse of the lung. III. Collapse of an entire lung or the major part thereof. Radiology 45:23, 1945c

Robbins LL, Hale CH: The roentgen appearance of lobar and segmental collapse of the lung. IV. Collapse of the lower lobes. Radiology 45:120, 1945d

Robbins LL, Hale CH: The roentgen appearance of lobar and segmental collapse of the lung. V. Collapse of the right middle lobe. Radiology 45:260, 1945e

Robbins LL, Hale CH: The roentgen appearance of lobar and segmental collapse of the lung. VI. Collapse of the upper lobes. Radiology 45:347, 1945f

Robbins LL, Hale CH, Merrill OE: The roentgen appearance of lobar and segmental collapse of the lung. I. Technic of examination. Radiology 44:471, 1945

Schaner EG, Chang AE, Doppman JL et al.: Comparison of computed and conventional whole lung tomography in detection pulmonary nodules: a prospective radiologic-pathologic study. AJR 131:51, 1978

Schneider HJ, Felson B, Gonzalez LL: Rounded atelectasis. AJR 134:225, 1980

Scott IR, Muller NL, Miller RR et al.: Resectable stage III lung cancer: CT, surgical and pathologic correlation. Radiology 166:75, 1988

Shah HR, Buckner CB, Purnell GL, Walker CW: Computed tomography and magnetic resonance imaging in the diagnosis of pulmonary thromboembolic disease. J Thorac Imaging 4:58, 1989

Shioya S, Haida M, Ono Y et al.: Lung cancer: differentiation of tumor, necrosis, and atelectasis by means of T1 and T2 values measured in vitro. Radiology 167:105, 1988

Sider L, Horejs D: Frequency of extrathoracic metastases from bronchogenic carcinoma in patients with normal-sized hilar and mediastinal lymph nodes on CT. AJR 151:893, 1988

Siegelman SS, Khouri NF, Leo FP et al.: Solitary pulmonary nodules: CT assessment. Radiology 160:307, 1986a

Siegelman SS, Khouri NF, Scott WW Jr et al.: Pulmonary hamartoma: CT findings. Radiology 160:313, 1986b

Siegelman SS, Zerhouni EA, Leo FP et al.: CT of the solitary pulmonary nodule. AJR 135:1, 1980

Silverman PM, Godwin JD: CT/bronchographic correlations in bronchiectasis. J Comput Assist Tomogr 11:52, 1987

Staples CA, Muller NL, Miller RR et al.: Mediastinal nodes in bronchogenic carcinoma: comparison between CT and mediastinoscopy. Radiology 167:367, 1988

Stark DD, Ferderle MP, Goodman PC et al.: Differentiating lung abscess and empyema: radiography and computed tomography. AJR 141:163, 1983

Stein MG, Mayo J, Muller N et al.: Pulmonary lymphangitic spread of carcinoma: appearance on CT scans. Radiology 162:371, 1987

Stevens GM, Jackman RJ: Outpatient needle biopsy of the lung: its safety and utility. Radiology 151:301, 1984

Strickland B, Strickland NH: The value of high definition, narrow section computed tomography in fibrosing alveolitis. Clin Radiol 39:589, 1988

Swensen SJ, Ehman RL, Brown LR: Magnetic resonance imaging of the thorax. J Thorac Imaging 4:19, 1989

Swensen SJ, Harms GF, Morin RL, Myers JL: CT evaluation of solitary pulmonary nodules: value of 185-H reference phantom. AJR 156:925, 1991

The PIOPED Investigators: Value of the ventilation/perfusion scan in acute pulmonary embolism: results of the Prospective Investigation of Pulmonary Embolism Diagnosis (PIOPED). JAMA 263:2753, 1990

Tobler J, Levitt RG, Glazer HS et al.: Differentiation of proximal bronchogenic carcinoma from postobstructive lobar collapse by magnetic resonance imaging comparison with computed tomography. Invest Radiol 22:538, 1987

Tolly TL, Feldmeier JE, Czarnecki D: Air embolism complicating percutaneous lung biopsy. AJR 150:555, 1988

Tumeh SS, Rosenthal DS, Kaplan WD et al.: Lymphoma: evaluation with Ga-67 SPECT. Radiology 164:111, 1987

Vanel D, Henry-Amar M, Lumbroso J et al.: Pulmonary evaluation of patients with osteosarcoma: roles of standard radiography, tomography, CT, scintigraphy, and tomoscintigraphy. AJR 143:519, 1984

vanSonnenberg E, Casola G, Ho M et al.: Difficult thoracic lesions: CT-guided biopsy experience in 150 cases. Radiology 167:457, 1988

Ward HB, Pliego M, Diefenthal HC, Humphrey EW: The impact of phantom CT scanning on surgery for the solitary pulmonary nodule. Surgery 106:734, 1989

Webb WR: Radiologic evaluation of the solitary pulmonary nodule. AJR 154:701, 1990

Webb WR: Plain radiography and computed tomography in the staging of bronchogenic carcinoma: a practical approach. J Thorac Imaging 2:57, 1987

Webb WR, Gatsonis C, Zerhouni EA et al.: CT and MR imaging in staging non-small cell bronchogenic carcinoma: report of the radiologic diagnostic oncology group. Radiology 178:705, 1991

Webb WR, Jensen BG, Sollitto R et al.: Bronchogenic carcinoma: staging with MR compared with staging with CT and surgery. Radiology 156:117, 1985

Webb WR, Muller NL, Naidich DP: High-resolution CT of the Lung. Raven Press, New York, 1992

Webb WR, Sostman HD: MR imaging of thoracic disease: clinical uses. Radiology 182:621, 1992

Weisbrod GL: Transthoracic percutaneous lung biopsy. Radiol Clin North Am 28:647, 1990

Weisbrod GL: Percutaneous fine-needle aspiration biopsy of the mediastinum. Clin Chest Med 8:27, 1987

Weisbrod GL, Lyons DJ, Tao LC, Chamberlain DW: Percutaneous fine-needle aspiration biopsy of mediastinal lesions. AJR 143:525, 1984

Wellner LJ, Putnam CE: Imaging of occult pulmonary metastases: state of the art. CA Cancer J Clin 36:48, 1986

Wernecke K, Vassallo P, Peters PE, von Bassewitz DB: Mediastinal tumors: biopsy under US guidance. Radiology 172:473, 1989

Westcott JL: Percutaneous transthoracic needle biopsy. Radiology 169:593, 1988

Westcott JL: Transthoracic needle biopsy of the hilum and mediastinum. J Thorac Imaging 2:41, 1987

Westcott JL: Percutaneous needle aspiration of hilar and mediastinal masses. Radiology 141:323, 1981

Westcott JL: Direct percutaneous needle aspiration of localized pulmonary lesions: results in 422 patients. Radiology 137:31, 1980

Westcott JL, Cole C: Plate atelectasis. Radiology 155:1, 1985

Whittlesey D: Prospective computed tomographic scanning in the staging of bronchogenic cancer. J Thorac Cardiovasc Surg 95:876, 1988

Woodring JH: Determining the cause of pulmonary atelectasis: a comparison of plain radiography and CT. AJR 150:757, 1988

Woodring JH, Fried AM: Significance of wall thickness in solitary cavities of the lung: a follow-up study. AJR 140:473, 1983

Woodring JH, Fried AM, Chuang VP: Solitary cavities of the lung: diagnostic implications of cavity wall thickness. AJR 135:1269, 1980

Wursten HU, Vock P: Mediastinal infiltration of lung carcinoma (T4N0-1): the positive predictive value of computed tomography. Thorac Cardiovasc Surg 35:355, 1987

Zerhouni EA, Boukadoum M, Siddiky MA et al.: A standard phantom for quantitative analysis of pulmonary nodules by computed tomography. Radiology 149:767, 1983

Zerhouni EA, Spivey JF, Morgan RH et al.: Factors influencing quantitative CT measurements of solitary pulmonary nodules. J Comput Assist Tomogr 6:1075, 1982

Zerhouni EA, Stitik FP, Siegelman SS et al.: CT of the pulmonary nodule: a cooperative study. Radiology 160:319, 1986

Ziskind MM, Weill H, Rayzant AR: The recognition and significance of acinus-filling processes of the lung. Am Rev Respir Dis 87:551, 1963

Zwirewich CV, Muller NL, Lam SCT: Photodynamic laser therapy to alleviate complete bronchial obstruction: comparison of CT and bronchoscopy to predict outcome. AJR 151:897, 1988

19

CONGENITAL ANOMALIES

Michael P. La Quaglia

Congenital anomalies of the lung represent a spectrum of closely related abnormalities that arise during an early stage of embryonic foregut maturation. Therefore, they have been referred to as lung bud anomalies or congenital bronchopulmonary foregut abnormalities. They may present during the early neonatal period with acute symptoms of increased intrathoracic pressure or rarely with congestive heart failure. Less severe problems can be associated with milder forms of these developmental abnormalities, which result in partial obstruction of secondary bronchi. They may be asymptomatic until later in childhood or early adulthood when they appear as radiopaque areas within normal pulmonary tissue. At this point symptoms and signs of recurrent pulmonary infection and eventually localized bronchiectasis may be evident. These congenital bronchopulmonary anomalies include congenital lobar emphysema, bronchogenic cyst, cystic adenomatoid malformation, and pulmonary sequestration. Because the development of the pulmonary circulation is an intimate component of lung development, I have also chosen to discuss pulmonary arteriovenous malformations in this context.

HISTORICAL NOTE

Congenital lobar emphysema was described by Nelson (1932) in 1932, and the pathologic features, in particular the deficiency of bronchial cartilage, were defined by Overstreet (1939) in 1939. Gross and Lewis (1945) performed a successful lobectomy for this condition in 1945, and the term *congenital lobar emphysema* was first used in 1951 (Lewis, Robertson and James, 1951).

The initial description of bronchogenic cysts of the mediastinum was by Meyer (1859) in 1859, and the first English language description was by Blackader and Evans (1911) in 1911. The first successful resection was performed in 1948 by Maier (1948). At the time of a report of a series by Eraklis, et al. (1969) in 1969, consisting of 10 patients, only 25 previous cases had been described in the literature.

Congenital cystic adenomatoid malformation of the lung was first recognized as a distinct entity by Ch'in and Tang (1949) in 1949.

Huber, in 1777, described an aberrant artery arising from the aorta and supplying a normal right lower lobe. Rokitansky (1861) and also Rektorzik (1861), both in 1861, described cases of what appears to be extralobar pulmonary sequestration. Pryce, in 1946, originated the term *pulmonary sequestration* and defined the anatomy.

The first lucid description of an abnormal connection between an artery and vein is attributed to Hunter (1757), who described a traumatic arteriovenous malformation in 1757 (Young, 1988). Hunter made the first clinical correlation between a palpable thrill and this lesion. Osler (1901) described a syndrome of hereditary telangiectasias of the skin and mucous membranes in 1901. He also noted that it had first been reported by Rendu in 1896. A further report by Parkes Weber (1907) followed. The disease, which now is called Rendu-Osler-Weber syndrome or hereditary hemorrhagic telangiectasia, is inherited as a mendelian dominant and is characterized by numerous spider angiomas of the skin and mucous membranes along with the development arteriovenous malformations of the liver and lungs. Arteriographic embolization of arteriovenous malformations was first applied to spinal cord lesions and subsequently adapted for use in visceral and pulmonary locations (Djindjian, et al., 1973).

HISTORICAL READINGS

Blackader AD, Evans DJ: A case of mediastinal cyst producing compression of the trachea, ending fatally in an infant of nine months. Arch Pediatr 28:194, 1911

Ch'in KY, Tang MY: Congenital adenomatoid malformation of one lobe of a lung with general anasarca. Arch Pathol 48:221, 1949

Djindjian R, Cophignon J, Théron J et al: Embolization by superselective arteriography from the femoral route in neuroradiology. Review of 60 cases: I. Technique. indications, complications. Neuroradiology 6:20, 1973

Eraklis AJ, Griscom NT, McGovern JB: Bronchogenic cysts of the mediastinum in infancy. N Engl J Med 281:1150, 1969

Gross RE, Lewis JE: Defect of the anterior mediastinum. Surg Gynecol Obstet 80:549, 1945

Huber JJ: Observationes aliquot de arteria singulari pulmoni concessa. Acta Helvet 8:85, 1777

Hunter W: The history of an aneurysm of the aorta with some remarks on aneurysms in general. Obs Soc Phys (Lond) 1:323, 1757

Lewis JE Jr: Pulmonary and bronchial malformations. In Holder T, Ashcraft KE (eds): Pediatric Surgery.

Maier HC: Bronchogenic cysts of the mediastinum. Ann Surg 127:476, 1948

Meyer H: Über angeborene blasige Missbildung der Lungen nebst einigen Bemerkungen über Cyanose aus Lungenleiden. Arch Pathol Anat 16:78, 1859

Nelson RL: Congenital cystic disease of the lung. J Pediatr 1:233, 1932

Osler W: On a family form of recurring epistaxis associated with multiple telangiectases of skin and mucous membrane. Bull Johns Hopkins Hosp 12:333, 1901

Overstreet RM: Emphysema of a portion of the lung in the early months of life. Am J Dis Child 57:861, 1939

Parkes Weber F: Multiple hereditary developmental angiomata of the skin and mucous membranes associated with recurring haemorrhages. Lancet 2:160, 1907

Pryce DM: Lower accessory pulmonary artery with intralobar sequestration of lung. A report of seven cases. J Pathol Bacteriol 48:457, 1946

Rektorzik E: Ueber accessorischen Lungenlappen. Woch Z Aerzte 17:4, 1861

Rendu M: Epistaxis répétées chez un sujet porteur de petits angiomes cutanes et muqueux. Bull Soc Med Hop Paris 13:731, 1896

Robertson R, James ES: Congenital lobar emphysema. Pediatrics 8:795, 1951

Rokitansky C: Lehrbuch der pathologischen Anatomie. 3rd Ed. Vienna, 1861

Young AE: Arteriovenous malformations. p. 228. In Mulliken JB, Young AE (eds): Vascular Birthmarks (Hemangiomas and Malformations). WB Saunders, Philadelphia, 1988

BASIC SCIENCE

Pulmonary Embryology

The steps in the development of the respiratory system from the primitive foregut are depicted in Figure 19-1. The respiratory tract is represented by a groove in the ventral wall of the foregut at the fourth week of gestation (Gray and Skandalakis, 1972; Langman, 1969; Sorokins, 1965; Willis, 1962). The groove itself will become the a portion of the pharynx and the retrotracheal portion of the esophagus. However, the pulmonary groove soon forms a diverticulum with an elongated slitlike opening into the pharyngoesophageal part of the foregut (Fig. 19-1A). The slit, itself, is gradually reduced in length by posteroanterior ingrowth and fusion of its lateral lips, thus forming a partition that separates the trachea from the upper esophagus. Finally, only the upper end remains patent as the definitive laryngeal orifice. This mechanism forms a basis for understanding the various forms of esophageal atresia and tracheoesophageal fistulae.

During the second month of gestation, the pulmonary diverticulum grows rapidly downward and forms the larynx, trachea, bronchi, and lungs. The pharyngeal diverticulum, or bud, elongates, and its tip swells, finally dividing to form the precursors of the primary bronchus of each lung (Fig. 19-1B). In turn, these lung buds elongate, swell, and subdivide, as do their descendants, until a large interbranching network of tubules is formed. This constitutes the early bronchial tree (Fig. 19-1C and D).

From the outset branching is not strictly dichotomous; the left primary bronchus forms a more obtuse angle with the trachea compared with the right. As the epithelium pushes out from the pharyngeal floor, it is accompanied by mesenchyme that originated beneath the laryngotracheal groove (Ham and Baldwin, 1941). This mesenchyme gradually condenses around the tracheobronchial tree and differentiates into cartilage, adventitial connective tissue, blood vessels, and lymphatic channels. The early fetal lung resembles an exocrine gland with numerous ducts ending in sac-shaped expansions that lie embedded in connective tissue. At this point they lack a rich blood supply, but in a second phase of lung development, the major blood vessels enlarge and the capillaries increase in number until the lung becomes the most highly vascularized organ in the body.

Alveolar formation is related to growth of the vasculature and is first observed in human fetuses at 18 weeks' gestation when angiogenesis is firmly underway in the mesenchyme (Loosli and Potter, 1951). Capillaries grow into the cuboidal endodermal lining (it has never been absolutely proved but is generally accepted that the lining of the lung arises from endoderm), and the loops push into the lumen of the airway. The interface of alveolar and endothelial cells is depicted in Figure 19-2. The capillaries become more abundant as gestation proceeds, and the lining epithelium is stretched over them while they are separated from the endothelium by

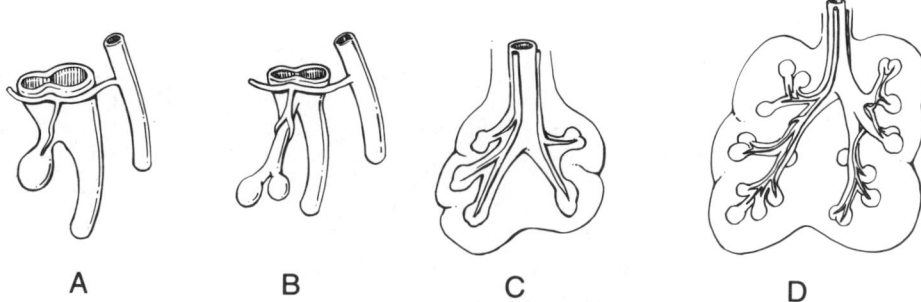

Figure 19-1. The progression of events in normal lung development. **(A)** Outpouching from the pharyngeal part of the primitive foregut has occurred. Branches from the aorta are also beginning their ingrowth. **(B)** The primitive anlagen of the right and left lungs have formed. **(C & D)** The subsequent subdivision of the lung forms the alveoli with their attendant vascular supply.

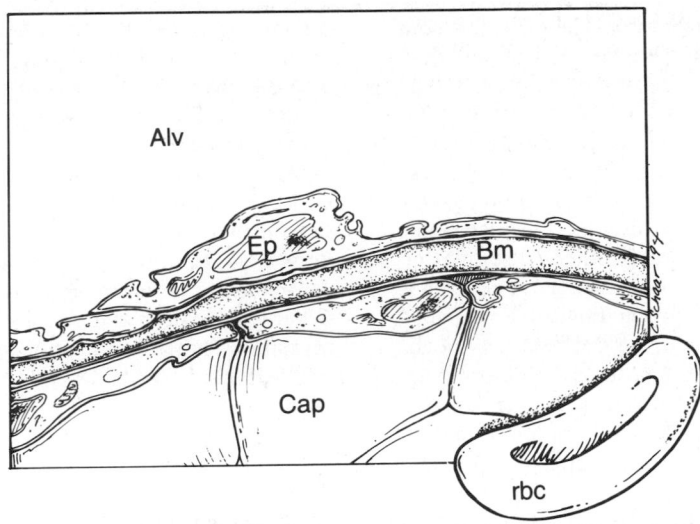

Figure 19-2. There is close proximity of alveolar and endothelial cells in the developing lung.

the basement membrane. The bodies of the cells are tucked into spaces between the capillary loops, becoming type I cells, while some of the fetal cuboidal epithelium differentiates into cytosome containing cubical or polygonal cells, which do not become drawn into thin sheets. These become the alveolar, or type II, cells.

The modification of the epithelium of the terminal air sacs into type I or II cells occurs during the twenty-fourth to twenty-eighth week of gestation. Because type II cells produce surfactant and do not develop before the twenty-fourth to twenty-eighth week, fetuses cannot survive the extrauterine environment if they are born at an earlier gestational age. Terminal budding continues to produce new alveolar regions. In newborns five or six generations of respiratory bronchioles are present at birth. In humans the number of alveoli continue to increase after birth up to the eighth year of life, and adults usually possess two generations of respiratory bronchioles (Engel, 1953). The dimensions of the pulmonary zones and segments may expand until the age of 40 years. Premature birth has no effect on subsequent lung development.

The blood vessels of the lung are derived from two sources: the plexiform network of vessels developing in the pulmonary mesenchyme and the heart. Like bronchi the vessels may vary in their course based on the selection of channels from the pre-existing mesenchymal network.

This short background on pulmonary embryology may help the reader visualize the mechanisms by which the following congenital anomalies arise.

Incidence of Various Malformations

Vogt-Moykopf, et al. (1992) did a survey of 59 hospitals performing thoracic surgery, of which 14 supplied data. Of the 1,347 anomalies diagnosed, 1,343 were treated surgically, and 5 patients died within the first 30 postoperative days (0.3 percent). In a retrospective study of 6,350 thoracotomies over a 10-year period (1978 to 1988), 198 pulmonary anomalies were identified (Vogt-Moykopf, et al., 1993). Table 19-1 illustrates the relative prevalence of the anomalies described.

CONGENITAL LABOR EMPHYSEMA

BASIC SCIENCE

Etiology

Congenital lobar emphysema is defined as a postnatal overdistension of one or more lobes of a histologically normal lung (Berlinger, et al., 1987; Haller, et al., 1979; Michelson, 1977; Monin, et al., 1979; Lacquet and Lacquet, 1977). Usually the upper and middle lobes are affected. In most patients

Table 19-1. Major Developmental Anomalies of the Lung

Anomaly	Prevalence	Associated Anomalies
Congenital lobar emphysema	Not uncommon	Bronchogenic cyst, PDH, tetralogy of Fallot, ventricular septal defect
Bronchogenic cyst	Uncommon	Abnormalities of the pulmonary artery
Cystic adenomatoid malformation	Rare	No significant association
Pulmonary sequestration	Not uncommon	No significant association
Pulmonary arteriovenous malformation	Rare	Rendu-Osler-Weber syndrome[a]
Congenital pulmonary hypoplasia or aplasia	Complete is extremely rare; unilateral is not uncommon	Microphthalmia, Potter's syndrome

[a] Fifteen percent of patients with Rendu-Osler-Weber syndrome have pulmonary arteriovenous malformations.

the process is confined to a single lobe. The cause of lobar emphysema may vary, depending on the clinical situation, but the common mechanism of action must involve a ball-valve obstruction of a lobar or segmental bronchus. This allows distal air trapping with resultant hyperinflation, causing further bronchial obstruction. In the acquired form of lobar emphysema, seen in infants with bronchopulmonary dysplasia, the obstruction may be caused by the occurrence of endobronchial granulation tissue. Another cause of bronchial obstruction in both the congenital and acquired form is absence or weakening of the supporting tracheal or bronchial cartilages. This allows the bronchus to collapse toward the lumen with expiration and results in progressive air trapping. In congenital lobar emphysema, cartilaginous malformation could result from absent or inadequate migration of mesenchyme into the endodermal pharyngeal pouch during the eighteenth week of gestation. Improper differentiation of mesenchyme into cartilaginous and fibrous supporting structures is also a mechanism that might ultimately cause congenital lobar emphysema.

Extrinsic bronchial obstruction may also play a role in some cases of congenital lobar emphysema. There are multiple reports of associated cardiac anomalies in infants with this lung anomaly (Borg, et al., 1975; Gordon and Dempsey, 1990; Keller, 1983; Roguin, et al., 1980). In one study, seven autopsied cases were shown to have developed lobar emphysema because of a check valve mechanism created by compression of the bronchi by a distended pulmonary artery (Isojima, et al., 1978). All these patients had clinical evidence of a severe left-to-right shunt prior to death. In the same report eight additional infants, also with left-to-right shunts and concurrent severe lobar emphysema, showed resolution of the emphysema after correction of the cardiac lesion. The authors concluded that resection of the emphysematous lobe should be avoided in favor of repair of the congenital heart defect in this subset of patients. In another report three patients with patent ductus arteriosus and respiratory failure were described (Toran, et al., 1989). Dilatation of the pulmonary arteries led to bronchial compression, which resulted in lobar emphysema. In this report the authors considered left-sided lobar emphysema to be a special group for which extrinsic compression may be the principal pathophysiologic factor. In addition to patent ductus arteriosus, double aortic arch, tetralogy of Fallot, ventricular septal defect, and congenital absence of the pulmonic valve have also been associated with lobar emphysema. Hasse, et al. (1975) reported on six patients with congenital lobar emphysema, three of whom had associated patent ductus arteriosus, with one of these also manifesting a double aortic arch. Two of the three with congenital cardiovascular anomalies responded to division of the obstructing vascular anomaly without the need for a lobectomy. It is estimated that congenital heart defects may be present in 20 percent of patients with lobar emphysema. Correction of the cardiac anomaly without a pulmonary lobectomy is recommended.

Rarely congenital lobar emphysema may arise because of a polyalveolar lobe (Tapper, et al., 1980). This entity is defined as a three- to fivefold increase in alveolar number, as determined by microscopic point counting of random lung sections. The airways and arteries are normal for age in number, size, and structure. Air may enter alveoli by collaterals but have no way to get out, resulting in lobar emphysema. The therapy is similar to that of other forms of the disease. Congenital lobar emphysema has also been associated with pectus excavatum, right-sided aortic arch, bilateral diaphragmatic eventration, and mediastinal bronchogenic cyst (Engel, et al., 1984; Fukumoto, et al., 1991; Gille, et al., 1979). Successful therapy of bilateral lobar emphysema has also been described (Ekkelkamp and Vos, 1987). Interestingly, there are a number of reports in the literature of lobar emphysema developing in dogs and cats and usually associated with malformations of the bronchial cartilages (Hoover, et al., 1992; La Rue, et al., 1990; Orima, et al., 1992; Voorhout, et al., 1986).

DIAGNOSIS

Clinical Features

Congenital emphysema most commonly affects newborns and small infants who present with varying degrees of respiratory distress. One-half of the cases present in the first 4 weeks of life, and most of the others are diagnosed before the sixth month of life. There are a number of patients who are older than 1 year at presentation, and rare cases of presentation in adulthood. Respiratory distress may be severe, with an infant presenting in the first hours or days with dyspnea, tachypnea, cyanosis, wheezing, coughing, thoracic or epigastric retractions, and nasal flare. The respiratory distress may be severe enough to require endotracheal intubation and urgent surgical intervention within the first 6 hours after birth (Canty, 1977; Keith, 1977; Senyuz, et al., 1989; Warner, et al., 1982). Later symptoms can include failure to thrive, faintness, psychomotor retardation, malformation of the thorax, and recurrent pulmonary infection (Al-Salem, et al., 1990).

On physical examination the chest wall on the involved side is more prominent but has decreased respiratory excursion. Breath sounds are paradoxically decreased over the affected lobe; the apical pulse is shifted away from the side of involvement. The diaphragm may also be depressed on the ipsilateral side.

Imaging and Other Diagnostic Studies

The plain chest radiograph is the best initial diagnostic tool. Typical findings include overinflation of a pulmonary lobe with mediastinal shift to the contralateral side (Fig. 19-3). The lobes most commonly affected are the left upper (43 percent), right upper (20 percent), and the right middle lobe (32 percent) (Man, et al., 1983). Bilateral involvement may occur in 20 percent of cases; solitary disease of a lower lobe is rare. Because of air trapping, the mediastinal shift can increase on expiration. In addition, the affected lobes may herniate across the mediastinum. The findings on chest radiography may be confused with atelectasis with compensatory emphysema, congenital cyst, postpneumonic pneumatocele, pneumothorax, infectious obstructive emphysema, pulmonary interstitial emphysema, unilateral hyperlucent lung (Swyer-James syndrome, Macleod's syndrome), congenital

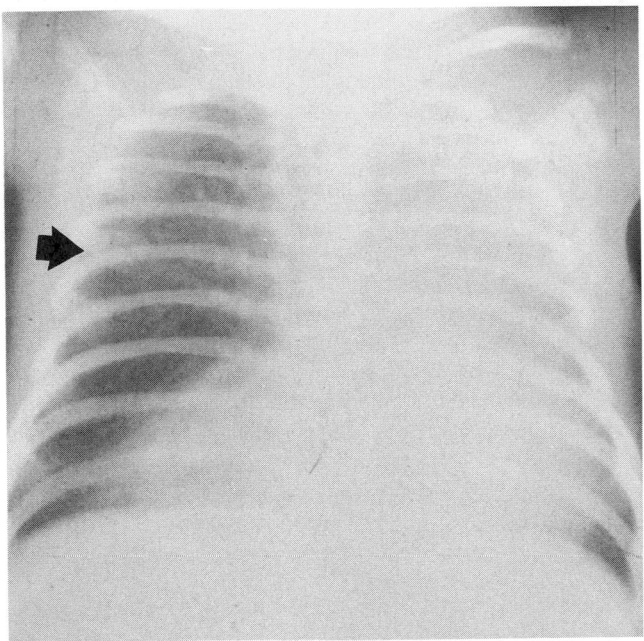

Figure 19-3. A plain chest radiograph of a newborn with congenital lobar emphysema. Hyperexpansion and mediastinal shift with contralateral atelectasis are noted.

cystic adenomatoid malformation, pneumomediastinum, and diaphragmatic hernia.

Computed tomography (CT) is a useful adjunct in the diagnosis of congenital lobar emphysema (Markowitz, et al., 1989; Pardes, et al., 1983). Mediastinal masses, especially bronchogenic cysts, bronchial anatomy down to the segmental level, and occasionally pulmonary artery slings can all be detected by CT. If the patient's condition allows it, CT of the chest should be performed soon after plain chest radiographs have raised a suspicion of congenital lobar emphysema (Fig. 19-4).

Bronchography is contraindicated. Because the bronchial tree is already severely compromised, intrabronchial admin-

istration of contrast agents may severely worsen the patient's clinical status.

Ventilation scintigraphy with a submicronic (0.2 to 0.8 μm in diameter) radioaerosol can show unventilated pulmonary segments and provide confirmatory data in patients suspected of having congenital lobar emphysema on chest radiographs (Loewy, et al., 1987). In this technique the child breathes radioactive (^{99m}Tc-sulfur colloid) aerosol through an anesthesia bag for 2 minutes followed by imaging. Children with murmurs, cyanosis, or other clinical findings that suggest congenital heart disease may require cardiac catheterization in a facility equipped to perform this and to undertake the repair of any cardiac anomalies.

Diagnostic bronchoscopy should be performed when there is a question of bronchial compression by vascular structures. Bronchoscopy can determine the sites of compression and might aid in planning future therapy. Fiberoptic bronchoscopy performed through a short endotracheal tube is suitable for this diagnostic procedure. Bronchoscopy has also shown evidence of tracheal stenosis in some of these patients.

MANAGEMENT

Therapy

The therapy for isolated congenital lobar emphysema is the prompt resection of the involved lobe (Haller, et al., 1979; Hill, et al., 1988; Michelson, 1977; Vogt-Moykopf, et al., 1992). Anesthesia management must take into consideration the underlying air-trapping obstruction, and high ventilatory pressure should be avoided (Cote, 1978; Goto, et al., 1987). In patients with congenital heart disease that causes a right-to-left shunt, a full cardiac evaluation is required. Repair of the heart defect might result in the relief of the lobar emphysema and should be given precedence. Some of these patients might also eventually require a lobectomy (Isojima, et al., 1978). Similar conclusions hold for patients with congenital vascular anomalies that cause lobar emphysema by vascular compression of the bronchus. Division of the compressing ductus arteriosus or vascular ring may obviate the need for

Figure 19-4. A CT scan of an infant with congenital lobar emphysema. This clearly demonstrates the hyperexpansion and mediastinal shift associated with this lesion.

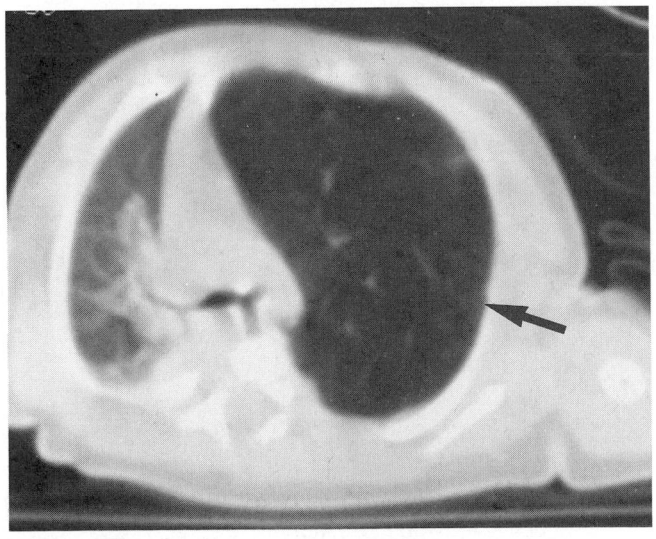

lobectomy and should be done first. If significant bronchomalacia was induced by the vascular compression, lobectomy may later be required.

The reported mortality rate associated with the surgical correction of congenital lobar emphysema is 10 to 28 percent and depends on the frequency of associated anomalies (Knoop, et al., 1984; Urban, et al., 1975). Complete clinical recovery should be expected for children without congenital heart defects. Long-term follow-up demonstrates that the development and physical performance in these patients is roughly equivalent to that of normal controls. The pulmonary volumes are about 90 percent of predicted, suggesting compensatory growth of the remaining lung tissue (Frenckner and Freychuss, 1982).

There is a subset of patients with congenital lobar emphysema but without serious or life-threatening symptoms who may not require surgical intervention. Kennedy, et al. (1991) in a retrospective study performed serial chest radiographs ($n = 12$) and follow-up ventilation/perfusion ($\dot{V}/\dot{Q}$) scans ($n = 6$) on 12 children treated without surgery. In all 12 improvement in symptoms was accompanied by improved appearance on plain chest radiographs. In the six that underwent V/Q scans, an increase in ventilation was more marked than was the improvement in perfusion. The indications for surgical intervention depend on the acuity of presenting symptoms. Usually, urgent thoracotomy with lobectomy must be performed, but as noted above, some patients may be observed if symptoms are less acute.

BRONCHOGENIC CYSTS

BASIC SCIENCE

Pathophysiology

Bronchogenic cysts originate before the bronchi are formed and may be either mediastinal or intrapulmonary. In children the majority of bronchogenic cysts are located in the mediastinum (65 percent), with the rest located in the following anatomic sites: 27 percent intraparenchymal and 8 percent in the inferior pulmonary ligament (DiLorenzo, et al., 1989). The mediastinal lesions can be in close proximity to the carina, mainstem bronchi, trachea, esophagus, or pericardium. Eraklis, et al. (1969) noted that obstructing carinal lesions that produced severe symptoms were difficult to locate until the mediastinal pleura had been divided and retracted anteriorly. Bronchogenic cysts comprise 10 to 15 percent of all mediastinal masses and occur in between 1 : 40,000 to 1 : 68,000 admissions.

Etiology

The precise embryologic steps leading to the development of a bronchogenic cyst are unknown. It is clear from the previous discussion of normal lung development that the respiratory system develops by pouching out from the primitive foregut. Most hypotheses regarding the development of bronchogenic cysts (and also cystic duplications of the esophagus) invoke a process of abortive pouching out and pinching off of a primitive lung bud from the foregut (Balquet,

1984; Letanche, et al., 1984). Because of its foregut origin, a bronchogenic cyst may be lined by ciliated columnar (respiratory) or squamous epithelium. Both linings possess mucus-secreting bronchial glands, which cause the cyst to fill under pressure. This in turn causes pressure on surrounding structures, particularly the membranous trachea or bronchi, and may lead to severe respiratory obstruction. Bronchogenic cysts may also contain focal intramural areas of hyaline cartilage and/or smooth muscle (Coselli, et al., 1987). They are most often found near the carina in the middle part of the mediastinum. The process of abnormal budding leads to centrally located cysts if they occur early in gestation; later occurrences may give rise to peripheral intraparenchymal lesions that may retain a bronchial communication to the airway.

DIAGNOSIS

Clinical Features

Bronchogenic cysts of the mediastinum can occur from infancy to late adulthood. Different presenting symptoms are observed in each group (Buckner, et al., 1989; Cartmill and Hughes, 1989; DiLorenzo, et al., 1989; Feketi, et al., 1988; Koskas, et al., 1992). Most newborns present with life-threatening respiratory distress and require urgent intervention for survival (Bower and Kiesewetter, 1977; Haller, et al., 1979). Older children and adults have milder symptoms or are diagnosed because of the incidental finding of a mediastinal mass or evidence of bronchial obstruction on imaging studies. This is illustrated in Table 19-2, in which the age range and presenting symptoms are cross-tabulated. In the report by St-Georges, et al. (1991), which deals with patients older than 16 years of age at diagnosis, cysts are categorized as mediastinal or pulmonary. There were 66 patients in the mediastinal group, of which 44 (66 percent) were symptomatic. The most common presenting complaints were chest pain, cough dyspnea, fever, purulent sputum, anorexia, and dysphagia. Also, patients with mediastinal lesions were more likely to have severe symptoms. Of the 20 patients with intrapulmonary cysts, 18 were symptomatic. These most commonly presented with cough, fever, dyspnea, and purulent sputum. In both sets hemoptysis was uncommon.

Bronchogenic cysts that cause airway obstruction have also been reported in the cervical area (Canty and Hendren, 1975; Cohen, et al., 1985; Park and Buford, 1955). These usually occur in infants and are associated with acute respiratory symptoms. Transdiaphragmatic bronchogenic cysts and a cyst presenting as a supraclavicular mass have also been reported (Amendola, et al., 1982; Dubois, et al., 1981).

In summary, bronchogenic cysts presenting in children younger than 1 year of age, especially newborns, usually cause severe airway obstruction with dyspnea, tachypnea, retractions, flaring, and air trapping with distal emphysema. In this age group, the lesion is almost always mediastinal. Bronchogenic cysts diagnosed later in childhood or in adulthood usually do not cause severe respiratory distress. Chest pain, cough, fever, and purulent sputum are more frequently observed. Up to 33 percent of older patients may also be asymptomatic.

Table 19-2.   Bronchogenic Cysts

Author (Year)	No. Patients	Ages	Symptoms	Size (cm)	Therapy	Follow-Up
Opsahl and Berman (1962)	1	20 days	Dyspnea, cough	3	Resection	Alive and well
Eraklis, et al. (1969)	10	Birth, 2 days, 6 mo, 6 mo, 23 mo, 1.5 yr	Dyspnea and respiratory distress in younger patients	2, 2, 3, 3.5, 4, 4,	Resection in eight	Three dead, two untreated, seven alive and well
Pokorny (1974)	11	Three before 5 mo, eight after 2 yr	Stridor, three with mild respiratory symptoms, five incidental	—	—	—
Canty, et al. (1975)	2	Birth, 10 days	Airway obstruction	—	Unroofing	Two alive and well
Haller, et al. (1975)	2	1 day, 6 weeks	Tachypnea, cyanosis	4, —	Resection	Two alive and well
Bower and Kiesewetter (1977)	6	Three < 1 yr, 3 yr, 6 yr, 10 yr	The three patients < 1 hr had respiratory symptoms	—	Resection	Six alive and well
Snyder (1985)	23	Range from 1 week to 14 yr	Younger patients present with pneumonia, stridor, cough	—	Resection	
St-Georges, et al. (1991)	86	Range from 16 to 19 yr	Chest pain, cough, dyspnea, fever	—	Resection	All alive and well

Imaging and Other Diagnostic Studies

Plain chest radiographs are the standard initial study for myriad intrathoracic conditions. Di Lorenzo, et al. (1989), in describing 26 children with bronchogenic cysts, reported that plain chest radiographs were accurately diagnostic in 20 (77 percent). Suen, et al. (1993), reporting on 42 patients ranging in age from 8 to 62 years (mean, 34.8 years), noted that the diagnostic accuracy of plain chest radiographs was 88 percent. Bronchogenic cysts most commonly presented as homogeneous water density shadows. Two of their patients had air-fluid levels, and both of these lesions were intrapulmonary. In the five patients not diagnosed by plain chest radiographs, all lesions were located in a subcarinal position. Plain chest radiographs alone can accurately diagnose approximately 80 to 90 percent of cases, and they are useful in initial screening (Figs. 19-5 and 19-6).

Experience with CT supports this imaging modality as the best confirmatory study at present. CT scans correctly identified the lesions in 100 percent of patients from the two studies discussed previously. The findings included a round, well-circumscribed, unilocular, or multilocular mass with a density ranging from that of water (0 to 20 Hounsfield units) to as high as 91 Hounsfield units. Occasionally the cyst is air filled, implying bronchial communication (Figs. 19-7 and 19-8). There is less experience with magnetic resonance imaging (MRI). Suen, et al. (1993) reported that six of their patients underwent magnetic resonance imaging, with definite findings noted in five. In one patient CT was required to differentiate the cystic contents from fat. The majority of bronchogenic cysts studied (five of six) imaged using this modality showed high signal intensity on both T_1- and T_2-weighted images.

Ultrasound has rarely been performed for this lesion. In two cases reported by Suen, et al. (1993), an anechoic lesion was identified. There are significant technical problems with routine thoracic ultrasound. Barium swallow was diagnostic in only two of six lesions in one report.

Bronchoscopy performed as part of the diagnostic workup for a bronchogenic cyst usually reveals extrinsic bronchial compression. Occasionally there is evidence of a fistulous communication between the cyst and the bronchial tree. This may appear as either a fistulous tract or the drainage of

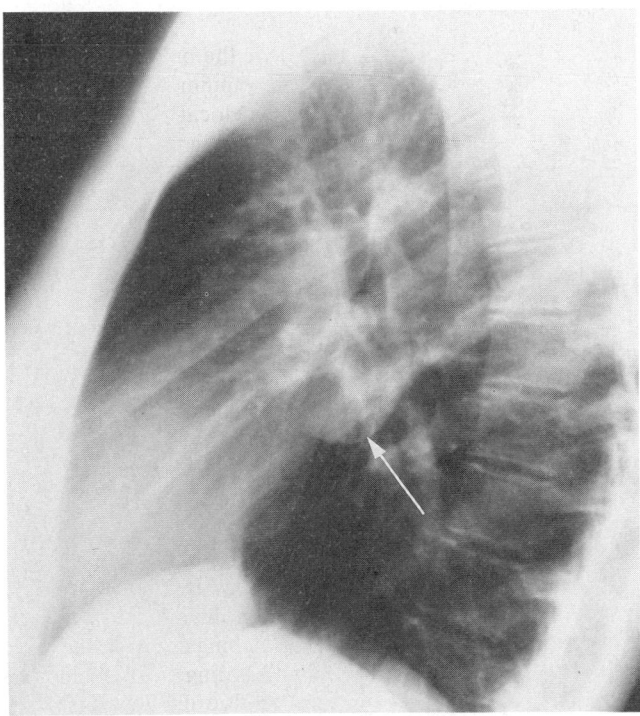

Figure 19-5.   A lateral chest radiograph demonstrating a mediastinal bronchogenic cyst.

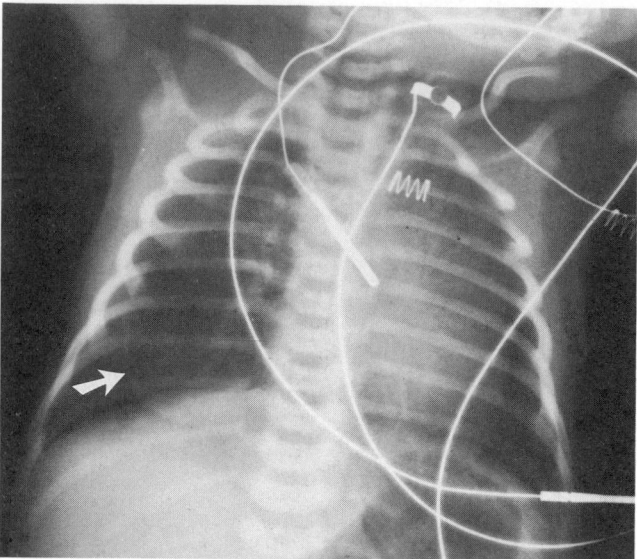

Figure 19-6. A plain chest radiograph demonstrating an intralobar bronchogenic cyst with bronchial communication.

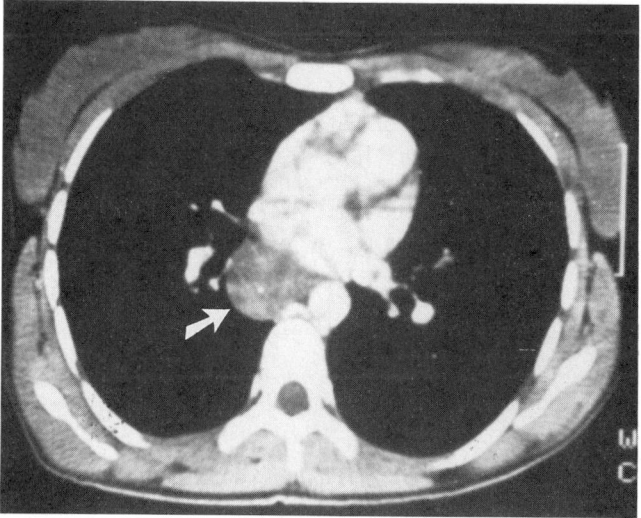

Figure 19-7. CT scan of the mediastinal bronchogenic cyst seen in Figure 19-5.

mucopurulent material into the bronchus. Reported bronchoscopic abnormalities varied from 1 of 4 (25 percent) to 9 of 26 (35 percent) patients in two reported series (DiLorenzo, et al., 1989; Suen, et al., 1993). In summary, patients who present with clinical findings suggesting bronchogenic cyst require a screening plain chest radiograph followed by axial CT of the chest. These studies should confirm the lesion and identify its anatomic location in almost 100 percent of patients. Bronchoscopy is not routinely indicated but will show evidence of external compression or cyst-bronchial fistulae in approximately one-third of patients.

MANAGEMENT

Therapy

Bronchogenic cysts have usually been treated by thoracotomy and excision of the cyst (Balquet, 1984; Eraklis, et al., 1969; Opsahl and Berman, 1962; Suen, et al., 1993). The anatomic location can be precisely determined using the plain chest radiograph and imaging studies. The cyst is usually approached by a posterolateral thoracotomy. Subcarinal lesions are normally approached from the right side. Exposure is facilitated by the placement of a double-lumen endotracheal tube and ipsilateral collapse of the lung. In younger patients a bronchial blocker can be used. The objective of the surgery is complete cyst removal, if feasible. This may be impossible or entail inordinate danger to the patient if there is adherence to the membranous portion of the trachea or mainstem bronchi or the cyst is inflamed. In these cases opening the cyst with removal of the mucus-secreting lining layer may be performed. Because removal of the inner layer prevents cyst distension with mucous secretions, the resultant airway compression is relieved. It is preferable to remove the cyst entirely if possible because rare cases of malignant degeneration have been reported.

Adults with bronchogenic cysts may be asymptomatic or have minimal complaints. Ginsberg and Kirby (1989) suggested that small, asymptomatic bronchogenic cysts in adult patients can be followed with serial chest radiographs, although larger or enlarging cysts should be removed. Several authors have also suggested that cyst aspiration, cyst wall biopsy, and possible removal of the cyst or intralesional instil-

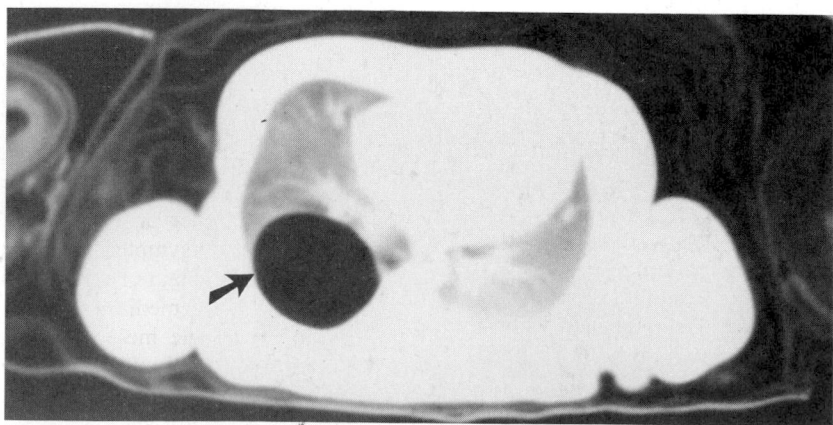

Figure 19-8. CT scan of the intralobar bronchogenic cyst seen in Figure 19-6.

lation of a sclerosant (i.e., tetracycline) could be accomplished mediastinoscopically (Carlens, 1959; Ginsberg, et al., 1972; Pursel, et al., 1966). Finally, Lewis, et al. (1992) reported on two cases of mediastinal bronchogenic cysts in adults (31 and 40 years old) who underwent thoracoscopic drainage and wall resection. A laser was used to ablate one of the cysts completely. Complete resection is preferable to cyst aspiration because it allows removal or ablation of the entire lesion, preventing the possibility of malignant degeneration.

CYSTIC ADENOMATOID MALFORMATION

BASIC SCIENCE

Pathophysiology

This condition is characterized by overgrowth of bronchioles. Defining histologic criteria include increased terminal respiratory structures appearing as cysts lined by cuboidal or pseudostratified columnar epithelium, an increase of elastic tissue within cyst walls along with polypoid mucosa, an absence of cartilage in the cyst wall, lining mucus-secreting cells, and no inflammatory process (Bale, 1979; Olson and Mendelsohn, 1978). Cystic adenomatoid malformation may occur as three distinct histologic subtypes. Type I is the most common (55 percent) and consists of large cystic spaces within a single pulmonary lobe. Type II (40 percent of cases) is composed of numerous small cysts measuring 1 to 10 mm in diameter. Type III is a solid mass without cysts consisting of adenomatoid hyperplasia or bronchial structures (Miller, et al., 1980; Rosado-de-Christenson and Stocker, 1991; Stocker, et al., 1977). In a large institutional series (34 cases) reported by Mentzer, et al. (1992), the malformation was unilateral in all cases and involved the left and right lungs with equal frequency. The majority (67 percent) were classified as Stocker type I cystic adenomatoid malformations; 24 percent were type II and 9 percent, type III. Most patients were treated by lobectomy or segmental/wedge resection, and only one patient in this series required pneumonectomy.

Etiology

In a study using postmortem bronchography or serial microscopic section of lungs in four patients with congenital cystic adenomatoid malformation, Moerman, et al. (1992) showed segmental bronchial absence or atresia to be present in each. These observations provide evidence that the primary defect in this condition is bronchial atresia. The morphologic subtype of congenital cystic adenomatoid malformation is thought to be dependent on the type of secondary dysplastic lung growth beyond the atretic segment. The authors suggest that the exact cause of the bronchial atresia may be heterogeneous, and possible mechanisms include primary disruption in cell growth or interruption of the fetal bronchial circulation. The simultaneous occurrence of congenital cystic adenomatoid malformation with pulmonary sequestration and polyalveolar lobe has been reported (Wagenvoort, et al., 1991; Yogasakaran and Sudhaman, 1991; Zangwill and Stocker, 1993). There is also a report of twins in which one fetus had

a cystic adenomatoid malformation and the other was normal (Rebarber and Mohan, 1992).

Recently, Boglino, et al. (1992) reported that cystic adenomatoid malformations from six patients showed significant reactivity with antibodies to the neuropeptide, neurotensin. This neuropeptide and others are thought to play a role in immune reactivity, especially the cytolytic activity of activated macrophages. Normal lung from the same patients was much less reactive. These data suggest that in utero infection is a possible cause of cystic adenomatoid malformation.

DIAGNOSIS

Fetal Diagnosis

During the last decade, there has been significant progress in fetal diagnosis based on improvements in fetal ultrasound (Boulot, et al., 1991; Deacon, et al., 1990; Heydanus, et al., 1993; Morris, et al., 1991; Sherer, et al., 1992; Taguchi, et al., 1993). Congenital cystic adenomatoid malformation is one such pulmonary process in which prenatal diagnosis is readily accomplished. Furthermore, it is now appreciated that a large fetal lung mass can cause mediastinal shift, pulmonary hypoplasia, polyhydramnios, and cardiovascular compromise, which leads to fetal hydrops and death (Adzick, et al., 1993; Heij, et al., 1990; Walker and Cudmore, 1990). The overall prognosis is dependent on the size of the mass and the extent of the secondary physiologic derangements caused by mediastinal compression. To complicate matters further, the Fetal Treatment Center at the University of California at San Francisco has reported three cases of congenital cystic adenomatoid malformation that decreased in size during pregnancy, with one of the lesions regressing almost entirely (Adzick, et al., 1993). The prenatal diagnosis of congenital cystic adenomatoid malformation is a clinical reality that has an impact on therapeutic alternatives.

Clinical Features

As is the case with bronchogenic cysts, congenital cystic adenomatoid malformations present in newborns and infants with tachypnea, cyanosis, retractions, and respiratory distress. The majority of patients present in the first month of life with acute respiratory symptoms. Air trapping may occur in cystic areas of the anomaly and result in a clinical and radiographic picture that is reminiscent of lobar emphysema. The cystic distension may rarely result in rupture, and the patient presents with a pneumothorax or tension pneumothorax (Bentur, et al., 1991; Hilpert and Pretorius, 1990; Kleinman, et al., 1982). Older children usually complain of cough and fever or have recurrent respiratory infections. They may be asymptomatic and their condition incidentally diagnosed by plain chest radiographs. Because air trapping with resultant mediastinal compression is the operative pathophysiologic mechanism, the patient's condition may deteriorate rapidly when the patient is intubated and placed on positive-pressure ventilation. The clinician must be aware of this possibility and be prepared to perform thoracotomy and resection rapidly.

Imaging and Diagnostic Studies

As noted previously ultrasound is able to diagnose cystic adenomatoid malformation in the fetus as early as the twentieth week of gestation (Morcos and Lobb, 1986; Nugent, et al., 1989; Scholz and Kuhnt, 1990). Simultaneous assessment for polyhydramnios and fetal hydrops can also be performed and is valuable to determine the prognostic risk. Some cystic adenomatoid malformations may also undergo spontaneous regression; therefore, serial ultrasound is helpful during follow-up and in planning either fetal or neonatal intervention.

After birth patients often present with respiratory distress, and plain chest radiographs are again the most important initial diagnostic study (Fig. 19-9). It is important to realize that congenital cystic adenomatoid malformation has been confused with congenital diaphragmatic hernia (foramen of Bochdalek), congenital lobar emphysema, bronchogenic cyst, and pneumothorax. The findings observed in plain chest radiographs include single or multiple large cysts, multiple small cysts of uniform size, and solid-appearing masses. Masses are typically intrapulmonary and contain scattered radiolucent areas. Some cysts within the malformation may contain air-fluid levels. In addition, a mediastinal shift away from the lesion is observed when the lesion is expanding because of air trapping. This also implies a bronchial communication. Cystic adenomatoid malformations that present with chronic symptoms (infection or cough) later in life do not usually communicate with the bronchus. Most cystic adenomatoid malformations are observed in the lower lobes.

After plain chest radiographs have revealed a unilateral multilocular density in one hemithorax, the next step diagnostically is the introduction of a small amount of water-soluble contrast material through a nasogastric tube to verify that the intestinal tract lies below the diaphragm and thus differentiate cystic adenomatoid malformation from diaphragmatic hernia.

The plain radiographic appearance of bowel loops in the thorax can be confused with cystic adenomatoid malformations. No further imaging studies are required after ruling out a foramen of Bochdalek hernia. If further information is required, CT of the chest may be helpful (Fig. 19-10).

MANAGEMENT

Therapy

Therapy may be divided into prenatal and postnatal categories. Because prenatal diagnosis and assessment of prognostic risk are both feasible with present technology, it is reasonable to consider prenatal intervention. Pioneering work in fetal therapy for this lesion was performed at the Fetal Treatment Center of the University of California at San Francisco (Adzick, et al., 1993, 1985; Adzick and Harrison, 1993; Harrison, et al., 1990). After first establishing a clinical protocol that allowed fetal operative intervention in humans, this group was able to report on their experience in nine cases of fetal intervention for cystic adenomatoid malformation. In six of these cases, resection of the massively enlarged lobe was performed; the other three underwent thoracoamniotic shunt. Four patients who underwent in utero resection are alive 6 to 21 months after birth. The authors note that ultrasound-guided percutaneous drainage results in only a temporary reduction in the size of the cyst, and reaccumulation with recurrent mediastinal compression occurs within 24 to 48 hours after thoracentesis. More recently other centers have reported their experience with antenatal intervention for congenital cystic adenomatoid malformation (Clark, et al., 1987; Dumez, et al., 1993; Nicolaides, et al., 1987). Because fetal surgery requires extensive scientific and clinical experience, it is appropriate for patients with prenatally diagnosed congenital cystic adenomatoid malformations to be referred to centers experienced with the myriad details of antenatal diagnosis and therapy.

Congenital cystic adenomatoid malformations that present postnatally are treated by posterolateral thoracotomy and resection of the involved lung tissue (Haller, et al., 1979; Nishibayashi, et al., 1981; Ribet, et al., 1990; Wesley, et al., 1986; Wolf, et al., 1980). Most commonly an entire lobe is replaced by the adenomatous process, and lobectomy is required. In certain cases diagnosed prenatally but with intrauterine regression, only a small residual is found at thoracotomy, and a more limited resection is possible. Furthermore, in some patients intrauterine regression of the cystic adenomatoid malformation may progress to a point at which no surgical intervention is required (Adzick, et al., 1985; Fine, et al., 1988; Hatjis and Wall, 1992; Saltzman, et al., 1988). When exploring these patients, it should be realized that the normal anatomic structures may be absent or grossly distorted. The best approach is a slow careful serial ligation of the vessels to the involved lobe followed by bronchial division. The results of surgical resection in postnatal disease are good, with resolution of the respiratory distress in the majority of patients.

Atkinson, et al. (1992) reported on three patients who developed pulmonary hypertension after postnatal resection of congenital cystic adenomatoid malformations. All three did

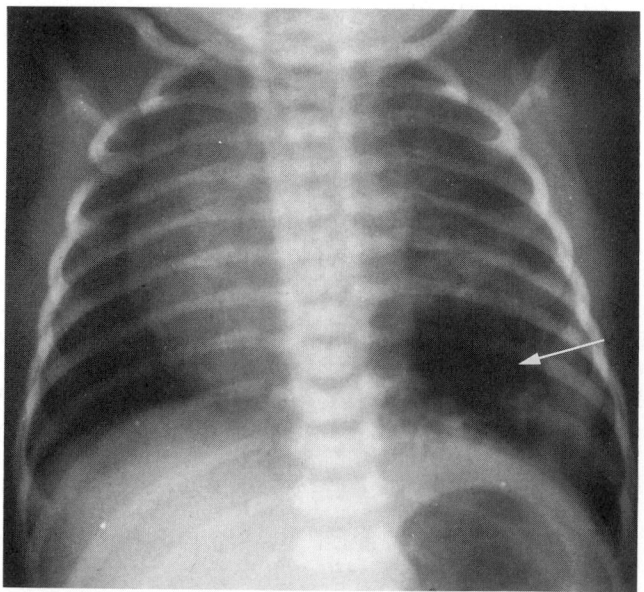

Figure 19-9. A plain chest radiograph demonstrating a congenital cystic adenomatoid malformation.

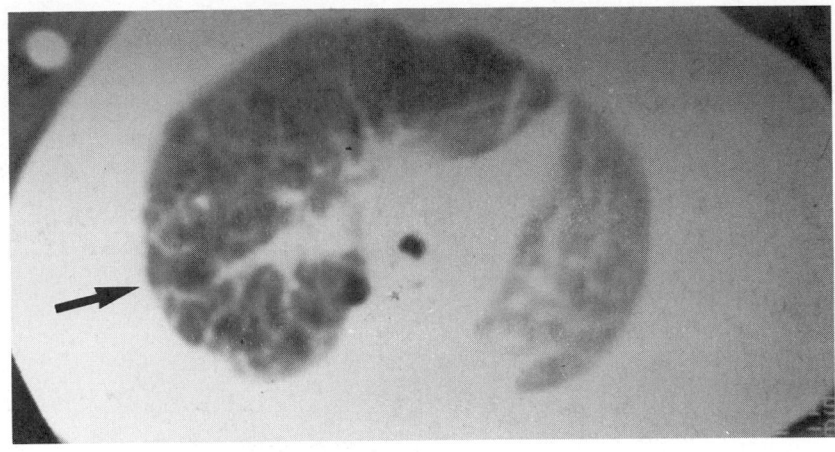

Figure 19-10. CT scan of a cystic adenomatoid malformation.

predictably well for a short period after the thoracotomy but required extracorporeal membrane oxygenator support for 66 to 112 hours for the subsequent development of pulmonary hypertension with hypoxemia and acidosis. All patients had the type I histologic subtype. The authors noted that, in one patient, histologic examination of the resected lung tissue showed marked smooth muscle thickening in a pulmonary arteriole. This was in contrast to the previously reported findings of normal pulmonary vasculature in all three histologic subtypes of cystic adenomatoid malformation.

PULMONARY SEQUESTRATION

BASIC SCIENCE

Pathophysiology

Pulmonary sequestrations are masses of nonfunctioning pulmonary tissue that lack a normal communication with the tracheobronchial tree (Gottrup and Lund, 1978; Sieber, 1986; Stocker and Kagan-Hallet, 1979). They may occur within the substance of the lung (intralobar) or originate in an extralobar location. They normally receive their arterial blood supply directly from the thoracic or abdominal aorta or from intercostal branches (Ferris, et al., 1983; Stocker, 1989). Sequestrations are differentiated from accessory pulmonary lobes, which are separated from the normal lung by pleural investments but maintain a normal communication with the trachea, bronchi, or foregut. Accessory pulmonary lobes are extralobar. The incidence of pulmonary sequestration is greater in male patients, by a ratio of 3:1 (Louie, et al., 1993).

Embryology

It is thought that these lesions arise as an accessory lung bud, which then migrates with the developing esophagus. This may account for the variable blood supply and occasional foregut communications observed with these lesions. Some have speculated that intralobar sequestrations may be acquired rather than congenital (Buntain, et al., 1977; Carter, 1969; Iwai, et al., 1973; Stocker and Malczak, 1984). Autopsy studies reveal inflammatory changes within intralobar se-

questrations in support of this concept. However, Nicolette, et al. (1993), in a series of four surgical specimens, were able to demonstrate progression from no inflammatory changes in a 3-week-old infant to severe bronchiectasis and marked acute and chronic inflammation in a patient operated on at 6 years of age (Holder and Langston, 1986). This progression of inflammatory changes supports a congenital cause for these intralobar sequestrations. Congenital cystic adenomatoid malformations (type II) have been observed within extralobar pulmonary sequestrations, suggesting similar etiologic factors (Nicolette, et al., 1993; Yogasakaran and Sudhamen, 1991). Other variations include a case of a bilateral sequestration with a bridging tunnel (horseshoe sequestration) (Zangwill and Stocker, 1993), pericardial sequestrations (Cerruti, et al., 1993; Levi, et al., 1990), and an association with congenital bronchoesophageal fistulae (Ahn, et al., 1991). In this latter case, the communication between the sequestration and the esophagus was identified by esophagogram and illustrated the possibility that pulmonary sequestrations can have abnormal communications with the foregut. Some of these foregut communications have been shown to contain pancreatic tissue (Evers, et al., 1990). Sixty to 90 percent of sequestrations are located in the left posteroinferior thorax close to the diaphragm and lower lobe. The posterobasal segment of the left lower lobe is a common site for intralobar sequestrations, but intralobar lesions have also been identified in the upper lobes and rarely in the middle lobe or bilaterally. There have also been multiple reports of sequestrations occurring below the diaphragm (Black and Welch, 1986; Lager, et al., 1991; Sargent, et al., 1992; Shih, et al., 1990; Stern, et al., 1990; Tilson and Touloukian, 1976).

As noted earlier, the blood supply to pulmonary sequestrations is systemic and consists of one large branch or multiple small branches from the thoracic aorta. The systemic arterial supply may be large enough to cause a severe left-to-right shunt, with resultant congestive heart failure or hemoptysis (Brus, et al., 1993; Levine, et al., 1992; Matzinger, et al., 1992). Aneurysmal degeneration has been reported in the abnormal sequestration vasculature. A rupture with hemothorax may occur, or the vessels may fistulize to the pulmonary artery (Hayakawa, et al., 1991). The venous drainage from a pulmonary sequestration may be through the pulmonary or azygos veins.

Extralobar sequestrations have the consistency of liver and do not contain air spaces; intralobar lesions may contain air spaces but have no normal communication with the normal tracheobronchial tree. Infected sequestrations can demonstrate air-fluid levels, implying communication to the tracheobronchial tree, probably caused by erosion and fistulization. There is a report of a sequestration containing a fungal mycetoma (Koyama, et al., 1992). Chronic inflammation in a sequestration may result in malignant change, as evidenced by a report of mesothelioma (Uppal, et al., 1993), or the development hundreds of neuroendocrine tumorlets in a chronically scarred intralobar sequestration (Paksoy, et al., 1992).

DIAGNOSIS

Clinical Features

Feeding difficulties, failure to thrive, dyspnea, cyanosis, and other signs of respiratory distress are frequent clinical findings in these patients (Pelosi, et al., 1992; Piccione and Burt, 1990). In older patients the sequestration may be asymptomatic and observed as an incidental finding on chest radiographs (Grove, et al., 1990). Older patients may also present with symptoms of chronic pulmonary infection or even bronchiectasis. All patients may have a continuous murmur, which radiates to the back. As noted earlier, there are also reports of aneurysmal degeneration of the systemic feeding artery to the sequestration with subsequent thrombosis and hemoptysis. Because a sequestration is a form of systemic-pulmonary shunt, some patients may also present with congestive heart failure. If the sequestration arises below the diaphragm, it may present as an abdominal mass.

Imaging and Diagnostic Studies

Antenatal ultrasound diagnosis has been reported. However, Dolkart, et al. (1992) noted that the definitive identification of pulmonary sequestrations is only made in 35 percent of cases, based on the typical ultrasonographic finding of a fetal mass (thoracic or sometimes infradiaphragmatic (Sugio, et al., 1992). When these lesions are noted with fetal hydrops, stillbirth or neonatal death is universal. Fetal hydrops is observed in 35 percent of cases. Associated findings included polyhydramnios, fetal pleural effusions, mediastinal shifts, and pulmonary hypoplasia. Preterm labor was also more frequently observed in the face of this in utero diagnosis. Matzinger, et al. (1992) reported finding a hyperechoic mass in the right upper quadrant of a fetus at 20 and 33 weeks' gestation. This was thought to be a neuroblastoma but on exploration was found to be an infradiaphragmatic pulmonary sequestration. Others have reported that fetal pulmonary sequestrations are echogenic on ultrasound but may have small hypoechoic areas.

After birth the usual initial imaging study is a plain chest radiograph (Fig. 19-11). In the case of extralobar sequestrations, the lung tissue has no connection with the bronchial tree and, therefore, has the consistency of liver. This appears

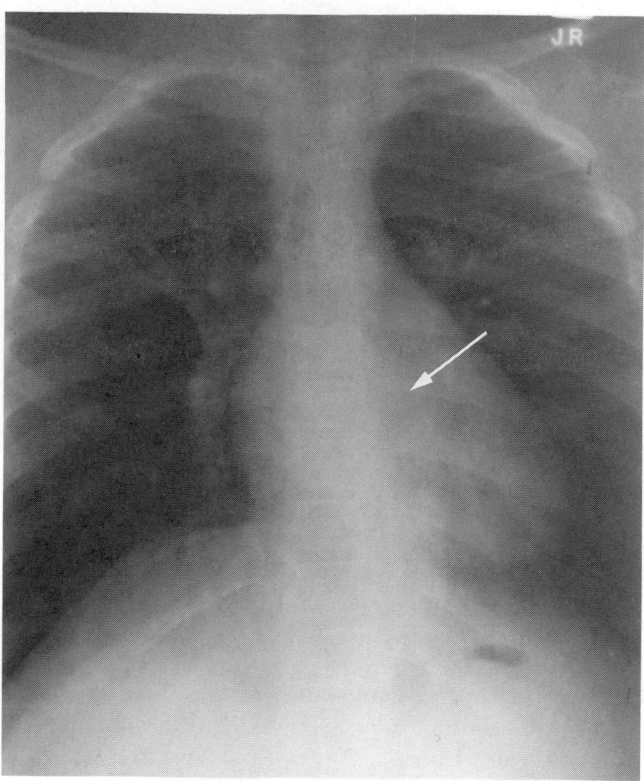

Figure 19-11. Plain chest radiograph of a left posterior pulmonary sequestration.

as a mass, usually between the lower lobe and the diaphragm, on plain chest films. Intralobar sequestrations may also present as a mass. Sometimes intralobar lesions contain air secondary to abnormal connections with the tracheobronchial tree and the radiographic picture is cystic. Rarely, both intra-

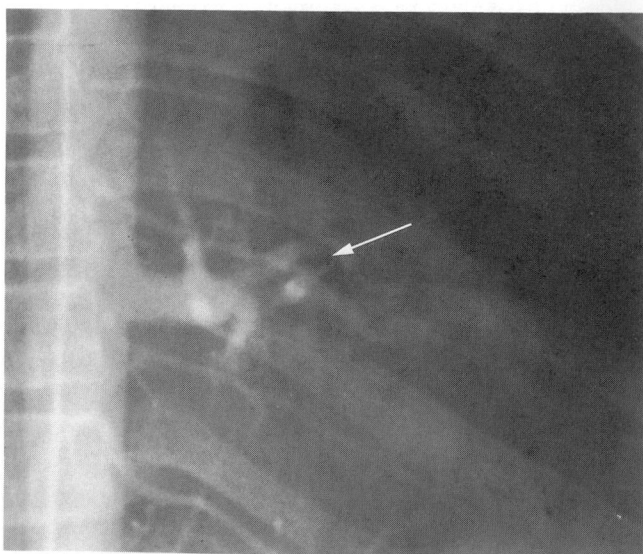

Figure 19-12. Aortography of the same patient whose sequestration is depicted in Figures 19-13 and 19-14. This shows a large feeding vessel *(arrow)* derived from the lower thoracic aorta with what appear to be four major subdivisions.

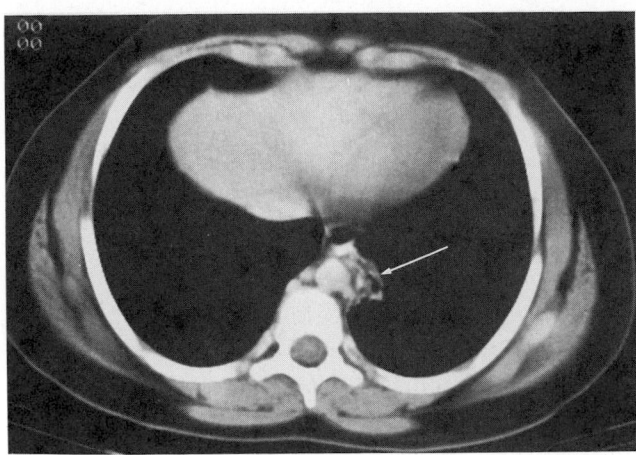

Figure 19-13. CT scan of a left posterior pulmonary sequestration. The arterial blood supply derived from the thoracic aorta is visible.

lobar and extralobar sequestrations have been observed in the same patient (Dolkart, et al., 1992). In the past, aortography with a demonstration of the abnormal systemic feeding vessel to the sequestration was used as a confirmatory procedure (Fig. 19-12). More recently, duplex Doppler ultrasound demonstrated the anomalous aortic branches without the morbidity (general anesthesia and risk of arterial injury or thrombosis) of aortography (Eisenberg, et al., 1992; Kim, et al., 1993). Abdominal vessels will not be clearly defined by plain radiographs, and CT or MRI images should be obtained to provide adequate anatomical detail. CT scans and magnetic resonance angiography may allow visualization of the arterial inflow and give information similar to contrast aortography (Hemanz-Schulman, et al., 1991; Kauczor, et al., 1992) (Figs. 19-13 and 19-14). In summary, a plain chest radiograph followed by Doppler ultrasound and magnetic resonance imaging to demonstrate systemic feeding vessels will give adequate diagnostic and anatomic information for surgery in

the case of thoracic sequestrations. More detailed imaging studies are required when an infradiaphragmatic lesion is suspected.

MANAGEMENT

Therapy

The therapy of pulmonary sequestrations is resection, with the specific approach dependent on the location of the lesion. Lower interspace posterolateral thoracotomy is performed for thoracic lesions. Retroperitoneal or abdominal sequestrations may require a laparotomy or even a thoracoabdominal approach. In general it is preferable to identify and ligate the arterial supply to the sequestration as the initial maneuver in the resection (Fig. 19-15). Serious hemorrhage may occur if these feeders are not identified and ligated. Resection can usually be performed without major morbidity and is curative. Intralobar lesions almost always require lobectomy. Extralobar sequestrations that are invested with a separate layer of visceral pleura are simply resected.

CONGENITAL PULMONARY VASCULAR MALFORMATIONS

BASIC SCIENCE

Pathophysiology

These lesions are characterized by an abnormal communication between abnormal pulmonary arteries and pulmonary veins, which results in greater or lesser degrees of right-to-left shunting.

Embryology

As noted previously the ingrowth of mesenchyme into the foregut pharyngeal pouch brings with it the capacity for the development of the pulmonary vasculature. During blood

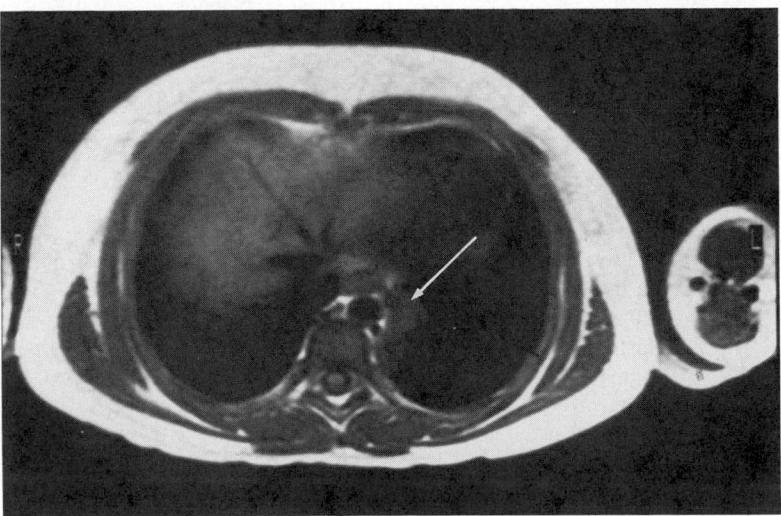

Figure 19-14. Magnetic resonance imaging scan of the same pulmonary sequestration imaged in Figure 19-13. Again, the systemic blood supply is evident.

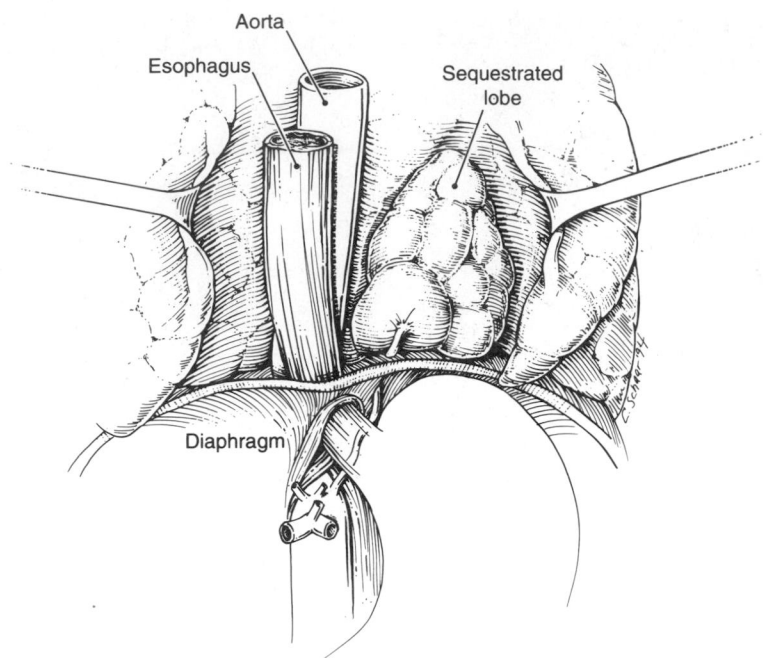

Figure 19-15. An illustration of a left posterior pulmonary sequestration showing the systemic arterial supply arising from below the diaphragm. Major hemorrhage can result from a failure to recognize this anomaly and inadvertent division of these vessels during resection.

vessel development, primitive arteriovenous connections form to initiate the flow of blood. Subsequent vascular remodeling results in normal vessel development. Arteriovenous malformations result from unknown stimuli during the stage of arteriovenous communication in the retiform plexus. The large friable sac that results can be the source of serious hemorrhage (Fig. 19-16).

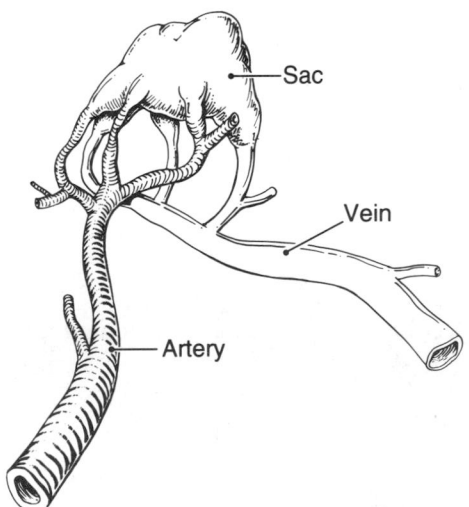

Figure 19-16. An illustration depicting the anatomic lesion in arteriovenous malformations. The saclike malformation is thin walled and easily ruptured or torn with resultant severe hemorrhage.

DIAGNOSIS

Clinical Features

Patients with pulmonary arteriovenous malformations may present with the Rendu-Osler-Weber syndrome (cutaneous and mucosal spider angiomas) (57 percent), hemoptysis, dyspnea on exertion (67 percent), congestive heart failure, or a major neurologic event, such as a stroke or intracerebral abscess (33 percent) (Djindjian, et al., 1973; Maruyama, et al., 1989; Puskas, et al., 1993). The degree of congestive heart failure is dependent on the size of the right-to-left shunt (Ribet and Denimal, 1991; Whyte, et al., 1992). A continuous murmur may be heard over the involved hemithorax. Because a thrombus may develop in the abnormal vessels constituting these lesions, some patients may present with evidence of systemic emboli, especially stroke, brain abscess, or multiple distant abscesses. There is also a reported association between multiple pulmonary arteriovenous malformations and polysplenia (Papagiannis, et al., 1993).

Imaging and Diagnostic Studies

Plain chest radiographs show a solid mass in the lung, and it may be difficult to differentiate an arteriovenous malformation from a lung tumor. In one reported case, an arteriovenous malformation closely simulated a bronchogenic carcinoma on plain chest radiographs, but no lesion was palpable at thoracotomy. The diagnosis was only made postoperatively (Kilgore and Chasen, 1983). In the past, pulmonary arteriograms have been diagnostic and also present the opportunity for therapeutic embolization. More recently, magnetic

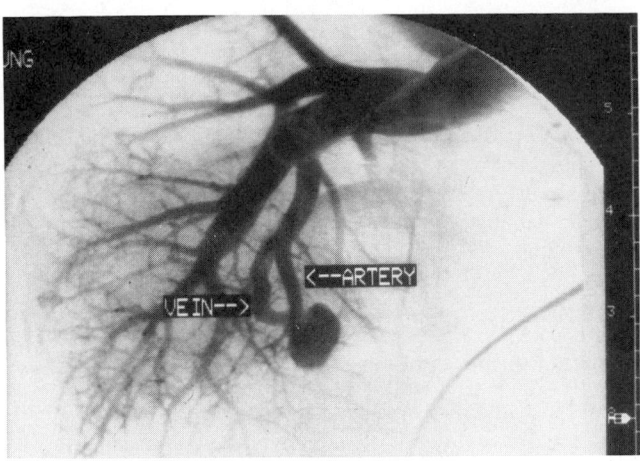

Figure 19-17. A pulmonary arteriogram demonstrating an arteriovenous malformation.

resonance imaging has been able to differentiate vascular malformations (hemangiomas or venous and arteriovenous malformations) with excellent accuracy (Gutierrez, et al., 1984; Dinsmore, et al., 1990; Webb, et al., 1984). Presently, MRI with the addition of magnetic resonance angiography is an adequate confirmatory test and gives good information concerning feeding vessels, multiple lesions, and anatomic localization. Other imaging modalities that have been used for the evaluation of pulmonary arteriovenous malformations include CT with contrast and contrast (agitated saline) echocardiograms (Barzilai, et al., 1991; Remy, et al., 1992).

MANAGEMENT

Therapy

The therapy for symptomatic congenital pulmonary arteriovenous malformations previously consisted of surgical resec-

tion when feasible. This is useful for localized and large lesions. More recently, there has been a trend to treat these lesions using angiographic embolization (Hartnell, et al., 1990; Hughes and Allinson, 1990; Jackson, et al., 1990). An assortment of balloons, springs, coils, and thrombogenic materials has been used with good initial success. Because embolization avoids the morbidity of thoracotomy and, at least in short-term follow-up, is effective in reducing the right-to-left shunt and ameliorating the symptoms of heart failure, it is now considered first-line therapy (Goergen and Sacharias, 1992; Pennington, et al., 1992) (Figs. 19-17 and 19-18). A pulmonary arteriovenous malformation is depicted in Figure 19-17, and its successful therapy by embolization is shown in Figure 19-18. Surgery should be reserved for localized lesions that have recurred or not responded to embolic therapy. In very large malformations, the combination of embolization followed by surgical removal may be advantageous in preventing infection in a large mass of infarcted lung tissue.

LUNG APLASIA AND HYPOPLASIA

BASIC SCIENCE

Pathophysiology

Pulmonary tissue may simply fail to develop totally or partially, giving rise to pulmonary aplasia or hypoplasia (Boxer, et al., 1978; Campanella and Odell, 1987; Chilvers, et al., 1990; Goergen and Sacharias, 1992; Gwinn, et al., 1976; Hofner, et al., 1979; Maltz and Nadas, 1968; Oran, et al., 1979; Oyamada, et al., 1953; Sbokos and McMillan, 1977; Shenoy, et al., 1979). An entire lung on one side may be missing or one or more lobes may be absent. Uncommonly agenesis of both lungs may also occur (Claireaux and Ferreira, 1958; Kaya and Dilmen, 1989; Ostor, et al., 1978). There is a reported association between bilateral pulmonary agenesis and microphthalmia (Toriello, et al., 1985).

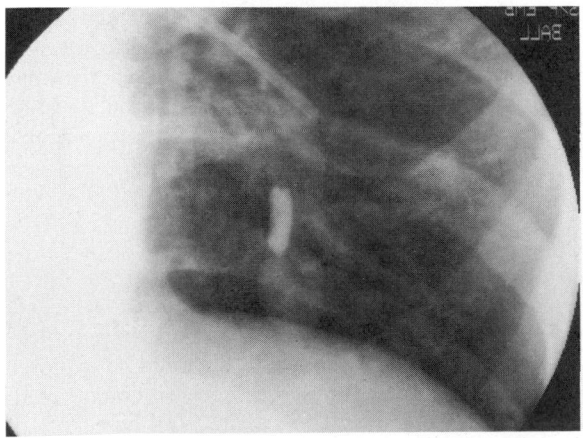
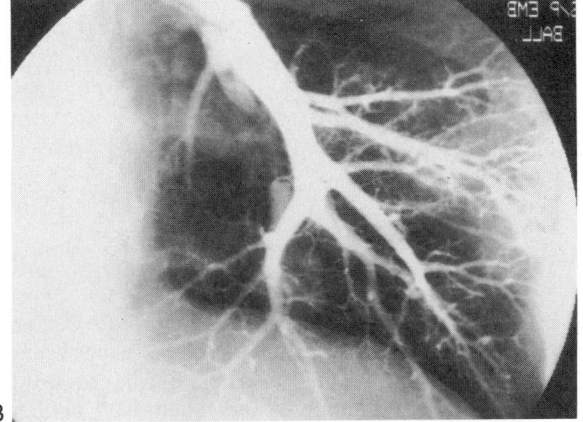

Figure 19-18. **(A)** A plain chest radiograph showing a detachable intravascular balloon positioned in the large feeding vessel to the arteriovenous malformation (AVM) depicted in Figure 19-17. **(B)** Successful obliteration of the AVM following detachment of the intravascular balloon. Assorted other devices (i.e., springs, Gelfoam, etc.) are now commonly used for this purpose.

Embryology

Potter's syndrome, which consists of bilateral renal agenesis associated with a typical appearance of the facies and pulmonary hypoplasia, suggests a connection between renal and pulmonary development (Gale and Stocker, 1987; Hislop, et al., 1979; Loendersloot, et al., 1978; Nakamura, et al., 1985; Ray, et al., 1975; Stechele and Straub, 1978; Spear, et al., 1987; Tinaztepe, et al., 1983). It is postulated that fetal lung development is controlled in utero by the kidneys, possibly through the secretion of growth factors. Brinsmead, et al. (1980), in a study on nephrectomized fetal lambs, showed that the fetal serum concentrations of placental lactogen and somatomedins was higher in the anephric animals (Greene, et al., 1986). The authors suggest that the kidney plays a role in the clearance of these hormones in the fetus. They speculate that the pulmonary growth retardation after fetal nephrectomy may be the result of increased binding of somatomedins by serum proteins or inhibition of somatomedin action by unidentified serum factors. Similarly, somatomedin-like receptor activity was greater in nephrectomized animals. These observations point to a feedback loop between the fetal lung and kidney, which is presently under intense investigation. In summary, renal maldevelopment is usually associated with pulmonary dysgenesis.

In other experiments of nature, complete tracheal or laryngeal obstruction has been associated with pulmonary hyperplasia (Brinsmead, et al., 1980; Scurry, et al., 1989). However, fetuses with incomplete tracheal or laryngeal obstruction (stenosis) usually develop pulmonary aplasia or hypoplasia (Harrison, et al., 1980; Konoshi, et al., 1986; Voland, et al., 1986; Wigglesworth, et al., 1987). For unknown reasons complete fetal airway obstruction stimulates lung growth, but incomplete obstruction suppresses it. There is also a strong reported association of pulmonary dysgenesis with tracheoesophageal fistula and/or esophageal atresia (Benson, et al., 1985; Black and Welch, 1986; Brereton and Rickwood, 1983; DeBuse and Morris, 1973; Ein, et al., 1989; Knowles, et al., 1988; McCormick and Kuhns, 1979; Takayanazi, et al., 1987). Pulmonary aplasia has also been associated with the absence of the phrenic nerve on the ipsilateral side (Hoffman, et al., 1989). Cardiac, vertebral, diaphragmatic, and rib anomalies have also been reported in conjunction with pulmonary dysgenesis (Chavalittamarong, et al., 1980; Courtney and MacKinnon, 1990; Gaziel, et al., 1983; Goldstein and Reid, 1980; Sbokos and McMillan, 1977; To-riello and Bauserman, 1985; Wigglesworth, et al., 1987), as have Frynn's and the scimitar syndrome and omphalocele (Osborne, et al., 1989; Vasquez Sanchez, et al., 1986).

A number of reports have cited the existence of cytogenetic abnormalities in patients with lung agenesis or hypoplasia (Hatanaka, et al., 1984; Hood, et al., 1990; Say, et al., 1980; Schober, et al., 1983). At present, however, there is no known specific genetic defect associated with aplasia or hypoplasia of the lung.

DIAGNOSIS

Clinical Features

Bilateral pulmonary agenesis or severe hypoplasia results in stillbirth or rapid death of the newborn. Other patients with severe hypoplasia may present with respiratory distress. Hemoptysis resulting from pulmonary artery hypertension is also reported (Cogswell and Singh, 1986; Hubsch, et al., 1987; Lopez-Majano, 1985; Mehta, et al., 1987; Pflueger, et al., 1984). Patients with slight degrees of hypoplasia or with aplasia of a single lobe may be asymptomatic and identified incidentally. Other patients may present with cough, wheeze, or pulmonary infection. The symptoms also depend on the extent and type of concomitant anomalies.

MANAGEMENT

Therapy

No therapy may be required for asymptomatic patients, and those with severe or bilateral dysplasia may not survive long enough for intervention to take place. In patients with severe symptoms who can be stabilized, pulmonary transplantation may offer hope of long-term survival.

MISCELLANEOUS LESIONS

Given the complexity of lung development, myriad other categories of congenital lesions can be imaged. Fortunately, other congenital pulmonary anomalies are even more uncommon than those discussed. There have been various reports of lymphangiomas or simple congenital cysts. With regard to the latter, there is controversy over whether they actually constitute a category separate from bronchogenic cyst. As always, the careful clinician must assess the lesion and direct therapy based on the severity of symptoms.

COMMENTS AND CONTROVERSIES

The role of fetal surgery and the use of endoscopic techniques in the treatment of congenital pulmonary anomalies remain controversial. Great strides have been made in antenatal diagnosis and intervention, but precise indications have not been elucidated for all lesions. Also, long-term follow-up to judge the results of therapy is not available. Finally, the cost of fetal intervention has not been weighed against its potential benefits. In the present climate of fiscal responsibility in medicine, these issues will have to be addressed. Nevertheless, this is a frontier of surgery and should be explored. It must be emphasized that fetal intervention is complicated and there are inherent risks, not only to the fetus, but also to the healthy mother. This type of surgery should be undertaken only in centers that have a record of excellence in both the technical and scientific aspects of prenatal intervention.

As more procedures are successfully performed with the

use of endoscopic techniques, it is logical to expect that pulmonary anomalies will be treated under certain circumstances videothoracoscopically. Again, the possibilities for endoscopic intervention should be explored, but only in experienced centers with a scientific approach, so that valid conclusions regarding toxicity and efficacy will be forthcoming.

M.P.L.Q.

The exciting developments occurring in antenatal diagnosis and fetal surgery presently reside within the province of pediatric surgeons. In large tertiary referral centers, pediatric cardiothoracic surgery is a subspecialty that almost certainly will be exploring this new field. Most adult cardiothoracic surgeons encounter congenital anomalies when they present in the young adult. This is especially true of pulmonary sequestration, bronchogenic cysts and AV malformations.

Unlike Dr. La Quaglia, I have always attempted to treat pulmonary sequestration by segmentectomy and have accomplished this quite successfully, thereby preserving the rest of the otherwise normal lobe. Bronchogenic cysts can develop late complications. A significant number of these patients, even when watched closely, will present with major complications including airways obstruction. For this reason, especially with the advent of simpler approaches such as video-assisted thoracoscopy, most bronchogenic cysts should be excised to avoid the complications of late rapid enlargement. This is especially true of mediastinal cysts, which can cause life-threatening airway compression.

There continues to be controversy concerning the best management of AV malformation. It is possible, with increasing expertise by interventional radiologists, that embolization will be the treatment of choice in all centers for this anomaly. However, there is a steep learning curve associated with this technique, meaning that it probably should be used only by those with significant expertise in angiographic embolization.

R.J.G.

REFERENCES

Adzick NS, Harrison MR: Management of the fetus with a cystic adenomatoid malformation. World J Surg 17:342, 1993

Adzick NS, Harrison MR, Flake AW et al: Fetal surgery for cystic adenomatoid malformation of the lung. J Pediatr Surg 28:806, 1993

Adzick NS, Harrison MR, Glick PL et al: Fetal cystic adenomatoid malformation. J Pediatr Surg 20:483, 1985

Ahn CM, Kim HJ, Cho HK et al: A case of intrapericardial extralobar pulmonary sequestration—first case in Korea. Korean J Intern Med 6:85, 1991

Al-Salem AH, Adu-Gyamfi Y, Grant CS: Congenital lobar emphysema. Can J Anaesth 37:377, 1990

Amendola MA, Shirazi KK, Brooks J et al: Transdiaphragmatic bronchopulmonary foregut anomaly: "dumbell bronchogenic cyst." Am J Radiol 138:1165, 1982

Atkinson JB, Ford EG, Kitagawa H et al: Persistent pulmonary hypertension complicating cystic adenomatoid malformation in neonates. J Pediatr Surg 27:54, 1992

Ayme S, Julian C, Gambarelli D et al: Fryns syndrome: report on 8 new cases. Clin Genet 35:191, 1989

Bale PM: Congenital cystic malformation of the lung. A form of congenital bronchiolar (adenomatoid) malformation. Am J Clin Pathol 71:411, 1979

Balquet P: Bronchogenic cysts compressing the trachea and main bronchus. Chir Pediatr 24:270, 1984

Barzilai B, Waggoner AD, Spessert C et al: Two-dimensional contrast echocardiography in the detection and follow-up of congenital pulmonary arteriovenous malformations. Am J Cardiol 68:1507, 1991

Benson JE, Olsen MM, Fletcher BD: A spectrum of bronchopulmonary anomalies associated with tracheoesophageal malformations. Pediatr Radiol 15:377, 1985

Bentur L, Canny G, Thorner P et al: Spontaneous pneumothorax in cystic adenomatoid malformation. Unusual clinical and histologic features. Chest 99:1292, 1991

Berlinger NT, Porto DP, Thompson TR: Infantile lobar emphysema. Ann Otol Rhinol Laryngol 96:106, 1987

Black MD, Bass J, Martin DJ, Carpenter BF: Intraabdominal pulmonary sequestration. J Pediatr Surg 26:1381, 1991

Black PR, Welch KJ: Pulmonary agenesis (aplasia), esophageal atresia, and tracheoesophageal fistula: a different treatment strategy. J Pediatr Surg 21:936, 1986

Blackader AD, Evans DJ: A case of mediastinal cyst producing compression of the trachea, ending fatally in an infant of nine months. Arch Pediatr 28:194, 1911

Blott M, Nicolaides K, Greenough A: Postnatal respiratory function after chronic drainage of fetal pulmonary cyst. Am J Obstet Gynecol 159:858, 1988

Boglino C, Inserra A, Serventi P et al: Neurotensin localization in adenomatoid cystic malformation versus normal lung: preliminary report of six consecutive cases. J Pediatr Surg 27:57, 1992

Borg SA, Young LW, Roghair GD: Congenital avalvular pulmonary artery and infantile lobar emphysema. A diagnostic correlation. AJR 125:412, 1975

Boulot P, Pages A, Deschamps F et al: Early prenatal diagnosis of congenital cystic adenomatoid malformation of the lung (Stocker's type I); a case report. Eur J Obstet Gynecol Reprod Biol 41:159, 1991

Bower RJ, Kiesewetter WB: Mediastinal masses in infants and children. Arch Surg 112:1003, 1977

Boxer RA, Hayes CJ, Hordof AJ, Mellins RB: Agenesis of the left lung and total anomalous pulmonary venous connection. Hemodynamic studies before and after complete surgical correction. Chest 74:106, 1978

Brereton RJ, Rickwood AM: Esophageal atresia with pulmonary agenesis. J Pediatr Surg 18:618, 1983

Brinsmead MW, Waters MJ, Thorburn GD et al: Increase in placental lactogen and somatomedins after nephrectomy. J Dev Physiol 2:205, 1980

Brus F, Nikkels PG, van Loon AJ, Okken A: Non-immune hydrops fetalis and bilateral pulmonary hypoplasia in newborn infant with extralobar pulmonary sequestration. Acta Paediatr 82:416, 1993

Buckner CB, Walker CW, Shah HR, Fitzrandolph RL: Bronchogenic cysts. Am Fam Physician 40:167, 1989

Buntain WL, Woolley MM, Mahour GH et al: Pulmonary sequestration in children: a twenty-five year experience. Surgery 81:413, 1977

Campanella C, Odell JA: Unilateral pulmonary agenesis. A report of 4 cases. South Afr Med J 71:785, 1987

Canty TG: Congenital lobar emphysema resulting from a bronchial sling around a normal right main pulmonary artery. J Thorac Cardiovasc Surg 74:126, 1977

Canty TG, Hendren WH: Upper airway obstruction from foregut cysts of the hypopharynx. J Pediatr Surg 10:807, 1975

Carlens E: Mediastinoscopy: a method for inspection and tissue biopsy in the superior mediastinum. Dis Chest 36:343, 1959

Carter R: Pulmonary sequestration: collective review. Ann Thorac Surg 7:68, 1969

Cartmill JA, Hughes CF: Bronchogenic cysts: a persistent dilemma. Aust NZJ Surg 59:253, 1989

Cerruti MM, Marmolejos F, Cacciarelli T: Bilateral intralobar pulmonary sequestration with horseshoe lung. Ann Thorac Surg 55:509, 1993

Chavalittamrong B, Podhipleux P, Pongpipat D: Agenesis of the left lung associated with vertebral anomalies, fusion of rib and sacralization: report of a case. J Med Assoc Thai 63:46, 1980

Chilvers ER, Whyte MK, Jackson JE et al: Effect of percutaneous transcatheter embolization on pulmonary function, right-to-left shunt, and arterial oxygenation in patients with pulmonary arteriovenous malformations. Am Rev Respir Dis 142:420, 1990

Ch'in KY, Tang MY: Congenital adenomatoid malformation of one lobe of a lung with general anasarca. Arch Pathol Lab Med 48:221, 1949

Claireaux AE, Ferreira HP: Bilateral pulmonary agenesis. Arch Dis Child 33:364, 1958

Clark SL, Vitale DJ, Minton SD et al: Successful fetal therapy for cystic adenomatoid malformation associated with second-trimester hydrops. Am J Obstet Gynecol 157:294, 1987

Cogswell TL, Singh S: Agenesis of the left pulmonary artery as a cause of hemoptysis. Angiology 37:154, 1986

Cohen SR, Thompson JW, Brennan LP: Foregut cysts presenting as neck masses. A report on three children. Ann Otol Rhinol Laryngol 94:433, 1985

Coselli MP, de Ipolyi P, Bloss RS et al: Bronchogenic cysts above and below the diaphragm: report of eight cases. Ann Thorac Surg 44:491, 1987

Cote CJ: The anesthetic management of congenital lobar emphysema. Anesthesiology 49:296, 1978

Courtney SP, MacKinnon AE: Pulmonary agenesis associated with fourteen other congenital abnormalities. Br J Clin Pract 44:291, 1990

Deacon CS, Smart PJ, Rimmer S: The antenatal diagnosis of congenital cystic adenomatoid malformation of the lung. Br J Radiol 63:968, 1990

DeBuse PJ, Morris G: Bilateral pulmonary agenesis, oesophageal atresia, and the first arch syndrome. Thorax 28:526, 1973

Di Lorenzo M, Collin PP, Vaillancourt R, Duranceau A: Bronchogenic cysts. J Pediatr Surg 24:988, 1989

Dinsmore BJ, Gefter WB, Hatabu H, Kressel HY: Pulmonary arteriovenous malformations: diagnosis by gradient-refocused MR imaging. J Comp Assist Tomogr 14:918, 1990

Djindjian R, Cophignon J, Théron J et al: Embolization by superselective arteriography from the femoral route in neuroradiology. Review of 60 cases: I. Technique, indications, complications. Neuroradiology 6:20, 1973

Dolkart LA, Reimers FT, Helmuth WV et al: Antenatal diagnosis of pulmonary sequestration: a review. Obstet Gynecol Surv 47:515, 1992

Doyle AJ: Demonstration of blood supply to pulmonary sequestration by MR angiography. AJR 158:989, 1992

Dubois P, Bèlanger R, Wellington JL: Bronchogenic cyst presenting as a supraclavicular mass. Can J Surg 24:530, 1981

Dumez Y, Mandelbrot N, Radunovic N et al: Prenatal management of congenital cystic adenomatoid malformation of the lung. J Pediatr Surg 28:36, 1993

Ein SH, Shandling B, Wesson D, Filler RM: Esophageal atresia with distal tracheoesophageal fistula: associated anomalies and prognosis in the 1980s. J Pediatr Surg 24:1055, 1989

Eisenberg P, Cohen HL, Coren C: Color Doppler in pulmonary sequestration diagnosis. J Ultrasound Med 11:175, 1992

Ekkelkamp S, Vos A: Successful surgical treatment of a newborn with bilateral congenital lobar emphysema. J Pediatr Surg 22:1001, 1987

Engel S: The structure of the respiratory tissue in the newly-born. Acta Anat (Basel) 19:353, 1953

Engle WA, Lemons JA, Weber TR, Cohen MD: Congenital lobar emphysema due to a bronchogenic cyst. Am J Perinatol 1:196, 1984

Eraklis AJ, Griscom NT, McGovern JB: Bronchogenic cysts of the mediastinum in infancy. N Engl J Med 281:1150, 1969

Evers WB, Vissers R, van Noord JA: Pulmonary sequestration with congenital broncho-oesophageal fistula. Eur Respir J 3:1067, 1990

Fekete F, Rongere C, Foulon JP, Molas G: Bronchogenic esophageal cysts in the adult. Four cases. Presse Med 17:851, 1988

Ferris EJ, Smith PL, Mirza FH et al: Intralobar pulmonary sequestration: value of aortography and pulmonary arteriography. Cardiovasc Intervent Radiol 4:17, 1981

Fine C, Adzick NS, Doubilet PM: Decreasing size of a congenital cystic adenomatoid malformation in utero. J Ultrasound Med 7:405, 1988

Frenckner B, Freychuss U: Pulmonary function after lobectomy for congenital lobar emphysema and congenital cystic adenomatoid malformation. A follow-up study. Scand J Thorac Cardiovasc Surg 16:293, 1982

Fukomoto K, Matsuzaki Y, Yoshioka M et al: Congenital bronchomalacia of the left main bronchus combined with lobar emphysema, pectus excavatum and right aortic arch—a case report. Nippon Kyobu Geka Gakkai Zasshi 39:943, 1991

Gale DH, Stocker JT: Cloacal dysgenesis with urethral, vaginal outlet, and anal agenesis and functioning internal genitourinary excretion. Pediatr Pathol 7:457, 1987

Gaziel Y, Hoek BB, van Niekerk CH: Agenesis of the right lung associated with hypoplasia of the fourth right rib. A case report. S Afr Med J 64:871, 1983

Gille P, Aubert D, Menget A, Thura JP: Bilateral congenital eventration of the diaphragm with giant lobar emphysema. Chir Pediatr 20:359, 1979

Ginsberg RJ, Atkins RW, Paulson DL: A bronchogenic cyst successfully treated by mediastinoscopy. Ann Thorac Surg 13:266, 1972

Ginsberg RJ, Kirby TJ: Bronchogenic cysts. p. 84. In Grillo HC, Austin WG, Wilkins EW Jr et al. (eds): Current Therapy in Cardiothoracic Surgery. BC Decker, Toronto, 1989

Goergen SK, Sacharias NR: Pulmonary arteriovenous malformations: pathology, clinical features and treatment with balloon and coil occlusion. Australas Radiol 36:222, 1992

Goldstein JD, Reid LM: Pulmonary hypoplasia resulting from phrenic nerve agenesis and diaphragmatic amyoplasia. J Pediatr 97:282, 1980

Gordon I, Dempsey JE: Infantile lobar emphysema in association with congenital heart disease. Clin Radiol 41:48, 1990

Goto H, Boozalis ST, Benson KT, Arakawa K: High-frequency jet ventilation for resection of congenital lobar emphysema. Anesth Analg 66:684, 1987

Gottrup F, Lund C: Intralobar pulmonary sequestration. A report of 12 cases. Scand J Respir Dis 59:21, 1978

Gray, Skandalakis: Embryology for Surgeons. WB Saunders, Philadelphia, 1972

Greene RA, Bloch MJ, Huff DS, Iozzo RV: MURCS association with additional congenital anomalies. Hum Pathol 17:88, 1986

Gross RE, Lewis JE: Defect of the anterior mediastinum. Surg Gynecol Obstet 80:549, 1945

Grove MK, Goodwin CD, Nanagas VN: Extralobar pulmonary sequestration. Cleve Clin J Med 57:88, 1990

Gutierrez FR, Glazer HS, Levitt RG, Moran JF: NMR imaging of pulmonary arteriovenous fistulae. J Comput Assist Tomogr 8:750, 1984

Gwinn JL, Lee FA, Davachi F, Rothberg M: Radiological case of the month. Agenesis of the left lung. Am J Dis Child 130:1121, 1976

Haller JA Jr, Golladay ES, Pickard LR et al: Surgical management of lung bud anomalies: lobar emphysema, bronchogenic cyst, cystic adenomatoid malformation, and intralobar pulmonary sequestration. Ann Thorac Surg 28:33, 1979

Haller JA Jr, Shermeta DW, Donahoo JS, White JJ: Life-threatening respiratory distress from mediastinal masses in infants. Ann Thorac Surg 19:364, 1975

Ham AW, Baldwin KW: A histological study of the development of the lung, with particular reference to the nature of alveoli. Anat Rec 81:363, 1941

Harrison MR, Adzick NS, Jennings RW et al: Antenatal intervention for congenital cystic adenomatoid malformation. Lancet 336:965, 1990

Harrison MR, Heldt GP, Brasch RC et al: Resection of distal tracheal stenosis in a baby with agenesis of the lung. J Pediatr Surg 15:938, 1980

Hartnell GG, Jackson JE, Allsion DJ: Coil embolization of pulmonary arteriovenous malformations. Cardiovasc Intervent Radiol 13:347, 1990

Hasse J, Lincoln JC, Paneth M: Differentiated surgical therapy in congenital lobar emphysema. Thoraxchir Vask Chir 23:250, 1975

Hatanaka K, Ozaki M, Suzuki M et al: Trisomy 16q13qter in an infant from a t(11;16)(q25;q13) translocation-carrier father. Hum Genet 65:311, 1984

Hatjis CG, Wall P: Type II congenital cystic adenomatoid malformation of the lung with a mediastinal shift. A case report. J Reprod Med 37:753, 1992

Hayakawa K, Soga T, Hamamoto K et al: Massive hemoptysis from a pulmonary sequestration controlled by embolization of aberrant pulmonary arteries: case report. Cardiovasc Intervent Radiol 14:345, 1991

Heij HA, Ekkelkamp S, Vos A: Diagnosis of congenital cystic adenomatoid malformation of the lung in newborn infants and children. Thorax 45:122, 1990

Hernanz-Schulman M, Stein SM, Neblett WW et al: Pulmonary sequestration: diagnosis with color Doppler sonography and a new theory of associated hydrothorax. Radiology 180:817, 1991

Heydanus R, Stewart PA, Wladimiroff JW, Los FJ: Prenatal diagnosis of congenital cystic adenomatoid lung malformation: a report of seven cases. Prenat Diagn 13:65, 1993

Hill RC, Mantese V, Spock A, Wolfe WG: Management of an unusual case of congenital lobar emphysema. Pediatr Pulmonol 5:252, 1988

Hilpert PL, Pretorius DH: The thorax. p. 276. In Nyberg DA, Mahony BS, Pretorius DH (eds): Diagnostic Ultrasound of Fetal Anomalies. Year Book Medical Publishers, Chicago, 1990

Hislop A, Hey E, Reid L: The lungs in bilateral renal agenesis and dysplasia. Arch Dis Child 54:32, 1979

Hoffman MA, Superina R, Wesson DE: Unilateral pulmonary agenesis with esophageal atresia and distal tracheoesophageal fistula: report of two cases. J Pediatr Surg 24:1084, 1989

Hofner W, Bardach G, Ferlitsch A, Kotscher E: Diagnosis of combined malformation of the lung and pulmonary vessels. Rontgenblatter 32:384, 1979

Holder PD, Langston C: Intralobar pulmonary sequestration. Pediatr Pulmonol 2:147, 1986

Hood OJ, Hartwell EA, Shattuck KE, Rosenberg HS: Multiple congenital anomalies associated with a 47,XXX chromosome constitution. Am J Med Genet 36:73, 1990

Hoover JP, Henry GA, Panciera RJ: Bronchial cartilage dysplasia with multifocal lobar bullous emphysema and lung torsions in a pup. J Am Vet Med Assoc 201:599, 1992

Huber JJ: Observationes aliquot de arteria singulari pulmoni concessa. Acta Helv 8:85, 1777

Hubsch P, Pichler W, Lang I, Mlczoch J: Isolated agenesis of the right pulmonary artery with late manifestation of pulmonary artery hypertension. Rontgenblatter 40:23, 1987

Hughes JM, Allison DJ: Pulmonary arteriovenous malformations: the radiologist replaces the surgeon. Clin Radiol 41:297, 1990

Hunter W: The history of an aneurysm of the aorta with some remarks on aneurysms in general. Obstet Soc Phys (London) 1:323, 1757

Isojima A, Yuasa H, Kusagawa M et al: Surgical treatment of infantile lobar emphysema in cardiovascular disease with left-to-right shunts. Jpn J Surg 8:57, 1978

Iwai K, Shindo G, Hajikano H et al: Intralobar sequestration with special reference to developmental pathology. Am Rev Respir Dis 107:911, 1973

Jackson JE, Whyte MK, Allison DJ, Hughes JM: Coil embolization of pulmonary arteriovenous malformations. Cor Vasa 32:191, 1990

Kauczor HU, Knopp MV, Branscheid D, Semmler W: Pulmonary sequestration: diagnosis based on MR angiographic findings. AJR 159:429, 1992

Kaya IS, Dilmen U: Agenesis of the lung. Eur Respir J 2:690, 1989

Keith HH: Congenital lobar emphysema. Pediatr Ann 6:36, 1977

Keller MS: Congenital lobar emphysema with tracheal bronchus. Can Assoc Radiol J 34:306, 1983

Kennedy CD, Habibi P, Matthew DJ, Gordon I: Lobar emphysema: long-term imaging follow-up. Radiology 180:189, 1991

Kilgore TL, Chasen MH: Pulmonary arteriovenous fistula simulating a vanishing tumor. South Med J 76:884, 1983

Kim HJ, Kim JH, Chung SK et al.: Coexistent intralobar and extralobar pulmonary sequestration: imaging findings. AJR 160:1199, 1993

Kleinman CS, Donnerstein RL, DeVore GR et al: Fetal echocardiography for evaluation of in utero congestive heart failure: a technique for study of nonimmune hydrops. N Engl J Med 306:568, 1982

Knoop U, Gharib M, Ewerback H, Ebel KD: Monatsschr Kinderheilkd 132:780, 1984

Knowles S, Thomas RM, Lindenbaum RH et al: Pulmonary agenesis as part of the VACTERL sequence. Arch Dis Child 63:723, 1988

Kolls JK, Kiernan MP, Ascuitto RJ et al: Intralobar pulmonary sequestration presenting as congestive heart failure in a neonate. Chest 102:974, 1992

Konoshi H, Nakamura H, Mizukami Y et al: A case of pulmonary agenesis associated with congenital tracheal stenosis and aberrant left pulmonary artery. Rinsho Hoshasen 31:741, 1986

Koskas M, Tournier G, Baculard A et al: Bronchogenic cysts in the carina. Rev Mal Respir 9:509, 1992

Koyama A, Sasou K, Nakao H et al: Pulmonary intralobar sequestration accompanied by aneurysm of an anomalous arterial supply. Intern Med 31:946, 1992

Lacquet LK, Lacquet AM: Congenital lobar emphysema. Prog Pediatr Surg 10:307, 1977

Lager DJ, Kuper KA, Haake GK: Subdiaphragmatic extralobar pulmonary sequestration. Arch Pathol Lab Med 115:536, 1991

Langman J: Medical Embryology. Williams & Wilkins, Baltimore, 1969

LaRue MJ, Garlick DS, Lamb CR, O'Callaghan MW: Bronchial dysgenesis and lobar emphysema in the adult cat. J Am Vet Med Assoc 197:886, 1990

Letanche G, Boyer J, Guibert B et al: Bronchogenic cysts and their atypical localizations. A case of pleurodiaphragmatic cyst. Rev Pneumol Clin 40:191, 1984

Levi A, Findler M, Dolfin T et al: Intrapericardial extralobar pulmonary sequestration in a neonate. Chest 98:1014, 1990

Levine MM, Nudel DB, Gootman N et al: Pulmonary sequestration causing congestive heart failure in infancy. Ann Thorac Surg 34:581, 1982

Lewis JE Jr: Pulmonary and bronchial malformations. In Holder TM, Ashcraft KW (eds): Pediatric Surgery.

Lewis RJ, Caccavale RJ, Sisler GE: Imaged thoracoscopic surgery: a new thoracic technique for resection of mediastinal cysts. Ann Thorac Surg 53:318, 1992

Loendersloot EW, Verjaal M, Leschot NJ: Bilateral renal agenesis (Potter's syndrome) in two consecutive infants. Eur J Obstet Gynecol Reprod Biol 8:137, 1978

Loewy J, O'Brodovich H, Coates G: Ventilation scintigraphy with submicronic radioaerosol as an adjunct in the diagnosis of congenital lobar emphysema. J Nucl Med 28:1213, 1987

Loosli CG, Potter EL: The prenatal development of the human lung. Anat Rec 109:320, 1951

Lopez-Majano V: Hemoptysis and pulmonary artery agenesis: case report. Eur J Nucl Med 11:91, 1985

Louie HW, Martin SM, Mulder DG: Pulmonary sequestration: 17-year experience at UCLA. Am Surg 59:801, 1993

Maier HC: Bronchogenic cysts of the mediastinum. Ann Surg 127:476, 1948

Maltz DL, Nadas AS: Agenesis of the lung. Presentation of eight new cases and review of the literature. Pediatrics 42:175, 1968

Man DW, Hamdy MH, Hendry GM et al.: Congenital lobar emphysema: problems in diagnosis and management. Arch Dis Child 58:709, 1983

Markowitz RI, Mercurio MR, Vahjen GA et al: Congenital lobar emphysema. The roles of CT and V/Q scan. Clin Pediatr 28:19, 1989

Maruyama J, Watanabe M, Onodera S et al: A case of Rendu-Osler-Weber disease with cerebral hemangioma, multiple pulmonary arteriovenous fistulas and hepatic arteriovenous fistula. Jpn J Med 28:651, 1989

Mashiach R, Hod M, Friedman S et al: Antenatal ultrasound diagnosis of congenital cystic adenomatoid malformation of the lung: spontaneous resolution in utero. J Clin Ultrasound 21:453, 1993

Matzinger MA, Matzinger FR, Matzinger KE, Black MD: Antenatal and postnatal findings in intra-abdominal pulmonary sequestration. Can Assoc Radiol J 43:212, 1992

McCormick TL, Kuhns LR: Tracheal compression by a normal aorta associated with right lung agenesis. Radiology 130:659, 1979

Mehta AC, Livingston DR, Kawalek W et al: Pulmonary artery agenesis presenting as massive hemoptysis—a case report. Angiology 38:67, 1987

Mentzer SJ, Filler RM, Phillips J: Limited pulmonary resections for congenital cystic adenomatoid malformation of the lung. J Pediatr Surg 27:1410, 1992

Meyer H: Über angeborene blasige Missbildung der Lungen nebst einigen Bemerkungen über Cyanose aus Lungenleiden. Arch Pathol Anat 16:78, 1859

Michelson E: Clinical spectrum of infantile lobar emphysema. Ann Thorac Surg 24:182, 1977

Miller RK, Sieber WK, Yunis EJ: Congenital adenomatoid malformation of the lung. A report of 17 cases and review of the literature.

p. 387. In Sommers SC, Rosen PP (eds): Pathology Annual, Part I. Appleton-Century-Crofts, East Norwalk, CT, 1980

Moerman P, Fryns JP, Vandenberghe K et al: Pathogenesis of congenital cystic adenomatoid malformation of the lung. Histopathology 21:315, 1992

Monin P, Didier F, Vert P et al: Giant lobar emphysema—neonatal diagnosis. Pediatr Radiol 8:259, 1979

Morcos SF, Lobb MO: The antenatal diagnosis by ultrasonography of type III congenital cystic adenomatoid malformation of the lung. Case report. Br J Obstet Gynaecol 93:1002, 1986

Morris E, Constantine G, McHugo J: Cystic adenomatoid malformation of the lung: an obstetric and ultrasound perspective. Eur J Obstet Gynecol Reprod Biol 40:11, 1991

Nakamura Y, Funatsu Y, Yamamoto I et al: Potter's syndrome associated with renal agenesis or dysplasia. Morphological and biochemical study of the lung. Arch Pathol Lab Med 109:441, 1985

Nelson RL: Congenital cystic disease of the lung. J Pediatr 1:233, 1932

Nicolaides KH, Blott M, Greenough A: Chronic drainage of fetal pulmonary cyst. Lancet 1:618, 1987

Nicolette LA, Kosloske AM, Bartow SA, Murphy S: Intralobar pulmonary sequestration: a clinical and pathological spectrum. J Pediatr Surg 28:802, 1993

Nishibayashi SW, Andrassy RJ, Wooley MM: Congenital cystic adenomatoid malformation: a 30-year experience. J Pediatr Surg 16:704, 1981

Nugent CE, Hayashi RH, Rubin J: Prenatal treatment of type I congenital cystic adenomatoid malformation by intrauterine fetal thoracentesis. J Clin Ultrasound 17:675, 1989

Olson JL, Mendelsohn G: Congenital cystic adenomatoid malformation of the lung. Arch Pathol Lab Med 102:248, 1978

Opsahl T, Berman EJ: Bronchiogenic mediastinal cysts in infants: case report and review of the literature. Pediatrics :372, 1967

Oran O, Caglar M, Kale G, Kanra G: Unilateral pulmonary agenesis—presentation of two new cases. Turk J Pediatr 21:16, 1979

Orima H, Fujita M, Aoki S et al: A case of lobar emphysema in a dog. J Vet Med Sci 54:797, 1992

Osborne J, Masel J, McCredie J: A spectrum of skeletal anomalies associated with pulmonary agenesis: possible neural crest injury. Pediatr Radiol 19:425, 1989

Osler W: On a family form of recurring epistaxis associated with multiple telangiectases of skin and mucous membrane. Bull Johns Hopkins Hosp 12:333, 1901

Ostor AG, Stillwell R, Fortune DW: Bilateral pulmonary agenesis. Pathology 10:243, 1978

Overstreet RM: Emphysema of a portion of the lung in the early months of life. Am J Dis Child 57:861, 1939

Oyamada A, Gasul BM, Holinger PH: Agenesis of the lung. Report of a case with review of all previously reported cases. Am J Dis Child 85:182, 1953

Paksoy N, Demircan A, Altiner M, Artvinli M: Localized fibrous mesothelioma arising in an intralobar pulmonary sequestration. Thorax 47:837, 1992

Papagiannis J, Kanter RJ, Effman EL et al: Polysplenia with pulmonary arteriovenous malformations. Pediatr Cardiol 14:127, 1993

Pardes JG, Auh YH, Blomquist K et al: CT diagnosis of congenital lobar emphysema. J Comput Assist Tomogr 7:1095, 1983

Park OK, Buford CH: Bronchogenic cyst of neck and superior mediastinum. Ann Surg 142:130, 1955

Parkes Weber F: Multiple hereditary developmental angiomata of the skin and mucous membranes associated with recurring haemorrhages. Lancet 2:160, 1907

Pelosi G, Zancanaro C, Sbabo L et al: Development of innumerable neuroendocrine tumorlets in a pulmonary lobe scarred by intralobar sequestration. Immunohistochemical and ultrastructural study of an unusual case. Arch Pathol Lab Med 116:1167, 1992

Pennington DW, Gold WM, Gordon RL et al: Treatment of pulmonary arteriovenous malformations by therapeutic embolization. Am Rev Respir Dis 145:1047, 1992

Pflueger SM, Scott CI Jr, Moore CM: Trisomy 7 and Potter's syndrome. Clin Genet 25:543, 1984

Piccione W Jr, Burt ME: Pulmonary sequestration in the neonate. Chest 97:244, 1990

Pryce DM: Lower accessory pulmonary artery with intralobar sequestration of lung. A report of seven cases. J Pathol 48:457, 1946

Pursel SE, Hershey EA, Day JC, Barrett RJ: An approach to cystic lesions of the mediastinum via the mediastinoscope. Ann Thorac Surg 2:752, 1966

Puskas JD, Allen MS, Moncure AC et al: Pulmonary arteriovenous malformations: therapeutic options. Ann Thorac Surg 56:253, 1993

Ray D, Hrudayanath P, Pulimood BM: Pulmonary agenesis associated with crossed renal ectopia. Indian J Chest Dis Allied Sci 17:90, 1975

Rebarber A, Mohan R: Prenatal diagnosis of cystic adenomatoid malformation of one fetus in a twin pregnancy: an unusual presentation. J Ultrasound Med 11:305, 1992

Rektorzik E: Ueber accessorischen Lungenlappen. Wochenschr Z Aerzte 17:4, 1861

Remy J, Remy-Jardin M, Wattinne L, Deffontaines C: Pulmonary arteriovenous malformations: evaluation with CT of the chest before and after treatment. Radiology 182:809, 1992

Rendu M: Epistaxis répétées chez un sujet porteur de petits angiomes cutanes et muqueux. Bull Soc Med Hôpitaux Paris 13:731, 1896

Ribet M, Denimal F: Pulmonary arteriovenous malformations. Chirurgie 117:533, 1991

Ribet M, Pruvot FR, Dubos JP et al: Congenital cystic adenomatoid malformation of the lung. Eur J Cardiothorac Surg 4:403, 1990

Robertson R, James ES: Congenital lobar emphysema. Pediatrics 8:795, 1951

Roguin N, Peleg N, Lemer J et al: The value of cardiac catheterization and cineangiography in infantile lobar emphysema. Pediatr Radiol 10:71, 1980

Rokitansky C: Lehrbuch der pathologischen Anatomie. 3rd Ed. Vienna, 1861

Rosado-de-Christenson ML, Stocker JT: Congenital cystic adenomatoid malformation. Radiographics 11:865, 1991

Saltzman DH, Adzick NS, Benacerraf BR: Fetal cystic adenomatoid malformation of the lung. Apparent improvement in utero. Obstet Gynecol 71:1000, 1988

Sargent MA, Liu PC, Smith CR, Daneman A: Infradiaphragmatic pulmonary sequestration. Can Assoc Radiol J 43:208, 1992

Say B, Carpenter NJ, Giacoia G, Jegathesan S: Agenesis of the lung associated with chromosome abnormality (46,XX, 2p+). J Med Genet 17:477, 1980

Sbokos CG, McMillan IKR: Agenesis of the lung. Br J Dis Chest 71:183, 1977

Schober PH, Muller WD, Behmel A et al: Pulmonary agenesis in partial trisomy 2p and 21q. Klin Padiatr 195:291, 1983

Scholz P, Kuhnt C: Congenital cystic malformation of the lung in a fetus. Zentralbl Gynakol 112:289, 1990

Scurry JP, Adamson TM, Cussen LJ: Fetal lung growth in laryngeal atresia and tracheal agenesis. Aust Paediatr J 25:47, 1989

Senyuz OF, Danismend N, Erdogan E et al: Congenital lobar emphysema—a report of 5 cases. Jpn J Surg 19:764, 1989

Shah VK, Marar UK, Gandhi MJ et al: Agenesis of lung with pulmonary hypertension. J Assoc Physicians India 34:819, 1986

Shenoy SS, Culver GJ, Pirson HS: Agenesis of lung in an adult. AJR 133:755, 1979

Sherer DM, Abramowicz JS, Metlay LA et al: Nonimmune fetal hydrops caused by bilateral type III congenital cystic adenomatoid malformation of the lung at 17 weeks gestation. Am J Obstet Gynecol 167:503, 1992

Shih SL, Lin JC, Chen BF et al: Extralobar pulmonary sequestration of the left retroperitoneum. Australas Radiol 34:356, 1990

Sieber WK: Lung cysts, sequestration, and bronchopulmonary dysplasia. p. 645. In Welch KJ, Randolph JG, Ravitch MM et al: (eds): Pediatric Surgery. Year Book Medical Publishers, Chicago, 1986

Sorokin S: Recent work on developing lungs. p. 467. In DeHaan RL, Ursprung H (eds): Organogenesis. Holt, Rhinehart and Winston, New York, 1965

Spear GS, Yetur P, Beyerlein RA: Bilateral pulmonary agenesis and microphthalmia. Am J Med Genet Suppl 3:379, 1987

Stechele U, Straub E: Potter-syndrome. Klin Padiatr 190:139, 1978

Stern E, Brill PW, Winchester P, Kosovsky P: Imaging of prenatally detected intra-abdominal extralobar pulmonary sequestration. Clin Imaging 14:152, 1990

St-Georges R, Deslauriers J, Duranceau A et al: Clinical spectrum of bronchogenic cysts of the mediastinum and lung in the adult. Ann Thorac Surg 52:6, 1991

Stocker JT: Pediatric Pulmonary Disease. Hemisphere, New York, 1989

Stocker JT, Kagan-Hallet K: Extralobar pulmonary sequestration: analysis of 15 cases. Am J Clin Pathol 72:917, 1979

Stocker JT, Madewell JE, Drake RM: Congenital cystic adenomatoid malformation of the lung. Classification and morphologic spectrum. Hum Pathol 8:155, 1977

Stocker JT, Malczak HT: A study of pulmonary ligament arteries: relationship to intralobar pulmonary sequestration. Chest 86:611, 1984

Suen HC, Mathisen DJ, Grillo HC et al: Surgical management and radiological characteristics of bronchogenic cysts. Ann Thorac Surg 55:476, 1993

Sugio K, Kaneko S, Yokoyama H et al: Pulmonary sequestration in older children and in adults. Int Surg 77:102, 1992

Taguchi M, Shimizu K, Ozaki Y et al: Prenatal diagnosis of congenital cystic adenomatoid malformation of the lung. Fetal Diagn Ther 8:114, 1993

Takayanagi K, Grochowska E, Abu-el Nas S: Pulmonary agenesis with esophageal atresia and tracheoesophageal fistula. J Pediatr Surg 22:125, 1987

Tapper D, Schuster S, McBride J et al: Polyalveolar lobe: anatomic and physiologic parameters and their relationship to congenital lobar emphysema. J Pediatr Surg 15:931, 1980

Tilson DD, Touloukian RJ: Mediastinal enteric sequestration with aberrant pancreas. A forme fruste of the intralobar sequestration. Ann Surg 176:669, 1976

Tinaztepe K, Balci S, Tinaztepe B, Dagli E: Potter's syndrome: bilateral renal agenesis (a report of two cases emphasizing associated malformations). Turk J Pediatr 25:179, 1983

Toran N, Ruiz de Miguel C, Reig J, Garcia-Bonafe M: Lobar emphysema associated with patent ductus arteriosus and pulmonary obstructive vascular disease. Pediatr Pathol 9:163, 1989

Toriello HV, Bauserman SC: Bilateral pulmonary agenesis: association with the hydrolethalus syndrome and review of the literature from a developmental field perspective. Am J Med Genet 21:93, 1985

Toriello HV, Higgins JV, Jones AS, Radecki LL: Pulmonary and diaphragmatic agenesis: report of affected sibs. Am J Med Genet 21:87, 1985

Uppal MS, Kohman LJ, Katzenstein AL: Mycetoma within an intralobar sequestration. Evidence supporting acquired origin for this pulmonary anomaly. Chest 103:1627, 1993

Urban AE, Stark J, Waterston DJ: Congenital lobar emphysema. Thoraxchir Vask Chir 23:255, 1975

Vasquez Sanchez J, Diaz de la Vega V, Lupi Herrera E et al: Scimitar syndrome. Arch Inst Cardiol Mex 56:157, 1986

Vogt-Moykopf I, Rau B, Branscheid D: Surgery for congenital malformations of the lung. Ann Chir 46:141, 1992

Vogt-Moykopf I, Rau B, Branscheid D: Surgery for congenital malformations of the lung. Ann Radiol 36:145, 1993

Voland JR, Benirschke K, Saunders B: Congenital tracheal stenosis with associated cardiopulmonary anomalies. Pediatr Pulmonol 2:247, 1986

Voorhout G, Goedegebuure SA, Nap RC: Congenital lobar emphysema caused by aplasia of bronchial cartilage in a Pekingese puppy. Vet Pathol 23:83, 1986

Wagenvoort CA, Zondervan PE: Polyalveolar lobe and congenital cystic adenomatoid malformation type II: are they related? Pediatr Pathol 11:311, 1991

Walker J, Cudmore RE: Respiratory problems and cystic adenomatoid malformation of the lung. Arch Dis Child 65:649, 1990

Warner JO, Rubin S, Heard BE: Congenital lobar emphysema: a case with bronchial atresia and abnormal bronchial cartilages. Br J Dis Chest 76:177, 1982

Webb WR, Gamsu G, Golden JA, Crooks LE: Nuclear magnetic resonance of pulmonary arteriovenous fistula: effects of flow. J Comput Assist Tomogr 8:155, 1984

Wesley JR, Heidelberger KP, DiPrieto MA et al: Diagnosis and management of congenital cystic disease of the lung in children. J Pediatr Surg 21:202, 1986

Whyte MK, Peters AM, Hughes JM et al: Quantification of right to left shunt at rest and during exercise in patients with pulmonary arteriovenous malformations. Thorax 47:790, 1992

Wigglesworth JS, Desai R, Hislop AA: Fetal lung growth in congenital laryngeal atresia. Pediatr Pathol 7:515, 1987

Willis RA: The Borderland of Embryology and Pathology. Butterworth, Washington, 1962

Wolf SA, Hertzler JH, Phillipart AI: Cystic adenomatoid dysplasia of the lung. Pediatr Surg 15:925, 1980

Yogasakaran BS, Sudhaman DA: Congenital cystic adenomatoid malformation of the lung in combination with a pulmonary sequestration. J Cardiovasc Vasc Anesth 5:368, 1991

Young AE: Arteriovenous malformations. p. 228. In Mulliken JB, Young AE (eds): Vascular Birthmarks (Hemangiomas and Malformations). WB Saunders, Philadelphia, 1988

Zangwill BC, Stocker JT: Congenital cystic adenomatoid malformation within an extralobar pulmonary sequestration. Pediatr Pathol 13:309, 1993

20

INFECTIONS

Bacterial Infections

Richard V. Hodder
Robert Cameron
Thomas R. J. Todd

PNEUMONIA AND RELATED CONDITIONS

DEFINITION

The term *pneumonia* refers to an infection of the lower respiratory tract that involves the respiratory bronchioles, alveolar ducts, and acini. Pneumonia can present with a variety of symptoms and clinical syndromes and is usually visualized as parenchymal opacities in either an air space (alveolar) or interstitial pattern on the chest radiograph. Pneumonia is thus distinguished from acute bronchitis, which may have a similar clinical presentation but refers to infective and noninfective causes of acute tracheobronchial inflammation without parenchymal opacities on the chest radiograph. The term *pneumonitis* is frequently used as a synonym for pneumonia but is probably best reserved for noninfectious causes, such as chemical, radiation-induced, and gastric acid aspiration pneumonitis, etc.

When a patient first presents with pneumonia, it is unusual for the causative pathogen(s) to be known with certainty. Therefore, initial antibiotic therapy must often be empiric. The physician's decision about which antibiotics(s) to use can be facilitated by viewing the patient's pneumonia from an epidemiologic perspective because this can help to suggest the most likely responsible organism(s). One such clinically useful classification is shown below. Community-acquired pneumonia (CAP) usually arises from a bacterial or viral infection and is most usefully further subclassified according to the mode of presentation and the nature of the host. The traditional practice of classifying CAP into so-called typical and atypical syndromes can no longer be considered valid because this approach lacks both sensitivity and specificity for the causative microorganisms (see below). Nosocomial or "hospital-acquired" pneumonia is usually defined as pneumonia arising 48 to 72 hours after admission to the hospital. It most commonly occurs when the host's respiratory defense mechanisms become compromised and, for the most part, is bacterial in nature, although fungal infections may be seen, particularly in the immunocompromised patient. A third major classification of pneumonia, is aspiration pneumonia, which may occur in either the community or hospital setting. It is further subclassified into either chemical pneumonitis from aspiration of gastric contents or primary (bacterial) aspiration pneumonia. A fourth category of pneumonia, pneumonia in the immunocompromised host, is also justifiable because of the particular epidemiologic and microbiologic features that characterize this syndrome and this patient population.

This chapter deals with those aspects of lower respiratory tract infection that are most relevant to the thoracic surgeon, namely, the syndromes of CAP and nosocomial pneumonia. The special circumstances of aspiration pneumonia, lung abscess, bronchiectasis, concurrent esophageal disease, and acute bronchitis and the infective exacerbation of chronic obstructive pulmonary disease (COPD) are also discussed. The particular problems of the immunocompromised patient are discussed in the last section of this chapter.

Although it is difficult to obtain accurate statistics on the true incidence of pneumonia because it is not a reportable disease, it is estimated to be the sixth most common cause of death in the United States and the most common cause of infection-related death (Garibaldi, 1985). It causes four times as many annual deaths as asthma (MacFarlane, 1987). The problem is much greater in developing countries, where pneumonia is the single most common disease that requires medical attention and where the mortality rate for childhood pneumonia is 30 times greater than that in developed countries (MacFarlane, 1987).

The population at greatest risk for CAP is now the age 65 and older segment of the population. Nursing-home-acquired pneumonia in particular is becoming an increasingly preva-

---

Epidemiologic Classification of Pneumonia

CAP

    Age < 60 years, previously well

    Age > 60 years and/or coexisting illness

    Severe or rapidly progressive pneumonia

Nosocomial pneumonia

    VAP

    Non–VAP

Aspiration pneumonia

    Chemical pneumonitis

    Infective pneumonia

Pneumonia in the immunocompromised host

    AIDS

    Patient undergoing chemotherapy

    Transplant recipient

    Other immunocompromised patients

---

lent and difficult problem (Marrie, et al., 1986; Marrie, 1992). The increasing use of organ transplantation, the phenomenon of the acquired immunodeficiency syndrome (AIDS), and the expanding use of radiotherapy and chemotherapy for bronchogenic carcinoma have also led to a high prevalence of pneumonia in the so-called compromised host. These are additional reasons for the persistence of pneumonia as an important clinical health care problem. For these reasons, the thoracic surgeon will frequently be called on to assess and treat patients who present with pneumonia both in and out of the hospital, and a rational approach to this entity in all of its common forms is thus essential.

HISTORICAL NOTE

Despite the fact that pneumonia has been recognized as a common health problem for centuries and is described in ancient medical writings (Castiglioni, 1947; McGehee, 1990), the central role of bacteria as etiologic factors was not fully appreciated until the late nineteenth century (Friedlander, 1882). In that same preantibiotic era, the high mortality rate then associated with pneumonia prompted Sir William Osler (1901) to refer to pneumonia as the "Captain of the Men of Death." However, beginning with the initial use of sulfonamides in the 1930s and penicillin in the 1940s, there has been a veritable explosion in the number of antimicrobial agents available. Specific therapy now exists for virtually every type of bacterial pneumonia. Indeed, in the century after Osler's statement about pneumonia-related mortality, there has been a dramatic and gratifying fall in the death rate associated with bacterial pneumonia, particularly for infections acquired outside the hospital (Hall, 1959). However, despite such advances in our understanding and therapy of this entity, pneumonia remains an important health problem that still carries a significant mortality rate, variously quoted to be in the range of 1 to 25 percent (Niederman, et al., 1993).

HISTORICAL READINGS

Castiglioni A: A History of Medicine. 2nd Ed. Krumbhaar EB, ed Knopf, New York, 1947

Friedlander C: Uber die Schizomyceten bei der acuten fibrosen Pneumonie. Virchows Arch B Cell Pathol 87:319, 1882

McGehee JL: A brief history of pneumonia. J Tenn Med Assoc 83:455, 1990

Osler W: The Principles and Practice of Medicine. 4th Ed. Appelton and Co., New York, 1901

COMMUNITY-ACQUIRED PNEUMONIA

CAP originates by definition outside the hospital setting and presents to the thoracic surgeon as a problem in diagnosis, either when it persists or when it results in rapid respiratory compromise. Thoracic surgeons should also be familiar with CAP because many patients referred for a thoracic surgery consultation are elderly with coexisting illness, such as chronic cardiopulmonary disease, and are predisposed to have CAP develop (Niederman, et al., 1993). The possibility of proximal airway obstruction or concurrent esophageal disease must frequently be considered.

Pathophysiology

Infectious agents may gain access to the lower airways by one of the following three main routes: (1) the inhalational route, (2) aspiration of upper airway and oropharyngeal microbial flora, and (3) the hematogenous route through the pulmonary and bronchial arteries. Contiguous spread from adjacent infected tissues can also occur but is rare. Pneumonia can also occur if a quiescent or dormant infection, such as tuberculosis or histoplasmosis, is reactivated, usually when the host's cell-mediated immunity becomes compromised.

Although it might be expected that the inhalational route would account for most cases of CAP, this mechanism appears to be clinically common only for pneumonia caused by respiratory viruses, *Mycoplasma pneumoniae, Chlamydia pneumoniae,* Legionella species, *Mycobacterium tuberculosis,* and some fungi, such as Histoplasma, etc.

Microaspiration of the endogenous oropharyngeal organisms that colonize the upper airways appears to account for most cases of CAP that require hospitalization. It has been shown that 50 percent of normal subjects and as many as 70 percent of subjects with impaired consciousness exhibit microaspiration of oropharyngeal secretions during sleep (Huxley, et al., 1978). This is potentially significant, particularly if the patient's lung defense mechanisms are compromised. Additional evidence to support this hypothesis comes from the observation of increased rates of upper airway colonization with gram-negative enteric bacilli in patient groups at risk for pneumonia, such as elderly (Granton and Grossman, 1993) and alcoholic patients and nursing home residents (Crossley and Thurn, 1989; Garb, et al., 1987; Marrie, et al., 1986). The reason for this increased colonization in these patient groups is uncertain but probably reflects compromised airway clearance mechanisms associated with malnutrition, cigarette smoking, and other variables, such as increased microbial adherence to respiratory epithelial surfaces, which may reflect the loss of cell surface fibronectin (Woods, et al., 1981a,b).

Hematogenous seeding of the lungs with microorganisms from an extrapulmonary site is an uncommon cause of CAP, and bacteremia is more likely to lead to the adult respiratory distress syndrome (ARDS) than to focal pneumonia. However, bacteremia or fungemia can lead to pneumonia, as occurs with infected thrombophlebitis and secondary pulmonary embolism and with right-sided infective endocarditis. The organisms most commonly associated with such hematogenous spread are *Staphylococcus aureus* and gram-negative enteric bacilli.

Despite the fact that the lungs are regularly exposed to large numbers of potentially pathogenic microorganisms through the inhalational and microaspiration routes, the healthy host with normal lung defenses maintains an essentially sterile lower respiratory tract (Reynolds, 1989). These intrinsic defense mechanisms consist of aerodynamic filtration by the upper airways, the cough reflex, mucociliary transport, specific humoral and cellular immunity, and phagocytosis by alveolar macrophages. Compromise of aerodynamic filtration is usually not a significant factor in the pathogenesis of CAP, although it can become an important mechanism in patients with chronic tracheostomies. On the other hand, a decreased ability to cough and clear secretions effectively may be a predisposing factor, particularly for patients with weak respiratory muscles. This can occur with long-standing severe COPD or after prolonged postthoracotomy convalescence. Persistent chest wall pain after surgery can also hinder an effective cough mechanism as can impaired consciousness secondary to analgesia sedative, or alcohol abuse. Mechanical clearance of bronchial secretions can also be compromised when there is endobronchial obstruction by a neoplasm or foreign body. Mucociliary transport itself can be impaired by ongoing cigarette smoking (Stanley, et al., 1986), by exposure to atmospheric pollutants and by coexisting illnesses, such as significant COPD, cystic fibrosis, the dysmotile cilia syndrome, and alcoholism, and after acute viral respiratory tract infections, particularly influenza A. All of these predispose to colonization of the lower respiratory tract and subsequent pneumonia (Fekety, et al., 1971; Louria, et al., 1959). The body's humoral and cell-mediated immunity can be compromised by malnutrition and aging and by immunosuppressive agents, for example, corticosteroids, which are often used in the population with COPD (Wiest, et al., 1989), and immunotherapy or radiotherapy given for bronchogenic carcinoma (Rosiello and Merrill, 1990). Patients with immunoglobulin deficiency are predisposed to have recurrent bacterial pneumonias, which can lead to bronchiectasis (Duncan and Raffin, 1992). Finally, the phagocytic function of pulmonary alveolar macrophages has been shown to be compromised by concomitant conditions, including hypoxia, exposure to tobacco smoke, uremia, alcohol, pulmonary edema, and viral infection.

Clinical and Etiologic Diagnosis

Pneumonia is suspected when patients have varying combinations of fever, chills, cough productive of purulent phlegm, and pleuritic chest pain. Between 10 and 30 percent of patients with CAP also complain of extrapulmonary symptoms, such as headache, nausea, diarrhea, myalgias, and arthralgias. Elderly patients tend to have fewer and more subtle symptoms (such as mental confusion) than do younger patients with CAP. Physical signs, such as crackles and wheezes, are not specific for pneumonia and can be present in patients with acute bronchitis or an acute exacerbation of COPD. A chest radiograph is therefore an essential diagnostic aid in the diagnosis and management of pneumonia (see below).

When a patient presents with suspected CAP, the immediate management priorities are to ensure cardiopulmonary stability, to treat acute respiratory failure if it exists, and to determine whether hospital admission will be necessary. The next most important goal is to achieve an accurate etiologic

---

Risk Factors for Severe CAP with Poor Outcome

Coexisting conditions

   Age > 60

   COPD (including bronchiectasis)

   Diabetes mellitus

   Chronic renal failure

   Congestive heart failure

   Chronic liver disease

   Alcohol abuse

   Malnutrition

   Postsplenectomy state

   Hospitalization in the preceding year

Physiologic derangements

   Respiratory rate > 30 breaths/min[a]

   Hypotension

      Systolic blood pressure < 90 mmHg

      Diastolic blood pressure < 60 mmHg[a]

   Temperature > 38.3°C (101°F)

   Tachycardia > 120 beats/min

Laboratory findings

   Leukocytosis > 30×10^9/L

   Leukopenia < 4×10^9/L

   Urea > 7 mMol/L (20 mg/dl)[a]

   Hemoglobin < 90 g/L

   PaO_2 < 60 mmHg

   $PaCO_2$ > 50 mmHg

   Multilobar or rapidly progressive radiographic opacities

Atypical presentation[b]

   Confusion

   Predominantly nonrespiratory complaints

   Absence of fever

---

[a] Factors predictive of mortality in CAP (Farr, et al., 1991).
[b] May lead to diagnostic confusion and subsequent therapeutic delay.

Table 20-1. Features of Typical Versus Atypical Pneumonia in the Normal Host[a]

Typical Pneumonia Syndrome	Atypical Pneumonia Syndrome
Abrupt onset of high fever and chills	Insidious onset, low fever, no chills
Cough productive of purulent phlegm	Spasmodic cough, usually nonproductive
Hemoptysis and pleuritic pain may occur	Hemoptysis and pleuritic pain uncommon
Abnormal findings on chest examination (crackles and/or consolidation)	Usually no crackles or consolidation on examination
Chest radiograph matches physical examination, often with lobar consolidation	Chest radiograph often demonstrates more extensive involvement than physical examination
Toxic-looking patient	Extrapulmonary manifestations may dominate the clinical picture
Middle-aged adults predominate	Young adults predominate
Sporadic occurrence	Close contacts often affected

[a] Overlap of features may occur, especially with Legionella species.

(microbiologic) diagnosis as quickly as possible so that specific antimicrobial therapy can be promptly initiated. Unfortunately a quick and specific microbiologic diagnosis is frequently not possible because neither the traditional presenting clinical syndromes (i.e., typical versus atypical) or the commonly used diagnostic tests (e.g., sputum smear are chest radiographs) are not specific or sensitive enough to identify the responsible pathogen(s) accurately in most patients (Fang, et al., 1990; Niederman, et al., 1993). Furthermore, data from sputum and blood cultures is generally not available for 24 to 48 hours, and serologic results taken even longer. These points were clearly demonstrated in a recent study of 154 patients hospitalized with CAP by Bates, et al. (1992). Despite extensive diagnostic testing, including viral and bacterial cultures of respiratory secretions and serologic testing for viruses, Legionella, Mycoplasma, and Chlamydia, responsible pathogens were identified in only 51 percent of patients. Other investigators (Fang, et al., 1990; Marrie, et al., 1989) have shown similar results. It therefore appears that many of the traditional clinical practices used in the workup of CAP, such as heavy reliance on Gram staining of expectorated sputum and extensive use of the laboratory for diagnostic testing, are based on relatively poor data and can no longer be justified for routine clinical use in uncomplicated cases of CAP (Fang, et al., 1990; Niederman, et al., 1993). Such detailed testing should probably be reserved only for patients at high risk of a poor outcome and for those who do not respond to initial therapy. The traditional syndromic approach of having the physician classify patients with CAP into either typical or atypical syndromes (Table 20-1) and then infer a microbial cause from this assignment is probably also apocryphal and thus of limited use. In a multicenter, prospective study of 359 patients admitted to the hospital with CAP, Fang, et al., (1990) observed that the clinical features of pneumonia caused by various pathogens were too similar for any clear clinically predictive patterns to emerge. In particular those findings considered classic for the so-called atypical pneumonia syndrome were completely nonspecific and therefore useless to predict the most likely in-

fecting organisms. It appears that for most patients hospitalized with CAP nowadays (namely elderly patients and those with coexisting illnesses) the popular typical versus atypical classification is obsolete and should be abandoned.

As a result of the above, initial antibiotic therapy must usually be chosen empirically. Fortunately in the past few years, several large prospective studies that used extensive diagnostic investigations to determine the most likely pathogens in CAP have provided the basis for this type of empiric approach. Three recent consensus conferences have reviewed the data from these multicenter studies and have published similar recommendations for the diagnosis and management of CAP (British Thoracic Society, 1987, 1993; Mandell and Niederman, 1993; Niederman, et al., 1993). Three major clinical variables appear to exert a significant influence on the spectrum of likely pathogens in the patient

---

Likely Pathogens in CAP Treated on an Outpatient Basis[a]

Age < 60 years without coexisting illnesses
  S. pneumoniae
  M. pneumoniae
  Respiratory viruses
  C. pneumoniae
  H. influenzae
  Miscellaneous
    Legionella spp.
    Staphylococcus spp.
    M. tuberculosis
    Endemic fungi
    Gram-negative bacilli

Age > 60 years and/or coexisting illnesses
  S. pneumoniae
  Respiratory viruses
  H. influenzae
  Aerobic gram-negative bacilli
  S. aureus
  Anerobes
  Miscellaneous
    M. catarrhalis
    Legionella spp.
    M. tuberculosis
    Endemic fungi

---

[a] Rank order of pathogen roughly reflects incidence in CAP. (Data from Niederman MS, Bass JB, Campbell GD et al: Guidelines for the initial management of adults with community-acquired pneumonia: diagnosis, assessment of severity, and initial microbial therapy. Am Rev Respir Dis 148:1418, 1993, and Mandell LA, Niederman MS: Antimicrobial treatment of community-acquired pneumonia in adults: a conference report. Can J Infect Dis 4:25, 1993.)

Likely Pathogens in Severe CAP Requiring Hospitalization[a]

Ward patients

  S. pneumoniae

  H. influenzae

  Polymicrobial (including anerobes, aspiration, and gram-negative bacteria)

  Legionella spp.

  S. aureus

  C. pneumoniae

  Respiratory viruses

  Miscellaneous

    M. pneumoniae

    M. catarrhalis

    M. tuberculosis

    Endemic fungi

Patients requiring ICU admission

  S. pneumoniae

  Legionella spp.

  Aerobic gram-negative bacilli (including P. aeruginosa)

  S. aureus

  M. pneumoniae

  Respiratory viruses

  Miscellaneous

    M. pneumoniae

    M. tuberculosis

    Endemic fungi

---

[a] Rank order of pathogens roughly reflects incidence in CAP. (Data from Niederman MS, Bass JB, Campbell GD et al: Guidelines for the initial management of adults with community-acquired pneumonia: diagnosis, assessment of severity, and initial microbial therapy. Am Rev Respir Dis 148:1418, 1993, and Mandell LA, Niederman MS: Antimicrobial treatment of community-acquired pneumonia in adults: a conference report. Can J Infect Dis 4:25, 1993.)

who presents with CAP and thus on the initial approach to therapy:

1. The patient's age (less than or greater than age 60).
2. The presence or absence of coexisting illness.
3. The severity of the illness at the initial presentation.

The analyses from these consensus conferences are summarized below. The relationships among these three clinical features and the most probable pathogens are illustrated. The rank order of the pathogens listed below roughly reflects their likely incidence in cases in which an etiologic diagnosis can be definitively made. Pneumococcus is still statistically the most likely responsible pathogen for CAP, with an incidence ranging from 11 to 76 percent (Fang, et al., 1990).

CAP Treated on an Outpatient Basis

In smokers *Haemophilus influenzae* is an important cause of CAP, perhaps because of the reported synergism between cigarette smoke and this organism in slowing mucociliary transport (Stanley, et al., 1986; Wilson, 1988). The epidemiology of CAP caused by *M. pneumoniae* and *C. pneumoniae* is similar, and these agents should be suspected during miniepidemics of CAP, particularly in the younger population, with frequent social contacts (families, schools, etc.). For patients 60 years of age or older or for those with important coexisting illnesses, although Pneumococcus is most likely, aerobic gram-negative bacilli, *S. aureus,* and *Moraxella catarrhalis* become more important considerations in the presence of coexisting illnesses, particularly COPD.

CAP Requiring Hospitalization

For patients sick enough to warrant hospitalization, but not ICU care, the mortality rate ranges from 5 to 25 percent, and there is a greater likelihood of anerobes (secondary to presumed aspiration), aerobic gram-negative pathogens, and Legionella spp. Patients with life-threatening CAP who require ICU admission have the highest mortality rate (up to 50 percent) and are more likely to have pneumonia caused by difficult gram-negative (bacilli (including Pseudomonas), *S. aureus,* or Legionella spp.

The cause of CAP in patients with AIDS is particular to that population. *Pneumocystis carinii* pneumonia occurs in most of these patients at some time during their clinical courses (Murray, 1992). In addition, infection with pneumococci, *H. influenzae,* cytomegalovirus, *M. tuberculosis,* and atypical mycobacteria must also be considered to be potentially important etiologic agents in these individuals.

CAP caused by Legionella species deserves separate mention, if only because of its popular mystique and the fact that difinitive diagnosis is often difficult or made only retrospectively from serologic testing. The Legionella species are ubiquitous aquatic bacteria. Hence most infections occur by spread of the organism through heat-exchange devices or other water distribution systems. Therefore, Legionella are frequently associated with epidemic outbreaks in large buildings (including hospitals) in association with water-cooling towers and fresh water supplies (Arnow, et al., 1982; Dondero, et al., 1980). Legionella species may also cause sporadic CAP, particularly in relationship to recent travel in the spring and fall (Fang, et al., 1989; Muder, et al., 1989). It may be the agent responsible for pneumonia in chronically ill and immunocompromised patients. One feature that suggests Legionnaires' disease is the fact that, although it may initially present as an atypical pneumonia syndrome, there is often rapid progression of both pulmonary symptoms and the chest radiograph, which shows progressive multifocal air space disease frequently complicated by pleural effusion (Mandell, et al., 1990).

Rarer causes of CAP may have more specific epidemiologic associations that can be elicited from the history. The thoracic surgeon should be aware of the greater likelihood of

CAP from encapsulated organisms, such as pneumococci and *H. influenzae*, in patients who are splenectomized as a result of multiple trauma.

Diagnostic Testing

As noted above, extensive diagnostic testing is not warranted on a routine basis for most patients who present with uncomplicated CAP and who are not severely ill. However, patients with CAP who have undergone thoracic surgery are often fragile with important coexisting illnesses and frequently abnormal chest radiographs. Thus the initial management of these patients should often include simple attempts to make an etiologic diagnosis on the day of presentation because an early specific diagnosis can be helpful.

Sputum Examination

Those situations in which sputum staining and culture are likely to be particularly helpful in the management of CAP are summarized below. Some authorities think that a Gram stain of a deep sample of lower airway secretions can be useful if it is examined according to strict criteria (Boerner

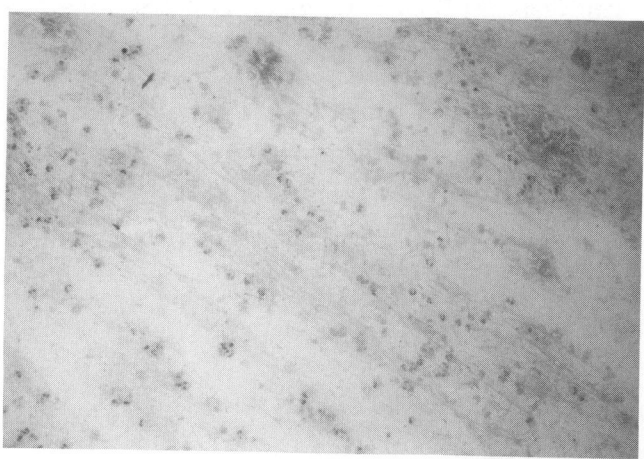

Figure 20-1. Microscopic examination of good-quality expectorated phlegm, with few squamous epithelial cells and many polymorphs.

and Zwadyle, 1982; Levy, et al., 1988; Marrie, 1994). However, others dispute its value when used routinely (Niederman, et al., 1993; Rein , et al., 1978; Woodhead, et al., 1991) (Fig. 20-1). In most epidemiologic studies and certainly in day-to-day practice under nonstudy conditions, however, sputum is frequently not available, or if it is produced, it is of such poor quality that it is not representative of the lower airways and therefore not useful for diagnosis (Fig. 20-2). The sensitivity and specificity of the sputum Gram stain results vary widely in its reported ability to predict the results of sputum culture. Prior to therapy with antibiotics is likely to be an important factor in this phenomenon.

Furthermore, Gram staining of sputum is also not able to detect certain frequent causes of CAP, such as *M. pneumoniae*, *C. pneumoniae*, respiratory viruses, and Legionella species. Direct fluorescent antibody (DFA) testing of sputum has been reported to be useful in the diagnosis of pneumonia Legionella caused by (Edelstein, et al., 1980). Although there

---

Value of Sputum Examination in CAP

Sputum smear and stain not helpful

M. pneumoniae

C. pneumoniae

Respiratory viruses

Sputum cultures not helpful

Normal or mixed oropharyngeal flora[a]

No growth observed[b]

Sputum smear and stain helpful

M. tuberculosis

Legionella spp. (direct fluorescent antibody staining)

Pneumocystis (special stains)

Sputum cultures helpful

Pure growth of suspected pathogen

M. tuberculosis

Legionella spp.

Endemic fungi

Organisms resistant to current antibiotics

Ampicillin-resistant *H. influenzae*

Resistant gram-negative bacteria

Penicillin-resistant pneumococci

---

[a] Usually reflects tracheobronchial colonization (e.g., in elderly patients or those with COPD). Often reported in cases of aspiration pneumonia caused by oral anerobes and/or gram-negative bacilli.

[b] Usually reflects prior treatment with broad-spectrum antibiotics.

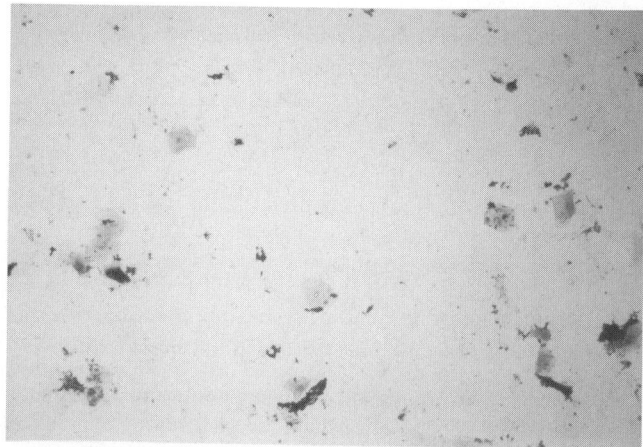

Figure 20-2. Microscopic examination of poor-quality expectorated phlegm, with too few polymorphs and too many epithelial cells.

is a high specificity (94 to 99 percent) for the test, the sensitivity is low (50 to 70 percent). Therefore, a negative DFA finding does not rule out Legionella pneumonia.

Invasive Diagnostic Techniques

Because of the difficulties in the interpretation of sputum stains and cultures, some authors recommend invasive procedures to obtain bronchial specimens for quantitative culture in patients with CAP (Bartlett, 1989; Tobin, 1987), although there have been few studies that directly compare the diagnostic accuracy of invasive versus noninvasive methods in this setting. A number of invasive diagnostic techniques are available to the thoracic surgeon, such as transtracheal aspiration, percutaneous fine-needle aspiration of the lung, bronchoscopy with protected specimen brushes, or bronchoalveolar lavage with protected and unprotected catheters (Middleton, et al., 1994).

Transtracheal aspiration (TAA) is rarely performed in this era of the flexible fiberoptic bronchoscope, but it has been reported to provide useful specimens to determine the cause of acute bacterial pneumonia (Ostergaard and Anderson, 1993). The potential for complications from TAA should not be underestimated and includes significant hemoptysis, subcutaneous and mediastinal emphysema, pneumothorax, and secondary soft tissue infection. Direct aspiration of the lung with a percutaneous fine-needle technique has also been used in the diagnosis of CAP (Bartlett, 1989).

If attempts at invasive diagnosis seem warranted in a particular patient with severe CAP, fiberoptic bronchoscopy with protected specimen brushes or bronchoalvcolar lavage with protected or unprotected aspiration catheters are the preferred techniques because they have a reasonable sensitivity and specificity and are safer and more comfortable for the patient than other invasive techniques (Bartlett, 1989; Middleton, et al., 1994).

More invasive techniques, such as transbronchial biopsy, open lung biopsy, and thorascopic lung biopsy, have all been used in the diagnosis of suspected pneumonia (Bartlett, 1989), but their role is also almost exclusively limited to radiographic opacities that occur in the immunocompromised patient who may have unusual or resistant pathogens and in whom it is often difficult to distinguish pneumonia from the underlying disease or the effects of chemotherapy or radiotherapy on the lung.

If pleural effusion complicates pneumonia, thoracentesis should be performed to examine the fluid for the presence of microorganisms, particularly if the patient is seriously ill from the infection (Sahn, 1993). When positive results are found, pleural fluid cultures are usually highly specific for the etiologic agent of the underlying pneumonia.

Chest Radiograph

Whenever the clinical presentation suggests the possibility of pneumonia, a chest radiograph should be obtained, partly to exclude the diagnosis of acute bronchitis (which may have a similar clinical presentation) and also because the observation of segmental or lobar alveolar (air space) opacities or pleural effusion has a good correlation with pyogenic bacteria as the most likely pathogen (Lynch and Armstrong, 1991).

Occasionally in the early stages of CAP, the chest radiograph may appear normal, and anecdotal evidence suggests that this may be more common in elderly, dehydrated patients. The chest radiograph may also reveal more extensive pneumonia than suspected clinically based on the physical examination of the chest, particularly in pneumonias caused by "granulomatous" microorganisms, such as Histoplasma (Figure 20-3). Such a situation can also occur in the immunocompromised neutropenic patient, in elderly debilitated patients, and in those in whom pneumonia presents as a focal mass, as can occasionally occur with many organisms, including pneumococci, *S. aureus,* and endemic fungi (Lynch and Armstrong, 1991).

Certain radiographic patterns of pneumonia may on occasion be of some help to narrow down the etiologic differential diagnosis. In particular the presence of a large pleural effusion, lobar consolidation (Fig. 20-4), or cavitation is highly suggestive of a bacterial cause. The presence of multiple nodular opacities with or without cavitation should suggest a hematogenous spread of *S. aureus* or necrotizing gram-negative organisms; this can occur among intravenous drug abusers (Fig. 20-5). When aspiration pneumonia occurs, there is a predilection for the dependent areas of the lung, which arc usually the superior segments of the lower lobes, more commonly on the right side, or the posterior segments of the upper lobes, depending on the position of the subject when the aspiration occurred (Fig. 20-6). Of particular importance to the thoracic surgeon is a radiographic pattern that suggests proximal endobronchial obstruction causing distal atelectasis

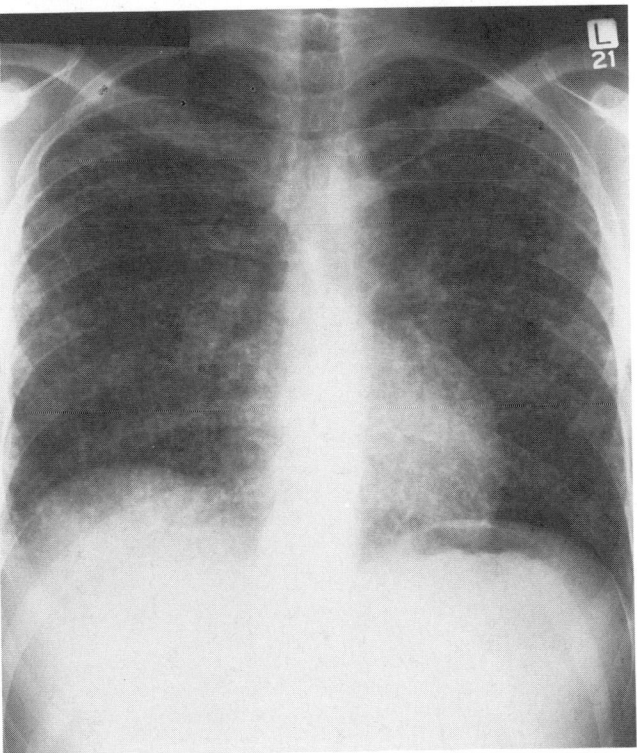

Figure 20-3. Histoplasma pneumonia in a patient with only minimal clinical findings on chest examination. Note nodular appearance suggesting a "granulomatous" infection.

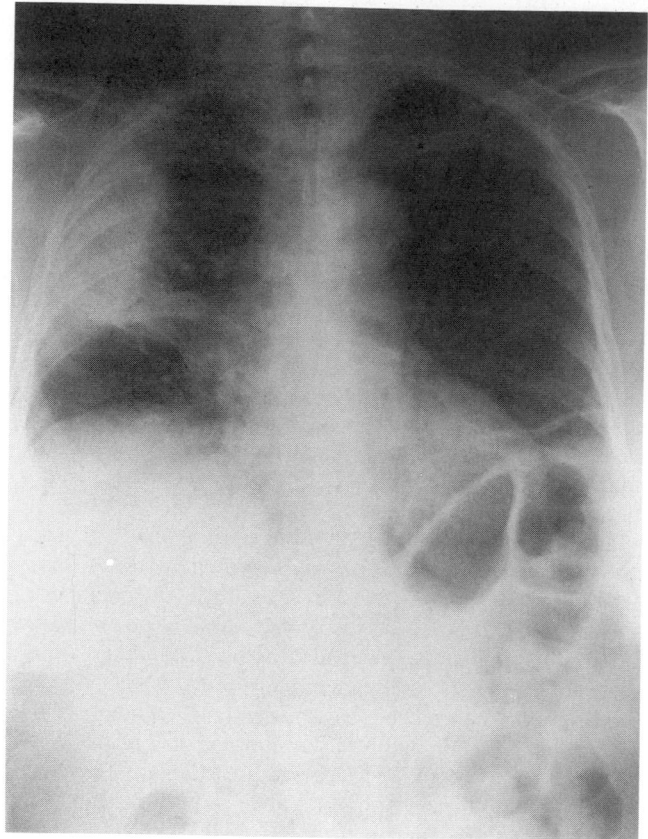

Figure 20-4. Right upper lobe consolidation caused by pneumococcal pneumonia. Crackles, dullness, and bronchial breath sounds were observed over the affected area.

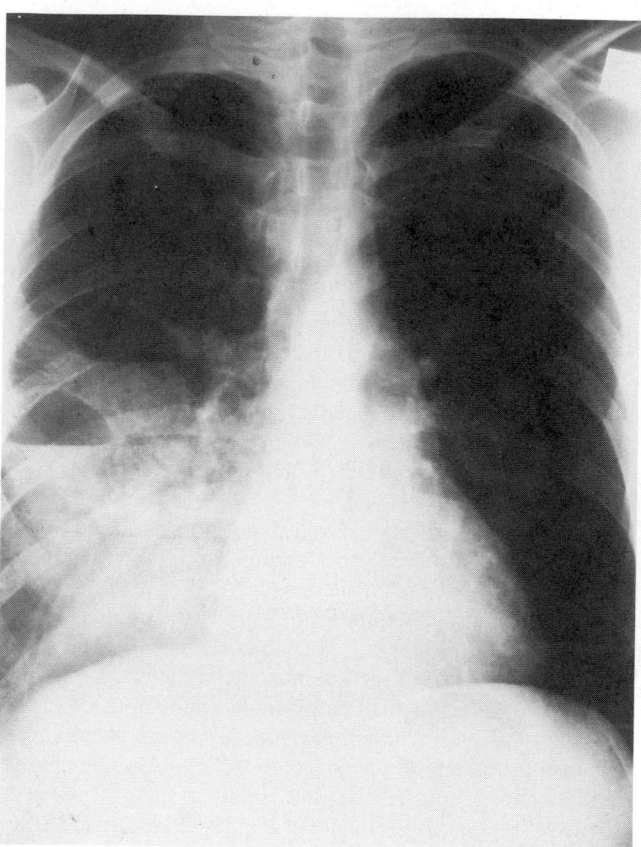

Figure 20-6. Aspiration pneumonia with abscess and numerous air-fluid levels in the right lower lobe.

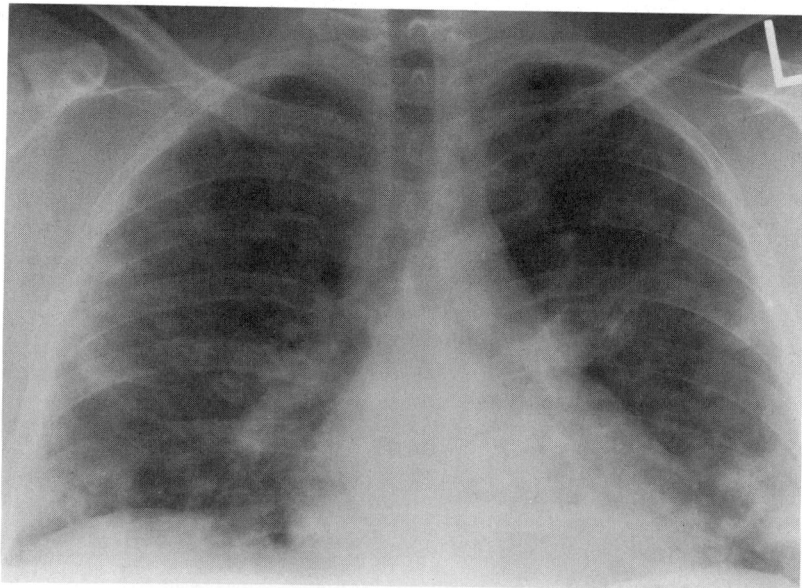

Figure 20-5. Radiograph of multiple cavities caused by *S. aureus* pneumonia in an intravenous drug abuser.

or postobstructive pneumonia. These findings should raise the possibility of an obstructing bronchogenic carcinoma (Fig. 20-7).

Blood Culture

Two sets of blood cultures should always be obtained from patients with CAP who are sick enough to be admitted to the hospital. Although only about 10 to 20 percent of patients with bacterial pneumonia are bacteremic, positive blood cultures will offer definitive proof of the cause of the disease.

Serologic and Other Blood Tests

Acute and convalescent phase serologic tests can be examined for antibodies to a variety of microbial agents (Campbell and Spika, 1988). However, these tests and tests for cold agglutinins are not very useful clinically and should not be performed routinely for CAP because they provide only delayed and retrospective information usually long after the course of the pneumonia has been determined. Serologic testing is primarily indicated for public health and epidemiologic purposes during acute outbreaks of pneumonia in which there is suspicion of pneumonias caused by Legionella, Coxiella, Mycoplasma, or Chlamydia.

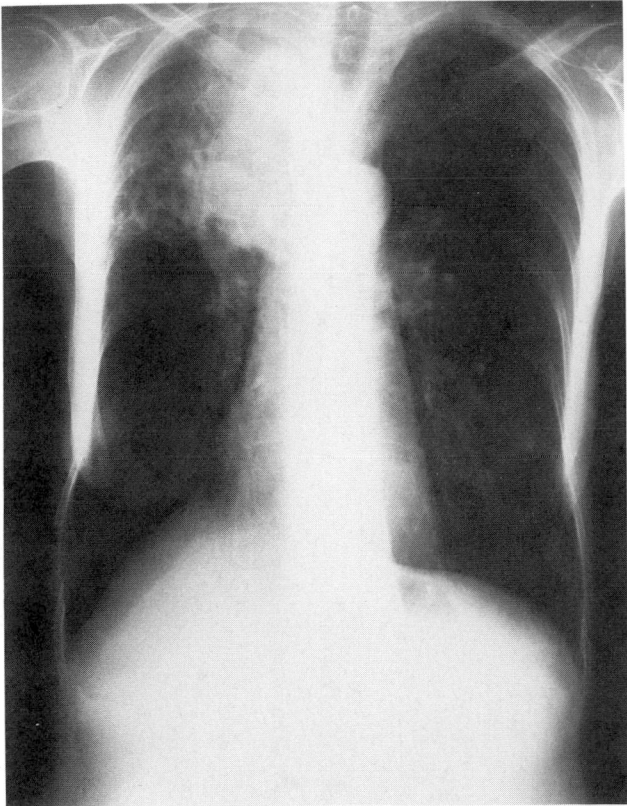

Figure 20-7. Right upper lobe pneumonia and partial atelectasis (note "tenting" of the hemidiaphragm) from endobronchial obstruction caused by carcinoma.

Therapy

Successful therapy of the patient with CAP includes both general supportive measures and specific antibiotic therapy.

Deciding on Hospitalization

Earlier those features were listed that have been shown to be associated with a poor outcome from CAP. When one or more of these factors are present, hospital admission should be strongly considered. Bacterial CAP after a recent influenza infection can be life threatening, especially in elderly patients (Louria, et al., 1959; Schwartzmann, et al., 1971). Typically patients become rapidly symptomatic with a sudden onset of chills, often pleuritic chest pain, and productive cough a few days to 2 weeks after apparent clinical resolution of the influenza. Recognition of this pattern of presentation should suggest elective admission to the hospital. Ultimately the decision to hospitalize the patient should not be based on rigid criteria but on clinical judgment. This point was clearly illustrated in a study by Fine, et al. (1990) in which 38 percent of patients with CAP who did not meet a set of predefined admission criteria subsequently experienced a complicated course that required inpatient care.

Supportive Therapy

Supportive therapy for patients with CAP includes maintenance of adequate hydration, either by increasing fluid intake at home or by use of intravenous hydration in the hospital, initial bed rest, maintenance of physiologic acid-base balance, and supplemental oxygen therapy as required. Patients managed at home should be encouraged strongly not to smoke because this can impair tracheobronchial clearance of secretions (Stanley, et al., 1986) and reduce arterial oxygen content by increasing carboxyhemoglobin levels. There is no evidence that chest physiotherapy is of any value during the acute phase of CAP, except for patients with significant chronic sputum retention, usually in the setting of bronchiectasis, or for severe chronic bronchitic patients who are having difficulty raising phlegm (Graham and Bradley, 1979). Patients with significant coexisting illnesses, such as COPD, coronary artery disease, or diabetes mellitus, may require specific therapy if these illnesses are also exacerbated because of concomitant pneumonia.

Specific Antibiotic Therapy

Guidelines for the initial selection of antibiotics to treat CAP are given in Figure 20-8. The recommendations for empiric therapy reflect many of the opinions from two recent consensus statements on CAP (Niederman, et al., 1993; Mandell and Niederman, 1993) and a recent authoritative review (Marrie, 1994). Also provided are therapeutic suggestions for other specific clinical settings, such as aspiration pneumonia and the therapy of CAP in the nursing home.

If sputum is available and is of good quality, a Gram stain should be performed. If one type of organism is clearly seen to predominate on the smear, this information should be used to guide initial antibiotic therapy, as indicated in Figure 20-8. Because of the potential problem of sputum contamination by oropharyngeal flora, the use of the Gram stain as described

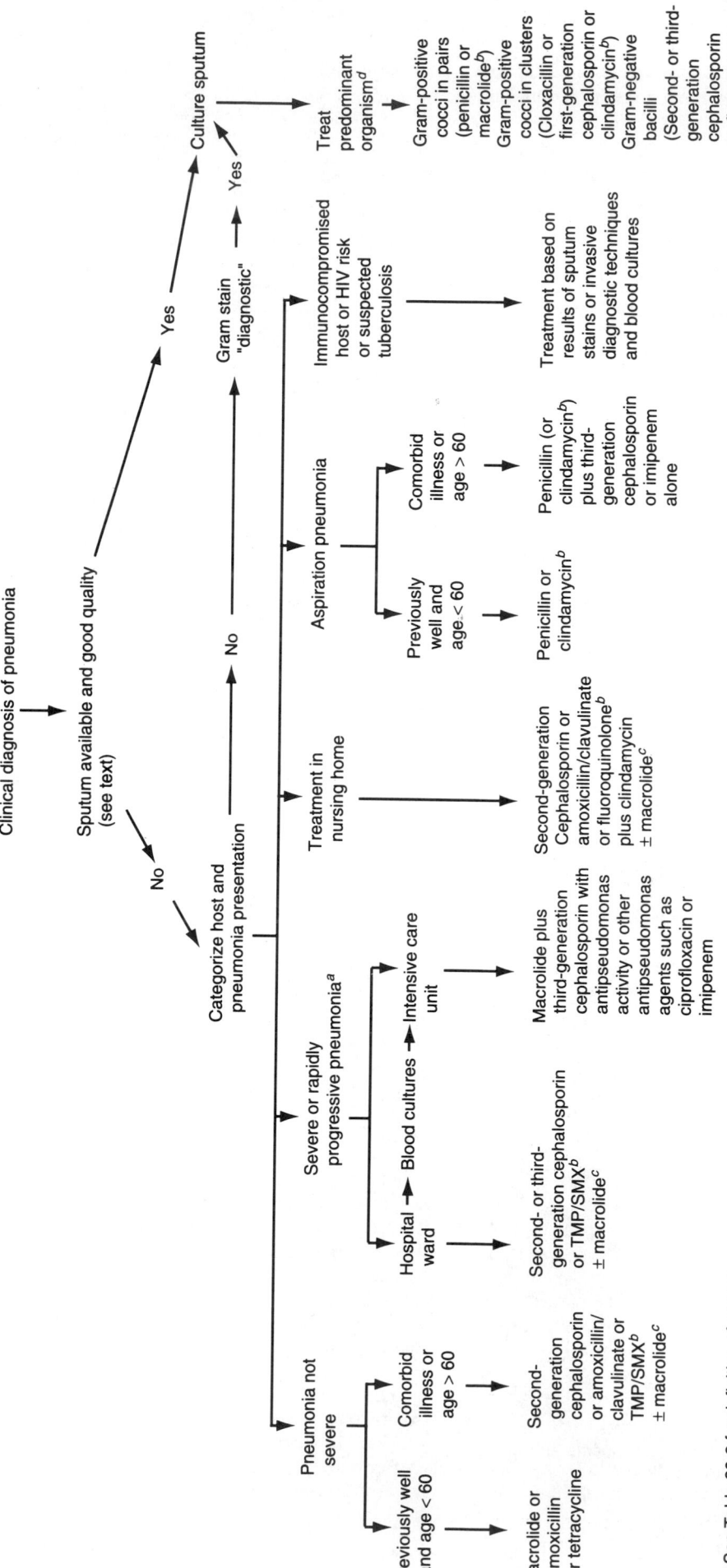

Figure 20-8. Antibiotic therapy dendogram for CAP (see text for details).

a See Table 20-2 for definition of *severe*.

b TMP/SMX, trimethoprim-sulfamethoxazole for penicillin-allergic patients.

c If Legionella is a concern (add rifampin if Legionella documented).

d Modify for severe pneumonia as indicated.

above should always be influenced by a careful consideration of the nature of the host and the presentation of the pneumonia, as outlined in Figure 20-8. Once sputum culture results are returned, it may be possible to "downgrade" the antibiotic choice to a less expensive and more specific agent.

The therapy for pneumonia in the immunocompromised host is addressed more fully in the last section of this chapter. In general because there is little margin for error in these compromised patients and in patients in whom there is a strong suspicion of tuberculosis, therapy should be based on the results of stains and cultures of sputum or other respiratory secretions often obtained with invasive diagnostic techniques.

If a bacterial aspiration pneumonia is suspected, coverage for the predominant oropharyngeal flora of the patient must be provided. Sputum smears findings in aspiration pneumonia usually indicate "mixed organisms" or "normal respiratory flora." Therefore, the character of the host must be used as a guide for antibiotic selection. In the young and previously well patient with suspected aspiration pneumonia, oral anerobes are likely to predominate. Penicillin is the drug of choice with clindamycin as a good alternative for patients who are allergic to penicillin. For patients who are older and those with coexisting illnesses, aspiration pneumonia may also be due to gram-negative organisms. Therefore, the antibiotic spectrum should be broader with a combination of penicillin or clindamycin plus a third-generation cephalosporin. Imipenem alone as monotherapy is also acceptable in this setting.

Because patients in nursing homes are elderly and usually have coexisting illnesses, a broad-spectrum approach is warranted, as reflected in the choices listed in Figure 20-8. Many of these elderly patients have oropharyngeal colonization with β-lactamase-producing organisms. Thus to provide good gram-positive and gram-negative coverage, a combination of amoxicillin plus clavulanic acid would be effective for most patients. Other options include an oral second-generation cephalosporin or, for penicillin-allergic patients, an oral fluoroquinolone plus clindamycin or trimethoprim-sulfamethoxazole (TMP/SMX).

For most patients presenting with CAP, the special circumstances noted above will not apply, and a specific microbial diagnosis will not be possible on the day of presentation. Therefore, initial therapy must be empiric. The choice can be simplified considerably by the physician noting the type of host, the severity of illness, and the clinical setting in which the pneumonia has occurred. This empiric approach is based on several epidemiologic studies that have identified the most likely responsible pathogens for various clinical presentations of CAP. Because only probabilities in regard to infecting organisms are used in this approach, the initial antibiotic choices suggested are relatively broad in spectrum to ensure that most of the likely pathogens will be effectively treated. A knowledge of the local microbial epidemiologic environment will also assist in the selection of a starting antibiotic regimen. For example, in areas where pneumonia caused by Legionella is relatively common, the initial antibiotic therapy should include a macrolide (Edelstein and Meyer, 1989).

For patients whose pneumonia is severe enough to require admission to the hospital or even to an ICU, additional organisms, including Legionella species, aerobic gram-negative bacteria, anaerobic bacilli, and S. aureus must be considered. For these reasons and because of the severity of the illness that affects these patients, the initial empiric antibiotic choices should be fairly broad-spectrum intravenous agents. For patients who can be managed in a hospital ward setting, a second- or third-generation cephalosporin or a penicillin with a β-lactamase inhibitor (e.g., ticarcillin and clavulanic acid) will usually be effective. For penicillin-allergic patients, TMP/SMX alone or with a macrolide is a reasonable alternative. For nonintubated patients with CAP, a second- or third-generation cephalosporin without antipseudomonal activity is usually sufficient because infection with Pseudomonas aeruginosa is unlikely unless the patient has structural abnormalities of the lungs, such as bronchiectasis, or has been treated with multiple courses of antibiotics or corticosteroids. On the other hand, for patients with CAP who have respiratory failure that necessitates intubation and therapy in an ICU from the outset, a third-generation cephalosporin with antipseudomonal activity should be chosen in addition to a macrolide because infection with pseudomonas and Legionella increases in likelihood in this patient group, depending on local microbial patterns. Another effective combination in this setting is a macrolide plus an intravenous fluoroquinolone with antipseudomonal activity, such as ciprofloxacin, or a macrolide plus imipenem.

Some caveats in regard to antibiotic use in the therapy of CAP in various clinical settings are worthwhile. In general the fluoroquinolones are not reliable enough against Streptococcus pneumoniae to be used as monotherapy for CAP. Therefore, they should be used in combination with a macrolide or a penicillin in patients in whom the responsible pathogen is not definitively known (Failla and Karam, 1993). The fluoroquinolones have excellent bioavailability when administered by the orgal or nasogastric routes and so offer the cost-saving potential of early stepdown therapy from the intravenous to the oral route (Gentry, et al., 1992; Kahn and Basin, 1989; Paladino, et al., 1991). Caution must be exercised, however, when fluoroquinolones are given orally or by the nasograstric route because decreased absorption has been noted when these drugs are administered concurrently with aluminum-, magnesium-, and calcium-containing antacids as a result of the formation of nonabsorbable chelates (Hooper and Wolfson, 1991).

Imipenem is the representative drug of a new class of β-lactams called carbapenems and has a broad antimicrobial spectrum, including methicillin-sensitive S. aureus, pneumococci, and most anerobes, including Bacteroides fragilis, Acinetobacter, and P. aeruginosa. Notably, however, other Pseudomonas species, including P. cepacia and P. maltophilia, and Enterococcus faecium are not covered.

Some caution is needed when certain antibiotics are administered to patients who are also receiving theophyllines for underlying COPD. The main concerns are ciprofloxacin and the macrolides (including the newer macrolides), both of which may increase serum theophylline levels by an inhibition of hepatic enzymes (Wijands, et al., 1986).

Several important but unanswered questions remain in regard to the use of antibiotics for the therapy of CAP. These issues include the duration of antimicrobial therapy and the question of when patients who are receiving intravenous antibiotics can safely be switched to oral therapy. Unfortunately there is little specific information available to address these questions definitively. In general, however, most uncomplicated cases of CAP should probably be treated for 7 to 10 days with antibiotics, although pneumonia caused by atypical organisms, such as *M. pneumoniae* and *C. pneumoniae,* may require longer therapy (14 to 21 days) (Marrie, 1994; Niederman, et al., 1993). Pneumonia caused by Legionella should probably be treated for 21 days (Marrie, 1994). Patients with structural lung disease, such as bronchiectasis, may require an even longer duration of antimicrobial therapy, particularly if *P. aeruginosa* is the offending pathogen. Intravenous antibiotic therapy is expensive, and every attempt should be made to step down to effective oral antimicrobial therapy whenever possible. Usually hospitalized patients with relatively uncomplicated CAP can be switched to oran antimicrobial therapy after 3 to 4 days of parenteral therapy or once they have been afebrile for 24 hours.

Failure to Respond to Initial Therapy

Most patients with CAP, whether treated in the hospital or as outpatients, will respond to initial empiric therapy and improve within 48 to 72 hours. Thus, the initial antibiotic therapy for CAP should probably not be changed for 2 to 3 days unless there has been a marked clinical deterioration, in which case invasive measures, such as bronchoscopy, may be necessary to guide further therapy. Appropriately treated patients usually defervesce, and the white blood cell count usually returns to normal within 2 to 4 days (Lehtomaki, 1988), although wheezes and crackles may persist longer than 1 week in up to 40 percent of patients who respond to therapy. If this expected improvement does not occur, several possibilities should be considered, including the following.

Was the Initial Antibiotic Selection Inadequate? The antibiotic options offered in Figure 20-8 are sufficiently broad spectrum to cover most likely pathogens in the clinical settings described. However, the problem of antibiotic resistance is growing worldwide, with an increasing prevalence observed for amoxicillin-resistant *H. influenzae* and penicillin-resistant *S. pneumoniae* (Marrie, 1994; Tremblay, et al., 1990). If *S. aureus* is suspected, the addition of an antistaphylococcal antibiotic, such as cloxacillin, would be reasonable.

Is There an Unusual Infection? Occasionally pneumonia is caused by uncommon organisms, usually in the context of a specific clinical setting, such as *Chlamydia psittaci* (psittacosis or bird exposure, treat with tetracycline); *Coxiella burnetii* (Q fever, exposure to cattle, sheep, goats, or parturient cats, treat with tetracycline), *M. tuberculosis* (elderly or immunocompromised patients, immigrants from endemic areas, treat with antituberculous agents), *Francisella tularensis* (Tularemia, exposure to rabbits or ticks, treat with streptomycin), *Yersinia pestis* (plague, exposure to rodents, or squirrels, treat with streptomycin), and fungi, such as Histoplasma, Cryptococcus, and Coccidioides (travel to endemic areas, treat with amphotericin B or newer antifungal agents if indicated).

Is This Infective Pneumonia? The differential diagnosis at this stage should reconsider the possibility of pulmonary thromboembolism with infarction, congestive heart failure, pulmonary vasculitis, bronchiolitis obliterans, eosinophilic pneumonia, atelectasis, neoplasm (e.g., bronchoalveolar cell carcinoma), etc., all of which can mimic pneumonia clinically and on the chest radiograph.

Has a Complication Developed? Here the physician should consider the possibility of atelectasis, pleural effusion, empyema, lung or brain abscess, meningitis, endocarditis, septic arthritis, drug fever, and antibiotic-induced pseudomembranous entercolitis.

Is There a Superinfection? This is most likely to be a problem when a secondary nosocomial pneumonia complicates a severe CAP that requires assisted ventilation in the ICU. Invasive diagnostic techniques are indicated.

Is There an Unrelated Infection? Subcutaneous abscesses, sinusitis, and urinary tract infections are the most likely possibilities.

Is There Intravenous Phlebitis? This development can complicate the picture by causing persistent fever and leukocytosis despite adequate therapy for the pneumonia.

Most pneumonias resolve sooner clinically than they do radiographically. Even for young, previously well patients, the chest radiograph will have returned to normal by 1 month in only 60 percent of patients (Jay, et al., 1975). Radiographic resolution is more likely to be delayed in elderly patients, particularly if COPD coexists. In this case only 25 percent of patients demonstrate radiographic resolution by 1 month, and complete clearing may require several months (Fein, et al., 1993; Jay, et al., 1975; Mittl, et al., 1994).

If pneumonia has cleared both clinically and radiographically but recurs, several possibilities, including postobstructive pneumonia from endobronchial obstruction, COPD, bronchiectasis, recurrent aspiration, immunocompromise, and malnutrition, should be considered (Geppert, 1990).

When patients with CAP do not respond to apparently appropriate antimicrobial therapy, particularly if the pneumonia is severe, extensive diagnostic procedures are indicated and include computed tomographic (CT) scanning of the thorax, serologic testing, and bronchoscopy to obtain deep lung specimens (Finesilver, et al., 1990; Ortqvist, et al., 1990). Difficulty often occurs in this situation, however, because patients are already receiving antibiotics. This has been known to cause a high false-negative rate for specimens obtained by fiberoptic bronchoscopy, regardless of the techniques used (Meduri, 1992). The value of CT scanning of the thorax for nonresolving pneumonia is primarily its ability to detect unsuspected pleural effusions, which should be tapped for diagnostic yield (Sahn, 1993).

Most patients hospitalized for CAP are ready for discharge after 7 to 10 days but may experience fatigue and some cough for 3 to 4 weeks. Most will have resumed normal activities after 6 weeks. Pulmonary function usually recovers completely after an episode of CAP unless there has been some complication that resulted in pulmonary fibrosis, bronchiectasis, bronchiolitis, lung abscess, or chronic empyema. In some patients with an underlying asthmatic diathesis, a persistent bronchial irritability syndrome, manifested by paroxysmal nonproductive cough, can be induced by pneumonia or acute bronchitis and may require temporary therapy with inhaled or even oral corticosteroids to regain control (Empey, et al., 1976).

Prevention

Important infective causes of acute respiratory disease include *S. pneumoniae, M. tuberculosis,* and influenza viruses, and effective preventative measures exist for all these infections.

The problem of recurrent pneumonia is of particular interest because it has been poorly studied, but recent data from Hedlund, et al. (1993) demonstrated that patients discharged from the hospital were five times more likely to suffer from recurrent pneumonia and three times more likely to die from pneumonia within 3 years of discharge. The causes of these recurrent pneumonias are not known, but because *S. pneumoniae* remains the most frequent cause of CAP, it would seem logical to consider prevention for such patients by the administration of the pneumococcal vaccine. Whether such prophylaxis would be effective is not known, but most patients with recurrent pneumonia are elderly with coexisting illnesses, and so current recommendations for pneumococcal vaccine use would be applicable in any case (Sims, et al., 1988).

Prognosis

Most patients with CAP are not severely ill and can be treated as outpatients. In this setting the prognosis of CAP remains good, with quoted mortality rates in the range of 1 to 5 percent (Niederman, et al., 1993). However, for patients with more severe pneumonia and for elderly patients with coexisting illnesses, hospitalization is often necessary. In this group the mortality rate from CAP approaches 25 percent, particularly if an intensive care unit (ICU) admission is necessary (Niederman, et al., 1993; Pachon, et al., 1990; Torres, et al., 1991). The prognosis of patients with CAP is determined both by the virulence of the infecting organism and by the presence or absence of coexisting illnesses. In the past few years, several studies have identified risk factors, which if present predict either an increased risk of death or a complicated course (Celis, et al., 1988; Farr, et al., 1991; Fine, et al., 1990; Ortqvist, et al., 1985; Torres, et al., 1991). When factors predictive of CAP are present, and particularly if more than one risk factor exists, hospital admission is the most prudent course. It is interesting that in several studies simple observation of the respiratory rate has been found to be one of the best predictors of death in CAP. Mortality rate rises rapidly once the respiratory rate rises above 30 breaths/min. In one study the mortality rate approached 50 percent in patients whose respiratory rate rose above 40 breaths/min (Van Eeden, et al., 1988). With a retrospective, historical cohort analysis of 245 patients with CAP, Farr, et al. (1991) analyzed mortality risk factors that had previously been identified in a British Thoracic Society epidemiologic study on CAP (British Thoracic Society, 1987). Although many potential risk factors were examined, only three were found to be clearly predictive of death in CAP, namely a respiratory rate above 30 breaths/min, a diastolic blood pressure less than 60 mmHg, and a blood urea concentration greater than 7 mMol/L. The overall mortality rate for CAP in this review was 8.2 percent, but when two or three predictive factors were present, the mortality rate was 28.6 percent.

Patients with overwhelming illness, including those with overt respiratory failure, those who require mechanical ventilation, those with signs of systemic sepsis, and those in whom the radiographic opacities are seen to progress rapidly within the first 24 to 48 hours of admission, are at high risk for death from CAP. It is important to note, however, that a poor prognosis and high mortality rate from CAP may also be seen in elderly patients who present with only vague signs of pneumonia. Such patients are often debilitated and respond poorly to infections. Despite the presence of significant pneumonia, cough may be minimal, fever may be absent, and extrapulmonary symptoms may predominate (e.g., confusion and fatigue) (Finkelstein, et al., 1983; Venkatesan, et al., 1990). Such a confusing presentation may result in the delayed recognition of CAP in elderly patients and a subsequent delay in starting appropriate antibiotic therapy.

NOSOCOMIAL PNEUMONIA

The term *nosocomial pneumonia* refers to the acquisition of pulmonary infection 48 to 72 hours after admission to an acute care facility. Given the unique bacterial colonization characteristics of the hospital environment and of hospital personnel, the epidemiologic factors and etiologic organisms are different from those seen in CAP. Nosocomial pneumonia is particularly common in patients who are undergoing elective thoracic or upper abdominal surgery (Horan, et al., 1986; Sanford, 1986).

Epidemiology and Pathophysiology

The thoracic surgeon is frequently called on to assess patients with nosocomial pneumonia. Most of these cases occur secondary to bacterial infection. Pneumonia is the second most common cause of nosocomial infection (Horan, et al., 1986) but is the most frequent cause of death secondary to hospital-acquired sepsis (Sanford, 1986; Gross, et al., 1980). Quoted mortality rates vary, depending on a number of factors, such as the underlying disease process. However, outcome appears to be particularly affected by the need for mechanical ventilation and the development of ventilator-associated pneumonia (VAP). Under such circumstances, mortality rates as high as 32 to 55 percent have been reported in longitudinal studies of large numbers of ICU patients (Craven, et al., 1986; Stevens, et al., 1974). The overall incidence of nosocomial pneumonia is greatly increased by the addition of mechanical ventilation, as reported by both Ribner (1986) and Torres, et al., (1990). Ribner (1986) reported that pneumonia occurred with 21 times the frequency in the ventilated patient; others have suggested that the incidence of this complication with mechanical ventilation may be as high as 10 to 24 percent (Stevens, et al., 1974; Torres, et al., 1990).

This incidence appears to be directly related to the duration of required ventilatory support and, according to some authors, may reach 68 percent in those individuals ventilated for more than 30 days, as suggested by the report of Langer et al. (1989). Additional risk factors for nosocomial pneumonia include old age (Hanson, et al., 1992), malnutrition, chronic lung disease, obesity, concurrent antibiotic use, and the performance of either thoracic or upper abdominal operative procedures (Haley, et al., 1981). With multivariate analysis in a prospective study of more than 300 ventilated patients, Torres, et al. (1990) determined that the main risk factors for VAP included the need for reintubation and the aspiration of gastric contents.

These associations do not explain completely the frequent occurrence of nosocomial pneumonia in the postoperative period and that noted coincident with the institution of mechanical ventilation. A general appreciation of the pathophysiologic factors and the number of interrelating factors as outlined in Figure 20-9. Surgery, particularly thoracic and major abdominal procedures, can be considered to have effects on host defenses and dramatic effects on the mechanical properties of the lung and chest wall. The effects of surgery on systemic host defense mechanisms have been studied extensively, and it is apparent that cell-mediated immunity is frequently impaired (Bartlett, 1977). In addition, intubation of the tracheobronchial tree decreases mucociliary clearance; at the same time, it dramatically increases the secretion of mucus and bypasses the normal barrier of the glottis. This sets the stage for aspiration of potentially pathogenic bacteria. The pain and discomfort generated by major truncal surgery results in patients who alter their normal pattern of breathing so that they breathe at low lung volumes and maintain minute ventilation by increasing their respiratory rates. As a consequence, functional residual capacity is decreased, airway closure occurs, and atelectasis results. In addition, the decreased functional residual capacity impairs the ability

to cough and effectively clear the secretions that are normally increased after surgery. Cough is further impaired by the pain and splinting of the chest wall and any abdominal distension that may have resulted from the surgical procedure.

Infection cannot occur without the presence of microorganisms. Intuitively we would suppose that colonization must precede the establishment of infection in any organ. Johanson, et al. (1969, 1972), in separate articles, showed that the rate of colonization of the oropharynx is associated with the severity of clinical illness and the duration of hospitalization. This same group (Johanson, et al., 1972) followed the clinical course of colonized patients and discovered that the incidence of pneumonia was much more frequent in the colonized group than in those whom they were unable to demonstrate colonization (23 percent in those who were colonized versus 3 percent in those who were not).

The microbiology of nosocomial pneumonia is different from that of CAP; most nosocomial pneumonia is caused by gram-negative enteric bacilli. This is especially the case for the patient population in ICU. This was shown by Johanson, et al. (1972) during their observational study of colonization rates. Organisms such as *P. aeruginosa, Serratia marcescens,* Acinetobacter, *Klebsiella oxytocia,* and Enterobacter species, which are rarely seen in the community, predominate in nosocomial pneumonia. *S. aureus* also occurs commonly (Rello, et al., 1990), and other unusual infections such as candidal pneumonia (Johnston, et al., 1991) occur with a frequency that suggests different pathophysiologic factors from those of CAP and operative factors other than simply an impairment in host defenses.

It has been of considerable interest on the part of surgeons and critical care physicians to speculate on the origin of the gram-negative bacilli that clearly dominate the clinical picture of nosocomial pneumonia. As suggested in Figure 20-10, both the oropharynx and the stomach appear to harbor these organisms in critically ill patients. There exist at present two

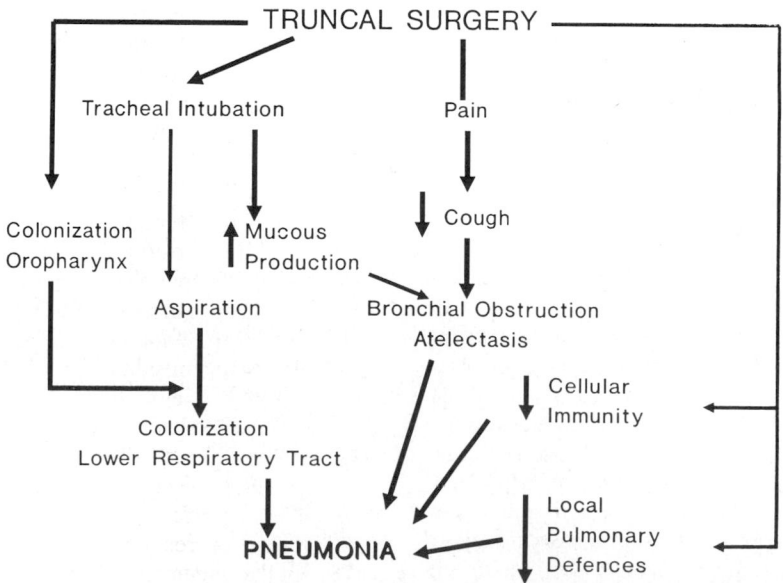

Figure 20-9. Dendrogram outlining the pathophysiology of nosocomial pneumonia (see text for details).

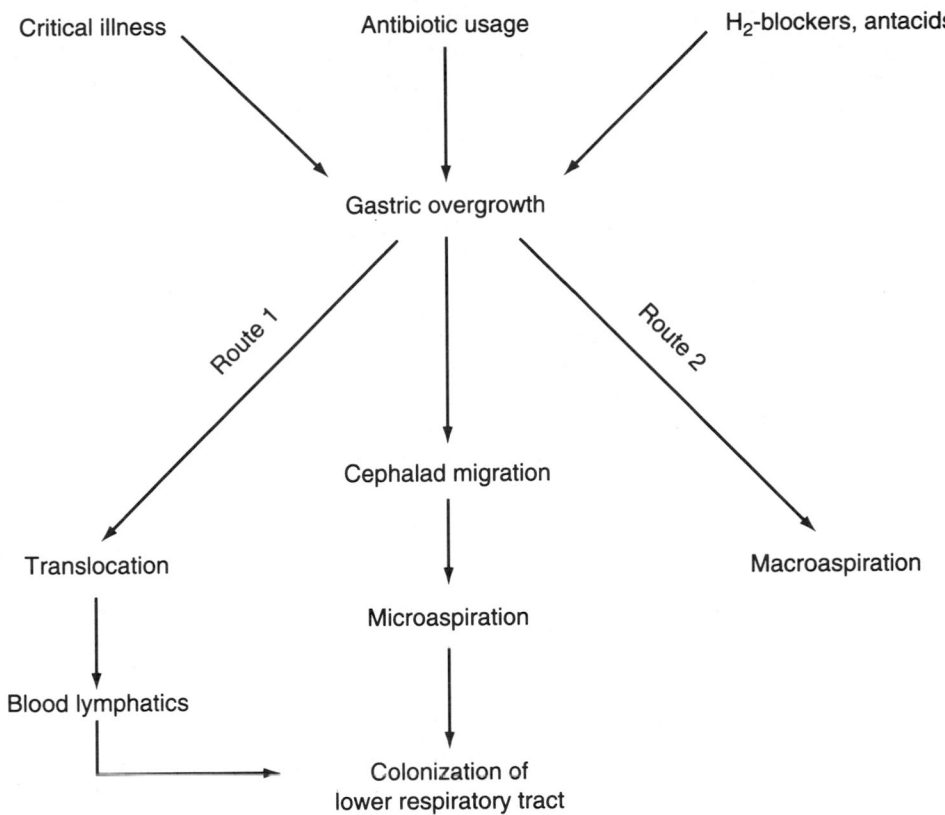

Figure 20-10. Dendrogram outlining the pathophysiology of gram-negative bacilli in the pathogenesis of nosocomial pneumonia (see text for details).

hypotheses in regard to how these microorganisms find their way into the distal bronchial tree. The first involves the overgrowth of bacteria in the stomach, associated with their subsequent migration cephalad through the gastrointestinal tract into the oropharynx. It is then postulated that the organisms find their way into the lower respiratory tract by micro- or macroaspiration. The second hypothesis suggests that bacteria in the small and large intestine undergo translocation into intestinal lymphatic channels and eventually into the circulation. It is postulated that such translocation is facilitated by a change in the intestinal barrier to bacterial movement and that this occurs secondary to a variety of conditions that are frequently present in the postoperative or critically ill patient.

Whether by aspiration or by gastric overgrowth secondary to decreased gastric acidity, the fact remains that the gastrointestinal tract appears to be a major source of infecting organisms. In some patients, colonization of the oropharynx appears to occur first, followed by colonization of the stomach and the tracheobronchial tree. The important point is that the airway is essentially contiguous with the oropharynx and the stomach. Therefore, changes in the microbial flora of the one will lead to similar changes in the other in short order.

If gastroesophageal reflux and tracheobronchial aspiration indeed play a vital role in the genesis of nosocomial pneumonia, then we must consider the effect that nasogastric feeding might have on the incidence of this problem Thurn, et al. (1990) maintained that rates of pneumonia were actually higher in patients who received enteral feeding through nasogastric tubes. Nonetheless a metanalysis conducted by Moore et al. (1991) demonstrated that the rates of pulmonary infection are reduced in patients who received enteral nutrition compared with those who received total parenteral nutrition. The specific mechanism to explain this salutory effect of early enteral feeding is not known but may reflect improved immunologic functioning of the gut.

Regardless of the point of origin, microorganisms are regularly aspirated into the tracheobronchial tree of hospitalized patients. When this occurs in normal hosts, the tracheobronchial tree usually remains sterile, whereas the airways are regularly colonized in critically ill patients. One explanation for this observation is that critically ill patients aspirate more often and in greater amounts than do healthy hosts. Another reason is that hospitalized seriously ill patients are more likely to have impaired antimicrobial defenses of the airways, which promote persistence and multiplication of organisms.

Environmental sources of potentially pathogenic bacteria should also be considered as possible factors in the problem of nosocomial pneumonia. Respiratory equipment, for example, can become contaminated and serve as a potential source for nosocomial pneumonia. This was more of a problem in the past. The development of new guidelines and the greater use of disposable equipment has significantly reduced the importance of respiratory devices in the pathogenesis of nosocomial pneumonia (Craven, 1989). The role of transmission of bacteria from the hands of health care workers has also been implicated. The routine use of hand washing between patients has been observed to be woefully inadequate. When comprehensive infection control programs have been enforced, the incidence of nosocomial pneumonia has been reduced.

Diagnosis

In the postoperative setting on the ward and especially in the ventilated patient, the reliability of the history and physical examination are often less secure. Furthermore, the normal signs of pulmonary infection are too often mimicked by processes other than pneumonia. Fever may be solely due to atelectasis. Purulent sputum and positive culture findings may be secondary to bronchial infection as a result of endotracheal intubation and contamination. Abnormal chest radiographs are the rule after thoracic surgery, and we may have difficulty discerning fluid overload from ARDS, atelectasis, pneumonia, etc. In the intubated ventilated patient, the clinical diagnosis of pneumonia is often in error for all the reasons noted above. The unreliability of the clinical diagnosis in this setting has led to the development of techniques designed to obtain distal airway secretions that are not contaminated from the proximal tracheobronchial tree. These include protected specimen brushing (PSB), bronchoalveolar lavage (BAL), and protected bronchoalveolar lavage (PBAL).

The brush for PSB (Fig. 20-11) sits in the inner cannula of a double-catheter system, the outer sleeve of which is blocked at its distal end with a plug of Gelfoam. As a result, the brush is protected from upper airway secretions when it is inserted through the suction port of a flexible bronchoscope. Once the fiberscope is positioned in the appropriate segmental orifice, the inner catheter is advanced, followed by the brush itself. The Gelfoam plug is extruded, and the brush is advanced into the distal airway of interest. With the use of quantitative bacterial culture techniques, several studies have shown that a growth of bacteria greater than 10^3 colony-forming units per milliliter (cfu/ml) is highly specific for the diagnosis of pneumonia (Moser, et al., 1982; DeCastro, et al., 1991), but when the results of brushing are ''negative,'' there is a significant chance that pneumonia may still be present. The high false-negative rate has led to the development of BAL as an alternative. BAL samples at least 100 times the lung area recovers 100 to 1,000 times more secretions than PSB. A significant quantitative culture for BAL is usually considered to be 10^4 cfu/ml. This procedure is not as free from upper airway contamination as PSB, and although it is very sensitive (low false-negative rate) in the

diagnosis of pneumonia, it is not terribly specific (high false-positive rate) (Chastre, et al., 1988; Kirkpatrick and Bass, 1989). As a result of all this investigation, it has been recommended that both BAL and PSB be used (Chastre, et al., 1989). The specificity of BAL can be greatly improved (up to 100 percent sensitivity) by an alteration in the technique described by Meduri and Chastre (1992), which uses a protected BAL catheter. Undertaken in this fashion, PBAL involves the passage of a balloon-tipped catheter either through a fiberscope or endotracheal tube (the latter under fluoroscopic control).

One problem inherent in the interpretation of the many articles published on these invasive techniques for sampling the lower airways is controversy over the definition of what is the procedure of choice for the presence of pneumonia itself. This is particularly an issue in VAP. Despite this uncertainty, nosocomial pneumonia should always be at least suspected whenever there are new or progressive opacities on the chest radiograph, which are accompanied by purulent secretions and may or may not be associated with fever or leukocytosis.

The performance of any of these techniques may not always be practical or cost effective. In the normal clinical situation, the presence of purulent secretions with a predominant organism on either Gram stain or culture and associated with a localized opacity on the chest radiograph should be sufficient evidence to commence appropriate antimicrobial therapy. Emphasis is placed on the localized radiographic opacity. This is not an unreasonable approach as long as the clinician realizes that there is considerable room for clinical error. More specific means of diagnosis (BAL, PBAL, or PSB) should be used as indicated in the algorithm illustrated in Figure 20-12. In particular, one of these specific means of sampling should be selected when the following conditions prevail:

1. A clinical suspicion of pneumonia in the face of generalized radiographic opacities. Such opacities may be secondary to ARDS, fluid overload, chemical pneumonitis, etc., but bacterial pneumonia can be a complicating event.

2. The failure to respond to what is considered appropriate initial treatment. This is especially true if initial therapy is based on cultures obtained from tracheal suctioning alone.

3. A new focal radiographic opacity in a severely ill patient in whom nevertheless a low clinical suspicion of pneumonia exists. Ruling out a pneumonia with a negative PSB, BAL, or PBAL finding may reduce the cost of needless antibiotic therapy and save the patient from unwanted drug side effects.

Therapy

There is no doubt that therapy for presumed bacterial nosocomial pneumonia is frequently initiated before a pathogen has been identified, and there are often good reasons for this. However, therapy should not be started before sputum or tracheobronchial secretions are obtained for Gram stain and culture, if this is possible. A Gram stain is particularly critical when the patient's condition warrants early and specific therapy. The choice of antimicrobials can then be based on the Gram stain findings, with any necessary alterations made

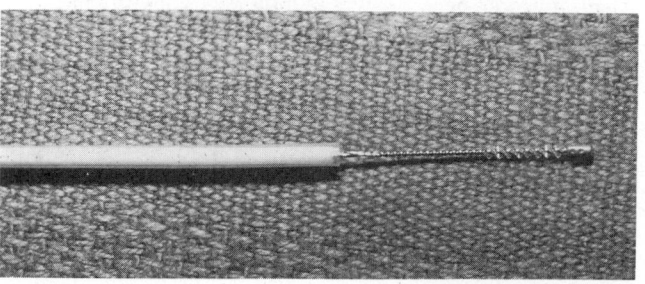

Figure 20-11. Protected specimen brush.

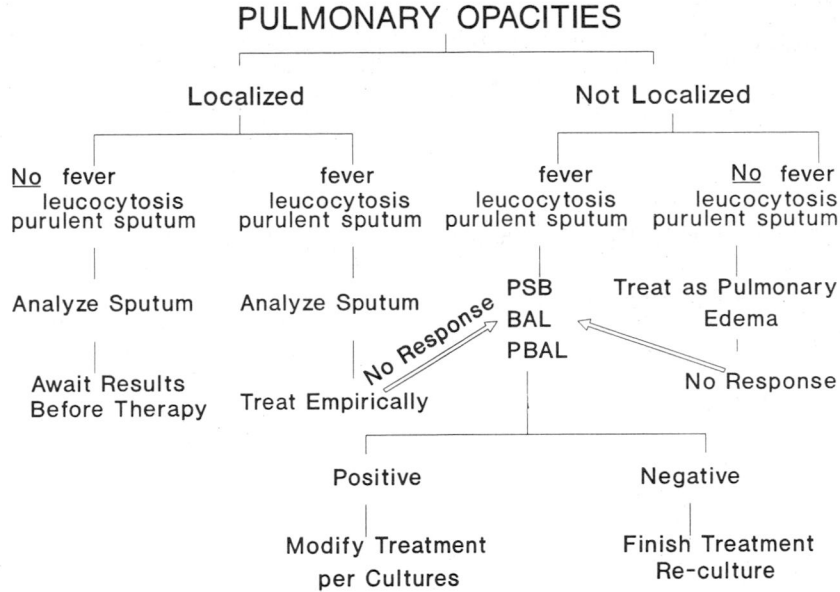

Figure 20-12. Algorithm for use of bronchoscopy in the diagnosis of pneumonia (see text for details).

when the final culture and sensitivity are available. The selection of antibiotics should also be influenced by the following:

1. The rapidity of onset of the pneumonic process.
2. The clinical condition of the patient (i.e., how much respiratory reserve exists and how severe is the attendant ventilation/perfusion mismatch and gas exchange abnormality, e.g., hypoxemia, or hypercarbia).
3. The epidemiologic characteristics of the particular surgical unit. What is the indigent microbial flora?
4. The immunocompetence of the patient. Patients who acquire pneumonia while they are leukopenic or receiving corticosteroids are likely to be infected with specific infecting organisms and to have a more fulminant process.

Empiric therapy for nosocomial pneumonia is different from that which is appropriate for CAP. Because hospital-acquired pulmonary infections frequently involve gram-negative enteric organisms, *S. aureus,* and/or anaerobes, coverage should take into account all three possibilities, particularly if the patient's condition is considered critical. Anaerobic infections are common after thoracic surgical procedures, particularly those on the esophagus and in patients in whom the cause is believed to be aspiration. A suitable regimen under such circumstances might consist of either an aminoglycoside or a third-generation cephalosporin combined with clindamycin for coverage of anaerobes and staphylococci. A Gram stain result with a predominance of gram-positive cocci would however demand that an antibiotic against potentially methicillin-resistant staphylococci (e.g., vancomycin) be used, especially for initial therapy in critically ill patients.

Initiation of appropriate antibiotics does not end the responsibility of the attending physician. It is imperative that the response to therapy be critically appraised frequently, by an assessment of the patient and the chest radiograph,

and the peak serum concentration of aminoglycosides when used. Peak concentrations of 8.0 mg/dl are desirable.

In recent years there has been considerable interest in the use of monotherapy instead of the combination approach noted above. Both third-generation cephalosporins and the synthetic β-lactam antibiotic imipenem have been shown to be as efficacious as multidrug therapy based on aminoglycosides (Laforce, 1989; Clissold, et al., 1987). The greatest interest in monotherapy currently is in imipenem because of its broad spectrum, including antianaerobic activity, and in ciprofloxacin, a fluorinated quinolone, because of its gram-negative and gram-positive spectrum and exceedingly good penetration into bronchial mucus (Clissold, et al., 1987). A recent multicentered randomized trial suggested that side effects were reduced with single-drug therapy, whereas therapeutic response was maintained (Fernandez-Guerrero, et al., 1991). As other antibiotics come on the market, it is anticipated that monotherapy will become the standard. However, monotherapy may not be the best choice when there is a clinical suspicion that pneumonia is due to *P. aeruginosa* because this organism is associated with higher mortality rates than the other gram-negative bacilli. Furthermore, synergism exists with the combination of a β-lactam antibiotic, such as imipenem, and an aminoglycoside in this setting.

SPECIAL CONSIDERATIONS

Aspiration Pneumonia

The term *aspiration pneumonia* has been used by various authors to describe different clinical syndromes, and this has often led to confusion in regard to the nature of the pulmonary insult (Bartlett and Gorbach, 1975). The three major aspiration syndromes are aspiration of gastric contents, pulmonary infection, and acute airway obstruction resulting from aspiration of inert material. This section deals only with aspiration

---

Pulmonary Aspiration Syndromes

Aspiration of gastric contents
  Acute chemical pneumonitis
  Bronchospasm
  Bronchial irritability syndrome
  Pulmonary fibrosis (chronic aspiration)
Primary aspiration pneumonia
  Anaerobic-aerobic bronchopneumonia
  Necrotizing pneumonia
  Lung abscess
  Empyema
Acute airway obstruction
  Large-volume liquid or particulate aspiration (e.g., "drowning")
  Obstructing food bolus (e.g., "café coronary")
  Foreign body aspiration

Conditions Predisposing to Pulmonary Aspiration

Loss of airway protective reflexes
  Depressed level of consciousness
  Old age
  Postextubation
  Neuromuscular disease
  Endotracheal tube
Structural/functional abnormalities
  Laryngeal pathology
  Tracheoesophageal fistula
  Esophageal achalasia
  Zenker's diverticulum
  Esophageal dysmotility
Factors promoting gastroesophageal reflux
  Gastroesophageal reflux disease
  Nasogastric and gastric lavage tubes
  Trendelenburg position
  Gastric distension from tube feeding
  Diabetic gastroparesis
  Gastric or small bowel obstruction
  Ileus
  Narcotics

---

of gastric contents and pulmonary infection, which may be primary from microaspiration of oropharyngeal microbial flora or occur as a secondary complication after acute chemical pneumonitis from gastric acid aspiration.

Pathophysiology

Several anatomic, neurophysiologic, and immunologic mechanisms exist to protect the lower airways from aspiration during swallowing or vomiting and to protect the pulmonary parenchyma and airways from infection secondary to silent aspiration of oropharyngeal microbial flora (De Paso, 1991). A number of pathologic conditions can disrupt these normal defense mechanisms and so predispose to the occurrence of pulmonary aspiration. The three most common predisposing conditions are (1) loss of physiologic airway protective reflexes, (2) structural and functional abnormalities of the upper airways and esophagus, and (3) gastroesophageal reflux. Probably the most common cause of the pulmonary aspiration syndrome is loss of airway protective reflexes as a result of a depressed level of consciousness. This is seen most commonly in the perioperative setting and is associated with surgical anesthesia (Blitt, et al., 1970; Culver, et al., 1951; Burgess, et al., 1979). Equally important factors are inappropriate use of postoperative analgesics or sedatives, intentional drug overdose, or central nervous system trauma. As has been noted above, there are several other predisposing factors to aspiration, including intubation itself, as well as advancing age (Pontopiddan and Beecher, 1960).

A number of structural and functional abnormalities can predispose to pulmonary aspiration. These include tracheobronchial fistulae and esophageal problems, such as dilatation, obstruction, and esophageal dysmotility caused by achalasia or carcinoma (Belsey, 1960). Pharyngeal and laryngeal dysfunction may increase the risk of gastric aspiration. It is seen after injuries or surgery to the neck with laryngeal nerve dysfunction and in association with tracheostomy and endotracheal and nasoenteric tubes (Alessi and Berci, 1986; Olivares, et al., 1974). Gastroesophageal reflux disease predis-

poses to pulmonary aspiration and is aggravated by such exogenous factors as ethanol and tobacco use, excessive caffeine intake, pregnancy, obesity, and the use of succinylcholine at intubation (Pelligrini, et al., 1979).

Aspiration of Gastric Contents. Aspiration of gastric contents can occur either silently or overtly. The report by Mendelson (1946) of chemical pneumonitis after aspiration of gastric contents complicating pregnancy remains the classic description; it emphasizes the role of hydrochloric acid in the pathogenesis of this syndrome. In general, both the amount (Greenfield, et al., 1989; Wynne, 1982) of gastric material aspirated and the pH (James, et al., 1984; Teabout, 1952; Wynne, et al., 1981) of the material are considered important in the pathogenesis of chemical pneumonitis. In an animal model of gastic aspiration, an aspirate with a pH of 1.5 was associated with immediate damage to the ciliated respiratory epithelium, which required several days for regeneration (Wynne, et al., 1981). Such damage to the respiratory mucosa and loss of the ciliated respiratory epithelial cells of the proximal airways leads to dysfunction of the normal pulmonary defense mechanisms and predisposes to secondary infectious pneumonia. Small-volume low-pH gastric aspiration commonly occurs in the immediate postoperative period and often goes unnoticed until secondary infection emerges 1 to 2 days later. For some patients, on the other hand, this type of aspiration, while unwitnessed (silent aspiration), may result in abrupt reflex bronchospasm and produce a syndrome indistinguishable from an acute asthmatic attack (Boyle, et al., 1985).

The more serious consequences of aspiration of gastric contents usually result from aspiration of material in volumes greater than 25 to 50 ml. These large-volume acid aspirates are quickly distributed throughout the lung within 12 to 18 seconds after aspiration (Hamelberg and Bosomworth, 1964; Dal Santo, 1986). When the pH is less than 2.5, the alveolar epithelial cells are rapidly destroyed along with all preformed surfactant. This type of aspiration is associated with the immediate onset of a profound local and systemic cardiorespiratory response, which can be life threatening and resembles an acute case of ARDS (Fig. 20-13) (Bynum and Pierce, 1976). The immediate acid-induced damage disrupts the alveolar capillary barrier, including the basement membranes and capillary endothelium. This causes a profound increase in the permeability of the pulmonary blood vessels, a so-called leaky alveolar-capillary state. Consequent to this can be a massive exudation of plasma from the pulmonary vasculature into the air spaces, which can be of such magnitude as to lead to tachycardia, intravascular volume depletion, and hypotension; on occasion it can culminate in cardiac and secondary cardiorespiratory collapse (Lewis, et al., 1971). The massive outpouring of plasma effectively neutralizes the gastric acid aspirate so that no further toxic damage occurs unless provoked by repeated gastric acid aspiration. There is usually profound arterial hypoxemia with respiratory alkalosis and hypocapnia; crackles, with or without wheezes, are heard throughout the lung fields. The chest radiograph is usually abnormal from the onset and shows widespread air space disease with no particular lobar predilection.

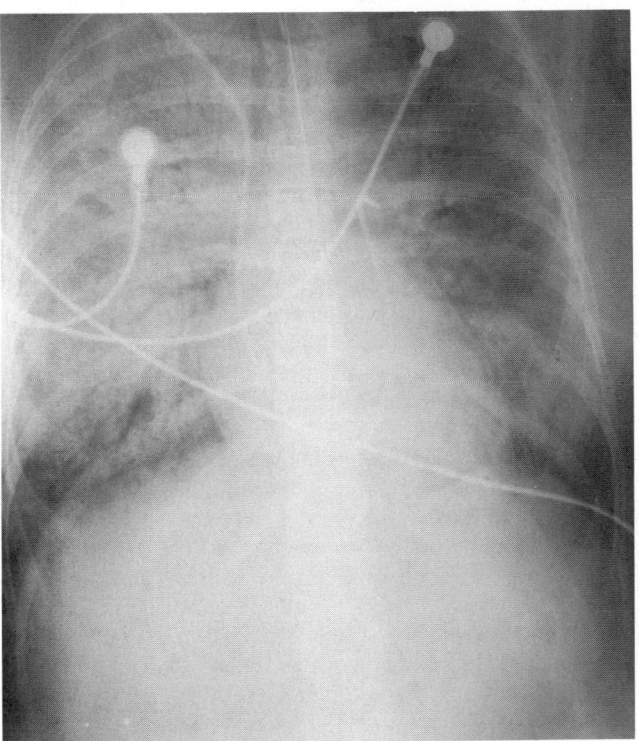

Figure 20-13. Chest radiograph showing ARDS from massive gastric acid aspiration. The patient is intubated and has a balloon-flotation catheter in place.

The natural history of this magnitude of gastric acid aspiration usually follows one of four relatively distinct outcomes (Bynum and Pierce, 1976; Hickling and Howard, 1988; De Paso, 1991).

1. Rapid death from refractory respiratory failure within days.
2. Progressive improvement to recovery within days.
3. Initial stabilization followed by secondary bacterial pneumonia.
4. Prolonged ARDS with multiple organ dysfunction syndrome.

Therapy.   The therapy of gastric acid aspiration is largely supportive; the maintenance of adequate oxygenation is of prime initial importance. Intubation and ventilation with positive end-expiratory pressure are frequently necessary. A considerable amount of intravascular volume loss can occur in the initial phases of large-volume gastric acid aspiration; therefore, aggressive restoration of intravascular volume may be required to achieve hemodynamic stability. However, this resuscitation may lead to an increase in pulmonary venous pressure, which can worsen alveolar-capillary leak and promote alveolar flooding. No specific resuscitation formula has been found to be more successful than any other; in particular the use of colloid resuscitation has not been shown to be any more effective or safer than standard crystalloid-based resuscitation (Pietzman, et al., 1982).

If significant particulate aspiration is suspected, a bronchoscopy, preferably with the rigid bronchoscope, is appropriate to obtain effective tracheobronchial toilet (Epstein, 1988). In the absence of significant particulate aspiration, there is little role for bronchoscopy, and in particular no role for lung lavage, not only because the gastric acid-induced aspiration damage is immediate but also because the gastric aspirate is rapidly neutralized by trachobronchial secretions (Dal Santo, 1986). For these reasons, the use of alkaline lavage is probably contraindicated and more likely to be harmful than beneficial (Bannister, et al., 1961).

Numerous investigations have demonstrated that there is no conclusive benefit for corticosteroids, either by the inhaled (Taylor and Pryse-Davies, 1968; Warriner, et al., 1981) or parenteral routes (Buchman, et al., 1984; Gates, et al., 1983; Glauser, et al., 1979; Sukumaran, et al., 1980; Wynne, et al., 1979). Therefore, they are not recommended for the routine therapy of gastric acid aspiration.

In the setting of small-volume aspiration, which causes acute bronchospasm, aerosolized adrenergic bronchodilators are frequently helpful. The addition of an anticholinergic-type bronchodilator may be valuable because there is evidence that some of the spasm is secondary to cholinergic-mediated irritant nerves in the airways (Boyle, et al., 1985). Although corticosteroids are not helpful in large-volume acid aspiration, they may on occasion be valuable in the therapy of bronchospasm associated with small-volume aspiration if aggressive bronchodilator therapy does not improve the air flow obstruction and symptoms quickly (Sukumaran, et al., 1980).

Some patients repeatedly experience small-volume gastric acid aspiration over months and years. This is often clinically silent, except for the consequences that may manifest as pulmonary fibrosis or more commonly as a bronchial irritability syndrome with chronic, usually nonproductive cough ("asthmatic cough") (DeMeester, et al., 1990).

Pneumonia Complicating Gastric Acid Aspiration. Infection usually plays no role in the early phase of gastric acid aspiration, which is largely a chemical pneumonitis, probably because the acid pH of the normal stomach renders it sterile (Gianella, et al., 1972; Murray, 1979). However, it is common practice in hospitalized critically ill patients to administer H_2-receptor antagonists and antacids to guard against so-called stress-induced gastritis. This practice may lead to overgrowth of bacteria in the stomach, a situation that may predispose to infectious complications of gastric aspiration (duMoulin, et al., 1982). Even so, postaspiration pneumonia is still not usually a problem in the otherwise normal host with intact pulmonary defense mechanisms because the aspirated organisms are usually cleared and neutralized effectively. However, in patients with impaired pulmonary defense mechanisms from any cause, either mechanical or immunologic, or in patients who are intubated and ventilated, the likelihood of postaspiration pulmonary infection may be as high as 40 percent (Bynum and Pierce, 1976; Murray, 1979).

Because infection does not appear to play an early role in the pathogenesis of gastric acid aspiration, there should be no role for early "prophylactic" broad-spectrum antibiotic therapy. To our knowledge, there are no controlled trials that examine the role of empiric antibiotics in this setting, and uncontrolled trials have not shown any benefit (Epstein, 1988; Murray, 1979).

When infective pneumonia complicates gastric acid aspiration, its onset is usually a few days after the aspiration event and is indicated by return of fever along with the production of purulent phlegm, new respiratory distress, and often worsening of radiographic opacities. Because these delayed postaspiration pneumonias are usually due to so-called physiologic microaspiration of oropharyngeal secretions and their indigent microbial flora, the likely pathogens involved depend on whether the aspiration occurred in a normal host or in a compromised host and whether the aspiration occurred in the community or in the hospital (Bartlett, 1974; Lorber and Swenson, 1974). Oral anerobes are therefore the most likely pathogens in CAP, whereas in the hospital setting, especially for in elderly or compromised hosts, gram-negative aerobic bacteria and *S. aureus* may also be important pathogens (Bartlett, et al., 1986). Appropriate antibiotics must therefore be selected empirically, and the approach is similar to that discussed in the next section, which deals with primary aspiration pneumonia.

Prevention of Aspiration. Many factors that predispose to gastric acid aspiration or primary aspiration pneumonia are not preventable. However, some predisposing causes can be modified (e.g., the use of small-bore nasoenteric feeding tubes rather than nasogastric suction tubes for feeding and the avoidance of overdistension of the stomach during nasogastric feeding; the residuals should be less than 30 percent of the hourly rate for continuous feeds). Meticulous care must also be taken when patients who have altered levels of con-

sciousness or swallowing difficulties are fed orally. Sucralfate instead of H_2-blockers or antacids might be used for the prevention of stress-induced gastritis (Driks, et al., 1987). The role of gastric motility agents, such as metoclopromide or cisapride, in the prevention of the incidence of gastric acid aspiration and subsequent pneumonia, although an appealing hypothesis, remains to be demonstrated (De Paso, 1991).

Patients who chronically aspirate because of pharyngeal or laryngeal dysfunction pose a particularly troublesome problem. If the laryngeal dysfunction is temporary, then intravenous alimentation may be all that is required for the period until airway protective function returns. For more chronic situations, an elective tracheostomy to provide ongoing access for tracheobronchial toilet may be necessary. Surgical feeding techniques with gastrostomy (Hassett, et al., 1988) or jejunostomy (Kaplan, et al., 1989) tubes do not guarantee protection against gastric aspiration, which may be related more to the degree of existing gastroesophageal reflux than any other variable. For these difficult situations, recourse to surgical therapies for aspiration may be appropriate (Blitzer, et al., 1988; Pelligrini, et al., 1979).

Primary Aspiration Pneumonia. The normal oral flora usually consist of predominantly anaerobic bacteria, including gram-positive cocci and gram-negative bacilli, such as Bacteroides and Fusobacterium species. Under certain conditions, this normal oral flora can be altered in favor of greater percentages of aerobic gram-negative bacilli, a transition most likely to be seen in elderly or alcoholic patients, those who reside in nursing homes, and in particular those in the hospital (Bartlett, et al., 1974). An awareness of this phenomenon is essential to select appropriate empiric antibiotic therapy when primary aspiration pneumonia is suspected.

In contrast to large-volume gastric acid aspiration, which usually causes widespread damage, primary aspiration pneumonia usually shows a strong predilection for dependent lung segments. Therefore, it most commonly occurs in the right lower lobe, particularly its superior segment, or in the posterior segment of the right upper lobe and much less commonly in the left upper lobe (Fig. 20-6). Also in contrast to gastric acid aspiration, which usually has a fairly florid and precipitous onset, primary aspiration pneumonia usually has an insidious onset over days to weeks, although an acute pneumonic picture may occur with relatively nonproductive cough and pleuritic chest pain (Bartlett and Finegold, 1974).

Therapy. Contrary to the regimen in gastric acid-induced aspiration pneumonitis, antibiotics are essential for successful therapy of primary aspiration pneumonia. Furthermore, therapy should usually be extended for several weeks to several months to prevent relapse (Bartlett and Finegold, 1974).

Antibiotics should be selected that will cover those organisms most likely to be responsible in any individual patient. For the normal host in the community setting, the main organisms to be covered are oral anerobes. Therefore, penicillin or clindamycin is usually the preferred drug. Cefoxitin may also be a useful agent, particularly if penicillin-resistant Bacteroides species (15 percent of cases) or *S. aureus* (not methicillin-resistant strains) are documented. For patients severely ill with aspiration pneumonia who require parenteral therapy and in regions where there is an appreciable incidence of *B. fragilis* that is resistant to clindamycin or cefoxitin, monotherapy therapy with imipenem is a logical choice, particularly in the setting of hospital-acquired aspiration pneumonia.

For patients with life-threatening necrotizing pneumonia or lung abscess, combination therapy is preferred; penicillin plus clindamycin or imipenem or metronidazole plus penicillin are effective regimens. If empyema complicates the illness, thoracostomy drainage should be promptly instituted (Sahn, 1993).

Concurrent Esophageal Disease

When patients present with recurrent pulmonary infections, several clinical situations may be responsible, and unrecognized esophageal disease should always be considered, even in the absence of specific symptoms. Such patients frequently do not spontaneously mention the presence of dysphagia, reflux, and coughing or choking during meals or at night, unless specifically asked. Conditions such as Zenker's diverticulum, gastroesophageal reflux with or without obstruction, achalasia, or even congenital tracheoesophageal fistula may be uncovered if the physician is sufficiently suspicious. For these reasons contrast studies should be performed whenever there is clinical suspicion of esophageal disease as the cause of recurrent pneumonia. These should be followed by endoscopy if indicated and certainly by esophageal function studies if there is a suggestion of gastroesophageal reflux. In particular, a 24-hour esophageal pH study provides evidence of problematic reflux throughout the entire day and at night. Lastly a nuclear aspiration examination may provide confirmatory evidence of aspiration as the basis for the recurrent pulmonary infection.

If a clear-cut cause of esophageal dysfunction is diagnosed, medical therapy (e.g., for reflux) or surgical repair of the esophageal defect usually corrects the recurrent problem.

Acute Bronchitis

Acute infective bronchitis in the normal host represents an airway manifestation of acute CAP; the infecting organisms for acute bronchitis are identical to those discussed earlier for CAP. Indeed, acute bronchitis may present with a clinical syndrome indistinguishable from CAP, and when CAP is ruled out, the diagnosis is made by inspection of the chest radiograph. Just as in CAP, therefore, consideration of the status of the host and the mode of onset of the acute bronchitis is helpful in suggesting the most likely etiologic agents and the preferred initial antibiotic therapy. For the young, previously well host, many episodes of acute bronchitis are due to respiratory viruses (Gwaltney, 1990; Verheij, et al., 1989), and unless a bacterial cause is strongly suspected or the patient is severely ill, it is reasonable to withhold antibiotic therapy for a few days and to treat the patient symptomatically. However, if the patient is particularly ill, if the symptoms persist beyond a few days, or if there is a second phase to the illness marked by a return of symptoms and purulent phlegm, bacterial bronchitis is likely. In this setting, empiric therapy

with a macrolide or penicillin should be adequate for most situations. As in CAP, heavy smokers should probably be treated with amoxicillin or one of the newer macrolides that is active against *H. influenzae*. If the patient is elderly or if there are coexisting illnesses, initial empiric therapy should include antibiotics with good gram-negative aerobic coverage, such as a second-generation cephalosporin, TMP/SMX, one of the newer macrolides, or amoxicillin/clavulanate.

It should be remembered that, in patients with an asthmatic predisposition, viral bronchitis can provoke an asthmatic exacerbation, which will require specific therapy. Just as in CAP, some patients who recover from the infective phase of acute bronchitis may be left with a nonspecific bronchial hyperirritability syndrome manifested by a largely nonproductive, irritative cough that may be paroxysmal and lead to loss of sleep, etc. In this situation exclusion of other causes of chronic cough and the institution of a short therapeutic trial of high-dose inhaled or even oral corticosteroids is usually sufficient to produce significant improvement in symptoms (Empey, et al., 1976).

Infective Exacerbation of COPD

COPD is usually characterized in its later stages by frequent exacerbations, manifested by increased cough, dyspnea, and deterioration in gas exchange. In those patients with the most severe degrees of air flow obstruction, such exacerbations may provoke acute respiratory failure that requires hospitalization and even the need for temporary assisted mechanical ventilation (Derenne, et al., 1988). Many patients with COPD exhibit significant bronchial hyper-responsiveness (Ramsdell, et al., 1982). Therefore, there are a number of noninfective triggering factors that may be associated with acute exacerbations of COPD. However, most authors believe that viral and/or bacterial infection is most commonly responsible for this problem (Anthonisen, et al., 1987; Murphy and Sethi, 1992; Tager and Speizer, 1975). Bacteria may be the primary cause of COPD exacerbation, or they may cause secondary infection after priming by an acute viral tracheobronchitis. A review of several studies indicates that on average about one-third of COPD exacerbations have been shown to be due to viral or on occasion mycoplasmal infection (Lamy, et al., 1973; McHardy, et al., 1980; Murphy and Sethi, 1992; Tager and Speizer, 1975). Whether repeated acute infectious exacerbations of COPD accelerate the natural age-related decline in lung function for patients with COPD remains controversial (Kanner, et al., 1979; Murphy and Sethi, 1992). Nevertheless, infective exacerbations of COPD can be associated with significant morbidity and mortality for these often elderly patients.

One of the difficulties in our determining the role of bacterial infection in the pathogenesis of COPD exacerbation is the fact that the organisms most commonly implicated, namely *H. influenzae*, *S. pneumoniae*, and *M. catarrhalis*, are common commensal colonizers of the normal upper respiratory tract and of the proximal lower airways for many patients with COPD. Thus the presence of these bacteria in the expectorated sputum of patients with COPD during periods of exacerbation does not clearly imply a cause-and-effect mechanism. Even the use of sophisticated serologic studies has not provided definitive answers to the colonization versus pathogen conundrum for COPD exacerbation (Murphy and Sethi, 1992). To date controlled clinical trials have examined antibiotic administered either prophylactically in an attempt to decrease the frequency of COPD exacerbations or therapeutically in an attempt to hasten the resolution of symptoms during an exacerbation. Results from several prospective, placebo-controlled studies suggest that antibiotic prophylaxis does in fact reduce the frequency of exacerbations in some patients, which indicates that bacterial infection probably has a pathogenetic role in some COPD exacerbations (Murphy and Sethi, 1992; Tager and Speizer, 1975). It appears that antibiotic prophylaxis is most effective for those patients with COPD who chronically produce purulent phlegm and experience several exacerbations each year. The methods of prophylaxis vary and have not been compared, but successful regimens have included one tablet daily of a broad-spectrum antibiotic with an antibiotic shift every few months or full-course therapy for the first week of every month.

A smaller number of prospective placebo-controlled randomized trials have been performed to investigate whether antibiotic therapy can accelerate recovery from acute COPD exacerbations; conflicting results were also found (Anthonisen, et al., 1987; Derenne, et al., 1988; Murphy and Sethi, 1992; Tager and Spiezer, 1975). About one-half of these studies suggest that, at least for some patients, particularly those with exacerbations characterized by increased cough and purulent sputum, bacterial infection plays an important role (Anthonisen, et al., 1987). However, even the severity of the COPD exacerbation does not indicate that a bacterial infection is the cause. In a recent study of 54 patients who were receiving mechanical ventilation for a COPD exacerbation, Fagon, et al. (1990), using bronchoscopy and PSB, could demonstrate a bacterial cause in only about 50 percent of patients, despite the fact that none had received prior antibiotic therapy.

Despite conflicting evidence in regard to the role of bacteria in the pathogenesis of COPD exacerbation, most clinicians continue to treat such exacerbations with broad-spectrum antibiotics. In this regard, antibiotics are usually chosen that treat those organisms most commonly believed to be associated with such exacerbations, namely *S. pneumoniae, H. influenzae,* and *M. catarrhalis.* Thus the tetracyclines, TMP/SMX, ampicillin, amoxicillin, amoxicillin/clavulanate, second-generation cephalosporins, fluoroquinolones, and the new macrolides are all reasonable choices for empiric therapy. Individual choices should be guided by patient tolerance and cost considerations.

The other important controversial area in the therapy of COPD exacerbation involves the role of corticosteroids, a question that has been debated for more than 30 years (Derenne, et al., 1988). Those studies that have demonstrated benefit for corticosteroids over placebo have shown more rapid improvement in pulmonary function (Albert, et al., 1980; Murata, et al., 1990). However, no study has yet shown that the addition of corticosteroids has a positive effect on the mortality rate for patients with COPD in the throes of acute exacerbation.

LUNG ABSCESS

DEFINITION

The word *abscess* is derived from the Latin *ab* or "away" and *cedere* meaning "to go." It refers to the natural progression of these lesions (i.e., they disappear once drainage, spontaneous or otherwise, has occurred). By definition, a lung abscess is a localized collection of pus that is contained in a cavity formed by the disintegration of the surrounding tissues (i.e., lung parenchyma). The pus is a characteristic liquid product of intense inflammation, which consists of leukocytes and a thin fluid referred to as "liquor puris." This definition of lung abscess excludes collections of infected fluid within pre-existing spaces (e.g., infected bronchogenic cysts, bullae, etc.), even though these are localized infected fluid collections within the lung. Lung abscesses can be either acute or chronic. An acute abscess has been defined arbitrarily as an abscess with a duration of less than 6 weeks. Most lung abscesses are solitary; however, multiple abscesses can occur, depending on the underlying disease process and the immune status of the patient. Although the incidence of lung abscesses dramatically decreased after the introduction of effective antibiotics in the late 1940s and 1950s, a recent explosion in the number immunodeficient patients as a result of successful organ transplantation, cancer chemotherapy, and spread of the human immunodeficiency virus (HIV) has led to a resurgence in the incidence of lung abscesses (Pappas, et al., 1970).

HISTORICAL NOTE

Historically, Brock, et al. (1942) were most responsible for elucidating the pathogenesis of most lung abscesses. They observed that most abscesses occurred in the posterior segment of the right upper lobe and the superior segment of the right lower lobe. These areas were termed *axillary* segments because of their close proximity to the lateral chest wall. Brock, et al. (1942) also noted that, in the recumbent position, the orifices to these segments were most directly in line with the upper respiratory passages. They hypothesized that aspiration of infected oropharyngeal secretions led, by gravity, to involvement of these areas. Subsequently, many investigators (Bernhard, et al., 1963; Shafron and Tate, 1968) have documented that Brock's et al. axillary segments, along with the superior segment of the left lower lobe, account for approximately 75 percent of all lung abscesses.

The therapy for lung abscesses dates back to the time of Hippocrates when the method was percutaneous drainage (Baker, 1985). By the late nineteenth century, the importance of pleural symphysis prior to any drainage procedure was appreciated to avoid collapse of the remaining lung and soilage of the pleural space (pyopneumothorax), a complication that was usually fatal. In the twentieth century, an Italian surgeon, V. Monaldi (1947, 1956), described a two-stage technique for endocavitary suction that avoided this obstacle. Monaldi drainage was initially applied to tuberculous cavities and only subsequently to lung abscesses. As an integral maneuver, Monaldi induced pleural symphysis, if not previously present, by the placement of a subpleural irritant (usually gauze) after a short rib resection. At a second operation 4 to 7 days later, the gauze was removed, and either further incision into the lung or tube drainage could be performed safely. Single-stage procedures, however, continued to be used in patients with previously fused pleura with increasing success (Neuhof, et al., 1941; Neuhof and Toaroff, 1942). Finally, after the introduction of the cuffed flexible endotracheal tube and the development of thoracic anesthesia, open thoracotomy and anatomic resection by segmentectomy, lobectomy, or pneumonectomy also became possible.

With the advent of the sulfonamides in 1938 and especially penicillin in 1941, the therapy of lung abscesses dramatically changed. Widespread use of antimicrobial medications for the first time provided effective therapy for early bacterial pneumonias and thus prevented progression to suppuration and abscess formation. Furthermore, if an abscess developed, antibiotic therapy combined with postural bronchial drainage ultimately led to resolution in most cases.

In the past 15 years, a resurgence in the practice of percutaneous drainage has led to a further reduction in thoracic surgical intervention for cases of lung abscesses. Most recently, however, increasing numbers of immunocompromised patients have had opportunistic lung infections and abscesses develop. These unusual and often aggressive infections provide a new challenge for the thoracic surgeon in the diagnosis and management of these diseases.

HISTORICAL READINGS

Brock RC, Hodgkiss F, Jones HO: Bronchial embolism and posture in relation to lung abscess. Guy's Hosp Rep 91:131, 1942

Monaldi V: Endocavitary aspiration in the treatment of lung abscess. Chest 29:193, 1956

Monaldi V: Endocavitary aspiration: its practical applications. Tubercle 28:223, 1947

Neuhof H, Touroff AS: Acute putrid abscess of the lung: hypreacute variety. J Thorac Cardiovasc Surg 12:96, 1942

Neuhof H, Touroff AS, Aufses AH: The surgical treatment, by drainage, of subacute and chronic putrid abscess of the lung. Ann Surg 113:209, 1941

PATHOPHYSIOLOGY

The cause of lung abscesses can be related to a number of different precipitating and predisposing factors. A classification system based on cause is outlined below. In general, lung abscesses may be divided into two major types: primary or secondary. The most common cause of primary bacterial lung abscesses is aspiration of oropharyngeal contents. This usually occurs during a period of impaired consciousness accompanied by a suppressed cough reflex. Conditions that frequently are associated with aspiration include anesthesia (both general and monitored anesthesia with intravenous sedation), neurologic disorders (cerebrovascular accidents, seizures, diabetic coma, trauma, etc.), drug ingestion (alcoholism, narcotics, etc.), and normal sleep. Poor oral hygiene

---

Etiologic Classification of Lung Abscesses

Primary
  Aspiration
    Impaired level of consciousness (alcoholism, seizures, drug overdose, stroke, general anesthesia, etc.)
    Poor oral hygiene (gingivodental sepsis)
    Esophageal diseases (motility disorders, gastroesophageal reflux, cancer, etc.)
  Necrotizing pneumonia
    Virulent organisms
      Acute pneumonia
        S. aureus
        K. pneumoniae
        Friedlander's bacillus
      Chronic pneumonia
        Fungi
        Tuberculosis
    Immunodeficiency (opportunistic infection)
      Immunosuppression (organ transplantation)
      Steroid therapy (inflammatory diseases)
      Cancer chemotherapy
      Diabetes
      Malnutrition and debilitation (ICU patients)
Secondary
  Bronchial obstruction
    Neoplasm
    Foreign body
    Lymphadenopathy
  Cavitating lesions
    Neoplasm
    Pulmonary infarct
  Direct extension
    Amebiasis (liver)
    Subphrenic abscess
  Hematogenous dissemination
    S. aureus
    E. coli
    Streptococcus spp.
    Salmonella spp.
Congenital or acquired cysts (not true abscesses)
  Bronchogenic cyst
  Hydatid cyst
  Traumatic cyst
  Bullae
  Tuberculosis

also contributes to the development of lung abscesses because oral, gingival, and dental sepsis increases the bacterial load in aspirated oropharyngeal contents. Finally an often overlooked source of acute and chronic aspiration is esophageal disease. Motor disturbances, particularly pharyngoesophageal diverticulae and achalasia, gastroesophageal reflux, and obstruction (usually caused by cancer or stricture) frequently are associated with aspiration.

Primary necrotizing pneumonias (not related to aspiration) also can lead to lung abscess formation. This may occur due to the virulence of the offending organism or due to the immunocompromised state of the host. Recently with the increasing number of patients with immunodeficiencies secondary to a variety of etiologic factors and patients with severe life-threatening illnesses who require intensive care unit management, an escalation in the incidence of opportunistic lung abscesses has been noted.

Secondary causes of lung abscesses include myriad congenital and acquired lesions. By far the most common secondary cause of lung abscess is bronchial obstruction from bronchogenic carcinoma and less frequently foreign bodies. Neoplasms and pulmonary infarcts can also cavitate, become secondarily infected, and present in a manner similar to a primary lung abscess. Rarely amebic liver abscesses, subphrenic abscesses, and hematogenous seeding result in pulmonary involvement and a secondary lung abscess. Secondary infection of congenital or acquired cystic lesions of the lung, as noted earlier, do not constitute true lung abscesses because the infection occurs in a preformed space. They are included for completeness because many other authors include this category in the discussion of lung abscess.

The anatomic location of most lung abscesses is determined by the segmental anatomy of the bronchial tree. Because most lung abscesses are related to aspiration that occurs with the patient in the supine position, those segments with dependent bronchial orifices in that posture are most affected, specifically, the posterior segments of the right upper lobe and the superior segments of the lower lobes [Brock, et al. (1942)'s axillary segments]. Many studies have documented the relative frequencies of lung abscesses in different areas of the lung. These can be summarized as follows: right upper lobe, 25 percent; right middle lobe, 10 percent; right lower lobe, 33 percent; left upper lobe, 12 percent; and left lower lobe, 20 percent (Chidi and Mendelsohn, 1974; Hagan and Hardy, 1983). The size of giant lung abscesses can reach more than 6 to 8 cm at times (Mengoli, 1985; Lawrence and Rubin, 1978).

The bacteriologic findings of lung abscesses depend somewhat on the underlying cause. For instance certain pathogens in particular have been associated with the development of lung abscesses secondary to aspiration. Classically aerobic gram-positive cocci and facultative gram-negative bacilli have been implicated, including *S. aureus, Streptococcus pyogenes, Klebsiella pneumoniae, Escherichia coli,* and Pseudomonas (Frieden, et al., 1991; Gorbach and Bartlett, 1974; Knight, et al., 1975; Kaye, et al., 1990). More recent studies, however, indicate that these organisms, which are also part of the normal oropharyngeal flora, may simply represent contamination of sputum specimens by passage through the oral cavity. With improved anaerobic culture techniques

and samples obtained through transtracheal aspiration, BAL, and percutaneous needle aspiration, newer data have revealed a predominance of anaerobic bacteria, such as *Fusobacterium nucleatum, Bacteriodes melaninogenicus* and *B. fragilis, Clostridium ramosum,* peptostreptotocci, and peptococci in more than 85 percent of cultures (Gorbach and Bartlett, 1974; Bartlett, et al., 1974; Lee, et al., 1991; Henriquez, et al., 1991). Similar organisms have been documented in necrotizing pneumonias in immunocompetent individuals (Bartlett, et al., 1974) and in children (Lee, et al., 1991). In cases of nosocomial lung abscess, gram-negative facultative organisms predominate (60 to 70 percent), although mixed flora are common (30 to 40 percent). In immunocompromised patients, however, opportunistic infection with more unusual organisms (e.g., *Candida albicans, Legionella micdadei, Legionella pneumophila,* and *P. carinii* (Naidich, et al., 1991; Pohlsan, et al., 1985) are more prevalent.

DIAGNOSIS

Clinically patients with lung abscesses complain of cough, fever, dyspnea, and occasionally pleuritic chest pain. The symptoms often are insidious without a clear date of onset and are associated with malaise and weight loss (if chronic). If the abscess ruptures into a bronchus, the patient relates a history of sudden hemoptysis followed by the production of purulent, foul-smelling sputum that is variable in color. Although the hemoptysis usually abates, a severe life-threatening pneumonia may occur from aspiration of the purulent material into areas of normal lung. Rarely massive hemoptysis may be the presenting complaint and may necessitate emergent surgical resection. Another emergent life-threatening complication is rupture into the pleural space, which produces a pyopneumothorax that usually is a catastrophic event typically presenting as septic shock. If the patient is fortunate enough to survive this disaster, the resulting empyema if untreated can erode through the chest wall, manifesting as an "empyema necessitans."

A detailed history should be obtained from all patients with suspected lung abscesses to place particular emphasis on the predisposing and precipitating factors noted above. A history of alcoholism, loss of consciousness, seizure, diabetes mellitus, poor oral hygiene, immunosuppression, possible foreign body aspiration, and bronchogenic neoplasm are specific details that must be explored. The existence of one of these factors in the presence of even minimal pulmonary findings requires that appropriate studies be obtained to exclude the possibility of a lung abscess.

The physical examination findings in patients with lung abscesses can be variable. Early in the disease process, signs of lobar consolidation and pneumonia may predominate; chronic lung abscesses may produce clubbing, signs of a pleural effusion, cachexia, and rarely a draining chest wound (empyema necessitans).

Lung abscesses may mimic other pulmonary pathologic processes and must be differentiated from them. Included in the differential diagnosis are other thoracic infections, such as tuberculosis, fungal infections, actinomycosis, and bronchiectasis, although tuberculous and fungal cavities rarely present with an air-fluid level. Three additional disorders deserve special comment. First a cavitating neoplasm (particularly squamous cell carcinoma) can be easily confused with a lung abscess; however, an irregular thick-walled cavity that does not respond to antibiotic therapy suggests the presence of a neoplasm that requires further diagnostic and therapeutic intervention. Second, a loculated or interlobar empyema closely resembles an abscess. A lenticular shape, obtuse angle with the chest wall, compression of neighboring bronchovascular structures, smooth inner wall margins, and a "split pleura" sign signifies the presence of pleural fluid rather than a lung abscess (Stark, et al., 1983; Freidman and Hellekant, 1977). Finally as noted above infected cysts and bullae are not considered lung abscesses but may be confused with the latter. Smooth contours, extremely thin walls, little surrounding inflammation, and eosinophilia or a positive Casoni skin test result (hydatid cysts) are characteristic of infected cysts rather than intraparenchymal lung abscesses.

Although occasionally the diagnosis of lung abscess can be made on the basis of history and physical examination alone, most require radiographic confirmation. Plain chest radiographs initially may demonstrate an area of intense consolidation, particularly in those segments prone to aspiration pneumonia. Later a rounded density with or without an air-fluid level may be detected (Fig. 20-14). Swenson, et al. (1991) noted that, unlike a loculated hydropneumothorax, abscesses typically have equal air-fluid level widths on both posteroanterior (PA) and lateral chest radiographs. Characteristically

the abscess has a relatively thin wall, which helps distinguish it from a cavitating neoplasm. CT is useful to confirm the plain radiographic findings (Fig. 20-14) and is particularly helpful to identify points of proximal bronchial obstruction and areas of cavitation within regions of dense consolidation. Certain features seen with either CT or plain radiographs suggest the possibility of recent or threatened hemoptysis. These include (1) emptying and refilling of the cavity on serial films, particularly if episodes of emptying correlate with clinical hemoptysis; (2) a persistent radiodensity associated with patchy radiolucencies, which indicates a clot-filled abscess cavity; and (3) mobile radiodensities within the fluid in the abscess cavity (Takaro, 1977).

Additional diagnostic procedures that should be performed in all patients include a complete blood count with differential white blood cell count, sputum culture, and bronchoscopy. The latter excludes the presence of a proximal obstructing neoplasm or foreign body and can be used to obtain adequate cultures through bronchoalveolar lavage (Henriquez, et al., 1991) and to establish drainage of the abscess. In some institutions the use of angiographic catheters has improved the ability to establish bronchial drainage of lung abscesses during rigid bronchoscopy (Connors, et al., 1975). Attempts at transbronchial drainage of large lung abscesses during bronchoscopy, however, can result in disastrous flooding of the tracheobronchial tree with purulent secretions, and this hazard must be considered in the decision to use this approach.

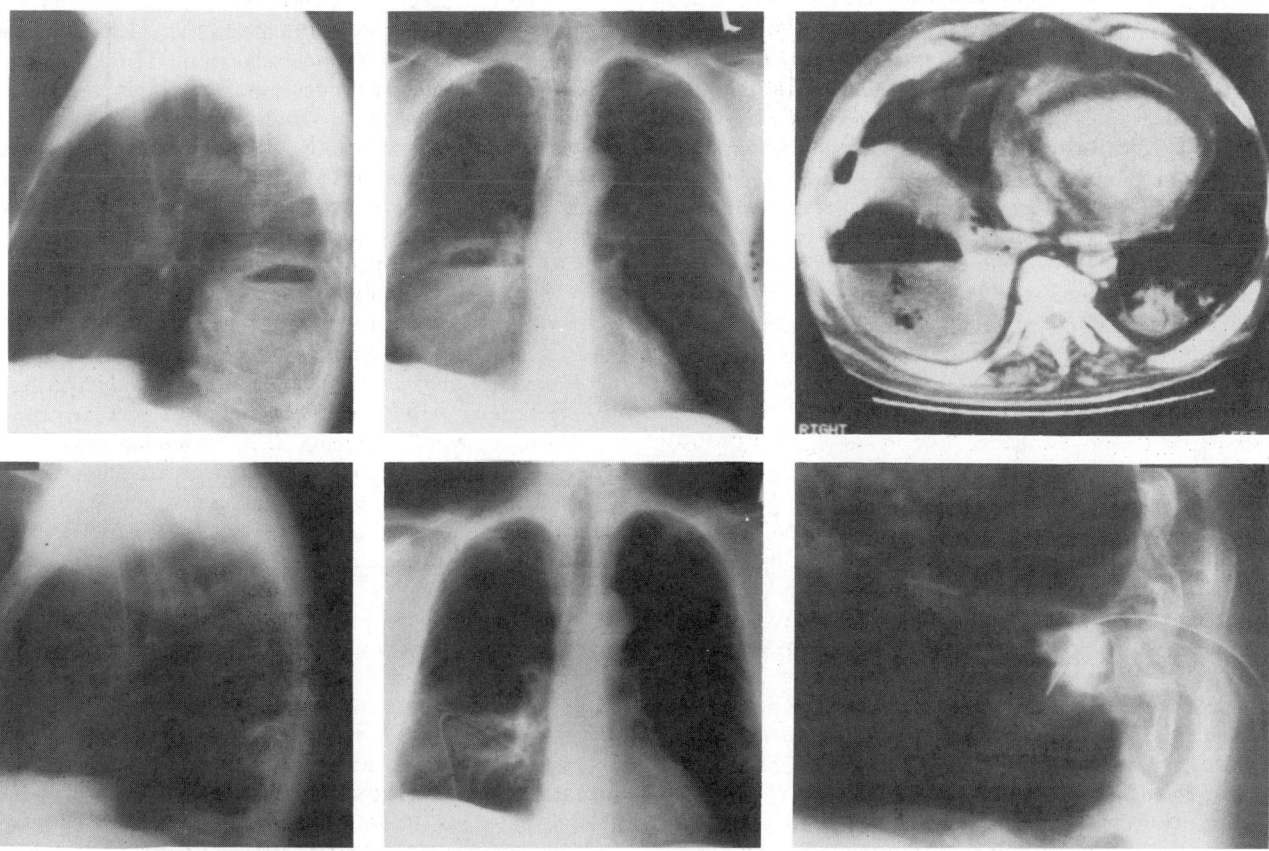

Figure 20-14. Lateral and PA views and CT scan of a large acute lung abscess (upper panels). Resolution of the CT scan with simple percutaneous drainage followed by chest tube insertion using the percutaneous tract (lower panels).

Fine-needle aspiration (FNA) of the abscess cavity for diagnostic culture has been advocated in both adults and neonates as an accurate method to obtain culture specimens (Lee, et al., 1991; Yang, et al., 1991). Recent data reported by Yang, et al. (1991) demonstrated a 94 percent success rate in the culture of pathogens from FNA compared with only 11 percent from sputum culture and 3 percent from BAL. The FNAs were performed safely under ultrasound guidance with a pneumothorax rate of only 6 percent (none required chest tube placement). Yang et al.'s data also compares favorably with the 82 percent bacteriologic accuracy and 14 percent pneumothorax incidence achieved by Grinan, et al. (1990). More importantly, however, the culture results led to a change in the antibiotic regimen in 43 percent of patients. In immunocompromised patients, FNA affords early and reliable identification of the often unusual offending organisms, which potentially can be life saving (Davidson, et al., 1976). In addition, the catastrophic flooding of the tracheobronchial tree with purulent material can be avoided with the percutaneous drainage technique.

MANAGEMENT

Medical

Since the appearance of the sulfonamides in the late 1930s and especially penicillin in the early 1940s, antibiotic administration has been the mainstay in the management of lung abscesses. For most cases, including those associated with aspiration, penicillin (up to 20 million units/day IV) administered over a prolonged period (up to 20 weeks) is sufficient and cost-effective therapy. Once the acute toxic febrile response subsides (up to 2 weeks), the patient's therapy often can be changed to an oral outpatient regimen for the remaining therapeutic period with equal efficacy (Weiss and Cherniack, 1974). Most lung abscesses respond promptly and resolve completely in 3 to 5 months. For patients with a suspected allergy to penicillin, specific skin testing, which usually requires only 30 to 60 minutes, should be performed. If a true allergy is confirmed, an alternative antibiotic, such as clindamycin (2,400 to 2,700 mg/day), should be used. Clindamycin has been shown to be particularly effective in anaerobic lung abscesses, even when compared with penicillin (Bartlett and Gorback, 1975; Gudiol, et al., 1990). In the setting of a nosocomial lung abscess, an aminoglycoside, a third-generation celphalosporin, or imipenem may be appropriate, depending on the responsible organism and institutional sensitivities. Furthermore, in immunosuppressed individuals, TMX/SMX or pentamidine, erythromycin, and amphotericin B may be indicated for cases of *P. carinii,* Legionella spp., and Candida spp. involvement, respectively.

Specific supportive measures are important adjuncts to antibiotic therapy. These include chest physiotherapy, bronchoscopy, and health maintenance measures. Chest physiotherapy consists of a prescribed system of breathing and coughing exercises, chest percussion, and postural drainage. Together these lay the foundation for successful antibiotic management. In patients with inadequate results from chest physiotherapy, therapeutic bronchoscopy may be required to remove tenacious secretions and establish bronchial drainage, and it may need to be repeated. Finally general health measures often must be addressed (e.g., nutrition; dental and gingival hygiene; drug, alcohol, and tobacco dependency; and overall medical health).

Surgical

Although the earliest accounts that describe percutaneous drainage of lung abscesses date back to the time of Hippocrates, only recently has this approach gained popularity. A surfeit of reports have appeared in the literature, most within the last 10 years, including those by Weissberg (1984); Yellin (1985); Kosloske (1986); Crouch, et al. (1987); Parker (1987); Rice (1987); Ball, et al. (1989), Cuestas (1989); vanSonnenberg (1991); Yang, et al. (1991); and Lambiase (1992). Percutaneous drainage procedures have now been applied in a variety of clinical settings, including in patients who are intubated in the intensive care unit with positive pressure ventilation (Rice, 1987). Localization techniques include fluoroscopy, CT, and ultrasound, and all appear to be equally reliable in most circumstances, although ultrasound may be superior to demonstrate lesion-pleural adhesions (Yang, et al., 1991). Ultrasound also can be performed as a bedside procedure, which eliminates the need to transport potentially unstable patients to the radiology department. The exact timing and indications for percutaneous drainage have not been defined, but the overall experience suggests that early drainage is beneficial in patients who do not respond to initial medical management and who do not have other surgical indications (see below). Specific proposed indications for immediate percutaneous catheter drainage include (1) an abscess under tension, as evidenced by mediastinal shift, displacement of fissures, or downward movement of the diaphragm (Fig. 20-14); (2) radiographic verification of contralateral lung contamination; (3) unremitting signs of sepsis after 72 hours of antibiotic therapy; (4) abscess size greater than 4.0 cm; (5) increase in abscess size; (6) rising fluid level despite therapy; and (7) persistent ventilatory dependency. Eleven recent reports of percutaneous catheter drainage are summarized in Table 20-2. Overall the cure rate was 89 percent after 4 to 59 days of drainage in 65 patients. The morbidity and mortality rates were low (overall 10.6 percent and 1.5 percent, respectively), and no cases of empyema or pyopneumonthorax were reported. These data are consistent with the findings reported by Mengoli (1985). In fact, Mengoli first pointed out that the incidence of empyema after tube drainage was less than that after surgical resection. All deaths in this current group were reported by Rice (1987) and occurred in critically ill patients in the ICU.

Thoracic surgical intervention in uncomplicated cases of lung abscesses today is rare, except in the presence of other contributing factors, such as large size (greater than 6 cm), massive hemoptysis, empyema, bronchial obstruction, a clinical suspicion of cancer, or failure of more conservative medical therapy. Furthermore, acute rupture into the pleural space that produces a pyopneumothorax continues to be a rare surgical emergency. When surgery is indicated, lobectomy is the preferred procedure rather than the Monaldi technique of drainage.

Table 20-2. Results of Percutaneous Drainage of Lung Abscesses

Reference	Patients	Mortality Rate	Morbidity Rate	Empyema	Drainage[a]	Cure Rate	Follow-Up[a]
Weissberg, 1984	7	0%	0%	0%	4–24 (10) days	100%[b]	3–36 (15) mo
Mengoli, 1985	3	0%	0%	0%	14–28 days	100%	2–4 mo
Yellin, 1985	7	0%	0%	0%	6–25 (11) days	100%	2–5 yr
Kosloske, 1986	1	0%	0%	0%	Less than 28 days	100%	NS
Crouch, et al., 1987	4	0%	NS	0%	NS	100%	NS
Parker, 1987	6	0%	16.7%	0%	10–59 (13) days	83.4%	2–24 (6) mo
Rice, 1987	11	9%	18%	0%	NS	73%	NS
Ball, et al., 1989	3	0%	0%	0%	19–24 (20) days	100%	3 mo
Cuestas, 1989	2	0%	0%	0%	23–41 days	100%	4 mo
vanSonnenberg, 1991	19	0%	21%	0%	4–38 days	84%	6 mo
Lambiase, 1992	2	0%	0%	0%	11–18 days	100%	NS

Abbreviation: NS, not stated.

[a] Drainage and follow-up are reported as a range, with median in parentheses, if available.

[b] Although all patients were clinically cured, one patient had a small residual "cyst" on the chest radiograph.

Several specific risks are important to consider if operative intervention is planned. Protection of the airway is paramount. The possibility of blood or pus contaminating the healthy contralateral lung is significant; therefore, the use of tracheal separation techniques with a double-lumen endotracheal tube (Carles or Robertshaw), contralateral mainstem bronchial intubation, or a bronchial blocker (Fogarty catheter) placed in the draining segment is recommended to prevent this intraoperative catastrophe. If these are not possible, the patient may be positioned either prone or supine as an alternative, albeit less satisfactory, prophylactic measure. Patients with massive hemoptysis are particularly likely to benefit from rapid airway control and lobectomy, which reduces the mortality rate from 54 percent to only 18 percent (Gourin and Garzon, 1974). Additional technical points for the surgeon to consider during the operation include keeping manipulation of the involved lung to a minimum, clamping the involved bronchus as soon as possible, and exercising great care in the dissection in and around the hilar bronchovascular structures because they frequently are involved with the inflammatory process and difficult to identify.

Results

Prior to the antibiotic era, lung abscesses carried a 30 to 50 percent mortality rate. With the introduction of antibiotics, however, approximately 75 to 88 percent of patients are cured with medical therapy alone, and the mortality rate has decreased to 5 to 20 percent (Delarue, et al., 1985). Furthermore, Delarue, et al. reported surgical cure in almost 90 percent of patients who underwent operations with only a 1 percent mortality rate. In an article that reviewed the literature, Mengoli (1985) collected 694 cases of external drainage and 689 cases of pulmonary resection, both with a 10 to 13 percent mortality rate. With the growing population of ICU and immunosuppressed patients, however, the incidence of lung abscess appears to be rising again. Furthermore, the mortality rate in these patients is substantially increased; it was reported recently to be as high as 28 percent (Hagan and Hardy, 1983). It is in this patient population that the management of lung abscesses poses a particular challenge for thoracic surgeons in the future.

BRONCHIECTASIS

DEFINITION

The term *bronchiectasis* is derived from the Greek *bronchos* or "windpipe" and *ektasis* meaning "dilatation." Therefore, strictly defined, bronchiectasis refers to the abnormal dilatation of bronchi. Commonly, however, bronchiectasis refers to the clinical syndrome marked by chronic dilatation of bronchi, a paroxysmal cough that produces variable amounts of fetid mucopurulent sputum, and recurrent pulmonary infections. Although formerly a prevalent pulmonary problem frequently complicated by hemoptysis, lung and brain abscesses, empyema, respiratory failure, and death, bronchiectasis has become dramatically less prominent as a clinical entity since the introduction of vaccination programs, antibiotics, and antituberculous medications. Today it is only reported commonly in certain geographic locations and certain ethnic groups [i.e., New Zealand (Hinds, 1958), Nigeria (Grillo, 1972), Australia (Maxwell, 1972), and India (Charan and Sinha, 1973) and among Polynesians (Wakefield and Waite, 1980) and Alaskan natives (Wilson and Decker, 1982)]. Although bronchiectasis provided much of the impetus for the development of thoracic surgical techniques (it affected at one time approximately 0.5 percent of the population), it presently is associated only rarely with the need for thoracic surgical intervention.

HISTORICAL NOTE

The history of bronchiectasis parallels that of thoracic surgery itself and has been eloquently outlined by Lindskog (1986). Briefly bronchiectasis was first described in 1819 by Rene Laennec (1819) in his classic treatise *De l'Auscultation Mediate ou Traite des Maladies des Poumons et du Coeur.* At the Hôpital Necker, now renamed l'Hôpital des Enfants, and with his new invention, a tubular wooden stethoscope, this former laboratory assistant of Guillaume Dupuytren described normal and abnormal ascultative findings present in various pulmonary and cardiac diseases and correlated them with anatomic and pathologic characteristics. In Chapter II of his historic work, entitled "De la Dilatation des Bronches," Laennec details two types of bronchial dilatation (i.e., cylindrical and saccular), which continue to be recognized by modern pathologists as two major forms of bronchiectasis (Laennec, 1826).

Therapy was not addressed, however, until Killian (1898) and Chevalier Jackson (1907) introduced innovations in the removal of aspirated foreign bodies, which thereby prevented subsequent bronchiectasis. Although a successful partial lobectomy for bronchiectasis was performed in 1901 by Heidenhain at Worms in Hesse, Samuel Robinson (1917) reported the first substantial attempt to remove the diseased segments of lung, including five staged (subtotal) lobectomies with en masse ligation of the hilar structures. Subsequently, Graham (1923), Whittemore (1927), and Sauerbruch (1928) described different approaches to staged resections. Shortly thereafter, however, Harold Brunn (1929) reported on five successful, single-stage lobectomies that used constant suction by intercostal catheters postoperatively to maintain drainage of the pleural space and complete expansion of the remaining lung. In the same year, Guedel and Waters (1929) invented the cuffed flexible endotracheal tube, which revolutionized thoracic surgery. After this Rudolph Nissen (1931) and Cameron Haight (1934) performed successful pneumonectomies for advanced bronchiectasis, and surgery for bronchiectasis in general soon flourished with Churchill and Belsey (1939) who described segmental resection and presented one of the earliest large series (86 cases). Detailed treatises on bronchopulmonary segmental anatomy by Jackson and Huber (1943) and subsequently by Boyden (1955) inspired the adoption of anatomic methods of dissection and individual ligation of the hilar bronchovascular structures, thereby markedly decreasing postoperative complications.

Since 1940 the principles of segmental resection for localized bronchiectasis have been published by numerous authors, including Churchill and Belsey (1939); Overholt and Langer (1947); Kergin (1950); Sealy et al. (1966); and more recently Dogan (1989). However, with the discovery of the sulfonamides in 1938, the production of penicillin in 1941, the availability of streptomycin in 1947 (and subsequently other antituberculous medications), the effectiveness of modern vaccines, and the prompt removal of foreign bodies, bronchiectasis has decreased in both its frequency and severity. With current medical therapy, the need for thoracic surgical intervention has become limited.

HISTORICAL READINGS

Brunn H: Surgical principles underlying one-stage lobectomy. Arch Surg 18:490, 1929

Churchill ED, Belsey R: Segmental pneumonectomy in bronchiectasis; the lingula segment of the left upper lobe. Ann Surg 109:481, 1939

Guedel AE, Waters RM: A new intratracheal cannula. Anesth Analg 7:238, 1929

Laennec RTH: Traite de l'Auscultation Mediate et des Maladies des Poumons et du Coeur. 2nd Ed. Chaude, Paris, 1826

Laennec RTH: De l'Auscultation Mediate ou Traite des Maladies des Poumons et du Coeur. Brosson et Chaude, Paris, 1819

Lindskog GE: Bronchiectasis revisited. Yale J Biol Med 59:41, 1986

PATHOPHYSIOLOGY

Both congenital and acquired disease processes can lead to the development of bronchiectasis. Most cases of bronchiectasis, however, are related to acquired disorders and are caused by two factors: infection and bronchial obstruction. In the past viral and bacterial pneumonias in infancy and childhood, such as pertussis, measles, influenza, tuberculosis, and bronchopneumonia, were common predisposing conditions that led to the development of bronchiectasis. A single severe pneumonia or repeated moderate infections caused destruction of bronchial cilia, mucosa, musculoelastic tissue, and occasionally even cartilage. Healing and replacement of these tissues with fibrosis resulted in loss of elasticity; contraction of the peribronchial tissues, which produced traction on the bronchial structures; and ultimately bronchial dilatation. Initial bronchial dilatation and destruction of normal mucociliary action led to secretion retention and secondary bouts of infection, which resulted in progressive fibrosis, loss of lung volume, and continued bronchial dilatation. Destruction of mucociliary function appears to be of particular importance in the pathogenesis of chronic infection and bronchiectasis (Isawa, et al., 1990). Other pathologic findings include squamous metaplasia, peribronchial pneumonitis with microabscesses, peribronchial lymphandenopathy, and bronchial artery enlargement, which increase the likelihood of hemoptysis and significant left-to-right arteriovenous shunting. The presence of true established bronchiectasis must be distinguished from pseudobronchiectasis. This phenomenon was first described by Blades and Dugan (1944) and is characterized by cylindric bronchial dilatation that is associated with acute bronchopneumonia and completely reverses after a period of weeks to months.

Bronchial obstruction from either endobronchial pathologic conditions or extrinsic compression can also cause bronchiectasis. Aspirated foreign bodies or endobronchial neoplasms can lead to endobronchial obstruction, retention of secretions, secondary infection, and bronchiectasis by a mechanism similar to that described above. Aspiration of a wide range of foreign bodies (e.g., peas, peanuts, coins, gastric contents, etc.) has been associated with the development of bronchiectasis. Extrinsic bronchial compression and obstruction from enlargement of peribronchial lymph nodes, which is commonly seen with neoplasms and chronic lung infections (e.g., histoplasmosis, coccidioidomycosis, and tuberculosis), also has been known to produce secretion retention, chronic infection, and bronchiectasis.

Congenital and familial diseases are an uncommon cause of bronchiectasis. The strongest association is that with the autosomal recessive dysmotile cilia syndrome (Kartagener's syndrome) which often presents with the classic triad of situs inversus, pansinusitis, bronchiectasis, and immotile sperm. Aberrant production, assembly, or attachment of dynein arms, which frequently can be verified on electron microscopy, results in impaired cilial function and poor clearance of secretions that presumably leads to chronic secondary infections and in 20 to 25 percent of patients ultimately to bronchiectasis (Eliasson, et al., 1977). Other congenital disorders that are associated with the development of bronchiectasis include (1) cystic fibrosis, an autosomal recessive disorder marked by tenacious bronchial secretions and abnormal ciliary function (di Sant'Agnese and Talamo, 1967); (2) the Williams-Campbell syndrome, an autosomal recessive disease characterized by congenital bronchomalacia caused by the absence of bronchial cartilage (Wayne and Taussig, 1976); (3) Mounier-Kuhn syndrome, a connective tissue disorder similar to Ehlers-Danlos syndrome distinguished by gross dilatation of the trachea and mainstem bronchi (Bass, 1974); (4) immunoglobulin (Ig) deficiencies (IgA or IgG), a heterogeneous group of diseases that predispose those patients to chronic lower respiratory tract infections and bronchiectasis (Takaro, et al., 1977); and (5) α_1-antitrypsin deficiency, an autosomal recessive condition that is associated with emphysema and occasionally bronchiectasis (Longstreth, et al., 1975). Finally an isolated familial clustering of right middle lobe bronchiectasis has been reported that involved four of five siblings in a single family (Danielson, et al., 1967).

Bronchiectasis most commonly involves the second- to fourth-order branches of the segmental bronchi because this portion of the proximal bronchial tree characteristically contains the least cartilagenous support. As originally described by Laennec (1819), bronchiectasis can be classified by the appearance of the dilated bronchi into cylindric and saccular forms. The cylindric type often is associated with post-tuberculous bronchiectasis; the saccular variety constitutes most postinfectious and postobstructive bronchiectases. A third type, frequently referred to as mixed or varicose, is sometimes included and is distinguished by alternating areas of saccular and cylindric dilatations.

The distribution of bronchiectasis, to a great extent, is characteristic of the underlying cause. For instance, the bronchiectasis associated with congenital and familial disorders, such as the dysmotile cilia syndrome (Kartagener's syndrome), hypogammaglobulinemia, and cystic fibrosis, is usually bilateral and diffuse and involves multiple segments from both upper and lower lobes. Tuberculosis and other granulomatous diseases, however, are marked by either unilateral or bilateral disease, most commonly limited to the upper lobes and superior segments of the lower lobes. Bronchiectasis after pyogenic and viral infections frequently is limited to the basal segments, middle lobe, and lingula. Bronchiectasis secondary to aspirated foreign objects normally is limited to those segments associated with the obstructive process, although some involvement of neighboring segments can occur. A specific syndrome (middle lobe syndrome) occurs if peribronchial lymph nodes enlarge (usually from tuberculosis or other granulomatous infection) and compress the right middle lobe bronchus. This causes localized obstruction, infection, and bronchiectasis. The middle lobe is most commonly affected because of the acute angle and slender, elongated configuration of its bronchus and the relative completeness of the adjacent fissures, which lead to poor collateral ventilation (Bradham, et al., 1966).

DIAGNOSIS

The clinical features of bronchiectasis can be characteristic but often may vary significantly. Patients frequently complain of a chronic or intermittent cough that is productive of a variable amount of foul-smelling, mucopurulent sputum, occasionally as much as 500 ml/day. Patients typically present with a history of recurrent febrile episodes, which are corre-

lated with increased volume of their sputa. Although usually a minor characteristic, hemoptysis may occur in up to 41 percent of localized and 66 percent of diffuse bronchiectases (Sealy, et al., 1966); rarely it may be massive. Bronchiectasis associated with tuberculosis and granulomatous disease, primarily involving the upper lobes, may not be associated with a productive cough (so-called dry bronchiectasis), and hemoptysis alone may be the primary complaint. Complaints of sinus problems and other chronic infections, infertility, and a family history of similar problems may indicate the presence of an inherited disorder associated with bronchiectasis. Patients with known bronchiectasis may experience exacerbations manifested by complaints of worsening cough, fever, dyspnea, or more subtle symptoms, such as increasing fatigue. Physical examination may reveal only early inspiratory rales along with relatively high-pitched expiratory rales (Piirila, et al., 1991). However, coarse expiratory rhonchi and localized dullness over involved areas frequently are noted, particularly during periods of acute exacerbations.

Without proper therapy, the disease may progress to an advanced form that is characterized by complaints of marked dyspnea, anorexia, and weight loss. In addition to these findings, the physical examination may reveal central cyanosis, pulmonary osteoarthropathy with marked clubbing, evidence of malnutrition and emaciation, and distant metastatic abscesses (particularly in the brain). Ultimately in extreme cases, evidence of cor pulmonale may develop.

The most important items to exclude in the differential diagnosis of patients with suspected bronchiectasis include neoplasms (bronchogenic and metastatic) and bronchial foreign bodies. The presence of these two are easily evaluated by flexible fiberoptic bronchoscopy. Today, however, a more common error is to fail to include bronchiectasis in the differential diagnosis of patients who present with a chronic cough or recurrent pulmonary infections. Failure to obtain a diagnostic study (see below) to exclude bronchiectasis in this setting results in the recent tendency to underdiagnose this disease (Monie, 1989).

Although bronchiectasis may be suspected on the basis of history, physical examination, and even bronchoscopy, an imaging study is usually obtained to confirm the diagnosis. Plain radiographs of the thorax are usually not helpful; they demonstrate only nonspecific findings (e.g., atelectasis, fibrosis, and pleural thickening). Occasionally, however, peribronchial inflammation produces curvilinear or paired bronchial shadows (tram lines) characteristic of saccular bronchiectasis (Fig. 20-15). Before the advent of CT, bronchograms were the definitive radiographic method that was used to confirm the diagnosis of bronchiectasis. These studies, however, required meticulous postural drainage and intensive antibiotic therapy for a period prior to the study and careful topical anesthesia (general anesthesia in children) during the procedure to obtain adequate visualization of the bronchial tree (Fig. 20-16).

High-resolution, fine-cut (1.5 to 5 mm) CT scans now represent the new procedure of choice for the diagnosis of bronchiectasis (Grenier, et al., 1986; Joharjy, et al., 1987; Gamsu and Klein, 1989; Munro, 1991; McGuiness, 1993). These detailed images demonstrate not only bronchial dilatation but also peribronchial inflammation and parenchymal disease (Fig. 20-17). Although the diagnosis can be made with only a 2

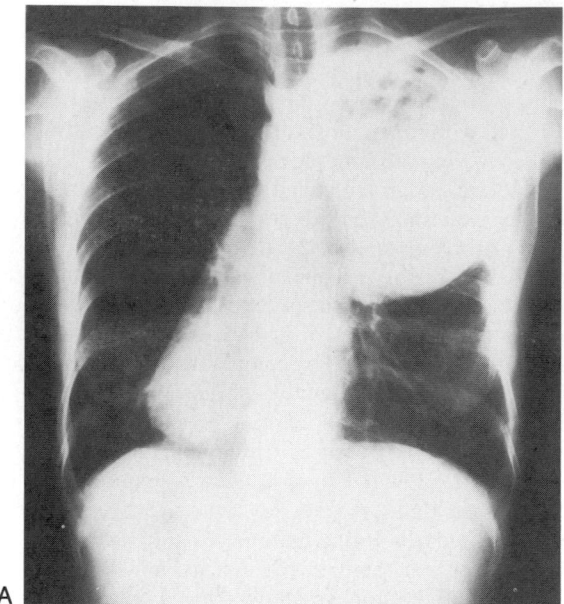

A

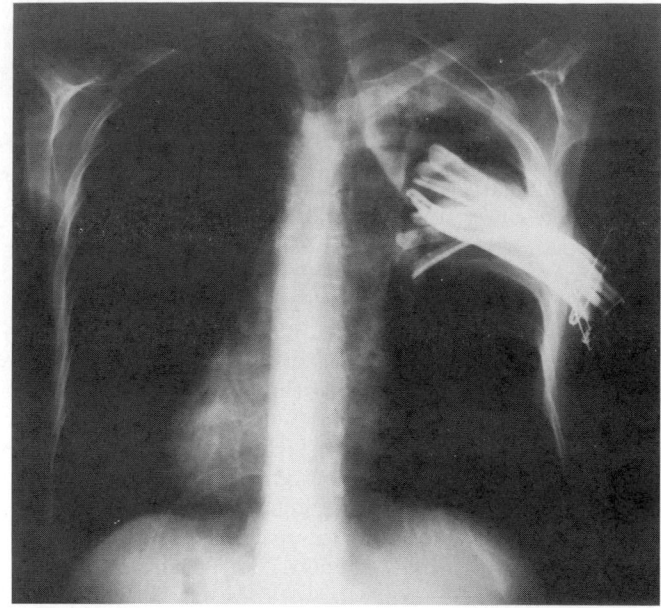

B

Figure 20-15. (A&B) Chest radiographs showing lung abscess and results of catheter drainage.

percent false-negative and a 1 percent false-positive rate (Young, et al., 1991), some thoracic surgeons still prefer standard bronchograms in preoperative patients to provide a more recognizable "road map" to aid in planning the resection. CT is also not as sensitive in the detection of cylindric

and varicose bronchiectasis as it is in the documentation of saccular disease (Muller, et al., 1984). Furthermore, bronchograms may be superior to demonstrate diffuse, crowded, cylindric bronchiectasis that is more suggestive of chronic bronchitis (or "reversible" bronchiectasis) than of truly localized "surgical" bronchiectasis (Blades, 1944).

MANAGEMENT

Medical

After a diagnostic flexible bronchoscopy to exclude the presence of bronchial obstruction by direct vision and an inherited mucociliary disorder by mucosal biopsy, the initial management for nearly all patients with suspected bronchiectasis should be conservative medical therapy. This includes intravenous broad-spectrum antibiotics, bronchodilators (usually given by nebulizer), humidification, expectorants, mucolytics and postural drainage. To be truly effective, postural drainage requires specific training and routine performance (Jaffe and Katz, 1973). If coughing and postural drainage are ineffective, endotracheal aspiration may be required. Once culture results are obtained, the antibiotic regimen should be tailored to the offending organisms. Common bacteria in patients with bronchiectasis include *H. influenza, S. aureus, K. pneumoniae, E. coli,* and in the chronic setting *Pseudomonas spp.* (Takaro, et al., 1977). Furthermore, infections caused by mycobacteria, fungi, Legionella, and other atypical organisms should be investigated. In patients with continued infection, bronchoscopy with BAL and PSB may provide more meaningful culture results. This conservative therapeutic approach should be continued for a period of several months, if necessary. This will generally suffice in most patients. Some recurrent infections may be avoided by annual injections of influenza and pneumococcal vaccines, and in some patients a trial of chronic "prophylactic" antibiotic administration

Figure 20-16. Chest radiograph showing typical appearance of bronchiectasis.

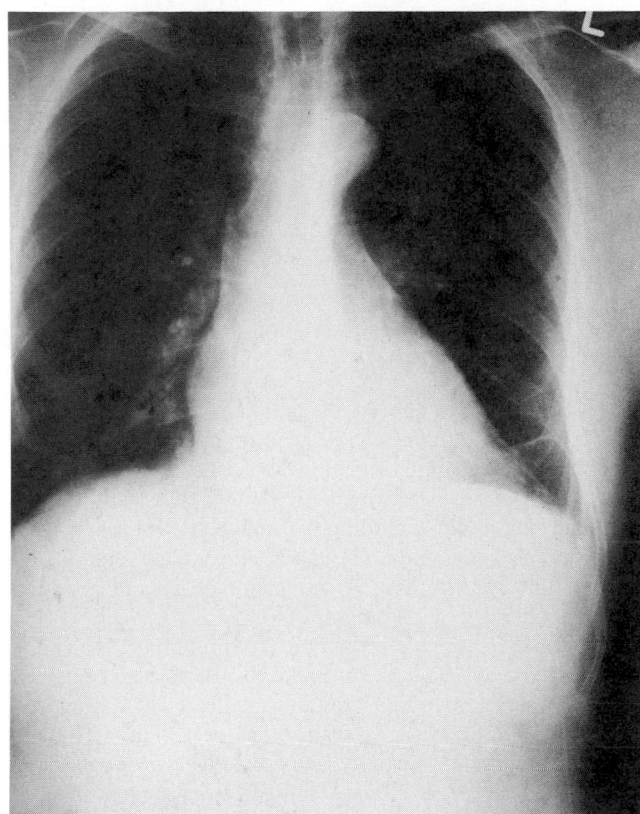
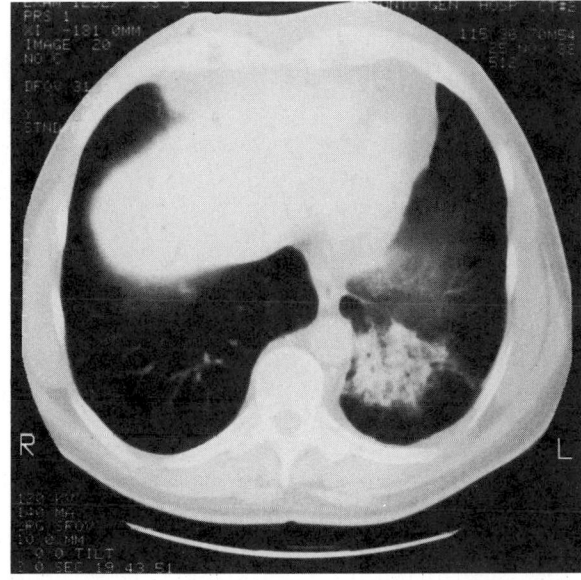

Figure 20-17. **(A)** A normal chest radiograph in a patient with suspected of bronchiectasis. **(B)** High-resolution CT scan of the same patient confirming the diagnosis of bronchiectasis.

with TMP/SMX, erythromycin, or ciprofloxacin twice daily for several months may be beneficial.

Surgical

The goal of surgical therapy is to remove all active disease and simultaneously to preserve as much functioning lung parenchyma as possible. Patients who are candidates for surgical resection must fulfill the following criteria: (1) have a localized bronchiectasis that is completely resectable; (2) have adequate pulmonary reserve to tolerate the proposed resection (normally two lobes or six segments must remain intact); (3) have an irreversible process and not a early treatable condition (i.e., pseudobronchiectasis, foreign body, bronchial stricture, etc.); (4) have significant symptoms with a continued chronic productive cough, significant hemoptysis, or recurring major episodes of pneumonia to justify surgery; and (5) have failed an adequate trial of medical management (see above).

A high-resolution, fine-cut CT scan currently is required for preoperative evaluation and provides the essential information that is necessary for planning the extent of the resection (Breatnach, et al., 1985). Depending on the preferences of the surgeon, preoperative studies also may include bronchography and pulmonary function testing, although generally the latter is not helpful because the segments involved with advanced bronchiectasis are usually nonfunctional and represent areas of arteriovenous shunting. The surgical approach involves segmental resection of all involved areas. Most commonly resection of all basal segments (unilaterally or bilaterally) with either the middle lobe or lingula is required. With tuberculous bronchiectasis, however, removal of the right and/or left upper lobe and superior segment of the lower lobe is more likely. For the rare patient with bilateral disease and valid indications for surgery, the side with the most severe disease is addressed first. If the disease is limited to a single lobe, lobectomy is a valid option. Regardless of the anatomy, a complete resection of all disease must be accomplished to avoid recurrence. Removal of only the most extensively involved segments of the lung virtually always is a prescription for failure.

The technical aspects of surgery for bronchiectasis can be at times challenging. First airway management must be carefully considered. Because of copious mucopurulent secretions, particular attention should be focused on meticulous maintenance of a clear airway to avoid soiling the remaining normal lung. Furthermore, some patients with bronchiectasis present with massive hemoptysis, which requires aggressive measures, including rigid bronchoscopy to identify the bleeding source, endobronchial suction, and on occasion balloon tamponade and bronchial artery embolization to control the airway. A Carlens-type double-lumen endotracheal tube frequently is helpful in the management of these difficult airway problems.

A second challenge to the thoracic surgeon is dissection of the inflamed and indurated hilum. Although it is a simple

Table 20-3. Results of Surgical Resection for Bronchiectasis[a]

Reference	Patients	Mortality Rate	Morbidity Rate	Asymptomatic	Improved
Sealy, et al., 1966	140	1.4%	3%	58%[a]	95%
Ripe, 1971	66	NS	NS	41%	60%
Sanderson, et al., 1974	242	0.4%	33%	31%	85%
Annest, et al., 1982	24	8.3%	13%	46%	83%
Vejlsted, et al., 1982	41	2.4%	17%	50%	100%
Wilson and Decker, 1982	84	0%	11%	77%	96%
Dogan, 1989	487	3.5%	11%	71%	NS

Abbreviation: NS, not stated.

[a] Overall 58% were asymptomatic; 80% of patients with localized disease and 36% of patients with multisegmental disease were asymptomatic.

procedure to perform, mass ligature of the hilar structures previously led to an unacceptably high incidence of postoperative fistula, pyopneumothorax, and empyema (Lindskog, 1986). With adoption of the practice of individual ligation of the bronchovascular structures, the results of surgery for bronchiectasis improved. However, dissection of the bronchus and pulmonary vessels in patients with bronchiectasis remains difficult and occasionally fraught with danger.

Results

The recent success of medical management of bronchiectasis with intensive postural drainage and broad-spectrum antibiotics has dramatically decreased the role of the thoracic surgeon in the care of these patients. An occasional patient, however, does not respond to medical therapy and requires surgical intervention. The results of surgery for bronchiectasis depend on the cause and type of lung involvement. Limited localized disease is associated with the best results; 80 percent of patients are rendered asymptomatic by surgical resection compared with only 36 percent of those patients with diffuse multisegmental involvement (Sealy, et al., 1966). Ripe (1971) identified several prognostic factors that predicted a favorable outcome, including (1) unilateral disease restricted to the basal segments, (2) young chronologic age, (3) absence of sinusitis/rhinitis, (4) no major airway obstruction, and (5) a history of pneumonia.

Complications after surgery for bronchiectasis can include a prolonged air leak, bronchopleural fistula, empyema, and pneumonia secondary to intraoperative contamination of the normal lung with mucopurulent secretions. The reported morbidity and mortality rates, however, are surprisingly low considering the intense inflammatory reaction associated with this disease. Generally the mortality rate is less than 1 percent, and the risk of major morbidity is only 3 to 5 percent (Takaro, et al., 1977). The overall results of surgical resection in the therapy of bronchiectasis over the last 30 years are summarized in Table 20-3.

COMMENTS AND CONTROVERSIES

The role of the surgeon in the management of chronic bacterial infections of the lung has certainly changed over the past few decades in North America. The incidence of bronchiectasis that requires surgical resection has diminished such that it is a relatively rare indication for surgical resection in most practices. Undoubtedly this is related to improved infant care, diminishing incidence of whooping cough, and appropriate antibiotic management of pulmonary infections.

Similarly lung abscess as a surgical problem has decreased dramatically since the introduction of percutaneous drainage. It is rare for a chronic or acute bacterial lung abscess to require surgical resection.

With the age of our population increasing, many more elderly patients undergo major surgical resections. Unfortunately these are the same patients who may have occult aspiration as a result of reflux disease, impaired nutrition, or impaired defense mechanisms. We must always be wary of nosocomial pneumonias that occur especially in the postoperative period. As this chapter points out, monotherapy is often worthwhile and can avoid the problems of superinfection so often seen in ICUs.

There is no doubt that the thoracic surgeon plays an important role in the therapy of all of these patients, despite the fact that major surgical intervention is rarely indicated for the management of these conditions.

R.J.G.

KEY REFERENCES

Fang GD, Fine M, Orloff J et al: New and emerging etiologies for community-acquired pneumonia with implications for therapy: a prospective multicentre study of 359 patients. Medicine (Baltimore) 69:307, 1990
This is a major contribution to our understanding of the epidemiology and cause of CAP. Discussing one of the largest patients populations ever studied, this article clearly demonstrates that the traditional splitting of patients into typical versus atypical pneumonia syndromes provides no useful diagnostic information and is therefore obsolete.

Niederman MS, Bass JB, Campbell GD et al: Guidelines for the initial management of adults with community-acquired pneumonia: diagnosis, assessment of severity, and initial antimicrobial therapy. Am Rev Respir Dis 148:1418, 1993

This in-depth summary of an international consensus conference on CAP provides a definitive statement on the initial management of the patient presenting with a pneumonia of unknown cause.

REFERENCES

Pneumonia and Related Conditions

Albert RK, Martin TR, Lewis SW: Controlled trial of methylprednisolone in patients with chronic bronchitis and acute respiratory insufficiency. Ann Intern Med 92:753, 1980

Alessi DM, Berci G: Aspiration and nasogastric intubation. Otolaryngol Head Neck Surg 94:486, 1986

Anthonisen NR, Manfredo J, Warren CPW et al: Antibiotic therapy in exacerbations of chronic obstructive pulmonary disease. Ann Intern Med 106:196, 1987

Arnow PM, Chou T, Weil D et al.: Nosocomial Legionnaire's disease caused by aerosolized tap water from respiratory devices. J Infect Dis 146:460, 1982

Bannister WK, Sattilaro AJ, Otis RD: Therapeutic aspects of aspiration pneumonitis in experimental animals. Anesthesiology 22:440, 1961

Bartlett JG: Invasive diagnostic techniques in pulmonary infections. In Pennington JE (ed): Respiratory Infections: Diagnosis and Management. 2nd Ed. Raven Press, New York, 1989

Bartlett JG: Diagnostic accuracy of transtracheal aspiration bacteriologic studies. Am Rev Respir Dis 115:777, 1977

Bartlett JG: The bacteriology of pulmonary infections following aspiration. West J Med 121:395, 1974

Bartlett JG, Finegold SM: Anaerobic infections of the lung and pleural space. Am Rev Respir Dis 110:56, 1974

Bartlett JG, Gorbach SL: The triple threat of aspiration pneumonia. Chest 68:560, 1975

Bartlett JG, Gorbach SL, Finegold SM: The bacteriology of aspiration pneumonia. Am J Med 56:202, 1974

Bartlett JG, O'Keefe I, Tally FP et al: The bacteriology of hospital-acquired pneumonia. Arch Intern Med 146:868, 1986

Bates JH, Campbell GD, Barron AL et al: Microbial etiology of acute pneumonia in hospitalized patients. Chest 101:1005, 1992

Belsey R: The pulmonary complications of oesophageal disease. Br J Dis Chest 54:342, 1960

Blitt CD, Gutman HL, Cohen DD et al: Silent regurgitation and aspiration during general anesthesia. Anesth Analg 49:707, 1970

Blitzer A, Krespi YP, Oppenheimer RW et al: Surgical management of aspiration. Otolaryngol Clin North Am 21:743, 1988

Boerner DF, Zwadyk P: The value of the sputum Gram's stain in community-acquired pneumonia. JAMA 247:642, 1982

Boyle JT, Tuchman DN, Altshulter SM et al: Mechanisms for the association of gastroesophageal reflux and bronchospasm. Am Rev Respir Dis 121(suppl):S16, 1985

British Thoracic Society: Guidelines for the management of community-acquired pneumonia in adults admitted to hospital. Br J Hosp Med 49:346, 1993

British Thoracic Society: Community-acquired pneumonia in adults in British hospitals in 1982–1983: a survey of aetiology, mortality, prognostic factors and outcome. Q J Med 62:195, 1987

Buchman SR, Sugarman JH, Tatum JL et al: Failure of methylprednisolone, ibuprofen or prostacyclin to reduce HCl induced pulmonary albumin leak in dogs. Surgery 92:163, 1984

Burgess GE, Cooper JR, Marino RJ et al: Laryngeal competence after tracheal extubation. Anesthesiology 51:73, 1979

Bynum LJ, Pierce AK: Pulmonary aspiration of gastric contents. Am Rev Respir Dis 114:1129, 1976

Campbell JF, Spika JS: The serodiagnosis of non-pneumococcal bacterial pneumonia. Semin Respir Infect 3:123, 1988

Castiglioni A: A History of Medicine. 2nd Ed. Knopf, New York, 1947

Celis R, Torres A, Catell JM et al: Nosocomial pneumonia: a multivariate analysis of risk and prognosis. Chest 93:318, 1988

Chastre J, Fagon JV, Soles P et al: Diagnosis of nosocomial bacterial pneumonia in intubated patients undergoing ventilation: comparison of the usefulness of BAL and PSB. Am J Med 85:498, 1988

Chastre J, Fagon JY, Gilbert DC: Diagnosis of nosocomial pneumonia in ICUs. Eur J Clin Microbiol Infect Dis 8:35, 1989

Clissold SP, Todd PA, Campoli-Richards DM: Imipenem/cilastatin—a review of its antibacterial activity, pharmacokinetic properties, and therapeutic efficacy. Drugs 33:183, 1987

Coonrod JD: Pneumococcal pneumonia. Semin Respir Infect 4:4, 1989

Craven DE, Kunches LM, Kilinsky V et al: Risk factors for pneumonia and fatality in patients receiving continuous mechanical ventilation. Am Rev Respir Dis 133:792, 1986

Crossley KB, Thurn JR: Nursing-home acquired pneumonia. Semin Respir Infect 4:64, 1989

Culver GA, Makel HP, Beecher HK: Frequency of aspiration of gastric contents by lungs during anesthesia and surgery. Ann Surg 133:289, 1951

Dal Santo G: Acid aspiration: pathophysiological aspects, prevention and therapy. Int Anesth Clin 24:31, 1986

DeCastro FR, Violan JS, Capuz BL et al: Reliability of the bronchoscopic protected catheter brush in the diagnosis of pneumonia in mechanically ventilated patients. Crit Care Med 19:171, 1991

DeMeester TR, Bonavina L, Iascone C et al: Chronic respiratory symptoms and occult gastroesophageal reflux: a prospective clinical study and results of surgical therapy. Ann Surg 211:337, 1990

De Paso WJ: Aspiration pneumonia. Clin Chest Med 12:269, 1991

Derenne JP, Fleury B, Pareinte R: Acute respiratory failure of chronic obstructive pulmonary disease. Am Rev Respir Dis 138:1006, 1988

Dondero TJ, Rendtorff RC, Mallison GF et al: An outbreak of Legionnaire's disease associated with a contaminated air-conditioning cooling tower. N Engl J Med 302:365, 1980

Driks MR, Craven DE, Celli BR et al: Nosocomial pneumonia in intubated patients given sucralfate as compared with antacids or histamine type 2 blockers. The role of gastric colonization. N Engl J Med 317:1376, 1987

duMoulin GC, Hedley-Whyte J, Paterson DG et al: Aspiration of gastric bacteria in antacid-treated patients: a frequent cause of postoperative colonization of the airway. Lancet 1:242, 1982

Duncan SR, Raffin TA: Pulmonary complications of immunosuppressive diseases other than human immunodeficiency virus infection. In Murray JF (ed): Pulmonary Complications of Systemic Disease. Marcel Dekker, New York, 1992

Edelstein PH, Meyer RD: Legionella pneumonias. In Pennington JE (ed): Respiratory infections: Diagnosis and Management. 2nd Ed. Raven Press, New York, 1989

Edelstein PH, Meyer RD, Finegold SM: Laboratory diagnosis of Legionnaire's disease. Am Rev Respir Dis 121:317, 1980

Empey DW, Laitinen LA, Jacobs L et al: Mechanisms of bronchial hyperreactivity in normal subjects after upper respiratory tract infection. Am Rev Respir Dis 113:131, 1976

Epstein DE: Aspiration diseases of the lungs. In Fishman AP (ed): Pulmonary Diseases and Disorders. 2nd Ed. McGraw-Hill, New York, 1988

Fagon JY, Chastre J, Trouillet JL et al: Characterization of distal bronchial microflora during acute exacerbation of chronic bronchitis: use of the protected specimen brush technique in 54 mechanically ventilated patients. Am Rev Respir Dis 142:1004, 1990

Failla P, Karam GH: The appropriate role of new antibiotics in the therapy of pulmonary infections. Clin Pulmon Med 1:11, 1993

Fang GD, Yu VL, Vickers RM: Disease due to Legionellaceae (other than Legionella pneumophila): historical, microbiological, clinical and epidemiological review. Medicine (Baltimore) 68:116, 1989

Farr BM, Sloman AJ, Fisch MJ: Predicting death in patients hospitalized for community-acquired pneumonia. Ann Intern Med 115:428, 1991

Fein AM, Feinsilver SH, Niederman MS: Non-resolving and slowly resolving pneumonia: diagnosis and management in the elderly patient. Clin Chest Med 14:555, 1993

Fekety FR, Caldwell J, Gump D et al: Bacteria, viruses, and mycoplasmas in acute pneumonia in adults. Am Rev Respir Dis 104:499, 1971

Fernandez-Guerrero M, Gudiol F, Rodriguez-Torres A et al: Nosocomial pneumonia—a comparative multicentre trial between monotherapy and cefotaxime and treatment with antibiotic combinations. Infection 6:5320, 1991

Fine MJ, Smith DN, Singer DE: Hospitalization decision in patients with community-acquired pneumonia: a prospective cohort study. Am J Med 89:713, 1990

Finesilver SH, Fein AM, Niederman MS et al: Utility of fiberoptic bronchoscopy in non-resolving pneumonia. Chest 98:1322, 1990

Finkelstein MS, Petkun WM, Freedman ML, Antopol SC: Pneumococal bacteremia in adults: age-dependent differences in presentation and outcome. J Am Geriatr Soc 31:19, 1983

Friedlander C: Uber die Schizomyceten bei der acuten fibrosen Pneumonie. Virchows Arch B Cell Pathol 87:319, 1882

Garb JL, Brown RB, Garb JR, Tuthill RW: Differences in etiology of pneumonias in nursing home and community patients. JAMA 240:2169, 1978

Garibaldi RA: Epidemiology of community-acquired respiratory tract infections in adults: incidence, etiology, and impact. Am J Med 78:32S, 1985

Gates S, Huang T, Cheney FW: Effects of methylprednisolone on resolution of acid aspiration pneumonitis. Arch Surg 118:1262, 1983

Gentry LO, Rodriguez-Gomez G, Kohler RB et al: Parenteral followed by oral ofloxacin for nosocomial pneumonia and community-acquired pneumonia requiring hospitalization. Am Rev Respir Dis 145:31, 1992

Geppert EF: Recurrent pneumonia. Chest 98:739, 1990

Gianella RA, Broitman SA, Zancheck N: Gastric acid barrier to ingested microorganisms in man. Gut 13:251, 1972

Glauser FL, Millen JE, Falls R: Increased alveolar epithelial permeability with acid aspiration. The effects of high dose steroids. Am Rev Respir Dis 120:1119, 1979

Graham WGB, Bradley DA: Efficacy of chest physiotherapy and intermittent positive-pressure breathing in the resolution of pneumonia. N Engl J Med 299:624, 1979

Granton JT, Grossman RF: Community-acquired pneumonia in the elderly patient. Clin Chest Med 14:537, 1993

Greenfield LJ, Singelton RP, McCaffree DR et al: Pulmonary effects of experimental graded aspiration of hydrochloric acid. Ann Surg 170:74, 1989

Gross PA, Neer HC, Aswapoker G et al: Deaths from nosocomial

infections. Experience in a university hospital and a community hospital. Am J Med 68:219, 1980

Gwaltney JM Jr: Acute bronchitis. In Mandell GL, Douglas RG Jr, Bennett JE (eds): Principles and Practice of Infectious Diseases. 3rd Ed. Churchill Livingstone, New York, 1990

Haley RW, Hooten TM, Culver D et al: Nosocomial pneumonia in US hospitals 1975–1976: estimated frequency by selected characteristic of patients. Am J Med 70:947, 1981

Hall WH: The specific diagnosis and treatment of the pneumonias. Med Clin North Am 43:191, 1959

Hamelberg W, Bosomworth PP: Aspiration pneumonitis: experimental studies and clinical observations. Anesth Analg 43:669, 1964

Hanson LC, Weber DJ, Rutala WA: Risk factors for nosocomial pneumonia in the elderly. Am J Med 92:161, 1992

Hassett JM, Sunby C, Flint LM: No elimination of aspiration pneumonia in neurologically disabled patients with feeding gastrostomy. Surg Gynecol Obstet 167:383, 1988

Hedlund JU, Ortqvist AB, Kalin ME, Granath F: Factors of importance for the long-term prognosis after hospital treated pneumonia. Thorax 48:785, 1993

Hickling KG, Howard R: A restrospective survey of treatment and mortality in aspiration pneumonia. Intensive Care Med 14:617, 1988

Honeybourne D, Nadrews JM, Ashby JP et al: An evaluation of the penetration of ciprofloxacin and amoxicillin in bronchial mucus. Thorax 43:715, 1988

Hooper DC, Wolfson JS: Fluoroquinolone antimicrobial agents. N Engl J Med 324:384, 1991

Horan TC, White JW, Jarvis WR et al: Nosocomial infection surveillance. MMWR CDC Surveill Summ 35:17S, 1986

Huxley EJ, Viroslav J, Gray WR et al: Pharyngeal aspiration in normal adults and patients with depressed consciousness. Am J Med 64:564, 1978

James CF, Modell JH, Gibbs CP et al: Pulmonary aspiration: effects of volume and pH in the rat. Anesth Analg 63:665, 1984

Jay SJ, Johanson WG, Pierce AK: The radiologic resolution of Streptococcus pneumoniae pneumonia. N Engl J Med 293:798, 1975

Johanson WG, Pierce WK, Sanford JP et al: Nosocomial respiratory infections with gram negative bacilli. Ann Intern Med 77:701, 1972

Johanson WG, Pierce AK, Sanford JP: Changing bacterial flora of hospitalized patients. Emergence of gram negative bacilli. N Engl J Med 281:1137, 1969

Johnston BL, Forward K, Marrie TJ: Nosocomial pneumonia in critical care in general thoracic surgery. Chest Surg Clin North Am 1:81, 1991

Kahn FA, Basir R: Sequential intravenous-oral administration of ciprofloxacin vs ceftazidime in serious bacterial respiratory treat infections. Chest 96:528, 1989

Kanner RE, Renzetti AD Jr, Klauber MR et al: Variables associated with changes in spirometry in patients with obstructive lung disease. Am J Med 67:44, 1979

Kaplan DS, Murthy VK, Linsheer WG: Percutaneous endoscopic jejeunostomy: long-term follow-up of 23 patients. Gastrointest Endosc 35:403, 1989

Kirkpatrick MB, Bass JB: Quantitative bacterial cultures of BAL fluids and protected brush catheter specimens from normal subjects. Am Rev Respir Dis 139:546, 1989

Laforce FM: Systemic antimicrobial therapy of nosocomial pneumonia; monotherapy vs combination therapy. Eur J Clin Microbiol Infect Dis 8:61, 1989

Lamy ME, Pouthier-Simon F, Debacker-William E: Respiratory viral infections in hospital patients with chronic bronchitis. Chest 63:336, 1973

Langer M, Mosconi P, Cigada M et al: Long term respiratory support and risk of pneumonia in critically ill patients. Am Rev Respir Dis 140:302, 1989

Lehtomaki K: Clinical diagnosis of pneumococcal, adenoviral, mycoplasmal and mixed pneumonias in young men. Eur Respir J 1:324, 1988

Levy M, Dromer F, Brion N et al: Community-acquired pneumonia: importance of initial non-invasive bacteriologic and radiographic investigations. Chest 92:43, 1988

Lewis RT, Burgess JH, Hampson LG: Cardiorespiratory studies in critical illness: changes in aspiration pneumonitis. Arch Surg 103:335, 1971

Lorber B, Swenson RM: Bacteriology of aspiration pneumonia: a prospective study of community and hospital-acquired cases. Ann Intern Med 81:329, 1974

Louria DB, Blumenfeld HL, Ellis JT et al: Studies on influenza in the pandemic of 1957–58 II: pulmonary complications of influenza. J Clin Invest 38:213, 1959

Lynch DA, Armstrong JD II: A pattern-oriented approach to chest radiographs in atypical pneumonia syndromes. Clin Chest Med 12:203, 1991

MacFarlane J: Community-acquired pneumonia. Br J Dis Chest 81:116, 1987

Mandell GL, Douglas RG, Bennett JE (eds): Principles and Practice of Infectious Diseases. 3rd Ed. Churchill Livingstone, New York, 1990

Mandell LA, Niederman MS: Antimicrobial treatment of community-acquired pneumonia in adults: a conference report. Can J Infect Dis 4:25, 1993

Marrie TJ: Community-acquired pneumonia. Clin Infect Dis 18:501, 1994

Marrie TJ: Pneumonia. Clin Geriatr Med 8:721, 1992

Marrie TJ, Durant H, Kwan C: Nursing home-acquired pneumonia. A case-control study. J Am Geriatr Soc 34:697, 1986

Marrie TJ, Durant H, Yates L: Community-acquired pneumonia requiring hospitalization: 5-year prospective study. Rev Infect Dis 11:586, 1989

McGehee JL: A brief history of pneumonia. J Tenn Med Assoc 83:455, 1990

McHardy VU, Inglis JM, Calder MA et al: A study of infective and other factors in exacerbations of chronic bronchitis Br J Dis Chest 74:228, 1980

Meduri GU, Chastre J: The standardization of bronchoscopic techniques for ventilator-associated pneumonia. Chest 102(suppl): 557S, 1992

Mendelson CL: Aspiration of stomach contents into the lungs during obstetric anesthesia. Am J Obstet Gynecol 52:191, 1946

Middleton RM, Kirkpatrick MB, Bass JB: Invasive techniques for the diagnosis of lower respiratory tract infections. In Niederman MS, Sarosi G, Glassroth J (eds): Respiratory Infections: A Scientific Basis for Management. WB Saunders, Philadelphia, 1994

Mittl RL, Schwab RJ, Duchin JS et al: Radiographic resolution of community-acquired pneumonia. Am J Respir Crit Care Med 149:630, 1994

Moore FA, Feliciano DV, Andrassy RJ et al: Early enteral feeding compared with parenteral reduces post-operative septic complications. The results of a meta-analysis. Ann Surg 216:172, 1991

Moser KM, Maurer J, Jassi L et al: Sensitivity, specificity and risk of diagnostic procedure in a clinical model of Streptococcus pneumoniae pneumonia. Am Rev Respir Dis 125:436, 1982

Muder RR, Yu VL, Fang GD: Community-acquired Legionnaire's disease. Semin Respir Med 4:32, 1989

Murata GH, Gorby MS, Chick TW, Halperin AK: Intravenous and oral corticosteroids for the prevention of relapse after treatment of decompensated COPD: effect on patients with a history of multiple relapses. Chest 98:845, 1990

Murphy TF, Sethi S: Bacterial infection in chronic obstructive pulmonary disease. Am Rev Respir Dis 146:1067, 1992

Murray HW: Antimicrobial therapy in pulmonary aspiration. Am J Med 66:188, 1979

Murray JF: Pulmonary complications of human immunodeficiency virus infection. In Murray JF (ed): Pulmonary Complications of Systemic Disease. Lung Biology in Health and Disease. Vol. 59. Marcel Dekker, New York, 1992

Olivares L, Segovia A, Revuetta R: Tube feeding and lethal aspiration in neurological patients: a review of 720 autopsy cases. Stroke 5:654, 1974

Ortqvist A, Kalin M, Lejdeborn L, Lundberg B: Diagnostic fiberoptic bronchoscopy and protected brush culture in patients with community-acquired pneumonia. Chest 97:576, 1990

Ortqvist A, Sterner G, Nilsson JA: Severe community-acquired pneumonia: factors influencing need of intensive care treatment and prognosis. Scand J Infect Dis 17:377, 1985

Osler W: The Principles and Practice of Medicine. 4th Ed. Appelton and Co., New York, 1901

Ostergaard L, Anderson PL: Etiology of community-acquired pneumonia: evaluation by transtracheal aspiration, blood culture or serology. Chest 104:1400, 1993

Pachon J, Prados MD, Capote F et al: Severe community-acquired pneumonia: etiology, prognosis and treatment. Am Rev Respir Dis 142:369, 1990

Paladino JA, Sperry HE, Backes JM et al: Clinical and economic evaluation of oral ciprofloxacin after an abbreviated course of intravenous antibiotics Am J Med 91:462, 1991

Peitzman AB, Shires GT III, Iuner H et al: Pulmonary acid injury: effects of positive end expiratory pressure and crystalloid versus colloid fluid resuscitation. Arch Surg 117:662, 1982

Pelligrini CA, DeMeester TR, Johnson LF et al: Gastroesophageal reflux and pulmonary aspiration: incidence, functional abnormality and results of surgical therapy. Surgery 86:110, 1979

Pontopiddan H, Beecher HK: Progressive loss of protective reflexes in the airway with the advance of age. JAMA 174:2209, 1960

Ramsdell JW, Nachtwey FJ, Moser KM: Bronchial hyperreactivity in chronic obstructive bronchitis. Am Rev Respir Dis 126:829, 1982

Rein MF, Gwaltney JM, O'Brien WM et al: Accuracy of Gram's stain in identifying pneumococci in sputum. JAMA 239:2671, 1978

Rello J, Quintana E, Ausman V et al: Risk factors for Staphylococcus aureus nosocomial pneumonia in critically ill patients. Am Rev Respir Dis 142:1320, 1990

Reynolds HY: Normal and defective respiratory host defenses. In Pennington JE (ed): Respiratory Infections: Diagnosis and Management. 2nd Ed. Raven Press, New York, 1989

Ribner B: Pneumonia: primary and nosocomial. In Dantzker DR (ed): Cardiopulmonary Critical Care. Grune & Stratton, Orlando, 1986

Rosiello RA, Merrill WW: Radiation-induced lung injury. Clin Chest Med 11:1, 1990

Sahn SA: Management of complicated parapneumonic effusions. Am Rev Respir Dis 148:813, 1993

Sanford JP: Lower respiratory tract infections In Bennett JV, Brachman PS (eds): Hospital Infections. Little, Brown, Boston, 1986

Schwartzmann SW, Adler JL, Sullivan RJ et al: Bacterial pneumonia during the Hong Kong influenza epidemic of 1968–1969. Experience in a city-county hospital. Arch Intern Med 127:1037, 1971

Sims RV, Steinman WC, McConville JH et al: The clinical effectiveness of pneumococcal vaccine in the elderly. Ann Intern Med 108:653, 1988

Stanley PJ, Wilson R, Greenstone MA et al: Effect of cigarette smoking on nasal mucociliary clearance and ciliary beat frequency. Thorax 41:519, 1986

Stevens RM, Teres J, Skillman JJ, Feingold DS: Pneumonia in an intensive care unit—a 30 month experience. Arch Intern Med 134:106, 1974

Sukumaran M, Granada MJ, Berger HW et al: Evaluation of corticosteroid treatment in aspiration of gastic contents: a controlled clinical trial. Mt Sinai J Med 47:335, 1980

Sutherland JE, Persky VW, Brody JA: Proportionate mortality trends: 1950 through 1986. JAMA 264:3178, 1986

Tager I, Speizer FE: Role of infection in chronic bronchitis. N Engl J Med 292:563, 1975

Taylor G, Pryse-Davies J: Evaluation of endotracheal steroid therapy in acid pulmonary aspiration syndrome. Anesthesiology 29:17, 1968

Teabout JR II: Aspiration of gastric contents: an experimental study. Am J Pathol 28:51, 1952

Thurn J, Crossley K, Gerdts A et al: Enteral hyper-alimentation as a source of nosocomial infection. J Hosp Infect 15:203, 1990

Tobin MJ: Diagnosis of pneumonia: techniques and problems. Clin Chest Med 8:513, 1987

Torres A, Aznar B, Gatell JM et al: Incidence, risks and prognosis of nosocomial pneumonia in mechanically ventilated patients. Am Rev Respir Dis 142:523, 1990

Torres A, Serra-Batlles J, Ferrar A et al: Severe community-acquired pneumonia: epidemiology and prognostic factors. Am Rev Respir Dis 144:312, 1991

Tremblay LD, Ecuyer JL, Provencher P, Bergeron MG: Susceptibility of Haemophilus influenzae to antimicrobial agents used in Canada. Can Med Assoc J 143:895, 1990

Van Eeden SF, Coetzee AR, Jorbert JR: Community-acquired pneumonia: factors influencing intensive care admission. S Afr Med J 73:77, 1988

Venkatesen P, Gladman J, MacFarlane JT et al: A hospital study of community-acquired pneumonia in the elderly. Thorax 45:254, 1990

Verheij TJM, Kaptein AA, Mulder JD: Acute bronchitis: aetiology, symptoms and treatment. Fam Pract 6:66, 1989

Warriner CB, Brooks L, Pare PD: The effect of inhalation of nebulized steroid on the acid aspiration syndrome. Can J Anaesth 28:436, 1981

Wiest PM, Flanigan T, Salata RA et al: Serious infectious complications of corticosteroid therapy for COPD. Chest 95:1180, 1989

Wijands WJA, Vree TB, van Herwaarden CLA: The influence of quinolone derivatives on theophylline clearance. Br J Clin Pharmacol 22:677, 1986

Wilson R: Secondary ciliary dysfunction. Clin Sci 75:113, 1988

Woodhead MA, Arrowsmith J, Chamberlain-Webber R et al: The value of routine microbial investigation in community-acquired pneumonia. Respir Med 85:313, 1991

Woods DE, Straus DC, Johanson WG, Bass JA: The role of salivary protease activity in adherence of gram-negative bacilli to mammalian buccal epithelial cells in vivo. J Clin Invest 68:1435, 1981a

Woods DE, Straus DC, Johanson WA, Bass JA: Role of fibronectin in the prevention of adherence of Pseudomonas aeruginosa to buccal cells. J Infect Dis 143:784, 1981b

Wynne JW: Aspiration pneumonitis: correlation of experimental models with clinical disease. Clin Chest Med 3:25, 1982

Wynne JW, Ramphal R, Hood CI: Tracheal mucosal damage after aspiration: a scanning electron microscope study. Am Rev Respir Dis 124:728, 1981

Wynne JW, Reynolds JC, Hood IC et al: Steroid therapy for pneumonitis induced in rabbits by aspiration of foodstuff. Anesthesiology 51:11, 1979

Lung Abscess

Baker RB: The treatment of lung abscess: current concepts. Chest 87:709, 1985

Ball WS, Bisset GS, Towbin RB: Percutaneous drainage of chest abscesses in children. Radiology 171:431, 1989

Bartlett JG, Gorbach SL: Treatment of aspiration pneumonia and primary lung abscess: penicillin G vs clindamycin. JAMA 234:935, 1975

Bartlett JG, Gorbach SL, Tally FP, Finegold SM: Bacteriology and

treatment of primary lung abscess. Am Rev Respir Dis 109:510, 1974

Bernhard WF, Malcolm JA, Wylie RH: Lung abscess: a study of 148 cases due to aspiration. Dis Chest 43:620, 1963

Brock RC, Hodgkiss F, Jones HO: Bronchial embolism and posture in relation to lung abscess. Guy's Hosp Rep 91:131, 1942

Chidi CC, Mendelsohn HJ: Lung abscess, a study of the results of treatment based on 90 consecutive cases. J Thorac Cardiovasc Surg 68:168, 1974

Connors JP, Roper, CL, Ferguson TB: Transbronchial catheterization of pulmonary abscesses. Ann Thorac Surg 19:254, 1975

Crouch JD, Keagy BA, Delany DJ: "Pigtail" catheter drainage in thoracic surgery. Am Rev Respir Dis 136:174, 1987

Davidson M, Tempest B, Palmer DL: Bacteriologic diagnosis of acute pneumonia: comparison of sputum, transtracheal aspirates, and lung aspirates. JAMA 235:158, 1976

Delarue NC, Pearson FG, Nelems JM, Cooper JD: Lung abscess: surgical implications. Can J Surg 23:297, 1985

Frieden TR, Biebuyck J, Hierholzer WJ: Lung abscess with group A beta-hemolytic streptococcus: case report and review. Arch Intern Med 151:1655, 1991

Friedman PJ, Hellekant CA: Radiographic recognition of bronchopleural fistula. Radiology 124:289, 1977

Gorbach SL, Bartlett JG: Anaerobic infections (second of three parts). N Engl J Med 290:1237, 1974

Gourin A, Garzon AA: Operative treatment of massive hemoptysis. Ann Thorac Surg 18:52, 1974

Grinan NP, Lucena FM, Romero JV et al: Yield of percutaneous needle lung aspiration in lung abscess. Chest 97:69, 1990

Gudiol F et al: Clindamycin vs penicillin for anaerobic lung infections. Arch Intern Med 150:2525, 1990

Hagan JL, Hardy JD: Lung abscess revisited: a survey of 184 cases. Ann Surg 197:755, 1983

Henriquez AH, Mendoza J, Gonzalez PC: Quantitative culture of bronchoalveolar lavage from patients with anaerobic lung abscesses. J Infect Dis 164:414, 1991

Kaye MG, Fox MJ, Bartlett JG et al: The clinical spectrum of Staphylococcus aureus pulmonary infection. Chest 97:788, 1990

Knight L, Fraser RG, Robson HG: Massive pulmonary gangrene: a severe complication of Klebsiella pneumonia. Can Med Assoc J 112:196, 1975

Lawrence GH, Rubin SL: Management of giant lung abscess. Am J Surg 136:134, 1978

Lee SK, Morris RF, Cramer B: Percutaneous needle aspiration of neonatal lung abscesses. Pediatr Radiol 21:254, 1991

Mengoli L: Giant lung abscess treated by tube thoracostomy. J Thorac Cardiovasc Surg 90:186, 1985

Monaldi V: Endocavitary aspiration in the treatment of lung abscess. Chest 29:193, 1956

Monaldi V: Endocavitary aspiration: its practical applications. Tubercle 28:223, 1947

Naidich DP et al: Pulmonary manifestation of AIDS. CT and radiographic correlations. Radiol Clin North Am 29:999, 1991

Neuhof H, and Touroff AS: Acute putrid abscess of the lung: hyperacute variety. J Thorac Cardiovasc Surg 12:96, 1942

Neuhof H, Touroff AS, Aufses AH: The surgical treatment, by drainage, of subacute and chronic putrid abscess of the lung. Ann Surg 113:209, 1941

Pappas G, Schroter, G Brettschneider L et al: Pulmonary surgery in immunosuppressed patients. J Thorac Cardiovasc Surg 59:882, 1970

Pohlsan EC et al: Lung abscess: a changing pattern of disease. Am J Surg 150:97, 1985

Shafron RD, Tate CF: Lung abscesses: a five-year evaluation. Dis Chest 53:12, 1968

Stark DD, Federle MP, Goodman PC et al: Differentiating lung abscess and empyema: radiography and computed tomography. AJR 141:163, 1983

Swenson SJ, Peters SG, LeRoy AJ et al: Radiology in the intensive-care unit. Mayo Clin Proc 66:396, 1991

Weiss W, Cherniack NS: Acute nonspecific lung abscess: a controlled study comparing orally and parenterally administered penicillin G. Chest 66:348, 1974

Yang PC, Luh KT, Lee YC et al: Lung abscesses: US examination and US-guided transthoracic aspiration. Radiology 180:171, 1991

Bronchiectasis

Annest LS, Kratz JM, Crawford FA: Current results of treatment of bronchiectasis. J Thorac Cardiovasc Surg 83:546, 1982

Bass EM: Tracheobronchomegaly: the Mounier-Kuhn syndrome. S Afr Med J 48:1718, 1974

Blades B, Dugan DJ: Pseudobronchiectasis. J Thorac Cardiovasc Surg 13:40, 1944

Boyden EA: Segmental Anatomy of the Lungs. McGraw-Hill, New York, 1955

Bradham RR, Sealy WC, Young WG: Chronic middle lobe infection: factors responsible for its development. Ann Thorac Surg 2:612, 1966

Breatnach ES, Nath PH, McElvin RB: Pre-operative evaluation of bronchiectasis by computed tomography. J Comput Assist Tomogr 9:949, 1985

Brunn H: Surgical principles underlying one-stage lobectomy. Arch Surg 18:490, 1929

Charan A, Sinha K: Clinical pattern and role of surgery in bronchiectasis. J Indian Med Assoc 60:412, 1973

Churchill ED, Belsey R: Segmental pneumonectomy in bronchiectasis; the lingula segment of the left upper lobe. Ann Surg 109:481, 1939

Danielson GK, Hanson CW, Cooper EC: Middle lobe bronchiectasis: report of an unusual familial occurrence. JAMA 201:111, 1967

di Sant'Agnese PA, Talamo SA: Pathogenesis and physiopathology of cystic fibrosis of the pancreas: fibrocystic disease of the pancreas (mucoviscidosis). N Engl J Med 277:1399, 1967

Dogan R: Surgical treatment of bronchiectasis: a collective review of 487 cases. Thorac Cardiovasc Surg 37:183, 1989

Eliasson R, Mossberg B, Camner P, Afzelius BA: The immotile-cilia syndrome: a congenital ciliary abnormality as an etiologic factor in chronic airway infections and male sterility. N Engl J Med 297:1, 1977

Gamsu G, Klein JS: High resolution computed tomography of diffuse lung disease. Clin Radiol 40:554, 1989

Graham EA: The surgical treatment of bronchiectasis. Arch Surg 6:321, 1923

Grenier P, Maurice F, Musset D et al: Bronchiectasis: assessment by thin-section CT. Radiology 161:95, 1986

Grillo IA: Bronchiectasis in Nigerians. Afr J Med Sci 3:213, 1972

Guedel AE, Waters RM: A new intratracheal cannula. Anesth Analg 7:238, 1929

Haight C: Total removal of the left lung for bronchiectasis. Surg Gynecol Obstet 58:768, 1934

Hinds JR: Bronchiectasis in the Maori. N Z Med J 57:328, 1958

Isawa T, Teshima T, Hirano T et al.: Mucociliary clearance and transport in bronchiectasis: global and regional assessment. J Nucl Med 31:543, 1990

Jackson C: Tracheo-Bronchoscopy, Esophagoscopy and Gastroscopy. Laryngoscope Co., St. Louis, 1907

Jackson CL, Huber JF: Correlated applied anatomy of the bronchial tree and lungs with a system of nomenclature. Dis Chest 9:319, 1943

Jaffe HJ, Katz S: Current ideas about bronchiectasis. Am Fam Physician 7:69, 1973

Joharjy IA, Bashi SA, Adbullah AK: Value of medium-thickness CT in the diagnosis of bronchiectasis. AJR 149:1133, 1987

Kergin RG: The surgical treatment of bilateral bronchiectasis. J Thorac Cardiovasc Surg 19:257, 1950

Killian G: Ueber direkte Bronchoskopie. Munch Med Wochenschr 45:844, 1898

Laennec RTH: Traite de l'Auscultation Mediate et des Maladies des Poumons et du Coeur. 2nd Ed. Chaude, Paris, 1826

Laennec RTH: De l'Auscultation Mediate ou Traite des Maladies des Poumons et du Coeur. Brosson et Chaude, Paris, 1819

Lewiston NJ: Bronchiectasis in childhood. Pediatr Clin North Am 31:865, 1984

Lindskog GE: Bronchiectasis revisited. Yale J Biol Med 59:41, 1986

Longstreth GF, Weitzman SA, Browning RJ, Lieberman J: Bronchiectasis and homozygous alpha$_1$-antitrypsin deficiency. Chest 67:233, 1975

Maxwell GM: Chronic chest disease in Australian aboriginal children. Arch Dis Child 47:897, 1972

Monie R: Underdiagnosis of bronchiectasis. Practitioner 233:163, 1989

Muller NL, Bergin CJ, Ostrow DN, Nichols DM: Role of computed tomography in the recognition of bronchiectasis. AJR 143:971, 1984

Nissen R: Exstirpation eines ganzen Lungenflugels. Zentralbl Chir 58:3003, 1931

Overholt RH, Langer LA: A new technique for pulmonary segmental resection and its application in the treatment of bronchiectasis. Surg Gynecol Obstet 84:257, 1947

Piirila P, Sovijarvi ARA, Kaisla T et al: Crackles in patients with fibrosing alveolitis, bronchiectasis, COPD, and heart failure. Chest 99:1076, 1991

Ripe E: Bronchiectasis I. A followup study after surgical treatment. Scand J Respir Dis 52:96, 1971

Robinson S: The surgery of bronchiectasis, including a report of five completed resections of the lower lobes of the lungs. Surg Gynecol Obstet 24:194, 1917

Sanderson JM, Kennedy MC, Johnson MF, Manley DC: Bronchiectasis: results of surgical and conservative management. A review of 393 cases. Thorax 29:407, 1974

Sauerbruch F: Chirurgie der Brustorgane. 3rd Ed. Springer, Berlin, 1928

Sealy WC, Bradham RR, Young WG: The surgical treatment of multisegmental and localized bronchiectasis. Surg Gynecol Obstet 123:80, 1966

Takaro T, Scott SM, Bridgman AH, Sethi GK: Suppurative diseases of the lungs, pleurae, and pericardium. Curr Probl Surg 14:9, 1977

Vejlsted H, Hjelms E, Jacobsen O: Results of pulmonary resection in cases of unilateral bronchiectasis. Scand J Thorac Cardiovasc Surg 16:81, 1982

Wakefield SJ, Waite D: Abnormal cilia in Polynesians with bronchiectasis. Am Rev Respir Dis 121:1003, 1980

Wayne KS, Taussig LM: Probable familial congenital bronchiectasis due to cartilage deficiency (Williams-Campbell syndrome). Am Rev Respir Dis 114:15, 1976

Whittemore W: The treatment of such cases of chronic suppurative bronchiectasis as are limited to one lobe of the lung. Ann Surg 86:219, 1927

Wilson JF, Decker AM: The surgical management of childhood bronchiectasis: a review of 96 consecutive pulmonary resections in children with nontuberculous bronchiectasis. Ann Surg 195:354, 1982

Young K, Aspestrand F, Kolbenstvedt A: High resolution CT and bronchography in the assessment of bronchiectasis. Acta Radiol 32:439, 1991

Pulmonary Tuberculosis

Marvin Pomerantz
J. Gordon Scannell
Robert J. Ginsberg

DEFINITION

Pulmonary tuberculosis is broadly defined as involvement of the lungs with infecting mycobacterial organisms. The *M. tuberculosis* organism produces the standard form of pulmonary tuberculosis; however, mycobacteria other than tuberculosis (MOTT) can produce similar pulmonary pathologic conditions. In this section, those infections caused by *M. tuberculosis* will be called *tuberculosis;* those caused by other organisms will be called *MOTT infections.*

HISTORICAL NOTE

Hippocrates wrote about a disease characterized by weight loss and wasting or phthisis. Consumption, another term for pulmonary tuberculosis, is also descriptive of these symptoms (Moran, 1990).

In the late nineteenth century, Koch (1891), a German general practitioner, developed a culture method for the isolation of the tubercle bacillus. By the early twentieth century, a system of sanitariums had been created for the therapy of tuberculosis. Their development corresponded closely with the development of thoracic surgery in the United States. It was in a sanitarium, while recuperating from tuberculosis, that John Alexander began his monumental works on the role of surgery in the therapy of tuberculosis (Meyer, 1991). It was Alexander's (1925, 1937) influence that helped to pioneer the surgical approach to pulmonary tuberculosis, and his aggressive approach to collapse therapy for pulmonary tuberculosis marked the beginning of thoracic surgery as a separate specialty.

The surgical management of pulmonary tuberculosis today is a far cry from that of 50 years ago when pulmonary tuberculosis was the entity that defined thoracic surgery as a surgical specialty. Gone are the debates over the merits of various forms of collapse therapy, collapse therapy as an alternative to bed rest and sanitarium care, resection versus collapse therapy, and if resection is done, how extensive should it be and when should it be performed. The changed scenario in tuberculosis, as in other forms of bronchopulmonary suppuration, is attributable principally to the development of effective antibiotic therapy and chemotherapy rather than to specific technical advances, adjuvant support systems, or increased understanding of the disease. Indeed, there is probably less understanding and appreciation of the objectives of surgical therapy of tuberculosis now than in the past, but in spite of enormous changes in the social, national, and international aspects of tuberculosis, it remains a disease to be reckoned with.

The traditional objective of surgery in the therapy of pulmonary tuberculosis has been to promote stable healing or to remove an irreversibly damaged, infected focus of disease (i.e., either a residual pulmonary cavity or a rigid-walled empyema space). These objectives remain valid, but we now concentrate on the removal of destroyed lung or lobe distal to an irreversibly damaged bronchus and subject to repeated tuberculous or pyogenic infections and use excision or pleuropneumonectomy plus "empyemectomy" rather than drainage and thoracoplastic collapse of the cavity. Residual pulmonary cavities after a course of chemotherapy that has rendered the sputum free of acid-fast organisms, the so-called open negatives, are no longer considered indications for surgery, even for segmental resection, except under special circumstances.

Indications for resection have gone through an interesting cycle. Before effective chemotherapy became available, avoidance of cutting into infected tissue was mandatory, and thus indications for resection were so strict that few were done. In a second phase, the age of Max Chamberlain (Chamberlain and Klopstock, 1950), cutting through contaminated but otherwise viable tissue under the protection of chemotherapy was considered safe, and so limited, often multiple, resections became popular. In the present (and, we hope, final) phase, long-term follow-up has shown that chemotherapy alone does as well as, or better than, resection for anatomically resectable disease; therefore, surgery is rarely indicated, except in certain circumstances, when it becomes a matter of judgment or when complications that require surgical intervention ensue.

HISTORICAL READINGS

Alexander J: The Collapse Therapy of Pulmonary Tuberculosis. Charles C Thomas, Springfield, IL, 1937

Alexander J: The Surgery of Pulmonary Tuberculosis. Lea & Febiger, Philadelphia, 1925

Chamberlain JM, Klopstock R: Further experiences with segmental resection in pulmonary tuberculosis. J Thorac Cardiovasc Surg 20:843, 1950

Churchill ED, Klopstock R: Lobectomy for pulmonary tuberculosis. Ann Surg 117:641, 1943

Koch R: The aetiology of tuberculosis (translated by B. Pinner). Bull Int Union Tuberc Lung Dis 56:87, 1891

Meyer JA: Tuberculosis and the coming of age for thoracic surgery. Ann Thorac Surg 20:881, 1991

Moran JF: Surgery of the Chest. 5th Ed. Vol. 1. WB Saunders, Philadelphia, 1990

Sarot IA: Extrapleural pneumonectomy and pleurectomy in pulmonary tuberculosis. Thorax 4:173, 1949

BASIC SCIENCE

Mycobacteria are obligate aerobic bacilli. The term *acid fast* in relation to these organisms derives from the fact that they retain dye despite exposure to the potent decolorizing agent, acid alcohol (Iseman, 1992). Except for some MOTT, these organisms are characteristically slow growing and take additional time to obtain sensitivities to drugs with standard techniques. Newer techniques, such as the BACTEC system (Goble, 1986), allow for a more rapid determination of sensitivities and therefore permit an earlier institution of drug-specific therapy.

MOTT infections, recognized for more than 50 years, are often named for their source or site of origin. The infecting organisms are characterized by their distinctive growth patterns in culture and response to antimycobacterial agents.

Both tuberculosis and MOTT infections induce tubercle production in infected tissue and therefore appear the same microscopically. *M. tuberculosis* is extremely virulent and is capable of invading normal tissue (Ahn, et al., 1982). Tuberculosis is transmitted from infected individuals by airborne particles, and even a small inoculum can produce significant parenchymal damage. MOTT organisms are found free in the environment, and it is assumed that their transmission is from environmental sources, not from other infected humans (Iseman, 1992). It is also believed that MOTT organisms more often invade abnormal tissue, although clinically these infections can range from indolent to a rapidly progressive, destructive pneumonic disease (Iseman, 1992).

Pulmonary tuberculosis is classically thought of as a staged disease.

Stage I, primary or childhood tuberculosis, consists of initial infection by organisms carried in fine droplets or dust into the bronchial tree and out into the peripheral tissues. The critical size of the infecting dose and the virulence of the infecting organisms will influence the intensity and extent of the host's reaction, which may vary from a trivial, undetected pneumonitis to a rapidly spreading pneumonia, as occurs in infants, malnourished children in war-torn or desperately impoverished environments, native populations traditionally free of tuberculosis, and immunosuppressed individuals. In stage I the patient's tuberculin skin test result is negative. In the absence of tuberculin sensitivity, stage I disease does not progress to the intense, necrotizing process we find in stage III, the abscess or cavity. It is probable that stage I disease ultimately produces the sensitivity to specific components of the acid-fast organism we recognize as a positive tuberculin test reaction. The disease usually resolves spontaneously as an insignificant scar or Ghon complex. In the circumstances noted earlier, however, the primary infection may progress to overwhelm the individual, even to become epidemic in a community. Finally in a certain number of patients, stage I disease may progress to stage II. Stage I disease is not cavitary, has no surgical implications unless there is pleural involvement, and is managed by chemotherapy in individuals and populations at risk.

Stage II disease, chronic infection of the lymphatic and hematogenous system, has as its most striking and lethal manifestation, miliary tuberculosis, which involves all organ systems. Usually there are specific targets of hematogenous spread, for example, tendon sheaths, bones and joints, kidneys, meninges, peritoneum, pleura (effusion and tuberculous empyema), lymph nodes (scrofula), and soft tissues (cold abscesses and Pott's disease), and pulmonary infiltrates without cavities, except terminally, as seen in immunocompromised patients. This stage is also treated with chemotherapy and surgical drainage of the abscesses or empyemas. For reasons not entirely clear, many patients never progress beyond stage II but manage to survive well clinically for many years in the shelter of chemotherapy and an improved hygienic environment.

Stage III disease, destructive cavitary disease, or adult tuberculosis, is the main object of our concern as thoracic surgeons. In this stage the patient has acquired a marked tissue sensitivity to the tubercle bacillus so that reinfection of the lung, whether from an exogenous or endogenous source, results in inflammatory fixation and intense tissue destruction (i.e., an abscess or cavity surrounded by an inflammatory infiltrate). The extent of the destructive process is the result of many factors: the size of the reinfection dose, whether inhaled (exogenous) or endogenously spread from another cavity or caused by erosion of a peribronchial lymph node into a bronchus. Other factors, such as the physical, nutritional, physiologic, and immunologic competence of the host and the invasive and destructive capability of the infecting strain, are important modifiers.

CLINICAL FEATURES

The symptoms of mycobacterial pulmonary infection may be subtle or fulminant. Nonspecific chest symptoms of cough, persistent cold, chest pain, and fever are common. Weight loss, hemoptysis, easy fatigability, and night sweats also commonly occur. Patients with these symptoms who have a history of exposure to individuals with tuberculosis should elicit a high degree of suspicion in the physician. Immunosuppressed individuals or those with diabetes are also at higher risk. Drug abusers and homeless or migrant persons also have a higher incidence of tuberculosis. Patients with previous pulmonary infections, particularly those that resulted in bronchiectasis, are especially prone to MOTT infections and standard tuberculosis.

If left untreated tuberculosis can be a rapidly fatal disease. MOTT infections, as noted earlier, can be indolent to rapidly progressive. Currently there are more than three million tuberculosis deaths worldwide each year. The rising number of multidrug-resistant infections, which now average about 9 percent of all tuberculosis cases in the United States (Iceman and Madsen, 1989), has renewed interest in the development of new drugs. In some countries resistant strains account for up to 56 percent of tuberculosis cases, making this an even more important health hazard (Iceman and Madsen, 1989). The immunologic features of mycobacterial disease (Edwards and Kirkpatrick, 1986) are an area of current investigation. Immunomanipulation has the potential to be a valuable tool in the therapy of tuberculosis and MOTT infections.

DIAGNOSIS

The efficient diagnosis of tuberculosis requires a high index of suspicion so that specimens can be obtained for bacteriologic and histologic examination. The source of these specimens depends on the exact location of disease. Sputum examination and cultures, bronchial washings, lymph node aspiration or biopsy, percutaneous transthoracic needle aspiration, thoracentesis, and pleural biopsy all may be used.

Although tuberculin skin testing is recommended for all individuals suspected of having clinically active tuberculosis, false-negative reactions are common, especially in immunosuppressed individuals. Conversion from negativity to positivity indicates a recent infection. The standard tuberculin test is the intracutaneous administration of 5 units of purified protein derivative tuberculin (Mantoux test).

A chest radiograph is paramount in the diagnosis of pulmonary or pleural tuberculosis. Abnormalities encountered on the chest radiograph require confirmation by histologic staining and preferably micobacterial culture of the sputum or other specimens. Drug sensitivities should be performed routinely.

INFECTION CONTROL

Tuberculosis is a highly catagious infection and is a function of the concentration of infectious droplet nuclei in room air and the duration of exposure. Health care workers who treat patients with tuberculosis are at risk. While treating patients with suspected or diagnosed tuberculosis, health care providers should wear well-fitting disposable masks with appropriate filtration properties. Similarly when diagnostic procedures are performed, appropriate gowns and gloves should be worn. Bronchoscopes and respiratory and anesthetic equipment should all be disinfected appropriately (American Thoracic Society, 1992).

THERAPY

Medical

The initial therapeutic strategy in reinfection is control of the infiltrative, invasive component. Before the advent of chemotherapy, this meant undergoing "the cure," that is, bed rest, sanitarium care, nutritional therapy, social service support, fresh air, sunshine, and hope. The cure took time. Chemotherapy's greatest impact was in its potential to reduce the time and the environmental demands necessary for cure enormously, to the point where sanitariums were eliminated

---

Antimycobacterial Drugs
INH
RMP
PZA
Ethambutol
Streptomycin
Ethionamide
Cycloserine
Para-aminosalicylate
Capreomycin
Kanamycin
Amikacin
Rifabutin
Ofloxacin
Ciprofloxacin

and the frustrations of failure (i.e., unhealed, infective cavities that persisted even after the surrounding infiltrate had virtually disappeared) were reduced.

The primary therapy for tuberculosis or MOTT infection is chemotherapy. Once an infection is suspected, therapy can be started empirically with any of a number of drug regimens. The usual first-line agents include isoniazid (INH), ethambutol, rifampin (RMP), and pyrazinamide (PZA). The exact amount and type of therapy is currently undergoing revision. However, the 1986 recommendations include an initial three-drug regimen (INH, RMP, and PZA) for 2 months and INH and RMP for an additional 6 months. Specific therapy with multidrug regimens is begun as soon as sensitivities are obtained. It is not uncommon to begin with four- to six-drug regimens, particularly when resistant organisms are suspected (Medical Section of the American Lung Association, 1986).

Unstable healing of cavities can result from blockage of the cavitary-bronchial junction followed by the formation of a tuberculoma, a mass composed of inspissated caseous material. When tuberculomas are multiple, the process is called nodular or fibronodular tuberculosis, and the concern is that at some future time the drainage of the blocked cavity may lead to reinfection or progression.

A third method of cavity healing, without closure, is the extension of healthy epithelium from the bronchial connection to line the residual cavity, which results in an open negative. Prior to the introduction of chemotherapy, it had been repeatedly demonstrated that viable tubercle bacilli might persist for years in the walls of such cavities. Now chemotherapy effectively controls the organisms until dense scar tissue encloses them.

Surgical

In that cavities represent destruction of tissue, the formation of a dense, linear, avascular scar in which organisms cannot survive or are densely encapsulated is called stable healing. These scars are familiar findings in routine autopsies and in patients who have been cured or are so-called good chronics.

To hasten the production of such scars was the strategy of collapse therapy (phrenicectomy, artificial pneumothorax, internal pneumolysis, extrapleural pneumothorax and plombage, or thoracoplasty). Prevention of scar contracture through relaxation of elastic tissue in the lung was the rationale for collapse therapy. John Alexander (1937) was the apologist and historian of collapse therapy; his book on the subject is a medical classic. Collapse therapy at present is limited to thoracoplasty plus drainage of chronic empyema cavities; conceivably it might be resurrected in conjunction with chemotherapy.

Indications

Surgery is usually limited to management of the complications of these infections, which include massive hemoptysis (loss of greater than 600 ml of blood in a 24-hour period), bronchopleural fistula, suspected cancer, trapped lung, and most commonly the development of resistant or persistent infection despite chemotherapy. Cavitary disease itself is not an indication for surgery unless it is associated with one of these complications. Bronchostenosis as a result of endobronchial tuberculosis is an uncommon finding in North America, but one that may necessitate removal of distal lung. Resection of the stenosis alone is extremely difficult but occasionally possible.

The relative indications for resection include the following:

1. Destroyed lung or lobe distal to an irrevocably damaged bronchus and subject to repeated tuberculous or pyogenic infection.

2. An open negative cavity of significant size (greater than 2 to 3 cm) in a young person who may be subject to future major stress (e.g., persons about to embark on careers that will prevent their making concessions to illness). This indication should probably be extended to the immunologically compromised host.

3. Demonstrable atypical multidrug-resistant organisms in cavitary disease that can be resected cleanly by lobectomy.

4. Recurrent, sputum-positive infection in a given segment or lobe even though no macroscopic cavity has been clearly demonstrated. Phthisiologic dogma holds that positive sputum is a manifestation of cavitary disease whether the cavity can be demonstrated or not. Demonstration of cavities with the old technique of tomography, no matter how sophisticated, is far inferior to present-day imaging techniques, such as CT.

5. The finding of an asymptomatic peripheral nodule, usually a tuberculoma, is still the most common indication for resection, even in the era of fine-needle biopsy. Limited resection (wedge or segment) is usually curative, even without postoperative chemotherapy.

6. Finally there are clear-cut indications for an operation in the management of tuberculous empyema (a) in the absence of a communicating bronchopleural fistula, decortication, and reexpansion of the underlying healthy or minimally involved lung are usually possible; and (b) in the presence of a significant bronchopleural fistula with destroyed lung and secondary infection, pleuropneumonec-

tomy or pleurolobectomy is indicated after an appropriate period of supportive therapy if the state of the contralateral lung permits.

Technical Considerations

In the unusual situation in which resection is indicated, there are several technical considerations. First, if the offending organism has become resistant, resection should be covered by chemotherapy beyond the first-line agents whenever possible. Second, bronchoscopically there should be minimal or no evidence of active inflammation that might compromise healing at the level of the proposed bronchial resection. Third a maximal amount of uninvolved lung tissue should be preserved. Segmental resection requires precise, painstaking dissection of hilar structures anatomically distorted by dense scar. Finally, the axiom that primary healing is the objective of tuberculosis surgery translates into meticulous use of electrocautery and fine ligatures and the pleuralization of raw surfaces to avoid persistent air leaks. Resection for pulmonary tuberculosis is highly selective and irreversible; therefore, technical misadventures that result in unplanned, extensive excisions are most unfortunate.

Presurgical Investigation

The workup includes complete pulmonary function tests, standard chest radiography, and CT. Ventilation/perfusion scans have been extremely useful to determine the amount and type of resection to be done. Often relatively normal-appearing lung has been found to have diminished or absent ventilation or perfusion and requires more extensive resection than had been planned (Fig. 20-18). Based on previous work (Pomerantz, et al., 1991), in those patients who require surgery, 3 months of drug-specific therapy is given whenever possible prior to operative intervention. Many patients who undergo surgery for tuberculosis or MOTT infection are extremely debilitated. These patients may require preoperative hyperalimentation in an attempt to establish an anabolic state prior to surgery. To be considered a surgical candidate, the patient must have localized disease and adequate pulmonary function.

Principles of Tuberculosis Surgery

Double-lumen endobronchial tubes are used to avoid cross-contamination. Resection often requires extrapleural dissection, and muscle flaps should be used liberally to bolster the bronchial closure and fill a contaminated space. This is thought to decrease the number of bronchial disruptions and infected spaces by the use of healthy muscle as an aid to the healing process. The latissimus dorsi is most commonly used; however, the serratus anterior or pectoralis major can also be used. In our opinion this lessens postoperative complications and the development of bronchopleural fistulae. Positive sputum, pre-existing bronchopleural fistulae, extensive polymicrobial contamination, and expected space problems after lobectomy have all been considered by us to be indications for the use of these muscle flaps (Pomerantz, et al., 1991). Because surgery is often a last resort for these patients, resection of all grossly involved lung is mandatory. It is better

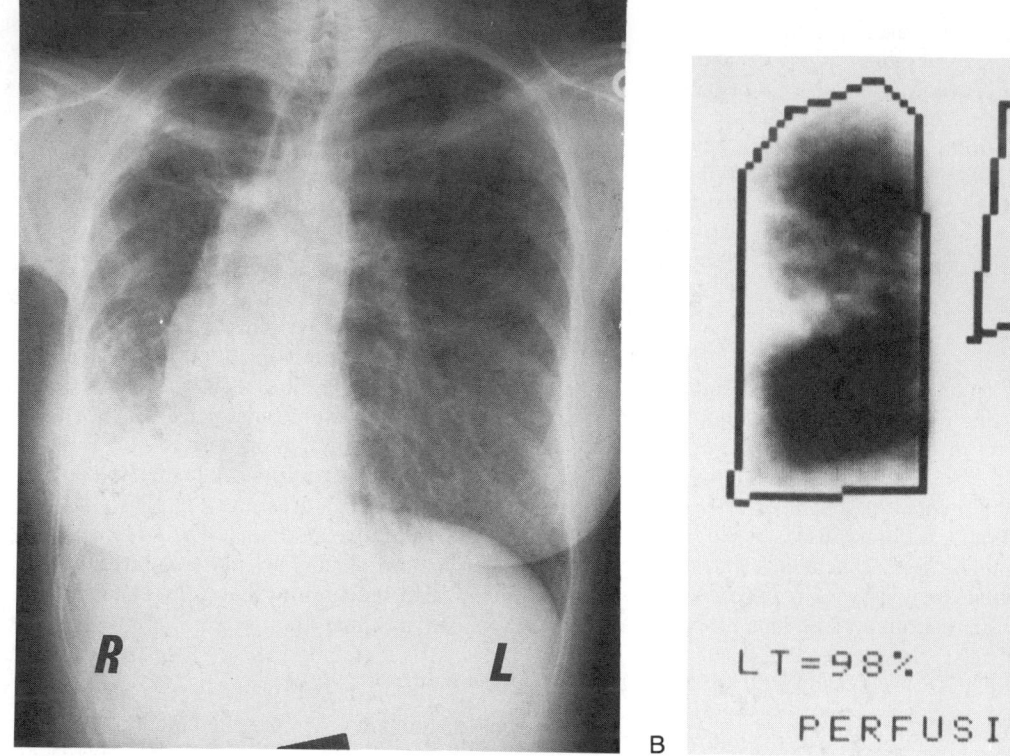

Figure 20-18. **(A)** Radiograph showing relatively normal-appearing residual right lung after right upper lobectomy. **(B)** Ventilation/perfusion scan in same patient showing a nonfunctioning residual right lung.

to err on the side of greater resection, if there is adequate pulmonary reserve, than to leave obviously diseased tissue. These patients have uniformly responded poorly to chemotherapy, and if the disease is not cleanly resected, a higher reactivation rate will occur.

It has been observed that, for patients who undergo resection for resistant tuberculosis, a pattern of left lung versus right lung destruction predominates. The exact reason for

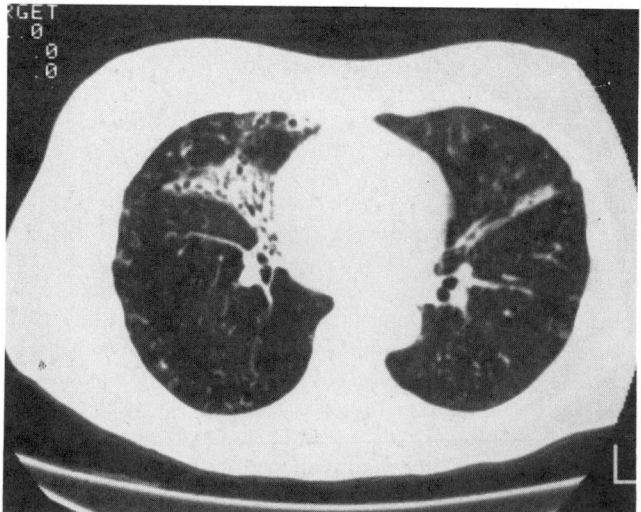

Figure 20-19. Patient with MOTT infection and bronchiectasis of middle lobe and lingula, as noted in CT scan.

this has not been determined (Pomerantz, et al., 1991). A pattern of middle lobe, with or without lingula, involvement has been observed in some MOTT-infected patients who do not respond to chemotherapy. These patients, in our experience, have all been women with saccular bronchiectasis in these areas (Fig. 20-19). Consolidation of the middle lobe and/or lingula is frequently found, and the infection can often not be eradicated until resection of these areas is carried out.

Surgery for Tuberculous Empyema

There is still a place for surgery in the management of a tuberculous empyema, an uncommon but important manifestation of the disease. Few such empyemas have no evident bronchopleural fistulae and lend themselves to thoracotomy, evacuation, decortication, and expansion of the underlying lung if it is not badly damaged by previous disease. Most patients with tuberculous empyemas have an associated bronchopleural fistula with a secondary invasive infection and an irrevocably damaged lung. These individuals are likely to be chronically ill, malnourished, and depleted. The first step, therefore, is to be certain there is adequate dependent drainage of the empyema to minimize further aspiration of its contents into the bronchial tree with consequent insult to the contralateral side and to concentrate on the nutritional and physical state of the patient. This stage must not be hurried.

When a plateau of well-being is reached, pleuropneumonectomy or pleurolobectomy is the procedure of choice. Sarot (1949) defined the rationale and technique of this operation in 1949, just as bacteriologic control became a reality, although the concept of excision and primary closure had been long established in surgery for tuberculosis.

The procedure requires a generous posterolateral thoracotomy that includes the previous drainage site, and the development of the extrapleural space to detach and excise as completely as possible the empyema cavity from the chest wall and diaphragm. Dissection is then carried into the mediastinum to isolate and divide the hilar structures. Contrary to what might be expected, the hilar dissection is usually not particularly difficult because the major pulmonary vessels are reduced in size and the peribronchial tissues, unless there has been an associated mediastinitis, are relatively avascular. Closure of the bronchus must be done with great care as close as is safely possible to the carina; the suture line is reinforced by viable mediastinal tissue or an intercostal pedicle flap. The chest is then closed without drainage or at most intercostal suction drainage for 8 to 12 hours to monitor bleeding. The use of local antibiotics in the pleura is a matter of choice, and systemic and appropriately chosen preoperative chemotherapy is a must.

This formidable operative procedure is surprisingly well tolerated if there is reasonable reserve on the contralateral side and the patients are in reasonable balance with their disease. Under these conditions, the long-term results are equally good. The ''Achilles heel'' is primary healing of the bronchial stump.

Postoperative Care

The perioperative care is similar to that given after any major thoracic resection. Suction drainage of the subcutaneous space from which the muscle flap was taken is mandatory. Premature removal of drains results in troublesome seroma formation and wound breakdown. Hyperalimentation should be continued postoperatively in those debilitated patients who have undergone resectional surgery in a continued attempt to maintain an anabolic state.

Results

The results after resection for resistant tuberculosis have been gratifying. With relatively localized disease, surgery plus continued long-term medical therapy has resulted in better than a 90 percent cure rate. The most serious complication has been the development of bronchopleural fistulae. Other complications include Horner syndrome, recurrent nerve injury, and wound complications. Respiratory disability in most cases is relative to the remaining good, functioning lung.

Patients who have undergone resections for MOTT infections have not done as well as those with tuberculosis. Those who have undergone right pneumonectomy have had a high percentage of bronchopleural fistulae develop in the early and late postoperative periods. This right-sided predilection for bronchopleural fistula formation has been commented on previously (Pomerantz, et al., 1991) and may be due to the frequent polymicrobial contamination found, the extent of infection in the bronchus at the level of resection, or anatomic considerations. Patients with MOTT infections of the middle lobe and/or lingula, however, have had excellent results after resection as have other patients who required lobectomies despite the presence of infection at the bronchial closure.

COMMENTS AND CONTROVERSIES

Tuberculosis is once again on the rise. Unfortunately, many of the new cases are resistant to first-line drugs or, as in some MOTT infections, are also poorly responsive to chemotherapy (Busillo, 1992). The increasing number of immunosuppressed individuals who contract these infections also adds to this health hazard. Until new drugs become available, or new techniques, such as immunotherapy, become practical, surgery will play an important role in the therapy of these infections. Surgical techniques must be meticulous to prevent bronchopleural fistula formation, particularly after right pneumonectomy for MOTT infection. Continued emphasis should be placed on preoperatively improvement of the nutritional aspects in the debilitated patient with tuberculosis and/or MOTT. For the near future, tuberculosis and MOTT infections will remain a medical and surgical problem that requires our attention.

M.P.
J.G.S.

The role of the thoracic surgeon in managing pulmonary tuberculosis has decreased remarkably since the advent of effective antimicrobial agents. The practice of thoracic surgery, however, has its foundations and early development based on the management of infectious diseases, such as tuberculosis and empyema. The recent resurgence of resistant forms of tuberculosis, especially in the immunocompromised host, makes this infection a common presentation to thoracic surgeons both for diagnosis and management of complications. This is especially true in Third-World countries. We must always remember that tuberculosis and other microbacterial infections must be considered when unusual infections or masses in the lung are encountered, especially in the immunocompromised host.

The reader is referred to further chapters in this text that discuss this entity (see the section on the immunocompromised patient at the end of this chapter and Ch. 39).

R.J.G.

KEY REFERENCES

Iceman MD: Infectious Diseases. WB Saunders, Philadelphia, 1992

This is a thorough review of the status of MOTT. The different patterns of infection and the different infecting organisms are thoroughly reviewed. The results of therapy are reviewed, and specific drug usage is discussed.

Pomerantz M, Madsen L, Goble M, Iceman M: Surgical management of resistant mycobacterial tuberculosis and other mycobacterial pulmonary infections. Ann Thorac Surg 52:1108, 1991

REFERENCES

Ahn CH, McLarty JW, Ahn SS et al.: Diagnostic criteria for pulmonary disease caused by Mycobacterium kansasii and Mycobacterium intracellulare. Am Rev Respir Dis 125:388, 1982

Alexander J: The Collapse Therapy of Pulmonary Tuberculosis. Charles C Thomas, Springfield, IL, 1937

Alexander J: The Surgery of Pulmonary Tuberculosis. Lea & Febiger, Philadelphia, 1925

American Thoracic Society: Statement. Am Rev Respir Dis 146:1623, 1992

Busillo CP, Lessnau KD, Sanjana V et al: Multidrug resistant Mycobacterium tuberculosis in patients with human immunodeficiency virus infection. Chest 102:797, 1992

Chamberlain JM, Klopstock R: Further experiences with segmental resection in pulmonary tuberculosis. J Thorac Cardiovasc Surg 20:843, 1950

Churchill ED, Klopstock R: Lobectomy for pulmonary tuberculosis. Ann Surg 117:641, 1943

Edwards D, Kirkpatrick: The immunology of mycobacterial disease. Am Rev Respir Dis 134:1062, 1986

Goble M: Drug-resistant tuberculosis. Semin Respir Infect 1:220, 1986

Isman MD, Madsen L: Drug-resistant tuberculosis. Clin Chest Med 10:341, 1989

Koch R: The aetiology of tuberculosis (translated by Pinner B, Pinner M) Bull Int Union Tuberc Lung Dis 56:87, 1891

Medical Section of the American Lung Association: Treatment of tuberculosis and tuberculosis infection in adults and children (joint statement of the American Thoracic Society and the Centers for Disease Control). Am Rev Respir Dis 134:355, 1986

Meyer JA: Tuberculosis and the coming of age for thoracic surgery. Ann Thorac Surg 52:881, 1991

Moran JF: Surgery of the Chest. 5th Ed. Vol. 1. WB Saunders, Philadelphia, 1990

Sarot IA: Extrapleural pneumonectomy and pleurectomy in pulmonary tuberculosis. Thorax 4:173, 1949

Mycotic Infection

Frederick L. Grover
Alan R. Hopeman

DEFINITION

Fungal infection of lung results from inhalation of the infectious agent. In cases of systemic fungal infection remote from the lung, the portal of entry with rare exceptions is the airway. In all probability asymptomatic or mild pulmonary infection occurs and clears spontaneously in such patients.

In earlier years these infections were most commonly due to primary pathogens, such as *Histoplasma capsulatum, Coccidioides immitis, Blastomyces dermatitidis, Sporothrix schenckii,* and *Paracoccidioides brasiliensis.* These were thought to arise de novo, and it was only after the development of more sophisticated knowledge of the immune system that it was recognized that some of these earlier cases presented in immunocompromised individuals. In recent years a large number of cases have presented that are caused by secondary or opportunistic pathogens, such as *Cryptococcus neoformans, Torulopsis glabrata,* and species of Candida, Mucor, and Aspergillus (Medoff and Kobayashi, 1980).

The major fungi that produce pulmonary manifestations were all first described nearly a century ago. Better understanding of these conditions began to accumulate with the development of satisfactory antituberculous drugs and the emergence of resectional surgery for the therapy of tuberculosis in the early 1950s. As resectional therapy came into common use, it became apparent that some of the patients whose conditions were diagnosed as tuberculosis on the basis of chest radiographic findings were indeed suffering from deep-seated fungal infections, particularly chronic cavitary histoplasmosis (Furcolow and Brasher, 1956).

Major impetus to rational therapy for pulmonary fungal infections came with the isolation of amphotericin B from a soil actinomycete, which provided for the first time an effective antifungal agent to be used in primary therapy of most of the major fungal diseases or as adjunctive support to surgical therapy in the management of fungal infection (Gold et al., 1955–1956).

Clear understanding of the nature of fungal infections in humans included the knowledge that during primary fungal infections millions of people have sustained subclinical infections with modification of skin test or serologic findings but with little evidence that clinical infection ever existed or will ever develop. Many more patients show a slight evidence of clinical disease, which clears rapidly and has no long-lasting effects. Serious fungal infection thus represents the small tip of a large iceberg. In addition, it is now recognized that some of the most difficult and rapidly advancing fungal infections are those caused by secondary or opportunistic pathogens in immunocompromised patients; this is found in an increasingly lethal pattern. The enlarging pool of these patients has been defined through the widespread use of corticosteroids to treat many conditions, of immunosuppressive agents after organ transplantation, of the use of chemotherapy to treat neoplasms, and of the discovery and description in the 1980s of AIDS. The old concept of pathogenic and nonpathogenic fungi is no longer clear (Van Trigt, 1990).

HISTORICAL NOTE

In this time of increasing knowledge and awareness of pulmonary fungal infection, it is interesting to trace the early discovery and understanding that progressed at a snail's pace in most instances. Histoplasmosis serves as an example. The first two cases were discovered in two adult young laborers from Martinique who died within 6 months of their arrival to work on the Panama Canal (Darling, 1906). Eight months later Darling found a third case in a 55-year-old Chinese worker who had lived in Panama for 15 years but had lived and worked in the Canal Zone for only 6 months. Although Darling remained in Panama until 1915, he attributed the fact that he could not find another case to the sanitation efforts of Colonel William E. Gorgas. Not until 15,000 autopsies (autopsy rate, 80 percent) and 45 years had passed was another case found in Panama (Draheim, et al., 1951) although a later article (Zimmerman, 1954) reported another Panamanian case that occurred in 1931 and was found in the autopsy files in 1954. The first clinical case recognized in the United States was reported from Minnesota (Riley and Watson, 1926).

Darling had incorrectly identified the offending organism as a protozoan. The first accurate determination that it was indeed a fungus came from cultures of a clinical case (DeMonbreum, 1934).

In a 1951 survey 138 cases of histoplasmosis were found in the literature, 65 of them pulmonary. Two additional cases of pulmonary parenchymal involvement confined to a lobe were treated by lobectomy, apparently the earliest example of pulmonary resection for this condition (Hodgson, et al., 1951).

At about this time improved antituberculous drugs were developed, and resectional surgery for tuberculosis was extended. A number of solitary nodules from the lung that had been designated as tuberculomas on the basis of their granulomatous appearance on microscopic examination were restudied with the then-new periodic acid-Schiff stain (Kligman and Mescon, 1950) and were confirmed to be due to *H. capsulatum*. The organism was also identified in hilar nodes (Puckett, 1953).

Surgical resection of chronic cavitary progressive disease developed after the observation that this condition was a problem in tuberculosis sanitoriums, either by being misdiagnosed and treated as tuberculosis or coexisting was acid-fact infection (Furculow and Brasher, 1956).

Other manifestations of infection with *H. capsulatum* soon came to light, and surgical therapy was proposed for the diagnosis or therapy for the complications of this disease, such as superior vena caval obstruction and prophylactic resection of mediastinal granuloma, in the hope of averting caval obstruction, mediastinal fibrosis, bronchial obstruction, or esophageal involvement.

In recent years with the development of immunosuppression from modern therapeutic methods and the description of AIDS by Gottlieb, et al. (1981), a number of fungal infections, including histoplasmosis, have played a prominent role as determinants of survival in this group of seriously ill patients, and the role of the surgeon in obtaining tissue for prompt diagnosis and therapy has been accentuated in those cases that defy less invasive diagnostic procedures (Trachiotis, et al., 1992).

Although histoplasmosis was described in 1906, only sporadic cases were documented during the next 30 years, and the impression was that it was a uniformly fatal disease. The true picture of a disease that affected large numbers of people, most of them in a benign manner, emerged as skin and serologic testing became available. A rather effective albeit toxic antifungal agent (amphotericin B) was discovered by Gold, et al. (1955–1956). A number of series assessed surgical therapy of chronic progressive (cavitary) hisoplasmosis. With refinement of the antifungal agent and careful studies, the role of surgery in this condition has diminished, but there remain surgical roles in the diagnosis and therapy of certain complications of histoplasmosis.

The evaluation of these changes spans nearly a century and closely parallels discoveries in the other major fungal infections. Blastomycosis in the cutaneous form was described as a protozoan infection at the turn of the century (Gilchrist, 1894). The systemic form was reported a few years later from a fatal case (Walker and Montgomery, 1902). Coccidioidomycosis was first described from Buenos Aires (Wernicke, 1892). This author also incorrectly identified the organism found in the tumors as a protozoan. *S. schenckii* was named for its discoverer (Schenck, 1898) and later redesignated *Sporotrichum schenckii*. Stoddard and Cutter (1916) described the pathologic and clincal features of cryptococcosis in humans. It was called torulosis. Sluyter was the first to describe aspergillosis (Sluyter, 1847). French pigeon handlers and hair manipulators were observed to suffer from this infection toward the end of the nineteenth century (Takaro, 1969). Sporadic cases of pulmonary mucormycosis were reported from Germany after the initial report by Furbringer (1876). Central nervous system and orbital cases were reported in the United States in 1943, but the first case of pulmonary mucormycosis in this country occurred in San Antonio in 1947 (Baker and Severance, 1948). Baker (1956) subsequently reported five more pulmonary cases and added three more cases from the literature. In his analysis he grouped the earlier German cases separately because the fungal hyphae were different from those seen in the later U.S. cases and concluded that, although they appeared acceptable as instances of mucormycosis, they were probably due to other forms of Phycomycetes.

Factors that certainly contributed to our improved knowledge of pulmonary fungal infections include greatly improved anatomic knowledge of the lung to facilitate surgical resection, the availability of adjunctive streptomycin to allow surgical resection of tuberculosis and thus advance the knowledge and practice of pulmonary surgery, and improved staining and culture methods to define the cause of pulmonary pathologic conditions more accurately. All these developments occurred in the decade 1940 to 1950.

HISTORICAL READINGS

Gold W, Stout HA, Pagano JF, Donovich R: Amphotericins A & B, antifungal antibiotics produced by a streptomycete. I. In vitro studies. Antibiot Annu 3:579, 1955–1956

Hodgson CH, Weed LA, Clagett OT: Pulmonary histoplasmosis. JAMA 145:807, 1951

Klingman AM, Mescon H: The periodic acid Schiff stain for the demonstration of fungi in animal tissues. J Bacteriol 60:415, 1950

Melick DW: Excisional surgery in pulmonary coccidioidomycosis. J Thorac Cardiovasc Surg 20:66, 1950

Takaro T: Mycotic infections of interest to thoracic surgeons. Ann Thorac Surg 3:72, 1967

DIAGNOSIS

Mycotic lung infections present a wide spectrum of clinical manifestations from the asymptomatic patient to the immunosuppressed patient with an opportunistic life-threatening fungal infection.

In the present era a careful history is important in regard to the possibility of fungal infection. Malnourished, debilitated, or diabetic patients; those who are receiving intensive antibiotic therapy; those with blood dyscrasias; and those

with Hodgkin's disease have all had an increased incidence of fungal infections. Although pulmonary or meningeal cryptococcosis has been most commonly associated with AIDS, all of the major fungal infections are now found to infect patients who have this syndrome (Ampel, et al., 1989; Chuck and Sande, 1989; Chechani, 1989; Clark, 1990; McKinsey, et al., 1989). In addition, it has long been recognized that patients with the pulmonary manifestations of tuberculosis, sarcoidosis, and lung cancer have commonly acquired pulmonary fungal infections.

The geographic nature of the three major pulmonary fungal diseases (histoplasmosis, coccidioidomycosis, and blastomycosis) has been well defined (Takaro, 1967). A geographic history may be useful in patients with new symptoms who have recently traveled to an endemic area. Histoplasmosis occurs most commonly in those states that border the Missouri, Ohio, and Mississippi River valleys. Blastomycosis is most common in the southeastern states. Coccidioidomycosis is found in California, Nevada, Arizona, New Mexico, and Texas in the lower Sonoran life zone.

When the patient presents with upper or lower respiratory symptoms of fever, cough, sputum production, hemoptysis, or pleuritic pain, a chest radiograph is commonly obtained. In most instances it will offer some indication of pulmonary, mediastinal, or pleural involvement.

It is to be emphasized that a firm diagnosis of fungal infection is only made after the demonstration of the organism in body exudates or tissues. Growth in culture is preferred, but recognition in smear, fresh mounts, or tissue sections sometimes is sufficient (Buechner, et al., 1973). Specific immunologic changes in host response may give a strong indication of the diagnosis and often lead to therapy before actual isolation of the organism can be achieved (Seabury, et al., 1971).

Once a pulmonary site is identified, specific diagnostic methods can be applied. Sputum retrieval is best accomplished by the induction of sputum production with warm aerosol treatments. Single sputum obtained in this manner should be promptly submitted to the laboratory. Twenty-four-hour sputum collections are of no value because of overgrowth by bacteria and saprophytic yeasts. A minimum of six induced sputum specimens obtained on successive mornings is recommended (Seabury, et al. 1971).

Bronchial washings or brushings may be useful, but in most instances sputum specimens are more reliable. Prompt delivery to the laboratory must again be emphasized if growth of fungi is to be successful. BAL of a bronchus that serves the involved area of the lung holds promise. Malabonga (1991) notes that lavage plus bronchial washings have a combined sensitivity on the smear equal to transbronchial biopsy and superior to that of transbronchial biopsy on the fungal culture in a small series of patients with AIDS and cryptococcal disease. Although open lung biopsy was previously the procedure of choice to identify pulmonary processes with certainty, the improvement of transbronchial techniques for diagnosis and the addition of transthoracic needle biopsy or radiographic insertion of a pigtail catheter into an abscess cavity or effusion in most cases will suffice to make the diagnosis with less risk to the patient.

Bonfils-Roberts, et al. (1990) outlined the precipitous drop in the use of open lung biopsy in seriously ill patients with

AIDS and noted that in only 1 of 66 cases was a successful therapeutic change initiated based on open lung biopsy findings. In this group 22 patients with severe respiratory failure died within 1 month, 3 during operation. Only 3 of the 66 had fungal infections.

Other diagnostic procedures include sampling of lymph nodes by scalene node biopsy or by mediastinoscopy for examination and culture, direct needle biopsy of an involved area of the lung, and the analysis of prostatic secretions. Ten to 15 percent of patients with blastomycosis have involvement of the genitourinary tract, and prostatic secretions contain the organism (Seabury, et al., 1971). In patients with AIDS and cryptococcal meningitis who have relapses after apparent successful primary therapy recurrent infection can most often be diagnosed by urine obtained after prostatic massage (Larsen, et al., 1989). Of 12 patients with urine cultures positive for *C. immitis,* fractional urine samples helped identify the prostate as the site of infection in four (Peterson, et al., 1976). The authors stress the importance of a rectal examination with the collection of prostatic secretions for culture. The epididymis and the upper urinary tract were also involved. Most patients were immunosuppressed. Spinal fluid analysis has been especially useful in meningitis induced by Cryptococcus, Coccidioides, and more rarely Histoplasma.

Occasionally blood, bone marrow, joint fluid, skin biopsy specimens that include ulcerative lesions or draining sinus tracts, and biopsy samples of mucous membranes may lead to the diagnosis in extrapulmonary mycotic infections.

Although the search for the etiologic agent in tissues or secretions continues, serologic or immunologic tests may be an aid to diagnosis, and skin tests may be useful in epidemiologic studies. Skin tests as a rule should not be used for diagnosis because (1) their value is limited, (2) cross-reactions occur in histoplasmosis, coccidioidomycosis, and blastomycosis, (3) a positive skin test result indicates that infection has occurred sometimes in the past but does not clarify the present clinical situation, (4) the skin test is of no use in early disease because skin test result positivity develops only after several weeks, and (5) the skin test elevates the level of serologic titers and interferes with their use in the establishment of a diagnosis or in the interpretation of disease progress by changing serologic titers. This interference may seriously affect the ability of the clinician to assess the progress or lack thereof with therapy and can add far more confusion than enlightenment.

Culturing of Clinical Specimens

Once clinical specimens have been obtained and promptly delivered to the laboratory, the growth of the culture is the responsibility of the laboratory, but a basic knowledge of the useful media enhances the possibility of the physician reaching a correct diagnosis. The basic culture media are Sabouraud's dextrose agar, brain-heart infusion agar, and Sabouraud's heart infusion agar. These may be prepared with plain blood or with 5 percent sheep blood. The sheep blood preparation is useful for tissue, bone marrow, or cerebrospinal fluid culture. All these media can be prepared with inhibitory agents, such as chloramphenicol or cycloheximide, and inhibitory agar is most effective for the culture of any speci-

men that may be contaminated with bacteria or saprophytic fungi the rapid overgrowth of which may prevent the growth of the true pathogen. Examples of such specimens are sputum, bronchial washings, nose and nasal sinus, skin, and mucous membranes. Spinal fluid does not require inhibitory media because it is rarely contaminated (Sarosi, et al., 1985). Prior to the culture the laboratory will apply techniques such as the selection of purulent parts of a specimen, homogenization, filtration, or centrifugation to concentrate the suspected organism and enhance the rate of successful culture. Useful culture methods for specific fungal infections will be indicated in the sections on specific diseases. In general, fungi grow slowly in culture, and cultures must be kept for a minimum of 30 days before the results are reported to be negative (Sarosi, et al., 1985). Some fungi may require up to 8 weeks for specific isolation and identification (Seabury, et al., 1971).

Serologic Diagnosis of Fungal Infections

The two types of serologic tests that are useful in the diagnosis of myocotic disease detect specific antibodies against fungal antigens or specific circulating fungal antigens (Sarosi, et al., 1985). Antibody testing is most common. IgM antibodies detected by a tube percipitin test appear early after infection and usually are not detectable after 6 months. Their presence suggests recent infection. IgG antibodies appear somewhat later, peak at 6 to 12 weeks, and may be present for months or years. These are usually found by a complement fixation test. Immunodiffusion tests also detect serum antibodies, usually of the types detected by IgG antibodies. Immunodiffusion is much easier to perform than complement fixation but is less sensitive (Sarosi, et al., 1985). Other serologic tests that detect fungal antibodies include counterimmunoelectrophoresis, enzyme-linked immunosorbent assay, passive hemagglutination assay, latex agglutination, and radioimmunoassay (Penn, et al., 1983).

Single-specimen serologic testing is much less effective than serial examinations that allow the physician to follow the titers. Titers vary between laboratories and within the same laboratory. When serial testing is desired, specimens should be obtained with part analyzed for screening and the remainder frozen to be sent in along with later specimens for simultaneous analysis. In general, serial examinations with intervals less than 3 weeks are not useful (Seaburg, et al., 1971).

Direct detection of specific circulating fungal antigens indicates the presence of a fungus and that the infection is active. Detection of cryptococcal polysaccharide capsular antigen by the latex agglutination test is the best example of antigen determination and the most important serologic test in the diagnosis of cryptococcosis (Penn, et al., 1983). The most useful serologic tests in specific fungal infections are outlined in the sections that describe each disease.

INDIVIDUAL FUNGAL INFECTIONS

Much of our knowledge about fungal disease stems from an era in medicine and surgery when methods of diagnosis were inadequate. Although the physician must be ever vigilant in the handling of specimens from transbronchial biopsies, bronchial washings, percutaneous lung biopsies, and routine sputum or induced sputum specimens, the availability of these methods has sharply reduced the need for surgical therapy in fungal infections with a few notable exceptions. A discussion of individual fungal infections highlights the current knowledge of these conditions. The individual drugs used in management are shown in Table 20-4.

Although it is difficult to establish the frequency of the fungal infections because of the large numbers of subclinical cases, a reasonable estimate of the frequency can be made. The infections are discussed in the order of their frequency of appearance in the United States: (1) histoplasmosis, (2) coccidioidomycosis, (3) blastomycosis, (4) cryptococcosis, (5) aspergillosis, (6) sporotrichosis, (7) mucormycosis, (8) candidiasis, and (9) paracoccidioidomycosis.

Paracoccidioidomycosis (South American blastomycosis) is the most prominent systemic fungal disorder in Latin America (Restrepo, et al., 1987). A 1974 review found only eight cases in the United States (Littman, 1974). All patients had lived in South American or Mexico and had long latent periods after leaving the endemic areas before their illnesses were diagnosed in the United States.

Histoplasmosis

Clinical Features

Histoplasmosis is induced by a dimorphic saprophytic fungus. The portal of entry is the airway. First described by Darling (1906) from the Panama Canal Zone and thought to be a rare infection, it is now evident that millions of people have been infected, especially in endemic areas along the great river valleys of the United States. This infection is usually an acute respiratory infection that is self-limited and requires no therapy (Saag, 1988). Large numbers of patients

Table 20-4. Antifungal Agents in Fungal Infections

Fungal Disease	Presentation	Drug Choice	Alternative	Possibly Effective (Insufficient Data)
Aspergillosis	Invasive	AMB (+flucytosine?)	—	Itraconazole
	ICH	AMB (+flucytosine?)	—	Itraconazole
Blastomycosis	Usual case	Observe for progression	AMB if further progression	Itraconazole
	Severe, meningeal, GU, ventilator-dependent, ICH	AMB		—
Candidiasis	Oral, esophageal	Fluconazole	AMB, oral ketoconazole	—
	Deep seated	AMB (+flucytosine?)	—	Fluconazole
Coccidioidomycosis	Acute pulmonary	None	—	
	Acute pulmonary +ICH	AMB	—	Fluconazole, itraconazole
	Disseminated	Ketoconazole (AMB if progresses)	—	Fluconazole, itraconazole
	Meningeal	AMB (IV and intrathecal)	—	Fluconazole, itraconazole
	AIDS			
	Initial	AMB (IV and intrathecal)	—	Fluconazole, itraconazole
	Maintenance	AMB	—	
Cryptococcosis	Pulmonary	None	AMB	—
	Pulmonary progression	AMB + flucytosine	—	—
	Disseminated	AMB (+flucytosine?)	—	—
	Meningeal	AMB + flucytosine	—	Fluconazole, itraconazole
	AIDS			
	Meningeal	AMB (+flucytosine?)[a]	—	Fluconazole, itraconazole
	Acute maintenance	Fluconazole	AMB	Itraconazole
Histoplasmosis	Acute pulmonary	None	AMB, is progressive	—
	Pneumonia, ventilator dependent, ICH	AMB	—	—
	Chronic pulmonary	Ketoconazole	AMB	Itraconazole
	AIDS			
	Initial	AMB	—	Itraconazole
	Maintenance	AMB	Ketoconazole	Itraconazole
Mucormycosis	Rhinocerebral	AMB + surgery	—	—
	Pulmonary	AMB + early surgery	—	—
	Disseminated	AMB	—	—
Paracoccidioidomycosis	Stable patient	Ketoconazole	Itraconazole	—
	Unstable patient	AMB (with or without sulfadiazine)	—	—
Sporotrichosis	Lymphocutaneous	Potassium iodide	—	Itraconazole, fluconazole
	Pulmonary	AMB	Ketoconazole	Itraconazole

Abbreviations: ICH, immunocompromised host; AMB, amphotericin B; GU, genitourinary; IV, intravenous.

[a] Sarosi (1990) noted that most patients with cryptococcosis and AIDS present with marginal bone marrow reserves and are likely to incur severe myelosuppression from flucytosine.

remain asymptomatic and are unaware of their illness. In the past this was called primary histoplasmosis, but Goodwin, et al (1981) point out that this is not an appropriate term because in histoplasmosis the infection often dies out completely and patients may be later infected or reinfected.

Acute pulmonary infections may present a radiographic piuctre of soft patchy infiltrates, smaller nodular infiltrates, and miliary infiltrates. Most clear spontaneously, but a few patients have an acute pulmonary disease with prolonged fever, cough, and persistent radiographic change. Antifungal drugs may be necessary if the condition is severe (Saag, 1988).

As the pulmonary infiltrates clear, the infiltrates may consolidate into a solitary nodule, and this granuloma often can-

not be distinguished from an early bronchogenic carcinoma that requires thoracotomy and surgical removal. Antifungal therapy is not required. If the active central portion of the nodule is obtained by FNA, it may allow the surgeon to avert thoracotomy. Such nodules often grow gradually by elaborating collagen, which also leads to consideration of a malignant process in the differential diagnosis.

In a few patients chronic cavitary histoplasmosis develops. This commonly occurs in patients with long-standing patterns of cigarette smoking, underlying chronic lung disease, or both. The lesions are most commonly in the upper lobes at the apex of the lung and are often bilateral (Dively and McCracken, 1966; Ahn, et al., 1969) (Fig. 20-20).

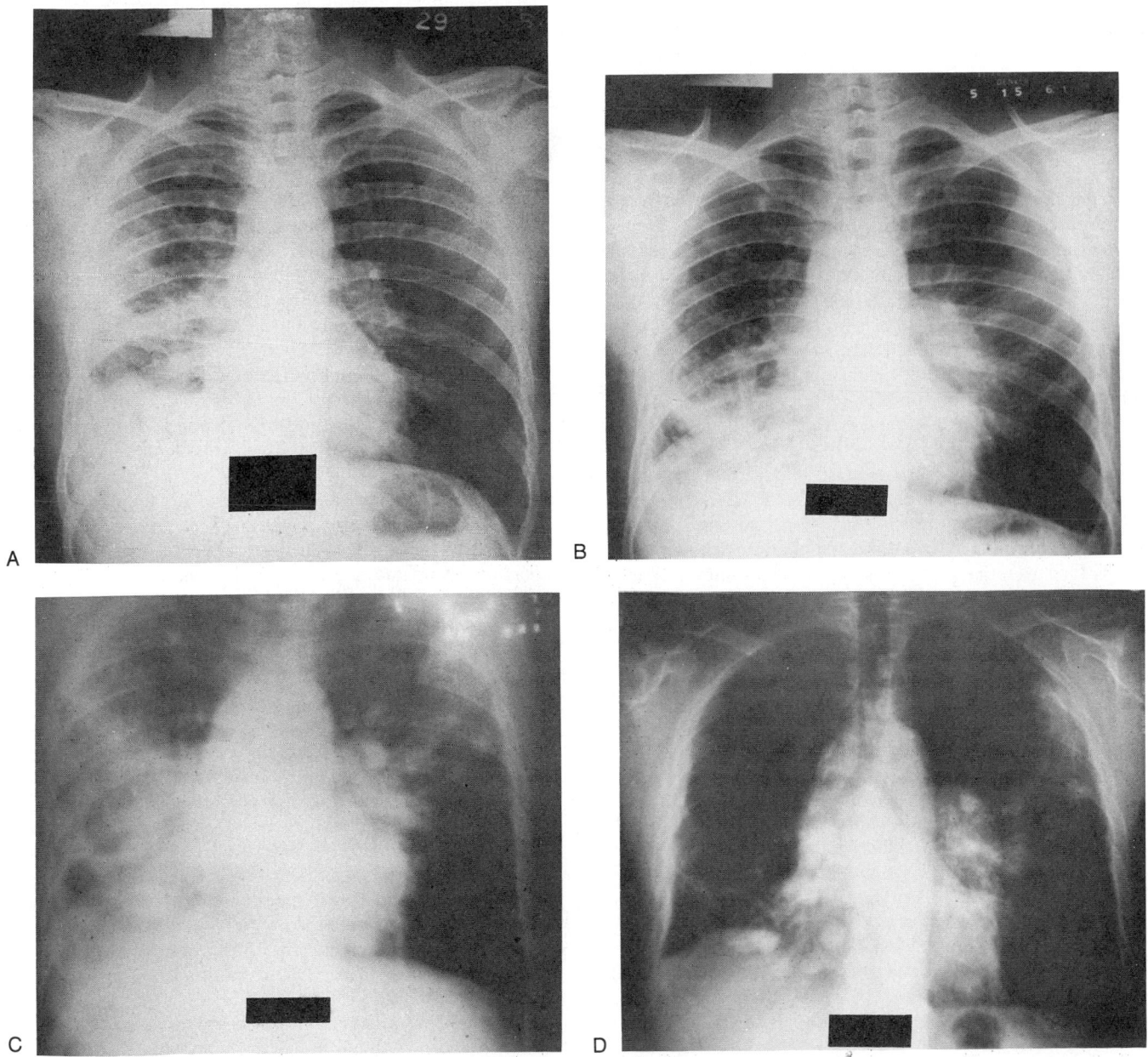

Figure 20-20. Chronic histoplasmosis: a 32-year documentation. This 57-year-old man had coronary artery bypass surgery at a Veterans Affairs facility with no evidence of pericardial disease. Serial chest radiographs from **(A)** 1954, **(B)** 1961, **(C)** 1982, and **(D)** 1986 and many intervening ones (not shown) show a constantly shifting pattern of pulmonary disease with calcification of pulmonary and mediastinal masses on the most recent radiograph.

Furculow and Brasher (1956) found a large number of patients with histoplasmosis confined to tuberculosis hospitals with a tentative diagnosis of tuberculosis because of the similar clinical presentations of the disease. Furcolow, et al. (1961) reported that 25 percent of patients with proved chronic cavitary histoplasmosis had concomitant tuberculosis.

Presentations of histoplasmosis of no concern to surgeons other than in the making of the diagnosis are the mild acute cases that require no therapy and the severe acute cases that are treated with antifungal drugs. Other clearly nonsurgical presentations of the disease are progressive disseminated histoplasmosis, which may appear in the immunocompetent patient but more commonly is seen with immunosuppression, AIDS, central nervous system disease, or a combination of these factors (Sarosi, 1988. Terrill and Hughes, 1992).

Takaro (1989) has emphasized that three presentations of histoplasmosis commonly are seen by thoracic surgeons. The first is the chronic granuloma which presents as a solitary pulmonary nodule after a mild acute infection or often remotely after the acute infection in an asymptomatic patient and is discovered on a routine chest radiograph. The second is chronic cavitary histoplasmosis, which must be distinguished from pulmonary tuberculosis, other pulmonary mycoses, or more rarely a pulmonary malignancy. The final form of histoplasmosis that commonly requires surgical attention is mediastinal granulomatous disease. As Takaro (1989) points out, in some patients histoplasmosis produces an intense granulomatous and fibrous reaction. The manifestations are numerous and include fibrosing mediastinitis with bronchial, tracheal, esophageal, or superior vena caval obstruction and pericarditis with tamponade. Other presentations are related to the lymph node enlargement or calcification common in long-term disease and are seen as middle lobe syndrome, tracheoesophageal, or bronchoesophageal fistula or as broncholithiasis with hemoptysis and "stone spitting."

A rare but clinically important presentation of histoplasmosis is fungal septicemia and endocarditis presenting on a native or prosthetic heart valve (Kanawaty, et al., 1991).

Diagnostic Modalities

Direct microscopic examination of sputum or other body fluids for *H. capsulatum* is rarely useful and has a low diagnostic yield. Smears of bone marrow or peripheral blood stained with Wright or Giemsa stains, however, are useful and may provide an early diagnosis.

Growth of the fungus on culture media at 30°C is usually slow, but growth may be identified as early as 5 days when the specimen contains large numbers of organisms. With a small number of organisms, growth may not appear for as long as 45 days (Sarosi, et al., 1985).

Complement fixation tests that use histoplasmin (or mycelial-phase) antigen and yeast-phase antigen have been useful in the diagnosis of histoplasmosis for more than 30 years. A serum complement fixation titer of 1:32 or more or a fourfold rise in titer during illness is highly suggestive of active histoplasmosis. Complement fixation titers of 1:8 or 1:16 are seen in chronic cavitary histoplasmosis but occur in up to 25 percent of normal blood donors.

Radioimmunoassay and immunodiffusion tests are quicker and simpler but are more sensitive. Thus negative test results are more useful in ruling out active disease.

Because skin testing for histoplasmosis evidences cross-reactions with blastomycosis and coccidioidomycosis and may in itself induce an elevation in the complement fixation titer, the use of histoplasmin skin testing has been denounced as a diagnostic hindrance (Levin, 1970).

A definitive diagnosis is made by the isolation or identification of *H. capsulatum* from clinical specimens. This may require weeks of incubation, such specimens may not be readily available for culture, and in some forms of infection, this is rarely accomplished. The proper use and interpretation of serologic test results is of major importance in the management of patients with histoplasmosis (Buechner, et al., 1973; Penn, et al., 1983; Sarosi, et al., 1985).

Therapy

Chronic Cavitary Histoplasmosis. In several surgical series reported by Dively and McCracken (1966); Ahn, et al. (1969); Sutaria, et al. (1970); and Prager, et al. (1980), it is apparent that there were significant morbidity and mortality rates from difficult surgery in this complex group of patients with underlying lung disease and often with diminished pulmonary reserve. An occasional pneumonectomy was as often done for technical difficulties with upper lobe or mediastinal disease as it was for involvement of the lung with histoplasmosis.

The 29 cases reported by Dively and McCracken (1966) were done without amphotericin B coverage. Three patients required pneumonectomy, six had limited thoracoplasty for space problems, and four had recurrent disease. Ahn, et al. (1969) presented a series of 42 patients and emphasized the apical and upper lobe nature of the disease. Only one patient had lower lobe involvement. Operations were carried out in 12 of the 42 patients, and the authors recommended pre- and postoperative amphotericin B coverage to produce superior results to amphotericin B or surgical therapy alone.

Sutaria, et al. (1970) applied a surgical approach to 110 of 530 patients diagnosed with pulmonary histoplasmosis. Thirteen patients had pulmonary infiltrative disease; 21, a solitary nodule; and 76, cavitary disease divided equally between those who also received amphotericin B and those who had surgery alone. Surgical complications occurred in 18 percent. Ten patients required postoperative thoracoplasty. The authors concluded that amphotericin B offered little protection against immediate postoperative complications but reduced the mortality and recurrence rates.

Prager, et al. (1980) presented a subset of 27 patients operated on for cavitary histoplasmosis. Twenty-two of the 27 had lobectomy with four segmental resections and one pneumonectomy. Three patients required postoperative thoracoplasty, and recurrent cavitary disease was observed in four patients. Because of marginal respiratory reserve, none underwent reoperations. Two were treated with amphotericin B. Recent developments in the therapy of chronic cavitary histoplasmosis with improved antifungal drugs suggests that drug therapy will supersede surgical therapy in this type of patient who as a rule has chronic underlying lung disease and diminished pulmonary reserve. The practice of rapid administration of amphotericin B has reduced the toxicity of the drug and allowed outpatient therapy. The availability of oral azole drugs, some not yet released, which are less toxic than amphotericin B, shows further promise of useful therapy. Takaro (1967) indicated that surgical resection of chronic cavitary histoplasmosis should be carried out if the lesions are sufficiently localized, maximal improvement with antifungal drug therapy has been attained, and the patient's pulmonary function is not seriously impaired by pulmonary fibrosis and emphysema. Takaro (1988) proposed that a patient with sputum-positive cavitary histoplasmosis should be treated with amphotericin B and not surgery because evidence in controlled studies did not promise a lowering of relapse rates or a prolongation of life. He also noted that some surgeons still advocate resection in these cases and in that event recommended 1 month of drug therapy both pre- and postoperatively.

Parker, et al. (1970) in a cooperative study reported that 235 or 238 patients had initial resolution of their chronic cavitary disease when they were treated with at least 2 g of amphotericin B. Fifteen percent had relapses within 5 years, and this was attributed to an older age group and a lower total dose of amphotericin B.

The National Institute of Allergy and Infectious Diseases Mycosis Study Group (1985) showed that ketoconazole is an effective alternative to amphotericin B for the therapy of chronic cavitary disease. On the basis of this study, it is recommended that patients be started on a regimen of 400 mg/day, increased to 600 to 800 mg/day if a favorable clinical response is not achieved (Saag, 1988). Patients who do not do well during ketoconazole therapy by reason of inadequate response or toxicity and immunocompromised patients should receive amphotericin B. Disseminated disease, even with appropriate therapy, may still have a mortality rate of 10 to 30 percent. Amphotericin B is required for disseminated histoplasmosis in the immunocompromised patient and in the rare patient with central nervous system disease. Patients who have a competent immune system and who appear less sick and do not have meningitis may benefit from a trial of ketoconazole therapy.

Patients with AIDS require amphotericin B as the drug of choice. Saag (1988) notes that a current but unsubstantiated recommendation for disseminated histoplasmosis in this group is to administer an induction course of amphotericin B of 500 to 1,000 mg followed by suppressive therapy of ketoconazole or weekly amphotericin B for life.

Fibrosing Mediastinitis. Mediastinal histoplasmosis and its aftermath, fibrosing mediastinitis, have presented major surgical challenges in the past. It is possible that the advances in drug therapy for pulmonary disease will carry over into improved results in mediastinal disease, but findings are not yet available in this smaller subgroup of patients. It is believed that mediastinal disease begins with lymph node involvement by *H. capsulatum,* which produces central necrosis. There is a prominent fibroblastic response according to Goodwin, et al. (1981), which in healing leaves encapsulated caseous foci that are often multiple and often calcified. The scarring associated with healing periadenitis affects adjacent mediastinal structures.

Gillespie (1956) first described superior vena caval obstruction in a 7-year-old farm girl 3 years after an episode of viral pneumonia. Histoplasmosis skin test findings were strongly positive, and the tuberculin test was negative. Salyer, et al. (1959) reported four more cases in which exploration yielded tissue that resembled cutaneous keloid. *H. capsulatum* was clearly identified in one case, two were negative, and one was suggestive of histoplasmosis on the tissue examination (Figs. 20-21 and 20-22).

As pointed out by Dines, et al. (1979) and others, it is difficult to prove that all cases of fibrosing mediastinitis are caused by histoplasmosis because the results of stains and cultures are often negative. The two other major diseases that cause mediastinal adenopathy, tuberculosis and sarcoidosis, have not produced this pattern of disease, and positive identification in some cases along with cases in which the serologic findings are positive or that demonstrate other features common to histoplasmosis lend credence to the belief that mediastinal histoplasmosis is responsible (Hewlett, et al., 1966).

Consolidated granulomatous masses of lymph nodes may in themselves cause obstruction of adjacent mediastinal structures by simple compression, as reported by Strimlan, et al. (1975) and Prager, et al. (1980). With rupture of such a granuloma into the mediastinum, a dense fibrous reaction ensues, and fibrosing mediastinitis develops (Figs. 20-23 and 20-24).

Removal of granulomatous masses in the early stages has been recommended by Ferguson and Burford (1965); Zaijtchuk, et al. (1973); Strimlan, et al. (1975); and Dines, et

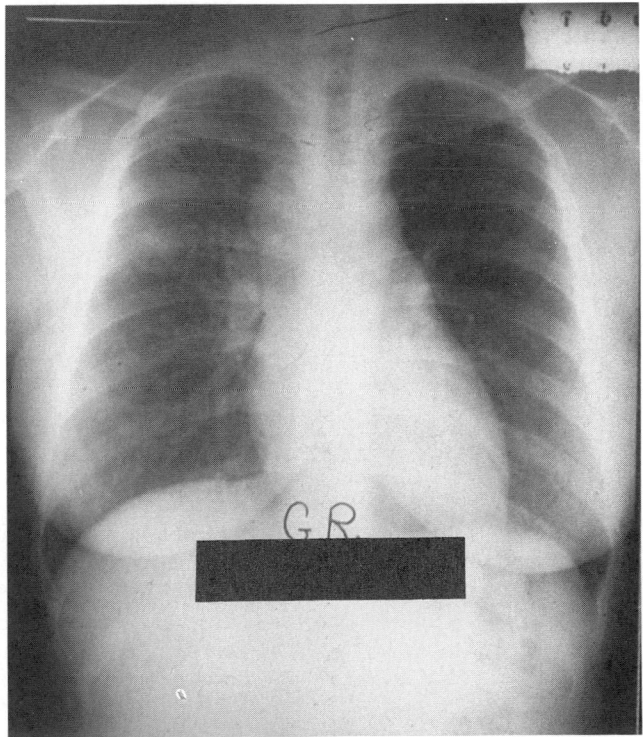

Figure 20-21. Superior vena cava obstruction. Right superior mediastinal mass and a round infiltrate in the right midlung field in a 24-year-old woman.

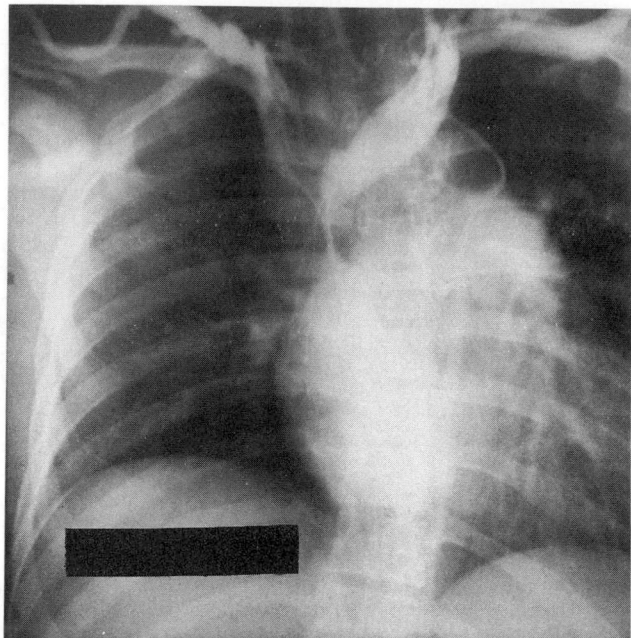

Figure 20-22. Bilateral upper extremity venogram demonstrates marked narrowing of the superior vena cava.

al. (1979) as a corrective measure for the compression of surrounding structures and as a preventive measure to avert fibrosing mediastinitis. Although this has not been proved, 10 of 11 patients treated by Zaijtchuck, et al. (1973) were followed for 3 to 15 years, and all were asymptomatic. Garrett and Roper (1986) found mediastinoscopy useful in diagnosing

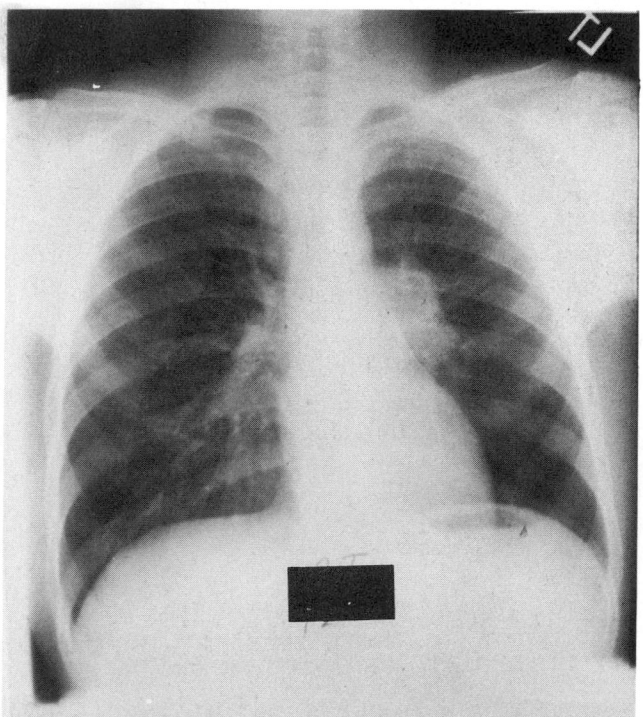

Figure 20-23. Fibrosing mediastinitis in a chest radiograph in this 15-year-old boy shows a prominent left hilar mass.

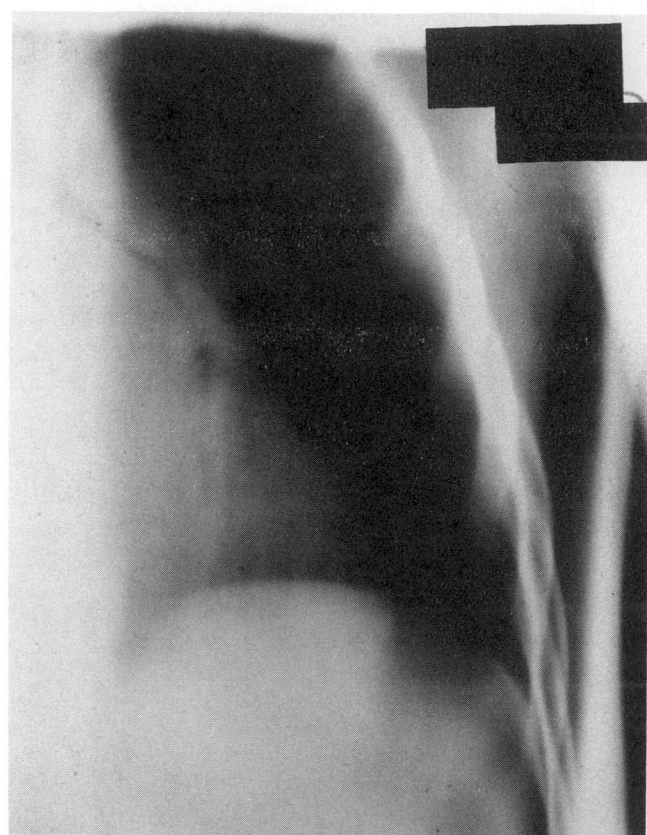

Figure 20-24. Tomograms demonstrate narrowing of the distal left main bronchus.

the conditions of 11 of 16 patients, thus avoiding thoracotomy to rule out carcinoma.

Broncholithiasis. One manifestation of mediastinal histoplasmosis commonly seen with significant adenopathy is broncholithiasis. According to Faber, et al. (1975) the spitting of stones was described by Aristotle in about 300 B.C. *H. capsulatum* was described as causative by Bhagavan, et al. (1971). Several authors have found it difficult to establish the cause from stains and cultures. Tuberculosis, silicosis, aspirated calculi, and rarely actinomycosis have been suggested as alternative causes by Faber, et al. (1975). Urschel (1990) emphasized that many patients with mediastinal disease, although they appear to have burned out infection, may in fact have a subacute phase of active disease and that this may be detected during observation and therapy by a determination of the erythrocyte sedimentation rate and complement fixation titers.

Schwarz, et al. (1976) reported that this group demonstrated *H. capsulatum* in every instance in the stones in more than 24 cases of broncholithiasis. Although fatal hemorrhage has been associated with broncholithiasis and hemoptysis as a frequent symptom, the bleeding is usually self-limited. The bleeding is caused by erosion of a calcification from a large node into the bronchus from a coalesced nodal mass, which may be in contact on its opposite wall with a major vascular structure.

Current surgical management, as described by Faber, et al. (1975) and Trastek, et al. (1985), favors thoracotomy as the preferred therapy. Trastek, et al. (1985) reported on 52 patients of whom 40 were treated initially by thoracotomy. Although all were successfully treated, 32 of the 40 had pulmonary resection at the time of thoracotomy. There were five complications (12.8 percent) and one postoperative death. Twelve patients had attempted bronchoscopic removal, and this was successful in 8. Two had significant complications from the procedure, and 3 of the 8 successful cases had recurrences. Of the 4 who did not respond to therapy, 3 underwent a later thoracotomy.

Cole, et al. (1986) proposed that attempts at the bronchoscopic removal of stones that extend well into the bronchial lumen should be made prior to thoracotomy and emphasized avoidance of excessive force or traction. Removal of stones succeeded in 8 of 40 patients. Twenty-five patients underwent thoracotomy with emphasis on preservation of lung function. Resections in 22 cases were evenly divided between segmental resection and lobectomy. Three patients had removal of broncholiths by bronchotomy, and one patient had repair of an acquired tracheoesophageal fistula. Faber, et al. (1975); Dines, et al. (1979); Cole, et al. (1986); and Urschel (1990) have all reported tracheoesophageal or bronchoesophageal fistulae in 5, 2, 1, and 1 cases, respectively. This condition apparently results from erosion of disease from an involved lymph node into both the esophagus and trachea or bronchus. In a review of the literature, Nelson and Benfield (1970) emphasized the importance of correction before respiratory infection destroys the lung and added two cases. The infectious origin of this condition is emphasized, with histoplasmosis playing only a small role.

Although compression has been reported in a few of the cases of granuloma, most of the cases with severe compromise of adjacent organs were found in patients with fibrosing mediastinitis. Common problems in this condition are vascular, airway, esophageal, and pericardial, and fistulization occurs between the airway and the esophagus as tracheoesophageal and tracheobronchial fistulae.

Superior Vena Cava Obstruction.   Superior vena cava obstruction has been described by nearly all authors, beginning with Gillespie (1956). Thirteen cases were observed by Urschel (1990), seven by Garrett and Roper (1986), and six by Dines, et al. (1979) among the larger series. Numerous attempts at superior vena caval bypass have been attempted with various materials. There has been little success in the long term. Doty (1982) reported significant success in the use of a spiral vein graft prepared from saphenous vein. Urschel (1990) reported three long-term successes with this technique, as did Garrett and Roper (1986).

Many patients survive superior vena cava narrowing or total occlusion with mild or moderate symptoms because extensive collateral venous drainage develops around the obstruction. The symptoms moderate as the collateral flow increases. Airway narrowing or obstruction in cases of fibrosing mediastinitis present a formidable problem (Hewlett, et al., 1966). Surgical release of the trachea or main bronchi may be possible, but relentless fibrosis usually continues. Garrett and Roper (1986) reported on lobectomy and pneumonectomy in two patients with recurrent postobstructive pneumonitis. Urschel (1990) was able to decompress the trachea in two of three patients successfully. A third responded to antifungal therapy.

Other Manifestations.   Esophageal involvement has been reported in 10 cases of mediastinal granuloma by Dukes, et al. (1976). Release of the constriction may be successful, but restenosis may occur. Conservative therapy may succeed as the acute disease subsides.

Pericarditis is a rare occurrence in histoplasmosis. It is more likely to occur in the granulomatous stage of mediastinal disease as pericardial effusion or acute tamponade. Prager, et al. (1980) and Urschel (1990) have reported such cases. In fibrosing mediastinitis the pericardial presentation is more likely to be constriction, as reported by Strimlan, et al. (1975) and Garrett and Roper (1986).

In a case report Kanawaty, et al. (1991) describes a patient with Histoplasma endocarditis on a prosthetic heart valve treated successfully without replacing the valve. Of 33 published cases, the author found only 4 on prosthetic valves, and none survived. There have been eight survivors among the patients with infection of a native valve, and all received amphotericin B.

In therapy for mediastinal histoplasmosis, there are some suggestions that surgical therapy may play even a smaller role than previously thought. Urschel (1990) indicated that in 12 of his 22 patients complement fixation studies showed an increasing titer over time, which suggested activity in what was presumed to be burned out disease without active infection. Six patients in this group were treated with ketoconazole, and in 2 failure of surgical decompression of the trachea and the superior vena cava was reversed by this therapy.

Garrett and Roper (1986) reported on healing of a blind esophageal tract and successful therapy of severe airway compromise in a child with the use of ketoconazole.

Negroni, et al. (1989) reported on the use itraconazole in a group of 31 patients with chronic disseminated disease and chronic pulmonary involvement. Clinical cure occurred in all disseminated cases, and significant improvement was found in the pulmonary cases. The course of therapy was for 6 months. In the 23 patients followed for more than 1 year, there were no recurrences.

These cases suggest that the newer azole compounds, which have significantly lower toxicity compared with amphotericin B, may be effective antifungal agents and give room for optimism. Long-term results of such therapy in large numbers of patients are not yet available.

Coccidioidomycosis

Clinical Features

Coccidioidomycosis occurs primarily in the southwestern portion of the United States and in northern Mexico. It is often seen in patients in other parts of the country who have traveled in the Southwest and have been exposed to *C. immitis*. Pathologic examination of human tissue demonstrates the dimorphic nature of the fungus. The endospores congregate in spherules or are free in the tissue if the spherule has ruptured, or mycelial forms may exist. Large numbers of people apparently contract the disease, although many of them are entirely asymptomatic, with skin test conversion as the only manifestation. In military populations new to the Southwest, the skin test conversion rate is 10 percent per year.

The portal of entry is the airway. In symptomatic patients cough, weight loss, fever, hemoptysis, and chest pain are common. The chest radiograph shows an infiltrate that may disappear over a short period or resolve to a solitary nodule or a cavitary lesion in the lung. In other patients the symptoms may persist, and the pulmonary infiltrate may increase. This persistent pulmonary form of the disease is defined if symptoms or radiographic abnormalities continue after 6 to 8 weeks. Drutz and Catanzaro (1978) note that these patients are often very ill and that their symptoms of fever, prostration, chest pain, productive cough, and occasionally hemoptysis may continue for months unless treated. Chronic progressive coccidioidal disease is defined in those patients who have a continuation of these symptoms, often for months or years, and have biapical fibronodular pulmonary lesions with cavitation.

Cavitation may present within the first 10 days of the pneumonic process of coccidioidomycosis, but more commonly it occurs later. Hemoptysis is seen in 70 percent of cases during cavitation. Ninety percent of cavities are single, 70 percent are in upper lung fields, and 5 percent cross fissures.

Major complications of coccidioidal cavities include secondary infection with either pyrogenic organisms and the development of a lung abscess or the formation of a fungus ball or mycetoma. Fungus balls are most commonly due to Aspergillus, but they may be composed of mycelial elements of *C. immitis*. Other complications are cavity rupture with bronchopleural fistula and empyema and hemoptysis, which is common but rarely massive (Drutz and Catanzaro, 1978).

Another pulmonary presentation of coccidioidal mycosis is the miliary form, which may present either acutely or chronically. As Catanzaro (1980) points out, it is an ominous sign because it clearly indicates that there has been hematogenous dissemination.

Ampel, et al. (1989) summarizes the distribution of coccidioidomycosis in the disseminated cases. The most common sites of spread are the skin, musculoskeletal system (bones, joints, and tendon sheaths), and the meninges where involvement is invariably fatal if not treated. Genitourinary manifestations include epididymitis, prostatitis, endometritis, and urethroscrotal or colovesical fistula. Peritonitis is sometimes seen, and tracheal, laryngeal, and cervical lymphadenopathy and acute thyroiditis have been reported.

Pappagianis (1988) reviewed the epidemiology of the disease and noted that the evidence from older articles clearly suggests that social differences exist, with an increased incidence of serious disease in blacks, Hispanics, Native Americans, and Filipinos. Sievers (1980) suggested that the methods used in some of the earlier reviews were faulty and that environmental factors play such a significant role that racial differences cannot be identified. Drutz (1980) counters that the most prudent course is to consider that these races may be more likely to have a severe infection, and once the condition is diagnosed, they should be followed closely for evidence of disseminated disease.

The role of pregnancy as a risk factor has also been challenged, although Ampel, et al. (1989) pointed out that, of 10 cases of coccidioidomycosis found in 47,120 pregnancies in Tucson, 3 progressed to disseminated disease.

Dissemination is also accelerated in patients undergoing hemodialysis, patients with blood type B or AB, and male patients. Dissemination may be either acute or chronic, and therapy with antifungal agents is indicated. Fatality rates remain high, even with long-term therapy.

Diagnostic Modalities

Skin testing is useful in epidemiologic studies but is of little value in clinical situations. Coccidioidin and spherulin are available from the mycelial phase and the tissue phase of the fungus, respectively. Because a positive skin test result indicates either past or recent exposure to the fungus, it reveals no clues as to whether the skin test finding relates to current or remote exposure. In patients with severe pulmonary or disseminated disease, the skin test result is often negative (Sarosi, 1988).

Complement fixation and tube precipitin tests for coccidioidomycosis were among the earliest serologic tests developed for pulmonary mycoses, and they continue to be useful (Buechner, et al., 1973; Penn, et al., 1983). Precipitins (serum IgM) may be detected in the first 1 to 3 weeks but are transitory and may disappear after 4 to 6 weeks. They may reappear with spreading or relapse of the disease. Complement fixation (serum IgG) develops slowly, appearing at 4 to 6 weeks and attaining maximum levels after 2 or 3 months. The severity of disease and the prognosis for the patient are reflected by high or rising titers (Buechner, et al., 1973; Penn, et al., 1983; Sarosi, et al., 1985).

The early diagnosis of coccidioidomycosis can easily be made from sputum or other clinical specimens stained with 10 percent potassium hydroxide and examined for endospores or spherules. A wet preparation can be repeatedly examined to identify hyphae that develop from the spherules. These preparations present a major biohazard. Currently a safer method is to examine the supernatants of both cultures for antigens with an immunodiffusion test, which is safer because less handling of the cultures is required (Sarosi, et al., 1985).

Complement fixation antibody is present in the spinal fluid of 70 percent of patients with meningeal involvement and in nearly all patients as the disease progresses (Sarosi, et al., 1985).

Petersen, et al. (1976) emphasized the importance of centrifugal concentration of urine specimens before the first morning urine underwent culture for coccidioidomycosis. Expressed prostatic secretions, however, were directly cultured. In this group of 12 patients, 8 had severe associated systemic disease, which impaired immunity. Nine of 11 tested with coccidioidin 1:10 were anergic. One patient in the group with Coccidioides isolated to the urinary tract, epididymis, and prostate had no dissemination to other organs in 15-year follow-up.

Therapy

Primary pulmonary disease requires no therapy. Catanzaro (1980) suggests that patients with significant toxicity, fever, or weight loss; an immunosuppressed state; a high titer complement fixation test result; or a poor skin test reaction to coccidioidin may be considered for drug therapy because of the increased risk of an unsatisfactory outcome.

Amphotericin B remains the drug of choice for serious coccidioidal disease. The total dose of amphotericin B is higher than that for other fungal infections. Graybill (1988) notes that the drug's toxicity is higher in this disease because of the long and repetitive courses often required. Intrathecal therapy is the only effective method to treat coccidioidal meningitis.

Ketoconazole was at first thought to be an extremely valuable adjunct to the therapy of coccidioidomycosis and was used for disseminated disease because it could be administered orally, had little nephrotoxicity, and could be used on an outpatient basis for prolonged periods, but controlled studies have demonstrated benefit in only about one-third of patients, according to Sarosi (1990). It is now used to treat stable immunocompetent patients with nonmeningeal disseminated disease and may be used up to 1 year. If the patient does not respond to therapy or a relapse occurs, Sarosi (1990) recommends amphotericin B be begun at once to a total dose of 2.5 to 3.0 g.

Two other azoles in clinical trial are fluconazole and itraconazole. Fluconazole is not dependent on gastric acid for its absorption as is ketoconazole, and because it is highly water soluble, it can be administered intravenously and orally. It also enters the spinal fluid very well. It is excreted unchanged in the urine, and the dose must be adjusted in patients with renal insufficiency, according to Terrell and Hughes (1992). Studies in coccidioidomycosis have shown good early responses, but some early failures and significant relapses. Because of the low toxicity, Catanzaro (1990) suggests that a trial at higher doses is justified.

Itraconazole has only recently been approved for clinical use in the United States but has been available for clinical trials for some time. Its toxicity is lower than that of the other triazoles. Some preliminary studies have shown it to be effective in patients with disease that is not responsive to amphotericin B therapy as in the enthusiastic report of Diaz, et al. (1991). Unfortunately therapeutic failure occurred in one patient and recurrences in 4 of 16 cases. Its use in coccidioidomycosis, including the meningeal form, is promising, but the final effects cannot be assessed (Graybill, et al., 1990; Terrell and Hughes, 1992).

Amphotericin B thus remains the drug of choice for serious infections with *C. immitis*. This includes pulmonary disease that is progressing during therapy, miliary disease, and any serious coccidioidal infection in an immunosuppressed patient.

Takaro (1967) stated that surgical therapy may be an important adjunct to medical therapy, although coccidioidomycosis is not primarily a surgical disease. Surgical experience since midcentury has confirmed this, and surgical therapy currently plays a diminishing role. There are concerns about the increasing immunosuppressed population. Kelly, et al.

(1985) reported that, in a recent series of patients treated for disseminated coccidioidal disease, eight of nine were immunosuppressed. Graybill (1988) reported that informal inquiries at that time suggested approximately 40 patients with coccidioidomycosis had AIDS, a growing population.

Greer and Grow (1949) reported 10 pulmonary resections for primary pulmonary coccidioidomycosis. Two previous resections were cited from the literature, one by Peers who feared dissemination and one by Blades for persistent hemoptysis. The surgical indications were spontaneous pneumothorax with a nonexpansile lung and a coccidioidal empyema, solid tumor in the lung, and malaise, fatigue, chest pain, or hemoptysis in the presence of a persistent cavity.

Melick (1950) surveyed all members of the American Association for Thoracic Surgery plus other individuals who might have occasion to carry out excisional surgery in this disease. Two hundred twenty-four individuals from 38 states, nine places in Canada, and Sweden, responded and submitted 109 instances of pulmonary resection for this disease. The complications were few, and they included empyema, bronchopleural fistula, and recavitation in other areas. There were three deaths.

During the 1950 to 1962 period, Forsee and Perkins (1954); Cogswell, et al. (1955); Cotton and Birsner (1959); Cotton, et al. (1955); Melick (1950); Aronstam and Hopeman (1961); and Rivkin, et al. (1962) all reported sizable series of surgical resections. Although the results were not uniform, the general tenor suggests that there was a higher rate of complications than were being experienced in patients with operations for pulmonary tuberculosis and that most of these complications (bronchopleural fistula, empyema, and recurrence of cavitary disease) occurred in the operations on cavitary disease. In the later articles a few patients received adjunctive therapy with amphotericin B. Winn (1959) reported dramatic success with this first antifungal agent in treating coccidioidal meningitis.

Hyde (1958,1968) proposed that cavitary disease should rarely be operated on, except in the case of repeated and severe hemoptysis, citing a high rate of bronchopleural fistula and empyema (29 percent) and disability as a result of the operation. He also found a 20 percent rate of development of new cavities in the operated cases. In his nonoperated cases, one-half of the cavities closed spontaneously, with a median closure time of 2 years.

There is clearly a role for surgical excision of solitary nodules in the lung that cannot be distinguished from malignancy, and antifungal therapy is not required.

Chronic pulmonary coccidioidomycosis has been attacked surgically in the past with some success but with high complication rates and probably is best treated with antifungal agents because many of these patients have diminished pulmonary reserve and complications are significant in operated cases. Sarosi, et al. (1970) described a group of 20 patients with coccidioidomycosis alone who were found in a search for fungal infections by the National Communicable Disease Center in tuberculosis hospitals over a period of 12 years. In this small group of patients, the best results were obtained when the patients received a total dose of amphotericin B of at least 30 mg/kg. Twenty other patients had culture-proved tuberculosis and coccidioidomycosis. A later report (Sarosi,

1988) suggests that drug therapy is problematic for chronic pulmonary disease.

Coccidioidal cavities in the past have aroused the most controversy. Grant and Melick (1967) indicated that the use of amphotericin B perioperatively and a change in surgical philosophy toward lobectomy over segmental or wedge resection had reduced complication rates in resections for coccidioidomycosis from 20 to 4 percent. Rivkin, et al. (1961) had earlier recommended lobectomy as the preferred resection. Examination of resected surgical specimens demonstrates significant numbers of satellite nodules around nodular disease or infiltrative disease, and these may account for local recurrences.

The observation by Beard, et al. (1960) and others that the administration of amphotericin B often converts sputum results to negative suggested that amphotericin B would be a useful surgical adjuvant therapy, but the American Thoracic Society official statement (1988) indicates that there are no data to compare this therapy with cases in which no drug is given. Takaro (1989) indicates that pre- and postoperative amphotericin B should be used in all patients with diabetes, significant other medical problems, bilateral or other unresected disease, and in cases with cavity rupture in which surgical therapy has been delayed.

Despite a diminished enthusiasm for surgical intervention, Salomon, et al. (1980) reported on 50 resections in coccidioidal disease. Twenty-two of the 50 were diagnostic, including 16 nodules. Six undiagnosed infiltrative lesions were in patients immunosuppression secondary to chemotherapy, leukemia, or both. The diagnosis of coccidioidomycosis in these six patients led to the administration of amphotericin B, and four of the six died within 1 month of their primary disease. Therapeutic resections were carried out in 28 patients. Twenty-four had cavitary disease, and six of these presented with severe hemoptysis. Three of the 28 presented with pyopneumothorax, and a bronchopleural fistula with a cavity ruptured into the pleural space. One of these patients died of sepsis and disseminated intravascular coagulation within 1 week. One patient in the cavitary group required early secondary thoracotomy for bleeding from an intercostal artery. This series presented acceptable complications. Even though amphotericin B was available throughout this 8-year period, only 11 patients were treated preoperatively with amphotericin B, which suggests that improved selection or improved surgical care was responsible for the low complication rate rather than antifungal therapy.

Baker, et al. (1978) described resectional therapy in 52 diabetic patients, of whom 36 were insulin dependent. A special subgroup of 10 patients had negative skin test results and extensive disease. One underwent an operation without resection and subsequently died of the disease. Nine of the 10 had total extirpation of the disease and were clinically stable, 7 of the 9 for more than 4 years. Several recent reviews addressing coccidioidal infection by Drutz and Catanzano (1978); Catanzaro (1980); Graybill (1988); Ampel, et al. (1989); and Takaro (1989) have made recommendations in regard to the role of surgical intervention. The diagnosis of pulmonary nodules of unknown cause is an acceptable surgical indication for most authors. Forseth, et al. (1986) demonstrated that needle biopsies of solitary pulmonary nodules in 348 patients established a diagnosis of coccidioidal disease in 29 percent; 43 percent had malignant disease. In the remaining undiagnosed lesions, surgical removal should be recommended. Catanzaro (1980) notes that occasionally a mass-like pulmonary lesion with hilar adenopathy may require a diagnostic thoracotomy.

Cavitary disease should be resected if the cavity is enlarging significantly, if it is thick walled, or if it is secondarily infected with evidence of a lung abscess or mycetoma. The original definition of a giant cavity exceeding 5 cm in diameter as a clear-cut indication for an operation is commonly disregarded. Hemoptysis is only regarded as an indication for an operation if it is life threatening or severe and repetitive, and this degree of bleeding occurs only rarely.

A special problem-type cavitary disease is the peripheral cavity that ruptures to the pleural space, creating a pyopneumothorax, bronchopleural fistula, and occasionally a trapped lung. Such cases have been specifically mentioned by Greer and Grow (1949); Forsee, et al. (1953); Aronstam and Hopeman (1961); Salomon, et al. (1980); and Cunningham and Einstein (1982). The report by Cunningham and Einstein indicates that 16 of 23 cases had no history of disease and no known cavity prior to rupture. All cases had elevated complement fixation titers, and 21 of the cases had positive cultures from the pleural fluid. Therapy should not wait for these results. Seven patients had lobectomy; 13, partial lobectomy; and 1 who was diabetic and required multiple pulmonary wedges, a pneumonectomy. There were no deaths. Adjuvant amphotericin B was used in 10 patients but is not recommended for patients with well-controlled pulmonary disease and a ruptured cavity who undergo early surgical therapy. Takaro (1989) and Cunningham and Einstein (1982) both suggested that early resection of cavitary disease located against the pleural surface should be encouraged in patients with negative skin test findings. If such a patient is seropositive, severely compromised immunity can be predicted.

Blastomycosis

Clinical Features

Blastomycosis exposure occurs in a clearly defined geographic area that encompasses the southeastern United States (Takaro, 1967). With the increased mobility of the population and the chronicity of some cases of blastomycosis, patients may often be identified in areas remote from the area of primary exposure.

The disease presents in either acute or chronic forms. Saag and Dismukes (1988) emphasize that, when the infection occurs acutely in immunocompetent individuals, it is usually self-limited and requires no therapy. In immunocompromised patients, acute and life-threatening infections with dissemination to other organ systems may occur and require prompt therapy. Patients often have central nervous system, genitourinary tract, skin, or bone involvement with or without evidence of pulmonary blastomycosis.

Chronic pulmonary blastomycosis presents with fever, malaise, weight loss, cough, and night sweats. Cutaneous lesions are common, along with skeletal or genitourinary involvement, and nearly one-half of the patients with disseminated disease do not have pulmonary involvement. Although central nervous system disease is uncommon, the mortality rate is high unless it is promptly diagnosed and treated.

Diagnosis

Blastomycosis (North American) requires an accurate diagnosis. Of all the fungal infections of the lung, it is the one that most closely duplicates the radiographic picture of bronchogenic carcinoma. The offending organism is identified as large budding yeast cells with double refractile walls, and the buds are broad based. Demonstration of the organism provides the definitive diagnosis and is accomplished in sputum studies or in material from skeletal lesions, skin lesions, mucous membranes, prostatic secretions, urine, lymph nodes, and direct organ biopsies (Takaro, 1967). Study of the sputum by the Papanicolaou method provides important assistance in making the diagnosis (Trumbull and Chesney, 1981; Takaro, 1982).

Identification of the organism with hematoxylin and eosin stains is sometimes difficult. Visualization is enhanced with periodic acid-Schiff or methenamine silver stains (Sarosi, et al., 1985).

Skin tests are largely useless because they have been reported to be negative in more than one-half of the patients with active disease and cross-react with skin tests for histoplasmosis and coccidioidomycosis (Buechner, et al., 1973).

Serologic tests are unreliable. A positive complement fixation test is found in fewer than one-half of the patients with confirmed disease (Penn, et al., 1983). Despite early enthusiasm for the immunodiffusion test, there are conflicting reports on its efficacy (Sarosi, et al., 1985).

Identification by culture methods is helpful, but because growth on media is related to the size of the inoculum and may require from 3 days to 3 weeks, this modality may not play a role in determining therapy in an acute case.

Therapy

Modest pulmonary infections do not require therapy unless they progress under observation in which case ketoconazole (400 to 800 mg/day) is prescribed (Sarosi, 1990). All patients with meningitis, critical respiratory state, or immunodeficiency syndromes should receive amphotericin B to a total dose of 2 g. In patients who are achlorhydric or require therapy with cimetidine or antacids, antifungal therapy should include amphotericin B because ketoconazole requires gastric acidity to facilitate its absorption from the gastrointestinal tract (Takaro, 1989). Itraconazole therapy has resulted in cure after failure with ketoconazole therapy (Terrell and Hughes, 1992).

Hiebert, et al. (1989) reviewed failures of ketoconazole therapy and concluded that most failures occurred when patients received only 400 mg/day rather than the 800 mg/day recommended by a national study. Patients who cannot tolerate the recommended dose should be treated with amphotericin B. Although Takaro (1983) indicated that blastomycosis remained a serious disease with a 5-year mortality rate of 20 percent, a more recent study by Sarosi (1990) noted that patients with meningeal involvement and those who were critically ill with ventilator dependence or hypoxia on room air who survived the first week of amphotericin B therapy always recovered completely and remained disease free for at least 2 years. This underscores the importance of early diagnosis and prompt therapy.

Saag and Dismukes (1988) observed that blastomycosis is uncommon in immunosuppressed patients. The reasons are unclear. Therapy with amphotericin B is recommended for any immunosuppressed patient, whereas the immunocompetent patient should receive ketoconazole. Itraconazole may be equally effective with lower toxicity (Terrell and Hughes, 1992).

Takaro (1967) emphasized that the indications for resective pulmonary surgery were rarely encountered because effective medical therapy had become available, noting the efficacy of amphotericin B and the usefulness of 2-hydroxystilbamidine in which there were only two therapeutic failures in 23 cases (Lockwood, et al., 1962). Standard therapy for the disease is now antifungal drugs, although surgical therapy of bronchopleural fistula or empyema is occasionally indicated.

Most early surgical series emphasized the use of surgical therapy because of inability to diagnose a pulmonary infiltrate (Newsom, 1982) or to rule out bronchogenic carcinoma clinically (Takaro, 1967). With improved diagnostic methods, these indications rarely apply.

Cryptococcosis

Clinical Features

The etiologic agent for cryptoccosis is *C. neoformans,* an encapsulated yeastlike budding saprophyte found in soul and avian excreta, especially that of the pigeon. There is no geographic distribution for the disease. First described under the name torulosis by Stoddard and Cutter (1916), the lung is believed to be the portal of entry.

Pulmonary symptoms may be absent or unrecognized, and the first clinical manifestation is often the development of a subacute or chronic meningitis. Prior to the availability of an effective antifungal agent, Kuykendall, et al. (1957) reported four cases apparently localized to the lung and regional lymph nodes treated by surgical excision. Literature review showed more than 300 cases with only 27 of these thought to be localized to the lung.

In the earlier years sporadic cases of cryptococcosis were seen in which no compromise of the immune system was recognized. Most cases, especially those with meningeal involvement, have serious coexisting diseases (Spickard, et al., 1963; Campbell, 1966). Corticosteroid therapy was also noted to increase susceptibility to cryptococcosis (Bennington, et al., 1964). Diabetes, lymphoma, chronic lung disease, tuberculosis, sarcoidosis, chronic hepatitis, and lung cancer have been reported as associated conditions by Spickard, et al. (1963); Lewis, (1972); Utz, et al. (1995); Bennett, et al. (1979); and others. More recently those conditions resulting in a severely immunocompromised host have become most important.

With the marked increase in the number of patients undergoing transplantations of various organs and chemotherapy for malignancy, the pool of immunosuppressed patients has become larger. Gottlieb, et al. (1981) described AIDS in previously healthy homosexual men. Although it is not the intent of this chapter to deal specifically with the immunosuppressed patient, the impact of this disease has been so great in the patient with AIDS that a brief comment is necessary.

It is estimated that 10 percent of patients with AIDS have cryptococcal meningitis, and nearly 60 percent of these die of this infection. Prompt antifungal therapy is necessary, and therapeutic failures and relapses are common.

Diagnosis

When *C. neoformans* is isolated from the sputum, a decision must be made to determine whether this represents simple colonization of the airway or true cryptococcal disease.

Reiss and Szilazyi (1965) found *C. neoformans* in the sputum of 6 of 92 patients with malignant disease. None of this group showed evidence of overt cryptococcal disease, which suggests that a carrier state exists in humans.

Hammerman, et al. (1973) in a group of 80 patients with cryptococci in pulmonary tissue or sputum had 16 patients whose conditions were diagnosed from tissue obtained at operation or autopsy. Only four had positive sputum results. Twelve patients were thought to have clinical cryptococcosis and had positive sputum isolates. Forty other patients had no evidence of cryptococcal disease but had positive sputum findings and were not treated. Twenty-seven of these patients had other pulmonary disease. This group of 40 patients was thought to be colonized with Cryptococcus and not to have invasive disease. Such patients should undergo an active search for extrapulmonary lesions by examination of cerebrospinal fluid and biopsy of skin or bone lesions. If any extrapulmonary lesions are found, a full course of antifungal therapy should be given.

In a 4-year period, Duperval (1977) found 65 patients with positive sputum culture findings for Cryptococcus. Twenty-two patients had meningitis or nonmeningeal disseminated disease. Forty-three patients with positive sputum culture results were not treated for Cryptococcus. Fourteen of 15 patients with a normal chest radiograph or with a pleural effusion only and 18 of 28 patients with a lung infiltrate survived at the time of the report without progressive pulmonary disease or dissemination. Of 11 deaths, none could be attributed to cryptococcal disease.

It is apparent that the clinical setting in which sputum positivity presents assists the physician in assessing whether colonization of the respiratory tract has occurred or whether true cryptococcal infection is present.

The diagnostic value of serologic tests for cryptococcosis is in question. Hatcher, et al. (1971) indicated that, by using the serum latex agglutination, indirect fluorescent antibody, and tube agglutination tests concurrently, a high level of diagnostic accuracy was attained. Kaufman and Blumer (1968) placed that presumptive diagnostic accuracy at 90 percent.

Despite such enthusiasm Duperval (1977) emphasized the value of cultures of blood and urine in the diagnosis of meningeal and nonmeningeal forms of disseminated cryptococcal disease. The latex agglutination test was positive only in patients with meningitis and in only 37.5 percent of that group.

Therapy

Cryptococcosis sometimes presents with solitary lung nodules or localized infiltrates in the lung when the diagnosis is made at thoracotomy. If the lesion in the lung is small and has been resected with an adequate margin, some authors would argue against further therapy because the patient can expect to be cured. Hammerman, et al. (1973) reported that in 3 of 92 such patients meningitis developed in the follow-up period. Of 36 patients treated with amphotericin B alone, 1 did not respond, and 2 died of progressive pulmonary disease. Fifteen patients who underwent surgery and were treated with amphotericin B did well, but a group of 28 whose conditions were diagnosed but had no specific therapy did less well. In 2, meningitis developed, 1 died of progressive pulmonary disease, and 2 subsequently required therapy.

At thoracotomy if the lesion cannot be excised in toto and only an incisional biopsy is done, Hatcher, et al. (1971) and Smith, et al. (1976) would recommend intravenous antifungal therapy. Thus it would seem that any time a pulmonary tissue diagnosis of cryptococcosis is obtained, antifungal therapy should follow. Sampling of the spinal fluid is mandatory with stain and culture for cryptococcosis in any patient with pulmonary disease.

If the diagnosis is made prior to the operation, as is increasingly frequent with transtracheal biopsy or direct needle aspiration, combined therapy with amphotericin B with flucytosine may obviate the need for surgery (Takaro, 1989).

Disseminated cryptococcosis with meningeal involvement should be treated with antifungal therapy.

In the immunocompetent patient Utz, et al. (1975) demonstrated that a combination of flucytosine given orally and intravenous amphotericin B was useful in the therapy of cryptococcal meningitis. This combination was based on in vitro studies that demonstrated synergistic or additive effect in a few cultures. A 6-week regimen of amphotericin B 2 mg daily and flucytosine 150 mg/kg in four divided doses was effective, and it has been widely used. The combination allowed lower doses to be given of amphotericin B to reduce toxicity and a shorter therapeutic period to reduce the hospital stay. It appeared to be superior to therapy with amphotericin B alone, and this dosing regimen has become standard. Creatinine clearance should be monitored and maintained above 50 ml/min, and flucytosine levels must be measured and kept below 100 μg/ml. Bennett, et al. (1979) reported a comparison study between amphotericin B alone and amphotericin B combined with flucytosine and concluded that the combined therapy was the regimen of choice for cryptococcal meningitis.

In severely immunocompromised patients, Sarosi (1990) recommended significantly increased doses of amphotericin B for the therapy of meningitis or invasive pulmonary disease. Flucytosine is potentially toxic to bone marrow, particularly in patients with AIDS, and therapy may induce severe granulocytopenia.

Initial therapy with amphotericin in immunocompromised patients shows good results, but therapeutic failures and relapses have led to proposals for suppressive therapy on a life-long basis. Twice-weekly amphotericin B combined with fluconazole or itraconazole is currently being studied. Chuck and Sande (1989) noted improved survival with long-term suppressive therapy in AIDS and also noted that, contrary to the experience in immunocompetent patients, those patients with AIDS and nonmeningeal cryptococcal infections fared as poorly as those with meningitis, which suggests that a full course of amphotericin B followed by suppressive therapy is justified. Larsen, et al. (1989) implicated the prostate as a likely site for silent persistent infection.

Although antifungal therapy is effective in all patients with disseminated disease, the significant underlying medical conditions often militate against long-term success.

Aspergillosis

Clinical Features

Three major clinical forms of aspergillosis are recognized (Takaro, 1967; Daly, et al., 1986): (1) allergic or bronchitic, (2) invasive or disseminated, and (3) saprophytic or aspergilloma. Allergic aspergillosis presents as an acute bronchitic form of hypersensitivity disease usually associated with asthma and treated with glucocorticoids (American Thoracic Society, 1988). Invasive or disseminated disease occurs almost exclusively in immunosuppressed, malnourished, or debilitated patients and may present as a necrotizing bronchopneumonia, hemorrhagic infarction, abscess formation, or bloodstream infection (Takaro, 1983). Saprophytic disease or aspergilloma occurs frequently in patients with underlying cavitary lung disease, including tuberculosis, sarcoidosis, lung cancers, bacterial abscess, or other cystic or cavitary lung disease. Daly, et al. (1986) reported that 92 percent of such patients had identifiable other lung disease. In a resected series of 15 patients, 5 had tuberculosis, 3 had sarcoidosis, and all but two of the remainder had serious coexisting medical illnesses (Battaglini, et al., 1985). In a 10-year experience with mycetomas in pulmonary tuberculosis, Butz, et al. (1985) identified 33 patients. Nineteen underwent surgical resection, and 17 had aspergillosis. Two had other fungal diseases. Surgical articles have further subdivided the aspergillomas into two groups identified by radiographic appearance and operative findings. Simple aspergillomas occur in an epithelium-lined cyst without severe surrounding parenchymal disease. Complex aspergillomas are thick walled with surrounding parenchymal disease. This is an important differentiation because morbidity and mortality rates are significantly higher in the complex cases (Battaglini, et al., 1985; Daly, et al., 1986). Of these three classes of disease, the aspergilloma is the only one with surgical significance.

Pleural infection with Aspergillus is a rare event in most series. Massard, et al. (1992) reports 16 of 77 cases were in a pleural location, with all but 2 in previously operated patients.

Diagnosis

Aspergilli are ubiquitous. They are identified in the oral cavity and sputum in both healthy persons and patients with chronic pulmonary disorders. Although they are easy to identify directly in secretions and grow readily on culture, it falls to the physician to assess the importance of their presence and to decide whether they are behaving as a pathogen (Buechner, et al., 1973).

When the organism can be identified in infected tissue with the potassium hydroxide preparation, the diagnosis is secure. The hyphae of Aspergillus stain well with methenamine silver, periodic acid-Schiff, and hematoxylin and eosin stains. Vascular invasion is prominent (Sarosi, et al., 1985).

Immunodiffusion tests detect precipitins in 90 percent of patients with aspergillomas and 70 percent of patients with allergic bronchopulmonary aspergillosis, but they are unreliable in the invasive variety of the disease (Penn, et al., 1983). The immunosuppressed status of these patients may account for the lack of identifiable precipitins (Sarosi, et al., 1985). Repeated positive culture results and changing serologic test findings are useful adjuncts to diagnosis and may support the clinical impression when the risks of biopsy are prohibitive.

In both types of aspergillomas, the air crescent radiographic sign is nearly diagnostic. This is a moon-shaped radiolucency that caps the fungus ball within the cavity and shifts with the patient's position (Henderson, et al., 1975). The fungus ball is a matted mass of hyphae, fibrin, and inflammatory cells (Takaro, 1987). Massard, et al. (1992) observed this sign to be positive in 42 of 55 patients. Marked predominance of the upper lobe location has been documented by several authors and is partially related to the upper lobe location of the underlying pulmonary disease (Soltanzadeh, et al., 1977; Rafferty, et al., 1983; Battaglini, et al., 1985).

Griepp, in a discussion of the article by Henderson, et al. (1975), recommended direct needle aspiration of pulmonary lesions suspected of representing aspergillosis. In a series of 84 heart transplants, 18 cases of premortem-diagnosed pulmonary aspergillosis were found. In 14 cases needle aspiration was used, and a positive diagnosis resulted in all and avoided the diagnostic or therapeutic modalities involving thoracotomy in these immunocompromised patients.

Therapy

Acute allergic aspergillosis is most effectively treated with glucocorticoids, and no antifungal agents are needed in this hypersensitivity disease (American Thoracic Society, 1988).

Amphotericin B has long been used in the therapy of invasive aspergillosis with only limited success. In limited numbers of patients with this form of the disease, itraconazole shows promise (American Thoracic Society, 1988; Terrell and Hughes, 1992).

Surgical therapy is appropriate in some aspergillomas. Virtually all authors report difficult technical surgical aspects in this fungal disease (Battaglini, et al., 1985; Daly, et al., 1986). The first surgical resection for pulmonary aspergillosis was reported in 1948 (Gerstl, et al., 1948). A review of the surgical experience from the literature in 1960 documented 42 cases, and the authors added 3 more cases and noted that bronchopulmonary aspergillosis was first described by Virchow in 1856 (Pecora and Toll, 1960).

Despite the ominous implication that major hemoptysis may occur in such patients, routine surgical resection is not undertaken in most centers. A significant proportion of the patient population will have advanced chronic lung disease to a degree that eliminates the surgical option. Most of the controversy about the resection of pulmonary aspergillomas hinges on the threat to life posed by the bleeding episodes in patients in which the operation is feasible with the promise of preserving sufficient pulmonary function. Some articles (Faulkner, et al., 1978; Butz, et al., 1985) suggest that bleeding can be stopped by bed rest, postural drainage, and antibiotic therapy for the associated pulmonary infection seen with most episodes of hemoptysis. Other authors (Solit, et al., 1971; Karas, et al., 1976; Battaglini, et al., 1985; Daly, et al., 1986) favor surgical resection for this indication. Butz, et al. (1985) also favors surgical resection but has not had to apply it until after cessation of bleeding in seven cases that were suitable for operation. Although prophylactic resection of fungus balls in asymptomatic patients has been proposed (Solit, et al., 1971; Massard, et al., 1992), most surgeons have not thought this to be justified (Battaglini, et al., 1985). Other surgical indications in this group of patients are indeterminate mass, severe cough, and disease progression.

Jewkes, et al. (1983) found systemic antifungal therapy without benefit in 18 patients and reported improved 5-year survival rates in patients with frank or major hemoptysis treated surgically over those treated medically. They observed, however, that the surgical group was selected for better pulmonary function and more localized disease and recommended resection in only those patients with severe hemoptysis and adequate pulmonary function.

Faulkner, et al. (1978) noted that a literature review of patients with aspergillomas treated nonoperatively revealed an increased risk of fatal pulmonary hemorrhage in patients with aspergillosis and underlying tuberculosis as opposed to patients with histoplasmosis or COPD as the underlying pulmonary condition. Although this group recommends resection of aspergillomas only in patients with recurrent episodes of severe hemorrhage and finds this rarely necessary, they raise the question of modifying the indications in the patient with tuberculosis and aspergillosis.

Surgical resection may be technically difficult and may lead to postoperative space problems because of the presence of dense fibrous tissue around the cavity wall, the obliteration of the pleural space and fissures, disease in the surrounding lung parenchyma, and the nonexpansile nature of the residual lung (Battaglini, et al., 1985; Massard, et al., 1992). Resection may require concomitant or subsequent thoracoplasty to prevent space problems and the possible development of empyema (Massard, et al., 1992; Shirakusa, et al., 1989).

In a recent series Massard, et al. (1992) applied surgical therapy aggressively, even in asymptomatic patients, in an effort to avoid repeated hemoptysis, conversion to invasive aspergillosis (Rafferty, et al., 1983), and rapid growth of the mycetoma in a group of 77 patients. Sixty-three patients underwent operations with an overall mortality rate of 9.5 percent, bleeding (defined by blood loss greater than 1,500 ml) in 37 patients, space problems in 24, respiratory failure in 6, and postpneumonectomy empyema in 4. The mortality rate for lobar or segmental resection was 6 percent and for thoracoplasty, 15 percent. The recommendation of segmental resection or lobectomy for localized disease followed by thoracoplasty if a space problem ensues and for pleuropneumonotomy with immediate thoracoplasty when lobectomy is not feasible emphasizes the difficult nature of operative therapy. This series reported pleural aspergillomas in 16 patients, which were spontaneous in 2 patients; residual

to lobectomy for cancer, tuberculosis, or aspergillosis (one patient) in 10 patients; and exploratory thoracotomy and collapse therapy in 1 and 3 patients, respectively. Because pleuropneumonectomy in six patients produced one operative death, five major operative bleeds, and four empyemas, the authors recommend avoidance of these procedures and suggest a generous thoracoplasty as the most judicious procedure for pleural disease.

Empyema from Aspergillus has been treated in various ways. Krakowka, et al. (1970) used intrapleural nystatin and Grow in discussing the article by Henderson, et al. (1975) reported the use of intrapleural amphotericin as did Irani, et al. (1971). Herring and Pecora (1976) reported success with decortication, although nonexpansile lung may not produce a satisfactory outcome. Shirakusa, et al. (1989) treated pleural empyema with open window thoracostomy, daily gauze dressing changes, and instillation of amphotericin B for 3 to 6 months followed by omental or muscle flap plombage over the surface of the exposed lung. Thoracoplasty may be required to obliterate the space and effect a cure.

Battaglini, et al. (1985) and Daly, et al. (1986) emphasized the surgical importance of differentiating simple aspergillomas from complex aspergillomas and the difficulty of this surgery and the poor expansion of remaining lung. In 15 cases Battaglini, et al. (1985) reported two deaths and four major postoperative complications, all in patients with complex aspergillomas. In 68 operated cases Daly, et al. (1986) found 15 cases of invasive aspergillosis at thoracotomy. All patients were immunosuppressed from nonpulmonary disease and had symptomatic pulmonary infiltrates, and most died soon after the diagnosis was made. Twenty-one of the remaining patients had simple aspergillomas, and 32 had complex lesions. One-third of the simple cases had complications compared with 78 percent of the complex group. There was 1 death in the simple group and 11 deaths in the complex group, and 84 percent of the simple group were alive and well at follow-up compared with 43 percent of the patients with complex mycetomas.

In the patient with a cavitary aspergilloma who has insufficient pulmonary reserve for resection, cavernostomy has been proposed and used (Eguchi, et al., 1971; Battaglini, et al., 1985; Shirakusa, et al., 1989). Jewkes, et al. (1983), on the other hand, reported four deaths after cavernostomy and instillation of antifungal agents in nine patients and suggested the possibility of an adverse reaction to the antifungal drug natamycin in two of the patients. Shirakusa, et al. (1989) used muscle and omental flap plombage after cavernostomy with daily gauze dressings and instillation of amphotericin B for 3 to 6 months prior to the flap procedure. This is the same protocol proposed for open window thoracostomy therapy of empyema.

Jewkes, et al. (1983) reported no benefit from systemic antifungal therapy in 18 patients with aspergillomas. Earlier authors had indicated that there was no penetration of the cavity in the lung by systemic amphotericin B.

Adelson and Malcolm (1968) first proposed and used intracavitary therapy in mycetomas. Griepp, in discussing the article by Henderson, et al. (1975), cited a heart transplant case that had not responded to systemic amphotericin B systemic therapy for aspergilloma and developed renal toxicity. The patient promptly recovered after a 30-day course of intracavitary amphotericin B. Hargis, et al. (1980) reported significant improvement in four of six patients treated with percutaneous intracavitary amphotericin B.

Magilligan, et al. (1981) reported the control of massive hemoptysis by transcatheter bronchial artery embolization in seven patients, two of whom had aspergillosis. Both had had tuberculosis and, over 4- and 11-month follow-ups, had only minor further bleeding. None were surgical candidates because of poor pulmonary reserve. Hughes, et al. (1986) used embolization of the bronchial circulation as a preliminary to resection in a patient with massive hemoptysis who had had two major bleeding episodes 7 years earlier for which she had refused hospital care.

Shapiro, et al. (1988), on the other hand, suggested that bronchial artery embolization was not effective in permanently controlling massive hemoptysis in patients with aspergillosis probably because of massive collateral circulation through pleural adhesions induced by the underlying pulmonary disease. Six episodes of acute hemoptysis in four patients have been controlled by intracavitary instillation of amphotericin B, acetylcysteine, and aminocaproic acid.

Itraconazole, an orally active triazole, has been used extensively in other countries and recently became available in the United States. It has a greater action against aspergillosis than either ketoconazole or fluconazole and demonstrates low toxicity. Responses have been documented in patients with invasive aspergillosis and aspergillomas, but total resolution of the processes is rare. It is unknown whether the agent can adequately penetrate the chronic cavity and be effective against the fungus.

In summary surgical therapy in Aspergillus infection is confined to the aspergilloma or the pleural manifestations of the disease. The operation is difficult and is often not permitted by the patient's pulmonary reserve or the finding of diffuse or bilateral disease. The major complications of the infection are hemoptysis, which may be major; progression to invasive infection; or enlargement of the aspergilloma. Most surgeons would operate only in symptomatic cases where there is localized disease and adequate pulmonary reserve. Hemoptysis may be major but is rarely life threatening. Aspergillosis occurs almost exclusively in patients with underlying pulmonary disease, such as tuberculosis, histoplasmosis, and sarcoidosis and in immunocompromised individuals. New drugs may be useful.

Sporotrichosis

Clinical Features

The causative agent of sporotrichosis is *S. schenckii*. It is a biphasic fungus and is found worldwide in soil. Because it regularly inhabits plants and thorned bushes, the cutaneous form is usually seen in gardeners and florists. Pulmonary infection is rare, and Van Trigt (1990) noted that it mimics tuberculosis in its manifestations in the lung. Hilar adenopathy, a persistent pulmonary infiltrate, and cavitary disease are the most common radiographic findings (Fig. 20-25).

The rarity of pulmonary infection is emphasized by the early article of Ridgeway, et al. (1962) who reported successful resection of cavitary disease in two patients. They could find only 10 other cases in the literature, none of which had

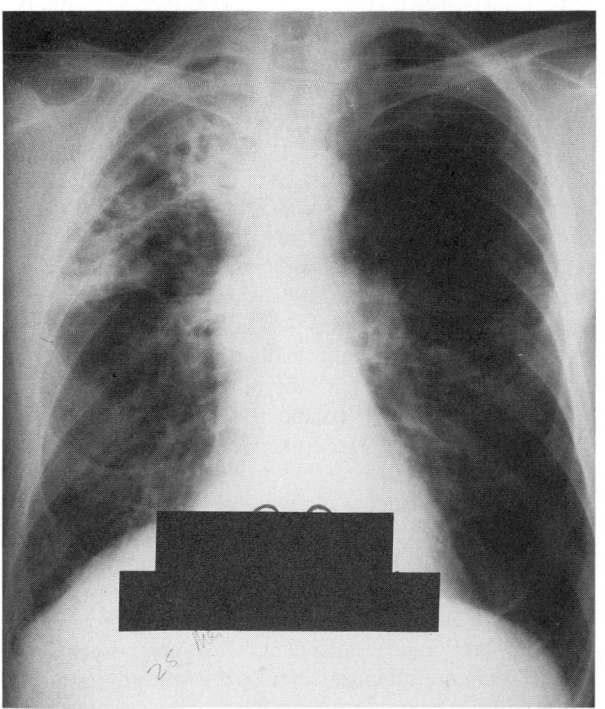

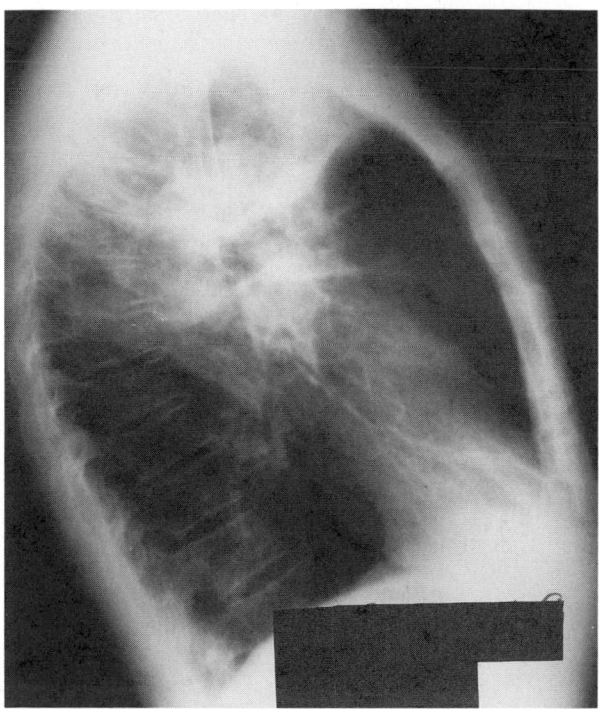

Figure 20-25. Sporotrichosis. **(A)** PA and **(B)** lateral chest films of a 54-year-old man who underwent exploration for suspicion of malignancy and left upper lobectomy done. Specimen demonstrated sporotrichosis. Postoperative space problem required tailoring thorocoplasty.

been operated on. Scott, et al. (1961) found 20 cases in a literature search, but only six were adequately documented.

Diagnosis

Suspicion of pulmonary sporotrichosis should be aroused in the physician when a patient presents with a chronic respiratory illness who works in gardening activities. The onset is insidious. Low-grade fever and gradual weight loss are common. Chest radiographs show a picture of chronic pneumonitis with fibrosis and cavitation and most closely resemble the films of histoplasmosis or tuberculosis. Serologic tests are not usually used, although a tube agglutination test is useful in diagnosing the rare extracutaneous infection (Sarosi, et al., 1985).

The organism is commonly found in the sputum and may be easily grown in culture within 3 to 5 days. Culture at 37°C yields the yeast form in 1 or 2 more days, and this evidence of dimorphism is also diagnostic (Sarosi, et al., 1985). Recognition of the characteristic yeast cell in pathologic specimens is accomplished only with difficulty (Baum, et al., 1969) even with the use of special stains (Sarosi, 1988).

Therapy

Although potassium iodide has been used effectively for antifungal therapy in the cutaneous form for many years, amphotericin B is effective and should be used in the pulmonary variety. Mohr, et al. (1979) observed cases that were not cured by amphotericin B but responded to iodide therapy. Baum, et al. (1969). Takaro (1989), and Van Trigt (1990) recommend combined surgical and amphotericin B therapy. Pluss and Opal (1986) also concluded that pulmonary disease should be resected with adjuvant pre- and postoperative amphotericin B and that imidazoles in a few patients have been ineffective. They do not completely dismiss the use of iodide as adjuvant therapy.

Terrell and Hughes (1992) indicate that itraconazole is effective against cutaneous and lymphangitic forms of the disease and suggest from isolated case reports that deep-seated infections might also respond to this agent.

The American Thoracic Society (1988) report suggests that the response to a saturated solution of potassium iodide, amphotericin B, and ketoconazole has been variable and that itraconazole is effective in a small number of cases. Because early authors (Takaro, 1967; Michelson, 1967) noted that surgical resection of localized pulmonary infection had been done with successful outcome, the role of the adjuvant use of any antifungal agent is difficult to assess in the rare patient with pulmonary infection. No nonsurgical form of therapy is clearly effective; therefore, resectional therapy should be used in localized pulmonary infection.

Mucormycosis

Clinical Features

Mucormycosis is a rare fungal infection presenting in either rhinocerebral or pulmonary forms. The rhinocerebral type is best treated by aggressive surgical debridement and high-dose amphotericin B therapy and will not be discussed fur-

ther. Pulmonary mucormycosis is induced by exposure to fungi of the class Zygomycetes and order Mucorales, which are saprophytic fungi found widely in soil.

Pulmonary infection is rare, although increasing numbers are seen with the growing population of patients receiving immunosuppression therapy or with diabetes, leukemia, lymphoma, neutropenia, agammoglobulinemia, and other hematologic disorders. Corticosteroid therapy and antibiotic administration have also been implicated by Bigby, et al. (1986) and Lehrer, et al. (1980). The infection is almost never seen in normal individuals.

The first pulmonary case in this country was reported by Baker and Severance (1948), although rhinocerebral disease had been reported earlier in that decade and is by far the most frequent form of the disease. A later review article by Baker (1956) found three case reports in the literature and added five cases seen in 1.5 years in North Carolina and South Carolina alone. None of these patients survived. Baker found a number of reports in the early German literature extending back to 1876 but after careful review tabulated them separately because the fungi were similar to Mucor in some respects but presented club-shaped excrescences on the hyphae unlike Mucor.

Diagnosis

An important aid to diagnosis is recognition by the attending physician that the disease occurs in patients with predisposing clinical factors and almost never occurs in their absence (Fig. 20-26). Pulmonary infection is heralded by the onset of fever, cough, sputum production, and respiratory distress, which is often severe. Hemoptysis is an ominous sign. Other opportunistic fungi (Aspergillus and Candida) may colonize the same respiratory tract and confuse the picture. Culture results are often negative but if positive strongly suggest invasive disease. Histologic evidence of tissue invasion provides the definitive diagnosis (Bigby, et al., 1986) (Fig. 20-27).

The diagnosis of mucormycosis is based on the presence of broad, nonseptate, right-angled branching hyphae, which are easily identified by hematoxylin and eosin or indigo carmine stain (Baker, 1956). The organisms are also easily seen in an aqueous potassium hydroxide preparation (Lehrer, et al., 1980). It was observed that in the lung the fungus penetrated bronchial walls and had a propensity for penetrating artery and vein walls with the fungus invading living rather than necrotic tissue. Thromboarteritis followed with the production of infarcts. Reliable serologic tests are not available (Sarosi, et al., 1985).

Early surgical successes were reported by Dillon, et al. (1958) who performed lobectomy for cure and Blankenberg and Verhoeff (1959) who followed right bilobectomy with drug therapy (sulfisoxazole and nystatin). The latter patient had no significant predisposing factors but 14 months later diabetes was diagnosed. Except for the early report by Baker (1956), there are no case series in the literature, only single-case reports gathered into reviews.

McBride, et al. (1960) found 55 cases in the literature and added 2. Twenty-three had pulmonary involvement, and in 13 the lungs were solely involved. Lehrer, et al. (1980) ob-

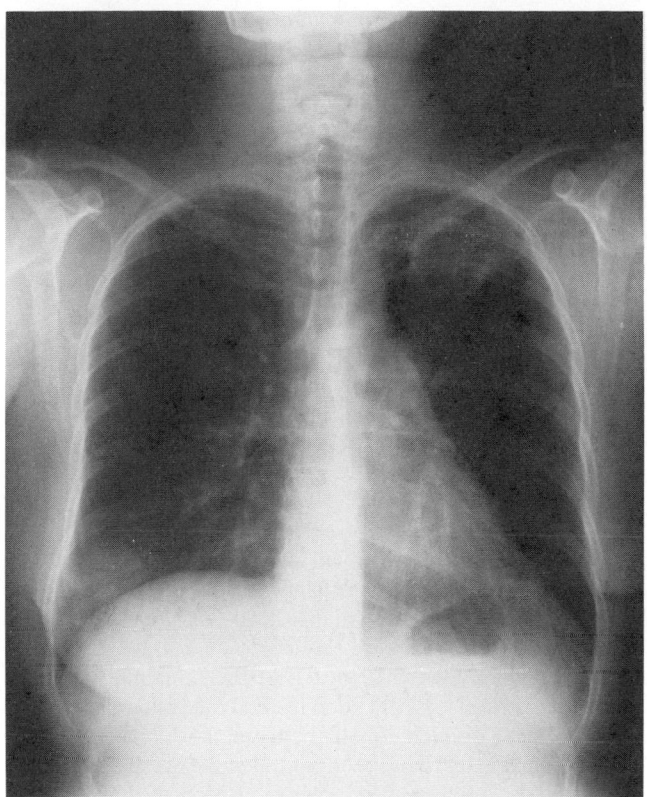

Figure 20-26. Mucormycosis. This 37-year-old woman postmastectomy presented for bone marrow rescue chemotherapy with a cavitating lesion left upper lobe, left hilar fullness, and a right lower lobe infiltrate.

served that there were only 13 known survivors of pulmonary mucormycosis to that date.

Bigby, et al. (1986) identified 18 cures from the literature, of which 11 patients underwent surgery alone and 6 received only amphotericin B. In 2 of these 6, however, the diagnostic biopsy removed a large portion of the involved lung. In addition, Bigby, et al. described 11 cases from the literature of primary major airway involvement with invasive mucormycosis. Nine of these 11 patients were diabetic. In 9 the diagnosis was made antemortem, 8 of these by bronchoscopic examination. Seven of the 9 died, all secondary to massive hemoptysis. Diagnostic clues are hoarseness, gross hemoptysis, and mediastinal widening on the chest radiograph.

Brown, et al. (1992) addressed the problem of bronchovascular mucormycosis in the diabetic patient. From the literature he collected 21 cases. Nine surgical cases survived lobectomy or segmental resection. Three received amphotericin B. Twelve patients were not operated on, and three survived. All of the survivors and 3 nonsurvivors were treated with amphotericin B. Five of 8 patients in this group underwent bronchial biopsy a few days before death. Marchevsky, et al. (1980) suggested transthoracic needle biopsy for diagnosis, and Hsu, et al. (1989) used this in a case of Rhizopus infection. In a recent case of mucormycosis we obtained a diagnosis by this method.

Therapy

The most important concepts in successful therapy of pulmonary mucormycosis are to entertain the diagnosis of fungal infection, make a prompt diagnosis, and begin therapy at once. Lehrer, et al. (1980); Digby, (1986); and Terrell and

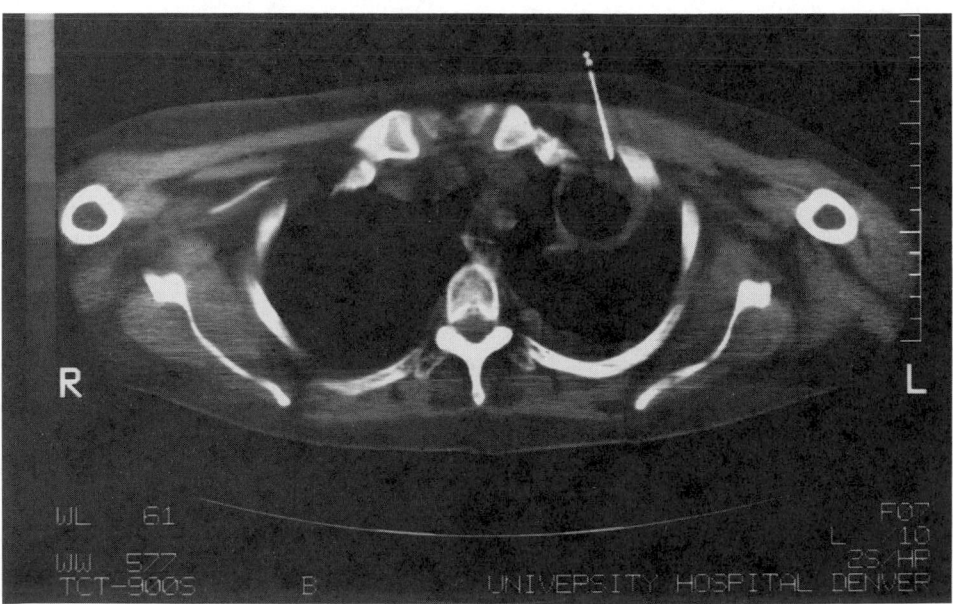

Figure 20-27. CT-guided needle biopsy produced the nonseptate right-angled branching hyphae of Mucor. Prompt left upper lobectomy and a later diagnosis of invasive aspergilloma at the lung hilum necessitated completion pneumonectomy.

Hughes (1992) confirm that amphotericin B is the only effective antifungal agent at this time. Terrell and Hughes note that mucormycosis is often unresponsive to amphotericin B in standard doses and therapy should be at a level of 1.0 to 1.5 mg/kg/day.

Because of the pathologic changes induced in the lung with blood vessel invasion, thrombosis, and infarction, the fungus propagates in a rich medium. Lehrer, et al. (1980); Takaro (1983); Digby (1986); Rozick, et al. (1989); Terrell and Hughes (1992); and the statements of the therapy of fungal disease from the American Thoracic Society (1979,1988), all support the philosophy that the proper therapy of mucormycosis in most instances is to treat promptly with amphotericin B and resect the involved pulmonary tissue promptly.

Candidiasis
Clinical Features

Although Candida is one of the most prevalent fungi, candidiasis is an uncommon problem for the thoracic surgeon. These opportunistic fungi usually infect the immunocompromised host or long-term hospitalized patients who are receiving prolonged antibiotic therapy, allowing fungal overgrowth, and have indwelling urinary catheters, intravenous tubes, or endotracheal tubes (Penn, et al., 1983).

Special clinical situations seen by the thoracic surgeon are the rare Candida pneumonia, esophagitis, and endocarditis. Candida meningitis also may be seen.

Diagnosis

Diagnosis of invasive candidiasis presents special problems. Species of Candida are present in 50 to 60 percent of respiratory secretions from uninfected patients. Cultures cannot separate colonization from tissue invasion. Positive blood culture findings for Candida require a careful search for the source. Vascular catheters should be removed or moved. Candidemia should be treated to improve survival and abort late metastatic Candida infections (Terrell and Hughes, 1992). Positive central nervous system cultures are diagnostic because that is a normally sterile site (Sarosi, et al., 1985).

Although reports of useful serologic tests have been common, no reliable serologic test is available. Assessment of Candida metabolites may be useful in the future.

Therapy

Candidemia should be treated with amphotericin B to a total dose of 250 to 1,000 mg. Candida pneumonia requires a lung biopsy before therapy because the tracheobronchial tree in hospitalized patients is usually colonized with Candida (American Thoracic Society, 1979).

Mild cases of esophagitis may be treated with oral nystatin. Ketoconazole and itraconazole are useful in this situation, but fluconazole may be the best form of therapy for significant esophageal candidiasis. Failure to respond promptly should lead to therapy with amphotericin B alone or in synergy with flucytosine.

Candida endocarditis has been described by Nordenberg, et al. (1975). Fungal endocarditis on a prosthetic valve is usually caused by Aspergillus or Candida and requires inten-sive amphotericin B therapy and prompt valve replacement (Cowgill, et al., 1986). Because of the tendency for vegetations from Candida to be bulky, there is always a risk that a large fungal thrombus will be released into the blood stream as an embolus. Special care must be exercised in such cases to avoid this occurrence when the patient is undergoing cardiopulmonary bypass for replacement of the infected valve.

Paracoccidioidomycosis (South American Blastomycosis)
Clinical Features

First described by Lutz (1908) in a Brazilian patient with severe oral lesions, this disease, which is endemic in South and Latin America, is rarely reported in the United States. Murray, et al. (1974) observed that all the reported U.S. cases had resided or traveled in endemic areas, albeit many years previously in a few cases.

Preliminary entry is believed to be by the respiratory tract. In a large consecutive series from South America, Machado and Lisboa (1960) reported that 292 of 338 patients had pulmonary lesions. When 41 were eliminated who also had tuberculosis, carcinoma, or sarcoidosis, of the remaining 235 with lung lesions nearly all (90 percent) had micronodular or infiltrative lesions divided equally between these two types. The lesions were usually bilateral and symmetric. In 58 percent all pulmonary areas were involved; 33 percent showed areas of cavitation. In decreasing order of frequency, the primary diagnosed lesions are in the oral cavity, lung, larynx, and skin.

Diagnosis

Most clinical cases occur in men, usually older than age 30 and commonly in the fourth and fifth decades. Rural workers predominate, which suggests that contact with soil is a factor in the disease. Urban workers and professionals have also been identified with the illness, however, who had no history of soil contact (Murray, et al., 1974).

Common symptoms of pulmonary paracoccidioidomycosis are cough, sputum production, dyspnea, and hemoptysis. Because only about one-quarter of the patients have infections confined to the lung, involvement of the skin, mucous membranes, lymph nodes, and adrenal glands may modify the symptomatic picture. Ulcerations may appear around the mouth, and dysphonia may be prominent with laryngeal involvement. Addison's disease has been diagnosed in a number of patients with advanced adrenal involvement. Tender cervical lymph node masses are common. Dissemination of the bowel, spleen, liver, pancreas, testes, bone, heart, and central nervous system is seen more rarely. Altered consciousness, increased intracranial pressure, hemiplegia, meningeal signs, or cord compression may all be found (Restrepo, et al., 1987; Murray, et al., 1974; Negroni, et al., 1987).

The diagnosis is commonly made by identification of the organism in tissue sections. Tissue culture is slightly less reliable. Agar gel immunodiffusion and high titers of complement fixation to specific antigens confirm the diagnosis. Serial complement fixation titers are of great prognostic value

(Buechner, et al., 1973; Negroni, et al., 1987; Restrepo, et al., 1987).

Therapy

Reasonable success from therapy with amphotericin B and more recent good reports of therapy with ketoconazole by Restrepo, et al. (1983) and even more favorable reports on irradication of the disease by Restrepo, et al. (1987) and Negroni, et al. (1987) using itraconazole indicate that there is no indication for surgical therapy of this disease. An official statement from the American Thoracic Society (1988) presents ketoconazole as the therapy of choice for paracoccidioidomycosis.

COMMENTS AND CONTROVERSIES

It is clear that an increasing number of patients will be exposed to the ravages of fungal diseases as new means to assault the immune system are developed. Trends over the 50 years since the surgical removal of foci of fungal infection became technically feasible were first toward increasing application of surgical methods. Then with the development of more effective antifungal drugs, attempts were made to treat these infections with drugs alone or with operative removal as an adjunct to the resectional therapy. As this section of this chapter documents, excessively vigorous attempts to remove the fungal infection, especially in central areas of the lung, often resulted in unplanned pneumonectomy with significant morbidity and mortality rate.

Improved therapy for pulmonary fungal infection can be expected from several quarters. Simplified diagnostic procedures, such as the demonstration that bronchial lavage and bronchial washings give equal diagnostic accuracy to those obtained by transbronchial biopsy, should shorten the interval to the institution of therapy. Culture media and methods are being continuously improved, and refinements in serologic testing are leading to more rapid diagnoses. Abandonment of skin testing because of its unfavorable effects on serologic testing may be contested by some but is generally accepted.

Major improvements in therapy are already at hand in the development of new antifungal agents, and this progress continues both here and abroad. Better therapeutic effect and less toxicity are the hallmarks of these improved agents.

The tenuous relationship between fungal infections and the at-risk population is epitomized by two recent events. The AIDS crisis is particular important. In the less than 15 years since the recognition of this syndrome and because of the high incidence of fungal infection in this immunosuppressed population and the urgency of attempts to deal with the disease, much has been learned in this short period about specific fungal infections, such as cryptococcosis. The January 1994 Los Angeles earthquake has already spawned reports of numerous cases of coccidioidomycosis in newspaper and television reports, presumably from spores in the dust stirred up in the aftermath of this ground-shaking event. Much will be learned from medical reports as this story unfolds.

Sporadic reports suggest that cavitary pulmonary lesions and areas in the pleural space are often treated beneficially by intracavitary irrigation with antifungal agents. Application of this method through transthoracic catheters should clarify whether this is truly beneficial in a large number of patients. Similarly the use of intravascular coils in cases of severe hemorrhage may be found to terminate hemorrhage and convert a desperate life-saving surgical event into a more ordered resection. In patients with widespread or bilateral disease in whom surgical resection is not indicated, this procedure may indeed by life saving in itself. Only the application of the procedure to larger numbers of cases can establish its true role in the management of such difficult cases.

F.L.G.
A.R.H.

Pulmonary mycotic infections continue to plague surgeons, especially when they deal with their complications. Some of the most challenging problems addressed by thoracic surgeons are those in regard to the ravages of histoplasmosis and aspergillosis.

The authors correctly point out the importance of diagnosis before therapy because most of these infections can be treated without surgical intervention. With the improved techniques of transbronchial brushings and biopsies and fluoroscopically or CT-guided transthoracic needle aspiration, it is rarely necessary to resort to either wedge resection or open thoracotomy for the diagnosis of these infections.

In my own experience, most eroded broncholiths can be easily managed bronchoscopically unless a tracheoesophageal fistual has developed. More recently there has been renewed interest in aggressively treating the early invasive aspergillosis by early surgical resection and antifungal therapy.

The increasing incidence of immunocompromised hosts as a result of chemotherapy, immunosuppression for transplantation, and AIDS has increased the awareness and diagnosis of these infections. For further information the reader is referred to the last section in this chapter on immunocompromised hosts.

R.J.G

KEY REFERENCES

American Thoracic Society Statement: Chemotherapy of the pulmonary mycoses. Am Rev Respir Dis 138:1078, 1988

This statement updates a similar statement from the American Thoracic Society made in 1974 and emphasizes new developments, such as the changes in fungal therapy occasioned by the introduction of the new oral agent, retoconazone. Furthermore continued study of the natural history of these diseases has improved knowledge of when to treat fungal diseases. Therapeutic agents are described and the management of specific mycoses is outlined.

Ampel NM, Wieden MA, Gagliani JN: Coccidioidomycosis: clinical update. Rev Infect Dis 11:897, 1989

Formerly a regional disease, coccidioidomycosis is now a major fungal infection of national interest because of travel and migration patterns through and to the Southwest. The decreased but important role of surgery is well defined.

Sarosi GA: Amphotericin B: still the "gold standard" for antifungal therapy. Postgrad Med 88:152, 1990

This how-to article emphasizes the myths surrounding the use of amphotericin B and offers valuable hints to minimize its adverse effects. In specific fungal infections the author makes useful recommendations concerning when and how to treat.

Takaro T: Fungal infection. p. 161. In Grillo HG, Austin WG, Wilkins EW Jr et al (eds): Current Therapy in Cardiothoracic Surgery. BC Decker, Philadelphia, 1989

This is a succinct description of the major fungal infections, and it identifies the role of surgery in diagnosing and treating these patients. It describes the limits of surgical therapy.

Terrell CL, Hughes CE: Antifungal agents used for deep-seated myotic infections. Mayo Clinic Proc 67:69, 1992

The most up-to-date current therapies available are found in this comprehensive review. Additional information about agents not yet available in the United States but available in other countries or to therapeutic protocol studies suggests that new agents soon to be released will be very effective.

REFERENCES

Adelson HT, Malcolm JA: Intracavitary treatment of pulmonary mycetomas. Am Rev Respir Dis 98:87, 1968

Ahn C, Kilman JW, Vasko JS, Andrews NC: The therapy of cavitary pulmonary histoplasmosis. J Thorac Cardiovasc Surg 57:42, 1969

American Thoracic Society, Ad Hoc Committee: Treatment of fungal diseases. Am Rev Respir Dis 120:1393, 1979

Aronstam EM, Hopeman AR: Surgical experiences with pulmonary coccidioidomycosis. J Thorac Cardiovasc Surg 42:200, 1961

Baker RD: Pulmonary mucormycosis. Am J Pathol 32:287, 1956

Baker EJ, Hawkins JA, Washow EA: Surgery for coccidioidomycosis in 52 diabetic patients with specific reference to immunologic factors. J Thorac Cardiovasc Surg 75:680, 1978

Baker RD, Severance AO: Mucormycosis with report of acute mycotic pneumonia (abstract). Am J Pathol 24:716, 1948

Battaglini JW, Murray GF, Keagy B et al: Surgical management of symptomatic pulmonary aspergilloma. Ann Thorac Surg 39:512, 1985

Baum GL, Donnerberg RL, Stewart D et al: Pulmonary sporotrichosis. N Engl J Med 280:410, 1969

Beard HW, Richert JH, Taylor RR: The treatment of deep mycotic infections with amphotericin B. Am Rev Respir Dis 81:43, 1960

Bennett JE, Dismukes WE, Duma RJ et al: The comparison of amphotericin B alone and combined with flucytosine in the treatment of cryptococcal meningitis. N Engl J Med 301:126, 1979

Bennington JH, Hober SL Morgenstern NL: Increased susceptibility to cryptococcosis following steroid therapy. Dis Chest 45:262, 1964

Bhagavan BS, Rao DRG, Weinberg T: Histoplasmosis producing broncholithiasis. Arch Pathol Lab Med 91:577, 1971

Bigby TD, Serota ML, Tierney LM Jr, Matthay MA: Clinical spectrum of pulmonary mucormycosis. Chest 89:435, 1986

Blackenberg HW, Verhoeff D: Mucormycosis of the lung. Am Rev Respir Dis 79:357, 1959

Bonfils-Roberts EA, Nickodem A, Nealon TF Jr: Retrospective analysis of the efficacy of open lung biopsy in acquired immunodeficiency syndrome. Ann Thorac Surg 49:115, 1990

Borelli D: A clinical trial of itraconazole in the treatment of deep mycoses and leishmaniasis. Rev Infect Dis 9(suppl):557, 1987

Borgers M, Vandenbossche H, Couwenbergh G: The pharmacology of agents used in the treatment of pulmonary mycoses. Clin Chest Med 7:439, 1986

Brown RB, Johnson JH, Kessinger JM, Sealy WC: Bronchovascular mucormycosis in the diabetic: an urgent surgical problem. Ann Thorac Surg 53:854, 1992

Buechner HA, Seabury JH, Campbell CC et al: The current status of serologic, immunologic, and skin tests in the diagnosis of pulmonary mycoses. Report of the Committee on Fungus Diseases and Subcommittee on Criteria for Clinical Diagnosis—American College of Chest Physicians. Chest 63:259, 1973

Butz RO, Acetina JR, Leininger BJ: Ten-year experience with mycetomas in patients with pulmonary tuberculosis. Chest 87:356, 1985

Catanzaro A: Pulmonary coccidioidomycosis. Med Clin North Am 64:461, 1980

Catanzaro A, Fierer J, Friedman PJ: Fluconazole in the treatment of persistent coccidioidomycosis. Chest 97:666, 1990

Cauwenbergh G, DeDoncker P, Stoops K et al: Itraconazole in the treatment of human mycoses: review of three years of clinical experience. Rev Infect Dis 9(suppl)5:146, 1987

Chan CS, Tuazon CU, Lessin LS: Amphotericin B induced thrombocytopenia. Ann Intern Med 96:332, 1982

Chuck SL, Sande MA: Infections with Cryptococcus neoformans in the acquired immunodeficiency syndrome. N Engl J Med 321:794, 1989

Cleary JD, Weisdorf D, Fletcher CV: Effect of infusion rate on amphotericin B-associated febrile reactions. DICP 22:769, 1988

Cogswell HW, Czerny EW, Fritz JM: Surgical lesions of coccidioidomycosis. Arch Surg 70:633, 1955

Cole FH, Cole FH Jr, Khandekar A, Watson DC: Management of broncholithiasis: is thoracotomy necessary? Ann Thorac Surg 42:255, 1986

Cotton BH, Birsner JW: Surgical treatment of pulmonary coccidioidomycosis. J Thorac Surg 38:435, 1959

Cotton BH, Paulsen GA, Birsner JW: Surgical considerations in pulmonary coccidioidomycosis: report of 100 cases. Am J Surg 90:101, 1955

Cowgill LD, Addonizio VP, Hopeman AR, Harken AH: Prosthetic valve endocarditis. Curr Probl Cardiol 11:617, 1986

Cunningham RT, Einstein H: Coccidioidal pulmonary cavities with rupture. J Thorac Cardiovasc Surg 84:172, 1982

Daly R, Pairolero PC, Piehler JM et al: Pulmonary aspergilloma: results of surgical treatment. J Thorac Cardiovasc Surg 92:981, 1986

Darling ST: A protozoan general infection producing pseudotubercles in the lung and focal necrosis in liver, spleen, and lymph nodes. JAMA 46:1283, 1906

DeMonbreum WA: The cultivation and cultural characteristics of Darling's Histoplasma capsulatum. Am J Trop Med 14:93, 1934

Diaz M, Puente R, de Hoyos LA et al: Itraconazole in the treatment of coccidioidomycosis. Chest 100:682, 1991

Dillon ML, Sealy WC, Fetter BF: Mucormycosis of the bronchus successfully treated by lobectomy. J Thorac Cardiovasc Surg 35:464, 1958

Dines DE, Payne WS, Bernatz PE, Pairolero PC: Mediastinal granuloma and fibrosing mediastinitis. Chest 75:320, 1979

Dismukes WE: Cryptococcal meningitis in patients with AIDS. J Infect Dis 157:624, 1988

Dively W, McCracken R: Cavitary pulmonary histoplasmosis treated by pulmonary resection. Ann Surg 163:921, 1966

Doty DB: Bypass of superior vena cava. J Thorac Cardiovasc Surg 83:326, 1982

Draheim JH, Mitchell JR, Elton NW: Histoplasmosis: fourth case report from the Canal Zone. Am J Trop Med 31:753, 1951

Drutz D: Racial susceptibility to coccidioidomycosis (letter). N Engl J Med 302:59, 1980

Drutz DJ, Catanzaro A: Coccidioidomycosis I & II. Am Rev Respir Dis 117:559, 1978

Drutz DJ, Fan JH, Tai TY et al: Hypokalemia, rhabdomyolysis and myoglobinemia following amphotericin B therapy. JAMA 211:824, 1970

Dukes RR, Strimlan CV, Dines DE et al: Esophageal involvement with mediastinal granuloma. JAMA 236:2313, 1976

Eguchi S, Endo S, Sakashita I et al: Surgery in the treatment of pulmonary aspergillosis. Br J Dis Chest 65:111, 1971

Faber LP, Jensik RJ, Chamla SK, Kittle CF: The surgical implication of broncholithiasis. J Thorac Cardiovasc Surg 70:779, 1975

Faulkner SL, Rowland V, Brown P et al: Hemoptysis and pulmonary aspergilloma: operative versus nonoperative treatment. Ann Thorac Surg 25:389, 1978

Ferguson TB, Burford TH: Mediastinal granuloma. Ann Thorac Surg 1:125, 1965

Forsee JH, Perkins RB: Focalized pulmonary coccidioidomycosis: a surgical disease. JAMA 155:1223, 1954

Forsee JH, Puckett TF, Hagmann FE: Surgical consideration in focalized pulmonary histoplasmosis. J Thorac Surg 26:131, 1953

Forseth J, Rohwedder JJ, Levine BE, Saubolle MA: Experience with needle biopsy for coccidioidal lung nodules. Arch Intern Med 146:319, 1986

Furbringer P: Beobochtungen uber Lungenmycose beim Menschen. Virchows Arch A Pathol Anat Histopathol 66:330, 1876

Furculow ML, Brasher CA: Chronic progressive (cavitary) histoplasmosis as a problem in tuberculosis sanitoriums. Am Rev Respir Dis 73:609, 1956

Furculow ML, Doto IL, Tosh FE, Lynch HJ: Course and prognosis of untreated histoplasmosis. JAMA 177:292, 1961

Garrett HE, Roper CL: Surgical intervention in histoplasmosis. Ann Thorac Surg 42:711, 1986

Gerstl B, Weidman WH, Newmann AV: Pulmonary aspergillosis: report of two cases. Ann Intern Med 28:662, 1948

Gilchrist TC: Protozoan dermatitis. J Cutan Genitourin Dis 12:496, 1894

Gillespie JG: Superior vena caval obstruction in childhood: report of a case secondary to histoplasmosis. J Pediatr 49:320, 1956

Gold W, Stout HA, Pagano JF, Donovich R: Amphotericins A & B, antifungal antibiotics produced by a streptomycete. I. In vitro studies. Antibiot Annu 3:579, 1955–1956

Goodwin RA Jr, Loyd JE, DesPrez RM: Histoplasmosis in normal hosts. Medicine (Baltimore) 60:231, 1981

Gottlieb MS, Schroff R, Shanker HM et al: Pneumocystis carinii pneumonia and mucosal candidiasis in previously healthy homosexual men: evidence of a newly acquired cellular immunodeficiency. N Engl J Med 305:1425, 1981

Grant AR, Melick DW: The surgical treatment of cavitary pulmonary coccidioidomycosis. Arch Surg 94:559, 1967

Graybill JR: Treatment of coccidioidomycosis. Ann N Y Acad Sci 554:481, 1988

Graybill JR, Stevens DA, Gagliani JN et al: Itraconazole treatment of coccidioidomycosis: NIAID mycosis study group. Am J Med 89:282, 1990

Greer JS, Grow JB: The surgical lesions of pulmonary coccidioidomycosis. Dis Chest 16:336, 1949

Hammerman KJ, Powell KE, Christianson CS et al: Pulmonary cryptococcosis: clinical forms and treatment. Am Rev Respir Dis 108:1116, 1973

Hargis JL, Bone RC, Stewart J et al: Intracavitary amphotericin B in the treatment of symptomatic pulmonary aspergillosis. Am J Med 68:389, 1980

Hatcher CR Jr, Sehdeva J, Waters WC III et al: Primary pulmonary cryptococcosis. J Thorac Cardiovasc Surg 61:39, 1971

Henderson RD, Deslauries J, Ritcey EL et al: Surgery in pulmonary aspergillosis. J Thorac Cardiovasc Surg 70:1088, 1975

Herring M, Pecora D: Pleural aspergillosis: a case report. Ann Surg 42:300, 1976

Hewlett TH, Steer A, Thomas DE: Progressive fibrosing mediastinitis. Ann Thorac 2:245, 1966

Hiebert CA, King JW, George RB: Late dissemination of pulmonary blastomycosis during ketoconazole therapy. Chest 95:240, 1989

Hodgson CH, Weed LA, Clagett OT: Pulmonary histoplasmosis. JAMA 145:807, 1951

Hsu J, Clayman JA, Gcha AS: Survival of a recipient of renal transplantation after pulmonary phycomycosis. Ann Thorac Surg 47:617, 1989

Hughes CF, Waugh R, Lindsay D: Surgery for pulmonary aspergilloma: preoperative embolization of the bronchial circulation. Thorax 41:324, 1986

Hyde L: Coccidioidal pulmonary cavitation. Dis Chest 54(suppl):273, 1968

Hyde L: Coccidioidal pulmonary cavitation. Am J Med 25:890, 1958

Irani FA, Dolovich J, Newhouse MT: Bronchopulmonary and pleural aspergillosis. Am Rev Respir Dis 103:552, 1971

Jewkes J, Kay PH, Paneth M, Citron KM: Pulmonary aspergilloma: analysis of prognosis in relation to hemoptysis and survey of treatment. Thorax 38:572, 1983

Jung JY, Almond CH, Campbell CD et al: Role of surgery in the management of pulmonary sporotrichosis. J Thorac Cardiovasc Surg 77:234, 1979

Kanawaty DS, Stalker MJB, Munt PW: Nonsurgical treatment of Histoplasma endocarditis involving a bioprosthetic valve. Chest 99:253, 1991

Karas A, Hankins JR, Attar S et al: Pulmonary aspergillosis: an analysis of 41 patients. Ann Thorac Surg 22:1, 1976

Kaufman L, Blumer S: Value and interpretation of serological tests for the diagnosis of cryptococcosis. Appl Environ Microbiol 16:1907, 1968

Kelly PC, Thomas AR, Sazie ESM: The outcome of disseminated coccidioidomycosis. p. 360. In Einstein HE, Catanzaro A (eds): Coccidioidomycosis: Proceedings of the Fourth International Conference. National Foundation for Infectious Diseases, Washington, D.C., 1985

Klingman AM, Mescon H: The periodic acid Schiff stain for the demonstration of fungi in animal tissues. J Bacteriol 60:415, 1950

Kovacs JA, Kovacs AA, Polis M et al: Cryptococcosis in the acquired immunodeficiency syndrome. Ann Intern Med 103:533, 1985

Krakowka P, Rowinska E, Halweg H: Infection of the pleura by Aspergillus fumigatus. Thorax 25:245, 1970

Kuykendall SJ, Ellis FH, Weed LA, Donoghue FE: Pulmonary cryptococcosis. N Engl J Med 257:1009, 1957

Larsen RA, Bozzette S, McCutchan JA et al: Persistent Cryptococcus neoformans infection of the prostate after successful treatment of meningitis. Ann Intern Med 111:125, 1989

Lehrer RI, Howard DH, Sypherd PS et al: Mucormycosis. Ann Intern Med 93:93, 1980

Levin S: The fungal skin test as a diagnostic hindrance (editorial). J Infect Dis 122:343, 1970

Lockwood WR, Busey JF, Batson BE, Allison F Jr: Experiences in the treatment of North American blastomycosis with 2-hydroxystilbamidine. Ann Intern Med 57:553, 1962

Machado FJ, Lisboa MJ: Consideracoes relativas a blastomycose sud-americana. De participacao pulmonar entre 338 casas consecutivas. O Hospital 58:431, 1960

Magilligan DJ, Ravipati S, Zayat P et al: Massive hemoptysis: control by transcatheter bronchial artery embolization. Ann Thorac Surg 32:392, 1981

Marchevsky AM, Bottone EJ, Geller SA, Giger DK: The changing spectrum of disease, etiology, and diagnosis of mucormycosis. Hum Pathol 11:457, 1980

Massard G, Roeslin N, Wihlm J-M et al: Pleuropulmonary aspergilloma: clinical spectrum and results of surgical treatment. Ann Thorac Surg 54:1159, 1992

McBride RA, Corson JM, Dammin GH: Mucormycosis. Am J Med 28:832, 1960

McKinsey DS, Gupta MR, Riddler SA et al: Long term amphotericin B therapy for disseminated histoplasmosis in patients with the acquired immunodeficiency syndrome (AIDS). Ann Intern Med 111:655, 1989

Medical Letter editors: Drugs for treatment of systemic fungal infections. Med Lett Drugs Ther 28:41, 1986

Medoff G, Kobayashi GS: Strategies in the treatment of systemic fungal infections. N Engl J Med 302:145, 1980

Melick DW: Excisional surgery in pulmonary coccidioidomycosis. J Thorac Cardiovasc Surg 20:66, 1950

Michelson E: Primary pulmonary sporotrichosis. Ann Thorac Surg 24:83, 1977

Mohr JA, Griffiths W, Long H: Pulmonary sporotrichosis in Oklahoma and susceptibilities in vitro. Am Rev Respir Dis 119:961, 1979

Murray HW, Littman ML, Roberts RB: Disseminated paracoccidioidomycosis (South American blastomycosis) in the United States. Am J Med 56:209, 1974

National Institute of Allergy and Infectious Diseases Mycosis Study Group: Treatment of blastomycosis and histoplasmosis with ketoconazole: results of a prospective randomized clinical trial. Ann Intern Med 103:861, 1985

Negroni R, Palmieri D, Koren F et al: Oral treatment of paracoccidioidomycosis and histoplasmosis with itraconazole in humans. Rev Infect Dis 9(suppl)1:547, 1987

Negroni R, Robles AM, Arechavala A, Taborda A: Itraconazole in human histoplasmosis. Mycoses 32:123, 1989

Nelson AR: The surgical treatment of pulmonary coccidioidomycosis. Curr Probl Surg (October):1, 1974

Nelson RJ, Benfield JR: Benign esophagobronchial fistula. Arch Surg 100:685, 1970

Norenberg R, Sethi GK, Scott SM, Takaro T: Opportunistic endocarditis following open heart surgery. Ann Thorac Surg 19:592, 1975

Pappagianis D: Epidemiology of coccidioidomycosis. Curr Top Med Mycol 2:199, 1988

Parker JD, Sarosi GA, Doto IL et al: Treatment of chronic pulmonary histoplasmosis: a National Communicable Disease Center Cooperative Mycosis Study. N Engl J Med 283:225, 1970

Pecora DV, Toll MW: Pulmonary resection for localized aspergillosis. N Engl J Med 263:785, 1960

Penn RL, Lambert RS, George RB: Invasive fungal infections. The use of serologic tests in diagnosis and management. Arch Intern Med 193:1215, 1983

Perfect JR, Durock DT: Penetration of imidazoles and triazoles into cerebrospinal fluid of rabbits. J Antimicrob Chemother 16:81, 1985

Petersen EA, Friedman BA, Crowder EO, Rifkind D: Coccidioiduria: clinical significance. Ann Intern Med 85:34, 1976

Pluss JL, Opal SM: Pulmonary sporotrichosis: review of treatment and outcome. Medicine (Baltimore) 65:143, 1986

Prager RL, Burney DP, Waterhouse G, Bender HW Jr: Pulmonary mediastinal and cardiac presentations of histoplasmosis. Ann Thorac Surg 30:385, 1980

Puckett TF: Pulmonary histoplasmosis. Ann Rev Tuberc 67:453, 1953

Rafferty PR, Biggs BA, Crompton GK, Grant IWB: What happens to patients with pulmonary aspergilloma? Analysis of 23 cases. Thorax 38:579, 1983

Ramirez RJ: Pulmonary aspergillosis: endobronchial treatment. N Engl J Med 271:1281, 1964

Ratcheson RA, Ommaya AK: Experience with the subcutaneous cerebrospinal fluid reservoir—preliminary report of 60 cases. N Engl J Med 279:1025, 1968

Reiss F, Szilazyi G: Ecology of yeast like fungi in a hospital population. Detailed investigation of Cryptococcus neoformans. Arch Dermatol 91:611, 1965

Restrepo A, Gomez I, Cano LE et al: Treatment of paracoccidioidomycosis with ketoconazole: a three year experience. The Second Annual International Symposium on Ketoconazole. Am J Med 74(suppl):48, 1983

Restrepo A, Gomez I, Robledo J et al: Itraconazole in the treatment of paracoccidioidomycosis. A preliminary report. Rev Infect Dis 9(suppl):S51, 1987

Restrepo A, Robledo J, Gomez I et al: Itraconazole therapy in lymphangitic and cutaneous sporotrichosis. Arch Dermatol 122:413, 1986

Ridgeway NA, Whitcomb FC, Erickson EE, Law SW: Primary pulmonary sporotrichosis. Am J Med 32:153, 1962

Riley WA, Watson CJ: Histoplasmosis of Darling with report of a case originating in Minnesota. Am J Trop Med 6:271, 1926

Rivkin LM, Winn DF Jr, Salyer JM: The surgical treatment of pulmonary coccidioidomycosis. J Thorac Cardiovasc Surg 42:402, 1961

Rozick J, Oxendine D, Heffner J, Brezinski W: Pulmonary zygomycosis: a cause of positive lung scan diagnosed by bronchoalveolar lavage. Chest 95:238, 1989

Salomon NW, Osborne R, Copeland JG: Surgical manifestations and results of treatment of pulmonary coccidioidomycosis. Ann Thorac Surg 30:433, 1980

Salyer JM, Harrison HN, Winn DJ Jr, Traylor RR: Chronic fibrous mediastinitis and superior vena cava obstruction due to histoplasmosis. Dis Chest 35:364, 1959

Sarosi GA, Armstrong D, Davies SF et al: Laboratory diagnosis of mycotic and specific fungal infections. Official statement—American Thoracic Society. Am Rev Respir Dis 132:1373, 1985

Sarosi GA, Parker JD, Doto IL, Tosh F: Chronic pulmonary coccidioidomycosis: a National Communicable Disease Center Cooperative Mycoses Study. N Engl J Med 283:325, 1980

Schwarz J, Schaen MD, Picardi JL: Complications of the arrested primary histoplasmic complex. JAMA 236:1157, 1976

Scott SM, Peasley ED, Aymes TP: Pulmonary sporotrichosis. N Engl J Med 265:453, 1961

Seabury JH, Buechner HA, Busey JF et al.: The diagnosis of pulmonary mycoses. Report of the Committee on Fungus Diseases and Subcommittee on Criteria for Clinical Diagnosis, American College of Chest Physicians. Chest 60:82, 1971

Shapiro MJ, Albelda SM, Mayock RL, McLean GK: Severe hemoptysis associated with aspergilloma. Chest 94:1225, 1988

Shirakusa T, Ueda H, Saito T et al: Surgical treatment of pulmonary aspergilloma and Aspergillus empyema. Ann Thorac Surg 48:779, 1989

Sievers ML: Racial susceptibility to coccidioidomycosis (letter). N Engl J Med 302:58, 1980

Smith FS, Gibson P, Nicholls TT, Simpson JA: Pulmonary resection for localized lesions of cryptococcosis (torulosis): a review of eight cases. Thorax 31:121, 1976

Solat RW, McKeoun JJ, Smullens S et al: The surgical implications of intracavitary mycetomas (fungus balls). J Thorac Cardiovasc Surg 62:411, 1971

Soltanzadeh H, Wychulis AR, Sadr F et al: Surgical treatment of pulmonary aspergilloma. Ann Surg 186:13, 1977

Spickard A, Butler WT, Andriole V, Utz JP: The improved prognosis of cryptococcal meningitis with amphotericin B therapy. Ann Intern Med 58:66, 1963

Stamm AM, Diasio RB, Dismukes WE et al: A National Institute of Allergy and Infectious Diseases Mycoses Study Group: toxicity of amphotericin B plus flucytosine in 194 patients with cryptococcal meningitis. Am J Med 83:236, 1987

Stoddard JL, Cutler EC: Torula infection in man: studies from the Rockefeller Institute for Medical Research. 6:1, 1916

Strimlan CV, Dines DE, Payne WS: Mediastinal granuloma. Mayo Clinic Proc 50:702, 1975

Strutz GM, Rossi NP, Ehrenhaft JL: Pulmonary aspergillosis. J Thorac Cardiovasc Surg 64:963, 1972

Sugar AM, Alsip SG, Galgiani JN et al: Pharmacology and toxicity of high dose ketoconazole. Antimicrob Agents Chemother 31:1874, 1987

Sugar AM, Saunders C: Oral fluconazole as suppressive therapy of disseminated cryptococcosis in patients with acquired immunodeficiency syndrome. Am J Med 85:481, 1988

Sutaria MK, Polk JW, Reddy P, Mohanty SK: Surgical aspects of pulmonary histoplasmosis. Thorax 25:31, 1970

Takaro T: Fungal infections of the lungs. p. 553. In Sabiston DC Jr, and Spencer FC (eds): Gibbon's Surgery of the Chest. 4th Ed. WB Saunders, Philadelphia, 1983

Takaro T: The lungs: suppurative and fungal diseases. In Gibbon JH Jr, Sabiston DC Jr, Spencer FC (eds): Surgery of the Chest. 2nd Ed. WB Saunders, Philadelphia, 1969

Takaro T: Mycotic infection of interest to thoracic surgeons. Ann Thorac Surg 3:71, 1967

Timmes JJ, Baum GL: Surgery in pulmonary coccidioidomycosis. Am Rev Respir Dis 77:17, 1958

Trachiotis GD, Hofner GH, Hix WR et al: Role of open lung biopsy in diagnosing pulmonary complications of AIDS. Ann Thorac Surg 54:898, 1992

Trastek VF, Pairolero PC, Ceithaml EL: Surgical management of broncholithiasis. J Thorac Cardiovasc Surg 90:842, 1985

Trumbull ML, Chesney RM: The cytological diagnosis of pulmonary blastomycosis. JAMA 245:836, 1981

Utz JP, Bennett JE, Brandriss MW et al: Amphotericin B toxicity. Am Intern Med 61:334, 1964

Utz JP, Garriques IL, Sande MA et al: The therapy of cryptococcosis with a combination of flucytosine and amphotericin B. J Infect Dis 132:368, 1975

Van den Bossche H, Willemsens G, Cools W et al: In vivo and in vitro effects of the antimycotic drug ketoconazole on sterol synthesis. Antimicrob Agents Chemother 17:922, 1980

Van Trigt P: Fungal infections of the lung. p. 624. In Sabiston DC Jr, Spencer FC, (eds): Gibbon's Surgery of the Chest. 5th Ed. WB Saunders, Philadelphia, 1990

Viamonte M, Martinez I: Selective bronchial arteriography in man. Radiology 83:830, 1964

Walker JW, Montgomery FH: Further report of a previously recorded case of blastomycosis of the skin; systemic infection with blastomyces; death; autopsy. JAMA 58:867, 1902

Wenicke R: Uber einen protozoenbefund Beimycosis fungoides. Zentralb Mikobiol 12:859, 1892

Williams KR, Burford TH: Surgical treatment of granulomatous paratracheal lymphadenopathy. J Thorac Cardiovasc Surg 48:13, 1964

Winn WA: The use of amphotericin B in the treatment of coccidioidal disease. Am J Med 17:617, 1959

Zajtchuk R, Strevey TE, Heydorn WH, Treasure RL: Mediastinal histoplasmosis. J Thorac Cardiovasc Surg 66:300, 1973

Zimmerman LE: A missing link in the history of histoplasmosis in Panama. U.S. Armed Forces Med J 5:1569, 1954

Appendix: Drugs for Therapy for Systemic Fungal Infections

AMPHOTERICIN B

Amphotericin B is a polyene antibiotic isolated from a streptomycete from the soil of the Orinoco Valley in Venezuela (Gold, et al., 1955–1956). Although widely used in experimental protocols over the next few years, it was first released commercially in 1960 and was the first drug specific for a number of fungal infections. This agent has been variously described as the "mainstay," the "cornerstone," the "gold standard," the "most potent," the "standard," and the "most effective" therapy for most systemic mycoses. Despite intensive research activities toward the development of less toxic antifungal drugs, amphotericin B remains the best available substance for the therapy of deep-seated fungal infections. Investigations into its antifungal properties show that amphotericin B has a great affinity for ergosterol, which is a major component of fungal cell membranes. This results in an increase in membrane permeability and induces potassium leakage from the cells with eventual cell death. In low concentrations the effect is fungistatic; at higher concentrations, the drug is fungicidal according to Medoff and Kobayashi (1980). Animal studies suggest that amphotericin B is also a potent immunoadjuvant and that it augments cell-mediated immunity, thus increasing host resistance to infection.

The usual upper limits of the suggested daily dose are 0.5 to 1.0 mg/kg of body weight, although Medoff and Kobayshi (1980) indicate that more than 0.5 mg is rarely used, and the maximum dose recommended by Sarosi (1990) is 50 mg per day.

Because the drug is excreted by the liver into the bile, the urinary concentration is low, and bladder fungal infections are best treated by local irrigations. Central nervous system fungal infections, especially coccidioidal meningitis, are often treated by intrathecal injection or by intracysternal or intraventricular therapy through an Ommaya reservoir (Ratcheson and Ommaya, 1968). This device allows the administration of amphotericin B two or three times weekly with simultaneous intravenous therapy for fungal meningitis. Amphotericin B produces renal dysfunction in nearly all treated patients. The glomerular filtration rate falls about 40 percent shortly after the onset of therapy, and during the course of therapy, it stabilizes at 20 to 60 percent of normal. Medoff and Kobayashi (1980) indicate that further progression of this unfavorable event may be averted by discontinuing therapy for 2 to 5 days, after which therapy can be reinstituted at the same dosage. Potassium loss and hydrogen ion wasting is a result of this renal dysfunction. Severe potassium loss has been reported to induce hypokalemic rhabdomyolysis (Drutz, et al., 1970). This additional component of renal failure may be overlooked or attributed to amphotericin B therapy. It is mandatory that serum potassium levels be carefully monitored and appropriate replacement be carried out (Sarosi, 1990).

Anemia that develops during therapy with this drug is due to bone marrow depression. Thrombocytopenia caused by decreased platelet production occurs occasionally. Hepatic dysfunction and allergic reactions rarely occur.

The most distressing adverse effect of amphotericin B therapy is the febrile response to the infusion. The fever may be accompanied by chills, anorexia, nausea, vomiting, headache, photophobia, malaise, and weight loss. Hypotension and shock were initially reported after beginning doses (Utz, et al., 1964). Subsequently such patients were found to have disseminated fungal infection with adrenal involvement, and the hypotension resulted from an Addisonian crisis induced by the elevation of body temperature (Sarosi, 1990). Because most of these reports were generated early in the use of the drug, it is presumed that the commercial product has been refined and extraneous components removed.

This distressing patient response to therapy has been modified by the prophylactic use of aspirin administered prior to therapy, the use of codeine or meperidine with the infusion, accompanying the infusion with parenteral hydrocortisone in the rare severe disabling response, and the use of a rapid infusion technique over 45 minutes to 2 hours rather than 6 to 8 hours (Cleary, et al., 1988). This has the added advantage of allowing convenient outpatient administration of the drug.

Monitoring amphotericin B toxicity allows prompt management of side effects and may permit prevention of some adverse effects. Hematocrit, serum potassium, blood urea nitrogen, creatinine, and carbon dioxide values and urinalysis should be obtained before therapy, twice weekly for the first 4 weeks and then weekly as long as the drug is given (Medoff and Kobayashi 1980).

FLUCYTOSINE

Flucytosine is a fluorinated pyrimidine developed as an antimetabolic drug for use in cancer chemotherapy and approved in 1972 for antifungal therapy. Its spectrum of antifungal activity is narrow. Susceptible fungi contain cytosine deaminase, which converts flucytosine to 5-fluorouracil within the cell, which inhibits the synthesis of DNA and RNA.

Resistant organisms emerge frequently during therapy with this agent. For this reason the agent is not used alone to treat fungal disease. The agent is given orally and is well tolerated, although rash, hepatitis, severe diarrhea, and bone marrow depression are reported. Leukocyte and platelet counts should be monitored, with serum concentrations of flucytosine, especially in patients with renal insufficiency because the drug is excreted in the urine. Flucytosine is useful in the therapy of candidiasis, cryptococcosis, and chromomycosis. The usual dose of flucytosine is 150 mg/kg/dy administered in four divided doses because of its half-life in the serum of 3 to 5 hours (Medoff and Kobayashi, 1980). If creatinine clearance drops below 50 mg/min and serum flucytosine levels rise above 100 μg/ml, the dosage must be reduced, or the drug must be discontinued.

When flucytosine and amphotericin B are given in combination, the dose of amphotericin B should not exceed 0.3 mg/kg to reduce the depression of renal function (Stamm, et al., 1987). Suppression of the bone marrow is most likely to occur when blood levels of flucytosine exceed 100 μg/ml for 2 or more weeks. This combination is commonly used in cryptococcal disease.

IMIDAZOLES AND TRIAZOLES

Miconazole

Miconazole was the first effective alternative antifungal drug that could be given intravenously. Although it is effective experimentally, it is rarely used because its short half-life requires frequent administration, it penetrates the cerebrospinal fluid poorly, and there were numerous reports of toxicity. Its only current uses are topical or in patients who cannot tolerate or in whom amphotericin B has not been effective (Medoff and Kobayashi, 1980).

Ketoconazole

Ketoconazole, an oral agent, was approved for use in 1981. It has a broad antifungal spectrum. Along with other azole compounds, it interferes with the synthesis and permeability of fungal cell membranes by inhibiting the conversion of lanosterol to ergosterol, which is the chief sterol in the membranes (Van den Bossche, et al., 1980). Its wide use will be seen as the major fungal infections are discussed. Absorption from the gastrointestinal tract depends on the presence of gastric acid so that the agent cannot be reliably used in achlorhydric patients or in patients who require H_2-blockers or antacids. It is metabolized by the liver. Unfortunately this excellent drug has significant adverse effects. The most common are gastrointestinal symptoms (anorexia, nausea, and vomiting), rash and pruritus, and an increase in serum transaminase levels, all of which may abate while the drug is continued. Symptomatic hepatitis may develop and requires cessation of the drug as does the rare development of sustained hypertension (Terrell and Hughes, 1992). Most of the adverse effects of this drug occur with daily doses of 800 mg or more, and 25 percent of patients receiving 1,200 mg and more than one-half of those who have received 1,600 mg each day have discontinued therapy.

Fluconazole

Fortunately fluconazole, another broad-spectrum triazole agent that was approved in 1990, appears to exhibit much less toxicity. This oral agent shows high bioavailability and does not rely on gastric acid for absorption. It is widely distributed in the body. To a large extent it is excreted unchanged in the urine and has a long serum half-life, allowing once-a-day dosing, which must be reduced in renal insufficiency. Recent reports suggest an important role for fluconazole to prevent relapses of cryptococcal meningitis in the patient with AIDS (Sugar and Saunders, 1988).

Itraconazole

Another orally active triazole, itraconazole, has only recently become available in the United States. Because it has previously been approved for clinical use in other countries and has been available to mycosis study group panels for controlled studies, a great deal of information about its effectiveness is known (Restropo, et al., 1987; Negroni, et al., 1987; Terrell and Hughes, 1992).

Itraconazole is metabolized by the liver and excreted mainly in the feces. Only a minimal amount can be found in the urine or cerebrospinal fluid (Medical Letter editors, 1986). Absorption is improved when there is food in the stomach. The toxicity is low. It is more active than ketoconazole against sporotrichosis, aspergillosis, and chromomycosis. Despite low spinal fluid levels it has been effective in meningitides produced by cryptococcosis and coccidioidomycosis and in disseminated histoplasmosis. A particular role in suppressive long-term therapy of cryptococcal meningitis in the presence of immunodeficiency syndrome to prevent relapse is promising (Terrell and Hughes, 1992).

Almost all current studies of itraconazole relate to the early results of therapy. Exact doses and long-term results, including late relapse of infection, are not yet available.

In general antifungal agents are more toxic than other agents used to treat human disease and require constant surveillance during therapy for evidence of adverse effects, which are sometimes severe. In addition, many fungal infections are found in the increasing population of patients who have depression of their immune systems, either from basic immune system-altering diseases or from therapies for serious conditions by methods that are detrimental to the protective systems.

Hydatid Disease

José J. P. Camargo

DEFINITION

The word *hydatid* comes from the Latin *hydatis,* meaning a drop of water. It implies a cyst-shaped structure that contains waterlike fluid. Although *hydatid* and *cyst* have the same meaning and the expression *hydatid cyst* is redundant, its use is "consecrated" in the medical literature.

HISTORICAL NOTE

Hydatid disease, or echinococcosis, is certainly one of the oldest human diseases. Hippocrates stated that "when the liver is filled with water and bursts into the epiploon, in this case the belly is filled with water and the patient dies" (Adams, 1946). Galen, in the first century A.D., also made reference to this disease. During the Middle Ages it was thought that the lesions were manifestations of some other morbid condition, but in the seventeenth century, Francesco Redi, an Italian physician, recognized the animal origin of hydatid cysts. A few years later Edward Tyson (1650–1708), who had studied the common ascaris worm, came to suspect the parasitic nature of the disease (Dew, 1928).

In 1782 Goeze accurately described the cyst of the tapeworm and its head with suckers and hooklets; he called it *Taenia visceralis socialis granulosa*. In 1786 Batsch recognized the small larva armed with a crown of hooklets under the microscope. Finally in 1808 Rudolphi studied the adult worm in the intestines of the dog and published a large treatise on the parasite, giving it the name Echinococcus (Dew, 1928).

In 1853 von Siebold, in a classic series of experiments, infected dogs with larvae of the parasite obtained from typical hydatid cysts of sheep, thereby establishing conclusively the relationship between the adult worm in the dog and the cystic larval form in the sheep (Saidi, 1976).

In the middle nineteenth century, the position of humans in the parasite's life cycle was defined as being identical to that of sheep (i.e., transmission through food of larvae derived from human sources to dogs and recovery of the mature worms in this animal's intestine).

The first report in medical literature of hydatid cyst in humans is attributed to Bremser in 1821 (Romero-Torres and Campbell, 1965).

HISTORICAL READINGS

Dew H: Hydatid Disease—Its Pathology, Diagnosis and Treatment, Australasian Medical Publishing, Sydney, 1928

Romero-Torres R, Campbell JR: An interpretative review of the surgical treatment of hydatid disease. Surg Gynecol Obstet 104:851, 1965

Saidi F: Surgery of Hydatid Disease. WB Saunders, Philadelphia, 1976

BASIC SCIENCE

Parasite and Its Cycle

The Echinococcus belongs to the phylum Platyhelminthes and the family Taeniidae. *Echinococcus granulosus* is the most common among the four best known species. When we consider the other species, only the *Echinicoccus multilocularis* produces disease in humans and has a highly aggressive behavior, but it is a much rarer form. *E. granulosus* as an adult parasite measures abouts 4 to 6 mm in length, and it is formed of four segments: the head with transverse diameter of 0.5 mm and three proglottids (Fig. 20-28).

The head (Fig. 20-28A) has a double crown of hooklets that serves to fix the parasite in the intestinal wall of its definite host, the dog or any other related canine. The first proglottid (Fig. 20-28B) is not a well-defined segment; the second one (Fig. 20-28C) contains the required equipment for sexual reproduction of this true hermaphrodite; and the

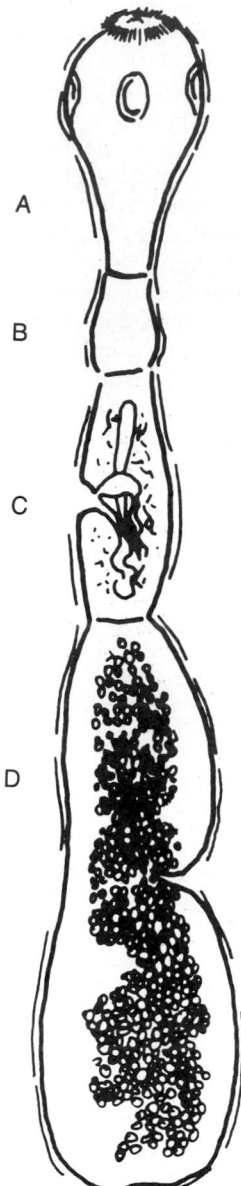

Figure 20-28. The adult parasite with **(A)** head, **(B)** indefinite proglottid, **(C)** the proglottid, which contains the sexual organs, and **(D)** the pregnant proglottid, which contains the eggs.

third (Fig. 20-28D), also called the pregnant proglottid, contains the eggs, varying in number from 400 to 800. When this last proglottid reaches maturity, it gets loose and is eliminated in the excrement of the infected animal, therefore infesting the environment. After this segment is discharged, the anterior becomes pregnant for reproduction later on. The detached eggs (Fig. 20-29) are highly resistant to physical and chemical agents and survive in adverse conditions for several weeks or months. The use of various agents supposed to be harmful in vitro to the egg has not been successful and has discouraged the use of any kind of treatment of food potentially contaminated.

Humans, similar to sheep and cattle, become an intermediate host. They are infected by ingestion of contaminated food

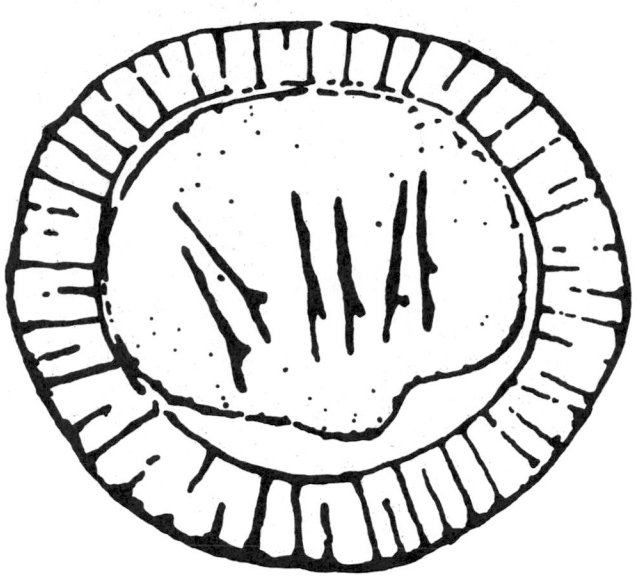

Figure 20-29. The egg eliminated by the adult worm.

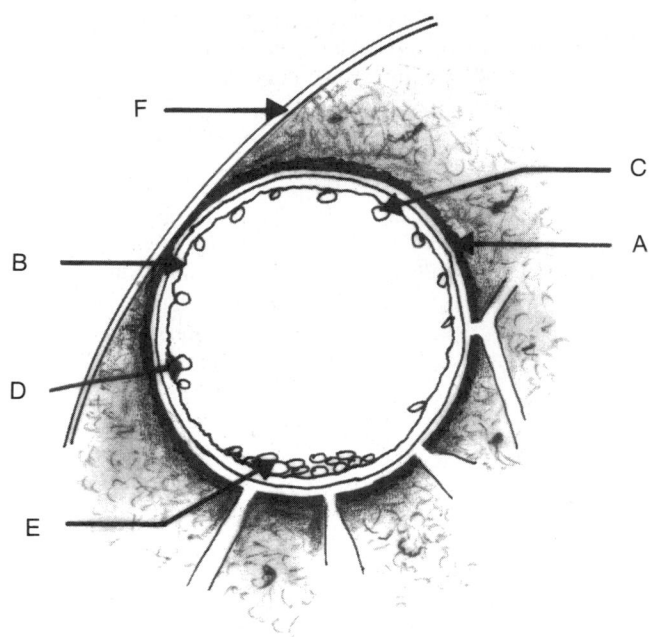

Figure 20-30. The hydatid cyst and its components: **(A)** host membrane or pericyst, **(B)** chitinous membrane or ectocyst, **(C)** germinal layer or endocyst, **(D)** the scolex, **(E)** the hydatid sand, and **(F)** the visceral pleura.

or, more frequently, by coming into close contact with an infested dog. In the duodenum or in the upper part of the jejunum of the intermediate host, the resistant chitinous membrane that covers the egg is ruptured by the action of the digestive enzymes. This allows the release of the hexacant embryo (Fig. 20-29), which is ready to migrate through the intestine wall to the portal venous system, theoretically to the "chyle cisterna" through the lymphatic route of the intestine wall. This embryo (25 μm) can be retained by the sinusoid capillaries of the liver (30 μm), or if they escape they can remain in the lung where capillaries prevent further migration. Rarely embryos can bypass the pulmonary barriers through precapillary anastomoses. They are responsible for the sporadic cases of extrapulmonary and extrahepatic hydatidosis.

The rate of organ involvement is variable, but generally the liver is involved in 55 percent of cases and the lung in 40 percent. In the remaining 5 percent there is distribution to other organs, mainly the kidney, spleen, and bones.

After capillary embolization, many embryos are destroyed by phagocytosis, but some reach the larval stage of the Echinococcus—the hydatid cyst (Fig. 20-30). This is formed by two components (1) the parasite itself and (2) the adventitia (host reactional layer), also called the pericyst (Fig. 20-30A). The parasite has a vesicle filled with a waterlike fluid with a two-layer wall. The thick acellular outer layer is called the chitinous membrane or ectocyst (Fig. 20-30B), and the nucleated inner one is called the germinal layer or endocyst (Fig. 20-30C). The cellular mass is formed in this, ultimately resulting in the development of scolices (Fig. 20-30D). The scolices contain the head of the Echinococcus. They often detach from the vesicle's inner wall and float in the fluid, which constitutes the so-called hydatid sand (Figs. 20-30E and Fig. 20-31).

Each scolex is a potential parasite that remains invaginated until proper development conditions occurs. Such conditions are usually optimal when the scolex reaches the intestine of

the dog. This animal ingests the viscerae from other infected animals, completing the cycle. The common practice of feeding dogs with the lungs from sheep and cattle completes the cycle of the parasite. The scolex can develop a secondary hydatid cyst (the so-called daughter vesicle) in the intermediate host tissue if the contamination of this tissue happens by fluid spillage from a living cyst, a fact that should be remembered by the surgeon during surgical manipulation.

The hydatid cyst promotes the formation of a membrane of variable thickness in different organs, with the host attempting to isolate the parasite from the rest of the adjacent structures. This membrane, the pericyst, is formed by thick

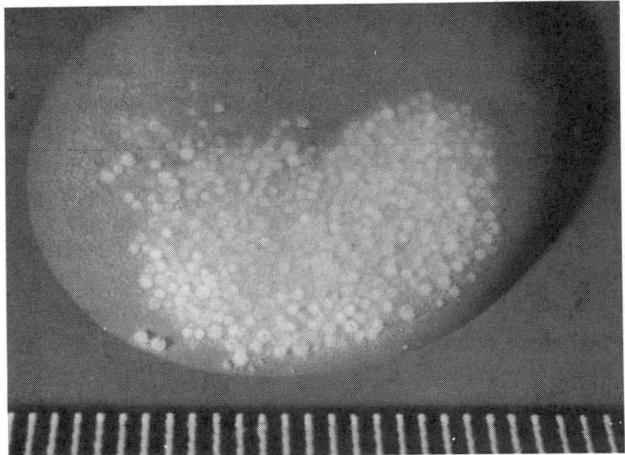

Figure 20-31. A drop of hydatid fluid after centrifugation viewed under a dissecting microscope showing hydatid sand.

connective tissue and in part by parenchymal tissue collapsed by compression. The parasite is nourished by osmosis, and its death depends on the breakdown of the equilibrium condition of the host.

Epidemiology

The countries considered to be highly infested include Uruguay, Argentina, Chile, Algeria, Tunisia, Cyprus, Turkey, Greece, Iran, the Balkans, Australia, and New Zealand. Moderate infestation is found in Peru, Brazil, Canada, Morocco, Alaska, Spain, France, and Italy. All others have minimal infestation. In Chile, for example, the echinococcal disease is prevalent with a rate of occurrence of 8.2 per 100,000 (Burgos, et al., 1991). In Tunisia hydatid disease is responsible for 10 percent of the country's surgical activity and costs approximately $80,000 per patient (Chaouachi, et al., 1989).

Many factors contribute to the development of hydatidosis, including poor hygienic conditions, lack of education, the population of animals such as dogs and sheep that transmit the disease, and physicochemical conditions of the soil, such a temperature (38 to 39°C), pH (6.8 to 7.6), low concentration of sodium chloride, and humidity (Karpathois, et al., 1985).

Pathologic Features

The lung is the second perferential site for the larval stage of the *E. granulosus* in humans. The pulmonary cysts that result from hematologic dissemination grow slowly; they are located below the visceral pleura and rarely in other intrathoracic sites. Because the usual entrance of the hydatid embryo into the lung occurs by hematologic dissemination, the implantation sites are almost invariably peripheral; they usually cause bulging of the visceral pleura. However, during its growth, the cyst tends to assume a more central position and, after a certain size is attained causes compression on adjacent bronchi. The sustained compression can result in ischemia and subsequent erosion of the bronchial wall (Fig. 20-32).

The space between the cyst's membrane and its adventitia is nonexistent, only becoming real by the time of the cyst's death, which is always related to an interruption in the parasite's nutritional equilibrium.

Clinical Features

The clinical and radiologic manifestations and the therapy for the hydatid cyst in the lung depend basically on its integrity, that is, intact (uncomplicated) or ruptured (complicated), as follows.

Intact Hydatid Cyst

Many cases are discovered as radiologic findings in asymptomatic patients or in the presence of an irrelevant clinical picture. The growth of the cyst is slow and it is symptomatic only when the cyst is large enough to cause compression. At this point an irritant cough becomes frequent; sometimes it is accompanied by chest pain.

Although it is rare, significant compression of adjacent structures may occur, which leads to less common manifesta-

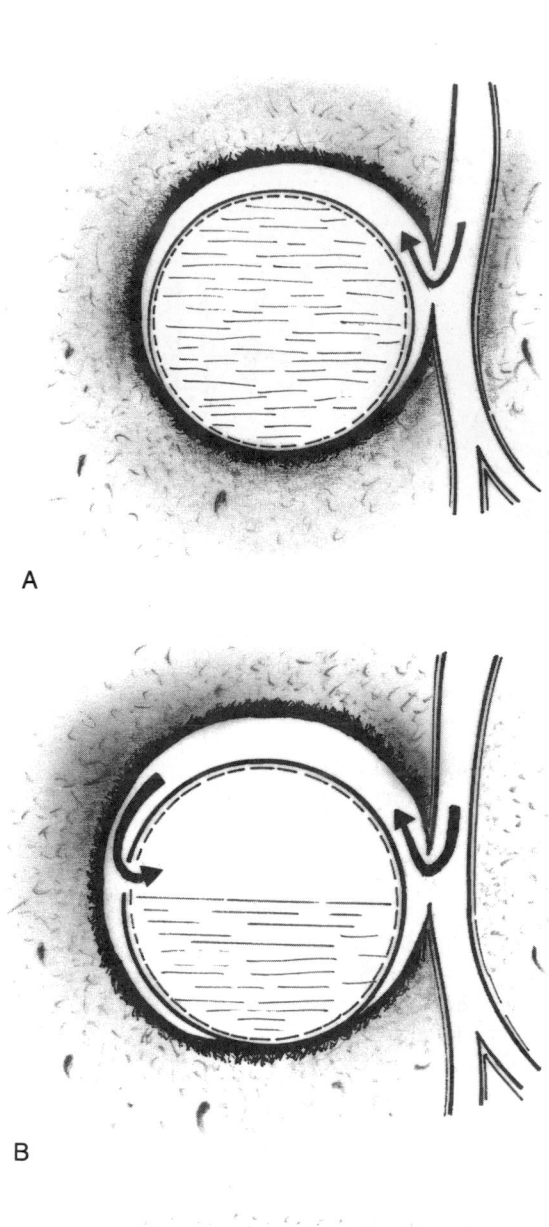

A

B

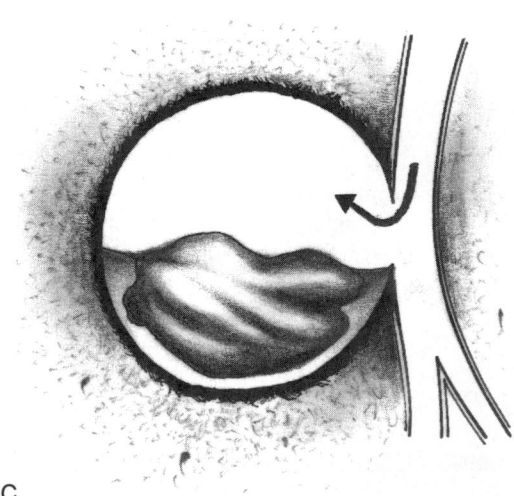

C

Figure 20-32. **(A)** Illustration of the initial mechanism of the cyst's death (detachment of the cyst's membrane). **(B)** The partial elimination of the fluid content of the cyst. **(C)** The cyst's membrane is not eliminated and persists in the lung cavity.

tions, such as superior vena cava syndrome and superior sulcus symptoms (Stathatos, et al., 1969).

The history of bloody sputum or, less frequently, frank hemoptysis is typical and announces the death of the cyst. By the time patients experience bloody sputum, the chest radiographs demonstrate a thin layer of air between the membrane of the host and the wall of the cyst (meniscus sign) (Fig. 20-33). The typical radiologic finding at this stage is a mass that measures more than 6 cm in diameter, is more prevalent in the periphery of the lower lobes, and has a smooth edge without signs of infiltration. The presence of an air lamina between the cyst and its adventitia is considered a pathognomonic radiologic finding of this disease. The changes in the fluid contents within the cyst are observed by the radiologist comparing radiographs in maximum inspiration and expiration or by simply changing the patient's position (e.g., decubitus and standing). Sometimes multiple cysts are found. Ocasionally an image that simulates a teardrop may suggest there is fluid inside the lesion, which contributes to the differential diagnosis of solid masses (Fig. 20-34). CT, magnetic resonance imaging (MRI) scans and the less costly ultrasound are valuable to confirm the diagnosis of a cystic lesion. If the diagnosis of hydatid cyst is suspected, needle aspiration is contraindicated because of the risk of pleural contamination.

Ruptured Hydatid Cyst

Rupture is the usual consequence of the death of the pulmonary cyst, whereas multivesiculation expresses the same phenomenon in the hepatic cyst. It is not known whether the death of the cyst occurs by separation of its membranes from the adventitia, which hinders its nourishment or the membranes separate because of the death of the cyst. Regardless of the mechanism involved, there is a sequence of clinical, radiologic, and anatomopatholgic events that are common in this stage of pulmonary echinococcosis. The loss of the cystic volume, with the appearence of gas in its cavity, and the membrane folding over onto itself into the cavity characterize the cyst's death. Bacterial contamination from bronchial involvement can simulate a chronic lung abscess, with the chitinous membrane included in the purulent fluid.

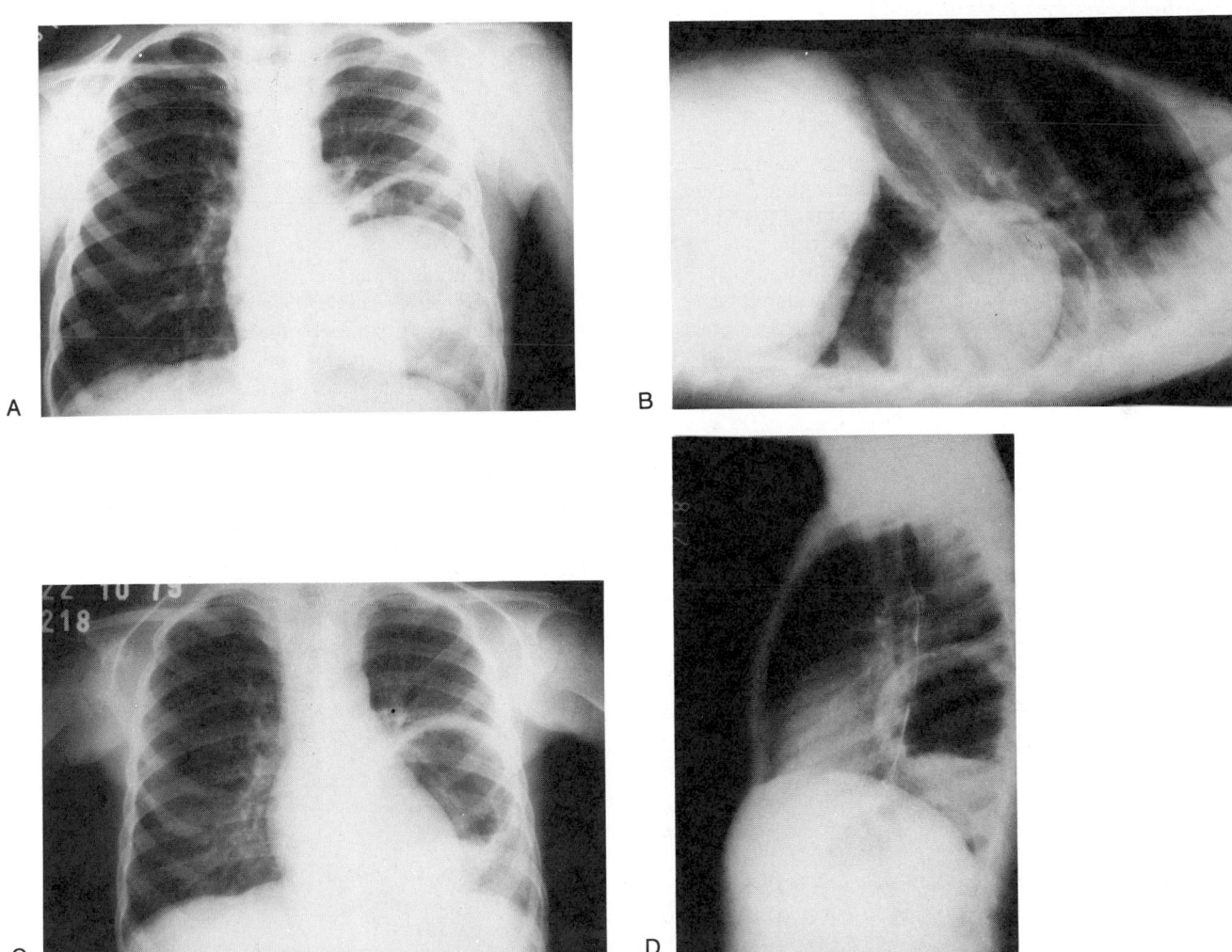

Figure 20-33. **(A & B)** Large cyst of the left lower lobe with meniscus sign. The only clinical complaint was bloody sputum. **(C & D)** Lung cavity almost empty after an expectoration. The cyst membrane lies on the bottom of the cavity.

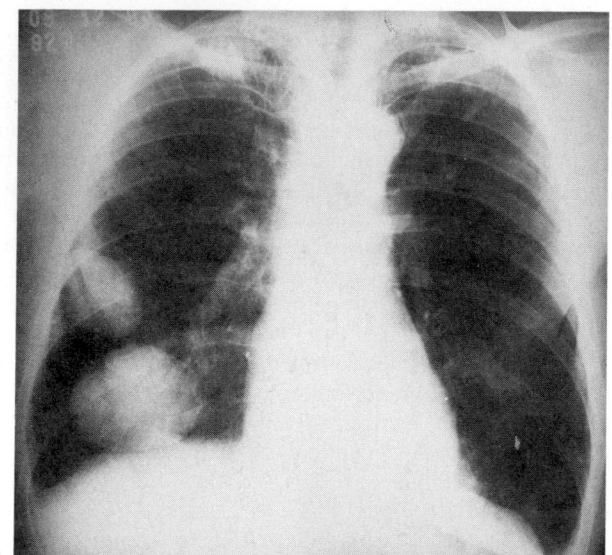
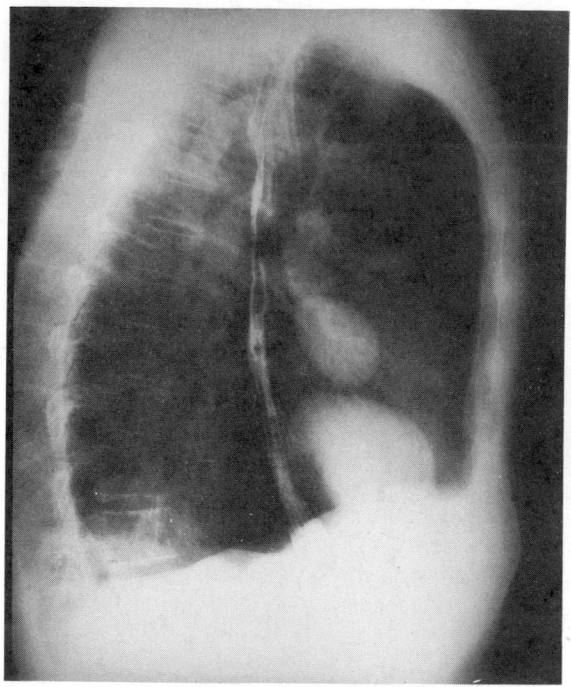

Figure 20-34. **(A & B)** This patient presents three cysts in the right lung; two are alive and one is dead. **(B)** The teardrop shape of live cysts in lateral radiograph is characteristic.

The intense inflammatory response that surrounds the cyst results in unresponsiveness to conservative therapy because of the inability to eliminate the membrane of the cyst (Sadrieh, et al., 1967) (Fig. 20-35).

The diagnostic possibility of a ruptured hydatid cyst with a retained membrane should always be considered when the surgeon is confronted with a chronic abscess that is unresponsive to usual therapy, especially if an irregular fluid level is seen in the cavity (water lily sign) (Fig. 20-36).

DIAGNOSIS

Clinical Presentation

The typical clinical picture for the diagnosis of pulmonary hydatidosis is represented by a young man (younger than 30 years of age in 75 percent of cases) who comes from an endemic region (85 percent) and presents with bloody sputum, chest pain, irritant cough, and radiograph of the chest

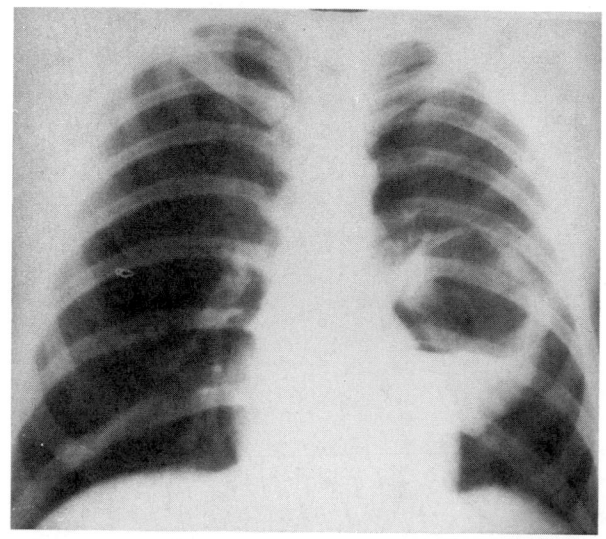
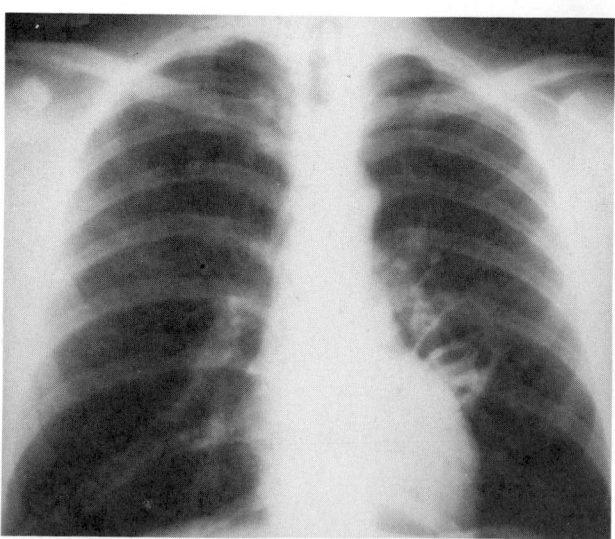

Figure 20-35. **(A)** The dead cyst with an irregular air-fluid level (water lily sign). **(B)** After elimination of fluid, the membrane folds in on itself.

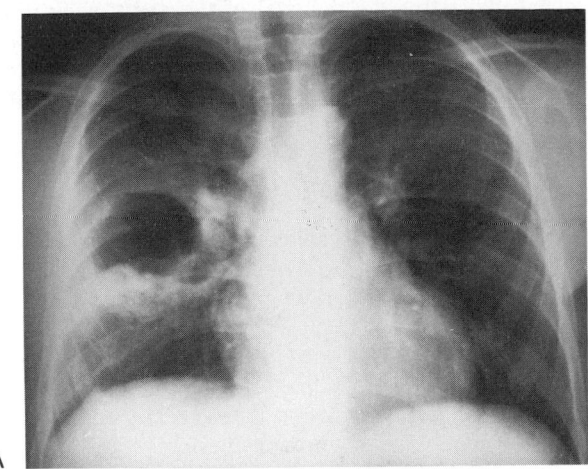
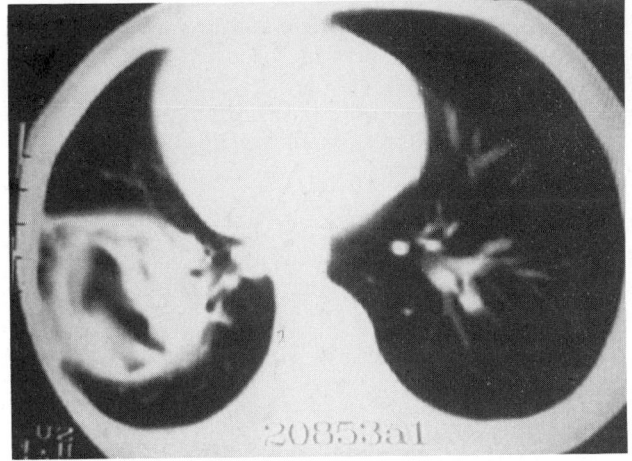

Figure 20-36. **(A)** The water lily sign is highly suggestive of a hydatid abscess. **(B)** The corresponding image in the CT scan.

showing single or multiple cystic lesions that predominate in the lower lobes. A history of a chronic abscess that is clinically untreatable and associated with the classic radiologic water lily sign also represents a frequent clinical presentation. Coughing up salty material occurred only in 10 percent of our patients. Many patients describe events compatible with hypersensitivity reactions, such as rash, urticaria, fever, rigor, and bronchospasm. At this stage the finding of eosinophilia has been often described (Marsden, 1979).

A history of pulmonary or hepatic hydatidosis is also a relevant fact for diagnosis. The coexistence of hepatic and pulmonary lesions should always be suspected. In 15 percent of our cases there was simultaneous involvement of the liver and lung. Inclusion of abdominal ultrasound or CT scan in the protocol of investigation of a lung lesion that is suspicious of hydatid origin is obviously important (Fig. 20-37). This investigation is especially worthwhile in the preoperative

evaluation of lesions that affect the right lung because it is possible to treat both the lung and the liver cyst in the same surgical procedure (Eren and Ozgen, 1990).

Laboratory Tests

Sputum Examination

Membranes, vesicles, scolices, and hooklets colored by the Best carmine are rarely identified but when present absolutely confirm only the diagnosis preoperatively.

Intradermal Testing (Casoni Test)

The Casoni test uses sterilized hydadid fluid as the antigen, and it is performed by injecting 0.20 or 0.25 ml into the anterior side of the forearm, similar to the procedure used for the tuberculin test. At the same time a control test with

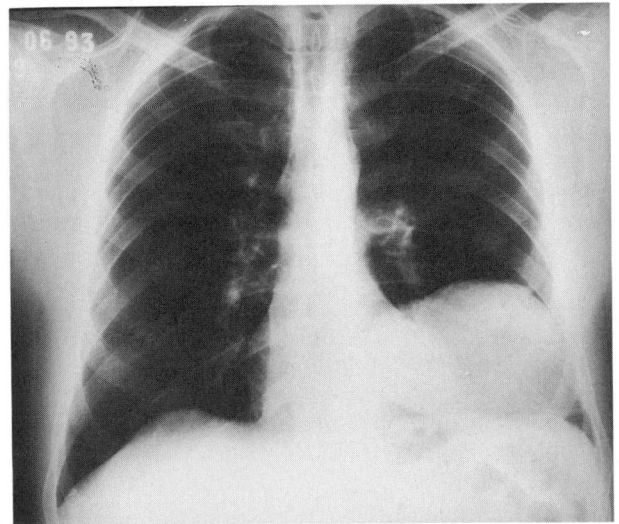
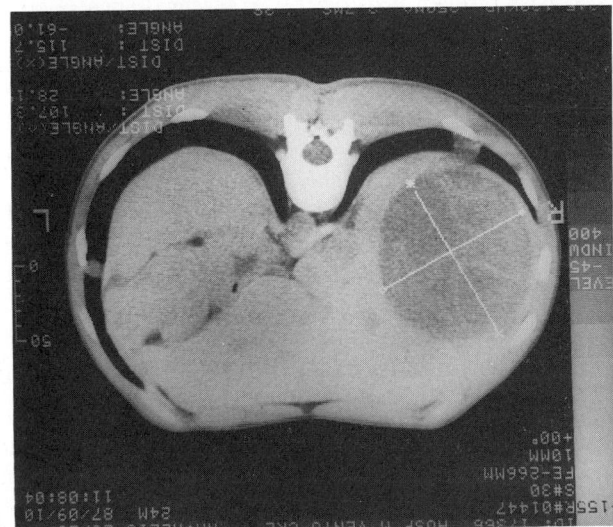

Figure 20-37. **(A)** A large hydatid cyst in the left lower lobe. **(B)** CT scan reveled a large hepatic cyst.

saline solution should be performed in the other forearm. The response is considered positive if the antigen produces a wheal with erythema, which may occur within the first hour after the injection. After 24 hours it is observed again. The positivity is variable and depends on the series; the rates range from between 70 to 95 percent. However, cross reactions with other kinds of parasites may occur, including Schistosoma and Taenia. According to Susman (1953), the immediate response is valuable before the first operation; it is postive in 75 percent of the uncomplicated cases and in 92 percent of the complicated or ruptured ones. The apersistently positive Casoni test result after surgical resection does not necessarily mean reinfection or the presence of residual cysts. On the other hand, the return to normal parameters means cure.

Complement Fixation (Weinberg Reaction)

The Weinberg reaction is positive in 75 percent of the cases and consists of the detection of IgM. In the cases in which the cysts are completely enclosed by a fibrous thick membrane, the reaction may be negative. A persistent positive test after surgical removal of a cyst indicates the absence of other living cysts.

Hemagglutination Test

The hemagglutination test was introduced in 1957 by Garabedian (Saidi, 1976). It has a low nonspecific reaction rate. Most investigators, using high titers of 1 : 400, regard it as diagnostic of the infection.

MANAGEMENT

Since the 1980s medical therapy has been attempted to treat hydatidosis because benzomidazolic drugs demonstrated some encouraging results. Gil-Grande (1983) reported partial or complete clinical responses in 36 to 94 precent of the patients treated with mebendazole. Morris (1985), using albendazole (10 mg/kg/day), obtained some remissions in 15 of 22 patients. The effectiveness of these drugs is apparently dependent on the thickness of the cyst wall because the drug has to pass through it to reach the germinal layer. Young patients and those with small cysts that have thin walls appear to benefit most from this medical therapy (Aletras and Symbas, 1989). The lack of response in many cases, the high rate of recurrence when therapy is not completed, and the intensity of the side effects of these drugs have restricted their use to selected cases that can be closely observed.

Although small cysts can be spontaneously eliminated, surgery is still the most effective therapy. Regardless the surgical methods adopted, the removal of the entire parasite, prevention of its dissemination, maximal preservation of pulmonary function, and the immediate obliteration of the remaining cavity are the basis for effective therapy.

In most cases in intact cysts, simple removal fulfills all these requirements and certainly is the ideal approach. The host membrane is widely opened by a short incision that surrounds the most superficial part of the cyst in the visceral pleura (Fig. 20-38). The cyst is then pushed out of its chamber with the aid of high-pressure ventilation provided by manual inflation of the corresponding arm of a double-lumen tube.

Immediately after the removal of the cyst, while positive pressure is maintained in the airway, the residual cavity is evacuated by continuous aspiration or is compressed to prevent contralateral aspiration of blood or other secretions. Until hemostasis is secured the enucleation method, originally described by Ugon (1947) and Barret (1949), is the most adequate technique to remove intact small and medium pulmonary cysts.

Peschiera (1972) suggested that the live contents should initially be evacuated to prevent the risk of contamination by rupture of the cyst during removal. During evacuation of the contents of large cysts, a scolicidal solution is used to avoid contamination of the operative field. Formaldehyde solution or pure formaldehyde have been suggested by many authors, but leakage of these substances is harmful to the pericystic tissues and therefore interferes with the healing process and increases the incidence of bronchopleural fistula (Saidi, 1976). The use of hypertonic saline is less harmful to the tissues and is recommended by many surgeons (Aletras and Symbas, 1989). The injection of scolicides into the cyst has been suggested by Peschiera (1972), or they can be inserted into the pericyst after the removal of the cyst, which is the technique adopted in our hospital. When we aspirate the cyst, we perfer to clamp the corresponding lobar bronchus to prevent bronchial contamination. A 10-gauge needle is directly connected to the suction apparatus and introduced into the most superficial part of the cyst. As the fluid is aspirated, an immediate retraction of the pericyst is observed. With the suction system still connected, the pericyst is opened, and the membrane is removed after division of its weak fibrinous adhesions.

Saidi (1976) enthusiastically recommended the aspiration of the cysts, pulmonary or hepatic, using cryogenic surgery, a creative procedure unknown in most countries.

After the removal of the cyst, the remaining cavity can be treated in a variety of ways. In 1948, Perez-Fontana (1948) from Uruguay suggested the resection of the host membrane as routine to prevent the infectious complications that result from residual cavities with walls that are too thick to collapse spontaneously. The resection of the host membrane identifies bronchial leaks into the parasitic chamber. They are sutured, and then the cyst is closed with a spiral suture that approximates the walls surrounding the wound left in the pulmonary parenchyma caused by the removal of the cyst and its adventitia.

In Perez-Fontana's (1948) pericystectomy, there is more bleeding and air leakage (Aletras and Symbas, 1989). In most cases, especially in young adults and children, the pericyst is thin, and the remaining cavity can be obliterated by simply approximating its walls by means of multiple absorbable sutures (Vicryl or chromic catgut).

Pulmonary hydatid cysts of 10 cm or more should be evacuated before removal to avoid the risk of rupture during the surgical procedure. This recommendation is based on the fact that the thickness of the wall of the cystic membrane is not proportional to its volume, which results in greater risks of rupture in large cysts with thin walls. The evacuation of the cyst should be preceded by bronchial clamping to prevent the leakage of hydatid fluid by gravity into the contralateral lung, which would result in serious perioperative complica-

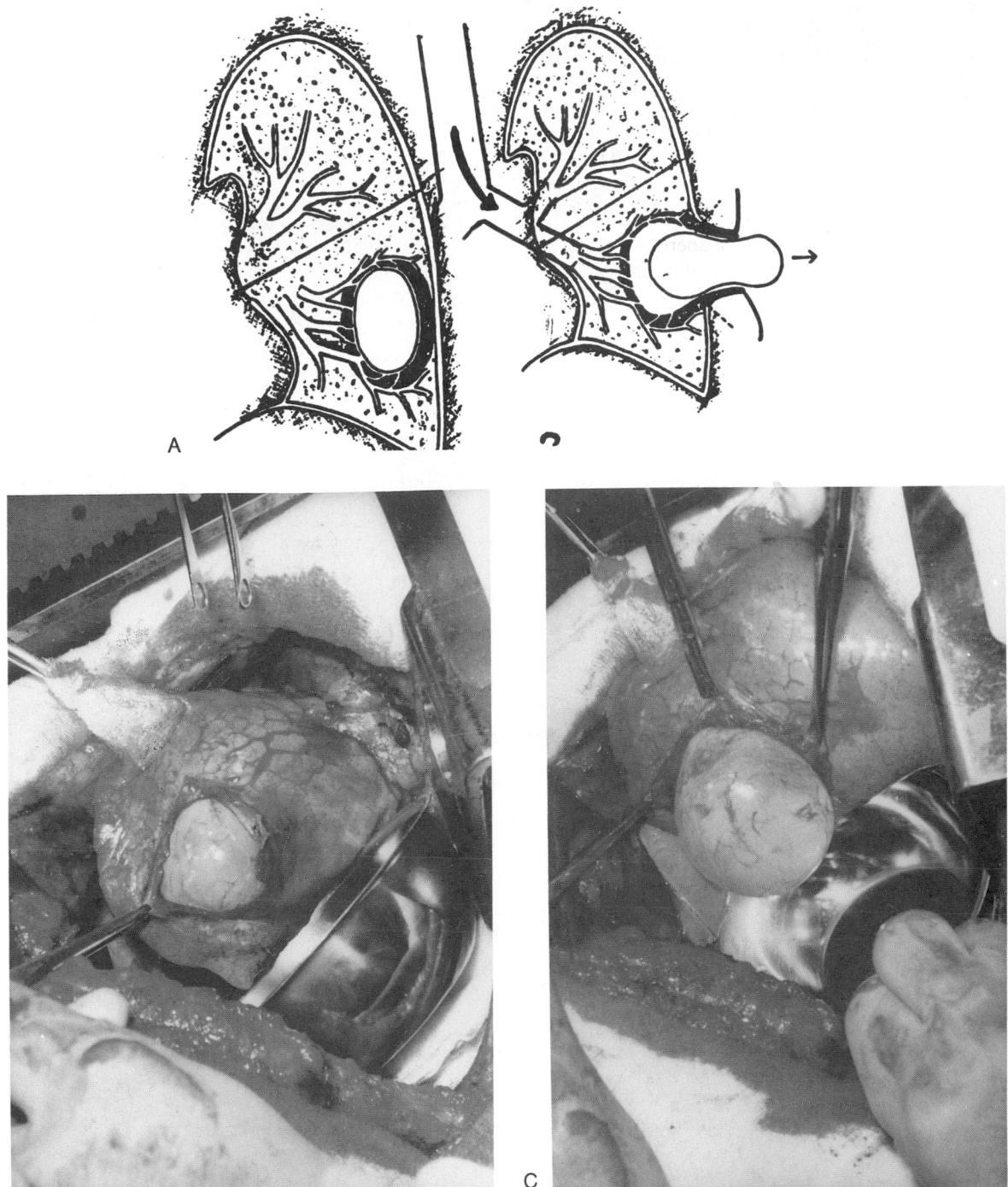

Figure 20-38.   **(A)** Schematic illustration of cyst enucleation. **(B)** The host membrane is broadly opened. **(C)** Lung inflation pushing out the cyst into the receptacle.

tions, including the possibility of massive dissemination to the opposite lung.

Large live cysts usually destroy the surrounding tissues by compression of the pulmonary parenchyma, and a segmental or more frequently a lobar resection is mandatory (Fig. 20-39).

A similar circumstance is often observed in cysts located in the middle lobe because of its relative lack of surrounding

parenchyma. In these cases lobectomy is the safest procedure. Recently ruptured cysts can be treated more conservatively because pericystectomy has already occured. An old dead cyst behaves as a chronic pulmonary abscess and can be treated by pulmonary resection, mostly lobectomy.

If intraoperative pleural contamination occurs, flooding the cavity with scolicidal agents is worthwhile. The use of hypotonic (distilled water) or hypertonic (10 percent saline) solu-

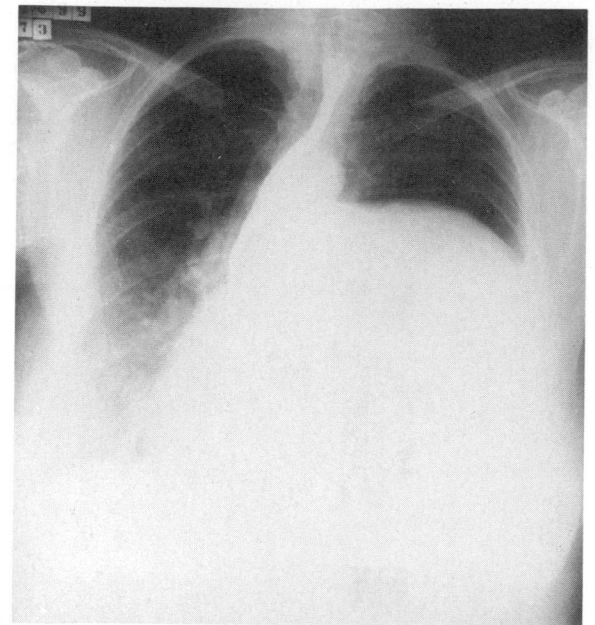

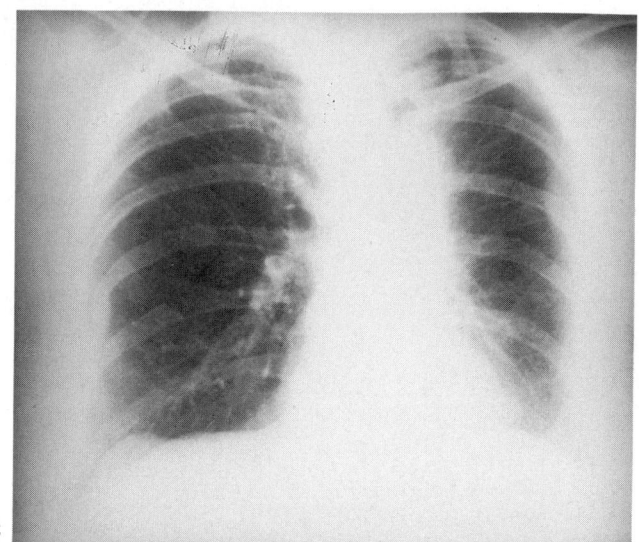

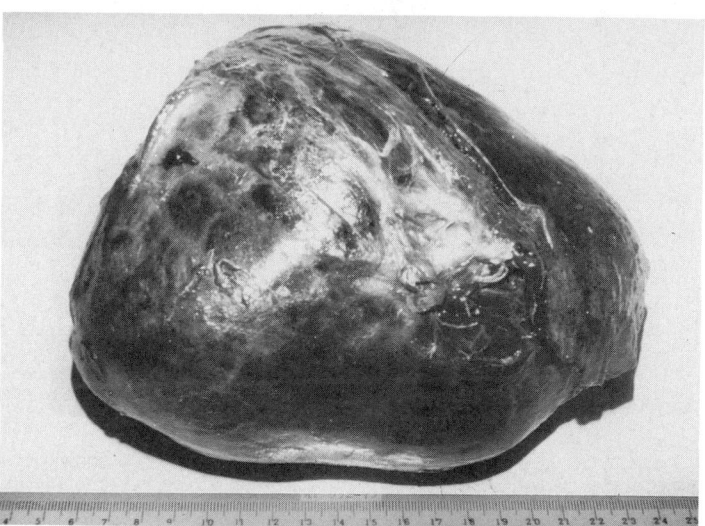

Figure 20-39. **(A)** A large hydatid cyst in the left lower lobe. **(B)** Surgical specimen, the entire lobe including the cyst. **(C)** Postoperative radiograph.

tions, or 10 percent formaldehyde solution has been suggested.

The potential complications associated with spillage of hydatid cysts include anaphylatic shock, pleural contaimination with resulting secondary hydatidosis, and contralateral bronchial dissemination (Katsas, 1957).

These operations have a low mortality rate, around 1 percent (Saidi, 1976; Aletras and Symbas, 1989).

Multiple Pulmonary Hydatidosis

This is defined as the presence of two or more primitive pulmonary hydatid cysts. It represents about 17 percent of the primary pulmonary presentations; in 75 percent of the cases, the cysts are bilateral (Tomalino, 1961).

Three or more cysts occur in 25 percent of these cases and result from massive contamination. They are frequently associated with the involvement of other viscera, especially, the liver (Fig. 20-40).

Unilateral multiple cysts are not difficult to excise. Bilateral ones are generally removed by staged posterolateral thoracotomies, performed on separate occasions. The procedure begins in the hemitorax with the dead cysts or, when they are all alive, on the side that contains the larger cysts or the greater number of cysts. When there is a concomitant liver cyst, the priority is right thoracotomy because this procedure allows the simultaneous removal of the liver and lung cysts by the surgeon simply adding a phenotomy to the procedure (Peleg et al., 1985; Eren and Ozgen, 1990).

At the end of the first thoracotomy, if the patient's general

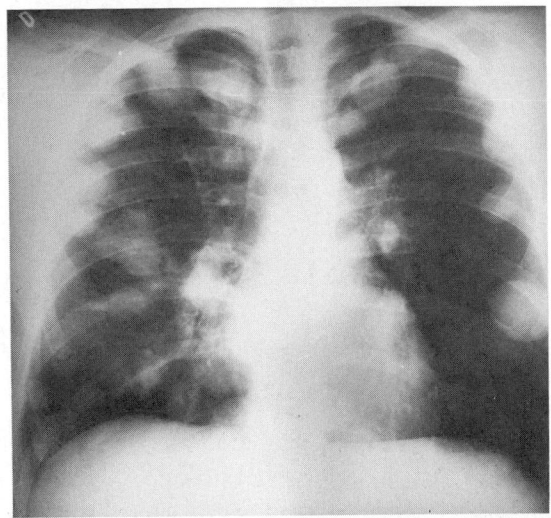

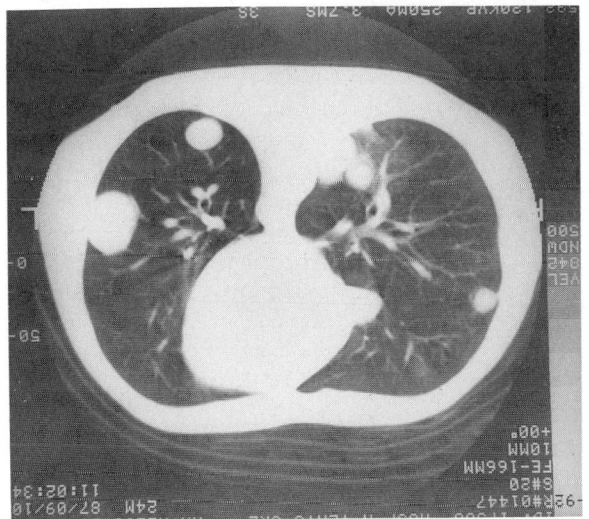

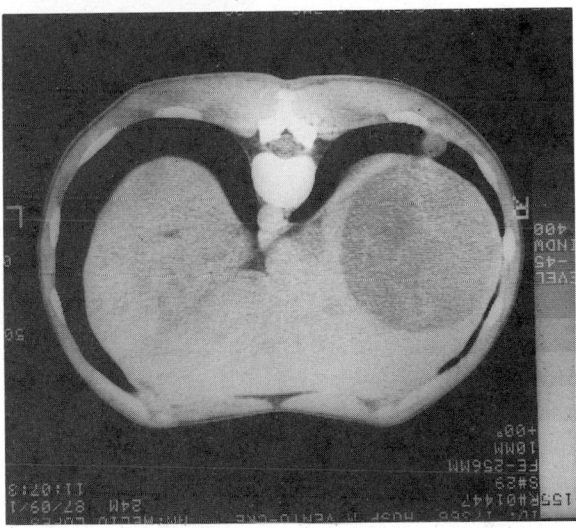

Figure 20-40. **(A)** Multiple bilateral pulmonary hydatid cysts. **(B)** CT scan showing the cysts of varying sizes. **(C)** The mother hepatic cyst that is responsible for hematologic dissemination.

condition permits, a contralateral thoracotomy can be performed during the same anesthesia. Young patients, with low surgical risks, are able to cope with sequential bilateral thoracotomies, which have psychological and economic advantages and a shorter hospital stay.

Several surgeons have used a median sternotomy for bilateral lesions (Cetin, et al., 1988). Although it carries less morbidity than the standard posterolateral thoracotomy, the sternotomy approach can pose a technical challenge, especially when the cysts are prevalent in the dorsal pulmonary segments.

When the number of cysts is great, it is important to distinguish between two different entities: multiple hydatidosis and metastatic pulmonary dissemination. In multiple hydatidosis, surgical therapy focuses on the excision of all lesions, similar to the approach used for malignant metastatic lesions, such as sarcomas. In these cases the clinical symptoms are often minimal, and many patients are assymptomatic, despite the great number of cysts. In metastatic pulmonary dissemination, pulmonary vascular involvement is characteristic, and the clinical picture is different. The patient presents with persistent cough, dyspnea, and early signs of cor pulmonale. Generally the cyst that causes hematologic dissemination is located in the liver and rarely in the heart. In these latter cases, the removal of all cysts is technically impossible, considering the location and frequent vascular involvement.

Most surgeons recommend the removal of the mother cyst (hepatic or cardiac) and observation. Occasionally after repeated episodes of expectoration, several vesicles are eliminated. The use of antihelminthic drugs has not been successful, and the tendency to have early cor pulmonale identifies a bad prognosis of these patients.

Although it has not been performed, bilateral lung transplantation appears to be a viable alternative for these unfortunate patients.

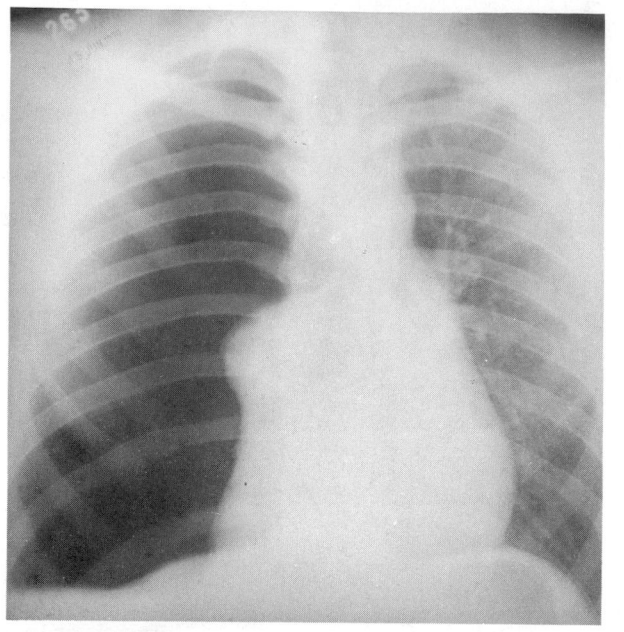
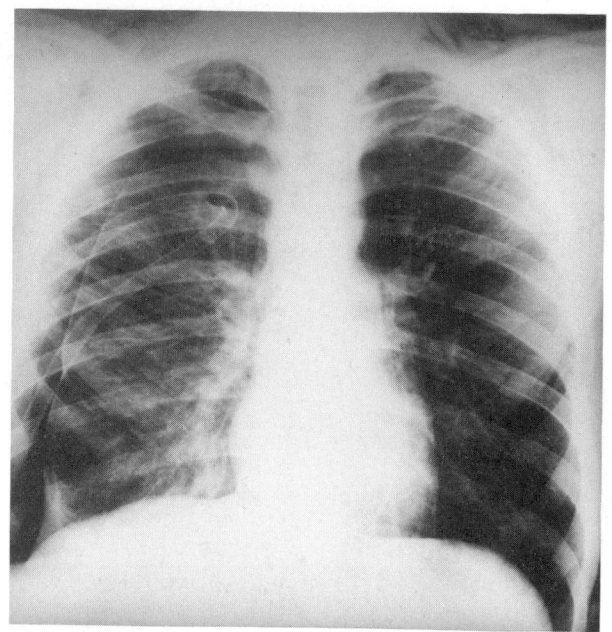

Figure 20-41. **(A)** A right spontaneous pneumothorax, with complete collapse of the lung. **(B)** An incomplete lung reexpansion and continuous air leakage.

Complications of Hydatidosis

The pleural complications of hydatid disease are relatively common (Tomalino, 1959). Rupture of a hydatid cyst into the pleura results in a pneumothorax followed quickly by a hydropneumothorax as a result of the intensity of the pleural reaction (Jesiotr and Romanoff, 1972). Occasionally surgical exploration detects a live cyst, entirely in the pleural cavity (Scremini and Rosa, 1970).

The pneumothorax is often massive; it is occasionally under tension and, when submitted to pleural drainage, presents a massive air leak with incomplete pulmonary expansion (Fig. 20-41). A pneumothorax that is unresponsive to pleural drainage in a young patient who comes from an endemic area

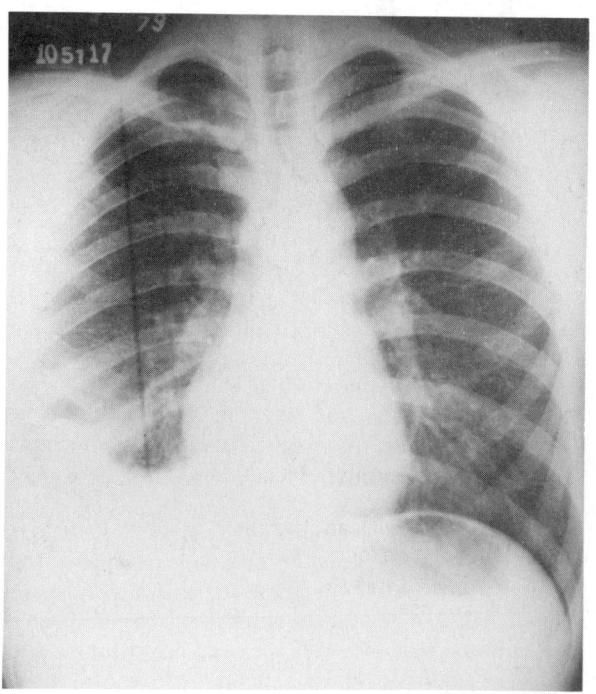
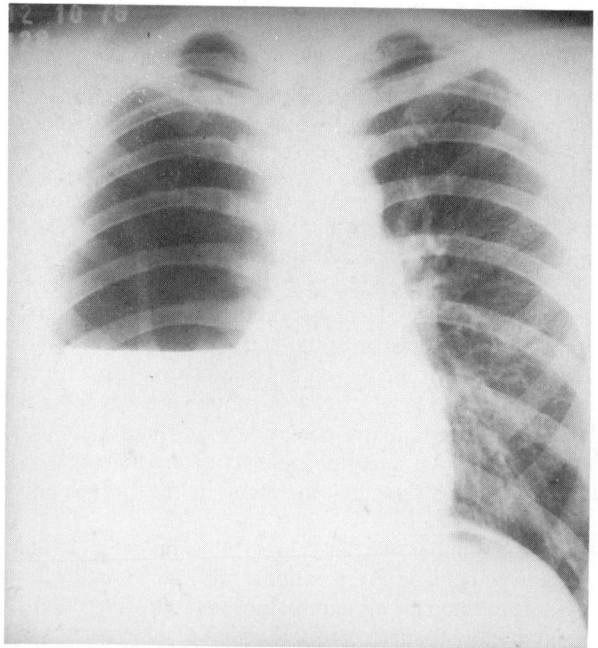

Figure 20-42. **(A)** A cavitated lesion in the right lower lobe. **(B)** One week later the patient presents with a hydropneumothorax. Thoracoscopy revealed the hydatid membrane floating in the empyema fluid.

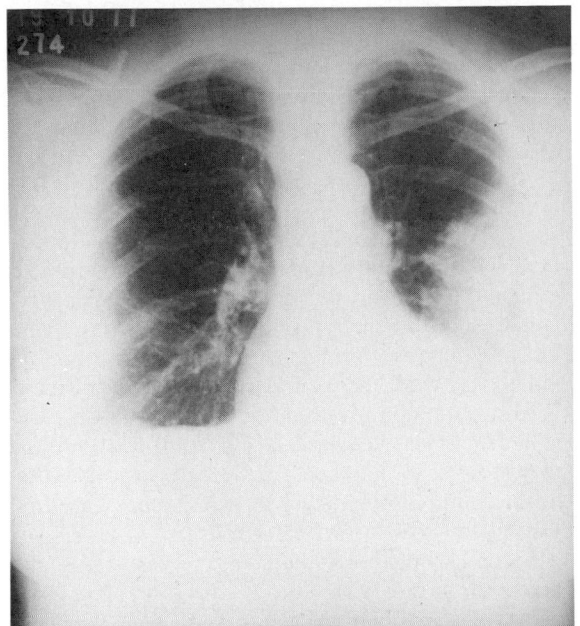

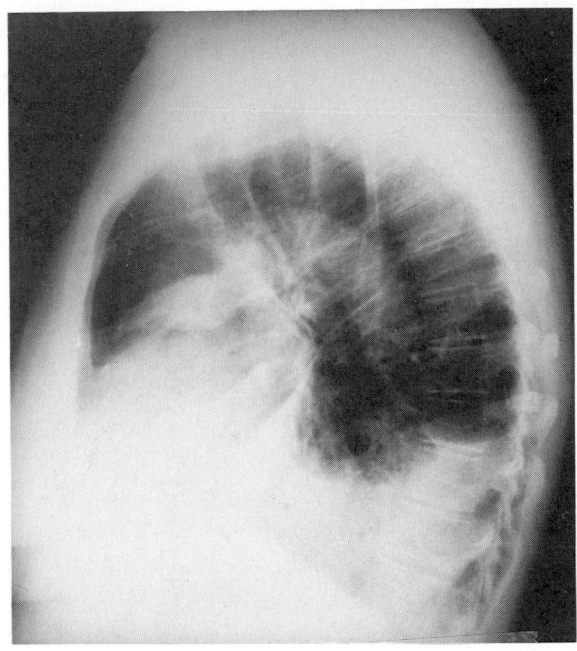

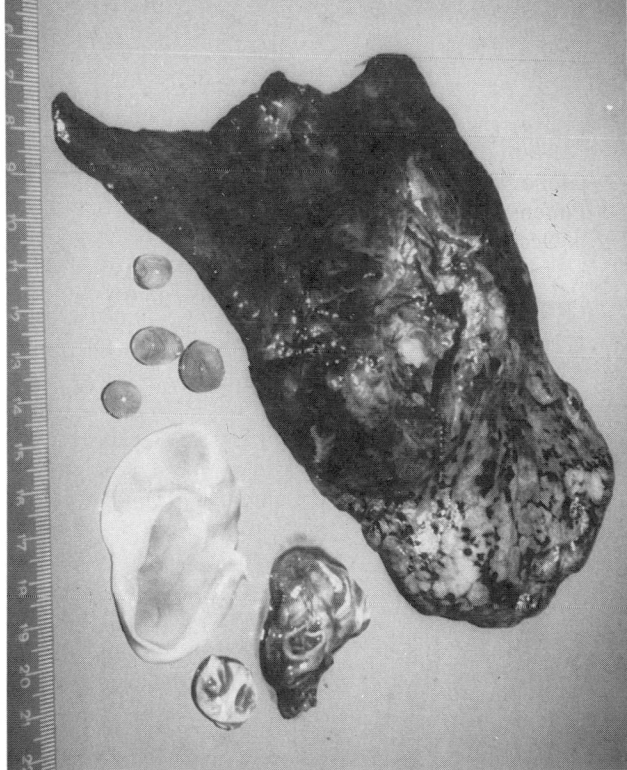

Figure 20-43. **(A & B)** A 66-year-old woman, a heavy smoker, who presented with an irregular left upper lobe mass and bloody pleural effusion. Cytologic and pleuroscopic test results were negative for malignancy. During thoracotomy a hydatid cyst was found in the anterior segment. **(C)** Surgical specimen of a large cyst and several small vesicles. The multiple vesiculation is an uncommon finding in pulmonary hydatid disease.

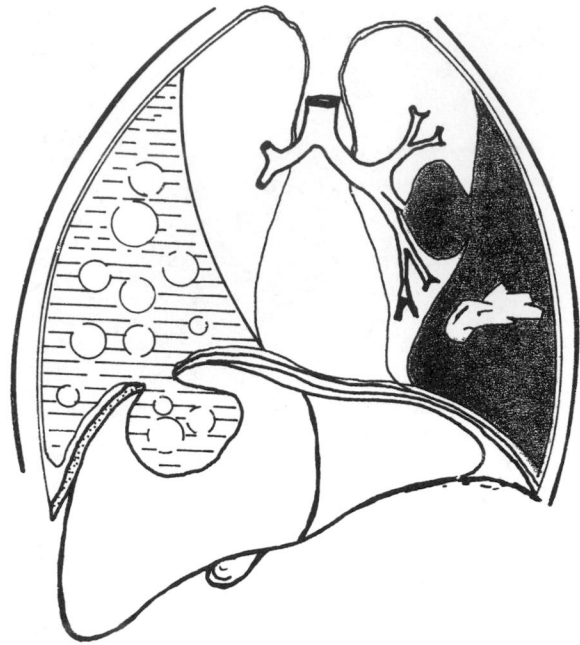

Figure 20-44. Two causes of spontaneous pleural contamination are the pulmonary hydatid cyst or the hepatic cyst. In both situations the cysts can be alive or dead.

should raise the surgeons suspicion of hydatid disease. Many times the definite diagnosis is an unexpected surgical finding in a patient who is undergoing exploratory thoracotomy for therapy of a pneumothorax that is unresponsive to closed-chest tube drainage. Segmental or wedge resection is usually required in these cases.

The large bronchopleural communication that results from the rupture of an hydatid cyst to the pleura contributes to

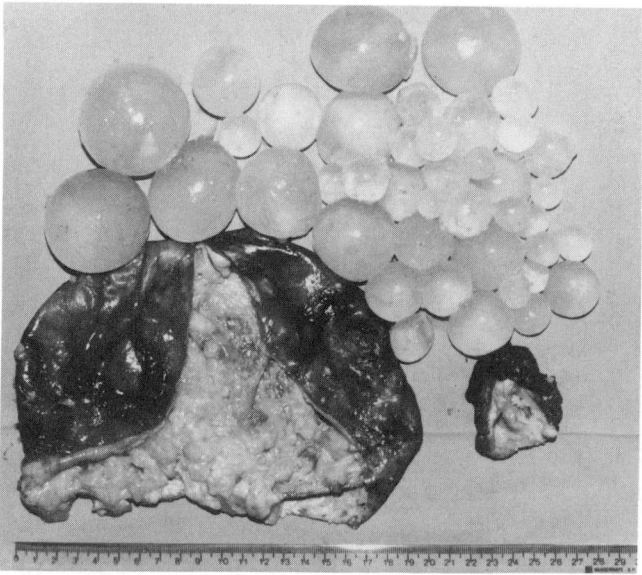

Figure 20-45. A large hepatic cyst removed entirely, showing the countless small vesicles characteristic of the cyst in liver hydatid disease. (Courtesy of Roberto Koch, M.D.)

the evolution of an empyema if the correct therapy is delayed. Many times when open drainage is performed to treat a chronic empyema, fragments of hydatid membranes can be recognized in the aspirated material (Fig. 20-42). Most of these cases require a segment or lobar resection with associated decortication.

An unusual presentation of pleural hydatidosis is attributed to an allergic reaction with recurrent serosanguineous effusions similar to neoplasic pleural effusions (Fig. 20-43). The cytologic results are negative for malignant cells, but these effusions present an intense eosinophilia, which when associated with the parenchymal lesions, which are apparently cystic, may lead to the correct diagnosis with removal of the pulmonary cyst, the pleural effusion does not recur.

An uncommon presentation is the hydatithorax. This results from massive leakage of hydatid fluid into the pleura; many vesicles are present. In these cases besides the removal of the ruptured pulmonary cyst, it is necessary to clean the pleural cavity with scolicidal solution.

Secondary pleural hydatidosis can result from the spontaneous rupture of a hepatic or live pulmonary cyst into the pleura (Fig. 20-44) or more frequently from surgical contamination when the cyst is removed. It is a serious complication of hydatidosis because of the pleural involvement (often massive) and the extreme difficulty of the complete removal of all cysts.

Thoracic extension of a hepatic cyst located in the superior aspects of the liver is on the whole uncommon. Crausaz (1967) found this in 3 percent of cases, but Toole, et al. (1953) reported an incidence of only 1 percent in 1,250 liver cysts. They believed that intrathoracic rupture is usually a consequence of suppuration within the liver cyst, which causes destruction of the pericyst and the surrounding tissues. It is also my impression that secondarily infected subdiaphragmatic hydatid cysts are more prone to break down the anatomic integrity of the diaphragm than are bacteriologically sterile ones.

The diaphragm acutally resists rupture of the cyst into the thoracic cavity to a remarkable degree, but when the migration occurs, the pleural adhesions that result from the intense inflammatory reaction may contain the rupture site and prevent dispersion of cystic contents into the pleural space. The only course open to the parasite is to penetrate the lung parenchyma. Rarely supradiaphragmatic adhesions do not form or are small. Then extrusion of the liver cyst is diverted into the free pleural space, and the lung is saved from invasion by the parasite.

The pulmonary parenchyma, once it is involved, undergoes an intense inflammatory reaction, and two lung lesions can be identified—a sinuous track that establishes a communication between the biliary and the bronchial system and a true intrapulmonary cavity. In the early stages there is only an asymtomatic elevation of the hemidiaphragm seen on the chest radiograph. At the other extreme the patient presents the rare but grave clinical picture of bronchobiliary fistula. The pulmonary lesion or the uncommon secondary pleural hydatidosis that results from transdiaphragmatic migration are invariably multivesicular (Fig. 20-45).

In most cases is possible to treat this complication with a low thoracotomy. The associated surgical procedures depend on the intraoperative findings. Pulmonary decortication and suturing of the small bronchial fistula in the lung surface are usually sufficient. Sometimes a minor resection, and rarely a lobectomy, is necessary. The multiple vesicles are removed as is the host membrane of the liver cyst, the diaphragm is sutured, and both cavities are drained separately.

A rare and little known complication of primary hydatid cyst of the lung is a secondary bronchogenic hydatid disease, which is even refuted by some authors, but occurs as a complication after surgical cure of a hydatid cyst that had ruptured into the bronchi. Sporadically this can occur spontaneously in immunosupressed patients (Kilani, et al., 1992).

COMMENTS AND CONTOVERSIES

Eradication of infestation of the intermediate host by controlling the primary host in high-incidence countries is paramount in dealing with this disease.

The following elements are considered fundamental for the prophylaxis of hydatidosis:

1. Sanitary education, mainly in the rural schools
2. Supervision of the butchery of animals for human consumption
3. Care in the disposal of the viscera of infested animals, including burning or deep disposal of the viscera, prolonged boiling, submitting the viscera to longitudinal and transversal deep cuts before submerging them in 30 percent saline solution between the first two steps (after this it can be given to the dogs) and control of infestation in the population of dogs with periodic administration of a vermifuge.

The eradication of hydatidosis has occurred in countries such as Iceland and New Zealand through adequate control. In these countries the presence of dogs in cities was prohibited and in rual areas their numbers were reduced.

J.J.P.C.

In North America nearly all cases of this disease are seen in immigrants with the classic syndromes outlined in this section. This is colloquially referred to as the "pastoral" variety of hydatid disease. The "sylvatic" form is most frequently seen in indigenous North Americans, mostly in northern Canada and Alaska. In this type a different strain of the tape worm is implicated, and the dog, deer, and moose are the usual intermediate hosts. In this form lung cysts occur more frequently than the liver cysts.

Other infesting metazoans include the round worm (Ascaris), hookworm (Ancylostoma), Strongyloides, Trichinella, and pulmonary larva migrans, most of which present with diffuse pulmonary infiltrations and eosinophilia. Often the surgeon's only responsibility in these diseases is to make the diagnosis by lung biopsy. On the other hand Paragonimus infestation can present as a nonsuppurative chronic granulomatous nodule that requires resection for diagnosis and Schistosomas infestation as Loeffler's syndrome, which requires bronchoscopy alone.

Protozoan infestations that occur in the lung include amebiasis, which like hydatid disease often presents as a lower lobe lung abscess that has perforated through the diaphragm by extension from the liver; toxoplasmosis, which with systemic involvement can present with a pneumonitis; and *P. carinii*, which is dealt with in more detail in the last section of this chapter.

Except for pneumocystis, hydatid disease continues to be the most common parasitic infestation that occurs in the thoracic cavity other than in those areas in which amebiasis is endemic. Because of the availability of worldwide travel, all thoracic surgeons must be aware of this disease and its management approaches.

R.J.G.

REFERENCES

Aletras H, Symbas P: Hydatid disease of the lung. p. 831. In Shields TW (ed): General Thoracic Surgery, 3rd Ed. Lea & Febiger, Philadelphia, 1989

Barret NR: Removal of simple univesicular pulmonary hydatid cyst. Lancet 2:234, 1949

Burgos L, Baquerizo A, Munoz W et al: Experience with the surgical treatment of 331 patients with pulmonary hydatidosis. J Thorac Cardiovasc Surg 102:427, 1991

Cetin G, Dogan R, Yuksel M et al: Surgical treatment of bilateral hydatid disease of the lung via median sternotomy: experience in 60 consecutive patients. Thorac Cardiovasc Surg 36:114, 1988

Chaouachi B, Ben-Sala S. Lakhoua R et al: Hydatid cysts in children. Diagnostic and therapeutic aspects. Apropos of 1195 cases. Ann Pediatr (Paris) 36:441, 1989

Crausaz PH: Surgical treatment of the hydatid cyst of the lung and hydatid disease of the liver with intrathoracic evolution. J Thorac Cardiovasc Surg 53:116, 1967

Dew H: Hydatid Disease—Its Pathology, Diagnosis and Treatment. Australasian Medical Publishing, Sydney, 1928

Eren N, Ozgen G: Simultaneous operation for right pulmonary and liver echinococcosis. Scand J Thorac Cardiovasc Surg 24:131, 1990

Gil-Grande LA: Treatment of liver hydatid disease with mebendazole: a prospective study of thirteen cases. Am J Gastroenterol 78:584, 1983

Jesiotr M, Romanoff H: Pneumothorax following rupture of a primary pleural hydatid cyst. J Thorac Cardiovasc Surg 43:594, 1972

Karpathois T, Fretzayas A, Nicolaidou P et al: Statistical aspects of hydatid disease in Greek adults. Am J Trop Med Hyg 34:124, 1985

Katsas GG: Morts subites ou rapides par kystes d'echinocoques. Arch Intern Hidatidosis 16:495, 1957

Kilani T, Horchani H, Daoues A: Secondary bronchogenic hydatidosis. Ann Radiol (Paris) 35:564, 1992

Morris DL: Albendazole: objective evidence of response in human hydatid disease. JAMA 253:2053, 1985

Peleg H, Best LA, Gaitini D: Simultaneous operation for hydatid cysts of right lung and liver. J Thorac Cardiovasc Surg 90:783, 1985

Perez-Fontana V: Nuevo metodo de operar en el quiste hidatico del pulmon. Arq Pediatr Uruguay 19:5, 1948

Peschiera CA: Hydatid cyst of the lung. In Shields TW (ed): General Thoracic Surgery. Lea & Febiger, Philadelphia, 1972

Romero-Torres R, Campbell JR: An interpretative review of the surgical treatment of hydatid disease. Surg Gynecol Obstet 104:851, 1965

Sadrieh M, Dutz W: Navabpoor MS: Review of 150 cases of hydatid cyst of the lung. Dis Chest 52:662, 1967

Saidi F: Surgery of Hydatid Disease. WB Saunders, Philadelphia, 1976

Scremini AP, Rosa F: Equinococosis pleural heterotopica. Torax 211, 1970

Stathatos C, Kontaxis AN, Zafiracopoulos P: Pancoast's syndrome due to hydatid cysts of the thoracic outlet. J Thorac Cardiovasc Surg 58:764, 1969

Susman MP: Hydatid disease as it affects the thoracic surgeon. J Thorac Cardiovasc Surg 26:111, 1953

Tomalino D: Equinococosis pulmonar multiple. Estudio sobre 100 observaciones. Torax 10:75, 1961

Tomalino D: Complicaciones pleurales de la hidatidosis. Torax 8:73, 1959

Toole H, Propatoridis J, Pangalos N: Intrapulmonary rupture of hydatid cysts of the liver. Thorax 8:274, 1953

Ugon CVA: Técnica de la extirpacion del quiste hidatico de pulmon. Bol Soc Cir Uruguay 18:167, 1947

Pulmonary Infections and the Immunocompromised Host

Diane E. Stover
M. Patricia Rivera

DEFINITION

Immunosuppression can be defined as a relative or absolute defect in antigen processing or effector cell (B-lymphocyte, T-lymphocyte, macrophage, or neutrophil) function. Clinically it is defined by the susceptibility to infection of certain populations rather than by specific laboratory tests of white blood cell or antibody function. These populations include patients with cancer, those who are receiving chemotherapeutic or immunosuppressive agents, those with AIDS, and those who have undergone organ transplantation.

HISTORICAL NOTE

Over the past several decades the number of immunosuppressed patients and the spectrum of disorders that they develop have markedly expanded. The reasons for this increase in both patients and diseases include more effective yet more intensive therapy for patients with cancer, the great success and widespread use of organ transplantation, and the AIDS epidemic. Radiotherapy and/or chemotherapy most likely have an impact on the natural defense mechanisms of the lung, thereby increasing susceptibility to pulmonary infections. The multiple quantitative and functional abnormalities of the cellular and humoral immune systems that occur in patients with HIV account for the marked increase in incidence of routine and opportunistic infections in the lungs of patients with AIDS.

With the expanding immunosuppressed population and often with the need to make a specific diagnosis urgently, physicians must choose the test or procedure that is most likely to yield a diagnosis quickly and at the lowest cost in morbidity. Probably the single most important technique that has revolutionized the diagnosis of pulmonary infections in the immunocompromised host is fiberoptic bronchoscopy. In 1967 Shigeto Ikeda of the National Cancer Institute in Tokyo designed and standardized the instrument that is now known as the flexible fiberoptic bronchoscope. This instrument has vastly expanded our ability to diagnose pulmonary infections in all patient populations, and it is well tolerated with few complications. It is particularly important in the immunocompromised host because it can be performed safely in the setting of mechanical ventilation, thrombocytopenia, and/or platelet dysfunction.

HISTORICAL READINGS

Fanta CH, Pennington JE: Pulmonary infections in the transplant patient. p. 207. In Morris PJ, Tilney NL (eds): Progress in Transplantation. Vol. 2. Churchill Livingstone, New York, 1985

Martin WJ, Smith TF, Sanderson DR et al: Role of bronchoalveolar lavage in the assessment of opportunistic pulmonary infections: utility and complications. Mayo Clin Proc 62:549, 1987

Pizzo PA, Robichaud KJ, Gill FA et al: Empiric antibiotic and antifungal therapy for cancer patients with prolonged fever and granulocytopenia. Am J Med 72:101, 1982

Stover DE: Diagnosis of pulmonary disease in the immunocompromised host. Semin Respir Med 10:89, 1989

Stover DE, Zaman MB, Hajdu SI et al: Bronchoalveolar lavage in the diagnosis of diffuse pulmonary infiltrates in the immunocompromised host. Ann Intern Med 101:1, 1984

EPIDEMIOLOGY

Classically textbooks divide infectious diseases that immunosuppressed patients acquire according to their underlying disease and in vitro immunologic abnormalities. However, not only intrinsic B- or T-cell immunologic defects but also other factors, such as environmental exposure, travel history, iatrogenic procedures, recent antibiotic therapy, and specific organ transplantation, must be considered when we try to identify a likely causative agent of pulmonary infection in the immunocompromised host (Shelhamer, et al., 1991).

Adults with HIV infection in the United States are primarily homosexual or bisexual men. Intravenous drug abuse is the second largest risk factor for the development of AIDS, and it is the primary source for heterosexual and perinatal transmission in the United States and Europe. A smaller percentage of total AIDS cases are due to transfusion of infected blood or blood products, especially in hemophiliac patients.

Although some epidemiologic features of HIV disease are common to all patients with AIDS, geographic variability in disease patterns occurs. For example, in the United States, *P. carinii* pneumonia (PCP) is the most common HIV-related pulmonary disease, whereas in Africa tuberculosis is seen with much greater frequency. Tuberculosis is also considerably more common in intravenous drug abusers, blacks, Hispanics, and patients from nonindustrialized countries than in white homosexual men. Some of these differences in infectious patterns may be explained by environmental and/or geographic exposure and the prevalence of infection among different patient populations, but other poorly defined and unknown risk factors appear to influence the pulmonary manifestations of HIV infection throughout the world.

CLINICAL FEATURES

General Considerations

The magnitude of pulmonary problems in the immunocompromised host is broad (Williams, et al., 1976; Murray and Mills, 1990). A listing of common pulmonary disorders found in this patient population is shown below.

The purpose of this section of this chapter is not only to discuss the most common infections that occur in the immunocompromised host but also to provide a framework for approaching the diagnosis of pulmonary infections, especially with regard to the selection of available diagnostic tests, procedures, and therapeutic interventions.

Common Causes of Pulmonary Infiltrates in the Immunocompromised Host

Infectious causes
  Bacterial
    S. pneumonia
    H. influenza
    S. aureus
    Gram-negative bacilli
    Legionella species
    Nocardia species
  Mycobacterial
    M. tuberculosis
    Atypical mycobacteria
  Fungal (opportunistic)
    Aspergillus species
    Mucor
    Candida species
    C. neoformans
    (Pathogenic)
    H. capsulatum
    C. immitis
  Viral
    Cytomegalovirus
    Herpes simplex
    Varicella-zoster
  Parasitic
    P. carinii
Noninfectious causes
  Pulmonary edema (cardiogenic and noncardiogenic)
  Neoplastic disorders
  Toxic lung injury (drug and radiation induced)
  Leukostasis
  Leukoagglutinin reaction
  Pulmonary hemorrhage
Unknown causes
  Nonspecific interstitial pneumonia
  Chronic organizing pneumonia

When the diagnosis of specific pulmonary diseases is considered in this population, several factors should be evaluated. The underlying immunocompromising condition and the immunologic defect that it imparts are important features (Singer, et al., 1979; Matthay and Greene, 1980) (Table 20-5). For example, patients with cell-mediated immune deficiencies, such as occur in lymphomas, organ transplantation, and/or high-dose corticosteroid therapy, are prone to infections, such as pneumocystosis, cytomegalovirus infection (CMV), tuberculosis, and cryptococcosis, and pathogenic (endemic) fungal infections, such as histoplasmosis and coccidioidomycosis. On the other hand, patients immunocompromised by virtue of granulocytopenia are susceptible to infections with gram-negative bacilli, *S. aureus,* and opportunistic fungi such as Aspergillus. A patient with breast carcinoma who is receiving high-dose corticosteroid therapy because of central nervous system metastases and then has diffuse bilateral pulmonary infiltrates develop is suspected of having PCP. The neutropenic patient with leukemia, who is receiving a course of empiric broad-spectrum antibiotics for a fever and then has a new pulmonary infiltrate develop, is more likely to have a fungal pneumonia, especially caused by Aspergillus (Pizzo, et al., 1982).

The radiographic pattern is helpful to focus the differential diagnosis on a certain subset of likely agents and estimate the urgency of making a specific diagnosis. A distinction is often made between processes localized to a lobe or segment and those that involve multiple lobes bilaterally, commonly described as diffuse. The presence of segmental or lobar infiltrates with a clinical history that suggests an acute illness would favor the diagnosis of bacterial pathogens, whereas diffuse infiltrates suggest opportunistic infections (such as PCP) or noninfectious processes (such as drug toxicity or lymphangitic spread of tumor) (Tenholder and Hooper, 1980).

Radiographic Appearance Associated with Pulmonary Infections in the Immunocompromised Host

Localized infiltrates (segmental or lobar)
  Bacteria
  Mycobacteria (especially tuberculosis)
  Fungi
Diffuse infiltrates
  P. carinii
  Viral pneumonia
  ARDS (sepsis with bacteria or fungus)
Hilar or mediastinal adenopathy
  Tuberculosis and atypical mycobacteria
  Pathogenic fungi
  Cryptococcus (occasionally)
Cavitation
  Bacteria (gram-negative bacilli, anaerobes, Nocardia, Actinomyces, and Legionella)
  Tuberculosis and atypical mycobacteria
  Septic emboli (bacterial and fungal)
Pleural effusion
  Bacteria
  Tuberculosis
  Fungi (occasionally)
Nodules
  Nocardia and Actinomyces
  Atypical mycobacteria
  Opportunistic fungi (especially Aspergillus)

Table 20-5. Relationship of Immune Defects to Pulmonary Infections

Immune Defect[a]	Examples of Disease with Immune Defect	Organisms Commonly Seen with Immune Defect

B-cell defect (decreased quantity or impaired function)	Some lymphoproliferative disorders (especially acute and chronic lymphatic leukemia)	Common
		  S. pneumonia
		  H. influenzae
		  Other gram-negative bacilli

	Multiple myeloma	
	Some drugs (especially corticosteroids antimetabolites and alkylating agents)	Less common P. carinii

T-cell defect (impaired cell-mediated immunity)	Some lymphoproliferative disorders (especially Hodgkin's disease)
	Renal insufficiency
	Some drugs (especially corticosteroids)
		Common
		  P. carinii
		  Mycobacteria
		  Cryptococcus and other pathogenic fungi
		  Herpesviruses (especially cytomegalovirus)

		Less common
		  Legionella
		  Nocardia

Granulocytes defect (decrease in number or impaired function)	Myeloproliferative disorders (especially acute myelogenic leukemia)
	Most chemotherapeutic agents
		Common
		  S. aureus
		  Gram-negative bacilli
		  Enteric bacilli
		  Opportunistic fungi (especially Aspergillus)

[a] During organ transplantation the immune defect that develops depends on the organ transplanted, the underlying disease, and the drugs used pre- or post-transplant. Pulmonary infections often have a predictable time for their appearance after certain transplants.

The presence of pleural-based, wedged-shaped infiltrates, cavitation, nodules, hilar adenopathy, or pleural effusions can also be helpful in focusing the physician's attention on certain disorders.

The seriousness of the illness and the rate of the patient's deterioration can help make decisions such as whether there is time to wait for a response to empiric therapy or whether an invasive procedure should be performed. Consideration of the disease's tempo can also narrow the differential diagnosis. Bacterial infections particularly in the neutropenic host can be acute in onset and heralded by fever with shaking chills. The acute, often fulminant onset of PCP is notorious in the non-HIV-infected patient. CMV pneumonia more often evolves over a period of weeks, a tempo similar to that for Aspergillus or Mucor. Nocardiosis, tuberculosis, and some fungal infections, such as cryptococcosis, usually follow an insidious course; their development over weeks to months may mimic noninfectious processes, such as metastatic disease, drug-induced lung injury, or radiation-induced fibrosis.

Other important considerations in the differential diagnosis of pulmonary disorders include the temporal relationship of the pulmonary disease to the underlying disease. For example, the HIV-infected patient in whom a pulmonary disorder develops early in the course of illness (i.e., when the CD4 lymphocyte count is greater than 500 cells/mm^3) is unlikely to have PCP and more likely to have either bacterial pneumonia or tuberculosis (Masur, et al., 1989). A patient who has undergone a bone marrow transplant and has pulmonary disease within the first month after the transplant is more likely to have bacterial or fungal pneumonia rather than CMV pneumonia, which usually develops several months after the bone marrow transplant (Fanta and Pennington, 1985) and almost always after engraftment occurs.

Prophylactic measures are being used to prevent pulmonary infections among patients who receive solid organ and bone marrow transplants or have HIV. Low intermittent doses of TMP/SMX or aerosolized pentamidine are commonly administered to these patients with a consequent marked reduction in the incidence of PCP. As a result the differential diagnosis of new pulmonary infiltrates is strongly influenced by the history of previous antibiotic prophylaxis.

Patient History

Besides these considerations other points in the clinical history that are worthy of emphasis include the travel history of the patient, an evaluation of the activity of the underlying disease, and a careful evaluation of the patient's fluid balance. If an HIV-infected patient with a CD4 lymphocyte count less than 100 cells/mm^3 recently traveled to the San Joaquin Valley, an area highly endemic for *C. immitis,* fungal disease with this organism should be strongly considered in the differential diagnosis of any pulmonary disorder. With such severe immunosuppression, this patient would be at high risk to have invasive disease develop. The female patient with breast cancer whose bibasilar interstitial infiltrates appear in combination with new hepatic and bony lesions should be suspected of having lymphangitic spread of her cancer, whereas in a woman whose breast cancer is responding to therapy, the

appearance of the same infiltrates should prompt a search for a different cause. Pulmonary edema occurs in any patient regardless of age. Large fluid volumes are often given with certain chemotherapeutic agents or for resuscitation of the hypotensive septic patient. Abnormal renal function and other poorly defined factors impair the body's ability to compensate for large fluid loads. Pulmonary edema can develop, which may be difficult to differentiate radiographically from PCP or viral pneumonia.

Fever is a nonspecific sign of infection. Many noninfectious processes, including malignancy, radiation pneumonitis, cytotoxic drug-induced lung disease, and nonspecific interstitial pneumonitis, cause fever as part of the inflammatory response. However, because fever is the most common sign of pulmonary infection, its absence strongly argues against infectious pneumonia. Cough and dyspnea are the common symptoms in both infectious and noninfectious processes.

Physical Examination

Although the physical examination in the immunocompromised host with pneumonia may be unrevealing, in the face of life-threatening dyspnea, hypoxemia, and diffuse infiltrates, to conclude that it is inconsequential would be an error. Rales can be heard before infiltrates appear. In addition, when the chest radiograph shows a unilateral infiltrate, the physical examination may reveal the presence of bilateral disease, which would alter diagnostic considerations. A pleural friction rub with a pulmonary infiltrate suggests a virulent bacterial or fungal (usually Aspergillus) infection. Localized wheezing suggests a partially obstructed bronchus, which may be due to a neoplasm, mucus, fungal bronchitis (especially caused by Aspergillus), or a blood clot. The presence of wheezing or a pleural friction rub is also strong evidence against certain diagnoses such as PCP and CMV. Finally, the physical examination is often superior to the findings on the chest radiograph in suggesting the overall severity of the illness. Quantitation of the respiratory rate alone may provide critical information about the seriousness of the illness and can help direct the timing and course of the diagnostic evaluation.

Occasionally extrapulmonic manifestations may be the best clue to the cause of the pulmonary disease. Of particular importance is a detailed examination of the skin, eye, and neurologic system. Finally and most importantly in the patient with diffuse bilateral pulmonary infiltrates, fluid balance should be evaluated. A physical examination that shows peripheral edema, jugular venous distension, and an early diastolic gallop could lead to the diagnosis of congestive heart failure and spare a patient an unnecessary lung biopsy. In our experience this is a commonly missed diagnosis.

Noninvasive Procedures

Laboratory Diagnoses

In the immunologically competent patient with pneumonia, sputum smear and culture, blood culture, and at times acute and convalescent antibody titers are the standard tools for diagnosis. Making an etiologic diagnosis in the immunocompromised host is more complex. The spectrum of potential infectious pathogens is broader, sputum is often not available, and antibody titers are insensitive. Furthermore, the utility of sputum analysis to diagnose bacterial pneumonia in this patient population is controversial. Although many experts believe that sputum cultures are inaccurate, others believe the Gram stain is helpful (Sickles, et al., 1973).

Besides the routine Gram and acid-fast stains, special preparations can be applied to sputum that occasionally can give immediate diagnostic information. India ink staining of a wet preparation of sputum can show the encapsulated budding yeast forms of Cryptococcus; a wet mount of sputum, the parasitic larvae of Strongyloides; and methenamine silver nitrate, Gram-Weigert, and toluidine blue 0 stains of air-dried smears, the cyst walls of Pneumocystis (Fig. 20-46). Sputum with the inhalation of hypertonic saline by ultrasonic nebulization gives up to a 90 percent diagnostic yield for Pneumocystis in HIV-infected patients with this type of pneumonia (Zaman, et al., 1988; Kovacs, et al., 1988). DFA staining provides a specific means of identifying Legionella, but the

organisms are not often expectorated into the sputum, and antibodies to all serotypes are not widely available. If metastatic cancer is suspected, it is always worthwhile to submit sputum for cytologic examination.

Sputum cultures that grow Cryptococcus and Nocardia are almost always pathogenic in the immunocompromised host; other organisms, such as Staphylococcus, gram-negative bacilli, and Candida may represent contamination or colonization of the upper respiratory tract rather than true pulmonary infections.

In summary although sputum collection for direct examination and culture has limited value and its results must be interpreted with caution, in any patient with pulmonary disease, sputum should be examined because the procedure is simple and safe and can give valuable information.

Skin Tests and Serology

In general skin testing is of little value in the diagnosis of acute infections in the immunocompromised host. However, when tuberculosis is suspected, a tuberculin skin test with

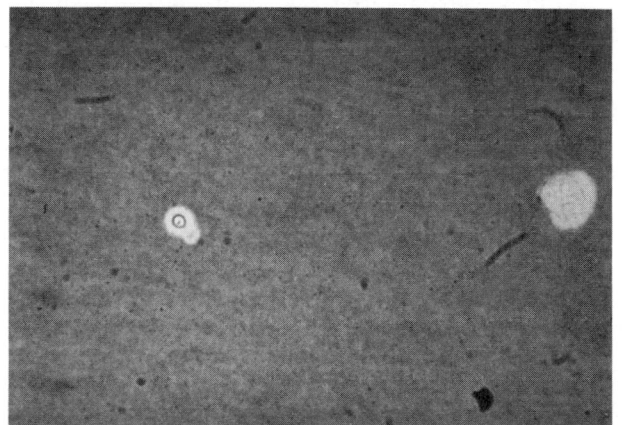

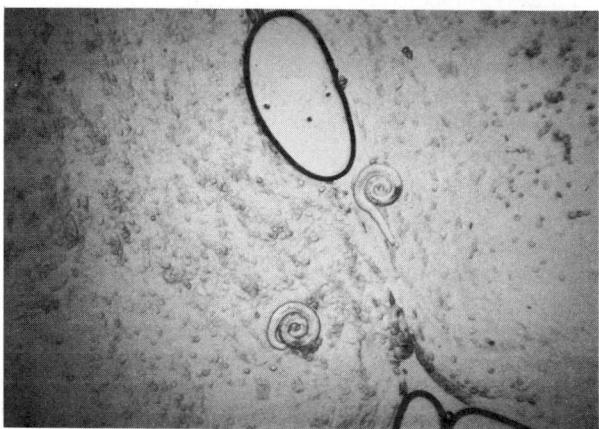

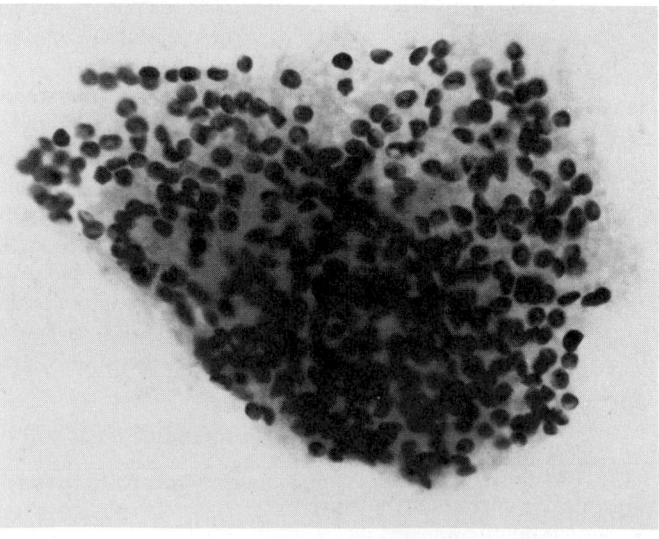

Figure 20-46. **(A)** India ink staining of a wet preparation of sputum showing the budding yeast form of *C. neoformans*. **(B)** A wet mount of sputum containing the larvae of *S. stercoralis*. **(C)** A Gram-Weigert stain of an air-dried smear of induced sputum demonstrating the typical crescent-shaped cysts of *P. carinii*.

controls should always be placed. Similarly serologic tests have not been useful in the diagnosis of pulmonary infections in these patients. Exceptions to this include the presence of serum cryptococcal antigen, which is considered highly useful in the diagnosis of disseminated and meningeal cryptococcosis (Goodman, et al., 1971). It is also helpful in the diagnosis of isolated cryptococcal pneumonia (Jensen, et al., 1985; Baugham, et al., 1992). The detection of Aspergillus antigenemia by radioimmunoassay is highly specific and moderately sensitive in the diagnosis of invasive aspergillosis; however, a reliable test kit is not commercially available (Weiner, et al., 1983).

Imaging Techniques

Although chest radiographs and other radiologic techniques used to evaluate pulmonary disease in the immunocompromised host are nonspecific, they may be helpful to narrow the diagnosis to a certain subset of likely agents. Occasionally the radiographic pattern of pulmonary infiltrates is so characteristic that the cause is apparent. Examples of this phenomenon include radiation pneumonitis and/or fibrosis, which causes infiltrates with linear margins that defy anatomic boundaries and are confined to the radiation portals. Another example is the "air crescent sign," which is a radiographic finding that is highly suggestive for pulmonary aspergillosis. This finding is caused by fungal invasion of blood vessels, which leads to necrosis of lung tissue and the creation of an ovoid mass (a sequestrum of devitalized tissue) within a cavity. A distinctive pattern of air crescents surrounding a central mass, which is referred to as a mycetoma or fungus ball, is created. CT scans of the chest can show a similar finding, called the "halo sign," weeks before the chest radiograph becomes abnormal (Kulhman, et al., 1985).

Common causes of pleural effusions in immunocompromised patients include congestive heart failure, malignancy, pulmonary embolism, and bacterial pneumonia. It is worth emphasizing that pulmonary edema is frequently mistaken for an opportunistic infection. The radiographic features that favor the diagnosis of congestive heart failure include cardiomegaly, engorgement of the pulmonary arteries and blurring of vascular markings, redistribution of blood flow to upper lung zones, the presence of Kerley B lines (horizontal lines of septal edema usually seen at the bases), and pleural effusions, including fluid in the fissure.

Gallium scanning of the lungs is a sensitive technique to detect active inflammatory lung disease, but it is nonspecific. It is especially helpful when the patient has pulmonary symptoms with a normal chest radiograph (Siemsen, et al., 1978). This situation can be seen with infection, especially Pneumocystis; drug toxicity; or lymphangitic spread of a tumor (Turbiner, et al., 1978).

Pulmonary Function Testing

Pulmonary function testing, especially measurement of the diffusing capacity and exercise arterial blood gases, provides a sensitive indicator of diffuse pulmonary disease and is useful to evaluate the immunocompromised patient with pulmonary symptoms and a normal chest radiograph (Stover and Meduri, 1988). A positive gallium lung scan or abnormal diffusing capacity in an immunocompromised patient with a normal chest radiograph necessitates further investigation.

Invasive Techniques

Invasive investigation often becomes necessary in those cases in which establishing a specific diagnosis is mandated to optimize the patient's management. The invasive techniques that are available to obtain respiratory secretions or lung tissue include TTA, transthoracic needle aspiration or biopsy, bronchoscopy with transbronchial biopsy and BAL, and thoroscopic or open lung biopsy (Table 20-6) (Stover, 1989). Of these bronchoscopy is the most commonly used procedure, followed by needle aspiration and open lung biopsy (Levine and Stover, 1991; Cunningham, et al., 1977; Stover, et al., 1984; Davidson, et al., 1976; Castellino and Blank, 1979; Zavala and Schoell, 1981; Toledo-Pereya, et al., 1990). TTA and transthoracic needle biopsy have become obsolete because of nonspecific results and/or high complication rates.

Table 20-6. Results of Various Invasive Procedures for the Diagnosis of Pulmonary Infiltrates in the Immunocompromised Host

| Procedure | No. Patients[a] | Specific Diagnosis | | Complications | | | |
| | | | | Pneumothorax | | Hemorrhage | |
		No.	%	No.	%	No.	%
Bronchoscopy							
Transbronchial biopsy	584	265	45	29	4.9	20	3.4
Bronchial brushings/washings	328	98	30	NA		NA	
Bronchoalveolar lavage	327	173	55	0		0	
Needle aspirate	178	116	65	35	20	10	6
Needle biopsy	147	85	58	42	29	16	11
Open lung biopsy[b]	334	238	71	32	10	6	2

Abbreviations: NA, not available; AIDS, acquired immunodeficiency syndrome.

[a] Excludes patients with AIDS.

[b] Other complications of open lung biopsy include hemothorax, pleural effusion or empyema, subcutaneous emphysema, wound infection or hematoma, and bronchopleural fistula. These are seen in 2–9% of the patients.

(Data from Davidson M, Tempest B, Palmen DL: Bacteriologic diagnosis of acute pneumonia. JAMA 235:158, 1976, and DeSouza R, MacKinnon S, Spagnola SV et al: Treatment of localized pulmonary phycomycosis. South Med J 72:609, 1979.)

Bronchoscopy

The most frequent indication for fiberoptic bronchoscopy in the immunocompromised host is to determine the cause of diffuse pulmonary infiltrates, which often occur in association with fever and new respiratory symptoms. Fiberoptic bronchoscopy with transbronchial biopsy, bronchial washings, brushings, and BAL has a relatively high yield in the diagnosis of diffuse pulmonary infiltrates in the non-HIV-immunosuppressed patient population (Stover, 1989; Levine and Stover, 1991) (Table 20-6). In fact when infections other than bacterial pneumonia are suspected, investigators have reported the sensitivity and specificity of this procedure to range from 80 to 90 percent (Stover, et al., 1984; Meduri, et al., 1991; Martin, et al., 1987). The most common infections diagnosed with bronchoscopy include PCP (Stover, et al., 1984; Meduri, et al., 1991; Martin, et al., 1987); viral pneumonia, especially caused by CMV (Emanuel, et al., 1986); and mycobacterial disease (Willcox, et al., 1987; Sarkar, et al., 1982). The bronchoscopic yield for the diagnosis of infection in HIV-infected patients is greater than 90 percent because of the high prevalence of PCP in this group (Ognibene, et al., 1984; Stover, et al., 1984; Broaddus, et al., 1985). Bronchoscopy may also be diagnostic for *L. pneumophila,* and when appropriate Legionella DFA staining should be done on BAL fluid (Kohorst, et al., 1983).

The development of a sheathed sterile brush (PSB) may improve the yield by allowing accurate aerobic and anaerobic bacterial cultures of bronchial secretions to be obtained without oropharyngeal microbial contamination (Fagon, et al., 1988; Wimberly, et al., 1982). The problem of reaching a localized lesion may also be alleviated with the development of needles that can be placed transbronchially (Wang, et al., 1984).

Despite the variability in yield from fiberoptic bronchoscopy with transbronchial biopsy, especially for noninfectious processes, its extremely low morbidity supports its use as the initial invasive procedure in immunocompromised patients with pulmonary infiltrates. Its major complications are pneumothorax, which is infrequent, and hemorrhage, which is rarely a cause of significant morbidity (Table 20-6).

BAL is a relatively new and effective technique that is used to diagnose diffuse pulmonary disease by fiberoptic bronchoscopy. The procedure involves the physician wedging the tip of the bronchoscope into a subsegmental bronchial lumen and then instilling approximately 90 to 120 ml of normal saline in 30 to 50-ml aliquots and aspirating the lavage fluid after each aliquot. Approximately one-half of the instilled volume is retrieved. A testament to the sampling of distal bronchioles and alveoli is the predominance of pulmonary alveolar macrophages in the lavage fluid. It is estimated that as many as 1 million alveoli are sampled by this method, as opposed to 20 to 50 alveoli that are included in a successful transbronchial forceps biopsy. Another advantage of BAL over fiberoptic bronchoscopy with transbronchial biopsy is that it is safe in the thrombocytopenic patient and in those who require mechanical ventilation (Stover, 1989; Levine and Stover, 1991; Stover, et al., 1984). It is most helpful in the diagnosis of opportunistic infections, especially *P. carinii* (Stover, et al., 1984; Meduri, et al., 1991; Martin, et al.,

1987; Ognibene, et al., 1984; Broaddus, et al., 1985), CMV pneumonia (Emanuel, et al., 1986), and intraparenchymal pulmonary hemorrhage (Stover, et al., 1984; Drew, et al., 1977). Stover, et al. (1984) reported making a specific diagnosis by analysis of BAL fluid alone in 66 percent of 97 non-HIV-immunosuppressed patients with diffuse pulmonary infiltrates. Thirty-eight of the 46 opportunistic infections (83 percent) were correctly diagnosed by examination and culture of the BAL fluid. Complications of the procedure are few; the most common is arterial oxygen desaturation, which can be effectively monitored by means of oximetry (Meduri, et al., 1991). The incidence of respiratory failure after bronchoscopy is about 1.6 percent; whether this is cause and effect is difficult to ascertain from the data available (Levine and Stover, 1991).

Transthoracic (Percutaneous) Needle Aspiration

Fluoroscopically guided needle TTA is particularly valuable for the diagnosis of peripheral nodular or cavitary infiltrates. The main advantages of percutaneous needle aspiration are that it directly samples the pathologic area and a small core of lung tissue or lung fluid is obtained, which can be examined microbiologically and cytologically (Castellino and Blank, 1979; Zavala and Schoell, 1981). A drawback of this technique is that the size of the sample is small, which limits the number of studies that can be done. It is particularly useful in pediatric cases and in recipients of heart transplants. The safety of percutaneous needle aspiration has been enhanced by the recent trend toward the use of thinner needles, for example, 22-gauge spinal needles. The major complications of the procedure include hemoptysis, especially with centrally located lesions, and pneumothorax with peripheral lesions.

Open Lung Biopsy and Thoracoscopic Lung Biopsy

When open lung biopsies are performed on immunosuppressed patients, tissue is obtained in 100 percent of the cases, and a definite diagnosis is made in 65 to 75 percent of patients with a 5 to 8 percent morbidity rate and a 0.5 to 2 percent mortality rate (Satterfield and McLaughlin, 1979; Rossiter, et al., 1979; Cockerill, et al., 1985). This technique has been used with a low complication rate in critically ill and thrombocytopenic patients (Table 20-6). The major complications are pneumothorax, hydrothorax, atelectasis, subcutaneous emphysema, and hemorrhage (Stover, 1989; Levine and Stover, 1991). The greatest advantage of an open lung biopsy in the immunocompromised patient is the rapidity with which a diagnosis can be achieved. A major drawback, however, is that, if respiratory diseases recur or occur sequentially, multiple operations with their attendant discomfort and morbidity are undesirable. Furthermore, the effect of an open lung biopsy on the course of the underlying pulmonary disease is difficult to assess.

Thoracoscopic surgery permits excellent visualization of the entire lung and the ability to take parenchymal biopsy specimens from specific areas or lesions through minimal incisions with diminished postoperative pain. Recently Lewis, et al. (1992) reported that 11 patients underwent lung biopsy with this procedure. All procedures were successful in obtaining adequate tissue. Each patient was extubated in the recovery room; in 10 of the 11 patients, chest tubes were removed by the third postoperative day with no subsequent air leaks. The patients resumed their preoperative activity levels within 1 week of discharge. Although there is little if any information in regard to the use of this technique in the immunocompromised host, we can only speculate that it appears promising. Further studies are necessary to evaluate its diagnostic yield and complication rate in this patient population.

PULMONARY INFECTIONS IN THE IMMUNOCOMPROMISED HOST

Many of the infections are presented in more detail by other authors in earlier sections of this chapter. The purpose of this discussion will be to review the presentation, diagnosis, and therapy of the most common infectious disorders as they apply to the immunosuppressed patient.

Bacteria

Common Bacterial Pneumonias

S. pneumoniae and *H. influenzae* are common CAPs, not only in the immunocompetent patient but also in those who are immunocompromised by B-cell defects, such as those found in multiple myeloma. Other patients who are immunocompromised by virture of granulocyte defects commonly get bacterial pneumonias caused by gram-negative organisms, including *P. aeruginosa*, *E. coli*, and Klebsiella species, and by certain gram-positive organisms, especially *S. aureus*. *S. marcescens* and Enterobacter and Proteus species occasionally cause pneumonia in these patients.

The clinical signs and symptoms of pneumonia in the immunocompromised host may be typical with an acute onset of shaking chills, fever, and productive cough. This type of presentation often accompanies bacterial pneumonia in the HIV-infected patient (Polsky, et al., 1986). In the setting of granulocytopenia, clinical signs and symptoms of pneumonia may be atypical or absent (Sickles, et al., 1975). Cough is usually present, but 30 percent of cases report no cough. Sputum production is seen in less than 60 percent, and in patients with absolute neutrophil counts less than 100 cells/mm³, purulent sputum has been reported in only 8 percent (Sickles, et al., 1973). The most sensitive sign of bacterial pneumonia, although nonspecific, is the presence of fever, which is seen in almost 100 percent of cases; rales and signs of consolidation are inconsistently present (Sickles, et al., 1973). The chest radiograph, however, is abnormal in 93 to 97 percent of cases; most show localized infiltrates (Singer, et al., 1979; Tenholder and Hooper, 1980). The incidence of bacteremia is higher as is the mortality rate in HIV-infected patients and patients with absolute neutrophil counts less than 100 cells/mm³ compared with immunocompromised hosts with pneumonia (Sickles, et al., 1973; Singer, et al., 1977); Gerberding, et al., 1986).

Because bacterial pneumonias in immunocompromised patients may progress rapidly, empiric broad-spectrum antibiotic coverage should be initiated as soon as the diagnosis is suspected. In non-neutropenic immunosuppressed hosts (e.g., HIV-infected patients), a second-generation cephalosporin or ampicillin is usually adequate. In those individuals who are neutropenic and have CAP or nosocomial bacterial pneumonia, an aminoglycoside together with a third-generation cephalosporin, an extended-spectrum penicillin (β-lactam), or imipenem are choice combinations because gram-negative organisms and *S. aureus* are common. In patients with renal insufficiency, aztreonam may be substituted for an aminoglycoside; however, the known synergistic killing of many bacteria by an aminoglycoside together with either a third-generation cephalosporin or β-lactam penicillin has not been demonstrated with aztreonam.

The duration of antibiotic therapy in the immunocompromised host for the therapy of bacterial pneumonias is controversial. A 2-week course of broad-spectrum antibiotics may be sufficient in many patients, especially if there is rapid clinical improvement and white blood cell recovery. When prolonged neutropenia is present, longer courses may be required.

Aspiration pneumonia is a term used to described anaerobic bacterial infections of the lung and pulmonary disease resulting from aspiration of gastric juice or solid particles. Dysphagia related to surgery and radiotherapy for head and neck tumors or mucositis caused by infection, chemotherapy, or radiotherapy places immunocompromised patients; especially those with cancer, at risk for aspiration (Logemann, 1985).

The acute complications of aspiration include bronchospasm and clinical pneumonitis, which presents with fever, tachypnea, cough, hypoxemia, and leukocytosis. Pulmonary infections after aspiration usually occur days after the acute event. Anaerobes are the most common isolates from "out-of-hospital" aspiratoin; nosocomial aspirations include anaerobes, gram-negative bacilli, and *S. aureus* (Rotstein, et al., 1988).

The diagnosis of infection shortly after the aspiration of gastrointestinal contents is often difficult because fever, leukocytosis, and pulmonary infiltrates can be due to the chemical injury. Persistent fever, radiographic abnormalities, or any other sign of infection after aspiration warrants prompt use of empiric antibiotic therapy in the immunocompromised host. At least two antibiotics directed toward coverage of anaerobes, *S. aureus,* and gram-negative bacilli should be used. Recommended regimens include ticarcillin/clavulanate for gram-positive organisms and anaerobic coverage and an aminoglycoside for gram-negative bacilli. Other regimens include combinations of clindamycin or metronidazole for anaerobic coverage and vancomycin or a semisynthetic penicillin for gram-positive coverage in combination with an aminoglycoside. Ten to 14 days of therapy is indicated in immunosuppressed patients, which preferably should be continued until myelosuppression has resolved.

Less Common Bacterial Pneumonias

Legionnaires' disease and *M. pneumoniae* are atypical bacterial pneumonias that can occur in immunocompromised patients. Sporadic cases and community-acquired outbreaks of Legionnaires' disease have been reported in these patients, but infection is more often acquired from a nosocomial source. Few studies have evaluated this disease in the immunosuppressed patient population. A study by Saravoltz, et al. (1979) reported fever and malaise in all their immunocompromised patients, a productive cough in 66 percent, and hemoptysis in 38 percent. Interestingly gastrointestinal complaints were infrequent. Radiographically a unilateral patchy alveolar infiltrate was seen, which progressed to consolidation and involved contiguous and noncontiguous areas of the lung. The presence of bilateral infiltrates and cavitation is relatively frequent. The diagnosis of Legionella infection is difficult to make in immunocompromised patients. Although culture of the organism from the respiratory tract, blood, tissue, or pleural fluid is diagnostic, DFA tests are quicker and clinically more applicable in this patient population (Winn, et al., 1980; Kohorst, et al., 1983). The use of DFA tests has certain drawbacks, which include serogroup dependence, limited sensitivity, and the need to have an expert interpret the slides (Winn, et al., 1980). The therapy for Legionella requires the use of antibiotics than can kill intracellularly by entering alveolar macrophages, and erythromycin is the mainstay (Edelstein and Meyer, 1988, Kirby, et al., 1980).

Although infections with *M. pneumoniae* in normal adults are common and relatively mild, severe pulmonary disease has been described in patients with antibody deficiencies and in those with malignancy (Perez and Leigh, 1991). The clinical manifestations include headache, fever, myalgias, malaise, and anorexia followed by sore throat and a dry, protracted cough, which at times may yield nonpurulent sputum (Murray, et al., 1975). Radiographic findings are variable, but most often show lower lobe patchy or reticular interstitial infiltrates. Because few laboratories culture for Mycoplasma, the diagnosis is usually not made, and patients are treated empirically. The antibiotics with proved efficacy are tetracycline and erythromycin (Murray, et al., 1975).

Although Nocardia species can occur in immunocompetent patients, the immunocompromised host, particularly one with impairment of cell-mediated immunity, is most susceptible to this type of infection (Palmer, et al., 1974). The lung is the primary site of infection; other organs commonly involved include the brain, skin, spleen, liver, kidney, bones, and lymph nodes. The symptoms and chest radiographs are nonspecific; however, chest pain may be present because of an extension of infection to the pleura or chest wall (Simpson, et al., 1981). Although simple colonization and subclinical infection can occur, isolation of Nocardia from the sputum of an immunocompromised host should always be considered diagnostically significant. Sulfonamides are the mainstay of therapy. Because relapse is common, prolonged therapy for at least 6 to 12 months is indicated, and parenteral therapy should be continued for at least 4 to 8 weeks.

M. catarrhalis (formerly called *Neisseria catarrhalis* and *Branhamella catarrhalis*) occasionally causes pulmonary infections in patients with HIV infection and γ-globulin dyscrasias (Polsky, et al., 1986; Diamond and Locber, 1984). The infection can vary from an acute febrile tracheobronchitis to a rapidly fatal pneumonia. Cephalosporins, erythromycin, tetracycline, and TMP/SMX are the antibiotics of choice because 75 percent of isolates are penicillin resistant (Doern, et al., 1980). Infections caused by Chlamydia, *Rhodococcus*

equi (formerly known as *Corynebacterium equi*), and group B streptococci are infrequent causes of pulmonary infections in the immunocompromised host.

Mycobacteria

The genus Mycobacterium includes the tubercle bacilli (*M. tuberculosis* and *Mycobacterium bovis*), Hanson's bacillus (*Mycobacterium leprae*), and the nontuberculous (or atypical) mycobacteria.

Tuberculosis

The prevalence of tuberculosis is reported to be higher in immunocompromised patients, particularly those with lung cancer, head and neck cancer, lymphoproliferative disorders, and HIV infection (Ortbals and Marr, 1978; Selwyn, et al., 1989). Because tuberculosis in the HIV-infected patient is unique, this is discussed later. In most immunocompromised patients, tuberculosis develops from reactivation of a latent pulmonary infection. The symptoms and signs are nonspecific, and the fever and constitutional symptoms that usually accompany tuberculosis are often attributed to the underlying neoplasm, which delays the diagnosis.

Immunocompromised patients are at increased risk to have rapidly progressive pulmonary tuberculosis. In a series of 201 patients with cancer and tuberculosis, 9 had tuberculous pneumonia, which was uniformly fatal (Kaplan, et al., 1974). Thirty-four patients in the same series had disseminated tuberculosis, with a mortality rate of 91 percent. Patients at greatest risk for severe tuberculosis were those who were receiving antineoplastic therapy.

Chest radiographs can show the typical upper lobe cavitation; however, masses or nodules that mimic cancer and complicate both the diagnosis and staging of the existing neoplastic disease can occur (Kaplan, et al., 1974). In addition, opportunistic infections, such as histoplasmosis, nocardiosis, and cryptococcosis, are diagnostic possibilities in presents with tuberculosis and nodular infiltrates or a solitary cavitary lesion. Pulmonary tuberculosis can be confirmed in most cases by sputum examination; in miliary tuberculosis, however, sputum cultures are positive in only two-thirds of cases and smears, in less than one-third (Munt, 1971). In some patients bronchoscopy may be necessary, and this technique has been reported to have a diagnostic yield of more than 90 percent for the diagnosis of tuberculosis in immunocompromised hosts (Willcox, et al., 1987; Sarkar, et al., 1982).

There are no control studies on the therapy of tuberculosis in these patients. Although the combination of INH and RMP administered for 9 months has been successful in patients with cancer (Dutt, et al., 1988) and those who are receiving corticosteroid therapy, some authorities recommend that a third drug (ethambutol, PZA, or streptomycin) be added for the first 2 months of therapy and then continue INH and RMP for an additional 7 to 10 months (Kuritzkes and Simon, 1991).

Although the anergy caused by the underlying disease may interfere with the purified protein derivative tuberculin test, it is reported to be positive in 60 to 75 percent on non-HIV-infected immunocompromised hosts. To increase sensitivity tuberculin skin tests should be performed before immunosuppressive therapy is instituted, and a reaction size of 5 mm of induration should be used to define a positive reaction. Immunocompromised patients with positive tuberculin reactions should receive 12 months of prophylaxis with INH (300 mg/day). Bacillus Calmette-Gúerin, an attenuated vaccine strain of *M. bovis,* is not recommended for tuberculosis prophylaxis because disseminated disease and death have been reported in these patients.

Tuberculosis in HIV-Infected Patients

Tuberculosis in HIV-infected persons results primarily from reactivation of latent infection. The highest incidence of active tuberculosis occurs in those with a positive tuberculin skin test or known tuberculosis exposure and in groups with a high background prevalence of tuberculosis, such as immigrants from countries with endemic tuberculosis, blacks, Hispanics, and intravenous drug users (Pitchenik, et al., 1987; Sunderam, et al., 1986).

Because *M. tuberculosis* is a more virulent organism than opportunistic pathogens, it tends to occur earlier in the course of HIV disease, often preceding or coinciding with the diagnosis of AIDS. If it occurs at a time when cell-mediated immunity is relatively intact, clinically the disease presents in a similar manner to tuberculosis in the immunocompetent patient (Hopewell, 1989). Tuberculosis that develops later in the course tends to present atypically, which may cause a delay in the diagnosis and initiation of appropriate therapy (Pitchenik, et al., 1984; Chaisson, et al., 1987).

The signs, symptoms, and physical examination in HIV-infected patients with tuberculosis are nonspecific. A chronic wasting syndrome may be the sole presenting sign of the disease. Fever is the most common symptom; it occurs in approximately 90 percent of cases. Night sweats, cough, sputum production, and dyspnea are also common; hemoptysis and pleuritic chest pain occur less frequently. Extrapulmonary disease (involving the lymph nodes, bone marrow, and central nervous system with or without pulmonary involvement) has been found in up to 70 percent of patients, particularly in those with more advanced immunosuppression (Pitchenik and Fertel, 1992).

In patients with higher T-helper cell counts and intact tuberculin skin reactivity, the classic findings of upper lobe infiltrates with or without cavitation are common. In the more severely HIV-infected immunosuppressed patient, radiographs reveal diffuse infiltrates, intrathoracic adenopathy with or without infiltrates, and pleural effusions. Cavitary lesions in patients with advanced HIV disease are rare, and these patients may even present with a normal chest radiograph (Barnes, et al., 1991).

The finding of acid-fast bacilli in body secretions or tissue is sufficient evidence to begin empiric therapy in an HIV-infected person suspected of having tuberculosis. However, confirmation by culture is necessary because many cases have nontuberculous mycobacterial disease. Furthermore, the results of drug susceptibility studies are useful in planning definitive therapy. Sputum smears have been reported to be positive for acid-fast bacilli in 30 to 100 percent of HIV-infected patients, and the yield is higher in the less severely immunocompromised patients. Positive sputum cultures for tuberculosis occur in 60 to 100 percent of cases. The overall positive yield by acid-fast staining and culture of bronchoscopic washings and lavage appears to be approximately 90 percent (Baugham, et al., 1991). Because granulomas may not be present in the severely immunocompromised patient, transbronchial biopsy is helpful in only a small percentage of HIV-infected patients. The use of the polymerase chain reaction test appears to be a rapid means to detect *M. tuberculosis* in clinical specimens, but the sensitivity and specificity of finding *M. tuberculosis* in sputum by this technique need to be determined (DeWitt, et al., 1990).

Generally therapy for tuberculosis caused by susceptible or single-drug-resistant organisms is similar and as effective in the HIV-infected host as it is in the normal population. In contrast no drug combination is effective in the therapy of recently identified multidrug-resistant strains of tuberculosis (Fischl, et al., 1992b). In this setting persistently positive acid-fast stains, disease dissemination, and high mortality rates have been observed. Although antituberculous medications are well tolerated in the general population, adverse reactions, mostly to RMP are frequent in HIV-infected patients. The drugs should not be discontinued for mild symptoms and/or laboratory abnormalities.

The initial evaluation of all HIV-infected patients should include tuberculin skin testing with 5 TU of purified protein derivative and at least two recall antigens (Candida, mumps, or tetanus toxoid). Any HIV-positive individual with a positive tuberculin test (i.e., 5 mm or more of induration) should be given prophylaxis, regardless of age (Centers for Disease Control, 1989).

Atypical Mycobacteria

The nontuberculous or atypical mycobacteria (MOTT) are widely distributed in nature and easily isolated from various environmental sources. Infection is not acquired by person-to-person spread as it is with *M. tuberculosis.* Pulmonary infection with MOTT can occur in those with lung cancer, head and neck cancer, hairy cell leukemia, and less commonly AIDS (Ortbals and Marr, 1978; Rolston, et al., 1985; MacDonnell and Glassroth, 1989).

A chronic pulmonary disease that resembles tuberculosis is the most important clinical problem associated with MOTT in the non-HIV-infected immunosuppressed host. *Mycobacterium avium-intracellulare* (also called *Mycobacterium avium complex*), *Mycobacterium kansasii,* and *Mycobacterium fortuitum* are the most commonly isolated organisms in patients with cancer (Ortbals and Marr, 1978; Rolston, et al., 1985). The clinical signs and symptoms are often nonspecific and include cough, dyspnea, and weight loss; fever and hemoptysis are less common. The chest radiograph may show nodules, thin-walled cavities in the upper lobes (anterior and apical segments), infiltrates, and intrathoracic adenopathy. The therapy of these organisms when they occur in the non-HIV-infected immunocompromised patients is the same as in the immunocompetent patient.

In contrast to the localized pulmonary disease seen in non-HIV-infected patients, MOTT species cause disseminated infection and only rarely cause clinically significant pulmonary disease, even when isolated from lung secretions in patients with AIDS (MacDonnell and Glassroth, 1989). HIV-infected patients with disseminated *M. avium-intracellulare* have a syndrome characterized by fever, weakness, diarrhea, abdominal pain, and general debilitation. It is usually seen late in the course of HIV infection when the CD$_4$ lymphocyte counts are less than 200 cells/mm^3, and blood cultures usually grow the organism. Although antimicrobial therapy has been ineffective in eradicating this infection or in significantly prolonging life in the HIV-infected patient, other MOTT infections, such as *M. kansasii,* may respond to therapy.

Fungi

Those patients with neutropenia as their primary immunologic defect (e.g., those with acute myelogenous leukemia) more commonly develop infections with Aspergillus and less commonly Candida and Phycomycetes (*Mucormycoses*). These organisms are called opportunistic fungi because they generally infect only those patients with abnormalities in host defenses. Patients who primarily have T-cell defects (e.g., those patients with Hodgkin's disease or those who are receiving corticosteroid therapy) more often have infections with Cryptococcus and the endemic fungi, such as Histoplasma, Coccidioides, and Blastomyces. These organisms are called pathogenic fungi because they also comonly infect immunologically normal individuals.

Opportunistic Fungi

Opportunistic fungal species are a major cause of complicating infection in immunocompromised patients. These infections are difficult to diagnose antemortem and to treat effectively. Early diagnosis and therapy may improve the outcome, although the overall prognosis remains poor.

Aspergillosis. Aspergillus, a ubiquitous fungus, is commonly found in soil, water, and decaying vegetable matter. Common species that cause disease in humans are *Aspergillus fumigatus* and *Aspergillus flavus*. Immunosuppressed patients at risk for invasive pulmonary aspergillosis include those with prolonged neutropenia; those who are receiving chronic corticosteroids, antibiotic therapy, and/or chemotherapy; and those with a prior history of Aspergillus pneumonia.

Aspergillus infection commonly presents in immunocompromised patients as an invasive necrotizing pneumonitis or a pulmonary infarct because of its propensity to erode blood vessels. The clinical features of pulmonary aspergillosis include fever, dyspnea, nonproductive cough, and acute pleuritic chest pain with or without a friction rub. Although the chest pain may be severe enough to require therapy with narcotics, the simultaneous chest radiograph may appear normal. Massive hemoptysis is a rare complication and tends to occur during the stage of bone marrow recovery and cavity formation (Albelda, et al., 1985). Often the only evidence of Aspergillus is prolonged fever with pulmonary infiltrates that do not respond to antibiotics.

Generally chest radiographs become abnormal as the symptoms escalate. Often the earliest radiographic manifestation of invasive aspergillosis is the presence of single or multiple nodules. The chest radiograph may then progress to show cavitation of these nodules, progression and enlarge-ment of the nodules to produce single or multiple areas of homogeneous consolidation, or the rapid development of large wedge-shaped pleural-based lesions that mimic pulmonary infarction. Cavitation may occur with or without a mycetoma, and CT can show the halo sign weeks before the chest radiograph becomes abnormal.

Because noninvasive tests lack specificity and sensitivity, invasive techniques are the mainstay to establish a diagnosis of pulmonary aspergillosis. The success rate of fiberoptic bronchoscopy is about 50 percent, and transbronchial biopsy adds little to the yield of bronchial washings, brushings, and lavage (Freeberg, et al., 1990). However, if the results are positive, transbronchial biopsy can establish the diagnosis of tissue invasion rather than simple colonization. Although open lung biopsy is the reference standard for the diagnosis of pulmonary aspergillosis, correlation with autopsy findings indicates that up to 25 percent of leukemic patients with pulmonary aspergillosis have negative findings on lung biopsy (Crawford, et al., 1988). Because of the difficulty in the diagnosis of aspergillosis and because of its frequency in neutropenic patients, empiric therapy for aspergillosis in the proper setting has become commonplace (Pizzo, et al., 1982).

Amphotericin B is the drug of choice for invasive aspergillosis with dosages in the range of 0.6 to 1.25 mg/kg/day, depending on the severity of the infection. Surgical resection should be considered in patients with acute aspergillosis in whom hemoptysis develops or in leukemic patients and bone marrow transplant recipients who, after therapy have residual disease, especially with mycetomas. Flucytosine appears to have additive or synergistic effects with amphotericin B against Aspergillus. Because its main adverse effect is bone marrow suppression, it is usually avoided. Most of these patients are granulocytopenic. More studies are needed to determine if RMP is synergistic or additive to amphotericin B in the therapy of human pulmonary aspergillosis.

Of the azoles itraconazole appears to be promising in animal studies (Longman and Martin, 1987). Another promising drug innovation is liposomal amphotericin B. This is produced by attaching amphotericin B to a liposomal vehicle, and higher drug doses can be given with enhanced efficacy and reduced toxicity (Lopez-Berenstein, et al., 1989). In patients who do not respond to or cannot tolerate continual amphotericin B, the liposomal form may be an alternative. The clearest correlation with survival in invasive aspergillosis seems to be remission of the underlying malignancy with recovery of functioning neutrophils. The role of neutrophil transfusions and granulocyte colony-stimulating factors for the therapy of pulmonary aspergillosis in neutropenic patients in uncertain (Roilides and Pizzo, 1992).

Mucormycoses. Although fungi of the order Mucorales (which include Mucor, Absidia, and Rhizopus) share several common clinical and histologic features with Aspergillus species, especially their predilection to infect the lung and vasculature, these fungi are uncommon in immunocompromised patients (Meyer, et al., 1972). Antemortem diagnosis of mucormycosis is difficult to confirm. Sputum cultures are rarely positive; however, if these fungi are found in sputum, invasive disease is likely. As with Aspergillus the only reliable antifungal therapy for mucormycoses is amphotericin B. The patient's response to therapy depends largely on early diagnosis, aggressive surgical debridement, remission of the underlying disease, and high accumulative doses of amphotericin B (DeSouza, et al., 1979).

Candidiasis. Interestingly, despite the high incidence of oral and pharyngeal Candida, Candida pneumonia is rare, even in the severely neutropenic patient. The reason is probably due to the fact that the alveolar macrophage is the major lung defense against Candida rather than the neutrophil (Baccari, et al., 1985). Because the isolation of this fungus from respiratory secretions is so common, a conclusive diagnosis of invasive disease requires confirmation with lung biopsy. The drug of choice for pulmonary candidiasis is amphotericin B.

Cryptococcosis. *C. neoformans* is ubiquitous, worldwide, and commonly recoverable from the environment. The fungi appear to grow best in desiccated pigeon feces. Because most patients with Cryptococcus give no history of contact with pigeons, it is most likely acquired as a airborne pollutant. Less than 25 years ago, 50 percent of the cases of disseminated cryptococcosis occurred in patients who were immunologically intact. Now the disease is more commonly associated with patients who have defects in cell-mediated immunity, such as those who are receiving chronic corticosteroid therapy and those patients with chronic lymphocytic leukemia, chronic myelogenous leukemia, Hodgkin's disease, and AIDS (Kaplan, et al., 1977; Chuck and Sande, 1989).

Disseminated cryptococcosis, clinically dominated by the occurrence of meningitis, is the most frequent presentation in immunocompromised patients. Although pulmonary involvement occurs in up to 50 percent of patients with disseminated infection, isolated pulmonary cryptococcosis is less frequent (Drutz, 1991).

The clinical manifestations of pulmonary cryptococcosis are usually minimal or absent; when symptoms do occur they include fever, cough, dyspnea, and pleuritic pain. Hemoptysis occurs infrequently, and occasionally acute cryptococcosis can mimic ARDS.

Radiographically cryptococcal pneumonia usually presents as a single well-defined mass that ranges from 2 to 10 cm in diameter and resembles primary lung cancer. Multiple nodules or miliary densities may also be found on chest radiographs. Cavitation, intrathoracic adenopathy, and pleural effusions are rare in the patient without AIDS; however, in HIV-infected patients, hilar and/or mediastinal adenopathy and pleural effusions, with or without parenchymal involvement, are common features (Kovacs, et al., 1985).

Because the disease is usually disseminated, cerebral spinal fluid, blood, and urine cultures provide excellent sources of diagnosis. Although only 20 percent of immunosuppressed patients with pulmonary cryptococcosis have sputum cultures that are positive, invasive disease should be considered present if the organism is retrieved from the sputum. In this setting the patient should be fully evaluated for disseminated infection, including a lumbar puncture.

The latex agglutination test for cryptococcal polysaccharide antigen is one of the most useful of all fungal serologic tests. It is highly sensitive and specific for invasive *C. neoformans* in patients with and without AIDS (Goodman, et al.,

1971; Chuck and Sande, 1989). Both serum and cerebrospinal fluid cryptococcal antigen should be followed to measure the efficacy of therapy.

Amphotericin B is the mainstay of therapy for cryptococcal infection, and flucytosine is synergistic with this drug. This combination is recommended for most patients with cryptococcal meningitis. In immunocompromised patients with pulmonary cryptococcosis, a course of drug therapy is indicated, but there is no agreement as to its nature or duration. Itraconazole and fluconazole are azoles with promising profiles, especially for long-term outpatient management of patients with AIDS. The prognosis of disseminated cryptococcal infection in immunocompromised hosts is poor. Of 46 patients with cancer and disseminated cryptococcosis, none survived for more than 2 years (Kaplan, et al., 1977). In patients with AIDS because relapses are common, life-long suppressive therapy is usually required. As maintenance therapy fluconazole at a dose of 200 mg/day is favored over both amphotericin B and ketoconazole.

Pathogenic Fungi

Histoplasmosis. *H. capsulatum,* a fungus endemic in the river valleys of central and southeastern United States, causes pulmonary and disseminated infections in patients whose cell-mediated immunity is impaired, such as those with Hodgkin's disease, acute and chronic lymphocytic leukemia, and AIDS. In such patients histoplasmosis is characterized by a progressive illness with evidence of extrapulmonary spread of infection. The clinical manifestations include fever, weight loss, malaise, hepatosplenomegaly, and cough. In disseminated disease bone marrow cultures have the highest yield. They are reported to be positive in 75 percent of cases, and blood cultures may be positive in more than 50 percent of cases (Wheat, 1989). BAL and transbronchial biopsy have disclosed the presence of *H. capsulatum* in 25 to 75 percent of cases; most of these represent patients with AIDS (Prechter and Prakash, 1989). A diagnosis of fungemia can be quickly established in up to 30 percent of patients with AIDS and disseminated histoplasmosis by visualization of the characteristic organisms on the buffy coat of peripheral blood smears after Wright or Giemsa staining. Radioimmunoassay of *H. capsulatum* antigen also offers a rapid method to diagnose disseminated histoplasmosis. Antigen can be detected in the blood in 50 percent and in the urine in 90 percent of patients with disseminated histoplasmosis (Wheat, et al., 1986). In the immunosuppressed patient with cancer who is undergoing histoplasmosis therapy with amphotericin B, a total dose of at least 35 mg/kg is indicated. Because relapse is so common, particularly in patients with AIDS, maintenance suppressive therapy with amphotericin B (100 to 500 mg weekly) is currently recommended (Daar and Meyer, 1992). Although ketoconazole is not recommended in the immunocompromised host, other azoles (e.g., itraconazole and fluconazole) may be helpful in this patient population.

Coccidioidomycosis. *C. immitis* is a fungus that is endemic in the southwestern United States, northern Mexico, and portions of Central and South America. Most infections occur in endemic areas by inhalation. Because the fungus does not colonize tissues, isolation of the organism signifies active infection. In the immunocompromised HIV- and non-HIV-infected host, disseminated coccidioidomycosis is the most common manifestation of the disease and may occur as a complication of the primary illness or as a result of reactivation of latent disease. The presenting symptoms are often nonspecific, but pulmonary symptoms, including cough and dyspnea, and chest radiographic abnormalities occur in up to 40 percent of patients. Sputum smears or cultures are positive in only 20 to 30 percent of patients, and fiberoptic bronchoscopy has a diagnostic yield of about 50 percent (Wallace, et al., 1981). Serologic tests are generally positive during an active infection and, in the immunocompromised host, may be valuable not only in the diagnosis but also in the management of coccidioidomycosis because the titers usually fall with successful therapy. Amphotericin B is recommended for all forms of coccidioidomycosis in these patients. In HIV disease relapses are common, and maintenance therapy is recommended (Galgiani and Ampel, 1990). The drug of choice for maintenance therapy is less clear and currently the subject of extensive research.

Uncommon Endemic Fungi. Blastomycosis (caused by *B. dermatitidis*) and paracoccidioidomycosis (caused by *P. brasiliensis*) have occurred sporadically in the immunocompromised patient with impaired cell-mediated immunity. The former organism is commonly found in the Mississippi and Ohio River valleys, and the latter is principally found in Central and South America and Mexico. The diagnosis of these organisms depends on visualization of the fungi on smear and tissue culture, and ketoconazole has been successful in the therapy of these organisms. However, severely immunocompromised patients should be treated with amphotericin B (Druta, 1991).

Viruses

Herpesviruses

In patients who are immunocompromised, especially those with deficiencies of cellular immunity, severe morbidity and death can occur during either primary infection or reactivation of herpesviruses. CMV pneumonia is the major cause of viral morbidity and death in bone marrow transplant recipients (Neiman, et al., 1977). CMV may be reactivated in the host, or it may be transmitted in the donor marrow or by transfusion of CMV-infected blood products. It is clinically manifested by interstitial pneumonitis that begins 8 to 12 weeks after bone marrow transplantation and after engraftment has taken place.

The clinical signs, symptoms, and radiographic findings of CMV pneumonia are nonspecific and indistinguishable from those of other common pneumonias seen in this patient population, such as idiopathic interstitial pneumonitis and PCP. Because of the ubiquity of the organism, CMV pneumonia is often difficult to document. The diagnosis can be reasonably made if the following criteria are met: clinical and radiographic evidence of interstitial pneumonia, demonstration of CMV antigen or nucleic acids in alveolar macrophages and/or epithelial cells obtained by BAL or open lung biopsy, isolation of CMV by culture from BAL fluid or lung tissue, and the absence of any other pathogens that might cause

interstitial pneumonia (Emanuel, et al., 1986). Recently we showed that BAL fluid provides an excellent source of cells that are representative of the lower respiratory tract to detect CMV antigens by monoclonal antibodies (Emanuel, et al., 1986). For most bone marrow transplant patients with CMV pneumonia, this technique has replaced the need to obtain tissue samples through closed or open lung biopsies.

Until recently therapy for CMV pneumonia in allogeneic bone marrow transplant recipients was unsuccessful. However, two relatively small uncontrolled studies suggested that the combined use of ganciclovir and intravenous Ig is associated with a significant decrease in the mortality rate from CMV pneumonia (Reed, et al., 1988; Emanuel, et al., 1988). With this regimen at our institution, the mortality rate from CMV pneumonia has decreased from 90 to 30 percent.

The incidence and severity of pulmonary involvement with CMV among recipients of solid organ transplants are considerably lower that those in allogeneic bone marrow recipients (Dummer, et al., 1984). Unlike the situation in bone marrow transplantation, the degree to which solid organ recipients experience CMV-associated illness is related to whether the infection is primary or a reactivation of a previous infection. In those with reactivation of CMV, the incidence of symptomatic disease is much lower than in those with a primary CMV infection. The approach to diagnosis is similar to that recommended for bone marrow transplants; however, the mainstay of therapy involves decreasing the amount of exogenous immunosuppression as much as the clinical situation allows. There are insufficient data available to recommend ganciclovir and/or intravenous Ig as standard therapy in solid organ allografts.

Although CMV is a well-documented pathogen in the eyes and gastrointestinal tract of patients with HIV infection, it is an uncommon pulmonary pathogen in these patients (Jacobson, et al., 1991).

In the immunocompromised host, both primary and reactivation of varicella can be a devastating illness and is associated with hematogenous visceral dissemination in up to 20 percent of cases. Although the histologic and cytologic features of varicella pneumonia are identical to those of herpes simplex virus, the diagnosis of varicella pneumonia is usually straightforward because the symptoms of pneumonia usually occur 3 to 7 days after the onset of the cutaneous lesions. Therapy of varicella pneumonia is recommended in both immunocompetent and immunocompromised patients because of the high mortality rate. Acyclovir is effective in both groups and is preferred over lymphoblastoid interferon or vidarabine because it has the lowest toxicity (Shepp, et al., 1986). Because untreated primary varicella and shingles may rapidly disseminate and cause death in immunocompromised patients, prompt therapy for this entity without any evidence of pneumonia is also highly recommended. In addition, a reduction in the level of immunosuppressive therapy may hasten the resolution of lesions and limit dissemination. Several studies show that postexposure prophylaxis (before signs of disease occur) with varicella-zoster Ig is highly effective in decreasing the morbidity rate in such patients (Centers for Disease Control, 1984).

Herpes simplex virus is a frequent cause of mucocutaneous disease in these patients, but lung involvement is uncommon.

Pulmonary disease with herpesvirus type I and II has varied from tracheobronchitis to bronchopneumonia. The presence of facial, oral, or esophageal herpetic lesions may be clues to the diagnosis because in one study mucocutaneous lesions occurred in 85 percent of patients with pulmonary disease (Ramsey, et al., 1982). Cough, dyspnea, and fever are common symptoms. Chest radiographs can show focal lesions, which often denote oropharyngeal aspiration of organisms into the lung. Diffuse infiltrates correlate with hematogenous spread to the lung (Ramsey, et al., 1982). The diagnosis of pulmonary herpes simplex virus infection depends on the isolation of the organism from respiratory specimens in the absence of contamination by oral or upper airway lesions. Bronchoscopy may suggest the diagnosis when a necrotizing tracheitis is noted. Acyclovir is the drug of choice.

Other Viruses

Influenza has not been well studied in the immunocompromised host. Some centers have reported a higher incidence of influenza A among children with cancer; others have reported a more prolonged illness, especially in the HIV-infected patient, and an excess mortality rate among patients with a variety of neoplasms. In the immunocompromised patient, the differential diagnosis may be wide, and laboratory studies usually are necessary for a specific diagnosis (Dowdle, et al., 1979). Influenza can be isolated from respiratory secretions, pulmonary tissue, or throat cultures within 1 to 2 days after they are obtained. To detect viruses sooner, immunofluorescent techniques can be used in tissue culture or directly in exfoliated nasopharyngeal cells. Antiviral therapy with amantadine or rimantadine has a beneficial effect on the symptoms of influenza A infections. However, their effectiveness in influenza pneumonia has not been studied. Prevention of influenza A and B involves the use of inactivated influenza vaccines, and although the immune response in these patients is variable, it is recommended that such patients receive vaccination (Centers for Disease Control, 1988). Adenovirus is uncommon in the immunocompromised adult patient population as is respiratory syncytial virus.

Protozoans

Pneumocystosis

P. carinii has been recognized since the 1940s as a cause of severe pneumonia in the immunocompromised host (Vanek, 1951). It occurs in patients with both B-cell and more commonly T-cell deficiencies, especially those with Hodgkin's disease, acute or chronic lymphatic leukemia, organ transplantation, HIV infection, and solid tumors who are receiving high doses of corticosteroids. The organism is global; it occurs in all climates and in all mammalian species. Controversy surrounds the issue of whether *P. carinii* is a protozoa or a fungus (Edman, et al., 1988). Extensive study of these organisms has been hampered by an inability to grow them in vitro. Based entirely on morphology, three forms have been identified: the cyst (which is the most commonly identified form in human tissue), the sporozoite (which is an intracystic structure), and the free-floating trophozoite. Although asymptomatic infection is thought to occur in the normal host early in life, active disease with pneumonia occurs only when

an infected individual becomes immunosuppressed months or years after the primary infection (Pifer, et al., 1978). Reports of person-to-person spread and cluster outbreaks in hospitals suggest that horizontal transmission may also occur (Singer, et al., 1975). The natural history of PCP in the immunocompromised host is characterized by progressive involvement of the lungs, culminating in death if untreated.

Nonproductive cough, dyspnea, and fever are the typical symptoms of PCP. It can be subclinical or chronic in HIV-infected patients or rapidly progressive in patients with cancer or transplants (Kovacs, et al., 1984; Levine and White, 1988). Examination of the lungs is often normal, but dry rales can be present. Wheezing and signs of consolidation are unusual. If they are present, other causes of pulmonary disease should be entertained. Routine laboratory and radiographic studies do not provide specific information about the diagnosis of PCP. Measurement of lactate dehydrogenase, arterial blood gases, or oxygen saturation with rest and exercise, and measurement of the diffusing capacity provide sensitive but nonspecific markers for the disease (Mazur, 1991; Jules-Elysee, et al., 1992).

The typical radiographic appearance of PCP is one of diffuse bilateral symmetric interstitial infiltrates, which characteristically progress to fluffy alveolar infiltrates as the disease worsens (Forrest, 1972; Naidich and McGuinness, 1991). Ten to 15 percent of patients have normal chest radiographs. In HIV-infected patients who are receiving aerosolized pentamidine, there have been increasing reports of atypical radiographic manifestations, most commonly the predominance of upper lobe infiltrates, cavitary lesions, and pneumothoraces (Jules-Elysee, 1990). These atypical findings have been attributed to the deposition patterns of aerosolized pentamidine (Jules-Elysee, et al., 1990). Pneumothoraces associated with aerosolized pentamidine and PCP are difficult to manage, usually require surgical intervention, and are associated with a high mortality rate (Tietjen, et al., 1989; Sepkowitz, et al., 1991).

The diagnosis of PCP can only be established by demonstrating the organism in respiratory secretions or body tissues (Fig. 20-46C). Although induced sputum has been shown to have a high yield for the diagnosis of PCP in the HIV-infected patient, is usefulness in other immunosuppressed populations has been limited to a few centers (Zaman, et al., 1988; Kovacs, et al., 1988; Masur, et al., 1988). The use of the polymerase chain reaction applied to sputum samples for the diagnosis of PCP may eventually enhance the yield (Wakefield, et al., 1991). At present bronchoscopic diagnosis is more sensitive than induced sputum and it remains the procedure of choice for the diagnosis of PCP in the non-HIV-infected patient when the suspicion is high for PCP (Martin, et al., 1987). The introduction of BAL has increased the sensitivity to detect *P. carinii* to more than 80 percent in the immunocompromised host, and the use of bilateral lavage has been shown to have an even higher yield (Stover, et al., 1984; Meduri, et al., 1991). In HIV-infected patients, an induced sputum should be done first.

There are two conventional drugs for the therapy of PCP, TMP/SMX and parenteral pentamidine (Hughes, et al., 1978). Some clinicians are reluctant to use TMP/SMX in neutropenic patients because of the possibility of worsening or prolonging neutropenia. Intravenous pentamidine is a reasonable therapeutic choice in this setting, although it is not clear whether TMP/SMX really causes neutropenia. Therapy in the non-HIV-infected patient is usually given for a total of 2 weeks; the success rate varies from 50 to 70 percent in the nonimmunocompromised host (Sepkowitz, et al., 1992). In patients with AIDS TMP/SMX (15 to 20 mg/kg/day of trimethoprim) or pentamidine (3 to 4 mg/kg/day) for a total of 3 weeks is recommended. The success rate with both of these agents in patients with AIDS is around 75 to 80 percent. Unfortunately the adverse reaction rate in such patients can be up to 80 percent with either drug (Sattler, et al., 1988). Promising alternatives with less toxicity include the combination of dapsone-trimethoprim (Medina, et al., 1990), clindamycin-primaquine, and the investigational quinolone, hydroxynapthoquinone 566C80, which appears to kill pathogens rather than suppress them. Aerosolized pentamidine has not been shown to be highly effective in the therapy of PCP (Falloon, et al., 1991; Soo Hoo, et al., 1990; Conte, et al., 1990).

In HIV-infected patients with PCP and an arterial partial oxygen pressure less than 70 mmHg during room-air breathing, the addition of corticosteroids to antimicrobial agents has been shown to decrease the likelihood of respiratory failure, mechanical ventilation, and/or death (Bozzette, et al., 1990). Although controlled randomized trials that add corticosteroids to conventional agents are not available in the non-HIV-infected population, it has been our experience that adding or increasing the dose of corticosteroids has a beneficial effect. Effective prophylaxis against PCP can be achieved by the administration of TMP/SMX orally in two daily doses, three consecutive days per week (Hughes, et al., 1987). In patients with AIDS aerosolized pentamidine has been show to offer protection against PCP but appears to be less effective than TMP/SMX (Leong, et al., 1990; Hardy, et al., 1992). Other disadvantages to the use of aerosolized pentamidine include breakthrough Pneumocystis infection with atypical persentations, an increase in the incidence of extrapulmonary Pneumocystis because the aerosol affords no protection outside the lung, and because of the vigorous coughing associated with its administration, the spread of tuberculosis has occurred and continues to be of great concern (Pearson, et al., 1992; Fischl, et al., 1992a).

Other Parasites

Strongyloides stercoralis and *Toxoplasma gondii* are other parasites that uncommonly affect the lung in immunocompromised patients. Disseminated strongyloidiasis usually occurs in patients with cellular immune defects who come from endemic areas and develop the so-called hyperinfection syn-

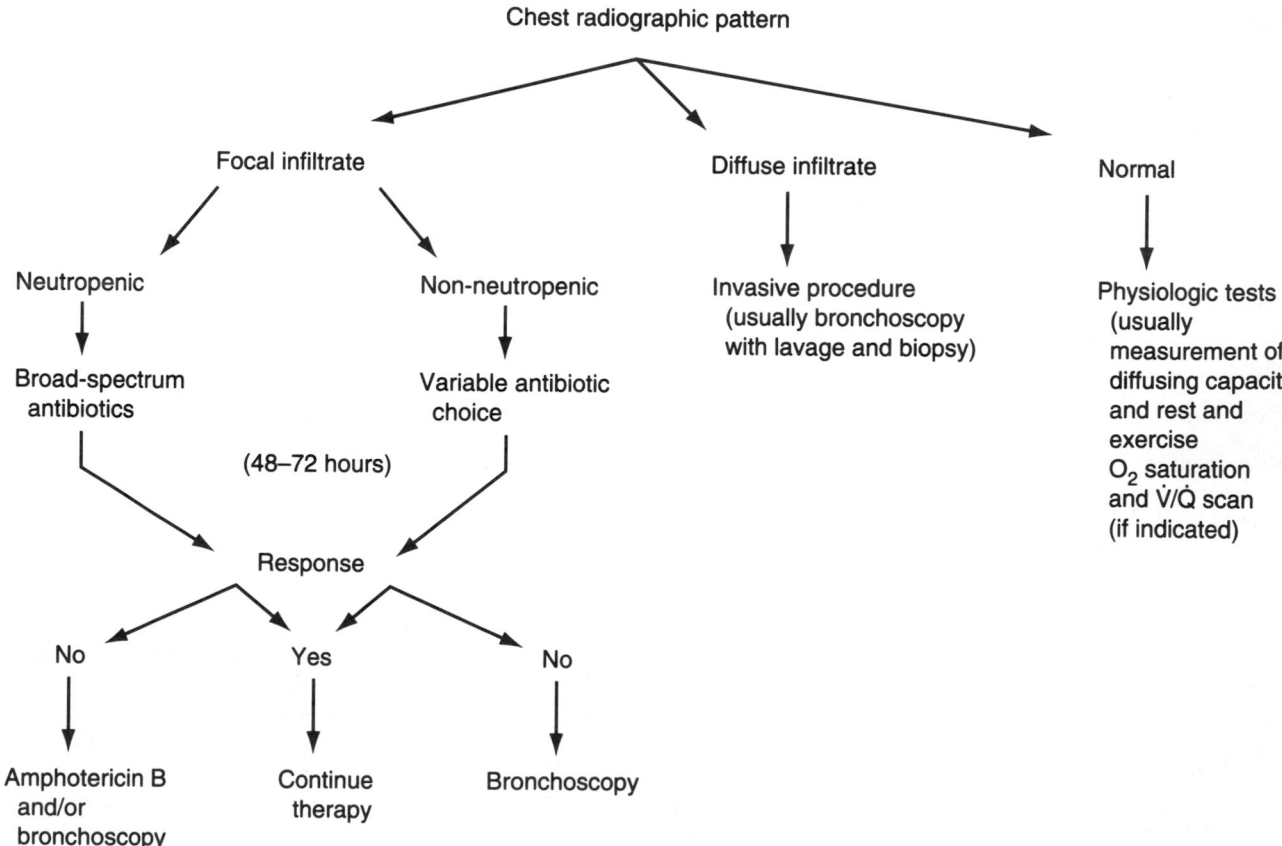

Figure 20-47. Algorithm for approach to immunocompromised patients with pulmonary infections based on presenting chest radiograph.

drome (Ingra-Siegman, et al., 1981). Although the pulmonary signs and symptoms of disseminated strongyloidiasis are non-specific, the diagnosis should be entertained in an immuno-suppressed patient who comes from an endemic area and has vague abdominal symptoms of pain, diffuse tenderness, and/or distension and then pneumonia. The diagnosis is made by demonstrating the larvae either in sputum or other respiratory secretions, especially BAL (Fig. 20-46B). The therapy for hyperinfection syndrome is thiabendazole. In our experience toxoplasmosis is an uncommon cause of pulmonary infiltrates in these patients. When it does occur it is usually in the setting of HIV infection or organ transplantation.

CONCLUSIONS

Although the spectrum of infectious pathogens that occur in the lungs of immunocompromised patients is broad, a general strategy for management of these patients is possible. An algorithm that illustrates these diagnostic and therapeutic options appears in Figure 20-47.

COMMENTS AND CONTROVERSIES

Frequently surgeons are called on to aid in the diagnosis of these dreaded pulmonary complications in the immunocom-promised host. In many patients severe hypoxemia has al-ready occurred. In such instances when transbronchoscopic techniques do not yield a diagnosis, open lung biopsy is the only rational option. Video-assisted techniques require uni-lateral collapse of the lung, which is frequently contraindi-cated in patients in extremis. An open lung biopsy (see Ch. 32) is simple, safe, and effective. A major thoracotomy is not required.

Less frequently the surgeon is called on to participate in therapy including the resection of localized lesions, in some instances before the induction of immunosuppression (e.g., high-dose chemotherapy with bone marrow rescue) lest these lesions proliferate as a result of immunosuppression. On oc-casion even in progressive infections, lesions isolated to one lobe (e.g., progressive aspergillosis) can only be successfully treated by pulmonary resection, albeit with an increased risk to the patient.

With the increasing prevalence of AIDS, immunosuppres-sion caused by transplantation and high-dose chemotherapy, etc., there is no doubt that surgeons will become increasingly involved in the management of these patients.

R.J.G.

KEY REFERENCES

Levine SJ, White DA: Pneumocystis carinii. Clin Chest Med 9:395, 1988

The biology of the organism and the epidemiology, pathology, clinical presentation, course and outcome, diagnosis, and therapy of Pneumocystis pneumonia in the HIV-infected patient are pre-sented in detail.

Murray JF, Mills J: Pulmonary infectious complications of human immunodeficiency virus infection: parts 1 and 2. Am Rev Respir Dis 5:1356, 1990

A comprehensive review of the infectious complications found in HIV-infected patients is presented.

Shelhamer J, Pizzo PA, Parrillo JE, Masur H: Respiratory Disease in the Immunosuppressed Host. JB Lippincott, Philadelphia, 1991

To date this book is the most comprehensive material on pulmo-nary disease in the immunocompromised host. A general prospec-tive on pulmonary host defenses, the utility of different diagnostic procedures, disease processes that occur in specific patient popula-tions (e.g., transplants and patients with HIV and cancer) and presentations of respiratory disease in these patients are discussed in detail.

Williams DM, Krick JA, Remington JS: Pulmonary infection in the immunocompromised host. Parts 1 and 2. Am Rev Respir Dis 114:359, 1976

A comprehensive review of infectious complications in the non-AIDS-infected immunocompromised host is presented.

REFERENCES

Albelda SM, Talbot GH, Gerson SL et al: Pulmonary consolidation and massive hemoptysis in invasive pulmonary aspergillosis. In-fluence of bone marrow recovery in patients with acute leukemia. Am Rev Respir Dis 131:115, 1985

Baccari MA, Bistoni F, Lohmann-Mathes ML: In vitro natural and cell-mediated cytotoxicity against Candida albicans: macrophage precursors as effector cells. J Immunol 134:2658, 1985

Barnes PF, Bloch AB, Davidson PT et al: Tuberculosis in patients with human immunodeficiency virus infection. N Engl J Med 324:1644, 1991

Baugham RP, Dohn MN, Loudon RG et al: Bronchoscopy with bronchoalveolar lavage in tuberculosis and fungal infections. Chest 99:92, 1991

Baugham RR, Rhodes JC, Dohn MN et al: Detection of cryptococcal antigen in bronchoalveolar lavage fluid: a prospective study of diagnostic utility. Am Rev Respir Dis 145:1226, 1992

Bozzette SA, Sattler FA, Chiu J et al: A controlled trial of early adjunctive treatment with corticosteroids for Pneumocystis carinii pneumonia in the acquired immunodeficiency syndrome. N Engl J Med 323:1451, 1990

Broaddus C, Dake MD, Stulberg MS et al: Bronchoalveolar lavage and transbronchial biopsy for the diagnosis of pulmonary infections in the acquired immune deficiency syndrome. Ann Intern Med 102:747, 1985

Castellino RA, Blank N: Etiologic diagnosis of focal pulmonary infection in immunocompromised patients by fluoroscopically guided percutaneous needle aspiration. Radiology 132:563, 1979

Centers for Disease Control: Tuberculosis and human immunodeficiency virus infection: recommendation of the advisory committee for the elimination of tuberculosis (ACET). Morb Mortal Wkly Rep 38:235, 1989

Centers for Disease Control: Prevention and control of influenza. MMWR Morb Mortal Wkly Rep 37:361, 1988

Centers for Disease Control: Varicella-zoster immune globulin for the prevention of chicken pox: recommendations of the Immunization Practices Advisory Committee. Ann Intern Med 100:859, 1984

Chaisson RE, Schecter GR, Theuer CP et al: Tuberculosis in patients with the acquired immunodeficiency syndrome. Clinical features, response to therapy and survival. Am Rev Respir Dis 136:570, 1987

Chuck SL, Sande M: Infections with Cryptococcus neoformans in the acquired immunodeficiency syndrome. N Engl J Med 321:794, 1989

Cockerill FR, Wilson WR, Carpenter HA et al: Open lung biopsy in immunosuppressed patients. Arch Intern Med 145:1398, 1985

Conte JE Jr, Chernoff D, Feigal DW Jr et al: Intravenous or inhaled pentamidine for treating Pneumocystis carinii pneumonia in AIDS. Ann Intern Med 113:203, 1990

Crawford SW, Hackman RC, Clark JG: Open lung biopsy diagnosis of diffuse pulmonary infiltrates after bone marrow transplantation. Chest 94:949, 1988

Cunningham JH, Zavala DC, Corry RJ, Keim LW: Trephine air drill, bronchial brush and fiberoptic transbronchial lung biopsies in immunosuppressed patients. Am Rev Respir Dis 115:213, 1977

Darr ES, Meyer RD. Bacterial and fungal infections. Med Clin North Am 76:173, 1992

Davidson M, Tempest B, Palmen DL: Bacteriologic diagnosis of acute pneumonia. JAMA 235:158, 1976

DeSouza R, MacKinnon S, Spagnola SV et al: Treatment of localized pulmonary phycomycosis. South Med J 72:609, 1979

DeWitt D, Steyn L, Shoemaker S et al: Direct detection of Mycobacterium tuberculosis in clinical specimens by DNA amplification. J Clin Microbiol 28:2437, 1990

Diamond LA, Lorber B: Branhamella catarrhalis pneumonia and immunoglobulin abnormalities: a new association. Am Rev Respir Dis 129:876, 1984

Doern CV, Siebers KG, Hallick LM et al: Antibiotic susceptibility of beta-lactamase-producing strains of Branhamella (Neisseria) catarrhalis. Antimicrob Agents Chemother 17:24, 1980

Dowdle W, Kendal AP, Noble GR: Influenza viruses. p. 585. In Lennette EH, Schmidt NJ (eds): Diagnostic Procedures for Viral, Rickettsial and Chlamydial Infections. APHA, Washington, D.C., 1979

Drew WL, Finely TN, Golde DW: Diagnostic lavage and occult pulmonary hemorrhage in the thrombocytopenic immunocompromised patients. Am Rev Respir Dis 116:215, 1977

Drutz DJ: Pneumonia due to endemic fungi. p. 335. In Shelhamer J, Pizzo PA, Parrillo JE, Masur H (eds): Respiratory Disease in the Immunosuppressed Host. JB Lippincott, Phila, 1991

Dummer JS, White LT, Ho M et al: Morbidity of cytomegalovirus infection in recipients of heart or heart-lung transplants who received cyclosporine. J Infect Dis 152:1182, 1984

Dutt AK, Moers D, Stead W: Short-course chemotherapy of tuberculosis in patients with associated disease. Chest 78(suppl):514, 1988

Edelstein PH, Meyer RD: Legionella pneumonias. p. 381. In Pennington JE (ed): Respiratory Infections: Diagnosis and Management. Raven Press, New York, 1988

Edman JC, Kovacs JA, Masur H et al: Ribosomal RNA sequences show Pneumocystis carinii to be a member of the fungi. Nature 334:519, 1988

Emanuel D, Cunningham I, Jules-Elysee K et al: Cytomegalovirus pneumonia after bone marrow transplantation successfully treated with the combination of ganciclovir and high-dose intravenous immune globulin. Ann Intern Med 109:777, 1988

Emanuel D, Peppard J, Stover DE et al: Rapid immunodiagnosis of cytomegalovirus (CMV) pneumonia by bronchoalveolar lavage using human and murine monoclonal antibodies. Ann Intern Med 104:476, 1986

Fagon J, Chastre J, Hance AJ et al: Detection of nosocomial lung infection in ventilated patients. Am Rev Respir Dis 138:110, 1988

Falloon J, Kovacs J, Hughes W et al: A preliminary evaluation of 566C80 for the treatment of Pneumocystis pneumonia in patients with the acquired immunodeficiency syndrome. N Engl J Med 325:1534, 1991

Fanta CH, Pennington JE: Pulmonary infections in the transplant patient. p. 207. In Morris PJ, Tilney NL (eds): Progress in Transplantation. Vol. 2. Churchill Livingstone, New York, 1985

Fischl MA, Daikos GL, Uttamchandandi RB et al: Clinical presentation and outcome of patients with HIV infection and tuberculosis caused by multiple drug resistant bacilli. Ann Intern Med 117:184, 1992b

Fischl MA, Uttamchandani RB, Daikos GL et al: An outbreak of tuberculosis caused by multiple drug resistant tubercle bacilli among patients with HIV infection. Ann Intern Med 117:177, 1992a

Forrest JV: Radiological findings in Pneumocystis carinii pneumonia. Radiology 103:539, 1972

Freeberg G, Stover DE, Levine S et al: Spectrum of pulmonary aspergillosis in immunocompromised hosts. Chest 98:31S, 1990

Galgiani JN, Ampel NM: Coccidioidomycosis in human immunodeficiency virus infected patients. J Infect Dis 162:1165, 1990

Gerberding JL, Krieger J, Sande MA: Recurrent bacteremic infection with S. pneumoniae in patients with AIDS virus (AV) infection (abstract). p. 177. In Program and Abstracts of the 26th Interscience Conference on Antimicrobial Agents and Chemotherapy. American Society for Microbiology, 1986

Goodman JS, Kaufman L, Koenig MG: Diagnosis of cryptococcal meningitis: value of immunologic detection of cryptococcal antigen. N Engl J Med 285:434, 1971

Hardy WD, Feinberg J, Finkelstein DM et al: A controlled trial of trimethoprim-sulfamethoxazole or aerosolized pentamidine for secondary prophylaxis of Pneumocystis carinii pneumonia in patients with the acquired immunodeficiency syndrome—AIDS Clinical Trials Group protocol 021. N Engl J Med 327:1842, 1992

Hopewell PC: Tuberculosis and the human immunodeficiency virus infection. Semin Respir Infect 4:11, 1989

Hughes WT, Feldman S, Chaudhary SC et al: Comparison of pentamidine isethionate and trimethoprim-sulfamethoxazole in the treatment of Pneumocystis carinii pneumonia. J Pediatr 92:285, 1978

Hughes WT, Rivera GK, Schell MJ et al: Successful intermittent chemoprophylaxis for Pneumocystis carinii pneumonitis. N Engl J Med 316:1627, 1987

Ingra-Siegman Y, Kapila R, Sen P et al: Syndrome of hyperinfection with Strongyloides stercoralis. Rev Infect Dis 3:397, 1981

Jacobson MA, Mills J, Rush J et al: Morbidity and mortality of patients with AIDS and first episode Pneumocystis carinii pneumonia unaffected by concomitant pulmonary cytomegalovirus infection. Am Rev Respir Dis 144:6, 1991

Jensen WA, Rose RM, Harmmer SM, Karchmen AW: Serologic diagnosis of focal pneumonia caused by Cryptococcus neoformans. Am Rev Respir Dis 132:189, 1985

Jules-Elysee JK, Stover DE, Zaman MB et al: Effect of aerosolized pentamidine: effect on diagnosis and presentation of Pneumocystis carinii. Ann Intern Med 112:750, 1990

Jules-Elysee K, Santamauro J, Vander Els N et al: Use of noninvasive tests in the diagnosis of PCP in non-AIDS patients. Am Rev Respir Dis 145:A543, 1992

Kaplan MH, Armstrong D, Rosen P: Tuberculosis complicating neoplastic disease. Cancer 33:850, 1974

Kaplan MH, Rosen PP, Armstrong D: Cryptococcosis in a cancer hospital. Clinical and pathological correlates in 46 patients. Cancer 39:22, 1977

Kirby BD, Snyder KM, Meyer RD et al: Legionnaires' disease: report of sixty-five nosocomial acquired cases and review of the literature. Medicine (Baltimore) 59:188, 1980

Kohorst WR, Schonfeld SA, Macklin JE, Whitcomb ME: Rapid diagnosis of Legionnaires' disease by bronchoalveolar lavage. Chest 84:186, 1983

Kovacs JA, Hiemenz JW, Macher AM et al: Pneumocystis carinii pneumonia: a comparison between patients with the acquired immunodeficiency syndrome and patients with other immunodeficiencies. Ann Intern Med 100:663, 1984

Kovacs JA, Kovacs AA, Polis M et al: Cryptococcosis in the acquired immunodeficiency syndrome. Ann Intern Med 103:533, 1985

Kovacs JA, Ng VL, Masur H et al: Diagnosis of Pneumocystis carinii pneumonia: improved detection in sputum with use of monoclonal antibodies. N Engl J Med 318:589, 1988

Kulhman JE, Fishman EK, Siegelman SS: Invasive pulmonary aspergillosis in acute leukemia: characteristic findings on CT. The CT halo sign, and the role of CT in early diagnosis. Radiology 157:611, 1985

Kuritzkes, DR, Simon HB: Pneumonia due to M. tuberculosis and to atypical mycobacteria. p. 312. In Shelhammer J, Pizzo PA, Parrillo JE, Masur H (eds): Respiratory Diseases in the Immunosuppressed host. JB Lippincott, Philadelphia, 1991

Leong GS, Feigal DW KR, Montgomery AB et al: Aerosolized pentamidine for prophylaxis against Pneumocystis carinii pneumonia. The San Francisco Community Prophylaxis Trial. N Engl J Med 323:769, 1990

Levine SJ, Stover DE: Bronchoscopy and related techniques. p. 73. In Shelhamer J, Pizzo A, Parrillo JE, Masur H (eds): Respiratory Disease in the Immunocompromised Host. JB Lippincott, Philadelphia, 1991

Lewis RJ, Caccavale RJ, Sisler GE: Imaged thoracoscopic lung biopsy. Chest 102:60, 1992

Logemann J: Aspiration in head and neck surgical patients. Ann Otol Rhinol Laryngol 94:373, 1985

Longman LP, Martin MV: A comparison of the efficacy of itraconazole, amphotericin B and 5 fluorocytosine in the treatment of Aspergillus fumigatus endocarditis in the rabbit. J Antimicrob Chemother 20:719, 1987

Lopez-Berenstein G, Bodey GP, Fainstein V et al: Treatment of systemic fungal infections with liposomal amphotericin B. Arch Intern Med 149:2533, 1989

MacDonnell KB, Glassroth J: Mycobacterium avium complex and other nontuberculous mycobacteria in patients with HIV infection. Semin Respir Infect 4:123, 1989

Martin WJ, Smith TF, Sanderson DR et al: Role of bronchoalveolar lavage in the assessment of opportunistic pulmonary infections: utility and complications. Mayo Clin Proc 62:549, 1987

Masur H, Gill VJ, Ognibene FP et al: Diagnosis of Pneumocystis pneumonia by induced sputum technique in patients with immunologic disorders other than acquired immunodeficiency syndrome. Ann Intern Med 109:755, 1988

Masur H, Ognibene FP, Yarchoan R et al: CD$_4$ cells are predictors of opportunistic pneumonias in human immunodeficiency virus (HIV) infection. Ann Intern Med 111:223, 1989

Matthay RA, Greene WH: Pulmonary infections in the immunocompromised patient. Med Clin North Am 64:529, 1980

Mazur H: Pneumocystis carinii pneumonia: p. 409. In Shelhamer J, Pizzo PA, Parrillo JC, Masur H (eds): Respiratory Disease in the Immunocompromised Host. JB Lippincott, Philadelphia, 1991

Medina I, Mills J, Leoung G et al: Oral therapy for Pneumocystis carinii pneumonia in the acquired immunodeficiency syndrome. N Engl J Med 323:776, 1990

Meduri GU, Stover DE, Greeno RA et al: Bilateral bronchoalveolar lavage in the diagnosis of opportunistic pulmonary infection. Chest 100:1272, 1991

Meyer RD, Rosen P, Armstrong D: Phycomycosis complicating leukemia and lymphoma. Ann Intern Med 77:871, 1972

Munt PW: Miliary tuberculosis in the chemotherapy era: with a clinical review of 69 American daults. Medicine (Baltimore) 51:139, 1971

Murray HW, Masur H, Senterfit LB et al: The protean manifestations of Mycoplasma pneumoniac infection in adults. Am J Med 58:229, 1975

Naidich DP, McGuinness G: Pulmonary manifestations of AIDS: CT and radiographic correlations. Radiol Clin North Amer 29:999, 1991

Neiman PE, Reeves W, Ray G et al: A prospective analysis of interstitial pneumonia and opportunistic viral infection among recipients of allogeneic bone marrow grafts. J Infect Dis 136:754, 1977

Ognibene FP, Shelhamer J, Gill V et al: The diagnosis of Pneumocystis carinii in patients with the acquired immune deficiency syndrome using subsegmental bronchoalveolar lavage. Am Rev Respir Dis 129:933, 1984

Ortbals DW, Marr JJ: A comparative study of tuberculosis and other mycobacterial infections and their associations with malignancy. Am Rev Respir dis 117:39, 1978

Palmer DL, Harvey RL, Wheeler JK: Diagnostic and therapeutic considerations in Nocardia asteroides infection. Medicine 53:391, 1974

Pearson ML, Jereb JA, Frieden TR et al: Nosocomial transmission of multidrug-resistant Mycobacterium tuberculosis. Ann Intern Med 117:191, 1992

Perez CR, Leigh MW: Mycoplasma pneumoniae as the causative agent for pneumonia in the immunocompromised host. Chest 100:860, 1991

Pifer LL, Hughes WT, Stagno S, Woods D: Pneumocystis carinii infection: evidence for high prevalence in normal and immunosuppressed children. Pediatrics 61:35, 1978

Pitchenik AE, Burr J, Suarez M et al: Human T-cell lymphotropic virus-III (HTLV-III) seropositivity and related disease among 71 consecutive patients in whom tuberculosis was diagnosed. Am Rev Respir Dis 135:875, 1987

Pitchenik AE, Cole C, Russell BW et al: Tuberculosis, atypical mycobacteriosis and the acquired immunodeficiency syndrome among Haitian and non-Haitian patients in South Florida. Ann Intern Med 101:641, 1984

Pitchenik AE, Fertel D: Tuberculosis and nontuberculosis mycobacterial disease (medical management of AIDS patients). Med Clin North Am 76:121, 1992

Pizzo PA, Robichaud KJ, Gill FA et al: Empiric antibiotic and antifungal therapy for cancer patients with prolonged fever and granulocytopenia. Am J Med 72:101, 1982

Polsky B, Gold JW, Whimbey E et al: Bacterial pneumonia in patients with the acquired immunodeficiency syndrome. Ann Intern Med 140:38, 1986

Prechter GC, Prakash VBS: Bronchoscopy in the diagnosis of pulmonary histoplasmosis. Chest 95:1033, 1989

Ramsey PG, Fife KH, Hackman RC et al: Herpes simplex virus pneumonia: clinical, virologic and pathologic features in 20 patients. Ann Intern Med 97:813, 1982

Reed EC, Bowden RA, Dandliker PS et al: Treatment of cytomegalovirus pneumonia with ganciclovir and intravenous cytomegalovirus immunoglobulin in patients with bone marrow transplants. Ann Intern Med 15:783, 1988

Roilides E, Pizzo PA: Modulation of host defenses by cytokines: evolving adjuncts in prevention and treatment of serious infections in the immunocompromised host. Clin Infect Dis 15:508, 1992

Rolston KVI, Jones PG, Fainstein V et al: Pulmonary disease caused by rapidly growing mycobacteria in patients with cancer. Chest 87:503, 1985

Rossiter SJ, Miller DC, Churg AM et al: Open lung biopsy in the immunosuppressed patient: is it really beneficial? J Thorac Cardiovasc Surg 77:338, 1979

Rotstein C, Cummings K, Nicolaou A et al: Nosocomial infection rates at an oncology center. Infect Control Hosp Epidemiol 9:13, 1988

Saravoltz LD, Burch KH, Fisher E et al: The compromised host and Legionnaires' disease. Ann Intern Med 90:533, 1979

Sarkar SK, Sharma TN, Puroket SD et al: The diagnostic value of routine culture of bronchial washings in tuberculosis. Br J Dis Chest 76:358, 1982

Satterfield JR, McLaughlin JS: Open lung biopsy in diagnosing pulmonary infiltrates in immunosuppressed patients. Ann Thorac Surg 28:359, 1979

Sattler FR, Cowan R, Nielsen DM et al: Trimethoprim-sulfamethoxazole compared with pentamidine for treatment of Pneumocystis carinii pneumonia in the acquired immunodeficiency syndrome. Ann Intern Med 109:200, 1988

Selwyn PA, Hartel D, Lewis VA et al: A prospective study of the risk of tuberculosis among intravenous drug users with human immunodeficiency virus infection. N Engl J Med 320:545, 1989

Sepkowitz KA, Brown AE, Telzak EE et al: Pneumocystis carinii pneumonia among patients without AIDS at a cancer hospital. JAMA 267:832, 1992

Sepkowitz KA, Telzak EE, Gold JW et al: Pneumothorax in AIDS. Ann Intern Med 114:455, 1991

Shepp DH, Dandliker PS, Meyers JD: Treatment of varicella zoster virus infection in severely immunocompromised patients: a randomized comparison of acyclovir and vidarabine. N Engl J Med 314:208, 1986

Sickles EA, Greene WH, Wiernik PH: Clinical presentation of infection in granulocytopenic patients. Arch Intern Med 135:715, 1975

Sickles EA, Young VM, Greene WH et al: Pneumonia in acute leukemia. Ann Intern Med 79:528, 1973

Siemsen JK, Grebe SF, Waxman AD: The use of gallium-67 in pulmonary disorders. Semin Nucl Med 8:235, 1978

Simpson GL, Stinson EB, Egger MJ et al: Nocardial infections in the immunocompromised host: a detailed study in a defined population. Rev Infect Dis 3:492, 1981

Singer C, Armstrong D, Rosen PP et al: Diffuse pulmonary infiltrates in immunocompromised patients: prospective study of 80 cases. Am J Med 66:110, 1979

Singer C, Armstrong D, Rosen PP et al: Pneumocystis carinii pneumonia: a cluster of eleven cases. Ann Intern Med 82:772, 1975

Singer C, Kaplan MH, Armstrong D: Bacteremia and fungemia complicating neoplastic disease: a study of 364 cases. Am J Med 62:731, 1977

Soo Hoo GW, Mohenifar Z, Meyer RD: Inhaled or intravenous pentamidine therapy for Pneumocystis carinii pneumonia in AIDS. Ann Intern Med 113:195, 1990

Stover DE: Diagnosis of pulmonary disease in the immunocompromised host. Semin Respir Med 10:89, 1989

Stover DE, Meduri GU: Pulmonary function tests. Clin Chest Med 9:473, 1988

Stover DE, White DA, Romano PA et al: Diagnosis of pulmonary disease in acquired immune deficiency syndrome (AIDS): role of bronchoscopy and bronchoalveolar lavage. Am Rev Respir Dis 130:659, 1984

Stover DE, Zaman MB, Hajdu SI et al: Bronchoalveolar lavage in the diagnosis of diffuse pulmonary infiltrates in the immunosuppressed host. Ann Intern Med 101:1, 1984

Sunderam G, McDonald RJ, Maniatis T et al: Tuberculosis as a manifestation of the acquired immunodeficiency syndrome (AIDS). JAMA 256:362, 1986

Tenholder MF, Hooper RG: Pulmonary infiltrates in leukemia. Chest 78:468, 1980

Tietjen PA, Jules-Elysee K, Stover DE: Increased incidence of pneumothoraces with aerosolized pentamidine. Chest 96:1875, 1989

Toledo-Pereya LH, De Miester TR, Kinealy A et al: The benefits of open lung biopsy in patients with previous nondiagnostic transbronchial lung biopsy. Chest 77:647, 1990

Turbiner EG, Yeh SD, Rosen PP et al: Abnormal gallium scintigraphy in Pneumocystis carinii pneumonia with a normal chest radiograph. Radiology 127:437, 1978

Vanek J: Atypical interstitial pneumonia of infants produced by Pneumocystis carinii. Cas Lek Cesk 90:1121, 1951

Wakefield AE, Guiver L, Miller RF et al: DNA amplification on induced sputum samples for diagnosis of Pneumocystis carinii pneumonia. Lancet 337:1370, 1991

Wallace JM, Cantanzaro A, Moser KM et al: Flexible fiberoptic bronchoscopy for diagnosing pulmonary coccidioidomycosis. Am Rev Respir Dis 123:286, 1981

Wang KP, Haponik EF, Britt EJ et al: Transbronchial needle aspiration of peripheral pulmonary nodules. Chest 86:819, 1984

Weiner MH, Talbot GH, Gerson SL et al: Antigen detection in the diagnosis of invasive aspergillosis. Utility in controlled blinded trials. Ann Intern Med 99:777, 1983

Wheat LJ: Histoplasmosis. Infect Dis Clin North Am 3:843, 1989

Wheat LJ, Kohler RB, Tewari RP: Diagnosis of disseminated histoplasmosis by detection of Histoplasma capsulatum antigen in serum and urine specimens. N Engl J Med 314:83, 1986

Willcox PA, Benatar SR, Potgieter PD: Use of the flexible fiberoptic bronchoscope in diagnosis of sputum-negative pulmonary tuberculosis. Thorax 37:598, 1987

Wimberly NW, Bass JB, Boyd BW et al: Use of bronchoscopic protected catheter brush for the diagnosis of pulmonary infections. Chest 81:556, 1982

Winn WC, Cherry WB, Frank RO et al: Direct immunofluorescent detection of Legionella pneumophilia in respiratory specimens. J Clin Microbiol 11:59, 1980

Zaman MK, Wooten OJ, Suprahmanya B et al: Rapid noninvasive diagnosis of Pneumocystis carinii pneumonia from induced liquified sputum. Ann Intern Med 109:7, 1988

Zavala DC, Schoell JE: Ultrathin needle aspiration of the lung in infectious and malignant disease. Am Rev Respir Dis 123:123, 1981

21

INTERSTITIAL LUNG DISEASE

Ronald F. Grossman
Andrea J. Cohen

DEFINITION

Interstitial lung disease (ILD) is a generic term for almost 200 heterogeneous lung diseases with several features in common. These disorders are called ILD because, on histologic examination, the interstitium is usually thickened secondary to infiltration with inflammatory cells and fibrosis. This term, however, is misleading because patients can demonstrate both interstitial, alveolar wall, vascular, and/or air space involvement secondary to their disease process; therefore, an alternative name is "diffuse infiltrative lung disease" (Crystal, et al., 1981).

BASIC SCIENCE

Epidemiology

The prevalence of ILD has been estimated to be 5 to 10 per 100,000 population in the United States (Crystal, et al., 1984). The most common conditions are sarcoidosis, idiopathic pulmonary fibrosis (IPF), drug-induced disease, pneumoconiosis secondary to inhalation of inorganic dust, ILD associated with collagen-vascular disease, and extrinsic allergic alveolitis.

There are several methods of classification of the ILDs. The most common of these are by

1. Known and unknown cause
2. Acute and chronic causes
3. Pathologic reaction

In this chapter, we classify ILD by known and unknown causes.

Anatomy and Pathogenesis

The walls of the alveoli are lined by a layer of epithelial cells lying on a thin basement membrane. Type 1 epithelial cells comprise 95 percent of these cells, and the rest are type 2 pneumocytes, the surfactant-producing epithelial cell (Murray, 1976). In the gas-exchanging areas of the alveolus, the capillaries are in close approximation to the basement membrane of the type 1 cell and are lined by a single layer of endothelium that rests on its own basement membrane. The area between the endothelial and epithelial basement membranes is the interstitium and contains structures such as fibroblasts, collagen, elastic fibers, and glycoproteins. The normal alveolar wall is only 5 to 10 μm wide but increases with disorders characterized by cellular infiltration (Fulmer, 1982a).

The mechanism for the production of interstitial pneumonitis is not well understood. The inflammation may be initiated by an agent or agents that injure the epithelial wall and activate inflammatory cells. With the release of mediators by inflammatory cells, an inflammatory reaction (an alveolitis) is initiated and perpetuated (Keogh and Crystal, 1982).

Normally approximately 80 cells can be identified per alveolus, and of these, about 90 percent are macrophages, 10 percent are lymphocytes, and less than 1 percent are neutrophils and eosinophils (Reynolds, 1987). In ILD there is a general increase in the number of the inflammatory cells and an alteration in their proportions (Daniele, et al., 1985). For example in sarcoidosis, there is T-helper cell alveolitis (Hunninghake and Crystal, 1981). These cells secrete factors that cause the chemotaxis of monocytes to the alveolus. The distortion of cell walls secondary to cell infiltration and granuloma formation usually occurs but without permanent damage (Rosen, et al., 1978). Macrophages can release factors that cause proliferation of fibroblasts and deposition of connective tissue, which ultimately distort the architecture (Bitterman, et al., 1982). Reduction of surfactant may contribute to alveolar collapse in these disorders, leading to distortion of lung architecture and impairment of healing (Burkhardt, 1989).

DIAGNOSIS

Clinical Features

The patient with ILD presents a problem of diagnosis and management because there are numerous conditions associated with ILD and the majority are rare. There are few therapeutic modalities available, and controlled clinical trials are infrequent because of the rarity and slowly progressive nature of these disorders. A practical approach is to obtain a careful history and physical examination, study the chest radiograph, and then determine the best approach to further diagnostic testing (Raghu, 1987). Acute disorders that can mimic ILD should be ruled out, such as viral or bacterial infections, *Pneumocystis carinii* infection, aspiration, or pulmonary edema. The tests with the best diagnostic yield can be selected for the suspected disease.

History

Most patients with ILD seek medical advice because of pulmonary symptoms or abnormal routine chest radiographs. The most common symptom is progressive shortness of breath on exertion and fatigue (Dill, et al., 1975). Other common presenting symptoms include cough, pleuritic pain, and less commonly, hemoptysis. Fever and weight loss may also be present. Chest pain and ankle swelling may occur late in the disease with the development of right heart failure.

A careful occupational and drug ingestion history is then obtained to ascertain clues to the cause. The patient's hobbies should be reviewed to determine whether they have been exposed to environmental agents, such as toxins or animal danders. The duration and severity of exposure should be documented. A full functional inquiry must be taken to reveal the presence of a systemic disorder. The family history may expose hereditary disorders, such as tuberous sclerosis or familial pulmonary fibrosis.

Physical Examination

The vital signs are frequently normal, but patients may demonstrate tachypnea and tachycardia. Clubbing of the fingers and toes is common, especially in IPF and asbestosis; cyanosis if present typically occurs late (Scadding and Hinson, 1974). Chest expansion is classically reduced, reflecting the reduction in the total lung capacity. The lung volumes may be normal or paradoxically increased in sarcoidosis, lymphangioleiomyomatosis (LAM), or tuberous sclerosis. Fine end-inspiratory crackles are audible at the posterior lung bases. Wheezes may be heard if there is a coincident obstructive component, as is often seen in sarcoidosis. Coarse crackles and bronchial breathing are less commonly heard. Perfectly normal chest examination results in the presence of diffuse pulmonary infiltrates seen radiographically suggest sarcoidosis (Baughman, et al., 1991).

The general physical examination may reveal evidence of uveitis or cutaneous lesions in sarcoidosis, malar rash in systemic lupus erythematosus (SLE), or the cutaneous findings of dermatomyositis. The cardiac examination is typically normal early in the course of the disease, but pulmonary hypertension may develop later. Signs of pulmonary hypertension include an audible and palpable second component of the second heart sound (increased P2), right ventricular heave, hepatic enlargement, and/or peripheral edema.

Laboratory Studies

The blood count and differential are not usually contributory, except in the presence of eosinophilic lung disease. The sedimentation rate may be elevated in many of these disorders and is not specific. A liver and renal screen should rule out systemic disease involving these organs. Rheumatoid factor, antinuclear antibody (ANA), and complement levels may be strikingly abnormal in connective tissue disease, but low titers of ANA and rheumatoid factor are common in patients with IPF (Holgate, et al., 1983). The serum angiotensin-converting enzyme (ACE) level is elevated in a majority of patients with sarcoidosis but is not pathognomonic of this disease (Studdy, et al., 1978). Antibodies against specific organic antigens may be elevated in cases of clinically suspected extrinsic allergic alveolitis, but these antigens are not specific and may simply indicate past exposure to the antigen (Reynolds, 1982). Antinuclear cytoplasmic antibodies (ANCA) are elevated in the majority of patients with Wegener's granulomatosis, and antibasement membrane antibodies levels may be present in patients with Goodpasture's syndrome (Nolle, et al., 1989; Briggs, et al., 1979).

Radiologic Findings

Chest Radiograph. The routine chest radiograph is limited in the etiologic diagnosis of ILD. As many as 10 percent of patients with biopsy-proved ILD have a normal presenting chest radiograph (Epler, et al., 1978). The normal pulmonary interstitium is ordinarily not visible by chest radiography. However, in the presence of fibrosis or edema of the interstitium, the attenuation of the interstitium increases, and it becomes detectable on the radiograph. Early involvement may manifest as perivascular or peribronchial thickening. A typical radiograph of a patient with ILD shows a linear or reticular and/or nodular interstitial pattern that is characteristically more prominent at the bases (Fig. 21-1). The infiltrate

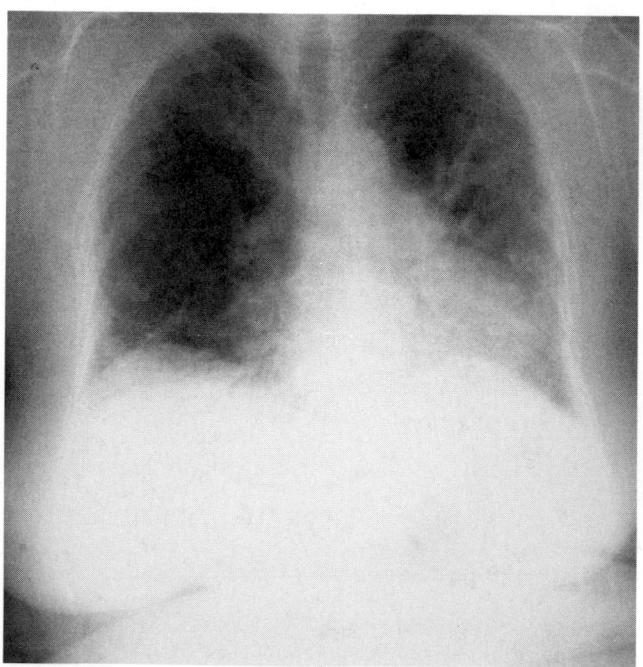

Figure 21-1. PA chest radiograph of a patient with idopathic pulmonary fibrosis. There are reticular nodular infiltrates present diffusely with predominance at the lung bases.

becomes coarser as the disease progresses, and finally, cysts and honeycombing develop. Thickening of the interstitium and the interlobular septa can produce a linear pattern on chest radiography.

A specific diagnosis is difficult to make on the basis of the chest radiograph alone. The appearance and distribution of the lung infiltrate may be helpful. For example, nodular disease is seen in Wegener's granulomatosis. A predominantly upper lobe distribution is seen with eosinophilic granuloma, sarcoidosis, and the fibrosis associated with ankylosing spondylitis (Fig. 21-2). The presence of lymphadenopathy or pleural involvement may help further to characterize a specific ILD. For example pleural effusions are often seen in association with pulmonary edema, malignancy, or rheumatoid arthritis. Chylous effusions may be present in patients with LAM. Patients with eosinophilic granuloma or LAM may present with a spontaneous pneumothorax. Bilaeral hilar lymphadenopathy favors a diagnosis of sarcoidosis or lymphoma. It is important that previous radiographs be examined to document the progression of disease. In many cases, the appearance on plain radiography is nonspecific and may mislead the clinician. The recent introduction of 1-mm collimation computed tomographic (CT) scans has highlighted the limitations of the routine chest radiograph (Zerhouni, et al., 1985).

Despite these problems, the chest radiograph is valuable in the detection of ILD. It is the radiographic procedure of choice for the initial assessment of the patient with suspected ILD and is a simple and practical way of following the course of the disease.

Computed Tomography. Computed tomography (CT) and high-resolution CT scans are useful adjuncts. The conventional CT scan is performed by imaging 8- to 10-mm thick slices at 10-mm intervals. The combination of 1 to 2-mm collimation and a high-frequency resolution algorithm is referred to as a high-resolution CT scan. This technique improves spatial resolution by 40 percent. High-resolution CT scanning can identify abnormalities of lung parenchyma better than does the chest radiograph (Muller and Ostrow, 1991). This is possible because CT eliminates superimposition of pulmonary structures. High-resolution CT can show the details of normal pulmonary anatomy, such as pulmonary vessels, bronchi, and secondary lobules. In addition because these diseases are often patchy in distribution, the CT scan can be a useful guide to the best biopsy site. Certain abnormalities on CT scan support the diagnosis of ILD, including irregular linear opacities, thickened interlobular septa, nodules, abnormal interfaces between vessels, bronchi, the visceral pleura, and air space opacification (Muller, et al., 1986). The specific diagnosis is made by noting the distribution and the description of the specific abnormalities. CT scan interpretations are most accurate in silicosis, IPF, lymphangitic carcinomatosis, and sarcoidosis (Muller et al., 1986; Mathieson, et al., 1989).

Gallium Scanning. Noninvasive tests that can evaluate the "activity" of ILD include ^{67}Ga citrate lung scanning and ^{99m}Tc diethylenetriamine pentaacetic acid (^{99m}Tc-DTPA) clearance studies. In addition ^{67}Ga scintography can be useful diagnostically. For example, Figure 21-3 illustrates intrathoracic and extrathoracic lymph node uptake characteristic of sarcoidosis. Right paratracheal and para- and infrahilar uptake have been noted only in sarcoidosis (Heshiki, et al.,

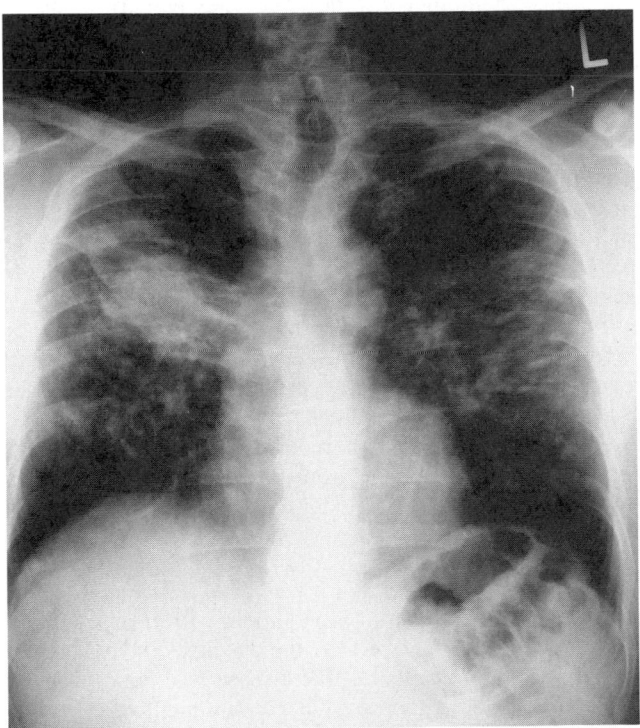

Figure 21-2. PA chest radiograph of a patient with sarcoidosis. There are reticular nodular infiltrates present with upper zone predominance.

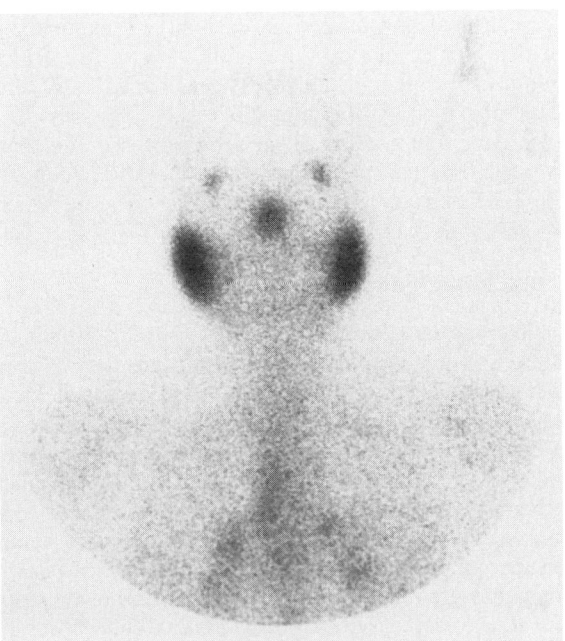

Figure 21-3. Gallium scan of a patient with sarcoidosis. Note the increased uptake of gallium in the conjunctival tissue, parotid glands, and hilar and mediastinal lymph nodes.

1974). The pattern of symmetrical parotid, lacrimal, and submandibular salivary gland localization is strongly associated with sarcoidosis (Beaumont, et al., 1982). Except for sarcoidosis, the pattern of gallium uptake is of limited diagnostic value. The gallium scan may be useful for follow-up of some patients receiving therapy for their disease, and it is a sensitive indicator of response. However repeat testing is limited because of the relatively high radiation exposure with each test.

In patients with IPF, the gallium scan is positive in 70 percent of cases (Line, et al., 1978). In some patients, quantitative scans may be useful in the staging of the disease and in evaluating the reponse to therapy. However, the quantity of gallium uptake is not predictive of which patient's condition will ultimately deteriorate (Pantin, et al., 1988). Gallium scanning may also be positive in drug-induced lung damage, as seen with bleomycin or amiodarone (Zhu, et al., 1988). These changes are not specific for drug-induced disease. Because the changes on gallium scanning are usually not specific for any disorder and the predictive value of the gallium scan has not been established, some investigators advocate the abandonment of this test as a routine investigation for ILD (Whitcomb and Dixon, 1984).

^{99m}Tc-DTPA, Lung Scanning. Aerosols labeled with ^{99m}Tc-DTPA are used to assess lung injury by measuring the increased permeability to solutes that results from rupture of the alveolar-epithelial boundary (Rinderknecht, et al., 1980). The measure of injury is the rate of clearance from the lung of the radiolabeled aerosol. Most centers use ^{99m}Tc-DTPA as the tracer element in the aerosol. The clearance is highly sensitive to virtually any kind of lung injury but is inherently nonspecific (Kramer and Divgi, 1991).

Magnetic Resonance Imaging. Magnetic resonance imaging (MRI) is not routinely used in the assessment of ILD because of its high cost and limited accessibility. Preliminary data show that high-resolution CT scan is superior to MRI in the anatomic assessment of the lung parenchyma. However, the contrast provided by MRI may allow superior assessment of the presence and grading of air space disease and thereby allow assessment of the disease's activity (McFadden, et al., 1987). MRI may ultimately be useful in serial examination of patients with ILD because of the lack of ionizing radiation.

Invasive Investigations

Bronchoscopy and Bronchoalveolar Lavage. Patients with ILD are usually investigated with bronchoscopy and bronchoalveolar lavage (Strumpf, et al., 1981). The flexible fiberoptic bronchoscope is wedged in a peripheral segment where the alveolitis is expected. Typically 100 ml of sterile saline is injected through the bronchoscope in 20-ml aliquots, and then samples of the alveolar fluid are recovered. Specimens are sent for cell count, cytologic examination, lymphocyte subtyping, and microbiologic studies. In cases in which eosinophilic granuloma is suspected, electron microscopy can be done to detect typical intracellular X bodies (Basset, et al., 1977). The finding of lipoproteinaceous material indicates alveolar proteinosis in appropriate patients, and iron-laden macrophages can be highly suggestive of pulmonary hemor-

rhage (Martin, et al., 1980; Drew, et al., 1977). The finding of oil-laden macrophages in large number corroborates a diagnosis of mineral oil aspiration (Corwin and Irwin, 1985). Alternatively in cases of suspected occupational lung disease, the lavage sample can be analyzed for particles of inorganic material or by electron probe analysis for dust particles (Davison, et al., 1983).

Bronchoscopy can rule out malignant or infectious processes. The lavage can be useful in detecting and classifying the alveolitis by cell type (Hunninghake, et al., 1979). This may narrow the differential diagnosis because certain ILDs are associated with a specific increase in cell type. For example, an increased percentage of lymphocytes is seen in sarcoidosis, extrinsic allergic alveolitis, and tuberculosis. The type of alveolitis may also help determine the prognosis of a specific disease and indicate the response to therapy in some patients. For example, T cell subtyping has revealed that there are increased T-helper cells in sarcoidosis (Hunninghake and Crystal, 1981). There is little evidence to suggest that the cell count and differential obtained from bronchoalveolar lavage are useful in predicting clinical response to therapy or the natural history of the disease in the majority of patients (Helmers and Hunninghake, 1989). It is generally not used to guide therapy and should be regarded as a research tool.

Biopsy. Transbronchial biopsy through the bronchoscope may provide sufficient tissue for the diagnosis of sarcoidosis, carcinoma, infections, or alveolar proteinosis. The diagnostic yield in sarcoidosis approaches 80 percent, but this procedure is less helpful in the other disorders (Thrasher and Briggs, 1982). The samples are generally too small to make a definitive diagnosis in other disorders, but they can give clues to the disease's cause. Mediastinoscopy with biopsy of enlarged mediastinal lymph nodes may be worthwhile in patients with diffuse infiltrates, especially in sarcoidosis, tuberculosis, lymphoma, and histoplasmosis. Thoracoscopic or open lung biopsies are usually required to obtain sufficient tissue in the ILDs (Flint, 1982). Samples should be sent from the operating room to the microbiology laboratory for assessment of bacteria, fungi, viruses, and parasites. Other specimens should be fixed for light and electron microscopy and immunofluorescence testing. Tissue should also be frozen, pending further investigations, such as viral studies or flow cytometry. It is important to discuss with the referring physician the tests required prior to the operative procedure. It is best to take at least two biopsies from areas with early and intermediate disease. In most cases, it is recommended that the lingula be avoided because tissue from this area tends to exhibit end-stage changes.

Patient Assessment

A functional assessment of each patient with ILD is mandatory. It is often performed after the diagnosis of ILD is confirmed and an assessment of the disease's activity has been made. This is best done by the measurement of complete pulmonary function studies (lung volumes, flow rates, and diffusing capacity), arterial blood gases, and in selected cases, exercise studies. In most instances, a restrictive ventilatory pattern is identified that is associated with a decrease in diffusing capacity (Fulmer, 1982b). In a subset of patients, the physiologic abnormalities suggest an obstructive ventilatory defect, despite the presence of a diffuse pulmonary infiltrate (Sharma and Johnson, 1988). This narrows the differential diagnosis to such disorders as sarcoidosis, eosinophilic granuloma, LAM, tuberous sclerosis, and ILD secondary to intravenous drug abuse. Arterial blood gases typically demonstrate hypoxemia with a mild respiratory alkalosis. Exercise studies reveal a pattern of rapid shallow breathing associated with oxygen desaturation, which may be profound (Crystal, et al., 1976).

Information from the bronchoalveolar lavage, gallium scan, and open lung biopsy may add important information on the disease's activity. After this information is reviewed, the physician can determine whether therapy is indicated. The age and general health of the patient should be considered prior to sending the patient for a lung biopsy or embarking on a long course of therapy. If possible it is advantageous to make a definitive tissue diagnosis prior to commencing toxic therapy. Therapy is usually offered to patients whose conditions demonstrate clear clinical deterioration after a short period of observation. In the absence of clinical deterioration, a period of close observation is required, and therapy is often withheld.

INTERSTITIAL LUNG DISEASES OF UNKNOWN CAUSE

Idiopathic Pulmonary Fibrosis

IPF (also called cryptogenic fibrosing alveolitis) occurs most commonly in patients between the ages of 50 and 60 years. A rapidly progressive fatal illness was originally described by Hamman and Rich (1944), but the syndrome was renamed IPF when the heterogeneous nature of the disorder was identified. Liebow, et al., (1965) later subdivided these disorders into usual interstitial pneumonitis (UIP), desquamative interstitial pneumonitis (DIP), lymphocytic interstitial pneumonitis (LIP), and giant cell interstitial pneumonitis. UIP and DIP are now referred to as IPF. In UIP there is alveolar wall invasion by inflammatory cells and fibrosis, with a variable macrophage alveolitis (Fig. 21-4). In DIP there is an accumulation of some inflammatory cells and mild fibrosis and a significant macrophage alveolitis. Originally these cells were thought to represent desquamated pneumocytes, but more recently, they have been clearly identified as macrophages. DIP may remit more often than does UIP, and it appears to be more responsive to the administration of corticosteroids (Carrington, et al., 1978).

Patients present with progressive dyspnea and a nonproductive cough. Physical examination may reveal fine crackles at the lung bases and finger clubbing (Scadding, 1974). The chest radiograph typically shows decreased lung volumes, bilateral interstitial infiltrates, and honeycombing in advanced disease. A reduced diffusion capacity and a restrictive ventilatory defect are found on pulmonary function testing. There are no specific blood tests that are diagnostic of IPF. The sedimentation rate may be elevated, and mild increases in rheumatoid factor and ANA titers are common. There also

---

Interstitial Lung Diseases of Unknown Origin

Idiopathic pulmonary fibrosis
Bronchiolitis obliterans organizing pneumonia
Sarcoidosis
Lymphangioleiomyomatosis
Eosinophilic granuloma
Pulmonary vasculitis
    Wegener's granulomatosis
    Churg-Strauss vasculitis
    Lymphomatoid granulomatosis
Interstitial lung disease associated with connective tissue disease
    Rheumatoid arthritis
    Systemic sclerosis
    Sjögren's syndrome
    Systemic lupus erythematosus
    Polymyositis/dermatomyositis
    Ankylosing spondylitis
Pulmonary renal syndromes
    Goodpasture's syndrome
    Idiopathic pulmonary hemosiderosis
Eosinophilic pneumonia
Alveolar proteinosis
Inherited disorders
    Tuberous sclerosis
    Neurofibromatosis
    Familial idiopathic pulmonary fibrosis
    Gaucher's disease
    Niemann-Pick disease
    Hermansky-Pudlak syndrome
Amyloidosis
Lymphocytic disorders
    Pseudolymphoma
    Lymphocytic interstitial pneumonitis
    Immunoblastic lymphoma
Bronchocentric granulomatosis
Pulmonary veno-occlusive disease
Graft-versus-host disease
Sequelae of adult respiratory distress syndrome

---

may be elevated levels of immune complexes (Dreisen, et al., 1978). The median survival of all patients is less than 5 years (Stack, et al., 1972).

IPF is a difficult condition to manage because the prognosis is unpredictable and therapeutic responses are unusual (Scadding and Hinson, 1967). Assessment and therapeutic protocols therefore differ in content between centers. A large sample of tissue, such as that obtained in an open lung biopsy, is essential for both a confident diagnosis and staging. It is

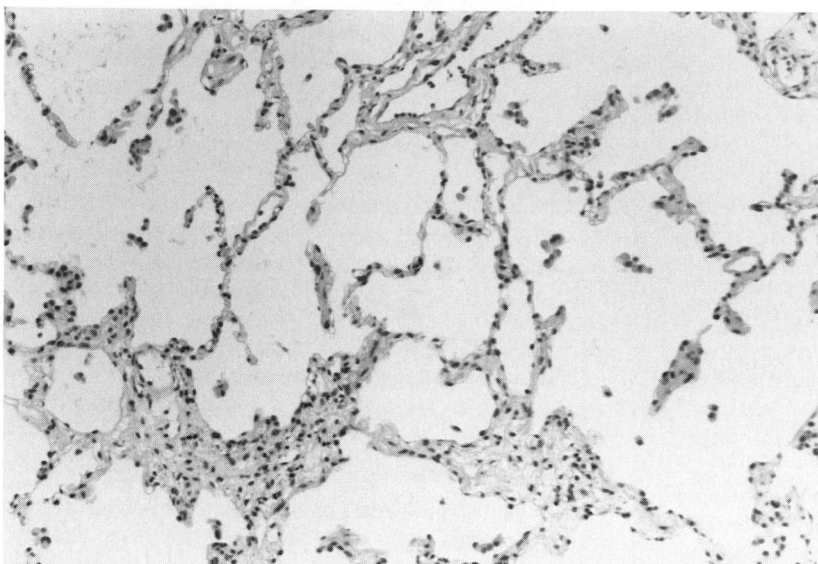

Figure 21-4. Open lung biopsy of a patient with idiopathic pulmonary fibrosis. Note the interstitial fibrosis with architectural restructuring (H&E, × 100).

important to document a definitive diagnosis and rule out other possible causes for fibrosis prior to committing the patient to a course of corticosteroids and/or immunosuppressants. Prior to commencing therapy, the patient should be staged for the level of the disease's activity. Symptoms, progression of radiographic abnormalities, gallium scan positivity, and reduction in pulmonary function over a follow-up period have all been used to determine activity. Those whose diseases are classified as inactive are generally followed at regular intervals. Patients whose diseases are deemed to be active are started on a course of corticosteroids. Those who do not respond to a 3-month trial may benefit by the addition of azathioprine and/or cyclophosphamide. Two randomized trials showed that the long-term survival rate may be improved by the early addition of immunosuppressants, such as azathioprine or cyclophosphamide, and early treatment for affected patients was advocated by some investigators (Raghu, et al., 1991; Johnson, et al., 1989). Success was also reported with cyclosporine in a limited number of patients, but there are no clinical trials to support its usage (Moolma, et al., 1991). Characteristics that support a better prognosis include the female gender, younger age, cellular biopsy (DIP), less symptoms on first consultation, and an increased amount of type 3 collagen in the biopsy (Raghu, 1987). Recently it was proposed that all patients start therapy at diagnosis to ensure a survival advantage; some physicians even prescribe corticosteroids for patients with IPF, independent of the disease's activity. Transplantation was successful in a select group of patients, and appropriate patients can be referred for assessment for a single lung transplant (Grossman, et al., 1990).

Bronchiolitis Obliterans Organizing Pneumonia

Bronchiolitis obliterans organizing pneumonia (BOOP) is associated with a short period (less than 2 months) of progressive dypsnea, cough, fever, and weight loss (Epler, et al.,

1985). Physical examination typically reveals bibasilar crackles but may show clubbing, bronchial breathing, and fever. Arterial blood gases reveal a widened alveolar-arterial gradient, and chest radiographs show interstitial and/or alveolar opacities. The main feature of BOOP is patchy air space consolidation with small nodular opacities. The distribution of air space disease is subpleural in 50 percent of patients. Bronchial wall thickening, dilatation, and pleural effusions may also be seen. The sedimentation rate is elevated, and pulmonary function tests show a restrictive ventilatory defect. Pathologic examination of the lungs shows young fibrous plugs in the respiratory bronchioles, alveoli, and alveolar sacs and an associated chronic interstitial pneumonitis dominated by lipid-laden macrophages (Fig. 21-5). Open lung biopsy is usually required to establish the diagnosis. It is important to distinguish this illness from IPF because the majority of patients with BOOP recover from their illness. Prednisone is given in a dosage of 1 mg/kg/day for about 3 months until a clinical response is obtained. Then the drug is slowly tapered to a maintenance dose of 20 mg on alternate days. However, no comparative dosing trials have been performed. Prednisone should be tapered slowly because recurrances have been observed. A subset of patients with BOOP develops progressive disease, which may ultimately be fatal despite therapy with high-dose corticosteroids, immunosuppressive therapy, and mechanical ventilation (Cordier, et al., 1989).

Sarcoidosis

Sarcoidosis, a multisystem granulomatous disease, can develop in most organ systems and lead to varied clinical presentations (Fig. 21-6). It was first recognized as a dermatologic disorder in 1878 by Sir Jonathan Hutchinson (1877), a British dermatologist, and the pathologic condition was described in 1899 by Caesar Boeck (1899), a Norwegian dermatologist. Almost 40 years after the first description of the

Figure 21-5. Open lung biopsy demonstrating bronchiolitis obliterans with organizing pneumonia. Note the presence of loose connective tissue obliterating the small airways with microscopic lipoid pneumonia (H&E, × 50).

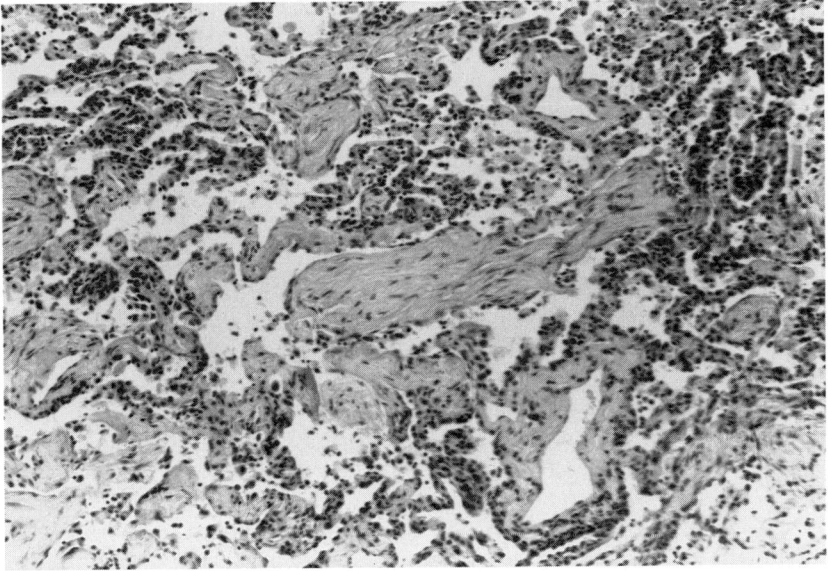

disease, the true systemic nature and the associated pulmonary involvement was clearly described (Kuznitsky and Bittorf, 1915).

The cause of the disease is unknown. Many putative agents have been identified, but none so far has withstood rigorous scrutiny. The most recent candidate is once again Mycobacteria because some investigators detected minute quantities of mycobacterial DNA in clinical samples from patients with sarcoidosis (Saboor, et al., 1992). However, even these provocative findings cannot be confirmed by other investigators (Bocart, et al., 1992).

There is an increased prevalence and severity of the disease in the black population (Johns, 1989). The organs that are most commonly involved include the lungs, skin, eyes, nervous system, heart, kidneys, and musculoskeletal system.

Specific syndromes of sarcoidosis include Lofgren's syndrome (1953), which is characterized by the abrupt onset of hilar lymphadenopathy, fever, and erythema nodosum, and Heerfordt's syndrome (1909) or uveoparotid fever, which is distinguished by fever, parotid gland swelling, uveitis, and cranial nerve palsies. The lungs are the most commonly involved organ in sarcoidosis, but up to one-third of patients with pulmonary sarcoidosis are asymptomatic. Their disease is discovered by routine chest radiography (Maycock, et al., 1963). The symptoms, if present, include dyspnea on exertion, wheezing, and a nonproductive cough.

Traditionally patients are staged radiographically. Stage 0 reveals no chest radiographic abnormalities. Stage 1 radiographs show hilar adenopathy alone. Stage 2 has hilar adenopathy and diffuse interstitial infiltrates. Stage 3 is denoted by

Figure 21-6. Open lung biopsy showing sarcoidosis. Note the granuloma present in the microvascular bundle (H&E, × 50).

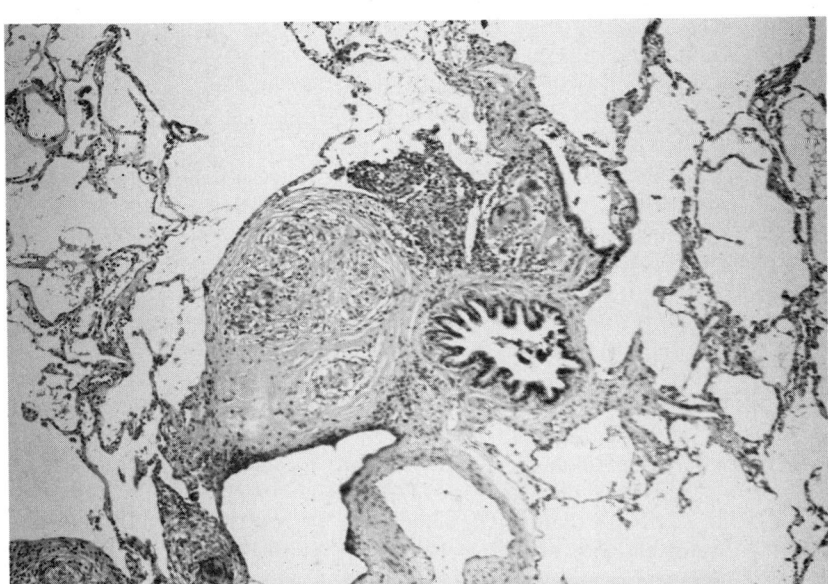

interstitial infiltrates without adenopathy. Stage 4 disease demonstrates advanced chronic changes with coarse interstitial markings, honeycombing, and hilar retraction (Geraint James, 1984). Radiographic findings when present commonly appear as diffuse reticular nodular infiltrates with a predilection for the lung apices but occasionally as a fluffy alveolar pattern. Infrequent findings include large nodules, which rarely cavitate, bullous disease, pleural effusions, eggshell calcification of lymph nodes, pneumothorax, and mycetomas in areas of advanced disease (Rockoff and Rohatgi, 1985). The value of radiographic staging is that the rate of radiographic resolution is inversely related to the radiographic stage at presentation; the mortality rate is directly correlated with the radiographic stage (DeRemee, 1983).

A CT scan can clearly demonstrate anterior mediastinal and subcarinal lymph node enlargement. The usual abnormality on the CT scan is nodules along the bronchovascular bundles, interlobar septa, major fissures, and subpleural region (Muller, et al., 1989). The nodules can be focal or diffuse or smooth or irregular, and they are less than 5 mm in diameter. The granulomas can cause thickening of the interlobar septa, pulmonary vessels, and bronchial vessels. If fibrosis develops, linear opacities appear that are usually peribronchovascular. Hazy increases in pulmonary densities correlate with active alveolitis, as assessed by gallium scanning (Line, et al., 1978).

Pulmonary function test results may be normal or demonstrate a restrictive and/or obstructive ventilatory defect and a reduction in the diffusing capacity (Boushy, et al., 1965). The pulmonary function tests, although defining the level of functional impairment, correlate poorly with the presence and intensity of the alveolitis (Lin, et al., 1985). There may be evidence of hypoxemia at rest or with exercise.

The diagnosis of sarcoidosis is often made clinically, especially in an asymptomatic patient with negative physical examination findings and bilateral hilar adenopathy (Winterbauer, et al., 1973). Many clinicians prefer to obtain tissue confirmation in all cases of possible sarcoidosis to avoid the possibility of missing a potentially treatable condition other than sarcoidosis, such as tuberculosis. A bronchoscopy with transbronchial lung biopsy is the preferred diagnostic test, with a yield of noncaseating granulomata in 70 to 90 percent of cases (Gilman and Wang, 1980; Rothe, et al., 1980). Cutaneous lesions and enlarged lymph nodes or lacrimal glands may be biopsied preferentially, if easily accessible (Sharma, 1985). Mediastinoscopy and open lung biopsy are reserved for the most difficult cases when other measures have not yielded the diagnosis.

The serum ACE levels are often elevated in sarcoidosis and can be used to follow disease activity in those patients in whom the test result is abnormal (Lieberman, 1975). Serum ACE concentrations may also be elevated in tuberculosis, leprosy, and Gaucher's disease (Studdy and Bird, 1989). Changes in serum ACE levels correlate poorly with changes in routine clinical parameters, such as chest radiographs or pulmonary function (Hollinger, et al., 1985). The pretreatment serum ACE level does not predict improvement in pulmonary function with therapy (Baughman, et al., 1984). In the majority of patients, serum ACE levels cannot be used to make therapeutic decisions.

Bronchoalveolar lavage was advocated as a tool to predict the clinical response to therapy (Keogh, et al., 1983). Unfortunately other studies have not confirmed the initial observations, and the clinical utility of this investigation is limited (Foley, et al., 1989; Turner-Warwick, et al., 1986).

Over a 3-year period, many patients with sarcoidosis have a spontaneous remission (Smellie and Hoyle, 1960). Patients with Lofgren's syndrome or hilar lymphadenopathy alone have the highest rates of spontaneous remission. It is rare for the disease to recur if it has regressed spontaneously. Untreated the disease can stop at moderate fibrosis or progress to end-stage lung disease. Therapy is usually reserved for patients with symptomatic pulmonary disease; systemic symptoms; hypercalcemia; or involvement of the eyes, kidneys, heart, or central nervous system (Muthiah and Macfarlane, 1990). In patients with stage I disease, therapy is withheld unless evidence of clinical, radiographic, or physiologic deterioration is documented. In patients with stages II or III disease and normal pulmonary function, therapy is usually withheld and introduced when deterioration is documented. In patients with stages II or III disease with abnormal lung function, therapy is usually started immediately. Prednisone in a dose of 0.5 to 1.0 mg/kg of body weight is initiated until an appropriate clinical response is reached, and then, it is tapered gradually. We have found that the best monitors to follow include serum ACE levels, chest radiographs, pulmonary function tests, gallium scans, and lung permeability scans, although not all these tests are helpful in every patient. There is currently no role for the use of inhaled steroids in the therapy of sarcoidosis. Other therapeutic modalities that have been tried include chloroquine, chlorambucil, methotrexate, and cyclosporine (O'Leary, et al., 1986; Kataria, 1980; Lower and Baughman, 1990; Martinet, et al., 1988). Few controlled clinical trials have been performed, and the role of these medications is uncertain. Transplantation is an option for the patient with end-stage disease.

Lymphangioleiomyomatosis

In 1937 von Stossel (1937) described diffuse cystic changes in the lung and lymphadenopathy in a women who died of respiratory failure. He commented on the proliferation of smooth muscle throughout the lung and called the process muscular cirrhosis of the lungs. LAM occurs typically in women of reproductive age. The presenting symptoms include cough, slowly progressive dyspnea, and hemoptysis; affected women may develop spontaneous pneumothorax with chylous pleural effusion. Chest radiographs show normal or increased lung volumes with reticulonodular shadows and small cystlike areas.

The lung's surface is covered with tiny cysts, which are found throughout the lung substance. Smooth muscle cells proliferate in the lung tissue throughout lymphatic, vascular, and bronchial structures. These lesions can cause (1) local airway obstruction, leading to air flow obstruction and cyst formation; (2) blood vessel obstruction, leading to venular congestion and bleeding; and (3) lymphatic obstruction, leading to chylothorax. With high-resolution CT, there is a combination of normal lung tissue and areas filled with numerous thin-walled cystic air spaces of multiple sizes (Merchant,

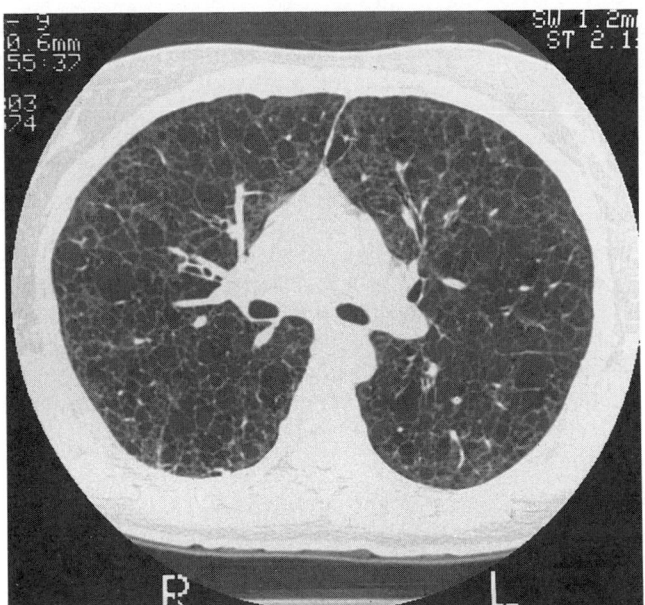

Figure 21-7. Lung window of a high-resolution CT scan of the thorax in a patient with lymphangioleiomyomatosis. Note the presence of cystic spaces throughout the lung parenchyma.

et al., 1985; Fig. 21-7). The cysts are made by muscle cell proliferation in the bronchioles and subsequent air trapping. LAM can be distinguished from IPF on CT scans because IPF has abnormalities in the subpleural areas and the bases, unlike LAM, which has diffuse abnormalities. In addition, the majority of cysts in LAM are surrounded by areas of normal lung, whereas the honeycombing in IPF is surrounded by abnormalities in the parenchyma.

Although the natural history of this disorder is not known, the general view is that most patients die within 10 years of the onset of disease (Corrin, et al., 1975). This view was challenged recently, and hormonal manipulation may lead to prolonged survival in some patients (Taylor, et al., 1990). Progesterone and/or oophorectomy appear to produce remissions in about 50 percent of patients; however, it is difficult to assess the response because the disease's course is variable (Eliasson, et al., 1989). Other therapy with androgens and tamoxifen is less successful. There is currently an ongoing trial with interferon-α_1 for treatment of LAM. Successful lung transplants have been done in a select group of patients.

Eosinophilic Granuloma

Eosinophilic granuloma is one of three disorders (Letterer-Siwe disease and Hand-Schüller-Christian disease are the other two) that traditionally have been called Histiocytosis X. The latter two are diseases of children and are not discussed further here. Eosinophilic granuloma is a rare condition of unknown cause that is characterized by histiocytic infiltration of the lung. In a minority of patients, there are also lesions of the bone, posterior pituitary, and skin.

The disease is usually diagnosed in the third decade, and most series report a male predominance (Friedman, et al., 1981). More than 90 percent of patients report a smoking history. Patients present with cough, dyspnea on exertion, fever, and weight loss. Spontaneous pneumothorax is common. The physical examination findings can be normal or reveal wheezing. Despite the name, there is no peripheral eosinophilia in this condition. Patients with systemic involvement can develop diabetes insipidus, diffuse lymphadenopathy, rashes, or bone lesions. Chest radiographs show preserved or enlarged pulmonary volumes with reticular nodular and nodular interstitial infiltrates involving the upper and middle lobes and sparing the costophrenic angles (Lacronique, et al., 1982). The nodules typically have a stellate shape and a tendency to cavitate when enlarged. The cavitated nodules can progress to honeycombing and bullae. A frequent finding is fine honeycombing of the central portions of the upper lobes. High-resolution CT scanning can identify small and large cysts and micronodules that are not apparent by chest radiography (Brauner, et al., 1989). CT findings correlate better with physiologic abnormalities than do radiographic findings (Moore, et al., 1989).

Histiocytes containing X bodies (i.e., pentalaminar rods 40 to 45 nm in width with central striations that resemble a tennis racket) can be seen with electron microscopic examination of bronchoalveolar lavage fluid (Basset, et al., 1977). The identification of X bodies is not pathognomonic for eosinophilic granuloma because they are found in Langerhans cells in the skin, lung cancer, and pulmonary fibrosis. In the appropriate clinical setting, they may be diagnostic. The course of disease is variable and can spontaneously regress or progress rapidly to death (Basset, et al., 1978). Features of the illness that suggest a progressive downhill course include extremes of age, multiple pneumothoraces, multisystem generalized disease, prolonged constitutional disturbance, extensive initial pulmonary radiologic involvement with formation of cysts, and a low carbon monoxide diffusing capacity. Corticosteroids and immunosuppressants have been used, but there is no evidence that they alter the course of the disease (Prophet, 1982). Large compressive masses were reduced with radiation therapy. Pleurodesis can prevent recurrent pneumothoraces. Lung transplantation is an option for selected patients with end-stage disease.

Pulmonary Vasculitis

Wegener's Granulomatosis

Wegener's granulomatosis was first described in the 1930s by Klinger (1931) and then Wegener (1936) as a form of periarteritis in which granulomatous inflammation of the nose and paranasal sinuses was prominent. It is characterized by granulomatous vasculitic inflammation of the nose, paranasal sinuses, and lungs and necrotizing glomerulitis. A limited form of the disease, in which there is no evidence of renal disease, was described by Carrington and Liebow (1966). Presenting symptoms include sinusitis, arthralgias, fever, otitis, cough, nasal symptoms, hemoptysis, and weight loss. Other less common presentations include ocular inflammation, rash, epistaxis, chest discomfort, malaise, dyspnea, hearing loss, or headache (Fauci, et al., 1978). Initially affected individuals may show pulmonary infiltrates, sinus tenderness, renal failure, proptosis, oral ulcers, or pleural effusions. At presentation pulmonary disease occurs in 94 percent of patients; renal disease is apparent in 85 percent (Fauci, et al., 1983).

Laboratory results are nonspecific, but the sedimentation rate may be markedly evaluated. A positive test for ANCA supports the diagnosis of Wegener's granulomatosis, but a negative result does not rule out the disease (van der Woude, et al., 1985). The chest radiograph most commonly demonstrates bilateral multiple nodules with cavitation. Up to 40 percent of patients present with a solitary nodule. Other radiographic patterns include atelectasis secondary to endobronchial lesions, pleural effusions, and diffuse interstitial or alveolar patterns (Cordier, et al., 1990). The diagnosis is made from tissue obtained at open lung biopsy. The classic pathologic findings are a necrotizing granulomatous vasculitis involving the small and medium-sized veins and arteries. The histologic finding of capillary inflammation distinguishes Wegener's granulomatosis from Goodpasture's syndrome in the case of acute pulmonary hemorrhage. Biopsies of the nose or sinuses tend not to be useful because they often demonstrate nonspecific granulomatous inflammation without frank vasculitis. Furthermore, biopsy of the kidneys does not reveal specific pathologic findings; a glomerulitis rather than graulomatous vasculitis is usually seen.

Prior to the introduction of cytotoxic drug therapy, more than 90 percent of patients with Wegener's granulomatosis died within 2 years. Currently standard therapy for Wegener's includes high-dose corticosteroids and cyclophosphamide. Therapy is continued until 1 year after recovery and then tapered over the following year. A rise in ANCA titers often precedes the clinical relapse, and it has been proposed to base therapeutic decisions on the results of this test (Cohen Tervaert, et al., 1990). Trimethoprim-sulfamethoxazole has been reported to improve the clinical course of patients with Wegener's granulomatosis. However, the data are not conclusive, and further evaluation is necessary (DeRemee, et al., 1985). Recently high-dose pooled intravenous immunoglobulin was used to treat systemic vasculitis, but its exact role has yet to be defined (Jayne, et al., 1991).

Churg-Strauss Vasculitis

Allergic angiitis and granulomatosis is a systemic vasculitis first described by Churg and Strauss (1951), involving the lung, skin, heart, and gastrointestinal tract. The pulmonary syndrome that affects most patients consists of atopy, asthma, and diffuse pulmonary infiltrates. The peripheral eosinophil count and sedimentation rate are often markedly elevated. The diagnosis is made on tissue from an open lung biopsy, and the histologic findings characteristically show granulomas, eosinophilic infiltrates, and necrotizing vasculitis. Most patients respond with steroids; a subgroup requires immunosuppressant drugs.

Lymphomatoid Granulomatosis

Lymphomatoid granulomatosis, originally described by Liebow, et al., (1972) is a disease characterized by infiltration of various organs with a polymorphic infiltrate consisting of atypical lymphocytoid and plasmacytoid cells with granulomatous inflammation in an angiocentric pattern. Although

the lung is most frequently involved, cutaneous, renal, and central nervous system involvement is common (Fauci, et al., 1982). The clinical manifestations are nonspecific and include cough, dyspnea, chest pain, fever, and weight loss. Spontaneously clearing multiple bilateral nodules that may cavitate characterize the radiographic findings (Israel, et al., 1977). Open lung biopsy shows invasion of small and medium-sized vessels by atypical lymphocytes, monocytes, and granulomas. Many classify lymphomatoid granulomatosis as a lymphoproliferative disorder rather than an inflammatory disease because of the tendency to transform into lymphoma. The lung disease usually responds to steroids and cyclophosphamide; however some patients require therapy with chemotherapeutic agents. Patients must be closely followed to detect the development of lymphoma.

Interstitial Lung Disease Associated with Connective Tissue Disease

Rheumatoid Arthritis

Until the early 1980s, rheumatoid arthritis was associated with five pulmonary complications: (1) pleurisy with or without effusion, (2) necrobiotic nodules (rheumatoid nodules), (3) Caplan's syndrome (rheumatoid pneumoconiosis), (4) interstitial pneumonitis and fibrosis, and (5) pulmonary arteritis (Hunninghake and Fauci, 1979). More recently bronchiolitis obliterans, whether occurring de novo or secondary to drugs used in the treatment of rheumatoid disease, such as penicillamine or gold, was described (Penny, et al., 1982; Holness, et al., 1983). Ellman and Ball (1948) first noticed the association of rheumatoid disease and ILD. Patients with rheumatoid arthritis develop an ILD similar to IPF. Beween 1.6 and 4.5 percent of patients have radiographic evidence of diffuse pulmonary fibrosis, but up to 40 percent of patients show pulmonary function abnormalities compatible with this syndrome (Jurik, et al., 1982; Roschmann and Rothenberg, 1987). Patients present with dyspnea and cough, and examination reveals basal crackles without clubbing. Pulmonary findings may precede the development of rheumatologic manifestations of the disease by several years. Pulmonary involvement is associated usually with seropositive, erosive, nodular rheumatoid disease (Walker and Wright, 1969). Bibasilar interstitial infiltrates are found on the radiograph, which may eventually progress to honeycombing. Patients with upper lobe bullous disease without basilar infiltrates have been reported, but this presentation is rare. Pulmonary function studies reveal a restrictive ventilatory pattern with an abnormality of gas transfer. Exercise studies indicate a pattern of rapid shallow breathing and exercise-induced oxygen desaturation. The disease may be progressive, but few patients with rheumatoid arthritis die of progressive respiratory failure. In those patients hospitalized for rheumatoid ILD, the prognosis is poor, with a median survival of 3.5 years and a 5-year survival rate of 39 percent (Hakala, 1988). There is no established therapy for this disease. There are occasional reports of treatment success with corticosteroids, penicillamine, methotrexate, and azathioprine. However, ILD can infrequently develop as a result of methotrexate therapy.

Systemic Sclerosis

Systemic sclerosis is a generalized disease of connective tissue that is characterized by inflammation and degeneration, leading to fibrosis. Shortly after the description of the original disease, pulmonary involvement was noted (Day, 1870). The organs that are most commonly affected include the skin, blood vessels, synovium, skeletal muscles, lungs, gastrointestinal tract, and kidneys. Women are affected three to four times more frequently than are men. Patients present with Raynaud's phenomenon, swelling and puffing of the fingers, or arthritis of the small joints of the hand. Many patients have esophageal involvement, and recurrent aspiration may play a role in the pathogenesis of the lung disease. Up to 70 percent of patients with scleroderma develop pathologic evidence of lung disease, although a minority are clinically symptomatic (Owens and Follansbee, 1987). The pathologic findings are similar to those in IPF. ILD is the most common manifestation and is seen as bibasilar linear or nodular infiltrates. Bronchoalveolar lavage shows an intense alveolitis with macrophages and granulocytes (neutrophils and eosinophils) in about one-half of patients (Silver, et al., 1990). Pulmonary function testing first reveals a reduction in the diffusing capacity and then a reduction in vital capacity. The relative risk for the development of pulmonary fibrosis in patients with systemic sclerosis is increased more than 16 times if the major histocompatibility class DR3/DRw52a or the autoantibody to topoisomerase I (Scl-70 autoantibody) is present (Briggs, et al., 1991). A small proportion of patients develop pulmonary arterial hypertension, and most of these patients have little or no evidence of fibrosis by chest radiography. These patients complain of marked dyspnea and fatigue, and a striking reduction in the diffusing capacity is usually found (Owens, et al., 1983). Most patients have a gradually progressive course, but the occasional patient may have a rapid onset and progression (Schneider, et al., 1982). There is no single agent that has been shown to be effective in clinical trials. Penicillamine interferes with the crosslinking of mature collagen. Two studies using this agent have indicated a trend toward improvement, but their design flaws render a definitive statement regarding the efficacy of this agent impossible (Steen, et al., 1985; de Clerck, et al., 1987). Patients with pulmonary arterial hypertension may respond to vasodilator therapy. There may be an increased frequency of lung cancer, especially bronchoalveolar and small cell carcinoma, in patients with scleroderma, but this remains controversial (Wiedemann and Matthay, 1989).

Sjögren's Syndrome

Sjögren's syndrome is an autoimmune chronic inflammatory disease the main features of which are xerostomia and keratoconjunctivitis sicca; a secondary form of the disease includes other connective tissue disease. Diffuse interstitial lung disease occurs in up to 25 percent of patients (Constantopoulos, et al., 1985). There may be diffuse bilateral reticular or nodular infiltrates on the chest radiograph. Occasionally the pathologic findings reveal LIP (Strimlan, et al., 1976). The course of ILD in patients with Sjögren's syndrome is unpredictable, and the condition can stabilize or progress to severe disease.

Corticosteroids appear to be efficacious in about one-half of the patients treated. LIP can transform to "pseudo-lymphoma" or malignant lymphoma, which appear as mass lesions on the chest radiograph.

Systemic Lupus Erythematosus

SLE is a disease of unknown cause characterized by multiorgan inflammation. It is associated with the production of autoantibodies against nuclear, cytoplasmic, and cell membrane antigens. The clinical manifestations of SLE include fatigue, anemia, rashes, fever, pericarditis, pleurisy, nephritis, vasculitis, and central nervous system disease. The pulmonary manifestations of SLE were recognized by Osler (1904), who reported a persistent lung infiltrate that varied with the clinical activity of the underlying disease. The respiratory system is involved more commonly in SLE than in the other collagen-vascular diseases. SLE can affect the pleura, interstitium, vasculature, larynx, airways, and respiratory musculature (Hunninghake and Fauci, 1979). Unlike rheumatoid arthritis and scleroderma, ILD is uncommon, occurring in less than 3 percent of patients (Eisenberg, et al., 1973). The pathologic findings in SLE include interstitial fibrosis, vasculitis, hematoxylin bodies, and interstitial pneumonitis. Other findings (including pulmonary hemorrhage, edema, and hyaline membranes), although reported, are often related to coincident illnesses (Haupt, et al., 1981). Electron microscopic evaluation of lung biopsies from patients with SLE and ILD reveal intracellular tubuloreticular structures within pulmonary vascular endothelial cells that may represent evidence of previous viral infection (Fraire, et al., 1971). It is highly probable that the pulmonary fibrosis in patients with SLE represents the sequelae of episodes of acute pneumonitis because most patients who survive the acute phase have functional abnormalities (Matthay, et al., 1974). Corticosteroids are the recommended therapy for ILD in SLE, and the response is variable.

Polymyositis/Dermatomyositis

Polymyositis is an inflammatory myopathy of unknown cause to which the term *dermatomyositis* is applied in the presence of the characteristic rash. Pulmonary involvement was first noted in 1956 by Mills and Matthews (1956). Traditionally three types of pulmonary involvement have been described: (1) aspiration pneumonia, (2) ventilatory insufficiency, and (3) ILD (Hepper, et al., 1964). Involvement of the posterior pharyngeal muscles can lead to dysphonia and dysphagia. Interstitial pneumonitis occurs in 5 percent of patients and precedes the muscular disease in one-third of patients (Schwarz, et al., 1976). The ILD in polymyositis/dermatomyositis can be asymptomatic; insidious, with the gradual development of dyspnea and ILD; or acute in onset, with dyspnea and lung infiltrates (Frazier and Miller, 1974). On lung biopsy, patients with extensive fibrosis fare poorly; those with evidence of active inflammation respond well to corticosteroids (Duncan, et al., 1974). Overall, corticosteroids are helpful in 50 percent of affected patients (Schwarz, et al., 1976).

Ankylosing Spondylitis

Ankylosing spondylitis is a chronic disease that can result in progressive stiffening of the sacroiliac joints and spine. Significant pulmonary disease is uncommon, with a reported incidence of 1.3 percent (Rosenow, et al., 1977). Common pulmonary manifestations include chest wall restriction and fibrobullous disease. Upper lobe fibrobullous disease develops in 1 percent of the population. Cavities may form and become superinfected with Aspergillus or atypical mycobacterial species. In the late stages, patients may develop hemoptysis and recurrent pneumothorax. There are no effective medications for this disease.

Pulmonary-Renal Syndromes

Goodpasture's Syndrome

In 1919 Goodpasture described the occurrence of pulmonary hemorrhage and glomerulonephritis 6 weeks after influenza. The term *Goodpasture's syndrome* was not introduced until 1958 (Stanton and Tange, 1958). Goodpasture's syndrome is an autoimmune disorder in which antiglomerular basement membrane autoantibody is implicated. The patients typically present with pulmonary hemorrhage and glomerulonephritis and show linear deposits of immunoglobulin along renal basement membrane (Wilson and Dixon, 1979). Antiglomerular basement membrane antibodies recognize an epitote in the α3(IV) chain of type 4 collagen (Saus, et al., 1988). Upper respiratory tract infections and exposure to volatile hydrocarbons precede the illness in some patients (Bierne and Brennan, 1972). Male patients predominant, and the majority of cases occur in patients between 20 and 50 years of age. Sixty to 80 percent of patients have clinically observed pulmonary and renal disease; in 10 percent the disease is limited to the lung (Rees, 1984). In the majority of patients, hemoptysis is the presenting complaint. Less commonly the patients present with nonspecific symptoms of renal failure. Laboratory examination reveals iron-deficiency anemia, mildly elevated sedimentation rate, and evidence of renal impairment. Urinalysis shows proteinuria, hematuria, and red blood cell casts. The single breath diffusing capacity may be elevated because intra-alveolar blood binds inhaled carbon monoxide; an elevation of this test finding may precede the onset of clinical pulmonary hemorrhage (Addleman, et al., 1985). Chest radiographs typically demonstrate a bilateral acinar filling pattern, but they can show a mixed interstitial-alveolar pattern or a reticulonodular pattern in persistent disease. In the appropriate clinical setting, a positive test for circulating antiglomerular basement membrane antibodies establishes the diagnosis (Young, 1989). If the diagnosis is in question, a renal biopsy should be performed and the biopsy specimen stained for light microscopy, immunofluorescent studies, and electron microscopy. Focal nephritis or crescentic glomerulonephritis is usually seen on light microscopy. Direct immunofluorescence testing stains linear deposits of immunoglobulin (usually IgG) along the glomerular basement membrane. The recommended therapy for Goodpasture's syndrome includes plasma exchange, high-dose parenteral corticosteroids, and cyclophosphamide. Plasma exchange reduces the level of antibody to the glomerular basement membrane, and immunosuppression inhibits its further synthesis, although it is not established that plasma exchange affects survival (Shumak and Rock, 1984). The use of pulse corticosteroid therapy has also been proposed, but its efficacy compared with standard doses of corticosteroids has not been examined (Leatherman, 1987).

Idiopathic Pulmonary Hemosiderosis

Idiopathic pulmonary hemosiderosis refers to alveolar hemorrhage that occurs in the absence of hemodynamic abnormality, infection, coagulopathy, or systemic disorders, such as SLE, antiglomerular basement membrane antibody disease, or vasculitis. This rare disease occurs mainly in children younger than 10 years of age and adults in their 20s and 30s. Adult male patients are affected more than are female patients. The most common presentations include hemoptysis and iron-deficiency anemia (Leatherman, et al., 1984). Other symptoms include dyspnea, cough, malaise, pallor, and fever. Transient alveolar opacities develop during the acute phase of the illness, and with repetitive episodes, an interstitial pattern develops with progressive dyspnea, crackles, clubbing, and pulmonary hypertension. Antiglomerular basement membrane antibodies are usually not present. Bronchoalveolar lavage fluid supports the diagnosis if hemosiderin-laden macrophages are demonstrated. On open lung biopsy, the alveoli are filled with blood and hemosiderin-filled macrophages, with nonspecific septal thickening and alveolar lining cell hyperplasia. Immunoglobulin deposition along the alveolar capillary basement membrane has not been demonstrated. Corticosteroids and immunosuppressants have been anecdotally reported to be successful in some patients (Leatherman, 1987).

Chronic Eosinophilic Pneumonia

Historically chronic eosinophilic pneumonia was described in the group of diseases characterized by pulmonary infiltrates and eosinophilia (Crofton, et al., 1952). Women are twice as likely as men to be affected with the disorder, and they present with asthmatic symptoms and systemic features, such as fever, night sweats, and weight loss (Jederlinic, et al., 1988). Laboratory investigations show marked eosinophilia, an elevated sedimentation rate, and high levels of IgE. The chest radiograph shows a characteristic pattern of peripheral infiltrates, the photographic negative of pulmonary edema (Gaensler and Carrington, 1977). Open lung biopsy is usually not required, but if performed, it reveals an alveolitis with eosinophils and macrophages, multinucleated giant cells, and angiitis with diffuse pulmonary fibrosis. The diagnosis is often made on clinical information, and steroid therapy is usually successful, although relapses are common (Pearson and Rosenow, 1978).

Pulmonary Alveolar Proteinosis

Pulmonary alveolar proteinosis (PAP), first described by Rosen, et al. (1958), is characterized by the accumulation of periodic acid-Schiff-positive phospholipid-rich material in the alveolar spaces, with minimal fibrosis and inflammation of the interstitium. Pulmonary macrophages exhibit morphologic abnormalities, including excessive lipid accumulation and giant secondary lysosome formation and function abnormally (Golde, et al., 1976; Gonzalez-Rothi and Harris, 1986). PAP has been associated with silica and aluminum dust, malignancy, fungi, and parasitic disease. There have been several cases of PAP reported with *P.carinii* infection (Israel and Magnussen, 1989). The patient typically presents with dyspnea on exertion. The chest radiograph reveals interstitial and fine alveolar densities. The serum lactic dehydrogenase level is frequently elevated in this disorder (Martin, et al., 1978). Bronchoalveolar lavage and transbronchial biopsy usually are diagnostic, but open lung biopsy may be required (Martin, et al., 1980). The recommended treatment for PAP is whole lung lavage under general anesthesia. The course of disease is unpredictable; it may resolve spontaneously or alternatively progress, ultimately leading to death (Claypool, et al., 1984).

Inherited Lung Disorders

Neurofibromatosis (von Recklinghausen's Disease)

Neurofibromatosis is an autosomal dominant disorder characterized by café au lait spots and neurofibroma of the nervous system and skin. Interstitial fibrosis occurs in up to 20 percent of patients.

Tuberous Sclerosis

Tuberous sclerosis is an autosomal dominant disorder associated with the development of multiple tumors of ectodermal and mesodermal origin. They have been described in the retina, skin, kidneys, brain, gingiva, heart, thyroid, pancreas, ovaries, uterus, and spleen. In 0.1 to 1.0 percent of patients, there is pulmonary involvement, which pathologically is identical to that seen in patients with LAM (Dwyer, et al., 1971). Chest radiographs show normal or large lung volumes, with a diffuse microreticulonodular pattern and/or honeycombing, and occasionally pneumothorax. Pulmonary function testing typically reveals airway obstruction with gas trapping and a decreased single breath carbon monoxide diffusing capacity (Slingerland, et al., 1989). The course is usually progressive, with death from respiratory failure quite common.

Familial Idiopathic Pulmonary Fibrosis

Familial IPF is an autosomal dominant disorder that is identical to IPF.

Amyloidosis

Three distinct forms of pulmonary amyloidosis have been described: (1) focal deposits of amyloid within the mucosa and adventitia of the major airways, (2) single or multiple parenchymal nodules, and (3) diffuse parenchymal infiltrates involving the alveolar septa and the walls of small blood vessels. Patients present with dyspnea, wheezing, chronic cough, or hemoptysis, and a restrictive ventilatory defect is found on pulmonary function testing. The chest radiograph typically shows diffuse reticulonodular infiltrates, but various different radiographic appearances may be present (Himmelfarb, et al., 1977). There is no treatment for systemic amyloidosis, and the disease is usually fatal.

Human Immunodeficiency Virus Disease and Interstitial Lung Disease

ILD was described in patients with human immunodeficiency virus (HIV) disease. *P. carinii* pneumonia and viral pneumonitis are the most common reasons for ILD. Kaposi's sarcoma and LIP, two causes of ILD occasionally seen in the HIV population, are discussed next.

Kaposi's Sarcoma

Kaposi's sarcoma occurs in 10 to 30 percent of patients with the acquired immunodeficiency syndrome, and pulmonary involvement occurs in 21 to 40 percent of those with cutaneous involvement (White and Matthay, 1989). Common presenting symptoms are cough, dyspnea, stridor, fever, hoarseness, or hemoptysis. Arterial blood gas measurements reveal a reduction in the partial pressure of oxygen and a widened alveolar-arterial gradient. The chest radiograph is usually abnormal and shows four major patterns: interstitial, alveolar, mixed alveolar-interstitial, or nodular disease. Mediastinal, hilar, and paratracheal adenopathy may also be present in Kaposi's sarcoma, and up to 30 percent of patients have unilateral or bilateral effusions. Nodular lung infiltrates accompanied by pleural effusions and intrathoracic lymphadenopathy in the right clinical setting is highly predictive of pulmonary Kaposi's sarcoma (Davis, et al., 1987). Thoracentesis and pleural biopsy do not contribute to the diagnosis of Kaposi's sarcoma. The CT scan may define the distribution of the tumor and demonstrate nodules, lymphadenopathy, and pleural disease, but these findings are not specific. Bronchoscopy may reveal the characteristic lesions of Kaposi's sarcoma in the tracheobronchial tree. The lesion appears as

---

Interstitial Lung Disease Associated with Human Immunodeficiency Virus

Infections
  Viral
      Cytomegalovirus
      Herpes
  Fungal
  Pneumocystis carinii
  Mycobacterium tuberculosis
  Mycobacterium avium-intracellulare
Lymphocytic interstitial pneumonitis
Nonspecific interstitial pneumonitis
Kaposi's sarcoma
Lymphoma
Bronchogenic carcinoma
Alveolar proteinosis

a flat or raised plaque with a violaceous color, but the absence of endobronchial lesions does not exclude the disease (Gill, et al., 1989). Bronchial washings do not contribute information to the diagnosis. Transbronchial biopsy is not recommended because the diagnostic yield is low. Crush artifact, hemorrhage, granulation tissue, and fibrosis may mimic the histologic findings of Kaposi's sarcoma. Open lung biopsy has the highest diagnostic yield but is not 100 percent sensitive because lesions have been found at autopsy that were not seen by open lung biopsy (Ognibene, et al., 1985). The histologic findings of Kaposi's sarcoma consist of swollen endothelial cells in vascular lumina, loose aggregations of spindle cells, hemorrhage, and stromal hemosiderin deposits with interstitial inflammation. There is no known effective treatment for Kaposi's sarcoma; however, short-term palliation can be produced with interferon-α, radiotherapy, or combined chemotherapy (White and Matthay, 1989). A high incidence of infections occurs in patients with Kaposi's sarcoma; therefore, new symptoms should be investigated.

Lymphocytic Interstitial Pneumonia

LIP is so common as a complication of HIV infection in children that its presence is used as an acquired immunodeficiency syndrome-defining illness, but it is less prevalent in adults (Centers for Disease Control, 1985). Clinical features include cough, dyspnea, fever, and bilateral reticulonodular or micronodular infiltrates that are either diffuse or predominate in the lower lobes on the chest radiograph (Fig. 21-8; Oldham, et al., 1989). Bronchoalveolar lavage demonstrates increased lymphocytes in patients with LIP, but this finding is not specific for this condition (Turner-Warwick and Haslam, 1987). Open lung biopsy is usually necessary for establishing the diagnosis. Typical histologic findings include a diffuse infiltration of the interstitium with lymphocytes and plasma cells. Immunologic stains show a predominance of T lymphocytes, without necrosis or evidence of vasculitis. The course of LIP is variable, and some patients recover without therapy. The results of therapy with steroids have been disappointing, and responders ultimately die with other conditions. LIP is not limited to HIV-positive patients and may be seen in other patients, such as those with Sjögren's syndrome.

DISEASES OF KNOWN ORIGIN

Extrinsic Allergic Alveolitis

The term extrinsic allergic alveolitis (EAA, or hypersensitivity pneumonitis) refers to a group of disorders characterized by a response of the lung to fine dusts of organic origin that penetrate into the distal lung parenchyma (Reynolds, 1982). EAA has acute, subacute, and chronic forms, which are determined by the frequency and intensity of exposure. In the acute disease, chills, fever, dyspnea, and malaise occur 4 to 6 hours after exposure. A careful history should be taken to determine whether the patient has been exposed to an offending antigen at work (hay, sugar cane, or malt) or at home (air conditioning or sauna) or has special hobbies (parakeet or pigeon breeding). Examination classically reveals crackles in the bases and, in severe cases, fever and cyanosis. In the subacute form of this disease, there is an insidious onset of malaise, cough, sputum production, dyspnea, fatigue, and anorexia, with weight loss. The patient with the chronic form of disease may develop respiratory failure. Patients with EAA typically exhibit precipitating antibodies against the organic dust or antigen. Bronchoalveolar lavage may reveal a lymphocytic alveolitis with a predominance of T-suppressor cells the function of which may be impaired (Hughes, et al., 1984). Biopsies show both alveolar and interstitial inflammation with lymphocytes, plasma cells, and macrophages with a foamy cytoplasm. Common histologic findings include granulomas, foreign-body material, and bronchiolitis obliterans (Reyes, et al., 1982). High-resolution CT scan may define subacute disease by demonstrating areas of hazy increased density (Silver, et al., 1989). In 50 percent of patients, small ill-defined nodules are seen in the areas of air space disease. Treatment of EAA consists of recognizing the offending antigen and eliminating patient contact. This may involve wearing protective masks, alteration in handling the antigen, or changes in occupation. Moderate and severely ill patients should be treated with high-dose corticosteroids.

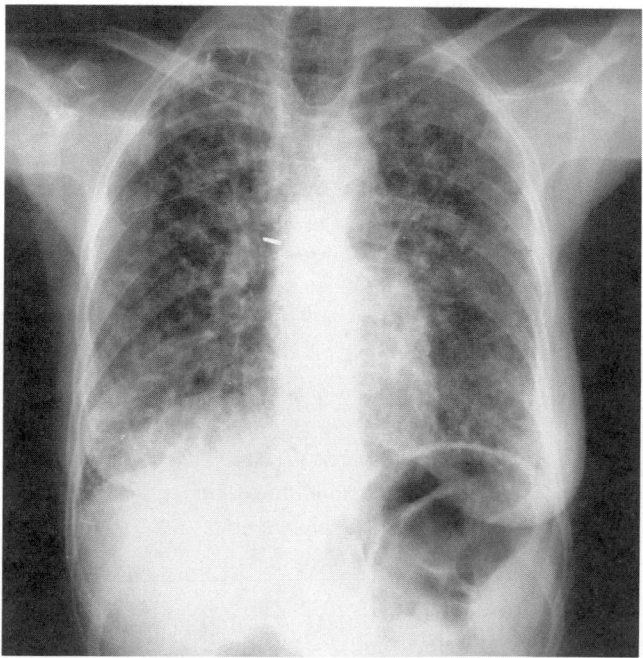

Figure 21-8. PA chest radiograph in a patient with lymphocytic interstitial pneumonitis.

Interstitial Lung Diseases of Known Cause

Extrinsic allergic alveolitis (hypersensitivity pneumonitis)

Radiation-induced lung disease

Drug-induced lung disease

Pneumoconiosis

Lymphangitic carcinomatosis

Examples of Diseases Caused by Inhaled Organic Dusts

Bird-breeder's lung
Air-conditioner lung
Farmer's lung
Cheese worker's lung
Malt-worker's lung
Bagassosis
Sequoiosis
Maple bark stripper's lung
Sauna taker's disease
Pituitary snuff lung
Paprika splitter's lung
Wood pulp worker's disease
Detergent worker's lung
Dry rot disease
Mummy unwrapper's disease
Mushroom worker's lung

Examples of Inorganic Dusts that Cause Interstitial Lung Disease

Silicates
  Talc
  Asbestos
  Aluminum silicates
  Mica
  Kaolin
  Diatomaceous earth
Silica
Metals
  Aluminum
  Beryllium
  Iron
  Barium
  Cadmium
  Tungsten
  Titanium
  Hafnium
  Cobalt
  Niobium
  Titanium oxide
  Tin
Rare earths
  Scandium
  Cerium
  Yttrium
  Lanthanum

Radiation-Induced Lung Disease

The first cases of radiation-induced lung injury were published in the 1920s (Hines, 1922). Radiation-induced lung injury presents as ILD in the patient with cancer and is difficult to differentiate from malignancy. Radiation-induced lung injury is classified into two clinical syndromes: radiation-induced pneumonitis and radiation-induced fibrosis, which follows it. Radiation-induced pneumonitis, which is reported as early as 2 weeks following the completion of therapy, occurs typically 2 to 6 months following the last dose. Radiographic changes can be expected 8 weeks after 4,000 cGy and 1 week earlier for each 1,000-cGy increment above 4,000 (Libshitz and Southard, 1974). Radiographic changes consistent with radiation-induced pneumonitis can be seen in 50 to 70 percent of patients who receive radiotherapy for carcinoma of the breast, but symptoms develop in less than 10 percent (Fleming, et al., 1961). The symptoms include a nonproductive cough, progressive dyspnea on exertion, low-grade fever, and pleuritic pain. An intractable cough may develop, with thick sputum production. Examination of the lungs is usually normal. The first abnormality noted on chest radiography is often a diffuse haze that quickly progresses to patchy alveolar opacities (Gross, 1977). Later the opacities form sharp boundaries to redefine the treated areas. In some cases, the changes may extend outside the radiation field, and abnormalities in the contralateral lung were reported. Bronchoalveolar lavage demonstrates an increase in total cells and a marked lymphocytosis in both relative and absolute terms (Gibson, et al., 1988). The acute pneumonitis can resolve or alternatively progress to respiratory failure.

Radiation-induced fibrosis develops in most patients with the radiation-induced pneumonitis syndrome within 1 year of therapy. Although most patients are asymptomatic, the condition in a minority of patients progresses to chronic respiratory failure. Chemotherapeutic agents, such as bleomycin, vincristine, cyclophosphamide, and dactinomycin increase the toxicity of radiation-induced injury. Pulmonary function tests show a decline in all lung volumes and a reduction in the diffusing capacity for carbon monoxide (Cudkowitz, et al., 1969). Lymphangitic spread can mimic radiation damage but can be distinguished by certain characteristics; lymphangitic disease involves the lung bases and shows prominent septal lines with symptoms more severe than the radiographic abnormality would indicate. Corticosteroids are used in severe cases of pneumonitis, although there are no clinical trials to validate their use in humans. During episodes of severe pneumonitis, prednisone (1 mg/kg/day) should be started (Gross, 1977). After a complete response has been documented, a slow taper is advised to prevent recurrent pneumonitis.

Drug-Induced Lung Disease

More than 50 drugs have been reported to cause pulmonary fibrosis (Rosenow, et al., 1992). Some drugs injure the lung in an idiosyncratic and sporadic fashion; others cause dose-dependent injury to the lung. Drugs may injure the lung through both direct and indirect mechanisms. The direct effects on the pulmonary parenchyma include oxidant injury,

Examples of Drugs and Other Agents that Cause Interstitial Lung Disease

Antibiotics
    Penicillin
    Sulfonamides
    Nitrofurantoin
    Tetracycline
    Erythromycin
    Isoniazid
    Para-aminosalicylic acid

Cardiac Drugs
    Amiodarone
    Hydralazine
    Procainamide
    Tocainamide
    β-Blockers
    Hydrochlorothiazide

Neurologic drugs
    Phenytoin
    Carbamazapine
    Chlorpromazine
    Imipramine
    Dantrolene
    Amitriptyline
    Methylphenidate
    Pentolinium
    Mecamylamine
    Hexamethonium

Rheumatologic drugs
    Phenylbutazone
    Corticosteroids
    Gold
    Naproxyn
    Penicillamine
    Cromolyn sodium
    Allopurinol

Endocrine drugs
    Tolbutamide
    Chlorpropamide

Oncologic drugs
    Bleomycin
    Cyclophosphamide
    Azathioprine
    Busulfan
    Chlorambucil
    Methotrexate
    Nitrosoureas

(Continues)

    Melphalan
    Procarbazine
    Mitomycin C
    Mercaptopurine
    Thioguanine

Other drugs/agents
    Mineral oil
    Talc (intravenous drug abuse)
    Silicon
    Nose drops
    Paraquat
    Radiation
    Oxygen
    Sulfur dioxide
    Chlorine gas
    Fats/oils
    Vinyl chloride
    Metal fumes
    Hydrocarbon or mercury vapors

cytotoxic effects on the capillary endothelial cells, deposition of phospholipids, and immune injury. Drugs may indirectly damage the pulmonary parenchyma by altering antioxidant defenses or by amplification of endogenous inflammatory responses. No laboratory tests exist that are diagnostic for drug-induced pulmonary disease. If a drug is suspected of causing disease, it should be discontinued. Most drug reactions are reversible; however, fatalities are not uncommon. Therapy with corticosteroids may be necessary in severe disease. Amiodarone, paraquat, and bleomycin are drugs that induce damage by different mechanisms; they are discussed in detail next.

Amiodarone-Induced Disease

Amiodarone is an antiarrhythmic agent useful in the treatment of serious ventricular arrhythmias. About 6 percent of patients who receive more than 400 mg/day for 2 or more months develop pulmonary toxicity (Martin and Rosenow, 1988). Symptoms of toxicity include exertional dyspnea, cough, fever, and chest pain. Malaise and weight loss have been recorded. Patients may present in two ways. There is a subacute illness characterized by cough, dyspnea, weight loss, and diffuse pulmonary infiltrates. There is also an acute syndrome with diffuse alveolar opacities that mimics pulmonary edema and pneumonia. Pleural effusions and localized infiltrates may be present. Physical findings of amiodarone-induced toxicity include fever, tachypnea, and inspiratory crackles. The presence of abnormalities on chest radiography may predict a higher risk for pulmonary toxicity. Routine pulmonary function testing reveals an impairment of the carbon monoxide diffusing capacity. Gallium scans may also be positive in amiodarone-induced pulmonary toxicity; however, they lack sensitivity and specificity (Zhu, et al., 1988). Bronchoalveolar lavage may reveal foamy alveolar macrophages containing intracytoplasmic lamellar inclusions. These cells are markers of amiodarone exposure and not diagnostic of toxicity. In most cases, discontinuation of therapy results in the complete reversal of the pulmonary abnormalities (Cooper, et al., 1986).

Bleomycin-Induced Disease

Bleomycin is a chemotherapeutic agent derived from a strain of *Streptomyces verticillus,* with a potential to produce pulmonary toxicity. Pulmonary fibrosis, the most common manifestation, can lead to respiratory failure and death. The true incidence of bleomycin toxicity is between 2 and 5 percent. There is a dose-toxicity relationship, such that, with doses exceeding 400 to 450 units of bleomycin, there are significant numbers of cases (Ginsberg and Comis, 1982). There is evidence that suggests that the combination of radiation or oxygen with bleomycin increases the risk of pulmonary toxicity (Goldiner, et al., 1978). Symptoms of toxicity occur at 4 to 10 weeks following therapy but have been reported up to 6 months later. The most prevalent symptoms are nonproductive cough, dyspnea, and fever. Fine crackles are commonly heard at the lung bases. As the disease advances, the crackles coarsen and occupy the lower two-thirds of the lung. Monitoring of total lung capacity seems to be a more specific indicator of toxicity than does the carbon monoxide diffusing capacity (Wolkowicz, et al., 1992). The chest radiograph demonstrates bibasilar reticular or nodular infiltrates. An early change is a triangular infiltrate in the costophrenic angles. With advanced disease, the infiltrates may progress to the middle and upper areas of the lungs. Some patients show a peripheral distribution of infiltrates in a subpleural allocation. Bilateral, focal, and asymmetric patterns and normal radiographs may be seen. A common finding is elevation of the diaphragm secondary to the loss of lung volume. Occasionally large nodules may be visualized, and this can present difficulties in the differentiation from metastatic disease. CT scans commonly show changes that were not seen on plain radiographs, especially subpleural ill-defined nodular densities at the posterior lung bases (Bellamy, et al., 1985). The evaluation of these nodules discovered on CT presents a diagnostic dilemma, and each patient must be evaluated on an individual basis. In patients with mild toxicity, discontinuation of the bleomycin may reverse the pulmonary disease, but corticosteroid therapy may be necessary. A smaller group will have progressive disease, and a fulminant course leading to death has been reported.

Talc Granulomatosis

Talc granulomatosis occurs in intravenous drug abusers who inject crushed tablets. Talc (magnesium silicate) deposits in the pulmonary arterioles, arteries, and interstitium. Patients present with cough, dyspnea, cor pulmonale, or sudden death. The chest radiograph may be normal in one-half of the affected patients, or it may show 1-mm micronodules. The nodules eventually coalesce, and extensive midlung zone fibrotic changes, as in progressive massive fibrosis, can de-velop. The lower lobes become relatively translucent, often with bullous formation (Pare, et al., 1989). Many of these patients demonstrate an obstructive ventilatory defect (Pare, et al., 1979). At a late stage, pathologic examination of the lung reveals emphysema, granulomatous inflammation, and fibrosis surrounding the talc particles.

Oxygen Toxicity

Oxygen in high concentrations is toxic to human lung. The mechanism of damage is postulated to be the inability of antioxidant enzymes to rid the lung of toxic free radicals from the oxygen therapy (Deneke and Fanburg, 1980). Damage occurs acutely (exudative phase) with an increase in alveolar-capillary permeability, which may be reversible, and chronically (proliferative phase) (Davis, et al., 1983). An ILD may develop with hyperplasia of type 2 cells and deposition of collagen in the interstitium.

Paraquat Toxicity

Ingestion of only one teaspoonful of liquid concentrate of the herbicide paraquat can be fatal. One to 5 days after paraquat poisoning, there is an acute syndrome of fever, dyspnea, fatigue, and gastrointestinal problems. Paraquat can induce an ILD because toxic oxygen radicals are generated, which causes a secondary alveolitis and subsequent fibrosis (Schoenberger, et al., 1984). Ultimately there is respiratory failure. In acute cases, the paraquat should be removed by gastric lavage, charcoal, and hemoperfusion. Vitamin E is often given as antioxidant therapy; however, there are no clinical trials to support its use. Oxygen should be kept at low concentrations because hyperoxia may accelerate injury.

Pneumoconiosis

Pneumoconiosis is defined by the International Labor Organization as the accumulation of inorganic dust in the lungs and the reactions of tissue to its presence. The type of injury depends on the type of inorganic dust and the length and strength of exposure. The most common syndromes include silicosis, coalworker's pneumoconiosis, asbestosis, and beryllium-induced disease.

Silicosis is caused by inhalation of silicon dioxide or crystalline silica. Patients characteristically present with dyspnea on exertion and an abnormal chest radiograph (Graham, 1992). Miners, foundry workers, tunnelers, casters, and ceramic molders are at risk. In simple silicosis, chest radiographs typically show rounded opacities with an upper lobe predominance. These nodules can progress and form large lung masses (progressive massive fibrosis) and destroy lung tissue. Eggshell calcification of the intrapulmonary, hilar, or mediastinal lymph nodes is common. Patients with silicosis are at increased risk for the development of tuberculosis, which often causes an increase in the opacities or cavitation.

Another common occupational ILD is asbestosis, which is characterized by interstitial pulmonary fibrosis manifested by dyspnea, cough, basal crepitations, clubbing, and ultimately right-sided heart failure (Mossman and Gee, 1989). Patients at risk include shipbuilders, boiler makers, miners, and brake-lining installers. Bronchoalveolar lavage or biopsies may reveal evidence of dust deposition, which can support the diagnosis (Sebastien, et al., 1988). In the patient with an appropriate occupational history, an abnormal chest radiograph has been accepted as evidence of asbestosis. The findings of asbestosis on high-resolution CT scans resemble those of UIP, including subpleural lines, parenchymal bands, thickening of the interlobular septal lines, thickening of structures in the secondary pulmonary lobule, and honeycombing.

Pulmonary Lymphangitic Carcinomatosis

Pulmonary lymphangitic carcinomatosis can mimic ILD. In pulmonary lymphangitic carcinomatosis, there is tumor growth along the pulmonary lymphatic channels. The major lymph vessels are found in the bronchovascular bundles, interlobular septa, and subpleural regions of the lung. There is a pathognomonic appearance of uneven thickening of bronchovascular bundles and the interlobular septa, giving these structures a beaded appearance. The thickening may be seen extending to the pleural surfaces, or it may form a polygonal arcade. The chest radiograph is normal in 50 percent of patients with biopsy-proved disease (Trapnell, 1964). The high-resolution CT scan shows characteristic polygonal lines that are not seen on conventional 10-mm cuts (Stein, et al., 1987). The diagnosis can usually made by bronchoalveolar lavage or transbronchial biopsy (Levy, et al., 1988). Open lung biopsy should be done if these tests are not diagnostic. Because the disease is focal in about 50 percent of patients, the CT scan can be used to guide the biopsy by the surgeon. Occasionally the diagnosis may be made by determining the cytologic characteristics of blood drawn through a wedged pulmonary artery catheter (Masson, et al., 1989).

COMMENTS AND CONTROVERSIES

Thoracic surgeons continually encounter ILD in their practices. The need for a definitive diagnosis often requires the expertise of a thoracic surgeon to perform an open lung biopsy. These patients frequently present with hemoptysis, pneumothorax, or focal lesions requiring attention. Because of the underlying pulmonary disease and the frequency of a restrictive component, postoperative management of such patients can be difficult. In the terminal phase of certain diseases, patients can now be considered for pulmonary transplantation, usually single lung transplantation.

R.J.G.

KEY REFERENCES

Cooper JAD Jr, White DA, Matthay RA: Drug induced pulmonary disease. Am Rev Respir Dis 133:321, 1986

This is a comprehensive review of the complications in the lung induced by a wide variety of therapeutic agents.

Crystal RG, Gadek JE, Ferrans VJ et al.: Interstitial lung disease: current concepts of pathogenesis, staging and therapy. Am J Med 70:542, 1981

This is a review of the proposed pathogenesis of interstitial lung disease, including the role of bronchoalveolar lavage and gallium scanning.

DeRemee RA: The roentgenographic staging of sarcoidosis: historical and contemporary perspectives. Chest 83:128, 1983

The author offers a defense of the traditional approach to the classification of patients with sarcoidosis.

Epler G, Colby T, McLoud T et al.: Bronchiolitis obliterans organizing pneumonia. N Engl J Med 312:152, 1985

A description of the clinical, radiographic, physiologic, and pathologic features of a large series of patients with BOOP. This article emphasizes the importance of the pathologic diagnosis because the prognosis of this disorder is different from IPF, with which it is commonly confused.

Fauci AS, Haynes BF, Costa J et al.: Lymphomatoid granulomatosis—prospective clinical and therapeutic experience over 10 years. N Engl J Med 306:68, 1982

A landmark article, this describes the response to chemotherapy and the development of lymphoma in patients who do not respond to therapy.

Grossman RF, Frost A, Zamel N et al.: Improvement in pulmonary function, graft profusion and exercise tolerance following single lung transplantation for pulmonary fibrosis. N Engl J Med 322:727, 1990

A description of the results in patients receiving single lung transplantation for IPF. The improvement in lung function and exercise tolerance is well documented.

Johnson MA, Kwan SK, Snell NJC et al.: Randomised controlled trial comparing prednisolone alone with cyclophosphamide and low dose prednisolone in combination in cryptogenic fibrosing alveolitis. Thorax 44:280, 1989

Prednisolone given in a dose of 60 mg/d for 1 month followed by a tapering regimen to 20 mg on alternate days was compared with cyclophosphamide 100 to 120 mg/day plus prednisolone 20 mg on alternate days. Many patients did not respond to either regimen, but there were responders in each group. It does not appear from this study that the cyclophosphamide regimen was significantly better than was the prednisolone alone.

Raghu G, Depaso WJ, Cain K et al.: Azathioprine combined with prednisone in the treatment of IPF. A prospective double-blind, randomized, placebo-controlled trial. Am Rev Respir Dis 144: 291, 1991

This study compared prednisone combined with azathioprine to prednisone alone in a prospective, double-blind, randomized, placebo-controlled trial. The number of patients enrolled was small, but there appeared to be a slight advantage for the azathioprine-prednisone group.

Raghu G: Idiopathic pulmonary fibrosis. A rational clinical approach. Chest 92:148, 1987

A reasonable approach to the management of a difficult group of patients is offered. The author is conservative with respect to the use of immunosuppressive agents.

Taylor JR, Ryu J, Colby TV, Raffin TA: Lymphangioleiomyomatosis. Clinical course in 32 patients. N Engl J Med 323:1254, 1990

The Stanford group followed a large number of patients with a rare disease. The survival of these patients was better than had been previously understood.

Wiedenmann HP, Matthay RA: Pulmonary manifestations of collagen vascular diseases. Clin Chest Med 10:677, 1989

The spectrum of disease caused by systemic lupus erythematosus, rheumatoid arthritis, scleroderma, polymyositis—dermatomyositis, mixed connective tissue disease, ankylosing spondylitis, relapsing polychondritis, and Sjögren's syndrome is reviewed.

Young KR Jr: Pulmonary-renal syndromes. Clin Chest Med 10: 655, 1989

This is an extensive review article on a heterogeneous group of disorders.

REFERENCES

Addleman M, Logan AS, Grossman RF: Monitoring intrapulmonary hemorrhage in Goodpasture's syndrome. Chest 87:119, 1985

Basset F, Corin B, Spencer H et al.: Pulmonary histiocytosis X. Am Rev Respir Dis 118:811, 1978

Basset F, Soler P, Jaurand MC et al.: Ultrastructural examination of bronchoalveolar lavage for diagnosis of pulmonary histiocytosis X: preliminary report on 4 cases. Thorax 32:303, 1977

Baughman RP, Fernandez M, Bosken CH et al.: Comparison of gallium-67 scanning, bronchoalveolar lavage, and serum angiotensin-converting enzyme levels in pulmonary sarcoidosis. Am Rev Respir Dis 129:676, 1984

Baughman RP, Shipley RT, Loudon RG, Lower EE: Crackles in interstitial lung disease. Comparison of sarcoidosis and fibrosing alveolitis. Chest 100:96, 1991

Beaumont D, Herry JY, Sapene M et al.: Gallium-67 in the evaluation of sarcoidosis: correlations with serum angiotensin-converting enzyme and bronchoalveolar lavage. Thorax 37:11, 1982

Bellamy EA, Husband JE, Blaquiere RM, Law MR: Bleomycin-related lung damage: CT evidence. Radiology 156:155, 1985

Bicrne GJ, Brennan JT: Glomerulonephritis associated with hydrocarbon solvents: Mediated by antiglomerular basement membrane antibody. Arch Environ Health 25:365, 1972

Bitterman PB, Rennard SI, Hunninghake GW, Crystal RG: Human alveolar macrophage growth factor for fibroblasts. Regulation and partial characterization. J Clin Invest 70:806, 1982

Bocart D, Lecossier D, De Lassence A et al.: A search for mycobacterial DNA in granulomatous tissues from patients with sarcoidosis using the polymerase chain reaction. Am Rev Respir Dis 145: 1142, 1992

Boeck C: Multiple benign sarcoid of the skin. J Cutan Genitourin Dis 17:543, 1899

Boushy SF, Kurtzman RS, Martin ND et al.: The course of pulmonary function in sarcoidosis. Ann Intern Med 62:939, 1965

Brauner MW, Grenier P, Mouelhi MM et al.: Pulmonary histiocytosis X: evaluation with high-resolution CT. Radiology 172:255, 1989

Briggs DC, Vaughan RW, Welsh KI et al.: Immunogenetic prediction of pulmonary fibrosis in systemic sclerosis. Lancet 338:661, 1991

Briggs WA, Johnson JP, Teichman S et al.: Antiglomerular basement membrane antibody-mediated glomerulonephritis and Goodpasture's syndrome. Medicine 58:348, 1979

Burkhardt A: Alveolitis and collapse in the pathogenesis of pulmonary fibrosis. Am Rev Respir Dis 140:513, 1989

Carrington CB, Gaensler EA, Coutu RE et al.: Natural history and treated course of usual and desquamative interstitial pneumonia. N Engl J Med 298:801, 1978

Carrington CB, Liebow AA: Limited forms of angiitis and granulomatosis of Wegener's type. Am J Med 41:497, 1966

Centers for Disease Control: Revision of case definitions of acquired immunodeficiency syndrome for national reporting—United States. MMWR Morb Mortal Wkly Rep 34:373, 1985

Churg J, Strauss L: Allergic granulomatosis, allergic angiitis and periarteritis nodosa. Am J Pathol 27:277, 1951

Claypool WD, Rogers RM, Matuschak GM: Update on the clinical diagnosis, management, and pathogenesis of pulmonary alveolar proteinosis (phospholipidosis). Chest 85:550, 1984

Cohen Tervaert JW, Huitema MG, Hene RJ et al.: Prevention of relapses in Wegener's granulomatosis by treatment based on antineutrophil cytoplasmic antibody titre. Lancet 336:709, 1990

Constantopoulos SH, Papadimitriou CS, Moutsopoulos HM: Respiratory manifestations in primary Sjogren's syndrome. A clinical, functional and histologic study. Chest 88:226, 1985

Cooper JAD Jr, White DA, Matthay RA: Drug-induced pulmonary disease. Am Rev Respir Dis 133:321, 1986

Cordier JF, Loire R, Brune J: Idiopathic bronchiolitis obliterans organizing pneumonia. Definition of characteristic clinical profiles in a series of 16 patients. Chest 96:999, 1989

Cordier JF, Valeyre D, Guillevin L et al.: Pulmonary Wegener's granulomatosis. A clinical and imaging study of 77 cases. Chest 97:906, 1990

Corrin B, Liebow AA, Friedman PJ: Pulmonary lymphangiomyomatosis: a review. Am J Pathol 79:348, 1975

Corwin RW, Irwin RS: The lipid-laden alveolar macrophage as a marker of aspiration in parenchymal lung disease. Am Rev Respir Dis 132:576, 1985

Crofton JW, Livingstone JL, Oswald NC, Roberts ATM: Pulmonary eosinophilia. Thorax 7:1, 1952

Crystal RG, Bitterman PB, Rennard ST et al.: Interstitial lung diseases of unknown cause. Disorders characterized by chronic inflammation of the lower respiratory tract. N Engl J Med 310: 154, 1984

Crystal RG, Fulmer JD, Roberts WC et al.: Idiopathic pulmonary fibrosis. Clinical, histologic, radiographic, physiologic, scintigraphic, cytologic, and biochemical aspects. Ann Intern Med 85:769, 1976

Crystal RG, Gadek JE, Ferrans et al.: Interstitial lung disease: current concepts of pathogenesis, staging and therapy. Am J Med 70:542, 1981

Cudkowitz L, Cunningham M, Haldane EV: Effects of mediastinal irradiation upon respiratory function following mastectomy for carcinoma of breast; a five-year follow-up study. Thorax 24: 359, 1969

Daniele RP, Elias JA, Epstein PE, Rossman MD: Bronchoalveolar lavage: role in the pathogenesis, diagnosis and management of interstitial lung disease. Ann Intern Med 102:93, 1985

Davis SD, Henschke CI, Chamides BK, Wescott JL: Intrathoracic Kaposi sarcoma in AIDS patients: radiographic-pathologic correlation. Radiology 163:495, 1987

Davis WB, Rennard SI, Bitterman PB, Crystal RG: Pulmonary oxygen toxicity. Early reversible changes in human alveolar structures induced by hyperoxia. N Engl J Med 309:878, 1983

Davison AG, Haslam PL, Corrin B et al.: Interstitial lung disease and asthma in hard-metal workers: bronchoalveolar lavage, ultrastructural, and analytic findings and results of bronchial provocation tests. Thorax 38:119, 1983

Day W: Case of scleroderma or sclerema with the autopsy and results. Am J Med Sci 59:350, 1870

de Clerck LS, Dequeker J, Francx L et al.: D-penicillamine therapy and interstitial lung disease in scleroderma. Long-term followup study. Arthritis Rheum 3:643, 1987

Deneke SM, Fanburg BL: Normobaric oxygen toxicity of the lung. N Engl J Med 303:76, 1980

DeRemee RA: The roentgenographic staging of sarcoidosis: historical and contemporary perspectives. Chest 83:128, 1983

DeRemee RA, McDonald TJ, Weiland LH: Wegener's granulomatosis: observations on treatment with antimicrobial agents. Mayo Clin Proc 60:27, 1985

Dill J, Ghose T, Landrigan P, MacKeen AD, Macneil AR: Crytogenic fibrosing alveolitis. Chest 67:411, 1975

Dreisen RB, Schwarz MI, Theofilopoulos AN, Stanford RE: Circulating immune complexes in the idiopathic interstitial pneumonias. N Engl J Med 298:353, 1978

Drew WL, Finley TN, Golde DW: Diagnostic lavage and occult pulmonary hemorrhage in thrombocytopenic immunocompromised patients. Am Rev Respir Dis 116:215, 1977

Duncan PE, Griffin JP, Garcia A, Kaplan SB: Fibrosing alveolitis in polymyositis. A review of histologically confirmed cases. Am J Med 57:621, 1974

Dwyer JM, Hickie JB, Garvan J: Pulmonary tuberous sclerosis. Report of three patients and a review of the literature. Q J Med 40:115, 1971

Eisenberg H, Dubois EL, Sherwin RP, Balchum OJ: Diffuse interstitial lung disease in systemic lupus erythematosus. Ann Intern Med 79:37, 1973

Eliasson AH, Phillips YY, Tenholder MF: Treatment of lymphangioleiomyomatosis. A meta-analysis. Chest 196:1352, 1989

Ellman P, Ball RE: "Rheumatoid disease" with joint and pulmonary manifestations. BMJ 2:816, 1948

Epler GR, McLoud TC, Gaensler EA et al.: Normal chest roentgenogram in chronic diffuse infiltrative lung disease. N Engl J Med 298:934, 1978

Fauci AS, Haynes BF, Katz P: The spectrum of vasculitis: clinical, pathologic, immunologic, and therapeutic considerations. Ann Intern Med 89:660, 1978

Fauci AS, Haynes BF, Katz P, Wolff SM: Wegener's granulomatosis: Prospective clinical and therapeutic experience with 85 patients for 21 years. Ann Intern Med 98:76, 1983

Fleming JA, Filbee JF, Wiernik G: Sequelae to radical irradiation in carcinoma of the breast. Br J Radiol 34:713, 1961

Flint A: The interstitial lung diseases. A pathologist's view. Clin Chest Med 3:491, 1982

Foley NM, Coral AP, Tung K et al.: Bronchoalveolar lavage cell counts as a predictor of short term outcome in pulmonary sarcoidosis. Thorax 44:732, 1989

Fraire AE, Smith MN, Greenberg SD et al.: Tubular structures in pulmonary endothelial cells in systemic lupus erythematosus. Am J Clin Pathol 56:244, 1971

Frazier RA, Miller RD: Interstitial pneumonitis in association with polymyositis and dermatomyositis. Chest 65:403, 1974

Friedman PJ, Liebow AA, Sokoloff L: Eosinophilic granuloma of lung: clinical aspects of pulmonary histiocytosis in the adult. Medicine 60:385, 1981

Fulmer JD: An introduction to the interstitial lung diseases. Clin Chest Med 3:457, 1982a

Fulmer JD: The interstitial lung diseases. Chest 82:172, 1982b

Gaensler EA, Carrington CB: Peripheral opacities in chronic eosinophilic pneumonia: the photographic negative of pulmonary edema. AJR 128:1, 1977

Geraint James D: Sarcoidosis. Postgrad Med J 60:234, 1984

Gibson PG, Bryant DH, Morgan GW et al.: Radiation-induced lung injury: a hypersensitivity pneumonitis? Ann Intern Med 109:288, 1988

Gill PS, Akil B, Colletti P et al.: Pulmonary Kaposi's sarcoma: clinical findings and results of therapy. Am J Med 87:57, 1989

Gilman MJ, Wang KP: Transbronchial lung biopsy in sarcoidosis: an approach to determine the optimal number of biopsies. Am Rev Respir Dis 122:721, 1980

Ginsberg SJ, Comis RL: The pulmonary toxicity of antineoplastic agents. Semin Oncol 9:34, 1982

Golde DW, Territo M, Finley TN, Cline MJ: Defective lung macrophages in pulmonary alveolar proteinosis. Ann Intern Med 85:304, 1976

Goldiner PL, Carlon GC, Cvitkovic E et al.: Factors influencing postoperative morbidity and mortality in patients treated with bleomycin. BMJ 1:1664, 1978

Gonzalez-Rothi RJ, Harris JO: Pulmonary alveolar proteinosis. Further evaluation of abnormal alveolar macrophages. Chest 90:656, 1986

Goodpasture EW: The significance of certain pulmonary lesions in relation to the etiology of influenza. Am J Med Sci 158:863, 1919

Graham WCB: Silicosis. Clin Chest Med 13:253, 1992

Gross NJ: Pulmonary effects of radiation therapy. Ann Intern Med 86:81, 1977

Grossman RF, Frost A, Zamel N et al.: Improvement in pulmonary function, graft perfusion, and exercise tolerance following single lung transplantation for pulmonary fibrosis. N Engl J Med 322:727, 1990

Hakala M: Poor prognosis in patients with rheumatoid arthritis hospitalized for interstitial lung disease. Chest 93:114, 1988

Hamman L, Rich AR: Acute diffuse interstitial fibrosis of the lungs. Bull Johns Hopkins Hosp 74:177, 1944

Haupt HM, Moore GW, Hutchins GM: The lung in systemic lupus erythematosus. Analysis of the pathologic changes in 120 patients. Am J Med 71:791, 1981

Heerfordt CF: Uber eine "Febris uveoparotidae subchronica." Graefes Arch Clin Exp Ophthalmol 70:254, 1909

Helmers RA, Hunninghake GW: Bronchoalveolar lavage in the non-immunocompromised patient. Chest 96:1184, 1989

Hepper NG, Ferguson RH, Howard FM: Three types of pulmonary involvement in polymyositis. Med Clin North Am 48:1031, 1964

Heshiki A, Schatz SL, McKusick KA et al.: Gallium-67 citrate scanning in patients with pulmonary sarcoidosis. AJR 122:744, 1974

Himmelfarb E, Wells S, Rabinowitz JG: The radiologic spectrum of cardiopulmonary amyloidosis. Chest 72:327, 1977

Hines LE: Fibrosis of the lung following roentgen-ray treatments for tumor. JAMA 79:720, 1922

Holgate ST, Haslam P, Turner-Warwick M: The significance of antinuclear and DNA antibodies in cryptogenic fibrosing alveolitis. Thorax 38:67, 1983

Hollinger WM, Staton GW Jr, Fajman WA et al.: Prediction of therapeutic response in steroid-treated pulmonary sarcoidosis. Evaluation of clinical parameters, bronchoalveolar lavage, gallium-67 scanning and serum angiotensin-converting enzyme levels. Am Rev Respir Dis 132:65,1985

Holness L, Tenenbaum J, Cooter NBE, Grossman RF: Fatal bronchiolitis obliterans associated with chrysotherapy. Ann Rheum Dis 42:593, 1983

Hughes DA, Haslam PL, Townsend PJ, Turner-Warwick M: Blood and bronchoalveolar lavage T-subsets in sarcoidosis and extrinsic allergic alveolitis. Thorax 39:708, 1984

Hunninghake GW, Crystal RG: Pulmonary sarcoidosis: a disorder mediated by excess helper T-lymphocyte activity at sites of disease activity. N Engl J Med 305:429, 1981

Hunninghake GW, Fauci AS: Pulmonary involvement in the collagen vascular diseases. Am Rev Respir Dis 119:471, 1979

Hunninghake GW, Gadek JE, Kawanami O et al.: Inflammatory and immune processes in the human lung in health and disease: evaluation by bronchoalveolar lavage. Am J Pathol 97:149, 1979

Hutchinson J: Anomalous disease of the skin of the fingers: papillary psoriasis. In: Illustrations of Clinical Surgery. J and A Churchill, London, 1877

Israel HL, Patchefsky AS, Saldana MJ: Wegener's granulomatosis, lymphomatoid granulomatosis, and benign lymphocytic angiitis and granulomatosis of lung. Recognition and treatment. Ann Intern Med 87:691, 1977

Israel RH, Magnussen CR: Are AIDS patients at risk for pulmonary alveolar proteinosis? Chest 96:641, 1989

Jayne DRW, Davies MJ, Fox CJV et al.: Treatment of systemic vasculitis with pooled intravenous immunoglobulin. Lancet 337:1137, 1991

Jederlinic PJ, Sicilian L, Gaensler EA: Chronic eosinophilic pneumonia. A report of 19 cases and a review of the literature. Medicine 67:154, 1988

Johns CJ: Sarcoidosis. Annu Rev Med 40:353, 1989

Jurik AG, Davidsen D, Graudal H: Prevalence of pulmonary involvement in rheumatoid arthritis and its relationship to some characteristics of the patients. A radiological and clinical study. Scand J Rheumatol 11:217, 1982

Kataria YP: Chlorambucil in sarcoidosis. 78:36, 1980

Keogh BA, Crystal RG: Alveolitis: the key to the interstitial lung disorders. Thorax 37:1, 1982

Keogh BA, Hunninghake GW, Line BR, Crystal RG: The alveolitis of pulmonary sarcoidosis: evaluation of natural history and alveolitis-dependent changes in lung function. Am Rev Respir Dis 128:256, 1983

Klinger H: Grenzformen der Periarteritis nodosa. Frankfurt Z Path 42:455, 1931

Kramer EL, Divgi CR: Pulmonary applications of nuclear medicine. Clin Chest Med 12:55, 1991

Kuznitsky E, Bittorf A: Boecksches sarkoid mit beteiligung innerer organe. Munch Med Wochenschr 62:1349, 1915

Lacronique J, Roth C, Battesti JP et al.: Chest radiological features of pulmonary histiocytosis X: a report based on 50 adult cases. Thorax 37:104, 1982

Leatherman JW: Immune pulmonary hemorrhage. Chest 91:891, 1987

Leatherman JW, Davies SF, Hoidal JR: Alveolar hemorrhage syndromes: diffuse microvascular lung hemorrhage in immune and idiopathic disorders. Medicine 63:343, 1984

Levy H, Horak DA, Lewis MI: The value of bronchial washings and bronchoalveolar lavage in the diagnosis of lymphangitic carcinomatosis. Chest 94:1028, 1988

Libshitz HI, Southard ME: Complications of radiation therapy: the thorax. Semin Roentgenol 9:41, 1974

Lieberman J: Elevation of serum angiotensin-converting-enzyme (ACE) level in sarcoidosis. Am J Med 59:365, 1975

Liebow AA, Carrington CRB, Friedman PJ: Lymphomatoid granulomatosis. Hum Pathol 3:457, 1972

Liebow AA, Steer A, Billingsley JG: Desquamative interstitial pneumonia. Am J Med 39:369, 1965

Lin YH, Haslam PL, Turner-Warwick M: Chronic pulmonary sarcoidosis: relationship between lung lavage cell counts, chest radiograph and results of standard lung function tests. Thorax 40:501, 1985

Line BR, Fulmer JD, Reynolds HY et al.: Gallium-67 citrate scanning in the staging of idiopathic pulmonary fibrosis: correlation with physiologic and morphologic features and bronchoalveolar lavage. Am Rev Respir Dis 118:355, 1978

Lofgren S: Primary pulmonary sarcoidosis. Acta Med Scand 145:424, 1953

Lower EE, Baughman RP: The use of low dose methotrexate in refractory sarcoidosis. Am J Med Sci 299:153, 1990

Martin RJ, Coulson JJ, Rogers RM et al.: Pulmonary alveolar proteinosis: the diagnosis by segmental lavage. Am Rev Respir Dis 121:819, 1980

Martin RJ, Rogers RM, Myers NM: Pulmonary alveolar proteinosis. Shunt fraction and lactic acid dehydrogenase concentration as aids to diagnosis. Am Rev Respir Dis 117:1059, 1978

Martin WJ II, Rosenow EC III: Amiodarone pulmonary toxicity: recognition and pathogenesis. Chest 93:1067, 1988

Martinet Y, Pinkston PA, Saltini C et al.: Evaluation of the in-vitro and in-vivo effects of cyclosporine on the lung T-lymphocyte alveolitis of active pulmonary sarcoidosis. Am Rev Respir Dis 138:1242, 1988

Masson RG, Krikorian J, Lukl P et al.: Pulmonary microvascular cytology in the diagnosis of lymphangitic carcinomatosis. N Engl J Med 321:71, 1989

Mathieson JR, Mayo JR, Staples CA et al.: Chronic diffuse infiltrative lung disease: comparison of diagnostic accuracy of CT and chest radiography. Radiology 171:111, 1989

Matthay RA, Schwarz MI, Petty TL et al.: Pulmonary manifestations of systemic lupus erythematosus: review of twelve cases of acute lupus pneumonitis. Medicine 54:397, 1974

Maycock RL, Bertrand P, Morrison CE et al.: Manifestations of sarcoidosis. Am J Med 35:67, 1963

McFadden RG, Carr TJ, Wood TE: Proton magnetic resonance imaging to stage activity of interstitial lung disease. Chest 92:31, 1987

Merchant RN, Pearson MG, Rankin RN, Morgan WKC: Computerized tomography in the diagnosis of lymphangioleiomyomatosis. Am Rev Respir Dis 131:295, 1985

Mills ES, Matthews WH: Interstitial pneumonitis in dermatomyositis. JAMA 160:1467, 1956

Moolma JA, Bardin PG, Rossouw DJ, Joubert JR: Cyclosporin as a treatment for interstitial lung disease of unknown aetiology. Thorax 46:592, 1991

Moore ADA, Godwin JD, Muller NL et al.: Pulmonary histiocytosis X: comparison of radiographic and CT findings. Radiology 172:249, 1989

Mossman BT, Gee JBL: Asbestos-related diseases. N Engl J Med 320:1721, 1989

Muller NL, Mawson JB, Mathieson JR et al.: Sarcoidosis: correlation of extent of disease at CT with clinical, functional and radiographic findings. Radiology 171:613, 1989

Muller NL, Miller RR, Webb WR et al.: Fibrosing alveolitis: CT-pathologic correlation. Radiology 160:585, 1986

Muller NL, Ostrow DN: High resolution computed tomography of chronic interstitial lung disease. Clin Chest Med 12:97, 1991

Murray JF: The Normal Lung. WB Saunders, Philadelphia, 1976

Muthiah MM, Macfarlane JT: Current concepts in the management of sarcoidosis. Drugs 40:231, 1990

Nolle B, Specks U, Ludemann J et al.: Anticytoplasmic autoantibodies: their immunodiagnostic value in Wegener granulomatosis. Ann Intern Med 111:28, 1989

Ognibene FP, Steis RG, Macher AM et al.: Kaposi's sarcoma causing pulmonary infiltrates and respiratory failure in the acquired immunodeficiency syndrome. Ann Intern Med 102:471, 1985

Oldham SAA, Castillo M, Jacobson FL et al.: HIV-associated lymphocytic interstitial pneumonia: radiologic manifestations and pathologic correlation. Radiology 170:83, 1989

O'Leary TJ, Jones G, Yip A et al.: The effects of chloroquine on serum 1,25-dihydroxyvitamin D and calcium metabolism in sarcoidosis. N Engl J Med 315:727, 1986

Osler W: On the visceral manifestations of the erythema group of skin diseases. Am J Med Sci 27:1, 1904

Owens GR, Fino GJ, Herbert DL et al.: Pulmonary function in progressive systemic sclerosis. Comparison of CREST syndrome varient with diffuse scleroderma. Chest 84:546, 1983

Owens GR, Follansbee WP: Cardiopulmonary manifestations of systemic sclerosis. Chest 91:118, 1987

Pantin CF, Valind SO, Sweatman M et al.: Measures of the inflammatory response in cryptogenic fibrosing alveolitis. Am Rev Respir Dis 138:1234, 1988

Pare JAP, Fraser RG, Hogg JC et al.: Pulmonary mainline granulomatosis: talcosis of intravenous methadone abuse. Medicine 58:229, 1979

Pare JP, Cote G, Fraser RS: Long-term follow-up of drug abusers with intravenous talcosis. Am Rev Respir Dis 139:233, 1989

Pearson DJ, Rosenow EC: Chronic eosinophilic pneumonia (Carrington's): a follow-up study. Mayo Clin Proc 53:73, 1978

Penny WJ, Knight RK, Rees AM et al.: Obliterative bronchiolitis in rheumatoid arthritis. Ann Rheum Dis 41:469, 1982

Prophet D: Primary pulmonary histiocytosis X. Clin Chest Med 3:643, 1982

Rees AJ: Pulmonary injury caused by antibasement membrane antibodies. Semin Respir Med 5:264, 1984

Reyes CN, Wenzel FJ, Lawton BR, Emanuel DA: The pulmonary pathology of farmer's lung disease. Chest 81:142, 1982

Reynolds HY: Bronchoalveolar lavage. Am Rev Respir Dis 135:250, 1987

Reynolds HY: Hypersensitivity pneumonitis. Clin Chest Med 3:503, 1982

Rinderknecht J, Shapiro L, Krauthammer M et al.: Accelerated clearance of small solutes from the lungs in interstitial lung disease. Am Rev Respir Dis 121:105, 1980

Rockoff SD, Rohatgi PK: Unusual manifestations of thoracic sarcoidosis. AJR 144:513, 1985

Roschmann RA, Rothenberg RJ: Pulmonary fibrosis in rheumatoid arthritis: a review of clinical features and therapy. Semin Arthritis Rheum 52:174, 1987

Rosen SH, Castleman B, Liebow AA: Pulmonary alveolar proteinosis. N Engl J Med 258:1123, 1958

Rosen Y, Athanassiades TJ, Moon S et al.: Nongranulomatous interstitial pneumonitis in sarcoidosis. Relationship to development of epitheloid granulomas. Chest 74:122, 1978

Rosenow E, Strimlan CV, Muhm JR et al.: Pleuropulmonary manifestations of ankylosing spondylitis. Mayo Clin Proc 52:641, 1977

Rosenow EC III, Myers JL, Swensen SJ, Pisani RJ: Drug-induced pulmonary disease. An update. Chest 102:239, 1992

Rothe RA, Fuller PB, Byrd RB et al.: Transbronchoscopic lung biopsy in sarcoidosis: optimal number and sites for diagnosis. Chest 77:400, 1980

Saboor SA, Johnson NM, McFadden J: Detection of mycobacterial DNA in sarcoidosis and tuberculosis with polymerase chain reaction. Lancet 339:1012, 1992

Saus J, Wieslander J, Langeveld JPM et al.: Identification of the Goodpasture antigen as the $\alpha 3(IV)$ chain of collagen IV. J Biol Chem 263:13374, 1988

Scadding JG: Diffuse pulmonary alveolar fibrosis. Thorax 29:271, 1974

Scadding JG, Hinson KFW: Diffuse fibrosing alveolitis (diffuse interstitial fibrosis of the lungs). Correlation of histology at biopsy with prognosis. Thorax 22:291, 1967

Schneider PD, Wise RA, Hochberg MC, Wigley FM: Serial pulmonary function in systemic sclerosis. Am J Med 73:385, 1982

Schoenberger CI, Rennard SI, Bitterman PB et al.: Paraquat-induced pulmonary fibrosis. Role of the alveolitis in modulating the development of fibrosis. Am Rev Respir Dis 129:168, 1984

Schwarz MI, Matthay RA, Sahn SA et al.: Interstitial lung disease in polymyositis and dermatomyositis: analysis of six cases and review of the literature. Medicine 55:89, 1976

Sebastien P, Armstrong B, Monchaux G, Bignon J: Asbestos bodies in bronchoalveolar lavage fluid and in lung parenchyma. Am Rev Respir Dis 137:75, 1988

Sharma OP: Sarcoidosis: clinical, laboratory and immunologic aspects. Semin Roentgenol 20:340, 1985

Sharma OP, Johnson R: Airway obstruction in sarcoidosis. A study of 123 nonsmoking black American patients with sarcoidosis. Chest 94:343, 1988

Shumak KH, Rock GA: Therapeutic plasma exchange. N Engl J Med 310:762, 1984

Silver RM, Scott Miller K, Kinsella MB et al.: Evaluation and management of scleroderma lung disease using bronchoalveolar lavage. Am J Med 88:470, 1990

Silver SF, Muller NL, Miller RR et al.: Computed tomography in hypersensitivity pneumonitis. Radiology 173:441, 1989

Slingerland JM, Grossman RF, Chamberlain D, Tremblay CE: Pulmonary manifestations of tuberous sclerosis in first degree relatives. Thorax 44:212, 1989

Smellie H, Hoyle C: The natural history of pulmonary sarcoidosis. Q J Med 29:539, 1960

Stack BHR, Choo-Kang FJ, Heard BE: The prognosis of cryptogenic fibrosing alveolitis. Thorax 27:535, 1972

Stanton MC, Tange JD: Goodpasture's syndrome (pulmonary hemorrhage associated with glomerulonephritis). Aust N J Med 7:132, 1958

Steen VD, Owens GR, Redmond C et al.: The effect of D-penicillamine on pulmonary findings in systemic sclerosis. Arthritis Rheum 28:882, 1985

Stein MG, Mayo J, Muller N et al.: Pulmonary lymphangitic spread of carcinoma: appearance on CT scans. Radiology 162:371, 1987

Strimlan CV, Rosenow EC III, Divertie MB, Harrison EG Jr: Pulmonary manifestations of Sjogren's syndrome. Chest 70:354, 1976

Strumpf IJ, Feld MK, Cornelius MJ et al.: Safety of fiberoptic bronchoalveolar lavage in evaluation of interstitial lung disease. Chest 80:268, 1981

Studdy P, Bird R, Geraint James D: Serum angiotensin-converting enzyme (SACE) in sarcoidosis and other granulomatous disorders. Lancet 2:1331, 1978

Studdy PR, Bird R: Serum angiotensin converting enzyme in sarcoidosis—its value in present clinical practice. Ann Clin Biochem 26:13, 1989

Thrasher DR, Briggs DD Jr: Pulmonary sarcoidosis. Clin Chest Med 3:537, 1982

Trapnell DH: The radiological appearance of lymphangitic carcinomatosa of the lung. Thorax 19:251, 1964

Turner-Warwick M, Haslam PL: Clinical applications of bronchoalveolar lavage. Clin Chest Med 8:15, 1987

Turner-Warwick M, McAllister LR, Britten A, Haslam PL: Corticosteroid treatment in pulmonary sarcoidosis: do serial lavage lymphocyte counts, serum angiotensin converting enzyme measurements and gallium-67 scans help management? Thorax 41:903, 1986

van der Woude FJ, Rasmussen N, Lobatto S et al.: Autoantibodies against neutrophils and monocytes: tool for diagnosis and marker of disease activity in Wegener's granulomatosis. Lancet 1:425, 1985

von Stossel E: Uber muskulare cirrhose der lunge. Beitr Klin Tuberk 90:432, 1937

Walker WC, Wright V: Diffuse interstitial pulmonary fibrosis and rheumatoid arthritis. Ann Rheum Dis 28:252, 1969

Wegener F: Uber generalisierte, septische Gefasserkrankungen. Verh Dtsch Ges Pathol 29:202, 1936

Whitcomb ME, Dixon GF: Gallium scanning, bronchoalveolar lavage, and the national debt. Chest 85:719, 1984

White DA, Matthay RA: Noninfectious pulmonary complications of infection with the human immunodeficiency virus. Am Rev Respir Dis 140:1763, 1989

Wilson CB, Dixon FJ: renal injury from immune reactions involving antigens in or of the kidney. p. 46. In Brenner BM, Stein J (eds): Contemporary Issues in Nephrology. Vol. 3. Churchill Livingstone, New York, 1979

Winterbauer RH, Belic N, Moores KD: A clinical interpretation of bilateral hilar lymphadenopathy. Ann Intern Med 78:65, 1973

Wolkowicz J, Sturgeon J, Rawji M, Chan CK: Bleomycin-induced pulmonary function abnormalities. Chest 101:97, 1992

Zerhouni EA, Naidich DP, Stitik FP et al.: Computed tomography of the pulmonary parenchyma II: interstitial disease. J Thorac Imaging 1:54, 1985

Zhu YY, Botvinick E, Dae M et al.: Gallium lung scintigraphy in amiodarone pulmonary toxicity. Chest 93:1126, 1988

22

EMPHYSEMA AND BULLOUS DISEASE

Melvyn Goldberg

The surgical treatment for bullous disease in emphysema has been redefined over the past four decades. The indications for surgical intervention, the types of surgical procedures, and the objectivity of the results have been questioned repeatedly. This chapter defines the current practical pathophysiologic findings of bullous disease formation, the specific indicators for surgical intervention, the current operative procedures, and those studies that show definite functional improvement postoperatively. To date this has been an area of intense clinical activity.

HISTORICAL NOTE

Benfield (1969) summarized the operative procedures in the past that were devised to treat bullous emphysema. These include procedures to increase or decrease the size of the thoracic cavity, to increase the flow of pulmonary arterial blood, to denervate the lung, and to stabilize the tracheobronchial tree.

Early in this century, Freund (1906) and Seidel (1908) devised chest wall operations to reverse rib cage restriction. This was performed by resecting several costal cartilages and a transverse sternotomy to allow greater pulmonary expansion.

Allison (1947) and Carter, et al. (1950) corrected the hyperinflated state of the chest by reducing the volume of the thorax with a thoracoplasty, pneumoperitoneum, and phrenic nerve division. These procedures are of historic value only, and neither approach was of any value. Gaensler, et al. (1953), Pearson (1935), Becklake, et al. (1954), and Mann and Murphy (1954) demonstrated that in all instances the aforementioned procedures were detrimental to pulmonary function postoperatively.

Operations have been performed to reverse the abnormal expansion and contraction of airways caused by the exaggerated flaccidity of the pars membranacea (functional tracheobronchial malacia). Guest, et al. (1965). Herzog (1954), Nissen (1954), and Rainer, et al. (1963) described procedures to accomplish this that included various types of tracheoplas-

ties, and ultimately tracheostomy, to allow access for tracheal toilet, ventilation, and a decrease of dead space.

Floyer (1717) was the first individual to apply surgery specifically to the abnormal air spaces of bullous emphysema, and he selectively aspirated air cysts, followed by the instillation of astringents in horses.

> "The cure of the broken Wind cannot easily be projected any other way, but by a Paracentesis in the Thorax for if the external Air be admitted, it will compress the flatulent Tumour and through the same hole a Styptic and Carminative Hydromel may be injected, to restore by its Stypticity the Tone of the Membranes, and discuss by its Aromatic Acrimony the windy Spirits or Air retain'd in the Lungs."

FitzPatrick and Crenshaw (1957) attempted to stimulate collateral circulation by pleurodesis from the chest wall to the visceral pleura and to poorly vascularized emphysematous areas below. In addition, Nakayama (1961), Overholt (1963), and Phillips (1964) suggested denervation of the pulmonary tissue by resection of the carotid body to decrease the bronchospasm concomitant with emphysema and thereby prevent secretional retention.

Brantigan, et al. (1959) and Kress, et al. (1968) advocated extensive multiple pulmonary parenchymal plications, presuming that the resection of peripheral lung tissue would increase the lung function of central areas by relieving peripheral compression of airways and vessels if the peripheral tissue was devoid of function. During the operation attempts were made to remove or plicate peripheral lung tissue, which was presumably functionless, and create a new lung volume that approached normal size in its expiratory phase (1,000 to 1,200 ml of lung volume). The resection would thereby restore the impaired physiologic mechanism of circumferential pull on the smaller airways and vessels. The bronchioles are collapsible tubes that contain no cartilage and are held open by an elastic lung field held in an expanded state by a rigid closed chest wall. A circumferential pull on the bronchioles holds them open. In panlobular emphysema, the lung volumes are large, and there is a loss of the circumferential pull to hold the bronchioles open. As the lung enlarges, a progressive increase in airway obstruction occurs during expiration. By reducing lung volume surgically by removing functionless lung at the periphery, restoration of normal circumferential pull occurs. Recently the hypotheses of the proponents of these procedures have been refuted and laid aside by Knudson and Gaensler (1965) and Gaensler and Muller (1964).

HISTORICAL READINGS

Benfield JR, Cree FM, Pellett JR, et al: Current approach to the surgical management of emphysema. Arch Surg 93:59, 1966
Brantigan OC, Mueller, E Kress MB: Surgical approach to pulmonary emphysema. Am Rev Respir Dis 80:195,1959
Fiore D, Biondetti PR, Sartori F, Calabrio F: The role of computed tomography in the evaluation of bullous lung disease. J Comput Assist Tomogr 6:105, 1982
FitzGerald MX, Keelan PJ, Cugall DW, Gaensler EA: Long-term results of surgery for bullous emphysema. J Thorac Cardiovasc Surg 68:566, 1974
Jensen KM, Miscall L, Steinberg I: Angiocardiography in bullous emphysema: its role in selection of the case suitable for surgery. AJR 85:229, 1961
Knudson RJ, Gaensler EA: Surgery for emphysema: collective review. Ann Thorac Surg 1:332, 1965
Monaldi V: Endocavitary aspiration: its practical applications. Tubercle 28:223, 1947

BASIC SCIENCE

Pathology

Cysts

Congenital bronchogenic cysts are lined with cuboidal respiratory epithelium. Acquired cysts of the lung are thin-walled spaces that remain as an area of lung destruction. They may result from a check valve obstruction of the small bronchioles that distends the distal lung to form a coalescent space or from inflammatory necrosis of the bronchial wall, resulting in the compression of adjacent pulmonary parenchyma to form a large pneumatocele.

Blebs

A bleb is a subpleural collection of air within the layers of the visceral pleura caused by a ruptured alveolus. The air dissects through the interstitial tissue into the thin fibrous layer of the visceral pleura, where it enlarges to form a bleb. It may produce a pneumothorax.

Blebs characteristically occur at the lung apices. Small blebs may coalesce to form larger ones, or they may be multiple and discrete, scattered diffusely over the upper surfaces of the lungs.

Bullae

A bulla is an air-filled space within the lung parenchyma, resulting from a deterioration of alveolar tissue. Bullae have fibrous walls and are trabeculated by the remnants of alveolar septa. Cooke and Blades (1952) described the following sequence. As the process continues, the cystlike space is limited at the lung periphery by the visceral pleura. If the visceral pleura is opened over a bulla, the air space beneath it will not be lined by squamous cells but by a disintegrating lung parenchyma, making up the walls and base of the bulla. Fine blood vessels completely stripped of supporting parenchyma cross the air space. Strands of connective tissue and fine denuded bronchioles crisscross the bulla. Multiple small communications with the adjacent bronchi are apparent. Bullae are almost always multiple, but they may be confined to a segment or lobe. The upper lobes are most frequently involved.

Cavities

If the cyst, bleb, or bulla is thicker than 3 mm, it can be called a cavity. This almost always occurs after the space has become infected. A thickening of the wall represents a specific or nonspecific inflammatory reaction.

Air Space

The air space abnormalities may or may not be associated with underlying lung disease. Such air space abnormalities were precisely defined by Klingman, et al. (1991).

The anatomic classification of emphysema that is based on acinar involvement was defined by FitzGerald, et al. (1974) and Hugh-Jones and Whimster (1978) (Fig. 22-1). As agreed by the World Health Organization and the American Thoracic Society, pulmonary emphysema is characterized by an increase beyond normal in the size of air spaces distal to the terminal nonrespiratory bronchiole that arises from the destruction of their walls (Fig. 22-1B).

Proximal Acinar Emphysema. Proximal acinar emphysema (centrilobular) (Fig. 22-1C) involves the respiratory bronchioles, which are enlarged and destroyed. It is commonly associated with smoking and distal airway inflammation.

Panacinar Emphysema. Panacinar emphysema (panlobular) (Fig. 22-1D) involves the entire acinus uniformly. This form is commonly associated with α_1-antitrypsin deficiency. This association was first described by Laurell and Eriksson (1963).

This type of emphysema is less benign than is distal acinar emphysema and may progress irregularly throughout the lungs. Routine chest radiographic studies identify the stigmata of diffuse emphysema, and the dyspnea that the patient experiences is usually much worse than the radiograph might suggest. Pride, et al. (1970) identified its association with a low diffusion capacity, and Jensen, et al. (1961) demonstrated the typical attenuation and pruning of the peripheral vasculature angiographically.

Distal Acinar Emphysema. Distal acinar emphysema (paraseptal) (Fig. 22-1E) involves the distal part of the acinus, ducts, and alveoli. It is usually associated with fibrosis and is subpleural in location. It is frequently associated with the formation of bullae and pneumothorax. This is the form of bullous disease that surgeons most commonly deal with and fortunately those that have the best results after surgical intervention.

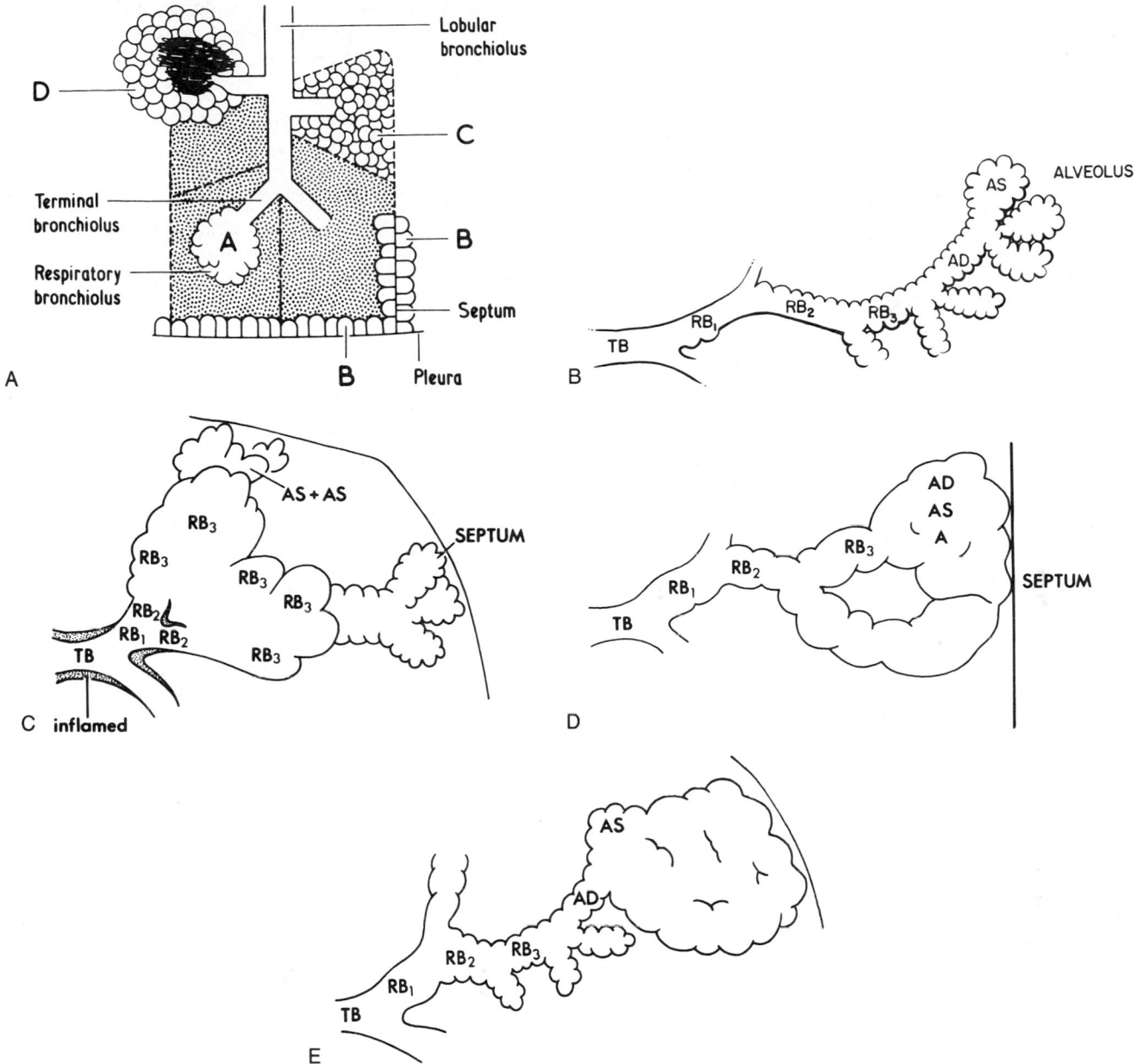

Figure 22-1. **(A)** Schematic showing various forms of emphysema: A, centriacinar (centrilobular emphysema); B, periacinar or paraseptal emphysema; C, panacinar emphysema; and D, irregular (scar) emphysema. **(B)** Component parts of acinus. **(C–E)** Specific forms of emphysema: **(C)** proximal acinar (centrilobular) emphysema, **(D)** panacinar (panlobular) emphysema, and **(E)** distal acinar (paraseptal) emphysema. Periacinar or paraseptal emphysema is probably the most common type among patients referred for surgery for bullous emphysema. The peripheral disruption of the acinus **(B)** is of little consequence deep within the lung, but in acini bordering the pleura, there is coalescence of the tiny spaces, and eventually the lung tissue separates from the visceral pleura to form bullae. (Fig. A from Gaensler EA, Cugell DW, Knudson RJ, FitzGerald MX: Surgical management of emphysema. Clin Chest Med 4:443, 1983; Figs. B–E from Thurlbeck WM: Morphology of Emphysema and Emphysema-Like Conditions in Chronic Airflow Obstructions in Lung Disease. p. 181. WB Saunders, 1976, with permission.)

This particular type of emphysema is usually benign and confined to the cortex of the lung. It seldom recurs after surgery, and only rarely will this disease progress, allowing the medulla of the lung to retract everywhere with partial obstruction of the communicating airways, air trapping, and resultant giant bulla and adjacent lung compression.

Clinical Classification

A clinical classification of pulmonary emphysema was reported by Dikjman (1986), identifying three distinct entities: compensatory emphysema, diffuse obstructive emphysema, and bullous emphysema. Compensatory emphysema is not

Table 22-1. Classification of Bullous Emphysema

Group	Bullae	Underlying Lung
I	Large, single	Normal
II	Multiple	Normal
III	Multiple	Diffuse emphysema
IV	Multiple	Other lung diseases

(From DeVries WC, Wolfe WG: The management of spontaneous pneumothorax and bullous emphysema. Surg Clin North Am 60:851, 1980, with permission.)

true emphysema because destruction of the acinus does not occur. It may represent hyperinflation of a portion of the lung to fill a large hemithorax secondary to atelectasis or resective surgery. Diffuse obstructive emphysema is otherwise described as chronic obstructive pulmonary disease. This can be further differentiated into a pathophysiologic classification, which was described by Knudson and Gaensler (1965) as types A and B. Bullous emphysema is found with relatively normal underlying tissue and characterized either by bulla or bleb formation.

A practical classification of bullous emphysema was defined by DeVries and Wolfe (1980) (Table 22-1). Group I identifies emphysema with a large single bulla in a normal underlying healthy lung. Group II identifies multiple bullae of the lung, also with an underlying normal lung. Groups III and IV identify bullous disease in the lung in generalized emphysema (group III) and in patients with other diffuse lung diseases (group IV), such as scleroderma, histoplasmosis, pulmonary fibrosis, eosinophilic granuloma, tuberous sclerosis, pneumoconiosis, and talcosis. Groups I and II are amenable to surgical extirpation with predictably good functional results, whereas the predicted value of surgery is less accurate in groups III and IV.

Pathophysiology

Many mechanisms for the pathophysiology of bullous formation have been described. Cooke and Blades (1952) suggested three mechanisms for bullous formation. First, a ball-valve mechanism between the cyst and the bronchus is responsible for progressive enlargement of the bulla. Second, the cyst enlarges because the intracystic pressure increases progressively and thereby collapses the unsupported adjacent pulmonary tissue. Third, inflammation and partial occlusion of the smaller airways produce further breakdown of the bullae with progressive enlargement and further occlusion of the smaller airways. Therefore, the effects of the bulla are to produce an enlarging cyst and a space-occupying lesion (which is poorly ventilated with no perfusion), decrease the diaphragmatic and chest wall movements, displace the mediastinum, and compress the underlying functional lung bilaterally.

Baldwin, et al. (1950) demonstrated that large bullae can act as space-occupying lesions that relax or even compress contiguous lung tissue. With the thorax open, either at operation or autopsy, such bullae expand and collapse instantaneously with positive pressure ventilation. Reid (1967) classified such lesions as "nonobstructive emphysema." The functional residual capacity (FRC) is large, nitrogen washout from the bullae (measured during Monaldi drainage) is slow, physi-

ologic dead space is reduced rather than increased, and ventilation scans show slow turnover within the bullae, as demonstrated by Hugh-Jones, et al. (1966). FitzGerald, et al. (1974) and Pride, et al. (1970) elegantly confirmed the following pathophysiologic schema.

1. When the thorax is open, positive pressure allows the lung behind the bulla to expand and radial tension on the airways to be restored. Therefore, bronchial connections leading to bullae become widely patent.

2. When the thorax is closed, surrounding lung tissue is relaxed on positive ventilation, radial tension on the airways is reduced, and all airways (including those connecting with the bullae) have high resistance to flow.

3. After the excision of peripheral bullae, lung tension is restored, and the lesion (diffuse obstruction) disappears.

4. The situation in the pulmonary vasculature is similar. Therefore, decreased elastic recoil causes increased vascular resistance in relatively normal regions of the lungs, and pulmonary hypertension is common in patients with giant bullae. There may be as much restoration of the vasculature when the lung tension is reestablished by surgical excision as there is in the pulmonary parenchyma.

Morgan, et al. (1989) looked carefully at four bullae undergoing resection. He studied intracystic partial pressures of oxygen (PO_2) and carbon dioxide (PCO_2) intracystic pressures, and postresection pathologic findings for bronchial communications. His results showed that bullae are not under pressure, there is no obstructive ball-valve effect, and as a result of parenchymal weakness, bullae are preferentially ventilated (Laplace's law). The elastic recoil of the adjacent lung retracts the lung away from the bulla, thus enlarging it. His conclusion was that the effect of surgery was not so much to ablate the space as to reconstruct the parenchyma of the lung, restoring its architecture and mechanical linkage with the chest wall while allowing the deflated lung to regain its elastic properties. The specific cause of bullous emphysema remains ill defined, although the contributions of smoking and α_1-antitrypsin deficiency were well recognized by Anenback, et al. (1972), Hutchison (1978), and Laurell and Eriksson (1963).

The most recent updated version of the pathophysiologic hypothesis of the formation of bullae was proposed by Klingman, et al. (1991). Mrogan, et al. (1989) suggested that, during the operation or in resected specimens, there are widely patent bronchi in the floor of the bullae with no valvular mechanisms. The probability of bullae containing gas under positive pressure with resultant compression of adjacent lung is unlikely. The cause of progression is continued intrinsic destruction of lung tissue locally and preferential inflation.

Morgan, et al. (1986 and 1989) observed that bullae, as observed by computed tomography, during inspiration and expiration do not change to any appreciable degree in size and the change that does occur is always in phase with the rest of the lung during respiration. The overall gas flow in and out of bullae is small but unimpeded. When bullae and the lung are exposed to the same negative intrapleural pressure, the bullae fill preferentially and always completely before the remainder of the lung is filled. This was confirmed in vitro by Ting, et al. (1963). The force of elastic recoil produces retraction of the surrounding lung away from the air space and enlarges it. Even though the bulla remains in free communication with the airway, it does not participate to any important extent in ventilation (because of its large volume) or in gas exchange (because of its relatively small and avascular internal surface area).

The degree to which bullae contribute to dyspnea depends on the amount of lung they displace and the extent of the underlying disease. Compression is of little subsequence.

Patient Selection for Surgical Treatment

Pathology

Knudson and Gaensler (1965) classified chronic obstructive pulmonary disease clinicopathologically into types A and B, respectively identified in the past by Dornhorst (1955) as pink puffers and blue bloaters (Table 22-2). Type A has specific air space abnormalities with better operative results. These patients have severe dyspnea, little sputum, increased residual volume (RV), and decreased carbon monoxide diffusing capacity. Type B has diffuse parenchymal abnormalities with much poorer operative results. These patients have severe bronchitis, excess sputum production, and perhaps cor pulmonale.

Although thought to be important decades ago by Baldwin, et al. (1950) and Siebens, et al. (1957), the differentiation of bullae into those that do and do not communicate with underlying airways plays little value in selecting patients for surgery with bullous disease. The only pathologic finding that is important is the size of the cysts and the status of the underlying lung. It has been disproved that cysts in situ in a closed chest are under any tension whatsoever, even when the mediastinum is displaced contralaterally. Siebens, et al. (1957) identified the importance of the underlying lung in the classification of bullae, with normal underlying lung producing much better functional results than those produced with an underlying emphysematous lung. Wesley, et al. (1972) pointed out that the type of emphysema is not as important as whether it significantly embarrasses the function of the adjacent lung tissue.

Clinical Presentation

Since the introduction of elective bullectomy in the early 1950s to reduce dyspnea in patients with bullous emphysema, several reports have stressed the importance of careful preoperative selection of patients (Billig, et al., 1968; FitzGerald, et al., 1974; Gunstensen and McCormack, 1973; Knudson and Gaensler, 1965; Pride, et al., 1970; Wesley, et al., 1972; and Laros, et al., 1986). All patients should be symptomatic with dyspnea. Prophylactic bullectomy in patients with asymptomatic giant bulla, at the moment, cannot be justified. A somewhat quantitative assessment for dyspnea should be used on a consistent basis in preoperative patient analysis. A modified Hugh-Jones and Lambert (1952) grading system for dyspnea is one of several such assessments (Table 22-3). Throughout the recent literature, there has been uniform agreement that a bulla must occupy greater than 30 percent of a hemithorax before surgery is advised. There is excellent subjective and objective data to suggest that anything less than this produces little if any functional improvement after surgery. Clinical improvement and rehabilitation occur in

Table 22-2. Types of Chronic Obstructive Bronchopulmonary Disease

	Parameter	Type A	Type B
Synonyms		Emphysematous	Bronchitic
		Pink puffer	Blue bloater
		Diffuse	Centrilobular
Subjective	Dyspnea	Severe	Usually severe
	Cough	Occasional	Severe
	Sputum	Scant	Copious
Physical	Breath sounds	Distant	Rales, wheezes
	Cyanosis	None	Frequent
Radiographic findings		Emphysema	Often normal
		Bullae	Fibrosis
Airway resistance		Severely increased	Severely increased
MBC and FEV$_1$		Severely reduced	Severely reduced
Lung volumes	VC	Normal, reduced	Severely reduced
	RV	Severely increased	Moderate, increased
	TLC	Usual increase	Normal, reduced
Blood gases	PO$_2$	Normal, reduced	Severely reduced
	PCO$_2$	Normal, reduced	Increased
Diffusing capacity		Severely decreased	Slightly decreased
Polycythemia		Rare	Frequent
Cor pulmonale		Rare	Frequent
Prognosis		Good	Poor

Abbreviations: FEV$_1$, forced expiratory volume in 1 second; MBC, maximum breathing capacity; PCO$_2$, partial pressure of carbon dioxide; PO$_2$, partial pressure of oxygen; RV, residual volume; TLC, total lung capacity; VC, vital capacity.
(From Knudson RJ, Gaensler EA: Surgery for emphysema: collective review. Ann Thorac Surg 1:332, 1965, with permission.)

Table 22-3. Hugh-Jones Criteria for Dyspnea (Modified)

Grade	Definition
0	No dyspnea on exertion
I	Dyspnea on running or climbing two flights of stairs
II	Dyspnea while walking or cycling against the wind
III	Unable to walk or cycle more than 1,000 m
IV	Unable to walk more than 100 m
V	Dyspnea on walking in the house, dressing, and washing

(From Hugh-Jones P, Lambert AV: A simple exercise test and its use for measuring exertion dyspnea. Br Med J 12:65, 1952, with permission.)

almost all moderately to severely symptomatic patients with bullae occupying more than 30 percent of a hemithorax (Wesley, et al., 1972; Iwa, et al., 1981; Billig, et al., 1968; Boushy, et al., 1969; Foreman, et al., 1968; and Sung, et al., 1973).

Extreme breathlessness in the presence of a giant bulla is still the best indication for an operation with resultant success (Baldwin, et al., 1950; Pride, et al., 1970; Wesley, et al., 1972; FitzGerald, et al., 1974; Eschapasse, et al., 1980; Weitzenbaum, 1980; and Witz and Roeslin, 1980). Pulmonary hypertension is not a contraindication to surgery, as outlined by FitzGerald, et al. (1974) and Pierce and Growdon (1962). Indeed, the pathophysiologic effect of the bulla on the vasculature of the underlying restricted lung tissue is the same as the effect on the lung tissue itself. With the relief of the space-occupying lesion, the underlying lung expands, the vasculature reopens, and the resistance in both the airway and the vessels may be sizably reduced.

Other criteria for patient selection are important:

1. Progressively enlarging nonfunctioning pulmonary units are detected (Spear, et al., 1961; Sung, et al., 1973; and Iwa, et al., 1981).

2. Bullae should be compressing (and rendering nonfunctional) a significant volume of potentially functional lung parenchyma (Sung, et al., 1973; Wesley, et al., 1972; Connolly and Wilson, 1989; and FitzGerald, et al., 1974).

3. Best results are found in patients with a minimal inflammatory component to the disease process (cough and sputum) (Wesley, et al., 1972; FitzGerald, et al., 1974; and Connolly and Wilson, 1989).

4. Patients with diffuse emphysema do not tolerate surgical procedures well, and best results occur in patients with localized bullous disease.

5. Removal of a bulla should eliminate the functionless unit and result in reexpansion and return to function of a significant volume of lung.

6. Recurrent pneumothorax is detected.

7. Persistent pneumothorax with bronchopleural fistula is found (Gaensler, et al., 1983).

8. The type of bulla is not as important as whether it significantly embarrasses the function of the adjacent lung tissue.

Functional Status

Much has been written about the differentiation between closed (noncommunicating) and open (communicating) bullae. A differentiation between these two types of bullae can

be made based on radiologic and functional studies, which has been described by Billig, et al. (1968), Billig (1976), Gunstensen and McCormick (1973), Boushy, et al. (1969), Laros, et al. (1986), and Weisel and Slotnick (1950). Both open and closed bullae are operable, and little or no differentiation between the two must be made preoperatively. The assessments are of academic value only.

In closed bullae a small inspiratory vital capacity (VC) is present because bullae do not contribute to the change in volume. The loss is located on the affected side, which also has only a moderately elevated RV by bronchospirometric assessment. No helium peaks appear on this side with deep expiration at the end of unilateral helium washout. The chest radiograph demonstrates no change in the size of the bulla at maximum expiration.

Open bullae demonstrate a normal VC with spirometry and a normal VC with bronchospirometric assessment of the affected side. The RV is high, and a typical helium peak appears at maximal expiration.

Pride, et al. (1973) and Dollery and Hugh-Jones (1963) demonstrated that ventilated cysts are extremely uncommon and they may function as respiratory dead space. Nonventilated cysts behave as space-occupying lesions, but they seldom produce active positive compression of the adjacent lung.

Jordanogiou and Pride (1968) showed that there is a loss of the elastic recoil pressure, leading to airway collapse during expiration and hyperinflation, as measured by the total lung capacity (TLC) and FRC. Ogilvie and Catterall (1959) suggested that overall this increases the work of breathing. Brantigan, et al. (1959) and Boushy, et al. (1968) concluded that elastic recoil can be increased if emphysematous bullae are removed.

Gaensler, et al. (1986) demonstrated that, with localized bullae, there is good correlation between their size and the forced expiratory volume in 1 second (FEV_1). Therefore, a reduction in FEV_1 disproportionate to the size of the bulla suggests significant diffuse disease. There are two indications that the impairment is caused by bullae compressing good lung tissue: (1) a reduction in the FVC almost equal to the reduction in FEV_1, and (2) FRC and TLC that are increased but not to the degree suggested by the lung volume on the chest radiograph.

The difference between the FRC determined by body plethysmographic assessment and that assessed by helium rebreathing indicates accurately the trapped gas volume. FitzGerald, et al. (1974) and Gaensler, et al. (1983) suggested that a large discrepancy is a good indication for surgical improvement. O'Brien, et al. (1986) emphasized that it is the nonbullous lung that determines the patient's postoperative function. Vishnevsky and Nickoladge (1990) have shown that a decrease in expiratory flow rates and high respiratory resistance suggests compression of the bronchial tree by bullous areas, the removal of which can cause an increase in FEV_1 and a decrease in bronchial resistance.

The capacity of bullae is assessed from the difference of the RV measured by body box testing and by lung helium dilution (Laros, et al., 1986; and Ichitani, 1985). After removal of the bullae, the decrease of RV by body box testing indicates a decrease of dead space (FitzGerald, et al., 1974;

Gaensler, et al., 1983; Laros, et al. 1986; and Ichitani, 1985). Normal values of diffusing capacity before and after the operation indicate the absence of generalized diffuse emphysema. If the diffusing capacity is reduced preoperatively, it is a good objective test for minimal improvement postoperatively (FitzGerald, et al., 1974; and Gaensler, et al., 1983 and 1986).

Sung, et al. (1973) and Parker (1974) showed that, in the majority of instances, patients with resting hypoxia or resting hypercapnia are not good candidates for surgery. Patients with pulmonary hypertension may also be poor candidates for surgery with resultant poor functional improvement (Fitzpatrick, 1958; Laforet, 1972; and Gunstensen and McCormack, 1973). The criteria of hypoxia, hypercapnia, and pulmonary hypertension are not absolute. Harris (1976) has shown that in selected instances, patients indeed can benefit from bullectomy, with the underlying lung function providing the basis for this improvement.

More recently Tenholder, et al. (1980) described progressive incremental exercise testing as a preoperative prognosticator for postoperative improvement. Foreman, et al. (1968), Fain, et al. (1967), and others have shown little correlation postoperatively between the clinical improvements and the results of pulmonary function studies. Progressive incremental exercise testing may provide an accurate method for correlating subjective improvement in dyspnea, objective improvement in gas exchange, and increased functional work capacity postoperatively. Progressive incremental exercise testing can identify the physiologic mechanisms of maximum exercise limitation and abnormal physiologic responses at submaximal exercise levels, as shown by Jones, et al. (1975) and Wasserman and Whipp (1975). The future use of this particular assessment has yet to be determined. The following pulmonary function studies should be performed preoperatively and postoperatively, but there are no magic rules to be derived from the literature to identify the patient who will benefit or who should be refused an operation (FitzGerald, et al., 1974; Pride, 1973; and Sung, et al., 1973). The tests include spirometric volumes, lung volumes, single breath diffusing capacity of carbon monoxide, constant volume body plethysmography for airway resistance, specific conductance and FRC, helium alveolar volume, static elastic recoil pressure of the lung, and arterial blood gases.

Clinical assessment in the selection of patients remains problematic. No one lung function test can adequately assess the mechanical and physiologic effects of this disease. Hugh-Jones and Whimster (1978) stated that an overall assessment of the patient preoperatively using many parameters is necessary to determine the candidacy of the patient for surgical intervention.

Imaging

Imaging techniques are used to identify (with as much accuracy as possible) the size, location, and extent of space-occupying lesions. In addition, the technique used identifies the character of the adjacent lung parenchyma that will or should provide improvement in lung function postoperatively.

When an elective operation for bullous emphysema is considered, differentiation between a single giant bulla and vanishing lobes or cysts is important (Billig, et al., 1968; Billig, 1976; FitzGerald, et al., 1974; Potgieter, et al., 1981; and Boushy et al., 1969).

When simple bullae appear to be present, surgery should not be considered if the bullae occupy one-third or less of a hemithorax because, in such instances, an operation seldom improves pulmonary function and validity (FitzGerald, et al., 1974; Laros, et al., 1986; Boushy, et al., 1969; Foreman, et al., 1968; and Pearson and Ogilvie, 1983).

Chest Radiography. Burke (1937), a radiologist, coined the term *vanishing lung syndrome*. This expression defines a condition in which bullous disease completely replaces the lung ipsilaterally on the chest radiograph. FitzGerald, et al. (1974) graded lung areas for signs of diffuse emphysema. Each hemithorax was divided into three horizontal zones and the character, size, and demarcation of the bullae were graded and coded. Vascular crowding, mediastinal shift, and herniation were measured and recorded. Stone, et al. (1960) showed that such radiographic findings, including severe hernation of the diaphragm on the affected side, mediastinal herniation, and herniation of a bulla to the contralateral side, did not correlate at all with a patient's symptoms. There was also no identifiable uniformity as to the rate of progression of the bullae over time. No correlation, in addition, was found between the size of the bulla and the symptoms (Fig. 22-2).

Old radiographs might be helpful in so far as they define with some accuracy the natural history and progression of the bullous disease. If the bullous lesion is progressing rapidly, surgical intervention may be more rational than a wait-and-see policy (Gaensler, et al., 1986).

Inspiratory and expiratory views are often obtained to differentiate between diffuse emphysema and localized bullous disease. With diffuse emphysema, expiration does not decrease the volume of the hemithorax substantially, whereas with localized bullous disease, expiration dramatically decreases the volume as a result of deflation of the crowded underlying normal lung. For the most part, large well-demarcated bullae are an absolute indication for surgery, with predictable results postoperatively (FitzGerald, et al., 1974; Capel and Belcher, 1957; and Sung, et al., 1973).

Bullous lesions occupying more than 50 percent of a hemithorax with normal compressed underlying parenchyma have the best results (Morgan and Strickland, 1984; Morgan, et al., 1986; Pearson and Ogilvie, 1983; Gaensler, et al., 1983 and 1986; and Laros, et al., 1986). Small bullae occupying one-third or less of the radiographic volume with normal lungs have no measurable effect on either lung volume or flow. Ogilvie and Catterall (1959) demonstrated that excision does not improve function or symptoms postoperatively, including in patients with underlying diffuse emphysema.

Bronchography. Prior to the advent of computed tomography, bronchography was used by several investigators, including Potgieter, et al. (1981) (Fig. 22-3). This assessment was used preoperatively to identify bronchiectasis and compression of the bronchi by adjacent bullous disease.

Angiography. Prior to computed tomography, the most accurate definition of areas of functioning lung tissue could only be made by pulmonary angiography. The alveolar "blush"

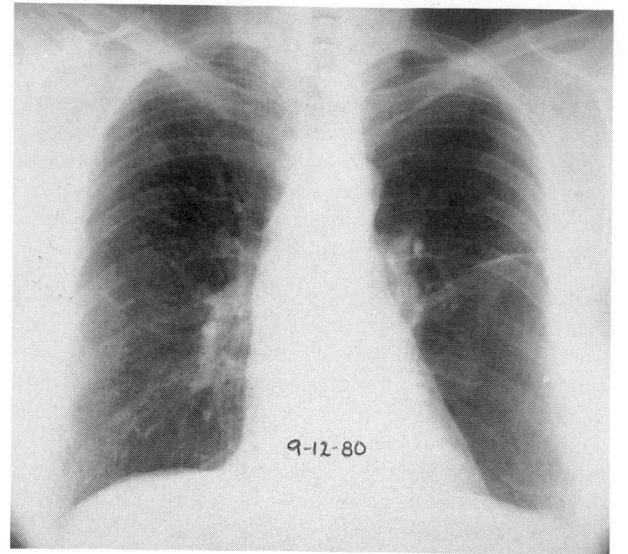
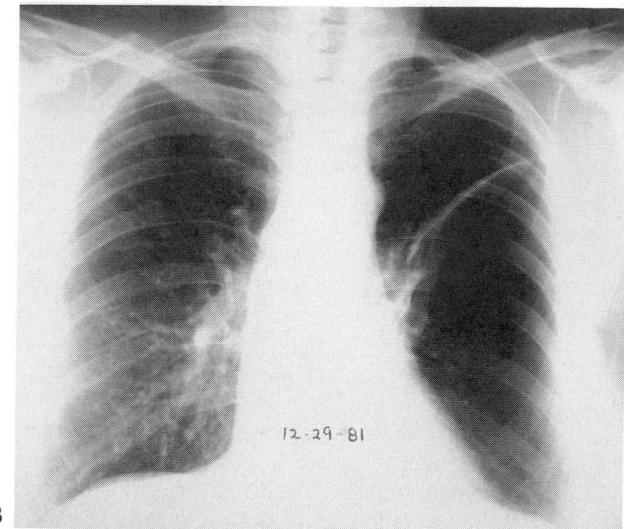
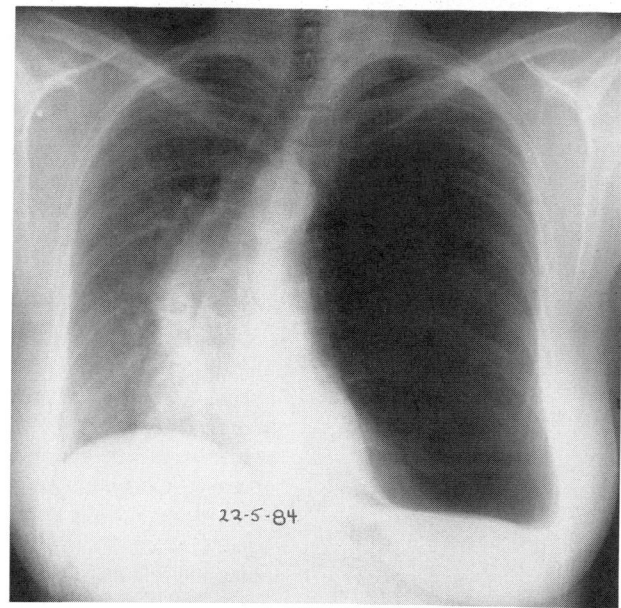

Figure 22-2. **(A–C)** Chest radiographs showing enlargement serially of a solitary bulla in the left lower lobe over 3.5 years. Ultimately this produced severe dyspnea and displacement of the diaphragm and mediastinum with additional compromise of the contralateral lung.

in peripheral lung tissue was the most reliable indicator of persisting capillary circulation. Preservation of vascularity was invariably associated with unimpaired local air flow. Delarue, et al. (1977) suggested that pulmonary angiography was the single most important investigation in determining the feasibility of surgical treatment. Angiographic crowding must be present and can readily be distinguished from a nonreversible effect of diffuse disease and localized emphysema (Chaves, et al., 1968; FitzGerald, et al., 1974; Jensen, et al., 1961; Sung, et al., 1973; Parker, 1974; and Wesley, et al., 1972).

Billig (1976) identified the importance of pulmonary angiography in assessing pulmonary hypertension and the value of inhaling 100% oxygen during the assessment. If the pulmo-nary artery pressure fell toward normal by improving the PO_2 with inhalation of 100 percent oxygen, this might show that local factors, which can be corrected by bullectomy, are functional in producing the pulmonary hypertension.

Miscall and Duffy (1953), Steinberg, et al. (1950), and Jensen, et al. (1961) described the effects of bullae on the underlying vasculature. The vasculature may demonstrate the effects of generalized emphysema, which produce a "winter tree" pattern in which arteriolar branches taper abruptly in the midzone and continue in a wiry constricted pattern, causing delayed blood flow to the periphery. Bullae are avascular, and they distort and compress the pulmonary arterial tree. The degree of functional impairment of the surrounding parenchyma can thereby be assessed.

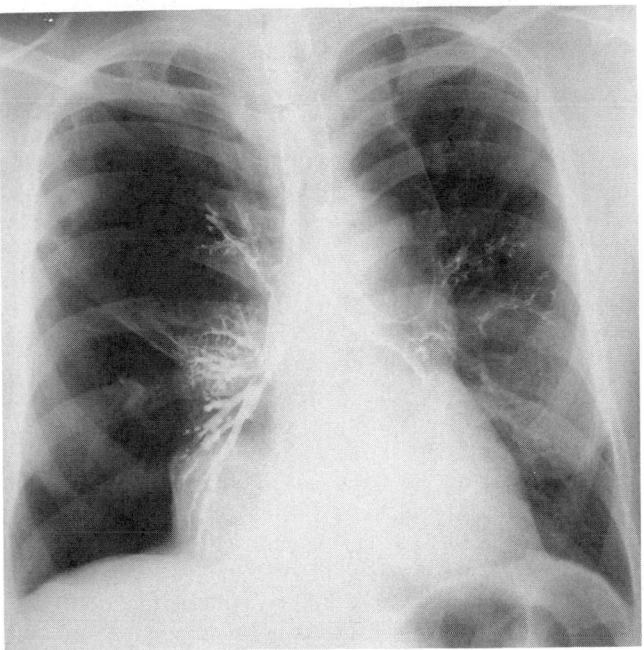

Figure 22-3. A bilateral pulmonary bronchogram in a patient with multiple bullae and underlying diffuse disease. The major bullae are on the right, with severe crowding of the bronchi (and presumably vessels) paramediastinally. Excellent symptomatic relief was obtained by multiple right bullectomies.

In summary, angiography may be useful when resection of multiple bullae is considered to determine the following:

1. The amount of lung parenchyma destroyed by the associated emphysematous process
2. The areas of functioning lung tissue identified by zones of functioning capillary circulation, seen as a vascular blush in the capillary phase of the angiogram
3. The bullae with respect to size, multiplicity, bilaterality, and avascularity
4. The degree of associated hypertension

Ventilation-Perfusion Scanning.   Regional function studies are important in patients with bilateral disease. Asymmetry of function indicates that surgery on the more impaired side entails less risk and is more likely to improve function. Gaensler, et al. (1983) demonstrated that perfusion scans are useful to estimate split function but they do not aid in localization because the deflects they show generally are already known from ordinary chest radiographs. The routinely observed slow entry and poor washout of bullae is predictable without this particular procedure.

However, combined ventilation-perfusion scans, as described by Poe, et al. (1973), Polga, et al. (1984), and Wesley, et al. (1972) provides a means to evaluate regional pulmonary parameters and may distinguish primary vascular from parenchymal disease. The regional pulmonary function can be identified both in the abnormal and normal lung, preoperatively, and as a basis for improvement postoperatively.

Computed Tomography.   The first description of the use of computed tomography in assessing surgical bullous disease was by Fiore, et al. (1982). In three cases, this group showed that computed tomography can (1) differentiate a pneumothorax from a large bulla, (2) identify the extensive nature of the bullous disease in other locations not seen by chest radiography or tomography, and most importantly, (3) assess the characteristics of the underlying lung relative to the compression and status of the vasculature (Fig. 22-4).

With its recent refinements, computed tomography has become the ultimate imaging technique for assessing patients before surgery who have bullous emphysema. The technique demonstrates the size, location, and extensiveness of bullous disease with increased sensitivity compared with older techniques, such as routine chest radiography, tomography, and angiography. It also provides increased sensitivity and resolution of the pulmonary vasculature and its crowding and the status of the tracheobronchial tree. Computed tomography gives useful anatomic information, which should be supplemented by physiologic and functional studies of regional and overall lung function (Carr and Pride, 1984).

Computed tomography was used to assess 43 patients preoperatively. Twenty of these patients had generalized emphysema, and 23 had defined bullous disease only. Operations were performed in 12 patients only with true bullae, with 5 undergoing thoracotomies and 7 undergoing Monaldi procedures. Computed tomography was used to assess the distribution, characteristics, size, location, and extent of the bullae; the vasculature of the remaining lung; and the function of the bullae with respect to volume and ventilation. Most bullae were found not to contribute to ventilation, and only patients with true bullae on computed tomography were offered operations (Morgan, et al., 1986).

A reduction in dead space ventilation or a release of lung compression may be unimportant in symptom relief following

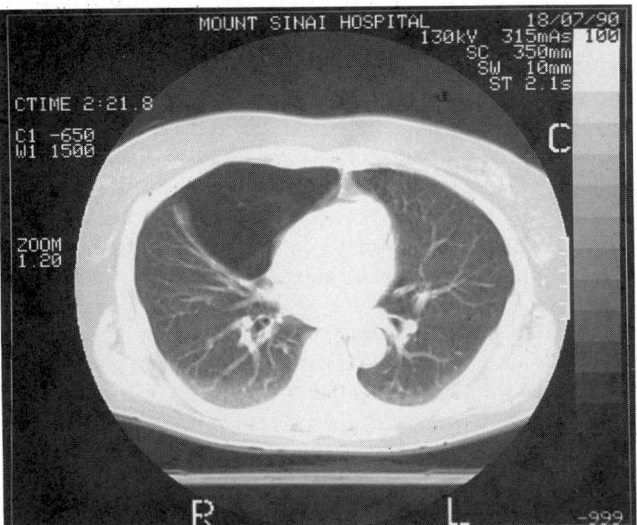

Figure 22-4.   Computed tomography of the chest with a large solitary bulla in the anterior right hemithorax and crowding of the vasculature in the adjacent normal lung.

bullectomy. Practically it may not be important to demonstrate that compressed or dead spaced ventilation is present to justify surgery. Morgan, et al. (1986) and Gaensler, et al. (1983 and 1986) have stated that the mere demonstration by computed tomography that an appreciable space exists may be the only grounds necessary for expecting improvement postoperatively.

MANAGEMENT

Current Surgical Modalities

Patients who benefit from the surgical excision of bullae have space-occupying nonfunctioning air spaces or localized nonfunctioning parenchymal areas encroaching on normal or near-normal adjacent lung. Excision removes the space-occupying lesions, allows the compressed lung to expand, permits better ventilation and perfusion similar to the remaining lung, and decreases both dead space and residual volume (Gaensler, et al., 1983 and 1986; and Benfield, 1969).

The surgeon must maximize the preservation of functioning lung tissue or potentially functioning lung tissue by avoiding major resections, such as lobectomies. This is extremely important in patients with diffuse lung disease who have limited overall lung function after bullectomy (DeVries and Wolfe, 1980).

The general indications for surgical intervention are as follows:

1. Moderate to severe dyspnea
2. A bulla occupying more than one-third of the lung field
3. A pulmonary angiogram demonstrating reduced blood flow to the involved lung field, as defined by Jensen, et al. (1961) and Miscall and Duffy (1953).
4. Complications of bullous disease, for example, pneumothorax, infection in a bulla, or massive hemoptysis (Berry and Ochsner, 1972)

Monaldi Procedures

Monaldi (Monaldi and Tentativi, 1938; and Monaldi, 1947) introduced a technique using intracavitary drainage for six cases of refractory tuberculous cavitary disease with success. Hennell (1936) and Field and Rosenberg (1937) reported the cure of solitary cysts of the lung by chemical cauterization using the injection of iodized oil or silver nitrate into cysts.

Head and Avery (1949), Head, et al. (1960), and Cooke and Schaff (1953) treated several cases of bullous disease successfully with the Monaldi technique in poor risk patients. The first large series was reported by MacArthur and Fountain (1977) with 31 patients undergoing such a procedure and an operative mortality of 6.5 percent in poor risk patients. Radiographic improvement occurred in 97 percent, pulmonary function improvement occurred in 83 percent (FEV_1 and VC), and symptomatic improvement occurred in 90 percent of patients.

The technique for bullous disease was originally described by John Alexander (1946). A two-stage procedure was initially designed to avoid the risk of pneumothorax and entailed the creation of pleural adhesions over the cyst wall by the insertion of an iodine pack extrapleurally at the first stage and drainage of the cyst 3 weeks later.

Presently one-stage procedures are used. A small portion of rib is excised subperiostally over the underlying bulla. A purse-string suture is inserted into the parietal pleura, picking up the visceral pleura and underlying cyst wall. Pleurae and cysts are then opened within the purse-string suture, and a large Foley catheter is inserted. The balloon is inflated with air, the purse-string suture is tightened, and the catheter end is placed underwater to seal and suction. A chest tube is inserted into the free pleural space. Pleurodesis (talc) of both the contents of the bulla and the pleural cavity may aid in the treatment (Venn, et al., 1988; Uyama, et al., 1988). Rice, et al. (1987) showed that this technique was excellent in compromised patients and safe with patients whose breathing was supported by ventilators for intracavitary drainage of lung abscesses or expanding cysts.

Venn, et al. (1988) accumulated a series of 20 patients in whom this technique was used for 22 bullae. It was demonstrated that sizable increases in pulmonary function study results postoperatively occurred with subjective improvement in almost all instances and follow-up of more than 2 years. Based on these data, patients can be operated on with hypercapnia but not with an FEV_1 less than 500 ml. These authors also recommend the use of talc in the interior of the bulla and the pleural cavity. The rationale for this is based on the reports of Stone, et al. (1960), Rubin and Buchberg (1968), and Harada, et al. (1984), who identified the resolution of bullae after they accumulated fluid spontaneously, whether infected or not.

In an editorial, Ginsberg (1988) described five patients with seen bullae treated in this fashion, all successfully. It was his suggestion that perhaps this technique would replace all other types of procedures performed by open thoracotomy.

Bullectomy

Most bullectomies are performed through a standard posterolateral approach through the fifth or sixth intercostal space. Recently, video-assisted thoracoscopy has developed as an alternative to open thoracotomy. Pedunculated bullae are easily treated through suture ligation of the pedicle and excision of the bulla. For patients with diffuse disease, the basic technique of plication is simple (Fig. 22-5). The development of surgical staplers has made this procedure even easier, and a modification of the method of Naclerio and Langer (1947), as reported by Nelems (1980), is now used routinely.

The largest bulla is opened longitudinally, and the cavity is explored from within. Strands of fibrous septae are excised (Fig. 22-6), and long forceps are applied from inside so that they grasp the pleura at the reflection of relatively normal parenchyma with the cyst cavity. The visceral pleura (cyst wall) is then folded back over the remaining raw surface of the lung, and the stapler is applied along the base of the bulla. The stapler is applied as many times as necessary until the raw surfaces of the entire base of the cyst are closed. This double layer of pleura acts as a buttress for the staples and reduces and prevents air leakage from the stapled margin. Parmar, et al. (1987) suggested that a Teflon pledget incorpo-

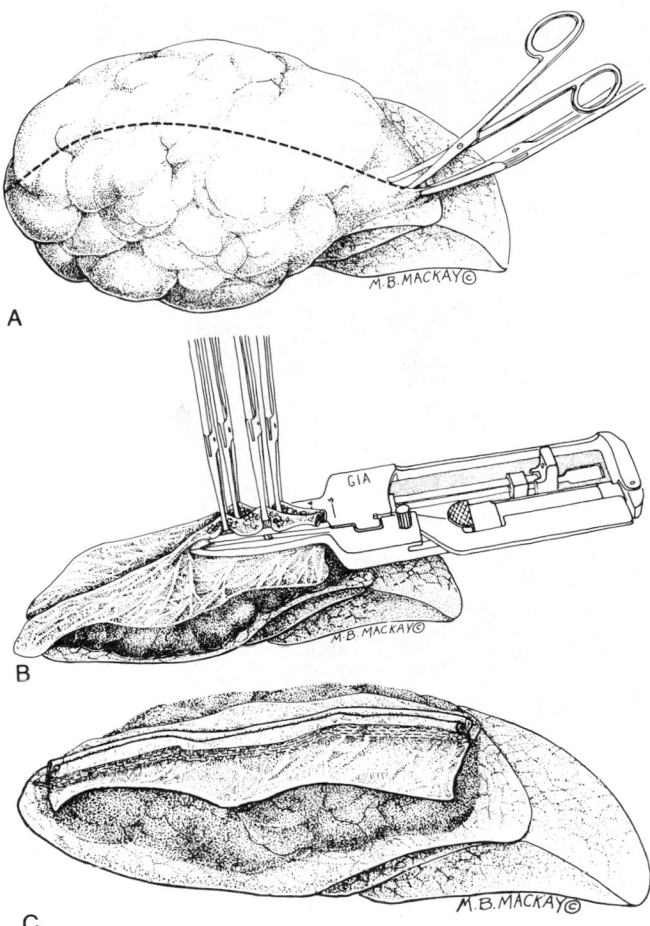

Figure 22-5. Operative technique. **(A)** Longitudinal opening of the bulla. **(B)** Folding of the visceral pleura over the raw surface of the lung and stapling of the entire base of the cyst. **(C)** Complete bullectomy. (From Deslauriers J, Leblanc P, McClish A: General Thoracic Surgery, 3rd Ed. p. 740. Lea & Febiger, Philadelphia, 1989, with permission.)

rated into the bullectomy staple line ensures pneumostasis postoperatively.

Following bullectomy pleural symphysis by poudrage (Cooke and Schaff, 1953), abrasion of the pleural surfaces, introduction of irritating chemicals (Brock, 1948), or parietal pleurectomy (Cabiran and Ziskind, 1964; Gaensler, 1956) were advocated. It is important to realize that chemical or mechanical pleurodesis is contraindicated, unless there is certainty that, immediately after the procedure, parietal-visceral contact is ensured. This suggests that bronchopleural fistulae must be closed before pleurodesis is attempted, a condition that is rarely satisfied after excision of a bulla in emphysema.

Median sternotomy has been advocated for bilateral pulmonary operations, including bilateral pleurodesis for spontaneous pneumothorax (Kalnins, et al., 1973; Mercier, et al., 1976), resection of bilateral metastatic tumors to the lungs (Takita, et al., 1977; Meng, et al., 1980), an other bilateral conditions (Lima, et al., 1981; Copper, et al., 1978). All these authors show that adequate exposure is obtained with a midline sternotomy for successful completion of most pulmonary procedures. This technique also provides quick exposure and closure, minimizing the operating time and the complication rate.

Cooper, et al. (1978), Peters, et al. (1969), and Ikeda, et al. (1988) demonstrated that midline sternotomy (compared with staged thoracotomies) produces slightly better pulmonary function study results postoperatively with a more rapid restoration over the course of the first week postoperatively. Previous studies were performed by Haughton (1968) and Mattila, et al. (1967) that showed little if any difference in postoperative lung function when these two types of thoracotomies were compared. Criticisms of the sternotomy include the development of sternal osteomyelitis and mediastinitis, and in some instances, the technical difficulty of the operation itself. The first two complications occur more frequently during cardiac surgery because of the prolonged procedures, poor perfusion, and hypoxia. This was demonstrated by Iwa, et al. (1981); Lee, et al. (1983); and Meng, et al. (1980). The technical difficulties are easily solved, as described by Urschel and Razzuk (1986). Connolly and Wilson (1989), is a review of 19 patients, preferred staged posterolateral thoracotomies at 4- to 6-week intervals. They suggested that the prolonged air leaks after simultaneous bilateral procedures (sternotomy) are morbid problems that are compounded when the bilateral procedure is performed. Deslauriers, et al. (1989) also prefer bilateral staged operations in which the functional results of the first procedure can be evaluated before proceeding with a contralateral thoracotomy.

Pulmonary Resection: Lobectomy/Segmental Resection

Pulmonary resection is rarely performed for bullous disease, but it may be the procedure of choice when a whole lobe has been replaced by bullae. This may be the initial impression at the thoracotomy when in fact there is merely separation of the lung from the visceral pleura, resulting in a large air space with relatively normal, but atelectatic, lung beneath. FitzGerald, et al. (1974); Gaensler, et al. (1983), and Shaw (1952) showed that, in such cases, lobectomy has had disappointing results because the lung tissue that could have been expanded following bullectomy had in fact been removed. Potgieter, et al. (1981) performed lobectomies in 3 patients of 21 undergoing thoracotomy for bullous disease. All patients with bullectomy had major complications postoperatively, and none of the three had functional or symptomatic improvement postoperatively.

Thoracoscopy

With the popularity of thoracoscopy, both in the diagnosis and treatment of intrathoracic disease, Wakabayashi, et al. (1991) described the use of thoracoscopy and carbon dioxide laser therapy for bullous emphysema in 22 poor-risk patients. Patients had either diffuse emphysema or multiple bullae. Defocused carbon dioxide laser beams were applied to the external surface of the bullae. Thick intraparenchymal bullae were opened, and the laser beams were applied to the internal surface of the bullae. After complete retraction of all visible

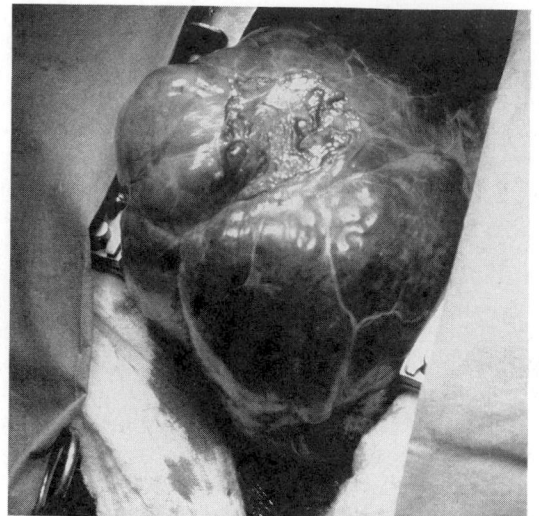

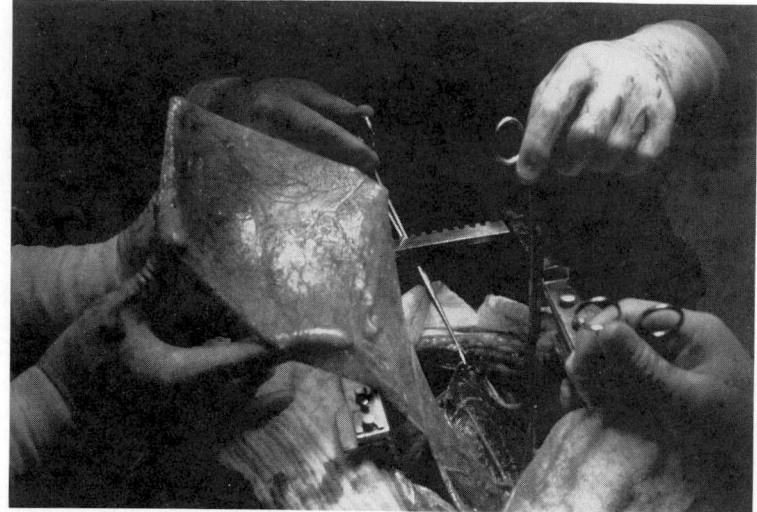

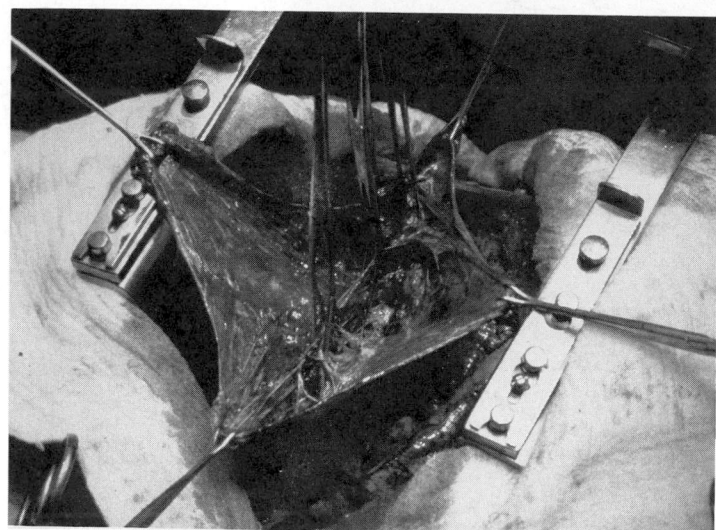

Figure 22-6. **(A)** A large bulla exposed at thoracotomy, occupying 50 percent of the hemithorax. **(B)** The largest bulla is opened longitudinally, and the cavity is explored from within. The bulla is deroofed, and denuded fibrous strands and vessels are present in its base. **(C)** Long Duval forceps are applied from within the bulla so that they grasp the base, which is withdrawn and incorporated into the stapled margin with the folded reflection of the remaining visceral pleura.

bullae, the lung was reexpanded. In contrast to most reports, patients who had less than 50 percent of the hemithorax replaced by bullae improved after laser ablation. This technique has also been used in Russia by Smoljar and Vertianov (1985) and most recently by Lewis (personal communication, 1991) who treats bullous disease by thoracoscopy resection and/or argon laser beam coagulation. Video-assisted thoracoscopy photoablation is appropriate therapy for single or multiple superficial bullae because the penetration of the energy source is seldom greater than 2 to 3 mm. Solitary cysts on narrow bases or pedicles can be excised after thoracoscopic ligation or endostapling, but bullae that are more extensive with broad bases and deep parenchymal involvement should be formally excised and/or plicated by thoracotomy. With this rapidly expanding field, more information on this particular mode of therapy will be available over the next several years.

Lung Transplantation

End-stage chronic obstructive lung disease with secondary vascular and bullous parenchymal changes long awaited the availability of organ transplantation. Reitz, et al. (1982) performed the first successful heart-lung transplantation for vascular disease. After this, transplantation offered a therapeutic option to treat end-stage pulmonary parenchymal and vascular disease that was otherwise fatal. The Toronto Lung Transplantation Group (1986) extended this pioneering work, reporting long-term survival with single- and double-lung transplantations (Cooper, et al., 1987; Patterson, et al., 1988).

As a result of these advances, transplantation therapy is now available for intractable end-stage pulmonary disease of many causes.

Cooper, et al. (1989) reported on six patients who were alive and well 5 to 15 months after bilateral pulmonary transplantation for end-stage chronic obstructive airway disease. It was suggested that cardiac transplantation in conjunction with bilateral lung transplantation is unnecessary and avoids the complications associated with the cardiac portion of the transplantation procedure, such as acute and chronic rejection and the development of advanced coronary artery disease. It also eliminates the need to secure a suitable donor with a combination of suitable cardiac and pulmonary functions and increases the supply of donor organs. Following this Emery, et al. (1991) described six patients who underwent double-lung transplantation for chronic obstructive lung disease with four moderately good functional results and who were followed up 8 to 24 months postoperatively. The conclusions of this short series were that these patients required prolonged hospitalization, the procedure was time intensive, and there were numerous complications at great expense.

Single-lung transplantation has been considered physiologically inappropriate for patients with chronic obstructive lung disease. It has been postulated that the high static compliance and elevated pulmonary vascular resistance of the native lung, functioning in parallel with the more normal allografted lung, could cause unacceptable ventilation-perfusion mismatching and/or overinflation of the native lung with encroachment on the expansion of the transplanted lung (Toronto Lung Transplant Group, et al., 1988; Stevens, et al., 1970). Because of these concerns, double-lung transplantation developed for patients with chronic obstructive lung disease. Trulock, et al. (1989) reported a single lung transplantation in a patient with chronic obstructive lung disease. They claimed that a significant disruption in gas exchange did not occur, unless a complication, such as rejection or infection, occurred in the graft. Recently a renewed interest has developed in single-lung transplantation for emphysema, as reported by Vanderhoeft, et al. (1971) and Mal, et al. (1989). More studies are required in the future to validate the indications and feasibility of single-lung transplantation for diffuse emphysema (see Ch. 33).

Surgery for Complications

Carcinoma in a Bulla

Tsutsui, et al. (1988) have thoroughly reviewed the subject of carcinoma in a bulla. Three patterns of development occur radiographically in the bulla containing the tumor: (1) nodular opacity within or adjacent to the bulla, (2) partial or diffuse thickening of the bulla wall, and (3) secondary signs of the bulla (diameter change, fluid retention, or pneumothorax).

The incidence of bullae in association with bronchogenic carcinoma is 2.5 percent and is highest in the sixth decade of life (51.6 percent). Stoloff, et al. (1971), Korol (1953), Goldstein, et al. (1968), and Aronberg, et al. (1980) have reported this association.

Peabody, et al. (1957) reinforced the necessity for accurate early radiographic assessment because, in most instances, the diagnosis is made late and is difficult to diagnose. The tumor is seen when it is in an advanced stage in 58.3 percent of cases.

Infected Bulla

Bullae commonly become infected because they do communicate in most instances with the tracheobronchial tree. Fortunately most can be managed medically, and surgery is limited only to refractory cases that might require surgical drainage or excision. This was the experience of Fain, et al. (1967), Ellison and Ellison (1964), and Stone, et al. (1960). The natural history of a bulla that contains fluid (infected or not) has been described by Lloyd (1949) and Rothstein (1954). Infection in the bulla results in a reduction in its size as a result of fibrotic contraction. The production of fluid produces closure of the connections with the airway and results in the absorption of air and the disappearance of the air spaces.

Hemoptysis

Patients with hemoptysis should undergo manditory bronchoscopy to rule out endobronchial lesions. The majority can be treated medically and are commonly associated with infected bullae. With resolution of the bulla and its infection, the hemoptysis usually resolves. FitzGerald, et al. (1974) and Berry and Ochsner (1972) recommended that surgery should be contemplated in those patients who have prolonged, recurrent, or extensive hemoptysis, and the therapy should be bulectomy.

Pneumothorax

Pneumothorax in bullous disease is seldom controlled by thoracotomy tube drainage alone. It commonly produces a persistent chronic bronchopleural fistula and a non-fully inflated underlying lung. Therefore, resection of the bulla and closure of the air leaks frequently is the only satisfactory solution. Joress (1956) and others agree that, after a short trial of 5 days of closed chest tube drainage and suction, thoracotomy should be performed and the bulla and leak treated directly.

Preoperative Management

Patients with bullous emphysema usually undergo elective surgery, which allows time for the optimization of pulmonary function. All patients should be required to stop smoking. An active chest physical therapy program is initiated, including deep breathing exercises, coughing exercises, and incentive spirometry. In many centers, a rehabilitation program is available, and a 4-week involvement would be worthwhile in patients who have severely compromised pulmonary function. It has been well established that the objective parameters of the pulmonary function are not improved after rehabilitation, but certainly, both mentally and subjectively, patients are much improved.

These patients commonly experience episodes of bronchospasm and the formation of excess secretions, which can be treated medically. High airway resistance and bronchospasm should be reduced maximally with appropriate bronchodilators, and antibiotics should be prescribed for intercurrent infections. On occasion my associates and I give patients corticosteroids, 5 days preoperatively, to optimize their pulmonary function and bronchodilation. With rehabilitation the patient's nutrition should be supplemented to provide a positive anabolic effect and an increase in muscle mass.

Anesthesia

Ting, et al.(1963) showed that, in bullous emphysema, Laplace's law, which relates the expanding force in a hollow structure to the cross-sectional area, applies. The pressure within a bulla equals the mural tension of the bulla divided by its radius multiplied by two. If positive pressure is applied to the airway, a large bleb tends to increase in size even more.

Isenhower and Cucchiara (1976) suggested that premedication be omitted to prevent preoperative pulmonary depression. The patient's intubation is performed awake to omit positive pressure ventilation during induction. A double-lumen tube is used on a routine basis to achieve split airway control and to ventilate contralateral isolated lung intraoperatively because most of the ventilation occurs in the bullous lung if both lungs are ventilated simultaneously. Eger and Saidman (1965) suggested that increased concentrations of oxygen be added only after intubation because preoperative increases in oxygen may remove the drive for spontaneous ventilation. These authors showed that the use of nitrous oxide in the presence of an air-filled cavity must be judicious to prevent a further increase in the size of the air space intraoperatively.

Munson (1974) emphasized the need to avoid nitrous oxide and stressed that patients should be breathing spontaneously during the procedure with manual assistance when required. He suggested no positive ventilation and no jet ventilation, and avoided inhalant anesthetics. Patients were managed only with intravenous anesthetics to minimize circulatory and ventilatory depressions.

Hasenbos and Gielen (1985) emphasized the value of intraoperative epidural lidocaine at the T3–T4 level and postoperative epidural morphine at least 3 days postoperatively. Most of the afferent nervous input from lungs and airways enters the central nervous system along the sympathetic nerves to the upper four thoracic segments. Brombage (1978), Widdicombe (1963), and Dohi, et al. (1982) have shown that afferent blockade with epidural lidocaine at the T3–T4 level can prevent and cure bronchospasm intraoperatively. This also allows intraoperative bronchial toilet to be accomplished with little circulatory depression. Postoperative epidural morphine at the T3–T4 level has been shown by Pinckaers, et al. (1981) and Dirksen, et al. (1984) to produce a rapid onset of analgesia without affecting muscle power or producing ventilatory depression, despite the high position of the thoracic epidural catheter.

Obviously pain control is of the utmost importance postoperatively to allow patients with chronic pulmonary disease and retained secretions to expectorate efficiently with adequate chest physical therapy and minimal pain.

Postoperative Management

Postoperatively patients may have large-volume bronchopleural fistulae and some difficulty fully aerating the underlying lung and obliterating the pleural space. On returning to the recovery room, an immediate postoperative chest radiograph is obtained to determine the completeness of lung expansion and obliteration of the pleural space. If this problem exists, endotracheal intubation and positive ventilation should be continued at least overnight. If the surgeon can predetermine large air leaks postoperatively, then more than two chest tubes should be used when closing the chest to gain better control of the pleural space. Chest tubes of course must be drained to underwater sealing, and negative suction must be applied to 20 to 30 cmH$_2$O. Pain is controlled with epidural morphine for 2 to 3 days postoperatively, which directly promotes effective physical therapy and the removal of retained bronchial secretions. We prophylactically prescribe antibiotics perioperatively to minimize the occurrence of postoperative infection.

Results

Fitzpatrick (1958), Tabakin, et al. (1959), Fain, et al. (1967), Capel and Belcher (1957), and Baldwin, et al. (1950) demonstrated that in most instances it is difficult to correlate postoperative subjective findings with postoperative quantitative objective data. Benfield (1969) suggested that one evaluation, which is not done frequently, seems to correlate better than do other parameters, that is, the measurement of the work of breathing. This represents the closest assessment to a patient's subjective dyspnea, which is relied on for subjective assessment of success.

Billig (1976) and Boushy, et al.(1969) showed that the values of postoperative pulmonary function depend on the following.

1. The extent to which the bullae contribute to the tests used; therefore, the appropriate test must be performed, and few have value
2. The extent to which ventilated bullae contribute to ventilated space and VC; resection and replacement by more normal tissue may cause little change in the VC.
3. The extent to which unventilated bullae are resected, producing an increase in VC by filling of the previously compressed lung
4. The extent to which the intrathoracic space occupied by the bullae is replaced by lung tissue
5. The presence of generalized disease

Boushy, et al. (1969) and Ogilvie and Catterall (1959) demonstrated that in general after bullectomy, pulmonary function changes toward normal and such alterations are only marked in patients with bullae that occupy most of a hemithorax.

FitzGerald, et al. (1974) related early and late pulmonary function to various preoperative assessments (Fig. 22-7). Early functional improvement was related to (1) resection of large bullae (FEV$_1$ and maximum voluntary ventilation);

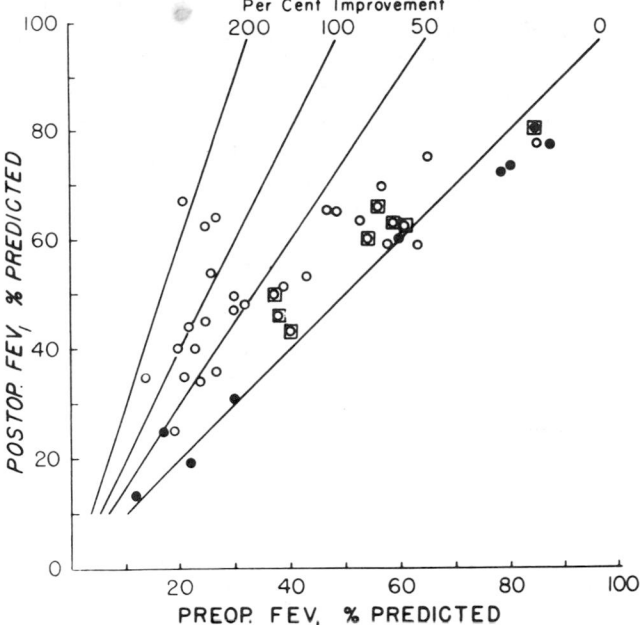

Figure 22-7. A comparison of preoperative with postoperative FEV$_1$ percentages in 42 patients with largely unilateral disease. Resection of small bullae, indicated by black dots, caused little improvement whether overall function initially was severely impaired or nearly normal. Resection of larger bullae, indicated by open circles, generally caused 50 to 200 percent improvement. Patients who had lobectomies, indicated by squares, showed little increase in FEV$_1$ after surgery. (From Gaensler EA, Cugell DW, Knudson RJ, FitzGerald MX: Surgical management of emphysema. Clin Chest Med 4:443, 1983, with permission.)

(2) marked asymmetry of function, with the involved side contributing little, which showed greater improvement (bronchospirometry); and (3) trapped air. The difference between FRC by body box testing and helium rebreathing postoperatively indicates trapped air resected. Pride, et al. (1979) suggested that the large difference preoperatively between FRC by these two measurements favor surgery. In addition, bullectomy for involvement of less than one-third of the hemithorax has little benefit as does bullectomy for diffuse disease. Hughes, et al. (1984) followed 11 patients who had undergone bullectomy for greater than 4 years postoperatively with yearly pulmonary function tests. Postoperative smokers had a pulmonary function decline, whereas nonsmokers postoperatively had slow, if any, decline in pulmonary function. Pride, et al. (1970) and Reid (1967) showed that the beneficial effects on symptoms poorly correlated with the objective change.

Iwa, et al. (1981) performed sternotomy and bilateral resections in 12 patients with bullous disease and showed a good correlation betwen postoperative subjective and objective results. Nine of 12 patients improved by two functional grades of dyspnea, and 7 of 12 patients had a marked increase in FEV$_1$ and VC. Improvement was also identified in patients who had preoperative hypoxia and hypercapnia.

Benfield, et al. (1966) followed 11 of 19 patients who had undergone bullectomy for greater than 1 year postoperatively. Initial improvement was seen in all 11, but after 1 year, only 5 had subjective improvement. Eleven of the 19 had increased exercise tolerance several months postoperatively, but this was subjective improvement only.

FitzGerald, et al. (1974) reported on 95 operations in 84 patients with bullous disease and found that the best results occurred in localized disease with little generalized obstructive airways disease.

Laros, et al. (1986) performed bullectomies for single giant bullae in 27 patients in whom more than 50 percent of the hemithorax was involved. Open communicating bullae were associated with increases in FEV$_1$ postoperatively, and the therapy of closed communicating bullae caused increases in VC postoperatively. No difference was identified in those with open or closed bullae, and patients who have chronic purulent bronchitis uniformly do poorly.

Pearson and Ogilvie (1983) concluded that successful surgery does not increase the rate of decline of background lung disease or encourage the growth of new bullae. This study also showed that, if patients are selected who have greater than 30 percent of the hemithorax involved with bullae, both objective and subjective benefits occur for greater than 5 years in most instances. Six of 12 patients had a FEV$_1$ of less than 1 L preoperatively.

Potgieter, et al. (1981) concluded that lobectomy should be avoided at all costs and operations should not be offered to bronchitic patients. All patients who had undergone bullectomy with bronchiectasis had major postoperative complications, including empyema, chronic fistula, and chronic collapse. Four of 6 patients with hypercapnia survived.

Wesley, et al. (1972) performed bullectomies in 14 patients with 11 long-term follow-ups 2 to 8 years postoperatively. Based on FEV$_1$, VC, and the transfer factor for carbon monoxide, there was a good correlation between subjective and objective data at the yearly follow-up. Long-term follow-up identified good improvement in 6 of 11, fair improvement in 3 of 11, and no improvement in 2.

Fitzpatrick (1958) and Tabakin, et al. (1959) understood that specific criteria for surgical intervention are still lacking. The postoperative results are unpredictable, and the most careful studies have shown few favorable changes and little correlation between subjective and objective improvement.

Laros, et al. (1986), Billig (1976), Billig, et al. (1968), FitzGerald, et al. (1974), Wesley, et al. (1972), and Pearson and Ogilvie (1983) demonstrated that any improvement shown by spirometric data postoperatively persists for several years and then gradually returns to normal preoperative values and beyond.

Mortality and Morbidity Rates

Mortality Rates

Data from carefully selected patient studies show that the operative mortality rate for bullous emphysema should be no greater than 5 percent. In reports of mortality rates of 21 percent (Delarue, et al., 1977; Head and Avery, 1960), most of the deaths occurred in patients who had generalized diffuse underlying obstructive airways disease, multifocal bullous disease, advanced age, or the presence or absence of pulmonary hypertension (Witz and Roeslin, 1980). The overall mortality rate in a series of 95 patients was 2.1 percent, with a 1.5 percent mortality rate occurring in localized disease and a 9.0 percent mortality rate occurring in generalized diffuse disease. In a smaller study of 50 patients by Head and Avery (1960), no deaths occurred in 31 patients with focal disease, and a 21 percent mortality rate was found in 19 patients with either multifocal disease or diffuse emphysema.

Morbidity Rates

Fifty percent of complications are related to either poor remaining lung expansion and pleural space problems, as defined by Delarue, et al. (1977). FitzGerald, et al. (1974) subclassified complications into those that were serious or minor. Serious complications occurred in 10.5 percent of this series, and these included acute respiratory failure, empyema, and chronic bronchopleural fistulae secondary to prolonged air leaks. The incidence of minor complications was 13.6 percent. Laros, et al. (1980) described severe subcutaneous emphysema postoperatively in 12 of 27 cases and also a prolonged air leak greater than 14 days in 12. Potgieter, et al. (1981) demonstrated that 100 percent of patients with bronchiectasis who had undergone bullectomy had major postoperative complications in the form of empyema, chronic pneumothorax, or chronic collapse of the remaining lung. This was associated with a mortality rate of 9.5 percent. A patient's postoperative care should be optimal, with aids in expectoration of retained secretions and cardiovascular maintenance. This procedure should be reserved only for those patients who develop prolonged respiratory failure.

SUMMARY

The present clear indications for surgery are mainly large or increasing bullae that result in compression of apparently good lung tissue and the complications of bullous disease, such as pneumothorax and infection.

The results of local resection of localized giant bullae are dramatic. Lobectomy should not be done until bullae have been removed locally and the remaining lung has been tested by positive ventilation. The resection of small bullae generally has little effect on lung function.

The indications for the resection of large bullae in the presence of diffuse emphysema require careful individual study. In such instances, small increments of function may be of great benefit.

Finally Monaldi-type intracavitary drainage may be indicated in those instances in which open thoracotomy cannot be tolerated. There is some evidence to date that perhaps this particular form of therapy is the procedure of choice in all instances of bullous disease requiring surgical resolution. With time more bullae electively will be treated in this particular fashion. In general, asymptomatic patients, those whose disease is not localized, and those without radiographic evidence of compression should not undergo an operation.

Pulmonary function tests are mandatory, but computed tomography is the single most useful method of assessing the extent of the bullous disease and the underlying lung disease. If the underlying lung architecture is diffusely cystic, then any surgical option is of a palliative nature only. Nevertheless, these patients should not be precluded from surgical consideration.

Potentially functional lung tissue must not be sacrificed during the operation. Limited resections that preserve all functioning lung tissue ensure maximal improvement. Postoperative complications can be minimized with postoperative intensive care, including tracheobronchial toilet, adequate pain control, and excellent chest physical therapy.

COMMENTS AND CONTROVERSIES

The exact indications and long-term results of surgery for bullous disease are still not completely clear. A patient with an expanding solitary bulla that compresses the lung and produces pulmonary symptoms is certainly helped by bullectomy. The value of surgery in diffuse noncompressive bullous disease is less clear. Lung transplantations have provided another method of treating such terminally ill patients, but the very long term results are unknown. There has been a growing interest in "lung shaving" procedures to decrease the volume of the hemithorax, thereby improving the respiratory mechanics of the chest wall and diaphragm. Such surgical approaches are now being investigated, using open thoracotomies and videothoracoscopic techniques (e.g., stapling or laser ablation of tissue). Whether or not this physiologic approach to the management of bullous disease will have any impact in the future is totally unknown.

The reader is referred to the chapter on pneumothorax (see Ch. 38) for further information on the management of blebs and bullae complicated by a spontaneous or traumatic pneumothorax.

R.J.G.

KEY REFERENCES

Cooper JD, Patterson GA, Grossman R, Maurer J: Double lung transplantation for advanced chronic obstructive lung disease. Am Rev Respir Dis 139:303, 1989

This classic paper describes six patients undergoing double-lung transplantation for end-stage emphysema and is a credit to the Toronto Lung Transplantation Group for devising the operation and then clinically testing its validity. It includes an excellent review of the problems associated with single-lung transplantation for this disease and the resultant ventilation and perfusion mismatches.

Klingman RR, Angelillo A, DeMeester TR: Cystic and bullous lung disease. Ann Thorac Surg 52:576, 1991

A recent review that successfully resolves many of the controversies related to the pathophysiologic findings and surgery of bullous lung disease. The review is current and represents a summation and the basis for four decades of interest and ambiguity. It is an excellent source for state-of-the-art information.

Morgan MDL, Denison DM, Strickland B: Value of computed tomography for selecting patients with bullous lung disease for surgery. Thorax 41:855, 1986

This is the first large series of 43 patients assessed preoperatively with computed tomography for bullous lung disease. The volume and ventilation of the true bullae were measured by computed tomography, and it was confirmed that most did not contribute to ventilation. Computed tomography is able to predict accurately the functional improvement in patients postbullectomy and is a desired preoperative assessment in selecting appropriate candidates for surgery.

Morgan MDL, Edwards CW, Morris J et al: Origin and behaviour of emphysematous bullae. Thorax 44:533, 1989

A long-believed hypothesis was that giant bullae produce symptoms of pulmonary compression and collapse by containing gas under pressure that has been generated through valvular feeding airways. This article disproves this postulate and suggests that bullae develop after retraction and collapse of surrounding lung away from a region of weakness produced by the pathologic process associated with emphysema.

Venn GE, Williams PR, Goldstraw P: Intracavitary drainage for bullous emphysematous lung disease: experience with the Brompton technique. Thorax 43:998, 1988

This article reports on a series of 20 patients undergoing a modern Monaldi procedure for bullous disease in high-risk patients with low mortality rates. The technique is described in detail, and a recommendation is made that in future all bullae might electively be treated by this minimally invasive procedure.

REFERENCES

Allison PR: Giant bullous cysts of the lung. Thorax 2:169, 1947

Anenback O, Hammond EC, Garfinkel L, Benante C: Relation of smoking and age to emphysema. N Engl J Med 286:853, 1972

Aronberg DJ, Sagel SS, LeFrak S: Lung cancer associated with bullous lung disease in young men. AJR 134:249, 1980

Baldwin E, Harden KA, Greene DG et al.: Pulmonary insufficiency. IV. A study of 16 cases of large pulmonary air cysts or bullae. Medicine 29:169, 1950

Becklake MR, Goldman HI, McGregor M: Effects of pneumoperitoneum on lung function in pulmonary emphysema. Thorax 9:222, 1954

Benfield JR, Cree FM, Pellett JR et al.: Current approach to the surgical management of emphysema. Arch Surg 93:59, 1966

Benfield JR: Clinical Cardiopulmonary Physiology. 3rd Ed. Grune and Stratton, New York, 1969

Bergin CJ, Muller NL, Miller RR: CT with qualitative assessment of emphysema. J Thorac Imaging 1:94, 1986

Berry BE, Ochsner A: Massive hemoptysis associated with localized pulmonary bullae requiring emergency surgery. J Thorac Cardiovasc Surg 63:94, 1972

Billig DM: Surgery for bullous emphysema. Chest 70:572, 1976

Billig DM, Boushy SF, Kohen R: Surgical treatment of bullous emphysema. Arch Surg 97:744, 1968

Boushy SF, Billig DM, Kohen R: Changes in pulmonary function after bullectomy. Am J Med 47:916, 1969

Boushy SF, Kohen R, Billig DM, Heiman MJ: Bullous emphysema. Clinical, roentgenologic and physiologic study of 49 patients. Chest 54:327, 1968

Brantigan OC, Mueller E, Kress MB: Surgical approach to pulmonary emphysema. Am Rev Respir Dis 80:195, 1959

Brock RC: Recurrent and chronic spontaneous pneumothorax. Thorax 3:88, 1948

Brombage PR: Epidural Analgesia. 1st Ed. WB Saunders, Philadelphia, 1978

Burke RM: Vanishing lungs. A case report of bullous emphysema. Radiology 28:367, 1937

Cabiran LR, Ziskind MM: Spontaneous pneumothorax in pulmonary emphysema. Dis Chest 46:571, 1964

Capel LH, Belcher JR: Surgical treatment of large air cysts of the lung. Lancet 272:759, 1957

Carr DH, Pride NB: Computed tomography in preoperative assessment of bullous emphysema. Clin Radiol 35:43, 1984

Carter MG, Gaensler EA, Kyllonen A: Pneumoperitoneum in the treatment of pulmonary emphysema. N Engl J Med 243:549, 1950

Chaves CM, Fain WR, Conn JH: Angiography in giant cystic disease of the lung. J Thorac Cardiovasc Surg 55:638, 1968

Connolly JE, Wilson A: The current status of surgery for bullous emphysema. J Thorac Cardiovasc Surg 97:351, 1989

Cooke FN, Blades BB: Cystic disease of lungs. J Thorac Surg 23:546, 1952

Cooke FN, Schaff B: Surgical management of emphysematous blebs and bullae. South Med J 46:474, 1953

Cooper JD, Nelems JM, Pearson FG: Extended indications for median sternotomy in patients requiring pulmonary resection. Ann Thorac Surg 26:413, 1978

Cooper JD, Pearson FG, Patterson GA et al.: Technique of successful lung transplantation in humans. J Thorac Cardiovasc Surg 93:173, 1987

Culliford AT, Cunningham JN Jr, Zeff RH: Sternal and costochondral infections following open heart surgery. J Thorac Cardiovasc Surg 72:714, 1976

Davies GM, Simon G, Reid L: Pre and post-operative assessment of emphysematous bullae. Br J Dis Chest 60:120, 1966

Delarue NC, Woolf CR, Sanders DF et al.: Surgical treatment for pulmonary emphysema. Can J Surg 20:222, 1977

Deslauriers J, Leblanc P, McClish A: General Thoracic Surgery. 3rd Ed. Lea & Febiger, Philadelphia, 1989

DeVries WC, Wolfe WG: The management of spontaneous pneumothorax and bullous emphysema. Surg Clin North Am 60:851, 1980

Dikjman JH: Morphological aspects, classification and epidemiology of emphysema. Bull Eur Physiopathol Respir 22:241, 1986

Dirksen R, Pinckaers JWM, VanEgmond J: Indicators for perispinal opiates. p. 397. In Gomez DJ, Egay LM, de la Cruz-Odi MF (eds): Anesthesia—Safety for All. Elsevier Science Publishing, New York, 1984

Dohi S, Nishikowa T, Ujike Y, Mayumi T: Circulatory responses to airway stimulation and cervical epidural blockade. Anesthesiology 57:359, 1982

Dollery G, Hugh-Jones P: Gas and blood distribution in lung disease. Br Med Bull 19:59, 1963

Dornhorst AC: Respiratory insufficiency. Lancet 1:1185, 1955

Eger EI, Saidman LJ: Hazards of nitrous oxide anesthesia with bowel obstruction and pneumothorx. Anesthesiology 26:61, 1965

Ellison LT, Ellison RG: Surgery of bullae, blebs and cysts of the lung. A six year review. Am Surg 30:774, 1964

Emergy RW, Graif L, Hale K et al.: Treatment of end-stage chronic obstructive pulmonary disease with double lung transplantation. Chest 99:533, 1991

Eschapasse H, Fabre J, Joffa R: Intérêt de la pleurectomie comme complement des resections de bulles d'emphysème. Rev Mal Respir 8:155, 1980

Fain WR, Conn JH, Campbell GD et al.: Excision of giant pulmonary emphysematous cysts: report of 20 cases without deaths. Surgery 62:552, 1967

Field W, Rosenberg L: Cystic disease of the lung. Cure of a solitary cyst by chemical cauterization. J Thorac Surg 7:218, 1937

Fiore D, Biondetti PR, Sartori F, Calabrio F: The role of computed tomography in the evaluation of bullous lung disease. J Comput Assist Tomogr 6:105, 1982

FitzGerald MX, Keelan PJ, Cugell DW, Gaensler EA: Long-term results of surgery for bullous emphysema. J Thorac Cardiovasc Surg 68:566, 1974

Fitzpatrick MJ: Prolonged observation of patients with cor pulmonale and bullous emphysema after surgical resection. Am Rev Respir Dis 77:387, 1958

Fitzpatrick MJ, Crenshaw CR: Some physiologic changes associated with surgical excision of emphysematous bullae. Am Med 22:534, 1957

Floyer A: Treatise of the asthma. 2nd Ed. London, 1717

Foreman S, Weil H, Duke R: Bullous disease of the lung. Physiologic improvement after surgery. Ann Intern Med 69:757, 1968

Freund WA: Zur operativen Behandlung gewissen Lungenkrankheiten insbesondere des auf starrer Thoraxdilatation beruhenden alveolaren Emphysems. Z Exp Pathol Ther 3:479, 1906

Gaensler EA: Parietal pleurectomy for recurrent spontaneous pneumothorax. Surg Gynecol Obstet 102:293, 1956

Gaensler EA, Cugell DW, Knudson RJ, FitzGerald MX: Surgical management of emphysema. Clin Chest Med 4:443, 1983

Gaensler EA, Jederlinic PJ, FitzGerald MX: Patient workup for bullectomy. J Thorac Imaging 1:75, 1986

Gaensler EA, Muller B: Aging of the lung after pneumonectomy. p. 322. In: Cander L, Moyer JH (eds): Aging of the Lung. Grune & Stratton, New York, 1964

Ginsberg RJ: Tube thoracostomy drainage. Chest 94:1125, 1988

Goldstein MJ, Snider GL, Liberson M, Poske RM: Bronchogenic carcinoma and giant bullous disease. Am Rev Respir Dis 97:1062, 1968

Guest JL, Yeh TS, Ellison LT, Ellison RG: Pulmonary parenchymal air space abnormalities. Ann Thorac Surg 1:102, 1965

Gunstensen J, McCormack RJM: The surgical management of bullous emphysema. J Thorac Cardiovasc Surg 65:920, 1973

Harada K, Shimada Y, Saoyama N et al.: Postinflammatory reduction of giant bullae and changes of the opposite lung bullae after unilateral bullectomy. Rinsho Geka 39:377, 1984

Hasenbos MAWM, Gielen MJM: Anaesthesia for bullectomy. Anaesthesia 40:977,1985

Haughton V: Changes in pulmonary compliance in patients undergoing cardiac surgery. Dis Chest 53:617, 1968

Head JR, Avery EF: Intracavitary suction (Monaldi) in the treatment of emphysematous bullae and blebs. J Thorac Surg 18:761, 1949

Head JM, Head LR, Hudson TR, Head JR: The surgical treatment of emphysematous blebs and localized vesicular and bullous emphysema. J Thorac Cardiovasc Surg 40:443, 1960

Hennell H: Acquired giant air cysts of the lung. Mt Sinai J Med 3:155, 1936

Herzog H: Erschlaffung und expiratorische Invagination der Membranosen Teile der intrathorakalen Luftrohre und der Hauptbronchien als Ursache der asphyktischen Anfalle beim Asthma bronchiale und bei der chronischen asthmoiden Bronchitis des Lungenemphysems. Schweiz Med Wochenschr 84:217, 1954

Hugh-Jones P, Lambert AV: A simple exercise test and its use for measuring exertion dyspnea. BMJ 12:65, 1952

Hugh-Jones P, Ritchie BC, Dollery CT: Surgical treatment of emphysema. BMJ 1:1133, 1966

Hugh-Jones P, Whimster W: The etiology and management of disabling emphysema. Am Rev Respir Dis 117:343, 1978

Hughes JA, MacArthur AM, Hutchinson DCS, Hugh-Jones P: Long-term changes in lung function after surgical treatment of bullous emphysema in smokers and ex-smokers. Thorax 39:140, 1984

Hutchison DCS: Alpha-1-antitrypsin deficiency and pulmonary emphysema: the role of proteolytic enzymes and their inhibitors. Br J Dis Chest 67:171, 1978

Ichitani Y: The pathophysiology and surgical indications of gigantic bullae. Nippon Kyobu Shikkan Gakkai Zasshi 132:1055, 1985

Ikeda M, Uno A, Yamane Y, Hagiwara N: Median sternotomy with bilateral bullous resection for unilateral spontaneous pneumothorax, with special reference to operative indications. J Thorac Cardiovasc Surg 96:615, 1988

Isenhower N, Cucchiara RF: Anesthesia for vanishing lung syndrome. Anesth Analg 55:750, 1976

Iwa T, Watanabe Y, Fukatani G: Simultaneous bilateral operations for bullous emphysema by median sternotomy. J Thorac Cardiovasc Surg 81:732, 1981

Jensen KM, Miscall L, Steinberg I: Angiocardiography in bullous emphysema: its role in selection of the case suitable for surgery. AJR 85:229, 1961

Jones NL, Campbell ESM, Edwards RHT: Clinical Exercise Testing. WB Saunders, Philadelphia, 1975

Jordanogiou J, Pride NB: A comparison of maximum inspiratory and expiratory flow in health and in lung disease. Thorax 23:38, 1968

Joress MH: Pulmonary cystic disease: observations in cases treated by exploratory thoracotomy. Dis Chest 35:256, 1956

Kalnins I, Torda TA, Wright JS: Bilateral simultaneous pleurodesis by median sternotomy for spontaneous pneumothorax. Ann Thorac Surg 15:202, 1973

Knudson RJ, Gaensler EA: Surgery for emphysema: collective review. Ann Thorac Surg 1:332, 1965

Korol E: Correlation of carcinoma and congenital cystic emphysema, 10 cases. Dis Chest 23:403, 1953

Kress MB, Goco RV, Brantigan OC: The role of surgery in the management of generalized pulmonary emphysema without blebs or bullae. Dis Chest 53:427, 1968

Kuwabara M, Taki T, Hatakenaka R et al.: The surgical treatment of bullous emphysema. A new method for management of giant bullae. Broncho-Pneumologie 30:202, 1980

Laforet EG: Current concepts in surgical management of chronic obstructive lung disease. N Engl J Med 287:175, 1972

Laros CD, Gelissen JH, Bergstein PG: Bullectomy for giant bullae in emphysema. J Thorac Cardiovasc Surg 91:63, 1986

Laurell CB, Eriksson S: The electrophoretic alpha-1-globulin pattern of serum in alpha-1-antitrypsin deficiency. Scand J Clin Lab Invest 15:132, 1963

Lee M, Prisco DL, Berger HW, Lajam F: One-stage surgery for bilateral bullous emphysema via median sternotomy: report of three cases. Mt Sinai J Med 50:522, 1983

Lima O, Ramos L, Biasi PD et al.: Median sternotomy for bilateral resection of emphysematous bullae. J Thorac Cardiovasc Surg 82:892, 1981

Lloyd MS: Bullous emphysema. Case report. J Thorac Surg 18:532, 1949

MacArthur AM, Fountain SW: Intracavity suction and drainage in the treatment of emphysematous bullae. Thorax 32:668, 1977

Mal H, Pariente R, Andreassian B: Unilateral lung transplantation in severe panacinar emphysema. Am Rev Respir Dis 139:A268, 1989

Mann B, Murphy EA: The treatment of hypertrophic emphysema by pneumoperitoneum. Thorax 9:87, 1954

Mattila T, Laustela E, Tala P: On the effect of sternotomy and thoracotomy incision on pulmonary function after open-heart operations. Ann Chir Gynaecol 56:58, 1967

Mattingly WT Jr, Dillon ML, Burki NK, Todd EP: Giant bullous emphysema: a surgical disease. J Ky Med Assoc 79:421, 1981

Meng RL, Jensik RJ, Kittle F, Penfield Faber L: Median sternotomy for synchronous bilateral pulmonary operations. J Thorac Cardiovasc Surg 80:1, 1980

Mercier G, Page A, Verdant A et al.: Outpatient management of intercostal tube drainage in spontaneous pneumothorax. Ann Thorac Surg 22:163, 1976

Miscall L, Duffy RW: Surgical treatment of bullous emphysema: contributions of angiocardiography. Dis Chest 24:489, 1953

Monaldi V: Endocavitary aspiration: its practical applications. Tubercle 28:223, 1947

Monaldi V, Tentativi D: Aspirazione endocavitaria nelle caverne tuberculari del pulmone. Lotta Contra la Tuberculosi 9:910, 1938

Morgan MDL, Strickland BS: Computed tomography in the assessment of bullous lung disease. Br J Dis Chest 78:10, 1984

Munson ES: Transfer of nitrous oxide into body air cavities. Br J Anaesth 46:202, 1974

Naclerio E, Langer L: Pulmonary cysts: special reference to surgical treatment of emphysematous blebs and bullae. Surgery 22:516, 1947

Nakayama K: Surgical removal of the carotid body for bronchial asthma. Dis Chest 40:595, 1961

Nelems JMB: A technique for controlling bullous cysts of lungs (abstr). In: Postgraduate Course in General Thoracic Surgery. University of Toronto, Toronto, May 1980

Nissen R: Tracheoplastik zur Beseitigung der Erschlaffung des membranosen Teils der intrathorakalen Luftrohre. Schweiz Med Wochenschr 84:219, 1954

O'Brien CJ, Hughes CF, Gianoutsos P: Surgical treatment of bullous emphysema. Aust N Z J Surg 56:241, 1986

Ogilvie C, Catterall M: Patterns of disturbed lung function in patients with emphysematous bullae. Thorax 14:216, 1959

Overholt RH: Glomectomy for asthma. N Y J Med 63:3372, 1963

Parker JP: Surgery in chronic lung disease. Surg Clin North Am 54:1193, 1974

Parmar JM, Hubbard WG, Matthews HR: Teflon strip pneumostasis for excision of giant emphysematous bullae. Thorax 42:144, 1987

Patterson GA, Copper JD, Goldman B et al.: Technique of successful clinical double lung transplantation. Ann Thorac Surg 45:626, 1988

Peabody, JW Jr, Katz S, Davis EW: Bronchial carcinoma arising in a lung cyst. AJR 77:1048, 1957

Pearson EF: Cystic disease of the lungs. Illinois Med J 67:28, 1935

Pearson MG, Ogilvie C: Surgical treatment of emphysematous bullae: late outcome. Thorax 38:134, 1983

Peters RM, Wellons HA, Htwe TM: Total compliance and work of breathing after thoracotomy. J Thorac Cardiovasc Surg 57:348, 1969

Pierce JA, Growdon JH: Physical properties of the lungs in giant cysts: report of a case treated surgically. N Engl J Med 267:169, 1962

Pinckaers JWN, Nijhuis GMM, Dirksen R: Postoperative nicomorphine analgesia by spinal or epidural application. p. 16. In Bruckner JB (ed): Anesthesiology and Intensive Medicine. Vol. 153. Springer Verlag, Heidelberg, 1981

Phillips JR: Removal of the carotid body in the treatment of asthma and obstructive emphysema. South Med J 57:1278, 1964

Poe PH, Wellman HN, Berke RA et al.: Perfusion-ventilation scintiphotography in bullous disease of the lung. Am Rev Respir Dis 107:946, 1973

Polga JP, Spencer RP, Raman TK, Sherman M: Radionuclide demonstration of improvement of spatial distribution of pulmonary function after removal of bullous lesion. Clin Nucl Med 9:725, 1984

Potgieter PD, Benatar SR, Hewitson R, Ferguson AD: Surgical treatment of bullous lung disease. Thorax 36:885, 1981

Pride NB, Barter CE, Hugh-Jones P: Ventilation of bullae and the effect of their removal on thoracic gas volumes and tests of overall pulmonary function. Am Rev Respir Dis 107:83, 1973

Pride NB, Hugh-Jones P, O'Brien E, Smith LA: Changes in lung function following surgical treatment of bullous emphysema. Q J Med 153:49, 1970

Rainer WG, Hutchinson D, Newby JP et al.: Major airway collapsibility in the pathogenesis of obstructive emphysema. J Thorac Cardiovasc Surg 46:559, 1963

Reid L: The Pathology of Emphysema. Year Book Medical Publishers, Chicago, 1967

Reitz BA, Wallwork JL, Hunt SA et al.: Heart-lung transplantation: successful therapy for patients with pulmonary vascular disease. N Engl J Med 306:557, 1982

Rice TW, Ginsberg RJ, Todd TRJ: Tube drainage of lung abscesses. Ann Thorac Surg 44:356, 1987

Rothstein E: Infected emphysematous bullae, 5 cases. Am Rev Respir Dis 69:287, 1954

Rubin EH, Buchberg AJ: Capricious behaviour of pulmonary bullae developing fluid. Dis Chest 54:546, 1968

Rubin LJ, Peter RH: Oral hydralazine therapy of primary pulmonary hypertension. New Engl J Med 302:69, 1980

Seidel H: Bemerkungen zur Chondrektomie bei Emphysem infolge starrer Thoraxdilatation. Beitr Klin Chir 58:808, 1908

Shaw RR: Localized hypertrophic emphysema. Pediatrics 9:220, 1952

Siebens AA, Grant AR, Kent DC et al.: Pulmonary cystic disease: physiologic studies and results of resection. J Thorac Surg 33:185, 1957

Smoljar VA, Vertianov VA: Laser photocoagulation in the treatment of bullous lung disease. Grud Serdechnososudistaia Khir 5:44, 1985

Spear HG, Daughty DC, Chesney JG, Marks A: The surgical management of large pulmonary blebs and bullae. Am Rev Respir Dis 84:186, 1961

Steinberg I, Dotter CT, Andrus DeW: Angiocardiography in thoracic surgery. Surg Gynecol Obstet 90:45, 1950

Stevens PM, Johnson PC, Bell RL et al.: Regional ventilation and perfusion after lung transplantation in patients with emphysema. N Engl J Med 282:245, 1970

Stoloff IL, Kanofsky P, Magilner L: The risk of lung cancer in males with bullous disease of the lungs. Arch Environ Health 22:163, 1971

Stone DJ, Schwartz A, Feltman JA: Bullous emphysema: a long-term study of the natural history and effects of therapy. Am Rev Respir Dis 82:493, 1960

Sung DT, Payne S, Black LF: Surgical management of giant bullae associated with obstructive airway disease. Surg Clin North Am 53:913, 1973

Tabakin BS, Adhikari PK, Miller DB: Objective long term evaluation of the surgical treatment of diffuse obstructive emphysema. Am Rev Respir Dis 80:825, 1959

Takita H, Merrin C, Didolkar MS et al.: The surgical management of multiple lung metastases. Ann Thorac Surg 24:359, 1977

Tenholder F, Jones PA, Matthews JI, Hooper RG: Bullous emphysema: progressive incremental exercise testing to evaluate candidates for bullectomy. Chest 77:802, 1980

Thurlbeck WM: Overview of the pathology of pulmonary emphysema in the human. Clin Chest Med 4:337, 1983

Thurlbeck WM: Morphology of Emphysema and Emphysema-Like Conditions in Chronic Airflow Obstructions in Lung Disease. p. 181. WB Saunders, Philadelphia, 1976

Ting EY, Klopstock R, Lyons HA: Mechanical properties of pulmonary cysts and bullae. Am Rev Respir Dis 87:538, 1963

Toronto Lung Transplant Group: Experiences with single lung transplantation for pulmonary fibrosis. JAMA 259:2258, 1988

Toronto Lung Transplant Group: Unilateral lung transplantation for pulmonary fibrosis. New Engl J Med 314:1140, 1986

Trulock EP, Egan TM, Kouchoukas NT et al.: Single lung transplantation for severe chronic obstructive pulmonary disease. Chest 96:738, 1989

Tsutsui M, Araki Y, Shirakusa T, Inutsuka S: Characteristic radiographic features of pulmonary carcinoma associated with large bullae. Ann Thorac Surg 46:679, 1988

Urschel HC, Razzuk A: Median sternotomy as a standard approach for pulmonary resections. Ann Thorac Surg 41:130, 1986

Uyama T, Monden Y, Harada K et al.: Drainage of giant bulla with balloon catheter using chemical irritant and fibrin glue. Chest 94:1289. 1988

Vanderhoeft PJ, Rocmans P, Nemry C et al.: Left lung transplantation in a patient with emphysema. Surgery 103:505, 1971

Vishnevsky AA, Nickoladze GD: One-stage operation for bilateral bullous lung disease. J Thorac Cardiovasc Surg 99:30, 1990

Wakabayashi A, Brenner M, Kayalek RA et al.: Thoracoscopic carbon dioxide laser treatment of bullous emphysema. Lancet 337:881, 1991

Wasserman K, Whipp BJ: Exercise physiology in health and disease. Am Rev Respir Dis 112:219, 1975

Weisel W, Slotnick I: Emphysematous bullae complicated by hemorrhage and infection. Am Rev Respir Dis 61:742, 1950

Weitzenbaum E: Physiopathologie de l'emphysème diffus et de l'emphysème bulleux. Rev Mal Respir 8:109, 1980

Wesley JR, MacLeod WM, Mullard KS: Evaluation and surgery of bullous emphysema. Thorac Cardiovasc Surg 63:945, 1972

West JP, Van Schoonhoven PV: Carcinoma of the lung developing in a congenital cyst. Surgery 42:1071, 1957

Widdicombe JG: Regulation of tracheobronchial smooth muscle. Physiol Rev 43:1, 1963

Wildevuur CRH, Benfield JR: A review of 23 human lung transplantations by 20 surgeons. Ann Thorac Surg 9:489, 1970

Witz JP, Roeslin N: La chirurgie de l'emphysème bulleux chez l'adulte: ses résultats éloignés. Rev Mal Respir 8:121, 1980

23

MASSIVE HEMOPTYSIS

Carlos Alberto Guimarães

DEFINITION

Massive bleeding into the airways is an imminent threat to life because asphyxiation occurs as the tracheobronchial tree fills with blood. Exsanguination itself is rarely the cause of death (Conlan, 1985).

Massive hemoptysis has been variably defined as 100 to more than 1,000 ml of blood expectorated from the lung over 24 to 48 hours. Many patients cough up only small amounts of blood and yet aspirate massively. Expectorated blood is often swallowed and cannot be measured. In evaluating these patients, our experience has led us to emphasize the presence or risk of aspiration rather than the volume of blood expectorated. Many patients with hemoptysis have compromised lung function, and even a small quantity of blood in the bronchial tree can lead to acute airway obstruction and asphyxiation.

In spite of this, the pivotal study of Crocco, et al. (1968) showed that the greater the rate of bleeding is, especially when greater than 600 ml in 16 hours, the higher the mortality rate is.

Therefore, I propose the division of massive hemoptysis into two groups: (1) quantitative massive hemoptysis, expectoration of volume of 400 ml or more of blood over 24 hours; and (2) qualitative massive hemoptysis, expectoration of any volume of blood in a patient with poor lung function related to a previous disease or to the hemoptysis itself.

The incidence of massive hemoptysis is difficult to ascertain in the medical literature. Amirana, et al. (1968) reported 17 patients with significant hemoptysis among 150 cases of hemoptysis in a group of 722 patients with tuberculosis. Crocco, et al. (1968) studied 67 patients with massive hemoptysis, which represented 1.5 percent of the 4,331 admissions to a pulmonary division.

I have experience with 284 patients seen at the Institute of Phthisiology and Pneumology of the Federal University of Rio de Janeiro who had expectorated blood in a volume of 400 ml or more over 24 hours, excluding 12 patients who had undergone palliative or diagnostic surgical procedures (Tables 23-1 and 23-2).

The etiologic diagnosis of massive hemoptysis is shown in Table 23-3. Pulmonary tuberculosis was the cause of bleeding in 216 (82.1 percent) patients; of them 127 (48.3 percent) had acid-fast bacilli recovered from the sputum. There were 25 cases of multi–drug-resistant tuberculosis. In 20 (7.6 percent) patients, bronchiectasis was the source of bleeding, 11 patients had pulmonary carcinomas, and 16 more patients had miscellaneous conditions (6, pneumonia; 4, atypical mycobacteriosis; 3, lung abscess; 1, aortic aneurysm; 1, benign tumor; and 1, chronic bronchitis).

HISTORICAL NOTE

At the time of Hippocrates (c. 460 to 375 B.C.), hemoptysis was pathognomonic of advanced phthisis. The Hippocratic aphorism, "The spitting of pus follows the spitting of blood, consumption follows the spitting of this and death follows consumption," gives ancient documentation to the significance of hemoptysis in intrathoracic disease. Although Aretaeus and the Greek physicians recognized many causes as early as 1,800 years ago, the expectoration of blood was for centuries regarded as etiologic in tuberculosis (Pursel and Lindskog, 1961).

At the twentieth annual meeting of the American Association for Thoracic Surgery, Eloesser (1938) read observations on sources of pulmonary hemorrhage and attempts at its control. He performed mass ligation at the hilum of seven patients, and only two recovered. He expressed discouragement with this technique and stated that it might be less dangerous to remove the lobe from which the hemorrhage comes.

Pitkin (1941) reported the first pneumonectomy for massive hemoptysis in a bronchiectatic patient, who was operated on April 5, 1941 by Dr. Samuel Freedlander. Ryan and Lineberry (1950) related the first pneumonectomy for tuberculosis associated with massive hemoptysis, and Feldman and Gusmão (1954) described a successful right upper lobectomy in a case of pulmonary tuberculosis. Bracco (1956) studied a series of five patients operated on for massive hemoptysis. They underwent three lobectomies (one for bronchiectasis, one for hydatidosis, and one for tuberculosis) and two pneumonectomies (both for tuberculosis). There was one postoperative death after a pneumonectomy.

Table 23-1. Patients with Massive Hemoptysis by Sex

	Group 1[a]	Group 2[b]	Total[c]
Male	131	64	195 (71.7%)
Female	54	23	77 (28.3%)
Total	185 (68.0%)	87 (32.0%)	272 (100.0%)

[a] Patients underwent no surgery at all.
[b] Patients underwent curative surgeries.
[c] $P > 0.05$ (not significant).

Remy, et al. (1973) reported for the first time bronchial artery embolization in four patients with massive or repeated hemoptysis. In all patients, the bleeding stopped. Hiebert (1974) described the successful use of a Fogarty balloon catheter through a rigid bronchoscope to tamponade bleeding in a patient with massive bronchial hemorrhage. Sahebjami (1976) mentioned the first iced-saline lavage during bronchoscopy to treat active (but not massive) bleeding during fiberoptic bronchoscopic examination, and Yang and Berger (1978) documented the first important series of conservative management of life-threatening hemoptysis. They treated 17 patients and found a mortality rate of 17.6 percent. Shneerson, et al. (1980) reported the first case of massive hemoptysis and aspergilloma treated successfully with radiotherapy.

HISTORICAL READINGS

Eloesser L: Observations on sources of pulmonary hemorrhage and attempts at its control. J Thorac Surg 7:671, 1938

Hiebert CA: Balloon catheter control of life-threatening hemoptysis. Chest 66:308, 1974

Pitkin CE: Repeated severe hemoptysis necessitating pneumectomy. Ann Otol Rhinol Laryngol 50:914, 1941

Remy J, Voisin C, Ribet M et al: Traitement, par embolisation, des hémoptysies graves ou répétées liées à une hypervascularisation systémique. Presse Med 2:2060, 1973

Sahebjaimi H: Iced saline lavage during bronchoscopy. Chest 69:131, 1976

BASIC SCIENCE

Anatomy

Cauldwell, et al. (1948) studied the bronchial arteries in 150 human cadavers. They originate, with few exceptions, from the proximal part of the thoracic aorta. The right bronchial

Table 23-2. Patients with Massive Hemoptysis by Age[a]

Age (years)	Group 1[b]	Group 2[c]	Total
10–29	35	21	56 (20.6%)
30–49	82	41	123 (45.2%)
50–69	54	25	79 (29.1%)
70–89	14	—	14 (5.1%)
Total	185 (68.0%)	77 (32.0%)	272 (100.0%)

[a] Mean = 43 years.
[b] Patients underwent no surgery at all.
[c] Patients underwent curative surgeries.

Table 23.3. Cause of Massive Hemoptysis

Diagnosis	Group 1	Group 2	Total (%)
Tuberculosis			
Active	93	34	127 (48.3%)
Inactive	48	41	89 (33.8%)
Bronchiectasis	13	7	20 (7.6%)
Carcinoma	9	2	11 (4.2%)
Others	13	3	16 (6.1%)
Total[a]	176 (66.9%)	87 (33.1%)	263 (100.0%)

[a] Nine patients had no diagnosis.

arteries arise from the lateral or dorsolateral aspect of the aorta, frequently in common with an intercostal artery (intercostobronchial trunk). The left bronchial arteries usually originate from the anterior surface of the thoracic aorta or from the concavity of the aortic arch. They pursue a rather tortuous course along the surface of the bronchi. Even peripherally it is common to see two bronchial arteries for each bronchus (Pump, 1972). Uflacker, et al. (1985) studied bronchial angiograms and encountered 10 different anatomic patterns.

Furuse, et al. (1987) conducted a study to determine the visibility of the bronchial arteries with dynamic computed tomography (CT). They believe that a bronchial artery larger than 2 mm is highly suggestive of an abnormality.

Remy-Jardin and Remy (1990) published a review about the nonbronchial systemic circulation of the lung in relation to lung diseases and hemoptysis. A common point in the majority of situations that lead to nonbronchial systemic arterial hypervascularization is the existence of a pleural symphysis, allowing the pulmonary penetration of these thoracic parietal vessels. In addition to the contribution of the transpleural nonbronchial systemic vessels, they discussed the role of the arteries of the pulmonary ligament. This third circulation can be the source of hemoptysis in a proportion similar to that of the pulmonary circulation (7 percent of all cases of massive hemoptysis).

Etiology

Inflammatory Disease

Tuberculosis. Descriptions of abnormalities of the lung vasculature in pulmonary tuberculosis derive from the original observations by Rasmussen in 1868 of aneurysmal dilatations of pulmonary arteries (Rasmussen aneurysms) (Yeoh, et al., 1967). Rasmussen analyzed 11 deaths from hemoptysis; 8 patients had suffered a rupture of a vessel in the wall of a tuberculous cavity. The Rasmussen aneurysm may be unique or multiple. They are false aneurysms, corresponding to dilatations of branches of the pulmonary artery, or most frequently of the bronchial artery, that cross the wall of a tuberculous cavity.

Cudkowicz (1968) studied the vasculature of tuberculous lungs in five postmortem examinations. The most uniform feature observed was the tortuosity and proliferation of the bronchial arteries to diseased areas. The tuberculous cavities have a rich bronchial blood supply. The pumonary artery branches have no part to play in the blood supply of caseating tuberculous areas because they undergo thrombosis in the early stages of the disease; this can be easily demonstrated by angiography. The presence of extensive arterial capillaries in the adhesions between the pleural surfaces and the tendency of these capillaries to recanalize the obliterated pleural arteries indicate that a profuse quantity of arterial blood is presented in the neighborhood of tuberculous foci in the periphery of such lungs.

In tuberculosis the mechanism of bleeding varies with the stage, type, and location of the disease. First to be considered is hemoptysis, which occurs in the acute exudative lesion. As a result of the softening of the lung tissue, bleeding results from necrosis of a small branch of the pulmonary artery or vein. A second type of hemorrhage in tuberculosis is the one that occurs in the chronic fibroulcerative type of the disease. This type of bleeding often results from the rupture of a pseudoaneurysm of an artery traversing the wall of a thick-walled cavity. A third type of hemorrhage occurs when a healed and calcified lymph node impinges on the wall of a bronchus. By the pressure of the calcific mass, erosion of the bronchus takes place, with ulceration into the lumen. An acute ulceration of the bronchial mucosa constitutes another cause for hemoptysis. Tracheobronchial tuberculosis may be part of a widespread parenchymal involvement, or it may occur more rarely as a primary bronchial infection. Finally, repeated small episodes of hemoptysis occur in patients whose radiographs show small fibrotic or calcific areas.

Aspergillosis. An intracavitary fungal ball is one of the most important causes of systemic hypervascularization. Various hypotheses try to explain the mechanism of hemorrhage, for example, friction of the fungal ball against the hypervascularized walls of the cavity, toxins and/or fibrinolytic enzymes elaborated by the fungus, and antigen-antibody reactions in the cavity wall. The fungal ball complicates the chronic pulmonary, pleural, or bronchial cavities, or it may appear during the evolution of aspergillosis, that is, invasive allergic bronchopulmonary or chronic necrotizing pulmonary aspergillosis. Because the majority of the cavities are situated in the posterior portions of the upper lobes, there is a great contribution of blood from the branches of axillary or subclavian arteries.

Bronchiectasis. In bronchiectasis there is evidence of proliferation and enlargement of the bronchial arteries, and precapillary bronchopulmonary anastomoses were demonstrated. These communications were most widespread near the diseased third- or fourth-order bronchi and the bronchiectatic sacs. At these levels of the bronchial tree, the bronchial arteries are normally small and can just be recognized in the adventitial coat of the pulmonary arteries as vasa vasorum, which do not communicate with the lumen of the pulmonary artery. There are also large bronchopulmonary anastomoses (Cudkowicz, 1968).

Necrotizing Pneumonitis. Patients with chronic necrotizing pneumonitis can bleed massively, with alcoholism often being a predisposing factor. Conlan, et al. (1983) reported 11 cases of chronic necrotizing pneumonitis in a group of 123 patients with massive hemoptysis.

Cystic Fibrosis. Patients with cystic fibrosis are prone to hemoptysis for a number of reasons. The lungs are focally and diffusely involved with retained secretions, bronchiolar obstruction, pulmonary abscesses, pneumonias, and bronchiectasis. The increased bronchial circulation is tortuous and dilated. There are also bronchiopulmonary artery shunts in areas of bronchiectasis.

Lung Abscess. Hemoptysis is a complication in 11 to 15 percent of patients with lung abscesses. Of these patients, 20 to 50 percent develop massive hemoptysis. The bacterial infection that is the cause of the abscess heals only if the cavity is adequately drained. The bacterial infection destroys lung tissue by the process of suppuration and necrosis. In the healing of the abscess, there is the formation of granulation tissue and leukocytic infiltration. When necrosis involves vascular granulation tissue, the capillaries bleed into the cavity of the abscess, and a clot forms, blocking the communicating bronchus. This poor drainage allows the infection to go unchecked, and further necrosis of the wall of the abscess and epithelial lining results. When this necrosis involves the larger tertiary branches of the pulmonary arteries, severe hemorrhage occurs, either filling the cavity rapidly or causing an episode of massive hemoptysis. These pathologic descriptions of the necrosis of capillaries in the wall of the abscess and focal necrosis of tertiary pulmonary arteries explain the gradual refilling of abscessed cavities with blood clots during periods of lesser hemoptysis and episodes of massive hemoptysis (Thoms, et al., 1972).

Neoplasm

There is proliferation of the bronchial arteries in primary pulmonary neoplasms, and this systemic vascularization is regarded as responsible for the frequency of hemoptysis associated with bronchial carcinomas. Some authors state that metastatic lung tumors show no such pattern; others believe that the blood supply of metastases in the lungs is similar.

Miller and McGregor (1980) published a retrospective analysis of 877 cases of lung cancer. Massive terminal hemoptysis (29 cases) was found to be significantly associated with cavitated squamous cell carcinoma, arising in either the right or left main bronchi. Radiotherapy, although used more frequently in the population with massive hemoptysis, did not appear to be causally related to bleeding of any degree.

Trauma

The adjacent main bronchus and the main trunk of the pulmonary artery may be injured in thoracic trauma. There is little time for management when there is a resulting hemorrhage into the tracheobronchial tree (Conlan, 1985).

Iatrogenic

The introduction of the Swan-Ganz catheter has allowed rapid catheterization of the pulmonary artery at the bedside in the critically ill patient. Of the serious complications, perforation of the pulmonary artery with associated hemorrhage has been reported by several groups. Barash, et al. (1981) evaluated the mechanisms by which perforaion of the pulmonary artery occurs. Anticoagulation, hypothermia, and pulmonary hypertension place the patient at higher risk. One or more of three separate mechanisms can be responsible for vascular perforation. First, the balloon can disrupt the pulmonary artery. Second, balloon inflation (eccentric or distorted) can cause the tip to be propelled through the vessel wall. Third, the catheter tip (with the balloon deflated) can be advanced too far distally and perforate the vessel.

Boyd, et al. (1983) developed a technique of catheter insertion and reported on a prospective study of complications of pulmonary artery catheterizations in 500 patients. After the tip of the catheter was positioned in the superior or inferior vena cava, its balloon was inflated with 1.5 ml of air and advanced while the distal pressure and the electrocardiograph were being monitored. Fluoroscopic guidance was used in only 24 instances. The catheter was advanced with the balloon until a wedge pressure was obtained. Then the balloon was deflated, the pulmonary artery pressure was identified, and the catheter was fixed in this position. Whenever the balloon was reinflated, the pressure tracing was carefully observed. If a wedge pressure appeared with a volume of less than 1 ml, distal migration was assumed to have occurred. The balloon was immediately deflated, the catheter was withdrawn centrally, and the balloon was reinflated and rewedged. This technique would minimize the occurrence of pulmonary artery injury by ensuring that the catheter tip was located as centrally as possible. Only one patient had hemoptysis following inflation of the balloon. After it was promptly deflated and the catheter was withdrawn, hemoptysis stopped.

Massive hemorrhage occurring as a complication of bronchoscopy is uncommon. However, there are few experienced endoscopists who have not faced this problem. Because the patient's cough reflex has been abolished by anesthesia, the tracheobronchial tree fills quickly with blood, and respiration is no longer possible. The massive hemoptysis usually causes death in a few minutes.

Pulmonary Embolism

Ligation of the main pulmonary artery does not cause pulmonary necrosis because of anastomosis between the bronchial and the pulmonary artery system. Infarction following distal pulmonary embolism, however, is common. After impaction of the embolus, hemorrhage and alveolar edema occur followed by necrosis and true infarction. A rapid influx of bronchial arterial blood, through anastomoses, into a small segment of peripheral lung can cause extravasation of blood. The resulting hemoptysis may assume massive proportions because of systemic heparinization. Reversal of the heparinization usually stops the bleeding (Conlan, 1985).

Arteriovenous Fistulae

Arteriovenous fistulae constitute a rare cause of massive hemoptysis, accounting for approximately 2 percent of instances in a large series (Conlan, 1985). Pulmonary arteriovenous fistulae were recently recognized as a manifestation of hereditary hemorrhagic telangiectasis (Rendu-Osler-Weber disease). In cases of pulmonary arteriovenous fistulae, 60 percent had associated telangiectasias of the skin or superfi-

cial mucous membranes. The precapillary pulmonary arteriovenous fistula communicates with the pulmonary arteries and veins, giving rise to a right to left shunt. The walls of these vascular structures are thin and may rupture. An angiodysplastic disorder that may involve any vessel appears to be the pathologic basis for the clinical findings.

Cardiac Valve Disease

Hemoptysis is a well-known complication of mitral stenosis, and probably it is related to the rupture of smaller vessels as a result of extreme congestion and hypertension in the pulmonary vessels. With increased pulmonary pressure, the gradient of blood flow is reversed through the bronchopulmonary venous connections; therefore, the submucosal bronchial veins dilate and are liable to rupture. Bland or septic embolization of the lungs from tricuspid valve vegetations, which are common in drug abusers, may produce pulmonary infarction and hemoptysis or a more chronic form, which may itself develop into a massive hemoptysis.

Bronchovascular Fistulae

Bronchovascular communications may be preceded by minor warning hemorrhages before the final engulfing fatal bleeding, and they may be caused by trauma, neoplasm, or intrinsic disease of large vascular structures adjacent to the tracheobronchial tree (Conlan, 1985).

Aortobronchial fistula is a rare but highly lethal condition. If not diagnosed, it is uniformly fatal, with death caused by massive hemoptysis. Demeter and Cordasco (1980) reviewed 30 cases of the world's literature. Seventy-nine percent of the patients had massive hemoptysis.

DIAGNOSIS

Clinical Features

As in other conditions, a thorough history is imperative. Hematemesis from a peptic ulcer or esophageal varices is rarely confused with hemoptysis, but epistaxis and bleeding from the gums or nasopharynx may be. The history should include (1) the amount and appearance of blood and clots; (2) the duration of bleeding; (3) chest pain; (4) the relationship of bleeding to rest, exertion, position, or cough; (5) localized wheezing or bubbling; (6) previous lung and heart diseases; and (7) cigarette smoking.

In our series of massive hemoptysis, 158 (58.0 percent) patients gave a history of previous pulmonary tuberculosis. About two-thirds of the patients with massive hemoptysis had an episode of hemoptysis before the onset of massive hemoptysis (Table 23-4). The chief clinical manifestations of

Table 23-4. Previous Hemoptysis in Patients with Massive Hemoptysis

Previous Hemoptysis	Nonsurgical	Surgical	Total (%)
Yes	124	59	183 (67.3)
No	61	28	89 (32.7)
Total	185 (68.0%)	87 (32.0%)	272 (100.0)

the 272 patients with massive hemoptysis at admission were hemoptysis (46.6 percent), cough (25.9 percent), expectoration (15.0 percent), and weight loss (12.5 percent).

A complete physical examination is equally essential, but frequently the bleeding has stopped before the patient is examined. The workup in an emergency situation may be limited to hematocrit, blood smear, leukocyte count, a coagulation study, and blood gases.

Imaging Studies

Radiography

A good quality chest radiograph, even with portable equipment, should be obtained. Localized pulmonary infiltration, atelectasis, cavitation, cyst formation, or a mass may indicate the source of bleeding, especially if it is unique. The mitral configuration of the heart shadow and Kerley B lines may also be helpful (Boren, et al., (1966). Massive pulmonary hemorrhage may occur from an area that appears normal by routine chest radiograph (McCollum, et al., 1975).

Special radiographic studies must not be neglected. Tomograms can demonstrate both cavities and solid lesions not clearly outlined on posteroanterior and lateral films. The pattern of an "air bronchogram" can be most helpful. Bronchograms or CT scans (after bleeding has ceased for several days) can help identify an obstruction, stenosis, and signs of chronic bronchitis or bronchiectasis. In certain instances, angiographic or perfusion scanning studies may confirm the location of a pulmonary embolus.

In our experience with 272 cases of massive hemoptysis, the patients had the following more common chest radiographic abnormalities at admission: cavities (28.5 percent), destroyed lung or lobe (26.2 percent), infiltrates (21.2 percent), fibroatelectasis (16.8 percent), and condensation (7.3 percent). Of these radiologic alterations, 67.8 percent were unilateral. There was a statistically significant difference ($P < 0.05$) between groups 1 and 2 in relation to the proportions of patients with uni- or bilateral radiologic abnormalities. In group 1, 36.6 percent of patients had bilateral lesions, and in group 2, 23.3 percent had the same changes.

Even before bleeding has subsided, the clinician can proceed with appropriate skin testing (tuberculin); sputum cultures for fungi, mycobacteria, and pyogens; and Papanicolaou smears. Chest radiographs are useful, not only because they help in locating the site of hemoptysis, but also because they may demonstrate the presence of aspiration. The physical findings may be misleading and must be interpreted with caution when there is aspiration. All too frequently, localized wheezes, rales, or rhonchi reflect the presence of aspirated blood, whereas the primary lesion may remain clinically silent (Amirana, et al., 1968). The radiologic abnormality of aspiration is usually seen first in the lobe or area that is causing the hemorrhage. Therefore, it occurs ipsilateral to the site of origin but may become bilateral (Bobrowitz, et al., 1983).

Thoms, et al. (1972) discussed the radiologic findings in massive hemoptysis in primary lung abscesses. They looked for clues in the radiographs that would predict recurrent bleeding. If such clues could be found, they would then have a sound basis for resecting the involved lobe before the second episode of bleeding. In some cases, the chest radiographs showed abscessed cavities that were emptying and refilling. The cavities emptied during an episode of massive hemoptysis and partially or completely refilled prior to the next and more severe episode of hemoptysis. The radiographs gave evidence that bleeding was continuing into the abscessed cavity even when there was no evidence of it in the sputum, and so we must recognize this emptying and refilling pattern (Fig. 23-1). There was another feature when a patient showed a cavity with an air-fluid level. As the hemoptysis progressed, the air-fluid level became a rounded density that moved around with changes in position. This change of the air-fluid level to movable mass consisted of another radiologic pattern. The third radiographic characteristic was one of persistent radiodensity. Thoms, et al. (1972) called it a persistent radiodensity pattern. All these signs were recognized as "possessing all the dangers of a time bomb."

Bronchial Arteriography

With selective catheterization of the bronchial arteries, arteriograms of high quality may be obtained, and a precise anatomic diagnosis is possible (Fig. 23-2). In tuberculosis there is hyperplasia of the bronchial artery, with numerous branches reaching the tuberculous lesions, especially the walls of the cavities and the adjacent regions; the angiogram may depict bronchopulmonary communications. In bronchiectasis there is an enlargement of the proximal portion of the bronchial artery, which winds around the ectatic bronchi, running in a twisting course and giving off numerous branches. On arteriography a pulmonary carcinoma has a characteristic pattern. Enlargement of the main bronchial artery is relatively slight, but many irregular branches develop within and surrounding the tumor.

Bronchoscopy

Beyond plain chest radiography, bronchoscopy is the key to localizing the lesion. Our experience shows no ill effects from bronchoscopy in patients with hemoptysis. Indeed it was helpful in the localization of the site of bleeding, especially in bilateral disease.

Questions have been raised regarding two concerns with this procedure: (1) what type of bronchoscope to use, and (2) the optimum time for endoscopy. Some clinicians claim that in massive hemoptysis only the rigid bronchoscope can provide adequate clearing of the blood from the tracheobronchial tree and maintain a satisfactory airway. Others noted the safety of evaluation of hemoptysis with fiberoptic bronchoscopy. We agree with Garzon, et al. (1982) that, if it is possible to see the site of the bleeding with the flexible bronchoscope, the patient probably is not bleeding massively.

We think that the most valuable procedure to localize the site of hemorrhage is the rigid bronchoscopy during active bleeding. The rigid bronchoscope is a wide conduit that allows ventilation, suction of blood and clots, and good vision. It allows the passage of suction cannulas, balloon-bearing catheters, or cold infusion solutions, and snug cannulation of the bronchus of the nonbleeding lung for ventilation. Bron-

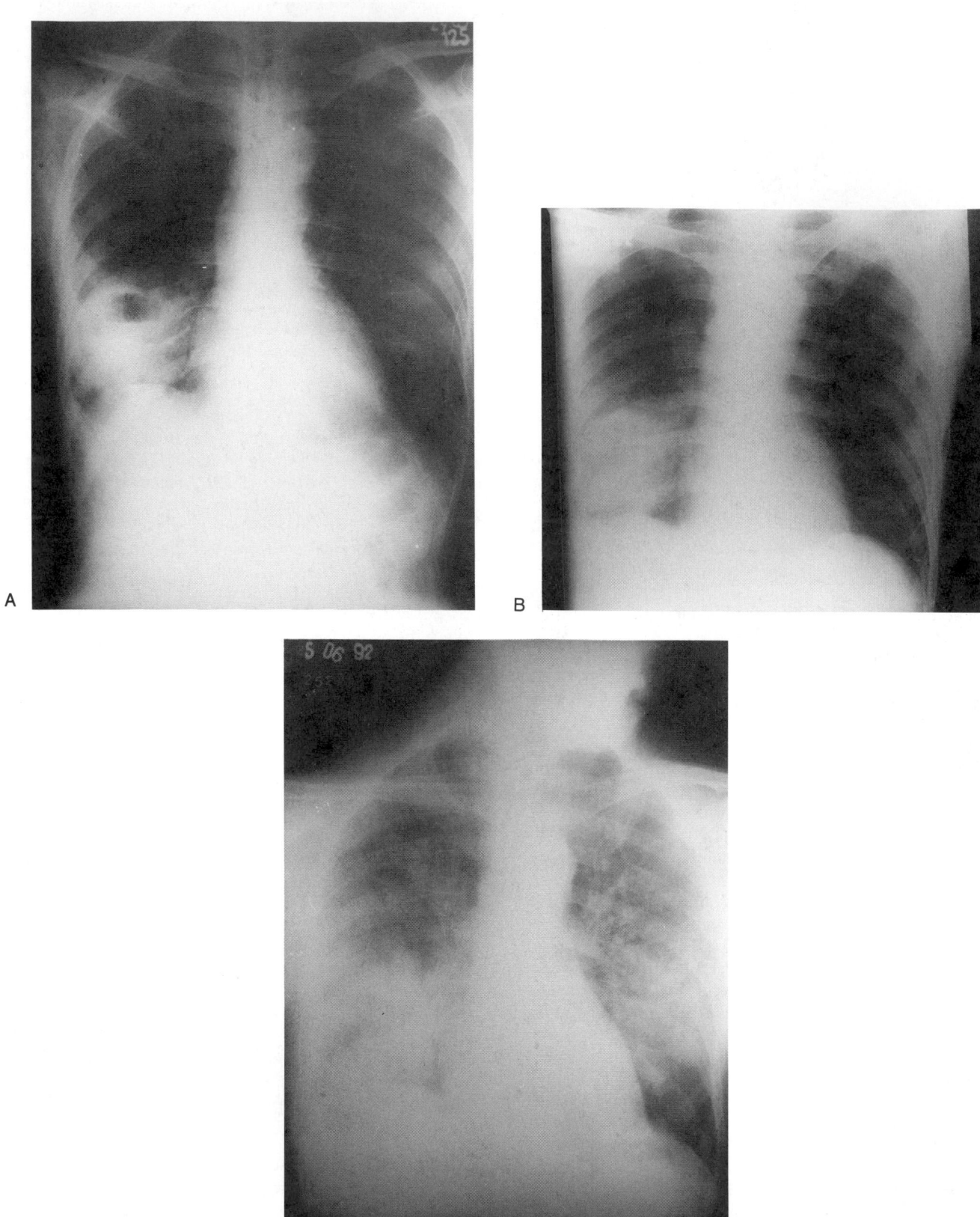

Figure 23-1. A lung abscess **(A)**, filling **(B)** and then emptying **(C)**, producing bilateral massive aspiration of blood.

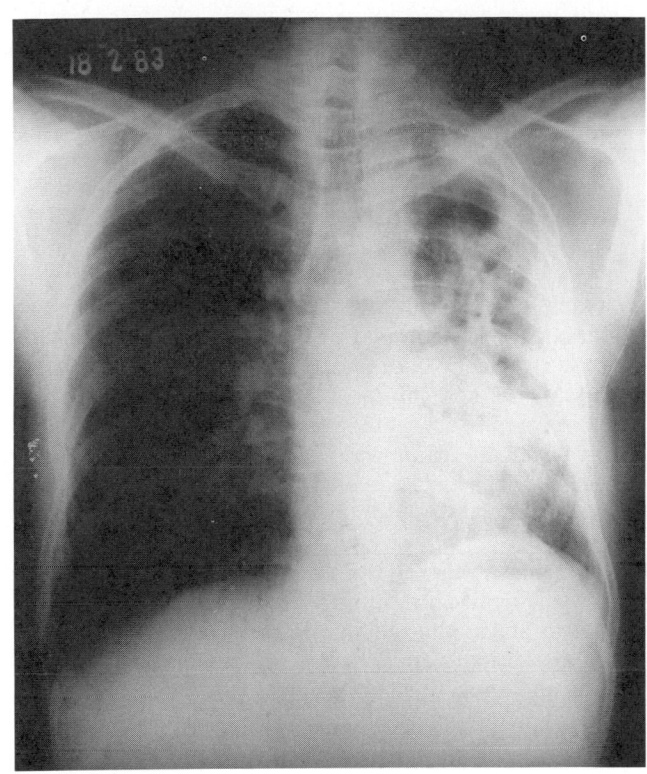

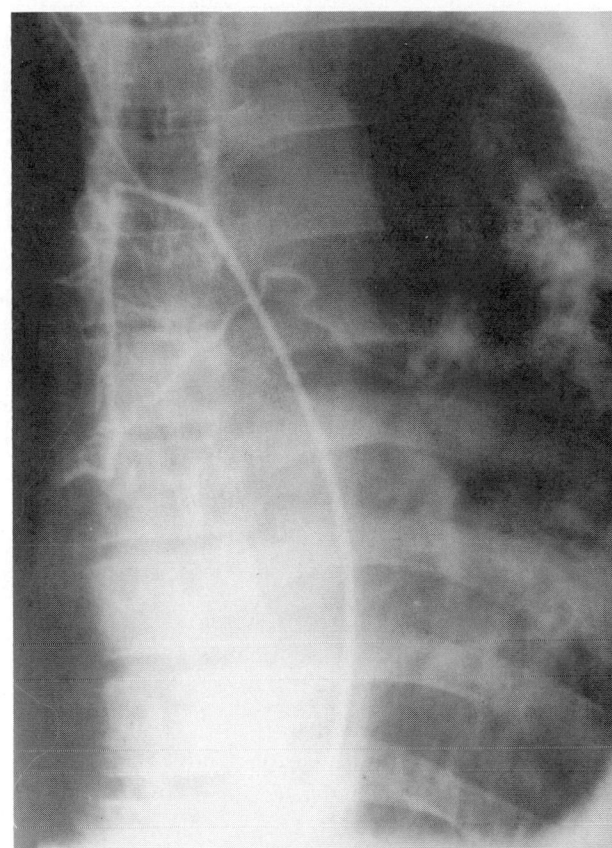

Figure 23-2. **(A)** A left lung destroyed by tuberculosis. **(B)** A bronchial arteriogram demonstrating the bleeding site.

choscopy enables the clinicians to decide whether or not a patient should receve medical therapy, an endoscopic control measure, or surgical treatment. Bronchoscopy is the procedure of choice in the management of massive hemoptysis and should be carried out by an endoscopist skilled in the use of both types of bronchoscopes (Conlan, 1985). We performed rigid bronchoscopy during massive hemoptysis in 148 patients, localizing the site of bleeding in 139 (93.9 percent).

It may be difficult at times to differentiate blood that has spilled over into a bronchus from blood originating distally, but repeated suctioning and careful observation often identifies the segment from which the bleeding originated (Boren, et al., 1966). We agree with Garzon and Gourin (1978), who advise the use of two sets of suction machines during bronchoscopy of a patient with massive hemoptysis to prevent suffocation.

When bronchoscopy is performed, the hemorrhage occasionally is so rapid that the site of origin cannot be identified immediately. Under these circumstances, the bronchoscope should not be removed but should be used to clear blood from the tracheobronchial tree. Light sedation without depressing the cough reflex and topical oropharyngeal anesthesia are used, and the Trendelenburg position may be helpful for adequate evacuation of blood (McCollum, et al., 1975).

MANAGEMENT

The management of patients with massive hemoptysis has five main objectives: (1) to prevent asphyxiation, (2) to localize the site of bleeding, (3) to arrest the hemorrhage, (4) to determine the cause of the hemoptysis, and (5) to treat the patients definitively (Jones and Davides, 1990). The care of a patient with massive hemoptysis demands an intensive care unit. Modalities used in the treatment of massive hemoptysis are listed below.

Medical Therapy

Before the bleeding is considered uncontrolled, medical therapy should be promptly initiated. If therapy is successful, even massive hemoptysis will steadily decrease. After 4 days, 87 percent of patients have decreased hemorrhages (Bobrowitz, et al., 1983).

Position the patient in bed with the head lower than the chest and the side of the bleeding dependent to prevent asphyxiation and aspiration. A wide-bore intravenous cannula is inserted (we use the internal jugular vein), and whole blood is kept on standby. Arterial blood gases are monitored.

Sedatives, such as diazepam 5 to 10 mg q6h, and antitus-

Modalities Used in Treatment of Massive Hemoptysis

Medical treatment

    Bed rest (position)

    Wide intravenous line

    Arterial blood gas monitoring

    Sedatives

    Cough suppressants (antitussives)

    Oxygen

    Broad-spectrum antibiotics

    Antituberculosis drugs

    Blood transfusion

    Reversal of anticoagulation (embolism)

    Corticosteroids (immunologic diseases)

    Pulmonary function tests

Methods of control

    Endobronchial control measures

        Ice-cold saline lavage (tracheostomy)

        Balloon tamponade

        Pulmonary separation

        Tamponade with vasoconstrictive substances

        Selective coagulative treatment

    Artery embolization

    External tubular drainage

    Positive end-expiratory pressure

    Pneumoperitoneum

    Pneumothorax

    Intravenous angiotensin

    Radiotherapy

Surgical therapy

sives (small doses of codeine) may be used to depress the excessive or violent coughing that keeps aggravating or stimulating the hemoptysis. However, if the cough reflex is completely suppressed, blood will be retained, and aspiration can occur, promoting pneumonitis and atelectasis (Bobrowitz, et al., 1983). If the partial arterial pressure of oxygen is less than 60 mmHg, supplemental oxygen should be used.

Some clinicians recommend that all patients with massive hemoptysis be given broad-spectrum antimicrobial agents empirically to limit possible complications or infections caused by aspiration. Others advise antibiotics if there is a history of bronchitis or chronic obstructive pulmonary disease, evidence of leukocytosis, or any suggestion of a bacterial complication (Bobrowitz, et al., 1983). Pursel and Lindskog (1961) stated that all patients with continuing hemoptysis of significant proportions should receive antimicrobials empirically to limit the possible infectious complications of aspiration into the uninvolved lung. We use penicillin with genta-

micin for all patients, hoping to reduce the incidence of pneumonia and sepsis from the aspiration of blood.

In patients with tuberculosis, it is imperative to initiate antituberculosis therapy with drugs to which the bacilli are sensitive. This is an effective measure in controlling the hemoptysis of active tuberculosis because such lesions are reversible. For each day that the patient receives new effective drugs, the prognosis improves. If surgery becomes necessary, the morbidity and mortality rates are minimized. We advocate the use of streptomycin with the standard drugs, especially when there is a cavitary lesion. In our exerience, most patients with active pulmonary tuberculosis and massive hemoptysis stop bleeding within 1 week after the onset of antituberculous drugs; none bled after the tenth day.

Blood transfusions may be required to keep the hematocrit above 30 percent, but excessive transfusion to raise the blood pressure to "normal" levels may actually promote bleeding.

Bronchodilators should not be administered because these may have vasodilator actions and precipitate renewed bleeding (Wedzicha and Pearson, 1990). An assessment of pulmonary function should be promptly carried out, even at the bedside.

Teklu and Felleke (1982) reported an interesting series of cases of massive hemoptysis in tuberculosis. They studied 74 patients at a sanatorium in Addis Ababa that had no surgical facilities. There were 17 deaths. All patients who died, except one who was operated on at another hospital, where managed conservatively (mortality rate of 16 of 73 or 21.9 percent).

Methods of Control

Endobronchial Control Measures

The introduction and spread of endobronchial control measures revolutionized the management of massive hemoptysis. The measures may be combined with either surgical or medical management, and they buy time for the restoration of clinical stability and the performance of essential diagnostic and management procedures (Conlan, 1985).

Ice-Cold Saline Lavage.   The mural musculature of the bronchial vessels is identical to that of peripheral vessels, and it responds to cold by vasoconstriction. The systematic lavage of the bleeding lung with large volumes of ice-cold saline solution can induce slowing and ultimate cessation of the bleeding by hypothermic vasospasm of the bronchial arterial branches that supply it (Conlan, 1985). We use a similar technique to the one reported by Conlan, et al. (1983). The requirements are as follows: (1) a rigid bronchoscope, (2) a large-bore suction catheter (which allows rapid suctioning of blood, clots, and irrigation fluid; it is better to use two separate sets of suction catheters), (3) ice-cold saline solution with ice blocks floating in it, and (4) an effective light source. We use topical anesthesia or no anesthesia at all in cases of respiratory arrest. Sedation when necessary can be achieved with 10 to 20 mg diazepam IV. The rigid bronchoscope is rapidly inserted with 100 percent oxygen pumped through it. All blood and clots are suctioned from the trachea and major bronchi. The bleeding side is identified, and the nonbleeding main bronchus is snugly cannulated with the rigid bronchoscope; ventilation is begun. The Trendelenburg position is used to facilitate the evacuation of blood from the trachea. After clinical stability is evident, the bleeding bronchus is cannulated, blood and clots are suctioned out, and 50-ml aliquots of iced-saline solution are injected into the endobronchial tree on that side. The iced solution is allowed to remain in contact for approximately 15 seconds and then is rapidly suctioned back. The nonbleeding lung is recannulated, and gas exchange is begun. Using this method, the process of ice-cold irrigation, alternating with periods of ventilation, can proceed quickly. After bleeding has slowed, it is possible to withdraw the bronchoscope into the trachea between periods of irrigation and use both lungs for ventilation. More than 1 L of ice-cold saline solution may be used for irrigation. We used ice-cold saline lavage in 129 patients with massive hemoptysis and the bleeding stopped in 125 (96.9 percent). At this point we then may use the flexible bronchoscope to increase the accuracy of the diagnosis. After the bleeding lobe or segment has been identified, appropriate pathologic and bacteriologic specimens or biopsies can be taken.

After termination of the irrigation procedure, the patient is placed with the bleeding lung dependent and returned to the intensive care unit where medical therapy is continued. We think it is important to repeat flexible or rigid bronchoscopy in the next 2 days, even if the bleeding has stopped, to aspirate old clots in the tracheobronchial tree. Ice-cold saline lavage buys time to evaluate the disease, to localize the bleeding, to perform the necessary pulmonary function tests, and to facilitate the planning of a safe and precise resection, if necessary. It remains, however, a transitory holding procedure, and if necessary, definitive therapy should not be delayed. Ice-cold saline lavage should be included as part of the rigid bronchoscopic technique initially used in all patients with massive hemoptysis. Nevertheless, it is not appropriate therapy for a bronchovascular fistula, for which other methods of endobronchial control should be used. At the end of the endoscopy, we decide whether to perform a tracheostomy. This procedure is valuable in cases of bilateral aspiration or for patients with minimal pulmonary reserve.

Balloon Tamponade.   Massive hemoptysis can be controlled by the placement of Fogarty-type embolectomy catheters and subsequent balloon inflation in the bleeding segmental bronchus, using the flexible fiberoptic bronchoscope. Since 1974 this technique has been applied to patients with bleeding from nonsurgical causes (bilateral extensive pulmonary disease; terminal malignant disease; severe associated cardiac, renal, hepatic, or metabolic diseases; and severe cystic fibrosis). It can be used preoperatively in surgical candidates. It allows an accurate localization of disease and subsequent appropriate and concise pulmonary resections. The limitations of the flexible fiberoptic bronchoscope in massive hemoptysis have already been emphasized, and most actively hemorrhaging patients require rigid bronchoscopy. If flexible endoscopy is carried out during a fortuitous pause in the bleeding or when bleeding has slowed spontaneously, it is indeed valuable. It can localize bleeding to the subsegmental bronchus level, especially in upper lobe disease. Saw, et al. (1976) described their experience in 10 patients with massive hemoptysis, using selective endobronchial tamponade with the Fogarty balloon through the flexible bronchoscope. Tamponade was achieved in all cases.

One of my colleagues (Marsico, 1991) created an endobronchial blocker that can be made in few minutes for an adult. He uses a 6-Fr. Foley catheter and an 8-Fr. nasogastric tube. The nasogastric tube is cut distally above the side holes and about 3 cm apart from the proximal end. From the Foley catheter, he uses the proximal end and the distal end (approximately 5 cm above the balloon). The proximal end of the Foley catheter is connected to the proximal end of the nasogastric tube. The distal end of the Foley catheter is inserted into the distal end of the nasogastric tube. The exterior surface of the proximal end of the Foley catheter can be smoothed with sandpaper and thus easily passed through the rigid bronchoscope. All connections are reinforced with glue, which is also used, to close the distal hole of the Foley catheter. In this way, the balloon can be filled with contrast medium (Fig. 23-3). The Marsico blocker has the following advantages: (1) it is cheap, (2) it is resistant, (3) there is a good adaptation to various diameters of the tracheobronchial tree, and (4) it is available in all hospitals.

We infrequently use the Marsico blocker as an endobronchial balloon tamponade because almost all patients stop bleeding with the ice-cold saline lavage. We always use it as a bronchial blocker during operations (see Surgical Therapy).

Pulmonary Isolation.   Isolation of the bleeding lung from the healthy one can be achieved by the use of either a double-lumen tracheal tube of the Carlen type or an ordinary balloon-bearing endotracheal tube to intubate selectively the nonbleeding lung. Both procedures should be preceded by rigid bronchoscopy to allow correct localization or lateralization of the source of bleeding and the suctioning of blood and all its products. The inner diameter of the double-lumen endotracheal tube is small and not suitable for the removal of large volumes of blood and clots from the airways. Selective intubation of the main bronchus of either lung with an ordinary endotracheal tube (8 mm in diameter and left long) is an attractive and useful option. It can be used for either right-

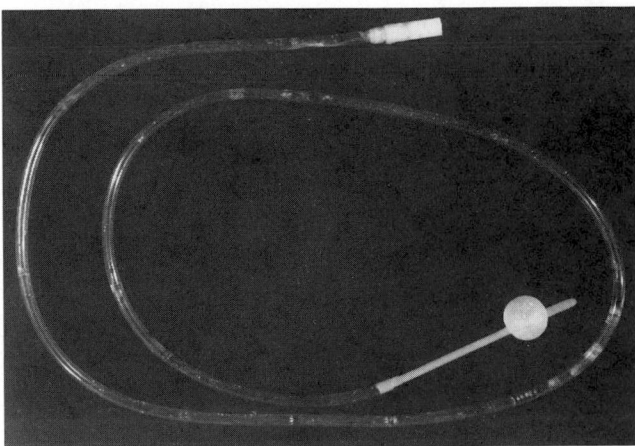

Figure 23-3.   An example of a homemade endobronchial blocker, as described by Marsico.

or left-sided bleeding. Rigid bronchoscopy should precede tube introduction. The techniques for each lung are different because of the variation in anatomy of the main bronchi (Conlan, 1985) (see Surgical Therapy).

Tampons with Vasoconstrictor Drugs. Packing of the bronchus with swabs or tampons soaked in vasoconstrictive drugs can be used in emergency circumstances when other effective therapy is not available. However, the dangers of an uncontrolled mobile endobronchial foreign-body mass must be weighed against the possible benefits (Conlan, 1985). We did not use pulmonary separation or vasoconstrictive drugs as methods of endobronchial control in our series of patients with massive hemoptysis.

Selective Coagulative Treatment. Bense (1990) reported on three patients with hemoptysis, in which fibrin precursors were sprayed into the bronchus selectively to the site of bleeding. The immediate formation of a fibrin clot, which plugged the bronchus, was observed; hemoptysis ceased promptly. The pressure of the propellant (20 to 30 millibar) is higher than the intracapillary pressure, a fact that might also have a favorable effect on hemoptysis by compressing these small vessels if they are the source of bleeding. Another indirect mode of action of this treatment should also be considered. Total occlusion of a bronchus by plugging causes regional hypoxic vasoconstriction. This decreases the regional blood flow at the site of the vascular damage and thus promotes the arrest of bleeding.

Arterial Embolization

Remy, et al. (1977) published a study of 104 patients presenting with either massive or repeated hemoptysis who were treated by embolization of the bronchial arteries with a resorbable material (Spongel). The procedure was performed by selective catheterization of the abnormal arteries. Forty-nine patients were treated during (and 55, after) hemoptysis. Of the 49 patients treated during hemoptysis, an immediate arrest of bleeding was achieved in 41, but 6 of these patients had relapses 2 to 7 months after the procedure. There was no recurrence of bleeding in the remaining 35 patients.

Remy, et al. (1984) believed that hemoptysis treatable only by embolization must be approached from the standpoint that most bronchial bleeding has a systemic origin, and consequently the bronchial arteries and the nonbronchial transpleural systemic arteries of the lung must be investigated and occluded. Persistence of the bleeding after a technically good embolization suggests an origin from vessels other than those previously obstructed, and the pulmonary circulation should be studied. A destructive process of the lung, whatever its pathogenesis, can erode any vessel in its vicinity, be it a pulmonary or systemic vessel. Jardin and Remy (1988) studied a group of seven patients in whom bronchial bleeding persisted despite previous bronchial embolization. In five cases, arrest of bleeding was only obtained when the internal mammary arteries and other systemic nonbronchial arteries were occluded. In two cases, the internal mammary artery was the only systemic nonbronchial vessel that was embolized percutaneously, followed by the immediate and complete cessation of bleeding. They stated that recognition of

the numerous collateral vessels and anastomoses of the internal mammary arteries is essential for successful percutaneous embolization for hemoptysis.

Uflacker, et al. (1985) reported on 35 patients with massive bleeding treated by bronchial artery embolization with absorbable gelatin sponge (Gelfoam) particles. Immediate control of hemoptysis was achieved in 31 patients (87.0 percent). Bronchial artery embolization alone caused long-term control of bleeding in 13 of 17 patients (76.5 percent) with massive bleeding. These authors do not consider the presence of anterior and posterior radicular arteries and posterior spinal arteries on the angiogram to be an absolute contraindication for bronchial artery embolization. However, when the anterior spinal artery is demonstrated, embolization should be avoided, or special care should be undertaken to avoid obstruction of this vessel by using larger particles for embolization.

A recurrence of hemoptysis after bronchial artery embolization may have several causes. Achieving only partial embolization is an obvious cause of recurrence. Progression of the basic disease is a major problem, and this shows why the approach to the patient must be multidisciplinary. Bronchial artery embolization is ineffective in treating diffuse pulmonary involvement. Occasionally persistent recurrent bleeding arises from the pulmonary artery, and examination of this arterial system is mandatory when other possibilities are excluded. The presence of a fungal ball in a pulmonary cavity is a main cause of rebleeding and a major drawback in the interventional therapy for massive hemoptysis. In most patients, acute bleeding stops after bronchial artery embolization, but most rebleed after some time if they are not treated surgically. Bronchial artery embolization is, therefore, a temporary treatment for massive hemoptysis in patients with aspergilloma.

Rabkin, et al. (1987) studied a group of 306 patients with acute pulmonary hemorrhage by means of bronchial arteriography who were treated with transcatheter embolization. In 120 patients, the hemoptysis was massive, with volumes exceeding 500 ml/day. The majority (n = 225) were treated during peak hemorrhages. Effective hemostasis was obtained initially in 278 (90.8 percent) patients, including 87.5 percent of those treated during peak hemorrhages. In 26 of 28 cases without an initial response, the pulmonary artery was the source of bleeding. Recurrent bleeding within 1 to 4 days, which required surgery, was observed in 39 patients who had initially successful hemostasis. Of 158 patients who were treated without surgery, subsequent episodes of hemoptysis occurred in 36.

Remy, et al. (1988) reviewed the technique for management of hemoptysis caused by arteriovenous aneurysms of the lung. They termed it "vaso-occlusion" of the pulmonary artery, and defined it as ". . . an angiographic technique which involves the voluntary and precise obstruction, temporary or permanent, of one or several branches of the pulmonary artery, utilizing coil springs or detachable balloons." They stated that this could not be called "embolization" because, with embolization, the migration of emboli is uncontrolled and depends on the blood flow.

In our series, bronchial artery embolization was attempted in 30 patients as a control method for massive hemoptysis.

In only one patient was the catheterization technically impossible. Among the 29 patients who underwent bronchial artery embolization, 27 (93.1 percent) stopped bleeding immediately, however, 18 patients (66.6 percent) had recurrences.

Percutaneous Abscess Drainage

There are relatively few indications for urgent percutaneous tube drainage of a cavitary pulmonary lesion in a patient with massive hemoptysis. We use this type of drainage when any cavity shows the radiologic patterns described by Thoms, et al. (1972) (see Imaging Studies) and the patient has a contraindication to thoracotomy (Fig. 23-1).

Mechanical Ventilation with Positive End-Expiratory Pressure

Some authors believe that all patients with massive hemoptysis should have an endotracheal tube in place to clean the tracheobronchial tree and, if necessary, to use mechanical ventilation with positive end-expiratory pressure. This not only enhances oxygenation but also increases the intrathoracic pressure, which serves as a tamponade for the site of bleeding.

Pneumoperitoneum and Pneumothorax

Collapse therapy with pneumoperitoneum or pneumothorax may be used in selected cases. In the collapsed lung, there is a great decrease in blood flow. Pneumothorax is contraindicated when there are pleural adhesions, which happens in many cases of massive hemoptysis. The most efficient collapses with pneumoperitoneum are obtained with elastic cavities located in pulmonary bases.

Vasoactive Drugs

Bilton, et al. (1990) reported a conservative measure to control profuse hemoptysis in a critically ill patient with poor lung function who had cystic fibrosis. He was given an intravenous infusion of vasopressin 20 units over 15 minutes, with immediate cessation of the bleeding. In view of this success, an infusion of vasopressin 0.2 units/min was started and continued for 36 hours. The site of action is probably arteriolar smooth muscle, through an increase in the intracellular concentration of inositol phosphates, which mobilize intracellular calcium, causing contraction. We do not have personal experience with this method of control, but it seems simple and reliable enough to be recommended.

Radiotherapy

Shneerson, et al. (1980) reported on a patient with massive hemoptysis and fungal ball. He was irradiated with a ^{60}Co mobaltron unit with a single anterior field to a total dose of 2000 cGy in 5 fractions over 7 days. His bleeding ceased completely 3 days after radiotherapy was started. However, 8 weeks later, he had three episodes of hemoptysis, totaling about 150 ml, for which he received a further 1,000-cGy midline dose with opposing fields to the left upper zone in five fractions over 7 days. He has had no further bleeding during 8 months of follow-up. The fungal ball did not change in size after therapy. Presumably the radiation had no net effect on the growth of the fungus but was acting on the vascular lining of the cavity. The early effects of radiation on small blood vessels include swelling, necrosis, and possibly hyperplasia of the endothelial cells, resulting in thrombosis and compression of the vessels by perivascular edema. Eventually perivascular and medial fibrosis occludes the vessels and impairs the capacity of the microcirculation to regenerate and remodel in the presence of injury or infection. These effects are dose dependent. The radiation may have acted similarly in this patient.

Surgical Therapy

The surgical management of massive hemoptysis has been extensively described in the medical literature over the past few decades. Pulmonary resection has been shown to be the most effective method for the control and prevention of recurrent bleeding in most patients. Several patient series have shown that surgical rather than medical methods are effective in reducing mortality rates from massive hemoptysis. In most reports concerning massive hemoptysis, the recommendation is made that an aggressive surgical approach with immediate or early pulmonary resection is the definitive therapy. However, more recently there have been reports emphasizing the role of conservative treatment in massive or life-threatening hemoptysis (Amirana, et al., 1968; Bobrowitz, et al., 1983; Bracco, 1956; Espinosa, et al., 1983; Conlan, et al., 1983; Garzon, et al., 1982; McCollum, et al., 1975; Thoms, et al. 1972; Yang and Berger, 1978; and Yeoh et al. 1967).

Emergency surgical therapy still carries substantial mortality and morbidity rates compared with elective pulmonary resection. The mortality rate is related to ongoing bleeding at the time of the operation. The spillage of blood, pus, or infected material into the dependent lung during an operation is the prime cause of death and postoperative respiratory morbidity. Likewise, the performance of a pulmonary resection in patients with poor lung function is a major contributory factor to postoperative mortality rates. Operations performed on nonbleeding patients whose disease and lung function are known is the ideal situation. Delaying surgical treatment until a spontaneous resolution of the hemorrhage occurs is not a reliable or ethical choice of management. However, the preoperative control of bleeding in every patient undergoing surgical treatment for massive hemoptysis is possible today. The use of endobronchial control techniques and the accurate identification of disease and its extent allow the precise planning of pulmonary resection to conserve functioning lung tissue (Conlan, 1985).

Patient Selection and Choice of Surgical Technique

Our criteria for selecting surgical therapy include (1) localized site of bleeding, (2) adequate pulmonary function, (3) no medical contraindications, (4) resectable carcinoma without distant metastases, and (5) no mitral disease (required of cardiac surgery). We select patients for pulmonary resection based on the volume expired in the first second of the forced vital capacity maneuver (FEV_1). Patients having a minimum FEV_1 of 2 or 1.7 L are considered fit for pneumonectomy or lobectomy, respectively. We do not perform any resection when the FEV_1 is less than 850 ml. With the FEV_1 is between 850 ml and 2 L, we use perfusion pulmonary scanning to calculate the predicted postoperative FEV_1 (Kristersson formula). With a predicted FEV_1 of less than 850 ml, no resection is done. With a predicted FEV_1 of more than 1.2 L, even pneumonectomy may be performed. Finally, when the predicted FEV_1 is between 850 ml and 1.2 L, we verify the mean pulmonary artery pressure; if the pressure is more than 25 mmHg, we believe no resection is advisable.

With the introduction of ice-cold saline lavage and arterial embolization, we can control almost all cases of massive hemoptysis. Despite this we perform urgent surgery (i.e., within 24 to 48 hours after initial control) only in the following circumstances.

(1) Fungal ball (almost all cases will rebleed after any control method)
(2) Lung abscess (generally an erosion of a large vessel)
(3) Failure of the control method (rare)
(4) Presence of a cavity with the following radiologic patterns: emptying and refilling, a movable mass, or a persistent radiodensity (rare)
(5) Obstruction of the main or lobar bronchus with a clot that cannot be suctioned during rigid bronchoscopy (rare)

In cases of urgent surgery for continuing bleeding, we try to avoid major resections. We give preference to a method of collapse (plombage and thoracoplasty), cavernostomy, parietopleuropulmonary devascularization, or even simple bronchial artery ligature. In our series, 19 (21.8 percent) patients were bleeding at the time of the pulmonary surgery, 30 (34.5 percent) patients were operated on up to 30 days after the episode of massive hemoptysis, and 38 patients (43.7 percent) were operated on after 30 days.

The surgical procedures may be classified into four groups as follows: (1) pulmonary resections (pneumonectomy, lobectomy, or segmentectomy); (2) collapse therapy (thoracoplasty or plombage); (3) cavernostomies; and (4) intrathoracic vascular ligatures. In our series, four patients underwent wedge resection in association with lobectomies. One patient underwent a two-stage left thoracoplasty and a right upper lobectomy at different times. Two patients underwent bronchial artery ligature, one of them as the sole procedure and another concomitantly with a contralateral pneumonectomy. Finally one patient had recurrent hemoptysis after bronchial and pulmonary artery embolization; he underwent a thoracotomy, and the lung was mobilized in the same way as for a resection with ligature of all the vessels between the lung and the chest wall and the vessels of the pulmonary ligament. We called this procedure "parietopleuropulmonary devascularization."

Technique

The basic principle of excisional surgery, maximal elimination of disease with minimal sacrifice of functional lung tissue, must be observed. We use posterolateral incision. In most cases, there is extensive pleural disease coexisting with parenchymal disease, frequently necessitating pleuropneumo-

nectomy. We develop a plane of cleavage between the endothoracic fascia and the parietal pleura and free the pleura and the lung as one from the chest wall, diaphragm, and mediastinal structures down to the hilus. From this stage on, the vessels and bronchus are managed as in a standard pneumonectomy. In some cases, when the adhesions between the lung and the chest wall are firm, we perform the procedure described by Ribeiro-Netto (1988), which consists of liberating the pleura and lung from the chest wall by the extrafascial route, creating a space between the ribs and thoracic fascia, or the freed periosteal and intercostal musculature, similar to a plombage thoracoplasty. We always cover the bronchial stump with intercostal muscle.

We performed six cavernostomies in patients with large cavities and blood aspiration. Four patients had active tuberculosis, and two had inactive tuberculosis (fungal ball). Two patients underwent cavernostomies during massive bleeding. There were no postoperative deaths. One patient had a prolonged bronchocutaneous fistula and another, respiratory insufficiency.

Various techniques have been advocated to facilitate anesthesia for emergency thoracotomy in the patient with endobronchial bleeding. Gauze tamponade of the bleeding bronchus through the bronchoscope, the use of endobronchial blocking devices, and the use of occlusive double-lumen tubes, such as the Carlen type, have been advised (Boren, et al., 1966).

Various methods may be used to control aspiration of blood during the surgery. We use the Marsico endobronchial blocker, which is introduced under direct vision through a bronchoscope. After the Marsico blocker is positioned properly, the balloon is inflated (Fig. 23-4). This blocker does not cause any problem during removal of the bronchoscope. After the bronchoscope is removed, an endotracheal tube is placed, and its cuff is inflated. This helps to hold the Marsico blocker against the wall of the trachea and avoid displacement of the balloon. The patient is then given general anesthesia and positioned for a thoracotomy. We do not routinely take a chest radiograph at this time to check the proper position of the balloon; however, the anesthesiologist should be aware of the possibility of displacement of the blocker. Displacement of the inflated balloon blocker can produce obstruction of the trachea; if this occurence is suspected, the balloon should be deflated immediately.

Complications related to one-lung ventilation may be technical or physiologic. Because of the shape and large size of double-lumen tubes, the incidence of difficult tracheal intubation is higher than with the use of single-lumen tubes. Unsuccessful or difficult intubation has been our only technical complication; we have had no cases of trauma, improper positioning, or tube dislodgment. The physiologic complication of hypoxemia may be the result of increased venous admixture, alteration of hypoxic pulmonary vasoconstriction, increased intra-alveolar pressure, decreased cardiac output, or atelectasis of the dependent lung.

We perform flexible bronchoscopy at the end of the surgical procedure and have found the postoperative course to be smoother if the aspirated blood clots and secretions are removed completely from the tracheobronchial tree immediately after surgery.

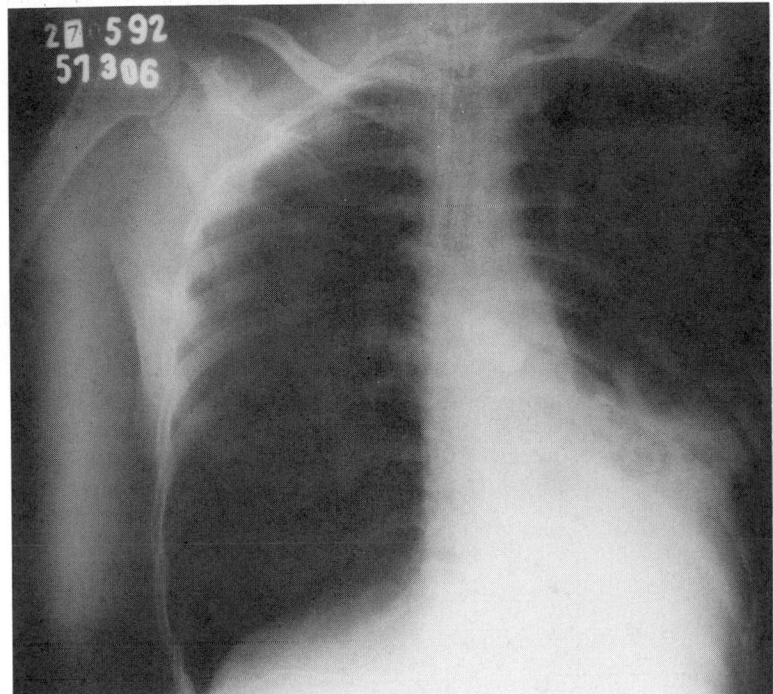
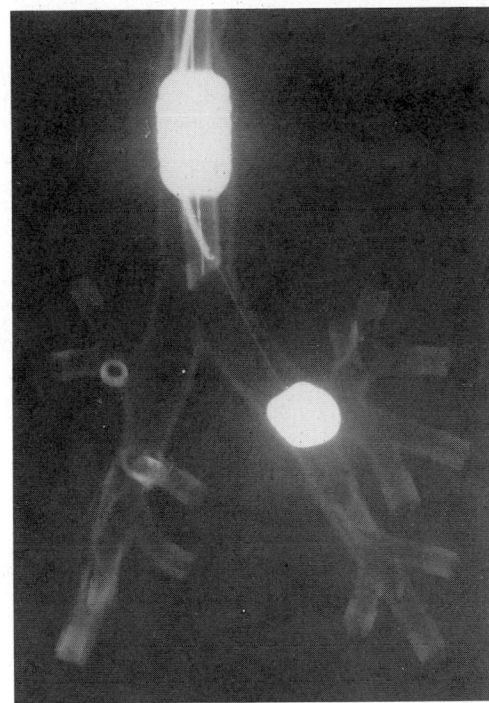

A B

Figure 23-4. **(A)** Marsico endobronchial blocker in left main bronchus. **(B)** Diagrammatic representation of Marsico endobronchial blocker in left mainstem bronchus.

Early Results

In a series of 272 patients with massive hemoptysis, 19 of 87 (21.8 percent) patients treated surgically died during the hospitalization period; of the 185 patients treated medically, 45 died (24.3 percent) (Table 23-5).

The 87 surgically treated patients underwent 94 procedures (Table 23-6). Postoperative complications occurred in 52 patients (59.8 percent). The major complication was pleural empyema (occurring in 19 patients), followed by respiratory failure (occurring in 18 patients) (Table 23-7). There were no complications in 35 of the operated patients (40.2 percent).

Among the 39 patients who underwent pneumonectomy, 11 (28.2 percent) had no postoperative complications; 13 (33.3 percent) had pleural empyema, 10 (25.6 percent) had respiratory insufficiency, and 15 (38.5 percent) had miscellaneous complications. In the lobectomy group, 12 patients (46.2 percent) had no postoperative complications. Five (19.2 percent) patients had pleural empyema; 4 (15.4 percent) respiratory failure; and 13 (50.0 percent) other complications (Table 23-8).

Table 23.6. Surgical Procedures in 87 Patients with Massive Hemoptysis

Type of Procedure	Patients (No.)	%
Pneumonectomy	39	41.5
Lobectomy	26	27.7
Plombage	9	9.6
Cavernostomy	6	6.4
Wedge resection	4	4.2
Segmentectomy	4	4.2
Thoracoplasty	3	3.2
Bronchial artery ligature	2	2.1
Devascularization	1	1.1
Total	94	100.0

Table 23.7. Postoperative Complications in 52 Patients with Massive Hemoptysis

Type of Complication	Patients (No.)	%
Pleural empyema	19	24.1
Respiratory failure	18	22.8
Pneumonia	8	10.1
Bronchopleural fistula	6	7.6
Intracavitary clot syndrome	6	7.6
Hypovolemia	4	5.0
Pulmonary edema	3	3.8
Misellaneous	15	19.0
Total	79	100.0

Table 23.5. Mortality Rate in 272 Patients with Massive Hemoptysis

Type of Treatment	Patients (No.)	Mortality Rate (%)
Medical	185	45 (24.3)
Surgical	87	19 (21.8)
Total	272	64 (23.5)

Table 23.8. Mortality Rates and Types of Operations in Massive Hemoptysis

		Mortality Rates	
Type of Operation	Patients (No.)	Patients (No.)	%
Pneumonectomy	39	13	33.3
Lobectomy	26	3	11.5
Segmentectomy	4	—	
Plombage	9	3	33.3
Thoracoplasty	2	—	
Cavernostomy	6	—	
Bronchial artery ligature	1	—	
Total	87	19	21.8

When we analyzed the surgical mortality rates in relation to the timing of the operation, we found that, when the type of surgery is a pneumonectomy, there was a statistically significant difference ($P < 0.05$) in mortality rates between the patients operated on during or after the massive hemoptysis. Among nine patients who underwent pneumonectomies during bleeding, the mortality rate was 66.7 percent, and among 30 patients who underwent pneumonectomies after the bleeding, the mortality rate was 23.3 percent (Table 23-9).

Among the 39 patients who underwent pneumonectomy, 11 (28.2 percent) had no postoperative complications; 13 (33.3 percent) had pleural empyema, 10 (25.6 percent) had respir"-quired surgery. The mortality rate in the medical group was 12.5 percent and in the surgical group, 31.8 percent (a statistically significant difference with $P < 0.05$).

In the group with multi–drug-resistant tuberculosis ($n = 25$), 12 patients (48.0 percent) underwent surgery. The medical mortality rate was 53.8 percent, and the surgical mortality rate was 33.3 percent during the period of observation.

Among the 89 patients with inactive tuberculosis and massive hemoptysis, 48 (53.9 percent) were in group 1, and 41 (46.1 percent) were in group 2. The mortality rate in the medical group was 6.3 percent, and in the surgical group it was 17.1 percent.

Late Results

An attempt was made to follow all patients after discharge, but clinic records were available only for 205 (75.3 percent). A follow-up period of 1 to 24 months was obtained in 127 (62.0 percent) cases; 42 (20.4 percent) had a follow-up of more than 48 months.

Table 23.9. Surgical Mortality Rates Among 39 Patients Undergoing Pneumonectomy

Death	Surgery During Bleeding	Surgery After Bleeding	Total (%)
Yes	6	7	13 (33.3)
No	3	23	26 (66.7)
Total[a]	9 (23.1%)	30 (76.9%)	39 (100.0)

[a] $P < 0.05$.

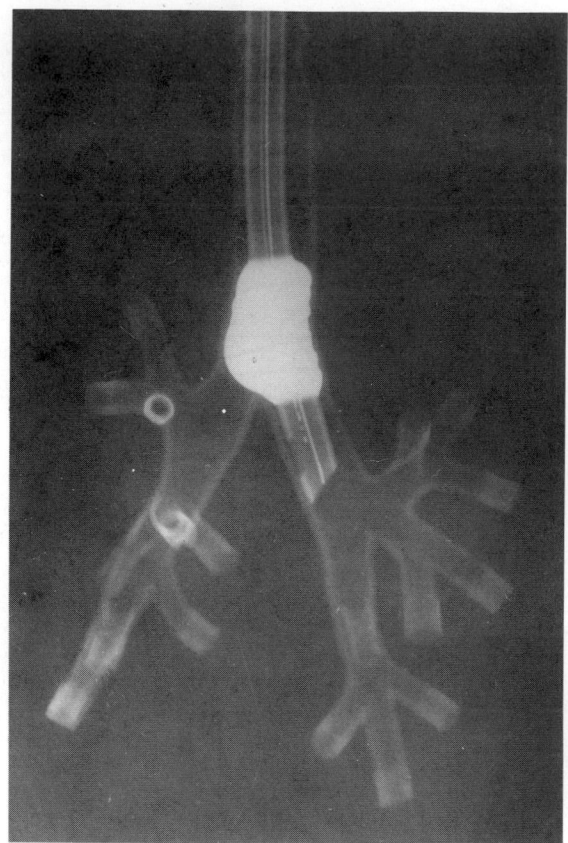

Figure 23-5. Use of long endotracheal tube in left mainstem bronchus to protect left airway from right-sided massive hemorrhage.

There was a statistically significant difference ($P < 0.05$) between the surgical and nonsurgical groups in relation to the proportions of patients who re-bled. In the nonsurgical group, 33.8 percent of the patients had another episode of hemoptysis, and in the surgical group, only 10.6 percent did.

There was also a statistically significant difference ($P < 0.05$) between the groups in relation to the proportions of patients who had as a cause of death an episode of massive hemoptysis. In the nonsurgical group, 40 patients died during the follow-up period, 34 (85.0 percent) with massive hemoptysis. In the surgical group, 24 patients died, only 7 (29.20 percent) with an episode of massive hemoptysis. With the experience of this series, we now manage massive hemoptysis as shown in Fig. 23-5.

SUMMARY

We believe that endobronchial control measures and artery embolization have radically changed the management of patients with massive hemoptysis. With the control of the hemorrhage, the clinician is able to identify nonsurgical patients and assess surgical candidates accurately. We await improved techniques of embolization of the nonbronchial system to avoid failures in the follow-up period.

COMMENTS AND CONTROVERSIES

Dr. Guimarães has unique experience in the management of massive hemoptysis because of his affiliation with an institute that still treats a significant number of patients with tuberculosis.

The thoracic surgeon must be well versed in rigid bronchoscopy, the placement of endobronchial blockers, and the use of double-lumen endotracheal tubes to manage the patient with significant hemoptysis. The clinician must always remember that, even though massive hemoptysis is defined as greater than 600 ml of blood per 24 hours, after 200 ml of blood per hour is lost by hemoptysis, this is a life-threatening situation. Patients do not die of exsanguination, but of suffocation; 200 ml of blood can completely fill the major and minor airways.

In other difficult, hopeless situations, bronchial arteriography and embolization has been extremely beneficial in arresting such major bleeding. The reader should be well advised to reread the technique of endobronchial ice-cold saline lavage, which can be extremely helpful. On occasion when resection is impossible and arteriography is unavailable, thoracotomy and ligation of the entire systemic blood supply without pulmonary resection can be life saving.

R.J.G.

KEY REFERENCES

Cauldwell EW, Siekert RG, Lininger RE, Anson BJ: The bronchial arteries. An anatomic study of 150 human cadavers. Surg Gynecol Obstet 48:395, 1948

This is the most complete anatomic study about bronchial arteries. It is an always up-to-date reference for physicians interested in massive hemoptysis.

Conlan AA: Massive hemoptysis—diagnostic and therapeutic implications. Surg Annu 17:337, 1985

This is the most in-depth article available about the causes, diagnostic procedures, and management methods in massive hemoptysis.

Crocco JA, Rooney JJ, Fankushen DS et al.: Massive hemoptysis. Arch Intern Med 121:495, 1968

These are the first authors to correlate the rate of bleeding to the mortality rate.

Remy J, Arnaud A, Fardou H et al.: Treatment of hemoptysis by embolization of bronchial arteries. Radiology 122:33, 1977

This is the first large series of patients undergoing embolization of the bronchial arteries in massive hemoptysis.

Remy-Jardin M, Remy J: La vascularisation systémique non bronchique du poumon. Rev Mal Respir 7:95, 1990

This is a general review of the nonbronchial systemic arterial circulation of the lung and its pathologic significance as an important source of hemoptysis.

REFERENCES

Amirana M, Frater R, Tirschwell P et al.: An aggressive surgical approach to significant hemoptysis in patients with pulmonary tuberculosis. Am Rev Respir Dis 97:187, 1968

Barash PG, Nardi D, Hammond G et al.: Catheter-induced pulmonary artery perforation. Mechanisms, management, and modifications. J Thorac Cardiovasc Surg 82:5, 1981

Bense L: Intrabronchial selective coagulative treatment of hemoptysis. Report of three cases. Chest 97:990, 1990

Bilton D, Webb AK, Foster H et al.: Life threatening haemoptysis in cystic fibrosis: an alternative therapeutic approach. Thorax 45:975, 1990

Bobrowitz I, Ramakrishna S, Shim Y: Comparison of medical v. surgical treatment of major hemoptysis. Arch Intern Med 143:1343, 1983

Boren J, Busey J, Corpe RF et al.: The management of hemoptysis. Am Rev Respir Dis 93:471, 1966

Boyd KD, Thomas SJ, Gold J, Boyd AD: A prospective study of complications of pulmonary artery catheterizations in 500 consecutive patients. Chest 84:245, 1983

Bracco AN: Resecciones pulmonares urgentes por hemoptisis incoercibles. Bol Soc Cir Bs As 40:107, 1956

Conlan AA, Hurwitz SS, Krige L et al.: Massive hemoptysis. Review of 123 cases. J Thorac Cardiovasc Surg 85:120, 1983

Cudkowicz L: The Human Bronchial Circulation in Health and Disease. Williams & Wilkins, Baltimore, 1968

Demeter SL, Cordasco EM: Aortobronchial fistula: keys to successful management. Angiology 31:431, 1980

Eloesser L: Observations on sources of pulmonary hemorrhage and attempts at its control. J Thorac Surg 7:671, 1938

Espinosa JIC, Fernandez JAC, Perez CN, Perrusquia JG: Cirugia en tuberculosis pulmonar por hemoptisis incoercible (analisis de 200 casos). Cirugia y Cirujanos 51:269, 1983

Feldman J, Gusmão RH: Lobectomia de urgência no tratamento de hemoptise causada por tuberculose pulmonar (urgent lobectomy in treatment of hemoptysis caused by pulmonary tuberculosis). Rev Bras Tuber 22:119, 1954

Furuse M, Saito K, Kunieda E et al: Bronchial arteries: CT demonstration with arteriographic correlation. Radiology 162:393, 1987

Garzon AA, Cerruti MM, Golding ME: Exsanguinating hemoptysis. J Thorac Cardiovasc Surg 84:829, 1982

Garzon AA, Gourin A: Surgical management of massive hemoptysis. A ten-year experience. Ann Surg 187:267, 1978

Hiebert CA: Balloon catheter control of life-threatening hemoptysis. Chest 66:308, 1974

Jardin M, Remy J: Control of hemoptysis: systemic angiography and anastomoses of the internal mammary artery. Radiology 168:377, 1988

Jones DK, Davies RJ: Massive haemoptysis. Medical management will usually arrest the bleeding. BMJ 300:889, 1990

Marsico GA: Controle da hemoptise maciça com broncoscopia e soro gelado (control of massive hemoptysis with bronchoscopy and ice-cold saline lavage) (thesis). Universidade Federal Fluminense, Rio de Janeiro, 1991

McCollum WB, Mattox KL, Guinn GA, Beall AC Jr: Immediate operative treatment for massive hemoptysis. Chest 67:152, 1975

Miller RR, McGregor DH: Hemorrhage from carcinoma of the lung. Cancer 46:200, 1980

Pitkin CE: Repeated severe hemoptysis necessitating pneumonectomy. Ann Otol Rhinol Laryngol 50:914, 1941

Pump KK: Distribution of bronchial arteries in the human lung. Chest 62:447, 1972

Pursel SE, Lindskog GE: Hemoptysis. A clinical evaluation of 105 patients examined consecutively on a thoracic surgical service. Am Rev Respir Dis 84:329, 1961

Rabkin JE, Astafjev VI, Gothman LN, Grigorjev YG: Transcatheter embolization in the management of pulmonary hemorrhage. Radiology 163:361, 1987

Remy J, Lemaitre L, Lafitte JJ et al.: Massive hemoptysis of pulmonary arterial origin: diagnosis and treatment. Radiology 143:963, 1984

Remy J, Remy-Jardin M, Wallaert B, Lafitte JJ: La vaso-occlusion de l'artère pulmonaire. Rev Mal Respir 5:429, 1988

Remy J, Voisin C, Dupuis C et al.: Traitement, par embolisation, des hémoptysies graves ou répétées liées à une hypervascularisation systémique. Presse Med 2:2060, 1973

Ribeiro-Netto A: A ressecção extramusculoperiostal "em gaiola de passarinho" (procedimento de Ribeiro-Netto) dos tumores pulmonares malignos invasores da face costal da parede torácica, dos tumores primários ou secundários da parede torácica, dos tumores primários ou secundários da parede torácica, do pulmão patológico e dos empiemas pleurais crônicos (extramusculo periosteal resection "en cage d'oiseau" or "bird-cage"—Ribeiro-Netto procedure) (thesis). Universidade Estadual do Rio de Janeiro, Rio de Janeiro, 1988

Ryan TC, Lineberry WT Jr: Pneumonectomy for pulmonary hemorrhage in tuberculosis. Am Rev Respir Dis 61:426, 1950

Sahebjami H: Iced saline lavage during bronchoscopy. Chest 69:131, 1976

Saw EC, Gottlieb LS, Yokoyama T, Lee BC: Flexible fiberoptic bronchoscopy and endobronchial tamponade in the management of massive hemoptysis. Chest 70:589, 1976

Shneerson JM, Emerson PA, Phillips RH: Radiotherapy for massive haemoptysis from an aspergilloma. Thorax 35:953, 1980

Teklu B, Felleke G: Massive haemoptysis in tuberculosis. Tubercle 63:213, 1982

Thoms NW, Wilson RF, Puro HE, Arbulu A: Life-threatening hemoptysis in primary lung abscess. Ann Thorac Surg 14:347, 1972

Uflacker R, Kaemmerer A, Picon PD: Bronchial artery embolization in the management of hemoptysis: technical aspects and long-term results. Radiology 157:637, 1985

Wedzicha JA, Pearson MC; Management of massive haemoptysis. Respir Med 84:9, 1990

Yang CT, Berger HW: Conservative management of life-threatening hemoptysis. Mt Sinai J Med 45:329, 1978

Yeoh CB, Hubaytar RT, Ford JM, Wylie RH: Treatment of massive hemorrhage in pulmonary tuberculosis. J Thorac Cardiovasc Surg 54:503, 1967

24

CHRONIC PULMONARY EMBOLISM

Pat O. Daily

DEFINITION

Chronic pulmonary embolism is characterized by persistent elevation of pulmonary vascular resistance secondary to pulmonary arterial obstruction from unresolved chronic pulmonary emboli. The cause of chronic pulmonary embolism remains insufficiently defined. Possible contributors are a hypercoagulable state, compromise of the fibrinolytic system, embolization of organized thrombi, and multiple episodes of pulmonary embolism. Similarly the incidence of patients developing chronic pulmonary embolism is not established. It is estimated that 0.1 to 4.0 percent of patients with acute pulmonary embolisms develop chronic pulmonary embolisms. The symptoms and survival vary according to the degree of pulmonary vascular obstruction. Although some patients may be asymptomatic, typically dyspnea is present with minimal exertion. With lesser degrees of pulmonary vascular obstruction, survival may be compromised only slightly. Greater levels of obstruction result in significantly shortened longevity.

HISTORICAL NOTE

As related by Chitwood, et al. (1984), the first description of some of the clinical characteristics associated with chronic pulmonary emboli was reported by Ljungdahl in 1928. However, some time elapsed before the first successful attempt at surgical relief of chronically occluded pulmonary arteries was reported by Snyder, et al. (1963). The presumptive diagnosis was a pulmonary neoplasm. The authors encountered thrombotic occlusion of the right pulmonary artery and removed the obstructions, at least in part, using endarterectomy spoons. Furthermore, the authors emphasized that the pulmonary alveolar membrane was not irreversibly damaged, and therefore, future surgical attempts were feasible because there was functional return of the affected pulmonary parenchyma.

In 1980 our group reported the results of four patients undergoing bilateral pulmonary thromboendarterectomy with median sternotomy (Daily, et al., 1980). Endaraterectomy in the first patient was performed without deep hypothermia and circulatory arrest. Severe bronchial backbleeding during endarterectomy was encountered in the three subsequent patients, necessitating periods of circulatory arrest so that visualization could be maintained during the process of thromboendarterectomy.

Reidel, et al. (1982) reported the only natural history study of chronic pulmonary embolism that correlated the degree of pulmonary vascular obstruction, as evidenced by mean pulmonary artery pressure, with the duration of survival. This information is essential before recommendation of pulmonary thromboendarterectomy can be considered. By 1984 Chitwood, et al. (1984) were able to find only 85 reported cases of surgical procedures for chronic pulmonary embolism in an extensive review of the world literature. Most of these patients had undergone lateral thoracotomy with only one lung approached. The overall operative mortality rate was 22 percent.

In 1987 we described modifications of the procedure reported in 1980 (Daily, et al., 1987). These modifications included the use of a cooling jacket to maintain myocardial temperatures at or below 10°C throughout the aortic cross-clamp period and especially provide protection of the right ventricle. In addition, dissection was carried out completely within the pericardial and pulmonary hylar tissues. Thus the possible accumulation of pleural effusions and the dissection of potential vascular adhesions were eliminated by avoiding entrance into the pleural spaces. We reported an operative mortality rate of 9 percent (3 of 33) in the 33 patients who underwent pulmonary thromboendarterectomy with this method. Saline slush, contained in a laparotomy pad, was used in seven patients (group B) for myocardial hypothermia and identified as a major risk factor for phrenic nerve paresis. This surgical approach is used currently (1993) with only minor modifications.

HISTORICAL READINGS

Chitwood WR, Sabiston DC, Wechsler AS: Surgical treatment of chronic unresolved pulmonary embolism. Clin Chest Med 5:507, 1984

Daily PO, Dembitsky WP, Peterson KL, Moser KM: Modifications of techniques and early results of pulmonary thromboendarterectomy for chronic pulmonary embolism. J Thorac Cardiovasc Surg 93:221, 1987

Daily PO, Johnston GG, Simmons CJ, Moser KM: Surgical management of chronic pulmonary embolism. J Thorac Cardiovasc Surg 79:523, 1980

Reidel M, Stanek V, Widimsky J, Preroesky I: Long-term follow-up of patients with pulmonary thromboembolism. Late prognosis and evolution of hemodynamic and respiratory data. Chest 81:151, 1982

Snyder WA, Kent DC, Baisch BF: Successful endarterectomy of chronically occluded pulmonary artery. J Thorac Cardiovasc Surg 45:482, 1963

BASIC SCIENCE

Surgical Anatomy

Visualization of the origin of each bronchopulmonary segmental artery is essential to perform relatively complete thromboendarterectomy. Thus, placing incisions distally in the pulmonary arteries by extending the incisions beyond the pericardial reflections on both the right and left sides is necessary in most cases. The superior vena cava anterior to the right pulmonary artery must be mobilized extensively to allow exposure of the right pulmonary artery.

Another consideration is the division of the pericardial reflection over the right pulmonary artery as it passes posterior to the right phrenic nerve. The line of incision through the pericardium should be placed immediately anterior to the right pulmonary artery to avoid the course of the right phrenic nerve. The incision is extended inferiorly 2 to 3 cm over the pulmonary veins and superiorly 2 to 3 cm to allow the frequently necessary distal extension of the right pulmonary artery incision. In some patients, the right middle lobe arterial branches may arise from the upper lobe branch rather than from the main trunk of the pulmonary artery. In this case, a separate incision is usually required in the right pulmonary artery 1 to 2 cm proximal to the origin of the right upper lobe branch with extension of the incision into the upper lobe artery to its trifurcation.

The primary incision is initiated in the right pulmonary artery somewhat more inferiorly and 3 to 4 cm proximal to the pericardial reflection. This incision is extended laterally until it reaches the right superior pulmonary vein, which crosses anterior to the pulmonary artery. The superior pulmonary vein can be retracted inferiorly and to the right to allow further extension of the incision. Through these two incisions, it is possible to visualize each of the origins of the bronchopulmonary segmental arteries. At all times, the path of the right phrenic nerve must be kept in mind because it courses a few millimeters anterior to the area of dissection. Furthermore, retraction in the area of the right phrenic nerve must be minimized to avoid injury and possible paresis. On the left side, the dissection is simpler because of the need to divide only the pericardial reflection over the left pulmonary artery as it exits the pericardium. Again the incision is extended from inferiorly over the pulmonary veins, immediately over the pulmonary artery, and superiorly a distance of 1 to 2 cm. As on the right side, the phrenic nerve passes anteriorly approximately 1 cm to the pulmonary artery. Again, its courses must be kept in mind and injury avoided.

The incision on the left side is initiated 4 to 5 cm within the pericardium in the pulmonary artery and extended distal to the pericardial reflection. The left upper lobe bronchus on the left side crosses anterior to the left pulmonary artery and essentially limits the distal extent of the incision. Through this single incision, it is possible to visualize all the bronchopulmonary segmental arteries, except perhaps the anteromedial segment, which is variably visualized.

Physiology

Chronic obstruction of the pulmonary arteries, resulting in elevated pulmonary vascular resistance, is the primary consideration with respect to physiologic findings. It has been demonstrated by Gibbon, et al. (1932) that more than 60 percent of the pulmonary vasculature must be occluded before measurable increases in pulmonary vascular resistance occur. Initially, pulmonary physiologic disturbances may be minimal. Relatively normal gas exchange is maintained as is pulmonary function. With worsening obstruction of the pulmonary vasculature, variable degrees of hypoxemia occur. A decrease in diffusion capacity may result, and progressive imbalance of perfusion and ventilation may occur.

The initial cardiac change is right ventricular hypertrophy secondary to the progression of pulmonary hypertension. As pulmonary hypertension worsens, right heart failure may ensue. In addition, hepatic congestion occurs along with the association of ascites, peripheral edema, and end-stage development of anasarca. In some patients, the persistence of deep venous thrombosis may contribute to lower extremity edema.

Pathology

The great majority of patients experience substantial resolution of emboli without significant residual pulmonary vascular obstruction after an acute embolic episode (Dalen, et al., 1969). However, major pulmonary vascular obstruction persists when resolution is deficient. In the absence of resolution, there is a rapid ingrowth of fibrous and elastic tissue into the embolus, which results in attachment of the embolus to the pulmonary arterial wall. This may occur within 1 week. Significant ingrowth of elastic and fibrous tissue at 2 weeks is seen in Figure 24-1. It is this attachment of embolic material to the pulmonary arterial wall that necessitates endarterectomy rather than simple embolectomy. Establishing the correct plane of dissection is essential to facilitate removal of the pulmonary arterial obstruction and avoid perforation of the relatively thin residual pulmonary arterial wall. The embolus and intima with some media are removed together. This plane of dissection is seen in Figure 24-2. The inner media of the pulmonary arterial wall shows the embolic material along with the initima and inner media of the pulmonary arterial wall. After endarterectomy the remaining pulmonary arterial

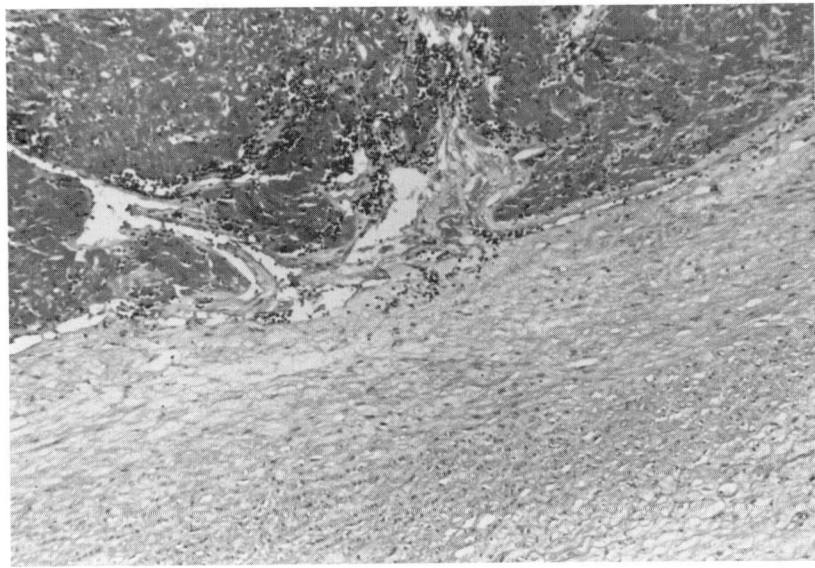

Figure 24-1. Cross-section of a pulmonary artery approximately 2 weeks after embolization. Significant ingrowth of fibrous tissues from the arterial wall into the embolus can be seen. Consequently, embolectomy by simple removal is no longer possible and thromboendarterectomy techniques are necessary. (H&E.) (From Daily PO: Chronic pulmonary embolism. p. 25. In Karp RB (ed): Advances in Cardiac Surgery. Mosby-Year Book, Chicago, 1993, with permission.)

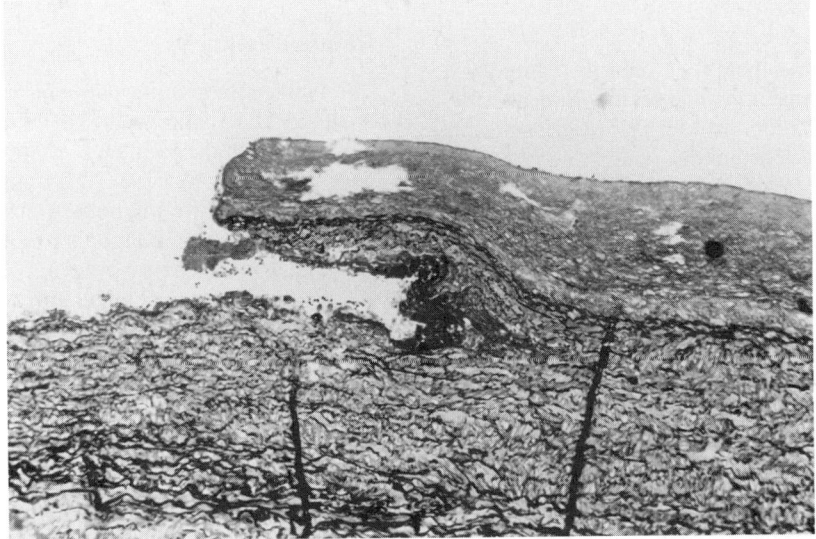

Figure 24-2. When the correct plane of dissection is established, the embolus is intimately attached to the media. The plane of dissection occurs in the superficial layer of the media. Consequently, a small amount of media and intima are removed with the embolus.

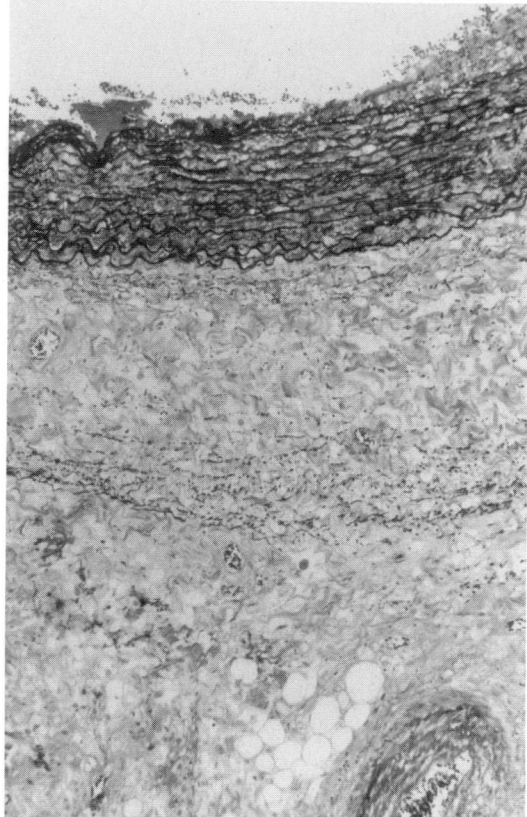

Figure 24-3. Endarterectomized pulmonary artery. The pulmonary artery after endarterectomy consists of most of the media. The embolus along with the intima and inner media have been removed.

wall consists of most of the media, as seen in Figure 24-3. Additional pathologic changes include medial hypertrophy, plexiform lesions, formation of webs, arteriosclerotic plaques, and superimposed thrombus.

Infrequently there may be considerable distension, possibly to aneurysmal proportions, of the more proximal pulmonary arteries, especially the main pulmonary artery and the proximal right and left pulmonary arteries, before the obstructing material is found. It is important to recognize that total occlusion from pulmonary embolism of either the left or right pulmonary artery may be mistaken for agenesis of the pulmonary artery. Also the syndrome of atrial septal defect with pulmonary hypertension and subsequent thrombosis—rather than embolization—of the pulmonary artery must be distinguished and surgical treatment avoided because the underlying pathologic condition may be Eisenmenger's syndrome.

DIAGNOSIS

Clinical Features

Approximately 80 percent of patients present with an established diagnosis of one or more episodes of pulmonary embolism. Associated evidence of deep vein thrombosis occurs in about 50 percent of patients. However, 20 percent have absolutely no history of either pulmonary embolism or deep vein thrombosis. The most prevalent symptom in both groups of patients is dyspnea with relatively minimal degrees of exertion. In most cases, the severity of the dyspnea has been progressive. Another associated complaint is that of easy fatiguability. Lesser numbers of patients experience near syncope with exertion, and about 25 percent have angina with exertion. Other less frequent symptoms include hemoptysis and chest pain. About 50 percent of patients have received anticoagulation at some point in the past.

The physical examination usually reveals normal chest findings. Occasionally there are decreased breath sounds in the lower chest, which are consistent with pleural effusions. Infrequently rales may be heard. Another less frequent but distinctive finding is that of murmurs over the lung fields, best heard posteriorly. These murmurs are most obvious during periods of breath holding and are analogous to those associated with pulmonary branch stenosis. It is important to note that these murmurs are *not* present in primary pulmonary hypertension.

Cardiac examination frequently reveals right ventricular hypertrophy. Right ventricular failure, characterized by elevated jugular venous pressure, left parasternal heave, a third heart sound, and a loud P_2 is present in more severe cases. In addition, a murmur of tricuspid regurgitation may be present. Patients with more severe pulmonary vascular obstruction may have hepatojugular reflux, liver enlargement with tenderness, and ascites. The lower extremities may be normal but often reveal evidence of chronic venous thrombosis with bilateral lower extremity edema. In other patients, evidence of chronic venous stasis, including brownish discoloration of the skin with bilateral ankle edema, is present.

Natural History

The incidence of acute pulmonary embolism has been estimated by Dalen and Alpert (1975) to exceed 500,000 patients per year. Both the incidence and the cause of chronic pulmonary embolism, however, are unknown. The percentage of patients with acute pulmonary embolism whose conditions progress to chronic pulmonary embolism has been reported to range from 0.1 to 4.0 percent (Moser, 1990; Chitwood, et al., 1984), with the lower figure probably being more accurate, resulting in 500 patients per year in the United States with chronic pulmonary embolism. However, this number is discrepant with the 85 cases of pulmonary thromboendarterectomy reported by Chitwood et al. (1984) in their review of the world literature because more surgical cases would be expected. Possible reasons for this discrepancy are failure to establish the correct diagnosis of chronic pulmonary embolism, rather than primary pulmonary hypertension, and the lack of awareness that pulmonary thromboendarterectomy is an effective procedure (Tilkian, et al., 1967). The cause of chronic pulmonary embolism likewise is ill defined. This subset of patients may have a hypercoagulable state, which may be associated with decreased levels of proteins C and S and antithrombin III. Incomplete resolution may be caused by some defect in the fibrinolytic system, or possibly, the nature of the emboli may play a role. Some emboli are of relatively recent formation, and therefore, they are more subject to fibrinolysis. Other emboli may be fibrotic and more resistant to resolution. Controversy continues as to whether single massive pulmonary embolism can lead to chronic pulmonary embolism or whether multiple episodes are required.

The survival rate of individuals with severe pulmonary hypertension is shortened significantly. There has been one natural history study to date relating survival to the level of pulmonary vascular obstruction, as evidenced by the mean pulmonary artery pressure (Reidel, et al., 1982). Patients with mean pulmonary artery pressures less than 30 mmHg remained relatively stable with respect to progression and had a 5-year survival rate of 90 percent or greater. However, patients with mean pulmonary artery pressures more than 30 mmHg had a 5-year survival rate of only 50 percent. When the mean pulmonary artery pressure was 50 mmHg or greater, the survival rate was only 10 percent. Furthermore, patients who had levels of pulmonary artery pressure above 30 mmHg tended to have progressive pulmonary hypertension (Table 24-1). The significance of these data is that patients who have mean pulmonary artery pressures less than 30 mmHg, which correlates with pulmonary vascular resistance of 300 dynes/sec/cm^{-5} or less, are usually not considered surgical candidates because of the mortality rates associated with the procedure of pulmonary thromboendarterectomy.

Differential Diagnosis

The differential diagnosis of chronic pulmonary embolism is essentially a distinction of this entity from other causes of pulmonary hypertension. It is convenient to divide causes of pulmonary hypertension into several categories. These include hypoxic vasoconstriction, pulmonary vascular occlusion, pulmonary parenchymal disease, and primary pulmonary hypertension. Hypoxic vasoconstriction of the pulmonary arteries may be secondary to chronic bronchitis, emphysema, cystic fibrosis, chronic hypoventilation, and/or high-altitude exposure. The most common causes of pulmonary vasoconstriction, emphysema, and chronic bronchitis account for more than 50 percent of all pulmonary hypertension cases.

Pulmonary vascular obstruction may be the result of pulmonary thromboemboli or embolic occlusion secondary to parasitic ova or tumors. Additional causes are secondary to pulmonary angiitis associated with collagen-vascular disorders or certain drugs. Parenchymal pulmonary disease may result in pulmonary hypertension by virtue of the destruction of pulmonary vascular surface. These diseases include chronic bronchitis, emphysema, bronchiectasis, and cystic fibrosis. Also, diffuse interstitial disease may be caused by

Causes of Pulmonary Hypertension
Hypoxic vasoconstriction
 Chronic bronchitis
 Emphysema
 Cystic fibrosis
 Chronic hypoventilation
 High altitude exposure
Pulmonary vascular occlusion
 Pulmonary thromboemboli
 Embolic occlusion
  Parasitic ova
  Tumor
 Pulmonary angiitis
  Collagen-vascular disorders
  Certain drugs
Pulmonary parenchymal disease
 Destruction of pulmonary vascular surface
  Chronic bronchitis
  Emphysema
  Bronchiectasis
  Cystic fibrosis
 Diffuse interstitial disease
  Pneumoconiosis
  Sarcoidosis
  Tuberculosis
  Chronic fungal diseases
  Adult respiratory distress
Primary pulmonary hypertension
 Exclusion of the foregoing

pneumoconiosis, sarcoidosis, tuberculosis, chronic fungal diseases, and adult respiratory distress syndrome. The diagnosis of primary pulmonary hypertension therefore remains one of exclusion, by the elimination of the foregoing potential causes of pulmonary hypertension.

Investigative Techniques

The chest radiograph usually reveals clear lung fields. However, there may be areas of hypoperfusion and other small areas of increased perfusion of the pulmonary vasculature. Significant right ventricular enlargement is often present (Fig. 24-4) and can be associated with dilatation of the proximal pulmonary arteries in the hilar areas bilaterally. The electrocardiogram is occasionally normal but can reveal changes characteristic of right ventricular enlargement and hypertrophy with right axis deviation. In advanced stages of chronic pulmonary embolism, diffuse ST segment and T wave changes may be representative of myocardial ischemia. Routine blood chemical study findings are typically normal. However, the presence of proteins C and S and antithrombin III deficiencies should be evaluated, and at times, "lupus anticoagulant" is found.

Pulmonary function study results at rest are within normal limits in approximately 80 percent of patients. When abnormal, the usual changes are characteristic of restrictive de-

Table 24-1. Pulmonary Arterial Pressure in Relation to Survival

Mean Pulmonary Arterial Pressure (mmHg)	5-Year Survival (%)
≤30	>90
31–40	45
41–50	35
≥50	10

(Data from Reidel M, Stanek V, Widimsky J, Preroesky I: Long-term follow-up of patients with pulmonary thromboembolism. Late prognosis and evolution of hemodynamic and respiratory data. Chest 81:151, 1982.)

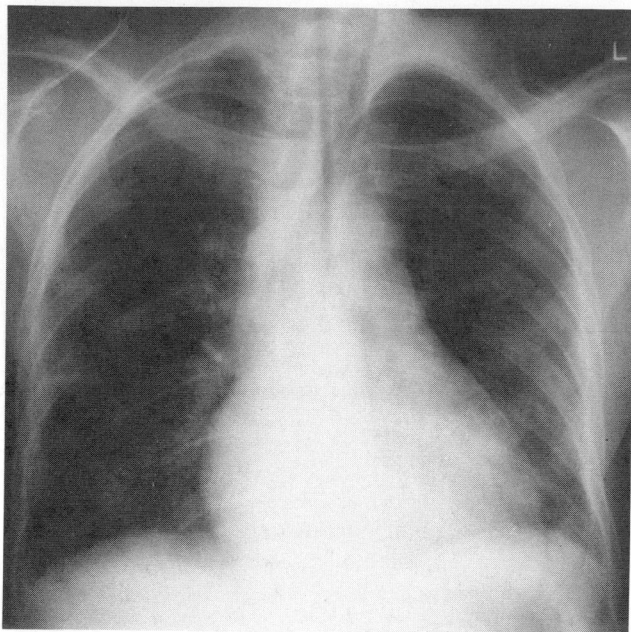

Figure 24-4. Chest radiograph taken 4 weeks preoperatively. There is significant enlargement of the right ventricle and pulmonary hilar regions.

fects; that is, there is a reduction in vital capacity, total lung capacity, and the forced expiratory volume in 1 second (FEV_1). Also, carbon monoxide diffusion may be reduced. Frequently arterial gas levels are normal at rest. With only moderately increased levels of exercise, arterial desaturation typically occurs.

Echocardiography has been used recently as a routine diagnostic study. The findings of echocardiography that suggest pulmonary hypertension include right ventricular enlargement along with abnormal motion of the interventricular septum. It is possible to estimate the level of pulmonary artery systolic pressure by Doppler techniques.

Pulmonary perfusion scanning is an important screening study. In virtually all patients with significant chronic pulmonary embolisms, there are multiple segmental or even lobar defects in perfusion, which are present bilaterally. Ventilation scanning reveals a "mismatch" with the perfusion defects. However, in primary pulmonary hypertension, the perfusion defects are much smaller and do not occur at the lobar or even segmental level. It should be emphasized that the perfusion scan may underestimate the degree of pulmonary vascular obstruction. Consequently, in patients with significant perfusion defects, pulmonary arteriography should be performed to further define the degree and cause of obstruction.

The technique of the pulmonary arteriogram is important in obtaining essential diagnostic information and, at the same time, minimizing risk. Nicod, et al. (1987) described the technique of positioning the catheter in the right pulmonary artery beyond the upper lobe branch. Large "cut-films" are taken in the anteroposterior projection. On the left side, the catheter is positioned similarly, but the preferred plane is the left anterior oblique. With this method, complications have been minimal, and no deaths have occurred in more than 400 patients to date. The pulmonary arteriogram is critical in diagnosing the presence or absence of intra-arterial obstructions and determining whether these obstructions are proximal enough to allow pulmonary thromboendarterectomy. If the obstructions begin in the pulmonary arteries proximally in the lobar branches, pulmonary thromboendarerectomy is feasible. Patients with obstructions that begin only at the orifices of the bronchopulmonary artery possibly are operative candidates, but it is highly likely that endarterectomy will be less complete than with more proximally located obstructions.

Other potential diagnostic entities that can simulate obstructions to the pulmonary arteries (as seen by pulmonary arteriography) include fibrosing mediastinitis, tumor invasion of the major pulmonary arteries, and primary tumors of the pulmonary arteries, such as leiomyosarcomas. Also Takayasu's disease may cause pulmonary artery obstructions. Fibrosing mediastinitis is ordinarily evaluated by computed tomography (CT). Frequently surgery must be undertaken to distinguish neoplastic from thrombotic obstructions. Systemic arterial obstructions may suggest Takayasu's disease.

Right heart catheterization is performed with pulmonary angiography to determine the elevation of pulmonary vascular resistance based on the pulmonary artery pressures and cardiac output. If the foregoing studies suggest operative candidacy, left heart catheterization with coronary arteriography is performed in all patients older than 35 years of age to delineate associated coronary artery disease or other cardiac defects (i.e., congenital and valvular lesions). Correction of associated defects is performed during cooling or rewarming.

Angioscopy is of diagnostic value when thrombotic material can be visualized in the pulmonary arteries. However, frequently chronic pulmonary obstructions are not associated with visible thrombus. In these instances, angioscopy does not distinguish whether or not the patient is a suitable candidate for pulmonary thromboendarterectomy. Lung biopsies, in spite of previous comments to the contrary, unfortunately do not sufficiently differentiate primary pulmonary hypertension from chronic pulmonary embolism. Specifically, plexiform lesions, thought to rule out chronic pulmonary embolisms (Kay, 1990), have been identified in patients with chronic pulmonary embolisms (Moser, et al. 1990b). Bronchial arteriography has been recommended for evaluating patients with chronic pulmonary embolism, especially to determine operability. However, complications such as paraplegia have been reported with this procedure. Furthermore, a negative finding would not rule out pulmonary thromboendarterectomy. Therefore, in our clinical experience, this procedure has not been performed.

MANAGEMENT

Principles

After the diagnosis of chronic pulmonary embolism is established as the cause of pulmonary hypertension, it is necessary to select which patients might benefit from pulmonary thromboendarterectomy. Three criteria have been defined to determine operability. The first is significant symptoms, primarily dyspnea or exertion with minimal levels of exertion or dyspnea at rest, requiring oxygen and typically associated with a New York Heart Association function classification III or IV. The second criterion incorporates the results of Reidel, et al. (1982) regarding the natural history of this disorder based on the level of pulmonary vascular obstruction. Specifically, patients with a mean pulmonary artery pressure less than 30 mmHg, which approximates a pulmonary vascular resistance less than 300 dynes/sec/cm^{-5}, generally are not surgical candidates. However, in rare instances, patients with lower levels of pulmonary vascular resistance elevation may be candidates for pulmonary thromboendarterectomy if their pulmonary vascular resistance rises substantially above 300 dynes/sec/cm^{-5} with relatively minimal exercise. The third, and essential, criterion is the pulmonary angiographic demonstration of the degree and location of pulmonary arterial obstructions. These obstructions must be located at least as proximal as the origin of the bronchopulmonary segmental artery and preferably at the lobar or even main pulmonary artery level.

The presence of irreversible entities, including various malignant neoplasms or other end-stage diseases, such as diabetes, severe myocardial dysfunction of an irreversible nature, and chronic renal failure requiring dialysis, represent contraindications to pulmonary thromboendarterectomy. Renal failure in some patients may be secondary to right heart failure and thereby reversible with pulmonary thromboendarterectomy. It is also important to evaluate lower extremity venous status by impedance plethysmography or, in some instances, venography. Patients with evidence of peripheral venous disease should undergo insertion of an inferior vena caval device to minimize the probability of recurrent pulmonary embolism. This can be done either before or during pulmonary thromboendarterectomy.

Operative Technique

Pulmonary Artery Dissection Plane

In a substantial percentage of patients, direct visualization of the pulmonary arterial lumen does not reveal apparent thrombotic material. Often it appears that the pulmonary arterial wall is essentially normal although perhaps thickened slightly. It must be recognized that obstruction exists even though at first glance there may be no apparent obstruction. This material cannot be removed by embolectomy techniques, including simple extraction and/or balloon methods. It is necessary to begin dissection in the wall of the pulmonary artery to establish the correct plane of dissection.

Circulatory Arrest

After the correct plane for endarterectomy has been determined, backbleeding associated with bronchial artery hyperplasia is seen in virtually all patients with significant obstruction of their pulmonary vasculature secondary to chronic pulmonary embolism. Because endarterectomy can be performed more completely and accurately with direct visualization, it is necessary to use deep hypothermia and periods of circulatory arrest. In anticipation of circulatory arrest, sodium thiamylal, methylprednisolone, and phenytoin are given.

Controversy exists regarding tolerable circulatory arrest times, but it is usually agreed that in adults periods in excess of 50 minutes at 20°C or less are associated with significant irreversible neurologic damage (Kirklin and Barrett-Boyes, 1993). We use intermittent periods of circulatory arrest of 20 minutes followed by periods of 10 minutes of reperfusion with blood at less than 20°C (Daily, et al., 1989). An alternative is to reperfuse until the mixed venous oxygen saturation has been restored to the prearrest level, which usually takes 8 to 10 minutes. With this method total circulatory arrest times of 120 minutes were reached without permanent neurologic damage (Daily, et al., 1990b).

Myocardial Protection

In many instances, although the relief of pulmonary vascular resistance is significant, it usually is not complete. Therefore, it is necessary to optimize protection of the right ventricle during aortic cross-clamping. Our current approach for myocardial protection consists initially of administering 1 L of cold blood cardioplegic solution and then maintaining myocardial hypothermia at 10°C or less with a myocardial cooling jacket (Daily and Kinney, 1991a). A typical temperature curve is seen in Figure 24-5. With this approach, early postoperative myocardial dysfunction has been minimal, as evidenced by an adequate cardiac index with minimal need for inotropic agents.

Associated Diseases

Concomitant coronary artery bypass grafting and/or correction of aortic and mitral valvular lesions may be performed during the process of cooling or rewarming. Management of tricuspid regurgitation is problematic. We evaluate tricuspid regurgitation intraoperatively after discontinuation of cardiopulmonary bypass. Even with severe tricuspid regurgitation, a specific tricuspid procedure, such as valvuloplasty, is not performed if the cardiac index is adequate. Dittrich, et al. (1989) reported significant resolution of tricuspid regurgitation relatively early in the postoperative period. If compromise of the cardiac index is associated with severe tricuspid regurgitation, valvuloplasty is performed. Inspection of the atrium and atrial septum is essential because thrombi that could embolize may be found within the atrium. Any atrial septal defect requires closure to preclude significant arterial desaturation secondary to right to left shunting and to eliminate the possibility of paradoxic embolization.

Surgical Technqiue

Patients undergoing pulmonary thromboendarterectomy are positioned supinely on the operating table on a mattress that allows both cooling and rewarming. The entire chest and upper abdomen are prepared and draped in the typical fashion for a median sternotomy. The lower extremities are prepared and draped free to allow access to the groin for the potential removal of a saphenous vein for coronary bypass grafting. After median sternotomy and pericardiotomy, caval cannulas are placed through the right atrial wall and directly into the

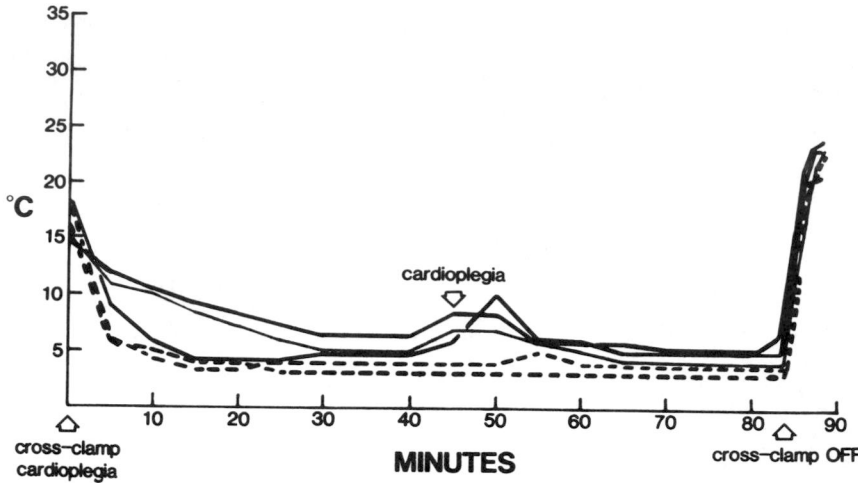

Figure 24-5. Myocardial temperature curves during cardiac ischemia, with cardioplegia and cooling jacket in use during pulmonary thromboendarterectomy. All myocardial temperatures are consistently maintained at 10°C or less; note the relative lack of temperature difference between curves. Curves shown are right ventricular epicardium, left ventricular epicardium, right ventricular myocardium, left ventricular myocardium, and septal.

superior and inferior vena cavae. Caval tapes are always used (Daily and Kinney, 1991a). An arterial cannula is placed in the ascending aorta. Just prior to initiating cardiopulmonary bypass, the left atrial pressure is measured directly, and the cardiac output is determined to calculate the pulmonary vascular resistance. During the process of cooling, the superior vena cava is mobilized superiorly and anteriorly as far as the innominate vein and posteriorly as far cephalad as the azygous vein. The superior vena cava is dissected free posteriorly and inferiorly to the level of the right atrium. This allows sufficient mobilization of the vena cava and exposure of the right pulmonary artery. Additional dissection is carried out over the right pulmonary artery, starting intrapericardially. The dissection is extended distally to the pericardial reflection; at this point, the pericardium is incised both inferiorly and superiorly, immediately anterior to the pulmonary artery. This allows further extension of the incision and, at the same time, minimizes the risk of damage to the right phrenic nerve. At this phase, it is feasible to open the right atrium, correct any septal defects, and remove any atrial thrombi. After ventricular fibrillation occurs secondary to hypothermic perfusion, a 14-mm sump tube is placed in the pulmonary artery, and a second similar sump tube is inserted through the left superior pulmonary vein and directed into the left ventricle to minimize left ventricular distension and to remove excessive bronchial artery flow. Before reaching 20°C, as mentioned previously, phenytoin, methylprednisolone, and thiamylal sodium are given intravenously. A cooling jacket is placed around the right and left ventricles, and the aorta is cross-clamped. One liter of cold blood cardioplegic solution is delivered through the ascending aorta.

An incision is started in the right pulmonary artery proximal to the pericardial reflection and extended beyond the pericardial reflection. Pathologic findings are noted. It is possible to perform limited dissection during the final stages of cooling if adequate visualization can be maintained. A separate incision may be necessary in the right pulmonary

artery with extension into the upper lobe branch to facilitate endarterectomy of more distally located obstructions in the right upper lobe. When a 20°C core temperature (as manifested by bladder and nasopharyngeal temperature) is reached, circulatory arrest occurs with exsanguination of the patient into the cardiopulmonary bypass reservoir. Several hyperinflations of the lungs during exsanguination facilitate the removal of blood from the pulmonary parenchyma, thus minimizing pulmonary backbleeding. Even so substantial backbleeding does occur in the early stages of endarterectomy because of residual blood.

Using a Penfield elevator or a scalpel, dissection is started away from the incision site in the pulmonary artery to avoid compromising arteriorrhaphy. The correct plane is that which allows relatively easy distal dissection and leaves most of the media intact. Direct visualization of the adventitia indicates the plane of dissection is too deep. After the correct plane is established, the dissection is performed circumferentially with aspirating dissectors in 360 degrees before distal extension is obtained. It is necessary to always dissect 360 degrees circumferentially simultaneously with distal extension. Otherwise the obstructing material may not be completely removed. When subsegmental branches are reached, endarterectomy is directed out through each of these until the specimen can be removed. The same procedure is carried out for the middle and upper lobe branches. If necessary an incision can be made separately in the upper lobe, as indicated previously. After the specimen has been removed or after 20 minutes of circulatory arrest, reperfusion is initiated with blood temperatures of 16 to 18°C, and the pulmonary arteriotomy is closed with two rows of continuous 6–0 polypropylene. After reperfusion an incision is made in the left pulmonary artery intrapericardially with extension beyond the pericardial reflection down to the left upper lobe bronchus. The same procedure is carried out to identify the correct plane and distal extension of the dissection.

On the left side, the anteromedial segment is particularly

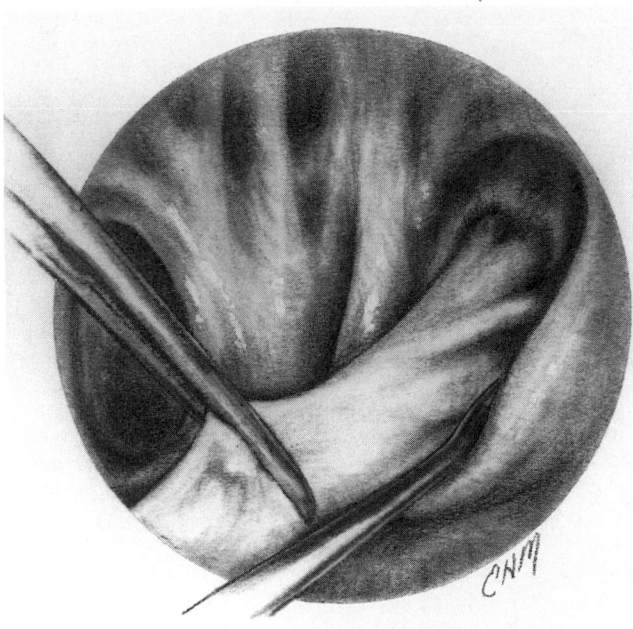

Figure 24-6. An endoscope has been passed through the pulmonary arteriotomy to demonstrate the appearance of the endarterectomy process. A vascular forceps is used to grasp material obstructing the bronchopulmonary segmental artery, and an aspirating dissector is passed distally 360 degrees circumferentially. The specimen is grasped more distally, and the process is repeated. It is necessary to use a hand-over-hand technique with the forceps alternating with dissection to remove the material completely. (From Daily PO, Dembitsky WP, Iversen S: Technique of pulmonary thromboendarterectomy for chronic pulmonary embolism. J Cardiovasc Surg 4:10, 1989, with permission.)

difficult to visualize directly. Otherwise the orifices of the bronchopulmonary segmental arteries can be seen. Figure 24-6 demonstrates the endarterectomy procedure being performed. Figure 24-7 illustrates an endarterectomized pair of bronchopulmonary segmental arteries. A typical specimen is seen in Figure 24-8. To facilitate simultaneous dissection and removal of bronchial backbleeding, dissectors have been elaborated that contain small suction ports at the tips (Fig. 24-9). The tips are spherical in shape and allow simultaneous dissection and suction as seen in Figures 24-10 and 24-11.

When endarterectomy of the left pulmonary artery is complete, rewarming is initiated, and closure, as previously described, is performed of the left pulmonary arteriotomy. Associated defects that were not addressed during cooling are corrected during rewarming. After discontinuation of cardiopulmonary bypass and correction of any surgical bleeding, sternotomy closure is routine. Just prior to sternotomy closure, a left atrial pressure line is placed, and the intraoperative pulmonary vascular resistance is determined.

Perioperative Care

Perioperative care centers around the maintenance of adequate cardiac function and sufficient oxygenation. The adequacy of cardiac function is evaluated by the cardiac index

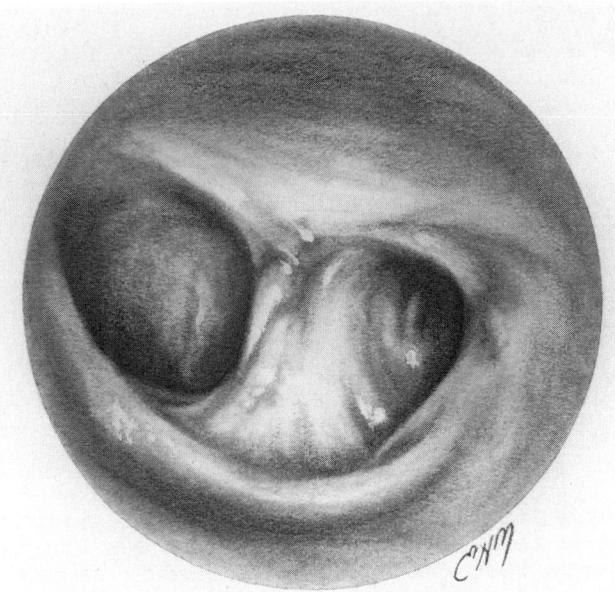

Figure 24-7. An endoscopic view of the previous location in Figure 24-6 after endarterectomy reveals the relatively glistening smooth wall of the bronchopulmonary segmental arterial branch and a previously endarterectomized branch to the viewer's left. (From Daily PO, Dembitsky WP, Iversen S: Technique of pulmonary thromboendarterectomy for chronic pulmonary embolism. J Cardiovasc Surg 4:10, 1989, with permission.)

and the level of left atrial pressure. Because significant residual pulmonary vascular obstruction frequently is present after pulmonary thromboendarterectomy, pulmonary artery wedge pressure is not always indicative of left heart filling pressure. Therefore, direct measurement of left atrial pres-

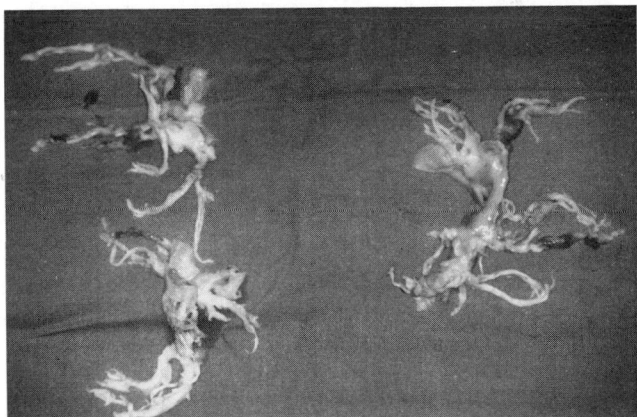

Figure 24-8. Surgical specimen from pulmonary thromboendarterectomy of both pulmonary arteries. This specimen is oriented with the patient's right side to the viewer's left. Essentially all the bronchopulmonary segmental arteries have been endarterectomized, resulting in a cast of the pulmonary arterial tree. (From Daily PO: Surgical treatment of acute and chronic pulmonary embolism. p. 1006. In Ernst CB, Stanley JC (eds): Current Therapy in Vascular Surgery—II. BC Decker, Philadelphia, 1991, with permission.)

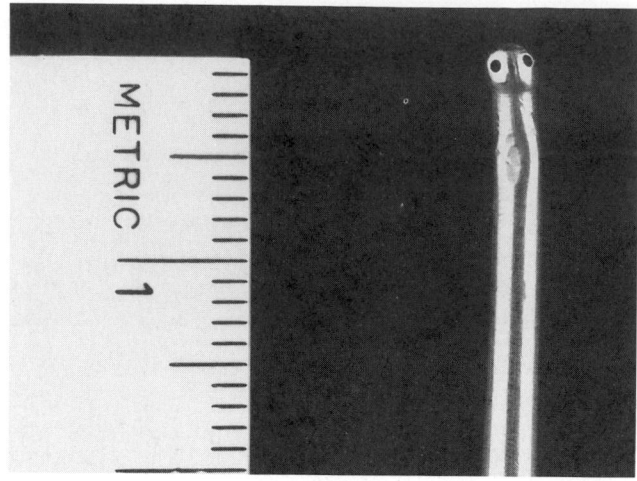

Figure 24-9. Detail of dissector tips. The tip of the dissector is spherical and 2 mm in outside diameter. Four holes, 0.5 mm in diameter, are drilled at 90 degrees to each other to permit simultaneous aspiration of blood during dissection. (From Daily PO, Dembitsky WP, Daily RP: Dissection for pulmonary thromboendarterectomy. Ann Thorac Surg 51:842, 1991b, with permission.)

sure allows a more precise determination of the need for volume expansion. An inadequate cardiac index is first managed by expansion of the volume to optimal levels, as evidenced by the mean left atrial pressure. After it is optimized, additional incremental improvement in myocardial function can be obtained by the use of inotropic agents, including dopamine, dobutamine, and amrinone.

The most significant pulmonary problem during perioperative period is reperfusion pulmonary edema, which occurs in essentially all patients. The severity of reperfusion pulmonary edema may vary from minimal evidence on a chest radiograph with no measurable hypoxemia to severe pulmonary edema with marked hypoxemia (Daily, et al., 1990a). In

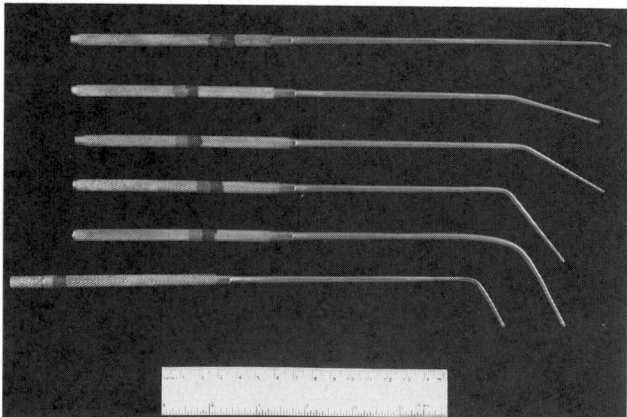

Figure 24-10. Array of dissectors. The various angles of the dissectors and tip lengths facilitate dissection of all bronchopulmonary segmental arteries. (From Daily PO, Dembitsky WP, Daily RP: Dissection for pulmonary thromboendarterectomy. Ann Thorac Surg 51:842, 1991b, with permission.)

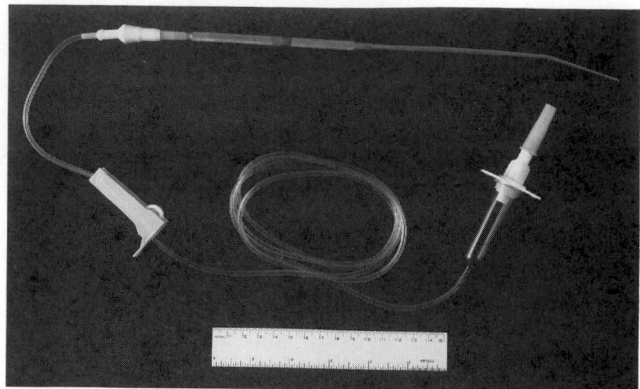

Figure 24-11. Connection to intravenous tubing. Standad intravenous tubing is inserted into the end of the handle. The opposite end can be connected to wall suction, a cell saver device, or cardiotomy suction to conserve blood. (From Daily PO, Dembitsky WP, Daily RP: Dissection for pulmonary thromboendarterectomy. Ann Thorac Surg 51:842, 1991b, with permission.)

the most severe form, actual hemorrhagic pulmonary edema may result in exsanguination of the patient (Daily, et al., 1990a and 1990b). Pathologic examination after this entity does not reveal any gross defects in the pulmonary vasculature. It is caused by an apparent breakdown in the alveolar capillary membrane, allowing hemorrhagic pulmonary edema to occur. The cause of this problem has not been elucidated but may be related to the reperfusion-caused release of anaphlytoxins and the damage associated with oxygen free radicals. Currently there is no direct therapeutic approach to minimize the effect of oxygen free radicals or prevent the release of anaphlytoxins. Frequent determinations of arterial oxygen tension levels allow an assessment of the adequacy of pulmonary function. When necessary ventilator settings are optimized to minimize reperfusion edema and facilitate oxygenation. In particular, prostaglandin E_1 (PGE_1) is routinely given to decrease pulmonary vascular resistance further. It is also important to determine pulmonary hemodynamics frequently. An unexplained rise in pulmonary vascular resistance may be associated with pulmonary artery thrombosis. On two occasions, postoperative patients were successfully treated by surgical exploration and removal of in situ pulmonary artery thromboses. Inflatable pneumatic boots are used in all patients to minimize lower extremity venous stasis. Attempts at early extubation are resisted until the patients meet all criteria for extubation to minimize the severity of reperfusion pulmonary edema.

Early Results

Prior to 1984, the results associated with pulmonary thromboendarterectomy were essentially anecdotal, as manifested by several series of 12 patients or less. However, Chitwood, et al. (1984), in an extensive review of the world literature, described results in 85 patients. The overall operative mortality rate was 22 percent, and in most patients, unilateral thoracotomy with endarterectomy of a single lung was performed. Dor, et al. (1981) reported a 25 percent mortality rate in a series of 12 patients undergoing unilateral pulmonary throm-

Table 24-2. Hospital Mortality and Morbidity Rates

	No. Patients	Hospital Mortality Rate[a]	Phrenic Nerve Paresis	Mean No. Days on Respirator
Group A (02/01/75–10/20/83)	16	3 (18.7%)	0 (0%)	8.4
Group B (03/12/84–09/11/84)	7	1 (14.3%)	5 (71%)	32.2
Group C (10/01/84–09/18/89)	149	17 (11.4%)	2 (1.34%)	4.5

[a] All deaths within 30 days or during hospitalization.

(Data from Daily PO, Dembitsky WP, Peterson KL, Moser KM: Modifications of techniques and early results of pulmonary thromboendarterectomy for chronic pulmonary embolism. J Thorac Cardiovasc Surg 93:221, 1987, and Daily PO, Dembitsky WP, Iversen S et al.: Current early results of pulmonary thromboendarterectomy for chronic pulmonary embolism. Eur J Cardiothorac Surg 4:117, 1990.)

boendarterectomy. Jault and Cabrol (1989) added 17 cases to the original 16 reported by Cabrol, et al. (1978). The overall mortality rate was 20 percent. In the first series, Cabrol, et al. (1978) recommended unilateral thoracotomy and endarterectomy, but currently, this group prefers median sternotomy with normothermic cardiopulmonary bypass and a beating heart (Jault and Cabrol, 1989). All other previous reports contained 12 or fewer patients.

In 1987 we reported (Daily, et al., 1987) our current results and modifications of the procedure described in 1980. A review of our patient series, extending from February 1, 1975, until September 9, 1989, revealed three distinct groups of patients with respect to the methods of myocardial protection and pulmonary artery dissection (Daily, et al., 1990b). In the first group of 16 patients, myocardial protection consisted of the initiation of cardiac arrest and myocardial hypothermia with crystalloid cardioplegia and maintenance of myocardial

hypothermia with saline irrigated into the pericardial cavity, as described by Shumway, et al. (1959). In the next group of seven patients, the methods of dissection and exposure of the pulmonary arteries were the same as in the first group. Myocardial protection was obtained by initiating cardiac arrest with cold blood cardioplegia, but myocardial hypothermia was maintained by the use of saline slush in a laparotomy pad placed around the heart. It was assumed that the laparotomy pad would minimize the risk of phrenic nerve paresis. However, five of these seven patients sustained paresis of one or both phrenic nerves. In a third cohort of patients, group C, myocardial protection consisted of the use of cold blood cardioplegic solution and maintenance of myocardial hypothermia with a cooling jacket. This resulted in the maintenance of myocardial temperatures at 10 to 11°C, or less, throughout the duration of aortic cross clamping. Table 24-2 summarizes these cohorts. We emphasize that the use of saline slush, even if contained in a laparotomy pad, should be rigorously avoided to minimize or eliminate the risk of phrenic nerve paresis. As seen in Table 24-2, phrenic nerve paresis was associated with a mean number of 32.2 days on a respirator, which represents an unacceptable and preventable complication.

Intraoperative hemodynamic changes in a consecutive series of 13 patients are seen in Figure 24-12. Postoperative

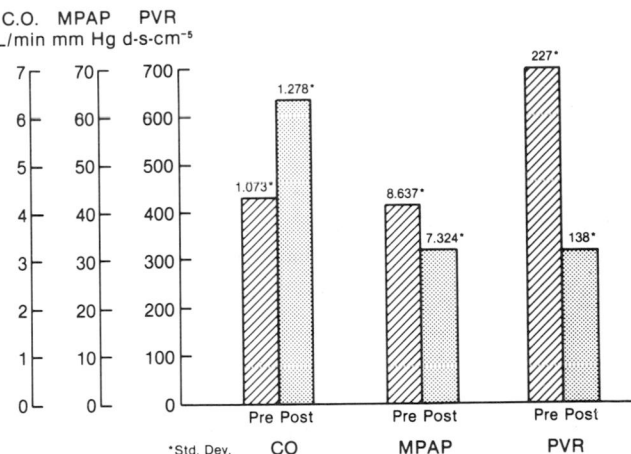

Figure 24-12. Intraoperative hemodynamic changes in group C (n = 13). A concomitant increase in cardiac output and decrease in mean pulmonary artery pressure account for a greater net decrease in pulmonary vascular resistance (mean decrease, 59 percent).

$$PVR = \frac{PAP\ mean - LAP\ mean \times 80}{CO}$$

CO, cardiac output; MAP mean, mean pulmonary artery pressure; PVR, pulmonary vascular resistance. (From Daily PO, Dembitsky WP, Peterson KL, Moser KM: Modifications of techniques and early results of pulmonary thromboendarterectomy for chronic pulmonary embolism. J Thorac Cardiovasc Surg 93:221, 1987, with permission.)

Table 24-3. Postoperative Complications (n = 124[a])

Total number of blood components (units)	14.5 ± 37.0	(0–300)	n = 118
Average number of days on ventilator	4.7 ± 5.7	(1–35)	
	No. Patients	%	
New myocardial infarction	2	1.6	
Reintubation	12	9.7	
Tracheostomy	6	4.8	
Phrenic nerve paresis (transient)	1	0.8	
Pneumonia (positive culture)	19	15.3	
Sternal wound infection	6	4.8	
Sepsis (positive blood culture)	9	7.3	
Bleeding requiring reoperation	7	5.6	
Postoperative low cardiac output (cardiac index <2.0 >6 h)	6	4.8	
Focal cerebral deficit	5	4.0	
Requiring dialysis	5	4.0	
No. days in hospital (hospital survivors)	19.8 ± 12.5	(2–71)	

[a] Intraoperative deaths excluded.

Table 24-4. Causes of Death

	No. Patients	%	Postoperative Day(s) Before Death
Respiratory and multiorgan failure	10	58.8	19.9 (range, 4–47)
Pulmonary hemorrhage[a]	3	17.6	1 (range, 0–3)
Acute myocardial infarction	1	5.9	3
Right heart failure[a]	1	5.9	0
Pulmonary artery thrombosis	1	5.9	6
Late cardic tamponade	1	5.9	17

[a] Intraoperative deaths.

(Data from Daily PO, Dembitsky WP, Iversen S et al.: Current early results of pulmonary thromboendarterectomy for chronic pulmonary embolism. Eur J Cardiothorac Surg 4:117, 1990.)

complications are included in Table 24-3 and causes of death in Table 24-4. Hospital mortality rates for the three cohorts of patients are seen in Table 24-2.

In a separate study, various preoperative and operative factors were considered to be potential determinants of hospital mortality rates and ventilator dependency (Daily, et al., 1990a). Ventilator dependency was defined arbitrarily as the need to ventilate a patient for 5 or more days postoperatively. Ventilator dependency occurred in 31.5 percent (39 of 124 patients), and the hospital mortality rate was 12.6 percent (16 of 127). Multivariate analysis revealed independent predictors of ventilator dependency to be the preoperative presence of ascites, the need for four or more units of blood or blood products, and increased cardiopulmonary bypass time. Predictors of death in the hospital were increased cardiopulmonary bypass time and a failure to decrease pulmonary vascular resistance by 50 percent of more. Potential predictors of ventilator dependency, which did not reach statistical significance but suggested trends, were the duration of symptoms, the New York Heart Association functional classification, and the presence of associated diseases. Potential preoperative predictors associated with death in the hospital also included the New York Heart Association functional classification IV, the presence of associated diseases, and advanced age.

A complication of circulatory arrest is the occurrence of postoperative delirium. A study reported by Wragg, et al. (1988) suggested that 77 percent of patients (18 of 22) developed delirium, defined as confusion, disorientation, agitation, and somnolence. An analysis of independent risk factors suggested that the most significant predictor of postoperative delirium was a circulatory arrest time of 55 minutes or more. However, in essentially all patients, delirium had disappeared by the time of discharge, and no permanent neurologic defects were observed in this group. At the May 1992 meeting of the American Association of Thoracic Surgery, Jamieson, et al. reported an additional cohort of 100 patients with an operative mortality rate of 9 percent. This rate was not significantly different from that in the 149 patients (17 of 149, 11.4 percent) previously described in Table 24-2. The surgical approach described in 1987 has remained essentially unchanged (Daily, et al., 1987).

Late Results

Most patients are able to return to a level of activity appropriate for their ages. Some younger patients have engaged in competitive sports. Moser, et al. (1990a) updated the late results of pulmonary thromboendarterectomy. A group of 79 patients were evaluated for a change in the New York Heart Association functional classification, as seen in Table 24-5. Hemodynamic data for 34 patients are illustrated in Table 24-6. Pulmonary vascular resistance decreased from a mean level of 997 dynes-sec-cm^{-5} preoperatively to 272 dynes-sec-cm^{-5} in the follow-up period. The decrease in pulmonary vascular resistance is usually associated with a substantial increase in pulmonary arterial flow, as seen by comparing preoperative (Fig. 24-13) and late postoperative (Fig. 24-14)

Table 24-5. New York Heart Association Functional Classification ($n = 79$)

Class	Before Surgery	After Surgery
IV	48	0
III	30	3
II	1	16
I	0	60

(Data from Moser KM, Auger WR, Fedullo PF: Chronic major-vessel thromboembolic pulmonary hypertension. Circulation 81:1735, 1990.)

Table 24-6. Hemodynamics ($n = 34$)

	Preoperative	Immediate Postoperative	Follow-Up
Mean pulmonary arterial pressure (mmHg)	48.5 ± 12.4	26.6 ± 7.5	24.3 ± 10.0
Cardiac output (L/min)	3.82 ± 1.29	5.92 ± 1.15	4.85 ± 1.01
Pulmonary vascular resistance, (dynes/sec/cm^{-5})	997 ± 624	230 ± 110	272 ± 256

(Data from Moser KM, Auger WR, Fedullo PF: Chronic major-vessel thromboembolic pulmonary hypertension. Circulation 81:1735, 1990.)

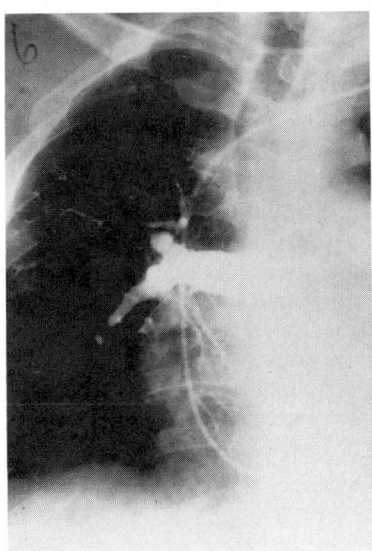
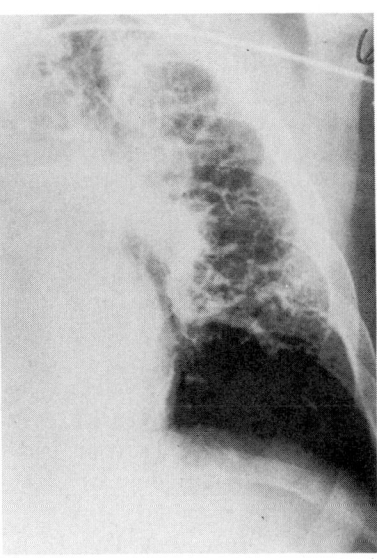

Figure 24-13. Preoperative pulmonary arteriogram. The pulmonary arteriogram of the right lung is to the viewer's left. There is diffuse obstruction of all the bronchopulmonary segmental arteries, except the left upper lobe and lingula, representing more than 60 percent total obstruction of the pulmonary vasculature. (From Daily PO, Dembitsky WP, Peterson KL, Moser KM: Modifications of techniques and early results of pulmonary thromboendarterectomy for chronic pulmonary embolism. J Thorac Cardiovasc Surg 93:221, 1987, with permission.)

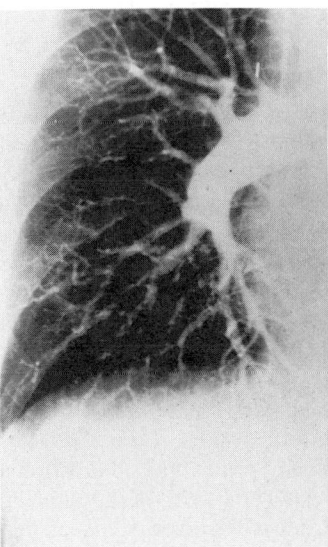
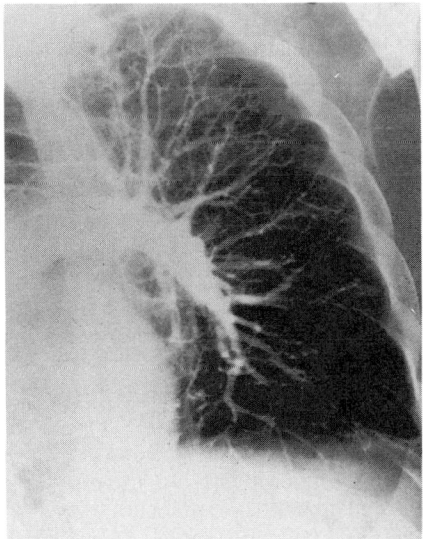

Figure 24-14. Postoperative pulmonary arteriogram at 8 months. There is significantly increased perfusion, but some bronchopulmonary subsegmental arterial defects persist. (From Daily PO, Dembitsky WP, Peterson KL, Moser KM: Modifications of techniques and early results of pulmonary thromboendarterectomy for chronic pulmonary embolism. J Thorac Cardiovasc Surg 93:221, 1987, with permission.)

pulmonary arteriograms. This reduction in pulmonary vascular resistance suggests that late survival should be significantly enhanced if pulmonary vascular resistance has the same implications after pulmonary thromboendarterectomy as in the natural history of chronic pulmonary embolism, as reported by Reidel, et al. (1982).

COMMENTS AND CONTROVERSIES

Pulmonary thromboendarterectomy continues to be a relatively infrequently performed procedure. Undoubtedly the lack of a high index of suspicion of the diagnosis is at least in part responsible. The diagnosis of chronic pulmonary embolism should be considered in all patients with pulmonary hypertension until chronic pulmonary embolism has been specifically eliminated. An additional factor related to the relative rarity of pulmonary thromboendarterectomy is a lack of awareness of this procedure and its effectiveness and the current level of risk.

One of the most significant continuing problems is the inability to predict accurately which patients will have enough obstructive thromboembolic material removed to cause a significant reduction in pulmonary vascular resistance. In our experience to date, 3 to 5 percent of patients have inadequate relief, as evidenced by a less than 50 percent reduction in pulmonary vascular resistance or failure to reduce pulmonary vascular resistance to less than 300 dynes/sec/cm^{-5}.

The operative mortality rates substantially increase in these patients and approach 100 percent when pulmonary vascular resistance remains at 800 dynes/sec/cm^{-5} or more. It was anticipated that endoscopy could eliminate this small group of patients in whom operability could not be accurately determined. To date that has not been the case. Perhaps with the development of other techniques, such as intravascular echo and Doppler sonography, more precise diagnoses can be obtained. It should be emphasized that, although long-term functional capability and survival results are excellent when a significant reduction in pulmonary vascular resistance is obtained, there is a smaller cohort of patients in whom lesser degrees of reduction of pulmonary vascular resistance are associated with persistent significant symptoms. We hope a detailed analysis of a larger data base will allow the preoperative identification of patients, usually with more distally located obstructions, who are likely to have an inadequate reduction of pulmonary vascular resistance.

Severe reperfusion pulmonary edema in some patients during the early postoperative period is another major problem. In three patients, severe hemorrhagic pulmonary edema occurred intraoperatively, resulting in their deaths on the operating table. To date neither predictors nor treatment of this disastrous complication have been defined. Perhaps therapeutic attempts to decrease the formation of oxygen free radicals and chemical blockage of anaphlytoxins will be beneficial.

The choice of pulmonary thromboendarterectomy rather than pulmonary transplantation as the primary therapeutic approach is worthy of some discussion. In the majority of patients in whom sufficient relief of pulmonary vascular resistance can be obtained, pulmonary thromboendarterectomy is the treatment of choice. The operative mortality rate is lower, and the long-term survival is significantly improved compared with both lung and heart-lung transplantation (Registry of the International Society for Heart and Lung Transplantation, 1992). However, those patients deemed inoperable or at especially high risk by virtue of the distal location of their pulmonary obstructions with high pulmonary vascular resistance findings (800 dynes-sec-cm^{-5} or more) should be considered for transplantation as their primary therapeutic approach.

Potential future trends in managing pulmonary thromboendarterectomy include the development of endoscopic techniques to remove more distally located pulmonary vascular obstructive material. To date the use of an endoscope for visualization of the distal pulmonary arteries suggests that this might be an effective avenue of approach. However, this method is in the early developmental stage. It is also conceivable that the future development of transvenous methods of pulmonary thromboendarterectomy are within the realm of possibility.

P.O.D.

Dr. Daily is one of the world experts in the surgical management of chronic pulmonary embolism. Few surgeons have significant experience in the surgical management of this entity. This is a frequently undiagnosed or misdiagnosed condition, and as the author rightly points out, a high index of suspicion is often required. A patient with signs of pulmonary hypertension or right ventricular failure should be investigated appropriately to avoid missing this potentially reversible problem.

In the future prospective studies will be necessary to define the respective roles of pulmonary thromboendarterectomy and lung transplantation in regard to the most effective therapeutic approach. Future developments in angioscopy and fluoroscopically guided ablation techniques may allow a less invasive effective therapy for this disease.

In most instances in this textbook, surgical techniques have been separated from the discussion of disease entities. However, in this instance, we thought that this unique disease and its surgical approach was best treated by combining the disease entity and its surgical therapy into one chapter.

The entity of acute pulmonary embolism is discussed in the introductory chapter on perioperative management (see Ch. 6), and readers are referred to this chapter for its discussion.

R.J.G.

KEY REFERENCES

Chitwood WR, Sabiston DC, Wechsler AS: Surgical treatment of chronic unresolved pulmonary embolism. Clin Chest Med 5:507, 1984

In this publication, the authors extensively reviewed the literature concerning chronic pulmonary embolism and its surgical management prior to 1984. They identified 85 patients undergoing pulmonary thromboendarterectomy with an overall mortality rate of 22 percent.

Daily PO, Dembitsky WP, Iversen S: Technique of pulmonary thromboendarterectomy for chronic pulmonary embolism. J Cardiovasc Surg 4:10, 1989

This article represents the most complete and detailed description of the technique of pulmonary thromboendarterectomy. In addition, several important perioperative considerations are described. Sufficient illustrations are included to facilitate comprehension of the steps for exposure of the distal pulmonary arteries. Also, the technique of endarterectomy itself is described in detail.

Daily PO, Dembitsky WP, Iversen S et al.: Risk factors for pulmonary thromboendarterectomy. J Thorac Cardiovasc Surg 99:670, 1990a

In this article, various factors are defined related to the operative mortality rate and/or the development of respiratory failure, as characterized by the need for mechanical ventilator use for 5 days or more.

Moser KM, Auger WR, Fedullo PF: Chronic major-vessel thromboembolic pulmonary hypertension. Circulation 81:1735, 1990a

In this publication, the natural history, diagnosis, and patient selection are discussed in detail. In addition, the late follow-up is presented in which the functional classification change is described in 79 patients and late cardiac catheterization data are presented in 34 patients.

Reidel M, Stanek V, Widimsky J, Preroesky I: Long term follow-up of patients with pulmonary thromboembolism. Late prognosis and evolution of hemodynamic and respiratory data. Chest 81:151, 1982

This is a critical article with regard to recommending whether or not pulmonary thromboendarterectomy should be performed because it correlates long-term survival with the level of pulmonary vascular obstruction, as manifested by the mean pulmonary artery pressure.

REFERENCES

Cabrol C, Cabrol A, Acar J et al.: Surgical correction of chronic postembolic obstructions of the pulmonary arteries. J Thorac Cardiovasc Surg 76:620, 1978

Daily PO, Dembitsky WP, Iversen S et al.: Current early results of pulmonary thromboendarterectomy for chronic pulmonary embolism. Eur J Cardiothorac Surg 4:117, 1990b

Daily PO, Dembitsky WP, Peterson KL, Moser KM: Modifications of techniques and early results of pulmonary thromboendarterectomy for chronic pulmonary embolism. J Thorac Cardiovasc Surg 93:221, 1987

Daily PO, Johnston GG, Simmons CJ, Moser KM: Surgical management of chronic pulmonary embolism. J Thorac Cardiovasc Surg 79:523, 1980

Daily PO, Kinney TB: Optimizing myocardial hypothermia: II. Cooling jacket modifications and clinical results. Ann Thorac Surg 51:284, 1991a

Daily PO, Dembitsky WP, Daily RP: Dissection for pulmonary thromboendarterectomy. Ann Thorac Surg 51:842, 1991b

Dalen JE, Alpert JS: Natural history of pulmonary embolism. Prog Cardiovasc Dis 17:259, 1975

Dalen JE, Banas JS, Brooks HL et al.: Resolution rate of acute pulmonary embolism in man. N Engl J Med 280:194, 1969

Dittrich HC, Chow LC, Nicod PH: Early improvement in left ventricular diastolic function after relief of chronic right ventricular pressure overload. Circulation 80:823, 1989

Dor V, Jourdan J, Schmitt R et al.: Delayed pulmonary thrombectomy via a peripheral approach in the treatment of pulmonary embolism and sequelae. Thorac Cardiovasc Surg 29:227, 1981

Gibbon JH Jr, Hopkinson M, Churchill ED: Changes in the circulation produced by gradual occlusion of the pulmonary artery. J Clin Invest 11:543, 1932

Jault F, Cabrol C: Surgical treatment for chronic pulmonary thromboembolism. Herz 14:192, 1989

Kay JM: Risk and benefit of lung biopsy in primary pulmonary hypertension (letter). Circulation 81:2029, 1990

Kirklin JW, Barrett-Boyes BG: Cardiac Surgery. 2nd Ed. Churchill Livingstone, New York, 1993

Moser KM: Venous thromboembolism. Am Rev Respir Dis 141:235, 1990

Moser KM, Nicod PH, Bloor CM: Risk and benefit of lung biopsy in primary pulmonary hypertension (letter). Circulation 81:2030, 1990b

Nicod P, Peterson KM, Levine MS et al.: Pulmonary angiography in severe chronic pulmonary hypertension. Ann Intern Med 107:565, 1987

Registry of the International Society for Heart and Lung Transplantation: Ninth official report—1992. J Heart Lung Transplant 11:599, 1992

Shumway NE, Lower RR, Stofer RC: Selective hypothermia of the heart in anoxic cardiac arrest. Surg Gynecol Obstet 109:750, 1959

Snyder WA, Kent DC, Baisch BF: Successful endarterectomy of chronically occluded pulmonary artery. J Thorac Cardiovasc Surg 45:482, 1963

Tilkian AG, Schroeder JS, Robin ED: Chronic thromboembolic occlusion of main pulmonary artery or primary branches. Am J Med 60:563, 1967

Wragg RE, Dimsdale JE, Moser KM et al.: Operative predictors of delirium after pulmonary thromboendarterectomy. A model for postcardiotomy delirium? J Thorac Cardiovasc Surg 96:524, 1988

25

BENIGN LUNG TUMORS

Larry R. Kaiser
Joseph E. Bavaria

DEFINITION

Benign tumors of the lung are extremely rare neoplasms. Although many of these lesions present as solitary pulmonary nodules and occasionally as multiple nodules, somewhat less than 15 percent of such nodules are benign neoplasms (Oldham, 1980). The classification of benign tumors remains somewhat controversial because of disagreement regarding the origin and prognosis of some of the more common lesions. A modification of the classification proposed originally by Liebow (1952) seems to be the simplest and most elegant scheme and should serve our purposes well. This proposal classifies lesions according to their presumed origin, whether epithelial or mesodermal. A number of the benign lesions must be classified as unknown in origin and some as inflammatory. Electron microscopy provides more accurate detail concerning ultrastructure, and the availability of this technique led to a revision in the classification of several lesions previously thought to be benign. Intravascular bronchoalveolar tumor, also known as sclerosing hemangioendothelioma, and pulmonary blastoma were both considered benign but now are known to behave in a malignant fashion. Hemangiopericytoma is another tumor that probably straddles the line between benign and malignant and should perhaps be labeled as "benignant." The names themselves imply the benignity originally attributed to these tumors. The situation with the lesion formerly known as pseudolymphoma is slightly more complex. This is discussed below. In this chapter we discuss the diagnosis and management of the benign neoplasms encountered in the lung and focus particularly on the influence that thoracoscopic excision may play now that it has become firmly established in the armamentarium of the general thoracic surgeon.

HISTORICAL NOTE

The history of the surgical treatment of pulmonary neoplasms encompasses less than 60 years, and the greatest attention has been paid to malignant neoplasms, which account for the overwhelming majority of lesions. In a landmark report published in 1963, Steele, writing on behalf of the Veterans

Administration–Armed Forces Cooperative Study of Resected Asymptomatic Solitary Pulmonary Nodules, presented the data obtained from 887 resected lesions collected beginning in 1959. There were 316 malignant tumors, 65 hamartomas, 474 granulomas, and 32 miscellaneous lesions, which included 1 hemangiopericytoma and 5 benign pleural mesotheliomas, a 12.5 percent incidence of benign lung tumors if the mesotheliomas are included. Most patients in this study (61 percent) were older than age 50 years, and all patients were male. The incidence of primary carcinoma was 39 percent in Veterans Administration patients; the incidence of granulomas was 78 percent in the patients in the Armed Forces hospitals. The author concluded that the data presented confirmed the then generally accepted fact that most

---

Classification of Benign Lung Tumors

Origin unknown
    Hamartoma
    Clear cell ("sugar") tumor
    Teratoma
Epithelial tumors
    Papilloma
    Polyps
Mesodermal tumors
    Fibroma
    Lipoma
    Leiomyoma
    Chondroma
    Granular cell tumor
    Sclerosing hemangioma
Other
    Plasma cell granulomas (histiocytoma)
    Xanthoma
    Amyloid
    Mucosa-associated lymphoid tumor—formerly pseudolymphoma (probably not a benign neoplasm)

Table 25-1. Spectrum of Benign Lung Tumors and Their Relative Frequency of Occurrence

Tumor	No. (%)
Hamartoma	101 (76.9)
Benign mesothelioma	16 (12.3)
Xanthomatous and inflammatory pseudotumors	7 (5.4)
Lipoma	2 (1.5)
Leiomyoma	2 (1.5)
Hemangioma	1 (0.8)
Adenoma of mucous glands	1 (0.8)
Mixed tumor	1 (0.8)

solitary pulmonary nodules must be resected if cancer is to be ruled out. Radiographic evidence of dense or concentric calcification was thought to be the only finding that eliminated the possibility of malignancy. Little has changed, although the advent of computed tomographic (CT) scans and the refinement of needle biopsy (both percutaneous and transbronchial) have resulted in fewer patients being operated on for non-neoplastic lesions. The basic principle, however, remains intact; that is, unless a nodule can be proved to be benign, it should be removed. The development of video thoracoscopic techniques of pulmonary resection may result in the resection of a few more benign lesions, but it should also eliminate the reluctance to refer a patient for surgical treatment because of hesitation over the possibility of a thoracotomy. In a review of a 10-year experience of 1,822 cases at the Mayo Clinic, Clagett, et al. (1964) found only 86 (4.7 percent) benign pulmonary tumors, most of which (66) were hamartomas. Included in this series were 11 benign mesotheliomas, or solitary benign fibrous tumors of the pleura, which we do not currently include in the spectrum of benign parenchymal lesions. A subsequent 10-year period at the same institution yielded 130 patients who underwent surgical resection of benign lung tumors (Arrigoni, et al., 1970). The spectrum of benign lung tumors seen and their relative frequency of occurrence is seen in Table 25-1. Hamartomas account for the striking majority of these benign lesions, a finding that seems to be true in all series. It is safe to say that, in any series of resected lesions, there is an incidence of resection of benign neoplasms. These lesions grow over time, often do not have characteristic calcification, were not present on a previous radiograph, and either the patient or the referring physician (or both) were anxious enough to seek a surgical opinion. When there is any doubt, the safest course to follow classically has been to remove the lesion.

HISTORICAL READINGS

Arrigoni MG, Woolner LB, Bernatz PE et al: Benign tumors of the lung: a ten-year surgical experience. J Thorac Cardiovasc Surg 60:589, 1970

Clagette OT, Allen TH, Payne WS, Woolner LB: The surgical treatment of pulmonary neoplasms: a 10-year experience. J Thorac Cardiovasc Surg 48:391, 1964

Steele JD: The solitary pulmonary nodule: report of a cooperative study of resected asymptomatic solitary pulmonary nodules in males. J Thorac Cardiovasc Surg 46:21, 1963

SPECIFIC BENIGN TUMORS OF THE LUNG

Hamartoma

The most common benign tumor of the lung is the hamartoma, found in about 0.25 percent of patients at autopsy. It accounts for about 8 percent of pulmonary neoplasms (McDonald, et al., 1954). These lesions are basically an abnormal mixing of the normal components of the lung. On histologic section they are composed mainly of cartilage and glandlike formations and may include a significant amount of fat (Fig. 25-1). Most hamartomas are asymptomatic and come to clinical attention because they must be differentiated from carcinomas following their identification on a routine chest radiograph. They occur most commonly in male patients (2 to 3 : 1 predominance) and are distributed across a spectrum of age ranges, but most are seen in patients between 30 and 60 years of age (Hansen, et al., 1992). Hamartomas occur in all parts of the lung, but most commonly, they are found in the periphery and rarely at the hilum. Often they present as parenchymal lesions but occasionally occur as endobronchial lesions with manifestations of obstruction, such as volume loss.

Radiographically, the majority present as solitary pulmonary nodules and rarely as multiple nodules. They tend to be well-circumscribed lesions, ranging usually between 1 and 2 cm in diameter, although larger ones, in the 5- to 6-cm range, are occasionally seen. Calcification may be present but may not be obvious on the plain chest radiograph. The CT scan may be more useful for demonstrating calcification, and in up to 50 percent of cases may also show fat (Siegelman, et al., 1986). The presence of fat density in a well-demarcated lesion is certainly suggestive of a benign neoplasm. In an older patient, it might conclude the diagnostic evaluation and prompt the clinician to follow the patient with serial chest radiographs. In the past, needle aspiration biopsies were done with great frequency. It has been our experience, however, that rarely are positive findings obtained from an aspiration biopsy of a hamartoma, but this varies between institutions. Many radiologists and cytopathologists are extremely comfortable diagnosing a hamartoma; the use of a larger needle designed to obtain a core biopsy certainly facilitates this. The clinician must obtain cartilage or fat to make a definitive diagnosis, but the patient would be spared an operation (Ramzy, 1976).

Slow growth is the norm for these tumors. In the series reported by Hansen, et al. (1992), tumor growth was observed in 48 percent of patients during a mean observation period of 4.1 years with an average increase in diameter of 3.2 ± 2.6 mm/year. Based on this finding, it is not unreasonable to watch these lesions if the clinician is fairly certain that a lesion is a hamartoma. Malignancy is rare, if it occurs at all, and only a few cases have been reported (Poulsen, et al., 1979).

Endobronchial hamartomas occur in 3 to 20 percent of

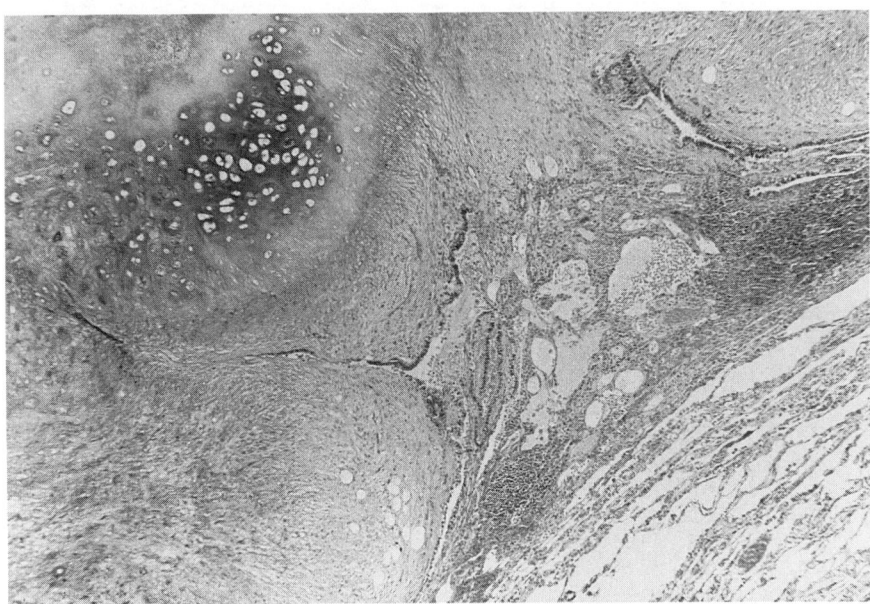

Figure 25-1. Microscopic section of a hamartoma demonstrating a mixture of cartilage, fat cells, and undifferentiated mesenchymal cells. There are clefts lined by a single layer of cuboidal epithelial cells.

cases (Mateson, 1965; Bergh, et al., 1967). In the series recently reported by Hansen, et al. (1992), only 1 patient in a series of 89 had an endobronchial hamartoma, but lesions in this location would be expected to be symptomatic. Figure 25-2A is the chest radiograph of a young woman presenting with dyspnea and cough who was found to have a hamartoma in the left main bronchus at bronchoscopy. Note the volume loss on the left with a mediastinal shift and hyperinflation of the right lung. Figure 25-2B, a perfusion lung scan, demonstrates a paucity of perfusion to the left lung, probably secondary to hypoxic vasoconstriction. Following bronchoscopic removal of the lesion, the chest radiograph returns to normal (Fig. 25-2C).

Hemangiopericytoma

Hemangiopericytoma is a difficult diagnosis in any site because the histologic pattern is often consistent with that of other sarcomas. Pulmonary hemangiopericytoma can occur at almost any age, and these tumors are similar in appearance to lesions that are found in multiple other sites. The name was originally suggested for a vascular tumor composed of capillary pericytes. They can be of any size, and in Meade, et al.'s (1974) report, they ranged from 2 to 15 cm in diameter. Approximately one-half were asymptomatic at the time of presentation. The signs and symptoms included hemoptysis dyspnea, and chest pain. Pathologically the tumor is characterized by its vascularity and the peritheliomatous arrangement of the tumor cells (Meade, et al., 1974). There are well-preserved vascular channels, although in larger tumors, there may be significant central necrosis. These vascular channels are surrounded by sheets of rounded or spindle-shaped cells that have pale cytoplasms and large vesicular nuclei. Mitoses

are infrequently seen. This tumor may behave in a benign or malignant fashion, and complete excision is the treatment of choice. The prognosis seems to be best in female patients with small tumors. Meade, et al. (1974) found 25 cases in the world literature with 4 deaths in 16 female patients and 6 deaths in 9 male patients. Whether this tumor should even be considered in a discussion of benign lung lesions is questionable.

Sclerosing Hemangioma

Sclerosing hemangioma was first described by Liebow and Hubbell (1974). This is an uncommon benign lung tumor that occurs most frequently in middle-aged women who are usually asymptomatic. The lesion presents as a solitary, peripheral, well-circumscribed nodule, which may be partially calcified (Fig. 25-3). Grossly the lesion may appear hemorrhagic. In a recent study by Sugio, et al. (1992), this tumor was the second most common neoplasm seen among the benign lesions ($n = 45$) resected from a cohort of 919 patients over a 17-year period. Ten patients (22.2 percent) had sclerosing hemangiomas compared with 22 with hamartomas. The tumors ranged in size from 1.3 to 8 cm in diameter. Radiographically these lesions appeared to be well-defined, homogeneous, round or oval masses in all patients.

The histologic features of sclerosing hemangioma vary, and four major patterns may be found in the same tumor: solid, papillary, vascular (Fig. 25-3A), and sclerotic (Fig. 25-3B).

As Yousem (1992) points out in his invited commentary following Sugio, et al.'s (1992) article, there has been a significant evolution in our understanding of this tumor. There may be malignant variants of this tumor that present as multi-

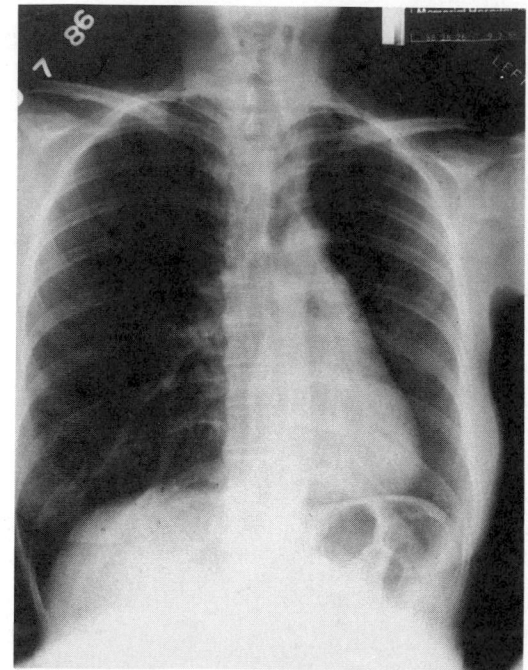

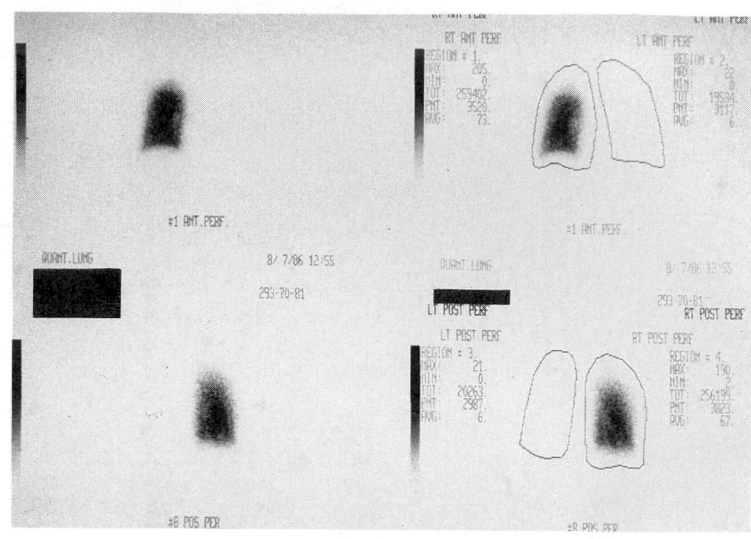

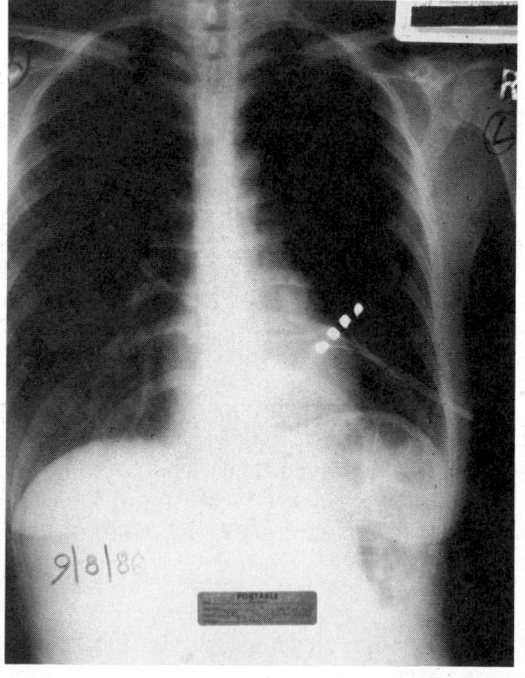

Figure 25-2. **(A)** Preoperative chest radiograph of a young woman with a hamartoma in the left mainstem bronchus. Note the loss of volume evident on the left as manifested by the mediastinal shift and the hyperinflation of the right lung. **(B)** Perfusion lung scan of the same patient demonstrating significantly diminished blood flow to the left lung. **(C)** Following bronchoscopic removal of the hamartoma, the chest radiograph returns to a completely normal appearance.

ple nodules in contradistinction to the benign form, which presents as a solitary nodule. The cell of origin, as suggested by immunohistochemical studies, is most likely a primitive respiratory epithelial cell, not a mesenchymal cell. The tumor should perhaps be more appropriately labeled as an alveolar pneumocytoma, based on this recent information. Surgical resection would be expected to result in a cure in the overwhelming majority of cases no matter what the cell of origin is.

Granular Cell Tumor

Granular cell tumors, formerly called myoblastomas and now perhaps more appropriately called schwannomas, may present as solitary pulmonary nodules or occur in the trachea or mainstem bronchi, occasionally as multiple lesions (Schuster, et al., 1975; Thomas, et al., 1984). Despite the name, skeletal muscle cells are not identified in most myoblastomas. Pearse (1950) proposed that the cells represent granular degeneration

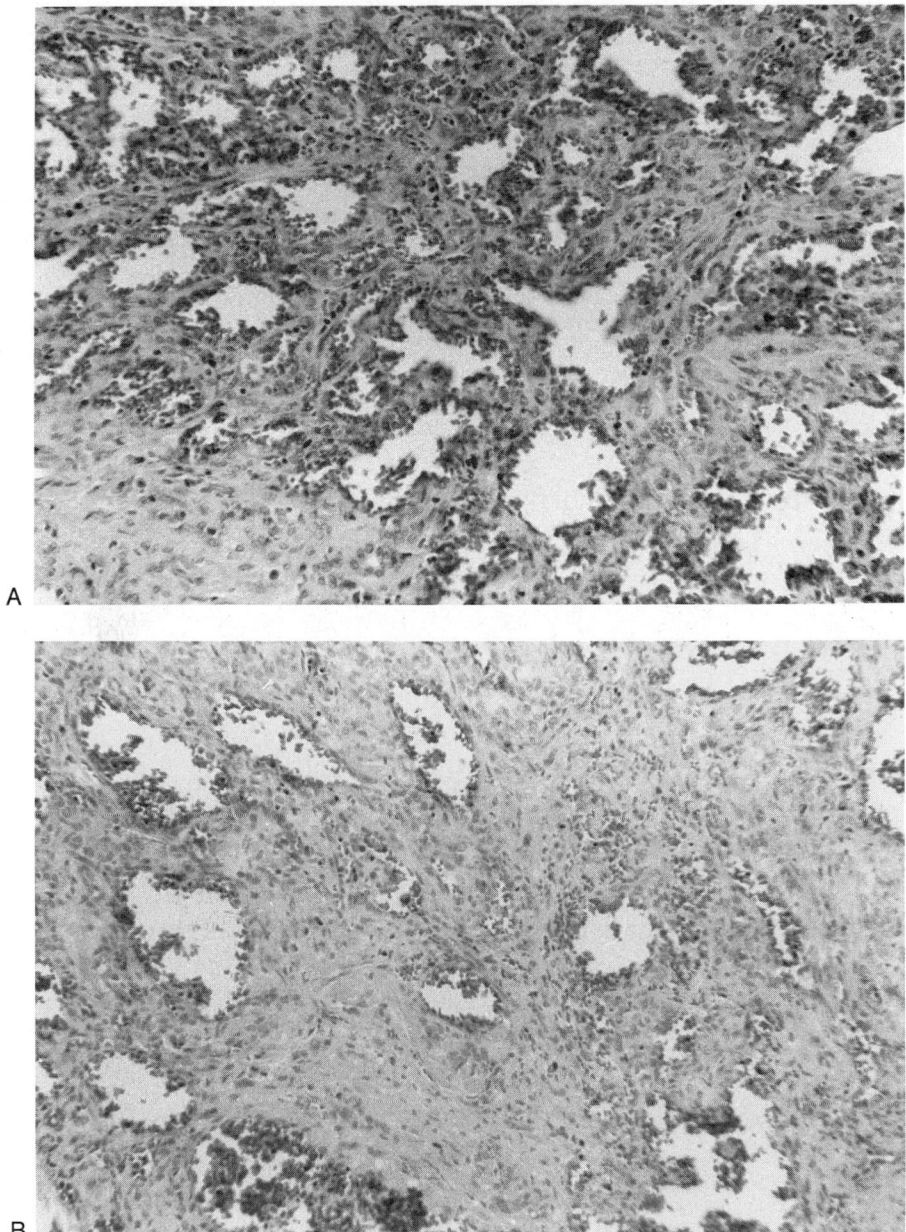

Figure 25-3. **(A)** Histologic section of a sclerosing hemangioma demonstrating the vascular pattern marked by the finding of multiple dilated vascular spaces often filled with blood cells and surrounded by tumor cells or fibrous tissue. **(B)** Sclerosing hemangioma showing a pattern more consistent with the fibrous type.

of perineural fibroblasts. They occur with equal frequency in both sexes, and the median age of patients with these tumors is 38 years, younger than that typically seen in patients with endobronchial malignancies. Patients typically present with cough or other symptoms suggestive of bronchial obstruction; hemoptysis occasionally may occur. Valenstein and Thurer (1978) reported only one recurrence in 46 cases of granular cell tumor.

Pseudolymphoma (Mucosa-Associated Lymphoid Tumor)

Pseudolymphomas are fascinating lesions that for many years were thought to be benign. Most present as asymptomatic incidental pulmonary nodules noted on a routine chest radiograph. Grossly they appear to be well-demarcated masses with a smooth, soft, pale cut surface (Fig. 25-4A). A minority

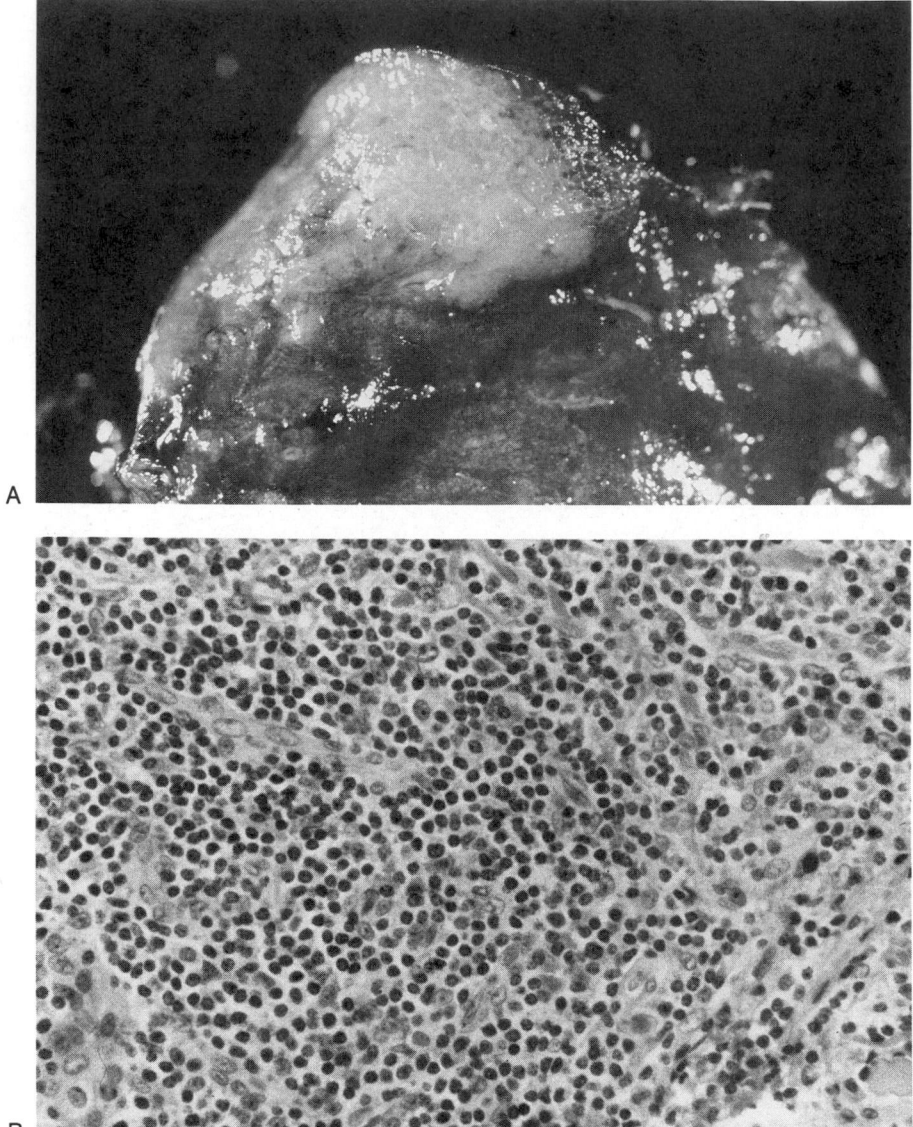

Figure 25-4. **(A)** Gross appearance of the cut surface of a bronchial-associated lymphoid tumor (BALT) demonstrating a clear demarcation from the surrounding lung tissue. **(B)** Microscopic appearance of a BALT showing the small lymphoid cells interspersed among clusters of plasma cells. These cells tend to localize around lymphoid follicles, often replacing the mantle zone and invading the follicle's center.

of patients may complain of chest pain or fever. In their original report of pseudolymphoma of the lung, Hutchinson, et al. (1964) commented on the radiographic finding of air bronchograms within the lesion that resulted from this presumed inflammatory mass surrounding a small bronchus but not constricting it. This is not a consistent finding, however, and there are no distinct radiologic criteria to distinguish these lesions from any other neoplasm.

There is a growing body of evidence based on immunohistochemical, molecular, and cytogenetic study that these lesions actually may be low-grade primary B-cell lymphomas of mucosa-associated lymphoid tissue (MALT). Microscopically the lesion consists of small lymphoid cells interspersed among clusters of plasma cells (Fig. 25-4B). Tumor cells

infiltrate along the alveolar septa, resulting in the characteristic lymphoepithelial lesion. The tumor usually has a nodular appearance because of its tendency to localize around lymphoid follicles. Wotherspoon, et al. (1990) recently described a case of a lung lesion with the definitive histologic features of a pseudolymphoma in which cytogenetic studies revealed an abnormal karyotype with a translocation t(1;14) characteristic of B-cell lymphomas.

Following excision we carry out a complete lymphoma staging workup to rule out the presence of systemic lymphoma. If no other evidence of lymphoma exists, we recommend follow-up only, fully recognizing that a percentage of these patients may develop disseminated lymphoma over a period of years. Despite Saltzstein's (1963) contention that these were reactive lesions, most are probably bona fide lymphomas, albeit low grade, and the term *pseudolymphoma* has probably outlived its usefulness.

Fibroma

Bronchopulmonary fibromas may present in either the tracheobronchial tree or within the pulmonary parenchyma. Pure fibromas are infrequently diagnosed in the lung, as is the case in the soft tissues. There may be myxomatous elements intermixed in these lesions. An endobronchial fibroma would be expected to produce atelectasis and may be associated with other signs and symptoms of obstruction (Corona and Okeson, 1974). Lesions of this type in this location lend themselves to easy removal through the rigid bronchoscope, or they may be excised with the laser. Similar to other benign tumors, fibromas presenting in the pulmonary parenchyma usually are asymptomatic and appear as well-circumscribed nodules without specific characteristics to differentiate them from other lesions. Wedge excision is both diagnostic and curative and may be undertaken thoracoscopically as the procedure of choice. Histologically these lesions show an abundance of collagen and bland spindle cells, which are typical of fibromas seen elsewhere in the body.

Lipoma

Most lipomas are bronchial in origin, arising from the submucosal fat present between cartilaginous rings of the bronchus. Parenchymal lipomas are rare. In the classic study of 130 benign lung tumors from the Mayo Clinic, only 2 were bronchopulmonary lipomas (Arrigoni, et al., 1970). The symptoms and signs associated with this lesion depend on the lesion's size and location. Because most are endobronchial in origin, manifestations of obstruction predominate with the larger lesions. Cough is especially common, and few patients with endobronchial lesions are asymptomatic. Endobronchial lipomas are usually pedunculated tumors with a narrow stalk that are covered by normal respiratory mucosa (Jensen and Petersen 1970). If there is significant destruction of lung tissue distal to one of these lesions, lobectomy or segmentectomy may be required, despite the ability to remove the lipoma bronchoscopically. Lipomas of both the visceral and parietal pleura may also be seen but are much less common than are the endobronchial variety (Politis, et al., 1979).

Leiomyoma of the Lung

Although rare, leiomyoma is the most common soft tissue tumor of the lung, and it is composed essentially of smooth muscle fibers (Gal, et al., 1989). Women account for two-thirds of the affected patients, and the mean age of all reported cases is 35 years (Orlowski, et al., 1978). Approximately one-third of patients are younger than 20 years of age. Similar to other benign tumors, the location of the lesion dictates the symptoms. Most of these lesions are solitary peripheral pulmonary nodules and therefore asymptomatic. They are found as incidental findings on plain chest radiographs or CT scans of the chest. There are no specific characteristics that distinguish this lesion from other pulmonary nodules. A small minority of patients present with symptoms secondary to endobronchial involvement.

There is substantial controversy regarding the origin of these tumors of the lung. Hypotheses include origination from the bronchial wall smooth muscle or the wall of bronchial arteries. On histologic section, they look like the smooth muscle tumors seen in multiple other sites. There is some support for the hypothesis that these tumors are metastatic myomas of uterine origin, despite their bland cytologic appearance (Mackay, et al., 1991). These so-called benign metastasizing leiomyomas have a bland histologic pattern with minimal mitoses or necrosis and look identical to myomas found in the uterus. By virtue of the fact that they have disseminated by a hematogenous route, many would argue against the designation of benign, no matter how bland the histologic appearance is.

Clear Cell (Sugar) Tumor of the Lung

Clear cell tumors of the lung are exceedingly rare neoplasms originally described by Liebow and Castleman (1963). In a detailed review of this tumor, Gaffey, et al. (1990) added 8 additional cases to the 21 cases of this tumor that had previously been reported. The patients were usually asymptomatic and presented with a peripheral solitary pulmonary nodule found incidentally on a plain chest radiograph. There was no predilection according to sex, and the majority of patients were in their 40s or 50s. Until recently these tumors were universally considered benign, but a report by Sale and Kulander (1988) describes a patient who died of metastatic clear cell tumor of the lung.

These tumors bear a striking microscopic resemblance to metastatic renal cell carcinoma, and the report by Gaffey, et al. (1990) attempts to clarify the pathologic distinctions between clear cell tumors of the lung and renal cell carcinomas by using clinical, histologic, immunohistochemical, and ultrastructural features. They are characterized by sheets and cords of polygonal cells separated by a prominent fibrovascular stroma. The "clear cells" may indeed have a clear cytoplasm, but they often have a granular eosinophilic cytoplasm. Based on their intense periodic acid-Schiff positivity, the granules are most likely glycogen, and the eosinophilic appearance to the cytoplasm is imparted when granules are present in large numbers. The nuclei are characteristically bland and vary in size; mitoses are usually absent. The chromatin is finely granular, and occasional intranuclear cytoplasmic invaginations are seen. Although not distinctly encapsulated, the lesions easily "shell out" of the surrounding lung tissue, usually are peripherally located, and generally are 2.0 cm or less in size. Immunohistochemical analysis now allows for the definitive diagnosis of clear cell tumors of the lung and their distinction from renal cell carcinomas.

Germ Cell Tumors

Benign teratomas presenting in the lung are distinctly uncommon, but they have been reported (Holt, et al., 1976). Some of the reported cases may be mediastinal lesions that involve contiguous lung.

DIAGNOSIS

Most benign tumors present as asymptomatic nodules found on a routine chest radiograph, which leads to further workup. This is almost universally the case with lesions located in the peripheral lung parenchyma. The presence of multiple nodules most commonly is metastatic disease as was the case in 73 percent of 114 patients reported by Gross, et al. (1985). A small percentage of benign lesions, however, present in an endobronchial location and may be manifested by lobar or whole lung collapse, hyperinflation secondary to a ball valvelike mechanism, cough, pneumonia, and occasionally hemoptysis. Infrequently a wheeze may be audible. These symptoms and signs occur when a lesion is located more centrally in the airway. In a series of 130 benign lung tumors, Arrigoni, et al. (1970) noted only 8 endobronchial lesions. A definitive diagnosis may be made only by obtaining tissue. This is easily accomplished by bronchoscopy when there is an endobronchial lesion, but peripheral lesions present more of a challenge. Sometimes their appearance on the chest radiograph is so characteristic, such as the "popcorn" calcification occasionally present in a hamartoma, that the diagnosis may be suggested. Other radiologic features, such as well-rounded edges or slow growth, are not specific for benign lesions and may be associated, as is calcification at times, with a malignant lesion. Needle biopsy, in our opinion, has little use in the diagnosis and management of patients with benign lung lesions, although some authors report a high incidence of diagnostic fine-needle aspiration biopsies in patients with lesions that are hamartomas (Steen-Hansen, 1987). A definitive diagnosis of hamartoma allows thoracotomy to be avoided, although some of these lesions may become large. There is a great deal of variation among clinicians regarding the use of a needle biopsy in the diagnosis of a solitary pulmonary nodule.

The evaluation of the solitary pulmonary nodule, almost since the advent of chest radiography, has occupied a considerable amount of time and energy expenditure on the part of radiologists, pulmonologists, and thoracic surgeons. Starting with a review of any previous chest radiographs, the aim of each is to save the patient from having to undergo an operation by using noninvasive or at least less invasive techniques in an attempt to prove that a lesion is benign. A negative needle biopsy finding is not helpful in managing a patient, and the clinician must obtain a positive diagnosis of benignity before dismissing the patient. The practitioner may choose to follow a lesion over a period of time, but a specific end point for the observation period must be defined. Patients must be reliable enough to return at appropriate intervals for reevaluations. Unfortunately, neither CT nor magnetic resonance imaging (MRI) provides definitive proof that a lesion is benign, although certain characteristics, notably dense calcification within a lesion seen on CT scan, may strongly suggest benignity and specifically a granuloma. Often the use of thinly collimated images (usually 1.5 to 2.0 mm) taken after a nodule is identified on CT may help to delineate the presence of calcification. The slice thickness for such images must be less than one-half the diameter of the nodule being evaluated. There are a number of technical problems that limit the usefulness of this technique, and the use of an external standard of a known density measurement, the anthropomorphic reference phantom devised by Zerhouni, et al. (1983), may add additional information. Using this technique, approximately 17 percent (range, 9 to 30 percent) of small nodules not seen to be definitely calcified on plain films can be diagnosed as benign when their attenuation values are equal to or higher than that of the reference nodule (Zerhouni, et al., 1986). A phantom study suggestive of benign pathologic findings may lead the clinician to follow serial chest radiographs for a period of time and, if no change in the size of the lesion is evident, to do nothing further.

Alternatively, percutaneous or transbronchial needle aspiration biopsy may be performed, but as mentioned earlier, the practitioner must obtain "positive" information to reach any definitive conclusions. Positive findings would include cartilage or fat suggestive of a hamartoma or fungal elements indicative of an infectious process. Only infrequently would benign tumors be expected to yield diagnostic positive results on an aspiration biopsy.

MANAGEMENT

In general simple excision of a benign lesion is curative. Often excision may be done without the need for an anatomic resection, although the type of resection is obviously dependent on the location of the lesion. The guiding principle, however, when dealing with a benign lesion is conservation of lung tissue. This includes the use of segmental resections and bronchoplastic procedures. Bronchoscopic excision may suffice for some lesions.

Recent advances in minimally invasive techniques for the removal of these lesions makes it less important to look for ways to avoid removing a lesion that may be benign. The advent of video-assisted thoracoscopy has changed significantly our thinking regarding solitary pulmonary nodules (Landreneau, et al., 1992). No longer must a patient be subjected to a formal posterolateral thoracotomy to make a diagnosis or definitively treat a benign lesion. Wedge excision through a thoracoscopic approach provides adequate therapy for benign pathologic conditions without the attendant morbidity of a thoracotomy. Patients leave the hospital sooner and return to normal activities in a shorter period compared with that following thoracotomy. Unless there is evidence of calcification suggestive of a granuloma, it is perhaps better to recommend thoracoscopic excision than to wait and watch. In the long run, it is probably easier on the patient.

The therapy for parenchymal hamartomas is guided more by the fact that the diagnosis usually cannot be definitively established until the lesion is removed. It is easy to visualize these lesions at the time of thoracoscopy, and either perform a wedge excision or enucleate them, as has been classically done during an open procedure. These lesions do not invade the surrounding parenchyma and shell out with ease following incision into the visceral pleura. Benign pulmonary lesions presenting in an endobronchial location often may be definitely treated with bronchoscopic excision. This usually requires performing rigid bronchoscopy to ensure complete removal of the lesion. With complete excision recurrence is unusual; repeat bronchoscopic removal is indicated for recurrence. Pulmonary resection is occasionally indicated for benign endobronchial lesions when there is significant destruction of pulmonary parenchyma distal to an obstructing

lesion or when the lesion occurs in a more peripheral endobronchial location.

COMMENTS AND CONTROVERSIES

Compared with carcinomas of the lung, benign tumors deserve only the slightest bit of attention, at least relative to their incidence. Yet, they are fascinating lesions, and some may not be as benign as we once thought. Video-assisted thoracoscopy provides an opportunity to excise a lesion completely with a minimally invasive approach, which in the case of a benign pulmonary lesion, is both diagnostic and therapeutic and saves the patient from having to undergo a thoracotomy. Ironically, surgeons may begin to see more of these benign neoplasms because pulmonologists, in our experience, are readily referring cases for operations that in

the past they might have watched indefinitely. This increase in referrals is due entirely to the development of video-assisted thoracoscopy and the recognition that therapy may, in many instances, be carried out satisfactorily without thoracotomy. However, notwithstanding this new technology, surgeons must still make a reasoned judgment, based on all the material available, as to whether a patient should undergo a surgical procedure, even a minimally invasive one.

R.J.G.

KEY REFERENCES

Hansen CP, Holtveg H, Francis D et al: Pulmonary hamartoma. J Thorac Cardiovasc Surg 104:674, 1992

The authors report a series of 89 cases of pulmonary hamartoma, of which 75 patients underwent operations. This is an excellent review on the topic of hamartoma, by far the most common benign lung tumor encountered. The authors obtained a diagnostic result in 34 of 40 patients (85 percent) who underwent needle biopsy, a higher percentage than would be expected.

Liebow AA: Tumors of the lower respiratory tract. In Atlas of Tumor Pathology, Section V. Fascicle 17. Armed Forces Institute of Pathology, Washington, D.C., 1952

This includes the classic description of the pathologic findings of benign and malignant tumors of the lung and bronchi. A classification scheme, essentially still in use today, is proposed in this monumental work.

Mackay B, Lukeman JM, Ordonez NG: Tumors of the lung. In Major Problems in Pathology. Vol. 24. WB Saunders, Philadelphia, 1991

This is an outstanding monograph on both benign and malignant tumors of the lung based on the authors' experience at M.D. Anderson Cancer Center in Houston, Texas. An excellent discussion on the pathologic findings of the benign lung tumors is included in the chapter on uncommon lung tumors, which also has an excellent up-to-date bibliography.

Oldham HN: Benign tumors of the lung and bronchus. Surg Clin North Am 60:825, 1980

This is an excellent overview of the topic that deals with the entire spectrum of benign lung tumors.

Zerhouni EA, Stitik FP, Siegelman SS et al: CT of the pulmonary nodule: a cooperative study. Radiology 160:319, 1986

This is the definitive study detailing the computed tomographic findings of the solitary pulmonary nodule, which includes criteria for establishing or at least suspecting benignity.

REFERENCES

Arrigoni MG, Woolner LB, Bernatz PE et al: Benign tumors of the lung: a ten-year surgical experience. J Thorac Cardiovasc Surg 60:589, 1970

Bergh NP, Hafstrom LO, Schersten T: Hamartoma of the lung: with special reference to the endobronchial localization. Scand J Respir Dis 48:201, 1967

Clagett OT, Allen TH, Payne WS, Woolner LB: The surgical treatment of pulmonary neoplasms: a 10-year experience. J Thorac Cardiovasc Surg 48:391, 1964

Corona FE, Okeson GC: Endobronchial fibroma: an unusual cause of segmental atelectasis. Am Rev Respir Dis 110:350, 1974

Gaffey MJ, Mills SE, Askin FB et al: Clear cell tumor of the lung: a clinicopathologic, immunohistochemical, and ultrastructural study of eight cases. Am J Surg Pathol 14:248, 1990

Gal AA, Brooks JS, Pietra GG: Leiomyomatous neoplasms of the lung: a clinical, histologic, and immunohistochemical study. Mod Pathol 2:209, 1989

Gross BH, Glazer GM, Bookstein FL: Multiple pulmonary nodules detected by computed tomography: diagnostic implications. J Comput Assist Tomogr 9:880, 1985

Holt S, Deverall PB, Boddy JE: A teratoma of the lung containing thymic tissue. J Pathol 126:85, 1976

Hutchinson WB, Friedenberg MJ, Saltzstein S: Primary pulmonary pseudolymphoma. Radiology 82:42, 1964

Jensen MS, Petersen AH: Bronchial lipoma. Three cases and review of the literature. Scand J Thorac Cardiovasc Surg 4:131, 1970

Landreneau RJ, Mack MJ, Hazelrigg SR et al: Video-assisted thoracic surgery: basic technical concepts and intercostal approach strategies. Ann Thorac Surg 54:800, 1992

Liebow AA, Castleman B: Benign clear cell tumors of the lung. Am J Pathol 43:13a, 1963

Liebow AA, Hubbell DS: Sclerosing hemangioma (histiocytoma, xanthoma) of the lung. Thorax 29:1, 1974

Mateson EM: Relationship between intrapulmonary and endobronchial cartilage-containing tumors (so-called hamartoma). Thorax 20:447, 1965

McDonald JR, Harrington SW, Clagett OT et al: Solitary circumscribed lesions of the lung. Arch Intern Med 93:842, 1954

Meade JB, Whitwell F, Bickford BJ, et al: Primary haemangiopericytoma of lung. Thorax 29:1, 1974

Orlowsk TM, Stasiak K, Kolodziej J: Leiomyoma of the lung. J Thorac Cardiovasc Surg 76:257, 1978

Politis J, Funahashi A, Gehisen JA et al: Intrathoracic lipomas: report of three cases and a review of the literature with emphasis on endobronchial lipoma. J Thorac Cardiovasc Surg 77:550, 1979

Poulsen JT, Jacobsen M, Francis D: Probable malignant transformation of a pulmonary hamartoma. Thorax 34:557, 1979

Ramzy I: Pulmonary hamartomas: cytologic appearance of fine needle aspiration biopsy. Acta Cytol 20:15, 1976

Sale GE, Kulander BG: "Benign" clear-cell tumor (sugar tumor) of the lung with hepatic metastases ten years after resection of pulmonary primary tumor. Arch Pathol Lab Med 112:1177, 1988

Saltzstein SL: Pulmonary malignant lymphomas and pseudolymphomas: classification, therapy, and prognosis. Cancer 16:928, 1963

Schuster PL, Khan FA, Azueta V: Asymptomatic pulmonary granular cell tumor presenting as a coin lesion. Chest 68:256, 1975

Siegelman SS, Khouri NF, Scott WW et al: Pulmonary hamartoma: CT findings. Radiology 160:313, 1986

Steele JD: The solitary pulmonary nodule: report of a cooperative study of resected asymptomatic solitary pulmonary nodules in males. J Thorac Cardiovasc Surg 46:21, 1963

Steen-Hansen E: The diagnostic value of chest x-ray combined with fine-needle aspiration biopsy in patients suspected for pulmonary hamartomas. Rontgenblatter 40:321, 1987

Sugio K, Yokoyama H, Kaneko S et al: Sclerosing hemangioma of the lung: radiographic and pathological study. Ann Thorac Surg 53:295, 1992

Thomas L, Risbud M, Gabriel JB et al: Cytomorphology of granular cell tumor of the bronchus: a case report. Acta Cytol 28:129, 1984

Valenstein SL, Thurer RJ: Granular cell myoblastoma of the bronchus: case report and literature review. J Thorac Cardiovasc Surg 76:465, 1978

Wotherspoon AC, Soosay GN, Diss TC et al: Low-grade primary B-cell lymphoma of the lung: an immunohistochemical, molecular, and cytogenetic study of a single case. Am J Clin Pathol 94:655, 1990

Yousen SA: Invited commentary of Sugio, et al. Ann Thorac Surg 53:300, 1992

Zerhouni EA, Boukadoum MA, Siddiky MA et al: A standard phantom for quantitative CT analysis of pulmonary nodules. Radiology 149:767, 1983

26

BRONCHIAL GLAND TUMORS

Dov Weissberg

HISTORICAL NOTE

The original description of what was probably a bronchial carcinoid is attributed to Laennec (1831); the term *adenoma* was first used by Müller in 1882. The misnomer *bronchial adenoma* has persisted for more than a century, incorrectly implying benignity and creating a false impression of a single pathologic entity. In fact five tumors comprise this disparate group: bronchial carcinoid, adenoid cystic carcinoma, mucoepidermoid carcinoma, bronchial mucous gland adenoma, and pleomorphic mixed tumor of the bronchial gland type. These neoplasms arise from different cell types, and each one is biologically, pathologically, and clinically different from all the others. The historic reason for grouping them together was a one-time wrong assumption of their benignity, hence the term *adenoma*. Because each one represents a separate entity, they are discussed under separate headings.

HISTORICAL READINGS

Engelbreth-Holm J: Benign bronchial adenomas. Acta Chir Scand 90:383, 1944

Heschl R: Über ein Zylindrom der Lunge. Wien Med Wochenschr 17:385, 1877

Laennec RTH: Traité de L'Auscultation Médiate et des Maladies des Poumons et du Coeur. 3rd Ed. Chaud, Paris, 1831

Müller H: Zur Entstehungsgeschichte der Bronchialerweiterungen. Vol. 15. Inausg. Diss. Univ. Halle. A. Busch, Ermsleben am Halle, Germany, 1882

BRONCHIAL CARCINOID

Clinical Features

Bronchial carcinoid constitutes 85 percent of this group of neoplasms. Because 90 percent of bronchial carcinoids are located in the main stem or the lobar bronchi, symptoms of obstruction occur relatively early. The obstruction results in emphysema, atelectasis, and secondary inflammatory changes in the unventilated parts of the lung, ranging from pneumonitis to lung abscess, with cough in 90 percent of patients, dyspnea in 60 percent, and hemoptysis in 50 percent. Wheezing is common, and pleural pain occurs frequently. These symptoms, particularly minimal hemoptysis, may have been present for years at the time of diagnosis (Table 26-1). Carcinoid syndrome occurs in 2 to 3 percent of patients. Peripheral tumors may remain asymptomatic for many years and grow to large sizes. Eventually the neoplasm may be detected through a routine radiograph. In the experience of McCaughan, et al. (1985), such was the case in 63 of 124 patients with bronchial carcinoids or 51 percent of their series. Radiographs show a mass in 16 percent of patients or changes secondary to bronchial occlusion, such as an infiltrate, distension radiolucency, or atelectasis, in 30 percent (Altman, 1973) (Figs. 26-1 and 26-2). Computed tomography (CT) helps to delineate the tumor and to determine the extent of penetration beyond the bronchus (Fig. 26-3).

In 1954, Thorson, et al. described a clinical syndrome—carcinoid syndrome—characterized by attacks of flushing, tachycardia and faintness, abdominal pain and diarrhea, bronchospasm, and valvular disease of the right heart. After years of recurrent flushing, erythema and telangiectasias may develop on the face and the upper trunk. These features have been attributed to the effects of 5-hydroxytryptamine (serotonin), its precursor 5-hydroxytryptophan, its breakdown product 5-hydroxyindoleacetic acid, kallikrein, bradykinin, and various catecholamines released by the tumor. Carcinoid syndrome is most commonly associated with intestinal carcinoids; less commonly it has been described in association with a variety of other neoplasms, including bronchial carcinoid and small cell lung cancer. In a series of 76 patients with bronchial carcinoid reported by Todd, et al. (1980), carcinoid syndrome occurred in two instances, an incidence of 2.6 percent. It is more common in the presence of massive metastatic involvement of the liver, presumably because of a diminished ability to inactivate the vasoactive substances, particularly serotonin, by the liver. However, a large bronchial carcinoid (5 cm or greater in diameter) or multiple lesions may cause these symptoms by synthesizing enough hormone to overcome the mechanisms of hepatic degradation. Accordingly, liver metastases are not an essential prerequisite for the occurrence of this syndrome in patients with bronchial carcinoid (Wareing and Sawyers, 1983).

Table 26-1. Symptoms and Signs in 47 Patients with Bronchial Carcinoids

Symptoms and Signs	No. Patients
Respiratory infection	24
Hemoptysis	16
Routine radiographic finding	15
Mass	4
Changes secondary to bronchial occlusion	11
Cough	14
Atelectasis	4
Pleural pain	4
Sputum	3
Dyspnea	3
Stridor	1

The lung is also capable of detoxifying serotonin because of its high content of monoamine oxidase (Ginsberg, et al., 1989). Because some patients with carcinoids, not necessarily those associated with the carcinoid syndrome, have been found to have high serum levels of serotonin and the products of its metabolism in their urine, it has been suggested that patients with suspected bronchial carcinoids be screened for the presence of these substances in their blood and urine (Ginsberg, et al., 1989). Our experience with such screening has been totally negative, albeit limited (and so has mine!—R.J.G.)

Pathology

Bronchial carcinoid belongs to the neuroendocrine group of tumors, the amine precursor uptake decarboxylase (APUD)

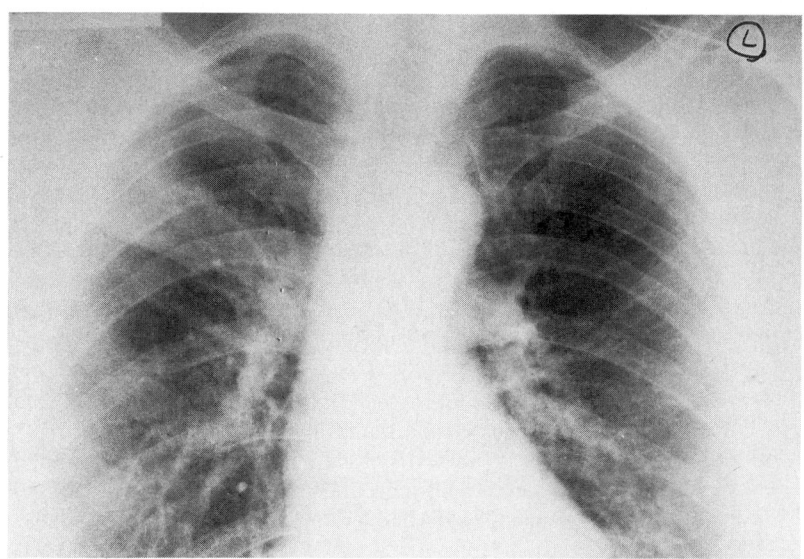

Figure 26-1. Radiograph of a 41-year-old man with typical carcinoid in the right upper lobe, causing pneumonitis, which was treated by sleeve lobectomy.

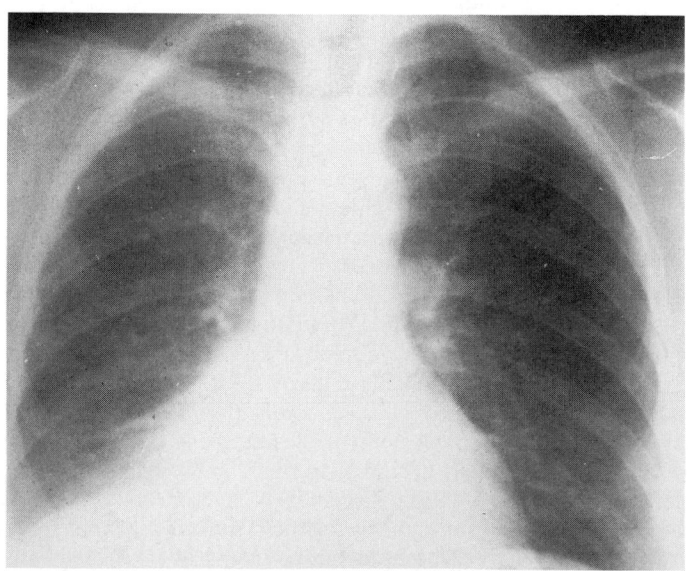

Figure 26-2. Typical carcinoid causing obstruction and atelectasis of the right lower lobe in a 33-year-old woman, which was treated by lobectomy.

Figure 26-3. CT of a 42-year-old man showing carcinoid of the trachea, just above the carina, which was treated by sleeve resection of three tracheal rings.

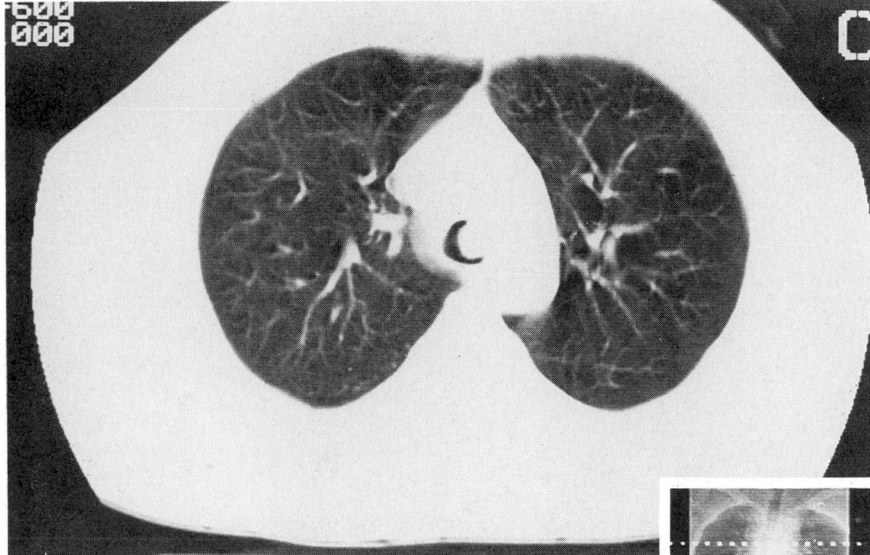

tumors, and it arises from the Kulchitzky cell of the respiratory epithelium. Most bronchial carcinoids are covered by an intact mucosa, with only a small part of the tumor protruding into the bronchial lumen, resembling the distribution found in an iceberg. A major part of the tumor grows extraluminally and penetrates the surrounding lung tissue (Fig. 26-4). More than 90 percent are located in the lobar or mainstem bronchi; less than 10 percent are peripheral (Fig. 26-5). Engelbreth-Holm (1944) and von Albertini (1951) recognized a group of carcinoids with atypical histologic features and introduced a concept of atypical bronchial carcinoid. This concept was later expanded when it was shown that carcinoids and small cell lung cancers belong to the same group of APUDomas arising from Kulchitzky cell of the bronchial mucosa (Bensch, et al., 1968; Toker, 1966). According to Yessner (1983), "the carcinoid should be considered a sibling of the small cell carcinoma, slow and mild-mannered, but occasionally packing a mean gene." Paladugu, et al. (1985) named this group of neoplasms Kulchitzky cell

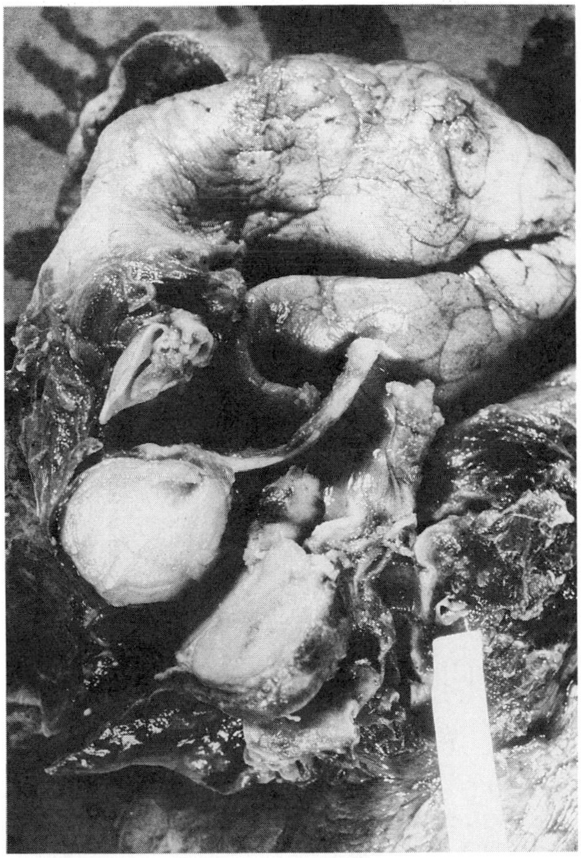

Figure 26-4. Resected bronchial carcinoid. The main bulk of the tumor is extraluminal.

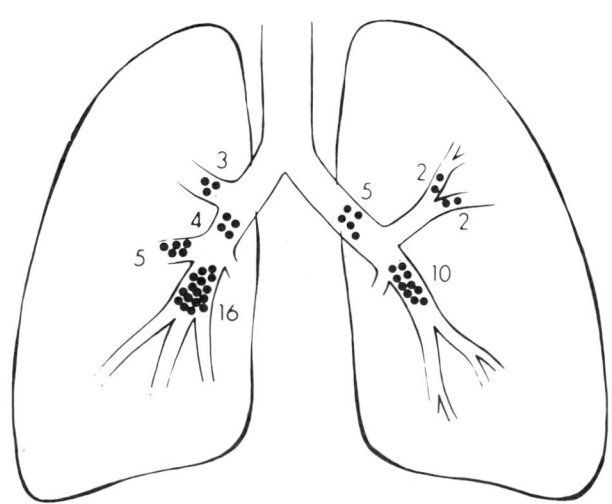

Figure 26-5. Anatomic distribution of 47 bronchial carcinoids.

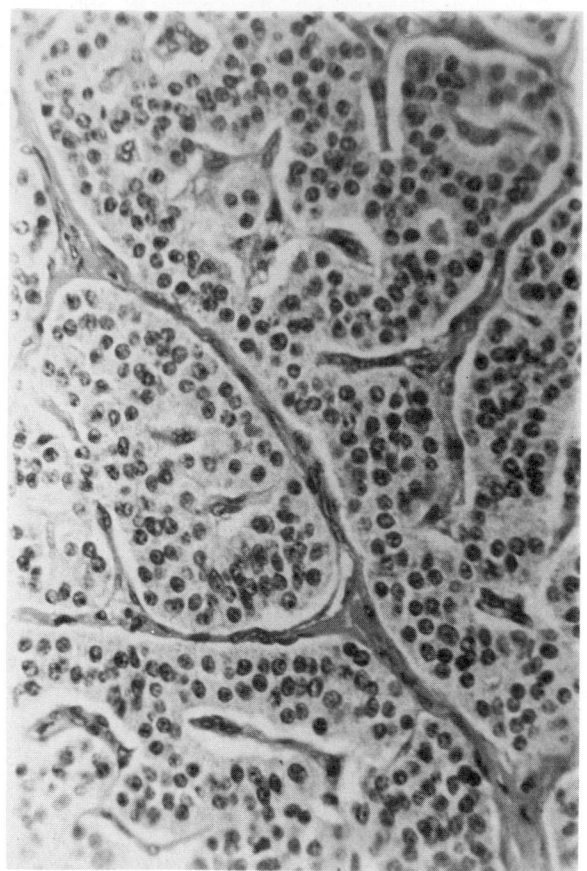

Figure 26-6. Carcinoid of the typical variety, or KCC-I. Uniform polyhedral cells are separated by a thin fibrovascular stroma.

carcinomas (KCC) and, to indicate their spectrum of malignancy, classified them into three groups, designating the typical carcinoid as KCC-I, the atypical carcinoid as KCC-II, and the small cell lung carcinoma as KCC-III. This classification reflects well the relationship among carcinoids of various degrees of malignancy and small cell undifferentiated carcinoma of the lung (Benfield, 1990).

The more common "typical" carcinoid or KCC-I (90 percent of bronchial carcinoids) has a low malignant potential (Fig. 26-6). It is composed of round or polygonal cells that exhibit little pleomorphism. The nuclei are relatively small and contain stippled or finely dispersed chromatin. Mitoses are rare. The cells are arranged in cords or solid clusters (Warren, et al., 1989). Although local invasion is common, it metastasizes in only 5 to 6 percent of instances, and the 5-year survival rate is more than 80 percent (Arrigoni, et al., 1972; Jensik, et al., 1974; O'Grady, et al., 1970) (Fig. 26-7).

The more aggressive atypical variant or KCC-II (10 percent) is characterized by increased cellularity, variability in the size and shape of the cells, a polymorphous nuclear configuration, and moderate mitotic activity with an average of one mitosis per one or two high-power fields (Fig. 26-8). According to Arrigoni, et al. (1972), this tumor metastasizes in 70 percent of patients, and the 5-year survival rate is 57 percent. In their series 30 percent of patients died as a result of the tumor; they survived an average of 27 months after resection. Accordingly, the carcinoid cannot be properly referred to as an adenoma. Even the KCC-I grade is a cancerous growth, albeit slow growing, but subject to recurrence and metastasis. Referring to such lesions as carcinomas reflects their true nature and serves a useful clinical purpose (Benfield, 1990).

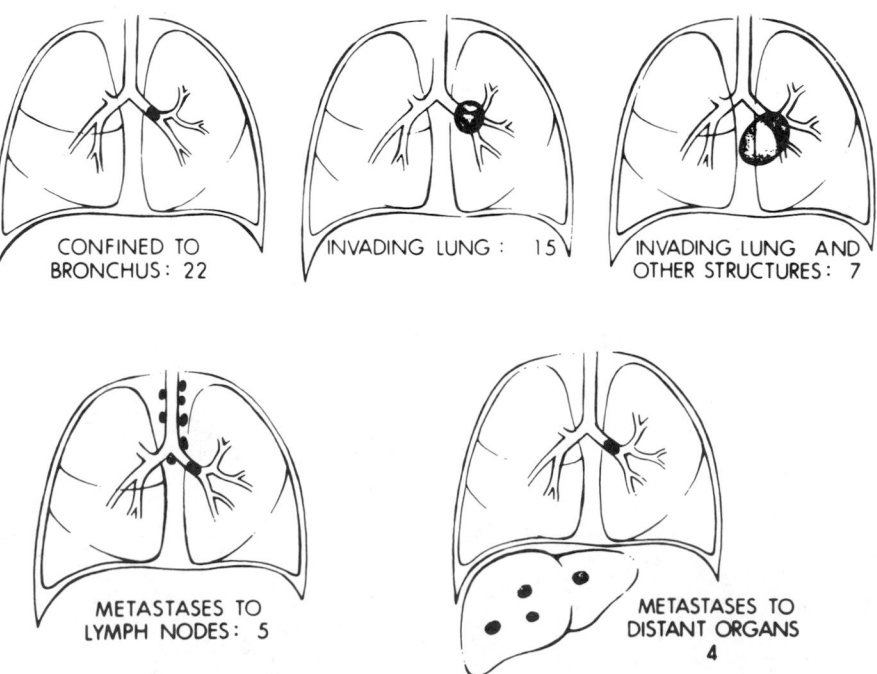

Figure 26-7. Pattern of dissemination in 47 patients with bronchial carcinoid.

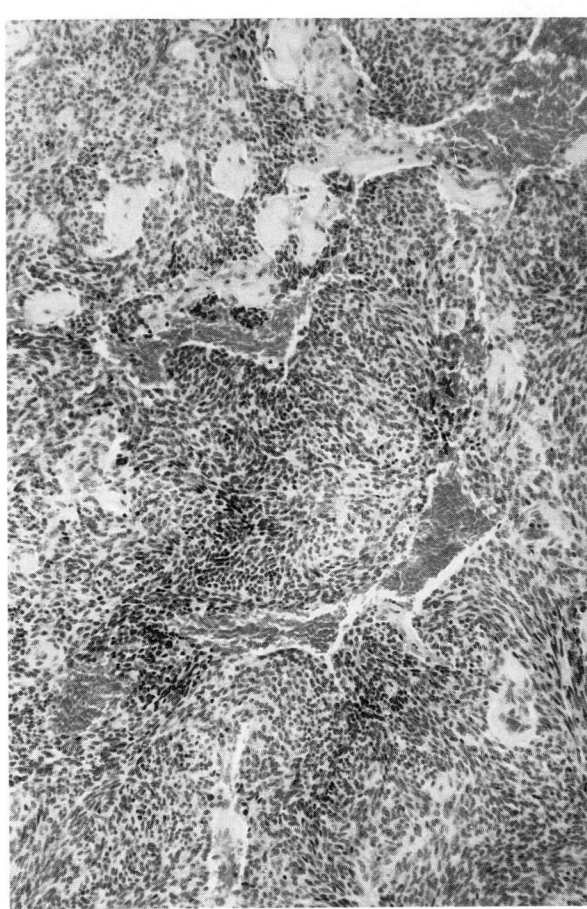

Figure 26-8. Atypical carcinoid (KCC-II). The cellular pleomorphism predominates. Nuclei are hyperchromatic and irregular (Grimelius stain, positive for argentaffin granules.)

Diagnosis

For intelligent planning of the most appropriate operation, a precise histologic diagnosis should be obtained ahead of time. Unfortunately, the diagnostic yield from the cytologic examination of bronchial washings or brushings is generally low, even in the presence of endobronchial disease (Chapleau, et al., 1991). Carcinoids located peripherally are rarely diagnosed prior to a thoracotomy unless needle aspiration biopsy is performed, and the examination of frozen sections of resected specimens differentiates carcinoid tumors from carcinomas in only 60 percent of cases (McCaughan, et al., 1985). A reliable tissue diagnosis is obtained at bronchoscopy. Most of these tumors are within the reach of the bronchoscope. The mucosa is usually intact and smooth, and the rich vascularity is not always apparent (Todd, et al., 1980). However, bleeding is frequent, and the biopsy specimen must be taken with caution. In my experience, moderate bleeding occurred in about 25 percent of patients, and I always have epinephrine spray on hand. Blood transfusion or emergency thoracotomy resulting from a biopsy has not been necessary in any of our patients; however, such catastrophes have been reported (Mark, 1980).

In discussing bronchoscopy, various authors stressed the superiority of either the rigid or the flexible bronchoscope (Todd, et al., 1980; McCaughan, et al., 1985). Both instruments are useful; each has advantages and limitations. The flexible bronchoscope reaches further into the bronchial tree, enabling the inspection and biopsy of peripheral lesions that are beyond the reach of the rigid intrument. Through the rigid bronchoscope, larger biopsy specimens can be obtained, a difference that may be of crucial importance. Bleeding is also easier to control through the open-tube instrument, should it occur.

Therapy and Prognosis

Resection

Resection is the only effective therapy for bronchial carcinoids. All neoplastic tissue must be excised, with the relief of the airway obstruction and the preservation of as much normal pulmonary parenchyma as possible.

Endoscopic Resection. Endoscopic resection, common in the past and still tempting because of the relatively slight trauma that it inflicts, does not fulfill these conditions. Most of these tumors are largely extraluminal, and endobronchial resection leaves the main bulk of the neoplasm behind. McCaughan, et al. (1985) performed six endobronchial resections, all in elderly patients with limited pulmonary reserve and a centrally located tumor. The resections were supplemented by transbronchoscopic implantation of radioactive seeds in three instances; one patient also received chemotherapy. There were local recurrences in four of the six patients, and one of these subsequently developed hepatic metastases and the carcinoid syndrome. Thus endobronchial resection cannot be recommended as a curative procedure. An exception to this rule is a small, pedunculated, and entirely intraluminal tumor. Such cases, however, are very rare. Another exception is a patient with contraindications to a thoracotomy. Any patient with a major bronchial occlusion caused by a carcinoid tumor who cannot tolerate a thoracotomy should have the airway opened, even if the resection is not complete. However, it must be remembered that the rich vascularity of carcinoids renders the piecemeal removal of these tumors through the bronchoscope extremely hazardous and may result in catastrophic bleeding. In these cases transbronchoscopic destruction of the neoplastic tissue, using diathermy fulguration (McCaughan, et al., 1985) or modern laser techniques (Brutinel, et al., 1987; Goldberg, et al., 1986; Personne, et al., 1986) opens the airway with much greater safety, but a cure would be most unusual.

Bronchotomy. Because bronchial carcinoids are locally invasive, resection aimed at a cure must encompass the tumor in its entirety. As a result of their slow-growing potential and low incidence of metastatic spread, conservative lung-saving operations should be used whenever possible. With the chest open, palpation of the bronchus permits a determination of the extent of growth. If the neoplasm is entirely endobronchial and pedunculated, bronchotomy with local excision may suffice, provided the frozen sections show that the resection was indeed complete (Goldman, 1958).

To ensure the completeness of resection, we are not satisfied with the transsection of the pedicle but always excise

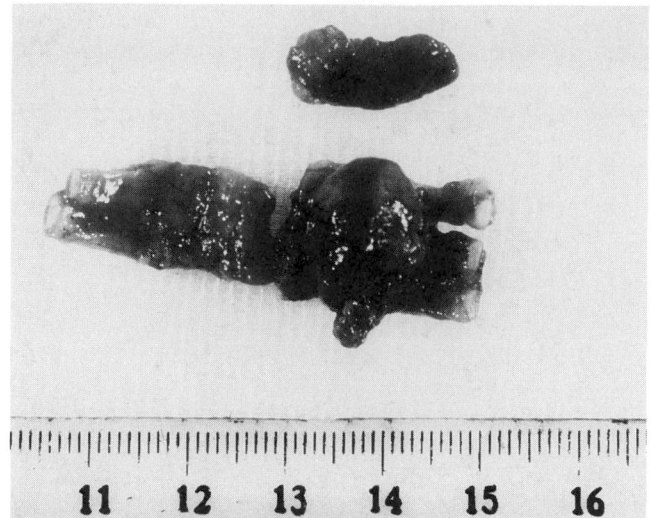

Figure 26-9. Small intraluminal carcinoid resected with a sleeve of bronchus.

such limited growths with a part of the bronchial wall, usually segments of one or two cartilage rings ("window" resection), and close the window by an approximation of the edges. The main bronchi render themselves amenable to such local excisions. Of the 22 patients in whom the tumor was confined to the bronchus, 6, who had pedunculated tumors, underwent this type of window resection; 16 others, all with sessile tumors, were treated by resection of a bronchial sleeve, without lung tissue (Fig. 26-9). During a follow-up period ranging from 2 to 19 years, there were no recurrences in this group of patients (Table 26-2).

Formal Resection. Most carcinoids are not limited to the bronchial wall. The location of the tumor and its extent, particularly its invasion of extrabronchial tissues and the presence of metastases in the lymph nodes, dictate the magnitude and type of resection, always done while attempting to conserve normal lung tissue.

Segmental or wedge resections are indicated for small nodules located peripherally, usually beyond the origins of the tertiary bronchi (Ginsberg, et al., 1989). These as a rule are easily palpable under the visceral pleura. To qualify for such a limited resection, the nodule should not exceed 3 cm in diameter. McCaughan, et al. (1985) noted that excision of larger carcinoids by the same conservative method increases the probability of recurrence markedly. They also pointed

Table 26-2. Type of Resection in 47 Patients with Bronchial Carcinoids

Resection	No. Patients
Window	6
Sleeve	16
Wedge or segment	6
Lobectomy	13
Sleeve lobectomy	3
Pneumonectomy	3

to a higher incidence of recurrence for atypical carcinoids and when lymph node metastases were present. In these patients segmental or wedge resections are contraindicated, and a formal lobectomy should be performed. Applying these principles to our patients, we performed segmental or wedge resections in six patients only, all for typical carcinoids (KCC-I) less than 3 cm in diameter (Table 26-2).

Lobectomy, considered by most authorities the standard resection for the majority of carcinoids (Attar, et al., 1985; McCaughan, et al., 1985; Okike, et al., 1976; Ginsberg, et al., 1989; Todd, et al., 1980) was performed in 13 patients. Certainly no lesser procedure should be considered for a KCC-II atypical carcinoid. We treated three such patients in the lobectomy group. Sleeve lobectomy was performed in three patients in whom the tumor was adjacent to the orifice of the lobar bronchus.

The indications for a pneumonectomy are exceptional, and this operation should be avoided, whenever possible. Nevertheless, we performed pneumonectomy on three occasions as follows: in two patients, because of extensive damage to the lung tissue distal to the lesion, and in one, because the extrabronchial extension of the neoplasm with invasion of the pulmonary artery precluded sleeve resection.

The merits of bronchoplastic operations for carcinoid are controversial. One extreme view was expressed by Åberg, et al. (1981), who presented evidence that, although the results of parenchyma-saving operations initially equaled those of a standard lobectomy, the prognosis deteriorated precipitously after 7 years, and 20 years postoperatively, the actuarial survival rate was only 15 percent. These authors concluded that lung-saving operations cannot be said to be radical, and in a choice between a bronchoplastic procedure and pneumonectomy, the latter is better. Not as radical a view was presented by McCaughan, et al. (1985), who recommended the more conservative procedures only when a preoperative pulmonary assessment precluded conventional resection. On the other hand, Jensik, et al. (1974) performed bronchoplastic procedures in 23 (70 percent) of a series of 33 patients with bronchial carcinoids. The recurrence rate was extremely low, and the survival rate by the life-table method was 86 percent at 5 years. Likewise, Okike, et al. (1978) performed conservative bronchoplastic operations on 16 of 181 patients with typical (KKC-I) carcinoids, with no recurrences. The merits of parenchyma-saving conservative operations have been stressed also by many others (Spencer, 1974; Weisel, 1974). More recently, Pairolero, et al. (1989) stated in support of this view, that in contrast to resections of bronchogenic carcinoma, a margin of resection of as little as 0.5 cm beyond the gross lesion is satisfactory.

Accumulating experience confirms that conservative sleeve resections are adequate for the complete removal of all disease; they permit the preservation of distal functioning pulmonary parenchyma. More often than not, sleeve resection is an alternative to pneumonectomy and should be performed whenever feasible (Okike, et al., 1978; Todd, et al., 1980; Ginsberg, et al., 1989). However, frozen-section examination of the resection margins is mandatory in every case. It must not be dismissed lightly just because gross findings seem to indicate the adequacy of the resection. Surgeons have used such shortcuts in the past, only to discover later that malignant cells were left behind. The use of a pleural flap to wrap around the anastomosis adds to the safety by helping to prevent dehiscence.

Conservatism notwithstanding, the operation for a potentially malignant tumor should be radical. The incidence of metastases to the regional lymph nodes in patients with bronchial carcinoid ranges from 5 percent (Todd, et al., 1980) to 18 percent (Turnbull, et al., 1972). McCaughan, et al. (1985) reported disease-free survival rates of 74 percent and 53 percent at 5 and 10 years, respectively, in patients with nodal metastases, compared with 96 percent and 84 percent, respectively, in those without metastatic disease. They also listed lymphatic metastases as one of the three most important risk factors influencing prognosis. Accordingly lymph node examination by frozen section should be done at the time of the operation, followed by a complete nodal dissection if metastases are found (Ginsberg, et al., 1989). Smith (1969) advocated complete nodal dissections as a matter of routine.

Although typical bronchial carcinoid may grow to 6 cm in diameter or more, the prognosis of this tumor following complete resection is excellent. According to Jensik, et al. (1974), Todd, et al. (1980), and Warren, et al. (1989), the tumor can be resected with less than 5-mm bronchial margins without the risk of local recurrence. Chapleau, et al. (1991) reported on 41 patients with bronchial carcinoids. There were 37 resections with 1 early postoperative death and 1 major surgery-related complication. The mean follow-up was 8 years, with the probability of survival being 97 percent at 5 years and 92 percent at 10 years. None of the patients treated for a peripheral tumor died, but there were two deaths among patients who had centrally located tumors with both transbronchial invasion and lymph node metastases. There was no relationship between the tumor's size and the prognosis.

Although distant metastases of a typical bronchial carcinoid are not common, they do occur. Warren and Gould (1990) studied 27 patients with typical bronchial carcinoids. The resection was conservative in 15 patients. Lymph node metastases were identified at surgery in two instances. Distant metastases were confirmed in two patients. After adjuvant radiotherapy and chemotherapy, one patient died of unrelated causes 10 years after the operation, and the other was alive at the 19-year follow-up. Thus, the presence of distant metastases does not preclude long-term survial. This contrasts sharply with the prognosis of the atypical bronchial carcinoid (KCC-II). This neoplasm metastasizes in 70 percent of patients, and the average survival after resection is only 27 months, with the 5- and 10-year survival rates of 69 percent and 52 percent, respectively, compared with 100 percent and 87 percent for KCC-I (Arrigoni, et al., 1972; McCaughan, et al., 1985).

Radiotherapy

Bronchial carcinoids are not sensitive to radiotherapy. Although favorable responses to irradiation in three patients were reported by Baldwin and Grimes (1967) one-quarter of a century ago, there is no other evidence that radiotherapy is of any value. In the absence of other reports on the radiosensitivity of these tumors, it is difficult to repress doubts about the correctness of the diagnosis in those three patients.

Thus, only palliative radiotherapy may be considered for nonresectable carcinoids or after incomplete resections.

Chemotherapy

Metastatic carcinoid tumors are uniformly fatal, and the experience with chemotherapy is limited. Goodwin (1980) reported an average survival of 2 years from the time of diagnosis of hepatic metastases. Ajani, et al. (1983) reported a 38 percent response rate with combinations of 5-fluorouracil, doxorubicin, and cyclophosphamide and a 22 percent response rate with combinations of doxorubicin, mitomycin C, and semustine. Engstrom, et al. (1984) reported a 32 percent response rate with streptozocin, 5-fluorouracil, and doxorubicin, with an overall survival of 21 months. A 40 percent symptom-free response rate with the subcutaneous administration of interferon for 1 year was observed by Hansen, et al. (1989). When interferon was combined with the embolization of hepatic metastases, the symptom-free response was 85 percent. Unfortunately, all these responses were short-lived, and overall chemotherapy for metastatic carcinoids appears disappointing (Moertel and Hanley, 1979; Moertel, 1983).

Therapy for Carcinoid Syndrome

Drug treatment of the carcinoid syndrome is applicable at three levels:

1. Inhibitors of serotonin synthesis, which include parachlorophenylalanine and α-methyldopa
2. Inhibitors of the release or the action of serotonin and of histamine, which include methysergide, methotrimeprazine, chlorpromazine, cyproheptadine, and somatostatin
3. Inhibitors of kallikrein, which include aprotonin and corticosteroids

However, the most effective treatment of the carcinoid syndrome is the resection of all resectable tumor-bearing tissue. This should be done whenever possible, even in the presence of metastases.

ADENOID CYSTIC CARCINOMA

In 1859 Theodor Billroth described a new tumor of the lacrimal gland and, because of the peculiar tubular arrangement of the cords of cells, coined the term *cylindroma*. The first description of the same neoplasm in the bronchus was that of Heschl in 1877. The unfortunate term *cylindroma* persisted for more than a century, causing much confusion by ignoring its malignant potential.

This tumor is encountered most commonly in the trachea and major bronchi, arising from mucus-secreting cells. Its occurrence in the peripheral parts of the lung is exceptional (Reddy, 1977; Inouse, et al., 1991).

Pathology

The cause of adenoid cystic carcinoma is unknown. The neoplasm is composed of small darkly staining cells arranged in cords or nests, separated from one another by a stroma of relatively acellular and avascular connective tissue with areas of vacuolization, producing a cribriform appearance (Fig. 26-10). It extends locally by direct infiltration into the submucosa, far beyond the visible and palpable confines, and into the perineural lymphatic channels (Collis, et al., 1976; Spencer, 1985; Mark, 1983). At the time of diagnosis, local spread has already taken place in the majority of patients. Adjacent organs may be invaded directly. However, the rate of growth is slow, and distant metastases occur late, most often to the liver, bone, kidneys, lungs, brain, and skin (Cleveland, et al., 1977; Ladefoged, et al., 1984; Spencer, 1985).

Diagnosis

The symptoms are related to upper airway obstruction, with wheezing, stridor, and hoarseness reported most frequently, followed by cough, hemoptysis, and recurrent pulmonary infection. Symptoms suggestive of asthma are often simulated, contributing to the diagnostic delays (Hajdu, et al., 1970; Cleveland, et al., 1977; Grillo, 1983). When the tumor is located in the trachea, the symptoms may occur late because the large lumen of the trachea prevents early occlusion. Belsey (1950) determined that 75 percent of the trachea must be occluded before symptoms occur (Fig. 26-11).

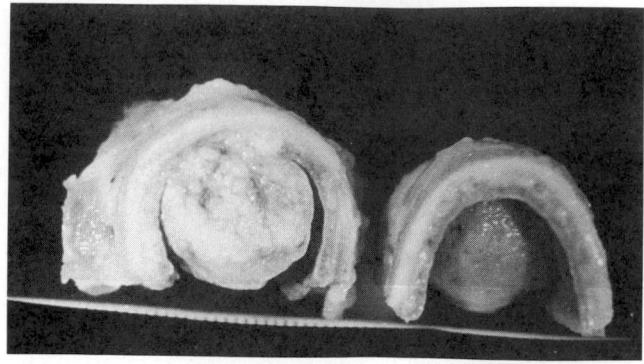

Figure 26-11. Resected specimen of the trachea occluded almost totally by adenoid cystic carcinoma. The patient breathed until his operation, albeit with difficulty. If necessary, preoperative laser ablation is preferable to intraluminal stenting.

At bronchoscopy, adenoid cystic carcinoma appears to be a circumscribed mass covered with pink epithelium, which is usually intact but occasionally ulcerated. The biopsy findings provide the diagnosis. Excessive bleeding is not a problem. CT helps to determine the extent of extraluminal growth. However, it is not entirely reliable because it does not reveal

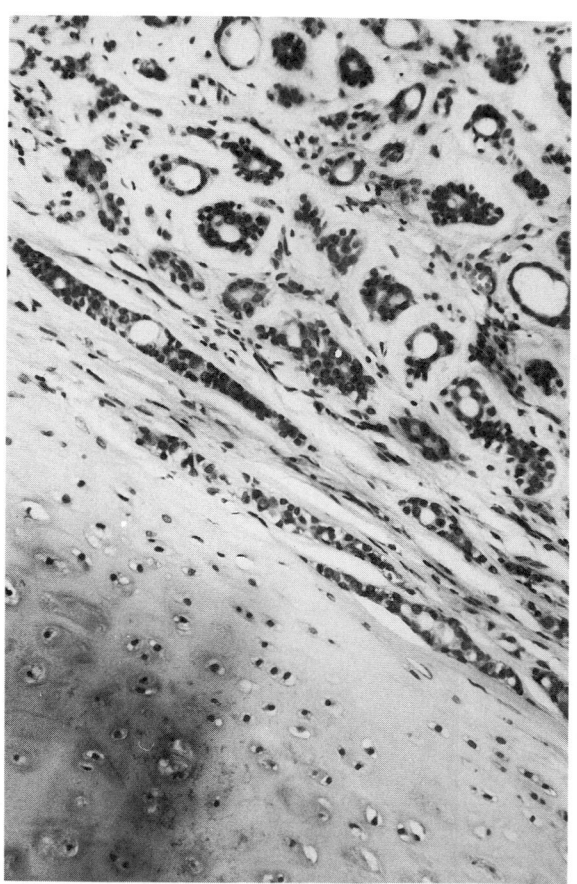
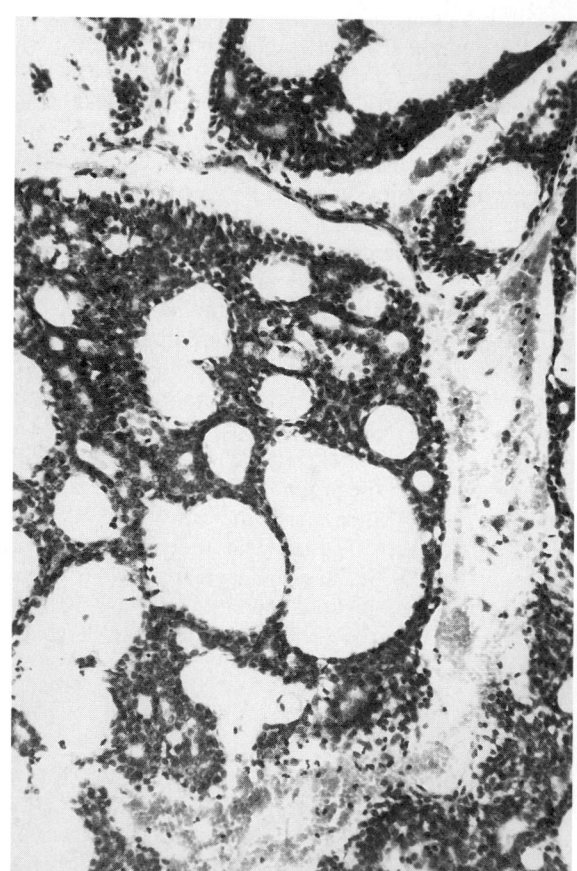

A

B

Figure 26-10. Microscopic appearance of adenoid cystic carcinoma. **(A)** Low-power magnification. **(B)** High-power magnification.

submucosal and perineural spread. This can be determined only by frozen-section examination of the resected specimen.

Therapy

Resection

Only complete surgical resection provides the chance of a cure. Assessment of the cardiovascular and pulmonary status is indicated, particularly in elderly patients and in those in whom major pulmonary or tracheal resection is contemplated. The completeness of the excision must be verified by frozen-section examination of the surgical margins, with special attention paid to the submucosa and perineural lymphatic channels, in which invasion is notorious (Conlan, et al., 1978).

The extent of resection depends on the location and extent of the tumor. Frist, et al. (1987), Lowe, et al. (1982), Pearson, et al. (1974), and many others reported successful resections of the trachea and carina. They achieved excellent results using direct anastomoses. The insertion of prosthetic materials to replace segments of the trachea resulted commonly in erosions of the innominate artery, leading to death, and these materials should be avoided whenever possible (Pearson, et al., 1974, 1984). With adequate mobilization of the trachea, we have resected segments up to 6 cm in length, with primary anastomosis; segments up to 8 cm without the use of prosthetic materials have been resected by Grillo and Mathisen (1990) and by Pearson (personal communication, 1992). For tumors arising in lobar or mainstem bronchi, lobectomy, sleeve resection of the bronchus, or a sleeve lobectomy are appropriate and should be planned ahead of time to preserve functioning lung tissue.

The presence of metastases in the regional lymph nodes does not preclude long-term survival and even cure, if the resection is complete. For this reason, dissection of the regional lymph nodes must be performed routinely.

Metastatic spread or the cardiorespiratory status of the patient may render a complete resection of the neoplasm impossible. In this situation, incomplete resection aimed at debulking and opening the airways, supplemented by radiotherapy for residual disease, may prolong the patient's life for several years. An alternative palliative treatment is bronchoscopic removal of the obstructing lesion, using biopsy forceps, or destruction of the tumor, using diathermy or the new laser techniques. Neither treatment is curative, but the prolongation of life and improvement in the quality of life can be significant (Brutinel, et al., 1987; Conlan, et al., 1978; Goldberg, et al., 1986; Leonardi, et al., 1978; Personne, et al., 1986). These endoscopic techniques may play a role also in the treatment of a locally recurrent tumor following prior resection or radiotherapy (Stuart-Harris and McCaughan, 1988).

As an alternative endotracheal and endobronchial stents may be used for palliation. Such stents should be biologically inert and easily tolerated by the patient. Spiral-reinforced models may offer an advantage by permitting flexibility and patency for many months. Various methods of their introduction have been pioneered by Clarke (1980), Orlowski (1987), Orlowski and Kolodziej (1986), Westably, et al. (1982), Wes-

taby (1983), and others. As a general rule, these prostheses are introduced endoscopically and should be stabilized in place to prevent early or late displacement.

Radiotherapy

The radiosensitivity of adenoid cystic carcinoma is low, but it has been shown that radical radiotherapy may induce tumor regression. Rarely cures have been reported. Vieta and Maier (1957) noted that the 5-year survival rates were nearly identical in patients treated surgically and those irradiated. Pearson, et al. (1974) used radiotherapy preoperatively to ablate small microscopic foci of the tumor that otherwise might remain after resection; Grillo (1982) advocated postoperative radiotherapy when there was tumor close to the resection margins and in presence of local lymphatic or perineural invasion.

Radiotherapy should be used in patients in whom a complete resection is not possible and for recurrences. Irradiation alone is indicated only in those patients who for medical reasons are considered inoperable (Turnbull, et al., 1972).

Chemotherapy

Of various chemotherapeutic regimens tried for adenoid cystic carcinoma, none is known to be effective (Jakobsson and Eneroth, 1970; Spiro, et al., 1974).

Prognosis

The prognosis depends on complete gross and microscopic clearance of all neoplastic tissue. Only when this is achieved, can cure be expected. Otherwise, local recurrence is the rule. The malignant potential of adenoid cystic carcinoma is reflected by the poor survival rates. In the series of Enterline and Schoenberg (1954), of 49 patients with adequate follow-up information, only 34 percent were living and apparently cured. Of 65 patients reported by Smout and French (1961), 51 were either dead or alive with disease. Because of the slow-growing potential, the 5-year survival rates of adenoid cystic carcinoma are not a reliable indicator of cure (Conlan, et al., 1978). Long-term survival with persistent disease is not unusual, and recurrences have been reported as late as 25 years after seemingly adequate resection (Grover, 1974). According to Grillo (1982), 10 to 15 years of observation are needed to establish final results.

MUCOEPIDERMOID CARCINOMA

Mucoepidermoid carcinoma of the tracheobronchial tree is an uncommon tumor. Conlan, et al. (1978) collected 55 cases from the literature up to 1973 and added 12 patients of their own. More recently Yousem and Hochholzer (1987) found 58 cases in the files of the Armed Forces Institute of Pathology, and Heitmiller, et al. (1989) reported on 18 patients from the Massachusetts General Hospital. Thus, the rarity of this neoplasm may have been exaggerated in the past. It has been reported in all age groups, from children 6 to 7 years old (Archer, et al., 1987; El-Jabbour, et al., 1986) to elderly patients, with the majority of patients in the fourth and fifth decades of life. The sex distribution is equal.

Pathology

The tumor arises from the minor salivary glands lining the tracheobronchial tree. It has a smooth well-circumscribed appearance, growing from a localized area into the bronchial lumen and gradually causing its occlusion (Conlan, et al., 1978). The overwhelming majority of these neoplasms have been found in the proximal tracheobronchial tree, down to the lobar bronchi. In a series of 67 mucoepidermoid tumors collected by Breyer, et al. (1980), only 3 lesions were located in the more distal airways. A single case of a peripheral mucoepidermoid tumor, not associated with an airway, was reported recently by Green, et al. (1991). Mucoepidermoid tumors arise from a single cell type but are differentiated along either the squamous or glandular type or both (Heitmiller, et al., 1989). In their final form, they are composed of a mixture of cell types, which includes squamous cells with keratinization, mucin-producing cells lining cystic spaces, and intermediate cells arranged in nests or cords. Their mitotic activity ranges from none detectable to 20 mitoses per 10 high-power fields (Heitmiller, et al., 1989). On the basis of mitotic activity, cellular necrosis, and nuclear pleomorphism, they were classified by Conlan, et al. (1978) into three grades of malignancy. Heitmiller, et al. (1989) advocated a simpler division into low- and high-grade tumors, which is now more widely accepted. This division correlates better with the operative assessment of tumor agressiveness and the prognosis. The high-grade variant metastasizes to regional lymph nodes and by hematogenous spread. The low-grade tumor can infiltrate the bronchial wall but does not invade vessels and does not metastasize (Ginsberg, et al., 1989).

The differential diagnosis includes adenosquamous carcinoma with which mucoepidermoid tumors are most easily confused (Heitmiller, et al., 1989; Yousem and Hochholzer, 1987).

Diagnosis

The most common symptoms are those of bronchial irritation and obstruction and include coughing, wheezing, hemoptysis, pneumonia, and atelectasis. Weight loss, malaise, and pain reflect the aggressiveness of the high-grade variant (Heitmiller, et al., 1989; Turnbull, et al., 1972).

Chest radiographs may show a pulmonary nodule or mass or postobstruction pneumonia or atelectasis; they may appear normal if the neoplasm is centrally located and does not cause an obstruction. The central location of most mucoepidermoid carcinomas facilitates bronchoscopic assessment. The usual appearance is that of a circumscribed and polypoid tumor. Biopsy is safe, usually diagnostic, and of great importance. It enables a correlation between the histologic grade of the neoplasm and its clinical behavior (Breyer, et al., 1980). A histologic diagnosis of a low-grade tumor points to a localized lesion without metastases; a diagnosis of a high-grade neoplasm should alert the surgeon to the probability of an invasive tumor necessitating an extensive resection. CT is valuable in determining the extent of extraluminal growth.

Therapy and Prognosis

Low-grade mucoepidermoid carcinomas should be completely excised, preserving as much normal lung tissue as possible. For most patients this usually means a lobectomy; however, the final decision regarding the extent of resection depends on the operative findings. For a small polypoid lesion, simple bronchotomy with local excision may suffice. The use of bronchoplastic lung-saving resections is of great value; however, the completeness of resection must never be sacrificed for the sake of conservatism. Various bronchoplastic procedures were used in 9 of 16 patients reported by Heitmiller, et al. (1989) and in 4 of 5 patients described by Breyer, et al. (1980) with excellent results. Lymph nodes should always be sampled. If the resection is complete, the prognosis is excellent, and no other treatment is indicated. However, a long-term follow-up is essential.

High-grade tumors should be treated as bronchogenic carcinomas. The prognosis in these patients depends on the tumor's invasiveness and the surgeon's achieving tumor-free surgical margins. Of 13 patients with high-grade tumors treated by resection by Yousem and Hochholzer (1987), 4 patients died, and 1 had a recurrence, for which a second resection had to be performed. The series of Heitmiller, et al. (1989) included 3 patients with high-grade invasive tumors. They all died within 11 to 16 months after their operations. Turnbull, et al. (1972) treated 12 patients with various stages of mucoepidermoid carcinomas. Excluding 2 patients who were admitted with terminal disease, the average survival of the 10 treated patients was 5.3 months.

Radiotherapy and chemotherapy were used for nonresectable lesions (Heitmiller, et al., 1989; Turnbull, et al., 1972) but were not shown to be of any value.

BRONCHIAL MUCOUS GLAND ADENOMA

Mucous gland adenoma of the bronchus is a rare tumor, with only 20 cases reported in the English literature (Allen, et al., 1974; Emory, et al., 1973; Key and Pritchett, 1979).

Pathology

This is a truly benign neoplasm that merits the term *adenoma*. The tumor is nearly always confined to the major bronchi and is easily accessible at bronchoscopy. It arises from mucous glands of the main or lobar bronchi, grows into the lumen of the airway, and is covered by intact bronchial epithelium. The neoplasm may cause bronchial obstruction; however, it does not penetrate the bronchial cartilage and does not invade surrounding tissues. The cut surface of the tumor is soft, with numerous microcysts exuding thick mucoid material. The glandular spaces are lined by well-differentiated cuboidal or columnar cells similar to the bronchial mucous glands from which the tumor originates. There are no mitoses.

Diagnosis

The radiographs may appear normal, there may be nodular density, or in the case of bronchial obstruction, distal atelec-

Figure 26-12. Computed tomographic scan (upper chest section) showing pleomorphic adenoma (mixed tumor) in the trachea. The tumor was resected with a short sleeve of the trachea.

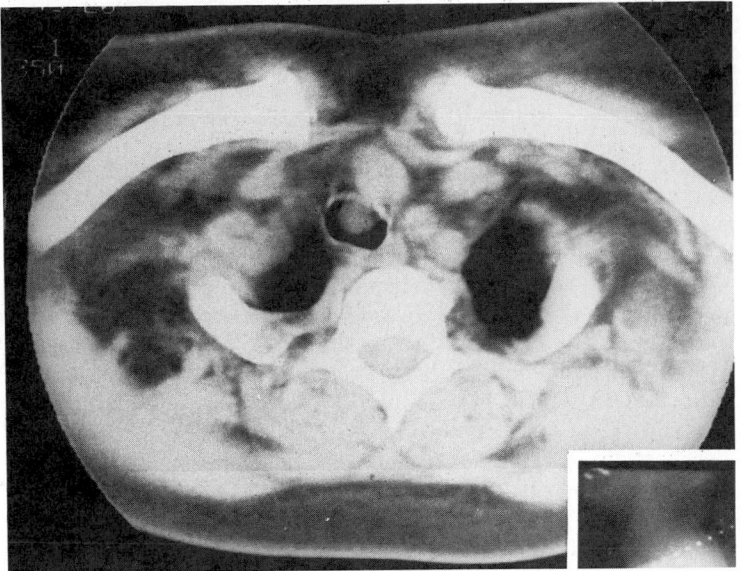

tasis with secondary inflammatory changes may be seen. Bronchoscopy with biopsy is diagnostic.

Therapy

The tumor should be resected with maximum preservation of the functioning lung tissue. Depending on its location and size, lobectomy, sleeve resection, or local excision through a bronchotomy are most commonly indicated. Resection is curative, and the prognosis is excellent.

PLEOMORPHIC MIXED TUMOR

This neoplasm is similar to the pleomorphic adenoma of the salivary glands. In 1965, Payne, et al. described two such neoplasms in the bronchi. Both tumors were invasive. One recurred 8 years after resection and was treated by the excision of local recurrences. The patient was well 3 years later. The second patient was treated by a lobectomy and was well 11 years later. Pleomorphic mixed tumors of bronchi were also described by Davis, et al. (1972); Spener (1979); and Wright, et al. (1983). Ma, et al. (1979), in their review of the literature extending from 1922 to 1978, documented 13 such tumors in the trachea, where they appear to be more common. We encountered one such lesion in the trachea. It was not invasive (Figs. 26-12 and 26-13).

These neoplasms appear as polypoid or sessile masses; some show a tendency to invade. Microscopically they consist of epithelial and stromal components with varying degrees of differentiation. The epithelial cells are arranged in tubules or clusters of cells. Mitoses are infrequent.

Pleomorphic mixed tumors should be treated by wide surgical excision.

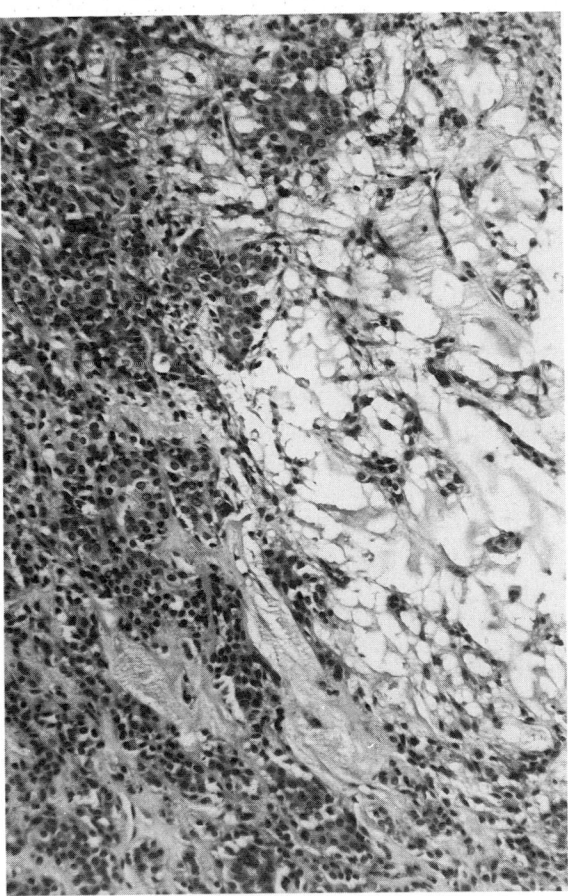

Figure 26-13. Photomicrograph of the tumor depicted in Figure 26-12 shows a mixture of glandular and squamoid elements.

COMMENTS AND CONTROVERSIES

These interesting group of tumors, previously designated as "bronchial adenomas," are, as Dr. Weissberg points out, best described as bronchial gland tumors. Other than mucous gland adenomas and pleomorphic adenomas, they all have malignant potential.

Bronchial carcinoids are by far the most common tumors and should be treated by conservative resection wherever possible. I have found that bronchoscopy can in many instances identify the fact that although the tumor presents itself in a major bronchus, in reality, its attachments are in a lobar bronchus, allowing for lobectomy rather than a more extended resection. Frozen-section analysis of the resection margin is imperative. Atypical carcinoids behave much like bronchogenic carcinoma with a similar prognosis. However, typical carcinoids—even with lymph node metastases—have an excellent prognosis as long as a complete lymph node dissection is performed. The KCC nomenclature only adds to the confusion and should be abolished. Carcinoids are not related to smoking, whereas "mean gene" SCLC is!

Adenoid cystic carcinomas belie their endoscopic appearance, often spreading along perineural lymphatics far beyond what can be appreciated endoscopically. They are one of the few tumors where an incomplete resection will afford excellent palliation when combined with postoperative radiotherapy, allowing a long-term survival despite tumor persistence. The reader is refered to Chapter 15 for further information regarding adenoid cystic carcinomas.

Mucoepidermoid tumors are rare. Frequently, pathologists will confuse these tumors with adenosquamous carcinomas. Despite this confusion, both tumors are malignant and should be treated in a similar fashion to nonsmall cell lung carcinoma.

Bronchial gland adenomas are really the only tumors in this group that can be considered for bronchoscopic removal.

R.J.G.

KEY REFERENCES

Paladugu RR, Benfield JR, Pak HY et al.: Bronchopulmonary Kulchitzky cell carcinomas. A new classification scheme for typical and atypical carcinoids. Cancer 55:1303, 1985

This is a classic work that puts in proper perspective the three neoplasms originating from the Kulchitzky cell. The name Kulchitzky cell carcinoma (KCC) reflects the overlap among these cancers; the division into KCC-I, -II, and -III indicates their spectrum of aggressiveness.

Thorson Å, Biörck G, Björkman G, Waldenström J: Malignant carcinoid of the small intestine with metastases to the liver, valvular disease of the right side of the heart (pulmonary stenosis and tricuspid regurgitation without septal defects), peripheral vasomotor symptoms, bronchoconstriction, and an unusual type of cyanosis. A clinical and pathological syndrome. Am Heart J 47;795, 1954

This is the first description of the full-blown carcinoid syndrome.

Yousem SA, Hochholzer L: Mucoepidermoid tumors of the lung. Cancer 60:1346, 1987

This is an extensive review of 58 patients with mucoepidermoid tumors confined to the lung, the largest series ever reported from a single institution. The useful histologic classification of the tumors into low- and high-grade variants correlates well with their clinical behavior.

REFERENCES

Åberg T, Blöndal T, Nõu E, Malmaeus J: The choice of operation for bronchial carcinoids. Ann Thorac Surg 32:19, 1981

Ajani JA, Legha SS, Karlu DA, Hill CS: Combination chemotherapy of metastatic tumors with 5-FU vs Adriamycin, Cytoxan and 5-FU vs Adriamycin, mitomycin C and methyl CCNU. Proc Am Assoc Clin Oncol 24;124,1983

Allen MS Jr, Marsh WL Jr, Geissinger WT: Mucous gland adenoma of the bronchus. J Thorac Cardiovasc Surg 67:966, 1974

Altman RC: Radiographic appearance of bronchial carcinoid. Thorax 28:443, 1973

Archer RL, Grogg SE, Sanders SP: Mucoepidermoid bronchial adenoma in a 6-year-old girl. J Thorac Cardiovasc Surg 94:452, 1987

Arrigoni MG, Woolner LB, Bernatz PE: Atypical carcinoid tumors of the lung. J Thorac Cardiovasc Surg 64:413, 1972

Attar S, Miller JE, Hankins J et al: Bronchial adenoma: a review of 51 patients. Ann Thorac Surg 40:126, 1985

Baldwin JN, Grimes OF: Bronchial adenomas. Surg Gynecol Obstet 124:813, 1967

Belsey R: Resection and reconstruction of the intrathoracic trachea. Br J Surg 38:200, 1950

Benfield JR: Neuroendocrine neoplasms of the lung. J Thorac Cardiovasc Surg 100:628, 1990

Bensch KG, Corrin B, Parients R, Spencer H: Oat-cell carcinoma of the lung. Its origin and relationship to bronchial carcinoid. Cancer 22:1163, 1968

Billroth T: Beobachtungen über Geschwulste der Speicheldrusen. Virchows Arch A Pathol Anat Histopathol 17:357, 1859

Breyer RH, Dainauskas JR, Jensik RJ, Faber LP: Mucoepidermoid carcinoma of the trachea and bronchus: the case for conservative resection. Ann Thorac Surg 29:197, 1980

Brutinel WM, Cortese DS, McDougal JC et al.: A two-year experience with the neodymium-YAG laser in endobronchial obstruction. Chest 91:159, 1987

Chapleau D, Pagé A, Verdant A et al.: Bronchial carcinoids: long-term prognostic factors. Can J Surg 34:111, 1991

Clarke DB: Palliative intubation of the trachea and main bronchi. J Thorac Cardiovasc Surg 80:736, 1980

Cleveland RH, Nice CM, Ziskind J: Primary adenoid cystic carcinoma (cylindroma) of the trachea. Radiology 122:597, 1977

Collis JL, Clarke DB, Smith RA: d'Abreu's Practice of Cardiothoracic Surgery. 4th Ed. Edward Arnold, London, 1976

Conlan AA, Payne WS, Woolner LB, Sanderson DR: Adenoid cystic carcinoma (cylindroma) and mucoepidermoid carcinoma of the bronchus. J Thorac Cardiovasc Surg 76:369, 1978

Davis PW, Briggs JC, Seal RM, Starring FK: Benign and malignant mixed tumours of the lung. Thorax 27:657, 1972

El-Jabbour JN, Slim MS, Bekdash B et al.: Bronchial mucoepidermoid tumor in childhood. Pediatr Surg Int 1:63, 1986

Emory WB, Mitchell WT Jr, Hatch HB Jr: Mucous gland adenoma of the bronchus. Am Rev Respir Dis 108:1407, 1973

Engelbreth-Holm J: Benign bronchial adenomas. Acta Chir Scand 90:383, 1944

Engstrom PF, Lavin PT, Moertel CG et al: Streptozocin + 5-FU vs doxorubicin therapy for metastatic carcinoid tumor. J Clin Oncol 2:1255,1984

Enterline HT, Schoenberg HW: Carcinoma (cylindromatous type) of trachea and bronchi and bronchial adenoma, a comparative study. Cancer 7:663, 1954

Frist WH, Mathisen DJ, Hilgenberg AD, Grillo HC: Bronchial sleeve resection with and without pulmonary resection. J Thorac Cardiovasc Surg 93:350, 1987

Ginsberg RJ, Shennib H, Paulson DL: Bronchial adenoma. p. 875. In Shields TW (ed): General Thoracic Surgery. 3rd Ed. Lea & Febiger, Philadelphia, 1989

Goldberg M, Ginsberg RJ, Basiuk JP: Endobronchial carbon-dioxide laser therapy. Can J Surg 29:180, 1986

Goldman A: Additional experiences in bronchotomy for bronchial adenoma. Ann Otol 67:1207, 1958

Goodwin JD: Carcinoid tumors: an analysis of 2837 cases. Cancer 45:104, 1980

Green LK, Gallion TL, Gyorkey F: Peripheral mucoepidermoid tumour of the lung. Thorax 46:65, 1991

Grillo HC: Tracheal tumors: diagnosis and management. p. 271. In Choi NC, Grillo HC (eds): Thoracic Oncology. Raven Press, New York, 1983

Grillo HC: Management of tracheal tumors. Am J Surg 143:697, 1982

Grillo HC, Mathisen DJ: Primary tracheal tumors: treatment and results. Ann Thorac Surg 49:69, 1990

Grover F: Discussion of Pearson et al. (1974). Ann Thorac Surg 18:27, 1974

Hajdu SI, Huvos AG, Goodner JT et al.: Carcinoma of the trachea. Clinicopathological study of 41 cases. Cancer 25:1448, 1970

Hansen LE, Schrumpf E, Klobenstvedt AN et al.: Recombinant alpha-2 interferon with or without hepatic artery embolization in the treatment of midgut carcinoid tumours. A preliminary report. Acta Oncol 28:439, 1989

Heitmiller RF, Mathisen DJ, Ferry JA et al.: Mucoepidermoid lung tumors. Ann Thorac Surg 47:394, 1989

Heschl R: Über ein Zylindrom der Lunge. Wien Med Wochenschr 17:385, 1877

Inoue H, Iwashita A, Kanegae H et al.: Peripheral pulmonary adenoid cystic carcinoma with substantial submucosal extension to the proximal bronchus. Thorax 46:147, 1991

Jakobsson PA, Eneroth CM: Variations in radiosensitivity of various types of malignant salivary-gland tumour. Acta Otolaryngol 263(suppl):186, 1970

Jensik RJ, Faber LP, Brown CM, Kittle CF: Bronchoplastic and conservative resectional procedures for bronchial adenoma. J Thorac Cardiovasc Surg 68:556, 1974

Key BM, Pritchett PS: Mucous gland adenoma of the bronchus. South Med J 72:83, 1979

Ladefoged C, Bisgaard C, Petri J: Solitary renal metastasis 23 years after extirpation of a bronchial adenoid cystic carcinoma. Scand J Thorac Cardiovasc Surg 18:245, 1984

Laennec RTH: Traité de L'Auscultation Médiate et des Maladies des Poumons et du Coeur. 3rd Ed. Chaud, Paris, 1831

Leonardi HK, Jung-Legg Y, Legg MA, Neptune WB: Tracheobronchial mucoepidermoid carcinoma: clinicopathological features and results of treatment. J Thorac Cardiovasc Surg 76:431, 1978

Lowe JE, Bridgman AH, Sabiston DC: The role of bronchoplastic procedures in the management of benign and malignant pulmonary lesions. J Thorac Cardiovasc Surg 83:272, 1982

Ma CK, Fine G, Lewis J, Lee MW: Benign mixed tumors of the trachea. Cancer 44:2260, 1979

Mark EJ: Pathology of tracheal neoplasms. In Choi NC, Grillo HC (eds): Thoracic Oncology. Raven Press, New York, 1983

Mark JBD: Discussion of Todd et al. J Thorac Cardiovasc Surg 79:535, 1980

McCaughan BC, Martini N, Bains MS: Bronchial carcinoids. J Thorac Cardiovasc Surg 89:8, 1985

Moertel CG: Treatment of the carcinoid tumor and the malignant carcinoid syndrome. J Clin Oncol 1:727, 1983

Moertel CG, Hanley JA: Combination chemotherapy trials for metastatic carcinoid tumor and the malignant carcinoid syndrome. Cancer Clin Trials 2:327, 1979

Müller H: Zur Entstehungsgeschichte der Bronchialerweiterungen. Vol. 15. Inausg Diss Univ Halle. A. Busch, Ermsleben a. H., 1882

O'Grady WP, McDivitt RW, Holman CW, Moore SW: Bronchial adenomas. Arch Surg 101:558, 1970

Okike N, Bernatz PE, Payne WS et al.: Bronchoplastic procedures in the treatment of carcinoid tumors of the tracheobronchial tree. J Thorac Cardiovasc Surg 76:281, 1978

Okike N, Bernatz PE, Woolner LB: Carcinoid tumors of the lung. Ann Thorac Surg 22:270, 1976

Orlowski TM: Paliatywne Intubacje Drzewa Oskrzelowego (Palliative Intubations of the Bronchial Tree). Akademia Medyczna we Wroclawiu, Wroclaw, 1987

Orlowski TM, Kolodziej J: Palliative intubation of the trachea and main bronchi. Lung Cancer 2:102, 1986

Pairolero PC, Trastek VF, Payne WS, Bernatz PE: Carcinoid tumors of the lung. p. 258. In Martini N, Vogt-Moykopf I (eds): International Trends in General Thoracic Surgery. Vol. 5. Thoracic Surgery: Frontiers and Uncommon Neoplasms. CV Mosby, St. Louis, 1989

Payne WS, Schier J, Woolner LB: Mixed tumors of the bronchus (salivary gland type). J Thorac Cardiovasc Surg 49:663, 1965

Pearson FG, Thompson DW, Weissberg D et al.: Adenoid cystic carcinoma of the trachea. Ann Thorac Surg 18:16, 1974

Pearson FG, Todd TRJ, Cooper JD: Experience with primary neoplasms of the trachea and carina. J Thorac Cardiovasc Surg 88:511, 1984

Personne C, Colchen A, Leroy M et al.: Indications and technique for endoscopic laser resections in bronchology. J Thorac Cardiovasc Surg 91:710, 1986

Reddy JP: Adenoid cystic carcinoma. J Thorac Cardiovasc Surg 74:329, 1977

Smith RA: Bronchial carcinoid tumors. Thorax 24:98, 1969

Smout MS, French AJ: Prognosis of pseudoadenomatous basal-cell carcinoma. Arch Pathol 72:121, 1961

Spencer FC: Discussion of Jensik. J Thorac Cardiovasc Surg 68:65, 1974

Spencer H: Pathology of the Lung. 4th Ed. Vol. 2. Pergamon Press, Oxford, 1985

Spencer H: Bronchial mucous gland tumors. Virchows Arch A Pathol Anat Histopathol 383:101, 1979

Spiro RH, Huvos AG, Strong EW: Adenoid cystic carcinoma of salivary gland origin: a clinicopathologic study of 242 cases. Am J Surg 128:512, 1974

Stuart-Harris R, McCaughan BC: Bronchial gland tumors ("bronchial adenomas"). p. 399. In Williams CJ, Krikorian JG, Green MR, Raghavan D (eds): Textbook of Uncommon Cancer. John Wiley & Sons, Chichester, 1988

Todd TR, Cooper JD, Weissberg D et al.: Bronchial carcinoid tumors. J Thorac Cardiovasc Surg 79:532, 1980

Toker C: Observations on the ultrastructure of a bronchial adenoma (carcinoid-type). Cancer 19:1943, 1966

Turnbull AD, Huvos AG, Goodner JT, Beattie EJ Jr: The malignant potential of bronchial adenoma. Ann Thorac Surg 14:453, 1972

Vieta JO, Maier HC: The treatment of adenoid cystic carcinoma (cylindroma) of the respiratory tract by surgery and radiation therapy. Dis Chest 31:493, 1957

von Albertini A: Pathologisch-anatomisches Kurzreferat zum Thema Lungenkrebs. Schweiz Med Wochenschr 81:659, 1951

Wareing TH, Sawyers JL: Carcinoids and the carcinoid syndrome. Am J Surg 145:769, 1983

Warren WH, Faber LP, Gould VE: Neuroendocrine neoplasms of the lung. J Thorac Cardiovasc Surg 98:321, 1989

Warren WH, Gould VE: Long-term follow-up of classical bronchial carcinoid tumors. Scand J Thorac Cardiovasc Surg 24:125, 1990

Weisel W: Discussion of Jensik. J Thorac Cardiovasc Surg 68:66, 1974

Westaby S: A silastic stent for palliation of extrinsic tracheal compression or unresectable tracheobronchial obstruction. Br J Surg 70:259, 1983

Westaby S, Jackson JW, Pearson FG: A bifurcated silicone rubber stent for relief of tracheobronchial obstruction. J Thorac Cardiovasc Surg 83:414, 1982

Wright ES, Pike E, Couves CM: Unusual tumors of the lung. J Surg Oncol 24:23, 1983

Yessner R: Small cell tumors of the lung. Am J Surg Pathol 7:775, 1983

27

CANCER

Biology

Jack A. Roth

DEFINITION

Lung cancer is generally classified into two major types: non-small cell lung cancer (NSCLC) and small cell lung cancer (SCLC). NSCLC is further subdivided into three major histologic types: squamous carcinoma, adenocarcinoma, and large cell carcinoma. This classification has been useful because the therapeutic approach to these two types is different. SCLC is usually disseminated at the time of presentation and, therefore, requires systemic therapy. It is highly responsive to chemotherapy, although most patients relapse within 1 year following treatment. Conventional therapy for localized NSCLC consists of treatment of the local tumor with either surgery or radiation therapy. It responds poorly to chemotherapy, and surgical resection is the preferred treatment. The biologic basis for these differences in natural history and responsiveness to therapy is one of the topics discussed in this chapter.

HISTORICAL NOTE

Primary carcinoma of the lung was an uncommon cancer until the 1930s. At this time a dramatic increase in the incidence of lung cancer began that has not yet abated. Lung cancer is now the most common cause of cancer death in both men and women. As described by Hoover (1978), the positive association between cigarette smoking and lung cancer was first suspected more than 60 years ago by Muller, Ochsner, and DeBakey. Recent epidemiologic studies confirm these observations. Lung cancer is one of the few human cancers in which the carcinogen is known. However, only recently have the molecular events in lung carcinogenesis been identified. The long time period between the initial exposure to

tobacco carcinogens and the development of clinical lung cancer suggests that multiple steps are required for the expression of the malignant phenotype.

It is generally thought that the carcinogenic effects of tobacco are the result of the polycyclic aromatic hydrocarbons from tars produced during combustion. Tobacco also contains specific carcinogens related to nicotine. Nicotine can form nitrosamines, such as 4-(N-methyl-N-nitrosamino)-1-(3-pyridyl)-1-butanone (NNK), which was identified in tobacco smoke by Hoffmann and Hecht (1974). This substance is a strong carcinogen in rodents.

The observation that the genes responsible for carcinogenesis were altered forms of genes normally present in eukaryotic cells, reported by Stehelin, et al. (1976), initiated many of the advances in molecular biology that have increased our understanding of lung carcinogenesis at the molecular level (Bishop, 1991; Cross and Dexter, 1991; Vinacour and Minna, 1989). Shih, et al. (1981) and Murray, et al. (1981) were among the first to identify and sequence human cancer genes (oncogenes). Subsequently, as discussed in this chapter, many of these genes have been implicated in the development of human cancer.

Supported by National Cancer Institute grants CA 45187-01 and Thoracic Training Grant CA09611-01 and in part by gifts to the Division of Surgery from Tenneco and Exxon for the core laboratory facility, by The Cancer Center Support grant (CA16672), and by the Mathers Foundation.

HISTORICAL READINGS

Hoffmann D, Hecht SS: N'nitrosonornicotine in tobacco. Science 186:265, 1974

Hoover R: Epidemiology: tobacco and geographic pathology. p. 3. In Harris CC (ed): Pathogenesis and Therapy of Lung Cancer. Marcel Dekker, New York, 1978

Murray MJ, Shilo BZ, Shih C et al: Three different human tumor cell lines contain different oncogenes. Cell 25:355, 1981

Shih C, Padhy LC, Murray MJ, Weinberg RA: Transferring genes of carcinomas and neuroblastomas introduced into mouse fibroblasts. Nature 290:261, 1981

Stehelin D, Varnus HE, Bishop JM, Vogt PK: DNA related to the transforming gene(s) of avian sarcoma viruses is present in normal avian DNA. Nature 260:170, 1976

LUNG CARCINOGENESIS

Models of multistep carcinogenesis were most extensively studied in the mouse skin and rat liver models by Stehelin, et al. (1976) and Goldsworthy, et al. (1986). A series of well-defined events occurs in these models. Cells exposed to a carcinogen undergo an initiation event. Following exposure to a carcinogen, the cells are irreversibly altered in their heritable structure. Exposure to a second agent or promoter causes a reversible expansion of the initiated cells. Further changes may cause the cells to enter the progression stage, with expression of features of the malignant phenotype, including metastatic potential.

The formation of metastases is a complex phenomenon that requires multiple steps, including growth and invasion of the primary malignant cells, penetration of the cells into the blood and lymphatic circulation, implantation into distant tissues, and proliferation in their new environment, as described by Nicolson (1988). Recently a metastasis suppressor gene was identified. The absence of this gene correlates with increased metastasis formation in murine tumors. The locus of this gene was deleted in 42 percent of lung cancers in a recent study by Leone, et al. (1991).

Studies in mice with carcinogen-induced lung cancers implicate genes of the *ras* family in the carcinogenic process, as reviewed by Malkinson (1989). Mouse lung tumors induced by tetranitromethane contained mutated K-*ras* genes. Mice harboring the mutated H-*ras* transgene developed tumors exclusively in the lungs, within weeks following birth. Belinsky, et al. (1989) induced lung tumors in mice with the tobacco-specific nitrosamine NNK or nitrosodimethylamine. Ninety percent of these tumors had transforming genes in the NIH 3T3 mouse assay, and in all lung tumors, this was K-*ras*. The mutations were generally guanine-cytosine to adenine-thymine transitions, indicating that DNA methylation is the most likely pathway to the induction of neoplasia by these carcinogens. This model is of interest because *ras* mutations are commonly found in human lung cancers.

CELL BIOLOGY

The cell of origin for lung cancers is controversial. The NSCLC histologic types all have phenotypic features of the differentiated cell types in normal or injured bronchial epithelium. SCLC cells have neuroendocrine markers, including high levels of the polypeptide hormones (e.g., gastrin-releasing peptide and calcitonin), creatine kinase isoenzyme BB, L-dopa decarboxylase, and neuron-specific enolase. Endocrine cells can be found in normal bronchial mucosa. Thus, one possibility is that each of the four major histologic types arises from alterations in its pre-existing normal counterpart.

As described by Mabry, et al. (1991), an alternative hypothesis is that the four types of lung cancer arise from a common stem cell and are related through a common differentiation pathway of the normal bronchial epithelium. This is supported by the clinical observation that SCLC tumors can contain mixtures of SCLC and NSCLC histologic types. These transitions have been observed in vitro following insertion of the appropriate oncogene. For example, insertion of a mutated H-*ras* oncogene in SCLC cells with overexpression of c-*myc* causes transition to the large cell undifferentiated phenotype.

GENETIC FACTORS

It is surprising that only 15 percent of cigarette smokers, including heavy smokers, develop lung cancer, as described by Hoover (1978). This suggests an inherited predisposition or cofactors, such as additional carcinogens, may predispose some individuals to the development of lung cancer. Lynch, et al. (1986) evaluated 254 individuals with lung cancer and 231 individuals with other smoking-related cancers. There was a lack of increased risk of developing lung cancer when only lung cancer in relatives was considered. However, there was a significant excess of cancers at all sites for relatives of the patients with lung cancer. This suggests a heritable variation in response to carcinogens. A familial risk for lung cancer was found in studies by Ooi, et al. (1986) and Samet, et al. (1986). Respiratory diseases also predispose to the development of lung cancer, as described by Samet, et al. (1986) and Skillrud, et al. (1986). Sellers, et al. (1990) analyzed 337 families, each of which was ascertained through a proband with lung cancer. The development of lung cancer in young individuals (50 years of age or younger) was compatible with mendelian codominant inheritance or a rare autosomal gene. This gene was not involved for older persons, reflecting the noncarriers who had long-term exposure to tobacco. The aryl hydrocarbon hydroxylase gene product can metabolize promutagenic and procarcinogenic compounds in cigarette smoke. McLemore, et al. (1990) showed that the aromatic hydrocarbon-inducible cytochrome P4501A1 gene is highly expressed at the RNA level in the normal lungs from active cigarette smokers but not in the normal lungs from nonsmokers. The ability to metabolize debrisoquin is genetically determined and is associated with susceptibility to lung cancer, as described by Caporaso, et al. (1990). This group showed that the ability to metabolize debrisoquin is independently associated with a susceptibility to lung cancer in a case-control study.

ONCOGENE ACTIVATION

Numerous genetic alterations have been identified in human lung cancer (Table 27-1). The relative importance of individual genetic lesions, the preferred order (if any) for genetic events, and the pathways by which altered genes mediate their action are not known for lung cancer. SCLC is the most extensively studied of all lung cancer histologic types. This is the result in part of the availability of many established

Table 27-1. Lung Cancer Oncogenes and Tumor Suppressor Genes

Dominant	Tumor Suppressor
K-*ras*	p53
myc family	3p
c-*jun*	rb
Growth factor	Protein tyrosine phosphatase-γ
Transforming growth factor-α	nm23
Epidermal growth factor receptor	
c-erbB2	

SCLC cell lines, which can be grown in serum-free chemically defined media, as described by Gazdar, et al. (1986); Gazdar and Oie (1985); and Carney, et al. (1981, 1985). The biologic behavior of SCLC is distinct from that of NSCLC. SCLC disseminates early in its course and exhibits a marked sensitivity to chemotherapy, followed by early recurrence. It is possible that genetic events may differ between SCLC and NSCLC. Recent studies, which are discussed below, indicate that differences exist at the molecular level. Thus molecular mechanisms may not be generalizable among the different forms of lung cancer.

The genes altered in cancer cells can be classified as having a positive or negative influence on cell growth. Genes with a positive influence on cell growth are designated as proto-oncogenes in their unaltered form. Once activated a single altered allele is sufficient to transform cells, and thus these genes are considered dominant in their action. Potential mechanisms of activation include mutation, amplification, and translocation (Fig. 27-1). Genes of this family may also encode for growth factors and their receptors. Genes that negatively influence cell growth and proliferation are called tumor-suppressor genes. The retinoblastoma gene is the most extensively characterized of this group. The loss or inactivation of both alleles are required for tumor formation, and therefore these are called recessive genes.

ONCOGENES MEDIATING STIMULATION OF GROWTH

Growth Factors and Their Receptors

Growth factors mediate their action by specific binding to cell receptors (Fig. 27-2). A signal is transduced from the extracellular domain of cell surface receptors to the cytoplasmic domain, usually resulting in the phosphorylation of this region of the receptor. This triggers a cascade of events that may include binding of other cytoplasmic molecules to the receptor and activation of protein kinase C. This in turn may activate "early" genes, such as c-*fos* and c-*jun*. The cell is then stimulated to proceed through the cell cycle.

Tumor cells that make a growth factor and express the receptor for that growth factor may stimulate their own growth (autocrine growth). Cells that have an autocrine loop

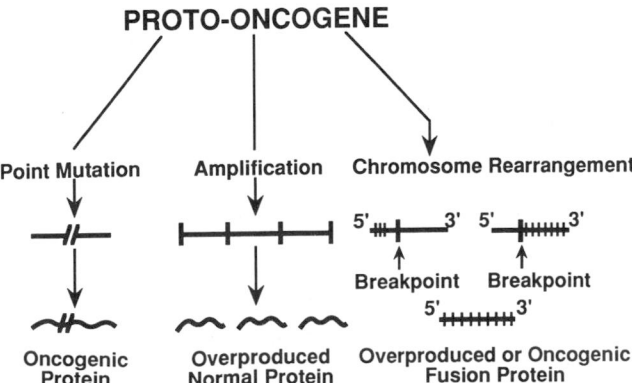

Figure 27-1. Mechanisms of gene activation for dominant oncogenes.

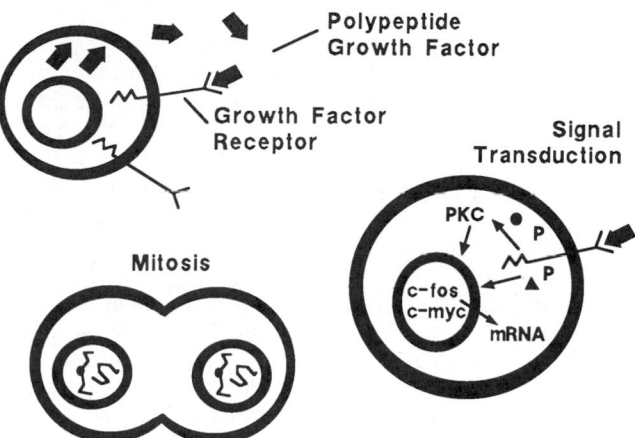

Figure 27-2. Schematic representation of growth factor ligand and receptor interaction and the possible effects of this interaction on the cell.

have several features. They secrete a biologically active growth factor and demonstrate increased proliferation to that factor. Antibodies that bind specifically to the growth factor inhibit cell growth. Growth factors may act to stimulate growth in adjacent cells in a paracrine manner. The interaction of ligand and receptor in the cytoplasm of the cell may form an internal autocrine loop, as described by Browder, et al. (1989).

Autocrine growth factors have been implicated in the stimulation of SCLC cell growth. The majority of SCLC cell lines produce bombesin, as described by Carney, et al. (1987). This 14-amino acid peptide is identical to a carboxy-terminal heptapeptide sequence of a mammalian analog, gastrin-releasing peptide. SCLC cell lines express a single class of high-affinity, saturable binding receptors for bombesin. Bombesin is also a potent stimulator of clonal growth for human SCLC. Bombesin receptors are not present on NSCLC.

Epidermal Growth Factor Receptor

Oncogene products that phosphorylate tyrosine residues (tyrosine kinases) are implicated in retrovirally induced neoplasia. For example v-*erb*B, the transforming gene of avian erythroblastosis virus, codes for a truncated version of the epidermal growth factor receptor (EGFR). Activation of the overexpressed normal receptor gene is sufficient for transformation of NIH 3T3 cells, as described by Riedel, et al. (1988). NSCLC, but not SCLC, cells express high levels of functional EGFR and have amplification of the EGFR gene, as described by Haeder, et al. (1988) and Sakiyama, et al. (1986). This suggests that growth factors and their receptors may play an important role in the development and maintenance of the malignant phenotype.

Schneider, et al. (1988, 1990a) investigated the EGFR (*erb*B1) structure in fresh NSCLC cells. Southern analysis showed amplification (more than twofold) of the EGFR gene in 6 of 60 tumors. However, 24 of 60 tumors showed an absence of a 4.2-kilobase EcoRI restriction enzyme fragment that was present in all normal lung specimens. This was detected specifically by a probe that recognizes the intracellular tyrosine kinase domain of *erb*B1. The absence of the fragment in tumor specimens did not correspond to the appearance of new lower molecular weight fragments detected by a complementary DNA probe, suggesting the fragment corresponds to a genomic region, possibly at an intron-exon junction. Schneider, et al. (1988, 1990a) showed that an alteration is present that leads to an increased cleavage efficiency of the restriction endonuclease EcoRI for a specific EcoRI site in this 4.2-kilobase fragment. Samples of lymphocyte DNA from 13 normal donors did not show the 4.2-kilobase fragment. The fragment was present in normal muscle DNA samples and could be cleaved with 40 U of enzyme/μg DNA with spermidine, in contrast to corresponding normal lung, which was not completely digested. Thus, this phenomenon is tissue specific. A possible explanation for this is the existence of tissue-specific methylation differences at the restriction enzyme cleavage site. The methylation of one base in a recognition sequence may inhibit cleavage.

The expression of EGFR by lung cancer cells suggests that the production of a ligand by these cells could mediate an autocrine or paracrine growth stimulation loop. The lung cancer cell lines studied did not produce EGF. However, they did produce transforming growth factor-α (TGF-α), which binds to the EGFR. TGF-α is a single polypeptide of 50 amino acids that is derived from a 160-amino acid transmembrane precursor by proteolytic cleavage. It is structurally and functionally related to EGF and binds to the EGFR. TGF-α alone does not transform NRK cells.

Anchorage-independent growth is seen when TGF-α and TGF-β are added together. TGF-α is a candidate autocrine growth factor for NSCLC. Previous studies indicated that medium conditioned from A549-1 lung carcinoma cells can promote the growth of human NSCLC cells in culture. This conditioned media is known to contain TGF-α; exogenous TGF-α added to cultures increased colony formation, as described by Siegfried, et al. (1988).

TGF-α does not need to be cleaved from its conserved integral membrane glycoprotein to have biologic activity. Wong, et al. (1989) transfected BHK cells with an expression vector containing altered sequences such that the cells did not secrete TGF-α but expressed the pro-TGF-α on the cell surface, as described by Bringmann, et al. (1989). The membrane-bound pro-TGF-α bound to EGFR on A431 cells and induced receptor autophosphorylation. Brachmann, et al. (1989) solubilized pro-TGF-α and found that it induced tyrosine autophosphorylation of EGFR in intact receptor-expressing cells and stimulated anchorage-independent growth of NRK fibroblasts. Thus both pro-TGF-α and TGF-α could function as autocrine growth factors. The possibilities include interactions of pro-TGF-α with a cytoplasmic form of the EGFR and EGFR expressed on adjacent cells.

The presence of EGFR on lung cancer cells suggests an autocrine-paracrine growth mechanism may be operative. This was investigated in vitro with cloned NSCLC cell lines by Putnam, et al. (1992). Four NSCLC cell lines expressed the EGFR. None of the cell lines expressed EGF by northern analysis. However, all cell lines expressed TGF-α messenger RNA, which can bind to the EGFR. Therefore the investiga-

tors studied the biologic response to and production of TGF-α by these cell lines. Each cell line expressed EGFR by ^{125}I-labeled EGF competitive binding and Scatchard analysis and by phosphorylation. The receptors were functionally active, as determined in immune complex kinase assays. The cells showed stimulated ^{3}H-labeled thymidine uptake in response to both TGF-α and EGF. Exogenously added TGF-α increased colony formation in soft agar for three of the four cell lines in media containing serum. All cell lines expressed some TGF-α messenger RNA, although to differing degrees. Possible differences were observed in the mechanism of autocrine growth stimulation among the four cell lines. Two cell lines were specifically growth inhibited by the anti-TGF-α monoclonal antibody AB-3 at a low cell density, suggesting the antibody blocks an autocrine growth loop. However, the AB-3 antibody did not alter the growth of two of the cell lines, even though these cells expressed EGFR and secrete TGF-a. Suramin, which blocks the binding of ligands to receptors in other autocrine systems, inhibited the growth of both cell lines, as described by Keating and Williams (1988) and Browder, et al. (1989). The addition of TGF-α, but not platelet-derived growth factor, specifically reversed the inhibition by suramin. This suggests that autocrine activation for this cell line occurred exclusively in the intracellular compartment between unprocessed receptor and unsecreted ligand. TGF-α appears to be an autocrine growth factor for NSCLC cells of both squamous and adenocarcinoma histologic types.

erb*B2*

The gene *erb*B2 is a member of the EGFR family. This family includes three genes with a receptorlike structure, including an external ligand-binding domain, a transmembrane domain, and a cytoplasmic tyrosine kinase domain. Drebin, et al. (1984) and Schechter, et al. (1984) first identified the *neu/erb*B2 oncogene in an ethylnitrosourea-induced rat neuroblastoma. The rat oncogene is activated by a point mutation, but the mechanism in human cells appears to be overexpression, as described by Di Fiore, et al. (1987) and Slamon, et al. (1987). The gene has homology with the EGFR gene, and the gene product (molecular weight, 185 kilodalton) is a tyrosine kinase. Although the structure of this protein is receptorlike, a functional ligand has not yet been conclusively identified by Lupu, et al. (1990). Schneider, et al. (1989, 1990b) in our laboratory were the first to identify activation of *erb*B2 in NSCLC. Amplification of *erb*B2 occurred in 10 percent of 60 paired samples of NSCLC and normal lung. However, adenocarcinomas showed high messenger RNA levels of *erb*B2. In contrast, SCLC cells did not express *erb*B2. A study of freshly excised surgical specimens confirmed and extended these findings, as described by Schneider, et al. (1990b). NSCLC specimens showed high levels of *erb*B2 RNA expression in 6 of 16 samples compared with those in paired normal lung samples. Increased expression occurred in both early and advanced stages. Fresh SCLC showed minimal or no expression. Kern, et al. (1990) found that the expression of the *erb*B2 gene product, p185, occurred at higher levels in the tumor than in the bronchiolar epithelium. They found that *erb*B2 expression in adenocarcinomas was independently correlated with diminished survival.

Insulinlike Growth Factor

Studies by Minuto, et al. (1988) and Natale, et al. (1988) suggest that insulinlike growth factor-I (IGF-I) may participate in autocrine growth stimulation. Shigematsu, et al. (1990) observed IGF-I immunostaining in primary NSCLC tumors removed at surgery. ^{125}I-labeled IGF-I competitive binding studies showed the presence of IGF-I receptors. The secretion of IGF-I by SCLC cell lines was shown by Macaulay, et al. (1990). Two classes of IGF-I receptors were identified by Scatchard analysis. Cell lines and fresh SCLC cells showed increased ^{3}H-labeled thymidine uptake in response to IGF-I, and this was specifically inhibited by an anti-IGF-I monoclonal antibody.

Dominant Oncogenes

ras Family

Oncogenes of the *ras* family (homologous to the rat sarcoma virus) have three primary members (H-*ras*, K-*ras*, and N-*ras*), and they are among the most common activated oncogenes found in human cancer, as described by Bos (1989). The *ras* genes code for a protein that is located on the inner surface of the plasma membrane, has guanosine triphosphatase activity, and may participate in signal transduction. The *ras* oncogenes are activated by point nucleotide mutations that alter the amino acid sequence of the protein p21. The presence of a single mutated allele is sufficient to transform some immortalized cell lines, such as NIH 3T3 cells, or other cells, such as rat primary embryo fibroblasts, in the presence of a cooperating oncogene.

Amplification of *ras* oncogenes is uncommon in lung cancer. Heighway and Hasleton (1986) found no amplification of K-*ras* in 25 primary specimens. A lymph node metastasis showed 30-fold amplification of K-*ras*. Expression of p21, as measured by binding of the monoclonal antibody rp-35, increased with the increasing size of the primary tumor, as described by Dosaka, et al. (1988).

Activation of the K-*ras* oncogene by point mutation occurs in lung cancer cell lines, as described by Yamamoto, et al. (1985) and Shimizu, et al. (1983). A mutation in codon 12 (glycine to cysteine) occurs in Calu-1 cells and in codon 61 in PR310 cells (glutamine to histidine). Restriction fragment length polymorphism analysis for a codon 12 mutation (glycine to arginine) did not show any mutations in 24 primary NSCLC lung cancers, as described by Milici, et al. (1986). Rodenhuis, et al. (1987, 1988) detected other mutations in the 12th K-*ras* codon by using a highly sensitive technique based on amplification with the polymerase chain reaction and detection with a panel of oligonucleotide probes. The K-*ras* mutations were confined to adenocarcinomas of the lung and occurred in 9 of 35 tumors. Mutations were not observed in adenocarcinomas from nonsmokers. A recent study by the same group showed that K-*ras* mutations were an independent prognostic factor, indicating a poor prognosis (Rodenhuis, et al., 1990). In all patients mutations occurred in a single allele. Reynolds, et al. (1991), using a NIH 3T3 cotransfection-nude mouse tumorigenicity assay, found activated proto-oncogenes of the *ras* family in 86 percent of lung cancers from smokers. Activated *ras* genes were present in 8 of 10 metastatic adenocarcinomas. No *ras* mutations have been identified in any SCLC tumors or cell lines, as described by Gazdar, et al. (1991). Infection of SCLC cell lines with the Harvey murine sarcoma virus altered the phenotype of the variant but not the classic cells, as described by Mabry, et al. (1988). Following infection the variant SCLC cell line developed features of a large cell undifferentiated lung carcinoma, including increased carcinoembryonic antigen and keratin expression.

Studies done to date favor the interpretation of *ras* activation as a progression factor in lung cancer. It apparently is activated in about one-third of adenocarcinomas arising in patients with a heavy smoking history. However, studies of premalignant lung lesions have not been done to determine whether such mutations exist at the precancerous stage, as is the case for adenocarcinoma of the colon, as described by Vogelstein, et al. (1988).

Any therapy aimed at the reversal of oncogene function must be highly specific. However, many oncogenes are members of multigene families, the function of which is critical for cell viability. Techniques that globally inhibit the expression of all family members are lethal to the cell. Both tumor and normal cells are affected, as described by Debus, et al. (1990). In our laboratory, Mukhopadhyay, et al. (1990, 1991b) used antisense technology to find the effects of eliminating expression of a mutant K-*ras* oncogene in NSCLC cells. A homozygous mutation at codon 61 was identified in the NCI-H460a large cell undifferentiated NSCLC cell line clone with a normal glutamine residue (cytosine-adenine-adenine) substituted by histidine (cytosine-adenine-thymine), using hybridization with specific oligonucleotide probes and direct polymerase chain reaction DNA sequencing. An antisense K-*ras* RNA construct selectively blocked the production of mutant p21 so the contribution of the mutated p21 protein to the malignant phenotype could be studied. A recombinant plasmid clone was constructed by using a wild-type 2-kilobase K-*ras* genomic DNA segment carrying second and third exons with flanking intron sequences subcloned into an Apr-1-neo expression vector in the antisense orientation. The intron sequence used has a low degree of homology, with other *ras* genomic sequences, so that specific inhibition of K-*ras* with preservation of H-*ras* and N-*ras* expression would occur. Previous studies with the uptake of *ras* antisense oligonucleotide by cancer cells resulted in cell death instead of regulated growth. This is probably because functioning p21 is necessary for cell viability, and the oligonucleotide blocked all p21 expression. Blockade of oncogene expression, which is not selective, can therefore be toxic to both normal and cancer cells. An additional novel feature of this construct was the use of a β-actin promoter that can constitutively direct synthesis of RNA in a human tumor cell.

The 2-kilobase DNA insert was stably integrated into H406a cells by Southern hybridization, and northern blot analysis detected the expression of antisense RNA. Western blot analysis showed a 95 percent reduction in specific K-*ras* p21 protein synthesis in the clones expressing the antisense RNA; H460a cells and sense K-*ras* clones showed unchanged levels of the K-*ras* p21 protein. The total p21 detected with a pan-*ras* monoclonal antibody showed only a slight decrease in the antisense clones, suggesting other *ras* genes were not affected. Antisense transfectants showed a threefold reduction in growth compared with sense transfectants and parental H460a cells but continued to grow in culture. The expression of antisense K-*ras* RNA significantly reduced the growth rate of H460a tumors in nu/nu mice. These experiments show that, in H460a cells engineered to synthesize antisense K-*ras* RNA, the level of K-*ras* messenger RNA and K-*ras* p21 protein were dramatically reduced. Therefore constructs can be made that distinguish among members of the *ras* family. Inhibition of K-*ras* reduced the growth rate of H460a cells but did not alter cell viability or continued growth in culture. This suggests that redundancy in p21 expression may compensate for an absense of expression by one member of this family so that functions essential for maintenance of cell viability are preserved. These observations raise the intriguing possibility of specific molecular therapy for cancer. Sequences could be delivered to tumor cells through viral vectors that specifically would inhibit expression of the oncogenes activated in the cancer cell. Such constructs would be relatively nontoxic because, as in the example cited above, they could target a single gene whose function might be subsumed by other redundant genes of the same family. Thus repeated infusions of immunologically distinct vectors could be performed. Retroviral vectors have the added advantage of being incorporated in the genome only of cells that replicate, thus favoring integration in cancer cell DNA.

Sporadic alterations in a variety of other oncogenes are described by Shiraishi, et al. (1989). Cline and Battifora (1987) found amplification of c-*erb*B-1, c-*myc*, and c-*myb* and deletions in c-H-*ras* and c-*myb*. The expression of proto-oncogenes in SCLC was determined by Kiefer, et al. (1987) using northern analysis. An increased expression of *myc* family genes was confirmed. The *ras* family and c-*raf*1 were expressed in all cell lines. Other oncogenes, including c-*fes*, c-*fos*, c-*erb*B-1, c-*mos*, c-*sis*, c-*erb*A, c-*src*, and c-*abl*, were expressed weakly or not at all.

myc *Family*

A subgroup of SCLC cell lines have an amplified c-*myc* gene, as described by Little, et al. (1983). The SCLC cell lines with an amplified c-*myc* gene are morphologic and biochemical variants of SCLC (SCLC-V). SCLC-V have a rapid doubling time, higher cloning efficiency, increased tumorigenicity, and increased resistance to radiation compared with SCLC, as described by Carney, et al. (1985). In addition, SCLC-V do not express L-dopa decarboxylase or peptide hormones. They do have elevated levels of the bombesin (BB) isoenzyme or creatine kinase and neuron-specific enolase, which distinguishes them from NSCLC, as described by Gazdar, et al. (1980). Little, et al. (1983) reported that five SCLC-V cell lines showed high levels of c-*myc* amplification and c-*myc* messenger RNA levels. Only one NSCLC cell line of five showed c-*myc* amplification. The c-*myc* gene was transfected into the H209 classic SCLC cell line, as described by Johnson, et al. (1986). One of the transfectants expressing high levels of c-*myc* had an increase in doubling time and increased cloning efficiency, but L-dopa decarboxylase levels and bombesinlike immunoreactivity were unchanged. Kiefer, et al. (1987) observed amplification of c-*myc* in both classic and variant SCLC cell lines. However, c-*myc* messenger RNA levels were more elevated in the variant cell lines. Three classic lines had amplification of N-*myc* messenger RNA and one variant line had amplification of N-*myc* and *myb*. Three SCLC-V cell lines showed high levels of a v-*fms*-related transcript, which is related but not identical to the colony stimulating factor (CSF)-1 receptor. Bepler, et al. (1989) identified a subpopulation of SCLC with intermediate neuroendocrine differentiation. The cell lines expressed some neuroendocrine markers, such as L-dopa decarboxylase, but not others, such as bombesin and neurotensin. These cell lines also had high levels of c-*myc* protein. Expression of c-*myc* protein was seen for two cell lines in which c-*myc* expression was low or not detectable. Expression of c-*raf*1 protein was low in 11 of the 12 cell lines. Four of five NSCLC cell lines expressed c-*myc* protein at high levels, and these were all of the large cell undifferentiated morphology. Cline (1984) and Cline and Battifora (1987) found 3 of 27 NSCLC cell DNA from primary tumors had amplification of the c-*myc* gene. Yoshimoto, et al. (1986) identified high levels of c-*myc* messenger RNA in a NSCLC cell line in the absence of DNA amplification. Run-on transcription studies showed the transcriptional rate for c-*myc* was high.

Analysis of SCLC cell lines for c-*myc* amplification revealed additional EcoRI restriction fragments, suggesting *myc*-related genes. A third gene in the *myc* family, L-*myc*, was cloned and showed homology to c-*myc* and N-*myc*, as described by Nau, et al. (1985). Four SCLC cell lines had amplified L-*myc* genes. The L-*myc* gene was cloned and sequenced and consists of three exons and two introns spanning 6.6 kilobases of human DNA, as described by Kaye, et al. (1988). There is homology with discrete regions of N-*myc* and c-*myc*. The L-*myc* gene encodes a series of nuclear phosphoprotein that arise by alternative messenger RNA processing, as described by Kaye, et al. (1988). L-*myc* can cooperate with an activated c-Ha-*ras* to transform primary rat embryo fibroblasts. However, Birrer et al. (1988) revealed the transforming efficiency was 1 to 10 percent of that seen with c-*myc*. One study by Kawashima, et al. (1988) found a correlation between restriction fragment length polymorphisms of the L-*myc* gene and lymph node metastases in NSCLC. The presence of either the S band (6-kilobase) or the S and L (10-kilobase) bands was associated with lymph node metastases.

Amplification and increased expression of the N-*myc* gene occurs in SCLC and NSCLC. Funa, et al. (1987) measured the expression of N-*myc* in SCLC biopsies by in situ hybridization. Increased expression was associated with a poor response to chemotherapy and short survival. Amplification of N-*myc* gene sequences, ranging from 5- to 170-fold, was observed in SCLC cell lines by Nau, et al. (1986). Both c-*myc* and N-*myc* were amplified, but only one member of the *myc* family was amplified in any one cell line. Saksela, et al. (1986) reported amplification of N-*myc* in an adenocarcinoma. Ibson, et al. (1987) found amplification of one of the *myc* family in 2 of 12 SCLC cell lines. Again only one member of the family was amplified in each cell line. All cell lines had deletions of chromosome 3. When fresh tumor specimens were analyzed by Yokota, et al. (1987), amplification and rearrangement of *myc* genes was heterogeneous. N-*myc* or

L-*myc* amplification was noted in 4 of 17 small cell cancers. Amplification of c-*myc* was seen in 3 of 12 NSCLC specimens. In some cases amplification was seen in the primary tumor but not in the metastases. In two cases amplification was seen only in cell lines but not in the original tumors. Expression of *myc* family genes was demonstrated in SCLC cell lines and nude mouse xenografts by using in situ hybridization techniques by Gu, et al. (1988).

The molecular mechanisms regulating the expression of each of the *myc* family genes are complex, as described by Krystal, et al. (1988). Both c-*myc* and L-*myc* messenger RNA showed a loss of transcriptional attenuation, which correlated with the overexpression seen in cell lines without gene amplification. Regulation of N-*myc* expression correlated with promoter activity and gene amplification. Sausville, et al. (1988) found an interesting association between responsiveness to bombesin and *myc* family expression. SCLC cell lines responsive to bombesin showed constitutive expression of L-*myc*. Nonresponsive cell lines expressed N-*myc* or c-*myc*.

The significance of increased expression in *myc* family genes remains uncertain. Initially c-*myc* amplification was described in SCLC cell lines with variant morphology. This variant morphology is also called small cell/large cell carcinoma and is thought to indicate an unfavorable prognosis. Cell lines with the variant morphology have relatively more resistance to chemotherapy and radiation therapy, as described by Carney, et al. (1983). However, the study of Aisner, et al. (1990), reviewing pathologic specimens of patients with extensive-disease SCLC, showed that the variant cell type was rare, occurring in only 4.4 percent of 550 specimens. There were no significant differences in response rates to chemotherapy or prognosis for patients with classic compared with variant morphology. Amplification of the c-*myc* gene was more frequent in cell lines from patients with SCLC who had tumor relapses compared with that in untreated patients, as described by Johnson, et al. (1987). Amplification of c-*myc* was associated with shorter survival in patients who had relapses. Brennan, et al. (1991) found that c-*myc* amplification was more frequent in tumors from treated (28 percent) compared with untreated (8 percent) patients with SCLC.

It is likely that increased *myc* expression leads to the progression of SCLC. It appears unlikely to be a primary event because it is detected in a minority of tumors. Its association with the variant cell type and the significance of this cell type requires additional study. Increased expression may occur by several mechanisms and is not always associated with gene amplification. Alterations in *myc* expression in NSCLC have not been extensively studied, but in one case several NSCLC showed increased expression of c-*myc* (Bepler, et al., 1989).

TUMOR-SUPPRESSOR GENES

The presence of certain gene products appears necessary for the maintenance of controlled cell growth. The inactivation or loss of certain genes may thus contribute to tumor growth. Both copies of the gene must be eliminated or inactivated to eradicate the growth suppressive function of the gene in the classic model. Because both copies must be eliminated, the tumor-suppressor gene is called "recessive." The retinoblastoma (*rb*) gene was one of the first tumor-suppressor genes to be identified. Patients with the familial predisposition have a germ line inactivation of one copy of the *rb* gene. The tumor develops when the wild-type allele is either inactivated or deleted. Sporadic retinoblastoma cases have somatic mutations or deletions, which eliminate the expression of the gene product. This model has stimulated studies searching for consistent chromosomal deletions in human tumors.

Deletions in the short arm of chromosome 3 (p14-p23) are frequently present in SCLC. Cytogenetic studies of fresh tumors confirmed the observations on cell lines, as described by DeFusco, et al. (1989). Allelic loss in this region was documented with polymorphic DNA probes, as described by Naylor, et al. (1987). Specific suppressor genes at the 3p locus have not yet been identified. A loss of heterozygosity for alleles on chromosomes 3, 11, 13, and 17 occurs in NSCLC, as was described by Kok, et al. (1987); Yokota, et al. (1987); Weston, et al. (1989); and Skinner, et al. (1990). The frequency of 3p deletions in NSCLC is controversial. Kok, et al. (1987) and Brauch, et al. (1987) found this deletion in all SCLC and NSCLC specimens; others found it in a minority of NSCLC specimens. The high frequency of deletions for both SCLC and NSCLC suggests that loss of specific gene function may be a critical step in the development of lung cancer. Two candidate suppressor genes are the nuclear oncogenes p53 and *rb*.

Loss of heterozygosity on chromosome 13q suggests the *rb* locus, located at 13q14, may be deleted. Harbour, et al. (1988) found that 60 percent of SCLC and 75 percent of carcinoid cell lines did not express *rb* messenger RNA. However, 90 percent of NSCLC cell lines expressed *rb*. Horowitz, et al. (1990) and Hensel, et al. (1990) confirmed the absence of *rb* protein expression by SCLC cell lines. Hensel, et al. (1990) confirmed that the inactivation of the *rb* gene is frequent in SCLC. Six of six patients who were informative had lost one *rb* allele. Of 13 SCLC cell lines, only 3 expressed more than a trace amount of *rb* messenger RnA. Xu, et al. (1991) found that the *rb* protein was absent by immunostaining in 10 of 36 primary NSCLC tumors.

p53

The p53 gene encodes a 375-amino acid phosphoprotein that can form complexes with viral proteins, such as large T antigen and E1B as described by Lane and Benchimol (1990). Missense mutations are the most common gene mutation yet identified for lung cancer. The mechanism of p53 transformation is controversial. The wild-type p53 gene may directly suppress or indirectly activate genes that suppress uncontrolled cell growth. The wild-type p53 is dominant over the mutant form and thus suppresses the transformed phenotype, as described by Baker, et al. (1990) and Chen, et al. (1990). Thus the absence of the wild-type p53 or inactivation of wild-type p53 may therefore contribute to transformation. However, some studies indicate the presence of the mutant p53 may be necessary for full expression of the transforming potential of the gene. The presence of the mutant p53 gene can confer a growth advantage to some cells, as described by Chen, et al. (1990) and Finlay, et al. (1989). Studies by Mukhopadhyay, et al. (1991a) and Roth, et al. (1991) in our laboratory show that absence of p53 is not sufficient for transformation of NSCLC cells. A lung cancer cell line expressing only the mutant p53 was transfected with an antisense p53 construct. A marked reduction in colony formation occurred compared with that in control transfections with vector alone or sense p53. The only colonies isolated continued to express p53. This suggests that the presence of the mutant p53 contributed to the maintenance of the transformed phenotype. The wild-type p53 also suppressed colony formation in cell lines expressing mutant p53.

Mutations of p53 are common in a wide spectrum of tumors. These mutations occur in both NSCLC and SCLC cell lines and fresh tumors, as described by Nigro, et al. (1989); Takahashi, et al. (1989); and Chiba, et al. (1990). Hollstein, et al. (1991) and Jones, et al. (1991) showed that two types of mutations occur as follows: transitions, in which a purine is substituted for a purine or a pyrimidine for a pyrimdine, and transversions, in which a purine is substituted for a pyrimidine or vice versa. Transversions have been identified in association with carcinogens such as benzo[a]pyrene. Transitions that have a predilection for cytosine paired with guanine (CpG) dinucleotides (frequently having 5-methylcytosine residues) are indicative of the spontaneous mutation rate. The majority of mutations in lung cancer are guanine-cytosine to thymine-adenine transversions distributed over 10 codons. This suggests a strong influence of tobacco carcinogens as the cause of these mutations.

Two other genes are candidates for tumor-suppressor genes in lung cancer. Expression of the *nm*23 gene is reduced in rodent tumor cells with the highly metastatic phenotype. The *nm*23 gene is located near the centromere of chromosome 17. Allelic deletion was shown in 5 of 12 informative cases, all of which were adenocarcinomas, as described by Leone, et al. (1991). The protein, tyrosine phosphatase-γ, maps to 3p21, a region frequently deleted in lung cancers (LaForgia, et al., 1991). Five of 10 lung cancers studied had evidence of allelic deletion of this gene. These studies suggest a possible role for both genes as tumor suppressors. A definitive demonstration of this will require reversal of the malignant phenotype following insertion of these genes into human lung cancer cells.

COMMENTS AND CONTROVERSIES

An understanding of the molecular mechanisms underlying the development and progression of lung cancer may allow the development of rational approaches to prevention, early diagnosis, and therapy. Molecular markers of bronchial epithelial cells may allow the identification of individuals at highest risk for lung cancer. These markers could improve the accuracy of diagnosis by sputum cytologic examination and provide intermediate end-point markers for chemoprevention trials. Molecular markers of prognosis may allow a better selection of patients for aggressive multimodality therapy.

Although much has been learned about molecular events in lung cancer, our knowledge about the mechanism of carcinogenesis is still fragmentary. Many more genetic abnormalities are probably present in lung cancer cells. The nature of these changes and their biologic significance is unknown. A major area of controversy is whether there is a necessary or preferred order for these genetic changes. One theory by Fearon and Vogelstein (1990) proposes that it is an accumulation of genetic alterations rather than a specific order that is critical. The identification of the pathways by which these genes mediate their effects is critical. This may allow the identification of accessible target molecules for prevention and therapy. It is important to know if it is necessary to reverse all or many of these genetic changes to alter the malignant phenotype of the cell. The evidence presented in this chapter suggests that it may be necessary to reverse only one or two abnormalities to have a profound effect on tumor cell growth and tumorigenicity. This is promising from the perspective of applying these findings to therapy. For example, the tracheobronchial tree is readily accessible to direct therapeutic manipulation. Thus a high-priority research area is the identification of genetic alterations in premalignancy and early malignancy. The development of viral vectors with a high efficiency of gene transduction given regionally in the tracheobronchial tree is one possible approach to altering oncogene expression in high-risk individuals. The potential low toxicity and specificity of this type of therapy makes this an exciting field for future study.

J.A.R.

An understanding of the biology of lung cancer is becoming increasingly important for the surgeon. Not only does it appear to impact on prognosis but soon may impact on therapy strategies. The field is growing rapidly and the understanding of the biology of lung cancer increases logarithmically every year.

It is hoped that all these advances in our understanding will convert to improved methods of prevention, early identification, estimation of prognosis, and ultimately therapeutic intervention. For all these reasons, thoracic surgeons managing patients with lung cancer must have a basic understanding of the biology of the disease.

R.J.G.

KEY REFERENCES

Bishop JM: Molecular themes in oncogenesis. Cell 64:235, 1991

This comprehensive review discusses the major molecular mechanisms implicated to date in the development of cancer. The topics include dominant oncogenes and tumor-suppressor genes.

Cross M, Dexter TM: Growth factors in development, transformation, and tumorigenesis. Cell 64:271, 1991

This article reviews the molecular aspects of growth factors. It discusses the biologic responses of cells to growth factors and their role in the development of malignancy.

Vinocour M, Minna JD: Cellular and molecular biology of lung cancer. In Roth JA, Ruckdeschel JC, Weisenburger TH (eds): Thoracic Oncology. WB Saunders, Philadelphia, 1989

This chapter presents a comprehensive review of molecular biology as it applies to lung cancer.

REFERENCES

Aisner SC, Finkelstein DM, Ettinger DS et al: The clinical significance of variant-morphology small-cell carcinoma of the lung. J Clin Oncol 8:402, 1990

Baker SJ, Markowitz S, Fearson ER et al: Suppression of human colorectal carcinoma cell growth by wild-type p53. Science 249:912, 1990

Belinsky SA, Devereux TR, Maronpot RR et al: Relationship between the formation of promutagenic adducts and the activation of the K-ras protooncogene in lung tumors from A/J mice treated with nitrosamines. Cancer Res 49:5305, 1989

Bepler G, Bading H, Heimann B et al: Expression of p64c-myc and neuroendocrine properties define three subclasses of small cell lung cancer. Oncogene 4:45, 1989

Birrer MJ, Segal S, DeGreve JS et al: L-myc cooperates with ras to transform primary rat embryo fibroblasts. Mol Cell Biol 8:2668, 1988

Bos JL: Ras oncogenes in human cancer: a review. Cancer Res 49:4682, 1989

Brachmann R, Lindquist PB, Nagashima M et al: Transmembrane TGR-alpha precursors activate EGF/TGF-alpha receptors. Cell 56:691, 1989

Brauch H, Johnson B, Hovis J et al: Molecular analysis of the short arm of chromosome 3 in small cell and non-small cell carcinoma of the lung. N Engl J Med 317:1109, 1987

Brennan J, O'Connor T, Makuch RW et al: Myc family DNA amplification in 107 tumors and tumor cell lines from patients with small cell lung cancer treated with different combination chemotherapy regimens. Cancer Res 51:1708, 1991

Bringman TS, Lindquist PB, Derynck R: Different transforming growth factor-alpha species are derived from a glycosylated and palmitoylated transmembrane precursor. Cell 48:429, 1989

Browder TM, Dunbar CE, Nienhuis AW: Private and public autocrine loops in neoplastic cells. Cancer Cells 1:9, 1989

Caporaso NE, Tucker MA, Hoover RN et al: Lung cancer and the debrisoquine metabolic phenotype. J Natl Cancer Inst 82:1264, 1990

Carney DN, Bunn PA Jr, Gazdar AF et al: Selective growth in serum-free hormone-supplemented medium of tumor cells obtained by biopsy from patients with small cell carcinoma of the lung. Proc Natl Acad Sci USA 78:3185, 1981

Carney DN, Cuttitta F, Moody TW, Minna JD: Selective stimulation of small cell lung cancer clonal growth by bombesin and gastrin-releasing peptide. Cancer Res 47:821, 1987

Carney DN, Gazdar AF, Bepler G et al: Establishment and identification of small cell lung cancer cell lines having classic and variant features. Cancer Res 45:2913, 1985

Carney DN, Mitchell JB, Kinsella TJ: In vitro radiation and chemotherapy sensitivity of established cell lines of human small cell lung cancer and its large cell morphological variants. Cancer Res 43:2806, 1983

Chen P-L, Chen Y, Bookstein R, Lee W-H: Genetic mechanisms of tumor suppression by the human p53 gene. Science 250:1576, 1990

Chiba I, Takahashi T, Nau MM et al: Mutations in the p53 gene are frequent in primary, resected non-small cell lung cancer. Oncogene 5:1603, 1990

Cline MJ, Battifora H: Abnormalities of proto-oncogenes in non-small cell lung cancer. Cancer 60:2669, 1987

Cline MJ, Slamon DJ, Lipsick JS: Oncogenes: implications for the diagnosis and treatment of cancer. Ann Intern Med 101:223, 1984

Debus N, Berdichevsky FB, Gryasnov SM: Effects of antisense oligodeoxyribonucleotides complementary mRNA of the human c-Harvey-ras oncogene on cell proliferation (abstr). J Cancer Res Clin Oncol 116(suppl, part 1):S-162, 1990

DeFusco PA, Frytak S, Dahl RJ et al: Cytogenetic studies in 11 patients with small cell carcinoma of the lung. Mayo Clin Proc 64:168, 1989

De Fiore PP, Pierce JH, Kraus MH et al: ErbB-2 is a potent oncogene when overexpressed in NIH/3T3 cells. Science 237:178, 1987

Dosaka H, Harada M, Kizumaki N et al: The relationship of clinical classification to ras p21 expression in human non-small cell lung cancer. Oncology 45:396, 1988

Drebin J, Stern DF, Link VC et al: Monoclonal antibodies identify a cell surface antigen associated with an activated cellular oncogene. Nature 312:545, 1984

Fearon ER, Vogelstein B: A genetic model for colorectal tumorigenesis. Cell 61:759, 1990

Finlay CA, Hinds PW, Levine AJ: The p53 proto-oncogene can act as a suppressor of transformation. Cell 57:1083, 1989

Funa K, Steinholtz L, Nou E, Bergh J: Increased expression of N-myc in human small cell lung cancer biopsies predicts lack of response to chemotherapy and poor prognosis. Am J Clin Pathol 88:216, 1987

Gazdar AF, Carney DN, Nau MN, Minna JD: Characterization of variant subclasses of cell lines derived from small cell lung cancer having distinctive biochemical, morphological, and growth properties. Cancer Res 45:2924, 1985

Gazdar AF, Carney DN, Russell EK et al: Establishment of continuous clonable cultures of small-cell carcinoma of the lung which have amine precursor uptake and decarboxylation cell properties. Cancer Res 40:3502, 1980

Gazdar AF, Giaccone G, Mitsudomi T: The association between drug resistance of lung cancer cell lines and neuroendocrine differentiation and oncogene activation. J Cell Biochem 15F(Suppl):16, 1991

Gazdar AF, Oie HK: Cell culture methods for human lung cancer. Cancer Genet Cytogenet 19:5, 1986

Goldsworthy TL, Hanigan MH, Pitot HC: Models of hepatocarcinogenesis in the rat: contrasts and comparisons. Crit Rev Toxicol 17:61, 1986

Gu J, Linnoila RI, Seibel NL et al: A study of myc-related gene expression in small cell lung cancer by in situ hybridization. Am J Pathol 132:13, 1988

Haeder M, Rotsch M, Bepler G et al: Epidermal growth factor receptor expression in human lung cancer cell lines. Cancer Res 48:1132, 1988

Harbour JW, Lai S-L, Whang-Peng J et al: Abnormalities in structure and expression of the human retinoblastoma gene in SCLC. Science 241:353, 1988

Heighway J, Hasleton PS: c-Ki-ras amplification in human lung cancer. Br J Cancer 53:285, 1986

Hensel CH, Hsieh CL, Gazdar AF et al: Altered structure and expression of the human retinoblastoma susceptibility gene in small cell lung cancer. Cancer Res 50:3067, 1990

Hoffmann D, Hecht SS: N'nitrosonornicotine in tobacco. Science 186:265, 1974

Hollstein M, Sidransky D, Vogelstein B, Harris CC: P53 mutations in human cancers. Science 253:49, 1991

Hoover R: Epidemiology: tobacco and geographic pathology. p. 3. In Harris CC (ed): Pathogenesis and Therapy of Lung Cancer. Marcel Dekker, New York, 1978

Horowitz JM, Park SH, Bogenmann E et al: Frequent inactivation of the retinoblastoma anti-oncogene is restricted to a subset of human tumor cells. Proc Natl Acad Sci U S A 87:2775, 1990

Ibson JM, Waters JJ, Twentyman PR et al: Oncogene amplification and chromosomal abnormalities in small cell lung cancer. J Cell Biochem 33:267, 1987

Johnson BE, Battey J, Linnoila I et al: Changes in the phenotype of human small cell lung cancer cell lines after transfection and expression of the c-myc proto-oncogene. J Clin Invest 78:525, 1986

Johnson BE, Ihde DC, Makuch RW et al: Myc family oncogene amplification in tumor cell lines established from small cell lung cancer patients and its relationship to clinical status and course. J Clin Invest 79:1629, 1987

Jones PA, Buckley JD, Henderson BE et al: From gene to carcinogen: a rapidly evolving field in molecular epidemiology. Cancer Res 51:3617, 1991

Kawashima K, Shikama H, Imoto K et al: Close correlation between restriction fragment length polymorphism of the L-myc gene and metastasis of human lung cancer to the lymph nodes and other organs. Proc Natl Acad Sci U S A 85:2353, 1988

Kaye F, Battey J, Nau M et al: Structure and expression of the human L-myc gene reveal a complex pattern of alternative mRNA processing. Mol Cell Biol 8:186, 1988

Keating MT, Williams LT: Autocrine stimulation of intracellular PDGF receptors in v-sis-transformed cells. Science 239:914, 1988

Kern JA, Schwartz DA, Nordberg JE et al: P185-neu expression in human lung adenocarcinomas predicts shortened survival. Cancer Res 50:5184, 1990

Kiefer PE, Bepler G, Kubasch M, Havemann K: Amplification and expression of proto-oncogenes in human small cell lung cancer cell lines. Cancer Res 47:6236, 1987

Kok K, Osinga J, Carritt B et al: Deletion of a DNA sequence at the chromosomal region 3p21 in all major types of lung cancer. Nature 330:578, 1987

Krystal G, Birrer M, Way J et al: Multiple mechanisms for transcriptional regulation of the myc gene family in small-cell lung cancer. Mol Cell Biol 8:3373, 1988

LaForgia S, Morse B, Levy J et al: Receptor protein-tyrosine phosphatase gamma is a candidate tumor suppressor gene at human chromosome region 3p21. Proc Natl Acad Sci U S A 88:5036, 1991

Lane DP, Benchimol S: P53: oncogene or anti-oncogene? Genes Dev 4:1, 1990

Leone A, McBride OW, Weston A et al: Somatic allelic deletion of nm23 in human cancer. Cancer Res 51:2490, 1991

Little CD, Nau MM, Carney DN et al: Amplification and expression of the c-myc oncogene in human lung cancer cell lines. Nature 306:194, 1983

Lupu R, Colomer R, Zugmaier G et al: Direct interaction of a ligand for the erbB2 oncogene product with the EGF receptor and p185erbB2. Science 249:1552, 1990

Lynch HT, Kimberling WJ, Markvicka SE et al: Genetics and smoking-associated cancers. Cancer 57:1640, 1986

Mabry M, Nakagawa T, Nelkin BD et al: V-Ha-ras oncogene insertion: a model for tumor progression of human small cell lung cancer. Proc Natl Acad Sci U S A 85:6523, 1988

Mabry M, Nelkin BD, Falco JP et al: Transitions between lung cancer phenotypes—implications for tumor progression. Cancer Cells 3:53, 1991

Macaulay VM, Everard MJ, Teale JD et al: Autocrine function for insulin-like growth factor I in human small cell lung cancer cell lines and fresh tumor cells. Cancer Res 50:2511, 1990

Malkinson AM: The genetic basis of susceptibility to lung tumors in mice. Toxicology 54:241, 1989

McLemore TL, Adelberg S, Liu MC et al: Expression of CYP1A1 gene in patients with lung cancer: evidence for cigarette smoke-induced gene expression in normal lung tissue and for altered gene regulation in primary pulmonary carcinoma. J Natl Cancer Inst 82:1333, 1990

Milici A, Blick M, Murphy E, Gutterman JU: c-K-ras codon 12 GGT-CGT point mutation. An infrequent event in human lung cancer. Biochem Biophys Res Commun 140:699, 1986

Minuto F, DelMonte P, Barreca et al: Evidence for autocrine mitogenic stimulation by somatomedin-C/insulin-like growth factor I on an established human lung cancer cell line. Cancer Res 48:3716, 1988

Mukhopadhyay T, Cavender A, Tainsky M, Roth JA: Expression of antisense K-ras message in a human lung cancer cell line with a spontaneous activated K-ras oncogene alters the transformed phenotype. Proc Am Assoc Cancer Res 31:304, 1990

Mukhopadhyay T, Cavender AC, Branch CD, Roth JA: Expression and regulation of wild type p53 gene (wtp53) in human non-small cell lung cancer (NSCLC) cell lines carrying normal or mutated p53 gene. J Cell Biochem 15F(Suppl):22, 1991a

Mukhopadhyay T, Tainsky M, Cavender AC, Roth JA: Specific inhibition of K-ras expression and tumorigenicity of lung cancer cells by antisense RNA. Cancer Res 51:1744, 1991b

Murray MJ, Shilo BZ, Shih C et al: Three different human tumor cell lines contain different oncogenes. Cell 25:355, 1981

Natale RB, Cuttitta F, Nakanishi Y et al: IGF-I can stimulate proliferation of non-small cell lung cancer cell lines in vitro (abstr). Proc Am Soc Clin Oncol 7:197, 1988

Nau MM, Brooks BJ, Battey J et al: L-myc, a new myc-related gene amplified and expressed in human small cell lung cancer. Nature 318:69, 1985

Nau MM, Brooks BJ, Carney DN et al: Human small-cell lung cancers show amplification and expression of the N-myc gene. Proc Natl Acad Sci U S A 83:1092, 1986

Naylor SL, Johnson BE, Minna JD, Sakaguchi AY: Loss of heterozygosity of chromosome 3p markers in small-cell lung cancer. Nature 329:451, 1987

Nicolson GL: Cancer metastasis: tumor cell and host organ properties important in metastasis to specific secondary sites. Biochim Biophys Acta 948:175, 1988

Nigro JM, Baker SJ, Preisinger AC et al: Mutations in the p53 gene occur in diverse human tumor types. Nature 342:705, 1989

Ooi WL, Elston RC, Chen VW et al: Increased familial risk for lung cancer. J Natl Cancer Inst 76:217, 1986

Putnam EA, Yen N, Gallick GE et al: Autocrine growth stimulation by transforming growth factor alpha in human non-small cell lung cancer. Surg Oncol 1:49, 1992

Reynolds SH, Anna CK, Brown KC et al: Activated protooncogenes in human lung tumors from smokers. Proc Natl Acad Sci U S A 88:1085, 1991

Riedel H, Massoglia S, Schlessinger J, Ullrich A: Ligand activation of overexpressed epidermal growth factor receptors transforms NIH 3T3 mouse fibroblasts. Proc Natl Acad Sci U S A 85:1477, 1988

Rodenhuis S, Slebos FJC, Kibbelaar RE et al: Mutational activation of the Kirsten-ras oncogene is associated with early relapse and poor survival in adenocarcinoma of the lung. Proc Am Soc Clin Oncol 9:228, 1990

Rodenhuis S, Slebos RJC, Boot AJM et al: Incidence and possible clinical significance of K-ras oncogene activation in adenocarcinoma of the human lung. Cancer Res 48:5738, 1988

Rodenhuis S, Van De Wetering ML, Mooi WJ et al: Mutational activation of the K-ras oncogene. N Engl J Med 317:929, 1987

Roth JA, Mukhopadhyay T, Yen N et al: Molecular approach to lung cancer therapy. J Cell Biochem Suppl 15F:4, 1991

Sakiyama S, Nakamura Y, Yasuda S: Expression of epidermal growth factor receptor gene in cultured human lung cancer cells. Jpn J Cancer Res 77:965, 1986

Saksela K, Bergh J, Nilsson K: Amplification of the N-myc oncogene in an adenocarcinoma of the lung. J Cell Biochem 31:297, 1986

Samet JM, Humble CG, Pathak DR: Personal and family history of respiratory disease and lung cancer risk. Am Rev Respir Dis 134:466, 1986

Sausville EA, Moyer JD, Heikkila R et al: A correlation of bombesin-responsiveness with myc-family gene expression in small cell lung carcinoma cell lines. Ann N Y Acad Sci 547:310, 1988

Schechter AL, Stern DF, Vaidyanathan L et al: The neu oncogene: an erb-B-related gene encoding a 185,000-Mr tumour antigen. Nature 312:513, 1984

Schneider PM, Hung M-C, Ames RS et al: Novel alteration in the epidermal growth factor receptor gene is frequently detected in human non-small cell lung cancer. Lung Cancer 6:65, 1990

Schneider PM, Hung M-C, Chiocca SM et al: Differential expression of the c-erbB-2 gene in human small cell and non-small cell lung cancer. Cancer Res 49:4968, 1989

Schneider PM, Hung M-C, Tainsky MA et al: Epidermal growth factor receptor gene abnormalities in human non-small cell lung cancer. J Cell Biochem Suppl 12A:113, 1988

Schneider PM, Praeuer HW, Fink U et al: Comparison of neu (c-erbB2) gene expression in small cell lung cancer (SCLC), non-small cell lung cancer (NSCLC), and normal lung. Proc Am Assoc Cancer Res 31:312, 1990b

Sellers TA, Bailey-Wilson JE, Elston RC et al: Evidence for mendelian inheritance on the pathogenesis of lung cancer. J Natl Cancer Inst 82:1272, 1990

Shigematsu K, Kataoka Y, Kurihara M et al: Partial characterization of insulin-like growth factor-I in primary human lung cancers using immunohistochemical and receptor autoradiographic techniques. Cancer Res 50:2481, 1990

Shimizu K, Birnbaum D, Ruly MA et al: Structure of the Ki-ras gene of the human lung carcinoma cell line Calu-1. Nature 304:497, 1983

Shiraishi M, Noguchi M, Shimosato Y, Sekiya T: Amplification of protooncogenes in surgical specimens of human lung carcinomas. Cancer Res 49:6474, 1989

Siegfried JM, Owens SE: Response of primary human lung carcinomas to autocrine growth factors produced by a lung carcinoma cell line. Cancer Res 48:4976, 1988

Skillrud DM, Offord KP, Miller RD: Higher risk of lung cancer in chronic obstructive pulmonary disease. Ann Internal Med 105:503, 1986

Skinner MA, Vollmer R, Huper G et al: Loss of heterozygosity for genes on 11p and the clinical course of patients with lung carcinoma. Cancer Res 50:2303, 1990

Slamon DJ, Clark GM, Wong SG et al: Human breast cancer correlation of relapse and survival with amplification of the HER-2/neu oncogene. Science 235:177, 1987

Stehelin D, Varnus HE, Bishop JM, Vogt PK: DNA related to the transforming gene(s) of avian sarcoma viruses is present in normal avian DNA. Nature 260:170, 1976

Takahashi T, Nau MM, Chiba I et al: P53: a frequent target for genetic abnormalities in lung cancer. Science 246:491, 1989

Vogelstein B, Fearon ER, Hamilton SR et al: Genetic alterations during colorectal-tumor development. N Engl J Med 319:525, 1988

Weston A, Willey JC, Modali R et al: Differential DNA sequence deletions from chromosomes 3, 11, 13, and 17 in squamous-cell carcinoma, large-cell carcinoma, and adenocarcinoma of the lung. Proc Natl Acad Sci U S A 86:5099, 1989

Wong ST, Winchell LF, McCune BK et al: The TGF-alpha precursor expressed on the cell surface binds to the EGF receptor on adjacent cells leading to signal transduction. Cell 56:495, 1989

Xu H-J, Hu S-X, Cagle PT et al: Absence of retinoblastoma protein expression in primary non-small cell lung carcinomas. Cancer Res 51:2735, 1991

Yamamoto F, Nakano H, Neville C, Perucho M: Structure and mechanisms of activation of c-K-ras oncogenes in human lung cancer. Prog Med Virol 32:101, 1985

Yokota J, Wada M, Shimosato Y et al: Loss of heterozygosity on chromosomes 3, 13, and 17 in small-cell carcinoma and on chromosome 3 in adenocarcinoma of the lung. Proc Natl Acad Sci U S A 84:9252, 1987

Yoshimoto K, Hirohashi S, Sekiya T: Increased expression of the c-myc gene without gene amplification in human lung cancer and colon cancer cell lines. Jpn J Cancer Res 77:540, 1986

Epidemiology

Anthony B. Miller

DEFINITION

Epidemiology is the science that identifies the distribution and determinants (causes) of disease. Descriptive epidemiology documents the changes in the incidence of and mortality rate from disease with time and the differences in the rates of disease in different populations. Analytic epidemiology evaluates disease determinants, mainly using two types of studies, case-control and cohort. In case-control studies, the histories of cases (patients with the disease) and controls (those without the disease), who are drawn from the same population as the cases, are compared. In cohort studies, the status of large numbers of individuals is ascertained, and they are followed to determine the subsequent incidence and/or mortality rate from the disease. Case-control studies usually consider one cancer site, but they can simultaneously evaluate the effect of multiple exposures to different hazards. Cohort studies usually consider limited numbers of exposures (e.g., occupation or tobacco use), but they can evaluate the effect of these exposures on many different diseases.

In this chapter I refer to two different measures of the risk of disease in humans, derived from analytical epidemiology: the relative and attributable risk. The relative risk is the multiple of disease risk in one group (e.g., smokers of cigarettes) relative to that in a referent group (e.g., nonsmokers of cigarettes). When the risk is increased, the relative risk is greater than one; when the risk is less than that in the referent group, the relative risk is less than one. A relative risk of 1.0 means no increased risk; one of 1.5 is a 50% increase in risk; one of 2.0 is a doubling of risk; and one of 10.0 is a 10-fold increase in risk. In a well-conducted study, a finding of a relative risk of more than 2.0 is very suggestive of a causal association; one greater than 5.0 is almost certainly causal. The attributable risk is the amount of disease attributable to (or caused by) a factor. In a cohort study, the amount of disease attributable to a factor can be directly determined. In a population-based case-control study, the amount of disease in that population attributable to the exposure can be estimated.

HISTORICAL NOTE

In the nineteenth century, lung cancer was a rare disease. Throughout most of this century, the incidence of and mortality rate from lung cancer in men in North America and Europe has been rising, as it is now in the rest of the world. The rates started rising in women about 30 years later than in men. Initially there was confusion as to the cause of this epidemic. Although some suspected tobacco, the potential causes also under consideration in the late 1940s were increased automobile exhaust fumes and general air pollution. However, the early case-control studies published in the 1950s (Doll and Hill, 1952; Wynder and Graham, 1950), followed by several cohort studies in Britain and North America (Doll and Peto, 1976; Hammond and Horn, 1958; Kahn, 1966), confirmed that the cause is tobacco, largely cigarette smoking. In the British doctors study (Doll and Peto, 1976), after a 20-year follow-up, the mean annual death rate from lung cancer in nonsmokers was 10 per 100,000; that in smokers of 15 to 24 cigarettes/day was 127 per 100,000. The risk in these smokers relative to the nonsmokers was therefore 12.7. The amount of deaths from lung cancer attributable to smoking 15 to 24 cigarettes/day among those with this intensity of smoking is derived by subtracting the rate of death from lung cancer in the nonsmokers from that in the smokers, under the assumption that the smokers would have had the same death rate as the nonsmokers if they had not smoked. In this instance the attributable risk is 127 minus 10 per 100,000 = 117 (i.e., $117/127 \times 100$ percent, or 92 percent). Numerous studies confirmed that 80 to 90 percent of the lung cancer in developed countries is attributable to tobacco use. The risk of lung cancer is dependent on the age at which smoking starts, the intensity of smoking, and the duration of the habit. Of these factors duration is the most important.

HISTORICAL READINGS

Doll R, Hill AB: A study of the aetiology of carcinoma of the lung. BMJ 2:1271, 1952

Doll R, Peto R: Mortality in relation to smoking: 20 years observations on male British doctors. BMJ 2:1525, 1976

Hammond EC, Horn D: Smoking and death rates—report on forty-four months of follow-up of 187,783 men. II. Death rates by cause. JAMA 166:1294,1958

Kahn HA: The Dorn study of smoking and mortality among US veterans. Report on eight and one-half years of observation. Monogr Natl Cancer Inst 19:1, 1966

Wynder EL, Graham EA: Tobacco smoking as a possible etiologic factor in bronchiogenic carcinoma. A study of six hundred and eighty-four proved cases. JAMA 143:329, 1950

DESCRIPTIVE EPIDEMIOLOGY

It is well recognized that lung cancer is now the most important cancer in men in terms of both incidence and mortality rate, and although it is not the most important cancer in women in terms of incidence (breast cancer still holds this position), it is now the number one cancer in terms of mortality rate in the United States and will shortly become so in Canada. The American Cancer Society estimated that there were 101,000 new cases of lung cancer diagnosed in men in the United States in 1991 and 60,000 in women, with the number of deaths being 92,000 and 51,000, respectively (Boring, et al., 1991). With the decline in the cardiovascular disease mortality rate, there is now good evidence that lung cancer is the number one cause of death attributable to tobacco in the United States (Shopland, et al., 1991), having supplanted coronary heart disease as the leading cause of death among smokers in about 1987.

For most of this century, lung cancer rates have been rising in men, with the rise in women occurring largely in the latter half of the century. An analysis of trends in smoking and projections of resulting long-term (to 2025) lung cancer mortality rates in men and women was attempted for the United States (Brown and Kessler, 1988). Although the age-adjusted rates in women are expected to almost reach those in men during this time period, they are not expected to exceed them. However, unless a substantial reduction in smoking occurs in women by the year 2000, the age-standardized rate in women will not begin to decline until about 2020. Within age groups, the decline in the lung cancer mortality rate for men is already occurring for all ages up to 55 years, but for women, the rate declines only up to age 45 years. The decline in the age-specific mortality rate for women is expected to remain about 20 years behind that for men. With declining smoking rates (Marcus, et al., 1989), there has been anticipation that a downturn of the male rates might be about to

occur. An analysis by birth cohort of U.S. data confirms this (Devesa, et al., 1989). Because of the dominance of smoking habits established when people are young on their subsequent risk of lung cancer, translating the declining lung cancer rates in patients younger than age 45 years into lifetime predictions for those born during the same period (birth cohorts) shows that the overall lung cancer rates in men will begin to decline in the 1990s and in women after the year 2000.

In populations where the full effect of smoking is seen (i.e., when there has been sufficient time for maximum smoking prevalence to have occurred and for the effect of the duration of smoking to be seen, as will shortly be the case in men in North America), lung cancer rates rise throughout life, most steeply at ages older than 50 years (Fig. 27-3). In women in North America, the age-specific incidence of lung cancer does not yet express the full effect of smoking, hence the downturn in rates at older ages and the continuing increase in age-standardized rates as the rates within older age groups continue to increase. Even so, with the age-standardized mortality rate of lung cancer in women now exceeding that of breast cancer, it is possible to appreciate the difference between the age-specific death rates from these two cancers at different ages (Fig. 27-4). At ages younger than about 65 years, breast cancer is a more important cause of death than is lung cancer. It is only at about age 65 years that there is a reversal in relative positions. (Figure 27-4 indicates a further reversal at age 80 years.) This occurs because the death rates from lung cancer are still increasing at the oldest ages. After about one decade or so, we can expect lung cancer in women in North America to be a more important cause of death than breast cancer is because of the delayed impact of cigarette smoking.) These differences in age-specific effects at younger ages are likely to persist, even with continuing increases in age-standardized mortality rates of lung cancer in women. Thus as a cause of premature death in younger women, breast cancer will remain number one.

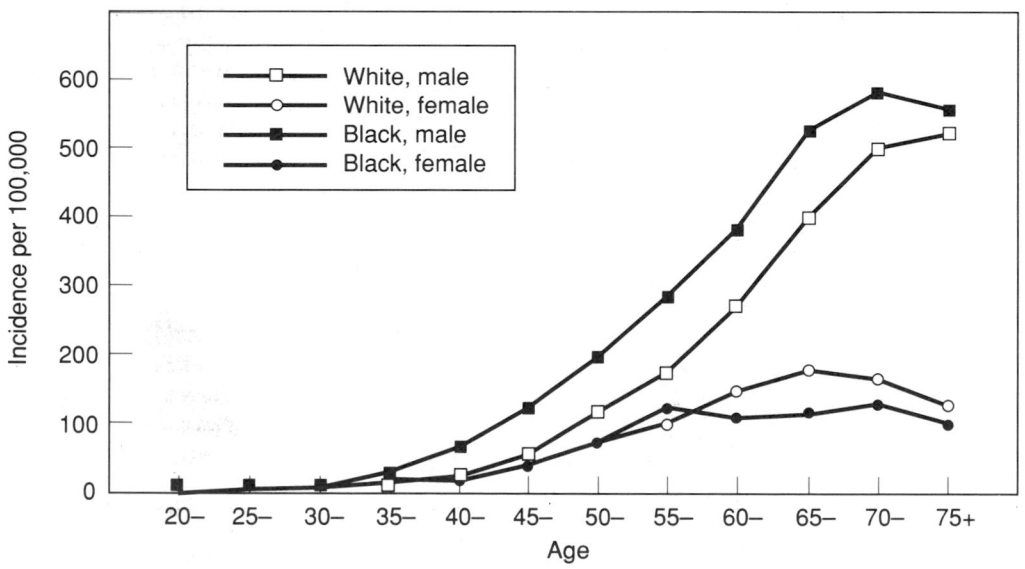

Figure 27-3. Age-specific incidence rates per 100,000 of lung cancer for whites and blacks, Los Angeles County, California, 1978 to 1982. (Data from Muir C, Waterhouse J, Mack T et al: Cancer Incidence in Five Continents. Vol. V. Lyon, IARC Scientific Publication, no. 88, 1987.)

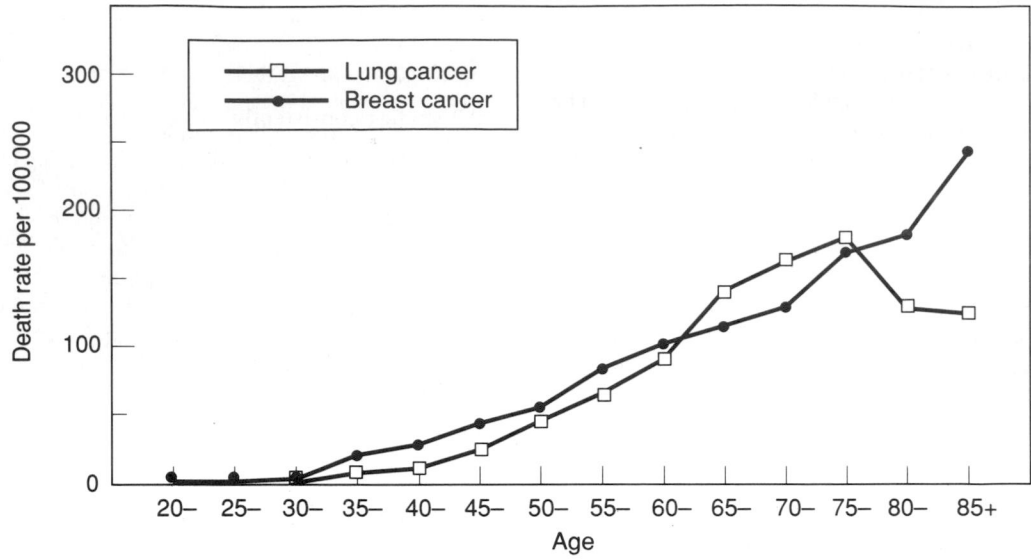

Figure 27-4. Age-specific death rates per 100,000 from breast cancer and lung cancer in women in Canada, 1988. (Data from Cause of death tabulations, Health Reports. Suppl 11. Canadian Centre for Health Information. Vol. 2. 1990.)

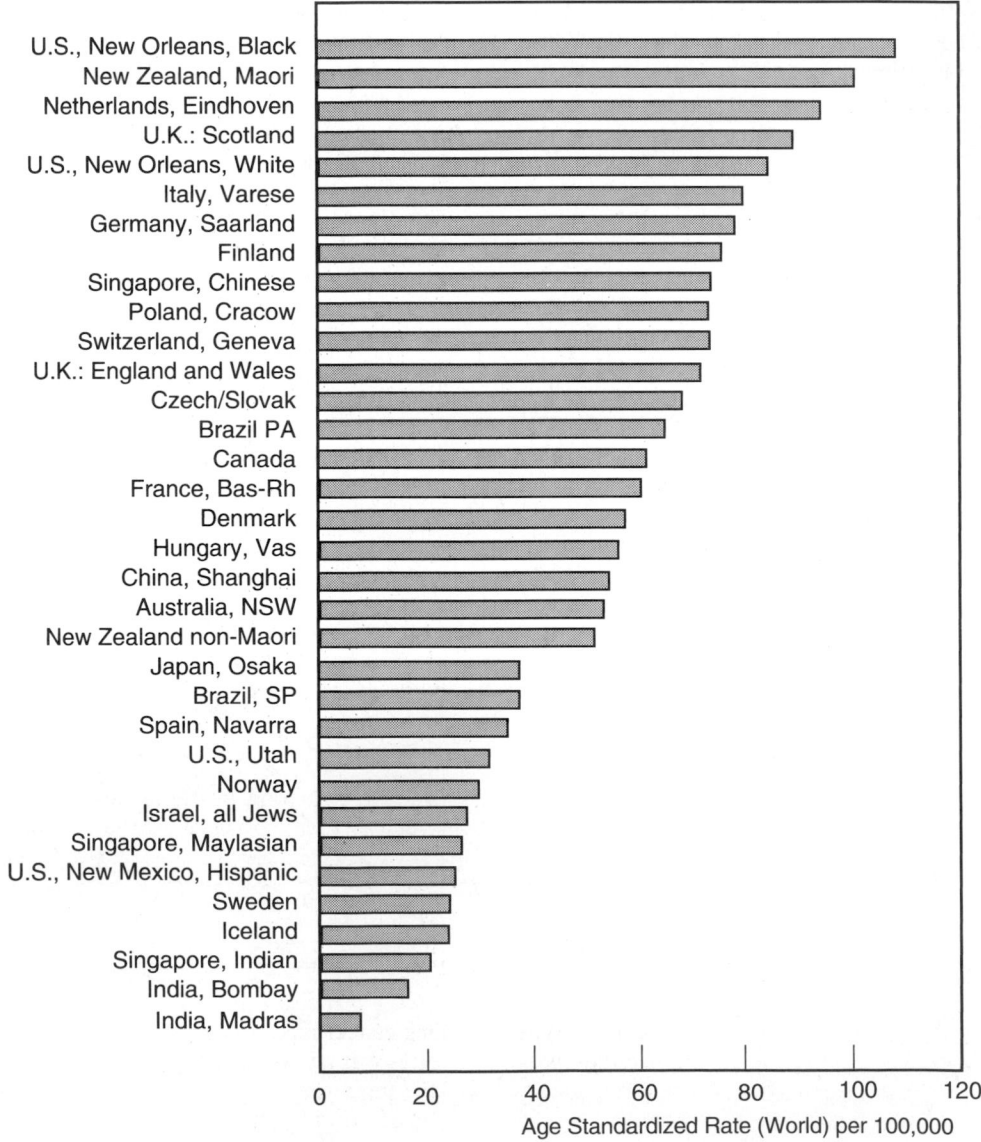

Figure 27-5. Age-standardized incidence rates (world standard population) per 100,000 of lung cancer in men for various registries that contribute to the data in Muir C, Waterhouse J, Mack T et al: Cancer Incidence in Five Continents. Vol. V. Lyon, IARC Scientific Publications, no. 88, 1987 (approximate time period 1978 to 1982).

Internationally as for other cancers, there are substantial differences in the incidence of lung cancer (Fig. 27-5). The highest rates in the world in the early 1980s were recorded in U.S. blacks in New Orleans with the Maoris of New Zealand in second place. The lowest were recorded from cancer registries in India. Nearly all of these differences reflect differences in the prevalence of cigarette smoking about 40 years ago. As the smoking prevalence changes, international differences will change, with a similar delay. It seems probable that, if present trends continue, in the next century the country with the highest rates will be China, with possibly Japan not far behind; the numbers of lung cancers diagnosed each year in many other countries of Asia, Africa, and South America will increase substantially, with falls continuing in Europe and North America. Thus lung cancer will have been the predominant cancer in the developed world in the 20th century, but it will become the predominant cancer in the developing world in the 21st century.

Within countries there are substantial differences by race and ethnicity (Fig. 27-5). Thus rates in U.S. blacks now exceed those in U.S. whites, although only at younger ages in women (Fig. 27-3). Again these differences largely reflect differences in earlier smoking rates, although for the black-white United States comparison, there may be a contribution from occupational factors. The Singapore cancer registry reports rates for Chinese, Malays, and Indians. The rates for the Singapore Chinese were higher than in Shanghai and nearly four times as high as the other ethnic groups in Singapore. Within the United States the highest rates were reported from New Orleans and the lowest in whites from Utah, presumably because of the low rates of smoking among members of the Mormon church.

LUNG CANCER AND ACTIVE SMOKING

More evidence is available on tobacco smoking as a cause of lung cancer than for any other complex mixture of carcinogens, such as is present in mainstream tobacco smoke (IARC, 1986). The evidence relating to exposure to sidestream or environmental tobacco smoke is reviewed in a later section of this chapter. The risk varies according to the type of tobacco smoked, amount of tobacco smoked, duration of smoking, and tar content of the tobacco smoked. The risk remains relatively constant, however, when individuals stop smoking. The evidence increasingly shows that women are at least as great a risk as men per amount smoked. This evidence is now reviewed.

Type of Tobacco Smoked

The risk is greater for cigarette smoking than for smoking any other type of tobacco. For example, in the British doctors cohort study, the risk for pipe and/or cigar smokers relative to nonsmokers who had never previously smoked cigarettes was 5.8; that for pipe and/or cigar smokers who also smoked cigarettes, 8.2; and that for cigarette smokers, only 14.0 (Doll and Peto, 1976). Similar differences in the risk with the type of tobacco were found in the other major cohort studies, with the risk consistently higher for smokers of cigarettes only (IARC, 1986, Table 54, p. 205).

Amount of Tobacco Smoked

All studies consistently show a dose-response relationship, that is the risk of lung cancer increases with the amount smoked, usually expressed as the number of cigarettes smoked per day. In the Canadian veterans study, for example, the risk for those who smoked 1 to 9 cigarettes per day was 10.0 relative to nonsmokers, 16.4 for those who smoked 10 to 20 per day, and 17.3 for those who smoked 21 or more cigarettes per day (Lossing, et al., 1966). Even higher risks for heavy smokers relative to nonsmokers have been found in some studies. For example, a risk of 25.1 for smokers of 25 or more cigarettes per day was found in the British doctors study (Doll and Peto, 1976) and a risk of 23.7 for smokers of 40 or more cigarettes per day in the U.S. veterans study (Rogot and Murray, 1980). The IARC (1986) report summarized the findings from the major cohort studies (Table 61, pp. 215 to 216).

Duration of Smoking

One of the key features of the relationship between cigarette smoking and lung cancer is the relevance of the duration of regular cigarette smoking to the lung cancer risk (Doll and Peto, 1976). Thus using a statistical model fitted to data from the British doctors study, Peto and Doll (1984) estimated that the excess annual lung cancer incidence rates after about 45, 30, and 15 years of cigarette smoking were in the ratio of approximately 100 : 20 : 1. The long delay that is seen between an increase in cigarette smoking and its full effect on national lung cancer rates is caused by this critical dependence on the duration of smoking (Doll and Peto, 1981). One effect of this dependence on duration is that the lifetime risk of lung cancer varies substantially according to whether cigarette smoking starts at the age of 15 years (or earlier) or is delayed until 20 or 25 years of age (IARC, 1986).

Effect of Different Levels of Tar

There are two major difficulties in assessing the risk of cigarettes of different tar contents (and the risk of filter versus nonfilter cigarettes). The first relates to the relatively recent reduction in the tar content in the last 30 years in North America and Europe. Most people currently developing lung cancer started smoking with much higher tar level cigarettes than are generally available now. The second relates to the fact that the main driving force for individuals in the amount they smoke is the level of nicotine to which they are addicted (Surgeon General, 1988). Nicotine reduction usually accompanies a reduction in the tar levels in cigarettes. Thus on switching to lower tar-level brands, smokers compensate by adopting smoking practices that have the effect of increasing the amount of nicotine absorbed, and hence the amount of tar inhaled, and by increasing the numbers of cigarettes smoked per day (Gritz, 1988). Nevertheless, both the Surgeon General (1982) and the IARC Working Group (1986) concluded that reduced tar levels were followed by a reduced lung cancer risk, although the risk for smoking low-tar cigarettes was still substantially greater than that in nonsmokers. One large case-control study of 7,804 cases of lung cancer and 15,207 hospital-based controls, which demonstrated this reduction in risk, was conducted in seven centers in western Europe (Lubin, et al., 1984). The results of this study suggest that lifetime smokers of nonfiltered cigarettes were at nearly twice the risk of lung cancer compared with lifelong filtered cigarette smokers, after controlling for the duration of cigarette use and the number smoked per day. The same study indicated that male smokers of high-tar cigarettes had about 1.7 times the risk of smokers of low-tar brands. For women the corresponding estimate was 7.7. It seems probable that the changes in tobacco content of cigarettes beginning about the mid 1950s have contributed to the decline in tar level and to the decline in the lung cancer mortality rate (Walker and Brin, 1988). Nevertheless in one study in the United States, careful control for differences in age and total amount smoked resulted in an insignificant risk reduction for smokers of low-tar cigarettes (Wilcox, et al., 1988). It was noted that cases who smoked low-tar cigarettes had compensated by increasing the number of cigarettes they smoked by almost one-half pack; a similar effect was not noted in the controls or in cases who smoked high-tar cigarettes.

Effect of Cessation of Smoking

The risk among exsmokers is usually compared with that of continuing smokers or nonsmokers. On the basis of the former comparison, it is usually concluded that the risk among exsmokers decreases the longer the time that smoking has been given up. However, this comparison has to take cognizance of the fact that continuing smokers incur a substantial increase in risk the longer they continue to smoke. Once this is appreciated, it is clear that the risk among exsmokers does not fall but stays at approximately the same level it had reached at the time smoking ceased, the level of that risk being determined by the duration of smoking up to the time of cessation and the intensity of smoking (Miller, 1984; IARC, 1986). This relationship was most clearly seen from the analyses of the British doctors study because there was a longer period of follow-up than that in other cohort studies and the investigators sought information on smoking habits at 5-year intervals during the course of the study and were thus able to classify more precisely than in other studies the changes of cigarette smoking that occurred with time. The study also demonstrated that the risk among exsmokers exceeded the risk among nonsmokers throughout the 20-year follow-up period (Doll and Peto, 1976). There were similar findings in the U.S. Veterans study (Rogot and Murray, 1980). Although in the American Cancer Society study the risk among exsmokers appeared to fall to the same level as that for nonsmokers 10 or more years after the cessation of smoking (Freedman and Navidi, 1990), this was based on only five deaths from lung cancer in exheavy smokers and one in former light smokers (Hammond, 1966). Furthermore, the data on cessation of smoking were based only on those obtained on enrollment in the study.

LUNG CANCER AND OTHER RISK FACTORS

Female Gender

Although most of the earlier studies of lung cancer involving women suggested lower risks from cigarette smoking than in men, the study of female British doctors suggested that, for

equivalent amounts smoked, women had as great a risk of lung cancer as did men (Doll, et al., 1980). However, the earlier studies showing lower risks in women than in men were conducted in populations in which women had not been smoking long enough to show the full effect of smoking, a problem largely avoided in the female British doctors study, which had a 22-year follow-up.

A case-control study in Los Angeles County enabled risks to be assessed in relation to the main histologic types of lung cancer in women (Wu, et al., 1985). About two-thirds of the cases had adenocarcinomas, and the risks for cigarette smokers relative to nonsmokers were increased 6.5-fold for those who smoked more than 20 cigarettes/day and 8-fold for those who began smoking at 18 years of age or earlier. For the patients with squamous cell carcinoma (well recognized as largely caused by smoking in men; IARC, 1986), the corresponding relative risks were 94.4 and 115.7, respectively. A similar differential effect was found in a French case-control study (Benhamou, et al., 1987). However, the estimated risks were substantially lower, perhaps because French women only recently began to smoke in heavy numbers, and at that time, lung cancer in women in France was rare.

In the Surgeon General's (1989) report, preliminary findings from the new large American Cancer Society Cancer Prevention Study II (CPS-II), based on more than 1.2 million American men and women followed from 1982 to 1986, are presented. This study, conducted in all 50 states, had the same design and methods as did the earlier large American Cancer Society cohort study of more than 1 million men and women conducted in 25 states, beginning in 1959 (Hammond, 1966). This earlier study is now called the Cancer Prevention Study I (CPS-I) and is directly comparable to CPS-II. It is clear that there has been a substantial increase in the risk of lung cancer in women as a result of the increased proportion of women in the population who have smoked for long periods. For example, the risk for female current smokers in CPS-II relative to nonsmokers (11.94) is now similar to that for men in CPS-I (11.35) (Surgeon General, 1989, Tables 4 and 7, pp. 148 and 151).

In a study done in New Jersey, particularly high risks were found for small cell carcinoma of the lung (Schoenberg, et al., 1989). Compared with that in nonsmokers, the risk was increased 62-fold for small cell carcinoma, 11-fold for squamous cell, and 4-fold for adenocarcinoma. Similar risk levels were found in a study of lung cancer in women in Sweden (Svensson, et al., 1989). This reminds us that although the risks are lower for adenocarcinoma with smoking than for other histologic types, in both sexes now, the majority of such cancers are caused by cigarette smoking (Brownson, et al., 1987).

In a recent case-control study in southern Ontario, 469 female cases of lung cancer were interviewed (315 in person and 154 by proxy) as were 472 male cases matched to the female cases by age and selected at random from the larger pool of male cases (335 in person and 137 by proxy). A matched population control was interviewed for each case. The risk of lung cancer per 10 pack-years relative to that in nonsmokers was 9.77 for the women and 7.18 for the men. The risk was higher for the women within each smoking intensity category and for each histologic type of carcinoma, except large or giant cell and unspecified carcinomas (Risch, et al., 1992).

Passive Smoking

The first studies to indicate a possible increased risk of lung cancer from passive smoking came from Japan and Greece, countries with a larger proportion of female nonsmokers than in North America. Hirayama (1981) reported a relative risk of 1.8 for female nonsmokers married to husbands who smoked relative to those whose husbands did not smoke from a large cohort study, which included a total of 108,906 women, 346 of whom died from lung cancer during a 14-year follow-up period, with 17,366 cigarette smokers, 69,645 nonsmokers married to smoking husbands and 21,895 nonsmokers married to nonsmoking husbands. Although the relative risk for female smokers was 3.8, the amount of lung cancer attributable to passive smoking in women was potentially greater than that from active smoking in Japan because of the four times as many women exposed to passive smoke than active smoking women. Analysis of the amount of smoking by the husbands suggested a dose-response relationship. Trichopoulos, et al. (1981), in a hospital-based case-control study, had almost identical findings. Thus the risk for nonsmoking women married to smoking husbands was 3.4 for husbands who smoked 20 or more cigarettes a day, 2.4 for those who smoked 1 to 19, and 1.8 for those married to exsmokers, relative to nonsmoking women married to nonsmoking husbands.

These early studies were greeted with some skepticism because of the potential for misclassification of smoking status. It would only be necessary for a few active female smokers to be misclassified as nonsmokers for the effects observed to be produced. The potential for this was particularly great in Hirayama's (1981) study because it was not as socially acceptable for women to smoke in Japan in 1966, when the data were collected, than it became later. Interestingly, a case-control study based on the atomic bomb survivors in Japan and performed later showed similar findings (Akiba, et al., 1986). Thus, the risk for nonsmoking women married to husbands who smoked 30 or more cigarettes a day relative to women married to nonsmoking husbands was 2.1 (95 percent confidence interval, 0.7, 2.5). There was also a suggestion of a dose-response relationship (P for trend, 0.06).

The publication of the early results led to a succession of studies. Some were largely negative (Garfinkel, 1981; Kabat and Wynder, 1984; Koo, et al., 1985). Part of the difficulty is related to the overwhelming importance of active smoking as a cause of lung cancer, even in women, and the rarity of lung cancer in nonsmokers. Thus to obtain sufficient subjects in a case-control study, Garfinkel, et al. (1985) had to identify cases from four hospitals over an 11-year period. Patients with colorectal cancer served as controls. A significantly increased doubling in risk was found for nonsmoking women with husbands who smoked 40 or more cigarettes a day or 20 or more at home, relative to nonsmoking women with nonsmoking husbands. This excess risk was largely restricted to cases with squamous cell carcinoma.

Excess risk for cases with histologic types recognized as being smoking related, such as squamous or small cell carcinomas, as distinct from adenocarcinomas, which is well recognized as being the most common type found in nonsmokers., was found in a number of other studies, adding to the biologic plausibility of the association. Thus Dalager, et al. (1986), in a joint analysis of the results of two case-control studies in the United States, found that the relative risk for the occurrence of squamous and small cell carcinomas in nonsmoking women married to smoking husbands was 2.88 (95 percent confidence interval, 0.91, 9.10); for adenocarcinoma, 1.02 (0.33, 3.16); and for other histologic types, 1.31 (0.48, 3.57), with women married to nonsmoking husbands as the reference group. A similar effect was found in a nested case-control study set within a cohort of 27,409 nonsmoking Swedish women identified from questionnaires mailed in 1961 and 1963 (Pershagen, et al., 1987). In this study it was possible to examine the effect of both the intensity of husbands smoking and histologic type simultaneously. The relative risk for the occurrence of squamous or small cell carcinoma among nonsmoking women married to husbands who smoked 15 or more cigarettes a day was 6.4 (95 percent confidence interval, 1.1, 34.7). The risk for the occurrence of other histologic types with similar intensity of the husbands' smoking was 2.4 (0.6, 8.7), relative to nonsmoking women married to non-smoking husbands.

Wald, et al. (1986) published the results of a metaanalysis (or conjoint analysis) of the 13 studies with the results then available that had been contributed to a report of the National Research Council (1986) on passive smoking. There was a consistent tendency for an excess risk to be seen from passive exposure to environmental tobacco smoke. The conjoint risk from 10 case-control studies was 1.27 (95 percent confidence interval, 1.05, 1.53) and from 3 cohort studies, 1.44 (1.20, 1.72), the latter heavily influenced by Hirayama's (1981) results. For all 13 studies, the combined estimate of relative risk was 1.35 (1.19, 1.54). An adjustment for misclassification reduced this risk to 1.30, but adjustment for the fact that the referents (largely nonsmoking women married to nonsmoking husbands) were in fact exposed to some environmental tobacco smoke from others raised the relative risk to 1.53. Since this analysis, the results of a further case-control study from Hong Kong have been reported (Lam, et al., 1987). This included a larger number of subjects than the earlier negative studies in Hong Kong did (Koo, et al., 1985, 1987), and a significant positive association was found among never-smoking women for passive smoking caused by a smoking husband (relative risk, 1.65; 95 percent confidence interval, 1.16, 2.35). In a more recent study of lung cancer in women in Sweden (Svennson, et al., 1989), an attempt was made to evaluate the role of passive smoking. However, the study was not large, and therefore the number of lung cases in nonsmokers was small. Thus although the risk estimates for passive smoking were of a similar order to those found in studies elsewhere (about a twofold increase in risk for nonsmokers exposed for long durations to heavy smoking in others), the findings were not statistically significant. Passive smoking was further evaluated in a case-control study of nonsmoking women in Greece (Kalandidi, et al., 1990). The marriage of a nonsmoking woman to a smoker was associated with a doubling of the risk of lung cancer. In a study of 191 patients with lung cancer who had never smoked in New York State (Janerich, et al., 1990), no effect of exposure to a spouse's smoking was found, but household exposure to 25 or more smoker-years during childhood and adolescence doubled the risk of lung cancer. This is an important observation because for some time it has been recognized that, as the duration of exposure to active smoking was such a critical variable, anything that lengthened this could increase the risk of lung cancer substantially. Although other positive and negative studies have been reported (Gao, et al., 1987; Humble, et al., 1987; Holowaty, et al., 1991; Lee, et al., 1986), it seems probable that the earlier combined estimate of risk still stands. Indeed a review conducted for the Environmental Protection Agency (1990) produced a pooled estimate of risk from 22 studies of 1.41 (95 percent confidence interval, 1.26, 1.57). Furthermore a preliminary report of the largest case-control study yet conducted in nonsmoking women of the relationship of environmental tobacco smoke to lung cancer confirmed the previous estimates of risk (Fontham, et al., 1991).

Passive smoking may also increase the risk of lung cancer in active smokers. A possibly particularly critical time may be exposure in childhood. Correa, et al. (1983) attempted to evaluate the effect of parental smoking adjusting for active smoking. There was no increased risk if the father was a smoker (relative risk, 0.83), but the relative risk was 1.36 if the mother was a smoker ($P < 0.05$). Sandler, et al. (1985) also found evidence of a greater cancer risk for individuals with household exposure to cigarette smoke during both childhood and adulthood than for individuals with exposures during only one period. These are plausible results that need evaluation in other studies. Given the importance of the duration of active smoking in the risk of lung cancer, as discussed in the previous section, it is conceivable that parental smoking could have a greater effect on the induction of lung cancer than would passive smoke exposure in adults, especially if followed by active smoking. The carcinogenic process could be initiated 10 or more years earlier, with an additive effect on subsequent lung cancer incidence.

In a report of a metanalysis of nine studies conducted in America, apparently financed by the tobacco industry, a nonsignificant combined estimate of risk of 1.12 (95 percent confidence interval, 0.95, 1.30) was derived (Fleiss and Gross, 1991). This was lower than the earlier estimates (National Research Council, 1986; Wald, et al., 1986), which the authors criticize. The different estimate is in part because the other estimates incorporated studies from other countries in which the effects of passive smoking may be easier to demonstrate, but also because the analysis of Fleiss and Gross (1991) also included four U.S. studies not available in 1986. One of these, however, was a 1987 doctoral dissertation, which at that time, reported negative findings but which, on further analysis, was found to show significant risks for household exposure to passive smoke (Janerich, et al., 1990), a report which may have appeared after the analysis of Fleiss and Gross (1991) was completed. It is of interest that the doctoral dissertation just referred to was the only unpublished study cited as justification for the claim in a commentary (Butler, 1991), supported by the RJR Nabisco Company, that the Working Group on Passive Smoking (1990) (itself supported by the tobacco industry) failed to cite unpublished relevant studies. The Working Group on Passive Smoking (1990) concluded that passive smoke was hazardous to health and significantly increased the risk of lung cancer in nonsmokers.

Lung Cancer in Asia

One of the largest cohort studies ever performed was initiated in 1966 in Japan by Hirayama (1982). This has been a fruitful source of data, largely confirming the findings from the studies in the West that implicate cigarette smoking as the major cause of lung cancer. A recent report from Japan of a large case-control study of the lung cancer risk in exsmokers largely confirms previous reports from cohort and case-control studies (Sobue, et al., 1991). The risks of lung cancer in exsmokers compared with those in continuing smokers diminished progressively with an increasing duration after a cessation of smoking. Although this study confirms what we know, it has to be carefully interpreted. The absence of a comparison with rates in lifelong nonsmokers means that we cannot assess whether the risk returns to the rates of nonsmokers.

China is also one of the countries in Asia where smoking rates are now high and where lung cancer is becoming more and more frequent as a consequence. Until recently, however, there was a widespread disbelief that smoking was hazardous. A series of studies are underway in China, and the results of a few are now available. In a study among Chinese women, cigarette smoking was a strong risk factor, but it accounted for only about one-quarter of the cases (Gao, et al., 1987). The remainder were adenocarcinomas, with various factors associated, including previous chest diseases and cooking with rapeseed oil at high temperatures. Cigarette smoking was found to be the principal cause of lung cancer in Shenyang, an industrial city in northeastern China, accounting for 55 percent of the lung cancers in men and 37 percent in women (Xu, et al., 1989). Increased risks were also found among those who reported exposure to smoky outdoor environments from air pollution and those with many years exposure to sleeping on beds heated by coal-burning stoves. In a further case-control study involving 965 female patients with lung cancer and 959 population controls conducted in two industrial cities of northeast China, cigarette smoking was found to be the main causal factor, accounting for about 35 percent of the cases (Wu-Williams, et al., 1990). Other factors found to be relevant in this population included air pollution from coal-burning stoves and exposure to indigenous smoky heating stoves and prior chronic bronchitis. An effect of passive smoking could not be demonstrated.

Radon Exposure

A series of studies in uranium miners in the United States, Canada, and Czechoslovakia confirmed that radon daughters released in poorly ventilated uranium mines increase the risk of lung cancer, with an approximate doubling of risk after a 5- to 10-year latent period (Committee on the Biological Effects of Ionizing Radiation, 1988). The risk levels were considerably raised for those with substantial cumulative exposure (Howe, et al., 1986; Woodward, et al., 1991), although there is some evidence that the effect is greatest at low dose rates (Howe, et al., 1987). Because the joint effect of smoking and radon exposure has been rather difficult to quantify (L'Abbé, et al., 1991), there has been residual suspicion that part of the radon effect may be really the result of smoking. This suspicion was put to rest with a study of lung cancer deaths in nonsmoking uranium miners from Colorado (Roscoe, et al., 1989). Fourteen deaths from lung cancer were observed during a 34-year observation period of 516 never-smoking uranium miners; only 1.1 such deaths were expected, giving a standardized mortality ratio of 12.7. This confirms that, in the absence of cigarette smoking, radon daughter exposure increases the risk of lung cancer.

There is increasing interest in indoor radon exposure as a possible risk factor for lung cancer (Edling, et al., 1986; Samet, 1989). Elevated lung cancer rates have been noted in U.S. counties with Precambrian granite deposits, known to result in raised radon daughter concentrations in homes (Archer, 1987). In a study in China, the opportunity was taken to evaluate the effect of indoor radon (Blot, et al., 1990). No relationship was found. However, in tin miners in a different area of China, lung cancer was found to be related to both water-pipe smoking and radon exposure in the mines (Qiao, et al., 1989). A quantitative analysis of the effect of radon showed that a long duration of exposure at a low rate may be more deleterious than a short duration of exposure at a high rate, a finding which replicates that of Howe, et al. (1987); the joint effects of water-pipe smoking and radon exposure were intermediate between additive and multiplicative (Lubin, et al., 1990).

In a case-control study of lung cancer among New Jersey women, a significant trend of increasing lung cancer risk with increasing radon exposure was found (Schoenberg, et al., 1990). The risk gradient was similar to that estimated for uranium miners. Even so, the risk was largely related to the highest exposure levels, which were measured in the homes of only 6 of the 433 cases, and 2 of the 402 controls with measurements. Because of this in this population, it can be calculated that high levels of radon exposure account for less than 2 percent of the cases of lung cancer.

Diet

Interest in diet and lung cancer began with a cohort study in Norway, which showed that an index of vitamin A intake was negatively associated with the incidence of lung cancer (Bjelke, 1975; Kvale, et al., 1983). Others had similar findings (Mettlin, et al., 1979; Gregor, et al., 1980).

With the finding of a negative association of β-carotene but not preformed vitamin A with the incidence of lung cancer (Shekelle, et al., 1981) and some understanding on how β-carotene might be protective (Peto, et al., 1981), attention shifted to β-carotene. Several authors found evidence of the protective effects of β-carotene (Hinds, et al., 1984; Samet, et al., 1985; Wu, et al., 1985; Ziegler, et al., 1986; Byers, et al., 1987). Furthermore some of the strongest associations in earlier work were with "vitamin A" indices derived from plant foods. Others also found evidence of a protective effect of vegetables on lung cancer (Ziegler, et al., 1986; Maclennan, et al., 1979; Hirayama, 1986). A study in Toronto did not find a protective effect of β-carotene, retinol, or total vitamin A consumption, but a protective effect for nitrate ingestion was found, considered as an index of the consumption of a number of vegetables (Jain, et al., 1990). Additional evidence came from a study in Athens where a protective effect of a high consumption of fruits but not carotenoids was found (Kalandidi, et al., 1990). In Hawaii, although a protective effect of β-carotene intake was found, the protective effect of all vegetables, including dark green vegetables, cruciferous vegetables, and tomatoes, was stronger than that for β-carotene (Le Marchand, et al., 1989). The studies in Hawaii and Toronto used quantitative dietary questionnaires, and therefore they may more accurately compute the relative importance of various dietary factors than do simpler frequency-based instruments. In a small study in Australia, a protective effect of fish consumption was noted but not one for foods containing retinol or β-carotene (Pierce, et al., 1989).

Studies of Californian Seventh-Day Adventists (who have low rates of smoking and alcohol consumption) have been productive in our understanding of diet and cancer associations. An analysis of data from a cohort study with a 6-year follow-up period showed associations both with smoking and dietary factors, which are independent (Fraser, et al., 1991). Fruit consumption was the factor with a strong statistically significant protective association. The authors were not able to assess the role of β-carotene but noted that foods included in their data set that have a substantial content of β-carotene showed no consistent association. However, in a small case-control study in England, there was some confirmation that dietary carotene was protective for lung cancer, with a nonsignificant protective effect for carotene-rich fruits and vegetables (Harris, et al., 1991). The serum β-carotene level was also lower in lung cancer cases than that in controls.

All investigators have been careful to adjust their analyses for smoking. Several also attempted to evaluate the interaction with smoking. In one study the reduced relative risk of lung cancer associated with vitamin A was most evident among men who smoked heavily (Kvale, et al., 1983). Hirayama (1986) suggested that green-yellow vegetable consumption might hasten the effect of the cessation of cigarette smoking and might also affect the risk caused by passive smoking. Samet, et al. (1985) found effects only in whites rather than in Hispanics and only in former rather than current cigarette smokers. Ziegler, et al. (1986) found the protective effect of vegetables was limited to current and recent cigarette smokers. Pisani, et al. (1986) found an increased risk of lung cancer for smokers who did not consume carrots, but no corresponding effect for ex- or nonsmokers. Byers, et al. (1987) found the risk reduction associated with vitamin A from fruits and vegetables was most evident for light or exsmokers. Bond, et al. (1987) found the strongest inverse association of a vitamin A index with the lung cancer risk among cigarette smokers.

Some investigators also attempted to evaluate the differential risks for dietary factors, according to histologic type. Several found associations that were strongest for squamous cell cancer (Gregor, et al., 1980; Ziegler, et al., 1986; Byers, et al., 1984, 1987). Byers, et al. (1984) also found associations with small cell cancer and Ziegler, et al. (1986), with adenocarcinoma for current and recent smokers.

Three correlation studies demonstrated an association between lung cancer mortality rates and per capita consumption of dietary fat (Carroll and Khor, 1975; Wynder, et al., 1987; Xie, et al., 1991). Two of these attempted to adjust for the consumption of tobacco (Wynder, et al., 1987; Xie, et al., 1991). Both found independent contributions from smoking and dietary fat consumption. The most recent (Xie, et al., 1991) found that animal but not vegetable fat contributed significantly to the risk. The interaction between cigarette smoking and animal fat consumption was significant, pointing toward a role for animal fat as a promoter of lung cancer. Some studies found increased risks for dietary cholesterol (Hinds, et al., 1983; Jain, et al., 1990).

In summary, although it is clear that cigarette smoking is far and away the most important risk factor for lung cancer, there appear to be modulating factors in plant foods and perhaps risk factors in animal foods. It cannot be assumed that all, if any, of the protective effect comes from β-carotene because many inhibitors of carcinogenesis come from vegetables. Whether or not vegetable consumption rather than pure β-carotene consumption is protective will be clarified when the results from several ongoing chemoprevention trials are available.

Occupational Factors

Occupational factors have long been recognized as increasing the risk of lung cancer (Tomatis, et al., 1990). The classic factors (other than uranium mining) unequivocally related to an occupational risk of lung cancer include exposure to asbestos (both in mining and manufacturing and insulating); occupations involving the inhalation of polycyclic aromatic hydrocarbons; iron and steel founding; and exposure to arsenic, chromates, and bis-chlormethyl ether. Although confounding by smoking has often been suspected as explaining some of the occupational associations, the difference in smoking prevalence between the occupational group and the comparison group must be large to explain the associations observed (Blair, et al., 1985).

Recently attention has shifted to try and identify new and possibly unexpected causes for lung cancer risk in occupational groups. A large international study evaluated the risk of exposure to human-made mineral fibers (Simonato, et al., 1987). The lung cancer mortality rate increased with the time since the first exposure, both in rock wool, slag wool, and glass wool production, but only the rock wool and slag wool excess was seen when local referent populations were substituted for national reference populations. In northern Sweden a case-control study largely found excess risks in occupations with exposures to known carcinogens (radon daughters, arsenic, and asbestos) (Damber and Larsson, 1987). In Sweden as a whole, a special register enabled trends of occupationally induced lung cancer to be assessed (Carstensen, et al., 1989). Decreasing trends for blacksmiths and members of the armed forces and increasing trends for foundry workers and construction machine operators were noted. In a recent case-control study within a cohort of Swedish smelter workers, strong associations were found for both estimated arsenic exposure and cigarette smoking (Järup and Pershagen, 1991). Both exposures appeared to increase the risk with an interaction between additive and multiplicative. The relationship with arsenic was strongest for the estimated average expo-

sure, less strong for cumulative exposure, and absent for the duration of exposure. There was some suggestion of a weaker effect of arsenic among heavy smokers than among light and medium smokers. The possibility that occupational lung cancer might be identified through specific histologic types was evaluated in a large census-derived data base in Finland (Sankila, et al., 1990). In general this was not confirmed, although miners and quarriers had a high risk of small cell carcinoma compared with other economically active men. In a combined analysis of three U.S. case-control studies, 10 years or more exposure to motor exhaust-related occupations was found to increase the lung cancer risk by 50 percent (Hayes, et al., 1989). Among specific occupations, the risk was elevated for truck drivers. Diesel exhaust exposure was further evaluated in another large U.S. study (Boffetta, et al., 1990). Although a 30 percent increase in the risk for probable exposure was found, this was accounted for by an adjustment for smoking and other confounders. Another potential risk exposure for lung cancer recently evaluated is formaldehyde, assessed in a cohort study of 26,561 workers employed in 10 facilities (Blair, et al., 1990). Although a 30 percent excess had been noted, this did not appear to be consistent within plants, nor could a dose-response relationship to formaldehyde be found. It appeared that other substances to which the workers were also exposed (including phenol, melamine, urea, and wood dust) might have been responsible for the excess number of lung cancer cases in the cohort. In contrast occupational exposure to silica is being recognized more and more frequently as increasing the risk of lung cancer. In Quebec, Canada, men who had received compensation for silicosis had more than three times the risk of death from lung cancer than that expected from population rates in Quebec (Infante-Rivard, et al., 1989). A doubling of the lung cancer risk was also found in a cohort of men in a silicosis register in Hong Kong (Ng, et al., 1990). Although there is some selection bias in relation to the inclusion of workers in such registers (Spivack, 1990; Abraham, 1990), the degree of elevation of risk found, especially in the Quebec study, seems unlikely to be the result of such factors (Infante-Rivard, et al., 1990ab).

Excess deaths from lung cancer were found in the melting department of two Ontario steel manufacturers (Finkelstein and Wilk, 1990; Finkelstein, et al., 1991). In the second plant (Finkelstein, et al., 1991), the excess risk was confined to men who had worked in the pouring pit department. No polycyclic aromatic hydrocarbons were detected in the environment of the work process. Indeed no definitive cause of the excess lung cancer risk in these two plants has yet been identified. In an investigation of lung cancer risk in three midwestern U.S. plants that manufactured heavy equipment, no significant excess risk was found for either welders or nonwelders of mild steel compared with that in the general population; neither was there an increased risk in welders compared with nonwelders (Steenland, et al., 1991). Although reassuring this contrasts with a finding of an increased risk of lung cancer of 2.43 (95 percent confidence interval, 1.56, 3.79) among workers in the ferrous primary metal manufacturing industry in an Occupational Cancer Incidence Surveillance study in metropolitan Detroit (Burns and Swanson, 1991). This large case-control study, which was based on data collected by the Detroit cancer registry, was designed to evaluate the lung cancer risk, and it also found an excess risk among furnace and steel workers (and in several other occupational groups). As was reported first many years ago for coke plant workers (Lloyd, 1971), it is clear that iron and steel refining and manufacturing have several component groups in which an excess lung cancer risk can be identified. The causal factors are likely to be diverse, probably do not include iron itself, but rather additives, contaminants, and other substances in the work environment (including arsenic, silica, and polycyclic aromatic hydrocarbons) that will have to be specifically identified in the relevant plants for appropriate preventive actions to be taken.

Attempts have been made to quantify the amount of lung cancer attributable to occupation. In two industrialized areas of northern Italy (Ronco, et al., 1988), when only occupations known to be causally associated with lung cancer were included in the estimate of the attributable risk, the percentage was 12 percent in one area and 5 percent in the other. When suspect occupations were also included, the attributable risks rose to 36 and 12 percent. In the United States, occupational data from five case-control studies were considered by Vineis, et al. (1988). The percentage of lung cancer attributable to occupations with potential exposure to well-recognized carcinogens ranged from 3 to 17 percent by study area. It was believed by the authors that errors in exposure classification made these estimates conservative.

Air Pollution

In the early stages of the investigations concerning the reasons for the increase in lung cancer, air pollution was strongly suspected as a possible cause. Over the years, however, it has become clear that general air pollution adds only a small component to the effect of individual air pollution through tobacco use. One of the earliest studies to demonstrate this was conducted in heavily polluted areas in the north of England. The risk of lung cancer, adjusted for smoking, was at most increased twofold in the heavily polluted areas compared with the less polluted areas (Dean, et al., 1978). A similar differential was found in an analysis of lung cancer mortality rates in a Scottish town that was related to degrees of pollution from two iron foundries (Smith, et al., 1987). However, in most studies, it has been difficult to exclude the effects of occupation, social class, and differential smoking, which seemed to be more likely to explain area differences in Contra Costa County, California, in spite of exposure to emissions from petroleum and chemical plants (Kaldor, et al., 1984). Indeed such factors may have explained the findings in the other studies. A similar effect was noted in a study in Texas (Buffler, et al., 1988) in which air pollution accounted for less than 5 percent of the total variation in the intraurban lung cancer mortality rate; a study in the heavily polluted town of Hamilton, Ontario, showed little effect of air pollution in increasing the risk after smoking was taken into account (Shannon, et al., 1988).

Nevertheless, when local air pollution is extreme, an increased risk of lung cancer appears to be related to it. This is the case for an area of China with severe exposure indoors to the emissions of smoky coal (Mumford, et al., 1987), as has also been noted for external air pollution in other areas of China (Xie, et al., 1989; Wu-Williams, et al., 1990). These findings are compatible with the conclusion of Tomatis, et al. (1990) that "it seems probable that, in heavily polluted areas, air pollution may contribute to mortality from lung cancer."

Familial Aspects of Lung Cancer and the Role of Genetics

Two reports recently confirmed the previously noted association of lung cancer with a positive family history (Tokuhata and Lilienfeld, 1963). In one from a study in the Texas Gulf Coast region, a risk of 2.8 for lung cancer in two or more relatives was reported (Shaw, et al., 1991). However, the association was stronger for the histologic types associated with smoking. A similar finding arose from a study in Canada in which a family history of any neoplastic disease was evaluated (McDuffie, 1991). Most of the sites with the highest elevations of risk were smoking associated, supporting an ecogenetic cause of cancer within the affected families (i.e., a strong influence of smoking, possibly superimposed on some genetic base, but requiring the environmental factor [smoking] to induce the disease).

For some time there has been a suspicion that a genetic susceptibility to certain carcinogens may play a role in the cause of lung cancer (Minna, et al., 1987). Markers for a susceptibility to lung cancer related to drug metabolism have been described (Ayesh, et al., 1984). Law (1990) reviewed the evidence and concluded that genetic factors must contribute to the lung cancer risk because it is the metabolites of environmental carcinogens that usually initiate a cancer and the metabolic pathways are genetically controlled. One of the metabolic pathways identified is associated with the drug debrisoquin, with fewer lung cancer cases than controls being poor metabolizers of debrisoquin, although the proportions of poor metabolizers in both groups was low in one study (1.9 versus 8.7 percent; Law, et al., 1989). The association seems stronger in those occupationally exposed to asbestos and polycyclic aromatic hydrocarbons. In such individuals extensive metabolizers of debrisoquin had a fourfold increase in the risk of lung cancer in comparison with poor metabolizers (Caporaso, et al., 1989). Another possible genetic marker that has been identified is the class mu phenotype of glutathione transferase, which appears to be more frequent in noncancer-affected smokers than in patients with lung cancer (Seidegard, et al., 1990). Perhaps more convincing, however, is the fact that evidence for mendelian inheritance of lung cancer was obtained through a segregation analysis of 337 families ascertained through lung cancer probands (Sellers, et al., 1990). The data were compatible with codominant inheritance of a rare autosomal gene that produces an earlier age of onset of lung cancer in individuals exposed to the appropriate carcinogenic stimulus, particularly smoking.

CONCLUSION

It is perhaps surprising that we continue to learn of etiologically relevant factors for what is the most important potentially preventable cancer in the world. Smoking remains pre-eminent, but factors that interact with smoking, such as occupation, diet, genetics, and possibly radon, are relevant. Much of the emerging knowledge can be incorporated into cancer control programs, especially the protective effect of smoking cessation. Indeed it is important that increased understanding of the possible effect of other factors (e.g., as for other cancers, the protective effect of plant foods) not result in diverting attention from smoking control policies. In this respect the almost unanimous agreement that passive smoking increases the risk of lung cancer in nonsmokers has moved smoking control out of the realm of individual action

into general public health. Occupational factors that increase the risk of lung cancer should continue to be sought and controlled. For radon daughter exposure in homes, however, the public health significance seems slight.

Internationally the most important action that could be taken to halt the epidemic of lung cancer would be to agree on appropriate smoking control policies, even though they sometimes seem to be in conflict with international trade. It is reprehensible that short-term financial gain should take precedence over long-term health.

COMMENTS AND CONTROVERSIES

It is almost unbelievable that it has been only 35 years since smoking was definitely implicated in the etiology of lung cancer. Since that time, there has been a rapid assimilation of knowledge concerning the epidemiology of this disease. There is no doubt that most cases of lung cancer are preventable, having developed due to manmade environmental alterations. The greatest impact on disease control will be made

when these environmental changes are reversed, confirming the assertion that our largest efforts should be directed toward prevention.

Previous exposure (e.g., breast, lymphoma) also increases the risk of lung disease, as does radon exposure.

R.J.G.

KEY REFERENCES

Committee on the Biological Effects of Ionizing Radiations of the National Research Council: BEIR IV. Health Risks of Radon and Other Internally Deposited Alpha-Emitters. National Academy Press, Washington, DC, 1988

This is the most important recent review of the health risks from radon daughters. Although most clearly relevant to the risks from uranium mining, it has substantial implications on the possible adverse effect of radon daughter exposure in homes.

Doll R, Peto R: Mortality in relation to smoking: 20 years observations on male British doctors. BMJ 2:1525, 1976

This is the report on the 20-year follow-up of the male British doctors cohort study. Probably one of the best known cohort studies ever conducted, it has the considerable advantage that information on current smoking was collected every 5 years after the cohort was established.

IARC: Tobacco Smoking. In IARC (eds): IARC Monographs on the Evaluation of the Carcinogenic Risk of Chemicals to Humans. Vol. 38. International Agency for Research on Cancer, Lyon, France, 1986

This is the most detailed and authoritative compilation of the carcinogenicity of tobacco yet available. It contains an extensive

literature review of the data available on the epidemiology of tobacco and lung (and other) cancers up to 1985.

Surgeon General: Reducing the health consequences of smoking: 25 years of progress. US Department of Health and Human Services, Rockville, MD, 1989

This is the 25-year anniversary issue of the annual Surgeon General's reports on the health consequences of tobacco since the series commenced in 1964. It contains an extensive review of changes in smoking rates in the United States and an update on lung cancer and tobacco epidemiology, including the preliminary results of the large American Cancer Society CPS-II.

Tomatis L, Aitio A, Day NE et al. (eds): Cancer: Causes, Occurrence and Control. IARC Scientific Publications. No. 100. International Agency for Research on Cancer, Lyon, 1990

This is an extensive review of the causes of cancer and the approaches available for its control. It contains summaries of the effects of many different factors on the risk of lung and other cancers. It provides for the world what Doll and Peto (1981) attempted to do for the United States, that is, a summary of the principal causes of cancer and the amount of disease attributable to these causes.

REFERENCES

Abraham JL: Silicosis and lung cancer. Lancet 335:1163, 1990

Akiba S, Kato H, Blot WJ: Passive smoking and lung cancer among Japanese women. Cancer Res 46:4804, 1986

Archer VE: Association of lung cancer mortality with Precambrian granite. Arch Environ Health 42:87, 1987

Ayesh R, Idle JR, Ritchie JC et al.: Metabolic oxidation phenotypes as marker for susceptibility to lung cancer. Nature 312:169, 1984

Benhamou E, Benhamou S, Flamant R: Lung cancer and women: results of a French case-control study. Br J Cancer 55:91, 1987

Bjelke E: Dietary vitamin A and human lung cancer. Int J Cancer 15:561, 1975

Blair A, Hoar S, Walrath J: Comparison of crude and smoking-adjusted standardized mortality ratios. J Occup Med 27:881, 1985

Blair A, Stewart PA, Hoover RN: Mortality from lung cancer among workers employed in formaldehyde industries. Am J Ind Med 17:683, 1990

Blot WJ, Xu ZY, Boice JD et al.: Indoor radon and lung cancer in China. J Natl Cancer Inst 82:1025, 1990

Boffetta P, Harris RE, Wynder EL: Case-control study on occupational exposure to diesel exhaust and lung cancer risk. Am J Ind Med 17:577, 1990

Bond GG, Thompson FE, Cook RR: Dietary vitamin A and lung cancer: results of a case-control study among chemical workers. Nutr Cancer 9:109, 1987

Boring CC, Squires TS, Tong T: Cancer Statistics, 1991. CA Cancer J Clin 41:19, 1991

Brown CC, Kessler LG: Projections of lung cancer mortality in the United States: 1985–2025. J Natl Cancer Inst 80:43, 1988

Brownson RC, Reif JS, Keefe et al.: Risk factors for adenocarcinoma of the lung. Am J Epidemiol 125:25, 1987

Buffler PA, Cooper SP, Stinnett S et al.: Air pollution and lung cancer mortality in Harris county, Texas, 1979–1981. Am J Epidemiol 128:683, 1988

Burns PB, Swanson GM: The Occupational Cancer Incidence Surveillance Study (OCISS): risk of lung cancer by usual occupation and industry in the Detroit metropolitan area. Am J Ind Med 19:655, 1991

Butler WJ: Commentary on "Links between passive smoking and disease: a best evidence synthesis—A report of the Working Group on Passive Smoking." CIM Vol. 13 no. 1:17–42, 1990. Clin Invest Med 14:484, 1991

Byers TE, Graham S, Haughey BP et al.: Diet and lung cancer risk: findings from the Western New York diet study. Am J Epidemiol 125:351, 1987

Byers T, Vena J, Mettlin C et al.: Dietary vitamin A and lung cancer risk: an analysis by histologic subtypes. Am J Epidemiol 120:769, 1984

Caporaso N, Hayes RB, Dosemeci M et al.: Lung cancer risk, occupational exposure, and the debrisoquine metabolic phenotype. Cancer Res 49:3675, 1989

Carroll KK, Khor HT: Dietary fat in relation to tumorigenesis. Prog Biochem Pharmacol 10:308, 1975

Carstensen JM, Pershagen G, Eklund G: Time trends in occupational risks of lung cancer among Swedish men from 1961–1979. Am J Ind Med 15:441, 1989

Correa P, Pickle LW, Fontham E et al.: Passive smoking and lung cancer. Lancet 2:595, 1983

Dalager NA, Pickle LW, Mason TJ et al.: The relation of passive smoking to lung cancer. Cancer Res 46:4808, 1986

Damber LA, Larsson LG: Occupation and male lung cancer: a case-control study in Northern Sweden. Br J Ind Med 44:446, 1987

Dean G, Lee PN, Todd GF, Wicken AJ: Report on a second retrospective mortality study in north-east England. Part II. Changes in lung cancer and bronchitis mortality and in other relevant factors occurring in areas of north-east England 1963–72. Research Paper 14, Part II. Tobacco Research Council, London, 1978

Devesa SS, Blot WJ, Fraumeni JF: Declining lung cancer rates among young men and women in the United States: a cohort analysis. J Natl Cancer Inst 81:1568, 1989

Doll R, Gray R, Hofner B, Peto R: Mortality in relation to smoking: 22 years observations on female British doctors. BMJ 1:967, 1980

Doll R, Hill AB: A study of the aetiology of carcinoma of the lung. BMJ 2:1271, 1952

Doll R, Peto R: The causes of cancer: quantitative estimates of avoidable risks of cancer in the United States today. J Natl Cancer Inst 66:1191, 1981

Edling C, Wingren G, Axelson O: Quantification of the lung cancer risk from radon daughter exposure in dwellings—an epidemiological approach. Environ Int 12:55, 1986

Environmental Protection Agency: Health effects of passive smoking: assessment of lung cancer in adults and respiratory disorders in children. U.S. Environmental Protection Agency, Washington, D.C., 1990

Finkelstsin MM, Boulard M, Wilk N: Increased risk of lung cancer in the melting department of a second Ontario steel manufacturer. Am J Ind Med 19:183, 1991

Finkelstsin MM, Wilk N: Investigation of a lung cancer cluster in the melt shop of an Ontario steel producer. Am J Ind Med 17:483, 1990

Fleiss JL, Gross AJ: Meta-analysis in epidemiology, with special reference to studies of the association between exposure to environmental tobacco smoke and lung cancer: a critique. J Clin Epidemiol 44:127, 1991

Fontham ETH, Correa P, Wu-Williams A et al.: Lung cancer in nonsmoking women: a multicenter case-control study. Cancer Epidemiol Biomarkers Prev 1:35, 1991

Fraser GE, Beeson WL, Phillips RL: Diet and lung cancer in Seventh-Day Adventists. Am J Epidemiol 133:683, 1991

Freedman DA, Navidi WC: Ex-smokers and the multistage model for lung cancer. Epidemiology 1:21, 1990

Gao YT, Blot WJ, Zheng W et al.: Lung cancer among Chinese women. Int J Cancer 40:604, 1987

Garfinkel L: Time trends in lung cancer mortality among nonsmokers and a note on passive smoking. J Natl Cancer Inst 66:1061, 1981

Garfinkel L, Auerbach O, Joubert L: Involuntary smoking and lung cancer: a case-control study. J Natl Cancer Inst 75:463, 1985

Gregor A, Lee PM, Roe FJC et al.: Comparison of dietary histories in lung cancer cases and controls with special reference to vitamin A. Nutr Cancer 2:93, 1980

Gritz ER: Cigarette smoking: the need for action by health professionals. CA Cancer J Clin 38:194, 1988

Hammond EC: Smoking in relation to the death rates of one million men and women. Monogr Natl Cancer Inst 19:127, 1966

Hammond EC, Horn D: Smoking and death rates—report on forty-four months of follow-up of 187,783 men. II. Death rates by cause. JAMA 166:1294, 1958

Harris RWC, Key TJA, Silcocks PB et al.: A case-control study of dietary carotene in men with lung cancer and in men with other epithelial cancers. Nutr Cancer 15:63, 1991

Hayes RB, Thomas T, Silverman DT et al.: Lung cancer in motor exhaust-related occupations. Am J Ind Med 16:685, 1989

Hinds MW, Kolonel LN, Hankin HJ et al.: Dietary vitamin A, carotene, vitamin C and risk of lung cancer in Hawaii. Am J Epidemiol 119:227, 1984

Hinds MW, Kolonel LN, Lee J, Hankin JH: Dietary cholesterol and lung cancer risk among men in Hawaii. Am J Clin Nutr 37:192, 1983

Hirayama T: Nutrition and cancer—a large scale cohort study. p. 299. In Knudsen I (ed): Genetic Toxicology of the Diet. Alan R Liss, New York, 1986

Hirayama T: Smoking and cancer in Japan. A prospective study on cancer epidemiology based on census in Japan. Results of 13 years follow up. p. 2. In Tominaga S, Aoki K (eds): The UICC Smoking Control Workshop, Nagoya, Japan. The University of Nagoya Press, Nagoya, 1982

Hirayama T: Non-smoking wives of heavy smokers have a higher risk of lung cancer: a study from Japan. BMJ 282:183, 1981

Holowaty EJ, Risch HA, Miller AB, Burch JD: Lung cancer in women in the Niagara region, Ontario: a case-control study. Can J Public Health 82:304, 1991

Howe GR, Nair RC, Newcombe HB et al.: Lung cancer mortality (1950–80) in relation to radon daughter exposure in a cohort of workers at the Eldorado Port Radium uranium mine: possible modification of risk by exposure rate. J Natl Cancer Inst 79:1255, 1987

Howe GR, Nair RC, Newcombe HB et al.: Lung cancer mortality (1950–80) in relation to radon daughter exposure in a cohort of workers at the Eldorado Beaverlodge uranium mine. J Natl Cancer Inst 77:357, 1986

Humble CG, Samet JM, Pathak DR: Marriage to a smoker and lung cancer risk. Am J Public Health 77:598, 1987

Infante-Rivard C, Armstrong B, Petitclerc M et al.: Response to Dr. Spivack. Lancet 335:1163, 1990a

Infante-Rivard C, Armstrong B, Petitclerc M et al.: Response to Dr. Abraham. Lancet 335:854, 1990b

Infante-Rivard C, Armstrong B, Petitclerc M et al.: Lung cancer mortality and silicosis in Québec, 1938–85. Lancet 2:1504, 1989

Jain M, Burch JD, Howe GR et al.: Dietary factors and risk of lung cancer: results from a case-control study, Toronto, 1981–1985. Int J Cancer 45:287, 1990

Janerich DT, Thompson WD, Varela LR et al.: Lung cancer and exposure to tobacco smoke in the household. N Engl J Med 323:632, 1990

Jårup L, Pershagen G: Arsenic exposure, smoking, and lung cancer in smelter workers—a case-control study. Am J Epidemiol 134:545, 1991

Kabat GC, Wynder EL: Lung cancer in nonsmokers. Cancer 53:1214, 1984

Kahn HA: The Dorn study of smoking and mortality among US veterans. Report on eight and one-half years of observation. Monogr Natl Cancer Inst 19:1, 1966

Kalandidi A, Katsouyanni K, Voropoulou N et al.: Passive smoking and diet in the etiology of lung cancer in non-smokers. Cancer Causes Control 1:15, 1990

Kaldor J, Harris JA, Glazer E et al.: Statistical association between cancer incidence and major-cause mortality, and estimated residential exposure to air emissions from petroleum and chemical plants. Environ Health Perspect 54:319, 1984

Koo LC, Ho JHC, Lee N: An analysis of some risk factors for lung cancer in Hong Kong. Int J Cancer 35:149, 1985

Koo LC, Ho JHC, Saw D, Ho CY: Measurements of passive smoking and estimates of lung cancer risk among non-smoking Chinese females. Int J Cancer 39:162, 1987

Kvale G, Bjelke E, Gart JJ: Dietary habits and lung cancer risk. Int J Cancer 31:397, 1983

L'Abbé KA, Howe GR, Burch JD et al.: Radon exposure, cigarette smoking, and other mining experience in the Beaverlodge uranium miners cohort. Health Phys 60:489, 1991

Lam TH, Kung ITM, Wong CM et al.: Smoking, passive smoking and histological types in lung cancer in Hong Kong Chinese women. Br J Cancer 56:673, 1987

Law MR: Genetic predisposition to lung cancer. Br J Cancer 61:195, 1990

Law MR, Hetzel MR, Idle JR: Debrisoquine metabolism and genetic predisposition to lung cancer. Br J Cancer 59:686, 1989

Lee PN, Chamberlain J, Alderson MR: Relationship of passive smoking to risk of lung cancer and other smoking-associated diseases. Br J Cancer 54:97, 1986

Le Marchand L, Yoshizawa CN, Kolonel LN et al.: Vegetable consumption and lung cancer risk: a population-based case-control study in Hawaii. J Natl Cancer Inst 81:1158, 1989

Lloyd JW: Long-term mortality study of steelworkers. V. Respiratory cancer in coke plant workers. J Occup Med 13:53, 1971

Lossing EH, Best EWR, McGregor JT et al.: A Canadian Study of Smoking and Health. Department of National Health and Welfare, Ottawa, 1966

Lubin JH, Blot WJ, Berrino F et al.: Patterns of lung cancer risk according to type of cigarette smoked. Int J Cancer 33:569, 1984

Lubin JH, Qiao YL, Taylor PR et al.: Quantitative evaluation of the radon and lung cancer association in a case-control study of Chinese tin miners. Cancer Res 50:174, 1990

MacLennan R, Da Costa J, Day NE et al.: Risk factors for lung cancer in Singapore Chinese, a population with high female incidence rates. Int J Cancer 20:854, 1979

Marcus AC, Shopland DR, Crane LA, Lynn WR: Prevalence of cigarette smoking in the United States: estimates from the 1985 current population survey. J Natl Cancer Inst 81:409, 1989

McDuffie HH: Clustering of cancer in families of patients with lung cancer. J Clin Epidemiol 44:69, 1991

Mettlin C, Graham S, Swanson MJ: Vitamin A and lung cancer. J Natl Cancer Inst 62:1435, 1979

Miller AB: The information explosion—the role of the epidemiologist. Cancer Forum 8:67, 1984

Minna JD, Battey JF, Birrer MJ et al.: Genetic changes involved in the pathogenesis of human lung cancer including oncogene activation, chromosomal deletions, and autocrine growth factor production. p. 155. In Fortner JG, Rhoads JE (eds): Accomplishments in Cancer Research, 1987. JB Lippincott, Philadelphia, 1988

Mumford JL, He XZ, Chapman RS et al.: Lung cancer and indoor air pollution in Xuan Wei, China. Science 235:217, 1987

National Research Council: Environmental Tobacco Smoke: Measuring Exposures and Assessing Health Effects. National Academy Press, Washington, D.C., 1986

Ng TP, Chan SL, Lee J: Mortality of a cohort of men in a silicosis register: further evidence of an association with lung cancer. Am J Ind Med 17:163, 1990

Pershagen G, Hrubec Z, Svensson S: Passive smoking and lung cancer in Swedish women. Am J Epidemiol 125:17, 1987

Peto R, Doll R: The control of lung cancer. p. 1. In Mizell M and Correa P (eds): Lung Cancer, Causes and Prevention. Verlag Chemie International, New York, 1984

Peto R, Doll R, Buckley JD et al.: Can dietary beta-carotene materially reduce human cancer rates? Nature 290:201, 1981

Pierce RJ, Kune GA, Kune S et al.: Dietary and alcohol intake, smoking pattern, occupational risk, and family history in lung cancer patients: results of a case-control study in males. Nutr Cancer 12:237, 1989

Pisani P, Berrino F, Macaluso M et al.: Carrots, green vegetables and lung cancer; a case-control study. Int J Epidemiol 15:463, 1986

Qiao YL, Taylor PR, Yao SX et al.: Relation of radon exposure and tobacco use to lung cancer among tin miners in Yunnan Province, China. Am J Ind Med 16:511, 1989

Risch HA, Howe GR, Jain M et al: Are female smokers at higher risk for lung cancer than male smokers? A case-control analysis by histologic type. Am J Epidemiol 138:281, 1993

Rogot E, Murray JL: Smoking and causes of death among US veterans: 16 years of observation. Public Health Rep 95:213, 1980

Ronco G, Ciccone G, Mirabelli D et al.: Occupation and lung cancer in two industrialized areas of northern Italy. Int J Cancer 41:354, 1988

Roscoe RJ, Stennland K, Halperin WE et al.: Lung cancer mortality among nonsmoking uranium miners exposed to radon daughters. JAMA 262:629, 1989

Samet JM: Radon and lung cancer. J Natl Cancer Inst 81:745, 1989

Samet JM, Skipper BJ, Humble CG et al.: Lung cancer risk and vitamin A consumption in New Mexico. Am Rev Respir Dis 131:198, 1985

Sandler DP, Wilcox AJ, Everson RB: Cumulative effects of lifetime passive smoking on cancer risk. Lancet 1:312, 1985

Sankila RJ, Karjalainen ES, Oksanen HM et al.: Relationship between occupation and lung cancer as analyzed by age and histologic type. Cancer 65:1651, 1990

Schoenberg JB, Klotz JB, Wilcox HB et al.: Case-control study of residential radon and lung cancer among New Jersey women. Cancer Res 50:6520, 1990

Schoenberg JB, Wilcox HB, Mason TJ et al.: Variation in smoking-related lung cancer risk among New Jersey women. Am J Epidemiol 130:688, 1989

Seideguard J, Pero RW, Markowitz MM et al.: Isoenzyme(s) of glutathione transferase (class mu) as a marker for the susceptibility to lung cancer: a follow up study. Carcinogenesis 11:33, 1990

Sellers TA, Bailey-Wilson JE, Elston RC et al.: Evidence for mendelian inheritance in the pathogenesis of lung cancer. J Natl Cancer Inst 82:1272, 1990

Shannon HS, Hertzman C, Julian JA et al.: Lung cancer and air pollution in an industrial city—a geographical analysis. Can J Public Health 79:255, 1988

Shaw GL, Falk RT, Pickle LW et al.: Lung cancer risk associated with cancer in relatives. J Clin Epidemiol 44:429, 1991

Shekelle RB, Lepper M, Lui S et al.: Dietary vitamin A and risk of cancer in the Western Electric study. Lancet 2:1185, 1981

Shopland DR, Eyre HJ, Pechacek TF: Smoking-attributable cancer mortality in 1991; is lung cancer now the leading cause of death among smokers in the United States? J Natl Cancer Inst 83:1142, 1991

Simonato L, Fletcher AC, Cherrie JW et al.: The International Agency for Research on Cancer historical cohort study of MMMF production workers in seven European countries: extension of the follow-up. Ann Occup Hyg 31:603, 1987

Smith GH, Williams FLR, Lloyd OL: Respiratory cancer and air pollution from iron foundries in a Scottish town: an epidemiological and environmental study. Br J Ind Med 44:795, 1987

Sobue T, Suzuki T, Fujimoto I et al.: Lung cancer risk among ex-smokers. Jpn J Cancer Res 82:273, 1991

Spivack SD: Silica and lung cancer. Lancet 335:854, 1990

Steenland K, Beaumont J, Elliot L: Lung cancer in mild steel welders. Am J Epidemiol 133:220, 1991

Surgeon General: The health consequences of smoking. Nicotine addiction. U.S. Department of Health and Human Services, Rockville, MD, 1988

Surgeon General: The health consequences of smoking. Cancer. U.S. Department of Health and Human Services, Rockville, MD, 1982

Svensson C, Pershagen G, Klominek J: Smoking and passive smoking in relation to lung cancer in women. Acta Oncol 28:623, 1989

Tokuhata GK, Lilienfeld AM: Familial aggregation of lung cancer in humans. J Natl Cancer Inst 30:289, 1963

Trichopoulos D, Kalandidi A, Sparros L, MacMahon B: Lung cancer and passive smoking. Int J Cancer 27:1, 1981

Vineis P, Thomas T, Hayes RB et al.: Proportion of lung cancers in males, due to occupation, in different areas of the USA. Int J Cancer 42:851, 1988

Wald NJ, Nanchahal K, Thompson SG, Cuckle HS: Does breathing other people's tobacco smoke cause lung cancer? BMJ 293:1217, 1986

Walker WJ, Brin BN: U.S. lung cancer mortality and declining cigarette tobacco consumption. J Clin Epidemiol 41:179, 1988

Wilcox HB, Schoenberg JB, Mason TJ et al.: Smoking and lung cancer: risk as a function of cigarette tar content. Prev Med 17:263, 1988

Woodward A, Roder D, McMichael AJ et al.: Radon daughter exposures at the Radium Hill uranium mine and lung cancer rates among former workers, 1952–87. Cancer Causes Control 2:213, 1991

Working Group on Passive Smoking: Links between passive smoking and disease: a best-evidence synthesis. Clin Invest Med 13:17, 1990

Wu AH, Henderson BE, Pike MC et al.: Smoking and other risk factors for lung cancer in women. J Natl Cancer Inst 74:747, 1985

Wu-Williams AH, Dai XD, Blot W et al.: Lung cancer among women in northeast China. Br J Cancer 62:982, 1990

Wynder EL, Graham EA: Tobacco smoking as a possible etiologic factor in bronchiogenic carcinoma. A study of six hundred and eighty-four proved cases. JAMA 143:329, 1950

Wynder EL, Hebert JR, Kabat GC: Association of dietary fat and lung cancer. J Natl Cancer Inst 79:631, 1987

Xie J, Lesaffre E, Kesteloot H: The relationship between animal fat intake, cigarette smoking, and lung cancer. Cancer Causes Control 2:79, 1991

Xu, ZY, Blot WJ, Xiao HP et al.: Smoking, air pollution, and the high rates of lung cancer in Shenyang, China. J Natl Cancer Inst 81:1800, 1989

Ziegler RG, Mason TJ, Stemhagen A et al.: Carotenoid intake, vegetables, and the risk of lung cancer among white men in New Jersey. Am J Epidemiol 123:1080, 1986

Pathology

Muhammad B. Zaman

DEFINITION

Benign and malignant neoplasms of the lung constitute one of the most varied and interesting group of tumors. Approximately 95 percent of all lung tumors are malignant and a vast majority of them can be classified into one of four major types as follows: (1) squamous cell carcinoma, (2) adenocarcinoma, (3) large cell carcinoma, and (4) small cell carcinoma.

The pathologic findings of these and other unusual lung tumors have been the subject of many publications, including two Armed Forces fascicles (Liebow, 1952; Carter and Eggleston, 1980); excellent reviews by Melamed (1968), Matthews

(1976), and Matthews and Gordon (1977); books by Spencer (1985), Glenn, et al. (1975), and Shimosato, et al. (1982); and chapters by Gmelich (1975), Millard (1977), and McDowell, et al. (1978). The first World Health Organization (WHO) classification of lung tumors, edited by Kreyberg, et al. (1967) appeared in 1967. As the incidence of lung cancer increased all over the world, more and more histologic material became available for diagnoses and classification; additional refinement and simplification occurred in the second edition of the classification (World Health Organization, 1981). Of the many different types and subtypes identified in this classification, the aforementioned four account for more than 90 percent of the cases. It is these four that most concern us clinically.

SQUAMOUS CELL (EPIDERMOID) CARCINOMAS

Squamous cell (epidermoid) carcinomas were once the most common type of lung cancer, accounting for perhaps one-half of all cases. Although the total number of lung cancer cases has increased dramatically each year for the last 75

Classification Scheme for Carcinoma of the Lung

   I. Squamous cell carcinoma (epidermoid carcinoma) variant:
      a. Spindle cell (squamous) carcinoma
  II. Small cell carcinoma
      a. Oat cell carcinoma
      b. Intermediate cell type
      c. Combined oat cell carcinoma
 III. Adenocarcinoma
      a. Acinar adenocarcinoma
      b. Papillary adenocarcinoma
      c. Solid carcinoma with much secretion
      d. Bronchioloalveolar carcinoma
  IV. Large cell (undifferentiated) carcinoma variants
      a. Giant cell carcinoma
      b. Clear cell carcinoma
   V. Adenosquamous carcinoma
  VI. Carcinoid tumors
 VII. Bronchial gland carcinomas
      a. Adenoid cystic carcinoma
      b. Mucoepidermoid carcinoma
VIII. Miscellaneous tumors
      a. Pulmonary blastoma
      b. Sarcomas of various types
      c. Lymphomas
      d. Melanomas
  IX. Mesotheliomas

(Modified from World Health Organization: Histological typing of lung tumors. In World Health Organization (ed): International Histological Classification of Tumors. No. 1. 2nd Ed. World Health Organization, Geneva, 1981, with permission.)

Table 27-2. Histologic Types of Lung Cancers in 10,040 Participants of the Memorial Sloan-Kettering Lung Cancer Screening Study

Type	No. Patients (%)
Squamous cell (epidermoid)	111 (31)
Small cell	55 (16)
Adenocarcinoma	164 (46)
Large cell (undifferentiated)	23 (6)
Carcinoid	1
Total	354

years, the increase in the rate of squamous cell carcinoma, at least recently, has not kept pace with that of adenocarcinoma, which is now the most common tumor type (Melamed, et al., 1987). In the population of male smokers from metropolitan New York, studied by us, 111 of the 354 lung cancers (31 percent) were of the squamous cell type (Table 27-2). Other large reviews of histologic types show a similar incidence of squamous cell carcinoma (Vincent, et al., 1977; Rosenow and Carr, 1979).

Morphogenesis

Squamous cell carcinomas arise from malignant transformation of hyperplastic (Fig. 27-6A) and sometimes metaplastic bronchial basal cells. Early squamous cell carcinomas are typically located in major bronchi, usually the lobar or first segmental bronchus of the upper lobes or the superior segment of the lower lobes (Shimosato, et al., 1982). In its earliest recognizable form, carcinoma in situ, the normally delicate, translucent columnar epithelium of the bronchial mucosa is replaced by a thickened, stratified squamous epithelium composed of malignant squamous cells (Fig. 27-6B).

Grossly the mucosa is granular to nodular and opaque or waxy. Rugal folds are effaced, and pits of bronchial gland orifices are obscured (Fig. 27-7). Squamous cancer cells exfoliate readily at this stage and are expectorated in cough specimens of sputum. They can be detected by cytologic examination. This stage is asymptomatic, except occasional patients have hemoptysis. As the carcinoma grows within the bronchial lumen and into and through the bronchial wall, it obstructs the bronchus (Fig. 27-8). The patient invariably becomes symptomatic with lobar or segmental collapse and distal endogenous lipid pneumonia. Superimposed bacterial pneumonia can also develop. These carcinomas may grow to a relatively large size locally before metastasizing, and even then metastases are limited for some time to peribronchial or hilar lymph nodes. Thus early-stage squamous cell carcinomas, even when large and ominous on chest radiographs, are highly amenable to treatment by resection.

Histology

Histologically invasive squamous cell carcinomas are graded as well, moderately, and poorly differentiated. Well-differentiated squamous cell carcinomas are relatively rare in the lung (10 percent). They exhibit distinct stratification and extensive keratin production, the latter in layers of parallel array and forming keratin pearls (Fig. 27-9). Individual cells are huge

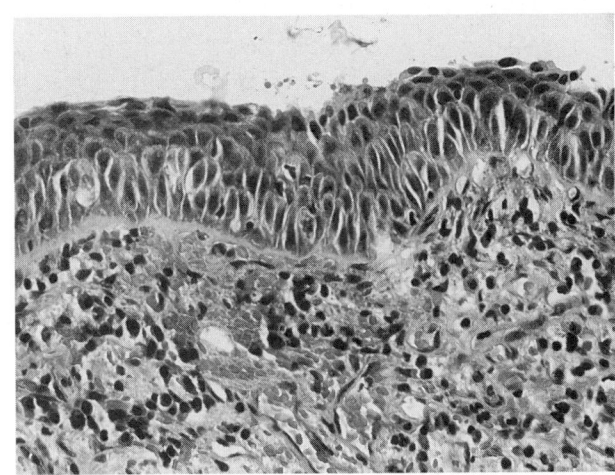
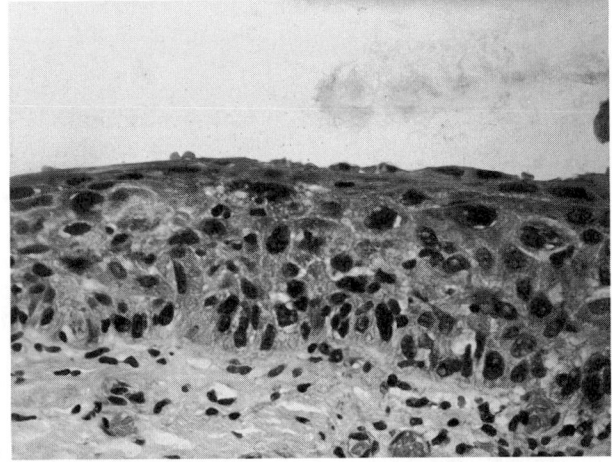

Figure 27-6. **(A)** Hyperplastic and atypical bronchial basal cells with surface squamous metaplasia. This is a precursor of the carcinoma in situ seen in Figure B. **(B)** Squamous cell carcinoma in situ. Note the nuclear pleomorphism, hyperchromasia, and loss of polarity of the cells.

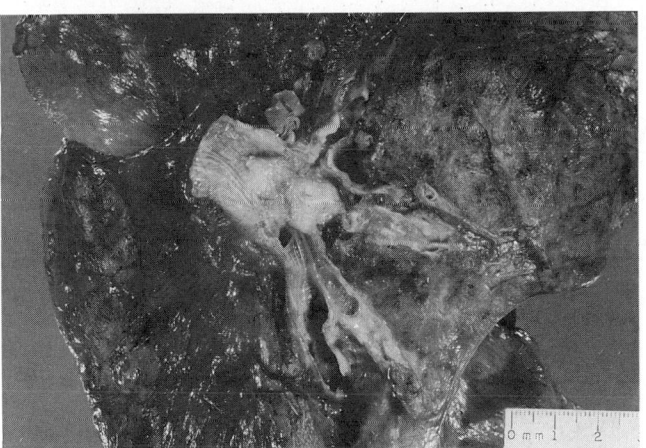

Figure 27-7. Squamous cell carcinoma in situ in the left lower lobe bronchus. The tumor is seen as waxy-white nodules 1 cm from the resection margin and extending to the subsegmental orifices.

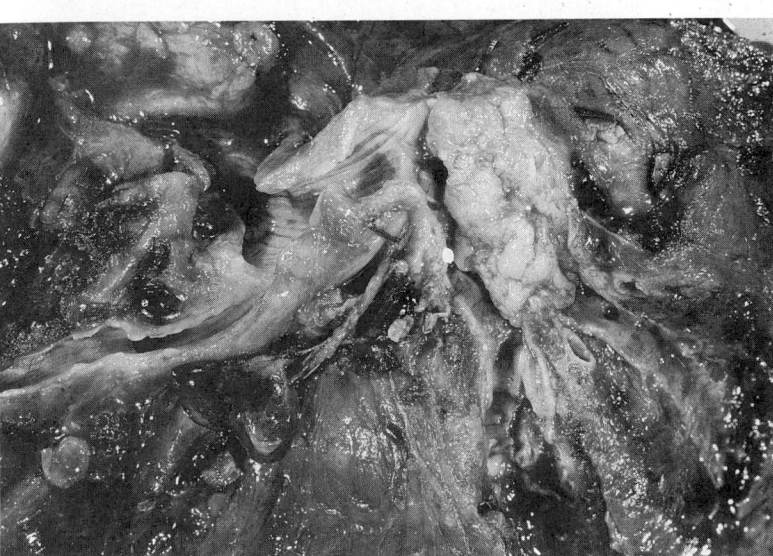

Figure 27-8. Squamous cell carcinoma obstructing the superior segment of the left lower lobe. Invasive carcinoma was present beyond the bronchial cartilage; the lymph nodes were free of tumor.

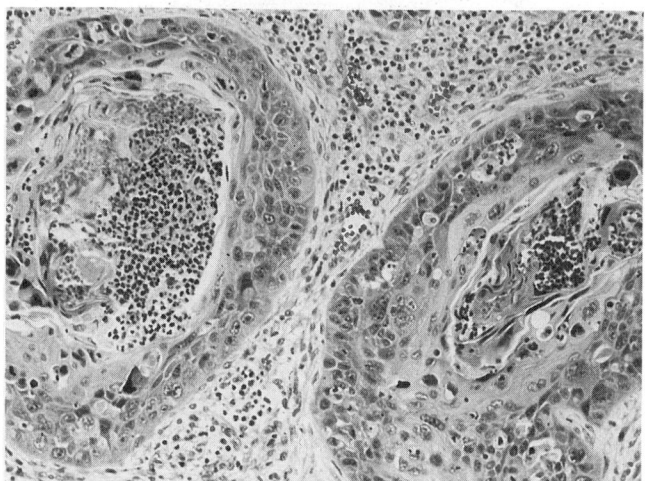

Figure 27-9. Well-differentiated squamous cell carcinoma. This highly keratinizing tumor is indistinguishable from oropharyngeal or laryngeal tumors at this metastatic site.

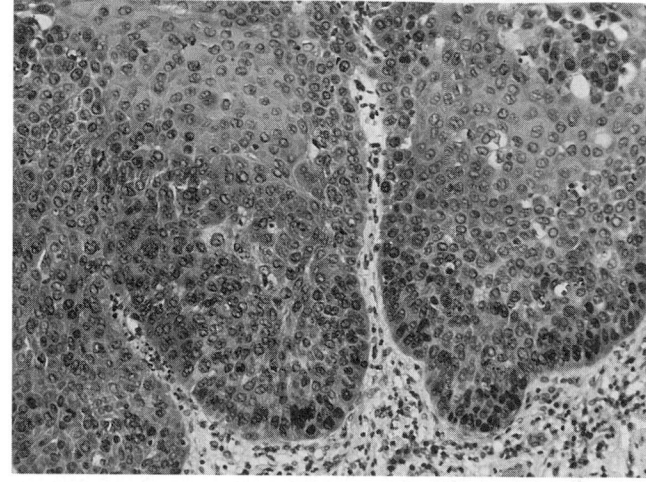

Figure 27-10. Moderately differentiated squamous cell carcinoma with focal keratinization in the upper left corner. This tumor was in situ in the right upper lobe anterior bronchus (RB₃).

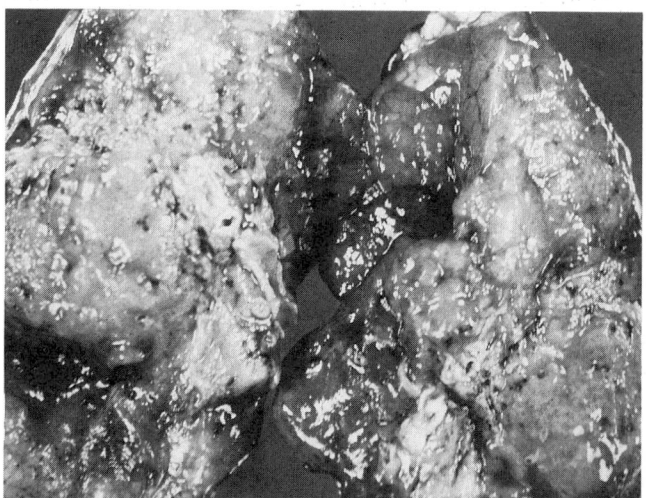

Figure 27-11. Bronchiolar adenocarcinoma involving the entire right upper lobe. The lobe is bisected, revealing a moist mucoid appearance, indistinguishable grossly from a *Klebsiella pneumoniae* infection.

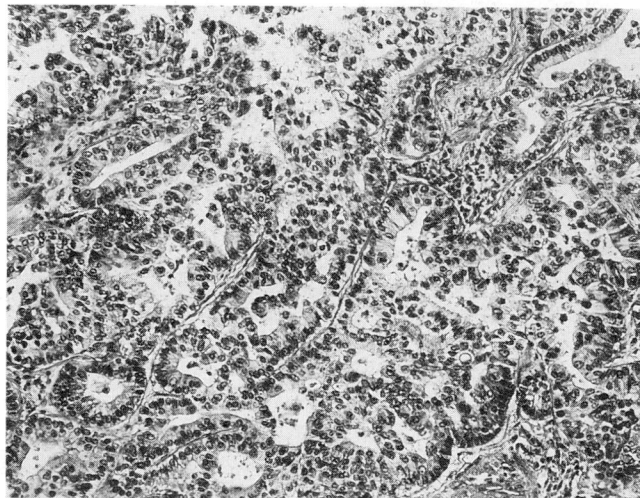

Figure 27-12. Acinar adenocarcinoma. Part of this 3-cm peripheral tumor was papillary and focally showed a bronchiolar pattern; not an uncommon finding in adenocarcinoma.

and pleomorphic with abundant cytoplasm and hyperchromatic angulated nuclei. The diagnosis is relatively easy to make in cytologic specimens with the characteristic cytoplasmic orangephilia seen with the Papanicolaou stain. Neck nodes with highly keratinizing squamous cell carcinoma found by fine-needle aspiration or biopsy are more likely to be of oropharyngeal or laryngeal origin rather than primary lung origin.

In moderately differentiated squamous cell carcinoma, there is much less evidence of keratinization. Approximately 20 percent of tumor cells should show glassy pink cytoplasm, with the remaining 80 percent being composed of undifferentiated cells (Fig. 27-10). Approximately 20 percent of squamous cell carcinomas are peripheral tumors that do not communicate with major bronchi. These tumors are generally poorly differentiated and composed of medium-sized undifferentiated cells with intercellular bridges and prominent nucleoli. Single cells and groups in cytologic specimens mimic adenocarcinoma, although there are differentiating features (Zaman, 1991).

All three grades of squamous cell carcinoma when large enough show central necrosis with superimposed inflammation and central cavitation. However, well-differentiated tumors are more inclined to do so, and stage for stage, they have the best prognosis.

Diagnosis

Fully 80 percent of squamous cell carcinomas have an endobronchial component (Shimosato, et al., 1982). Thus sputum and/or bronchial cytologic examination is rewarding. The peripheral tumors are amenable to percutaneous fine-needle aspiration or transbronchial biopsy. Rarely an open thoracotomy is necessary to make the diagnosis.

ADENOCARCINOMA

Adenocarcinoma and bronchiolar (bronchioloalveolar) carcinoma of the lung constitute the largest group of pulmonary carcinomas, about 46 percent. The WHO recognizes four subtypes of adenocarcinoma (see box above). Except for the jaagziekte type of bronchiolar carcinoma, which has a characteristic gross and histologic appearance (Fig. 27-11) and is often multicentric in origin, it is not always possible, nor is it necessary to subclassify adenocarcinomas because these tumors often exhibit a mixed pattern of acinar, papillary, or even bronchiolar differentiation in the same histologic section (Fig. 27-12).

Morphogenesis

Unlike squamous cell and small cell carcinomas, a majority of adenocarcinomas arise from peripheral bronchioles, rather than major bronchi. All begin as a solitary nodule, and only rarely can an adenocarcinoma be documented in an in situ stage (Fig. 27-13). The acinar and papillary adenocarcinomas grow by destruction and invasion of tissue, much like adenocarcinomas of other organs. They form glandular patterns, may produce mucin, and in some cases, may be difficult to distinguish from metastatic adenocarcinoma to the lung.

Because they are peripheral in origin, these tumors do not exfoliate cancer cells into the bronchus and are not likely to be identified by sputum cytologic examination until they are relatively large and have invaded into one of the larger bronchial branches. On the other hand, their position within aerated pulmonary tissue facilitates radiographic detection. They are the most frequently diagnosed by percutaneous needle aspiration or transbronchial biopsy.

The solid growth pattern is another variant, and the presence of intracellular mucin separates them from undifferentiated large cell carcinomas. Many of these glandular carcinomas metastasize first to regional lymph nodes, much like squamous cell carcinomas. However, a significant number of them, approximately 20 percent, reach distant sites (e.g., brain, bone, adrenal gland, and liver) by blood-borne spread, although regional lymph nodes are free of metastatic disease. Adenocarcinomas that are subpleural in origin can spread through the pleural lymphatic channels and are likely to generate an effusion containing cancer cells.

Bronchiolar carcinoma is unique because of the way it grows along alveolar septi (Fig. 27-14), frequently presenting multifocally. The tumor cells closely resemble the columnar or cuboidal mucinous or nonmucinous bronchial epithelium and spread throughout the lung by aerogenous dissemination. Tumors that are composed of cuboidal or low columnar cells, which are peg shaped, are of either clear cell or type II alveolar epithelial cell origin (Fig. 27-15). A rare subtype of bronchiolar adenocarcinoma is ciliated (Fig. 27-16).

The gross appearance and radiographic presentation are those of a consolidated or pneumonic lung (Fig. 27-11). Because there is little destruction of pre-existing bronchi, a characteristic air bronchogram is seen radiographically. Lymph node metastases are common, but death is usually the result of respiratory insufficiency from intrapulmonary spread.

LARGE CELL (UNDIFFERENTIATED) CARCINOMA

Large cell (undifferentiated) carcinoma has been subdivided into solid clear cell and giant cell variants. Together they comprised only 6 percent of tumors in our series (Table 27-2). The percentage is higher in most other large series and is a reflection of noncompliance with the strict criteria set by WHO for this diagnosis; many of such tumors are adenocarcinomas.

These are undifferentiated carcinomas, and we believe that they are anaplastic adenocarcinomas. However, they are separately classified because there is no consensus on their histogenesis and they have a more aggressive clinical behavior. The clear cell variant histologically closely resembles renal cell carcinoma but may show intracellular mucin.

The exception is giant cell carcinoma, which is considered a variant of large cell carcinoma. This aggressive but rare tumor contains a prominent component of highly pleomorphic, multinucleated cells characterized by a lack of intercellular cohesion. The nucleoli are large, acidophilic, and may be multiple (Fig. 27-17). Adenocarcinomas with some giant cells should not be included in this category. Metastatic giant cell carcinomas of the thyroid or pancreas have similar cyto-

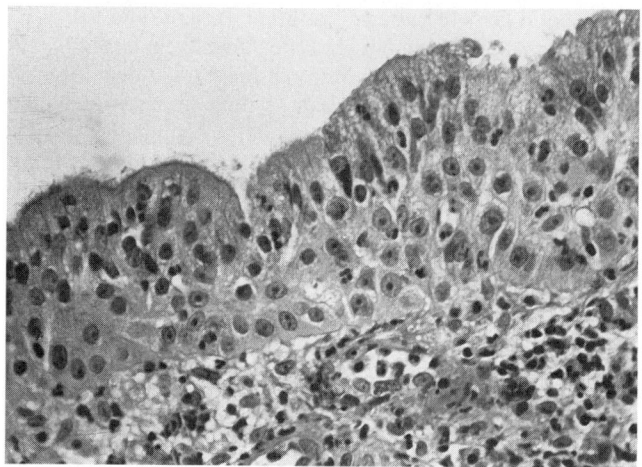

Figure 27-13. Adenocarcinoma in situ in a segmental bronchus. Note that the hyperplastic basal cells have a glandular differentiation with uniform cells, ovoid nuclei, prominent nucleoli, and transparent cytoplasm. Also note the normal ciliated cells at the surface. Compare with the tumor in Fig. 27-6A, which has progressed to become a squamous cell carcinoma in situ.

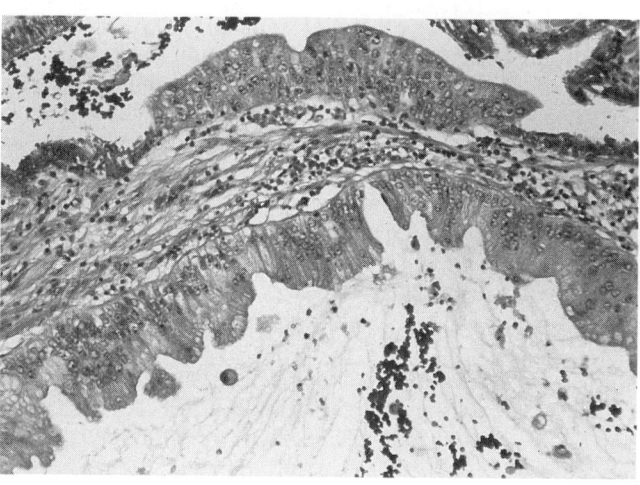

Figure 27-14. Bronchiolar carcinoma in situ. The lower bronchiole is completely lined by tall columnar mucinous neoplastic cells. The upper bronchiole is only partly replaced, meaning that the tumor is primary in the lung and not a metastatic mucinous adenocarcinoma.

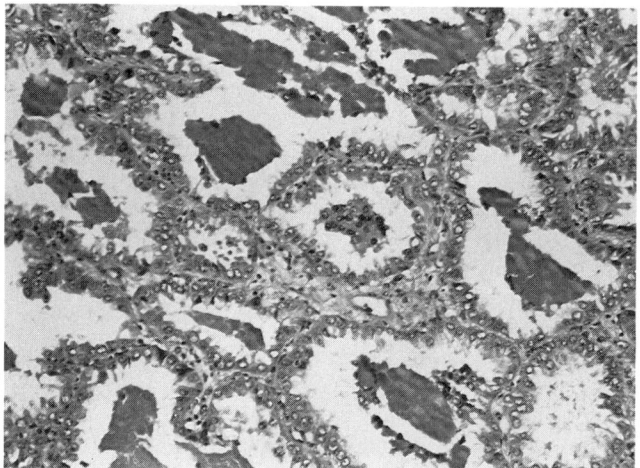

Figure 27-15. Bronchiolar adenocarcinoma of either clear cell or type II alveolar epithelial cell origin. The proteinaceous material in the lumen of the acini is mucin negative.

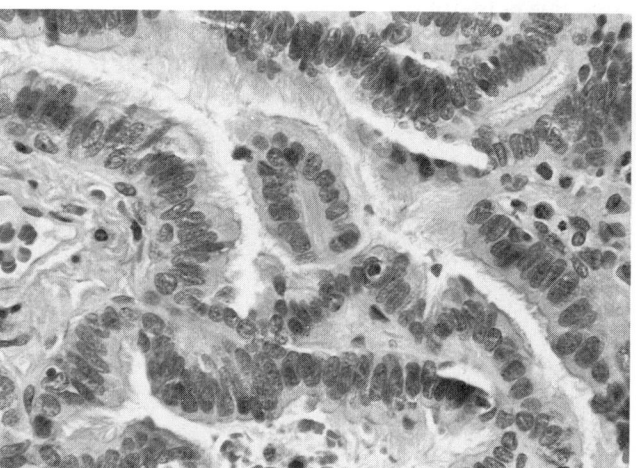

Figure 27-16. A rare example of ciliated bronchiolar adenocarcinoma. I have seen only one example in reviewing more than 1,500 lung cancer cases.

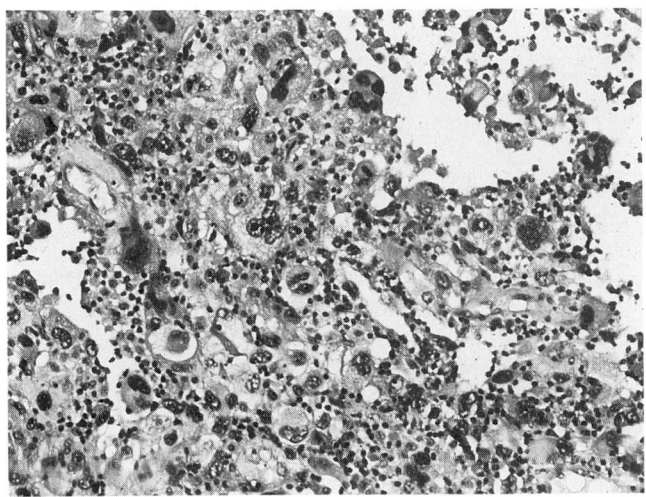

Figure 27-17. Giant cell carcinoma of the lung. Note the highly pleomorphic multinucleated cells without cohesion and infiltrated by leukocytes.

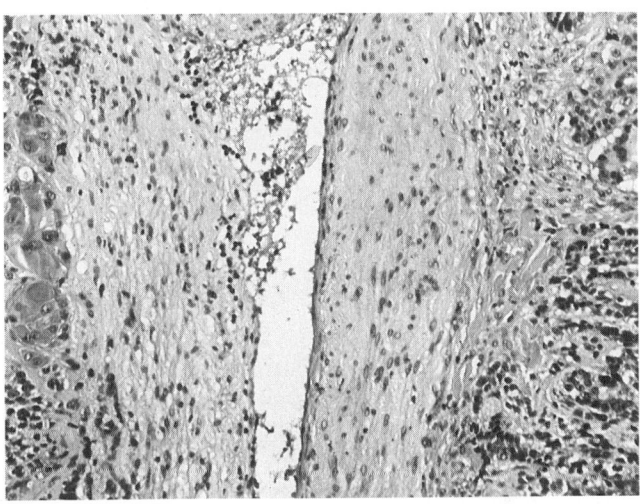

Figure 27-18. Combined oat cell carcinoma. In this selected field, small cell carcinoma is in the right lower, and adenocarcinoma in the upper, corner. Keratinizing squamous cell carcinoma is seen at the left margin. The bulk of the remaining tumor was the small cell type.

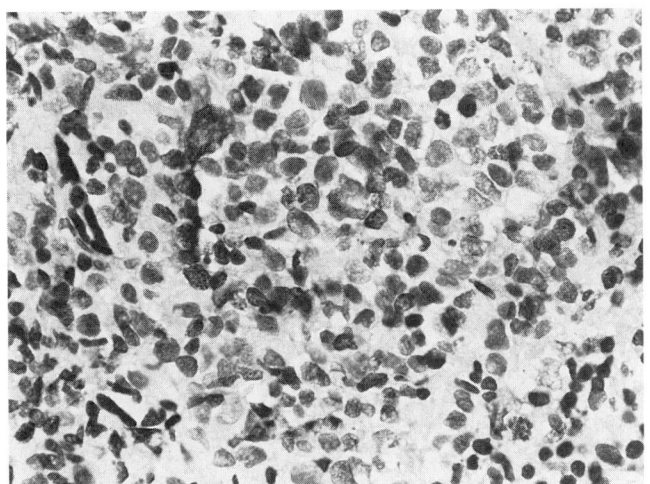

Figure 27-19. Small cell carcinoma, oat cell type. The compact growth pattern with nuclei in contact with each other denotes the lack of appreciable cytoplasm.

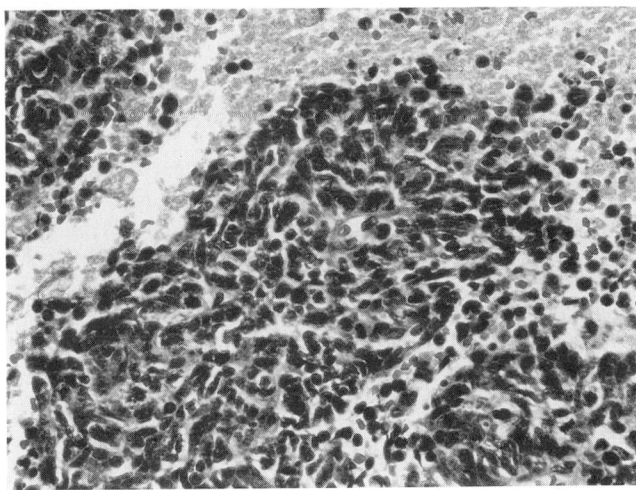

Figure 27-20. Small cell carcinoma, intermediate cell type. The cells are ovoid or fusiform. Necrosis and nuclear pyknosis are evident.

Table 27-3. Small Cell Carcinomas of the Lung: Incidence

	Total Lung Cancer	Small Cell Cancer (%)
National Lung Program (male smokers older than 45 years of age)	354	55 (16)
New York State (Male and female smokers all ages[a])	421	105 (25)
New York State (Male and female nonsmokers and former smokers of all ages[a])	432	33 (8)

[a] Data from Janerich DT et al: Lung cancer and exposure to tobacco smoke in the household. N Engl J Med 323:632, 1990, the New York State Department of Health, Albany, NY, and unpublished data.)

morphologic findings and are indistinguishable without a clinical correlation.

SMALL CELL CARCINOMAS

Small cell carcinomas constitute approximately 20 percent of all primary lung carcinomas, although in a screening population of ambulatory and presumably asymptomatic population of male smokers, they are under-represented (16 percent). Table 27-3 compares the incidence of small cell carcinomas in a hospital-based patient populatoin of smokers and nonsmokers or former smokers with this screening population.

Since the estimated 1993 incidence of lung cancer in the United States is 170,000 (American Cancer Society, 1993), approximately 35,000 of these most rapidly growing, widely disseminating, and aggressive variants of lung carcinoma will be encountered. Squamous cell carcinomas and small cell carcinomas are most closely related to cigarette smoking; conversely these two histologic types seldom occur in pure nonsmokers (Rosenow and Carr, 1979).

Morphogenesis

Small cell carcinomas, like squamous cell carcinomas, arise from a malignant transformation of hyperplastic bronchial basal cells. However, a majority of these neoplastic basal cells remain small in size and undifferentiated. When a small cell carcinoma is widely sampled and examined microscopically, the finding of focal areas of squamous or glandular differentiation is common (Fig. 27-18); these are called combined oat cell carcinomas. The small cell component of these tumors are exquisitely sensitive to combination chemotherapy and radiotherapy. However, the disease generally recurs, and at autopsy, the residual tumor is often a nonsmall cell carcinoma. This phenomenon is neither maturation nor differentiation of the small cell carcinoma under therapy; rather the nonsmall cell component of the combined oat cell carcinoma has multiplied unopposed (Mathews, et al., 1978a).

The hypothesis that small cell carcinomas are neuroendocrine in origin and related to carcinoid tumors (Spencer, 1985) can be refuted epidemiologically, histogenetically, ultrastructurally, immunohistologically, therapeutically, and prognostically (Table 27-4).

Small cell carcinomas also arise in major lobar or segmental bronchi, and only about 25 percent occur in peripheral lung. Many of these tumors present with metastases, which are both lymphatic and blood borne and which can be assumed to be present at diagnosis, even if not apparent. An asymptomatic diagnosis of small cell carcinoma is rarely possible by screening; an incidental chest radiograph can detect an occasional case as a coin lesion. Approximately 50 percent of these lesions show mediastinal lymph node metastases.

Histology

Histologically small cell carcinomas are subdivided into oat cell and intermediate cell types, but this subdivision is of interest primarily to the pathologist and has little or no real clinical significance (Mathews, et al., 1978b). The oat cell carcinomas are made up of small round to ovoid cells with little appreciable cytoplasm. The tumor is devoid of stroma and appears highly cellular with many of the nuclei pushing each other; a molding artifact is created. Areas of necrosis and pyknosis are a constant feature as are frequent mitoses. Nuclear chromatin is coarse and abundant. Thus the cells are darkly stained, and the nucleoli are inconspicuous (Fig. 27-19). This tumor must be differentiated from lymphoma, preferably by immunocytochemical analysis.

Table 27-4. Factors Differentiating Small Cell Carcinoma and Carcinoid Tumors

Small Cell Carcinoma	Carcinoid Tumors
Related to smoking or other environmental carcinogen	Not related to smoking, no known carcinogen
Occurs in old age	All ages
Arises from hyperplastic basal cells	Arises from Kulchitsky cells
Few dense-core neurosecretory granules	Numerous neurosecretory granules
Chromogranin and Grimelius stains[a] are negative	Both stains positive
Radio- and chemosensitive	Does not respond to radio- or chemotherapy
5-Year survival rate anecdotal	70–90% 5-year survival after resection

[a] Stains neurosecretory granules.

The intermediate cell variety of small cell carcinoma has nuclear characteristics similar to those of oat cell variety, but the cells are considerably larger, less regular in appearance, and have more abundant cytoplasm. The cells may be polygonal or fusiform in shape. Thin fibroconnective strands divide the tumor into compartments and may closely mimic poorly differentiated squamous cell carcinoma (Fig. 27-20). In fact there is no objective method or stain to separate them. This type of cancer is less common than oat cell carcinoma is and tends to occur more in the periphery of the lung.

A third type, combined oat cell carcinoma, is recognized when foci of squamous cell carcinoma or adenocarcinoma are present in an oat cell carcinoma (Fig. 27-18). This variety is underdiagnosed in bronchial biopsy material. Open biopsy or attempted resection of specimens of small cell carcinoma would show approximately 25 percent combined oat cell carcinoma on adequate sampling.

Diagnosis

Most small cell carcinomas are diagnosed from cytologic specimens, either endoscopic brushings or percutaneous aspiration. Bronchial biopsies often show crush artifacts and must be distinguished from lymphoma, carcinoid, and poorly differentiated squamous cell carcinoma. A biopsy of nodal disease or distant metastases also confirms the diagnosis.

ULTRASTRUCTURAL FEATURES AND IMMUNOHISTOCHEMISTRY

Many reports describe the ultrastructural features of the four major types of lung carcinomas described in this chapter. In well-differentiated squamous cell carcinomas, bundles of tonofilaments (keratin), numerous prominent desmosomes, widened intercellular spaces bridged by the apposing cell processes (intercellular bridges), and keratohyaline granules are characteristic. In poorly differentiated variants, none of these features are prominent. Adenocarcinomas and large cell carcinomas show ultrastructural features of cellular secretions (e.g., presence of extra- and/or intracellular lumen containing mucosubstance, extensive rough endoplasmic reticulum, large Golgi apparatus, and numerous mitochondria).

Small cell carcinomas, like squamous cell carcinomas, show tonofilaments, small desmosomes, and possibly a few small dense-core granules. McDowell, et al. studied large numbers of lung tumors (Shimosato, et al., 1982) ultrastructurally and observed the presence of mucus, dense-core granules, and tonofilaments in tumors of all categories, confirming the light morphologic observations that, when enough sections are studied, more than one morphologic pattern can be seen in any individual tumor (Fig. 27-18).

The same findings of heterogeneity are manifested in immunohistochemical analysis; antigens of many different specifications are shared by all primary epithelial lung tumors. The exception is carcinoid tumors, described earlier (Table 27-4), which stain positive for chromogranin. However, immunohistochemical testing is extremely helpful in distinguishing among mesenchymal tumors (sarcomas), melanomas, and lymphomas, and ultrastructural studies are no longer routinely done for undifferentiated tumors. In conclusion, both electron microscopy and immunohistochemical analysis indicate that the four major types of lung tumors arise from a common stem cell with a tendency to differentiate along one or more pathways.

CONCLUSION

The great variety of tumors that can arise in the human lung reflects the complex histologic composition of this organ. Most of these tumors, perhaps 95 percent, arise from the bronchial basal epithelial cells and submucosal glands.

The fact that many nonsmall cell lung cancers have mixed histologic findings and combined oat cell carcinomas are often seen in the resected material leads many authorities to the conclusion that all squamous cell carcinomas and small cell carcinomas and the majority of solid adenocarcinomas (WHO IIIC) and undifferentiated large cell carcinomas arise from multipotential basal reserve cells. When neoplastic reserve cells remain small and undifferentiated, we call them small cell carcinoma. When they become enlarged and metaplastic, we call them squamous cell carcinoma. When they enlarge and produce mucin, we call them large cell or adenocarcinoma. However, all too often the hyperplastic and neoplastic reserve cells show a mixed differentiation.

COMMENTS AND CONTROVERSIES

A knowledge of basic pathologic findings as they relate to lung cancer is of supreme importance to the clinician. Practically speaking, the most important differentiation is whether or not the tumor is a small cell or nonsmall cell carcinoma because the investigation and management differ considerably. With increasing frequency, pathologists are identifying more than one cell type in a given tumor. This is not surprising, considering the common stem cell hypothesis of the origin of bronchogenic carcinomas. When considering therapeutic approaches to such tumors, the tumor with the worst prognosis (e.g., small cell lung cancer) should dominate the therapeutic attack.

Although it is less important clinically to distinguish the various types of nonsmall cell lung cancer, electron micros-

copy and immunohistochemical tests are important when attempting to differentiate thoracic tumors in which the site of origin (e.g., mediastinum versus lung) is in doubt.

Although the tumor-node-metastasis (TNM) classification and cell type remain the most important prognostic factors, much still has to be learned about pathologic subtypes, electron microscopic appearance, immunohistochemical analyses, and genetic factors with regard to their prognostic significance.

This chapter section is an overview of the pathologic findings in lung cancer. Interested readers should consult the publications outlined by the author in his introduction for more detailed information.

R.J.G.

KEY REFERENCES

Melamed MR, Flehinger BJ, Zaman, MB: Impact of early detection on the clinical course of lung cancer. Surg Clin North Am 67:909, 1987

Three hundred fifty-four lung cancers were found in 10,000 male smokers by periodic scanning (chest radiography and sputum cytologic examination) for 5 to 8 years. Many of the resected early tumors were studied by serial step sections of the bronchial tree and special stains. This and other original studies are the basis for the views on the histogenesis of common types of lung cancers detailed in this chapter.

Shimosato Y, Melamed MR, Nettesheim P (eds): Morphogenesis of Lung Cancer. Boca Raton, CRC Press, FL, 1982

Much of this text concerns the morphogenesis of human lung cancer, especially the four major types. The contributors present recent original work on the histology, ultrastructure, growth characteristics, and function of various types of lung cancers in relation to their histogenesis. The text is appropriately illustrated with unique gross photomicrographs and numerous light microscopic and ultrastructural images.

World Health Organization: Histological typing of lung tumors. In World Health Organization (ed): International Histological Classification of Tumors. No. 1. 2nd Ed. World Health Organization, Geneva, 1981

This is an updated histologic classification of tumors and tumorlike lesions of the pulmonary parenchyma, based on light microscopy, and developed by an expert panel of more than 30 pathologists from as many countries.

Zaman MB: Pulmonary Cytology. Clin Lab Med 11:293, 1991

Most lung tumors are presently diagnosed by examining one or more types of cytologic specimens. This article describes the optimal specimen and illustrates the morphocytologic features of various types of primary and metastatic intrathoracic tumors. There are a handful of limitations. The author shares his experience, which was accumulated and refined over the course of 15 years in a large cancer hospital.

REFERENCES

American Cancer Society: 1993 Cancer Facts and Figures. American Cancer Society, Atlanta, 1993

Carter D, Eggleston JC: Tumors of the lower respiratory tract. In: Atlas of Tumor Pathology. Series 2. Part 17. Armed Forces Institute of Pathology, Washington, D.C., 1980

Glenn WWL, Liebow AA, Lindskog GE: Thoracic and Cardiovascular Surgery with Related Pathology. 3rd Ed. Appleton-Century-Crofts, New York, 1975

Gmelich JT: The pathology of cancer of the lung. p. 17. In Seydel HG, Chait A, Gmelich JT (eds): Cancer of the Lung. John Wiley & Sons, New York, 1975

Janerich DT et al: Lung cancer and exposure to tobacco smoke in the household. N Engl J Med 323:632, 1990

Kreyberg L, Liebow AA, Uehlinger EA: Histological Typing of Lung Tumors. World Health Organization, Geneva, 1967

Liebow AA: Tumors of the lower respiratory tract. In Atlas of Tumor Pathology. Section 5. Part 17. Armed Forces Institute of Pathology, Washington, DC, 1952

Mathews MJ et al: Effects of chemotherapy on the histology of small cell carcinoma of the lung (SCCL)—a postmortem study of 54 cases. Proc Am Soc Clin Oncol 19:397, 1978a

Mathews MJ et al: Histologic subtypes of small cell carcinoma of the lung (SCCL) and their clinical significance. Proc Am Soc Clin Oncol 19:397, 1978b

Matthews MJ, Gordon PR: Morphology of pulmonary and pleural malignancies. p. 49. In Straus MJ (ed): Lung Cancer: Clinical Diagnosis and Treatment. Grune & Stratton, New York, 1977

Matthews MJ: Problems in morphology and behavior of bronchopulmonary malignant disease. p. 23. In Israel L, Chahinian AP (eds): Lung Cancer: Natural History, Prognosis and Therapy. New York, Academic Press, New York, 1976

McDowell EM, Becci PJ, Barrett LA et al: Morphogenesis and classification of lung cancer. p. 445. In Harris CC (ed): Pathogenesis and Therapy of Lung Cancer. Marcel Dekker, New York, 1978

Melamed MR: Pathology. p. 35. In Watson WL (ed): Lung Cancer: A Study of Five Thousand Memorial Hospital Cases. CV Mosby, St. Louis, 1968

Millard M: Lung, pleura and mediastinum. p. 1038. In Anderson WAD, Kissane JM, (eds): Pathology. 7th Ed. CV Mosby, St. Louis, 1977

Rosenow EC III, Carr DT: Bronchogenic carcinoma. CA Cancer Clin 29:233, 1979

Spencer H: Pathology of the Lung. 4th Ed. Pergamon Press, New York, 1985

Vincent RG, Pickren JW, Lane WW et al: The changing histopathology of lung cancer: a review of 1682 cases. Cancer 39:1647, 1977

Diagnosis and Staging

Michael Maddaus
Robert J. Ginsberg

HISTORICAL NOTE

The staging of lung cancer began with the development of the TNM classification system by Denoix in 1946. Although modified, it remains the basis of staging systems for many tumors, including lung cancer. In 1959 the American Joint Committee for Cancer Staging and End Results Reporting (AJCC) was formed by several organizations, including the American College of Surgeons, National Cancer Institute, the American Cancer Society, and others. Their goal was to develop staging systems for different cancers by assigning task forces to each particular cancer. Mountain, et al. (1974) described the AJCC lung cancer staging system (based on the original TNM descriptors devised by Denoix [1946]) that had been developed by the lung cancer task force.

Although the AJCC staging system functioned well, several problems became apparent when significant survival differences were noted between subsets of the same clinical stage. For example, stage I included one subset with N1 disease, a group subsequently shown to have a poorer prognosis than those with N0 disease, and stage III included an array of subsets consisting of all patients with disease more advanced than N1 nodal involvement. Thus stage III included patients with isolated mediastinal nodal disease, patients with chest wall involvement and no nodal disease, and patients with metastatic disease; it did not separate operative from nonoperative candidates.

The AJCC lung cancer staging system was used until 1985 when Mountain (1986) presented the new international staging system developed by members of the AJCC task force on lung cancer in conjunction with the International Union Against Cancer. The new international staging system was developed to correct problems with the AJCC system, and since 1985, it has been adopted worldwide.

Surgical exploration of the mediastinum as a staging procedure was first developed by Harken, et al. (1954). Through a supraclavicular incision, a Jackson laryngoscope was inserted into the mediastinum, and lymph node biopsies were performed. Cervical mediastinoscopy, through a pretracheal suprasternal notch incision, was developed by Carlens (1959) in Sweden and was subsequently popularized by F. G. Pearson in North America.

HISTORICAL READINGS

Carlens E: Mediastinoscopy: a method for inspection and tissue biopsy in the superior mediastinum. Dis Chest 36:343, 1959
Denoix PF: Enquete permanent dans les centres anticancereux. Bull Inst Nat Hyg (Paris) I:70, 1946
Harken DE, Black H, Clauss R, Ferrand RE: Simple cervicomediastinal exploration for tissue diagnosis of intrathoracic disease. N Engl J Med 251:1041, 1954
Mountain CF, Carr DT, Anderson WAD: A system for the clinical staging of lung cancer. AJR 120:130, 1974

CLINICAL PRESENTATION

Ninety-five percent of patients with lung cancer are symptomatic at the time of diagnosis. Of these, 27 percent have symptoms secondary to the primary tumor, 32 percent have symptoms of metastatic spread, and 34 percent have systemic symptoms (malaise, weight loss, and anorexia) (Carbone, et al., 1970). Thus at presentation, a high percentage of patients already have clinical evidence of systemic spread and are inoperable. Only 5 percent or less are asymptomatic with an abnormal chest radiograph, and still fewer have occult carcinomas with a normal chest radiograph.

The clinical presentation of lung cancer is one of the most varied and unpredictable in all of medicine. Such a wide range of symptoms and signs is related to several factors as follows: (1) tumor histologic findings, which determine, to a significant degree, biologic activity and anatomic location; (2) intrinsic tumor biology, leading to differing growth rates and the production of a variety of paraneoplastic syndromes; (3) the anatomic location, which determines the tumor's mechanical effects; and (4) the stage at presentation, ranging from asymptomatic to widely disseminated metastatic disease.

The impact of tumor histologic findings on the clinical presentation of lung cancer must be emphasized. In general squamous cell and small cell carcinoma, because they are centrally located tumors, arise in the proximal bronchi and often produce symptoms of airway irritation or obstruction. The common symptoms include cough, hemoptysis, wheezing (because of high-grade airway stenosis), dyspnea secondary to bronchial occlusion (with or without postobstructive atelectasis), and postobstructive pneumonia (caused by secretion retention and atelectasis).

In contrast adenocarcinoma and its variant, large cell carcinoma, are often peripherally located and rarely cause the airway symptoms seen with squamous and small cell carcinomas. Instead they often present as asymptomatic peripheral nodules on the chest radiograph or, when symptomatic, with parietal pleural or chest wall invasion (resulting in pleuritic or chest wall pain). Pleural seeding and development of a malignant effusion (with progressive dyspnea) can also occur. Because of their peripheral location, adenocarcinoma and large cell carcinoma are often not visible on flexible bronchoscopic examination.

Bronchoalveolar carcinoma is a highly variable tumor. It may present as a solitary nodule, as multifocal nodules, or

as a diffuse infiltrating process easily confused with a consolidating pneumonia (Donaldson, et al., 1978). In the diffuse infiltrating or pneumonic form, marked shortness of breath and hypoxia may develop, and occasionally extreme bronchorrhea with expectoration of massive volumes (more than 1 L/day) of light tan fluid can lead to dehydration and electrolyte imbalance. Unlike adenocarcinoma, chest wall invasion is unusual. A unique radiologic feature of bronchoalveolar carcinoma is the presence of air bronchograms, resulting from the tendency of the tumor to fill alveolar air spaces instead of destroying and compressing the surrounding normal lung.

Pulmonary Manifestations

The pulmonary symptoms result from bronchus and/or lung involvement by the primary tumor (Fig. 27-21).

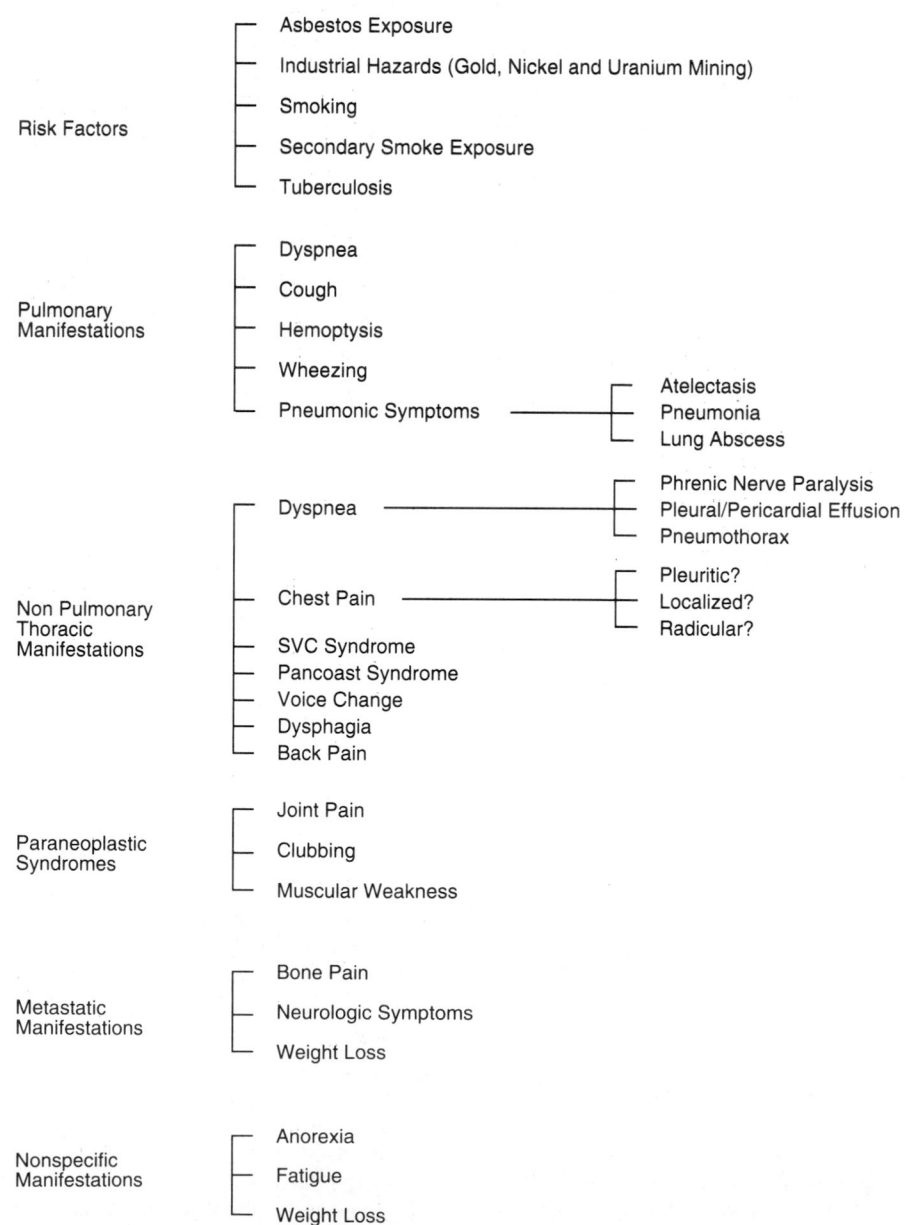

Figure 27-21. Risk factors and symptoms to be evaluated in patients with suspected or proved lung cancer.

Cough

Cough from bronchial irritation, the most common pulmonary symptom, occurs in 75 percent of patients (Cromartie, et al., 1980). Initially attributed (in smokers) to a chronic cigarette cough, with persistence or worsening, it eventually defines itself as significant. The cough is caused by inflammation or compression (extraluminal or intraluminal) of a bronchus.

Dyspnea

Dyspnea, the second most frequent pulmonary symptom, occurs in 50 to 60 percent of patients (Cromartie, et al., 1980). With central tumors, dyspnea results from partial or complete bronchial occlusion with or without postobstructive atelectasis, whereas with peripheral tumors, dyspnea (if present) is usually the result of pleural effusion or lymphatic spread.

Wheezing

Wheezing is seen with partial occlusion of a proximal bronchus and occurs when the airway diameter is narrowed to less than 50 percent of its diameter.

Hemoptysis

Hemoptysis occurs in 25 to 40 percent of patients, usually simple blood streaking of sputum and almost exclusively with centrally located tumors, which are degenerating or invading and ulcerating surrounding bronchial tissue. Massive hemoptysis is rare.

Pneumonic Symptoms

Pneumonic symptoms occur as a result of bronchitis, atelectasis, or postobstructive pneumonia. With postobstructive atelectasis and/or pneumonia, a combination of symptoms may occur: cough, sputum production, fever, and pleuritic chest pain (caused by contact of inflamed lung with parietal pleura).

Lung Abscess

Lung abscess results from secondary infection of a necrotic tumor cavity or postobstructive pneumonia. This occurs most frequently with squamous or large cell anaplastic cancer.

Nonpulmonary Thoracic Manifestations

When the primary tumor invades contiguous structures (e.g., chest wall, diaphragm, pericardium, phrenic nerve, recurrent laryngeal nerve, superior vena cava, or esophagus) or when enlarged tumor-bearing lymph nodes mechanically compress a structure (e.g., superior vena cava), specific signs and symptoms evolve (Fig. 27-21).

Diaphragm Invasion

Invasion of the diaphragm leads to diaphragmatic dysfunction with an enhanced sense of dyspnea on exertion and/or a pleural effusion. The diaphragm's extensive lymphatic plexus (which normally drains fluid from the peritoneal cavity) with invasion can lead to early lymphatic spread. Visceral pleural involvement may lead to pneumothorax (infrequent), more commonly pleural effusion secondary to occlusion of pulmonary lymphatic channels, or shedding of tumor cells into the pleural space. Pleural effusions may also be caused by mediastinal lymphatic obstruction, atelectasis, or pneumonitis. Regardless of the cause, pleural effusions produce dyspnea by restricting lung expansion, leading to decreased ventilation and atelectasis.

Chest Wall Involvement

Chest wall involvement from extension of the tumor into the parietal pleural surface or deeper structures (intercostal muscles, ribs, and neurovascular bundle) most often occurs with peripherally located adenocarcinomas. Pleuritic pain results from parietal pleural irritation and is usually transitory. Growth beyond the parietal pleura into rib and/or muscle produces a gnawing localized pain; invasion of the neurovascular bundle produces radicular chest wall pain. A unique syndrome occurs with extension of apical lung tumors superiorly into the thoracic outlet (Fig. 27-22). Superior sulcus tumors present with variable combinations of shoulder pain (from direct invasion of the ribs and muscles), radicular arm pain (from invasion of the C8 and T1 nerve roots of the brachial plexus), and Horner's syndrome (unilateral enophthalmos, ptosis, myosis, and anhidrosis of the face from invasion of the stellate sympathetic ganglion). The total symptom complex referred to is the Pancoast syndrome.

Tumors located on the medial lung surface may invade mediastinal structures. Phrenic nerve involvement leads to diaphragmatic paralysis and/or hiccups with dyspnea on exertion. The diagnosis is usually confirmed by plain chest radiography (showing elevation of one diaphragm, Fig. 27-23) or fluoroscopic examination of the diaphragm with breathing and sniffing maneuvers. Invasion of the recurrent laryngeal nerve ocurs predominantly on the left side because of the proximity of the left recurrent laryngeal nerve to the pulmonary hilum and the left upper lobe as it passes under the aortic arch. Paralysis occurs with extension of a primary left upper lobe tumor into the vagus nerve or from invasion or compression of the vagus nerve by aortopulmonary and anterior mediastinal lymphatic metastases (stations 5 and 6, Fig. 27-24). Recurrent laryngeal nerve involvement produces voice changes, ranging from subtle tone changes to distinct hoarseness.

Pericardial Involvement

Pericardial involvement can produce benign or malignant pericardial effusions occasionally associated with pericardial tamponade. Tamponade often presents subtly with increasing dyspnea or with a new arrhythmia (sinus tachycardia or atrial fibrillation). The diagnosis is made by having a high index of suspicion based on the primary tumor's location, by evidence of increased cardiac size on the chest radiograph, and ultimately, by echocardiography. Because a pleural effusion is often simultaneously present, there is often a delay in recognizing a pericardial effusion. Such as effusion should be considered when there is persistent dyspnea or cough, particularly if the dyspnea persists after successful management of a pleural effusion.

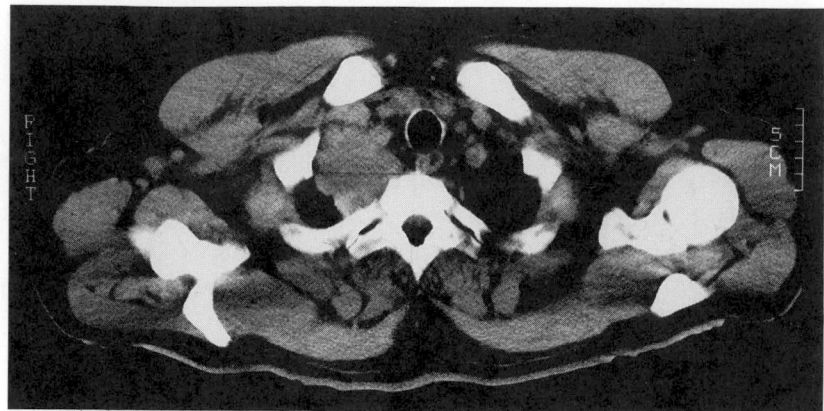

Figure 27-22. CT scan demonstrating a right apical Pancoast tumor.

Esophageal Invasion

Esophageal invasion is rare. Dysphagia occurs primarily from extrinsic esophageal compression by enlarged tumor-bearing subcarinal or posterior mediastinal lymph nodes. This occurs primarily with lower lobe tumors and indicates advanced disease. With time tumor-bearing lymph nodes may erode through the esophagus and trachea, creating a tracheoesophageal fistula, leading to recurrent aspiration pneumonitis.

Superior Vena Cava Syndrome

Superior vena cava syndrome can occur from invasion of the superior vena cava by a right upper lobe tumor or more commonly from extrinsic compression of the superior vena cava by enlarged tumor-bearing mediastinal lymph nodes. Small cell carcinoma, with its propensity to early and wide-spread lymphatic dissemination, is the predominant cause. Overall it occurs in 4 percent of patients with lung cancer. Although up to one-third of patients have secondary thromboses of the vena cava, with time the majority develop sufficient venous collaterals, allowing at least partial decompression with a relief of symptoms.

Direct extension of a tumor in any lobe can occur to a vertebral body, with the development of a persistent, gnawing, and often severe localized back pain. Growth into the epidural space can produce symptoms of spinal cord compression.

Paraneoplastic Syndromes

Paraneoplastic syndromes related to lung cancer are unusual (occurring in approximately 2 percent of patients) but are some of the most dramatic and interesting syndromes seen.

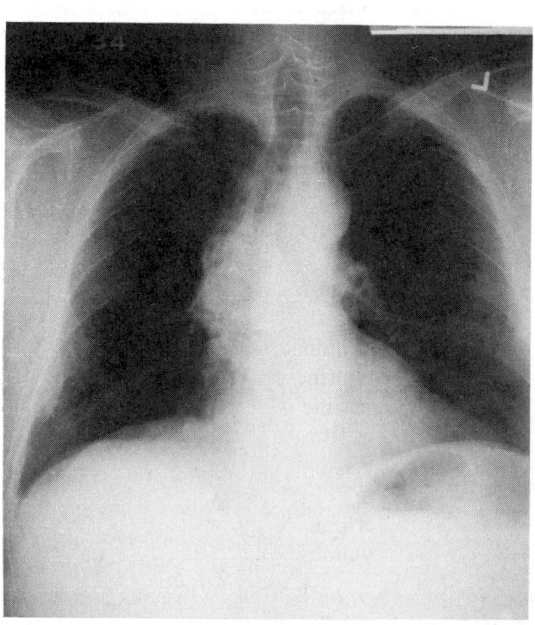
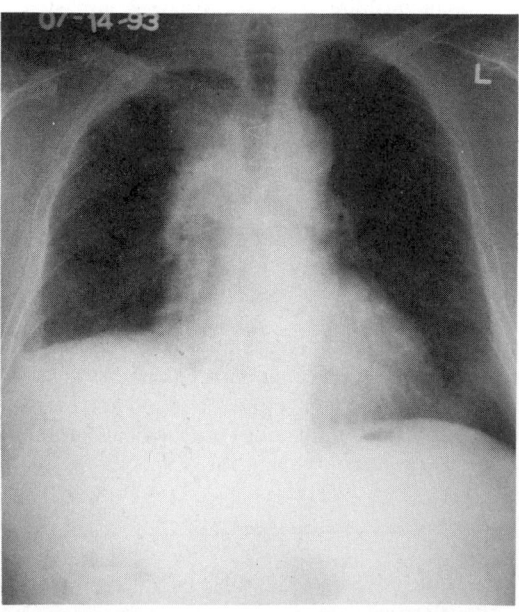

Figure 27-23. Phrenic nerve paralysis. The left chest radiograph shows a previously normal right hemidiaphragm. The right chest radiograph shows an elevated right hemidiaphragm secondary to invasion of the right phrenic nerve by a hilar tumor.

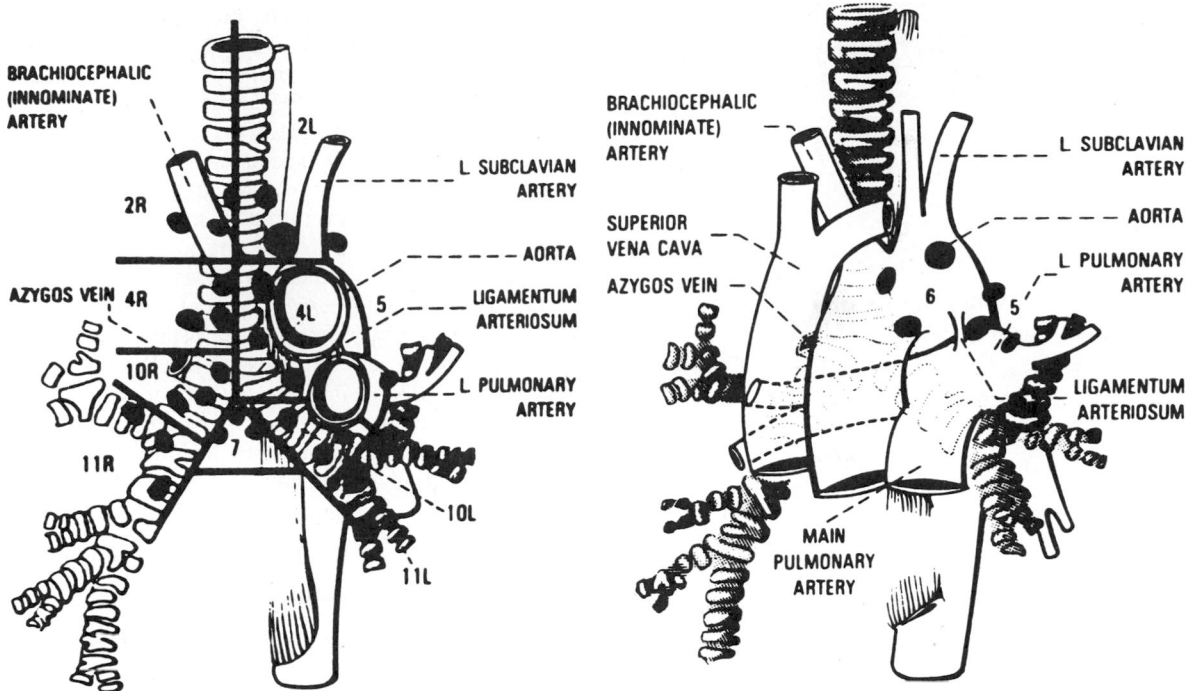

Figure 27-24. American Thoracic Society lymph node mapping schema showing anatomic boundaries of each lymph node station. (From American Thoracic Society: Clinical staging of primary lung cancer. Am Rev Respir Dis 127:659, 1983, with permission.)

Although occurring with other tumors, lung cancer is the most frequent cause, with small cell and squamous cell carcinoma predominating. A paraneoplastic syndrome may be the first indication of a tumor's presence. Thus the clinician must recognize the symptoms of a paraneoplastic syndrome to diagnose an early surgically treatable lung cancer. Unfortunately the symptoms are often attributed to metastatic or advanced disease (particularly with neurologic symptoms), with a delay in the recognition and treatment of the primary tumor. The many paraneoplastic syndromes seen with lung cancer are listed below. The following highlights important features of the more commonly seen syndromes.

Clubbing of the fingers and/or toes may occur independently or may be associated with hypertrophic pulmonary osteoarthropathy. As in other paraneoplastic syndromes, hypertrophic pulmonary osteoarthropathy may precede the diagnosis of the primary lung tumor by many months. Unlike the endocrinopathies, it is rare in small cell lung cancer.

Hypertrophic Pulmonary Osteoarthropathy

Hypertrophic pulmonary osteoarthropathy is a proliferating periostitis involving the distal ends of the long bones, particularly the tibia, fibula, and radius. Periostitis leads to tenderness and swelling and with progression may involve the metacarpals and metatarsals. There may also be an associated acute polyarthritis. Always associated with hypertrophic pulmonary osteoarthropathy (but not vice versa) is the presence of clubbing of the fingers and toes. Thus patients present with bone and joint pain (which at times can be incapacitating) and with clubbing of the digits. Alkaline phosphatase levels are often elevated, but serum hepatic enzyme levels are nor-

mal. Plain radiographs of the affected bones demonstrate periosteal inflammation and elevation, and radionuclide bone scans reveal an intense and symmetrical generalized uptake, particularly in the long bones. The symptoms often respond dramatically to aspirin and nonsteroidal anti-inflammatory agents. However, treatment is directed at the primary tumor, with complete symptomatic relief often being obtained immediately after resection of the primary tumor. In unresectable cases vagotomy proximal to the pulmonary hilum has occasionally been of some benefit.

Syndrome of Inappropriate Antidiurectic Hormone Secretion

As with Cushing's syndrome, elevated levels of antidiuretic hormone are common (up to 70 percent of patients with lung cancer), but patients are infrequently symptomatic. Symptoms are seen primarily with small cell cancer (Odell and Wolfsen, 1978), which because it secretes larger quantities of antidiuretic hormone, leads to hyponatremia, low serum osmolality, and a urine osmolality greater than 500 mOsm/kg. The symptoms include anorexia, nausea and vomiting, and progression of the hyponatremia, increasing neurologic dysfunction (confusion, lethargy, and seizures). The therapy is fluid restriction in mild cases and, with severe neurologic symptoms, hypertonic saline infusion. On a more chronic basis, demeclocycline may be effective.

Hypercalcemia

Although approximately 10 percent of patients with lung cancer develop hypercalcemia during the course of their disease, only 15 percent of cases are secondary to production of para-

---

Paraneoplastic Syndromes in Patients with Lung Cancer

Endocrine
    Hypercalcemia (ectopic parathyroid hormone)
    Cushing's syndrome
    Syndrome of inappropriate antidiuretic hormone
    Carcinoid syndrome
    Gynecomastia
    Hypercalcitonemia
    Elevated growth hormone
    Elevated prolactin, follicle-stimulating hormone, luteinizing hormone
    Hypoglycemia
    Hyperthyroidism

Neurologic
    Encephalopathy
    Subacute cerebellar degeneration
    Progressive multifocal leukoencephalopathy
    Peripheral neuropathy
    Polymyositis
    Autonomic neuropathy
    Eaton-Lambert syndrome
    Optic neuritis

Skeletal
    Clubbing
    Pulmonary hypertrophic osteoarthropathy

Hematologic
    Anemia
    Leukemoid reactions
    Thrombocytosis
    Thrombocytopenia
    Eosinophilia
    Pure red cell aplasia
    Leukoerythroblastosis
    Disseminated intravascular coagulation

Cutaneous
    Hyperkeratosis
    Dermatomyositis
    Acanthosis nigricans
    Hyperpigmentation
    Erythema gyratum repens
    Hypertrichosis lanuginosa acquista

Other
    Nephrotic syndrome
    Hypouricemia
    Secretion of vasoactive intestinal peptide with diarrhea
    Hyperamylasemia
    Anorexia or cachexia

---

thyroid hormone or other humoral substances, including prostaglandin E_2 (Cryer and Kissaine, 1979). Secretion of ectopic parathyroid hormone occurs most often with squamous cell carcinoma. Support for the diagnosis of ectopic parathyroid hormone secretion is provided by the presence of hypophosphatemia (secondary to the action of parathyroid hormone on renal tubules). Serum levels of parathyroid hormone can be measured to confirm the diagnosis. However, the clinician must also rule out concurrent metastatic bone disease by bone scan and/or skeletal survey. Because of its more chronic nature, the hypercalcemia of ectopic parathyroid hormone secretion causes primarily neurologic symptoms (lethargy and a depressed level of consciousness) and dehydration. Most importantly patients with ectopic parathyroid hormone secretion often have resectable tumors, and after complete resection, the calcium level normalizes. Unfortunately tumor recurrence is extremely frequent and may manifest as recurrent hypercalcemia.

Myopathic and Neurologic Syndromes

Neuromyopathies are the most common paraneoplastic syndromes of lung cancer. Up to 16 percent of patients with lung cancer have evidence of neuromuscular disability; of these 56 percent have small cell carcinoma, 22 percent have squamous cell carcinoma, 16 percent have large cell carcinoma, and 5 percent have adenocarcinoma (Morton, et al., 1966). Unlike the endocrinopathies they occur later in the course of the disease and tend to occur in patients who already have significant weight loss. A difficulty arises in differentiating neuromuscular weakness secondary to a neuromyopathy from the generalized disability secondary to metastatic disease. Thus, in patients with neurologic and/or muscular symptoms, it is important to rule out evidence of central nervous system (CNS) metastases with computed tomography (CT) or magnetic resonance imaging (MRI) of the head and other evidence of metastatic disease, which could lead to general disability.

Carcinomatous Myopathies

The carcinomatous myopathies are the most frequently seen paraneoplastic syndromes. Eaton-Lambert syndrome (most frequently seen in small cell lung cancer) is a myasthenia-like syndrome related to a defect in neuromuscular conduction, and it is associated with proximal muscle weakness and fatigability, particularly of the thighs. Eaton-Lambert syndrome can occur before the onset of any symptoms of the primary tumor, even before it is visible on a chest radiograph. The syndrome is produced by an immunoglobulin IG antibody that interferes with neuromuscular conduction at the motor end plate. Therapy is directed at the primary tumor, with either resection, radiation, and/or chemotherapy. Many patients have dramatic improvement postresection or with successful medical therapy. Patients with refractory symptoms may improve with the administration of guanidine hydrochloride. Neostigmine, used in myasthenia gravis, is usually ineffective.

Neuropathies

Neuropathies are primarily peripheral and are combined sensory-motor neuropathies. They can vary from mild sensory loss or weakness to complete sensory loss and/or paralysis. CNS abnormalities are unusual but can be severe. They include cortical cerebellar degeneration with ataxia, vertigo, nystagmus, and dysarthria. An encephalomyelopathy may occur with a wide range of CNS symptoms dominated by psychiatric manifestations.

Cushing's Syndrome

Cushing's syndrome occurs primarily with small cell carcinoma and is secondary to production of an adrenocorticotropic hormonelike substance, which is indistinguishable from the normal hormone. The adrenocorticotropic hormone production is autonomous and not supressible by dexamethasone. Although a high percentage of patients with small cell carcinoma have elevated adrenocorticotropic hormone levels by radioimmunoassay, less than 2 percent have symptoms of Cushing's syndrome (Richardson, et al., 1978). Because of the rapid onset of elevated hormone levels, the symptoms are primarily metabolic (severe hypokalemic alkalosis with progressive weakness or hyperglycemia) with few physical signs of Cushing's syndrome. The diagnosis is made by demonstrating elevated plasma cortisol levels, which lack the normal diurnal variation, elevated blood adrenocorticotropic hormone levels, or elevated urinary 17-hydroxycorticosteroids, all of which are not suppressible by administration of exogenous dexamethasone.

Metastatic Symptoms

Metastases occur most commonly in the CNS, spinal cord, bones, liver, adrenal glands, lungs, and skin and soft tissues.

Central Nervous System Metastases

CNS metastases are present in 10 percent of patients at diagnosis with another 10 to 15 percent developing CNS metastases over the course of their disease. The symptoms are primarily caused by increased intracranial pressure, leading to headache, nausea and vomiting, and changes in the level of consciousness. Focal neurologic signs, such as weakness, seizures, etc., are less common.

Bone Metastases

Bone metastases occur in up to one-fourth of all patients, with the spine, pelvic bones, and femur being the most common sites of involvement. The metastases are primarily osteolytic, producing localized pain; thus any localized skeletal complaints in a patient with lung cancer warrants evaluation with plain bone radiographs, bone scans, and/or CT scan.

Hepatic and Adrenal Metastases

Hepatic metastases are usually an incidental finding on routine CT scans or, when symptomatic, are part of a premorbid state. Adrenal metastases are also primarily asymptomatic findings on routine CT scans and rarely lead to adrenal hypofunction. Although biochemical tests of hepatic function are routinely obtained, because of its simplicity, upper abdominal CT scans should be performed as a routine part of all chest CT scans to detect asymptomatic hepatic and adrenal metastases.

Skin and Soft Tissue Metastases

Skin and soft tissue metastases occur in approximately 1 percent of patients and present as painless subcutaneous or intramuscular masses. Occasionally the tumor erodes through the overlying skin, with necrosis and creation of a chronic wound. They may require excision for both mental and physical palliation.

Nonspecific Symptoms

As in other types of tumors, lung cancer may produce a variety of nonspecific symptoms, such as anorexia, weight loss, fatigue, and malaise. The cause of these symptoms is unclear, but they obviously should trigger a concern for the presence of distant spread of the tumor with an appropriate metastatic evaluation.

STAGING SYSTEM

Staging is the measurement of the extent of the tumor in any given patient. Assigning patients to a particular clinical TNM subset and stage allows the most appropriate individual therapeutic decisions to be made, which are based on the reported results of various forms of therapy previously used in different stages of the disease. Staging also provides prognostic information and allows a comparison of data between studies. Also the impact of new therapeutic interventions can be evaluated for efficacy and a comparison of the expected survival curves can be made.

The staging process is a continuous one: First a clinical estimate of the stage of disease (cTNM) is determined based on the history, physical examination, and radiologic and invasive studies. Subsequently during surgery, the stage is either confirmed or revised based on the operative findings. After surgery a final pathologic stage is determined, based on the pathologic results (pTNM).

The new international staging system, which is based on the TNM system of classifying tumor and lymph node status was developed in 1986 (Mountain, 1986) and has since been adopted worldwide. To understand the nodal descriptors N1, N2, and N3 used in the new international staging system, it is necessary to be fully conversant with the lymph node mapping schema devised by Naruke, et al. (1978) and modified by the American Thoracic Society in 1983. In this system lymph nodes are placed into well-defined stations based on clearly defined anatomic boundaries (Figs. 27-24 and 27-25). Diagramatic representations of different stages are shown in Figures 27-26 through 27-29.

The new international staging system was applied (based on clinical estimates of the extent of disease) to a data base of more than 3,000 patients from the M. D. Anderson Hospital and the Lung Cancer Study Group (Mountain, 1986). From this a series of 5-year survival curves was obtained for each stage (Fig. 27-30), which verified the significant survival differences between each stage. This was confirmed by other investigators (Naruke, et al., 1988, 1978; Watanabe, et al., 1991; Martini, et al., 1983).

Despite the improvements of the new international staging system, it is important to realize that within each stage there may be marked differences in postoperative 5-year survival rates. For example, within stage I, T2N0M0 tumors have been shown by Mountain (1986); Naruke, et al. (1988); and Watanabe, et al. (1991) to have 5-year survival rates that are 10 percent or more below those for T1N0M0 tumors. Also within stage IIIa (potentially completely resectable), there are extreme differences in 5-year survival rates after complete resection, that is, T3N0 tumors have a 5-year survival rate

---

New International Staging System: TNM Classification

Primary tumor (T)

TX: Tumor proved by the presence of malignant cells in bronchopulmonary secretions but not visualized radiographically or bronchoscopically, or any tumor that cannot be assessed as in a retreatment staging

T0: No evidence of primary tumor

Tis: Carcinoma in situ

T1: A tumor that is 3.0 cm or less in greatest dimension, surrounded by lung or visceral pleura, and without evidence of invasion proximal to a lobar bronchus at bronchoscopy[a]

T2: A tumor more than 3.0 cm in greatest diameter or a tumor of any size that either invades the visceral pleura or has associated atelectasis or obstructive pneumonitis extending to the hilar region. At bronchoscopy the proximal extent of demonstrable tumor must be within a lobar bronchus or at least 2.0 cm distal to the carina. Any associated atelectasis or obstructive pneumonitis must involve less than an entire lung

T3: A tumor of any size with direct extension into the chest wall (including superior sulcus tumors), diaphragm, or the mediastinal pleura or pericardium without involving the heart, great vessels, trachea, esophagus, or vertebral body, or a tumor in the main bronchus within 2.0 cm of the carina without involving the carina

T4: A tumor of any size with invasion of the mediastinum or involving the heart, great vessels, trachea, esophagus, vertebral body, or carcina or the presence of malignant pleural effusion[b]

Nodal involvement (N)

N0: No demonstrable metastasis to regional lymph nodes

N1: Metastasis to lymph nodes in the peribronchial or the ipsilateral hilar region, or both, including direct extension

(Continues)

N2: Metastasis to ipsilateral mediastinal lymph nodes and subcarinal lymph nodes

N3: Metastasis to contralateral mediastinal lymph nodes, contralateral hilar lymph nodes, and ipsilateral or contralateral scalene or supraclavicular lymph nodes

Distant metastasis (M)

M0: No (known) distant metastasis

M1: Distant metastasis present; specific site(s).

---

[a] An uncommon superficial tumor of any size with its invasive component limited to the bronchial wall, which may extend proximal to the major bronchus, is classified at T1.

[b] Most pleural effusions associated with lung cancer are caused by tumor. There are, however, some patients in whom cytopathologic examination of pleural fluid (on more than on specimen) is negative for tumor, and the fluid is nonbloody and not an exudate. In such instances in which these elements and clinical judgment dictate that the effusion is not related to the tumor, the patient should be staged as T1, T2, or T3, excluding effusion as a staging element.

---

of 40 to 50 percent, whereas T1 to T3 tumors with N2 nodal involvement have a 5-year survival rate of 5 to 25 percent. The variable survival rate after resection within the group with N2 nodal involvement (5 to 25 percent) demonstrates that, even within what appears to be a uniform stage of disease, there can be significant variation in postoperative survival. In the case of N2 disease, the number and location of nodal stations involved and whether the metastatic tumor within the node has grossly replaced the node and/or is growing into surrounding tissues all probably have an impact on the postoperative prognosis. Future advances in molecular biology will likely allow certain biologic markers or cellular functions to be a component of staging, and these (as with the presence or absence of nodal involvement) may allow clinicians to identify patients at high risk for disease recurrence. They will likely play an important role in guiding pre- and postoperative therapy.

DIAGNOSIS AND STAGING

The diagnosis and clinical staging of lung cancer are two processes that occur simultaneously, beginning with the history and physical examination. Based only on this, an accurate initial clinical estimate of the extent of disease can often be made. Directed radiologic and invasive studies can be performed to obtain a tissue diagnosis and to determine further the clinical stage of the disease (Fig. 27-31). Many of these studies (e.g., chest radiography, CT scan, bronchoscopy, and mediastinoscopy) serve both purposes.

History and Physical Examination

The history and physical examination are the most important initial steps in the evaluation of a patient with lung cancer. Several features of the history deserve special emphasis. A history of tobacco smoking defines an increased risk of developing lung cancer, based on the number of years of

New International Staging System: Stage Grouping

TX N0 M0: An occult carcinoma with bronchopulmonary secretions containing malignant cells but without other evidence of the primary tumor or evidence of metastasis to the regional lymph nodes or distant metastasis

Stage 0

Tis N0 M0: Carcinoma in situ

Stage I

T1 N0 M0, T2 N0 M0: A tumor that can be classified T1 or T2 without any metastasis to nodes or distant metastasis

Stage II

T1 N1 M0, T1 N1 M0: Any tumor classified as T1 or T2 with metastasis to the lymph nodes in the peribronchial or ipsilateral hilar region only

Stage IIIA

T3 N0 M0, T3 N1 M0, T1 N2 M0, T2 N2 M0, T3 N2 M0: A tumor that can be classified as T3 without nodal metastasis or with metastasis limited to the peribronchial, ipsilateral hilar, and ipsilateral mediastinal lymph nodes; T1 and T2 tumors that have metastasized to the level of the ipsilateral mediastinal lymph nodes only are also included

Stage IIIB

Any T, N3 M0; T4 and N, M0: Any tumor more extensive than T3, any tumor with supraclavicular or contralateral mediastinal lymph node involvement, or any tumor with a malignant pleural effusion but without evidence of distant metastasis

Stage IV

Any T, and N, M1: Any tumor with distant metastatic spread

Proposed Definitions of Regional Nodal Stations for Prethoracotomy Staging

X: Supraclavicular nodes.

2R: Right upper paratracheal (suprainnominate) nodes: nodes to the right of the midline of the trachea between the intersection of the cudal margin of the innominate artery with the trachea, and the apex of the lung. (Includes highest R mediastinal node.) (Radiologists may use the same caudal margin as in 2L.)

2L: Left upper paratracheal (supra-aortic) nodes: nodes to the left of the midline of the trachea between the top of the aortic arch and the apex of the lung. (Includes highest L mediastinal node.)

(Continues)

4R: Right lower paratracheal nodes: nodes to the right of the midline of the trachea between the cephalic border of the azygos vein and the intersection of the caudal margin of the brachiocephalic artery with the right side of the trachea. (Includes some pretracheal and paracaval nodes.) (Radiologists may use the same cephalic margin as in 4L.)

4L: Left lower paratracheal nodes: nodes to the left of the midline of the trachea between the top of the aortic arch and the level of the carina, medial to the ligamentum arteriosum. (Includes some pretracheal nodes.)

5: Aortopulmonary nodes: subaortic and para-aortic nodes, lateral to the ligamentum arteriosum or the aorta or left pulmonary artery, proximal to the first branch of the left pulmonary artery.

6: Anterior mediastinal nodes: nodes anterior to the ascending aorta or the innominate artery. (Includes some pretracheal and preaortic nodes.)

7: Subcarinal nodes: nodes rising caudal to the carina of the trachea but not associated with the lower lobe bronchi or arteries within the lung.

8: Paraesophageal nodes: nodes dorsal to the posterior wall of the trachea and to the right or left of the midline of the esophagus. (Includes retrotracheal, but not subcarinal nodes.)

9: Right or left pulmonary ligament nodes: nodes within the right or left pulmonary ligament.

10R: Right tracheobronchial nodes: nodes to the right of the midline of the trachea from the level of the cephalic border of the azygos vein to the origin of the right upper lobe bronchus.

10L: Left peribronchial nodes: nodes to the left of the midline of the trachea between the carina and the left upper lobe bronchus, medial to the ligamentum arteriosum.

11: Intrapulmonary nodes: nodes removed in the right or left lung specimen plus those distal to the mainstem bronchi or secondary carina. (Includes interlobar, lobar, and segmental nodes.)[a]

---

[a] Post-thoracotomy staging: nodes could be divided into stations 11, 12, 13 according to the AJCC classification. (From American Thoracic Society: Clinical staging of primary lung cancer. Am Rev Respir Dis 127:659, 1983, with permission.)

---

smoking. Recent evidence also implicates secondary exposure to tobacco smoke, particularly in children raised with tobacco-smoking relatives, as a risk for the development of lung cancer. Asbestos exposure is also a risk factor for the development of lung cancer; the risk increases with the length and intensity of the exposure. A history of both asbestos exposure and tobacco smoking actually has a multiplicative rather than an additive effect on the risk of developing lung

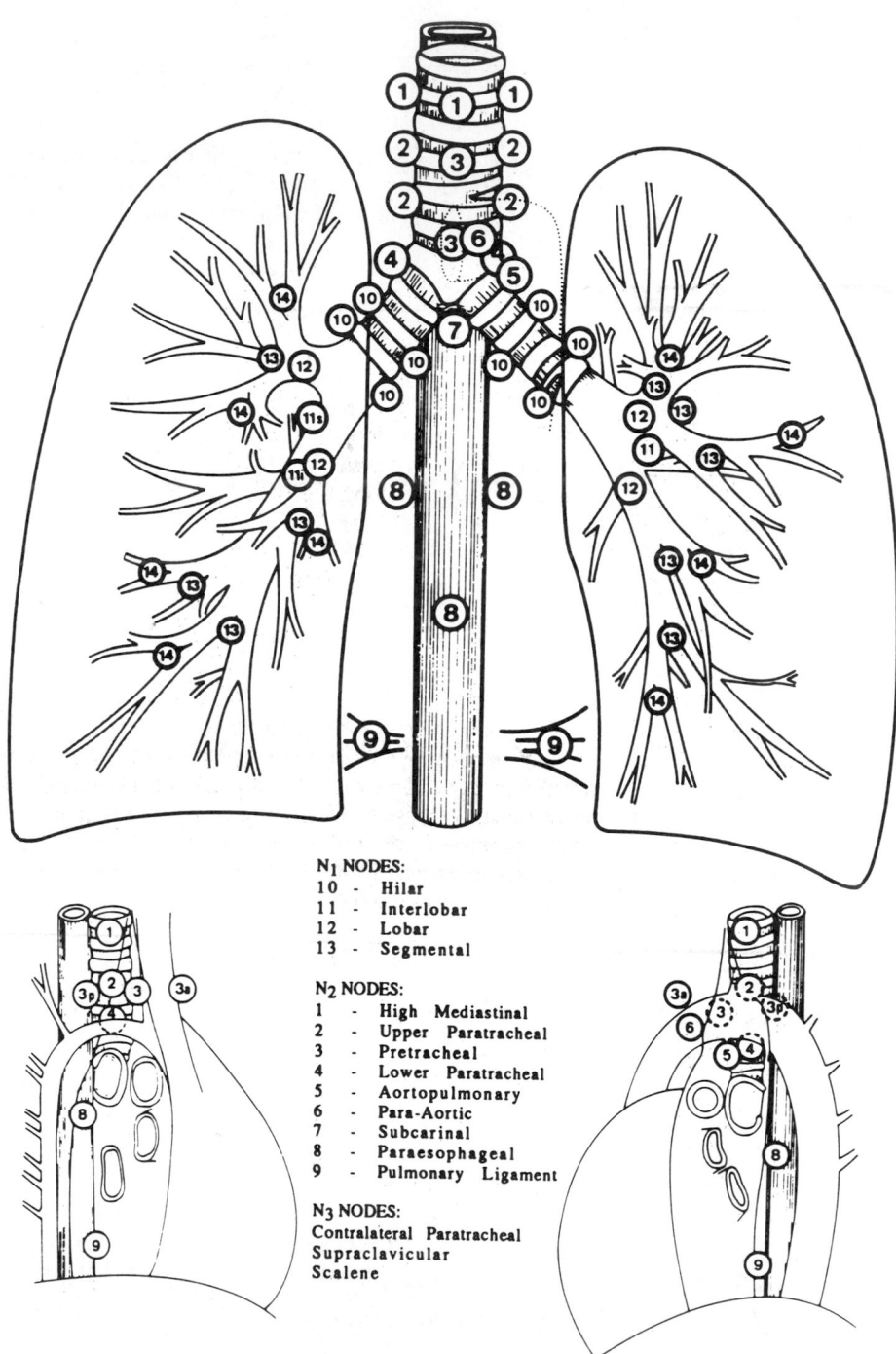

N₁ NODES:
10 - Hilar
11 - Interlobar
12 - Lobar
13 - Segmental

N₂ NODES:
1 - High Mediastinal
2 - Upper Paratracheal
3 - Pretracheal
4 - Lower Paratracheal
5 - Aortopulmonary
6 - Para-Aortic
7 - Subcarinal
8 - Paraesophageal
9 - Pulmonary Ligament

N₃ NODES:
Contralateral Paratracheal
Supraclavicular
Scalene

Figure 27-25. Sites of pulmonary lymph node drainage with numeric designations for each site. (From Naruke T, Suemasu K, Ishikawa S: Lymph node mapping and curability at various levels of metastasis in resected lung cancer. J Thorac Cardiovasc Surg 76:832, 1978, with permission.)

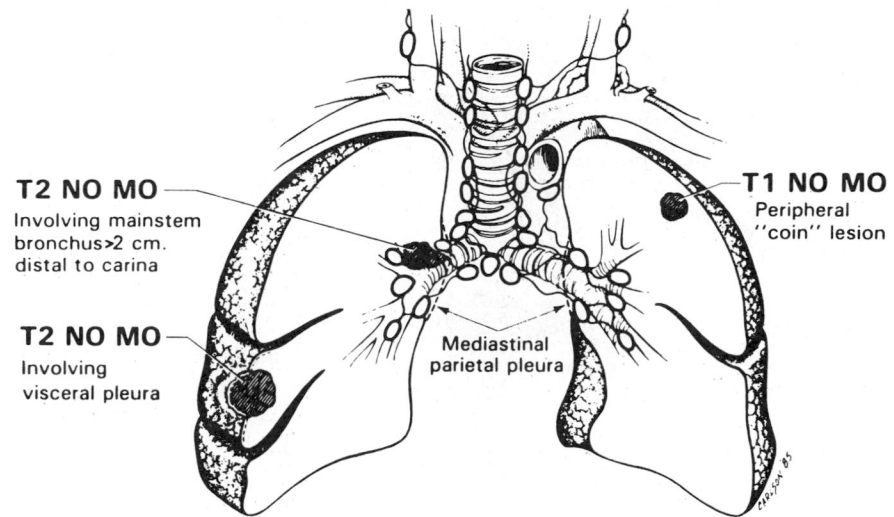

Figure 27-26. Stage I disease: no lymph node involvement. (From Mountain CF: A new international staging system for lung cancer. Chest 89(suppl):225S, 1986, with permission.)

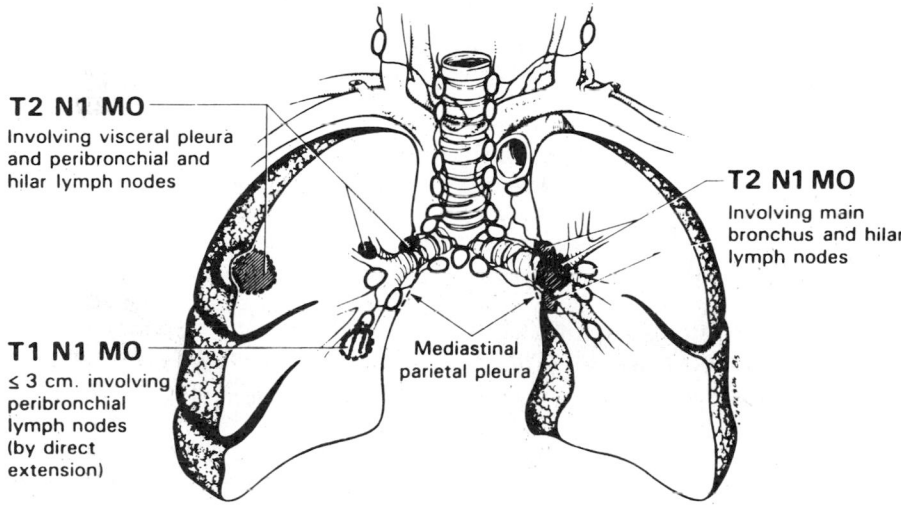

Figure 27-27. Stage II disease: intrapulmonary and/or hilar nodes involved. (From Mountain CF: A new international staging system for lung cancer. Chest 89(suppl):225S, 1986, with permission.)

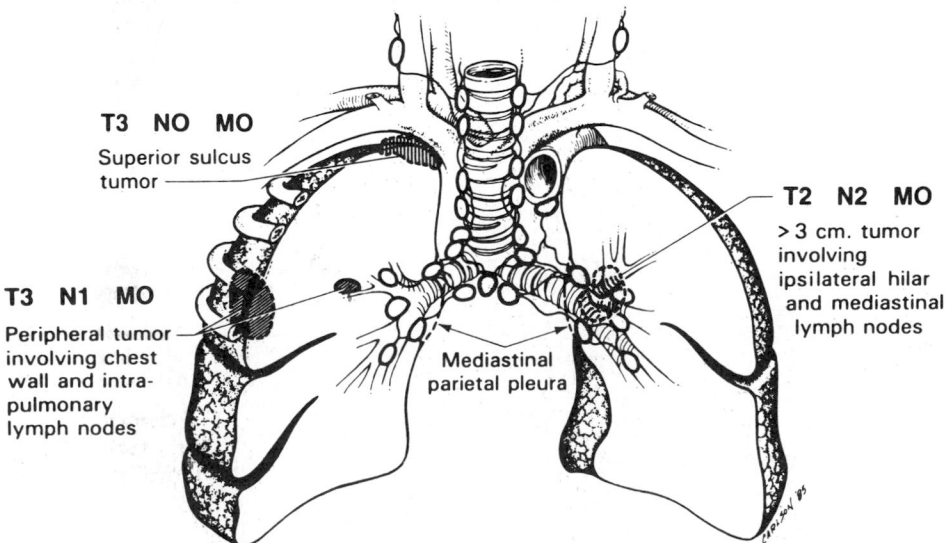

Figure 27-28. Stage IIIa disease. (From Mountain CF: A new international staging system for lung cancer. Chest 89(suppl):225S, 1986, with permission.)

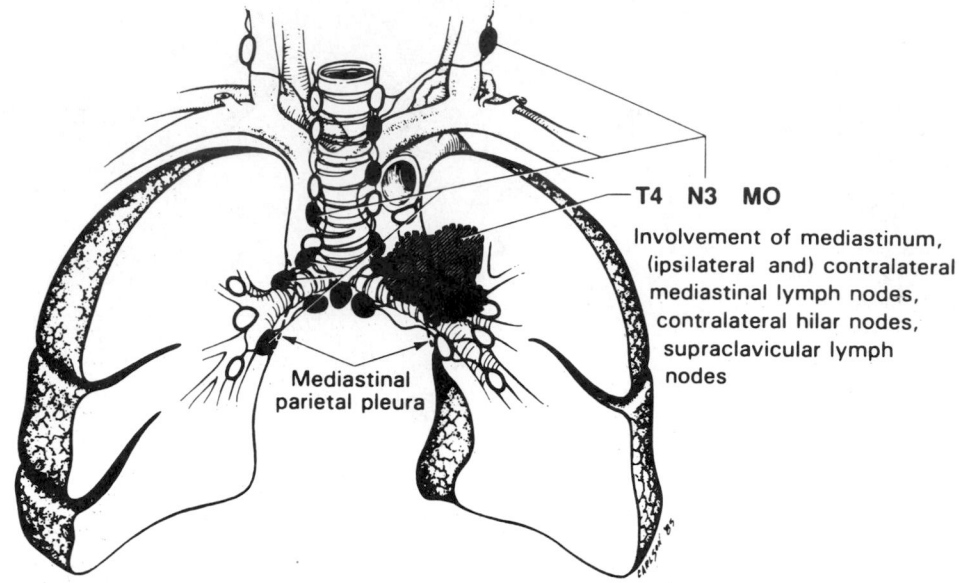

T4 N3 MO

Involvement of mediastinum,
(ipsilateral and) contralateral
mediastinal lymph nodes,
contralateral hilar nodes,
supraclavicular lymph
nodes

Mediastinal
parietal pleura

Figure 27-29. Stage IIIb disease. (From Mountain CF: A new international staging system for lung cancer. Chest 89(suppl):225S, 1986, with permission.)

cancer. Other industrial exposures (gold, nickel, and uranium mining) have a similar cocarcinogenic effect. Weight loss of greater than 5 percent of body weight is significant and should alert the clinician to the possible presence of locally advanced disease or metastatic spread, as do specific symptoms suggestive of metastases.

The physical examination first assesses the overall status of the patient. Is the patient vigorous or debilitated? Is there evidence of weight loss with muscle wasting? Further examination focuses on the oropharynx, for evidence of other tumors associated with tobacco use; the neck and supraclavicular areas, for evidence of lymph node metastases; the lungs, to detect areas of consolidation, pleural effusion, or localized chest wall discomfort; and the digits, for evidence of clubbing.

Sputum Cytology

Microscopic examination of the sputum for tumor cells is a simple and effective diagnostic technique. However, with the availability of bronchoscopy and percutaneous needle biopsy, sputum cytologic examination is infrequently used and in fact even forgotten. The diagnostic yield depends on several factors as follows: sputum production, tumor location, tumor size, tumor histologic type, and the ability and experience of the cytopathologist. The optimal method of sputum collection is to pool early morning sputum samples from 3 consecutive days and preserve them in Saccamano's solution or other similar preservatives.

In a consecutive series of 449 cases of lung cancer, Ng and Horack (1983) demonstrated the overall diagnostic sensitivity of the sputum examination to be 82.8 percent (85 percent for small cell, squamous, and large cell carcinoma and 75 percent for adenocarcinoma, bronchoalveolar carcinoma, and adenosquamous carcinoma). In addition, there was a correlation between the number of specimens collected and the diagnostic yield, that is, 83 percent for three and 90 percent for five or more specimens. Both Pilloti, et al. (1982) and Liang (1989) confirmed that the number of specimens necessary for optimal diagnositc sensitivity is three; increasing the number to five or more does not significantly improve the diagnostic yield.

Other factors influencing diagnostic sensitivity are tumor location, size, and histologic type. Because of their proximal

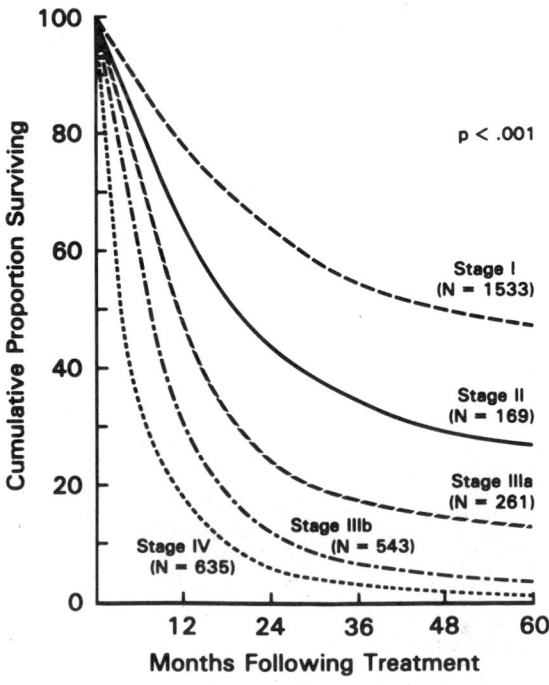

Figure 27-30. Cumulative proportion of patients surviving 5 years by clinical stage of disease (From Mountain CF: A new international staging system for lung cancer. Chest 89(suppl):225S, 1986, with permission.)

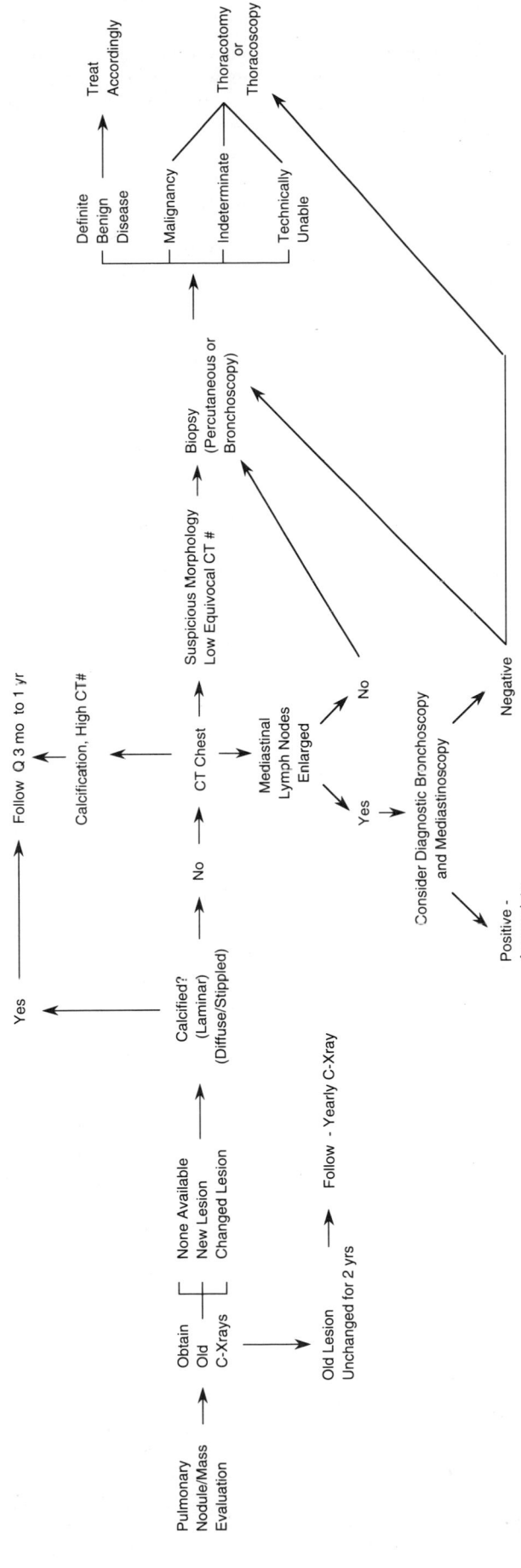

Figure 27-31. Algorithm for evaluation of a pulmonary nodule or mass.

bronchial location and endobronchial site, central tumors have a higher probability of shedding tumor cells into the sputa that will be expectorated. Kato, et al. (1983) demonstrated a diagnostic yield of 77 percent for central tumors versus 47 percent for peripheral tumors. They also found that large tumors and those associated with collapse or consolidation and a lower lobe location had higher diagnostic yields. The poorest diagnostic yield occurs with small peripheral tumors, as low as 20 percent for those less than 3.0 cm. Histologic findings influence the diagnostic yield less. In general squamous cell tumors are more frequently diagnosed than are adenocarcinomas or large cell carcinomas, most likely because of their central location.

Potentially premalignant dysplastic cells can also be detected in the sputum. Risse, et al. (1988), on follow-up of 46 patients with dysplastic sputum cytologic findings but no other evidence of lung cancer, found that 21 (46 percent) developed lung cancer. Patients with dysplastic changes should undergo bronchoscopy, with brushing and biopsy of any abnormalities in addition to segmental bronchial washings. Tockman, et al. (1988) appear to have improved the sensitivity of detection of malignancy in dysplastic cells by staining with monoclonal antibody (not yet commercially available) to neoplastic antigens. Using this technique tumor antigens were detected up to 2 years prior to the development of lung cancer. If proved to be accurate, such techniques may allow early resection if the site of such changes can be localized.

Finally false-positive sputum cytologic findings occur in 1 to 3 percent of examinations. The primary causes (Truong, et al., 1985) are viral infections (which can produce cellular changes difficult to distinguish from malignancy, particularly adenocarcinoma) or any acute inflammatory process (e.g., asthma, tuberculosis, or bronchitis). Thus clinical correlation is always necessary.

Chest Radiograph

High-quality posteroanterior and lateral chest radiographs are the single most important examinations in the diagnosis of lung cancer. These localize the site of peripheral or central pulmonary lesions and detect evidence of hilar and mediastinal enlargement (suggestive of lymphatic spread), pleural effusions, and areas of atelectasis or consolidation. A completely normal chest radiograph essentially rules out the presence of lung cancer, except in the rare instance of an occult tumor.

The presence of a pleural effusion on chest radiography (or CT scan) is not synonymous with the presence of a malignant pleural effusion. A malignant pleural effusion can only be diagnosed by finding malignant cells in a sample of pleural fluid examined microscopically. A pleural effusion associated with a peripherally based tumor, particularly one that abuts the visceral or parietal pleural surface, does have a higher probability of being malignant. Pleural effusions are often secondary to the atelectasis or consolidation seen with central tumors. Thus no pleural effusion can be assumed to be malignant until proved to be so by cytologic examination.

The spread of the tumor to hilar or mediastinal lymph nodes is in general unreliably detected by plain chest radiograph. Despite the presence of mediastinal lymph node enlargement,

mediastinoscopy or other methods of lymph biopsy is still necessary to prove the presence of metastatic spread.

Elevation of a hemidiphragm can be the result of volume loss (from atelectasis) or paralysis of the hemidiaphragm secondary to involvement of the phrenic nerve by the primary tumor, particularly those abutting the mediastinum. With paralysis a paradoxical motion of the diaphragm is seen thoracoscopically with sniffing. Finally evidence of rib destruction (caused either by direct invasion by a peripheral tumor contiguous with the chest wall or by metastasis) or vertebral body involvement by metastasis may be seen.

Computed Tomography

CT scanning of the chest and upper abdomen is now virtually a routine part of the evaluation of any patient either suspected of having or documented to have lung cancer, especially in developed countries.

CT provides information about the primary lesion, including the size and presence of signs of benignity (calcification, density, etc.), the relationship to surrounding structures, and invasion of contiguous structures. However, it must be strongly emphasized that, without unequivocal evidence of invasion of a contiguous structure (e.g., rib or vertebral body destruction), no conclusion can be made. In general thoracotomy should not be denied based on presumptive evidence of invasion of chest wall, vertebral body, or mediastinal structures; proof of invasion may require thoracotomy.

CT also provides detailed information about the remaining lung parenchyma and pleural space. Other pulmonary nodules (unseen by chest radiography), bullae, pleural thickening or masses, and unsuspected pleural effusions may be identified. When chest CT includes the upper abdomen, unsuspected metastases may be found in the liver or adrenal gland, which, as shown by Pagani (1984), occur in the liver in 3 to 6 percent (with normal hepatic function) and the adrenal glands in 3 to 7 percent of patients. Therefore we think that scanning of the upper abdomen should be a routine part of every chest CT.

Finally the greatest value of CT in evaluating lung cancer is in assessment of the mediastinal lymph nodes for the possible presence of metastatic tumor. At present CT is the most effective noninvasive method available to assess the mediastinal lymph nodes for enlargement (McCloud, et al., 1992).

Because a positive CT result (nodal diameter more than 1.0 cm) predicts actual metastatic involvement in only about 70 percent of cases, patients should not be denied attempted curative resection based only on a positive CT scan. The histologic evaluation must always be performed if the finding of metastatic nodal involvement would determine inoperability.

A negative CT result (lymph nodes less than 1.0 cm) in general is much more accurate. With a negative CT result and a T1 or T2 lesion, in general there will be a false-negative rate of less than 10 percent, and mediastinoscopy is omitted by many surgeons. However, as demonstrated by Daly, et al. (1987) the false-negative rate increases to 28 percent with central T3 tumors; in this situation mediastinoscopy is recommended. In addition, Vallieres and Waters (1987) demonstrated that T1 adenocarcinomas or large cell carcinomas have a higher rate of early micrometastatic spread; therefore we think that all such patients should undergo mediastinoscopy.

Radionuclide Scanning of Mediastinum

The ability of radionuclide scans to diagnose and stage lung cancer is limited by its lack of specificity. Routine nuclide scanning with gallium citrate or cobalt-bleomycin has been used mainly for detecting unsuspected mediastinal spread after the diagnosis has been made. However, the rate of incorporation of the radioisotope by the primary tumor and its metastatic foci is variable and thus has limited its clinical use in either diagnosis or staging (Kies, et al., 1978; Little, et al., 1986). More recently isotope-labeled monoclonal antibodies have been investigated as a technique for staging and diagnosing this disease. Specific monoclonal antibodies that are directed at lung cancer cells in the future may be valuable as diagnostic and staging modalities.

Magnetic Resonance Imaging

MRI of pulmonary lesions and mediastinal nodes has been disappointing and in general has offered no improvement over CT. There are, however, specific situations in which it is of value. Neurogenic paravertebral tumors and lung cancers suspected of invading either the vertebral body or spinal canal are best assessed with magnetic resonance imaging because it provides superior detail of the spinal canal and detects changes in the bone marrow suggestive of involvement by carcinoma with greater accuracy than does CT. Heelan, et al. (1985) found MRI to be more accurate than CT in assessing possible invasion of mediastinal structures, but as demonstrated by Stiglbauer, et al. (1991), this enhanced ability may also overdiagnose mediastinal invasion with a high incidence of false-positive results. Because of its superb imaging of vascular structures, MRI may be useful to define a tumor's relationship to a major vessel. Finally it is particularly useful when contrast material is contraindicated. Thus routine use of MRI in lung cancer is unnecessary and should be reserved for patients with contrast allergies or with suspicion of mediastinal, vascular, or vertebral body invasion.

Transthoracic Needle Aspiration

Fine-needle aspiration biopsy of pulmonary nodules is an excellent method of obtaining cytologic and/or histologic material for a positive identification of malignancy. This is performed by using fluoroscopic or CT-guided techniques. The positive yield in experienced hands can be as high as 95 percent. The accuracy of cytologic examination in identifying histologic subtypes, however, is only 75 percent. However, an indeterminate biopsy result cannot be accepted as negative. False-negative examinations are frequent and must be considered indeterminate unless a positive benign diagnosis (e.g., hamartoma or tuberculosis) can be made (Wescott, 1980). An algorithm for investigating a solitary pulmonary nodule is presented in Figure 27-31.

Bronchoscopy

Visualization of the tracheobronchial tree with the rigid or flexible bronchoscope is, in addition to chest radiography and CT, a standard part of the evaluation of patients suspected or known to have lung cancer. Flexible fiberoptic bronchoscopy

with video-imaging capabilities has replaced rigid bronchoscopy, except in select circumstances. Flexible bronchoscopy allows visualization of the proximal tracheobronchial tree up to the second, and occasionally the third, subsegmental bronchus. In general bronchoscopy serves three invaluable purposes as follows: (1) diagnostic, (2) staging, and (3) assessment of the remaining bronchial tree.

The diagnosis of lung cancer by bronchoscopy can be pursued by one of five techniques: direct biopsy; transbronchial needle aspiration; brushing; saline lavage (for cytologic testing); and fluoroscopically guided transbronchial biopsy, brushing, or transbronchial needle aspiration. Using more than one technique often improves the diagnostic yield; in particular after performing any biopsies, routine brushing and washing of the area should be done to retrieve cells ''liberated'' by the biopsy. In addition, following any diagnostic bronchoscopic procedure, the yield of sputum cytologic testing appears to increase, making this technique of value as an added diagnostic tool.

In general three findings may be encountered at bronchoscopy. In 25 to 50 percent of patients, usually with small cell and squamous tumors because of their central location, an obvious endobronchial tumor or a suspicious lesion is seen. If three or four biopsies are always obtained followed by brushings and washings, the diagnostic yield for endobronchial tumors should be greater than 90 percent.

Bronchial distortion (usually thickening or blunting of a minor carina or evidence of extrinsic compression) secondary to the tumor or enlarged lymph nodes extrinsic to the airway may be all that is evident. Transbronchial needle aspiration (Wang and Terri, 1983; Harrow et al., 1989) can be useful in this circumstance.

Seen most often with peripheral lesions is a normal bronchoscopic examination. In this situation transbronchial biopsy, brushing, and/or needle aspiration with the aid of fluoroscopic localization is often useful, particularly for lesions more than 2.0 cm in diameter. The value of transbronchial needle aspiration in the diagnosis of peripheral lung cancers was confirmed by Schenk, et al. (1987) who found that it increased the diagnostic yield to 71 percent from 64 percent with biopsy, brushing, and washing, further emphasizing the point that in general a combination of techniques should be used to ensure the best chance of making a diagnosis.

Bronchoscopy is also an important staging tool and can potentially provide information in two areas. The first is general information about tumor location, the length of the normal bronchus proximal to the tumor, the tumor's relationship to the tracheal carina (T3 versus T2 or T1), whether there is evidence of extrinsic compression of proximal airways (by extrinsic tumor or enlarged lymph nodes), and finally as noted by Shure and Fedullo (1985), about the presence or absence of submucosal or peribronchial spread. They found that concentric bronchial narrowing, bronchial indentation, and either absent mucosal markings or a hypervascular-appearing mucosa on bronchoscopy were findings suggestive of such spread.

Second, bronchoscopy can detect lymphatic metastases by transbronchial needle aspiration of mediastinal lymph nodes (usually subcarinal). Shure and Fedullo (1984) evaluated transbronchial needle aspiration of the subcarinal lymph nodes in 134 patients with suspected lung cancer. In 110 patients subsequently proved to have lung cancer, the diagnosis was made by subcarinal node aspiration in 16, demonstrating that this is another potential way of making a primary diagnosis. They also found a positive subcarinal lymph node aspirate to be the only evidence of unresectability in 11 of the 16 patients. Care must be taken before excluding patients from surgery, however, because as noted by Cropp, et al. (1984), false-positive results can occur from incorporation of tumor cells into the needle from the epithelial surface. In addition, differentiation between resectable N2 versus unresectable N2 or N3 disease cannot be determined by needle aspiration alone. A more invasive approach (mediastinoscopy or thoracoscopy), which can determine the number of nodal stations involved and the presence or absence of extracapsular extension, may be required.

Cervical Mediastinoscopy

Cervical mediastinoscopy is the most accurate way (short of thoracotomy) to stage superior mediastinal lymph nodes. A thoroughly performed cervical exploration has several advantages over CT, that is, (1) a histologic diagnosis may be made, (2) it accurately determines the presence or absence of N2 disease with a precise anatomic mapping by nodal station, (3) the identification of extranodal extension of the tumor and whether such extension involves contiguous structures (trachea or aorta) can be made, and (4) it can identify N3 disease. Because the presence of mediastinal lymphadenopathy may affect treatment decisions, accurate assessment is important.

The indications for mediastinoscopy are debated. In general lymph nodes larger than 1.0 cm on CT should undergo biopsy through a mediastinoscopy because the accuracy of CT for predicting metastatic involvement in enlarged nodes is only 70 percent. Conversely a negative CT result (lymph nodes less than 1.0 cm) is, in many centers, sufficient to prove operability. Mediastinoscopy is omitted, and pulmonary resection with mediastinal lymph node dissection are performed, yielding a high rate of complete resection. Because of the poor prognosis (even with complete resection) conferred by the presence of either high paratracheal (station 2) node involvement, multiple sites of N2 disease, or N3 disease, others believe that mediastinoscopy is routinely indicated to avoid unnecessary thoracotomy.

The results of routine application of mediastinoscopy as a staging procedure were examined by Luke, et al. (1986) in a prospective analysis of 1,000 consecutive mediastinoscopies. Positive lymph nodes were found in 296 (29.6 percent) and negative lymph nodes in 704 (70.4 percent) examinations, rates consistent with other large series of mediastinoscopy. Of 590 patients with a negative mediastinoscopy result who underwent thoracotomy, 93 percent were resected (85 percent curative and 7 percent palliative). Unsuspected N2 disease was found in 52 patients, for a false-negative rate of 8.9 percent. However, most of these were at sites inaccessible by mediastinoscopy, posterior subcarinal, periesophageal, and anterior mediastinal, regions that allow complete resectability.

What then are the current indications for mediastinoscopy in the staging of lung cancer? This depends on the training,

experience, and philosophy of the thoracic surgeon. Most agree that the absolute indications for mediastinoscopy are (1) lymph node enlargement more than 1.0 cm on CT and (2) all patients being evaluated for entry into neoadjuvant therapy protocols. Relative indications include patients with a negative CT result and (1) T2 or T3 primaries or (2) T1 adenocarcinoma or large cell carcinoma (Vallieres and Waters, 1987).

The issue of the routine application of mediastinoscopy to patients with negative CT scans is the one most dependent on philosophy. Proponents of routine mediastinoscopy cite the low complication rate, the 10 to 15 percent false-negative rate of CT, the ability to select patients with N2 disease most likely to benefit from resection without neoadjuvant therapy (single station, ipsilateral, lower paratracheal, and no extracapsular extension), and the higher rate of thoracotomies that lead to curative resection. Proponents of a selective application of mediastinoscopy cite the high rate of negative mediastinoscopy examinations (70 percent) and the ability to resect patients with unsuspected N2 disease completely (assuming routine performance of a mediastinal lymph node dissection). Although both approaches have merit and are supported by available data, our practice, for the reasons outlined earlier, with rare exceptions, is to perform routine mediastinoscopy during the same general anesthetic as the thoracotomy.

Left Anterior Mediastinotomy or Extended Mediastinoscopy

These techniques, when applied to lung cancer staging, are used to evaluate lymph node stations 5 and 6 in patients with left hilar or left upper lobe tumors. In general if enlargement of station 5 or 6 lymph nodes is detected on CT, cervical mediastinoscopy should precede mediastinotomy (or extended mediastinoscopy), even in the absence of paratracheal lymph node enlargement. If negative results are found, left anterior mediastinotomy or extended cervical mediastinoscopy (Ginsberg, 1987) may be done. The indications for prethoracotomy assessment of station 5 and 6 are (1) potential entry into an adjuvant therapy protocol for N2 disease preoperatively; (2) a CT suggestion of bulky nodal metastases or extracapsular spread, which may preclude complete resection; and (3) to make a tissue diagnosis in the occasional patient with recurrent laryngeal nerve paralysis caused by extracapsular nodal extension with contiguous involvement of the nerve. Alternatively if cervical mediastinoscopy gives negative results, the surgeon may proceed directly to thoracotomy with the intent of resection of the primary and all enlarged lymph nodes in stations 5 and 6; even if nodal metastases are present, a reasonable 5-year survival rate is possible (Patterson, et al., 1987).

Scalene Node Biopsy

Routine scalene node biopsy of nonpalpable lymph nodes, previously the only available nodal staging procedure, is no longer used. However, palpable cervical lymph nodes should be assessed, preferably by needle aspiration biopsy. Scalene node biopsy is valuable to rule out N3 disease in patients with proved N2 disease, and this can be performed at the time of mediastinoscopy of this latter examination give positive findings. In our experience (Ginsberg, unpublished data), approximately 5 to 10 percent of patients have unsuspected N3 disease and are discovered using this approach.

Thoracoscopy

More recently video-assisted thoracoscopy has been used in the diagnosis and staging of lung cancer. Peripheral nodules can be identified and undergo biopsy or be excised using video-assisted, minimally invasive techniques. Mediastinal lymph nodes (most notably stations 5 and 6) can be sampled for histologic examination (Lewis, et al., 1992; Mack, et al., 1992; Miller, et al., 1992). In addition, this technique identifies suspected pleural disease, and the status of pleural effusions can be accurately assessed. The exact indications and use of this developing minimally invasive technique awaits prospective studies and remains an investigative tool at present. This approach, however, does not exclude the need for superior mediastinal node assessment (mediastinoscopy).

Thoracotomy

Diagnostic thoracotomies are still occasionally necessary in the diagnosis and staging of lung cancer. However, with less invasive procedures, more than 95 percent of tumors can be accurately diagnosed and staged without thoracotomy. Despite this there is a small minority of patients in whom there is a high suspicion of cancer without a diagnosis prior to thoracotomy. At the time of thoracotomy, a diagnosis can be made by fine-needle aspiration, Tru-Cut biopsy, or (preferably) an excisional biopsy with frozen-section analysis. All these techniques can provide tissue, which can be rapidly assessed by pathologists. As noted earlier, a determination that a tumor is either T3 or T4 often cannot be made until the thoracotomy. If a diagnosis of lung cancer is made at the time of thoracotomy, further staging by mediastinal lymph node sampling or complete lymph node dissection is mandatory.

Evaluation for Metastatic Disease

In patients considered to be potential operative candidates, the surgeon must determine preoperatively whether metastatic disease is present, which would confer inoperability (Fig. 27-32). This assessment is critical to avoid major surgical intervention when there is no hope for a curative resection. By far the most useful assessment of M status is a complete history and physical examination. Significant weight loss or general debility is usually a sign of metastatic disease. Similarly focal symptoms of metastatic involvement, such as headache or localized bone pain, require investigation. Biochemical estimates of hepatic function (serum glutamic oxaloacetic transaminase or alkaline phosphatase levels) and calcium (to detect bone metastases) regardless of symptoms are routinely obtained in all patients with lung cancer.

Whether the indication is symptoms or elevated biochemical levels, the noninvasive techniques most valuable to detect metastases include abdominal CT (liver and adrenal), liver ultrasound, brain CT or MRI, and ^{99}Tc radionuclide bone scan.

Routine organ scanning (bone, brain, and abdomen) is not required in every potentially operable patient whose disease is well established. Ramsdell, et al., (1977) Grant, et al., (1988) Sider and Horejs (1988), and other have shown that, in patients who are operative candidates with early-stage disease (I or II), the positive yield of routine organ scanning is small and is frequently confounded by many false-positive results (particularly with bone scans). Some advocate routine brain CT or MRI in patients with adenocarcinoma because of their well-documented higher incidence of failure in this site. The value of this, however, is unproved.

In patients with potentially operable but locally advanced (clinical stage IIIa) disease, routine organ scanning yields many more true-positive results in otherwise asymptomatic patients. Quinn, et al. (1986) reviewed 53 patients who were evaluated with liver scanning (followed by ultrasound or CT when positive), bone scanning, and brain CT. Clinical evidence of metastases was present in 30 patients; of these 9 had positive scans (7 bone and 2 brain). In 20 asymptomatic patients, only 3 had positive scans (all bone scans), and each had evidence of mediastinal nodal metastasis on chest CT. Sider and Horejs (1988) confirmed this finding in a study of 114 patients with potentially operable nonsmall cell lung cancer. Metastatic disease was found in 12 patients with evidence of mediastinal nodal metastasis on chest CT. Thus in potentially operable patients with mediastinal lymph node enlargement, complete organ scanning may eliminate the need for invasive mediastinal staging.

The use of multiorgan scanning to evaluate for asymptomatic metastatic disease in other patients should be done on a selective basis. We think that the general indications are (1) patients with clinical stage I or II disease who are marginally acceptable candidates, based on poor pulmonary function or other medical illness; (2) patients with a recent weight loss of greater than 5 percent of body weight; (3) patients with clinical stage IIIa disease who are potentially operative candidates; and (4) patients with stage IIIa disease who, although not operative candidates, would be candidates for either chemotherapy or curative intent radiotherapy.

A positive metastatic scan in general requires histologic confirmation, other than for brain metastases or destructive bone lesions. This is best done by radiologic, radionuclide, or ultrasound-guided fine-needle aspiration biopsy. On rare occasions laparoscopy or laparotomy is required to ensure that a positive liver CT indeed represents metastatic disease if the patient is otherwise considered operable. Special note needs to be made about the potential dilemma posed by adrenal masses or enlargement. Although the incidence of benign adenomas 1 to 5 cm in diameter in the general population is approximately 2 percent, in patients with lung cancer, this assumption may be incorrect. Pagani (1984) found unsuspected adrenal metastases in 7.8 percent of the patients thought to have only local chest disease. Therefore percutaneous biopsy of any significant adrenal mass or enlargement (greater than 1.5 or 2 cm) is necessary if the patient has no

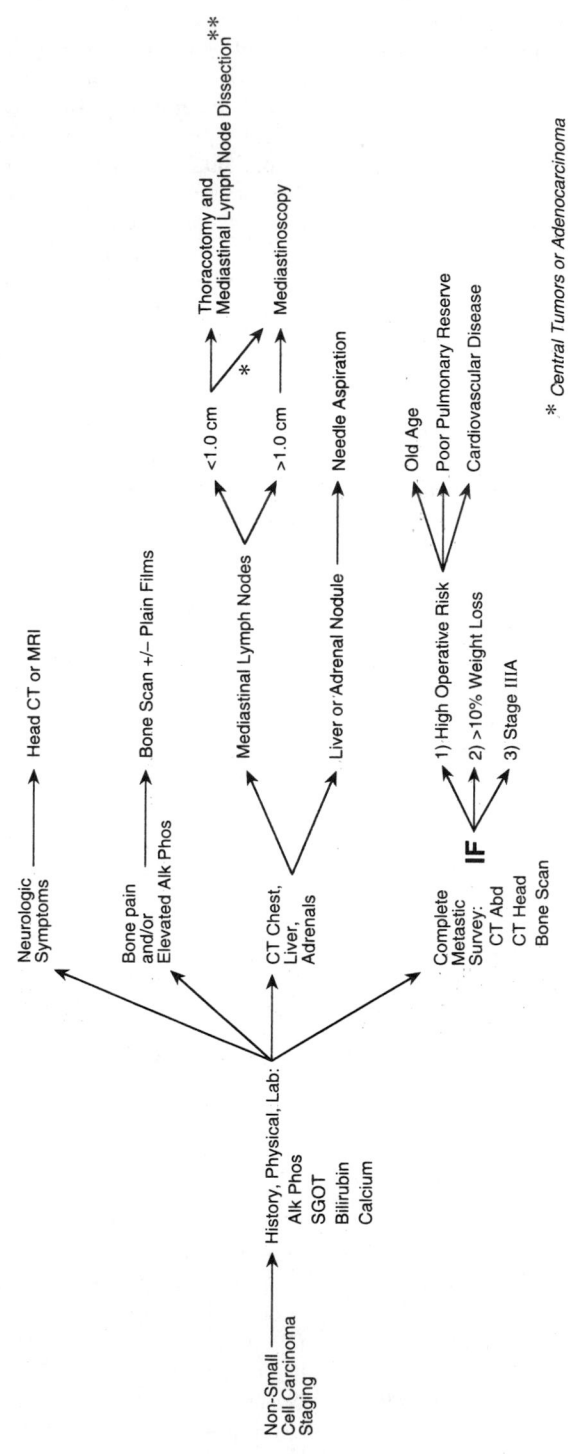

Figure 27-32. Algorithm for metastatic screening.

evidence of other metastases. If aspiration results are negative for malignancy and adrenal cells have been obtained, the clinician should assume the lesion is benign. Magnetic resonance imaging differentiation of benign versus malignant has not been proved to be valuable.

CONCLUSIONS

The diagnosis and staging of lung cancer use similar noninvasive and invasive techniques. Accurate treatment planning necessitates a diagnosis (small cell versus nonsmall cell) and a clinical estimate of stage before planning treatment.

KEY REFERENCES

Cooper JD, Ginsberg RJ: The use of mediastinoscopy in lung cancer: preoperative evaluation. In Current Controversies in Thoracic Surgery. WB Saunders, Philadelphia, 1986

This is an in-depth review of the debate about the role of mediastinoscopy and CT scanning in staging the mediastinum. The accompanying chapter by Shields should also be read.

McCloud TC, Bourgouin PM, Greenberg RW et al: Bronchogenic carcinoma. Analysis of staging in the mediastinum with CT by correlative lymph node mapping and sampling. Radiology 182:319, 1992

This is an excellent prospective study comparing CT scanning and

mediastinoscopy. Particularly interesting is the comparison of CT and mediastinoscopy by nodal stations.

Miller JD, Gorenstein LA, Patterson GA: Staging: the key to rational management of lung cancer. Ann Thorac Surg 53:170, 1992a

This is an up-to-date review of the new international staging system and the radiologic and invasive techniques used in staging.

Mountain CF: A new international staging system for lung cancer. Chest 89(suppl):225S, 1986

The original description of the new international staging system is given.

REFERENCES

Carbone PP, Frost JK, Feinstein AR et al: Lung cancer: perspective and prospects. Ann Intern Med 73:1024, 1970

Carlens E: Mediastinoscopy: a method for inspection and tissue biopsy in the superior mediastinum. Dis Chest 36:343, 1959

Cromartie RS, Parker EF, May JE et al: Carcinoma of the lung: a clinical review. Ann Thorac Surg 30:30, 1980

Cropp AJ, DiMarco AF, Lankerani M: False-positive transbronchial needle aspiration in bronchogenic carcinoma. Chest 85:696, 1984

Cryer PE, Kissaine JM: Clinicopathologic conference: malignant hypercalcemia. Am J Med 65:486, 1979

Daly BDT, Faling LJ, Bite G et al: Mediastinal lymph node evaluation by computed tomography in lung cancer. J Thorac Cardiovasc Surg 94:664, 1987

Denoix PF: Enquete permanent dans les centres anticancereux. Bull Inst Nat Hyg (Paris) I:70, 1946

Donaldson JC, Kaminsky DB, Elliot RC: Bronchiolar carcinoma. Report of 11 cases and review of the literature. Cancer 41:250, 1978

Ginsberg RJ: Extended cervical mediastinoscopy: a single staging procedure for bronchogenic carcinoma of the left upper lobe. Thorac Cardiovasc Surg 94:673, 1987

Grant D, Edwards D, Goldstraw P: Computed tomography of the brain, chest, and abdomen in the preoperative assessment of nonsmall cell lung cancer. Thorax 43:883, 1988

Harken DE, Black H, Clauss R, Ferrand RE: Simple cervicomediastinal exploration for tissue diagnosis of intrathoracic disease. N Engl J Med 251:1041, 1954

Harrow EM, Oldenburg FA, Lindenfelter MS, Smith AM: Transbronchial needle aspiration in clinical practice: a five year experience. Chest 96:1268, 1989

Heelan R, Martini N, Westcot JW et al: Carcinomas involving the hilum and mediastinum: computed tomographic and magnetic resonance evaluation. Radiology 156:111, 1985

Kato H, Konako C, Ono J et al: Cytology of the Lung: Techniques and Interpretation. Igaku-Shoin, Tokyo, 1983

Kies MS, Baker AW, Kennedy PS: Radionuclide scans in staging of carcinoma of lung. Surg Gynecol Obstet 147:175, 1978

Lewis RJ, Caccavale RJ, Sisler GE, Mackenzie JW: One hundred consecutive patients undergoing video-assisted thoracic operations. Ann Thorac Surg 54:421, 1992

Liang XM: Accuracy of cytologic diagnosis and cytotyping of sputum in primary lung cancer: analysis of 161 cases. J Surg Oncol 40:107, 1989

Little AG, DeMeester TR, Ryan JW: The use of radionuclide scans in lung cancer: gallium-67 scanning for preoperative staging. p. 122. In Current Controversies in Thoracic Surgery. WB Saunders, Philadelphia, 1986

Luke WP, Pearson FG, Todd TRJ et al: Prospective evaluation of mediastinoscopy for assessment of carcinoma of the lung. J Thorac Cardiovasc Surg 91:53, 1986

Mack MJ, Aronoff RJ, Acuff TE et al: Present role of thoracoscopy in the diagnosis and treatment of diseases of the chest. Ann Thorac Surg 54:403, 1992

Martini N, Flehinger BJ, Nagasaki F, Hart B: Prognostic significance of N1 disease in carcinoma of the lung. J Thorac Cardiovasc Surg 86:646, 1983

Miller DL, Allen MS, Trastek VF et al: Videothoracoscopic wedge excision of the lung. Ann Thorac Surg 54:410, 1992b

Morton DL, Itabashi HH, Gromes OF: Nonmetastatic neurologic complications of bronchogenic carcinoma: the carcinomatous myopathies. J Thorac Cardiovasc Surg 51:14, 1966

Mountain CF, Carr DT, Anderson WAD: A system for the clinical staging of lung cancer. AJR 120:130, 1974

Naruke T, Goya T, Tsuchya R et al: Prognosis and survival in resected lung cancer based on the new international staging system. J Thorac Cardiovasc Surg 96:440, 1988

Naruke T, Suemasu K, Ishikawa S: Lymph node mapping and curability at various levels of metastasis in resected lung cancer. J Thorac Cardiovasc Surg 76:832, 1978

Ng A, Horak GC: Factors significant to the diagnostic accuracy of lung cytology in bronchial washing and sputum samples. II. Sputum samples. Acta Cytol 27:397, 1983

Odell WD, Wolfsen AR: Humoral syndromes associated with cancer. Annu Rev Med 29:379, 1978

Pagani JJ: Non-small cell lung carcinoma adrenal mestastases: computed tomography and percutaneous needle biopsy in their diagnosis. Cancer 53:1058, 1984

Patterson GA, Piazza D, Pearson FG et al: Significance of metastatic disease in subaortic lymph node. Ann Thorac Surg 43:155, 1987

Pilotti S, Rilke F, Gribaudi D et al: Sputum cytology for the diagnosis of carcinoma of the lung. Acta Cytol 26:649, 1982

Quinn DL, Ostrow LB, Porter DK et al: Staging of non-small cell bronchogenic carcinoma: relationship of the clinical evaluation to organ scans. Chest 89:270, 1986

Ramsdell JW, Peters RM, Taylor AT Jr et al: Multi-organ scans for staging lung cancer. J Thorac Cardiovasc Surg 73:653, 1977

Richardson RI, Greco FA, Oldham RK et al: Tumor products and potential markers in small cell lung cancer. Semin Oncol 5:253, 1978

Risse EKJ, Vooijis GP, Van't Hof MA: Diagnostic significance of "severe dysplasia" in sputum cytology. Acta Cytol 32:629, 1988

Schenk DA, Bryan CL, Bower JH et al: Transbronchial needle aspiration in the diagnosis of bronchogenic carcinoma. Chest 92:83, 1987

Shure D, Fedullo PF: Transbronchial needle aspiration in the diagnosis of submucosal and periobronchial bronchogenic carcinoma. Chest 88:49, 1985

Shure D, Fedullo F: The role of transcarinal needle aspiration in the staging of bronchogenic carcinoma. Chest 86:5819, 1984

Sider L, Horejs D: Frequency of extrathoracic metastases from bronchogenic carcinoma in patients with normal-sized hilar and mediastinal lymph nodes on CT. AJR 151:893, 1988

Stiglbauer R, Schurawitzki H, Klepetko W et al: Contrast-enhanced MRI for the staging of bronchogenic carcinoma: comparison with CT and histopathologic staging—preliminary results. Clin Radiol 44:293, 1991

Tisi GM, Friedman PJ, Peters RM et al: Clinical staging of primary lung cancer. Am Rev Respir Dis 127:659, 1983

Tockman MS, Gupta PK, Myers JD et al: Sensitive and specific monoclonal antibody recognition of human lung cancer antigen on preserved sputum cells. J Clin Oncol 6:1685, 1988

Truong L, Underwood R, Greenberg S et al: Diagnosis and typing of lung carcinomas by cytopathologic methods. Acta Cytol 29:379, 1985

Vallieres E, Waters PF: Incidence of mediastinal node involvement in clinical T1 bronchogenic carcinomas. Can J Surg 30:341, 1987

Wang JP, Terri TB: Transbronchial needle aspiration in the diagnosis of staging of bronchogenic carcinoma. Am Rev Respir Dis 127:344, 1983

Watanabe Y, Shimizu J, Oda M et al: Proposals regarding some deficiencies in the new international staging system for non-small cell lung cancer. Jpn J Clin Oncol 21:160, 1991

Wescott JL: Direct percutaneous needle aspiration of localization pulmonary lesions: results in 422 patients. Radiology 137:31, 1980

Surgical Management

Nael Martini
Robert J. Ginsberg

Surgical treatment in lung cancer is still regarded as the most effective method of controlling the primary tumor, provided it is resectable for cure and the risks of the procedure are low. Radiation therapy, when used alone or with chemotherapy, has been effective in palliation and has resulted in occasional cures but has not achieved the success rate of surgery. Except for small cell lung cancer, chemotherapy is reserved for palliation of advanced tumors because no cures have been reported unless it is combined with surgery or irradiation.

The incidence of lung cancer is still at epidemic proportions. The American Cancer Society (1994) projected a lung cancer incidence of 172,000 new cases for 1993, with a male to female ratio of 1.4:1. Unfortunately, 89 percent of these cases are expected to die ultimately of their disease despite the fact that 30 percent of such patients are surgical "candidates."

HISTORICAL NOTE

Surgery for lung cancer was first reported in the literature before the turn of the century. Sauerbruch (1926) reported that Heidenhan had performed a partial resection for lung cancer using cautery with the patient surviving 2 months. Pean (1895) also reported the successful removal of a lung cancer by partial excision, including the chest wall, the actual operation having been performed 30 years previously. In

1912, Hugh Morriston Davies (1913–1914) completed the first dissection lobectomy for lung cancer, with the patient unfortunately dying 8 days later from empyema.

The modern area of a surgical resection for lung cancer required the development of underwater drainage. The first one-stage lobectomy was reported by Brunn (1929), followed by Allan and Smith (1932) who used a two-stage resection in 1930. The production of adhesions by pleural abrasion was followed by lobectomy and mass ligature. Following Graham's (Graham and Singer, 1933) historic pneumonectomy in 1932, surgical resection quickly became prevalent, with pneumonectomy being the procedure of choice (Churchill, 1933). The technique of segmentectomy was described by Churchill and Belsey (1939). Radical pneumonectomy with en bloc removal of mediastinal lymph nodes was first proposed by Alison in 1946. Subsequent to this, more refined techniques were developed including: sleeve resection by Price-Thomas (1956) in 1947, carinal resection by Mathey, et al. (1966) and Thompson (1966) independently in 1966, en bloc resection of the chest wall by Coleman (1947) and for a superior sulcus tumor in 1956 (Chardak and MacCallun, 1956), although this was only popularized in 1961 by Shaw and Paulson (Shaw, et al., 1961). Although lesser resections had been performed as compromised procedures in patients with poor pulmonary function by a variety of authors, Jensik, et al. (1973) reported the first series of segmental resections as intentional curative procedures.

HISTORICAL READINGS

Alison PR: Intrapericardial approach to the lung root in the treatment of bronchial carcinoma by dissection pneumonectomy. J Thorac Surg 15:991, 1946

Allan CI, Smith FJ: Primary carcinoma of the lung with report of case treated by operation. Surg Gynecol Obstet 55:151, 1932

Brunn HB: Surgical principles underlying one-stage lobectomy. Arch Surg 18:490, 1929

Chardak WM, MacCallun JD: Pancoast tumor (5 yr survival without recurrence or metastases following radical resection and postoperative irradiation). J Thorac Surg 31:535, 1956

Churchill E, Belsey HR: Segmental pneumonectomy in bronchiectasis. Ann Surg 109:481, 1939

Churchill ED: The surgical treatment of carcinoma of the lung. J Thorac Surg 2:254, 1933

Coleman FP: Primary carcinoma of the lung with invasion of ribs: pneumonectomy and simultaneous block resection of chest wall. Ann Surg 126:156, 1947

Davies HM: Recent advances in the surgery of the lung and pleura. Br J Surg 1:228, 1913–1914

Graham EA, Singer JJ: Successful removal of the entire lung for carcinoma of the bronchus. JAMA 101:1371, 1933

Jensik RJ, Faber LP, Milloy FJ, Monson DO: Segmental resection for lung cancer. A fifteen year experience. J Thorac Cardiovasc Surg 66:563, 1973

Mathey J, Binet JP, Galey JJ et al: Tracheal and tracheobronchial resections: technique and results in 20 cases. J Thorac Cardiovasc Surg 51:1, 1966

Pean J: Chirurgie des poumons. Discussion Ranc Chir Proc Verh Paris 9:72, 1895

Price-Thomas C: Conservative resection of the bronchial tree. J R Coll Surg Edinb 1:169, 1956

Sauerbruch F: Die Operation Entfernung von Lungengesch-wulste. Zentralbl Chir 53:852, 1926

Shaw RR, Paulson DL, Kee JL Jr: Treatment of the superior sulcus tumor by irradiation followed by resection. Ann Surg 154:29, 1961

Thompson DT: Tracheal resection with left lung anastomosis following right pneumonectomy. Thorax 21:560, 1966

PREOPERATIVE ASSESSMENT

It is now standard practice to stage all cancers of the lung carefully at the time of their initial diagnosis (see preceding section). Since 1986 the international TNM staging system has been adhered to by most oncologists (Mountain, 1987). Briefly stated tumors confined to the lung without any metastases, regional or distant, are classified as stage I and tumors associated with only hilar or peribronchial lymph node involvement (N1), as stage II. Locally advanced tumors with mediastinal or cervical lymph node metastases and those with extension to chest wall, mediastinum diaphragm, or carina are classified as stage III tumors, and tumors presenting with distant metastases are classified as stage IV tumors.

The 5-year survival rate following complete resection of a lung cancer is stage dependent (Table 27-5). Incomplete resection invariably does not cure the patient. Many recent series show that about 70 percent of patients with stage I resected lung cancer survive 5 years, and 80 percent never have recurrences (almost 20 percent of patients dying within 5 years of resection die of unrelated causes without recurring tumor) (Martini, et al., 1986; Williams, et al., 1981). At the other extreme, only a handful (less than 10 percent) of patients resected with stage IIIb disease are ever cured.

SURGICAL PRINCIPLES AND MANAGEMENT OF LUNG CANCER

It is no longer acceptable for lung cancer to be treated by a slapdash resection without regard to oncologic principles. The following guidelines of oncologic surgery must be adhered to:

1. Whenever possible the tumor and all intrapulmonary lymphatic drainage must be removed completely, most frequently by lobectomy or pneumonectomy.

2. Care must be taken not to transgress the tumor during the resection to avoid tumor spillage.

Table 27-5. 5-Year Survival Rates by Stage Following Complete Resection in Lung Cancer

Stage		Survival (%)
Stage I (n = 539)		76
T1N0		84
T2N0		68
Stage II (n = 214)		47
Stage IIIa		
T3N0 (chest wall)		56
T3N0 (carina)		36
T3N0 (mediastinum)		29
N2 (surgery)	(n = 151)	30
N2 (chemotherapy + surgery)	(n = 89)	26

3. En bloc resection of closely adjacent or invaded structures is preferable to a discontinuous resection.

4. Resection margins should be assessed by frozen-section analysis whenever possible; this includes bronchial, vascular, and any other margins with close proximity to the tumor. Re-excision is preferred whenever possible if positive resection margins are encountered.

5. All accessible mediastinal lymph nodes should be removed for pathologic evaluation, preferably by mediastinal lymph node dissection, and should be identified and properly labeled by the surgeon.

Surgical resection is the therapy of choice for early-stage nonsmall cell lung cancer. Surgical therapy alone is generally offered to all patients with stage I and II disease and also to specific groups of patients with stage III disease.

Nonsmall Cell Lung Cancer

Stage I Lung Cancer

Occult Lung Cancer

Localization. Few patients have lung carcinoma before it becomes apparent radiographically, accounting for less than 1 percent of the lung cancer population. They include individuals who participate in early lung cancer detection programs and patients who present to institutions with hemoptysis in the absence of any abnormal findings on routine chest radiographs. Prior to considering therapy, occult carcinomas presenting in this fashion need a careful investigation to localize the site of the cancer. The fact that the patient has a normal chest radiograph and a positive sputum on cytologic examination does not necessarily indicate that the patient has lung carcinoma, let alone an early lung carcinoma. In most instances the cytologic examination indicates a squamous cell cancer. A careful aerodigestive examination is essential to rule out carcinoma in that region. It has been our experience that one of three patients who have positive sputum cytologic results and negative chest radiographs have a carcinoma in the head and neck region (Martini and Melamed, 1980). Following a detailed examination of the head and neck, a careful diagnostic bronchoscopy is performed initially under local anesthesia to examine the proximal airway. With the use of the modern fiberoptic bronchoscope, it has become possible to extend the inspection of the tracheobronchial tree from the mainstem and lobar bronchi to segmental and subsegmental bronchi. By this method alone, the clinician can usually identify the specific site of a radiographically occult lung cancer. If the lesion is located centrally in a main or lobar bronchus, it is readily visualized, and a biopsy can be easily obtained. However, in instances in which the tracheobronchial tree appears normal at bronchoscopy, a meticulous sampling of each segmental bronchus by endoscopic brushings and cytologic analysis becomes necessary, unless a tumor has been identified in the head and neck region. Careful attention to detail to avoid cross contamination has resulted in localizing even these peripheral tumors in nearly all instances. Only repeated positive brushings from an isolated segment is acceptable for such localization. Recently more sophisticated techniques of in vivo fluorescent staining of mucosal malignancy with hematoporphyrin derivatives or laser-induced fluorescence excitation have enhanced the sensitivity and specificity of the bronchoscopic localization (Hayata, et al., 1984; Edell and Cortese, 1989; Lam, et al., 1993). These techniques are helpful in identifying and localizing occult malignancy that is not apparent to the naked eye during bronchoscopy. The clinician must always be wary of "field cancerization" with multiple in situ aerodigestive tumors.

Therapy. Following localization the therapy of choice for a radiographically occult carcinoma of the lung is surgical extirpation of the primary tumor by segmentectomy, lobectomy, or pneumonectomy, with or without a sleeve resection as necessary. Because most occult lung cancers are relatively central in position, lesser resections usually are not possible. Photodynamic therapy, using transbronchoscopic laser-induced photoexcitation of hematoporphyrin derivative, has been shown to be effective by Hayata, et al. (1984) and Cortese, et al. (1983) to eradicate occult in situ endobronchial lung cancer, and the short-term follow-up has been encouraging. After invasive carcinoma has been identified, resection is necessary.

The median survival of patients treated surgically for a radiographically occult carcinoma is long. Recurrences are rare, but new lung primaries are frequently observed in this group of patients. As high as 45 percent of these patients develop new carcinomas, the majority of which are new endobronchial squamous cell cancers (Martini and Melamed 1980). It becomes essential therefore that a continued surveillance of these patients be carried out at 6- to 12-month intervals.

Stage I Disease (T1N0, T2N0)

Therapy. This is the most common form of early lung cancer seen by most physicians. Many cases in this category are detected on routine chest radiographs in patients that present for unrelated medical conditions. Most are discrete peripheral tumors, presenting as a coin lesion. Computed tomographic (CT) scans are routinely done on these patients to assess the mediastinum, the liver, and the adrenal glands. Full-organ scanning beyond the CT scan has not been shown to be cost effective. Routine mediastinoscopy remains controversial if the CT scan is negative. If no mediastinal involvement is suspected, these patients are recommended to undergo surgical therapy. At the time of thoracotomy, a systematic lymph node dissection or sampling is carried out to ensure that no hilar or mediastinal nodal metastasis is present.

Lesser resections by wedge excision or segmentectomy have been advocated by some for small peripheral tumors. Jensik (1987) and Kulka and Forai (1985) reported on a large series of patients with stage I carcinoma treated in this conservative fashion. Recently the Lung Cancer Study Group completed a randomized clinical trial of lobectomy versus a lesser resection by wedge or segmentectomy in stage I carcinomas presenting as small peripheral tumors (Ginsberg, 1991). Preliminary reports of this study suggest an increased incidence of local recurrence in patients treated by lesser resections than lobectomy. This was confirmed by an analysis of the Rush-Presbyterian segmental resection data by Warren, et al. (1993). Although the apparent advantage of a lesser resection is the conservation of lung tissue, this was not evident in the long-term pulmonary function assessment. An important disadvantage is the 10 to 15 percent risk of local recurrence in the locoregional area. We confine this form of therapy only to patients with a limited lung reserve (McCormack and Martini, 1980). In more central nodules, therapy necessarily requires lobectomy or pneumonectomy.

The role of mediastinal lymph node dissection (versus lymph node sampling) in this early stage of disease remains to be decided. However, there is no doubt that the formal type of complete dissection provides the most accurate postsurgical staging, unless preoperative mediastinoscopy is combined with complete intraoperative lymph node sampling. A randomized comparative trial of these two modalities (Izibicki, et al., 1994) demonstrated no survival or local recurrence advantage to either therapeutic arm in stages I and II disease if mediastinoscopy was used in conjunction with intraoperative sampling.

For tumors protruding from a lobar orifice into the main bronchus, particularly in patients with limited pulmonary reserve, a sleeve lobectomy should be considered. This procedure conserves the pulmonary parenchyma and offers lower morbidity and mortality rates than a pneumonectomy, with comparable curability when a complete resection is done (Gaissert, et al., 1993).

Survival.   Patients with small peripheral tumors (T1N0M0) that are 3 cm or less in diameter and confined to the lung parenchyma without evidence of regional lymphatic metastases or extension to chest wall, diaphragm, or pleura have a 5-year disease-free survival rate of 83 percent when treated by primary surgical resection (McCormack and Martini, 1980). Tumors greater than 3 cm in diameter that are still confined to lung without metastasis to nodes or distant sites also have a favorable prognosis with a 5-year disease-free survival rate in 65%. The overall 5-year survival rate in stage I carcinoma of the lung, whether T1 or T2 in size, that is surgically treated in our institution is currently 76 percent at 5 years (Figure 27-33). This was confirmed by other investigators (Naruke, et al., 1988a; Lung Cancer Study Group, 1987; Mountain, 1988).

No adjuvant treatment is recommended for patients with stage I disease following resection. Patterns of recurrence at this stage of disease suggest that, of the 20 percent of patients who ultimately do have recurrences, the majority have re-

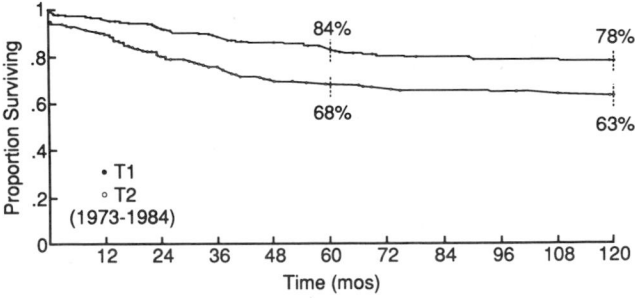

Figure 27-33. Survival following complete resection in stage I nonsmall cell lung cancer (T1N0M0–T2N0M0).

lapses at distant sites, with more than 20 percent of all recurrences being solitary brain metastases. However, because of the paucity of such patients, no firm recommendation can be made concerning adjuvant treatment. Close follow-up for the detection of solitary recurrences or second primaries is advised.

Stage II Disease

Tumors confined to the lung or bronchus with involvement of hilar or bronchopulmonary lymph nodes as the sole site of tumor spread (T1-2N1 disease) make up less than 5 percent of the lung cancer population and less than 10 percent of all resected lung cancers. We recently reviewed our experience at Memorial Sloan-Kettering Cancer Center on the surgical treatment of stage II lung cancer (Martini, et al., 1992). From 1973 to 1989, 214 patients had undergone a complete resection of their stage II lung cancer with a mediastinal lymph node dissection. Of these 35 patients had T1N1 lesions and 179, T2N1 tumors. The male to female ratio was 2 : 1, and the median age was 62 years. Eighty-three percent of the patients with T1 lesions had adenocarcinomas, whereas this difference in histologic findings was not apparent in T2 lesions in which adenocarcinomas and squamous cancers were of equal frequency.

Lobectomy is the procedure of choice in most patients. In our series 68 percent of our patients had a lobectomy; 31 percent, a pneumonectomy; and only 1 percent, a wedge resection or segmentectomy. A lobectomy was sufficient to encompass all disease in 34 of 35 T1 lesions. Of interest was the fact that one-half of the patients had a single N1 node involvement, and 85 percent of the patients had nodal involvement at a single N1 level. At this stage of disease, we believe it is imperative to perform a complete lymph node dissection because occult mediastinal metastases occur with increasing frequency.

The overall survival rate following resection, calculated by the Kaplan-Meier method and considering all deaths, was 39 percent at 5 years. There was no difference in survival between T1 or T2 lesions. However, there was a distinct difference in survival between tumors that were 3 cm and smaller in size and those that were 5 cm or greater. There was a trend in the survival rate by histologic type that favored epidermoid carcinoma over adenocarcinoma with a *P* value of 0.07. The location of the primary tumor, the location of the N1 nodes, the extent of the surgical resection, and the presence or absence of visceral pleural involvement had no appreciable impact on the survival rate. Importantly the number of lymph nodes involved was significant. The survival rate following resection in patients with involvement of a single lymph node was 45 percent compared to 31 percent in patients with multiple lymph node involvement (Fig. 27-34).

The patterns of recurrence differed by histologic type. There were more local or regional recurrences in patients with squamous cancers and more distant metastases in patients with adenocarcinomas. The incidence of local or regional recurrence was reduced by the administration of postoperative radiation therapy. However, there was no impact on survival by the addition of postoperative radiation therapy in this group of patients, and this confirms the Lung Cancer

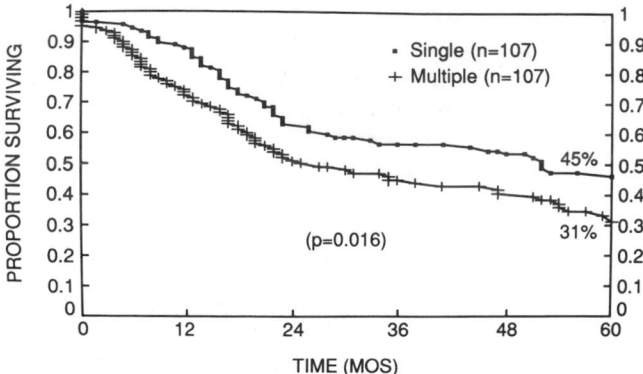

Figure 27-34. Survival by number of N1 nodes involved following complete resection in stage II nonsmall cell lung cancer.

Study Group (1986) report. Recurrence rates were high despite resection. Favorable prognostic factors included the number of involved nodes and the size of the lesion.

Most patients who did not respond to the initial therapy developed distant metastases, suggesting the need for an effective systemic treatment, but the specific regimens that might benefit this group of patients are still under study. The Lung Cancer Study Group, in another trial comparing postoperative irradiation with chemoirradiation, reported some advantages in the time to recurrence of combined adjuvant radiation and chemotherapy in adenocarcinoma (Holmes, et al., 1986). However, this latter study did not compare or assess adjuvant treatment with chemotherapy alone and with no adjuvant treatment in stage II adenocarcinoma. More data are necessary to assess the role and type of adjuvant treatment in these patients.

Because 60 percent of patients have recurrences following surgical resection, mostly at distant sites, early effective systemic treatment is needed if we wish to improve the results of surgical therapy. Postoperative adjuvant trials of chemotherapy, immunotherapy, or combinations of the two have had little effect on the survival rate in randomized studies (Lung Cancer Study Group, 1986; Holmes, et al., 1986). Induction (neoadjuvant and preoperative) chemotherapy was not tested in this subset of patients.

Stage III Disease

The majority of lung cancers presenting for therapy are advanced tumors. When distant metastases are absent, they are classified as stage III disease with extension of the primary tumor to chest wall, mediastinum, and diaphragm (T3 or T4 disease) or mediastinal and cervical lymph node involvement (N2 or N3 disease). Many of these locally advanced tumors are amenable to surgical or combined modality therapy that includes surgery, particularly T3 and/or N2 disease (stage IIIa). At this stage of disease, it is important to rule out distant metastases with preoperative organ scanning.

Tumors Invading Chest Wall. Cancers of the lung that invade the chest wall are usually peripheral in position. Hilar or mediastinal lymph node metastases are less likely to occur in this group of patients. These tumors extend to invade the parietal pleura, but some involve the muscles and ribs of the chest wall. Even with chest wall invasion, significant numbers of these patients are amenable to treatment by resection. Factors that influence survival in this group of patients are (1) complete resectability of the tumor, (2) the extent of invasion of the chest wall, and (3) the presence or absence of regional lymph node metastases. We reviewed 111 patients with carcinoma of the lung invading the chest wall who were treated surgically (McCaughan, et al., 1985). Of these, 77 percent had a complete resection with an overall 5-year survival rate of 40 percent in those completely resected. In those in whom resection was incomplete (macroscopic or microscopic disease) or not possible, the survival time did not extend beyond 2.5 years. Postoperative radiation therapy in this group of patients did not have an impact on their ultimate survival. This was confirmed by the Mayo experience (Piehler, et al., 1982) and others.

The extent of chest wall involvement by the tumor also affected survival. In patients in whom the tumor extended to the parietal pleura but did not penetrate beyond the parietal pleura into the soft tissues of the chest wall and the ribs, the 5-year survival rate following complete resection was better than in patients with deeper involvement of the chest wall (62 versus 35 percent in patients with T3N0M0 disease).

Our series suggested that a significant number of patients whose tumors are confined to involvement of the parietal pleura can be treated by an extrapleural mobilization of the tumor without necessarily resecting en bloc the adjoining segments of ribs as long as the resection margins are negative. On the other hand, Pairolero and Arnold (1985) stressed the need for a routine chest wall resection whenever adherence of a peripheral tumor to the chest was identified at thoracotomy. However, many of their patients did not demonstrate any involvement beyond the parietal pleura. Whether or not en bloc resection of chest wall (versus parietal pleura only) is required in every instance remains a contentious issue.

We favor chest wall reconstruction with a Marlex mesh-methylmethacrylate sandwich technique whenever there is a suspicion of chest wall instability, but we rarely find this necessary with the resection of fewer than three contiguous rib segments. For such smaller defects, Marlex mesh patch closure ensures acceptable cosmetic results and chest wall stability (McCormack, et al., 1981; McCormack, et al., 1987). Others prefer a Gor-Tex patch for larger defects (Pairolero and Arnold, 1985). Very small defects may require no reconstruction, especially if situated posteriorly beneath large muscles or scapula.

The presence of hilar or mediastinal nodes adversely affects survival in this group of patients despite a complete resection. The survival rate following a complete resection in the presence of nodal disease is only 20 percent at 5 years. Unlike our experience, some investigators believe that, in patients who have chest wall invasion and concurrent mediastinal nodal metastasis, the salvage rate is essentially nonexistent. Many of these patients are currently being offered neoadjuvant treatment with re-evaluation following a response. There is no evidence that preoperative radiation therapy benefits patients with tumors invading the chest wall. Postoperative radiation therapy in patients who have evidence of mediastinal lymph node metastases or residual disease is usually advised in an attempt to decrease the incidence of local recurrence (Patterson, et al., 1982), although the efficacy of this treatment is unknown. A randomized trial by the Lung Cancer Study Group to assess the value of postoperative radiotherapy in this group of patients was abandoned because of low accrual.

Superior Sulcus Tumors. Superior sulcus tumors (Pancoast tumors) represent a subset of carcinomas of the lung invading the chest wall. By reason of their location in the pleural apex, they invade adjoining tissues early. The patients are generally symptomatic from the outset. Early invasion of the lower brachial plexus, especially the T1 nerve root, is common. Shoulder and arm pain radiating to the inner aspect of the upper arm (T1) and the ulnar distribution in the fourth and fifth fingers of the hand (C8) is a common presenting symptom. Extension to the stellate ganglion with a consequent Horner's syndrome is seen in at least one-third of the patients. Extension to the ribs or vertebrae is common.

Most superior sulcus tumors are initially diagnosed histologically or cytologically by a transcutaneous needle biopsy performed under fluoroscopic or CT guidance. Diagnostic bronchoscopy is less helpful in establishing a tissue diagnosis in this group of patients because of the peripheral position of the lesion, although transbronchoscopic biopsy using image intensification has been done. The majority of tumors are squamous carcinomas or adenocarcinomas, but 3 to 5 percent are small cell carcinomas with vastly different therapeutic implications, hence the importance of a tissue diagnosis before treatment.

Shaw, et al., (1961) and Paulson (1982, 1985) first advocated the combined use of preoperative radiation and resection and demonstrated a 31 percent 5-year survival rate. They also noted that, in a small percent of these patients, mediastinal lymph node metastases (N2) may coexist and few patients in this group survive longer than 1 year. Mediastinoscopy was consequently recommended in the preoperative evaluation of these patients to rule out the presence of N2 disease.

The current standard therapy for this group of patients is a combination of preoperative radiation followed by resection whenever possible. Therapy begins by a preoperative course of external radiation therapy to a dose of 3,000 to 4,000 cGy to the tumor (Hilaris, et al., 1987; Hilaris and Martini, 1982). This can be given in 300-cGy fractions over 2 weeks or 1,000 cGy/week for a period of 4 weeks. The radiation portal includes the primary tumor, the adjacent mediastinum, and the ipsilateral supraclavicular area. Following a rest period of 1 month, these patients are assessed for surgical treatment. If no distant disease is evident, these patients are then offered surgical exploration for removal of the residual tumor. In our opinion, the presence of a Horner's syndrome or ipsilateral supraclavicular node involvement is not an absolute contraindication for combined preoperative radiation and surgery; 20 percent of patients considered for this therapeutic approach have Horner's syndrome, and 17 percent present with supraclavicular lymph nodes (Hilaris, et al., 1987). The standard resection described by Paulson encompasses en bloc removal of the affected lobe and chest wall, including the entire first rib and posterior segments of ribs two, three, and often four; transverse processes of the contiguous thoracic vertebrae;

nerve roots C8 and T1 to 3; the lower trunk of the brachial plexus; and the dorsal sympathetic chain with mediastinal node dissection. Paulson's (1982, 1985) latest series suggests that nearly 90 percent of the patients explored have undergone complete resection. At Memorial Sloan-Kettering, we also combined preoperative radiation therapy with surgery but observed that only 21 percent of all patients surgically explored after irradiation had a complete resection of their tumor (Hilaris, et al., 1987).

The determinants of unresectability have generally been involvement of the subclavian artery or the vertebral body with or without cord compression or widespread invasion of the major divisions of the brachial plexus. We found magnetic resonance imaging to be extremely valuable for this assessment. In most patients in whom the tumor is incompletely resected or found unresectable, interstitial implantation of radioisotopes (brachytherapy) is used to complete the radiation therapy of the tumor. The 5-year survival rate results obtained by us and others following complete resection were similar to that reported by Shaw, et al. (1961) and Paulson (1982, 1985) and were confirmed by many others. Whether preoperative irradiation adds to surgical therapy has been questioned. Shahian, et al. (1987) reported improved results with "sandwich irradiation," that is, adding postoperative therapy to full therapeutic doses. The adverse prognostic factors we identified included N1 or N2 disease, incomplete resection, and wedge (versus lobectomy) resection of the pulmonary component (Dartevelle, et al., 1993).

Tumors in Proximity to Carina. Another subset of stage III carcinomas that benefits from surgical management includes patients with central tumors that extend within 2 cm of the carina. In many instances the carina itself is not involved despite a T3 presentation, and in many instances surgical extirpation of the tumor is possible. In some no lymphatic metastases are evident at the time of the resection. In patients in whom resection can be undertaken despite the proximity of the lesion to the carina but without its involvement, the 5-year anticipated survival rate following resection is currently reported to be 36 percent (Martini, et al., 1988a).

The presence of tumor at a major lobar orifice and the need to conserve lung tissue are the main indications for sleeve resection. A pneumonectomy may be required to encompass all of a tumor protruding from a lobar orifice into the main bronchus and to provide a clear margin of resection. This may not be possible because of a compromised pulmonary reserve. In such situations a sleeve lobectomy is a worthwhile alternative and has lower morbidity and mortality rates than does pneumonectomy (Vogt-Moykopf, et al., 1986). When a complete excision is possible, the curability rate by sleeve lobectomy appears comparable to that obtained by pneumonectomy. Faber, et al. (1984) performed 101 sleeve lobectomies over a 21-year period, with only two postoperative deaths in the entire series. The survival rate in this group of patients was 30 percent at 5 years and 22 percent at 10 years. Unfortunately peribronchial lymphatic invasion is present in many instances, and this precludes considerations for sleeve resection. Mehran, et al., (1993) reported on the adverse effect of nodal disease managed by sleeve lobectomy. In this latter group, when pneumonectomy cannot be considered, interstitial implantation of radioisotopes without resection has been a rewarding alternative in our experience (Hilaris and Martini, 1979), although primary external beam radiotherapy is also a valid therapeutic alternative.

Tumors Invading Mediastinum. Patients presenting with invasion of the primary tumor into the mediastinum generally do poorly if treated by surgery alone. Two-thirds of these patients also have mediastinal lymph node metastases. Few centers have reported their results in this subset of patients. From 1974 to 1984, 225 patients underwent thoracotomy at Memorial Sloan-Kettering Cancer Center for nonsmall cell carcinoma invading only the mediastinum (T3) (Burt, et al., 1987). Of these only 49 patients (22 percent) underwent complete resection of all intrathoracic disease. The 5-year survival rate in this group of patients was only 9 percent. Partial resection, implantation of isotopes to the residual disease, plus external radiation therapy was carried out in 33 patients (15 percent) with a 3- and 5-year survival rate of a surprising 22 percent. Partial resection without implantation was done in 42 patients (19 percent) and implantation without resection in 101 patients (45 percent). There were no 5-year survivors in the latter two groups.

Pulmonary resection combined with implantation and postoperative radiation therapy appears to offer some survival advantage in this specific subset of patients. Even then only a few benefit from this combined approach. This group of patients could potentially benefit from a new approach with combined modality therapy that includes induction chemo- or radiotherapy to improve the probability of complete resection.

N2 Disease

"Resectable." Metastasis to mediastinal lymph nodes (N2 disease) is probably the most frequent deterrent to cancer cure despite a localized presentation. Mediastinal metastasis is noted in nearly one-half of all patients at presentation with nonsmall cell lung carcinoma. Many view this large group of patients as having incurable disease despite the best efforts of surgery and radiation therapy (Paulson, and Urschel, 1971; Pearson, 1985) because the majority probably have occult micrometastatic disease already present elsewhere.

We believe that selected patients with ipsilateral N2 disease can benefit from effective management by surgery, usually combined with radiation or chemotherapy. From 1974 to 1981, 1,598 patients with nonsmall cell lung cancer were seen; 706 of them had mediastinal lymph node metastases. Of these 151 (21 percent) were completely resectable (Martini, et al., 1983). Mediastinoscopy was not routinely performed as part of staging before thoracotomy. Clinical evidence of N2 disease was based largely on radiographic and bronchoscopic findings. Patients with a normal-appearing mediastinum on routine chest radiographs and a normal carina at bronchoscopy without compression or distortion of the trachea or main bronchi were classified as having N0 or N1 disease. Patients who had an abnormal mediastinum on chest radiographs, which was suggestive of N2 disease, and those with findings at bronchoscopy suggestive of carinal involvement were considered to have clinically manifested N2 disease.

These were histologically documented by mediastinoscopy or by bronchoscopic biopsies.

Of 151 patients treated by complete resection (10 percent of the entire group), 94 had adenocarcinomas, 46 had squamous cancers, and 11 had large cell carcinomas. The overall 5-year survival rate was 30 percent (Martini and Flehinger, 1987).

We compared survival rates with respect to histologic type and showed no difference in survival at 5 years between patients with adenocarcinomas (30 percent) and those with epidermoid carcinomas (32 percent). However, the survival rate was affected by tumor size. Better survival rates at 5 years were noted in patients with small tumors (T1, 46 percent) compared with those with large tumors (T2, 27 percent) or those with extension outside the lung or in proximity to the carina (T3, 14 percent; $P = 0.003$).

The survival rate was also calculated by nodal size and the number of involved nodes. When nodal involvement was present, the size per se did not affect the survival rate because patients with normal-sized nodes, nodes of 2 cm or less in size, and nodes greater than 2 cm had essentially similar survival rates ($P = 0.17$). This suggests that patients with encapsulated lymph nodes, regardless of their size, can have prolonged survival if the nodes are completely removed. However, the number of nodes affected was significant. Patients with a single involved N2 node did better than those with multiple nodal involvement at one or more levels ($P = 0.005$).

The survival rate by the level of involved nodes was also calculated. Prolonged survival was observed with nodal involvement in all major mediastinal compartments (paratracheal, subcarinal, and aorticopulmonary window).

The survival rate was also compared by the extent of N2 involvement. Patients presenting with radiologic or endoscopic evidence of clinical N2 disease had a poor survival rate. Only 18 percent of these patients had resectable disease, and only 9 percent of those treated by resection survived 5 years.

There is benefit from resection in a small select group of patients presenting with carcinoma of the lung and mediastinal nodal involvement because the long-term survival time of 5 or more years after complete resection is noted in 30 percent of the patients. However, for the resection to be effective, it must be complete. It must encompass all detectable disease in the lung and mediastinum. Most importantly the resection must be offered to good-risk patients to avoid or minimize undue surgical complications and deaths. Similar survival rates are seen when patients are selected following mediastinoscopy with single-level encapsulated lymph node involvement and N2 disease discovered at thoracotomy despite a negative mediastinoscopy result (Pearson, 1985; Martini and Flehinger, 1987).

"Unresectable." CT scanning has now become an integral part of the staging and presurgical evaluation of the mediastinum (Ferguson, et al., 1986; Graves, et al., 1985; Martini, et al., 1985). CT scanning correlates well (80 to 90 percent accuracy) with negative nodes less than 1 cm in diameter. Many centers accept this as evidence of mediastinal "negativity" and proceed with surgical resection based on this nega-

tive result. Enlarged mediastinal lymph nodes (greater than 1 cm in shortest diameter) detected on CT scans should be confirmed to be positive by mediastinoscopy or other invasive staging before embarking on therapy because 30 percent of such cases do not contain tumors in the mediastinal nodes and can be offered primarily surgical therapy. Other patients have minimal mediastinal disease, which is amenable to immediate surgical therapy, whereas most have more extensive disease than anticipated and may require combined modality or nonsurgical primary therapy.

The patients with N2 disease that benefit best from surgery as their primary therapy are those that present with peripheral tumors, an apparently normal mediastinum on plain chest radiographs and at bronchoscopy, and a normal mediastinum on CT scan, with a single, but encapsulated, discrete ipsilateral lymph node involvement, discovered either at surgery or mediastinoscopy.

The importance of CT scanning and mediastinoscopy, we believe, is to identify significant mediastinal disease (i.e., involvement in multiple levels of N2 nodes, invasion of mediastinal structures by nodal disease, or contralateral [N3] nodal disease). Unfortunately neither CT scan nor plain radiography correlates well with N2 disease when the tumor in the lung is central or hilar in location or extends to the mediastinum, making it difficult to separate T3 from N2 disease. In these groups of patients, invasive mediastinal evaluation by mediastinoscopy is helpful. We defined these patients as having bulky N2 disease. Neither postoperative radiotherapy, postoperative chemotherapy, or a combination of both has significantly improved the survival times of these patients (Lung Cancer Study Group, 1986; Holmes, et al., 1986).

The role of preoperative radiation therapy alone for N2 disease has been extensively evaluated in the past, and there is general agreement that preoperative irradiation does not improve survival (Warram, collaborative study, 1975; Shields, et al., 1970). This is so despite a reported increase in resectability, locoregional control, and apparent sterilization of some of the tumors, as evidenced in the resected specimens following preoperative radiation therapy, because most patients die of distant metastases.

Efforts are now under way in several centers to assess the benefit of preoperative therapy by chemotherapy or combined chemo- and radiation therapy in locally advanced lung carcinoma that is incurable at present by conventional methods with surgery and irradiation (Taylor, et al., 1987; Burkes, et al., 1989), comparing this approach with nonsurgical therapy. Phase II studies suggest an improved survival compared with that in historical controls, and two recent randomized trials confirm the benefit of induction therapy compared with immediate surgery (Kris, et al., 1987, 1985ab).

Regimens containing cisplatin have had the highest and most reproducible response rates, specifically (mitomycin, vindesine or vinblastine, and cisplatin (MVP) combinations and regimens with 5-fluorouracil infusions plus cisplatin (Taylor, et al., 1987; Kris, et al., 1987; Gralla, et al., 1987).

In January 1984 we began using chemotherapy preoperatively in patients with N2 disease (Martini, et al., 1988b). From 1984 to 1991, 136 patients with histologically confirmed nonsmall cell lung cancer and stage IIIa (N2) disease received two to three cycles of MVP chemotherapy (Martini, et al., 1993). All patients had clinical N2 disease, defined as bulky mediastinal lymph node metastases or multiple levels of lymph node involvement in the ipsilateral mediastinum or subcarinal space on chest radiographs, CT scans, or mediastinoscopy. The overall major response rate to chemotherapy was 77 percent (105 of 136). Thirteen patients had a complete response, and 92 patients had a partial but major response (more than 50 percent). The overall complete resection rate was 65 percent (89 of 136) with a complete resection rate of 78 percent (82 of 105) in patients with a major response to chemotherapy. There was no histologic evidence of tumor in the resected specimens of 19 patients. The overall survival was 28 percent at 3 years and 17 percent at 5 years (median, 19 months). For patients who had a complete resection, the median survival time was 27 months, and the 3- and 5-year survival rates were 41 percent and 26 percent, respectively (Fig. 27-35). There were seven therapy-related deaths. To date 33 patients, all of whom had complete resections, have had no recurrence after treatment. These results demonstrate that (1) preoperative chemotherapy with MVP produces high response rates in stage IIIa (N2) disease, (2) high complete resection rates occur after a response to chemotherapy, and (3) survival times are longest in patients who have a complete resection after a major response to chemotherapy.

The role of surgeons in managing such patients must begin prior to any induction therapy and must include preoperative assessment of the T (bronchoscopy) and N (mediastinoscopy) stages and a predetermination of the expected resection that might follow the induction therapy. After completion of such preoperative treatment, a careful reassessment is required to determine whether the patient's disease is potentially resectable and the patient has the cardiopulmonary capabilities of tolerating such a resection, keeping in mind the adverse cardiopulmonary toxicities of specific agents (e.g., mitomycin, doxorubicin, and bleomycin) and radiotherapy. Following induction therapy, resection is possible in most responders, and complete mediastinal lymph node dissection is essential in all those with complete resections. Despite the intensive preoperative regimens, surgical morbidity and mortality rates have not exceeded those expected following resection of locally advanced stage III lung cancer.

More than 30 different preoperative trials with chemotherapy or combined chemotherapy and irradiation for locally advanced nonsmall cell lung cancer have been reported, encompassing a total of more than 1,000 patients (Kris, et al., 1987; Burkes, et al., 1992; Faber and Bonomi 1990; Strauss, et al., 1992; Lynch, et al., 1992; Pass, et al., 1992). The rationale for combining preoperative radiation therapy with chemotherapy in some studies is based on the expectations of additive or synergistic effects (Faber, et al., 1989; Rowland, et al., 1988; Yashar, et al., 1992; Rusch, et al., 1993).

All reports on preoperative treatment to date can only be viewed as feasibility studies because of the small number of patients studied in each report, but all demonstrate high responses to induction treatment with increased resectability in responders. The early survival data of these trials are sufficiently encouraging to support the initiation of large-scale randomized studies, which are currently in progress to

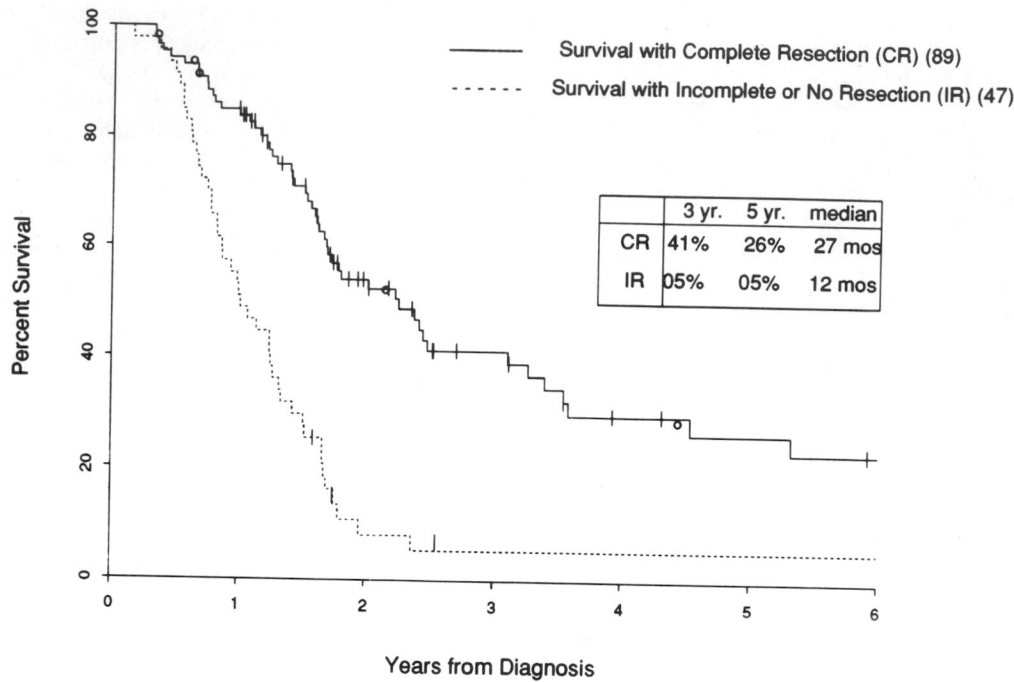

Figure 27-35. Survival by the extent of resection following induction chemotherapy in stage IIIA (N2) nonsmall cell lung cancer ($P = 0.00002$.)

assess fully the role of induction therapy and surgery versus the current standard therapy, radiotherapy (with or without chemotherapy), in these "unresectable" N2 patients. Recent reports suggest up to a 15 percent 5-year survival rate with chemoradiotherapy as the primary treatment (Dillman, et al., 1990; Schaake-Koning, et al., 1992). Two such randomized trials have recently been reported (Rosell, et al., 1994; Roth, et al., 1994).

Stage IIIb Disease (T4 or N3). Patients presenting with (1) supraclavicular or contralateral mediastinal lymph node metastases (N3); (2) invasion of the spine, trachea, carina, esophagus, aorta, or heart (T4); or (3) malignant pleural effusion (T4) are currently grouped under stage IIIb disease and are considered inoperable. Most of these patients are candidates for irradiation, chemotherapy, or both. Few at present are considered for surgical therapy, even after a response to these nonsurgical modes. Currently phase II clinical trials are assessing the potential role of combined modality therapy, including surgery for this subset of patients. Occasionally patients are found at thoracotomy to have completely resectable disease, which is resected. These comprise most of the reported long-term survivors.

T4 Disease. Lesions that extend to and invade the carina have a much poorer prognosis than those in the mainstem bronchi. Some authors advocate aggressive pneumonectomy with tracheal sleeve resection and direct reanastomosis of the trachea to the contralateral mainstem bronchus in young patients who are good surgical risks with up to a 20 percent 5-year survival rate, often in the face of 13 to 30 percent operative mortality rates (Deslauriers, 1985; Jensik, et al., 1982). The therapy (sleeve pneumonectomy) should be reserved for young healthy patients with clinical stage N0 dis-

ease, as determined by mediastinoscopy, who have completely resectable disease. We prefer at present to treat all other patients with combined interstitial (brachytherapy) and external irradiation without resection. Transbronchoscopic laser or photodynamic therapy with and without a hematoporphyrin derivative may play an important adjuvant role in the future management of such localized tracheal invasion (Oho, et al., 1983). Other T4 lesions can be completely resected in selected instances, offering an occasional cure. Unfortunately local recurrence ultimately develops in most patients. This includes also direct invasion of the vertebra, superior vena cava, esophagus, and atrium.

N3 Disease. Contralateral mediastinal lymph node metastases are considered by most surgeons to be an absolute contraindication to surgery because long-term survival with surgery is rare and anecdotal. However, the Southwest Oncology Group has completed a phase II induction chemo- and radiotherapy program followed by surgery for this group of patients. The early results of this trial suggest a complete resection rate similar to that seen with induction therapy for N2 disease (Rusch, et al., 1993). Long-term results, including survival rates, in patients treated for N3 disease by this aggressive fashion are still unknown. Many centers in Japan use a median sternotomy to accomplish an extended lymph node dissection to include contralateral mediastinal and ipsilateral or bilateral neck node dissection for patients with N3 involvement. There are occasional long-term survivors using this aggressive approach (Naruke, et al., 1988b; Hata, et al., 1988; Watanabe, et al., 1988). Although unlikely to provide substantial long-term benefit, these approaches are worthy of well-constructed clinical trials.

Solitary Metastases (M1)

Brain. Brain metastases constitute nearly one-third of all observed recurrences in patients with resected nonsmall cell lung cancer, and twice that incidence is found at autopsy of all patients dying with lung cancer. Most brain metastases occur in those patients with a histologic diagnosis of adenocarcinoma as opposed to squamous or large cell carcinoma.

Therapy. When local and regional control are achieved but brain metastases develop as the sole site of recurrence, the therapy for the brain metastasis determines the ultimate survival. Untreated patients with brain metastases have a median survival of less than 3 months. When brain metastases are multiple or advanced systemic disease is also present, the therapy of choice is whole-brain irradiation. However, one-third of the patients presenting with brain metastases have solitary lesions. Therapy with combined surgery and radiation can be effective (Martini, 1986; Patchell, et al., 1986). Those most likely to receive long-term benefit from surgical resection are patients with a single surgically accessible brain metastasis and no other evident systemic disease. However, a recent randomized trial suggests that surgery offers the best form of palliation despite other noncerebral metastases (Patchell, et al., 1990).

High-dose corticosteroid therapy reduces edema, causing regression of neurologic symptoms that is sometimes complete. It is the initial treatment prescribed for all patients. Surgery or radiation therapy are usually initiated after 3 to 4 days of steroid therapy.

Magilligan, et al., (1986) reported on 41 patients treated surgically for their brain metastases. All had solitary metastases, and in 14 of 41 or one-third of the patients, the neurologic symptoms preceded the diagnosis of lung cancer, which is in keeping with our experience. Improvement in neurologic symptoms was noted in most patients, the operative mortality rate was low, and there was a clear survival advantage over patients treated by nonsurgical means, all of which is also in accord with the findings of most recent reports.

Two studies now have demonstrated conclusively that surgical extirpation followed by whole-brain irradiation is superior to whole-brain irradiation alone in managing solitary cerebral metastases with regard to survival and quality of life.

Our current view on the management of solitary brain metastases is as follows. When the brain lesion is detected first and the search for the primary tumor is negative, resection of the cranial metastasis is the therapy of choice (Martini, 1986; Burt, et al., 1992). When the brain metastasis presents subsequent to the resection of the lung carcinoma and no other site of recurrence is present or the patient has minimal disease elsewhere, resection of the intracranial lesion is again the therapy of choice. When both brain and lung lesions are detected simultaneously, if both lesions are resectable, craniotomy is done first and thoracotomy shortly thereafter, unless extenuating circumstances (e.g., massive hemoptysis) dictate otherwise. If either the lung or brain lesion is suspected to be unresectable, surgical therapy is directed first to the site where resectability is questioned most; otherwise therapy by nonsurgical means is recommended.

We favor postoperative whole-brain irradiation for all patients who have had resected brain metastases because of its potential ability to sterilize the tumor bed, even in patients who have had an apparent complete surgical excision. An American cooperative group randomized trial is currently assessing the value of postresection whole-brain irradiation compared with no further treatment.

Survival. The 1-year survival of 55 percent, and the mean survival of 2.3 years reported by Magilligan, et al. (1986) was similar to ours (Burt, et al., 1992). The overall 5-year survival rate for such patients approaches 20 percent. Surgical therapy should be offered to patients with single surgically accessible brain metastases, no evident systemic disease elsewhere, and a primary cancer confined to the lung.

Other Metastatic Sites. Frequently patients with surgically resectable lung cancer have a solitary distant metastasis on routine preoperative surveys. Frequent sites of such solitary lesions include the lung, adrenal glands, and bone.

Lung. Despite the possibility of a second lesion being a metastatic deposit, many of these second lesions represent synchronous primary tumors and should be considered as such, considering resection of both tumors whenever possible. The long-term results of those patients with solitary lung metastases suggests that many patients are salvaged. Deslauriers, et al. (1989a) reviewed the solitary metastatic lesions identified in resected specimens and reported a 22 percent 5-year survival rate. Similarly in those patients with synchronous primary pulmonary metastases, about 25 percent have long-term survival when treated surgically.

Adrenal Gland. Solitary adrenal metastases are being detected with increasing frequency because of the routine upper abdominal CT scanning in the preoperative workup (Sandler, et al., 1982; Nielsen, et al., 1982; Burt, et al., 1993; Allard, et al., 1990). We and others have offered resection of the primary tumor and the solitary metastatic focus if both are complete resectable (Twomey, et al., 1982; Raviv, et al., 1990; Reyes, et al., 1990). The long-term results of such aggressive therapy are unknown, although 5-year survivors have been reported, whereas none have been reported with nonsurgical therapy.

Bone and Other Sites. It is rare for truly solitary metastases to occur in the bone, liver, and other common metastatic sites, such as the skin. However, if thorough preoperative staging procedures do not reveal any other sites of metastases and if both lesions (primary and solitary metastatic focus) are completely resectable, surgical therapy is offered if the risks are low.

Small Cell Lung Cancer

It is now well accepted that surgical resection used alone is not curative in most patients with small cell lung cancer. However, patients with small peripheral lesions without lymph node metastases (T1N0 and T2N0) benefit from resection. In most retrospective analyses, postoperative chemotherapy appears to improve this result. A small number of patients with more locally advanced tumors are also inadvertently treated surgically at the outset because of unknown or mistaken histologic types. This group should receive postoperative chemotherapy and irradiation, according to standard protocols for the therapy of small cell lung cancer. The overall survival rate of these patients is at least equivalent to that seen in nonoperated patients treated by chemotherapy and irradiation alone, if not somewhat improved (Shepherd, et al., 1991; Shah, et al., 1992).

The rationale for surgery in limited small cell carcinoma stems from the fact that 85 percent of patients present with a recurrence following standard nonsurgical treatment, 50 percent of these in the chest despite mediastinal irradiation. However, the role of surgery in such patients, in those who do not respond to chemotherapy, or in those who have recurrences locally after an initial response is still unclear. There is no evidence to date that surgery in these patients has any survival advantage, and further study is necessary.

We believe adjuvant systemic therapy is indicated in all patients with resected tumors to eradicate residual micrometastases. In all the adjuvant chemotherapy trials reported by the Veterans Administration Surgical Adjuvant Group (Higgins, 1972), patients who received postresection chemotherapy appear to have done better than those who did not.

There is no clear benefit from surgery in the presence of clinically evident regional lymph node metastases. Eleven patients with involvement of the mediastinal lymph nodes (N2) were treated surgically by Meyer (1987). All patients had relapses and died of their disease. Others, however, reported success with induction therapy plus surgery (Shepherd, et al., 1989; Salazar and Creech, 1980).

Initial chemotherapy appears not to provide any more benefit than does initial surgery. The experience of the Toronto Lung Oncology Group with primary surgical therapy followed by chemotherapy and irradiation in 44 patients with N1 or N2 disease demonstrated no significant survival advantage in this group of patients when compared with patients treated by chemotherapy followed by surgery (Ginsberg, 1989). Osterlind, et al. (1989) also showed no influence on survival of surgical resection prior to chemotherapy in operable patient. Surgery does not seem to be beneficial in patients who do not respond to chemotherapy, unless the tissue diagnosis is questioned.

A combined intergroup prospective trial (Lung Cancer Study Group, Eastern Cooperative Oncology Group, and European Organization for the Research and Treatment of Lung Cancer) is currently evaluating, in a randomized fashion, the survival advantage of chemotherapy and radiation versus neoadjuvant chemotherapy plus surgery in potentially resectable limited small cell carcinoma (Ginsberg, 1989). Approximately 150 patients have been entered and randomized into the study; early analyses suggest no benefit for surgical resection for clinically evident N2 small cell lung cancer. Neoadjuvant chemotherapy followed by surgery or irradiation and surgery for local recurrence are currently reserved for highly selected patients with minimal local disease.

Palliative Resections

For surgery to be effective in controlling lung cancer, it must be complete and potentially curative. The role of surgery for the palliation of patients with unresectable tumors is debatable. There are specific situations, such as an unremitting lung abscess distal to an obstructing tumor, massive hemoptysis, or painful invasion of the chest wall (ribs or vertebrae) that have led surgeons to consider and perform palliative or incomplete resections in the hope of improving the patient's symptoms.

Lung Abscess

An unresolving lung abscess, either caused by a necrotizing tumor (usually a squamous cell carcinoma) or a lung abscess distal to an obstructing tumor, rarely requires surgical resection. Other options, such as endobronchial laser therapy to relieve the proximal obstruction followed by external radiotherapy or percutaneous drainage of the abscess, usually suffice to alleviate the symptoms. However, if complete resection is probable, a surgical approach should be considered. Otherwise the lesser measures described may relieve all symptoms and result in satisfactory palliation without noncurative surgery.

Massive Hemoptysis

Massive uncontrolled hemoptysis is a rare feature of untreated lung cancer. Most frequently it is the result of the development of a vascular-bronchial fistula following radiotherapy. In most of these instances, exsanguination and/or suffocation lead to the instantaneous death of the patient. On occasion persisting but significant hemoptysis allows time to control the situation. Bronchoscopic treatment by laser coagulation or the placement of an endobronchial blocker or bronchial artery embolization by percutaneous angiography may relieve the problem. Rarely a thoracotomy is indicated, despite the tumor's unresectability. In completely unresectable cases, hilar stripping of all vessels from the bronchi may relieve the problem. Occasionally a palliative resection is required to control the bleeding.

Chest Wall Invasion

When a patient with an otherwise unresectable tumor as a result of extensive nodal involvement or distant metastases presents with excruciating chest wall pain caused by invasion of the ribs or vertebrae, consideration is occasionally given to resection of the primary tumor for palliative purposes, combining incomplete resections with brachytherapy. In most cases it is preferable to use other nonsurgical measures, such as external beam irradiation or narcotics and even a rhizotomy if necessary. However, on rare occasions, when thoracic vertebrae are invaded and destroyed, causing extradural compression, attempts at resection of the primary tumor invading the vertebra together with vertebral body resection have been used, with or without the addition of brachytherapy, to protect the spine from high-dose external irradiation. Short-term pain relief can be obtained in this fashion. Unfortunately, in most instances, the tumor recurs within 3 to 6 months. The palliative benefit obtained by these surgical approaches has never been prospectively compared with that of less aggressive alternatives for pain control.

In summary palliative resections should be avoided when less aggressive nonsurgical approaches are available that provide similar palliative results.

POSTOPERATIVE MORBIDITY AND MORTALITY RATES

Because most reported cures in carcinoma of the lung have occurred in patients treated surgically, it is natural to want to expand the role of surgery, either alone or combined with radiation, chemotherapy, or both. Many physicians are justifiably concerned with the postoperative mortality figures of 5, 10, and 25 percent quoted in the literature, along with an equally high incidence of nonfatal complications.

Proper case selection and careful preoperative and perioperative management can minimize postoperative complications. Major complications occur in nearly 10 percent of the patients with stage I or II disease and in 20 percent of those requiring extended resections for the treatment of locally advanced tumors (stage III) (Deslauriers, et al., 1989b).

A review of our own case material was undertaken to find out what the complication rates of surgery were. The records of 961 consecutive patients treated surgically for carcinoma of the lung were reviewed (Nagasaki, et al., 1982). The effect of various factors on the incidence of postoperative complications was assessed. The variables evaluated included age, sex, cardiopulmonary status, cell type, stage of disease, and type of procedure performed.

The postoperative course was uneventful in 81 percent of the patients, 8 percent had minor complications, 9 percent had major complications, and 2 percent died. Most of the complications were cardiorespiratory. The high-risk factors identified included old age, a restricted pulmonary reserve, and the need for pneumonectomy. The low incidence of mortality and morbidity observed was attributed to careful preoperative evaluation, selection of the appropriate surgical procedure, and the use of routine preoperative physiotherapy for all patients.

The Lung Cancer Study Group analyzed 2,000 consecutive resections for lung cancer and reported an overall postoperative mortality rate of 3.3 percent (Ginsberg, et al., 1983). More recent retrospective analyses confirm that pneumonectomy carries an overall 6.7 percent mortality rate, whereas lobectomy and lesser resections should not exceed a 2 percent postoperative mortality figure. To minimize complications a lesser resection may be considered in elderly patients and in all physiologically compromised persons who present an increased risk for surgery.

Specific Considerations

Intraoperative Tumor Spillage

Transgression of the tumor with spillage of cells intraoperatively theoretically could lead to pleural implants and local recurrence. If such tumor spillage occurs, the hemithorax should be copiously irrigated with large quantities of saline. Whether cell lysing agents (e.g., hypertonic saline, water, absolute alcohol, or chemotherapeutic agents) have any role to play in such irrigations is unknown.

Positive Resection Margins

Bronchial, vascular, and close-proximity margins should be always monitored by frozen-section analysis at the time of surgery. Reresection to negative margins is advised whenever a positive margin is identified. Although a 2-cm bronchial resection margin is ideal, we accept a negative margin, no matter the distance from the tumor. In situ disease at the resection margin carries a much better prognosis than that caused by invasive disease or submucosal or adventitial lymphatic involvement (Kaiser, et al., 1989).

Perioperative Blood Transfusion

Retrospective data has not confirmed the adverse prognostic effect of perioperative blood transfusions in the long-term survival of patients with resected lung cancers. Tartter, et al. (1984) reported that perioperative blood transfusion adversely affects the prognosis after the resection of stage I nonsmall cell lung cancer. In 165 patients with stage I disease, using disease-free survival rates as the end point, they found a significantly decreased disease-free survival rate in transfused patients. Hyman, et al. (1985) also reported a significantly increased relative risk of dying in transfused patients among their 105 patients stage I or II resected lung cancer.

To determine the impact of perioperative transfusion on the recurrence-free interval, the status of 352 patients treated by resection for stages I and II nonsmall cell lung cancer at Memorial Sloan-Kettering Cancer Center was investigated (Keller, et al., 1988). The recurrence rate was not significantly different in transfused patients compared with those who received no blood, even when stratified for stage. Furthermore the number of units transfused was not associated with the time to tumor recurrence. Our results did not support the contention that perioperative blood transfusion is associated with a decreased recurrence-free interval. Despite this we avoid unnecessary blood transfusions and encourage autologous blood donations whenever possible.

Lobectomy Versus Pneumonectomy

Intraoperatively, especially with central lesions by virtue of the primary tumor or involved lymph nodes, a decision has to be made whether a lobectomy or pneumonectomy should be performed. Incomplete resections never cure. Before considering a lobectomy complete, all resection margins should be confirmed by frozen-section analysis. The "sump" lymph nodes lying on the pulmonary artery between the upper and lower lobes should be examined. If there is any question that these contain tumor, indicating that a larger resection (e.g., pneumonectomy) is required, frozen-section analysis of such lymph nodes should be performed. When performing an upper lobectomy, involvement of the sump lymph nodes between the upper and lower lobes necessitates a completion pneumonectomy. Following right lower lobectomy, involvement of the sump nodes around the middle lobe requires the addition of a middle lobectomy, necessitating a bilobectomy with reresection. Any lymph involvement proximal to the upper lobe takeoff along the mainstem bronchi necessitates pneumonectomy, as does involvement of the lymph nodes around the main pulmonary artery. In all instances the surgeon must remember that there is one good chance to cure the patient, and a complete resection is required for this.

Local Recurrence Following Initial Pulmonary Resection

Occasionally when patients have recurrences, their disease relapses only in the local site, either by virtue of a previous incomplete resection or occult intrapulmonary lymph node disease in the remaining lung. Close follow-up of resected patients is required to detect such local recurrences. Whenever these occur, the patient should be reinvestigated. If no evidence of distant metastatic spread is present and mediastinal lymph node involvement is absent, completion pneumonectomy is the best possible treatment if the patient has sufficient pulmonary reserve and the lesion is suitable for this treatment. Gregoire, et al. (1993) recently analyzed the results of such completion pneumonectomy. Although the operative mortality rate was higher than expected for standard pneumonectomy (10 versus 5 to 7 percent), a significant number of patients can be salvaged with this approach.

COMMENTS AND CONTROVERSIES

Role of Thoracoscopic Surgery

The role of video-assisted thoracoscopic surgery in the management of lung cancer is still being investigated in many centers. Certainly it appears that limited resections (less than lobectomy) should be reserved for severely compromised patients. Whether thoracoscopic surgery allows an adequate resection is as yet unknown. We are extremely concerned that local recurrence will be a significant problem if this technique is used. We certainly prefer segmentectomy rather than wedge resection whenever possible.

Whether or not video-assisted thoracoscopic surgery has value versus open thoracotomy in performing lobectomy and adequate mediastinal nodal staging has yet to be determined. The cost effectiveness of this approach has not as yet been demonstrated.

Surgery for T4 and N3 Disease

Surgeons continue to explore the limits of potential resection and the curability of lung cancer. There is no doubt that the occasional selected individual with a T4 tumor can be totally cured if a complete resection can be performed. Despite many attempts by surgeons to extend the limits of resection for T4 disease, it does not appear that more than a few patients with such locally advanced tumors will benefit from surgical resection. Whether or not "downstaging" by using induction chemo- or radiotherapy may be of value in this stage of disease has yet to be defined.

Induction Chemotherapy in Patients with Earlier Stage, Poor Prognostis Disease

The result of surgical resection for stage II and patients with poor prognostis stage I disease (e.g., T2N0 greater than 5-cm lesions) led investigators to determine the role of adjuvant chemotherapy and radiotherapy for these patients. Neither approach appears to be beneficial, although postoperative radiotherapy decreases local recurrence rates. The long-term survival of such patients is not affected by adjuvant treatment. With the encouraging results of induction therapy in more advanced disease, it would be worthwhile to investigate the role of such treatment in these poor prognosis, earlier stage tumors. An aborted attempt was made at a nationwide study to investigate this approach, but it failed because of lack of accrual. We think it is warranted for individual institutions to develop phase II trials to investigate this combined modality therapy.

Mediastinal Lymph Node Dissection

There is no doubt that routine mediastinal lymph node dissections provide the best surgical staging at the time of operation and may on occasion contribute to long-term survival in patients with occult N2 disease. The role of extending this lymph node dissection in patients with N3 disease to include two-field lymphadenectomies (mediastinal and cervical) is being explored by our Japanese colleagues. On occasion it does appear that, with occult N3 disease, long-term survival using this approach is possible. Most patients, however, are also treated with adjuvant chemoradiotherapy. Whether or not surgical treatment of N3 disease by either induction chemotherapy, chemoradiotherapy, and/or extended lymphadenectomy will ever be proved to be beneficial for patients is unknown.

N.M.
R.J.G.

KEY REFERENCES

Cortese DA, Pairolero PC, Bergstralh EJ et al: Roentgenographically occult lung cancer. A ten-year experience. J Thorac Cardiovasc Surg 86:373, 1983

Ginsberg RJ: Limited resection in the treatment of stage I non-small cell lung cancer; An overview. Chest 96(suppl):50S, 1989

Martini N, Burt ME, Bains MS et al: Survival after resection in stage II non-small cell lung cancer. Ann Thorac Surg 54:460, 1992

Martini N, Kris MG, Flehinger BJ et al: Preoperative chemotherapy for stage IIIa(N2) lung cancer. The Sloan-Kettering experience with 136 patients. Ann Thorac Surg 55:1365, 1993

McCaughan BC, Martini N, Bains MS, McCormack P: Chest wall invasion of carcinoma of the lung: therapeutic and prognostic implications. J Thorac Cardiovasc Surg 89:836, 1985

These key references summarize the current state of the art in the surgical treatment of lung cancer. They include the best treatment by stage and focus on multimodality therapy in the more advanced stages of disease. They should be valuable references for the practicing clinician.

REFERENCES

Alison PR: Intrapericardial approach to the lung root in the treatment of bronchial carcinoma by dissection pneumonectomy. J Thorac Surg 15:99, 1946

Allan CI, Smith FJ: Primary carcinoma of the lung with report of case treated by operation. Surg Gynecol Obstet 55:151, 1932

Allard P, Yankaskas BC, Fletcher RH et al: Sensitivity and specificity of computed tomography for the detection of adrenal metastatic lesions among 91 autopsied lung cancer patients. Cancer 66:457, 1990

American Cancer Society: Cancer Facts and Figures—1994. American Cancer Society, Atlanta, 1994

Brunn HB: Surgical principles underlying one-stage lobectomy. Arch Surg 18:490, 1929

Burkes R, Ginsberg RJ, Shepherd M et al: Neo-adjuvant trial with MVP (mitomycin-C + vindesine + cisplatin) chemotherapy for stage III (T1-3, N2 M0) unresectable non-small cell lung cancer (NSCLC). Proc Am Soc Clin Oncol 8:221, 1989

Burkes RL, Ginsberg RJ, Shepard FA et al: Induction chemotherapy with mitomycin, vindesine, and cisplatin for stage III unresectable non-small-cell lung cancer: results of the Toronto phase II trial. J Clin Oncol 10:580, 1992

Burt M, Wronski M, Arbit E et al: Resection of brain metastases from non-small cell lung carcinoma: results of therapy. J Thorac Cardiovasc Surg 103:399, 1992

Burt ME, Heelan R, Coit D et al: Prospective evaluation of unilateral adrenal metastases in patients with operable non-small cell lung cancer: impact of magnetic resonance imaging. J Thorac Cardiovasc Surg 107:584, 1994

Burt ME, Pomerantz AH, Bains MS et al: Results of surgical treatment of stage III lung cancer invading the mediastinum. Surg Clin North Am 67:987, 1987

Chardak WM, MacCallun JD: Pancoast tumor (5 yr survival without recurrence or metastases following radical resection and postoperative irradiation). J Thorac Surg 31:535, 1956

Churchill E, Belsey HR: Segmental pneumonectomy in bronchiectasis. Ann Surg 109:481, 1939

Churchill ED: The surgical treatment of carcinoma of the lung. J Thorac Surg 2:254, 1933

Coleman FP: Primary carcinoma of the lung with invasion of ribs: pneumonectomy and simultaneous block resection of chest wall. Ann Surg 126:156, 1947

Warram J (collaborative study): Preoperative irradiation of cancer of the lung: final report of a therapeutic trial. Cancer 36:914, 1975

Dartevelle TG, Chapelier AR, Macchiarini P et al.: Anterior transcervical-thoracic approach for radical resection of lung tumors invading the thoracic inlet. J Thorac Cardiovasc Surg 105:1025, 1993

Davies HM: Recent advances in the surgery of the lung and pleura. Br J Surg 1:228, 1913–1914

Deslauriers J: Involvement of the main carina. p. 139. In Delarue NC, Eschapasse H (eds): International Trends in General Thoracic Surgery. WB Saunders, Philadelphia, 1985

Deslauriers J, Brisson J, Cartier R et al: Carcinoma of the lung: evaluation of satellite nodules as a factor influencing prognosis after resection. J Thorac Cardiovasc Surg 97:504, 1989a

Deslauriers J, Ginsberg RJ, Dubois P et al: Current operative morbidity associated with elective surgical resection for lung cancer. Can J Surg 32:335, 1989b

Dillman RO, Seagran SL, Propert KJ et al: A randomized trial of induction chemotherapy plus high-dose radiation versus radiation alone in stage III non-small-cell lung cancer. N Engl J Med 323:940, 1990

Edell ES, Cortese DA: Bronchoscopic localization and treatment of occult lung cancer. Chest 96:919, 1989

Faber LP, Bonomi PD: Neoadjuvant treatment in locally advanced non-small cell lung cancer. Semin Surg Oncol 6:255, 1990

Faber LP, Jensik RJ, Kittle CF: Results of sleeve lobectomy for bronchogenic carcinoma in 101 patients. Ann Thorac Surg 37:279, 1984

Faber LP, Kittle CF, Warren WH et al: Preoperative chemotherapy and irradiation for stage III non-small cell lung cancer. Ann Thorac Surg 47:669, 1989

Ferguson MK, MacMahon H, Little AG et al: Regional accuracy of computed tomography of the mediastinum in staging of lung cancer. J Thorac Cardiovasc Surg 91:498, 1986

Gaissert HA, Mathisen DJ, Grillo HC et al: Comparison of survival and lung function following sleeve lobectomy and pneumonectomy for lung cancer. Presented at the 73rd Annual Meeting of the American Association for Thoracic Surgery, Chicago, April 25–28, 1993

Ginsberg RJ: Surgery and small cell lung cancer—an overview. Lung Cancer 5:232, 1989

Ginsberg RJ, Hill LD, Eagan RT et al: Modern thirty-day operative mortality for surgical resections in lung cancer. J Thorac Cardiovasc Surg 86:498, 1983

Ginsberg R, Rubinstein L, Lung Cancer Study Group: A randomized trial of lobectomy versus limited resection in patients with T1N0 non-small cell lung cancer (abstr). Lung Cancer 7:83, 1991

Graham EA, Singer JJ: Successful removal of the entire lung for carcinoma of the bronchus. JAMA 101:1371, 1933

Gralla RJ, Kris MG, Martini N et al: Adjuvant chemotherapy approaches in non-small cell lung cancer. p. 147. In Salmon SE (ed): Adjuvant Therapy of Cancer. Grune & Stratton, Orlando, 1987

Graves WG, Martinez MJ, Carter PL et al: The value of computed tomography in staging bronchogenic carcinoma: a changing role for mediastinoscopy. Ann Thorac Surg 40:57, 1985

Gregoire J, Deslauriers J, Guojin L, Rouleau J: Indications, risks, and results of completion pneumonectomy. J Thorac Cardiovasc Surg 105:918, 1993

Hata E, Hayakawa K, Miyamoto H et al: The incidence and prognosis of the contralateral mediastinal node involvement of the left lung cancer patients who underwent bilateral mediastinal dissection and pulmonary resection through a median sternotomy (abstr). Lung Cancer 4:A87, 1988

Hayata Y, Kato, Konaka C et al: Photoradiation therapy with hematoporphyrin derivative in early and stage I lung cancer. Chest 86:169, 1984

Higgins GA: Use of chemotherapy as an adjuvant to surgery for bronchogenic carcinoma. Cancer 30:1383, 1972

Hilaris BS, Martini N: Multimodality therapy of superior sulcus tumors. p. 113. In Bonica J (ed): Advances in Pain Research and Therapy. Raven Press, New York, 1982

Hilaris BS, Martini N: Interstitial brachytherapy in cancer of the lung: a 20-year experience. Int J Radiat Oncol Biol Phys 5:1951, 1979

Hilaris BS, Martini N, Wong GY, Nori D: Treatment of superior sulcus tumors (pancoast tumor). Surg Clin North Am 67:965, 1987

Holmes EC, Gail M, Lung Cancer Study Group: Surgical adjuvant therapy for stage II and III adenocarcinoma and large cell undifferentiated carcinoma. J Clin Oncol 4:710, 1986

Hyman NH, Foster RS Jr, DeMeules JE, Costanza MC: Blood transfusions and survival after lung cancer resection. Am J Surg 149:502, 1985

Izibicki JR, Thetter O, Habekost M et al: Radical systematic mediastinal lymphadenectomy in non-small cell lung cancer: a randomized trial. B J Surg 81:229, 1994

Jensik RJ: Miniresection of small peripheral carcinomas of the lung. Surg Clin North Am 67:951, 1987

Jensik RJ, Faber LP, Kittle CF et al: Survival in patients undergoing tracheal sleeve pneumonectomy for bronchogenic carcinoma. J Thorac Cardiovasc Surg 84:489, 1982

Jensik RJ, Faber LP, Milloy FJ, Monson DO: Segmental resection for lung cancer. A fifteen year experience. J Thorac Cardiovasc Surg 66:563, 1973

Kaiser LR, Fleshner P, Keller S, Martini N: The significance of extramucosal residual tumor at the bronchial resection margin. Ann Thorac Surg 47:265, 1989

Keller SM, Groshen S, Martini N, Kaiser LR: Blood transfusion and lung cancer recurrence. Cancer 62:606, 1988

Kris M, Cohen E, Gralla R: An analysis of 134 phase II trials in non-small cell lung cancer (abstr). p. 39. In Proceedings of the IV World Conference on Lung Cancer, Toronto, Canada, 1985a

Kris MG, Gralla RJ, Clark RA et al: Consecutive dose finding trials adding lorazepam to the combination of metoclopramide plus dexamethasone: improved subjective effectiveness over the combination of diphenhydramine plus metoclopramide plus dexamethasone. Cancer Treat Rep 69:1257, 1985b

Kris MG, Gralla RJ, Martini N et al: Preoperative and adjuvant chemotherapy in patients with locally advanced non-small cell lung cancer. Surg Clin North Am 67:1051, 1987

Kulka F, Forai I: The segmental and apical resection of primary lung cancer. p. 81. In Proceedings of the IV World Conference on Lung Cancer, Toronto, Canada, 1985

Lam S, MacAulay C, Hung J et al: Detection of dysplasia and carcinoma in situ with a lung imaging fluorescence endoscopic device. J Thorac Cardiovasc Surg 105:1035, 1993

Lung Cancer Study Group: Postoperative T1N0 non-small cell lung cancer. Squamous versus nonsquamous recurrences. J Thorac Cardiovasc Surg 94:349, 1987

Lung Cancer Study Group: Effects of postoperative mediastinal radiation on completely resected stage II and stage III epidermoid cancer of the lung. N Engl J Med 315:1377, 1986

Lynch TJ Jr, Clark JR, Kalish LA et al: Continuous-infusion cisplatin, 5-fluorouracil, and bolus methotrexate in the treatment of advanced non-small cell lung cancer. Cancer 70:1880, 1992

Magilligan DJ Jr, Duvernoy C, Malik G et al: Surgical approach to lung cancer with solitary cerebral metastasis: twenty-five years' experience. Ann Thorac Surg 42:360, 1986

Martini N: Rationale for surgical treatment of brain metastasis in non-small cell lung cancer. Ann Thorac Surg 42:357, 1986

Martini N, Bains MS, McCormack PM et al: Surgical Treatment in non-small cell carcinoma of the lung: the Memorial Sloan-Kettering experience. p. 111. In Hoogstraten B, Addis BJ, Hansen HH et al (eds): (UICC) Current Treatment of Cancer, Lung Tumors. Springer-Verlag, Heidelberg, 1988a

Martini N, Flehinger BJ: The role of surgery in N2 lung cancer. Surg Clin North Am 67:1037, 1987

Martini N, Flehinger BJ, Zaman MB, Beattie EJ Jr: Results of resection in non-oat cell carcinoma of the lung with mediastinal lymph node metastases. Ann Surg 198:386, 1983

Martini N, Heelan R, Westcott J: Comparative merits of conventional, computed tomographic and magnetic resonance imaging in assessing mediastinal involvement in surgically confirmed lung carcinoma. J Thorac Cardiovasc Surg 90:639, 1985

Martini N, Kris MG, Gralla RJ et al: The effects of preoperative chemotherapy on the resectability of non-small cell lung carcinoma with mediastinal lymph node metastases (N2M0). Ann Thorac Surg 45:370, 1988b

Martini N, McCaughan BC, McCormack P, Bains MS: Lobectomy for stage I lung cancer. p. 171. In Kittle CF (ed): Current Controversies in Thoracic Surgery. WB Saunders, Philadelphia, 1986

Martini N, Melamed MR: Occult carcinomas of the lung. Ann Thorac Surg 30:215, 1980

Mathey J, Binet JP, Galey JJ et al: Tracheal and tracheobronchial resections: Technique and results in 20 cases. J Thorac Cardiovasc Surg 51:1, 1966.

McCormack PM, Bains MS, Beattie EJ Jr, Martini N: New trends in skeletal reconstruction after resection of chest wall tumors. Ann Thorac Surg 31:45, 1981

McCormack PM, Bains MS, Martini N et al: Methods of skeletal reconstruction following resection of lung carcinomas invading the chest wall. Surg Clin North Am 67:979, 1987

McCormack P, Martini N: Primary lung cancer. N Y State J Med 80:618, 1980

Mehran R, Deslauriers J, Guojin L et al: Survival related to nodal status after sleeve resection for primary lung cancer. J Thorac Cardiovasc Surg 107:1087, 1994

Meyer JA: Indications for surgical treatment in small cell carcinoma of the lung. Surg Clin North Am 67:1103, 1987.

Mountain CF: Prognostic implication of the international staging system for lung cancer. Semin Oncol 15:236, 1988.

Mountain CF: The new international staging system for lung cancer. Surg Clin North Am 67:925, 1987.

Nagasaki F, Flehinger BJ, Martini N: Complications of surgery in the treatment of carcinoma of the lung. Chest 82:25, 1982.

Naruke T, Goya T, Tsuchiya R, Suemasu K: Prognosis and survival in resected lung carcinoma based on the new international staging system. J Thorac Cardiovasc Surg 96:440, 1988a

Naruke T, Goya T, Tsuchiya R, Suemasu K: Extended radical operation for N2 left lung cancer through median sternotomy (abstr). Lung Cancer 4(suppl):A87, 1988b

Nielsen ME Jr, Heaston DK, Dunnick NR, Korobkin M: Preoperative CT evaluation of adrenal glands in non-small cell bronchogenic carcinoma. AJR 139:317, 1982

Oho K, Ogawa I, Amemiya R et al: Indications for endoscopic Nd-YAG laser surgery in the trachea and bronchus. Endoscopy 15:302, 1983

Osterlind K, Hansen M, Hansen HH, Dombemowsky P: Influence of surgical resection prior to chemotherapy on long-term results in small cell lung cancer. A study of 150 operable patients. Eur J Cancer 5:589, 1989

Pairolero PC, Arnold PG: Chest wall tumors. Experience with 100 consecutive patients. J Thorac Cardiovasc Surg 90:367, 1985

Pass HI, Pogrebniak HW, Steinberg SM et al.: Randomized trial of neoadjuvant therapy for lung cancer: interim analysis. Ann Thorac Surg 53:992, 1992

Patchell RA, Cirrincione C, Thaler HT et al: Single brain metastases: surgery plus radiation or radiation alone. Neurology 36:447, 1986

Patchell RA, Tibbs PA, Walsh JW et al: A randomized trial of surgery in the treatment of single metastases to brain. N Engl J Med 322:494, 1990

Patterson GA, Ilves R, Ginsberg RJ et al: The value of adjuvant radiotherapy in pulmonary and chest wall resection for bronchogenic carcinoma. Ann Thorac Surg 34:692, 1982

Paulson DL: The "superior sulcus" lesion. p. 121. Delarue NC, Eschapasse H (eds): International Trends in General Thoracic Surgery. WB Saunders, Philadelphia, 1985

Paulson DL: Combined preoperative irradiation and extended resection for carcinoma in the superior pulmonary sulcus. p. 47. In Bonica JJ, et al (eds): Advances in Pain Research and Therapy. Raven Press, New York, 1982

Paulson DL, Urschel HC Jr: Selectivity in the surgical treatment of bronchogenic carcinoma. J Thorac Cardiovasc Surg 62:554, 1971

Pean J: Chirurgie des poumons. Discussion Ranc Chir Proc Verh Paris 9:72, 1895

Pearson FG: Mediastinal adenopathy—the N2 lesion. p. 104. In

Delarue NC, Eschapasse H (eds): International Trends in General Thoracic Surgery. WB Saunders, Philadelphia, 1985

Piehler JM, Pairolero PC, Weeland LH et al.: Bronchogenic carcinoma with chest wall invasion: factors affecting survival following en-bloc resection. Ann Thorac Surg 34:684, 1982

Price-Thomas C: Conservative resection of the bronchial tree. J R Coll Surg Edinb 1:169, 1956

Raviv G, Klein E, Yellin A et al.: Surgical treatment of solitary adrenal metastases from lung cancer. J Surg Oncol 43:124, 1990

Reyes L, Parvez Z, Nemoto T et al.: Adrenalectomy for adrenal metastasis from lung carcinoma. J Surg Oncol 44:32, 1990

Rosell R, Gomez-Codina J, Camps C et al: A randomized trial comparing preoperative chemotherapy plus surgery with surgery alone in patients with non-small cell lung cancer. N Engl J Med 330:153, 1994

Roth JA, Fosella F, Komaki R et al: A randomized trial comparing perioperative chemotherapy and surgery with surgery alone in resectable Stage IIIA non-small-cell lung cancer. J Nat Cancer Inst 86:673, 1994

Rowland K, Bonomi P, Taylor SG IV et al: Phase II trial of etoposide, cisplatin, 5-FU and concurrent split course radiation in stages 3A and 3B non-small cell lung cancer (NSCLC) (abstr). Proc Am Soc Clin Oncol 7:203, 1988

Rusch VW, Albain KS, Crowley JJ et al: Surgical resection of stage IIIA and stage IIIB non-small cell lung cancer after concurrent induction chemoradiotherapy: a Southwest Oncology Group trial. J Thorac Cardiovasc Surg 105:97, 1993

Salazar OM, Creech RH: "The state of the art" toward defining radiation therapy in the management of small cell bronchogenic carcinoma. Int J Radiat Oncol Biol Phys 6:1103, 1980

Sandler MA, Paerlberg JL, Madrazo BL et al: Computed tomographic evaluation of the adrenal gland in the preoperative assessment of bronchogenic carcinoma. Radiology 145:733, 1982

Sauerbruch F: Die Operation Entfernung von Lungengesch-wulste. Zentralbl Chir 53:852, 1926

Schaake-Koning C, Van Den Bogaert W, Dalesio O et al: Effects of concomitant cisplatin and radiotherapy on inoperable non-small-cell lung cancer. N Engl J Med 326:524, 1992

Shah SS, Thompson J, Goldstraw P: Results of operations without adjuvant therapy in the treatment of small cell lung cancer. Ann Thorac Surg 54:498, 1992

Shahian DM, Neptune WB, Ellis FH: Pancoast tumors: improved survival with preoperative and postoperative radiotherapy. Ann Thorac Surg 43:32, 1987

Shaw RR, Paulson DL, Kee JL Jr: Treatment of the superior sulcus tumor by irradiation followed by resection. Ann Surg 154:29, 1961

Shepherd FA, Ginsberg RJ, Feld R et al: Surgical treatment for limited small-cell lung cancer. J Thorac Cardiovasc Surg 101:385, 1991

Shepherd FA, Ginsberg RJ, Patterson GA et al: A prospective for adjuvant surgical resection after chemotherapy for limited small cell lung cancer. J Thorac Cardiovasc Surg 97:177, 1989

Shields TW, Higgins GA, Lawton R et al: Preoperative x-ray therapy as an adjuvant in the treatment of bronchogenic carcinoma. J Thorac Cardiovasc Surg 59:49, 1970

Strauss GM, Herndon JE, Sherman DD et al: Neoadjuvant chemotherapy and radiotherapy followed by surgery in stage IIIA non-small cell carcinoma of the lung: report of a Cancer and Leukemia Group B phase II study. J Clin Oncol 10:1237, 1992

Tartter PE, Burrows L, Kirschner P: Perioperative blood transfusion adversely affects prognosis after resection of stage I (subset N0) non-oat cell lung cancer. J Thorac Cardiovasc Surg 88:659, 1984

Taylor SG IV, Trybula M, Bonomi PD et al: Simultaneous cisplatin-fluorouracil infusion and radiation followed by surgical resection in regionally localized stage III, non-small cell lung cancer. Ann Thorac Surg 43:87, 1987

Thompson DT: Tracheal resection with left lung anastomosis following right pneumonectomy. Thorax 21:560, 1966

Twomey P, Montgomery C, Clark O: Successful treatment of adrenal metastases from large-cell carcinoma of the lung. JAMA 248:581, 1982

Vogt-Moykopf I, Fritz TH, Meyer G et al: Bronchoplastic and angioplastic operation in bronchial carcinoma: long-term results of a retrospective analysis from 1973 to 1983. Int Surg 71:211, 1986

Warren WH, Faber LP: Segmentectomy vs. lobectomy in patients with stage I pulmonary carcinoma: five year survival and patterns of intrathoracic recurrence. J Thorac Cardiovasc Surg 107:1087, 1994

Watanabe Y, Ichihashi T, Iwa T: Median sternotomy as an approach for pulmonary surgery. Thorac Cardiovasc Surg 36:227, 1988

Williams DE, Pairolero PC, Davis CS et al: Survival of patients surgically treated for stage I lung cancer. J Thorac Cardiovasc Surg 82:70, 1981

Yashar J, Weitberg AB, Glicksman AS et al: Preoperative chemotherapy and radiation therapy for stage IIIa carcinoma of the lung. Ann Thorac Surg 53:445, 1992

28

NON-SMALL CELL LUNG CANCER

Chemotherapy

Frances A. Shepherd

DEFINITION

Lung cancer is now the leading cause of cancer-related death for both men and women in North America (Boring, et al., 1992). Adenocarcinoma, squamous cell carcinoma, and large cell anaplastic carcinoma, referred to collectively as non-small cell lung cancer (NSCLC), together represent more than three-quarters of all pulmonary neoplasms. The relative proportion of these three histologic cell types has changed during the last two decades, and currently, adenocarcinoma is seen most frequently (in approximately 35 percent of patients), followed by squamous (30 percent), and large cell (10 to 15 percent). At the time of initial diagnosis, almost 50 percent of patients with tumors of these cell types have clinically detectable spread beyond the thorax, and a further 10 to 15 percent have locally advanced unresectable tumors. Furthermore, more than 50 percent of patients who undergo surgical resection have recurrences with either localized unresectable disease or hematogenous metastases. This means that more than 80 percent of patients with NSCLC are potential candidates for systemic chemotherapy at some time during the course of their disease. This represents more than 100,000 patients per year in North America.

HISTORICAL NOTE

As the twentieth century draws to a close and we pause to assess the contribution that chemotherapy has made to the management of this disease, the practicing oncologist may be chastened to observe that little, if any, improvement in the survival rate has occurred in the last three to four decades, despite the introduction of many new chemotherapeutic agents during that time. In fact, a recent review of cancer therapy in the United States suggested that the increasing age-adjusted death rate for patients with lung cancer is having a significant negative effect on the rate of cancer-free survival overall (Bailor and Smith, 1986).

Despite the large patient base for clinical trials, the role of systemic chemotherapy in the management of NSCLC remains one of the most controversial issues in medical oncology today (Vokes, et al., 1991). The therapeutic philosophy varies from one extreme of chemotherapy for all patients (Buccheri, 1991) to outright therapeutic nihilism and the view that chemotherapy is unjustified outside a clinical trial (Haskell, 1991). Although this controversy was applied initially only to patients with advanced unresectable tumors, the incorporation of chemotherapy into combined-modality therapeutic programs in early-stage resectable disease has broadened the debate to include virtually all stages of NSCLC.

The application of chemotherapy to NSCLC was reviewed almost a decade ago by Bakowski and Crouch (1983) and Joss, et al. (1984). These authors identified ifosfamide, vindesine, cisplatin, and mitomycin C as the most active agents against NSCLC. Ten years later, these agents still form the nucleus for all combination chemotherapeutic regimens. The first reports of single-agent activity against NSCLC appeared in the 1960s (Green, et al., 1969). These observations quickly led to trials of combination chemotherapy, and in the mid-1970s, encouraging response rates of more than 40 percent were being reported with a variety of regimens (Bitran, et al., 1976; Chahinian, et al., 1979; Eagan, et al., 1977). Sadly, little has changed since that time, and the overall contribution of chemotherapy to the prolongation of a patient's survival is modest in those with NSCLC.

HISTORICAL READINGS

Bailor JC, Smith EM: Progress against cancer! N Engl J Med 314:1226, 1986

Vokes EE, Bitran JD, Vogelzang NJ: Chemotherapy for non-small cell lung cancer. The continuing challenge. Chest 99:1326, 1991

PROGNOSTIC FACTORS

The stage is one of the most important determinants of both prognosis and survival in NSCLC. Several staging systems have been used during the past 30 years, but recently, a new system was proposed jointly by the American Joint Committee on Cancer, the International Union Against Cancer, and the Japanese Cancer Committee (Mountain, 1986). In this staging system, patients with T1N1 tumors are now included in stage II rather than stage I because the survival of all patients with N1 nodal involvement is significantly inferior to that of patients with T1–2N0 tumors. One of the most important improvements in the new system is the subdivision of stage III into stage IIIA (tumors that are potentially surgically resectable for cure) and stage IIIB (unresectable tumors). These new stage groupings provide important prognostic information because they clearly define groups of patients with differing survival rates (Ferguson, 1990).

Although it is clear that stage is an important determinant of survival in NSCLC, several other prognostic factors have been identified that may have a significant influence on the natural history of the disease, the response to therapy, the therapeutically related morbidity and mortality rates, and the overall survival rates. In all studies of chemotherapy for NSCLC, it is crucial, therefore, to define clearly the patient population in the trial and to identify the prognostic variables that may have a significant impact on the results obtained. This is particularly important for the reporting of phase II trials, which represent the most common type of clinical trials in NSCLC published in the literature.

Twenty studies of prognostic factors in NSCLC have been reviewed recently (Maki and Feld, 1991). Direct comparisons between studies are difficult to make for several reasons. Some of the studies focused only on surgical patients, whereas others were restricted only to patients with advanced inoperable disease. The variables chosen for analysis were not uniform between studies, and although all studies used univariate analysis, multivariate analyses were carried out in only 13. Various statistical methods were applied for both univariate and multivariate analyses. Furthermore, four of the seven studies that contained more than 100 patients included patients with small cell histologic types.

Prognostic factors in operable patients will be more important for future trials because chemotherapy is now being applied to earlier stages of NSCLC, as either adjuvant therapy following surgical resection or as preoperative induction therapy in locally advanced disease. An analysis of patients with stage I (including T1N1) disease from the Lung Cancer Study Group (LCSG) trials showed that pathologic subtype and tumor-node-metastasis (TNM) stage were the strongest predictors for recurrence, whereas preoperative performance status and postoperative infection added importantly to the histologic type and TN status with respect to the prediction of overall survival (Gail, et al., 1984). Some, but not all, retrospective reviewers have suggested that the need for postoperative blood transfusions may have a negative effect on recurrence and survival (Keller, et al., 1988).

Most studies of prognostic factors have focused on inoperable patients who have participated in chemotherapy trials and have included patients with locally advanced disease (M0) and hematogenous metastases (M1). It is important to recognize that the patients with stage IV disease in these studies represent a preselected subgroup of those with stage IV disease overall in that they have been considered eligible for clinical chemotherapeutic trials. Patients with adverse prognostic factors, such as poor performance status, severe derangements in hepatic or renal function, brain metastases, etc., have usually been excluded from clinical studies.

A metanalysis of 6,247 patients entered in chemotherapeutic trials in NSCLC identified several variables that were important for the response to therapy (Donnadieu, et al., 1991). The overall and complete response rates correlated strongly with stage or disease extent (limited disease, 39 percent; extensive disease, 25 percent). The response rates were significantly lower for single-agent chemotherapy than for combination chemotherapy, and the best results were obtained when combination chemotherapy included cisplatin, a vinca alkaloid, mitomycin C, or ifosfamide. A review of chemotherapeutic trials in 699 patients with stage IV disease treated by Eastern Cooperative Oncology Group (ECOG) protocols demonstrated lower response rates in patients with liver, bone, and bone marrow involvement and a poor initial performance status (Bonomi, et al., 1989).

With respect to survival, almost all studies have confirmed that the extent of disease (stage) and performance status have a statistically significant impact on the survival rate. Weight loss and an elevated lactic dehydrogenase (LDH) level have also been found to be significant, whereas age and histologic subtype do not seem to alter the survival rate significantly (Maki and Feld, 1991). Female sex has been associated with a longer survival in several studies (Maki and Feld, 1991; Ferguson, et al., 1990). In a retroprospective study of 478 men and 294 women with primary lung cancer, the survival time of women was found to be longer than that of men for all histologic subtypes and all stages of disease at presentation (Ferguson, et al., 1990).

Most large series evaluating prognostic factors have focused on the clinical characteristics of the patients at presentation and the histologic subtypes of their tumors. For patients undergoing surgical resection, adequate tissue is frequently available for more sophisticated in vitro testing, and several laboratory parameters have now been identified that may provide prognostic information in certain subsets of patients. In a retrospective analysis of DNA content and ploidy in 146 cases of resected NSCLC, patients with diploid squamous cell carcinomas survived significantly longer than did those with aneuploid tumors ($P = 0.002$), irrespective of stage (Sahin, et al., 1990). The tumor's proliferative activity, as measured by thymidine labeling index was found to be prognostic in univariate analysis, although in multivariate analysis, stage was found to be significantly more important (Alama, et al., 1990). In some, but not all, studies, the presence of neuroendocrine markers (Berendsen, et al., 1989) and the ability to establish tumor cell lines in vitro have both been associated with an adverse prognosis (Stevenson, et al., 1990; Carney, 1991, 1992). The identification of K-*ras* mutations in tumor cell lines has also been associated with shortened survival times, irrespective of the extent of disease

(Mitsudomi, et al., 1991). Enhanced *ras* expression, which was identified in surgical resection specimens analyzed immunohistochemically, was also found to correlate with shortened survival times (Harada, et al., 1992). It has been observed recently that the survival time of patients with blood type A or AB who had primary tumors that were negative for the blood group antigen A was significantly shorter than that of patients with antigen A-positive tumors (Lee, et al., 1991).

It is clear, therefore, that many variables other than the therapy selected may influence both the response and survival rates in patients with NSCLC.

SINGLE-AGENT THERAPY

With the exception of one study (Bonomi, et al., 1989), all reviews of single-agent chemotherapy for NSCLC have demonstrated a lower response rate and shorter survival time than those for combination chemotherapy (Bakowski and Crouch, 1983; Joss, et al., 1984; Donnadieu, et al., 1991). Nonetheless, the continued evaluation of single agents is crucial for the identification of new active compounds that may have the potential to be incorporated into combination chemotherapeutic regimens. Although several dozen single agents have been evaluated during the last three decades, less than 12 have demonstrated adequate activity to justify their continued use in combination regimens.

Cisplatin and Other Platinum Analogs

Although other chemotherapeutic drugs have demonstrated higher single-agent activity than cisplatin, it remains an im-

---

Single Agents that Have Demonstrated Activity in Non-Small Cell Lung Cancer

Agents with response rates > 15%
  Cisplatin
  Epirubicin (high dose)
  Ifosfamide
  Mitomycin C
  Vinblastine
  Vindesine
Agents with response rates < 15%
  Carboplatin
  Cyclophosphamide
  Doxorubicin
  Etoposide
  5-Fluorouracil
  Methotrexate
Promising new investigational agents
  Camptothecin-11
  Docetaxel
  Edatrexate
  Fotemustine
  Gemcitabine
  Navelbine
  Paclitaxel
  Zeniplatin

---

portant drug in combination chemotherapeutic protocols. In phase II trials, response rates from 6 to 32 percent (average, 20 percent) were achieved when cisplatin was used alone in varying dosing schedules (Bakowski and Crouch, 1983). It may be administered in divided doses over 3 to 5 days or as a single large dose of up to 120 mg/m^2 on a single day. The optimal dose and schedule remain controversial. At least two studies suggest that the high dose (100 to 120 mg/m^2) is superior with respect to both the response (Donnadieu, et al., 1991) and the duration of the response (Gralla, et al., 1981), but this was not confirmed in a recent study undertaken by the Southwest Oncology Group (SWOG) (Gandra, et al., 1991). Cisplatin is one of the most important agents in the therapy of NSCLC, not only because of its significant single-agent activity, but also because it is associated with only modest myelosuppression and has demonstrated both in vivo and in vitro synergy with several other chemotherapeutic agents that are active against NSCLC. For these reasons, it forms the backbone of most combination regimens. Recently it has also been recognized that cisplatin can be administered concurrently with thoracic radiotherapy without undue toxicity (Soresi, et al., 1988).

Other platinum analogs have been evaluated, including carboplatin and iproplatin (Bunn, 1989a; Bonomi, et al., 1989; Green, et al., 1992). Both of these agents have response rates of less than 10 percent in previously untreated patients. Despite a response rate of only 9 percent however, a prospective randomized ECOG study demonstrated significantly prolonged survival for a cohort of patients with stage IV disease who were treated with carboplatin alone compared with other combination regimens (Bonomi, et al., 1989). Carboplatin is associated with less gastrointestinal toxicity, neurotoxicity, and nephrotoxicity, although it is more myelosuppresive than is cisplatin, and this may limit its usefulness in combination regimens.

Zeniplatin is a third-generation platinum complex that has demonstrated greater cytotoxicity to some solid tumor xenographs in vivo than does cisplatin. In a phase II trial of previously untreated patients with advanced NSCLC, zeniplatin 145 mg/m^2 was administered every 21 days with intravenous hydration over 24 hours without mannitol. One patient achieved a complete response, and there were five partial responses (33 percent). The dose-limiting toxicity was neutropenia, which seems to be more severe than that seen with cisplatin (Jones and Smith, 1991).

Ifosfamide

Cyclophosphamide has limited usefulness in the treatment of NSCLC. As a single agent, it has demonstrated response rates of less than 15 percent, and it is seldom used in combination regimens any longer. Ifosfamide is an alkylating agent that can be used in significantly higher doses than its parent compound cyclophosphamide. Although it has been available for clinical use since the early 1970s, hemorrhagic cystitis, which was identified as the dose-limiting toxicity in phase I trials, limited the usefulness of ifosfamide until the introduction of the uroprotective agent mesna. The role of ifosfamide in the therapy of lung cancer was reviewed recently (Johnson, 1990; Eberhardt and Niederle, 1992). It has been evaluated in varying doses and schedules, and as a single agent, it produces responses in more than 20 percent of patients. In lung cancer trials, the administration of ifosfamide at a dose of 1.2 to 2.0 g/m² for 5 consecutive days did not appear to result in response rates higher than those produced by therapy with bolus doses of 4.0 to 5.0 g/m² on day 1 only, despite the higher total dose delivered in the 5-day schedules. Bolus therapy may, however, be associated with slightly greater toxicity.

Vinca Alkaloids

Both vindesine and vinblastine are active against NSCLC. Although in single-therapeutic arm phase II trials, vindesine, which is a semisynthetic analog of vinblastine, has shown slightly higher response rates, it has not been licensed for general use in the United States, and so vinblastine remains the vinca alkaloid most frequently used in combination chemotherapeutic regimens for NSCLC. A recent study comparing the relative usefulness of chemotherapeutic agents used in combination with cisplatin showed no added benefit for vindesine, but there was a significant benefit ($P > 0.001$) for vinblastine (Donnadieu, et al., 1991).

Mitomycin C

Mitomycin C has demonstrated reproducible single-agent activity of 15 to 20 percent when given at maximal single-agent doses. Unfortunately, however, at these high doses, this drug has been associated with pulmonary fibrosis, cumulative marrow suppression, prolonged thrombocytopenia, and the hemolytic uremic syndrome in a small number of patients. Pulmonary toxicity may be reduced by the administration of a steroid with mitomycin (Spain, 1988), and bone marrow toxicity may be avoided by reducing the dose and prolonging the interval between therapeutic courses.

Etoposide

The epipodophyllotoxin etoposide has only modest activity when used as a single agent (Bakowski and Crouch, 1983; Donnadieu, et al., 1991), but because of in vivo and in vitro synergy, it has been used extensively in combination with cisplatin. Recent observations in the therapy of patients with small cell lung cancer (SCLC) suggest that the optimal dose, schedule, and route of administration for etoposide has yet to be determined. A prospective randomized trial demonstrated convincingly that a 5-day schedule was superior to a 1-day schedule of equal doses of etoposide given to patients with SCLC (Slevin, et al., 1989). There is now evidence to suggest that the chronic daily administration of oral etoposide may be better still (DeVore, 1992). Although most studies to date have been in patients with SCLC, at least one trial suggested that similar results may be obtained in NSCLC (Waits, et al., 1992). Five of 25 patients (20 percent) achieved partial responses after two courses of oral etoposide 50 mg/m²/day for 21 consecutive days. Further trials are ongoing in this area.

Other Agents

Other agents with single-agent activity less than 10 percent include cyclophosphamide, lomustine, 5-fluorouracil (5-FU), methotrexate, doxorubicin, and epirubicin. Response rates up to 19 percent may be achieved with epirubicin in a high dose (135 to 150 mg/m²), but this is at the expense of greater myelosuppresion and potentially greater cardiotoxicity. These doses would not be suitable for incorporation into most combination chemotherapeutic regimens (Feld, et al., 1992).

Promising New Single Agents

Edatrexate

Edatrexate is a new water-soluble antifole that reaches higher intracellular concentrations than methotrexate through passive transfer across the cell membrane and undergoes greater conversion to polyglutamate forms within neoplastic cells. In a phase II trial of 20 patients with stage III or IV NSCLC treated with edatrexate 80 mg/m² once weekly for 5 weeks, a 32 percent major objective response rate was observed. Mucositis was the most frequent and dose-limiting toxicity. In contrast, however, another study of 47 patients revealed a response rate of only 11 percent and a similar toxicity profile (Souhami, et al., 1991). Because edatrexate causes minimal myelosuppression, it is a promising agent for use in combination with other chemotherapeutic agents, and comparative trials are currently ongoing (Shum, et al., 1988).

Gemcitabine

Gemcitabine, a pyrimidine antimetabolite, is a new deoxycytidine analog that was synthesized initially as an antiviral agent. In two phase II studies using gemcitabine 800 to 1000 mg/m² week for three doses, conflicting results were obtained. In a North American study, only 1 of 31 patients achieved a partial response, whereas in a similar European study, 15 of 58 (26 percent) of patients achieved partial responses. The differences in these two studies may be explained by differences in the patient populations with respect to histologic type, performance status, age, distribution, and history of prior radiotherapy (Anderson, et al., 1991; Lund, et al., 1991). Because dose-limiting toxicity was not seen at 1000 mg/m², further single-agent studies assessing higher doses are currently ongoing.

Navelbine (Vinorelbine)

Navelbine is a semisynthetic vinca alkaloid that is the only one that is modified at the catharanthine ring rather than the vindoline ring of the molecule (Depierre, et al., 1991). Like other vinca alkaloids, it acts by inhibiting microtubule assembly, and its dose-limiting toxicity is leukopenia and neutropenia. It appears to be significantly less neurotoxic than the other vinca alkaloids are. In a phase II trial of 78 untreated patients with NSCLC, of which 70 were evaluable for response, a partial remission was observed in 23 patients (33 percent). The patients were treated on a weekly schedule, starting at 30 mg/m², and at this dose, approximately one-third of cycles were delayed because of granulocytopenia. An oral formulation is also available, and early phase I studies are active at this time.

Taxanes (Paclitaxel and Docetaxel)

The taxanes exert their antitumor activity by inducing excessive polymerization of tubulin, which interferes with normal mitotic activity. Phase II trials of Paclitaxel have shown single-agent response rates greater than 20 percent in previously untreated patients with NSCLC. Doses ranging from 175 to 250 mg/m^2 infused over 3 to 24 hours every three weeks have been evaluated (Murphy, 1992), but at the higher doses growth factors have been used to reduce myelosuppression. Phase I to II trials of Paclitaxel in combination with other agents are currently ongoing. Docetaxel, a semi-synthetic taxane, has also demonstrated significant single-agent activity against NSCLC (Rigas, 1993; Fossella, 1994) with response rates as high as 21 percent reported, even for patients who have received prior treatment with cisplatin-containing chemotherapy.

Camptothecins (Irinotecan)

The camptothecins are a new family of natural products that exert their anticancer activity through the inhibition of the enzyme topoisomerase I. These compounds form complexes with the enzyme that lead to single-strand breaks in DNA and the inhibition of DNA and RNA synthesis. In a recently reported phase II trial of camptothecin-11 (CPT-11), 150 mg/m^2 weekly in previously untreated patients with NSCLC, 23 of 72 patients (31.9 percent) achieved partial responses (Fukuoka, et al., 1992). The dose-limiting toxicities observed were leukopenia and diarrhea. In a similar study of CPT-11 100 to 125 mg/m^2 weekly, 31.8 percent of 44 patients achieved partial responses (Asakawa, et al., 1991).

Fotemustine

Fotemustine is a new nitrosourea compound that demonstrated activity against squamous cell lung cancer in early phase I trials. In a phase II trial in NSCLC, fotemustine 100 mg/m^2 on days 1 and 8 followed by a 5-week rest period resulted in a 16 percent response rate. This degree of response is encouraging because only patients with poor prognostic factors, including a relapse after prior chemotherapy or brain metastases, were included in the study. Four of 36 previously treated patients responded to therapy, as did 6 of 29 untreated patients (23 percent). The dose-limiting toxicity was thrombocytopenia, and three patients required platelet transfusions (Monnier, et al., 1991).

COMBINATION CHEMOTHERAPY

As is the case in other tumor types, response rates in NSCLC are higher when combination chemotherapy is used compared with single-agent therapy. Before any combination chemotherapeutic regimen can be evaluated, the patient population under study must be assessed carefully. The response rate for patients with locally advanced disease may be as much as twofold higher than that seen when the same regimen is administered to patients with stage IV disease and hematogenous metastases. Even within stage IV, there is a hierarchy of response, with metastatic deposits in the liver or bone much less likely to respond than those in the lung or lymph glands. Finally, other prognostic indicators, such as performance status, sex, degree of weight loss, LDH level, etc., should be assessed. It should also be noted that the response in most patients is a partial response. A complete clinical response is seen in only 10 to 15 percent of patients with

localized disease and less than 5 percent of patients with hematogenous metastases.

Although many chemotherapeutic regimens result in significant responses, the contribution of such therapy to the prolongation of survival remains controversial. In general, survival gains have been small in both locally advanced and disseminated disease trials. Even in the trials that have demonstrated a statistically significant prolongation of survival, it is questionable whether the short weeks or months gained are clinically relevant in view of the potential toxicity and cost of the therapy involved. In advanced disease, chemotherapy is never curative, and the survival curves remain exponential, with no sign of a "plateau" or "tail" on the curve." As chemotherapy is administered in earlier stages of NSCLC, combined modality therapeutic programs should not be considered successful if they result merely in a shift of the survival curve to the left, with the prolongation only of the median survival but without an accompanying increase in the level of the plateau and cure rate.

At this time, it is fair to say that cisplatin forms the cornerstone of most combination chemotherapeutic regimens that are active against NSCLC. The approximate response rates for the common cisplatin-containing regimens and some other current regimens are shown in Table 28-1. The response rates should not be compared directly because most reported trials are nonrandomized phase II studies and contain heterogeneous patient populations with many variations in prognostic variables that may have significant effects on response and survival rates. For individual regimens, the response and survival rates are presented in more detail in the following sections, which discuss the application of chemotherapy to various stages of NSCLC.

ADJUVANT CHEMOTHERAPY FOLLOWING SURGICAL RESECTION FOR STAGES I, II, AND IIIA

The poor survival rates following surgical resection for patients with stage II and III disease has led several groups to investigate the usefulness of adjuvant chemotherapy after complete or partial resection of NSCLC. In general, to be effective in the adjuvant setting, combination chemotherapeutic regimens should result in response rates of greater than 50 percent in patients with advanced disease, and a significant proportion of patients should achieve complete clinical responses. The most active regimens result in responses in only 30 to 40 percent of patients with advanced disease, and complete clinical responses are rare. It is not surprising, therefore, that a major survival advantage has not been seen in most of the prospective randomized trials of adjuvant therapy to date.

The results from several prospective trials of adjuvant chemotherapy are summarized in Table 28-2. The LCSG was formed in 1977 to evaluate the role of adjuvant therapy after surgery for NSCLC. The trials undertaken by this group are particularly important because all patients underwent meticulous mediastinal node sampling at the time of surgery to allow for precise staging. The first chemotherapy trial of the LCSG evaluated postoperative cyclophosphamide, doxorubicin, and cisplatin (CAP) or immunotherapy with bacillus Calmette-Guérin (BCG) in patients with completely resected

Table 28-1. Active Chemotherapeutic Combinations for the Treatment of Non-Small Cell Lung Cancer

Chemotherapeutic Regimen	Range of Response (%)	Reference
Cisplatin or carboplatin-containing regimens		
CAP: Cyclophosphamide, doxorubicin, cisplatin	15–25	Rapp, et al., 1988
BEP: Bleomycin, etoposide, cisplatin	20–40	Osoba, et al., 1985
PV: Cisplatin and a vinca alkaloid, either vinblastine or vindesine	15–30	Bunn, 1989b
MVP: Mitomycin C, vindesine or vinblastine, cisplatin	30–60	Bunn, 1989b
EP: Etoposide, cisplatin	20–30	Bunn, 1989b
FPV: 5-Fluorouracil, cisplatin	15–25	Richards, et al., 1991
FOMi/CAP: 5-Fluorouracil, vincristine, mitomycin C, cyclophosphamide, doxorubicin, cisplatin	10–20	Weick, et al., 1991
CE: Carboplatin, etoposide	10–30	Bunn, 1989a
Ifosfamide-containing regimens		
IM: Ifosfamide, mitomycin C	25–30	Gurney, et al., 1991
IE: Ifosfamide, etoposide	27	Drings, 1989
IP: Ifosfamide, cisplatin	18–35	Drings, 1989
MIP: Mitomycin, ifosfamide, cisplatin	35–50	Cullen, et al., 1988
ICE: Ifosfamide, carboplatin, etoposide	43	Van Zandwijk, et al., 1990
ICE: Ifosfamide, cisplatin, etoposide	35–40	Shepherd, et al., 1992a

stage II or III adenocarcinoma or large cell undifferentiated carcinoma (Holmes, et al., 1986). The recurrence rate was significantly lower in the chemotherapeutic arm. The median survival was approximately 7 months longer, and the 2-year survival rate was also greater, although this did not reach statistical significance by the two-sided log-rank test. This trial has been criticized because it did not have a no-therapy control arm.

In another trial, the LCSG also observed a benefit in patients with incompletely resected tumors who received postoperative CAP and radiotherapy compared with those treated with radiotherapy alone (Lad, et al., 1988). Once again, the median survival time was prolonged by approximately 7 months, but the 3-year survival rate was equal in both therapeutic arms. The last LCSG study evaluated the usefulness of CAP chemotherapy following complete resection of early-stage tumors (T1N1 and T2N0) compared with no additional therapy. This study was disappointing because no improvement was seen for patients treated with CAP with respect to either the median survival or long-term survival time (Feld, 1993). The Finnish lung cancer group has recently completed a similar adjuvant trial of CAP chemotherapy in patients with early stage (T1-3N0) NSCLC (Niirinen, et al., 1992). In contrast to the last LCSG study reported by Feld et al., this study *did* demonstrate a survival advantage for patients in the chemotherapy arm at 5 and 10 years ($P = 0.5$). The

greatest benefit was seen in patients with T2N0 tumors, but because of the small number of patients in this subgroup, the difference did not reach statistical significance (72.5 percent versus 50.3 percent; $P = 0.15$).

When the LCSG trials were initiated more than one decade ago, CAP chemotherapy was believed to be one of the most active regimens for the therapy of NSCLC. A recent study by the National Cancer Institute of Canada (NCIC) demonstrated a higher response rate and longer survival times for patients with extensive disease treated with vindesine and high-dose cisplatin compared with CAP (Rapp, et al., 1988). The results of the NCIC trial led the Montreal Group to evaluate adjuvant vindesine and cisplatin in an attempt to build on the previous LCSG trials. Following resection, patients without lymph node involvement were randomized to the chemotherapy or control group, and patients with nodal disease (N1 and N2) were randomized to receive chemotherapy and radiation or radiation alone (Ayoub, et al., 1991). An interim analysis at a median follow-up time of 22 months showed significant prolongation of disease-free survival only for the patients who achieved 50 percent or more of their intended chemotherapeutic dose intensity ($P = 0.05$). The median survival of this group was approximately 6 months longer than that of the no-chemotherapy group, a result that is similar to that seen in the early LCSG trials (Ayoub, personal communication, 1992). Other platinum-based regimens have

Table 28-2. Randomized Trials of Adjuvant Chemotherapy After Surgical Resection for Non-Small Cell Lung Cancer

Reference	Stage	Therapy	No. Patients	Median Survival	% Survival 1 yr	2 yr	3 yr
Holmes, et al., 1986	II and III completely resected	CAP	62	23 mo	75	41	—
		BCG	68	16 mo	64	30	—
Lad, et al., 1988	I, II, III incompletely resected	CAP-RT	78	20 mo	60	41	24
		RT	86	13 mo	54	32	20
Feld, et al., 1992	T2N0	CAP	136	76 mo	89	80	60 (5 yr)
	T1N1 completely resected	No Rx	133	83 mo	88	73	52 (5 yr)
Niirinen, et al., 1992	T1-3N0 completely resected	CAP	54	NR	95	90	67 (5 yr)
		No Rx	56	NR	90	80	56 (5 yr)

Abbreviations: CAP, cyclophosphamide, doxorubicin, cisplatin; BCG, bacillus Calmette-Guérin; RT, radiotherapy; No Rx, no-therapy control arm, NR, not reached.

been evaluated by the National Kyushu Cancer Centre in Japan, but no improvement in median or overall survival rate was seen in their trial (Ichinose, et al., 1991). Finally, ECOG and the Radiation Therapy Oncology Group (RTOG) are currently conducting a trial of postoperative etoposide and cisplatin plus radiotherapy versus radiotherapy alone in patients with completely resected stages II and IIIA NSCLC.

Although some of these studies have demonstrated a definite biologic effect for adjuvant chemotherapy, the survival gains have been modest at best. At this time, adjuvant chemotherapy should not be considered standard therapy for NSCLC, but future trials with some of the newer regimens are definitely indicated.

CHEMOTHERAPY FOR LOCALLY ADVANCED (STAGE IIIA AND IIIB) DISEASE

Between one-quarter and one-third of patients with NSCLC present with disease that has not spread outside the thorax but is too extensive for surgical resection. The standard management for these patients with locally advanced stages IIIA and IIIB tumors is thoracic irradiation, which results in objective tumor regression in a significant proportion of patients. This is frequently associated with a palliation of symptoms, but few patients are cured. The 5-year survival rate is usually less than 10 percent.

The poor long-term results for patients with stage III disease at presentation clearly indicates an urgent need for the development of clinical research protocols to identify new therapeutic strategies that may prolong the patient's survival and increase the cure rate. The observation that death for most patients with stage III tumors is caused by distant metastases has led to a reevaluation of the role of combined modality therapeutic approaches, which include chemotherapy. The intent of such therapy is to eradicate the micrometastatic deposits that are obviously present at the time of the initial diagnosis, even though they are undetectable clinically. Chemotherapy has the potential to be very active against these small deposits because their growth kinetic parameters should theoretically be faster than those of the primary tumor, with a resultant heightened sensitivity to the effects of these drugs. Furthermore, chemotherapy is likely to be most active against the primary tumor when it is administered at this early stage of the disease before drug-resistant clones have had a chance to emerge. This is confirmed by the observation that the response to chemotherapy is almost twofold higher in patients with locally advanced disease compared with that in patients with clinically detectable hematogenous metastases.

In addition to its systemic effects, there are several ways in which chemotherapy may improve local control. The response to therapy may render a technically unresectable tumor resectable, although this should not be considered the primary end point of such therapy because other therapies may achieve local control without the need for surgery. Chemotherapeutic agents may act as radiation sensitizers when given concurrently with radiotherapy, and radiation has the potential to be more effective when administered sequentially to smaller tumors that have responded to induction chemotherapy.

Sequential Chemotherapy and Radiotherapy

Several trials were initiated in the early 1980s to determine whether the sequential administration of combination chemotherapy and thoracic irradiation could prolong the survival of patients with locally advanced NSCLC. The results of four of these trials are summarized in Table 28-3. In the trial reported by Morton, et al. (1991), a cisplatin-containing regimen was not used, and in the trial of Mattson, et al. (1988) the CAP regimen with low-dose cisplatin was used. Only in the studies of Dillman, et al. (1990) and Le Chevalier, et al. (1992) was cisplatin used at doses of 100 to 120 mg/m^2.

It is disappointing to note that, even in the studies that used high-dose cisplatin, the median survival was just slightly longer than 1 year. Furthermore, despite significant prolongation of the median survival the actual survival gain was less than 1 month for two studies, 2 months for one, and 4 months for the other. The 2-year survival rate was similar in all studies and ranged from 12 to 15 percent for the radiotherapy-alone arms and 20 to 26 percent for the radio- and chemotherapy arms. No survival benefit was seen at 3 years and 5 years

Table 28-3.   Randomized Trials of Radiotherapy with or Without Chemotherapy in Locally Advanced Non-Small Cell Lung Cancer

Reference	Radiotherapeutic Dose (Gy)	Chemotherapeutic Regimen	No. Patients	Median Survival (mo)	% Survival		
					1 yr	2 yr	3 yr
Mattson, et al., 1988	55	—	119	10.3	41	15	11
	55	CAP	119	11.0	41	20	7
Morton, et al., 1991	60	—	58	9.6	43	12	7 (5 yr)
	60	MACC	56	10.4	47	23	5 (5 yr)
Dillman, et al., 1990	60	—	77	9.7	40	13	11
	60	PV	79	13.8	55	26	23
Le Chevalier, et al., 1992	65	—	177	10.0	41	14	4
	65	VCPC	176	12.0	51	21	12
Soresi, et al., 1988	50	—	50	11.0	48	40	?
	50	Weekly P	45	16.0	73	25	?
Schaake-Koning, et al., 1992	55	—	108	?	46	13	2
	55	Weekly P	98	?	44	19	13
	55	Daily P	102	?	54	26	16

Abbreviations: CAP, cyclophosphamide, doxorubicin, cisplatin; MACC, methotrexate, doxorubicin, cyclophosphamide, lomustine; PV, cisplatin, vinblastine; VCPC, vindesine, cyclophosphamide, cisplatin, lomustine; P, cisplatin.

in the Mattson, et al. (1988) and Morton, et al. (1991) studies, respectively, and only the Dillman, et al. (1990) and Le Chevalier, et al. (1992) studies continued to show a small survival advantage beyond the 2-year mark. The Dillman trial was reported by the RTOG and ECOG, and early observations suggest a similar advantage to combination therapy. Only 1- and 2-year results are available at this time, so the long-term benefit of the addition of cisplatin and vinblastine to radiation awaits confirmation from this trial (Sause, 1994).

At this time, therefore, it is still not possible to state conclusively that chemotherapy adds significantly to the long-term survival time and cure rate of patients treated with radiotherapy for locally advanced NSCLC, even though all of the trials demonstrated modest improvements in both median and 2-year survival rates. The studies to date have been small, and investigators should be encouraged to continue this form of research with larger trials as more effective agents and regimens are developed. As has been so clear in the evolution of adjuvant therapy for breast cancer, it will be necessary to undertake large multicenter trials to identify the subgroups of patients who have the potential to benefit most from such combined modality therapy.

Concurrent Chemotherapy and Radiotherapy

The optimal sequence for the administration of chemotherapy and radiation in locally advanced NSCLC has not yet been determined. In the trials described above, chemotherapy was administered before radiation in all trials, and in some, it was continued for responding patients after the radiotherapy had finished. The concurrent administration of chemo- and radiotherapy offers all the benefits of the early administration of systemic therapy with the added potential benefit of improved local control as a result of synergy between the chemotherapeutic agents and the radiotherapy.

Several trials designed primarily to assess the feasibility of the concurrent administration of chemo- and radiotherapy are summarized in Table 28-4. The earliest agent to be evaluated was 5-FU. It was initially administered as a bolus, but in recent studies, it has been administered as a continuous infusion over 72 to 120 hours based on the in vitro observation that the exposure of cells to 5-FU continuously for 24 hours followed by radiation increases cell kill significantly (Byfield, et al., 1982). A similar potentiation of radiation effects has been seen with cisplatin (Douple and Richard, 1982), but the mechanism by which these drugs potentiate radiotherapy has not been established conclusively. Phase II trials of the concurrent administration of radiation and either single-agent 5-FU or cisplatin have demonstrated that combined modality therapy is feasible. The hematologic toxicity is modest and never dose limiting. Radiation-induced esophagitis may be increased and may be severe enough to require hospitalization and parenteral fluid administration, although this degree of toxicity is seen in only a small proportion of patients. Late toxicity, including radiation caused pneumonitis and myelitis, has also been reported in some trials.

These two drugs have also been used together or in combination with other agents, such as etoposide or vinblastine and concurrent radiotherapy (Table 28-4). These trials have shown that combination chemotherapy is associated with a higher degree of bone marrow suppression, neutropenia-associated sepsis, and even a small percentage of deaths, but the incidence and severity of radiation-induced esophagitis and pneumonitis does not differ significantly from that seen with single-agent chemotherapy. These phase II trials should not be compared directly because there was considerable variation in the dose and schedule of the radiotherapy; drug selection, dose, and schedule; and the patient populations studied. Some patients also underwent surgical resection after chemo- and radiotherapy. Although response rates were high and ranged from 50 to 80 percent, the median survival time for all studies was disappointingly low (16 months of less).

There have been only two randomized trials that have compared radiotherapy alone with radio- and concurrent chemotherapy (Soresi, et al., 1988; Schaake-Koning, et al., 1992). In a study at the National Tumor Institute of Milan, patients were randomized to receive radiotherapy alone at a dose of 50 Gy in 28 fractions, or the same radiation dose with cisplatin 15 mg/m^2 weekly. Patients in the combination thera-

Table 28-4. Phase II Trials of Concurrent Chemotherapy and Thoracic Radiotherapy for Locally Advanced Non-Small Cell Lung Cancer

References	Radiotherapeutic Dose (Gy)	Chemotherapeutic Regimen	Response (CR + PR)	Median Survival
Byfield, et al., 1983	Split course: 25 × 5; 20 × 18–20	5–FU 20–35 mg/kg per day over 120 hr × 2 courses	36% (CR)	10 mo
Schaake-Koning, et al., 1986	Split course: 30 × 10; 25 × 10	Cisplatin 10–35 mg/m^2 weekly × 4 courses	80%	Not reported
Soresi, et al., 1988	18 × 30	Cisplatin 15 mg/m^2 weekly × 6	64%	16 mo
Taylor, et al., 1987	Split course: 20 × 5 for 4–6 courses	Cisplatin 60 mg/m^2, day 1 5–FU mg/m^2 over 120 h monthly × 4–6	56%	16 mo
Weiden and Piantadosi, 1991	20 × 15	Cisplatin 75 mg/m^2 days 1 and 29 5–FU 1 g/m^2 over 16 h days 1–4, 29–32	57%	10.5 mo
Rowland, et al., 1988	20 × 5	Cisplatin 60 mg/m^2, day 2 Etoposide 60 mg/m^2, days 1–4 5–FU 800 mg/m^2, over 96 h	74%	16 mo
Strauss, et al., 1988	20 × 15 × 2 courses	Cisplatin 100 mg/m^2, days 1 + 29 Vinblastine 3 mg/m^2, days 1, 3, 29, 31 5–FU 30 mg/kg, days 1–3 and 29–31	62%	Not reported
Friess, et al., 1987, 1989	18 × 25 plus 10–15 boost	Cisplatin 50 mg/m^2, days 1 + 8 Etoposide 50 mg/m^2, days 1–5 × 4 courses	80%	16 mo

Abbreviations: CR, complete response; PR, partial response; 5-FU, 5-fluorouracil.

peutic arm had a higher response rate (64 versus 50 percent), but no statistical differences were observed in disease-free or overall survival rates (Soresi, et al., 1988). In a recent European trial, patients were randomized to receive split-course radiotherapy (55 Gy in 20 fractions) alone or the same therapy with cisplatin either 30 mg/m^2 per week or 6 mg/m^2 daily. There were no significant differences with respect to the response rate among the three therapeutic arms, but the daily-cisplatin group had significantly longer survival times than did the no-chemotherapy group ($P = 0.009$). The weekly cisplatin group was intermediate between the other two groups and not significantly different from either (Schaake-Koning, et al., 1992).

Induction Chemo(radio)therapy and Surgery

Although radiation is the standard therapy for unresectable locally advanced disease, there has been recent interest in combined modality therapeutic programs of chemotherapy followed by surgery. Neoadjuvant or induction chemotherapy before surgery has a theoretic appeal for several reasons. The response to chemotherapy may allow an otherwise unresectable tumor to be surgically resected. This should not be viewed as the primary goal of therapy, however, because it must be remembered that other therapeutic modalities can achieve local control and most patients die of distant failure. If this form of combined modality therapy is to result in a significant prolongation of the long-term survival time, it will likely be caused by the eradication of micrometastatic disease. Surgical resection following chemotherapy provides a true pathologic assessment of the response to induction therapy, which may be used to guide subsequent therapy. In a sense the preoperative therapy may be viewed as an "in vivo chemosensitivity test," and postoperative chemotherapy may be recommended only for those patients who demonstrate a response to their initial therapy.

There have been several phase II feasibility trials of induction chemotherapy or chemoradiotherapy, which are summarized in Tables 28-5 through 28-7. It is impossible to draw firm conclusions from these trials because they represent a mixed population of patients with stage IIIA and IIIB disease and include even some patients with earlier stage tumors. Chemotherapeutic regimens have not been standardized, and some patients have had both combination chemo- and radiotherapy before surgical resection.

Important observations may be made from these studies, however. The response rates achieved in these early-stage good-performance-status patients were significantly higher than those seen with the same combinations when they were administered to patients with advanced stage IV tumors. The response rates ranged from 39 percent to as high as 76 percent, and a complete pathologic response was documented in up to 15 percent of patients (predominantly the squamous pathologic type).

The median survival time ranged from 9 to 30+ months, with an average of approximately 18 months. On the surface, this might appear to be better than the median survival time of approximately 1 year that is achieved with radiotherapy alone, but it should be emphasized that all of these studies represent a select subgroup of patients with stage III disease and that most patients with poor prognostic findings, such as superior vena cava obstruction, involvement of mediastinal structures, etc., were excluded from these trials. The long-term survival and cure rates are much more difficult to interpret from the literature. The most optimistic interpretation would be approximately 25 to 35 percent survival at 3 to 5 years.

It is not possible to draw firm conclusions with respect to the optimal chemotherapeutic regimen to be used as induction therapy before surgery. No single combination chemotherapeutic regimen nor any of the trials that administered both

Table 28-5. Phase II Trials of Induction Chemotherapy and Surgery for Locally Advanced Non-Small Cell Lung Cancer Induction Chemotherapy Alone

Reference	Drugs	Chemotherapy Courses Preoperative	Postoperative	Response (%) CR	PR	Surgery (%) Thoracotomies	Complete Resection	Survival Median	Long Term
Gralla, 1988	Cisplatin Mitomycin Vinblastine or vindesine	2–3	2	12	63	72	57	19.5 mo	34% 3 yr
Burkes, et al., 1992	Cisplatin Mitomycin Vinblastine	2–3	2	8	56	56	46	18.6 mo	25% 3 yr
Lad, et al., 1991 (LCSG-881)	Cisplatin Mitomycin Vinblastine	2	0		54	54	46	12.0 mo	?
Fosella, et al., 1991	Cyclophosphamide Cisplatin Etoposide	3	3	8	17	75	58	?	75% 1 yr
Johnson, et al., 1991	Cisplatin Vinblastine	2	2		54	54	7	12.0 mo	11% 3 yr

Abbreviations: CR, complete response; PR, partial response.

Table 28-6. Phase II Trials of Induction Chemotherapy and Surgery for Locally Advanced Non-Small Cell Lung Cancer Induction Chemotherapy and Radiotherapy

| | | Chemotherapy | | Radiation Dose (Gg) | | Response (%) | | Surgery (%) | | Survival | |
| | | Courses | | | | | | | | | |
Reference	Drugs	Preoperative	Postoperative	Preoperative	Postoperative	CR	PR	Thoracotomies	Complete Resection	Median	Long Term
Spain, 1988	Cisplatin Mitomycin Vinblastine infusion	3–4	0	55–60	—	23	50	?	?	19 mo	31% 4 yr 26% 6 yr
Vokes, et al., 1989	Cisplatin Etoposide Vindesine	2	0	—	20		45	15	15	8 mo	?
Skarin, et al., 1989	Cyclophosphamide Doxorubicin Cisplatin	2	4	30	25	5	24	90	88	32.3 mo	31% 5 yr
Strauss, et al., 1986	Cisplatin Vindesine	2	2	30	25–30	11	58	59	55	>13 mo	?

Abbreviations: CR, complete response; PR, partial response.

Table 28-7. Phase II Trial of Induction Chemotherapy and Surgery for Locally Advanced Non-Small Cell Lung Cancer Induction Chemotherapy and Concurrent Radiotherapy

| | | Chemotherapy | | Radiation Dose (Gg) | | Response (%) | | Surgery (%) | | Survival | |
| | | Courses | | | | | | | | | |
Reference	Drugs	Preoperative	Postoperative	Preoperative	Postoperative	CR	PR	Thoracotomies	Complete Resection	Median	Long Term
Eagen, et al., 1987	Cyclophosphamide Doxorubicin Cisplatin	3	0	30	—	5	46	49	33	11 mo	8% 2 yr
Weiden and Piantadosi, 1991	Cisplatin 5-FU by continuous infusion for 96 h	2	0	30	—	2	54	64	34	13 mo	
Faber, et al., 1989	Cisplatin 5-FU by continuous infusion for 120 h ± etoposide	4	0	40	—	?	?	73	68	22 mo	40% 2 yr
Weitberg, et al., 1990	Etoposide Cisplatin by continuous infusion for 96 h	2	2	50	—	14	71	61	48	15.7 mo	32% 2 yr
Albain, et al., 1991	Etoposide Cisplatin	2	0	45	—	1	68	84	73	15 mo	32% 2 yr

Abbreviations: CR, complete response; PR, partial response; 5-FU, 5-fluorouracil.

chemo- and radiotherapy demonstrated significant superiority with respect to the response, complete resection, or median or long-term survival rates.

These studies have all demonstrated that induction therapy before surgical resection is feasible, but the absence of standards with respect to patient selection, induction regimens, and the reporting of results makes it impossible to compare these studies with historical survival data. It is clear, therefore, that prospective randomized trials of induction chemotherapy must be undertaken to compare this form of combined modality therapy with other more standard forms of therapy for locally advanced NSCLC.

CHEMOTHERAPY FOR ADVANCED DISEASE

The role of chemotherapy in advanced (stage IV) disease remains a topic of considerable controversy to this day. Affected patients are not curable at this stage of their disease, and so the primary goals of therapy must be the palliation of symptoms and the prolongation of survival. A high rate of response is an inadequate measure of the usefulness of combination chemotherapy. The response must be accompanied by a *meaningful* prolongation of survival without unacceptable toxicity.

There seems to be little doubt that a response to chemotherapy is associated with a prolongation of survival. Despite this, the overall contribution that chemotherapy makes to survival remains modest. There have been seven prospectively randomized trials of chemotherapy versus best supportive care for patients with advanced NSCLC (Table 28-8). In only the studies of Rapp, et al. (1988) and Cormier, et al. (1982) was a *statistically significant* prolongation of survival achieved with chemotherapy, although in the Cormier trial, the patients in the best supportive care therapeutic arm had a very short median survival time of only 8.5 weeks. In the Rapp, et al., study, the median survival time for patients in the high-dose cisplatin and vindesine therapeutic arm was less than 4 months longer than that of patients

in the control arm, with most of that time spent on therapy with the attendant toxicity of high-dose cisplatin. This study focused on the duration of survival but did not assess palliation or analyze the quality of life for the patients in the three therapeutic arms. Because of concerns that the small survival benefit seen in the combination chemotherapeutic arms might be associated with an unacceptable financial cost, a formal economical evaluation of this study was undertaken (Jaakkimainen, et al., 1990). It is interesting, and perhaps surprising, that this evaluation demonstrated that the use of combination chemotherapy was cost effective because of the high costs of supporting patients on the supportive care therapeutc arm, who actually spent more time in the hospital than did patients on either of the chemotherapeutic arms. Therefore, economic factors should not be a major factor in the decision to treat or not to treat with chemotherapy.

Although it is clear that chemotherapy exerts a biologic effect in patients with advanced NSCLC, broad generalizations cannot be made for the therapy of this group of patients as a whole. Whenever possible, patients should be treated during clinical trials of either new agents or new combinations of drugs. Continued research in patients with advanced disease is essential to identify regimens that may have sufficient activity to justify their future use in patients with earlier stages of disease. At this time, chemotherapy is sufficiently active to justify its use in patients who want therapy and who understand its limitations. The therapy must be individualized and should be offered to patients who have the greatest chance to benefit from it and the least potential to develop toxicity.

BIOLOGIC RESPONSE MODIFIERS

Interferon and Interleukin

The interferons (IFN) are a family of naturally occurring products that are produced by lymphocytes and have antiviral, immunomodulatory, and antitumor effects. IFN used

Table 28-8. Randomized Trials of Chemotherapy Versus Supportive Care for Patients with Advanced Non-Small Cell Lung Cancer

Reference	Therapy	No. Evaluable Patients	Median Survival (wk)	P Value
Rapp, et al., 1988	VP	44	32.6	}0.01
	CAP	43	24.7	
	BSC	50	17.0	}0.05
Ganz, et al., 1989	VblP	22	18.6	0.26
	BSC	26	14.4	
Woods, et al., 1990	VP	97	27.0	0.33
	BSC	91	17.0	
Cellerino, et al., 1991	CEP/MEC	58	34.3	0.135
	BSC	57	21.1	
Cormier, et al., 1982	MACC	20	30.5	
	BSC	19	8.5	0.0005
Kassa, et al., 1991	VP	44	22.0	0.29
	BSC	43	16.5	
Quoix, et al., 1991	VP	28	27	0.33
	BSC	10	17	

Abbreviations: BSC, best supportive care; VP, vindesine and cisplatin; CAP, cyclophosphamide, doxorubicin, and cisplatin; VblP, vinblastine and cisplatin; CEP, cyclophosphamide, epirubicin, and cisplatin; MEC, methotrexate, etoposide, and lomustine; MACC, methotrexate, doxorubicin, cyclophosphamide, and lomustine.

alone has not demonstrated significant activity against NSCLC, but synergy has been demonstrated between IFN-α and chemotherapy in some experimental models. This observation led to prospective trials of combination chemotherapy with or without IFN (Smyth, et al., 1990). In a trial of cyclophosphamide, epirubicin, and cisplatin alone or the same drugs combined with IFN-α, the response rate in the IFN therapeutic arm was 22 percent compared with 11 percent in the chemotherapy-alone one ($P = 0.14$), but the median survival was 6 months in both ($P = 0.75$) (Rosso, et al., 1991). IFN did not seem to contribute significantly to chemotherapeutic toxicity, but the IFN dose had to be reduced or suspended in 20 percent of patients because of toxicity. A similar trial of combination chemotherapy with cisplatin and etoposide given alone and in combination with IFN-α or IFN-γ is currently ongoing, and an interim analysis has revealed no significant difference between the therapeutic arms with respect to response or toxicity (Maasilta, et al., 1991). Phase II trials have also suggested that IFN may be combined safely with radiotherapy, but randomized trials to assess the usefulness of such combined modality therapy have not been undertaken (Chang, et al., 1990). The role of IFN as adjuvant therapy is under investigation currently for patients with SCLC. Whether it might also be useful following surgical resection in NSCLC is unknown at this time.

Interleukin-2 (IL-2) is another naturally occurring lymphokine that is being assessed in patients with NSCLC. In an ECOG trial, IL-2 was administered alone or with IFN-β. Three of 73 patients had a response, and the median survival time of the group was 35.6 weeks. The combined IL-IFN therapeutic arm did not seem to be superior to IL alone (Krigel, et al., 1991).

The National Biotherapy Study Group assessed the usefulness of adoptive immunotherapy with IL-2 and lymphokine-activated peripheral blood mononuclear (LAK) cells as an adjunct to chemotherapy. In a small pilot trial of 14 patients, two patients achieved complete remissions, and four patients had partial remission (Barth, et al., 1990).

At this time, the use of biologic response modifiers, such as IFN or IL-2 must be considered highly experimental and should not be contemplated outside a clinical trial (see Biologic Therapy later in this chapter).

Colony-Stimulating Factors

The dose-limiting toxicity for most chemotherapeutic agents is bone marrow suppression. Several clinical studies have demonstrated that the new recombinant colony-stimulating factors can accelerate the recovery of myelopoeisis by reducing both the degree and the duration of neutropenia after cytotoxic chemotherapy. The colony-stimulating factors have been evaluated extensively in patients with SCLC treated with standard-dose chemotherapy (Bronchud, et al., 1987; Crawford, et al., 1991). The primary objective of these studies was to ameliorate toxicity and to reduce the incidence of neutrophenia-associated sepsis. These studies demonstrated that patients treated with standard-dose chemotherapy have fewer episodes of febrile neutropenia when they are given colony-stimulating factors, but other trials show that it may not be possible to increase the chemotherapeutic dose substantially over prolonged periods even with colony-

stimulating factor support (Shepherd, et al., 1992b). In NSCLC, one trial suggested that it may be possible to administer combination chemotherapy with mitomycin C, vindesine, and cisplatin every 21 days rather than every 28 days with the addition of granulocyte colony-stimulating factor (Takada, et al., 1990).

The true role of hematopoeitic growth factors in lung cancer chemotherapy remains to be determined. Further trials are indicated to assess new colony-stimulating factors; to compare their efficacy to prophylactic antibiotics; and to address the issues of dose, schedule, and cost.

Monoclonal Antibodies

Radiolabeled monoclonal antibodies with activity directed against specific cell surface antigens on malignant cells have the potential to be useful as diagnostic imaging and therapeutic tools in many malignancies. The epidermal growth factor receptor is expressed in many epithelial tissues and has increased expression in squamous malignancies, including squamous cell carcinoma of the lung. Monoclonal antibodies have been developed that bind to the epidermal growth factor receptor, and in vitro studies have demonstrated synergistic effects against squamous carcinoma cell lines when doxorubicin and antiepidermal growth factor were used together (Baselga, et al., 1991). Phase I toxicity trials are ongoing at this time in patients with metastatic NSCLC, but it is too early to draw any conclusions regarding the usefulness of this or other monoclonal antibodies (see Biologic Therapy).

Modifiers of Drug Resistance

Because NSCLC demonstrates relative resistance to chemotherapy, various agents, such as verapamil and cyclosporine, which have the potential to overcome multidrug resistance, are under study. In a recent trial, 72 patients were randomized to receive chemotherapy alone with ifosfamide and vindesine or the same chemotherapy with oral verapamil (Millward, et al., 1991). The response rate was 21 percent for chemotherapy alone and 42 percent for chemotherapy and verapamil ($P < 0.05$), and the median survival times were 22 and 40 weeks, respectively ($P < 0.025$). The degree of neurotoxicity was greater in the combination therapeutic arm, but other toxicities did not seem to be increased.

Cyclosporine was assessed in combination with cisplatin and etoposide (Cho, et al., 1991). In a small phase I-II trial, four of nine patients achieved partial responses, and the toxicity did not seem to be increased. Further dose escalations of cyclosporine are being studied.

Retinoids

Retinoids are differentiating agents that play an important role in the maintenance of the normal epithelium. It is thought that they control differentiation through their effects on oncogene expression and peptide growth factors. In vitro studies have demonstrated that retinoic acid can cause terminal differentiation of fully neoplastic cells in both murine and cell culture systems. Much of the clinical experience with retinoids has been in patients with head and neck cancer. In a prospective randomized trial of 103 patients with squamous cell cancer of the head and neck, patients treated with 13-*cis*-retinoic acid had a significantly reduced incidence of second primary tumors ($P = 0.005$) compared with those treated with placebo (Hong, et al., 1990). A similar trial of adjuvant retinoic acid after resection of NSCLC is about to start in North America.

There is in vitro evidence to suggest that the combination of retinoids and IFN may be synergistic. This observation has led to phase II trials of retinoids and IFN in a variety of malignancies, including refractory squamous cell carcinoma of the skin, malignant melanoma, and mycosis fungoides. All of these preliminary trials have demonstrated activity for the combination, with complete clinical responses seen in patients with mycosis fungoides and skin cancer (Lippman, et al., 1991). These observations led two groups to initiate Phase II trials of 13-cis-retinoic acid and α-INF for patients with advanced NSCLC. In a study limited to patients with squamous cell tumors, only one response was observed (Rinaldi, 1993), and in a similar study of the NCIC in which patients with both squamous cell carcinoma and adenocarcinoma were evaluated, an identical response rate was observed (Arnold, personal communication, 1994).

COMMENTS AND CONTROVERSIES

New Drugs

Unfortunately, with the exception of analogs, there are few new agents on the horizon that are likely to have a significant impact on the therapy of NSCLC. Gemcitabine is perhaps one of the most promising new drugs. It has demonstrated good single-agent activity and is associated with only mild bone marrow suppression, which should allow its incorporation into multiple-drug regimens. The taxanes navelbine and irinotecan have also demonstrated good single-agent activity, but all are associated with significant myelosuppression. Phase I and II trials of these agents in combination are underway at this time.

Combined Modality Therapy

It is clear that no single therapeutic modality, be it surgery, radiotherapy, or chemotherapy, is able to achieve cure for most patients with NSCLC. Whether combined modality therapy will be able to improve survival and cure rates still remains controversial. The addition of systemic chemotherapy to radiotherapy for patients with locally advanced disease has resulted in modest, but statistically significant, prolongation of survival times in some, but not all, trials. Because the magnitude of the survival benefit has been so small, combined modality therapy has not been adopted as standard practice in most centers. Nonetheless, future trials in this area are clearly indicated. The results from the Schaake-Koning, et al. (1992) trial of concomitant daily cisplatin and radiotherapy are intriguing and deserve further study. Other agents, such as oral etoposide, may be administered on a daily basis and may also be suitable for prolonged administration with radiotherapy.

Many phase II pilot studies have now confirmed the feasibility of induction chemotherapy followed by surgical resection for patients with locally advanced disease. The time has now come to stop doing phase II trials and to proceed to phase III studies. The SWOG, RTOG, and EGOG have initiated an intergroup trial in which patients with stage IIIA and IIIB disease are randomized to receive etoposide and cisplatin administered concurrently with local radiotherapy or the same therapy followed by surgery. This trial is asking a local control question, that is, is radiotherapy or surgery superior with respect to local disease control and can this translate into a prolongation of survival? The NCIC has initiated a trial in which patients are randomized to receive radiotherapy only or induction chemotherapy with cisplatin and vinblastine followed by surgery. This trial is designed to assess whether agressive systemic and local therapy is superior to the standard therapy, which at this time in Canada, is radiation alone without systemic chemotherapy.

Investigational Therapy

It is clear that colony-stimulating factors can reduce the degree and duration of nadir neutropenia and the incidence of neutropenia-associated sepsis after chemotherapy. The ability of growth factors to permit significant dose escalation is as yet unproved. Furthermore, it is not at all clear whether modest increases in dose will result in a significant prolongation of survival. Future studies are indicated, and they should be designed to identify significant improvements in response and survival rates and should not focus on secondary end points, such as the nadir granulocyte count or incidence of fever. An economic analysis should form part of all such future trials.

The biologic response modifiers and retinoids will probably not play a significant role in the advanced disease setting. Nonetheless, it is important to undertake phase I and II trials of these agents in patients with incurable tumors to determine toxicity profiles and optimal doses and schedules and to evaluate the possibility of combined modality therapy. There are clues from other tumor types that these agents may play a role in the adjuvant setting. Mattson, et al. (1991) reported a prolongation of survival in patients with SCLC treated with IFN after chemotherapy. Hong, et al. (1990) has reported a reduction in second primary cancers in patients with head and neck cancer treated with 13-*cis*-retinoic acid. Whether similar effects will be seen in NSCLC remains speculative, but sufficient data now exist to justify the initiation of clinical trials in this area.

F.A.S.

As Dr.Shepherd outlines, the chemotherapy for NSCLC has made great strides in the past 20 years. There are now effective agents that occasionally produce complete responses in early-stage lung cancer, and there is reasonable evidence that patients benefit from chemotherapy in disseminated disease. Despite this optimism, the results of chemotherapy in the management of NSCLC pale in comparison with the results achieved in recent years in treating other tumors, such as lymphomas, breast carcinomas, and germ cell tumors.

Unfortunately, few really new drugs have been developed in the management of NSCLC in the past decade. However, more recently, newer agents (e.g., the taxanes and gemcitabine) and modifications of toxic agents (e.g., navelbine and edatrexate) have demonstrated their effectiveness in producing responses in this disease.

Future developments and improvements in treatment will depend on developing combination drug therapies that are more effective than the ones we have available. The continued efforts in phase II and phase III trials we hope, in the future, will ultimately develop therapeutic strategies that are more effective than presently available.

Combined modality therapies, utilizing chemotherapy in combination with radiotherapy and/or surgery have demonstrated some improved therapeutic effects. Further investigations are warranted.

The use of chemotherapy as adjuvant therapy following completely resected lung cancer has yet to demonstrate anything more than some delay in the time to the recurrence of the disease. Improved survival has rarely been demonstrated in these randomized trials. On the other hand, induction chemotherapy followed by surgery for locally advanced disease has now been shown to improve the median survival and, most probably, long-term survival in locally advanced disease that is still resectable (e.g., preoperatively identified N2 disease).

Despite the lack of the development of a "magic bullet," there has been an improvement in the management of NSCLC through the use of combination chemotherapy. In the future, similar small improvements may ultimately lead to significant changes in the outlook of patients with locally advanced or disseminated disease and possibly in patients with completely resected disease. To improve the therapy of this disease, such advances are required because, following complete surgical resection, most patients have recurrences at distant sites that are only amenable to early systemic therapy.

R.J.G.

KEY REFERENCES

Dillman RO, Seagren SL, Propert KJ et al: A randomized trial of induction chemotherapy plus high-dose radiation vs. radiation alone in stage III non-small cell lung cancer. N Engl J Med 323:940, 1990

Holmes EC, Gail M, Lung Cancer Study Group: Surgical adjuvant therapy for stage II and stage III adenocarcinoma and a large-cell undifferentiated carcinoma of the lung. Cancer 50:1713, 1986

Jaakkimainen L, Goodwin PJ, Pater J et al: Counting the costs of chemotherapy in a National Cancer Institute of Canada randomized trial in non-small cell lung cancer. J Clin Oncol 8:1301, 1990

The prospectively randomized trial reported by Rapp et al., for the NCIC is a landmark trial documenting a survival benefit for patients with advanced NSCLC treated with systemic chemotherapy. The economic analysis of this trial reported by Jaakkimainen, et al., demonstrates that financial considerations should not be of primary concern in the decision to treat patients with advanced NSCLC because the costs for patients who do not receive therapy may actually be greater. Such patients spend more time in the hospital receiving palliative care.

Lad T, Rubinstein L, Fadeghi A: The benefit of adjuvant treatment for resected locally advanced non-small cell lung cancer. J Clin Oncol 6:9, 1988

The Holmes and Lad articles are important because they report the results of two LCSG trials of adjuvant chemotherapy for NSCLC. Although the survival benefits were modest at best, these two well-designed prospectively randomized studies provide us with the suggestion that adjuvant chemotherapy after surgical resection may be of benefit for some patients. They also suggest that further trials with more aggressive chemotherapeutic regimens may be indicated.

Maki E, Feld R: Prognostic factors in patients with non-small cell lung cancer. A critique of the world literature. Lung Cancer 7:27, 1991

This article provides an excellent review of the clinical factors that are important for response and survival. An understanding of these factors is critical to the interpretation of clinical trials at all stages of NSCLC.

Rapp E, Pater J, Willan A et al: Chemotherapy can prolong survival in patients with advanced non-small cell lung cancer. A report of the Canadian multicenter trial. J Clin Oncol 6:633, 1988

Schaake-Konig C, van den Bogaert W, Dalesio O et al: Effects of concomitant cisplatin and radiotherapy on inoperable non-small cell lung cancer. N Engl J Med 326:524, 1992

The Dillman and Schaake-Konig articles provide the most compelling evidence that the administration of chemotherapy with local radiotherapy may result in superior survival for patients with locally advanced NSCLC. In the Dillman study, chemo- and radiotherapy were administered sequentially, and in the Schaake-Koning trial they were given concurrently. In addition, the Schaake-Koning study evaluated a novel daily schedule for cisplatin administration.

REFERENCES

Alama A, Costantini M, Repetto L et al: Thymidine labelling index as prognostic factor in resected non-small cell lung cancer. Eur J Cancer 25:622, 1990

Albain K, Rusch V, Crowley J et al: Concurrent cisplatin (DDP, VP-16 and chest irradiation (RT) followed by surgery for stages IIIA and IIIB non-small cell lung cancer (N-SCLC): A Southwest Oncology Group (SWOG) study # 8805 (abstr). Proc Am Soc Clin Oncol 10:241, 1991

Anderson H, Lund B, Hansen HH et al: Phase II study of gemcitabine in non small cell lung cancer (NSCLC) (abstr). Proc Am Soc Clin Oncol 10:247, 1991

Asakawa M, Fujita A, Fukuoka M et al: Phase II study of CPT-11, a new camptothecin derivative in previously untreated non-small cell lung cancer (abstr). Lung Cancer 7:125, 1991

Ayoub J, Vigneault J, Hanley A et al: The Montreal Multi-Centre Trial. Inoperable non-small cell lung cancer (NSCLC): A multivariate analysis of the predictors of relapse (abstr). Proc Am Soc Clin Oncol 10:247, 1991

Bailor JC, Smith EM: Progress against cancer! N Engl J Med 314:1226, 1986

Bakowski MT, Crouch JD: Chemotherapy of non-small cell lung cancer: a reappraisal and a look to the future. Cancer Treat Rev 10:159, 1983

Barth N, West W, Oldham R et al: A phase II trial of adoptive immunotherapy (AIT) and sequential chemotherapy with cisplatin (CP), VP-16 in advanced non-small cell lung cancer (NSCLC). (NBSG87-14) (abstr). Proc Am Soc Clin Oncol 9:235, 1990

Baselga J, Miller W, Norton L et al: Synergistic effects of chemotherapy and anti-epidermal growth factor receptor (EGFr) monoclonal antibodies (MAb) (abstr). Lung Cancer 7(suppl):17, 1991

Berendsen HH, de-Leij L, Popperma S et al: Clinical characterization of non-small cell lung cancer tumors showing neuroendocrine differentiation features. J Clin Oncol 11:1614, 1989

Bitran JD, Desser RK, DeMeester TR et al: Cyclophosphamide, Adriamycin, methotrexate and procarbazine (CAMP)—effective four-drug combination chemotherapy for metastatic non-oat cell bronchogenic carcinoma. Cancer Treat Rep 60:1225, 1976

Bonomi PD, Finkelstein DM, Ruckdeschel JD et al: Combination chemotherapy versus single agents followed by combination chemotherapy in stage IV non-small cell lung cancer: a study of the Eastern Cooperative Oncology Group. J Clin Oncol 17:1602, 1989

Boring CC, Squires TS, Tong T: Cancer statistics 1992. CA Cancer J Clin 42:19, 1992

Bronchud MH, Scarffe, JH, Thatcher N et al: Phase I-II study of recombinant human granulocyte colony-stimulating factor in patients receiving intensive chemotherapy for small cell lung cancer. Br J Cancer 56:809, 1987

Buccheri G: Chemotherapy and survival in non-small cell lung cancer. The old vexata questio. Chest 99:1328, 1991

Bunn PA: Review of therapeutic trials of carboplatin in lung cancer. Semin Oncol 16(suppl 5):27, 1989a

Bunn PA: The expanding role of cisplatin in the treatment of non-small cell lung cancer. Semin Oncol 16(suppl 6):10, 1989b.

Burkes R, Ginsberg R, Shepherd F et al: Induction chemotherapy with mitomycin, vindesine, and cisplatin for stage III unresectable non-small cell lung cancer: results of the Toronto phase II trial. J Clin Oncol 10:580, 1992

Byfield JE, Calabro-Jones PM, Klisak I et al: Pharmacologic requirements for obtaining sensitization of human tumor cells in vitro to combined 5-Fluorouracil or Ftorafur and x-rays. Int J Radiat Oncol Biol Phys 8:1923, 1982

Byfield JE, Stanton W, Sharp TR et al: Phase I-II study of 120-hour infused 5-FU and split course radiation therapy in localized non-small cell lung cancer. Cancer Treat Rep 67:933, 1983

Carney DN: The biology of lung cancer. Curr Opin Oncol 4:292, 1992

Carney D: Lung cancer biology. Curr Opin Oncol 3:288, 1991

Cellerino R, Tummarello D, Guidi F: A randomized trial of alternating chemotherapy versus best supportive care in advanced non-small cell lung cancer. J Clin Oncol 9:1453, 1991

Chahinian AP, Mandel EM, Holland JK et al: MACC (methotrexate, Adriamycin, cyclophosphamide, and CCNU) in advanced lung cancer. Cancer 43:1590, 1979

Chang A, McDonald S, Kim IS et al: Combination treatment of radiation (XRT) and recombinant interferon BETA$_{ser}$ (betaseron) in patients with inoperable or metastatic non-small cell lung cancer (NSCLC) (abstr). Proc Am Soc Clin Oncol 9:247, 1990

Cho J, Hurtado N, Wong S et al: Phase I-II trial of cyclosporin A (CsA), cisplatinum (CDDP) and VP-16 in non-small cell lung cancer (NSCLC) (abstr). Proc Am Soc Clin Oncol 10:251, 1991

Cormier Y, Bergeron D, La Forge J et al: Benefits of polychemotherapy in advanced non-small-cell bronchogenic carcinoma. Cancer 50:845, 1982

Crawford J, Ozer H, Stoller R et al: Reduction by granulocyte colony-stimulating factor of fever and neutropenia induced by chemotherapy in patients with small-cell lung cancer. N Engl J Med 325:164, 1991

Cullen MH, Joshi R, Chetiyawardna A: Mitomycin, ifosfamide and cisplatin in non-small cell lung cancer: treatment good enough to compare. Br J Cancer 9:359, 1988

Depierre R, Lemarie E, Dabouis G et al: A phase II study of navelbine (vinorelbine) in the treatment of non-small cell lung cancer. Am J Clin Oncol 14:115, 1991

DeVore R, Hainsworth J, Greco FA et al: Chronic oral etoposide in the treatment of lung cancer. Semin Oncol 19(suppl. 14):28, 1992

Donnadieu N, Paesmans M, Sculier J-P: Chemotherapy of non-small cell lung cancer according to disease extent: a meta-analysis of the literature. Lung Cancer 7:243, 1991

Douple EB, Richmond RC: Enhancement of the potentiation of radiotherapy by platinum drugs in a mouse tumour. Int J Radiat Oncol Biol Phys 8:501, 1982

Drings P: European experience with ifosfamide in non-small cell lung cancer. Semin Oncol 26:294, 1989

Eagan RT, Ingle JN, Frytak S et al: Platinum-based polychemotherapy versus dianhydrogalacitol in advanced non-small cell lung cancer. Cancer Treat Rep 61:1339, 1977

Eagan RT, Rudd C, Lee RE et al: Pilot study of induction therapy with cyclophosphamide, doxorubicin and cisplatin (CAP) and chest irradiation prior to thoracotomy in initially inoperable stage III M0 non-small cell lung cancer. Cancer Treat Rep 71:895, 1987

Eberhardt W, Niederle N: Ifosfamide in non-small cell lung cancer: a review. Semin Oncol 19(suppl 1): 40, 1992

Faber LP, Kittle CF, Warren WII et al: Preoperative chemotherapy and irradiation for stage III non-small cell lung cancer and also thoracic surgery. Ann Thorac Surg 47:669, 1989

Feld R, Wierzbicki R, Walde D et al: Phase I-II study of high dose epirubicin in advanced non-small cell lung cancer. J Clin Oncol 20:297, 1992

Feld R, Rubenstein L, Thomas P (Lung Cancer Study Group): Adjuvant chemotherapy with cyclophosphamide, doxorubicin, and cisplatin in patients with completely resected Stage I non-small cell lung cancer. J Natl Cancer Inst 85:299, 1993

Ferguson MK: Diagnosing and staging of non-small cell lung cancer. Hematol Oncol Clin North Am 4:1053, 1990

Ferguson MK, Skosey C, Hoffman PC, Golomb HM: Sex-associated differences in presentation and survival in patients with lung cancer. J Clin Oncol 8:1402, 1990

Fossella F, Ryan B, Dhingra H et al: Interim report of a prospective randomized trial of neo-adjuvant chemotherapy plus surgery versus surgery only for IIIA non-small cell lung cancer (NSCLC) (abstr). Proc Am Soc Clin Oncol 10:256, 1991

Fossella F, Lee J, Shin D et al: Taxotere™ (Docetaxel: DTXL), an active agent for platinum-refractory non-small cell lung cancer (NSCLC): preliminary report of a phase II study. Proc Am Soc Clin Oncol 13:336, abstracted, 1994

Friess GG, Balkadi M, Harvey WH: Simultaneous cisplatin and etoposide with radiation therapy in locoregional non-small cell lung cancer. Final results of a pilot trial. p. 121. In Gralla RJ, Einhorn LH (eds): Small Cell Lung Cancer and Non-Small Cell Lung Cancer. Royal Society of Medicine Services Limited, London, 1989

Friess GG, Balkadi M, Harvey WH: Concurrent cisplatin and etoposide with radiotherapy in locally advanced non-small cell lung cancer. Cancer Treat Rep 71:681, 1987

Fukuoka M, Niitani H, Sizuki A et al: A phase II study of CPT-11, a new derivative of camptothecin, for previously untreated non-small cell lung cancer. J Clin Oncol 10:16, 1992

Gail MH, Eagan RT, Feld R et al: Prognostic factors in patients with resected stage 1 non-small cell lung cancer: a report from the Lung Cancer Study Group. Cancer 54:1802, 1984

Gandara DR, Tanaka MT, Crowley J, Livingston RB: Comparison of standard dose cisplatin, high dose cisplatin and high dose cisplatin plus mitomycin in metastatic non-small cell lung cancer: preliminary results of a phase III study (abstr). Proc Am Soc Clin Oncol 10:246, 1991

Ganz PA, Figlin RA, Haskell CM: Supportive care versus supportive care and combination chemotherapy in metastatic non-small cell lung cancer. Cancer 63:1271, 1989

Gralla RJ: Pre-operative and adjuvant chemotherapy in non-small cell lung cancer. Semin Oncol 15(suppl 7):8, 1988

Gralla RJ, Casper ES, Kelsen DP et al: Cisplatin and vindesine combination chemotherapy for advanced carcinoma of the lung: a randomized trial investigating two dosage schedules. Ann Intern Med 95:414, 1981

Green M, Kreisman H, Soll D et al: Carboplatin in non-small cell lung cancer: an update on the Cancer and Leukemia Group B experience. Semin Oncol 19(suppl 2):44, 1992

Green R, Humphrey E, Close H, Patno M: Alkylating agents in bronchogenic carcinoma. Am J Med 46:516, 1969

Gurney H, de Campos ES, Dodwell D et al: Ifosphamide and mitomycin in combination of the treatment of patients with progressive advanced non-small cell lung cancer. Eur J Cancer 27:565, 1991

Harada M, Dosaka-Akita H, Miyamoto H et al: Prognostic significance of the expression of ras oncogene product in non-small cell lung cancer. Cancer 69:72, 1992

Haskell CM: Chemotherapy and survival of patients with non-small cell lung cancer. A contrary view. Chest 99:1325, 1991

Hong WK, Lippman S, Itri L et al: Prevention of second primary tumors with isotretinoin in squamous-cell carcinoma of the head and neck. N Engl J Med 323:795, 1990

Ichinose Y, Hara N, Ohta M et al: Postoperative adjuvant chemotherapy in non-small cell lung cancer: prognostic value of DNA ploidy and post-recurrent survival. J Surg Oncol 46:15, 1991

Johnson DH: Overview of ifosphamide in small cell and non-small cell lung cancer. Semin Oncol 17(suppl 4):24, 1990

Johnson DH, Strupp J, Greco FA et al: Neoadjuvant cisplatin plus vinblastine chemotherapy in locally advanced non-small cell lung cancer. Cancer 68:1216, 1991

Jones AL, Smith IE: Zeniplatin (CL286,558), an active new platinum analog in advanced non-small cell lung cancer (NSCLC): a phase II study (abstr). Proc Am Soc Clin Oncol 10:268, 1991

Joss RA, Cavalli F, Goldhirsch A et al: New agents in non-small cell lung cancer. Cancer Treat Rev 11:205, 1984

Kassa S, Lund E, Thorud E et al: Symptomatic treatment versus combination chemotherapy for patients with extensive non-small cell lung cancer. Cancer 67:2443, 1991

Keller S, Groshen S, Martini N, Kaiser L: Blood transfusion and lung cancer recurrence. Cancer 62:606, 1983

Krigel R, Lynch K, Kucuk O et al: Interleukin 2 (IL-2) therapies prolong survival in metastatic non-small cell lung cancer (NSCLC) (abstr). Am Soc Clin Oncol 10:246, 1991

Lad T, Wagner H, Piantadosi S: Randomized phase II evaluation of pre-operative chemotherapy alone and radiotherapy alone in stage IIIA non-small cell lung cancer (abstr). Proc Am Soc Clin Oncol 10:258, 1991

Le Chevalier T, Arriagada R, Tarayre M et al: Significant effect of adjuvant chemotherapy on survival in locally advanced non-small cell lung cancer. J Natl Cancer Inst 84:58, 1992

Lee JS, Ro JY, Sahin AA et al: Expression of blood-group antigen A: a favorable prognostic factor in non-small cell lung cancer. N Engl J Med. 324:1084, 1991

Lippman SM, Parkinson Dr, Weber RS et al: Isotretinoin plus α-interferon: effective therapy of advanced squamous cell carcinoma

(SCC) of the skin (abstr). Proc Am Soc Clin Oncol 10:197, 1991

Lund B, Anderson H, Walling J et al: Phase II study of gemcitabine in non-small cell lung cancer (NSCLC). Proceedings of the 6th World Conference on Lung Cancer (abstr). Lung Cancer 7:121, 1991

Maasilta P, Holsti L, Pyrhonen S et al: Augmentation of cytotoxicity of chemotherapy by cytokines in non-small cell lung cancer (abstr). Lung Cancer 7:126, 1991

Mattson K, Holsti LR, Holsti P et al: Inoperable non-small cell lung cancer: radiation with or without chemotherapy. Eur J Clin Oncol 24:477, 1988

Mattson K, Nilranen A, Holsti LR et al: Natural alpha interferon as maintenance therapy for small cell lung cancer. Proceedings of the 6th World Conference on Lung Cancer, Melbourne, November 10-14 (abstr). Lung Cancer 7(suppl):127, 1991

Millward MJ, Munro N, Cantwell BMJ et al: Randomized trials of oral verapamil with chemotherapy for non-small cell lung cancer (NSCLC). Proceedings of the 6th World Conference on Lung Cancer, November 10-14, 1991, Melbourne, Australia (abstr). Lung Cancer 7:107, 1991

Mitsudomi T, Steinberg SM, Oieltk et al: Rat gene mutations in non-small cell lung cancer are associated with shortened survival irrespective of treatment intent. Cancer Res 51:4999, 1991

Monnier A, Poujol J, Cerrina M et al: Potemustine in non-small cell lung cancer: phase II study in 32 patients with poor prognostic factors (abstr). Proc Am Soc Clin Oncol 10:248, 1991

Morton RF, Jett JR, McGinnis WL et al: Thoracic radiation therapy alone compared with combined chemoradiotherapy for locally unresectable non-small cell lung cancer. Ann Intern Med 115:681, 1991

Mountain C: A new international staging system for lung cancer. Chest 89:225S, 1986

Murphy WK, Winn RJ, Fossella FV: A phase II study of Taxol in patients with non-small cell lung cancer (abstr). Proc Am Soc Clin Oncol 11:294, 1992

Niiranen S, Niitamo-Korhonen, Kouri A et al: Adjuvant chemotherapy after radical surgery for non-small-cell lung cancer: a randomized study. J Clin Oncol 10:1927, 1992

Osoba D, Rusthoven JJ, Turnbull KA et al: Combination chemotherapy with bleomycin, etoposide and cis-platinum in metastatic non-small cell lung cancer. J Clin Oncol 3:1478, 1985

Quoix E, Dietemann A, Charbonneau J et al: La chimiotherapie comportant du cisplative est-elle utile dans le cancer bronchique non microcelluleve au stad IV? Resultats d'une étude randomisée. Bull Cancer 78:341, 1991

Richards F, Perry DJ, Goutsou M et al: Chemotherapy with 5-fluorouracil (5-FU) and cisplatin or 5-FU, cisplatin, and vinblastine for advanced non-small cell lung cancer. Cancer 67:2974, 1991

Rigas J, Francis P, Kris M et al: Phase II trial of Taxotere in non-small cell lung cancer (NSCLC). Proc Am Soc Clin Oncol 12:336, abstracted, 1993

Rinaldi DA, Lippman SM, Burris HA et al: Phase II study of 13-cis-retinoic acid in patients with advanced squamous cell lung cancer. Proc Am Soc Clin Oncol 12:348, abstracted, 1993

Rosso R, Ardizzoni A, Salvati F et al: Combination chemotherapy and recombinant (R) alpha interferon (IFN) for metastatic non-small cell lung cancer (NSCLC): a randomized FONICAP trial (abstr). Lung Cancer 7:131, 1991

Rowland KM Jr, Bonomi P, Taylor SG IV et al: Phase II trial of etoposide, ciplatin, 5-FU and concurrent split course radiation in stage IIIA and IIIB non-small cell lung cancer. Proc Am Soc Clin Oncol 7:203, 1988

Sahin AA, Ro JY, el-Naggar AK et al: Flow cytometric analysis of the DNA content of non-small cell lung cancer. Ploidy as a significant prognostic indicator in squamous cell carcinoma of the lung. Cancer 65:530, 1990

Sause W, Scott C, Taylor S et al: RTOG 8808 ECOG 4588 preliminary analysis of a phase III trial in regionally advanced non-small cell lung cancer. Proc Am Soc Clin Oncol 13:325, abstracted, 1994

Schaake-Koning C, Bartelink H, Hara Adema B et al: Radiotherapy and cisdiamminedichloroplatinum (II) as a combined treatment modality for inoperable non-small cell lung cancer, a dose finding study. Int J Radiat Oncol Biol Phys 12:379, 1986

Shepherd FA, Evans WK, Goss PE et al: Ifosfamide, cisplatin and etoposide (ICE) in the treatment of advanced non-small cell lung cancer. Semin Oncol 19(suppl 1):54, 1992a

Shepherd FA, Goss PE, Rusthoven J, Eisenhauer EA: Phase I trial of granulocyte-macrophage colony-stimulating factor with high-dose cisplatin and etoposide for the treatment of small cell lung cancer: a study of the National Cancer Institute of Canada Clinical Trials Group. J Natl Cancer Inst 84:59, 1992b

Shum KY, Kris MG, Gralla RJ et al: Phase II study of 10-ethyl-10-deaza-aminopterin in patients with stage III and IV non-small cell lung cancer. Semin Oncol 6:446, 1988

Skarin A, Jochelson M, Sheldon T et al: Neo-adjuvant chemotherapy in marginally resectable stage III MO non-small cell lung cancer: long-term follow-up in 41 patients. J Surg Oncol 40:266, 1989

Slevin ML, Clark PI, Joel SP et al: A randomized trial to evaluate the effect of schedule on the activity of etoposide in small cell lung cancer. J Clin Oncol 7:1333, 1989

Smyth JF, Bowman A, Fergusson RJ, Allan SG: Potentiation of cisplatin by alpha-interferon in advanced non-small cell lung cancer (NSCLC): a phase II study. Ann Oncol 1:351, 1990

Soresi E, Clerici M, Grilli R et al: A randomized clinical trial comparing radiation therapy versus radiation therapy plus cis-dichlorodi-ammine-platin (II) in the treatment of locally advanced non-small cell lung cancer. Semin Oncol 15(suppl 7):20, 1988

Souhami R, Hartley J, Allen R et al: Phase II study of 10-EdAm (10-ethyl-10-deazaaminopterin) in untreated advanced non-small cell lung cancer (NSCLC) (abstr). Proc Am Soc Clin Oncol 10:252, 1991

Spain RC: Neo-adjuvant mytomycin C, cisplatin and infusion vinblastine in locally and regionally advanced non-small cell lung cancer: problems and progress from the perspective of long-term follow-up. Semin Oncol 15(suppl 4):6, 1988

Stevenson H, Gazdar A, Phelp S et al: Tumor cell lines established in vitro, an independent prognostic factor for survival in non-small cell lung cancer. Ann Intern Med 113:764, 1990

Strauss G, Sherman L, Matthiesen O et al: Concurrent chemotherapy and radiotherapy followed by surgery in marginally resectable stage IIIA non-small cell lung carcinoma of the lung. A Cancer and Acute Leukemia Group B study (abstr). Proc Am Soc Clin Oncol 7:203, 1988

Strauss G, Sherman D, Schwartz J et al: Combined modality therapy for regionally advanced stage III non-small cell carcinoma of the lung employing neo-adjuvant chemotherapy, radiotherapy, and surgery (abstr). Proc Am Soc Clin Oncol 5:172, 1986

Takada M, Fukuoka M, Furuse K et al: Recombinant human G-CSF (rG0-CSF) in patients with non-small cell lung cancer (NSCLC) treated with combination chemotherapy (CT) of mitomycin, vindesine and cisplatin (MVP) (abstr). Proc Am Soc Clin Oncol 9:224, 1990

Taylor SG IV, Trybula M, Bonomi P et al: simultaneous cisplatin-fluorouracil infusion and radiation followed by surgical resection in regionally localized stage III non-small cell lung cancer. Ann Thorac Surg 43:87, 1987

Van Zandwijk N, Tenbokel W, Anders J et al: Dose-finding studies with carboplatin, ifosfamide, etoposide and mesna in non-small cell lung cancer. Semin Oncol 17:16, 1990

Vokes EE, Bitran JD, Hoffman PC et al: Neo-adjuvant vindesine, etoposide and cisplatin for locally advanced non-small cell lung cancer. Chest 86:110, 1989

Vokes EE, Bitran JD, Vogelzang NJ: Chemotherapy for non-small cell lung cancer. The continuing challenge. Chest 99:1326, 1991

Waits TM, Johnson DH, Hainsworth JD et al: Prolonged administration of oral etoposide in non-small cell lung cancer: a phase II trial. J Clin Oncol 10:292, 1992

Weick JK, Crowley J, Natale R et al: A randomized trial of five cisplatin-containing treatments in patients with metastatic non-small cell lung cancer: a Southwest Oncology Group study. J Clin Oncol 9:1157, 1991

Weiden PL, Piantadosi S: Cisplatin and 5FU infusion chemotherapy for non-small cell lung cancer. A phase II study of the Lung Cancer Study Group. J Natl Cancer Inst 83:266, 1991

Weitberg A, Posner M, Yashar J et al: A combined modality therapy for stage IIIA non-small cell carcinoma of the lung (NSCLC) (abstr). Proc Am Soc Clin Oncol 9:226, 1990

Woods RL, Williams CJ, Levi J et al: A randomized trial of cisplatin and vindesine versus supportive care only in advanced non-small cell lung cancer. Br J Cancer 61:608, 1990

Radiotherapy

Thomas H. Weisenburger

DEFINITION

Cancer of the lung, a rare disease in the early part of this century, has become the leading cause of cancer-related death in men and women in the United States. Approximately 164,000 cases were expected to be diagnosed in 1992 (Boring, et al., 1992), of which 80 percent will have NSCLC. Approximately 55 percent of these patients will have distant metastases, 30 percent will have regional lymphatic involvement, and 15 percent will have the tumor confined to the lung (Paulson, 1968; LaRoux, 1968). Only 15 percent of patients can be offered resection for cure (Shields and Robinette,

1973). The remainder of the patients who present without clinically apparent distant metastatic disease (approximately 45,000 to 50,000 patients per year) are candidates for definitive and potentially curative radiotherapy. Unfortunately, the overall cure rate in this population is low, however, and there has been a continuing debate about whether radiotherapy should be offered to all patients in this category (Krant, 1966; Rubin, et al., 1970; Berry, et al., 1977; Phillips and Miller, 1978; Brashear, 1978; Cox, et al., 1983; Cohen, 1983; Pett, et al., 1986; Payne, 1988).

Radical radiotherapy for lung cancer has some associated morbidity, and it should not be considered a "soft alternative to surgery" (Ash, 1984). Physicians caring for these patients must base their decisions regarding therapeutic recommendations on their clinical assessment of the many prognostic factors pertaining to each individual patient and on their understanding of the benefits and morbidities of the various therapeutic modalities.

> To cure sometimes,
> To relieve often,
> To comfort always.

> — Anonymous
> (quoted in Lee, 1974)

HISTORICAL NOTE

In 1940 Leddy and Moersch (1940) reported one of the first series documenting long-term survival with radiotherapy. Of 250 patients with primary lung cancer, 125 were followed without therapy, and 125 received orthovoltage radiotherapy. None of the untreated patients survived 1 year. Twenty-five of the treated group survived 1 year, and 5 (4 percent) survived 5 years. Smart and Hilton (1956) treated 40 patients with orthovoltage radiotherapy alone following biopsy. These were selected patients who had localized lesions with no radiographic or clinical evidence of lymph node metastases. They were in good general condition and were considered operable. Nine patients (22.5 percent) were alive at 5 years and 3 (7.5 percent) at 10 years. This clearly established radiotherapy as a potentially curative modality in selected patients. Morrison, et al. (1963) compared surgery versus radiotherapy in 37 patients who had epidermoid carcinomas. Patients undergoing radiotherapy received 45 Gy in 4 weeks delivered with 8-MeV photons. The 4-year survival rate was 30 percent versus 6 percent for surgery and radiotherapy, respectively, establishing early that surgery is the therapy of choice for operable patients and also demonstrating again, despite the low dose, that radiotherapy can provide a small but real opportunity for cure. Since these pioneering articles, much work has been, and continues to be, done to define the optimum dose and fractionation scheme and to integrate radiotherapy with surgery and/or chemotherapy. The difficulty has been the high rate of pre-existing occult metastatic disease in locally advanced NSCLC, which often obscures any effect of local therapy either surgical or radiotherapeutic, and the lack of comparability of the treated population in many reported combined modality series (Cox, et al., 1990; Holmes, 1990).

HISTORICAL READINGS

Cox JD, Azarnia N, Byhart RW et al: A randomized phase I/II trial of hyperfractionated radiation therapy with total doses of 60.0 Gy to 79.2 Gy: possible survival benefit with ≥ 69.6 Gy in favorable patients with Radiation Therapy Oncology Group stage III non-small-cell lung carcinoma: report of Radiation Therapy Oncology Group 83-11. J Clin Oncol 8:1543, 1990

Holmes EC: Adjuvant therapy of non small cell lung cancer. p. 119. In Salmon SE (ed): Adjuvant Therapy of Cancer. Vol. IV. WB Saunders, Philadelphia, 1990

Leddy E, Moersch HJ: Roentgen therapy for bronchiogenic carcinoma. JAMA 15:2239, 1940

Morrison R, Deeley TJ, Cleland WP: The treatment of carcinoma of the bronchus. A clinical trial to compare surgery and supervoltage radiotherapy. Lancet 1:683, 1963

Smart J, Hilton G: Radiotherapy of cancer of the lung: results in a selective group of cases. Lancet 1:880, 1956

BASIC SCIENCE

An understanding of the lymphatic pathways of the lung is necessary when evaluating patients with lung cancer for radiation therapy. The lymphatic channels of the left upper lobe drain to the nodes between the aortic arch and the pulmonary artery (Lee, 1977). Metastatic nodes in this area may cause paralysis of the left vocal cord by involving the recurrent nerve. The right upper lobe drains to the mediastinal node at the junction of the superior vena cava and the azygos vein. The inferior portions of the lungs drain to nodes in the inferior pulmonary ligaments, communicating with the subcarinal nodes superiorly and the nodes near the cisterna chyli inferiorly (Weinberg, 1972), perhaps explaining the worse prognosis for lower lobe carcinoma described by Deeley (1974). The remaining portions of the lung drain to the hilar lymph nodes. Involvement of the parietal pleura allows the direct spread to regional lymph nodes outside the thorax (axillary, supraclavicular, or subdiaphragmatic lymph nodes, depending on location). The location of the primary tumor and lymphatic metastases, if present, must be determined in relation to the sensitive structures of the thorax. The arrangement of treatment portals is usually designed to include the primary tumor and the lymph node regions at risk while limiting the dose delivered to normal tissues (normal lung, heart, esophagus, and spinal cord) to tolerable levels.

Each fraction of radiotherapy eliminates a percentage of the tumor cells treated, leaving a surviving fraction of cells. The goal of therapy is to reduce the probability of survival of the last clonogenic cell to as low a level as possible. The effect of radiotherapy on the tumor cells depends on the basic radiosensitivity of the cells and the biologic factors that influence the response to fractionated radiotherapy. These include *repair* from radiation damage, *reoxygenation* of the tumor during the course of treatment, *redistribution* of the cells in the cell cycle, and *repopulation* of the cells between fractions (the four Rs of radiobiology). Withers, et al. (1988) noted that there is *accelerated* repopulation of clonogenic cells in response to therapy that occurs during it. Delays in completing a course of therapy once started (as in split-course therapy) are to be avoided. They also noted that chemotherapy prior to radiotherapy may induce the same effect, which could decrease the likelihood of local control with radiotherapy.

The actual dose required in the clinical setting is determined by the number of sites at risk, the number and sensitivity of the clonogens present, and the control rate desired (Fletcher, 1984; Marks, 1990). Doses of 45 to 50 Gy will eliminate nearly 100 percent of occult disease in surgically undisturbed lymphatic channels (Fletcher, 1984). Doses in a postoperative patient with a potentially greater population of hypoxic cells may need to be higher (Marks, 1990). Clinically apparent disease with a greater number of cells will require even higher doses.

DIAGNOSIS AND STAGING

Following histologic confirmation of the diagnosis of NSCLC, the patient must be carefully evaluated for the anatomic extent of both local and distant disease and for the prognostic indicators important in selecting candidates for radiotherapy. A computed tomographic (CT) scan of the chest and upper abdomen, including the adrenal glands and liver, should be performed. If adrenal enlargement is noted, a biopsy is recommended because of the high false-positive rate. Nielson, et al. (1982) reported that only 4 of 15 adrenal masses seen on a CT scan in 84 patients were confirmed by biopsy. Oliver, et al. (1984) noted 32 adrenal masses on CT scans in 330 patients with NSCLC, and only 8 of the 25 that underwent biopsy were positive (32 percent). CT scans of the brain have a low yield in asymptomatic patients. Hooper, et al. (1984) observed that none of 28 asymptomatic patients with NSCLC had a positive brain scan. They noted that, as the number of clinical and laboratory indicators of disease increased, the likelihood of a positive scan increased. Salvatierra, et al. (1990) reported the results of whole-body bone scanning and CT scans of the brain and upper abdomen in 146 patients with NSCLC who had potentially resectable disease. Metastatic disease was found in 44 patients (30 percent). Brain metastases were found in 19 patients (13 percent), only 4 of whom (2.7 percent) were asymptomatic. Bone scans were positive in only 3.4 percent of asymptomatic patients. They found that, if head CT scans in symptomatic patients with squamous cell carcinomas and all patients with adenocarcinomas and large cell carcinomas, bone scans in symptomatic patients, and abdominal CTs on all patients had been performed, only one patient would have been understaged, and 80 percent of bone scans and 53 percent of brain scans would have been avoided.

Evaluation of patients for the presence of various prognostic factors identified with survival may help in deciding whether radical radiotherapy is indicated, although none of the negative indicators alone should preclude the decision to proceed. Patients with good performance status, inoperability because of medical reasons, unresectability determined at thoracotomy, no significant weight loss, and more limited disease stage had a better prognosis (Stanley, 1980; Komaki, et al., 1985). In a Stanford series evaluating prognostic factors in 269 patients treated with radiotherapy, the presence of pain or hemoptysis or the requirement of fields larger than 200 cm^2 was associated with lower survival rates (Caldwell

and Bagshaw, 1968). None of the 34 patients with vocal cord paralysis survived 2 years.

Selection criteria for radical radiotherapy have included evidence of adequate pulmonary function based on a forced expiratory volume at 1 second of 700 ml, ability to climb one flight of stairs without severe dyspnea, no evidence of hypercapnea at rest, and a maximum breathing capacity of at least 50 percent of predicted (Lee, 1974). The hemoglobin level should be above 10 g/dl (Lee, 1977). The presence of a malignant pleural effusion is a contraindication to radical therapy (Ash, 1984).

MANAGEMENT

Radiotherapy for patients with NSCLC can be used as an adjunct to surgery, as primary therapy in the medically inoperable or unresectable patient (either alone or combined with chemotherapy), as "prophylactic" therapy of subclinical disease to prevent the development of clinical disease, or as palliative therapy.

Surgical Adjuvant Radiotherapy

Preoperative Radiotherapy

Prospective studies of preoperative radiotherapy in clinically resectable patients have not shown an increase in survival compared with surgery alone (Komaki, 1985). Bromley and Szur (1955) found 47 percent of 66 patients had no tumors after preoperative radiotherapy, but the mortality rate was high (15 percent). There were significant complications. Bloedorn, et al. (1961) studied 37 patients who received doses up to 60 Gy, with a finding of 46 percent sterilization at the time of surgery. The operative mortality rate of 22 percent exceeded the 5-year survival rate of 20 percent. Shields (1972) reported on 300 clinically resectable patients who were randomized to surgery alone or preoperative radiotherapy. The 4-year survival rate of the surgery-alone group was 21 percent compared with the combined modality group rate of only 13 percent. In addition, postoperative complications were more frequent in the combined therapy group. A Collaborative Study (1975) of the National Cancer Institute (NCI) reported on 550 patients who were randomly assigned to surgery alone or preoperative radiotherapy plus surgery with survival rates of 14 and 16 percent, respectively, at 5 years. Despite the lack of definitive benefit with preoperative therapy for resectable patients, preoperative irradiation is routinely considered in the therapy of patients with superior sulcus tumors.

Postoperative Radiotherapy

The role of postoperative radiotherapy has been controversial for many years. Analysis of the various nonrandomized and randomized studies of postoperative radiotherapy demonstrates the significant heterogeneity of the patient populations and therapeutic parameters studied, including stage, mediastinal evaluation, radiation fields, and doses delivered, which makes it difficult to draw definitive conclusions (Table 28-9) (Weisenburger, 1991). Postoperative radiotherapy in patients without evidence of lymphatic metastasis has no significant

Table 28-9. Selected Studies of Postoperative Radiotherapy for Lung Cancer

Reference (yr treated)/ No. Patients	Histologic Type	N Stage (No. Patients)	Mediastinal Staging	Dose[a] (Gy)	Survival[b] S	S + RT	Comments
Retrospective reviews							
Green, et al., 1975 (1954–66), 219	Adenocarcinoma Epidermoid carcinoma	N0 (123) N1 (64) N2 (32)	If suspicious	44 30–60	0% 6%	62% 21%	Increased survival only in N+ patients with both adenocarcinoma and epidermoid carcinoma
Kirsh and Sloan, 1982 (1959–75), 136	Adenocarcinoma Epidermoid carcinoma	N2 (136)	All Patients	50–60	0% 0%	12% 34%	Increased survival for both adenocarcinoma and epidermoid carcinoma patients with N2 disease
Choi, et al., 1980 (1971–77), 166	Adenocarcinoma Epidermoid carcinoma	N0 (6) N1 (95) N2 (34)	If suspicious	50 40–56	8% 33%	43% 33%	Increased survival in N+ patients with adenocarcinoma only Most recurrences noted at ≤50 Gy
Randomized trials							
Paterson and Russell, 1962 (1955–58), 202	All	Not stated	Not stated	45	41%	31%	Fields too small No stratification for T and N stage 3-Yr Survival
Bangma, 1972 (1958), 73	All	N0 (55) N1 (11) N2 (7)	Not stated	46 44	74%	62%	1-Yr results
Van Houtte, et al., 1980 (1966–1975), 224	All	N0	Not stated	60	43%	24%	Detrimental effect of radiotherapy because of fields used and dose to the lung
LCSG 773 Weisenburger and Gail, 1986 (1978–1985), 210	Epidermoid carcinoma	N0 (9) N1 (157) N2 (44)	All Patients	50	38%	38%	Significant decrease in local recurrence rate with RT No survival benefit with RT Decreased overall recurrence rate but no increase in survival in N2 patients but number of N2 patients small

Abbreviations: S, surgery; RT, postoperative radiotherapy.

[a] Average or median and range, if given.

[b] 5 yr unless otherwise stated.

(Modified from Weisenburger T: Postoperative radiotherapy for non-small-cell lung cancer. Chest Surg Clin North Am 1:71, 1991, with permission.)

survival benefit (Paterson and Russell, 1962; Bangma, 1972; Green, et al., 1975; Van Houtte, et al., 1980).

Retrospective studies by Green, et al. (1975) and Kirsh and Sloan (1982) reported that postoperative radiotherapy significantly increased the survival rate for patients with lymph node metastases from epidermoid carcinoma. Choi, et al. (1980) did not show an increase in survival rate with postoperative radiotherapy, but the groups were not comparable because the postoperative radiotherapy group included 52 percent of patients with T3 or N2 involvement versus 24 percent in the surgery-only group. In addition, systematic mediastinal lymph node evaluation had not been performed, leading to a potential bias in the distribution of patients with an uneven distribution of subclinical N2 involvement. The randomized prospective trial by the LCSG (LCSG 773) (Weisenburger and Gail, 1986) showed a substantial decrease in local recurrences as the first site of recurrence, indicating that the desired effect of control of intrathoracic disease had been achieved but without a significant increase in the survival time. The study, however, only contained 44 patients with mediastinal metastatic disease, and as stated by the authors, this is a subgroup in which irradiation may be beneficial. They reported a higher number of deaths caused by cardiac or respiratory causes in the treated group (11 of 108 versus 5 of 108 in the control group), but the difference was not statistically significant. It should also be noted that these patients had complete resections, as defined by negative mar-

gins and thorough mediastinal sampling, and that the most proximal lymph node was not involved. The conclusions from this study apply to similarly staged patients.

Several retrospective studies have also shown increased survival rates in patients with adenocarcinoma with node-positive (Green, et al., 1975; Choi, et al., 1980) or N2 disease (Kirsh and Sloan, 1982) who have received postoperative radiotherapy. There has not been a prospective randomized trial in patients with adenocarcinomas who have had adequate presurgical evaluation and extensive mediastinal staging. The LCSG in their study 772 (Holmes and Gail, 1986) evaluated patients with stage II and III adenocarcinomas and large cell undifferentiated carcinomas, comparing chemotherapy versus levamisole. They noted 17 percent of the first recurrences were exclusively local compared with 41 percent of the first recurrences in patients with epidermoid carcinoma in LCSG 773 who were in the control group. This would make a beneficial effect of radiotherapy on survival more difficult to demonstrate (Weisenburger and Gail, 1987).

Postoperative radiotherapy probably significantly reduces the risk of locoregional relapse in patients who have lymph node metastases to either hilar or mediastinal lymph nodes. There will be no significant increase in the survival time in patients with negative lymph nodes, and any increase in survival in those patients with positive nodes is likely to be small because of the tendency of these patients to develop disseminated disease (Tubiana, 1989). Until the results of a

Table 28-10. Selected Studies of Radiotherapy for Non-Small-Cell Lung Cancer

Reference	No. Patients	Patient Category	5-Yr Survival
Caldwell and Bagshaw (1968)	269	Inoperable	6%
Cox, et al. (1980)	92	Inoperable/unresectable, high performance status	11%
Smart and Hilton (1956)	40	Operable	23%
Haffty, et al. (1988)	43	Stage I, technically operable, medically inoperable	21%
Zhang, et al. (1989)	44	Early-stage, technically operable, medically inoperable	32%
Talton, et al. (1990)	77	T1–3 N0, technically operable, medically inoperable	17%

(From Cox JD, Komaki R, Eisert D et al: Irradiation for inoperable carcinoma for the lung and high performance status, JAMA 244:1931, 1980, with permission.)

number of current studies are available, it seems reasonable in view of the definite decrease in local recurrence and possible survival benefit to consider postoperative radiotherapy in patients with positive mediastinal nodes. Care must be exercised, however, in the selection and therapy of these patients because the additional loss of pulmonary volume after the lung resection may make a critical difference in clinical pulmonary performance (see Complications of Radiotherapy).

Primary Radiotherapy Alone

Primary radical radiotherapy for NSCLC provides long-term survival in approximately 6 percent of patients with unresectable disease (Caldwell and Bagshow, 1968), 11 percent in patients with more favorable prognostic indicators (Cox, et al., 1980), and as high as 17 to 32 percent (Smart and Hilton, 1956; Haffty, et al., 1988; Zhang, et al., 1989; Talton, et al., 1990) when early-stage resectable patients are treated (Table 28-10; Fig. 28-1).

Despite the numerous studies that have been reported using many varied dose and time combinations, the optimal fractionation schedule has not yet been determined (Perez, 1985). Several conclusions can be drawn, however, concerning radiotherapy as primary therapy. The RTOG protocol 73-01 compared 40-Gy continuous and split-course therapy with 50- and 60-Gy continuous course. Higher doses and the use of a continuous as opposed to a split course were associated with greater local control (Perez, et al., 1982). The survival time was longer in those patients who achieved local control, but there was no significant difference in the overall survival rate between the groups. The RTOG studies have since used a course of radiotherapy with 2.0-Gy fractions to a dose of 60 Gy in 6 weeks, limiting the spinal cord dose to approximately 45 Gy as their standard therapeutic arm in studies of altered fractionation schemes. This schedule results in local control of approximately 60 percent as indicated by clinical evaluation. A recent report by Arriagada, et al. (1991) that incorporated aggressive restaging with bronchoscopy yielded a much lower incidence of local control of 17 percent in patients with stage III disease who were treated with radiotherapy alone.

Altered fractionation schemes have been evaluated by several groups. The RTOG (Cox, et al., 1990) reported increased survival rates using a hyperfractionated course of radiotherapy delivering doses of 69.2 Gy with a 1.2-Gy twice a day schedule compared with the results from previous RTOG studies using 60 Gy in 30 daily fractions over 6 weeks. The 3-year survival rate was 20 percent compared with 7 percent

in the standard fractionation arm ($P = 0.002$). A phase III randomized study is underway comparing these two therapeutic arms. Saunders, et al. (1991) reported on 62 patients treated with continuous hyperfractionated accelerated radiotherapy (CHART) consisting of 1.4- or 1.5-Gy fractions given every 6 hours over 12 consecutive days. They compared the results with those in an earlier series of similar patients treated with radiotherapy and misonidazole at their institution and noted a better radiographic complete response rate of 42 versus 15 percent and an improved 2-year survival probability of 34 versus 12 percent. A randomized trial comparing CHART with 60 Gy in 6 weeks at 2 Gy per day is in progress.

Intraoperative radiotherapy (IORT) using an electron beam has been evaluated by several investigators clinically (Abe, et al., 1980; Pass, et al., 1987; Juettner, et al., 1990; Calvo, et al., 1990) and in the laboratory setting (Tochner, et al., 1992). The experience with IORT is too limited at this time to draw conclusions about its usefulness in combination with or instead of more conventional therapy.

Radiotherapy Combined with Chemotherapy

The combination of chemotherapy and primary radiotherapy has been and continues to be actively investigated and is considered by some (Turrissi, 1991) to be the standard of care. Dillman, et al. (1990) studied 180 patients comparing radiotherapy alone with radiotherapy preceded by a course of cisplatin on days 1 and 29 and five weekly cycles of vinblastine (neoadjuvant chemotherapy). There was a significant increase in the median survival time (13.8 versus 9.7 months) and 2-year survival rate (26 versus 13 percent) for the neoadjuvant group compared with those in the conventional radiotherapy-alone group ($P = 0.006$). If early deaths within 15 weeks of entry into the study were eliminated, there was only a trend toward better survival ($P = 0.059$). There were no differences in the pattern of failure, but uniform reevaluations were not performed at the time of recurrence (Cox, 1991). Arriagada, et al. (1991) reported a randomized trial of 353 patients who either received radiotherapy alone, consisting of 65 Gy in 26 fractions of 2.5 Gy each over 45 days, or induction chemotherapy with vindesine, cyclophosphamide, cisplatin, and lomustine for three cycles followed by the same radiotherapy followed by the same chemotherapy for three more cycles if there was no progression. The 2-year survival rates of 14 and 21 percent for the control and experimental groups, respectively, were not statistically significantly different ($P = 0.08$). Schaake-Koning, et al. (1992) compared a split-course of radiotherapy alone, giving 30 Gy in 10 frac-

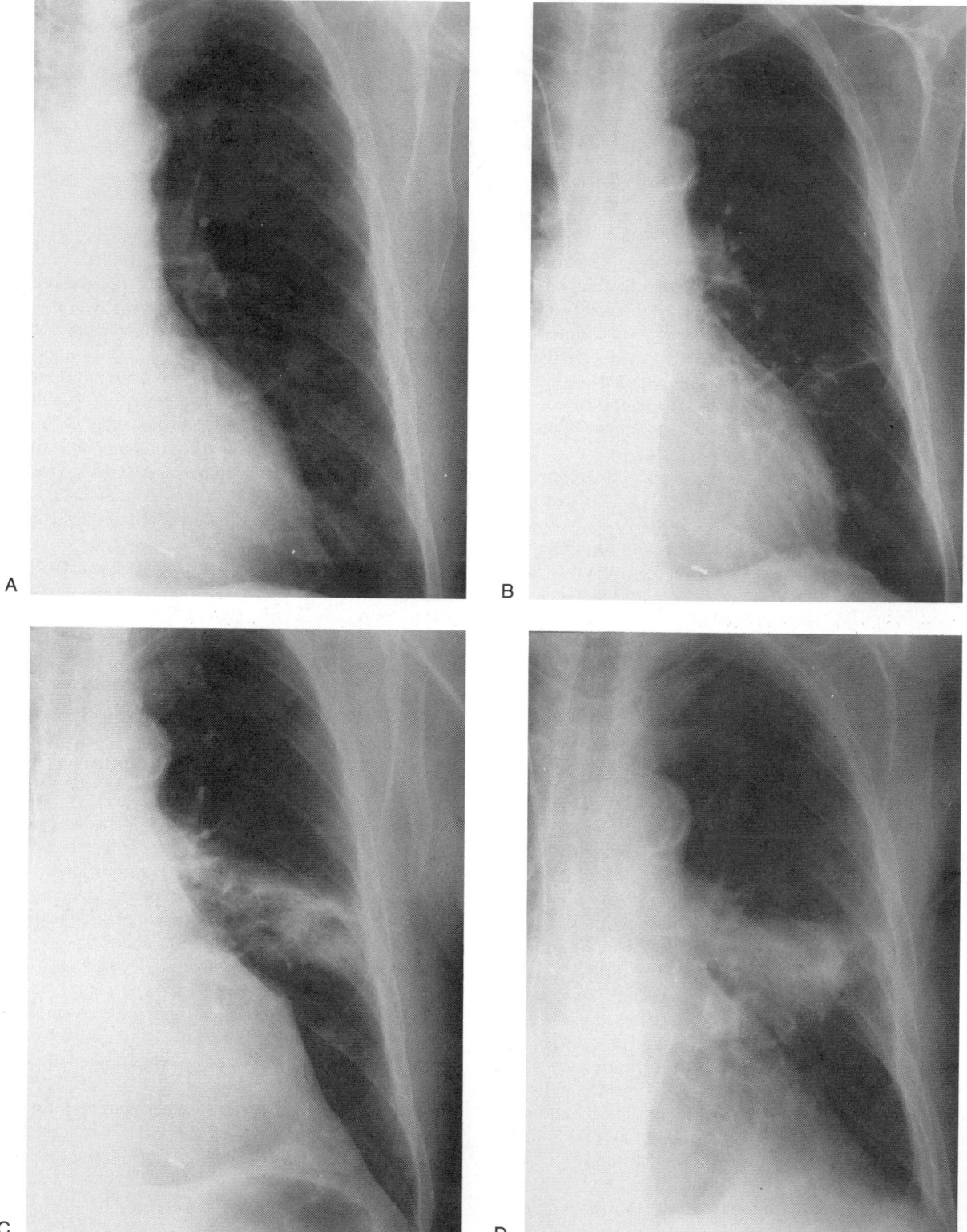

Figure 28-1. Radiographs from a 79-year-old patient with squamous cell carcinoma noted in the left lung field treated with radiotherapy alone. **(A)** Prior to radiotherapy. **(B)** Two months after therapy, the lesion is less visible. **(C)** Four months later, radiographic changes in the lung are noted. **(D)** Four years later, fluid has collected in the major fissure (pseudotumor) overlying the area of radiation-induced fibrosis. The patient remained free of disease until his death 5 years after therapy of heart failure. The heart was excluded from the treatment volume. (Courtesy of M. Northrop, M.D.)

tions of 3 Gy, followed by a 3-week rest, and then 25 Gy given in 10 2.5-Gy fraction over 2 weeks to the same regimen combined with cisplatin either weekly or daily with the irradiation. The 2-year survival rates in the daily cisplatin plus radiotherapy group was increased compared with those in the radiotherapy-alone group (26 versus 13 percent, $P = 0.009$); the survival rate of the weekly cisplatin group of 19 percent was not different from either group. They reported a significant decrease in local failure in the daily-cisplatin group. The authors note that the split course may have been suboptimal because of the possibility of accelerated repopulation during the rest period but point out that the daily cisplatin did increase local control in spite of the split-course regimen.

Prophylactic Cranial Irradiation

Brain metastases from NSCLC are frequent, developing in 16 percent of patients with squamous cell carcinomas and 30 percent of those with adenocarcinomas and large cell carcinomas, according to RTOG data (Perez, et al., 1987). Russell, et al. (1991) reported a delay in the appearance of metastatic disease but no significant difference in the incidence of brain metastases or survival in a randomized study of elective brain irradiation for patients with adenocarcinomas or large cell carcinomas. Prophylactic cranial irradiation is not considered routine practice in NSCLC.

Palliative Radiotherapy

Radiotherapy can provide effective palliation of the symptoms produced by lung cancer in the majority of patients. Slawson and Scott (1979) reported a 61 percent response rate overall in 330 patients who had symptoms. Hemoptysis was relieved in 84 percent (95 of 113), chest pain in 61 percent (66 of 108), dyspnea in 60 percent (51 of 85), superior vena cava syndrome in 86 percent (36 of 42), and vocal cord paralysis in only 6 percent (3 of 54). Reddy and Marks (1991) reported complete or partial reexpansion of the lung in 74 percent of 48 patients with malignant obstructions. Patients treated within 2 weeks of onset had a complete response rate of 71 percent as opposed to 23 percent if treated after that time.

The doses and fields of radiotherapy that are prescribed will depend on the individual circumstances surrounding the need for palliation. The expected survival, the extent of disease, the severity of symptoms, the expected side effects of therapy, and a desire to deliver the therapy as efficiently as possible all factor into the decision regarding the dose, time, and field management. A dose of 30 Gy in 10 fractions of 3 Gy each over 2 weeks is frequently initially prescribed, with the reevaluation for additional therapy depending on the patient's condition and response. Rapidly progressive symptoms in a patient with a limited life expectancy may be treated with larger fractions over a shorter time (20 Gy in five daily fractions of 4 Gy), with a consideration of additional therapy as noted above. Patients with a longer life expectancy may benefit from higher doses. The RTOG reported on the response of patients treated for painful bone metastases and noted that, although short intense courses of radiotherapy (15 to 25 Gy in 1 week) can give meaningful palliation, more highly fractionated schemes using higher total doses (30 to 40 Gy in 2 to 3 weeks) produced more pain relief (Tong, et al., 1982; Blitzer, 1985). Patients with superior vena cava syndrome without evidence of metastatic disease may benefit from a course of radical radiotherapy even when the intent is palliative (Lokich and Goodman, 1975).

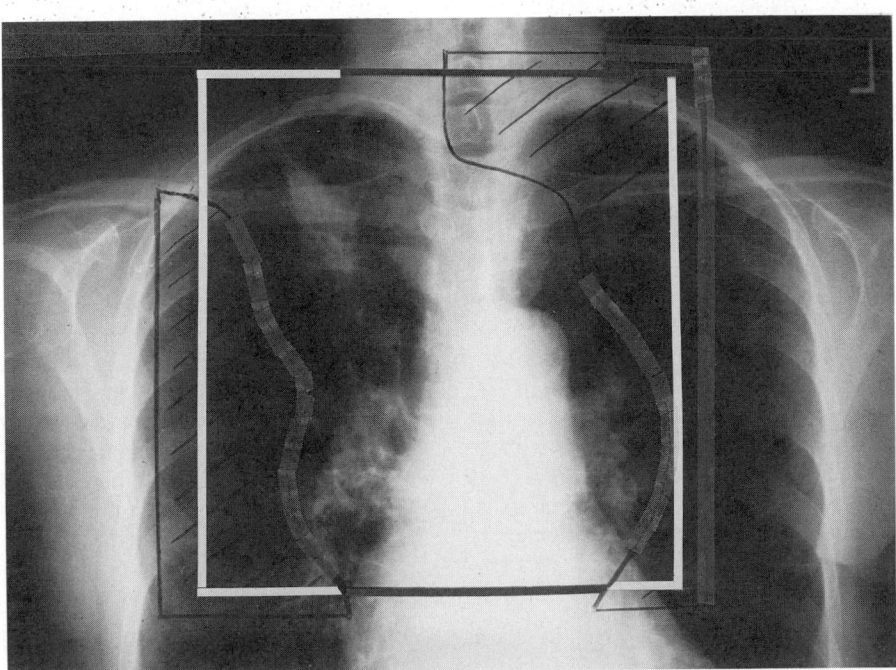

Figure 28-2.   Simulation radiograph for anterior beam. The shaded areas will be blocked.

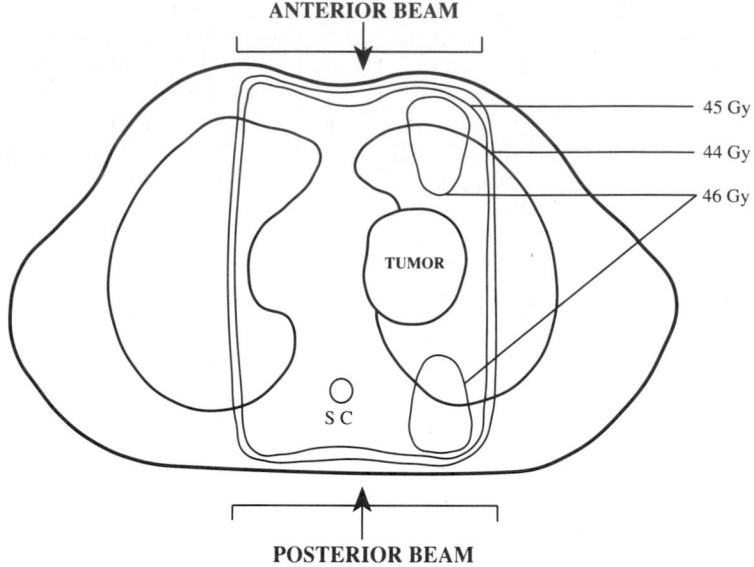

ANTERIOR BEAM

45 Gy

44 Gy

46 Gy

TUMOR

S C

POSTERIOR BEAM

Figure 28-3. Computerized therapeutic plan output utilizing CT scan input for the contours of the anatomic structures for anterior and posterior beams. SC, spinal cord.

Technical Aspects of Radiotherapy

CT scans of the chest have become established in the management of patients with NSCLC when they are treated with radiotherapy. Mira, et al. (1982) compared chest CT with conventional radiographs for therapeutic planning in 45 patients. Eleven of 14 patients whose radiographs were considered to demonstrate the tumor volume satisfactorily had greater tumor extension on CT scan. Of the 31 patients whose radiographs did not show the tumor volume, 21 (68 percent) could be defined by CT scan. There are limitations to CT scans because atelectasis cannot always be distinguished from a tumor and the resolution of the best scanners is 0.5 mm, allowing for undetected subclinical involvement outside the irradiation portals.

CT scans can provide the attenuation characteristics of the tissues being irradiated. Correcting for the decreased attenuation as the beam passes through aerated lung can result in doses 5 to 28 percent higher than those calculated without correction (van't Reit, et al., 1985). The clinical usefulness of this correction has not yet been demonstrated.

The therapeutic volume should have a 2-cm margin around the appreciable tumor and should include the entire mediastinum (Figs. 28-2 and 28-3) (Bleehen and Cox, 1985). The inferior border should be at least 5 cm below the carina. If the lower lobe is involved, the field should extend to the diaphragm. Both hilar regions should be included, with a 1-cm margin around the contralateral hilar region (Perez, et al., 1982). The ipsilateral supraclavicular region is generally included if the tumor is poorly differentiated or in the upper lobe or there is significant mediastinal adenopathy. This reduces the incidence of supraclavicular metastases but has not been shown to influence survival (Cox, 1985). In patients with marginal pulmonary function, it is reasonable to exclude the supraclavicular fossae. The superior portion of the anteroposterior/posteroanterior fields is usually thinner because of

the slope of the chest wall (Fig. 28-4A) (Lambert, 1978), and a wedge or compensating filter may be necessary to provide a uniform distribution of dose (Fig. 28-4B). The fields are reduced to exclude the spinal cord at approximately 45 Gy with the aid of a simulator and CT-guided therapeutic planning (Fig. 28-5). The fields of radiotherapy are usually delineated by individual focused blocks that are fashioned for each portal used (Figs. 28-6 and 28-7). Spinal cord blocks placed in the posterior field to limit the dose to the cord also limit the dose to the mediastinum and are to be avoided (Cox, 1985).

Complications of Radiotherapy

The most frequent symptomatic side effect is esophagitis, which occurs in 50 percent of the patients (Lee, 1977). This usually begins 2 weeks after the initiation of therapy and subsides 1 to 2 weeks after its completion. Radiographic evidence of radiation-induced pneumonitis occurs in almost all patients treated for lung cancer with radiation therapy (Figs. 28-1C & D). Hellman, et al. (1964) reported a 100 percent incidence of radiographic evidence of radiation-induced pneumonitis but only a 5 percent incidence clinically. More recent data from the RTOG indicates a risk of 2.7 percent of life-threatening pneumonitis with doses of 60 Gy (Cox, et al., 1990). The severity of the symptoms of dry cough, dyspnea, chest tightness, and occasionally a mild fever depends on the dose and volume of the lung treated. If a small volume was treated, the symptoms usually subside. However, as the volume increases, the cough can be productive of thick whitish to uniformly pink sputum, and the dyspnea can become severe and life threatening. The differential diagnosis includes bacterial or viral infection, recurrent cancer, lymphangitic spread, or metastatic disease (Roswit and White, 1977). A review of the chest radiographs with the radiation therapy portal films is necessary to determine if the

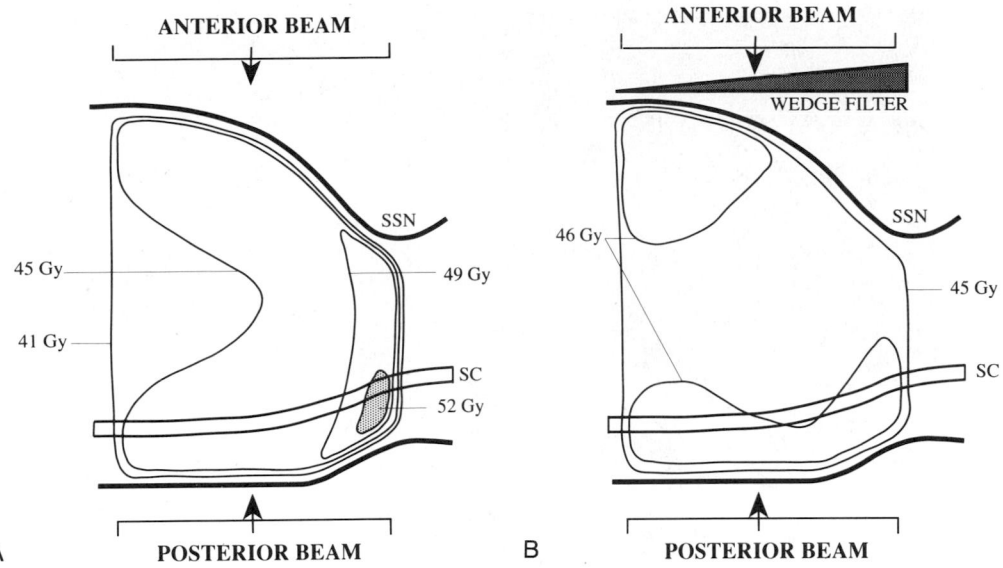

Figure 28-4. **(A)** Because the diameter of the chest wall at the suprasternal notch (SSN) is thinner than at the field center, the dose to the spinal cord (SC) can be 15 percent higher than the central axis dose. **(B)** A wedge or compensating filter can reduce this difference to an acceptable level.

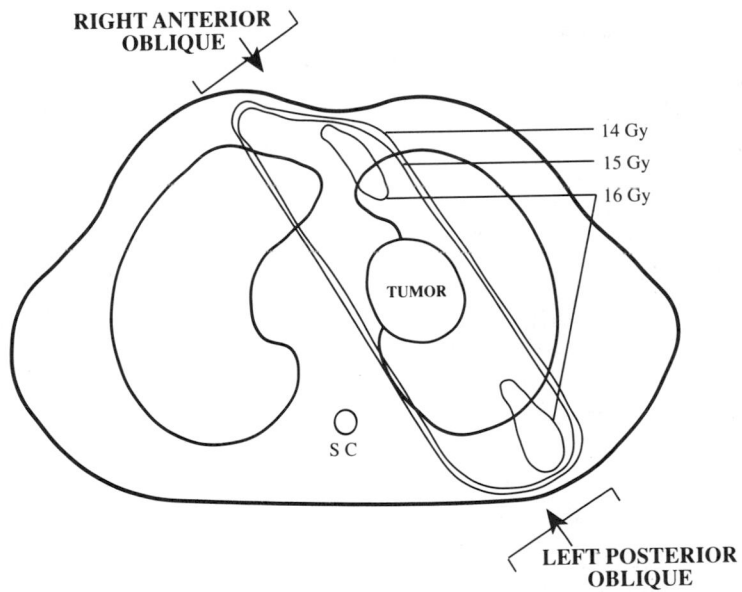

Figure 28-5. Computerlized therapeutic plan output for possible arrangement of off-cord boost beams. SC, spinal cord.

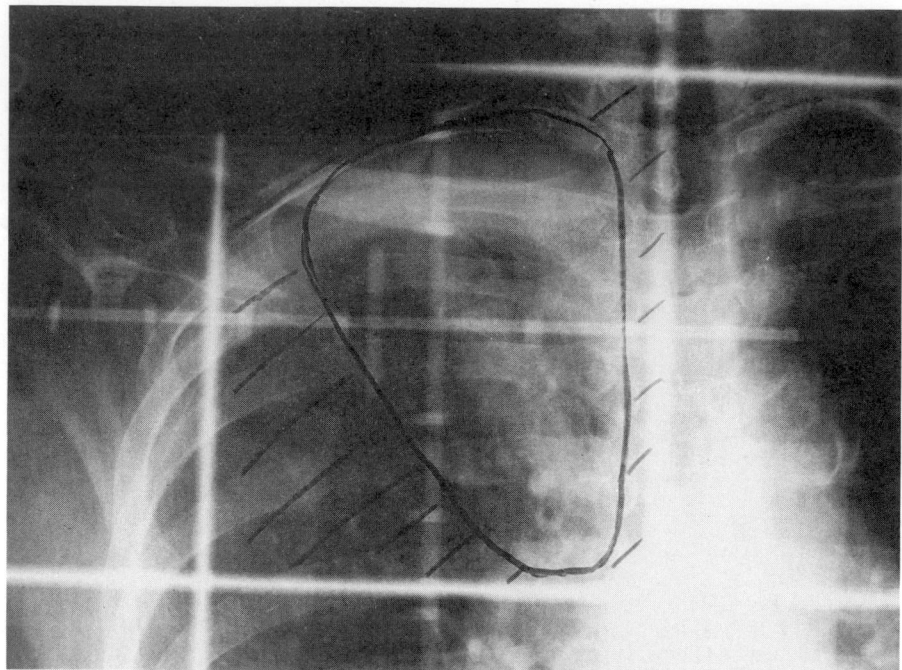

Figure 28-6. Simulation film for off-cord boost field. See Figure 28-7.

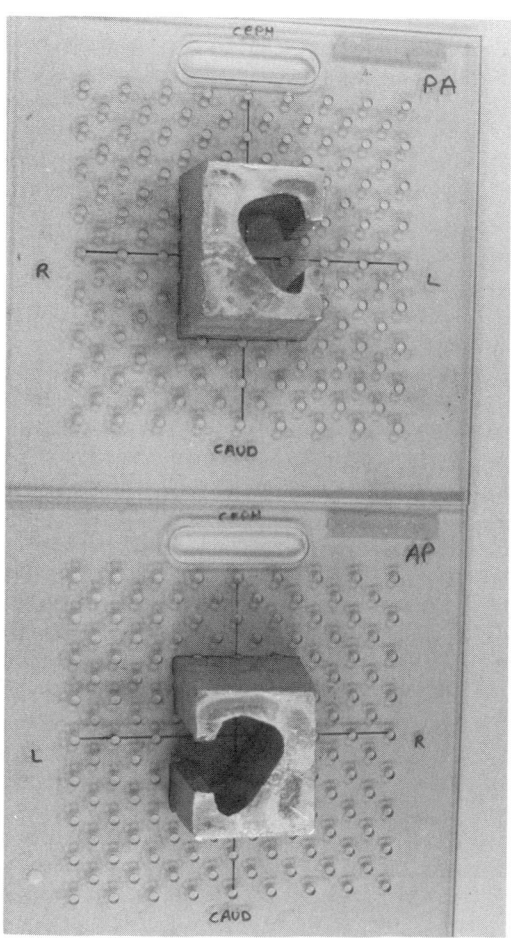

involved lung was in the treated volume. The risk of radiation-induced myocarditis and pericarditis relate directly to the volume of the heart treated (Ruckdeschel, et al., 1975). Lawson, et al. (1972) reported a 4 percent incidence if one-half of the heart received 45 to 50 Gy in 4 to 5 weeks. With respect to acute effects, Lagrange, et al. (1992) demonstrated a temporary decrease of approximately 10 percent in the left ventricle ejection fraction 2 weeks after mediastinal radiation with the recovery of pretherapy function within 2 months. Radiation-induced myelitis is the most devastating complication from thoracic radiotherapy and can be avoided with a careful administration of the radiotherapy. Doses to the cord of 45 Gy in 4.5 to 5 weeks in a continuous course of 1.8 to 2 Gy per day are generally considered safe (Phillips and Buschke, 1969; Wara, et al., 1975).

Figure 28-7. Focused blocks used for the anterior and posterior fields, as defined by the simulator film in Figure 28-6.

COMMENTS AND CONTROVERSIES

Radiotherapy is the best single agent, aside from surgery, in the management of NSCLC. It is a curative modality in patients with locoregional disease, but only in a small minority, and it is an effective palliative therapy in a majority of patients with symptomatic disease. Despite advances in the delivery of therapy using CT scans, computer-generated dosimetry, and therapeutic simulators, local control remains an elusive goal in the majority of patients. The optimal delivery of radiotherapy alone or in combination with surgery and/or chemotherapy remains to be defined and is the subject of active investigation.

The controversies that remain include the selection criteria for radical radiotherapy in unresectable patients and for postoperative radiotherapy in patients with nodal metastases. After local control is achievable in the majority of patients, it may be reasonable to reconsider the question of prophylactic cranial irradiation.

Areas of active investigation include the aforementioned hyperfractionation studies, which may lead to increased local control. Because the majority of patients develop metastatic disease, however, improved systemic chemotherapeutic agents are needed before there can be substantial improvements in overall survival rate in NSCLC.

T.H.W.

Like surgery, radiotherapy is effective only as a local therapy. In patients with potentially curable localized disease, when surgery cannot be offered, primary radiotherapy remains the therapy of choice. The addition of concomitant or induction chemotherapy may improve the ultimate results of this nonsurgical therapy.

The role of adjuvant radiotherapy is still debated. Other than decreasing the incidence of local recurrence, adjuvant radiotherapy, even in locally advanced disease or in completely resected disease, does not appear to improve the ultimate survival rate. This is not unexpected considering the fact that the preponderant type of recurrence following resection for lung cancer is systemic. The destructive complications related to postoperative radiotherapy and the long-term effects on pulmonary function have not been well delineated. The cost benefit, therefore, of adjuvant radiotherapy following surgical resection is extremely questionable.

The use of external beam irradiation for palliation is unquestioned. Focal areas that cause symptoms can certainly be managed effectively by radiotherapeutic means. Whether or not full-dose radiotherapy is required for this palliative therapy is still unknown.

R.J.G.

KEY REFERENCES

Bleehen N, Cox JD: Radiotherapy for lung cancer. Int J Radiat Biol Phys 11:1001, 1985

This is a summary article from the International Association for the Study of Lung Cancer meeting in Cambridge, England, that describes current standard therapy and discusses prospects for the future.

Cox JD, Azarnia N, Byhart RW et al: N2 (clinical) non-small cell carcinoma of the lung: prospective trials of radiation therapy with total doses ≥ 60 Gy by the Radiation Therapy Oncology Group. Int J Radiat Oncol Biol Phys 20:7, 1991

This is a review of the most recent fractionation studies by the RTOG, including comparisons with current combined modality studies.

Perez CA, Stanley K, Grundy G et al: Impact of irradiation technique and tumor extent in tumor control and survival of patients with unresectable non-oat cell carcinoma of the lung: report of the Radiation Therapy Oncology Group. Cancer 50:1091, 1982

This report of RTOG 73-01 compares various fractionation schemes.

REFERENCES

Abe M, Takehishi M, Yabumoto E et al: Clinical experiences with intraoperative radiotherapy of locally advanced cancers. Cancer 45:40, 1980

Arriagada R, le Chevalier T, Quoix E et al: ASTRO Plenary: effective chemotherapy on locally advanced non-small cell lung cancer: a randomized study of 353 patients. Int J Radiat Oncol Biol Phys 20:1183, 1991

Ash D: Role of radiotherapy. Recent results. Cancer Res 92:99, 1984

Bangma PJ: Postoperative radiotherapy. p. 163. In Deeley TJ (ed): Modern Radiotherapy: Carcinoma of the Bronchus. Appleton-Century-Crofts, New York, 1972

Berry RJ, Laing AH, Newman CR et al: The role of radiotherapy in treatment of inoperable lung cancer. Int J Radiat Oncol Biol Phys 2:443, 1977

Blitzer P: Reanalysis of the RTOG study of palliation of symptomatic osseous metastases. Cancer 55:1468, 1985

Bloedorn FG, Cowley RA, Cuccia CA et al: Combined therapy: irradiation and surgery in the treatment of bronchogenic carcinoma. AJR 85:175, 1961

Boring CC, Squires TS, Tong T: Cancer statistics, 1992. CA Cancer J Clin 42:19, 1992

Brashear RE: Should asymptomatic patients with inoperable bronchogenic carcinoma receive immediate radiotherapy? No. Am Rev Respir Dis 117:411, 1978

Bromley LI, Szur L: Combined radiotherapy and resection of carcinoma of the bronchus: experiences with 66 patients. Lancet 2:937, 1955

Caldwell WL, Bagshaw MA: Indications for end results of irradiation for carcinoma of the lung. Cancer 22:99, 1968

Calvo FA, Ortiz de Urbina D, Abuchaibe O et al: Intraoperative radiotherapy during lung cancer surgery: technical description and early clinical results. Int J Radiat Oncol Biol Phys 19:103, 1990

Choi NCH, Grillo HC, Gardiello M et al: Basis for new strategies in postoperative radiotherapy of bronchogenic carcinoma. Int J Radiat Oncol Biol Phys 6:31, 1980

Cohen MH: Is immediate radiation therapy indicated for patients with unresectable non-small cell cancer? No. Cancer Treat Rep 67:333, 1983

Collaborative Study: Preoperative irradiation of cancer of the lung: final report of a therapeutic trial. Cancer 36:914, 1975

Cox JD: Induction chemotherapy for non-small cell carcinoma of the lung: limitations and lessons. Int J Radiat Oncol Biol Phys 20:1375, 1991

Cox JD: Current role of radiation therapy for inoperable carcinoma of the lung. p. 55. In Cox JD (ed): A Categorical Course in Radiation Therapy of Lung Cancer. Radiologic Society of North America, New York, 1985

Cox JD, Azarnia N, Byhart RW et al: A randomized phase I/II trial of hyperfractionated radiation therapy with total doses of 60.0 Gy to 79.2 Gy: possible survival benefit with ≥ 69.6 Gy in favorable patients with Radiation Therapy Oncology Group stage III non-small-cell lung carcinoma: report of Radiation Therapy Oncology Group 83-11. J Clin Oncol 8:1543, 1990

Cox JD, Komaki R, Byhardt RW: Is immediate chest radiotherapy obligatory for any or all patients with limited-stage non-small cell carcinoma of the lung? Yes. Cancer Treat Rep 67:327, 1983

Cox JD, Komaki R, Eisert D et al: Irradiation for inoperable carcinoma of the lung and high performance status. JAMA 244:1931, 1980

Deeley TJ: Radiotherapy for carcinoma of the bronchus. Cancer Treat Rev 1:39, 1974

Dillman RO, Seagren SL, Propert K et al: A randomized trial of induction chemotherapy plus high dose radiation versus radiation alone in stage III non-small cell lung cancer. N Engl J Med 323:942, 1990

Fletcher GH: Subclinical disease. Cancer 53:1274, 1984

Green N, Kurohara SS, George FW III, Crews QE Jr: Post resection irradiation for primary lung cancer. Radiology 116:405, 1975

Haffty BG, Goldberg MB, Gerstley J et al: Results of radical radiation therapy in clinical stage I technically operable non-small cell lung cancer. Int J Radiat Oncol Biol Phys 15:69, 1988

Hellman S, Kligerman MM, von Essen CF et al: Sequelae of radical radiotherapy of carcinoma of the lung. Radiology 82:1055, 1964

Holmes EC, Gail MH (for the Lung Cancer Study Group): Surgical adjuvant therapy for stage II and III adenocarcinoma and large cell undifferentiated carcinoma. J Clin Oncol 4:710, 1986

Holmes EC: Adjuvant therapy of non small cell lung cancer. p. 119. In Salmon SE (ed): Adjuvant Therapy of Cancer. Vol. IV. WB Saunders, Philadelphia, 1990

Hooper RG, Tenholder MF, Underwood GH et al: Computed tomographic scanning of the brain in the initial staging of bronchogenic carcinoma. Chest 85:774, 1984

Juettner FM, Arian-Schad K, Porsch G et al: Intraoperative radiation therapy combined with external irradiation in non-resectable non-small cell lung cancer: preliminary report. Int J Radiat Oncol Biol Phys 18:1143, 1990

Kirsh MM, Sloan H: Mediastinal metastases in bronchogenic carcinoma: influence of postoperative irradiation, cell type and location. Ann Thorac Surg 33:459, 1982

Komaki R: Preoperative and postoperative irradiation for cancer of the lung. J Belge Radiol 68:195, 1985

Komaki R, Cox J, Hartz AJ et al: Characteristics of long-term survivors after treatment for inoperable carcinoma of the lung. Am J Clin Oncol 8:362, 1985

Krant MJ: The question of irradiation therapy in lung cancer. JAMA 195:177, 1966

Lagrange JL, Darcourt J, Benoliel J et al: Acute cardiac effects of mediastinal irradiation: assessment by radionuclide angiography. Int J Radiat Oncol Biol Phys 22:897, 1992

Lambert PM: Radiation myelopathy of the thoracic spinal cord in long-term survivors treated with radical radiotherapy using conventional fractionation. Cancer 41:1751, 1978

Lawson RAM, Ross WM, Gold RJ et al: Post radiation pericarditis: report on four more cases with special reference to bronchogenic carcinoma. J Thorac Cardiovasc Surg 63:841, 1972

LaRoux BT: Bronchial carcinoma. Thorax 23:136, 1968

Leddy E, Moersch HJ: Roentgen therapy for bronchiogenic carcinoma. JAMA 15:2239, 1940

Lee RE: Radiotherapy for lung cancer. p. 163. In Strauss MJ (ed): Lung Cancer Clinical Diagnosis and Treatment. Grune and Stratton, New York, 1977

Lee RE: Radiotherapy of bronchogenic carcinoma. Semin Oncol 1:245, 1974

Lokich J, Goodman R: Superior vena cava syndrome. JAMA 231:58, 1975

Marks LB: A standard dose of radiation for "microscopic disease" is not appropriate. Cancer 66:2498, 1990

Mira JG, Potter JL, Thorton GD et al: Advantages and limitations of computed tomography scans for treatment planning of cancer. Int J Radiat Oncol Biol Phys 8:1617, 1982

Morrison R, Deeley TJ, Cleland WP: The treatment of carcinoma of the bronchus. A clinical trial to compare surgery and supervoltage radiotherapy. Lancet 1:683, 1963

Nielson ME, Heiston DK, Dunnick NR: Preoperative CT evaluation of adrenal glands in non-small cell bronchogenic carcinoma. AJR 139:317, 1982

Oliver TW Jr, Bernardino ME, Miller JI et al: Isolated adrenal masses in non-small cell bronchogenic carcinoma. Radiology 153:217, 1984

Pass HI, Sindelar WF, Kinsella TJ et al: Delivery of intraoperative radiation therapy after pneumonectomy: experimental observations and early clinical results. Ann Thorac Surg 44:14, 1987

Paterson R, Russell MH: Clinical trials in malignant disease IV: lung cancer: value of postoperative radiotherapy. Clin Radiol 13:141, 1962

Paulson DL: A philosophy of treatment for bronchogenic carcinoma. Ann Thorac Surg 5:289, 1968

Payne DG: Non-small cell lung cancer: should unresectable stage III patients routinely receive high-dose radiation therapy? J Clin Oncol 6:552, 1988

Perez CA: Non-small cell carcinoma of the lung: dose-time parameters. Cancer Treat Symp 2:131, 1985

Perez CA, Pajak TF, Rubin P et al: Long-term observations of the patterns of failure in patients with unresectable non-oat cell carcinoma of the lung treated with definitive radiotherapy. Cancer 59:1874, 1987

Pett SB Jr, Wernly JA, Akl BF: Lung cancer—current concepts and controversies. West J Med 145:52, 1986

Phillips TL, Buschke F: Radiation tolerance of the spinal cord. AJR 105:659, 1969

Phillips TL, Miller RJ: Should asymptomatic patients with inoperable bronchogenic carcinoma receive immediate radiotherapy? Yes. Am Rev Respir Dis 117:404, 1978

Reddy SP, Marks JE: Total atelectasis of the lung secondary to malignant airway expansion. Am J Clin Oncol 13:394, 1991

Roswit B, White DC: Severe radiation injuries of the lung. AJR 129:127, 1977

Rubin P, Ciccio S, Setisarn B: Controversial status of radiation therapy in lung cancer. p. 855. In Proceedings of The Sixth National Cancer Conference. JB Lippincott, Philadelphia, 1970

Ruckdeschel JC, Chang P, Morton RG et al: Radiation related pericardial effusions in patients with Hodgkin's disease. Medicine 54:245, 1975

Russell AH, Pajak TE, Selim HM et al: Prophylactic cranial irradiation for lung cancer patients at high risk for development of cerebral metastasis: results of a prospective randomized trial conducted by the Radiation Therapy Oncology Group. Int J Radiat Oncol Biol Phys 21:637, 1991

Salvatierra A, Baamonde C, Llamas JM et al: Extrathoracic staging of bronchogenic carcinoma. Chest 97:1052, 1990

Saunders MI, Dische S, Grosch EJ et al: Experience with CHART. Int J Radiat Oncol Biol Phys 21:871, 1991

Schaake-Koning C, Van den Bogaert W, Dalesio O et al: Effects of concomitant cisplatin and radiotherapy on inoperable non-small cell lung cancer. N Engl J Med 326:524, 1992

Shields TW: Preoperative radiation therapy in the treatment of bronchial carcinoma. Cancer 30:1388, 1972

Shields TW, Robinette CD: Long term survivors after resection of bronchial carcinoma. Surg Gynecol Obstet 136:759, 1973

Slawson RG, Scott RM: Radiation therapy in bronchogenic carcinoma. Radiology 132:175, 1979

Smart J, Hilton G: Radiotherapy of cancer of the lung: results in a selective group of cases. Lancet 1:880, 1956

Stanley KE: Prognostic factors for survival in patients with inoperable lung cancer. J Natl Cancer Inst 65:25, 1980

Talton BM, Constable WC, Kersh CR: Curative radiotherapy in non-small cell carcinoma of the lung. Int J Radiat Oncol Biol Phys 19:1521, 1990

Tochner ZA, Pass HI, Sindelar WF et al: Long term tolerance of thoracic organs to intraoperative radiotherapy. Int J Radiat Oncol Biol Phys 22:65, 1992

Tong C, Gillick L, Hendrickson FR: The palliation of symptomatic osseous metastases: final results of the study by the Radiation Therapy Oncology Group. Cancer 50:893, 1982

Tubiana M: Radiotherapy in non-small cell lung cancer. Chest 96(suppl):85s, 1989

Turrissi AT: The integration of platinum and radiotherapy in the treatment of lung cancer. Semin Oncol 18(suppl 3):81, 1991

Van Houtte P, Rockmans P, Smets P et al: Postoperative radiation therapy in lung cancer: a controlled trial after resection of curative design. Int J Radiat Oncol Biol Phys 6:983, 1980

van't Reit A, Stam HC, Mak ACA et al: Implications of lung corrections for dose specification in radiotherapy. Int J Radiat Oncol Biol Phys 11:621, 1985

Wara WM, Phillips TL, Sheline GE et al: Radiation tolerance of the spinal cord. Cancer 35:1558, 1975

Weinberg JA: The intrathoracic lymphatics. p. 231. In Haagensen CD, Feind CR, Herter FP et al. (eds): The Lymphatics in Cancer. WB Saunders, Philadelphia, 1972

Weisenburger T: Postoperative radiotherapy for non-small-cell lung cancer. Chest Surg Clin North Am 1:71, 1991

Weisenburger T, Gail M: Postoperative mediastinal radiation for cancer of the lung (letter). N Engl J Med 316:1476, 1987

Weisenburger T, Gail M (for the Lung Cancer Study Group): Effects of postoperative mediastinal radiation on completely resected stage II and III epidermoid carcinoma of the lung. N Engl J Med 315:1377, 1986

Withers HR, Taylor JMG, Maciejewski B: The hazard of accelerated tumor clonogen repopulation during radiotherapy. Acta Oncol 27:131, 1988

Zhang HX, Yin WB, Zhang LJ et al: Curative radiotherapy of early operable non-small cell lung cancer. Radiother Oncol 14:89, 1989

Brachytherapy and Intraoperative Radiotherapy

John G. Armstrong

DEFINITION

The principal types of radiation used for the therapy of tumors are external beam and brachytherapy. With external beam radiotherapy, the source of radiation is outside the patient and must pass through superficial tissues to arrive at its destination. Examples of external beam machines include linear accelerators that can produce photons or electrons and isotopic cobalt-based machines that produce photons. IORT is delivered during the operative procedure. While still anesthetized and draped, the patient is transported to the linear accelerator (as described above), and the machine is pointed directly into the operative field and is oriented toward the tumor bed. Retractors can be used to remove normal tissues from the pathway of the radiation. Brachytherapy is the therapy of tumors by the direct application of radioactive sources, either into a tumor (interstitial) or into a naturally occurring cavity (intracavitary) such as the airways. In contrast to external beam radiotherapy, the source of radiation is an isotope that emits radiation in a localized manner and delivers a high dose to the tissues from within (*Brachy* meaning *short*).

HISTORICAL NOTE

The interstitial implantation of radioactive isotopes for lung cancer began in 1941 at Memorial Sloan-Kettering Cancer Center in New York (Henschke, 1958). Initially encapsulated ^{222}Rn was used. Radioactive isotopes encapsulated in metal seeds were placed through hollow needles into tumors, one seed at a time. There was no mechanism to calculate the optimal distribution of seeds or to ensure that the seeds could be evenly distributed throughout the tumor. In addition, the dose to the tumor could not be calculated, and therapy was prescribed solely in terms of the total amount of "activity" of the radioisotope. Subsequently, encapsulated radioactive ^{125}I seeds were used. The development of the Mick applicator permitted accurate spacing of the ^{125}I seeds evenly distributed throughout the tumor. An intraoperative nomogram was devised to permit the delivery of uniform doses to tumors of varying sizes and shapes. By measuring the tumor intraoperatively, a nomogram could be used to calculate the total activity required, the optimal placement of the Mick applicator needles, and the spacing of the individual seeds along the needles. Dose calculations are now computerized and reflect the actual dose delivered to the tumor, which can be displayed in a three-dimensional format.

Intracavitary brachytherapy for lung cancer consists of intraluminal therapy of cancers in the major airways. Under bronchoscopic guidance, catheters are positioned in the lumen of the bronchus beyond the site of the tumor in the airway. The radioactive source is then placed in the catheter and is positioned at the site of the tumor. Initially, the source used was an iridium wire, which was of sufficient length to span the tumor with several additional centimeters on either side. After the removal of the bronchoscope, the catheter containing the wire was left in place for 1 day or more. The typical dose 1 cm from the center of the source was 30 to 40 Gy over 1 to 2 days. The disadvantages of this technique were its duration, discomfort for the patient, and the need to protect the staff from the radiation exposure associated with this prolonged therapy. The development of high-activity remote afterloading machines removed these practical disadvantages and led to a great interest in the use of this technology for the palliation of obstructing airway malignancies.

HISTORICAL READINGS

Henschke UK: Interstitial implantation in the treatment of primary bronchogenic carcinoma. AJR 79:981, 1958

Hilaris BS, Martini N: The current state of intraoperative interstitial brachytherapy in lung cancer. Int J Radiat Oncol Biol Phys 15:1347, 1988

Nori D, Hilaris B, Martini N: Intraluminal irradiation in bronchogenic carcinoma. Surg Clin North Am 67:1093, 1987

BASIC SCIENCE

Radiobiology

Radiobiology is the study of the action of ionizing radiation on living cells. The effect is mediated indirectly by the formation of chemically reactive free radicals that attack the base pairs of DNA, leading to chemical changes and biologic damage. The interval between the chemical damage and the expression of biologic effects may be hours, days, months, or even years. A number of factors contribute to the timing and magnitude of the biologic effect and are described as the "4 Rs" of radiobiology.

The impact of a given dose of radiation on the target cell is related to the cells ability to *repair* radiation damage. Although the biologic mechanisms of repair have not been elucidated, they have been quantified mathematically. It appears that a minimum of 4 to 6 hours is required for the optimal repair of damage to normal tissues. Tumor cells may repair radiation damage less well than do normal cells, hence, the preferential killing of malignant cells. If the repair is complete before cell division occurs, then there is no untoward effect on the cell or its progeny. However, if the repair is incomplete or severe, the damage is lethal, and the cell dies on attempting division. Because radiation-induced death occurs when mitosis is attempted, the response to radiation may occur a long time after the therapy. In the interval between two fractions of radiation exposure, both tumor and normal cells *repopulate*. This has an adverse effect on the potential to control a tumor (particularly, if it is rapidly growing). In contrast, this allows compensatory proliferation of actively dividing normal tissues (e.g., mucuosal membrane) but has no beneficial effect on slowly dividing normal tissues (such as spinal cord).

Because molecular oxygen is required to stabilize radiation damage, large tumors with central hypoxic zones are relatively radioresistant. It has been shown that these hypoxic areas disappear throughout a course of fractionated radiotherapy, and this phenomenon (described as *reoxygenation*) explains why large tumors can be cured despite the presence of hypoxic areas. The most radiosensitive phases of the cell cycle are G2 and M. As a fractionated course of radiotherapy proceeds, the tumor's cells tend to accumulate in these phases (perhaps because sublethal radiation-induced damage has not been repaired and control mechanisms prevent mitosis), and therefore, they become radiosensitive. This is referred to as *redistribution*.

Physics

The physical characteristics of isotopes determine their biologic effects. The typical energy of radiation emitted from isotopes ranges from a high of 1.25 MeV from ^{60}Co to a low of 0.028 MeV for [125]I. At the high end of the energy spectrum, the emitted radiation penetrates tissue well, to such an extent that ^{60}Co can be used as the radiation source for external beam radiotherapy machines. In contrast, the low-energy emissions penetrate tissue poorly. In addition, the dose decreases in proportion to the square root of the distance from the source. Therefore, the majority of the dose is released into the immediately adjacent tissues. Because of this physical advantage of brachytherapy, high activities of isotope can be placed directly into the tumor with a powerful localized antitumor effect.

Radioactive [125]I

The rate of radioactive decay of an isotope is indicated by its half-life, which is the time required for it to decay to one-half of its original activity. Radioactive ^{125}I has a half-life of 60 days. It can be calculated that it will decay to 1.5 percent of its original activity by 1 year after a permanent implant. Thus, the majority of the biologic effect is delivered in the first 2 months, and ^{125}I is safe to use as a permanent interstitial implant. The disadvantage of this low-dose rate (8 cGy/h) is that it facilitates complete repair of radiation-induced damage, in theory negating the antitumor effect. In addition, if the tumor contains rapidly cycling cells (such as a histologically high-grade neoplasm), they may repopulate during this protracted therapy. In defense of ^{125}I, the low-dose rate may facilitate redistribution and increase tumor cell death. The reality is that tumors respond in a heterogeneous manner, and ^{125}I can permanently eradicate some tumors. Another disadvantage of ^{125}I is that the poor penetrance of the beam requires that the seeds be placed in (or in close proximity to) the tumor.

[192]Ir

[192]Ir is the other important isotope used for lung cancer brachytherapy. Unlike ^{125}I, the emitted radiation has a higher energy (0.38 MeV). Consequently, the radiation from this isotope penetrates more deeply and can effectively treat to a distance of 1 cm from the location of the source. In addition, the dose rate from this isotope is higher, and it can be used for temporary brachytherapy. The most common use of this isotope is in high-dose-rate machines that use a source of 10 Ci, which can deliver a dose of 500 cGy at 1 cm from the source in a matter of minutes. Thus ^{192}Ir is used for repeated intraluminal therapy of tumors accessible by bronchoscopy. This approach appears to have a greater antitumor effect than do numerically similar total doses of fractionated external beam radiotherapy. This is probably because the large fraction size (500 cGy versus 180 to 200 cGy with external beam) exceeds the repair potential of tumor cells. In addition, there are components of the tumor (closer than 1 cm to the source) that receive much higher doses than the prescription dose of 500 cGy.

MANAGEMENT

Permanent Interstitial Implants

Indications

Permanent interstitial implants have been used if the patient has an early-stage technically resectable tumor but cannot tolerate the required resection. In addition, they are used as adjuncts in incompletely resectable tumors or as primary therapy for unresectable tumors.

Technique

A permanent implant is performed at thoracotomy under general anesthesia. The unresected tumor is measured, and the area or volume to be covered is identified. This includes a margin around the clinically evident tumor. If the tumor is a palpable mass, the appropriate nomogram for volume implants is consulted to determine the total activity required and the separation of the needles. The lesion is then firmly grasped, and the Mick needle is inserted into the tumor. The hand grasping the tumor is used to palpate the deepest extent of the tumor and determine the depth of insertion. The required number of needles are inserted into the tumor and are usually placed 1 cm apart. The Mick applicator is then used to deposit the seeds in the tissue at predetermined intervals along the track of the needle as it is withdrawn. Plaques of residual disease or areas of possible microscopic disease are covered with a planar implant, attached either by direct suturing of ^{125}I seeds encapsulated in Vicryl or by evenly spacing suture seeds in a premeasured Dexon mesh and suturing the

mesh directly onto the area at risk (Hilaris, et al., 1988). The latter technique is well suited to areas such as the major vessels or paraspinal region (Armstrong, et al., 1991). Postoperatively, when the chest tubes are removed, plain radiographs are taken to determine the location of the seeds and produce computerized dose distribution calculations. The typical dose delivered with ^{125}I is 16,000 cGy minimal peripheral dose. When done by experienced practitioners, this approach is remarkably safe. It has not increased postoperative morbidity or mortality rates to any appreciable extent. In one instance at Memorial Hospital, a seed migrated into the pulmonary vein and eventually lodged in the circle of Willis, with ensuing neurologic sequelae.

The majority of patients treated with permanent ^{125}I implants have also received supplemental postoperative external beam radiotherapy. The usual dose is 5,040 cGy in conventional fractions (180 to 200 cGy). An example of a patient with a T4N0 unresectable squamous cancer is presented in Figure 28-8.

Results

Medically Inoperable Tumors.   Some patients with T1-2-N0-1 resectable disease have medical contraindications or refuse surgery. For such patients, external beam radiotherapy alone is a potentially curative therapy (Armstrong and Minsky, 1989). An alternative approach has been reported by the Memorial Sloan-Kettering group. They used brachytherapy for 55 patients with borderline pulmonary function test results (Hilaris, et al., 1987b). Preoperatively the tumors were considered resectable by lobectomy or a lesser procedure. At the time of surgery, however, a more radical procedure that the patient could not tolerate was considered necessary. Consequently, the gross tumor was implanted with ^{125}I seeds intraoperatively. Following brachytherapy, 24 patients received a median dose of 44 Gy of external beam radiotherapy. The actuarial 5-year survival rate was 32 percent, suggesting that this approach is reasonable for patients whose conditions are found to be medically inoperable at the time of surgery. Fleischman, et al. (1992) also treated early-stage tumors with permanent ^{125}I implants. The patients were selected for this therapy if they had node-negative technically resectable tumors that were medically inoperable, as described above. The survival rate of the 14 patients was approximately 32 percent at 2 years. Local control was obtained in 10 of 12 patients with tumors 5 cm or less in maximum dimension. Both patients with larger tumors had locally recurrences.

Pancoast Tumors.   The management of Pancoast tumors is controversial. Radiotherapy is considered to be an essential component of therapy, either as sole therapy, as preoperative therapy, postoperatively, or as intraoperative brachytherapy (Paulson, 1985; Neal, et al., 1991; Anderson, et al., 1986; Miller, et al., 1979; Attar, et al., 1979; Komaki, et al., 1981). Preoperative radiotherapy, pioneered by Shaw, et al. (1961) is used to reduce the volume of the tumor, thus facilitating complete resection. Subsequent reports of preoperative radiotherapy demonstrated 5-year survival rates in the range of 20 to 30 percent. Hilaris, et al. (1987a) treated 82 patients

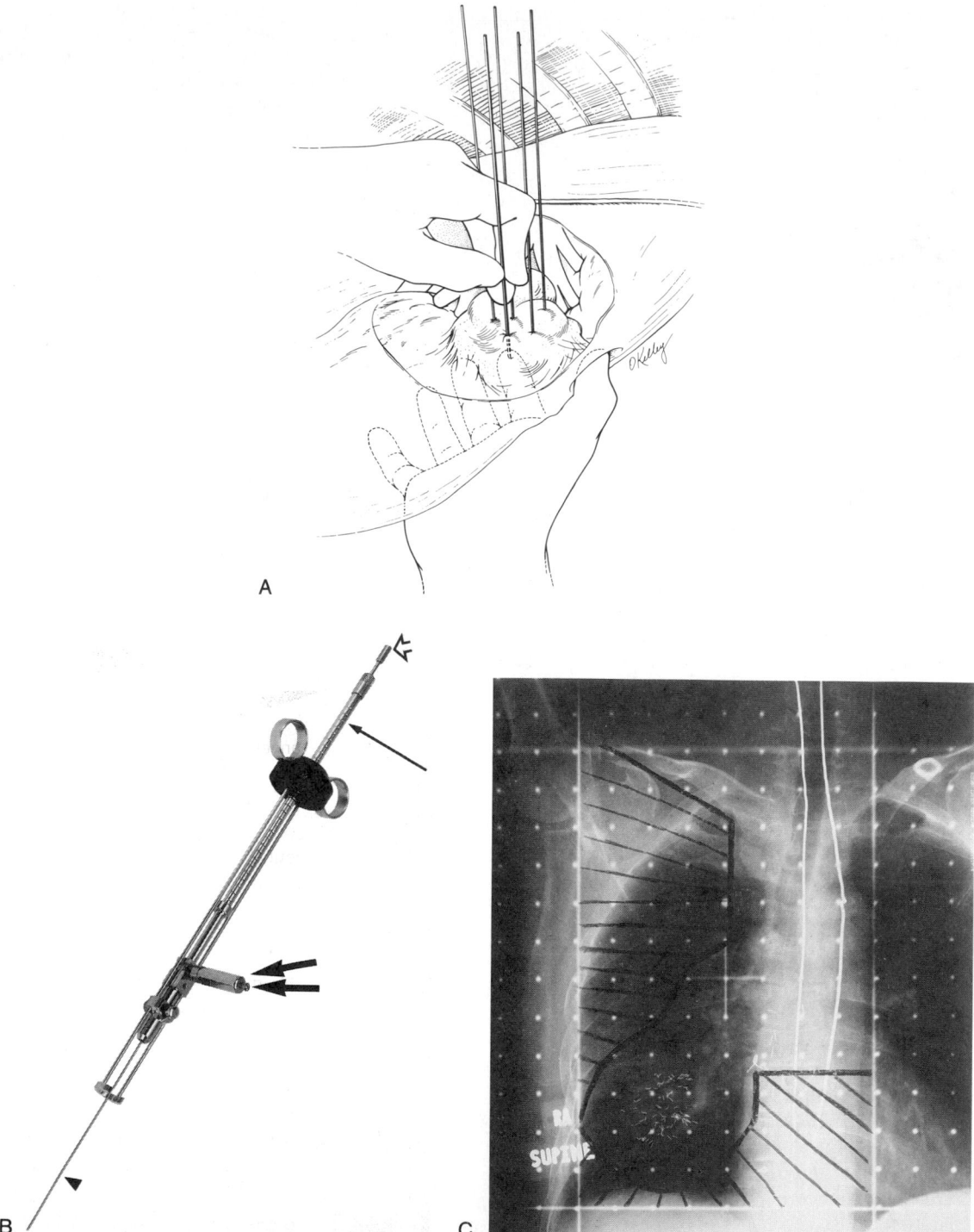

Figure 28-8. A NSCLC invading the right pulmonary artery was unresectable because the patient's pulmonary function tests were too poor to permit pneumonectomy. The implant was performed with ^{125}I. **(A)** At thoracotomy, the afterloading trochars are placed in the tumor one at a time, spaced approximately 1 cm apart (see text). When all the trochars are inserted, the Mick afterloader is used, and the radioactive seeds are deposited along the length of each trochar as it is withdrawn by the applicator (see Fig. B). **(B)** The Mick applicator. The cartridge of radioactive ^{125}I seeds (*double arrows*) is inserted into the applicator. The plunger is used to advance the seeds (one by one) into the tumor, withdrawing the central applicator (*long slender arrow*) to space the seeds. **(C)** After recovery from surgery, the patient received external beam radiotherapy, consisting of 5,040 cGy to the primary tumor, ipsilateral hilum, mediastinum, and ipsilateral supraclavicular area. The radioactive seeds are seen within the tumor on the simulation radiograph.

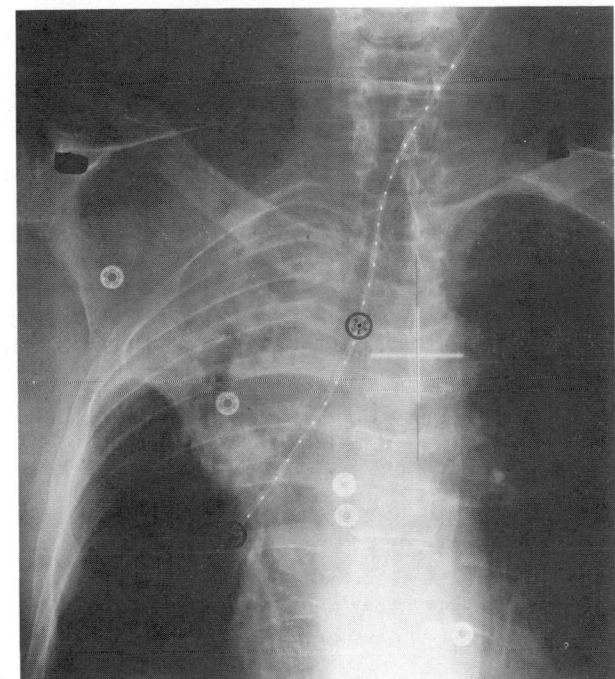 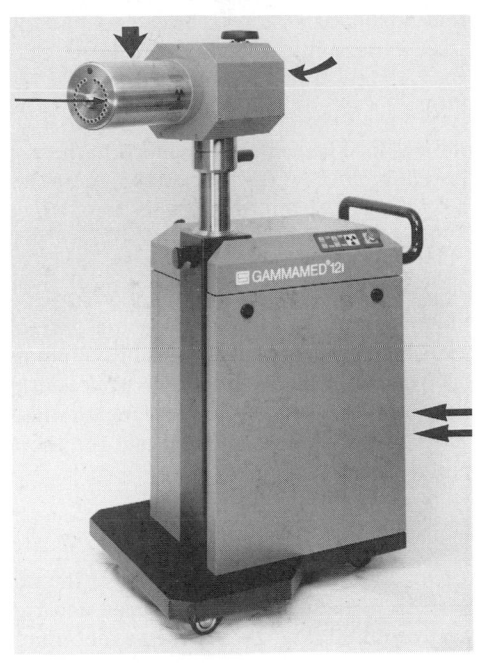

A   B

Figure 28-9. **(A)** A 68-year-old man with medically inoperable (poor pulmonary function) T2N0 squamous cancer of the right mainstem bronchus who was treated with primary external beam radiotherapy to a total dose of 5,960 cGy. Seven months later, the tumor had progressed. The localization radiograph shows the afterloading catheter. **(B)** A remote afterloading device. The main portion of the device (*double arrows*) contains a power supply, electronics, and most of the cables. The radioactive source is kept in the safe (*single thick arrow*) when not in active use. Cable-driving devices (*curved arrow*) are used to propel both a dummy cable and source and the real cable and source. The cable controls the location of the real source, which exits the machine through any one of 24 channels (*long slender arrow*) and enters the catheter (applicator), which is situated in the airway.

with 2,000 to 4,000 cGy of preoperative radiotherapy followed by resection and permanent interstitial implantation of ^{125}I in the majority. The fatal complication rate was 1 percent, and the 5-year survival rate was 29 percent. In addition to this experience with preoperative radiotherapy, this group (Hilaris, et al., 1987b) also employed initial surgery with intraoperative brachytherapy for 36 patients, followed by postoperative radiotherapy and reported 20 percent 5-year survival rates. Although the results achieved with combined brachytherapy, surgery, and external beam radiotherapy are impressive, they are not strikingly different from the survival rates reported in series without brachytherapy.

Locally Advanced Lung Cancer.   Hilaris and Martini (1988) reported on 101 patients with unresectable primary tumors invading the major vessels, pericardium, or esophagus who were treated with biopsy only, brachytherapy, and external beam radiotherapy. These patients had no evidence of mediastinal metastases at thoracotomy. The median survival time was 11 months, and the 2-year survival rate was 21 percent. A contemporary group of 44 patients with locally advanced primary tumors and a clinically negative mediastinum were treated with external beam radiotherapy (with or without chemotherapy) and had a median survival time of 8 months and 2-year survival rate of 10 percent. In 100 patients with stage III NSCLC, ^{125}I implants were used for unresected or incompletely resected primary tumors and ^{192}Ir implants were placed in the mediastinum for N2 disease. The local control

rate was more than 70 percent at 5 years, and the survival rate was 22 percent (Hilaris, et al., 1985). Lewis, et al. (1990) treated 82 patients with intraoperative brachytherapy as an adjunct to surgical resection. In general, temporary implants with ^{192}Ir were used for microscopic residual disease, and permanent ^{125}I implants were used for gross disease. Supplemental external beam radiotherapy was used (approximately 50 Gy). The techniques of the Memorial group were used. The tumor stage was IIIA or IIIB in 89 percent of cases, and the implanted volume was 6 cm or less in maximum dimension. The overall survival rate was 40 percent at 2 years. The survival rate at 2 years was 50 percent if microscopic residual disease was implanted and 30 percent if gross residual disease was implanted.

Intraluminal Brachytherapy

Direct permanent implantation of ^{125}I seeds into endobronchial tumors was also pioneered at Memorial-Sloan Kettering Cancer Center in the 1960s. Relief of symptoms was achieved in about 60 percent of patients, but there was significant morbidity as a result of perforation of the airway, hemorrhage, and ventilatory arrest (Nori, et al., 1987). Subsequent workers avoided direct implantation into tissues (interstitial) and used temporary intraluminal placement of ^{60}Co or ^{192}Ir to deliver one or more large fractions over a few days (Schray, et al., 1985; Mehta, et al., 1989) High-dose-rate fractionated intraluminal therapy was developed to avoid such prolonged therapeutic times, which were uncomfortable for the patient and required hospitalization with its attendant expense and radiation risk to personnel (Macha, 1987).

Indications

The use of high-dose-rate intraluminal brachytherapy (HDR-ILBRT) is relatively new. Consequently, there are insufficient data to answer several basic questions about patient selection, optimal techniques, and dose-fractionation schemes. The generally accepted criteria for the use of HDR-ILBRT are previous external beam radiotherapy, pathologically documented recurrence in the bronchus or trachea with an intraluminal component, and significant symptoms caused by the local disease. If the obstruction is the result predominantly of extrinsic disease, the high-dose region will be superficial to the cause of the obstruction, and the therapy may be less helpful.

Technique

If endobronchial laser resection is planned at the time of the first HDR-ILBRT, then general anesthesia and rigid bronchoscopy are required (Fig. 28-9). When endobronchial laser resection is not used, the bronchoscopy is performed as an outpatient procedure with sedation, local anesthesia, cardiac monitoring, and pulse oximetry. The bronchoscope is inserted transnasally, and a routine examination of the airway is performed. The brachytherapy catheter is placed through the working channel of the bronchoscope and is lodged at least 3 cm distal to the obstruction. Leaving the catheter in place, the bronchoscope is withdrawn, and the catheter is taped to the nose, thus securing it in position. Another useful technique is to pass a guidewire through a cannula through the midline of the neck into the upper trachea and a Seldinger-type dilator over this wire. The brachytherapy catheter can be passed through the dilator into the airway. When the position of the catheter in the trachea is verified by the bronchoscope, the dilator can be withdrawn and peeled off the catheter, leaving it in the airway. Using fiberoptic bronchoscopy, the catheter is then manipulated into position and secured to the overlying skin.

A "dummy" source is placed in the catheter and pushed to its distal end. The dummy is a wire that has radiopaque beads located at 0.25- to 1-cm intervals, which can be occupied by the radiation source. Radiographs are taken to verify the location of the catheter and decide which potential source locations are to be treated. It is important to treat the entire tumor and a margin of 3 cm proximally and distally. Computerized planning is used to calculate the dwell time of the source at the various locations along the treated length of airway. (The newer machines can use a number of catheters and can be programmed to modify dwell times to create an envelope of dosing volume around the tumor.) The therapeutic time is calculated to give the prescribed dose at a distance of 1 cm from the source. When the planning is complete, the catheter is connected to the afterloading machine, which contains a high-activity ^{192}Ir source (10 Ci), which travels along the catheter and is programmed to remain at specific locations to deliver a precisely controlled dose over several minutes.

The optimal radiotherapeutic parameters for HDR-ILBRT are far from clear. The variables include the use of initial laser debulking, external radiotherapy, number of brachytherapy procedures, dose per fraction, depth of prescribed dose, interval between procedures, and total dose. The various permutations of these variables are described in Table 28-11. The most commonly used approach is to deliver a total of three courses spaced 1 week apart. The dose per fraction is prescribed at 1 cm from the source and varies between 5 and 10 Gy. Doses in the low range of this scale may be more appropriate for patients previously treated with high doses of external radiotherapy (60 Gy or more).

Table 28-11. A Summary of Reported Results with Intraluminal Brachytherapy[a]

Reference	No. Patients	Laser Resection	Fraction Size (Gy)	No. Fractions Mean	Mean Total Dose (Gy)	Endoscopic Response	Toxicity	Survival
Hatlevoll, et al., 1991 (Norway)	14	13	6–8	3	18–24	—[e]	35% (5/14) fatal hemorrhage	—[e]
Grafton, et al., 1991 (Vancouver)	105	No	30	1	30	—[e]	3% (3/105)[b] hemoptysis	—[e]
Burt, et al., 1990 (Manchester)	50	No	15–30	1	15–20	88% (15/17)	4% (2/50)[c] hemoptysis	—[e]
Bedwinek, et al., 1991 (St. Louis)	38	24% 9/38	6	3	18	87% (22/27)	32% (12/38)[d] hemoptysis	6.5 mo median
Seagren and Harrell, 1990 (San Diego)	50	72% (36/50)		3 1	20 10	—[e]	6% (3/50)	—[e]
Fass, et al., 1990 (New York)	15	No	5–6	1–6	5–30	—[e]	20% (3/15)	—[e]
Miller and Phillips, 1990 (Georgia)	88	24%	10	3	30	90% (+ laser) 75% (− laser)	1% (1/88) hemoptysis	91% > 6 mo

[a] Most patients had previously received up to 60 Gy of external beam radiotherapy. Where cited, 50–80% of patients had a good symptomatic response.

[b] All three presented with hemoptysis.

[c] Not considered to be related to therapy.

[d] Three of 12 had hemoptysis before therapy.

[e] No data supplied.

Results

The results of several series are detailed in Table 28-11. HDR-ILBRT is a relatively simple procedure in experienced hands and is well tolerated. The overall therapeutic time is short, and hospitalization can be avoided. This approach can be a cost-effective method to palliate disease in patients who have few alternative options.

HDR-ILBRT is an effective method to palliate lung cancer that is causing airway obstruction or other problems related to intraluminal disease. Relief of hemoptysis is achieved in 38 to 90 percent of patients, cough is relieved in 50 to 66 percent of patients, and dyspnea is relieved in 43 to 64 percent of patients. The median duration of symptomatic response is often not well documented but would appear to be in the 4- to 5-month range, which is a significant proportion of the expected survival time in this group of patients with such a bad prognosis.

An objective assessment of the response using bronchoscopy after HDR-ILBRT is difficult because of the inability of conventional bronchoscopic video equipment to measure visible disease or to assess the response of extrinsic disease. Using subjective visual criteria, the typical range of responses observed is 75 to 90 percent.

Endobronchial laser resection provides immediate relief of symptoms, facilitates catheter placement beyond the obstruction, and may increase response rates and duration of response. In one series in which laser resection was used for some patients, bronchoscopic responses occurred in 90 percent (19 of 21) of the patients receiving laser resection with HDR-ILBRT compared with 75 percent (50 of 67) of those treated with HDR-ILBRT alone ($P = 0.08$) (Miller and Phillips, 1990). Seagren and Harrell (1990) reported significantly improved response rates among a population of 36 patients who underwent laser resection versus 14 who did not.

The serious complications include hemorrhage, fistula formation, pneumonitis, tracheal perforation, and radiation-induced bronchitis. These are fortunately rare, with the exception of hemorrhage, which has been reported to occur in 0 to 36 percent of patients. Only two series report an incidence above 6 percent (Bedwinek, et al., 1991; Hatlevoll, et al., 1991. These high figures are difficult to explain and may be a result of a statistical fluke or tumor progression. Alternatively, as proposed by Bedwinek, et al., the majority of these complications occurred in upper lobe tumors in which the catheters may have been close to the main pulmonary arteries.

Because of the heterogeneity of current reports, in the future, it will be important to define prognostic factors accurately (e.g., clinical characteristics, previous therapy, extrinsic versus intrinsic obstruction, degree of obstruction, and primary versus nodal obstruction), which will facilitate the ability of trials to develop prospectively optimal therapeutic parameters and optimal combinations with external beam radiotherapy and laser therapy.

Intraoperative Radiotherapy

IORT using linear accelerators with modified cones has been described by a number of investigators (Abe, et al., 1980). The cone is applied to the area of unresected residual tumor, and normal structures that are not involved by the cancer are retracted or covered with custom-made blocks. Electron energies are selected to cover the required depth appropriately. Doses in the range of 10 to 25 Gy are given in a single fraction in the operating room. The NCI ran a phase I trial and reported that two of four patients died as a result of complications and the other two had life-threatening fistulae (Pass, et al., 1987). In Austria 21 patients with negative nodes after mediastinal dissection received 10 to 20 Gy IORT to unresected primary tumors. Postoperatively this was supplemented by 45 to 46 Gy external beam radiotherapy. The authors report CT scan-documented responses as early as 4 weeks, which improved with time, eventually leading to a 33 percent complete response rate and a disease-free survival rate of 90 percent (19 of 21) at a median follow-up of 1 year. The good results in this group of patients may be caused by the negative nodes and the fact that a lot of the tumors were resectable early-stage tumors in medically unfit patients. Only one patient died as a result of therapy (Juettner, et al., 1990). Less favorable results were obtained in Spain where 34 patients with unresected or incompletely resected primary or nodal tumors received an intraoperative dose of 10 to 15 Gy followed by 46 to 50 Gy of external beam radiotherapy postoperatively (Calvo, et al., 1990). Acute pneumonitis occurred in 35 percent (12 of 34), the median survival time was only 12 months, and the freedom from thoracic progression rate was only 30 percent. In conclusion, the relatively limited experience with IORT added to external beam radiotherapy for NSCLC did not demonstrate that it is superior to radical external beam radiotherapy alone. In view of its frequent toxicity, its use must be regarded as experimental.

COMMENTS AND CONTROVERSIES

Despite the large experience at Memorial Sloan-Kettering, intraoperative interstitial brachytherapy has not been widely adopted. The series reported have good local control and survival for the various disease categories. Although it is a theoretically attractive technique, its superiority to external beam radiotherapy alone has not been clearly demonstrated. An attempt to conduct a randomized trial of external beam radiotherapy with and without brachytherapy for incompletely resected NSCLC was closed because of accrual failure (Armstrong, unpublished data).

J.G.A.

The use of intraoperative brachytherapy remains controversial and has never been tested in a prospective randomized trial that would compare it with routine postoperative irradiation. Its main indications are for residual gross tumor, residual microscopic tumor, or "close" resection margins. Its theoretic advantages include less pulmonary toxicity and the application of higher doses to areas close to vital structures (e.g., spinal cord). A recent analysis that I performed at Memorial Sloan-Kettering suggests no distinct advantage for the use of intraoperative brachytherapy in the management of superior sulcus tumors for the above reasons.

The role of intraoperative external beam radiotherapy to either supplement or treat unresectable tumors has also not been tested in a controlled fashion. The initial reports have been less than encouraging.

Brachytherapy used intraluminally for the palliation of obstructing tumors of the airway and for augmentation of primary radiotherapy for the management of lung cancer appears to be the best use of this type of therapy. It has certainly been proved to have a distinct advantage in palliating previously irradiated obstructing tumors.

At Memorial Sloan-Kettering Cancer Center, we are currently embarking on an investigation of IORT using high-dose brachytherapy in an attempt to provide local control for patients with malignant mesotheliomas that are undergoing an attempt at total surgical removal of the disease.

R.J.G.

KEY REFERENCES

Henschke UK: Interstitial implantation in the treatment of primary bronchogenic carcinoma. AJR 79:981, 1958

This is a report of the initial experience with interstitial implantation at Memorial Sloan-Kettering.

Hilaris BS, Martini N: The current state of intraoperative interstitial brachytherapy in lung cancer. Int J Radiat Oncol Biol Phys 15:1347, 1988

This is a review of the long-term experience with interstitial implantation at Memorial Sloan-Kettering.

REFERENCES

Abe M, Takahishi M, Yabumoto E et al.: Clinical experiences with intraoperative radiotherapy of locally advanced cancers. Cancer 45:40, 1980

Anderson T, Moy P, Holmes E: Factors affecting survival in superior sulcus tumors. J Clin Oncol 4:1589, 1986

Armstrong JG, Minsky BD: Primary radiation therapy for stage I and II medically inoperable non-small cell lung cancer. Cancer Treat Rev 16:247, 1989

Armstrong JG, Fass DE, Bains M et al.: Paraspinal tumors: techniques and results of brachytherapy. Int J Radiat Oncol Biol Phys 20:787, 1991

Attar S, Miller J, Satterfield J et al.: Pancoast's tumor: irradiation or surgery? Ann Thorac Surg 28:578, 1979

Bedwinek J, Petty A, Bruton C et al.: The use of high dose rate endobronchial brachytherapy to palliate symptomatic endobronchial recurrence of previously irradiated bronchogenic carcinoma. Int J Radiat Oncol Biol Phys 22:23, 1991

Burt P, O'Driscoll R, Notley M et al.: Intraluminal irradiation for the palliation of lung cancer with the high dose rate Micro-Selectron. Thorax 45:765, 1990

Calvo F, Ortiz de Urbina D, Abuchaibe O et al.: Intraoperative radiotherapy during lung cancer surgery: technical description and early clinical results. Int J Radiat Oncol Biol Phys 19:103, 1990

Fass DE, Armstrong JG, Harrison LB, Nori D: Fractionated high dose endobronchial treatment for recurrent lung cancer. Endocuriether Hyperthermia Oncol 6:211, 1990

Fleischman E, Kagan R, Streeter O et al.: Iodine-125 interstitial brachytherapy in the treatment of carcinoma of the lung. J Surg Oncol 49:25, 1992

Grafton C, Lam S, Voss N et al.: High dose rate endobronchial brachytherapy using the Microselection. Lung Cancer 7(suppl 1):97, 1991

Hatlevoll R, Karlsen K, Aamdal S, Bohman T: Endobronchial radiotherapy for malignant bronchial obstruction or recurrence. Lung Cancer 7(suppl 1):95, 1991

Hilaris B, Gomez J, Nori D et al.: Combined surgery, intraoperative brachytherapy, and postoperative external radiation in stage III non-small cell lung cancer. Cancer 55:1226, 1985

Hilaris B, Martini N, Wong G, Nori D: Treatment of superior sulcus tumor (Pancoast tumor). Surg Clin North Am 67:965, 1987a

Hilaris BS, Nori D, Anderson LL: Brachytherapy techniques. p. 46. In Hilaris BS, Nori D, Anderson LL (eds): Atlas of Brachytherapy. Macmillan, New York, 1988

Hilaris BS, Nori D, Martini N: Intraoperative radiotherapy in stage I and II lung cancer. Semin Surg Oncol 3:22, 1987b

Juettner FM, Arian-Schad K, Porsch G et al.: Intraoperative radiation therapy combined with external irradiation in nonresectable non-small-cell lung cancer: preliminary report. Int J Radiat Oncol Biol Phys 18:1143, 1990

Komaki R, Mountain C, Holbert J et al.: Superior sulcus tumors: treatment selection and results for 85 patients without metastases (M0) at presentation. Int J Radiat Oncol Biol Phys 19:31, 1990

Komaki R, Roh J, Cox J, Lopes da Conceicao A: Superior sulcus tumors: results of irradiation of 36 patients. Cancer 48:1563, 1981

Lewis J, Ajlouni M, Kvale P et al.: Role of brachytherapy in the management of pulmonary and mediastinal malignancies. Ann Thorac Surg 49:728, 1990

Macha H, Coch K, Stadler M et al.: New technique for treating occlusive and stenosing tumors of the trachea and main bronchi: endobronchial irradiation by high dose iridium-192 combined with laser utilization. Thorax 42:511, 1987

Mehta M, Shahabi S, Jarjour N, Kinsella T: Endobronchial irradiation for malignant airway obstruction. Int J Radiat Oncol Biol Phys 17:847, 1989

Miller J, Mansour K, Hatcher C: Carcinoma of the superior pulmonary sulcus. Ann Thorac Surg 28:44, 1979

Miller J, Phillips T: Neodymium-YAG laser and brachytherapy in the management of inoperable bronchogenic carcinoma. Selectron Brachytherapy J Suppl 1:23, 1990

Neal C, Amdur R, Mendenhall W et al.: Pancoast tumor: radiation therapy alone versus preoperative radiation plus surgery. Int J Radiat Oncol Biol Phys 21:651, 1991

Nori D, Hilaris B, Martini N: Intraluminal irradiation in bronchogenic carcinoma. Surg Clin North Am 67:1093, 1987

Pass HI, Sindelar W, Kinsella T et al.: Delivery of intraoperative radiation therapy after pneumonectomy: experimental observations and early clinical results. Ann Thorac Surg 44:14, 1987

Paulson D: The "superior sulcus" lesion. p. 121. In Delarue N, Eschapasse H (eds): International Trends in General Thoracic Surgery. Vol. 1. WB Saunders, Philadelphia, 1985

Schray M, McDougall J, Martinez A et al.: Management of malignant airway obstruction: clinical and dosimetric considerations using an iridium-192 afterloading technique in conjunction with the neodymium-YAG laser. Int J Radiat Oncol Biol Phys 11:403, 1985

Seagren S, Harrell J: Prospective trial of palliative high dose rate endobronchial irradiation with or without laser for recurrent non-small cell lung cancer. Proc Am Soc Clin Oncol 9:224, 1990

Shaw R, Paulson D, Kee J: Treatment of the superior sulcus tumor by irradiation followed by resection. Ann Surg 154:29, 1961

Biologic Therapy

Helen W. Pogrebniak
Harvey I. Pass

With our improvement in understanding normal host immune responses, including defense mechanisms against cancer, a new fourth modality of anticancer therapy became feasible—biologic therapy.

DEFINITIONS

Immunotherapy refers to a therapy that elicits an immune response that augments the host's antitumor defenses. Biologic therapy can be specific or nonspecific and active or passive. Specific immunotherapy is therapy with specific reactivity to tumor-associated antigens, such as monoclonal antibody therapy, tumor cell vaccines, or the use of tumor-infiltrating lymphocytes (TIL). Nonspecific immunotherapy is therapy that augments or restores the host's immune system but is lacking tumor specificity, such as immune adjuvants and cytokines. Active immunotherapy refers to therapy that actively elicits an immune response, such as tumor cell vaccines, adjuvants, and cytokines, whereas passive immunotherapy is the transfer of immunologic reagents that mediate tumor regression to the host. Biologic therapy, initially synonymous with immunologic, now must include the emerging field of gene therapy (see Comments and Controversies).

HISTORICAL NOTE

William B. Coley (1893), a surgeon, was one of the earliest physicians to make a substantial attempt at treating malignancies with biologic therapy. Prompted by a report of the regression of an unresectable sarcoma after a severe infection of erysipelas, Coley purposely attempted to induce erysipelas in patients with cancer by injecting live microorganisms. Coley's toxins, as they became known, did induce responses in some patients; however, with the introduction of radiotherapy, this early crude biologic therapy fell into disuse.

Interest in the response of lung cancer to immunotherapies was initiated when Takita (1970) and then Ruckdeschel, et al. (1972) reported an improved survival rate in patients with lung cancer who survived postoperative empyemas versus uninfected patients. The improvement in survival was thought to be the result of the adjuvant immunostimulatory effect of the bacterial products.

HISTORICAL READINGS

Coley WB: The treatment of malignant tumors by repeated inoculations of erysipelas: with report of ten original cases. Am J Med Sci 105:487, 1893

Ruckdeschel JC, Codish SD, Stranahan A, McKneally MF: Postoperative empyema improves survival in lung cancer. N Engl J Med 287:1013, 1972

Takita H: Effect of postoperative empyema on survival of patients with bronchogenic carcinoma. J Thorac Cardiovasc Surg 59:642, 1970

BASIC SCIENCE

The early observations that malignancies occasionally spontaneously regress suggests that tumors evoke an immune response (Fig. 28-10). Tumor specific immunity was demonstrated in a series of classic experiments conducted in the 1950s. Foley (1953), Prehn and Main (1957), and Klein, et al. (1960) demonstrated that, after strangulation or excision of a tumor, the formerly tumor-bearing mouse would reject the same tumor when it was reimplanted.

Mediators of Tumor Cytolysis

A variety of immune processes can mediate tumor lysis, including subsets of T lymphocytes, B lymphocytes, macrophages, and natural killer (NK) cells. Cytotoxic T-lymphocytes (CTL) are the best characterized cytolytic immune cells. CTL-mediated tumor cell lysis requires direct cell contact through the T-cell receptor and is limited to those cells that have the same major histocompatibility complex (MHC) class I or II loci (MHC restricted). After adhesion to the tumor antigen occurs, lysis is initiated within minutes. Alternatively, CTL can bind to the tumor target through an antibody bound to the immune cell rather than through the T-cell receptor, a lytic process that is termed antibody-dependent cellular cytotoxicity (ADCC). TILs are CTL that are obtained from tumor specimens and that can be activated and expanded in vitro with IL-2. They are specific and have lytic activity, primarily for autologous tumor or MHC-compatible allogeneic tumor.

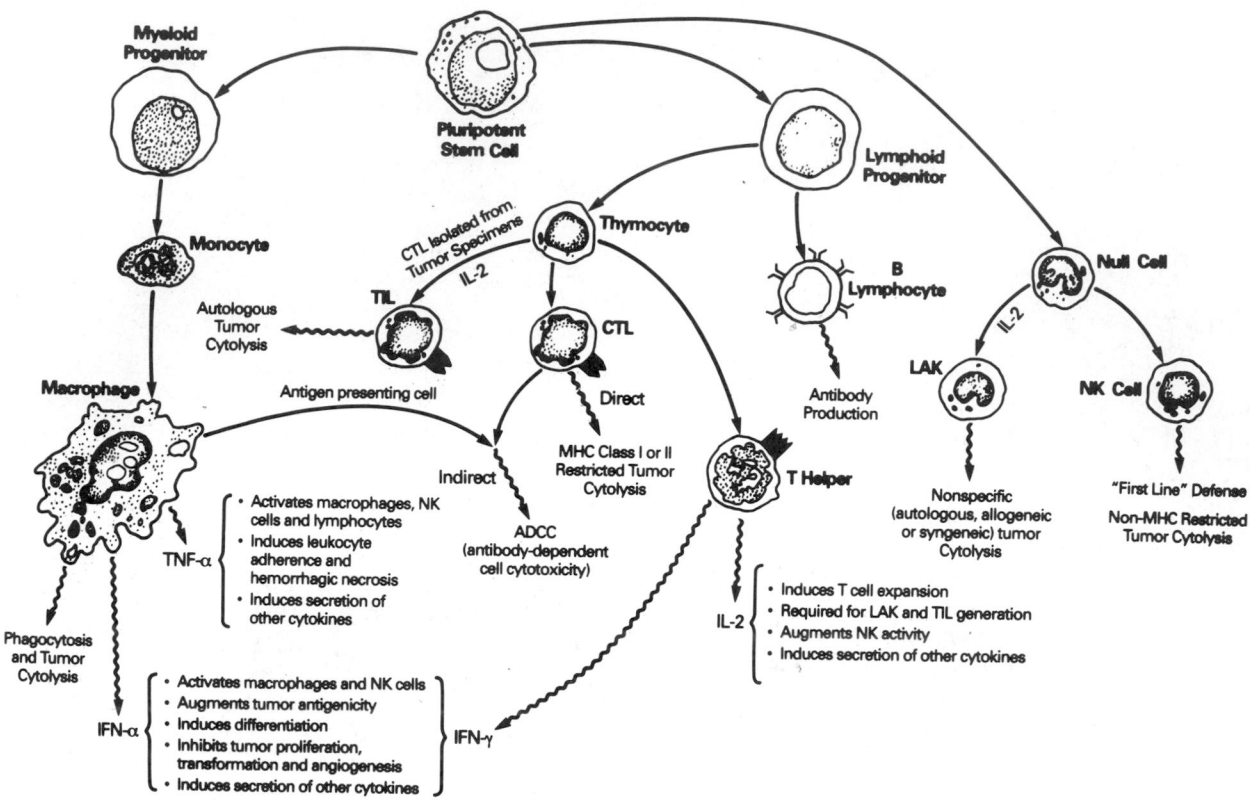

Figure 28-10.   Immune mechanisms involved in the immunotherapy of lung cancer.

Antibodies mediate cytolysis by binding complement or by functioning as an ''opsonin'' to facilitate phagocytosis (see under Monoclonal Antibody Therapy). B lymphocytes indirectly promote tumor cytolysis through the production of antibodies. LAK cells are null lymphocytes (separate from the T and B categories) that can acquire the ability to lyse tumor cells following incubation with IL-2.

Activated macrophages have a dual role in mediating tumor cell destruction. They can directly phagocytize and lyse tumor cells over a 48- to 72-hour period, and they also serve as antigen-presenting cells to other effectors, especially CTLs. The role of NK cells in tumor cytolysis has not been completely defined. Theoretically, NK cells may represent a first line of defense because NK tumor cell lysis is not MHC restricted (i.e., less specific) and does not require prior immune activation; however, NK cells demonstrate low lytic activity to fresh tumor cells in vitro. Immune cells can also mediate cytolysis by the release of secretory products. Cytokines, such as IL-2, IFN, and tumor necrosis factor (TNF); proteases; and other soluble proteins produced by immune cells can directly or indirectly (by the induction of an inflammatory response) cause tumor lysis.

Pathogenesis of Cancer Immunosuppression

To appreciate the rationale behind immunotherapy and to design specific therapies, we must have an understanding of the cause of the impaired immunoregulation in patients with cancer. Either a very large or a very small tumor inoculum may result in tumorigenesis. Small numbers of tumor cells bearing tumor antigens can ''sneak through'' immunosurveillance. This results in the recognition of the tumor-associated antigens as ''self,'' permitting further tumor proliferation. However, more often in animal tumor models, a large inoculum that overwhelms the host's defenses is necessary for tumor allografting.

It has been well documented in animal and human studies that the tumor-bearing host has a suppressed immune system. Both humoral (antibody) and cellular (lymphocytes and macrophages) immunity can be affected. The tumor itself may also release immunosuppressive factors, such as transforming growth factor-β, prostaglandins, acute-phase reactants, and other factors that have not yet been identified. In addition, circulating suppressor T lymphocytes may also contribute to a lack of efficacy of the anticancer therapy. In an attempt to eliminate these suppressive factors, some adoptive immunotherapy protocols incorporate pretherapy with irradiation or cyclophosphamide (North, 1982).

To complicate the issue further, not only are the etiologic agents that are implicated in the pathogenesis of cancer immunosuppressive themselves, but also anticancer therapy in and of itself is immunosuppressive. Hematopoietic cells are exquisitely sensitive to the effects of radio- and chemotherapy. In addition, these therapies are mutagenic and carcinogenic, and this may explain the occurrence of second malignancies following the therapy of a first malignancy (Harris, 1979) and the increased incidence of cancers in patients receiving transplant immunosuppressive chemotherapy (Penn, 1988).

Further indirect evidence that impaired immunoregulation is implicated in carcinogenesis is that the incidence of most cancers, including lung cancer, increases with age, and many immune responses decrease with age (Makinodan and Kay, 1980). However, because carcinogenesis requires many steps and a long latency period, these two observations may not be causally related.

Lung Cancer as an Immunosuppressive Disease

Many studies have documented that patients with lung cancer have a decrease in circulating lymphocytes and depressed cellular immunity (Krant, et al., 1968; Han and Takita, 1972; Brugarolas and Takita, 1973; Anthony, et al., 1974; Liebler, et al., 1977). Those with lung cancer have a decreased delayed-type hypersensitivity (DTH) reaction to dinitrochlorobenze and decreased lymphocyte stimulation with phytohemagglutinin, concanavalin A, and pokeweed mitogen. Moreover, the degree of immunosuppression has been demonstrated to correlate with stage, resectability, degree of differentiation, response to therapy, and survival. It is these immunologic findings in patients with lung cancer that prompted investigators to manipulate the immune response with biologic therapies.

MANAGEMENT

The Adjuvants

Adjuvants are nonspecific stimulators of the immune response and are therefore designated as a form of active nonspecific immunotherapy. Almost 100 years after Coley treated many patients with his toxins, interest in nonspecific immunotherapy was rejuvenated when Mathé, et al. (1969) reported that the addition of another organism, the BCG to standard chemotherapy prolonged remission in children with acute lymphoblastic lymphoma. Since then, numerous clinical trials have been conducted with the immunomodulators BCG, *Corynebacterium parvum,* and levamisole.

Adjuvant therapies attempt to overcome the immunosuppressive effects of malignancies in a generalized nonspecific manner. BCG stimulates both the cellular and humoral mediated immune responses, whereas *C. parvum* primarily augments cell-mediated immunity. Unlike BCG and *C. parvum,* the anthelmintic drug levamisole only restores the immune response to normal and does not stimulate it above the normal level (Davis, et al., 1982). Levamisole augments T-cell function and number and enhances the phagocytosis and chemotaxis of macrophages and neutrophils.

Bacillus Calmette-Guérin

BCG is a nonspecific adjuvant isolated by Calmette and Guérin through progressive attenuation of a virulent strain of *Mycobacterium bovis.* Many of the clinical trials evaluating BCG in patients with lung cancer have had contradictory results (Table 28-12), possibly as a result of differences in the strain, viability, concentration, dose, or route of the BCG administration. The modes of delivery include the Heaf gun (multiple simultaneous application), scarification, and intralesional or intracavity administration (intrapleural delivery). As can be seen from Table 28-12, the basic problem with comparing the BCG studies is the lack of standardization of dose, site, and strategy of BCG used and the heterogeneity of the populations. Moreover, only one randomized study (McKneally, et al., 1976; Maver, et al., 1982; McKneally, et al., 1981) favored BCG therapy with corroboration only by a nonrandomized, yet substantial, study from Japan (Yamamura, et al., 1979). Most interestingly, however, is the failure of the LCSG study (Mountain and Gail, 1981; Oldham, et al., 1982) in 1981 and the Ludwig Lung Cancer Study Group (1986) to reproduce McKneally, et al.'s results. We should also note that two randomized studies with increased BCG-related empyemas did not show a survival difference (Ludwig Lung Cancer Study Group, 1986; Law, et al., 1982).

Corynebacterium parvum

C. parvum has not been studied as extensively as BCG, and many of the trial results have been contradictory. Although intrapleural instillation of *C. parvum* has been used successfully to treat malignant effusions (Millar, et al., 1979), most clinical trials have failed to demonstrate a survival benefit with *C. parvum* therapy (Table 28-13). The largest trial, in fact, conducted by the Ludwig Lung Cancer Study Group (1985) demonstrated a decreased survival in the *C. parvum*-treated group.

Levamisole

Levamisole has no antineoplastic effect alone and must be used as an adjuvant to conventional therapy. As with the other immunologic adjuvant trials, the results with levamisole have been disappointing (Table 28-14). Although Amery et al.'s (1979) initial levamisole lung cancer trial was promising at the 1- to 2-year interim analysis, after 4 years of maturation, no difference in survival was noted between the levamisole-treated and the placebo groups. Moreover, the LCSG trials by Holmes, et al. (1985), Anthony, et al. (1979), and the Veteran's Administration Lung Cancer Group Study (Davis, et al., 1982) reported significant decreases in the disease-free interval and survival in the patients who received levamisole therapy.

Tumor Cell Vaccines

Tumor cell vaccines are a form of active specific immunotherapy whereby the antigenic tumor-derived products are administered in an attempt to elicit an immune reaction against tumor-specific antigens. After it was demonstrated that immunization with bacterial and mycobacterial products could successfully protect from infectious diseases, a similar quest was begun in the early 1900s to identify anticancer vaccines.

Early efforts to identify cancer-specific antigens and heteroimmune sera were disappointing because the immune reaction was often not directed at the tumor product but at the adjuvants included in the crude tumor homogenates. Nevertheless, throughout the 1960s and early 1970s many attempts

Table 28-12. Bacillus Calmette-Guérin Trials

Reference	No. Patients (R vs. NR[a])	Patient Population	Study Design	Strain and Dose	Follow-Up	Results
McKneally, et al., 1976	60 (R)	Stage I NSCLC	Surgery + BCG vs. surgery alone	Tice strain; 1 × 10^7 viable organisms plus isoniazid intrapleurally	~ 1 yr	Early results. Improved survival and fewer recurrences with BCG; P = 0.003. 1-Yr survival rate 100% with BCG vs. 77% for controls
1981	6 (R)		Long-term follow-up		4–7 yr	Improved survival and fewer recurrences with BCG only in patients with stage I disease; P = 0.003
Pines, 1976	48 (R)	Inoperable squamous cell	Radiotherapy + BCG vs. radiotherapy alone	Glaxo strain; 25–125 × 10^6 organisms per application by Heaf gun	2–5 yr	No difference in survival (P > 0.02)
Pouillart, et al., 1976	39	Resectable squamous cell	Surgery + BCG vs. surgery alone	Pasteur Institute BCG; 75 mg of living organisms by scarification	2 yr	Because of small numbers, statistical analysis not possible but a trend toward improved survival with BCG (chance for 2-yr survival, 66% with BCG vs. 38% for controls)
Holmes, et al., 1977	7 (NR)	Resectable NSCLC	Resection and intralesional BCG	Glaxo strain; 0.5–1.0 ml BCG intralesionally preoperatively	—	Well tolerated, feasible form of therapy
Roscoe, et al., 1977	92 (R)	Resectable NSCLC	Surgery + Heaf gun vs. surgery + intradermal BCG vs. surgery alone	Glaxo strain; Heaf gun: 50–250 × 10^6 viable units. Intradermal: 0.4–0.9 × 10^6 viable units at 1, 2, 5, 9, 13, + 26 wk; then every 26 wk	15–33 mo	No difference in survival
Bjornsson, et al., 1978	76 64[b] (R)	Stage III bronchogenic	Chemotherapy + BCG vs. chemotherapy + C. parvum vs. chemotherapy alone	Methanol-extracted residue; 1 mg monthly intradermally	>8 mo	No difference in survival
Edwards and Whitwell, 1978	120 (NR)	Resectable bronchogenic	Surgery + BCG vs. surgery alone	Glaxo strain; 5 × 10^6 organisms subdermally	5 yr	No difference in survival
Jansen, et al., 1978	29 (R)	UICC stage II squamous cell	Surgery + BCG vs. surgery alone	RIV strain; 5 × 10^6 by scarification	3–13 mo	Trend toward increased disease-free interval. Cannot comment on survival because patients received other therapies after recurrence
Sarna, et al., 1978	79 (R)	Unresectable, metastatic, or recurrent bronchogenic	Chemotherapy + BCG vs. chemotherapy alone	Chicago Research strain; 1 × 10^6 live organisms per site. Tine application to four quadrants every week × 12, then biweekly	30-wk median	No difference in survival
Miller, et al., 1979	325 308[b] (R)	Stage I–III bronchogenic	Surgery + BCG vs. surgery only	Strain not specified; 10–15 × 10^6 live attenuated organisms, 120 mg orally	3–5 yr	No difference in survival, time to recurrence, development of metastatic disease

Study	No. of Patients[b]	Stage	Treatment	BCG Strain and Dose	Follow-up	Results
Miyazawa, et al., 1979	126 40[b] (NR)	Stage I–III NSCLC	Surgery + cyclophosphamide + BCG vs. surgery + cyclophosphamide Patients with involved mediastinal lymphadenopathy received mitomycin C bronchial artery infusion and patients with residual disease postoperatively received radiotherapy	Japan BCG Institute strain; $2–4 \times 10^6$ viable organisms or 5.4 mg tine administration; preoperatively, one dose postoperatively every month × 4 doses	10–28 mo	Improved survival with BCG $P < 0.05$ for all patients $P < 0.02$ for the 40 patients who completed all therapy (100% survival with BCG vs. 63% for controls)
Yamamura, et al., 1979	455 (NR)	Stage I–IIIb bronchogenic	Conventional therapy plus BCG vs. controls	Oil-attached BCG cell wall Induction: 200–400 μg weekly or maintenance biweekly, 100 or 200 μg every month; usually given intradermally, but in unresectable tumors also given intralesionally; given intrapleurally for malignant effusions	—	Improved survival with BCG vs. historical controls; $P < 0.0001$ Improved survival in IIIb disease ($n = 5$, $P = 0.016$)
Lowe, et al., 1980	92 (R)	Resectable bronchogenic	Surgery + BCG vs. surgery alone	Glaxo strain; 1×10^6 viable units intrapleurally plus isoniazid	14–36 mo	No difference in survival
Mountain and Gail, 1981	473 425[b] (R)	Stage I NSCLC	Surgery + BCG vs. surgery alone	Tice strain; 1×10^7 viable units intrapleurally plus isoniazid	1.5 yr	No difference in survival or incidence of recurrence
Law, et al., 1982	78 (R)	Stage I–III NSCLC	Surgery + BCG vs. surgery alone	Tice strain; 1×10^7 viable organisms intrapleurally one-half of patients received isoniazid	13 mo	No difference in survival
Little, et al., 1986	29 (R)	Stage I NSCLC	Surgery + BCG vs. surgery alone	Strain not specified; dose not specified; scarification	5 yr	Small sample size but trend toward improved survival in the BCG-treated group ($P = 0.075$) 5-yr survival rate, 86% with BCG vs. 64% for controls)
Ludwig Lung Cancer Study Group, 1986	441 407[b] (R)	Stage I and II NSCLC	Surgery + BCG vs. surgery + vehicle	Tice strain; 1×10^7 colony-forming units intrapleurally plus isoniazid	4.7 yr mean	No difference in survival Prolongation of disease-free interval with BCG ($P = 0.044$)

Abbreviations: NSCLC, non-small cell lung cancer; UICC, International Union on Against Cancer; BCG, bacillus Calmette-Guérin

[a] Randomized versus nonrandomized.

[b] Number of evaluable patients.

Table 28-13. C. parvum Trials

Reference	No. Patients (R vs. NR[a])	Patient Population	Study Design	Dose	Follow-Up	Results
Bjornsson, et al., 1978	76 64[b] (R)	Stage III bronchogenic	Chemotherapy + BCG vs. chemotherapy + C. parvum vs. chemotherapy only	0.25 mg escalating to 3 mg intravenously monthly	> 8 mo	Prolonged survival with C. parvum (P < 0.05)
Sarna, et al., 1978	79 (R)	Unresectable, metastatic, or recurrent bronchogenic	Chemotherapy + BCG vs. chemotherapy + C. parvum vs. chemotherapy alone	2.5 mg/m² intravenous infusion weekly × 12 then biweekly	30 wk median	No difference in survival > 50% of C. parvum-treated patients refused further therapy
Woodruff and Waldbaum, 1983	49 (R)	Resectable bronchogenic	Surgery + C. parvum vs. surgery alone	20 mg of dry weight killed intravenously one time 10–12 days postoperatively	6 yr	Trend toward increased survival with C. parvum (5-yr survival rate, 52% with C. parvum vs. 20% control)
Ludwig Lung Cancer Study Group, 1985	475 405[b] (R)	Stage I or II NSCLC	Surgery + C. parvum vs. surgery alone	7 mg intrapleurally	4.6 yr	Decreased survival with C. parvum (P = 0.02)

Abbreviations: NSCLC, non-small cell lung cancer; BCG, bacillus Calmette-Guérin.
[a] Randomized versus nonrandomized.
[b] Number of evaluable patients.

Table 28-14. Levamisole Trials

Reference	No. Patients (R vs. NR[a])	Patient Population	Study Design	Dose	Follow-Up	Results
Study Group for Bronchogenic Cancer, 1975	111 (R)	Resectable bronchogenic	Surgery + levamisole vs. surgery alone	50 mg 2 times per month orally	~ 1 yr	Trend toward improved survival with levamisole
Wright, et al., 1978	100 (R)	Resectable NSCLC	Surgery + levamisole vs. surgery + BCG vs. surgery alone	Levamisole: 2.5 mg/kg 3 days preoperatively and 2 days per week × 18 mo BCG: Tice strain, 1 × 10[7] viable units intrapleurally plus isoniazid	245 days	No difference in survival
Amery, et al., 1979, 1980	211 (R)	Resectable bronchogenic	Surgery + levamisole vs. surgery alore	50 mg orally three times a day 3 days per 2 wk × 2 yr	4yr	No difference in survival
Anthony, et al., 1979	328 217[b] (R)	Resectable NSCLC	Surgery + levamisole vs. surgery alone	2 mg/kg orally 3 days per week × 2 yr	> 2 yr	Decreased survival with levamisole but an excess of non-cancer-related deaths.
van Houtte, et al., 1980	73 51[b] (R)	Stage I-II NSCLC	Surgery + mediastinal radiation + levamisole vs. surgery + mediastinal radiotherapy alone	100 mg/m[2] orally 2 × per week for 2 yr	> 1 yr	No difference in survival
Davis, et al., 1982	446 381[b] (R)	Unresectable bronchogenic	Chemotherapy + levamisole vs. chemotherapy alone	150 mg/m[2] orally 3 × per week	~ 4 yr	Trend toward decreased survival with levamisole ($P = 0.084$)
Krauss, et al., 1984	251 139[b] (R)	Unresectable NSCLC	Radiotherapy + levamisole vs. radiotherapy alone	2.5 mg/kg orally 2 days per week × 1 yr	~ 4 yr	No difference in survival
Holmes, et al., 1985	130 (R)	Stage II-III NSCLC	Surgery + chemotherapy vs. surgery + levamisole + intrapleural BCG	Levamisole: 2.5 mg/kg orally 3 days per 2 wk × 18 mo BCG: Tice strain 1 × 10[7] viable organisms plus isoniazed	4 yr	Decreased survival with levamisole ($P = 0.005$) (33% survival with levamisole vs. 54% for control patients)
Herskovic, et al., 1988	74 64[b] (R)	Stage II or III lymph node-positive NSCLC	Radiotherapy + levamisole vs. radiotherapy alone	2.5 mg/kg orally 2 days per week × 1 yr	> 4 yr	No difference in survival

Abbreviations: VALG, Veteran's Administration Lung Cancer Group Study; SECSG, Southeastern Cancer Study Group; LCSG, Lung Cancer Study Group; RTOG, Radiation Therapy Oncology Group; NSCLC, non-small cell lung cancer; BCG, bacillus Calmette-Guérin.

[a] randomized versus nonrandomized.
[b] Number of evaluable patients.

were made to treat patients with blood or blood products that were thought to possess anticancer activity. The donors were usually patients who had regression of their cancers, either spontaneously or through therapy. There were only anecdotal reports of responses.

The search for tumor-specific antigens, however, led to the identification of novel cell surface differentiation antigens (the cluster of differentiation or CD antigens), which are used to identify different lymphocyte populations, and the identification of transplant antigens (the MHC antigens). With the identification of MHC restriction, it was realized that the regression of transplanted tumors in noninbred mice was not the result of an immune reaction against tumor-specific antigens but rather the rejection of a foreign graft.

The first success at demonstrating tumor-specific antigens was in 1943 when Gross (1943) reported that inbred mice could be immunized against a tumor that developed in an inbred mouse of the same strain. In 1970, Morton, et al. (1970) demonstrated the development of specific immunity during their trial of intralesional BCG in the therapy of patients with melanoma. The rejection of noninjected metastatic lesions in some patients suggested that BCG primed the immune system to recognize tumor antigens at distant sites.

Successful therapy with tumor vaccines depends on the identification of antigens on tumors not normally found on the tissue of origin or the overexpression of normal tissue antigens. Tumors are antigenic for a variety of reasons. Malignant transformation may result in the expression of previously silent genes, resulting in the production of new proteins. In addition, rapidly dividing tumor cells may improperly produce proteins, and these mutant proteins may be recognized as foreign. Finally, tumor cells may induce antigenicity by overproducing normal proteins that were previously present at too low a concentration to be immunologically recognized and induce self-tolerance. In fact, tumor-associated antigens have been demonstrated in both SCLC and NSCLC (Hollinshead, et al., 1975).

Tumor cell vaccines require two components: the antigen plus an adjuvant. The antigen consists of autologous or allogeneic tumor cells or cell extracts that are viable or inactivated by disruption or irradiation. To increase the immunogenicity, a process termed xenogenation is used. The antigenic expression of membrane proteins is increased by treating the cells with viruses; chemical therapy with mutagens or enzymes; or physical therapy with ultraviolet light, heat, or freeze-thaw manipulations.

Several trials have attempted to determine if tumor vaccines have a significant antitumor effect (Table 28-15); however, as with the other immunotherapy trials, the results have been conflicting. The earliest study, conducted by Newman, et al. (1977), accrued too few patients for statistical analysis. Nevertheless, there was a trend toward an improved survival rate in resected patients with bronchogenic cancer who received chemotherapy plus autologous antiserum compared with that in control patients who were treated with surgery and chemotherapy (81 versus 59 percent survival, respectively). Because therapy with autologous tumor products is cumbersome and time consuming, and thereby limits the number of patients that can be treated, some investigators have prepared the tumor vaccine from allogeneic tumor cells

pooled from multiple patients, often matched for histologic subtype. Takita, et al. (1985) used such a vaccine in resected patients with stage I and II squamous cell lung cancers and demonstrated an increase in the 5-year survival rate from 33 percent in control patients to 63 percent in tumor vaccine plus complete Freund's adjuvant (CFA)-treated patients ($P = 0.003$). This trial initially had a third arm, surgery plus CFA. These patients, however, received skin tests with tumor cells up to five times throughout the course of the trial, and their data were combined with those of the patients who received the tumor vaccine for analysis. A similarly designed, but larger, trial, consisting of 234 patients with stage I or II bronchogenic lung cancers by Hollingshead, et al. (1987) confirmed the earlier results. The median survival time in the patients treated with resection only was 46 months, whereas at the 5-year follow-up, the median survival time had not yet been reached in patients treated with surgery plus the tumor cell vaccine ($P = 0.002$). Despite these encouraging results, an equal number of trials have had negative results. Given the equivocal results and the burdensome nature of tumor vaccine therapy, other forms of biologic therapy are being explored more vigorously.

Cytokine Therapy

The discovery that immune cells produce cytokines, secretory products that regulate the immune response, greatly expanded the potential number of anticancer agents. To date, the effect of the IFN, TNF-α, and IL-2 against lung cancer has been studied.

The IFNs were the first cytokines discovered when Isaacs and Lindenmann (1957) identified a new polypeptide secreted by virally infected cells. Clinically, IFN-α is the most extensively studied cytokine and the first to be successfully cloned and mass produced by recombinant DNA technology. Interest in IFN-α as an anticancer agent was generated when Strander, et al. (1984) demonstrated that leukocyte IFN therapy delayed the dissemination of osteogenic sarcoma.

There are three types of IFNs. IFN-α (produced by leukocytes) and IFN-β (produced by fibroblasts) together are termed type I IFNs. They have considerable similarities in amino acid sequence and are both elicited in response to viral infections. IFN-γ or type II IFN has little homology to the type I IFNs and is produced by T lymphocytes in response to antigenic or mitogenic stimuli.

IFN may have anticancer activity through direct or host-mediated mechanisms. It has direct antitumor activity by inhibiting tumor cell growth, by suppressing transformation, by inhibiting angiogenesis, and by inducing differentiation. Equally important is IFN's immunomodulatory activities. IFN enhances host-mediated anticancer activity through upregulation of tumor-associated antigens, NK cell function, and macrophage activity.

Since its discovery by Morgan, et al. (1976), IL-2 has been identified as a critically important molecule in immune regulation. IL-2 has a variety of functions, including selective expansion of T lymphocytes, enhancement of NK activity, generation of LAK cells (see Adoptive Immunotherapy), and induction of the release of a variety of other cytokines. Because T lymphocytes, NK cells, and LAK cells are all in-

Table 28-15. Tumor Vaccine Trials

Reference	No. Patients (R vs. NR[a])	Patient Population	Study Design	Vaccine	Follow-Up	Results
Newman, et al., 1977	72 69[b] (R)	Resectable bronchogenic	Surgery + chemotherapy + antiserum vs. surgery + chemotherapy	Autologous antiserum 3–6 g antitumor immunoglobulin ½ of available antiserum × 4	49 wk mean (antiserum patients) 56 wk mean (control patients)	Too few patients for statistical analysis, trend toward improved survival with the antiserum (81% vs. 55% for controls
Perlin, et al., 1980	51 (R)	Stage I + II NSCLC	Surgery only vs. surgery + BCG vs. surgery + BCG + tumor vaccine	Autologous irradiated tumor cells 5 × 10[7] cells intradermally and subcutaneously BCG, Pasteur Institute strain, 3–5 × 10[6] cells viable organisms via Heaf gun, 2 × per month × 2 yr	2–51 mo	Short follow-up and many statistical manipulations, trend toward increased disease-free survival with tumor vaccine therapy
Hollinshead and Stewart, 1981	52 (R)	Stage I bronchogenic	Surgery alone vs. surgery + chemotherapy vs. surgery + tumor vaccine vs. surgery + chemotherapy + tumor vaccine	Allogeneic tumor-associated antigens matched for histologic type in Freund's complete adjuvant ~ 1500 µg intradermally	> 5 yr	Improved survival with tumor vaccine (P < 0.001) (tumor vaccine plus tumor vaccine and chemotherapy, 78% survival vs. 46% for control and chemotherapy only)
Souter, et al., 1981	95 80[b] (R)	Stage I + II NSCLC	Surgery only vs. surgery + tumor vaccine	Autologous irradiated tumor cells 20 × 10[6] cells intradermally given with 30 µg C. parvum	~ 2 yr	No difference in survival
Stack, et al., 1982	83 (R)	Resectable bronchogenic	Surgery only vs. surgery + tumor vaccine	Autologous irradiated tumor cells intradermally every week × 3 given with 50–250 × 10[6] Glaxo strain BCG via Heaf gun	> 6 yr	No difference in survival except for patients with positive skin tests (P = 0.04) (5-yr survival rate, 68% with tumor vaccine vs. 25% for control patients)
Lachman, et al., 1985	25 22[b] (R)	Stage I squamous cell	Surgery only vs. surgery + tumor vaccine	Autologous irradiated tumor cells 5 × 10[7] cells intradermally given with 1 × 10[6] Tice strain BCG intradermally	~ 3 yr	No difference in survival
Takita, et al., 1985, 1991	85 81[b] (R)	Stage I + II squamous cell	Surgery only vs. surgery + adjuvant vs. surgery + tumor vaccine	Pooled allogeneic tumor cells; 500 µg intradermally every month × 3; given with Freund's complete adjuvant	5 yr	Significant improvement in survival with tumor vaccine (P = 0.003) with 63% 5-year survival rate vs. 33% for controls
Price-Evans, 1987	120 (R)	Resectable bronchogenic	Surgery + BCG + adjuvant vs. surgery + BCG + tumor vaccine	Autologous irradiated tumor cells intradermally days 3, 10, 17, 24, 31 given with BCG and Freund's incomplete adjuvant	5 yr	No difference in survival
Hollinshead, et al., 1987	234 (R)	Stage I + II bronchogenic	Surgery alone vs. surgery + adjuvant vs. surgery + tumor vaccine	Pooled histologically matched tumor cells intradermally every month × 3 given with Freund's complete adjuvant	5 yr	Improved survival in tumor vaccine group (P = 0.0002) with median survival not yet achieved vs. 46 month median survival in control groups
Schulof, et al., 1988	82 18[b] (R)	Resectable NSCLC	Surgery + tumor vaccine ± radiotherapy	Autologous irradiated tumor cells 1 × 10[7] cells intradermally every week × 3 given with 1 × 10[7] Tice strain BCG	—	No correlation between the development of delayed-type hypersensitivity and recurrences

Abbreviations: NSCLC, non-small cell lung cancer; BCG, bacillus Calmette-Guérin.

[a] Randomized vs. nonrandomized
[b] Number of evaluable patients

volved in the immune responses mediating tumor regression, the anticancer effects of IL-2 have been extensively studied in a number of malignant histologic types.

A large number of clinical trials have been performed with IL-2 alone or in combination with LAK cells. Birdon, et al. (1983) was the first to administer IL-2 to patients with cancer. Two patients with melanomas were treated with partially purified IL-2. The performance of large-scale clinical trials, however, required the availability of large quantities of IL-2, which became a reality with the development of recombinant DNA technology. Using recombinant IL-2, Rosenberg, et al. (1985) at the NCI demonstrated objective responses in patients with cancer who received IL-2 alone and with LAK cells. These landmark studies sparked the enthusiasm for other immunotherapy trials.

TNF was originally described in 1975 by Carswell, et al. (1975) as an endotoxin-derived serum factor that caused the regression of meth-A sarcomas in experimental animals. The mechanisms of TNF's antitumor action are unknown. It is both an activator and a cytotoxic product of macrophages. In addition, it activates lymphocytes and NK cells, promotes leukocyte adherence, disrupts vascular integrity, and induces the secretion of other cytokines, specifically IL-1 and IL-6.

Clinically, TNF has failed to meet expectations when administered as a single agent. In human phase I trials, systemic side effects, including hypotension, fevers, rigors, thrombocytopenia, and neutropenia, have been dose limiting. The maximum tolerated dose of TNF (10 μg/kg) is 40-fold less on a per-kilogram basis than the dose (400 μg/kg) that is required to generate a significant antitumor response in mice (Asher, et al., 1987, 1991). Thus, current trials are exploring the use of TNF in combination with other cytokines.

IFN, TNF, and IL-2 have been evaluated alone and in combination in a limited number of patients with lung cancer. Since 1981, these phase I trials have demonstrated that cytokine therapy can be administered safely, and occasionally it may mediate the regression of lung cancer (Table 28-16). The best results were obtained by Mattson, et al. (1985) who achieved objective responses with both low- and high-dose IFN given in combination with radio- or chemotherapy. This study, however, must take into account the histologic types studied (i.e., SCLC, which itself is chemo- radiotherapy responsive). Indeed, after initial IFN therapy, radiotherapy was added for progressive localized disease or cranial metastases. Likewise, extrathoracic dissemination mitigated the use of systemic chemotherapy. This study achieved complete responses of 50 to 62 percent with radiotherapy and 44 to 50 percent with chemotherapy. These studies have provided the impetus for further ongoing trials. However, the contribution of IFN to these dramatic results is unclear, and unfortunately, a phase III design was not used.

Adoptive Immunotherapy

Adoptive immunotherapy refers to the transfer of autologous immune cells with antitumor activity to the tumor-bearing host. Landsteiner and Chase (1942) accomplished the first successful transfer of cellular immunity in 1942. They demonstrated that the transfer of peritoneal exudate cells from mice

sensitized to a variety of compounds induced DTH in the naive recipient mouse to the immunogen. Throughout the 1950s and 1960s, several investigators were able to cause tumor regression in animals by the adoptive transfer of immune cells; nevertheless, the clinical studies that followed in the 1960s and 1970s were unsuccessful because of the requirement for the transfer of large numbers of lymphocytes. The discovery, cloning, and ultimate availability of T-cell growth factor (now termed IL-2) permitted the continuous culture and expansion of T cells in vitro (Morgan, et al., 1976; Gillis and Smith, 1977). Subsequently, novel cytotoxic lymphocyte populations could be identified. LAK cells and TIL currently are the effector populations that are most often used in current adoptive immunotherapy trials.

LAK cells are generated by the culture of lymphoid precursors, such as peripheral blood lymphocytes, thymocytes, splenocytes, lymph node, or bone marrow cells in the presence of IL-2. In the clinical situation, this is performed by plasmapheresis of lymphocytes from peripheral blood followed by IL-2 exposure ex vivo. LAK cells do not require prior sensitization to tumor antigens for activation. IL-2 is the sole stimulus for LAK-mediated cytolysis. Thus, LAK cell cytolysis is nonspecific in that LAK cells lyse many targets, including autologous, allogeneic, or syngeneic tumor cells. LAK cells, however, do not lyse normal fresh tissue targets. They are known to recognize and bind to the tumor target and release cytotoxic substances, such as perforin, from cytoplasmic granules, mediating target cell death. They are also able to kill tumor targets by ADCC. In 1980, Yron, et al. (1980) isolated LAK cells from murine splenocytes cultured in IL-2 and demonstrated that these cells lysed tumors but not normal cells.

TIL and CTL are T cells that have been isolated from tumor specimens and expanded ex vivo in IL-2. TIL are thought to be specifically activated because of their intimate association with the antigenic tumor cells. Ex vivo expansion of TIL not only generates sufficient number of cells for therapy but also theoretically removes the CTL from any suppressive effect of the tumor. Unlike LAK cells, TIL lysis is MHC restricted and therefore specific for autologous or MHC-matched allogeneic tumor. Similar to other CTL, TIL-mediated lysis also requires cell-to-cell contact. TIL may also indirectly mediate tumor regression because TIL have been demonstrated to secrete cytokines, such as TNF and IFN, in response to tumor exposure. Klein, et al. (1980) examined and characterized the lymphoid cells that infiltrate tumors (TIL) in humans.

These findings provided the basis for the LAK and TIL cell trials that followed. Rosenberg, et al. (1985, 1988) demonstrated the feasibility and potential utility of LAK cell therapy in 1985 and TIL cell transfer in 1988, thereby generating enthusiasm for subsequent adoptive immunotherapy studies.

The generation of patient-specific LAK or TIL is labor and resource intensive, and hence, only a few patients with lung cancer have received adoptive immunotherapy (Table 28-17) in a phase II setting. Both West, et al. (1987) and Friedman, et al. (1989) evaluated the efficacy of continuous infusion IL-2 plus LAK in patients with advanced cancers. Their trials included five and three patients, respectively, with lung cancer, and one responder was noted in each study. A slightly

Table 28-16. Cytokine Trials

Reference	No. Patients	Study Design	Patient Population	Agents	Dose and Route	Results
Hill, et al., 1981	29	Phase I	Mixed histologic types	IFN-α	$0.5–2.0 \times 10^6$ U/kg IV	In the two patients with squamous cell cancer, one had complete resolution of his pleural effusion, and the other had no response
Jones, 1983	10	Phase II	Small cell	IFN-α	$50–100 \times 10^3$ U/m^2 × 5 days then 3 × 10^3 U/m^2 × 3 weeks via continuous IV infusion	No efficacy
Grunberg, 1985	16, 12[a]	Phase II	NSCLC	IFN-α	50×10^6 U/m^2 IM 3 × per week	No efficacy
Mattson, et al., 1985	9(high dose), 6(low dose)	Phase II IFN ± chemoradiotherapy	Small cell	IFN-α	High dose, 800×10^6 units continuous IV infusion × 5 days followed by 6×10^6 units IM 3 times daily	No efficacy as a single agent; however, with multimodality therapy, very high response rates ?IFN contribution
Krigel, et al., 1986		Phase I	Multiple histologic types	IFN-β; IL-2	$2–30\ 10^6$ U/m^2 IV 3 times per week × 4 wk; $1–500 \times 10^4$ U/m^2 subcutaneously 3 times per week × 4 wk	Defined maximal tolerated doses IFN-β = not reached IL-2 5×10^6 U/m^2 Stabilization of disease in one patient with NSCLC
Yang, et al., 1990, 1991a	16, 12[a]	Phase I	Stage IIIb or IV NSCLC	IL-2; TNF-α	Continuous low-dose infusion at 1×10^6 U/m^2 IV × 5 days; 25, 50, or 100 μg/m^2 IM daily × 5 Both every 3 weeks	Maximal tolerated dose, IL-2 plus 50 μg/m^2 TNF 1 PR and 3 MR
Yang, et al., 1991b	8	Phase I	Stage IIIb or IV NSCLC	OKT3; IL-2; TNF	27–103 μg/m^2 IV over 48 h; 6×10^6 U/m^2 IV infusion every day × 5; 25 μg/m^2 IM daily × 5	Well tolerated 1 CR and 1 MR

Abbreviations: NSCLC, non-small cell lung cancer; CR, complete response; PR, partial response; MR, minor response; IFN, interferon; IL, interleukin; TNF, tumor necrosis factor

[a] Number of evaluable patients.

Table 28-17. Adoptive Immunotherapy Trials

Reference	No. Patients	Patient Population	Therapy	Results
Krandin, et al., 1987	7	Unresectable metastatic adeno-carcinoma of the lung	TIL (no IL-2)	5/7 some tumor shrinkage
				0/7 PR or CR
West, et al., 1987	5	Lung cancer, histologic type not specified	IL-2 + LAK	1/5 PR
Friedman, et al., 1989	3	Unresectable NSCLC	IL-2 + LAK	1/3 MR
Barth, et al., 1990	16	Metastatic NSCLC	IL-2 + LAK + chemotherapy	2/14 CR
	14[a]			4/14 PR

Abbreviations: CR, complete response; PR, partial response; MR, minor response; NSCLC, non-small cell lung cancer; TIL, tumor-infiltrating lymphocytes; IL, interleukin; LAK, lymphokine-activated killer cells.

[a] Number of evaluable patients.

higher response rate was noted by Barth, et al. (1990) with combination therapy consisting of conventional chemotherapy (cisplatin and etoposide) plus IL-2 and LAK in 14 evaluable patients with NSCLC. The study by Krandin, et al. (1987) is the only trial to date to evaluate the efficacy of TIL in patients with lung cancer. Seven patients with unresectable metastatic adenocarcinomas of the lung received autologous TIL. Although five of seven patients had tumor shrinkage, no patient achieved a partial response. It is probable that an enhanced response would have been seen if IL-2 had been administered concomitantly because TIL growth is IL-2 dependent.

Monoclonal Antibody Therapy

Monoclonal antibodies are immunoglobulins derived from the progeny of a single cell. Antibodies are generated when an antigen binds with a cell surface receptor on a B lymphocyte. This triggers proliferation and clonal expansion, generating a large number of cells bearing the same receptor. These cells shed a soluble receptor (immunoglobulin) specific for the original antigen. In vivo, this reaction is much more complex because most immunogens have more than one antigenic determinant. Therefore, although the response of a single B cell to an antigen is *monoclonal,* the response of an individual to an antigen is *polyclonal.*

The fact that hyperimmune sera is polyclonal hampered the isolation and development of effective antibodies until the advent of hybridoma technology. In 1975, Köhler and Milstein (1975) described the methodology for monoclonal antibody production and were awarded the Nobel Prize for their work. They fused an immortal cell, a myeloma, with an antibody-producing cell, creating a hybridoma. Despite the availability of monoclonal antibodies for the past 15 years, their use has not become part of the standard therapy of patients with cancer to date. Nevertheless, monoclonal antibodies have been invaluable in the immunologic characterizations necessary for tumor biology research.

There are many consequences of the specific binding of an antigen and an antibody. The most important in tumor cell destruction is the initiation of ADCC, the mechanism whereby CTL (and occasionally neutrophils and macrophages) cause cytolysis. In ADCC, an antibody binds to the target cell that expresses the antigen. This complex binds to the effector cell, resulting in the activation of the cytotoxic

mechanism and the destruction of the target cell. Antigen-antibody binding also activates the complement cascade, resulting in cell lysis. Furthermore, antibodies enhance and promote phagocytosis by binding to both the antigenic particle and the phagocytic cell (a process termed opsonization). Finally, antibodies may mediate tumor regression by binding to and blocking receptors for autocrine growth factors.

A significant number of antibodies have been generated against lung cancer antigens. In one recent review, greater than 50 antibodies to NSCLC alone were identified (Stein and Goldenberg, 1991). Nevertheless, the use of monoclonal antibodies is still in its infancy, with phase I trials predominating.

Monoclonal antibodies are under investigation for their ability to mediate tumor regression as single agents. In a phase I study, Stahel, et al. (1991) evaluated SDZ ABL364, which recognizes the Le^Y hapten in patients with SCLC that have relapsed. No tumor responses were noted.

Monoclonal antibodies are also being evaluated as carriers of toxic compounds. Dinehart, et al. (1990), in a phase I study, used KC-4, an antibody that recognizes the human milk fat globule antigen, to augment host immunity by stimulating ADCC. Patients also received KC-4 bound to a radiolabel to evaluate the efficacy of tumor imaging. The diagnostic accuracy of this immunoconjugate was approximately 80 percent for tumors at least 3 cm in diameter; however, no antitumor effect was observed. Elias, et al. (1990a,b) compared the toxicity of the antibody KS1/4 alone versus KS1/4-methotrexate conjugate in patients with stage IIIb or IV NSCLC. The gastrointestinal toxicity was dose limiting. One patient who had previously received radiotherapy had tumor shrinkage and may have responded to the antibody-conjugate therapy.

Antibodies to other growth factors, such as transferrin and insulin growth factor, which are implicated as autocrine factors in lung cancer, are also under investigation. Mulshine, et al. (1988, 1990) evaluated antigastrin-releasing peptide therapy in patients with SCLC. Divgi, et al. (1989) used antiepidermal growth receptor therapy in patients with squamous cell lung cancers. In both phase I studies, no tumor responses were noted.

Despite the absence of antitumor responses in these phase I trials, progress has been made in the characterization, isolation, and delivery of antitumor antibodies, and phase II trials that would be better able to address the issues of efficacy are ongoing. Moreover, other novel applications of monoclonal antibodies are currently under investigation, such as the use of antibodies ex vivo to purge bone marrow cells prior to autologous bone marrow transplantation in vivo (Humblet,

et al., 1989; Okahe, et al., 1985). Another novel use of monoclonal antibodies has been their conjugation to light-sensitive compounds to enhance the efficacy of porphyrin-based photodynamic therapy (Pogrebniak, et al., 1991).

COMMENTS AND CONTROVERSIES

The use of biologic therapy for the specific therapy of thoracic malignancies is still in its infancy. As can be seen from the previous discussion, the number of truly evaluable trials using the most current of the biologic response modifiers is small at this time, and most of the pioneering work is still restricted to in vitro and in vivo models and, therefore, not yet in the clinical realm. Thus, the therapy of patients with lung cancer with biologic response modifiers remains experimental. To date, no large-scale trial has confirmed the positive findings from small single-institution trials. Neither the administration of biologic response modifiers alone or in conjunction with chemo- or radiotherapy has consistently improved response or survival rates compared with those in controls. In the future, the greatest concentration of effort will be in the use of cytokines, adoptive therapy, and innovative molecular biologic approaches and in the use of monoclonal antibodies for site-directed therapy.

We must realize, however, the difficulties encountered by the clinicians conducting these trials. Until the discovery of recombinant DNA methods, many biologic response modifiers were available only in limited quantities and were impure. Similarly, the isolation and preparation of patient- or tumor-specific antibodies, vaccines, or TIL still remains cumbersome and limiting. Even after the reagent is available, the clinician needs to design a rational therapeutic strategy; however, the mechanism of action of these biologic response modifiers and the complex interrelationships in vivo are still being elucidated. Thus, the optimal dose, route, and timing of many of these therapies have been empirically selected. Additional problems arise with patient selection and therapy. Because this is the beginning of biologic therapy, most of the studies done thus far were phase I or II. Unfortunately, most of these patients did not respond to other forms of therapy, including radio- and chemotherapy, possibly rendering the patient's tumor more resistant to further therapeutic attempts. These previous therapies could also have an impact on the patient's functional reserve, which may already be compromised if there was a previous pulmonary resection, thereby limiting the tolerance of these patients to the experimental regimen. The cytokines and adoptive immunotherapy are associated with significant toxicity. IL-2 administered alone, or with LAK cells or TIL, is associated with the development of a generalized capillary leak, resulting in hypotension, pulmonary infiltrates, weight gain, respiratory dysfunction, and mental confusion. In addition, the observed toxicities include renal and hepatic dysfunction and thrombocytopenia. Moreover, IL-2 has been associated with a small number of myocardial events, including myocarditis, infarction, and arrhythmia. Patients with lung cancer, because of their underlying smoking history or advanced age, will require careful screening, possibly including pulmonary func-

tion testing and thallium stress testing. Careful evaluation will be crucial to select patients able to complete these proposed therapies safely.

IL-2 is not the only agent associated with toxicity. Long-term IFN therapy is associated with excessive fatigue, anorexia, nausea, fever, chills, and rigors. Although most patients will become tolerant to these effects with time, the toxicity can be magnified when the IFN is given with other agents. Hepatic toxicity, necessitating dose modification, can also occur with IFN.

Monoclonal antibody therapy also will require refinement. Tumor heterogeneity, poor antigenic expression, and antigenic modulation have hampered the identification of unique antigenic targets. Therefore, the isolation and characterization of antibodies has been difficult. The amount of antibody required in vivo to effect therapeutic changes is large. Moreover, the development of human antimouse antibodies, when the antibody is derived from murine sources, can limit monoclonal antibody therapy.

Certainly, the role of thoracic surgeons and their familiarity with novel biologic therapies will expand in the future. Presently, some institutions have involved the thoracic surgeon in performing thoracotomies for the purpose of removing pulmonary lesions from patients who do not have a curative option to procure tumor-associated macrophages or lymphocytes. We can predict that, in a select group of good performance status individuals, this approach may be attempted in patients with primary lung cancers.

Thoracic surgeons, however, should begin to participate in the development of data bases with regard to the malignancies they excise. It is increasingly important that tissue specimens that are removed be snap frozen at $-70°C$ so they may be submitted for further analysis. Furthermore, collaboration between thoracic surgeons and benchwork investigators can lead to the development of cell lines in culture. The availability of frozen tumor specimens and cell lines is an absolute requisite for the future of biologic therapy because the analysis of these specimens may give insight regarding differences in expression of the transcripts for growth factors, cytokines, and differentiation products compared with each other and normal tissue.

As described by Takahashi (1989), lung cancer is associated with mutations in dominant and recessive oncogenes, such as ras and the p53 genes. By identifying the protein abnormalities produced by these genes, it may be possible to inoculate the immune response such that certain lymphocytes can be primed to kill cancer cells that contain these mutant peptides. Moreover, with the use of presently available molecular biologic techniques, the synthesis of ribonucleic acids that block the construction of the mutant protein could be prepared. The in vitro and in vivo bases for such experiments have been described (Georges, et al., 1993; Roth, 1992; Roth, et al., 1992; Mukhopadhyay, et al., 1991). The *ras* oncogene can be frequently mutated in lung cancer and may then result in growth promotion. Roth's group (1992) showed that, by downregulating the production of the mutated peptide that is coded for by the *ras* oncogene, the growth of lung cancer cells in vitro and in vivo was inhibited. The chosen strategy to downregulate the uninibited growth was the construction of a segment of the *ras* oncogene nucleic acids in an antisense orientation, which when incorporated, will shut down translation. The intratracheal instillation of such antisense constructs, using a retrovirus as the vector to tranfect cells and produce viral supernatants with high titers of the antisense, downregulated growth in a nude mouse tumor model in 90 percent of the animals. Similar experiments have been performed by manipulating mutated tumor-suppressor genes (i.e., p53). Phase I clinical trials evaluating the efficacy of such an approach with genetic therapy are underway at the M. D. Anderson Cancer Center.

There are a number of ongoing clinical trials that are investigating novel forms of biologic therapy for lung cancer, including cytokine prevention of neutropenia during standard chemotherapy and bone marrow transplantation; IFN therapy combined with combination chemotherapy; IL-2 and LAK cells for lung cancer; and the targetting of autocrine growth factor receptors with monoclonal antibodies alone or as immunoconjugates. The reader is urged to be aware of such programs through use of the Physicians Data Query (301)-496-7403 or 1-800-638-8480 because the demonstration of the utility of biologic response modifiers depends on the successful completion of well-controlled phase I–III trials with sufficient numbers of patients.

In the future, an increased understanding of tumor immunology, with further characterization of previously identified biologic response modifiers and the discovery of new potent biologics with anticancer activities, will revolutionize immunotherapy.

H.W.P.
H.I.P.

Despite the disappointing results obtained in the 1970s and 1980s using a variety of nonspecific immunostimulants (e.g., BCG, *C. parvum,* and levamisole) and the failure of tumor vaccines to have any impact in managing lung cancer, especially using those agents in postoperative adjuvant therapy, biologic modification of a tumor and/or host in the therapy of lung cancer is now showing exciting promise. Although this therapy is in its infancy, rapid progress has been made in understanding the antigenic properties of malignant cells and the genetic aberrations that occur in malignant transformation. Because of this exciting research, we now have hope that, within the next decade or two, biologic therapy may play a role in the management of this disease. Especially exciting is the field of oncogene therapy, which now is actively being investigated in many centers. Ultimately, it is hoped that tumors will be modified genetically and self-destruct, that monoclonal antibodies will be used to direct antineoplastic therapy, and that host defenses will be improved by immunomodulation. Because lung cancer presents at a relatively advanced stage in almost 80 percent of patients, this type of systemic therapy will be crucial if we are to have any impact on the curability of this disease.

R.J.G.

KEY REFERENCES

Carswell EA, Old LJ, Kassel RL et al.: An endotoxin-induced serum factor that causes necrosis of tumors. Proc Natl Acad Sci U S A 72:3666, 1975

The discovery of TNF revolutionized the concept that cytokines in themselves could cause tumor regression in vivo. Since the discovery of this cytokine, a whole cascade of cytokines have been studied for antitumor efficacy, and the relationship, possibly to empyema-related tumor cytolysis, becomes inescapable.

McKneally MF, Maver C, Kausel HW: Regional immunotherapy of lung cancer with intrapleural BCG. Lancet 1:377, 1976

This is a landmark extraordinarily controversial prospective randomized study using intrapleural BCG after resection of lung cancer. The survival benefits reported in early-stage disease, unfortunately, were not reproduced in two other well-controlled much larger trials.

Morgan DA, Ruscetti FW, Gallo RG: Selective in vitro growth of T-lymphocytes from normal bone marrows. Science 193:1007, 1976

This is the original description of T-cell growth factor, now known as IL-2. This agent, associated with lymphocyte expansion and the development of activated NK cells, is crucial to the future of adoptive immunotherapy for many histologic types of cancer.

Rosenberg SA, Lotze MT, Muul LM et al.: Observations on the systemic administration of autologous lymphokine-activated killer cells and recombinant interleukin-2 to patients with metastatic cancer. N Engl J Med 313:1485, 1985

This is the first large-scale report on the use of IL-2-based immunotherapy in 25 patients with cancer. Objective regression was observed in 11 of the 25 patients. The original description of potential IL-2-related complications is also reported.

Rosenberg SA, Packard BS, Aebersold PM et al.: Use of tumor infiltrating lymphocytes and interleukin-2 in the immunotherapy of patients with metastatic melanoma. A preliminary report. N Engl J Med 319:1676, 1988

The "second-generation" initial report explains the use of TIL for the therapy of metastatic melanoma concomitantly with IL-2. The cells were removed from the harvested tumors, expanded ex vivo, and then adoptively transferred back to the patients.

REFERENCES

Amery WK: Adjuvant levamisole in the treatment of patients with resectable lung cancer. Ann Clin Res 12:1, 1980

Amery WK, Cosemans J, Gooszen HC et al.: Adjuvant immunotherapy with levamisole in resectable lung cancer. Cancer Immunol Immunother 7:191, 1979

Anthony HM, Mearns AJ, Mason MK et al.: Levamisole and surgery in bronchial carcinoma patients: increase in deaths from cardiorespiratory failure. Thorax 34:4, 1979

Anthony HM, Templeman GH, Madsen KE, Mason MK: The prognostic significance of DHS skin tests in patients with carcinoma of bronchus. Cancer 34:1901, 1974

Asher AL, Mulé JJ, Kasid A et al.: Murine tumor cells transduced with the gene for tumor necrosis factor-α. Evidence for paracrine immune effects of tumor necrosis factor against tumors. J Immunol 146:3227, 1991

Asher AL, Mulé JJ, Reichert CM et al.: Studies on the anti-tumor efficacy of systemically administered recombinant tumor necrosis factor against several murine tumors in vivo. J Immunol 138:963, 1987

Barth N, West W, Oldham R et al.: A phase II trial of adoptive immunotherapy (AIT) and sequential chemotherapy with cisplatin (CP), VP-16 in advanced non-small cell lung cancer (NSCLC). Proc Am Soc Clin Oncol 9:235, 1990

Birdon C, Czerniecki M, Ruell P et al.: Clearance rates and systemic effects of intravenously administered interleukin-2 (IL-2) containing preparations in human subjects. Br J Cancer 47:123, 1983

Bjornsson S, Takita H, Kuberka N et al.: Combination chemotherapy plus methanol extracted residue of bacillus Calmette-Guérin or Corynebacterium parvum in stage III lung cancer. Cancer Treat Rep 62:505, 1978

Brugarolas A, Takita H: Immunologic status in lung cancer. Chest 64:427, 1973

Coley WB: The treatment of malignant tumors by repeated inoculations of erysipelas: with report of ten original cases. Am J Med Sci 105:487, 1893

Davis S, Mietlowski W, Rohwedder JJ et al.: Levamisole as an adjuvant to chemotherapy in extensive bronchogenic carcinoma. Cancer 50:646, 1982

Dinehart DG, Schmelter RF, Lear JL: Imaging of non-small cell lung cancers with a monoclonal antibody, KC-4G3, which recognizes a human milk fat globule antigen. Cancer Res 50:7068, 1990

Divgi CR, Welt S, Yeh, SDJ et al.: Phase I and imaging trial with radiolabeled anti-EGF receptor monoclonal antibody 225(mAb) in squamous cell lung cancer. Proc Am Soc Clin Oncol 8:183, 1989

Edwards FR, Whitwell F: Use of BCG as an immunostimulant in the surgical treatment of carcinoma of lung: a five-year follow-up report. Thorax 33:250, 1978

Elias DJ, Horschowitz L, Kline LE et al.: Phase I clinical comparative study of monoclonal antibody KS1/4 and KS1/4-methotrexate immunoconjugate in patients with non-small cell lung carcinoma. Cancer Res 50:4154, 1990a

Elias DJ, Kline LE, Dillman RO et al.: Monoclonal antibody (MOAB) KS1/4-methotrexate (MTX) conjugate in patients with non-small cell lung carcinoma. Proc Am Soc Clin Oncol 9:249, 1990b

Foley EJ: Antigenic properties of methylcholanthrene-induced tumors in mice of the strain of origen. Cancer Res 13:835, 1953

Friedman N, Bernstein Z, Goldrosen M et al.: Phase II trial of IL-2/LAK therapy for patients with Hodgkin's disease (HD), non-Hodgkin's lymphoma (NHL) and non-small cell (NSC) lung cancer. Proc Am Soc Clin Oncol 8:194, 1989

Georges RN, Mukhopadhyay T, Zhang Y et al.: Prevention of orthotopic human lung cancer growth by intratracheal instillation of a retroviral antisense K-ras construct. Cancer Res 53:1743, 1993

Gillis S, Smith K: Long term culture of tumor specific cytotoxic T-cells. Nature 268:154, 1977

Gross L: Intradermal immunization of C3H mice against a sarcoma that originated in an animal of the same line. Cancer Res 3:326, 1943

Grunberg SM, Kempf RA, Itri LM et al.: Phase II study of recombinant alpha interferon in the treatment of advanced non-small cell lung carcinoma. Cancer Treatment Reports 69:1031, 1985

Han T, Takita H: Immunologic impairment in bronchogenic carcinoma: a study of lymphocyte response to phytohemagglutinin. Cancer 30:616, 1972

Harris CC: A delayed complication of cancer therapy—cancer. J Natl Cancer Inst 63:275, 1979

Herskovic A, Baver M, Seydel HG et al: Post-operative thoracic irradiation with or without Levamisole in non-small cell lung cancer: results of a Radiation Therapy Oncology Group Study. Int J Radiat Oncol Bio Phys 14:37, 1988

Hill NO, Pardue A, Khan A et al.: Phase I human leukocyte interferon trials in cancer and leukemia. J Clin Hematol Oncol 11:23, 1981

Hollinshead A, Stewart THM, Takita H et al.: Adjuvant specific active lung cancer immunotherapy trials. Cancer 60:1249, 1987

Hollinshead AC, Sega S, Stewart THM: Comparison of lung cancer antigens. Tumori 61:125, 1975

Hollinshead AC, Stewart THM: Specific and nonspecific immunotherapy as an adjunct to curative surgery for cancer of the lung. Yale J Biol Med 54:367, 1981

Holmes EC, Mink J, Ramming KP et al.: New Method of immunotherapy for lung cancer. Lancet 2:586, 1977

Holmes EC, Hill LD, Gail M: A randomized comparison of the effects of adjuvant therapy on resected stages II and III non-small cell carcinoma of the lung. Ann Surg 202:335, 1985

Humblet Y, Feyens A-M, Agaliotis D et al.: Immunological and pharmacological removal of small cell lung cancer cells from bone marrow autografts. Cancer Res 49:5058, 1989

Isaacs A, Lindenmann J: Virus interference: I. The interferon. Proc R Soc Lond 147:258, 1957

Jansen HM, The TH, DeGast GC et al.: Adjuvant immunotherapy with BCG in squamous-cell bronchial carcinoma. Immune-reactivity in relation to immunostimulation (preliminary results in a controlled trial). Thorax 33:429, 1978

Jones DH, Bleehen NM, Slater AJ et al.: Human lymphoblastoid interferon in the treatment of small cell lung cancer. Br J Cancer 47:361, 1983

Klein E, Vanky F, Galili V et al.: Separation and characteristics of tumor infiltrating lymphocytes in man. p. 79. In Witz IP, Hanna MG (eds): Contemporary Topics in Immunobiology. Plenum, New York, 1980

Klein G, Sjögren HO, Klein E, Hellström KE: Demonstration of resistance against methylcholanthrene-induced sarcomas in the primary autochthonous host. Cancer Res 20:1561, 1960

Köhler G, Milstein C: Continuous cultures of fused cells secreting antibody of predefined specificity. Nature 256:495, 1975

Krandin RL, Boyle LA, Preffer FI et al.: Tumor-derived interleukin-2-dependent lymphocytes in adoptive immunotherapy of lung cancer. Cancer Immunol Immunother 24:76, 1987

Krant MJ, Manskopf G, Brandrup CS, Madoff MA: Immunologic alterations in bronchogenic cancer. Cancer 21:623, 1968

Krauss S, Comas F, Perez C et al.: Treatment of inoperable non-small cell carcinoma of the lung with radiation therapy, with or without levamisole. Am J Clin Oncol 7:405, 1984

Krigel R, Poiesz B, Comis R et al.: A phase I study of recombinant interleukin-2 (rIL-2) plus recombinant beta SER 17 interferon (IFN-βSER). Proc Am Soc Clin Oncol 5:225, 1986

Lachmann PJ, Grant RM, Freedman LS et al.: A preliminary trial of a novel form of active immunotherapy in squamous cell carcinoma of the lung. Br J Cancer 51:415, 1985

Landsteiner K, Chase MW: Experiments on transfer of cutaneous sensitivity to simple compounds. Proc Soc Exp Biol Med 49:688, 1942

Law MR, Lam WK, Studdy PR et al.: Complications of intrapleural BCG in the treatment of operable non-small cell bronchial carcinoma. Br J Dis Chest 76:151, 1982

Liebler GA, Concannon JP, Magovern GJ et al.: Immunoprofile studies for patients with bronchogenic carcinoma I. Correlation of pretherapy studies with survival. J Thorac Cardiovasc Surg 74:506, 1977

Little AG, DeMeester TR, Ferguson MK et al.: Modified stage I ($T_1N_0M_0$, $T_1N_0M_0$), nonsmall cell lung cancer: treatment results, recurrence patterns, and adjuvant immunotherapy. Surgery 100:621, 1986

Lotze MT, Chang AE, Seipp CA et al.: High-dose recombinant interleukin-2 in the treatment of patients with disseminated cancer. JAMA 256:3117, 1986

Lowe J, Shore DF, Iles PB et al.: Intrapleural BCG in operable lung cancer. Lancet 1:11, 1980

Ludwig Lung Cancer Study Group: Immunostimulation with intrapleural BCG as adjuvant therapy in resected non-small cell lung cancer. Cancer 58:2411, 1986

Ludwig Lung Cancer Study Group: Adverse effect of intrapleural Corynebacterium parvum as adjuvant therapy in resected stage I and II non-small cell carcinoma of the lung. J Thorac Cardiovasc Surg 89:842, 1985

Makinodan T, Kay MMB: Age influence on the immune system. Immunology 29:287, 1980

Mathé G, Amiel JL, Schwartzenberg L et al.: Active immunotherapy for acute lymphoblastic leukemia. Lancet 2:697, 1969

Mattson K, Holsti LR, Niiranen A et al.: Human leukocyte interferon as part of a combined treatment for previously untreated small cell lung cancer. J Biol Response Modifiers 4:8, 1985

Maver C, Kausel H, Lininger L, McKneally M: Intrapleural BCG immunotherapy of lung cancer patients. Cancer Res 80:227, 1982

McKneally MK, Lininger L, McIlduff JB, Foster ED: Four-year follow-up on the Albany experience with intrapleural BCG in lung cancer. J Thorac Cardiovasc Surg 81:485, 1981

Millar JW, Hunter AM, Horne NW: Intrapleural immunotherapy with Corynebacterium parvum in recurrent malignant pleural effusions. Thorax 35:856, 1979

Miller AB, Taylor HE, Baker MA et al.: Oral administration of BCG as an adjuvant to surgical treatment of carcinoma of the bronchus. Can Med Assoc J 121:45, 1979

Miyazawa N, Suemasu K, Ogata T et al.: BCG immunotherapy as an adjuvant to surgery in lung cancer: a randomized prospective clinical trial. Jpn J Clin Oncol 9:19, 1979

Morton DL, Eilber FR, Malmagren RA et al.: Immunologic factors which influence response to immunotherapy in malignant melanoma. Surgery 68:158, 1970

Mountain CF, Gail MH: Surgical adjuvant intrapleural BCG treatment for stage I non-small cell lung cancer. J Thorac Cardiovasc Surg 82:649, 1981

Mukhopadhyay T, Tainsky M, Cavender AC, Roth JA: Specific inhibition of K-ras expression and tumorigenicity of lung cancer cells by antisense RNA. Cancer Res 51:1744, 1991

Mulshine J, Avis I, Carrasquillo J et al.: Phase I study of an anti gastrin releasing peptide (GRP) monoclonal antibody in patients with lung cancer. Proc Am Soc Clin Oncol 9:230, 1990

Mulshine JL, Avis I, Treston AM et al.: Clinical use of a monoclonal antibody to bombesin-like peptide in patients with lung cancer. Ann N Y Acad Sci 547:360, 1988

Newman CE, Ford CHJ, Davies DAL, O'Neill GJ: Antibody-drug synergism: an assessment of specific passive immunotherapy in bronchial carcinoma. Lancet 2:163, 1977

North RJ: Cyclophosphamide-facilitated adoptive immunotherapy of an established tumor depends on elimination of tumor-induced suppressor T cells J Exp Med 55:1063, 1982

Okabe T, Kaizu T, Ozawa K et al.: Elimination of small cell lung cancer cells in vitro from human bone marrow by a monoclonal antibody. Cancer Res 45:1930, 1985

Oldham RK, Gail MH, Baker MA et al.: Immunological studies in a double blind randomized trial comparing intrapleural BCG against placebo in patients with resected stage I non-small cell lung cancer. Cancer Immunol Immunother 13:164, 1982

Penn I: Cancer is a long-term hazard of immunosuppressive therapy. Autoimmunity 1:545, 1988

Perlin E, Oldham RK, Weese JL et al.: Carcinoma of the lung: immunotherapy with intradermal BCG and allogeneic tumor. Int J Radiat Oncol Biol Phys 6:1033, 1980

Pines A: A 5-year controlled study of BCG and radiotherapy for inoperable lung cancer. Lancet 1:380, 1976

Pogrebniak HW, Matthews W, Black et al.: Targeted phototherapy with sensitizer-monoclonal antibody and light. Surg Forum 42:447, 1991

Pouillart P, Mathé G, Palangie T et al.: Trial of BCG immunotherapy in the treatment of resectable squamous cell carcinoma of the bronchus (stages I and II). Cancer Immunol Immunother 1:271, 1976

Prehn RT, Main JM: Immunity to methylcholanthrene-induced sarcomas. J Natl Cancer Inst 18:769, 1957

Price-Evans DA, Roberts HL, Hewitt S et al.: A trial of adjuvant immunotherapy for bronchial carcinoma with irradiated autochthonous tumour cells. Int J Immunother 3:293, 1987

Roscoe P, Pearce S, Ludgate S, Horne NW: A controlled trial of BCG immunotherapy in bronchogenic carcinoma treated by surgical resection. Cancer Immunol Immunother 3:115, 1977

Roth JA: Molecular surgery for cancer. Arch Surg 127:1298, 1992

Roth JA, Mukhopadhyay T, Tainsky MA et al.: Molecular approaches to prevention and therapy of aerodigetive tract cancers. Monogr Natl Cancer Inst 13:15, 1992

Ruckdeschel JC, Codish SD, Stranahan A, McKneally MF: Postoperative empyema improves survival in lung cancer. N Engl J Med 287:1013, 1972

Sarna GP, Lowitz BB, Haskell CM et al.: Chemo-immunotherapy for unresectable bronchogenic carcinoma. Cancer Treat Rep 62:681, 1978

Schulof RS, Mai D, Nelson MA et al.: Active specific immunotherapy with an autologous tumor cell vaccine in patients with resected non-small cell lung cancer. Mol Biother 1:30, 1988

Souter RG, Gill PG, Gunning AJ, Morris PJ: Failure of specific active immunotherapy in lung cancer. Br J Cancer, 44:496, 1981

Stack BHR, McSwan N, Stirling JM et al.: Autologous x-irradiated tumor cells and percutaneous BCG in operable lung cancer. Thorax 37:588, 1982

Stahel RA, Lacroix H, Sculier JP et al.: Phase I/II study of monoclonal antibody SDZ ABL364 in relapsed small cell lung cancer. Proc Am Assoc Cancer Res 32:189, 1991

Stein R, Goldenberg DM: Prospects for the management of non-small-cell carcinoma of the lung with monoclonal antibodies. Chest 99:1466, 1991

Strander Y, Aparisi T, Bronstrom LA et al.: Adjuvant treatment of osteosarcoma with human IFN. p. 247. In Zoon KC, Noguchi PD, Lui TY (eds): Interferon: Research, Clinical Application, and Regulatory Consideration. Elsevier North Holland, New York, 1984

Study Group for Bronchogenic Carcinoma: Immunopotentiation with levamisole in resectable bronchogenic carcinoma: a double-blind controlled trial. BMJ 3:461, 1975

Takahashi T, Nau MM, Chiba I et al.: P53: a frequent target for genetic abnormalities in lung cancer. Science 246:491, 1989

Takita H: Effect of postoperative empyema on survival of patients with bronchogenic carcinoma. J Thorac Cardiovasc Surg 59:642, 1970

Takita H, Hollinshead A, Hart T Jr et al.: Adjuvant specific immunotherapy of resectable squamous cell lung carcinoma: analysis at the eighth year. Cancer Immunol Immunother 20:231, 1985

Takita H, Hollinshead AC, Adler RH et al.: Adjuvant, specific, active immunotherapy for resectable squamous cell lung carcinoma: a 50 year survival analysis. J Surg Oncol 46:9, 1991

van Houtte P, Bondue H, Rocmans P et al.: Adjuvant immunotherapy by levamisole in resectable lung cancer: a control study. Eur J Cancer 16:1597, 1980

West WH, Tauer KW, Yannelli JR et al.: Constant-infusion recombinant interleukin-2 in adoptive immunotherapy of advanced cancer. N Engl J Med 316:898, 1987

Woodruff M, Walbaum P: A phase-II trial of *Corynebacterium parvum* as adjuvant to surgery in the treatment of operable lung cancer. Cancer Immunol Immunother 16:114, 1983

Wright PW, Hill LD, Peterson AV Jr et al.: Preliminary results of combined surgery and adjuvant bacillus Calmette-Guérin plus levamisole treatment of resectable lung cancer. Cancer Treat Rep 62:1671, 1978

Yamamura Y, Sakatani M, Ogura T, Azuma I: Adjuvant immunotherapy of lung cancer with BCG cell wall skeleton (BCG-CWS). Cancer 43:1314, 1979

Yang SC, Grimm EA, Parkinson DR et al.: Clinical and immunomodulatory effects of combination innumotherapy with low-dose interleukin 2 and tumor necrosis factor α in patients with advanced non-small cell lung cancer: a phase I trial. Cancer Res 51:3669, 1991a

Yang SC, Grimm EA, Roth JA: Immunotherapy of lung cancer. Chest Surg Clin North Am 1:191, 1991b

Yang SC, Owen-Schaub L, Mendiguren-Rodriguez A et al.: Combination immunotherapy for non-small cell lung cancer. J Thorac Cardiovasc Surg 99:8, 1990

Yron I, Wood TA, Spiess PJ et al.: In vitro growth of murine T-cells the isolation and growth of lymphoid cells infiltrating syngeneic solid tumors. J Immunol 125:238, 1980

Postresection Follow-Up

Nael Martini
Robert J. Ginsberg

Complete resection is the therapy of choice for localized NSCLC and certain selected small cell tumors. However, despite a potentially curative resection, tumor recurrence does occur with all stages of presentation. The rate is estimated to be 20 to 30 percent following complete resection for stage I tumors, 50 percent for stage II, and 70 to 80 percent for resected N2 disease (Martini, 1990). Less frequently, second primary lung cancers occur. In our experience, the incidence of second primary lung cancers following complete resection for stage I tumors is 11 percent. Local recurrences also occur despite a complete resection, particularly following wedge resection or segmentectomy (Ginsberg, 1985). Both second primary lung cancers and local recurrences may be amenable to further surgical resection with curative intent. Following surgical resection for lung cancer, it is therefore important to maintain close supervision of the patient to identify and treat recurrent or new primary disease as early as possible.

TUMOR RECURRENCE

Local Recurrence

A resection is considered complete and potentially curative when the primary tumor and all accessible mediastinal lymph nodes are removed, no gross disease is left behind, and all margins of resection are reported histologically clear of tumor. The extent of pulmonary resection necessary to achieve a complete resection is influenced by the size and location of the tumor. Lobectomy is preferred for peripheral tumors (Martini, et al., 1986). For centrally located tumors, bilobectomy, pneumonectomy, or sleeve lobectomy may become necessary to encompass all disease. When the tumor is small and peripheral, a lesser resection may be performed, particularly if the pulmonary reserve of the patient is limited. Although long-term survival may be achieved by lesser resections, the risks of local recurrence are high (10 to 15 percent) (Martini, et al., 1985). We define local recurrence as evidence of tumor within the same lung or at the bronchial stump, regional recurrence as clinically manifest disease in the mediastinum despite mediastinal lymph node dissection, and distant recurrence as disease in the contralateral lung or elsewhere outside the hemithorax.

Patients with incomplete resection of their primary tumor develop local recurrence and do poorly even when the residual disease is only microscopically evident at the bronchial margin of resection (Pairolero, et al., 1984). Recurrence at the bronchial stump, in the chest wall, or in the remaining portion of a lobe when a lesser resection than lobectomy is done is the result of inadequate initial excision. Thus we consider local recurrence and regional lymph node metastasis

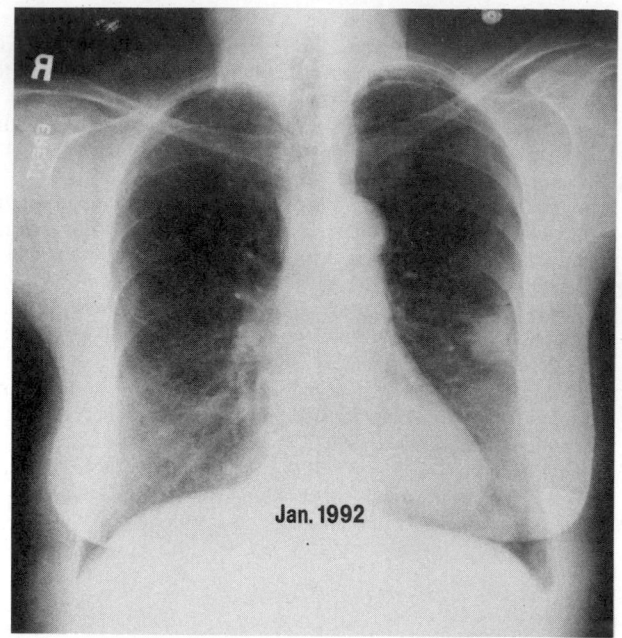
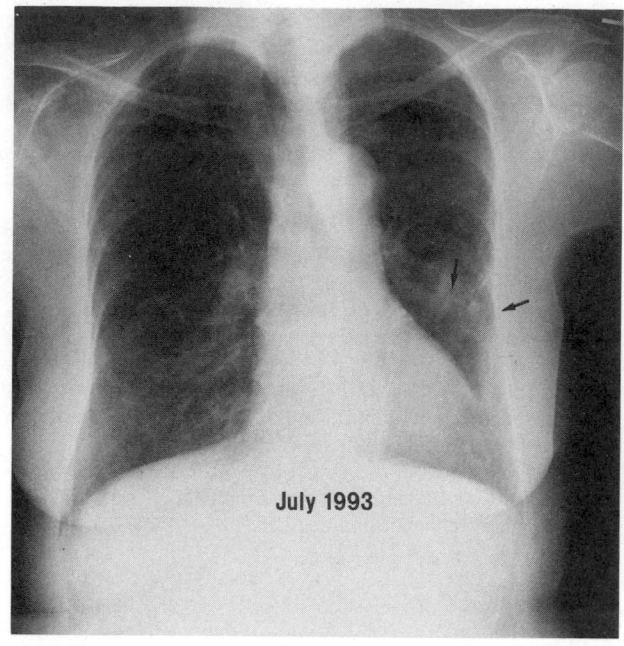

Figure 28-11. **(A)** Chest radiograph demonstrating a 2-cm lesion of the left lung in an 80-year-old woman. She was treated by wedge resection, using a thoracoscopic approach. **(B)** Eighteen months later, a local recurrence was evident on the routine follow-up radiograph. This lesion was amenable to complete resection by lobectomy. The arrows indicate the proximity of the recurrence to the staple line used in the wedge resection.

after resection to represent persistent disease, which cannot be termed a second carcinoma (Fig. 28-11).

The determinants of survival in lung cancer are the stage and resectability. The 5-year survival rate following complete resection is 70 percent in stage I disease, 40 percent in stage II disease, and 25 to 30 percent in stage III disease, whereas long-term survival in the face of distant disease is essentially nonexistent (Gail, et al., 1984; McCaughan, et al., 1985; Martini, 1990; Martini, et al., 1992). Careful follow-up becomes necessary in all patients following resection to identify recurrence or a new primary lung cancer.

Local or regional recurrence and distant metastases, if they occur, most commonly are detected within the first year after

therapy, and the rate diminishes with time. Although recurrent lung cancer manifests itself most frequently within the first 2 to 3 years of initial therapy, and rarely beyond 5 years (Table 28-18), second primary lung cancers may occur at any time following resection. For this reason, patients with resected lung cancer require lifetime follow-up.

When a complete potentially curative resection of a primary carcinoma of the lung is performed, when the margins are clear, and when lymph node metastasis is absent, any new lesion—even if in the same lung—may represent a new and separate primary tumor. The diagnosis is most convincing when the new lesion is in the contralateral lung and the histologic type of the new tumor is different. More importan-

Table 28-18. Incidence of Recurrence Postresection by Stage

Stage	No. Patients	Overall Recurrence		Cumulative Recurrence (%)			
		No.	%	Year 1	Year 2	Year 3	Year 5
I	598	162	(27)	55 (34)	94 (58)	121 (71)	144 (89)
II	214	112	(52)	63 (56)	86 (77)	93 (83)	107 (96)
I + II	812	274	(34)	118 (43)	180 (66)	214 (78)	251 (92)
IIIa							
N2 (S)	151	113	(75)	64 (57)	94 (83)	104 (92)	110 (97)
N2 (C + S)	89	53	(60)	28 (53)	40 (75)	51 (90)	53 (100)
T3 (Med)	46	26	(56)	16 (62)	20 (77)	24 (92)	25 (96)
T3 (CW)	77	37	(48)	29 (78)	34 (92)	35 (95)	36 (97)
All N2	240	166	(69)	92 (55)	134 (81)	155 (93)	163 (98)
All IIIa	363	229	(63)	137 (60)	188 (82)	214 (93)	224 (98)

Abbreviations: S, surgery; C, chemotherapy; Med, mediastinum; CW, chest wall.

tly, new lesions of the lung of a benign nature can also develop. Tissue diagnosis is therefore essential whenever a new solitary lesion appears after adequate resection of a primary lung cancer.

In a recently completed review, we identified 118 patients from our tumor registry who had been treated at Memorial Sloan-Kettering Cancer Center for primary lung cancer and were alive 10 years from their initial diagnosis and therapy (Temeck, et al., 1984). Nineteen of the 118 patients (16 percent) developed new cancers of the lung 6 to 22 years after therapy of their first lung cancer. Of the 19 patients, 13 had a different histologic type from their original tumor, and 6 had the same histologic type.

Metastatic Disease

A small subgroup of patients has solitary sites of metastatic disease following completely resected lung cancer. Occasionally, these solitary metastatic sites can be effectively treated, allowing the patient a possibility of long-term survival. No matter the stage, approximately two-thirds of patients have recurrences distantly as the first evidence of recurrence (Martini, et al., 1993). In descending order of frequency, these sites include brain, bone, liver, and adrenal glands. A solitary brain metastasis may be treated by surgical excision with an expected 15 to 20 percent 5-year survival rate (Burt, et al., 1992). There are no data regarding other solitary sites of metastases treated in this aggressive fashion, but isolated instances of long-term survival have been cited in the literature. For this reason, in following completely resected patients, it is important to direct the history and physical examination to potential metastatic sites amenable to therapy.

METHODS OF FOLLOW-UP

History and Physical Examination

After the immediate recovery period, a status-check visit is recommended every 3 months for the first year, every 4 months for the second year, and once to twice a year thereafter; most physicians recommend only a yearly checkup after 5 years. The incidence of recurrence after 5 years ranges from less than 5 to 15 percent depending on the stage of the disease at the initial presentation. The risks of developing new primaries persists at a rate of 1 to 3 percent per year of survival. Although late recurrences are reported to occur sporadically after 10 years (1 to 3 percent), a yearly checkup is considered sufficient thereafter.

At least 50 percent of all patients are symptomatic at the first manifestation of recurrent or metastatic disease. Locoregional recurrence often produces recurrent or new chest pain, persistent cough, hoarseness caused by recurrent laryngeal nerve palsy, or symptoms of superior vena caval obstruction. Nonspecific signs, such as continued weight loss or anorexia, often herald hepatic metastases. Intracranial metastatic disease is frequently the first site of recurrence and is usually associated with neurologic signs (i.e., visual disturbances, mental changes, and speech or gait disturbances). New and unremitting skeletal pain suggests bony metastases.

Chest Radiograph

The most useful examination to detect locoregional recurrence or a second primary tumor is a posteroanterior and lateral chest radiograph. At each follow-up visit, a chest radiograph is taken, the patient is seen, and the general condition is assessed. If the patient is feeling well and is asymptomatic, the physical examination is generally confined to the surpraclavicular region to rule out any adenopathy and to the upper abdomen to assess any hepatomegaly. The chest radiographs are reviewed and always compared with previous ones. If no interval change is identified and no pulmonary pathologic condition is suspected, no further testing is usually necessary. Any additional tests are generally prompted by either symptoms, signs, or radiographic changes.

Following a resection of a lung cancer, most patients generally quit smoking on their own accord. If no complications occur and no recurrence ensues, most patients have no cough, and therefore, routine sputum examinations are unrewarding if the patient is totally asymptomatic and the chest radiographs show no new findings. An exception to this rule is a patient whose initial diagnosis was based on hemoptysis; a histologic finding of squamous cell carcinoma on bronchial washings, brushings, or biopsy; and a radiographic occult lung cancer (Melamed, et al., 1984).

Biochemical Studies

Elevated serum calcium, alkaline phosphatase, serum glutamic oxalate transaminase, and LDH levels are nonspecific markers of recurrent cancer. Whether biochemical determinations should be included in the routine follow-up examination of postsurgical patients is judgmental. We do not use these general screening tests routinely but advise our patients to remain under the care of their internist or family practitioner for their comprehensive screening of non-neoplastic disorders, which usually includes an electrocardiogram and hematologic and biochemical studies.

The carcinoembryonic antigen (CEA) level seems to be valuable as a follow-up test only in those patients in whom the antigen was elevated prior to surgery. In such instances, a repeat CEA level is measured shortly after surgery because most elevated CEA levels preoperatively generally return to normal values. If this occurs, serial CEA assessment becomes worthwhile.

Presently, no specific tumor marker for carcinoma of the lung has been detected. It is to be hoped that, in time, this will become available and will increase our ability, not only to detect early lung cancer, but also to detect early treatable recurrences.

Bronchoscopy

An unexplained cough of recent onset may necessitate a consideration of a diagnostic bronchoscopy despite a negative chest radiographic findings. Repeated bronchoscopy on a regular basis is not indicated. However, in special circumstances, this examination should be considered, including (1) patients in whom the tumor is near or at the bronchial resection margin, (2) patients with severe dysplasia or in situ changes at the resection margin, and (3) patients with known multiple bronchial epithelial tumors.

The introduction of fiberoptic bronchoscopy makes the examination simple and extremely well tolerated without the need for general anesthesia. It should be advised when symptoms, signs, or radiologic or cytologic findings suggest recurrent local disease.

Computed Tomographic Scanning

Routine CT scanning of the chest and upper abdomen and brain and bone scanning do not appear to be helpful and should only be done when clinical features suggest that recurrent disease is likely and requires confirmation; however, no prospective study of their usefulness and cost effectiveness in follow-up has been performed.

It is often difficult to detect locoregional recurrence in patients, especially following pneumonectomy, because of the failure of a chest radiograph to penetrate the hemithorax or mediastinum. We have been impressed with the ability of CT scanning of the chest to detect recurrences in those patients with symptoms that suggest this problem but relatively normal chest radiographs. Patients frequently present with recurrent ipsilateral chest pain or a dry hacking cough, which is suggestive of recurrent disease. Previously, especially in postpneumonectomy patients, the symptoms remained enigmatic for months. However, with the use of CT scanning, recurrent disease in the ipsilateral hemithorax or mediastinum is more easily detected.

COMMENTS AND CONTROVERSIES

Most practitioners are convinced of the value of routine follow-up of patients following surgical therapy for lung cancer, although its effectiveness has never been measured. Despite the availability of expensive laboratory and imaging studies, it has never been demonstrated that these added tests improve the management of patients with recurrent disease, despite the fact that earlier detection of selected cases may occur.

Unfortunately, at present, there are no biochemical or serologic tumor markers of value in follow-up. We hope that, in the future, the development of such tumor markers will allow earlier detection of solitary treatable sites of metastases. The value of routine expensive imaging tests (e.g., CT scans) in the follow-up of such patients requires a prospective analysis. Although follow-up sputum cytologic analysis, even in patients with squamous cell carcinomas, has not been accepted as a routine study, the significant incidence of second aerodigestive tumors occurring in such patients makes this examination of potential value. Tockman, et al. (1988) recently identified an antigen with monoclonal antibody staining that suggests a potential earlier identification of such recurrent or new primary tumors. This is presently being tested in a prospective national study.

N.M.
R.J.G.

KEY REFERENCES

Gail MH, Egan RT, Feld R et al.: Prognostic factors in patients with resected stage I non-small cell lung cancer: a report from the Lung Cancer Study Group. Cancer 54:1802, 1984

Ginsberg RJ: Follow-up supervision after resection for lung cancer. p. 274. In Delarue NC, Eschapasse H (eds): International Trends in General Thoracic Surgery: Lung Cancer. WB Saunders, Philadelphia, 1985

Martini N, Ghosn P, Melamed MR: Incidence of local recurrence-new primary carcinoma following resection of bronchogenic tumors. p. 164. In Delarue NC, Eschapasse H (eds): International Trends in General Thoracic Surgery. WB Saunders, Philadelphia, 1985

Pairolero PC, Williams DE, Bergstralh MS et al.: Post-surgical stage I bronchogenic carcinoma: morbid implications of recurrent disease. Ann Thorac Surg 38:331, 1984

Few articles in the literature have addressed specifically how best to follow-up patients with lung cancer postresection. These key references address this subject in part and focus on the frequency of recurrences or new primary cancers and on the benefits of periodic surveillance.

REFERENCES

Burt M, Wronski M, Arbit E et al.: Resection of brain metastases from non-small-cell lung carcinoma. Results of therapy. J Thorac Cardiovasc Surg 103:399, 1992

Martini N: Surgical treatment of non-small cell lung cancer by stage. Thoracic neoplasms. Semin Surg Oncol 6:248, 1990

Martini N, Burt ME, Bains MS et al.: Survival after resection in stage II non-small cell lung cancer. Ann Thorac Surg 54:460, 1992

Martini N, Flehinger BJ: The role of surgery of N2 lung cancer. Surg Clin North Am 67:1037, 1987

Martini N, Kris MJ, Flehinger BJ et al.: Preoperative chemotherapy of stage IIIa(N2) non-small cell lung cancer: the Memorial Sloan-Kettering experience with 136 patients. Ann Thorac Surg 55:1365, 1993

Martini N, McCaughan BC, McCormack P, Bains MS: The extent of resection for localized lung cancer: lobectomy. p. 171. In Kittle FC (ed): Current Controversies in Thoracic Surgery. WB Saunders, Philadelphia, 1986

McCaughan BC, Martini N, Bains MS, McCormack P: Chest wall invasion of carcinoma of the lung: therapeutic and prognostic implications. J Thorac Cardiovasc Surg 89:836, 1985

Melamed MR, Flehinger BJ, Zaman MB et al.: Screening of early lung cancer detection: results of the Memorial Sloan-Kettering study in New York. Chest 86:44, 1984

Temeck BK, Flehinger BJ, Martini N: A retrospective analysis of 10 year survivors from carcinoma of the lung. Cancer 53:1405, 1984

Tockman MS, Gupta PK, Myers JD et al.: Sensitive and specific monoclonal antibody recognition of human lung cancer antigen on preserved sputum cells: a new approach to early lung cancer detection. J Clin Oncol 6:1685, 1988

Late Complications

Jean Deslauriers
Pasquale Ferraro

When patients are discharged from the hospital after pulmonary resections, they are still at risk of developing late complications related to their operations. These are uncommon events that, for the most part, become apparent during the first year of follow-up. Although late complications are seldom life threatening, delayed diagnosis or mismanagement often leads to chronicity and prolonged disability.

HISTORICAL NOTE

Although the first successful resection for lung cancer was in 1932, complications following partial lung resections for pulmonary disease prior to this were common. The first successful anatomic resection depended on solving technical problems leading to major complications.

Very early on, problems related to the bronchial closure had been identified. Kummel (1911) performed a pneumonectomy, clamping the pedicle and leaving the clamps in situ since individual ligation was unknown at the time. The patient died of complications after only 6 days. In 1912, Davies performed the first lobectomy for lung cancer. Prior to this, the only resections were very primitive operations that included exteriorization of the tumor, suturing the visceral and parietal pleura together, and ultimately cauterizing the eviscerated mass (Pean, 1895). Following Brunn's 1929 description of intercostal drainage and underwater seal, lobectomy became a distinct possibility. But, unfortunately, empyema and bronchopleural fistula continued to be major problems. Prevention of these complications due to technical problems awaited the development of individual ligation, pioneered by the efforts of Hinz (1923), Churchill (1933), Rienhoff (1933) and Churchill and Belsey (1939).

It was not until these techniques had been developed that patients survived long enough to be followed and the late complications of pulmonary resection slowly became evident.

HISTORICAL READINGS

Brunn HB: Surgical principles underlying one-stage lobectomy. Arch Surg 18:490, 1929

Churchill ED: The surgical treatment of carcinoma of the lung. J Thorac Surg 2:254, 1933

Churchill E, Belsey HR: Segmental pneumonectomy in bronchiectasis. Ann Surg 109:481, 1939

Davies HM: Recent advances in the surgery of the lung and pleura. Brit J Surg 1:228, 1913–1914

Hinz R: Totale extirpation der linken lunge wegen bronchial carcinoma. Arch Klin Chir 124:104, 1923

Kummel H: Proceedings of the 40th Congress, Berlin, April 19–22, 1911. Verh Dtsch Ges Chir 40:147, 1911

Pean J: Chirurgie des poumons. Discussion Ranc Chir Proc Verh Paris 9:72m, 1895

Rienhoff WF: Pneumonectomy. A Preliminary report of operative technique in two successful cases. Bull Johns Hopkins Hosp 53:390, 1933

INFECTIONS AND SPACE COMPLICATIONS

Persistent Spaces After Lobectomy or Lesser Resections

Persistent pleural air spaces following lobectomies or lesser resections are common, and for many years, they were thought to lead inevitably to infection if left untreated (Rainer and Newby, 1967; Kirsh, et al., 1975). Consequently, numerous intraoperative and postoperative prophylactic measures, such as tailoring thoracoplasty, pleural tent, pneumoperitoneum, phrenoplasty, and high postoperative intrapleural suction, were designed to prevent such spaces from occurring (Kirsh, et al., 1975).

In 1959, Shields, et al. (1959) published a classic article on the fate of persistent pleural air spaces following resection for pulmonary tuberculosis. A review of 584 pulmonary resections revealed an incidence of 128 (21.9 percent) persistent pleural air spaces postoperatively. Of these spaces, 86 (67.1 percent) were asymptomatic, and 42 (32.9 percent) were symptomatic. The asymptomatic spaces were benign with respect to the patient's course; the symptomatic spaces were hazardous and accounted for complications of varying severity in all 42 patients, with eventual death of 3. It was concluded that prophylaxis with careful dissection in the intersegmental or interlobar plane and closure of any major leaks at the time of stripping, was the best management.

In 1966, Barker, et al. (1966) questioned the then accepted concept that all postresectional thoracic spaces represented frank bronchial leaks that required active surgical intervention. It was assumed that bronchopleural fistulae constituted a prelude to empyemas, and hence, active prophylaxis and therapy of these spaces should be initiated early. In this series, 730 partial lung resections were performed for pulmonary tuberculosis, and 86 patients had postresection spaces (Table 28-19). Fifteen patients had persistent spaces for longer than 4 weeks after their operations, and of these, five closed spontaneously within 1 year. Only two patients had evidence of a major pleuropulmonary communication, and in both cases, long-term follow-up did not turn up important complications. In a similar study, Silver, et al. (1966) concluded that most postresectional residual spaces resolve without complications or major surgical intervention.

Normally, the space after lobectomy or lesser resection is obliterated by the shift of adjacent dynamic structures, such as the heart, mediastinum, and diaphragm; the approximation of ribs with internal bulging of the intercostal muscles; the hyperinflation of the remaining lung; and the intrapleural accumulation of blood and serum in recesses and fissures. This obliteration is facilitated by the negative intrapleural pressure, the lack of air leakage from the lung and/or bronchus, and the unimpaired expansibility of the lung.

Table 28-19. Fate of 86 Postresection Spaces

Fate	No. Patients (%)
Spontaneous obliteration	76 (88)
Less than 4 wk	71
4 wk to 1 yr	5
Persistent for 1–10 yr	10 (11)
Uninfected	8
With bronchopleural fistula	2

(From Barker WL, Langston HT, Naffah P: Post-resectional thoracic spaces. Ann Thorac Surg 2:299, 1966, with permission.)

Risk factors for the development of persistent spaces are the inability of the lung to fill the hemithorax, such as occurs in patients with underlying fibrosis or the presence of a bronchopleural fistula either at the alveolar or bronchial level. On the basis of their studies, Barker, et al. (1966) classified persistent postresection spaces as benign or malignant. A benign space is characterized as one that is small and getting smaller on serial radiographs, is thin walled, and has no or minimal and decreasing fluid. It occurs in a patient who has no fever or leukocytosis and who has no major symptoms (Fig. 28-12). Most of these spaces have no bronchial or alveolar communications and have an intraspace pressure that is negative and will disappear without therapy over a period of weeks or months (Fig. 28-13).

In contradistinction with benign spaces, patients with malignant spaces have fever and leukocytosis, and they are generally ill (Barker, et al., 1966). These spaces are large and getting larger, have a thick wall, and contain fluid in increasing amounts. These infected spaces are usually obvious during the early postoperative period, but sometimes they are only diagnosed at the time of the first or second postoperative visit (Fig. 28-14). Clinically, these patients present with a failure to thrive, purulent bronchorrhea with or without hemoptysis, unresolving chest pain, and sometimes spiking temperature.

After lung cancer surgery, most residual air spaces are not infected and should be observed until their complete resolution. Investigation by thoracentesis or other procedures is not indicated and may in fact be contraindicated because of the risks of infecting a previously sterile space. These recommendations apply to all asymptomatic spaces whether they have an air fluid or not and whether they persist for only a few weeks postoperatively or for years. However, if the patient develops systemic or local symptoms of infection or if the space is enlarging, appropriate therapy should be instituted promptly.

Late Empyema and Bronchopleural Fistula

Definition and Incidence

Although late empyemas and bronchopleural fistulae may occur separately, they generally are associated with one another and thus are discussed together in this chapter.

Late-onset postpneumonectomy empyema has been arbitrarily defined by Kerr (1977) as an empyema occurring 3 months after surgery in a patient with an uneventful postoperative course. The overall incidence of postoperative empyemas is between 2 and 13 percent after pneumonectomy (Leroux, et al., 1986) and less than 1 percent after lobectomy. The exact incidence of late-onset empyemas, however, is unknown, although it is likely to represent a rare complication.

In their original article on open drainage and irrigation for postpneumonectomy empyemas, Clagett and Geraci (1963) make one of the first references to the occurrence of late empyema. In a series also from the Mayo Clinic (Pairolero, et al., 1990), the interval between pneumonectomy and the diagnosis of subsequent empyema ranged from 1 week to 33 years (median, 4 weeks). The complication was apparent within 4 months of pneumonectomy in 32 patients (71 percent)

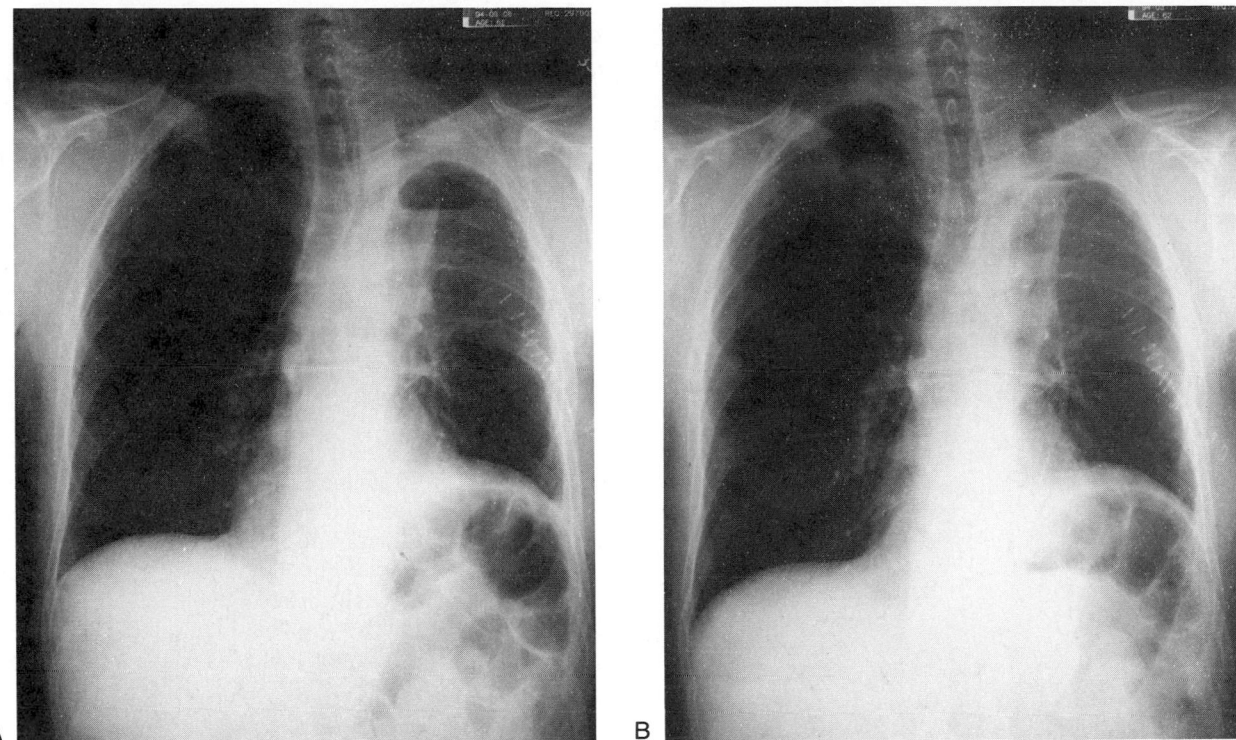

Figure 28-12. Asymptomatic benign space following left upper lobectomy. **(A)** Early postoperative chest radiograph showing a thin-walled air space located anteriorly and at the apex. **(B)** Near-complete disappearance of the space 10 days postoperatively.

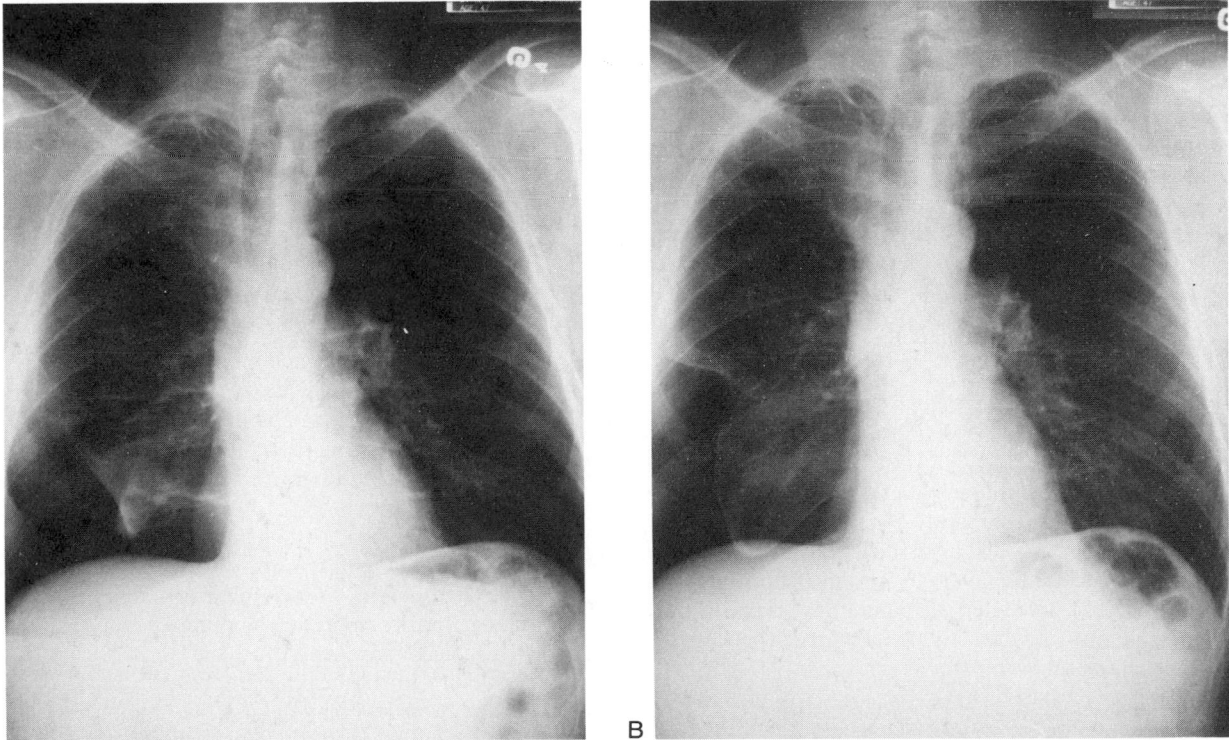

Figure 28-13. Asymptomatic benign space following right lower lobectomy. **(A)** Postoperative posteroanterior chest radiograph taken 3 weeks postoperatively and showing a large basal space. **(B)** Four weeks later, the space is smaller, and the patient has remained asymptomatic.

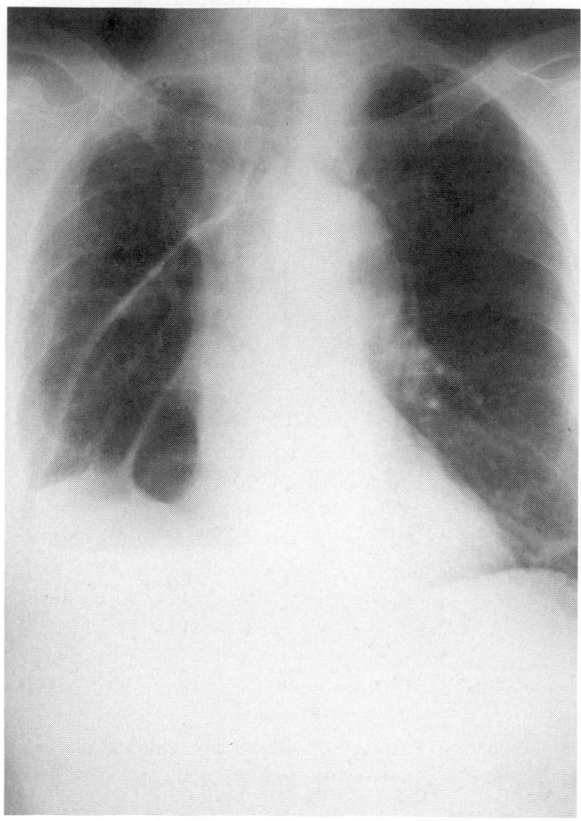

Figure 28-14. Symptomatic malignant space following lower and middle lobectomy. Posteroanterior chest radiograph showing a large thick-walled air space with multiple air-fluid levels diagnosed 5 months postoperatively.

and later than 4 months in 13 patients (29 percent). In three patients, the empyema developed after 5 years (10.5, 13, and 33 years). In the Toronto series (Shamji, et al., 1983), the complication was apparent within 12 weeks of the operation in 23 cases (74.2 percent) and after 3 months in the remaining 8 individuals (25.8 percent).

The overall incidence of postresectional bronchopleural fistulae is 1 to 3 percent (Boyd and Spencer, 1972; Williams and Lewis, 1976; Vester, et al., 1991), but precise data on the occurrence of late fistulae is lacking because most occur in association with empyemas. In 1984, Steiger and Wilson (1984) reported six cases of late fistulae in a series of 11 patients, and Vester, et al., (1991) described 14 late cases from a series of 35 patients with postoperative fistulae. The latter group also showed that in patients who received preoperative irradiation, a significantly longer time (average, 48 days) elapsed before the diagnosis of bronchopleural fistula than in the other patients (average, 18 days). In 1992, Asamura, et al. (1992) presented 13 patients with late fistulae among 52 patients with bronchopleural fistulae developing after pulmonary resection.

Pathophysiology

The exact pathophysiology of late-onset empyema is not completely understood. As suggested by Witz and Roeslin (1981), two possibilities exist. In most cases, the empyema results

---

Pathogenesis of Late Postresection Empyemas

Secondary to late bronchopleural or esophagopleural fistula
Contamination of the space during the initial surgery
Seeding through the hematogenous route
Direct spread through the esophageal hiatus or diaphragm

---

from a bronchopleural or an esophagopleural fistula with contamination of the postpneumonectomy space. In Kerr's series (1977), fistulae (two bronchial and two esophageal) were found in four of nine patients presenting with empyemas 8 months to 13 years after pneumonectomies. The second possible mechanism of infection involves the contamination of the pleural cavity during the initial surgery. Microorganisms may lodge in small pockets or loculations of fluid and lie dormant for months or years before producing an empyema. Although plausible, this hypothesis cannot be verified with any certainty.

In theory, seeding of the postpneumonectomy space may also occur by the hematogenous route, as is the case with bacterial endocarditis. This mechanism is supported by a number of authors. In five cases of late-onset empyema (Kerr, 1977), patients had signs of infection in the contralateral lung, and pneumococal and streptococcal agents were isolated from the empyema. In 1983, Model (1983) described a case of empyema occurring 10 years after pneumonectomy in a patient receiving therapy for pneumonia. Bellamy, et al. (1991) also reported three cases of late empyema (7, 10, and 30 months after resection) with organisms of blood-borne origin. The bacteria isolated were *Pasteurella multocida*, *Campylobacter fetus*, and various anaerobes in the third patient. Rogiers, et al. (1991b) described a case of empyema 4 years after pumonary resection for carcinoma in which *Mycobacterium tuberculosis* was cultured. In all these reports, the authors concluded that the pleural space had been contaminated by blood-borne agents because no evidence of bronchial or esophageal fistulae could be found. A final theory was proposed by Holden, et al. (1972) in the discussion of a case of late postpneumonectomy empyema occurring in a patient soon after appendiceal peritonitis. The same Bacteriodes species were isolated in the cultures of the empyema and of the intra-abdominal contents. In this case, spread probably occurred through the esophageal hiatus or the diaphragm.

Although the exact pathogenesis of late bronchopleural fistulae is unknown, different hypotheses exist. In the early postoperative period, bronchopleural fistulae are secondary to technical errors in bronchial stump closure. Intermediate fistulae, such as those seen 8 to 10 days after resection, result from a failure in the healing process. Extensive dissection around the bronchus may damage its blood supply and lead to ischemia and impaired healing. Other factors may also be involved. In a multivariate analysis of risk factors in 1360 patients, Asamura, et al. (1992) showed that wider resections, such as pneumonectomies, residual carcinoma, preoperative irradiation, and diabetes, significantly increased the risk of postoperative bronchopleural fistulae. Late occurring bronchopleural fistulae are generally believed to be caused by an underlying empyema because the presence of an infectious process in the pleural cavity impairs healing and may lead to the breakdown of the stump. Other possible factors are the presence of an occult bronchopleural fistula, which was undetected early postoperatively; the presence of residual cancer at the bronchial margin (Soorae and Stevenson, 1979); and a long stump (Lynn, 1958), which can lead to infection and dehiscence.

Clinical Features and Diagnosis

The clinical features associated with late-onset empyemas vary greatly and often are nonspecific. Patients may be asymptomatic; may show mild symptoms of pulmonary sepsis with fever, productive cough, and dyspnea; or may present with severe toxemia. If undetected, the empyema may rupture into the bronchus, flooding the contralateral lung and causing respiratory distress. Factors, such as the size of the empyema, the bacterial agent involved, the presence of an underlying bronchopleural fistula, and the patient's general condition, usually determine the extent of the symptoms.

In Kerr's (1977) report, five of nine patients presented with an empyema necessitatis (Fig. 28-15). In Stafford and Clagett's (1972) series of 18 cases of postpneumonectomy empyema, 10 patients had late-onset empyemas (6 weeks to

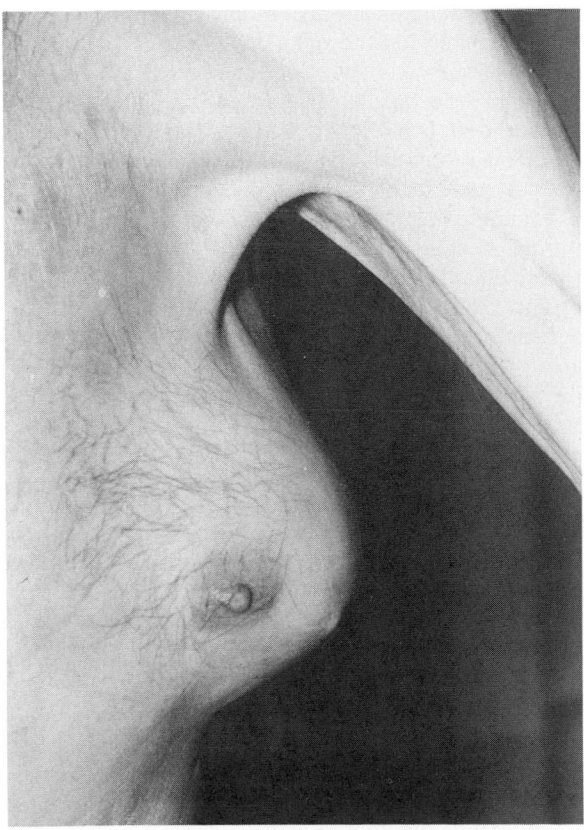

Figure 28-15. A patient presenting with an empyema necessitatis secondary to a postpneumonectomy empyema.

26 years after surgery). The diagnosis was overlooked in these cases, and 6 of 10 patients presented with an empyema necessitatis. In one other case of late empyema (Rogiers, et al. 1991a), the patient presented with respiratory failure secondary to tracheal compression by the empyema, and he was quickly relieved of his symptoms by thoracentesis.

Late bronchopleural fistulae may present with signs and symptoms of an empyema, or affected patients may develop sudden dyspnea, subcutaneous emphysema, and contralateral deviation of the trachea. Expectoration of purulent material associated with these symptoms is virtually diagnostic of the complication. Khargi, et al. (1993) also showed that, in rare cases, bleeding can occur from the pulmonary artery stump in patients with a postpneumonectomy bronchopleural fistula.

The diagnosis of late-onset empyema may be difficult and is usually delayed (Kerr, 1977; Rogiers, et al., 1991a). The history and physical examination are often unrewarding unless signs of a bronchopleural fistula are present. A standard chest radiograph alone, however, may lead to the diagnosis. The physician must specifically look for a fall in the fluid level (more than 1.5 cm) or a new fluid level, the presence of loculated intrapleural gas, or a mediastinal shift to the nonoperated side (Friedman and Hellekant, 1977). Also recommended in the workup are chest CT scans and bronchoscopy, which are useful to exclude associated or recurrent carcinomas. This workup also documents the presence or absence of a bronchopleural fistula and evaluates the pleural cavity in regard to its size and the exact site of the empyema. A diagnosis of empyema must always be confirmed by thoracentesis with appropriate cultures and biochemical and cytologic examinations being carried out on the aspirated fluid or pus. A suspected bronchopleural fistula may be demonstrated by the use of a xenon gas ventilation-isotope scan (Lowe and Siddiqui, 1984; Moote, et al., 1987). Although seldom required, bronchography with Lipiodol instillation in the bronchial stump and methylene blue injection into the pleural space with subsequent appearance of colored sputum may be valuable.

Management

The management of late empyemas or bronchopleural fistulae is similar to that of these complications occurring early during the postoperative period. Initially, it includes control of respiration, tube thoracostomy, appropriate systemic antibiotics, and nutritional support (Grégoire, et al., 1987; Erola, et al., 1988; Pairolero, et al., 1992). Although open window thoracostomy may only be necessary in selected cases refractory to closed chest drainage, some authors (Virkkula and Kostiainen, 1970; Stafford and Clagett, 1972; Goldstraw, 1979; Lemmer, et al., 1985) recommend open pleural drainage in all patients.

Long-term management is individualized and varies according to the success of the initial measures, the patient's condition, the presence of an associated bronchopleural fistula, and the surgeon's experience. The objectives are sterilization of the space, closure of the fistula, and obliteration of the remaining pleural cavity (Allen, et al., 1992). A Clagett procedure may be sufficient for a late empyema without a bronchopleural fistula (Kerr, 1977; Bellamy, et al., 1991). If unsuccessful, an intrathoracic muscle transposition (Pairolero, et al., 1990; Erola, et al., 1988; Miller, et al., 1984) or a space-reducing thoracoplasty (Hopkins, et al., 1985; Grégoire, et al., 1987) may be required. The management of an empyema associated with a bronchopleural fistula requires open chest drainage. Persistent fistulas necessitate the use of a muscle transposition and/or thoracoplasty procedure. If basic surgical principles are respected and if there is no recurrent carcinoma, the results are generally satisfactory, with success rates of 70 to 90 percent.

Persistent Spaces After Pneumonectomy

Pathogenesis and Clinical Features

In 1965, Christiansen, et al. (1965) studied the chest radiographs of 60 pneumonectomized patients and calculated that filling of the pleural space is a phenomenon that requires 3 weeks to 7 months to take place. They suggested that the pleural space fills progressively with serosanguineous fluid and plasma and that the gradual organization of the fluid completely obliterates the hemithorax. In 1969, Suarez, et al. (1969) reviewed autopsy protocols in 37 cases in which pneumonectomy had been performed at the Mayo Clinic (average time between pneumonectomy and death, 46.7 months). Of the patients studied, 10 had specific evidence of total obliteration, and 27 exhibited some degree of residual space. The amount and character of the fluid found in such spaces were not related to the postoperative interval.

Like obliteration of the postlobectomy space, obliteration of the postpneumonectomy space is aided by the shift of adjacent mediastinal structures, elevation of the diaphragm, approximation of the ribs with internal bulging of the intercostal muscles, intrapleural collection of blood and serum, and negative intrapleural pressure. In a study by Suarez et al. (1969), most cases of complete obliteration demonstrated an extensive shift of the mediastinal structures and a diaphragmatic leaf located at or above the fourth rib posteriorly.

Not unlike what can be observed after partial resection, some patients without a demonstrable fistula never fill their postpneumonectomy spaces; other empty their spaces during the early period of follow-up. This syndrome is called "postpneumonectomy pneumothorax" or persistent space after pneumonectomy.

All these patients have a microscopic fistula, which is often impossible to document, either because it is too small or because it is only intermittently patent. Classically, these individuals are asymptomatic. However, on the chest radiograph (Fig. 28-16), the fluid level in the pneumonectomy space is lower than it was previously, and the mediastinum has shifted contralaterally toward the remaining lung. In these cases, the pleural fluid is probably reabsorbed by the parietal pleural because of pressure changes from negative to atmospheric in the space.

Management

When the patient with this complication is asymptomatic, management should be conservative, and approximately 75 percent either reaccumulate pleural fluid (Fig. 28-17) or maintain an empty space without further complications. The patient should be told about the problem and be instructed to watch for signs and symptoms of empyema or bronchopleural fistula. If a fistula is identified or an empyma develops, the management should be the same as previously described.

Late Esophagopleural Fistula

The occurrence of an esophagopleural fistula following pneumonectomy is an uncommon event, and in early reports (Takaro, et al., 1960; Dumont and DeGraef, 1961) most were seen after pulmonary resections done for tuberculosis or suppurative diseases. The diagnosis of an esophagopleural fistula may be difficult and overlooked; patient management still represents an important challenge for the thoracic surgeon.

Incidence and Pathogenesis

The incidence of postpneumonectomy esophagopleural fistula is estimated to be 0.4 to 0.6 percent by Takaro, et al. (1960); Evans (1972); and more recently, Shama and Odell (1985). Although these fistulae were thought to occur more frequently after surgery for tuberculosis, this may not be the case. The incidence in Takaro, et al.'s series (1960) of 934 resections for tuberculosis was similar to that of Evans (1972) who reported on 1,389 pneumonectomies done for carcinomas. Thus, the large number of esophagopleural fistulae reported after tuberculosis surgery probably only reflects the greater prevalence of the disease at the time.

Following pneumonectomy, esophagopleural fistulae occur predominantly on the right side (75 to 88 percent of all cases) (Takaro, et al., 1960; Engelman, et al., 1970) because, on that side, the esophagus lies close to the hilum and carinal nodes. In the left hemithorax, the aorta is interposed between the esophagus and pleural cavity and therefore protects against the development of esophagopleural fistulae. The most common sites of fistula formation are the carinal and subcarinal regions (Takaro, et al., 1960; Dumont and DeGraef, 1961; Benjamin, et al., 1969). As described by Dumont and DeGraef, the blood supply to the esophagus in these locations is segmental and often deficient, thus creating an area of vulnerability.

The pathophysiology of esophagopleural fistula formation is multifactorial and may vary depending on the onset of the fistula. In Takaro, et al.'s review (1960) of 33 cases, the esophagopleural fistula developed within 3 months of surgery in 16 patients. In the remaining 17 patients, the fistula occurred from 3 months to 6 years after the pneumonectomy. Shama and Odell (1985) reported three cases of early-onset esophagopleural fistula and four cases of fistulae occurring 3 years, 6 years, 17 years, and 25 years postoperatively.

Most authors agree that, in cases of early esophagopleural fistulae (less than 3 months), direct trauma and devascularization of the esophagus are responsible for the development of the fistula (Takaro, et al., 1960; Dumont and DeGraef, 1961; Engelman, et al., 1970; Benjamin, et al., 1969; Shama and Odell, 1985). Other possible etiologic factors include the presence of caseating lymph nodes adherent to the esophageal wall or direct inflammatory involvement of the esophagus by a suppurative process. These conditions make the

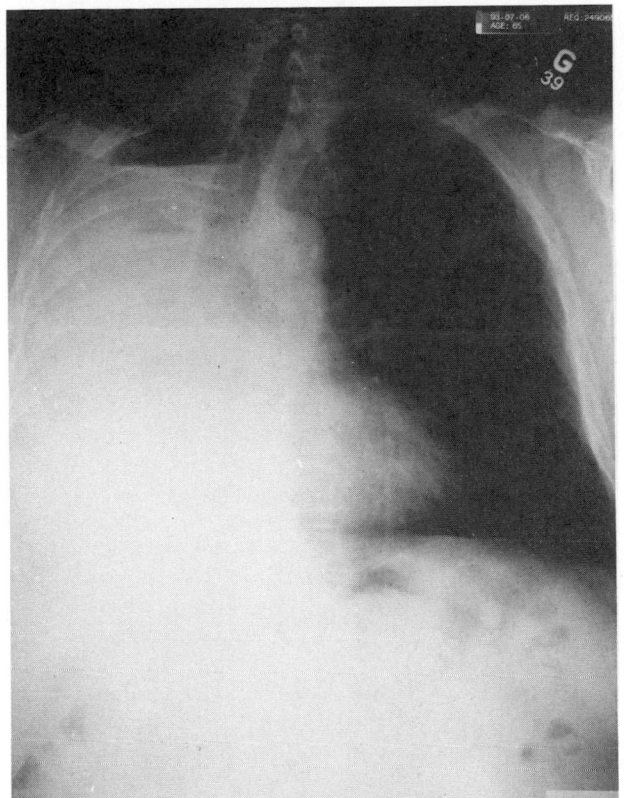

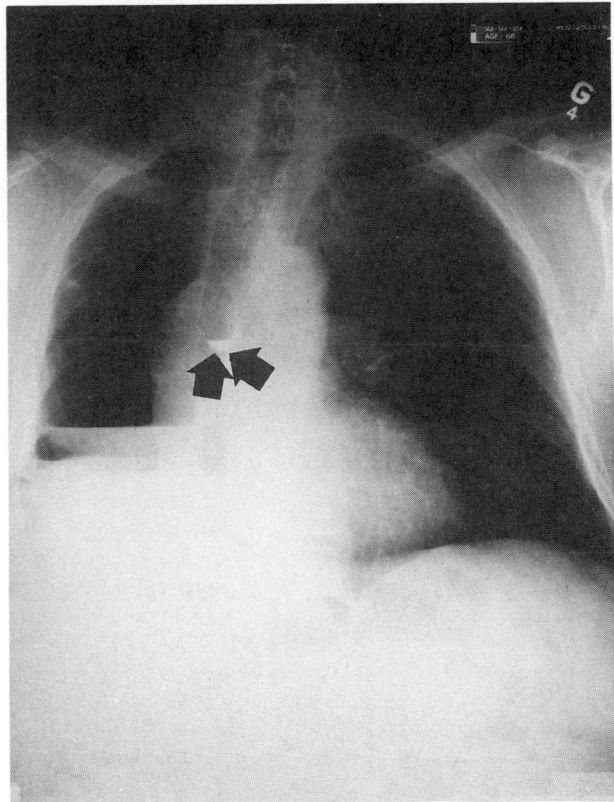

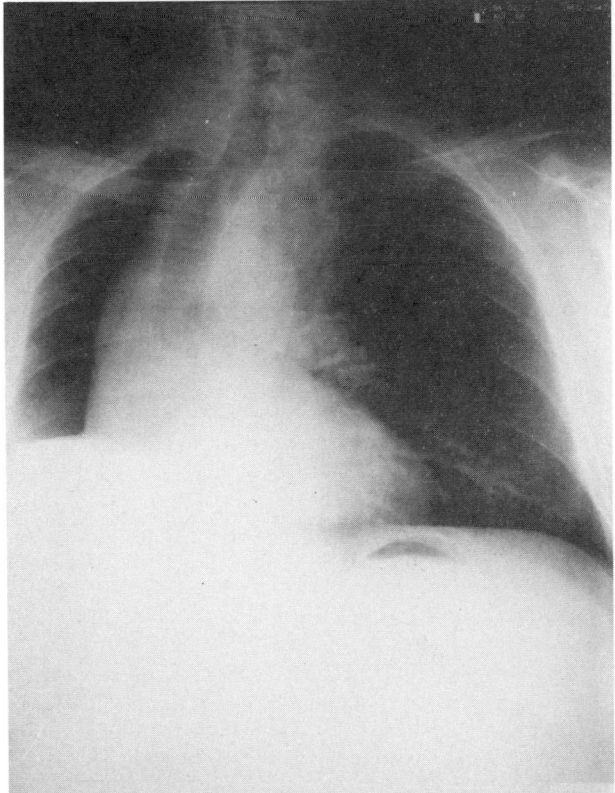

Figure 28-16. Persistent space after pneumonectomy. Posteroanterior chest radiographs taken **(A)** 2 weeks, **(B)** 1 month, and **(C)** 6 months after right pneumonectomy. The patient is completely asymptomatic and being followed conservatively. Several bronchoscopies have failed to demonstrate a bronchopleural fistula. Note that Lipiodol instillation in the bronchus does not show a fistula (*arrows*, Fig. B) and that the mediastinum has remained shifted toward the operated side.

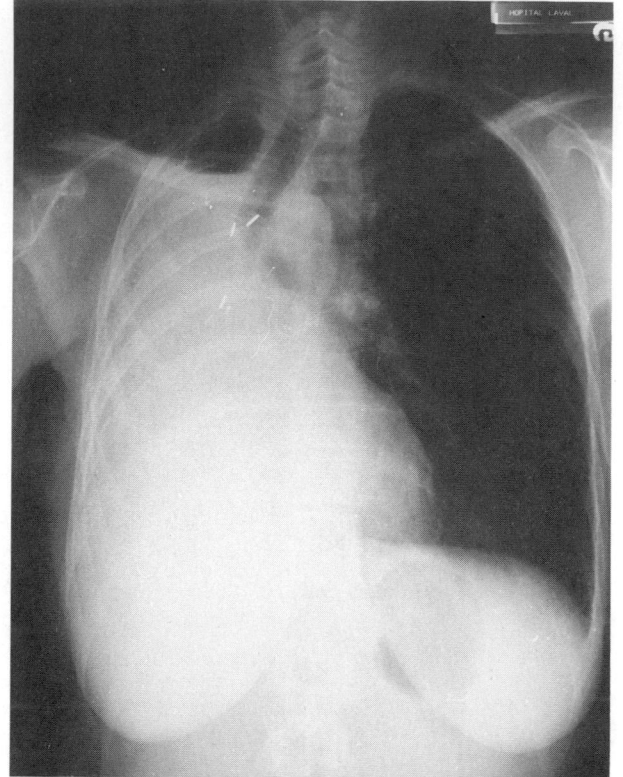

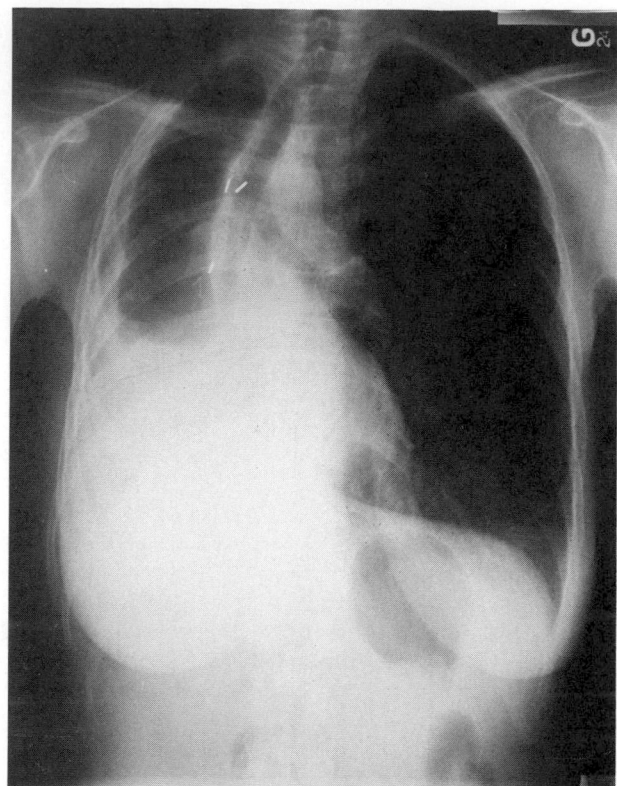

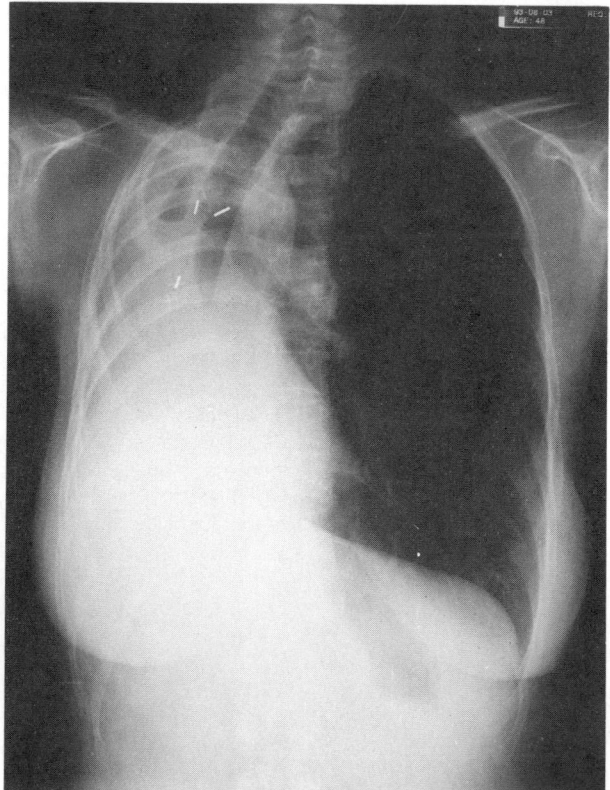

Figure 28-17. Persistent space after pneumonectomy. Posteroanterior chest radiograph taken **(A)** 4 weeks, **(B)** 8 weeks, and **(C)** 6 months after pneumonectomy. Note that the pleural fluid decreased initially in the space but later reaccumulated. No bronchopleural fistula was ever demonstrated.

pulmonary resection more difficult and increase substantially the risk of inadvertent injury to the esophagus.

In contrast to early esophagopleural fistulae, the pathogenesis of late-onset fistulae remains unclear. Takaro, et al. (1960) and Benjamin, et al. (1969) suggested that a chronic infectious process, such as an empyema, a periesophageal abscess, or a peribronchial abscess, may rupture into the esophagus and create a fistula. In a report on three patients and a review of 49 collected cases from the literature, Van den Bosch, et al. (1980) also believe that an infectious process may be responsible for late-onset esophagopleural fistula. Evans (1972) found that a bronchopleural fistula was present in seven of eight patients with an esophagopleural fistula, and all patients presented an empyema for a period of 1 to 22 months prior to the diagnosis of the esophagopleural fistula.

In 1961, Dumont and DeGraef (1961) suggested that a mechanical process, such as traction on the esophageal wall, creates an inflammatory reaction, which leads to the formation of a fistula between the esophageal lumen and pleural cavity. According to this hypothesis, the empyema is the result and not the cause of the fistula.

Symes, et al. (1972) proposed a different mechanism to explain the pathogenesis of esophagopleural fistulae. They presented the case of a 62-year-old man in whom a left pneumonectomy had been performed for a bronchogenic carcinoma. Sixteen months later, the patient developed an esophagopleural fistula that was attributed to recurrent lung carcinoma because there were no signs of empyema or bron-

chopleural fistula. Esophagopleural fistula may thus occur as a result of recurrent local disease.

Clinical Features and Diagnosis

Early diagnosis of an esophagopleural fistula is essential to reduce the rates of patient morbidity and mortality. The clinical features are often those of an empyema and/or bronchopleural fistula, but the diagnosis of an esophagopleural fistula must be considered when a suspected bronchopleural fistula has been ruled out. These patients may present with varying degrees of toxicity, fever, dyspnea, chest pain, and possible subcutaneous emphysema. On occasion, however, they will present with malnutrition, weight loss, and fatigue, a clinical picture that may be difficult to distinguish from that of a locally recurrent or disseminated carcinoma. On thoracentesis, the finding of food particles or gastric juices confirms the diagnosis. The presence of desquamated epidermoid cells in the pleural fluid is pathognomonic, as reported by Eriksen (1964).

The diagnostic workup must include standard chest radiographs, CT scan, and a bronchoscopy to eliminate recurrent disease and the commonly associated bronchopleural fistula. A contrast esophagogram (Fig. 28-18) and esophagoscopy establish the diagnosis, locate the site of the fistula, and help estimate its size. In selected cases, ingestion of methylene blue or the helium test (Van den Bosch, et al., 1980) may also be useful.

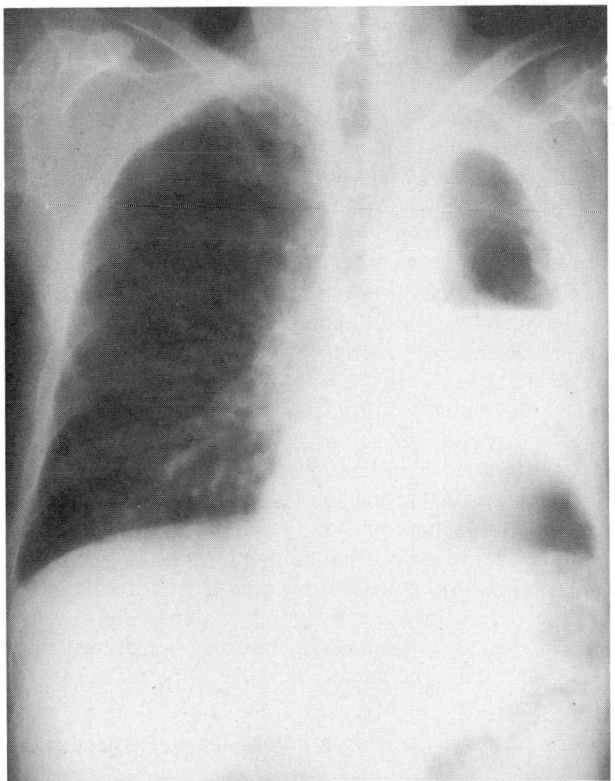 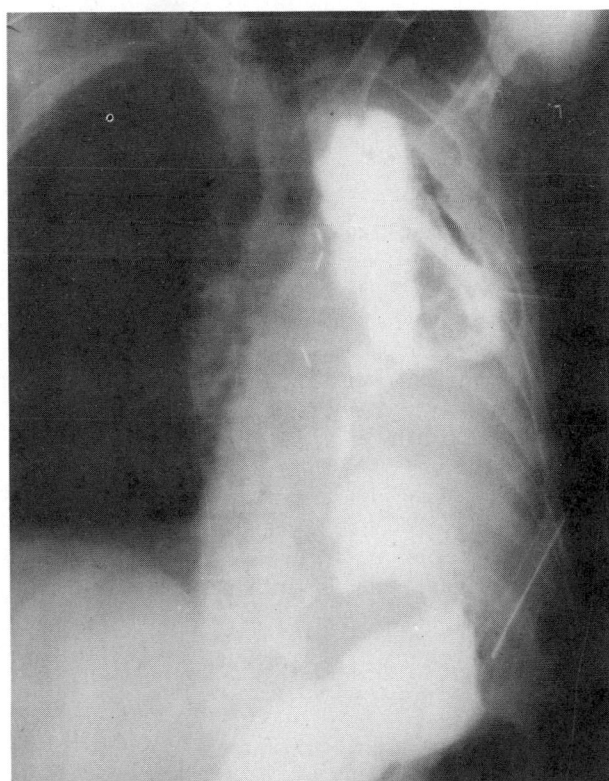

Figure 28-18. Esophagopleural fistula. **(A)** Posteroanterior chest radiograph showing a fluid level in a left pneumonectomy space 3 months following incomplete resection of lung cancer followed by radiation. **(B)** Constrast esophagogram established the diagnosis of a late esophagopleural fistula.

Management

Although a variety of procedures exist, the management of esophagopleural fistulas must be individualized, and both the patient's condition and the specific characteristics of the fistula must be considered. In Takaro, et al.'s (1960) series, 8 patients were treated by direct repair of the fistula (1 death); 4 patients, by gastric or colonic interposition (4 deaths); 10 patients, by chest wall surgery, including drainage and Schede thoracoplasty (2 deaths); and 10 patients, by conservative measures (9 deaths). Overall, 21 percent of patients were cured, and a mortality rate of 49 percent was reported. These authors concluded that therapy of these fistulae is complicated and unsatisfactory.

Successful management of patients must include adequate nutritional support and effective therapy of the associated empyema. Sethi and Takaro (1978) and Van den Bosch, et al. (1980) recommend total parenteral nutrition; others, such as Shama and Odell (1985) and Faber, et al. (1990), advocate enteral feeding. Closed or open pleural drainage with irrigation is required to treat the empyema (Takaro, et al. 1960; Dumont and DeGraef, 1961; Banjamin, et al., 1969; Shama and Odell, 1985). After the infectious process is under control and the patient is stable, attention can be turned to the fistula.

Complicated reconstructions, such as gastric or colonic interposition, are not suitable in these frail patients. We agree with those who recommend direct primary repair of the fistula reinforced with pleura, omentum, or a pedicled chest wall or intercostal muscle flap (Benjamin, et al., 1969; Engelman, et al., 1970; Efthimidis, et al., 1974; Richardson, et al., 1976; Mud, et al., 1987). An 86 percent success rate is reported with this procedure from a literature review (Sethi and Takaro, 1978). A space-reducing thoracoplasty may be added if the postpneumonectomy space is large and shows signs of residual infection (Evans, 1972; Richardson, et al., 1976).

Shama and Odell (1985) offer an interesting alternative to the therapy of these fistulae. Although condemned by Evans (1972) and Sethi and Takaro (1978), Shama and Odell recommend open drainage of the empyema and prolonged nasogastric feeding. After the fistula has healed, attempts are made at sterilizing the cavity by irrigation. These authors successfully treated five of seven patients in this fashion and believe that treating the empyema is the key to the problem and that the fistula will heal by itself after the empyema is under control. This approach is valid and justified in elderly patients who cannot tolerate more extensive procedures.

When the esophagopleural fistula is secondary to recurrent carcinoma, only palliative therapy can be offered. As reported by Symes, et al. (1972), an endoluminal esophageal prosthesis may occlude the fistula and alleviate the patient's symptoms.

LATE BRONCHIAL COMPLICATIONS OTHER THAN FISTULA

Bronchial Stump Suture Granulomas

Granulations at the bronchial suture line are almost always caused by the use of highly reactive suture material, such as silk or Tevdec. In a report from Stanford (Baumgartner and Mark, 1981), all eight patients with bronchial margin granula-

tions had their bronchus closed with Tevdec, which is a multifilament plastic nonabsorbable suture material. The median time between the resection and the development of respiratory symptoms was 18 months (8 to 57 months).

Scott, et al. (1975, 1976) addressed the problem of healing of the bronchial stump when different methods of closure were used. They compared closure and inflammatory reactions when silk, chromic catgut, and stainless steel staples were used for bronchial closure in experimental animals. They concluded that, compared to silk and nylon, the onset of the exudative reaction is delayed and at all times minimal with staples. Because most surgeons currently use staple closure for bronchi, granulation tissue is now seldom seen as a complication of surgery. When it occurs, it is almost always caused by relative ischemia or impaired healing of the bronchus.

Patients with bronchial stump suture granulomas nearly always complain of a dry irritative cough. This symptom may be intermittent and relieved by the spontaneous expectoration of granulation tissue or suture material. Hemoptysis is not uncommon but is seldom of a life-threatening nature.

The diagnosis of bronchial stump suture granulomas can be made at bronchoscopy by which both granulations and suture material can be seen. A local inflammatory reaction can also be seen. Bronchoscopy is also useful to rule out the presence of locally recurrent carcinoma.

Management consists of removing all exposed sutures with the flexible or rigid bronchoscope, and in Baumgartner, et al. (1981) series, immediate and subtained relief was obtained in seven of eight patients.

Long Stump Syndrome

Lynn (1958) was one of the first surgeons to recognize that one of the most important sources of breakdown of the bronchus stump was the failure to observe high division of the bronchus. He made the following observation, "If the bronchus is not divided almost flush with the trachea during pneumonectomy or as close to the parent bronchus as possible during segmental resection or lobectomy, then a sump for the accumulation of secretions is left. This is the greatest source of post operative infection, delayed healing and breakdown."

Long stump syndromes are uncommon and mostly seen after left pneumonectomy (Fig. 28-19) or middle and lower lobectomies. The clinical presentation is usually that of recurring infection, chronic purulent bronchorrhea, and hemoptysis. At bronchoscopy, the stump is markedly inflamed with suture granulomas often being present.

The management can be conservative, with respiratory hygiene, postural physiotherapy, and antibiotics, or when necessary, granulomas can be removed by bronchoscopy. Occasionally, the stump will have to be reresected.

Anastomotic Strictures After Sleeve Resection

The incidence of granuloma formation at the anastomosis after sleeve resection has been reduced to virtually 0 percent with the use of absorbable sutures. Nevertheless, if they should occur and be symptomatic with stridor, hemoptysis,

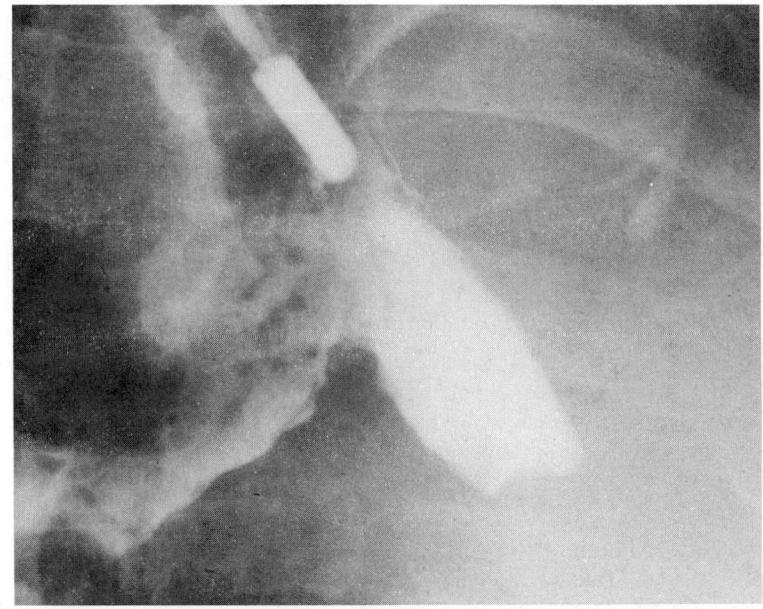

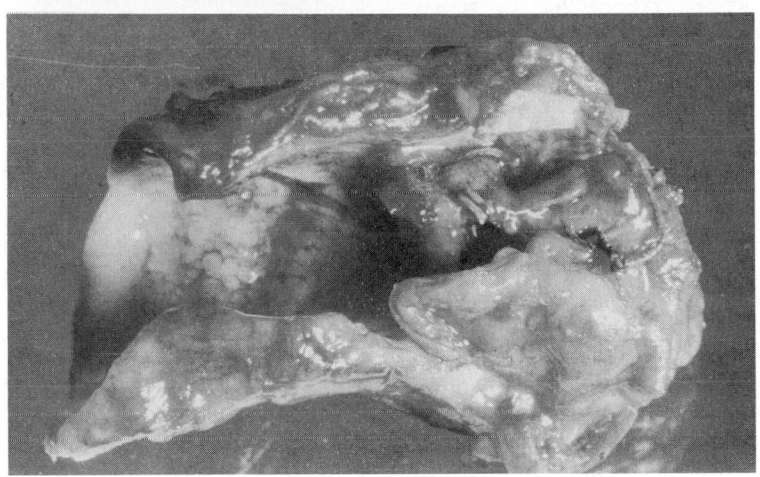

Figure 28-19. Long stump syndrome. **(A)** Bronchogram showing a long stump after left pneumonectomy. This patient was symptomatic and underwent reresection through a median sternotomy. **(B)** The resected specimen showing large amounts of granulation tissue in the stump.

or recurrent pneumonia, granulomas can be removed, sometimes with the adjacent sutures, through the bronchoscope.

Late anastomotic strictures are caused by an interrupted blood supply or anastomotic dehiscence with secondary healing and stricture formation. In most reported series, the incidence of this complication ranges from 2 to 5 percent. Therapy consists of repeated dilatations and removal of granulation tissue, reresection, and anastomosis or completion pneumonectomy. In a recent series of 142 patients who underwent sleeve resection for lung cancer (Mehran, et al., 1994), 4 patients had a late complication at the site of the bronchial anastomosis. Among these, two had granulation tissue that was successfully removed with a bronchoscope, and two had a fibrous stricture that was dilated in one but necessitated completion pneumonectomy in the other. Tsang and Goldstraw (1989) showed that endobronchial stenting

with a Silastic prosthesis may also be a valid option in the therapy of this complication.

POST-THORACOTOMY CHEST PAIN

Definitions and Incidence

The concepts of post-thoracotomy pain and of its management are complex and fascinating. Over the years, great advances have been made in the therapy of pain in the early postoperative period with developments in pre-emptive analgesia, postoperative maintenance therapy, and patient-controlled analgesia. Unfortunately, compared with early post-thoracotomy pain, much less is known about chronic pain, which is an unnecessary source of anxiety and discomfort for a patient who has undergone a thoracotomy and curative resection for a malignancy. Generally, surgeons find the therapy of these pain syndromes frustrating because the results are often unsatisfactory.

Post-thoracotomy pain is important because it is usually more severe and of longer duration than that of pain following other surgical procedures (Loan and Morrison, 1967; Conacher, 1990). The post-thoracotomy pain syndrome refers to pain in the area of the surgical incision that linger beyond the expected postoperative course (Jackson, 1993). The International Association for the Study of Pain (1986) defines this syndrome as pain that recurs or persists along a thoracotomy scar at least 2 months following the surgical procedure. Other authors, such as Sutton (1993), consider post-thoracotomy pain chronic only if it lasts for more than 6 months postoperatively and is unrelated to the underlying pathologic condition.

Following thoracotomy, mild chest pain without repercussions on daily life is common, with an incidence of 44 to 54 percent, as reported by Kalso, et al. (1992) and Dajczman, et al. (1991). The presence of severe disabling chronic pain is, however, less common, with an estimated incidence of 5 percent (Conacher, 1992; Sutton, 1993). It is often described as a sensation of continuous burning or aching in the scar with a dysesthetic or lancinating component extending beyond the immediate area of the incision (Jackson, 1993). Patients may complain of a dull or stabbing pain, numbness, or hyperesthesia or of secondary features, such as frozen shoulder or back pain. Conacher (1992) describes post-thoracotomy pain syndrome more specifically as a post-thoracotomy neuralgia, which is a benign pain condition unrelated to the underlying pathologic condition.

Pathophysiology and Clinical Features

The exact cause of chronic post-thoracotomy pain is unknown. Following surgery, nociceptive stimuli arise from the skin incision, damaged costovertebral structures, fractured or excised ribs, and parietal pleura. These injuries cause direct mechanical and thermal damage to nerve endings and sensitization of primary afferent nociceptors (Sabanathan, et al., 1993). The stimuli from the chest wall structures and pleura are conducted to the central nervous system by the intercostal nerves, those from the diaphragmatic pleura by the phrenic nerve, and those from the lung and mediastinum by the vagus nerve (Conacher, 1990). Although these events are important in the development of acute post-thoracotomy pain, their role in chronic pain is unclear. Furthermore, psychological factors affecting the patient's personality and emotional status may also influence the occurrence and severity of chronic pain (Loan and Morrison, 1967; Jackson, 1993).

Different causes of chronic post-thoracotomy pain have been described, and it is important to distinguish pain as the "symptom" from pain as the "disease" (Jackson, 1993). In the presence of recurrent carcinoma, infectious process, or fractured ribs, pain results from an identifiable source, and this is the symptom of an underlying problem. In a study by Kanner, et al. (1982), a recurrent cancer or infectious complication was found in 29 of 32 patients evaluated for persistent post-thoracotomy pain. Thus, all patients presenting with chronic chest pain must be thoroughly evaluated by clinical history, complete physical examination, and a

workup, which includes a chest radiograph, a CT scan (or magnetic resonance imaging), and a bone scan. If the cause of pain is identified, it can be appropriately treated.

When no cause is found, the chronic pain should be dealt with as a disease process. These forms of post-thoracotomy pain syndrome are considered benign and are either neurogenic or musculoskeletal in origin. A number of phenomena are associated with post-thoracotomy neurogenic pain. The pain may first result from entrapment of nerve fibers in the scar tissue (intercostal neuralgia). In these patients, light touch produces intense radiating pain, accompanied by a burning sensation if a reflex sympathetic dystrophy is associated. The relief of pain with injection of a local anesthetic is virtually diagnostic of this condition. Another cause of neurogenic pain is a neuroma. A palpable mass in the wound, the loss of pinprick sensation over the skin, and pain on palpation lead to this diagnosis. Third, sympathetic dystrophy presents as a burning pain associated with hyperpathia, decreased skin temperature, and increased sweeting (Ramamurthy, 1986).

Benign musculoskeletal post-thoracotomy pain syndromes are less common than pains of neurogenic origin. As discussed previously, recurrent tumor and metastatic disease must first be ruled out, and associated conditions, such as shoulder bursitis or tendinitis, must also be looked for. Unrecognized rib fractures at the time of thoracotomy may be involved in the production of pain. Section of the richly innovated chest wall muscles produces extensive soft tissue injury and inflammation, which may also generate musculoskeletal pain syndromes through a variety of chemical mediators (Conacher, 1990).

It has been shown that muscle-sparing thoracotomy incisions are associated with less pain in the early postoperative period (Lemmer, et al., 1990; Hazelrigg, et al., 1991). Their impact on chronic chest pain, however, is unknown. A specific type of musculoskeletal post-thoracotomy pain, known as myofascial pain syndrome, has been described (Jackson, 1993). Patients have trigger points or localized areas in thoracic muscles, such as the serratus anterior or latissimus dorsi, which produce pain that is referred to distant sites when palpated.

How does the severity of early postoperative pain correlate with the development of chronic chest pain? In Kalso, et al.'s (1992) study, patients who had persistent pain had significantly more pain during the first postoperative week compared with those without chronic pain. However, no difference was found in the amounts of opioids given or in the nurses' comments when comparing the patients. It seems that patients with persistent pain are inclined to remember more pain. As shown by Eich, et al. (1985), memory about the intensity of past physical pain depends on the intensity of present pain.

Management

The management of patients with post-thoracotomy pain syndrome is difficult and benefits from a multidisciplinary approach. A hospital pain "team" can play a key role in developing an appropriate therapeutic plan. In a review of 73 cases of post-thoracotomy neuralgia (more than 3 months' duration), Conacher (1992) found that more than 70 percent of patients received three or more different therapeutic modalities. These included analgesics (narcotics or nonsteroidal anti-inflammatory drugs [NSAID]), local anesthetics, and/or local steroids; transcutaneous electric nerve stimulation (TENS); cryotherapy; surgical or chemical neurolysis; and acupuncture. Despite the great number and variety of therapies, no patients admitted to being relieved of all symptoms.

It has been shown that peripheral nerve injuries may produce central changes in the dorsal root ganglia and that, after such central processes are established, pain may persist independent of peripheral stimulation (Melzack and Loeber, 1978). This hypothesis may explain why local therapy of post-thoracotomy pain syndrome is often frustrating and unsuccessful.

When dealing with benign neurogenic or musculoskeletal chronic chest pain, local measures may nonetheless be valuable, and they represent first-line therapy. Intercostal neuralgias or nerve entrapment are initially treated with intercostal nerve blocks using a local anesthetic (e.g., bupivacaine) with or without steroids. A thoracic epidural infusion or paravertebral blocks may be useful. In 1992, Kirvela and Antila (1992) reported on the use of paravertebral nerve blocks in 32 patients with chronic chest pain. Although 58 percent of patients were relieved, only 8 percent were relieved for more than 4 months.

Cryoanalgesia has also been recommended for neuralgia. First described by Lloyd, et al. (1976), cyroanalgesia uses extreme cold ($-75°C$) to cause temporary disruption of nerve conduction and thus alleviate pain. A number of recent reports, however, have condemned its use (Orr, et al., 1981; Conacher, 1986; Roxburgh, et al., 1987; Berrisford and Sabanathan, 1990). In Conacher's (1986) study on cryotherapy for post-thoracotomy neuralgia, 21 percent of patients showed no improvement, and 29 percent were actually worse after therapy.

When a neuroma is found or suspected, a small amount (less than 1 ml) of anesthetic may be infused into it. If the pain is relieved, the procedure is repeated with a neurolytic phenol solution (Jackson, 1993). Wound exploration and surgical excision are also possible but carry the risk of creating further damage. The presence of a sympathetic dystrophy requires paravertebral sympathetic blocks, nerve root blocks, or an epidural infusion (Ramamurthy, 1986).

The therapeutic options for musculoskeletal chronic chest pain include physical therapy to strengthen muscle tone and improve shoulder mobilization. Heat massages and ultrasound may also be valuable (Jackson, 1993), and NSAIDs may be added to the physical therapy. The use of TENS is also recommended, especially in the presence of myofascial pain syndrome. Oral and systemic medication (narcotics, NSAIDs, and tricyclic antidepressants) and different neuroablative techniques are available and important adjuncts to the local therapeutic measures described.

In all cases of post-thoracotomy pain syndrome, it is essential and important foremost to exclude the presence of recurrent cancer, metastatic disease, or an infectious complication. The patient must then be reassured as to the benign nature of the problem. Understanding the underlying pathophysiology and obtaining a working diagnosis are crucial to provide adequate and successful patient management. Although they often only offer temporary relief, local therapeutic measures continue to represent the mainstay of therapy for chronic chest pain.

LATE PHYSIOLOGIC COMPLICATIONS

Postpneumonectomy Syndrome

Definitions and Incidence

The postpneumonectomy syndrome is caused by airway obstruction, which is itself secondary to the extreme mediastinal shift and rotation after pneumonectomy. In this situation, the mainstem bronchus becomes compressed between the spine and aorta posteriorly and the pulmonary artery anteriorly. This syndrome mainly occurs in younger patients in whom the bronchus is softer and more compressible, and has been described almost exclusively after right pneumonectomy (Grillo, et al., 1992).

The exact incidence of the postpneumonectomy syndrome is unknown, although Jansen, et al (1992) reported only 1 case among 640 patients who had undergone pneumonectomies (incidence of 0.2 percent). This low incidence likely reflects the older age of the patients undergoing pneumonectomy for lung cancer.

Pathogenesis

In a classic review, Grillo, et al. (1992) reported on 11 patients with the postpneumonectomy syndrome and concluded that the airway obstruction clearly results from mediastinal displacement.

After right pneumonectomy, the mediastinum moves counterclockwise to the right and posteriorly (Shepard, et al., 1986). The realignment of intrathoracic structures results in tracheal displacement to the right and compression of the left main bronchus, and sometimes the distal trachea, as it angles beneath the aorta and is flattened against the vertebral column or against the descending aorta (Grillo, et al., 1992) (Fig. 28-20). Szarnicki, et al. (1978) also showed the same findings in a child in whom the lower trachea was compressed by the arch of the aorta after right pneumonectomy.

Although Grillo, et al. (1992) and others (Quillin and Shackleford, 1991) reported the same syndrome after left pneumonectomy, all these patients had a right-sided aortic arch. In Quillin and Shackelford's case, the right-sided descending aorta and ligamentum arteriosum played a central role in the bronchial obstruction. In the cases that occurred after left pneumonectomy, Grillo, et al. (1992) showed that, because the right main bronchus is so much shorter than the left, it is not uncommon to find that the right upper lobe bronchus and the bronchus intermedius are also compressed against the vertebral column.

These observations may not be entirely true because we now have seen four cases of postpneumonectomy syndrome occurring after left pneumonectomy and a normally located left-sided aortic arch (Daniel, et al., personal communication, 1994) (Fig. 28-21). In these cases, the right main bronchus, right upper lobe bronchus, and right bronchus intermedius

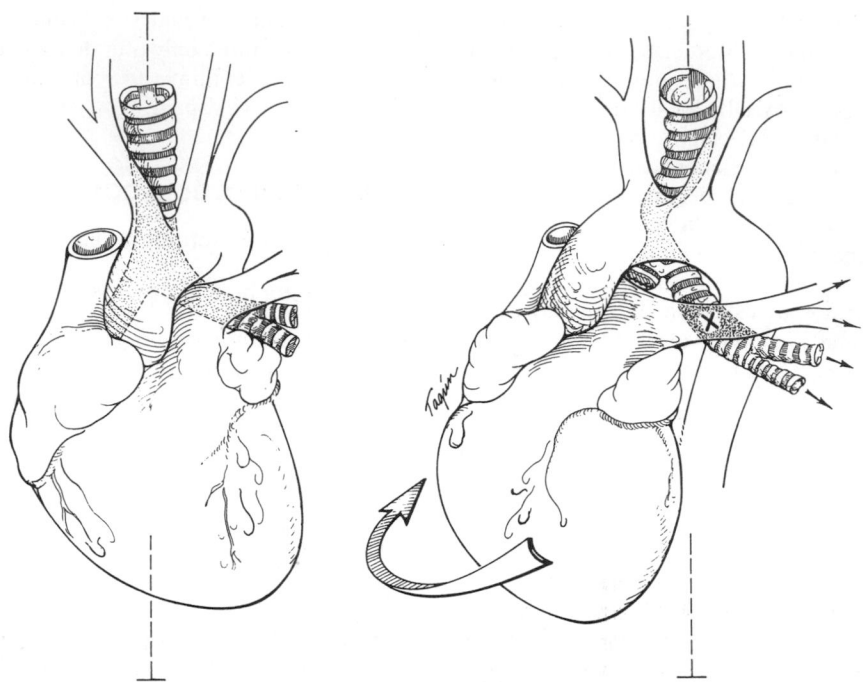

Figure 28-20. Postpneumonectomy syndrome after right pneumonectomy with left-sided arch. This diagram shows that the trachea and carina are displaced to the right with left main bronchus compression between the left pulmonary artery and descending aorta or against the spine. The dashed vertical line indicates the midline. (From Grillo HC, Shepard JAO, Mathiesen DJ, Kanorck DJ: Post-pneumonectomy syndrome. Diagnosis, management, and results. Ann Thorac Surg 54:638, 1992, with permission.)

are stretched, tented, and compressed between the spine posteriorly and pulmonary artery anteriorly.

Rusch, et al. (1990) and others (Powell, e al., 1979) showed that these syndromes are more likely to develop in infants and young children, presumably because of increased mobility of the mediastinum, increased elasticity and compliance of the remaining lung (which allows overdistension), and greater compressibility of the trachea and bronchi (which have less cartilaginous support).

Clinical Features and Diagnosis

Patients can present with an acute onset of dyspnea and airway obstruction, or they can present with a more insidious onset of symptoms, such as repeated bouts of pulmonary infection, persistent cough, and stridor. The interval between the pneumonectomy and the onset of symptoms is variable, and in Grillo, et al.'s (1992) series, it ranged from 5 months to 17 years. Shepard, et al. (1986) also presented the case of one patient who developed the syndrome 37 years after pneumonectomy. In many patients, the symptoms are well tolerated until a critical point of airway obstruction is reached, which brings about acute respiratory failure.

The diagnosis of postpneumonectomy syndrome is based on a high index of suspicion and a methodical multimodality investigation in which CT scanning and bronchoscopic examination are the most important. Conventional radiographic examination always show extreme posterior mediastinal displacement, anterior lung herniation, and stretching of the remaining main bronchus over the spine. CT of the chest is essential to demonstrate the rotation of the heart and great vessels and the exact site and extent of bronchial obstruction against the spine (Grillo, et al., 1992). Confirmation of bronchial narrowing can finally be obtained by bronchoscopy, which can also demonstrate the presence or absence of bronchomalacia.

Management

Surgical therapy of the postpneumonectomy syndrome is directed toward correcting the tracheobronchial compression and diminishing the extreme mediastinal shift and rotation (Riveron, et al., 1990). Relieving the obstruction by way of lysis of adhesions (Wasserman, et al., 1979); suspension of the mediastinum, pericardium, and pulmonary artery to the anterior chest wall (Adams, et al., 1972); division of the aortic arch with placement of a Dacron prosthesis (Szarnicki, et al., 1978); and phrenectomy have all been reported to have variable and unpredictable results.

Using the concept that Lucite balls can prevent overexpansion of the remaining lung after pneumonectomy (Johnson, et al., 1949), Silastic breast implants (Wasserman, et al., 1979), and more recently tissue expanders, such as those used by plastic surgeons, have been successfully used to reposition and maintain the mediastinum toward the midline. These prostheses are inserted in the pleural space and filled with the necessary amount of fluid to replace the mediastinum in the midline, a motion that can be monitored by measuring the central venous pressure. The operation is fairly simple, and the improvement is often immediate and dramatic.

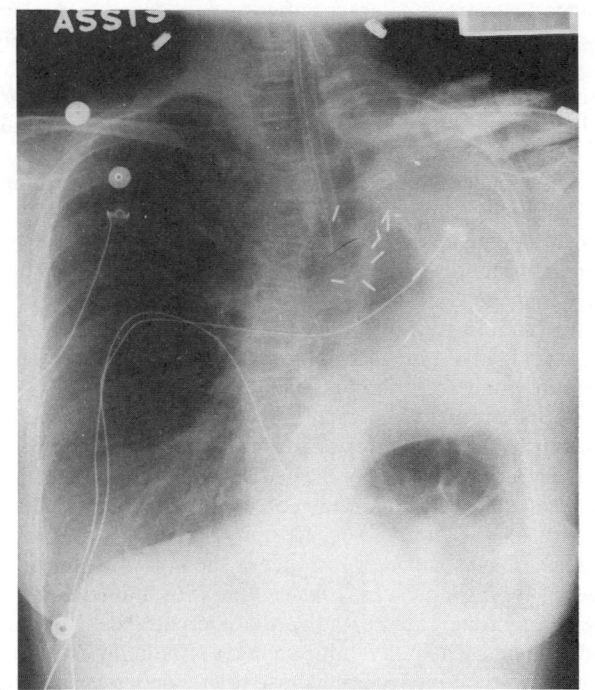

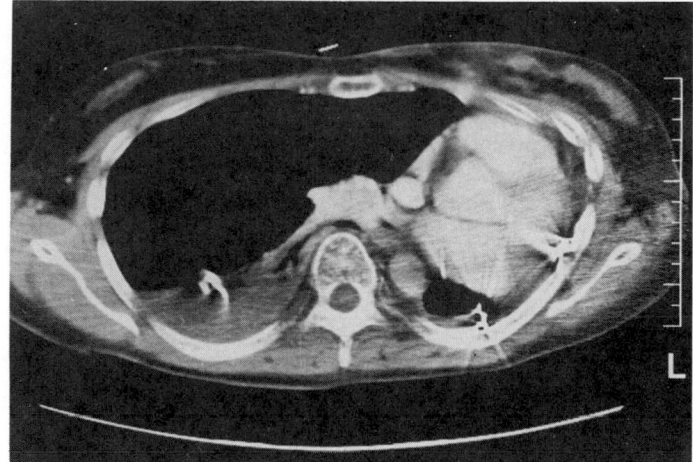

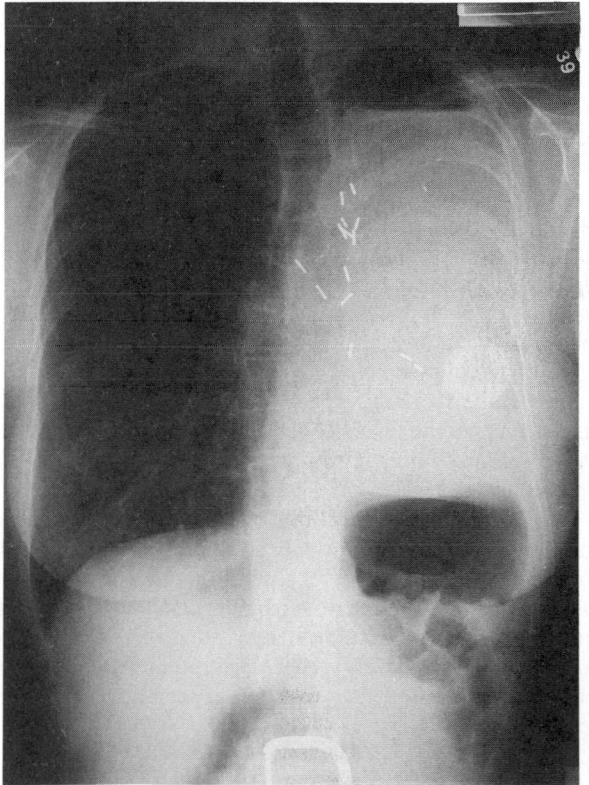

Figure 28-21. Postpneumonectomy syndrome after left pneumonectomy and left-sided arch. **(A)** Standard chest radiograph taken 1 year after left pneumonectomy and showing extreme mediastinal shift. There is an infiltrate in the right lower lung, and the patient had to be intubated. **(B)** CT scan showing the mediastinal shift and severe narrowing of the right main bronchus. **(C)** The mediastinum has been repositioned in a central position by the insertion of a Silastic expander. The patient has remained well 2 years after the insertion of the prosthesis.

One of the problems associated with the correction of this syndrome is the presence of bronchomalacia in the involved bronchus. In these patients, simple mediastinal replacement and fixation by filler material seems to be insufficient, and Grillo, et al. (1992) proposed the placement of bronchial stents, which are either internal or specially constructed T tubes.

Late Respiratory Failure

As pneumonectomy became the standard of care for the therapy of bronchogenic carcinoma in the 1940s, attention was drawn to the functional changes in the remaining lung, and pulmonary insufficiency was recognized as a potential late complication. Gaensler, et al. (1955), in an early report on 460 patients found dyspnea with severe or total disability postoperatively in 7.8 percent of patients. This group also recognized respiratory failure as an important cause of late death. A number of studies on respiratory and circulatory alterations following pulmonary resection appeared thereafter in the literature (Gorlin, et al., 1957; Harrison, et al., 1958; Burrows, et al., 1960; De Graff, et al., 1965).

How do we explain the occurrence of respiratory insufficiency several months or years after a pneumonectomy? It is well known that several structural and physiologic changes develop in the remaining lung parenchyma. Experimental studies in animals subjected to pneumonectomy have shown overdistension and emphysematous changes in the contralateral lung. The lung also has histologic evidence of hyperplasia with fragmentation of the alveoli and loss of elastic tissue (Longaire and Johansmann, 1940). Harrison, et al. (1958) believed that these changes could cause an increase in airway resistance with abnormal alveolar gas mixing and arterial oxygen desaturation, eventually leading to late pulmonary failure. The destructive changes in the alveolar walls following surgery were termed "compensatory emphysema" by Phillips, et al. (1941), but other authors did not demonstrate such changes in the remaining lung after pneumonectomy (Birath, et al., 1947; Jones, et al., 1960; Burrows, et al., 1960).

A number of hypotheses concerning hemodynamic and circulatory alterations have also been proposed. In a patient who has undergone pneumonectomy, the blood flow through the remaining lung is substantially increased, but the total capillary bed available for gas exchange remains unchanged. When the oxygen requirements and pulmonary blood flow increase on exertion, the capillary bed cannot accommodate the demand, and this may result in pulmonary hypertension and arterial oxygen desaturation (Harrison, et al., 1958). Burrows, et al. (1960) also suggested that exercise may have an active vasomotor effect on the lung, thus creating pulmonary artery hypertension, which could in turn lead to progressive pulmonary failure. In a study of postpneumonectomy patients, De Graff, et al. (1965) found a reduction in maximal oxygen intake on exercise, and neither a reduced ventilation nor a lower diffusing capacity was responsible for the changes. These authors believed a decrease in cardiac output was the limiting factor.

In these early reports, the investigational methods were few, and thus, a correlation between structural and physiologic changes and clinical outcome could not be demonstrated. The more recent development of dynamic respiratory studies and of sophisticated hemodynamic monitoring apparatuses has provided a wealth of information. Boushy, et al. (1971), in a study of 62 patients who had undergone preoperative and postoperative pulmonary function tests, found that changes in exercise tolerance after resection were not related to morphologic emphysema or bronchitis in the remaining lung. Lobectomies were shown to have little effect on exercise capacity and late respiratory failure (Berend, et al., 1980; Vejlsted and Halkier, 1982). After surgery, there are generally no alterations in the distribution of ventilation or the diffusing capacity, and modifications in pulmonary function simply reflect changes in pulmonary volumes.

Van Meighem and Demedts (1989) reported on cardiopulmonary function following lung resections for carcinoma. They found a decrease in vital capacity (15 percent for lobectomies and 35 to 40 percent for pneumonectomies) and a decrease in static lung compliance (increase in elastic recoil pressures and transdiaphragmatic pressures). At rest, patients had normal pulmonary artery pressures and vascular resistances; during exercise, an increase in pulmonary artery pressure and an absence of the physiologic decrease in pulmonary vascular resistance were noted. In postpneumonectomy patients, these authors suggest that there may be a relative increase in vasoactive substances, such as angiotensin II, leading to systemic vasoconstriction with a secondary decrease in stroke volume and cardiac output. These vascular and pulmonary hemodynamic changes alter pulmonary function and may in theory predispose to late pulmonary failure.

Mossberg, et al. (1976) studied working capacity and exercise limitation in pneumonectomized patients. They found a reduction in ventilatory function (increase in static pulmonary volumes and decrease in dynamic volumes), a decrease in diffusing capacity, impaired gas exchange, a low stroke volume, and an elevated left atrial pressure and pulmonary artery pressure during exercise, all of which contributed to a lower working capacity. In a more recent comprehensive study, Pelletier, et al. (1990) reported a 25 percent decrease in maximal working capacity following pneumonectomy. Dyspnea increased significantly for a given workload after pneumonectomy, whereas no significant change was found following lobectomy. In this report, the reduction in forced expiratory volume could explain only 30 percent of the change in the working capacity. A number of other mechanisms, such as the characteristics of the respiratory muscles and different hemodynamic parameters, are thus probably also involved.

Late respiratory failure following pulmonary resection is an important cause of patient morbidity and death, and its pathophysiology is complex, multifactorial, and not completely understood. Hemodynamic and ventilatory factors and parenchymal structural changes are involved. A thorough preoperative evaluation is therefore required in all patients with a limited pulmonary reserve, especially if they are 70 years of age or older.

COMMENTS AND CONTROVERSIES

As can be seen from the review, late complications of pulmonary surgery are rare events, but when they occur, they usually are difficult to diagnose and treat. They should be distinguished from recurrent carcinoma, and it is not unusual for patients to be told that they are terminally ill with tumor when the problem is a postpneumonectomy empyema or a postpneumonectomy syndrome.

It is for these reasons that we recommend a close follow-up for at least the first 2 years after the operation. All patients should be seen and have a chest radiograph 1 month postoperatively and again every 3 months for the following 2 years. In our unit, each patient is also given a pamphlet that lists and explains symptoms, such as fever, chest pain, or purulent sputum, which may be indicative of a pending late complication.

J.D.
P.F.

Late-appearing empyema following lobectomy or pneumonectomy can be a daunting problem. The initial management by tube thoracostomy and ultimately open drainage is a standard technique. In most instances, open window thoracostomy is required to effect better mechanical debridement. My associates and I prefer repeated daily packing of saline or hypochlorite impregnated gauze. Ultimately, tailoring thoracoplasty and/or muscle transposition may be necessary to closer the space. However, we have found that repeated packing, especially with situations less than pneumonectomy in the lower regions of the chest, can close the space by progressive fibrosis and contraction.

In late-appearing fistulae, we firmly believe in the initial strategy of tube thoracostomy and closed chest drainage. Following this, open thoracotomy is performed once it is determined that the patient can ventilate with an open chest wound as determined by releasing the thoracostomy tube from its underwater position. Open-window thoracostomy is often successful in closing the fistula and cleaning the contaminated space. We prefer a large window (2 to 3 ribs, 6- to 7-cm length being removed) and repeated packing of the cavity to effect mechanical debridement. In a significant number of such patients, the fistulae will close. Once open-window thoracostomy is performed, the patient can be treated as an outpatient.

For persisting fistulae, a variety of approaches have been suggested including: ipsilateral thoracotomy and direct closure using a vascularized flap of transposed muscle (intercostal, chest wall, rectus abdominis) or a vascularized pedicle of omentum. If a fistula is not present, attempts at sterilization of a persisting cavity (the Claggett procedure) can be very successful if particular attention is directed toward mechanical debridement of the cavity and replacement of the empyema wall with healthy granulation tissue before sterilization.

Anastomotic strictures following sleeve resections can occasionally be treated by laser resection if the stricture is extremely short. This is best done using a carbon dioxide laser, incising the stricture radically in quadrants over 4 or 5 sessions.

I have found, on occasion, that post-thoracotomy pain is caused by cross-union of ribs inadvertently fractured at thorcotomy. This malunion can be identified by specific rib x-rays or tomograms. Surgical removal of the cross-union and freeing of the entrapped nerve can relieve the problem. Prevention of late post-thoracotomy pain may be related to amelioration of the early post-thoracotomy pain, which appears to be almost inevitable. A recent development is the use of "preemptive analgesia," which appears to be extremely effective in diminishing early postoperative pain. This includes preoperative institution of analgesia by percutaneous paravertebral block or epidural analgesia.

The postpneumonectomy syndrome has only recently been described. The procedure of choice appears to be repositioning of the mediastinum. On occasion, this has been sucessfully treated by intrabronchial insertion expandable metallic stents. However, results of the late follow-up of such stents is unavailable.

The occurrence of late respiratory failure, especially following right pneumonectomy, is a disappointing result. This whole area remains a challenge, in being able not only to predict this complication, but also to prevent its occurrence and manage it once it is manifest. We require more reports on its incidence, especially following pneumonectomy, and more reports of very long term follow-up of pulmonary function in resected patients. This is an area worthwhile of further study.

R.J.G.

KEY REFERENCES

Gaensler EA, Cugell DW, Lindgren I et al.: The role of pulmonary insufficiency in mortality and invalidism following surgery for pulmonary tuberculosis. J Thorac Surg 29:163, 1955

Classic analysis of pulmonary function after pneumonectomy by a physiologist-surgeon.

Grillo HC, Shepard JAO, Mathisen DJ, Kanorek DJ: Post-pneumonectomy syndrome. Diagnosis, management, and results. Ann Thorac Surg 54:638, 1992

Best article on the postpneumonectomy syndrome, with clear descriptions and pathogenesis, pathophysiology, and principles of management.

Lynn RB: The bronchial stump. J Thorac Surg: 36:70, 1958

A good overview of the principles involved in bronchial stump closure and healing.

Pairolero P, Arnold PG, Trastek VF et al.: Post-pneumonectomy empyema—the role of intrathoracic muscle transposition. J Thorac Cardiovasc Surg 99:958, 1990

The results of a large series of early and late postpneumonectomy empyemas treated by muscle filling of the space.

Shama DM, Odell JA: Esophageal fistula after pneumonectomy for inflammatory disease. J Thorac Cardiovasc Surg 89:77, 1985

Discussion of the pathophysiology and principles of management of patients with esophagopleural fistula.

Shields TW, Lees WMM, Fox RT, Salazar G: Persistent pleural air space following resection for pulmonary tuberculosis. J Thorac Cardiovasc Surg 38:523, 1959

Excellent review of the incidence and rate of postresectional spaces. Provides guidelines as to the strategy of management.

REFERENCES

Infectious and Space Complications

Allen MS, Deschamps C, Trastek VF, Pairolero PC: Bronchopleural fistula. Chest Surg Clin North Am 2:823, 1992

Asamura M, Naruke T, Tsuchiya R et al.: Bronchopleural fistulas associated with lung cancer operations. J Thorac Cardiovasc Surg 104:1456, 1992

Barker WL, Langston HT, Naffah P: Post-resectional thoracic spaces. Ann Thorac Surg 2:299, 1966

Bellamy J, Saada J, Dang QD: Pyothorax tardifs d'origine hématogène après pneumonectomie. Ann Chir 45:182, 1991

Benjamin I, Olsen AM, Ellis FH: Esophagopleural fistula. A rare post-pneumonectomy complication. Ann Thorac Surg 7:139, 1969

Boyd AD, Spencer FC: Bronchopleural fistulas. How often should they occur? Ann Thorac Surg 13:195, 1972

Brunn HB: Surgical principles underlying one-stage lobectomy. Arch Surg 18:490, 1929

Christiansen KH, Morgan SW, Karich AF, Takaro T: Pleural space following pneumonectomy. Ann Thorac Surg 1:298, 1965

Churchill ED: The surgical treatment of carcinoma of the lung. J Thorac Surg 2:254, 1933

Churchill E, Belsey HR: Segmental pneumonectomy in bronchiectasis. Ann Surg 109:481, 1939

Clagett OT, Geraci JE: A procedure for the management of post-pneumonectomy empyema. J Thorac Cardiovasc Surg 45:141, 1963

Davies HM: Recent advances in the surgery of the lung and pleura. Brit J Surg 1:228, 1913–1914

Dumont A, De Graef J: La fistule esophagopleurale, complication tardive de la pneumonectomie. Lyon Chir 57:481, 1961

Efthimiadis M, Xanthakis D, Primikyrios N et al.: Late esophagopleural fistula after pneumonectomy for bronchial carcinoma. Chest 65:579, 1974

Engelman RM, Spencer FC, Berg P: Post-pneumonectomy esophageal fistula. Successful one-stage repair. J Thorac Cardiovasc Surg 59:871, 1970

Eriksen KR: Esophagopleural fistula diagnosed by microscopic examination of pleural fluid. Acta Chir Scand 128:771, 1964

Erola S, Virkkula L, Varstela E: Treatment of post-pneumonectomy empyema and associated bronchopleural fistula. Scand J Thorac Cardiovasc Surg 22:235, 1988

Evans JP: Post-pneumonectomy oesophageal fistula. Thorax 27:674, 1972

Faber C, Kartheuser A, Buche M et al.: Fistules oesophago-respiratoires traitées par suture primaire. À propos de deux observations de fistule oeso-pleurales et de deux observations de fistules oeso-bronchiques. Ann Chir 44:290, 1990

Friedman PJ, Hellekant CAG: Radiologic recognition of bronchopleural fistula. Radiology 124:289, 1977

Goldstraw P: Treatment of post-pneumonectomy empyema: the case of fenestration. Thorax 34:740, 1979

Grégoire R, Deslauriers J, Beaulieu M, Piraux M: Thoracoplasty: its forgotten role in the management of non-tuberculous post-pneumonectomy empyema. Can J Surg 30:343, 1987

Hinz R: Totale extirpation der linken lunge wegen bronchial carcinoma. Arch Klin Chir 124:104, 1923

Holden MP, Wooler GH: Pus somewhere, pus nowhere else, pus above the diaphragm: post-pneumonectomy empyema necessitatis. Am J Surg 124:669, 1972

Hopkins RA, Ungerleider RM, Staub EW et al.: The modern use of thoracoplasty. Ann Thorac 40:181, 1985

Kerr WF: Late onset post-pneumonectomy empyema. Thorax 32:149, 1977

Khargi K, Duurkens VAM, Knaepen PJ, de la Rivière AB: Hemorrhage due to inflammatory erosion of the pulmonary artery stump in post-pneumonectomy bronchopleural fistula. Ann Thorac Surg 56:357, 1993

Kirsh MM, Rotman H, Behrendt DM et al.: Complications of pulmonary resection. Ann Thorac Surg 20:215, 1975

Kummel H: Proceedings of the 40th Congress, Berlin, April 19–22, 1911. Verh Dtsch Ges Chir 40:147, 1911

Lemmer HJ, Botham MJ, Orringer MB: Modern management of adult thoracic empyema. J Thorac Cardiovasc Surg 90:849, 1985

Leroux BT, Mohlala ML, Odell JA, Whitton FD: Suppurative disease of the lung and pleural space. Part I: Empyema thoracis and lung abscess. Curr Probl Surg 23:1, 1986

Lowe RE, Siddiqui AR: Scintimaging of bronchopleural fistula: a simple method of diagnosis. Clin Nucl Med 9:10, 1984

Miller JI, Mansour KA, Nahai F et al.: Single stage complete muscle flap closure of the post-pneumonectomy empyema space: a new method and possible solution to a disturbing complication. Ann Thorac Surg 38:227, 1984

Model D: Occult empyema presenting ten years after pneumonectomy. Lancet 22:192, 1983

Moote D, Ehrlich L, Martin RH: Post-pneumonectomy bronchopleural fistula imaged by ventilation lung scanning. Medicine 12:337, 1987

Mud HJ, Van Houten H, Slingerland R et al.: A modified pectoralis muscle flap for closure of post-pneumonectomy esophagopleural fistula: technique and results. Ann Thorac Surg 43:359, 1987

Pairolero P, Deschamps C, Allen MS, Trastek MS: Postoperative empyema. Chest Surg Clin North Am 2:813, 1992

Pean J: Chirurgie des poumons. Discussion Ranc Chir Proc Verh Paris 9:72m, 1895

Rainer WG, Newby JP: Prevention of residual space problems after pulmonary resection. Am J Surg 114:744, 1967

Richardson JD, Campbell D, Trinkle JK: Esophagopleural fistula after pneumonectomy. Chest 69:795, 1976

Rienhoff WF: Pneumonectomy. A preliminary report of operative technique in two successful cases. Bull Johns Hopkins Hosp 53:390, 1933

Rogiers PH, Van Mieghem W, Engelaar D, Demedts M: Late onset post-pneumonectomy empyema manifesting as tracheal stenosis with respiratory failure. Respir Med 85:333, 1991a

Rogiers PH, Verschakelen J, Knockaert D, Vanneste S: Occult tuberculous post-pneumonectomy space empyema four years after lung resection. Postgrad Med J 67:672, 1991b

Sethi GK, Takaro T: Esophagopleural fistula following pulmonary resection. Ann Thorac Surg 25:74, 1978

Shamji FM, Ginsberg RJ, Cooper JD et al.: Open window thoracostomy in the management of post-pneumonectomy empyema with or without bronchopleural fistula. J Thorac Cardiovasc Surg 86:818, 1983

Silver AN, Epinas EE, Byron FX: The fate of the post-resection space. Ann Thorac Surg 2:311, 1966

Soorae AS, Stevenson HM: Survival with residual tumor on the bronchial margin after resection for bronchogenic carcinoma. J Thorac Cardiovasc Surg 78:175, 1979

Stafford EG, Clagett OT: Post-pneumonectomy empyema. Neomycin instillation and definitive closure. J Thorac Cardiovasc Surg 63:771, 1972

Steiger Z, Wilson RF: Management of bronchopleural fistulas. Surg Gynecol Obstet 158:267, 1984

Suarez J, Clagett OT, Brown AL: The post-pneumonectomy space:

factors influencing its obliteration. J Thorac Cardiovasc Surg 57:539, 1969

Symes JM, Page AJF, Flavell G: Esophagopleural fistula: a late complication after pneumonectomy. J Thorac Cardiovasc Surg 63:783, 1972

Takaro T, Walkup HE, Okano T: Esophagopleural fistula as a complication of thoracic surgery. A collective review. J Thorac Cardiovasc Surg 40:179, 1960

Van den Bosch JMM, Swierenga J, Gelissen HJ, Laros CD: Post-pneumonectomy oesophagopleural fistula. Thorax 35:865, 1980

Vester SR, Faber LP, Kittle CF et al.: Bronchopleural fistula after stapled closure of bronchus. Ann Thorac Surg 52:1253, 1991

Virkkula L, Kostiainen S: Post-pneumonectomy empyema in pulmonary carcinoma patients. Scand J Thorac Cardiovasc Surg 4:267, 1970

Williams NS, Lewis CT: Bronchopleural fistula: a review of 86 cases. Br J Surg 63:520, 1976

Witz JP, Roeslin N: Les empyèmes et fistules bronchiques après pneumonectomie. Résultat d'une enquête à propos de 444 observations. Ann Chir 35:669, 1981

Late Bronchial Stump Complications Other than Fistulae

Baumgartner WA, Mark JBD: Bronchoscopic diagnosis and treatment of bronchial stump suture granulomas. J Thorac Cardiovasc Surg 81:553, 1981

Lynn RB: The bronchus stump. J Thorac Surg 36:70, 1958

Mehran RJ, Deslauriers J, Piraux M et al.: Survival related to nodal status after sleeve resection for lung cancer. J Thorac Cardiovasc Surg 107:576, 1994

Scott RN, Faraci RP, Goodman DG et al.: The role of inflammation in bronchial stump healing. Ann Surg 181:4, 1975

Scott RN, Faraci RP, Hough A, Chrétien PB: Bronchial stump closure techniques following pneumonectomy. A serial comparative study. Ann Surg 184:205, 1976

Tsang V, Goldstraw PL: Endobronchial stenting for anastomotic stenosis after sleeve resection. Ann Thorac Surg 48:568, 1989

Post-Thoracotomy Chest Pain

Berrisford RG, Sabanathan SS: Cryoanalgesia for post-thoracotomy pain (letter). Ann Thorac Surg 49:509, 1990

Conacher ID: Therapists and therapies for post-thoracotomy neuralgia. Pain 48:409, 1992

Conacher ID: Pain relief after thoracotomy. Br J Anaesth 65:806, 1990

Conacher ID: Percutaneous cryotherapy for post-thoracotomy neuralgia. Pain 25:227, 1986

Dajczman E, Gordon A, Krelsman M, Wolkove N: Long term post-thoracotomy pain. Chest 99:270, 1991

Eich E, Reeves JL, Jaeger B, Graff-Radford SB: Memory for pain: relation between past and present pain intensity. Pain 23:375, 1985

Hazelrigg S, Landreneau RJ, Boley TM et al.: The effect of muscle sparing versus standard posterolateral thoracotomy on pulmonary function, muscle strength and postoperative pain. J Thorac Cardiovasc Surg 101:394, 1991

International Association for Study of Pain: Post-thoracotomy pain syndrome (XVII-14), classification of chronic pain. Pain 3(suppl):S138, 1986

Jackson KE: Postthoracotomy pain syndromes. p. 201. In Granlee, Rauck (eds): Pain Management in Cardiothoracic Surgery. JB Lippincott, Philadelphia, 1993

Kalso E, Perttunen K, Kaasinen S: Pain after thoracic surgery. Acta Anaesthesiol Scand 36:96, 1992

Kanner RM, Martin N, Foley KM: Nature and incidence of post-thoracotomy pain (abstr). Proc Am Soc Clin Oncol 2:152, 1982

Kirvela O, Antila M: Thoracic paravertebral block in chronic postoperative pain. Reg Anesth 17:348, 1992

Lemmer J, Gromez MN, Symreng T et al.: Limited lateral thoracotomy improved postoperative pulmonary function. Arch Surgery 125:873, 1990

Lloyd JW, Barnard JDW, Glynn CJ: Cryoanalgesia, a new approach to pain relief. Lancet 2:932, 1976

Loan WB, Morrison TD: The incidence and severity of post-operative pain. Br J Anaesth 39:695, 1967

Melzack R, Loeber JD: Phantom body pain in paraplegics: evidence for a central pattern generating mechanism for pain. Pain 4:195, 1978

Orr JA, Keeman DJ, Dundee NN: Improved pain relief after thoracotomy: use of cryophobe and morphine infusion. BMJ 283:945, 1981

Ramamurthy S: Thoracic and low back pain. p. 464. In Raj P (ed): Practical Management of Pain. Year Book Medical Publishers, Chicago, 1986

Roxburgh JC, Markland CG, Ross BA, Kerr WF: Role of cryanalgesia in the control of pain after thoracotomy. Thorax 42:292, 1987

Sabanathan S, Richardons T, Mearns AJ: Management of pain in thoracic surgery. Br J Hosp Med 50:114, 1993

Sutton BA: Post-operative management and the provision of pain relief. p. 122. In Gothard JWW (ed): Anaesthesia for Thoracic Surgery. Blackwell Scientific Publications, Oxford, 1993

Late Physiologic Complications

Adams HD, Junod FL, Aberdeen E, Johnson J: Severe airway obstruction caused by mediastinal displacement after right pneumonectomy in a child: case report. J Thorac Cardiovasc Surg 63:534, 1972

Berend N, Woolcock AJ, Marlin GE: Effects of lobectomy on lung function. Thorax 35:145, 1980

Birath G, Crafoord G, Rudstron P: Pulmonary function after pneumonectomy and lobectomy. J Thorac Surg 16:492, 1947

Boushy SF, Billig DM, North LB, Helgason AH: Clinical course related to pre-operative and post-operative pulmonary function in patients with bronchogenic carcinoma. Chest 59:383, 1971

Burrows B, Harrison RW, Adams WE et al.: The post-pneumonectomy state. Clinical and physiologic observations in thirty-six cases. Am J Med 28:281, 1960

De Graff AC, Taylor HF, Ord JW et al.: Exercise limitation following extensive pulmonary resection. J Clin Invest 44:1514, 1965

Gorlin R, Knowles JH, Storey FS: Effects of thoracotomy on pulmonary function. J Thorac Surg 34:242, 1957

Harrison RN, Adams WE, Long ET et al.: The clinical significance of cor pulmonale in the reduction of cardiopulmonary reserve following extensive pulmonary resection. J Thorac Surg 36:352, 1958

Jansen JP, de la Rivière AB, Carpentier-Alting MP et al.: Post-pneumonectomy syndrome in adulthood. Surgical correction using an expandable prosthesis. Chest 101:11, 1992

Johnson J, Kirby CK, Lazatin CS, Cooke JA: The clinical use of a prosthesis to prevent overdistention of the remaining lung following pneumonectomy. J Thorac Surg 18:164, 1949

Jones JJ, Robinson JL, Meyer BW, Motley HL. Primary carcinoma of the lung. A follow-up study including pulmonary function studies of long-term survivors. J Thorac Cardiovasc Surg 39:144, 1960

Longaire JJ, Johansmann R: An experimental study of the fate of the remaining lung following total pneumonectomy. J Thorac Surg 10:131, 1940

Mossberg B, Bjök VO, Holmgren A: Working capacity and cardiopulmonary function after extensive lung resections. Scand J Thorac Cardiovasc Surg 10:247, 1976

Pelletier C, Lapointe L, Leblanc P: Effects of lung resection on pulmonary function and exercise capacity. Thorax 45:497, 1990

Phillips FJ, Adams WE, Hrdina LS: Physiologic adjustment in sublethal reduction of lung capacity in dogs. Surgery 9:25, 1941

Powell RW, Luck SR, Raffensperger JG: Pneumonectomy in infants and children: the use of a prosthesis to prevent mediastinal shift and its complications. J Pediatr Surg 14:231, 1979

Quillin SP, Shackelford GD: Post-pneumonectomy syndrome after left lung resection. Radiology 179:100, 1991

Rasch DK, Grover FL, Schnapf BM: Right pneumonectomy syndrome in infancy treated with an expandable prosthesis. Ann Thorac Surg 50:127, 1990

Riveron FA, Adams C, Lewis JW et al.: Silastic prosthesis plombage for right post-pneumonectomy syndrome. Ann Thorac Surg 50:465, 1990

Shepard JA, Grillo HC, McLoud TC et al.: Right pneumonectomy syndrome: radiologic findings and CT correlation. Radiology 161:661, 1986

Szarnicki R, Maurseth K, de Leval M, Stark J: Tracheal compression by the aortic arch following right pneumonectomy in infancy. Ann Thorac Surg 25:231, 1978

Van Mieghem W, Demedts M: Cardiopulmonary function after lobectomy or pneumonectomy for pulmonary neoplasm. Respir Med 83:199, 1989

Vejlsted H, Halkier E: Pre- and post-operative lung function after pulmonary resection. Scand J Thorac Cardiovasc Surg 16:87, 1982

Wasserman K, Jamplis RW, Lash H et al.: Post-pneumonectomy syndrome: surgical correction using Silastic implants. Chest 75:78, 1979

29

SMALL CELL LUNG CANCER

Ronald Feld
Robert J. Ginsberg

HISTORICAL NOTE

Although chemotherapy is the major form of therapy in small cell lung cancer (SCLC) and is discussed in detail, it is often useful to review how therapy evolved to its present approach. Initially surgery was the therapy of choice for patients with all types of lung cancer, but in SCLC, it was abandoned following the results of a randomized trial carried out in the United Kingdom by the Medical Research Council, which compared radiotherapy alone with surgery alone in patients with limited disease (Miller, et al., 1969; Fox, et al., 1973). Even though the mean survival time for all these patients was short (10 months) with only 5 percent of patients alive at 5 years, the fact that all surviving patients were being treated in the radiation therapy arm made this the standard form of therapy from that point on.

Green, et al. (1969) demonstrated the activity of cyclophosphamide against SCLC compared with placebo. They showed that the median survival for patients with extensive disease who were receiving placebo was approximately 6 weeks and for patients with limited disease, only 12 weeks. These data must be remembered when attempting to put into perspective the modest improvements observed in the treatment of this disease during the 1970s, 1980s, and early 1990s.

Many single agents have been tested in patients with SCLC and have shown response rates of 20 percent or more (Feld, et al., 1988). A recent review of all studies from 1970 to 1990 identified 11 active drugs (Grant, et al., 1992). Newer agents were found to be active in recent years, adding more drugs to earlier lists. When active drugs were combined, an improved response rate was observed with complete response rates ranging from 20 to 50 percent and rising even higher in patients with limited disease (Minna, et al., 1989). Retrospective reviews of the median survival of patients treated with either single agents or combination chemotherapy showed that those receiving combinations survived longer. Randomized trials comparing single agents with combination chemotherapy with or without chest irradiation have demonstrated a benefit for the combinations.

Bergsagel, et al. (1972) showed that the addition of cyclophosphamide to standard thoracic irradiation in patients with limited disease resulted in a survival benefit. This was confirmed by others and led to the use of combined modality therapy in the early 1970s (Smyth, 1984). Most frequently, thoracic irradiation is added to combination chemotherapy in patients with limited disease, but it is not usually given to patients with extensive disease. Some groups are now adding thoracic irradiation in patients with extensive disease who achieve a complete response.

When it was noted that a large number of patients had relapses in the central nervous system, prophylactic cranial irradiation (PCI) was tested in randomized trials and showed a reduced failure rate in the brain without any survival advantage (Feld, et al., 1988). Subsequently, it became standard to add PCI routinely for all patients with SCLC, regardless of stage. In the 1980s, signs of neurologic toxicity associated with either the radiation therapy or the combined treatment (radiotherapy and chemotherapy) were noted, and more stringent criteria for the use of PCI have been advocated since that time. In particular, it has been recommended that PCI should be limited to patients who have shown a complete response because they are the most likely to benefit. In this subpopulation, the potential disadvantage of PCI, that is, central nervous system (CNS) toxicity (not observed in all studies) (Lishner, et al., 1990), is probably worth risking.

Although still controversial in some circles, it would appear that, based on the results of a metanalysis of recent randomized trials (Arriagada, et al., 1991), thoracic irradiation adds to combination chemotherapy in patients with limited SCLC, and this is discussed later. Most centers therefore treat patients who achieve a complete response, and many treat patients who achieve at least a partial response with this therapeutic modality. There are also arguments on how best to give thoracic irradiation. The issues include dose, fractionization, portal size, and at what point the radiation therapy

* We gratefully acknowledge the assistance provided by Anne Burrows Faulkner in the careful preparation of this manuscript.

should be given in reference to the beginning of combination chemotherapy. These questions are discussed in more detail later.

There has also been significant interest in the use of surgery in this disease. Most groups recommend operating on peripheral lesions in early-stage disease (stages I and II). Often these patients receive thoracic irradiation and possibly PCI with or without chemotherapy along with their surgery. In patients with more advanced disease, the only well-designed randomized trial carried out by the Lung Cancer Study Group did not, unfortunately show a benefit from the addition of surgery to radiation and chemotherapy (Lad, et al., 1991a). Consequently, this is not a standard approach, although some centers around the world still use it as part of their therapy in selected patients.

In general, immunotherapy (biologic responsive modifiers) have not shown any major benefit in this disease. One study using thymosin fraction V (Cohen, et al., 19779) did show a survival benefit, but this was not confirmed (Shank, et al., 1983). More recently a study by Mattson, et al. (1991) from Finland suggested a benefit to maintenance therapy with interferon-α in patients responding to standard therapeutic modalities. Cooperative groups in the United States have attempted to confirm this information, but the final analysis of these data is not yet available. At the present time, this form of therapy should not be considered standard.

HISTORICAL READINGS

Albain KS, Crowley JJ, LeBlanc M et al: Determinants of improved outcome in small-cell lung cancer: an analysis of the 2,580-patient Southwest Oncology Group data base. J Clin Oncol 8:1563, 1990

Arriagada R, Pignon JP, LeChevalier TL: Thoracic radiotherapy in small cell lung cancer: rationale for timing and fractionation. Lung Cancer 5:237, 1989

Campling B, Quirt IC, DeBoer G et al: Is bone marrow examination in small-cell lung cancer really necessary? Ann Intern Med 105:508, 1986

Carney DN: The biology of lung cancer. Curr Opin Oncol 4:292, 1992

Crawford J, Ozer H, Stoller R et al: Reduction by granulocyte colony-stimulating factor of fever and neutropenia induced by chemotherapy in patients with small-cell lung cancer. N Engl J Med 325:164, 1991

Ettinger DS: Evaluation of new drugs in untreated patients with small-cell lung cancer: its time has come. J Clin Oncol 8:390, 1990

Feld R: Late complications associated with the treatment of small-cell lung cancer. Cancer Treat Res 45:301, 1989

Fukuoka M, Furuse K, Saijo N et al: Randomized trial of cyclophosphamide, doxorubicin and vincristine versus cisplatin and etoposide versus alternation of these regimens in small cell lung cancer. J Natl Cancer Inst 83:855, 1991

STAGING

Staging plays a key role in the choice of therapeutic modalities for the treatment of SCLC. Although chemotherapy is the main therapeutic modality used in SCLC, thoracic irradiation or surgery may also be valuable, depending on the stage of the tumor before therapy. The most important reason for staging, however, is its potential effect on prognosis.

As would be expected, less advanced cases of SCLC have better long-term survival rates than more advanced cases. Although in non-SCLC tumor-node-metastasis (TNM) staging with the relatively recent International Union Against Cancer–American Joint Committee on Cancer classification (Mountain, 1986) is used routinely, this has not been found to be the most useful approach for staging patients with SCLC. Most patients with this disease have stage III or IV disease at the time of diagnosis, making the TNM staging system less likely to be predictive of long-term survival. Most therapeutic trials in the treatment of SCLC have used a very simple two-stage system, as originally suggested by the Veterans Administration Lung Cancer Study Group. This divides patients into those with limited and those with extensive disease. Limited disease is defined as a tumor confined to one hemithorax and its regional lymph nodes, including the ipsilateral mediastinal, ipsilateral supraclavicular, and contralateral hilar nodes, and it should all be easily encompassed within a tolerable radiotherapy portal (Zelen, 1973). Ipsilateral pleural effusions, left laryngeal nerve involvement, and superior vena caval obstruction are considered limited; pericardial involvement and bilateral pulmonary involvement are considered extensive because they would require too large a radiotherapy portal. Unfortunately, some confusion occurs when considering how to stage patients with contralateral mediastinal or supraclavicular lymph node metastases and patients with ipsilateral pleural effusions. These are often handled differently by different investigators. A recent consensus report prepared at the International Association for the Study of Lung Cancer Workshop on SCLC in 1989 suggested that limited disease should include patients with disease restricted to one hemithorax with regional lymph node metastases (including hilar, ipsilateral, and contralateral mediastinal, ipsilateral, and contralateral supraclavicular nodes) and with ipsilateral pleural effusions independent of whether cytologic findings are positive or negative (Stahel, et al., 1989). The inclusion of contralateral mediastinal and supraclavicular metastases and ipsilateral pleural metastases in limited disease is recommended because the prognosis of patients with these sites of disease (which includes ipsilateral pleural effusions) is superior to that of patients with distant sites of metastases.

One other variation in staging among investigators results because of the number and type of staging procedures used. If one investigator carries out more exhaustive staging than another does, a higher yield of patients with extensive disease results, but surprisingly, the outcome in both groups of patients (limited and extensive disease) improves, while not affecting the overall survival. This has usually been termed "stage migration" or the "Will Rogers phenomenon" (Pfister, et al., 1990). Although it is virtually impossible to correct for this effect, the clinician must be aware of its possibility when unusually good results are reported.

The two-stage system generally separates patients with different outcomes well. Those with limited disease have a higher objective regression rate, a higher complete response rate, and significantly longer disease-free and long-term survival rates compared with patients who have extensive disease. Patients who achieve complete response in either stage do relatively well.

Staging Procedures for Patients with Small Cell Lung Cancer Not on Clinical Trials

Complete physical examination
Chest radiograph
Routine hematologic tests (CBC, differential, and
   platelet count)
Liver function tests
Alkaline phosphatase (for bony metastases)
Serum electrolytes (looking for low sodium)
Ultrasound or CT abdomen (for liver and adrenals)
Radionuclide bone scan
Skeletal radiographic examinations if bone scan
   not definite
CT or MRI brain (if symptoms)
Bone marrow aspiration and biopsy (only if abnormal
   hematologic results)

Abbreviations: CBC, complete blood count; CT, computed tomography; MRI, magnetic resonance imaging.

The Toronto group has identified a subgroup called "very limited disease." This arose during a retrospective study of 180 patients with limited disease in which the 33 without mediastinal involvement, supraclavicular node involvement, or pleural effusions had a projected 25 percent 5-year survival rate (Shepherd, et al., 1984).

Subgroups may also be important for patients with extensive disease. Patients with single sites of extensive disease have longer survival times than do patients with multiple sites of metastases and in fact are not dissimilar from those with limited disease (Ihde, et al., 1981). Patients with specific sites of involvement, including the liver and brain, do particularly poorly (Ihde, 1985). In most series 50 to 65 percent of patients who turn out to have extensive diseases are to some degree dependent on how exhaustive the staging is at a particular center. The staging procedures that are most appropriate and necessary for patients who are not being treated in clinical trials are shown below. Excessive staging procedures in this setting can be a burden for individual patients and can also unnecessarily increase the cost of medical care. More exhaustive staging is probably indicated only in clinical trials, as shown below. These are similar to that noted in a recent review on staging of patients with SCLC (Stahel, 1991). A recent study suggests that a simpler approach to staging may be as good and cheaper (Richardson, et al., 1991). This requires confirmation.

Areas of Controversy

Intrathoracic Tumors

Although chest radiographs are useful for the evaluation of disease in the lungs, chest wall, and mediastinum, they may still underestimate the extent of disease in these sites. Computed tomographic (CT) scanning of the thorax may be more accurate in detecting tumors within the lung itself, and it is useful for radiation therapy planning, although it probably adds little to the evaluation of the mediastinum, unless the findings are negative (Hirsch, 1989; Lewis, et al., 1990). Enlarged nodes in the mediastinum may not be indicative of tumor and may mislead the investigator into raising the stage of the patient being evaluated. CT scans of the thorax are often extended to include the abdomen, which, of course, may help in defining metastases in the liver or the adrenal glands. Abnormalities in the adrenal glands are not infrequent, but available data have not clearly established that a patient with abnormalities (metastases or adenoma) at this site has a worse outcome than do patients with limited disease. Magnetic resonance imaging (MRI) does not to date show any benefit in patients with SCLC or non-SCLC over CT scanning (Hirsch, 1989). Fiberoptic bronchoscopy is not necessarily beneficial unless surgery is being contemplated. A baseline may be useful if reevaluation is to be considered following a possible response to therapy (Stahel, 1991).

Hepatic Metastases

Hepatic metastases are common in patients with SCLC. Liver function tests alone are not useful unless the results are completely normal, in which case there is rarely evidence for a tumor at this site (Hirsch, 1989). Ultrasound or CT scans of the liver are usually the preferred approaches because both these techniques may also detect adrenal metastases. Some investigators also recommend an ultrasound-guided needle

---

Possible Staging Procedures for Patients with Small Cell Lung Cancer Being Treated in Clinical Trials

CT of thorax (for mediastinum and measurement
   of primary lesion)
Ultrasound or CT of abdomen (for liver and adrenals)
Routine bone marrow aspiration and biopsy
   (? multiple sites)
Liver biopsy (by peritoneoscopy or possibly with
   ultrasound guidance)
Routine CT scans of brain (? MRI)
Total body MRI (including bone marrow)
Fiberoptic bronchoscopy
Mediastinoscopy (rarely necessary)
^{67}Ga scanning of mediastinum
Serum carcinoembryonic antigen level
Serum lactic dehydrogenase level
Neuron-specific enolase (serum and ? cerebrospinal
   fluid)
Serum arginine-vasopressin level
Lumbar puncture for cytologic examination
Growth pattern of tumor cells in culture (i.e., classic
   versus variant)

Abbreviations: CT, computed tomography; MRI, magnetic resonance imaging.

biopsy. The use of peritoneoscopy, with its potential morbidity, to prove involvement of the liver is probably unnecessary in most patients.

Bone Marrow

It has been customary during clinical trials to do bone marrow aspirates and biopsies in patients with SCLC. Usually single iliac crest aspirations and biopsies are carried out, but in some series, this has been done bilaterally. Even more sophisticated techniques increase the likelihood of finding bone marrow involvement by the tumor, for example, using specific monoclonal antibodies in (Stahel, et al., 1985; Berendsen, et al., 1988). The latter approach may be very important for the screening of patients being considered for potential autologous bone marrow transplantation along with intensive chemotherapy but is probably of far less importance for patients who are not undergoing this type of aggressive therapy. Even MRI has been used with early data, suggesting this method may be more sensitive (Carney, et al., 1989).

A more controversial issue is whether bone marrow involvement should be sought or not. Some studies have found very few patients with metastases at this site (less than 10 percent), and even less frequently, it is the only site that classifies the patient as having extensive disease and therefore potentially changes the prognosis (Hirsch, 1989; Campling, et al., 1986). Some investigators found that lactic dehydrogenase (LDH) might also give similar information without a relatively uncomfortable invasive procedure (Hirsch, 1989; Sagman, et al., 1991a). This is still controversial, and consequently for the time being, bone marrow aspirates and biopsies (usually unilateral) continue to remain a part of the standard pretreatment investigation at most academic centers, despite real questions about their value.

Central Nervous System Metastases

Central nervous system metastases occur at presentation in approximately 10 percent of the patients with SCLC but may occur at autopsy in up to 65 percent (Hirsch, 1989; Klastersky, 1990). The standard investigation for this site has been CT scanning, although MRI is probably superior to CT, as it is for most brain abnormalities. The role of positron emission tomographic (PET) scans is as yet unknown (Klastersky, 1990). Carcinomatous meningitis is a rare presenting feature of this disease. When symptoms occur, a sample of cerebrospinal fluid is used to demonstrate malignant cells, usually by cytocentrifugation (Feld, et al., 1988). Nodular filling defects along the root sleeves may be seen by myelography or with MRI of the cord when spinal cord compression is present.

Biomarkers

Many biomarkers have been studied in this disease and are usually measured before, during, and after treatment. Adrenocorticotropic hormone (ACTH), calcitonin, neuron-specific enolase, plasma neurophysins, and antidiuretic hormone have not been clearly useful prognosticators in these patients (Feld, et al., 1988; Hansen, 1990). Pretreatment carcinoembryonic antigen (CEA) levels correlate with the stage of the disease and may actually be an independent prognostic factor (Sculier, et al., 1985). Their disadvantage is that the antigen concentration is only elevated in approximately one-third of patients, thereby making it a less valuable indicator. Pretreatment LDH levels may be a useful prognostic factor, based on a number of recent publications (Sagman, et al., 1991a; Rawson and Peto, 1990; Albain, et al., 1990; Stahel, 1992).

Several groups reported that rising levels of biomarkers sometimes precede clinical evidence of tumor relapse by weeks or months (Feld, et al., 1988; Biran, et al., 1991). Currently, good therapy is usually unavailable for relapses of this disease; therefore, the value of an early knowledge about the relapse of these tumors is questionable. The consensus at the moment is that biomarkers are probably of little value for the pretreatment prognosis or as early evidence of relapse; however, further research is ongoing on the subject. A relatively new biomarker is the C-terminal flanking peptide of human gastrin-releasing peptide (Holst, et al., 1989), which may indicate a worse prognosis, but again, further data are required.

Restaging

This is a definite area of controversy. A retrospective study recently carried out by the National Cancer Institute of Canada found that routine restaging in patients with limited disease who had responded was probably of little value (Feld, 1992b). Although a small survival benefit was demonstrated in a subgroup of patients who had negative rebronchoscopic results compared with those patients with positive ones, the investigators recommended that this approach only be considered in a clinical trial. Economic analysis also supported the concept of not proceeding with restaging. Others still recommend restaging, especially rebronchoscopy (Stahel, et al., 1989; Stahel, 1991).

Prognostic Factors

Prognostic factors may be useful for individual patient prognosis and for proper stratification in clinical trials. The factors that have been documented by most groups as important include the stage of disease (limited versus extensive), performance status, and whether patients have received previous chemotherapy (Stahel, et al., 1989; Ihde, 1971; Stahel, 1991; Rawson, et al., 1990; Albain, et al., 1990). A large number of other prognostic factors have been noted by different investigators (Table 29-1). Female gender has recently become an accepted good prognostic factor by a number of investigators (Stahel, 1992). Consensus is yet to be reached on which factors are the most important; however, the information derived from staging and prognostic factors must be carefully considered when comparing the results of therapy in published articles on clinical trials in this disease. Newer methods, such as recursive partitioning and amalgamation, may be useful, as evidenced by two recent articles (Albain, et al., 1990; Sagman, et al., 1991b).

CHEMOTHERAPY

Single Agents

Chemotherapy is presently the mainstay of therapy for all stages of SCLC. Green, et al. (1969) demonstrated improved survival rates in patients with extensive SCLC after three

Table 29-1. Possible Prognostic Factors for Survival in Treated Patients with Small Cell Lung Cancer

	Effect on Survival	
Prognostic Factors	Positive Effect	Negative Effect
Increasing stage (limited versus extensive)		X
Worsening poorer performance status		X
Weight loss		X
Prior treatment		X
Gender (sex; female patients do better)	X	
Increased number of sites of distant metastases		X
Site of metastases (liver or brain versus others)		X
Site of primary tumor (TNM staging)—smaller	X	
Age >70 years		X
Mediastinal involvement (TNM staging)		X
Increased serum CEA, LDH, neuron-specific enolase levels		X
Histologic subtypes intermediate versus other		? X
Hypouricemia		X
Alkaline phosphatase		X
Hypoalbuminemia		X
Immune defects		X
Classic growth pattern (versus variant)	X	
Pericardial involvement		X

Abbreviations: CEA, carcinoembryonic antigen; LDH, lactic dehydrogenase; TNM, tumor-node-metastasis.

courses of cyclophosphamide compared with placebo. Since that time, many active drugs have been identified. A partial list of the most active single agents in SCLC is shown in Table 29-2. The most frequently used include etoposide, cisplatin, cyclophosphamide, doxorubicin, and vincristine. New agents that look promising include gemcitabine and paclitaxel and its derivatives.

Single-agent chemotherapy produces objective responses but rarely complete regression, even in previously untreated

Table 29-2. Established Active Single Agents in the Treatment of Small Cell Lung Cancer

Active Single Agents	Approximate Single-Agent Activity (%)
Carmustine	20
Carboplatin[a]	40
Lomustine	15
Cisplatin[a]	15
Cyclophosphamide[a]	40
Doxorubicin[a]	30
Epirubicin (high dose)	50
Etoposide intravenous[a]	40–50
Etoposide oral[a]	50
Hexamethylmelamine	30
Ifosfamide	40–50
Methotrexate	35
Nitrogen mustard	35
Teniposide	40–50
Vincristine[a]	35
Vindesine	30

[a] Agents most commonly used today.

patients with SCLC. Based on studies carried out by the National Cancer Institute of Canada and the Eastern Cooperative Oncology Group, it would appear that it is both ethical and appropriate to treat previously untreated patients with extensive SCLC by using an experimental agent (Ettinger, 1990; Evans, et al., 1990). The evaluation should occur early if this is done, and if no response is observed, patients should be switched to an active regimen before their condition is irretrievable. This may be less of a problem when the clinician uses derivatives of known active agents, such as anthracyclines (Blackstein, et al., 1990) and platinum compounds. Both previously mentioned cooperative groups have had experiences with both active and inactive agents and observed reasonable response and survival rates, irrespective of the activity of the new drug. Treating previously treated patients may result in prematurely negative data with potentially useful drugs. A recent review suggesting the use a lower response rate (10 percent) as evidence of activity in previously treated patients may still be a useful approach (Grant, et al., 1992). In addition to the active agents mentioned, a large number of phase II trials have unfortunately found that many agents show little or no activity (Table 29-3) in patients with SCLC (Grant, et al., 1992).

Combination Chemotherapy

Despite partial responses and occasional complete responses, the relatively poor results with single-agent chemotherapy led to attempts at combining these agents in patients with SCLC, as has been done with other malignancies. Just under 20 percent of 753 patients given single-agent chemotherapy had an objective response, and less than 3 percent obtained a complete response in a study carried out by Bunn and

Table 29-3. Activity of Recently Tested Single Agents in Small Cell Lung Cancer

Active Agents[a]	Possibly Active Agents[b]	Inactive Agents[c]
Epirubicin (high dose)	Iproplatin	Mitoguazone
Carboplatin	Gemcitabine	Mitomycin C
Hexamethylmelamine	Lonidamine	Aclarubicin
Ifosfamide	Paclitaxel	Diaziquone
Vindesine		Bisantrene
Teniposide		Cytarabine
		Idarubicin
		Mitoxantrone
		Vinblastine
		PCNU
		Esorubicin

[a] At least 20% single-agent activity.
[b] 10–20% single-agent activity.
[c] < 10% single-agent activity.

Ihde (1981). In contrast among 1,236 patients who received combination chemotherapy, a 70 percent objective response rate was seen, with 31 percent being complete. In addition, those who received combination chemotherapy survived longer than did those who received single agents. A number of randomized trials compared single agents versus combination chemotherapy, with or without chest radiotherapy, and demonstrated a slight benefit from combination chemotherapy in both objective tumor response and median survival (Minna, et al., 1989). Bunn and Ihde (1981) also reviewed the literature regarding the appropriate number of drugs to be included in combinations for this disease. They found that there was no significant difference in the complete response rate or long-term disease-free survival rate when more than three drugs were used in patients with limited disease.

The most commonly used and highly active combinations for the treatment of this disease worldwide are shown in Table 29-4. Although these are among the most common, virtually any combination of the most active agents has been used with reasonable results. It can be expected that any of these regimens should result in response rates in excess of 80 percent (50 to 60 percent complete response) in patients

Table 29-4. Frequently Used Chemotherapeutic Combinations for Small Cell Lung Cancer[b]

Chemotherapeutic Combination	Possible Abbreviation
Cyclophosphamide, Adriamycin (doxorubicin)	CA
Adriamycin (doxorubicin), etoposide (VP-16)	AE
Etoposide (VP-16), cisplatin	V$_P$P
Cyclophosphamide, Adriamycin (doxorubicin) Vincristine etoposide [VP-16])	CAVE
Cyclophosphamide, Adriamycin (doxorubicin), vincristine	CAV
Etoposide (VP-16), carboplatin	V$_P$CP[a]
Ifosfamide, cisplatin (Etoposide (VP-16))	ICE (VIP)
Cisplatin, vincristine (Oncovin), doxorubicin, etoposide	CODE[a]

[a] Recently found to be active in several studies and will probably increase in popularity in the near future.
[b] All regimens give response rates of 70–90% in patients with limited disease and 55–75% in patients with extensive disease.

with limited disease and 65 to 70 percent in patients with extensive disease (10 to 20 percent complete response) (Feld, et al., 1988). If adequate staging procedures are done, the median survival for patients with limited disease should be 12 to 15 months or more. In recent trials of combined modality therapy, median survival times in excess of 18 to 20 months occurred (Murray, et al., 1991a; Johnson, 1990; Johnson, et al., 1991; Tourani, et al., 1991). Unfortunately the median survival time for patients with extensive disease is still approximately 10 months or less, with a range of 8 to 12 months (Ihde, et al., 1991; Kristjansen, 1991). Approximately 15 to 20 percent of patients with limited disease and less than 5 percent of those with extensive disease remain disease free for more than 2 years. Those patients who achieve a complete response usually live longer than do those who show only a partial response, the former being the only group with the potential for long-term disease-free survival. Patients with limited disease usually live significantly longer than do those with extensive disease, as do patients who have a better performance status at presentation.

Intensity of Chemotherapy

Cohen, et al. (1977) showed that, when comparing low-dose intensive induction therapy consisting of cyclophosphamide, CCNU (lomustine), and methotrexate (CCM), the more intensive therapy resulted in a higher response rate and a longer median survival. In a review of nonrandomized trials by Morstyn, et al. (1984), there was a suggestion of benefit for more intense regimens, but this was a relatively minor increment. Despite being retrospective, the review did not show a major improvement in survival. In fact the more intensive regimens often increased toxicity. An Eastern Cooperative Oncology Group study confirmed that, using cyclophosphamide, methotrexate, and etoposide without dosage reductions for myelosuppression, showed results to be similar to those of other series but with both increased hematologic and pulmonary toxicity (Bonomi, et al., 1985). An attempt at testing both intensity and the more recent "dose intensity," as it is frequently called by the Canadian investigator Hrynuik, et al. from the Hamilton Cancer Centre, was recently completed and reported by Ihde, et al. (1991). They compared the outcome in patients with either low- or high-dose etoposide and cisplatin and unfortunately found no benefits for the high-dose regimen. They did find an increase of toxicity. Attempts at using autologous bone marrow transplantation along with very high doses of agents, such as cyclophosphamide or combinations, gave results similar to those achieved with standard dose combination chemotherapy (Souhami, et al., 1982; Souhami, 1985). This might be the result of the emergence of early drug-resistant clones of SCLC.

In summary, it can be stated that moderate-dose therapy using presently available drugs is necessary to achieve a response and reasonable survival in patients with SCLC. Although there seems to be a dose-response curve for some drugs (e.g., cyclophosphamide) with this disease, administering very high doses of the most active drugs does not seem to be beneficial. The issue of dose intensity has been addressed in a number of tumors, and to date, no prospective trials have shown a clear benefit for a more dose-intensive approach, although retrospective studies have certainly shown a benefit for this approach (Hryniuk, et al., 1987).

Different pharmacologic approaches with known active drugs may be exemplified by the recent interest in the use of relatively low-dose oral etoposide on a continuous 14- or 21-day schedule with approximately 1 week off and then restarting this therapy. This was pioneered by Johnson and Greco from Nashville (Johnson, 1990; Johnson, et al., 1991), Einhorn, et al. (1990) from Indiana University, and Clark, et al. (1990, 1991) from the United Kingdom. The toxicity in previously untreated patients seems tolerable and makes this a reasonable approach in elderly patients in whom an aggressive approach with a more standard regimen is contraindicated or refused by the patient (Carney, et al., 1990). In addition, there are instances of responses in patients who received previous injectable etoposide and who have either responded in the past or not responded at all. This information suggests we have a lot of work to do to learn how to use presently available drugs properly. In addition to looking at new agents, oral etoposide was combined with cisplatin and carboplatin, but preliminary data do not suggest a major benefit over the oral etoposide alone by continuous daily treatment (Murphy, et al., 1991; Evans, et al., 1991).

One of the reasons that intensive therapy has not been extensively studied is because of the severe myelosuppression associated with aggressive approaches to this disease. With the availability of colony-stimulating factors (granulocyte [G-CSF] and granulocyte-macrophage [GM-CSF]), studies have been carried out to see if this approach might also be useful in patients with SCLC and allow for greater dose escalation and possibly improved results. A landmark study in patients with extensive SCLC, which allowed Food and Drug Administration approval of G-CSF (Amgen) in the United States, compared the regimen CAE (cyclophosphamide, Adriamycin [doxorubicin], and etoposide), a seldomly used combination in the 1990s, with or without G-CSF. The study documented the biologic effects of the growth factor, with a marked reduction in febrile episodes, patient days in the hospital, granulocytopenia, etc., and no negative effect on survival (Crawford, et al., 1991). An almost identical study was carried out by a European group and reported in abstract form, showing virtually identical results (Green, et al., 1991). Studies are ongoing with GM-CSF but at present are not yet as optimistic as the data observed with G-CSF (Bishop, et al., 1991; Anderson, et al., 1991a).

The issue of whether this is an advance in the treatment of SCLC can certainly be questioned. The survival in the various studies that show a clear biologic effect of the growth factor is not any better than those achieved by far less toxic regimens currently available to all practitioners in the community. These regimens include alternating cyclophosphamide, doxorubicin, and vincristine with etoposide and cisplatin or just etoposide and cisplatin, to name but two. To establish real value for these new growth factors in this disease, studies must either demonstrate a major reduction in toxicity by using a standard regimen with or without growth factors, or when testing a much more dose-intensive regimen compared with a non-dose-intensive regimen with growth factors used along with the dose-intensive regimen, they must

end up by reducing the likelihood of serious toxicity and improving survival. As previously mentioned, without growth factors, etoposide and cisplastin used in a more dose-intense way was not superior (Ihde, et al., 1991). One wonders whether most of the benefits of febrile episode reduction and decreased days in the hospital can be achieved by using only oral prophylactic antibiotics, such as cotrimoxazole or a fluoroquinolone antibiotic. Unfortunately, further studies need to be done to address these issues. As previously mentioned, standard-dose regimens without growth factor would still seem to be reasonable for community-based physicians to use in their practice.

Late Intensification Therapy

Based on data acquired from patients with acute leukemia, it has been assumed that more aggressive therapy might be better tolerated when patients were in remission than when a large tumor burden was present (Thomas, et al., 1979). Therapy at that point (after an initial response) might include the same agents used for induction or totally different chemotherapy. Although a number of studies have been done looking at this approach in this disease, the results are not strikingly different from those obtained in trials using conventional doses of chemotherapy along with thoracic irradiation where appropriate in patients with SCLC. A Belgian study is more optimistic (Prignot, et al., 1985). Patients were randomized in this study at week 18 to receive late intensification therapy or not. The 2-year survival rate with intensification was 17 percent and only 4 percent without it, although the overall survival from the time of randomization was not significantly improved. A review of other studies on this subject was less optimistic (Feld, et al., 1988). It is interesting that, in many of these studies, most patients are not eligible for randomization (at least if patients with extensive disease are included in sufficient numbers) because they must achieve complete response even to be considered for this approach. Even in limited disease, in most studies less than one-half of the patients achieve a complete response. The major difficulties with this approach may be the large tumor burden present in patients with SCLC, even after initial induction therapy. It may also be caused by the relative ineffectiveness of the agents currently used, the relative unimportance of high doses of moderately active agents, and the possible infusion of tumor cells when autologous marrow is used, even when the best purging approaches are employed.

Alternating Non-Cross-Resistant Chemotherapy

Tumor resistance to chemotherapy is probably a significant cause of therapeutic failure in SCLC (Goldie and Coldman 1984). This resistance may be present at the start of therapy or it may be acquired during it. During the 1980s, the Goldie-Coldman hypothesis, which is an approach to early resistance, became popular. The authors proposed a mathematic model based on the hypothesis that tumor cell kill displays a logarithmic pattern and tumors continuously develop resistant mutations during therapy. Their assumption was that alternating two combinations of non-cross-resistant drugs early in the course of therapy might decrease the development of drug-resistant clones and increase the chance of cure (Goldie and Coldman, 1984; Goldie, et al., 1982). In their model it was necessary that the combinations tested be truly clinically non-cross-resistant and that both non-cross-resistant combinations be active as initial treatment of the disease being evaluated. Most frequently, the benefit of this approach was noted in the treatment of Hodgkin's disease, in which it appeared that treatment with MOPP (mechlorethamine (nitrogen mustard), vincristine (Oncovin), procarbazine, and prednisone) alternating with ABVD (Adriamycin [doxorubicin], bleomycin, vinblastine, and dactinomycin [DTIC]) was superior to MOPP alone (Bonadonna, 1982). However, there are studies showing that ABVD may be superior to MOPP, which may mean that another explanation for the observation is still necessary (Santoro, et al., 1987). In addition, preliminary data may actually suggest that ABVD is equivalent to alternating MOPP and ABVD (Canellos, 1990) again, emphasizing the difference in the two regimens rather than the superiority of the alternating approach.

Because of the encouraging data in Hodgkin's disease and the availability of many active agents, resulting in possible non-cross-resistant combinations to test, this approach has been used frequently in the treatment of patients with SCLC. A review by Elliott, et al. (1984) pointed out some of the shortfalls in some of the trial designs but also showed that in general there were not a lot of clearly positive studies. A Canadian study compared cyclophosphamide, Adriamycin, vincristine (CAV) alone with alternating CAV and etoposide-cisplatin for a total of six courses in previously untreated patients with extensive SCLC. In this large trial, a 6-week difference in median survival was observed (Evans, et al., 1987) and was believed to be cost effective (Goodwin, et al., 1988). A second study in patients with limited disease carried out across Canada compared three courses of CAV followed by three courses of etoposide and cisplatin with six courses of the alternating regimen. No difference in outcome was found (Feld, et al., 1987). However, it may be difficult to detect the small potential benefit of different approaches to alternating therapy. On the other hand, etoposide and cisplatin may be the superior combination so that no differences could be observed between the two therapeutic arms. Other studies, such as those carried out by the Southeast Cooperative Oncology Group (Roth, et al., 1992) and a Japanese cooperative group (Fukuoka, et al., 1991) do not totally support the concept that alternating combination chemotherapy is superior to standard regimens, although the Japanese study shows a significant survival advantage to alternation in patients with limited disease. A more recent review on this subject (Havemann, 1990) supports the view that there are conflicting results in the literature, but no clear superiority to alternating chemotherapy can be demonstrated.

Some believe that the results from the Canadian study (Evans, et al., 1987) mean that alternating chemotherapy should be standard treatment. Most investigators worldwide think that the alternating approach is reasonable but not necessarily superior to other approaches. Further studies should be done to clarify this issue.

Another Canadian study testing the timing of thoracic irradiation (Murray, et al., 1991a), which was previously alluded to, showed that giving the thoracic irradiation early seemed to result in survival superior to that seen when saving it until the end of therapy. This may also argue for the use of more aggressive therapy early in an attempt to try to avoid resistance.

Another approach came from the pioneering efforts of the Vancouver group. Murray, et al. (1991b) showed that the use of a four-drug intense regimen, such as CODE (cisplatin, vincristine [Oncovin], doxorubicin, and etoposide—the majority of the major active agents) for a short time (9 to 12 weeks) gave apparent superior results in patients with extensive SCLC and also possibly in non-SCLC (Murray, et al., 1989). This includes additional prophylactic supportive agents, such as corticosteroids, oral antifungals, and oral antibiotics. The results to date are promising in SCLC but may in part be caused by selection bias. To address this issue, an intergroup study between the Southwest Oncology Group, Eastern Cooperative Oncology Group, and the National Cancer Institute of Canada has begun to test the CODE regimen against a more standard approach in patients with extensive SCLC. Only when these results are available will it be clear whether this very intense and difficult regimen given over a short period is at least equal, if not superior, to some of the more prolonged and potentially more toxic approaches to this disease. If this regimen is found to be an advance, this should also improve the quality of life of these patients.

Duration

Up to the middle or late 1980s, it was not uncommon to treat patients with chemotherapy for a minimum of 12 to 24 months. More recently there has been more concern about the quality of life of patients receiving such treatments.

A number of retrospective studies, including a large one from Toronto (Feld, et al., 1984), suggested no benefit to prolonged therapy. A very large randomized trial carried out by the European Organization for Research on the Treatment of Cancer (EORTC) Lung Group showed no benefit in survival, at least in patients with limited disease, although there may have been the suggestion of a benefit in patients with extensive disease (Splinter, et al., 1986; Splinter, 1988, 1989). A recent update of a French trial also testing this hypothesis showed a small survival benefit in patients with SCLC maintained on therapy (LeBeau, et al., 1991). Few studies support the use of prolonged therapy in this disease. In addition, a recent update on a United Kingdom's Medical Research Council trial showed no benefit of six courses of therapy over three courses (Girling, 1991).

It appears that at this point four to six courses of chemotherapy for patients who show a complete response should be adequate and that presently available maintenance chemotherapy is not of any additional benefit. It is still unclear whether maintenance with long-term interferon-α will be beneficial or not in this disease, as suggested by the Finnish trial (Mattson, et al., 1991), and therefore until this is confirmed, it should not be part of standard care.

New Drug Development

One of the most important approaches in the treatment of SCLC is the procurement of new active agents for managing the disease and defining better ways of using presently available therapy, as already described with the recent interest in using daily oral etoposide. We reemphasize the concept of using new agents in previously untreated patients. As previously mentioned, this seems to be safe as long as a crossover design is used with early crossover to an established regimen to avoid patients being too ill to receive potentially valuable treatment after waiting too long. Lower response rates are expected in previously treated patients (Grant, et al., 1992).

Although a large number of new agents have become available for testing in this disease, few have appeared promising. High-dose epirubicin was found by a number of groups to be active in both SCLC and non-SCLC (Blackstein, et al., 1990; Meyer, et al., 1982; Banham, et al., 1990; Johnson, 1989; Feld, et al., 1992a; Eckhardt, et al., 1990; Wils, et al., 1990). It probably should replace doxorubicin in SCLC. Although not used routinely, carboplatin has been established as an active agent in this disease (Grant, et al., 1992; Johnson, 1989; Thatcher and Lind, 1990). It is unclear whether it is as active as cisplatin, but certainly it is a reasonable alternative to prevent or reduce neurotoxicity and nephrotoxicity in selected patients at high risk (e. g., patients with pre-existing kidney or hearing problems). Ifosfamide is also active in SCLC (Johnson, 1989, 1990), but its superiority to cyclophosphamide has not yet been proved. Expense, the required use of mesna, and its usual requirement for administration in a hospital all make it a somewhat more difficult agent to use in SCLC than are most of the other available active agents. The only other agents that look promising at this stage of development are gemcitabine and paclitaxel (taxol) and perhaps its derivatives. Gemcitabine appears to be active in non-SCLC (Anderson, et al., 1991b; Lund, et al., 1991). In preliminary as yet unreported data, both agents appear active in SCLC, but larger phase II trials are required to determine their relative activity compared with other available agents. Derivatives of paclitaxel are also likely to be tested in the near future and are likely to be active. No other obvious chemotherapeutic agents are on the horizon for this disease. Agents that attempt to bypass established drugs resistance, such as verapamil, have to date not been proved to be helpful in patients with SCLC (Figueredo, et al., 1990; Milroy, et al., 1991). A correlation of in vitro drug sensitivity with potentially active agents may turn out to be useful. Preliminary data from the National Cancer Institute are not overly encouraging but show that this approach is feasible (Gazdar, et al., 1990a).

RADIATION THERAPY

Although it was hoped that chemotherapy would be adequate to control this disease, patients with SCLC frequently relapse first in the thorax. In initial trials it was hoped that thoracic irradiation in patients with limited disease would reduce local failure and result in improved median and long-term disease-free overall survival.

As previously mentioned the Medical Research Council Trial carried out in the United Kingdom (Miller, et al., 1969; Fox, et al., 1973) showed that thoracic irradiation was superior to surgery, and as a result, it became the standard therapy. When chemotherapeutic regimens were developed that resulted in significant prolongation of survival, it became unclear as to whether radiation therapy added to the benefi-

cial effects of combination chemotherapy. There was also the potential for additional toxicity as a result of radiotherapy to the thorax, bone marrow, esophagus, and cardiovascular system. A number of randomized trials were carried out in patients with limited disease, comparing combination chemotherapy alone to combination chemotherapy plus radiotherapy. Details of the major trials are shown in Table 29-5 with references and a recent metanalysis carried out by Warde and Payne (1992) and one by Arriagada, et al. (1991), which both show a significant but small survival benefit to combined modality therapy. A detailed discussion of these data is beyond the scope of this chapter.

From these metanalyses, it may be concluded that combining chemotherapy and radiation therapy, using current approaches, only have a modest impact on long-term survival. More aggressive approaches, as exemplified by a trial carried out by the National Cancer Institute (Bunn, et al., 1987), unfortunately resulted in a number of therapy-related deaths, which were sufficient to offset some of the survival advantage of the combined modality regimen that otherwise might not have been seen (Brooks, et al., 1986). In addition to decreased failure in the lung, resulting in a slight prolongation of survival, there is also likely to be an improvement in the quality of life (in patients receiving this modality of therapy). Newer fractionation schemes, particularly multiple daily fractions, as initially piloted by Turrisi (1991), may actually show even more benefit for the addition of radiation therapy to combination chemotherapy in the future. Randomized trials, using more standard fractionation versus multiple daily fractions, are presently ongoing in the United States. The results of these trials are anxiously awaited because they may result in a major improvement in outcome in this serious disease.

Timing, Dose, and Volume of Thoracic Irradiation

Although the Cancer and Leukemia Group B study did not show any clear benefit to early thoracic irradiation (Perry, et al., 1987), a large multicenter Canadian trial carried out by the National Cancer Institute of Canada found an advantage to early thoracic irradiation (Murray, et al., 1991a). This trial used standard alternating chemotherapy with CAV, alternating with etoposide and cisplatin. The thoracic irradiation was either given early (concurrently with the second course of etoposide and cisplatin) or late with the sixth (final) course of chemotherapy and again with etoposide and cisplatin. Thoracic irradiation was given with the cisplatin-containing regimen because it was believed there would not be any enhancement of pulmonary toxicity. The survival results were impressive, with 25 percent 4-year survival rates in the early treatment versus a 15 percent in the late treatment (Murray, et al., 1991). Even more encouraging was the fact that these differences appeared to be getting larger with the passage of time. Obviously this study may need to be confirmed before this approach is adopted as standard therapy, but this appears to be an observation that reflects benefits for early thoracic irradiation in this disease. If multiple daily fractions are superior, such a regimen should probably be tested early in therapy to maximize its possible beneficial effect.

Although a dose-response effect probably exists, a Canadian randomized study comparing 25 versus 37.5 Gy in re-

Table 29-5. Randomized Trials of Thoracic Radiotherapy in Limited Small Cell Lung Carcinoma[a] Treated by Chemotherapy: Design and Results

Author (Year)	Radio-CT Sequence	Chemotherapeutic Regimen	Beginning of RT (Days)[b]	Chest (Gy/fraction)	Radiotherapy	No. Randomized	No. Analyzed	Median Survival Time (Weeks)	2-Year Survival Rates (%)	No. of Lethal Toxicities
Bunn, et al. (1987)	C	CYC, MTX, CCNU alt VCR, ADR, PCB	D1–3	40/15	No	49	49	50	12	4
					Yes					—
Greco, et al. (1986)	C	CYC, ADR, VCR[c]	D1	45/15 split	No	373	210	54	—	—
					Yes			64	—	—
Osterlind, et al. (1986)	C	CYC, VCR, MTX, CCNU	D43	40/10	No	148	76	52	12	0
					Yes		69	44	4	6
Perry et al. (1987)	C	CYC, VCR, VP-16 alt CYC, ADR, VCR	D1 or D64	50/24	No	426	129	102	15	2
					Yes (D1)		125	98	24	3
					Yes (D64)		145	110	30	1
Stevens, et al. (1979)	C	CYC, ADR, VCR alt CYC, MTX	D22	35/10 split	No	18	18	50	—	—
					Yes	14	14	56	—	—
Perez, et al. (1984)	A	CYC, ADR, VCR	D29[d]	40/14 split	No	148	142	49	19	—
					Yes	156	146	60	28	—
Fox, et al. (1980, 1981)	S	CYC, ADR, VCR	D63	40/20	No	44	44	64	—	—
					Yes	40	40	63	—	—
Kies, et al. (1987)	S	VCR, MTX, VP16 alt CYC, ADR, VCR	D85+	48/22 split	No	56	53	68	28	0
					Yes	47	40	68	33	2
Nou, et al. (1988)	S	CYC, ADR, VCR, MTX alt CYC, VCR, MTX, CCNU	D77	40/20	No	31	31	64	15	2
					Yes	25	25	67	26	2
Ohnoshi, et al. (1986)	S	CYC, VCR, MTX, PCB alt VP-16, ADR, CCNU	D30	40/20	No	26	26	65	16	0
					Yes	24	24	52	25	2
Souhami, et al. (1984)	S	VCR, ADR alt CYC, MTX	D85[f]	40/20	No	139	73	41	—	2
					Yes		57	46	—	2
Creech, et al. (1988)	S	CYC, CCNU, MTX[e]	D43	50/?	No	243	243	62[g]	—	3
					Yes			75	—	

Abbreviations: CT, chemotherapy; RT, chest radiotherapy; PCI, prophylactic cranial irradiation; C, concurrent chest RT and CT; S, sequential; A, alternating; alt, alternating chemotherapy; CYC, cyclophosphamide; MTX, methotrexate; CCNU, lomustine; VCR, vincristine; ADR, doxorubicin; PCB, procarbazine; VP-16; etoposide.

[a] Only results obtained in patients with limited disease (even if extensive disease patients included in the trial).

[b] D1, beginning of chemotherapy.

[c] Second randomization of patients in CR or PR: intensification CT (etoposide + cisplatin) versus no CT—significant result on survival preliminary report.

[d] In the radiotherapy group, only patient with complete, partial response or with stable disease after chemotherapy were treated by radiotherapy.

[e] In responders to induction chemotherapy: CYC, MTX, CCNU alternating with ADR, VP-16.

[f] In the chemotherapy group, some nonresponders received thoracic RT.

[g] Median survival in responders.

(Adapted from Arriagada R, Pignon JP, LeChevalier TL: Thoracic radiotherapy in small cell lung cancer: rationale for timing and fractionation. Lung Cancer 5:237, 1989, with permission.)

Table 29-6. Randomized Prophylactic Cranial Irradiation Trials

Author (Year)	Patients PCI −	Patients PCI +	Stage of Disease	PCI Time/Dose Fraction	CNS Relapse (No./%) −PCI	CNS Relapse (No./%) +PCI	Sole Brain Relapse (No./%) −PCI	Sole Brain Relapse (No./%) +PCI	Systemic Treatment	Observation Time	Survival
Jackson, et al. (1977)	15	14	All	Day 1: 30 Gy/10	4 (27)[a]	0 (0)[a]	NR		VAC or LM	NR	NS
Cox, et al. (1978)	21	24	LD	Day 1: 20 Gy/10	5 (24)[b]	4 (17)[b]	NR		None	NR	NR
Beiler, et al. (1979)	31	24	LD	Week 3: 24 Gy/8	5 (16)[a]	0 (0)[a]	NR		LMCV	NR	NS
Maurer, et al. (1980)	84	79	All	Week 9: 30 Gy/10	15 (18)[a]	3 (4)[a]	NR		C, CVM, CVMx, or CM	NR	NS
Hansen, et al. (1980)	55	54	LD	Week 12: 40 Gy/20	6/20 (30)[b]	4/26 (15)[b]	2 (4)	2 (4)	LMC	> 18 mo.	NS
Eagan, et al. (1981)	15	15	LD	Week 20: 36 Gy/10	11 (73)[a]	2 (13)[a]	NR		CAVED	16 mo.	NS
Katsenis, et al. (1982)	18	17	All	Day 1: 40 Gy/25	8 (44)[a]	2 (12)[a]	NR		CVM, CAM, or LMC	> 10 mo.	NS
Seydel, et al. (1983)	112	107	LD	Day 1: 30 Gy/10	22 (20)[a]	5 (5)[a]	NR		LC (50%)	> 24 mo.	NS
Aroney, et al. (1983)	15	18	All	At CR: 30 Gy/10	4 (27)[b]	0 (0)[b]	NR		ACE/CLVP	NR	NS
Total	366	350			80 (22)	20 (6)					

Abbreviations: NS, not significant; NR, not reported; A, doxorubicin; C, cyclophosphamide; D, cisplatin; E, etoposide; L, lomustine; LD, limited disease; P, procarbazine; V, vincristine

[a] $P < 0.05$.

[b] Not significant.

(Adapted from Kristjansen PEG: The role of cranial irradiation in the managements of patients with SCLC. Lung Cancer 5:148, 1989, with permission.)

sponding patients showed only a modest delay in intrathoracic progression and no overall survival benefit for the higher dose (Coy, et al., 1988). Despite this study most practitioners tend to use higher doses of at least 40 Gy within 3 weeks or higher doses if the fractionation scheme is prolonged over 5 to 6 weeks.

Prophylactic Cranial Irradiation

A large number of randomized trials comparing PCI with no additional treatment have been carried out, and although most of them show a significant reduction in CNS relapse for patients receiving PCI, none shows a survival advantage. A summary of these radiation studies is shown in Table 29-6. Kristjansen (1989) from Cophenhagen recently reviewed this subject extensively.

The clinician must also take into consideration the morbidity of the therapy because acute effects are probably more severe with regimens using larger fractions and those given with concurrent chemotherapy, particularly when they contain an anthracycline. Some studies of PCI show significant toxicities, including a virtual incapacity to carry out the activities of daily living; others do not (Lishner, et al., 1990; Fleck, et al., 1990) produce this effect. As a result it is believed by many that this issue has not been settled, and consequently a large number of trials aimed at testing the value of this therapeutic modality are ongoing internationally. Better measures of toxicity, quality of life, etc. are being measured in many of these studies, and it is hoped that a consensus on the use of this modality will be available in the not too distant future. Most authorities would at this time recommend PCI for patients with limited disease who achieve a complete response; other patients with SCLC would not normally receive this modality of therapy.

Palliation

A major role for radiation therapy in patients with SCLC is palliation of symptoms (Klastersky, 1990). A situation in which radiation therapy is used palliatively includes superior vena caval obstruction. This may be given as the first and only form of therapy, or it may be given after chemotherapy. The latter is more common. In addition, radiation therapy may be used to treat recurrent laryngeal or phrenic nerve palsy, hemoptysis, esophageal compression, pleural effusions, and painful bony lesions. Standard therapy for spinal cord compression is usually radiation therapy, although surgery may be used in selected cases. The use of concomitant steroid therapy has largely supplanted escalating-fraction sizes during therapy. Cerebral metastases are often treated with radiation therapy. Patients with meningeal disease may benefit occasionally from craniospinal irradiation. Other localized masses in unusual sites may benefit from local radiation therapy, either to unblock a hollow organ, such as the ureter, bronchus, etc., or to relieve pain, etc. Appropriate palliative radiotherapy may make a marked difference to the quality of life of these patients when the tumor progresses and a cure is not a reasonable possibility.

SURGERY

As previously suggested in the historical perspective, surgery, once the main form of therapy for this disease until the United Kingdom's Medical Research Council trial changed its place in this disease, remains a controversial and as yet undecided issue despite re-examination of its role over the past 15 years (Miller, et al., 1969; Fox, et al., 1973). Chemotherapy is the present standard therapy for limited-stage SCLC (Livingston, 1986). The Veterans Administration Lung Group recommended that SCLC that presents as a solitary pulmonary nodule be treated by pulmonary resection (Higgins, et al., 1975). This is standard therapy around the world and is often combined with a number of courses of combination chemotherapy with or without thoracic irradiation and PCI (Ginsberg, 1989; Ginsberg and Karrer 1989). It is mainly carried out in patients with peripheral T1N0 lesions found at pathologic review to be SCLC. Reports in the late 1970s and early 1980s demonstrated that surgery alone could provide curative therapy in up to 25 percent of such patients (Mountain, 1978; Shields, et al., 1982). With the addition of postoperative chemotherapy, even better long-term survival in this early stage of disease were reported. In a retrospective analysis of patients receiving postoperative chemotherapy with only stage I disease, especially with a T1N0 disease, there was an up to 80 percent survival rate for more than 5 years (Myer, et al., 1982). Postoperative thoracic irradiation is usually only given in situations in which the lesion is classified as N1. Five-year survival rates in the range of 20 to 30 percent have also been reported in patients with more advanced stages I, II, and IIIa SCLC when the lesions were totally excised and treated with postoperative chemotherapy. Some of these patients do extremely well with just chemotherapy and radiotherapy in this setting (Shepherd, et al., 1984). In fact, this led to a randomized study in patients with limited SCLC by the Lung Cancer Study Group in conjunction with the Eastern Cooperative Oncology Group and EORTC, which compared chemotherapy plus radiation to the chest and brain with and without surgery. Unfortunately, as previously mentioned, the results of this study suggest no benefit to the addition of surgery in that setting (Lad, et al., 1991b, 1991c). In addition, the North American Lung Cancer Study Group recently reported the results of a randomized trial comparing the nonsurgical with the adjuvant surgical approach in limited disease (Bunn, 1991). Although most of the 144 patients randomized were preoperatively staged as having limited (versus very limited) disease, the results of this randomized trial show no difference in either therapeutic arm and no difference when a subset analysis attempted to isolate the very limited group. Other authors confirmed these equivalent results in nonrandomized retrospective analyses. It would probably be impossible for another large-scale trial to be carried out to evaluate this issue critically. There may in fact be a benefit for patients with less disease in the chest. This is especially important because the trial referred to previously included patients with locally advanced disease, which may have skewed the results and may partially account for the negative outcome. However, at present it is not recommended that surgery be used routinely in this group of patients with SCLC. There does not appear to be a role for surgery in preoperatively identified N2 disease, except as part of clinical trials (Myer, et al., 1982); however, it is our opinion that it is still appropriate to investigate adjuvant surgery in a prospective randomized trial confined to this very limited SCLC group.

Another important point is that, although a histologic biopsy or cytologic analysis may demonstrate SCLC in certain cases, this may be inaccurate or there may be mixed cell types. Some patients who have limited disease and do not respond to chemotherapy may still have a non-SCLC tumor that may benefit from surgical resection, even possibly resulting in cure. This is also a major issue to be addressed when there are isolated recurrences more than 18 months to 2 years beyond the original presentation of limited SCLC. Again these may be second primaries and should be totally evaluated for the possibility of curative resection.

The role of surgery in multimodality therapy to improve the control of the primary site was investigated more recently by using induction chemotherapy prior to surgical resection. These programs also included consolidation chemotherapy and mediastinal radiotherapy with or without PCI.

The final role that has been suggested for surgery in the treatment of SCLC is that of salvage therapy when primary chemoirradiation does not control the local disease or when there are recurrences and only the primary site is affected. In this instances surgical therapy after reinduction chemotherapy has been used as a salvage procedure.

Primary Surgery

SCLC that has been resected, usually without prior knowledge of the cell type, results in significant 5-year survival rates in completely resected patients. The most recent series reporting their data suggest that postoperative chemotherapy is a necessary part of treatment (Table 29-7). In most centers, following surgical resection, a minimum of five to six courses of an adequate two- or three-drug regimen chemotherapy is

advised. If hilar and mediastinal lymph node disease is found at the time of surgery, postoperative mediastinal irradiation is also advised. The role of PCI is yet to be decided.

It is difficult to compare this multimodality surgical approach to chemoradiation alone because medical oncologists on the whole do not classify these very limited tumors as a separate entity (Shepherd, et al., 1984); however, some retrospective analyses have been performed despite this. Osterlind, et al. (1985), in their retrospective analysis, did not demonstrate any beneficial effect for surgical resection. On the other hand, Shepherd, et al. suggested a twofold improvement in survival by using surgery as part of therapy and by improving control of the primary site (Salzer, et al., 1990a).

Induction Chemotherapy plus Adjuvant Surgery

The role of surgery in more proximal tumors with clinical N1 or minimal N2 disease (but still resectable by non-SCLC critera) is less apparent. Few induction chemotherapeutic trials have been reported. The experience of the Toronto Group (Shepherd, et al., 1989) and the Innsbruck Group (Salzer, et al., 1990) suggest that, with this combined modality therapy using surgery as an adjuvant, 5-year survival rates in the range of 40 percent can be obtained (Table 29-8). Those tumors with good responses to chemotherapy that were downstaged by the time of surgery to the N0 level have as high as a 60 to 70 percent 5-year survival rate. Persisting nodal disease yields a less satisfactory 20 to 30 percent 5-year survival rate. An interesting sidelight of such therapy is the fact that many of the resected tumors contain no remaining SCLC, but they do contain persisting elements of non-SCLC.

Salvage Surgery

The Toronto Group promulgated the concept of salvage surgery for SCLC persisting in the primary site after induction treatment or recurring only in the primary site following a complete response. In both instances, mediastinoscopy is used to eliminate patients with unresectable disease (Shepherd, et al., 1991). Although this salvage type of operation has led to only a handful of long-term survivors, it is rare for reinduction chemotherapy and radiotherapy in locally recurrent or persistent disease even results in long-term disease-free survival.

Table 29-7. Results of Primary Surgery for Small Cell Lung Cancer

Authors (Year)	No. Patients	Mean Survival Time (mo.)	5-Year Survival Rates (%)
Surgery + chemotherapy			
Karrer and Shields (1991)	183	26	45
Shepherd, et al. (1991)	79	21	40
Ohta, et al. (1986)	25		31
Osterlind, et al. (1989)	52		23[a]
Surgery ± chemotherapy			
Merkle, et al. (1986)	170		18
Maassen and Greschuchna (1986)	124		20[a]
Surgery			
Sorensen, et al. (1986)	76		12
Miyazawa, et al. (1986)	25		8

[a] 3-year survival rate.

Table 29-8. Induction Chemotherapy Followed by Surgery for Small Cell Lung Cancer: the Toronto Results

Stage	No. Patients	Mean Survival Time (Years)	Estimated 5-Year Survival Rate
Overall	38	1.8	38%
N0	11	Not reached	45%
N1	13	1.3	30%
N2	14	1	40%

BIOLOGIC RESPONSE MODIFIERS

As Induction Therapy

In general a large number of agents, including bacillus Calmette-Guérin (BCG) or the methanol extraction residue of BCG and *Corynebacterium parvum* have been tested in all types of lung cancer, with no really clear evidence that they are beneficial (Shank and Sher, 1985). The only promising study, as previously mentioned, is from the U.S. National Cancer Institute, where a randomized trial using thymosin fraction V was carried out (Cohen, et al., 1979). A significant increase in survival was noted with the highest dose (60 mg/m²) but has not been confirmed (Shank, et al., 1983). Woll and Rozengurt (1989) recently reviewed the literature on this subject.

Antibodies directed against bombesin (a gastrinlike peptide hormone) were evaluated in phase I studies. Further work is being done with this approach, as recently reviewed by Carney (Carney, 1991, 1992), but so far, these antibodies are not clinically useful. Interferons, interleukins, etc., have not been found to be useful as therapy in lung cancer; therefore, to date, we can say that biologic responsive modifiers on their own have no place in the standard induction therapy of patients with SCLC. Future agents to be studied could be useful, but only time will tell.

As Maintenance Therapy

As previously mentioned, the only significantly positive study using maintenance therapy is the one by Mattson, et al. (1991) from Finland, who seemed to show a survival advantage with long-term interferon-α maintenance. This study was repeated by the Southwest Oncology Group, but the data are not yet available. The use of interferon-γ was tested by the North Central Oncology Group, but the data from this study are still unpublished.

In Combination with Other Therapies

The best example of using biologic response modifiers in combination with other therapy is using growth factors, such as G-CSF and GM-CSF. These were mentioned in detail in the previous section. In summary G-CSF seems to reduce myelosuppression, febrile episodes, and days of hospitalization, but to date, it has not been shown to have any survival benefit. GM-CSF may also do this, but it has a lot of other inherent toxicities, including the possibility of enhanced thrombocytopenia. In fact thrombocytopenia not dealt with by either G-CSF or GM-CSF may present serious difficulties. If the clinician wants to use myelosuppressive therapy, the dose-limiting hematologic toxicity will in fact be thrombocytopenia rather than granulocytopenia, as is the case when the presently available CSF preparations are used. New growth factors, alone or in combination, may be able to get around this problem in the future; however, it can be stated that in 1992 CSFs are not a required part of therapy in patients with SCLC treated with moderate-dose chemotherapy.

Another interesting concept that to date has only been tested in non-SCLC is looking at chemotherapy plus biologic response modifiers, such as cisplatin and interferon-α. A combination of cisplatin and interferon-α was shown to be active in a pilot study by Smyth, et al. (1990) in patients with non-SCLC and extensive disease. Similar results were observed in approximately 100 patients treated by an international cooperative group funded by Hoffman-LaRoche (Holdener E, personal communication, 1992). Randomized trials have yet to be presented or published regarding the clear value of interferon-α in this setting; however, this general principle requires further testing because it seems to have had a benefit in combination with 5-fluorouracil, with or without leucovorin, in patients with colon cancer (Wadler, et al., 1989, 1991). Whether this approach will be useful in SCLC has yet to be determined. Another potential use for one type of biologic response modifier (monoclonal antibodies to SCLC antigens) may be in the detection of these tumors. Imaging techniques are already available and look promising. The same monoclonal antibodies may be useful as possible therapeutic interventions in the future, as discussed in a recent review by Stahel (1992), but clinical studies are only just beginning.

COMPLICATIONS OF CHEMOTHERAPY IN SMALL CELL AND NON-SMALL CELL LUNG CANCER

Early Complications

All modalities of therapy can result in significant individual toxicities. Those associated with individual modalities of therapy are shown in Table 29-9, and these are divided into those that occur early following treatment and those that occur late. These must always be considered when offering such treatment to patients who have SCLC and should be discussed with the patient in detail. A detailed description of these problems is beyond the scope of this chapter but can be found elsewhere (Feld, 1981, 1990, 1992a; Feld, et al., 1989). Although these data come from studies in patients with SCLC; similar complications would be expected with non-SCLC.

Of importance is that new approaches and supportive care may offset many of these toxicities. For example, nausea and vomiting is a frequent and serious problem in patients with SCLC because cisplatin is a frequently used agent, along with other agents that cause moderate emesis. The use of dexamethasone in combination with serotonin antagonists, as exemplified by ondansetron and granisetron, has improved this situation substantially (Aaproms, 1991). Early nausea is virtually eliminated, although delayed-onset nausea is still a potential problem in some patients.

Myelosuppression with its potential for infection has been a serious problem in the treatment of SCLC. As previously discussed a common regimen used in the 1980s was CAE. This resulted in severe and prolonged myelosuppression, leading to as high as a 40 to 50 percent admission rate for febrile neutropenia for these patients. Therapeutic results were reasonable, but the complication rate was probably unacceptable. This regimen was supplanted by regimens, such as etoposide and cisplatin, which have less than 5 percent admission rates for this complication. Another approach to this problem was the use of growth factors, particularly G-CSF, to reduce the degree and length of neutropenia, hence

Table 29-9. Early and Possible Late Toxicities in Patients with Small Cell Lung Cancer

Therapy	Early Toxicities	Possible Late Toxicities

Chemotherapy	Nausea and vomiting
	Alopecia
	Peripheral neuropathy
	Myelosuppression with possible resulting
	bleeding (cisplatin)
	Anemia
	Constipation
	Electrolyte disturbances
	Cardiotoxicity
	Nephro- and ototoxicity
	Hemorrhagic cystitis
	Mucositis
	Hypo- or hypertension (etoposide)
	Bronchoesophageal fistulae
		Unusual infections (e.g., herpes zoster)
		Anthracycline-induced cardiomyopathy
		Pulmonary fibrosis
		Central nervous system toxicity (especially in conjunction
		with prophylactic cranial irradiation)
		Second malignancies:
		    Second lung primaries
		    Other solid tumors
		    Acute leukemia

Radiotherapy Thoracic	Esophagitis ± stricture Pneumonitis Cardiac toxicity	Pulmonary fibrosis Late cardiac effects Myelitis ? Predisposition to second primary
Cranial	Erythema of the scalp Otitis externa Prolongation of chemotherapy-induced myelosuppression	Somnolence, confusion, problems with concentration, and memory deficits Tremor, dysarthria, slurred speech, and ataxia Frank dementia
Surgery	Immediate postoperative problems (can be fatal) Pain at thoracotomy incision site Bronchopleural fistulae	Continued long-term pain at incision site Bronchopleural fistulae Respiratory failure secondary to removal of functioning lung

reducing the infection and hospitalization rate. In addition, patients in the hospital are discharged sooner. A landmark study discussed previously was carried out with the previously mentioned regimen (CAE) compared with the same regimen with G-CSF. The addition of the CSF substantially reduced the myelosuppressive and subsequent infectious complications (Crawford, et al., 1991), and this result was confirmed in a similarly designed European study (Green, et al., 1991). This is a costly approach to dealing with this problem. The other options include less myelosuppressive but equally effective chemotherapy, as previously suggested, or possibly using oral prophylactic antibiotics, such as cotrimoxazole or various marketed fluoroquinolones.

Cardiotoxicity can usually be avoided by the use of less cardiotoxic anthracyclines, such as epirubicin, which is active in both SCLC (Blackstein, et al., 1990; Eckhardt, et al., 1990) and non-SCLC (Feld, et al., 1992). In addition, the use of only four to six courses of therapy, which is now standard throughout the world, reduces the frequency of this problem and many of the other side effects, thereby improving the quality of life of these patients. The use of mesna, especially when combined with ifosfamide, has virtually eliminated the problem of hemorrhagic cystitis associated with this agent (Johnson, 1990). It also can be used with high-dose cyclophosphamide to avoid this complication. If nephrotoxicity, ototoxicity, or emesis is a problem, the cisplatin-containing regimen can be switched to one with carboplatin. This usually either prevents or stabilizes these side effects but will of course cause more myelosuppression. Carboplatin is also far more expensive and possibly less active in this disease (Green, et al., 1992).

Peripheral neuropathy remains a frequent problem. Of particular concern is the late-onset neuropathy associated with cisplatin. This can come on even a few months after the final course of cisplatin and can be disabling. New approaches to this problem are needed.

Modern radiotherapy planning despite higher doses can usually avoid many of the complications of this treatment. Radiation myelitis can occur in 1 to 5 percent of patients within 5 years after a spinal cord dose of 50 Gy in 25 fractions over 5 weeks (Rubin and Casarett 1972). Because large fractions may increase this risk, an increased number of smaller fractions is frequently used.

PCI is frequently used in patients with SCLC, although it is not usually used in patients with non-SCLC. It is controversial whether long-term toxicities are a serious and common problem. The Toronto experience of PCI in SCLC was relatively positive, with a low incidence of significant abnormalities, which were similar to those in patients who do not receive PCI (Lishner, et al., 1990). The same issue of the *Journal of Clinical Oncology* contains a study from Indiana University with serious long-term complications (Fleck, et al., 1990). In an editorial Turrisi (1990) tries to rationalize why this might be and indicates that it may be related to the fractionation schemes used. Large trials are ongoing worldwide, both to test the efficacy and the toxicity of this modality. The design of these trials is prospective and randomized and should result in definitive answers to both issues in the near future.

Late Complications

Although a large number of late complications of therapy are shown in Table 29-8, the one that is potentially of most concern is the development of second malignancies in potentially cured patients. In patients with SCLC, second lung primaries are relatively frequent complications if patients survive long enough (Sagman, et al., 1992). These may go unnoticed or be assumed to be a relapse of the initial tumor. This may prevent possible surgical removal with the potential for cure. A second primary must always be considered when new lesions are seen in patients, certainly beyond 2 years from diagnosis and even less in some cases. Other solid tumors also occur with reasonable frequency as second primaries, probably partly related to therapy but more likely associated with the patients' age (median, 60+ years). Acute leukemia, fortunately, is a rare event and will become less common with the discontinued use of nitrosoureas and procarbazine for SCLC in recent years and the far shorter duration of treatment. Second lung primaries and even acute leukemia are occasionally seen in patients with non-SCLC but are less of a problem.

FUTURE DIRECTIONS IN THERAPY

Unfortunately there is a paucity of new agents that appear potentially active in these diseases. Two promising drugs that already appear active include gemcitabine and paclitaxel, but published data are not yet available. In addition, there are a number of paclitaxel derivatives that are also likely to be effective. Let us hope that these new agents can be added to our already useful armamentarium. The recent addition of ifosfamide to the list of active agents may be helpful, but its neurotoxicity and its usual requirement for inpatient administration to prevent hemorrhagic cystitis may make it a less desirable agent than are some of the others already in common use (Eberhardt and Niederle, 1992). Because of these inherent problems, real evidence that it is superior to other agents, particularly cyclophosphamide, is needed before it becomes part of standard therapy.

An interesting new development is the better use of established drugs. It has been known for some time that the administration of etoposide over a somewhat prolonged time of 3 to 5 days is superior to single-day administration (Slevin, et al., 1989). As already discussed a number of studies suggested that daily oral etoposide for 14 to 21 days may significantly enhance its activity and possibly even reduce its toxicity. It may be better absorbed at low doses on a chronic basis than when given in high doses orally, as is usually the case at present. This may explain the activity that has been seen in patients who have had previous exposure to etoposide intravenously. It has been sufficiently nontoxic to be used as a single agent in elderly patients in whom less toxicity and improved quality of life are desirable (Carney, et al., 1990). As some have said, if this is the most active single agent when given in this way, combining it with other approaches may be an interesting new approach. In particular, it should probably be combined with cisplatin or carboplatin, although it is likely that other combinations will also be tried. Based on the unusual schedule dependency of this agent, there may even be an argument for multiple daily doses or continuous intravenous infusion.

As already noted, another significant observation was made by the Vancouver group. They used an intense combination for 9 to 12 weeks in patients with extensive SCLC and in patients with extensive non-SCLC (CODE regimen).

This regimen includes cisplatin, vincristine, doxorubicin, and etoposide. Although very toxic and requiring a high performance status population that is easily followed for potential toxicity, excellent results have been seen (Murray, et al., 1989, 1991b). The authors used additional supportive care approaches, including chronic steroid administration, antifungal and antibiotic prophylaxis, and close follow-up, to try to minimize the problems associated with this approach. It seems sufficiently encouraging that an intergroup study in extensive SCLC has been started by the Southwest Oncology Group and the National Cancer Institute of Canada. This trial compares CODE with CAV alternating with etoposide and cisplatin for a total of six courses, and the appropriate supportive care will be given in the experimental therapeutic arm. Only selected patients will be included in the trial to maximize the possibility of showing any benefit.

The use of early radiotherapy with concurrent chemotherapy was superior to late radiotherapy in the limited SCLC study carried out by the National Cancer Institute of Canada (Murray, et al., (1991a).) Some of the new chemotherapeutic agents and combinations discussed above should also be tested in conjunction with concurrent early radiotherapy in future trials, which should evaluate both single and multiple daily fractionation techniques. In both SCLC and non-SCLC, studies should be designed to confirm the European trial, which demonstrated superiority for daily low-dose cisplatin with concurrent radiation (Schaake-Koenig, et al., 1992). Consideration could also be given to the addition of chronic oral etoposide to the regimen to improve the antitumor effects of cisplatin.

The use of biologic response modifiers as maintenance therapy may be useful in both SCLC and non-SCLC. Interferon-α prolonged the survival of responding patients with SCLC in the study reported by the Finnish group (Mattson, et al., 1991). This study was repeated by the Southwest Oncology Group, but data are not yet available to confirm the results of Mattson, et al. Trials are now underway to evaluate the usefulness of adjuvant retinoids after complete resection of non-SCLC. If these trials result in either a prolongation of survival or a reduction in second primary tumors, future trials of retinoids in combination with interferon would be indicated to confirm the synergy for these two agents, which has been seen in vitro. Other possibilities include the use of agents that are antagonistic to antigen receptors on SCLC tumor cells, but these will probably take some time to develop.

The ability of growth factors to permit dose intensification without the need for autologous bone marrow transplantation will certainly be further explored in this disease. Future studies should be designed to identify significant survival benefits associated with dose-intense regimens and should not focus primarily on second end points, such as nadir granulocyte counts or the incidence of fever, as has been the case in most studies to date.

It may also be of interest to combine chemotherapy with biologic response modifiers. Our center explored this in patients with non-SCLC with a combination of cisplatin and interferon-α. The response rate in an international study including about 100 patients is approximately 30 percent. This is much higher than would be expected from the cisplatin alone. We wonder whether the response rate of standard chemotherapeutic regimens can be modified with other biologic agents. Further work in this area is indicated, based on the apparent benefit of adding interferon to 5-fluorouracil in colon cancer, as already noted by Waddler, et al. (1989, 1991). It is also hoped that further studies on the biology of SCLC and non-SCLC will result in major improvements in the 1990s and allow us to escape from the present plateau in advances that occurred during the 1980s.

Toxicity is a frequent problem in patients with lung cancer; however, if all the side effects are considered and appropriate management is initiated to either prevent or treat them, they are usually manageable, taking into account the seriousness of the disease being treated. Short-duration chemotherapy (four to eight courses), proper use of antiemetics, good radiation therapy planning, and rapid hospitalization and therapy for patients with febrile neutropenia or bleeding episodes will all help to alleviate this problem in the future.

COMMENTS AND CONTROVERSIES

Most of the controversies in the diagnosis and treatment of SCLC have already been addressed in some detail. Controversies that still exist in the staging of this disease include how best to stage intrathoracic disease and hepatic disease, whether to do a bone marrow aspirate and/or biopsy and the number of samples to take, and whether to look for asymptomatic meningeal disease. The value of biomarkers in SCLC, although extensively studied, still has advocates and those who believe it is a worthless endeavor. In addition, new biomarkers become available on a regular basis, and each needs to be looked at in turn, both as an initial prognostic factor and an indicator of relapse.

Although we do not routinely restage responding patients with limited SCLC, many centers still do, despite the morbidity and cost to the patient and health care system. We hope this will not be a controversy for much longer.

Prognostic factors in SCLC are still a major area of interest, and many questions exist on how best to use them. Although most investigators agree that some factors, such as stage (limited versus extensive), performance status, and gender, are critical, many of the other factors previously discussed remain controversial.

There are still major disagreements on how best to treat SCLC. Some of the issues include the dose and dose intensity of chemotherapy, the value of thoracic irradiation in limited disease (probably resolved by recent metanalyses), the bene-

fit of PCI irradiation with its potential serious late toxicities, and whether alternating chemotherapeutic combinations are really superior to sequential ones.

The timing, dose, and fractionation schemes for the administration of thoracic irradiation in patients with limited SCLC are the subjects of many ongoing clinical trials. We hope these will define the best ways to use this modality, which now seems to have a survival advantage in patients with SCLC. The place of biologic response modifiers, if any in this disease, needs to be defined.

The role for surgery in SCLC has yet to be clearly defined. There is no doubt that surgeons will continue to operate on peripheral nodules when the diagnosis is uncertain or in question. In addition, until the results of nonsurgical treatment for these peripheral tumors is known, surgery still offers the best hope of permanent cure. Following surgical excisions, postoperative chemotherapy appears to be advantageous.

The exact role of adjuvant surgery for central very limited disease clinically staged as I, II, or IIIa has yet to be fully defined. Certainly, the recent report of the North American Lung Cancer Study Group suggests no difference in survival benefit in those patients treated with the addition of surgery.

R.F.
R.J.G.

KEY REFERENCES

Evans WK, Feld R, Murray N et al: Superiority of alternating non-cross-resistant chemotherapy in extensive small cell lung cancer. A multicenter randomized clinical trial by the National Cancer Institute of Canada. Ann Intern Med 107:451, 1987

This article reports the results of a National Cancer Institute of Canada trial in patients with extensive non-SCLC. There were two arms of therapy: standard CAV or six courses of CAV alternating with etoposide and cisplatin for a total of six cycles. The best response was higher in the patients with alternating chemotherapy, and the progression-free survival time for patients receiving the alternating chemotherapy was significantly longer (median, 6 weeks). In addition, the overall survival was also significantly longer in this therapeutic arm, despite the fact that major toxicities were approximately equal. These results showed a modest superiority of alternating chemotherapy over standard therapy. This article is the basis for making alternating chemotherapy one of the standard approaches in extensive SCLC.

Feld R: Complications in the treatment of small cell carcinoma of the lung. Cancer Treat Rev 8:5, 1981

This article reviews the complications of the treatment of SCLC, primarily early, but some mention of late complications in all studies reported to that time. This is one of the classic articles on this subject. The conclusions were that combining radiation with chemotherapy containing doxorubicin may increase the incidence of esophagitis, radiation-induced pneumonitis, and skin toxicity. In general combined modality therapy is relatively safe, although it caused a slight increase in the frequency of infectious complications compared with chemotherapy alone. Chemotherapy adds significant toxicity to radiation but is a necessary part of therapy. Reporting of toxicity should be a key part of reporting data on studies involving this patient population.

Feld R, Evans WK, Coy P et al: Canadian multicentre randomized trial comparing sequential and alternating administration of two non-cross resistant chemotherapy combinations in patients with limited small cell carcinoma of the lung. J Clin Oncol 5:1401, 1987

This article describes the results of a randomized trial carried out by the National Cancer Institute of Canada comparing the use of alternating CAV with etoposide and cisplatin for six courses with three courses of initial CAV followed by three courses of etoposide and cisplatin in patients with limited disease. In addition, patients were randomized to two doses of thoracic irradiation. The data showed no difference in outcome between the two regimens.

Fox W, Scadding JG: Medical Research Council comparative trial of surgery and radiotherapy for primary treatment of small celled or oat celled carcinoma of the bronchus. Ten year follow-up. Lancet 2:63, 1973

This study reports the 10-year results of a controlled trial of surgery versus a policy of radical radiotherapy in the treatment of SCLC. The analysis included 144 patients with 71 patients allocated at random to surgery and 73 allocated to radiotherapy. There were no 10-year survivors in the surgical series, but on the radiotherapeutic series, 11 remained well. The mean survival for the surgical series was 199 days and the radical radiotherapeutic series was 100 days, which was statistically significant. This reinforced the 5-year report on the same study and became the basis for making radiotherapy standard treatment in this disease at the time of this trial.

Fukuoka M, Furuse K, Saijo N et al: Randomized trial of cyclophosphamide, doxorubicin and vincristine versus cisplatin and etoposide versus alternation of these regimens in small cell lung cancer. J Natl Cancer Inst 82:855, 1991

This article describes the multicenter randomized comparison of CAV alone versus etoposide and cisplatin alone versus an alternating regimen, starting with the CAV regimen. The alternating or the etoposide and cisplatin regimen gave a higher response rate, but the complete response rates were similar. The response duration on the alternating version was significantly longer than that noted with the CAV alone. The survival time was also of borderline significance, but it seemed to be longer with the alternating regimen than with the CAV alone in patients with limited disease. Survival in the alternating therapeutic arm was significantly superior to the CAV arm alone in patients with limited disease, although it was not in those with extensive disease. The authors concluded that alternating chemotherapy was superior to standard chemotherapy.

Gazdar AF, Steinberg SM, Russell EK et al: Correlation of in vitro drug-sensitivity testing results with response to chemotherapy in survival in extensive-stage small cell lung cancer: a perspective clinical trial. J Natl Cancer Inst 82:117, 1990

The article describes the results of a clinical protocol in which specimens were obtained from metastatic sites during routine staging procedures in a group of patients undergoing treatment for proven extensive SCLC. After initial staging procedures including biopsy, patients were treated with etoposide and cisplatin. During the initial 12 weeks of therapy, tumor cells from tumor-containing specimens and in vitro drug sensitivity were carried out. Where possible after 12 weeks, the patients were restaged, and where appropriate tissue was available, post-therapy samples were taken for in vitro sensitivity. If the in vitro drug sensitivity testing data was available, the patients with partial or no response and those who had relapses after complete response to primary therapy were switched to the best in vitro regimen. If these data were not available, an empiric combination of cyclophosphamide, doxorubicin, and vincristine was administered. The authors concluded that the selection of individual chemotherapy is labor intensive but feasible.

Ginsberg RJ: Surgery and small cell lung cancer—an overview. Lung Cancer 5:232, 1989

This article is an overview of the role of surgery in the management of SCLC. It attempts to look at surgery in very early disease and its role after neoadjuvant chemotherapy in patients who do not respond to induction chemotherapy.

Miller AB: Epidemiology, prevention and prognostic factors, and natural history of lung cancer. Curr Opin Oncol 4:286, 1992

This article describes recent data on active and passive smoking, occupational hazards as a causation of lung cancer, and diet and also looks at recent information on prognostic factors. The author concluded that passive smoking remains interesting, although further and larger studies are needed to prove its causation in this disease. However, the most reasonable conclusion remains that passive smoking is dangerous to health. It was believed that LDH is now proved to be a significant prognostic factor and that new markers should be looked for to add to the already known factors.

Perry MC, Eaton WL, Propert KJ et al: Chemotherapy with or without radiation therapy in limited small-cell carcinoma of the lung. N Engl J Med 316:916, 1987

This randomized controlled trial tried to clarify the role for thoracic radiotherapy in patients with limited SCLC. The chemotherapy they gave consisted of cyclophosphamide, etoposide, and vincristine with doxorubicin subsequently replacing etoposide in alternating cycles 7 through 18. Chemotherapy was given every 3 weeks for 18 months. Radiotherapy was either given initially (starting on day 1 of cycle 1), after three initial cycles of chemotherapy, or not at all. There was a significant survival benefit for those receiving radiotherapy but not for the order in which they received it. This is one of the classic articles describing a positive outcome from thoracic irradiation therapy, which proved to be the correct observation based on a metanalysis of many such studies.

Stahel RA: Morphology, surface antigens, staging and prognostic factors of small cell lung cancer. Curr Opin Oncol 4:308, 1992

This article looks at the advances in the field described, based on recent reports. He concludes that the morphologic and biologic properties of SCLC change with chemotherapy toward a non-SCLC and well-differentiated neural endocrine phenotype. This may in part be responsible for drug resistance. He emphasizes that the recent data suggest a benefit to radiating patients with limited disease, and therefore, it becomes important to focus on cost-effective ways of anatomic staging. He recommended that efforts to analyze pretreatment prognostic factors be continued.

Tsai CM, Ihde DC, Kadoyami C et al: Correlation of in vitro sensitivity testing of long-term small cell lung cancer cell lines with response and survival. Eur J Cancer 26:1148, 1990

The authors gave patients four 3-week cycles of etoposide and cisplatin and did in vitro sensitivity testing using the Weisenthal dye exclusion assay on material collected during pretherapy diagnostic staging procedures. The authors found that the in vitro sensitivity of long-term SCLC cell lines predicted the clinical response and survival. They concluded that the use of human tumor cell lines to screen for the in vitro sensitivity of new drugs might be done in a similar manner.

Turrisi AT: Brain irradiation and systemic chemotherapy for small-cell lung cancer: dangerous liaisons? J Clin Oncol 8:196, 1990

This editorial comments on two articles in this specific issue of the journal. One shows significant long-term toxicity from PCI in patients with SCLC and the other shows little compared with a similar aged population who did not receive such treatment. Turrisi attempts to identify reasons for the differences in the two articles. He suggests that the timing of the PCI may be the important variable. He also implicates the difference in the systemic agents used as possible causes of this problem. He concludes that PCI should probably be reserved for selected patients because it does not affect survival and recommends further randomized trials to address this subject.

REFERENCES

Aaproms: 5-HT[3] receptor antagonists—an overview of their present status and future potential in cancer therapy-induced emesis. Drugs 42:551, 1991

Albain KS, Crowley JJ, LeBlanc M et al: Determinants of improved outcome in small-cell lung cancer: an analysis of the 2,580-patient Southwest Oncology Group data base. J Clin Oncol 8:1563, 1990

Anderson H, Gurney H, Thatcher N et al: Recombinant human GM-CSF in small cell lung cancer: a phase I/II study. Recent Results Cancer Res 121:155, 1991a

Anderson H, Lund B, Hansen HH et al: Phase II study of gemcitabine in non small cell lung cancer (NSCLC) (abstr). Proc Am Soc Clin Oncol 10:247, 1991b

Aroney RS, Aisner J, Wesley MN et al: Value of prophylactic cranial irradiation in prevention of central nervous system metastases in small cell lung cancer. Potential benefit restricted to patients with complete response. Cancer Treat Rep 67:675, 1983

Arriagada R, Ihde DC, Johnson DH et al: Meta-analysis of randomized trials evaluating the role of thoracic radiotherapy in limited small cell lung carcinoma (SCLC) (abstr). Presented at the 6th World Conference on Lung Cancer, Melbourne, November 10–14. Lung Cancer 7(suppl):98, 1991

Arriagada R, Pignon JP, Le Chevalier TL: Thoracic radiotherapy in small cell lung cancer: rationale for timing and fractionation. Lung Cancer 5:237, 1989

Banham SW, Henderson AF, Bicknell S et al: High dose epirubicin chemotherapy in untreated poorer prognosis small cell lung cancer. Respir Med 84:241, 1990

Beiler DD, Kane RC, Bernath AM et al: Low dose elective brain irradiation in small cell carcinoma of the lung. Int J Radiat Oncol Biol Phys 5:941, 1979

Berendsen HH, de-Leij L, Postmus PE et al: Detection of small cell lung cancer metastases in bone marrow aspirates using monoclonal antibody directed against neuroendocrine differentiation antigen. J Clin Pathol 41:273, 1988

Bergsagel DE, Jenkin RDT, Pringle JF et al: Lung cancer: clinical trial of radiotherapy alone vs. radiotherapy plus cyclophosphamide. Cancer 30:621, 1972

Biran H, Feld R, Malkin A: Circulating arginine-vasopressin, calcitonin, carcinoembryonic antigen, neuron-specific enolase, and beta-2 microglobulin fluctuations during combined modality induction therapy for small-cell bronchogenic carcinoma. Association of postchemotherapy AVP surge with high tumor response rate and durable remission. Tumour Biol 12:131, 1991

Bishop JF, Morstyn G, Stuart-Harris R et al: Dose and schedule of granulocyte macrophage colony stimulating factor (GM-CSF) carboplatin and etoposide in small cell lung cancer (SCLC) (abstr). Proc Am Soc Clin Oncol 10:240, 1991

Blackstein M, Eisenhauer EA, Wierzbicki R et al: Epirubicin in extensive small-cell lung cancer: a phase II study in previously untreated patients: a National Cancer Institute of Canada Clinical Trials Group Study. J Clin Oncol 8:385, 1990

Bonadonna G: Chemotherapy strategies to improve the control of Hodgkin's disease: the Richard and Hinda Rosenthal Foundation Award Lecture. Cancer Res 42:4309, 1982

Bonomi P, O'Reilly WO, Vogl SE et al: Intensive induction treatment of small cell bronchogenic carcinoma with cyclophosphamide, methotrexate and etoposide. Cancer Treat Rep 69:1007, 1985

Brooks BJ Jr, Seifter EJ, Walsh TE et al: Pulmonary toxicity with combined modality therapy for limited stage small-cell lung cancer. J Clin Oncol 4:200, 1986

Bunn PA, Lichter AS, Makuch RW et al: Chemotherapy alone or chemotherapy with chest radiation therapy in limited stage small-cell lung cancer. Ann Intern Med 106:655, 1987

Bunn PA: Presented as part of a symposium at the 6th World Conference on Lung Cancer, Melbourne, Australia, November 10–14, 1991.

Bunn PA Jr, Ihde DC: Small cell bronchogenic carcinoma: a review of therapeutic results. p. 169. In Livingston BB (ed): Lung Cancer. 1. Boston, Martinus Nijhoff, 1981

Campling B, Quirt IC, DeBoer G et al: Is bone marrow examination in small-cell lung cancer really necessary? Ann Intern Med 105:508, 1986

Canellos GP: Can MOPP be replaced in the treatment of advanced Hodgkin's disease. Semin Oncol 17:2, 1990

Carney D: Lung cancer biology. Curr Opin Oncol 3:288, 1991

Carney DN: The biology of lung cancer. Curr Opin Oncol 4:292, 1992

Carney DN, Grogan L, Smit EF et al: Single-agent oral etoposide for elderly small cell lung cancer patients. Semin Oncol 17, (suppl 2):49, 1990

Carney DN, Redmond O, Harford P et al: Bone marrow involvement (BMI) by small cell lung cancer (SCLC) using magnetic resonance imaging (MRI) (abstr). Proc Am Soc Clin Oncol 9:228, 1989

Clark P, Cottier B, Joel S et al: Two prolonged schedules of single-agent oral etoposide of differing duration and dose in patients with untreated small cell lung cancer (SCLC) (abstr). Proc Am Soc Clin Oncol 10:268, 1991

Clark PI, Cottier B, Joel SP et al: Prolonged administration of single-agent oral etoposide in patients with untreated small cell lung cancer (SCLC) (abstr). Proc Am Soc Clin Oncol 9:226, 1990

Cohen MH, Chretien PB, Ihde DC et al: Thymosin fraction V and intensive combination chemotherapy. Prolonging the survival of patients with small cell lung cancer. JAMA 241:1813, 1979

Cohen MH, Creaven PJ, Fossieck BE Jr et al: Intensive chemotherapy of small cell bronchogenic carcinoma. Cancer Treat Rep 61:349, 1977

Cox JD, Petrovich A, Paig C et al: Prophylactic cranial irradiation in patients with inoperable carcinoma of the lung. Preliminary report of a cooperative trial. Cancer 42:1135, 1978

Coy P, Hodson I, Payne DG et al: The effect of dose of thoracic irradiation on recurrence in patients with limited stage small cell lung cancer. Initial results of a Canadian multicenter randomized trial. Int J Radiat Oncol Bio Phys 14:219, 1988

Crawford J, Ozer H, Stoller R et al: Reduction by granulocyte colony-stimulating factor of fever and neutropenia induced by chemotherapy in patients with small-cell lung cancer. N Engl J Med 325:164, 1991

Creech R, Richter M, Finkelstein D: Combination chemotherapy with or without consolidation radiation therapy (RT) for regional small cell carcinoma of the lung (abstr). Proc Am Soc Clin Oncol 7:196, 1988

Eagen RT, Frytak S, Lee RE et al: A case for preplanned thoracic and prophylactic whole brain irradiation therapy in limited small cell lung cancer. Cancer Clin Trials 4:261, 1981

Eberhardt W, Niederle N: Ifosfamide in non-small cell lung cancer: a review. Semin Oncol 19(suppl 1):40, 1992

Eckhardt S, Kolaric K, Vukas G et al: Phase II study of 4′epi-doxorubicin in patients with untreated extensive small cell lung cancer. Med Oncol Tumor Pharmacother 7:19, 1990

Einhorn LH, Pennington K, McClean J: Phase II trial of daily oral VP-16 in refractory small cell lung cancer: a Hoosier Oncology Group study. Semin Oncol 17(suppl 2):32, 1990

Elliott JA, Osterlind K, Hansen HH: Cyclic alternating "non-cross resistant" chemotherapy in the management of small cell anaplastic carcinoma of the lung. Cancer Treat Rev 11:103, 1984

Ettinger DS: Evaluation of new drugs in untreated patients with small-cell lung cancer: its time has come. J Clin Oncol 8:374, 1990

Evans WK, Eisenhauer EA, Cormier Y et al: Phase II study of amonafide: results of treatment and lessons learned from the study of an investigational agent in previously untreated patients with extensive small-cell lung cancer. J Clin Oncol 8:390, 1990

Evans WK, Feld R, Murray N et al: Superiority of alternating non-cross-resistant chemotherapy in extensive small cell lung cancer. A multicenter randomized clinical trial by the National Cancer Institute of Canada. Ann Lat Med 107:450, 1987

Evans WK, Stewart DJ, Maroun J et al: Oral VP-16 and carboplatin for small cell lung cancer (abstr). Proc Am Soc Clin Oncol 10:247, 1991

Feld R: Lung and mediastinum: editorial overview. Curr Opin Oncol 4:283, 1992a

Feld R: Complications associated with the treatment of small cell lung cancer. Lung Cancer (in press), 1992b.

Feld R: Lung and mediastinum: editorial overview. Curr Opin Oncol 2:309, 1990

Feld R: Late complications associated with the treatment of small-cell lung cancer. Cancer Treat Res 45:301, 1989

Feld R, Evans WK, DeBoer G et al: Combined modality induction therapy without maintenance chemotherapy for small cell carcinoma of the lung. J Clin Oncol 2:294, 1984

Feld R, Ginsberg R, Payne DG: Treatment of small cell lung cancer. p. 229. In Roth JA, Ruckdeschel JC, Weisenburger TH (eds): Thoracic Oncology. WB Saunders, Philadelphia, 1988

Feld R, Wierzbicki R, Walde D et al: Phase I-II study of high dose epirubicin in advanced non-small cell lung cancer. J Clin Oncol 20:297, 1992

Figueredo A, Arnold A, Goodyear M et al: Addition of verapamil and tamoxifen to the initial chemotherapy of small cell lung cancer. A phase I/II study. Cancer 65:1895, 1990

Fleck JF, Einhorn LH, Lauer RC et al: Is prophylactic cranial irradiation indicated in small-cell lung cancer? J Clin Oncol 8:209, 1990

Fox RM, Tattersall MHN, Woods RL: Radiation therapy as an adjuvant in small cell lung cancer treated by combination chemotherapy: a randomized study (abstr). Proc Am Soc Clin Oncol 22:502, 1981

Fox RM, Woods RL, Brodie GN et al: A randomized study: small cell anaplastic lung cancer treated by combination chemotherapy and adjuvant radiotherapy. Int J Radiat Oncol Biol Phys 6:1083, 1980

Ginsberg RJ, Karrer K: Surgery in small cell lung cancer. Lung Cancer 5:139, 1989

Girling DJ: Prospective randomised trial of 3 or 6 courses of etoposide, cyclophosphamide, methotrexate and vincristine and of 6 courses of etoposide and ifosfamide in small cell lung cancer (SCLC) (abstr). For the British Medical Research Council Lung Cancer Working Party. Presented at the 6th World Conference on

Lung Cancer, Melbourne, November 10–14. Lung Cancer 7(suppl):103, 1991

Goldie JH, Coldman AJ: The genetic origin of drug resistance in neoplasms: implications for systemic therapy. Cancer Res 44:3643, 1984

Goldie JH, Coldman AJ, Gudavskas GA: Rationale for the use of alternating non-crossresistant chemotherapy. Cancer Treat Rep 66:439, 1982

Goodwin PJ, Feld R, Evans WK: Cost-effectiveness of cancer chemotherapy: an economic evaluation of a randomized trial in small cell lung cancer. J Clin Oncol 6:1537, 1988

Grant SC, Gralla RJ, Kris MG et al: Single-agent chemotherapy trials in small-cell lung cancer, 1970 to 1990: the case for studies in previously treated patients. J Clin Oncol 10:484, 1992

Greco FA, Perez C, Eihnorn LH et al: Combination chemotherapy with or without concurrent thoracic radiotherapy (RT) in limited-stage (LD) small cell lung cancer (SCLC): a phase III trial of the Southeastern Cancer Study Group (SEG) (abstr). Proc Am Soc Clin Oncol 5:178, 1986

Green JA, Trillet VN, Manegold C: 4-MetHuG-CSf (G-CSF) with CDE chemotherapy (CT) in small cell lung cancer (SCLC): interim results from a randomized, placebo controlled trial (abstr). For the European G-CSF Lung Cancer Study Group. Proc Am Soc Clin Oncol 10:243, 1991

Green RA, Humphrey E, Close H et al: Alkylating agents and bronchogenic carcinoma. Am J Med 46:516, 1969

Hansen HH, Dombornowsky P, Hirsch FR et al: Prophylactic irradiation in bronchogenic small cell anaplastic carcinoma. Cancer 46:279, 1980

Hansen M: Paraneoplastic syndrome and tumor markers for small cell and non-small cell lung cancer. Curr Opin Oncol 2:345, 1990

Havemann MWK: Alternating chemotherapy in small cell lung cancer. Onkologie 13:157, 1990

Higgins GA, Shields TW, Keehn RJ: The solitary pulmonary nodule. Ten-year follow-up of Veterans Administration-Armed Forces Cooperative study. Arch Surg 110:570, 1975

Hirsch F: Staging and prognostic factors: 1. Staging procedures. Lung Cancer 5:152, 1989

Holst JJ, Hansen M, Bork E et al: Elevated plasma concentration of C-flanking gastrin-releasing peptide in small cell lung cancer. J Clin Oncol 7:1831, 1989

Hryniuk WM, Figueredo A, Goodyear M: Applications of dose intensity to problems of chemotherapy of breast and colorectal cancer. Semin Oncol 14:3, 1987

Ihde DC: Staging evaluation and prognostic factors in small cell lung cancer. p. 241. In Aisner J (ed): Lung Cancer. Contemporary Issues in Clinical Oncology. Vol. 3. Churchill Livingstone, New York, 1985

Ihde DC, Makuch RW, Carney DN et al: Prognostic implications of stage of disease and sites of metastases in patients with small cell carcinoma of the lung treated with intensive combination chemotherapy. Am Rev Respir Dis 123:500, 1981

Ihde DC, Mulshine J, Kramer B et al: Randomized trial of high vs. standard dose etoposide (VP16) and cisplatin in extensive small cell lung cancer (SCLC) (abstr). Presented at the 6th World Conference on Lung Cancer, Melbourne, November 10–14. Proc Am Soc Clin Oncol 10:240, 1991

Jaakkimainen L, Goodwin PJ, Pater J et al: Counting the costs of chemotherapy in a National Cancer Institute of Canada randomized trial in non-small cell lung cancer. J Clin Oncol 8:1301, 1990

Jackson DV, Richards F, Cooper R et al: Prophylactic cranial irradiation in small cell carcinoma of the lung. A randomized study. JAMA 237:2730, 1977

Johnson BE, Salem C, Nesbitt J et al: Limited (Ltd) stage small cell lung cancer (SCLC) treated with concurrent BID chest radiotherapy (RT) and etoposide cisplating (VP/PT) followed by chemotherapy (CT) selected by in vitro drug sensitivity testing (DST) (abstr). Presented at the 6th World Conference on Lung Cancer, Melbourne, November 10–14. Lung Cancer 7(suppl):152, 1991

Johnson DH: Overview of ifosphamide in small cell and non-small cell lung cancer. Semin Oncol 17(suppl 4):24, 1990

Johnson DH: New drugs in the management of SCLC. Lung Cancer 5:221, 1989

Johnson DH, Turrisi AT, Chang AY et al: Alternating chemotherapy (CT) and thoracic radiotherapy (TRT) in limited small cell lung cancer (LSCLC): A test of the Looney hypothesis. For the Eastern Cooperative Oncology Group. Proc Am Soc Clin Oncol 10 (abstr):243, 1991

Karrer K, Denck H, Karnicka-Mlofkowska H et al: Multi-modality treatment after surgery for cure of small cell lung cancer (SCLC) (abstr). Lung Cancer 4:A153, 1988

Karrer K, Shields T: The importance of complete resection in the multimodality treatment of SCLC (abstr). For ISC-Lung Cancer Study Group. Presented at the 6th World Conference on Lung Cancer, Melbourne, November 10–14. Lung Cancer 7(suppl): 71, 1991

Katsenis AT, Karpasitis N, Giannakakis J et al: Elective brain irradiation in patients with small-cell carcinoma of the lung: preliminary report. p. 277. In Lung Cancer International Congress Series. Excerpta Medica, 1982

Kies MS, Mira JC, Livingston RB et al: Multimodal therapy for limited small cell lung cancer: a randomized study of induction chemotherapy with or without thoracic radiation in complete responders and with wide field versus reduced volume radiation in partial responders. J Clin Oncol 5:592, 1987

Klastersky J: Diagnosis and staging in small cell lung cancer. Curr Opin Oncol 2:331, 1990

Kristjansen PEG: The role of cranial irradiation in the management of patients with SCLC. Lung Cancer 5:264, 1989

Kristjansen PEG, Osterland K, Dombernowsky P et al: A three-armed randomized trial in small cell lung cancer (SCLC) of two induction regimens with tenoposide and cisplatin or carboplatin followed by alternating chemotherapy versus alternating chemotherapy (abstr). Lung Cancer 7(suppl):121, 1991

Lad T, Thomas P, Piantadosi S: Surgical resection of small cell lung cancer—a prospective randomized evaluation (abstr). Presented at the 6th World Conference on Lung Cancer, Melbourne, November 10–14. Lung Cancer 7(suppl):162, 1991b

Lad T, Thomas P, Piantadosi S et al: Thoracotomy staging of small cell lung cancer (abstr). Presented at the 6th World Conference on Lung Cancer, Melbourne, November 10–14. Lung Cancer 7(suppl):53 1991a

Lad T, Wagner H, Piantadosi S: Randomized phase II evaluation of pre-operative chemotherapy alone and radiotherapy alone in stage IIIA non-small cell lung cancer (abstr). Proc Am Soc Clin Oncol 10:258, 1991c

LeBeau B, Chastang CL, Brechot JM: Small cell lung cancer (SCLC): long term results of a randomized trial assessing chemotherapy continuation in patients reaching complete remission after six courses (abstr). For the ''Petites Cellules'' Group (02PC 83 protocol). Presented at the 6th World Conference on Lung Cancer, Melbourne, November 10–14. Lung Cancer 7(suppl):130, 1991

Lewis JW Jr, Pearlberg JL, Beute GH et al: Can computed tomography of the chest stage lung cancer? Yes and no. Ann Thorac Surg 49:591, 1990

Lishner M, Feld R, Payne DG et al: Late neurological complications after prophylactic cranial irradiation in patients with small-cell lung cancer: the Toronto experience. J Clin Oncol 8:215, 1990

Livingston RG: Current chemotherapy of small cell lung cancer. Chest 89:2585, 1986

Lund B, Anderson H, Walling J et al: Phase II study of gemcitabine in non-small cell lung cancer (NSCLC) (abstr). Presented at the

6th World Conference on Lung Cancer Melbourne, November 10–14. Lung Cancer 7:121, 1991

Maassen W, Greschuchna D: Small cell carcinoma of the lung—to operate or not? Surgical experience and results. Thorac Cardiovasc Surg 34:71, 1986

Mattson K, Nilranen A, Holsti LR et al: Natural alpha interferon as maintenance therapy for small cell lung cancer (abstr). Presented at the 6th World Conference on Lung Cancer, Melbourne, November 10–14. Lung Cancer 7(suppl):127, 1991

Maurer LH, Tulloh M, Weiss RB et al: A randomized combined modality trial in small cell carcinoma of the lung. Comparison of combination chemotherapy-radiation therapy versus cyclophosphamide-radiation therapy. Effects of maintenance chemotherapy and whole brain irradiation. Cancer 45:30, 1980

Merkle NM, Mickisch GH, Kayser K et al: Surgical resection and adjuvant chemotherapy for small cell carcinoma. Thorac Cardiovasc Surg 34:39, 1986

Meyer JA, Comis RL, Ginsberg SJ: Selective surgical resection in small cell carcinoma of the lung. J Thorac Cardiovasc Surg 84:641, 1982

Meyer JA, Gullo JJ, Ikins PM et al: Adverse prognostic effect of N2 disease in treatment of small cell carcinoma of the lung. J Thorac Cardiovasc Surg 88:495, 1984

Miller AB, Fox W, Tall R: Five-year follow-up of the Medical Research Council's comparative trial of surgery and radiotherapy for the primary treatment of small celled carcinoma or oat celled carcinoma of the bronchus. Lancet 12:501, 1969

Milroy R, Paul J, Cram L et al: Randomised clinical study of verapamil in addition to chemotherapy in small cell lung cancer (SCLC) (abstr). Presented at the 6th World Conference on Lung Cancer, Melbourne, November 10–14. Lung Cancer 7(suppl):114, 1991

Minna JD, Pass H, Glatstein H et al: Cancer of the lung. p. 591. In De Vita VT Sr, Hellman S, Rosenberg S (eds): Cancer Principles and Practice of Oncology. 3rd Ed. JB Lippincott, Philadelphia, 1989

Miyazawa N, Tsuchiya R, Naruke T et al: A clinicopathological study of surgical treatment of small cell carcinoma of the lung. Jpn J Clin Oncol 16:297, 1986

Morstyn G, Ihde DC, Lichter AS et al: Small cell lung cancer 1973–1983: early progress and recent obstacles. Int J Radiat Oncol Biol Phys 10:515, 1984

Mountain C: A new international staging system for lung cancer. Chest 89: 225S, 1986

Mountain CV: Clinical biology of small cell lung cancer: relationship to surgical therapy. Semin Oncol 5:272, 1978

Murphy PB, Hainsworth JD, Greco FA et al: Cisplatin (P) and prolonged administration of oral etoposide (E) in extensive small cell lung cancer (ESCLC) patients (PT): a phase II trial (abstr). Proc Am Soc Clin Oncol 10:257, 1991

Murray N, Coy P, Pater J et al: The importance of timing for thoracic irradiation (TI) in the combined modality treatment of limited stage small cell lung cancer (LSCLC) (abstr). Proc Am Soc Clin Oncol 10:243, 1991a

Murray N, Shah A, Osoba D et al: Intensive weekly chemotherapy for the treatment of extensive-stage small-cell lung cancer. J Clin Oncol 9:1632, 1991b

Murray N, Shah A, Osoba D et al: Dose-intensive chemotherapy (CODE) for non-small cell lung cancer (NSCLC) (abstr). Proc Am Soc Clin Oncol 8:219, 1989

Myer JA, Comis RL, Ginsberg RJ et al: Phase II trial of extended indications for resection in small cell carcinoma of the lung. J Thorac Cardiovasc Surg 83:12, 1982

Nou E, Brodin O, Bergh J: A randomized study of radiation treatment in small cell bronchial carcinoma treated with two types of four drug chemotherapy regimens. Cancer 62:1079, 1988

Ohnoshi T, Hiraki S, Kawahara S et al: Randomized trial comparing chemotherapy alone and chemotherapy plus chest irradaition in limited stage small cell lung cancer: a preliminary report. Jpn J Clin Oncol 16:271, 1986

Ohta M, Hara N, Ichinose Y: The role of surgical resection in the management of small cell carcinoma of the lung. Jpn J Clin Oncol 16:289, 1986

Osterlind K, Hansen M, Hansen HH et al: Influence of surgical resection prior to chemotherapy on long-term results in small cell lung cancer. A study of 150 operable patients. Eur J Cancer Clin Oncol 5:589, 1989

Osterlind K, Hansen HH, Hansen HS et al: Chemotherapy versus chemotherapy plus irradiation in limited small cell lung cancer. Results of a controlled trial with 5 years follow-up. Br J Cancer 54:7, 1986

Osterlind K, Hansen M, Hansen HH et al: Treatment policy of surgery in small cell carcinoma of the lung: retrospective analysis of a series of 874 consecutive patients. Thorax 40:272, 1985

Perez CA, Einhorn L, Oldham RK et al: Randomized trial of radiotherapy to the thorax in limited chemotherapy and elective brain irradiation: a preliminary report. J Clin Oncol 2:1200, 1984

Pfister DG, Wells CK, Chan CK et al: Classifying clinical severity to help solve problems of stage migration in nonconcurrent comparisons of lung cancer therapy. Cancer Res 50:4664, 1990

Prignot J, Humblet Y, Francis C et al: A randomized trial for small cell lung cancer. Late intensification chemotherapy or not (abstr): Proceedings of the IV World Conference on Lung Cancer, Toronto, August 25–30, 1985

Rapp E, Pater J, Willan A et al: Chemotherapy can prolong survival in patients with advanced non-small cell lung cancer. A report of the Canadian Multicentre Trial. J Clin Oncol 6:633, 1988

Rawson NSB, Peto J: An overview of prognostic factors in small cell lung cancer: a report of prognostic factors in small cell lung cancer: a report of the Subcommittee for the Management of Lung Cancer in the United Kingdom, Co-ordinating Committee on Cancer Research. Br J Cancer 61:597, 1990

Richardson GE, Venzon DJ, Steinberg SM et al: An algorithm for staging patients (PTS) with small cell lung cancer (SCLC) can save 40% of the initial evaluation costs (abstr). Proc Am Soc Clin Oncol 10:242, 1991

Roth BJ, Johnson DH, Einhorn LH et al: Randomized study of cyclophosphamide, doxorubicin, and vincristine versus etoposide and cisplatin versus alternation of these two regimens in extensive small cell lung cancer: a Phase III trial of the Southeastern Cancer Study Group. J Clin Oncol 10:282, 1992

Rubin P, Casarett GI: A direction for clinical radiation pathology. Front Radiat Ther Oncol 6:1, 1972

Sagman U, Feld R, Evans WK et al: The prognostic significance of pretreatment serum lactate dehydrogenase in patients with small-cell lung cancer. J Clin Oncol 9:954, 1991a

Sagman U, Lishner M, Maki E et al: Second primary malignancies following the diagnosis of small cell lung cancer. J Clin Oncol 10:1525, 1992

Sagman U, Maki E, Evans WK et al: Small cell carcinoma of the lung: derivation of a prognostic staging system. J Clin Oncol 9:1639, 1991b

Salzer M, Muller LC, Huber H et al: Operation for N2 small-cell lung carcinoma. J Thorac Cardiovasc Surg 49:759, 1990

Santoro A, Bonadonna G, Valagussa P et al: Long-term results of combination chemotherapy-radiotherapy approach in Hodgkin's disease: superiority of ABVD plus radiotherapy versus MOPP plus radiotherapy. J Clin Oncol 5:27, 1987

Schaake-Konig C, van den Bogaert W, Dalesio O et al: Effects of concomitant cisplatin and radiotherapy on inoperable non-small cell lung cancer. N Engl J Med 326:524, 1992

Sculier JP, Feld R, Evans WK et al: Carcinoembryonic antigen: a useful prognostic marker in small cell lung cancer. J Clin Oncol 3:1349, 1985

Seydel JG, Creech R, Pagano M et al: Combined modality treatment of regional small cell undifferentiated cardinoma of the lung. A cooperative study of the RTOG and ECOG. Int J Radiat Oncol Biol Phys 9:1135, 1983

Shank B, Sher H: Controversies in treatment of small cell carcinoma of the lung. Cancer Invest 3:367, 1985

Shank B, Sher H, Hilaris B et al: Increased survival with high-dose multifield radiotherapy and intensive chemotherapy in limited small cell carcinoma of the lung. Int J Radiat Oncol Biol Phys 9(suppl 1):122, 1983

Shepherd FA, Ginsberg R, Evans WK et al: "Very limited" small cell lung cancer (SCLC): results of non-surgical treatment (abstr). Proc Annu Meet Am Soc Clin Oncol 3:223, 1984

Shepherd FA, Ginsberg RJ, Evans WK et al: Reduction in local recurrence and improved survival in surgically treated patients with small cell carcinoma of the lung. J Thorac Cardiovasc Surg 86:498, 1983

Shepherd FA, Ginsberg RJ, Feld R et al: Surgical treatment for limited small-cell lung cancer: the University of Toronto Lung Oncology Group Experience. J Thorac Cardiovasc Surg 1091:385, 1991

Shepherd FA, Ginsberg RJ, Patterson GA et al: A prospective study of adjuvant surgical ressection after chemotherapy for limited small cell lung cancer: a University of Toronto Lung Oncology Group study. J Thorac Cardiovasc Surg 97:177, 1989

Shields TW, Higgins GA, Matthews NJ et al: Surgical resection in the management of small-cell carcinoma of the lung. J Thorac Cardiovasc Surg 84:481, 1982

Slevin ML, Clark PI, Joel SP et al: A randomized trial to evaluate the effect of schedule on the activity of etoposide in small cell lung cancer. J Clin Oncol 7:1333, 1989

Smyth JF: The management of small cell anaplastic lung cancer. p.115. In Smyth JF (ed): The Management of Lung Cancer. Edward Arnold, London, 1984

Smyth JF, Bowman A, Fergusson RJ et al: Potentiation of cisplatin by alpha-interferon in advanced non-small cell lung cancer (NSCLC): a phase II study. Ann Oncol 1:351, 1990

Sorensen HR, Lund C, Alstrup P: Survival in small cell lung carcinoma after surgery. Thorax 41:479, 1986

Souhami RL, Geddes DM, Spiro SG et al: Radiotherapy in small cell cancer of the lung treated with combination chemotherapy: a controlled trial. B M J 288:1643, 1984

Souhami RL, Harper PG, Linch D et al: High-dose cyclophosphamide with autologous marrow transplantation as initial treatment of small cell carcinoma of the bronchus. Cancer Chemother Pharmacol 8:31, 1982

Souhami RL, Bradbury I, Geddes DM et al: Prognostic significance of laboratory parameters measured at diagnosis in small cell carcinoma of the lung. Cancer Res 45:2878, 1985a

Souhami RL, Finn G, Gregory WM et al: High-dose cyclophosphamide in small cell carcinoma of the lung. J Clin Oncol 3:958, 1985b

Splinter T, McVie J, Dalesio O et al: EORTC 08825 induction versus induction plus maintenance chemotherapy (CT) in small cell lung cancer (abstr). Proc Annu Meet Am Soc Clin Oncol 5:188, 1986

Splinter TAW: Chemotherapy of SCLC: duration of treatment. Lung Cancer 5:186, 1989

Splinter TAW: EORTC 08825 induction versus induction plus maintenance chemotherapy in small cell lung cancer. Definitive evaluation (abstr). For the EORTC Lung Co-operative Group. Proc Am Soc Clin Oncol 7:202, 1988

Stahel R, Aisner J, Ginsberg R et al: Staging and prognostic factors in small cell lung cancer. Lung Cancer 5:119, 1989

Stahel RA: Diagnosis, staging and prognostic factors of small cell lung cancer. Curr Opin Oncol 3:306, 1991

Stahel RA, Mabry M, Skarin AT et al: Detection of bone marrow metastasis in small cell lung cancer by monoclonal antibody. J Clin Oncol 3:455, 1985

Stevens E, Einhorn L, Sohn R: Treatment of limited small cell cancer (abstr). Proc Am Assoc Cancer Res 20:435, 1979

Thatcher N, Lind M: Carboplatin in small cell lung cancer. Semin Oncol 17(suppl 2):40, 1990

Thomas ED, Buckner CD, Clift RA et al: Bone marrow transplantation for acute non-lymphoblastic leukemia in first remission. N Engl J Med 301:597, 1979

Tourani JM, Levy R, Even P et al: Short intensive five drug chemotherapy (CT) followed by intensive irradiation for limited small cell lung cancer (LSCLC). Improved response rate and survival. A pilot study (abstr). Proc Am Soc Clin Oncol 10:245, 1991

Turrisi AT: The integration of cisplatin and radiotherapy in the treatment of lung cancer. Semin Oncol 18(suppl 3) 81, 1991

Wadler S, Lebersky B, Atkins M et al: Phase II trial of fluorouracil and recombinant interferon alpha-2a in patients with advanced colorectal carcinoma: an Eastern Cooperative Oncology Group study. J Clin Oncol 9:1806, 1991

Wadler S, Schwartz EL, Goldman M et al: Fluorouracil and recombinant alpha-2A-interferon: an active regimen against advanced colorectal carcinoma. J Clin Oncol 7:1769, 1989

Warde P, Payne D: Does thoracic irradiation improve survival or local control in limited stage small cell carcinoma of the lung—a meta analysis. J Clin Oncol 10:890, 1992

Wils J, Utama I, Sala L et al: Phase II study of high dose epirubucin in non-small cell lung cancer. Eur J Cancer 26:1140, 1990

Woll PJ, Rozengurt E: Therapeutic implications of growth factors in small cell lung cancer. Lung Cancer 5:287, 1989

Zelen M: Keynote address on biostatistics and data retrieval. Cancer Chemother Rep 4:31, 1973

30

RARE PRIMARY MALIGNANT NEOPLASMS

Michael Burt
Maureen Zakowski

Most primary pulmonary neoplasms are malignant. Of these, bronchogenic carcinomas comprise the great majority. However, other malignant neoplasms do arise in the lung but are extremely uncommon. Because these tumors are disparate in their histogenesis, there is no single accepted classification, and when discussed, these rare malignant neoplasms are dealt with individually.

CLINICAL FEATURES

Most patients with a rare primary pulmonary malignant tumor present with clinical features that mimic those in patients presenting with a nonsmall cell carcinoma of the lung. Except for those patients with intravascular bronchioalveolar tumors, most present with a solitary pulmonary nodule on chest radiograph. In general, the majority of patients (50 to 85 percent) are symptomatic, with the most common symptoms being cough, dyspnea, chest pain, and hemoptysis. Other less common symptoms include wheezing, fever, fatigue, and weight loss.

As the following sections demonstrate, the diagnosis in the majority of patients with any of the rare primary malignant tumors of lung is made during the operation for locoregional disease. In general the diagnosis, staging, and treatment of these rare malignant tumors of the lung should follow identical guidelines for those of patients with nonsmall cell cancer. As is illustrated, the natural history of most of these tumors mimics that of nonsmall cell lung cancer.

PULMONARY BLASTOMA

The first description of this tumor was by Barrett and Barnard (1945) in 1945. The patient described was a 40-year-old woman who presented in January 1943 with "influenza," fatigue, weight loss, anemia, and a chest radiograph demonstrating "a circumscribed opacity of even density in the middle of the right lung . . . about as large as a small grapefruit."

In August 1943 she underwent a right pneumonectomy. In 1952 a follow-up report by Barnard (1952) revealed that "the patient has had no further trouble attributable to the tumor since its removal in 1943." The microscopic appearance was described, and the tumor was labeled "embryoma of lung." In 1961 Spencer (1961) described three cases and coined the term "pulmonary blastoma" because of the similarity of this lesion to nephroblastoma (Wilms tumor).

Since the report of Spencer, the histogenesis of this tumor has been debated. In some cases the tumor bears a striking resemblance to fetal lung in the pseudoglandular stage at about 3 months' gestation (Kodama, et al., 1984; Manning, et al., 1985; Muller-Hermelink and Kaiserling, 1986).

Microscopically this tumor contains a mixture of epithelial and mesenchymal components, either of which may be dominant. Hemorrhage and necrosis are common features. The epithelial component may be arranged on branched tubules and surrounded by spindle or polygonal stromal cells. The stroma may show cartilaginous, osseous, or skeletal muscle (rhabdoid) differentiation, and metastases may be epithelial, stromal, or both (Fraser, et al., 1989; Mackay, et al., 1990). An association of pulmonary blastoma and cystic lung disease in children has been described (Weinblatt, et al., 1982). Fine-needle aspiration biopsy has been used to make this diagnosis preoperatively (Francis and Jacobsen, 1979). Figure 30-1 demonstrates the histologic features of this tumor.

Some of the confusion in the literature has to do with the similarities between pulmonary blastoma and carcinosarcoma. Ashworth (1983) recently formulated definitions of blastoma and carcinosarcoma that appear to be accepted as follows: (1) a blastoma is a tumor of variable malignant potential that reproduces, in a disorderly fashion, the embryonal structures of the organ of origin; and (2) carcinosarcoma is a malignant tumor composed of histologically malignant epithelial and stromal elements. Immunologic evidence was presented by Yousem, et al. (1990) that agrees with this definition of blastoma. They found a remarkable resemblance

---

Rare Primary Malignant Neoplasms of the Lung

Blastoma, pulmonary
Carcinosarcoma
IVBAT
Malignant lymphoreticular disorders
    Hodgkin's disease
    Non-Hodgkin's lymphoma
    Plasmacytoma
Malignant melanoma
Malignant germ cell tumors
    Malignant teratoma
    Choriocarcinoma
Sarcoma
    Chondrosarcoma
    Osteosarcoma
    Soft tissue sarcoma
Miscellaneous
    Ependymoma, malignant
    Ewing's sarcoma
    Lymphoepithelioma
    Pseudomesotheliomatous carcinoma

---

between the antigenic profile of blastoma and embryonic lung, as others have found between nephroblastoma (Wilms' tumor) and fetal kidney (Albeda, et al., 1989).

Pulmonary blastomas are uncommon. Jacobson and Francis (1980) reviewed their experience at one hospital in Sweden over the 8-year period from 1971 to 1978 and found 11 cases. This represented 0.5 percent of all lung neoplasms seen during that period.

In a review of the English literature from the first reported case in 1945 until now, 76 cases have been sufficiently de-

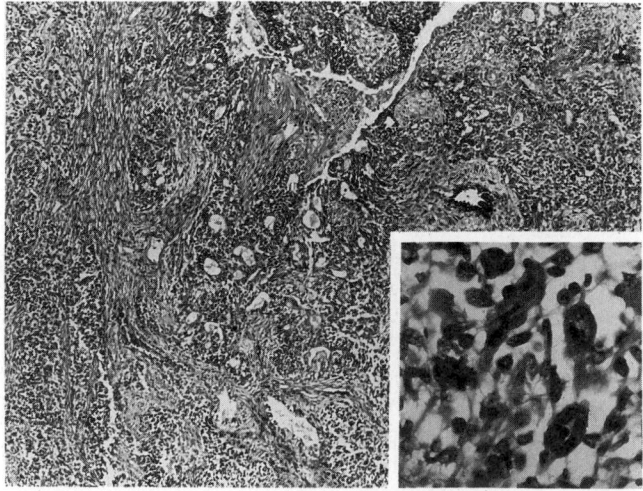

Figure 30-1. Pulmonary blastoma. Note the well-formed glands in a spindle cell stroma. The insert shows rhabdomyoblastic differentiation of the stroma.

scribed to allow a survival analysis. The number of cases per report varied from 1 to 11 (Barrett and Barnard, 1945; Barnard, 1952; Spencer, 1961; Yousem, et al., 1990; Jacobson and Francis, 1980; Parker, et al., 1966; Henry and Keal, 1966; Bauermeister, et al., 1966; Barson, et al., 1968; Stackhouse, et al., 1969; Cox, et al., 1970; Iverson and Straehley, 1973; Dixon and Breslow, 1973; Ghaffar, et al., 1975; Karcioglu and Someren, 1974; Kennedy and Prior, 1976; McCann, et al., 1976; Kern and Stiles, 1976; Fung, et al., 1977; Francis and Jacobsen, 1979; Tamai, et al., 1980; Gibbons, et al., 1981; Marcus, et al., 1982; Weinblatt, et al., 1982; Kummet and Doll, 1982; Medbery, et al., 1984; Jimenez, 1987; Manivel, et al., 1988; Jetley, et al., 1988; Ozkaynak, et al., 1990). The largest report from a single institution was by Koss, et al. (1991) from the Armed Forces Institute of Pathology (AFIP) who described 52 patients with pulmonary blastomas. The following discussion attempts to summarize the available information concerning presentation, therapy, and survival from the 76 case reports and the analysis of the 52 patients presented from the AFIP.

Of the 128 patients described in the literature, 74 (58 percent) were male, and 54 (42 percent) were female, a male to female ratio of 1.4. The age at diagnosis ranged from neonatal to 77 years (median, 40 years). Figure 30-2 demonstrates the age distribution of these 128 patients. The location of the tumor is listed in Table 30-1. The distribution of left (45 percent) versus right lung (54 percent) was as expected.

At presentation many patients (40 percent) are asymptomatic, but approximately 60 percent have symptoms. In the report from the AFIP, 33 percent presented with cough, 31

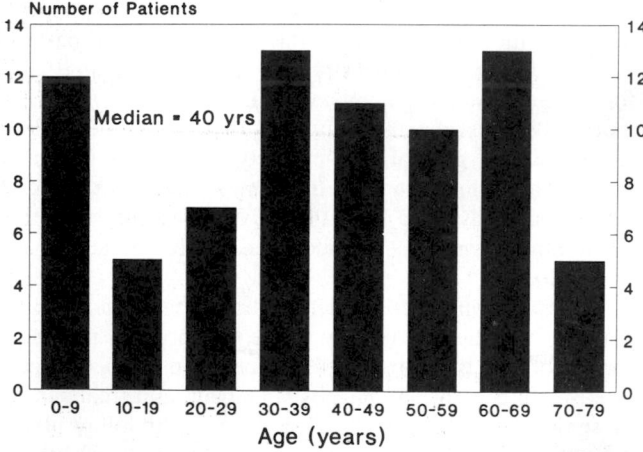

Figure 30-2. Age distribution of 128 patients with pulmonary blastomas. (Data from Barnard, 1952; Barson, et al, 1968; Barrett and Barnard, 1945; Bauermeister, et al, 1966; Cox, et al, 1970; Dixon and Breslow, 1973; Francis and Jacobsen, 1979; Fung, et al, 1977; Ghaffar, et al, 1975; Gibbons, et al, 1981; Henry and Keal, 1966; Iverson and Straehley, 1973; Jacobson and Francis, 1980; Jetley, et al, 1988; Jiminez, 1987; Karcioglu and Someren, 1974; Kennedy and Prior, 1976; Kern, et al, 1976; Koss, et al, 1984; Kummet and Doll, 1982; Manivel, et al, 1988; Marcus, et al, 1982; McCann, et al, 1976; Medbery, et al, 1984; Ozkaynak, et al, 1990; 1984; Parker, et al, 1966; Spencer, 1961; Stackhouse, et al, 1969; Tamai, et al, 1980; Weinblatt, et al, 1982; and Yousem, et al, 1990.)

Table 30-1. Location of Pulmonary Blastomas[a]

	No.	Percent
Left lung	34	45
Upper lobe	17	
Lower lobe	17	
Right lung	41	54
Upper lobe	15	
Middle lobe	6	
Lower lobe	20	
Bilateral	1	1
Total	76	

[a] Location available in 76 cases.

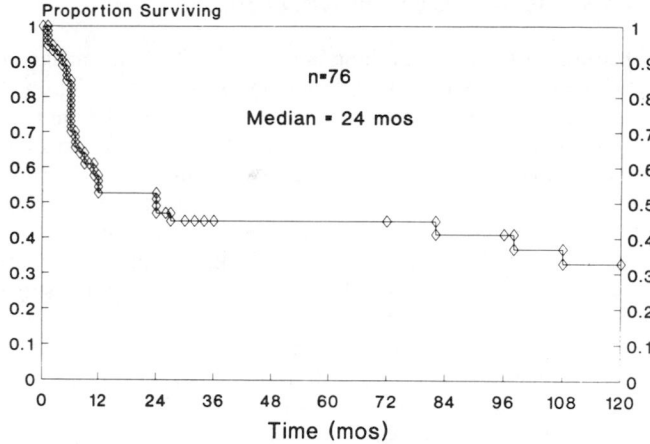

Figure 30-3. Overall actuarial survival of 76 patients with pulmonary blastomas. (Data from Barnard, 1952; Barson, et al, 1968; Barrett and Barnard, 1945; Bauermeister, et al, 1966; Cox, et al, 1970; Dixon and Breslow, 1973; Francis and Jacobsen, 1979; Fung, et al, 1977; Ghaffar, et al, 1975; Gibbons, et al, 1981; Henry and Keal, 1966; Iverson and Straehley, 1973; Jacobson and Francis, 1980; Jetley, et al, 1988; Jiminez, 1987; Karcioglu and Someren, 1974; Kennedy and Prior, 1976; Kern, et al, 1976; Koss, et al, 1984; Kummet and Doll, 1982; Manivel, et al, 1988; Marcus, et al, 1982; McCann, et al, 1976; Medbery, et al, 1984; Parker, et al, 1966; Spencer, 1961; Stackhouse, et al, 1969; Tamai, et al, 1980; Weinblatt, et al, 1982; and Yousem, et al, 1990.)

percent with chest pain, 20 percent with hemoptysis, 14 percent with dyspnea, 12 percent with weight loss, 8 percent with fever, and 4 percent with recurrent pneumonia. Most pulmonary blastomas are peripheral. They range in size from 1 to 28 cm in diameter (median, 7 to 8 cm).

Most patients (85 percent) presented with locoregional disease and underwent pulmonary resection (n = 109). Unlike most series of pulmonary resection for nonsmall cell lung cancer, a greater proportion of patients with pulmonary blastomas underwent pneumonectomy (Table 30-2). Of the 19 patients not undergoing resection, approximately one-half had advanced locoregional disease (i.e., pleural effusion, etc.), and the other half had distant disease. Because of the heterogeneous nature of the many reports in the literature, pathologic staging was not able to be summarized. However, there were more than a few reports describing hilar and a few describing mediastinal nodal metastases.

The overall survival rate of the 76 patients with sufficient information to be analyzed is depicted in Figure 30-3. The 5- and 10-year actuarial survival rates for this group were 45 and 33 percent, respectively, with a median of 24 months. These findings are similar to the overall 5-year survival rate of approximately 50 percent reported for the 52 patients from the AFIP.

Figure 30-4 depicts the survival of those patients undergoing resection versus those that did not. The resected patients did significantly better.

Most patients who experience recurrences after resection do so with distant metastases, many failing in the brain.

In summary pulmonary blastoma behaves much like a nonsmall cell lung carcinoma. The evaluation, indications for surgery, and pulmonary resection should be identical to those of a patient with suspected or proved nonsmall cell lung cancer.

Table 30-2. Operation Performed in Patients with Pulmonary Blastomas

	No.	%
Pneumonectomy	39	36
Lobectomy (or bilobectomy)	58	53
Wedge resection/segmentectomy	12	11
Total resections	109	

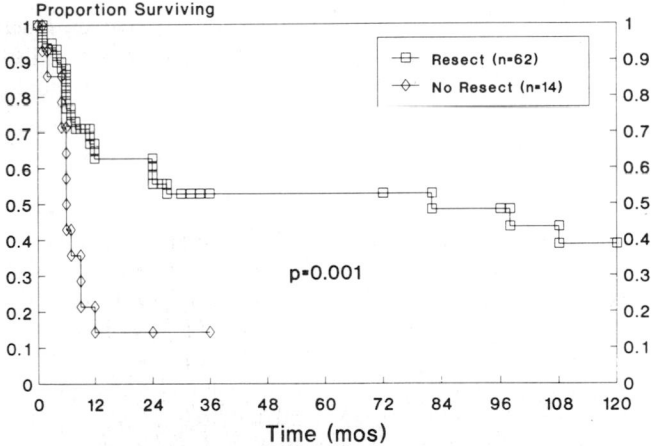

Figure 30-4. Survival of patients undergoing resection of pulmonary blastomas compared with those who did not (comparison by log-rank test). (Data from Barnard, 1952; Barson, et al, 1968; Barrett and Barnard, 1945; Bauermeister, et al, 1966; Cox, et al, 1970; Dixon and Breslow, 1973; Francis and Jacobsen, 1979; Fung, et al, 1977; Ghaffar, et al, 1975; Gibbons, et al, 1981; Henry and Keal, 1966; Iverson and Straehley, 1973; Jacobson and Francis, 1980; Jetley, et al, 1988; Jiminez, 1987; Karcioglu and Someren, 1974; Kennedy and Prior, 1976; Kern, et al, 1976; Koss, et al, 1984; Kummet and Doll, 1982; Manivel, et al, 1988; Marcus, et al, 1982; McCann, et al, 1976; Medbery, et al, 1984; Parker, et al, 1966; Spencer, 1961; Stackhouse, et al, 1969; Tamai, et al, 1980; Weinblatt, et al, 1982; and Yousem, et al, 1990.)

CARCINOSARCOMA OF THE LUNG

Carcinosarcoma of the lung is a tumor with both malignant epithelial and malignant mesenchymal components. Virchow considered carcinosarcoma a "manifestation of the multipotentially of the mother tissue," such that the "sarcoma and carcinoma grow side by side like two branches of the same tree" (Bergmann, et al., 1951). The simultaneous development of epithelial and stromal malignancy is another possibility, but it is less likely than differentiation of a malignant tumor into two or more divergent pathways from a single primitive neoplastic cell.

The first case report is attributed to Kika, as cited by Herxheimer and Reinke (1912), in 1908, but there is no information available concerning the patient. Bergman, et al. (1951) in 1951 reviewed eight cases of carcinosarcoma of lung and described the first two cases that were successfully resected. Both resections were by pneumonectomy, and both were performed by Dr. Evarts Graham.

In the report of Bergmann, et al. (1951), the authors noted that, of 258 resected bronchopulmonary tumors at one hospital in St. Louis, they found 2 patients with carcinosarcomas, an incidence of 0.8 percent.

The English literature was reviewed from 1908 to the present, and 91 patients with carcinosarcomas of the lung were reported (Bergmann, et al., 1951; Herxheimer and Reinke, 1912; Moore, 1961; Prive, et al., 1961; Jenkins, 1968; Chaudhuri, 1971; Kakos, et al., 1971; Razzuk, et al., 1971; Bull and Grimes, 1974; Roth and Elquezabal, 1978; Addis and Corrin, 1985; Ishida, et al., 1990; Meade, et al., 1991; Engel, et al., 1991; Davis, et al., 1984). Of these 91 patients, no clinical data were presented in 24, only autopsy data in 16, and in 34 there were sufficient data for summarization. The remaining 17 patients were summarized in the largest report from a single institution, the Mayo Clinic (Davis, et al., 1984).

Of the 34 patients with carcinosarcomas of lung, for whom there were sufficient data to analyze, 29 (85 percent) were men, and 5 (15 percent) were women, a male to female ratio of 5.8. Their ages ranged from 46 to 74 years (median, 64 years). These pooled data were comparable to those of the Mayo series. In that series 3 of 17 patients (18 percent) were asymptomatic, and the other patients presented with cough, hemoptysis, wheezing, dyspnea, or chest pain. Chest radiographs demonstrated well-circumscribed lesions in all 17 patients from the Mayo series and in all 34 patients pooled from the literature. Of these, 68 percent presented with upper lobe lesions (12 left and 11 right), and 32 percent had lower lobe lesions (5 left and 6 right). Endobronchial disease was present in 62 percent of patients by bronchoscopy.

Of the patients reported in the literature, 31 (91 percent) presented with local disease and underwent pulmonary resection. Of these 14 (45 percent) underwent pneumonectomy and 17 (55 percent), lobectomy. There was one postoperative death, a postoperative mortality rate of 3 percent. Of the three patients not resected, one received no therapy and died 1 month after diagnosis, and two received radiotherapy and were alive with disease at 3 months.

The overall survival rate of the 34 patients pooled from the literature is depicted in Figure 30-5. The 1- and 5-year actuarial survival rates were 46 and 19 percent, respectively,

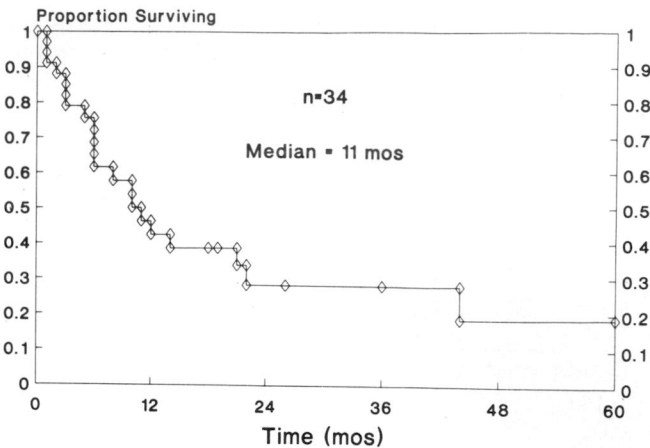

Figure 30-5. Overall actuarial survival of 34 patients with carcinosarcomas of the lung. (Data from Addis and Corrin, 1985; Bergmann, et al, 1951; Bull and Grimes, 1974; Chaudhuri, 1971; Davis, et al, 1984; Engel, et al, 1991; Herxheimer and Reinke, 1912; Ishida, et al, 1990; Jenkins, 1982; Kakos, et al, 1971; Meade, et al, 1991; Moore, 1961; Prive, et al, 1961; Razzuk, et al, 1971; and Roth and Elquezabal, 1978.)

with a median of 11 months. This is comparable to the median survival time of 12 months reported by the Mayo group.

Throughout the literature, two groups of carcinosarcoma of the lung have been described: (1) peripheral and (2) central, usually with endobronchial tumor. All reports that mention this division state that the peripheral tumors do significantly worse than the central tumors. Figure 30-6 demonstrates that, when the survival of the 34 patients from the literature was calculated based on location of the tumor, there was no significant difference demonstrated.

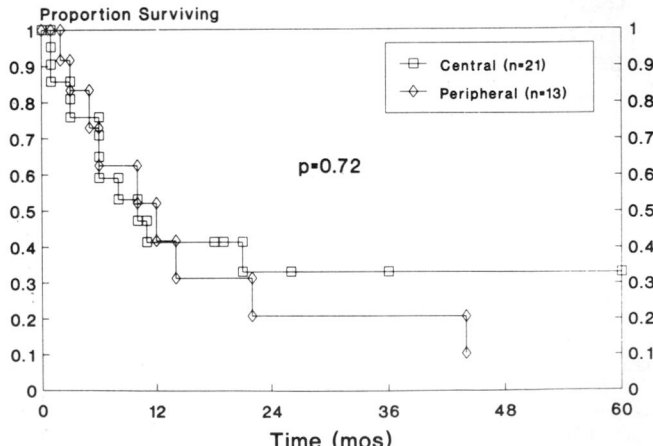

Figure 30-6. Survival of patients with central carcinosarcomas of the lung compared with those with peripheral lesions (comparison by log-rank test). (Data from Addis and Corrin, 1985; Bergmann, et al, 1951; Bull and Grimes, 1974; Chaudhuri, 1971; Davis, et al, 1984; Engel, et al, 1991; Herxheimer and Reinke, 1912; Ishida, et al, 1990; Jenkins, 1982; Kakos, et al, 1971; Meade, et al, 1991; Moore, 1961; Prive, et al, 1961; Razzuk, et al, 1971; and Roth and Elquezabal, 1978.)

Patients who have recurrences after resection, do so in a pattern similar to that of patients with nonsmall cell lung cancer, with distant metastases predominating. Metastases to the lung, liver, adrenal gland, brain, bone, and heart have all been described.

Histologically, carcinosarcomas can show much necrosis, especially when they are peripheral in location. The epithelial component of carcinosarcoma is usually squamous cell carcinoma and less often adenocarcinoma, with large cell undifferentiated carcinoma found with the lowest frequency. Small cell carcinoma has not been reported in these tumors (Fraser, et al., 1989). The mesenchymal component may be made up of undifferentiated spindle cells, but areas of cartilaginous, osteoid, or rhabdoid differentiation have been reported (Ishizuka, et al., 1988) and pleomorphic areas resembling malignant fibrous histiocytoma (Fraser, et al., 1989). Metastases, which may be present at the time of diagnosis, may be sarcomatous, epithelial, or both. Immunohistochemical staining is useful in demonstrating the presence of both mesenchymal and epithelial areas to distinguish carcinosarcomas from poorly differentiated ''sarcomatoid'' carcinomas, in which the ''sarcomatoid'' cells stain only for epithelial markers. The characteristic features of the tumor are seen in Figure 30-7.

In summary carcinosarcoma of the lung is a relatively uncommon tumor. It appears that its locoregional spread and pattern of distant metastasis mimics that of nonsmall cell lung cancer. As in pulmonary blastoma, the evaluation and treatment of carcinosarcoma of lung should be similar to that of nonsmall cell lung cancer.

INTRAVASCULAR BRONCHIOALVEOLAR TUMOR

Intravascular bronchioalveolar tumor (IVBAT) is an unusual, rare malignant tumor of the lung that was first described by Dail and Liebow (1975) in 1975 in an abstract and later in a full report (Dail, et al., 1983). In early reports, IVBAT was thought to be a peculiar form of bronchioloalveolar carcinoma with a high rate of vascular involvement. Although recent electron microscopic and immunologic studies (Dail, et al., 1983; Corrin, et al., 1979; Azumi and Churg, 1981; Sherman, et al., 1981; Weldon-Linne, et al., 1981) demonstrated that this tumor is of vascular endothelial origin and not alveolar cell origin, the acronym for the lung involvement was retained to indicate that these tumors growth in alveoli, bronchioles, and vessels.

This malignant tumor is typically multifocal, and there is some evidence to suggest that the multiple foci arise synchronously (Eggleston, 1985). Grossly, the well-demarcated pulmonary nodules of IVBAT have a firm cartilaginous cut surface, and microscopically the almost acellular central portion of the tumor is surrounded by a cellular periphery that consists of an intraalveolar collection of plump spindle cells and looser myxomatous tissue. The interstitial tissue can become hyalinized and sclerotic, and calcification and ossification can occur. The tumor can extend to adjacent alveoli and into peribronchial lymphatic channels. This tumor is probably best categorized as a low-grade sarcoma (Fraser, et al., 1989). The characteristic histologic appearance is demonstrated in Figure 30-8.

A review of the English literature yielded 33 patients with sufficient data to analyze the demographics and survival rates (Dail, et al., 1983; Corrin, et al., 1979; Azumi and Churg, 1981; Sherman, et al., 1981; Weldon-Linne, et al., 1981; Eggleston, 1985; Emery, et al., 1982; Marsh, et al., 1982; Sicilian, et al., 1983; Gledhill and Kay, 1984; Borlee-Hermans, et al., 1985; Sweeney, et al., 1986; Miettinen, et al., 1987).

Most patients (85 percent) are female, and 15 percent are male. The ages range from 12 to 69 years (median, 35 years). At presentation one-half of the patients are asymptomatic, with the diagnosis suspected by routine chest radiograph. Of those with symptoms, two-thirds have relatively minor complaints (such as mild cough or mild chest discomfort), and one-third have major symptoms (such as moderate to severe dyspnea or marked weight loss).

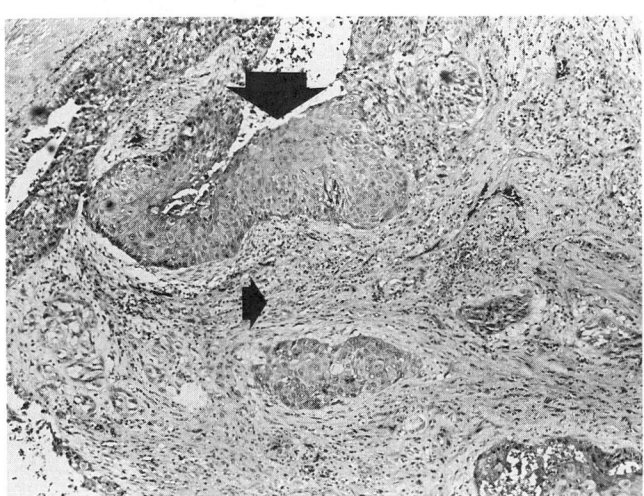

Figure 30-7. Primary carcinosarcoma of lung. This tumor is characterized by the presence of carcinoma, in this case, squamous cell carcinoma (*large arrow*), and sarcoma, here undifferentiated (*small arrow*).

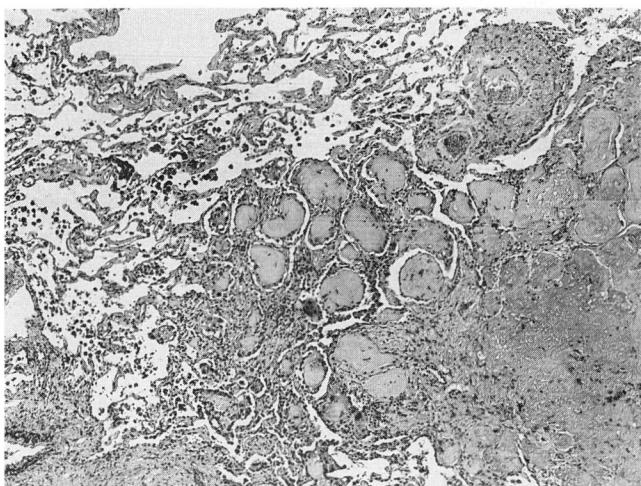

Figure 30-8. IVBAT. Note the eosinophilic nodules of hyalinized stroma surrounded by cells with an epithelial appearance. These nodular tumor masses fill the alveolar spaces.

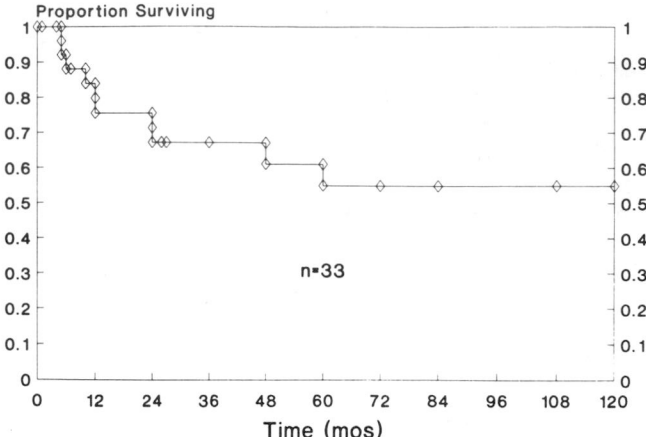

Figure 30-9. Overall actuarial survival of 33 patients with IVBAT. (Data from Azumi and Churg, 1981; Borlee-Hermans, et al, 1985; Corrin, et al, 1979; Dail, et al, 1983; Eggleston, 1985; Emery, et al, 1982; Gledhill and Kay, 1984; Marsh, et al, 1982; Miettinen, et al, 1987; Sherman, et al, 1981; Sicilian, et al, 1983; and Sweeney, et al, 1986.)

All but two patients presented with multiple, bilateral pulmonary nodules. One presented with unilateral multiple nodules, and another with a left lower lobe nodule. All patients underwent open lung biopsy (resection of the left lower lobe in one) to make the diagnosis. Of the 33 patients, 8 (24 percent) presented with or subsequently developed metastases (liver in six, retroperitoneum in one, and small bowel in one).

There is no specific therapy. Multiple chemotherapeutic regimens have been tried but usually only in symptomatic patients near death (Dail, et al., 1983). Radiation therapy was unsuccessful in one patient (Azumi and Churg, 1981). The disease tends to be indolent, with death usually resulting from slowly progressive pulmonary compromise secondary to replacement of the lung parenchyma by the tumor. Figure 30-9 depicts the overall actuarial survival rate for this group. The 5- and 10-year overall survival rates are 61 and 55 percent, respectively, with the median survival not reached at 10 years.

In summary IVBAT should be suspected in a young, asymptomatic woman who presents with multiple, bilateral pulmonary nodules. Biopsy is required to make the diagnosis. Patients should be offered therapy only if symptomatic because the natural history of this disorder may span 5 to 10 years, and as yet, there is no proved effective chemotherapeutic regimen.

PRIMARY MALIGNANT LYMPHORETICULAR DISORDERS OF THE LUNG

The term *lymphoreticular system,* as commonly used, refers to mobile and fixed cellular elements concerned with the body's defense: macrophages, reticuloendothelial elements, and functionally related lymphatic tissues. Because all these tissues are found in the normal lung, primary tumors of the lymphoreticular system can originate in the lung. Therefore although extremely uncommon, primary Hodgkin's disease, non-Hodgkin's lymphoma, and plasmacytoma of the lung do occur. Taken together these three malignant entities comprise approximately 0.5 percent of all primary lung tumors. Secondary involvement of the lung by a lymphoproliferative disorder is much more common, which in Hodgkin's disease and non-Hodgkin's lymphoma has been reported to be 40 percent (Kern, et al., 1961) and 49 percent (Risdall, et al., 1979), respectively. The following discussion concerns primary Hodgkin's disease, non-Hodgkin's lymphoma, and plasmacytoma of the lung.

Hodgkin's Disease

The first report of primary Hodgkin's disease of the lung was by Weber (1930) in 1930. The presentation of Hodgkin's disease as extranodal disease is extremely uncommon (Wood and Coltman, 1973). Primary extranodal Hodgkin's disease represented 0.6 percent of 155 patients with Hodgkin's disease seen at Yale from 1980 to 1987 (Radin, 1990) and 0.07% of 1,470 patients seen at Stanford from 1960 to 1980 (Johnson, et al., 1983). To be defined as primary pulmonary Hodgkin's disease, most authors accept the following criteria: (1) histologic features of Hodgkin's disease, (2) restriction of the disease to the lung with no nodal involvement (some authors accept "minimal" nodal involvement) (Radin, 1990), and (3) adequate clinical and/or pathologic exclusion of disease at distant sites (Johnson, et al., 1983; Yousem, et al., 1986; Zulian, et al., 1986). By this definition the staging of patients with primary pulmonary Hodgkin's disease, according to the Ann Arbor staging system (Carbone, et al., 1971), would be IE (involvement of a single extranodal site) or IIE (localized involvement of an extranodal site and its contiguous lymph node chain).

Because it is rare, few centers have seen more than a handful of patients. To summarize the presentation, therapy, and outcome, a literature search was performed, and from this 61 patients were found to have sufficient data to be analyzed (Kern, et al., 1961; Yousem, et al., 1986; Zulian, et al., 1986; Monahan, 1965; Guttman and Saavedra, 1968; Dhingra and Flance, 1970; Nelson, et al., 1983; van der Schee, et al., 1990). The excellent review of Radin (1990) was the source of much of the raw data analyzed.

Of 61 patients with primary Hodgkin's disease of lung, 39 percent were male, and 61 percent were female, a male to female ratio of 0.65. Their ages ranged from 12 to 82 years (median, 37 years). Fifteen percent were asymptomatic. Eighty-five percent were symptomatic with, in decreasing frequency, cough, weight loss, chest pain, dyspnea, hemoptysis, fatigue, rash, night sweats, and wheezing. Of those with symptoms, 52 percent had the B-type symptoms characteristic of Hodgkin's disease (weight loss, fever, and night sweats).

The location of the chest radiographic finding was unilateral in 46 patients (72 percent) and bilateral in 15 (25 percent). Two patients had a normal chest radiograph with endobronchial Hodgkin's disease diagnosed by bronchoscopy. All bilateral disease demonstrated multiple nodules; unilateral disease presented as a single nodule in 85 percent and multiple in 15 percent. Overall a solitary nodule was seen in 39 of 61 patients

(64 percent), and of these 12 (31 percent) demonstrated cavitation.

Intrathoracic Hodgkin's disease, either primary or with contiguous mediastinal spread, is most often of the nodular sclerosing type. The other subtypes are lymphocyte predominant, lymphocyte depleted, and mixed cellularity. The histologic appearance of primary pulmonary Hodgkin's disease is identical to that seen in lymph nodes at other sites, and the pattern varies with different histologic subtypes (Fraser, et al., 1989). This is characterized by the presence of Reed-Sternberg calls (or their variants), which are large pleomorphic cells that are binucleate and with prominent nucleoli and often called "mirror-image" cells. The Reed-Sternberg cells are present in the appropriate background of inflammatory cells (lymphocytes, plasma cells, histiocytes, and eosinophils). Granulomas may also be present. Immunohistochemical staining may be useful in the diagnosis of Hodgkin's disease, particularly in identifying lymphocyte predominant Hodgkin's disease, which is probably a different entity than the other subtypes. Figure 30-10 shows the histologic appearance of Hodgkin's disease primary in lung.

In this review all patients had tissue obtained by thoracotomy, with either open biopsy (59 percent) or resection (41 percent) by pneumonectomy ($n = 9$), lobectomy ($n = 11$), segmentectomy ($n = 2$), or wedge resection ($n = 3$). Whether a diagnosis of Hodgkin's disease can reliably be obtained by percutaneous transthoracic needle biopsy or bronchoscopy is debated among pathologists, although both methods have been used to make this diagnosis (Moralles and Matthews, 1987; Wisecarver, et al., 1989; Flint, et al., 1988). There are even reports of the diagnosis being made by sputum cytology (Reale, et al., 1983).

The therapy of patients with primary Hodgkin's disease of the lung has varied considerably by decade and institution. Of the 61 patients reviewed, 41 percent underwent complete resection of their intrathoracic disease, 39 percent underwent radiotherapy, and 47 percent received chemotherapy; obviously some received combination therapy. Figure 30-11 de-

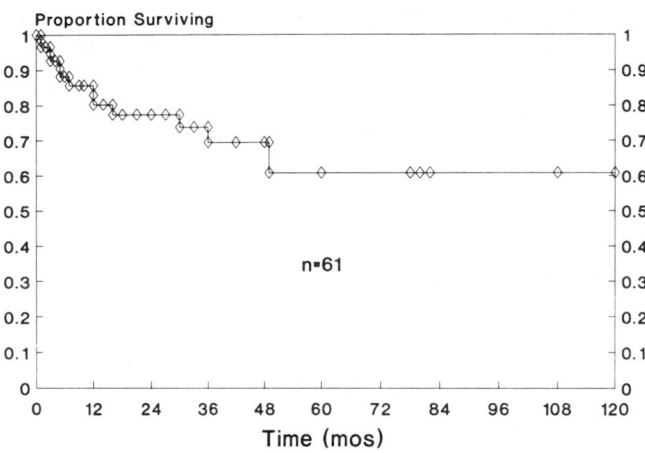

Figure 30-11. Overall actuarial survival of 61 patients with primary Hodgkin's disease of the lung. (Data from Dhingra and Flance, 1970; Guttman and Saavedra, 1968; Kern, et al, 1961; Monahan, 1965; Moralles and Matthews, 1987; Nelson, et al, 1983; Yousem, et al, 1986; and Zulian, et al, 1986.)

picts the overall actuarial survival of 61 patients with primary Hodgkin's disease of the lung; approximately 61 percent were alive at 5 and 10 years. The survival rates of patients with and without B symptoms were compared, and although no significant difference was found ($P = 0.15$), there was a distinct trend in which those who had B symptoms did worse (38 percent alive at 5 years) than those without B symptoms (83 percent alive at 5 years). With regard to therapy, Figure 30-12 is of interest because it depicts the 5-year actuarial survival rate of the 38 patients who received only single-modality therapy. Although limited by the small numbers and the retrospective nature of this review, the importance of local control of primary Hodgkin's disease is evident in this graph. Although there were no significant differences in

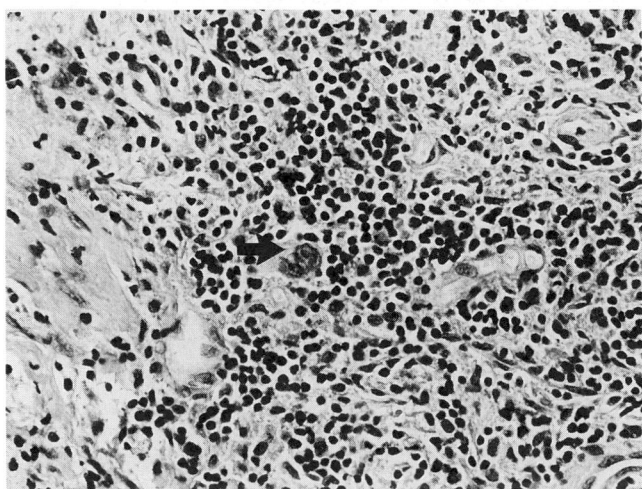

Figure 30-10. Primary Hodgkin's disease of the lung. The diagnosis of Hodgkin's disease anywhere rests on the identification of Reed-Sternberg cells (*arrow*).

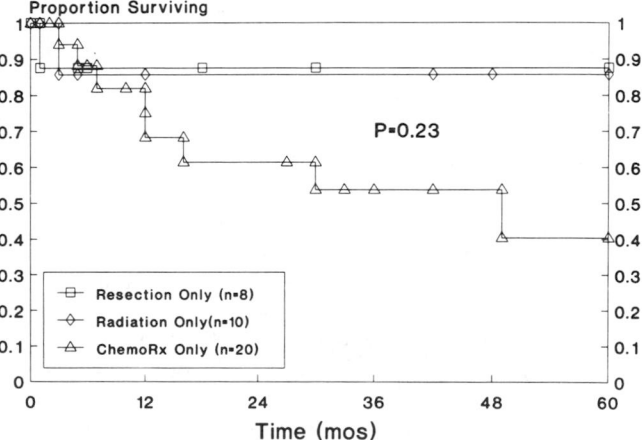

Figure 30-12. Overall actuarial survival of patients with primary Hodgkin's disease of the lung treated with single-modality therapy only. (Data from Dhingra and Flance, 1970; Guttman and Saavedra, 1968; Kern, et al, 1961; Monahan, 1965; Moralles and Matthews, 1987; Nelson, et al, 1983; Yousem, et al, 1986; and Zulian, et al, 1986.)

survival rates ($P = 0.23$) for those treated with surgery alone, radiation therapy alone, and chemotherapy alone, there was a distinct trend that, if chemotherapy was used alone, without effective local control, the patients did worse. Of note 75 percent of the 20 patients receiving chemotherapy received "modern chemotherapy," which is effective against Hodgkin's disease (mechlorethamine, vincristine, procarbazine, and prednisone and/or doxoubicin, bleomycin, vincristine, and decarbazine).

In summary many patients with primary Hodgkin's disease of the lung may have their disease diagnosed during thoracotomy for a "coin" lesion. These patients should undergo formal pulmonary resection with mediastinal lymph node dissection. Other patients may present the diagnostic problem of multiple bilateral or unilateral nodules. Although an attempt at diagnosis by less invasive methods should be made, most undergo open biopsy because transthoracic needle biopsy or bronchoscopy have not been sufficiently accurate in the past. After a diagnosis of pulmonary Hodgkin's disease has been made by biopsy or resection, a diligent search for other sites of disease should be performed. If no other disease is found and the patient's disease stage is confirmed to be IE or IIE, it is recommended that radiation therapy be offered. Whether chemotherapy should be offered to all patients with stage IE or IIE primary Hodgkin's disease of the lung is debatable. It could be argued that patients with bilateral disease in reality have stage IV disease and therefore should be offered chemotherapy as their best hope for long-term survival.

Non-Hodgkin's Lymphoma

The first case of primary non-Hodgkin's lymphoma of the lung was reported by Sugarbaker and Craver (1940) in 1940. Although primary extranodal non-Hodgkin's lymphoma of all sites is not uncommon, comprising 10 percent of 380 consecutive untreated patients with this disease seen at Tufts from 1966 to 1976 (Rudders, et al., 1978), primary non-Hodgkin's lymphoma of the lung is relatively uncommon. In the Tufts series there were no cases of primary extranodal non-Hodgkin's lymphoma arising in the lung, but another large series found that 3.6 percent of extranodal non-Hodgkin's lymphoma occurred in the lung (Freeman, et al., 1972), therefore, primary non-Hodgkin's lymphoma of the lung probably represents 0.4 percent of all patients with this lymphoma. The series from Memorial Sloan-Kettering Cancer Center (1949 to 1982) reported 36 cases of primary non-Hodgkin's lymphoma of the lung. During this period 5,030 patients with non-Hodgkin's lymphoma were seen; thus the estimated frequency of this lymphoma arising in the lung was 0.34 percent of all cases (L'Hoste, et al., 1984).

In a review of the literature from 1940 to 1991, 500 patients with primary non-Hodgkin's lymphoma of the lung were reported (Sugarbaker and Craver, 1940; L'Hoste, et al., 1984; Saltzstein, 1963; Papaiannou and Watson, 1965; Ellison, et al., 1964; Ehrenstein, 1966; Hilbun and Chavez, 1967; Rabiah, 1968; Rubin, 1968; Dahlgren and Ovenfors, 1969; Greenberg, et al., 1972; Mark, 1977; Sinclair, et al., 1978; Sakula, 1979; Marchevsky, et al., 1983; Koss, et al., 1983; LeTourneau, et al., 1983; Herbert, et al., 1984; Turner, et al., 1984; Peterson, et al., 1985; Baas and van Herwaarden,

1986; Reverter, et al., 1987; Asherson, et al., 1987; Ben-Ezra, et al., 1987; Davis and Gadek, 1987; Farquhar, et al., 1988; Tan, et al., 1988; Sprague and deBlois, 1989; Polish, et al., 1989; Hansen, et al., 1989; Poelzleitner, et al., 1989; McCormack and Martini, 1989; Wotherspoon, et al., 1990; Eliasson, et al., 1990; Schwaiger, et al., 1991; Bosanko, et al., 1991; Kennedy, et al., 1985). This included the 90 cases from the literature reviewed by Saltzstein (1963) and Papaiannou (1965) prior to 1963 and 1965, respectively. If these cases are excluded, there have been 410 patients with primary pulmonary non-Hodgkin's lymphoma reported in 36 articles from 1963 to 1991; the median number of patients per report was 2.

In the Memorial series ($n = 36$) (L'Hoste, et al., 1984), 44 percent were asymptomatic, with the abnormality detected by chest radiograph. Of the patients presenting with a complaint, 30 percent had cough, 11 percent had chest pain, 11 percent had malaise, and 7 percent had pneumonia. There were 18 male and 18 female patients (male to female ratio, 1) whose ages ranged from 12 to 75 years (mean, 53 years). The AFIP report (Koss, et al., 1983) listed the chest radiographic findings in 124 patients with primary non-Hodgkin's lymphoma of the lung as (1) solitary nodule in 58 percent, (2) solitary infiltrate in 27 percent, (3) multiple pulmonary nodules in 9 percent, and (4) multiple infiltrates in 6 percent. An occasional radiographic finding in the pulmonary nodules that suggests lymphoma is the presence of an air bronchogram.

Primary non-Hodgkin's lymphoma of the lung is uncommon; it is, however, reported more often in patients with acquired immunodeficiency syndrome (Gibson, et al., 1987). The majority of primary pulmonary non-Hodgkin's lymphoma are of the B-cell type as are the majority of these lymphomas in general. The diagnosis may be made by using fine-needle aspiration or bronchial cytologic examination. The origin of pulmonary non-Hodgkin's lymphoma is probably from the normally present bronchus-associated lymphoid tissue. Grossly the parenchymal lesions of lymphoma are white to tan in color and may be well defined or diffuse. The lymphoma cells are found predominantly in interstitial tissues (Fraser, et al., 1989), and extension into pleura can occur. Tumor necrosis is uncommon. Figure 30-13 shows the proliferation of neoplastic lymphoid cells adjacent to respiratory epithelium.

After a histologic diagnosis of non-Hodgkin's lymphoma is made, the patient should be thoroughly evaluated for any evidence of extrathoracic disease. Once this is completed, the patient's disease is then staged according to a modification of the Ann Arbor Staging Classification (Carbone, et al., 1971; L'Hoste, et al., 1984) as follows: (1) stage IE, lung only involved; (2) stage II1E, lung and hilar nodes involved; (3) stage II2E, lung and mediastinal nodes involved; and (4) Stage II2EW, lung and adjacent chest wall or diaphragm involved.

Although the disease in patients with primary non-Hodgkin's lymphoma of the lung can be histologically classified by one of the four classification systems [Rappaport (Rappaport, 1966), Lukes-Collins (Lukes and Collins, 1974), Kiel (Lennert) (Lennert, 1978), or the International Working Formulation (Non-Hodgkin's Lymphoma Pathologic Classification Project, 1982)], a simpler approach is to group the disease

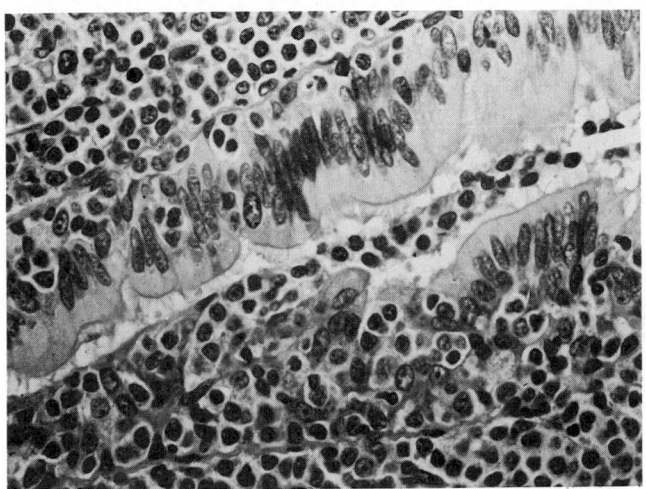

Figure 30-13. Primary non-Hodgkin's lymphoma of the lung. The round monotonous-appearing lymphoma cells are pushing up and infiltrating respiratory epithelium.

in patients with primary non-Hodgkin's lymphoma of the lung into small cell (lymphocytic) and large cell (histiocytic) lymphomas for simplicity and treatment planning. In the Memorial experience (L'Hoste, et al., 1984), 58 percent of the disease in these patients would be classified as small cell lymphoma and 42 percent, as large cell. Of those with small cell lymphomas, 90 percent had a complete resection, and 10 percent had a biopsy only. In this group 35 percent received chemotherapy. Of this group of small cell non-Hodgkin's lymphomas, only 40 percent recurred. In the large cell non-Hodgkin's lymphoma group, only 33 percent underwent resection, and 67 percent had biopsies only. However, 89 percent of this group received chemotherapy. The recurrence rate was 50 percent in this group. The overall survival rates for the 21 small and 15 large cell non-Hodgkin's lymphomas is shown in Figure 30-14. There was an 87 percent 5-year

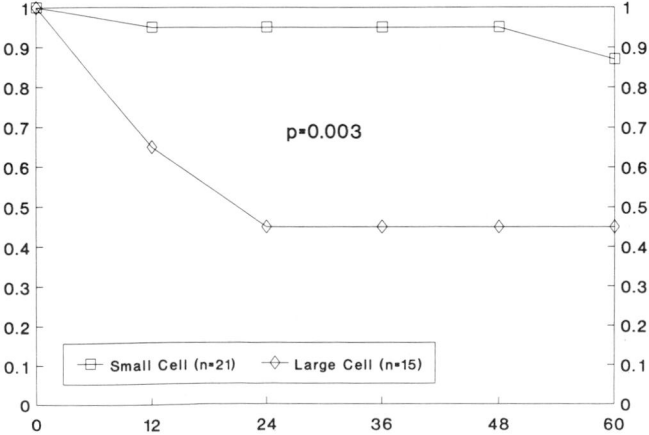

Figure 30-14. Survival of patients with primary small and large cell non-Hodgkin's lymphoma of the lung. (Adapted from L'Hoste RJ, Filippa DA, Lieberman PH, Bretsky S: Primary pulmonary lymphomas: a clinicopathologic analysis of 36 cases. Cancer 54:1397, 1984, with permission.)

survival rate for those patients with primary small cell non-Hodgkin's lymphoma of the lung compared with a 45 percent 5-year survival rate for the large cell type. Similar survival rates were documented by other authors (Freeman, et al., 1972; Saltzstein, 1963; Koss, et al., 1983; Turner, et al., 1984).

In summary primary non-Hodgkin's lymphoma of the lung usually presents in the 40- to 60-year-old patient with an asymptomatic pulmonary nodule. After the extent of the disease is evaluated, these patients should undergo resection. Patients with large cell non-Hodgkin's lymphoma should receive chemotherapy added to their therapeutic plan. Patients with stage IE small cell non-Hodgkin's lymphoma of the lung may be watched expectantly, but those with stage IIE should probably be offered chemotherapy.

Solitary Plasmacytoma

Malignant plasma cell neoplasms are a group of related disorders, each of which is characterized by the proliferation of plasma cells, which are immunoglobulin-secreting cells derived from B-cell immunocytes. The most common of these malignant plasma cell neoplasms is multiple myeloma, which represents approximately 1 to 2 percent of all malignant neoplasms in the United States. A small fraction of patients (4 percent) present with solitary malignant plasma cell neoplasms of soft tissues, which is termed extramedullary plasmacytoma (Woodruff, et al., 1979). Most extramedullary plasmacytomas present in the nasopharynx, upper respiratory tract, and oropharynx. Primary plasmacytoma of the lung is extremely uncommon. In a review of six collected series, only 4 percent (13 of 352 patients) of extramedullary plasmacytomas occurred in the lung (Woodruff, et al., 1979; Wiltshaw, 1976; Corwin and Lindberg, 1979; Knowling, et al., 1983; Meis, et al., 1987; Holland, et al., 1992).

The first reported case of an extramedullary plasmacytoma of the lung was by Gordon and Walker (1944) in 1944. In a review of the English literature since then, there have been 12 cases reported in which sufficient data were available for analysis (Childress and Adie, 1950; Hill and White, 1953; Kernen and Meyer, 1966; Mazumdar, et al., 1969; Wile, et al., 1976; Baroni, et al., 1977; Amin, 1985; Kennedy and Kneafsey, 1959; Cotton and Penido, 1952; Rozsa and Frieman, 1953). It appears that primary plasmacytoma of the lung occurs more frequently in men (male to female ratio, 2). The ages of these patients ranged from 3 to 72 years (median, 43 years). Eleven of these patients were treated with pulmonary resections (eight lobectomies and three pneumonectomies), and in three of these, radiation therapy was also added. In one chemotherapy was added. One patient underwent a biopsy followed by radiotherapy and chemotherapy. The actuarial survival curve is depicted in Figure 30-15. The overall 5-year survival rate was 40 percent, and this probably reflects the small number of patients and the limited follow-up reported (median, 11 months; range, 1 to 96 months) because nine are alive and well and the three who died did so of unrelated causes. Of note two patients (17 percent) developed multiple myeloma 7 and 26 months after resection.

Primary pulmonary plasmacytoma can present as a parenchymal, endotracheal, or endobronchial lesion. Endotracheal lesions can be responsible for airway obstruction, and endo-

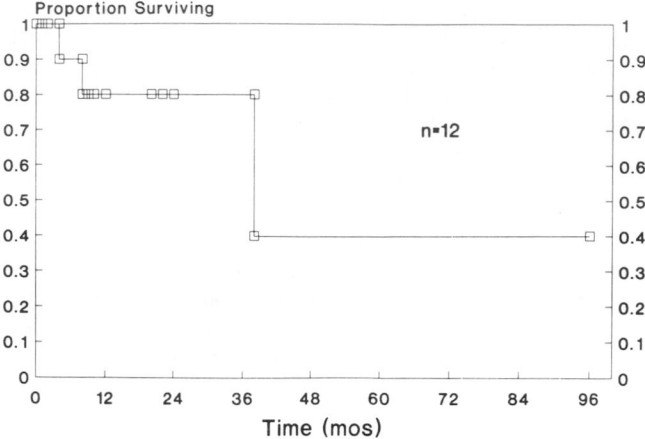

Figure 30-15. Overall actuarial survival of patients with primary extramedullary plasmacytomas of the lung. (Data from Amin, 1985; Baroni, et al, 1977; Childress and Adie, 1950; Cotton and Penido, 1952; Hill and White, 1953; Kennedy and Kneafsey, 1959; Kernen and Meyer, 1966; Mazumdar, et al, 1969; Rozza and Frieman, 1953; and Wile, et al, 1976.)

bronchial lesions can cause atelectasis or pneumonitis (Mazumder, et al., 1969). Microscopically the tumor consists of sheets of atypical plasma cells, identical to those of multiple myeloma. Ossification can occur (Kinare, et al., 1965). Amorphous eosinophilic material representing immunoglobulin or amyloid may be present (Morinaga, et al., 1987). This tumor must be distinguished from a plasmacytoid B-cell lymphoma, and immunohistochemical stains for immunoglobulins may be helpful. Most pulmonary plasmacytomas are not associated with abnormal serum or urine immunoglobulin levels (Fraser, et al., 1989). Figure 30-16 depicts the plasma cells and amorphous immunoglobulin deposits in plasmacytomas.

In summary extramedullary plasmacytoma of the lung is exceptionally rare. If found during thoracotomy, a resection

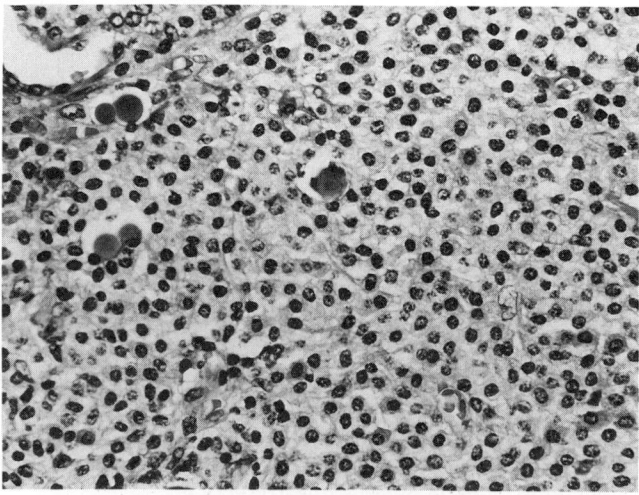

Figure 30-16. Primary plasmacytoma of the lung. Note the monomorphic plasma cells with a cartwheel chromatin pattern and the rounded deposits of immunoglobulin.

should be performed for local control. If no other sites of disease are found, if serum electrophoresis is normal, and if Bence Jones proteinuria is absent, these patients should be followed expectantly but closely. In a larger series of extramedullary plasmacytoma or solitary plasmacytoma of the bone, approximately 40 to 60 percent of patients eventually developed multiple myeloma (Woodruff, et al., 1979; Wiltshaw, 1976; Corwin and Lindberg, 1979; Knowling, et al., 1983; Meis, et al., 1987; Holland, et al., 1992) and then considered for systemic therapy with alkylating agents.

PRIMARY MALIGNANT MELANOMA OF THE LUNG

Primary malignant melanoma at any site except the skin, eye, juxtacutaneous mucous membranes, and leptomeninges is extremely uncommon. Primary malignant melanoma of the lung is truly rare. The generally accepted criteria for a primary pulmonary melanoma are (1) the absence of a current or previous primary melanoma elsewhere or the absence of a previously resected or cauterized cutaneous lesion of unknown type, (2) no ocular tumor resection, (3) a solitary tumor in the surgical specimen from the lung, (4) tumor morphology consistent with a primary melanoma, (5) no demonstrable melanoma in other organs at time of operation, and (6) autopsy findings without primary malignant melanomas being demonstrated elsewhere (Jensen and Egedorf, 1967).

The first reported case of primary malignant melanoma of the lung has often been attributed to Todd (1888) in 1888. Subsequent cases were then reported by Kunkel and Torrey (1916), Carlucci and Schleussner (1942), and Allen and Spitz (1953). Although some believe these cases were truly primary pulmonary melanomas, others believe that there was not enough evidence to support this and consider the first adequately documented case of primary melanoma of lung to be that reported by Salm (1963) in 1963.

During a search of the English literature since Salm's report in 1963, 12 cases of primary malignant melanoma of lung were found and analyzed (Jensen and Egedorf, 1967; Salm, 1963; Reed and Kent, 1964; Reid and Mehta, 1966; Allen and Drash, 1968; Taboada, et al., 1972; Robertson, et al., 1980; Cagle, et al., 1984; Alghanem, et al., 1987; Bagwell, et al., 1989). There were six men and six women (male to female ratio, 1), whose ages ranged from 40 to 80 years (median, 58 years). Approximately 25 percent were asymptomatic; the rest had cough, hemoptysis, chest pain, dyspnea, or pneumonia. No predilection for side or upper or lower lobes was present. The tumors ranged in size from 1.0 to 10.0 cm in diameter (median, 4.0 cm). Two (17 percent) were endobronchial. Eleven patients (92 percent) underwent complete resection (six by lobectomy, three by pneumonectomy, one by segmentectomy, and one by wedge resection); one received only radiation therapy after the biopsy. The overall actuarial survival curve for these 12 patients is depicted in Figure 30-17. The 5-year survival rate was 46 percent, with a median survival of 24 months. Those who died did so of distant metastases (brain, liver, bone, adrenal, heart, and/or lung).

Cutaneous or mucosal malignant melanoma can spontaneously regress (Mackay, et al., 1990), and some authors believe that the diagnosis of primary pulmonary melanoma of the lung cannot be made unless the lesion is located in the bronchial

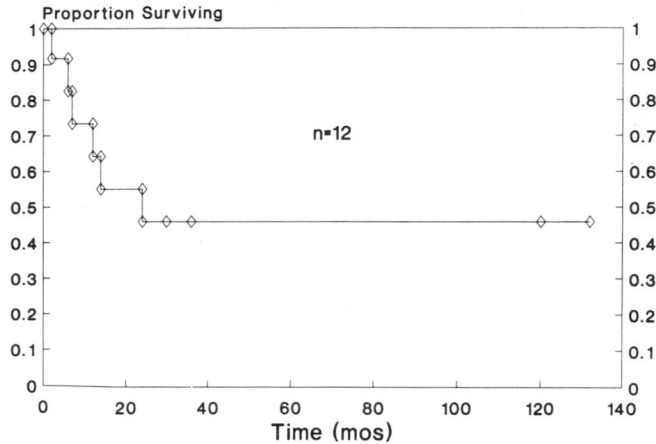

Figure 30-17. Overall actuarial survival of patients with primary malignant melanomas of the lung. (Data from Alghanem, et al, 1987; Allen and Drash, 1953; Cagle, et al, 1984; Carstens, et al, 1984; Jensen and Egedorf, 1967; Reed and Kent, 1964; Reid and Mehta, 1966; Robertson, et al, 1980; Salm, 1963; and Taboada, et al, 1972.)

epithelium only (Taboada, et al., 1972; Robertson, et al,. 1980; Cagle, et al., 1984; Bagwell, et al., 1989; Carstens, et al., 1984; Gepharat, 1981). Some investigators think that pulmonary melanoma may be derived from cells of the primitive foregut that migrate to the tracheobronchial tree in fetal life (Jensen and Egedorf, 1967; Salm, 1963; Robertson, et al., 1980; Cagle, et al., 1984).

The histologic appearance of malignant melanoma of the lung is identical to that of a metastatic melanoma at any site. Large pleomorphic cells, sometimes with prominent necleoli, can be seen. Intranuclear inclusions may be present, and a search for pigment should be made. Immunohistochemical stains and electron microscopy may be helpful. Figure 30-18 depicts the histologic appearance of primary pulmonary malignant melanoma.

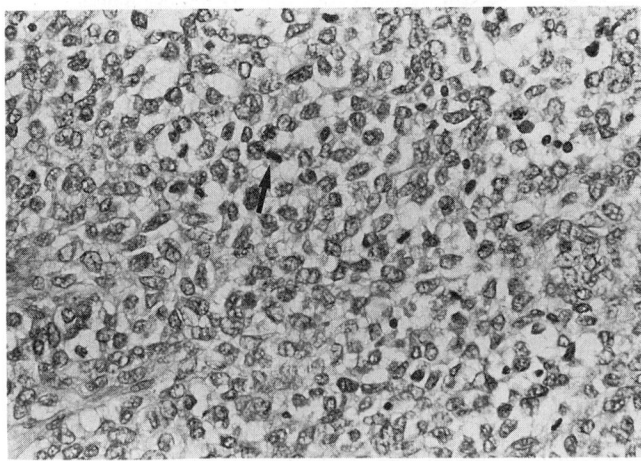

Figure 30-18. Primary malignant melanoma of the lung. This melanoma has a monotonous almost bland appearance with many mitotic figures (*arrow*). When melanoma cells are not pigmented, immunohistochemical stains are helpful in making the diagnosis.

In summary primary melanoma of the lung presents as a solitary nodule. The evaluation and therapy should be identical to those of a patient with nonsmall cell lung cancer, but an extensive examination of the skin, eyes, and mucosa, including the pharynx, vagina, esophagus, and anal canal, should be conducted in an attempt to locate a possible primary site elsewhere.

PRIMARY MALIGNANT GERM CELL TUMORS

Primary malignant germ cell tumors of the lung are exceedingly rare. Two types have been described: malignant teratoma and choriocarcinoma.

Malignant Teratoma

Benign intrapulmonary teratomas, some occurring endobronchially (Jamieson and McGowan, 1982), are exceedingly uncommon, with only 20 documented cases by 1978 (Day and Taylor, 1975; Holt, et al., 1978). Primary malignant teratoma of the lung is truly rare. A review of the literature yielded four patients with enough information to confirm the diagnosis of a malignant intrapulmonary teratoma (Ruland, 1956; Schiodt and Jensen, 1960; Gautam, 1969; Pound and Willis, 1969). The case of Barrett and Barnard (1945) has been recorded in multiple reviews as a malignant teratoma, but in actuality it has been classified by Spencer (1961) as a pulmonary blastoma. In the report of Ruland (1956), little clinical information is presented. The case of Schiodt and Jensen (1960) was a 66-year-old man who underwent an apicoposterior segmentectomy of the left upper lobe for a "walnut-sized" malignant teratoma. The patient had a recurrence locally and died approximately 1 year after the operation. The case of Gautam (1969) was a 68-year-old man who underwent a pneumonectomy for a 5-cm malignant teratoma with an endobronchial component completely obstructing the left upper lobe bronchus. No follow-up after discharge was presented. The case of Pound and Willis (1969) was a 10-month-old boy who presented with supraclavicular lymphadenopathy, which on biopsy revealed an undifferentiated large cell carcinoma. There was complete opacification of the right chest. He died 6 days after admission, and the autopsy revealed a 9-cm malignant teratoma within the right lower lobe with associated hilar and mediastinal lymph node metastases.

Pulmonary teratomas may represent extensions of a mediastinal tumor into the lung parenchyma. Intraparenchymal tumors are more common than endobronchial ones (Jamieson and McGowan, 1982). Histologically endodermal-, ectodermal-, and mesodermal-derived tissue is present, usually in a cystic mass, and pancreatic tissue may be identified.

In summary primary intrapulmonary malignant teratoma is exceptionally rare. Its presentation mimics that of a nonsmall cell lung cancer, and therapy should be directed similarly.

Choriocarcinoma

Although the secretion of human chorionic gonadotropin is not uncommon in primary bronchogenic carcinoma (Muggia, et al., 1975; Hattori, et al., 1979; Miyake, et al., 1987; Fukuda, et al., 1990), occurring in approximately 6 percent of lung cancers (Braunstein, et al., 1973), primary extragonadal choriocarcinoma of the lung is extremely uncommon. In a review of the literature in 1962, Fine, et al. (1962) could document no case of primary choriocarcinoma of the lung in the 109 reported cases of primary extragonadal choriocarcinoma in male patients.

The first reported case of primary choriocarcinoma of the lung was by Gerber (1935) in 1935. Since then, at least eight other cases have been reported (Berman, 1940; Kay and Reed, 1953; Gerin-Lajore, 1954; Zapatero, et al., 1982; Tanimura, et al., 1985; Pushchak and Farhi, 1987; Sullivan, 1989; Sridhar, et al., 1989). Of these nine cases, six were female patients, and three were male (male to female ratio, 0.33). Their ages ranged from 7 months to 67 years (median, 37 years). Of note, six patients (67 percent) presented with hemoptysis. Six patients underwent pulmonary resection (four by pneumonectomy and two by lobectomy). Two of the patients died postoperatively following pneumonectomy. Of note one patient died after a biopsy during bronchoscopy from profuse endobronchial bleeding. Of the remaining six patients, four died of disease at 1, 4, 4, and 15 months after the diagnosis, with metastases to the brain, liver, lung, and/or spleen. The remaining two patients are alive and well at 6 and 36 months after lobectomy. One patient, who later died of disease, had a partial response to chemotherapy (5-fluorouracil, etoposide, and cisplatin) (Sridhar, et al., 1989).

Choriocarcinoma may be misdiagnosed as adenocarcinoma, and the presence of immunohistochemical staining for human chorionic gonadotropin or α-fetoprotein (or the presence of the serum elevation of these proteins) may be necessary to make the diagnosis.

In summary primary extragonadal choriocarcinoma of the lung is exceptionally uncommon. It usually presents as a large, solitary lesion and appears to be a vascular tumor because 67 percent of patients presented with hemoptysis and one patient died of hemorrhage after a bronchoscopic biopsy.

PRIMARY SARCOMA OF THE LUNG

Primary malignant mesenchymal tumors (sarcomas), although rare, can arise in the lung, just as they do in all other anatomic sites. Most reports of primary sarcomas of the lung describe soft tissue sarcomas, but primary chondrosarcomas and osteosarcomas, although even rarer, do occur.

Chondrosarcoma

Primary extraskeletal chondrosarcoma of the lung is an extremely uncommon entity. Utilizing the rigid criteria of Morgan and Salama (1972), only 10 well-documented cases were available for review (Greenspan, 1933; Bini, 1942; Lowell and Tuhy, 1949; Sedlezky, 1955; Filho and Pasqualucci, 1963; Daniels, et al., 1967; Rees, 1970; Sun, et al., 1982; Yellin, et al., 1983). Of these there were four men and six women (male to female ratio, 0.7), whose ages ranged from 23 to 74 years (median, 44 years). The majority presented with cough. Two had hemoptysis, and two had chest pain. All presented with a solitary, usually large, pulmonary mass. Of those 10 patients, 3 received no therapy and died of locoregional disease

at 6, 6, and 20 months following the onset of symptoms. Seven patients underwent resection (two by pneumonectomy, three by lobectomy, one by wedge resection, and one by endobronchial resection). Of those resected one died of metastatic disease to the lung 24 months after the lobectomy. The remaining six patients were alive and well 1 to 48 months following resection. Of note two patients (20 percent) had metastases to their mediastinal lymph nodes.

As noted by Morgan and Salama (1972), primary extraskeletal chondrosarcoma of the lung presents as a solitary well-circumscribed slow-growing tumor that, if left untreated, may spread within the thorax and cause death. Distant metastases are uncommon (10 percent). If diagnosed preoperatively these tumors should be resected because resection appears to translate to long-term survival. Because 20 percent of these tumors have metastasized to mediastinal lymph nodes, a mediastinal lymph node dissection at the time of resection appears to be advisable.

Primary pulmonary chondrosarcoma may be derived from tracheobronchial cartilage, but an origin from bronchial chondroma or hamartoma is possible (Fraser, et al., 1989). Grossly the tumor may appear to be a round lobulated mass within the lung (Morgan and Salama, 1972). The histologic appearance is of plump, somewhat pleomorphic chondrocytes, some showing binucleation. Calcification or ossification may be present (Morgan and Salama, 1972).

Osteosarcoma

Primary osteosarcoma of the lung is extremely rare. In two of the largest series of extraosseous osteosarcomas, no cases of primary osteosarcoma of the lung were reported (Fine and Stout, 1956; Sordillo, et al., 1983). In a review of the literature, only seven cases were considered primary osteosarcoma of the lung (Yamashita, et al., 1964; Nosanchuk and Weatherbee, 1969; Reingold and Amromin, 1971; Nascimento, et al., 1982; Colby, et al., 1989). Of these seven patients, there were four men and three women, whose ages ranged from 51 to 77 years (median, 62 years). Most patients presented with cough; one had hemoptysis. All lesions were solitary by chest radiography, and most were greater than 4 cm in diameter. Of the seven reported patients, two received no therapy and with a follow-up of only 1 month, one died of disease, and one was alive with disease. One patient was treated with cyclophosphamide and died 6 months after the start of therapy secondary to neutropenia and sepsis. Of the four patients who underwent resection (one by pneumonectomy and three by lobectomy), one patient was alive and well at 6 months, one was alive with disease at 14 months, and two died of unrelated causes at 4 and 6 months. Of note three of the seven developed distant metastases (lung in two and liver in one). In addition, two patients developed hilar lymph node metastases, both of whom also had distant metastases.

Histologically spindle cells with myxoid, chondroid, or osteoid tissue are present. The osteoid must be cytologically malignant and must be present to make the diagnosis of osteosarcoma.

In summary primary osteogenic sarcoma of the lung presents as a large solitary lesion on chest radiography. If no distant disease is documented, resection appears to be the treatment of choice. Because 29 percent of these patients had hilar lymph node metastases, a mediastinal lymph node dissection appears advisable.

Soft Tissue Sarcoma

Primary soft tissue sarcomas of the lung are rare. In a review of the experience at Memorial Sloan-Kettering Cancer Center, Martini, et al. (1971) reported on 22 patients with primary soft tisue sarcomas who were evaluated over a 42-year period (1926 to 1968). During that time, 5,714 patients with primary lung cancer were seen, a relative incidence of primary pulmonary sarcoma to lung cancer of 0.4 percent. When reviewing the literature, the descriptions of patients with "primary sarcoma of the lung" prior to 1975 are confusing. Many reports, such as those of Hochberg and Crastnopol (1955), include the lymphoproliferative disorders under the term *sarcoma*. In Hochberg and Crastnopol's (1955) review of 77 "primary sarcomas of the bronchus and lung," 44 (57 percent) were soft tissue sarcomas, 26 (34 percent) were lymphoproliferative disorders (including Hodgkin's disease, lymphosarcoma, malignant lymphoma, and reticulum cell sarcoma), 5 (6 percent) were carcinosarcomas, and 2 (3 percent) werc chondrosarcomas. However, since 1931 at least 221 primary soft tissue sarcomas of lung have been reported (Nascimento, et al., 1982; Martini, et al., 1971; Hochberg and Crestnopol, 1955; Ball, 1931; Carswell and Kraeft, 1949; Neilson, 1958; Bartley and Arean, 1965; Conquest, et al., 1965; Caves and Jacques, 1971; Crane and Sutton, 1972; Guccion and Rosen, 1972; Kalus, et al., 1973; Meade, et al., 1974; Cameron, 1975; Ueda, et al., 1977; Bedrossian, et al., 1979; Kern, et al., 1979; Chowdhury, et al., 1980; Thomas, et al., 1981; Gebauer, 1982; Wick, et al., 1982; Eriksson, et al., 1982; Spragg, et al., 1983; Shuman, 1984; Lee, et al., 1984; Avagnina, et al., 1984; Silverman and Coalson, 1984; Van Assendelft, et al., 1984; Pedersen, et al., 1984; Goldthorn, et al., 1986; Venn, et al., 1986; Beluffi, et al., 1986; Capewell, et al., 1986; Yousem, 1986; Allan, et al., 1987; Ott, et al., 1987; Yousem and Hochholzer, 1987a, 1987b; McDonnell, et al., 1988; Shariff, et al., 1988; Pettinato, et al., 1989; Rusch, et al., 1989). The number of patients per report is small, ranging from 1 to 42 patients per report (median, 1). The largest single report was by McCormack and Martini (1989). The raw data from the 42 patients in this report from Memorial Sloan-Kettering Cancer Center were reanalyzed and, because they are representative of other reports in the literature, are presented below.

Of the 42 patients with primary soft tissue sarcomas of the lung, 19 were male, and 23 were female (male to female ratio, 0.8), whose ages ranged from 1.5 to 78 years (median, 52 years). Approximately 25 percent of patients were asymptomatic, and the lesions were detected by routine chest radiograph. Seven patients (17 percent) presented with hemoptysis. The remaining patients presented with cough, dyspnea, chest pain, and/or systemic symptoms, such as fatigue, malaise, fever, or weight loss. All lesions were solitary masses, the diameter of which ranged in size from 1 to 17 cm (median, 5.5 cm).

The histologic subtypes of soft tissue sarcomas in these 42 patients are listed in Table 30-3. Although not specified, the

Table 30-3. Primary Soft Tissue Sarcomas of the Lung

Histology	No.	%
Leiomyosarcoma	16	38
Spindle cell sarcoma	13	31
Rhabdomyosarcoma	5	12
Malignant fibrous histiocytoma	3	7
Angiosarcoma	2	5
Fibrosarcoma	2	5
Malignant hemangiopericytoma	1	2
Total	42	

(Adapted from McCormack PM, Martini N: Primary sarcomas and lymphomas of lung. p. 269. In Martini N, Vogt-Moykopf I (eds): Thoracic Surgery: Frontiers and Uncommon Neoplasms. Vol. 5. CV Mosby, St. Louis, 1989, with permission.)

spindle cell sarcomas probably contain a number of malignant peripheral nerve tumors.

Twenty-nine (69 percent) of these patients underwent resection of their primary pulmonary soft tissue sarcomas (15 by lobectomy, 7 by pneumonectomy, 6 by wedge resection, and 1 by segmentectomy). Of those not resected, five received no therapy, six received radiation therapy, and two received radiation and chemotherapy.

The overall survival curve for these 42 patients with primary soft tissue sarcomas of thc lung is depicted in Figure 30-19. The overall 1-, 3-, and 5-year survival rates were 55, 31, and 25 percent, respectively, with a median of 13 months. In the report from the Mayo Clinic (Nascimento, et al., 1982), size was thought to have an impact on survival. In the Memorial Sloan-Kettering Cancer Center experience, although not significant, there was a distinct trend in which survival was better in patients with tumors less than or equal to 5 cm compared with those with tumors greater than 5 cm (Fig. 30-20).

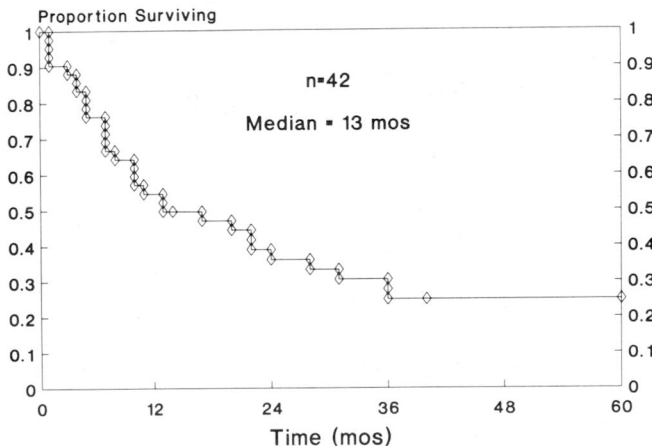

Figure 30-19. Overall actuarial survival of patients with primary soft tissue sarcomas of the lung. (Adapted from McCormack PM, Martini N: Primary sarcomas and lymphomas of lung. p. 269. In Martini N, Vogt-Moykopf (eds): Thoracic Surgery: Frontiers and Uncommon Neoplasms. Vol. 5. CV Mosby, St. Louis, 1989, with permission.)

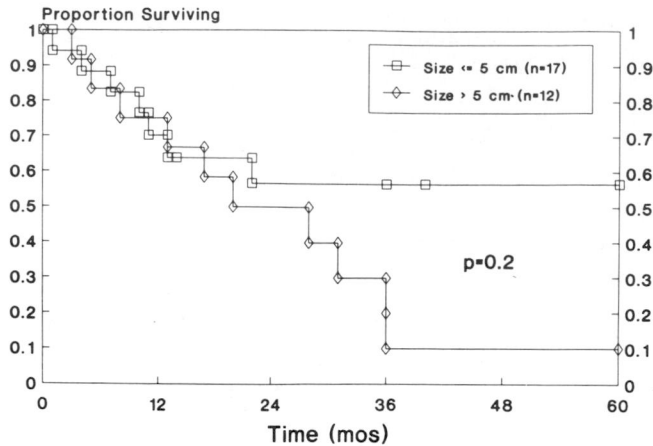

Figure 30-20. Actuarial survival of those patients with primary soft tissue sarcomas of the lung less than or equal to 5 cm compared with those with tumors greater than 5 cm. (Adapted from McCormack PM, Martini N: Primary sarcomas and lymphomas of lung. p. 269. In Martini N, Vogt-Moykopf (eds): Thoracic Surgery: Frontiers and Uncommon Neoplasms. Vol. 5. CV Mosby, St. Louis, 1989, with permission.)

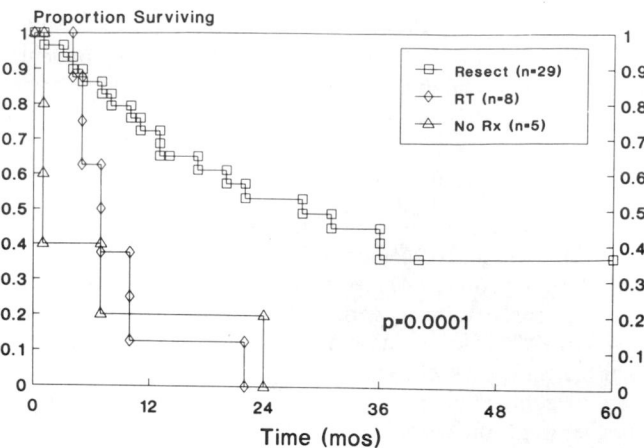

Figure 30-22. Actuarial survival of patients with soft tissue sarcomas undergoing resection, radiation therapy, or no therapy. (Adapted from McCormack PM, Martini N: Primary sarcomas and lymphomas of lung. p. 269. In Martini N, Vogt-Moykopf (eds): Thoracic Surgery: Frontiers and Uncommon Neoplasms. Vol. 5. CV Mosby, St. Louis, 1989, with permission.)

Malignant fibrous histiocytoma is the most common soft tissue sarcoma. The histologic classification of this sarcoma dates back only about 20 years, and it is possible that pulmonary sarcomas previously diagnosed as fibrosarcomas, leiomyosarcomas, myxosarcomas, or unclassified sarcomas would be called malignant fibrous histiocytomas today (Fraser, et al., 1989). Four histologic subtypes are described: (1) storiform pleomorphic, (2) myxoid, (3) giant cell, and (4) inflammatory (Weiss, 1982). Storiform pleomorphic is most common within the lung (Yousem and Hochholzer, 1987a). This consists of bundles of spindle cells arranged in a cartwheel or "storiform" pattern. Present in this background are pleomorphic, often giant cells, with many mitotic figures. The histologic appearance of this spindle cell neoplasm is demonstarted in Figure 30-21.

The most important predictor of survival is complete resection of the primary tumor. Figure 30-22 depicts the actuarial survival of the 29 patients undergoing resection of their primary soft tissue sarcomas of the lung compared with that of the 8 receiving radiation therapy (2 also had chemotherapy) and the 5 receiving no therapy. The patients undergoing resection survived significantly longer (36 percent alive at 5 years) than those receiving radiation therapy or no therapy (no one survived longer than 2 years).

In summary primary pulmonary soft tissue sarcomas may present in all decades of life as solitary pulmonary nodules. After they are diagnosed, it appears that complete resection translates into a survival benefit.

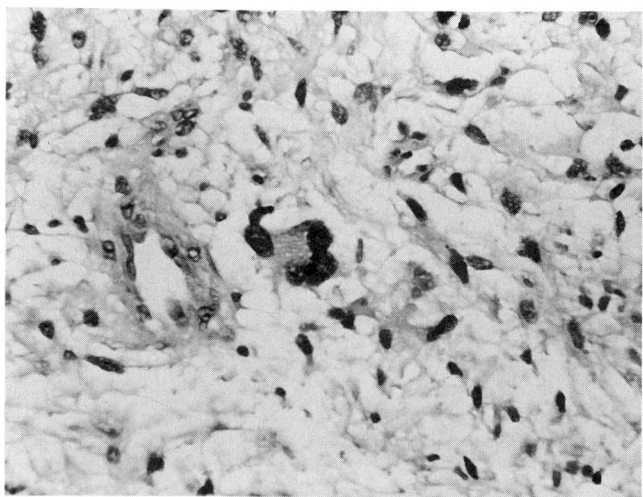

Figure 30-21. Primary malignant fibrous histiocytoma of the lung. Large pleomorphic cells are visible in a background of spindle cells.

MISCELLANEOUS MALIGNANT TUMORS

There have been case reports of primary ependymoma (Crotty, et al., 1992), Ewing's sarcoma (Palmer, et al., 1981), lymphoepithelioma-like carcinoma (Miller, et al., 1991), and pseudomesotheliomatous carcinoma (Dessy and Pietra, 1991) of the lung. Because of the scarcity of data on these extraordinarily rare primary malignant tumors of the lung, the reader is referred to these references for more information.

COMMENTS AND CONTROVERSIES

This indeed is the ultimate compendium of the rare primary malignant neoplasms that can be found in the lung. Dr. Burt has reviewed virtually the entire English literature on each tumor, thereby summarizing the knowledge to date. As with benign tumors, most of these lesions will be encountered very infrequently by any single thoracic surgeon. For this reason, the most effective therapy for each of these lesions has not been well documented. An example of this dilemma is seen in pulmonary lymphomas. Although we continue to offer resection to all patients diagnosed with pulmonary lymphomas, it is unknown whether surgical resection is required to effect curative therapy. Like lymphomas elsewhere, these tumors are chemoresponsive and also respond to radiotherapy. However, with the present state of knowledge, it appears that where possible, total surgical excision is still the mainstay of treatment for all of these unusual tumors.

R.J.G.

KEY REFERENCES

Amin R: Extramedullary plasmacytoma of the lung. Cancer 56:152, 1985

This report describes three patients with primary plasmacytomas of the lung and summarizes the literature in a succinct fashion.

Bagwell SP, Flynn SD, Cox PM, Davison JA: Primary malignant melanoma of the lung. Am Rev Respir Dis 139:1543, 1989

This is a case report of one patient with primary malignant melanoma of the lung. It is also the best review of the literature available.

Colby TB, Bilbao JE, Battifora H, Unni K: Primary osteosarcoma of lung: a reappraisal following immunohistologic study. Arch Pathol Lab Med 113:1147, 1989

This report from the Mayo Clinic describes three patients with primary osteosarcomas of the lung and reviews the limited literature in detail.

Dail DH, Liebow AA, Gmelich JT et al: Intravascular, bronchiolar, and alveolar tumor of the lung (IVBAT): an analysis of twenty cases of a peculiar sclerosing endothelial tumor. Cancer 51:452, 1983

This report summarizes the collected series of 20 patients with IVBAT from the AFIP. It is the largest report in the literature.

Davis MP, Eagan RT, Weiland LH, Pairolero PC: Carcinosarcoma of the lung: Mayo Clinic experience and response to chemotherapy. Mayo Clin Proc 59:598, 1984

This is the largest report about carcinosarcomas of the lung from a single institution. It describes the clinical findings of 17 patients from the Mayo clinic and details the clinical presentation, therapy, and outcome.

Koss MN, Hochholzer L, O'Leary T: Pulmonary blastomas. Cancer 67:2368, 1991

This is the largest report about pulmonary blastomas from a single institution. It describes the clinical and pathologic findings in a collected series of 52 patients from the AFIP.

L'Hoste RJ, Filippa DA, Lieberman PH, Bretsky S: Primary pulmonary lymphomas: a clinicopathologic analysis of 36 cases. Cancer 54:1397, 1984

This report, which is the largest reported series from a single institution, describes the presentation, therapy, and clinical outcome of 79 patients seen at Memorial Sloan-Kettering Cancer Center.

McCormack PM, Martini N: Primary sarcomas and lymphomas of lung. p. 269. In Martini N, Vogt-Moykopf I (eds): Thoracic Surgery: Frontiers and Uncommon Neoplasms. Vol. 5. CV Mosby, St. Louis, 1989

This report from Memorial Sloan-Kettering Cancer Center reviews the clinical presentation, therapy, and outcome of 42 patients with primary soft tissue sarcomas of the lung.

Pound AW, Willis RA: A malignant teratoma of the lung in an infant. J Pathol 98:111, 1969

This report reviews the literature on primary malignant teratoma of the lung, of which there are few reports.

Sridhar KS, Saldana MJ, Thurer RJ, Beattie EJ: Primary choriocarcinoma of the lung: report of a case treated with intensive multimodality therapy and review of the literature. J Surg Oncol 41:94, 1989

This report describes one patient with primary choriocarcinoma of the lung. It also is an excellent review of the sparse data available in the literature.

Yellin A, Schwartz L, Hersho E, Lieberman Y: Chondrosarcoma of the bronchus: report of a case with resection and review of the literature. Chest 84:224, 1983

This report describes a patient with a primary chondrosarcoma of the lung and reviews the limited literature available on this rare neoplasm.

Yousem SA, Weiss LM, Colby TV: Primary pulmonary Hodgkin's disease: a clinicopathologic study of 15 cases. Cancer 57:1217, 1986

This report from Stanford University is the largest single institutional series of primary Hodgkin's disease of the lung. The clinical data of 15 patients are reviewed, as is the literature.

REFERENCES

Addis BJ, Corrin B: Pulmonary blastoma, carcinosarcoma and spindle-cell carcinoma: an immunohistochemical study of keratin intermediate filaments. J Pathol 147:291, 1985

Albeda RW, Monenaar WH, deLey L, This-Ipema AH: Heterogene-ity of Wilms' tumor blastoma. An immunohistological study. Virchows Arch A Pathol Anat Histopathol 414:263, 1989

Alghanem AA, Mehan J, Hassan AA: Primary malignant melanoma of the lung. J Surg Oncol 34:109, 1987

Allan BT, Day DL, Dehner LP: Primary pulmonary rhabdomyosarcoma of the lung in children: report of two cases presenting with spontaneous pneumothorax. Cancer 59:1005, 1987

Allen AC, Spitz S: Malignant melanoma. A clinicopathological analysis of the criteria for diagnosis and prognosis. Cancer 6:1, 1953

Allen MS, Drash EC: Primary melanoma of the lung. Cancer 21:154, 1968

Amin R: Extramedullary plasmacytoma of the lung. Cancer 56:152, 1985

Asherson RA, Muncey F, Pambakian H et al: Sjögren's syndrome and fibrosing alveolitis complicated by pulmonary lymphoma. Ann Rheum Dis 46:701, 1987

Ashworth TG: Pulmonary blastoma, a true congenital neoplasm. Histopathology 7:585, 1983

Avagnina A, Elsner B, DeMarco L et al: Pulmonary rhabdomyosarcoma with isolated small bowel metastasis: a report of a case with immunohistochemical and ultrastructural studies. Cancer 53:1948, 1984

Azumi N, Churg A: Intravascular and sclerosing bronchioalveolar tumor: a pulmonary sarcoma of probable vascular origin. Am J Surg Pathol 5:587, 1981

Baas AAF, van Herwaarden CLA: Primary non-Hodgkin's lymphoma of the lung. Eur J Respir Dis 68:218, 1986

Ball HA: Primary pulmonary sarcoma: a review, with report of an additional case. Am J Cancer 15:2319, 1931

Barnard WG: Embryoma of lung. Thorax 7:299, 1952

Barrett NR, Barnard WG: Some unusual thoracic tumors. Br J Surg 32:447, 1945

Baroni CD, Mineo TC, Ricci et al: Solitary secretory plasmacytoma of the lung in a 14-year-old boy. Cancer 40:2329, 1977

Barson AJ, Jones AW, Lodge KV: Pulmonary blastoma. J Clin Pathol 21:480, 1968

Bartley TD, Arean VM: Intrapulmonary neurogenic tumors. J Thorac Cardiovasc Surg 50:114, 1965

Bauermeister DE, Jennings ER, Beland AH, Judson HA: Pulmonary blastoma, a form of carcinosarcoma: report of a case of 24 years' duration without treatment. Am J Clin Pathol 46:322, 1966

Bedrossian CWM, Verani R, Unger KM, Salman J: Pulmonary malignant fibrous histiocytoma. Chest 75:186, 1979

Beluffi G, Bertolotti P, Mietta A et al: Primary leiomyosarcoma of the lung in a girl. Pediatr Radiol 16:240, 1986

Ben-Ezra J, Winberg CD, Wu A et al: Concurrent presence of two clonal populations in small lymphocytic lymphoma of the lung. Hum Pathol 18:399, 1987

Bergmann M, Ackerman LV, Kemler RL: Carcinosarcoma of the lung: review of the literature and report of two cases treated by pneumonectomy. Cancer 4:919, 1951

Berman L: Extragenital chorioepithelioma with report of a case. Am J Cancer 38:23, 1940

Bini G: Osservazioni anatomiche ed istopatologiche sopra particolau forme de tumori polmonari maligni di natura mesenchimale. Pathologica 34:77, 1942

Borlee-Hermans G, Bury TH, Grand JL et al: Intravascular bronchioloalveolar tumour. Eur J Respir Dis 66:341, 1985

Bosanko CMM, Korobkin M, Fantone JC et al: Lobar primary pulmonary lymphoma: CT findings. J Comput Assist Tomogr 15:679, 1991

Braunstein GD, Vaitukaitis JL, Carbone PP, Ross GT: Ectopic production of human chorionic gonadotropin by neoplasms. Ann Intern Med 78:39, 1973

Bull JC, Grimes OR: Pulmonary carcinosarcoma. Chest 65:9, 1974

Cagle P, Mace ML, Judge DM et al: Pulmonary melanoma: primary vs. metastatic. Chest 85:125, 1984

Cameron EWJ: Primary sarcoma of the lung. Thorax 30:516, 1975

Capewell S, Webb JN, Crompton GK: Primary leiomyosarcoma of the lung presenting with a persistent pneumothorax. Thorax 41:649, 1986

Carbone PP, Kaplan HS, Musshof K et al: Report of the committee on Hodgkin's disease staging classification. Cancer Res 31:1860, 1971

Carlucci GA, Schleussner RC: Primary (?) melanoma of lung. A case report. J Thorac Surg 11:643, 1942

Carstens PHB, Kuhns JG, Ghazi C: Primary malignant melanomas of the lung and adrenals. Hum Pathol 15:910, 1984

Carswell J, Kraeft NH: Fibrosarcoma of the bronchus: report of a case diagnosed by bronchoscopy and treated by pneumonectomy. J Thorac Surg 19:117, 1949

Caves PK, Jacques J: Primary intrapulmonary neurogenic sarcoma with hypertrophic pulmonary osteoarthropathy and asbestosis. Thorax 26:212, 1971

Chaudhuri MR: Bronchial carcinosarcoma. J Thorac Cardiovasc Surg 61:319, 1971

Childress WG, Adie GC: Plasma cell tumors of the mediastinum and lung: report of two cases. J Thorac Cardiovasc Surg 19:794, 1950

Chowdhury LN, Swerdlow MA, Jao et al: Postirradiation malignant fibrous histiocytoma of the lung: demonstration of alpha-antitrypsin-like material in neoplastic cells. Am J Clin Pathol 74:820, 1980

Conquest HF, Thornton JL, Massie JR, Coxe JW III: Primary pulmonary rhabdomyosarcoma: report of three cases and literature review. Ann Surg 161:688, 1965

Corrin B, Manners B, Millard M, Weaver L: Histogenesis of the so-called "intravascular bronchioalveolar tumour." J Pathol 128:163, 1979

Corwin J, Lindberg RD: Solitary plasmacytoma of bone vs. extramedullary plasmacytoma and their relationship to multiple myeloma. Cancer 43:1007, 1979

Cotton BH, Penido JRF: Plasma cell tumors of the lung: report of a case. Dis Chest 21:218, 1952

Cox JL, Fuson RL, Daly JT: Pulmonary blastoma: a case report and review of the literature. Ann Thorac Surg 9:364, 1970

Crane M, Sutton JP: Primary sarcoma of the lung. South Med J 65:850, 1972

Crotty TB, Hooker RP, Swenson SJ et al: Primary malignant ependymoma of the lung. Mayo Clin Proc 67:373, 1992

Dahlgren SE, Ovenfors CO: Primary malignant lymphoma of the lung. Acta Radiol 8:401, 1969

Dail DH, Liebow AA: Intravascular bronchioalveolar tumor (abstr). Am J Pathol 78:6a, 1975

Dail DH, Liebow AA, Gmelich JT et al: Intravascular, bronchiolar, and alveolar tumor of the lung (IVBAT): an analysis of twenty cases of a peculiar sclerosing endothelial tumor. Cancer 51:452, 1983

Daniels AC, Conner GH, Straus FH: Primary chondrosarcoma of the tracheobronchial tree: report of a unique case and brief review. Arch Pathol Lab Med 84:615, 1967

Davis MP, Eagan RT, Weiland LH, Pairolero PC: Carcinosarcoma of the lung: Mayo clinic experience and response to chemotherapy. Mayo Clin Proc 59:598, 1984

Davis WB, Gadek JE: Detection of pulmonary lymphoma by bronchoalveolar lavage. Chest 91:787, 1987

Day DW, Taylor SA: An intrapulmonary teratoma associated with thymic tissue. Thorax 30:582, 1975

Dessy E, Pietra GG: Pseudomesotheliomatous carcinoma of the lung: an immunohistochemical and ultrastructural study of three cases. Cancer 68:1747, 1991

Dhingra HK, Flance IJ: Cavitary primary pulmonary Hodgkin's disease presenting as pruritus. Chest 58:71, 1970

Dixon DS, Breslow A: Pulmonary blastoma. Am Rev Respir Dis 108:968, 1973

Eggleston JC: The intravascular bronchioalveolar tumor and the sclerosing hemangioma of the lung: misnomers of pulmonary neoplasia. Semin Diagn Pathol 2:270, 1985

Ehrenstein F: Primary pulmonary lymphoma: review of the literature and two case reports. J Thorac Cardiovasc Surg 52:31, 1966

Eliasson AH, Rajagopal KR, Dow NS: Respiratory failure in rapidly progressing pulmonary lymphoma: role of immunophenotyping in diagnosis. Am Rev Respir Dis 141:231, 1990

Ellison RG, Bailey AW, Yeh TJ et al: Primary lymphosarcoma of the lung. Am Surg 30:737, 1964

Emery RW, Fox AL, Raab DE: Short reports: intravascular bronchioloalveolar tumour. Thorax 37:472, 1982

Engel AF, Groot G, Bellot S: Carcinosarcoma of the lung. A case history of disseminated disease and review of the literature. Eur J Surg Oncol 17:94, 1991

Eriksson A, Thunell M, Lundqvist G: Pendulating endobronchial rhabdomyosarcoma with fatal asphyxia. Thorax 37:390, 1982

Farquhar DL, Crompton GK, McIntyre MA, Leonard RCF: Non-Hodgkin's lymphoma of the lung. Scott Med J 33:243, 1988

Filho BG, Pasqualucci MEA: Sarcoma condroblastico primitivo do pulmao. Rev Bras Cir 45:293, 1963

Fine G, Smith RW, Pachter MR: Primary extragenital choriocarcinoma in the male subject. Am J Med 32:776, 1962

Fine G, Stout AP: Osteogenic sarcoma of the extraskeletal soft tissues. Cancer 9:1027, 1956

Flint A, Kumar NB, Naylor B: Pulmonary Hodgkin's disease: diagnosis by fine-needle aspiration. Acta Cytol 32:221, 1988

Francis D, Jacobsen M: Pulmonary blastoma: preoperative cytologic and histologic findings. Acta Cytol 23:437, 1979

Fraser RG, Paré JA, Fraser RS, Genereux GP: Diagnosis of Diseases of the Chest. 3rd Ed. WB Saunders, Philadelphia, 1989

Freeman C, Berg JW, Cutler SJ: Occurrence and prognosis of extranodal lymphomas. Cancer 29:252, 1972

Fukuda M, Sasaki Y, Morita M et al: Large cell carcinoma of the lung secreting human chorionic gonadotropin which responded to combination chemotherapy: case report. Jpn J Clin Oncol 20:299, 1990

Fung CH, Lo JW, Yonan TN et al: Pulmonary blastoma: an ultrastructural study with a brief review of literature and a discussion of pathogenesis. Cancer 39:153, 1977

Gautam HP: Intrapulmonary malignant teratoma. Am Rev Respir Dis 100:863, 1969

Gebauer C: The postoperative prognosis of primary pulmonary sarcomas: a review with a comparison of the histologic forms and the other primary endothoracal sarcomas based on 474 cases. Scand J Thorac Cardiovasc Surg 16:91, 1982

Gepharat GN: Malignant melanoma of the bronchus. Hum Pathol 12:671, 1981

Gerber IE: Ectopic chorioepithelioma. Mt Sinai J Med 7:135, 1935

Gerin-Lajoie L: A case of chorioepithelioma of the lung. Am J Obstet Gynecol 68:391, 1954

Ghaffar A, Vaidynathan SV, Elguezabal A, Levowitz BS: Pulmonary blastoma: report of two cases. Chest 67:600, 1975

Gibbons JRP, McKeown F, Field TW: Pulmonary blastoma with hilar lymph node metastases: survival for 24 years. Cancer 47:152, 1981

Gibson PG, Bryant DH, Harkness J et al: Pulmonary manifestations of the acquired immunodeficiency syndrome. Aust N Z J Med 17:551, 1987

Gledhill A, Kay JM: Hepatic metastases in a case of intravascular bronchioalveolar tumour. J Clin Pathol 37:279, 1984

Goldthorn JF, Duncan MH, Kosloske AM, Ball WS: Cavitating primary pulmonary fibrosarcoma in a child. J Thorac Cardiovasc Surg 91:932, 1986

Gordon J, Walker G: Plasmacytoma of the lung. Arch Pathol Lab Med 37:222, 1944

Greenberg SD, Heisler JG, Gyorkey F, Jenkins DE: Pulmonary lymphoma versus pseudolymphoma: a perplexing problem. South Med J 65:775, 1972

Greenspan EB: Primary osteoid chondrosarcoma of the lung: report of a case. Am J Cancer 18:603, 1933

Guccion JG, Rosen SH: Bronchopulmonary leiomyosarcoma and fibrosarcoma: a study of 32 cases and review of the literature. Cancer 30:836, 1972

Guttman RF, Saavedra JA: Primary Hodgkin's disease of the lung: report of a case. Dis Chest 53:660, 1968

Hansen LA, Prakash UBS, Colby TV: Pulmonary lymphoma in Sjögren's syndrome. Mayo Clin Proc 64:920, 1989

Hattori M, Imura H, Matsukura S et al: Multiple-hormone producing lung carcinoma. Cancer 43:2429, 1979

Henry K, Keal EE: Pulmonary blastoma with a striated muscle component. Br J Dis Chest 60:87, 1966

Herbert A, Wright DH, Isaacson PG, Smith JL: Primary malignant lymphoma of lung: histopathologic and immunologic evaluation of nine cases. Hum Pathol 15:415, 1984

Herxheimer G, Reinke F: Pathologie des krebses. Ergebn D Allg Path U Path Anat 16:280, 1912

Hilbun BM, Chavez CM: Lymphoma of the lung. J Thorac Cardiovasc Surg 53:721, 1967

Hill LD, White ML Jr: Plasmacytoma of the lung. J Thorac Cardiovasc Surg 25:187, 1953

Hochberg LA, Crastnopol P: Primary sarcoma of the bronchus and lung. Arch Surg 73:74, 1955

Holland J, Trenkner DA, Wasserman TH, Fineberg B: Plasmacytoma: treatment results and conversion to myeloma. Cancer 69:1513, 1992

Holt S, Deverall PB, Boddy JE: A teratoma of the lung containing thymic tissue. J Pathol 126:85, 1978

Ishida T, Tateishi M, Kaneko S et al: Carcinosarcoma and spindle cell carcinoma of the lung: clinicopathologic and immunohistochemical studies. J Thorac Cardiovasc Surg 100:844, 1990

Ishizuka T, Yoshitake J, Yamada T et al: Diagnosis of a case of pulmonary carcinosarcoma by detection of rhabdomyosarcoma cells in sputum. Acta Cytol 32:658, 1988

Iverson RE, Straehley CJ: Pulmonary blastoma: long term survival of juvenile patient. Chest 63:436, 1973

Jacobson M, Francis D: Pulmonary blastoma. A clinicopathologic study of 11 cases. Acta Pathol Microbiol Scand 88:151, 1980

Jamieson MPG, McGowan AR: Endobronchial teratoma. Thorax 37:157, 1982

Jenkins BJ: Carcinosarcoma of the lung: report of a case and review of the literature. J Thorac Cardiovasc Surg 55:657, 1968

Jensen OA, Egedorf J: Primary malignant melanoma of the lung. Scand J Respir Dis 48:127, 1967

Jetley NK, Bhatnagar V, Krishna A et al: Pulmonary blastoma in a neonate. J Pediatr Surg 23:1009, 1988

Jimenez JF: Pulmonary blastoma in childhood. J Surg Oncol 34:87, 1987

Johnson DW, Hoppe RT, Cox RS et al: Hodgkin's disease limited to intrathoracic sites. Cancer 52:8, 1983

Kakos GS, Williams TE, Assor D, Vasko JS: Pulmonary carcinosarcoma: etiologic, therapeutic, and prognostic considerations. J Thorac Cardiovasc Surg 61:777, 1971

Kalus M, Rahman F, Jenkins DE, Beall AC Jr: Malignant mesenchymoma of the lung. Arch Pathol Lab Med 95:199, 1973

Karcioglu ZA, Someren AO: Pulmonary blastoma: a case report and review of the literature. Am J Clin Pathol 61:287, 1974

Kay S, Reed WG: Chorioepithelioma of the lung in a female infant seven months old. Am J Pathol 21:555, 1953

Kennedy A, Prior AL: Pulmonary blastoma: a report of two cases and a review of the literature. Thorax 31:776, 1976

Kennedy JD, Kneafsey DV: Two cases of plasmacytoma of the lower respiratory tract. Thorax 14:353, 1959

Kennedy JL, Nathwani BN, Burke JS et al: Pulmonary lymphomas and other pulmonary lymphoid lesions: a clinicopathologic and immunologic study of 64 patients. Cancer 56:539, 1985

Kern WH, Crepeau AG, Jones JC: Primary Hodgkin's disease of the lung: report of 4 cases and review of the literature. Cancer 14:1151, 1961

Kern WH, Hughes RK, Meyer BW, Harley DP: Malignant fibrous histiocytoma of the lung. Cancer 44:1793, 1979

Kern WH, Stiles QR: Pulmonary blastoma. J Thorac Cardiovasc Surg 72:801, 1976

Kernen JA, Meyer BW: Malignant plasmacytoma of the lung with metastases. J Thorac Cardiovasc Surg 51:739, 1966

Kinare SG, Parulkar GB, Panday SR et al: Extensive ossification in a pulmonary plasmacytoma. Thorax 20:206, 1965

Knowling MA, Harwood AR, Bergsagel DE: Comparison of extramedullary plasmacytomas with solitary and multiple plasma cell tumors of bone. J Clin Oncol 1:255, 1983

Kodama T, Shimosato Y, Watanabe S et al: Six cases of well-differentiated adenocarcinoma simulating fetal lung tubules in pseudoglandular stage: comparison with pulmonary blastoma. Am J Surg Pathol 8:735, 1984

Koss MN, Hochholzer L, Nichols PW et al: Primary non-Hodgkin's lymphoma and pseudolymphoma of lung: a study of 161 patients. Hum Pathol 14:1024, 1983

Koss MN, Hochholzer L, O'Leary T: Pulmonary blastomas. Cancer 67:2368, 1991

Kummet TD, Doll DC: Chemotherapy of pulmonary blastoma: a case report and review of the literature. Med Pediatr Oncol 10:27, 1982

Kunkel OF, Torrey E: Report of a case of primary melanotic sarcoma of lung presenting difficulties in differentiating from tuberculosis. N Y State J Med 16:198, 1916

Lee JT, Shelburne JD, Linder J: Primary malignant fibrous histiocytoma of the lung: a clinicopathologic and ultrastructural study of five cases. Cancer 53:1124, 1984

Lennert K: Malignant Lymphomas Other than Hodgkin's Disease. Springer-Verlag, New York, 1978

Le Tourneau A, Audouin J, Garbe L et al: Primary pulmonary malignant lymphoma, clinical and pathological findings, immunocytochemical and ultrastructural studies in 15 cases. Hematol Oncol 1:49, 1983

Lowell LM, Tuhy JE: Primary chondrosarcoma of the lung. J Thorac Cardiovasc Surg 18:476, 1949

Lukes RJ, Collins RD: Immunologic characterization of human malignant lymphomas. Cancer 34:1488, 1974

Mackay B, Lukeman JM, Ordonez NG: Tumors of the Lung. WB Saunders, Philadelphia, 1990

Manivel JC, Priest JR, Watterson J et al: Pleuropulmonary blastoma: the so-called pulmonary blastoma of childhood. Cancer 62:1516, 1988

Manning JT, Ordonez NG, Rosenberg HS et al: Pulmonary endodermal tumor resembling fetal lung: report of a case with immunohistochemical studies. Arch Pathol Lab Med 109:48, 1985

Marchevsky A, Padilla M, Kaneko M, Kleinerman J: Localized lymphoid nodules of lung: a reappraisal of the lymphoma versus pseudolymphoma dilemma. Cancer 51:2070, 1983

Marcus PB, Dieb TM, Martin JH: Pulmonary blastoma: an ultrastructural study emphasizing intestinal differentiation in lung tumors. Cancer 49:1829, 1982

Mark LK: Primary lymphoma of the lung. JAMA 237:895, 1977

Marsh K, Kenyon WE, Earis JE, Pearson MG: Intravascular bronchioloalveolar tumour. Thorax 37:474, 1982

Martini N, Hajdu SI, Beattie EJ Jr: Primary sarcoma of the lung. J Thorac Cardiovasc Surg 61:33, 1971

Mazumdar P, Abraham S, Damodaran VN, Saha NC: Pulmonary plasmacytoma: a case report. Am Rev Respir Dis 100:866, 1969

McCann MP, Fu YS, Kay S: Pulmonary blastoma: a light and electron microscopic study. Cancer 38:789, 1976

McDonnell T, Kyriakos M, Roper C, Mazoujian G: Malignant fibrous histiocytoma of the lung. Cancer 61:137, 1988

Meade JB, Whitwell F, Bickford BJ, Waddington JKB: Primary haemangiopericytoma of lung. Thorax 29:1, 1974

Meade P, Moad J, Fellows D, Adams CW: Carcinosarcoma of the lung with hypertrophic pulmonary osteoarthropathy. Ann Thorac Surg 51:488, 1991

Medbery CA III, Bibro MC, Phares JC et al: Pulmonary blastoma: case report and literature review of chemotherapy experience. Cancer 53:2413, 1984

Meis JM, Butler JJ, Osborne BM, Ordonez NG: Solitary plasmacytomas of bone and extramedullary plasmacytomas: a clinicopathologic and immunohistochemical study. Cancer 59:1475, 1987

Miettinen M, Collan Y, Halttunen P et al: Intravascular bronchioloalveolar tumor. Cancer 60:2471, 1987

Miller B, Montgomery C, Watne AL et al: Lymphoepithelioma-like carcinoma of the lung. J Surg Oncol 48:62, 1991

Miyake M, Ito M, Mitsuoka A et al: Alpha-fetoprotein and human chorionic gonadotropin-producing lung cancer. Cancer 59:227, 1987

Monahan DT: Hodgkin's disease of the lung. J Thorac Cardiovasc Surg 49:173, 1965

Moore T: Carcinosarcoma of the lung. Surgery 50:886, 1961

Moralles FM, Matthews JI: Diagnosis of parenchymal Hodgkin's disease using bronchoalveolar lavage. Chest 91:785, 1987

Morgan AD, Salama FD: Primary chondrosarcoma of the lung: case report and review of the literature. J Thorac Cardiovasc Surg 64:460, 1972

Morinaga S, Watanabe H, Gemma A et al: Plasmacytoma of the lung associated with nodular deposits of immunoglobulin. Am J Pathol 11:989, 1987

Muggia FM, Rosen SW, Weintraub BD, Hansen HH: Ectopic placental proteins in nontrophoblastic tumors. Cancer 36:1327, 1975

Muller-Hermelink MK, Kaiserling E: Pulmonary adenocarcinoma of fetal type: alternating differentiation argues in favor of a common endodermal stem cell. Virchows Arch A Pathol Anat Histopathol 409:195, 1986

Nascimento NG, Unni UK, Bernatz PE: Sarcomas of the lung. Mayo Clin Proc 57:355, 1982

Neilson DB: Primary intrapulmonary neurogenic sarcoma. J Pathol 76:419, 1958

Nelson S, Prince D, Terry P: Primary Hodgkin's disease of the lung: case report. Thorax 38:310, 1983

Non-Hodgkin's Lymphoma Pathologic Classification Project. National Cancer Institute sponsored study of classifications of non-Hodgkin's lymphoma. Cancer 49:2112, 1982

Nosanchuk JS, Weatherbee L: Primary osteogenic sarcoma in lung: report of a case. J Thorac Cardiovasc Surg 58:242, 1969

Ott RA, Eugene J, Kollin J et al: Primary pulmonary angiosarcoma associated with multiple synchronous neoplasms. J Surg Oncol 35:269, 1987

Ozkaynak MF, Ortega JA, Laug W et al: Role of chemotherapy in pediatric pulmonary blastoma. Med Pediatr Oncol 18:53, 1990

Palmer RN, Saini N, Guccion J: Ewing's-like sarcoma appearing as a primary pulmonary neoplasm. Arch Pathol Lab Med 105:277, 1981

Papaiannou AN, Watson WL: Primary lymphoma of the lung: an appraisal of its natural history and a comparison with other localized lymphomas. J Thorac Cardiovasc Surg 49:373, 1965

Parker JC, Payne WS, Woolner LB: Pulmonary blastoma (embryoma): report of two cases. J Thorac Cardiovasc Surg 51:694, 1966

Pedersen VM, Schulze S, Madsen KH, Krogdahl AS: Primary pulmonary leiomyosarcoma: review of the literature and report of a case. Scand J Thorac Cardiovasc Surg 18:251, 1984

Peterson H, Snider HL, Yam LT et al: Primary pulmonary lymphoma: a clinical and immunohistochemical study of six cases. Cancer 56:805, 1985

Pettinato G, Manivel JC, Saldana MJ et al: Primary bronchopulmonary fibrosarcoma of childhood and adolescence: reassessment of a low-grade malignancy. Pathol 20:463, 1989

Poelzleitner D, Huebsch P, Mayerhofer S et al: Primary pulmonary lymphoma in a patient with the acquired immune deficiency syndrome. Thorax 44:438, 1989

Polish LB, Cohn DL, Ryder JW et al: Pulmonary non-Hodkin's lymphoma in AIDS. Chest 96:1321, 1989

Prive L, Tellem M, Meranze DR, Chodoff RD: Carcinosarcoma of the lung. Arch Pathol Lab Med 72:119, 1961

Pushchak MJ, Farhi DC: Primary choriocarcinoma of the lung. Arch Pathol Lab Med 111:477, 1987

Rabiah FA: Primary lymphocytic lymphoma (lymphosarcoma of the lung). Am Surg 34:275, 1968

Radin AI: Primary pulmonary Hodgkin's disease. Cancer 65:550, 1990

Rappaport H: Tumors of the hematopoietic system. In Atlas of Tumor Pathology. Fascicle 8. Armed Forces Institute of Pathology, Washington, DC, 1966

Razzuk MA, Urschel HC, Race GJ et al: Carcinosarcoma of the lung: report of two cases and review of the literature. J Thorac Cardiovasc Surg 61:541, 1971

Reale FR, Variakojis D, Compton J et al: Cytodiagnosis of Hodgkin's disease in sputum specimens. Acta Cytol 27:258, 1983

Reed RJ, Kent EM: Solitary pulmonary melanomas: two case reports. J Thorac Cardiovasc Surg 48:226, 1964

Rees GM: Primary chondrosarcoma of lung. Thorax 25:366, 1970

Reid JD, Mehta VT: Melanoma of the lower respiratory tract. Cancer 19:627, 1966

Reingold IM, Amromin GD: Extraosseous osteosarcoma of the lung. Cancer 28:491, 1971

Reverter JC, Coca A, Font J, Ingelmo M: Erythema nodosum and pulmonary solitary nodule as the first manifestations of a non-Hodgkin's lymphoma. Br J Dis Chest 81:397, 1987

Risdall R, Hoppe RT, Warnke R: Non-Hodgkin's lymphoma: a study of the evolution of the disease based upon 92 autopsied cases. Cancer 44:529, 1979

Robertson AJ, Sinclair DJM, Sutton PP, Guthrie W. Primary melanocarcinoma of the lower respiratory tract. Thorax 35:158, 1980

Roth JA, Elquezabal A: Pulmonary blastoma evolving into carcinosarcoma. Am J Surg Pathol 2:407, 1978

Rozsa S, Frieman H: Extramedullary plasmacytoma of the lung. AJR 70:982, 1953

Rubin M: Primary lymphoma of lung. J Thorac Cardiovasc Surg 56:293, 1968

Rudders RA, Ross ME, DeLellis RA: Primary extranodal lymphoma: response to treatment and factors influencing prognosis. Cancer 42:406, 1978

Ruland L: Malignant teratoblastoma of the lung. Thorac Cardiovasc Surg 4:119, 1956

Rusch VW, Shuman WP, Schmidt R, Laramore GE: Massive pulmonary hemantiopericytoma: an innovative approach to evaluation and treatment. Cancer 64:1928, 1989

Sakula A: Primary malignant lymphoma of lung. Postgrad Med J 55:46, 1979

Salm R: A primary malignant melanoma of the bronchus. J Pathol 85:121, 1963

Saltzstein SL: Pulmonary malignant lymphomas and pseudolymphomas: classification, therapy, and prognosis. Cancer 16:928, 1963

Schiodt T, Jensen KG: Malignant teratoid tumour of the lung: ? malignant hamartoma. Thorax 15:120, 1960

Schwaiger A, Prior C, Weyrer K et al: Non-Hodgkin's lymphoma of the lung diagnosed by gene rearrangement from bronchoalveolar lavage fluid: a fast and noninvasive method. Blood 77:2538, 1991

Sedlezky I: Malignant pulmonary lesion with calcification. Can Assoc Radiol J 6:65, 1955

Shariff S, Thomas JA, Shetty N, D'Cunha S: Primary pulmonary rhabdomyosarcoma in a child, with a review of literature. J Surg Oncol 38:261, 1988

Sherman JL, Rykwalder PJ, Tashkin DP: Intravascular bronchioalveolar tumor. Am Rev Respir Dis 123:468, 1981

Shuman RL: Primary pulmonary sarcoma and left atrial extension via left superior pulmonary vein: en bloc resection and radical pneumonectomy on cardiopulmonary bypass. J Thorac Cardiovasc Surg 88:189, 1984

Sicilian L, Warson F, Carrington CB et al: Intravascular bronchioalveolar tumor (IV-BAT). Respiration 44:387, 1983

Silverman JF, Coalson JJ: Primary malignant myxoid fibrous histiocytoma of the lung: light and ultrastructural examination with review of the literature. Arch Pathol Lab Med 108:49, 1984

Sinclair RA, Sullivan JR, McConchie I: Primary lymphoma of lung. Med J Aust 1:356, 1978

Sordillo PP, Hajdu SI, Magill GB, Golbey RB: Extraosseous osteogenic sarcoma: a review of 48 patients. Cancer 51:727, 1983

Spencer H: Pulmonary blastoma. J Pathol 82:161, 1961

Spragg RG, Wolf PL, Haghighi P et al: Angiosarcoma of the lung with fatal pulmonary hemorrhage. AM J Med 74:1072, 1983

Sprague RI, deBlois GG: Small lymphocytic pulmonary lymphoma: diagnosis by transthoracic fine needle aspiration. Chest 96:929, 1989

Stackhouse EM, Harrison EG, Ellis FH: Primary mixed malignancies of lung: carcinosarcoma and blastoma. J Thorac Cardiovasc Surg 57:385, 1969

Sugarbaker ED, Craver LF: Lymphosarcoma: study of 196 cases with biopsy. JAMA 115:17, 1940

Sullivan LG: Primary choriocarcinoma of the lung in a man. Arch Pathol Lab Med 113:82, 1989

Sun CCJ, Kroll M, Miller JE: Primary chondrosarcoma of the lung. Cancer 50:1864, 1982

Sweeney WB, Vesoulis Z, Blaum LC Jr: Intravascular bronchioloalveolar tumor: a distinctive surgical and pathological entity. Ann Thorac Surg 42:702, 1986

Taboada CF, McMurray JD, Jordan RA, Seybold WD: Primary melanoma of the lung. Chest 62:629, 1972

Tamai S, Kameya T, Shimosato Y et al: Pulmonary blastoma: an ultrastructural study of a case and its transplanted tumor in athymic nude mice. Cancer 46:1389, 1980

Tan TB, Spaander PJ, Blaisse M, Gerritzen FM: Angiotropic large cell lymphoma presenting as interstitial lung disease. Thorax 43:578, 1988

Tanimura A, Natsuyama H, Kawano M et al: Primary choriocarcinoma of the lung. Hum Pathol 16:1281, 1985

Thomas WJ, Koenig HM, Ellwanger FR, Lightsey AL: Primary pulmonary rhabdomyosarcoma in childhood. Am J Dis Child 135:469, 1981

Todd FW: Two cases of melanotic tumors in lungs. JAMA 11:53, 1888

Turner RR, Colby TV, Doggett RS: Well-differentiated lymphocytic lymphoma: a study of 47 patients with primary manifestation in the lung. Cancer 54:2088, 1984

Ueda K, Gruppo R, Unger F et al: Rhabdomyosarcoma of lung arising in congenital cystic adenomatoid malformation. Cancer 40:383, 1977

Van Assendelft AHW, Strengell-Usanov L, Kastarinen S. Pulmonary haemangiopericytoma with multiple metastases. Eur J Respir Dis 65:380, 1984

van der Schee AC, Dinkla BA, van Knapen A: Primary pulmonary manifestation of Hodgkin's disease. Respiration 57:127, 1990

Venn GE, Gellister J, DaCosta PE, Goldstraw P: Malignant fibrous histiocytoma in thoracic surgical practice. J Thorac Cardiovasc Surg 91:234, 1986

Weber H: Lungenlyphogranulome. Beitr Z Path Anat VZ Allg Path 84:1, 1930

Weinblatt ME, Siegel SE, Isaacs H: Pulmonary blastoma associated with cystic lung disease. Cancer 49:669, 1982

Weiss SW: Malignant fibrous histiocytoma. A reaffirmation. Am J Surg Pathol 6:773, 1982

Weldon-Linne CM, Victor TA, Christ ML, Fry WA: Angiogenic nature of the ''intravascular bronchioalveolar tumor'' of the lung: an electron microscopic study. Arch Pathol Lab Med 105:174, 1981

Wick MR, Scheithauer BW, Piehler JM, Pairolero PC: Primary pulmonary leiomyosarcomas. Arch Pathol Lab Med 106:510, 1982

Wile A, Olinger G, Peter JB, Dornfeld L: Solitary intraparenchymal pulmonary plasmacytoma associated with production of an M-protein: report of a case. Cancer 37:2338, 1976

Wisecarver J, Ness MJ, Rennard SJ et al: Bronchoalveolar lavage in the assessment of pulmonary Hodgkin's disease. Acta Cytol 33:527, 1989

Wiltshaw E: The natural history of extramedullary plasmacytoma and its relation to solitary myeloma of bone and myelomatosis. Medicine 55:217, 1976

Wood N, Coltman CA: Localized primary extranodal Hodgkin's disease. Ann Intern Med 78:113, 1973

Woodruff RK, Whittle JM, Malpas JS: Solitary plasmacytoma I: extramedullary soft tissue plasmacytoma. Cancer 43:2340, 1979

Wotherspoon AC, Soosay GN, Diss TC, Isaacson PG: Low-grade primary B-cell lymphoma of the lung: an immunohistochemical, molecular, and cytogenic study of a single case. Am J Clin Pathol 94:655, 1990

Yamashita T, Kiyota T, Ukishima G et al: Autopsy case of chondro-osteoid sarcoma originating in the lung. J Shonai Med Assoc 23:472, 1964

Yousem SA: Angiosarcoma presenting in the lung. Arch Pathol Lab Med 110:112, 1986

Yousem SA, Weiss LM, Colby TV: Primary pulmonary Hodgkin's disease: a clinicopathologic study of 15 cases. Cancer 57:1217, 1986

Yousem SA, Hochholzer L: Malignant fibrous histiocytoma of the lung. Cancer 60:2532, 1987a

Yousem SA, Hochholzer L: Primary pulmonary hemangiopericytoma. Cancer 59:549, 1987b

Yousem SA, Wick MR, Randhawa P, Manivel JC: Pulmonary blastoma: an immunohistochemical analysis with comparison with fetal lung in its pseudoglandular stage. Am J Clin Pathol 93:167, 1990

Zapatero J, Bellon J, Baamonde C et al: Primary choriocarcinoma of the lung. Presentation of a case and review of the literature. Scand J Thorac Cardiovasc Surg 16:279, 1982

Zulian GB, Jacot-des-Combes E, Aapro MS: Primary pulmonary Hodgkin's disease and the dilemma of E stage. Eur J Surg Oncol 12:307, 1986

31

PULMONARY METASTASES

E. Carmack Holmes

HISTORICAL NOTE

The lung is the most common site of metastases for all malignancies, with the possible exception of those that develop in the area of portal venous drainage. In the past the presence of pulmonary metastases was thought invariably to signify disseminated disease, and surgical intervention was believed to be contraindicated. The modern era of surgery for pulmonary metastases began with an intentional resection of a pulmonary metastases by Barney and Churchill (1939) in 1939. They resected a metastatic renal cell carcinoma, and their patient survived 23 years. A series of resections for pulmonary metastases were reviewed by Alexander and Haight (1947) in 1947. A significant number of these patients remained disease free for 3 years or longer. This review suggested that in certain cases resection of pulmonary metastases might be beneficial to the patient. Indeed in 1965, Thomford (Thomford, et al., 1965) reported a 5-year survival rate of 31 percent in a group of patients with multiple unilateral metastases. Subsequently, others (McCormack and Martin, 1979; Morton, et al., 1973; Huth, et al., 1980) expanded the indications for the resection of pulmonary metastases and included patients who had multiple bilateral pulmonary metastases. These larger series led to a more critical evaluation of the selection criteria that should be used in determining which patients can benefit from pulmonary resection.

HISTORICAL READINGS

Alexander J, Haight C: Pulmonary resection for solitary metastatic sarcomas and carcinomas. Surg Gyncol Obstet 85:129, 1947

Barney JD, Churchill EJ: Adenocarcinoma of the kidney with metastases to the lung cured by nephrectomy and lobectomy. J Urol 42:269, 1939

Huth JF, Holmes EC, Vernon SE et al.: Pulmonary resection for metastatic sarcoma. Am J Surg 140:9, 1980

McCormack PN, Martini N: The changing role of surgery for pulmonary metastases. Ann Thorac Surg 28:139, 1979

Morton DL, Joseph WL, Ketchan AS et al.: Surgical resection and adjuvant immunotherapy for selective patients with multiple pulmonary metastases. Ann Surg 178:360, 1973

Thomford NR, Woolner LB, Clagett OT: Surgical treatment of metastatic tumors in the lungs. J Thorac Cardiovasc Surg 49:357, 1965

DIAGNOSIS

Symptoms

Most patients with pulmonary metastases remain relatively asymptomatic for long periods. Pulmonary metastases lodge in the periphery of the lung in the subpleural location. For this reason direct bronchial involvement is relatively uncommon. Therefore bronchial obstruction, cough, and hemoptysis are not usually early symptoms. More often patients develop symptoms from pneumothorax, pleural effusion, or pleuritic chest pain. Certain tumors do have a tendency to metastasize occasionally to the bronchial submucosa and give rise to symptoms earlier. Melanomas, nonseminomatous germ cell tumors, and renal carcinomas can behave in this way. In the modern era, most patients who develop pulmonary metastases are known to have a history of a previous malignancy, and therefore most of these lesions are discovered on follow-up radiographs and computed tomographic (CT) scans.

Radiologic Techniques

Computed tomography (CT) is the most sensitive technique for picking up pulmonary metastases. In one series, CT scans detected 78 percent of all nodules greater than 3 mm in diameter. However, it should be appreciated that CT scans may also pick up lesions that eventually turn out to be benign at thoracotomy (Chang, et al., 1979). Subpleural lymph nodes are the most common CT-positive findings that subsequently prove to be benign.

In most patients known to have a previous history of a malignancy, the development of nodules on CT scans is found to be malignant. However, under some circumstances a solitary pulmonary nodule may represent a second independent lung primary tumor. This is particularly true in older patients with a history of smoking and in patients with head and neck carcinomas. Patients with a solitary pulmonary nodule and a history of melanoma have been reported to have a high incidence of second primary and benign tumors (Pogrebniak, et al., 1980).

Magnetic resonance imaging (MRI) has not improved the diagnosis of these lesions over that of conventional CT. However, in instances in which growth of the metastatic lesion into the pulmonary veins is suspected, MRI can be useful. Occasionally metastatic sarcomas grow within the lumen of the inferior pulmonary vein and protrude into the atrium (Fig. 31-1). When this is suspected, MRI is helpful in making the diagnosis, and this can be supplemented with transesophageal ultrasound.

In general bronchoscopy is nonrevealing in these patients. However, on occasion an unsuspected intraluminal metastasis is present. Although this is rare, it is important to use bronchoscopy in these patients after the induction of general anesthesia and prior to thoracotomy to rule out this possibility.

SELECTION CRITERIA FOR RESECTION

The traditional criteria for selecting patients for resection of pulmonary metastases include:

1. The primary lesion must be completely controlled.
2. The histologic type of the primary tumor must be determined.
3. The metastatic lesion must be limited to the lung without evidence of other distant metastatic disease.

4. The tumor must have a favorable tumor doubling time.
5. All the metastases must be resectable, with an acceptable operative risk and adequate residual pulmonary function.
6. In many instances it is believed that the length of the disease-free interval between the therapy of the primary tumor and the onset of the pulmonary metastases is an important prognostic factor.
7. Interestingly the number of pulmonary metastases and the bilaterality of the pulmonary metastases have not been a consistent predictor of survival.

Many investigators have analyzed these prognostic variables and selection criteria. There has not been general agreement on which factors are important in all instances. Certainly not all prognostic factors appear to be valid for all histologic types. The validity of these selection criteria depend to a great extent on the histologic type and the availability of effective chemotherapy. For instance many carcinomas tend to spread to sites other than the lung. Breast cancer has a propensity to involve the musculoskeletal system and the lungs. Colon cancer has a propensity to metastasize to the liver and the lungs, and melanoma has an affinity for brain metastases. Therefore, the selection criteria for these patients would be much different than for patients with soft tissue and bone sarcomas, in whom the lung is the sole site of pulmonary metastases in more than 70 percent of patients. In this latter group of patients, an aggressive surgical ap-

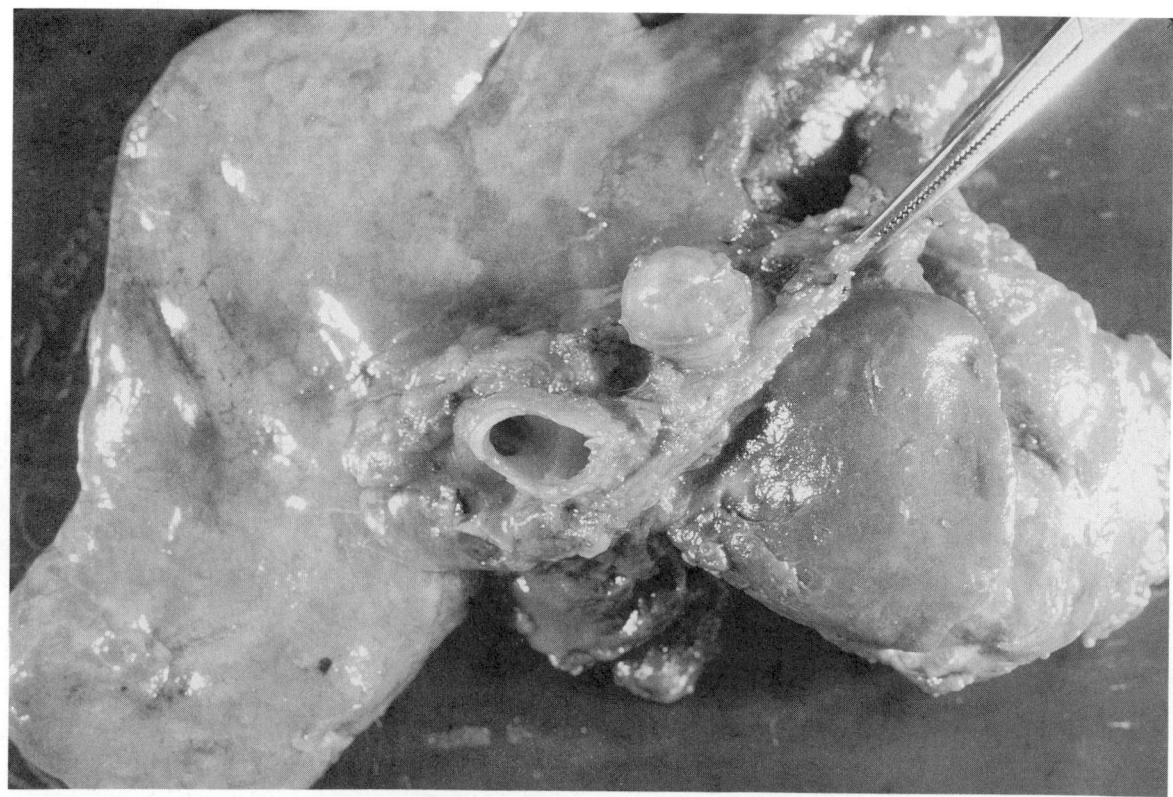

Figure 31-1. Pneumonectomy specimen from a patient with osteosarcoma protruding within the lumen of the inferior pulmonary vein into the left atrium. The MRI was helpful in identifying this problem preoperatively.

proach is indicated, and frequently many of these mentioned selection criteria do not apply to sarcomas.

For patients who have undergone recent chemotherapy or radiation therapy, it is important to consider the possibility of pulmonary toxicity. More and more multiple chemotherapeutic agents are being used in these patients and sometimes also in combination with radiation therapy. In this setting severe pulmonary damage may be present and may not be clinically apparent (Twohig and Matthay, 1979). As more experience is gained with these agents, a higher incidence of pulmonary toxicity is being appreciated. This is particularly true of patients treated with Vinca alkaloids in combination with other agents. It is well known that bleomycin and mitomycin C cause pulmonary toxicity. In addition, the clinician must be extremely careful in patients who have received doxorubicin and radiation therapy to the lungs. Doxorubicin and radiation therapy are synergistic in their pulmonary toxicity. When these conditions are unrecognized, surgery and general anesthesia may be life threatening. The postoperative picture is one of a fulminate acute respiratory distress syndrome, with a rapid decrease in pulmonary compliance in association with noncarcinogenic pulmonary edema. The condition can be rapidly fatal. The diagnosis of pulmonary injury can be made preoperatively by transbronchial biopsies, and this should be performed in situations in which there is any index of suspicion of subclinical pulmonary toxicity.

SURGICAL TECHNIQUE

Patients with pulmonary metastases generally have lesions that are in the periphery of the lung and in a subpleural location. These lesions should be resected by multiple wedge excisions whenever possible. The preservation of pulmonary tissue is important because these patients may require repeated thoracotomies. Occasionally lobectomy may be indicated and should be performed in patients with adequate pulmonary functions. Video-assisted thoracoscopic resections are not recommended, except for diagnostic purposes. Small lesions cannot be seen or palpated, and local recur-

rences are a major problem when video-assisted thoracoscopic techniques are used (Fig. 31-2).

The resection of pulmonary metastases may be accomplished through a thoracotomy, mediastinotomy, or staged bilateral thoracotomies. Most pulmonary metastases can be resected through a mediastinotomy. In some instances it is extremely difficult to resect left lower lobe lesions through this approach. When using lateral thoracotomies, we prefer the muscle-sparing incision that we have previously described (Bethencourt and Holmes, 1988). In this technique superior and inferior flaps are elevated, the latissimus dorsi is retracted posteriorly, the serratus is split in the direction of its fibers, and the chest can be entered through the appropriate intracostal space. Usually it is not necessary to divide a rib, and ample exposure using two retractors at right angles to one another can be obtained to perform virtually any resection. These incisions heal rapidly and allow patients to return to full activity fairly soon, and they require significantly less analgesia during their hospital stays. When it is necessary to perform staged bilateral thoracotomies, the use of the muscle-sparing incision permits the second procedure to be done in a shorter time interval than does a standard posteriolateral thoracotomy.

The mediastinotomy incision is generally less painful than the lateral incision, and the postoperative recovery is faster. Studies have also shown that there is a faster recovery of pulmonary function following a mediastinotomy than following a lateral thoracotomy. When performing a mediastinotomy, it is important to close the pleura at the completion of the operation. This allows for fewer adhesions and the easier performance of a re-exploration through the mediastinotomy incision. The division of the inferior pulmonary ligament assists in the exposure of the left lower lobe, and the use of an internal mammary artery external retractor can also give added exposure.

With both the muscle-sparing lateral thoracotomy and the mediastinotomy, it is important to use a double-lumen intracheal tube for selective lung collapse. The lung should be palpated both in the inflated and the deflated condition. The

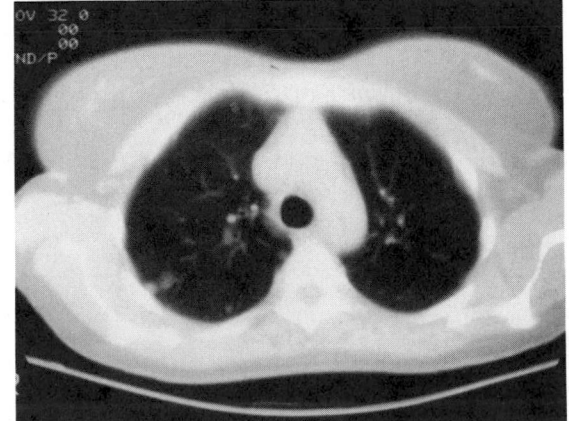
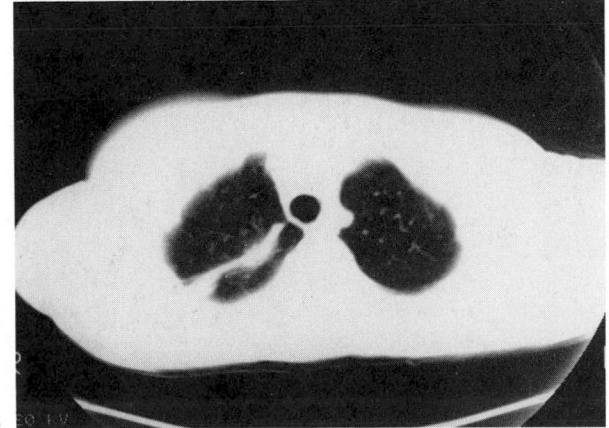

Figure 31-2.   **(A)** Two small metastatic nodules in a 26-year-old patient with osteosarcoma. **(B)** Massive suture line and chest wall recurrence 3 months following resection with a thoracoscopy.

mediastinal and hilar lymph nodes should be carefully inspected, and particular care should be paid to evaluating the chest wall and diaphragm. Not infrequently the surgeon may find small drop metastases in the posterior diaphragmatic sulcus, the lower chest wall, and the diaphragm. All metastases should be marked with an adjacent suture prior to resection because resection staple lines make palpation of other nodules difficult. Nodules can be resected using 30-, 55-, and 90-mm staplers. Frequently the gastrointestinal anastomosis stapler is useful for resecting deeper lesions. A margin of 0.5 cm is all that is required for these resections.

The operative morbidity rate should be low in both the lateral thoracotomy and the mediastinotomy. Deaths are unusual with either approach, and most series report few or no operative deaths in these patients.

RESULTS

When we talk about the results of resections of lung metastases, it is important to consider the histologic type of the primary tumor and also the availability of effective chemotherapy. There are certain tumors, such as carcinomas of the esophagus, stomach, pancreas, and prostate, in which the pattern of spread is such that resection of the pulmonary metastases has no effect whatsoever on the survival (Table 31-1). Therefore the resection of these pulmonary metastases is to be avoided.

Breast Cancer

There is another intermediate group of tumors in which occasionally the resection of pulmonary metastases may be indicated. In breast cancer the lung may occasionally be the first site of recurrent breast cancer. Resection for therapeutic purposes is usually not indicated because excellent chemotherapy is available for these patients. However, in some instances a single solitary pulmonary metastases may need to be resected to confirm the histologic type and to obtain tissue for estrogen and progesterone receptors. On rare occasions when the pulmonary metastases are limited to the lung, the disease-free interval is prolonged, and the tumor doubling time is sufficiently slow, therapeutic resection of breast metastases may be indicated.

Colon Cancer

Patients with colon cancer usually present with hepatic metastases or with both hepatic and pulmonary metastases simultaneously. Therefore, patients with colon cancer are not often candidates for the resection of pulmonary metastases. However, on infrequent occasions the lungs may be the sole site of metastases. In these instances if the disease-free interval is greater than 1 year, if the tumor doubling time of the fastest growing tumor is in excess of 40 days, and if there is no evidence of other metastatic disease, these patients may benefit from resection. Five-year survival rates under these

Table 31-1.   Characteristics of Nonsarcomatous Pulmonary Metastases by Primary Site

	5-Year Survival Rate (%)	Adverse Prognostic Factors	Comments	References
Head and neck	41–43	Primary in oral cavity Disease-free interval <13 months	Multiplicity of lesions, locoregional recurrence, and stage of primary unrelated to survival	Mazer, et al. (1988)
Testicular	59–70	Immature elements present Bilateral disease Multiple lesions	Resection indicated in absence of elevated markers Retroperitoneal disease should be resected at time of thoracotomy	Callery, et al. (1983) Mandelbaum, et al. (1980)
Renal cell	21–54	Disease-free interval Size >3.0 cm	Simultaneous resection of primary and pulmonary disease Most common primary site of resectable pulmonary metastasis Repeated resections beneficial in selected patients for assessing adjuvant response and harvesting tumor-infiltrating lymphocytes	Jett, et al. (1983), Schott, et al. (1988), Mountain, et al. (1978)
Colorectal	38–47	Disease-free interval <12 months Size >3.0 cm Multiple lesions or nodal involvement Elevated carcinoembryonic antigen level	Synchronous hepatic involvement limits number of potential candidates Age, sex, location, stage, and grade of primary unrelated to survival Repeated resections beneficial in selected patients	Phil, et al. (1992), Goya, et al. (1989), McAfee, et al. (1992)
Breast	15–49	Estrogen-receptor negative Disease-free intervals <1 year	Synchronous bone, mediastinal, or chest wall involvement limits number of potential candidates	Lanza, et al. (1992), Mountain, et al. (1984), McCormack (1990)
Melanoma	3–5	Incomplete resection pulmonary disease Shorter disease-free intervals Demonstrated lymphatic invasion More than two nodules	Late-appearing isolated nodules *without* locoregional recurrence may have >20% 5-year survival rate Resections used in selected patients for harvesting tumor-infiltrating lymphocytes	Harpole, et al. (1992), Gorenstein, et al. (1991)

circumstances range from 15 to 35 percent, and in one series a 52 percent 5-year survival rate for solitary metastases from primary colon cancer was reported (McCormack and Atti-yeh, 1977).

Melanoma

Melanoma presents a particularly vexing problem. It is such an unpredictable disease that it is difficult to interpret results without extremely large numbers of patients. Also in melanoma it is easy for the investigator to select the data and prove almost any point. However, most reports indicate that the resection of metastatic disease from malignant melanoma has extremely poor results. In some reports there are no significant differences in the mean survival rates between patients rendered disease free by pulmonary resection and those who had unresectable tumors (Pogrebniak, et al., 1980; Harpole, et al., 1992). Certainly an occasional long-term survivor has been observed. For this reason the selection criteria must be extremely rigorous. It should be re-emphasized that some patients presenting with a solitary pulmonary nodule and a history of melanoma have histologic types other than metastatic melanoma. Therefore, it is particularly important to investigate these patients thoroughly and rule out second primary lung tumors (Pogrebniak, et al., 1980).

Renal Tumors

Renal tumors commonly metastasize to the lung, and indeed patients presenting with solitary pulmonary nodules may harbor an occult renal carcinoma. It is one of the more common metastatic tumors that present with solitary pulmonary nodules. Many of these patients are candidates for pulmonary resection. Resections of the primary tumor and simultaneous resection of the pulmonary metastatic lesion are indicated. Five-year survival rates from the resection of renal carcinoma vary from 25 to 40 percent (Wilkins, 1978). In view of these results and also in view of the fact that renal cancers may have a relatively slow tumor doubling time, most surgical oncologists take an aggressive approach to resection. For many years there was no effective systemic chemotherapy for metastatic renal cancer. However, recently biologic therapy, including interferon, interleukin-2, tumor-infiltrating lymphocytes, and lymphocyte-activated killer cells have given response rates as high as 35 percent (Rosenberg, et al., 1989). When these therapies are used, frequently surgical resection is indicated to determine whether histologically viable disease remains. In this situation surgery becomes a staging procedure, and the results of surgery determine whether or not additional therapy is indicated.

Nonseminomatous Germ Cell Tumors

Nonseminomatous germ cell tumors frequently metastasize to the retroperitoneum and the lungs. The development of cisplatin-based chemotherapy has dramatically improved the survival of these patients. The surgical resection of pulmonary metastases in these patients has also been beneficial. Patients with nonseminomatous testicular tumors metastatic to the lung have a 65 percent cure rate after surgical resection (Callery, et al., 1983). In some instances only benign teratomas are found during surgery, and some have advised that these lesions should not be resected unless the serum markers are elevated. It has been our position that all of these should be resected regardless of the levels of the serum markers because immature elements can be found even when the markers are not elevated.

Soft Tissue Sarcomas

Soft tissue sarcomas frequently metastasize to the lung, and the lung is usually the only site of metastatic disease. For this reason many patients with metastatic soft tissue sarcomas are candidates for pulmonary resection. These patients are frequently younger and tolerate the resection well. Unfortunately soft tissue sarcomas do not respond to chemotherapy as well as osteogenic sarcomas do. However, some respond better than others. For instance Ewing's sarcomas have an excellent response to chemotherapy and radiation therapy, and reports indicate that the 5-year survival rate in these patients is 30 percent, which is similar to our experience (Burt et al., 1992). On the other hand, soft tissue sarcomas, such as leiomyosarcomas, liposarcomas, and mixoid and chrondrasarcomas have poor response rates to chemotherapy. However, in view of the fact that these tumors frequently metastasize to the lung and to the lung only, the best means for palliation and increasing the disease-free interval is by repeated surgical resection. Five-year survival rates for the resection of soft tissue sarcomas depend to a great extent on the selection criteria, and reports of survival rates vary between 25 and 45 percent. Those patients with fewer than four metastatic lesions, those with tumors with prolonged doubling times, and those with prolonged disease-free intervals in whom the primary tumor is completely controlled are likely to experience 5-year survival rates of 40 to 50 percent (Roth, et al., 1985; Putnam, et al., 1984). On the other hand, chemotherapy-resistant tumors and those with multiple bilateral nodules, those who have short disease-free intervals, and those whose tumors have rapid doubling times do not respond well to pulmonary resection.

Osteogenic Sarcoma

Osteogenic sarcoma has been a major success story over the past 15 years. In the prechemotherapy era, 95 percent of these patients developed pulmonary metastases, and the 5-year survival rate was less than 10 percent. At the University of California at Los Angeles prior to the development of effective chemotherapy, 92 percent of patients with primary osteosarcoma developed pulmonary metastases. Two hundred forty-seven patients with osteogenic sarcoma were treated between 1971 and 1991 (Skinner, et al., 1992).

When doxorubicin and high-dose methotrexate became available, the incidence of pulmonary metastases dropped from 92 to 63 percent. When bleomycin, cyclophosphamide, and dactinomycin were added to this regimen, the incidence of pulmonary metastases dropped from 63 to 48 percent. Most recently with the availability of doxorubicin, high-dose methotrexate, cisplatin, and ifosfamide, the incidence of pulmonary metastases have dropped to 31 percent. Therefore

Table 31-2. Osteogenic Sarcoma: University of California at Los Angeles Experience

Therapeutic Group	Percent with Lung Metastases (No.)	Disease-Free Interval (mo.)
I (no chemotherapy)	92 (12/13)	5
II (doxorubicin, high-dose methotrexate)	63 (33/52)[a]	10
III (doxorubicin, high-dose methotrexate, bleomycin, cyclophosphamide, dactinomycin)	48 (35/73)[a]	6
IV (doxorubicin, high-dose methotrexate, cisplatin, ±ifosfamide)	31 (34/109)[a]	7
Total	46 (114/247)	8

[a] $P < 0.05$.

over the 20-year period in which more effective chemotherapy was developed, the overall incidence of pulmonary metastases dropped from 92 to 31 percent (Table 31-2). Concomitantly during this time, the percentage of patients with metastases undergoing pulmonary resection rose from 17 percent in the prechemotherapy era to 82 percent over the last 5 years. The 5-year survival rate currently in patients undergoing resection for metastatic osteosarcoma ranges between 35 and 50 percent. The availability of effective chemotherapy has eliminated many of the standard selection criteria for these patients. In our studies the disease-free interval, number of nodules, and tumor doubling time has had no significant impact on survival (Table 31-3). This is almost certainly because these patients have been treated with chemotherapy and the chemotherapy has significantly altered the biology of the disease. It is now well documented that adjuvant therapy following the resection of primary osteogenic sarcoma significantly improves the survival rate from less than 10 percent to greater than 70 percent. The adjuvant chemotherapy also diminishes the incidence of pulmonary metastases. When patients do develop pulmonary metastases, the number of metastases are fewer, and the tumor doubling time is slower (Goorin, et al., 1991). Patients who have received chemotherapy are not uncommonly found to have eliminated malignant cells. It is generally believed that this finding is associated with a better survival rate. Currently our only selection criteria for operating on patients with osteogenic sarcomas is the presence of completely resectable disease and an adequate pulmonary reserve. Previously we did not operate on patients with a history of a malignant effusion. However, currently if the malignant effusion can be controlled with chemotherapy, these patients are operated on, and their tumors are completely resected, including resection of the diaphragm and chest wall if necessary. We have found that the use of intrapleural mitoxantrone (20 mg/m²) is effective in controlling recurrent effusions and sterilizing the intrapleural space.

Thus the only significant prognostic variable in these patients is whether or not the tumor can be completely resected. It must be emphasized that these patients may require repeated thoracotomies. However, it has been shown that patients who undergo multiple thoracotomies have as good a survival rate as those who require only one thoracotomy (Pastorino, et al., 1991).

Multiple thoracotomies for the resection of soft tissue and osteogenic sarcomas give survival rates of 20 and 40 percent. The survival rates for patients having one, two, or three thoracotomies were not significantly different in two different studies (Pastorino, et al., 1991; Casson, et al., 1991).

Chemotherapy has decreased the incidence of pulmonary metastases from osteosarcoma from 92 to 31 percent, and the proportion of patients undergoing resection has increased from 17 to 82 percent. Aggressive surgical management of pulmonary metastases has led to a 40 percent 5-year survival rate. Therefore pulmonary resection should be attempted in any patient with potentially resectable pulmonary metastases whose primary tumor is controlled and who has no extrapulmonary involvement.

Table 31-3. Univariate Analysis

Factor	P Value Overall Survival	P Value Post-Thoracotomy Survival
Age	0.143	
Sex	0.464	
Tumor site	0.559	
Amputation versus limb salvage	0.310	
No. of nodules	0.744	
Disease-free interval	0.013 ──────→	0.113
Bilateral disease	0.712	
No. of thoracotomies	0.589	

COMMENTS AND CONTROVERSIES

We have adopted an aggressive multimodality approach to patients with metastatic pulmonary disease. A long disease-free interval, effective chemotherapy, and slow tumor doubling times have been associated with favorable results following resection. The preoperative evaluation should include rigorous pulmonary function evaluation, including spirometry, diffusing capacity, and occasionally exercise testing, particularly in those who have received combined modality adju-

vant therapy and are at increased risk for postoperative adult respiratory distress syndrome.

Mediastinal or hilar lymphadenopathy identified preoperatively does not preclude pulmonary resection unless it is proved to be metastatic by mediastinoscopic, thoracoscopic, bronchoscopic, or fine-needle biopsy. "Debulking" or resection in the face of grossly residual disease to reduce the tumor load (i.e., to make chemotherapy more effective) has not been demonstrated to be effective and is not recommended.

Early postoperative mobilization, which is facilitated by the routine use of median sternotomy or muscle-sparing thoracotomy, and maximum preservation of pulmonary parenchyma are essential elements of the surgical technique in these patients who may eventually require multiple resections. We have found follow-up plain radiographs are not sensitive for recurrences secondary to postoperative changes; thus, CT scans are obtained at 4- to 6-month intervals for routine surveillance.

The role of the thoracoscopic resection of pulmonary malignancies is evolving and will undoubtedly have increasing utility in the treatment of secondary tumors. Because of the high incidence of multiple lesions and the difficulty in appreciating more deeply located nodules thoracoscopically, open resection with manual inspection and palpation of the involved lung is the preferred current therapy. Thoracoscopy is reserved for diagnostic biopsy and occasionally for post-chemotherapeutic tumor staging (e.g., renal cell and testicular cancers).

Surgical management of these lesions in the future will be further enhanced by the development of tumor markers for earlier serologic detection and tumor localization. The surgeon will work increasingly closely with the medical oncologist in the development of techniques of biologic immunotherapy.

E.C.H.

Pulmonary metastases are being treated surgically with increasing frequency, even when multiple metastases are present. In most series, complete resection of all metastases allows a 5-year disease-free survival of 30 to 40 percent, no matter the site of origin of the primary tumor. Although it is commonly accepted that more than four metastases results in a much poorer prognosis, even in these cases, 5-year survival can be significant.

I concur with Dr. Holmes in condemning video-assisted thoracoscopic approaches, even for solitary lesions, because of the significant incidence of undetected second lesions found on palpation of the collapsed lung at thoracotomy.

The role of adjuvant therapy following pulmonary metastasectomy in other than osteogenic sarcomas is unknown. The demonstration that adjuvant chemotherapy improves survival in resected carcinomas of the colon and breast suggests that after pulmonary metastasectomy for these conditions, adjuvant therapy should be considered and would be worthy of a randomized trial to assess its effectiveness.

Although traditionally breast carcinoma metastatic to the lung has not been considered a curable condition, recent reports suggest otherwise when treating solitary nodules. It should be remembered that of all solitary pulmonary nodules found in patients with breast carcinoma, over 50 percent are not metastases but primary tumors of the lung.

I have found great utility in the clam-shell (transverse sternotomy) approach for bilateral lesions.

R.J.G.

KEY REFERENCES

Casson AG, Putnam JB, Johnson D et al.: Efficacy of pulmonary metastastectomy for recurrent soft-tissue sarcoma. J Clin Oncol 47:1, 1991

The survival of 39 patients who underwent surgical resection for metastatic soft tissue sarcomas is reviewed. There was a significant increase in the survival in those patients who could be completely resected. Those with a single metastatic nodule had a much better survival than did those with multiple metastases. Other factors, such as disease-free interval and tumor doubling time, were not prognostic.

Harpole DH Jr, Johnson CM, Wolf WG et al.: Analysis of 945 cases of pulmonary metastatic melanoma. J Thorac Cardiovasc Surg 103:743, 1992

Pulmonary metastases were documented in 945 patients with melanoma with 1-, 3-, and 5-year survival rates of 30, 9, and 4 percent, respectively. Their data indicate that patients with one solitary metastasis do benefit from resection and have better survival rates than do those with multiple pulmonary nodules. They suggest the use of selective resection for isolated pulmonary metastasis in patients with malignant melanoma.

Lanza LA et al.: J Thorac Cardiovasc Surg 94:181, 1987

These investigators evaluated 19 patients with Ewing's sarcoma metastatic to the lung. Ten (53 percent) were made disease free by resection of the pulmonary metastases, six were found to have unresectable disease, and three were found to have benign pulmonary disease. The actuarial survival rate of the 10 patients who were completely resected was 15 percent, with a median survival of 28 months. Patients who underwent the resection of fewer than four metastatic lesions had a better prognosis. These authors emphasize that patients with metastatic Ewing's sarcoma to the lung may benefit from an aggressive surgical approach and warn that a significant proportion of these patients may have benign pulmonary disease.

Mandelbaum I, Williams SD, Einhorn LH: Aggressive surgical management of testicular carcinoma to the lungs and mediastinum. Ann Thorac Surg 30:224, 1980

Twenty-two patients with metastatic testicular carcinoma to the lung were evaluated. Five patients had nodules in the lungs that were fibrotic with no evidence of tumor, and nine showed embryonal cell carcinoma in the lung. All patients who had cystic teratomas are alive and free of disease. Cure rates following resection in these patients can be as high as 60 percent.

Pastorino U, Gasparin M, Tavecchio L et al.: The contribution of salvage surgery to the management of childhood osteosarcoma. J Clin Oncol 9:1357, 1991

These authors have extensive experience with 174 patients treated with metastatic osteosarcoma. The overall 5-year survival rate currently is 58 percent. The median survival is 33 months. During the period of observation, the proportion of patients who underwent complete resection of their pulmonary metastases rose from 17 to 55 percent. These excellent surgery and survival rates are achieved because of the excellent improvement in chemotherapy in this disease.

Skinner KA, Eilber MD, Holmes EC et al.: Surgical management and chemotherapy for pulmonary metastases from osteosarcoma. Arch Surg 127:1065, 1992

Two hundred forty-seven patients with stage I osteosarcomas were evaluated. The incidence of lung metastases in these patients decreased from 92 to 31 percent with the development of adequate and effective chemotherapy. With the development of adequate chemotherapy, the resection rate for pulmonary metastases increased from 17 to 82 percent. The overall 5-year cure rate currently with resection of metastatic osteosarcoma is 41 percent. Adjuvant chemotherapy and the resection of pulmonary metastases have transformed a uniformly fatal condition into one with a reasonable expectation of long-term survival.

REFERENCES

Alexander J, Haight C: Pulmonary resection for solitary metastatic sarcomas and carcinomas. Surg Gynecol Obstet 85:129, 1947

Barney JD, Churchill EJ: Adenocarcinoma of the kidney with metastases to the lung cured by nephrectomy and lobectomy. J Urol 42:269, 1939

Bethencourt DM, Holmes EC: Muscle sparing posterolateral thoracotomy. Ann Thorac Surg 45:337, 1988

Burt M, Martin K, Ozuru O, Ginsberg RJ: Medial tumors of the chest wall plasmacytoma and Ewing's sarcoma. Presented at the annual meeting of the American Association of Thoracic Surgery.

Callery CD, Holmes EC, Vernon S et al.: Resection of pulmonary metastases from non-seminomatous testicular tumors: correlation of clinical and histological features with treatment outcome. Cancer 51:1152, 1983

Chang AE, Schaner EG, Conkle DM et al.: Evaluation of computer tomography in the detection of pulmonary metastases. Cancer 43:193, 1979

Goorin AM, Jonathan JS, Baker A et al.: Changing pattern of pulmonary metastases with adjuvant chemotherapy in patients with osteosarcoma: results from the Institutional Osteosarcoma Study. J Clin Oncol 9:600, 1991

Gorenstein LA, Putnam JB, Natarajan et al.: Improved survival after resection of pulmonary metastases from malignant melanoma: see comments. Ann Thorac Surg 52:204, 1991

Goya T, Miyazawa N, Kondo H et al.: Surgical resection of pulmonary metastases from colorectal cancer. 10-Year follow-up. Cancer 64:1418, 1989

Huth JF, Holmes EC, Vernon SE et al.: Pulmonary resection for metastatic sarcoma. Am J Surg 140:9, 1980

Jett JR, Hollinger CG, Zinsmiester AR, Pairolero PC: Pulmonary resection of metastatic renal cell carcinoma. Chest 84:442, 1983

Lanza LA, Natarajan G, Roth JA, Putnam JB Jr: Long-term survival after resection of pulmonary metastases from carcinoma of the breast. Ann Thorac Surg 54:244, 1992

Mazer TM, Robbins KT, McMurtrey MJ, Byers RM: Resection of pulmonary metastases from squamous carcinoma of the head and neck. Am J Surg 156:238, 1988

McAfee MK, Allen MS, Trastek VF et al.: Colorectal lung metastases: results of surgical excision. Ann Thorac Surg 53:780, 1992

McCormack P: Surgical resection of pulmonary metastases. Semin Surg Oncol 6:297, 1990

McCormack PM, Attiyeh FF: Resected pulmonary metastases from colorectal cancer. Dis Colon Rectum 22:553, 1977

McCormack PM, Bains MS, Beattie Jr et al.: Pulmonary resection in metastatic carcinoma. Chest 73:163, 1978

McCormack PN, Martini N: The changing role of surgery for pulmonary metastases. Ann Thorac Surg 28:139, 1979

Morton DL, Joseph WL, Ketchan AS et al.: Surgical resection and adjuvant immunotherapy for selective patients with multiple pulmonary metastases. Ann Surg 178:360, 1973

Mountain CF, McMurtrey MJ, Hermes KE: Surgery for pulmonary metastases: a 20 year experience. Ann Thorac Surg 38:323, 1984

Phil E, Hughes ES, McDermott FT: Lung recurrence for curative surgery for colorectal cancer. Dis Colon Rectum 30:417, 1992

Pogrebniak HW, Stovroff M, Roth JA, Pass HI: Resection of pulmonary metastases from malignant melanoma: results of a 16 year experience. Ann Thorac Surg 46:20, 1980

Putnam JB, Roth JA, Wesley MN et al.: Analysis of prognostic factors in patients undergoing resection of pulmonary metastases from soft-tissue sarcomas. J Thorac Cardiovasc Surg 87:260, 1984

Rosenberg S, Lotze M, Yang JC et al.: Experience with the use of high dose interleukin-2 in the treatment of 652 cancer patients. Ann Surg 210:474, 1989

Roth JA, Putnam JB, Wesley MN, Rosenberg S: Differing determinants of prognosis following resection of pulmonary metastases from osteogenic and soft-tissue sarcoma patients. Cancer 155:1361, 1985

Schott G, Weissmuller J, Vecera E: Methods and prognosis of the extirpation of pulmonary metastases following tumor nephrectomy. Urol Int 43:272, 1988

Thomford NR, Woolner LB, Clagett OT: Surgical treatment of metastatic tumors in the lungs. J Thorac Cardiovasc Surg 49:357, 1965

Twohig KJ, Matthay RA: Pulmonary effects of cytotoxic agents other than bleomycin. Clin Chest Med 11:31, 1979

Wilkins EW Jr: The status of pulmonary resection from metastases: experience at Masschusetts General Hospital. In Weiss L, Gilbert HA (eds): Pulmonary Metastases. GK Hall, Boston, 1978

32

SURGICAL TECHNIQUES

INTRODUCTION

Thoracic surgery remains an exciting field for many reasons. It is one of the few surgical specialties where the complete care of the patient from diagnosis to investigation to therapy can remain within the realm of the practicing surgeon. The physician-surgeon must be an accomplished diagnostician, physiologist, and technician. This chapter is concerned with the latter area of expertise. It is fair to say that pulmonary surgery remains one of the most challenging areas of surgical endeavor. The accomplished thoracic surgeon must be an expert endoscopist, must have the capabilities of performing all surgical diagnostic interventions, and must be well versed in cardiopulmonary anatomy. The techniques of thoracic surgery continue to expand as evidenced by the burgeoning field of video-assisted thoracoscopy.

In the following chapter parts, we have requested that the authors not dwell on surgical techniques described in many operative surgical volumes. Instead, we have asked the authors to present their personal preferences and where possible to indicate the favorite "tricks" that they have honed to perfection over the years. The reader is well advised to refer to standard volumes of operative techniques for further instruction and illustration. A helpful adjunct for the readers of *Thoracic Surgery* is that of Urschel and Cooper (*Atlas of Thoracic Surgery,* Churchill Livingstone, New York, 1995). This chapter is not intended to be a compendium of operative pulmonary surgery but only an introduction to supplant that information already found in standard textbooks.

Those readers interested in surgery for chronic pulmonary embolus and the operative approaches for lung and heart-lung transplantation are referred to Chapters 24 and 33.

Mediastinoscopy

Thomas J. Kirby
Stanley C. Fell

HISTORICAL NOTE

Cervical mediastinal exploration was originally described by Harken and associates in 1954. Their technique was basically an extension of scalene node biopsy as developed by Daniels (1949) and was used to sample lymph nodes in the superior mediastinum and paratracheal areas. Carlens (1959) and Pearson (1965), using a specially designed mediastinoscope and

a suprasternal notch incision, developed and popularized the indications and techniques currently used. Lymph nodes in the aortopulmonary window can be sampled by an anterior mediastinotomy approach, a technique first described by McNeil and Chamberlain (1966). This technique can also be employed on the right side to explore and assess involvement of the anterior mediastinum, right hilum, and superior vena cava. Ginsberg and associates (1987) developed the technique of "extended" cervical mediastinoscopy as an alternative to left anterior mediastinotomy.

HISTORICAL READINGS

Carlens E: Mediastinoscopy: a method for inspection and tissue biopsy of the superior mediastinum. Chest 36:343, 1959

Daniels AC: Method of biopsy useful in diagnosing intrathoracic diseases. Dis Chest 16:360, 1949

Ginsberg RJ, Rice TW, Goldberg et al: Extended cervical mediastinoscopy, a single staging procedure for bronchogenic carcinoma of the left upper lobe. J Thorac Cardiovasc Surg 94:673, 1987

Harken DE, Black H, Clauss R, Farrand RE: A single cervical-mediastinal exploration for tissue diagnosis of intrathoracic disease. N Engl J Med 251:1041, 1954

McNeil TM, Chamberlain JM: Diagnostic anterior mediastinoscopy. Ann Thorac Surg 22:260, 1966

Pearson FG: Mediastinoscopy: a method of biopsy in the superior mediastinum. J Thorac Cardiovasc Surg 49:11, 1965

INDICATIONS AND DIAGNOSIS

Although mediastinoscopy and mediastinotomy are used primarily in the staging of lung carcinoma, they are also of value in biopsying mediastinal masses and lymph nodes to establish the diagnosis in diseases such as sarcoidosis, lymphoma, and mediastinal tumors. Bronchogenic carcinoma that has metastasized to mediastinal lymph nodes (stage IIIa or IIIb disease) is in most cases not resectable for cure. Neither adjuvant nor neoadjuvant treatment in the form of radiotherapy and/or chemotherapy has altered the dismal prognosis of stage III lung carcinoma (5-year survival <10 percent). Thus the importance of establishing involvement of mediastinal lymph nodes with metastatic disease (N2 or N3 disease) prior to thoracotomy is readily apparent. This information will avoid unnecessary thoracotomies in patients with incurable disease (N3 and multistation N2 disease, extracapsular invasion, extension into mediastinal structures (T4 tumors)) and also correctly stage patients who are potential candidates for neoadjuvant trials. Frozen section results of mediastinal nodes are accurate, allowing the surgeon to proceed immediately to thoracotomy if indicated.

Another staging procedure for assessing the status of mediastinal lymph nodes is transbronchial needle aspiration/biopsy as reported by Wang and associates (1983). This technique is of value in establishing a diagnosis of bronchogenic carcinoma or confirming inoperability in those patients with radiographically unresectable mediastinal lymph node involvement. Otherwise, all patients should be staged with mediastinoscopy and/or mediastinotomy. These techniques allow accurate assessment of mediastinal lymph node involvement, resulting in an informed and appropriate judgment as to resectability and possible treatment options.

Computed tomography (CT) and magnetic resonance imaging (MRI) are useful screening tests to detect enlargement of mediastinal lymph nodes and direct mediastinal invasion. Although Daly, et al. (1984) and Glazer, et al. (1984) reported sensitivities in the 90 percent range, Staples, et al. (1988) and McLoud, et al. (1992) and associates reported a sensitivity in the 60 percent range and a specificity of 50 percent, defining a lymph node size greater than 1 cm in the short axis as pathologically enlarged. As compared with the 90 percent sensitivity of mediastinoscopy, the relatively poor sensitivity of CT scanning would thus result in many unnecessary thoracotomies. In a patient with a normal CT scan and a T1 peripheral carcinoma, mediastinoscopy might be omitted, but otherwise all patients should be invasively staged. CT scans can also be of value in identifying enlarged mediastinal lymph nodes and mediastinal invasion by tumor. The surgeon is thus forewarned to pay particular attention to these areas during mediastinoscopy.

Cervical Mediastinoscopy

With a bolster under the patient's shoulders and the neck fully extended, a 3- to 4-cm skin incision is made one fingerbreadth above the suprasternal notch. Dissection is carried down directly in the midline, bluntly separating the strap muscles with the aid of small right angle retractors. The thyroid gland is retracted superiorly, with care taken not to avulse the inferior thyroid veins, which can be electrocoagulated or ligated with fine suture to avoid troublesome bleeding. The pretracheal fascia is exposed, opened, and bluntly dissected from the anterior aspect of the trachea by using the index finger. By direct palpation an attempt is made to identify mediastinal adenopathy, masses, or areas of direct mediastinal invasion. The fascia just inferior and anterior to the innominate artery should be entered to allow the anterior mediastinum and subinnominate space to be assessed. A mediastinoscope can now be introduced along the anterior surface of the trachea (Fig. 32-1). Mediastinal lymph nodes that are accessible to biopsy include the subcarinal (#7), subinnominate (#3a), ipsilateral and contralateral tracheobronchial (#4), and paratracheal (#2). Posterior subcarinal, paraesophageal (#8), and inferior pulmonary ligament (#9) lymph nodes cannot be biopsied through a standard cervical mediastinoscopy or anterior mediastinotomy.

A metal suction catheter is used as a dissecting instrument to further dissect fascial planes and identify lymph nodes and vascular structures. There is usually a firm layer of fascial tissue that has to be opened in order to gain access to the subcarinal space. If there is any question as to the vascular nature of a structure, it is wise to use a spinal needle mounted on a small syringe to aspirate the structure in question. It is not necessary to remove the entire lymph node to provide representative tissue. Small, bleeding vessels are easily coagulated by using the tip of the suction catheter and touching the proximal end of the catheter with an electrocautery tip. Vascular clips may also be applied through the mediastinoscope. As described by Deslauriers, et al. (1976), if there is a need to assess the pleural space (e.g., for the presence of an effusion or possible metastatic involvement), the mediastinal pleura just lateral to the trachea can be bluntly broken through and the mediastinoscope introduced to inspect the pleural space and obtain suitable tissue or fluid samples.

Anterior Mediastinotomy

Anterior mediastinotomy was developed by McNeil and Chamberlain (1966) to sample lymph nodes in the subaortic and periaortic regions that are not accessible through cervical

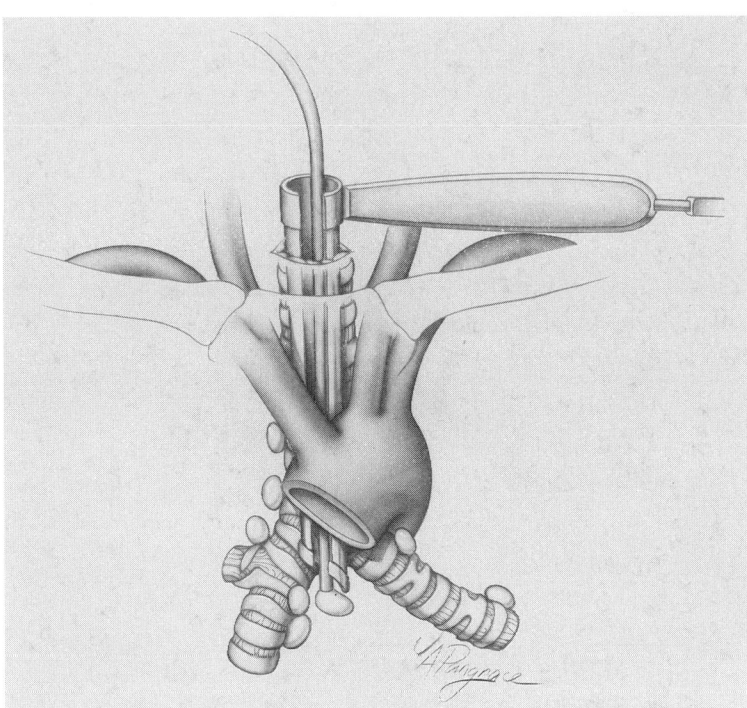

Figure 32-1. Cervical mediastinoscopy: a mediastinoscope is introduced through a suprasternal notch incision into the pretracheal space, where samples of paratracheal, tracheobronchial, subcarinal, and subinnominate lymph nodes can be obtained.

mediastinoscopy. Mediastinotomy is classically carried out through the second left intercostal space. The technique can also be employed on the right side to biopsy mediastinal masses and lymph nodes. In the technique as originally described, a vertical parasternal incision removing the second costal cartilage was used. A transverse incision directly over the second intercostal space, which does not remove a costal cartilage, is also effective.

A 3- to 4-cm skin incision is made directly over the second intercostal space just lateral to the sternal border. Dissection is carried down to the pectoralis major, separating its fibers. Electrocautery is used along the superior border of the second costal cartilage to divide the intercostal muscles, with care taken not to injure the internal mammary vessels. An attempt is made to bluntly dissect the mediastinal pleura with an index finger down to the aortopulmonary window without entering the pleural space. If the pleural space is entered, a pleural drainage catheter is placed at the end of the procedure, with the anesthesiologist's hand bagging the patient to evacuate all intrapleural air. Unless the underlying lung parenchyma has been injured, one should be able to remove the catheter at the end of the procedure or in the recovery room. If mediastinotomy is being carried out in conjunction with mediastinoscopy, the aortopulmonary window can be bimanually palpated by inserting one index finger through the neck incision and the other through the mediastinotomy incision. This will help in identifying adenopathy or tumor fixation in the area.

A mediastinoscope can now be safely introduced through the incision (Fig. 32-2). Care must be taken not to injure the phrenic or vagus nerves as they pass over the aortic arch. The superior pulmonary vein, aorta, and left main pulmonary artery as it passes under the aortic arch are all at risk of injury. If the proper technique is followed, regional lymph nodes are easily and safely identified and biopsied.

Extended Cervical Mediastinoscopy

Extended cervical mediastinoscopy as described by Ginsberg and associates (1987) can supplant left anterior mediastinotomy and carries the advantage of avoiding a separate incision. Blunt dissection with an index finger is used to open tissue between the innominate and carotid arteries, superior to the arch of the aorta. A mediastinoscope is then introduced anterior to the aortic arch and between the innominate and carotid arteries (Fig. 32-3). The mediastinoscope can then be advanced over top of the aorta to the aortopulmonary window. In addition to the innominate and carotid arteries, the same nerves and vessels as in mediastinotomy are at risk of injury.

Scalene Lymph Node Biopsy

The involvement of supraclavicular lymph nodes (stage IIIb disease) is obviously a grave prognostic sign. Enlarged nodes in this area may be simply needle-aspirated to confirm involvement, but a negative aspirate does not rule out metastatic disease and will have to be confirmed with an excisional biopsy. Enlarged lymph nodes may be locally excised, or a formal excision of the scalene fat pad may be performed.

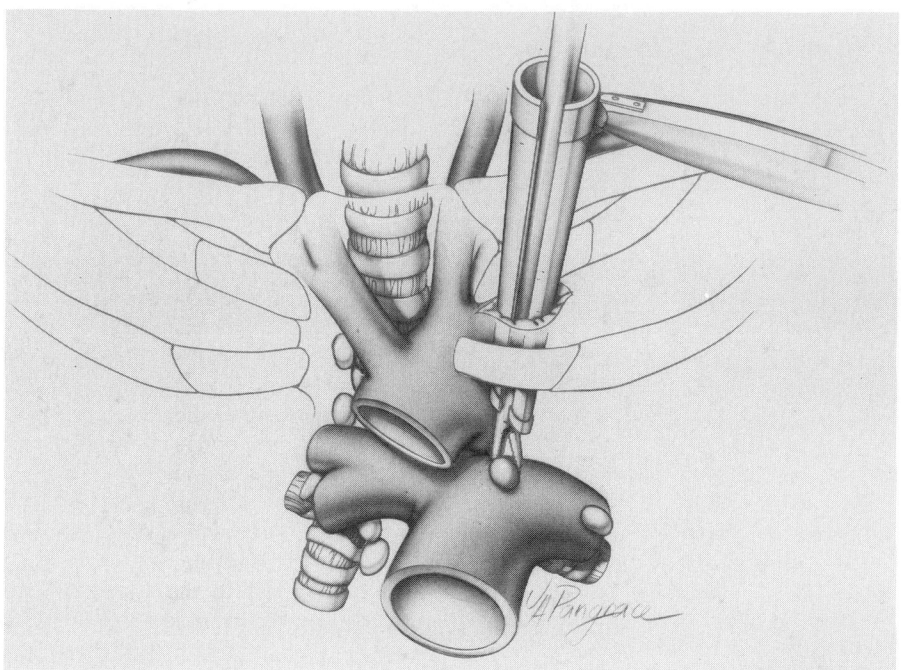

Figure 32-2. Anterior mediastinoscopy: a mediastinoscope is introduced through a parasternal incision placed in the second intercostal space. On the left side, this allows periaortic and aortopulmonary window lymph nodes to be sampled.

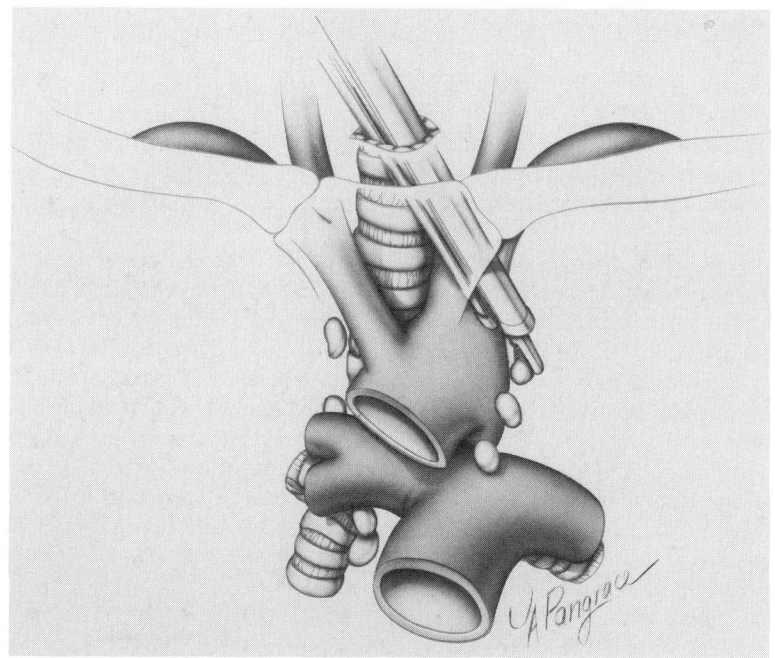

Figure 32-3. Extended cervical mediastinoscopy: by the same approach as for standard cervical mediastinoscopy, a mediastinoscope is introduced over the aortic arch and into the aortopulmonary window.

A small 3- to 4-cm incision is placed over the origin of the sternocleidomastoid muscle just above and parallel to the clavicle. Either dissection is carried down between the clavicular and sternal heads, or the entire muscle is retracted medially. This exposes the scalene fat pad, which lies on top of the anterior scalenus muscle medial to the internal jugular vein (Fig. 32-4). The fat pad is carefully dissected away from the internal jugular vein laterally and the scalenus anterior muscle posteriorly. Care must be taken not to injure the phrenic nerve, which is separated from the operative field by only a thin fascial sheath overlying the scalenus anterior. The transverse cervical artery, which usually enters inferiorly, is divided to allow complete excision of the fat pad, which should contain five or more lymph nodes for pathologic examination.

COMPLICATIONS

In experienced hands, the complications of mediastinoscopy and mediastinotomy are rare (1 to 2 percent), but the potential for catastrophic complications is apparent. Puhakka (1989) reported on 2,021 mediastinoscopies with a complication rate of 2.3 percent and no associated deaths. Only 10 (0.5 percent) of these complications were considered major; these were four cases of hemorrhage, three of tracheal rupture, and three of wound infection. Basca and colleagues (1974) reported on 11,623 mediastinoscopies from 15 different series. Bleeding that required operation was noted in 0.1 percent of cases, with pneumothorax occurring in 0.5 percent and vocal cord paralysis in 0.4 percent. In another series of 1,000 cases, Luke and associates (1989) from the University of Toronto reported a 2.3 percent complication rate. Only three complications were considered major, including two cases of hemorrhage and one of tracheal injury. Minor complications included six pneumothoraces, five wound infections, and nine other complications. There were no reported recurrent nerve injuries.

Major complications during mediastinoscopy are most commonly encountered at either tracheobronchial angle. On the right side, the azygos vein and anterior pulmonary arterial branch to the right upper lobe are at risk of injury. The azygos vein is easily mistaken for an anthracotic lymph node and inadvertently biopsied. Experience and the liberal use of a long aspirating needle prior to biopsy will prevent this complication. Lymph nodes in this area are often directly adherent to branches of the pulmonary artery, which are therefore at risk if deep biopsies are taken or if excessive traction is applied. The apical arterial branch can also be injured if the mediastinoscope is "levered" anteriorly, resulting in a traction injury to the artery. At the left tracheobronchial angle, the recurrent laryngeal nerve is in close proximity to regional lymph nodes and is easily traumatized if care is not taken. Again, the entire lymph node should not be sampled since the recurrent laryngeal nerve is usually directly adherent to nodes in this area. Bleeding is best handled with packing placed through the mediastinoscope rather than by electrocautery, which may cause permanent damage to the recurrent nerve.

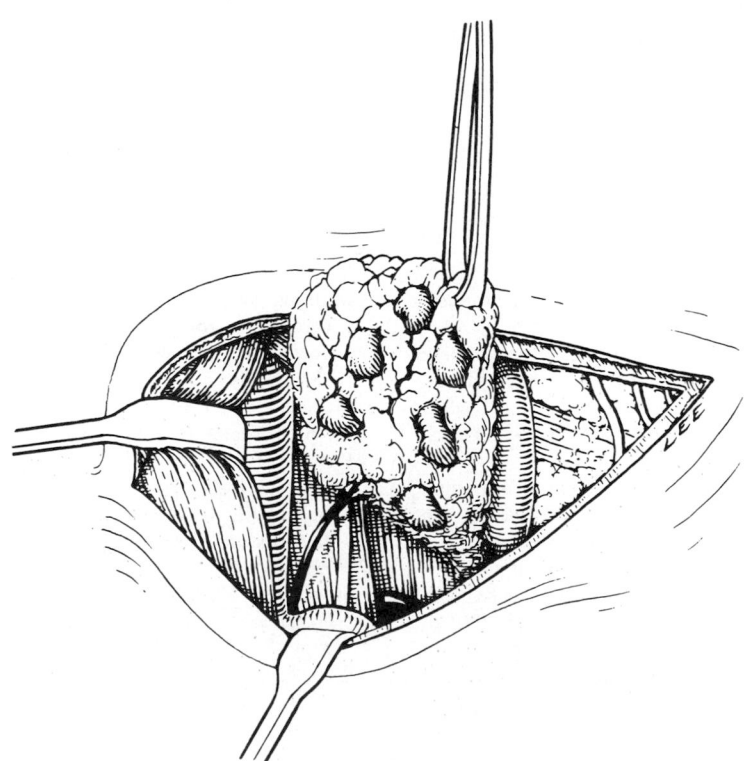

Figure 32-4. With the sternocleidomastoid muscle retracted medially, the scalene fat pad is mobilized off the internal jugular vein and the scalenus anterior muscle posteriorly. The phrenic nerve can be seen lying on the scalenus anterior with the transverse cervical artery entering the fat pad inferiorly.

In the event of massive bleeding, mediastinal packing will usually control the hemorrhage while blood is obtained and preparations are made for a possible thoracotomy or median sternotomy. Following 10 minutes of gauze tamponade, with the operating room prepared for a major procedure, the gauze packing is gently removed. In many cases the hemorrhage will have subsided or decreased so that the bleeding site can be identified. In the face of persistent uncontrollable hemorrhage, the mediastinum should be repacked and a decision made as to whether thoracotomy or median sternotomy offers the best approach to control of the hemorrhage. Median sternotomy is the most versatile incision and allows most injuries to be easily identified and controlled. It also allows the surgeon to expeditiously institute cardiopulmonary bypass to gain control of major vessel injuries. A disadvantage of sternotomy is the difficulty in carrying out a definitive pulmonary resection once the hemorrhage is controlled.

Injuries to the esophagus are extremely rare. As the esophagus lies directly posterior to the subcarinal space, most injuries occur during the exploration of this space and the biopsy of subcarinal lymph nodes. This injury is often not recognized at the time of surgery and often is only diagnosed postoperatively when the patient develops mediastinitis and an esophagogram is obtained. The detection of cervical or mediastinal air, pneumothorax, and/or pleural effusion in the early postoperative period should alert the surgeon to the possibility of this complication and lead to further investigation. These injuries are dealt with by the same principles applied to managing other forms of esophageal trauma (see Ch 64).

Tracheobronchial tree injuries are also rare. They are usually recognized at the time of surgery when an air leak is encountered. As reported by Puhakka (1989), most of these injuries can be controlled by packing of the area with absorbable cellulose gauze (Surgicel, Johnson & Johnson, New Brunswick, NJ). It is also prudent to leave a drain in the area. The positive pressure of mechanical ventilation makes even small injuries to the airway appear significant, but once the patient has been extubated and is breathing spontaneously, most of these injuries will seal. As reported by Schubach and Landreneau (1992), more extensive injuries will require a direct surgical approach and primary repair.

KEY REFERENCES

Carlens E: Mediastinoscopy: a method for inspection and tissue biopsy of the superior mediastinum. Chest 36:343, 1959

The initial report on cervical mediastinoscopy using a suprasternal notch incision as compared with the more cumbersome approach originally reported by Harken and associates (1949). This technique has withstood the test of time and is still employed today.

Luke WP, Pearson FG, Todd TRJ et al: Prospective evaluation of mediastinoscopy for assessment of carcinoma of the lung. J Thorac Cardiovasc Surg 91:53, 1986

This report on 1,000 mediastinoscopies performed in the staging of lung cancer demonstrates its high level of sensitivity, specificity, and overall accuracy combined with a low operative morbidity.

Pearson FG: Mediastinoscopy: a method of biopsy in the superior mediastinum. J Thorac Cardiovasc Surg 49:11, 1965

An excellent review of the initial experience of the surgeon responsible for popularizing mediastinoscopy in North America and demonstrating its value in staging bronchogenic carcinoma.

REFERENCES

Basca S, Czako Z, Vezendi S: The complications of mediastinoscopy. Panminerva Med 16:402, 1974

Daly BDT Jr, Faling LJ, Pugatch RD et al: Computed tomography: an effective technique for mediastinal staging in lung cancer. J Thorac Cardiovasc Surg 88:486, 1984

Daniels AC: Method of biopsy useful in the diagnosing certain intrathoracic diseases. Dis Chest 16:360, 1949

Deslauriers J, Beaulieu M, Dufour C et al: Mediastino-pleuroscopy: a new approach to the diagnosis of intra-thoracic diseases. Ann Thorac Surg 22:265, 1976

Ginsberg RJ, Rice TW, Goldberg et al: Extended cervical mediastinoscopy: a single staging procedure for bronchogenic carcinoma of the left upper lobe. J Thorac Cardiovasc Surg 94:673, 1987

Glazer GM, Orringer MB, Gross BH, Quint LE: The mediastinum in non-small cell cancer: CT-surgical correlation. AJR 142:1101, 1984

Harkens DE, Black H, Clauss R, Farrand RE: A single cervical-mediastinal exploration for tissue diagnosis of intrathoracic disease. N Engl J Med 251:1041, 1954

McLoud TC, Bourgouin PM, Greenberg RW et al: Bronchogenic carcinoma: analysis of staging in the mediastinum with CT by correlative lymph node mapping and sampling. Radiology 182:319, 1992

McNeil TM, Chamberlain JM: Diagnostic anterior mediastinotomy. Ann Thorac Surg 2:532, 1966

Puhakka H: Complications of mediastinoscopy. J Laryngol Otol 103:312, 1989

Schubach SL, Landreneau RJ: Mediastinoscopic injury to the bronchus: use of incontinuity bronchial flap repair. Ann Thorac Surg 93:1101, 1992

Staples CA, Muller NL, Miller RR et al: Mediastinal nodes in bronchogenic carcinoma: comparison between CT and mediastinoscopy. Radiology 67:367, 1988

Wang KP, Brower R, Haponik EF, Siegelman S: Flexible transbronchial needle aspiration for staging bronchogenic carcinoma. Chest 84:571, 1983

Open Lung Biopsy

Thomas J. Kirby
Stanley C. Fell

The thoracic surgeon is frequently required to obtain a specimen of lung tissue for diagnosis in patients, often critically ill, with respiratory symptoms associated with undiagnosed pulmonary fibrosis or infiltrates. With the refinement of transbronchial needle aspiration/biopsy and bronchoalveolar lavage, open lung biopsy is now less frequently performed but may be indicated if these investigations fail to yield a diagnosis.

PATIENT POSITION

Depending on the surgical approach there are two options in positioning the patient. For an anterolateral thoracotomy the patient is placed supine with a roll under the shoulders and hips to rotate the side to be biopsied by 30 degrees (Fig. 32-5). Alternatively, the patient can be placed in a full lateral position and the chest entered through the auscultatory triangle (Fig. 32-6). Ruskin and associates (1990) have shown that open lung biopsy can be safely performed in the intensive care unit (ICU), which avoids the logistics of transporting an often critically ill patient who can be difficult to ventilate. However, the operating room offers definite advantages over the ICU setting, including better lighting, full instrumentation, and the availability of appropriately trained personnel. Many open lung biopsies may be performed by a video-assisted thoracoscopic approach, as detailed in Chapter 9. However, the perceived advantages of this approach over a small anterolateral thoracotomy have yet to be demonstrated in a comparative study.

TECHNIQUE

If an anterolateral thoracotomy approach is selected, a 6- to 8-cm submammary thoracotomy is made and the chest entered through the fourth or fifth intercostal space, which enables biopsy specimens to be obtained from both the upper and lower lobes (Fig. 32-5). Alternatively, with the patient in the full lateral thoracotomy position, the incision can be placed over the auscultatory triangle and the chest entered by reflecting the latissimus dorsi anteriorly and the trapezius posteriorly (Fig. 32-6). At least two biopsies from different lobes should be performed to ensure that adequate and representative tissue is obtained. Careful review of the open lung biopsies and computed tomography (CT) scans will help direct the surgeon to the appropriate areas. Biopsy specimens should be taken from pulmonary parenchyma that appears to be involved by the underlying disease process as well as from areas that by inspection appear relatively normal. This should provide the pathologist with representative samples of the disease in various stages of its evolution, increasing the chance for an accurate diagnosis and perhaps aiding in determining the prognosis. Stapling instruments allow biopsies to be expeditiously carried out, providing a secure hemostatic and airtight closure (Fig. 32-7 and 32-8).

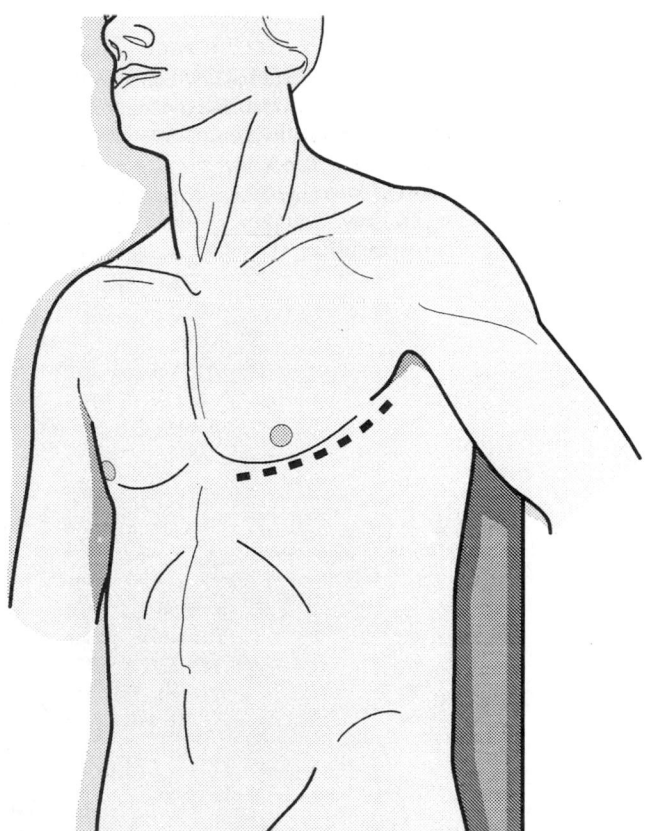

Figure 32-5. Positioning for an anterior lateral thoracotomy and open lung biopsy. The patient is placed supine with a roll under the operative side to rotate the chest by 30 degrees.

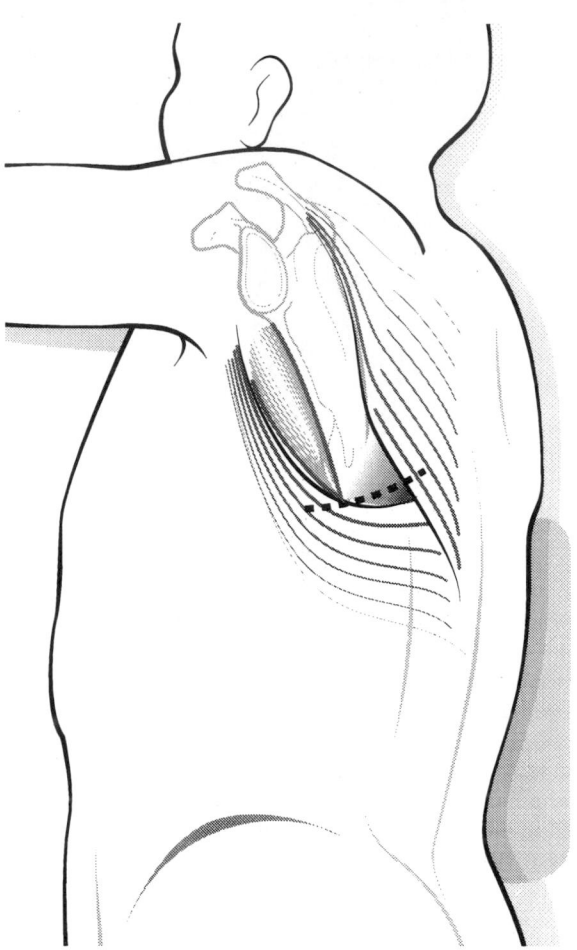

Figure 32-6. An alternative approach to an open lung biopsy is a full lateral position, placing the incision over the auscultatory triangle (as illustrated) and entering the chest between the trapezius and latissimus dorsi muscles.

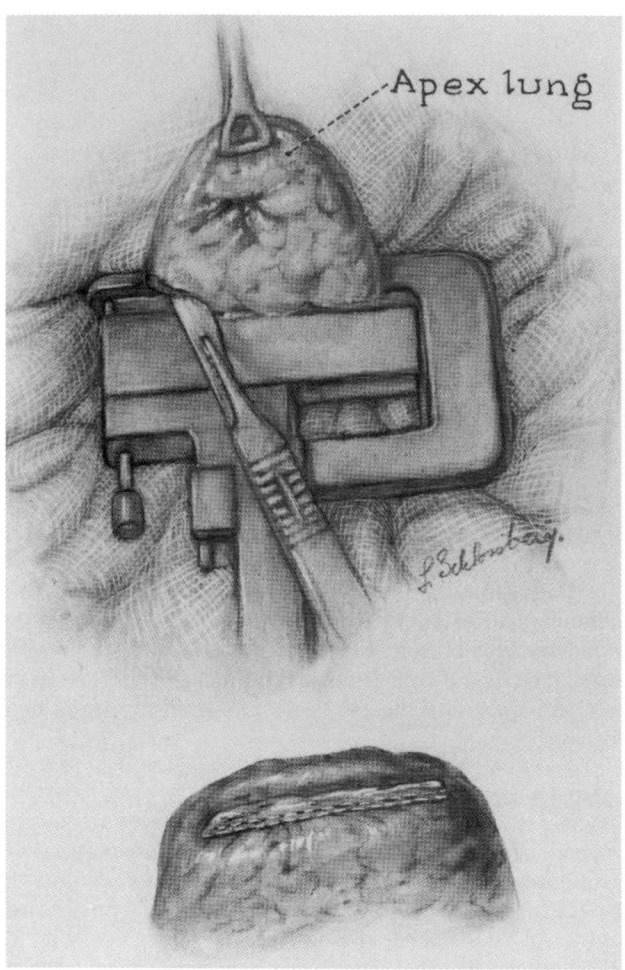

Figure 32-7. A linear stapler being used for a wedge biopsy.

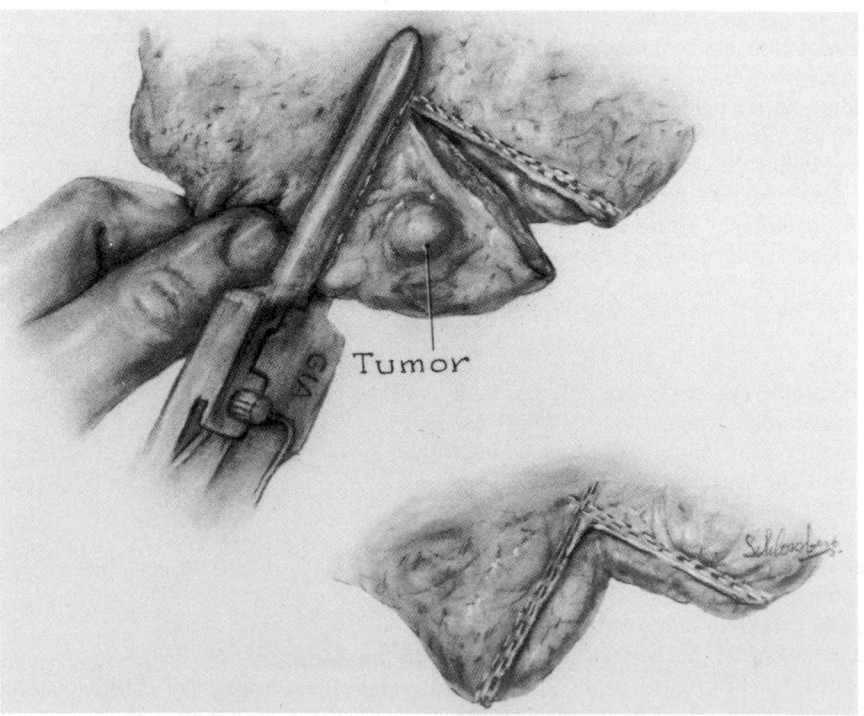

Figure 32-8. An alternative method using a linear stapler to obtain an open lung biopsy.

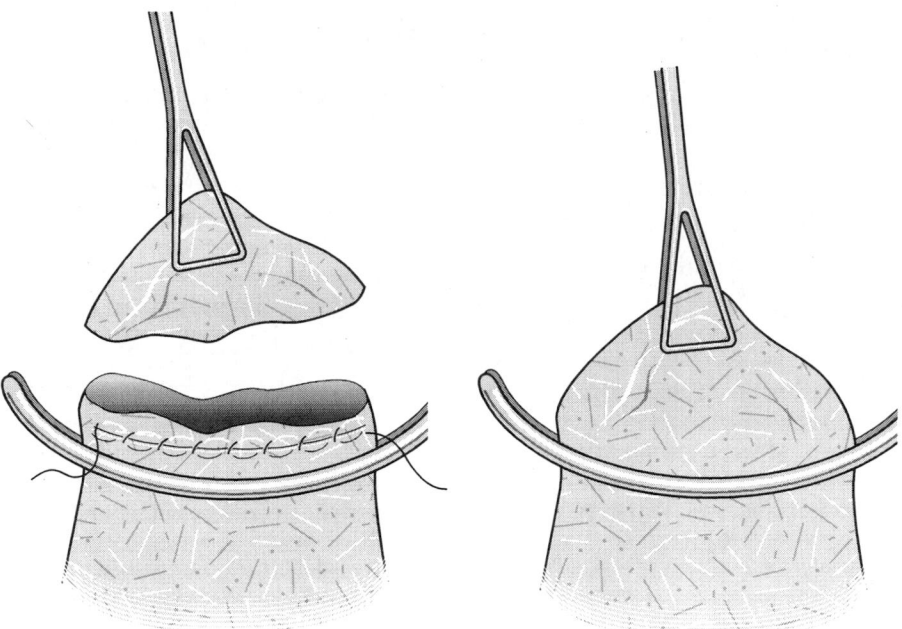

Figure 32-9. Prior to the introduction of stapling instruments, noncrushing clamps were used to obtain a lung biopsy, and the cut surface was simply oversewn.

Prior to the availability of stapling instruments a lung clamp was simply applied to the outer edge of the lung parenchyma, a specimen excised, and the cut surface oversewn (Fig. 32-9).

It is best to obtain a frozen section of the specimen to demonstrate that an adequate specimen has been obtained and to alert the pathologist if special investigations (e.g., electron microscopy, silver staining for pneumocystis) are necessary. In general, it is best to avoid biopsying the middle lobe and lingula, as these pulmonary segments occasionally have microscopic fibrosis and vascular changes even in the absence of underlying lung disease. However, it is still possible to obtain diagnostic tissue from these areas as shown by reports from Imoke, et al. (1983) and Weng, et al. (1980). If infection is a preoperative consideration, especially in an immunocompromised patient, a specimen should be sent for appropriate cultures.

RESULTS

Although there is some controversy regarding the value of open lung biopsy in influencing therapy and/or prognosis, there are reports in the literature that are encouraging. Nelems and colleagues (1976) reported that the working preoperative diagnosis in patients undergoing open lung biopsy was incorrect 55 percent of the time but that the diagnostic accuracy of the procedure was 96 percent. McKenna and associates (1984) reported a 90 percent accuracy of open lung biopsy, with 71 percent of patients having their therapy changed as a result. Cheson and colleagues (1985) found that in immunocompromised patients open lung biopsy led to a definitive diagnosis in 54 percent and a change of therapy in 38 percent.

Walker and associates (1989) reported on 61 patients who had undergone open lung biopsy, including 22 who were immunocompromised; open lung biopsy gave a specific diagnosis in 13 (59 percent) and resulting in a change in therapy in 17 (77 percent). In the 39 nonimmunocompromised patients, a specific diagnosis was only obtained in 8 (21 percent) and led in a change in therapy in 16 (41 percent). Warner and colleagues (1988) reported on 80 patients with diffuse pulmonary infiltrates and acute respiratory failure who underwent open lung biopsy. Open lung biopsy led to a specific diagnosis in 66 percent and a change in therapy in 70 percent. However, only 30 percent of these patients left hospital, with just 11 percent surviving for more than 1 year. Survival was best in young patients and those not requiring preoperative mechanical ventilation. Warner et al. concluded that although open lung biopsy was an accurate diagnostic tool, its utility is limited by the lack of therapy for the underlying disease process.

In properly selected cases, open lung biopsy should lead to a specific diagnosis and change in therapy in 50 to 70 percent of patients. Although in many cases there is no specific therapy for the underlying disease process, the fact that therapy may be added or subtracted on the basis of an accurate diagnosis would logically dictate that the procedure offers the best chance for recovery.

The mortality associated with open lung biopsy can be daunting. Saterfield and McLaughlin (1979) reported a 12 percent mortality and Nelems and colleagues (1976) 57 percent. Death is obviously related to the underlying disease process rather than to the operative procedure itself and occurs most frequently with ICU patients who are ventilator-dependent.

KEY REFERENCES

Warner DO, Warner MA, Divertie MB: Open lung biopsy in patients with diffuse pulmonary infiltrates and acute respiratory failure. Am Rev Respir Dis 137:90, 1988

A detailed report on 80 patients with diffuse pulmonary infiltrates and acute respiratory failure. This study shows the accuracy of open lung biopsy in establishing a diagnosis but also points out the limited therapeutic options for most of the underlying disease processes.

Walker WA, Cole HF, Khandekar A et al: Does open lung biopsy affect treatment in patients with diffuse pulmonary infiltrates? J Thorac Cardiovasc Surg 97:534, 1989

This retrospective review of 61 patients demonstrates the accuracy of open lung biopsy in both immunocompromised and noncompromised patients with diffuse pulmonary infiltrates and how the results of biopsy often lead to a change in therapy.

REFERENCES

Cheson BD, Samlowski WE, Tang TT, Spruance SL: Value of open lung biopsy in 87 immunocompromised patients with pulmonary infiltrates. Cancer 55:453, 1985

Daniels AC: Method of biopsy useful in the diagnosing of certain intrathoracic diseases. Dis Chest 16:360, 1949

Imoke E, Dudgeon DL, Colombana P et al: Open lung biopsy in the immunocompromised pediatric patient. J Pediatr Surg 10:816, 1983

McKenna RJ Jr, Mountain CF, McMurtrey MJ: Open lung biopsy in immunocompromised patients. Chest 86:671, 1984

Nelems JM, Cooper JD, Henderson RD et al: Emergency open lung biopsy. Ann Thorac Surg 22:260, 1976

Ruskin G, Brodman R, Condit D, Karpel J: Prospective evaluation of bedside open lung biopsy (abstr). Am Rev Respir Dis, suppl. 141:A596, 1990

Saterfield JR Jr, McLaughlin JS: Open lung biopsy in diagnosing pulmonary infiltrates in immunosuppressed patients. Ann Thorac Surg 28:359, 1979

Weng TR, Levinson H, Wentworth P et al: Open lung biopsy in children. Am Rev Respir Dis 97:673, 1980

Pneumonectomy

Paul F. Waters

HISTORICAL NOTE

The first successful one-stage pneumonectomy was performed by Graham and Singer in 1933 for a patient with bronchogenic carcinoma. This followed the first pneumonectomy in multiple stages in a patient with tuberculosis and empyema, achieved by Macewen in 1895. Earlier attempts had not met with success. In 1910 Kummel performed a pneumonectomy for lung cancer by clamping the pedicle and leaving the clamps in situ; that patient survived 6 days. The first individual hilar ligation was accomplished by Hinz in 1922, and that patient succumbed to heart failure on the third postoperative day. Churchill in 1930, Archibald in 1931, and Ivanissevich in 1933 had also attempted removal of a whole lung with no survival beyond a few days. Churchill left a tube in the residual bronchus, bringing it out through the chest wall. Reinhoff first described the modern-day technique of individual ligation of the pulmonary vessels and suturing of the bronchus. By the 1940s the standard operation for resectable lung cancer became pneumonectomy.

HISTORICAL READINGS

Abbey Smith R, Nigam BK: Resection of proximal left main bronchus carcinoma. Thorax 43:616, 1979

Graham EA, Singer JJ: Successful removal of an entire lung for carcinoma of the bronchus. JAMA 101:1371, 1933

Meade RH: A History of Thoracic Surgery. Charles C Thomas, Springfield, IL, 1961

INDICATIONS

Removal of an entire lung was the initial suggested therapy for bronchogenic carcinoma, although in many cases lesser resections such as lobectomy or segmentectomy are considered appropriate. It is generally accepted that with careful selection and staging, pneumonectomy is the correct treatment for lung cancer that cannot be treated by lobectomy. Pneumonectomy for inflammatory lung disease, bronchiectasis, tuberculosis, and other nonmalignant conditions is quite uncommon in modern-day pulmonary medicine following the advances in antibiotics (Sarot and Gilbert, 1949).

Incision

The most common incision used for the removal of the lung is the posterolateral thoracotomy with access to the pleural cavity via the fifth intercostal space. This approach allows access to all areas of the lung, both posterior and anterior and is the most popular. Although many surgeons routinely remove a rib, this is not necessary. If the rib is excised, then in the rare instance when empyema and infection cause dehiscence of the thoracotomy incision, it may be difficult to eventually close the incision because of the loss of tissue the rib represents.

Posterior thoracotomy with the patient in the prone position was popular in the early days of thoracic surgery, when control of airway secretions was a major problem in the removal of lungs for septic inflammatory diseases such as tuberculosis. In modern times the techniques of airway control with reliable endobronchial intubation and one-lung anesthesia are such that the prone position for this reason is not necessary. Moreover, access to the vascular structures of the hilum is less convenient, and so the posterior approach to a prone patient is very rarely employed. Anterior thoracotomy with the patient supine results in an incision that is poorly tolerated cosmetically, and access to the necessary hilar structures is suboptimal, so that this approach also is rarely employed for pneumonectomy.

Median sternotomy carries with it the advantage of less postoperative compromise of pulmonary function, and some practitioners favor it for that reason. It allows good access to the hilar structures for right pneumonectomy and in fact is used routinely for right single-lung transplant. It is quite difficult and sometimes impossible to perform left pneumonectomy through this approach because the heart prevents access to the inferior veins. There is also the theoretic risk of sternal infection, which might be increased when this approach is used for clean contaminated cases such as those involving pulmonary resection (Cooper, et al., 1978; Takita, et al., 1977).

ANESTHESIA

It is very important for the surgeon performing thoracic surgery and pulmonary resections to maintain very clear communication with the attending anesthesiologist. It is also important that the anesthesiologist be experienced in thoracic anesthesia and be comfortable with the various techniques of one-lung anesthesia. Careful monitoring of blood pressure using an arterial line, of blood gases, of end-tidal carbon dioxide, and of pulmonary arterial pressures with a Swan-Ganz line, as well as urine output measurement and pulse oximetry, will all be required depending on the preoperative condition of the patient.

Single-lung anesthesia is best provided with the use of a standard disposable Robert-Shaw double-lumen endotracheal tube. Some surgeons prefer to use either a bronchial blocker in combination with a standard endotracheal tube or one of the newer commercially available tubes that have a built-in blocker, especially for left pneumonectomy.

OPERATIVE TECHNIQUE

On many occasions the decision to perform pneumonectomy has been made preoperatively on basis of the type or location of the pathology. On other occasions the need for pneumonectomy is determined intraoperatively. In either situation, the possibility of performing a lesser resection without compromising the intended purpose of the procedure should always be kept in mind. It is not uncommon, for example, to find a situation in which a bronchoplastic sleeve resection can be performed instead of pneumonectomy. This determination may sometimes not be possible until intraoperative assessment is made.

Once thoracotomy has been performed, a determination of the extent of the disease, its resectability, and the suitable resection is made (Brock and Whitehead, 1955; Cahan, et al., 1951). If the need for pneumonectomy is confirmed, the approach to the resection should be flexible, depending on the circumstances of each particular case. In any event, the hilum is dissected to identify the pulmonary artery and the two (inferior and superior) pulmonary veins (Fig. 32-10).

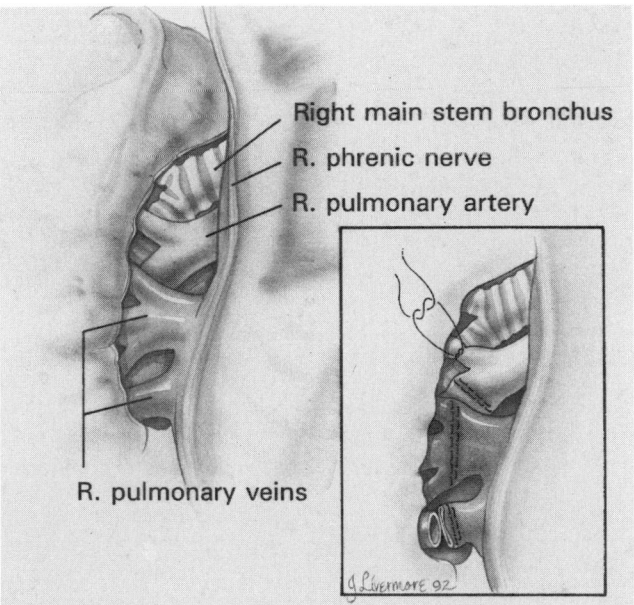

Right main stem bronchus
R. phrenic nerve
R. pulmonary artery

R. pulmonary veins

Figure 32-10. The hilum of the right lung has been dissected completely, demonstrating from an anterior view the right mainstem bronchus, right pulmonary artery, and pulmonary veins. Note that the veins have been stapled and the right anterior pulmonary artery has been stapled distal to a ligature on the first branch. This maneuver allows greater length on the mainstem pulmonary artery.

Pulmonary Veins

Although ideally the division of the veins should occur early in the procedure and before the division of the artery, this may not always be possible, depending on each intraoperative situation (Miller, et al., 1968). Much of the dissection is best performed bluntly with an "educated" finger to complete the vessel identification. The inferior pulmonary veins are usually dissected by retracting the lung anteriorly and superiorly. When not involved with tumor, they are easily dissected. I prefer to staple or oversew the main trunk. Other authors doubly ligate or suture-ligate branches separately. The superior pulmonary vein is in close proximity to the pulmonary artery anteriorly on both sides and is handled similarly to the inferior vein. The vessels may be handled in various ways. The most popular method seems to be the use of vascular staples, which are especially designed for this purpose. They are safe and extremely convenient.

Before the veins are manipulated in certain central tumors, the veins should be gently palpated to be sure they do not contain extension of the tumor. If tumor is present, a determination should be rapidly made as to its extent and resectability. Tumor released from such veins can result in a potentially disastrous tumor embolus. It is usually necessary to examine the intrapericardial portion of the veins to make this determination. Several millimeters of atrium may be encompassed in the resection if necessary. Again, as a clamp is applied to the atrium in such circumstances, venous return from the other lung may be compromised, rapidly resulting in hemodynamic instability required less central application. The clamp should be applied for 1 or 2 minutes before any incision in the vessels is made, so that if instability is noted, the clamp can be reapplied.

Pulmonary Artery

Where the tumor is close to the origin of the pulmonary artery, it may not be possible to obtain enough room to safely apply these staplers. In this situation use of a proximal atraumatic vascular clamp, with oversewing the vessel in a more traditional way, is perfectly acceptable. When possible, division of the first branch of the pulmonary artery on either the left or the right side allows greater length for ultimate division of the main trunk. With the more frequent use of Swan-Ganz catheters, it is important to be sure the device is not included in the artery when it is divided. The pulmonary artery is weakened by application of staples in continuity. It is therefore important to avoid traction on the vessel once it has been stapled but before it is divided.

Difficulty can occur when the tumor is "tight" on the pulmonary artery and obtaining sufficient length for safe control presents a problem. There are a few techniques available to deal with this. On either side the pericardium may be opened anterior to the pulmonary artery and the intrapericardial portion of the pulmonary artery identified (Allison, 1946). This maneuver will produce 1 or 2 cm of additional length. It is important to avoid injury to the phrenic nerve when doing this and also to ensure that adequate hemostasis on the pericardiotomy is secured. Postoperative bleeding from this area can be troublesome and result in unacceptable blood

loss requiring reexploration and even causing pericardial tamponade. The size of the pericardial defect should be considered at the end of the procedure and the necessary steps taken to prevent cardiac herniation and compromise to venous return.

On the left side, dissection may be continued proximally and the remnant of the ductus (ligamentum arteriosus) divided to obtain further length on the left main pulmonary artery (Fig. 32-11). The left recurrent laryngeal nerve is vulnerable here, and care should be taken to avoid injury to it, cautery nearby, or traction on it. As one proceeds centrally, it is possible to divide the left pulmonary artery at its origin (Fig. 32-12). Care should be taken to avoid compromise to the contralateral right pulmonary artery when the vessel is divided. It is also wise to have a vessel loop around the main right or left pulmonary artery during the dissection. This will allow control of a potentially lethal problem and salvage if the artery is entered or torn. Where extensive intrapericardial dissection is contemplated, the possibility of requiring cardiopulmonary bypass should be considered. This is exceedingly rare, but the question of how to institute it should have crossed the surgeon's mind.

On the right side, control of the intrapericardial artery may require mobilization of the superior vena cava and dissection of the artery medial to this, allowing a greater length of artery for control. One should remember that the pulmonary artery is unforgiving and does not tolerate undue traction or rough handling. The veins are much tougher, and inadvertent injury is less of a consideration.

On occasion, when the bulk of tumor is anterior and large, the vessels may be divided after the bronchus, first the vein and then the artery (Fig. 32-13). Resectability should be determined with certainty before this approach is used, although

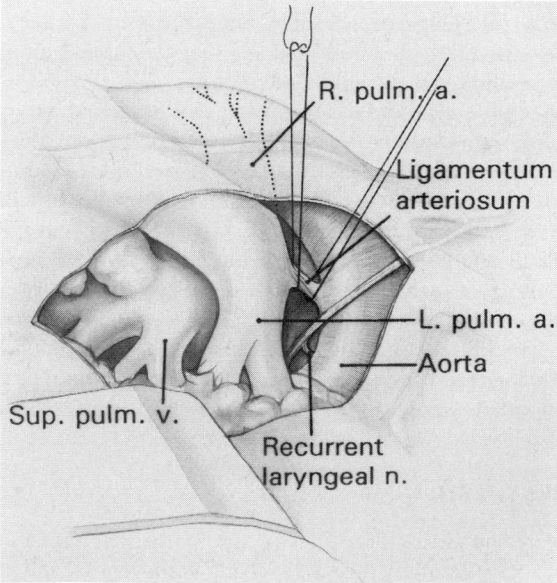

Figure 32-11. The left pulmonary hilum has been totally exposed intrapericardially. The ligamentum arteriosum is being divided to provide further length on the left main artery. The recurrent nerve must always be protected.

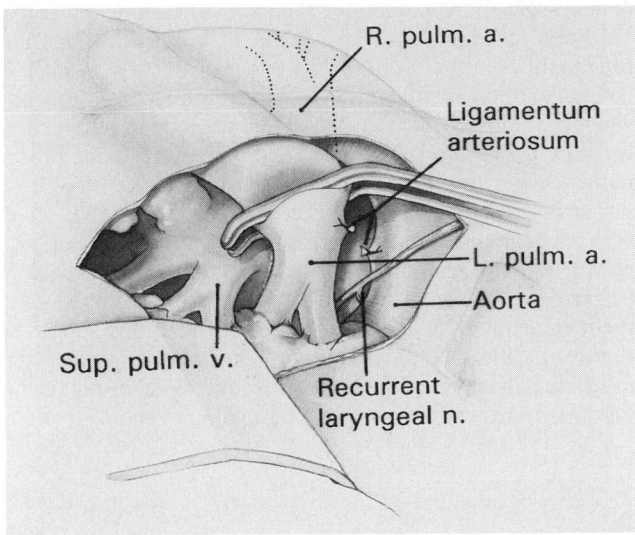

Figure 32-12. Following division of the ligamentum arteriosum, a Satinsky clamp is applied just distal to the pulmonary conus. Care must always be taken not to impinge upon the right pulmonary artery.

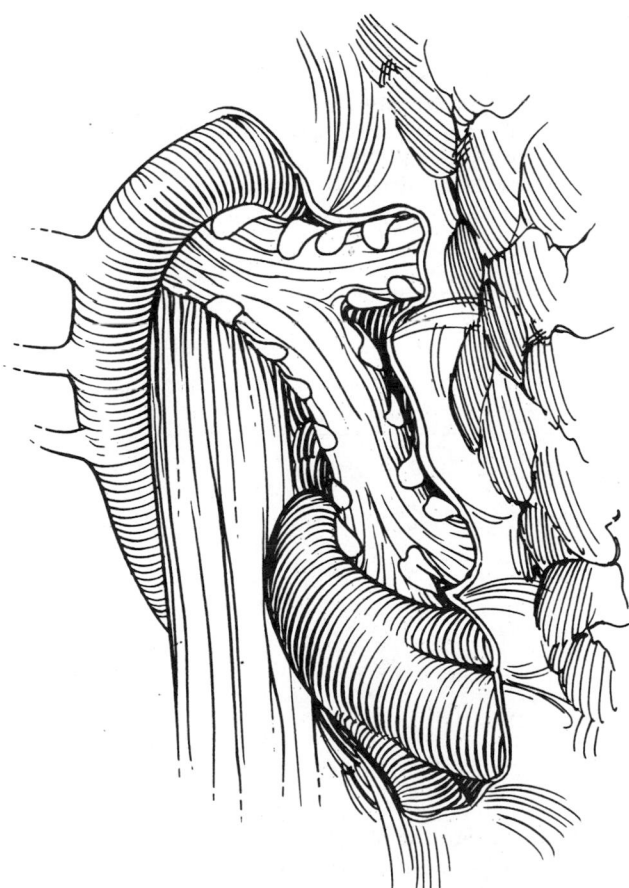

Figure 32-13. The right lung is retracted anteriorly, exposing the right mainstem bronchus. With difficult hilar dissection, often the bronchus can be dissected first and divided, exposing the pulmonary artery from behind.

this is sometimes a difficult judgment requiring considerable experience. Once the great pulmonary vessels have been divided, the suture lines are carefully examined for satisfactory hemostasis. Where the dissection has been very central, the site of division may retract, and small amounts of bleeding may not be readily apparent.

Bronchus

The handling of the bronchus is also a function of experience and personal preference. Dissection of the bronchus proximal to the resection margin should be kept to a minimum in order to preserve as much as possible of its blood supply intact. The goal of the process is to divide the mainstem bronchus as proximally as possible in order to avoid the problem of a long bronchial stump. On the right side it is very easy to judge the point of bronchial division in relation to the trachea and avoid a long stump. It is a little more difficult on the left side, so that particular care should be taken to follow the left main bronchus centrally to the carina. Sometimes this requires an initial resection, removal of the specimen, and a subsequent revision, taking the bronchus a little more proximally. If staplers are not available, possible, or desired, the bronchus may be closed by standard suturing techniques. It appears that nonabsorbable suture is to be avoided because of the incidence of suture granuloma and troublesome hemoptysis later. We have preferred to use Vicryl or similar suture. Sutures are interrupted, in an anterior-posterior orientation. They are placed about 1 mm apart, encompassing the first cartilaginous ring. At the completion of the bronchial closure, the suture line is tested underwater for air leak with the anesthesiologist's help. A Valsalva maneuver with about 30 to 35 cmH$_2$O static airway pressure is sufficient. If there are any air leaks, they should be dealt with and obliterated. This may require additional suture or additional tissue depending on the circumstances. Additional tissue implies the mobilization of neighboring tissues such as pleura, pericardium, pericardial fat, omentum, and intercostal bundle, to suggest a few possibilities. The routine use of additional tissue to patch the bronchial suture line is controversial. Some believe it is necessary in every case; others think that it provides an enclosed area to encourage local infection. I do not routinely cover the bronchus.

Postpneumonectomy Space

Before closure, the usual checklist should be covered: satisfactory hemostasis, the absence of air leak, the condition and size of any pericardial defect, and if applicable, an examination for possible esophageal or thoracic duct injuries. The phrenic should not be crushed or otherwise intentionally damaged.

The thoracotomy is closed in standard fashion, although it is desirable to consider the location of the mediastinum. If the incision has been a posterolateral thoracotomy, the mediastinum will fall away during the procedure with resulting compromise of contralateral lung function and even possible impairment of venous return. Once the chest is closed and the patient is supine, steps should be taken to evacuate air from the operated hemithorax to return the mediastinum to the midline (Suarez, et al., 1969). A sterile needle can be introduced into the chest in the operating room and air evacuated until the sensation of resistance to evacuation is obtained. We have left a 16-gauge soft catheter in the hemithorax during the closure, bringing it out through the front of the incision. The catheter is positioned and the closure conducted so as to allow immediate removal of the catheter without a defect in the chest wall. With the catheter in place, a member of the surgical team and the necessary equipment (a "Christmas tree," 50-ml syringe, and three-way stopcock) remain sterile while the patient is returned to the supine position. Sufficient air is then evacuated in a sterile fashion to accomplish the goal; this is usually about 1 L of air in the average adult patient. The changes in position may be accompanied by arrhythmia and hypotension, so that it

is necessary for a member of the surgical team to remain in the operating room for this. Some surgeons leave a chest tube in the hemithorax following pneumonectomy to achieve balancing of the mediastinum and to announce promptly any significant blood loss. This tube, if employed, should receive no more than 5 cmH_2O suction, and personnel caring for the patient should be warned that additional suction may have disastrous consequences. Alternatively, commercially available "pneumonectomy" drainage systems allow for balanced drainage, maintaining the pneumonectomy space at -1 cmH_2O. Other surgeons leave the tube clamped after the mediastinum has been repositioned. The tube should be removed within 12 to 24 hours of the surgery. I have not used a tube because of the risk of introducing microorganisms via this route, with subsequent infection.

REFERENCES

Abbey Smith R, Nigam BK: Resection of proximal left main bronchus carcinoma. Thorax 43:616, 1979

Allison PR: Intrapericardial approach to the lung root in the treatment of bronchial carcinoma by dissection pneumonectomy. J Thorac Surg 15:99, 1946

Brock R, Whytehead LL: Radical pneumonectomy for bronchial carcinoma. Br J Surg 43:8, 1955

Cahan GC, Watson WL, Pool JL: Radical pneumonectomy. J Thorac Surg 22:449, 1951

Cooper JD, Nelems JM, Pearson FG: Extended indications for median sternotomy in patients requiring pulmonary resection. Ann Thorac Surg 26:413, 1978

Graham EA, Singer JJ: Successful removal of an entire lung for carcinoma of the bronchus. JAMA 101:1371, 1933

Meade RH: A History of Thoracic Surgery. Charles C Thomas, Springfield, IL, 1961

Miller GE, Aberg THJ, Gerbode F: Effect of pulmonary vein ligation on pulmonary artery flow in dogs. J Thorac Cardiovasc Surg 55:668, 1968

Sarot IA, Gilbert L: Extrapleural pneumonectomy and pleurectomy in pulmonary tuberculosis. Thorax 4:173, 1949

Suarez J, Clagett OT, Brown AL Jr: The post-pneumonectomy space. J Thorac Cardiovasc Surg 57:539, 1969

Takita H, et al: The surgical management of multiple lung metastases. Ann Thorac Surg 24:359, 1977

Lobectomy

Nael Martini
Robert J. Ginsberg

HISTORICAL NOTE

The first proper dissection lobectomy was performed by Hugh Morriston Davies in 1912. Prior to this, most pulmonary resections were performed by hilar ligation and cautery dissection of the surrounding lung. Although the operation was technically successful, Davies' patient died 8 days later of

an empyema. For the next 15 years, surgeons continued to remove lung by nonanatomic means. In 1929 Brunn reported a one-stage lobectomy and demonstrated the value of underwater drainage in anticipation of a bronchopleural fistula. Despite these early successes with dissection lobectomy, pneumonectomy remained the treatment of choice following Graham's successful report in 1932. It was not until

Churchill's report of long-term survival following lobectomy for peripheral lung cancer in the early 1950s that this procedure became acceptable in the management of lung cancer. Before this lobectomy had been reserved for inflammatory diseases such as tuberculosis and bronchiectasis.

HISTORICAL READINGS

Brunn HB: Surgical principle underlying one stage lobectomy. Arch Surg 18:490, 1929.

Churchill ED: Lobectomy and pneumonectomy in bronchiectasis of cystic disease. J Thorac Surg 6:286, 1937

Churchill ED, Sweet RH, Sutter L, Scannel JG: The surgical management of carcinoma of the lung. A study of cases treated at the Massachusetts General Hospital from 1930-50. J Thorac Cardiovasc Surg 20:349, 1950

Davies HM: Recent advances in the surgery of lung and pleura. Br J Surg 1:228, 1913–1914

Lobectomy remains the preferred method for the surgical therapy of peripheral lung cancer. Pneumonectomy is reserved for the more centrally placed tumors, and resections less extensive than lobectomy are carried out in patients with compromised pulmonary function or less frequently, electively in those with small peripheral tumors. There continues to be a 10 to 15 percent risk of local recurrence within the remaining portion of the resected lobe when lesser resections are performed, particularly in patients with adenocarcinomas. Indications for lobectomy in benign disease includes pulmonary tuberculosis, chronic lung abscess and bronchiectasis, benign tumors, fungal infections, and congenital anomalies.

GENERAL CONSIDERATIONS

Although the techniques of lobectomy have been amply described, the main emphasis in modern-day lung cancer surgery has been focused on complete resection with node excision of lymphatic drainage for better staging and local control. We prefer complete mediastinal lymph node dissection (visa-vis lymph node sampling) to accomplish this.

Operative Positions

For lobectomy the lateral approach through a posterolateral incision is usually preferred. Entry into the pleural space is gained through the fifth intercostal space or through the periosteal bed of the fifth rib when an upper or middle lobectomy is contemplated and through the sixth intercostal space or the bed of the sixth rib when a lower lobectomy is planned. This is particularly true for tumors in the periphery of the lobes. In more centrally placed tumors, it may be advantageous to expose the pleural space through the fifth intercostal space to provide better access to the hilum for a safe dissection. More recently, muscle-sparing incisions have been increasingly used.

An anterior approach via a sternotomy, median or transverse, provides excellent access to the superior pulmonary veins and the main pulmonary arteries but poorer access to the major bronchi and the inferior pulmonary veins. Access for safe pulmonary resections via sternotomy has been facilitated by the use of double-lumen endobronchial intubation and one-lung anesthesia.

Initial Mobilization

After the pleural space is entered, adhesions, if present, are divided by either blunt or sharp dissection. Any free pleural fluid is aspirated for cytologic study and culture. The entire lung is then inspected and palpated to assess the extent of involvement, to identify other occult tumors, and to determine if lobectomy is possible. The mediastinum is inspected also to rule out the presence of any disease outside the lung that needs to be attended to or biopsied before any pulmonary resection is carried out. The mediastinal pleura is then completely incised to facilitate hilar and lymph node dissection.

Bronchial Closure

Additional aspects of modern-day resection include the liberal use of staplers instead of hand sewing, particularly for the bronchus and frequently also for the pulmonary artery and veins. Adequate closure can be achieved by the manual technique but closure by stapling is equally safe, clearly more expedient, and currently the most widely used form of bronchial closure. A few precautions can lead to safe stapling without consequent complications:

1. Avoid devascularizing the bronchial stump.
2. Make sure the right "leg length" of stapler is used. Although the 3.5-mm stapler is adequate for most bronchial stumps, in individuals in whom the bronchial wall is thick, larger staplers such as the 4.8-mm may be more appropriate.
3. Make sure that there is an adequate stump to staple to avoid impingement on the main bronchus or other lobar bronchi and also that the margins are clear of tumor and inflammatory tissues.

Adhesions and Fissures

Two problems, adhesions and incomplete fissures, are common to many lobectomies, especially when performed for inflammatory lesions, in which adhesions between the visceral and parietal pleurae are common. When the adhesions are thin and avascular, division with scissors or blunt dissection with the fingers or a sponge stick is a simple matter. For dense adhesions, sharp dissection by scalpel or electrocautery is required to develop intrapleural planes. Despite best efforts, it may be difficult to avoid injuring lung parenchyma, in which case dissecting extrapleurally is advisable. An incision is made in the parietal pleura adjacent to the adherent area, and an extrapleural fascial plane is developed by blunt dissection with the index finger or a sponge. The parietal pleura overlying the densely adherent area is then excised.

The lobar fissures are often not completely open from the periphery to the hilum. Incomplete fissures may be due to inflammatory adhesions, congenital failure of complete development, or extension of a tumor from one lobe to another. If the problem is solely that of inflammatory adhesions, blunt dissection should be tried first. If the adhesions are filmy, a gentle sweeping motion with a sponge stick will suffice. Dense adhesions and completely fused fissures require stapling. Classic anatomic stripping of the fissure, as with segmental resection, may be useful but results in significant oozing and air leakage. Division with a linear stapler, which staples and divides, is generally more secure and more efficient.

Hilar Dissection

Dissection of the secondary hilar structures for a lobectomy is more tedious and time-consuming than dissection of the hilar structures for a pneumonectomy. Anomalies are much more frequent, and in many cases the fissures between the lobes are incomplete. When the lobectomy is performed for inflammatory disease, adhesions are more often a problem.

In performing a lobectomy, ideally one first divides the artery, then the veins, then the bronchus. For lung cancer surgery, some surgeons have favored division of the veins first to prevent the escape of circulating tumor cells into the main bloodstream. In reality, this rarely if ever occurs. More importantly, when the veins are ligated first, the lobe may become more congested and retain blood that is unnecessarily sacrificed with the resected specimen.

Division of the bronchus before ligating the vessels is reserved for patients with associated lung abscesses, in which case spillage into the main bronchus and to the opposite lung is feared. This technique may also be used to advantage where vessel dissection is difficult. Once the bronchus has been divided, the interlobar vessels (e.g., involving the right upper and right lower lobes) are immediately in view.

In patients with central tumors, it is occasionally advantageous not to adhere to the recommended ligation sequence of artery, then vein, then bronchus but rather to remove that structure whose absence provides better exposure to the remaining vessels and/or bronchus.

SPECIAL CONSIDERATIONS

Right upper lobectomy

The pleura over the anterior aspect of the right hilum is incised to provide exposure to the pulmonary artery and its branches to the upper lobes. The mediastinal pleura is incised posterior to the phrenic nerve, and the incision is extended down to the superior pulmonary vein. Then the superior vein is exposed and mobilized by sharp and blunt dissection and encircled with a heavy ligature, which is not tied (Fig. 32-14). The anterior segmental artery is subsequently mobilized and also encircled but not tied with a heavy ligature. It is preferable not to ligate the vessels to be sacrificed until all have been identified and the surgeon is satisfied that a lobectomy will completely encompass all the diseased tissue to be removed.

The dissection is then directed toward the major or oblique fissure, where the interlobar portion of the pulmonary artery is identified and the ascending branch to the right upper lobe exposed (Fig. 32-15). It is often necessary to separate the upper and lower lobes by completing the dissection of the posterior aspect of the oblique fissure. This can be done by

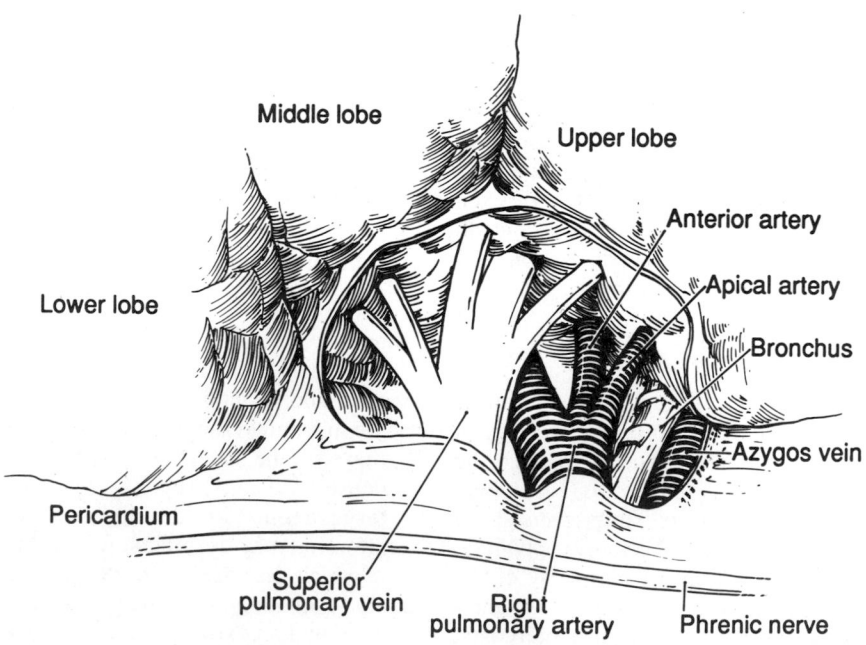

Figure 32-14. Anterior view of the right hilum. The patient is in a lateral thoracotomy position. The lung is retracted posteriorly. The mediastinal pleura is open widely posterior to the phrenic nerve, exposing the pulmonary artery with its branches to the right upper lobe, the superior pulmonary vein, and the azygos tributary of the superior vena cava. Dividing the apical segmental vein first will improve exposure to pulmonary artery branches. Note the middle lobe vein, which is to be protected during the upper lobectomy.

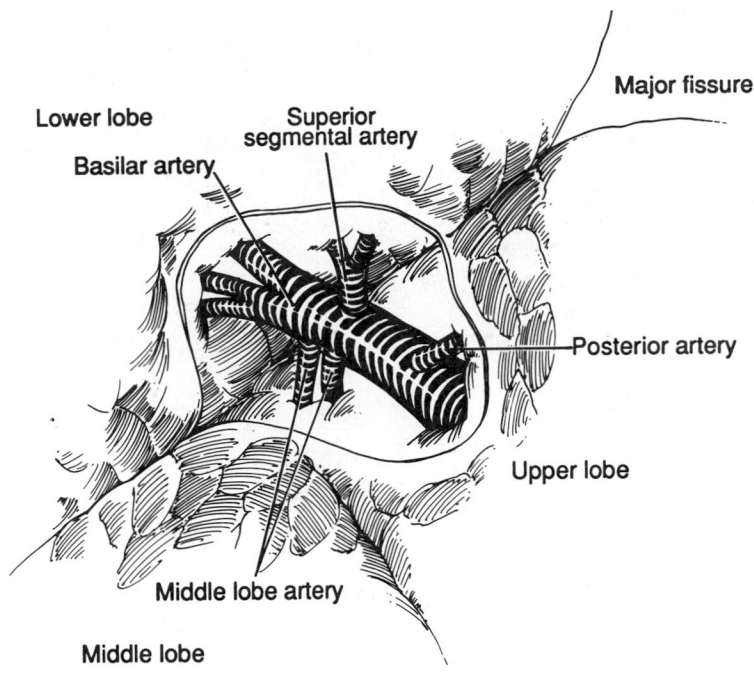

Figure 32-15. View into the right major fissure from in front. The fissure has been opened widely to expose and identify the segmental arteries to the upper, middle, and lower lobes. Anomalies of these vessels are common. The location of the posterior segmental artery to the right upper lobe is most variable, and this artery may be a branch of the superior segmental artery. Occasionally this segmental arterial branch is absent.

dividing the fused fissure between clamps or by stapling. Also, the minor or transverse fissure between the upper and middle lobes is rarely complete. The transverse fissure is dissected as previously described.

The right upper lobe bronchus is then exposed and mobilized to ascertain that no disease is at its margin that will preclude a lobectomy. Once that is done, the segmental arteries to the right upper lobe are individually doubly ligated, transfixed, and divided. The superior pulmonary vein is either doubly ligated, transfixed, and divided or secured by stapling or suturing. The right upper lobe bronchus is subsequently dissected, stapled at its takeoff, and divided distal to the staples, which completes the lobectomy. The inferior pulmonary ligament is then divided to release the middle and lower lobes. At the completion of the right upper lobectomy, care must be taken to reposition the middle lobe correctly. With a complete minor fissure, the middle lobe should be secured to the adjoining lobe to avoid volvulus by staple or suture. Hemostasis is secured, and two chest tubes are placed through separate incisions, one directed to the pleural apex and another over the diaphragm. The tubes are connected to water seal drainage and the thoracic incision is closed in layers in the usual fashion.

Right Lower Lobectomy

Dissection begins in the central portion of the major fissure to identify the arteries to the lower lobe and ensure that both middle and upper lobes can be separated and are free of disease. Dissection is carried out along the pulmonary artery, identifying its major basilar division and the superior segmen-

tal division (Fig. 32-16). The inferior pulmonary ligament is divided and the inferior pulmonary vein exposed and dissected out (Fig. 32-17). Once that is done, the two main arteries to the right lower lobe are doubly ligated, transfixed, and divided. The inferior pulmonary vein is also doubly ligated, transfixed, and divided or secured by stapling. The

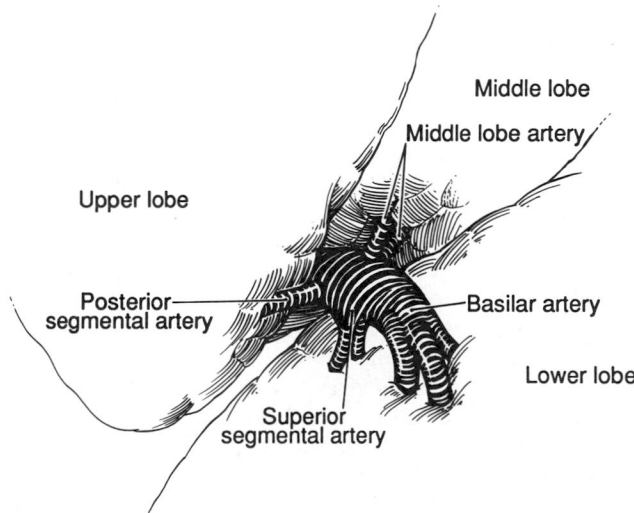

Figure 32-16. View of the lobar hilum from behind during the dissection of the middle lobe arteries. The major and minor fissures are opened widely to expose all three lobes. Meticulous attention to detail and familiarity with the vascular anatomy of the right hilum are paramount in avoiding injury to the lobar vessels to be preserved.

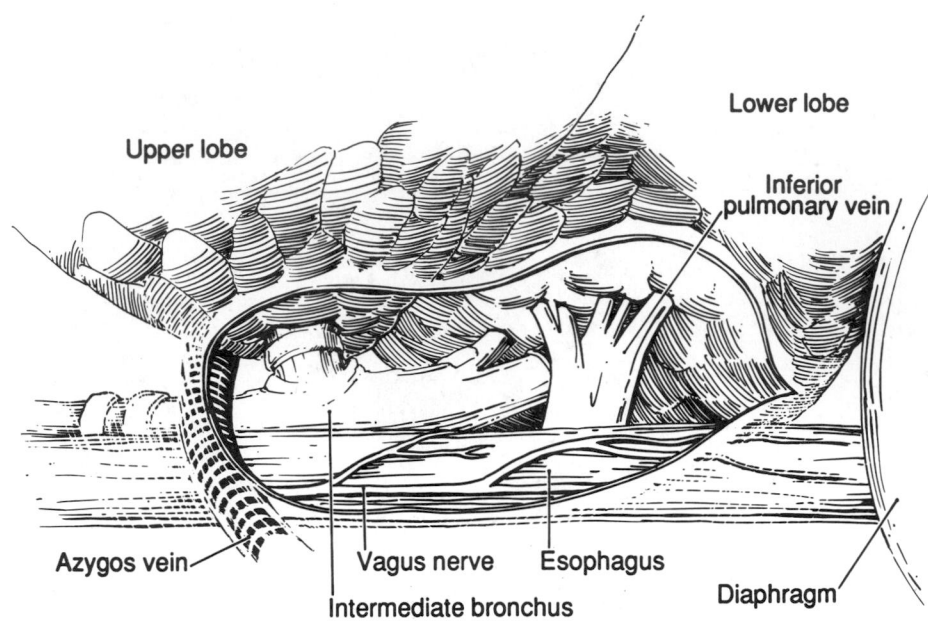

Figure 32-17. Posterior view of the right hilum. The patient is in a posterolateral thoracotomy position. The lung is retracted anteriorly to expose the main and lobar bronchi, the inferior pulmonary vein, and the esophagus.

lower lobe bronchus is then exposed and mobilized to ensure an adequate cuff for stapling distal to the right middle lobe bronchial takeoff. The lower lobe bronchus is stapled and divided distal to the stapled line, which completes the lobectomy. Occasionally, a high takeoff of the superior segmental bronchus requires separate closure of the basilar and superior segmental stumps to avoid impingement on the middle lobe. The mediastinal lymph node dissection, the placement of the chest tubes, and the closure of the chest remain unchanged.

Right Middle Lobectomy

Dissection begins at the minor or transverse fissure, which is often fused and necessitates division by electrocautery or by stapling. The arterial supply to the middle lobe is found at the junction of the transverse and oblique fissures. There are usually two middle lobe vessels supplying the medial and the lateral segments (Fig. 32-16). Exposure, mobilization followed by ligation, transfixion, and division of each of these vessels will lead to exposure of the middle lobe bronchus. As a rule, it is preferable to expose the venous branches to the middle lobe before dissecting the middle lobe bronchus. The middle lobe veins are easily accessed from the superior pulmonary vein; each is mobilized, doubly ligated, transfixed, and divided distal to the transfixion. The middle lobe bronchus is readily mobilized by blunt or digital dissection, stapled at its takeoff, and divided distal to the stapled line. Completion of the lobectomy usually necessitates completing the fissures to the upper and lower lobes by blunt dissection or by stapling the lung at the fissures. Occasionally with difficult fissures, division of all structures from the anterior approach is easier (i.e., divide vein, then bronchus, then arteries before dividing the fissures).

Bilobectomy

In diseases affecting the right lung, bilobectomy becomes necessary when the lesion is peripheral but crosses fissures. Involvement of the minor fissure will necessitate an upper and middle lobectomy to encompass all disease. Invasion of the posterior portion of the major fissure by tumor will necessitate a lobectomy and wedge resection or segmentectomy of the adjoining lobe. Involvement of the anterior portion of the major fissure will dictate the need for a middle and lower lobectomy.

Bilobectomy is also necessary also when a lesion is endobronchial at or near the takeoff of the midle or lower lobes, extending into the intermediate bronchus, or when lymph node involvement in lower lobe tumors dictates removal of the middle lobe as well. Some of these patients will benefit from a sleeve lobectomy if pulmonary compromise is at issue.

Left Upper Lobectomy

Two distinctive features of a left upper lobectomy include the presence of the recurrent laryngeal nerve at the aortopulmonary window and the arterial supply to the left upper lobe (Fig. 32-18).

Dissection is first directed to the aortopulmonary window, where the mediastinal pleura is divided beginning anterior to the descending aorta just past the arch. The incision is first directed toward the inferior pulmonary vein and then proximally below the arch, exposing the vagus nerve and identifying the recurrent laryngeal nerve. This exposes the main pulmonary artery. The dissection is then focused on the major fissure, and all arterial branches to the left upper lobe are sequentially exposed and mobilized. It is preferable to first

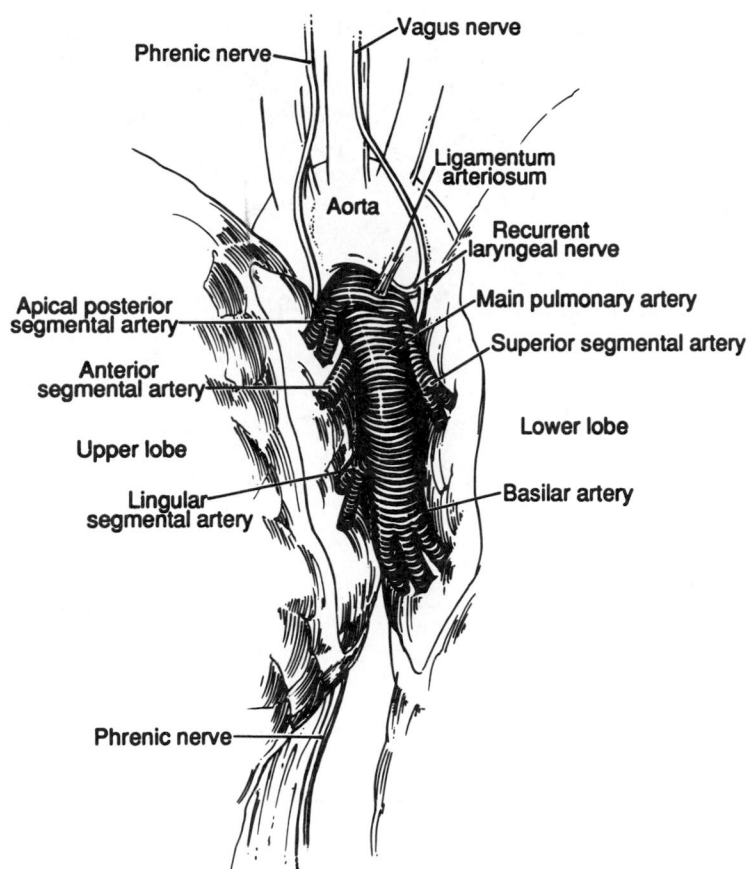

Figure 32-18. Exposure of the left hilum, interlobar view. The patient's head is to the top and the back to the right. The segmental arterial supply to both upper and lower lobes is detailed. Note the ligamentum arteriosum, which can be divided to facilitate difficult dissections.

identify the lingular vessels and then move cephalad to isolate the apicoposterior segmental and anterior segmental vessels.

By retracting the upper lobe downward, one can also provide access to the anterior segmental artery. Unless one is careful to avoid undue traction, injury by traction alone to that vessel at its takeoff from the main pulmonary artery may compel the surgeon to perform a pneumonectomy to control the bleeding. Moreover, the apicoposterior segmental vein often limits adequate exposure of this artery. For these two reasons, it is generally preferred to begin dissection of the lingular vessels and move proximally. Mobilization, ligation, transfixion, and division of the lingular arteries and the anterior segmental arteries are thus safely carried out. The upper lobe is retracted posteriorly to expose the pericardium and phrenic nerve and to provide access to the superior pulmonary vein. The latter is readily dissected out, its segmental veins are individually ligated, and the main pulmonary vein is stapled proximally or divided after placing a vascular clamp and oversewn. This usually provides excellent exposure to the anterior segmental artery and facilitates its dissection and safe division. The upper lobe bronchus is then easily visualized in the major fissure. It is skeletonized and stapled at its takeoff and divided distal to the staple line, which completes the lobectomy.

Left Lower Lobectomy

By contrast to the left upper lobe, considered to be technically the most difficult lobe to resect, the left lower lobe is viewed as the easiest lobe to remove. Dissection begins in the major fissure. The arterial supply to the superior and basilar segments is visualized and dissected out. Each of the branches is individually doubly ligated, transfixed, and divided. The mediastinal pleura anterior to the descending aorta is incised to the level of the inferior pulmonary ligament. Division of the ligament provides exposure to the inferior pulmonary veins. The left lower lobe bronchus lies immediately beneath the arterial branches and is easily exposed. Both vein and lobar bronchus are managed in a manner similar to that used in a right lower lobectomy, with avoidance of any impingement on the upper lobe bronchus.

Prevention of Postlobectomy Spaces

Frequently, the remaining lobe or lobes are considered insufficient to fill the ipsilateral hemithorax. This can be especially true in pulmonary fibrotic diseases or following left upper lobectomy. In such cases a variety of maneuvers can be used to attempt to decrease the hemithoracic space. These include temporary paralysis of the phrenic nerve by crushing or injection of local anesthetic; a ''soft thoracoplasty'' of the upper chest and mediastinum by mobilizing the apical pleura, allowing it to fall down over the remaining lobe (this produces an extrapleural space, which ultimately can fill with fluid); postoperative creation of a pneumoperitoneum gradually over a few days to elevate the diaphragm; insertion of more than two chest tubes with high postoperative suction; or as has been suggested in the past, repositioning of the diaphragm to a higher level. In most cases attention to detail, with closure of large leaking areas in the residual lobe, accurate placement of chest tubes, and fastidious attention in the postoperative period, will result in fewer problematic postoperative spaces.

KEY REFERENCES

Beattie EJ, Economou SG: An Atlas of Advanced Surgical Techniques. WB Saunders, Philadelphia, 1968

Hood RM: Techniques in General Thoracic Surgery. WB Saunders, Philadelphia, 1985

Ravitch MM, Steichen FM: Atlas of General Thoracic Surgery. WB Saunders, Philadelphia, 1988

Waldhausen JA, Pierce WS: Johnson's Surgery of the Chest. 5th Ed. Year Book Medical Publishers, Chicago, 1985

These key references encompass detailed descriptions and step-by-step illustrations of the techniques of the more common thoracic surgical procedures.

REFERENCES

Brunn HB: Surgical principals underlying one stage lobectomy. Arch Surg 18:490, 1929

Churchill ED: Lobectomy and pneumonectomy in bronchiectasis of cystic disease. J Thorac Surg 6:286, 1937

Churchill ED, Sweet RH, Sutter L, Scannell JG: The surgical management of carcinoma of the lung. A study of cases treated at the Massachusetts General Hospital from 1930–50. J Thorac Cardiovasc Surg 20:349, 1950

Davies HM: Recent advances in the surgery of lung and pleura. Br J Surg 1:228, 1913–1914

Segmental Resection

Stanley C. Fell
Thomas J. Kirby

DEFINITION

Anatomic segmental resection is the excision of one or more bronchopulmonary segments of a lobe, with individual ligation and division of the corresponding bronchovascular structures. Although portions of lobes may be excised by use of clamps, stapling devices, cautery, or lasers, these nonanatomic methods are properly classified as wedge resections.

HISTORICAL NOTE

Clinical application of the known detailed knowledge of human bronchovascular anatomy did not occur until Kramer and Glass originated the term *bronchopulmonary segment* in their study of lung abscess in 1932.

Segmental resection was first proposed and performed by Churchill and Belsey in 1939. These authors stated that ''the bronchopulmonary segment may replace the lobe as the surgical unit of the lung.'' The surgical and anatomic study of Blades and Kent in 1942 popularized the technique of individual ligation of hilar structures. Subsequently, Overholt and Langer (1949) systematized the operative methods for resection of all bronchopulmonary segments.

Segmental resection was developed for the surgical management of tuberculosis and bronchiectasis. Both are often multisegmental and bilateral diseases. Segmental resection made it possible to extirpate irreversible disease with minimal loss of functioning lung parenchyma. A further advantage claimed for segmental resection in resections for tuberculosis

The authors gratefully acknowledge the support of the Feldesman Fund for Thoracic Surgery at the Montefiore Medical Center, Bronx, New York, in the preparation of this chapter.

was that it minimized compensatory hyperinflation of the residual lung, a phenomenon believed (erroneously) in the preantibiotic era to accelerate the reactivation of quiescent residual disease. Segmental resection has more recently been applied to the surgical therapy of primary or metastatic lung cancer.

HISTORICAL READINGS

Churchill ED, Belsey R: Segmental pneumonectomy in bronchiectasis. Ann Surg 109:481, 1939

Kent EM, Blades B: The anatomic approach to pulmonary resection. Ann Surg 116:782, 1942

Kramer R, Glass A: Bronchoscopic localization of lung abscess. Ann Otol Rhinol Laryngol 41:1210, 1932

Overholt RH, Langer L: The Technique Of Pulmonary Resection. Charles C Thomas, Springfield, IL, 1951

PRINCIPLES OF SEGMENTAL RESECTION

General Considerations

Segmental resection is technically more difficult than lobectomy, requiring intimate three-dimensional knowledge of the relevant bronchoarterial relationships and possible arterial anomalies. Preoperative bronchoscopy is required to ensure that segmental bronchi are free of disease. Following thoracotomy, lysis of adhesions, and hemostasis, complete mobilization of the lung is required to facilitate the exposure required for resection and subsequent pulmonary reexpansion.

In cases of lung cancer, sampling of hilar and mediastinal lymph nodes with frozen section analysis is mandatory to determine the applicability of segmentectomy. Ideally, the tumor is 2 cm or less in diameter and deeply seated in the segment with surrounding normal lung tissue. Subpleural tumors near the edge of a lobe are generally amenable to generous wedge resection with a stapling device. Visual examination and palpation determine whether the residual segments are of sufficient volume to warrant their preservation. In surgery for inflammatory disease, a shrunken fibrotic basilar segment, for example, is usually associated with compensatory hypertrophy of the superior segment, which makes salvage of this segment worthwhile. In carcinoma this phenomenon is not noted.

The most reliable landmark of a segment is its bronchus, which is rarely anomalous. Identification of the segmental bronchus may be facilitated by repeated traction on the tumor and finger palpation in the hilar area for the resultant tautening of the segmental bronchus. The segmental bronchi of the right upper and lower lobes and left lower lobe are usually identifiable prior to the division of any segmental arteries. This situation does not obtain in the left upper lobe, in which the segmental bronchi are obscured by the segmental arteries.

The order of division of the segmental hilar structures may vary; generally the arterial branches are divided first, which allows for identification of the segmental bronchus. The segmental veins may then be identified. Since the venous drainage may not be readily apparent, venous ligation is best performed last, after the intersegmental plane has been delineated and developed. The *intersegmental* veins define the perimeter of a bronchopulmonary segment and drain contiguous segments. Dissection in the intersegmental plane, sparing the intersegmental vein and thus preserving the venous drainage of adjacent segments, is a stringent requirement of segmental resection if complications are to be avoided.

Identification and separation of the intersegmental plane is performed by differential inflation, in which occlusion of the segmental bronchus in a deflated lung is followed by expansion of the lung. The excluded segment remains airless and can be readily delineated. Occasionally collateral ventilation will fill the diseased segment. The reverse procedure may then be employed; the lung is expanded, and following occlusion of the segmental bronchus, the lung is deflated. The expanded diseased segment is thus demarcated. The bronchus is transected, leaving a stump of sufficient length so that closure will not occlude other segmental orifices. Manual closure of the segmental bronchus, using a few fine polyglactin or silk sutures, is preferred. Stapling devices are often difficult to apply at the tertiary hilum, and their application may compromise adjacent segmental orifices or leave a long stump.

A right-angled clamp is applied to the specimen end of the bronchus, elevated, and retracted under the left thumb (by a right-handed surgeon). Traction is applied to the clamp with the lung partially inflated. Dissection of the segmental plane by scissors is commenced inferior to the bronchus. Fine fibrous strands, possibly representing tiny bronchi or veins, that impede the development of the intersegmental plane are clipped and divided. Finger dissection along the path of least resistance completes the intersegmental plane to the pleura, using the intersegmental vein as a guide.

Alternatively, the bronchus clamp is held by the left thumb and the fingers of the left hand apply pressure to the pleural surface of the segment, thus everting the deep surface of the segment along the intersegmental plane. Again, the fibrous strands that impede the progress of the dissection are individually clipped and divided. The segmental vein, if not conveniently demonstrated and divided earlier in the procedure, is now readily identified and ligated.

Pressure applied with a gauze pad to the raw lung surface for several minutes will usually control bleeding; if not, cautery is used. Small air leaks are controlled with fine sutures. Air leaks may also be controlled by suturing the raw surface down to a contiguous segment, but this method may induce distortion and kinking of bronchi and thus limit reexpansion of the residual segments, a major goal of segmental resection. A pedicled pleural flap applied to the raw surface also may be useful, particularly following resection of apical or superior segments.

While the above description is that of segmental resection as classically performed, the development of stapling devices has added a new dimension to the technique. The prevalence of obstructive emphysema in cancer patients mandates stringent control of air leak, for which staples have no equal at this time. Biologic adhesives are not readily available and require further evaluation.

If stapling devices are to be used, they are best applied along the intersegmental plane in the partially inflated lung after division of the segmental artery and bronchus in order to avoid excessive distortion of the residual lobe. Stapling facilitates extending the resection into an adjacent subsegment if this is required to obtain an adequate margin about the tumor.

Two large-bore intercostal catheters are inserted prior to closure, one placed apical and anterior and the other posterolateral, lying on the diaphragm. The anterior tube should be sutured to the apical pleura to ensure continued evacuation of air leak. Suction of 20 cmH$_2$O is applied to the drainage apparatus. If necessary, nasotracheal suction and bronchoscopy are performed to achieve complete expansion of the residual lung, thus preventing late pleural space problems.

Prolonged air leak is the most common complication of segmental resection, occurring in approximately 10 percent of cases; its management depends on the severity of the leak, the extent of lung expansion, and the condition of the patient. Small alveolopleural fistulae may seal, leaving a "neutral air space," which usually reabsorbs with gradual lung expansion. If empyema supervenes, drainage and later obliteration of the space by muscle flap transposition or limited thoracoplasty will be required. A large air leak associated with radiographic evidence of opacification of the residual lobe suggests that completion lobectomy may be indicated.

Technical Considerations

Right Upper Lobe

Apical Segment. The mediastinal pleura is incised about the hilus of the right upper lobe, the incision extending from the superior pulmonary vein anteriorly and continuing about the branches of right upper lobe to its lower border. Anteriorly the superior pulmonary arterial trunk is demonstrated; the apical segmental artery is its uppermost branch (Fig. 32-19). The lower branch is the anterior segmental artery, which is crossed by the apical segmental vein. The apical segmental vein and artery are ligated and divided. If the artery is short, additional length may be obtained by dissecting with a right-angle clamp into the pulmonary parenchyma and dividing the parenchyma with cautery.

Scissors dissection exposes the posterior surface of the lobar bronchus. Several branches of the bronchial artery require division. Pledget dissection will demonstrate the posterior aspects of the segmental bronchi (Fig. 32-20). The apical segmental bronchus arises from the upper portion of the right upper lobe bronchus. Traction on the segment and palpation of the bronchus, as well as bronchial occlusion and differential inflation, confirm that the appropriate bronchus has been isolated. Closure of the bronchus and excision of the segment are performed as previously described (Figs. 32-21 and 32-22).

Posterior Segment. The posterior segment is often removed with the apical segment of the right upper lobe in resections for inflammatory disease. The posterior segmental bronchus arises from the midportion of the right upper lobe bronchus. The posterior portion of the major fissure is opened to demonstrate the origin of the posterior segmental artery from the anterior aspect of the interlobar artery, just above the origin of the superior segmental artery. Rarely, the superior segmental artery of the lower lobe gives rise to the posterior

segmental artery of the upper lobe. If it is not possible to complete the major fissure readily, the posterior segmental artery may be demonstrated after division of the posterior segmental bronchus. Dissection of the bronchus must be performed with great care since the artery lies directly anterior to it and is vulnerable to injury. Elevation of the stump of the divided bronchus will demonstrate the posterior segmental artery. Traction on the distal stump of the bronchus and differential inflation will demonstrate the line of demarcation between the posterior and anterior segments.

The posterior segmental vein is best identified and divided following completion of the retrograde dissection, so that injury to the anterior and inferior segmental veins is avoided.

Anterior Segment. Dissection of the anterior segment is the most technically difficult of all segmental resections. Its bronchus is not easily accessible from the posterior aspect, being obscured by the posterior segmental vein. Dissection of the arterial supply and preservation of the venous drainage of contiguous segments is tedious.

The mediastinal pleura is incised about the anterior aspect of the hilus of the right upper lobe to below the level of the middle lobe vein. The superior trunk of the pulmonary artery is identified; its lower branch crossed by the apical vein is the anterior segmental artery. The apical segmental vein joins the anterior segmental vein to form the upper trunk of the superior pulmonary vein and must be preserved. It is generally convenient to ligate and divide the anterior segmental vein prior to ligation and division of the segmental artery. The interlobar pulmonary artery is closely applied to the undersurface of the vein, and careless dissection may be disastrous. The middle lobe vein originating at the lower border of the superior pulmonary vein is identified and preserved. The inferior segmental vein is ligated and divided, while avoiding injury to the posterior segmental vein lying deep to it.

The horizontal fissure is then completed by using a stapling device. The interlobar pulmonary artery is visualized. Occasionally accessory arteries to the anterior segment are noted and require division. The anterior segmental bronchus, originating near the lower border of the lobar bronchus, is then divided and closed and the segment excised.

Given the setting of a voluminous anterior segment and small apical and posterior segments, lobectomy may be preferable to segmental resection. Lobectomy is technically easier, and the patient's postoperative course is likely to be smoother.

Right Lower Lobe

Superior Segment. The oblique fissure is opened to expose the interlobar pulmonary artery, which is deeply situated in the region where the oblique and horizontal fissures meet (Fig. 32-23). The middle lobe artery originates from the anteromedial surface of the interlobar artery, while the superior segmental artery originates posterolaterally at a slightly lower level. Rarely, the posterior ascending artery to the upper lobe originates from the superior segmental artery, and occasionally there are two superior segmental branches. The basal segmental arteries may have a short common trunk from

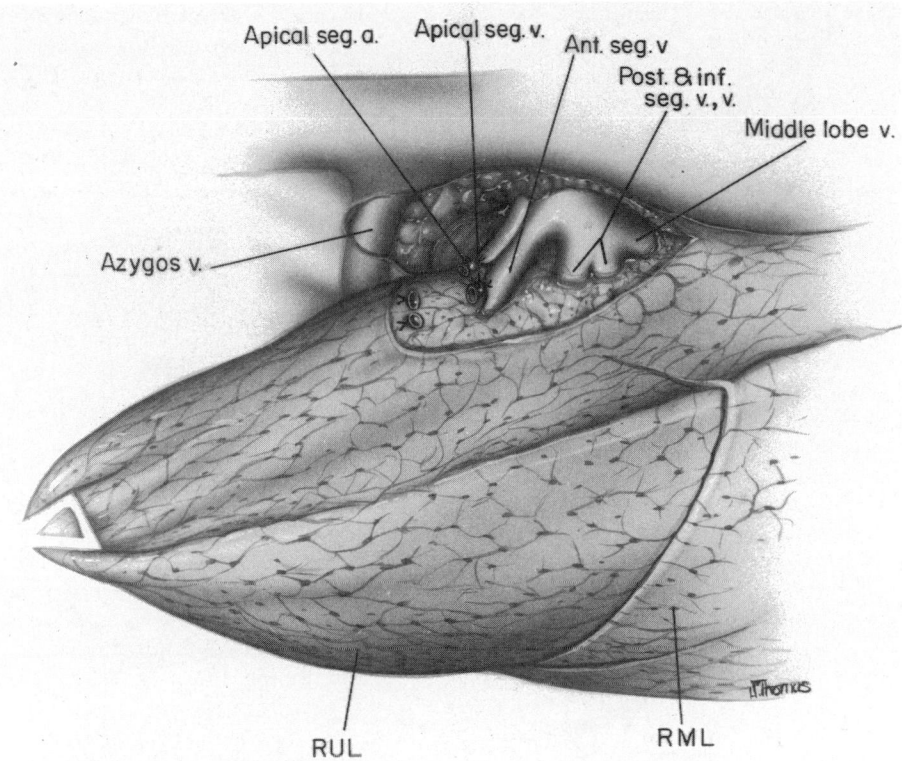

Figure 32-19. The apical segmental artery and vein have been ligated and divided.

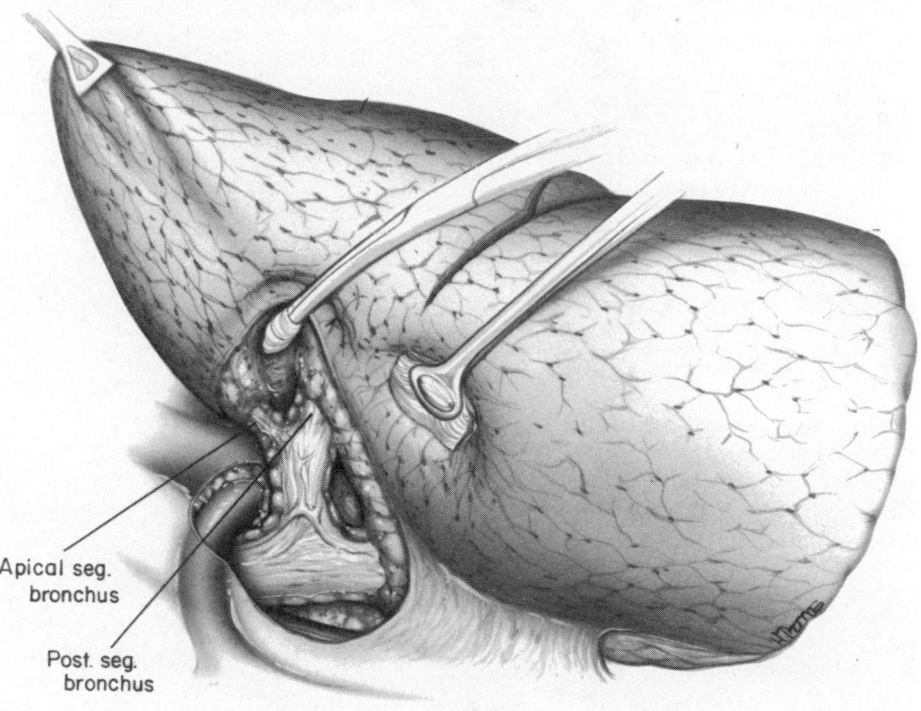

Figure 32-20. Following medial retraction of the right upper lobe, the apical segmental bronchus is dissected.

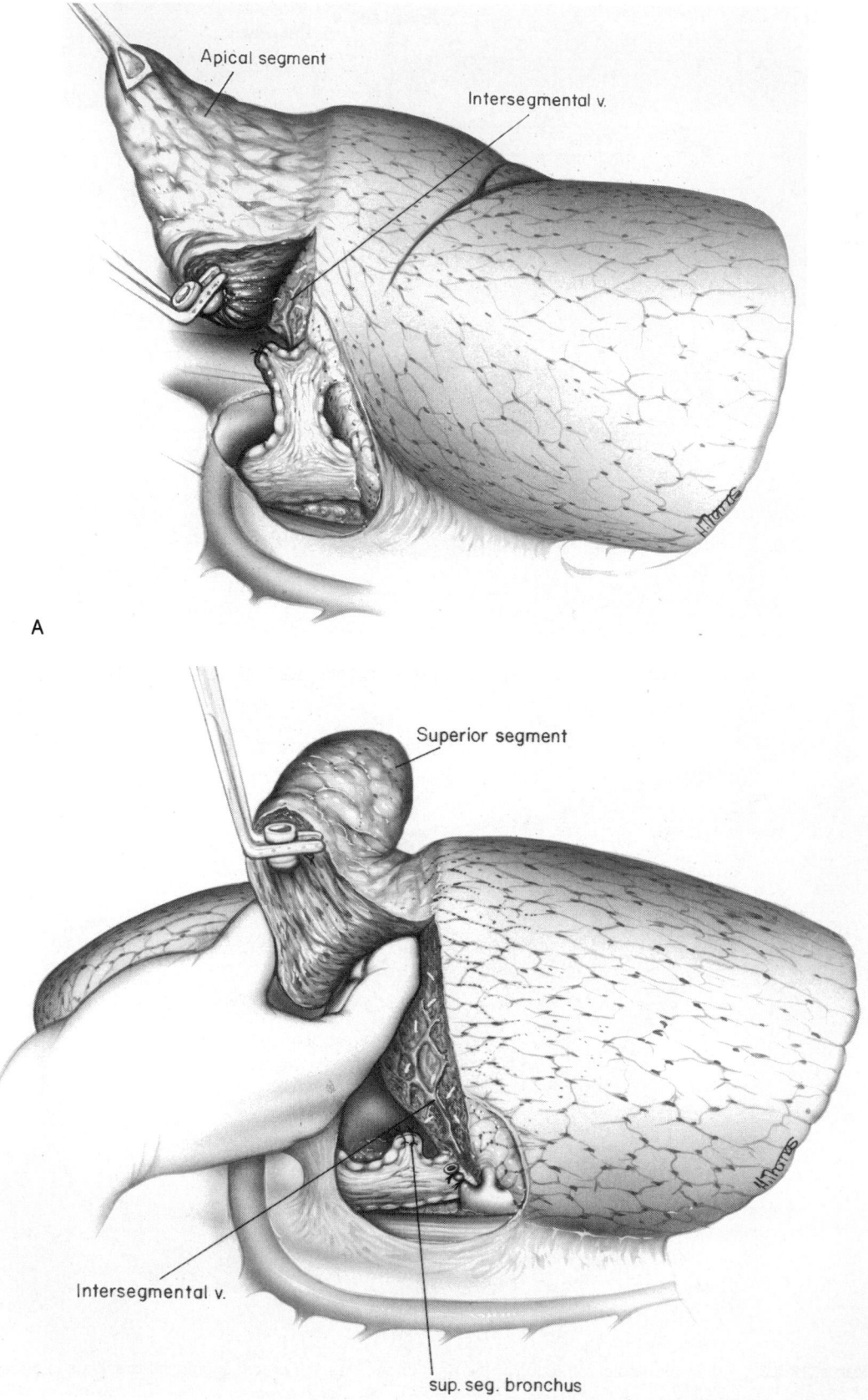

A

B

Figure 32-21. **(A)** Dissection of the intersegmental plane between apical and posterior segments is commenced. **(B)** Finger dissection of intersegmental plane, preserving the intersegmental vein.

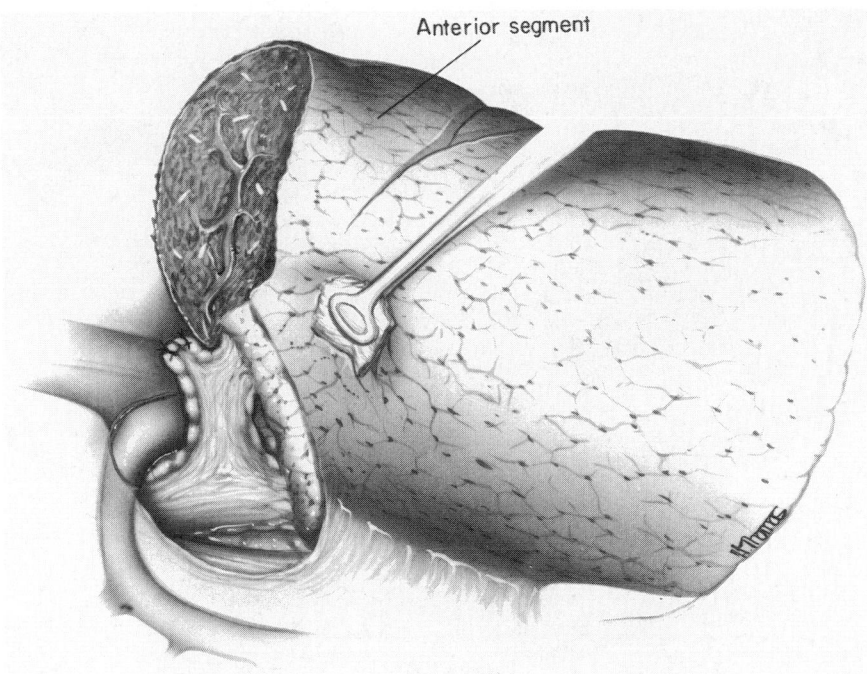

Figure 32-22. Completed apical segmentectomy.

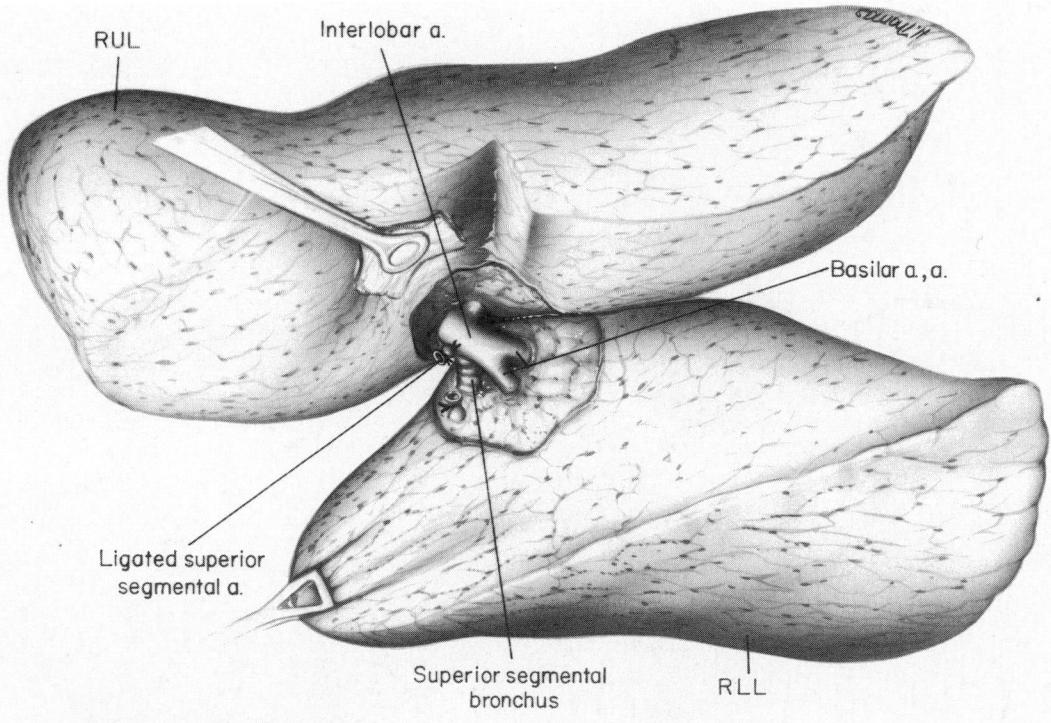

Figure 32-23. The oblique fissure has been opened and the interlobar pulmonary artery exposed. The superior segmental artery has been ligated and divided.

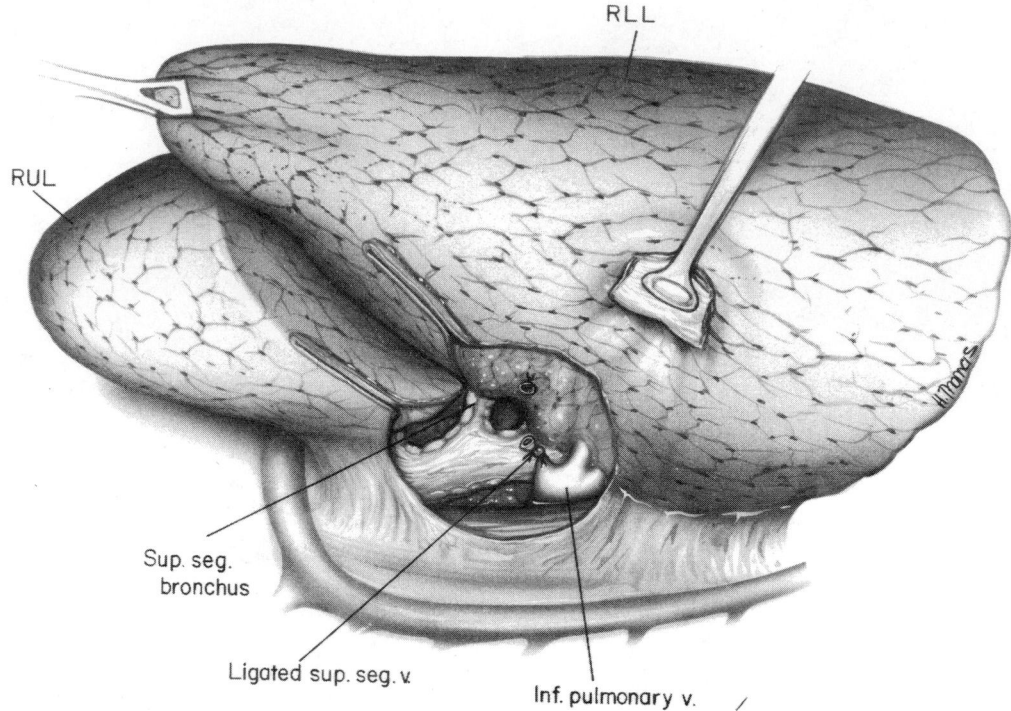

Figure 32-24. Posterior aspect of right lower lobe hilum. The superior segmental vein has been divided and the superior segmental bronchus identified.

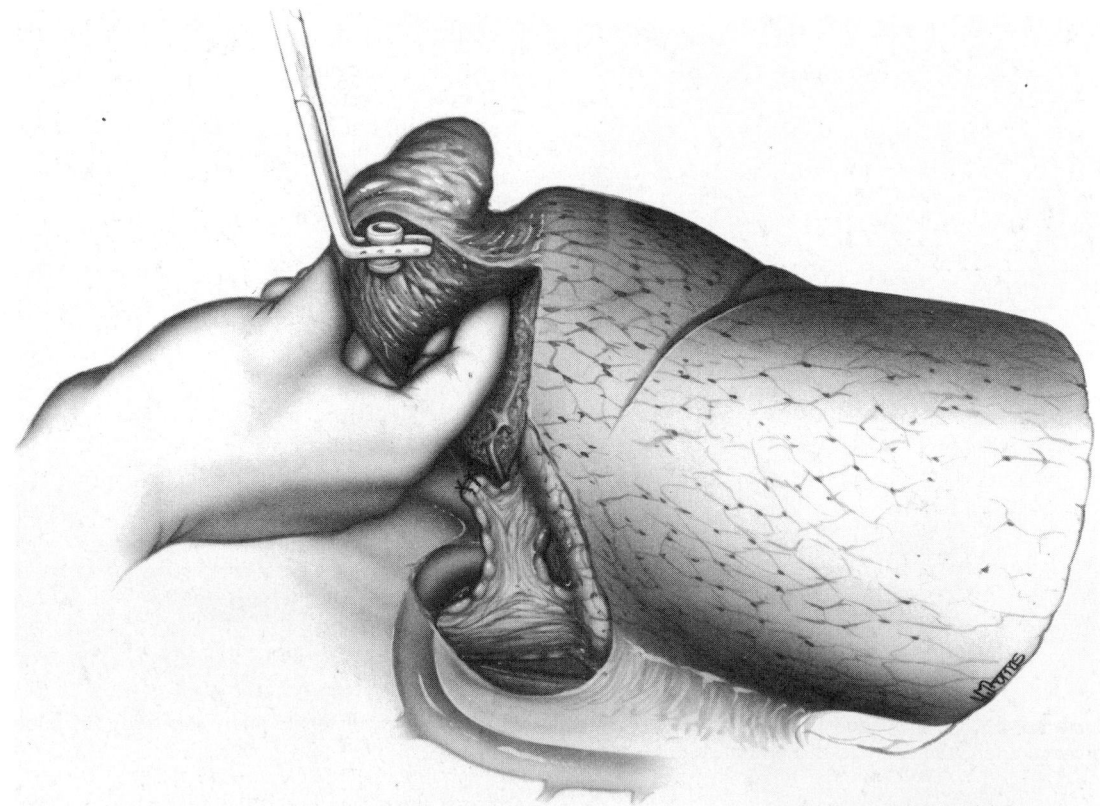

Figure 32-25. Traction on specimen bronchus and finger dissection of intersegmental plane, sparing the intersegmental vein.

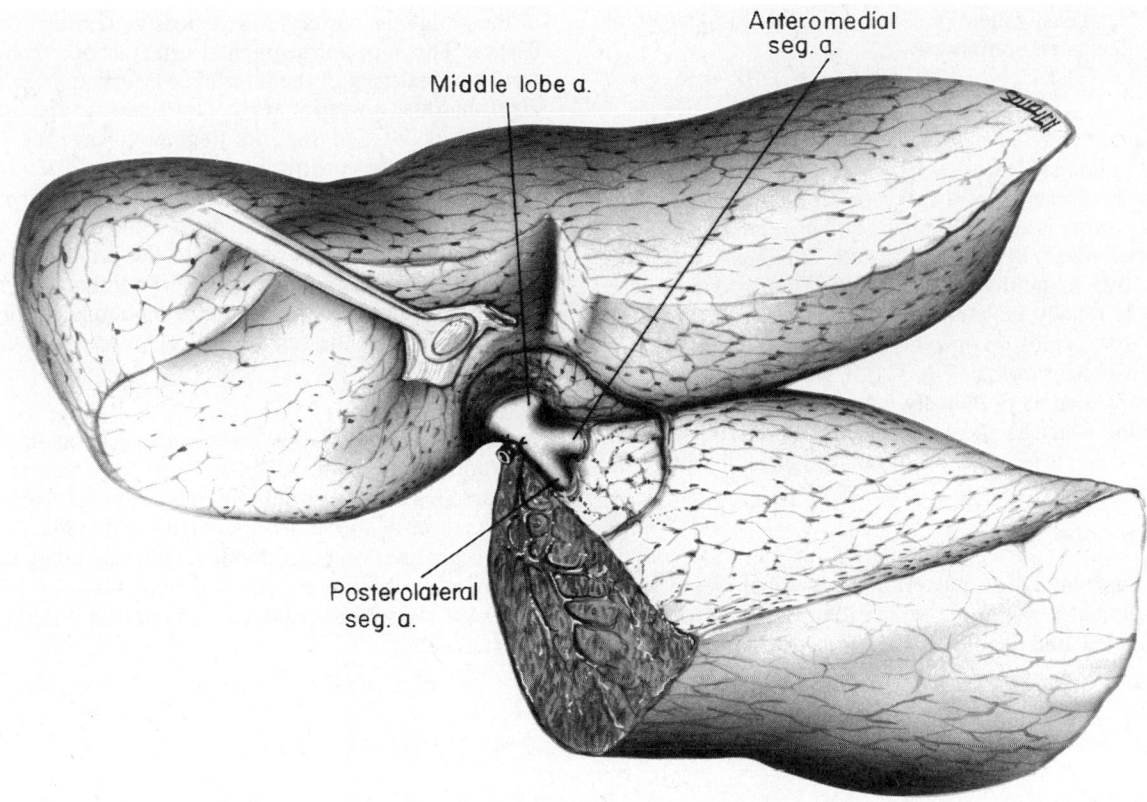

Figure 32-26. Completed superior segmentectomy.

which two branches originate, or all four basal segmental arteries may originate separately distal to the middle lobe artery. Following division of the superior segmental artery, the superior segmental vein, which is the uppermost tributary of the inferior pulmonary vein, is divided (Fig. 32-24). It lies at a slightly lower level than and posterior to the superior segmental bronchus. The superior segmental bronchus is divided, leaving a stump sufficiently long that ventilation of the middle lobe bronchus is not compromised. The segment is then excised as previously described (Figs. 32-25 and 32-26).

Basal Segments.   Exposure and anatomy are as described above. The basal segmental bronchi follow the arterial distribution closely, being situated posterior and medial to their respective segmental arteries.

Following division of the basal segmental arteries, the inferior pulmonary ligament is divided. Three or four basal segmental veins join the inferior pulmonary vein, either individually or via two trunks. Following division of the basal segmental veins, the basal bronchi are divided and sutured distal to the superior segmental bronchus, and the segment is excised.

Left Upper Lobe

Commonly performed segmental resections involving the left upper lobe are excision of the apicoposterior segment, upper division (apicoposterior and anterior segment) resections, and lingulectomy.

The key to segmental resection of the left upper lobe is control of the left pulmonary artery. It is best dissected in its subadventitial plane and encircled with a Silastic loop for proximal control. Isolation of the left pulmonary artery allows for easier dissection of its apical and anterior segmental branches, which are often short and broad and thus susceptible to injury. Anteriorly and inferior to the pulmonary artery, the superior pulmonary vein and its tributaries are demonstrated: the superior venous trunk drains the apicoposterior segment, the middle trunk drains the anterior segment, and the lowermost trunk drains the lingula.

The oblique fissure is completed by sharp dissection or with a stapling device with the pulmonary artery visualized. Dissecting the pulmonary artery from its perivascular sheath over the midpoint of its presenting surface as it enters the fissure facilitates this dissection. Additional posterior segmental arteries may be demonstrated, as well as the lingular arteries arising as terminal branches from the upper border of the interlobar pulmonary artery. The segmental bronchi of the left upper lobe are concealed by arteries. No arteries to the apicoposterior segment should be divided until all arteries to the left upper lobe have been demonstrated because of possible anatomic variations. Traction on the tumor and the distal bronchus will demonstrate which arteries require division. Division of the appropriate segmental arteries exposes the segmental bronchus, which is then divided and sutured. Traction is applied to the specimen end of the bronchus, and the intersegmental plane is delineated as previously described. The venous drainage is generally best divided when it is most easily identified—that is, after the segmental dissection has been completed.

Lingula

The oblique fissure is open for its entire length, and the interlobar pulmonary artery is exposed (Fig. 32-27). As noted above, in the presence of a fused or incomplete fissure the pulmonary artery is at risk of injury, and proximal isolation of the main pulmonary artery is indicated. The lingular arteries, generally two in number, are identified and divided. The bronchus is readily isolated and divided, leaving sufficient length so that its closure does not compromise ventilation of the upper division bronchi (Fig. 32-28). Retrograde dissection is then performed as previously described (Fig. 32-29). The lingula vein, which is the lowest tributary of the superior pulmonary vein, is identified and transsected as the final step (Fig. 32-30).

Left Lower Lobe

Superior Segment. The posterior mediastinal pleura is incised medial to the vagus nerve, the inferior pulmonary ligament is divided, and the oblique fissure is opened. Dissection of the pulmonary artery commences as it enters the oblique fissure. The superior segmental artery arises from the posterolateral surface of the interlobar artery at a slightly lower level than the posterior segmental artery to the upper lobe. There may be two superior segmental arteries. They are divided after demonstrating the lingula arteries originating anteriorly and the basal arterial trunks. The uppermost tributary of the inferior pulmonary vein is the superior segmental vein, which lies slightly inferior to the bronchus. It crosses the basal bronchus to enter the inferior pulmonary vein. Following division of the vein, the bronchus is readily divided and sutured, and the segment is removed as previously described.

Basal Segments. The dissection proceeds as described for the superior segment. After the superior segmental and lingula arteries have been demonstrated, the basal arterial trunk with its three branches are dissected and divided. Posteriorly, basal segmental veins are divided, with care taken to preserve the superior segmental vein. Following division of the vein, the basal bronchi are divided and sutured and the segment is excised.

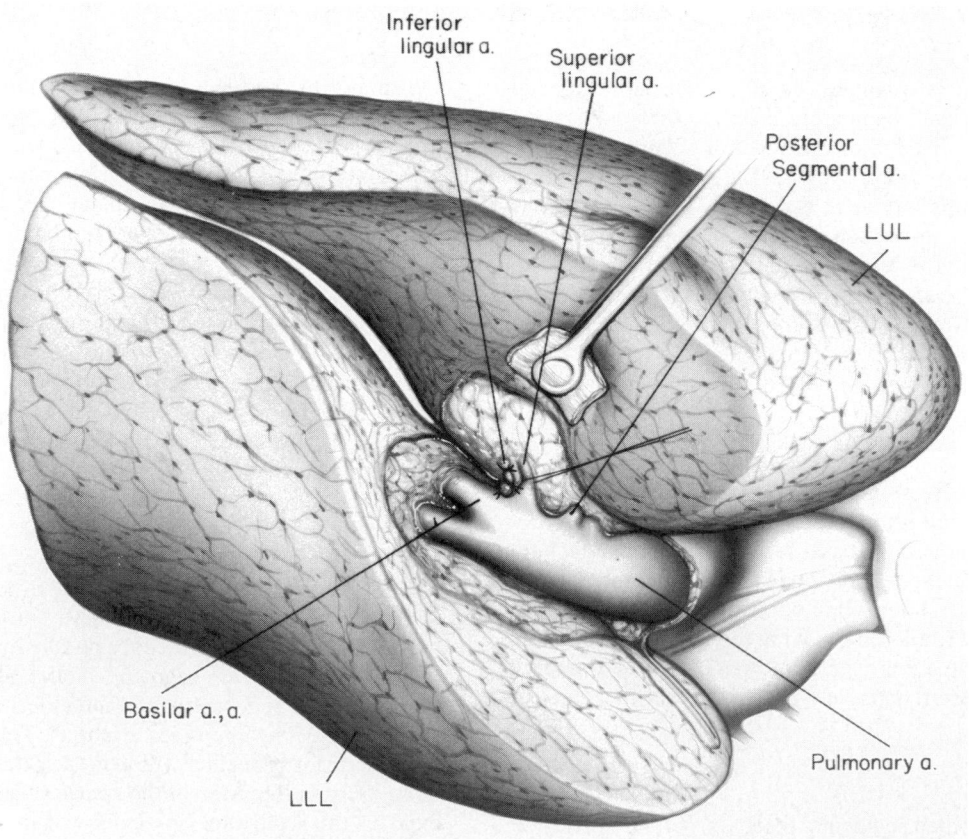

Figure 32-27. The oblique fissure has been opened, and the branches of the interlobar pulmonary artery have been demonstrated. One lingula artery has been ligated.

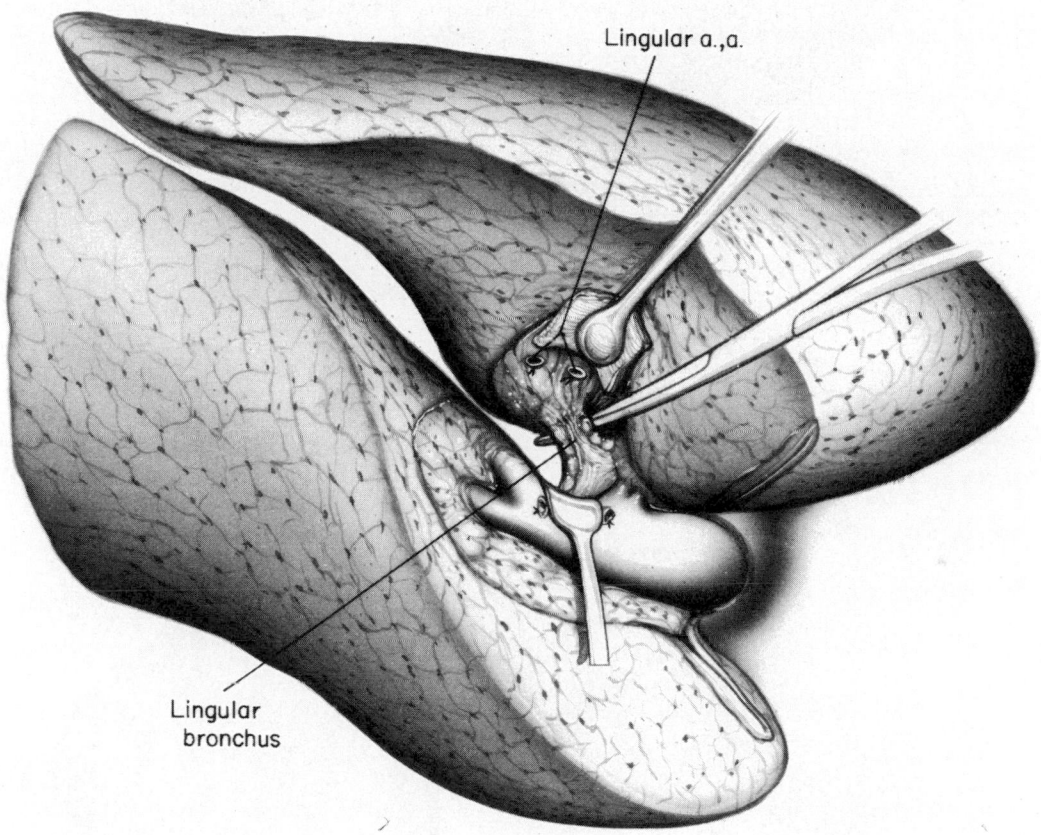

Lingular a.,a.

Lingular
bronchus

Figure 32-28.   Following the division of the lingula arteries, the lingula bronchus is dissected.

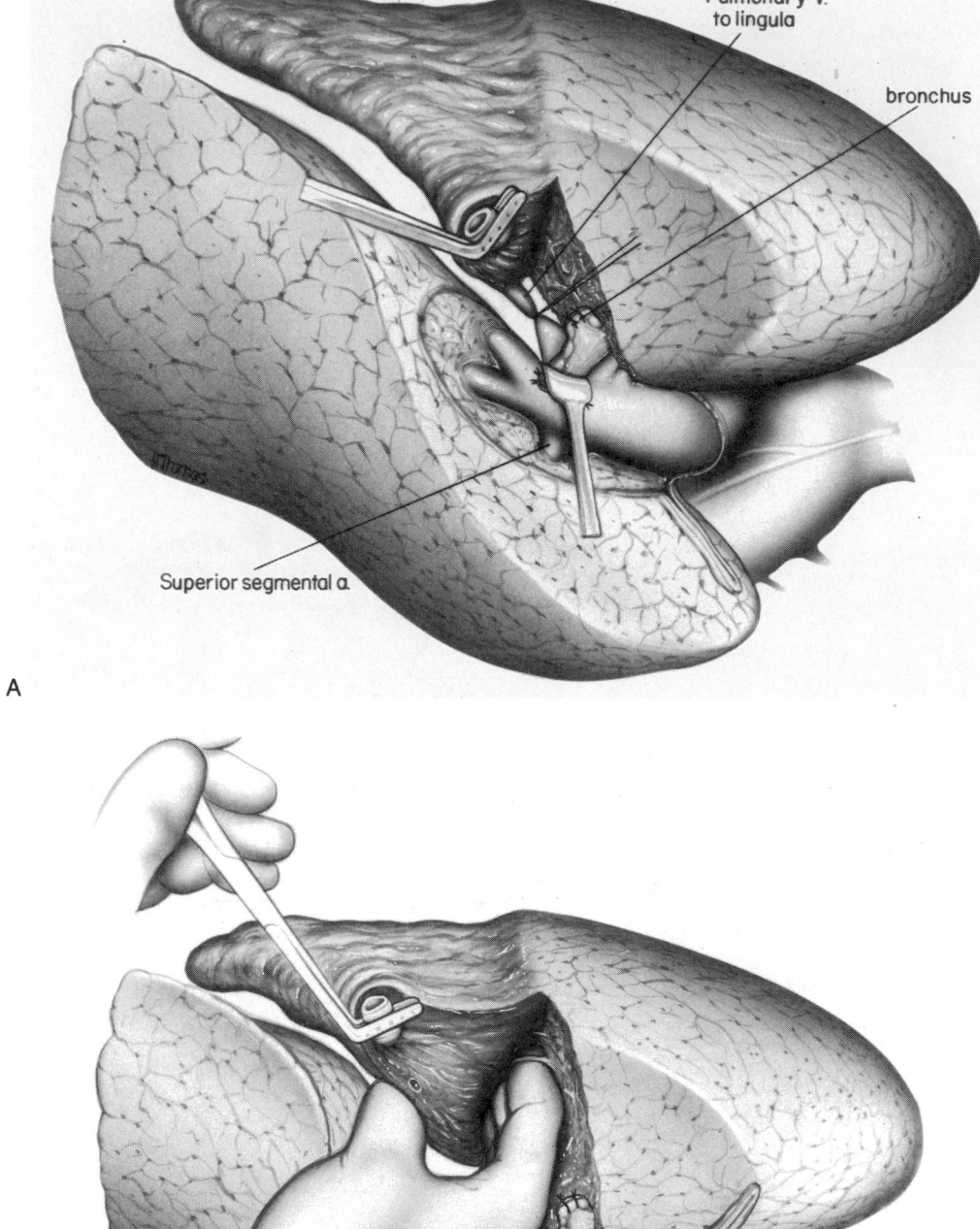

Pulmonary v.
to lingula

bronchus

Superior segmental a.

A

B

Figure 32-29.   **(A & B)** Traction on specimen bronchus and dissection of the intersegmental plane.

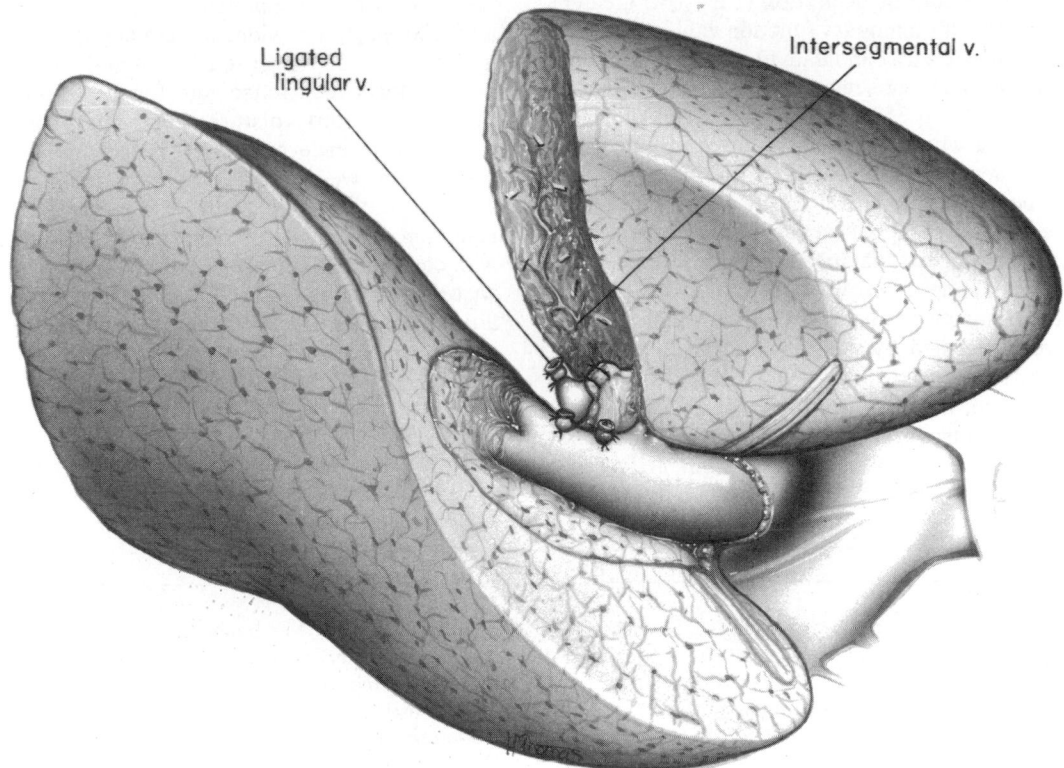

Figure 32-30. Completed lingulectomy. The divided lingula vein is demonstrated.

COMMENTS AND CONTROVERSIES

Segmental resection was designed for and is admirably suited to the surgical management of bronchiectasis and tuberculosis, benign diseases with multisegmental and bilateral distribution. Salvage of functional parenchyma is of paramount importance in such cases.

These diseases have largely disappeared from thoracic surgery services in developed nations by virtue of improvements in social hygiene and the availability of antibiotics. Considering also the dismal reality that thoracic surgery training is an atrophied appendage to many cardiothoracic programs and the attrition in the ranks of thoracic surgeons who have mastered segmental resection, McElvein's (1991) comment that "few of these resections are now being performed and many thoracic surgeons are not familiar with this method" is understandable. Fortunately, a few major teaching institutions have kept the technique of segmental resection alive and have employed it not only in patients with compromised respiratory reserve but also in patients who could tolerate lobectomy.

The development of single-lung anesthesia and improved stapling devices have made wedge resection an almost irresistible alternative to anatomic segmental resection. Huge wedges of parenchyma may be excised without regard to anatomic planes. Despite warnings that distortion of residual parenchyma might lead to pleural complications, such as

empyema and bronchopleural fistula, documentation of these events is lacking in the surgical literature. Commonly, the stapled residual lobe has a grotesque appearance in the open chest, but the postoperative radiograph is quite satisfactory (Kittle, 1989).

Ravitch and Steichen (1988) state that "with the advent of mechanical sutures, the classic anatomical segmental resection has become a technique of the past." They acknowledge, however, that preliminary ligation of the segmental artery and the bronchus may still be useful. It is our opinion that stapling devices are a useful adjunct to the classic technique of segmental resection, especially in patients with marginal pulmonary function. It is in this group that avoidance of prolonged air leak is critical. Careful sequential application of a stapler along the demonstrated intersegmental plane of a partially expanded lobe minimizes distortion and loss of volume of the remaining lobar segments. If air leak is controlled and the bronchi are patent, pleural space problems are unlikely to occur. There is general agreement that patients with compromised pulmonary function by reason of intrinsic lung disease or prior resection should be offered limited resection if this is feasible. Miller and Hatcher (1987) have defined the criteria: maximum breathing capacity greater than 35 percent of predicted, forced expiratory volume in 1 second (FEV_1) greater than 0.6 L, and forced expiratory volume between 25 and 75 percent of expiration (FEV_{25-75}) greater than or equal to 0.6 L. If pulmonary function values are less, the patient is not considered a candidate for limited resection.

Local recurrence following segmental resection has been reported to be from 12 to 35 percent, this latter incidence representing cases in which the tumor crossed an intersegmental plane. (Miller and Hatcher, 1987) Jensik (1986) reported a 55 percent 5-year survival with a 12 percent local recurrence rate. In some of these cases completion lobectomy was possible, which suggests that lobectomy could have been tolerated at the initial operation. Wain, et al. (1991) reported a 5 percent local recurrence rate in 128 cases in which limited resections were performed by choice—that is, in patients who could tolerate lobectomy.

The incidence of local recurrence following segmental resection has led to controversy regarding its applicability if lobectomy could be tolerated. Proponents of segmental resec-

tion reason that incomplete fissures between lobes do not afford lobectomy a wider margin about the tumor than segmental resection does (Jensik, 1986). Nevertheless, their 12 percent local recurrence rate for T1N0 lung cancer (with tumor size <3 cm) is disturbing. Martini, et al. (1986) reported a local recurrence rate of 19 percent following segmental resection or wedge excision and no local recurrences after lobectomy. We agree with those who state that segmental resection should be restricted to T1N0 tumors in patients with compromised pulmonary function who would not otherwise be surgical candidates. Segmental resection is, however, a useful method for excision of benign tumors, metastases, and inflammatory lesions.

S.C.F.
T.J.K.

REFERENCES

Jensik RJ: The extent of resection for localized lung cancer: segmental resection. p. 175. In Kittle CF (ed): Current Controversies in Thoracic Surgery. WB Saunders, Philadelphia, 1986

Kittle CF: Atypical resections of the lung: bronchoplasties, sleeve sections, and segmentectomies—their evolution and present status. Curr Probl Surg, 26:109, 1989

Martini N, McCaughan BC, McCormack PM et al: The extent of resection for localized lung cancer: lobectomy. p. 171. In Kittle CF (ed): Current Controversies in Thoracic Surgery. WB Saunders, Philadelphia, 1986

McElvein RB: Commentary on Landreneau SR, Johnson JA,

Hazelrigg SR: Neodymium:yttrium-aluminum garnet laser-assisted pulmonary resections. Ann Thorac Surg 51:973, 1991

Miller JI, Hatcher CR: Limited resection of bronchogenic carcinoma in the patient with marked impairment of pulmonary function. Ann Thorac Surg 44:340, 1987

Ravitch MM, Steichen FM: Atlas of General Thoracic Surgery. WB Saunders, Philadelphia, 1988, p. 200

Wain JC, Mathisen DJ, Hilgenberg AD et al: Wedge and segmental resection for primary lung carcinomas. Presented at Am Assoc Thorac Surg Meeting, May 1991

Limited Pulmonary Resections

Carolyn M. Dresler

DEFINITION

Limited pulmonary resection is removal of a portion of lung parenchyma in an amount smaller than a segmentectomy or lobectomy.

HISTORICAL NOTE

Technical limitations delayed the successful performance of limited or lesser resections until methods became available to control air leaks occurring when the lung parenchyma

was transected. The Perelman resection described below, developed by the Russian surgeon Mikhail Perelman in 1983, allowed the removal of lung nodules deep within the lung tissue. This technique immediately led to even newer technical advances utilizing lasers for cutting and coagulation.

Lesser resection (i.e., removal of less lung than a lobectomy or segmentectomy) is usually performed by an excisional biopsy technique. Benign tumors, granulomas, inflammatory lesions, metastatic disease, and the unknown primary lung cancer presenting as a peripheral lung nodule are appropriately removed by lesser resections. If the lesion is nonmalignant, no further resection is indicated and further treatment will depend on the pathology of this lung biopsy. If the diagnosis is one of malignancy, the medical status of the patient should dictate whether or not further resection is indicated. Because they preserve as much lung tissue as possible, these limited resections may be the maximally tolerated operation for patients with poor pulmonary reserve. If patients have borderline pulmonary function, (e.g., forced expiratory volume in 1 second [FEV$_1$] less than 800 to 900 cc, FEV$_1$ to forced vital capacity ratio [FEV$_1$/FVC] ≤50 percent, maximum voluntary ventilation [MVV] ≤35 to 40 percent) or have had a previous pulmonary resection, preservation of as much lung tissue as possible is indicated. Severe cardiac compromise also may limit the extent of lung resection possible.

Techniques for lesser resections are undergoing significant changes as technology for less invasive procedures improve. The most dramatic change is the advent of video-assisted surgery. This technique combines a thoracoscopic procedure first described by Jacobaeus (1922) with modern lighting and imaging instruments that allow a whole new approach to the thorax. The advantages, limitations, and possibilities are still being defined. At present, these smaller resections are increasingly performed by the video-assisted technique.

HISTORICAL READINGS

Jacobaeus HC: The practical importance of thoracoscopy in surgery of the chest. Surg Gynecol Obstet 34:289, 1922

Perelman M: Precision techniques for removal of pathological structures from the lungs. Surgery 11:12, 1983

WEDGE RESECTION

Wedge resection is a nonanatomic local excision used for diagnosis and therapy involving removal of the offending lesion plus a small amount of surrounding lung. The procedure is performed through a small open thoracotomy, either anteriorly or posteriorly, and the ribs are gently spread. The nodule to be resected is palpated, and the remaining lung is carefully examined to confirm no other abnormalities. When treating carcinoma, the regional lymph nodes—specifically, segmental, hilar, and mediastinal—should be sampled to confirm that no metastases are present. The nodule is usually peripherally based with no chest wall involvement and amenable to a wedge resection with an adequate margin. If the nodule is deep, toward the hilum, or near to central vessels, a wedge resection is not appropriate. The size of the nodule that can be resected by a wedge technique is dependent on how close it is to the periphery of the lung and on the adequacy of the margin.

Once it has been confirmed that a wedge resection is possible and indicated, the lung is inflated. Two Duvall lung clamps are placed on the edge of the pleura on each side of the lesion. A linear stapler is then placed in order to obtain approximately a 2-cm margin in all directions. Linear staples

are progressively applied until the lesion has been widely resected.

Prior to widespread use of staplers, the same resection was performed by a suture technique. Straight clamps, such as long tonsil or Swedish clamps, are placed surrounding the lesion, again with an appropriate margin. The wedge resection is then sharply dissected and removed. Chromic catgut or other absorbable suture is then used to seal the lung with a double row of sutures. The first row of horizontal mattress stitches is followed by a second row of whip stitches. After use of either technique, the closure is examined for hemostasis and air tightness, and the wedge resection is inspected for margins.

VIDEO-ASSISTED WEDGE RESECTION

If wedge resection is to be performed by the video-assisted technique, the patient is positioned in the same manner as if an open technique were to be performed. The incisions are made in order to facilitate visualization of the nodule and optimal manipulation of the instruments. This resection is performed with the lung made atelectatic with either a bronchial blocker or a double-lumen tube. Currently, we find that a standard sponge clamp or small Duvall clamp functions excellently as a lung forcep (Fig. 32-31). Again, the lung is explored and the nodule identified. The lung forcep positions the lung and suspect lesion into the jaws of the endoscopically placed linear stapler (Fig. 32-32). Care is taken to ensure appropriate placement of sequential staple lines. The endoscopically resected portion of lung can then be removed from one of the smaller incisions. The line of resection is then inspected for hemostasis, and the lung is reexpanded.

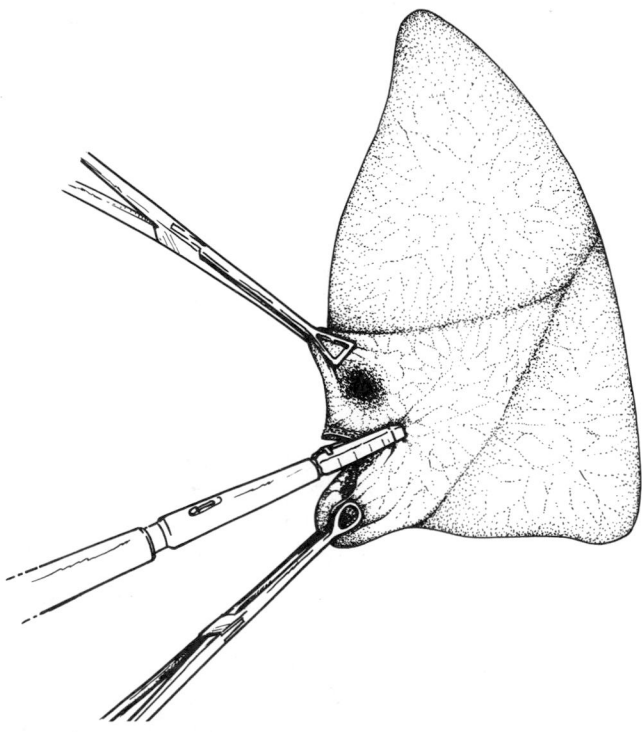

Figure 32-31. Application of stapler to begin excision of nodule.

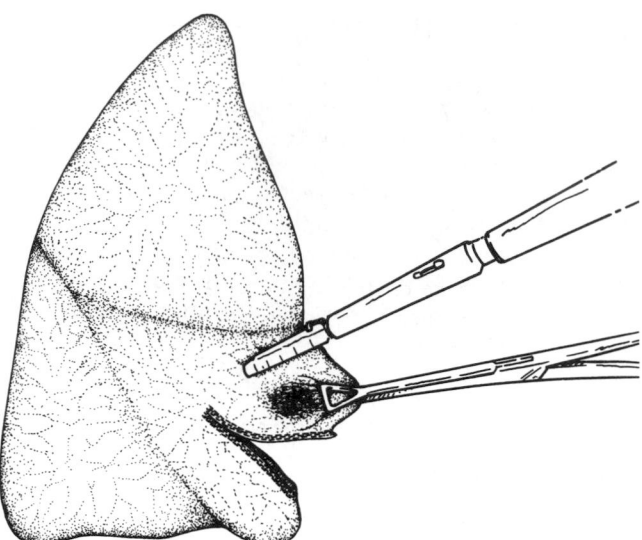

Figure 32-32. Second application of stapler, maintaining adequate margins.

Judgment is required in deciding whether nodules are appropriate for endoscopic versus open resection. As discussed elsewhere in this book, a wedge resection is not considered an adequate operation for primary lung carcinoma unless used as a compromise procedure. Therefore, although current technology allows removal of a peripheral carcinoma by a thoracoscopic technique, it cannot be considered an adequate cancer operation.

PRECISION RESECTION (PERELMAN RESECTION)

Perelman described his precision resection technique in 1983, and a confirmatory report was made by Cooper, et al. in 1986. Whereas the wedge resection may be appropriate for

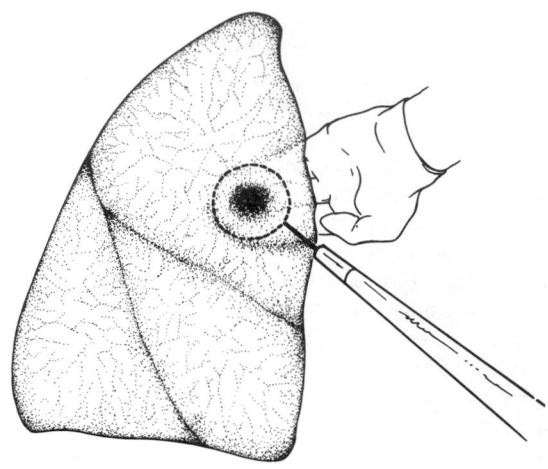

Figure 32-34. The cautery outlines the area of dissection.

peripheral lesions, the precision excision technique may be used in more central or deep-seated lesions. The same considerations regarding the appropriateness of the technique must be assessed as for wedge resection. This technique requires that the lung be inflated. The assistant positions the nodule with manual pressure so that it abuts the closest pleural surface (Fig. 32-33).

Electrocautery, preferably with the pencil or needle-point tip, is then used. In the original report Perelman described grasping the lung tissue with fine forceps and then using electrocautery. The area of dissection is outlined by cautery on the surface of the pleura (Fig. 32-34). The electrocautery dissection is then performed slowly in a circumferential manner, allowing an adequate margin. The assistant must be careful to maintain adequate manual pressure to continually "express" the nodule (Fig. 32-35). Care must be taken to maintain an adequate margin of normal lung tissue around the lesion, as it is not difficult to inadvertently begin to dissect into the nodule.

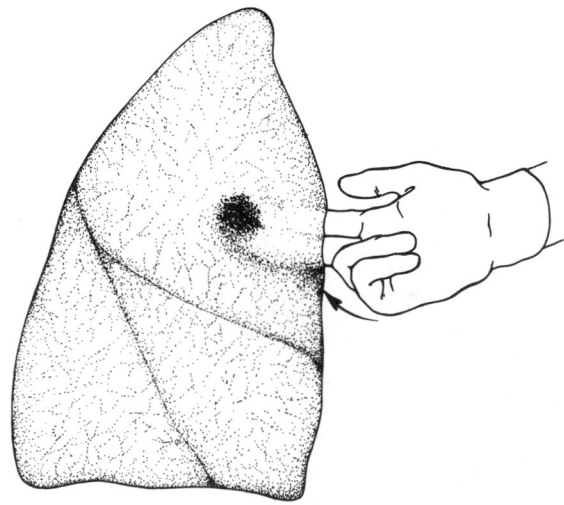

Figure 32-33. Manual pressure is applied to position nodule nearest the closest pleural surface.

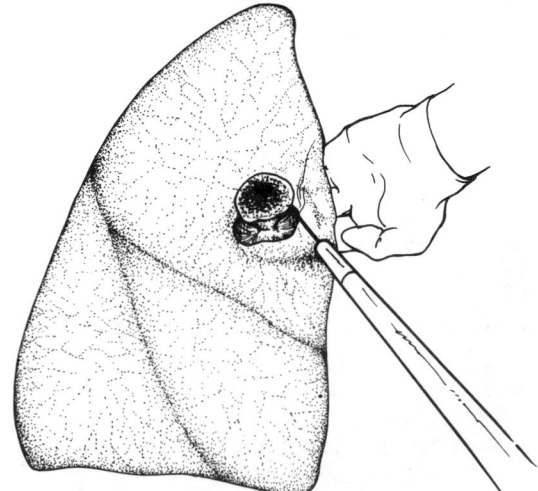

Figure 32-35. Continual pressure is applied to "express" the nodule.

When visible branches of the bronchial or vascular tree are encountered, they are secured with suture ligatures. Once the nodule has been widely circumferentially dissected, it is removed. A well charred cavity remains, which is inspected for air leaks and bleeding. These should be minimal and are controlled with suture ligatures of 4–0 Vicryl. The cavity can be left open without reapproximation of the edges, allowing for complete drainage. Other authors advocate closing the cavity with a spiral stitch or approximating the pleural surfaces, allowing the cavity to fill with blood and serum. The chest is then closed in standard fashion with chest tube drainage.

Postoperative chest x-rays will show the cavitary defect. This gradually resolves over a period of months as the lung heals. The minimal postoperative air leaks usually resolve within 2 to 3 days.

LASER RESECTION

Laser-assisted resections have become increasingly popular. The technique is exactly the same as the precision electrocautery procedure, except that the neodymium:yttrium-aluminum-garnet (Nd:YAG) laser is used. The virtues of the Nd:YAG laser include its ability to be focused and "defocused" in order to vary the intensity of the applied energy. The focused beam increases the power density and therefore facilitates vaporization. If the beam is withdrawn slightly, it is defocused, allowing for greater coagulation effects. As with the electrocautery, vessels or bronchi larger than 2 to 3 mm should be controlled with ligatures. The resulting charred, resected space is handled identically to that obtained in the electrocautery technique. As with any newer procedure, there is a learning curve before facile ease and speed are obtained.

Proponents of the laser technique such as Landreneau, et al. (1991) and Desai, et al. (1988) assert that they achieve good hemostasis, minimal blood loss, and appropriate operative time. However, lasers are expensive and require significant in-service education for support personnel and operators and strict attention to safety. The current advantages of laser-assisted minimal pulmonary excision rarely justify its preference over the older technique of electrocautery. Laser applications in video-assisted thoracoscopy for lung resection are still being explored and defined.

KEY REFERENCE

Perelman M: Precision techniques for removal of pathological structures from the lungs. Surgery 11:12, 1983

This short article is the first technical description of precision cautery excision of pulmonary lesions.

REFERENCES

Cooper JD, Perelman M, Todd TRJ et al: Precision cautery excision of pulmonary lesions. Ann Thorac Surg 41:51, 1986

Desai SJ, Mchta AC, Medendorp S et al: Survival experience following Nd:YAG laser photoresection for primary bronchogenic carcinoma. Chest 94:939, 1988

Ferguson MK, DeMeester TR, DesLauriers J et al: Diagnosis and management of synchronous lung cancers. J Thorac Cardiovasc Surg 89:378, 1985

Kittle CF, Penfield Faber L, Jensik RJ, Warren WH: Pulmonary resection in patients after pneumonectomy. Ann Thorac Surg 40:294, 1985

Jacobaeus HC: The practical importance of thoracoscopy in surgery of the chest. Surg Gynecol Obstet 34:289, 1922

Landreneau RJ, Hazelrigg SR, Johnson JA et al: Neodymium: yttrium-aluminum garnet laser-assisted pulmonary resections. Ann Thorac Surg 51:973, 1991

Martini N, Ghosn N, Melamed MR: International Trends in General Thoracic Surgery. Vol. 1. WB Saunders, Philadelphia, 1985

Miller JI, Hatcher CR: Limited resection of bronchogenic carcinoma in the patient with marked impairment of pulmonary function. Ann Thorac Surg 44:340, 1987

Moghissi K: Local excision of pulmonary nodular (coin) lesion with noncontact yttrium-aluminum-garnet laser. J Thorac Cardiovasc Surg 97:147, 1989

Bronchoplastic Bronchovascular Techniques

Ryosuke Tsuchiya

DEFINITION

Sleeve resection of the bronchus was described by Paulson and Shaw in 1955 as a bronchoplastic procedure. The combined procedure of bronchoplasty and resection and anastomosis of the pulmonary artery is known as *bronchovasculoplasty*.

HISTORICAL NOTE

In 1932 Bigger (1935) performed the first bronchotomy to remove a tumor of the left main bronchus in a 14-year-old boy; because the tumor could not be completely resected by the bronchotomy alone, a completion pneumonectomy was also performed. Unfortunately, the patient developed purulent pericarditis and died.

In 1939 Eloesser (1940) successfully removed an adenoma originating at the orifice of the lower left lobe bronchus. In 1944 Belsey (1946) removed an adenoma with segments of bronchus and successfully repaired the defects of the bronchial wall using fascia. In 1947 Price-Thomas (1955) performed the first sleeve resection of the bronchus to remove an adenoma originating in the right main bronchus; in 1949 D'Abreu and MacHale (1951) performed a similar operation for removal of an adenoma; and in 1951 Gebauer (1951) performed the first elective excision (sleeve resection) of a whole main bronchus with severe tuberculous stenosis.

In 1949 Carlens reported the development of a flexible double-lumen catheter for bronchospirometry, which was later used for one-lung anesthesia in bronchoplastic procedures.

Price-Thomas credited Allison with performing the first sleeve resection for therapy of lung cancer in 1952. In 1955 Paulson and Shaw who first used the term *bronchoplastic* to describe these operations, reported their results in treating a series of 16 patients, of including 4 with traumatic rupture, 3 with tuberculous bronchostenosis, 2 with bronchial adenoma, and 7 with bronchogenic carcinoma. Johnston and Jones (1959) and Paulson and Shaw (1960) reported the long-term results of lobectomy and sleeve resection of the main bronchus in the treatment of patients with bronchial carcinoma. Six years later Jensik (1966) recommended irradiation prior to bronchopulmonary sleeve resection for lung cancer to improve results. Many more reports on the results of bronchoplastic procedures for bronchogenic carcinomas, as well as for benign tumors and adenomas, of the proximal bronchi followed throughout the 1970s and 1980s (Jensik, et al., 1972; Naruke, et al., 1977; Bennett and Smith, 1978; Weisel, et al., 1979; Alp, et al., 1987; Low, et al., 1982; Rea, et at., 1989).

Hsieh, et al. (1988), reporting an experimental study on the influence of suture material in bronchial anastomosis in growing puppies, concluded that absorbable suture was superior to nonabsorbable suture in pediatric bronchoplasty.

HISTORICAL READINGS

Alp M, Ucanok D, Dogan R et al: Surgical treatment of bronchial adenomas: results of 29 cases and review of the literature. Thorac Cardiovasc Surg 35:290, 1987

Belsey R: Stainless steel wire suture technique in thoracic surgery. Thorax 1:39, 1946

Bennett WF, Smith RA: A twenty-year analysis of the results of sleeve resection for primary gronchogenic carcinoma. J Thorac Cardiovasc Surg 76:840, 1978

Bigger IA: The diagnosis and treatment of primary carcinoma of the lung. South Surg 4:401, 1935

Carlens E: A new flexible double-lumen catheter for bronchospirometry. J Thorac Cardiovasc Surg 18:742, 1949

D'Abreu AL, MacHale SJ: Bronchial ''adenoma'' treated by local resection and reconstruction of the left main bronchus. Br J Surg 39:355, 1951

Eloesser L: Transthoracid bronchotomy for removal of benign tumors of the bronchi. Ann Surg 112:1067, 1940

Gebauer PW: Reconstructive surgery of the trachea and bronchi: late results with dermal grafts. J Thorac Cardiovasc Surg 22:568, 1951

Hsieh C, Tomita M, Ayabe H et al: Influence of suture on bronchial anastomosis in growing puppies. J Thorac Cardiovasc Surg 95:998, 1988

Jensik RJ: Preoperative irradiation and bronchopulmonary sleeve resection for lung cancer. Surg Clin North Am 46:145, 1966

Jensik RJ, Faber LP, Milloy FJ, Amato JJ: Sleeve lobectomy for cacinoma. J Thorac Cardiovasc Surg 64:400, 1972

Johnston JB, Jones PH: The treatment of bronchial carcinoma by lobectomy and sleeve resection of the main bronchus. Thorax 14:48, 1959

Low JE, Bridgman AH, Sabiston DC Jr: The role of Bronchoplastic procedures in the surgical management of benign and malignant pulmonary lesions. J Thorac Cardiovasc Surg 83:227, 1982

Naruke T, Yoneyama T, Ogata T, Suemasu K: Bronchoplastic procedures for lung cancer. J Thorac Cardiovasc Surg 73:927, 1977

Paulson DL, Shaw RR: Results of bronchoplastic procedures for bronchogenic carcinoma. Ann Surg 151:729, 1960

Paulson DL, Shaw RR: Bronchial anastomosis and bronchoplastic procedures in the interest of preservation of lung tissue. J Thorac Cardiovasc Surg 29:238, 1955

Price-Thomas C: Conservative resection of the bronchial tree. J R Coll Surg Edinburgh 1:169, 1955

Rea F, Binda R, Spreafico G et al: Bronchial carcinoids: a review of 60 patients. Ann Thorac Surg Surg 47:412, 1989

Weisel RD, Cooper JD, Delarue NC et al: Sleeve lobectomy for carcinoma of the lung. J Thorac Cardiovasc Surg 78:839, 1979

BASIC SCIENCE

Surgical Anatomy of the Bronchi and Pulmonary Artery

Bronchi may be classified into two categories, extrapulmonary and intrapulmonary. Both main bronchi and the right intermediate bronchus are extrapulmonary. Structurally, the extrapulmonary bronchi are practically identical to the trachea, consisting of cartilaginous, horseshoe-shaped rings and a membranous portion (Fig. 32-36). In the intrapulmonary bronchi, the rings are replaced by irregularly shaped cartilaginous plates, which are distributed around the bronchus in a paving stone configuration (Fig. 32-37). These structural differences are important in the creation of the anastomosis in a sleeve resection, as adjustments must be made for the difference in luminal size of the two bronchial segments.

The right pulmonary artery gives rise to branches that supply the upper lobe and crosses in front of the intermediate

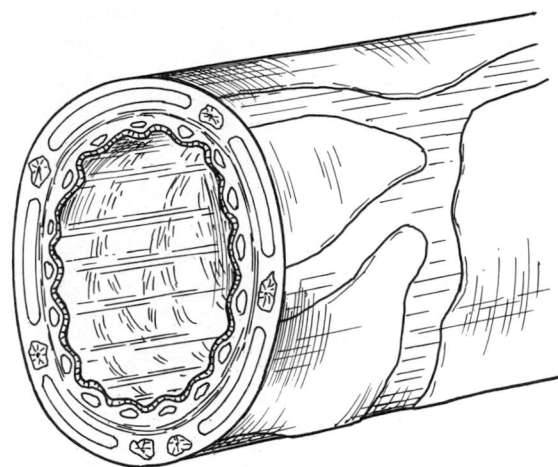

Figure 32-37. The intrapulmonary bronchus has cartilaginous plates distributed in a paving stone configuration but no membranous portion.

bronchus. The left pulmonary artery runs across the left main bronchus and the carina of the left upper lobe (Fig. 32-38). Therefore, a neoplasm in the upper division of the left lung that has invaded the upper lobe carina necessitates a sleeve lobectomy and possibly a sleeve resection of the pulmonary artery.

Blood Supply of the Bronchi

Cauldwell, et al. (1948), in a review of the bronchial arterial blood supply in 300 specimens, reported nine variations. Salassa, et al. (1977) examined the gross and microscopic blood supply of 21 tracheal specimens and found rich anastomoses in the paracarinal nodes which interconnected the circulation of the upper thoracic trachea with the superior, the middle, and possibly the inferior bronchial arteries. Inui, et al. (1990), in evaluating the healing of bronchial anastomosis by laser Doppler velocimetry, reported that the state of healing of the anastomosis site was closely related to bronchial mucosal blood flow. Excessive devascularization of the bronchus should be avoided to maintain a good blood supply at the bronchial anastomosis.

Bronchial Innervation

Both vagus nerves enter the thoracic cavity through the thoracic outlet along with the internal carotid artery. The right vagal nerve branches to the bronchi and lung extend along the bronchial artery at its crossing with the azygos vein. The left vagal nerve courses toward the root of the left subclavian artery and branches into the left recurrent nerve and then extends to the bronchi and lungs before exiting along the esophagus as the posterior vagus.

PREOPERATIVE ASSESSMENT

Preoperative assessment is very important, not only to determine the limit of the resection but also to estimate the functional status of the residual lung. The extent of bronchial

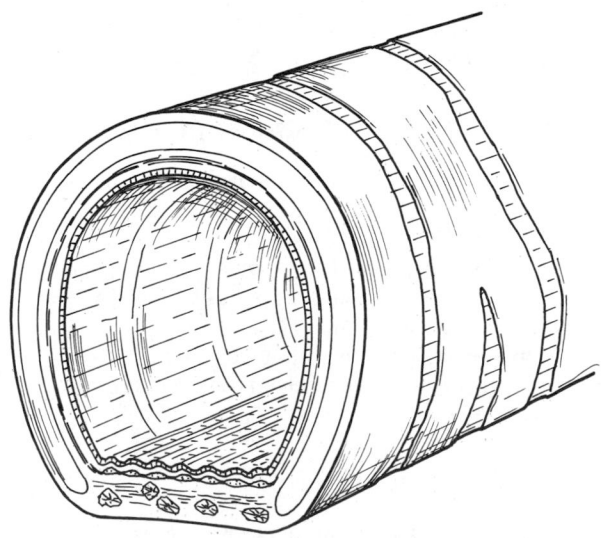

Figure 32-36. The extrapulmonary bronchus, like the trachea, consists of a horseshoe-shaped cartilaginous portion and a membranous portion.

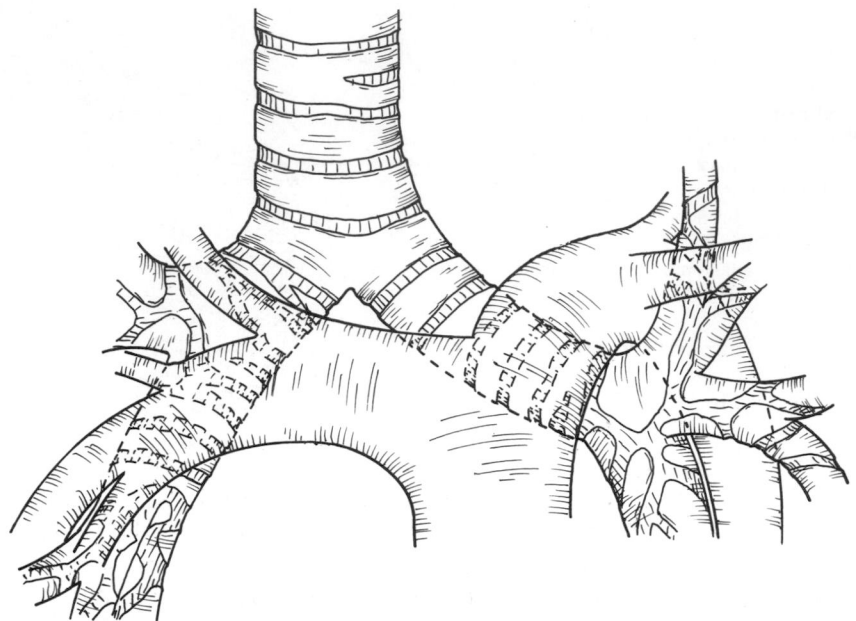

Figure 32-38.   The relationship between the bronchial tree and the pulmonary arteries. The right pulmonary artery branches to the right upper lobe bronchus and extends across the intermediate bronchus. The left pulmonary artery courses over the left upper lobe bronchus. A lung cancer located in the left upper lobe bronchus therefore has already invaded the left pulmonary artery by the time the tumor invades the left second carina. Such a tumor necessitates not only sleeve lobectomy but also sleeve resection of the pulmonary artery.

resection is usually determined by the bronchoscopic findings; computed tomography (CT), magnetic resonance imaging (MRI), and pulmonary arteriography may provide added information about the anatomic and functional status of each lobe of the lung.

Bronchoplastic procedures are most commonly performed for squamous cell carcinomas. The border of the central (hilar) type of squamous cell carcinoma can be easily recognized with the fiberoptic bronchoscope because the epithelial layer of the bronchus is usually involved. When the lesion only involved the epithelium, as in carcinoma in situ or intraepithelial spreading carcinoma, the luster of the epithelium disappears and the surface becomes cloudy. With further involvement, widening, fusion of longitudinal bundles, and surface irregularities appear. The border between the abnormal findings and normal tissue is usually very distinct. Preoperative bronchoscopic biopsies ensure accuracy in the endoscopic assessment. In cases of submucosal invasion by lymphatics, it is often difficult to determine the extent of invasion of the carcinoma, and intraoperative frozen section analysis is required.

Patients with carcinoid tumors or adenoid cystic carcinoma may also require bronchoplastic procedures. Central carcinoids and some adenoid cystic carcinomas grow as polypoid lesions with distinct borders. Removal of the polypoid lesion may be required to determine the distal limit of resection. Most adenoid cystic carcinomas, however, have ill-defined borders and spread submucosally along perineural lymphatics and extratracheally. In these cases the limit of resection of the bronchus cannot be determined grossly prior to surgery, or even during the operation, which mandates intraoperative frozen section analysis.

PREOPERATIVE MANAGEMENT

Preoperative administration of antibiotics and endoscopic removal of any bronchial obstruction will prevent the development of pneumonia, which often occurs as a result of retention of purulent sputum. Even if there is no evidence of infection, polypoid lesions should be removed if possible in order to facilitate assessment of the extent of invasion by the tumor. Although proximal and distal biopsies aid in assessing the extent of tumor invasion and in determining the procedure required, the final determination depends on intraoperative frozen section assessment of the cut surface of the surgical specimen.

INTRAOPERATIVE MANAGEMENT OF THE AIRWAY

There are several methods of managing the airway during bronchoplastic procedures. Right- and left-sided double-lumen tubes are widely used in bronchoplasty. Fogarty occlusion catheters may be used to produce endobronchial blockade, especially for left-sided surgery, as reported by Ginsberg (1981) and Tsuchiya, et al. (1981).

High-frequency jet ventilation can also be used with a conventional single-lumen tracheal tube (El-Baz, et al.; Kain and Smith, 1977).

OPERATIVE TECHNIQUE

A standard posterolateral thoracotomy is generally the most suitable incision for bronchoplasty, as it affords the best exposure for safe dissection of the proximal bronchus, tracheal carina, and pulmonary arteries and veins. Paulson, et al. (1970) and Bennett and Smith (1978), however, have emphasized the excellent exposure of the hilum achieved with a posterior approach. We usually resect the fifth rib from the transverse process to the cartilage, as well as 1-cm segments of the fourth and sixth ribs posteriorly to obtain a very wide operating field.

After the thorax has been opened, the surgeon must confirm the preoperative findings, including the location and extent of primary tumor, the status of the lymph nodes, and the presence of pleural dissemination, intrapulmonary metastasis, or lymphatic spread. Paulson, et al. (1970) and Weisel, et al. (1979) have stated that in general, the finding of extensive nodal involvement of the bronchial wall or extension of tumor across fissure lines should be considered a contraindication to bronchoplasty.

We then perform a complete mediastinal and hilar lymph node dissection and isolate pulmonary arteries and veins as for a pneumonectomy before resecting of the bronchus.

Right Upper Sleeve Lobectomy

The hilum of the right lung is dissected, and the branches of the superior pulmonary vein draining the right upper lobe of the lung, the superior trunk of the right pulmonary artery, and the ascending pulmonary artery are divided. The anterior surface of the main and intermediate bronchi and the interlobar lymph nodes are then dissected. The pulmonary ligament is divided by electrocautery, the subcarinal lymph nodes are dissected, and the posterior surfaces of both main bronchi, the intermediate bronchus, and the carina are exposed. The upper mediastinal lymph nodes are then dissected, with division of the azygos vein and exposure of the anterior and right lateral surfaces of the trachea and carina. Extensive

dissection of the left lateral wall of the trachea and separation of the trachea from the esophagus are avoided in order to preserve the vascular supply of the trachea. Incomplete fissures are separated by electrocautery or stapler. Interlobar lymph node dissection is performed to completely expose the bronchus and confirm the extent of invasion of the bronchial wall by tumor.

Stay sutures are placed in the right main and intermediate bronchi. Proper positioning of the bronchial cuts is confirmed by pulling the sutures toward each other. The site of dissection of the main bronchus is determined according to the spread of the tumor. The intermediate bronchus is usually cut at the orifice of the middle lobe bronchus to obtain bronchial ends of approximately the same caliber and to avoid having to use a long intermediate bronchus with a poor blood supply for the anastomosis even if the lower border of tumor invasion is more proximal.

The margins of the resected main and intermediate bronchi are examined by frozen section to confirm the border of tumor invasion. If cancerous tissue is found at the margin, further resection is performed whenever possible. We perform the anastomosis (Fig. 32-39) of the main and intermediate bronchi using subepithelial interrupted sutures for the cartilaginous portion and either full-layer or subepithelial interrupted sutures for the membranous portion (4–10 Prolene [Ethicon Inc., Somerville, NJ] or Maxon [Davis & Geck, Danbury, CT]) (Tsuchiya, et al., 1990). We find that a subepithelial interrupted suture affords the best coaptation of the bronchial epithelium at the anastomosis, preventing granuloma formation, ulcers, and deformity of the bronchial stumps. Double-needle sutures are used and passed exactly through the subepithelial layer from the cut surface to the adventitia of the bronchus (Fig. 32-40). Suturing is begun

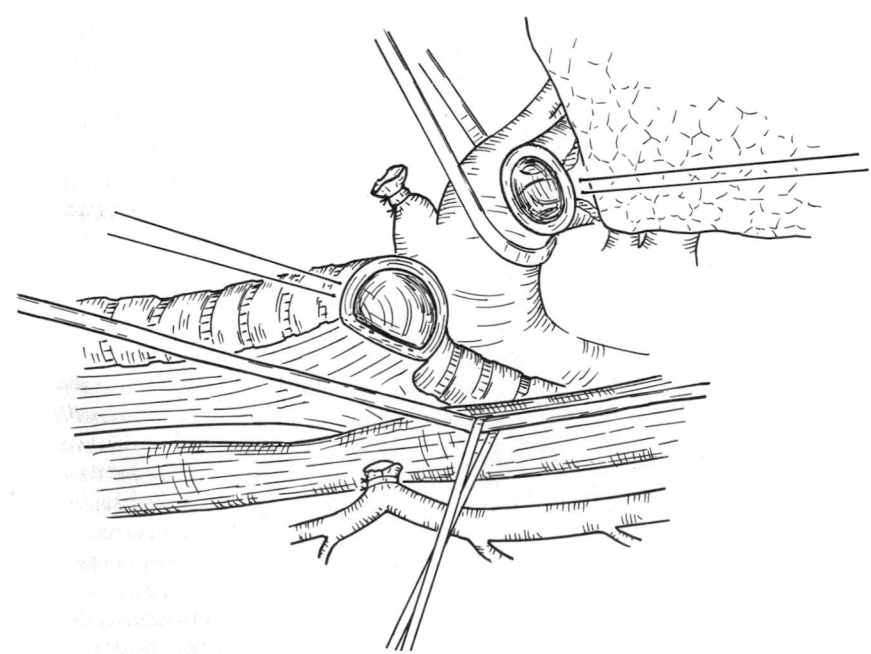

Figure 32-39. Right upper sleeve lobectomy is the most commonly performed bronchoplastic procedure. During reanastomosis, the pulmonary artery must be protected.

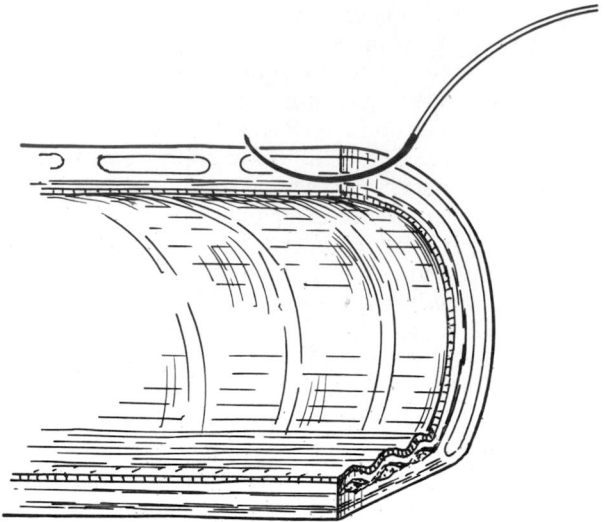

Figure 32-40. Double-needle technique is used to pass interrupted sutures through the subepithelial layer from the cut surface to the adventitia of the bronchus.

at the medial edge and stopped at the lateral edge of the cartilaginous portion. Suturing of the membranous portion is begun at the medial edges of the membranous portions of the main and intermediate bronchi. The membranous portion of the main bronchus is slightly gathered and that of the intermediate bronchus is slightly stretched by each suture to adjust for any difference in caliber.

Three methods are used to compensate for the difference in caliber between the larger central bronchus and the smaller peripheral bronchus. First, the interval between sutures of the central bronchus may be made slightly larger than that of the peripheral bronchus. A second technique is to adjust for the difference by gathering or stretching the membranous portions of both bronchi. The third method is used in right upper sleeve lobectomy; since both bronchi are extrapulmonary and thus have a structure similar to that of the trachea, suturing is started at the edge of the cartilaginous portion of the intermediate bronchus and 1 to 2 mm from the edge of the right main bronchus and is stopped at the other edge of

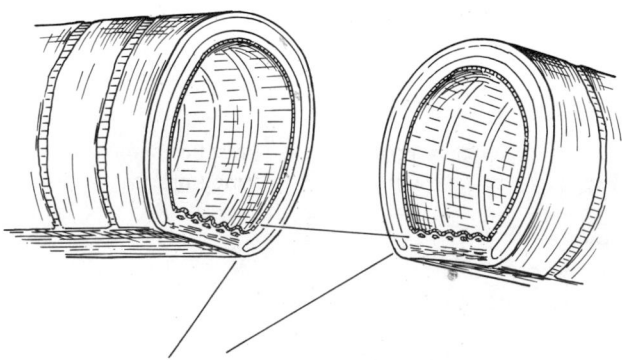

Figure 32-41. Adjusting for the difference in caliber of the bronchial segments. Suturing is started at the edge of the cartilaginous portion of the intermediate bronchus and 1 to 2 mm from the edge of the cartilaginous portion of the right main bronchus.

the cartilaginous portion of the intermediate bronchus and 1 to 2 mm from the edge of the cartilaginous portion of the right main bronchus (Fig. 32-41).

When the sutures are tied, the stay sutures are pulled toward each other to decrease tension on the anastomosis, and the lobes connected to the central bronchus by the bronchial anastomosis are pushed toward the central bronchus (Fig. 32-42). These procedures prevent cutting of the bronchial wall by decreasing tension (Fig. 32-43). Mobilization of the hilum by intrapericardial release can be helpful.

The anastomosis is examined for air leakage by a water seal test. The anastomosis is protected by a pedicled pericardial fat pad nourished by the internal thoracic artery and vein. Two chest tubes are inserted into the apicoanterior thoracic cavity: one is placed in the dead space created by the right upper lobe defect for the escape of air leaking from the interlobar cut surface of the lung, and the other is placed in the lower back thoracic cavity to allow pleural drainage.

Left Upper Sleeve Lobectomy with Resection of the Pulmonary Artery

A tumor located in the left upper lobe may infiltrate the arch of the left pulmonary artery before invading the left main bronchus or left upper lobe carina, depending on the anatomic relationship between the tumor and the pulmonary artery and bronchial tree. Therefore, left upper sleeve lobectomy combined with resection of the pulmonary artery is the most popular type of bronchovasculoplasty.

After a standard posterolateral thoracotomy has been performed, if the tumor is found to be suitable for bronchoplasty, the anterior hilum of the left lung is dissected, the superior pulmonary vein is ligated, and the anterior surface of the left main bronchus and the interlobar lymph nodes are dissected. A tape passed around the left main pulmonary artery will allow complete control. The anterior mediastinal lymph nodes are dissected to preserve the phrenic, vagal, and recurrent nerves. The ligamentum arteriosum is exposed by the upper mediastinal lymph node dissection and is divided to obtain clear access to the carina and proximal left main bronchus (Boyd, et al., 1970). The aortic arch is retracted, the recurrent nerve is taped and preserved, and the tracheobronchial lymph nodes are dissected. The inferior pulmonary ligament and the subcarinal and posterior hilar lymph nodes are dissected to expose the membranous and medial cartilaginous portions of the left main bronchus. Exposure of the pulmonary artery is continued until the superior segmental artery of the lower lobe can be identified. The anterior segmental pulmonary artery is exposed from the front or interlobar space. An incomplete fissure between the upper and lower lobes is separated by electrocautery or stapler.

A tape is passed around the interlobar pulmonary artery to facilitate retraction, and the degree of tumor invasion of the pulmonary artery and bronchus is assessed. After invasion of the pulmonary artery and bronchus has been confirmed, the root and interlobar segment of the pulmonary artery are clamped distal to all upper lobe branches, and after the lingular arteries have been divided, the artery is divided with the bronchus. The left main bronchus is divided proximal to the tumor, and the location of the double-lumen catheter or

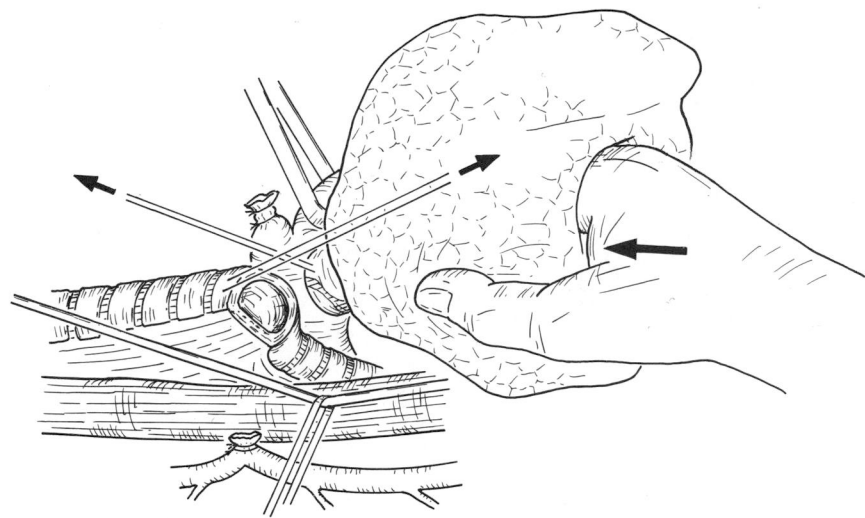

Figure 32-42. Mobilization of preserved middle and lower lobes. An assistant standing at the patient's back grasps the preserved right middle and lower lobes and pushes them toward the patient's head to decrease the tension of the anastomosis for right upper sleeve lobectomy.

blocker is adjusted through the open left main bronchus to maintain ventilation of the right lung. The lower bronchus of the left lung is then divided, and the tumor is removed along with the affected portions of the left upper lobe, pulmonary artery, main bronchus, and second carina (Fig. 32-44).

The bronchial (first) and arterial anastomoses are performed after the stumps of the bronchi and pulmonary artery have been determined by frozen section to be free of tumor invasion. After the medial portion of the bronchi is sutured, the stumps are ligated from the most medial portion of the bronchi laterally, so that the cartilaginous portion of the left

main bronchus from the medial edge to the anterolateral angle is approximated. The rest of the cartilaginous portion and finally the membranous portion are then sutured in order to adjust for any difference in caliber between the two segments. Because the left lower lobe bronchus is intrapulmonary, it has no membranous portion. After the anastomosis of the bronchi has been completed and tested for patency and leakage, the pulmonary arteries are approximated continuously with use of two or three stay sutures and monofilament nylon.

The anastomosis of the bronchi is usually covered by a pedicled fat pad, a pedicled muscle flap, or omentum. Omentum is the best covering material because a large amount is available and it has a good blood supply and good plasticity. However, an extra incision is required for this. We prefer a pedicled pericardial fat pad nourished by the intrathoracic artery and vein (Brewer and Bai, 1955), but when this cannot be used because of poor nutrition or invasion by tumor, a flap of latissimus dorsi muscle may be used. In the case of bronchovasculoplasty, the covering separates the bronchial anastomosis from the anastomosis or plasty of the pulmonary artery and is absolutely necessary to prevent bronchoarterial fistula.

POSTOPERATIVE CARE

To ensure success, bronchoplasty must be an uncomplicated, bloodless, and expeditiously performed procedure. Well-organized postoperative care is an important factor, as are a well-trained paramedical staff and a well-informed patient.

The condition of the anastomosis should be checked immediately after completion as well as postoperatively because bleeding from the bronchial stump and/or inadequate adaptation of the anastomosis is occasionally found. Even when the anastomosis has been performed adequately, sputum retention can be found beyond the anastomosis. Fiberoptic bronchoscopy should be performed in the morning of the first postoperative day to observe the anastomosis and to

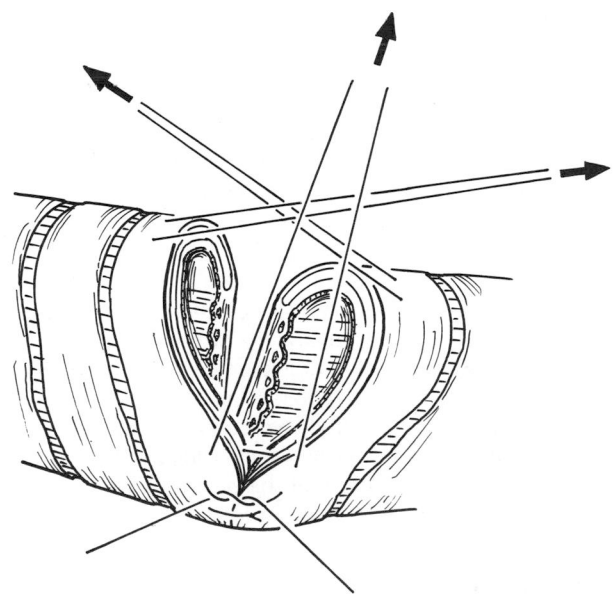

Figure 32-43. Cutting of the bronchial wall by sutures is avoided by using stay sutures to draw the segments toward each other and thus decrease tension on the anastomosis. Pulling up the next suture will also serve to decrease tension.

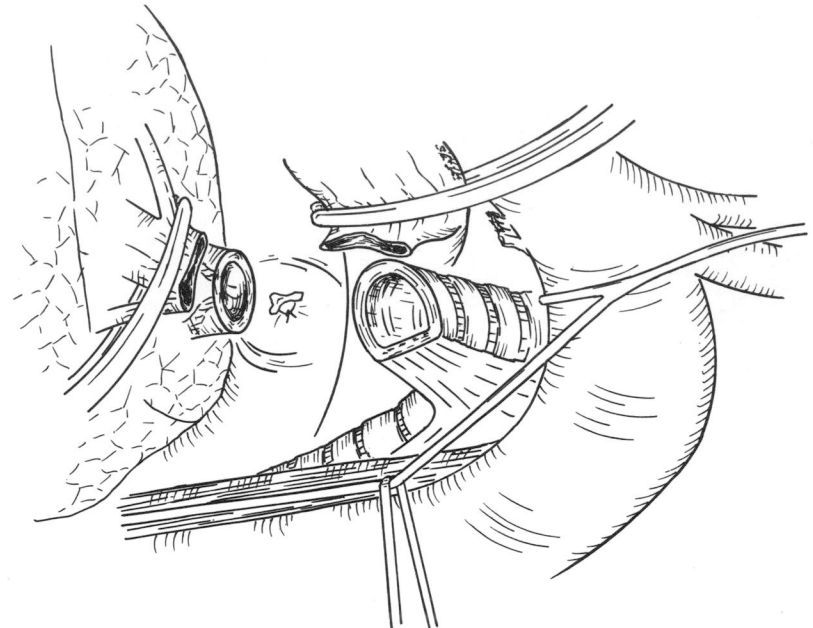

Figure 32-44. Left upper sleeve lobectomy. The left main bronchus and pulmonary artery are resected with the cancer, as in bronchovasculoplasty for lung cancer.

aspirate sputum even if the patient has no abnormal symptoms. Viscous sputum adhering to the bronchial wall cannot be detected by auscultation or chest radiography. The need for further fiberoptic bronchoscopic evaluation is determined by the findings of the examination performed on the first postoperative day. In elderly patients, bronchoscope-assisted tracheal toilet is usually needed by the end of the first postoperative week; however, in young patients it is performed once or twice to confirm the findings in the anastomosis and other bronchial lumina.

COMPLICATIONS AND RESULTS

Operative Mortality

In the first report involving a large number of cases, Johnston and Jones (1959) reported the results of 98 cases of lobectomy and sleeve resection of the main bronchus. Of the 98 patients, 8 died as a direct result of the operation. Two patients died of a combination of sputum retention, bronchopneumonia, and respiratory insufficiency. One patient died of hemoptysis; at necropsy a communication with the pulmonary artery at the bronchial suture line was found. Another patient died of a cause not related to the bronchoplasty. Many other reports have been published, with operative mortality rates ranging from 1.8 to 11.4 percent (Ree and Paneth, 1970; Paulson, et al., 1970; Jensik, et al., 1972; Naef, et al., 1974; Bennett and Smith, 1978; Weisel, et al., 1979; Van Den Bosch, et al., 1981; Van Schil, et al., 1991).

Early Complications

Postoperative bleeding is the most common early complication in lung cancer surgery with or without bronchoplasty. Intrabronchial bleeding from the anastomosis is a complica-

tion specific to bronchoplasty. Upon completion, the anastomosis should be examined intraoperatively by fiberoptic bronchoscopy to check not only its adaptation but also for any persistent bleeding. Bleeding may cause hemoptysis and/or aspiration pneumonia. Maladaptation of the anastomosis can cause granulation and stenosis of the bronchus. If bleeding and/or maladaptation is recognized intraoperatively, it should be corrected immediately by reanastomosis. Rehabilitation, early ambulation, and exercise are useful adjuncts to prevent postoperative pulmonary complications.

Ischemic changes of the peripheral bronchus of the anastomosis can occur when overaggressive lymph node dissection is performed or a long peripheral bronchus is preserved to decrease the tension on the anastomosis. Most of these changes are only temporary, but some may result in stenosis or bronchopleural fistula. Bronchovascular fistula occasionally occurs when an anastomosis exists near a stump or involves the pulmonary artery; covering the bronchus is therefore helpful.

Bronchoplasty shortens the bronchus and may cause bending and stenosis of the pulmonary artery, especially when the left pulmonary artery is not resected, which occasionally results in pulmonary infarction. While this is a rare occurrence, it is an important complication of bronchoplasty. When a radical sleeve resection of a long left bronchus is performed, sleeve resection of the pulmonary artery is also required to prevent this complication.

Late Complications

The most troublesome late complication is bronchopleural or bronchovascular fistula. Preoperative irradiation, chemotherapy, and ischemic changes caused by dissection of the bronchial artery are the major causes of such fistulae, which usually occur 3 to 4 weeks after operation; fistulae caused by technical failure usually occur within a few days of surgery. When a fistula occurs, surgical repair of the anastomosis is usually futile and completion pneumonectomy is required.

Stenosis of the anastomosis may occur as a late complication of bronchoplasty. Maladaptation of the anastomosis is considered the most common cause of stenosis. The stenosis may be dilated or, if granulations are the cause, managed by laser or cauterized. Stents may be of value. Occasionally surgical repair or completion pneumonectomy is required in recalcitrant cases.

Long-Term Results

Low, et al. (1982) summarized reports in the literature on 565 bronchoplastic procedures from 1947 to 1981. Of these, 504 were performed for lung cancer, 51 for adenoma, 6 for bronchial stenosis, and 4 for trauma. They also reported survival data among 480 patients undergoing sleeve lobectomy for lung cancer and found that operative mortality was about 7 percent (32 of 480), 1-year survival was 79 percent (129 of 162), a 5-year survival was 33 percent (53 of 159), and 10-year survival was 21 percent (15 of 71).

Vogt-Moykopf, et al. (1986) reported the results of the largest single series of patients undergoing bronchoplasty for lung cancer. Among the 248 patients the 5-year survival rates were as follows: stage N0 disease, 37 percent; stage N1 disease, 30 percent; stage N2 disease, none. Naruke (1989) reported the results of a series of 111 patients and found that the 5-year survival rates of patients with stage N0, N1, and N2 disease were 50, 46, and 33 percent, respectively. Van Schil, et al. (1991), reporting the results of a series of 112 patients, found 5-year survival rates of patients with stage N0, N1, and N2 disease of 59, 21, and 44 percent, respectively. These results are similar to those of patients treated by lobectomy reported by Naruke, et al. (1988).

COMMENTS AND CONTROVERSIES

Indications for Surgery

Squamous cell carcinoma and low-grade malignant tumors are the commonest indications for bronchoplasty. Squamous cell carcinomas with intraepithelial spread do better with bronchoplasty than carcinomas with submucosal spread, most of which are adenocarcinomas and have lymphatic permeation beyond the limits of resection. The preoperative diagnosis of histologic type and assessment of bronchial extent of cancer are therefore important to determine the usefulness of bronchoplasty in the individual patient.

Covering the Anastomosis

The anastomosis is covered with omentum, a fat pad, or a muscle flap in order to prevent bronchopleural or bronchovascular fistula formation. It cannot prevent early fistula caused by technical failure, however, nor can it decrease the frequency of anastomotic separation, because these complications occur before the omentum or flap can adhere to and nourish the bronchi. The main purpose of these coverings is to minimize the effect of such complications.

Technique and Materials

The time of onset of the bronchial fistula indicates whether it was caused by technical or predisposing factors. Hsieh, et al. (1988) concluded that absorbable suture was superior to nonabsorbable suture in pediatric bronchoplasty, and Inui, et al. (1990) reported that the state of healing of the anastomosis was closely related to bronchial mucosal blood flow. However, the difference in clinical course of the patients in whom absorbable and nonabsorbable materials were used is minimal. Maladaptation produced granulations, resulting in stenosis of the bronchial lumen. Ischemic changes in the peripheral bronchus affect wound healing and if prolonged, can result in fistula or stenosis. Therefore, sharp and straight cut edges, accurate adjustment for differences in caliber of the bronchial lumen, proper cutting position of the bronchus, and adequate dissection of lymph nodes around the bronchus are required to prevent bronchial fistula.

R.T.

KEY REFERENCES

Carlens E: A new flexible double-lumen catheter for bronchospirometry. J Thorac Cardiovasc Surg 18:742, 1949

A flexible double-lumen catheter was developed for bronchospirometry and later was used in one-lung anesthasia for bronchoplastic procedures. The construction of the catheter is shown.

Cauldwell EW, Siekert RG, Lininger, RE, Anson BJ: The bronchial arteries. Surg Gynecol Obstet 86:395, 1948

The origin, course and distribution of the bronchial arteries are described for a series of 150 cadavers. The specimens were classified into types (I to IX) in the order of decreasing frequency of occurrence and subclassified on the basis of arterial origin.

Jensik RJ, Faber LP, Milloy FJ, Amato JJ: Sleeve lobectomy for carcinoma. J Thorac Cardiovasc Surg 64:400, 1972

This is one of the early reports of results of sleeve lobectomy for lung cancer. Preoperative irradiation was used to a greater degree (66 percent of cases) than previously reported by others in the hope that with reduction in tumor size more sleeve resections could be carried out.

Tsuchiya R, Goya T, Naruke T, Suemasu K: Resection of tracheal carina for lung cancer. J Thorac Cardiovasc Surg 99:779, 1990

The suturing technique for anastomosis of bronchi, suture materials, and covering of the anastomosis are discussed. Anastomosis was performed with subepithelial interrupted sutures at the cartilaginous portion and full-layer or subepithelial interrupted sutures at the membranous portion with 3–0 or 4–0 polypropylene or Maxon.

Van Schil PE, de la Riviere AB, Knaepen PJ et al: TNM staging and long-term followup after sleeve resection for bronchogenic tumors. Ann Thorac Surg 52:1096, 1991

The results of sleeve resection for bronchogenic tumors are discussed. Survival is best for carcinoid tumors and squamous cell carcinoma with negative nodes. The presence of N1 or N2 disease significantly worsens prognosis, with no 10-year survivors and no difference between N1 and N2 status.

REFERENCES

Alp M, Ucanok K, Dogan R et al: Surgical treatment of bronchial adenomas: results of 29 cases and review of the literature. Thorac Cardiovasc Surg 35:290, 1987

Belsey R: Stainless steel wire suture technique in thoracic surgery. Thorax 1:39, 1946

Bennett WF, Smith RA: A twenty-year analysis of the results of sleeve resection for primary bronchogenic carcinoma. J Thorac Cardiovasc Surg 76:840, 1978

Bigger IA: The diagnosis and treatment of primary carcinoma of the lung. South Surg 4:401, 1935

Boyd AD, Spencer FC, Lind A: Why has bronchial resection and anastomosis been reported infrequently for treatment of bronchial adenoma? J Thorac Cardiovasc Surg 59:359, 1970

Brewer LA, Bai AF: Surgery of the bronchi and trachea. Am J Surg 89:331, 1955

D'Abreu AL, MacHale SJ: Bronchial "adenoma" treated by local resection and reconstruction of the left main bronchus. Br J Surg 39:355, 1951

El-Baz N, El-Ganzouri A, Ivankovich AD: One-lung high-frequency ventilation for intrathoracic surgery. In Scheck PA, Sjostrand UH, and Smith RB (eds): Perspectives in High-Frequency Ventilation.

Eloesser L: Transthoracic bronchotomy for removal of benign tumors of the bronchi. Ann Surg 112:1067, 1940

Gebauer PW: Reconstructive surgery of the trachea and bronchi: late results with dermal grafts. J Thorac Cardiovasc Surg 22:568, 1951

Gebauer PW: Plastic reconstruction of tuberculous bronchostenosis with dermal grafts. J Thorac Cardiovasc Surg 19:604, 1950

Ginsberg RJ: New technique for one-lung anesthesia using an endobronchial blocker. J Thorac Cardiovasc Surg 82:542, 1981

Hsieh C, Tomita M, Ayabe H et al: Influence of suture on bronchial anastomosis in growing puppies. J Thorac Cardiovasc Surg 95:998, 1988

Inui K, Wada H, Yokomise H et al: Evaluation of a bronchial anastomosis by laser Doppler velocimetry. J Thorac Cardiovasc Surg 96:614, 1990

Jensik RJ: Preoperative irradiation and bronchopulmonary sleeve resection for lung cancer. Surg Clin North Am 46:145 1966

Johnston JB, Jones PH: The treatment of bronchial carcinoma by lobectomy and sleeve resection of the main bronchus. Thorax 14:48, 1959

Klain M, Smith RB: High-frequency percutaneus transtracheal jet ventilation. Crit Care Med 5:280, 1977

Low JE, Bridgman AH, Sabiston DC Jr: The role of bronchoplastic procedures in the surgical management of benign and malignant pulmonary lesions. J Thorac Cardiovasc Surg 83:227, 1982

Naef AP, Schmid de Gruneck J: Right pneumonectomy or sleeve lobectomy in the treatment of bronchogenic carcinoma. Ann Thorac Surg 17:168, 1974

Naruke T: Bronchoplastic and bronchovascular procedures of the tracheobronhial tree in the management of primary lung cancer. Chest (suppl) 96:53S, 1989

Naruke T, Goya T, Tsuchiya R, Suemasu K: Prognosis and survival in resected lung carcinoma based on the new international staging system. J Thorac Cardiovasc Surg 96:440, 1988

Naruke T, Yoneyama T, Ogata T, Suemasu K: Bronchoplastic procedures for lung cancer. J Thorac Cardiovasc Surg 73:927, 1977

Paulson DL, Shaw RR: Results of bronchoplastic procedures for bronchogenic carcinoma. Ann Surg 151:729, 1960

Paulson DL, Shaw RR: Bronchial anastomosis and bronchoplastic procedures in the interest of preservation of lung tissue. J Thorac Cardiovasc Surg 29:238, 1955

Paulson DL, Urschel HC Jr, McNamara JJ, Shaw RR: Bronchogenic procedures for bronchogenic carcinoma. J Thorac Cardiovasc Surg 59:38, 1970

Price-Thomas C: Conservative resection of the bronchial tree. J R Coll Surg Edinburgh 1:169, 1955

Rea F, Binda R, Spreafico G et al: Bronchial carcinoids: a review of 60 patients. Ann Thorac Surg 47:412, 1989

Ree GM, Paneth M: Lobectomy with sleeve resection in the treatment of bronchial tumors. Thorax 25:160, 1970

Salassa JR, Pearson BW, Payne WS: Gross and microscopical blood supply of the trachea. Ann Thorac Surg 24:100, 1977

Tsuchiya R, Hiraga K, Tengan L, Suemasu K: Management of airway by Fogarty occlusion catheter in pulmonary resection. Jpn Ann Thorac Surg 1:642, 1981 (in Japanese, abstruct in English)

Van Den Bosch JMM, Laros CD, Schaepkens ALEMS, Wagenaar SJSC: Lobectomy with sleeve resection in the treatment of tumors of the bronchus. Chest 80:154, 1981

Vogt-Moykopf I, Fritz TH, Meyer G, et al: Bronchoplastic and angioplastic operation in bronchial carcinoma: long-term results of a retrospective analysis from 1973 to 1983. Int Surg 71:211, 1986

Weisel RD, Cooper JD, Delarue NC et al: Sleeve lobectomy for carcinoma of the lung. J Thorac Cardiovasc Surg 78:839, 1979

Superior Sulcus Tumor

Farid Shamji
Robert J. Ginsberg
Harold C. Urschel, Jr.

INTRODUCTION

A true superior sulcus tumor is usually a primary lung cancer, which early on, extends beyond the lung to invade important anatomic structures in the narrow, crowded thoracic inlet. Local tumor invasion may involve the lower trunk of the brachial plexus, including the roots of the eight cervical and first thoracic nerves, and also the sympathetic chain and the stellate ganglion. There may be local extension into adjacent upper ribs and thoracic vertebrae. The subclavian artery may become encased in the tumor mass as it extends into the root of the neck. Spread of the tumor through the adjacent intervertebral foramen may cause epidural spinal cord compression. Although superior pulmonary sulcus tumors were originally considered to be inoperable and incurable because of their relative inaccessibility and extensive local invasion in the thoracic inlet, in recent years it has become obvious that in selected patients the therapy that completely eradicates the local growth gives the most appreciable pain relief and survival in terms of both quality and duration.

HISTORICAL NOTE

Henry K. Pancoast, in his presidential address to the American Medical Association in 1932, described the clinical features of a lung cancer involving the apex of the chest, now known as a Pancoast tumor. The syndrome associated with this apical tumor includes Horner syndrome and radiologic destruction of ribs, as well as atrophy of the hand muscles. Until the reports by Chardack and MacCallum (1956) and Shaw, et al. (1961), there had been no curative resections of this disease. At present, any apical tumor with associated pain around the shoulder and extending down the arm is termed a *superior sulcus tumor*.

HISTORICAL READINGS

Chardack WM, MacCallum JD: Pancoast tumor: five year survival without recurrence or metastases following radical resection and postoperative irradiation. J Thorac Surg 31:535, 1956
Pancoast HK: Superior pulmonary sulcus tumors. Tumor characterized by pain, Horner's syndrome, destruction of bone and atrophy of hand muscles. JAMA 99:1391, 1932
Shaw RR, Paulson DL, Kee JL: Treatment of the superior sulcus tumor by irradiation followed by resection. Ann Surg 154:29, 1961

THERAPY

Preoperative radiotherapy to a moderate dose, 30 to 45 Gy followed by extended en bloc resection in selected patients is the most common therapeutic protocol for true superior sulcus tumors, although the value of preoperative versus postoperative radiotherapy has never been established. Resection is carried out 4 to 6 weeks after completion of radiotherapy. For local resection to be complete and curative, it usually includes the following:

1. Chest wall
   a. Entire first rib and posterior parts of other involved ribs, most often the second and third ribs
   b. Occasionally, portions of upper thoracic vertebrae (up to one-quarter of the body can be removed without undue instability), including their transverse processes if necessary
2. Corresponding thoracic nerve roots up to the intervertebral foramen
3. A portion of the lower trunk of the brachial plexus, with sacrifice of the first thoracic nerve and usually with preservation of the eighth cervical nerve root
4. A portion of the stellate ganglion and the thoracic sympathetic chain
5. A pulmonary resection, usually by lobectomy or occasionally by anatomic segmental or wedge resection, although the latter has recently been shown to yield a poorer ultimate survival rate
6. Radical mediastinal lymph node dissection

It is important to identify those patients who are most likely to benefit from the combined therapy. This requires proper patient selection, careful and thorough staging of the cancer by mediastinal node biopsy and distant organ scanning, and examination of the local findings from noninvasive assessment by computed tomography (CT) scanning and magnetic resonance imaging (MRI).

In most cases N2 disease discovered at mediastinoscopy, invasion of thoracic vertebral cancellous bone, and involvement of subclavian vessels have been considered to indicate inoperability. This has been questioned recently with the popularization of the anterior approach (see Dartevelle's discussion later in this chapter of the cervical approach to apical lesions).

OPERATIVE TECHNIQUE

Anesthesia and Patient Position

General anesthesia using a double-lumen endobronchial tube greatly facilitates exposure within the chest. Full monitoring capacity is established for continuous recording of arterial blood pressure, oxygen saturation, cardiac rhythm, central venous pressure, and urine output. The patient is placed in the full lateral position with the affected side uppermost. The upper arm rests on a support. Conventional draping with sheets provides satisfactory exposure from the nape of the neck to the costal arch and from the nipple to the spinous processes of the thoracic spine.

The Incision

Lateral Thoracotomy Incision for Initial Exploration

The skin incision (Fig. 32-45) is started 3 cm beneath the nipple or just lateral to the breast in women and extends in a gentle arc 2 cm below the inferior angle of the scapula.

The incision is carried deeper by use of electrocautery. The latissimus dorsi muscle is divided toward the lower margin of the incision. The fascia posterior to the serratus anterior muscle is incised along its posterior edge, and the muscle is divided along the lower part of the incision. In most cases the chest is entered through a normal intercostal space between the two highest ribs that have not been invaded by the tumor (usually the fourth or fifth interspace), as determined by the preoperative CT scan and/or MRI; this allows one intact rib to be removed below the lower extent of the tumor (Fig. 32-46). The chest is explored to determine tumor resectability and the extent of the resection (i.e., the number of ribs and the portions of vertebral bodies and the corresponding transverse processes to be removed (Fig. 32-47).

Parascapular Incision for Exposure of the Thoracic Inlet and Chest Wall Resection

Once resectability has been determined, the skin incision is extended posteriorly in a gentle arc from below the inferior angle of the scapula to a point midway between the spinous process and the medial border of the scapula. From this point the incision is carried vertically upward, ending opposite the level of the spinous processes of the seventh cervical vertebra and is then carried deeper with electrocautery, dividing the trapezius muscle for the full length of the incision. Deep to the trapezius are the levator scapulae and rhomboid minor and major muscles (from superior to inferior), which insert into the medial border of the scapula. The rhomboids are divided with care taken to avoid injury to the underlying dorsal scapular nerve (the nerve to the rhomboids) and the

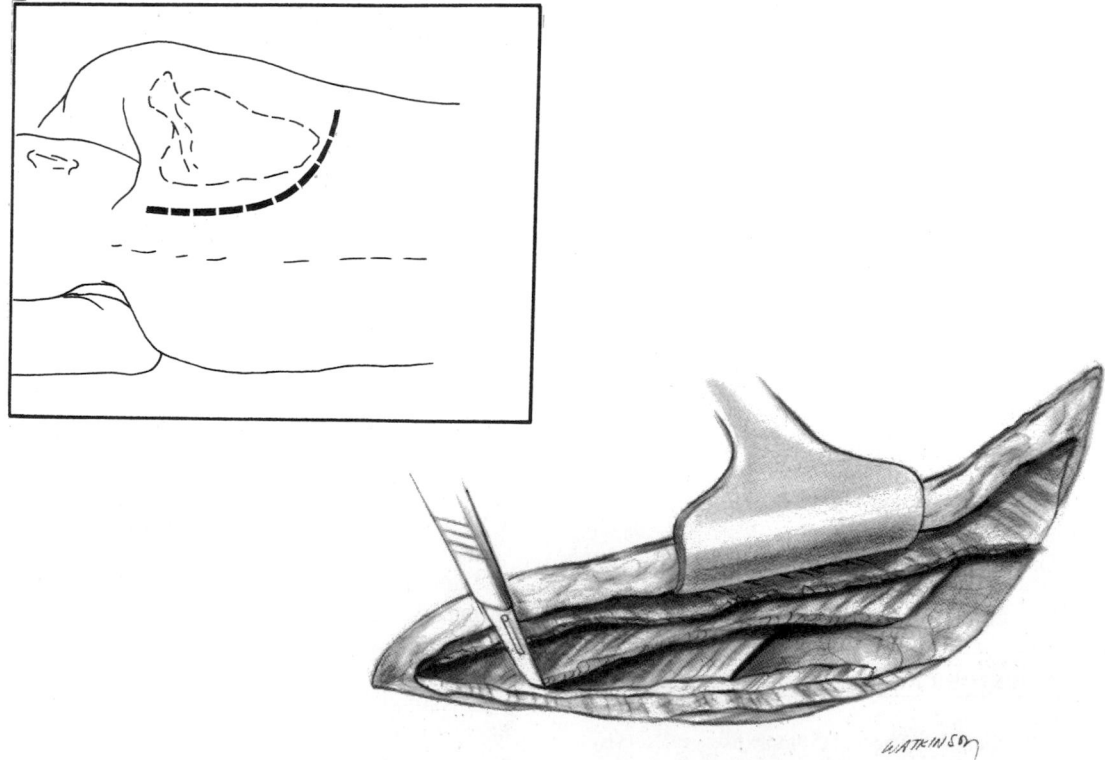

Figure 32-45. The posterolateral incision, which should extend proximally to the C7 spinous process. The trapezius has been divided and the rhomboids are in their final stage of division. (From Cooper JD, Urschel HC Jr: Superior pulmonary sulcus carcinoma resection: posterior approach. In Atlas of Thoracic Surgery. p. 181. Churchill Livingstone, New York, 1995, with permission.)

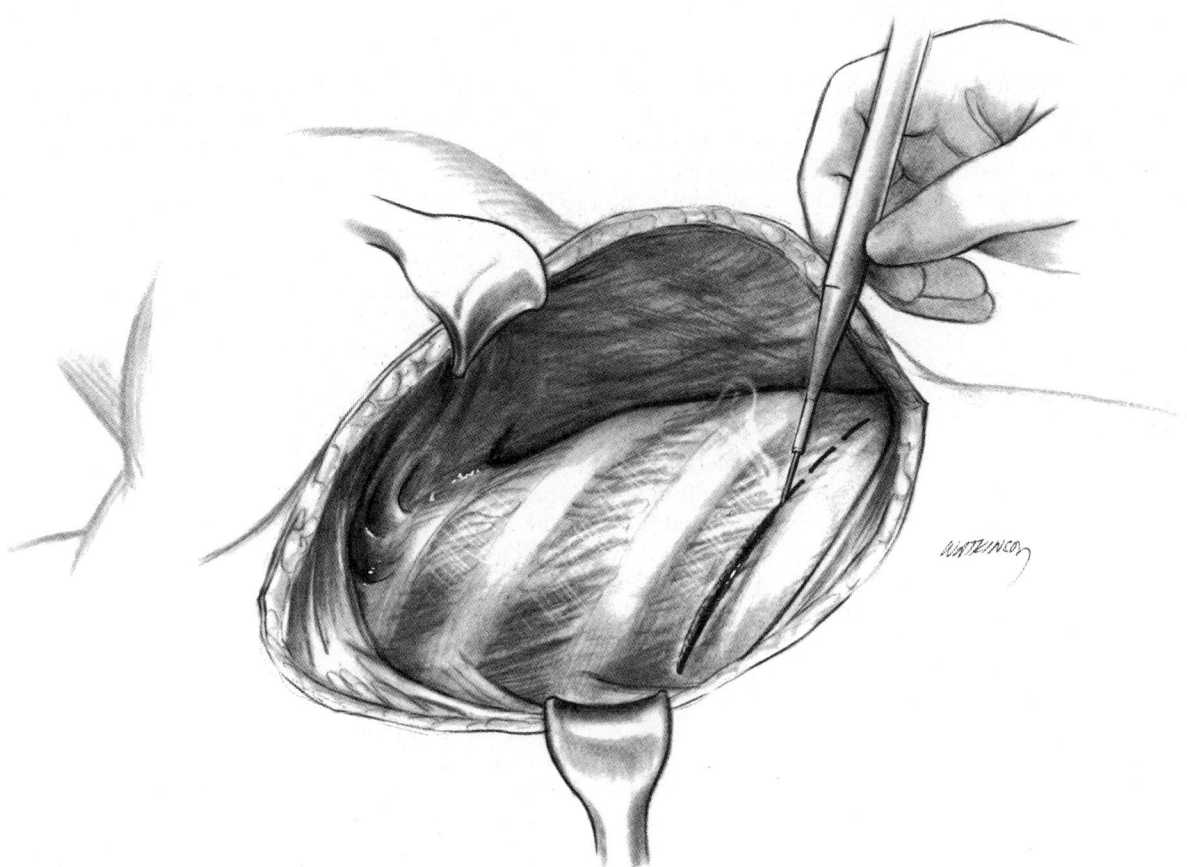

Figure 32-46. The interspace selected for initial exploration is opened. (From Cooper JD, Urschel HC Jr: Superior pulmonary sulcus carcinoma resection: posterior approach. In Atlas of Thoracic Surgery. p. 181. Churchill Livingstone, New York, 1995, with permission.)

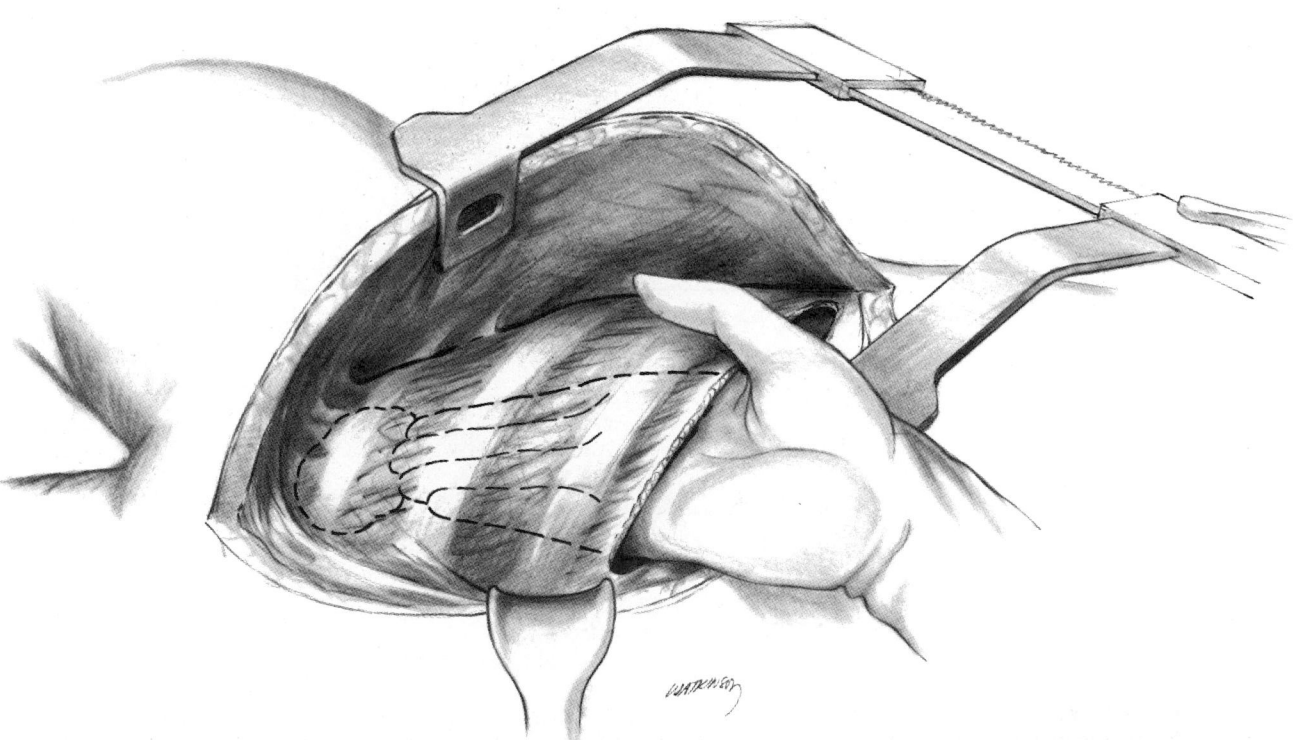

Figure 32-47. Palpation of the tumor assesses resectability. (From Cooper JD, Urschel HC Jr: Superior pulmonary sulcus carcinoma resection: posterior approach. In Atlas of Thoracic Surgery. p. 183. Churchill Livingstone, New York, 1995, with permission.)

accompanying descending scapular artery; the nerve and artery run down the medial border of the scapula. The division of the rhomboids allows the medial border of the scapula to be elevated from the chest wall, allowing access to the thoracic inlet and thus allowing en bloc chest wall resection before pulmonary resection.

En Bloc Chest Wall Resection

A rib-spreading retractor is placed in position to allow gentle elevation of the scapula with the lower blade outside the thoracotomy incision on the chest wall and the upper blade under the inferior angle of the scapula. Loose areolar tissue between the dense fascial covering of the subscapularis muscle and the chest wall is divided by a combination of sharp and blunt dissection to allow access to the first rib and the thoracic inlet. The chest wall excision is now outlined. An incision is made along the anterior border of the erector spinae muscle from the fifth to the first thoracic vertebra. The muscle is sharply dissected away from the angles of the ribs and the transverse processes in order to expose these bony structures for division later on. Hemostasis, deep to the dissected muscle mass, is obtained with temporary packing. The tumor is palpated from inside the chest, and the number of ribs requiring resection and the anterior margin of resection of the ribs and the intervening intercostal muscles are determined and marked on the outer surface of the chest wall by use of electrocautery. This margin should be at least 5 cm anterior to the growth and include one uninvolved rib inferiorly.

Attention is now directed to the thoracic inlet, and its important anatomic relationships are carefully examined in order to avoid inadvertent injury to the subclavian artery and vein and the brachial plexus during dissection around the first rib. The scalenus anterior and medius muscles are carefully divided with scissors, either at their insertion point on the first rib or higher if indicated by the extent of the tumor. The scalenus posterior muscle, which inserts into the second rib, is divided where it crosses the outer border of the first rib. The superior margin of the first rib is freed where there is no tumor attachment while the subclavian artery and vein and the brachial plexus are protected with the operator's index finger.

The division of the ribs is started anteriorly, along the previously outlined wide margin of resection, beginning with the normal rib immediately below the tumor (Fig. 32-48). Electrocautery is used to score the periosteum over a 1-cm width of all the ribs to be divided, except the first rib. By use of rib shears a short segment of each rib is removed in succession and labeled with adjacent soft tissue as the anterior margin of resection. The intervening intercostal muscles and their neurovascular bundles are suture-ligated and divided. Traction on the specimen side of the chest wall with a sharp towel clip helps to expose the anterior end of the first rib for transection. The lower trunk of the brachial plexus and its nerve roots from the eighth cervical and first thoracic nerves are now more clearly visible, as well as the relationship of the apical lung tumor to these structures.

The intercostal space below the lowest rib to be resected is entered and opened posteriorly to the angle of the rib. The

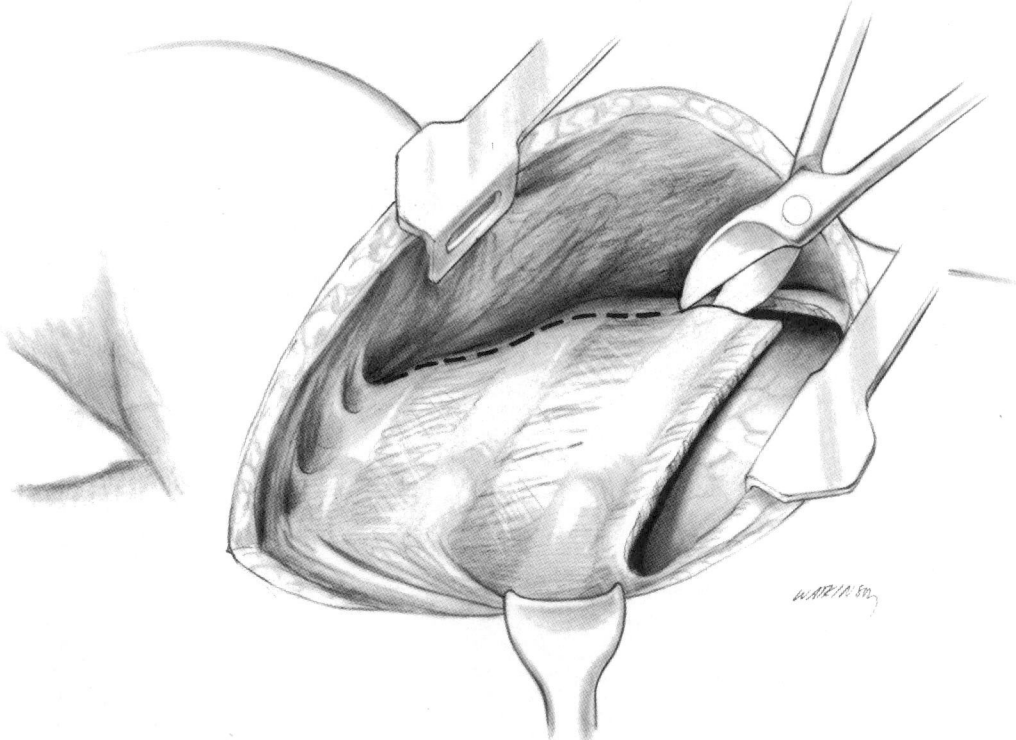

Figure 32-48. The resection of the en bloc specimen begins anteriorly by dividing the anterior margin of the rib, well away from the tumor. (From Cooper JD, Urschel HC Jr: Superior pulmonary sulcus carcinoma resection: posterior approach. In Atlas of Thoracic Surgery. p. 183. Churchill Livingstone, New York, 1995, with permission.)

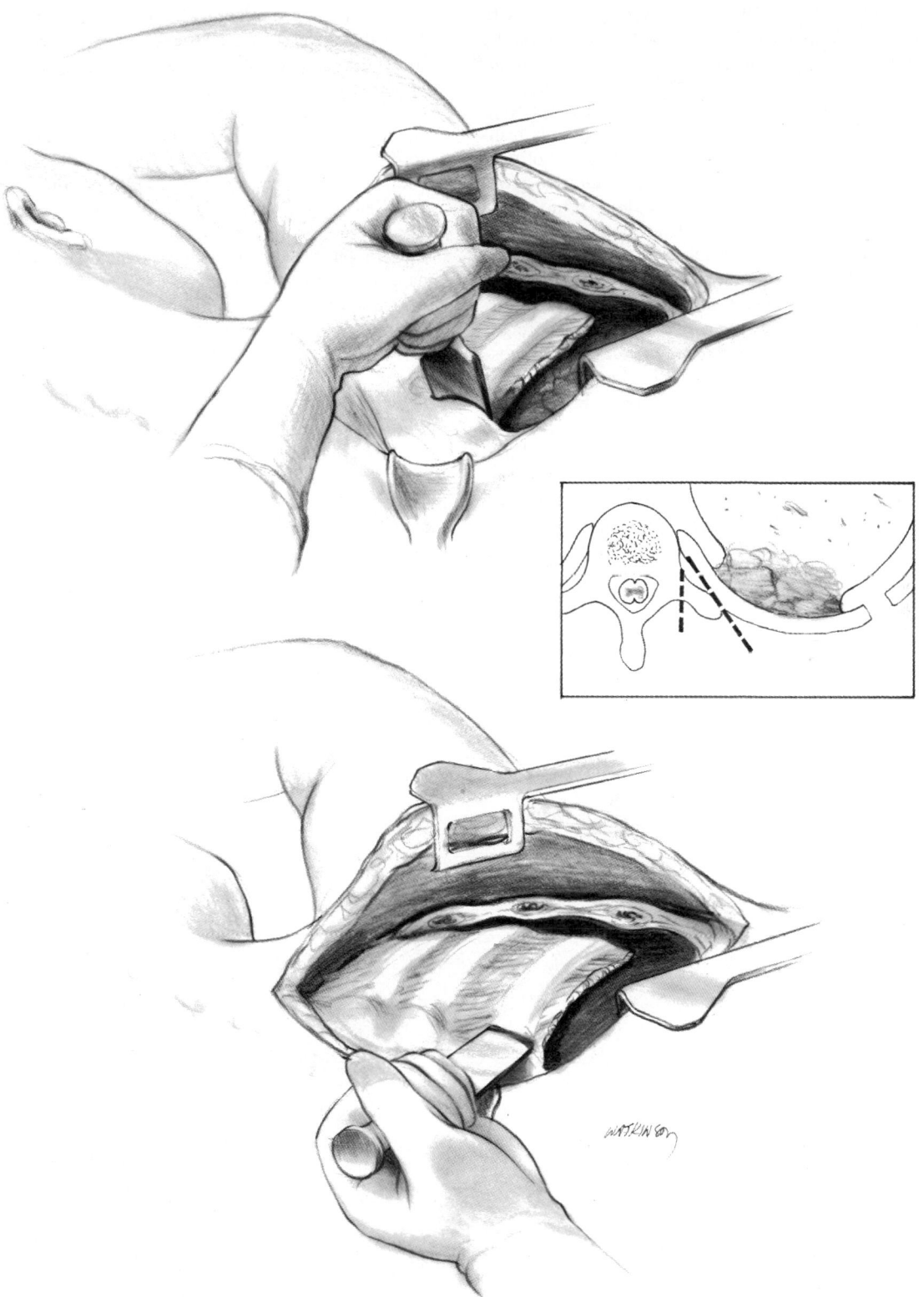

Figure 32-49. The rib is resected with or without the transverse process (see text).

chest wall resection is continued posteriorly, starting with the lowermost rib already divided anteriorly and proceeding upward. The erector spinae muscle is retracted to allow access to the transverse processes and the angles of the corresponding ribs. The rib is elevated with a sharp towel clip to improve the exposure, and the transverse process is transected flush with the lamina by use of a curved osteotome, which is held at right angles to the vertebral column to avoid entering the spinal canal (Fig. 32-49). If there is no rib or vertebral invasion, the rib may be disarticulated from the transverse process without transsecting the latter structure, preserving spinal stability. The head of the rib is disarticulated at the costovertebral joint with a periosteal elevator. The intervening intercostal nerve is divided after securing it with a hemoclip at the interverbral foramen, and the intercostal vessels are suture-ligated and divided. The posterior line of resection is continued upwards until finally the posterior end of the first rib is reached.

At this point the roots of the eighth cervical nerve above and the first thoracic nerve below the neck of the first rib, which join to form the lower trunk of the brachial plexus, are clearly seen, as is the extent of their involvement by tumor invasion (Fig. 32-50). The head of the first rib is disarticulated from the costovertebral joint after transecting the transverse process. The first thoracic nerve root is divided at the intervertebral foramen for completeness of tumor resection if

invaded by the tumor, in which case the tumor is shaved off from the lower trunk of the brachial plexus while keeping intact the eighth cervical nerve component (Fig. 32-51). Occasionally, the eighth cervical nerve root may also need to be divided because of invasion by the tumor, and in this case the lower trunk of the brachial plexus is also divided distal to the point of invasion. It is important to secure the nerve roots with hemoclips before dividing at the foramen to prevent leakage of cerebrospinal fluid (CSF); if this happens, the foramen should be lightly packed with a piece of free muscle and the erector spinae muscle sutured to the lateral aspect of vertebral bodies for tamponade of the leak. The dissection is continued into the root of the neck, where the tumor is gradually separated from the subclavian artery through the adventitial plane; rarely, the arterial wall is invaded, in which case resection and reconstruction will be necessary after obtaining proximal and distal control.

Posteriorly, the relationship of the tumor mass to the upper thoracic vertebral bodies is assessed. Depending on the degree of tumor attachment and the frozen section analysis of the periosteum, the tumor resection may require removal of a portion of the involved vertebral bodies; up to one-quarter of the body may be removed without affecting stability. The sympathetic chain is secured with hemoclips and divided both below and above the tumor mass, taking portion of the stellate ganglion (Fig. 32-52).

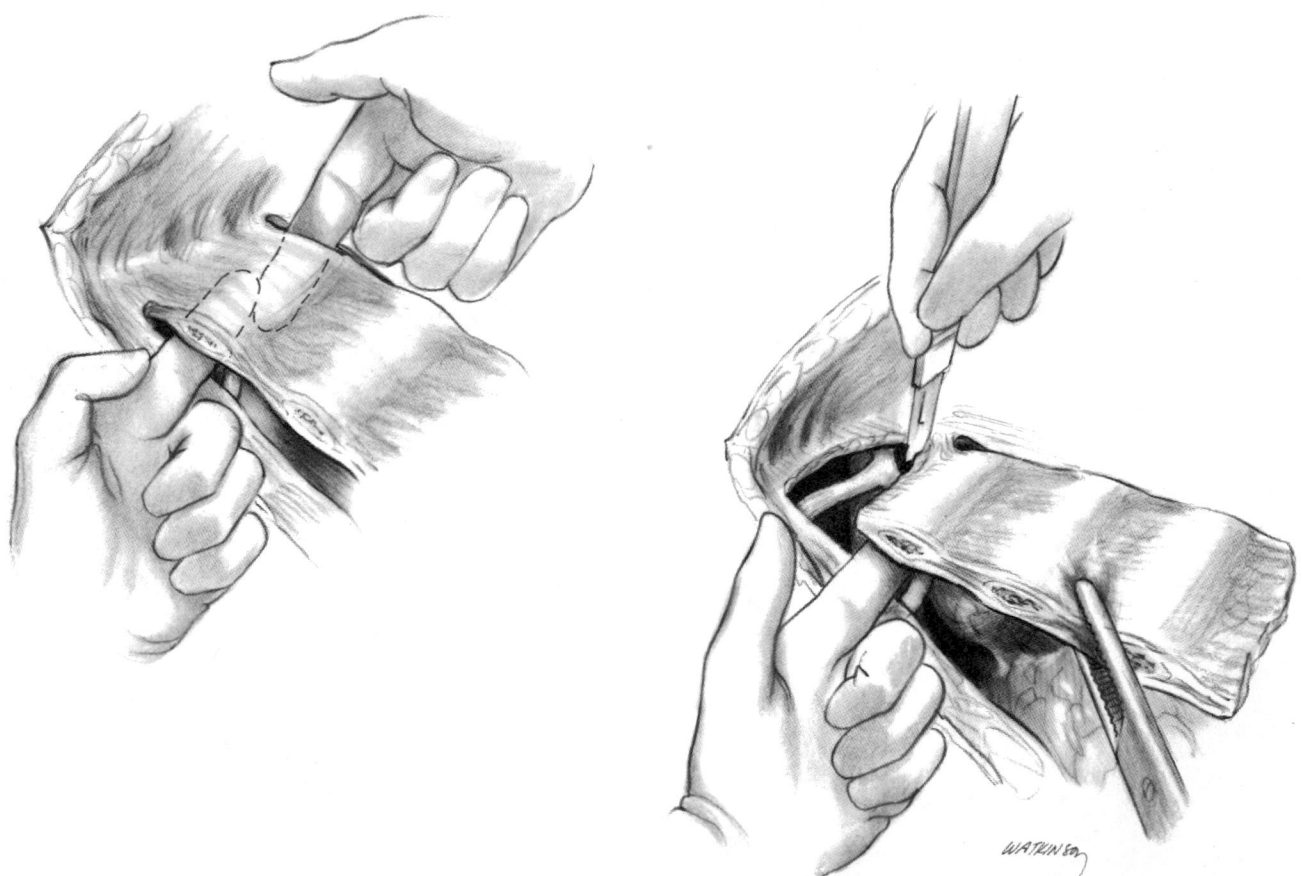

Figure 32-50. Removing the superior aspect of the first rib from the subjacent brachial plexus. (From Cooper JD, Urschel HC Jr: Superior pulmonary sulcus carcinoma resection: posterior approach. In Atlas of Thoracic Surgery. p. 185. Churchill Livingstone, New York, 1995, with permission.)

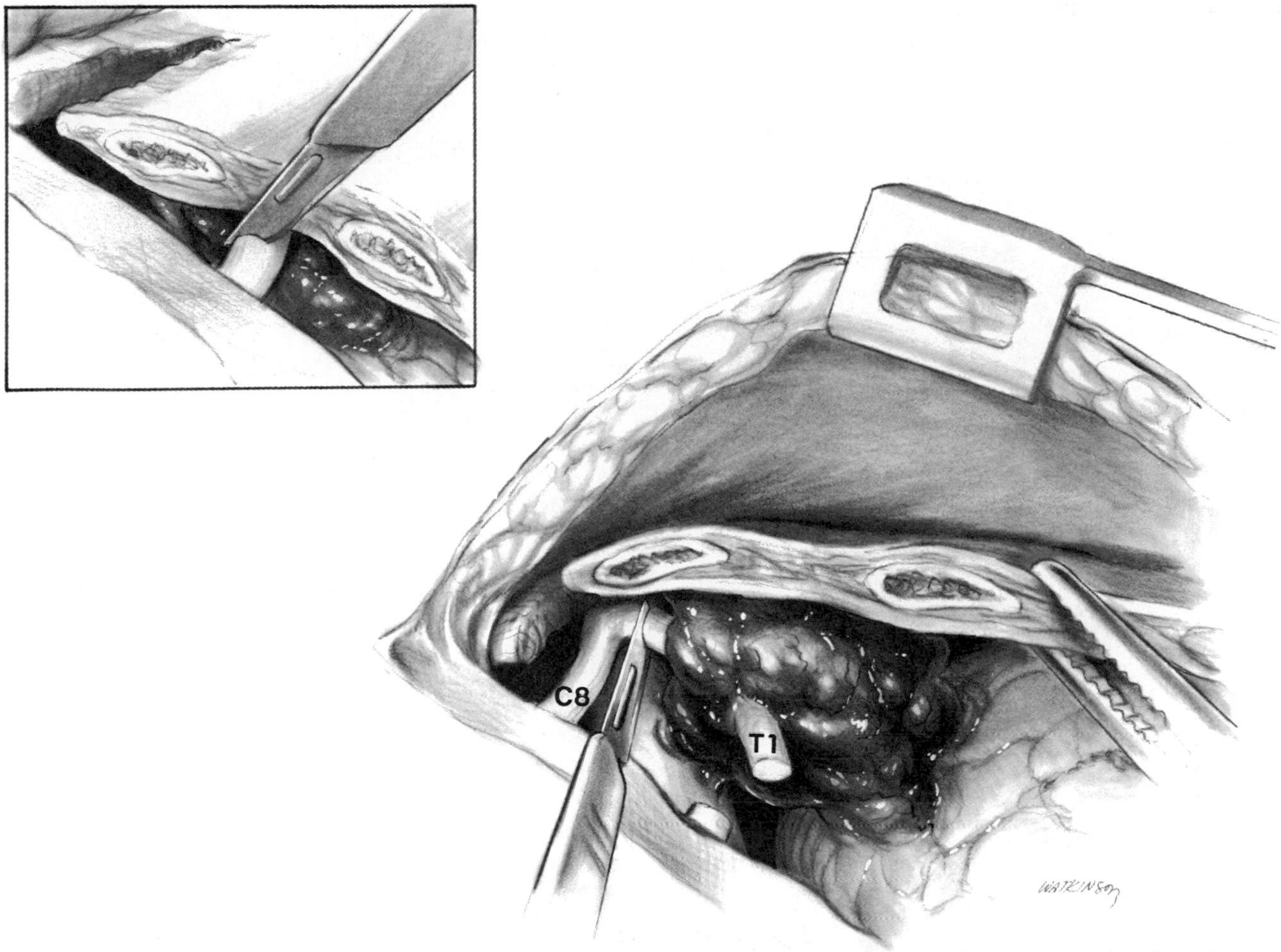

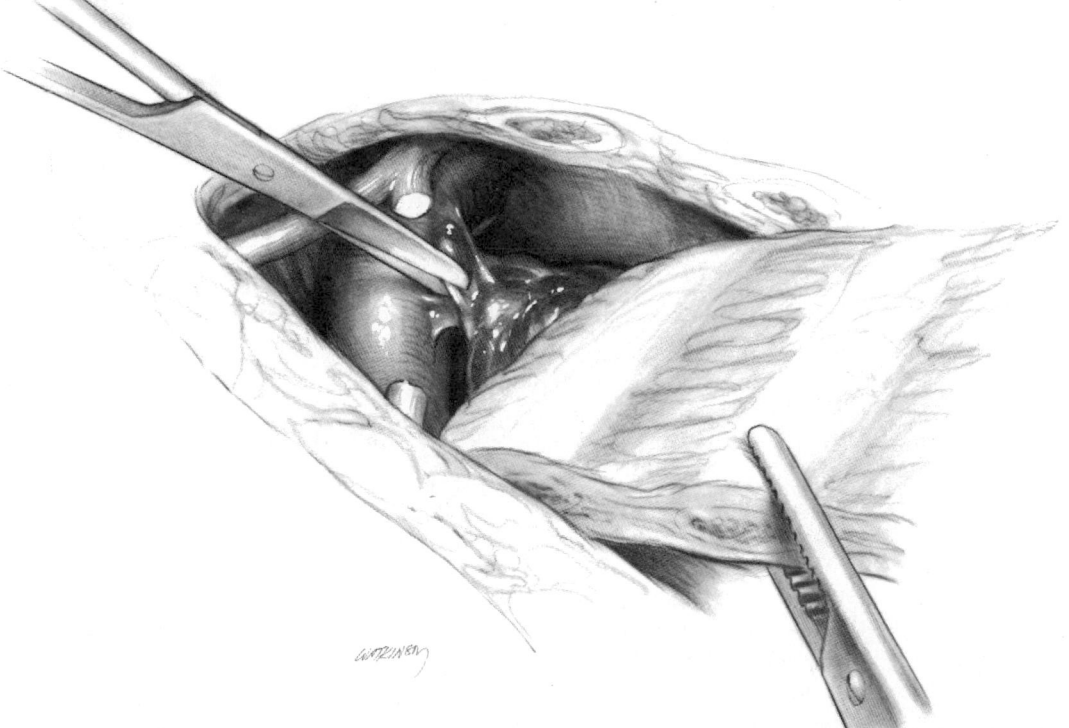

Figure 32-51. The T1 nerve root has been divided at the end of the vertebral foramen (inset) and is now being divided at a juncture with the C8 nerve root. (Figs. 32-51 and 32-52 from Cooper JD, Urschel HC Jr: Superior pulmonary sulcus carcinoma resection: posterior approach. In Atlas of Thoracic Surgery. p. 187. Churchill Livingstone, New York, 1995, with permission.)

Figure 32-52. The inferior half of the stellate ganglion is being dissected from the subclavian artery.

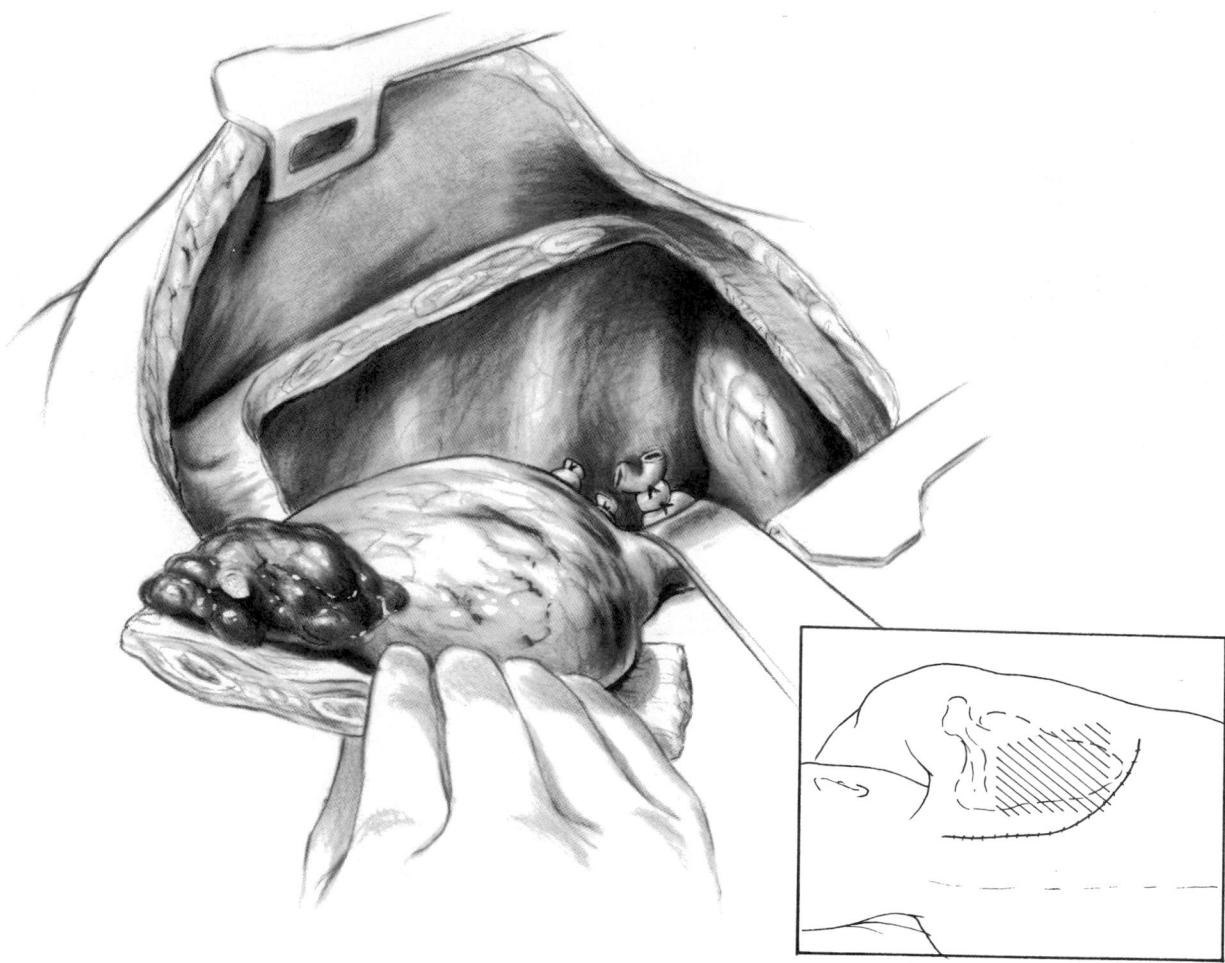

Figure 32-53. Following lobectomy, the en bloc specimen is being removed. (From Cooper JD, Urschel HC Jr: Superior pulmonary sulcus carcinoma resection: posterior approach. In Atlas of Thoracic Surgery. p. 189. Churchill Livingstone, New York, 1995, with permission.)

Once the chest wall resection is complete, the involved segment of the chest wall, still attached to the apical lung tumor, is allowed to drop into the chest cavity, and pulmonary resection is performed.

Pulmonary Resection

In most cases a dissection upper lobectomy is carried out with individual ligation of the blood vessels and the bronchus (Fig. 32-53). The superior mediastinal lymph nodes are resected en bloc through a vertical incision in the superior mediastinum. The posterior subcarinal, lobar, interlobar, and hilar lymph nodes are sampled separately for completeness of the intraoperative staging.

Chest Reconstruction

The erector spinae muscle mass is sutured to the lateral aspect of the vertebral bodies with interrupted sutures of 0 Vicryl. This provides good hemostasis and tamponades CSF leak

from the intervertebral foramina. When necessary, the chest wall defect is now reconstructed using a Marlex 2-mm Gore-Tex patch. The patch is tailored to the size of the defect and is secured and stabilized in place, under tension for a taut cover, with 2/0 Prolene sutures. The sutures are placed through the patch along all the margins of the defect except the superior margin, which is left free to allow free mobility of the plexus, artery, and vein. A continuous running suture along the three margins fixes the patch under tension. We only reconstruct larger defects, usually greater than three resected ribs.

Closure of the Thoractomy Incision

The chest is drained with two intercostal chest tubes inserted through separate stab incisions. The remaining lung is reinflated, with care taken to avoid torsion. Closure of the chest is then begun with using pericostal sutures of 1 Vicryl. The individual muscle layers are reapproximated. The subcutaneous tissue is closed, and the skin is closed with a subcuticular suture.

Cervical Approach to Apical Lesions

Philippe Dartevelle
Paolo Macchiarini

HISTORICAL NOTE

Because of their location within the narrow confines of the thoracic inlet, apical lung carcinomas are likely to involve, by direct extension, the structures of this target area. There are two distinct categories of apical tumors, those described by Pancoast (1932) as superior sulcus tumors and the more common extensive lesions presenting as apical chest tumors or tumors of the upper thorax, which in their advanced stage might invade the inlet structures (Paulson, 1973).

Superior sulcus tumors frequently are small neoplasms, situated at a definite location of the thoracic inlet (Pancoast, 1932), that evoke a characteristic clinical picture called the Pancoast syndrome (Teixeira, 1983; Tobias, 1931). Local nerve and bone involvement produces this syndrome at an early stage of the disease, often before the mass is well defined radiographically (Pancoast, 1932) and lymphatic and distant metastasis occur (Shahian, et al., 1987). For many years these tumors were considered inoperable, and therapy consisted of palliative radiation. However, during recent decades, it became evident that their best management consists of preoperative radiation therapy (30 Gy) followed by surgical resection (Pancoast, 1932; Shaw, et al., 1961; Paulson, 1989; Miller, et al., 1979; Attar, et al., 1979; Standford, et al., 1979; Devine, et al., 1986; Paulson, 1975). As reported by Shaw, et al. (1961), the operation consisted of an extended en bloc resection of the chest wall (usually including posterior portions of the first three ribs and their transverse processes), the intercostal nerves, and the lower trunk of the brachial plexus, together with the involved lung (resected usually by lobectomy or segmental resection), performed through a posterior interscapulovertebral approach. This combined modality usually results in long-term survivals (5-year rates of approximately 30 to 34 percent) and cure for selected patients (Attar, et al., 1979; Devine, et al., 1986; Miller, et al., 1979; Paulson, 1975, 1989; Shaw, et al., 1961; Standford, et al., 1979). Positive mediastinal lymph nodes and extensive vertebral body, brachial plexus, and subclavian vascular invasion represent poor prognostic factors and thus contraindications for surgical resection (Anderson, et al., 1985; Paulson, 1973, 1975, 1989).

In defining the precise location of superior sulcus tumors, Pancoast (1932) found it necessary to discard the term *apical chest tumors,* which he had used in his original paper (Pancoast, 1924) "because it has proved to be confusing and has permitted the inclusion of other more common tumors of the upper part of the thorax." Thus, the more common apical tumors of the upper lobes, which in their natural history ultimately invade the thoracic inlet and present with the Pancoast syndrome and other signs and symptoms of pulmonary, mediastinal, and inlet involvement, are different lesions, of greater extent and stage of involvement than the superior sulcus tumors (Paulson, 1973). Because of their locally advanced stage and impressive tendency to invade the structures lying in the thoracic inlet (Dartevelle et al., 1993), the difficulty and hazards of achieving a complete resection of the tumor-bearing inlet area (Macchiarini et al., 1993), and the surgery-related morbidity and mortality (Paulson, 1973, 1975; Wright et al., 1987), these apical tumors have represented so far an unresectable and an extremely dismal disease, the standard therapy for which has been palliation or best supportive care (Mountain, 1988).

The main problem in dealing with apical chest tumors is whether or not they invade the thoracic inlet. For those that do, a complete oncologic and safe surgical clearance of the entire tumor-bearing area is not achievable by the conventional approaches. We describe an anterior transcervical-thoracic technique, which allows radical resection of apical lung carcinomas invading the thoracic inlet and the structures lying above this area regardless of tumor location.

HISTORICAL READINGS

Anderson TM, Moy PM, Holmes EC: Factors affecting survival in superior sulcus tumors. J Clin Oncol 4:1598, 1985

Attar S, Miller JE, Satterfield J et al: Pancoast's tumor: irradiation or surgery? Ann Thorac Surg 28:578, 1979

Dartevelle P, Chapelier A, Macchiarini P et al: Anterior transcervical-thoracical approach for radical resection of lung tumors invading the thoracic inlet. J Thorac Cardiovasc Surg 105:1025, 1993

Devine JW, Mendenhall WM, Million RR, Carmichael MJ: Carcinoma of the superior pulmonary sulcus treated with surgery and/or radiation therapy. Cancer 57:941, 1986

Macchiarini P, Dartevelle P, Chapelier A et al: Technique for resecting primary or metastatic non-bronchogenic tumors of the thoracic outlet. Ann Thorac Surg 55:611, 1993

Macchiarini P, Fontanini G, Hardin M et al: Relation of neovascularization to metastasis in non-small cell lung cancer. Lancet 340: 145, 1992

Mathisen DJ, Grillo HC: Lung Cancer: A Comprehensive Treatise. Grune & Stratton, Orlando, 1988

Miller JI, Mansour KA, Hatcher CR: Carcinoma of the superior pulmonary sulcus. Ann Thorac Surg 28:44, 1979

Mountain CF: Prognostic implications of the international staging system for lung cancer. Semin Oncol 15:236, 1988

Pancoast HK: Superior sulcus tumors. JAMA 99:1391, 1932

Pancoast HK: Importance of careful roentgen-ray investigations of apical chest tumors. JAMA 83:1407, 1924

Paulson DL: General Thoracic Surgery, Lea & Febiger, Philadelphia, 1989

Paulson DL: Carcinomas in the superior pulmonary sulcus. J Thorac Cardiovasc Surg 70:1095, 1975

Paulson DL: The importance of defining location and staging of superior pulmonary sulcus tumors. Ann Thorac Surg 15:549, 1973

Shahian DM, Wildford BN, Ellis FH Jr: Pancoast tumors: improved survival with preoperative and postoperative radiotherapy. Ann Thorac Surg 43:32, 1987

Shaw RR, Paulson DL, Kee JL Jr: Treatment of the superior sulcus tumor by irradiation followed by resection. Ann Surg 154:29, 1961

Standford W, Barnes RP, Tucker AR: Influence of staging in superior sulcus (Pancoast) tumors of the lung. Ann Thorac Surg 29:406, 1979

Teixeira JP: Concerning the Pancoast tumor: what is the superior pulmonary sulcus? Ann Thorac Surg 35:577, 1983

Tobias JW: Sindrome apico-costo-vertebral-doloroso por tumor apexiano: su valor diagnostico en el cancer primitivo del pulmon. Thesis, Imp. Mercatali, Buenos Aires, 1931

Wright CD, Moncure AC, Shepard JOA et al: Superior sulcus lung tumors. J Thorac Cardiovasc Surg 94:69, 1987

SURGICAL ANATOMY

The insertion of the anterior, middle, and posterior scalenus muscles on the first and second ribs, respectively, divides the thoracic inlet into three compartments (Fig. 32-54). The anterior (prescalenus) compartment contains the platysma and sternocleidomastoid muscles, the external and anterior jugular veins, the inferior belly of the omohyoid muscle, the subclavian and internal jugular veins and their major branches, and the scalene fat pad. The middle (interscalenus) compartment contains the anterior scalenus muscle with the phrenic nerve lying on its anterior aspect, the subclavian artery with its primary branches except the posterior scapular artery, the trunks of the brachial plexus, and the middle scalenus muscle. The posterior compartment (extrascalenus), lies posterior to the middle scalenus muscles and includes the long thoracic and external branch of the accessorius spinalis nerves, the posterior scapular artery, the sympathetic chain and stellate ganglion, vertebral bodies, and spinal foramen.

According to the level of involvement of the first rib, apical tumors might be classified as anterior (invading the anterior part of the first rib, the subclavian vessels, the anterior scalenus muscle, and the phrenic nerve), middle (invading the middle part of the first rib, the middle scalenus muscle, and the trunks of the brachial plexus), and posterior (invading the vertebral bodies, the posterior part of the first ribs, the lower roots of the brachial plexus, and the posterior wall and posterior branches of the subclavian artery).

DIAGNOSIS

Clinical Features

The clinical features of apical tumors depend predominantly on the location of their invasion at the level of the thoracic inlet. Posterior tumors usually present with all signs and symptoms of the Pancoast syndrome (Teixeira, 1983; Tobias, 1931). Apical tumors invading the middle compartment of the thoracic inlet may present with signs and symptoms related to the compression or infiltration of the trunks of the brachial plexus. Anterior apical tumors generally present with severe pain related to the bony destruction of the first rib, the ipsilateral superior vena cava hemisyndrome, and phrenic nerve palsy.

Staging

Any patient presenting with signs and symptoms suggesting involvement of the thoracic inlet should undergo a careful and detailed preoperative workup to establish a diagnosis of apical carcinoma of the lung and to determine operability. The Pancoast syndrome (Teixeira, 1983; Tobias, 1931) may result from malignancies other than apical tumors (e.g., thyroid or laryngeal tumors, mesothelioma, or Hodgkin disease [McGoon, 1964], primary or metastatic nonbronchogenic neoplasms [Macchiarini et al., 1993], and benign diseases [Camelotte et al., 1984]).

The diagnosis is established by history and physical examination, chest x-ray, bronchoscopy and sputum cytology, fine-needle transthoracic and aspiration biopsy, and computed tomography (CT) of the chest. We share the opinion of Paulson (1985) on the usefulness of a histologic proof by open biopsy; however, in rare circumstances a thoracoscopy might be indicated for obtaining histologic confirmation when the other investigations are negative. If there is evidence of mediastinal lymphadenopathy on chest x-ray or CT scanning, mediastinoscopy is mandatory since patients with clinical N2 disease are not suitable candidates for operation. Neurologic examination, electromyography, and radiography are performed to delineate tumor extension to the brachial plexus, phrenic nerve, and spinal canal, whereas vascular invasion is studied by venous angiography, subclavian arteriography, and Doppler ultrasound (cerebrovascular disorders might contraindicate the sacrifice of the vertebral artery) and by magnetic resonance imaging (MRI). The initial workup also includes all investigative procedures delineating extrathoracic metastases.

Indications and Contraindications

Any patient presenting with an apical lung carcinoma of non-small cell histology invading the thoracic inlet might be considered for the cervical approach. Absolute contraindications to this surgical technique are the presence of extrathoracic

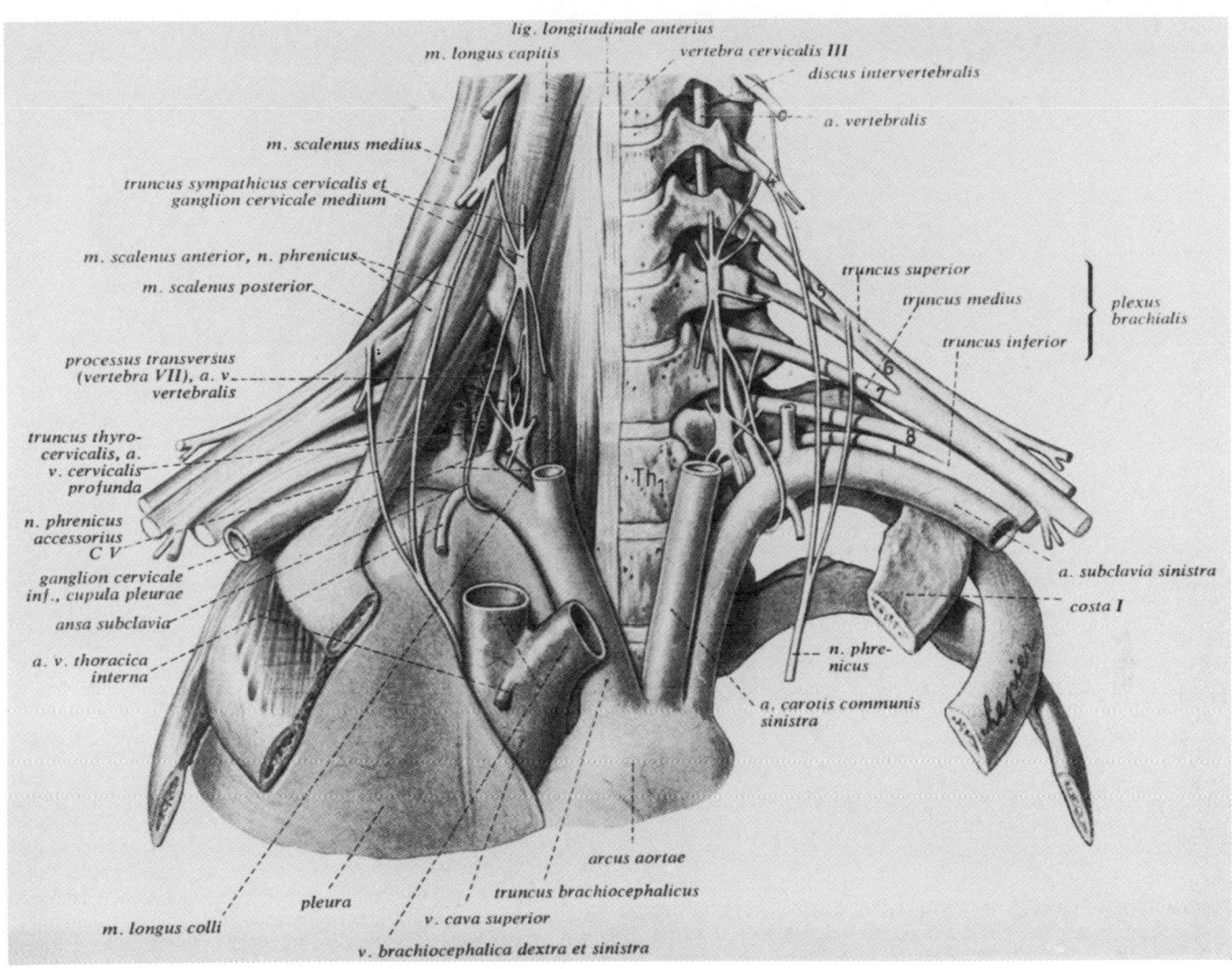

Figure 32-54. Illustrative view of the anatomy of the thoracic inlet. (From Sobotta-Becher: Atlas der Anatomie des Menschen, Urban & Schwarzenberg, Munich, 1973, with permission.)

sites of metastasis and clinical and histologically confirmed mediastinal lymph node involvement. Extensive involvement of the brachial plexus is a relative contraindication provided that a complete surgical resection may be anticipated. Patients whose tumors abut the vertebral body should not be deemed inoperable unless invasion of the cortex is confirmed.

MANAGEMENT

Operative Technique

One-lung anesthesia and measurements of central venous and arterial pressures and body temperature are necessary. A Foley catheter is inserted, and the patient is placed in the supine position with the neck hyperextended and the head turned away from the involved side. An L-shaped cervicotomy incision is made; the vertical and horizontal branches follow the anterior border of the sternocleidomastoid muscle and the inferior border of the internal half of the clavicle, respectively (Fig. 32-55). Division of the sternal attachment

of the sternocleidomastoid muscle allows adequate exposure of the superior border of the subclavian vessels. Once the inferior belly of the omohyoid muscle is transected, the scalene fat pad is dissected and pathologically examined to exclude scalene lymph node micrometastasis. The ipsilateral superior mediastinum is then inspected. The tumor's extension to the thoracic inlet is then carefully assessed, and if the tumor is deemed resectable, the internal half of the clavicle is removed.

The next operative procedures are carried out in three steps: (1) dissection of the subclavian veins; (2) dissection of the subclavian artery; and (3) exposure of the brachial plexus.

The jugular and subclavian veins are first dissected so that branches to the subclavian vein can eventually be divided. On the left side, ligation of the thoracic duct is required. Division of the distal part of the internal, external, and anterior jugular veins makes the approach of venous confluence at the origin of the innominate vein easier (Fig. 32-56). If the subclavian vein is involved, it can be easily resected after

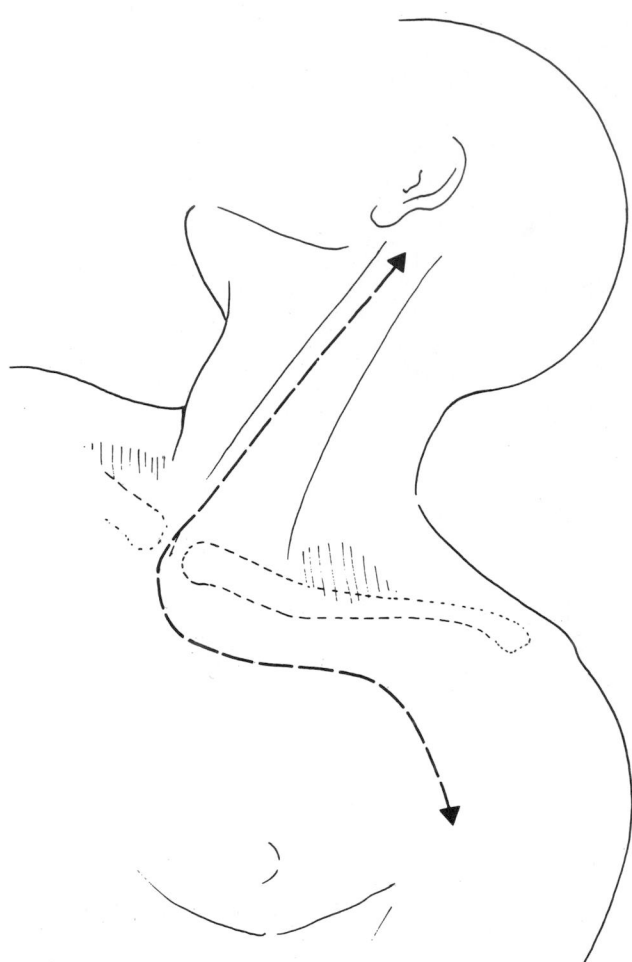

Figure 32-55. Left anterior transcervical incision. The patient is placed in the supine position with the neck hyperextended and the head turned away from the involved side. An L-shaped skin incision is made from the angle of the mandible down to the sternal notch, extended horizontally under the internal half of the clavicle, and eventually prolonged into the deltopectoral groove. (From Macchiarini P, Dartevelle P, Chapelier A et al: Technique for resecting primary or metastatic non-bronchogenic tumors of the thoracic outlet. Ann Thorac Surg 55:611, 1993, with permission.)

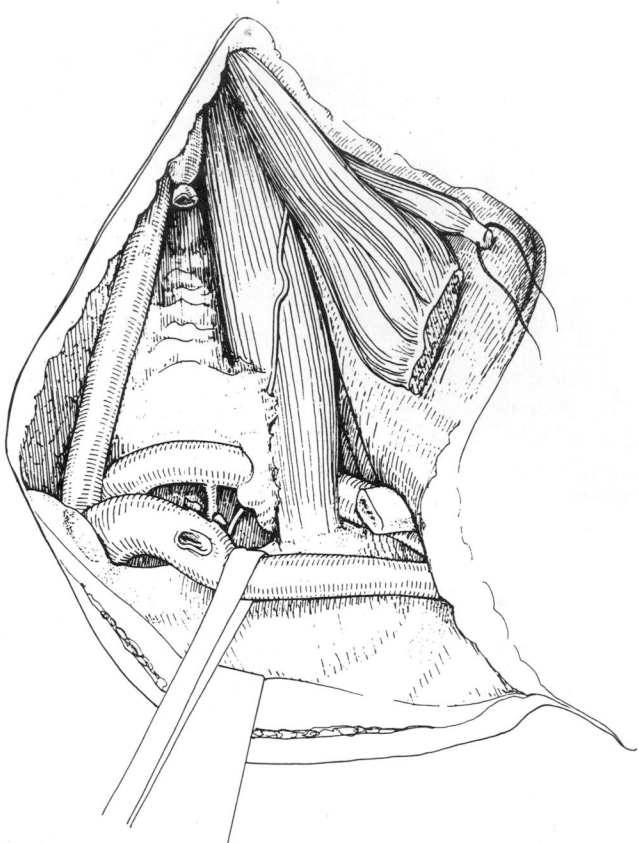

Figure 32-56. Illustrative view after having divided the sternal head of the sternocleidomastoid and the inferior belly of the omohyoid muscles and resected the scalene fat pad and the internal half of the clavicle. Thereafter, the exposure, dissection, and division of the external and internal jugular veins greatly facilitate exposure of the subclavian vein and permit assessment of tumor resectability. (From Dartevelle P, Chapelier A, Macchiarini P et al: Anterior transcervical approach for radical resection of lung tumors involving the thoracic inlet. J Thorac Cardiovasc Surg 105:1025, 1993, with permission.)

its proximal and distal control has been achieved. Direct extension of the tumor to the innominate vein does not preclude resection.

The subclavian artery is then dissected. Its distal part can be exposed after division of the anterior scalenus muscle over the first rib in tumor-free margins. The phrenic nerve must be clearly visualized and exposed on the anterior aspect of the scalenus muscle, and, depending on its involvement, it must be carefully protected or resected (Fig. 32-57). The eventual division of branches of the subclavian artery, if invaded by tumor, is simplified after proximal control of its origin has been achieved. The internal mammary artery and the ascending cervical artery are often divided, and the vertebral artery, when involved, can also be resected (Fig. 32-57). When the tumor rests against the wall of the subclavian artery, the artery can be freed by following a subadventitial

plane. Whenever the arterial wall is involved by tumor, resection of the artery in order to obtain tumor-free margins is necessary (Fig. 32-57); we strongly recommend dividing all branches (except the vertebral artery) of the subclavian artery, since this further exposes the subclavian artery. Revascularization is performed at the end of the cervical procedure, either with a polytetrafluoroethylene (PTFE) graft (no. 6 or 8 mm) or by end-to-end anastomosis. In middle-type tumors, the middle scalenus muscle can be extensively invaded, which requires its high division to obtain tumor-free margins.

Extension or compression of the brachial nerves by tumor requires an "outside-in" dissection. Secondary branches and then primary branches of the brachial plexus are freed. The lower trunk and C8 and T1 nerve roots can be dissected up to the spinal foramen. Although tumor spread to the brachial plexus may be high, neurolysis is usually achieved without the need for division of branches of the brachial plexus above T1 (Fig. 32-58). Thereafter, exposure of the vertebral bodies, dorsal sympathetic chain, and stellate ganglion (Fig. 32-59) is easily obtained, and tumor spread to these structures can be resected with tumor-free margins. Damage to the lateral and long thoracic nerves should be avoided, since this might result in winged scapula.

Once the first and second ribs are freed of all attachments from the transverse process of the vertebrae posteriorly to the costocartilage anteriorly, they are easily resected, either through the same cervical approach or by prolonging the horizontal incision into the deltopectoral groove. The resection of the first two ribs (Fig. 32-60) allows en bloc excision of the tumor and involved underlying parenchyma by either wedge resection (performed with a TA-55 or TA-90 stapler) (Fig. 32-61) or upper lobectomy (Fig. 32-62).

Meticulous hemostasis throughout the procedure will ensure clear visual exposure at all times. Careful inspection and verification of all vascular structures previously resected or ligated prevents postoperative hemorrhage and lymphatic leakage. If the entire tumor-bearing area is resected by the anterior approach alone, the cervical incision is closed in two layers after the sternal insertion of the sternocleidomastoid muscle is sutured and a conventional drainage of the ipsilateral chest cavity is placed. In posterior apical tumors involving the third rib, a complementary posterior thoracotomy as described by Shaw, et al., (1961) may be performed as a one-stage procedure.

Early and Late Results

Between January 1980 and July 1992, 31 patients of median age 58 years (range, 36 to 73) presented with apical tumors invading the thoracic inlet and were treated by the technique described above (Table 32-1). None of them received preoperative radiation therapy. All underwent a radical resection. There were no perioperative deaths. Postoperative complications paralleled those observed after major en bloc chest wall resections, particularly in those patients in whom the phrenic nerve was resected.

En bloc removal of the inlet tumor, first two ribs, and underlying lung was performed through the anterior transcervical approach alone in nine patients. An additional posterior thoracotomy was necessary in the remaining patients because of a chest wall involvement below the second rib. The operations performed in the 31 patients included 14 wedge resections, 16 lobectomies, and 1 pneumonectomy; the pneumonectomy was necessary because of metastatic lymph nodes in the aortopulmonary window and involvement of the intrathoracic vagus and phrenic nerves. All the remaining patients had normal mediastinal lymph nodes at pathologic examination. In 17 patients (55 percent), the inferior root (T1) of the brachial plexus was involved by the tumor and resected;

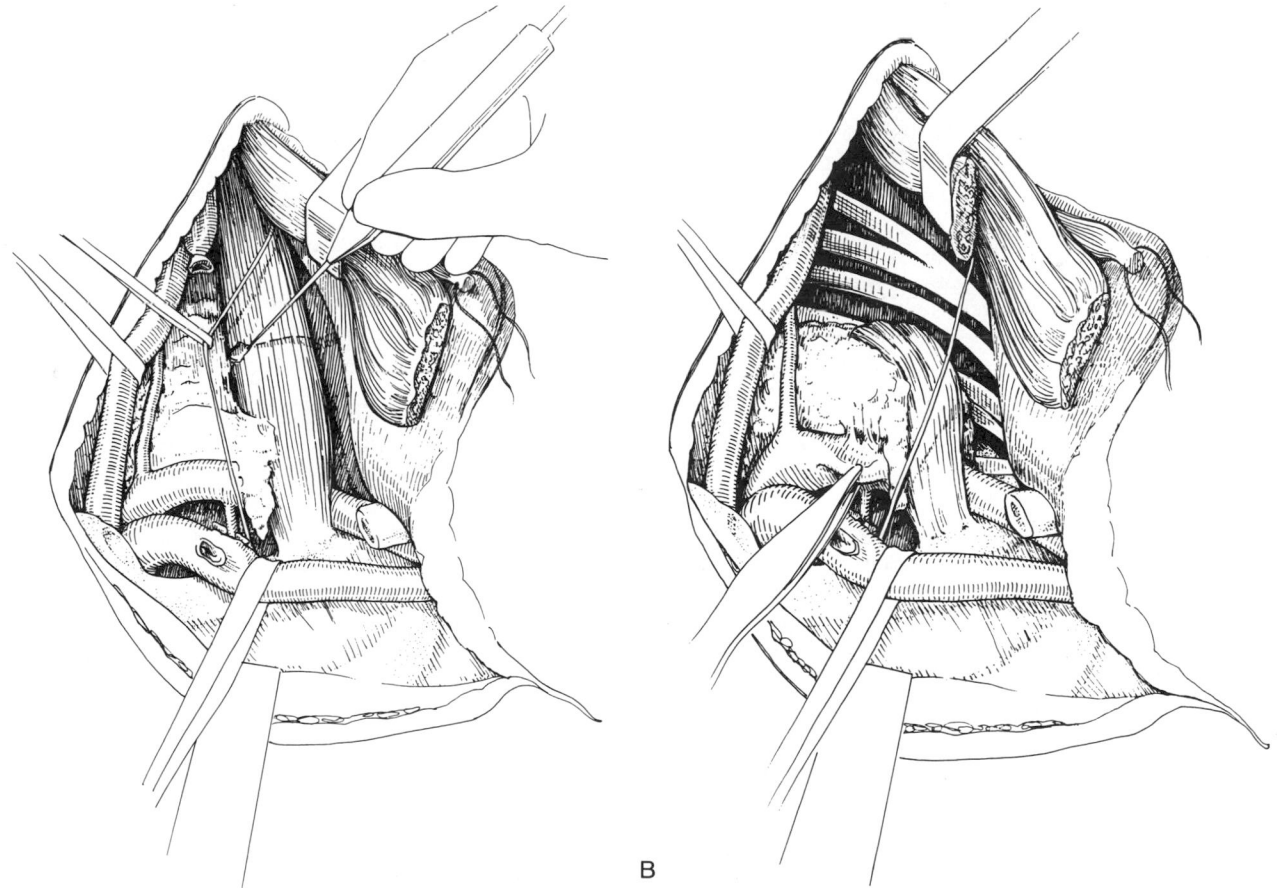

A   B

Figure 32-57. (**A**) The subclavian artery is exposed after division of the insertion of the anterior scalenus muscle on the first rib; the phrenic nerve is protected and preserved. (**B**) Retraction of the anterior scalenus muscles allows identification of the interscalene trunks of the brachial plexus; the subclavian artery might be gently freed from the tumor by dividing all collateral branches (the vertebral artery is generally preserved if not invaded). (*Figure continues.*)

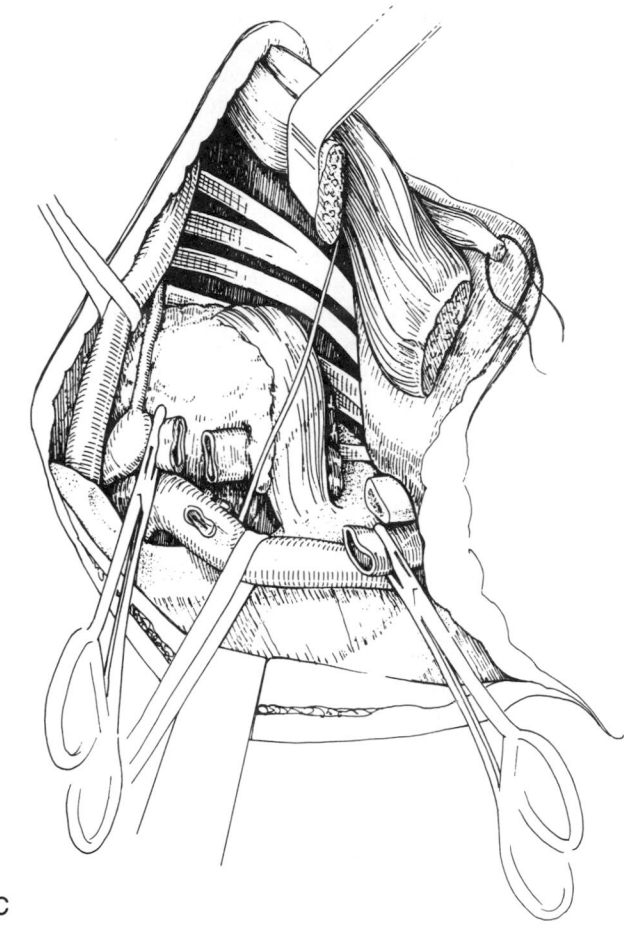

C

Figure 32-57 (*Continued*). (**C**) If involved by the tumor, the sub-clavian artery might be divided after its proximal and distal control have been achieved. (From Dartevelle P, Chapelier A, Macchiarini P et al: Anterior transcervical approach for radical resection of lung tumors invading the thoracic inlet. J Thorac Cardiovasc Surg 105:1025, 1993, with permission.)

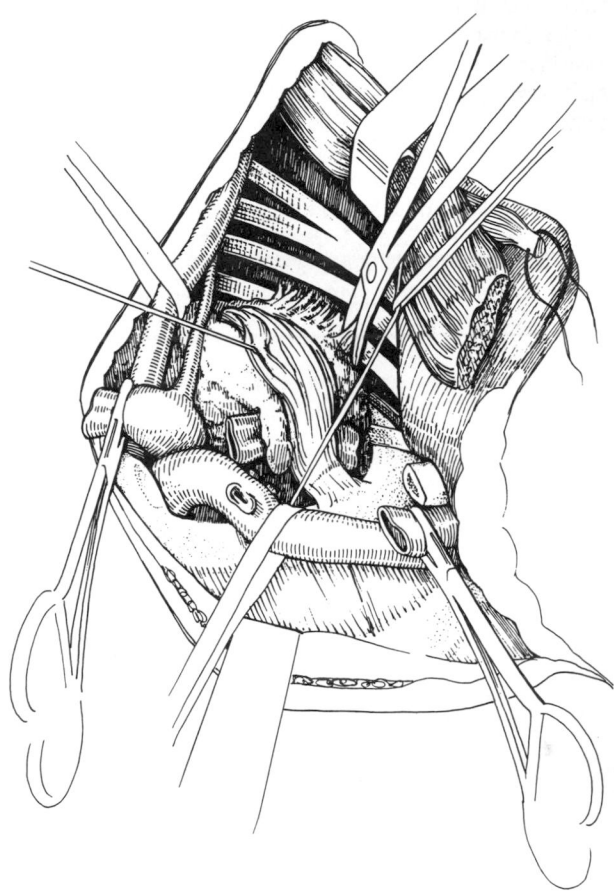

Figure 32-58. Tumor involvement of the brachial plexus requires an inside-out neurolysis if the upper trunks are involved or a resection of T1 if the lower trunk or nerve roots are involved. (From Dartevelle P, Chapelier A, Macchiarini P et al: Anterior transcervical approach for radical resection of lung tumors invading the thoracic inlet. J Thorac Cardiovasc Surg 105:1025, 1993, with permission.)

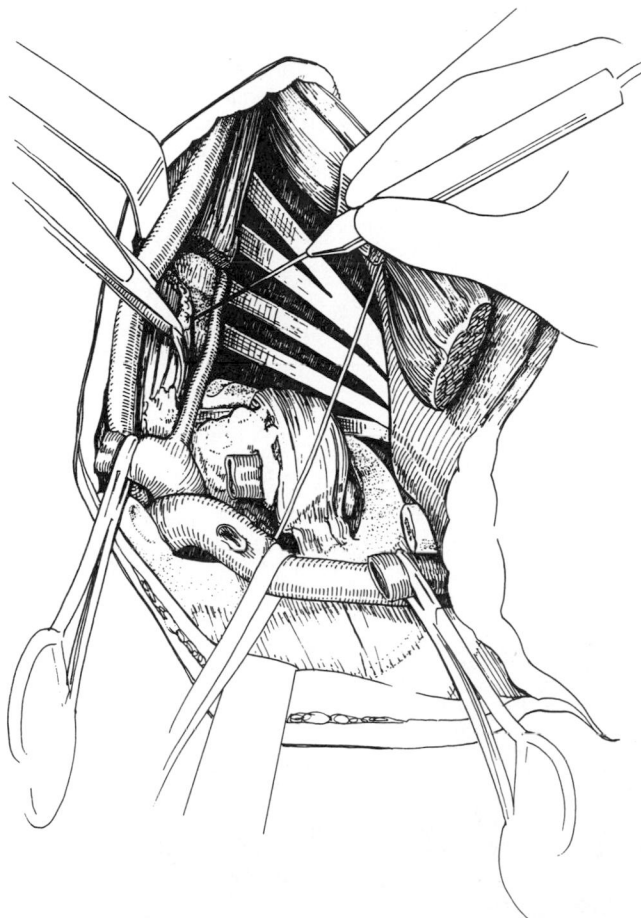

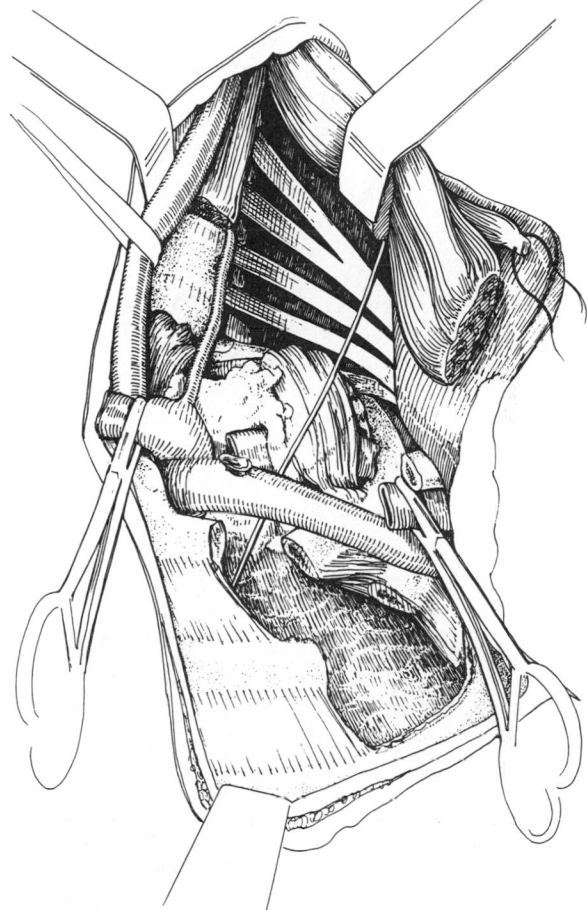

Figure 32-59. The prevertebral muscles are detached from the vertebral bodies and both the stellate ganglion and dorsal sympathetic chain are isolated and finally released from all surrounding attachments by use of raspatories. (From Dartevelle P, Chapelier A, Macchiarini P et al: Anterior transcervical approach for radical resection of lung tumors invading the thoracic outlet. J Thorac Cardiovasc Surg 105:1025, 1993, with permission.)

Figure 32-60. Once structures above the thoracic inlet are freed from the tumor, the first two ribs might be separated anteriorly at the chondrocostal junction and resected posteriorly in tumor-free margins. Prolonging the incision into the deltopectoral groove facilitates this maneuver. (From Dartevelle P, Chapelier A, Macchiarini P et al: Anterior transcervical approach for radical resection of lung tumors involving the thoracic outlet. J Thorac Cardiovasc Surg 105:1025, 1993, with permission.)

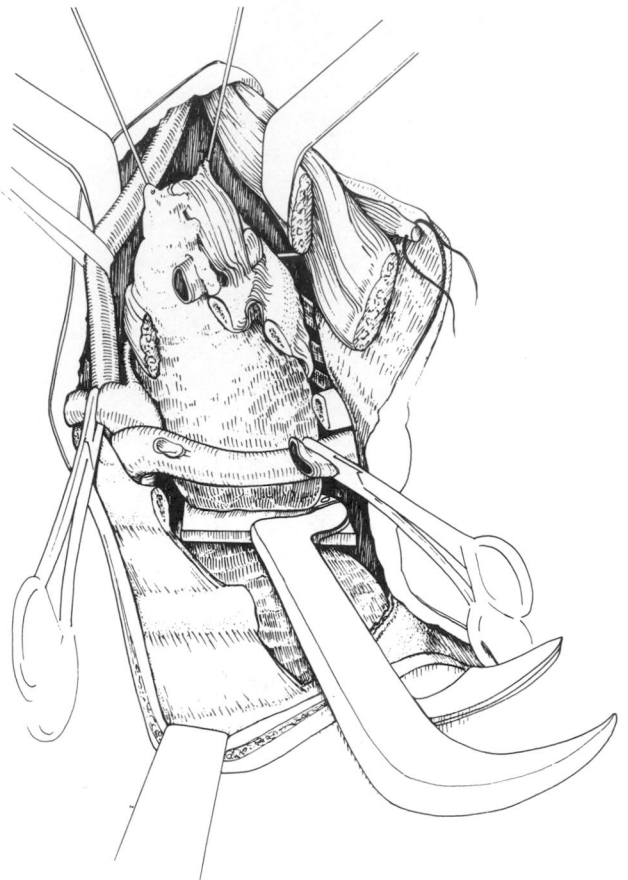

Figure 32-61. The thoracic inlet extension of the apical tumor, involved first two ribs, subclavian artery, and underlying lung parenchyma are resected with a stapler instrument (wedge resection). (From Dartevelle P, Chapelier A, Macchiarini P et al: Anterior transcervical approach for radical resection of lung tumors invading the thoracic outlet. J Thorac Cardiovasc Surg 105:1025, 1993, with permission.)

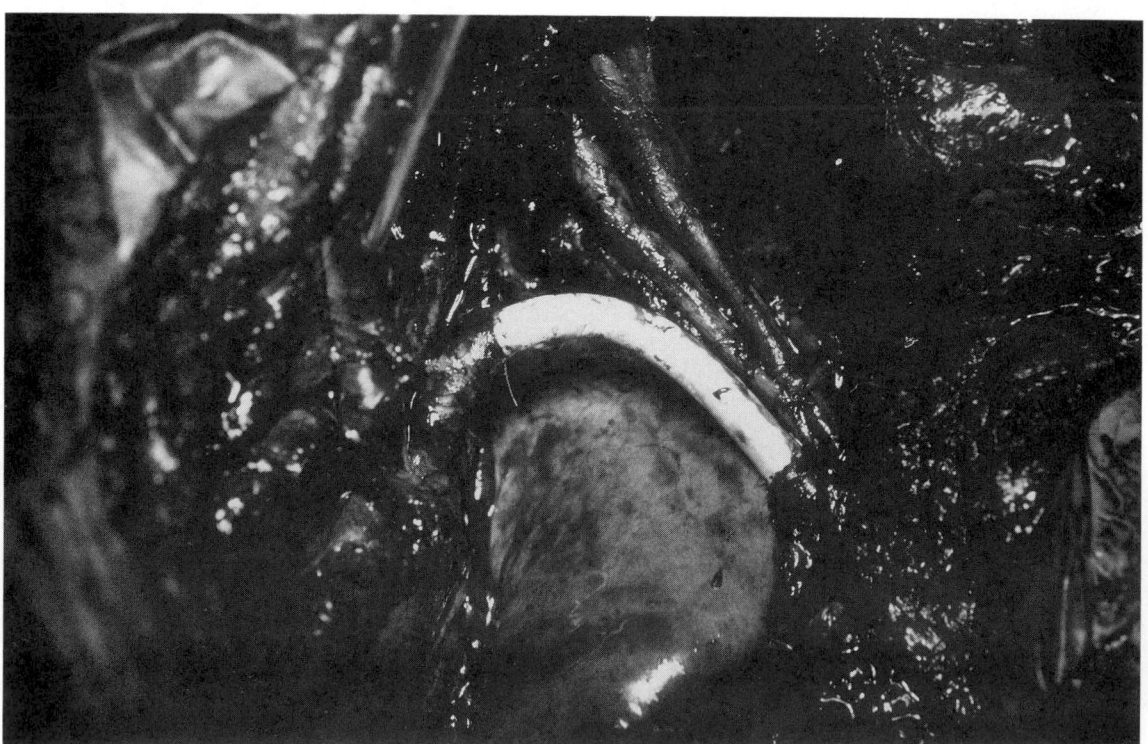

Figure 32-62. Operative view after transcervical approach for a left-sided apical tumor involving the thoracic inlet. As shown, the subclavian vein was resected, the subclavian artery revascularized with a 6-mm PTFE graft (the vertebral artery was preserved), the trunks of the brachial plexus were freed from the tumor, the first two ribs were resected, and the apical lung carcinoma was removed by an upper lobectomy.

Table 32-1. Tumor Characteristics of 31 Apical Non-Small Cell Lung Cancers Involving the Thoracic Inlet

Tumor Characteristics	Values
Site: right/left	20/11
Inlet location: anterior/middle/posterior	8/22/1
Histology: squamous/adenocarcinoma/mixed	11/17/3
Histologic grading (1 to 3 scale, median)	2
Tumor size (cm, median)	5.5

among these 17 patients, 5 also required removal of the phrenic nerve. Two other patients underwent resection of their phrenic nerve alone. Thirteen patients (42 percent) had extensive subclavian vessel involvement; their operative management included resection of the subclavian artery alone in four patients, subclavian artery and vein in three, subclavian and vertebral arteries in one, subclavian artery and vein and ver-

tebral artery in two, subclavian vein alone in one, vertebral artery alone in one, and both the subclavian vein and vertebral artery in one. The subclavian artery was revascularized with a prosthetic replacement in seven cases (a PTFE tubular ring graft being used in all but one patient) and an end-to-end anastomosis in three.

Postoperative radiotherapy was given to 27 patients (87 percent), being used alone in 16 and in combination with adjuvant chemotherapy in 11. With a median follow-up of 3.5 years, the overall projected 5-year survival rate was 29 percent. Twelve patients are currently alive and disease-free at 2 to more than 145 months; one patient died, disease-free, from a myocardial infarction 15 months after operation; and the remaining 16 patients died from recurrence of their primary tumor, locally in 2 cases and systemically in 14. We performed univariate and multivariate analysis but failed to identify clinical and pathologic factors predictive of survival.

COMMENTS AND CONTROVERSIES

The surgical technique presented has been used in a total of 31 patients over a 12-year period, and several positive technical and therapeutic inferences can be drawn from this experience.

The anterior transcervical approach offers a unique chance to adequately and directly assess tumor extension to all the structures of the thoracic inlet, the scalene fat pad, and the upper mediastinum before any crucial structure is needlessly resected. Unlike the classic posterior approach (Shaw, et al., 1961), it provides excellent exposure of the entire thoracic inlet and a safe dissection and complete surgical clearance of involved segments of the subclavian vein and artery and related branches, the phrenic nerve, the scalenus muscles, and the lower, middle, and upper trunk of the brachial plexus. This is particularly attractive since the major pitfalls in the posterior approach to superior sulcus tumors invading the subclavian vessels or extensively invading the brachial plexus has been the considerable difficulty in adequately and safely visualizing, manipulating, and resecting these structures. For instance, previous experiences with subclavian artery invasion and resection have been disappointing (Attar, et al., 1979; Paulson, 1975; Wright, et al., 1987), while extensive brachial plexus invasion (middle and upper trunks) has been usually considered to contraindicate surgical resection. Conversely, by using this anterior approach, one might anticipate a complete and safe resection of the tumor-bearing inlet area. Moreover, as experience has increased, it has become evident that prolongation of the horizontal incision into the deltopectoral groove allows a spectacular operative view and easily facilitates en bloc resection of the inlet extension of the apical tumor, underlying involved lung parenchyma, the pulmonary pedicle, and the first two ribs. This approach does not preclude a complementary posterior, one-stage thoracotomy if further chest wall and vertebral or major pulmonary resections are necessary. It is our opinion that once the inlet structures are detached by the transcervical approach, the posterior phase of the classical posterior thoracotomy (Shaw, et al., 1961) is markedly easier. There is no a priori reason

to hesitate to add the posterior approach if doubt remains about adequate margins.

The question arises as to whether this operation adds dangers or increases mortality or morbidity. This procedure needs to be performed by experienced surgeons knowledgable in this anatomic area and in all aspects of thoracic and vascular surgery. Indeed, the operation results in negligible morbidity, no mortality, and minimal discomfort. Its major disadvantage is the development of minimal shoulder discomfort in those patients requiring resection of both the clavicle and the external branch of the spinal accessory nerve. The postoperative sequelae related to the resection of the lower trunk of the brachial plexus and sympathetic chain are similar to those observed by Paulson (1975). Subclavian vein division usually results in an ispilateral but transient venous distension of the upper limb; however, revascularization of the subclavian artery by PTFE grafts is essential and mandatory to avoid fatal ischemic complications described by several authors (Miller, et al., 1979; Paulson, 1975) and mitigate the fibrotic changes inducible by radiation therapy.

The major therapeutic inference is that the availability of this technique might extend the indication of operation for apical lung carcinomas, irrespective of their location. In effect, while it offers the aformentioned technical advantages over the posterior approach for superior sulcus tumors invading the subclavian vessels, this operation appears to be the optimal approach for resecting apical tumors invading the thoracic inlet. Therefore, this operation may expand the pool of candidates with lung carcinomas for in whom surgery has been always considered to be contraindicated (Mountain, 1988). One has to keep in mind that absolute contraindications to this operation are the presence of extrathoracic sites of metastasis, clinical and histologically confirmed mediastinal lymph node involvement, and small cell histology. Extensive involvement of the brachial plexus is a relative contraindication if a complete surgical neurolysis may be anticipated. Involvement of the subclavian vessels should no longer be considered an operative contraindication; however, it should be kept in mind that while the subclavian vein can be either resected or ligated, the subclavian artery needs immediate revascularization. As suggested by Mathisen and Grillo (1988), unless invasion through the cortex of the vertebral body is documented, patients should not be deemed inoperable on the basis of minor deformity of the vertebral body.

It should be noted that, regardless of local control, a significant proportion of patients in our series developed and ultimately succumbed to distant metastases despite local control. Shahian, et al. (1987) stated that death of patients with superior sulcus tumors usually results from distant metastatic disease that is present at the time of operation although not detected by conventional screening methods; this indicates the need for more effective systemic therapy of this disease.

P.D.
P.M.

KEY REFERENCES

Dartevelle P, Chapelier A, Macchiarini P, et al: Anterior transcervical-thoracical approach for radical resection of lung tumors invading the thoracic inlet. J Thorac Cardiovasc Surg 105:1025, 1993

An original anterior transcervical technique is presented for the radical resection of apical chest tumors invading the thoracic inlet. The 5-year survival rate in 29 patients treated with this technique was 30 percent, demonstrating that subclavian vessel, extensive brachial plexus, and phrenic nerve invasion and tumor location (anterior versus middle versus posterior) do not represent surgical contraindications and poor prognostic factors.

Pancoast HK: Superior sulcus tumors. JAMA 99:1391, 1932

The first exhaustive description defining the superior sulcus tumor as occurring "at a definite location at the thoracic inlet, characterized clinically by pain around the shoulder and down the arm, Horner's syndrome and atrophy of the muscle of the hand and to present roentgengraphic evidences of a small, homogeneous shadow at the extreme apex, always more or less local rib destruction and often vertebral infiltration." By virtue of this exact description, it became evident that superior sulcus tumor are distinct entities from the more common apical chest tumors (Paulson, 1924).

Paulson DL: Carcinomas in the superior pulmonary sulcus. J Thorac Cardiovasc Surg 70:1095, 1975

This paper reports 5- and 10-year survivals of 34 and 29 percent, respectively, and provides evidence for the superiority of preoperative radiation therapy and surgical resection over radiation therapy alone. This landmark contribution also demonstrated that contraindications for operation are extensive vertebral bodies, brachial plexus, and subclavian artery involvement, as well as mediastinal lymph nodes and distant metastases.

Shaw RR, Paulson DL, Kee JL Jr: Treatment of the superior sulcus tumor by irradiation followed by resection. Ann Surg 154:29, 1961

This is the first paper reporting long-term survivals in patients with Pancoast tumors treated with preoperative radiation (30 Gy) and surgical resection. This approach still remains the therapy of choice for patients with pure superior sulcus tumors.

REFERENCES

Anderson TM, Moy PM, Holmes EC: Factors affecting survival in superior sulcus tumors. J Clin Oncol 4:1598, 1985

Attar S, Miller JE, Satterfield J et al: Pancoast's tumor: irradiation or surgery? Ann Thorac Surg 28:578, 1979

Camelotte A, Crinquette J, Callens J: Benign tumors of the bronchi causing Pancoast syndrome. J Sci Med Lille 82:719, 1964

Devine JW, Mendenhall WM, Million RR, Carmichael MJ: Carcinoma of the superior pulmonary sulcus treated with surgery and/or radiation therapy. Cancer 57:941, 1986

Macchiarini P, Dartevelle P, Chapelier A et al: Technique for resecting primary or metastatic non-bronchogenic tumors of the thoracic outlet. Ann Thorac Surg 55:611, 1993

Macchiarini P, Fontanini G, Hardin M et al: Relation of neovascularization to metastasis in non-small cell lung cancer. Lancet 340:145, 1992

Mathisen DJ, Grillo HC: Lung Cancer: A Comprehensive Treatise. Grune & Stratton, Orlando, 1988

McGoon DC: Transcervical technique for removal of specimen from superior sulcus tumor for pathologic study. Ann Surg 159:407, 1964

Miller JI, Mansour KA, Hatcher CR: Carcinoma of the superior pulmonary sulcus. Ann Thorac Surg 28:44, 1979

Mountain CF: Prognostic implications of the international staging system for lung cancer. Semin Oncol 15:236, 1988

Pancoast HK: Importance of careful roentgen-ray investigations of apical chest tumors. JAMA 83:1407, 1924

Paulson DL: General Thoracic Surgery, Lea & Febiger, Philadelphia, 1989

Paulson DL: Cervical approach for percutaneous needle biopsy of Pancoast tumors. Ann Thorac Surg 39:586, 1985

Paulson DL: The importance of defining location and staging of superior pulmonary sulcus tumors. Ann Thorac Surg 15:549, 1973

Shahian DM, Wildford BN, Ellis FH Jr: Pancoast tumors: improved survival with preoperative and postoperative radiotherapy. Ann Thorac Surg 43:32, 1987

Standford W, Barnes RP, Tucker AR: Influence of staging in superior sulcus (Pancoast) tumors of the lung. Ann Thorac Surg 29:406, 1979

Teixeira JP: Concerning the Pancoast tumor: what is the superior pulmonary sulcus? Ann Thorac Surg 35:577, 1983

Tobias JW: Sindrome apico-costo-vertebral-doloroso por tumor apexiano: su valor diagnostico en el cancer primitivo del pulmon. Thesis, Imp. Mercatali, Buenos Aires, 1931

Wright CD, Moncure AC, Shepard JOA et al: Superior sulcus lung tumors. J Thorac Cardiovasc Surg 94:69, 1987

Extended Pulmonary Resections

Patricia M. McCormack

DEFINITION

As neoplasms of the lung grow, they may infiltrate tissues or contiguous organs and structures. The most commonly invaded structures are the chest wall, vertebral bodies, diaphragm, pericardium, esophagus, and superior vena cava. In those situations in which invasion of lung carcinomas extends beyond the visceral pleura, the ability to resect the contiguous invaded structure or organ varies greatly. The prognosis is directly related to the completeness of the resection. Resection techniques for each structure are discussed below.

HISTORICAL NOTE

Carcinoma of the lung is the most frequent cause of cancer deaths in both men and women. Lung cancers invade the chest wall in 5 percent of cases, which amounted to 8,250 cases in 1992. Approximately 1 to 2 percent invade vertebral bodies, diaphragm, pericardium, esophagus, and superior vena cava.

In 1899 Parham was the first to describe a successful resection of a chest wall tumor in the American literature. He stressed leaving an intact parietal pleura, lest the normal respiratory function be interrupted and death result.

In 1943 Graham, et al. produced a thoracic surgical manual, which standardized the surgical approach for chest wall injuries, on the basis of experience gained during World War I. The gravity of a sucking chest wound was recognized, and immediate closure to maintian ventilation was urged. Surrounding soft tissues were used to close the defect. These authors also recommended tube thoracostomy for drainage and ventilation purposes.

Brewer (1983) chronicled his experience during World War II, applying these principles and improving their application. Resection of a portion of the lung in continuity with the chest wall invaded by the tumor is now commonplace. Early chest wall resections were performed when the resulting defect was small. This defect was bridged by a variety of materials, including dura mater, fascia lata, ox fascia, and more recently, Marlex mesh. Rigid materials, including autogenous ribs, metal struts, and Lucite, have also been used. If a large defect occurred, the Marlex mesh and fascia-like materials did not prevent a respiratory flail and patients remained on respirator support for prolonged periods. This changed in 1974 with the introduction of the Marlex mesh–polymethylmethacrylate prosthesis.

Reconstruction techniques using materials that are readily available, are adaptable to any size and contour needed, and are integrated by the body tissues with little reaction to their presence and low infection rates were reported by McCormack, and co-workers (1981) using a mesh with polymethylmethacrylate. Pairolero popularized the use of a plastic patch impermeable to air and liquids.

Sundaresan, et al. (1985) described the technique and results of resections of a vertebral body in continuity with a lung cancer. This requires collaboration among neurosurgeons and orthopedic and thoracic surgeons.

Complete sleeve resections of the vena cava, with reconstruction by varying techniques, uniformly failed until Chu, et al., in 1974 and Doty in 1982 described the construction of a spiral vein graft. Long-term patency rates improved, but the intrinsic complexity of this technique prevented widespread acceptance. Dartevelle, et al. in 1987 detailed the use of a polytetrafluoroethylene (Gore-Tex) graft with proven patency if used as a venous substitute when resecting the superior vena cava because of tumor.

Dartevelle, et al. (1991) used a Gore-Tex graft for vena cava reconstruction combined with a right pneumonectomy in six patients with lung cancer. Two of the six lived 16 and 51 months, respectively; the median survival of the four others was 13 months. All grafts remained patent in this series.

HISTORICAL READINGS

Brewer LA III: The contributions of the Second Auxiliary Surgical Group to military surgery during Word War II with special reference to thoracic surgery. Ann Surg 197:318, 1983

Chu CJ, Tazis H, MacRae ML: Replacement of superior vena cava with the spiral composite vein graft. Ann Thorac Surg 17:553, 1974

Dartevelle P, Chapelier A, Navajas M et al: Replacement of the superior vena cava with polytetrafluoroethylene grafts combined with resection of mediastinal-pulmonary malignancy: report of 13 cases. J Thorac Cardiovasc Surg 94:361, 1987

Dartevelle PJ, Chapelier AR, Pastorino U et al: Long-term follow-up after prosthetic replacement of the superior vena cava combined with resection of mediastinal-pulmonary malignant tumors. J Thorac Cardiovasc Surg 102:259, 1991

Doty DB: Bypass of superior vena cava: six year's experience with spiral vein graft for obstruction of superior vena cava due to benign and malignant disease. J Thorac Cardiovasc Surg 83:326, 1982

Graham EV, Bigger IA, Churchill EO, Eloesser L: Thoracic Surgery. WB Saunders, Philadelphia, 1943

McCormack PM, Bains MS, Beattie EJ et al: new trends in skeletal reconstruction after resection of chest wall tumors. Ann Thorac Surg 31:45, 1981

Parham DW: Thoracic resections for tumors growing from the bony chest wall. Trans South Surg Assoc 2:223, 1899

Sundaresen N. Bains MS, McCormack PM: Surgical treatment of spinal cord compression in patients with lung cancer. Neurosurgery 16:350, 1985

BASIC SCIENCE

Respiratory physiology relates to the process of ventilation, which is the transport of inspired air to and of expired air from the alveoli. This requires neuromuscular integrity of the chest wall, including the bony skeleton. The principal respiratory derangements after chest wall resection are the result of altered ventilation.

When there is a defect in the rigid chest wall during respiration, there is a paradoxic motion of that portion of the chest wall. During inspiration it is pulled inward, decreasing the volume on that side, and on expiration it expands, causing the expired air from the normal side to travel back and forth between the lungs rather than in and out the airway to exchange gases. This rapidly leads to decreased tidal volume, hypoxemia, hypercarbia, and increased airway resistance, with resulting fatigue and respiratory failure. Insertion of a prosthesis in the chest wall prevents such a flail.

DIAGNOSIS

Clinically the extension of carcinoma of the lung to contiguous structures is accompanied by pain at the site in the chest wall or vertebral body. Superior vena cava involvement produces the classic superior vena cava syndrome, with neovascularity over the thorax, as the edema of the face and upper extremities fades. It is usually asymptomatic, being suspected on imaging studies or discovered at surgery. Invasion into the pericardium and diaphragm is either asymptomatic or manifested by arrhythmia, hiccups, or referred pain. Esophageal involvement is unsuspected until almost complete obstruction leads to dysphagia.

In patients with superior sulcus tumors, it may take 6 months or longer—and a variety of erroneous diagnoses—before a chest x-ray is taken for a painful shoulder requiring ever more powerful analgesics for relief. The differential diagnosis of an apical lesion includes tuberculosis, but a computed tomography (CT) scan and a magnetic resonance imaging (MRI) scan delineate the extent of the tumor very clearly. Fine-needle aspiration will readily lead to a correct diagnosis.

In superior vena cava syndrome, a CT scan will show the presence of a mass compressing the vein. MRI clearly delineates the vascular involvement and the presence of collateral vessels. The absence of a mass suggests either an infectious or an inflammatory process. If a needle biopsy fails to lead to a diagnosis, an open biopsy is required. A venogram is sometimes helpful to show the extent of clot and involvement of proximal vessels. However, the extensive involvement required to produce the superior vena cava syndrome usually precludes a surgical approach for curative treatment.

Esophageal invasion must be suspected when dysphagia occurs. A barium swallow will pinpoint the site of obstruction, and esophagoscopy will confirm invasion. However, if the wall is thickened or edematous even in the absence of mucosal tumor, invasion of the esophageal wall is likely. Plans for treating this contingency must be made preoperatively.

SURGICAL TECHNIQUES

Chest Wall Invasion

Principles

The goal of surgery when lung cancer invades the chest wall is twofold: complete resection of all cancer with clear surgical margins and restoration of the rigid chest wall and of the soft tissues resected with the tumor. Maintenance of normal respiratory physiology is ensured by this operative technique.

The placement of the skin incision will vary with the site of the invasion. Superior sulcus tumors have already been discussed earlier in this chapter by Shamji and Ginsberg; invasion of ribs other than in the superior sulcus and sternum is considered below. In most cases the standard posterolateral incision is adequate. The skin and soft tissues are incised, always one tissue layer superficial to the invading cancer. Care must be taken in selecting the intercostal space for entry into the pleural cavity; usually this is one space below the invaded rib. Upon entering the pleural cavity, careful digital palpation will confirm the location and extent of the tumor. The intercostal incision is then lengthened to the appropriate interspace.

When pleurodesis is complete but tumor invasion beyond the parietal pleura is doubted, an extrapleural plane is developed by sharp dissection 2 to 3 cm away from the tumor. This place is continued by using careful finger dissection to peel the parietal pleura away from the chest wall. If the parietal pleura dissects away easily, tumor invasion further into the chest wall is usually not present. This should be confirmed by a frozen section biopsy of the parietal pleura. The area of the parietal pleura attached to the tumor is then cut free from the remaining pleura and resected en bloc with the lobe. However, whenever there is doubt, an en bloc excision of the chest wall should be performed.

When resistance is met during finger dissection, this approach is stopped. Invasion of the tumor into the rigid chest wall is presumed and chest wall resection is planned. When the amount of chest wall involvement is small, it is usually easier to resect the ribs first and then perform the lobectomy. If the amount of chest wall resection required is larger than 10 cm, it may be easier to perform the lobectomy first. In rare cases it may be easier to perform a wedge resection of the tumor-bearing portion of the lobe using the GIA stapler and allow the remainder of the lung to collapse away from the chest wall. The remainder of the lobe is resected later. Whatever the approach used, the entire tumor should be resected en bloc to prevent tumor spillage. Chest wall resection is then carried out. Margins are set one rib above and below the rib(s) involved and 3 to 5 cm laterally and medially. Whenever possible, frozen section confirmation of complete resection is desirable.

The periosteum is divided by using cautery. The neurovascular bundle is freed from the subcostal groove, the rib is cut, and the neurovascular structures are then clipped and divided. All soft tissue is divided by cautery up to the next rib. This technique is followed for each rib included in the resection. At the superior and inferior margins, the intercostal space is incised to join the lateral and medial resected margins. The amount of normal rib beyond the palpable tumor should be 5 cm if possible. When the tumor has invaded into the cancellous portion of the rib, some authors advocate total resection of this rib. My associates and I have not done so and others have not been able to prove that this more conservative resection detrimental to survival. When chest wall resection (Fig. 32-63A) is completed, attention is directed to the pulmonary resection. The technique for the usual dissection can now be followed, as the chest wall tumor is attached to the lung and freed from its prior position. It is sent to pathology as an en bloc specimen. After the remaining lung has been reexpanded, chest tubes are placed in the standard fashion. The intercostal space is reapproximated up to the area of the defect. If the defect is small (<5 cm) and/or is situated beneath the scapula, a rigid reconstruction with a prosthesis may not be necessary.

With larger defects reconstruction is now done. Two techniques using nonreinforced materials are in general use: (1) Marlex mesh, usually doubled crosswise at a 90-degree angle for added strength, is cut to size and sutured to the edges of the defect with strong nonabsorbable sutures; (2) 3-cm Gore-Tex patch specifically designed for chest wall reconstruction is used. With both these materials the repair results in a flat chest contour. Marlex mesh allows ingrowth of tissue and remains rigid. The Gore-Tex patch does not allow the ingrowth of body tissue and becomes flaccid with time.

Contour as well as rigidity can be restored by reinforcing Marlex mesh with methyl methacrylate; this method is especially suited for larger unsupported defects. First a pattern is made by placing a clean lap pad over the defect (Fig. 32-63B). A sheet of Marlex is placed on top of the pattern. The methyl methacrylate monomer is mixed until it is thick enough to remain on top of the mesh. It is spread over the mesh according to the outline of the pattern, leaving a 2-cm rim of mesh for the sewing ring. A second sheet of Marlex mesh is placed over the methyl methacrylate layer. This "sandwich" can then be shaped to the desired contour while the methyl methacrylate is setting (5 to 10 minutes) (Fig. 32-63B). When hard and cool enough to handle, it is sutured to the edges of the defect (Fig. 32-63C) with a heavy absorbable suture. Soft tissues (Fig. 32-63D) are then sutured in standard fashion to complete the closure of the incision.

When the resection includes overlying soft tissues as well as the bony parts of the chest wall, a suitable myocutaneous flap may be required for closure (Fig. 32-63E). The plastic surgeon should be consulted preoperatively in order to plan the procedure and to let the patient understand what to expect.

When the sternum is involved with tumor, part or all of the sternum can be removed. Clear margins are secured and the sternum is divided after the internal mammary artery (or arteries) and veins(s) are securely tied and cut. This Marlex sandwich technique can be used for sternal replacement. It is especially practical if ribs and sternum are removed en bloc.

When only a portion of the sternum is resected, an alternative method of replacement may be used. Following resection of lung and sternum and placement of chest tubes, one layer of mesh is sutured in place under the ribs. The methacrylate is mixed, and while it is still very thin, some is injected into the cut edge of the sternum with a piston syringe. The remainder is spread over the mesh in the shape of the resected sternum. This will bond firmly with the methacrylate in the sternal marrow. A second layer of mesh is sutured in place on top of the reconstruction. Caution is needed because setting of methyl methacrylate is an exothermic reaction in which the temperature reaches 140°F. The underlying structures must be protected with a folded towel or by constant irrigation with cold saline. Soft tissue replacement is by primary closure or myocutaneous flap, as planned preoperatively.

Perioperative Care

Respiratory insufficiency was the postoperative complication that precluded chest wall resection prior to the initiation of immediate reconstruction. Since 1974 no patient has required either a tracheostomy or respirator support when a large defect was repaired with mesh or the Marlex-methacrylate prosthesis. Good pulmonary toilet is essential and is assured by the presence of an experienced respiratory therapy team.

Seromas accumulate atop the prosthesis. Repeated aspiration is unnecessary and should *not* be done for fear of infection. The seroma will shortly be absorbed. It is prudent to ensure antibiotic coverage for 7 days until the incision heals.

Infection of the prosthesis is the most serious complication. With the Marlex mesh a seal quickly forms, walling off the infected space from the body. When infection is limited to the surface of the prosthesis, adequate drainage and irrigation may save the prosthesis.

If drainage and irrigation are not effective or if the infection is on the undersurface of the prosthesis, the prosthesis will have to be removed. Adequate drainage should be established and an antibiotic given. If the patient is not toxic, a delay of 6 weeks before removing the prosthesis allows a fibrous capsule to form. When the prosthesis is removed, this capsule will maintain chest wall stability without a resulting flail.

The Marlex prosthesis does not obscure the underlying lung for chest x-rays unless barium-impregnated methyl methacrylate is used. In the event of reoperation, the prosthesis will need to be removed entirely by cutting the mesh around the periphery. A bone cutter will be necessary to cut through the polymethylmethacrylate in order to remove a part of the prosthesis.

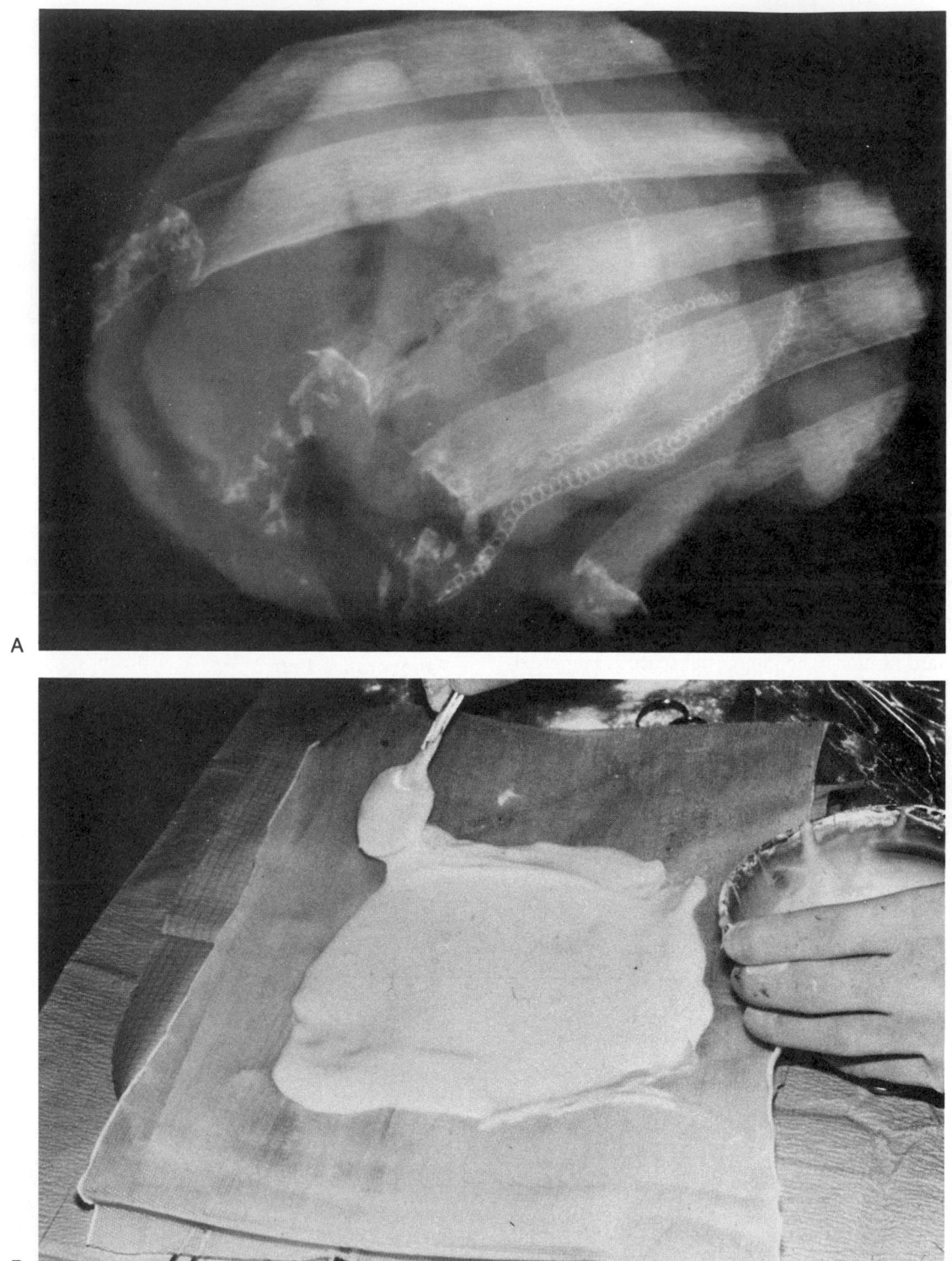

Figure 32-63.   Chest wall reconstruction. **(A)** X-ray of resected chest wall tumor. **(B)** Spreading methylmethacrylate over mesh. (*Figure continues.*)

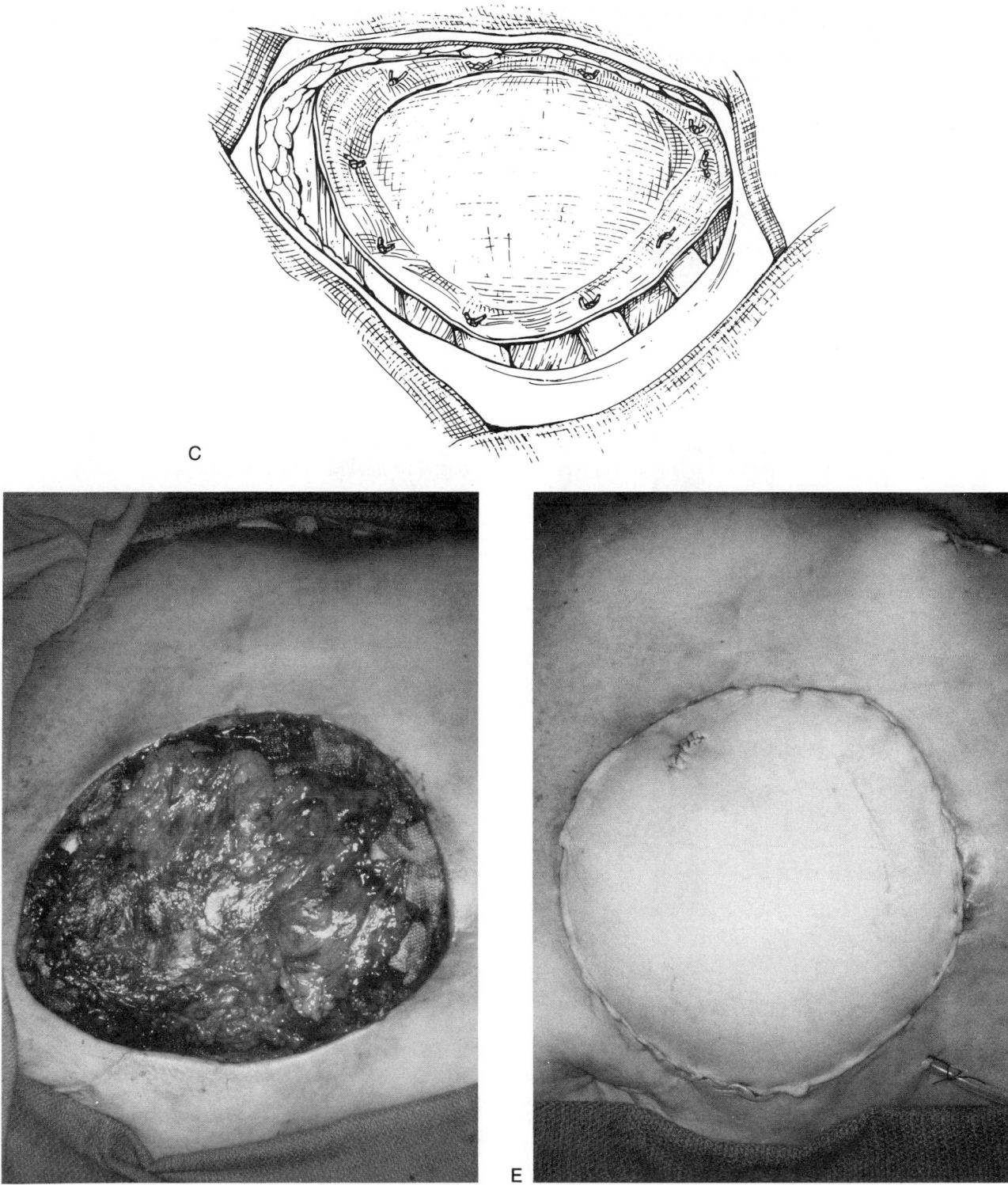

Figure 32-63 (*Continued*).   **(C)** Prosthesis sutured in place. **(D)** Omentum sutured over prosthesis. **(E)** Myocutaneous flap sutured to skin.

Results

Between 1974 and 1983, 125 patients underwent lung and chest wall resection for non-small cell lung cancer (McCaughan, et al., 1985). Of 48 patients who had no or incomplete resection, none survived 12 months. The operative mortality rate was 2 percent in those patients who had immediate reconstruction. Five-year survival was directly related to completeness of resection, (42 percent versus zero), the absence of lymph node metastases (56 versus 20 percent) and depth of chest wall invasion (50 versus 16 percent). However, in the absence of nodal metastases, the depth of chest wall invasion was not significant (Fig. 32-63). Trastek et al. (1984) and Riehlves (1982) reported 5-year survivals of 39.7 and 32.9 percent, respectively, following lung and chest wall resection.

COMMENTS AND CONTROVERSIES

With the ability to easily reconstruct any size defect with materials readily available in the operating room, surgery should be offered to any patient whose lung cancer invades the chest wall. The 58 percent survival in the absence of nodal metastases is better than that obtained with any other therapeutic modality. With the improved survival advantage following preoperative chemotherapy in the presence of N2 disease, surgery should be offered to this group of patients as well. The type of prosthetic material used in reconstruction depends on the surgeon's preference. A curved contour can only be achieved with the composite repair. The largest resection and reconstruction to date using the Marlex composite consisted of the second through tenth ribs from the sternum to the vertebral body along with the left upper lobe. The patient was extubated in the operating room and survived for 3½ years, leading a normal life.

The value of radiation therapy in chest wall invasion is controversial. Carrel, et al. (1990) reported an improved 5-year survival with preoperative irradiation, and Patterson, et al. (1982) a 56 versus 38 percent 5-year survival advantage with preoperative irradiation.

P.M.M.

Lung and Vertebral Body

Direct invasion of the vertebral body by a lung cancer (Fig. 32-64A) is a rare but grave complication of an already serious malignancy. Superior sulcus tumors have been discussed earlier in this chapter. Attention here will focus on invasive tumors below the third thoracic vertebra. Vertebral body invasion, in general, precludes curative therapy; surgery, however, affords excellent palliation in selected cases.

The diagnosis is suspected when back pain is present. However, it may be an incidental finding on CT scan in the absence of symptoms. The MRI scan has added coronal and sagittal views, which delineate clearly the extent of tumor encroachment and whether it involves the spinal canal. Such information is crucial in planning the surgical approach with the neurosurgeon (Sundaresan et al. 1985).

Nonsurgical therapy (Arnold and Pairolero, 1984)—chemotherapy or radiotherapy—provides short-term symptomatic relief only except in certain neoplasms (e.g., small cell carcinoma). Combined resection is indicated in properly selected patients under the following conditions: (1) no other disease is present or paralysis is impending; (2) the overall status of the patient is good; and (3) at least a 6-month survival is anticipated. Extensive involvement of mediastinal lymph nodes or disease outside the chest would make resection impractical.

When the neoplasm is localized to the lung and the adjacent vertebral body, a standard posterolateral thoracotomy has been the best approach. The chest is opened, with the incision placed to intersect the invaded vertebra and extending to the posterior midline. The lung resection is usually carried out first. When the arteries, veins, and bronchus have been secured, the tumor invading the vertebra is resected from the remainder of the lung and left in continuity with the vertebral body (Fig. 32-64B). One rib is severed above and below this tumor mass. Posterior paraspinous muscles are retraced medially and the costotransverse junction is disarticulated. Nerve roots are clipped at the intervertebral foramina. The tumor mass is mobilized with a margin of uninvolved chest wall including ribs. Vertebral bodies are totally excised with osteotomes, rongeurs, and curettes. Discs—intact if possible—above and below the resected bodies are removed. The dura is maintained intact. Steinman pins are placed in the normal vertebral bodies above and below the resection (Fig. 32-64C). Spinal stability is established by pouring methyl methacrylate into the defect, incorporating the Steinman pins, and allowing it to solidify in situ (Fig. 32-64D). This solidification is an exothermic reaction in which temperature may rise to 140°F, so a continuous stream of cold saline must be poured over the methacrylate until it cools in order to protect the spinal cord from excessive heat. The thoracotomy incision is closed in routine fashion with chest tubes in place (Fig. 32-64E).

Postoperative care is the same as for routine thoracotomy patients. This technique yields an immediately stabilized spine and obviates the need for prolonged bed rest or a back brace.

Palliation rather than cure is the goal of this procedure. Prevention of cord compression and resultant paralysis as well as amelioration of pain are very important elements in this palliation. Involvement of the vertebral body precludes obtaining a good free margin at surgery. Brachytherapy with iodine 125 can be used carefully around the spinal cord, but limited use of this modality precludes drawing a conclusion as to its value. Adding radiation postoperatively has not decreased the recurrence rate, so it is usually postponed until needed. This procedure in a select group of patients resulted in a 10 percent survival at 5 years. To date chemotherapy has not affected the survival of this group of patients, but it should certainly be investigated.

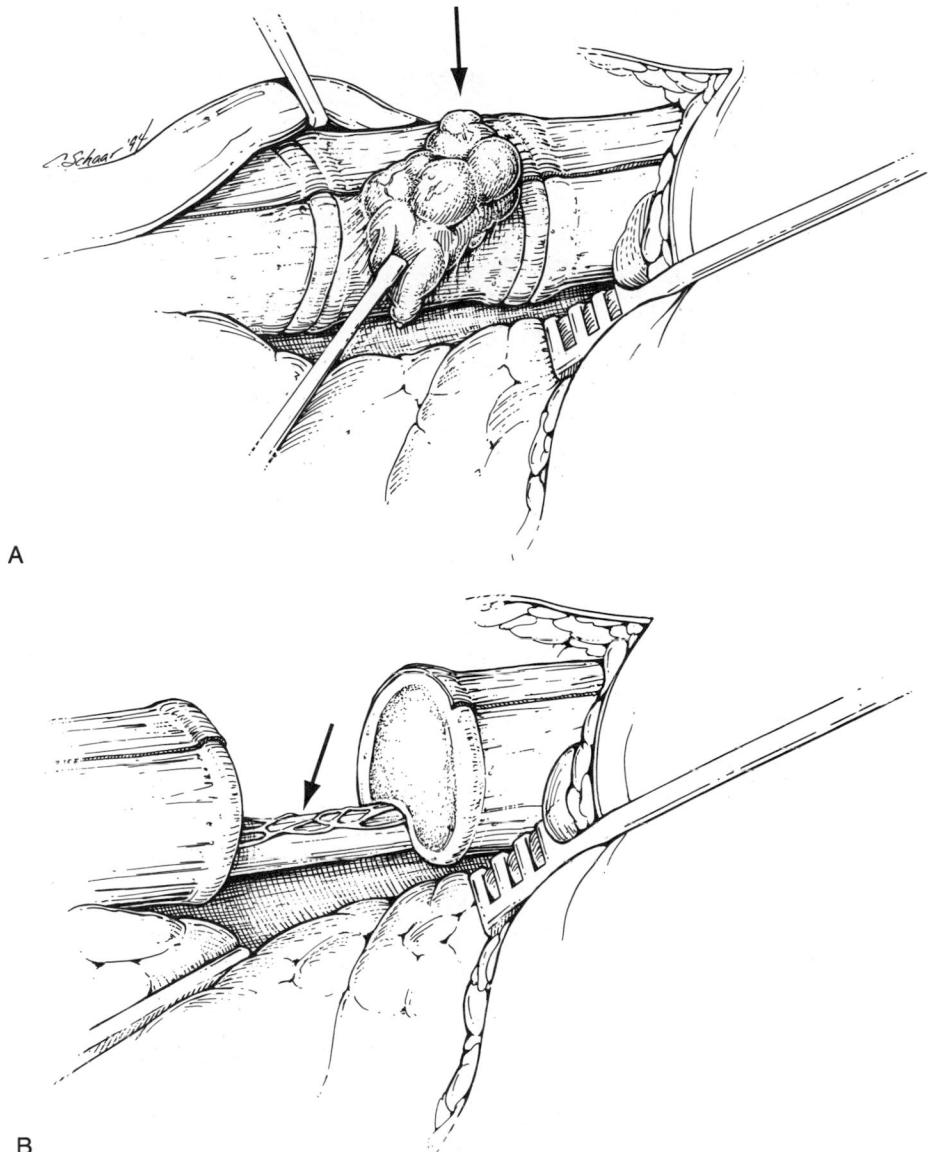

Figure 32-64.   Vertebral body reconstruction. **(A)** Tumor (*arrow*) invading vertebral body. **(B)** After resection of tumor and vertebral body (*arrow*, spinal cord). (*Figure continues.*)

Superior Vena Cava

Lung carcinoma rarely invades the superior vena cava. The most frequent manifestation of such invasion is the onset of the superior vena cava syndrome, manifested by edema of the head and upper extremities, with swelling, and venous engorgement (Fig. 32-65A). There follows a gradual emergence of tributary veins in the superficial tissues of the chest wall as the suffusion of the head subsides. CT and MRI scans will clearly define the extent of caval involvement. Careful selection of patients is mandatory before surgery, since this usually represents advanced disease with a very low likelihood of survival.

Minimal invasion of the superior vena cava in bronchogenic carcinoma may be by primary tumor or by mediastinal lymph node metastases. When the tumor or the involved nodes cannot be easily dissected free from the adventitia of the caval wall, resection should be considered. Most caval involvement allowing resection involves one wall, and partial resection may be sufficient. With more extensive invasion, complete caval replacement has been performed, with occasional long-term survivors reported. With respect to lung cancer, caval replacement is recommended only when no N2 disease is present.

A posterolateral thoracotomy is the preferred approach because the involvement of the superior vena cava is usually from the azygos vein. The amount of caval invasion is assessed and the resection is planned.

The decision to resect the lung first or the cava first relates to the location and size of the tumor. If the lung and the cava

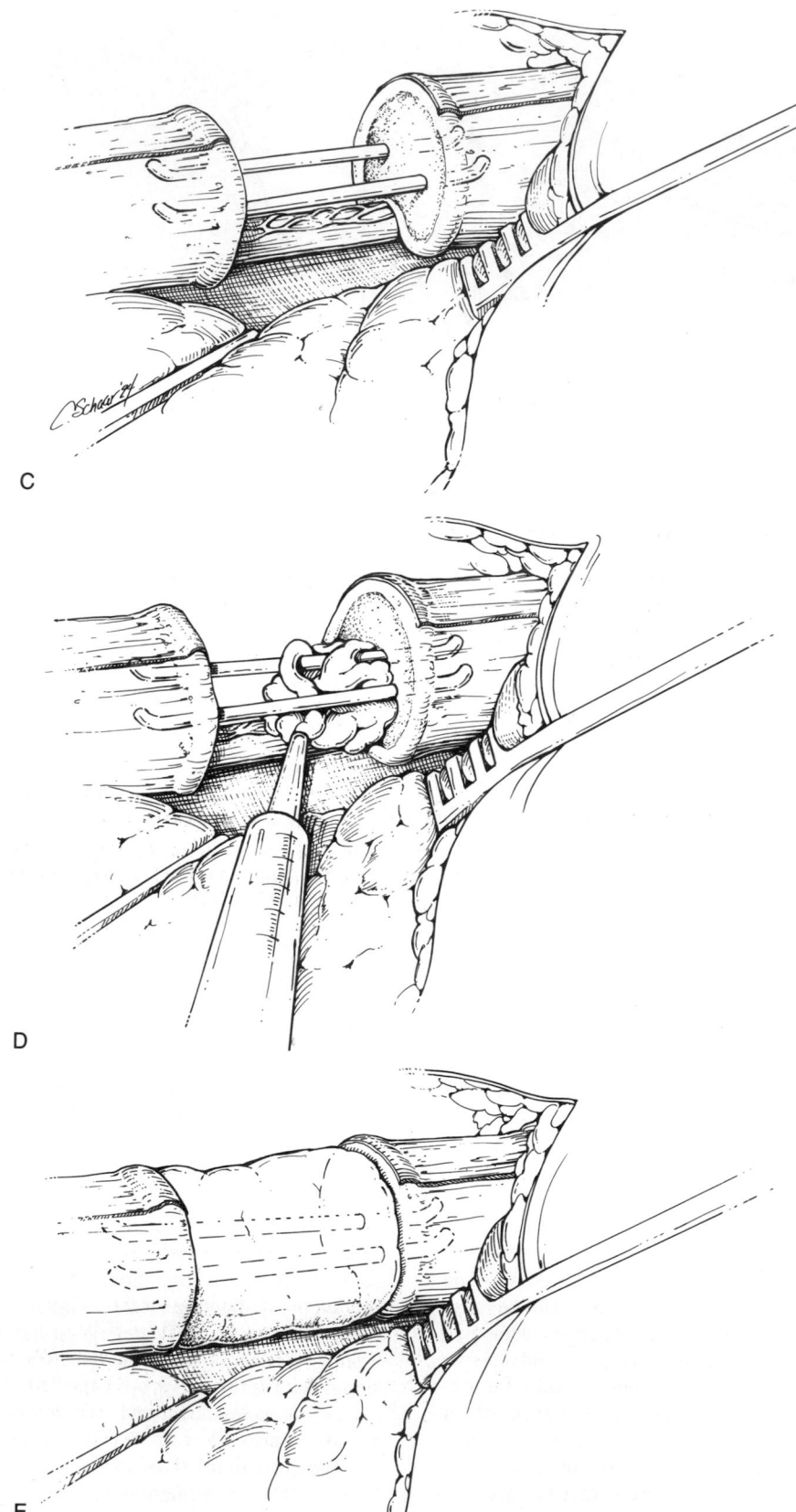

C

D

E

Figure 32-64 (*Continued*). **(C)** Steinman pins inserted into intact vertebral bodies above and below resection (spinal cord visible). **(D)** Methylmethacrylate injected around Steinman pins to replace resected vertebral body. **(E)** Completed reconstruction of resected vertebral body.

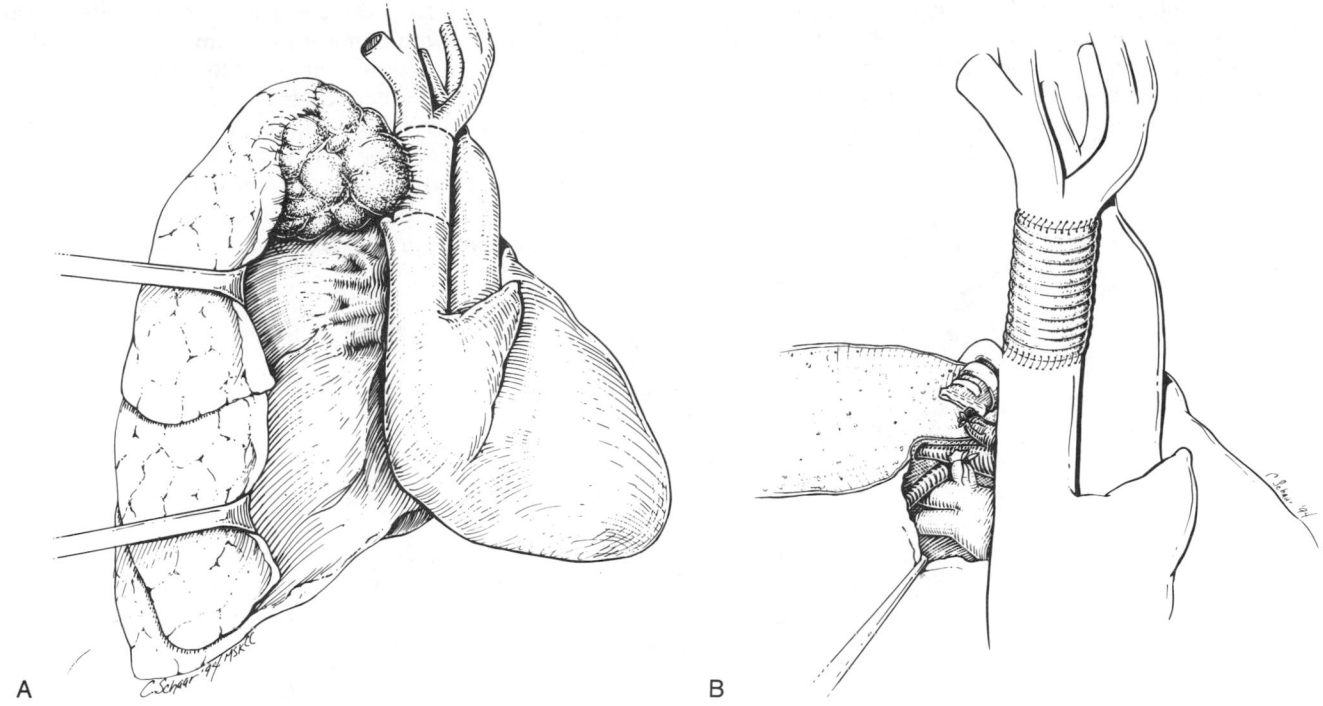

A   B

Figure 32-65.   Caval invasion. **(A)** Illustration of tumor invading superior vena cava. **(B)** Reconstruction with PTFE graft.

can be resected en bloc, it will obviate the need to transect the tumor and remove it in two pieces. The use of an intraluminal shunt or a bypass from innominate vein to atrial appendage is at the option of the surgeon. It has been advocated by some authors (Patterson, et al., 1982; Piccione, et al., 1990). Caval cross-clamping for 1 hour is usually well tolerated, if care is taken to replace blood volume with lower extremity intravenous lincs.

If the caval involvement allows clamping to be done for control, this is best done before the caval segment is resected. Easier access to the vasculature of the upper lobe is thus obtained. A standard upper lobectomy is then carried out and the specimen is removed en bloc; this normally can be done in less than 1 hour, during which time the cava is clamped. Careful attention to hemodynamics on the part of the anesthesiologist is mandatory during this period.

When the resection is completed, polytetrafluoroethylene (PTFE) graft is inserted by first attaching the end nearest the atrium (Fig. 32-65B). The superior end is next sutured, but before the last suture is tightened, it is filled retrograde with blood to force all air out of the graft. When that is accomplished, the clamp is removed. The use of heparin following caval resection is at the discretion of the surgeon. Reconstruction of the superior vena cava is contraindicated with extensive thrombosis or established collateral circulation. The presence of thrombosis risks an embolus postoperatively, and established collateral flow will decrease the amount of central flow and increase the chance of graft thrombosis. The (PTFE) graft should be large (i.e., 18 or 20).

The PTFE graft has proved successful and is now used with good results. Pericardium is the most widely used side patch. The spiral graft using saphenous vein is very tedious

and hence unpopular. Postoperatively, good central venous pressure must be maintained. Full blood volume will ensure a good flow through the graft to maintain potency. Dehydration is to be avoided. Some surgeons have continued to administer anticoagulants for 6 months. Antibiotic coverage for 1 week is advisable. Intravenous catheterization through the graft must be avoided, as it has led to graft thrombosis. Short-term results have been very gratifying.

A partial involvement of the superior vena cava was seen in 0.7 percent of the 2,554 patient with non-small cell lung cancer treated at Memorial Sloan-Kettering Cancer Center from 1974 to 1984. Of these patients 225 (8 percent) had mediastinal invasion. In those undergoing partial cavectomy, there were no 5-year survivors. In Dartevelle's group late evaluation by angiogram, CT scan, or autopsy showed potency despite radiation therapy (Dartevelle, et al., 1987).

Diaphragm

Lung tumors that directly invade the diaphragm can be totally resected. There is no report in the literature addressing exclusively this phase of tumor spread, and diffuse diaphragmatic involvement precludes resection.

Initially, the evaluation of complete resectability of the tumor is made. Dissection of the hilar structures is necessary to ensure clear margins of the bronchial artery and veins. Mediastinal nodes are removed. If complete tumor resection is deemed possible, attention is then directed to the last questionable area of resectability.

An incision is made through the full thickness of the diaphragm in an area at least 2 cm from the tumor edge. This is widened sufficiently to permit digital exploration of the inferior surface to assess the depth of tumor invasion, namely, full thickness of diaphragm and clearance of intraperitoneal organs. If the liver or other intra-abdominal organ is invaded, the value of resection, even though technically possible, is in doubt. When tumor infiltration is limited to the diaphragm, the involved area can be resected in continuity with the lung.

Incision of the diaphragm is completed with maintenance of a 2-cm margin around the palpable tumor where possible (Fig. 32-66A). If the tumor invades any rib(s), they are resected en bloc as described above. After the diaphragm with tumor is completely encircled, the pulmonary resection is carried out in routine fashion.

Reconstruction of the diaphragm is always done on the left side. On the right side, if a pneumonectomy has been carried out and the liver maintains the seal between the pleural and peritoneal cavities, replacement may not be needed.

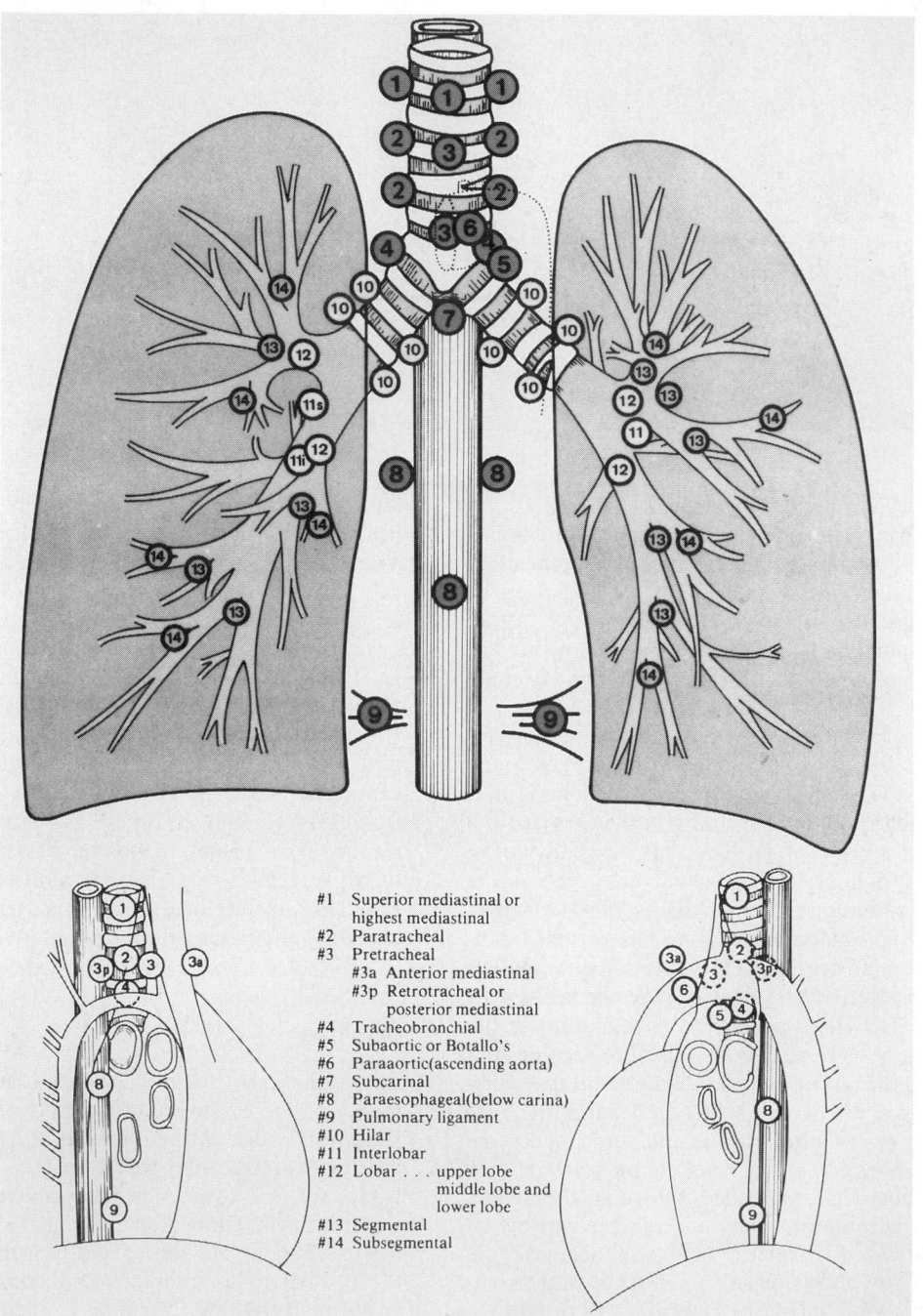

Figure 32-66.   Lymph node map showing the location, name, and number of the various regional lymph nodes. (From Naruke T, Suemasu K, Ishikawa S et al: Lymph node mapping and curability at various levels of metastasis in resected lung cancer. J Thorac Cardiovasc Surg 76:832, 1978, with permission.)

If a portion of the lung remains, an intact or repaired diaphragm will be an essential part of normal postoperative physiology (Fig. 32-66B).

When a small portion only is resected, reapproximation of the cut surfaces is easily managed with interrupted nonabsorbable sutures. When the defect is too large to permit the edges to be approximated, a plastic prosthesis is sutured in place to close the defect. Any strong mesh will suffice; however, a Gore-Tex patch is impervious to air and fluid and makes an excellent replacement.

Postoperatively, no special precautions are necessary for diaphragmatic resection. The survival rate is related not to the diaphragmatic resection but rather to the completeness of the resection and the incidence of mediastinal nodal involvement.

Other Mediastinal Structures

Pericardium

The pericardium is in contact with the lung over most of its surface. Invasion of the pericardium in resectable lung cancers remains unusual despite this anatomic approximation. When exploration of the pleural cavity demonstrates invasion into the pericardium, this aspect of resectability is addressed first.

Pericardiotomy is performed carefully, away from the phrenic nerve. This nerve should be spared if possible unless a pneumonectomy is done. Digital exploration of the pericardial cavity gives accurate assessment of the location of the normal anatomy and its relation to the invading tumor and thus provides assessment of resectability.

When resection is judged to be possible, the dissection is begun. If it makes hilar accessibility easier, the pericardium is usually dissected first and maintained en bloc with the lung, especially if a pulmonary vein or artery is involved. The pericardium should always be reconstructed to prevent extrusion of an atrial appendage or cardiac torsion, either of which results in disaster. Any of the synthetic meshes (Vicryl, Prolene, or Marlex) or a Gore-Tex patch can be sutured to the pericardial defect to prevent this from happening. A small pericardial defect or a complete left defect may not need repair.

Postoperative Care. When a 1-mm Gore-Tex patch is used, serial echocardiograms should be taken for indication of the onset of pericardial effusion. When any of the meshes are used, this not a problem. Prognosis relates not to extension into the pericardium but rather to the ability to achieve complete resection and to the status of the mediastinal lymph nodes. Invasion of the pericardium does not preclude complete resection, which can and should be performed when indicated.

Esophagus

Combined resections of esophagus and lung have been performed for cancers originating in either organ, but these cases are rare and reported anecdotally. In instances of primary lung cancer involving the esophagus, it is almost always by subcarinal lymph node spread rather than by extension of the primary tumor. The prognosis is dismal. When dysphagia is a predominant symptom an intraluminal esophageal stent will provide the best palliation. The esophagus should rarely be resected. When the esophagus is directly invaded by an adjacent tumor, en bloc resection of both tumors can be considered if there is no mediastinal lymph node involvement.

Very careful preoperative diagnostic studies, including barium swallow, esophagoscopy, and CT scan of thorax and abdomen, to rule out metastatic disease are imperative. Only if the disease is confined to the primary site should resection be considered. In right-sided lung tumors, the lobe is resected. A second incision is then needed. Either a throracoabdominal or a midline incision with the operating table tilted to the right is possible. Mobilization of the stomach is carried out and the anastomosis is performed in the right hemithorax. In left-sided tumors a thoracoabdominal approach may be considered. Another option is total esophagectomy with transportation of the stomach to the neck, thus avoiding an intrathoracic.

Postoperative Care. Antibiotic coverage and good respiratory toilet are essential after this extensive resection. A normal Gastrografin swallow on day 7 will allow all tubes to be removed. No survival data are available, as these cases are so few; occasionally long-term survivors have been reported. Careful patient selection is mandatory.

Miscellaneous

Other intrathoracic structures are only rarely invaded by lung carcinomas. The right atrium may have tumor from the pulmonary vein or from direct invasion by the primary. Intrapericardial invasion of the pulmonary artery or veins carries a grave prognosis and can only rarely be resected. The vagus and phrenic nerves are infrequently involved by direct invasion and can usually be sacrificed with impunity.

COMMENTS AND CONTROVERSIES

Surgical resection remains the sole modality with acceptable survival results in lung cancer. The extension of this technique beyond the usual boundaries to achieve a cure when none seems possible has been described above.

Some techniques are more risky than others. Chest wall resection and reconstruction is well within the capacity of a well trained general thoracic surgeon. Diaphragmatic and pericardial resections should be routinely performed when involvement is found. Vertebral body resection requires an interested, knowledgeable neurosurgeon and/or orthopedic surgeon. Superior vena cava and esophageal resection should be performed only by those whose interest in these problems has made them adept at treating them. In all cases selection of the proper candidate for the proposed resection is paramount.

Patient safety intra- and postoperatively, along with as much survival time as can be achieved, is the ultimate goal.

P.M.M.

KEY REFERENCES

Arnold PG, Pairolero PC: Chest wall reconstruction: experience with no consecutive patients. Ann Surg 199:725, 1984

Chu CJ, Tazis H, MacRae ML: Replacement of superior vena cava with the spiral composite vein graft. Ann Thorac Surg 17:553, 1974

Illustrated description of technique required for construction the spiral composite vein substitute for the vena cava.

Dartevelle P, Chapelier A, Navajas M et al: Replacement of the superior vena cava with polytetrafluoroethylene grafts combined with resection of mediastinal-pulmonary malignant: report of 13 cases. J Thorac Cardiovasc Surg 94:361, 1987

Long-term follow-up and detailed presentation of techniques.

McCaughan BC, Martini N, Bains MS, McCormack P: Chest wall invasion in carcinoma of the lung: therapeutic and prognostic implication. J Thorac Cardiovasc Surg 89:836, 1985

McCormack PM, Martini N: Tumors involving the diaphragm. p. 256. In Rob CG, Roe BB (eds): Paradiaphragmatic Surgery. Appleton Davies, Pasadena, 1991

Nakahara K, Ohno K, Mastumura A et al: Extended operation for lung cancer invading the aortic arch and superior vena cava. J Thorac Cardiovasc Surgery 97:428, 1989

Very extensive surgery was successfully carried out, but its value remains to be proved.

REFERENCES

Boyd AD, Shaw WW, McCarthy JG et al: Immediate reconstruction of full-thickness chest wall defects. Ann Thorac Surg 32:337, 1981

Brewer LA III: The contributions of the Second Auxilliary Surgical Group to military surgery during World War II with special reference to thoracic surgery. Ann Surg 197:318, 1983

Carrel T, Nachbur B, Veraguth P: En bloc resection for bronchogenic carcinoma with chest wall invasion: value of preoperative radiotherapy. Eur J Cardiothorac Surg 4:534, 1990

Dartevell PG, Chapelier AR, Pastorino U et al: Long term follow-up after prosthetic replacement of the superior vena cava combined with resection of mediastinal-pulmonary malignant tumors. J Thorac Cardiovasc Surg 102:259, 1991 p. 259–65.

DeMeester TR, Alertucci M, Dawson PJ et al: Management of tumor adherent to the vertebral column. J Thorac Cardiovasc Surg 97:373, 1989

Doty DB: Bypass of superior vena cava: six year's experience with spiral vein graft for obstruction of superior vena cava due to benign and malignant disease. J Thorac Cardiovasc Surg 83:326, 1982

Esato K, Shintani K, Yasutake S et al: Experimental replacement of vena cava with expanded polytetrafluroethylene graft. Int Surg 66:227, 1981

Graham EV, Beggie IA, Churchill EO, Eloesser L: Thoracic Surgery. WB Saunders, Philadelphia, 1943

Heelan RT, Demas BE, Caravelle JF et al: Magnetic resonance and computed tomography of superior sulcus tumors. Radiology 170:637, 1989

Hilaris P, Nori D: Intraoperative therapy for nonresectable disease. p. 207. In Eschapasse H, Delarue NC (eds): International Trends in General Thoracic Surgery. Vol. 1. Lung Cancer. WB Saunders, Philadelphia, 1985

McCormack PM, Bains MS, Beattie EJ Jr, Martini N: New trends in skeletal reconstruction after resection of chest wall tumors. Ann Thorac Surg 31:45, 1981

Parham DW: Thoracic resections for tumors growing from the bony chest wall. Trans South Surg Assoc 2:223, 1899

Patterson GA, Ilves R, Ginsberg RJ et al: The value of adjuvant radiotherapy in pulmonary and chest wall resection for bronchogenic carcinoma. Ann Thorac Surg 24:692, 1982

Piccione W Jr, Faber LP, Warren WH: Superior vena caval reconstruction using autologous pericardium. Ann Thorac Surg 50:417, 1990

Pickler JM, Pairolero PC, Weiland LM et al: Bronchogenic carcinoma with chest wall invasion: factors affecting surgical following en bloc resection. Ann Thorac Surg 34:684, 1982

Sundaresan N, Bains MS, McCormack PM: Surgical treatment of spinal cord compression in patients with lung cancer. Neurosurgery 16:350, 1985

Toty L, Bakdach H: Repair of loss of substance of the thoracic wall and pericardium using a net of resorbable material. Nouv Presse Med 11:3265, 1982

Tou Y, Isobe M, Tutina et al: Suspected primary tumor in the diaphragm revealing large cell carcinoma in the lung with sarcomatous change. Nippon Kyobu Geka Gakkai Zasshi 38:1083, 1990

Trastik VF, Pairolero PC, Piehler JM et al: En bloc (non-chest wall) resections for bronchogenic carcinoma with parietal fixation. J Thorac Cardiovasc Surg 87:352, 1984

Mediastinal Lymph Node Dissection

Tsuguo Naruke

HISTORICAL NOTE

Surgical therapy of lung cancer by pneumonectomy combined with mediastinal lymph node dissection was reported as early as the 1940s by Allison (1946) and Brock (1948). Others, including Cahan and co-workers (1951), Weinberg (1951), and Brock and Whytehead (1958), later reported on variations of this combined procedure.

Allison (1946) referred to intrapericardial pneumonectomy with dissection of mediastinal tissue and lymph nodes as *radical pneumonectomy*. This procedure involves opening the pericardium to remove the hilum and lung together. Brock (1948) suggested that the dissection of lymph nodes in an expanded area be termed *block dissection pneumonectomy*.

Initially, lobectomy was recommended only for elderly patients with poor cardiopulmonary reserve (Jonson, et al., 1958). In 1960 Cahan reported on radical lobectomy as an alternative to pneumonectomy. Radical lobectomy is an operation in which one or two lobes of an entire lung are excised in a block dissection with their hilar and mediastinal lymphatics. The number of cases in which a curative lobectomy can be performed has grown as a result of the improvements in early detection of lung cancer.

The technique of lymph node dissection was based on the lymphatic studies by Rouviere (1932), Nohl (1962), and Borrie (1965). My own work (Naruke, 1967) on the staging and mapping of the lymph nodes has further clarified staging and lymphatic dissection.

HISTORICAL READINGS

Allison PR: Intrapericardial approach to the lung root in the treatment of bronchial carcinoma by dissection pneumonectomy. J Thorac Surg 15:99, 1946

Borrie J: Lung Cancer: Surgery and Survival. Appleton & Lange, East Norwalk, CT, 1965

Brock RC: Bronchial carcinoma. Br Med J 2:737, 1948

Brock RC, Whytehead LL: Radical pneumonectomy for bronchial carcinoma. Br J Surg 43:8, 1958

Cahan WG: Radical lobectomy. J Thorac Surg 39:555, 1960

Cahan WG, Watson WL, Pool JL: Radical pneumonectomy. J Thorac Surg 22:449, 1951

Jonson JJ, Kirby CK, Blackmore WS: Should we insist on radical pneumonectomy as a routine procedure in the treatment of carcinoma of the lung? J Thorac Surg 36:309, 1958

Naruke T: The spread of lung cancer and its relevance to surgery. Jpn J Surg 68:1607, 1967

Nohl HC: The Spread of Carcinoma of the Bronchus. Lloyd-Luke Ltd., London, 1962

Rouviere H: Anatomie des lymphatiques de l'homme. Massonet, Paris, 1932

Weinberg JA: Identification of regional lymph nodes in the treatment of bronchogenic carcinoma. J Thorac Surg 22:517, 1951

LYMPH NODE NOMENCLATURE

Although there had been many earlier reports on the topography of mediastinal lymph nodes and on lymphatic routes, until 1967 there was no standard lymph node terminology. Analysis of lymph node dissection combined with lung resection for lung cancer cases led to the development of the nomenclature of lymph node sites (Naruke, 1967; Naruke and Suemasu, 1976). This map was adopted in 1976 by the American Joint Committee for Cancer Staging and End Results Reporting (AJC) to help in the classification of lung cancer (AJC, 1979; Martini, 1976; Mountain, 1976), and was published as the TNM classification of malignant tumors by the Union Internationale Contre le Cancer (UICC) in 1980 (Sellers, 1980). Other modified versions of this classification have been published; however, the original mapping as outlined below was authorized by the Japan Lung Cancer Society (1987) in 1980 and continues to be used by my institution (Figs. 32-66 and 32-67).

1. The superior nodes corresponding to the upper third of that part of the trachea within the thorax. These include the nodes located around the trachea, the site of which is defined by a horizontal line at the height of the upper rim of the subclavian artery and a horizontal line at the center point of the trachea, where the upper rim of the brachiocephalic vein ascends to the left, crossing in front of the trachea.

2. The paratracheal nodes which are between nodes 1 and 4 lateral to the trachea

3. The pretracheal nodes, including nodes posterior to the trachea, which are called retrotracheal nodes (3p), and

nodes arising posterior to the brachiocephalic vein and the superior vena cava, called anterior mediastinal nodes (3a)

4. The tracheobronchial nodes, located on or near the angle between the trachea and the main bronchi. The nodes on the right side are level with and inside the azygos vein, and those on the left are inside the subaortic nodes

5. The subaortic (Botallo's) nodes, occurring at the ligamentum arteriosum

6. The para-aortic nodes, which are lateral to the ascending aorta and aortic arch and anterior to the vagus nerve

7. The subcarinal nodes, located below the point at which the trachea divides into the main bronchi

8. The paraesophageal nodes, located posterior to the trachea and carina and adjacent to the esophagus

9. The pulmonary ligament nodes, which are within the pulmonary ligament and include those in the posterior wall and lower part of the inferior pulmonary vein

10. Nodes in the periphery of the trachea and main bronchus

11. Interlobar nodes and nodes between the lobar bronchi. On the right they are classified according to location between the upper and middle lobes (11s) or between the middle and lower lobes (11i).

12. Nodes around the lobar bronchus

13. Nodes in the periphery of the segmental bronchi

14. Nodes around the subsegmental bronchi or in the periphery of the bronchi

GENERAL PRINCIPLES

Operative Approach

A double-lumen endobronchial tube is recommended for pulmonary resection combined with lymph node dissection. After the tube has been inserted into the trachea and its proper position confirmed with the pediatric fiberoptic bronchoscope, the tube is fixed.

In right lung cancer cases it is possible to perform a partial dissection of left mediastinal nodes through a standard posterolateral thoracotomy. We prefer to use the fourth intercostal space. In left lung cancer cases, however, a complete mediastinal node dissection cannot be performed because of anatomic constraints. A left posterolateral thoracotomy is usually performed in these cases, and an additional median sternotomy is necessary when complete dissection of pretracheal and/or contralateral nodes is indicated.

Dissection Technique

Through skillful use of scissors and electrocautery, the hilum and mediastinal organs are exposed. The pulmonary vein is ligated first, after which the mediastinal and hilar nodes and the lung are dissected en bloc without interrupting the lymphatics. The order of these procedures may have to be changed depending on the location or extension of the tumor; the rule is to perform a complete dissection as quickly as possible.

Before dissection is begun, the mediastinal pleura is totally separated from the pulmonary ligament from diaphragm to hilum, and the inferior mediastinum is separated from the neighboring fatty tissue and the esophagus. For dissection of the upper mediastinum, the mediastinal pleura is incised vertically from the upper margin of the hilar pleura toward the apex of the thorax, and the incision is held open with traction sutures. The vagus and phrenic nerves are taped and preserved carefully. Special care must be taken to prevent injury to the recurrent nerve.

The fatty tissue including lymph nodes, held by Allis intestinal forceps, is separated from the surrounding structures, which exposes arteries, veins, trachea, bronchi, esophagus, and nerves. It is important to dissect only the tissue enclosing the nodes and to avoid damaging the nodes themselves; if the nodes are crushed, cancerous cells can disseminate into the operative field. Fine blood vessels and lymphatics are ligated to avoid postoperative bleeding and/or exudation of lymphatics.

SITE-SPECIFIC CONSIDERATIONS

Lymph node tumors of the right upper lobe metastasize to peribronchial, lobar, interlobar, hilar, and superior mediastinal nodes; retrograde metastasis to nodes in the middle and lower lobes is rare, and subcarinal spread is infrequent. Upper lobectomy is therefore combined with dissection of lymph nodes of the superior mediastinum, subcarinal area, and middle trunk only. With middle lobe tumors, metastases tend to occur to the hilum, the bifurcation of the trachea, and the superior mediastinum and particularly to sump nodes of the upper or lower lobe. If these sump nodes are involved, combined resection of the upper and lower lobes should be performed. Right lower lobe tumors tend to metastasize to middle lobe sump nodes and nodes around the main bronchus, the bifurcation of the trachea, and the upper mediastinum. In such cases bilobectomy, including sump nodes as far as the upper mediastinum, is necessary.

In left upper lobe tumors, metastases to the subaortic and para-aortic nodes occur in a high percentage of cases, while metastases to nodes in the superior mediastinum are less frequent. Resection of the left upper lobe combined with dissection of the upper mediastinum should be performed in cases of left upper lobe tumor. Since the probability of metastasis to subcarinal and subaortic nodes exists, complete dissection of lymph nodes around the upper lobe and main bronchus is necessary. When there are metastases to the superior mediastinum and/or subcarinal lymph nodes, it is necessary to carry out a dissection of the contralateral (right) mediastinal nodes.

Dissection of Right Mediastinal Lymph Nodes

After the hilar pleura has been opened and the phrenic nerve taped, the peripheral fatty tissue is dissected toward the right lobe, and the superior pulmonary vein is exposed. The azygos vein can be dissected at this time or it can be done after dissection of the mediastinal nodes. The azygos vein is divided whenever the lymph nodes are enlarged, metastases are suspected, perinodal invasion and adhesion are extensive, or an expansive tumor is apparent. If pretracheal (3) and tracheobronchial (4) nodes are small and soft, the upper medi-

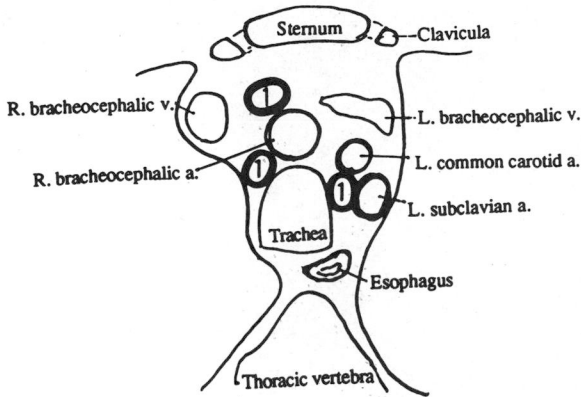

Transverse section through at the level of
the 2nd thoracic vertebra

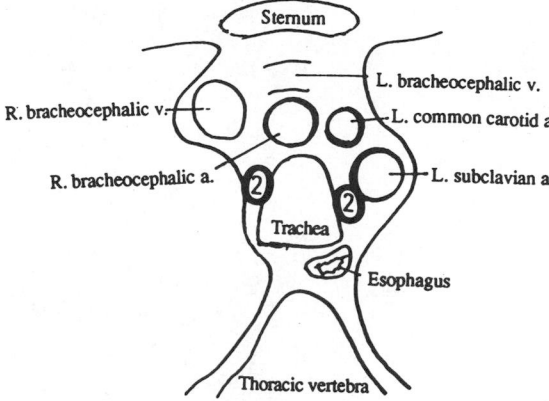

Transverse section through at the level of
the 3rd thoracic vertebra

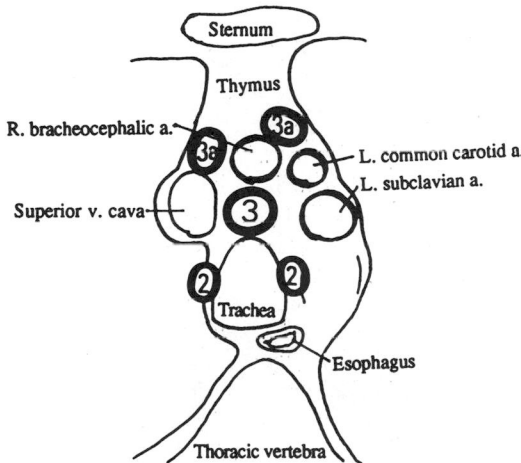

Transverse section through the upper part of
the 4th thoracic vertebra

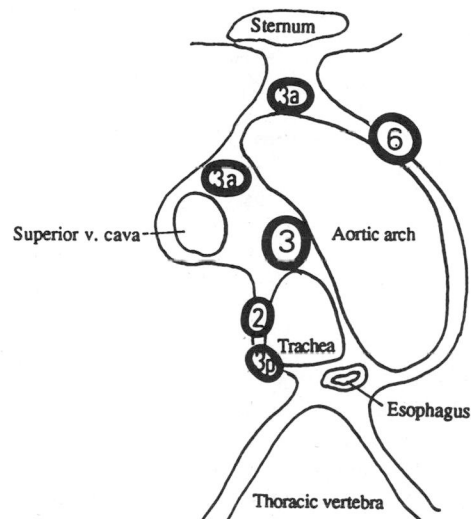

Transverse section through at the level of
the 4th thoracic vertebra

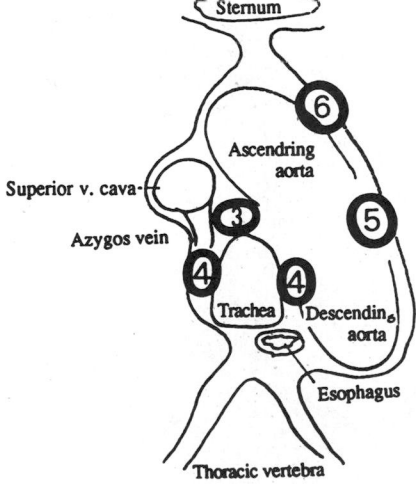

Transverse section through the upper part of
the 5th thoracic vertebra

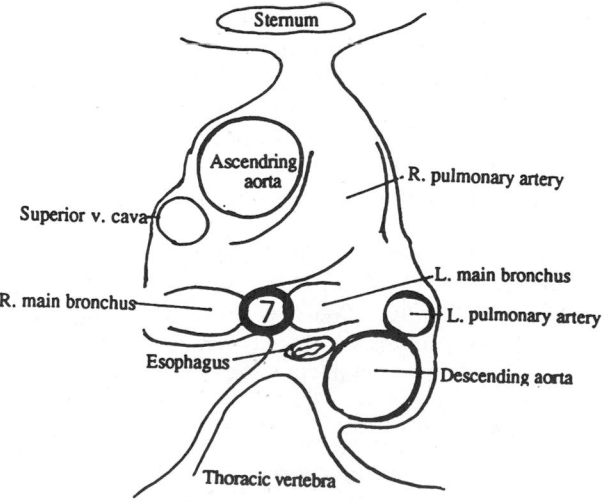

Transverse section through the lower part of
the 5th thoracic vertebra

Figure 32-67.   Sites of lymph nodes as seen on CT scan.

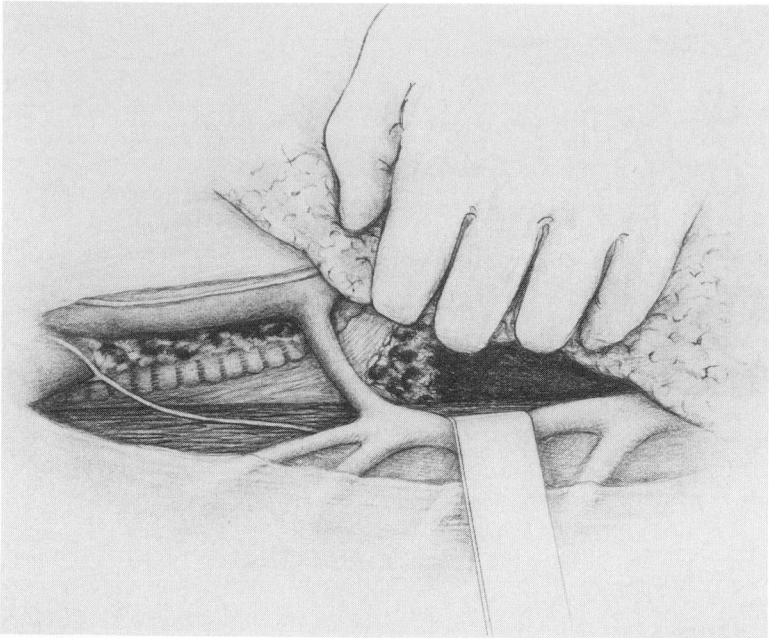

Figure 32-68. Exposure of subcarinal lymph nodes for dissection.

astinal nodes can be dissected clearly without dividing the azygos vein.

Posterior Mediastinum

The lung is retracted and the vagus nerve is exposed and taped. The pulmonary branch of the vagus nerve is then cut. Next, a flexible intestinal spatula is inserted into the bifurcation of the trachea in order to open it, with care to avoid injury to the descending aorta. After exposure of the pericardium, the lowest subcarinal (7) nodes are dissected, the contralateral left main bronchial (10) nodes are pulled by lymph node forceps, and the subcarinal (7) nodes are dissected. The branch of the bronchial artery that runs from the tracheal bifurcation to the posterior wall of the right main bronchus is ligated and divided. As the medial side of the left main bronchial cartilage is exposed, the contralateral left main bronchial (10) nodes are dissected, as are the subcarinal (7), right main bronchial (10), and upper right bronchial (12) nodes. As is seen during the dissection, these nodes are connected to the nodes of the right upper lobe bronchus (Fig. 32-68).

Dissection of lymph nodes in the pulmonary ligament (9) is started from the lowest part of the pulmonary ligament and continued with the dissection of paraesophageal (8) nodes. Regional anatomy for dissection of lymph nodes in the hilum and mediastinum in a right pneumonectomy is shown in Fig. 32-69.

Superior and Anterior Mediastinum

At the apex of the thorax, the subclavian and brachiocephalic arteries are exposed and the right recurrent nerve is identified. In dissecting the right superior mediastinum there is hardly ever a situation in which lymph node metastasis would

force one to sacrifice the recurrent nerve. This may be necessary, however, with metastasis to the left mediastinal lymph nodes and the left recurrent nerve. Further dissection contin-

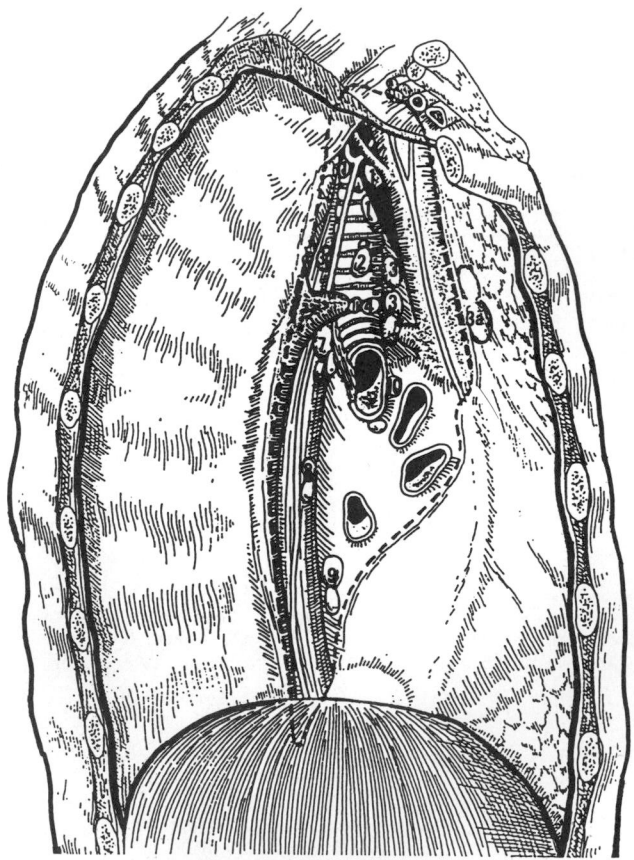

Figure 32-69. Regional anatomy for dissection of the right hilum and mediastinum.

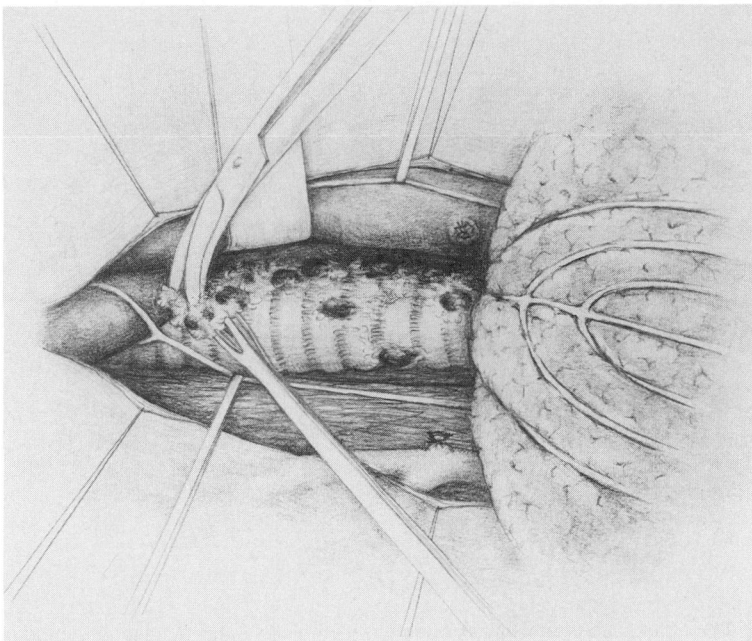

Figure 32-70.   Right upper mediastinal lymph node dissection.

ues downward, exposing the brachiocephalic artery, superior vena cava, pretracheal fascia, and right wall of the ascending aorta. The small veins that flow into the superior vena cava from mediastinal fatty tissue are ligated and transected.

Superior mediastinal (1), posterior mediastinal (3p), paratracheal (2), tracheobronchial (4), and paratracheal (3) nodes are dissected in order. The esophagus is thus exposed. This dissection is facilitated by retracting the innominate vein with a spatula (Fig. 32-70).

Dissection of the vagus nerve, which has been taped in advance, is begun toward the inferior side of the trachea, while tracheal dissection is begun posteriorly. Left tracheobronchial (4) nodes are dissected, and the trachea, bronchus, and pulmonary artery are totally exposed. Metastasis to anterior mediastinal (3a) nodes often occurs when metastases to the hilum and other mediastinal nodes are present. However, there are occasional cases in which the anterior mediastinal (3a) nodes are positive and the hilar and other mediastinal nodes are uninvolved (skip lesions). All these nodes should be removed.

Specific Considerations

Upper Lobe Tumors.   Following division of the superior pulmonary vein and mediastinal node dissection, interlobar separation is carried out and the ascending artery is ligated and divided. The lymph nodes between lobes are then dissected. These ''sump'' nodes have to be dissected as completely as possible, together with the upper lobe bronchial nodes.

In cases of upper lobe cancer in which it is suspected that dissection of superior interlobar (11s) nodes by lobectomy might have been insufficient, dissection of these nodes as well as peribronchial (12) nodes in the upper lobar bronchus requires bilobectomy with removal of the middle lobe. Pneu-

monectomy is indicated when there are large sump nodes and when involved nodes or the tumor itself infiltrates the bronchus and/or the pulmonary artery.

Once pretracheal (3) nodes are dissected, the right pulmonary artery is exposed. Upper lobectomy combined with dissection of mediastinal nodes is completed. After ligation and division of the right upper lobe artery, the lymph nodes attached to the upper lobe bronchus and the tracheobronchial (4) nodes are dissected (Fig. 32-71). In upper lobe tumors, it is not necessary to dissect paraesophageal (8) and pulmonary ligament (9) nodes.

Middle Lobe Tumors.   With middle lobe tumors, after the pulmonary vein has been ligated and divided, bilobectomy of middle and upper lobes or of middle and lower lobes is performed, depending on the extent of metastasis to the interlobar (11s or 11i) nodes. Some cases may require pneumonectomy depending on the extent of metastasis to lymph nodes.

Lower Lobe Tumors.   For tumors of the lower lobe, the pulmonary ligament (9) nodes are dissected and the pulmonary ligament is divided. The dissection is carried out in ascending order to include both and the pulmonary ligament (9) and paraesophageal (8) nodes. The inferior pulmonary vein is exposed, ligated, and divided.

The esophagus is retracted with a flexible intestinal spatula, to reveal the tracheal bifurcation. The nodes at the bifurcation of the trachea (7) and those in the periphery of the right main bronchus (10) are dissected, after which the fissures are separated. After dissection of the interlobar, lower lobe bronchus, subcarinal, and right main bronchus nodes, the inferior pulmonary artery is ligated and divided, and the lower lobe bronchus is transected and its stump closed. The upper mediastinal nodes are then dissected as described above.

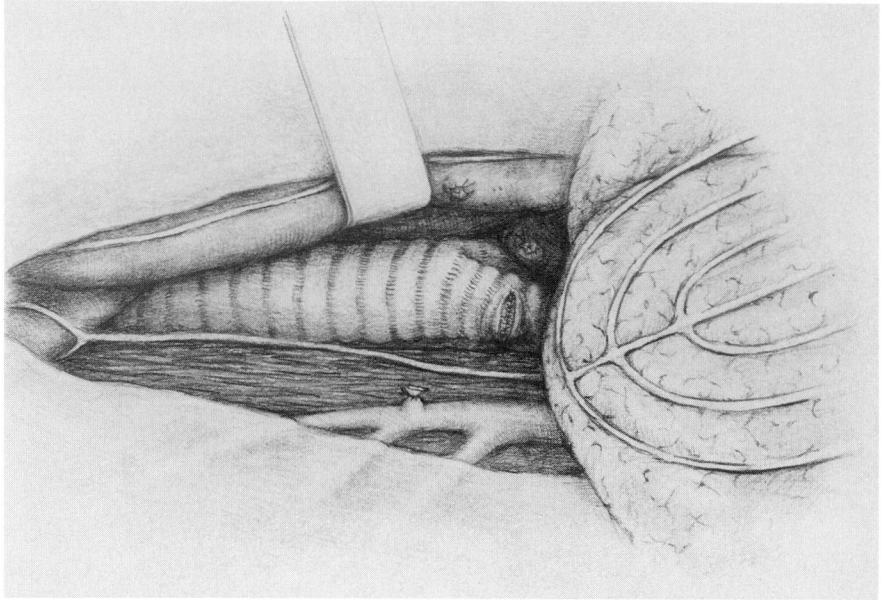

Figure 32-71. Status after right upper lobectomy combined with mediastinal lymph node dissection.

Dissection of Left Mediastinal Lymph Nodes

Posterior Mediastinum

In operations on the left mediastinum, dissection of subcarinal (7) nodes is also performed prior to dissection of the superior mediastinum. Good exposure of the subcarinal region is obtained by retracting the lung anteriorly. Following dissection of the pulmonary ligament (9) nodes, the mediastinal pleura is opened, and the vagus nerve is taped. The descending aorta and the esophagus are retracted posteriorly with a flexible intestinal spatula; the tracheal bifurcation is thus exposed (Fig. 32-72). The left lobar bronchus is exposed from the inferior side, lymph nodes around this bronchus are dissected, and the dissection is continued until it reaches the bifurcation of the left main bronchus, at which point the pulmonary branches of the vagus nerve are ligated and divided. The surgical visual field is widened by retracting the lung with the hand or with a lung retractor toward the surgeon. The subcarinal (7) nodes and then the left bronchial (10) nodes are dissected from the interior of the right main bronchus. At the carina the branch of the left bronchial artery is ligated and divided. Regional anatomy for dissection of hilar and mediastinal nodes in left pneumonectomy is shown in Fig. 32-73.

Anterior Mediastinum

The left superior mediastinum is different from the right superior mediastinum in that the limits of the right are not as well defined. It is most important to carry out the dissection of the subaortic (5) as well as the para-aortic (6) nodes. The wall of the left brachiocephalic vein, which runs from the top of the thoracic cavity to beneath the parietal pleura, is incised and exposed. The fatty tissue is identified and the incision is carried as far as the pleura; the dissection of fatty tissue is carried out further toward the hilum. The phrenic and the vagus nerves should be taped in advance. The posterior wall of the subclavian artery is then exposed. By exposing the side wall of the subclavian artery through the incision, it should be possible to dissect the superior mediastinal nodes between the common carotid and subclavian arteries. To make this procedure complete, however, it is necessary to mobilize the aortic arch or to use a transternal approach as well as to perform a complete pretracheal (3) node dissection. If the ligamentum arteriosum is divided, dissection of tracheobronchial (4) and subaortic (5) nodes becomes easy, and we prefer to divide this ligament routinely.

The upper mediastinal pleura is incised as far as the top of the thorax, and the phrenic and vagus nerves are taped. Four traction sutures are inserted in the mediastinal pleura, and the hemiazygos vein is ligated and divided.

After the fatty thymic tissue has been identified and the pericardium has been reached, the adipose tissue is removed,

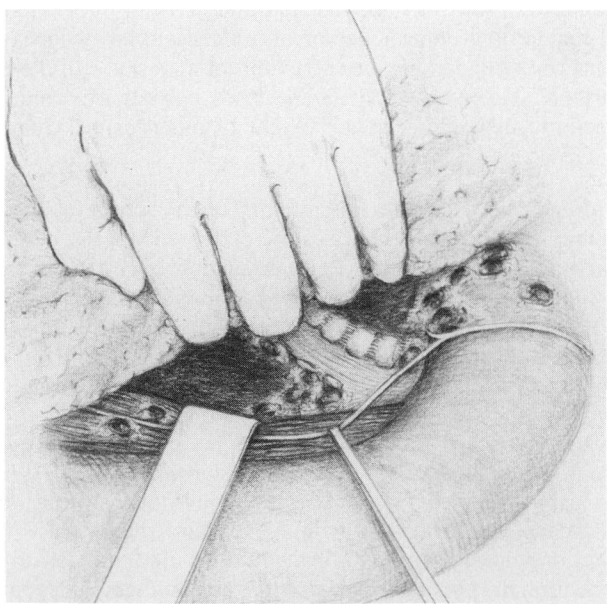

Figure 32-72. Exposure of subcarinal lymph nodes.

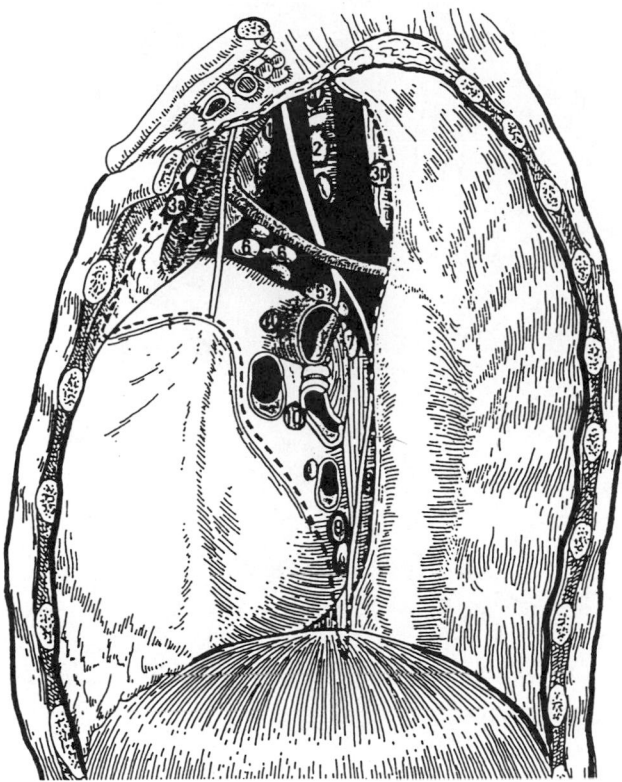

Figure 32-73. Regional anatomy for dissection of the left hilum and mediastinum.

the ascending aorta is exposed, and the para-aortic (6) nodes are dissected. The dissection is carried out toward the main pulmonary artery in the hilum. The left brachiocephalic (innominate) vein is also exposed. After this procedure, some of the anterior mediastinal (3) nodes can be dissected. Upon exposure of the left common carotid and left subclavian arteries, the dissection of the lymph nodes is carried out in a downward direction. Superior mediastinal (1) and paratracheal (2) nodes are then dissected (Fig. 32-74).

The thoracic duct, located at the deepest point between the left common carotid and left subclavian arteries, cannot

be seen. Damaging the mediastinal branches of the thoracic duct can cause chylothorax; therefore lymphatics and fine blood vessels should be ligated and divided.

Superior Mediastinum

When metastases are identified in subcarinal (7) and/or tracheobronchial (4) nodes, dissection of the superior mediastinal (1), paratracheal (2), pretracheal (3), and posterior mediastinal (3p) nodes and additional procedures are required to permit meticulous dissection. One of these procedures is mobilization of the aortic arch. The subclavian artery is taped and the pleura is incised posterior to the aorta. Intercostal arteries are ligated and divided as necessary, and the descending aorta is taped. The left subclavian artery and the aorta are thus moved anteriorly, and the left wall of the trachea and esophagus are exposed. The superior mediastinal (1), paratracheal (2), pretracheal (3) or retrotracheal (3p), and anterior mediastinal (3a) nodes are dissected (Fig. 32-75). At this time careful attention will prevent damage to the recurrent nerve, which runs upward along the side wall of the trachea. By division of the ligamentum arteriosum, tracheobronchial (4) nodes can be dissected easily, as previously described.

Another procedure to extend mediastinal lymph node dissection is through a median sternotomy by changing the position of the patient from lateral to supine (Figs. 32-76 and 32-77).

Specific Considerations

Upper Lobe Tumors. The phrenic nerve is taped, the lymph nodes in the periphery of the pulmonary vein are dissected, and the superior pulmonary vein is exposed, ligated, and divided. After dissection of the nodes between the upper and lower lobe bronchi, the lobes are separated and the branches of the pulmonary artery in the tissue are ligated and divided. After the upper lobe bronchus has been exposed together with the dissected nodes, it is divided, which completes the lobectomy and mediastinal lymph node dissection.

Lower Lobe Tumors. The pulmonary ligament (9) nodes are dissected, and the inferior pulmonary vein is exposed,

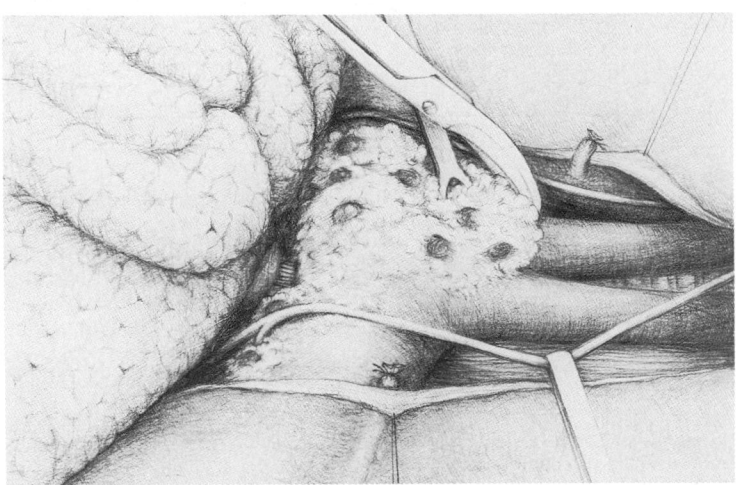

Figure 32-74. Left upper mediastinal lymph node dissection.

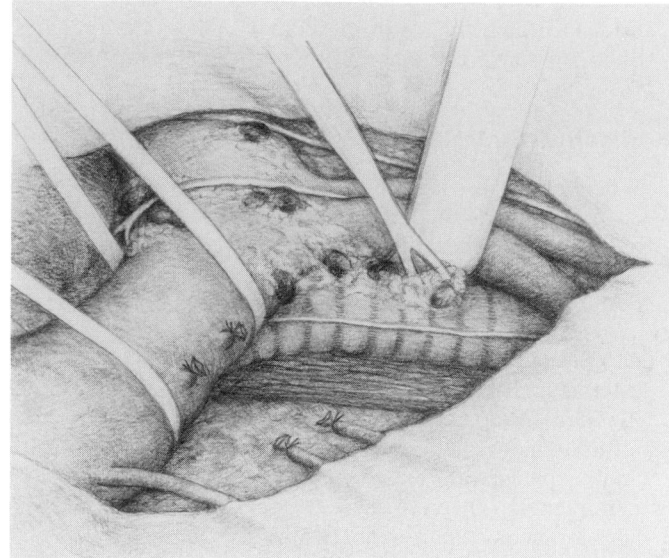

Figure 32-75. Pretracheal lymph node dissection by turning the aorta.

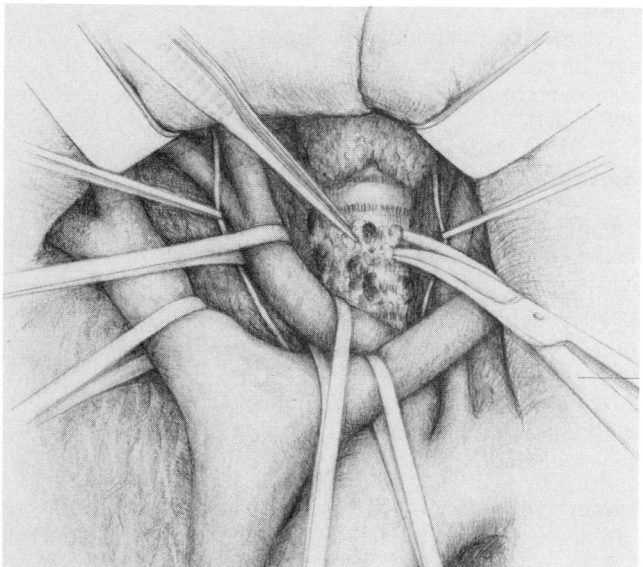

Figure 32-76. Upper mediastinal lymph node dissection through median sternotomy.

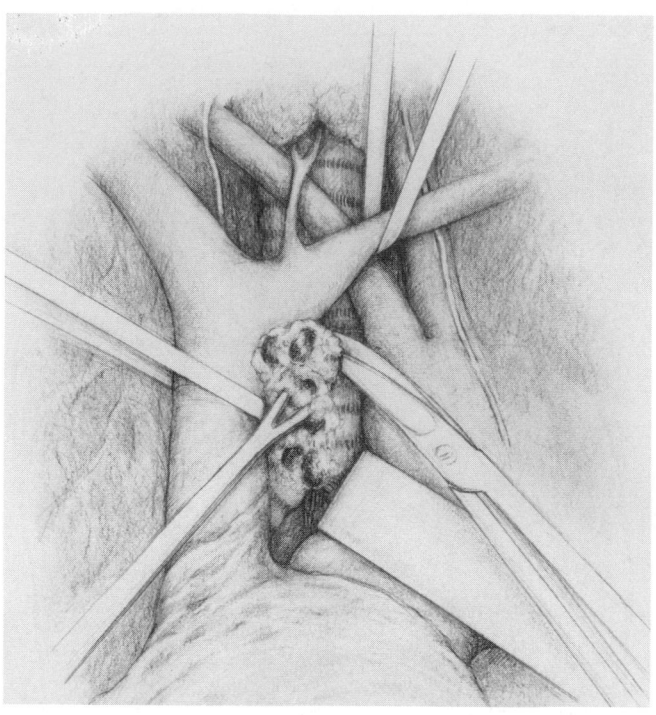

Figure 32-77. Pretracheal lymph node dissection through median sternotomy.

ligated, and divided. Next, the lung is retracted and contralateral hilar (10), subcarinal (7) nodes, and hilar (10) nodes are dissected. Then, after interlobar exposure and dissection of interlobar (11) nodes, lobectomy is completed by ligature and division of the pulmonary artery branches and division of the lower lobe bronchus.

Left Pneumonectomy. When left pneumonectomy is indicated, after dissection of the pulmonary ligament (9) nodes the dissection is continued in an upward direction as far as the inferior pulmonary vein, which is ligated and divided. Next, the superior pulmonary vein is ligated and divided. The dissection proceeds upward, and the paraesophageal (8) nodes, some of the hilar (10) nodes, and the subcarinal (7) nodes are dissected. The upper mediastinum is dissected, exposing the main pulmonary artery, which is then ligated and divided. Finally, by dividing the left main bronchus, the en bloc left pneumonectomy–lymph node dissection is completed.

KEY REFERENCES

Cahan WG: Radical lobectomy. J Thorac Cardiovasc Surg 39:555, 1960

Radical lobectomy is defined as an operation in which one or two lobes of the entire lung are excised en bloc, including regional hilar and mediastinal lymph nodes. The technical steps and clinical implication of the procedure are discussed on the basis of radical lobectomies successfully performed at the Memorial Sloan-Kettering Cancer Center.

Naruke T, Suemasu K, Ishikawa S et al: Lymph node mapping and curability at various levels of metastasis in resected lung cancer. J Thorac Cardiovasc Surg 76:832, 1978

The first paper using mapping classification to record all patients with lung cancer staged intraoperatively and with nodal metastases. The paper also discusses the spread of lung cancer and postoperative results. Lymph node sites are well classified and illustrated in color. Recognized worldwide for its contribution to radical operations for lung cancer.

Nohl, HC: The Spread of Carcinoma of the Bronchus. Lloyd-Luke, London, 1962

A detailed analysis of anatomy, pathology, and clinical behavior of the spread of lung cancer, especially lymphatic spread of resected cases of lung cancer.

REFERENCES

Allison PR: Intrapericardial approach to the lung root in the treatment of bronchial carcinoma by dissection pneumonectomy. J Thorac Cardiovasc Surg 15:99, 1946

American Joint Committee for Cancer Staging and End Results Reporting, Task Force on Lung Cancer: Staging of Lung Cancer, 1979

American Thoracic Society: Clinical staging of primary lung cancer. Am Rev Respir Dis 127:659, 1983

Borrie J: Lung Cancer: Surgery and Survival. Appleton & Lange, East Norwalk, CT, 1965

Brock RC: Bronchial carcinoma. Br Med J 2:737, 1948

Brock RC, Whytehead LL: Radical pneumonectomy for bronchial carcinoma. J Thorac Cardiovasc Surg 43:8, 1958

Cahan WG: Radical lobectomy. J Thorac Surg 39:555, 1960

Cahan WG, Watson WL, Pool JL: Radical pneumonectomy. J Thorac Cardiovasc Surg 22:449, 1951

Carr DT: The staging of lung cancer. Am Rev Respir Dis 117:819, 1978

Gary MG, Barry HG, Leslie EQ et al: Normal mediastinal lymph nodes: number and size according to American Thoracic Society mapping. AJR 144:261, 1985

International Union Against Cancer (Union Internationale Contre le Cancer [UICC]): TNM Atlas. Illustrated Guide to the TNM/p TNM Classification of Malignant Tumors. 3rd Ed., Geneva, 1989, p. 134

Japan Lung Cancer Society: General Rules for Clinical and Pathological Recording of Lung Cancer. 3rd Ed., 1987

Jonson JJ, Kirby CK, Blackmore WS: Should we insist on radical pneumonectomy as a routine procedure in the treatment of carcinoma of the lung? J Thorac Cardiovasc Surg 36:309, 1958

Martini N: Improved methods of recording data in lung cancer. Clin Bull Memorial Sloan-Kettering Cancer Center 6:93, 1976

Mountain CF: Cancer of the Lung: Classification and Staging of Lung Cancer by Site. American Joint Committee for Cancer Staging and End Results Reporting. 1976, p. 95

Naruke T: The spread of lung cancer and its relevance to surgery. Jpn J Surg 68:1607, 1967

Naruke T, Suemasu K: Surgical treatment for lung cancer with metastasis to mediastinal lymph nodes. J Thorac Cardiovasc Surg 71:279, 1976

Nohl HC: The Spread of Carcinoma of the Bronchus, Lloyd-Luke Ltd., London, 1962

Rouvière H: Anatomie des lymphatiques de l'homme. Massonet, Paris, 1932

Sellers AH: A Brochure of Checklists. International Union Against Cancer (UICC), Geneva, 1980

Weinberg JA: Identification of regional lymph nodes in the treatment of bronchogenic carcinoma. J Thorac Cardiovasc Surg 22:517, 1951

Video-Assisted Thoracic Surgery

Ralph J. Lewis
Robert J. Caccavale
Glenn E. Sisler

DEFINITION

Video-assisted thoracic surgery (VATS) is a minimally invasive technique that allows complex intrathoracic surgery to be performed without making a thoracotomy incision. By using an operating telescope with a micro camera, intrathoracic structures are visualized on a monitor and operated upon through small intercostal incisions. Numerous procedures previously requiring a formal thoracotomy can be performed safely, precisely, and expeditiously.

HISTORICAL NOTE

In 1910 H. C. Jacobaeus performed the first thoracoscopy using an electrified cystoscope. In 1925 he reported 120 cases of thoracoscopy in which pleural adhesions were divided (pneumonolysis) in the treatment of tuberculosis and discussed his experience in the diagnosis of pleural tumors (Jacobaeus, 1910, 1922, 1925). Pneumonolysis remained the primary use of thoracoscopy until the advent of antituberculous medication in the 1950s.

We described a technique called direct diagnostic thoracoscopy in 1976 (Lewis, et al., 1976). A mediastinoscope was used to obtain tissue biopsies and evaluate the extent of mesothelioma (Lewis, et al., 1981). In retrospect, this was minimally invasive surgery. The technique of direct diagnostic thoracoscopy was advanced and refined during the ensuing years, including the use of two mediastinoscopes simultaneously, which provided better visualization and allowed a wider range of procedures to be performed.

With the development of microcameras and reliable fiberoptic equipment, urologists, gynecologists, and orthopaedists developed surgical techniques and gained considerable experience with endoscopic surgery. As optics and instrumentation improved, more complex surgery was performed. In the late 1980s, several general surgery pioneers developed video-assisted laparoscopic cholecystectomy. This quickly revolutionized surgery of the gallbladder. During this period of time we began using a technique different from that used in the abdomen. It was eventually called VATS.

HISTORICAL READINGS

Jacobaeus HC: Die Thorakoskopie und ihre praktische Bedeutung. Ergebn Ges Med 7:112, 1925

Jacobaeus HC: The practical importance of thoracoscopy in surgery of the chest. Surg Gynecol Obstet 34:289, 1922

Jacobaeus HC: Über die Möglichkeit, die Zystoskopie bei Untersuchung seroser Hohlungen anzuwenden. Munch Med Wochenschr 40:2090, 1910

Lewis RJ, Caccavale RJ, Sisler GE: 100 consecutive cases of imaged thoracic surgery. Ann Thorac Surg 54:421, 1992.

Lewis RJ, Caccavale RJ, Sisler GE: Video-assisted thoracic surgical resection of malignant lung tumors. J Thorac Cardiovasc Surg 104:1679, 1992; 1992b

Lewis RJ, Kunderman PJ, Sisler GE, Mackenzie JW: Direct diagnostic thoracoscopy. Ann Thorac Surg 21:536, 1976

Lewis RJ, Sisler GE, Mackenzie JW: Diffuse, mixed malignant pleural mesothelioma. Ann Thorac Surg 31:53, 1981

Mack M, Aronoff R, Acuff T et al: The present role of thoracoscopy in the diagnosis and treatment of disease of the chest. Ann Thorac Surg 54:403, 1992

Early in 1990 we began to visualize the intrathoracic space by means of a rigid fiberoptic operating telescope and microcamera with transmission of images to a video monitor (Lewis, et al., 1991). A wide variety of diagnostic and therapeutic procedures have been performed by using conventional thoracic surgical instruments through small intercostal incisions in conjunction with one-lung ventilation.

Complex intrathoracic surgical procedures have been performed without the inherent morbidity associated with traditional thoracotomy (Lewis, et al., 1992; Mack, et al., 1992; Miller, 1991; Newman, et al., 1992). Postoperative pain is reduced, use of medical services is minimized, hospitalization is shortened, and recovery time is markedly decreased.

INDICATIONS AND PATIENT SELECTION

VATS is a technique used to enter the chest. Not every patient's anatomy or disease allows the use of this approach; therefore patient selection is extremely important when considering this technique.

Diagnostic evaluation of the pleura has traditionally been the most common indication for thoracoscopy, and with the advent of improved optics and instrumentation, numerous procedures have now become generally accepted (box below). These include lung biopsy, excision of pulmonary nodules, bleb resection, parietal pleurectomy, pleural biopsy, empyemectomy, chemical and mechanical pleurodesis, mediastinal lymph node biopsy, biopsy and excision of mediastinal tumors, sympathectomy, and pericardial window construction.

Even more complex procedures have been performed with excellent early results. These include esophageal myotomy for achalasia, excision of mediastinal cysts, ablation of simple and complex bullae, pleurectomy for malignant pleural disease, and resection of certain primary lung cancers. Broader experience will be required to determine the true value of these procedures. Although lobectomy, pneumonectomy,

---

Indications for Video-Assisted Thoracic Surgery
Pleura
Diagnostic evaluation
Mechanical/chemical pleurodesis
Pleurectomy
Pulmonary
Lung biopsy
Resection of lung mass/nodule
Bleb resection
Bullae ablation
Pericardium
Pericardial drainage
Pericardiectomy
Mediastinum
Lymph node biopsy
Biopsy/resection of mediastinal mass
Biopsy/excision of mediastinal cyst
Vagotomy
Esophageal myotomy
Benign esophageal tumor resection
Thoracic duct ligation
Miscellaneous
ACID placement
Evaluation of thoracic trauma

esophagectomy, and hiatal hernia repair are now possible with VATS, further development of instrumentation and technique will be needed before VATS is widely applied to these procedures.

CONTRAINDICATIONS

There are several contraindications to VATS (box below) including an obliterated pleural space and inability to tolerate one-lung ventilation. Patients who are likely to have an obliterated pleural space are those with a history of empyema, tuberculosis, or previous thoracotomy. If the pleural space cannot be identified, a standard thoracotomy is performed. Inability to tolerate single-lung ventilation is determined by an unacceptably low oxygen saturation or abnormally elevated airway pressures. Patients who are ventilator-dependent are generally considered poor candidates for VATS.

Contraindications to Video-Assisted Thoracic Surgery
Absolute
Pleural symphysis
Inability to tolerate single-lung ventilation
Respiratory insufficiency with high airway pressures
Contralateral pneumonectomy
Relative
Previous thoracotomy
Previous VATS

EQUIPMENT

During the early development of VATS, many of the instruments used were based on those used for laparoscopic surgery. Since these were not always appropriate or adequate, standard thoracic surgical instruments were used through small intercostal incisions. A standard thoracotomy set should always be available in the event a thoracotomy is needed. VATS instrumentation is currently being developed at a rapid pace. As instrumentation improves, so will the ability to safely perform a greater variety of complex thoracic procedures. Commonly used instruments and devices are briefly described below.

Endoscopes

A variety of rigid and hybrid scopes (the hybrid instrument has a rigid shaft with a flexible tip) are available. They include a lens system connected with fiberoptic light bundles incorporated into the shaft. The 10-mm panoramic view scope with a zero-degree field of vision is most commonly used. Instruments with a field of vision of 30 or 45 degrees are available and are occasionally useful to view oblique areas of the thoracic cavity.

Light Sources

A high-intensity light source operates in a temperature range of 5,600 to 6,000 K. The higher this rating, the whiter the light, thus allowing better color resolution. The lamp is metal halide or xenon. Low-intensity light operates at around 3,400 K, giving a more yellow light. Colors are not as well represented at this intensity. Lamps in this category are tungsten and halogen.

Ports

Ports are metal or plastic sleeves used to introduce and remove instruments from the thoracic cavity. The trocar (Fig. 32-78) is a sharp-tipped removable rod placed within the sleeve to aid in insertion and to prevent blood from filling the sleeve. Some models have a Luer lock valve to attach an insufflation device or smoke evacuator.

Hemostasis

The monopolar electrocautery is frequently used with its own tip as well as with instruments that are properly insulated for use with the cautery. These include scissors, graspers, and forceps. Provision must be made to evacuate the smoke generated. The argon beam coagulator is a noncontact electrocoagulation instrument that uses argon gas to deliver radiofrequency energy. The stream of argon gas clears blood from the tissue to be coagulated, thus allowing better visualization and hemostasis. Little smoke is generated.

Smoke Evacuator

The plume generated by the electrocautery or laser can obscure the surgeon's vision and presents a potential health hazard to the operating room staff. Dedicated smoke evacuators are available which use a closed-circuit suction system to filter the plume, preventing its escape into the ambient air.

Staplers

Several manufacturers have developed endoscopic stapling devices. They are available in 30- and 60-mm lengths, are

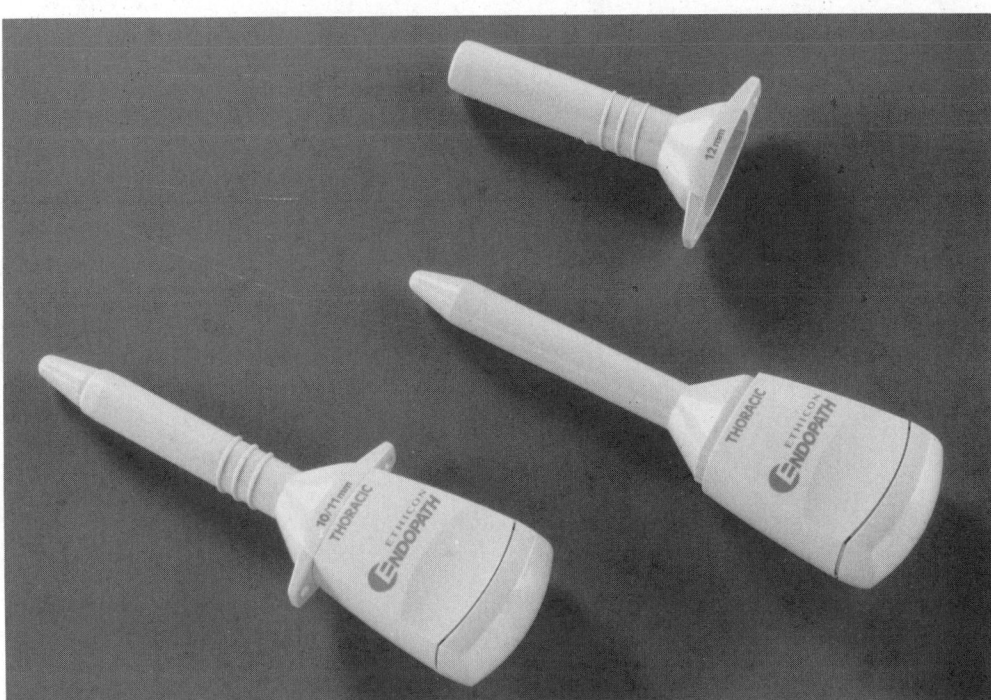

Figure 32-78. Thoracic trocar.

reloadable, place staggered rows of titanium staples, and simultaneously divide the tissue between the two inner rows of staples. These staplers can be placed through operating ports ranging in size to 18 mm. The ELC 60 and ELC 35 (Fig. 32-79) or Endo GIA 30 (Fig. 32-80) easily pass through 12-mm ports. When using small intercostal incisions, a variety of traditional staplers, such as the RL 30 and 60, can be used. Endoscopic clip appliers are available from several manufacturers as multifire devices with a rotating shaft and head (Fig. 32-81).

Instruments

Hand-held endoscopic instruments for VATS have been developed recently (Fig. 32-82). Graspers are instruments designed to hold tissue, which usually have a pistol grip with or without a ratchet mechanism. When grasping large structures such as the lung, we prefer standard ring forceps, as they are quite effective, easy to use, and atraumatic. Endoscopic scissors, particularly the disposable type, are effective and valuable instruments, since they remain sharp for the entire procedure. Nondisposable scissors tend to become dull. Long Metzenbaum and straight scissors can often be used effectively, particularly when dividing thick tissue.

OPERATING ROOM SETUP

Ideally, the operating team should consist of the surgeon, first assistant, camera operator, and scrub nurse. If personnel is limited, the scrub nurse can operate the camera. The rack of equipment, which usually includes the video monitor, the camera, the light source, and the video cassette recorder,

should be located at the end of the operating table perpendicular to the anticipated direction of the diagnostic telescope (Fig. 32-83). For most procedures the telescope is aimed toward the apex, and therefore the equipment should be positioned at the head of the table. To allow adequate space for the anesthesiologist, the table can be rotated 30 to 45 degrees.

While the patient is being prepared, the scrub nurse soaks the operating telescope in warm saline to minimize fogging of the lens when it is passed into the thoracic cavity. A complete thoracotomy tray should be in the operating room in the event a thoracotomy is required.

OPERATIVE TECHNIQUE

Patients undergoing VATS should be treated as are any patients undergoing thoracotomy. General anesthesia with split-lung ventilation and appropriate monitoring is essential. Monitoring should include arterial oxygen saturation, blood pressure, and end-tidal carbon dioxide concentration. An arterial line can be placed selectively. Proper airway management is essential when performing VATS. It is discussed in detail in Chapter 9.

Following establishment of general anesthesia and tube placement, the patient is placed in the lateral decubitus position. The table is flexed, which lowers the hips and allows unimpeded movement of the operating telescope (Fig. 32-84). The chest is then prepared and draped in the standard manner. The entire chest wall should be exposed to allow entry through any interspace, after which the ipsilateral lung is collapsed. An initial 1- to 2-cm long incision is made with a scalpel. The pleural space is entered, and a small clamp

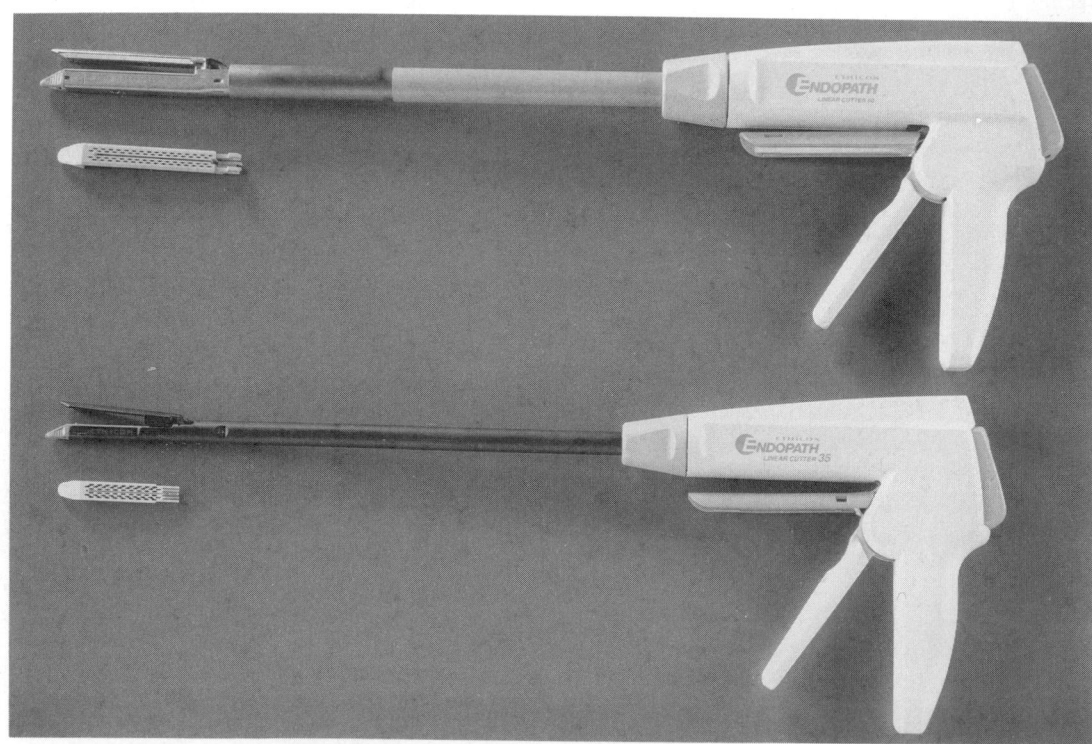

Figure 32-79. ELC 60 stapler (*top*) and ELC 35 stapler (*bottom*).

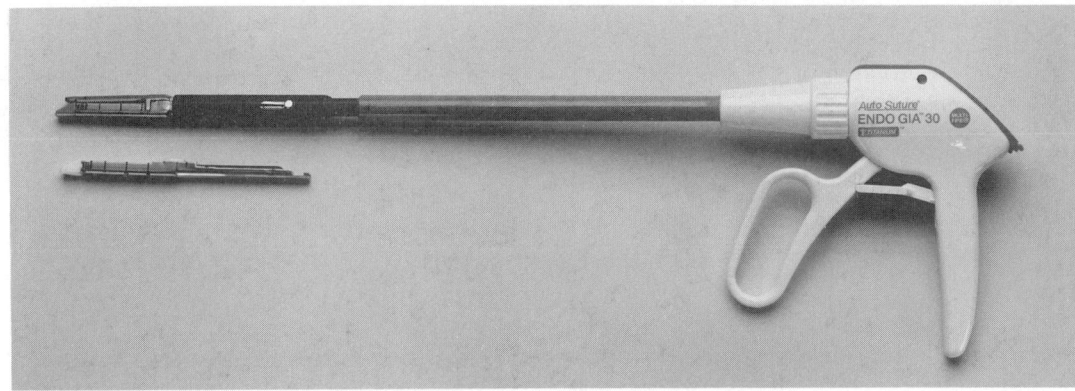

Figure 32-80.   Endo GIA 30 stapler.

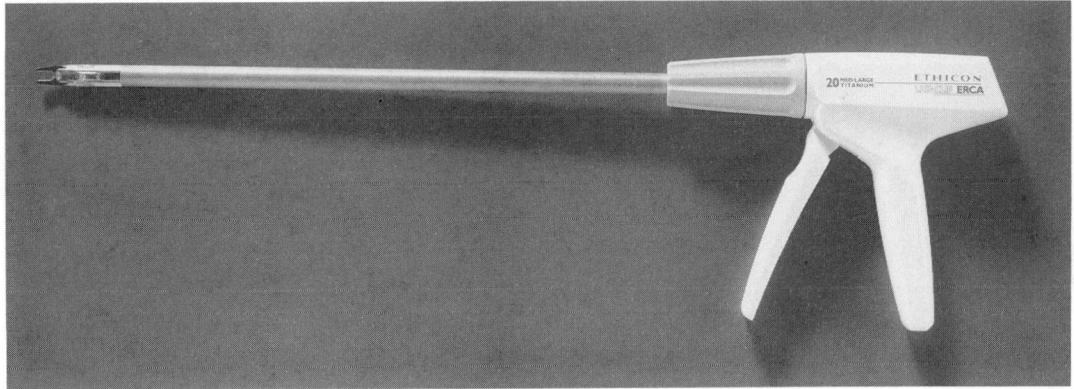

Figure 32-81.   Endoscopic clip applier.

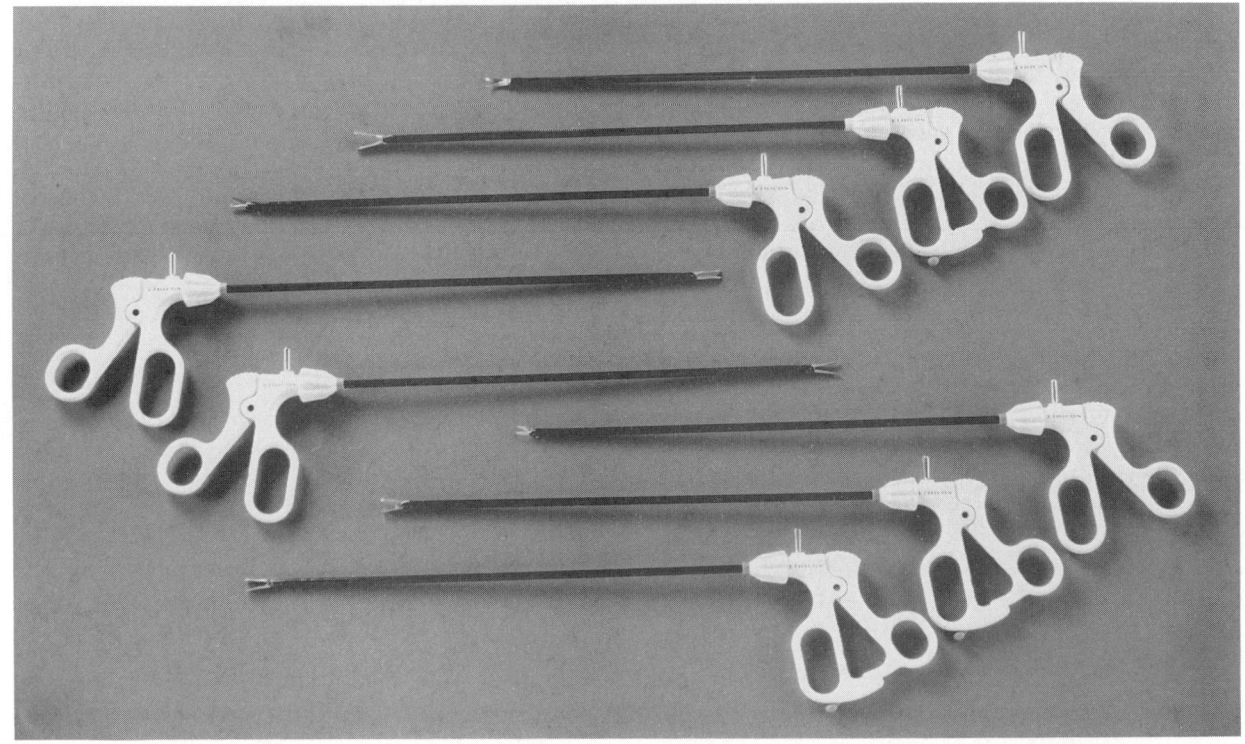

Figure 32-82.   Endoscopic instruments.

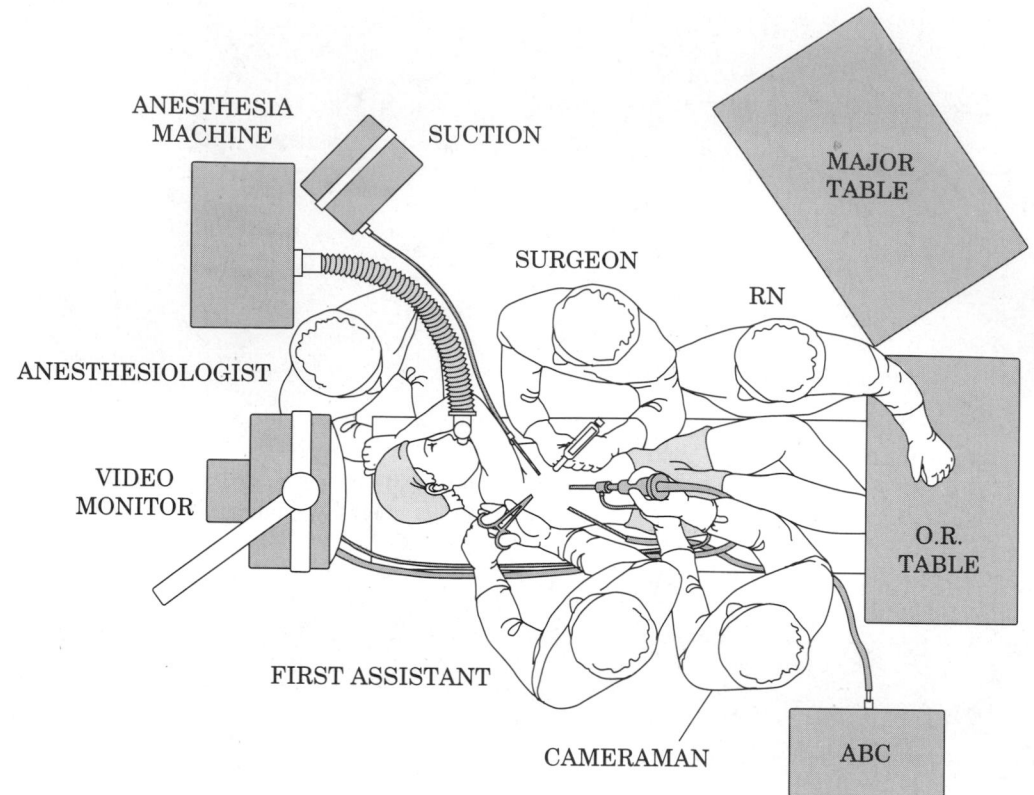

Figure 32-83. Operating room setup.

followed by digital exploration is used to confirm the presence or absence of adhesions. If the pleural space is free, a 12-mm trocar is inserted. The trocar is then removed from the sleeve, and the operating telescope is inserted through the sleeve into the thorax. If adhesions are present, an attempt is made to sweep them gently from the chest wall to create a space large enough to insert the telescope. If the adhesions are firm and not easily lysed, a thoracotomy is performed. The initial trocar location should be guided by the expected pathology.

The telescope is brought into the thorax over the dome of the diaphragm, which generally corresponds to the seventh or eighth intercostal space along the midaxillary line. The thorax is explored and the pathology identified. Two small intercostal incisions are made without spreading the ribs and used to perform the surgical procedures. These incisions are usually opposite each other, widely separated, and close to the pathology. The length of each incision is determined by the instruments being used. Usually a total of three incisions is required for most procedures; however, additional incisions may be necessary depending upon the degree of difficulty or the particular pathology (Landreneau, et al., 1992a).

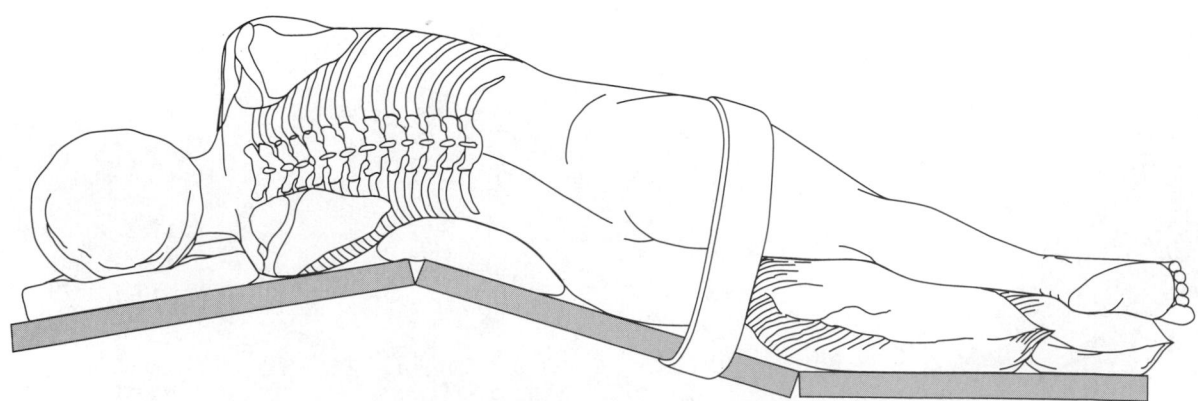

Figure 32-84. Patient position on operating table.

VIDEO-ASSISTED THORACIC SURGERY FOR PULMONARY DISEASE

Lung Biopsies

In properly selected patients who require lung biopsy, VATS offers several advantages over traditional anterior thoracotomy (Chechani, et al., 1992; Ferson, et al., 1993). There is excellent visualization of the entire lung, which allows multiple biopsy specimens to be taken safely from carefully selected areas of the lung (Fig. 32-85). With use of the endoscopic staplers, the incisions are less than 2 cm in length, which seems to cause little pain or disability. The diagnostic yield is high and the morbidity low. The procedure is carried out with the patient in the lateral decubitus position. The camera port is made through the seventh intercostal space at the midaxillary line. Two intercostal incisions are made, one through the fourth intercostal space along the anterior axillary line and the other through the fifth intercostal space in the auscultatory triangle. The portion of lung chosen for biopsy is grasped with an endoscopic lung clamp or a ring forceps. Through the opposite port an endoscopic stapler is introduced, positioned, and fired across the desired piece of lung. The specimen is then passed out of the chest through one of the intercostal incisions. The staple line is carefully examined for bleeding. Generally, two specimens are obtained from separate lobes. A single intercostal tube is placed, which is usually removed within 12 to 48 hours.

Although VATS lung biopsy offers numerous advantages, certain patients are poor candidates for this approach. These include acutely ill patients who require mechanical ventilator support, high fractional inspired oxygen concentrations, and positive end-expiratory pressure (PEEP), and who have high peak airway pressures. This type of patient has not tolerated single-lung ventilation and is probably better served by an anterior thoracotomy.

Lung Masses and Nodules

A wide variety of lung masses or nodules can be treated effectively by VATS (Landreneau, et al., 1992b; Lewis, et al., 1992b; Miller, et al., 1992; Wakabayashi, 1991). Initially, bronchoscopy and cervical mediastinoscopy are performed, and if these are negative, VATS exploration is carried out. The principles of patient positioning and port placement have been outlined in the operative technique section. All patients are positioned in a lateral decubitus position. The camera port is generally located through the seventh intercostal space in the midaxillary line. After the chest has been entered with the camera, the pathology is identified if possible, and then under intrathoracic visualization, the other two intercostal incisions are made. It is possible to palpate the lung to improve one's ability to find and confirm the lesion by inserting a finger through an intercostal incision and moving the lung to the finger with a ring forceps. If the lesion is small (<2 cm) and peripheral, it is resected with generous margins by use of an appropriate stapling device depending on the location and size of the lesion. Multiple staple lines are frequently required for proper resection. The neodymium: yttrium-aluminum-garnet (Nd:YAG) laser can also be used

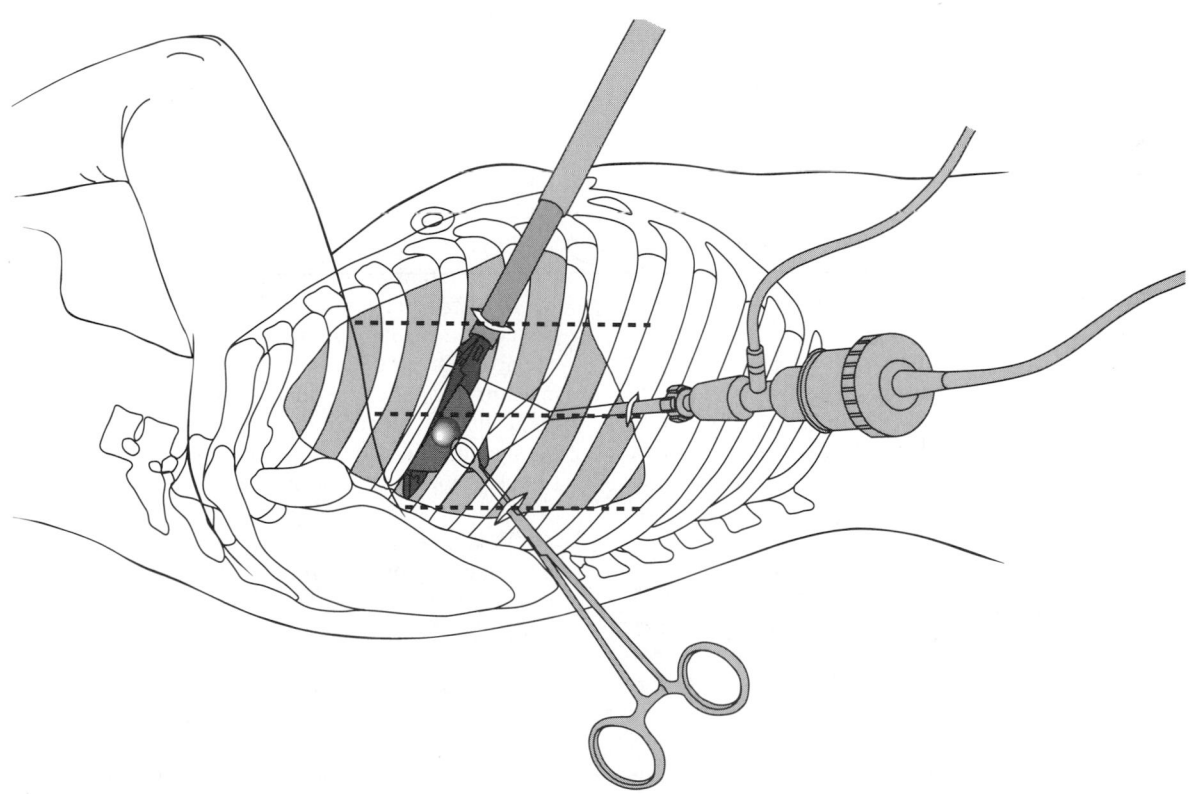

Figure 32-85. Video-assisted thoracic surgical lung biopsy.

effectively, alone or in conjuction with staplers (Landreneau, et al., 1991). The laser has the advantage of sparing the maximal amount of normal lung tissue, but its use is time-consuming and has certain inherent risks. A frozen section diagnosis is made. If benign, the line of resection is examined for hemostasis. An attempt is made to look for air leaks by partially inflating the lung and bathing the staple line with saline under direct vision. If the staple line is satisfactory, the procedure is terminated after one or two chest tubes have been inserted.

If the resected lesion is malignant, a thorough search is made for evidence of matastasis. VATS provides an excellent view of the pleura and mediastinum. The parietal pleura is examined for nodules. The fissures are opened with use of sharp and blunt dissection to search for lymph nodes. The pleura covering the hilum and mediastinum is incised with an endoscopic scissors and these areas are explored. Representative lymph nodes are biopsied by using endoscopic clips, endoscopic scissors, and biopsy forceps and sent for frozen section. If metastatic disease is present in the pleura or N_2 nodal stations, the procedure is terminated. If N_1 lymph nodes are found to contain metastatic tumor, a lobectomy is performed by either VATS or thoracotomy. In the absence of metastasis, a decision must be made either to accept the limited resection as curative or to perform a lobectomy. Many factors must be considered, including age, general medical condition, pre-existing pulmonary disease, and history of previous malignancies. Unfortunately, at this time there is no universally accepted standard for wedge resection of malignant lesions.

Currently, if a nodule less than 2 cm in diameter is located just below the visceral pleura and all lymph nodes are negative, a sublobar resection with adequate margins is considered curative by some authors (Pastorino, et al., 1991; Read, et al., 1990). If a nodule is larger than 2 cm or located more than 3 cm from the visceral pleura, a lobectomy is indicated. Obviously, procedures should be modified to meet the needs of the elderly, pulmonary-compromised, and debilitated. A high percentage of this latter group probably would not survive the disabling adverse effects of a traditional thoracotomy incision; yet even if this were done, they would still be candidates for only a very limited pulmonary resection.

By using VATS the trauma associated with the standard thoracotomy incision can be eliminated, and the necessary planned lung resection can still be performed. VATS has permitted wedge, subsegmental, segmental, and sublobar resections to be successfully completed with very acceptable margins. In selected patients VATS lobectomy has been satisfactorily accomplished by using anatomic dissection (Mack, et al., 1992).

If, however, VATS lobectomy is to become an acceptable and feasible procedure, new techniques specific for VATS must be developed. Isolation and ligation of individual hilar structures, a procedure borrowed from the open thoracotomy, has proved to be cumbersome, difficult and even dangerous for VATS.

A new technique called simultaneously stapled lobectomy permits stapling of all hilar structures in their natural and normal anatomic configuration. Simultaneously stapled lobectomy is not ''mass ligation'' or ''tourniquet'' lobectomy, both of which can crush and distort the hilar anatomy and result in ischemia. If VATS is to progress and develop safely and expeditiously, techniques such as simultaneously stapled lobectomy will be required.

With the patient in the lateral thoracotomy position, the first incision is made in the sixth intercostal space in the midaxillary line for the scope. The thorax is then carefully explored for metastatic implants of positive lymph nodes. A 2-cm incision is made next in the third intercostal space in the anterior axillary line. If the fissures are favorable, lymph nodes are absent, and the hilar area is pliable and elastic, a conjoint stapling lobectomy may be attempted in carefully selected patients.

By using sharp and blunt dissection and the ELC 35 or 60 stapler (Ethicon Endosurgery, Cincinnati, OH), the fissures are completed (Fig. 32-86). The base of the lobe is dissected, partially exposing the bronchus and pulmonary vessels, and any lymph nodes encountered are excised. The lobe to be resected is elevated with a ring clamp, and a red rubber catheter is passed around its hilar area. Each end is brought out through the 4-cm incision anteriorly. The large open end of the catheter is passed over the anvil of the stapler and is used to guide the TL 60 stapler into position around the hilum (Fig. 32-87). The catheter is next removed from the anvil of the stapler. The pin is closed, and the stapler is positioned at the base of the hilum. It is then fired for a 2-mm staple closure specifically for bronchial occlusion. This staple line, consisting of two rows of staples, is carefully evaluated for the integrity of the closure. The stapler is reloaded and passed around the hilum a second time but slightly distal to the first staple line. Again, it is fired to a 2-mm closure. The lobe is excised from the stapler, with a small cuff of tissue left. The lobe is placed in the apex of the chest. Two right-angle clamps are used to hold the cuff of tissue remaining on the stapler as the stapler is slowly released. If bleeding occurs, the stapler is closed to maintain hemostasis. The hilum can now be treated electively (i.e., with one to two sutures, or the argon beam coagulator if necessary). The staple line consisting of four rows of staples is carefully examined (Fig. 32-88). If the tumor is exposed or is too close to the surface, the lobe is placed in a plastic bag before removal from the chest.

The thorax is flooded with saline to test the bronchial closure as the lung is being expanded. Once the lesion is excised, it is removed from the thorax through the intercostal incision along the anterior axillary line. If the tumor extends to the visceral pleura or if any portion of the tumor is exposed, the specimen is placed in a plastic bag, such as an arthroscopy sleeve, prior to moving the specimen through the chest wall to minimize seeding. The removal of large lesions from the thorax is greatly facilitated by the use of a plastic bag. This has helped us remove entire lobes of the lung as well as large neurogenic tumors without spreading the ribs. If a lesion cannot be easily removed by VATS because of its location or size, careful staging is carried out by examining the pleura and N_2 nodal stations such as the aorta-pulmonary window and subcarinal lymph node stations. These are areas that are difficult, or in some cases even impossible, to explore by cervical mediastinoscopy. If all findings are negative, a conventional thoracotomy is performed. When findings are positive, the procedure is terminated and the patient referred for

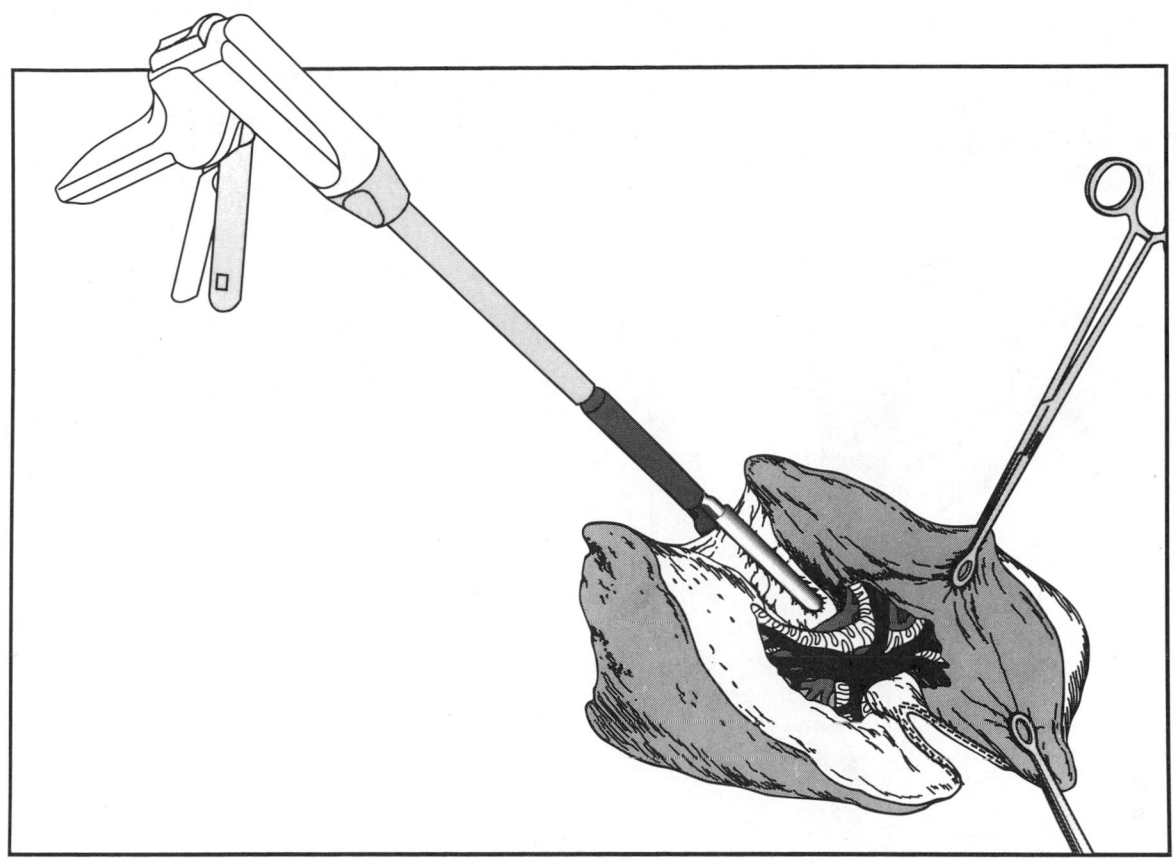

Figure 32-86. Fissure opened and completed by using the ELC 35 or 60 stapler.

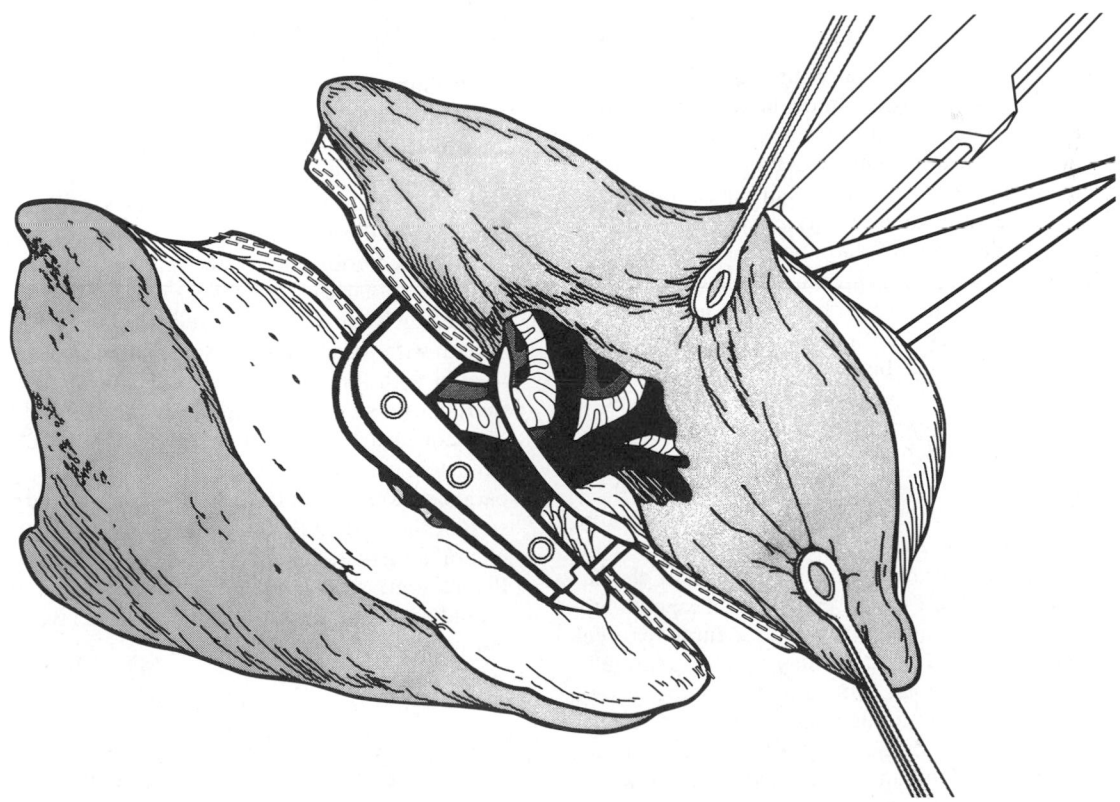

Figure 32-87. TL 60 stapler encompassing hilum, red rubber catheter in place.

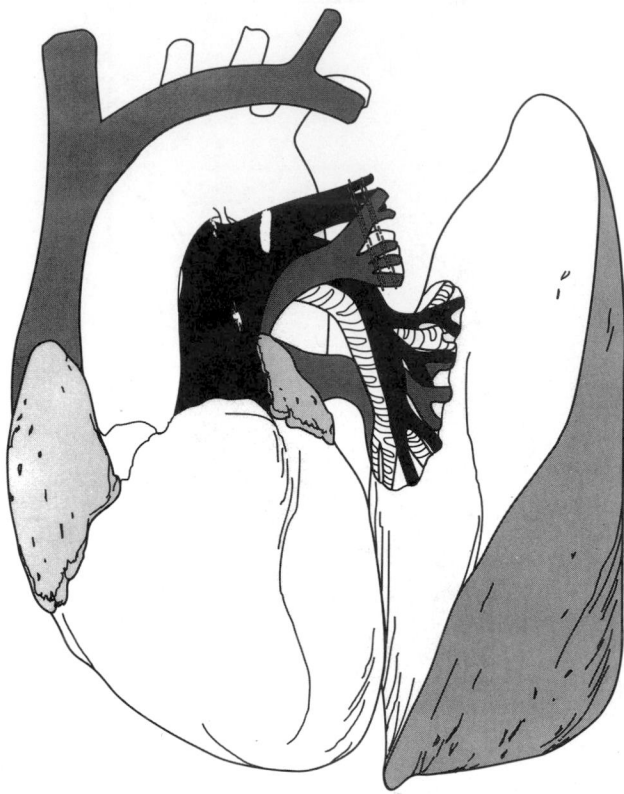

Figure 32-88. Hilar structures stapled in natural anatomic configuration.

neoadjuvant therapy. After completing a course of neoadjuvant therapy, these patients can easily undergo VATS exploration to determine resectability. Unfortunately, in our experience resectability is achieved in very few of these patients.

Thirty-eight patients in whom a traditional thoracotomy was considered inappropriate underwent a VATS lobectomy uneventfully. There was no mortality. Two persistent air leaks averaging 13 days healed spontaneously. All patients continue to do well without evidence of recurrent tumor, and all hilar tissues have healed without complications. The longest follow-up is now 26 months. A larger experience and longer follow-up period will be necessary before the true merits of conjoint stapling lobectomy can be determined.

Occasionally a lesion may be too small to be easily identified by VATS. preoperative needle localization using computed tomography (CT) greatly facilitates removal of these lesions (Miller, et al., 1992). Pulmonary metastases can be easily resected by VATS. This fact has been utilized to confirm metastases or to determine the effectiveness of chemotherapy. High-resolution CT can be employed preoperatively to identify and locate all lesions; however, for curative resections, some surgeons believe that the lung should be carefully palpated to delineate all small lesions that could be missed on preoperative imaging. Individual judgment must be used to determine if VATS or thoracotomy should be used, depending on the nature of the underlying malignancy, the age of the patient, the overall prognosis, and the information needed.

Recurrent Pneumothorax

Apical bullae and blebs that lead to spontaneous pneumothorax are easily treated by VATS (Hazelrigg, et al., 1993b; Nathanson, et al., 1991; Tore and Belloni, 1989; Wakabayashi, 1989; Wakabagashi et al., 1990). Our endoscopic technique is similar to the procedure performed at thoracotomy. This includes stapling of the apical bullae or blebs followed by resection of the diseased lung. A partial pleurectomy to the fifth rib is then performed. The patient is positioned in a lateral decubitus position, and the camera port is made at the seventh intercostal space. If the patient is tall and thin with a long thorax, the operating ports are made higher than usual, with the posterior incision at the fourth intercostal space along the lateral aspect of the pectoralis muscle. The endoscopic stapler can be brought in through either incision depending on the location and orientation of the diseased lung. The parietal pleurectomy is initiated by elevating the edge of the parietal pleura along the edge of the intercostal incison. By using a Kittner dissector and ring forceps for countertraction, the pleura is easily stripped from the chest wall from the fifth rib to the apex. We have had no bleeding complications from this procedure. One or two chest tubes are placed depending on the surgeon's preference.

Bullous Emphysema

A number of patients with chronic obstructive pulmonary disease associated with non functioning, compressive bullae have been treated by VATS with encouraging results. Most patients had progressive dyspnea despite aggressive medical management including the use of steroids and home oxygen. The preoperative evaluation consisted of arterial blood gas analysis, pulmonary function studies, including carbon monoxide diffusion capacity, and a graded exercise tolerance test. Interestingly, all patients tolerated single-lung ventilation. The lateral decubitus position was used, and the camera port was made through the seventh intercostal space at the midaxillary line. Two intercostal incisions, 1 to 2 cm in length, were made through the fourth and fifth intercostal spaces along the anterior and posterior axillary lines, respectively. Bullae with narrow bases were decompressed, twisted, stapled at their base, and excised. More commonly, complex bullae with broad bases were encountered, which were treated with the argon beam coagulator. The application of thermal energy readily tends to shrink and collapse the bullae but can lead to delayed necrosis of the bullous wall and persistent air leaks. Air leaks are common, particularly in patients taking steroids. Several techniques to promote adhesion of the lung to the chest wall have been tried, including pleural abrasion, talc insufflation, and parietal pleurectomy. Pleurectomy should not be used in any patient who may be a candidate for a future lung transplant. Two chest tubes are always placed.

PROBLEMS

Although the incisions are small, VATS is major, complex surgery that deserves all the care and attention normally given to patients undergoing thoracotomy. Intraoperative hemorrhage and inadvertent lung injury are the most common

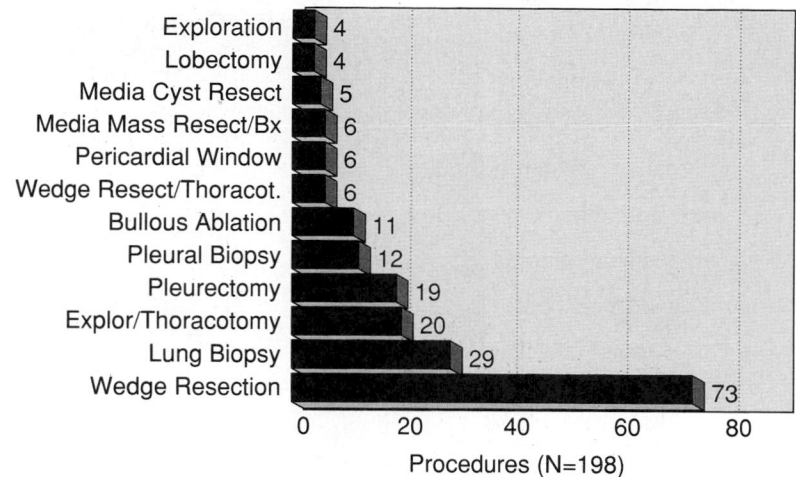

Figure 32-89. Video-assisted thoracic surgery procedures. (Data from The Surgical Institute for Minimally Invasive Procedures.)

complications. These can usually be adequately controlled with existing instruments and staplers, but if hemorrhage is significant, emergent thoracotomy may be required. It cannot be overemphasized that formal thoracotomy equipment should be in the operating room and readily available at all times during VATS. Postoperatively, persistent air leaks, atelectasis, pneumonia, empyema, and arrhythmia are the most common complications.

Chest tubes should be inserted in all patients to ensure complete lung expansion and maintain complete drainage of the pleural space. They should be managed and removed according to standard principles.

RESULTS

Assessing the results of any new procedure is difficult until appropriate clinical trials are performed and analyzed. The American Association for Thoracic Surgery (AATS) and So-

ciety of Thoracic Surgeons (STS) Joint Committee on Video-Assisted Thoracic Surgery has developed the VATS Study Group, a multi-institutional group created to collect data on VATS procedures (Hazelrigg, et al., 1993a). In addition, multiple prospective trials are in progress by the VATS Study Group to clearly define the role of VATS.

Landreneau and colleagues (1992b) reported a multi-institutional experience involving 467 patients who were successfully treated by VATS without mortality. A wide variety of procedures were performed, including 234 lung resections, 38 blebectomies, 112 procedures for pleural disease, 44 mediastinal mass resections and biopsies, 22 pericardiectomies, and 19 miscellaneous procedures.

We recently analyzed our first 175 patients who underwent 198 VATS procedures (Fig. 32-89). Indications for surgery included lung mass/nodule, lung infiltrates, pleural mass/effusion, bullous emphysema, mediastinal mass/cyst, pneumothorax and pericardial effusion (Fig. 32-90). There were

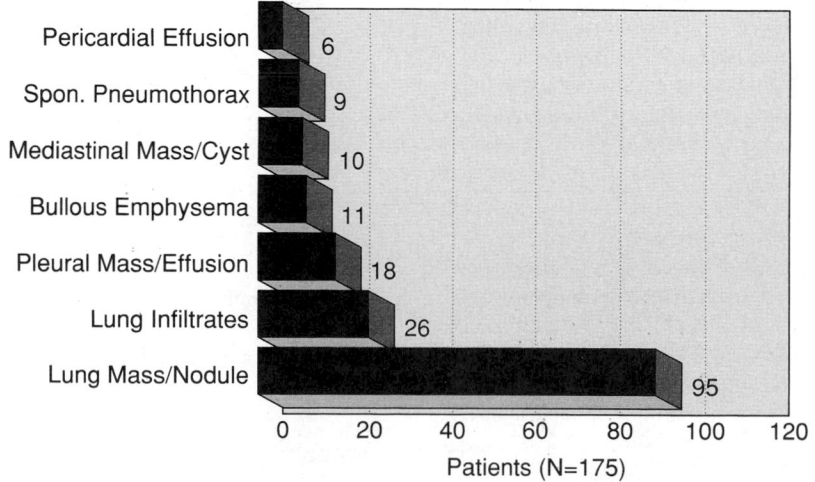

Figure 32-90. Indications for video-assisted thoracic surgery. (Data from The Surgical Institute for Minimally Invasive Procedures.)

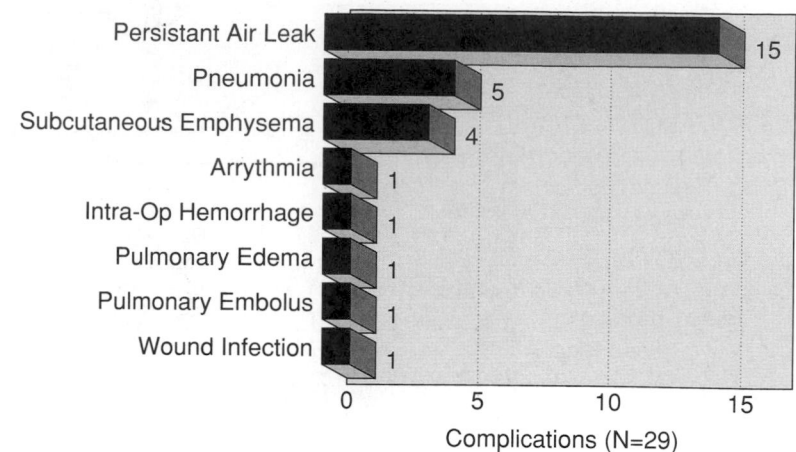

Figure 32-91.   Complications of video-assisted thoracic surgery (patient population, 175). (Data from The Surgical Institute for Minimally Invasive Procedures.)

29 complications (17 percent) and no deaths (Fig. 32-91). It is of interest to note that 13 (45 percent) of the complications occurred in the 11 patients (6 percent) who underwent bullous ablation for advanced, symptomatic bullous emphysema. The

second patient in our series required an urgent thoracotomy for bleeding when an endoloop slipped from the lung parenchyma. Staplers have been used exclusively since that case.

COMMENTS AND CONTROVERSIES

VATS has had a major impact on the field of thoracic surgery, but many issues remain unresolved. Patients with disease entities such as benign lung nodules, lung infiltrates, pericardial effusion, recurrent or persistent pneumothorax, and pleural disease seem to benefit from the reduced morbidity associated with VATS. The techniques used for these problems are similar whether the approach is VATS or thoracotomy. A variety of less common problems have been treated successfully by VATS, including excision of mediastinal cysts and masses, esophageal myotomy, sympathectomy, and automatic implantable cardioverter defibrillator (AICD) placement. Although experience with these procedures is small, the reported results are promising. It is primary carcinoma of the lung that has caused the most controversy regarding the use of VATS. Numerous reports, both favorable and unfavorable, on limited resection of stage 1 tumors exist in the literature. A standard for limited resection of bronchogenic

carcinoma does not exist today. Well-designed protocols and clinical trials are needed to answer these questions. The multi-institutional VATS study group, formed to collect data on VATS procedures, currently has a number of prospective trials in progress comparing VATS with traditional procedures.

VATS is a new and exciting technique with immense potential to reduce morbidity, decrease hospital stay, and accelerate recovery time. However, the established principles of thoracic surgery must be followed. Only through scientifically conducted trials will answers be found to many of the questions being raised by VATS.

R.J.L.
R.J.C.
G.E.S.

KEY REFERENCES

Hazelrigg SR, Nunchuck S, Lo Cicero III J et al: Video-Assisted Thoracic Surgery Study Group data. Ann Thorac Surg 56:1039, 1993a

The VATS Study Group has developed a registry from cases sent in by numerous thoracic surgeons throughout the United States. Statistics concerning types of cases being done, complications, and mortality are being compiled.

Landreneau RJ, Mack MJ, Hazelrigg SR et al: Video-assisted thoracic surgery: basic technical concepts and intercostal approach strategies. Ann Thorac Surg 54:800, 1992a

The technique of VATS, its applications, various approaches, and problems are discussed. Important basic concepts are presented.

Lewis RJ, Caccavale RJ, Sisler GE: 100 consecutive cases of imaged thoracic surgery. Ann Thorac Surg 54:421, 1992a

This paper describes how most intrathoracic surgical problems that usually require an open thoracotomy can be treated with VATS. Techniques for each diagnosis, instrumentation, operating room setups, postoperative recovery, and complications are discussed.

Lewis RJ, Caccavale RJ, Sisler GE. Special Report: video endoscopic thoracic surgery. N J Med 88:7:473, 1991

An early approach to lung biopsy for diffuse interstitial disease using VATS.

REFERENCES

Chechani V, Landreneau RJ, Shaikh SS: Open lung biopsy for diffuse infiltrative lung disease. Ann Thorac Surg 54:296, 1992

Coltharp WH, Arnold JH, Alford WC Jr et al: Videothoracoscopy: improved technique and expanded indications. Ann Thorac Surg 53:776, 1992

Ferson PF, Landreneau RJ, Dowling RD et al: Thoracoscopic vs. "open" lung biopsy for the diagnosis of infiltrate lung disease. J Thorac Cardiovasc Surg 105:194, 1993

Hazelrigg SR, Landreneau RJ, Mack MJ et al: Thoracoscopic stapled resection for spontaneous pneumothorax. J Thorac Cardiovasc Surg 105:389, 1993b

Jacobaeus HC: Die Thorakoskopie und ihre praktische Bedeutung. Ergeb Ges Med 7:112, 1925

Jacobaeus HC: The practical importance of thoracoscopy in surgery of the chest. Surg Gynecol Obstet 34:289, 1922

Jacobaeus HC: Über die Möglichkeit, die Zystoskopie bei Untersuchung seroser Hohlungen anzuwenden. Munch Med Wochenschr 40:2090, 1910

Landreneau RJ, Hazelrigg SR, Ferson PF et al: Thoracoscopic resection of 85 pulmonary lesions. Ann Thorac Surg 54:415, 1992b

Landreneau RJ, Herlan DB, Johnson JA et al: Thoracoscopic neodymium: yttrium-aluminum-garnet laser-assisted pulmonary resection. Ann Thorac Surg 52:1176, 1991

Lewis RJ, Caccavale RJ, Sisler GE: Video-assisted thoracic surgical resection of malignant lung tumors. J Thorac Cardiovasc Surg 104:1679, 1992b

Lewis RJ, Kunderman PJ, Sisler GE, Mackenzie JW: Direct diagnostic thoracoscopy. Ann Thorac Surg 21:536, 1976

Lewis RJ, Sisler GE, Caccavale RJ: Imaged thoracic lobectomy: should it be done? Ann Thorac Surg 54:80, 1992

Lewis RJ, Sisler GE, Mackenzie JW: Diffuse, mixed malignant pleural mesothelioma. Ann Thorac Surg 31:53, 1981

Mack M, Aronoff R, Accuff T et al: The present role of thoracoscopy in the diagnosis and treatment of disease of the chest. Ann Thorac Surg 54:403, 1992

Mack MJ, Gordon MJ, Postma TW et al: Percutaneous localization of pulmonary nodules for thoracoscopic lung resection. Ann Thorac Surg 53:1123, 1992

McKneally MF: Lobectomy without a rib spreader. Ann Thorac Surg 54:2, 1992

Miller DL, Allen MS, Deschamps C et al: Video-assisted thoracic surgical procedure: management of a solitary pulmonary nodule. Mayo Clin Proc 67:462, 1992

Miller JI Jr: Therapeutic thoracoscopy: new horizons for an established procedure. Ann Thorac Surg 52:1036, 1991

Nathanson LK, Shimi SM, Wood RAB, Cuschieri A: Videothoracoscopic ligation of bulla and pleurectomy for spontaneous pneumothorax. Ann Thorac Surg 52:316, 1991

Newman JH, Caccavale RJ, Sisler GE, Lewis RL: Video-assisted thoracic surgery. Hosp Phys 28:15, 1992

Pastorino U, Valente M, Bedini V et al: Limited resection for stage 1 lung cancer. Eur J Surg Oncol 17:42, 1991

Read RC, Yoder G, Schaeffer RC: Survival after conservative resection for $T_1N_0M_0$ non-small cell lung cancer. Ann Thorac Surg 49:391, 1990

Tore M, Belloni P. Nd:YAG laser pleurodesis through thoracoscopy: new curative therapy in spontaneous pneumothorax. Ann Thorac Surg 47:887, 1989

Wakabayashi A: Expanded applications of diagnostic and therapeutic thoracoscopy. J Thorac Cardiovasc Surg 102:721, 1991

Wakabayashi A: Thoracoscopic ablation of blebs in the treatment of recurrent or persistent spontaneous pneumothorax. Ann Thorac Surg 48:651, 1989

Wakabayashi A, Brenner M, Wilson AF et al: Thoracoscopic treatment of spontaneous pneumothorax using carbon dioxide laser. Ann Thorac Surg 50:786, 1990

33

TRANSPLANTATION

Lung Transplantation

G. A. Patterson
Joel D. Cooper

Since the first successful human lung transplant in 1983 (Toronto Lung Transplant Group, 1986), remarkable progress has been achieved. Lung transplantation is successfully used world-wide. Improved donor and recipient selection, technical advances, superior immunosuppression strategies, and newer antibiotic regimens have improved results dramatically. The operative mortality rate is now in the range of 10 percent. One and 2-year survival rates are 80 and 70 percent, respectively. However, problems remain, most notably chronic rejection, which is manifested in the pulmonary allograft as bronchiolitis obliterans.

HISTORICAL NOTE

In the early 1950s Metras (1950) in France and Hardin and Kittle (1954) in the United States demonstrated the technical feasibility of canine lung transplantation. The initial perception that pulmonary vascular resistance increased in the lung allograft was dispelled by reports that meticulous vascular anastomotic technique resulted in normal pulmonary artery pressures. Similar techniques are used today.

Hardy (1963) reported the first human lung transplantation in 1963. The patient died after 18 days. Nonetheless, this short-lived success not only demonstrated the technical feasibility of the operation but also stimulated worldwide interest in pulmonary transplantation.

During the subsequent 15 years, approximately 40 clinical lung transplants were performed in centers around the world. None of these procedures was successful. Only one recipient was actually discharged from the hospital, a 23-year-old patient (Derom, et al., 1971). This patient left the hospital 8 months following transplantation but died a short time thereafter as a result of chronic rejection, sepsis, and bronchial stenosis. Most patients died within the first 2 weeks of transplantation, as a result of primary graft failure, sepsis, or rejection. The most frequent cause of death beyond the second postoperative week was bronchial anastomotic disruption. The initial lung transplant in the Toronto experience was performed for a young ventilator-dependent patient with inhalation burns (Nelems, et al., 1980). The patient died during the third postoperative week after a bronchial anastomotic dehiscence. This problem of bronchial anastomotic dehiscence stimulated the interest of a number of surgical laboratories. Lima, et al. (1981), working with Cooper and his colleagues in Toronto, demonstrated that high-dose corticosteroid therapy (2 mg/kg/day, which at that time was necessary for adequate immunosuppression) had an adverse effect on bronchial anastomotic healing. That same group also demonstrated that the ischemic donor bronchus could be revascularized within a few days by a flap of abdominal omentum with a pedicle (Morgan, et al., 1983). Not only would the omental pedicle provide new collateral circulation to the ischemic bronchus, but also the omentum provided a potential benefit in containing anastomotic dehiscence in the event of partial disruption. During this same interval, it became apparent that cyclosporine had impressive immunosuppressive properties and could eliminate the routine need for high-dose corticosteroid immunosuppression. Furthermore, it was also demonstrated by the Toronto group that cyclosporine had no adverse effect on bronchial anastomotic healing (Goldberg, et al., 1983).

In 1981 the Stanford group reported their initial clinical experience with combined heart-lung transplantation in a group of patients with pulmonary vascular disease (Reitz, et al., 1982). The combined heart-lung transplant had been previously attempted without success by Cooley, et al. (1969) and then by Lillihei (1970) and Barnard, et al. (1981). The Stanford experience demonstrated conclusively that, with the new immunosuppressive drug cyclosporine, the transplanted lung would provide acceptable long-term function in patients with pulmonary hypertension and right ventricular failure. However, by 1983, successful isolated lung transplantation had not yet been achieved.

Satisfactory patient selection remained the final obstacle to successful clinical lung transplantation. We reasoned that end-stage respiratory failure from pulmonary fibrosis would provide the ideal condition for single-lung transplantation. The increased resistance to perfusion and ventilation in the native lung would preferentially direct perfusion and ventilation to the transplanted lung. A clinical lung transplant program at the University of Toronto was initiated in 1983. We maintained a policy of careful recipient selection and strict adherence to rigid donor criteria. Bronchial omentopexy was used in every transplant procedure, and early perioperative corticosteroids were avoided. With these strategies we achieved the first successful lung transplant in 1983 (Toronto Lung Transplant Group, 1986) in a 58-year-old man with idiopathic pulmonary fibrosis.

Subsequent development of an experimental (Dark, et al., 1986) and clinical (Patterson, et al., 1988) en bloc double-lung replacement technique enabled the application of bilateral lung replacement to patients for whom a single-lung transplant was not appropriate. Although this procedure did have the definite attraction of preservation of the recipient heart, it was a technically complex procedure. In addition, it was associated with a high incidence of complications, notably donor airway ischemia (Patterson, et al., 1990) and cardiac denervation (Schafers, et al., 1990).

A number of innovations have been achieved in recent years that have expanded the application of pulmonary transplantation. Patients with obstructive pulmonary disease were previously thought suitable only for bilateral lung replacement. It has now been conclusively shown that single-lung transplantation provides an attractive option for such patients (Mal, et al., 1989). Combined heart-lung transplantation was formerly thought to be the only option for patients with pulmonary vascular disease; however, recent experience has shown that single- (Pasque, et al., 1991) and bilateral lung transplantation (Bando, et al., 1994a) provide satisfactory functional results in this patient group.

A number of technical advances have been achieved, most notably the development of a simplified method for bilateral sequential lung replacement (Pasque, et al., 1990). An anterior transverse incision provides superior exposure for safe division of pleural adhesions. Sequential excision and replacement of both lungs often avoids the need for cardiopulmonary bypass. The shortened donor bronchial length of two single-lung allografts reduces the incidence of bronchial anastomotic complications. Direct bronchial artery revascularization for double- (Couraud, et al., 1992; Daly, et al., 1993) and single-lung transplants (Daly, et al., 1994) has been described and is currently used in a number of programs; other programs await the reports on long-term results.

Improved strategies of pulmonary preservation have enabled reliable long-distance procurement and satisfactory early allograft function in the majority of cases. We have also demonstrated that pharmacologic agents, such as prostaglandin E_1 (Aoe, et al., 1994), pentoxifylline (Okabayashi, et al., 1994), and nitric oxide (Triantafillou, et al., 1994) can also lessen reperfusion injury.

Advances have also been made in the prevention and therapy of postoperative sepsis. Bacterial infection, particularly troublesome in patients with cystic fibrosis, has been lessened by the routine use of broad-spectrum prophylactic antibiotics and inhaled aminoglycosides. Herpes simplex infections have been lessened by routine prophylactic use of acyclovir. Cytomegalovirus (CMV) infection, a potentially fatal complication in recipients of lung transplants, has been markedly reduced by appropriate matching of donor and recipient CMV serologic findings when possible and prophylactic use of ganciclovir.

HISTORICAL READINGS

Dark JH et al: Experimental en-bloc double-lung transplantation. Ann Thorac Surg 42:394, 1986

Derom F et al: Ten-month survival after lung homotransplantation in man. J Thorac Cardiovasc Surg 61:835, 1971

Goldberg M et al: A comparison between cyclosporin A and methylprednisolone plus azathioprine on bronchial healing following canine lung allotransplantation. J Thorac Cardiovasc Surg 85:821, 1983

Hardin CA, Kittle CF: Experience with transplantation of the lung. Science 119:87, 1954

Hardy JD: Lung homotransplantation in man. JAMA 186:1065, 1963

Lillehei CW: Discussion of Wildevuur CRH, Benfield JR: A review of 23 human lung transplantations by 20 surgeons. Ann Thorac Surg 9:489, 1970

Mal H et al: Unilateral lung transplantation in end stage pulmonary emphysema. Am Rev Respir Dis 140:797, 1989

Metras H: Note preliminaire sur la graffe totale du poumon chez le chien. Fr Acad Sci 1176, 1950

Morgan WE et al: Improved bronchial healing in canine left lung reimplantation using omental pedicle wrap. J Thorac Cardiovasc Surg 85:139, 1983

Patterson GA et al: Technique of successful clinical double-lung transplantation. Ann Thorac Surg 45:626, 1988

Reitz BA et al: Heart-lung transplantation: successful therapy for patients with pulmonary vascular disease. N Engl J Med 306:557, 1982

Toronto Lung Transplant Group: Unilateral lung transplantation for pulmonary fibrosis. N Engl J Med 314:1140, 1986

PATIENT SELECTION

Recipient

General Considerations

General selection criteria are listed below and are described in detail in a recent review by Trulock (1993b). We have maintained a policy of listing for pulmonary transplants only those patients whom we believe have a limited life expectancy (12 to 24 months) as a result of their underlying pulmonary disease. As discussed below, it has become apparent that the time course of deterioration and subsequent death is highly variable, depending on the specific disease. With the inherent risk of lung transplantation and the acute shortage of suitable donor lungs, we believe that it is not appropriate to offer lung transplantation to patients who are not in imminent

---

Recipient Selection Criteria

Clinically and physiologically severe disease

Medical therapy ineffective or unavailable

Substantial limitation in activities of daily living

Limited life expectancy

Adequate cardiac function without significant coronary artery disease

Ambulatory with rehabilitation potential

Acceptable nutritional status

Satisfactory psychosocial profile and emotional support system

---

danger of death from their underlying pulmonary disease. Patients who have coexisting dysfunction involving another organ system are not eligible for transplantation. This is, of course, a particular problem in considering patients in older age groups. In general we do not accept a patient older than age 60 years. Patients with a history of malignant disease within the past 5 years are not eligible for lung transplantation. An exception to this criterion is the rare patient with bilateral bronchoalveolar carcinoma without metastatic disease who might be eligible for lung transplantation in some programs. The occasional patient with a more recent malignancy that is judged to be cured might be considered, as are other potential candidates. Patients with serious psychological dysfunction are not able to meet the rigorous demands of patient compliance necessary for a successful lung transplantation. We do not evaluate patients who continue to smoke.

Previous thoracic surgery or pleurodesis is not a specific contraindication to lung transplantation. However, adhesions and the anatomic distortion of previous surgery complicate the conduct of a transplant procedure and allowance must be made for this in operative planning. Patients receiving high-dose corticosteroid therapy (e.g., prednisone $\geq$ 20 mg/day) are not eligible for lung transplantation. Such high doses of corticosteroids have a well-documented negative influence on bronchial healing and the patient's susceptibility to postoperative infection. However, patients receiving low- or moderate-dose steroid therapy (e.g., prednisone 10 mg/day or less) are candidates and have undergone pulmonary transplantation without an increased incidence of bronchial anastomotic complications. Ventilator dependency is not a contraindication to transplantation, however, most programs have a selective policy concerning such patients because they fear that waiting lists will fill with ventilated patients.

We insist that all patients listed for transplantation (excepting those with primary pulmonary hypertension or Eisenmenger's syndrome) participate in a progressive monitored exercise rehabilitation program while they await transplantation. Virtually all patients experience a marked improvement in strength and exercise tolerance without any measurable change in pulmonary function. We are convinced that this improved endurance enables patients to withstand the rigors

of a transplant procedure and subsequent convalescence better.

Specific Considerations

Obstructive Pulmonary Disease. Obstructive pulmonary disease, notably emphysema and α-antitrypsin deficiency, is the most common indication for lung transplantation. More than one-third of transplant procedures reported to the St. Louis International Lung Transplant Registry were performed for obstructive lung disease (Cooper, 1993). The general criteria for transplantation in these patients have been published (Trulock, 1993b). Most patients have deteriorated to a point at which oxygen supplementation is required. In our experience the mean supplemental oxygen requirement is slightly in excess of 4 L/min. The obstructive physiology in these patients results in a forced expiratory volume at 1 second (FEV_1) well below 1 L at approximately 15 percent of predicted normal values. Fortunately, this patient group has a relatively stable course during the inevitable long wait for a suitable donor.

Although obstructive pulmonary disease is the most common indication for which single-lung transplantation is performed, the ideal operative procedure for these patients is not yet defined. The functional outcomes of single- and bilateral-lung transplantation for these patients are discussed subsequently. In general, for young patients, particularly those with α-antitrypsin deficiency, we prefer to use bilateral sequential single-lung transplantations. The bilateral option is also more attractive in larger recipients for whom an oversized single donor lung would be difficult to obtain. On the other hand, for smaller recipients, single-lung transplantation offers a more attractive option, particularly when an oversized donor lung can be used. Finally, in the older patient, single-lung transplantation offers an attractive option because it is a technically simple procedure and is associated with a lower operative mortality rate.

Septic Lung Disease. Cystic fibrosis is the most frequently encountered condition in this category (Cooper, 1993). As the most common inherited disorder among whites, cystic fibrosis is a common disease, resulting in diffuse bronchiectatic destruction of both lungs. Without transplantation the overwhelming majority of patients die as a result of progressive respiratory failure in the second or third decade of life. The most reliable predictors of life expectancy in patients with cystic fibrosis have recently been published (Kerem, et al., 1992). A FEV_1 less than 30 percent of predicted, an elevated partial carbon dioxide pressure ($PaCO_2$), a requirement for supplemental oxygen, frequent admissions to the hospital for the control of acute pulmonary infections, and failure to maintain weight are reliable predictors of early death in these patients. These are the criteria that we use in selecting patients for lung transplantation. After reaching this stage of disease, patients with cystic fibrosis usually have a rapidly progressive downhill course. Indeed, in the Papworth experience, approximately one-third of patients with cystic fibrosis accepted for transplantation died while waiting for a suitable donor (Sharples, et al., 1993).

Fibrotic Lung Disease. Pulmonary fibrosis now represents one of the less common indications for single-lung transplantation. Specific selection criteria for patients with pulmonary fibrosis have not changed significantly since they were originally published by the Toronto Lung Transplant Group (1986) several years ago. In our experience, candidates for transplantation have had classic restrictive physiologic findings with a mean forced vital capacity (FVC) and FEV_1 of 1.35 and 1.14, respectively (Trulock, et al., 1991). All have required supplemental oxygen, have had marked impairment of exercise tolerance, and demonstrated oxygen desaturation with minimal exertion. Moderate and occasionally severe pulmonary hypertension is seen in these patients. In contrast to those with obstructive physiology (Trulock, 1993b), patients with pulmonary fibrosis who have deteriorated to the point of requiring consideration for a transplant generally have a rapid downhill course and will not survive a lengthy wait for a suitable donor lung.

Pulmonary Vascular Disease. The application of lung transplantation, particularly single-lung transplantation, in these patients is a particularly exciting development. These patients were formerly thought to require combined heart-lung transplantation. However, Fremes, et al. (1990), at the University of Toronto, reported the first successful single-lung transplant in a patient with patent ductus Eisenmenger's syndrome. Since this report a number of centers have demonstrated clearly that right ventricular function improves immediately following transplantation and that improvement is maintained in long-term follow-up (Cooper, 1993). There are reliable predictors of early death in patients with primary pulmonary hypertension (D'Alonzo, et al., 1991). Markedly elevated pulmonary artery pressures with mean pressures in excess of 60 mmHg, syncopal episodes, and clinical evidence of right ventricular failure, with significant elevation of central venous pressure and depression of the cardiac index, are predictors of death in patients with primary pulmonary hypertension. Among our first 22 patients undergoing single-lung transplant for pulmonary vascular disease, the mean New York Heart Association functional class pretransplant was 3.4. The risk of sudden death in this patient population is high.

In consideration of these factors, in our program, patients with primary pulmonary hypertension are listed and transplanted as soon as possible. In our Barnes Hospital experience, 57 patients with primary pulmonary hypertension have been listed on the active transplant list. Fourteen (25 percent) of these patients died before a suitable donor was identified. This is a much higher rate of death while waiting than for other disease categories. Unfortunately, as the number of potential recipients continues to surpass the number of available donors, this problem will remain. At the present time, in the United States, the time on the waiting list determines the priority for an available donor. There is no consideration given to the severity of disease or expected survival time.

Despite having equivalent degrees of pulmonary hypertension, patients with Eisenmenger's physiology have a less predictable rate of deterioration, and the appropriate timing for transplantation in these patients is correspondingly less certain. In these patients we rely on the development of intractable and progressive symptoms of right ventricular failure as the predominant selection criterion.

Donor

Rapid progress in transplantation has resulted in a shortage of suitable allografts for all organs. This is a particularly significant problem for lung transplantation insofar as at most only 20 percent of otherwise suitable organ donors have lungs that meet the standard donor lung criteria. Most of the conditions that result in brain death (trauma or spontaneous intracerebral hemorrhage) are associated with significant pulmonary parenchymal pathologic findings as a result of lung contusion, infection, aspiration, or neurogenic pulmonary edema.

Satisfactory gas exchange is imperative for donor lungs. This can be confirmed by a partial oxygen pressure (PaO_2) greater than 300 mmHg with an inspired oxygen concentration of 100 percent and 5 cmH_2O positive end-expiratory pressure (PEEP). A PaO_2 to fraction of inspired oxygen (FIO_2) ratio of 300 or greater provides adequate evidence of satisfactory gas exchange. A donor chest radiograph taken shortly prior to harvest must reveal clear lung fields. Bronchoscopic assessment at the donor institution often reveals mucopurulent secretions from which a variety of organisms might be cultured. This finding is commonly observed and is not a contraindication to lung transplantation if the donor is otherwise suitable. However, bronchoscopic evidence of aspiration or frank pus in the airway is a definite contraindication to transplantation.

Donor and recipient ABO compatibility is essential. At present donor and recipient histocompatibility antigen (HLA) matching is not performed. There is controversy regarding the impact of HLA matching. There are no data in the literature that suggest it may have any impact on subsequent graft function. Furthermore, any delay in donor harvest to conduct such matching places the donor lungs at risk of deterioration. Unfortunately, we do not have at our disposal satisfactory preservation strategies to permit "postharvest" tissue matching. We prefer to use cytomegalovirus (CMV)-negative donors for CMV-negative recipients whenever possible.

Standard Lung Donor Selection Criteria

Age less than 55 years

No history of pulmonary disease

Normal serial chest radiographs

Adequate gas exchange ($PaO_2 > 300$ mmHg on FIO_2 1.0 and PEEP 5 cmH_2O)

Normal bronchoscopic examination

Negative serologic screening for hepatitis B and human immunodeficiency virus (HIV)

Recipient matching for ABO blood group

Size matching

A significant consideration is the matching of size between the donor and recipient. Acceptable size matching depends on the nature of the recipient's pulmonary disease and the type of transplant planned. Size matching can be achieved by a comparison of vertical lung height, transverse chest diameter, and chest circumference. However, we have found these donor measurements are sometimes unreliable when made by busy and perhaps inexperienced donor coordinators in a remote donor hospital. Much more reliable are predicted donor and recipient pulmonary volumes, which are calculated using standard nomograms based on age, sex, and height.

In patients undergoing single-lung transplantation for obstructive pulmonary disease, we attempt to place allografts with 15 to 20 percent greater volume than the recipient predicted pulmonary volume. Implantation of such a large allograft is easily achieved in a patient with obstructive pulmonary disease because of the enormous size of the recipient pleural space. However, in patients with pulmonary fibrosis or pulmonary vascular disease, the pleural spaces are reduced or normal in size, respectively. It is therefore inadvisable to oversize these patients to an excessive degree. In patients undergoing bilateral lung replacement, we prefer to match the donor's pulmonary volumes to the pulmonary volume or anticipated pulmonary dimensions that the recipient would possess in the absence of pulmonary disease.

In certain circumstances the donor selection criteria can be somewhat relaxed. A minor degree of pulmonary infiltrate can be accepted in a donor being used for a bilateral transplantation. We have recently analyzed our most recent 100 donor lungs and determined that those with "marginal" quality, as judged by arterial blood gas analysis and radiographic assessment, provided postoperative function equivalent to those judged excellent (Sundaresan, et al., 1994) (Fig. 33-1). On occasion a donor is identified with marginal gas exchange and radiographic evidence of a unilateral pulmonary infiltrate. In a number of such situations, we have made an intraoperative donor assessment with ventilation and perfusion only to the seemingly normal donor lung, judged that lung to be acceptable, and conducted a successful unilateral transplantation (Puskas, et al., 1992a).

Other strategies have been adopted to increase the donor pool. Living related bilateral lobar transplantation has been successfully used in a highly selected small group of patients with cystic fibrosis (Cohen, et al., 1994). Although innovative and exciting, this procedure is not going to have any meaningful impact on the overall shortage of lung allografts. Xenografts offer the only potential hope for a large increase in the supply of suitable donor lungs.

LUNG PRESERVATION

Lung preservation has been the focus of intense laboratory interest for a number of years. Several detailed reviews of this subject have recently been published (Christie and Waddell, 1993; Novick, 1992). Clinical pulmonary preservation has progressed considerably since the Toronto group initially reported unilateral lung transplantation using donor lungs harvested in an atelectatic state and stored by topical hypothermic immersion (Todd, et al., 1988). There are minor differences in the preservation strategies of most clinical lung transplant programs, but the basic principles remain the same.

Following systemic donor heparinization and just prior to circulatory arrest, a pulmonary vasodilator is administered. We use prostaglandin E_1 (PGE_1) 500 μg as a direct bolus injection into the pulmonary artery. Pulmonary arterial flush is then achieved with the lungs in a state of moderate inflation at a FIO_2 greater than room air (usually 100 percent). Most programs use an intracellular flush solution, most commonly modified Euro-Collins solution (4 mEq mg SO_4 and 3 percent glucose) or University of Wisconsin solution. Following extraction, the lung allograft is immersed in iced crystalloid solution and maintained in a semi-inflated state during transport. This technique results in reliable allograft function following ischemic times of up to 6 hours. On occasion we have extended the ischemic time, particularly for the second lung of a bilateral sequential transplant in which the ischemic time has occasionally reached 8 to 10 hours with satisfactory subsequent function.

A detailed review of experimental pulmonary preservation is beyond the scope of this chapter, but there have been several interesting developments.

Inflation

The state of lung inflation during pulmonary artery flush and storage probably has a significant impact on post-transplant pulmonary function. Puskas, et al. (1992c) demonstrated that canine lungs flushed and stored in a hyperinflated state produce more reliable post-transplant lung function after a prolonged (30-hour) period of storage compared with lungs stored at low pulmonary volumes. Using the same model, our laboratory recently demonstrated that hyperinflation during storage and flush is necessary to achieve the maximum benefit. However, when we adopted a policy of donor hyperinflation in our clinical program, we noted a disturbing incidence of allograft dysfunction. Recent evidence from our laboratory utilizing a rabbit model suggests that hyperinflation produces increased pulmonary capillary permeability. We confirmed this finding in a recent series of canine allotransplants. For this reason we recommend that lungs be flushed and stored in a state of moderate inflation that is consistent with normal end-tidal inspiration.

Temperature of Flush and Storage

Virtually all clinical lung transplant programs use a pulmonary artery flush at 1 to 4°C. Following extraction lungs are immersed in crystalloid and packed in ice, resulting in their storage and transport at approximately 1°C. A number of investigators have shown that a more moderate degree of hypothermia (10°C) results in superior pulmonary function. This has been demonstrated in our own laboratory in an in vitro rabbit lung perfusion model (Wang, et al., 1993) and a standard model of canine left lung allotransplantation (Date, et al., 1992) and bilateral baboon lung transplantation (Sundaresan, et al., 1993a). However, in a previous canine allograft study, Mayer, et al. (1992) were unable to show a difference between storage at 4°C versus 10°C in canine left lung allografts.

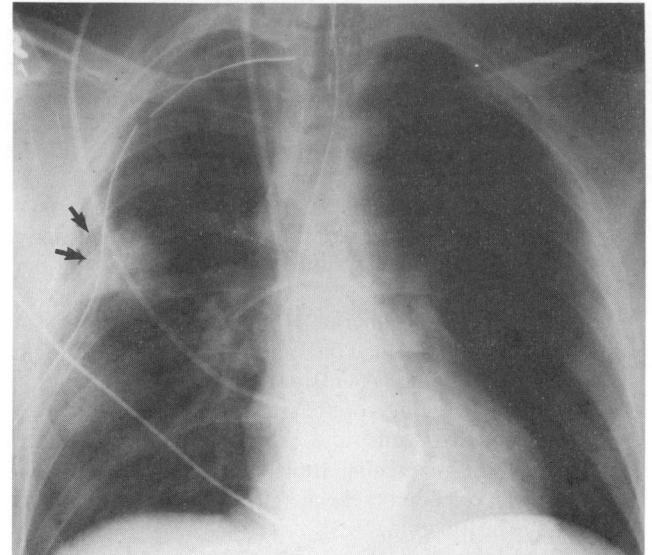
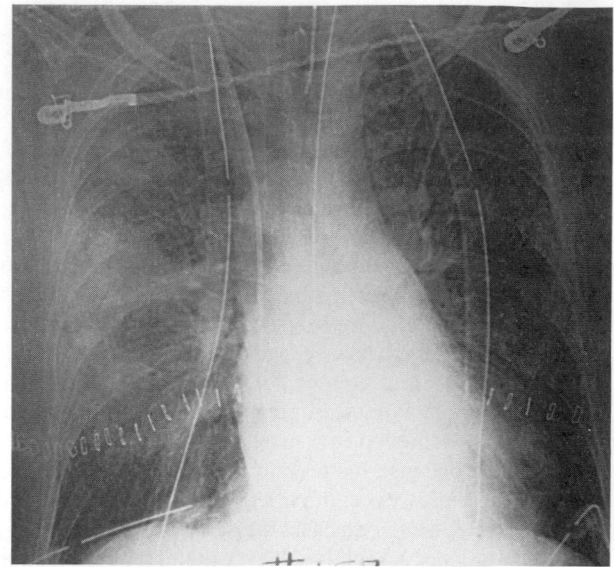
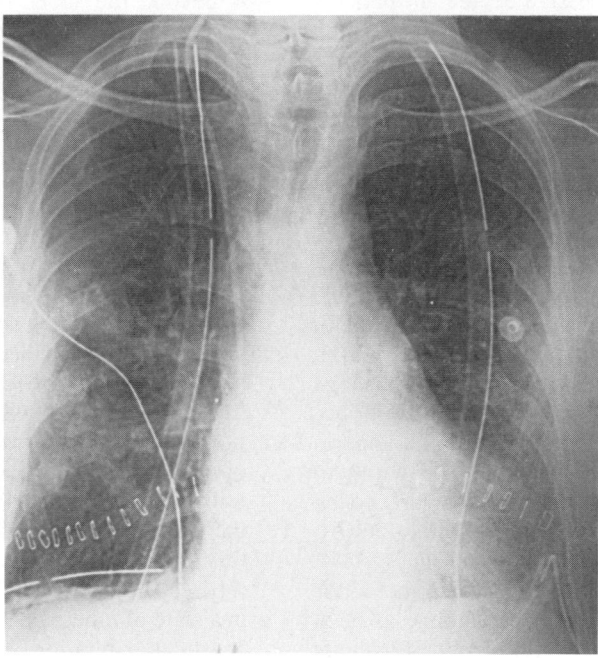

Figure 33-1. **(A)** Anteroposterior chest radiograph from a patient with brain death as a result of a motor vehicle accident. The right chest tube evacuated a 50 percent pneumothorax. The arrows point to a right upper lobe contusion. Several hours following this radiograph, both lungs were harvested for use as bilateral sequential allografts in a patient with obstructive lung disease. (From Shields TW: General Thoracic Surgery. Lea & Febiger, Philadelphia, 1994, with permission.) **(B)** Immediate postoperative recipient radiograph demonstrating some progression of the right upper lobe contusion. **(C)** Recipient chest radiograph taken 3 days following transplantation. Note the dramatic clearing of the right upper lobe contusion.

Composition of Flush Solution

There has been considerable controversy as to the optimal composition of the pulmonary flush solution. Various solutions are used clinically at present. Some groups advocate cardiopulmonary bypass to cool the donor, thereby essentially flushing the lungs with cooled autologous donor blood (Yacoub, et al., 1989). The Papworth group popularized the use of an extracellular solution supplemented with donor blood to achieve a flush hematocrit of approximately 10 percent (Hakim, et al., 1988). During the past several years, a number of experimental studies have demonstrated that an extracellular low-potassium dextran (LPD) solution provided superior function over the standard intracellular Euro-Collins solution (Keshavjee, et al., 1992). It was argued that this LPD solution induced less pulmonary vasoconstriction during flush. However, we have recently shown that, if pulmonary vasodilatation is achieved with prostaglandin E₁ prior to flush, Euro-Collins solution provides equivalent preservation to that achieved with LPD (Puskas, et al., 1992b).

A number of groups have used the intracellular University of Wisconsin solution and observed acceptable results. A number of earlier reports suggested that the intracellular University of Wisconsin solution was not an effective preservation solution in animal models. However, that information may not be directly applicable to humans. The Pittsburgh group (Hardesty, et al., 1993) recently conducted a retrospective review of their experience and concluded that the University of Wisconsin solution may actually provide superior preservation to that observed with the more commonly used modified Euro-Collins solution.

Pharmacologic Manipulation

In addition to their apparent benefit when administered prior to pulmonary artery flush (Mayer, et al., 1992), recent evidence suggests that vasodilator prostanoids may also have some beneficial effect in the early post-transplant period. Matsuzaki, et al. (1993) demonstrated that PGE_1 infusion ameliorated the reperfusion injury following 2 hours of warm ischemia in an in situ rabbit lung model. We continued this work, demonstrating that PGE_1 significantly improves canine lung allograft function following an 18-hour ischemic period (Aoe, et al., 1994). We continue to use it routinely during the postoperative period in our clinical program. Pentoxifylline also ameliorates canine lung allograft reperfusion injury as does the potent vasodilator nitric oxide.

There is a mounting body of evidence suggesting that oxygen free radicals are important in the genesis of ischemia reperfusion injury in the lung. This subject was concisely reviewed by Christie and Waddell (1993). A number of antioxidant interventions, including enzymatic (superoxide dismutase, catalase, or glutathione peroxidase) and nonenzymatic (allopurinol, glutathione, dimethylthiourea, and lazaroid) have shown impressive results in reducing lung reperfusion injury. Some of these agents have been used with success in clinical lung transplant programs.

Metabolism

Among solid organs harvested and preserved for transplantation, the lung is unique. Oxygen in the inflated alveoli and intracellular glucose augmented by glucose in the flushing solution allows the cooled lung to maintain aerobic metabolism and preserve its adinosine triphosphate (ATP) levels during extended periods of preservation (Date, et al., 1993). In fact it may be possible for the lung to maintain a state of aerobic metabolism within the cadaver for short periods following death. Egan, et al. (1993) demonstrated satisfactory gas exchange in canine lung allografts harvested from canine donors some hours after death.

TECHNIQUE

Donor Extraction

Our donor extraction technique was recently reported by Sundaresan, et al. (1993b). After arrival at the donor hospital, it is important for the lung extraction team to assess the chest radiographs and perform fiberoptic bronchoscopy. The final assessment is made by gross inspection of the lungs, exposed by a median sternotomy performed in conjunction with the midline laparotomy for the extraction of abdominal organs.

The abdominal organs are prepared for extraction by their respective surgical teams. It is important for the liver team to insert a large-caliber cannula in the inferior vena cava for liver flush effluent rather than planning to vent the hepatic flush into the chest through the divided inferior vena cava, thereby obscuring the view of the thoracic organ extraction team.

Both vena cavae are encircled within the pericardium. The aorta is mobilized and encircled. Care must be taken to avoid injury to the right main pulmonary artery lying immediately posterior to the superior vena cava and ascending aorta. The aorta is mobilized and encircled. It is not necessary to dissect the main pulmonary artery.

The donor is heparinized. A cardioplegia cannula is placed in the ascending aorta. A large-bore pulmonary flush cannula is then placed in the main pulmonary artery immediately proximal to its bifurcation. PGE_1 (500 μg) is administered directly into the main pulmonary artery. This produces an immediate fall in systemic pressure. At this point, venous inflow occlusion is achieved by double ligation of the superior vena cava and clamping of the inferior vena cava at the diaphragm. The aorta is then cross-clamped, and cardioplegia is initiated. Cardioplegia is vented through the inferior vena cava, which is divided immediately above the previously placed clamp. After cardioplegic arrest has been achieved, pulmonary flushing is initiated. With the lungs maintained in a state of moderate inflation, pulmonary artery flushing is achieved with 3 L of modified Euro-Collins solution delivered at a pressure of 30 cmH_2O. This solution is vented through the amputated tip of the left atrial appendage (Fig. 33-2). Cold effluent is allowed to collect in both pleural spaces. Topical hypothermia is supplemented by crushed ice.

It is our preference to extract the donor heart in situ. It should be stated emphatically that in every case satisfactory cardiac and bilateral lung grafts can be safely extracted. The superior vena cava is divided between the previously placed ligatures, again taking care not to injure the underlying right main pulmonary artery. The aorta is divided superiorly to the cardioplegia cannula. The main pulmonary artery is then divided through the cannulation site. The heart is then elevated and retracted to the right. The left atrium is opened midway between the coronary sinus and the inferior pulmonary vein. The left atrial incision is then continued toward the right. The right side of the left atrial wall is then divided, taking care to preserve a rim of atrial muscle on the pulmonary vein side (Fig. 33-3). This completes the cardiac excision.

Extraction of the lungs is then continued by mobilization and division of the trachea well above the carina. It is our preference to divide the trachea with a stapling instrument, leaving the lungs in a state of moderate inflation. The great vessels are divided at the apex of the chest, and the esophagus transsected with a stapling instrument. The entire thoracic contents are then extracted from the spine in a caudal direction. The thoracic aorta and esophagus are transsected at the diaphragm. The lung allografts are then immersed in cold crystalloid solution and transported semi-inflated. Should

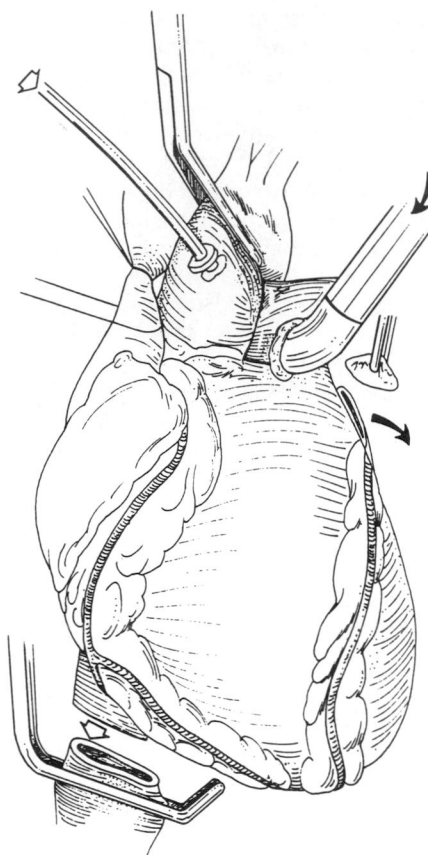

Figure 33-2. Cardioplegia is administered proximal to an aortic cross clamp and vented through the transsected inferior vena cava (*open arrow*). Pulmonary flush solution is administered through the main pulmonary artery and vented through the amputated tip of the left atrial appendage (*solid arrow*). (From Sundaresen S et al: Donor lung procurement: assessment and operative technique. Ann Thorac Surg 56:1409, 1993, with permission.)

each lung be used in different transplant centers, they are separated into separate allografts at the donor hospital. The donor left main bronchus is divided at its origin with a cutting stapling device to leave the airway to both lungs sealed (Fig. 33-4). Otherwise, the grafts should be transported en bloc for separation immediately prior to implantation. On arrival at the recipient hospital, the graft is exposed and kept cold during the remainder of its preparation. The esophagus and aorta are removed, leaving all other soft tissues on the specimen side, to maximize bronchial arterial collateral flow to the donor lung. If bronchial revascularization is to be attempted, the anterior wall of the proximal descending aorta is left on the specimen (Couraud, et al., 1992).

Viewing the double-lung block from its anterior aspect, the posterior pericardium is divided inferiorly to superiorly. The posterior left atrium is divided, leaving equal atrial cuffs on both sides. The remaining pericardium posterior to the left atrium is then divided. The pulmonary artery is divided at its bifurcation (Fig. 33-4). It is important to separate the pulmonary artery from its pericardial attachments on each side out to the first pulmonary arterial branch. This prevents

compromise of pulmonary artery's caliber distal to the pulmonary artery's anastomosis following implantation.

Subcarinal nodes are then divided, and the left main bronchus is transsected. The left main bronchus is then dissected from the nodal tissue and divided two rings proximal to the upper lobe orifice. On the right side, excision of the carina usually provides an adequate length (two rings proximal to the upper lobe origin) for subsequent bronchial anastomosis. It is important during dissection of the bronchus to minimize any nodal dissection at the site of bronchus transsection to maximize retrograde bronchial collateral blood flow to the donor bronchus after transplantation.

Recipient Anesthesia

A successful lung transplant program requires active involvement of expert anesthesiologists familiar with complex cardiothoracic anesthesia techniques, bronchoscopy, and cardiopulmonary bypass. Full hemodynamic monitoring is required in every patient. We routinely use a Foley catheter, central venous line, pulmonary artery Swan-Ganz catheter, and radial artery catheter. It is often useful to supplement the radial artery catheter with a femoral artery line, especially if cardiopulmonary bypass is anticipated. We routinely use a transesophageal echocardiographic probe and believe that it is especially critical in patients with severe pulmonary hypertension and coexisting right ventricular dysfunction.

The airway is routinely intubated with a left-sided double-lumen endobronchial tube, which enables independent ventilation of either or both lungs. A single-lumen tube with an endobronchial Fogarty catheter enables independent ventilation. However, this technique does not have the reliability of a double-lumen tube. A single-lumen tube can present difficulties, particularly in a bilateral transplant recipient in whom intraoperative maneuvering of the tube can be troublesome. In patients with cystic fibrosis, thick tenacious purulent secretions are continuously expressed into the bronchial lumen during manipulation of the lungs for extraction. In these patients we place a large-caliber single-lumen tube and, using a flexible fiberoptic bronchoscope, aspirate the airway completely prior to placement of the double-lumen tube and initiation of the procedure.

In patients of small stature, a single-lumen tube must be used. If a bilateral procedure is planned in such patients, cardiopulmonary bypass should be used routinely during extraction and implantation. This is the standard technique for bilateral transplantation in children (Spray, et al., 1993).

It has been our practice to use aprotinin routinely in patients in whom there is an anticipation of intrapleural adhesion (e.g., cystic fibrosis, bronchiectasis, or patients with previous thoracic surgery). This agent effectively reduces perioperative blood loss, especially when cardiopulmonary bypass is required in patients with extensive pleural or mediastinal adhesions (Westaby, 1993).

Single Lung Transplantation

Choice of Side. In general we prefer to transplant the side with the least pulmonary function, as judged by preoperative

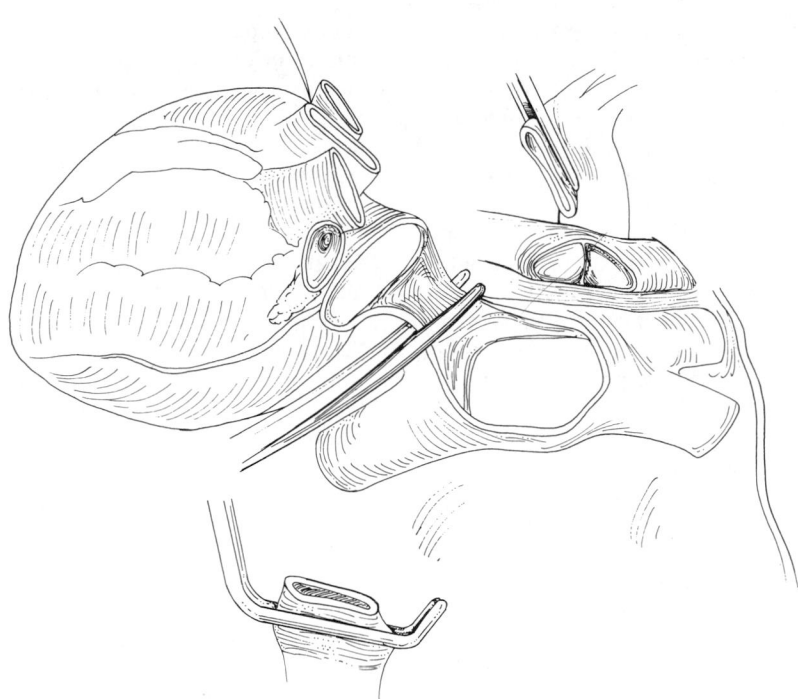

Figure 33-3.   The ascending aorta is divided. The main pulmonary artery has been transsected at its bifurcation. The heart is retracted upward and to the right to enable safe division of the left atrium leaving suitable cuffs on both cardiac and lung allografts. (From Sundaresen S et al: Donor lung procurement: assessment and operative technique. Ann Thorac Surg 56:1409, 1993, with permission.)

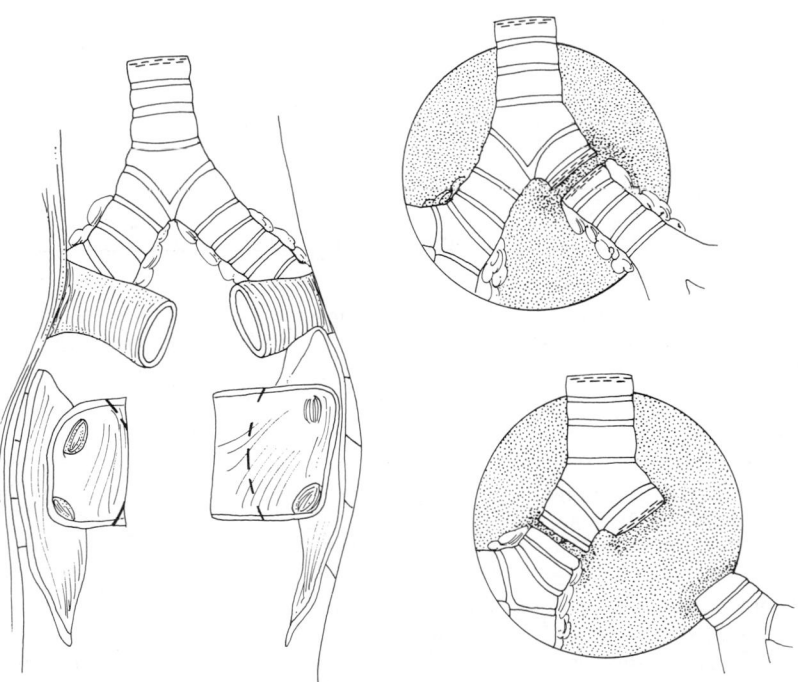

Figure 33-4.   The pericardium and left atrium are divided with the left atrium further trimmed (*dotted lines*). The airway is transsected and kept sealed by using a gastrointestinal anastomosis stapling device across the proximal left mainstem bronchus. The donor airway is further revised for implantation, as shown in the bottom right. (From Sundaresen S et al: Donor lung procurement: assessment and operative technique. Ann Thorac Surg 56:1409, 1993, with permission.)

quantitative nuclear perfusion scans. It was previously argued that the right side was preferable for patients with obstructive pulmonary disease. However, in our experience and that of others (Levine, et al., 1993), there is no difference in functional outcome among single-lung recipients, regardless of the transplanted side. If cardiopulmonary bypass is anticipated, as in patients with primary pulmonary hypertension or severe pulmonary fibrosis with associated pulmonary hypertension, the right side is the preferred transplant side. For patients with Eisenmenger's syndrome, we prefer the right side to facilitate closure of the coexisting atrial or ventricular septal defects. A patent ductus arteriosus can be repaired in association with a transplant on either side.

Exposure.   A generous posterolateral thoracotomy through the fifth interspace or bed of the excised fifth rib is the preferred approach. For right-sided transplants in which cardiopulmonary bypass is anticipated, cannulation of the ascending aorta is facilitated somewhat by the use of a fourth interspace incision. A median sternotomy can be used for right-sided transplants, especially if associated cardiac repair dictates an anterior approach, permitting access to the left side of the heart. The patients are always positioned with the ipsilateral groin in the operative field for subsequent cannulation if necessary. Femoral partial bypass was formerly our technique of choice. However, intrathoracic cannulation avoids a groin incision and the necessary arterial and venous repairs following decannulation. The ascending aorta and right atrium can be easily cannulated through the right chest. The cannulas are positioned in the anterior aspect of the incision and remain well out of the operative field throughout the procedure. Through a left posterolateral thoracotomy, the proximal left pulmonary artery and descending aorta can be easily cannulated.

Recipient Pneumonectomy.   Following adequate exposure of the pleural space, pleural adhesions are divided. These can be extensive in patients with fibrotic or septic lung disease and are ordinarily absent in patients with emphysema and primary pulmonary hypertension. Extreme care is taken not to injure the phrenic and recurrent laryngeal nerves. The inferior pulmonary ligament is divided. The pulmonary veins and main pulmonary artery are encircled outside the pericardium. During this dissection the need for cardiopulmonary bypass is determined. The ventilation of the contralateral lung and occlusion of the ipsilateral pulmonary artery determine whether the contralateral native lung provides adequate gas exchange and hemodynamics to tolerate pneumonectomy and implantation without cardiopulmonary bypass. Assessment of right ventricular contractility with the transesophageal echo probe is especially useful at this point (Triantafillou, et al., 1994).

Easily accessible upper lobe pulmonary artery branches are ligated and divided. This increases the length of pulmonary artery available for subsequent pulmonary artery anastomosis. It also decreases the caliber of the pulmonary artery to match the donor's size to the recipient's pulmonary artery, particularly when significant pulmonary hypertension is present. Furthermore, having a ligated recipient upper lobe branch helps with proper orientation of the donor and recipi-

ent pulmonary arteries. The pulmonary artery just distal to this branch is stapled proximally. A distal pulmonary artery clamp is placed, the vessel is divided, and its distal aspect is ligated to minimize back bleeding, which can be torrential if vigorous bronchial circulation is present.

Pulmonary veins are divided between the stapled lines or between silk ligatures placed on each venous branch at the hilum. This latter option increases the size of the subsequent left atrial cuff. Pulmonary artery division is often made easier after division of the superior pulmonary vein.

Peribronchial nodal tissue is divided, and bronchial arterial vessels are secured with ligatures. The bronchus is transsected just proximal to the upper lobe origin, and the lung is excised (Fig. 33-5). The recipient bronchus is then trimmed back up into the mediastinum, taking care to avoid any devascularization of the recipient bronchus at the site of anastomosis. The pericardium around the vein stumps is then widely opened, and hemostasis is achieved in the mediastinum.

Implantation.   The donor lung, wrapped in cold moist gauze, is then placed in the posterior portion of the thorax. In this position, manipulation of the lung can be avoided during the entire implantation. The lung is kept cold by using topical application of crushed ice. This topical hypothermia provides an extended period of cold preservation, giving additional time for meticulous anastomoses.

The bronchial anastomosis is performed first (Fig. 33-6). Various techniques have been described. Our preference is to close the membranous posterior wall initially, using a continuous suture of 4–0 absorbable monofilament suture. The anterior cartilaginous airway is then closed by using an interrupted suture of absorbable monofilament. Sutures are placed by using a modified mattress or figure-eight technique to intussuscept the smaller (usually the donor) into the larger bronchus for a distance of one cartilaginous ring. Small-caliber bronchi can be narrowed by this intussusception technique. In this circumstance, an end-to-end closure is obtained by using simple interrupted sutures of monofilament absorbable material. The bronchial anastomosis is covered by using either local peribronchial nodal tissue or a pedicle flap of pericardium or thymic fat. We no longer use bronchial omentopexy in routine transplant procedures.

A vascular clamp is then placed as proximal as possible on the ipsilateral main pulmonary artery. The donor and recipient arteries are trimmed to size, and an end-to-end anastomosis is created using 5–0 polyprophylene suture (Fig. 33-7). Care must be taken to excise an adequate length of donor and recipient pulmonary artery. Excessive length can result in kinking of the pulmonary artery after allograft inflation. Proper orientation of the donor and recipient pulmonary artery is also obviously important.

Lateral traction on the pulmonary vein stumps enables central placement of an angled atrial clamp. For right-sided transplants, it is occasionally necessary to open the interatrial groove to increase the length of recipient left atrium available for placement of the clamp. Pulmonary vein stumps are then amputated, and the bridge of tissue between the two is incised to create a suitable cuff for the left atrial anastomosis (Fig. 33-8). Following completion of this anastomosis, but

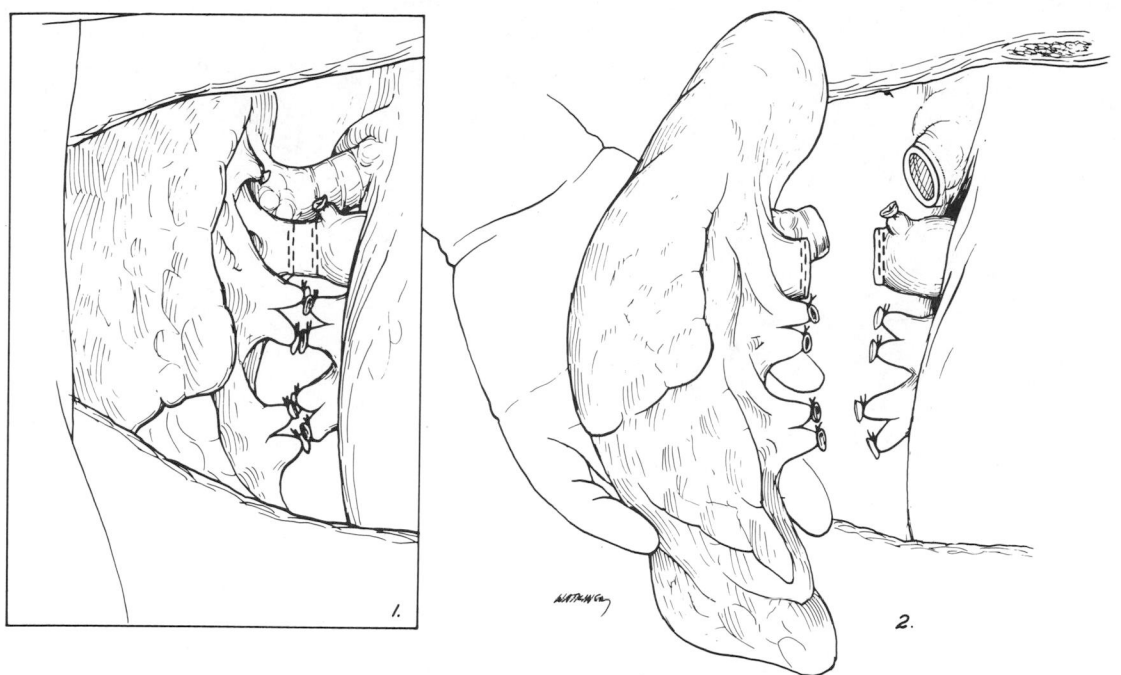

Figure 33-5. Excision of the native right lung is depicted. The pulmonary artery is stapled beyond its first upper lobe branch. Pulmonary veins are divided between ligatures, and the bronchus is transsected just proximal to the upper lobe orifice. (From Shields TW: General Thoracic Surgery. Lea & Febiger, Philadelphia, 1994, with permission.)

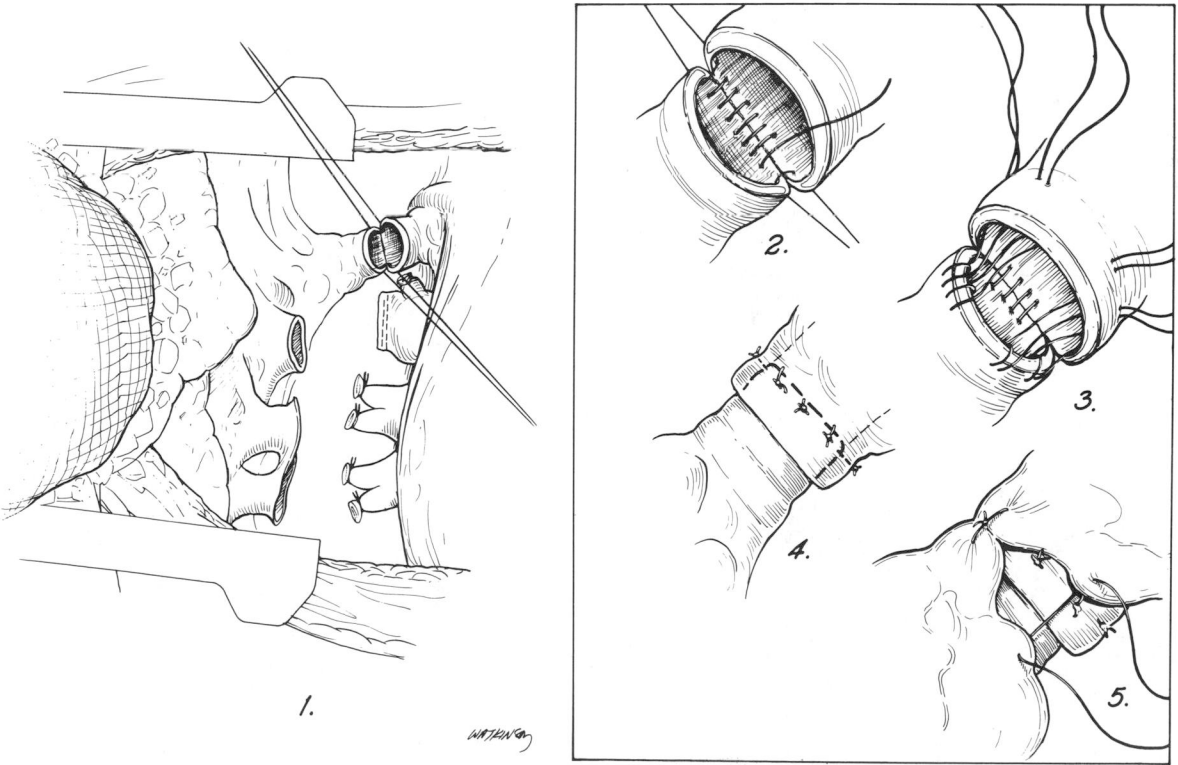

Figure 33-6. A right bronchial anastomosis is depicted with the lung cooled by topical crushed ice. The membranous wall is opposed first. The cartilaginous wall is intussuscepted, in this case donor into recipient bronchus, for one cartilaginous ring. Peribronchial nodal tissue covers the anastomosis.

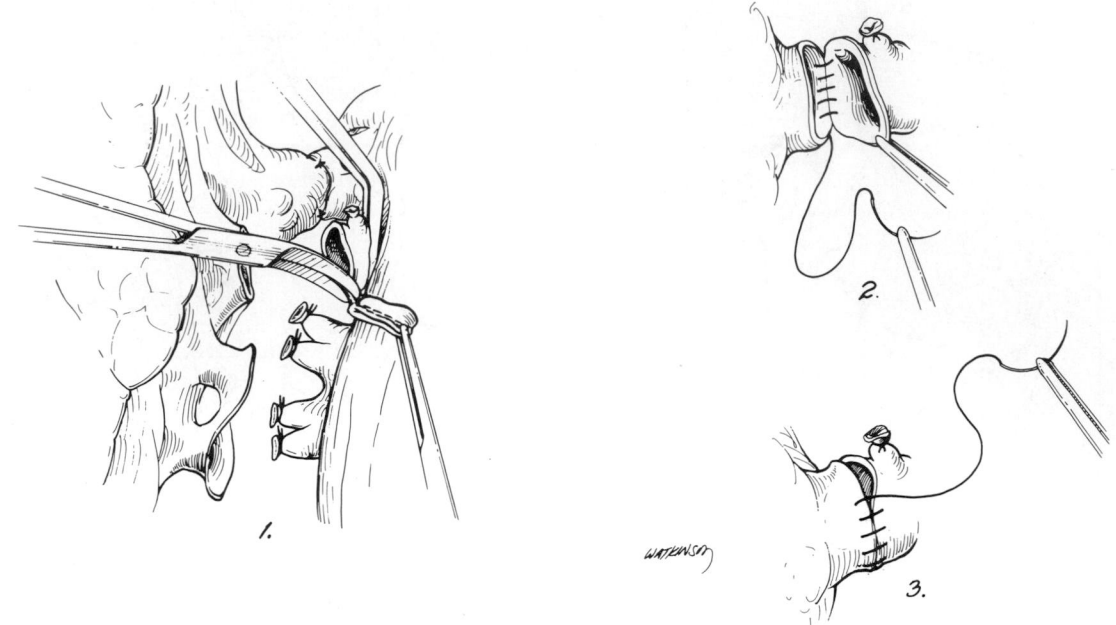

Figure 33-7. A central pulmonary artery clamp is placed, the staple line is excised, and an end-to-end anastomosis is constructed with 5–0 polypropylene. (From Shields TW: General Thoracic Surgery. Lea & Febiger, Philadelphia, 1994, with permission.)

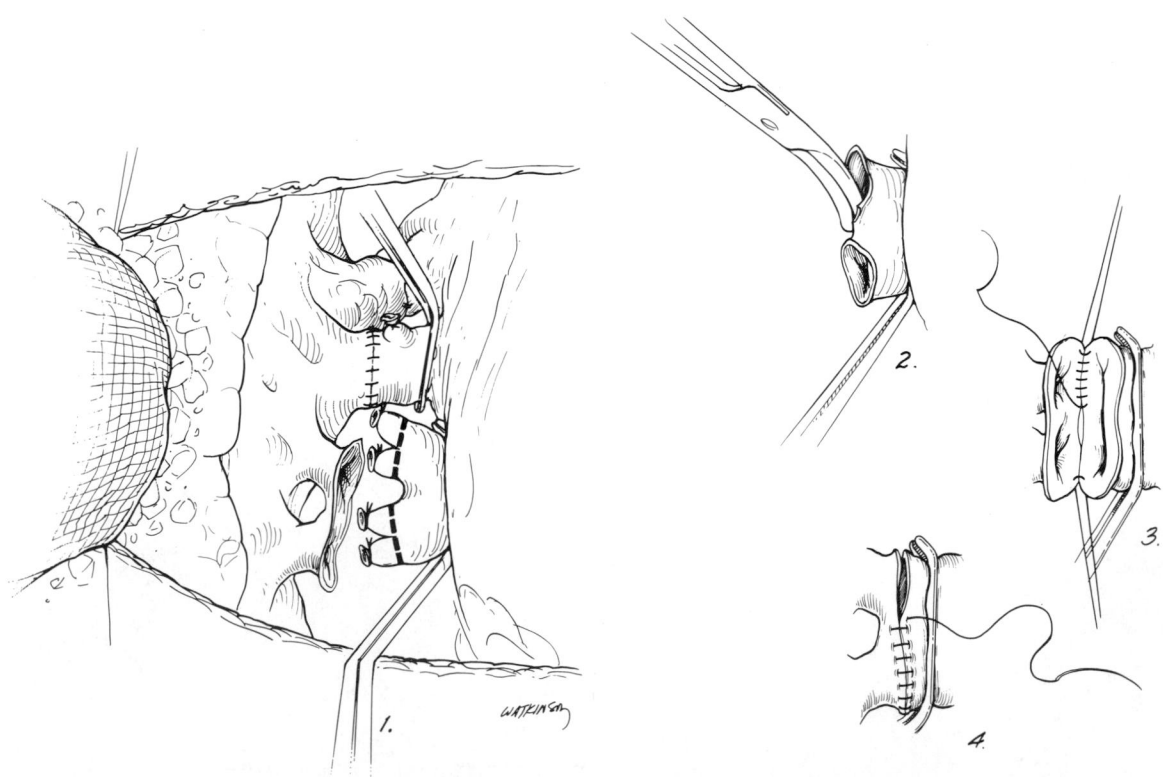

Figure 33-8. A central left atrial clamp is in place while the vein stumps are amputated and the bridge of atrial muscle is divided. Then 4–0 polypropylene suture is used to complete the anastomosis. (From Shields TW: General Thoracic Surgery. Lea & Febiger, Philadelphia, 1994, with permission.)

before tying the final stitch, the lung is gently inflated while the pulmonary artery clamp is temporarily removed, enabling the lung to be "deaired" through the open left atrial anastomosis. All suture lines are then secured and inspected, and the vascular clamps are removed. It is our practice to initiate reperfusion with the recipient receiving a continuous infusion of PGE_1. This infusion is continued for at least several days after the transplant. Two pleural drains are left in each pleural space, and routine closure is achieved using absorbable suture material. At the termination of the procedure, the double-lumen endotracheal tube is replaced with a large-caliber single-lumen tube. Flexible bronchoscopy is then performed to inspect the bronchial anastomosis and evacuate the airway of any blood or secretions.

Sequential Bilateral Lung Transplantation

Exposure. Bilateral sequential single-lung transplantations are conducted through bilateral anterolateral fourth or fifth interspace thoracotomies connected by a transverse sternotomy (Fig. 33-9). This "clam shell" incision provides adequate exposure for safe division of pleural adhesions. In patients with cystic fibrosis, these can be particularly dense at the apex and posterior aspect of the chest. In addition, this incision provides satisfactory exposure for institution of cardiopulmonary bypass by ascending aortic and right atrial cannulation.

Pneumonectomy and Implantation. The techniques of pneumonectomy and implantation are identical to those just described for single-lung transplantation. The side with the worse function (as predicted by preoperative ventilation and perfusion nuclear scans) is replaced first. If function is equivalent, the right lung is replaced first. Cardiopulmonary bypass may be necessary at several junctures during bilateral sequential transplant (Triantafillou, unpublished data, 1993). In patients with small airways not amenable to double-lumen tube placement, cardiopulmonary bypass is instituted following mobilization of both lungs and maintained during bilateral extraction and implantation. Occasionally, the remaining contralateral native lung does not enable satisfactory gas exchange or hemodynamics to occur during removal or replacement of the first lung. Cardiopulmonary bypass is instituted at this point. The most common situation wherein bypass is necessary occurs following implantation of the first lung. The transplanted lung may not support the recipient's circulation and gas exchange. This problem presents itself as a progressive increase in pulmonary artery pressure.

If increased pulmonary artery pressure is genuine and substantial, pulmonary edema will develop with associated hypoxemia. This is a typical clinical phenomenon, and its cause is not well understood. It may be the result of poor preservation. Alternatively, it may be caused by recipient systemic bacteremia, as it is most commonly observed following implantation of the first lung in patients with cystic fibrosis. It is prudent to institute cardiopulmonary bypass for the completion of the procedure as soon as clinical problems arise rather than waiting until an emergent situation develops in an unstable patient.

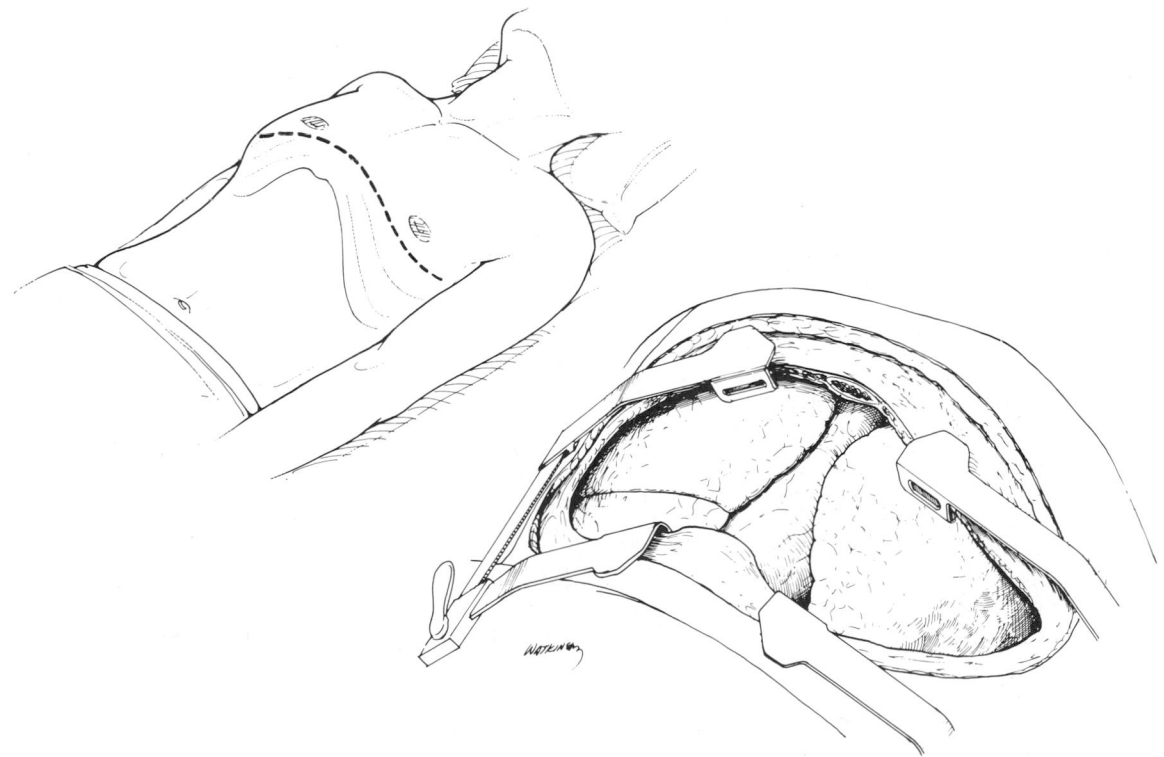

Figure 33-9. Bilateral anterolateral thoracotomies are performed through the fourth or fifth interspace with transverse division of the sternum. (From Shields TW: General Thoracic Surgery. Lea & Febiger, Philadelphia, 1994, with permission.)

En Bloc Bilateral Lung Transplantation

Some authors advocate a return to the originally described en bloc double-lung procedure (Patterson, et al., 1988) accompanied by revascularization of the bronchial circulation. In this circumstance, the aortic button mentioned in the donor dissection above is identified after reperfusion. A back-bleeding orifice is assumed to be of bronchial origin. Alternatively, at the time of allograft preparation, the suspected right bronchial arterial orifice can be marked by a fine suture. Revascularization is then achieved by internal mammary artery (Daly, et al., 1993) or saphenous vein graft to the aorta (Couraud, et al., 1992). Alternatively, should the length of the pedicle permit, direct connection of the patch to the ascending aorta is also possible.

POSTOPERATIVE MANAGEMENT

Ventilation

In general patients are ventilated with standard ventilatory techniques. The FIO_2 is kept at a level to maintain PaO_2 at greater than 70 mmHg. A tidal volume of 12 to 15 m/kg is usually sufficient, and a PEEP of 5 to 7.5 cmH_2O is used, except in patients who have had single-lung transplantations for obstructive pulmonary disease. Extubation is performed in accordance with standard requirements of satisfactory gas exchange and mechanics. The majority of patients are extubated within 24 to 48 hours following transplantation following a standard intermittent mandatory ventilation or pressure support wean. This type of ventilatory management is used in all bilateral lung transplant recipients and in single-lung recipients transplanted for pulmonary fibrosis.

However, patients who have undergone single-lung transplantation for chronic obstructive pulmonary disease and pulmonary vascular disease are managed differently. In the former condition, we generally make an effort to avoid the use of PEEP, and select tidal volumes that are somewhat lower than would ordinarily be used. These adjustments are made in an effort to reduce hyperinflation of the contralateral hypercompliant native lung and resultant compression of the less compliant transplanted lung. This can be a major problem. In some patients a volume reduction of the native lung by lobectomy or even pneumonectomy has been performed in an effort to decompress the contralateral transplanted lung. In patients with pulmonary vascular disease, we have elected to use a prolonged period (48 to 72 hours) of elective ventilation. Patients are kept heavily sedated and often paralyzed for that period. We choose to maintain these patients in a position with the native lung dependent to maintain inflation and appropriate drainage of the transplanted lung. Standard tidal volumes are used, but PEEP of 7.5 to 10 cmH_2O is applied. In occasional patients, early graft dysfunction, rejection, or infection will necessitate a prolonged period of postoperative mechanical ventilation. We have no hesitation about performing a tracheostomy. The tracheostomy improves patient comfort, facilitates mobilization, permits oral nutrition, and results in a more positive attitude in the ventilator-dependent patient.

Fluid Management

During the first few postoperative days, fluid management is carefully monitored by a determination of pulmonary capillary wedge pressure and daily weight. In spite of the vigilance of our anesthesiology colleagues, most patients return from the operating room with a significant positive fluid balance. Diuretics are used aggressively during the early postoperative period. On occasion, patients who have undergone single-lung transplants for primary pulmonary hypertension develop hemodynamic instability if their right heart filling pressures are excessively reduced.

Sepsis Prophylaxis

Bacterial

All patients are given routine prophylaxis, using ceftazidime and vancomycin. These agents are continued for several days. If indicated by cultures of bronchial secretions from the donor or recipient, adjustments in these antibiotics are made. In the cystic fibrosis population, aerosolized colistin or tobramycin is also used. These patients also require, in addition to the broad-spectrum antibiotics noted above, specific antipseudomonal coverage, as dictated by the sensitivities of their preoperative sputum cultures.

Viral

Herpes simplex was formerly a frequent cause of postoperative morbidity as a result of oral ulcerations and occasional pneumonitis. However, routine use of acyclovir prophylaxis has eliminated herpes infection as a frequent postoperative complication. CMV remains a significant problem in pulmonary transplant recipients. Most programs have adopted the strategy of matching seronegative donors with seronegative recipients whenever possible. The highest incidence of severe CMV infection occurs with donor-negative/recipient-positive transplants. In these patients, prophylaxis with intravenous ganciclovir is used routinely according to the following protocol.

Ganciclovir	5 mg/kg IV	twice daily	weeks 2–8
		once daily	weeks 8–12
		three times weekly	weeks 12–16

There is a reasonable argument for using this prophylactic regimen in any circumstance in which either the donor or recipient is seropositive. Although CMV infection or disease is uncommon during prophylaxis, there is a high rate of CMV disease after cessation of prophylactic therapy, especially in the donor-negative recipient-positive combination.

Fungal

It has been our practice not to use routine fungal prophylaxis. However, in the circumstance in which a heavy growth yeast is identified post-transplant in the donor's bronchial culture, prophylactic ketoconazole or low-dose amphotericin B is justified. There have been anecdotal reports of early systemic candidal septicemia in patients receiving lungs from donors whose bronchial cultures grew Candida.

Pneumocystis carinii

This parasite was formerly an occasional cause of postoperative pulmonary infection. However, routine use of cotrimoxazole prophylaxis has eliminated this as a significant pathogen. Alternative agents are used when an allergy to sulfa is present.

Immunosuppression

All clinical lung transplant programs rely on triple-agent immunosuppression, consisting of cyclosporine, azathioprine, and corticosteroid.

Azathioprine 1.5 mg/kg IV is administered immediately preoperatively. Cyclosporine 2 to 3 mg/kg is begun during the first few postoperative hours after satisfactory renal function is ensured. The dose is adjusted to maintain whole blood levels in the range of 350 to 400 ng/ml. This level often induces a significant increase in serum creatinine, necessitating a reduction in the cyclosporine dose. After several days, when an oral diet is initiated, oral cyclosporine can be started with twice-daily doses, as determined by the whole blood level. Azathioprine is continued at a dose of 1 to 2 mg/kg IV, and when an oral diet is initiated, the same dosing level can be administered by the oral route. The dose must be adjusted to maintain a white blood cell count in excess of 3,500/dl.

The early use of perioperative corticosteroids is controversial. Methylprednisolone 10 to 15 mg/kg IV is given intraoperatively just prior to graft perfusion. Most programs have adopted the use of moderate-dose corticosteroid therapy (methylprednisolone 0.5 to 1 mg/kg/day IV) for several days before initiating an oral dose of prednisone of 0.5 mg/kg/day. However, we have demonstrated (Miller, et al., 1993) that withholding this oral dose of prednisone has no adverse effect on bronchial healing and may in fact lessen the risk of perioperative sepsis.

A matter of considerable controversy is the use of postoperative cytolytic therapy (antithymocyte globulin or OKT3). These cytolytic agents are in use in a number of programs. The Pittsburgh group reported a reduced incidence of acute rejection in patients receiving rabbit antithymocyte globulin (Griffith, et al., 1992). In our own program, we use ATGAM (Upjohn, Kalamazoo, MI). It has been argued that these agents, particularly OKT3, predisposed patients to a higher incidence of CMV infection. However, this was an experience accumulated at a time when CMV matching was not widely practiced and CMV prophylaxis was not routinely used. It is probable that the early use of cytolytic therapy does reduce the frequency and severity of early postoperative rejection episodes.

For most patients, chronic immunosuppression consists of cyclosporine, prednisone, and azathioprine. After the first month post-transplant, the doses of cyclosporine are reduced to maintain blood levels in the range of 250 to 300 ng/me. Prednisone is also reduced to minimize the complications of long-term steroid use.

Infection and Rejection Surveillance

Acute rejection following lung transplantation is expected. Ninety-seven percent of recipients in our program have been treated for acute rejection on at least one occasion during the first 3 postoperative weeks. Early acute rejection episodes are characterized by dyspnea, low-grade fever, moderate leukocytosis, hypoxemia, and a diffuse perihilar interstitial infiltrate on the chest radiograph. This clinical picture most typically occurs for the first time on about the fifth to the seventh post-transplant day. All these clinical features are also consistent with infection. Clinical examination, radiographic assessment, and fiberoptic bronchoscopy are valuable tools in resolving the frequent dilemma of infection versus rejection in lung transplant recipients (Trulock, 1993a). During the first week or two postoperatively, if acute rejection is suspected, our usual strategy is to administer a trial bolus dose of methylprednisolone of 500 to 1000 mg and observe the clinical response. If rejection is the problem, a dramatic improvement in clinical findings, radiographic appearance, (Fig. 33-10), and PaO$_2$ will usually be observed within 8 to 12 hours. If this is the case, the patient receives two additional daily intravenous bolus doses of methylprednisolone in a somewhat reduced dose.

An alternative approach is to perform routine fiberoptic bronchoscopy whenever there is a clinical indication in the absence of recently identified untreated organisms identified by sputum culture. The advantage of routine flexible bronchoscopy is that it enables the performance of bronchoalveolar lavage and transbronchial biopsy. Although bronchoalveolar lavage has not been useful in the diagnosis of rejection, it is invaluable in the identification of opportunistic infections commonly encountered in transplant recipients. Transbronchial biopsy is the procedure of choice in the diagnosis of pulmonary rejection. We have used this modality frequently in patients with unexplained pulmonary infiltrates not responsive to corticosteroid therapy. Transbronchial biopsy is a highly sensitive and specific diagnostic tool for the evaluation of acute rejection. Routine bronchoalveolar lavage and transbronchial biopsies are performed at 3 weeks; 3, 6, 9, and 12 months; and on an annual basis thereafter.

COMPLICATIONS

Technical Error

As in any major operative intervention, a variety of technical complications may be encountered during the postoperative period. In former years hemorrhage was a frequent complication. In the early experience of some programs undertaking heart-lung and en bloc double-lung transplants, approximately 25 percent of patients required reoperation for postoperative hemorrhage. However, with currently used surgical techniques, such as the posterolateral thoracotomy for single-lung transplantation and the clam shell incision for bilateral lung replacement, surgical exposure is superb. In addition, aprotinin has dramatically reduced intraoperative and postoperative bleeding, especially in patients with extensive pleural adhesions requiring cardiopulmonary bypass. Among 105 bilateral sequential single-lung transplants performed by our group, only one patient (who required extracorporeal membrane oxygenation [ECMO] support) required reexploration for hemorrhage.

Anastomotic complications can also occur and result in postoperative graft dysfunction. Griffith, et al. (1994) recently reported their experience with anastomotic complications following lung transplantation and made a number of important technical points. An unsatisfactory bronchial anasto-

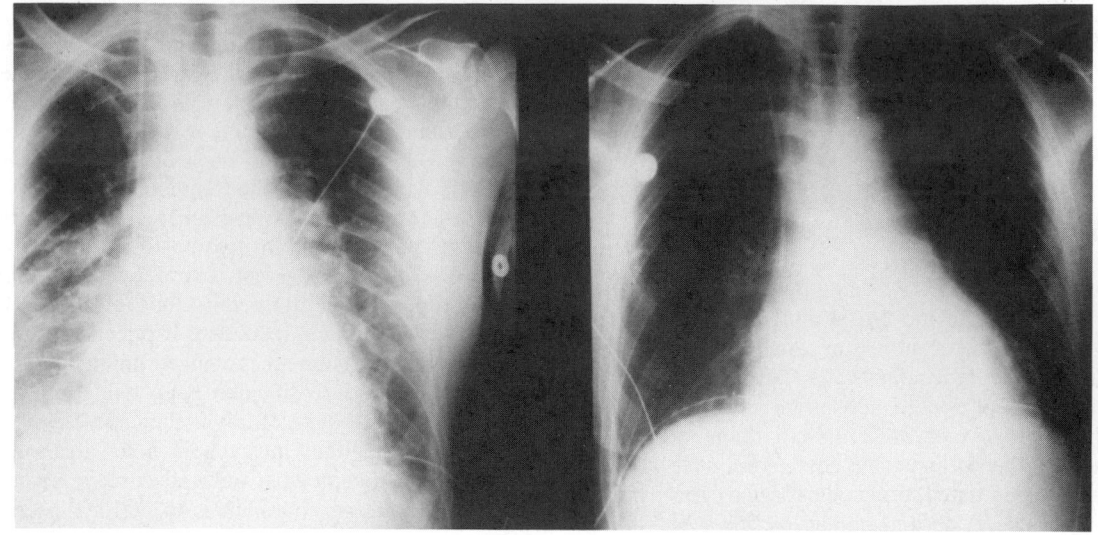

Figure 33-10. Posteroanterior chest radiographs from a patient 7 days following bilateral sequential single-lung transplantation. **(A)** On the morning of the seventh postoperative day, the radiograph shows a bilateral diffuse infiltrate. A clinical diagnosis of rejection was made, and the patient received methylprednisolone 1 g IV bolus. **(B)** Radiograph taken 8 hours later demonstrates a dramatic improvement in the infiltrate, which is consistent with the typical response of acute rejection to steroid bolus therapy. (From Shields TW: General Thoracic Surgery. Lea & Febiger, Philadelphia, 1994, with permission.)

mosis is routinely identified in the operating room during the postimplantation bronchoscopy. Inadequate anastomotic caliber dictates an immediate surgical revision.

Persistent pulmonary hypertension and unexplained hypoxemia can occur as a result of stenosis at the pulmonary artery anastomosis. This problem may be suggested by a nuclear perfusion scan, which will demonstrate less than the anticipated flow to a single-lung graft or unequal distribution of flow in a bilateral-lung recipient. Occasionally, a stenotic anastomosis can be visualized by transesophageal echocardiography. However, contrast angiography should be performed in any patient in whom there is a concern. At the time of angiography, the pressure gradient across the pulmonary artery anastomosis should be determined. A gradient of 15 to 20 mmHg is commonly encountered, especially in single-lung recipients in whom most of the cardiac output is directed to the transplanted lung or in bilateral recipients with a high cardiac output. The need for anastomotic revision is dictated by the clinical situation.

Compromise in flow across the atrial anastomosis can also occur as a result of unsatisfactory anastomotic technique. Compression of the anastomosis by a clot or an omental or pericardial flap brought anterior or posterior to the atrial anastomosis for purposes of bronchial anastomotic coverage can also impair ipsilateral pulmonary venous drainage. Impaired venous outflow results in elevated venous pressure and ipsilateral pulmonary edema. Pulmonary artery pressures remain unexpectedly high, and flow through the graft is less than expected. Transesophageal echocardiography can image the trial anastomosis clearly. Contrast studies may be helpful in demonstrating a reduced level of flow through the anastomosis. However, open exploration is occasionally necessary to confirm the diagnosis and conduct an appropriate repair.

Early Graft Dysfunction

Approximately 20 percent of patients have severe early graft dysfunction (Haydock, et al., 1992). This problem may arise as a result of unsuspected donor lung pathologic conditions, such as aspiration, infection, or contusion. Inadequate preservation can occur as a result of technical difficulties at the time of harvest or prolonged warm ischemia during implantation. It is imperative to exclude remedial technical problems. Most commonly, allograft dysfunction occurs unexpectedly with no obvious cause (Fig. 33-11). The development of immediate postoperative florid pulmonary edema, severe hypoxemia, persistent pulmonary hypertension, and reduced pulmonary compliance can present a formidable management problem.

The patient requires intensive supportive measures. These patients generally can be managed with aggressive intensive care unit (ICU) ventilatory and pharmacologic intervention. High levels of PEEP and vigorous diuresis are important strategies. However, severe graft dysfunction or coexisting cardiac failure may require ECMO support. In our entire experience with 215 lung transplant recipients, only 5 have required ECMO support (arteriovenous) during the immediate postoperative phase. Four of these five patients survived and were discharged from hospital. In most patients, early allograft dysfunction (as for other forms of diffuse alveolar damage) resolves over several days of intensive care support with patients obtaining satisfactory long-term allograft function (Haydock, et al., 1992).

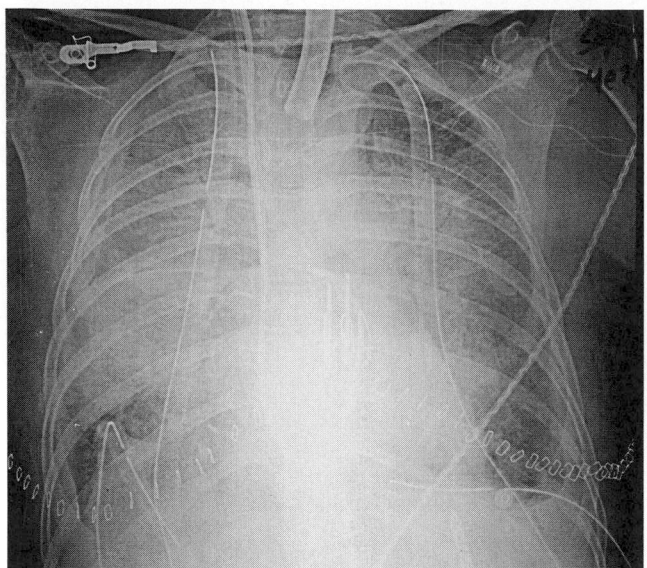

Figure 33-11. Anteroposterior chest radiograph taken immediately postoperatively in a patient who underwent bilateral sequential single-lung transplant. Despite satisfactory lung harvest, acceptable ischemic time (right, 4.5 hours; left, 6 hours) and only 3 hours of cardiopulmonary bypass time, severe allograft dysfunction occurred. All anastomoses were intact. Quantitative perfusion scan revealed 40 percent flow to the right lung and 60 percent to the left. The patient was euvolemic. The patient recovered from this severe lung injury over a period of 7 days.

Infection

Bacterial

Bacterial pneumonia is the most commonly encountered infection postlung transplantation. An aggressive approach is taken to identify the specific organism. Fiberoptic bronchoscopy with a protected brush should be undertaken if routine sputum cultures do not provide an identifiable organism. Routine intravenous antibiotic therapy is used, and in the majority of patients, the pneumonia rapidly clears. Patients with cystic fibrosis present a real management dilemma during the postoperative period because they are susceptible to recurrent pulmonary infections from the same Pseudomonas organisms harbored in the airway and upper airway sinuses post-transplant. This is particularly true of patients with highly resistent *Pseudomonas cepacia* (Snell, et al., 1993).

Lung abscess is occasionally encountered in lung transplant recipients. Patients with cystic fibrosis occasionally develop multifocal lung abscesses, presumably as a result of inhaled contamination from an upper airway or sinus infection. In single-lung recipients, the native lung is also susceptible to bacterial infection, which on occasion can cavitate, producing a lung abscess (Semenkovich, et al., 1994). These patients should be managed as is any other patient with a lung abscess. Appropriate broad-spectrum antibiotic therapy is administered, and bronchoscopy is performed to ensure that no airway obstruction is present. Occasionally, external drainage is required (Fig. 33-12).

Viral

Viral pneumonitis can occur during the postoperative period. During the early postoperative phase, herpes simplex infection was formerly encountered frequently. However, with the routine use of acyclovir, it is now an unusual complication. CMV infection is more commonly encountered when the donor, recipient, or both are CMV seropositive. Ettinger, et al. (1993) recently reviewed our experience at Washington University. Ninety-two percent of patients in their report developed CMV infection, with 75 percent of them having biopsy-proved CMV pneumonitis. A donor-negative recipient-positive combination resulted in more frequent and severe infections. No donor-negative recipient-negative patient developed an infection or disease. Biopsy-proved CMV pneumonitis was associated with radiographic infiltrate in less than 30 percent of cases. The detection of CMV in bronchoalveolar lavage was not always predictive of CMV pneumonitis. The high incidence of CMV infection and disease in our experience reflects the aggressive viral surveillance used in our program.

We do not treat CMV infection without biopsy proof of CMV disease. In this circumstance ganciclovir 5 mg/kg IV is administered twice daily for 2 to 3 weeks. In severe pneumonitis CMV hyperimmune globulin is also administered. The majority of patients respond promptly to this regimen.

Fungal

The most frequent cause of significant fungal infection posttransplant is Aspergillus. Unfortunately, after aspergillus has become a resident organism, it is difficult to clear. In patients without evidence of active invasive infection, we have administered ketoconazole with reasonable success. However, in patients whose infections do not clear with ketoconazole or who have developed an invasive infection, amphotericin B is required. Invasive Aspergillus infection usually is fatal.

A particularly interesting group of patients are those who have had single-lung transplants for pulmonary fibrosis and who develop Aspergillus infection in the diseased native lung. These patients should be treated aggressively, with the expectation that the Aspergillus will probably not clear from the native lung. In this circumstance, contralateral native lung pneumonectomy is warranted.

Pleural Space Complications

Pleural space complications occur frequently following pulmonary transplantation. Pneumothorax is encountered in two circumstances. It can occur as a result of airway dehiscence with communication into the pleural space (Fig. 33-13). However, this is not a frequent occurrence, and when present, it is usually readily managed by intercostal tube drainage with appropriate reexpansion of the underlying lung. A more common circumstance is the development of insignificant pneumothoraces in patients with obstructive pulmonary disease, either emphysema or cystic fibrosis, who have undergone bilateral replacement and received lungs much smaller than the pleural space into which they were implanted. Often a minimal degree of bilateral pneumothorax occurs subsequent to chest tube replacement. In general,

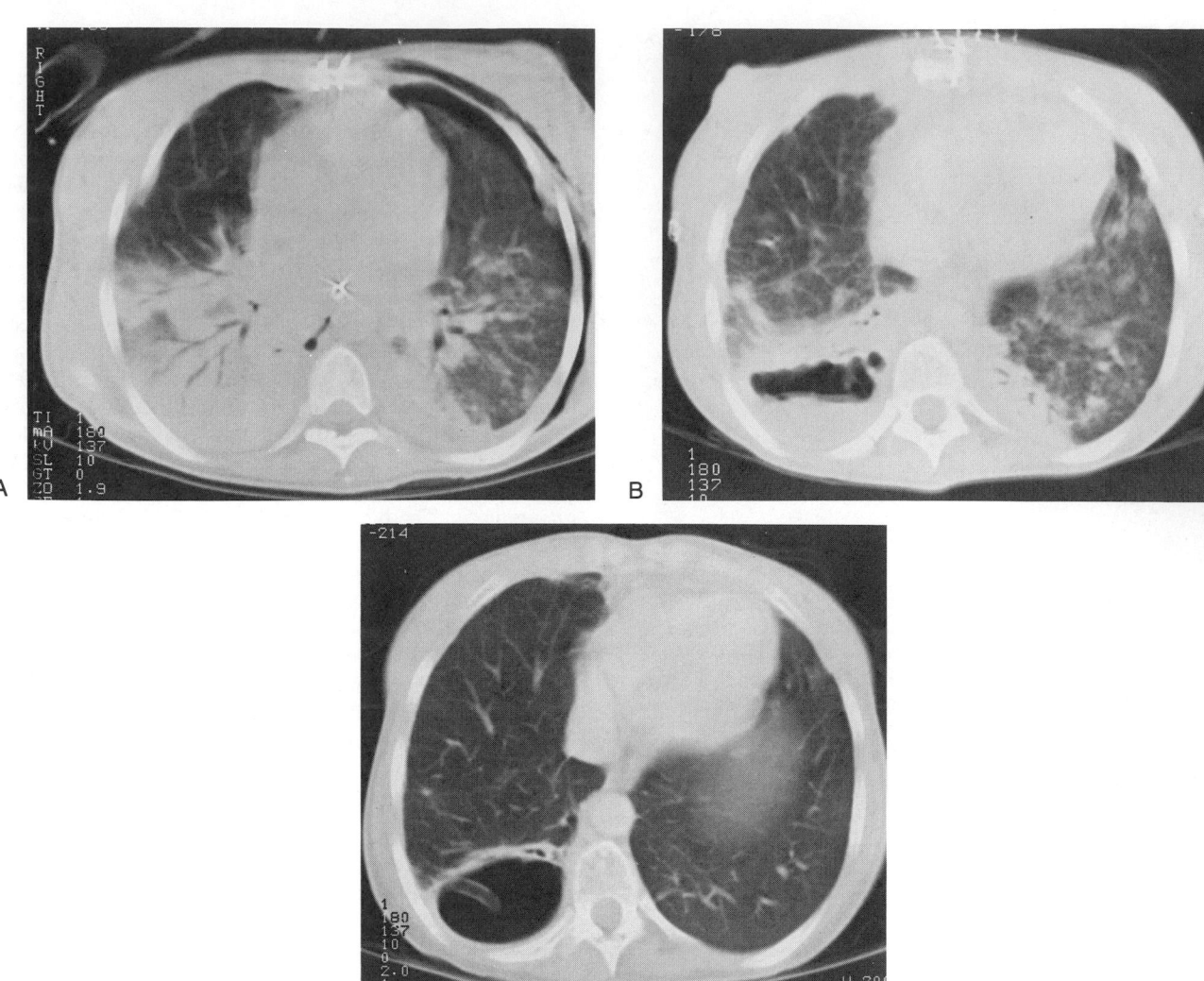

Figure 33-12. **(A)** Ten days following bilateral sequential single-lung transplantation for cystic fibrosis. The patient was noted to have a right lower lobe pneumonia and an incidental contralateral left pneumothorax with subcutaneous emphysema. **(B)** During the ensuing week, the right lower lobe pneumonia cavitated. An obvious air-fluid level was visible. **(C)** Tube thoracostomy achieved satisfactory drainage while the patient was convalescent. An elective rib resection was performed several months postoperatively.

these pneumothoraces can be ignored, the pleural air will eventually resorb, and any remaining space will fill with fluid.

Pleural effusions are commonly encountered, particularly in the group just noted in whom the pulmonary volume is somewhat smaller than the pleural space. A sympathetic effusion may occur in association with an underlying pulmonary infection or rejection. As with other effusions, these generally clear with appropriate therapy of the underlying parenchymal condition.

Empyema is infrequently encountered in lung transplant recipients. Spontaneous development of an empyema is rare. More commonly, an empyema develops following any prolonged air leak as a result of the open lung biopsy performed on a patient receiving high-dose corticosteroids. Persistent air leak, failure to achieve reexpansion of the lung, and subse-

quent pleurodesis result in a chronic pleural space that will eventually become infected. A number of these patients have been treated by open drainage, by rib resection, or by a formal creation of a Clagett window or Eloesser flap. Interestingly, an empyema rarely occurs as a result of bronchial dehiscence in communication with the pleural space. In the majority of these patients, satisfactory intercostal tube drainage with reexpansion of the underlying lung results in satisfactory anastomotic healing and the absence of any significant pleural space infection (Patterson, 1993).

Airway Complications

Airway complications were formerly a frequent cause of morbidity and mortality following pulmonary transplantation. Using standard methods of implantation, the donor bronchus

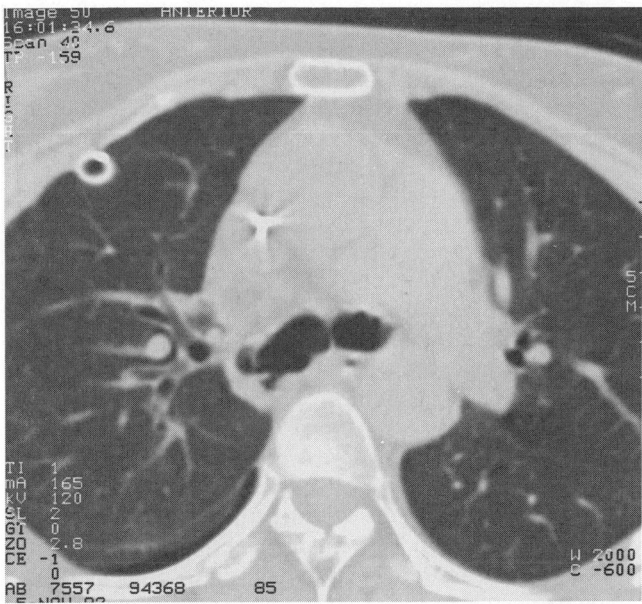

Figure 33-13. In a patient receiving bilateral sequential lung allografts for obstructive pulmonary disease, a small right main bronchial dehiscence developed. The dehiscence can be clearly seen in this CT image. A small pneumothorax is present. The anterior chest tube maintained satisfactory expansion of the lung until the membranous wall had healed completely and the air leak ceased.

is rendered ischemic, without reconstitution of its systemic bronchial artery circulation. The donor bronchus is thereby reliant on collateral pulmonary flow during the first few days following transplantation. It has been previously demonstrated that pulmonary collateral flow makes a substantial contribution to bronchial viability at the distal bronchus and lobar origin level. A shortened donor bronchial length (two rings proximal to the upper lobe takeoff) reduces the length of donor bronchus that is dependent on collateral flow. In addition, improved techniques of preservation have resulted in increased bronchial viability following transplantation. Post-transplant pulmonary parenchymal pathologic conditions also result in decreased collateral flow, rendering the ischemic donor bronchus at increased risk for necrosis and subsequent dehiscence. Superior preservation, improved sepsis prophylaxis, and immunosuppression have reduced the incidence of airway complications. The role of perioperative steroids is important in this regard. We recently demonstrated that epithelial regeneration and revascularization of rat heteroptic tracheal allografts (Davreux, et al., 1993) is improved by postoperative corticosteroid administration. In addition, the Hannover group (Inui, et al., 1993) recently demonstrated that postoperative corticosteroid therapy improves retrograde bronchial blood flow in porcine lung allografts.

In our own experience, healing problems of the airway anastomosis have been identified in 19 percent of patients. In one-half, endoscopic evidence of necrosis and/or partial anastomotic separation was identified at bronchoscopy, required no therapy, and healed with no complications. In the other half, a significant airway complication resulted, including death (1.5 percent); stricture of the malacia, requiring a stent (6 percent) or simple dilatation (1 percent); or bronchopleural fistula, requiring a chest tube (1.5 percent). At the present time, no correlation has been recognized between the technique of anastomosis, the length of ischemic time, or the type of immunosuppressive regimen and the subsequent development of an airway complication. Death as a result of airway complication has occurred in less than 2 percent of patients reported to the St. Louis International Lung Transplant Registry.

Airway complications are identified in a number of ways. Routine postoperative bronchoscopic surveillance, as used by most programs, generally provides early evidence that an anastomotic complication has occurred. On occasion, CT that is performed for some other indication demonstrates an unexpected airway stenosis or dehiscence. In fact, we have learned that the CT scan is a useful diagnostic tool in the evaluation of documented or suspected donor airway complications. Late airway stenoses are generally made manifest by symptoms of dyspnea, wheezing, or a decreased FEV_1. Bronchoscopic assessment confirms the diagnosis.

Most airway complications are identified early following transplantation. A normal bronchial anastomotic suture line demonstrates a narrow rim of epithelial sloughing, which ultimately heals. On occasion, patchy areas of superficial necrosis of the donor bronchial epithelium are observed. These are also of no concern and ultimately heal without incidence. Minor degrees of bronchial dehiscence are also of little long-term consequence. Membranous wall defects generally heal without any airway compromise, whereas cartilaginous defects usually result in some degree of late stricture. Significant dehiscence (greater than 50 percent of the circumference) may result in compromise of the airway. This problem should be managed expectantly by laser ablation or mechanical debridement of the area to maintain satisfactory airway patency. A word of caution should be issued to the laser enthusiasts who in their zealous attempts to maintain airway caliber can injure the vital normal distal donor airway into which a stent can only be placed if the distal main airway is intact. Occasionally, a significant dehiscence results in direct communication with the pleural space (Fig. 33-13) or pericardium. However, if the lung remains completely expanded and the pleural space is evacuated, the leak ultimately seals, and the airway usually heals without stenosis. A dehiscence may communicate directly with the mediastinum, resulting in mediastinal emphysema. If the lung remains completely expanded and the pleural space is filled, then adequate drainage of the mediastinum can be achieved by mediastinoscopy, placing a drain in close proximity to the anastomotic line. This also results in satisfactory healing of the anastomosis, often without stricture.

Surgical revision of the anastomosis is only possible if an adequate length of donor airway is available for resuturing. This type of reconstruction has been successfully performed (Kirk, et al., 1990). However, it is rarely possible if the donor bronchus was cut to an appropriate short length at the time of the initial procedure. Massive dehiscence of the airway with uncontrolled leak or mediastinal contamination has been treated by a successful retransplantation in a number of programs.

Chronic airway stenoses can present significant management problems. A right main bronchial anastomotic stricture is generally easily managed by repeated dilatation and ultimate placement of an endobronchial stent. The right main bronchus is easily dilated, and there is generally room for the placement of a right main bronchial orifice stent without impingement of the right upper lobe bronchus.

However, on the left side, strictures can be somewhat more difficult to manage. Dilatation of the distal left main bronchus is technicall more difficult because of its angulation. In addition, the lobar bifurcation immediately distal to the usual site of anastomosis does not provide a suitable length of bronchus distal to the stricture for the placement of large-caliber dilating bronchoscopes. Finally, stents placed across a left distal left main bronchial anastomotic stricture may occlude the upper or lower lobe orifice as it bridges the stricture.

We have used Silastic endobronchial stents preferentially. Straight bronchial stents have been used for main bronchial strictures. Y stents have been used for the occasional tracheal stricture seen following heart-lung transplantation or more commonly en bloc double-lung transplantation with tracheal anastomosis. We previously described the technique of insertion (Cooper, et al., 1989). Wire mesh (Gianturco) stents can only be used for malacic strictures completely lined by epithelium. If a wire stent is placed in a granulating stricture, the wires become embedded by granulation, and a stricture develops within the stent.

Silastic stents are tolerated exceptionally well. However, patients do require daily inhalation of N-acetyl cystine to keep the stents patent. Stents have resulted in dramatic improvements in pulmonary function (DeHoyos, et al., 1992). Fortunately, most of these stents have been required only temporarily. After a period of several months, most patients are able to maintain satisfactory airway patency without having the stent in place.

Finally, distal bronchial strictures on occasion can be unmanageable by dilatation or stent insertion. In these patients retransplantation is an option and has been used successfully (Novick, et al., 1993).

Rejection

Insofar as immunologic matching is crude (ABO blood group only) and immunosuppression strategies are imperfect, it is not surprising that rejection is a troublesome problem following lung transplantation. Acute rejection is encountered during the early postoperative period in almost all patients (Cooper, et al., 1994). This rarely presents a significant clinical problem. However, chronic rejection is the most common underlying cause of late death following lung transplantation. This is a particularly vexing problem because its pathogenesis is poorly understood and there is no effective means of therapy.

Acute rejection has a typical clinical presentation of dyspnea, low-grade fever, perihilar interstitial infiltrate, hypoxia, and increased white blood cell count. Typically, the first episode occurs within the first 5 to 7 postoperative days. Several episodes during the first 2 months are not unusual. In most circumstances, the diagnosis is confirmed by an abrupt response to a bolus dose of methylprednisolone (500 mg to 1 g). However, the above clinical picture can often be confused with infection.

At present the clinical parameters noted above are the most commonly used indicators of rejection. Intensive laboratory investigation is underway in a number of centers to try and identify some relatively noninvasive technique by which rejection might be identified. Nuclear scanning has little value. Various immunologic tests have also been advocated. The Pittsburgh group had initial enthusiasm for a primed lymphocyte test, which we have not found particularly useful. We recently demonstrated increased cytotoxicity of bronchoalveolar lavage lymphocytes in patients with biopsy-proved rejection. There is mounting evidence that various cytokines are important mediators in the development of rejection, and the manipulation of their expression may be of ultimate therapeutic importance.

The technique of choice in the diagnosis of rejection is transbronchial biopsy performed under fluoroscopic control. The Papworth group (Higenbottam, et al., 1988) deserves credit for demonstrating the safety and value of this technique in the lung transplantation population. The typical histologic appearance is that of perivascular lymphocytic infiltrate (Fig. 33-14). The internationally accepted classification for pulmonary rejection was reported by Yousem, et al. (1990).

The factors that predispose patients to an increased incidence of rejection are unclear. There is experimental evi-

---

Working Formulation for Classification and Grading of Pulmonary Rejection

A. Acute rejection
   0. Grade 0—no significant abnormality
   1. Grade 1—minimal acute rejection*
   2. Grade 2—mild acute rejection*
   3. Grade 3—moderate acute rejection*
   4. Grade 4—severe acute rejection*

B. Active airway damage without scarring
   1. Lymphocytic bronchitis
   2. Lymphocytic bronchiolitis

C. Chronic airway rejection
   1. Bronchiolitis obliterans, subtotal
      a. Active
      b. Inactive
   2. Bronchiolitis obliterans, total
      a. Active
      b. Inactive

D. Chronic vascular rejection

E. Vasculitis

---

*Grades 1 to 4 are subdivided according to bronchial inflammation:
   a. With evidence of bronchiolar inflammation
   b. Without evidence of bronchiolar inflammation
   c. With large airway inflammation
   d. No bronchioles are present

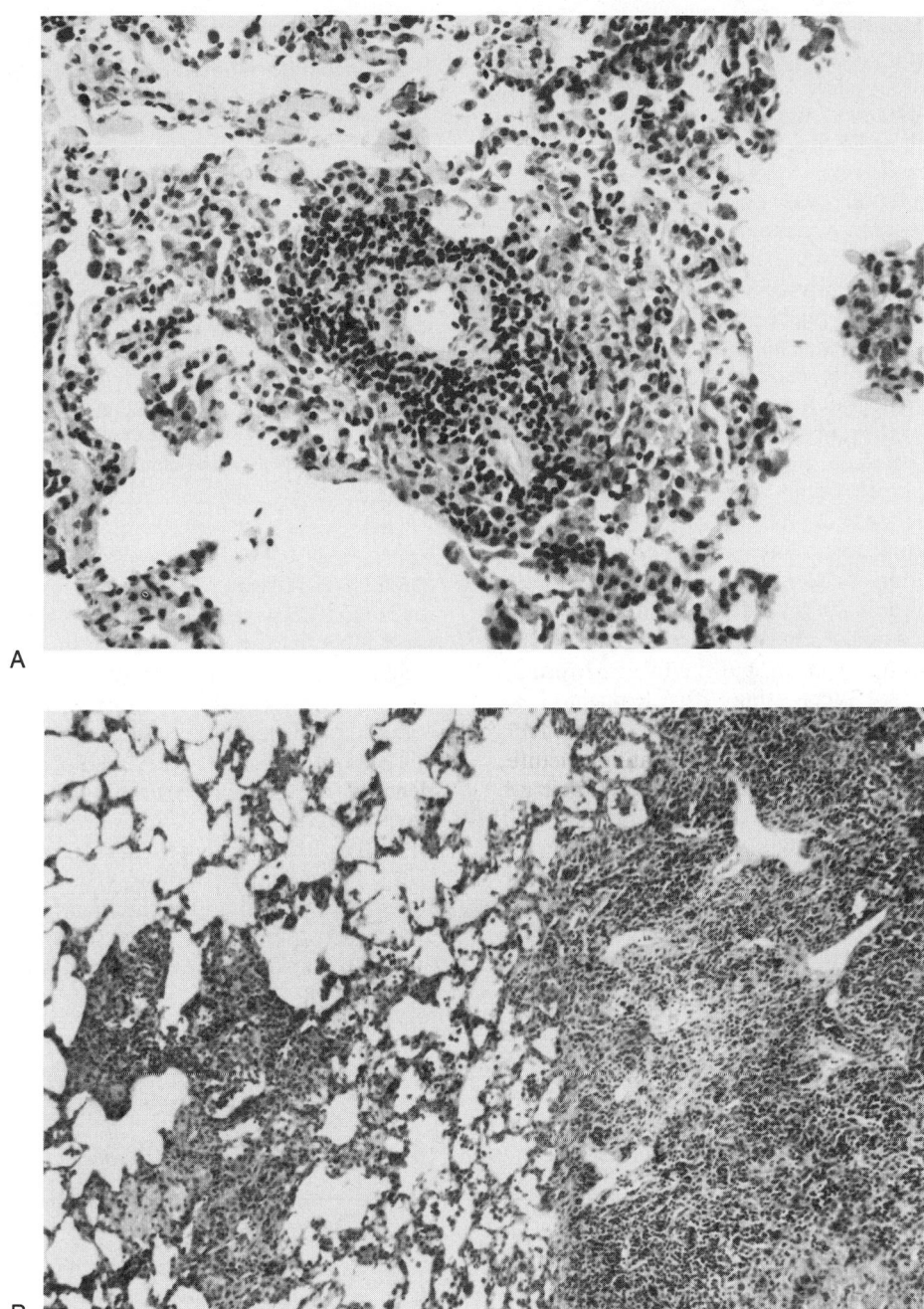

Figure 33-14. **(A)** A photomicrograph of a transbronchial biopsy specimen showing typical early (A1b) rejection. Isolated perivascular cuffs of lymphocytes are noted. **(B)** A more severe degree of rejection is evident in this photomicrograph of a transbronchial biopsy specimen. Perivascular and interstitial lymphoid infiltrates are present, which is consistent with grade 3 rejection (A3a). (From Shields TW: General Thoracic Surgery. Lea & Febiger, Philadelphia, 1994, with permission.)

dence that poorly preserved allografts are more likely to suffer subsequent rejection. There is some evidence that expression of major histocompatibility complex class II antigens on bronchial epithelium and pulmonary capillary endothelium is increased following extended periods of preservation. In addition, we recently demonstrated expression of the adhesion molecule I-CAM following extended preservation of human lung allografts (Hasagawa, et al.,

1993). Infection may also predispose to subsequent rejection. A number of groups have reported serious rejection episodes following close on the heels of established bacterial or viral infection.

Irrespective of its cause, in the majority of patients, acute rejection can be effectively controlled. Most patients respond promptly to the first course of methylprednisolone. Occasionally, a second course of steroid may be necessary to bring a serious rejection episode under control. Persistent rejection despite this intervention is distinctly unusual. In this circumstance, cytolytic therapy with ATGAM or OKT3 should be considered. Recent evidence suggests that alternative immunosuppressants, such as FK506, may be useful in this situation. There is increasing experimental (Hirai, et al., 1993) and clinical (Keenan, et al., 1993) evidence that FK506 may offer some advantages over cyclosporine as a first-line immunosuppressive agent.

It might be assumed that early rejection increases the likelihood of subsequent chronic rejection and allograft dysfunction. Our own experience suggests that there is no relationship between the number of early clinical acute rejection episodes and subsequent graft function (Cooper, et al., 1994). However, the Pittsburgh group (Bando, et al., 1994b) showed a clear relationship between the frequency and severity of biopsy-proved acute rejection and the subsequent development of chronic rejection.

Unfortunately, chronic rejection remains a major problem. The clinical presentation of chronic rejection is a progressive fall in FEV_1. This may actually precede the clinical symptoms of dyspnea. Despite advanced chronic rejection, chest radiographs and CT scans may be normal but should be performed to rule out other causes of a decreasing FEV_1. Bronchoscopy is necessary to ensure that there is no bronchial anastomotic compromise. Pulmonary function studies reveal obstructive physiologic findings. The pathologic hallmark of chronic rejection is obliterative bronchiolitis (Fig. 33-15). The term chronic rejection is often used interchangeably with bronchiolitis obliterans. However, this practice clouds the fact that not all post-transplant obliterative bronchiolitis is immunologically mediated. Various other etiologic factors, including aspiration or chronic infection, can result in obliterative bron-

---

Bronchiolitis Obliterans Syndrome Scoring System

0   No significant abnormality: FEV_1 > 80% of baseline value*

1   Mild obliterative bronchiolitis syndrome: FEV_1 66–80% of baseline value*

2   Moderate obliterative bronchiolitis syndrome: FEV_1 51–65% of baseline value*

3   Severe obliterative bronchiolitis syndrome: FEV_1 50% or less of baseline value*

*Grades 0 to 3 are subdivided into category a, without pathologic evidence of obliterative bronchiolitis, or category b, with pathologic evidence of obliterative bronchiolitis.

---

chiolitis. However, all transplant programs have come to realize that 25 percent of recipients will develop post-transplant allograft dysfunction caused by obstructive physiologic conditions. This problem appears to be unrelated to the underlying disease or the type of transplant.

A recent consensus conference sanctioned by the International Heart and Lung Transplant Society termed this chronic allograft dysfunction bronchiolitis obliterans syndrome (Cooper, et al., 1993). This clinical terminology was used to reflect the importance of clinical findings (i.e., diminished FEV_1 in its diagnosis). Biopsy is not required to make a diagnosis of bronchiolitis obliterans syndrome. Furthermore, the scoring system noted below reflects the fact that patients can move from one score to another. Although most patients'

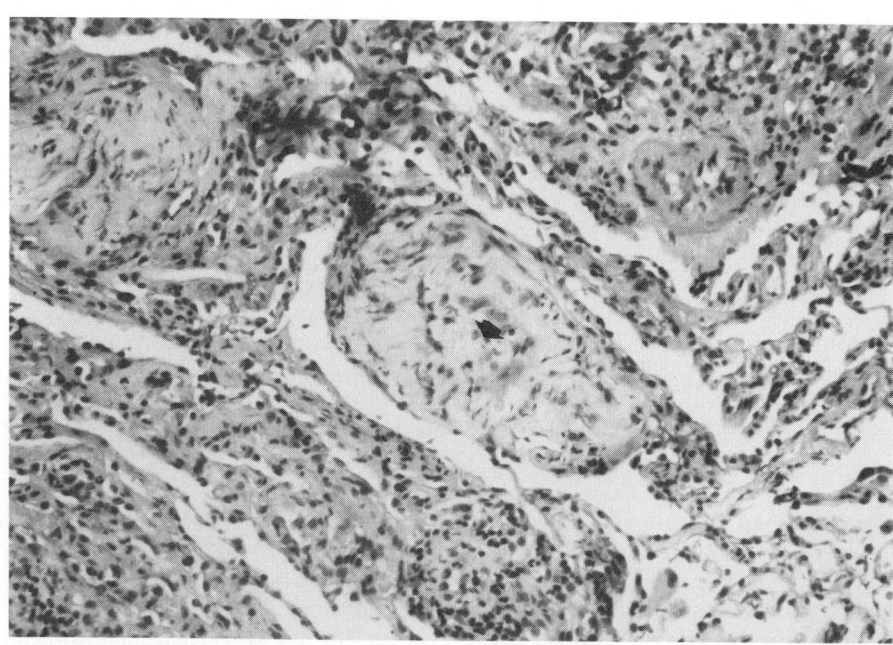

Figure 33-15. This photomicrograph of a transbronchial biopsy specimen reveals typical findings of bronchiolitis obliterans thought to be the result of chronic rejection. Mature fibrous obliteration of the bronchiolar lumen is evident (*arrow*). (From Shields TW: General Thoracic Surgery. Lea & Febiger, Philadelphia, 1994, with permission.)

conditions either stabilize or deteriorate, all programs have had patients with bronchiolitis obliterans syndrome who have improved (for whatever reason) with augmentation of immunosuppression (Cooper, et al., 1993).

Unfortunately, therapeutic options for established bronchiolitis obliterans are limited. Standard therapy consists of augmentation of immunosuppression, either by high-dose corticosteroid or cytolytic therapy. On occasion, the obliterative bronchiolitis can be arrested with maintenance of pulmonary function at the same level as when the immunotherapy was augmented. Unfortunately, the majority of patients either develop progressive obliterative bronchiolitis or, as a result of the augmented immunosuppression, contract some opportunistic infection, which is lethal.

Retransplantation has been offered to a large number of patients with chronic rejection bronchiolitis obliterans (Novick, et al., 1994). However, in the majority of such patients, the process reappears within a short period following retransplantation. Nonetheless, there are a small number of patients who have survived and obtained excellent long-term results following retransplantation for this devastating condition.

RESULTS

Operative Mortality

Improvements in selection, technique, and management have resulted in a dramatic reduction in the operative mortality rate. We recently reported an early mortality rate of only 8 percent in our initial 131 single and bilateral transplants (Cooper, 1993). Our updated survival data are illustrated in Figure 33-16. The Toronto group experience was reported by DeHoyos, et al. (1992). Operative mortality for single and double lung transplant was 13% and 21% respectively. Other large programs have reported equally impressive results. Spray, et al. (1992) at Washington University have reported exciting results of lung transplantation in children. This group of patients represents a particular challenge, especially those

with Eisenmenger's syndrome, in whom technically difficult operative procedures were undertaken with success.

There appears to be some difference in the early mortality rate, depending on the type of procedure or underlying disease (Fig. 33-17). Bilateral procedures are associated with higher early operative mortality than are single-lung transplantations. This reflects an increase in technical difficulty and the increased risk of septic complications in the cystic fibrosis group. The Toronto group (Ramirez, et al., 1992) reported a high incidence of postoperative death caused by sepsis. This was particularly frequent in those recipients harboring highly resistant *P. cepacia* organisms. In our program there does not appear to be a difference in perioperative mortality rates among the disease categories for which single-lung transplants are undertaken. However, other groups have reported increased mortality rate in patients undergoing single-lung transplantation for primary pulmonary hypertension in comparison with those suffering from emphysema. This is simply a reflection of the difficulties of the postoperative course of patients with pulmonary vascular disease.

The causes of operative death, as reported to the St. Louis Lung Transplant Registry (Cooper, 1993), are shown in Table 33-1.

Late Mortality

It is only during the last several years that large numbers of patients have undergone pulmonary transplantation. Although there are a few patients who have survived 6 to 8 years following lung transplantation, there are insufficient numbers to have reliable data on long-term survival. In Cooper's (1993) report of our own experience, 13 of 130 patients suffered late deaths, and 81 percent of patients were alive with a median follow-up of 19 months. In DeHoyos, et al.'s (1992) report of the Toronto experience, 4-year actuarial survival rates were 53 percent and 62 percent for single and bilateral transplants, respectively. In the Toronto experience, late deaths occurred in 28 percent of single-lung recipients and only 3 percent of bilateral recipients. Our experience is

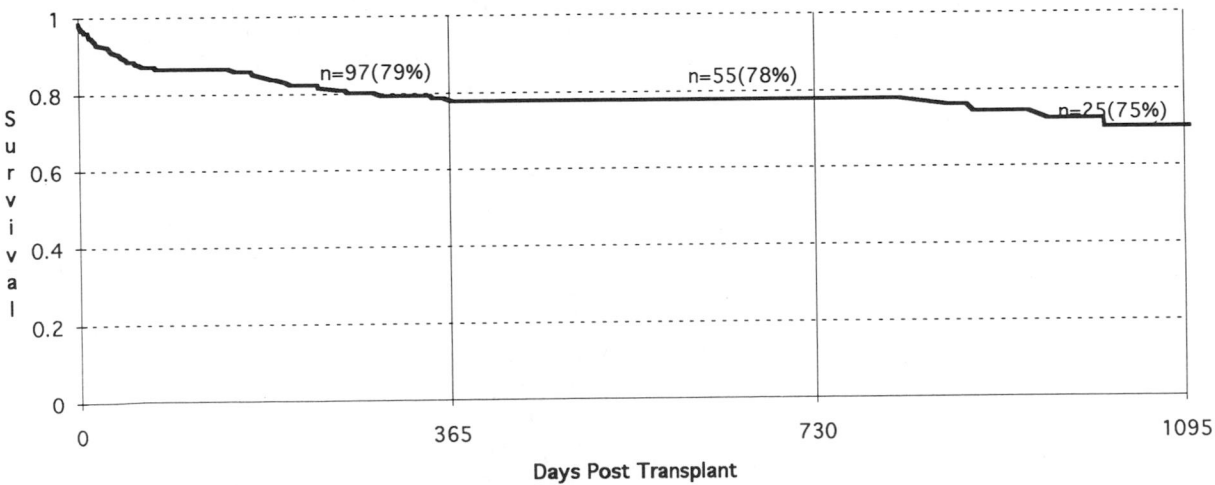

Figure 33-16.   Actuarial survival curve for the entire Washington University Barnes Hospital Lung Transplant Program.

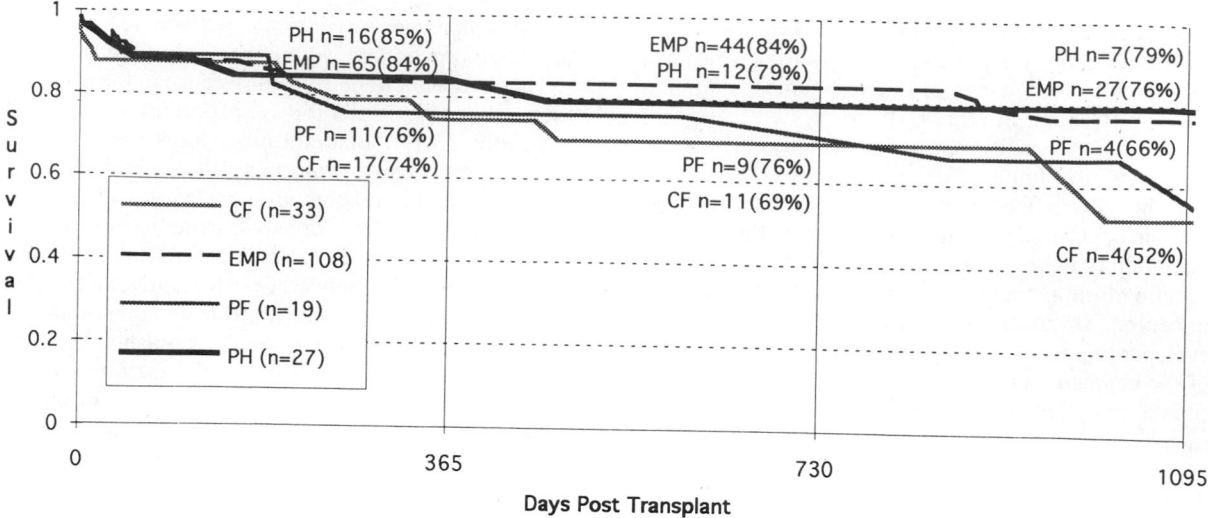

Figure 33-17. Actuarial survival curves for the Washington University Barnes Hospital Lung Transplant Program, according to major disease categories. Note the difference in late survival, according to disease. In our experience patients with emphysema and those undergoing single-lung transplant for pulmonary hypertension seem to have a survival advantage over patients with pulmonary fibrosis and cystic fibrosis.

similar. This suggests that long-term results, perhaps because of superior pulmonary reserve, are superior following bilateral lung replacement.

Survival data from the St. Louis International Lung Transplant Registry is shown in Figure 33-18. Considering that many of the programs reporting to the Registry have limited experience, the overall world wide results are impressive and improving steadily. Causes of late death, as reported to the St. Louis International Lung Transplant Registry, are shown in Table 33-2.

Functional Results

Among operative survivors the functional results are excellent. The usual patient can return to normal levels of exercise tolerance without oxygen supplementation within 6 to 8 weeks of transplantation.

Obstructive Pulmonary Disease

This is the most frequent indication for lung transplantation. Single- and bilateral-lung transplantations have been used

with success. Gas exchange, pulmonary function, and exercise tolerance are dramatically improved, as illustrated in Figures 33-19 to 33-21. Single and bilateral recipients achieve satisfactory postoperative lung volumes.

However, there is considerable controversy regarding the long-term functional advantages of bilateral-versus single-lung transplants for this disease. Early functional assessment suggests minimal difference between the two procedures. However, bilateral-lung replacement offers significant functional advantages long term. This may offset the increased operative risk of bilateral transplantation, especially in younger patients with emphysema.

Septic Pulmonary Disease

A number of centers have reported satisfactory results with the application of bilateral-lung transplantations in these patients. Ramirez, et al. (1992) from Toronto reported excellent gas exchange, pulmonary function, and exercise tolerance among operative survivors. Our Washington University experience is similar (Figs. 33-19 to 33-21). Dramatic improvement in chest contour was apparent (Fig. 33-22).

Table 33-1. Cause of Early (<90 Days) Postoperative Mortality ($n = 471$)

Causes of Death	No.	%
Sepsis	129	27
Primary organ failure	71	15
Heart failure	38	8
Airway dehiscence	30	6
Rejection	30	6
Hemorrhage	27	6
Cytomegalovirus	24	5
Multiorgan failure	23	5
Other	99	21

Table 33-2. Cause of Late (>90 Days) Postoperative Mortality ($n = 341$)

Causes of Death	No.	%
Sepsis	100	29
Bronchiolitis obliterans	54	16
Malignancy	27	8
Rejection	26	8
Respiratory failure	21	6
Cytomegalovirus	19	6
Hemorrhage	10	3
Heart failure	9	3
Other	75	22

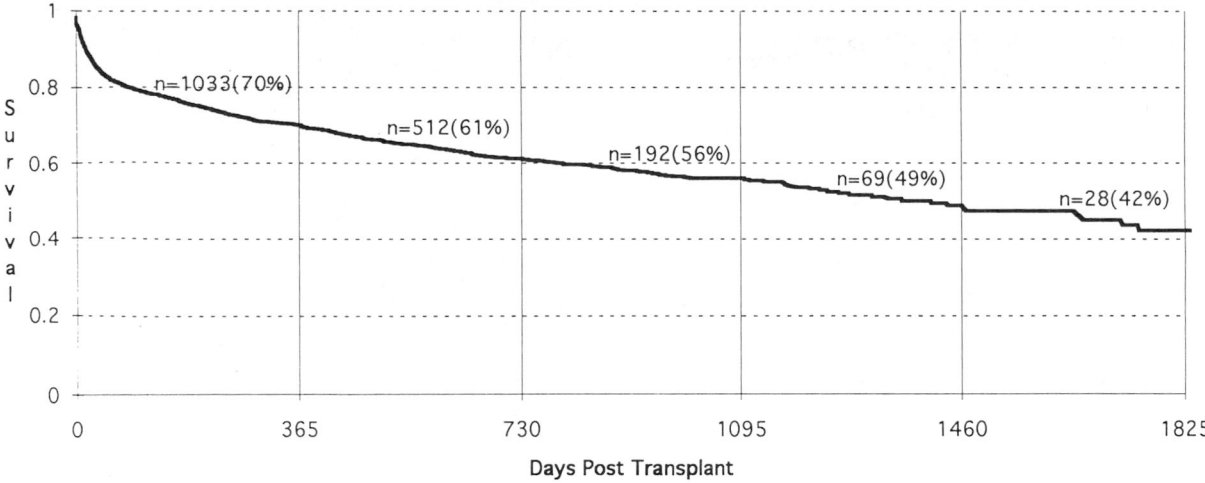

Figure 33-18. Overall actuarial survival among patients registered in the St. Louis International Lung Transplant Registry as of September 1993.

Fibrotic Pulmonary Disease

Whereas this condition was formerly the most frequent indication for pulmonary transplantation, it is now one of the less common indications. Nonetheless, enough data are available to realize that the long-term functional result in this group of patients is excellent. The longest surviving lung transplant recipient has lived 8.5 years following a right single-lung transplant for pulmonary fibrosis (Fig. 33-23). Single-lung transplantation provides satisfactory pulmonary volumes for these patients. Gas exchange and exercise tolerance are maintained during late follow-up (Figs. 33-19 to 33-21).

Pulmonary Vascular Disease

Our program has been particularly interested in single-lung transplantation for patients with primary pulmonary hypertension and Eisenmenger's syndrome (Pasque, et al., 1991). It is well documented that the cardiac function of these patients recovers promptly with the reduction in right heart afterload provided by a satisfactory lung allograft. However, the early postoperative course of these patients is complicated because of the impressive ventilation/perfusion mismatch, which can

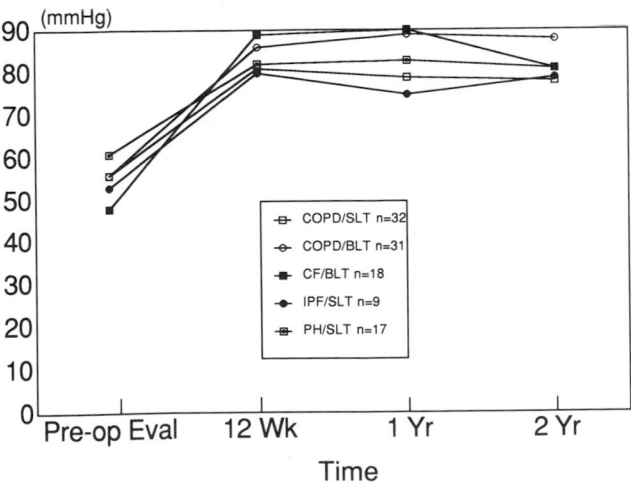

Figure 33-19. Pre- and postoperative room air PaO$_2$ values among adult recipients in the Washington University Barnes Hospital experience, according to disease categories. Note the dramatic and sustained increase in oxygenation in all patient groups. (From Shields TW: General Thoracic Surgery. Lea & Febiger, Philadelphia, 1994, with permission.)

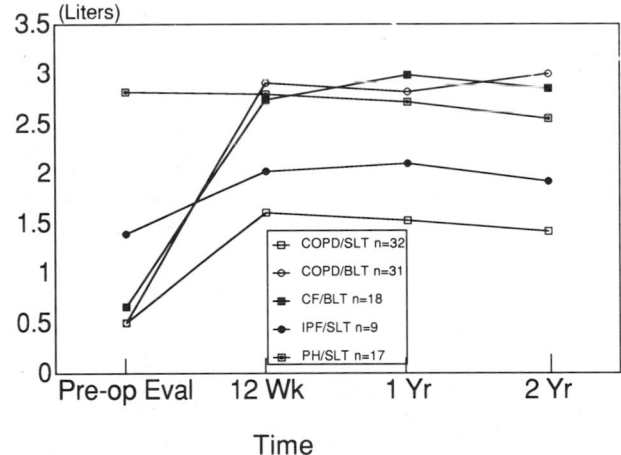

Figure 33-20. Pre- and postoperative FEV$_1$ among adult recipients in the Washington University Barnes Hospital experience, according to disease categories. Dramatic and sustained improvements are noted in bilateral (BLT) recipients with chronic obstructive pulmonary disease (COPD) or cystic fibrosis (CF). Less dramatic improvements in FEV$_1$ are noted in single-lung recipients (SLT) with COPD or idiopathic pulmonary fibrosis (IPF). Single-lung recipients with pulmonary hypertension (PH) and normal preoperative FEV$_1$ derived no improvement in that parameter following transplant. (From Shields TW: General Thoracic Surgery. Lea & Febiger, Philadelphia, 1994, with permission.)

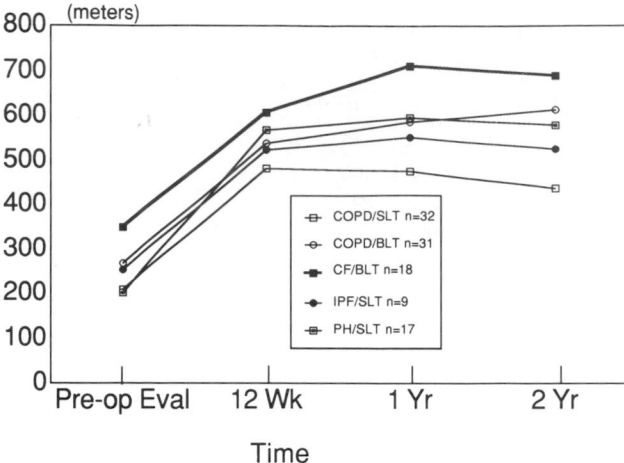

Figure 33-21. Preoperative (eval) and postoperative 6-minute walk distances (in meters) for adult recipients in the Washington University, Barnes Hospital program, according to various disease and transplant categories. Note the dramatic improvement in exercise tolerance in all patient groups. This improvement appears to be sustained, except perhaps in the COPD group who received single-lung transplantation, in which a slight decrease was noted in late follow-up. (From Shields TW: General Thoracic Surgery. Lea & Febiger, Philadelphia, 1994, with permission.)

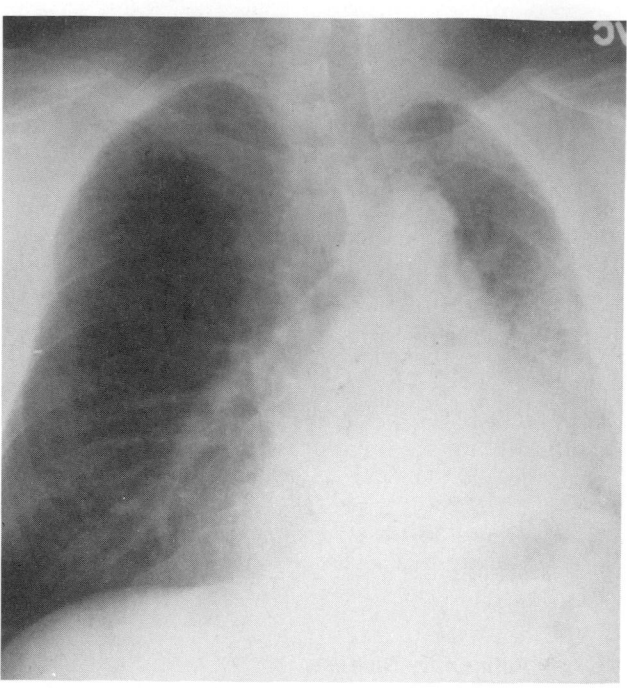

Figure 33-23. Chest radiograph from a patient who underwent right single-lung transplantation for idiopathic pulmonary fibrosis in February 1985. He continues to have an excellent functional result more than 8 years following transplantation.

occur because 90 to 95 percent of right heart output is directed to the transplanted lung and more than 50 percent ventilation is directed to the native lung. Our program has evolved a rigorous protocol for the early postoperative management of these patients, and our results have been gratifying. Of 22 patients undergoing transplantation for pulmonary vascular disease, there have been only 2 operative deaths and 3 late

deaths, resulting in a 91 percent operative mortality rate and a late survival rate of 77 percent. The mean New York heart functional class improved from a pretransplant mean value of 3.4 to a post-transplant mean value of 1.3. Gas exchange and exercise tolerance (depicted in Figs. 33-18 to 33-20) dem-

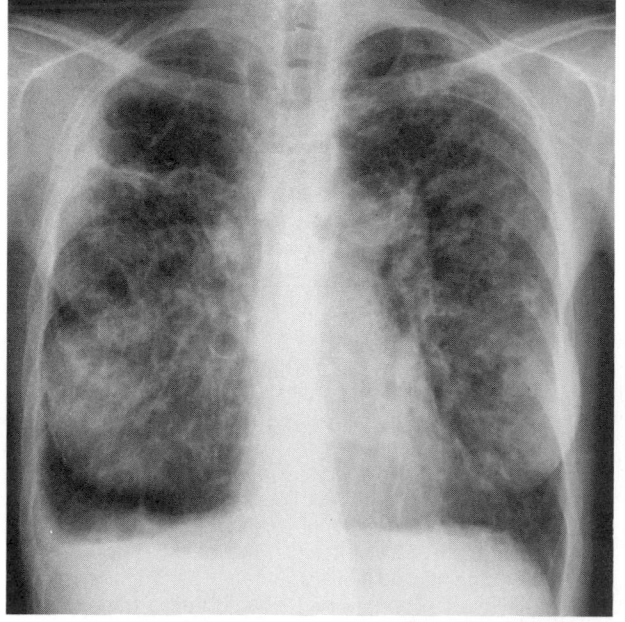

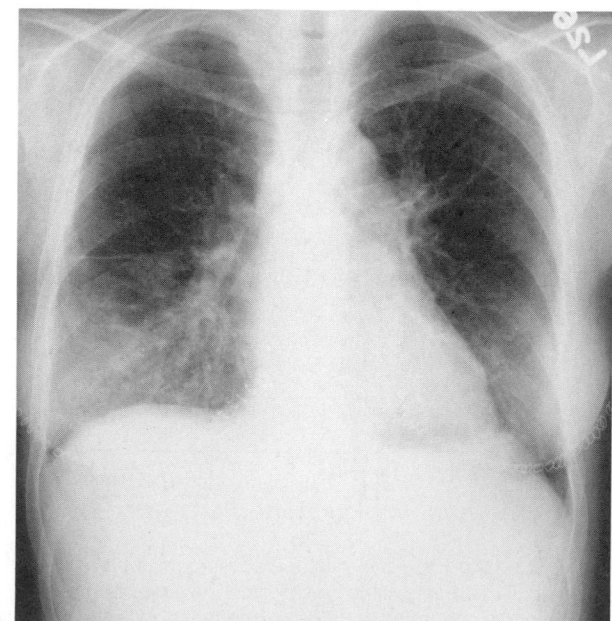

Figure 33-22. **(A)** Preoperative chest radiograph from a patient with cystic fibrosis. **(B)** Postoperative chest radiograph in the same patient following bilateral sequential single-lung transplants. Note the return of a normal chest contour.

onstrate that these patients have functional results equivalent to any other transplant group in our experience.

Notwithstanding our results, other groups have had significant difficulty with the application of single-lung transplantation in these patients. Bilateral-lung replacement has been advocated by a number of other programs (Bando, et al., 1994a). The standard operation previously offered these patients, combined heart-lung transplant, is still practiced widely, particularly in the United Kingdom. These bilateral-lung replacement procedures may have a long-term advantage over single-lung transplantations in this patient group. Patients who have undergone single-lung transplantation for pulmonary hypertension do exceedingly well as long as bronchiolitis obliterans can be avoided. However, when bronchiolitis obliterans syndrome develops in primary pulmonary hypertension or Eisenmenger's syndrome, patients who have received single-lung transplants have severe resultant functional impairment.

COMMENTS AND CONTROVERSIES

Lung transplantation has evolved into widely applied effective therapeutic option for a large number of patients with end-stage pulmonary disease. The successful lung transplant programs are those that have adopted a dedicated multidisciplinary team approach to the investigation and management of patients with a variety of such diseases. The ever increasing international experience is reflected in the proceeding pages. A number of major problems await solution, for example, inadequate donor supply, inferior strategies of allograft preservation, insufficient selectivity of immunosuppression, and chronic allograft rejection. Prospective trials are required to determine which of currently used therapeutic strategies is superior. Multi-institution cooperation will be required for their completion. Such a multi-institution group is in its formative stage.

It is apparent that the long-term survival will steadily decrease over time. We estimate the 5-year survival to be 50 to 60 percent. There is an urgent need for improved strategies for the management of bronchiolitis obliterans syndrome. The induction of specific tolerance, long the dream of transplant surgeons, may be possible. In the future, the era of routine xenografting may also occur, the ultimate solution to our current donor shortage. Until that time, the distribution of the limited donor supply and the management of chronic rejection will remain the most pressing problems of clinical lung transplantation.

G.A.P.
J.D.C.

During a 15-year period, human lung transplantation has progressed from repeated failures to a successful venture, now clinically applied worldwide. The key to this success was the introduction of cyclosporine and the persistence of many investigators, especially the Toronto Lung Transplant Group. Despite the rapid accumulation of experience, increasing indications for its use and the continually improving short- and long-term success rates, there is much still to be improvement needed, especially in the area of lung preservation, prevention of pulmonary sepsis, and avoidance of late bronchiolitis obliterans. The 50 percent 5-year survival for lung transplantation is the lowest rate of all organ transplantations because of the problems mentioned above. Especially worrisome is the increasing report of late recurrent sepsis in patients with cystic fibrosis who have undergone transplantation. Despite this, lung transplantation has provided a new life for countless patients suffering from chronic respiratory failure.

R.J.G.

KEY REFERENCES

Toronto Lung Transplant Group: Unilateral lung transplantation for pulmonary fibrosis. N Engl J Med 314:1140, 1986

The Toronto Lung Transplant Group describes the first successful lung transplantation with satisfactory functional results and long-term survival. The importance of a programmatic approach, rigorous recipient and donor selection criteria, and meticulous attention to operative and perioperative care are outlined. While there has been evolution in selection criteria and technical details, the basic principles outlined here manuscript have not changed.

DeHoyos AL et al: Pulmonary transplantation: early and late results. J Thorac Cardiovasc Surg 103:295, 1992

The Toronto Lung Transplant Group provides the first report of early and late results in a large series of single and bilateral lung recipients. The development experience of the Toronto group, the large number of cystic fibrosis patients, and use of en bloc double lung transplant explains the operative mortality, which is higher than that currently reported in other experienced centers. However, this report documents the excellent long-term functional results obtained by most patients. It also documents obliterative bronchiolitis as an important cause of late morbidity and mortality.

Mal H et al: Unilateral lung transplantation in end stage pulmonary emphysema. Am Rev Respir Dis 140:797, 1989

This paper represents the first report of successful single lung transplant in patients with emphysema. Subsequent to this report, unilateral lung transplantation has become the procedure of choice for emphysema in many programs. It represents the single most common lung transplant procedure worldwide.

Fremes SE et al: Single lung transplantation and closure of patent ductus arteriosus for Eisenmenger's syndrome. J Thorac Cardiovasc Surg 100:1, 1990

In this case report, the Toronto Lung Transplant Group reports the first successful cardiac repair and single lung transplant for Eisenmenger's syndrome. Prior to this report the standard transplant option for such patients was combined heart-lung transplantation. Subsequent reports from other centers have documented satisfactory early and late results following single lung transplant for patients with pulmonary vascular disease.

Pasque MK et al: Improved technique for bilateral lung transplantation: rationale and initial clinical experience. Ann Thorac Surg 49:785, 1990

This paper by the Washington University Group represents the initial description of the bilateral sequential single lung transplant technique. The previously employed en bloc double lung procedure was a tedious procedure requiring cardiopulmonary bypass and cardioplegic arrest. The simpler bilateral sequential single lung technique has become the procedure of choice, employed worldwide for bilateral lung replacement.

REFERENCES

Aoe M et al: Administration of prostaglandin E_1 following lung transplantation improves early graft function. Ann Thorac Surg 1994 (in press)

Bando K et al: Current results and indications of single, bilateral, and heart and lung transplantation for pulmonary hypertension. J Thorac Cardiovasc Surg 1994a (in press)

Bando K et al: Obliterative bronchiolitis after lung and heart-lung transplantation: an analysis of risk factors and management. J Thorac Cardiovasc Surg 1994b (in press)

Barnard CN et al: Clinical transplantation of the heart: a review of 13 years personal experience. J R Soc Med 74:670, 1981

Christie NA, Waddell TK: Lung preservation. Chest Surg Clin North Am 3:29, 1993

Cohen RG et al: Living related donor lobectomy for bilateral lobar transplantation in patients with cystic fibrosis. Ann Thorac Surg 1994 (in press)

Cooley DA et al: Organ transplantation for advanced cardiopulmonary disease. Ann Thorac Surg 8:30, 1969

Cooper JD: St. Louis International Lung Transplant Registry. 1993

Cooper JD et al: Use of silicone stents in the management of airway problems. Ann Thorac Surg 47:371, 1989

Cooper JD et al: A working formulation for the standardization of nomenclature and for clinical staging of chronic dysfunction in lung allografts. J Heart Lung Transplant 12:713, 1993

Cooper JD et al: Results of single and bilateral lung transplantation in 131 consecutive recipients. J Thorac Cardiovasc Surg 107:460, 1994

Couraud L et al: Bronchial revascularization in double-lung transplantation: a series of 8 patients. Ann Thorac Surg 53:88, 1992

D'Alonzo GE et al: Survival in patients with primary pulmonary hypertension: results from a national prospective registry. Ann Intern Med 115:343, 1991

Daly RC et al: Successful double lung transplant with direct bronchial artery revascularization. Ann Thorac Surg 1993 (in press)

Daly RC et al: Direct immediate revascularization for single-lung transplantation. Ann Thorac Surg 1994 (in press)

Dark JH et al: Experimental en-bloc double-lung transplantation. Ann Thorac Surg 42:394, 1986

Date H et al: In a canine model, lung preservation at 10°C is superior to that at 4°C. J Thorac Cardiovasc Surg 103:773, 1992

Date H et al: Evaluation of lung metabolism during successful twenty-four-hour canine lung preservation. J Thorac Cardiovasc Surg 105:480, 1993

Davreux CJ et al: Improved tracheal allograft viability in immunosuppressed rats. Ann Thorac Surg 55:131, 1993

Derom F et al: Ten-month survival after lung homotransplantation in man. J Thorac Cardiovasc Surg 61:835, 1971

Egan TM et al: Effect of a free radical scavenger on cadaver lung transplantation. Ann Thorac Surg 55:1453, 1993

Ettinger NA et al: Cytomegalovirus infection and pneumonitis. Impact after isolated lung transplantation. Am Rev Respir Dis 147:1017, 1993

Fremes SE et al: Single lung transplantation and closure of patent ductus arteriosus for Eisenmenger's syndrome. J Thorac Cardiovasc Surg 100:1, 1990

Goldberg M et al: A comparison between cyclosporin A and methylprednisolone plus azathioprine on bronchial healing following canine lung allotransplantation. J Thorac Cardiovasc Surg 85:821, 1983

Griffith BP et al: Anastomotic pitfalls in lung transplantation. J Thorac Cardiovasc Surg 107:743, 1994

Griffith BP et al: Acute rejection of lung allografts with various immunosuppressive protocols. Ann Thorac Surg 54:846, 1992

Hakim M et al: Selection and procurement of combined heart and lung grafts for transplantation. J Thorac Cardiovasc Surg 85:474, 1988

Hardesty RL et al: A clinical trial of University of Wisconsin solution for pulmonary preservation. J Thorac Cardiovasc Surg 105:660, 1993

Hardin CA, Kittle CF: Experience with transplantation of the lung. Science 119:87, 1954

Hardy JD: Lung homotransplantation in man. JAMA 186:1065, 1963

Hasegawa S et al: Changes in ICAM-1 expression during human lung preservation. Am Rev Respir Dis 147:A263, 1993

Haydock DA et al: Management of dysfunction in the transplanted lung: experience with 7 clinical cases. Ann Thorac Surg 53:635, 1992

Higenbottam T et al: Transbronchial lung biopsy for the diagnosis of rejection in heart-lung transplant patients. Transplantation 46:532, 1988

Hirai T et al: Prolonged lung allograft survival with a short course of FK506. J Thorac Cardiovasc Surg 105:1, 1993

Inui K et al: Bronchial circulation after experimental lung transplantation: the effect of long-term administration of prednisolone. J Thorac Cardiovasc Surg 105:474, 1993

Kerem E et al: Prediction of mortality in patients with cystic fibrosis. N Engl J Med 326:1187, 1992

Keshavjee SH et al: The role of dextran 40 and potassium in extended hypothermic lung preservation for transplantation. J Thorac Cardiovasc Surg 103:314, 1992

Kirk AJB et al: Successful surgical management of bronchial dehiscence after single-lung transplantation. Ann Thorac Surg 49:147, 1990

Levine SM et al: Graft position and pulmonary function after single lung transplantation for obstructive lung disease. Chest 103:444, 1993

Lillehei CW: Discussion of Wildevuur CRH, Benfield JR: A review of 23 human lung transplantations by 20 surgeons. Ann Thorac Surg 9:489, 1970

Lima O et al: Effects of methylprednisolone and azathioprine on bronchial healing following lung autotransplantation. J Thorac Cardiovasc Surg 82:211, 1981

Matsuzaki Y et al: Amelioration of post-ischemic lung reperfusion injury by PGE. Am Rev Respir Dis 148:882, 1993

Mayer E et al: Reliable eighteen-hour lung preservation at 4°C and 10°C by pulmonary artery flush after high-dose prostaglandin E_1. J Thorac Cardiovasc Surg 103:1136, 1992

Metras H: Note preliminaire sur la graffe totale du poumon chez le chien. Fr Acad Sci. 1176, 1950

Miller JD et al: An evaluation of the role of omentopexy and of early perioperative corticosteroid administration in clinical lung transplantation. J Thorac Cardiovasc Surg 105:247, 1993

Morgan WE et al: Improved bronchial healing in canine left lung reimplantation using omental pedicle wrap. J Thorac Cardiovasc Surg 85:139, 1983

Nelems IM et al: Human lung transplantation. Chest 78:569, 1980

Novick RJ: New trends in lung preservation: a collective review. J Heart Lung Transplant 11:377, 1992

Novick RJ et al: Redo lung transplantation: a North American-European experience. J Heart Lung Transplant 12:5, 1993

Novick RJ et al: Pulmonary retransplantation for obliterative bronchiolitis. J Thorac Cardiovasc Surg 107:755, 1994

Okabayashi K et al: Pentoxifylline reduces lung allograft reperfusion injury. Ann Thorac Surg (in press)

Pasque MK et al: Single-lung transplantation for pulmonary hypertension: three-month hemodynamic follow-up. Circulation 84:2275, 1991

Patterson GA: Airway complications. Chest Surg Clin North Am 3:157, 1993

Patterson GA et al: Technique of successful clinical double-lung transplantation. Ann Thorac Surg 45:626, 1988

Patterson GA et al: Airway complications after double lung transplantation. J Thorac Cardiovasc Surg 99:14, 1990

Puskas JD et al: Unilateral donor lung dysfunction does not preclude successful contralateral single lung transplantation. J Thorac Cardiovasc Surg 103:1015, 1992a

Puskas JD et al: Equivalent eighteen-hour lung preservation with low-potassium dextran or Euro-Collins solution after prostaglandin E_1 infusion. J Thorac Cardiovasc Surg 104:83, 1992b

Puskas JD et al: Reliable 30 hour lung preservation by donor hyperinflation. J Thorac Cardiovasc Surg 104:1075, 1992c

Ramirez JC et al: Bilateral lung transplantation for cystic fibrosis. J Thorac Cardiovasc Surg 103:287, 1992

Reitz BA et al: Heart-lung transplantation: successful therapy for patients with pulmonary vascular disease. N Engl J Med 306:557, 1982

Schafers HJ et al: Cardiac innervation after double lung transplant. J Thorac Cardiovasc Surg 99:22, 1990

Semenkovich JW et al: Complications in the native lung following single lung transplantation. Radiology 1994 (in press)

Sharples L et al: Prognosis of patients with cystic fibrosis awaiting heart and lung transplantation. J Heart Lung Transplant 12:669, 1993

Snell GI et al: Pseudomonas cepacia in lung transplant recipients with cystic fibrosis. Chest 103:336, 1993

Spray TL et al: Pediatric lung transplantation for pulmonary hypertension and congenital heart disease. Ann Thorac Surg 54:216, 1992

Spray TL et al: Pediatric lung transplantation: indications, techniques and early results. J Thorac Cardiovasc Surg 1993 (in press)

Sundaresan S et al: A primate model of sequential bilateral lung transplantation to evaluate lung preservation employing low potassium dextran solution. Ann Thorac Surg 1993a (in press)

Sundaresan S et al: Donor lung procurement: assessment and operative technique. Ann Thorac Surg 56:1409, 1993

Sundaresan S et al: Successful outcome of lung transplantation is not compromised by the use of marginal donor lungs. J Thorac Cardiovasc Surg 1994 (in press)

Todd TR et al: Separate extraction of cardiac and pulmonary grafts from a single organ donor. Ann Thorac Surg 46:356, 1988

Triantafillou AN et al: Cardiopulmonary bypass requirements in adult lung transplant recipients: The Washington University experience. Ann Thorac Surg 1994 (in press)

Trulock EP: Management of lung transplant rejection. Chest 103:1566, 1993a

Trulock EP: Recipient selection. Chest Surg Clin North Am 3:1, 1993b

Trulock EP et al: The Washington University-Barnes Hospital experience with lung transplantation. JAMA 266:1943, 1991

Wang LS et al: Influence of temperature of flushing solution on lung preservation. Ann Thorac Surg 55:711, 1993

Westaby S: Aprotinin in perspective. Ann Thorac Surg 55:1033, 1993

Yacoub MH et al: Distant organ procurement for heart and lung transplantation. Transplant Proc 21:2548, 1989

Yousem SA et al: A working formulation for the standardization of nomenclature in the diagnosis of heart and lung rejection: Lung Rejection Study Group. J Heart Transplant 9:593, 1990

Heart-Lung Transplantation

A. Haverich
H. G. Borst

DEFINITION

Heart-lung transplantation refers to the combined or en bloc allografting of the heart and both lungs for end-stage cardiopulmonary disease.

HISTORICAL NOTE

Alexis Carrel (1907) was the first to attempt transplantation of the heart and both lungs at the beginning of this century, although this involved only transplantation into the neck of a recipient cat. In 1946, Demikhov (1962) transplanted the heart and lungs of a dog, with the recipient surviving for 2 hours on the allografted organs alone. During the same period, other researchers, notably Marcus, et al. (1953) were also studying experimental heart-lung transplantation. Marcus, et al. developed a technique for transplanting the heart and both lungs into the abdomen and suggested the possibility of using a heterologous heart-lung preparation (xenograft) as an extracorporeal pump in open heart surgery. In 1953, Neptune, et al. reported the use of hypothermia to protect the recipient during orthotopic cardiopulmonary transplantation. Four years later, the use of a pump oxygenator to perform such operations in dogs was reported by Webb and Howard (1957). These authors found it possible to restore the heart to relatively normal function, and the animals lived from 75 minutes to 22 hours. However, their experimental animals were unable to breathe spontaneously; thus this group concluded that respiratory dysfunction, resulting from simultaneous bilateral pulmonary denervation, made cardiopulmonary transplantation impracticable. In 1958, Blanco, et al. (1958) also reported attempts at orthotopic heart and lung replacement using a pump oxygenator. Spontaneous respirations returned in two dogs after mechanical ventilation was discontinued. Similar findings were made by Lower, et al. (1961) 3 years later. Still, the respiratory pattern was reported to be altered with increased tidal volumes and slow respiratory rates. In a study of the working heart-lung preparation to examine heart viability after storage, Robicsek, et al. (1967) repeated Demikhov's experiments, with up to 37 hours of survival. Respiratory difficulties again prevented long-term survival. Superb experiments of Nakae, et al. (1967), who performed cardiopulmonary autotransplantation

in several species of animals suggested that denervation of both lungs did not prevent a return of adequate spontaneous respiration in primates, as it did in dogs. These experiments were followed by the studies of Castaneda, et al. (1972) and later of Reitz, et al. (1981) in monkeys to confirm long-term survival and a normal respiratory pattern in autotransplanted heart-lung grafts. Subsequent experiments using allotransplants in primates definitively confirmed the clinical applicability of combined heart-lung transplantation.

The first clinical attempt was made by Cooley, et al. (1969) on August 31, 1968 in a 2-month-old infant who died 14 hours after the operation. In December 1969, Lillehei (1970) performed the second human heart-lung transplantation in a 43-year-old patient with emphysema. The patient died 8 days later from pneumonia. Barnard (1981) was the third surgeon to try this operation in July 1971. The patient did well initially but died on the twenty-third day from disruption of the bronchial suture line. In this case, bilateral bronchial anastomoses rather than a tracheal suture line had been performed. Ten years later, a fourth transplant was reported by Reitz, et al. (1981) at Stanford University. The use of cyclosporine and the application of the surgical technique developed in this group's experimental program resulted in the first long-term survivor, a 45-year-old woman with primary pulmonary hypertension (Reitz, 1980, 1982b). Since then, more than 2,000 combined heart-lung transplantations have been performed worldwide (Kaye, 1992).

HISTORICAL READINGS

Cooley DA, Bloodwell RD, Hallman GL et al: Organ transplantation for advanced cardiopulmonary disease. Ann Thorac Surg 8:30, 1969

Reitz BA, Burton NA, Jamieson SW et al: Heart and lung transplantation. Autotransplantation and allotransplantation in primates with extended survival. J Thorac Cardiovasc Surg 80:360, 1980

Reitz BA, Wallwork J, Hunt SA et al: Heart-lung transplantation: successful therapy for patients with pulmonary vascular disease. N Engl J Med 306:557, 1982b

Webb WR, Howard HS: Cardio-pulmonary transplantation. Surg Forum 8:313, 1957

INDICATIONS

Following its first successful clinical application, heart-lung transplantation remained reserved for patients with primary and secondary pulmonary hypertension. This selection, based on Reitz, et al.'s (1982b) criteria, was made because of the poor results previously obtained in patients with parenchymal lung disease and an infected tracheobronchial tree. With increasing clinical experience, patients presenting with a number of pulmonary disorders, including restrictive and obstructive pathologic types, were accepted as candidates for the operation (Penketh, et al., 1987; Kaiser, et al., 1991; Khagani, et al., 1991). In fact, even patients with bronchiectasis and cystic fibrosis were considered for surgery (Leval, et al., 1991; Scott, et al., 1988a).

The established foreseeable results of heart-lung replacement during the first 5 years of its clinical application also resulted in an increasing number of operations being performed in patients who actually were not in need of replacement of the heart. In these patients heart-lung transplantation was performed, and the recipient's heart was given to another patient awaiting isolated heart transplantation (i.e., domino procedure; Yacoub, et al., 1988, 1990). Although this approach is still used by some surgeons, the majority of cardiothoracic transplant centers would now perform single- or double-lung transplantation in candidates with adequately preserved cardiac function (Levine, et al., 1990; Spray, et al., 1992). The heart of the respective organ donor may simultaneously be transplanted into a cardiac transplant recipient. This change in the indications for heart-lung transplantation has been grossly influenced by the lack of adequate numbers of organ donors for combined heart-lung transplantation. In most countries, the number of potential heart transplant recipients has grown to such an extent that cardiopulmonary allografts only rarely are offered for transplantation. This severe restriction in organ supply has recently resulted in two developments in thoracic organ transplantation. First, the number of heart-lung transplantations performed worldwide has reached a plateau since 1988 (Kaye, 1992). Second, increasing numbers of patients with "classic" indications for heart-lung transplantation (Reitz, 1982b), including primary and secondary pulmonary hypertension, are being treated by single- or double-lung transplantation. In cases with Eisenmenger's syndrome, simultaneous repair of the intra- or extracardiac shunt followed by single-lung implantation has been repeatedly reported.

As a result, we would currently consider potential recipients for heart-lung transplantation only if end-stage pulmonary disease coexisted with *irreversible* right or biventricular failure. Because this is rarely the case in parenchymal lung disease, present and probably future indications for en bloc replacement generally are reserved for end-stage pulmonary hypertension, Eisenmenger's syndrome (especially if combined with complex cardiac anomalies), and thromboembolic pulmonary disease.

DIAGNOSIS

Clinical Features

When the rare cases of parenchymal pulmonary disease that result in end-stage heart failure are excluded, the clinical features of the typical candidate for heart-lung transplantation, who has primary or secondary pulmonary hypertension, are predominant arterial hypoxemia, aggravated by exercise, and signs of chronic right heart failure (McGregor, et al., 1986). Accepted patients should have reached New York Heart Association class III or IV. Because of predominant right heart failure, clinical signs of tricuspid insufficiency, such as extended neck veins and hepatic enlargement, are usually present. Interestingly, peripheral edema is almost never seen in some patients, even in the late course of the disease. Jaundice caused by hepatic congestion may be an earlier clinical sign.

Natural History

The natural history of pulmonary hypertension may vary significantly, according to the pathogenesis in individual patients (Fuster, et al., 1984; Rozkovec, et al., 1986). We have performed heart-lung transplants in two patients older than 50 years of age with an Eisenmenger's complex (one with an atrioventricular canal and one with a ventricular septal defect) with a history of right heart failure of more than 20 years' duration. Primary pulmonary hypertension, by contrast, especially if occurring postpartum, may lead to a rapid clinical deterioration, sometimes resulting in death within 1 year after the first clinical signs. This large variation in survival after establishing the diagnosis makes it difficult to decide when the patient should be put on the waiting list. Anamnestic features, such as endobronchial bleeding or syncope, both of which suggest a dismal prognosis quo ad vitam, may be helpful in regard to this decision. Some candidates, however, may stay alive actively on a heart-lung waiting list for more than 2 years, reflecting the insecurities of the prognosis in such patients.

Differential Diagnosis

The differential diagnosis of the underlying disease is usually of no importance if transplantation is clearly indicated on account of arterial hypoxemia combined with end-stage right heart failure. However, thromboembolic pulmonary disease and congenital heart disease should be ruled out in all cases with borderline right ventricular function because either pulmonary thromboendarterectomy or repair of the defect followed by single-lung transplantation may be performed in such cases. If thromboembolic disease is expected, phlebography and pulmonary angiography should be performed to prove or exclude this pathologic condition and to assess the potential risk of recurrent thromboembolic events.

Systemic illness, such as collagen disease, systemic vasculitis, or rheumatoid arthritis, should be ruled out as the underlying disorder associated with pulmonary hypertension. Such entities represent contraindications for transplantation because the recurrence of pulmonary hypertension cannot be excluded and vasculitis per se may limit patient survival.

Investigative Techniques

Taking into account that the replacement of the heart and both lungs represents a major surgical intervention, comparably little has to be done in terms of preoperative investigations. After the exact diagnosis of pulmonary hypertension and right heart failure has been established by right heart catheterization and echocardiography, little has to be done with respect to cardiopulmonary functional assessment. Only in patients with borderline right ventricular function is a complete assessment of both left and right ventricular function necessary to exclude the option of single-lung transplantation. This assessment should include the right ventricular ejection fraction by echocardiography or multiple-gated blood scan, the degree of pulmonary and tricuspid valve regurgitation, the left ventricular ejection fraction, coronary angiography, and aortic and mitral valve function. If Eisenmenger's syndrome cannot be excluded, an angiocardiographic search for a potential intracardiac shunt should always be complemented by aortography to rule out a patent ductus arteriosus or an aortopulmonary window. In patients with thromboembolic pulmonary hypertension and only moderately impaired right ventricular ejection function (more than 20 percent as in mild to moderate tricuspid insufficiency or mild pulmonary valve regurgitation on echocardiography), pulmonary angiography is mandatory to exclude the indication for thromboendarterectomy.

Among the specific investigations with regard to the transplant procedure itself, the assessment of chest size by radiography (posteroanterior projection) and direct size measurements (Fig. 33-24) for comparison with the potential organ donor at the time of transplantation is necessary. Computed tomography of the chest is helpful to assess the anatomic position of the heart and great vessels and potential pleural and mediastinal thickening, especially in reoperated cases. Cranial computed tomography often shows signs of cortical atrophy of various degree. This investigation is believed to

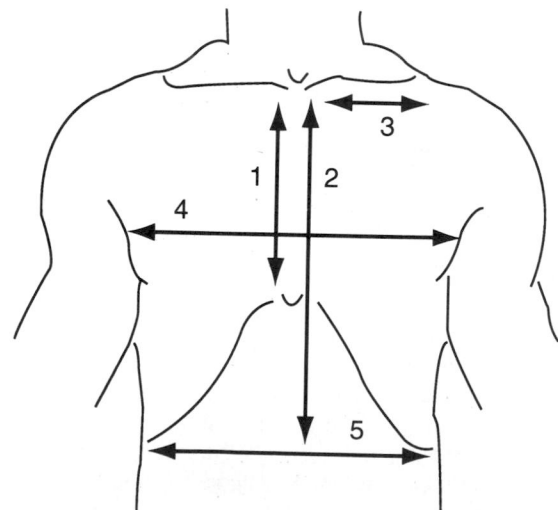

Figure 33-24. Thoracic chest measures that allow for a comparison between donor and recipient prior to explantation: 1, length of the sternum; 2, manubrium to lower thoracic circumference; 3, manubrium to acromion; 4, thoracic circumference at the level of the nipples; 5, at the level of the lower chest circumference. (From Haverich A: Herz- und Herz-Lungen-Transplantation. p. 551. In Borst HG, Klinner W, Oelert H (eds): Herzchirurgie. Springer-Verlag, Berlin, 1978, with permission.)

be mandatory in candidates with a history of cerebrovascular accidents. Abdominal sonography is always performed to assess the size and structure of the liver and the biliary system (gallstones), renal anatomy, and the status of the intra-abdominal blood vessels. Peripheral arterial disease is excluded clinically and by noninvasive methods (ultrasound techniques); phlebography is done in patients with histories of deep vein thromboses. Investigations of other organ systems, such as the central nervous system, peripheral nervous system, and gastrointestinal tract, and only indicated if substantiated by the medical history.

Blood is drawn to (1) verify the degree of cardiopulmonary failure, (2) assess the renal hepatic and hematologic status, and (3) document the immunologic baseline characteristics of the potential recipients.

1. An arterial blood gas analysis is performed at rest. If normal, it is repeated during exercise.

2. Renal and hepatic function are assessed by routine serologic and hematologic examinations (coagulation status). If abnormal, this study is complemented by specific studies (glomerular filtration rate, renal plasma flow, and direct/indirect bilirubin values). Hematologically, a differential white blood count, red blood count, and the hematocrit and platelet counts are performed. A full coagulation status report, including antithrombin III levels, is also ordered.

3. Blood group, rhesus factor, and preformed reactive antibodies must be known before placing the patient on the waiting list. If the percentage of preformed antibodies exceeds 10 percent, a direct cross-match between donor (lymphocytes) and recipient (plasma) will be necessary at the time of transplantation. At present, we do not perform histocompatibility antigen (HLA) typing preoperatively because the current supply of organs does not allow for organ allocation according to HLA criteria. The virologic history should be assessed by antibody screening, including Epstein-Barr and herpes simplex viruses. Transplantation-specific infections, most importantly cytomegalovirus (CMV); hepatitis A, B, and C; and human immunodeficiency virus (HIV) serologic testing, should be investigated. Some centers match donor and recipient according to the CMV status. Even if this policy is not followed, knowledge of the preoperative CMV status and potential conversions after the procedure may be helpful in the postoperative management.

MANAGEMENT

Principles of Management

Histocompatibility

Despite ample evidence for the positive influence of HLA matching on the long-term function of allotransplanted parenchymal organs, this strategy has not become a reality in thoracic organ transplantation. First, there are logistic problems in obtaining donor HLA typing prior to heart and lung retrieval, especially in distant organ procurement. Second, the number of potential recipients, according to blood groups,

---

Contraindications to Heart-Lung Transplantation

Major
- Active (nonpulmonary infection)
- Severe chest deformity
- Malignant disease
- Severe renal or hepatic disease
- Uncontrolled systemic disease
- Severe central nervous system disability
- Drug abuse or psychological instability
- Positive hepatitis or HIV serologic findings

Minor
- Advanced age >55 years
- Young age <6 years
- Previous thoracic surgery
- Diabetes mellitus
- Active peptic ulceration

---

type of transplantation (heart-lung versus single-lung versus double-lung transplantation, and size of the potential recipients leaves only a few options for HLA-compatible transplantation in most organ-procurement organizations. The current practice, therefore, remains to perform heart-lung transplantation irrespective of HLA typing. Reports on long-standing hemolysis in blood group A, B, or AB recipients of group O lungs, however, would suggest ABO identical transplantation is necessary.

To minimize hyperacute rejection by preformed cytotoxic antibodies (which is more often seen in postpartum female patients and in those who have undergone previous blood transfusions, e.g., following open heart surgery), the recipient's serum is tested against a random panel of lymphocytes from about 50 blood donors. If more than 10 percent of the lymphocytes are lysed, presensitization must be suspected, and repeat analysis (after 4 to 12 weeks) is obligatory. If still positive, a direct cross-match must be performed prior to transplantation. In any case, a retrospective cross-match should be initiated postoperatively to estimate the immunologic risk of the respective donor/recipient combination. It is our policy also to perform HLA typing of both donor and recipient at this time for potential future investigation and management.

Recipient Selection

After the pretransplant evaluation has confirmed both the correct diagnosis of the underlying disease and its degree of severity, the selection of a patient as a potential recipient only requires the exclusion of contraindications (above). Any of the criteria mentioned, however, may be a matter of discussion in the individual patient.

Specific considerations in regard to patient selection at the time of an organ becomes available should include basic immunologic and demographic criteria, such as sex, height, weight, and age. We try to avoid transplantation between genders because of its increased immunologic risk. Great

care must be taken to avoid any oversizing (more than 10 percent) of the donor's organs compared with the recipient's chest. In general, transplantation within one gender can be done according to donor/recipient heights only. In cases with doubtful intrathoracic volume estimates, such as in pediatric donors, the posteroanterior chest radiograph or measurements should be compared (see above).

Recipient Preparation

When a potential donor organ becomes available, any febrile illness must be excluded during the first contact with the potential recipient, which is usually made by phone. Transportation to the recipient hospital should be by the fastest mode available to ensure sufficient time for a final checkup. This includes preoperative instruction of the patient and obtaining the patient's consent for the procedure, chest radiograph, and immediate blood testing, such as white blood cell count, serum levels of creatinine and hepatic transaminases, coagulation parameters, an arterial blood gas analysis, and an order of blood for transfusions with the blood bank. Two units of whole blood, 4 units of concentrated red cells, and 10 units of fresh-frozen plasma should be readily available. If applicable, the recipient may receive the pretransplant dose of immunosuppression therapy; followed by a whole-body shave and scrub. We do not transfer a heart-lung transplant recipient to the operating room before the explanting surgeon has confirmed that the donor organs to be removed are suitable for implantation.

Donor Selection

Selection of the appropriate donor organs for heart-lung transplantation remains a critical issue in view of both the limited number of allografts available and their quality, especially of the lungs in the organ donor. Less than 20 percent of potential heart donors may be suitable for heart-lung donation (Jamieson, et al., 1984a; Harjula, et al., 1987). Pneumonic changes may occur in a brain-dead individual as a result of infection or aspiration, precluding donation of the lungs. Tracheal intubation, often performed emergently under less than optimal sterile conditions, and neurogenic pulmonary edema both may result in pulmonary dysfunction (Novitzky, et al., 1987). To minimize the risk of pulmonary failure or infection after transplantation, the potential donor should meet the following criteria.

Age.   Preferably, the donor should be younger than 40 years (male patient) or 45 years of age (female patient) to reduce the risk of coronary artery disease. With the present severe shortage of suitable donors, this age limit might be extended if the donor appears suitable in other respects. In cases of doubt, coronary angiography should be performed.

Medical History.   The donor should be a nonsmoker with no history of significant pulmonary or cardiac disease.

Cardiac and Pulmonary Function.   Normal cardiac function is essential, and adequate gas exchange should be present. With a positive end-expiratory pressure (PEEP) of 5 cmH$_2$O and a fraction of inspired oxygen (FiO$_2$) of 0.40 (40 percent O$_2$) or less, the partial oxygen pressure (PaO$_2$) should be greater than 100 mmHg. With a F_{IO_2} of 1 (100 percent O_2), the PaO_2 should be greater than 300 mmHg. The static pressure should not exceed 20 cmH_2O at an inspiratory volume of 15 ml/kg, indicating relatively normal lung compliance.

To achieve or maintain such function, fluid restriction may be necessary, especially with respect to crystalloid solutions. Close monitoring of central venous pressure and cautious administration of catecholamines are mandatory, as in cardiac donors. Prolonged artificial ventilation, a F_{IO_2} exceeding 0.5 (50 percent), and PEEPs greater than 10 mmHg should be avoided.

Pulmonary Infection. In view of the risk of nosocomial infections, mechanical ventilation in brain-dead subjects for more than 4 days generally precludes the use of the lungs for transplantation. The chest radiograph should be free of major pulmonary infiltrates, including post-traumatic opacities, suggesting contusion or infection. Minor infiltrates, however, in our experience, have not precluded donation. Frequent aseptic and thorough endotracheal suction and toilette is mandatory, and a broad-spectrum antibiotic should be administered before the donor undergoes the operation.

The presence of purulent sputum or definite signs of bronchial aspiration at the time of routine pre-explant bronchoscopy is considered a contraindication to donation; the presence of some pus cells without detectable pathogens on a Gram stain generally will not preclude donation. Postoperative antibiotic treatment must be based on the results of the bacterial culture.

Size Match. In contrast to orthotopic heart transplantation and single-lung transplantation, a close size match between the donor and recipient thoracic cavity is required for heart-lung transplantation because undue compression of the donor lungs within the recipient's thoracic cage will lead to cardiac compression and atelectasis. Although fewer problems result from the use of smaller donor organs, the donor thoracic cavity's dimensions should not be less than 20 percent of those of the recipient.

To compare the relative sizes of donor and recipient thoracic cavities, we believe that simple measurement of weight and height within sex-related transplants will suffice. Some surgeons, however, compare the radiographic dimension of the thorax or measurements of the chests of the donor and the recipient (Hakim, et al., 1988). Experience has shown that these techniques are only necessary in pediatric cases and in sex-unrelated cardiopulmonary transplantations. In routine adult male-to-male or female-to-female transplantation, the donor should not be taller than 5 cm or smaller than 10 cm compared with the recipient.

Donor Management. The donor is maintained on a PEEP of 5 cmH_2O with the lowest possible F_{IO_2} required to maintain a PaO_2 greater than 100 mmHg. The mean arterial blood pressure is maintained at a minimum of 60 mmHg. Because diabetes insipidus is present in most donors, the urinary output is usually excessive. Fluid replacement has to be kept at the minimum necessary to maintain normotension. Following blood volume correction, fluids will be administered to replace those lost by diuresis, but fluid overload must be prevented to avoid overhydration of the donor lungs. Therefore,

every effort should be made to maintain a relatively low central venous pressure (approximately 5 cmH_2O). Under these criteria, if an acceptable arterial pressure cannot be maintained, catecholamines (dopamine maximal dose, 8 μg/kg/min) or vasopressors (norepinephrine and α-adrenergic constrictors) should be administered (Fisher and Alexander, 1992; Okamoto, et al., 1992).

Excision of Donor Organs: Surgical Technique. The technique of excising the donor organs is described irrespective of the mode of graft preservation used. In multiorgan donors, the chest is usually opened at the same time as the abdominal surgeons are beginning explantation because this facilitates the dissection of the liver and enables the cardiothoracic surgeon to inspect the heart and lungs.

A median sternotomy is usually preferred. However, a bilateral anterior thoracotomy has also been also suggested by Hardesty and Griffith (1985), allowing for easier dissection of the posterior mediastinum and better control of bleeding. Following a median sternotomy, an anterior longitudinal pericardiotomy is performed, and the heart and aorta are exposed up to the innominate and left carotid arteries (Fig. 33-25). The pericardium, with adjacent pleura, is bilaterally excised. The presence of dense and extensive pleural adhesions usually is a contraindication for using the affected lung for transplantation. The superior vena cava (SVC), inferior vena cava (IVC), ascending aorta, and trachea (between the SVC and aorta) all are mobilized. The ascending aorta is dissected free from the main pulmonary artery. A tape is passed around the ascending aorta, and this structure is retracted to the left to expose the trachea. Minimal dissection is carried out around the trachea because it is important to preserve its blood supply through the coronary collaterals.

Two different principles of preservation of the thoracic organs are currently applied for clinical use: simple hypothermic flush perfusion and cooling by extracorporeal circulation, both followed by cold storage. The details are given below. For simple flush perfusion, a 14-Fr catheter is inserted into the main pulmonary artery, and a cardioplegic infusion line is placed in the ascending aorta. If donor cooling by extracorporeal circulation is preferred, aortic and right atrial cannulation is necessary. Both methods require prior full heparinization (300 IU/kg). For venting of the left heart, the tip of the left atrial appendage may be transsected (flush perfusion), or a vent catheter can be placed into the left atrium through its appendage or the right superior pulmonary vein. The vent catheter can also be placed in the apex of the left ventricle.

Cold (4°C) saline is poured into both pleural cavities to cool the lungs, which may or may not be maintained on mechanical ventilation (preferably using unheated room air) during this period. After satisfactory cooling of the organs has been achieved, both caval veins are transsected at the level of the pericardial reflections, the ascending aorta is divided as high as possible, and the trachea is transsected, preserving as much of its length as is available above the carina (Fig. 33-25) after central closure by a stapled line (remember the endotracheal tube!). The heart-lung graft is excised en bloc in a craniocaudal direction by dividing the posterior mediastinal tissue anterior to the esophagus and descending aorta (Fig. 33-26). To avoid subsequent post-

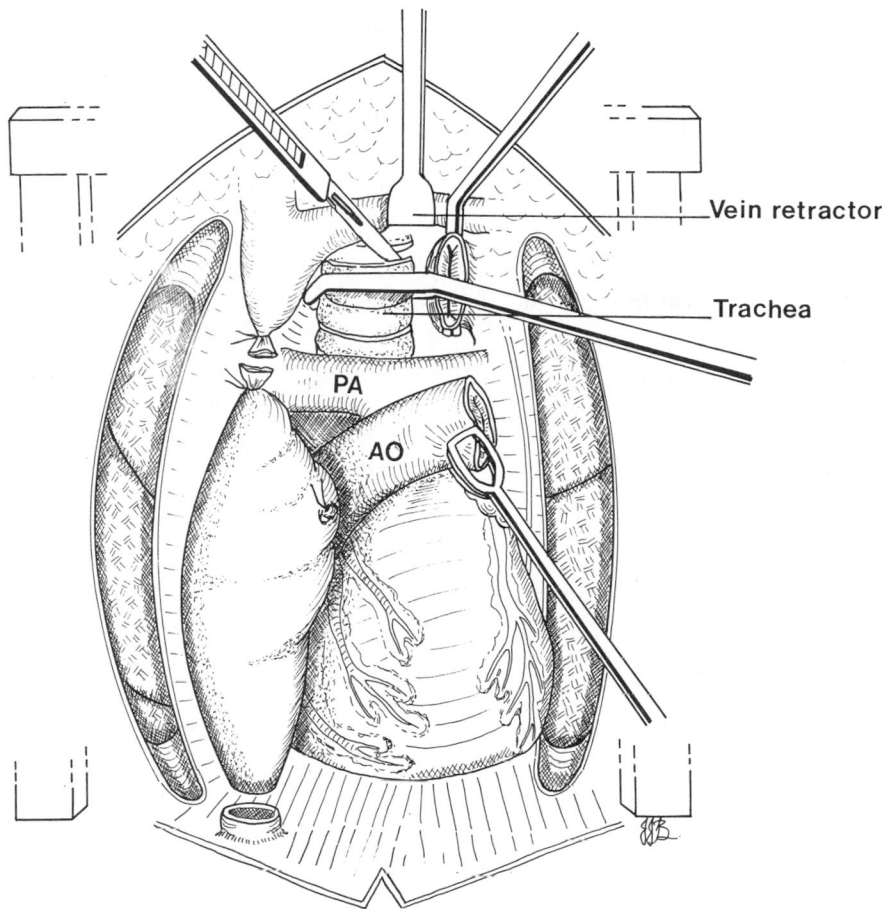

Figure 33-25. The ascending aorta has been retracted downward and to the left, exposing the trachea, which has been clamped and divided as high as possible (after withdrawal of the endotracheal tube). (From Haverich A: Selection of the donor. p. 277. In Cooper DKC, Novitzsky (eds): The Transplantation and Replacement of Thoracic Organs. Kluwer Academic Publishers, Dordrecht, the Netherlands, 1990, with permission.)

transplant bleeding in the recipient, electrocautery should be used wherever possible; the inferior pulmonary ligaments should be either stapled or suture ligated. During explantation, the lungs must be handled with maximal care to prevent trauma. Following excision, some surgeons prefer the lungs to remain partially inflated although others advocate deflation. We prefer partial inflation of the lungs to prevent prolonged post-transplant atelectasis. The heart-lung block is placed in a sterile container or a bag filled with cold (4°C) fluid (blood or Ringer's lactate solution), which in turn is placed in a box of appropriate size that is filled with ice. The organs are then transported to the recipient site.

The alternative to the craniocaudal dissection of the posterior mediastinum is caudocranial explantation. This approach allows for continued intubation of the trachea. In the presence of complete atelectasis, retraction of the heart and lungs is usually much easier. At the end of the procedure, the lungs are reinflated, and the trachea is stapled and dissected above.

Cardiopulmonary Preservation. Among the many techniques for pulmonary preservation evaluated experimentally and reviewed repeatedly in the literature (Haverich, et al., 1985b; Novick, et al., 1992), three methods have emerged

and are currently in clinical use. The concept of crystalloid flush perfusion is the method most often used in human lung and heart-lung transplantation (Bando, et al., 1989, 1990; Collins, et al., 1969; Jurmann, et al., 1990; Kennan, et al., 1991). The other two modalities include cooling of the lungs with cold blood by either pump oxygenator (Bando, et al., 1991; Wahlers, et al., 1986; Kontos, et al., 1987a,b; Ladowski, et al., 1984, 1985) or flush perfusion with cold donor blood (Hakim, et al., 1985; Hooper, et al., 1990; Jones, et al., 1985; Locke, et al., 1991). Another alternative, the autoperfusing heart-lung preparation, has been used clinically by only a few groups (Robicsek, et al., 1967, 1985; Hardesty and Griffith, 1985, 1987; Miyamoto, et al., 1987).

Hypothermic Flush Perfusion with Crystalloid Solutions. Hypothermic flush perfusion has been the basis of preservation of solid organs for the purpose of transplantation. Thus, most renal, hepatic, and cardiac allografts are harvested using simple perfusion with a crystalloid solution followed by cold storage. Although numerous biochemical compositions have been suggested for this purpose, buffered solutions with an intracellular ionic composition and slightly increased osmolarity compared with serum, such as the Euro-

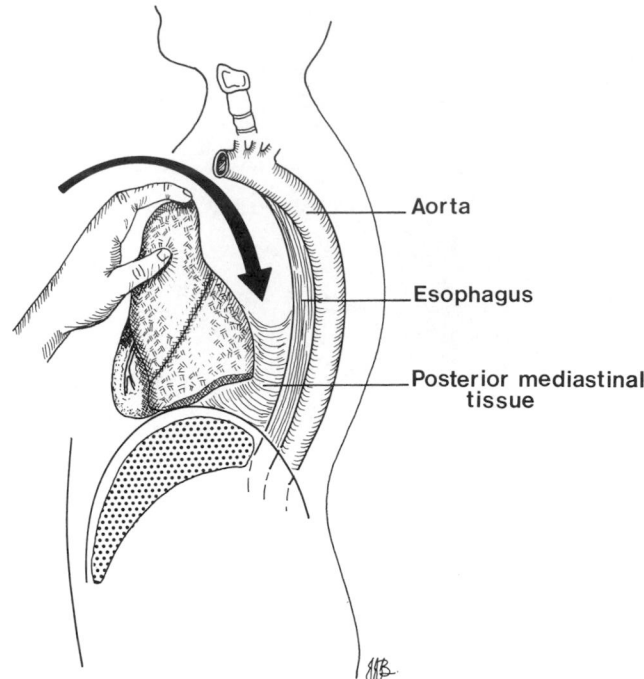

Figure 33-26. The plane of the dissection between the heart (and lungs) and posterior mediastinal structures (esophagus and descending aorta) is shown. (From Haverich A: Selection of the donor. p. 277. In Cooper DKC, Novitzsky (eds): The Transplantation and Replacement of Thoracic Organs. Kluwer Academic Publishers, Dordrecht, the Netherlands, 1990, with permission.)

Collins solution, are preferred by many centers. The ease of application and satisfactory graft function represent the chief advantages of this method. Euro-Collins solution, modified by the addition of magnesium sulfate (Table 33-3), is administered into the main pulmonary artery following aortic cross-clamping at 60 ml/kg over 4 minutes. For this purpose, a 14-Fr cannula is inserted into the main pulmonary artery. It is advisable to measure the pulmonary artery pressure during perfusion. The pressure should be kept above 15 mmHg but should not exceed 25 mmHg to facilitate the even distribution of the perfusate within both lungs. For the same purpose, pretreatment of the donor using a prostaglandin analog, such as PGE_1 or PGI_2, is used by many centers (Bonser, et al., 1990, 1991; Moncada, 1982). In our practice, PGI_2 is given

Table 33-3. Composition of Modified Euro-Collins Solution for Lung Preservation in Clinical Heart-Lung Transplantation

Component	Amount
KH_2PO_4	2.05 g/L
K_2HPO_4	7.40 g/L
KCl	1.12 g/L
$NaHCO_3$	0.84 g/L
$MgSO_4$	1.00 g/L
Glucose	38.5 g/L
pH	7.3–7.4

intravenously immediately prior to flush perfusion (500 to 1,000 μg until the systolic arterial pressure falls by 30 mmHg). In addition, PGI_2 may be added to the flush perfusate (100 ng/L).

Hypothermic Flush Perfusion with Blood. During procurement, the lungs may also be flushed with third-party donor blood, as advocated by the Cambridge group (Hakim, et al., 1985; Jones, et al., 1985). This approach may be as simple to perform as single crystalloid flush with respect to the technical and instrumental requirement and has also resulted in a predictably adequate lung function after transplantation.

Cooling by Extracorporeal Circulation. This mode of preservation for heart-lung transplantation was first described experimentally in 1984 (Ladowski, et al., 1984). It is now used by a number of transplant centers around the world. The major drawback of this technique is the need to transport a relatively large amount of equipment to the donor center. A roller pump, perfusion circuits, heat exchanger, and oxygenator constitute the minimum requirements for this purpose. Also, there is good experimental evidence of a reduced post-transplant gas exchange by lungs preserved with excorporeal circulation compared with those undergoing flush perfusion with Euro-Collins solution. The pulmonary vasculature, in contrast however, may be better preserved with the former method (Wahlers, et al., 1986; Locke, et al., 1991).

Both simple hypothermic flush and extracorporeal circulation offer simple and relatively efficient modes of pulmonary preservation. Heart and lung ischemic intervals of up to 3 to 4 hours have been shown to be safe with either method (Feeley, et al., 1986), although the typical reimplantation response (vide infra) may still occur on occasions.

Operative Technique

The induction of anesthesia includes oral tracheal intubation, placement of a peripheral arterial line, one or two central venous lines, a peripheral venous line, and a urinary catheter (Sale, et al., 1987). A peripheral oxymetric probe (finger tip) and rectal and nasopharyngeal temperature probes are also applied. The patient is then placed in a supine position, and a median sternotomy is performed. Following division of the thymus, the left innominate vein is exposed, and the pericardium is opened in the midline. This incision is extended caudally in a Y shape. Four pericardial stay sutures are placed. The ascending aorta is mobilized from the pulmonary arterial trunk, and the right pulmonary artery and purse-string sutures are placed in the aortic arch opposite the origin of the brachiocephalic artery. Following heparinization, the ascending aorta is cannulated. For venous return, two purse-string sutures are placed posteriorly in the right atrium just above the interatrial sulcus. The SVC and IVC cannulas are inserted, and cardiopulmonary bypass is initiated. The rectal temperature is reduced to 28°C. While cooling proceeds and with the heart empty, both the IVC and SVC are exposed, encircled with tapes, and snared for the total cardiopulmonary bypass. The aorta is cross-clamped proximal to the aortic cannula (Fig. 33-27).

Cardiectomy is first performed on the atrial level. The right and left atrium are divided close to the atrioventricular

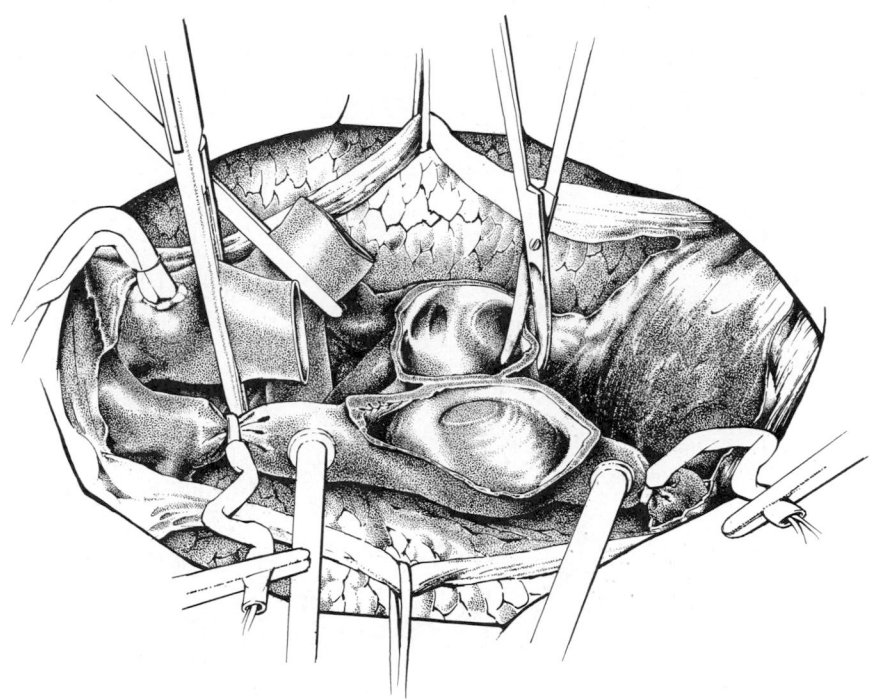

Figure 33-27. Operative view following explantation of the recipient's heart during heart-lung transplantation. Both phrenic nerves are isolated, including a pericardial flap. Both the aorta and the pulmonary artery are cross-clamped. To further mobilize both lungs, the dorsal remnant of the left atrium is transsected between left and right pulmonary veins. (From Haverich A: Herz- und Herz-Lungen-Transplantation. p. 551. In Borst HG, Klinner W, Oelert H (eds): Herzchirurgie. Springer-Verlag, Berlin, 1978, with permission.)

groove, leaving sufficient remnants of the left and especially the right atrial wall. For this purpose, the right atrium is incised first at its lateral aspect with the appendage included in the tissue removed. The interatrial septum is incised at the foramen ovale. The left atrial free wall is transsected along the coronary sinus with the apex of the heart lifted anteriorly and to the right. The great vessels are divided about 2 cm above the semilunar valves (leaving the opportunity to harvest them as homografts) (Fig. 33-27).

Following cardiectomy, the remnant of the pulmonary trunk is divided in the midline, separating the left and right main pulmonary arteries. This incision is extended posteriorly into the pericardium and downward until the posterior remnants of the left atrium are reached. These are also divided in the midline, including the underlying posterior pericardium. The atrial cuffs, including the attached pericardium, are further mobilized on both sides as far as possible toward the pulmonary hilum, taking care not to injure the vagus nerves at this level. Blood vessels arising from the posterior mediastinum are ligated or clipped.

Further dissection of the pulmonary artery includes full mobilization toward the lung hilum on both sides. On the left side, this is done on the left side by also excising a "button" that carries the ductus ligament, which is left in place (recurrent nerve!). On the right side, dissection of the right pulmonary artery includes its portion behind the aorta and the SVC.

The operative field now allows for a left-sided pneumonectomy (Fig. 33-28). In preparation for this, the anterior portion of the pericardium on the left is excised, including the anterior

pleura. A pedicle of the pericardium carrying the phrenic nerve is left behind by a careful incision 3 cm anterior and posterior to the nerve from the pulmonary artery to the diaphragm. The left lung is then mobilized; the pulmonary ligament is divided, with all bleeding carefully controlled; and the posterior portion of the hilum is dissected sharply close to the parenchyma of the lung. This dissection is carried out with careful control of collateral vessels until both the pulmonary artery and the remnants of the left atrium (including the adjacent pericardium) on the left side can be mobilized toward the pleural space. Then, again with careful control of bleeding, the left main bronchus is dissected free, closed by stapling, and divided distally. The left lung is then removed from the operating field.

On the right, the anterior pleura is opened from the brachiocephalic vein to the diaphragm. Under careful visualization of the right-sided phrenic nerve, the pericardium is incised 3 cm anterior to the nerve from the pulmonary artery toward the diaphragm. Here the anterior portion of the pericardium is divided at the diaphragm but left attached proximally as a pedicle. Again under constant visualization of the phrenic nerve, the pericardium is incised dorsally to the nerve in close proximity to the right hilar structures. This incision is made from the azygos vein to the diaphragm. No electrocautery should be used at this point; instead bleeding vessels are either clipped or ligated. Then an incision is made posterior to the interatrial grove (as in mitral valve replacement). With careful attention not to injure the SVC or IVC, this incision is directed posteriorly beneath the IVC until the right-sided

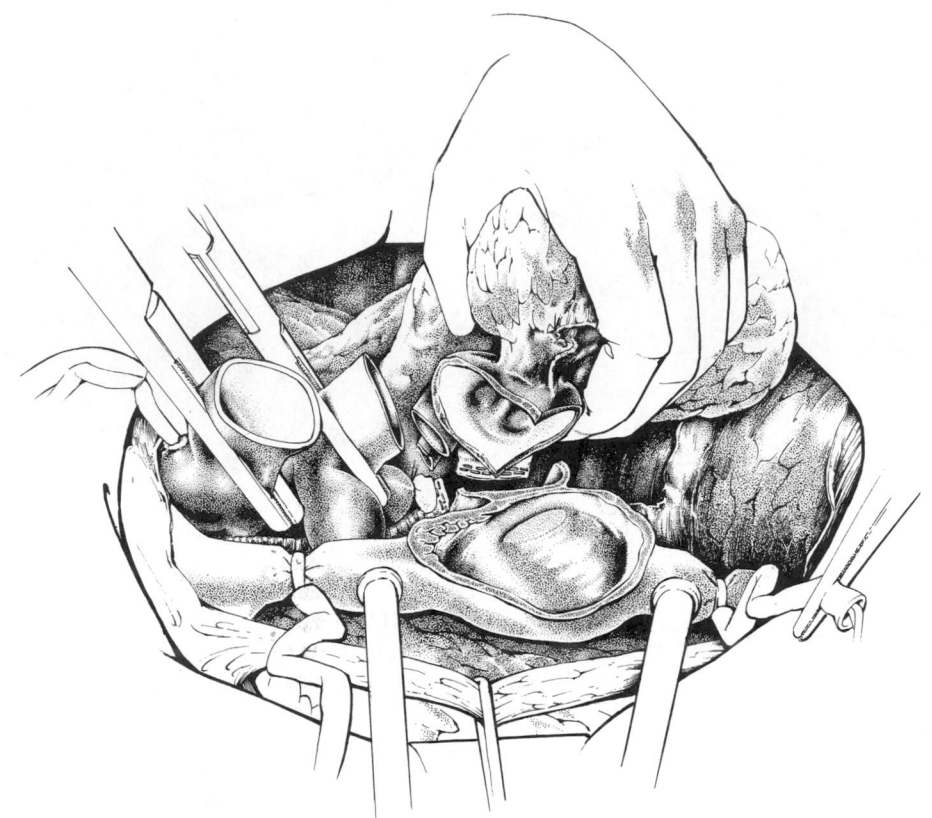

Figure 33-28. Following separation of the remnants of the left atrium and transsection of the left pulmonary artery and bronchus, the left recipient lung is removed. (From Haverich A: Herz- und Herz-Lungen-Transplantation. p. 551. In Borst HG, Klinner W, Oelert H (eds): Herzchirurgie. Springer-Verlag, Berlin, 1978, with permission.)

remnants of the left atrium can be mobilized toward the right pleura. Mobilization of the right lung is then carried out, according to the technique used on the left, followed by stapling and dividing the bronchus and removal of the right lung.

At this point, careful bleeding control in the posterior mediastinum should be secured with close attention to the course of both vagus nerves. Only then are remnants of both main bronchi grasped with Allis clamps and pulled caudally. With the aorta retracted to the left, further dissection of the tracheal carina is performed, carefully preserving the surrounding collateral-rich tissue. The trachea is then divided exactly one cartilage ring cephalad to the carina. Again bleeding must be controlled because this area will be inaccessible after implantation of the donor organs (Fig. 33-29).

The donor organs are brought to the surgical field with the trachea still closed by a row of staples or a clamp. The trachea is then divided one or two cartilage rings proximal to the carina. In doing so, the trachea should be dissected only in the area where the final division takes place. Mucous secretions are aspirated from both main bronchi. The suction device is then discarded to prevent subsequent contamination of the surgical field. The secretions are collected for bacteriologic culture.

Now the heart-lung block is transferred into the recipient's chest. The left lung is introduced into the left pleura cavity by passing it posteriorly to the phrenic nerve, and the right

lung is passed posteriorly to both the right atrial cuff and the phrenic nerve (Fig. 33-30). Proper positioning of the lungs at this stage is ensured by identifying each lung separately and excluding rotation of the organs. Cold laparotomy pads are applied over the heart and lungs to prevent rewarming.

A stay suture (3–0 polydioxanon [PDS]) is placed on each side of the recipient's trachea at the junction of the membranous and the cartilaginous portions. They are then passed through corresponding points of the recipient's trachea. The tracheal suture line can be accomplished by several different techniques. Our preference is described. A single running suture 4–0 (PDS) is used for the posterior (membranous) part of the trachea (Fig. 33-30). Both stay sutures also are tied down at this stage. The cartilaginous part is anastomosed with single 3–0 PDS sutures, which are tied outside the trachea. A total of six to eight of these sutures is required. Two- to three-mm bites of trachea spaced at similar intervals are thought to be adequate. The anastomosis is then tested under saline to rule out the presence of air leaks. Currently, we test the anastomosis to a maximum airway pressure of 20 cmH$_2$O.

It has been our preference to seal this anastomosis with a mixture of antibiotics and fibrin adhesive (Haverich, et al., 1989). For this purpose, 2 ml of fibrinogen (component I) and a mixture of neomycin and bacitracin (Nebacetin) and thrombin solution (component II) are applied circumferentially around the tracheal anastomosis. Then the right-sided pericardial patch is passed counterclockwise around this

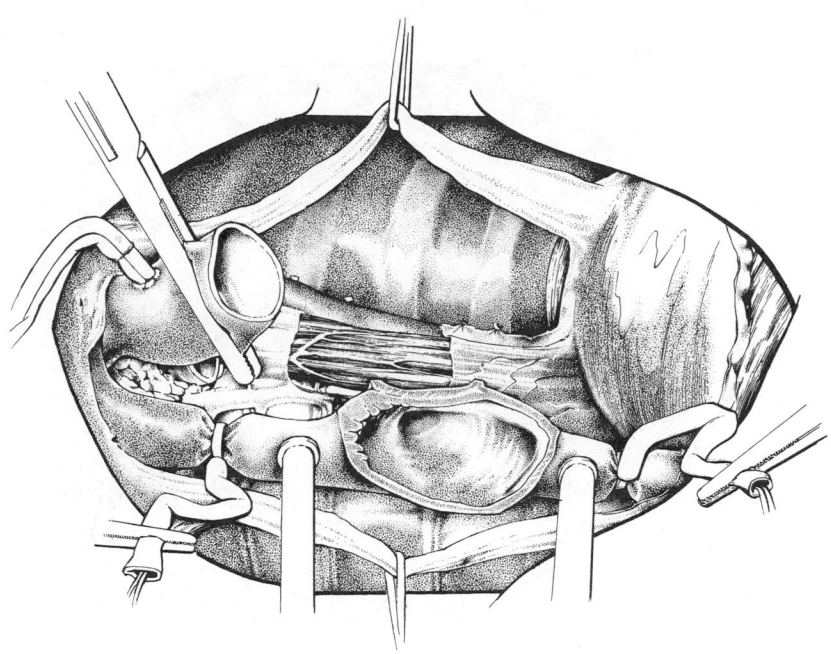

Figure 33-29. Operative, view following complete resection of the recipient heart-lung, including the main pulmonary artery and the tracheal carina. (From Haverich A: Herz- und Herz-Lungen-Transplantation. p. 551. In Borst HG, Klinner W, Oelert H (eds): Herzchirurgie. Springer-Verlag, Berlin, 1978, with permission.)

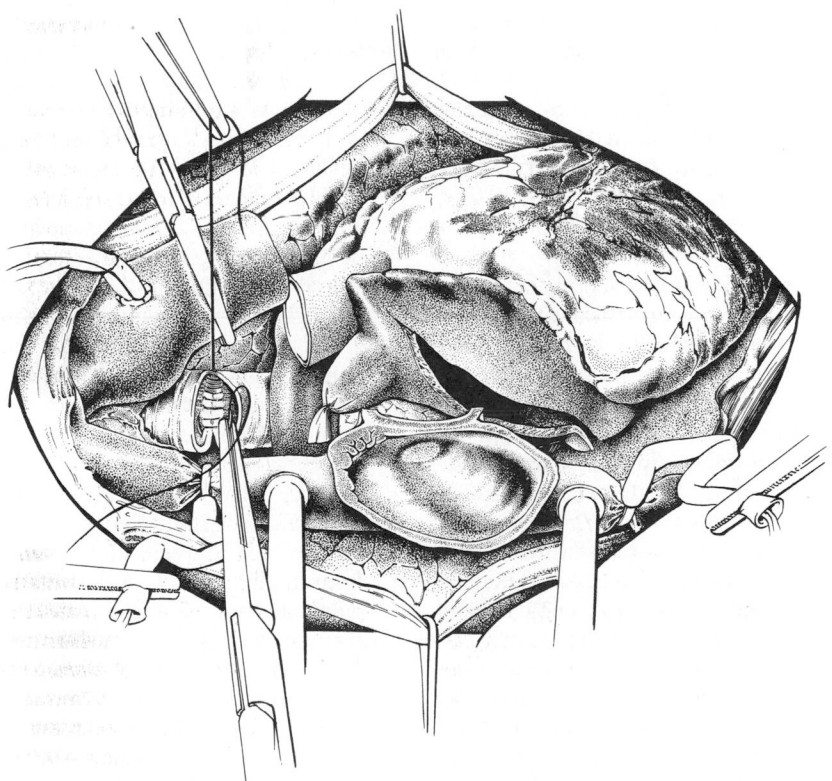

Figure 33-30. Implantation of the donor organs is initiated by end-to-end anastomosis of donor and recipient trachea. (From Haverich A: Herz- und Herz-Lungen-Transplantation. p. 551. In Borst HG, Klinner W, Oelert H (eds): Herzchirurgie. Springer-Verlag, Berlin, 1978, with permission.)

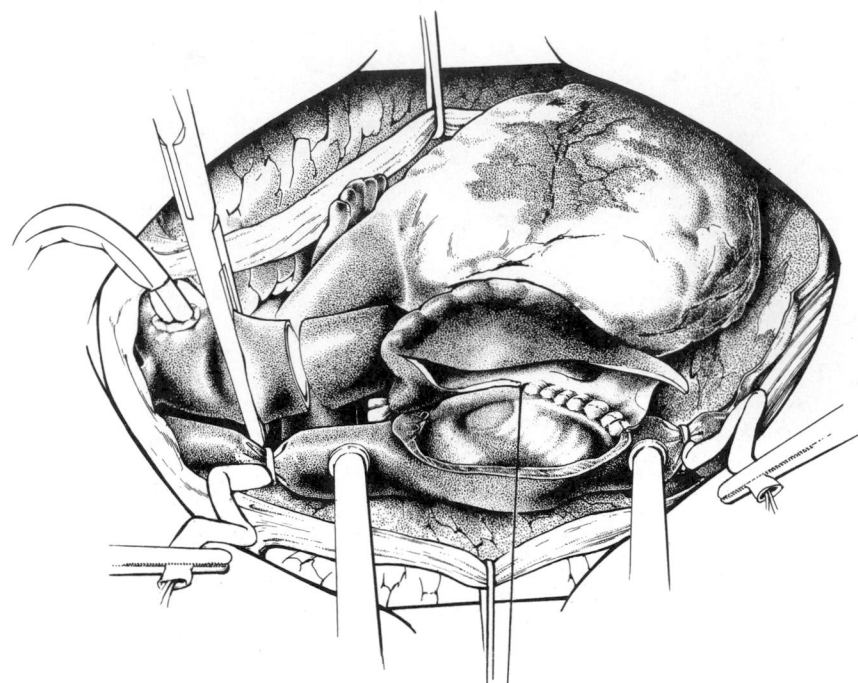

Figure 33-31. Side-to-side anastomosis between donor and recipient right atrium using running 3–0 polypropylene suture. The stumps of donor and recipient aorta have not been connected. (From Haverich A: Herz- und Herz-Lungen-Transplantation. p. 551. In Borst HG, Klinner W, Oelert H (eds): Herzchirurgie. Springer-Verlag, Berlin, 1978, with permission.)

anastomosis and again is secured with fibrin sealant and two stay sutures, one on the left and one on the right of the trachea.

The preparation for the right atrial anastomosis includes an oblique incision of the donor atrium from the lateral aspect of the IVC orifice toward the right atrial appendage, preserving the sulcus terminalis and the sinus node (Fig. 33-31). A patent foramen ovale in the recipient can be closed at this stage.

In the presence of a very thin interatrial septum or in cases with an atrial septal defect, the posterior wall of the right-sided left atrium may be pulled through behind the right atrium, serving as a reinforcement for the left lateral aspect of the right atrial suture line.

The right atrial anastomosis is accomplished with a continuous double-armed 3–0 polypropylene suture, starting at the midpoint of the medial wall of both right atria and corresponding to the remnant of the atrial septum on the recipient side. The right atrial suture line is continued first toward, then around the IVC, and finally cranially. If necessary, the incision in the donor right atrial wall can be lengthened to match the orifice of the recipient's right atrium. Thereafter, the sutures are carried along the lateral wall of the right atrium. They are tied only after deairing the right heart (see below). Prior to construction of the aortic suture line, the lengths of the donor and recipient vessels are assessed, and the excess tissue is trimmed from one or both ends. An end-to-end anastomosis is constructed with a continuous double-armed 4–0 polypropylene suture, which is terminated at the most superior aspect of the suture line to allow for deairing.

Before reperfusion of the heart and lungs, deairing is performed through the right atrial suture line following the release of SVC and IVC snares. The pulmonary artery is stabbed with a large-bore needle. Ventilation is then begun with the venous line of the extracorporeal circulation partially occluded to allow for filling of the pulmonary vasculature. Prior to release of the aortic cross-clamp, the ascending aorta and the apex of the left ventricle are stabbed, and any remaining air is removed by manual compression of the heart.

In many instances, the heart has to be electrically defibrillated. Temporary ventricular pacing may be required at this stage. Also, the "washout phenomenon" of the pulmonoplegic solution results in transient hyperkalemic effects when the coronary arteries are perfused with blood returning through the left atrium. The administration of calcium and catecholamines results in the restoration of normal sinus rhythm, usually within 15 minutes.

During rewarming, ventilation is maintained with 50 percent oxygen to avoid undue release of oxygen-free radicals from the lung tissue. Following stabilization of cardiac and pulmonary function, the patient can be weaned from extracorporeal circulation, usually after 30 minutes of reperfusion. At this stage, a PEEP of 6 cmH$_2$O should be maintained, and continuous spontaneous deairing of the left heart through the ascending aorta should be allowed. Following decannulation of the aorta and the right atrium and bleeding control, two pleural chest tubes are inserted into each side, one draining the apical portion of each pleura and the second, the costophrenic sinus. Normally, no mediastinal tubes are inserted. The sternal incision is closed in a routine fashion.

Perioperative Care

Intensive Care Unit

In general, the postoperative care of heart-lung transplant recipients on the intensive care unit does not differ significantly from that of other patients after major cardiac or thoracic interventions. The cardiac status is usually characterized by a high cardiac output at heart rates between 120 and 140 beats/min because denervation of the heart. Right and left ventricular function, unlike the situation after cardiac transplantation, is usually normal, and the requirement for inotropic support is minimal. In cases with doubtful cardiac status, a Swan-Ganz catheter is readily inserted to assess pulmonary artery pressure, cardiac output, and pulmonary capillary wedge pressure. The most common form of circulatory insufficiency in our heart-lung transplant patients has been high-output failure from low peripheral vascular resistance, especially in patients with preoperative hepatic insufficiency. This situation requires vasoconstrictor therapy.

Pulmonary function usually is adequate; thus routine postoperative respiratory therapy may be commenced (McGoldrick, et al., 1990). This includes ventilatory settings with a FIO_2 greater than 0.5 and a PEEP of 6 to 10 mmHg. At frequent intervals, arterial gas samples should be taken to ensure an arterial oxygen saturation greater than 95 percent. In rare cases with profound reperfusion injury, a higher FIO_2 may be required for variable time spans. In such cases, vigorous bronchial toilette by frequent endobronchial suction may be required for pulmonary edema. Extubation may be initiated at FIO_2 of 0.3 or less, when the patient is fully awake, cooperative, and able to cough with sufficient strength.

The chest tubes, initially connected to a underwater seal and a negative pressure of -15 to 20 cmH$_2$O, should be left in place for at least 5 days because small air leaks may persist or newly develop and the transplanted lungs show a tendency to produce fluid secretions because of the lack of lymphatic channels (as much as 500 to 1,000 ml/day).

Reversed isolation used to be the standard care regimen for heart-lung transplant recipients until 5 years ago. Since then, a number of reports demonstrated no significant differences regarding infectious episodes between patients with and without isolation procedures on the intensive care unit. Therefore, at our unit, one-to-one nursing and frequent changes of (nonsterile) gloves represent the only specific measures for organizational infectious prophylaxis after thoracic organ transplantation.

Immunosuppression

During the operation, the patient receives 1 g of methylprednisolone IV, followed by daily doses of methylprednisolone of 125 mg IV for the first 3 days. Azathioprine 5 mg/kg is the only drug administered prior to the operation, which is again given in a dose of 1.5 to 2.0 mg/kg after the patient has resumed an oral diet. Azathioprine therapy is continued as one therapeutic arm of the long-term triple-drug immunosuppressive regimen with the aim to suppress the white blood count to 4,000 to 5,000 cells/mm^3. Today, cyclosporine remains the mainstay of immunosuppressive therapy. We start intravenous administration of this drug as soon as the pa-

tient's renal function has recovered from surgery and extracorporeal circulation. This can usually be assessed 24 hours after surgery. The current criteria are a urine output greater than 1.5 ml/kg/h and a stable or decreasing serum creatinine level. The cyclosporine dose is adjusted to whole-blood trough levels (200 to 300 ng/ml by high-performance liquid chromatography). A matter of dispute has been early- and long-term administration of oral corticosteroids. The initial fear of precipitating tracheal healing complications when steroids are given during the first 2 weeks (Reitz, et al., 1982a) could not be substantiated by subsequent observations in larger patient series (Haverich, et al., 1989). Therefore, we continue corticosteroid treatment after the initial bolus therapy at a moderate oral dose of 0.5 mg/kg/day divided into two doses. The steroid dosage is then tapered by 2.5 mg every third day until the maintenance dose of 0.15 mg/kg/day has been reached. This protocol was adopted from our routine in heart transplantation and is believed to be justified by the registry results of the International Society for Heart Transplantation. This registry shows more favorable results of triple-drug therapy compared with those of other regimens.

Infection Prophylaxis and Therapy

Pulmonary infections represented the most common complication in allograft recipients. Following lung transplantation, a number of factors unique to this procedure increase the risk of intrathoracic infection (Dummer, et al., 1985, 1986; Duncan, et al., 1991). The tracheobronchial tree of organ donors usually is colonized by bacteria and is compromised as a result of aspiration, intubation, or nosocomial infections acquired during intensive care treatment. Moreover, CMV infection, toxoplasmosis, and tuberculosis may be transferred by the donor lung, potentially resulting in severe illness if reactivated in the recipient.

As in other forms of lung transplantation, the operative field in heart-lung transplantation must be considered potentially contaminated because the trachea has to be transsected. Accordingly, septic disruption of the tracheal anastomosis has been repeatedly reported (Griffith, et al., 1987b). Rupture of the ascending aortic suture line has also been observed in patients.

Postoperatively, the "reimplantation response" may occur during the first 4 to 6 days (Siegelman, et al., 1973; Jamieson, et al., 1984b; Prop, et al., 1984). This special form of pulmonary edema is thought to result from interruption of lymphatic drainage and may result in increased susceptibility of the transplanted lung to infection. The same findings are true for the diminished cough reflex because of denervation of the transplanted tracheobronchial tree (Dauber and Zeevi, 1988; Mancini and Tauxe, 1986).

The high risk of pulmonary infections resulting from the risk factors mentioned has been repeatedly reported (Dummer, et al., 1986; Gryzan, et al., 1988; Hakim, et al., 1985; Hutter, et al., 1989). With increasing experience, our institution has developed a sophisticated protocol of primary and secondary antimicrobial prophylaxis (Table 33-4). This regimen may not be applicable to all transplant units and may be adapted to local pharmacologic preferences or the endemic microbial environment.

Table 33-4. Antimicrobial Prophylaxis in Heart-Lung Transplantation

Type of Infection	Primary Prophylaxis	Secondary Prophylaxis (Positive Culture, No Clinical Signs of Infection)
Viral		
Herpes simplex	Acyclovir	Acyclovir
CMV	Hyperimmune globulin	Ganciclovir
Bacterial	Cefazolin (48 h)	According to antibiogram
	Cefotaxime/tobramycin (5 days)	
Tuberculosis	Isoniazid (6 mo)	
Candida albicans	—	Fluconazole or itraconazole
Aspergillus	—	Itraconazole
Pneumocystis	Cotrimoxazole (twice weekly)	Continue therapy

The details of therapy and the huge variety of potential bacterial, viral, protozoal, and fungal infections that may be identified in the postoperative course after heart-lung transplantation, including their management, is beyond the scope of this chapter. Suffice it to say that any suspected infection must result in prompt investigation by radiography, serology, and bronchoscopy with bronchoalveolar lavage. During the first 6 months after transplantation, we also recommend immediate administration of a broad-spectrum antibiotic and CMV hyperimmune serum following bronchoalveolar lavage in cases with clinical signs of infection (Erice, et al., 1987). The therapy is then modified after the infecting organism has been identified. Instantaneous exclusion of pulmonary infection is especially important because pulmonary rejection represents one differential diagnosis.

Other Prophylactic Measures

After the patient is able to leave the room, a mask and gloves should be worn while the patient is ambulatory in the hospital. Mobilization outside the room by regular bicycle exercise is performed, even if supplemental oxygen is required or the chest tubes still are in place. Intensive physical therapy, including regular postural drainage is maintained, with patients later taught to manage their own airway clearance.

Diagnosis and Therapy for Rejection

The diagnosis of allograft rejection is difficult after heart-lung transplantation (Reitz, et al., 1983; Veith and Hagstrom, 1972; Veith, et al., 1972). It is well known today that the transplanted heart is protected from acute rejection in this setting in that it usually does not reject at all or only subsequent to rejection of the lungs (Byers, et al., 1973; Cooper, et al., 1986; Griffith, et al., 1985; McGregor, et al., 1985; Novitzki, et al., 1986; Prop, et al., 1985a, 1987; Scott, et al., 1984; Wahlers, et al., 1987). Routine endomyocardial biopsy, therefore, has been abandoned from the surveillance protocols in most heart-lung transplant centers (Baldwin, et al., 1987; Glanville, et al., 1987b; Higenbottam, et al., 1988a). Instead, all diagnostic measures must concentrate on the pulmonary grafts. Physical signs, chest radiographs, pulmonary function testing, and transbronchial biopsy have all been reported to correlate with pulmonary rejection (Griffith, et al., 1987b; Herran, et al., 1984; Prop, et al., 1985b). Many centers perform transbronchial biopsies on a routine basis during any episode suspicious of lung rejection (Dauber and Zeevi, 1988; Higenbottam, et al., 1988b; Hutter, et al., 1988; Scott, et al., 1991). This approach has proved unsatisfactory in our patients because of the low sensitivity and specificity of the histologic findings in the specimens from transbronchial biopsy (Halasz, et al., 1973). A definite risk of bleeding and pneumothorax has also been reported, which may be lethal in patients with significantly impaired pulmonary function. Our approach has been to perform standard bronchoscopy and alveolar lavage in patients with clinical and functional signs of pulmonary deterioration (Clelland, et al., 1989; Duquesnoy, et al., 1985; Gryzan, et al., 1985; Prop, et al., 1988). As such, fever, a low peripheral oxygen saturation, a reduced vital capacity, and especially a diminished FEV_1 with an obstructive pattern on airflow analysis, are suggestive (Theodore, et al., 1984). Often, a "hilar flare" occurring around day 9 after transplantation represents the first sign of pulmonary rejection (Chiles, et al., 1985). The radiologic signs, however, may be less impressive in acute rejection episodes occurring in the later postoperative course (Millet, et al., 1989).

During bronchoscopy, the complete airway, including the tracheal anastomosis, is carefully inspected. Unlike purulent bacterial infections, acutely rejecting lungs often present with small amounts of ubiquitous nonliquid whitish secretions. The material obtained by bronchoalveolar lavage is analyzed for bacterial and viral organisms and fungi. In patients in poor clinical condition, in whom pulmonary infection is unlikely, methylprednisolone is initiated immediately after bronchoscopy. Otherwise, the therapy is withheld until the Gram stain and CMV early antigen test results (Gray, et al., 1987) are available to exclude an infectious episode as the cause of pulmonary deterioration.

In the presence of rejection, 1 g IV of methylprednisolone is given per day for 3 consecutive days. Only recipients with severe rejection refractory to steroids are subsequently treated by anti-T-cell antibodies, such as rabbit or horse antithymocyte globulin. Concomitant with this therapy, infectious prophylaxis is intensified with antibiotics (e.g., cephalosporins) and anti-CMV hyperimmune globulins. This prevents infection of the pulmonary graft secondary to rejection-induced damage. Whether this secondary prophylaxis is necessary or not has not been proved by controlled clinical studies.

Early Results

Data on 30-day mortality rates are available, both from the registry of the International Society for Heart and Lung Transplantation (ISHLT) (Kaye, 1992) and from single-center studies (Burke, et al., 1986; Couraud, et al., 1990). Prior to 1986, the 30-day mortality rate was reported to be about 30 percent worldwide (Reitz, 1982). Since then, significant improvement was seen with current mortality rates of about 20 percent. Of the 1,200 patients registered in the data base of the ISHLT, a total of 200 died early. The main cause of early death was bleeding and pulmonary failure (Jamieson, et al., 1984a). With improved techniques of donor lung preservation, the latter risk factor appears to be substantially reduced. Bleeding complications could also be significantly reduced, probably as a result of improved surgical technique and the beneficial effect of using aprotinin during the operation.

In our experience with 29 heart-lung transplants, no early deaths were related to pulmonary failure or bleeding. In fact, with the routine use of aprotinin from the start of our program, no reoperation for bleeding control has been necessary. Therefore, the high incidence of technical failures, amounting to 40 percent of the early deaths in the data base of the ISHLT, may be further reduced in the future. Infection, the second most important risk factor for early death, by contrast, will probably continue to be the major cause of death (Brooks, et al., 1985). Improved management of heart-lung transplant recipients in terms of prophylaxis of infection type and the dosing of immunosuppressive therapy will be necessary to allow for improved early survival rates (Beveridge, et al., 1984, Novick, et al., 1990).

Late Results

At present, 60 percent of heart-lung transplant recipients live 12 months postoperatively. Much better results than those reported by the ISHLT registry have been obtained in some single-center studies. Thus, Papworth Hospital reported a 1-year survival rate of 80 percent (Scott, 1988b), which matches our results of a 1-year survival rate of 79 percent. Therefore, 1-year success rates of 80 percent or more should be obtainable in the future.

Beyond the first 12 months, the death rate after heart-lung transplantation appears to be twice as high as that after heart transplantation alone. Late death occurs at an annual rate of 5 percent, for a 5-year survival rate of 40 percent (Kaye, 1992). This high rate of late lethal complications is also mirrored by the survival data after single- and double-lung transplantations. In the absence of detailed multicenter analyses of the causes of late death in heart-lung transplantation, chronic rejection most probably is the major lethal factor during the long-term follow-up (Burke, et al., 1985, 1986; Dawkins, et al., 1985; Jamieson, et al., 1985, Reichart, et al., 1987). Chronic pulmonary allograft rejection, or obliterative bronchiolitis (Epler and Colby 1983; Paradis, et al., 1988), is present in nearly one-half of the surviving patients 4 to 5 years postoperatively (Allen, et al., 1986; Griffith, et al., 1988). This entity is characterized by a chronic decrement of vital capacity and FEV_1. The abnormal airflow pattern suggests peripheral bronchial obstruction to be the primary mechanism of the disturbed pulmonary function, which ultimately leads to impaired gas exchange and death from respiratory failure (Burke, et al., 1984, 1985; Haverich, et al., 1985a; Scott, et al., 1989; Yousem, et al., 1985). No specific measures, other than retransplantation, are currently available to eliminate or treat this complication (Glanville, et al., 1987a). Compared with the magnitude of the problem, other causes of late death play a relatively minor role and occur at similar incidence rates after heart, kidney, and liver transplantation.

COMMENTS AND CONTROVERSIES

During the past 5 years, pulmonary allografting has undergone major changes. The limited availability of heart and lungs for en bloc transplantation has resulted in a worldwide stagnate number of operations. The simultaneous increase in surgical activities with respect to isolated lung grafting limits the application of combined cardiopulmonary transplantation to patients with truly irreversible pulmonary and cardiac failure, including those with uncorrectable congenital cardiac anomalies. All other disorders, including pulmonary hypertension of various causes and Eisenmenger's syndrome, will probably continue to be treated by lung transplantation alone. Currently available single-center results indicate that double-lung transplantation rather than single-lung transplantation represents the more successful approach in such patients. Early and late consequences of the "programmed" ventilation/perfusion mismatch in single-lung transplantation in severe pulmonary hypertension probably will induce a change in favor of double-lung transplantation.

The major impediment to true long-term survival after any type of allogeneic lung replacement and, in fact, any organ transplantation, remains chronic rejection. The high incidence of obliterative bronchiolitis after the first year post-transplantation must encourage intensive research to obviate its development or to formulate new regimens of drug therapy. At present, improved selection of donor/recipient pairs on immunologic grounds by HLA matching appears to be the sole prophylactic measure against chronic rejection. After the diagnosis of obliterative bronchiolitis is made, increased immunosuppression using currently available drugs has repeatedly resulted in a standstill of the course of the disease. True control of this complication in terms of restoration of normal lung function parameters, however, has not been achieved, signalling the utmost importance of further research in this field.

A.H.
H.G.B.

This detailed account of heart-lung transplantation also includes the technical aspects. It was thought that these techniques were best described within the context of this chapter rather than being included with other pulmonary techniques at the end of this section.

The authors correctly point out the current place of heart-lung transplantation. It should be emphasized that because of the chronic lack of suitable donors and the increasing number of suitable recipients, most transplant groups whenever possible will use a single-lung transplantation. Where indicated, double-lung transplantation is preferred to heart-lung transplants, thus allowing a more rational use of available organs. It is fair to say, however, that some groups still practice the "domino" operation in which a recipient with a normal heart but requiring two lungs will receive a heart-lung transplantation and the recipient's heart will then be used as the donor heart for another recipient.

Because of the aforementioned lack of donors worldwide, the number of heart-lung transplantations is decreasing, whereas heart, single-lung, and double-lung transplantations continue to increase. In most centers, patients requiring heart-lung transplantation have an extremely prolonged wait.

Initially, heart-lung transplantation carried an extremely high perioperative mortality rate because of postoperative bleeding. The techniques described in this chapter have resolved much of this problem. However, the perioperative mortality rate from heart-lung transplantation continues to exceed that of heart, single-lung, or double-lung transplantation, although the 1- and 2-year survival rates of this transplantation are similar to that seen with single organs.

R.J.G.

KEY REFERENCES

Haverich A, Aziz S, Scott WC et al: Improved lung preservation using EuroCollins solution for flush-perfusion. Thorac Cardiovasc Surg 34:368, 1986

This is the original article describing the experiments on a flush perfusion technique, resulting in successful distant organ procurement for heart-lung transplantation. The basic principles regarding pressure and volume requirements of the pulmonary vasculature during cold flush perfusion are presented.

Khaghani A, Banner N, Ozdogan E et al: Medium-term results of combined heart and lung transplantation for emphysema. J Heart Lung Transplant 10:15, 1991

Indications, techniques, complications, and results in 17 patients with (noninfected) pulmonary emphysema undergoing heart-lung transplantation are described.

McCarthy PM, Starnes VA, Theodore J et al: Improved survival after heart-lung transplantation. J Thorac Cardiovasc Surg 99:54, 1990

Changes in patient management, such as modified immunosuppression, routine bronchoscopy, and earlier recognition of infection and rejection, have resulted in an improved survival rate and a decrease in the severity of obliterative bronchiolitis in a series of 65 heart-lung transplantations.

Scott JP, Fradet G, Smyth RL et al: Management following heart and lung transplantation: five years experience. Eur J Cardiothorac Surg 4:197, 1990

Patient selection criteria, the use of transbronchial biopsies, and early and late postoperative management are described in a series of 70 patients who underwent heart-lung transplantation. The article gives a detailed description of how to differentiate between pulmonary rejection and infection.

Scott J, Higenbottam TW, Hutter J et al: Heart-lung transplantation for cystic fibrosis. Lancet 2:192, 1988a

An early series of six patients with cystic fibrosis undergoing heart-lung transplantation is described. Pre-, intra-, and postoperative management and results are reported in this special subset of transplant candidates with infectious pulmonary disease.

REFERENCES

Allen MD, Burke CM, McGregor CGA et al: Steroid-responsive bronchiolitis after human heart-lung transplantation. J Thorac Cardiovasc Surg 92:449, 1986

Baldwin JC, Oyer PE, Stinson EB et al: Comparison of cardiac rejection in heart and heart-lung transplantation. J Heart Lung Transplant 6:352, 1987

Bando K, Pillai R, Cameron DE et al: Leukocyte depletion ameliorates free radical-mediated lung injury after cardiopulmonary bypass. J Thorac Cardiovasc Surg 99:873, 1990

Bando K, Schüler S, Cameron DE et al: Twelve-hour cardiopulmonary preservation using donor core cooling, leukocyte depletion, and liposomal superoxide dismutase. J Heart Lung Transplant 10:304, 1991

Bando K, Tago M, Teraoka H et al: Extended cardiopulmonary preservation for heart-lung transplantation: a comparative study of superoxide dismutase. J Heart Lung Transplant 8:59, 1989

Beveridge T, Krupp P, McKibbin C: Lymphomas and lymphoproliferative lesions developing under cyclosporin therapy (letter). Lancet 1:788, 1984

Blanco G, Adam A, Rodriguez-Perez D, Fernandez A: Complete transplantation of canine heart and lungs. Arch Surg 76:20, 1958

Bonser RS, Fragomeni LS, Jamieson SW et al: Effects of prostaglandin E_1 in twelve-hour lung preservation. J Heart Lung Transplant 10:310, 1991

Bonser RS, Fragomeni LS, Harris K et al: Acute physiologic changes after extended pulmonary preservation. J Heart Lung Transplant 9:220, 1990

Brooks RG, Hofflin JM, Jamieson SW et al: Infectious complications in heart-lung transplant recipients. Am J Med 79:412, 1985

Burke CM, Glanville AR, Theodore J, Robin ED: Lung immunogenicity, rejection, and obliterative bronchiolitis. Chest 92:547, 1987

Burke CM, Morris AJR, Dawkins KD et al: Late airflow obstruction in heart-lung transplantation recipients. J Heart Lung Transplant 4:437, 1985

Burke CM, Theodore J, Baldwin JC et al: Twenty-eight cases of human heart-lung transplantation. Lancet 1:517, 1986

Burke CM, Theodore J, Dawkins KD et al: Post-transplant obliterative bronchiolitis and other late lung sequelae in human heart-lung transplantation. Chest 86:824, 1984

Byers JM, Sabanayagam P, Baker RR et al: Pathologic changes in baboon lung allografts. Ann Surg 178:754, 1973

Carrel A: The surgery of blood vessels. Bull Johns Hopkins Hosp 18:18, 1907

Castaneda AR, Arnar O, Schmidt-Habelman P et al: Cardiopulmonary autotransplantation in primates. J Cardiovasc Surg 13:523, 1972

Chiles C, Guthaner DF, Jamieson SW et al: Heart-lung transplantation: the postoperative chest radiograph. Radiology 154:299, 1985

Clelland CA, Higenbottam TW, Scott JA et al: Lymphocyte counts and T-cell phenotypes in bronchoalveolar lavage (BAL) in relation to transbronchial lung biopsy (TBB) in patients with heart-lung transplants. Thorax 44:873, 1989

Collins GM, Bravo-Shugarman M, Terasaki PI: Kidney preservation for transplantation: initial perfusion and 30 hours ice storage. Lancet 2:1219, 1969

Cooley DA, Bloodwell RD, Hallman GL et al: Organ transplantation for advanced cardiopulmonary disease. Ann Thorac Surg 8:30, 1969

Cooper DKC, Novitzky D, Rose AG, Reichart BA: Acute pulmonary rejection precedes cardiac rejection following heart-lung transplantation in a primate model. J Heart Lung Transplant 5:29, 1986

Couraud L, Baudet E, Velly J-F et al: Lung and heart-lung transplantation for end-stage lung disease. Eur J Cardiothorac Surg 4:318, 1990

Dauber JH, Zeevi A: Lung transplantation: lessons learned about local immune function and pulmonary defense mechanisms. p. 625. In Daniele RP (ed): Pulmonary Immunology. McGraw-Hill, New York, 1988

Dawkins KD, Haverich A, Derby GC et al: Long-term hemodynamics following combined heart and lung transplantation in primates. J Thorac Cardiovasc Surg 89:55, 1985

Demikhov VP: Experimental Transplantation of Vital Organs. Consultants' Bureau, New York, 1962

Dummer JS, Montero CG, Griffith BP et al: Infections in heart-lung transplant recipients. Transplantation 41:725, 1986

Dummer JS, White LT, Ho M et al: Morbidity of cytomegalovirus infection in recipients of heart or heart-lung transplants who received cyclosporin. J Infect Dis 152:1182, 1985

Duncan AJ, Dummer JS, Paradis IL et al: Cytomegalovirus infection and survival in lung transplant recipients. J Heart Lung Transplant 10:638, 1991

Duquesnoy RJ, Zeevi A, Fung J et al: Functional characterization of lymphocytes in bronchoalveolar lavages from heart-lung transplant patients. J Heart Lung Transplant 4:135, 1985

Epler GR, Colby TV: The spectrum of bronchiolitis obliterans. Chest 83:161, 1983

Erice A, Jordon MC, Chace BA et al: Ganciclovir treatment of cytomegalovirus disease in transplant recipients and other immunocompromised hosts. JAMA 257:3082, 1987

Feeley TW, Mihm FG, Downing TP et al: Hypothermic preservation of the heart and lungs with Collins solution: effect on cardiorespiratory function following heart-lung allotransplantation in dogs. Ann Thorac Surg 41:301, 1986

Fisher RA, Alexander JW: Management of the multiple organ donor. Clin Transpl 6:328, 1992

Fuster V, Steele PM, Edwards WD et al: Primary pulmonary hypertension: natural history and the importance of thrombosis. Circulation 70:580, 1984

Glanville AR, Baldwin JC, Burke CM et al: Obliterative bronchiolitis after heart-lung transplantation: apparent arrest by augmented immunosuppression. Ann Intern Med 107:300, 1987a

Glanville AR, Imoto E, Baldwin JC et al: The role of right ventricular endomyocardial biopsy in the long-term management of heart-lung transplant recipients. J Heart Lung Transplant 6:357, 1987b

Gray JJ, Alvey B, Smith DJ, Wreghitt TG: Evaluation of a commercial latex agglutination test for detecting antibodies to cytomegalovirus in organ donors and transplant recipients. J Virol Methods 16:13, 1987

Griffith BP, Durham SJ, Hardesty RL et al: Acute rejection of the heart-lung allograft and methods of its detection. Transplant Proc 19:2527, 1987a

Griffith BP, Hardesty RL, Trento A, Bahnson HT: Asynchronous rejection of heart and lungs following cardiopulmonary transplantation. Ann Thorac Surg 40:488, 1985

Griffith BP, Hardesty RL, Trento A et al: Heart-lung transplantation: lessons learned and future hopes. Ann Thorac Surg 43:6, 1987b

Griffith BP, Paradis IL, Zeevi A et al: Immunologically mediated disease of the airways after pulmonary transplantation. Ann Surg 208:371, 1988

Gryzan S, Paradis IR, Dauber JH et al: The role of bronchoalveolar lavage (BAL) in monitoring patients after heart-lung transplantation (H/LTx). J Heart Lung Transplant 4:134, 1985

Gryzan S, Paradis IL, Zeevi A et al: Unexpectedly high incidence of *Pneumocystis carinii* infection after lung-heart transplantation. Implications for lung defense and allograft survival. Am Rev Respir Dis 137:1268, 1988

Hakim M, Higenbottam T, Bethune D et al: Selection and procurement of combined heart and lung grafts for transplantation. J Thorac Cardiovasc Surg 95:474, 1988

Hakim M, Wreghitt TG, English TAH et al: Significance of donor-transmitted disease in cardiac transplantation. J Heart Lung Transplant 4:302, 1985

Halasz NA, Cantanzaro A, Trummer M et al: Transplantation of the lung: correlation of physiologic, immunologic, and histologic findings. J Thorac Cardiovasc Surg 66:581, 1973

Hardesty RL, Griffith BP: Autoperfusion of the heart and lungs for preservation during distant procurement. J Thorac Cardiovasc Surg 93:11, 1987

Hardesty RL, Griffith BP: Procurement for combined heart-lung transplantation. J Thorac Cardiovasc Surg 89:795, 1985

Harjula A, Baldwin JC, Starnes VA et al: Proper donor selection for heart-lung transplantation: the Stanford experience. J Thorac Cardiovasc Surg 94:874, 1987

Haverich A, Dawkins KD, Baldwin JC et al: Long-term cardiac and pulmonary histology in primates following combined heart and lung transplantation. Transplantation 39:356, 1985a

Haverich A, Frimpong-Boateng K, Wahlers T, Schäfers H-J: Pericardial flap-plasty for protection of the tracheal anastomosis in heart-lung transplantation. J Cardiac Surg 4:136, 1989

Haverich A, Scott WC, Jamieson SW: Twenty years of lung preservation—a review. J Heart Lung Transplant 4:234, 1985b

Herran JJ, Theodore J, van Kessel A et al: Appropriate ventilatory response to exercise in human heart-lung transplantation. Clin Res 31:417A, 1984

Higenbottam T, Hutter JA, Stewart S, Wallwork J: Transbronchial biopsy has eliminated the need for endomyocardial biopsy in heart-lung recipients. J Heart Lung Transplant 7:435, 1988a

Higenbottam TW, Stewart S, Penketh A, Wallwork J: Transbronchial lung biopsy for the diagnosis of rejection in heart-lung transplant patients. Transplantation 46:532, 1988b

Hooper TL, Locke TJ, Fetherston G et al: Comparison of cold flush perfusion with modified blood versus modified Euro-Collins solution for lung preservation. J Heart Lung Transplant 9:429, 1990

Hutter JA, Scott J, Wreghitt T et al: The importance of cytomegalovirus in heart-lung transplantation recipients. Chest 95:627, 1989

Hutter JA, Stewart S, Higenbottam T et al: Histologic changes in heart-lung transplant recipients during rejection episodes and at routine biopsy. J Heart Lung Transplant 7:440, 1988

Jamieson SW, Baldwin J, Stinson EB et al: Clinical heart-lung transplantation. Transplantation 37:81, 1984a

Jamieson SW, Dawkins KD, Burke C et al: Late results of combined heart-lung transplantation. Transplant Proc 17:212, 1985

Jamieson SW, Stinson EB, Oyer PH et al: Heart and lung transplantation for pulmonary hypertension. Am J Surg 147:740, 1984b

Jones KD, Cavarocchi N, Hakim M et al: A single flush technique for successful distant organ procurement in heart-lung transplantation. J Heart Lung Transplant 4:614, 1985

Jurmann MJ, Dammenhayn L, Schäfers H-J, Haverich A: Pulmonary reperfusion injury: evidence for oxygen-derived free radical mediated damage and effects of different free radical scavengers. Eur J Cardiothorac Surg 4:665, 1990

Kaiser LR, Cooper JD, Trulock EP et al: The evolution of single lung transplantation for emphysema. J Thorac Cardiovasc Surg 102:333, 1991

Kaye MP: The registry of the International Society for Heart and Lung Transplantation. Ninth Official Report 1992. J Heart Lung Transplant 11:599, 1992

Kennan RJ, Griffith BP, Kormos RL et al: Increased perioperative lung preservation injury with lung procurement by Euro-Collins solution flush. J Heart Lung Transplant 10:650, 1991

Kontos GJ, Adachi H, Borkos AM et al: A no-flush, core-cooling technique for successful cardiopulmonary preservation in heart-lung transplantation. J Thorac Cardiovasc Surg 94:836, 1987a

Kontos GJ, Adachi H, Borkos AM et al: Successful four-hour heart-lung preservation with core-cooling on cardiopulmonary bypass: a simplified model that assesses preservation. J Heart Lung Transplant 6:106, 1987b

Ladowski JS, Hardesty RL, Griffith BP: Protection of the heart-lung allograft during procurement. Cooling of the lungs with extracorporeal circulation or pulmonary artery flush. J Heart Lung Transplant 3:351, 1984

Ladowski JS, Kapelanski DP, Teodori MF et al: Use of autoperfusion for distant procurement of heart-lung allografts. J Heart Lung Transplant 4:330, 1985

Leval MR de, Smyth R, Whitehead B et al: Heart and lung transplantation for terminal cystic fibrosis. J Thorac Cardiovasc Surg 101:633, 1991

Levine SM, Gibbons WJ, Bryan CL et al: Single lung transplantation for primary pulmonary hypertension. Chest 98:1107, 1990

Locke TJ, Hooper TL, Flecknell PA, McGregor CGA: Preservation of the lung: comparison of flush perfusion with cold modified blood and core cooling by cardiopulmonary bypass. J Heart Lung Transplant 10:1, 1991

Lower RR, Stofer RC, Hurley EJ, Shumway NE: Complete homograft replacement of the heart and both lungs. Surgery 50:842, 1961

Mancini MC, Tauxe WN: Assessment of pulmonary clearance in heart-lung transplant recipients using technetium-99 minimicronized albumin colloid (MMAC). Am Rev Respir Dis 133:A11, 1986

McGoldrick JP, Scott JP, Smyth R et al: Early graft function after heart-lung transplantation. J Heart Lung Transplant 9:693, 1990

McGregor CGA, Baldwin JC, Jamieson SW et al: Isolated pulmonary rejection after combined heart-lung transplantation. J Thorac Cardiovasc Surg 90:623, 1985

McGregor CGA, Jamieson SW, Baldwin JC et al: Combined heart-lung transplantation for end-stage Eisenmenger's syndrome. J Thorac Cardiovasc Surg 91:443, 1986

Millet B, Higenbottam TW, Flower CD et al: The radiographic appearances of infection and acute rejection of the lung following heart-lung transplantation. Am Rev Respir Dis 140:62, 1989

Miyamoto Y, Lajos TZ, Bhayana JN et al: Physiologic constraints in autoperfused heart-lung preservation. J Heart Lung Transplant 6:261, 1987

Moncada S: Biology and therapeutic potential of prostacyclin. Stroke 14:157, 1982

Nakae S, Webb WR, Theodorides T, Sugg WL: Respiratory function following cardiopulmonary denervation in dog, cat, and monkey. Surg Gynecol Obstet 125:1285, 1967

Novick RJ, Menkis AH, McKenzie FN et al: Should heart-lung transplant donors and recipients be matched according to cytomegalovirus serologic status? J Heart Transplant 9:699, 1990

Novick RJ, Menkis AH, McKenzie FN: New trends in lung preservation: a collective review. J Heart Lung Transplant 11:377, 1992

Novitzky D, Cooper DKC, Rose AG, Reichart B: Acute isolated pulmonary rejection following transplantation of the heart and both lungs: experimental and clinical observations. Ann Thorac Surg 42:180, 1986

Novitzky D, Wicomb WN, Rose AG et al: Pathophysiology of pulmonary edema following experimental brain death in the Chacma baboon. Ann Thorac Surg 43:288, 1987

Okamoto K, Kinoshita Y, Yoshioka T et al: Myocardial preservation in brain-dead patients maintained with vasopressin and catecholamine. Clin Transpl 6:294, 1992

Paradis IL, Zeevi A, Duquesnoy R et al: Immunologic aspects of chronic lung rejection in humans. Transplant Proc 20(suppl I): 812, 1988

Penketh A, Higenbottam TW, Hakim M, Wallwork J: Heart and lung transplantation in patients with end-stage lung disease. BMJ 295:311, 1987

Prop J, Ehrie MG, Crapo JD et al: Reimplantation response in isografted rat lungs. Analysis of causal factors. J Thorac Cardiovasc Surg 87:702, 1984

Prop J, Kuijpers K, Petersen AH et al: Why are lung allografts more vigorously rejected than hearts? J Heart Lung Transplant 4:433, 1985a

Prop J, Tazelaar HD, Billingham ME: Rejection of combined heart-lung transplants in rats. Function and pathology. Am J Pathol 127:97, 1987

Prop J, Wagenaar-Hilbers JPA, Petersen AH, Wildevuur CHR: Characteristics of cells lavaged from rejecting lung allografts in rats. Transplant Proc 20:217, 1988

Prop J, Wildevuur CR, Nieuwenhuis P: Lung allograft rejection in the rat. II. Specific immunological properties of lung grafts. Transplantation 40:126, 1985b

Reichart B, Blaschke F, Cooper DKC et al: Transplantation of the heart and both lungs: initial experience of twelve operations in ten patients. Clin Transpl 1:231, 1987

Reitz BA: Heart-lung transplantation—a review. J Heart Lung Transplant 2:291, 1982

Reitz BA, Bieber CP, Raney AA et al: Orthotopic heart and combined heart and lung transplantation with cyclosporin-A immune suppression. Transplant Proc 13:393, 1982a

Reitz BA, Burton NA, Jamieson SW et al: Heart and lung transplantation. Autotransplantation and allotransplantation in primates with extended survival. J Thorac Cardiovasc Surg 80:360, 1980

Reitz BA, Gaudiani VA, Hunt SA et al: Diagnosis and treatment of allograft rejection in heart-lung transplant recipients. J Thorac Cardiovasc Surg 85:354, 1983

Reitz BA, Pennock JL, Shumway NE: Simplified operative method for heart and lung transplantation. J Surg Res 31:1, 1981

Reitz BA, Wallwork J, Hunt SA et al: Heart-lung transplantation:

successful therapy for patients with pulonary vascular disease. N Engl J Med 306:557, 1982b

Robicsek F, Lesage A, Sanger PW et al: Transplantation of "live" hearts. Am J Cardiol 20:803, 1967

Robicsek F, Master TN, Duncan GD et al: An autoperfused heart-lung-preparation: metabolism and function. J Heart Lung Transplant 4:334, 1985

Rozkovec A, Montanes P, Oakley CM: Factors that influence the outcome of primary pulmonary hypertension. Br Heart J 55:449, 1986

Sale JP, Patel D, Duncan B, Waters JH: Anaesthesia for combined heart and lung transplantation. Anaesthesia 42:249, 1987

Scott JP, Fradet G, Smyth RL et al: Prospective study of transbronchial biopsies in the management of heart-lung and single lung transplant patients. J Heart Lung Transplant 10:626, 1991

Scott JP, Higenbottam TW, Clelland C et al: The natural history of obliterative bronchiolitis in heart-lung transplant recipients. Transplant Proc 21:2592, 1989

Scott JP, Hutter JA, Higenbottam TW, Wallwork J: Combined heart and lung transplantation. Cardiol Pract 6:21, 1988b

Scott WC, Haverich A, Billingham ME: Lethal rejection of the lung without significant cardiac rejection in primate heart-lung transplants. J Heart Lung Transplant 4:33, 1984

Siegelman SS, Sinha SBP, Veith FJ: Pulmonary reimplantation response. Ann Surg 117:30, 1973

Spray TL, Mallory GM, Canter CE et al: Pediatric lung transplantation for pulmonary hypertension and congenital heart disease. Ann Thorac Surg 54:216, 1992

Theodore J, Jamieson SW, Burke C et al: Physiologic aspects of human heart-lung transplantation. Pulmonary function status of the post-transplanted lung. Chest 86:349, 1984

Veith FJ, Hagstrom JW: Alveolar manifestations of rejection: an important cause of the poor results with human lung transplantation. Ann Surg 175:336, 1972

Veith FJ, Sinha SBP, Blumcke S et al: Nature and evolution of lung allograft rejection with and without immunosuppression. J Thorac Cardiovasc Surg 63:509, 1972

Wahlers T, Haverich A, Fieguth HG et al: Flush perfusion using Euro Collins solution vs cooling by means of extracorporeal circulation in heart-lung preservation. J Heart Lung Transplant 5:89, 1986

Wahlers T, Khaghani A, Martin M et al: Frequency of acute heart and lung rejection after heart-lung transplantation. Transplant Proc 19:3537, 1987

Webb WR, Howard HS: Cardio-pulmonary transplantation. Surg Forum 8:313, 1957

Yacoub M, Khagani A, Aravot D et al: Cardiac transplantation from life donors. Am Coll Cardiol 11:102, 1988

Yacoub MH, Banner NR, Khaghani A et al: Heart-lung transplantation for cystic fibrosis and subsequent domino heart transplantation. J Heart Lung Transplant 9:459, 1990

Yousem SA, Burke C, Billingham M: Pathologic pulmonary alterations in long-term human heart-lung transplantation. Hum Pathol 16:911, 1985

34

ANATOMY AND PHYSIOLOGY

Jean Deslauriers
Reza John Mehran
Marc Desmeules

ANATOMY

The pleura is formed of two serosal membranes, one covering the lung (the visceral pleura) and one covering the inner chest wall (the parietal pleura). One surface glides over the other one, facilitating proper lung movements during the different phases of respiration. The pleural space is the space delimited by the two layers. Under normal conditions it contains only a small amount of liquid that functions as a lubricator. The total amount of the pleural fluids ranges between 0.1 and 0.2 ml/kg, with a thickness of about 10 μm (Staub, et al., 1985). The two pleural cavities are completely independent of each other, but in some conditions the parietal pleura of each side can be in contact anteriorly behind the sternum.

The transition between the parietal and visceral pleurae is at level of the pulmonary hilum. At this level the reflection covers the different constituents of the hilum, except inferiorly where the reflection extends down to the diaphragm. The overall shape of this reflection is a racquet, the handle of which forms the pulmonary ligament, also known as the triangular ligament of the lung. The limits of the triangular ligament are (1) medially on the right the esophagus, on the left the aorta, and the pericardium; (2) superiorly on the inferior pulmonary vein; and (3) inferiorly on the diaphragm. The ligament contains a few small arteries and veins of little clinical significance, tributaries of bronchial and esophageal arteries, and lymph nodes draining the inferior lobe.

EMBRYOLOGY

During the end of the third week of gestation, the embryonic mesoderm differentiates into the para-axial mesoderm, the intermediate mesoderm, and the lateral plate (Figs. 34-1 to 34-4). The lateral plate forms two different layers: (1) the somatic mesoderm or somatopleure and (2) the splanchnic mesoderm or splanchnopleure. Gradually, the somatic mesoderm progresses to meet in the midline, in the ventral portion of the embryo, closing the intraembryonic celom from the extraembryonic celom. The somatic mesoderm becomes the parietal layer and the splanchnic mesoderm, the visceral layer of the intraembryonic celomic sac.

By the end of the seventh week, the diaphragm separates the pleuropericardial and peritoneal spaces. Meanwhile the separation of the serosal cavities of the chest starts, with the medial growth of the pericardial folds. The folds contain the phrenic nerves and the common cardinal veins (Cuvier's duct), the precursors of the superior vena cava. The folds coalesce in the midline during the fifth week, separating the pericardial from the pleural space. During the same period, the pulmonary buds grow and contribute to the formation of the final shape of the pleural and pericardial cavities (Figs. 34-3 and 34-4). By the third month, the pleural cavities have expanded cranially, caudally, and ventrolaterally to surround the pericardium.

ADULT PLEURAL SAC

Visceral Pleura

The visceral pleura covers the surface of the lung and extends into the fissures. The visceral pleura is thin, transparent, and tightly adherent, by the way elastic fibers, to the underlying alveolar wall elastica (Fig. 34-5). It is the disruption of these elastic fibers that results in the formation of pleural blebs (Harley, 1987).

Parietal Pleura

The parietal pleura is more complex anatomically. This layer covers almost completely the inner surface of the thoracic wall and also the medial aspect of the mediastinum. The attachment of the parietal pleura to these structures is through a fibrous layer known as the endothoracic fascia (Fig. 34-5). The endothoracic fascia is a cleavage layer in which the parietal pleura can be separated from the chest wall. The

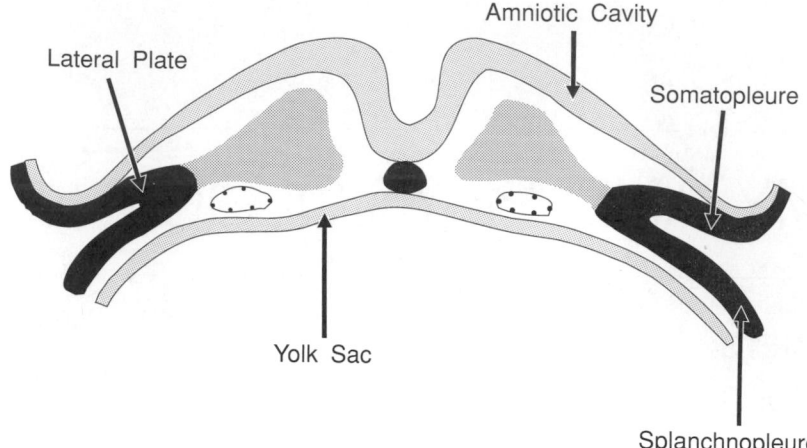

Figure 34-1. Differentiation of the lateral plate into the somatopleure and the splanchnopleure, the precursors of the parietal and visceral pleura, respectively (early third week of gestation).

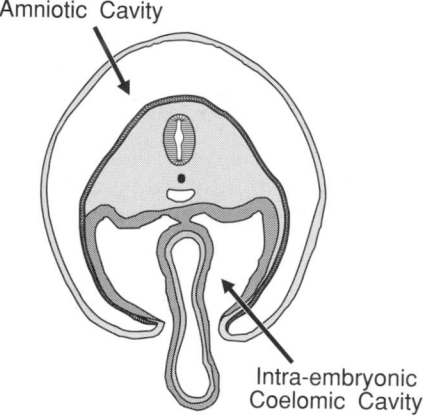

Figure 34-2. The creation of the intraembryonic celomic cavity by ventral migration of the somatopleure toward the midline.

thickness and strength of the endothoracic fascia varies with its location. The fascia is strongest over the inner surface of the ribs. Posterior to the sternum and in the pericardium, the endothoracic fascia is almost nonexistent. This makes the detachment of the pleura in these locations impossible. At the level of the thoracic inlet, the fascia is again very strong and forms a diaphragm called the fibrous cervicothoracic septum (Nebut, et al., 1982) or the cervicothoracic diaphragm of Bourgery (Bouchet and Cuilleret, 1974). This diaphragm is supported by a number of suspensory ligaments to surrounding structures.

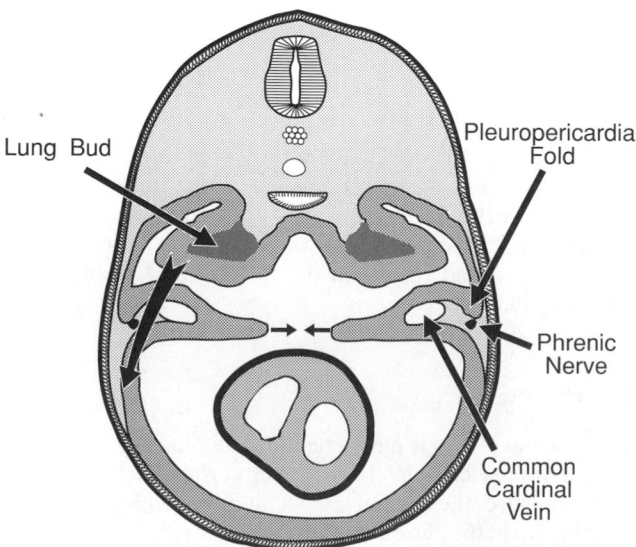

Figure 34-3. Creation of the lung bud and the pleuropericardial folds (around fifth week).

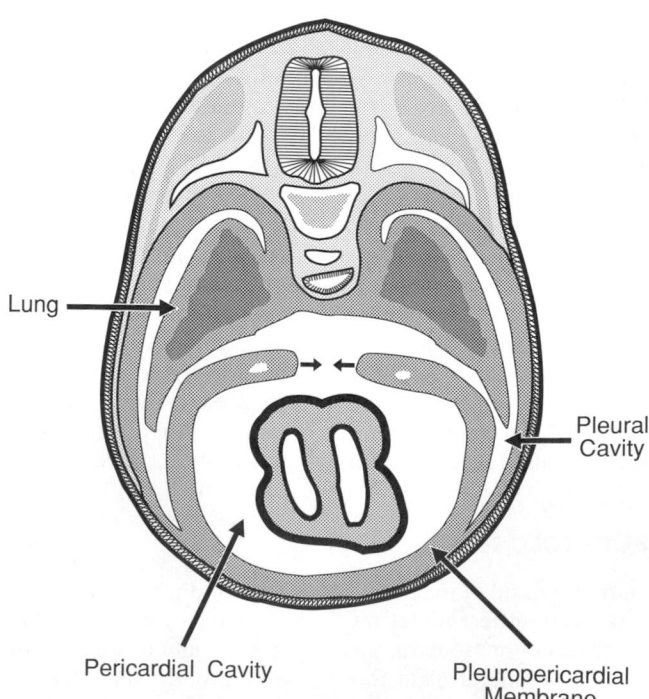

Figure 34-4. Midline fusion of the pleuropericardial folds, with separation of the pleural cavity from the pericardial sac. Expansion of the pleural cavity (fifth week to third month).

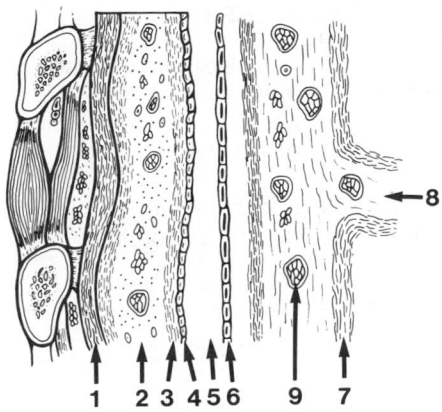

Figure 34-5. The different layers of the parietal and visceral pleurae: 1, endothoracic fascia; 2, subpleural connective tissue layer; 3, superficial elastic layer; 4, parietal mesothelial layer; 5, pleural space; 6, visceral mesothelial layer; 7, deep elastic layer; 8, interlobular septa; and 9, connective fiber.

Pleural Sinuses

The parietal pleura can be divided into the costal, mediastinal, and diaphragmatic pleura. The transition between each segment is done at the level of the pleural sinuses. The pleural sinuses are (1) the anterior and posterior costomediastinal sinuses, (2) the costophrenic sinus, and (3) the mediastinophrenic sinus. The parietal pleura in the sinuses, especially in the posterior costophrenic sinus, are in contact at rest, but the sinuses fill with lung during inspiration.

In only one order of mammal, the Proboscidea, which includes the elephant, are the fetal pleural cavities replaced by elastic tissue (Lawrence, 1983). In humans the capacity of the pleura is well seen after a pneumonectomy in which the remaining lung expands into the contralateral pleural space.

Pleural Topography

The projection of the pleural sinuses over the chest wall are fairly similar on the right and the left. Anteriorly the lung extends no lower than the sixth rib in the midclavicular line, whereas the pleurae costophrenic sinus extends to the seventh rib. Laterally in the midaxillary line, the lung descends to the eighth rib; the lateral costophrenic sinus descends to the ninth rib. Posteriorly the lung extends to the eleventh rib and the pleura, to the twelfth rib. The pleural space and the lung extends above the bony limits of the thoracic inlet.

Blood Supply

The blood supply of the parietal pleura comes exclusively from the systemic arteries. The costal pleura is supplied by intercostal arteries and branches from the internal mammary arteries; the mediastinal pleura is vascularized by bronchial, upper diaphragmatic, and internal mammary arteries. The blood supply to the cervical pleura (pleural dome) comes from subclavian arteries. For the most part, venous blood drains into peribronchial veins and/or directly into the venae cavae.

In contrast the visceral pleura is vascularized by both the systemic (through the bronchial arteries) and the pulmonary circulation. Venous blood is drained into the pulmonary venous system.

Lymphatic Drainage

The pleural space is located at the boundary of two different lymphatic systems, both of which play a major role in the removal of fluid, cells, and foreign particles from the pleural space.

In the subpleural space of the visceral pleura, large lymphatic capillaries form a meshed network that drains into the pulmonary lymphatic system. These capillaries are more abundant over the lower lobes and are connected to the deep pulmonary plexuses located in the interlobular and peribronchial spaces.

The lymphatic drainage of the parietal pleura is more elaborate, with direct communications between the pleural space and the parietal pleural lymphatic channels. These communications, called stomata, are 2 to 6 μm in diameter and predominate over the lower portions of the mediastinal, diaphragmatic, and costal pleura. They have endoluminal valves and drain into a network of submesothelial lymphatic lacunae. Over the costal pleura these collecting vessels run parallel to the ribs to reach the internal mammary nodal chain anteriorly and the intercostal nodal chain posteriorly. At the diaphragm the drainage is to the retrosternal, mediastinal, and celiac nodes. The transdiaphragmatic anastomoses allow for the passage of fluid and foreign particles from the peritoneal cavity into the pleural space.

Innervation

The visceral pleura is devoid of somatic innervation; in contrast the parietal pleura is innervated through a rich network of somatic, sympathetic, and parasympathetic fibers. At the costal pleura level, these fibers travel through the intercostal nerves. Pain stimuli at the diaphragm are transmitted through the phrenic nerve.

MICROSCOPIC ANATOMY

Pleural Membrane

The visceral and parietal pleural membrane is constituted of a single layer of mesothelial cells resting on connective tissue. Mesothelial cells are stretchable, and their size and shape may vary, depending on their location. Abundant microvilli cover their surface. The presence of a rich endoplasmic reticulum points to some secretory capacity. By expanding the cell surface, microvilli favor phagocytosis and fluid absorption (pinocytosis). They are also well adapted for deforming structure and help in sliding. Hills (1992) demonstrated recently that the pleural surface contains an adsorbed surface-active phospholipid coating. This graphitelike material exhibits remarkable antiwear properties comparable to the best lubricants.

The epithelium lies on a basal membrane with various amounts of collagen and elastic fibers. It contains blood vessels, nervous endings and lymphatic channels. In the visceral pleura, this underlayer is directly connected to the fibroelastic network of the lung and thus helps to distribute mechanical stress evenly throughout the structure. Arterial vascularization of the parietal pleura comes from the systemic circulation through the internal mammary and intercostal arteries. The arterial blood supply of the visceral pleura is mixed. It comes in part from the pulmonary circulation, but Gilbert and Hakim (1992) observed that the relative contribution of the systemic circulation through the branches from the bronchial arteries is increased at the subpleural level.

The parietal pleura contains two particular features not present in the visceral pleura. A rich network of lymphatic vessels is concentrated in the posteroinferior portion of the chest. These vessels communicate directly with the pleural space through openings or "stomata," as described by Wang (1975) in the parietal pleura. They are provided with valves and play an important role in the reabsorption of fluid and the removal of proteins, particles, and cells from the pleural space.

Kampmeier foci or milky spots are found in the lower portion of the mediastinal pleura and are covered with slightly different, cuboidal mesothelial cells. They consist of an aggregate of macrophages, lymphocytes, histiocytes, plasma cells, mast cells, and undifferentiated mesenchymal cells encircling thick blood capillaries and lymphatic channels. Kanazawa (1985) demonstrated that they participate in the defense of the pleural space in different ways. They exhibit phagocytic activity, trap macrophages and particles, appear to exert some focal suction, and have the capacity to produce leukocytes under the stimulus of inflammation, not unlike the lymphoid tissue in the tonsils.

Pleural Space

The thickness of the pleural space is not uniform. In some areas, both pleural surfaces are closely apposed; in others, such as at the junction of lung fissures, the thickness of the fluid is increased. The width of the pleural space varies between 10 and 20 μm. A thin film of pleural fluid and surface-active material prevents both pleural surfaces from rubbing against each other.

MECHANICAL PROPERTIES

The lung and the thorax are two elastic structures connected in series and acting in opposite directions. The mechanisms that hold the lung close to the chest wall are complex and depend mainly on two physiologic processes: (1) those ensuring a constant removal of pleural fluid and (2) those preventing the accumulation of free gas in the pleural space. These mechanisms involve the interplay of different pressures.

Pleural Pressure

The pressure at the surface of the pleura (P_{PL}) results from the mechanical properties of the respiratory system (Fig. 34-6) and can be described by the following equation:

$$P_{RS} = P_L + P_W$$

where P_{RS} is the pressure of the respiratory system, P_L is the pressure exerted by the lung, and P_W is the pressure developed in the chest wall.

The pressures measured at the boundaries of these structures are the alveolar pressure (P_{ALV}), the pleural pressure (P_{PL}), and the ambient barometric pressure (P_{BAR}). The pleural pressure is equal to the difference of the alveolar minus the transpulmonary pressure as shown in the following equations:

$$P_L = P_{ALV} - P_{PL}$$
$$P_{PL} = P_{ALV} - P_L$$

In static conditions, the alveolar pressure is equal to zero, and the equation becomes:

$$P_{PL} = -P_L$$

The latter equation demonstrates that the pleural pressure is proportional to the pressure developed in the lung. When the pulmonary volume is at its functional residual capacity, the elastic forces of the lung and thorax are in equilibrium, and the pleural pressure equals -2 to -5 cmH$_2$O. As the pulmonary volume increases during inspiration to the vital capacity, the pleural pressure becomes progressively more

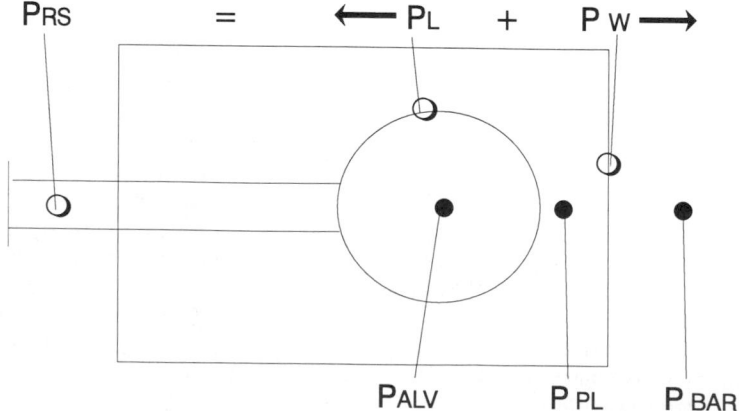

Figure 34-6. This model represents the pressures involved in the mechanics of the respiratory system. P_{RS} is the total respiratory system pressure and results of the sum of P_L, the pressure developed in the lung, plus P_W, the pressure developed in the chest wall. P_{ALV}, alveolar pressure; P_{PL}, pleural pressure; P_{BAR}, ambient barometric pressure.

negative, -25 to -35 cmH$_2$O. In any condition in which the elastic recoil of the lung is increased, for example, interstitial fibrosis, edema, atelectasis, or resection of the parenchyma of the lung, the pleural pressure becomes more subatmospheric. In situations in which airway resistance is increased such as chronic obstructive pulmonary disease, bronchial stenosis, or obstruction by a foreign body or secretions, the negativity of the pleural pressure increases further during inspiration.

Vertical Gradient of Pleural Pressure

The pleural pressure is not uniform all around the surface of the lung. Minor local variations of pleural liquid pressure occur in relation to variations in the thickness of the pleural space, but these are of no practical consequence. More importantly a vertical pleural pressure gradient exists from the top to the bottom of the thoracic cavity. The mechanisms responsible for this gradient have been reviewed by Agostoni (1986). The effect of gravity on the lung is one important determinant. Other factors include the size, volume, shape, and position of the lung. The pleural pressure changes by approximately 0.25 cmH$_2$O/cm of height and is more negative at the apex (-7 to -9 cmH$_2$O) than at the base (0 to -2 cmH$_2$O) of the lung in an upright subject. This is one reason why the upper portion of the lung usually collapses more in partial pneumothorax.

Gas Pressures

Given that the hydrostatic pleural pressure is subatmospheric, there is a theoretical risk that gases dissolved in the blood and interstitial fluid could be freed in the pleural space. The pleural space is influenced by the partial pressures of gas prevailing in the arterial and venous blood that irrigates the pleura. The cascade of changing partial pressures changes from the atmosphere to those of the venous blood are summarized in Table 34-1. Oxygen and carbon dioxide are exchanged during respiration. Nitrogen is not consumed or produced during respiration. However, because the respiratory quotient is less than 1, more oxygen is consumed than carbon dioxide is rejected in the alveoli. As a consequence nitrogen's partial pressure increases slightly from 563 mmHg in the inspired gas to 572 mmHg in the alveolar gas. The partial pressure of nitrogen in the blood equals 575 mmHg and is close to equilibrium with the alveolar gas (Cotes, 1979). The situation is different with oxygen and carbon dioxide. As a result of cellular respiration, the contents of the blood change at the capillary level. The oxygen content decreases,

and the carbon dioxide content increases. The repercussions of these gas exchanges are different on the partial pressures for both gases because the dissociation curves of oxygen and carbon dioxide in the blood are not the same. A partial oxygen pressure of 95 mmHg in arterial blood drops to 40 mmHg in venous blood, a 55-mmHg difference. The partial carbon dioxide pressure goes from 40 to 45 mmHg, a corresponding gain of only 5 mmHg. The total pressure of dissolved gases equals 757 mmHg in arterial blood and becomes 703 mmHg in venous blood, a drop of 54 mmHg (or 72 cmH$_2$O) compared with that in arterial blood and the pleural space. This pressure gradient protects the pleural space against the spontaneous formation of gas as long as the hydrostatic pressure does not exceed -72 cmH$_2$O. It ensures also that air collected in the pleural space, as in the pneumothorax, will be reabsorbed by the venous side of the circulating blood.

PLEURAL FLUID DYNAMICS

Normal Fluid

Only a small amount of fluid can be recovered from the pleural space under normal conditions. A volume of 0.1 to 0.2 ml/kg may be extrapolated from experimental data in

---

Composition of Normal Pleural Fluid

Volume: 0.1–0.2 ml/kg
Protein: 10–20 g/L
Albumin: 50–70%
Glucose: As in plasma
Lactic dehydrogenase: <50% of plasma level
Cells/mm^3: 4,500
  Mesothelial cells: 3%
  Monocytes: 54%
  Lymphocytes: 10%
  Granulocytes: 4%
  Unclassified: 29%
pH: 7.38 (mixed venous blood $+$ 0.02)
Partial pressure of carbon dioxide: 45 mmHg ($=$ mixed venous blood)
Bicarbonate: 25 mmol/L ($=$ mixed venous blood)

(From Agostini E: Mechanisms of pleural space. In American Physiological Society: Handbook of Physiology. Sec. 3. Vol. 3. Part 2. American Physiological Society, Bethesda, MD, 1986, with permission.)

Table 34-1. Partial Pressures of Gases in Air and Blood[a]

Partial Pressure	Atmosphere	Alveolar Gas	Arterial Blood	Pleural Space	Venous Blood
Water	47	47	47		47
Oxygen	150	102	95		40
Carbon dioxide	0	39	40		45
Nitrogen	563	572	575		575
Total	760	760	757		703
				⌊Gradient $+$ 54 mmHg⌋	

[a] All pressures in millimeters of mercury, assuming temperature at 37°C, saturated in water vapor.

animals. The protein content is low, 10 to 20 g/L, a fact that led Staub, et al. (1985) to question the mechanisms of fluid reabsorption. The composition of normal pleural fluid is presented below.

Pleural Fluid Turnover

Pleural fluid is constantly secreted, mostly by filtration from the microvessels in the parietal pleura. This was confirmed recently by Broaddus, et al. (1991). A quantitative assessment is difficult, however. Animal studies reviewed by Pistolesi, et al. (1990) yield a wide range of values from 0.02 to 2.0 ml/kg/h. Under pathologic conditions fluid may originate from other sources. In congestive (Wiener-Kronish, et al., 1984; Broaddus, et al., 1990) and in chemically induced lung edema (Miller, et al., 1989; Wiener-Kronish, et al., 1988), liquid may filtrate directly from the pulmonary interstitium into the pleural space. Under such conditions as much as 25 percent of pulmonary edema fluid may be cleared through the visceral pleura. Peritoneal fluid may also leak into the chest through pores in the diaphragm in patients with ascites or who are undergoing peritoneal dialysis.

Agostoni, et al. (1957) proposed that pleural fluid exchange could be entirely explained by the balance of hydrostatic and osmotic pressures. The Starling equation states that the flow of fluid through a semipermeable membrane like the pleura depends on three factors: (1) the permeability coefficient of the pleura, (2) the difference of hydrostatic pressures, and (3) the difference of osmotic pressures across the pleura. Application of this equation shows that, at the level of the parietal pleura, the net difference of pressures favors the

---

Starling's Equation Applied to Pleural Fluid Dynamics

$$F = K \times [(P_{CAP} - P_{PL}) - (\pi_{CAP} - \pi_{PL})]$$

where: F is fluid movement across the pleura; K is permeability coefficient; P_{CAP} is hydrostatic capillary pressure; P_{PL} is hydrostatic pleural pressure; π_{CAP} is osmotic capillary pressure; and π_{PL} is osmotic pleural pressure.

---

passage of fluid into the pleural space. The same principles apply to the visceral pleura, a tributary of the pulmonary circulation, where lower capillary pressures favor fluid resorption of pleural fluid.

However, ideas concerning fluid resorption have been revised recently. Indeed the visceral pleura is irrigated by capillaries from both the systemic and pulmonary circulation. According to Agostoni and Zocchi (1991), the Starling mechanism and solute-coupled absorption both contribute to the fluid resorption when the pleural osmotic pressure is low. In 1954, Courtice and Simmond (1954) produced evidence that respiratory movements were important for the resorption of pleural effusion and that the removal of proteins and particles from the pleural space went through the lymphatic channels of the chest wall. Evidence from recent animal studies confirms that the lymphatic circulation of the parietal pleura also plays a major role in the resorption of pleural fluid. The mechanisms of pleural fluid turnover are summarized in Figure 34-7.

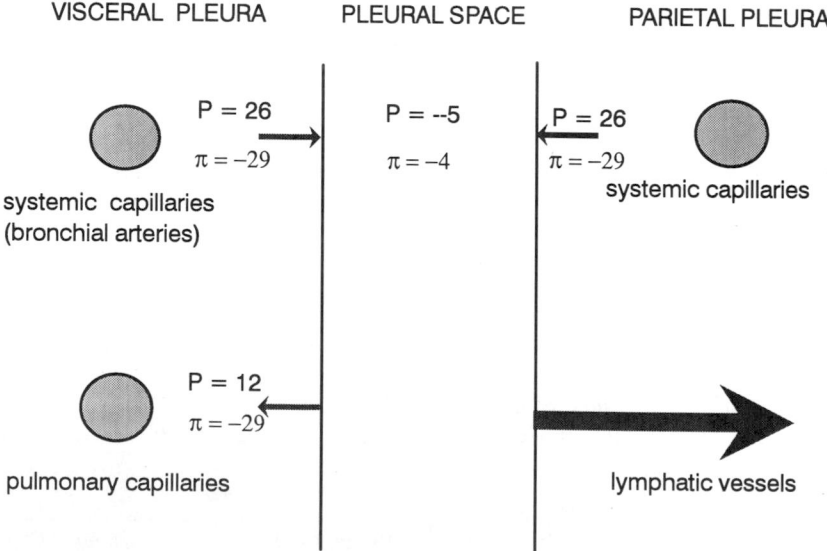

Figure 34-7. The mechanisms of pleural fluid exchanges at the level of the parietal and the visceral pleura. P is the hydrostatic pressure, and π is the osmotic pressure (both in centimeters of water). The arrows indicate the direction of flow. In areas in which the pleura is vascularized by the systemic circulation, the net balance of pressures, according to Starling's equation, favors the filtration of fluid toward the pleural space. Capillary hydrostatic pressures are lower in the capillaries of the pulmonary circulation, and the balance of pressures favors pleural fluid resorption through the visceral pleura. However, most of the resorption occurs through the lymphatic channels of the parietal pleura.

REFERENCES

Agostoni E: Mechanics of the pleural space. In American Physiological Society: Handbook of Physiology. Sec. 3. Vol. 3. Part 2. American Physiological Society, Bethesda, MD, 1986

Agostoni E, Taglietti A, Setnikar I: Absorption forces of the capillaries of the visceral pleura in determination of the intrapleural pressure. Am J Physiol 191:277, 1957

Agostoni E, Zocchi L: Starling forces and lymphatic drainage in pleural liquid and protein exchanges. Respir Physiol 86:271, 1991

Bouchet A, Cuilleret J: Anatomie topographique, le thorax. Simep, Villwurbanne, France, 1974

Broaddus VC, Araya M, Carlton DP, Bland RD: Developmental changes in pleural liquid protein concentration in sheep. Am Rev Respir Dis 143:38, 1991

Broaddus VC, Wiener-Kronish JP, Staub NC: Clearance of lung edema into the pleural space of volume-loaded anesthetized sheep. J Appl Physiol 68:2623, 1990

Cotes JE: Lung Function. Blackwell, London, 1979

Courtice FC, Simmonds WJ: Physiologial significance of lymph drainage of the serous cavities and lungs. Physiol Rev 34:419, 1954

Gilbert E, Hakim TS: Relative contribution of bronchial flow to subpleural region in dog lung. J Appl Physiol 73:855, 1992

Harley R: Anatomy of the pleura. Semin Respir Med 9:1, 1987

Hills BA: Graphite-like lubrication of mesothelium by oligolamellar pleural surfactant. J Appl Physiol 73:1034, 1992

Kanazawa K: Exchanges through the pleura. In Chrétien J, Bignon J, Hirsch A (eds): Pleura in Health and Disease. Marcel Dekker, New York, 1985

Lawrence GH: Considerations of the anatomy and physiology of the pleural space. p. 3. In Lawrence GH (ed): Problems of the Pleural Space. WB Saunders, Philadelphia, 1983

Miller KS, Russell AH, Sahn SA: Pleural effusions associated with ethchlorvynol lung injury result from visceral pleural leak. Am Rev Respir Dis 140:764, 1989

Nebut M, Hirsch A, Chrétien J: Embryology and anatomy of the pleura. p. 1. In Chrétien J, Hirsch A (eds): Diseases of the Pleura. Masson, Paris, 1982

Pistolesi M, Miniati M, Giuntini C: Pleural liquid and solute exchange. Am Rev Respir Dis 140:825, 1990

Staub NC, Wiener-Kronish JP, Albertine KH: Transport through the pleura. In Chrétien J, Bignon J, Hirsch A (eds): Pleura in Health and Disease. Marcel Dekker, New York, 1985

Wang NS: The preformed stomas connecting the pleural cavity and the lymphatics in the parietal pleura. Am Rev Respir Dis 111:12, 1975

Wiener-Kronish JP, Albertine KH, Licko V, Staub NC: Protein egress and entry rates in pleural fluid and plasma in sheep. J Appl Physiol 56:459, 1984

Wiener-Kronish JP, Broaddus VC, Albertine KH et al.: Relationship of pleural effusions to increased permeability pulmonary edema in anesthetized sheep. J Clin Invest 82:1422, 1988

35

DIAGNOSTIC PROCEDURES

Jean Deslauriers
Guy Carrier
Gilles Beauchamp

INTRODUCTION

Although pleural diseases are relatively common in the practice of thoracic surgery, their diagnosis is often problematic. Pleural effusions, for instance, can be secondary to a number of thoracic, abdominal, or systemic diseases, and their origin can still be unknown after thoracentesis or pleural biopsy.

In such patients clinical history and physical examination are important because most pleural effusions are a manifestation of extrapleural diseases. Imaging of the pleural space also represents first-line investigation, with conventional radiographs, computed tomography (CT), high-resolution CT, ultrasound, isotopic studies, and magnetic resonance imaging (MRI) often providing definitive clues to the etiology of the effusion.

More invasive techniques such as thoracentesis or percutaneous pleural biopsies have contributed substantially to the investigation of pleural diseases, and with them a diagnosis can be firmly established in 80 to 85 percent of cases with minimal morbidity. Patients may also benefit because those procedures will help to rule out specific and treatable diseases such as pleural tumors or tuberculosis. Recent advances in thoracoscopy and video-assisted thoracic surgery (VATS) have further improved the sensitivity and sensibility of these diagnostic procedures.

It has been said that the term "... *idiopathic pleural effusion* ... is idiotic from the standpoint of the physician and pathetic from that of the patient" (Branscomb and Harrison, 1966; Gaensler, 1970). This statement is even more true in the 1990s because modern diagnostic techniques have eased the access to the pleural space, where fluid and tissue can be sampled and sent for detailed biochemical, bacteriologic, and pathologic analysis.

HISTORICAL NOTE

Thoracocentesis is a procedure that involves thrusting a needle into the pleural space for the purpose of removing accumulated air or fluid. It was established as a diagnostic procedure by Bowditch (1852) and since then has been used extensively for the investigation of patients with pleural effusions of unknown origin.

In 1955 De Francis and colleagues reported the use of the Vim-Silverman needle to biopsy the pleura and establish a diagnosis of tuberculosis in two of six patients with pleural effusion. Between 1958 and 1961 Cope (1958), Abrams (1958), and others (Harvey and Harvey, 1958; Skowran, 1960; Carpenter and Lowell, 1961) introduced similar types of needles, which have proved capable of obtaining satisfactory specimens without damage to the lung. In 1958 Mestitz et al. reported their experience with the Abrams needle. There were no serious complications related to the procedure, and histologic proof was obtained in 104 (52 percent) of 200 patients.

Thoracoscopy was introduced by Jacobeus (1910) as a method to be used for the lysis of pleural adhesions. He also recommended the technique as a method for obtaining tissue for histologic examination (Jacobeus, 1921, 1925). Between 1925 and 1965 references to thoracoscopy as a diagnostic modality were rare and came mostly from the European literature (Sergent and Kourilsky, 1939; Delarue and DePierre, 1956). In 1942 Fabri and Parmeggiani reported the use of thoracoscopy to evaluate pleural exudates, and in 1943 Fourestier and Duret reported three cases of pleural malignancies in which the diagnosis was made by pleuroscopy. During the 1970s and early 1980s diagnostic thoracoscopy was repopularized by Boutin and associates (1981, 1984), who reported on 1,000 cases of chronic pleurisy in which the etiology had been still unknown after the usual investigation. In their series the diagnosis was still unknown after thoracoscopy in only 4 percent of patients.

Over the years thoracoscopy has been performed in a number of ways. The instrument could be a simple mediastinoscope, a flexible bronchoscope, a cystoscope, a rigid bronchoscope, or a specially designed thoracoscope with a cold light source. Currently, the thoracoscope is coupled to a microcamera system, which allows for the involvement of the whole surgical team in the procedure through video systems. Thoracoscopy has been performed through the neck or through the intercostal space and under local or regional as well as under general anesthesia.

HISTORICAL READINGS

Abrams LD: Pleural-biopsy punch. Lancet 1:30, 1958

Boutin C, Farisse P, Rey F et al.: La thoracoscopie doit-elle être un examen de routine en pratique pneumologique courante? Med Hyg 42:2992, 1984

Boutin C, Viallat JR, Cargnino P, Farisse P: Thoracoscopy in malignant pleural effusion. Am Rev Respir Dis 124:588, 1981

Bowditch HI: Paracentesis thoracis. Am J Med Sci 23:103, 1852

Carpenter RL, Lowell JR: Pleural biopsy and thoracentesis by new instrument. Chest 40:182, 1961

Cope C: New pleural biopsy needle. JAMA 167:1107, 1958

De Francis N, Kiosk E, Albano E: Needle biopsy of parietal pleura: preliminary report. N Engl J Med 252:948, 1955

Delarue J, De Pierre R: Contribution à l'étude des pleurésies cancéreuses cliniquement primitives. Intérêt de la biopsie sous pleuroscopie. J Fr Med Chir Thorac 6:653, 1956

Fabri G, Parmeggiani D: Observations on thoracoscopy in pleural exudates. Policlin Sez Prat 5:49, 1942

Fourestier M, Duret M: Nécessité de la biopsie pleurale pour le diagnostic de l'endothéliome de la plèvre. Presse Med 32:467, 1943

Harvey C, Harvey HPB: Subclavian lymph node, pleural and pulmonary biopsy in diagnosis of intra-thoracic disease. Postgrad Med J 34:204, 1958

Jacobeus HC: Possibility of the use of the cystoscope for investigation of serous cavities. Munch Med Wochenschr 57:2090, 1910

Jacobeus HC: The practical importance of thoracoscopy in surgery of the chest. Surg Gynecol Obstet 32:493, 1921

Jacobeus HC: Thoracoscopy and its practical applications. Ergeb Ges Med 7:122, 1925

Mestitz P, Purves MJ, Pollard AC: Pleural biopsy in diagnosis of pleural effusion: report of 200 cases. Lancet 2:1349, 1958

Sergent E, Kourilsky R: Contribution to the study of endothelioma. Presse Med 47:257, 1939

Skowran CA: Kerrison rongeur: Needle punch biopsy. Del Med J 32:294, 1960

INITIAL ASSESSMENT

The initial assessment of a patient with suspected or proven pleural disease is critical not only because history taking and physical examination may provide clues as to the diagnosis but also because they may be useful in suggesting the etiology of the underlying disease and the likelihood that this disease is related to the pleural effusion (Jay, 1985).

History and Physical Examination

In the medical history of a patient with a pleural effusion, the most important questions relate to the possibility of previous asbestos exposure, tuberculous contact, or malignancy. Also important to elucidate is a possible history of recent respiratory symptoms such as may be seen with pulmonary infection or bronchogenic carcinoma.

The typical symptoms associated with pleural diseases are dyspnea and "pleuritic" chest pain radiating to the shoulder and made worse by deep breathing and cough. It is worth noting that the severity of symptoms does not necessarily reflect the amount of disease or effusion. Patients can be relatively asymptomatic with large effusions or be very symptomatic with a smaller effusion associated with intense pleural inflammation. With respect to asymptomatic effusions, Smyrnios, et al. (1990) have shown that the spectrum of causes is similar to that for symptomatic effusions and that patients should be evaluated in the same fashion.

Chest pain is due to inflammation of the parietal and diaphragmatic pleura, distortion of the mediastinum with phrenic nerve stretching, or frank neoplastic invasion of the parietal pleura and/or chest wall. Pain stimuli radiating to the shoulder, back, or neck are carried through the sensory part of the phrenic nerve.

As shown by Jay (1985), the physical findings are generally related to the amount of pleural effusion, but again they lack sensitivity and specificity (Table 35-1). These include decreased breath sounds, decreased chest expansion, and tracheal shift. Other findings that should be looked for are palpable nodes in the neck, a thoracic mass, red or fluctuant areas in the chest wall, asymetry of the rib cage, and pain induced by palpation of specific areas of the chest. All these findings will help the planning of further investigation so that it may proceed in a methodical and controlled fashion.

IMAGING

Conventional Radiographic Examination

Conventional radiographic imaging represents the mainstay of the initial evaluation of patients with suspected pleural disease. It is simple, accessible, safe, cheap, and rapid, and in addition it allows bedside examination. It is also easy to reproduce, which thus makes it a useful tool for follow-up.

Pneumothorax is one of the commonest pleural abnormalities, and on an erect chest radiograph a few milliliters of air in the pleural space can usually be detected (Schabel, 1987). It is seen as a pure air lucency without bronchovascular

Table 35-1. Physical Signs of Pleural Effusion

Amount of Effusion	Respiratory Rate	Chest Expansion	Fremitus	Breath Sounds	Contralateral Tracheal Shift
Small (<300 ml)	N, ↑	N	N	V	O
Moderate (300–1,500 ml)	N, ↑–↑↑	N, ↓	N, ↓	↓, V	O
Large (>1,500 ml)	↑↑	↓↓	↓↓	↓↓BV, O	O, +

Abbreviations: N, normal; V, vesicular; BV, bronchovesicular; O, absent; +, present.

(From Jay SJ: Diagnostic procedures for pleural disease. Clin Chest Med 6:33, 1985, with permission.)

markings and is limited medially by a thin water density representing the visceral pleura. Small pleural effusions are often associated with pneumothoraces.

Radiographs taken during forced expiration may increase the relative volume and lucency of a pneumothorax and permit its detection when it cannot be seen on a standard radiograph. This, however, is unusual and does not justify the routine use of both inspiration and expiration films for the documentation of suspected pneumothoraces. On a supine or a portable film, a pneumothorax of small or even of moderate volume may not be visible (Tocico, et al., 1985), but it can be suspected on the basis of indirect signs such as an increased lucency of the affected hemithorax, a deep sulcus of increased lucency (Gordon, 1980) (air collected in the antero-inferior costophrenic sulcus), or extremely well defined diaphragmatic or cardiac contours (Rhea et al., 1979).

The diagnosis of tension pneumothorax cannot usually be made on a plain radiograph taken at total lung capacity (Fraser and Paré, 1977b). It should rather be documented fluoroscopically by a shift of the mediastinum toward the side of the pneumothorax during inspiration and by restricted inflation of the normal lung with limited movement of the ipsilateral hemidiaphragm during expiration. Standard chest radiographs may also be useful to determine the cause of the pneumothorax, as subpleural blebs, fibrotic lung, or metastatic disease may at times be clearly seen. Misplacement of a chest tube in an interlobar fissure may be definitively documented on lateral chest x-rays.

Normal pleural fluid in the amount of 1 to 5 ml (Black, 1972) is usually not detectable on standard chest x-rays. As shown by Moskowitz, et al. (1973), lateral decubitus films are more sensitive and may be able to detect 5 ml of fluid. The earliest sign of pleural effusion on an erect radiograph is the displacement of the normally sharp costophrenic angle away from the lateral chest wall, a feature that may be present with 25 ml of pleural fluid (Rudikoff, 1980). The presence of 200 ml of fluid usually leads to the blunting of the lateral costophrenic angle on posteroanterior (PA) erect films, but on occasion up to 500 ml may not cause any blunting of the costophrenic angle; such is the case with subpulmonic effusions, in which the fluid is located between the lung and the diaphragm. Collins, et al. (1972) have nicely described four radiologic signs associated with subpulmonic effusions: (1) the apex of the hemidiaphragm migrates laterally from its usual medial location; (2) the medial portion of the diaphragm appears flat, with accentuation on expiration; (3) the upper abdomen appears more dense, owing to the filling of the posterior costophrenic angle with pleural fluid; and (4) on the left side, the apparent distance between the diaphragm and the stomach bubble is increased.

On supine films large quantities of pleural fluid may be missed, especially if the effusion is bilateral. In those cases it may be suspected from a veiling density of one hemithorax associated with persistence of vascular markings or from the presence of an apical cap, a blunting of the costophrenic angle (Ruskin, et al., 1987; Woodring, 1984), or a liquid density in a scissural position. Occasionally pleural fluid will collect in atypical locations (Henschke, et al., 1989) such as the interlobar fissure, where it presents as a "pseudotumor" recognized by its biconvex lenticular shape and scissural

position. In cases of pseudotumors pleural fluid is often present elsewhere in the pleural space.

Standard chest radiographs cannot distinguish between the densities of a transudate, an exudate, an empyema, a hemothorax, and a chylothorax. Transudates associated with congestive heart failure are usually bilateral, but when they are unilateral, they are more common on the right side, a feature that is different from what is seen in constrictive pericarditis, in which the effusion is more often left-sided (Kreel, 1990). Parapneumonic effusions are usually serous exudates, which resolve spontaneously once the pneumonia is under control and resolving (Fraser and Paré, 1979b). Consequently, a rapid increase in the amount of pleural fluid with an associated pneumonia suggests an impending or established empyema. Exudates and empyemas tend to loculate and accumulate posteroinferiorly, producing the "pregnant lady" or "inverted D" sign (Kreel, 1990) on lateral chest x-ray.

Empyemas may be difficult to distinguish from lung abscesses on standard chest x-rays. Lung abscesses are usually more spherical, with an almost equal length of the air-fluid level in both frontal and lateral views. An empyema forms an obtuse angle as it apposes the chest wall, whereas a lung abscess forms an acute angle. Lung abscesses finally tend to respect lobar and segmental boundaries, which are frequently crossed by an empyema (Stark, et al., 1983a). Empyemas and hemothoraces may ultimately lead to pleural thickening, to distortion of the diaphragm, which may also lose its dome shape, to blunting of the costophrenic angles, and to unilateral pleural calcifications.

Pleural disease is the commonest manifestation of asbestos exposure. Pleural plaques, pleural calcifications, benign pleural effusions, and malignant mesotheliomas can all be seen. Pleural plaques are present in 20 to 60 percent of workers exposed to strong concentration of asbestos fibers (Schwartz, et al., 1990; Schwartz, 1991), and there is a latency period of over 20 years for radiographically visible calcified plaques to appear (Schwartz, 1991; Fletcher and Edge, 1970). These plaques are generally located posterolaterally, where they follow the contours of the seventh to the tenth rib. They are often bilateral but tend to be asymmetric (Gefter and Conant, 1988; Fisher, 1985). In 25 percent of cases pleural plaques are unilateral, and in those cases they tend to be more frequently left-sided (Gefter and Conant, 1988; Withers, et al., 1984). Pleural plaques are almost always located on the parietal pleura, although at times they can occur on the visceral pleura, usually within the interlobar fissures (Rockoff, et al., 1987).

The use of oblique views to detect pleural plaques is controversial (Baker and Greene, 1982; McLoud and Flower, 1985; Reger, et al., 1982) because the increased sensitivity of this view also increases the incidence of false positive results. Normal muscle and fat shadows may cause false images of pleural thickening, but these are usually more symetrical in distribution than pleural plaques. Hillerdal and Lindgren (1980) have shown that the presence of bilateral pleural plaques at least 5 mm thick or of bilateral calcified diaphragmatic plaques has a 100 percent positive predictive value for the diagnosis of asbestos-related pleural plaques. Up to 50 percent of pleural plaques are calcified (Fraser and Paré,

1979a), making this the second most common finding in asbestos-related disease.

Benign asbestos pleurisy is a less common manifestation of asbestos-related pleural disease. It is usually recurrent, bilateral, associated with chest pain (Gaensler, 1971), and less than 500 ml in total volume. Because pleural effusion is seldom associated with asbestos exposure alone, its mere presence should raise the possibility of another disease such as a mesothelioma (Fraser and Paré, 1979a).

Rounded atelectasis (Mintzer, et al., 1981) is a form of atelectasis associated with pleural disease and more commonly with asbestos-related pleural disease. It presents as a well circumscribed mass abutting on a pleura, which is always thickened. In those cases there is also crowding of adjacent bronchi and blood vessels, producing the so-called comet tail sign (Schneider, et al., 1980). The diagnosis of rounded atelectasis may be suspected on the basis of standard radiographs, but characteristic features are often difficult to appreciate.

Diffuse malignant mesotheliomas are uncommon neoplasms, associated in about 60 to 80 percent of cases with a history of asbestos exposure (Mossman and Gee, 1989). Although calcified pleural plaques may be seen with mesotheliomas, they are uncommon (Kawashima and Libshitz, 1990). A mesothelioma usually presents as an irregular or nodular thickening of the pleura with or without a pleura effusion (Fig. 35-1), and typically there is no contralateral shift of the mediastinum because of the constrictive effect produced by the tumor (Fraser and Paré, 1979) on the underlying lung.

Standard chest radiographs may allow detection of local pleural thickening or of localized pleura-based masses. Pleural apical thickening is a common finding, often representing nonspecific fibrous scarring of the lung apex. It is usually bilateral, and calcifications are seldom associated. Old tuberculosis may also be responsible for pleural apical thickening which in those cases is usually unilateral and associated with fibrosis and retraction of the lung parenchyma. Occasionally, Pancoast tumors can mimic benign pleural thickening, and this should be considered in the differential diagnosis, especially if the finding is unilateral and associated with pain.

Benign pleural tumors are rare, and most are incidental findings on chest x-ray. They present as broad-based masses with rounded margins forming an obtuse angle with the pleura. Tangential views may also demonstrate well defined medial margins and ill-defined lateral margins with the pleura. Accurate diagnosis is generally not possible unless one can appreciate such characteristic features as a change in location of the tumor, which is typical of benign fibrous mesotheliomas (Fig. 35-2) (Weisbrod and Yee, 1983).

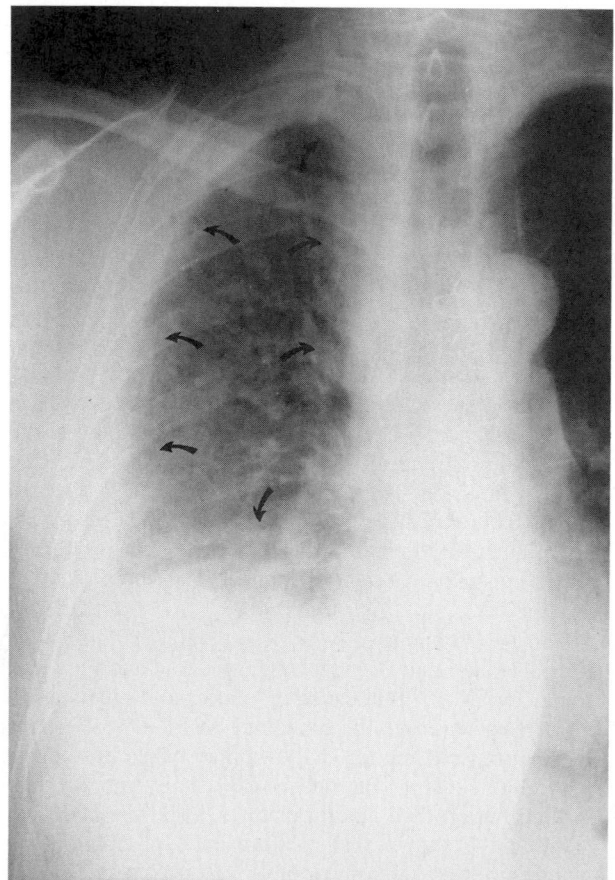

A

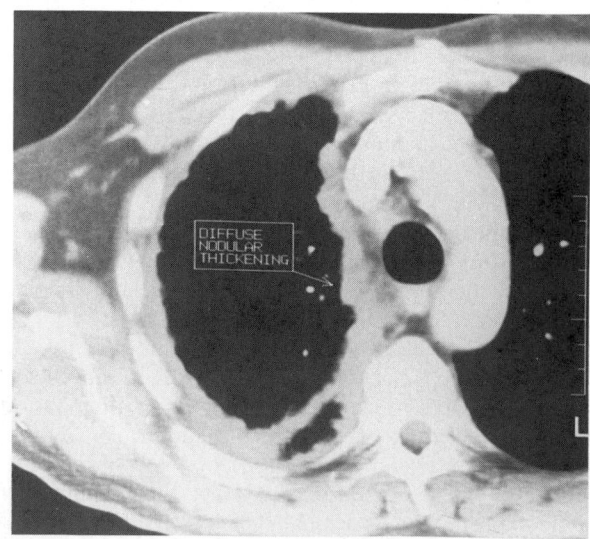

B

Figure 35-1. Malignant mesothelioma. **(A)** Standard chest radiograph demonstrating diffuse pleural nodular thickening and loss of volume of the right hemithorax; **(B)** same findings on CT scan, where thickening of the fissure can also be seen.

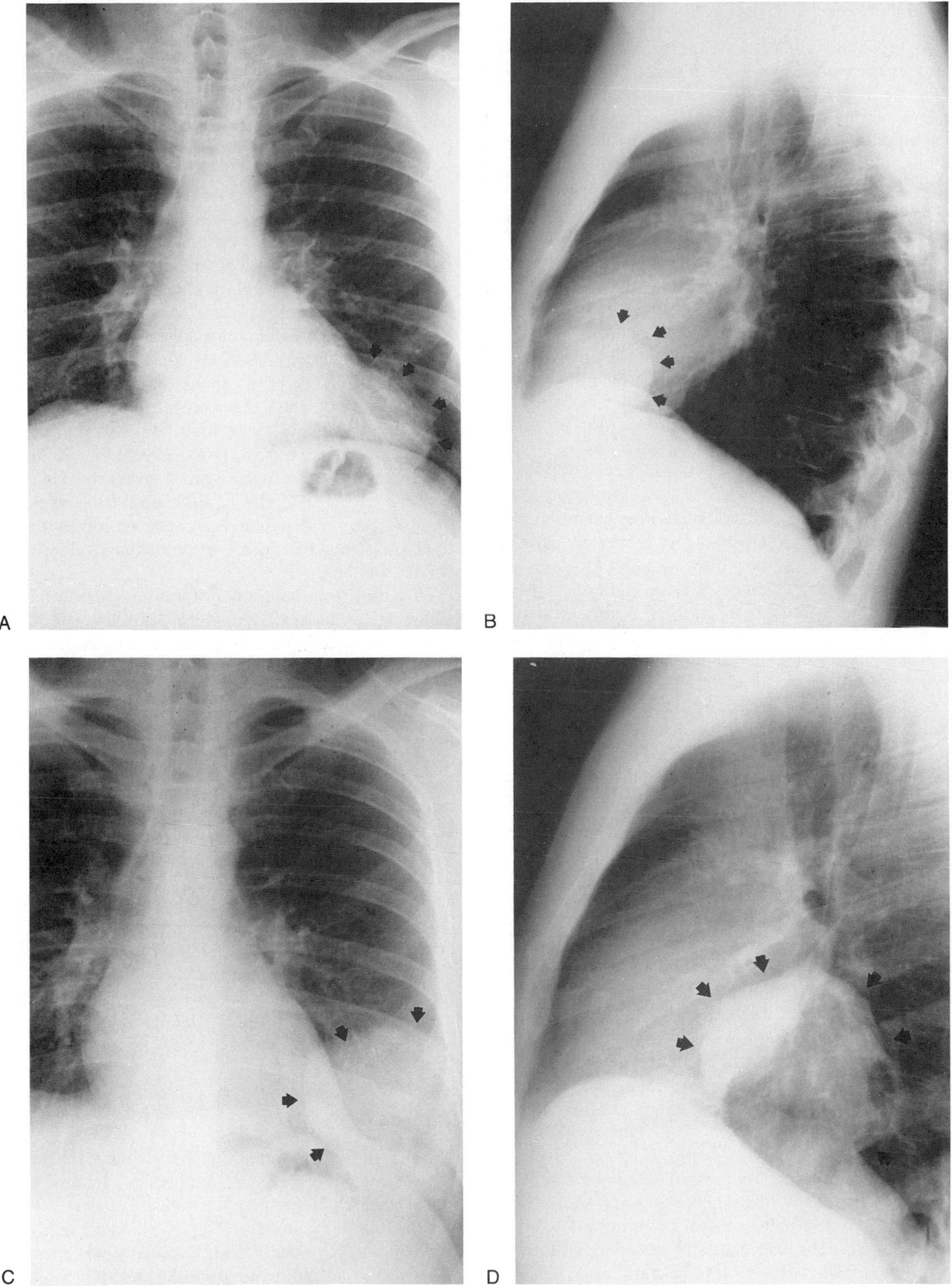

Figure 35-2. Benign mesothelioma. **(A)** PA and **(B)** lateral chest radiographs showing a well circumscribed left posterior paracardiac mass. **(C & D)** Three years later the lesion has increased in size and has moved to the left posterior paracardiac position. At surgery a benign pedunculated mesothelioma originating in the oblique fissure was seen.

Computed Tomography

High-contrast resolution and axial transverse slices eliminating confusing superposition of images have had a major impact on the use of the CT scan to evaluate pleural disease. CT may demonstrate disease at an earlier stage than other imaging techniques, and characterization of tissue density is also possible by the analysis of attenuation coefficient numbers (Hounsfield units). Pleural and parenchymal lesions can easily be separated. CT images can also be reproduced, allowing for accurate follow-up of pleural lesions (Rusch, et al., 1988).

CT scanning is able to detect small pneumothoraces sometimes not seen on chest x-ray, and it is also useful to demonstrate underlying parenchymal lesions such as interstitial disease, bullae, lung metastases, or other lesions causing the pneumothorax. It can be used to rule out a pneumothorax in a patient with a hyperlucent area on chest x-ray (Bourgouin, et al., 1985), and questions about the location of a chest tube can readily be answered.

Pleural fluid is easily seen on CT scan; however, CT is of limited value for differentiation between a transudate and a exudate (Müller, 1993). Hemothoraces can be diagnosed either by the presence of a fluid level or by an increased density of the pleural fluid (McLoud and Flower, 1991).

Differentiation between a pleural effusion and ascites may be a problem because both are in close proximity on axial images of the lower chest and upper abdomen. In such cases four radiologic signs may help to establish a correct diagnosis. The *interface sign* (Teplick, et al., 1982) refers to a sharp interface between fluid and spleen or liver with ascites or to an interface which is ill defined with a pleural effusion. The *displaced crus sign* (Dwyer, 1978) describes diaphragmatic crus displacement away from the spine in pleural effusions while ascites is seen anterior and lateral to the crus. The *diaphragm sign* (Müller, 1993) refers to the different position of pleural fluid and ascites in relation to the diaphragm; the pleural fluid usually lies peripheral to the diaphragm while the ascites is medial. Finally, the *bare area sign* (Halvorsen, et al., 1986) refers to the anatomy of the right lobe of the liver, which is attached to the posterior abdominal wall, and therefore ascites cannot extend behind the liver at this level; pleural effusions can be seen posterior to the liver.

Differentiation between an empyema and a sterile effusion may be possible by use of CT with intravenous injection of contrast agent. Enhancement of the parietal and visceral pleura, thickening of the extrapleural subcostal tissues, and increased attenuation of the extrapleural fat all favor the diagnosis of empyema over that of a sterile effusion (Waite, et al., 1990).

CT is more accurate than standard radiographs for differentiating an empyema from a lung abscess, since a CT scan usually sees the thin and uniform wall of empyemas while the wall of a lung abscess is thicker and irregular (Williford and Godwin, 1983). The *split pleural sign* (Stark, et al., 1983a) is associated with empyemas; it refers to fluid collected between the thickened parietal and visceral pleural membranes. Parenchymal compression seen with empyemas and the sharp boundaries between empyema and lung (Stark, et al., 1983a) are better demonstrated by CT scanning. Injection of contrast medium, especially by the bolus method, also facilitates the differentiation between an empyema and a lung abscess (Bressler, et al., 1987). A CT scan can demonstrate loculations unsuspected on chest x-ray, and it can also help to explain failure of tube drainage by showing either that the tube is out of the collection, that it is in the lung or in the fissure, or that it is kinked in its entry through the chest wall (Stark, et al., 1983b).

In the evaluation of asbestos-related disorders, CT and especially high-resolution CT have greater sensitivity than chest x-rays (Friedman, et al., 1988; Aberle, et al., 1988). Because of its high cost, however, CT is not recommended for screening (Müller, 1993) except to rule out a false positive diagnosis of pleural plaques due to intercostal muscles or extrapleural fat. CT allows for differentiation between pleural plaques and pulmonary lesions, and the diagnosis of rounded atelectasis is more easily made on CT scan than on chest x-ray. Contrast enhancement is present in rounded atelectasis, and this finding alone may facilitate its differentiation from a neoplasm (Blouin, et al., 1991) (Fig. 35-3).

CT can be used to diagnose and assess the extent of mesothelioma (Fig. 35-1) and is also helpful in the postsurgical follow-up of mesothelioma patients, as it may demonstrate tumor recurrence before it is clinically evident or seen on standard radiographs.

CT may also be useful to differentiate between benign and malignant processes (Leung, et al., 1990). Circumferential pleural thickening, nodular pleural thickening, parietal pleural thickening greater than 1 cm, and mediastinal pleural involvement all suggest the presence of malignant disease. Mesotheliomas are, however, difficult to differentiate from pleural metastatic disease (Leung, et al., 1990). Finally CT is recommended for the follow-up of patients with previous malignant thymomas treated by radiotherapy or surgery, because pleural seeding is often the first sign of recurrent disease (Zerhouni, et al., 1982) and this can easily be detected by CT examination.

In localized pleural tumors, CT can be used but there are no pathognomic features for differentiating a benign from a malignant lesion unless one can see a homogeneous fatty density typical of a subpleural lipoma (McLoud and Flower, 1991). In bronchogenic carcinoma, standard CT is not accurate for distinguishing between neoplastic contiguity with the pleura and frank invasion, but its accuracy may be increased with the use of artificial CT pneumothorax (Yokoi, et al., 1991).

Ultrasound

The superficial location of the pleura makes it easily accessible to ultrasound, a simple, noninvasive imaging technique, which is much less expensive than CT.

Ultrasound is complementary to standard radiographs for the detection of pleural fluid, especially when the presence of fluid is uncertain, as is often the case when an extensive pulmonary consolidation is present. It may help to characterize the effusion, and the demonstration of septae, sometimes not seen on CT, may suggest possible difficulties with tube drainage. Occasionally, pleural thickening or tumor may be very hypoechogenic and may be mistaken for pleural fluid.

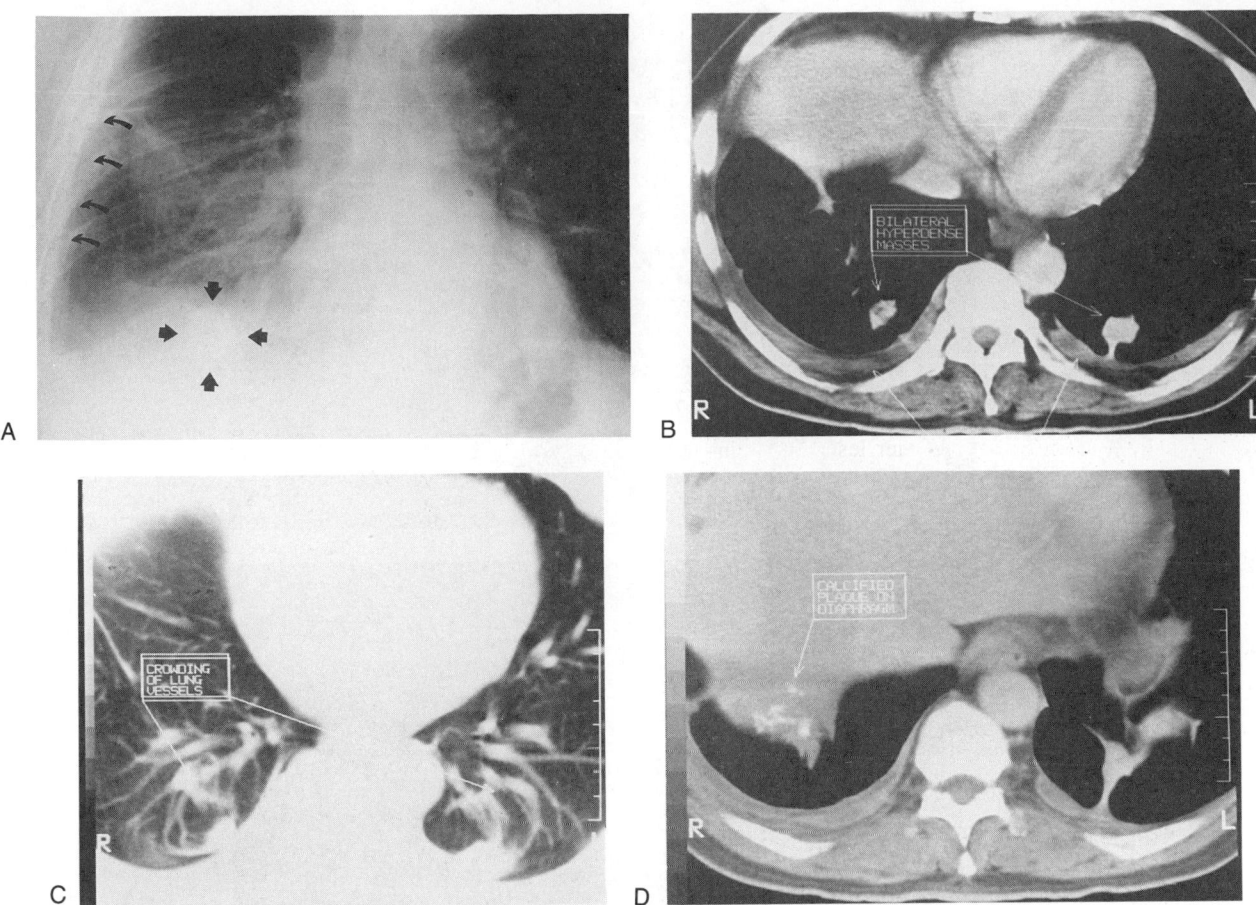

Figure 35-3. Asbestos-related disease. **(A)** Standard PA chest radiograph showing bilateral pleural thickening (*small arrows*) and a mass (rounded atelectasis) located behind the right hemidiaphragm (*large arrows*); **(B)** CT scan demonstration of pleural thickening and bilateral rounded atelectasis with typical enhancement after injection of contrast; **(C)** CT scan demonstration of crowding of lung vessels medially to rounded atelectasis and **(D)** diaphragmatic pleural calcifications.

Demonstration of highly reflective bronchi in consolidated lungs (McLoud and Flower, 1991) or of a sonographic "fluid bronchogram" (Dorne, 1986) allows differentiation between parenchymal and pleural disease.

Real-time ultrasound imaging usually demonstrates normal movement of the visceral pleura synchronous with that of the underlying lung during the respiratory cycle. Local invasion of the parietal pleura by a peripheral bronchogenic carcinoma can be therefore ruled out if one sees the sliding of the visceral pleura over the parietal pleura at the tumor site (Carrier, et al., 1987). In the evaluation of chest wall invasion by peripheral lung cancer, Suzuki, et al. (1993) demonstrated a sensitivity of 100 percent and a specificity of 98 percent in the presence of at least two of the three following ultrasound criteria: (1) disruption of the pleura, (2) fixation of the tumor during breathing, and (3) extension through the chest wall.

Multiple-plane imaging with ultrasound allows for easier assessment of the apical and diaphramatic pleura than does CT scanning. Subphrenic abscesses are readily distinguished from pleural effusions. Small Pancoast tumors can also be seen and biopsied under ultrasound guidance (Carrier, et al., 1987).

Ultrasound guidance of interventional pleural procedures is one of the most important contribution of ultrasound to the investigation of pleural diseases. Real-time and multiplane imaging allows safe and accurate procedures (Fig. 35-4), and the incidence of pneumothorax after ultrasound-guided biopsy is low because the short tract between skin and pleura helps in avoiding the adjacent lung (Carrier, et al., 1987). In pleural biopsies, the development of high-speed 18- and 20-gauge cutting needles combined with ultrasound guidance provides better histologic samples and helps to differentiate the pathologic processes.

Nuclear Medicine

Radionuclide studies may be useful in the evaluation of pleural diseases. Ventilation/perfusion isotope lung scans can be done when searching for pulmonary embolism as a cause for pleural effusion. Myelography with ^{111}In DTPA (diethylenetriaminepentaacetic acid) has been useful in the diagnosis of pleurosubarachnoid fistula after surgery or trauma (Krasnow, et al., 1989). Ventilation scanning may also be useful to demonstrate postpneumonectomy bronchopleural fistulae

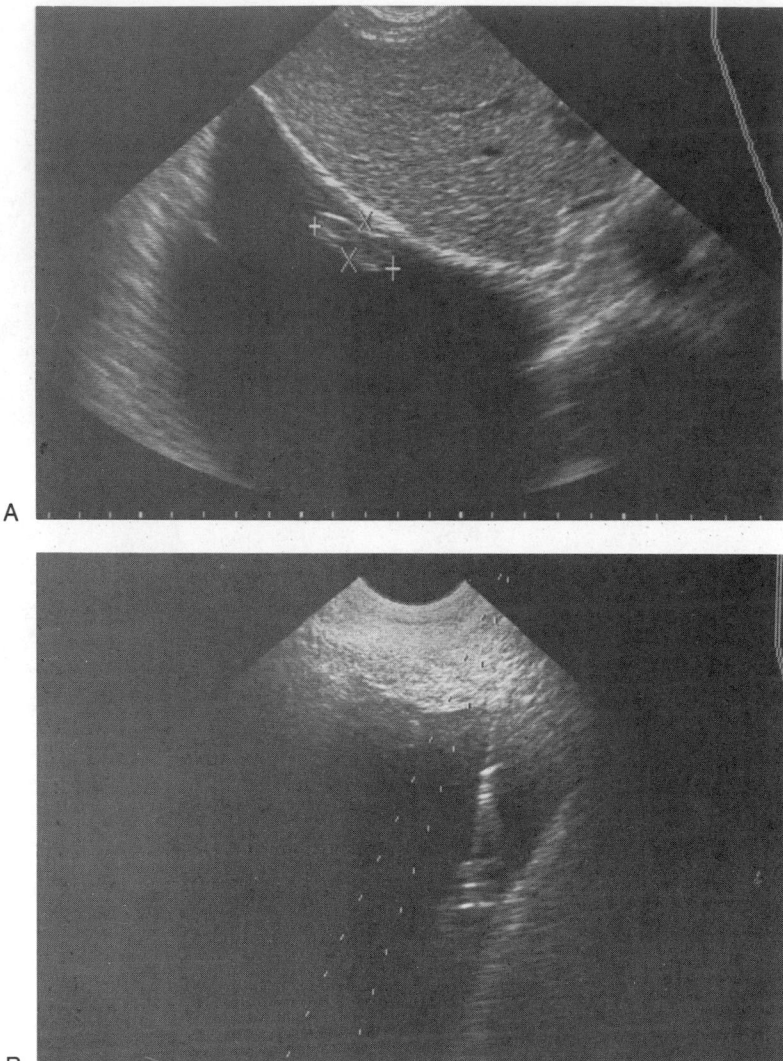

Figure 35-4. Diagnosis of malignant pleural effusion documented by ultrasound. **(A)** Pleural effusion with a small pleural nodule; **(B)** biopsy of the pleural nodule under sonographic guidance showed metastatic adenocarcinoma.

(Moote, et al., 1987), while ^{67}Ga scanning can document if the pleural fluid is purulent. Suspicion of peritoneopleural (Verreault, et al., 1986) communication may be evaluated with either technetium 99m sulfur colloid or technetium 99m macroaggregated albumin [99m]Tc (MAA) injected intraperitoneally (Fig. 35-5).

Magnetic Resonance Imaging

MRI, a noninvasive imaging technique, has a limited role in the evaluation of pleural diseases. It is expensive and does not allow for bedside examination. Although preliminary results suggest that MRI may help in the characterization of pleural fluid (Davis, et al., 1990), it is of little clinical significance at present.

Since MRI produces images in axial, coronal, and sagittal planes, it may be superior to CT scanning for the evaluation of the apical and diaphragmatic pleura (Fig. 35-6). This is

particularly interesting in the assessment of Pancoast tumors, for which invasion of the spinal canal and of the base of the neck or involvement of the brachial plexus may be demonstrated by MRI (McLoud and Flower, 1991). MRI may be also useful for patients with mesothelioma, especially to document mediastinal invasion or extension into the chest wall or below the diaphragm (McLoud and Flower, 1991).

BIOPSY PROCEDURES

Thoracentesis

Any alteration of the fluid transportation gradients, of the lymphatic drainage, or of the physical integrity of the pleural surfaces can result in accumulation of pleural fluid. Under those circumstances, thoracentesis with biochemical, microbiologic, and cytologic studies of the fluid is of great importance in evaluating the cause and nature of the effusion.

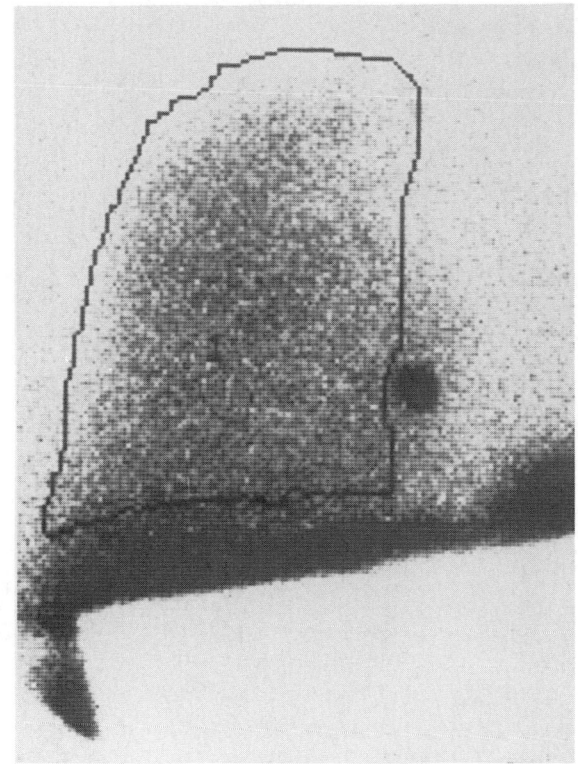

A

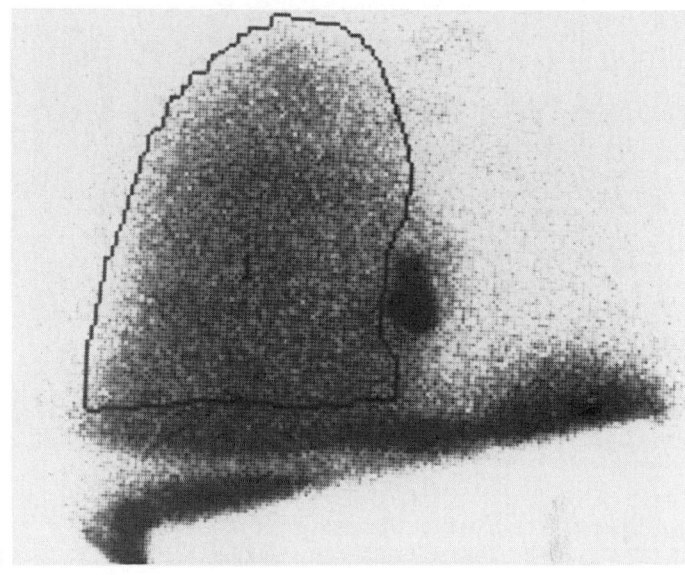

B

Figure 35-5. Peritoneopleural communication documented by nuclear medicine. **(A)** ^{99m}Tc MAA injected intraperitoneally flows in the pleural space in this patient with ascites and unilateral pleural effusion. **(B)** Same findings with ^{99m}Tc sulfur colloid isotope scan. (Courtesy of Jean Guimond, M.D.)

Thoracentesis is performed under local anesthesia, and other than a hemorrhagic diathesis, there are virtually no absolute contraindications to the procedure. Relative contraindications include an uncooperative patient, a small amount of fluid, and a clinically secure diagnosis (Sahn, 1987). The classic technique of thoracentesis involves good anesthesia of the parietal pleura, entry in the pleural space, aspiration of a small amount of fluid to confirm the proper location of the needle, and fluid removal with a larger needle. Approximately 50 ml of pleural fluid is sufficient to carry out most analyses. Kovarik (1970) and Krausz and Manny (1976) have described modified techniques of thoracentesis, in which they use an angiocath to provide greater safety for the patient and more flexibility for the physician. In many centers thoracentesis is now performed under ultrasound guidance, a technique that has the advantage of directing the needle into the effusion.

Thoracentesis is diagnostic in 50 to 60 percent of patients with a pleural effusion, and higher yields can be obtained for diseases, such as empyemas, hemothoraces, and chylothoraces, that rely less on cytology and biochemistry for their diagnosis. In 1987 Collins and Sahn reported the results of a prospective study of 129 consecutive thoracenteses in 86 patients. Pleural fluid analysis in conjunction with the clinical presentation placed 78 pleural fluids into diagnostic categories, and 92 percent of thoracenteses provided clinically useful information.

Cytologic analysis, even with repeated examination of large amounts of pleural fluid, is diagnostic in only 60 to 80 percent of patients with metastatic disease to the pleura (Light, 1983). It is higher in patients with ovarian or breast cancer and lower for patients with bronchogenic carcinoma or mesothelioma (Miguères, et al., 1981). When the cytology is positive for malignant cells, the histologic type of the primary tumor can sometimes be determined (Serre, et al., 1990), but up to 5 percent of patients may have a false positive cytology reading. In a study of 414 patients with pleural effusion, Prakash and Reiman (1985) were able to show that cytologic analysis has a higher sensitivity (P <0.001) than needle biopsy for diagnosing malignant pleural effusions. It is also important to note that it is virtually impossible to differentiate between a malignant mesothelioma and a metastatic adenocarcinoma by cytologic examination of the pleural fluid alone.

Although several complications of thoracentesis have been reported, most are minor. They include vasovagal reactions, hemothorax and/or pneumothorax, contamination of the pleural space, and improper placement of the needle in organs located below the diaphragm. In Collins and Sahn's series (1987), 34 objective complications occurred in 26 of 129 thoracenteses (20 percent), and 65 subjective complications occurred in 56 of 123 thoracenteses (46 percent), anxiety and site pain being the commonest of these events. In another study on the complications of thoracentesis (Seneff, et al.,

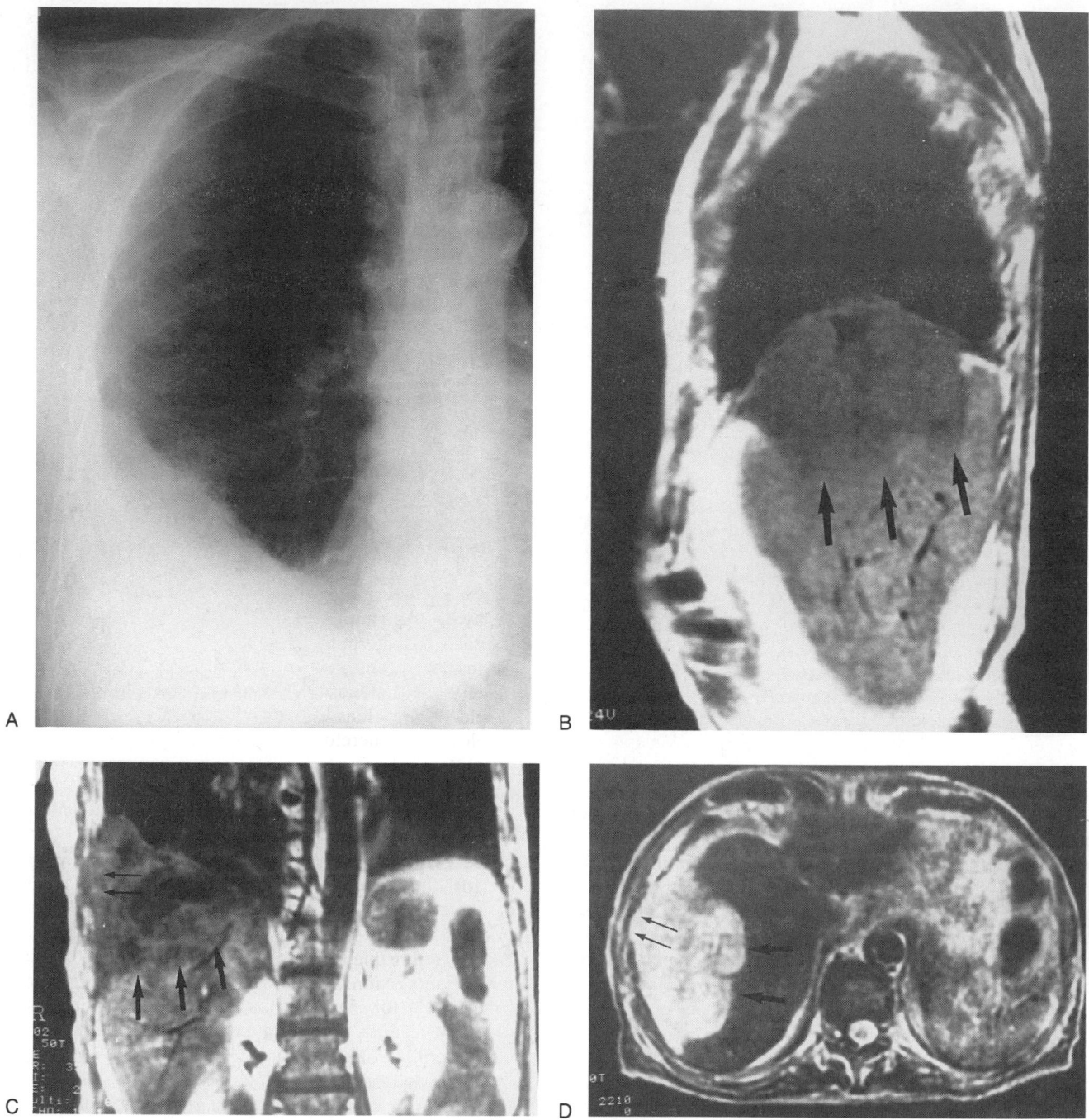

Figure 35-6. MRI imaging of diaphragmatic and chest wall neoplastic invasion by lung carcinoma. **(A)** Standard chest radiograph showing a density obscuring the right hemidiaphragm. Chest wall invasion (small arrows) and liver invasion (large arrows) as demonstrated by MRI: **(B)** sagittal T1 weighted magnetic resonance image (WMRI); **(C)** coronal T1 WMRI; **(D)** axial T2 WMRI. (Courtesy of Gilles Bouchard, M.D.)

1986), major complications occurred in 14 percent of patients and minor complications in 33 percent. These occurred even when a lecture and printed guidelines on performing thoracentesis had been given and experienced individuals were in attendance.

Other reported but unusual complications of thoracentesis are hypoxemia, which may worsen temporarily after fluid removal, and reexpansion pulmonary edema, which may fol-

low the development of marked negative pleural pressure during thoracentesis (Light, et al., 1980).

Closed Pleural Needle Biopsy

The conventional technique of closed pleural biopsy using an Abrams or a Cope needle provides a diagnosis in 37.5 to 67 percent of patients with malignancy of the pleura (Rao, et al., 1965; Cantó, et al., 1977) and in 54 to 75 percent of patients with tuberculous pleurisy (Tomlinson and Sahn, 1987). Cantó et al. (1977) have further shown that most tumors are located in the lower half of the thorax, and within that portion most are either located on the visceral, diaphragmatic, or mediastinal pleura, none of which is readily accessible by conventional techniques of needle biopsy.

Various needles can be used for biopsy of the parietal pleura, but at present the Vim-Silverman, Cope, and Abrams needles are the most extensively used. The Vim-Silverman needle is a puncture type of needle, the Cope a hook type cutting inside out, and the Abrams a guillotine type cutting laterally. In general, the results of pleural biopsy depend less on the type of needle than on the experience of the operator and pathologist.

In the series of Poe, et al. (1984), 211 patients underwent pleural biopsies, and adequate tissue was obtained in 207. Specificity was 100 percent and sensitivity 90 percent for tuberculosis and 68 percent for neoplasia. In another study, Salyer and colleagues (1975) showed that malignant neoplasms involving the pleura could be diagnosed in 90 percent of cases if both pleural fluid and tissues were examined. Contrary to what is seen with malignant effusions, the diagnosis of pleural tuberculosis is easier to make by pleural biopsy than by cytologic examination (Scharer, and McClement, 1967; Frist, et al., 1979). In a review of 14 papers from 1958 to 1985, reporting a total of 2,893 pleural biopsies, the diagnostic yield was 57 percent with carcinoma of the pleura and 75 percent with tuberculous pleurisy (Sahn, 1988; Tomlinson and Sahn, 1987).

Complications of closed pleural biopsy are infrequent if the procedure is performed by or under the direct supervision of a staff pulmonary disease specialist or a thoracic surgeon (Poe, et al., 1984). Pneumothorax is the commonest complication, having occurred 8.4 percent of patients in the series of Poe, et al. (1984). Fité, et al. (1989) also described the breakage and detachment of an Abrams needle in the pleural cavity during performance of a pleural biopsy.

Thoracoscopy

As a consequence of the relatively low yields of thoracentesis and pleural biopsies, in about 20 percent of patients with pleural effusion, no etiology can be found despite exhaustive and expensive testing (Gunnels, 1978; Poe, et al., 1984). Of much concern are the 50 percent of this group who will ultimately show evidence of malignancy. By thoracoscopy 90 to 100 percent of the surfaces of both visceral and parietal pleura can be explored. This allows direct access for biopsy of suspicious areas, and because the biopsy specimens are bigger and obtained from different sites, it significantly improves the yield of what is obtained by percutaneous blind biopsy.

Indications and Contraindications

Thoracoscopy is indicated for patients with a pleural effusion of still unknown etiology after conventional methods such as thoracentesis and needle biopsy have been tried and proved unsuccessful. It is especially indicated in patients with a known primary tumor at another site, a history of asbestos exposure, a combined pleural and pericardial effusion, or a family history of malignancy (Canto, et al., 1990). It may also be indicated for the diagnosis of pleura-based masses. In all those cases thoracoscopy is not a first-line diagnostic technique but, rather it should be performed after other methods have failed to provide a positive diagnosis. Diagnostic thoracoscopy can also be used to categorize patients with spontaneous pneumothoraces (Vanderschueren, 1990; Rivas de Andrès and Lanzas, 1993) at the time of the first episode.

Other than the usual contraindications to general anesthesia and surgery, the only true contraindication to diagnostic thoracoscopy is a fused pleural space, a condition seldom seen in patients with significant pleural effusions.

Technique and Instrumentation

General endotracheal anesthesia with a double-lumen tube is used in all cases, and patients are placed in a full thoracotomy position with the surgeon operating from the patient's back. A 0-degree camera-lens system with an incorporated working channel is used, and we find that the clarity of the field of vision is greatly improved if the lens tip is covered with a fine layer of an antifog material. One or two trocars are necessary to perform the procedure.

If one tries to aspirate the effusate through the working channel of the thoracoscope, the lung will inflate and obstruct the field, and the lens will often become foggy and covered with blood. It is therefore preferable to insert a second small (5-mm) trocar in order to allow the entry of air into the pleural space while suctioning. This second entry site usually located in the posterior axillary line in the seventh intercostal space can also be used to manipulate the biopsy forceps.

Once the cavity is dry, it is fully inspected with special attention to the lower half of the pleural space, particularly the costophrenic angles, which often are not readily visible. By using the biopsy forceps inserted through the smaller trocar, it is possible to manipulate the lung in order to complete the inspection. Any suspicious-looking pleural lesion or nodules over the lung surface are generously biopsied and the specimens sent for pathologic and bacteriologic analysis. We always do frozen section analyses of these tissues because additional sampling can be done when necessary. It is also important to send part of the specimen for electron microscopic analysis because this examination is essential to differentiate between malignant mesotheliomas and metastatic carcinomas.

In obvious neoplastic effusions or in those with an already documented diagnosis of malignant effusion, we terminate the procedure by sprinkling a fine layer of talc powder over the lung surface and inserting one or two 28 Fr chest tubes.

Occasionally thoracoscopy can be performed under local anesthesia (Rusch and Mountain, 1987). Under those conditions the procedure must be done quickly and in a pleural space without adhesions. In addition, the operation must always be carried out under anesthetic surveillance and with careful monitoring of both cardiac and lung function.

Operative Findings

One of the most common findings of diagnostic thoracoscopy is a nonspecific inflammation of the pleural membranes. With an acute inflammatory reaction, there is increased vascularization, redness, edema, and disappearance of the pleural transparence, all findings more often seen over the diaphragm and in the costovertebral gutters. When inflammation is more chronic, the pleura is thickened, opaque, and whitish gray in color. Specific benign pleural lesions such as granulomas or pleural plaques can usually be readily recognized. Metastatic lesions are often found over the lower half of the space and are recognized as small nodules, masses, or polypoid lesions. White, patchy lesions of the pleura may also be seen, and these must be differentiated from pleural plaques.

The diagnosis of malignant mesothelioma can be made by gross examination of the pleura. In the epithelial or mixed varieties, multiple small, friable, and vascular lesions, sometimes filled with viscous fluid, can be seen. These can be localized over the diaphragm, scattered over the whole space, or confluent in the more advanced stages of disease. In the sarcomatous and more localized variety, there may be only a thickened pleura although large nodules and masses can also be found. In a review of 35 cases of mesotheliomas, Boutin and colleagues (1979) showed that pleural biopsy was conclusive in only 40 percent of cases, while a positive diagnosis was obtained in 94 percent of cases by thoracoscopy. Sgro, et al. (1991) also obtained a yield of 85.7 percent after thoracoscopy in 21 cases of proven mesothelioma.

We have seen many cases in which the diagnosis of malignant mesothelioma was obtained by thoracoscopic biopsy of what appeared to be normal pleura or inoffensive pleural plaques often located over the diaphragm or in costophrenic angles. In those cases in which the diagnosis is made at an early stage, it is possible that radical resectional surgery will improve overall survival.

Morbidity

Diagnostic thoracoscopy should be considered a major procedure and should only be performed by operators familiar with pleural space anatomy. If the procedure is done for inspection and biopsy, complications are few and usually minor in nature. These consist of prolonged air leaks if the visceral pleura has been biopsied, failure to reexpand the lung, and pleural space infection. Contamination of the sites of incision or of the chest wall by malignant cells is often seen with diffuse malignant mesotheliomas.

Results

In 1971 Brandt and Mai reported on 1,130 diagnostic thoracoscopies, of which 414 were performed for an undiagnosed pleural effusion. When thoracoscopy was combined with cytologic and bacteriologic studies, only 2.5 percent of effusions were still of unknown etiology. In 1991 Wakabayashi reported 315 thoracoscopies performed under general anesthesia, with a mortality of 1 percent and a diagnostic accuracy of 99 percent.

In a collective review of 1,500 thoracoscopies from different centers, Menzies and Charbonneau (1991) found that the diagnostic accuracy of this technique was around 90 percent and morbidity, which included arrhythmias, bleeding and empyema, was under 3 percent. In their own series of 102 thoracoscopies performed under local anesthesia, the diagnostic accuracy was 96 percent, the sensitivity was 91 percent, the specificity was 100 percent, and the negative predictive value was 93 percent. Major operative complications occurred in 1.9 percent of cases. Other recent studies have presented similar data (Hucker, et al., 1991; Buchhotz, et al., 1990; Kimura, et al., 1990; Get'man, et al., 1989).

OTHER PROCEDURES

Open Thoracotomy

With the recent development of thoracoscopy techniques, there are very few circumstances in which open thoracotomy is necessary for the diagnosis of pleural diseases (Kirby and Ginsberg, 1990). In our opinion, it is only indicated when the pleural space is obliterated and thoracoscopy is not possible or when the surgeon wishes to proceed immediately with a surgical procedure such as decortication, pleurectomy or pleuropneumonectomy in the case of a malignant mesothelioma. In all other instances videothoracoscopy is far better than open thoracotomy to fully explore the pleural space.

In an interesting paper, Ryan, et al. (1981) studied the outcomes of 51 patients in whom the cause of a pleural effusion was still unknown after open thoracotomy. In 31 patients (60.8 percent), there was no recurrence of the effusion, and no cause became apparent during a follow-up period of $1\frac{1}{2}$ to 15 years. In 18 patients the cause of the effusion became apparent from 12 days to 6 years after thoracotomy. In 13 of these 18 patients, malignancy (6 patients with lymphoma, 4 with malignant pleural mesothelioma, and 3 with other malignancy) was ultimately diagnosed.

Bronchoscopy

Although the literature is somewhat controversial on the role of bronchoscopy in patients with undiagnosed pleural disease, it is our opinion that most of these patients, especially those who will undergo thoracoscopy or open thoracotomy, should have this examination. In the series of Feinsilver et al. (1986), 28 patients with unexplained pleural effusion, no mass on chest x-ray, and no lobar atelectasis underwent fiberoptic bronchoscopy. In this group the yield was only 4 percent (1 positive of 28 patients) despite a final diagnosis of tumor in 7. Based on these findings and on their own experience, Tomlinson and Sahn (1987) concluded that the key point for the indication of bronchoscopy appears to be the presence or absence of radiographic abnormalities in addition to the pleural effusion.

By contrast, Williams and Thomas (1981) also reported 28 patients who underwent fiberoptic bronchoscopy as part of the evaluation of an undiagnosed pleural effusion. In four patients the diagnosis was made by this examination, with three patients found to have bronchial carcinoma and one tuberculosis. Williams and Thomas concluded that bronchoscopic examination is of value in the workup of patients with undiagnosed pleural effusions without radiographic evidence of mass lesion or atelectasis.

In our experience most pleural effusions are caused by pulmonary diseases, and in those cases, especially if tuberculosis or malignancy is suspected, the importance of bronchoscopy cannot be overestimated.

CONCLUSION

From this review it is obvious that the cause of most pleural effusions or of other pleural diseases can be determined by the judicious use of available diagnostic methods. Imaging techniques can readily detect an effusion, but they generally are not very accurate in identifying its etiology. Thoracentesis and blind pleural biopsies are diagnostic in 80 percent of patients, while thoracoscopy has a yield of close to 100 percent.

When investigating a pleural effusion, it is important to have a methodical and structured approach to the use of these techniques. For instance, it is important to begin with simple methods such as careful history taking, standard chest radiographs, and thoracentesis rather than to proceed with thoracoscopy as the first line of investigation. This approach not only will reduce the cost of investigation but also will minimize patient morbidity.

KEY REFERENCES

Collins TR, Sahn SA: Thoracentesis: clinical value, complications, technical problems and patient experience. Chest 91:817, 1987

Excellent review on the role of thoracentesis in the diagnosis of pleural effusions. Critical evaluation of the complications associated with the procedure.

Jay SJ: Diagnostic procedures for pleural diseases. Clin Chest Med 6:33, 1985

This article reviews the role and results of all the techniques used for the diagnosis of pleural diseases.

Poe RH, Israel RH, Utell MV, et al.: Sensibility, specificity and predictive values of closed pleural biopsy. Arch Intern Med 114:325, 1984

Shows that closed pleural biopsy with simultaneous fluid analysis is a valuable diagnostic procedure.

Sahn SA: Pleural fluid analysis: narrowing the differential diagnosis. Semin Respir Med 9:22, 1987

Reviews the role and diagnostic yield of thoracentesis. Excellent discussion on pleural fluid cells.

Tomlinson JR, Sahn SA: Invasive procedures in the diagnosis of pleural diseases. Semin Respir Med 9:30, 1987

This excellent article analyzes the role of pleural biopsy, thoracoscopy, and open pleural biopsy.

REFERENCES

Aberle DR, Gamsu G, Ray CS: High-resolution CT of benign asbestos-related diseases: clinical and radiographic correlation. AJR 151:883, 1988

Abrams LD: Pleural-biopsy punch. Lancet 1:30, 1958

Baker EL, Greene R: Incremental value of oblique chest radiographs in the diagnosis of asbestos-induced pleural disease. Am J Ind Med 3:17, 1982

Black LF: The pleural space and pleural fluid. Mayo Clin Proc 47:493, 1972

Blouin O, Carrier G, Ferland S: Atélectasie ronde: nouveau critère diagnostique. Proc French Canadian Assoc Radiologists Ann Meeting, Montreal, Oct. 9-11, 1991, p. 20

Bourgouin P, Cousineau G, Lemire P, Hébert G: Computed tomography used to exclude pneumothorax in bullous lung disease. Can Assoc Radiol J 36:341, 1985

Boutin C, Farisse P, Rey F, et al.: La thoracoscopie doit-elle être un examen de routine en pratique pneumologique courante? Med Hyg 42:2992, 1984

Boutin C, Farisse P, Viallat P, et al.: La thoracoscopie dans le mésothéliome pleural. Intérêt diagnostique, pronostique at thérapeutique. Rev Fr Mal Respir 7:680, 1979

Boutin C, Viallat JR, Cargnino P, and Farisse P: Thoracoscopy in malignant pleural effusion. Am Rev Respir Dis 124:588, 1981

Bowditch HI: Paracentesis thoracis. Am J Med Sci 23:103, 1852

Brandt HJ, Mai J: Differential diagnosis of pleural effusions using thoracoscopy. Pneumologie (Stuttg) 145:192, 1971

Branscomb BV, Harrison TR: Diseases of the pleura, mediastinum and diaphragm. p. 946. In Fifth Edition. Harrison TR, RD Adams, IL Bennett Jr, et al. (eds): Principles of Internal Medicine. McGraw-Hill, New York, 1966

Bressler EL, Francis IR, Glazer GM, Gross BH: Bolus contrast medium enhancement for distinguishing pleural from parenchymal lung disease: CT features. J Comput Assist Tomogr 11:436, 1987

Buchhotz J, Mayer M, Giesekus D: The diagnosis of pleural effusion using thoracoscopy. Zentralb Chir 115:1565, 1990

Cantó A, Blasco E, Casillas M, et al.: Thoracoscopy in the diagnosis of pleural effusion. Thorax 32:550, 1977

Cantó A, Rivas J, Saumench J, et al.: Points to consider when choosing a biopsy method in cases of pleurisy of unknown origin. Chest 84:176, 1983

Cantó A, Saumench J, Moya J: Points to consider when choosing a biopsy method in cases of pleuritis of unknown origin with special reference to thoracoscopy. p. 49. In Deslauriers J, Lacquet LK (eds.) International Trends in General Thorac Surgery. CV Mosby, St. Louis, 1990

Carpenter RL, Lowell JR: Pleural biopsy and thoracentesis by new instrument. Chest 40:182, 1961

Carrier G: Used of ultrasonography, computed tomography, and nuclear magnetic resonance imaging in the diagnosis of pleural diseases. p. 25. In Delarue NC, Eschapasse H (eds): Thoracic Surgery: Surgical Management of Pleural Diseases. In Deslauriers J, Lacquet LK (eds): International Trends in General Thoracic Surgery. Vol. 6. CV Mosby, St. Louis, 1990

Carrier G, Mercier A, Bilodeau S: La place de l'échographie dans la sphère thoracique. Proc French Canadian Assoc Radiologists Ann Meeting, Montreal, Nov. 25–27, 1987, p. 64

Collins JD, Burwell D, Furmanski S, et al.: Minimal detectable pleural effusions. Radiology 105:51, 1972

Cope C: New pleural biopsy needle. JAMA 167:1107, 1958

Davis SD, Henschke CI, Yankelevitz DF, et al.: MR Imaging of pleural effusions. J Comput Assist Tomogr 14:192, 1990

De Francis N, Kiosk E, Albano E: Needle biopsy of parietal pleura: preliminary report. N Engl J Med 252:948, 1955

Delarue J, De Pierre R: Contribution à l'étude des pleurésies cancéreuses cliniquement primitives. Intérêt de la biopsie sous pleuroscopie. J Fr Med Chir Thorac 6:653–63, 1956

Dorne HL: Differentiation of pulmonary parenchymal consolidation from pleural disease using the sonographic fluid bronchogram. Radiology 158:41, 1986

Dwyer A: The displaced crus: a sign for distinguishing between pleural fluid and ascites on computed tomography. J Comput Assist Tomogr 2:598, 1978

Fabri G, Parmeggiani D: Observations on thoracoscopy in pleural exudates. Policlini Sez Prat 5:49, 1942

Feinsilver SH, Barrows AA, Braman SS: Fiberoptic bronchoscopy and pleural effusion of unknown origin. Chest 90:517, 1986

Fisher MS: Asymmetrical changes in asbestos-related disease. Can Assoc Radiol J 36:110, 1985

Fité E, Force L, Casarramowa F, Verdaguer A: Breakage and detachment of an Abrams needle in the pleural cavity during performance of a pleural biopsy. Chest 95:928, 1989

Fletcher DE, Edge JR: The early radiological changes in pulmonary and pleural asbestosis. Clin Radiol 21:355, 1970

Fourestier M, Duret M: Nécessité de la biopsie pleurale pour le diagnostic de l'endothéliome de la plèvre. Presse Med 32:467–8, 1943

Fraser RG, Paré JAP: Diagnosis of Diseases of the Chest. p. 1746. WB Saunders, Philadelphia, 1977

Fraser RG, Paré JAP: Diagnosis of Diseases of the Chest. p. 598. WB Saunders, Philadelphia, 1977

Friedman AC, Fiel SB, Fisher MS, et al.: Asbestos-related pleural disease and asbestosis: a comparison of CT and chest radiography. AJR 150:269, 1988

Frist B, Kahan AV, Koss LG: Comparison of the diagnostic value of biopsies of the pleura and cytological evaluation of pleural fluids. Am J Clin Pathol 72:48, 1979

Gaensler EA: Idiopathic pleural effusion. N Engl J Med 283:816, 1970

Gaensler EA, Kaplan AI: Asbestos pleural effusion. Ann Intern Med 74:178, 1971

Gefter WB, Conant EF: Issues and controversies in the plain-film diagnosis of asbestos-related disorders in the chest. J Thorac Imaging 3:11, 1988

Get'man VG, Kelemen LL, Kizimenko VM: The importance of thoracoscopy in the differential diagnosis of pleurisy. Vrach Delo 9:49, 1989

Gordon R: The deep sulcus sign. Radiology 136:25, 1980

Gunnels JS: Perplexing pleural effusion. Chest 74:390, 1978

Halvorsen RA, Fedyshin PJ, Korobkin M, et al.: Ascites or pleural effusion? RadioGraphics 6:135, 1986

Harvey C, Harvey HPB: Subclavian lymph node, pleural and pulmonary biopsy in diagnosis of intra-thoracic disease. Postgrad Med J 34:204, 1958

Henschke CI, Davis SD, Romano RM, Yankelevitz DF: Pleural effusions: pathogenesis, radiologic evaluation, and therapy. J Thorac Imaging 4:49, 1989

Hillerdal G, Lindgren A: Pleural plaques: correlation of autopsy findings to radiographic findings and occupational history. Eur J Respir Dis 61:315, 1980

Hucker J, Bhatnagar NK, Al-Jilaihawi AN, Forrester-Wood CP: Thoracoscopy in the diagnosis and management of recurrent pleural effusions. Ann Thorac Surg 52:1145, 1991

Jacobeus HC: Thoracoscopy and its practical applications. Ergeb Ges Med 7:122, 1925

Jacobeus HC: The practical importance of thoracoscopy in surgery of the chest. Surg Gynecol Obstet 32:493, 1921

Jacobeus HC: Possibility of the use of the cystoscope for investigation of serous cavities. Munch Med Wochenschr 57:2090, 1910

Kawashima A, Libshitz HI: Malignant pleural mesothelioma: CT manifestations in 50 cases. AJR 155:965, 1990

Kimura M, Nakamura J, Tomizawa S, et al.: The role of thoracoscopy in pleural biopsy in cases with pleural effusion. Nippon Kyobo Shikkan Gakkai Zasshi 28:882, 1990

Kirby TJ, Ginsberg RJ: Role of open thoracostomy in undiagnosed pleural effusions. p. 62. In Delarue NC, Eschapasse H (eds): Thoracic Surgery: Surgical Management of Pleural Diseases. In Deslauriers J, Lacquet LK (eds): International Trends in General Thoracic Surgery. Vol. 6. CV Mosby, St. Louis, 1990

Kovarik JL: Thoracentesis: a modified technic. Postgrad Med 48:96, 1970

Krasnow AZ, Collier BD, Isitman AT, et al.: The use of radionuclide cisternography in the diagnosis of pleural cerebrospinal fluid fistulae. J Nucl Med 30:120, 1989

Krausz M, Manny J: A safe method of thoracentesis. J Thorac Cardiovasc Surg 72:323, 1976

Kreel L: Conventional and new imaging techniques. p. 19. In Delarue NC, Eschapasse H (eds): Thoracic Surgery: Surgical Management of Pleural Diseases. In Deslauriers J, Lacquet LK (eds): International Trends in General Thoracic Surgery. Vol. 6. CV Mosby, St. Louis, 1990

Leung AN, Müller NL, Miller RR: CT in differential diagnosis of diffuse pleural disease. AJR 154: 487, 1990

Light RW: Pleural Diseases. Lea & Febiger, Philadelphia, 1983

Light RW, Jenkinson SG, Minh VD, George RB: Observations on pleural fluid pressures as fluid in withdrawn during thoracentesis. Am Rev Respir Dis 121:799, 1980

McLoud TC, Flower CDR: Imaging the pleura: sonography, CT and MR imaging. AJR 156:1145, 1991

McLoud TC, Woods BO, Carrington CB, et al.: Diffuse pleural thickening in an asbestos-exposed population: prevalence and causes. AJR 144:9, 1985

Menzies R, Charbonneau B: Thoracoscopy for the diagnosis of pleural disease. Ann Intern Med 114:271, 1991

Mestitz P, Purves MJ, Pollard AC: Pleural biopsy in diagnosis of pleural effusion: report of 200 cases. Lancet 2:1349, 1958

Miguères J, Jover A, Bouissou H, et al.: Place de la ponction-biopsie à l'aiguille et du cyto-diagnostic dans le diagnostic des pleurésies malignes. Poumon Coeur 37:29, 1981

Mintzer RA, Gore RM, Vogelzang RL, Holz S: Rounded atelectasis and its association with asbestos-induced pleural disease. Radiology 139:567, 1981

Moote D, Ehrlich L, Martin RH: Postpneumonectomy bronchopleural fistula imaged by ventilation lung scanning. Clin Nucl Med 12:337, 1987

Moskowitz H, Platt RT, Schachar R, Mellins H: Roentgen visualization of minute pleural effusion. Radiology 109:33, 1973

Mossman BT, Gee JBL: Asbestos-related diseases. N Engl J Med 320:1721, 1989

Müller NL: Imaging of the pleura. Radiology 186:297, 1993

Prakash UBS, Reiman HM: Comparison of needle biopsy with cytologic analysis for the evaluation of pleural effusion: analysis of 414 cases. Mayo Clin Proc 60:158, 1985

Rao NV, Jones PO, Greenberg SD, et al.: Needle biopsy of parietal pleura in 124 cases. Arch Intern Med 115:34, 1965

Reger RB, Ames RG, Merchant JA, et al.: The detection of thoracic abnormalities using posterior-anterior (PA) vs PA and oblique roentgenograms. Chest 81:290, 1982

Rhea JT, Van Sonnerberg E, McLoud T: Basilar pneumothorax in the supine adult. Radiology 133:593, 1979

Rivas de Andrès JJ, Lanzas JT: Thoracoscopy and spontaneous pneumothorax (letter). Ann Thorac Surg 55:811, 1993

Rockoff SD, Kagan E, Schwartz A, et al.: Visceral pleural thickening in asbestos exposure: the occurrence and implications of thickened interlobar fissures. J Thorac Imaging 2:58, 1987

Rudikoff JC: Early detection of pleural fluid. Chest 77:109, 1980

Rusch VW, Godwin JD, Shuman WP: The role of computed scanning in the initial assessment and the follow-up of malignant pleural mesothelioma. J Thorac Cardiovasc Surg 96:171, 1988

Rusch VW, Mountain C: Thorocoscopy under regional anesthesia for the diagnosis and management of pleural disease. Am J Surg 154:274, 1987

Ruskin JA, Gurney JW, Thorsen MK, Goodman LR: Detection of pleural effusions on supine chest radiographs. AJR 148:681, 1987

Ryan CJ, Rodgers RF, Unni KK, Hepper NGG: The outcome of patients with pleural effusion of indeterminate cause at thoracotomy. Mayo Clin Proc 56:145, 1981

Sahn SA: The pleura. Am Rev Respir Dis 138:184, 1988

Salyer WR, Eggleston JC, Erozan YS: Efficacy of pleural needle biopsy and pleural fluid cytopathology in the diagnosis of malignant neoplasm involving the pleura. Chest 67:536, 1975

Schabel SI: Radiologic techniques in pleural disease. Semin Respir Med 9:13, 1987

Scharer L, McClement JH: Isolation of tubercule bacilli from needle biopsy specimens of parietal pleural. Am Rev Respir Dis 97:466, 1967

Schneider HJ, Ferson B, Gonzales LL: Rounded atelectasis. AJR 134:225, 1980

Schwartz DA: New developments in asbestos-related pleural disease. Chest 99:191, 1991

Schwartz DA, Fuortes LJ, Galvin JR, et al.: Asbestos-induced pleural fibrosis and impaired lung function. Am Rev Respir Dis 141:321, 1990

Seneff MG, Corwin RW, Gold LH, Irwin RS: Complications associated with thoracentesis. Chest 90:97, 1986

Sergent E, and Kourilsky R: Contribution to the study of endothelioma. Presse Med 47:257, 1939

Serre G, Daste G, Vincent C, et al.: Diagnostic approach to the patient with pleural effusion: cytologic analysis of pleural fluid. p. 35. In Delarue NC, Eschapasse H (eds): Thoracic Surgery: Surgical Management of Pleural Diseases. In Deslauriers J, Lacquet LK (eds): In International Trends in Gen Thoracic Surgery. Vol. 6. CV Mosby, St. Louis, 1990

Sgro B, Gorla A, Tacchi G, et al.: Thoracoscopy in the diagnosis of pleural mesothelioma. Chir Ital 43:95, 1991

Skowran CA: Kerrison rongeur: Needle punch biopsy. Del Med J 32:294, 1960

Smyrnios NA, Jederlinic PJ, Irwin RS: Pleural effusion in an asymptomatic patient: spectrum and frequency of cases and management considerations. Chest 97:192, 1990

Stark DD, Federle MP, Goodman PC, et al.: Differentiating lung abscess and empyema: radiography and computed tomography. AJR 141:163, 1983

Stark DD, Federle MP, Goodman PC: CT and radiographic assessment of tube thoracotomy. AJR 141:253, 1983

Suzuki N, Saitoh T, Kitamura S: Tumor invasion of the chest wall in lung cancer: diagnosis with US. Radiology 187:39, 1993

Teplick JG, Teplick SK, Goodman L, Haskin ME: The interface sign: a computed tomographic sign for distinguishing pleural and intra-abdominal fluid. Radiology 144:359, 1982

Tocico IM, Miller MH, Fairfax WR: Distribution of pneumothorax in the supine and semirecumbent critically ill adult. AJR 144:901, 1985

Vanderschueren RGJRA: The role of thoracoscopy in the evaluation and management of pneumothorax. Lung 168(suppl):1122, 1990

Verreault J, Lepage S, Bisson G, Plante A: Ascites and right pleural effusion: demonstration of a peritoneo-pleural communication. J Nucl Med 27:1706, 1986

Waite RJ, Carbonneau RJ, Balikian JP, et al.: Parietal pleural changes in empyema: appearances on CT. Radiology 175:145, 1990

Wakabayaski A: Expanded applications of diagnostic and therapeutic thoracoscopy. J Thorac Cardiovasc Surg 102:721, 1991

Weisbrod GL, Yee AC: Computed tomographic diagnosis of a pedunculated fibrous mesothelioma. Can Assoc Radiol J 34:147, 1983

Williams T, Thomas P: The diagnosis of pleural effusions by fiberoptic bronchoscopy and pleuroscopy. Chest 80:566, 1981

Williford ME, Godwin JD: Computed tomography of lung abscess and empyema. Radiol Clin North Am 21:575, 1983

Withers BF, Ducatman AM, Yang WN: Roentgenographic evidence for predominant left-sided location of unilateral pleural plaques. Chest 95:1262, 1984

Woodring JH: Recognition of pleural effusion on supine radiographs: how much fluid is required? AJR 142:59, 1984

Yokoi K, Mori K, Miyazawa N, et al.: Tumor invasion of the chest wall and mediastinum in lung cancer: evaluation with pneumothorax CT. Radiology 181:147, 1991

Zerhouni EA, Scott WW, Baker RR, et al.: Invasive thymomas: diagnosis and evaluation by computed tomography. J Comput Assist Tomogr 6:92, 1982

36

PLEURAL EFFUSION: BENIGN AND MALIGNANT

Valerie W. Rusch

Pleural effusions are often treated empirically, even though they are a common and significant clinical problem. In the past 10 years, several advances have made possible a more systematic approach to the management of pleural effusions. Ongoing research, primarily based on animal models, has provided a better understanding of the pathophysiology of pleural effusions (Sahn, 1988; Kinasewitz and Fishman, 1981; Wiener-Kronish, et al., 1985, 1988; Broaddus and Light, 1992; Broaddus, et al., 1990). Characterization of the biochemical characteristics of pleural fluid has improved our ability to diagnose the cause of an effusion by using the relatively noninvasive approach of thoracentesis (Light, 1983). The advent of computed tomography (CT) in the late 1970s dramatically improved the noninvasive evaluation of pleural disease. Thoracoscopy, which was always a popular procedure in Europe (Deslauriers and Lacquet, 1990; Boutin, et al., 1991), is becoming widely practiced in North America for the diagnosis and treatment of pleural disease because of the recent application of video-assisted technology. Patients who previously were subjected to multiple thoracenteses and percutaneous pleural biopsies are now offered thoracoscopy if the initial noninvasive evaluation is not diagnostic. Finally pleurodesis for malignant pleural effusions, which was often a highly individualized procedure, is now being evaluated in carefully designed prospective trials.

A better understanding of pathophysiology, better imaging, faster and more accurate methods of diagnosis, and the careful assessment of therapy have improved the diagnosis and therapy of pleural effusions. This chapter covers the current approach to the management of pleural effusions, focusing on malignant pleural effusions, which are the most common problem seen by surgeons.

PATHOPHYSIOLOGY

The anatomy and physiology of the pleural space were described in detail in Chapter 34. Pleural effusions develop because of a disturbance in the mechanisms that normally move 5 to 10 L of fluid across the pleural space every 24 hours and resorb it, leaving only 5 to 20 ml present at any time (Kinasewitz and Fishman, 1981). Increased capillary permeability (inflammation or tumor implants), increased hydrostatic pressure (congestive heart failure), decreased oncotic pressure (hypoalbuminemia), increased negative intrapleural pressure (atelectasis), and decreased lymphatic drainage (lymphatic obstruction by a tumor or radiation-induced fibrosis) can all cause a pleural effusion. In patients with cancer, several different mechanisms often contribute to the formation of an effusion (Table 36-1). These mechanisms may relate directly to the presence of the tumor (e.g., obstruction of lymphatic channels), may reflect underlying medical problems (e.g., congestive heart failure or hypoalbuminemia), or be a combination of both.

CLINICAL PRESENTATION AND DIAGNOSIS

Small pleural effusions are asymptomatic. Larger pleural effusions cause dyspnea, cough, and chest discomfort. Dullness to percussion and diminished breath sounds are present on the physical examination. The clinical diagnosis is confirmed by chest radiograph (Felson and Vix, 1974). Small pleural effusions cause blunting of the costophrenic angle. If the pleural space is free, larger effusions produce the classic picture of a fluid level with a meniscus sign (Fig. 36-1). A lateral decubitus radiograph confirms the freely flowing nature of the fluid (Fig. 36-2). Massive effusions cause a complete opacification of the hemithorax. Rarely they present as a tension hydrothorax, with a mediastinal shift by radiography and a tracheal shift with severe respiratory distress and hemodynamic instability. Loculated pleural effusions are harder to diagnose on a standard chest radiograph. They present as opacities of varying sizes and shapes that can be hard to distinguish from a pulmonary parenchymal process, such as atelectasis or dense consolidation (Figs. 36-3). Lateral decubitus radiographs do not show layering of the fluid. Ultrasound detects a loculated fluid collection and determines the proper site for thoracentesis, but the most useful examination under these circumstances is a CT scan. This helps direct

Table 36-1. Interaction Among Pathogenetic Mechanisms and Contributing Factors Favoring the Accumulation of Pleural Fluid

Pathogenetic Mechanisms	Impared Lymphatic Drainage	Increased Pleural Osmotic Pressure	Increased Capillary Permeability	Increased Venous Pressure
Pleural implants	+	+	+	−
Lymphatic metastases				
Mediastinal nodes	+	+	−	−
Lymphangitis	+	+	−	−
Tumor cell suspension	+	+	+	−
Contributing syndromes				
Superior vena cava syndrome	+	+	−	+
Congestive heart failure	+	+	−	+
Pericarditis or effusion	+	+	−	−
Infection	+	+	+	−
Mediastinal irradiation	+	+	−	−
Ascites	+	+	−	+
Hypoalbuminemia	−	+	−	−

Symbols: +, contributes; −, does not contribute.

(Data from Roth JA, Ruckkdeschel JC, Weisenburger TH (eds): Thoracic Oncology. p. 596. WB Saunders, Philadelphia, 1989 and Harper GR: Pleural effusions in cancer. Clin Cancer Briefs 1:1, 1979.)

therapy by outlining the size and location of the fluid collections accurately and by distinguishing underlying parenchymal disease from pleural fluid and thickening (Fig. 36-4).

The clinical setting in which an effusion occurs influences the approach to diagnosis and therapy. A patient who develops a small effusion in conjunction with pneumonia but is improving while receiving antibiotics is likely to have a parapneumonic effusion and could be treated expectantly. The same would be true of a patient with known cirrhosis and long-standing ascites who has a small pleural effusion. In contrast, a woman who develops a new pleural effusion sev-

eral years after treatment for a node-positive breast cancer merits intensive investigation. Before any invasive workup is initiated, the patient with a pleural effusion should have a careful history and physical examination so that all subsequent evaluation is directed toward the clinically likely causes.

Knowledge of the most common causes of pleural effusions is also helpful in pinpointing the etiologic agent. Overall the four most common causes of pleural effusions in the United States are congestive heart failure, bacterial pneumonia, malignancy, and pulmonary emboli. Viral pneumonia, cirrhosis

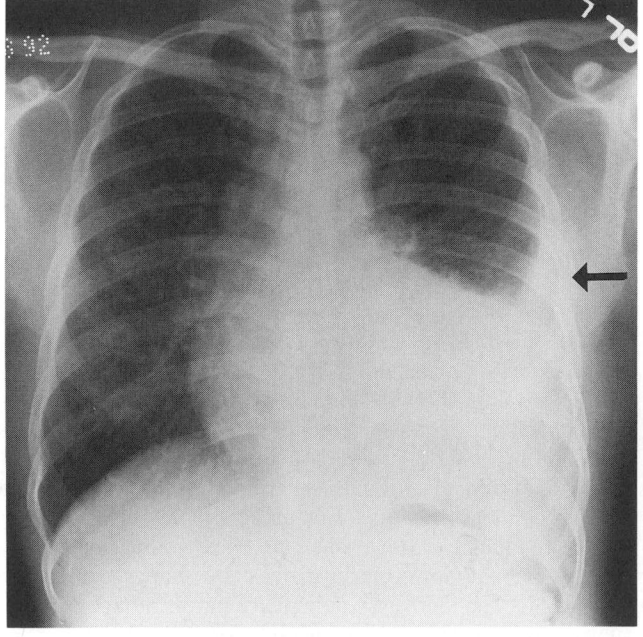

Figure 36-1. Posteroanterior chest radiograph of a patient with widely disseminated lung cancer and a left pleural effusion. The retrocardiac region is opacified, and there is a fluid level with a typical meniscus sign (*arrow*).

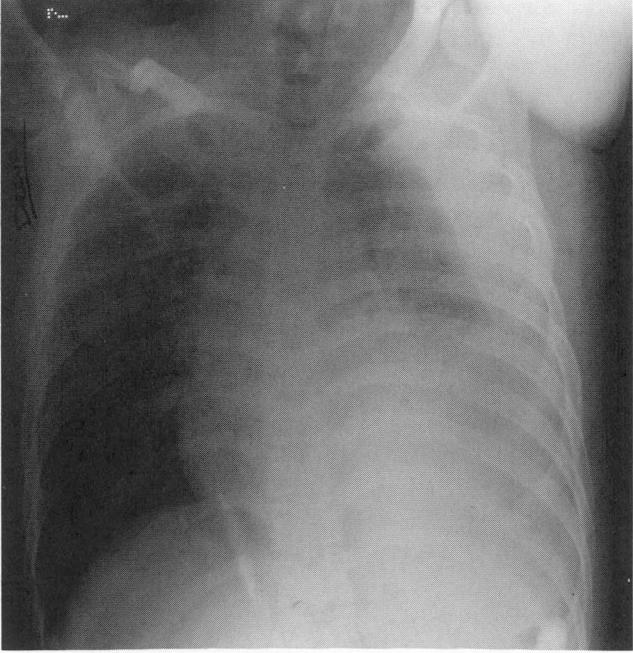

Figure 36-2. The lateral decubitus chest radiograph of the patient shown in Fig. 36-1 shows that the pleural effusion layers easily and is therefore free flowing.

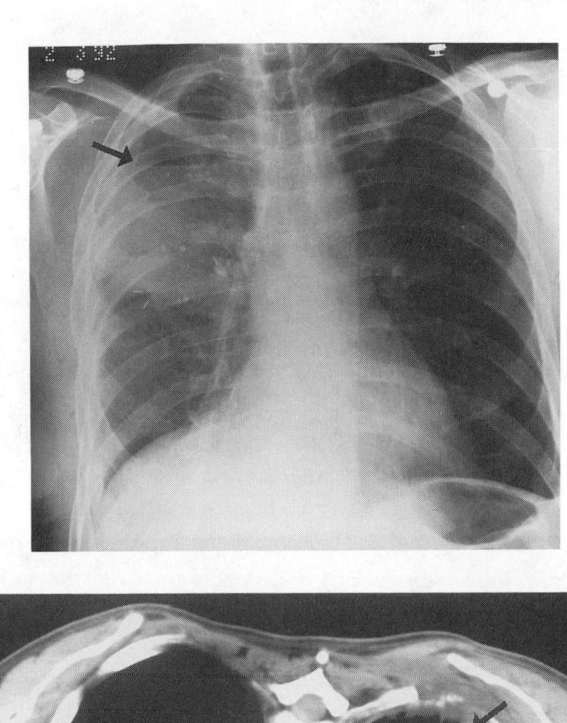

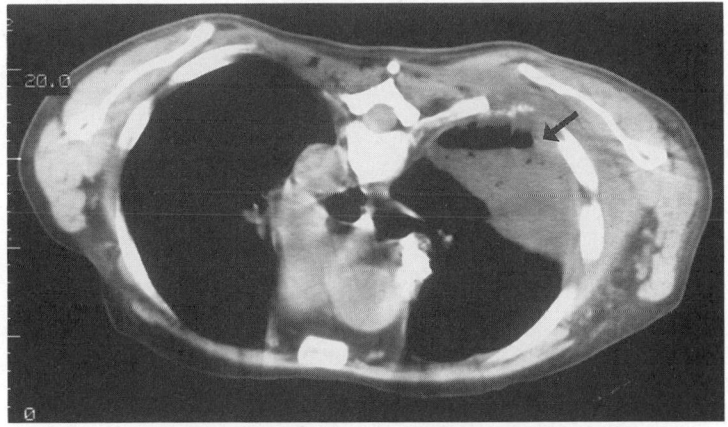

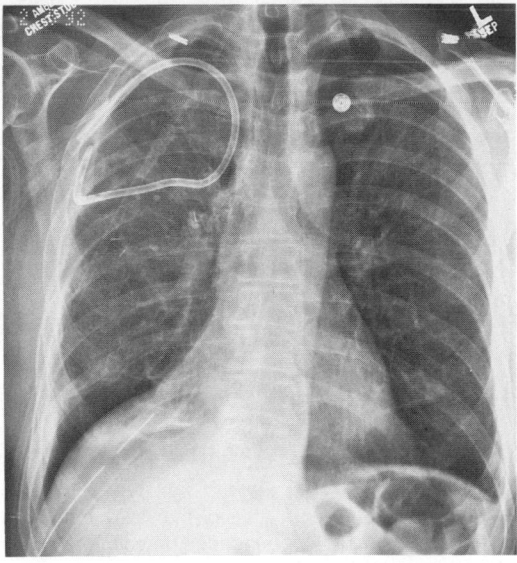

Figure 36-3. **(A)** Loculated right pleural effusion in patient status postdecortication of the right lung for empyema. There is a hazy density in the right midlung field with a fluid level at its upper margin (*arrow*). **(B)** CT scan of the patient shown in Figure A, taken in the prone position, demonstrates a loculated fluid collection with an air-fluid level (*arrow*). **(C)** Posteroanterior chest radiograph of the same patient following percutaneous catheter drainage of the fluid collection, shows clearing of the hazy density seen on the initial chest radiograph.

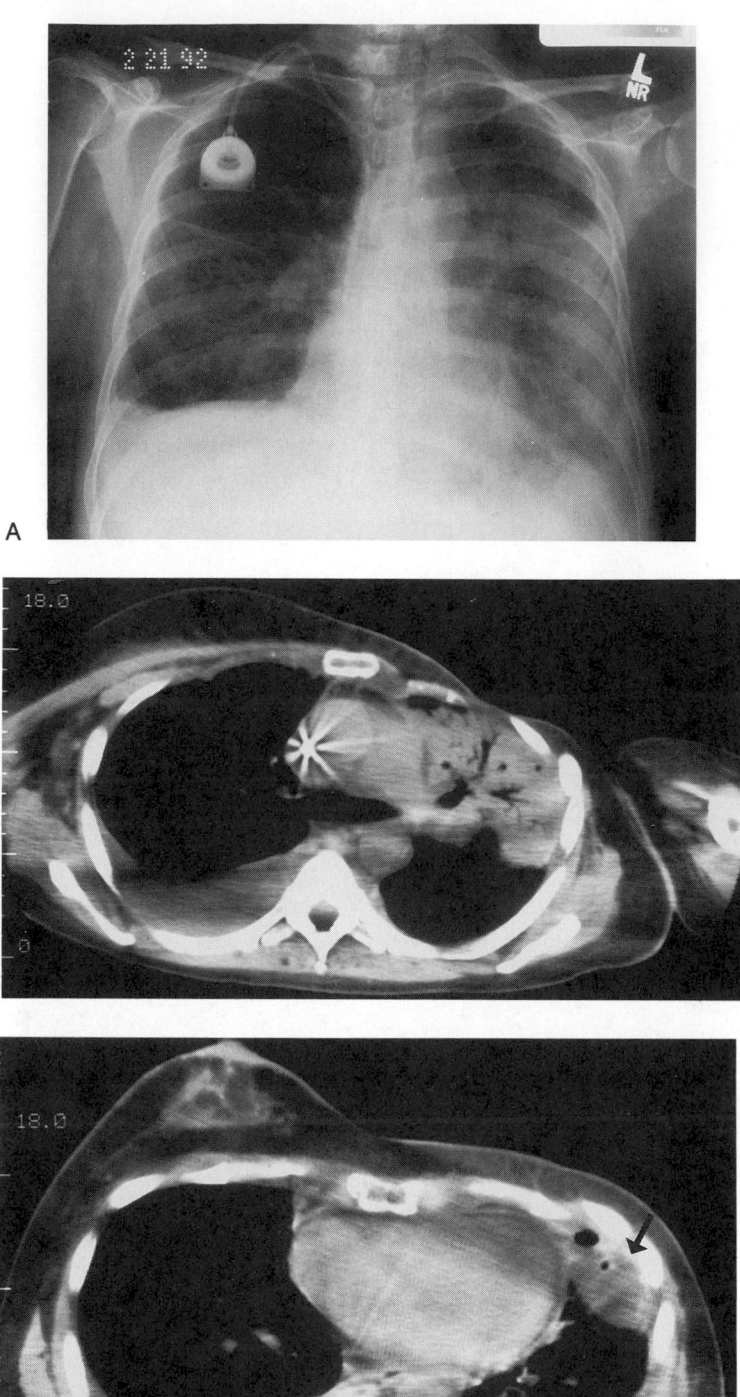

Figure 36-4. **(A)** Another example of a loculated pleural effusion that is extremely difficult to distinguish from underlying parenchymal disease in a patient who had severe radiation-induced fibrosis. The posteroanterior chest radiograph shows a hazy density in the mid and lateral aspect of the left lung with an underlying air bronchogram. **(B)** CT scan of this patient at the level of the carina shows dense consolidation of the left upper lobe with an air bronchogram. There is no pleural fluid present at this level. **(C)** CT scan of the same patient at the level of the midheart shows a large free-flowing right pleural effusion and a multiloculated left pleural effusion (*arrows*). This combination of parenchymal disease and multiloculated pleural effusion accounts for the abnormalities seen on the plain chest radiograph in Fig. A. It would be hard to interpret the chest radiograph and make a determination of whether drainage of the pleural effusion were appropriate without the aid of the CT scan.

Table 36-2. Primary Organ Site or Neoplasm Type in Male Patients with Malignant Pleural Effusions

Primary Site or Tumor Type	No. Male Patients	Percent Male Patients
Lung	140	49.1
Lymphoma/leukemia	60	21.1
Gastrointestinal tract	20	7.0
Genitourinary tract	17	6.0
Melanoma	4	1.4
Mesothelioma	3	1.0
Miscellaneous less common tumors	10	3.5
Primary site unknown	31	10.9
Total	285	100.0

(From Johnson WW: The malignant pleural effusion: a review of cytopathologic diagnoses of 584 specimens from 472 consecutive patients. Cancer 56:905, 1985, with permission.)

with ascites, gastrointestinal disease, collagen-vascular disease, and tuberculosis are less common etiologies (Light, 1983). The most common causes of malignant pleural effusion are lung cancer, breast cancer, and lymphoma. However, the frequency of the type of cancer responsible for a pleural effusion depends on the patient's gender. Lung cancer, lymphoma, and gastrointestinal cancers are the three most common causes in men; breast cancers, gynecologic cancers, and lung cancers are the most common ones in women (Tables 36-2 and 36-3).

If the diagnosis is not clinically obvious, a thoracentesis should be performed and the character of the fluid noted. Bloody fluid occurs with pulmonary emboli, malignancy, or trauma. Clear milky fluid is strongly suggestive of a chylothorax; turbid or purulent fluid is indicative of an empyema.

The pleural fluid should be sent for cytologic examination, culture, and cell count. Simultaneous pleural fluid and serum glucose, protein, and lactic dehydrogenase levels should be performed. Effusions are classified as exudative or transudative based on the protein and lactic dehydrogenase levels. An effusion is considered an exudate if the pleural fluid to serum ratio of protein is greater than 0.5, and the lactic dehydrogenase ratio is greater than 0.6. The most common

Table 36-3. Primary Organ Site or Neoplasm Type in Female Patients with Malignant Pleural Effusions

Primary Site or Tumor Type	No. Female Patients	Percent Female Patients
Breast	70	37.4
Female genital tract	38	20.3
Lung	28	15.0
Lymphoma/leukemia	14	8.0
Gastrointestinal tract	8	4.3
Melanoma	6	3.2
Urinary Tract	2	1.1
Miscellaneous less common tumors	3	1.6
Primary site unknown	17	9.1
Total	187	100.0

(From Johnson WW: The malignant pleural effusion: a review of cytopathologic diagnoses of 584 specimens from 472 consecutive patients. Cancer 56:905, 1985, with permission.)

cause of transudative effusions is congestive heart failure. There are many causes of exudative effusions, but the most common ones are malignancy, infection, and pulmonary emboli. The pleural fluid concentration of glucose is also helpful because a level less than 60 mg/dl is seen only in four conditions: malignancy, tuberculous pleuritis, parapneumonic effusions, and rheumatoid pleural effusion (Petterson and Riska, 1981; Smyrnios, et al., 1990; Vladutiu, et al., 1981). Thus a patient who has a bloody exudative effusion with a low glucose level is likely to have a malignancy.

Several other biochemical tests are helpful in specific clinical situations. The amylase level is elevated in three conditions: esophageal perforation, pancreatitis, and malignant effusions. A triglyceride level should be obtained if a chylothorax is suspected. A level above 110 mg/dl is considered diagnostic. Pleural fluid pH and glucose levels have been used in the evaluation of parapneumonic effusions. Light (1983) reported that a pH less than 7.00 in conjunction with a glucose level less than 60 mg/dl indicates that a parapneumonic effusion will progress to a frank empyema. However, other authors have not found the pH and glucose levels to be this reliable in the management of parapneumonic effusions. Complement, rheumatoid factor, and antinuclear antibody levels are often elevated in collagen-vascular disease and

---

Differential Diagnosis of Pleural Effusions

I. Transudative pleural effusions
   A. Congestive heart failure
   B. Cirrhosis
   C. Nephrotic syndrome
   D. Peritoneal dialysis
   E. Glomerulonephritis
   F. Myxedema
   G. Pulmonary emboli
   H. Sarcoidosis

II. Exudative pleural effusions
   A. Neoplasic diseases
     1. Metastatic disease
     2. Mesothelioma
   B. Infectious diseases
     1. Bacterial infections
     2. Tuberculosis
     3. Fungal infections
     4. Parasitic infections
     5. Viral infections
   C. Pulmonary embolization
   D. Gastrointestinal disease
     1. Pancreatitis
     2. Subphrenic abscess
     3. Intrahepatic abscess
     4. Esophageal perforation
     5. Diaphragmatic hernia
   E. Collagen-vascular diseases
     1. Rheumatoid pleuritis
     2. Systemic lupus erythematosus

(Continues)

3. Drug-induced lupus
4. Immunoblastic lymphadenopathy
5. Sjögren's syndrome
6. Familial Mediterranean fever
7. Wegener's granulomatosis
G. Drug-induced pleural disease
1. Nitrofurantoin
2. Dantrolene
3. Methysergide
4. Bromocriptine
5. Procarbazine
6. Methotrexate
7. Practolol
H. Miscellaneous diseases and conditions
1. Asbestos exposure
2. Postpericardiectomy or postmyocardial infarction syndrome
3. Meigs's syndrome
4. Yellow nail syndrome
5. Sarcoidosis
6. Uremia
7. Trapped lung
8. Radiation therapy
9. Electrical burns
10. Urinary tract obstruction
11. Iatrogenic injury
I. Hemothorax
J. Chylothorax

(From Light RW: Pleural Diseases. p. 62. Lea & Febiger, Philadelphia, 1983, with permission.)

should be obtained if this is being considered in the differential diagnosis (Light, 1983).

Other tests have been used to determine the cause of pleural effusions and particularly to distinguish whether or not an effusion is malignant. The carcinoembryonic antigen level has been the most widely used pleural fluid marker. Levels of this antigen above 5.0 ng/ml are a specific but relatively insensitive marker of malignancy (Asseo and Tracopoulos, 1982; Rittgers, et al., 1978; Sorensen, 1991; Tamura, et al., 1988). Creatine kinase isoenzyme BB, adenosine deaminase, and galactosyltransferase have been reported to distinguish benign from malignant effusions in small series of patients (Kim, et al., 1982; Pettersson, et al., 1984; Silverman, et al., 1979). Various immunohistochemical stains have been used to identify malignant cells and to distinguish them from reactive mesothelial cells (Herbert and Gallagher, 1982). Flow cytometry is relatively inaccurate in diagnosing malignancy because cytologically positive pleural effusions do not always contain aneuploid cells (Schneller, et al., 1987). Cytogenetic techniques can diagnose malignant pleural effusions, but they are labor intensive and do not consistently add to the standard cytologic examination (Dewald, et al., 1976, 1982; Falor, et al., 1982; Monif, et al., 1976). Uptake of ^{99m}TC phosphate in malignant pleural effusions has been anecdotally reported in patients undergoing bone scans to search for osseous metastases (Goldstein and Gefter, 1983; Kida, et al., 1984). Although this is not likely to be useful as a routine diagnostic test, its clinical significance as an incidental finding should be remembered.

The long list of tests that can be performed on pleural effusion to pinpoint a cause are of academic rather than practical interest. The character of the fluid (e.g., bloody versus serous), a determination of whether it is an exudate or a transudate, measurement of the glucose level, and culture and cytologic examination are the most important initial tests (Rodriguez-Panadero and Lopez Mejias, 1989; Roth, et al., 1990; Xaubet, et al., 1985). Additional biochemical analyses should be used selectively based on the clinical setting. If the examination of the pleural fluid is nondiagnostic, a percutaneous pleural biopsy should be considered. A pleural biopsy alone yields a diagnosis of malignancy in 40 to 69 percent of cases. When pleural fluid cytologic findings and pleural biopsy results are combined, the yield increases to 80 to 90 percent (Migueres, et al., 1981; Prakash and Reiman, 1985; Poe, et al., 1984; Winkelmann and Pfitzer, 1980). Pleural biopsy can also diagnose some benign diseases, such as tuberculous effusion or amyloidosis, in situations in which the pleural fluid analysis is uninformative (Chertow, et al., 1991; Kavuru, et al., 1990; Seibert, et al., 1991).

Patients whose effusions remain undiagnosed after a thoracentesis and percutaneous pleural biopsy should undergo a CT scan of the chest and abdomen, a bronchoscopy, and a thoracoscopy. If the effusion is large, the CT scan should be done after the fluid has been evacuated so that the lung can be imaged when it is fully expanded. The CT detects underlying pulmonary parenchymal and abdominal disease that may not be evident otherwise. Bronchoscopy diagnoses endobronchial tumors (primary or metastatic) that may be responsible for an effusion because of postobstructive atelectasis. Thoracoscopy is performed to obtain a tissue diagnosis by directed pleural biopsy and to do a pleurodesis, usually by talc poudrage. Several large series report a diagnostic accuracy of 80 to 100 percent for thoracoscopy, depending on the reasons for which thoracoscopy was performed. In almost all patients, it is the definitive way of diagnosing a malignancy involving the pleura (Boushy, et al., 1978; Faurschou, 1985; Faurschou, et al., 1985; Hucker, et al., 1991; Page, et al., 1989; Rusch and Mountain, 1987; Vanderscharen, 1981; Voellmy, 1981; Weissberg, et al., 1980). The exceptions are patients in whom thoracoscopy cannot be performed because of a fused pleural space. The recent development of video-assisted thoracoscopy has significantly expanded the diagnostic potential of this technique by making lung biopsies and more extensive nodal dissection possible (Lewis, et al., 1992; Oakes, et al., 1984). In the past patients often underwent multiple thoracenteses and percutaneous pleural biopsies in an effort to avoid a thoracotomy for diagnosis. Thoracoscopy, widely used in Europe for a long time, was a largely forgotten procedure in North America for the diagnosis of pleural disease (Thermann, et al., 1985). With the popularization of video-assisted thoracoscopy, patients with undiagnosed pleural effusions will probably be referred sooner for this minimally invasive but highly diagnostic procedure.

MANAGEMENT

General Principles

Transudative pleural effusions are managed by therapy of the underlying disease and usually resolve after this has been controlled (Light, 1983; Friedman and Slater, 1978). Occasionally, additive intervention is required, either because the effusion is symptomatic or because the underlying medical problem is refractory to maximal medical treatment. For example, tube thoracostomy might be necessary to drain a large effusion secondary to a pulmonary embolus, or a pleurodesis or pleuroperitoneal shunt might be required to control a symptomatic effusion in a patient with medically refractory ascites.

Some exudative effusions also resolve after therapy of the underlying disease. This is true of effusions caused by gastrointestinal disease, drugs, collagen, vascular disease, and nonbacterial infections (Light, 1983; Deslauriers and Lacquet, 1990; Seibert, et al., 1991). Some exudative effusions caused by malignancy are also best managed in this manner if the tumor is highly responsive to chemotherapy or radiation. The classic example is an effusion or chylothorax caused by a lymphoma, which usually resolves quickly after chemotherapy or radiation alleviates the lymphatic obstruction (Xaubet, et al., 1985). Effusions caused by solid tumors, such as breast cancer and ovarian cancer, for which effective chemotherapy is available, also often resolve spontaneously after chemotherapy is instituted (Deslauriers and Lacquet, 1990; Friedman and Slater, 1978; Reshad, et al., 1985).

The most difficult management problem is the malignant pleural effusion caused by a tumor that is refractory to chemotherapy. Traditionally these have been treated by some form of pleurodesis. Before proceeding with pleurodesis, however, it is important to make certain that the patient does not have "trapped" lung with a fixed pleural space. The lung is often encased by a peel of visceral pleural tumor that causes chronic collapse of the lung and prevents the parietal and visceral pleural surfaces from coming into apposition with each other. Effective pleurodesis under these circumstances is obviously impossible. Partial entrapment of the lung with smaller loculated effusions is also common in patients with cancer. Sometimes this is not caused by a pleural tumor but is the result of a chronic effusion that contains a lot of protein and fibrinous debris, which create a limited fibrothorax. A trapped lung is readily recognized by a lack of expansion of the lung after therapeutic thoracentesis or chest tube insertion (Fig. 36-5). Complete or near-complete expansion of the lung and evacuation of the pleural space should be documented on a chest radiograph before proceeding with pleurodesis.

Pleurodesis for Malignant Effusions

At one time it was believed that malignant pleural effusions could be controlled by serial thoracentesis or tube thoracostomy alone without pleurodesis. Although Lambert, et al. (1967) reported a recurrence rate of only 17 percent for effusions managed by tube thoracostomy alone, subsequent experience with this approach demonstrated that virtually all patients experienced a rapid reaccumulation of their effusion (Anderson, et al., 1974). Today drainage of the effusion without pleurodesis (usually by serial thoracentesis) is only considered appropriate for terminally ill patients who are unwilling or unable to tolerate other therapies.

A large number of agents have been used intrapleurally to try to control malignant pleural effusions. These agents can be classified in two broad categories, according to their modes of action: cytostatic agents (which presumably control the effusion by reducing the tumor volume) and sclerosants

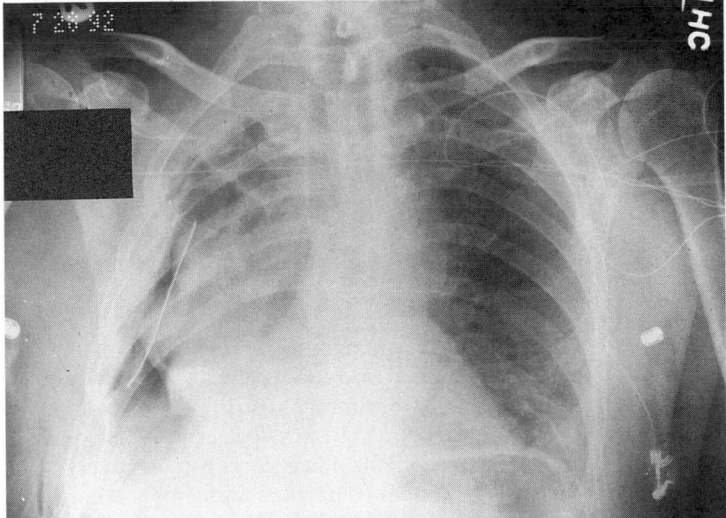
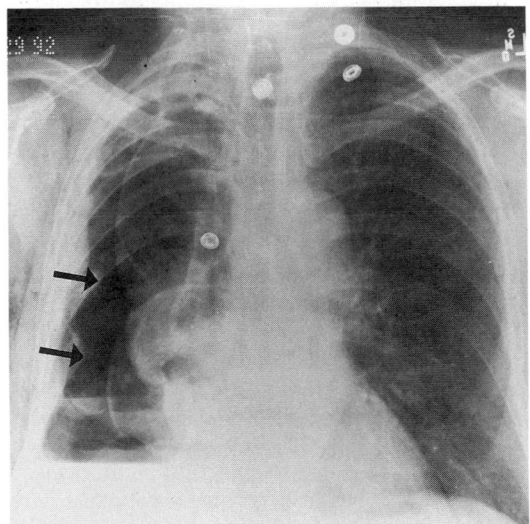

Figure 36-5. **(A)** Posteroanterior chest radiograph on a patient with malignant mesothelioma who underwent a thoracoscopy for diagnosis. The lung was clearly trapped at thoracoscopy. The initial postoperative portable chest radiograph shows evacuation of the pleural space with an unexpanded lung. **(B)** The chest radiograph obtained the following day after removal of chest tube shows this more clearly. There is a fixed pleural space (*arrows*) and lack of re-expansion of the underlying lung. This patient would not be an appropriate candidate for pleurodesis.

(which produce a chemical pleuritis that leads to the formation of adhesions and subsequent obliteration of the pleural space (Frankel, et al., 1961). Radioactive colloids and some chemotherapeutic agents (nitrogen mustard, doxorubicin, and bleomycin) may combine both modes of action when administered intrapleurally. However, with the exception of cisplatin and perhaps thiotepa and 5-fluorouracil, most chemotherapeutic drugs act predominantly as sclerosants.

The early experience with pleurodesis for malignant pleural effusions was comprehensively reviewed (Austin and Flye, 1979; Hausheer and Yarbro, 1985). Nitrogen mustard controls the effusion in approximately one-third of cases but causes significant pleuritic pain and fever and may be associated with bone marrow depression, depending on the dose used (Anderson, et al., 1974; Leininger, et al., 1969). Thiotepa and 5-fluorouracil have fewer side effects but are no better at controlling effusions (Friedman and Slater, 1978). Response rates as high as 80 percent have been reported for intrapleural doxorubicin, but the associated problems of pain, fever, and nausea and vomiting preclude its routine use (Ike, et al., 1991; Masuno, et al., 1991; Keeford, et al., 1980). Quinacrine is an effective sclerosant that controls effusion in up to 80 percent of patients but causes severe pleuritic pain, fever, nausea, and occasionally, hypotension, hallucinations, and seizures (Taylor, et al., 1977; Bayly, et al., 1978). These agents have been abandoned, either because of their ineffectiveness or because of their significant toxicity. Radioactive colloids including radioactive zinc (^{63}Zn), gold (^{198}Au), and chromium phosphate ($Cr^{32}PO_4$) were associated with little toxicity but were successful in only 50 to 60 percent of patients (Hausheer and Yarbro, 1985; Ariel, et al., 1966). They were also expensive and inconvenient because of the need to shield hospital personnel from the radioactivity and therefore are no longer routinely used. Experience with these agents, however, established that pleurodesis was more likely to be successful if the pleural space was fully evacuated by tube thoracostomy before instillation of the sclerosant and the chest tube was left in place after the pleurodesis until the drainage was minimal. This remains an important principle in performing a pleurodesis.

Tetracycline pleurodesis was introduced in 1972. It had the advantage of being inexpensive, easily available, and relatively nontoxic. Its major side effect was severe pleuritic pain, which was often difficult to control even with appropriate systemic premedication and the use of intrapleural lidocaine (Landvater, et al., 1988; Wallach, 1978; Zaloznik, et al., 1983). Success rates ranging from 39 to 83 percent have been reported with tetracycline in several prospective studies comparing it with other agents (Table 36-4). The effectiveness of tetracycline may be dose and technique related. Tetracycline had so many advantages over other sclerosants that it rapidly became the agent of choice, even though it did not always result in a successful pleurodesis.

Bleomycin has also become a popular sclerosant (Bitran, et al., 1981; Ostrowski, 1986; Paladine, et al., 1970). Its success rate is at least as good and perhaps better than that of tetracycline, and it may cause less pain (Ruckdeschel, et al., 1991). A recent prospective randomized trial that compared pleurodesis with 1 g of tetracycline to 60 units of bleomycin found that the median time to recurrence or progression of

Table 36-4. Results of Tetracycline Pleurodesis in Pleural Effusions

Patient Success (No.)	Success Rate (%)
10/12	83
7/7	100
10/12	83
53/60	80
15/25	60
101/108	94

(Adapted from Boutin C, Vaillat JR, Aeolony Y: Practical Thoracoscopy. p. 68. Springer-Verlag, Berlin, 1991, with permission.)

the effusion was 32 days for tetracycline and 46 days for bleomycin. The recurrence rate within 90 days of instillation was 30 percent with bleomycin and 53 percent with tetracycline. Toxicity was similar for the two agents. Although it usually is well tolerated, it can occasionally cause nephrotoxicity in patients with underlying renal insufficiency. Bleomycin is also expensive.

The manufacture of tetracycline was recently discontinued, and this has led to a resurgence in the use of talc, a sclerosant that was first used by Bethune (1935) in 1935 and has been especially popular in Europe. Because it is insoluble, talc has usually been administered as a powder by insufflation at thoracoscopy or thoracotomy. Several series, however, report instilling it as a suspension by tube thoracostomy (Adler and Sayek, 1976; Chambers, 1958; Webb et al., 1992). Experimentally talc was shown to cause an intense chemical pleuritis that exceeds that caused by other agents (Frankel, et al., 1961; Adler and Sayek, 1976). Table 36-5 summarizes most of the published experience with talc. Its reported success rate has consistently been 80 percent or better (Adler and Rappole, 1967; Aelony, et al., 1991; Boniface and Guerin, 1989; Camishion, et al., 1962; Daniel, et al., 1990; Hamed, et al., 1989; Harley, 1979; Ladjimi, et al., 1985, 1989, 1991; Migueres and Jover, 1981; Ohri, et al., 1992; Pearson and MacGregor, 1966; Scarbonchi, et al., 1981; Shedbalkar, et al., 1971; Srensen, et al., 1984; Todd, et al., 1980). Several randomized trials suggest that talc is superior to tetracycline or bleomycin (Boutin, et al., 1991, Fentiman, et al., 1986; Hamed, et al., 1988; Hartman, et al., 1992). Iodine has sometimes been added to the talc to keep the talc sterile and to intensify the pleuritis (Jones, 1969; Webb, et al., 1992), but this is clearly not necessary in light of the high success rate of noniodized talc.

Fever and pleuritic pain occur after the administration of talc, although pain seems to be far less common and less severe than that with tetracycline. There have been rare reports of adult respiratory distress syndrome developing after talc pleurodesis (Bouchama, et al., 1984; Rinaldo, et al., 1983), but given the hundreds of patients treated with talc over several decades, the risk of this complication appears to be minuscule. It has been hypothesized that the development of adult respiratory distress syndrome may be related to the amount of talc used or to contaminants within the talc preparation (Weissberg, 1984). However, published series report using widely varying amounts of talc (usually at least 5 to 10 g), and some do not specify the amount of talc used at

Table 36-5. Results of Studies of Talc Pleurodesis for Malignant Pleural Effusions

Author (Year)	Method of Administration	No. Effusions Controlled/No. Effusions Treated (%)
Chambers (1958)	Suspension, chest tube	17/20 (85)
Camishion, et al. (1962)	Poudrage, thoracotomy	30/31 (97)
Roche (1963)	Poudrage, thoracoscopy	6/6 (100)
Pearson and MacGregor (1966)	Poudrage, thoracotomy or trocar	17/19 (89)
Adler and Rappole (1967)	Poudrage, thoracoscopy	4/4 (100)
Jones (1969)	Poudrage, thoracoscopy	22/23 (96)
Shedbalkar, et al. (1971)	Not stated	22/28 (96)
Adler and Sayek (1976)	Suspension, chest tube	41/44 (93)
Harley (1979)	Poudrage, thoracoscopy	41/44 (93)
Austin and Flye (1979)	Suspension, chest tube	38/41 (91)
Todd, et al. (1980)	Poudrage, thoracotomy or trocar	158/163 (97)
Scarbonchi, et al. (1981)	Poudrage, thoracoscopy	70/77 (91)
Migueres et al. (1981)	Poudrage, thoracoscopy	15/26 (58)
Srensen, et al. (1984)	Suspension, chest tube	9/9 (100)
Ladjimi, et al. (1985)	Poudrage, thoracoscopy	66/78 (85)
Viallat, et al. (1986)	Poudrage, thoracoscopy	23/25 (92)
Fentiman, et al. (1986)	Poudrage, thoracoscopy	11/12 (92)
Boniface and Guerin (1989)	Poudrage, thoracoscopy	233/254 (92)
Ladjimi, et al. (1989)	Poudrage, thoracoscopy	192/218 (88)
Hamed, et al. (1989)	?Poudrage, thoracoscopy	10/10 (100)
Daniel, et al. (1990)	Poudrage, thoracoscopy	18/20 (90)
Ladjimi, et al. (1991)	Poudrage, thoracoscopy	18/21 (84)
Aelony, et al. (1991)	Poudrage, thoracoscopy	23/28 (82)
Engeler (1992)	Poudrage, thoracoscopy	19/20 (95)
Ohri, et al. (1992)	Poudrage, thoracoscopy	35/37 (95)
Webb, et al. (1992)	Suspension, chest tube	37/37 (100)
Hartman, et al. (1992)	Poudrage, thoracoscopy	22/25 (88)

all. Moreover when a talc poudrage is performed, it is hard to estimate the amount of talc remaining in the pleural space because some of it is dissipated into the air during the procedure. There has been some concern in the past that talc pleurodesis might lead to a significant decrease in pulmonary function and predispose to the development of malignancy. A mild restrictive defect was seen as a late sequela in patients who underwent talc pleurodesis for spontaneous pneumothorax (Lange, et al., 1988). Long-term follow-up (14 to 40 years) by the British Thoracic Association of 210 patients who underwent pleurodesis disclosed no increased incidence of lung cancer or mesothelioma (Chappel, et al., 1979). The risk of carcinogenesis from talc may have been related to contamination of the talc preparations with asbestos. Talc prepared for medical use today is asbestos free. Neither one of these issues is important for patients with malignant pleural effusions who usually have a life expectancy less than 1 year and who need pleurodesis to palliate their dyspnea.

Several collective reviews (Austin and Flye, 1979; Friedman and Slater, 1978; Hausheer and Yarbro, 1985) attempted to assess the relative merits of the various agents used as sclerosants (Table 36-6). This is difficult because many of the published series are retrospective and uncontrolled. Prospective trials have often been poorly designed because they are based on small numbers of patients and loosely defined eligibility and response criteria. Follow-up is usually short, and a central review of chest radiographs to verify the response data is rare (Rusch, 1991). In addition, patients with

malignant pleural effusions represent a difficult patient population in which to carry out clinical trials. They have a limited life expectancy, with about one-half of the patients dying within 3 months of therapy. Thus large numbers of patients must be entered into a study to have statistically adequate

Table 36-6. Results of the Principal Randomized, Controlled Studies of Pleurodesis in the Treatment of Pleurisy

Patients (No.)	Agents Used	Success Rates (%)
25	Quinacrine/Thiot	64/27
22	TCN/quinacrine	83/90
25	TCN/bleomycine	58/54
21	Cory/mustine	56/42
24	TCN/drainage	72/36
37	Mustard/talc	56/90
24	TCN/drainage	77/22
21	Talc/drainage	100/60
40	Talc/TCN	90/50
32	Cory/TCN	88/79
41	Talc/TCN	92/48
32	Cory/bleomycin	65/13
34	TCN/bleomycine	39/31
30	Talc/doxycycline	90/63

Abbreviations: Cory, Corynebacterium parvum; TCN, tetracycline; Thiot, thiotepa.

(Adapted from Boutin C, Vaillat JR, Aeolony Y: Practical Thoracoscopy. p. 68. Springer-Verlag, Berlin, 1991, with permission.)

numbers of patients available to analyze response rates and toxicity. Many patients require ongoing radiation or chemotherapy, which can make it hard to evaluate the effect and morbidity of pleurodesis. Underlying pleural or pulmonary disease and minor degrees of entrapment of the lung confuse the interpretation of the response on chest radiographs. Assessment of symptoms is rarely meaningful because patients often have multiple reasons to feel dyspneic (e.g., pleural effusion plus lymphangitic spread of the tumor). Only recently has there been an attempt to develop well-designed clinical trials that include an adequate number of patients.

Intrapleural Cytotoxic Agents

Several different agents have been used to try to control pleural effusions by cytotoxicity rather than sclerosis. Some of these are thought to act indirectly by immunomodulation; others exert direct cytotoxicity. *Corynebacterium parvum* enjoyed a period of popularity as an intrapleural agent after it was found to be antitumoral activity in an animal model (Casali, et al., 1988; Felletti and Ravazzoni, 1983; McLeod, et al., 1985). Success rates ranging from 56 to 100 percent were reported, but at least one study found the incidence of pain and fever to be greater than that with tetracycline (Leahy, et al., 1985). It is not used routinely because the same or better results can be achieved with sclerosants that are more easily available. Intrapleural interleukin-2 was found to control effusions in a small number of patients in whom it induced lymphokine-activated killer cells (Nagashima, et al., 1987; Yasumoto, et al., 1987). The expense and systemic toxicity of interleukin-2 limit its routine use, and its role outside of the research setting remains to be shown.

Cisplatin is the drug that has been the most widely used for intracavitary chemotherapy. Multiple studies of intraperitoneal cisplatin, primarily for the treatment of ovarian cancer, have shown that it acts by cytotoxicity rather than sclerosis and that the local pharmacologic advantage achieved by intracavitary administration can lead to tumor regression when systemic treatment has failed (Kirmani, et al., 1991; Markman, et al., 1991). The depth of penetration of drugs given by the intracavitary route appears to be 5 mm or less; therefore they are not effective in the setting of bulky tumor (Markman, 1986). Cisplatin-based chemotherapy was also administered intrapleurally (Markman, et al., 1984, 1985), and the pharmacokinetic properties were found to be analogous to the intraperitoneal route of administration (Rusch, et al., 1992b). There has been one study of cisplatin-based intrapleural chemotherapy for malignant pleural effusions, which reported a 49 percent response rate (Rusch, et al., 1991). Intrapleural cisplatin carries the potential of significant toxicity because a significant amount is absorbed systemically (Rusch, et al., 1992b) and therefore is unlikely to be used routinely for the management of malignant pleural effusions. Rather it may be useful in clinical trials designed to maximize the local intrathoracic effects of chemotherapy (Rusch, et al., 1992a).

Techniques of Administration

Administration of Sclerosing Agents by Tube Thoracostomy. Good and Sahn (1978) believed strongly that the technique of administration of tetracycline affected the likelihood of pleurodesis being successful. They recommended insertion of a chest tube in the eighth or ninth intercostal space in the posterior axillary line and drainage of the effusion for 24 hours. Complete drainage of the pleural effusion and full expansion of the lung was documented by chest radiography. A dose of 15 to 20 mg/kg of tetracycline mixed in 75 ml of sterile water is then instilled through the chest tube into the pleural space. This is followed by 200 ml of air to facilitate contact of the tetracycline with both visceral and parietal pleural surfaces. The chest tube is clamped, and the patient is rotated to the left and right lateral decubitus, prone, and supine positions every 30 minutes to disperse the solution of tetracycline throughout the pleural cavity. At the end of 2 hours, the chest tube is unclamped and placed back on suction. It is removed when the drainage is less than 150 ml per 24 hours.

The methods proposed by Good and Sahn (1978) became widely accepted guidelines for the administration of any sclerosing agent by tube thoracostomy. However, in practice there are some variations in the precise technique used. The dose of tetracycline sometimes is a fixed dose (most often 1 g) and sometimes is calculated according to body weight (15 to 20 mg/kg). The solution and the amount of fluid in which it is mixed vary. Some physicians administer lidocaine before or with the instillation of tetracycline; others do not (Wallach, 1978). The length of time that the chest tube is left to drainage before instillation of the intrapleural agent also varies. Some physicians believe that drainage should be allowed to decrease 100 to 150 ml per 24 hours before instillation of the intrapleural agent; others proceed with instillation as soon as the pleural space is completely evacuated, usually within 48 hours of inserting the chest tube. Some physicians remove the chest 24 hours after pleurodesis; others leave it in place until the drainage is less than 150 ml per 24 hours. However, the principles to be considered in performing a pleurodesis by tube thoracostomy remain as follows: First for a pleurodesis to be effective, the lung must be fully expanded so that the parietal and visceral pleural surfaces are in apposition. Second there must be good dispersion of the agent throughout the pleural space. This is less likely to occur if the chest tube has been in for several days and loculations have begun to form around the tube. Third the pleural surfaces must be kept in close apposition after instillation of the agent for the chemical pleuritis to progress to pleural symphsis. This is most likely to happen if the chest tube is left in place and on suction until drainage is minimal.

Talc Poudrage. Talc can be administered as a suspension through a tube thoracostomy, but it is most often insufflated by poudrage. Traditionally asbestos-free talc was dry heat sterilized by hospital pharmacies and stored in sterile glass containers (test tubes or Petri dishes) in 5- to 10-g aliquots. It was then transferred to a bulb syringe or to a powder blower and insufflated at thoracoscopy or thoracotomy. Attaching the bulb syringe to a red rubber catheter facilitates insufflation at thoracoscopy. Insufflation by a powder blower can also be done by attaching it to a source of pressurized air or oxygen, just as would be done with an atomizer. This produces a finer and more uniform coverage of the pleura than does hand insufflation with a bulb syringe, but either method seems to produce a satisfactory pleurodesis. A spray can containing 4 g of sterile asbestos-free talc is now commercially available. This eliminates many of the logistic problems previously faced by hospitals in the preparation of sterile talc. Talc produces a rapid pleural symphysis, and it is helpful to insert two chest tubes (28 Fr anterior and posterior tubes or 28 Fr anterior and 32 Fr right-angle diaphragmatic tubes) to prevent loculated fluid collections. If these do develop during the immediate postoperative period, they usually are resorbed over 1 to 2 months subsequently. Another method of administering talc at thoracotomy is to mix it with a small amount of water to create a paste that is then spread across the pleural surfaces. However, poudrage is a faster and more convenient technique.

Administration of Cytotoxic Agents. A technique similar to that described by Good and Sahn (1978) for tetracycline is used for the administration of cytotoxic agents intrapleurally, but different considerations apply for cytotoxic than for sclerosing agents. They are left in the pleural space longer to maximize contact with the pleural tumor. The length of instillation time is dictated by the pharmacokinetic properties of the individual drug. Cisplatin is left in the peritoneal or pleural space for 4 hours because after that time it has been near totally absorbed into the systemic circulation (Markman, 1986; Rusch, et al., 1992b). The chest tube can be immediately removed after instillation of a cytotoxic drug because there is no need to produce pleural symphysis. However, full expansion of the lung before instillation of the drug should be documented just as for sclerosing agents because an effusion caused by a trapped lung is no more effectively treated by cytotoxic than by sclerosing agents.

Management of an Effusion in Patients with a Trapped Lung

Patients who have a trapped lung are not candidates for therapy with sclerosants and are unlikely to benefit from intrapleural cytotoxic agents because they have bulky tumor. Even though they have a collapsed unexpandable lung, some of these patients experience a relief of dyspnea and chest discomfort when the effusion is evacuated, perhaps because this alleviates mediastinal compression. Some patients have a lung that can re-expand partially and experience a definite improvement in pulmonary function with drainage of the effusion. The insertion of a pleuroperitoneal shunt is one way to palliate such patients (Cimochowski, et al., 1986; Little, et al., 1988; Bang, et al., 1990; Weese and Schouten, 1982). The device used for this procedure, the Denver pleuroperitoneal shunt (Codman and Shurtleff, Inc., Randolph, MA) is a single-unit silicone rubber conduit consisting of a unidirectional valved pumping chamber located between fenestrated pleural and peritoneal catheters. One catheter is introduced into the pleural space by using a Seldinger technique, and directed toward the posterior costophrenic sulcus. The other catheter is placed into the peritoneal cavity by a small upper quadrant muscle splitting incision. The pumping chamber is positioned in a subcutaneous pocket created over the anterolateral costal margin that provides a stable base for shunt compression (Ponn, et al., 1991). Pleuroperitoneal shunting is also a therapeutic option for patients with pleural effusions secondary to intractable ascites and has sometimes been combined with peritoneovenous shunting for such patients. However, active participation by the patient or family is required for the shunt to function because the pumping chamber must be actively compressed approximately 25 times every 4 hours. Patients who are unable to cooperate with this routine should not have a shunt implanted. In properly selected patients, pleuroperitoneal shunting provides good palliation with minimal morbidity. The risk of infection is minimal, but shunt occlusion as a result of fibrin deposition over the ends of the catheter occurs occasionally and may require replacement of the shunt.

Pleurectomy

Pleurectomy with or without decortication was one of the early approaches used for malignant pleural effusions. Jensik, et al. (1963) reported a series of 52 pleurectomies, 15 of which were associated with decortication. The immediate mortality rate was 6 percent, and the 30-day mortality rate was 18 percent. Two patients developed recurrent effusions, and the average survival was only 10.4 months. Subsequently, Martini, et al. (1975) reported on a series of 106 patients whose malignant pleural effusion was treated by pleurectomy. Most patients required two to three units of blood transfusion intraoperatively, and the overall 30-day mortality rate was 10 percent. In both of these series, which antedate modern chemotherapeutic regimens, patients with breast cancer had the longest survival. The high operative mortality rates undoubtedly reflect the poor performance status and limited reserve of patients who have malignant pleural effusions. With far less morbid therapeutic options now available, pleurectomy for the palliation of malignant pleural effusions has largely been abandoned. Only a highly selected group of patients are candidates for a pleurectomy. This includes patients who have a trapped lung and still have an excellent performance status.

SUMMARY

Patients who present with a pleural effusion should first undergo a thorough clinical evaluation to try to identify the likely cause. The size and location of the effusion and the determination of whether or not it is free flowing should be made on posteroanterior, lateral, and lateral decubitus chest radiographs. CT is helpful in characterizing effusions that appear loculated and in detecting underlying pulmonary or intra-abdominal disease that may be responsible for the effusion. Thoracentesis with biochemical analysis of the pleural fluid, culture, and cytologic examination should then be performed to determine whether the effusion is a transudate or an exudate, whether it is malignant, and to direct further evaluation. Ultrasound and CT can localize loculated effusions for thoracentesis. If the cytologic findings are negative and malignancy is suspected, percutaneous pleural biopsy and repeat thoracentesis and/or thoracoscopy is indicated to establish a definitive tissue diagnosis.

Transudative effusions are managed by therapy of the underlying medical condition. Exudative effusions are also treated in this manner if they are not malignant. Patients with malignant effusions must have a determination made as to whether the lung will fully re-expand after evacuation of the effusion. If the lung expands completely, the effusion can be managed by sclerosis. Talc is probably the most effective sclerosant currently available, although tetracycline and bleomycin have also been popular. Intrapleural cytotoxic agents should still be considered investigational. If the lung is trapped and the patient is symptomatic, pleuroperitoneal shunting is an option. The diagnosis and therapy have often been empiric in the past. The increasing use of thoracoscopy and attempts to perform more carefully designed clinical trials are improving the approach to this often debilitating problem.

KEY REFERENCES

Boutin C, Viallat JR, Aelony Y: Practical Thoracoscopy. Springer-Verlag, Berlin, 1991

> This is a beautifully illustrated text describing the techniques and applications of thoracoscopy.

Deslauriers J, Lacquet LK: Thoracic Surgery: Surgical Management of Pleural Diseases. CV Mosby, St. Louis, 1990

> This is a multiauthored text that provides an in-depth review of the pathophysiology and management of pleural diseases.

Hausheer FH, Yarbro JW: Diagnosis and treatment of malignant pleural effusion. Semin Oncol 12:54, 1985

> This is a comprehensive review of the management of malignant pleural effusion.

Light RW: Pleural Diseases. Lea & Febiger, Philadelphia, 1983

> This is a comprehensive reference on the diagnosis and therapy of pleural effusions with emphasis on the biochemical characteristics of pleural fluid.

REFERENCES

Adler RH, Rappole BW: Recurrent malignant pleural effusions and talc powder aerosol treatment. Surgery 62:1000, 1967

Adler RH, Sayek I: Treatment of malignant pleural effusion: a method using tube thoracostomy and talc. Ann Thorac Surg 22:8, 1976

Aelony Y, King R, Boutin C: Thoracoscopic talc poudrage pleurodesis for chronic recurrent pleural effusions. Ann Intern Med 115:778, 1991

Anderson CB, Philpott GW, Ferguson TB: The treatment of malignant pleural effusions. Cancer 33:916, 1974

Ariel IM, Oropeza R, Pack G: Intracavitary administration of radioactive isotopes in the control of effusions due to cancer. Cancer 19:1096, 1966

Asseo PP, Tracopoulos GD: Simultaneous enzyme immunoassay of carcinoembryonic antigen in pleural effusion and serum. Am J Clin Pathol 77:66, 1982

Austin EH, Flye WS: The treatment of recurrent malignant pleural effusion. Ann Thorac Surg 28:190, 1979

Bayly TC, Kisner DL, Sybert A et al: Tetracycline and quinacrine in the control of malignant pleural effusions. Cancer 41:1188, 1978

Bethune N: Pleural poudrage—a new technique for the deliberate production of pleural adhesions as a preliminary to lobectomy. J Thorac Surg Cardiovasc 4:241, 1935

Bitran JD, Brown C, Desser RK et al: Intracavitary bleomycin for the control of malignant effusions. J Surg Oncol 16:273, 1981

Boniface E, Guerin JC: Value of talc administration using thoracoscopy in the symptomatic treatment of recurrent pleurisy. Apropos of 302 cases. Rev Mal Respir 6:133, 1989

Bouchama A, Chastre J, Gaudichet A et al: Acute pneumonitis with bilateral pleural effusion after talc pleurodesis. Chest 85:795, 1984

Boushy SF, North LB, Helgason AH: Thoracoscopy: technique and results in eighteen patients with pleural effusion. Chest 74:386, 1978

Broaddus VC, Light RW: What is the origin of pleural transudates and exudates? Chest 102:658, 1992

Broaddus VC, Wiener-Kronish JP, Staub NC: Clearance of lung edema into the pleural space of volume-loaded anesthetized sheep. J Appl Physiol 68:2623, 1990

Camishion RC, Gibbon JH, Nealon TF: Talc poudrage in the treatment of pleural effusion due to cancer. J Clin North Am 42:1521, 1962

Casali A, Gionfra T, Rinaldi M et al: Treatment of malignant pleural effusions with intracavitary *Corynebacterium parvum*. Cancer 62:806, 1988

Chambers JF: Palliative treatment of neoplastic pleural effusion with intercostal intubation and talc instillation. West J Surg Obstet Gynecol 66:26, 1958

Chappel AG, Johnson A, Charles J et al: A survey of the long-term effects of talc and kaolin pleurodesis. Br J Dis Chest 73:285, 1979

Chertow BS, Kadzielawa R, Burger AJ: Benign pleural effusions in long-standing diabetes mellitus. Chest 99:1108, 1991

Cimochowski GE, Joyner LR, Fardin R et al: Pleuroperitoneal shunting for recalcitrant pleural effusions. J Thorac Cardiovasc Surg 92:866, 1986

Daniel TM, Tribble CG, Rodgers BM: Thoracoscopy and talc poudrage for pneumothoraces and effusions. Ann Thorac Surg 50:186, 1990

Dewald G, Dines DE, Weiland LH, Gordon H: Usefulness of chromosome examination in the diagnosis of malignant pleural effusions. N Engl J Med 295:1494, 1976

Dewald GW, Hicks GA, Dines DE, Gordon H: Cytogenetic diagnosis of malignant pleural effusions: culture methods to supplement direct preparations in diagnosis. Mayo Clin Proc 57:488, 1982

Falor WH, Ward RM, Brezler MR: Diagnosis of pleural effusions by chromosome analysis. Chest 81:193, 1982

Faurschou P: Diagnostic thoracoscopy in pleuro-pulmonary infiltrates without pleural effusion. Endoscopy 17:21, 1985

Faurschou P, Francis D, Faarup P: Thoracoscopic, histological, and clinical findings in nine case of rheumatoid pleural effusion. Thorax 48:371, 1985

Felletti R, Ravazzoni C: Intrapleural *Corynebacterium parvum* for malignant pleural effusions. Thorax 38:22, 1983

Felson B, Vix VA: Roentgenographic recognition of pleural effusion. JAMA 229:695, 1974

Fentiman IS, Rubens RD, Hayward JL: A comparison of intracavitary talc and tetracycline for the control of pleural effusions secondary to breast cancer. Eur J Cancer 22:1079, 1986

Frankel A, Krasna I, Barnofsky ID: An experimental study of pleural symphysis. J Thorac Cardiovasc Surg 42:43, 1961

Friedman MA, Slater E: Malignant pleural effusion. Cancer Treat Rev 5:49, 1978

Goldstein HA, Gefter WB: Detection of unsuspected malignant pleural effusion by bone scan. AJR 10:556, 1983

Good JT, Sahn SA: Intrapleural therapy with tetracycline in malignant pleural effusions: the importance of proper technique. Chest 74:602, 1978

Hamed H, Fentiman IS, Chaudary MA, Rubens RD: Comparison of intracavitary bleomycin and talc for control of pleural effusions secondary to carcinoma of the breast. Br J Surg 76:1266, 1989

Harley HRS: Malignant pleural effusions and their treatment by intercostal talc pleurodesis. Br J Dis Chest 73:173, 1979

Harper GR: Pleural effusions in cancer. Clin Cancer Briefs 1:1, 1979

Hartman DL, Mathur PN, Gaither JM et al: Comparison of thoracoscopic talc pleurodesis with standard chest tube using tetracycline and bleomycin for control of malignant pleural effusion (abstr). Presented at the 72nd Annual Meeting of the American Association for Thoracic Surgery, 1992

Herbert A, Gallagher PJ: Interpretation of pleural biopsy specimens and aspirates with the immunoperoxidase technique. Thorax 37:822, 1982

Hucker J, Bhatnager NK, Al-Jilaihawa N, Forrester-Wood CP: Thoracoscopy in the diagnosis and management of recurrent pleural effusions. Ann Thorac Surg 42:1145, 1991

Ike O, Shimizu Y, Hitomi S et al: Treatment of malignant pleural effusions with doxorubicin hydrochloride-containing (L-lactic acid) microspheres. Chest 99:911, 1991

Jensik R, Cagloe J, Milloy F et al: Pleurectomy in the treatment of pleural effusion due to metastatic malignancy. J Thorac Cardiovasc Surg 46:322, 1963

Johnson WW: The malignant pleural effusion: a review of cytopathologic diagnoses of 584 specimens from 472 consecutive patients. Cancer 56:905, 1985

Jones GR: Treatment of recurrent malignant pleural effusion by iodized talc pleurodesis. Thorax 24:69, 1969

Kavuru MS, Adamo JP, Ahmad M et al: Amyloidosis and pleural disease. Chest 98:20, 1990

Keeford RF, Woods RL, Fox RM, Tattersall MHN: Intracavitary Adriamycin, nitrogen mustard and tetracycline in the control of malignant effusions. Med J Aust 2:447, 1980

Kida T, Hujita Y, Sasaki M, Inoue J: Accumulation of ^{99m}Tc methylene diphosphonate in malignant pleural and ascitic effusion. Oncology 41:427, 1984

Kim D, Weber GF, Tomita JT, Hirata AA: Galactosyltransferase variant in pleural effusion. Clin Chem 28,5:1133, 1982

Kinasewitz GT, Fishman AP: Influence of alterations in Starling forces on visceral pleural fluid movement. J Appl Physiol 51:671, 1981

Kirmani S, Lucas W, Kim S et al: A phase II trial of intraperitoneal cisplatin and etoposide as salvage treatment for minimal residual ovarian carcinoma. J Clin Oncol 9:649, 1991

Ladjimi S, Djemel A, Ben Youssef R, Ben Ayed F: Diagnostic and therapeutic thoracoscopy in 83 cases of chronic pleurisy. Rev Mal Respir 2:355, 1985

Ladjimi S, M'Raihi ML, Djemel A et al: Pleural talc treatment using thoracoscopy in lymphomatous pleurisy. Rev Mal Respir 8:75, 1991

Ladjimi S, M'Raihi L, Djemel A, Mathlouthi A: Results of talc administration using thoracoscopy in neoplastic pleurisies. Apropos of 218 cases. Rev Mal Respir 6:147, 1989

Lambert CJ, Shah HH, Urschel HC Jr: The treatment of malignant pleural effusion by closed trocar tube drainage. Ann Thorac Surg 3:1, 1967

Landvater L, Hix WR, Mills M et al: Malignant pleural effusion treated by tetracycline sclerotherapy: a comparison of single vs. repeated instillation. Chest 93:1196, 1988

Lange P, Mortensen J, Groth S: Lung function 22–35 years after treatment of idiopathic spontaneous pneumothorax with talc poudrage or simple drainage. Thorax 43:559, 1988

Leahy BC, Honeybourne D, Brear SG et al: Treatment of malignant pleural effusions with intrapleural *Corynebacterium parvum* or tetracycline. *Eur J Respir Dis* 66:50, 1985

Leininger BJ, Barker WL, Langston HT: A simplified method for management of malignant pleural effusion. J Thorac Cardiovasc Surg 58:758, 1969

Lewis RJ, Caccavale RJ, Sisler GE: Video assisted thoracic surgical resection of malignant lung tumors. J Thorac Cardiovasc Surg 104:1679, 1992

Little AG, Kadowaki MH, Ferguson MK et al: Pleuroperitoneal shunting: alternative therapy for pleural effusions. Ann Surg 208:443, 1988

Markman M: Intracavitary chemotherapy. In Hickey R (ed): Current Problems in Cancer. Year Book Medical Publishers, Chicago, 1986

Markman M, Cleary S, King ME, Howell SB: Cisplatin and cytarabine administered intrapleurally as treatment of malignant pleural effusions. Med Pediatr Oncol 13:191, 1985

Markman M, Hakes T, Reichman B et al: Intraperitoneal cisplatin and cytarabine in the treatment of refractory or recurrent ovarian carcinoma. J Clin Oncol 9:204, 1991

Markman M, Howell SB, Green MR: Combination intracavitary chemotherapy for malignant pleural disease. Cancer Drug Delivery 1:333, 1984

Martini N, Bains MS, Beattie EJ Jr: Indications for pleurectomy in malignant effusion. Cancer 35:734, 1975

Masuno T, Kishimoto S, Ogura T et al: A comparative trial of LC9018 plus doxorubicin and doxorubicin alone for the treatment of malignant pleural effusion secondary to lung cancer. Cancer 68:1495, 1991

McLeod DT, Calverley PMA, Millar JW, Horne NW: Further experience of *Corynebacterium parvum* in malignant pleural effusion. Thorax 40:515, 1985

Migueres J, Jover A: Indications for intrapleural talc under pleuroscopic control in malignant recurrent pleural effusions. Based upon 26 cases. Poumon Coeur 37:295, 1981

Migueres J, Jover A, Bouissou H et al: Place de la ponction-biopsie à l'aiguille et du cyto-diagnostic dans le diagnostic des pleurésies malignes. Poumon Coeur 37:29, 1981

Monif GRG, Steward BN, Block AJ: Living cytology: a new diagnostic technique for malignant pleural effusions. Chest 69:626, 1976

Nagashima A, Yasumoto K, Nakahashi H et al: Antitumor activity of pleural cavity macrophages and its regulation by pleural cavity lymphocytes in patients with lung cancer. Cancer Res 47:5497, 1987

Oakes DD, Sherck JP, Brodsky JB, Mark JBD: Therapeutic thoracoscopy. J Thorac Cardiovasc Surg 87:269, 1984

Ohri SK, Oswal SK, Townsend ER, Fountain SW: Early and late outcome after diagnostic thoracoscopy and talc pleurodesis. Ann Thorac Surg 53:1038, 1992

Ostrowski MJ: An assessment of the long-term results of controlling the reaccumulation of malignant effusions using intracavity bleomycin. Cancer 57:721, 1986

Page RD, Jeffrey RR, Donnelly RJ: Thoracoscopy: a review of 121 consecutive surgical procedures. Ann Thorac Surg 48:66, 1989

Paladine W, Cunningham TJ, Sponzo R et al: Intracavitary bleomycin in the management of malignant effusions. Cancer 38:1903, 1976

Pearson FG, MacGregor DC: Talc poudrage for malignant pleural effusion. J Thorac Cardiovasc Surg 51:732, 1966

Pettersson T, Ojala K, Weber TH: Adenosine deaminase in the diagnosis of pleural effusions. Acta Med Scand 215:299, 1984

Pettersson T, Riska H: Diagnostic value of total and differential leukocyte counts in pleural effusions. Acta Med Scand 210:129, 1981

Poe RH, Israel RH, Utell MJ et al: Sensitivity, specificity, and predictive values of closed pleural biopsy. Arch Intern Med 144:325, 1984

Ponn RB, Blancaflor J, D'Agostino RS et al: Pleuroperitoneal shunting for intractable pleural effusions. Ann Thorac Surg 51:605, 1991

Prakash UBS, Reiman HM: Comparison of needle biopsy with cytologic analysis for the evaluation of pleural effusion: analysis of 414 cases. Mayo Clin Proc 60:158, 1985

Reshad K, Inui K, Takeuchi Y et al: Treatment of malignant pleural effusion. Chest 88:393, 1985

Rinaldo JE, Owens GR, Rogers RM: Adult respiratory distress syndrome following intrapleural instillation of talc. J Thorac Cardiovasc Surg 85:523, 1983

Rittgers RA, Loewenstein MS, Feinerman AE et al: Carcinoembryonic antigen levels in benign and malignant pleural effusions. Ann Intern Med 88:631, 1978

Rodriguez-Panadero F, Lopez Mejias J: Low glucose and pH levels in malignant pleural effusions. Diagnostic significant and prognostic value in respect to pleurodesis. Am Rev Respir Dis 139:663, 1989

Roth BJ, O'Meara TF, Cragun WH: The serum-effusion albumin gradient in the evaluation of pleural effusions. Chest 98:546, 1990.

Roth JA, Ruckdeschel JC, Weisenburger TH (eds): Thoracic oncology. WB Saunders, Philadelphia, 1989

Ruckdeschel JC, Moores D, Lee JY et al: Intrapleural therapy for malignant pleural effusions. Chest 100:1528, 1991

Rusch V, Saltz L, Venkatraman E et al: A phase II trial of pleurectomy/decortication followed by intrapleural and systemic chemotherapy for malignant pleural mesothelioma. J Clin Oncol (in press)

Rusch VW: The optimal treatment of malignant pleural effusions: a continuing dilemma. Chest 100:1483, 1991

Rusch VW, Figlin R, Godwin D et al: Intrapleural cisplatin and cytarabine in the management of malignant pleural effusions: a Lung Cancer Study Group trial. J Clin Oncol 9:313, 1991

Rusch VW, Mountain C: Thoracoscopy under regional anesthesia for the diagnosis and management of pleural disease. Am J Surg 154:274, 1987

Rusch VW, Niedzwiecki D, Tao Y et al: Intrapleural cisplatin and mitomycin for malignant mesothelioma following pleurectomy: pharmacokinetic studies. J Clin Oncol 10:1001, 1992b

Sahn SA: The pleura. Am Rev Respir Dis 138:184, 1988

Scarbonchi J, Boutin C, Cargino P, Scarbonchi-Efimieff T: Intrapleural talc in malignant pleural effusions. Poumon Coeur 37:283, 1981

Schneller J, Eppich E, Greenebaum E et al: Flow cytometry and feulgen cytophotometry in evaluation of effusions. Cancer 59:1307, 1987

Seibert AF, Hynes J, Middleton R, Bass JB: Tuberculous pleural effusion: twenty-year experience. Chest 99:883, 1991

Shedbalkar AR, Head JM, Head LR et al: Evaluation of talc pleural symphysis in management of malignant pleural effusion. J Thorac Cardiovasc Surg 61:492, 1971

Silverman LM, Dermer GB, Zweig MH et al: Creatinine kinase BB: a new tumor-associated marker. Clin Chem 25:1432, 1979

Smyrnios NA, Jederlinic PJ, Irwin RS: Pleural effusion in an asymptomatic patient: spectrum and frequency of causes and management considerations. Chest 97:192, 1990

Sorensen PG: Carcinoembryonic antigenic malignant pleural effusions: a negative report. Eur J Respir Dis 62:138, 1991

Srensen PG, Svendsen TL, Enk B: Treatment of malignant pleural effusion with drainage, with and without instillation of talc. Eur J Respir Dis 65:131, 1984

Tamura S, Nishigaki T, Moriwaki Y et al: Tumor markers in pleural effusion diagnosis. Cancer 61:298, 1988

Taylor SA, Hooton NS, Macarthur AM: Quinacrine in the management of malignant pleural effusion. Br J Surg 64:52, 1977

Thermann M, Loddenkemper R, Schroder D: Thoracoscopy—a forgotten endoscopic procedure? Endoscopy 17:203, 1985

Todd TRJ, Celarue NC, Ilves R et al: Talc poudrage for malignant pleural effusion. Chest 78:542, 1980

Tsang V, Fernando HC, Goldstraw P: Pleuroperitoneal shunt for recurrent malignant pleural effusions. Thorax 45:369, 1990

Vanderschuren RG: Thorascopie sous anesthésie locale. Poumon Coeur 37:21, 1981

Viallat JR, Tubiana N, Boutin C, Farisse P: Pleurisy in blood diseases: value of thoracoscopic poudrage. Rev Pneumol Clin 42:274, 1986

Vladutiu AO, Brason JW, Adler RH: Differential diagnosis of pleural effusions: clinical usefulness of cell marker quantitation. Chest 79:297, 1981

Voellmy W: Résultats diagnostiques de la thoracoscopie dans les affections du poumon et de la plèvre. Poumon Coeur 37:67, 1981

Wallach HW: Intrapleural therapy with tetracycline and lidocaine for malignant pleural effusions. Chest 73:246, 1978

Webb WR, Ozmen V, Moulder PV et al: Iodized talc pleurodesis for the treatment of pleural effusions. J Thorac Cardiovasc Surg 103:881, 1992

Weese JL, Schouten JT: Pleural peritoneal shunts for the treatment of malignant pleural effusions. Surg Gynecol Obstet 154:391, 1982

Weissberg D: Talc and adult respiratory distress syndrome (letter to the editor). J Thorac Cardiovasc Surg 87:474, 1984

Weissberg D, Kaufman M, Zurkowski Z: Pleuroscopy in patients with pleural effusion and pleural masses. Ann Thorac Surg 29:205, 1980

Wiener-Kronish JP, Broaddus VC, Albertine KH et al: Relationship of pleural effusions to increased permeability pulmonary edema in anesthetized sheep. J Clin Invest 82:1422, 1988

Wiener-Kronish JP, Matthay MA, Callen PW et al: Relationship of pleural effusions to pulmonary hemodynamics in patients with congestive heart failure. Am Rev Respir Dis 132:1253, 1985

Winkelmann M, Pfitzer P: Blind pleural biopsy in combination with cytology of pleural effusions. Acta Cytol 25:373, 1981

Xaubet A, Diumenjo MC, Marin A et al: Characteristics and prognostic value of pleural effusion in non-Hodgkin's lymphomas. Eur J Respir Dis 66:135, 1985

Yasumoto K, Miyakai K, Nagashima A et al: Induction of lymphokine-activated killer cells by intrapleural instillations of recombinant interleukin-2 in patients with malignant pleurisy due to lung cancer. Cancer Res 47:2184, 1987

Zaloznik AJ, Oswald SG, Langin M: Intrapleural tetracycline in malignant pleural effusions. Cancer 51:752, 1983

37

EMPYEMA AND BRONCHOPLEURAL FISTULA

Jean Deslauriers

EMPYEMA

An empyema can be defined as a grossly purulent pleural effusion. Although this infection usually originates from the lung, the portal of entry may be through the chest wall or from sources located below the diaphragm or in the mediastinum. Infection occurs when the host reaction is overwhelmed by the number and virulence of the inoculum. Whereas the normal pleural space is resistant to infection, the abnormal space, such as one that already contains blood or fluid, is highly susceptible to empyema formation.

The therapy of empyemas depends on a clear understanding of the pathogenesis of pleural infection. More than 75 years ago, Graham and Bell (1918) described the basic principles of empyema management as they still apply today. These principles involved adequate drainage of the empyema cavity, with avoidance of pneumothorax in the acute stage, and early sterilization with obliteration of the infected space. When these guidelines are followed and careful attention is given to specific antibiotic therapy, thoracotomy drainage when necessary, and maintenance of adequate nutrition, most empyemas can be successfully treated, even in the poor-risk patient.

HISTORICAL NOTE

Hippocrates is credited with the first recorded drainage operation for empyema. He clearly understood the natural history of undrained empyemas when he (1953) wrote in a treatise on pleurisy and "peripneumonia": "Les pleurétiques qui dès le commencement rendent des crachats de différentes couleurs et consistance meurent au troisième jour ou au cinquième; s'ils réchappent, c'est différé au septième ou au neuvième; ou bien ils commencent à suppurer au onzième."* Hippocrates (1965) also wrote: "When empyemata are opened by the cautery or by the knife, and the pus flows pale and white the patient survives, but if is mixed with blood, muddy and foul smelling, he will die."

The nineteenth century saw the introduction of aspiration of acute pleural effusions and Wyman (Atwater, 1972) and his colleague Henry I. Bowditch (1852) are credited with permanently establishing this procedure in the practice of medicine. The description of the first therapeutic thoracentesis was given by Wyman (Atwater, 1972) in a letter to Sir William Osler as follows: "With Dr. Homans' advice and assistance, the chest was punctured with an exploring trocar and cannula between the sixth and seventh ribs about six inches from the spine, and twenty ounces of straw colored serum drawn off slowly with great relief of the urgent symptom." Commenting on pleural space infections, Osler (1892) wrote (Moran, 1988), "It is sad to think of the number of lives which are sacrified annually by the failure to recognize that empyema should be treated as an ordinary abscess by free incision." Historic records indicate that, in 1819, Sir William Osler himself underwent a rib resection at his home for drainage of a postpneumonic empyema (Barondess, 1974; Varkey, et al., 1981).

Thoracentesis was modified by the description of closed-tube thoracostomy by Playfair (1875) and Hewitt (1876) and of siphon drainage and irrigation by Von Bülau (1891). As

---

* Translation to English of the quote from Hippocrates: "Patients with pleurisy who, from the beginning, have sputum of different colors or consistencies die on the third or the fifth day. If they survive, death is delayed until the seventh or the ninth day, or they become "suppurative" by the eleventh day."

thoracic surgery developed rapidly during that period, other procedures, such as thoracoplasty (Schede, 1890; Estlander, 1879) and decortication (Fowler, 1893; Delorme, 1894), were introduced to obliterate the space, either by collapsing the chest wall over the lung or by reexpanding the lung. The results were not always good, but in 1901, Fowler (Yeh, et al., 1963) concluded that decortication was applicable to all patients with chronic non-tuberculous empyemas who could tolerate the operation. He further said that decortication could be used instead of Estlander's operation in most cases and should replace the Schede operation in all.

The consequences of open pneumothorax and the importance of closed-tube drainage of empyemas were not appreciated until a 1918 survey by the Surgeon General of the United States. The mortality rates reported averaged 30 percent for rib resection and open drainage of acute empyemas (Graham and Bell, 1918). Because of the creation of an open pneumothorax, death frequently occurred within 30 minutes of the procedure and was attributed to the pneumothorax and mediastinal instability rather than to the empyema. The Empyema Commission headed by Graham recommended closed drainage rather than open drainage in the early stages of empyema, and soon after the adoption of these changes, the mortality rate decreased to 5 to 10 percent. Essential to these new principles was the careful avoidance of open pneumothorax in the acute stage, prevention of chronicity by rapid sterilization and obliteration of the infected cavity, and careful attention to the nutrition of the patient (Graham, 1925; Peters, 1989).

With the onset of the antibiotic era, the incidence of pneumococcal and streptococcal empyemas fell dramatically, and the mortality rate from empyemas also declined sharply. More recently, the increasing significance of anaerobic infections, the development of new generations of drug-resistant organisms, and the increasing frequency of immunosuppression has led to new problems because patients are often unable to produce the inflammatory reaction necessary to localize the empyema and obliterate the space (Delarue, 1990).

HISTORICAL READINGS

Atwater EC: Morrill Wyman and the aspiration of acute pleural effusions, 1850. A letter from New-England. Bull Hist Med 36:235, 1972

Barondess JA: A case of empyema: notes on the last illness of Sir William Osler. p. 59. In Transactions of the American Clinical and Clinicopathological Association: The 87th Annual Meeting. Vol. 86. Waverly Press, Baltimore, 1975

Bowditch HI: On pleuritic effusions and the necessity of paracentesis for their removal. Am J Med Sci 22:320, 1852

Delarue NC: Empyema: principles of management—an old problem revisited. p. 178. In Deslauriers J, Lacquet LK (eds): International Trends in General Thoracic Surgery. Vol. 6. CV Mosby, St. Louis, 1990

Delorme E: Nouveau traitement des empyèmes chroniques. Gazette des Hôpitaux 67:94, 1894

Estlander JA: Résection des côtes dans l'empyème chronique. Rev Med Chir (Paris) 3:156, 1879

Fowler GR: A case of thoracoplasty for the removal of a large cicatricial fibrous growth from the interior of the chest, the result of an old empyema. Med Record 44:938, 1893

Fowler GR, quoted by Meade R: A History of Thoracic Surgery. Charles C Thomas, Springfield, IL, 1961

Graham EA: Some fundamental considerations in the treatment of empyema thoracis. CV Mosby, St. Louis, 1925.

Graham EA, Bell RD: Open pneumothorax: its relation to the treatment of acute empyema. Am J Med Sci 156:939, 1918

Hewitt CF: Thoracentesis: the plan of continuous aspiration. BMJ 1:317, 1876

Hippocrate: Oeuvres Médicales: d'Après l'Édition de Foês. Aux Éditions du Fleuve, Lyon, 1953

Hippocrates, quoted by: Major Classic Descriptions of Disease. Charles C Thomas, Springfield, IL, 1965

Moran JF: Surgical management of pleural infections. Semin Respir Infect 3:383, 1988

Osler W: The Principles and Practice of Medicine. D. Appleton, New York, 1892

Peters RM: Empyema thoracis: historical perspective. Ann Thorac Surg 48:306, 1989

Playfair GE: Case of empyema treated by aspiration and subquently by drainage: recovery. BMJ 1:45, 1875

Schede M: Die Behandlung der Empyema. Virh Dtsch Ges Inn Med 9:41, 1890

Varkey B, Rose HD, Kulty K, Politis J: Empyema thoracis during a ten-year period. Analysis of 72 cases and comparison to a previous study (1952 to 1967). Arch Intern Med 141:1771, 1981

Von Bülau G: Für die Heber Drainage bei Behandlung des Empyems. Z Klin 18:31, 1891

Yeh TJ, Hall DP, Ellison RG: Empyema thoracis: a review of 110 cases. Am Rev Respir Dis 88:785, 1963

DEFINITIONS AND PATHOLOGY

An empyema is a collection of pus in a natural body cavity. One of the most common varieties of empyema is the empyema thoracis, which can either be localized (e.g., encapsulated or subpulmonic) or involve the entire pleural space (le Roux, et al., 1986).

Stages of Empyema Progression

The American Thoracic Society (1962) divides the formation of an empyema into three distinct stages, which indicate disease progression in the pleural space. These occur over

---

Pathologic Findings of Empyemas

Stage 1: Exudative, with swelling of pleural membranes.

Stage 2: Fibrinopurulent with heavy fibrin deposits.

Stage 3: Organization with ingrowth of fibroblasts and deposition of collagen.

Complications: (1) Pulmonary fibrosis and contraction of the chest wall. (2) Spontaneous drainage: (a) through the skin—empyema necessitatis; (b) through, the bronchus—bronchopleural fistula. (3) Others: osteomyelitis, pericarditis, mediastinal abscess.

a 3- to 4-week period. For management purposes, two stages are recognized: an acute process and an organizing phase.

During the exudative phase (stage I), there is considerable swelling of the pleural membranes with outpouring of thin exudative fluid. Fibrin is deposited over all surfaces, and despite early angioblastic and fibroblastic proliferation that extends outward from the pleura, the peel is not thickened enough to prevent complete lung reexpansion once the space is emptied. During the fibrinopurulent phase (stage II, Fig. 37-1), there are heavy fibrin deposits over all pleural surfaces, more so over the parietal pleura than over the visceral pleura. The pleural fluid is turbid or frankly purulent. At this stage, the pleura is still relatively intact, and the lung, although less mobile, can be reexpanded. Loculations form during this stage.

Within 3 to 4 weeks, organization (stage III) begins with massive ingrowth of fibroblasts and formation of collagen fibers over both parietal and visceral surfaces. The pus is very thick, and the lung, which at this stage is virtually functionless, is imprisoned within a thick fibrous peel. It can no longer expand without being decorticated. Within 7 weeks, arterioles can also be demonstrated that infiltrate the peel.

Complications

Complications can occur at any time during the formation of an empyema, but they are more likely to develop during the chronic stage of disease. One of the most common complications is caused by increasing amounts of fibrosis and scar tissue in the lung that produce pulmonary fibrosis. Scar tissue can also penetrate the parietal pleura and reach the intercostal spaces, which become narrowed and contracted. This gives the chest wall the appearance of a carapace (le Roux, et al., 1986).

Empyema necessitatis (Fig. 37-2) is characterized by the dissection of pus through the soft tissues of the chest wall and eventually through the skin. Similarly, the sudden appearance of purulent sputum signals the onset of a bronchopleural fistula with spontaneous drainage of pus into the bronchial tree (Fig. 37-3). In a series of 77 patients with bronchopleural fistula presented by Hankins, et al. (1978), spontaneous fistulas ($n = 28$) were secondary to tuberculosis in 23 patients and to bacterial pneumonia or lung abscess in 5. Unusual complications include rib or spine osteomyelitis, pericarditis, mediastinal abscesses, or caudal transdiaphragmatic drainage of the empyema into the peritoneal cavity.

Parapneumonic Effusions

Patients with bacterial pneumonia may have an associated pleural effusion, which is called a parapneumonic effusion. Uncomplicated effusions are nonpurulent, have a negative Gram stain result and culture, and do not loculate in the pleural space. They resolve spontaneously with antibiotic therapy (Potts, et al., 1978). Complicated effusions are either empyemas or loculated parapneumonic effusions that require surgical drainage for adequate resolution. According to Light, et al. (1980), the pleural fluid pH and lactate dehydrogenase (LDH) and glucose levels appear to be useful to differentiate uncomplicated from complicated parapneumonic effusions.

PATHOGENESIS

Most empyemas are the result of bacterial suppuration in organs that are contiguous to the pleural surfaces. Among these, the lungs are the most commonly contaminated. In such cases, empyema occurs by direct bacterial spread across the visceral pleura or by free intrapleural rupture of microscopic and peripherally located lung abscesses. In a classic description of putrid empyemas, Maier and Grace (1942) showed that most were associated with bronchiectasis, pulmonary abscess, and suppurative pneumonia. In most other series, empyemas are secondary to bronchopulmonary infections in 50 to 60 percent of cases (Yeh, et al., 1963; Sherman, et al., 1977; Ali and Unruk, 1990), and most if not all of the so-called primary empyemas are due to subclinical pneumonic processes. Vianna (1971) also showed that most patients with postpneumonic empyemas have various underlying conditions, such as alcoholism or chronic pulmonary diseases. Inactive pulmonary tuberculosis, diabetes mellitus, long-term steroid therapy, and various malignancies comprise other common predisposing conditions. Substance abusers are also known to be at risk for bacterial and aspiration pneumonia and other pulmonary infections. These may lead to parenchymal destruction with subsequent contamination of the pleural space, which results in either simple empyema or complex infections, including bronchopleural fistulas (Hoover, et al., 1988).

There is little evidence that hematogenous infections of the pleural space can occur from a distant infection site (classically, osteomyelitis) without an intermediate peripheral lung abscess, which then ruptures in the pleural space (le Roux, et al., 1986). In Sherman et al.'s series (1977) of 102 patients, 4 cases represented metastatic hematogenous seeding of the pleural space from cellulitis of the left foot, multiple subcutaneous abscesses in a heroin addict, gram-negative sepsis secondary to decubitus ulcers, and pelvic abscess after vaginal hysterectomy.

Other potential sources of infections should be looked for when the cause of empyema is unclear. Rupture of the esophagus, for instance, nearly always results in empyema formation. A clear history of prior endoscopy is obtained in most

---

Pathogenesis of Thoracic Empyemas

Contamination from a source contiguous to the pleural space (50–60%)
  Lung
  Mediastinum (esophagus or nodes)
  Deep cervical
  Chest wall and spine
  Subphrenic paracolic abscesses
Direct inoculation of the pleural space (30–40%)
  Minor thoracic interventions
  Postoperative infections
  Penetrating chest injuries
Hematogenous infection of the pleural space (1%)

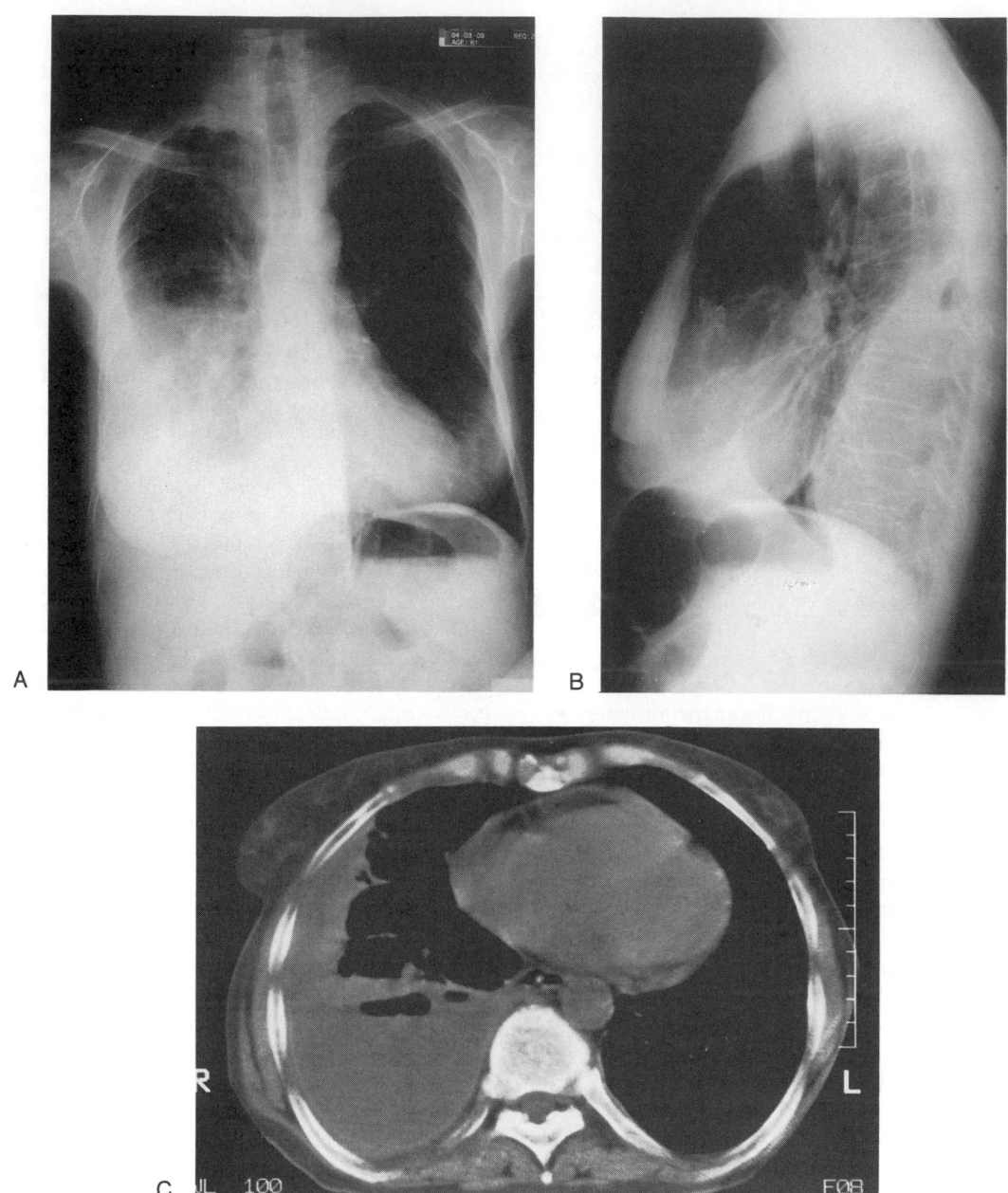

Figure 37-1. **(A)** PA and **(B)** lateral chest radiographs and **(C)** CT scan of a 62-year-old woman with postpneumonic empyema during the fibrinopurulent stage. Note the typical image of a posteriorly located inverted D-shaped density (pregnant lady sign). (*Figure continues*).

cases of instrumental perforation, but a high index of suspicion is often necessary to diagnose a spontaneous esophageal perforation. In those cases, empyema is the result of mediastinitis, with breach of the mediastinal pleura. Rare causes of contamination include infections in the deep posterior region of the neck and, more infrequently, infections in the chest wall or thoracic spine. Thoracic empyemas secondary to infected mediastinal nodes are highly unusual events.

Although subphrenic abscesses can occasionally contaminate the pleural space through direct transdiaphragmatic erosion, most effusions associated with these abscesses are ster-

ile exudates (Fig. 37-4). le Roux (1965) and Le Roux, et al. (1986) showed that lymph drainage from the subphrenic spaces is cephalad through the diaphragm, and this is the likely route of transferal of subphrenic infections to the pleural space. le Roux (1965) also noted that silent paracolic abscesses can occasionally erode through the diaphragm and infect the pleural space. Similarly, hepatic amebic (Whitton, 1990) or hydatic (Nin Vivo, et al., 1990) abscesses can erode through the diaphragm and produce secondary pleural empyemas.

Direct inoculation of the pleural space can occur as a result

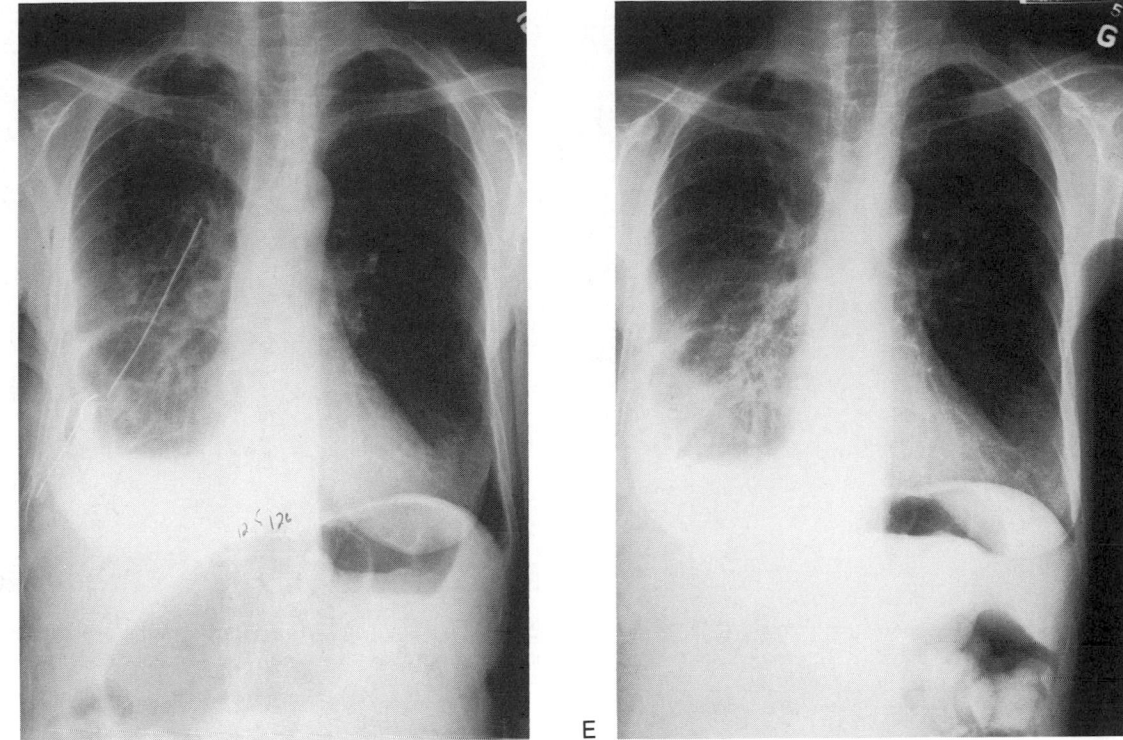

Fig. 37-1 (*Continued*).   **(D)** Chest radiograph taken after thoracoscopy drainage and **(E)** after complete resolution of the empyema.

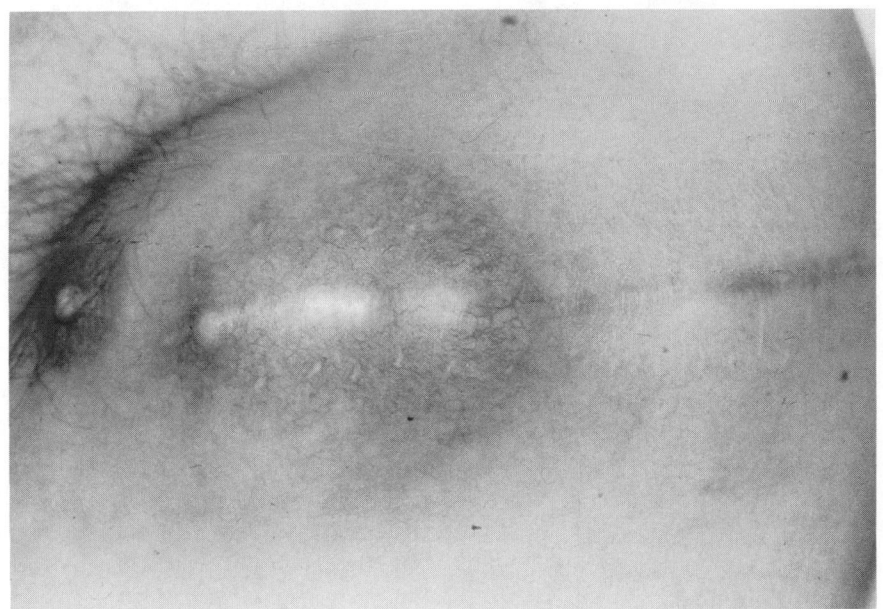

Figure 37-2.   Patient with an empyema necessitatis that has eroded through the soft tissues of the chest wall.

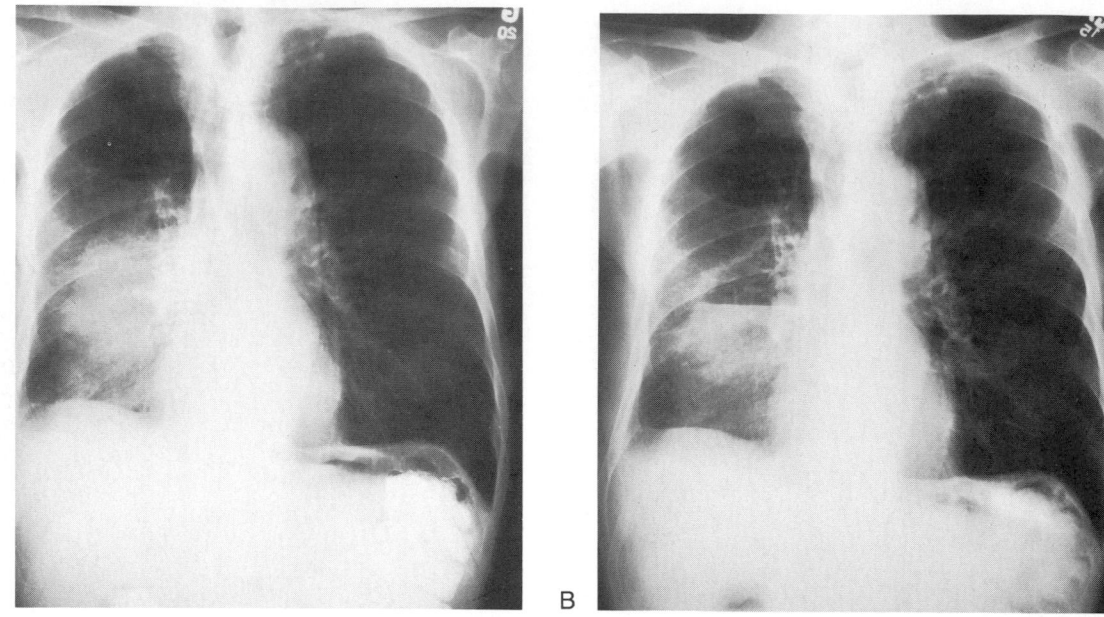

Figure 37-3. Bronchopleural fistula. **(A)** Chest radiograph of a 75-year-old man showing an empyema over the lower third of the right hemithorax. Three days later, the patient had sudden expectoration of abundant purulent material. **(B)** Repeated chest radiograph shows an air-fluid level containing space.

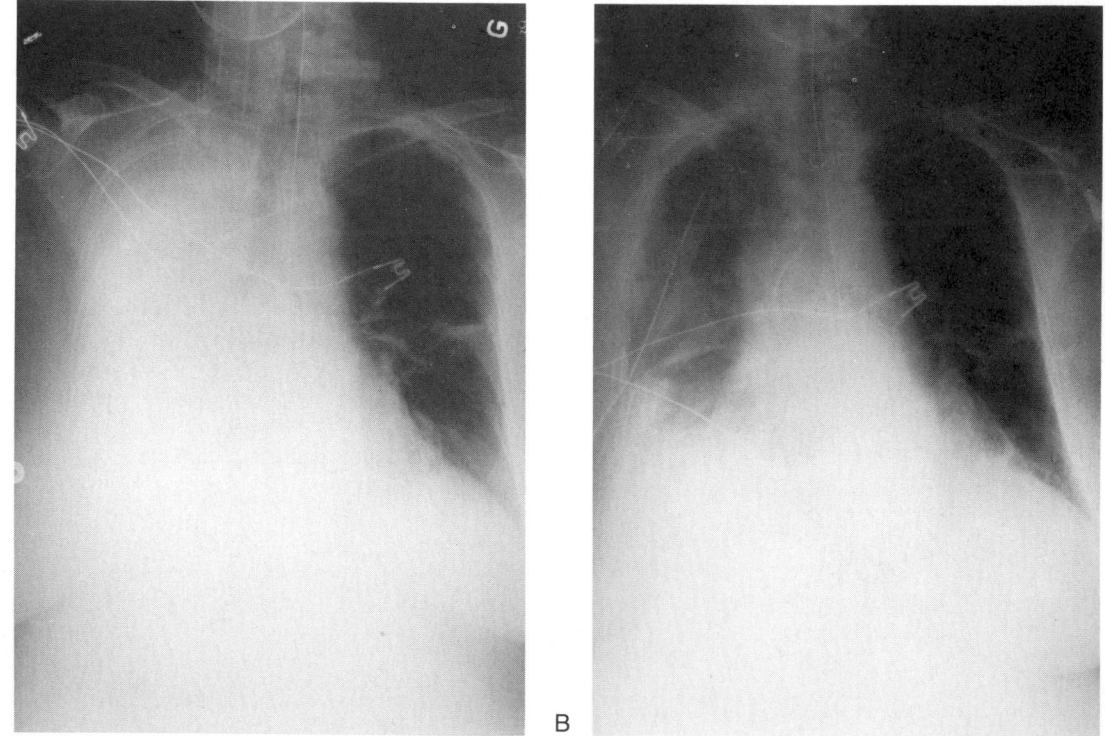

Figure 37-4. **(A)** PA chest radiograph of a 40-year-old patient with massive exudative effusion secondary to perforated Crohn's disease with multiple intra-abdominal abscesses. **(B)** Radiograph showing adequate drainage and lung re-expansion.

of minor thoracic interventions, such as thoracentesis, blind pleural biopsy, or chest tube drainage. In a series published in the early 1980s (de la Rocha, 1982), empyema secondary to minor procedures was identified in eight patients. The procedures that preceded the development of pleural sepsis were dilatation of the esophagus ($n = 2$), biopsy of the liver ($n = 1$), thoracentesis ($n = 3$), thoracoscopy ($n = 1$), and chest tube drainage ($n = 1$). Postoperative empyemas are almost exclusively seen after operations in which the esophageal or bronchial lumens have been entered. The incidence of this complication is in the range of 6 to 8 percent after pneumonectomy and 1 to 2 percent after lobectomy.

Virtually all post-traumatic empyemas are associated with penetration of the chest wall or the presence of a hemothorax. In the first instance, empyema formation is the result of organic foreign bodies being carried into the pleural space (Thurer and Palatinos, 1987). In an interesting study, Ogilvie (1950) showed that the nature of the missile (e.g., shell splinters, bullets, or bayonets) played little part in determining the rate of infection in empyemas secondary to penetrating injuries. In the second instance, the hemothorax becomes secondarily infected by way of contamination through the chest tube or from an infection in the adjacent lung. In 1977, Arom et al. (1977) made a distinction between post-traumatic empyemas and infected organizing hemothoraces (clotted hemothoraces) in which masses of blood clot became secondarily infected. It has also been shown by Ogilvie (1950) that air in the pleural space associated with blood is more likely to become secondarily infected than is a pneumothorax or a hemothorax alone. In an experimental model for empyema thoracis, Mavroudis, et al. (1985) showed that concomitant hemothorax increased the incidence of empyema and early death after *Staphylococcus aureus* was inoculated in the pleural space ($P < 0.05$).

In rarer cases, traumatic empyemas follow blunt esophageal rupture, acute diaphragmatic hernia with bowel strangulation and/or necrosis, or aspiration of a foreign body with perforation of lung tissue (Baethge, et al., 1990).

BACTERIOLOGY

In the preantibiotic era, the predominant organisms recovered from empyemas were pneumococci and *Streptococcus pneumoniae* (Brown, et al., 1956; Keefer, et al., 1941). While summarizing a total of 3,000 empyema cases reported from 1934 to 1939, Ehler (1941) noted that pneumococci were found in 63.9 percent of empyemas, *Streptococcus pyogenes* in 9.4 percent, and *S. aureus* in 6.5 percent. He concluded that other organisms were found so rarely as to be curiosities (Bartlett, et al., 1974). The incidence of empyema was greater (80 percent) with streptococcal pneumonia than with other types of pneumonia because of the greater lung destruction. In those cases, myriad tiny abscesses occurred along the lymphatic channels and discharged the infecting organisms into the effusion in great quantities; this converted the effusion into an empyema within a matter of hours (Thomas, et al., 1966).

The introduction and increasing use of antibiotics was accompanied, not only by a marked reduction in the incidence and mortality rates of empyemas, but also by a change in the

spectrum of causative organisms. In a study on the changing ecology of acute bacterial empyema, Finland and Barnes (1978) showed that streptococcal pneumonia declined from 1935 to 1953 but continued to occur in community-acquired empyemas. The incidence of *S. aureus*-related empyema increased, and it became the most frequent organism in 1955. It declined to its original levels after 1965, but gram-negative rods increased in importance. The predominant isolates in recent years have been *S. aureus* (29 to 69 percent of culture-positive cases) and enteric gram-negative bacilli (29 to 60 percent of culture-positive cases) (Bartlett, et al., 1974). In a report by Vianna (1971), 41 patients with bacterial pneumonia complicated by empyema were studied, and *S. aureus* was the most common causative organism isolated (14 of 41, 34 percent). Gram-negative bacteria were isolated in 64 percent of empyemas that complicated some other underlying disease, a feature interpreted as partly the result of previous antibiotic therapy. The incidence of *S. aureus*-induced empyemas has also increased in children. During the years 1955 to 1958, it was the causal organism in 92 percent of cases in children younger than 2 years, as reported by Ravitch and Fein (1961).

The recovery rates for anaerobes vary from 19 (Sullivan, et al., 1973) to 76 percent (Bartlett, et al., 1974). These microorganisms are normal inhabitants of the mouth, intestines, and female genital tract. They reach the lung by aspiration from the mouth or bacteremic spread from the intestines or areas of pelvic suppuration. In the series reported by Sullivan, et al. (1973), 226 culture-proved empyemas were analyzed, and anaerobes were isolated in 44 patients. More than 50 anaerobic bacteria were identified, but the most common was Peptostreptococcus. In that series, 41 deaths occurred among 184 patients with aerobes (22 percent), and 8 occurred among 42 patients with either anaerobes alone or a mixture of aerobes and anaerobes (14 percent mortality rate).

In the series of Bartlett's et al. (1974), 76 percent of patients with empyemas had either anaerobes alone (35 percent) or in combination with aerobic agents (Table 37-1). In most cases, the flora were complex, with an average of three different species of bacteria per case. According to Bartlett, et al., the paucity of anaerobic isolates in most reports of empyema is due to inadequate methods to preserve oxygen-sensitive forms during transfer to the laboratory and lack of adequate anaerobic culture techniques.

Often, a culture of empyema fluid does not establish a microbiologic diagnosis. In one series (le Roux, 1965) in which most patients had been treated elsewhere with various antibiotics before being referred for surgical management, a causal organism could not be isolated in 80 percent of patients.

DIAGNOSIS

The diagnosis of an empyema is made on clinical grounds, the presence of leukocytosis, characteristic findings on chest radiographs, and the recovery of purulent fluid from the pleural space.

The possibility of an empyema should always be raised in the presence of an acute illness with an associated pleural effusion. Typical symptoms, such as high fever, toxicity, or

Table 37-1. Bacteriologic Findings in 83 Cases of Empyema

	Total Cases	Anaerobes Only (%)	Anaerobes Plus Aerobes or Facultative Bacteria (%)	Aerobic or Facultative Bacteria only
Prospective cases	35	13 (37)	12 (34)	10
Retrospective cases	48	16 (33)	22 (46)	10
Total	83	29 (35)	34 (41)	20

(From Bartlett JG, Thadepalli H, Gorbach SL, Fingold SM: Bacteriology of empyema. Lancet 1:338, 1974, with permission.)

local tenderness, are often present. In the series of Varkey et al. (1981) of 72 cases of empyema, the most common initial manifestations were dyspnea (82 percent), fever (81 percent), cough (70 percent), and chest pain (67 percent). In addition, a major underlying disease was present in 45 patients. Because the symptoms are related to such factors as the cause and stage of the empyema, the amount of pus in the pleural space, the status of the host's defense mechanisms, and the virulence of the microorganisms involved, they may vary from only a few to those of severe toxicity. Symptoms may also vary in relation to the cause of the empyema. Patients with parapneumonic empyemas, for instance, often present with cough and purulent sputum; the symptoms of patients with empyemas secondary to subphrenic abscesses may be exclusively abdominal complaints. On the basis of the clinical history, Maier and Grace (1942) divided cases of putrid anaerobic empyemas into two groups. In the first group, expectoration of foul sputum indicated the presence of a pulmonary anaerobic suppurative process or of an anaerobic empyema with a bronchopleural fistula. In the second group, the foul sputum was absent, and the symptoms suggested ordinary pneumonia. Most patients with an empyema have leukocytosis, with a shift of the cell count to the left.

Chest radiographs show a pleural effusion with or without underlying pneumonia or lung abscess. On lateral radiographs, the empyemas are nearly always posterior and lateral, and most extend to the diaphragm. The classic image is that of a posteriorly located inverted D-shaped density (pregnant lady sign) as seen in the lateral chest film (Fig. 37-1B). Computed tomographic (CT) scanning is useful to differentiate between a lung abscess and an empyema, to ascertain the underlying pulmonary pathologic condition, to stage the empyema (as determined by the thickness of the fluid and the presence or absence of a trapped lung), and to assess the degree of loculations present.

Ultrasound may be used to document the presence of fluid or distinguish between pleural fluid, pleural thickening, or parenchymal consolidation. It is also useful for guided pleural needle aspiration of fluid, especially when the position of the diaphragm cannot be documented with certainty on standard radiographs. As described by Moran (1988) and Orringer (1988), an empyemogram can be done by injecting contrast material at the time of initial thoracentesis and then by obtaining posteroanterior (PA) and lateral chest films and decubitus views. This technique may provide information about the extent of the empyema cavity and the presence or absence of loculations within the space.

After the presence of pleural fluid has been confirmed, diagnostic thoracentesis should be carried out without delay.

Orringer (1988) showed that the gross appearance and odor of pleural fluid are among the most significant items of informations obtainable by thoracentesis. Thin fluid, even with positive bacteriologic findings may respond to selective antibiotherapy and thoracentesis; thick pus requires formal surgical drainage. Anaerobic pus is usually foul; aerobic pus has no offensive odor.

The aspirated fluid should be sent for Gram staining, aerobic and anaerobic cultures, and antibiotic sensitivity. Several authors have shown that careful attention to the technique is important to recover anaerobes. Varkey, et al. (1981) noted that the variability in the reported incidence of anaerobic empyemas may be due to differences in the methods of transportation and processing of the pleural fluid specimens. In addition to standard bacteriologic examinations, pleural fluid should also be sent for viral, tubercular, and fungal cultures. The percentage of negative cultures varies between 25 and 60 percent; this variation is caused by inappropriate culture techniques or the use of effective antimicrobial agents, which can penetrate the empyema fluid and prevent bacterial growth (Bergeron, 1990). In the presence of an empyema necessitatis, the microorganisms recovered from the cutaneous drainage may not be responsible for the disease because the fistula may be contaminated by skin flora or hospital pathogens.

The biggest controversy in pleural fluid analysis relates to its biochemistry. Some authors (Light, 1985, 1987; Houston, 1987) believe that pleural effusions with low fluid pH (less than 7.0), low glucose concentration (less than 50 mg/dl), and high LDH contents (more than 1,000 IU/L) should be drained because these parameters indicate a complicated effusion or impending empyema. These changes can be picked up before organisms are found on Gram staining or culture, and they usually occur concomitantly. In uncomplicated effusions, the pH is greater than 7.30, the glucose level is less than 60 mg/dl, and the LDH concentration is less than 1,000 IU/L (Sahn and Light, 1989), and these need not be drained. If the patient has free-flowing nonpurulent fluid with borderline biochemical parameters, Sahn and Light (1989) recommend appropriate antibiotic therapy and repeated thoracentesis 12 hours later. If the pleural fluid measurements are stable or improving, continued antibiotic therapy is warranted, but if there is a worsening of these measurements, chest tube drainage is generally necessary for resolution (Sahn and Light, 1989). In the series of Potts et al. (1976), three categories of parapneumonic effusions were characterized. A pH greater than 7.30 was present in all 10 benign effusions, and spontaneous resolution occurred in each case. All 10 empyemas and the 4 loculated effusions had a pH less than 7.30.

Regrouping of Patients with Empyema into Diagnostic Classes

Class I: Low pH pleural effusion. Postpneumonia effusion, pleural fluid pH less than 7.2, negative pleural fluid cultures.

Class II: Classic empyema. Positive pleural fluid cultures, absence of multiple loculations on chest radiograph.

Class III: Complicated empyema. Multiple loculations on chest radiograph, initially or subsequently, or trapped lung.

(From Van Way III C, Narrod J, Hopeman A: The role of early limited thoracotomy in the treatment of empyema. J Thorac Cardiovasc Surg 96:436, 1988, with permission.)

Physiologically, these biochemical changes are explained by an increased leukocytic activity and acid production in the pleural fluid.

Based on all these diagnostic parameters, Van Way, et al. (1988) proposed a useful method of regrouping patients with empyemas into diagnostic classes. Patients with class I empyemas ($n = 12$) were treated with short-duration chest tubes, and there were no deaths. Patients with class II empyemas ($n = 28$) were treated with chest tubes, and there were 2 deaths (7 percent). There were 40 patients with class III empyemas, and most required some form of surgical intervention.

During the investigation of patients with empyemas, it is also important to look for the causative process. Sullivan, et al. (1973), for instance, showed that carious teeth, retained roots, or advanced periodontal disease were present in 17 of 24 patients, with anaerobic empyemas of pulmonary origin. Bronchoscopy should always be done to rule out foreign bodies or endobronchial tumors.

MANAGEMENT

Acute Empyema

In acute empyemas, antibiotics are used to control the infection, and intercostal tube drainage is both simple and effective to drain and obliterate the space. Repeated thoracentesis, in conjunction with antibiotic therapy, may be indicated when the fluid is thin and the toxicity is well controlled. According to Moran (1988), antibiotics and thoracentesis can be curative in nearly all cases of parapneumonic effusions if the therapy is instituted early enough. By contrast, Personne (1990) indicated that thoracentesis alone is usually a mistake because the chances of complete success are minimal. It often leads to the formation of multiloculated pockets, which eventually become difficult to drain. Ferguson (1990) further noted that, "although simple drainage and antibiotic therapy remain the norm, an enlarging group of patients, particularly those with complicated or post operative empyema, will require aggressive surgical intervention. Early recognition of these patients and institution of surgical intervention as primary therapy rather than as a last resort will likely result in improved survival and shortened hospital stay." Open drainage plays no role in the therapy of acute empyemas.

Antibiotics

Several factors, such as the pathogen involved, the stage of the empyema, and the immune status of the host, determine the response to antibiotics. Concentrations of antibiotics in the infected pleural space must be high enough to neutralize the pathogens, a feature possible during the exudative phase of disease but less likely during the fibrinopurulent or organization stages (Bergeron, 1990). Initially and while awaiting for the results of antibiotic susceptibility, a semisynthetic penicillin, such as cloxacillin, or clindamycin should be given if the empyema has been acquired in the community or if the Gram staining reveals clusters of gram-positive cocci compatible with *S. aureus* (Bergeron, 1990). A guide to the choice of antibiotics is given in Table 37-2. In patients with anaerobic or gram-negative empyemas, penicillin is the antibiotic of choice; clindamycin can also be used. It is generally agreed that antibiotics should be continued for a period of 4 to 6 weeks.

Drainage

Surgical removal of pus by proper pleural space drainage remains the cornerstone of empyema management. This procedure not only evacuates the pus but also allows for the apposition of pleural surfaces, a feature that eventually leads to obliteration of the pleural space and resolution of the infection. The timing of surgical drainage and the choice of the drainage procedure must be tailored to the individual patient (Moran, 1988).

Pleural drainage can be accomplished by closed-tube thoracostomy, by open thoracotomy, or by thoracoscopy. Following proper ultrasound or CT delineation of the size, shape, and location of the collection, we now routinely use video thoracoscopic techniques to "clean out" the space and position the tube in the most dependent portion of the cavity (see Ch. 43). With this technique, the pus can be completely evacuated, the loculations can be broken down, and the fibrin peel can be removed from the surface of the lung. In patients too ill to tolerate a general anesthetic, drainage can be done under local anesthesia. In such cases, be careful not to penetrate the diaphragm, which is often retracted upward and indistinguishable from the caudal end of the empyema.

Drainage can also be accomplished by early open thoracotomy (Personne, 1990; Van Way, et al., 1988; Morin, et al., 1972, Hoover, et al., 1986), a procedure wrongly termed early decortication (Mandal and Thadepalli, 1987; Fishman and Ellertson, 1977; Frimodt-Moller and Vejlsted, 1985). Open thoracotomy is indicated when tube thoracostomy is unsuccessful because of multiple loculations or inaccessible purulent collections (Mavroudis, et al., 1981). Under general anesthesia, a small incision is made over the cavity, and a short segment of rib is resected. The empyema is then completely evacuated (Fig. 37-5). Through a separate incision, a large-bore chest tube is secured in the most dependent portion of the space. In Fishman and Ellertson's series (1977), six of

Table 37-2. Choice of Antibiotics in Empyemas

Organism	First Choice	Alternative
Gram-positive bacteria		
S. pneumoniae	Penicillin	Erythromycin, clindamycin
S. aureus (BL−)	Penicillin	Cefazolin, clindamycin
S. aureus (BL+)	Oxacillin	Cefazolin, clindamycin
S. aureus (methicillin resistant)	Vancomycin	Ciprofloxacin, aminoglycosides
Staphylococcus epidermidis (BL−)	Penicillin	Cefazolin, clindamycin
S. epidermidis (BL+)	Oxacillin	Cefazolin, clindamycin
S. epidermidis (methicillin resistant)	Vancomycin	Ciprofloxacin, aminoglycosides
Streptococcus fecalis	Ampicillin, gentamycin	Vancomycin
Gram-negative bacteria		
Pseudomonas aeruginosa	Ceftazidime	Imipenem, aminoglycosides, ticarcillin, ciprofloxacin
Escherichia coli, Proteus mirabilis	Cefazolin	Cefamandole, cefotixin, ampicillin (if sensitive)
H. influenzae	Cefamandole	Cefuroxime, ampicillin (if sensitive)
Bacteroides fragilis	Clindomycin or metronidazole	Cefotixin

Abbreviation: BL (+ or −), β-lactamase producer or nonproducer.
(From Bergeron MG: The changing bacterial spectrum and antibiotic choice. p. 197. In Deslauriers J, Lacquet LK (eds): International Trends in General Thoracic Surgery. Vol. 6. CV Mosby, St. Louis, 1990, with permission.)

eight immunosuppressed patients survived "early decortication" and were discharged 3 to 6 weeks after the operation. Morin, et al. (1972) also reported excellent results with early thoracotomy in 23 patients with posteriorly located D-shaped densities seen on the lateral chest radiograph. In Van Way, et al.'s series (1988), limited thoracotomy for drainage and placement of tubes was done in 22 patients, and all had resolution of their empyemas with no additional procedure. Miller (1990) also advocates early thoracotomy at 3 to 4 weeks when standard chest tube thoracostomy does not relieve the loculated fluid because the surgical risk in less than 1 percent and the expected outlook is good in more than 95 percent of patients. Of 52 reported patients, there were no operative deaths, and good results were obtained in 50 of 52. In substance abuse patients, exploratory thoracotomy is recommended within 24 to 48 hours if the patient has toxic manifes-

---

Principles of Therapy of Acute Empyemas

Appropriate selection of antibiotics

Drainage: closed-tube drainage, video-assisted thoracoscopic drainage, open "rib resection" drainage (early thoracotomy or early decortication)

Intrapleural fibrinolytic enzymes (streptokinase or urokinase)

Supportive measures: respiratory care, nutrition, therapy of associated medical conditions

Therapy of the underlying cause of empyema

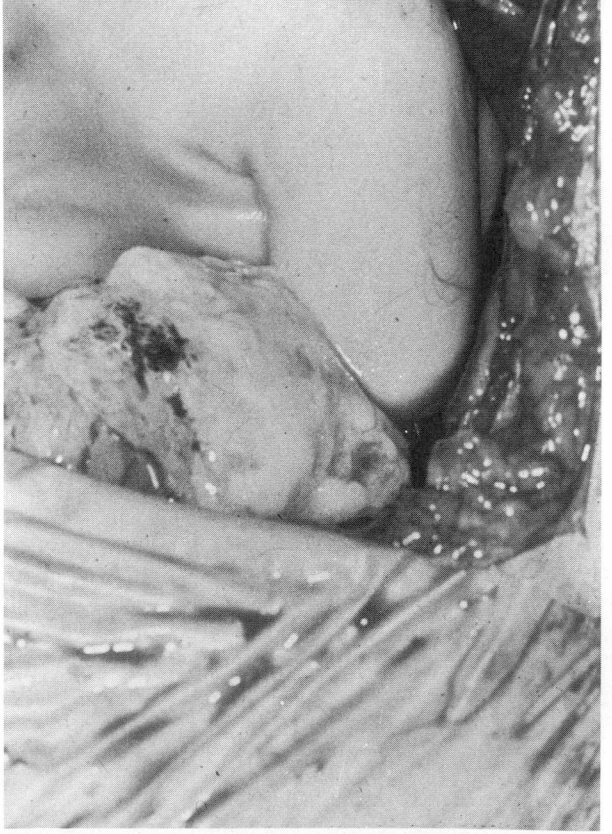

Figure 37-5. Operative photograph showing fibrin being removed from an empyema space through a rib resection thoracotomy. (Courtesy of Jean Morin, M.D.)

tations despite drainage, or if there is evidence of parenchymal destruction, multiple loculations, or trapped lung (Hoover, 1988).

In post-traumatic empyemas, the criteria for early decortication include residual air-fluid levels despite chest tube drainage, a clinically deteriorating course with evidence of infection or sepsis that arises from the pleura, pleural restriction with inadequate expansion of the lung, and failure of chest tubes to allow for resolution of pleural contamination within 14 days of injury (Coon and Shuck, 1975). Decortication is even more indicated in post-traumatic empyema because the infection occurs within a pleural clot the periphery of which is already well organized and fibrous (Pezzella, et al., 1983; Villalba, et al., 1979).

If the lung expands well, the chest tube (it is irrelevant how it was inserted) is left under suction drainage for a period of 2 to 3 weeks or until the space is permanently obliterated. This is likely to have occurred when the daily amount of drainage is low (less than 25 ml/day), when there are no up-and-down movements of fluid in the tubing, or when no pneumothorax develops if the tube is opened to atmospheric pressure. At this point, closed drainage can be changed to open drainage by cutting off the chest tube close to the chest wall. The tube is then shortened at the rate of about 1 inch/ week or until granulation tissue and fibrosis lead to its spontaneous expulsion from the pleural space (Fig. 37-6). When the lung expands well with tube drainage and there is no persistent empyema cavity, intrapleural irrigation of antibiotics, as suggested by Luizy, et al. (1966); Dieter, et al. (1970); and Rosenfeldt, et al. (1981) presents no additional advantages.

Intrapleural Enzymes

The use of intrapleural enzymes for the therapy of acute empyemas was described by Tillett and Sherry (1949). At the recommended dose of 250,000 units diluted in 100 ml of physiologic saline solution, streptokinase appears to be beneficial as a stimulant of the liquefaction of fibrin clots and facilitates the subsequent drainage of the pleural space (Bergh, et al., 1977). In some cases, it may also alleviate the need for decortication. These enzymes should not be given during the acute phase of empyema (Barrett, 1954) and they should be used with caution because they can be associated with severe allergic reactions. More recently, Robinson, et al. (1994) presented a series of 13 consecutive patients with fibrinopurulent empyemas who had incomplete drainage. Streptokinase (250,000 units in 100 ml of 0.9 percent saline solution) or urokinase (100,000 units in 100 ml of 0.9 percent saline solution) was instilled daily into the chest tube, and the tube was clamped for 6 to 12 hours, followed by suction. This regimen was completely successful in 10 of 13 patients (77 percent), with resolution of the empyema, eventual withdrawal of the chest tubes, and no recurrence.

The use of talc has also been described by Weissberg and Kaufman (1986). They reported on five patients with fibrino-purulent empyemas who did not respond to conventional therapy and in whom intrapleurally insufflated talc powder led to pleurodesis. Although no side effects were observed, this technique should clearly be restricted to a few selected patients.

Supportive Measures

Supportive measures, which include proper respiratory care with therapy of associated respiratory infection and obstructive pulmonary disease and maintenance of nutrition by enteral feedings, are essential for the successful management of early empyemas. Active chest physiotherapy is particularly important to promote lung reexpansion and prevent chest wall contraction. Because nearly 50 to 60 percent of patients with parapneumonic empyemas have a major associated medical illness, it is imperative that this condition be diagnosed and appropriately managed.

Chronic Empyemas

Usual causes of chronicity include a delay in diagnosis, improper drainage during the acute phase, continuing reinfection (such as occurs with a bronchopleural fistula or lung abscess), presence of a foreign body, or presence of a specific infection (such as tuberculosis or a fungal infection). In 1896, Paget (Holmes Sellors and Cruickshank, 1951) wrote, "One might add a score of cases to show that an unhealed empyema is, as a rule, the direct result of the patient's neglect, or of

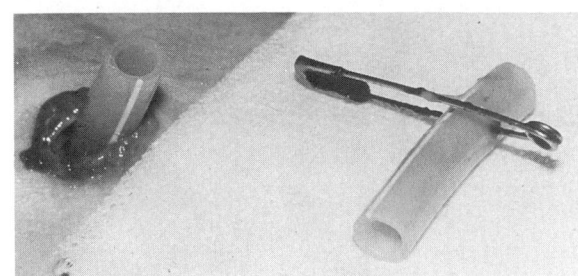
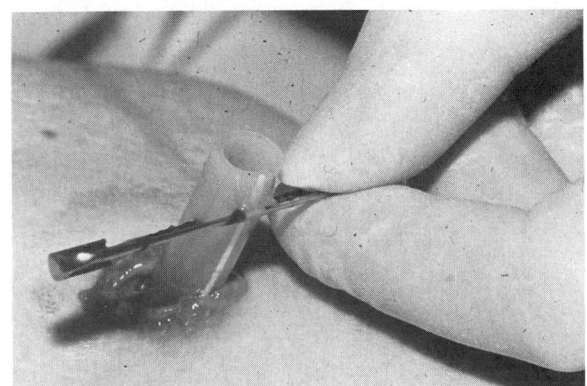

Figure 37-6. **(A)** Chest tube being shortened by about 1 inch. **(B)** Safety pin being used to prevent tube from falling back into the space.

the surgeon's delay, or of inadequate and useless surgery; but our business now is to inquire how we may most surely and safely cure it.'' Chronicity is diagnosed by persisting and/or increasing fever and chest pain, thick pleural fluid, unresolving radiologic findings, and incomplete reexpansion of the lung following closed drainage (Delarue, 1990). When the empyema has reached this stage, simple forms of therapy, such as rib resection, open drainage, or window thoracostomy, may be useful initially, but they are, as a rule, ineffective for definitive space obliteration. Decortication of the lung, space filling by muscle transplants, space collapse, or space sterilization are alternative therapeutic options that should be considered before a final decision is made.

Rib Resection Drainage and Open Thoracic Window

The first therapeutic priority is to provide adequate drainage of the empyema. In poor-risk patients, this can be accomplished either by inserting a large drainage tube or by the creation of an open thoracic window. Lemmer, et al. (1985) noted that early rib resection, especially for postoperative empyemas and for empyemas that have occurred in immunosuppressed patients, was likely to result in fewer therapeutic failures. In their series, control of the empyema was obtained in 10 of 11 patients treated by this method.

Rib resection drainage is a relatively minor procedure, but it should be done only a time at which sufficient adhesions have formed between the visceral and parietal pleura. It is primarily indicated for debilitated poor-risk patients and for patients with small residual spaces that are expected to obliterate early (Samson, 1971). The operation is performed under general anesthesia. It requires the resection of a short segment of rib over the most dependent part of the cavity, the opening and deloculation of the space, and the insertion of a large multifenestrated tube into the cavity. If the visceral pleural is thin and ''stretchable,'' space obliteration may eventually occur through lung reexpansion, contraction of the space, and filling by granulation tissue. With this technique, the recovery period is long, and frequent dressings and tube changes are usually needed. In Conlan, et al.'s series (1983), 50 patients with chronic empyemas without bronchopleural fistulas were treated with rib resection, closed tube drainage, and twice-daily instillation of 2 percent taurolidine solution into the empyema space through the drainage tube. Forty-one patients underwent further therapy, which consisted of drain removal, decortication, or open-window thoracostomy.

A more permanent form of drainage can be established by the creation of an open-window thoracostomy, a technique originally described by Eloesser (1935) as a drainage procedure for acute tuberculous empyemas (see elsewhere in this book). An open thoracic window is particularly useful for patients in whom long-term drainage may be required. The advantages of the technique are that the cavity can easily be irrigated and cleaned and the dressings can be changed daily on an outpatient basis. Given time, some of these windows close spontaneously, either by filling of the space with granulation tissue or by complete reepithelialization from the skin flaps (Fig. 37-7) (Virkkula and Eerola, 1974). In most patients, however, the space is too large for spontaneous closure to occur. In these cases, the window may have to be left open permanently, or it may be closed at a later stage with muscle transplant on a pedicle.

Space Sterilization

Sterilization of chronic persistent empyema cavities was originally described as a therapeutic option for parapulmonary empyema spaces. According to Virkkula, et al. (1990), Heuer (1920) first described space sterilization techniques when he discussed the therapy of 24 patients with chronic empyemas, some of which were of tuberculous origin. He used drainage

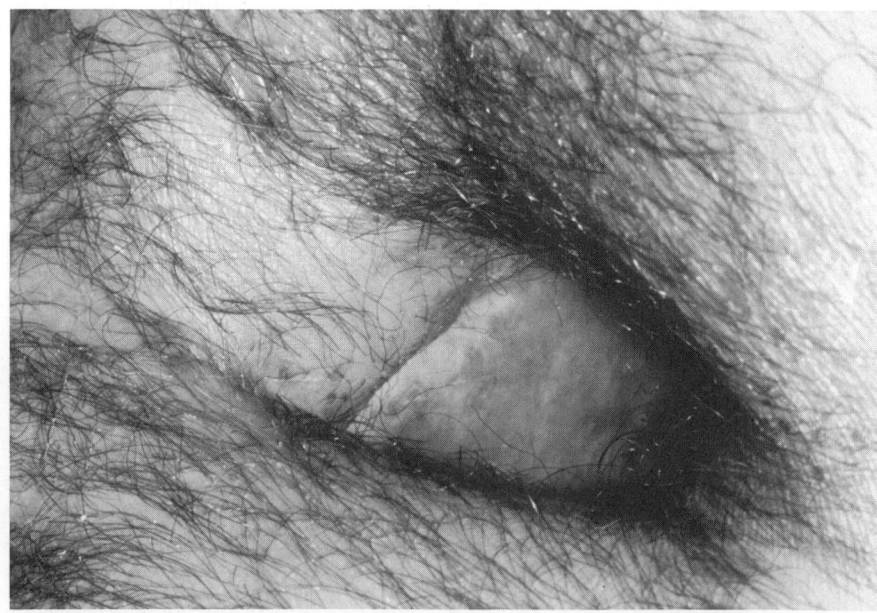

Figure 37-7.   Open thoracic window that closed spontaneously by reepithelialization from the skin flaps.

and sterilization of the empyema cavities with antiseptic chemicals. In a number of patients, he tried, in addition to space sterilization, operative maneuvers that involved the parietal pleura.

One of the most significant contributions to the therapy of chronic empyemas was made by Clagett and Geraci (1963) who, in 1963, reported a technique of space sterilization of postpneumonectomy empyemas (see elsewhere in this book). This technique was effective in 50 to 70 percent of patients who did not have an associated bronchopleural fistula (Stafford and Clagett, 1972; Goldstraw, 1979).

Space sterilization techniques can also be used in patients with empyemas without previous pneumonectomy (Weissberg, 1982; Bayes, 1987). In Weissberg's series, open-window thoracostomy was created in 12 patients with empyema and sepsis after conventional therapy with antibiotics and drainage had failed. Complete obliteration of the empyema cavity by granulation tissue occurred in 11 of 12 patients within 1 to 8 months; the time variation depended on the size of the space. Smolle-Jüttmer, et al. (1992) also showed that open-window thoracostomy is worthwhile because of its potential for rapid and low-risk control of severe life-threatening septic conditions in desperate cases of pleural empyema.

Space Filling

Decortication and Empyemectomy. Decortication is defined as the removal of a constricting peel and empyemectomy, as the complete excision of the empyema space and of its contents (see Ch. 42). Both of these procedures are done to encourage lung reexpansion in the hope of filling the residual space. The success rates depend on an intact visceral pleura, a lung that is expandable, and most importantly, a space that can be obliterated by pulmonary reexpansion. In a series of 94 patients reported on by Sensenig, et al. (1963), the results of decortication for chronic non-tuberculous empyema were as follows: good, 79; passable, 9; and poor, 2. Four patients died, all of them older than 45 years of age. To eradicate any potential source of chronic infection completely, it is occasionally necessary to resect a segment or lobe of the lung adjacent to the empyema. In a few cases, total pleuropneumonectomy may be necessary.

Muscle Transposition. Since it was first reported by Abrashanoff (1911), muscle flaps on pedicles have been used extensively (Miller, et al., 1984; Pairolero, et al., 1983) for the therapy of residual infected pleural spaces, whether closed or in the form of open-window thoracostomies. The indications for muscle transposition include obliteration of persistent pleural spaces and reinforcement of the bronchial stump following closure of an associated bronchopleural fistula (Deschamps, et al., 1990).

Viable tissue in the cavity is essential for successful surgery. The muscle selection should be based, not only on its availability, but also on the location, size, and shape of the empyema space. The blood supply, innervation, and bulk of the muscle must be preserved, and it must fill the entire space because empyema is likely to recur if a residual space is left. No attempt to close small bronchopleural fistulae (less than 2 mm) should be made; however, large fistulae must be de-brided and closed. Space drainage should always be used during the first 10 to 12 postoperative days.

The surgical procedure consists of mobilizing the appropriate muscle and inserting it in the empyema space by removing a portion of one or two ribs. For apical spaces, the pectoralis major is ideal; the latissimus dorsi or serratus anterior may be used for low posterior spaces. In some cases, a thoracoplasty may also be required to obliterate large cavities.

Space Collapse—Thoracoplasty

The concept of resecting ribs to decrease the size of the thorax and collapse an infected space was first described by Estlander (1879) and Schede (1980) (see Ch. 43). In 1937, Alexander (1937) reintroduced some of these principles. He proposed a posterior extramusculoperiosteal approach through which the residual spaces could be collapsed in most cases.

During the last 30 years, collapse therapy has lost much of its popularity because it is considered by many to be a mutilating and poorly tolerated operation. Two recent studies have shown, however, that extrapleural thoracoplasty is an excellent therapeutic option for selected patients. In the Hopkins, et al. (1985) series of 30 patients, the operative mortality rate was 10 percent, and permanent space closure was obtained in 82 percent of the survivors. Grégoire, et al. (1987) showed that, of 17 patients who underwent one-stage thoracoplasties for the therapy of postpneumonectomy empyemas, there were no operative deaths, and immediate control of the empyema was obtained in 15 (88 percent) patients.

In 1989, Nakaoka, et al. (1989) presented the cases of 22 patients with chronic empyema thoracis who underwent decortication. In 11 of them, decortication alone did not achieve sufficient lung reexpansion, and the parietal wall was collapsed, without rib resection, to contact the surface of the decorticated lung. All 11 patients had a one-stage cure, and in all, pulmonary function was well preserved.

BRONCHOPLEURAL FISTULA

Bronchopleural fistulae aggravate the clinical course of empyemas and constitute a major therapeutic challenge. The presence of a bronchopleural fistula indicates persistent contamination of the pleural space, difficulties in the reexpansion of the lung, and possible aspiration in the remaining lung. For most patients with empyemas, the presence or absence of a bronchopleural fistula makes the difference between recovery, chronicity, or death.

INCIDENCE AND PATHOGENESIS

Bronchopleural fistulae usually follow pulmonary resection. In the series of Malave et al. (1971), 1,307 pulmonary resections were done, and in 35 patients (2.7 percent), bronchopleural fistulae developed. Pertinent etiologic factors included endobronchial tuberculosis, drug-resistant organisms, contamination of the pleural space, concomitant illness, and surgical technique. In a more recent study (Vester, et al., 1991), the overall incidence of postresection fistulae was 1.6 percent (35 of 2,243 resections), and approximately two-thirds of the patients underwent preoperative radiotherapy, chemotherapy, or both. Postoperative bronchopleural fistulae can either be at the bronchial or at the peripheral level (alveolar peripheral air leak).

Patients are considered to have a spontaneous fistula if no previous pulmonary resection has been carried out (Hankins, et al., 1978). These usually occur in association with tuberculosis, bacterial pneumonia, or lung abscesses. They can also be seen with spontaneous pneumothoraces, especially those secondary to chronic obstructive pulmonary disease or to acquired immunodeficiency syndrome (AIDS) (Crawford, et al., 1992). In the series of Crawford et al., 44 patients with AIDS were treated for spontaneous pneumothorax, and in 14 of them, a persistent bronchopleural fistula for more than 10 days developed.

MANAGEMENT

The management of patients with postresection fistulae depends on why the bronchial stump or lung tissue has failed to hold the sutures (Perelman and Rymko, 1990). Primary failures result from poor closure technique, persistent pathologic changes in the bronchial wall, or impaired healing, such as that seen in patients who have undergone radiotherapy. In these cases, the therapy may be conservative with suction drainage of the pleural cavity and possible use of fibrin sealants applied over the lung surface (McCarthy, et al., 1988; Jørgensen, et al., 1984) or through the flexible fiberoptic bronchoscope (York, et al., 1990; Jensen and Sharna, 1985). In some cases, reclosure of the bronchus, reamputation of the stump, additional sealing of the pulmonary sutures, or additional resection may be advisable (Perelman and Rymko, 1990).

Secondary failures occur in empyemas in which the bronchial stump reopens because of local pressure by the purulent exudate (Perelman and Rymko, 1990). In this situation, drainage should be done initially followed by definitive management, which consists of bronchial reclosure, myoplasty, or thoracoplasty. These patients are usually very ill, and definitive therapy should be delayed until the empyema has become chronic and the patient's overall medical condition has improved. Puskas, et al. (1994) showed that direct surgical repair of chronic bronchopleural fistulae may be achieved in most patients by suture closure and aggressive transposition of vascularized flaps on pedicles.

EMPYEMA IN CHILDREN

Empyemas that occur in children are usually complications of upper or lower respiratory tract infections. As in adults, the pathologic response is divided into three phases, and the principles of therapy are based on appropriate antibiotic therapy, adequate drainage, and maintenance of lung expansion.

INCIDENCE, PATHOGENESIS, AND BACTERIOLOGY

Nearly all empyemas that occur in children are of the post-pneumonic type, although it is difficult to determine the exact incidence of this complication. Stiles, et al. (1970) reported on a series of 152 patients (1955 to 1969) with acute pneumonia that was accompanied by enough pleural fluid to be significant in regard to the clinical management. These patients were considered to have acute pneumonia with empyema. Most were secondary to staphylococcal pneumonia, and five deaths occurred, an overall mortality of 3.3 percent. By contrast, series published in the 1980s nearly always reported on less than 40 cases (Mayo, et al., 1982; Raffensperger, et al., 1982; Kosloske and Cartwright, 1988; Gustafson, et al., 1990). Raffensperger, et al. (1982) noted that "more effective antibiotics have practically eliminated the disease." This apparent decline in the incidence of empyemas in children not only is related to better physician education but to better and more specific medical management of the pneumonia and secondary pleural effusion. It is possible, however, that in future years, the incidence will be on the rise again, with the emergence of antibiotic-resistant microorganisms and of immunosuppression in children with AIDS or other related syndromes. In developing countries, pleural sepsis is still prevalent (Farpour and Sojedee, 1967; Anyanwa and Egbue, 1981). Factors such as malnutrition and poor hygiene complicate the clinical progress and management of children with pneumonia.

Not unlike what has been noted in the adult population, the bacteriologic findings of empyema in children have changed considerably over the years. In the preantibiotic era, pneumococci (Ravitch and Fein, 1961) and streptococci were the most frequent organisms isolated in postpneumonic empyemas (Gustafson, et al., 1990). After World War II, *S. aureus* became the most prevalent bacterium, and this is well documented in several reports (Henchen and Haggerty, 1958; Koch, et al., 1959). In a classic article on empyema written in 1961, Ravitch and Fein (1961) noted that there had not been any cases of empyema caused by *Haemophilus influenzae* since 1944 nor any as a result of streptococci since 1948. Furthermore, they had seen only five cases caused by pneumococci since 1947. In Cattaneo and Kilman's (1973) report, coagulase-positive staphylococci were the offending organisms in 80 percent of the positive pleural cultures; only three patients had pneumococci. Stiles, et al. (1970) also showed that, when a definite organism could be identified, staphylococci were recovered in 93 percent of cases (78 of 84). In recent years, *H. influenzae,* β-hemolytic streptococci, *S. pneumoniae,* and anaerobes have emerged as the leading offending organisms (Foglia and Randolph, 1987; Kosloske, 1988). In Kosloske and Cartwright's (1988) series of 22 patients treated by open drainage, streptococci ($n = 5$) and *H. influenzae* ($n = 3$) were the most common single pathogens.

In children, the bacteriologic findings of empyema are important because they affect the speed and severity of loculations that develop in the space. Anaerobic effusions, for instance, loculate quickly and often require aggressive surgical drainage because of a thick pleural peel not amenable to conventional therapy (Gustafson, et al., 1990). By contrast, staphylococcal effusions are often fibrinoid deposits with little actual fluid. If there is fluid, it is unilocular and amenable to adequate drainage by conventional tube thoracostomy.

CLINICAL PRESENTATION AND DIAGNOSIS

The most common presenting symptom of an empyema in children is fever. In a series of 42 patients with either parapneumonic effusion ($n = 21$) or empyema ($n = 21$) presented by Chonmaitree and Powell (1983), the clinical signs associated with effusion included fever (81 percent), tactile and vocal fremitus (81 percent), and respiratory difficulties (52 percent). For patients with empyema, the clinical signs were also fever (95 percent), tactile and vocal fremitus (62 percent), and respiratory difficulties (62 percent). In the series of McLaughlin et al. (1984) of 16 patients aged 1 month to 15 years, fever, cough, and dyspnea were the most common symptoms and signs; all three appeared in 12 of 16 patients (75 percent) on admission. Other clinical signs include decreased breath sounds, tachypnea (30 to 40 breaths/min), tachycardia, intercostal retractions, and lethargy (25 percent of patients in the series of McLaughlin et al. (1984). Middlekamp, et al. (1969) noted that symptoms of upper respiratory infection, cough, lethargy, anorexia, malaise, fever, abnormal respiratory rate, and grunting respiration were commonly associated with empyema.

The white blood cell count is nearly always elevated (15,000 to 20,000) with a shift to the left in the differential count. Radiographic findings include the presence of pleural effusion, pneumonic infiltrates, or pneumatoceles. In Chonmaitree and Powell's series (1983), pneumonic infiltrates associated with empyema were lobar in distribution in 52 percent of the patients, segmental in 33 percent, and bilateral patchy in 14 percent. Sometimes, it is not possible to distinguish between pulmonary infiltrates and pleural effusion or pleural fibrin deposits (fibrinous pleurisy). Foglia and Randolph (1987) showed the importance of using CT to ascertain more accurately the configuration of the fluid collections and lung compression and to differentiate parenchymal from pleural involvement.

Thoracentesis is a more definitive diagnostic procedure and should be done early in patients with a parapneumonic effusion. It may show frank pus or a positive Gram stain result, or biochemical findings that suggest an infectious process may be found.

MANAGEMENT

In 1982, Mayo, et al. (1982) described the goals of therapy of acute nontuberculosis empyemas in children, that is, "to save life with complete elimination of the empyema and the avoidance of recurrent empyema pockets; to return respiratory function promptly to normal by reexpansion of the trapped lung and restoration of mobility of the chest wall and diaphragm; to eliminate complications or chronicity and thereby any need for a crippling or debilitating surgical procedure; to reduce days of hospital stay." Despite these clearly outlined objectives, the management of empyema is still controversial in the pediatric literature.

Goals of Therapy in Acute Nontuberculous Empyema in Children

To save life
To eliminate the empyema
To reexpand the trapped lung
To restore mobility of the chest wall and diaphragm
To return respiratory function to normal
To eliminate complications or chronicity
To reduce the duration of hospital stay

(From Mayo P, Saha SP, McElvein RB: Acute empyena in children treated by open thoracotomy and decortication. Ann Thorac Surg 34:401, 1982, with permission.)

In 1987, Foglia and Randolph (1987) nicely showed that the specific therapy of empyema in children should be based on the stage of disease, the type of bacteria that predominate within the pleural fluid, the response to the therapy instituted, and the degree of lung trapping. Most children with empyema recover when treated with parenteral antibiotics that are selected on the basis of pleural fluid culture and appropriate tube drainage. Drainage may also be required for massive effusions with respiratory distress or when there is a pneumothorax associated with the empyema (pyopneumothorax).

If there is no resolution of the process, as evidenced by radiographs that show persistent fluid loculations or thick pleural shadows for several weeks, persistence of symptoms or leukocytosis, or progression of pulmonary infiltrates despite adequate drainage and antibiotics, open deloculation is recommended by many authors (Mayo, et al., 1982; Raffensperger, et al., 1982; Kosloske and Cartwright, 1988; Gustafson, et al., 1990). Gustafson, et al. (1990) showed that "early decortication in these highly select patients with symptomatic respiratory empyemas shortened the hospital stay, minimized the risks of long term use of antibiotics and prolonged chest tube drainage, completely reexpanded the trapped lung, and led to excellent long term results." In this series, the recover-

---

Factors Influencing Therapy in Nontuberculous Empyema in Children

Stage of disease
Specific bacteria isolated
Response to the therapy instiued
Degree of lung trapping

(From Foglia RP, Randolph J: Current indications for decortication in the treatment of empyema in children. J Pediatr Surg 22:28, 1987, with permission.)

ies in all such treated patients were rapid. The procedure consisted of breaking down loculations and establishing proper drainage, which can be done by minithoracotomy, full thoracotomy, or with the thoracoscope in older children. The use of thoracentesis alone with antibiotics parenterally and/or intrapleurally or of streptokinase solutions infused through the chest tube (Rodgers, 1987) is not recommended if a true empyema has been diagnosed.

The second factor of importance for the therapy of empyemas in children is the organism isolated from the pleural fluid (Foglia and Randolph, 1987). *S. aureus* or other gram-positive organisms usually induce unilocular empyemas that are amenable to good drainage by accurate placement of a large intercostal catheter (Kosloske, 1986). These almost never require early deloculation. By contrast, anaerobic empyemas tend to be loculated, and empyemas produced by β-hemolytic streptococci, *S. pneumoniae,* and *H. influenzae* cause a thick fibrous peel over the lung.

The third factor that may alter therapy is the degree of lung trapping, as documented on the CT scan. Foglia and Randolph (1987) showed that "when the empyema reaches an organized stage and no free fluid remains, there is little excuses for waiting for weeks to see if some resolution of the process will occur. In those instances, formal decortication should be carried out early because lung growth and function may be permanently adversely affected."

In modern days, there is little role for the conversion of closed-tube thoracotomy to open drainage because the failure rate is notoriously high and the morbidity and mortality rates are unacceptable (Mayo, et al., 1982).

CONCLUSION

Empyema thoracis has been a major clinical concern throughout recorded medical history. During the twentieth century, and particularly over the past two decades, management has been influenced by the identification of a spectrum of new and more virulent pathogens and by the increasing incidence of immunologically compromised hosts.

The introduction of new antibacterial agents has been a major advance in the therapy of these infectious problems. In many centers, deloculation by thoracoscopic or open thoracotomy techniques is also performed early to reexpand the lung and prevent the more serious complications associated with chronicity.

The overall mortality rate associated with empyemas currently ranges between 9 and 33 percent (Benfield, 1981; Grant and Finley, 1985; Jess, et al., 1984). Most deaths occur in elderly patients or depend as much on the condition that predispose the patient to the empyema as on the empyema itself.

KEY REFERENCES

Barrett NR: The treatment of acute empyema. Ann R Coll Surg Engl 15:25, 1954

This is an excellent discussion of various therapies that have been applied to acute empyemas over the years.

Bergeron MG: The changing bacterial spectrum and antibiotic choice. p. 197. In Deslauriers J, Lacquet LK (eds): International Trends in General Thoracic Surgery. Vol. 6. CV Mosby, St. Louis, 1990

This is an excellent review of the bacteriologic findings in empyemas and of the principles to follow while selecting antibiotic therapy.

Foglia RP, Randolph J: Current indications for decortication in the treatment of empyema in children. J Pediatr Surg 22:28, 1987

The authors present the principles of empyema management in children. This is a good discussion that highlights the controversies.

Light RW: Parapneumonic effusions and empyema. Clin Chest Med 6:55, 1985

This is a complete review from a medical standpoint of the pathophysiology, investigation, and management of empyemas.

Moran JF: Surgical management of pleural space infections. Semin Respir Infect 3:383, 1988

This is a good review article on the surgical management of empyemas. The authors analyze all surgical options to manage empyemas in the acute or chronic form.

Robinson LA, Moulton AL, Fleming WH et al.: Intrapleural fibrinolytic treatment of multiloculated empyemas. Ann Thorac Surg 57:803, 1994

This article analyzes the indications, techniques, and results of the intrapleural use of fibrinolytic agents. The authors provide an excellent review of the principles involved in empyema management.

REFERENCES

Abrashanoff: Plastishe Methode zur Schliessung von Fistel-gangen welche von inneren Organen kommen. Zentralbl Chir 38:186, 1911

Alexander J: The Collapse Therapy of Pulmonary Tuberculosis. Charles C Thomas, Springfield, IL, 1937

Ali I, Unruh H: Management of empyema thoracis. Ann Thorac Surg 50:355, 1990

American Thoracic Society, Medical Section of the National Tuber-culosis Association: Management of non tuberculous empyema. Am Rev Respir Dis 85:935, 1962

Anyanwu CH, Egbue M: Management of pleural sepsis in Nigerian children. Thorax 36:282, 1981

Arom KV, Grover FL, Richardson JD, Trinkle JK: Post traumatic empyema. Ann Thorac Surg 23:254, 1977

Atwater EC: Morrill Wyman and the aspiration of acute pleural effusions, 1850. A letter from New-England. Bull Hist Med 36:235, 1972

Baethge BA, Eggerstedt JM, Olash FA: Group F streptococcal empyema from aspiration of a grass inflorescence. Ann Thorac Surg 49:319, 1990

Barondess JA: A case of empyema: notes on the last illness of Sir William Osler. p. 59. In Transactions of the American Clinical and Clinicopathological Association: The 87th Annual Meeting. Vol. 86. Waverly Press, Baltimore, 1975

Bartlett JG, Thadepalli H, Gorbach SL, Finegold SM: Bacteriology of empyema. Lancet 1:338, 1974

Bayes AJ, Wilson JAS, Chiu RCJ et al.: Clagett open-window thoracostomy in patient with empyema who had and had not undergone pneumonectomy. Can J Surg 30:329, 1987

Benfield GFA: Recent trends in empyema thoracis. Br J Dis Chest 75:358, 1981

Bergh NP, Ekroth R, Larsson S, Nagy P: Intrapleural streptokinase in the treatment of haemothorax and empyema. Scand J Thorac Cardiovasc Surg 11:265, 1977

Bowditch HI: On pleuritic effusions and the necessity of paracentesis for their removal. Am J Med Sci 22:320, 1852

Brown B, Ory EM, Meads M et al.: Penicillin treatment of empyema: report of 24 cases and review of the literature. Ann Intern Med 24:343, 1956

Cattaneo SM, Kilman JW: Surgical therapy of empyema in children. Ann Surg 106:564, 1973

Chonmaitree T, Powell KR: Para pneumonic pleural effusion and empyema in children. Review of a 19-year experience, 1962-1980. Clin Pediatr 22:414, 1983

Clagett OT, Geraci JE: A procedure for the management of post-pneumonectomy empyema. J Thorac Cardiovasc Surg 45:141, 1963

Conlan AA, Abramor E, Delikaris O, Hurwitz SS: Taurolidine instillation as therapy for empyema thoracis. S. Afr Med J 64:653, 1983

Coon JL, Shuck JM: Failure of tube thoracostomy for post-traumatic empyema: an indication for early decortication. J Trauma 15:588, 1975

Crawford BK, Galloway AC, Boyd AD, Spencer FC: Treatment of AIDS-related bronchopleural fistula by pleurectomy. Ann Thorac Surg 54:212, 1992

de la Rocha AG: Empyema thoracis. Surg Gynecol Obstet 155:839, 1982

Delarue NC: Empyema: principles of management—an old problem revisited. p. 178. In Deslauriers J, Lacquet LK (eds): International Trends in General Thoracic Surgery. Vol. 6. CV Mosby, St. Louis, 1990

Delorme E: Nouveau traitement des empyèmes chroniques. Gazette des Hôpitaux 67:94, 1894

Deschamps C, Trastek VF, Arnold PG, Pairolero PC: Surgical approach to chronic empyema: decortication and muscle transposition. p. 233. In Deslauriers J, Lacquet LK (eds): International Trends in General Thoracic Surgery Vol. 6. CV Mosby, St. Louis, 1990

Dieter RA, Pifarré R, Neville WE et al.: Empyema treated with neomycin irrigation and closed-chest drainage. J Thorac Cardiovasc Surg 59:496, 1970

Ehler AA: Non-tuberculous thoracic empyema: a collective review of the literature from 1934 to 1939. Int Abstr Surg 72:17, 1941

Eloesser L: An operation for tuberculous empyema. Surg Gynecol Obstet 60:1096, 1935

Estlander JA: Résection des côtes dans l'empyème chronique. Rev Med Chir (Paris) 3:157, 1879

Farpour A, Sajedee M: Empyema in pediatric patients in Iran. Am J Surg 114:856, 1967

Ferguson MK: The healing hand. Chest 97:4, 1990

Finland M, Barnes MW: Changing ecology of acute bacterial empyema: occurrence and mortality at Boston City Hospital during 12 selected years from 1935 to 1972. Infect Dis 137:274, 1978

Fishman NH, Ellertson DG: Early pleural decortication for thoracic empyema in immunosuppressed patients. J Thorac Cardiovasc Surg 74:537, 1977

Fowler GR, quoted by Meade R: A History of Thoracic Surgery. Charles C Thomas, Springfield, IL, 1961

Fowler GR: A case of thoracoplasty for the removal of a large cicatricial fibrous growth from the interior of the chest, the result of an old empyema. Med Record 44:938, 1893

Frimodt-Moller PC, Vejlsted H: Early surgical intervention in non-specific pleural empyema. Thorac Cardiovasc Surg 33:41, 1985

Goldstraw P: Treatment of the post-pneumonectomy empyema. The case for fenestration. Thorax 34:740, 1979

Graham EA: Some Fundamental Considerations in the Treatment of Empyema Thoracis. CV Mosby, St. Louis, 1925

Graham EA, Bell RD: Open pneumothorax: its relation to the treatment of acute empyema. Am J Med Sci 156:839, 1918

Grant DR, Finley RJ: Empyema: analysis of treatment techniques. Can J Surg 28:449, 1985

Grégoire R, Deslauriers J, Beaulieu M, Piraux M: Thoracoplasty: its forgotten role in the management of non tuberculous post pneumonectomy empyema. Can J Surg 30:343, 1987

Gustafson RA, Murray GF, Warden HE, Hill RC: Role of lung decortication in symptomatic empyemas in children. Ann Thorac Surg 49:940, 1990

Hankins JR, Miller JE, Altar S et al.: Bronchopleural fistula. Thirteen-year experience with 77 cases. J Thorac Cardiovasc Surg 76:755, 1978

Henchen WH III, Haggerty RJ: Staphylococcic pneumonia in infancy and childhood JAMA 168:6, 1958

Heuer GA: Observations on the treatment of chronic empyema. Ann Surg 72:80, 1929

Hewitt CF: Thoracentesis: the plan of continuous aspiration. BMJ 1:317, 1876

Hippocrate: Oeuvres Médicales: d'Après l'Édition de Foës. Aux Éditions du Fleuve, Lyon, 1953

Hippocrates, quoted by: Major Classic Descriptions of Disease. Charles C Thomas, Springfield, IL, 1965

Holmes Sellors T, Cruickshank G: Chronic empyema. Br J Surg 38:411, 1951

Hoover EL, Hsu HK, Ross MJ et al.: Reappraisal of empyema thoracis. Surgical intervention when the duration of illness is unknown. Chest 90:511, 1986

Hoover EL, Hsu HK, Webb H et al.: The surgical management of empyema thoracis in substance abuse patients: a 5-year experience. Ann Thorac Surg 46:563, 1988

Hopkins RA, Ungerleider RM, Staub EN, Young WG: The modern use of thoracoplasty. Ann Thorac Surg 40:181, 1985

Houston MC: Pleural fluid pH: diagnostic, therapeutic and prognostic value. Am J Surg 154:333, 1987

Jensen C, Sharna P: Use of fibrin glue in thoracic surgery. Ann Thorac Surg 39:521, 1985

Jess P, Brynitz S, Moller AF: Mortality in thoracic empyema. Scand J Thorac Cardiovasc Surg 18:85, 1984

Jørgensen A, Møller IW, Johnsen A, Borgeskov S: Bronchopleural leakage treated with fibrin sealant and high-frequency positive-pressure ventilation. Scand J Thorac Cardiovasc Surg 18:130, 1984

Keefer CS, Rantz LA, Rammelkamp CH: Hemolytic streptococcal pneumonia and empyema, study of 55 cases with special reference to treatment. Ann Intern Med 14:1533, 1941

Koch R, Carson M, Donnell G: Staphylococcal pneumonia in children. J Pediatr 55:473, 1959

Kosloske AM: Infections of the lungs, pleura and mediastinum. In Welch KJ et al (eds): Pediatric Surgery. 4th Ed. Year Book Medical Publishers, Chicago, 1986

Kosloske AM, Cartwright KC: The controversial role of decortication in the management of pediatric empyema. J Thorac Cardiovasc Surg 96:166, 1988

Lemmer JH, Botham MJ, Orringer MB: Modern management of adult thoracic empyema. J Thorac Cardiovasc Surg 90:849, 1985

le Roux BT: Empyema thoracis. Br J Surg 52:89, 1965

le Roux BT, Mohlala ML, Odell JA, Whitton D: Suppurative diseases of the lung and pleural space. Part 1: Empyema thoracis and lung abscess. Curr Probl Surg 23:6, 1986

Light RW: Parapneumonic effusions and empyema. Clinics in Chest Medicine 6:55–62, 1985.

Light RW: Parapneumonic effusions and empyema. Semin Respir Med 9:37, 1987

Light RW, Girard WM, Jenkinson SG, George RB: Parapneumonic effusions. Am J Med 69:507, 1980

Luizy J, Mathey J, Le Brigand H, Galey JJ: Technique d'irrigation pleurale sous dépression continue dans le traitement des pyothorax. Rev Tubercul Pneumol 30:393, 1966

Maier AC, Grace EJ: Putrid empyema. Surg Gynecol Obstet 74:69, 1942

Malave G, Foster ED, Wilson JA, Munro DD: Bronchopleural fistula. Present day study of an old problem. Ann Thorac Surg 11:1, 1971

Mandal AK, Thadepalli H: Treatment of spontaneous bacterial empyema thoracis. J Thorac Cardiovasc Surg 94:414, 1987

Mavroudis C, Ganzei BL, Katzmark S, Polk HC: Effect of hemothorax on experimental empyema thoracis in the guinea pig. J Thorac Cardiovasc Surg 89:42, 1985

Mavroudis C, Symmonds JB, Minagi H, Thomas AN: Improved survival in management of empyema thoracis. J Thorac Cardiovasc Surg 82:49, 1981

Mayo P, Saha SP, McElvein RB: Acute empyema in children treated by open thoracotomy and decortication. Ann Thorac Surg 34:401, 1982

McCarthy PM, Trastek VF, Bell DG et al.: The effectiveness of fibrin glue sealant for reducing experimental pulmonary air leak. Ann Thorac Surg 45:203, 1988

McLaughlin FJ, Goldmann DA, Rosebaum DM et al.: Empyema in children: clinical course and long-term follow-up. Pediatrics 73:587, 1984

Middlekamp JN, Purkerson ML, Burford TH: The changing pattern of empyema thoracis in pediatrics. J Thorac Cardiovasc Surg 47:165, 1969

Miller JI: Empyema thoracis. Ann Thorac Surg 50:343, 1990

Miller JI, Mansour KA, Nahai F et al.: Single-stage complete muscle flap closure of the post-pneumonectomy empyema space: a new method and possible solution to a disturbing complication. Ann Thorac Surg 38:227, 1984

Morin JE, Munro DD, Maclean LD: Early thoracotomy for empyema. J Thorac Cardiovasc Surg 64:530, 1972

Nakaoka K, Nakalara K, Lioka S et al.: Post operative preservation of pulmonary function in patients with chronic empyema thoracis: a one-stage operation. Ann Thorac Surg 47:848, 1989

Nin Vivo J, Brandolino MV, Pomi JA et al.: Hydatid pleural disease. p. 427. In Deslauriers J, Lacquet LK (eds): International Trends in General Thoracic Surgery. Vol. 6. CV Mosby, St. Louis, 1990

Ogilvie AG: Final results in traumatic haemothorax: a report of 230 cases. Thorax 5:116, 1950

Orringer MB: Thoracic empyema—back to basics. Chest 93:901, 1988

Osler W: The Principles and Practice of Medicine. D. Appleton, New York, 1892

Paget S: Surgery of the Chest. John Wright and Sons, Bristol, 1896

Pairolero PC, Arnold PG, Piehler JM: Intrathoracic transposition of extrathoracic skeletal muscle. J Thorac Cardiovasc Surg 86:809, 1983

Perelman ME, Rymko LP: Management of empyemas: the problems of associated bronchopleural fistulas. p. 301. In Deslauriers J, Lacquet LK (eds): International Trends in General Thoracic Surgery. Vol. 6. CV Mosby, St. Louis, 1990

Personne C: Role of early thoracotomy in the treatment of empyema. p. 225. In Deslauriers J, Lacquet LK (eds): International Trends in General Thoracic Surgery. Vol. 6. CV Mosby, St. Louis, 1990

Peters RM: Empyema thoracis: historical perspective. Ann Thorac Surg 48:306, 1989

Pezzella AT, Walls JT, Curtis JJ: Non tuberculouis empyema: a clinical experience. Texas Heart Inst J 10:263, 1983

Playfair GE: Case of empyema treated by aspiration and subsequently by drainage: recovery. BMJ 1:45, 1875

Potts DE, Levin DC, Sahn SA: Pleural fluid pH in parapneumonic effusions. Chest 70:328, 1976

Potts DE, Taryle DA, Sahn SA: The glucose-pH relationship in parapneumonic effusions. Arch Intern Med 138:1378, 1978

Puskas JD, Mathisen DJ, Grillo HC et al.: Treatment strategies for bronchopleural fistula. Presented at the Annual Meeting of the American Association for Thoracic Surgery, New York, April 24–28, 1994

Raffensperger JG, Luck SR, Shkolnik A, Ricketts RR: Mini-thoracotomy and chest tube insertion for children with empyema. J Thorac Cardiovasc Surg 84:497, 1982

Ravitch M, Fein R: The changing picture of pneumonia and empyema in infants and chidlren: a review of the experience at the Harriet Lane home from 1934 through 1958. JAMA 175:1039, 1961

Rodgers BM: discussion of Foglia RP and Randolph J: Current indications for decortication in the treatment of empyema in children. J Pediatr Surg 22:32, 1987

Rosenfeldt FL, McGibney D, Braimbridge MV, Watson DA: Comparison between irrigation and conventional treatment for empyema and pneumonectomy space infections. Thorax 36:272, 1981

Sahn SA, Light RW: The sun should never set on a para pneumonic effusion. Chest 95:945, 1989

Samson PE: Empyema thoracis; essentials of present-day management. Ann Thorac Surg 11:210, 1971

Schede M: Die Behandlung der Empyeme. Verh Dtsch Ges Inn Med 9:41, 141, 1890

Sensenig DM, Rossi NP, Ehrenhaft JL: Decortication for chronic non-tuberculous empyema. Surg Gynecol Obstet 117:443, 1963

Sherman MM, Subramanian V, Berger RL: Management of thoracic empyema. Am J Surg 133:474, 1977

Smolle-Jüttner E, Beuster W, Pinter H et al.: Open-window thoracostomy in pleural empyema. Eur J Cardiothorac Surg 6:635, 1992

Stafford EG, Clagett OT: Post-pneumonectomy empyema. Neomycin instillations and definitive closure. J Thorac Cardiovasc Surg 63:771, 1972

Stiles QR, Lindersmith GG, Tucker BL, Meyer BW, Jones JC: Pleural empyema in children. Ann Thorac Surg 10:37, 1970

Sullivan KM, O'Toole RD, Fisher RH, Sullivan KN: Anaerobic empyema thoracis. The role of anaerobes in 226 cases of culture-proven empyemas. Arch Intern Med 131:521, 1973

Thomas DF, Glass JL, Baisch BF: Management of streptococcal pneumonia. Ann Thorac Surg 2:658, 1966

Thurer RJ, Palatinos GM: Surgical aspects of the pleural space. Semin Respir Med 9:98, 1987

Tillett WS, Sherry S: The effect in patients of streptococcal fibrinolysin (streptokinase) and streptococcal desoxyribonuclease on fibrinous, purulent and sanguineous pleural exudations. J Clin Invest 28:173, 1949

Van Way III C, Narrod J,k Hopeman A: The role of early limited thoracotomy in the treatment of empyema. J Thorac Cardiovasc Surg 96:436, 1988

Varkey B, Rose HD, Kesavan-Kutty CP, Politis J: Empyema thoracis during a ten-year period. Analysis of 72 cases and comparison to a previous study (1952 to 1967). Arch Intern Med 141:1771, 1981

Vester SR, Faber LP, Kittle F et al.: Bronchopleural fistula after stapled closure of bronchus. Ann Thorac Surg 52:1253, 1991

Vianna NJ: Non tuberculous bacterial empyema in patients with and without underlying diseases. JAMA 215:69, 1971

Villalba B, Lucas CE, Ledgerwood AM, Asfaw 1: The etiology of post-traumatic empyema and the role of decortication. J Trauma 19:414, 1979

Virkkula L, Eerola S: Treatment of post-pneumonectomy empyema. Scand J Thorac Cardiovasc Surg 8:133, 1974

Virkkula L, Eerola S, Varstela E: Surgical approach to the chronic empyema: space sterilization. p. 263. In Deslauriers J, Lacquet LK (eds): International Trends in General Thoracic Surgery. Vol. 6. CV Mosby, St. Louis, 1990

Von Bülau G: Für die Heber Drainage bei Behandlung des Empyems. Zklin Med 18:31, 1891

Weissberg D: Empyema and bronchopleural fistula. Experience with open window thoracotomy. Chest 82:447, 1982

Weissberg D, Kaufman M: The use of talc for pleurodesis in the treatment of resistant empyema. Ann Thorac Surg 41:143, 1986

Whitton I: Pleural amebiasis. p. 452. In Deslauriers J, Lacquet LK (eds): International Trends in General Thoracic Surgery. Vol. 6. CV Mosby, St. Louis, 1990

Yeh TJ, Hall DP, Ellison RG: Empyema thoracis: a review of 110 cases. Am Rev Respir Dis 88:785, 1963

York JEL, Lewall DB, Hirji M et al.: Endoscopic diagnosis and treatment of postoperative bronchopleural fistula. Chest 197:1390, 1990

38

SPONTANEOUS PNEUMOTHORAX AND PNEUMOMEDIASTINUM

Gilles Beauchamp

DEFINITION

A pneumothorax is defined as an accumulation of air in the pleural space with secondary lung collapse. This accumulation may come from different sources, but rupture of the visceral pleura with secondary air leak from the lung is the single most common cause. Free air in the pleural space may also originate from a ruptured esophagus or from the loss of integrity of the chest wall. Seldom is it produced by gas-forming organisms, which may be present in the pleural space.

In most instances pneumothoraces present with minor symptoms without any major physiologic changes. Rarely a simple pneumothorax can be progressive and give rise to significant hemodynamic and respiratory instability with hypoxia and shock. This clinical picture is seen with tension pneumothoraces, and it deserves emergency treatment.

Pneumothoraces can be classified according to their cause and clinical presentation. They can either be spontaneous, traumatic, or iatrogenic, the first category including both primary and secondary varieties (Killen and Gobbel, 1968). A primary spontaneous pneumothorax happens in individuals with no known pulmonary disease; a secondary pneumothorax occurs in patients with clinical or radiographic evidence of underlying lung disease. Traumatic pneumothoraces occur as the result of penetrating or blunt trauma disrupting the bronchus, the lung, or the esophagus. A traumatic pneumothorax is said to be open when there is associated disruption of the chest wall. Iatrogenic pneumothoraces include diagnostic and therapeutic pneumothoraces. Therapeutic pneumothoraces are no longer used as a method of therapy, but diagnostic pneumothoraces are occasionally required. Inadvertent iatrogenic pneumothoraces are relatively common in the hospital environment but these are not considered in this discussion.

HISTORICAL NOTE

The presence of air in the pleural cavity has been recognized since antiquity. According to Killen and Gobbel (1968), the understanding of the disease and of its therapy evolved from early observations during the seventeenth and eighteenth century to a better clinical description during the 19th century. During the 20th century, a greater knowledge of pleural physiology and the development of modern techniques of thoracic surgery led to a more scientific approach to both the diagnosis and therapy of this condition.

A pneumothorax was first identified by Boerhaave in 1724 (Emerson, 1903), and the first postmortem description of a tension pneumothorax is from Meckel in 1759 (Killan and Gobbel, 1968). The term pneumothorax was introduced by Etard in 1803, but Laennec in 1819 was the first to describe the signs and symptoms associated with this entity (Killen and Gobbel, 1968). At the time tuberculosis was considered to be the leading cause of pneumothorax, although De Villiers had reported in 1926 on a patient with spontaneous pneumothorax, which appeared to be secondary to the rupture of pulmonary blebs (Killen and Gobbel, 1968). A major step in the understanding of the pathophysiology of spontaneous pneumothorax was made in 1932 when Kjaergaard (1932) demonstrated that rupture of isolated lung blebs instead of tuberculosis was the most common cause of spontaneous pneumothoraces occurring in apparently healthy individuals.

For a long time the therapy of spontaneous pneumothorax relied solely on bed rest for several weeks. Although known since the late 19th century, intercostal tube thoracostomy was introduced gradually in the 1950s as a method of therapy to accelerate the re-expansion of the lung. In the early 1960s, it became clear that tube thoracostomy was the method of choice for the treatment of the first episode (Klaasen and Meckstroth, 1962). Lockwood (1928) suggested the possible

---

Classification of Pneumothorax

Spontaneous
  Primary (healthy individuals)
  Secondary (underlying pulmonary disease)
    Chronic obstructive pulmonary disease
    Infection
    Neoplasm
    Catamenial
    Miscellaneous
Traumatic
  Blunt
  Penetrating
Iatrogenic
  Inadvertent
  Diagnostic
  Therapeutic

---

role of surgery in the therapy of pneumothoraces, but Bigger (1937) was the first to carry out thoracotomy for the resection of blebs. In 1941 Churchill performed gauze abrasion of the pleura (Tyson and Crandall, 1941), and Tyson and Crandall (1941) also performed an elective thoracotomy with the excision of subpleural blebs. Gaensler (1956) and Thomas (1958) described the technique of parietal pleurectomy to prevent recurrences of pneumothoraces. Clagett (1968) in an editorial called attention to this somewhat too radical procedure and

---

Historical Highlights

Antiquity
  Hippocrates
Identification of the disease
  Boerhaave (1724): lung collapse and ruptured esophagus
  Meckel (1959): postmortem description of a tension pneumothorax
  Etard (1803): term *pneumothorax* coined (autopsy description)
  Laennec (1918): description of physical signs and symptoms
  Kjaergaard (1932): rupture of lung blebs as the most common cause of spontaneous pneumothorax
Evolution of therapy
  Noble (1873): chest canula, rubber tube, and water seal
  Lockwood (1928): surgery first suggested as a method of therapy
  Bigger (1937): thoracotomy, resection of blebs
  Churchill (1941): gauze abrasion
  Gaensler (1956): subtotal parietal pleurectomy
  Deslauriers, et al. (1980): axillary thoracotomy, bleb resection, and apical parietal pleurectomy

---

suggested the use of pleural abrasion instead of pleurectomy. Youmans, et al. (1970) provided clinical and experimental evidence of the efficacy of pleural abrasion for creating pleural adhesions and reducing recurrences. Deslauriers, et al. (1980) suggested a resection of the apical blebs associated with a limited apical pleurectomy through a small axillary incision as the method of choice for treating recurrent primary spontaneous pneumothoraces. More recently a renewed interest in the thoracoscopic approach suggests that it could become the method of choice for resecting apical subpleural blebs and performing an apical pleurectomy and/or a pleural abrasion.

HISTORICAL READING

Killen DA, Gobbel WG: Spontaneous Pneumothorax. Little, Brown, Boston, 1968

BASIC SCIENCE

Anatomy

The visceral pleura covers the surfaces of the lung but offers no cleavage plane with the parenchyma. The parietal pleura on the other hand is a serous membrane that covers the inner surface of the mediastinum, ribs, diaphragm, and pleural dome. The presence of the endothoracic fascia between the pleura and the chest wall provides a cleavage plane, which enables the surgeon to perform a parietal pleurectomy easily. The parietal pleura is vascularized by branches of the intercostal arteries, and the apical pleura is vascularized by branches of the subclavian arteries. The parietal pleura, contrary to the visceral pleura, has somatic innervation, and pain stimuli are transmitted through the intercostal and phrenic nerves (Desmeules, et al., 1990).

Physiology

When a patient is at rest and relaxed and thus at functional residual capacity, the elastic forces of the chest wall and lung tend to separate the parietal from the visceral pleura, therefore creating a negative pressure with respect to the atmospheric pressure. It is the so-called pleural pressure. The intrapleural pressure is also negative with respect to the alveolar pressure. The negative intrapleural pressure is not uniform throughout the pleural space, and a gradient can be measured between the apex and the base of the lung. At the apex the pressure is more negative than at the base, and this difference tends to favor a greater distension of the alveoli located at this site. The intrapleural gradient has been measured at $0.20\,cmH_2O/cm$ of vertical distance. In taller individuals this gradient may even be greater at the apex and contribute to the development of pneumothoraces.

When a communication develops between the lung's parenchyma and the pleural space, the positive intra-alveolar air flows from the lung into the pleural space until there is no pressure difference (Fig. 38-1). The same happens with a communication between the chest wall and the pleural cavity.

In patients with significant (more than 25 percent) pneumothoraces, hypoxemia can develop (Norris, et al., 1968), with

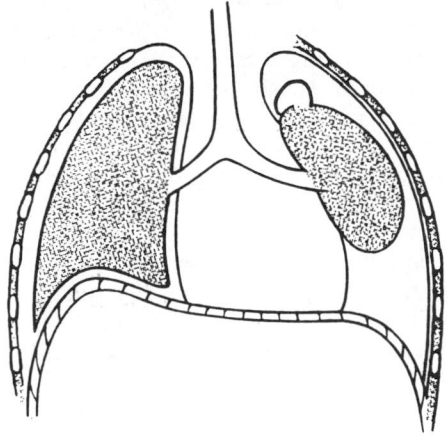

↓ Apex to base pressure gradient

↓ Lung compliance

↓ F.R.C.

↓ Ventilation

↓ Oxygenation

Slight shunt

Figure 38-1. Some of the physiologic characteristics of spontaneous pneumothorax. F.R.C., functional residual capacity.

alveolar hypoventilation. Moran, et al. (1977) showed that the reduction in arterial partial oxygen pressure was caused by an alteration of the ventilation-perfusion ratio. Anatomic shunting and alveolar hypoventilation (Dines, 1970) also contribute to the low arterial partial oxygen pressure. Anthonisen (1977) explained the ventilation maldistribution in pneumothoraces by the airway closure at low lung volumes. Besides oxygenation problems a pneumothorax can often lead to a reduction in the lung's compliance, vital capabity, total capacity, and functional residual capacity (Gilmartin, et al., 1985). The normal apex-to-base pleural pressure gradient also disappears (Agostini, 1986). When the air is evacuated from the pleural space, the arterial partial oxygen pressure return to normal baseline values (Moran, et al., 1977).

When a tension pneumothorax is present, the intrapleural pressure exceeds the atmospheric pressure throughout expiration. This type of pneumothorax develops because of a one-way valve mechanism. During inspiration air moves from the lung or from the outside into the pleural space because of an open communication, and it creates a positive pressure. During expiration the air cannot flow back because of the valve mechanism, and the pleural space is under tension.

For many years it was believed that in a tension pneumothorax air compression of the mediastinum decreased the cardiac output through a reduction of the venous return. In experimental studies, however, Rutherford, et al. (1968) showed that in such cases hypoxia is more the effect of increased pulmonary blood flow in the hypoventilated or nonventilated lung (shunt effect) than of mediastinal air compression. Gutsman, et al. (1983) also showed that in acute tension pneumothorax only part of the pleural pressure created by the pneumothorax was transmitted to the mediastinum. In an experimental model for acute tension pneumothorax, Hurewitz, et al. (1986) described a fall in the stroke volume and a progressive reduction in systemic oxygen transport and tissue oxygenation with a fixed cardiac output. Thus the alteration in cardiovascular function was postulated to be secondary to insufficient tissue oxygenation, which in turn resulted in an inability to increase the cardiac output. The cardiovascular collapse seen in these patients may therefore be more the result of respiratory failure because it is a direct mechanical effect of the increased intrathoracic pressure on the circulation (Fig. 38-2).

Resorption of Pleural Gas

The normal pleural space is free of gas, and it has a negative pressure. When air penetrates into this space, the pressure becomes positive and approximates that of the atmosphere.

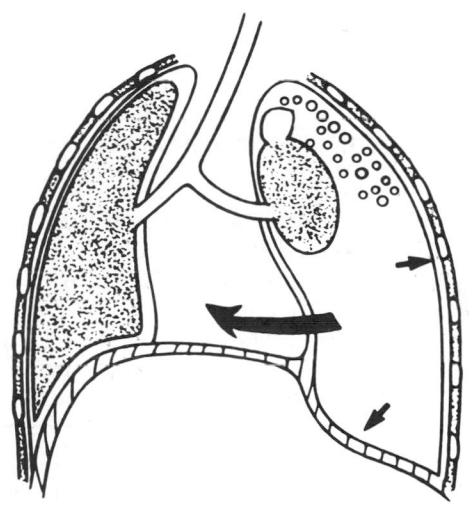

↑ Continuous air flow—one-way valve

↑ Intrapleural pressure

↑ Mediastinal shift: alteration of lung mechanic

↓ Ventilation

↑ Shunt

↓ Oxygenation

↓ Cardiac stroke volume

↑ Heart rate

Figure 38-2. Some of the physiologic characteristics of a tension pneumothorax.

In the surrounding tissues of the chest cavity, the pressure is subatmospheric, therefore favoring the resorption of oxygen, carbon dioxide, and nitrogen into the venous system. The pleura is known to be a semipermeable surface through which gases move by simple diffusion and equilibrate. The pressure gradient between gases in the pleural space and in the subpleural venous system is the driving pressure; each gas resorbs independently. The process of resorption of the intrapleural gas takes place gradually in successive phases.

The rate of resorption of a pneumothorax depends first on the quality of the pleural surface. For example, in the presence of a fibrotic pleura, the resorption is slower than in a normal pleura. The rate of resorption is also proportional to the total surface area of the pleura. The quantity of gas present in the pleural cavity is also a determinant. The greater the gas amount is, the longer it will take for resorption. Finally the composition of the gases in a pneumothorax can be a variable. For example, oxygen is more diffusible and soluble, and for this reason its transfer from the pleura to the circulation is faster in comparison with carbon dioxide or nitrogen.

In the process of resorption of a pneumothorax, two phases are identified. There is first an equilibration of the oxygen and carbon dioxide partial pressures between the pleural space and the blood. In the second phase there is a progressive resorption of the remaining intrapleural gases. Gradually the intrapleural pressure becomes more negative and favors re-expansion of the lung. When the lung does not re-expand, fluid enters by transudation and fills the cavity (Cormier, 1990).

Macroscopic Staging of Spontaneous Pneumothorax

Spontaneous pneumothorax is not a single well-defined entity, and at surgical exploration the surgeon may find different stages of the same disease. Swierenga, et al. (1974, 1977) and Vanderschueren (1981) contributed to the staging of spontaneous pneumothorax. According to these authors, any of four stages of the disease may be found. Stage I corresponds to a normal lung without evidence of a bleb or bullae. This happens in 30 to 40 percent of patients presenting with spontaneous pneumothorax. In stage II there is no evidence of bleb or bullae, but pleuropulmonary adhesions are present, suggesting previous pneumothoraces. This is found in 12 to 15 percent of patients. In stage III small bullae and blebs less than 2 cm in diameter are found (28 to 41 percent of patients). In stage IV multiple bullae more than 2 cm in diameter are identified in 17 to 29 percent of patients. The size of the bullous lesions correlates with age; most patients with stage IV disease are older than 40 years of age.

Histopathology

The terms *blebs* and *bullae* are frequently used in the surgical literature. Blebs are defined as small (less than 2 cm) subpleural collections of air contained within the visceral pleura, resulting from ruptured alveoli. The blebs are usually found at the apex of the upper lobe or the posterior apex of the lower lobe (Edge, 1966). These blebs are often accompanied by apical fibrosis (Lichter, 1974). Blebs are considered to be

a form of interstitial emphysema, which is called periacinar or paraseptal emphysema and occurs independently of widespread emphysema. It results from the rupture of paraseptal, subpleural, or peribronchial alveoli with dissection of air into the adjacent connective tissues. When air escapes from the lung, it makes its way between the lamina elastica interna and externa of the visceral pleura. Blebs are well demarcated from the remaining normal parenchyma and communicate with it by a narrow neck. Electron microscopic examination of their outer surface of the blebs shows a complete absence of the mesothelial cells, with naked collagen fibers and small pores, which cause the air leaks (Ohata and Suzuki, 1980). Eosinophilic pleuritis often accompanies the rupture of blebs into the pleural cavity. In this condition histiocytes, eosinophils, fibrin, multinucleated giant cells, and mesothelial cells are found.

Bullae are large air-filled spaces that can be associated with any form of emphysema. They can also occur in a normal lung. Bullae refer to air-filled spaces located within the lung's parenchyma, which are the result of alveolar wall destruction (Klingman, et al., 1990). They correspond to type I, II, and III bullae, as described by Reid (1966). In type I bullae thin walls, consisting of pleura and connective tissue with few blood vessels, are found. These bullae are located at the apex or at the edge of the lobes. They correspond to overinflation of a small volume of parenchyma and communicate with the lung by a narrow neck. In type II bullae the mesothelial cells on the surface are usually relatively well preserved; deteriorated alveolar structures are found at their base, corresponding to panacinar emphysema. The diseased alveoli are in continuity with the bullae through a broad neck (Ohata and Suzuki, 1980). In type III bullae the base is extremely large and extends deep into the lung. Their contents consist of panacinar emphysematous lung tissue.

The pathologic findings of secondary pneumothoraces are those associated with chronic obstructive palmonary disease, diffuse interstitial pulmonary disease, eosinophilic granuloma, sarcoidosis, pneumoconiosis, neoplasms, and different types of infections.

Pneumothoraces associated with acquired immunodeficiency syndrome (AIDS) are secondary to *Pneumocystis carini* pneumonia, cytomegaloviral pneumonia, tuberculosis, or mycobacterial pneumonia.

Physiopathology

Specific mechanisms by which the pneumothorax develops are still open to debate, and exertion is probably not a major factor. In a recent study Bense (1984) analyzed the variation in atmospheric pressure in relation to spontaneous pneumothoraces and found that the hospital admission rate for spontaneous pneumothorax was significantly increased 48 hours after a fall in atmospheric pressure. Scott, et al. (1989) also showed a relationship between spontaneous pneumothoraces and changes in atmospheric pressure but stated that numerous other factors contribute to the development of spontaneous pneumothorax. Studies done in flight personnel who had sustained previous episodes of pneumothorax showed that the small apical bullae increased in size when subjected to the decreasing atmospheric pressure in altitude chambers. This study suggests that ballooning and the rupture of bullae occur under variations of intrabronchial and intrathoracic pressure (Dermksian and Lamb, 1959).

PRIMARY SPONTANEOUS PNEUMOTHORAX

Clinical Features

The most likely cause of a primary spontaneous pneumothorax is the rupture of small subpleural blebs (Gaensler, 1956). This may occur at rest or during exercise, and it is seen most often in young tall male patients (Melton, et al., 1979) with smoking habits (Bense, et al., 1987). A familial tendency was described (Sugiyama, et al., 1986). In the North American population, the incidence varies from 6 to 7 per 100,000 men to 1 to 2 per 100,000 women (Melton, et al., 1979). Primary spontaneous pneumothorax is slightly more common on the right side (Brooks, 1973), and bilateral pneumothoraces occur in less than 10 percent of patients (Donovan, 1987). There are recurrences in approximately 25 percent of patients, usually within 2 years (Singh, 1982) and on the same side (Getz, 1983). After a second pneumothorax, the chances of having a third episode increase to more than 50 percent (Gobbel, et al., 1963).

Among the complications associated with primary spontaneous pneumothorax, tension pneumothorax occurs in 2 to 3 percent and significant hemothorax, in 5 percent. Fluid accumulation occurs in 20 percent of patients, but subcutaneous emphysema and pneumomediastinum, empyema, and chronicity are uncommon. In fact the most frequent complications of spontaneous pneumothorax are its recurrence or the persistent bronchopleural fistula. These two conditions are often indications for surgery.

Diagnosis

The clinical presentation is usually related to the degree of pulmonary collapse. Although some patients may have a pneumothorax that is asymptomatic, they most often present with acute chest pain and dyspnea. After a few hours, the intensity of the chest pain usually decreases, and it becomes more tolerable. Occasionally patients have a nonproductive cough (Devries and Woolfe, 1981). Physical findings may be totally absent if the collapse of the lung is minimal, but when a substantial collapse is present, there is a decrease in chest wall movement on the affected side. On percussion the chest cavity is hyperresonant and tympanic, and on auscultation breath sounds are decreased or absent. A pleural friction rub can sometimes be heard. Tachycardia is found in most patients.

The clinical diagnosis of a pneumothorax is best confirmed by erect posteroanterior and lateral chest radiographs (Fig. 38-3). Expiration posteroanterior chest radiography may also be useful to demonstrate a small pneumothorax not seen on a standard film. In a study of induced pneumothorax in cadavers, Carr, et al. (1992) showed that the lateral decubitus view is better to confirm the presence of a pneumothorax. Pseudopneumothoraces, such as skin folds, chest wall, or other abnormalities, must be ruled out. Occasionally pulmonary cysts or emphysematous bullae may also be mistaken for a pneumothorax. The radiologic diagnosis of a tension pneumothorax is suggested by a complete collapse of the lung with a contralateral shift of the heart and mediastinum and inversion of the hemidiaphragm (Fig. 38-4).

Quantitation of the size of a pneumothorax is always useful, but unfortunately the method for this quantitation varies greatly and lacks uniformity. The methods of Kircher and Swartzel (1954) and the one from Axel (1981) are based on measurements from a standard chest radiograph of the collapsed lung and of the hemithorax in an anterioposterior view. Light (1990), suggested the measurement of the average diameters of the collapsed lung and of the involved hemithorax, with the cubing of these diameters to estimate the percentage of collapsed lung. For example, if the diameter of a hemithorax is 10 cm and the diameter of the collapsed lung is 6 cm, the collapsed lung is estimated by the formula $100 - 6^3/10^3$. Thus the estimated size of the pneumothorax is 78 percent. Rhea et al. (1982) proposed the use of a nomogram to calculate the size of the pneumothorax. With this method one must first find the average interpleural distance by measuring the interpleural distance at the apex and at the midpoints of both upper and lower lungs. The average interpleural distance is then calculated and the number reported on a nomogram, which gives an estimate of the size of the pneumothorax. It is a simple and reproducible method for predicting the size of a pneumothorax. An example of these calculations is shown in Figure 38-5. The weakness of these methods is their

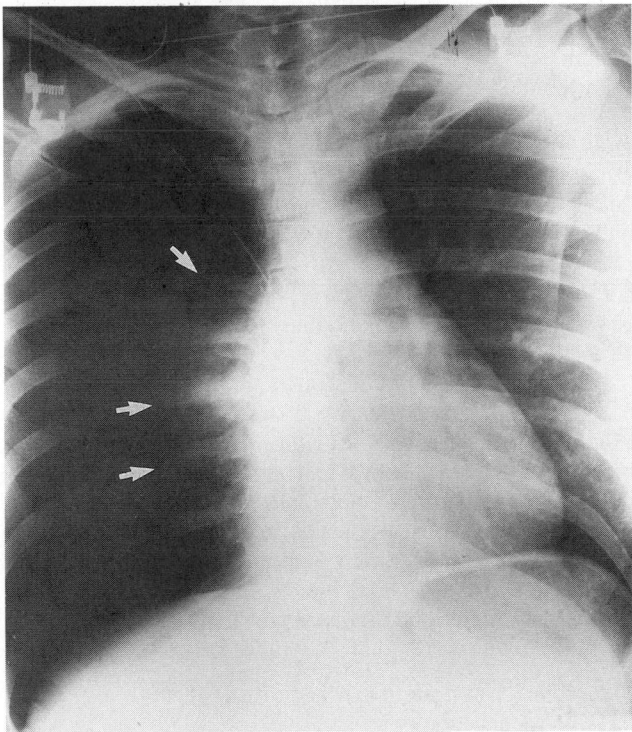

Figure 38-3.   A pneumothorax is identified by finding the location of the visceral pleura.

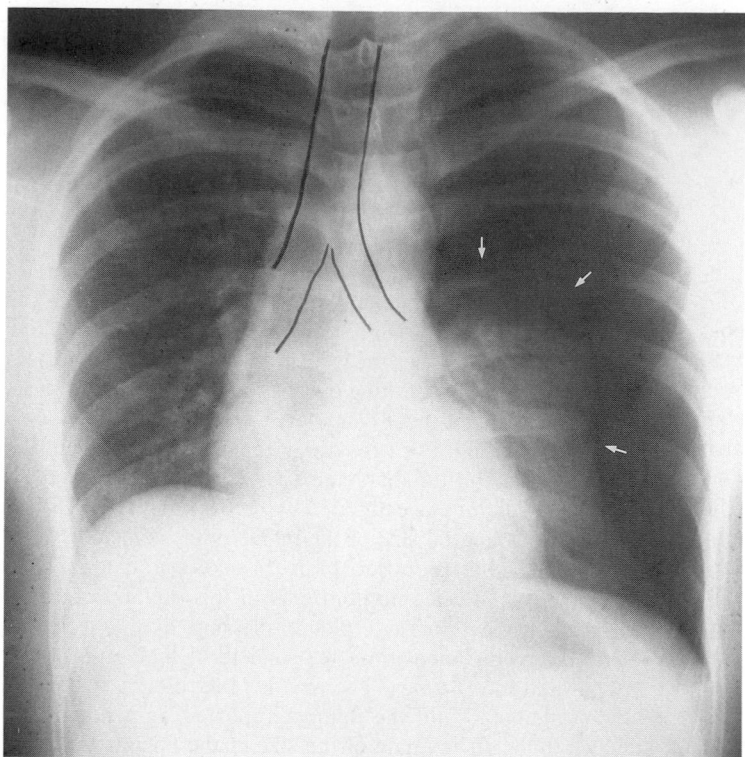

Figure 38-4. Chest radiograph showing a tension pneumothorax with mediastinal shift and deviated trachea.

dependence on a constant shape of the lung during collapse, and computed tomographic (CT) scans have shown that this is not always the case (Engdahl et al., 1993).

CT is now being used with increasing frequency to evaluate patients with spontaneous pneumothorax. Lesur, et al. (1990) reported diffuse but moderate central lobular emphysema in 12 young smoking patients with primary spontaneous pneumothorax. CT of the lung is more sensitive than conventional radiology to detect small early emphysematous changes. A detailed description of the number, size, and location of the blebs is often possible. A precise evaluation of the contralateral side can be carried out and is useful for predicting contralateral recurrences. Based on CT findings, it may eventually be possible to establish guidelines for treatment (Warner, et al. 1991) (Fig. 38-6).

In patients with left-sided pneumothorax, the electrocardiograph may show a rightward shift of the QRS axis, with a diminution of precordial R voltage, a decreased QRS amplitude, and a precordial T-wave inversion, which resolves with re-expansion of the lung (Walston, et al., (1974). When a large pneumothorax is present, the interposition of gas between the heart and the electrode may lead to a decrease of the QRS amplitude and the R and T waves and simulate an anterior myocardial infarction (Diamond and Estes, 1982).

Complications

Persistent Air Leak

Air leakage may persist for more than 48 hours after the therapy of a pneumothorax. Most often the air leak is seen in patients with secondary pneumothoraces, but occasionally patients with a primary spontaneous pneumothorax develop this complication. Most of the time a persistent air leak is associated with incomplete expansion of the lung. In this setting a second chest tube may become necessary before surgery is considered.

Tension Pneumothorax

A tension pneumothorax happens when alveolar air enters continuously into the pleural space but is not evacuated. Tension develops in the pleural space as the intrapleural pressure becomes greater than the atmospheric pressure. The patient shows signs of respiratory distress with tachycardia and appears anxious. Both dyspnea and pain are more important than in a simple pneumothorax. The patient may become hypotensive with peripheral cyanosis, tracheal deviation, and the physical signs of a large pneumothorax. In this situation immediate decompression of the pleural space with a needle, chest drain, or any other instrument is imperative before total circulatory collapse occurs (Rivarola, 1990).

Pneumomediastinum

Pneumomediastinum is secondary to the dissection of air along the bronchi and vascular sheets of pulmonary vessels and may complicate spontaneous pneumothorax. It is generally of no clinical consequence, but other causes of pneumomediastinum, such as injury to major airways or perforation of the esophagus, may need to be ruled out. Pneumoperitoneum secondary to a pneumothorax is rare, and it must be differentiated from a pneumoperitoneum associated with a perforated abdominal viscus (Maunders, et al., 1984). Interstitial and subcutaneous emphysema are usually of no consequence.

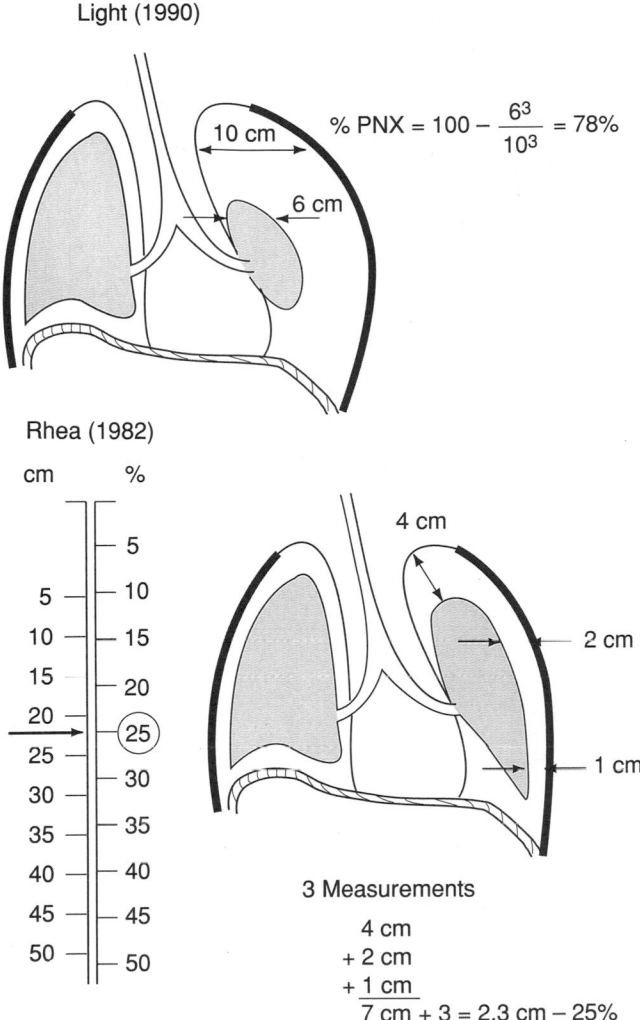

Light (1990)

$$\% \text{ PNX} = 100 - \frac{6^3}{10^3} = 78\%$$

10 cm

6 cm

Rhea (1982)

cm %

3 Measurements

4 cm
+ 2 cm
+ 1 cm

$$\overline{7 \text{ cm} \div 3 = 2.3 \text{ cm} - 25\%}$$

Figure 38-5. Estimation of the size of a pneumothorax according to the method described by Light (1990) and Rhea, et al. (1982).

Hemothorax

Hemothorax is a rare complication of pneumothorax and results most often from the rupture of a small vessel located in adhesions between the visceral and the parietal pleura. Often re-expansion of the lung with a chest tube helps to tamponade the bleeding point. Occasionally the patient becomes hypotensive and requires emergency surgery.

Bilateral Pneumothorax

Bilateral pneumothoraces happen in less than 1 percent of cases. They may be simultaneous but most often are sequential.

Management

In the management of spontaneous pneumothoraces, there are different clinical situations that may require different therapeutic approaches. The nonoperative approach includes observation, simple aspiration, and thoracostomy with ambu-latory tube drainage. Chemical pleurodesis with tetracycline or talc are options that can be added to tube thoracostomy to reduce the risk of recurrences. The operative therapy consist of apical bullectomy with or without pleurodesis by pleurectomy or gauze abrasion.

Observation

Asymptomatic patients in good health with small (less than 20 percent) pneumothoraces and no evidence of radiographic progression may be treated expectantly (Clague and El-Ansory, 1984). The rate of air resorption from the intrapleural space is estimated to be 1.25 percent of the volume of the pneumothorax per 24 hours (50 to 70 ml/day) (Kircher and Swarlzel, 1954). To ensure that no complications develop, it is recommended that these patients be observed in a hospital for a period of 24 to 48 hours, and before leaving the hospital, the patients must be instructed about the potential hazards of a tension pneumothorax. Weekly follow-up with a clinical examination and chest radiograph is carried out until the pneumothorax has completely resolved. The main inconvenience of this form of therapy is the duration of the pneumothorax, which far exceeds what it seen with pleural drainage by tube thoracostomy. O'Rourke and Yec (1989) reported a 5 percent mortality rate in patients treated by observation alone. In two patients of this group of 40 treated by observation alone, an unrecognized pleural air leak quickly led to a tension pneumothorax with sudden death. Nine other patients subsequently required insertion of a chest tube. In spite of this experience, observation remains a therapeutic option in certain specific situations. The clinician must be aware that prolonged observation (more than 14 days) may lead to the development of an entrapped lung and necessitate a surgical approach. Thus whenever the lung does not re-expand after 1 week, aspiration or chest tube drainage is indicated.

Aspiration and Small Chest Tube Drainage

Simple aspiration of air with a 16-gauge intravenous cannula connected to a three-way stopcock and a 60-ml syringe is an option (Bevelaqua and Aranda, 1982), and the success rate is estimated at 50 percent (Delius, et al., 1989).

Since the introduction by Sargent and Turner (1970) of the dart technique for emergency treatment of pneumothoraces, different drainage devices have been commercially developed. For example, the McSwain dart is a 16-Fr. polyethylene catheter, which is 15 cm in length, has a winged flange on its tips (Wayne and McSwain, 1980), and is attached to a flutter valve for drainage. Another device is the thoracic vent, which is a small-bore 13-Fr. urethane catheter trocar connected to a one-way valve. A valved aspiration cannula with a 60-ml syringe is also provided for the evacuation of air, and the device may be connected to a suction apparatus and water-seal system (Samuelson, et al., 1991).

Small 9-Fr. chest tubes with or without flutter valves have also been used as an alternative to larger and more conventional thoracostomy tubes (Conces, et al., 1988). The success rate is high, but there are problems associated with kinking and occlusion of the tube. The technique of aspiration remains limited by a 20 percent to 50 percent rate of recurrence (Seremetis, 1970).

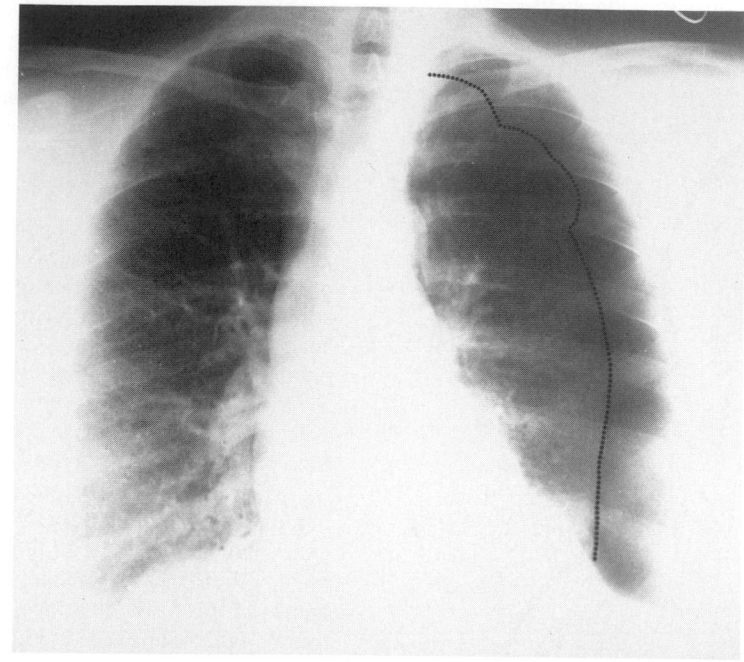

A

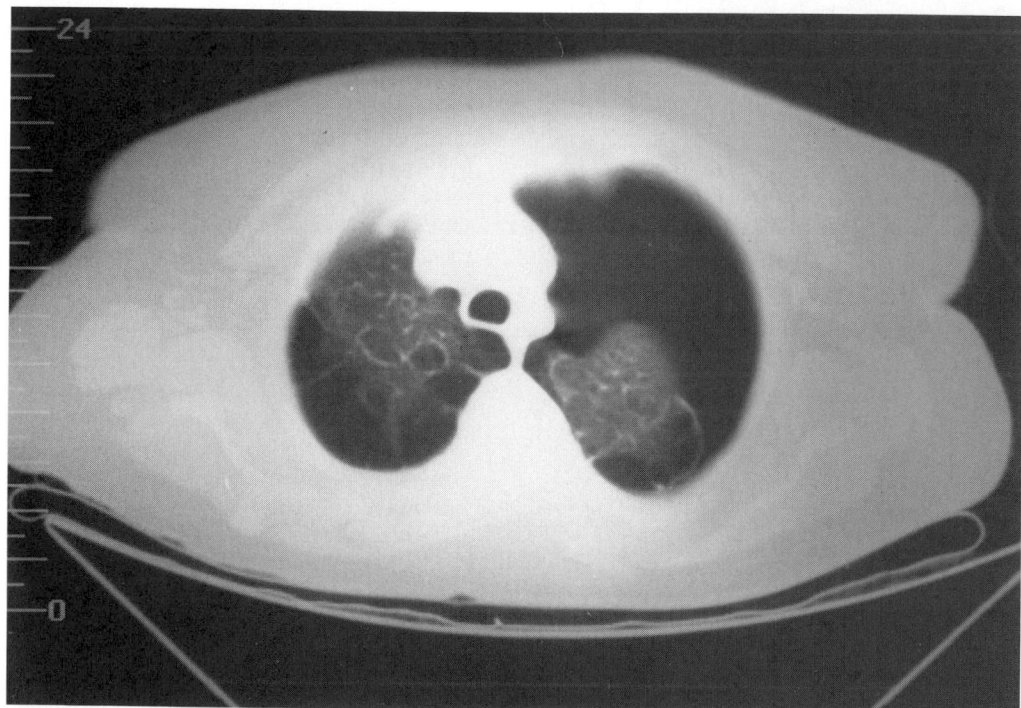

B

Figure 38-6. **(A)** Chest radiograph showing left-sided pneumothorax and normal right lung. **(B)** CT scan of the same patient showing ipsilateral and contralateral bullae with left-sided pneumothorax.

Conventional Tube Thoracostomy

Conventional tube thoracostomy remains the procedure of choice for the management of moderate to large pneumothoraces. The presence of symptoms, the radiographic progression of a pneumothorax, a tension pneumothorax, contralateral disease, and failure of re-expansion are all indications for tube thoracostomy, which allows for rapid and complete evacuation of air from the pleural space. With proper chest drainage, the lung re-expands rapidly, and the air leak stops in less than 48 hours in the majority of patients. Although underwater-seal drainage is sufficient for most cases of pneumothoraces (Sy and Dyc 1982), we prefer the use of negative intrapleural pressure to maintain lung re-expansion during the first hour. In spite of full lung re-expansion, immediate relapse after tube thoracostomy is not unusual (Seremetis, 1970).

Ambulatory Tube Drainage

The Heimlich (1968) flutter-valve system is a passive one-way chest drainage system, which was shown by Mercier, et al. (1976) to be safe, efficient, and economical in the outpatient management of primary spontaneous pneumothorax. In our experience it is more efficient when used after the lung is first re-expanded with underwater-seal drainage suction for at least 1 or two hours. If the lung maintains its re-expansion and if the air leak is minimal, a flutter valve can be installed and the patient discharged from the hospital. The chest tube is removed 24 hours after the air leak has stopped and the lung has maintained a good re-expansion.

In-Hospital Therapy

A patient must be admitted to the hospital if after tube thoracostomy a large air leak is present or the lung cannot maintain its re-expansion. The patient should be treated with underwater suction drainage until full expansion occurs and the air leak stops. The underwater-seal system can eventually be converted to a flutter valve and the patient discharged.

Nonsurgical Therapy of Recurrences

Some authors suggest chemical pleurodesis instead of surgery to prevent recurrences of spontaneous pneumothoraces. However, there is controversy about the role of chemical pleurodesis, and surgeons have generally been concerned about the liberal use of chemicals in the pleural space. Many agents, such as quinacrine (Larrieu, et al., 1979), autologous blood (Robinson, 1987), silver nitrate (Wied, et al., 1983), and bleomycin (Hnatiuk, et al., 1990) have been used in the past, but only tetracycline and talc are still currently in use.

Tetracycline was first used in the therapy of malignant pleural effusions (Robinson, 1987), and it is believed that the local irritating effect of the drug is related to its low pH (Sahn, et al., 1979). It can be instilled through the chest tube at a dose of 500 mg to 1 g diluted in 250 ml of normal saline, which disperses rapidly and completely into the pleural space (Lorch, et al., 1988). To reduce the amount of chest pain, lidocaine (250 mg of 1 percent solution) or ketamine (Stephenson, 1985) can be administered with the tetracycline. Almind, et al. (1989) reported recurrence rates of 13 percent after tetracycline instillation compared with 36 percent in patients with chest tube drainage alone. In a prospective multicenter randomized and controlled clinical trial, Light, et al. (1990) showed a recurrence rate as high as 25 percent at 5 years for the tetracycline group, and he stressed the inconveniences of intense chest pain associated with the instillation of tetracycline. Tetracycline injection should only be used in specific situations in which the patient refuses surgery or the operative risk is too high. The option of tetracycline injection may not be available in the future because the production of injectable tetracycline hydrochloride has been discontinued (Heffner and Unrush, 1992).

Talc was proved to be effective in the therapy of malignant pleural effusion, and it is now used in the therapy of spontaneous pneumothoraces. Talc is a powder of hydrous magnesium silicate that contains different contaminants. Purified talc is commercailly available and is free of asbestos. It is considered to be safe for therapeutic use (Selikoff, et al., 1987). Talc is effective in inducing pleural fibrosis and adhesions, but it has significant side effects, such as fever, pain, and impaired pulmonary function, and should be only used when the lung is completely re-expandable. It can be injected through a chest tube in a suspension form (2 g diluted in 50 ml of normal saline), or it can be sprinkled over the entire pleural surfaces with a syringe (Weisberg, 1986). It can also be aerolized as a powder throught he thoracoscope, as proposed by Gillet-Juvin and Guérin (1991) or with a talc insufflator (Deslauriers and Piraux, 1990). One major concern about the use of talc intrapleurally in spontaneous pneumothorax is the possible deleterious effect on the pulmonary function. However, Viskum, et al. (1989), in a group of 99 patients treated between 1954 and 1964, found no evidence of impaired pulmonary function. In a series of patients reported by Lange, et al. (1988), there was only mild restrictive impairment without clinical significance 22 to 25 years after talc insufflation. The effectiveness of talc insufflation to prevent the recurrence of pneumothoraces was reviewed by Boutin, et al. (1991). In 75 published series comparing different methods of therapy, patients had a recurrence rate of approximately 7 percent after talc insufflation.

Most surgeons are concerned about the routine use of chemopleurodesis in the therapy of spontaneous pneumothorax because it is a benign disease that occurs in young people who may require thoracotomy for other diseases at a later date. Because of the important symphysis that follows chemopleurodesis, such thoracotomies may be difficult and associated with high morbidity rates, especially if lung resection or transplantation is considered. Chemical pleurodesis should therefore be used only in selected cases.

Indications for Surgery

At First Episode. Surgery may be indicated at the time of the first episode when a pneumothorax is complicated by a persistence of an air leak for more than 3 days, hemothorax,

---

Indications for Surgery in Primary Spontaneous Pneumothorax

First episode
  Prolonged air leak
  Nonre-expansion of the lung
  Bilateral pneumothoraces
  Hemopneumothorax
  Occupational hazard (flight personnel, divers)
  Absence of medical facilities in isolated area
  Tension pneumothorax
  Associated single large bulla
Second episode
  Ipsilateral recurrence
  Contralateral recurrence after a first pneumothorax

failure to re-expand, bilaterality or tension or if the patient is at risk because of occupation. Today some authors like Murray, et al. (1993) suggest that all young patients with a significant spontaneous pneumothorax should be spared a tube thoracostomy to proceed immediately to a transaxillary thoracotomy with definitive therapy. This approach is not the standard therapy, and most patients are still operated on because of complications of their disease.

Most air leaks seal within 24 to 48 hours after chest tube drainage, and according to Seremetis (1970), only 3 to 5 percent of patients have a persistent fistula. If an air leak is persistent for more than 48 hours, however, continuing drainage with or without suction for periods of 8 to 10 days results in only a minimal increase in pulmonary healing (Schoennenberger, et al., 1991). Surgery should therefore be considered after 3 to 4 days of tube drainage (Granke, et al., 1986).

Despite proper tube drainage, the lung sometimes only partially re-expands either because of a bronchopleural fistula and/or of an associated pachypleuritis with a trapped lung. In those cases surgery is often necessary, and the best procedure is a decortication, re-expansion of the lung, and closure of the fistula. The occurrence of simultaneous bilateral pneumothoraces is rare, but when it occurs, bilateral tube thoracostomy is necessary and should be followed by surgery on one side. The occurrence of a first episode of a tension pneumothorax is an indication to proceed with surgery to avoid a second potential life-treating condition. Most of the time the patient asks for some type of definitive therapy.

When a patient presents with a first episode of pneumothorax with a single large bulla identified on the chest radiograph or the CT scan, we think surgery should be recommended to the patient. In those patients in which the CT scan has identified subpleural blebs, it is not clear whether surgery should be recommended at the time of the first episode.

Less than 5 percent of patients present with a spontaneous hemopneumothorax, although 20 to 25 percent of patients have a small pleural effusion. In those patients with significant bleeding, surgery may be required. Standard thoracotomy or thoracoscopy is often necessary for definitive control of the bleeding site and pleural drainage. Large hemothoraces (more than 1,000 me) are rare, but they can lead to late complications, such as empyema and fibrothorax, if not properly evacuated.

Patients at risk of developing pneumothoraces because of occupations such as flight personnel or scuba divers may be treated by surgery at the time of the first episode (Clarck, et al., 1972). Patients living in isolated areas or patients traveling frequently, especially those with evidence of air cysts on chest radiographs, may also be candidates for early surgery. The management of a pneumothorax that occurs in a pregnant woman during the first trimester or near parturition should be conservative, and a chest tube can be inserted without problems.

After Second Episode. Recurrence is the most common indication for surgery in patients with primary spontaneous pneumothoraces. When a second episode occurs on the opposite side, it is a clear indication to operate on at least one side. When there is a recurrence during pregnancy, Dhalla

and Teskey (1985) indicate that surgery can be performed safely. During the second trimester transaxillary thoracotomy or thoracoscopy and resection of the apex can be performed without significant morbidity. It seems to be a desirable approach to avoid problems at the time of delivery.

Surgical Therapy

The principles of the surgical therapy of spontaneous pneumothorax consist of resecting the blebs and bullae and obliterating the pleural space for the prevention of recurrences. In most patients wedge resection of the apical blebs is sufficient to control the air leak (Lichter, 1974). Multiple wedge resections may also be required when the disease is present at several sites (Brooks, 1973). Segmentectomy and lobectomy are usually unnecessary and contraindicated. Except for Ferguson, et al. (1981), who carry only an excision of bullae, the majority of authors combine apical resection or blebectomy with a procedure to obliterate the pleural space (Deslauriers, et al., 1980). The rate of recurrences after surgery is less than 1 percent (Caes, et al., 1987; Granke, et al., 1986).

Obliteration of the Pleural Space. Obliteration of the pleural space is thought to be necessary to prevent recurrences. It can be accomplished by chemical pleurodesis, by mechanical abrasion, or by parietal pleurectomy, which can be performed alone or in association with resection of the lung at the time of thoracotomy or thoracoscopy.

Parietal Pleurectomy. Parietal pleurectomy creates an inflammatory surface with secondary "fixation" of the lung to the endothoracic fascia. Gaensler (1956) was the first to describe the use of pleurectomy, and Thomas and Gebauer (1958) were the first to report its effectiveness to prevent recurrences. Askew (1976) and Deslauriers, et al. (1980) also described more limited apical pleurectomy to promote pleural space obliteration. Weeden and Smith (1983) reported a complication rate of 23 percent after subtotal pleurectomy and of 9.5 percent after a more limited apical pleurectomy; most authors report no operative deaths. The results of parietal pleurectomy are excellent, with few recurrences reported. In a review of 752 patients who had undergone apical or subtotal pleurectomy, Weeden and Smith (1983) had only 3 instances of recurrence (0.4 percent). Thus pleurectomy is highly effective, and because the blebs responsible for most spontaneous pneumothoraces are nearly always limited to the apex, apical pleurectomy with bleb excision is now considered the operation of choice for the definitive control of recurrences (Deslauriers, et al., 1980).

Gaensler (1956) showed no impairment of respiratory function after pleurectomy, and Singh (1982) and Weeden and Smith (1983) found no differences in pulmonary function between pre- and postpleurectomy values.

Pleural Abrasion. In 1968 Claggett (1968) suggested that pleural abrasion rather than pleurectomy should be used to prevent recurrences. According to Moores (1990) pleural abrasion produces obliteration of the pleural space with little reaction on the lung side, and it has the advantages of preserving an extrapleural plane and of being done with minimal morbidity (Pairolero and Payne, 1986). The recurrence rate following pleural abrasion is 2.3 percent in 9 reported series totaling 301 patients (Weeden and Smith, 1983).

Rate of Recurrences After Therapy.   The rate of recurrence of a primary spontaneous pneumothorax after various therapeutic modalities was reported by Boutin, et al. (1991) to vary from 2 to 30 percent, depending on the type of treatment (Table 38-1). Recurrences are definitely more frequent when patients are treated by observation, thoracostomy, or chemical pleurodesis. The recurrence rate is much lower when talc pleurodesis is used. Long-term results with low morbidity and mortality rates are still best achieved by surgery.

Surgical Approach.   *Thoracotomy.*   Full posterolateral thoracotomy is seldom required for the treatment of primary spontaneous pneumothorax in patients younger than 40 years of age. In most of these patients, the apex of the lung can be resected, and a pleurectomy or pleural abrasion can be performed through a short cosmetically acceptable axillary incision (Murray, et al., 1993), or a minimal thoracotomy done through the auscultatory triangle (Lau and Shawkat, 1982) or thoracoscope.

When entering the chest cavity, the apical blebs are identified, and a thorough search for other blebs in the superior segment of the lower lobe is carried out before performing the apical resection. The apical pleurectomy is started at the incision where the pleura is stripped from the endothoracic fascia until the apex is reached. Bleeding is controlled with miniclips and/or electrocautery. The rest of the parietal pleura can be abraded with a dry gauze sponge. A single apical 28-Fr. chest tube is left in the pleural place, and this tube is removed 48 hours later. The patient is sent home usually by the 3rd postoperative day. When bilateral disease is present, the surgeon can proceed with a median sternotomy (Ikeda, et al., 1988). However, we prefer and recommend bilateral axillary thoracotomies.

Thoracoscopy.   The use of thoracoscopy for the diagnosis and therapy of spontaneous pneumothorax has been known for a long time in Europe where an extensive experience has been accumulated (Swierenga, et al., 1974; Boutin, et al., 1991). With thoracoscopy a pneumothorax cannot only be assessed and staged, but the endoscopic threapy can be executed on the basis of these findings. Thoracoscopy can be performed routinely at the first episode (Verschoof, et al., 1988), and the findings allow for the classification of patients in one of three categories: (1) patients with no obvious abnormalities, (2) patients with small apical blebs, and (3) patients with more generalized bullous disease. The decision to perform chemical pleurodesis or surgery can then be made based on those findings. Patients with more generalized bullae or larger blebs are better treated with surgical resection (Wied, et al., 1983; Vanderschueren, 1990).

Gillet-Juvin and Guérin (1991) used thoracoscopic talc poudrage under local anesthesia for the therapy of pneumothorax associated with large emphysematous bullae in 71 patients, and the results were good to excellent in 93 percent of patients, with few complications. This technique may be useful for patients with chronic obstructive pulmonary disease. It can also be used for the therapy of pneumothorax associated with cystic fibrosis and for spontaneous pneumothorax (Daniel, et al., 1990). With the development of video-assisted thoracic surgery, endoscopic or laser ablation of blebs has become a surgical option. LoCicero, et al. (1985) showed, both in experimental and clinical studies, that the carbon dioxide and neodymium: yttrium aluminum garnet (Nd: YAG) lasers can be successfully used to seal pleural blebs. The carbon dioxide laser works better in a bloodless field; the Nd: YAG laser is more powerful and can be used in the presence of blood.

Torre and Belloni (1989) were the first to report a significant experience with Nd: YAG laser pleurodesis done through the thoracoscope. They treated 14 patients by coagulation of the apical blebs and scarification of the parietal pleura over the first five ribs. Thirteen of the 14 had no recurrences, with a follow-up averaging 29 months. Wakabayashi, et al. (1990) described the use of the carbon dioxide laser in the therapy of patients with apical blebs and diffuse bullous emphysema. The procedure is conducted under general anesthesia with a double-lumen tube in the presence of a collapsed lung. Two small openings are made over the anterior and posterior axillary lines at the level of the fifth interspace, and these are used to introduce the thoracoscope and one operating probe. Pleural adhesions are first divided with endoscopic scissors and electrocautery, and then the entire inner surface of the lung is exposed to the carbon dioxide laser. This is important because, without laser therapy of the inside of the blebs or bullae, this method will fail in 25 percent of patients. Wakabayashi (1989) and Wakabayashi, et al. (1990) now propose operative intervention in all cases of a first occurrence of pneumothorax with laser bleb coagulation and pleurodesis. This is not our opinion.

The use of the argon beam electrocoagulator was evaluated by Rusch, et al. (1990) who concluded that this method is effective to control blood loss and seal air leaks from the pulmonary parenchyma. This new instrumentation, which functions in a noncontact manner, is said to be both safe and efficient. It causes less tissue injury than standard electrocautery, and its use through the thoracoscope may become more popular in the future.

The resection of subpleural blebs and the obliteration of the pleural space by pleurectomy can also be performed under video-assisted thoracoscopy (Nathanson, et al., 1991). The operation is carried out under general anesthesia with a single- or double-lumen tube. Four thoracic openings are made, two for insertion of the 11-mm cannulas for the telescope and dissecting instruments and two others for the insertion of the 5.5-mm cannulas and the use of grasping forceps, scissors, and suturing materials. The lung is collapsed with or without carbon dioxide insufflation, and after the initial inspection, ligation of the blebs or bullae can be performed

Table 38-1. Recurrence of Primary Spontaneous Pneumothorax After Various Therapies

Therapy	Recurrences (%)
Expectant	30
Aspiration	20–50
Chest tube drainage	20–30
Pleurodesis (tetracycline)	25
Pleurodesis (talc)	7
Surgery	2

Cause of Secondary Spontaneous Pneumothorax

Airway and pulmonary disease
  Chronic obstructive pulmonary disease (bullous or diffuse emphysema)
  Asthma
  Cystic fibrosis
Interstitial lung disease
  Pulmonary fibrosis
  Sarcoidosis
Infectious disease
  Tubercular and other mycobacterial
  Bacterial
  P. carinii
  Parasitic
  Mycotic
  AIDS
Neoplasic
  Bronchogenic carcinoma
  Metastatic (lymphoma or sarcoma)
Catamenial (endometriosis)
Miscellaneous
  Marfan's syndrome
  Ehlers-Danlos syndrome
  Histiocytosis X
  Scleroderma
  Lymphangiomyomatosis
  Collagen disease

with the Endoloop (Ethicon, U.S.A.) or the endogastrointestinal anastomosis stapling device (Melvin, et al., 1992). Apical parietal pleurectomy can be easily performed with endoscissors and forceps. The diathermy probe can also be used to cauterize the pleura. The video-assisted thoracoscopic technique reproduces the bullectomy and parietal pleurectomy previously performed through a thoracotomy (Kleinmann, et al., 1991). Surgical exposure is often much better than what is seen through an axillary thoratocomy in which the posterior aspect of the lung cannot be reached easily. With the development of endothoracic stapling instruments, the operation is not only easier but also quicker to perform.

In 1992 Landreneau, et al. (1992) reported the same technique but with the use of only three thoracoscopic ports. Many advantages to this procedure were described, mainly complete inspection of the entire pleural surface, decreased postoperative pain, a shorter postoperative stay, and immediate and full expansion of the lung. Thoracoscopy allows for the nonmedical personnel to be involved in the procedure, and it optimizes the available assistance.

SECONDARY SPONTANEOUS PNEUMOTHORAX

Spontaneous pneumothorax can be secondary to a variety of pulmonary and nonpulmonary disorders. According to Schoenenberger, et al. (1991), most patients with secondary pneumothoraces are male and older than 45 years; most have documented or clinically apparent pulmonary disease (Lichter, 1974). Table 38-2 describes some of the differences between primary and secondary spontaneous pneumothoraces.

Pneumothorax Complicating Chronic Obstructive Pulmonary Disease

This is the most common variety of secondary pneumothorax. It occurs in patients older than 50 years of age and is the result of rupture of a bulla into the pleural space.

Most patients with chronic obstructive pulmonary disease and pneumothorax present with chest pain and acute sudden respiratory distress with hypoxia, hypercarbia, and acidosis. Because of their limited pulmonary function, these patients may show little tolerance to even a small pneumothorax. The diagnosis can be difficult because the physical findings are those of chronic obstructive pulmonary disease with hyperresonance on percussion and diminished breath sounds at

Table 38-2. Comparison Between Primary and Secondary Spontaneous Pneumothoraces

	Primary	Secondary
Age (yr)	< 40	> 50
Sex (male/female)	5:1	4:1
Smokers	75%	85%
Pathologic condition	Subpleural blebs	Diffuse emphysema, bullous emphysema
Duration of air leaks	< 48 h	> 48 h
Duration of hospital stay	< 6 days	1–15 days
Surgical approach	Axillary thoracotomy, thoracoscopy, minimal thoracotomy	Posterolateral thoracotomy
Surgical therapy	Resection of apical blebs, pleurodesis	Resection of leaking parenchyma, pleurodesis
Recurrences	< 1%	Depending on underlying disease
Mortality rate	0%	Up to 10%

auscultation. In most cases the diagnosis is made by chest radiographs, which may sometimes be difficult of interpret because of the increased radiolucency of the diseased lung. In these difficult cases, a CT scan may be necessary to confirm the diagnosis, localize the pneumothorax better (Bourgouin, et al., 1985), and distinguish between a large bulla and a pneumothorax.

The emergency therapy of patients with secondary pneumothoraces is similar to the one described for patients with primary spontaneous pneumothoraces, except that observation alone is seldom justified. The clinician should always try to re-expand the lung with tube drainage, which is often continued for a longer period than in primary pneumothoraces. Videm, et al. (1987) showed that, because of poor lung vascularization, these patients have a prolonged chest tube drainage with a higher incidence of in-hospital infections and empyemas. If the pleural space is adequately drained and the lung is maintained in a re-expanded state, the air leak eventually stops. In some patients, however, a bronchopleural fistula persist for 10 to 15 days, and open thoracotomy must be considered.

When surgery is required, the procedure must be individualized and based on the extent of disease and the localization of the air leak. Lobectomy or segmental resection is to be avoided, and ligation or stapling resection of the bullae should be carried out, followed by subtotal parietal pleurectomy or pleural abrasion. The mortality rate for surgery may reach 10 percent (Keszler, 1990; Martigne, et al., 1984), and the morbidity rate is significant (Weeden and Smith, 1983). In those individuals with a poor overall physical condition, surgery may be too risky, and other options, such as chemical pleurodesis (Almassi and Haasler, 1989), autologous blood injection (Robinson, 1987), and permanent drainage with fistula (Hood, et al., 1986), must be considered.

Pneumothorax and Cystic Fibrosis

Pneumothorax occurs in about 10 percent of patients with cystic fibrosis, and it may be a life-threatening condition in those patients with poor lung function. The outcome of conservative therapy is associated with a high rate of recurrences, and the advent of lung transplantation has complicated the decision for surgery (Tribble, et al., 1986). If a pleural abrasion is done, it may contraindicate future transplantation. The best solution is an axillary thoracotomy or a thoracoscopic approach with apical resection without pleurodesis (Noyes and Orenstein, 1992).

Pneumothorax Secondary to Infection

Pneumothorax can be secondary to lung infection (bacterial, viral, mycotic, or parasitic), pleural infection (empyema), or intra-abdominal infection (subphrenic abscess). Cavitary pulmonary infections are particularly prone to complication with a pneumothorax. Pulmonary tuberculosis is known to be associated with the development of pneumothoraces, which often require a prolonged period of chest drainage (Wilder, et al., 1962). In cases of tuberculosis, surgery should not be considered before the patient has received sufficient systemic antituberculosis therapy.

Pneumothorax and Acquired Immunodeficiency Syndrome

Since the early 1980s, there have been increasing numbers of reports describing the association between spontaneous pneumothorax and pneumomediastinum and AIDS (Byrnes, et al., 1989). Pneumothoraces associated with AIDS are usually secondary to *P. carini* pneumonia (Joe, et al., 1986) and De Lorenzo, et al. (1987) reported a 6 percent incidence of pneumothorax in these patients. Pneumothorax can also occur in patients with Kaposi's sarcoma or mycobacterial, cytomegaloviral, or pyogenic infections. Sometimes it is the initial pulmonary manifestation of AIDS (Kuhlman, et al., 1989). In patients with AIDS, a pneumothorax may remain small and asymptomatic, but it may also enlarge rapidly to become under tension, causing severe respiratory failure. There is also a predilection for synchronous bilateral pneumothoraces with associated significant bronchopleural fistulas and higher incidence rates of ipsilateral and contralateral recurrences.

The large number of pneumothoraces seen in patients with AIDS is likely to be secondary to the increased incidence of cystic disease in these patients. The lesions occur most often at the apex of both lungs and consist of subpleural air spaces filled with eosinophilic exudate, *P. carinii* organisms, fibrous material, and macrophages (Travis, et al., 1990). Histologic studies suggest that the cystic lesions found are the result of infection associated with tissue destruction and fibrosis (De Lorenzo, et al., 1987).

The initial management should be conservative whenever possible, and sometimes small pneumothoraces can resolve with observation alone. Most patients have, however, large and persistent air leaks, which will eventually require tube thoracostomy (Fleischer, et al., 1988; Byrnes, et al., 1989). Occasionally patients may be treated on an outpatient basis with a one-way flutter valve (Driver, et al., 1991). To prevent early recurrences, chemical pleurodesis with tetracycline has been used, but without effective results (Chechani, 1990). Surgery with resection of the diseased area and pleurectomy remains the most effective therapy. Although a high operative mortality rate was reported (Beers, et al., 1990), patients with AIDS usually tolerate surgery reasonably well, and most do not require mechanical ventilation during the postoperative period. CT scanning may be useful to demonstrate the presence of air cysts in the contralateral lung. When bilateral disease is identified, a median sternotomy can be done (Byrnes, et al., 1989) or a bilateral staged axillary thoracotomy.

Pneumothorax and Neoplasia

Occasionally bronchial obstruction by lung cancer may lead to a pneumothorax, or a pneumothorax may develop as a result of the rupture of an ischemic primary tumor or metastasis into the pleural space. Pneumothoraces may also develop during chemotherapy (Lote, et al., 1981) or radiotherapy. Although pneumothoraces are most commonly associated with metastatic sarcoma (Dines, et al., 1973; Smevik and Klepp, 1982), they have been described with teratomas; Wilms's tumors; melanomas; carcinomas of the kidney, pancreas, or cervix; gynecologic malignancies; (Helmkamp, et al., 1982); lymphomas (Yellin and Benfield, 1986); and chorio-carcinomas (Ouellette and Inculet, 1992). Although not always completely effective in preventing recurrences, closed chest tube drainage is the therapy of choice, and surgery is rarely indicated. Chemical pleurodesis may also be used to prevent recurrences (Rammohan, et al., 1986).

Catamenial (Monthly) Pneumothorax

Pneumothoraces associated with menstruation were described by Maurer, et al. (1958) and Lillington, et al. (1972). Recurrent pneumothoraces occur et al. within 48 to 72 hours of the onset of menses. To make the diagnosis the clinician must recognize the association of recurrent pneumothoraces in coincidence with the perimenstrual period.

Catamenial pneumothorax affects 3 to 6 percent of women between 20 and 30 years of age (Nakamura, et al., 1986). Most pneumothoraces occur on the right side, and the episodes may be recurrent over several years. The pneumothorax is usually small and presents clinically with chest pain and dyspnea.

The pathogenesis of catamenial pneumothorax is unclear, and many hypotheses have been proposed. Air may reach the pleural space from the cervix and abdomen through congenital diaphragmatic defects (Maurer, et al., 1958). Focal thoracic endometrial implants may be present on the visceral pleura or in the lung, with air leakage occurring during menstruation. Endometrial implants may also obstruct bronchioles, causing hyperinflation and alveolar rupture (Lillington, et al., 1972). Increased levels of the prostaglandin F_2 tromethamine level at the time of menses may also cause bronchial and vascular constriction, leading to alveolar rupture and subsequent pneumothorax. Finally several mechanisms may be involved simultaneously in the development of those pneumothoraces.

The management of catamenial pneumothoraces is similar to that of other types of pneumothoraces in which small and asymptomatic episodes may be treated conservatively and large and symptomatic episodes require tube drainage. The management of recurrences is more problematic, and many options are possible (Carter and Etten Sohn, 1990) as follows: (1) treat each episode with a chest tube, (2) administer oral contraceptives to suppress ovulation or give a weak androgen; (3) use chemical pleurodesis; (4) perform hysterectomy and bilateral oophorectomy, and (5) do a thoracotomy with pleural abrasion or pleurectomy. Fleisher, et al. (1990) pro-

posed an interesting treatment algorithm, taking into consideration whether hormonal therapy is contraindicated and/or pregnancy desired or not. In the opinion of this group, thoracotomy is indicated when pregnancy is desired or when laparoscopic tubal ligation is contraindicated.

MISCELLANEOUS

Other diseases have been associated with pneumothorax. These include Marfan's syndrome (Sensenig and Lamarche, 1980), Ehlers-Danlos syndrome, histiocystosis X, pulmonary infarction, interstitial fibrosis of the lung, eosinophilic granuloma, sarcoidosis, and tuberous sclerosis. This list does not claim to be exhaustive, and spontaneous pneumothorax can certainly happen in many other diseases.

PRIMARY SPONTANEOUS PNEUMOMEDIASTINUM

Primary spontaneous pneumomediastinum was first described by Hamman (1939). It is an uncommon and benign condition that occurs more frequently in men. Contrary to primary spontaneous pneumothorax, it is usually seen after physical effort or after an increase in intra-abdominal pressure (Yellin, 1983; McMahon, 1976). Asthmatic patients may also be more prone to developing primary spontaneous pneumomediastinum (Yellin, 1983).

Spontaneous pneumomediastinum is the result of the rupture of alveoli and alveolar septa, the interstitial air collection dissecting along the peribronchial and perivascular spaces, to reach the mediastinum and neck eventually through the mediastinocervical fascia (Keszler, 1988).

In most instances of pneumomediastinum, chest pain is a major symptom. Although rare incapacitating dyspnea or dysphagia and cough may also be present. On the physical examination subcutaneous emphysema can be felt over the neck or chest wall, and a continuous murmur may be heard over the apex of the heart (Hamman sign). The diagnosis is confirmed by a chest radiograph, and other examinations may also have to be done to rule out esophageal or tracheal perforation (Gray and Hanson, 1966).

After other causes of mediastinal emphysema have been excluded, primary spontaneous pneumomediastinum can be treated expectantly. Only rarely will it require emergency surgical decompression. If air dissects into the pleural space and creates a pneumothorax, tube thoracostomy may be necessary. Although uncommon, recurrences have been described (Abolnik, et al., 1991).

COMMENTS AND CONTROVERSIES

Primary spontaneous pneumothorax occurs in young patients with no evidence of coexisting lung disease while secondary pneumothorax is mostly seen in emphysema patients. Unless there is a complication, most surgeons will manage the first episode by conventional tube drainage. Recurrences have been treated by a great number of modalities but at present, the techniques of blebectomy with parietal pleurectomy appear to be the safest and they provide excellent long term results.

In patients with primary spontaneous pneumothorax, surgical access can be obtained through the axilla or by the newer technique of video assisted thoracic surgery (VATS). It is ironic to note that the earliest indication for thoracoscopy was the induction of pneumothorax and now, 75 years later, the almost same technique is used to manage spontaneous pneumothorax.

Both of these approaches are advantageous because they avoid the trauma and morbidity associated with conventional thoracotomy. Whether there is a difference in the individual's tolerance has yet to be determined. In VATS pleurectomy/blebectomy, for example, three thoraco parts are necessary and these are two more than the trans axillary technique, usually carried out through a 3.5–4.0 cm incision.

In my opinion, the real advantage of VATS surgery over conventional procedures is in the management of patients with pneumothoraces secondary to chronic obstructive lung disease. These individuals are at high risk for recurrence—50% in most series—and because of the patient's underlying lung condition each episode may be life threatening. In addition, such patients present high and often prohibitive operative risks. For these reasons, it is now our policy to recommend VATS surgery after the first episode of secondary spontaneous pneumothorax. The procedure consists of sub-total parietal pleurectomy with talc in sufflation over the surfaces of the diaphragm and pericardium. No attempt is made to remove blebs or bullae because this will often produce prolonged air leaks and substantially increase operative morbidity.

J.D.

KEY REFERENCES

Boutin C, Viallat JR, Aelony Y: Practical Thoracoscopy. Springer-Verlag, Berlin, 1991

This book contains an excellent chapter on the thoracoscopic management of pneumothoraces.

Deslauriers J, Lacquet LK: Surgical management of pleural diseases. In DeLarue NC, Eschapasse H: International Trends in General Thoracic Surgery. Vol. 6. CV Mosby, St. Louis, 1990

This volume is devoted to the pleural space, with special emphasis on its surgical approach and management, as seen by international experts.

Hood MR, Antman K, Boyd A et al: Surgical Diseases of the Pleura and Chest Wall. WB Saunders, Philadelphia, 1986

This is a book devoted to the surgical approach of pleural diseases, including a well-written chapter on pneumothoraces.

Killen DA, Gobbel WG: Spontaneous Pneumothorax. Little Brown, Boston, 1968

Although published more than 20 years ago, this book remains a classic in the understanding of pneumothoraces and is the most complete review of the history of pneumothoraces.

Light RW: Pleural Diseases. 2nd Ed. Lea & Febiger, Philadelphia, 1990

A complete review of the diagnosis and treatment of pleural diseases is provided with a good chapter on primary and secondary pneumothoraces.

REFERENCES

Abolnik I, Lossos IS, Brewer R: Spontaneous pneumomediastinum: a report of 25 cases. Chest 100:93, 1991

Agostini E: Mechanics of the pleural space. p. 531. In Fishman (ed): Handbook of Physiology. Section 3. Vol. 3. American Physiological Society, Bethesda, MD, 1986

Almassi GH, Haasler GB: Chemical pleurodesis in the presence of persistent air leak. Ann Thorac Surg 47:786, 1989

Almind H, Lange P, Viskun K: Spontaneous pneumothorax: comparison of simple drainage, talc pleurodesis and tetracycline pleurodesis. Thorax 44:627, 1989

Anthonisen NR: Regional lung function in spontaneous pneumothorax. Am Rev Respir Dis 115:873, 1977

Askew AR: Parietal pleurectomy for recurrent pneumothorax. Br J Surg 63:203, 1976

Axel L: A simple way to estimate the size of a pneumothorax. Invest Radiol 16:165, 1981

Beers MF, John M, Swartz M: Recurrent pneumothorax in AIDS patients with Pneumocystis pneumonia. Chest 98:266, 1990

Bense L: Spontaneous pneumothorax related to falls in atmospheric pressure. Eur J Respir Dis 65:544, 1984

Bense L, Eklund G, Wiman LG: Smoking and the increased risk contracting spontaneous pneumothorax. Chest 92:1009, 1987

Bevelaqua FA, Aranda C: Management of spontaneous pneumothorax with small lumen catheter manual aspiration. Chest 81:6, 1982

Bigger IA: Operative surgery. CV Mosby, St. Louis, 1937

Bourgouin P, Cousineau G, Lemire P, Hebert G: Computed tomography used to exclude pneumothorax in bullous lung disease. Can Assoc Radiol J 36:341, 1985

Brooks JW: Open thoracotomy in a management of spontaneous pneumothorax. Ann Surg 177:798, 1973

Byrnes TA, Brevig JK, Yeoh CB: Pneumothorax in patients with acquired immunodeficiency syndrome. J Thorac Cardiovasc Surg 98:546, 1989

Caes F, Cham B, Van den Brande P, Welch W: Transaxillary thoracotomy for treatment of spontaneous pneumothorax. Acta Chir Belg 87:137, 1987

Carr JJ Reed JC, Choplin RH et al: Plain and computed radiography for detecting experimentally induced pneumothorax in cadavers: implications for detection in patients. Radiology 183:193, 1992

Carter JE, Etten Sohn DB: Catamenial pneumothorax. Chest 98:713, 1990

Chechani V: Tetracyline pleurodesis for persistent air leak. Ann Thorac Surg 49:166, 1990

Clagett OT: The management of spontaneous pneumothorax (editorial). J Thorac Cardiovasc Surg 56:761, 1968

Clague H, El-Ansory E: Conservative management of spontaneous pneumothorax. Lancet 687:1, 1984

Clarck TA, Hutchinson DE, Deaner RM et al: Spontaneous pneumothorax. Am J Surg 124:728, 1972

Conces DJ, Tarver RD, Gray C et al: Treatment of pneumothoraces utilizing small caliber chest tubes. Chest 95:55, 1988

Cormier Y: Gas transfer in the pleural space. p. 10. In Deslauriers J, Lacquet LK (eds): International Trends in General Thoracic Surgery. Vol. 6. CV Mosby, St. Louis, 1990

Daniel TM, Tribble CG, Rodgers BM: Thoracoscopy and talc poudrage for pneumothoraces and effusions. Ann Thorac Surg 50:186, 1990

Delius RE, Obeid FN, Horst HM et al: Catheter aspiration for simple pneumothorax. Arch Surg 124:833, 1989

DeLorenzo LJ, Huang TC, Maguire JP, Stone DJ: Roentgenographic patterns of *Pneumocystis carinii* pneumonia in 104 patients with AIDS. Chest 91:323, 1987

Dermksian G, Lamb LE: Spontaneous pneumothorax in apparently healthy flying personnel. Ann Intern Med 51:39, 1959

Deslauriers J, Beaulieu M, Despres JP et al: Transaxillary thoracotomy for treatment of spontaneous pneumothorax. Ann Thorac Surg 30:35, 1980

Deslauriers J, Piraux M: Diagnosis and management of spontaneous pneumothorax in the young adult: role of parietal pleurectomy. p. 119. In Deslauriers J, Lacquet LK. (eds): International Trends in General Thoracic Surgery. Vol. 6. CV Mosby, St. Louis, 1990

Desmeules M, Deslauriers J, Beauchamp G: Surgical anatomy of the pleura. p. 13. In Deslauriers J, Lacquet LK (eds): International Trends in General Thoracic Surgery. Vol. 6. CV Mosby, St. Louis, 1990

Devries WC, Woolfe WG: The management of spontaneous pneumothorax in emphysema. Surg Clin North Am 60:851, 1981

Dhalla SS, Teskey J: Surgical management of recurrent spontaneous pneumothorax during pregnancy. Chest 88:201, 1985

Diamond JR, Estes MN: ECG changes associated with iatrogenic left pneumothorax simulating anterior myocardial infarction. Am Heart J 103:303, 1982

Dines DE, Clagett OT, Payne WS: Spontaneous pneumothorax in emphysema. Mayo Clin Proc 45:481, 1970

Dines DE, Cortese DA, Brennon MD et al: Malignant pulmonary neoplasia predisposing to spontaneous pneumothorax. Mayo Clin Proc 48:541, 1973

Donovan PJ: Bilateral spontaneous pneumothorax. Ann Emerg Med 16:1277, 1987

Driver GA, Peden JG, Adams HG, Rumley RL: Heimlich valve, treatment of *Pneumocystis carinii* associated pneumothorax. Chest 100:281, 1991

Edge J, Simon G, Reid L: Peri-acinar paraseptal emphysema: its clinical, radiological, and physiological features. Br J Dis Chest 60:10, 1966

Emerson CP: Pneumothorax: a historical, clinical and experimental study. Johns Hopkins Rep 11:1, 1903

Engdahl O, Torgil T, Boe J: Chest radiograph—a poor method for determining the size of a pneumothorax. Chest 103:26, 1993

Ferguson LJ, Imrie CW, Hutchison J: Excision of bullae without pleurectomy in patients with spontaneous pneumothorax. Br J Surg 68:214, 1981

Fleisher AG, Clement PB, Nelems B: Catamenial pneumothorax: pathophysiology and management. p. 132. In Deslauriers J, Lacquet LK (eds): International Trends in Gen Thoracic Surgery. Vol. 6. CV Mosby, St. Louis, 1990

Fleisher AG, McElvaney G, Lawson L et al: Surgical management of spontaneous pneumothorax in patient with acquired immunodeficiency syndrome. Ann Thorac Surg 45:21, 1988

Gaensler EA: Parietal pleurectomy for recurrent spontaneous pneumothorax. Surg Gynecol Obstet 102:293, 1956

Gaensler EA, Jederlinic PJ, Fitzgerald MY: Patient work-up for bullectomy. J Thorac Imaging 1:75, 1986

Getz SB, Beasely WE: Spontaneous pneumothorax. Am J Surg 145:823, 1983

Gillet-Juvin K, Guérin JC: Le talcage sous thoracoscopie des pneumothorax par rupture de bulles d'emphysème. Rev Mal Respir 8:289, 1991

Gilmartin JJ, Wright AJ, Gibson GJ: Effects of pneumothorax or pleural effusion on pulmonary function. Thorax 40:60, 1985

Gobbel WG Jr, Rhea WG Jr, Nelson IA et al: Spontaneous pneumothorax. J Thorac Cardiovasc Surg 46:331, 1963

Granke K, Fischer CR, Gago O et al: The efficacy and timing of operative intervention for spontaneous pneumothorax. Ann Thorac Surg 42:540, 1986

Gray JM, Hanson GG: Mediastinal emphysema: etiology, diagnosis and treatment. Thorax 21:325, 1966

Gutsman P, Yerger L, Wanner A: Immediate cardiovascular effects on tension pneumothorax. Am Rev Respir Dis 127:171, 1983

Hamman L: Spontaneous mediastinal emphysema. Bull Johns Hopkins Hosp 64:1, 1939

Heffner JE, Unrush LC: Tetracycline pleurodesis, adios, farewell, adieu. Chest 101:1, 1992

Heimlich HJ: Valve drainage of the pleural cavity. Dis Chest 53:282, 1968

Helmkamp BF, Beecham JB, Wandtke TJ, Keys H: Spontaneous pneumothorax in gynecologic malignancy. Am J Obstet Gynecol 142:706, 1982

Hnatiuk OW, Dillard TA, Oster CN: Bleomycin sclerotherapy for bilateral pneumothoraces in a patient with AIDS. Ann InternMed 113:988, 1990

Hurewitz AN, Sidhu EH, Bergofsky B et al: Cardiovascular and respiratory consequences of tension pneumothorax. Bull Eur Physiopathol Respir 22:545, 1986

Ikeda M, Akira U, Yamane Y, Hagiwala N: Median sternotomy with bilateral bullous resection in unilateral spontaneous pneumothorax with special reference to operative indications. Thorac Cardiovasc Surg 96:615, 1988

Joe L, Gorden F, Parker RH: Spontaneous pneumothorax with *Pneumocystis carinii* infection: occurrence in patients with acquired immunodeficiency syndrome. Arch Intern Med 146:1816, 1986

Keszler P: Management of pneumothorax in the emphysematous patient. p. 130. In Deslauriers J, Lacquet LK (eds): International Trends in General Thoracic Surgery. Vol. 6. CV Mosby, St. Louis, 1990

Keszler P: Surgical pathology of bullae with and without pneumothorax. Eur J Cardiothorac Surg 2:416, 1988

Kircher LT Jr, Swartzel RL: Spontaneous pneumothorax and its treatment. JAMA 155:24, 1954

Kjaergaard H: Spontaneous pneumothorax in the apparently healthy. Acta Med Scand Suppl 43:159, 1932

Klassen KP, Meckstroth CV: Treatment of spontaneous pneumothorax: prompt expansion with controlled thoracotomy tube suction. JAMA 182:1, 1962

Kleinmann P, Lévi JF, Debesse B: La pleurectomie pariétale percutanée par vidéo-endoscopie. Rev Mal Respir 8:459, 1991

Klingman R, Angellillo V, DeMeester T: Cystic and bullous lung disease. Ann Thorac Surg 52:576, 1990

Kuhlman JE, Knowles MC, Fishman EK, Siegelman SS: Premature bullous pulmonary damage in AIDS: CT diagnosis. Radiology 173:23, 1989

Landreneau RJ, Hazelrigg SR, Ferson PF et al: Thoracoscopic resection of 85 pulmonary lesions. Ann Thorac Surg 54:415, 1992

Lange P, Mortensen J, Groth S: Lung function 22-35 years after treatment of idiopathic spontaneous pneumothorax with talc poudrage or simple drainage. Thorax 43:559, 1988

Larrieu AJ, Tyers GFU, Williams EH et al: Intrapleural instillation of quinacrine for treatment of recurrent spontaneous pneumothorax. Ann Thorac Surg 28:146, 1979

Lau OJ, Shawkat S: Pleurectomy through the triangle of auscultation. Thorax 37:945, 1982

Lesur O, Delorme N, Fromaget JM et al: Computed tomography in the etiologic assessment of idiopathic spontaneous pneumothorax. Chest 98:341, 1990

Lichter I: Long term follow-up of planned treatment of spontaneous pneumothorax. Thorax 29:32, 1974

Light RW, O'Hara VS, Moritz TE et al: Intrapleural tetracycline for the prevention of recurrent spontaneous pneumothorax. JAMA 264:2224, 1990

Lillington GA, Mitchell SP, Wood GA: Catamenial pneumothorax. JAMA 219:1328, 1972

LoCicero J, Hartz RS, Frederiksen JA et al: New applications of the laser in pulmonary surgery: hemostasis and sealing of air leaks. Ann Thorac Surg 40:546, 1985

Lockwood CD: Discussion of paper by Watson EE, Robertson C: Recurrent spontaneous pneumothorax, report of three cases. Arch Surg 6:341, 1928

Lorch DG, Gordon L, Wooten S et al: Effect of patient positioning on distribution of tetracycline in the pleural space during pleurodesis. Chest 93:527, 1988

Lote K, Dahl O, Vigander T: Pneumothorax during combination chemotherapy. Cancer 47:743, 1981

Mahfood S, Hix WR, Aaron BL et al: Reexpansion pulmonary edema. Ann Thorac Surg 45:340, 1988

Martigne C, Velly JF, Levy F et al: La chirurgie du pneumothorax spontané chez l'insuffisant respiratoire chronique. Bordeaux Med 17:507, 1984

Maunders RJ, Pierson DJ, Hudson LD: Subcutaneous and mediastinal emphysema. Arch Intern Med 144:1447, 1984

Maurer ER, Schall JA, Mondez FL: Chronic recurrent spontaneous pneumothorax due to endometriosis of the diaphragm. Jama 168:2013, 1958

McMahon DJ: Spontaneous pneumomediastinum. Am J Surg 131:550, 1976

Melton LJ, Hepper NG, Offord KP: Incidence of spontaneous pneumothorax in Olmsted County, Minnesota: 1950 to 1974. Am Rev Respir Dis 120:1379, 1979

Melvin WS, Krasna MJ, McLaughlin JS: Thoracoscopic management of spontaneous pneumothorax. Chest 102:1875, 1992

Mercier C, Page A, Verdant A et al: Out-patient management of intercostal tube drainage in spontaneous pneumothorax. Ann Thorac Surg 22:163, 1976

Moores D: Pleurodesis by mechanical pleural abrasion for spontaneous pneumothorax. p. 126. In Deslauriers J, Lacquet LK (eds): International Trends in General Thoracic Surgery. Vol. 6. CV Mosby, St. Louis, 1990

Moran JF, Jones RH, Wolfe WG: Regional pulmonary function during experimental unilateral pneumothorax in the awake state. J Thorac Cardiovasc Surg 74:396, 1977

Murray KD, Matheny RG, Howanitz EP, Myerowitz PD: A limited axillary thoracotomy as primary treatment of recurrent spontaneous pneumothorax. Chest 103:137, 1993

Nakamura H, Konischiike J, Sugamura A et al: Epidemiology of spontaneous pneumothorax in women. Chest 89:378, 1986

Nathanson LK, Shermi SM, Wood RA, Cuschieri A: Video thoracoscopic ligation of bullae and pleurectomy for spontaneous pneumothorax. Ann Thorac Surg 53:316, 1991

Noble D: Some particulars of treatment in a case of pneumothorax. BMJ 2:425, 1873

Norris RM, Jones JG, Bishop JM: Respiratory gas exchange in patients with spontaneous pneumothorax. Thorax 23:427, 1968

Noyes BE, Orenstein DM: Treatment of pneumothorax in cystic fibrosis in the era of lung transplantation. Chest 101:1187, 1992

Ohata M, Suzuki H: Pathogenesis of spontaneous pneumothorax with special references to the ultrastructure of emphysematous bullae. Chest 77:771, 1980

O'Rourke JP, Yee ES: Civilian spontaneous pneumothorax: treatment options and long-term results. Chest 96:1302, 1989

Ouellette D, Inculet R: Unsuspected metastatic choriocarcinoma presenting as unilateral spontaneous pneumothorax. Ann Thorac Surg 53:144, 1992

Pairolero PC, Payne SW: The surgical management of recurrent or persistent pneumothorax: abrasive pleurodesis. p. 43. In Kittle FC (ed): Current Controversies in Thoracic Surgery. WB Saunders, Philadelphia, 1986

Rammohan G, Bonacini M, Dwek JH, Das A: Pleurodesis in metastatic pneumothorax. Chest 90:918, 1986

Reid L: Emphysema: classification and clinical significance. Br J Dis Chest 60:57, 1966

Rhea JT, DeLuca SA, Greene RE: Determining the size of pneumothorax in the upright patient. Radiology 144:733, 1982

Rivarola CH: Tension pneumothorax. p. 153. In Deslauriers J, Lacquet LK (eds): International Trends in General Thoracic Surgery. Vol. 6. CV Mosby, Philadelphia, 1990

Robinson CLN: Autologous blood pleurodesis in recurrent and chronic spontaneous pneumothorax. Can J Surg 30:428, 1987

Rusch VW, Schmidt R, Shoji Y, Fujimura Y: Use of the argon beam electrocoagulator for performing pulmonary wedge resections. Ann Thorac Surg 49:287, 1990

Rutherford RB, Hurt HH Jr, Brickman RD et al: The pathophysiology of progressive tension pneumothorax. J Trauma 8:212, 1968

Sahn SA, Good IT Jr, Potts DE: The pH sclerosing agents: a determinant of pleural symphysis. Chest 76:198, 1979

Samuelson SL, Golberg EM, Ferguson MK: The thoracic vent, clinical experience with a new device for treating simple pneumothorax. Chest 100:880, 1991

Sargent EM, Turner AF: Emergency treatment of pneumothorax: a single catheter technique for use in the radiology department. AJR 109:531, 1970

Schoenenberger RA, Haefeli EW, Weiss P, Ritz RF: Timing of invasive procedure in therapy for primary and secondary spontaneous pneumothorax. Arch Surg 126:875, 1991

Scott GC, Berger R, McKean HE: The role of atmospheric pressure variation in the development of spontaneous pneumothoraces. Am Rev Respir Dis 139:659, 1989

Selikoff IJ, Broder RA, Bader ME: Asbestosis and neoplasia. Am J Med 424:87, 1987

Sensenig DM, Lamarche P: Marfan syndrome and spontaneous pneumothorax. Am J Surg 139:601, 1990

Seremetis MG: The management of spontaneous pneumothorax. Chest 57:65, 1970

Singh SV: The surgical treatment of spontaneous pneumothorax by parietal pleurectomy. Scand J Thorac Cardiovasc Surg 16:75, 1982

Smevik B, Klepp O: The risk of spontaneous pneumothorax in patients with osteogenic sarcoma and testicular cancer. Cancer 49:1734, 1982

Stephenson LW: Treatment of spontaneous pneumothorax with intrapleural tetracycline. Chest 88:803, 1985

Sugiyama Y, Maeda H, Yotsumoto H et al: Familial spontaneous pneumothorax. Thorax 41:969, 1986

Swierenga J: Atlas of Thoracoscopy. Boehringer, Ingelheim, 1977

Swierenga J, Wagennar JPM, Gergstein PGM: The value of thoracoscopy in the diagnosis and treatment of diseases affecting the pleura and lung. Pneumologie 151:11, 1974

Sy SO, Dyc YU: Catheter drainage of spontaneous pneumothorax: suction or no suction, early or late removal. Thorax 37:46, 1982

Thomas PA, Gebauer PW: Pleurectomy for recurrent spontaneous pneumothorax. J Thorac Surg 35:117, 1958

Torre M, Belloni P: Nd: YAG laser pleurodesis through thoracoscopy: new curative therapy in spontaneous pneumothorax. Ann Thorac Surg 47:887, 1989

Travis WD, Pittaluga S, Lipschik GY et al: Atypical pathologic manifestations of *Pneumocystis carinii* pneumonia in the acquired immune deficiency syndrome Am J Surg Pathol 14:615, 1990

Tribble CB, Selden RF, Rogers BM: Talc poudrage in the treatment of spontaneous pneumothorax in patients with cystic fibrosis. Ann Surg 677:204, 1986

Tyson MD, Crandall WB: The surgical treatment of recurrent idiopathic spontaneous pneumothorax. J Thorac Surg 10:566, 1941

Vanderschueren RG: The role of thoracoscopy in the evaluation and management of pneumothorax. Lung (suppl):1122, 1990

Vanderschueren RG: Le talcage pleural dans le pneumothorax spontané. Poumon-Coeur 37:273, 1981

Verschoof GPM, Velde T, Greve LH et al: Thoracoscopic pleurodesis in the management of spontaneous pneumothorax. Respiration 53:197, 1988

Videm V, Pillgram-Larsen J, Ellingsen O et al: Spontaneous pneumothorax in chronic obstructive pulmonary disease: complications, treatment and recurrences. Eur J Respir Dis 71:365, 1987

Viskum K, Lange P, Mortensen J: Long term sequelae after talc pleurodesis for spontaneous pneumothorax. Pneumologie 43:105, 1989

Wakabayashi A: Thoracoscopic ablation of blebs in the treatment of recurrent or persistent spontaneous pneumothorax. Ann Thorac Surg 48:651, 1989

Wakabayashi A, Brenner M, Wilson A et al: Thoracoscopic treatment of spontaneous pneumothorax using carbon dioxide laser. Ann Thorac Surg 50:786, 1990

Walston A, Brewer DL, Kitchens CS et al: Electrocardiographic manifestation of spontaneous left pneumothorax. Ann Intern Med 80:375, 1974

Warner BW, Bailey WW, Shipley RT: Value of computed tomography of the lung in the management of primary spontaneous pneumothorax. Am J Surg 162:39, 1991

Wayne M, McSwain NE: Clinical evaluation of a new device for the treatment of tension pneumothorax. Ann Surg 191:760, 1980

Weeden D, Smith GH: Surgical experience in the management of spontaneous pneumothorax 1972-1982. Thorax 387:37, 1983

Weisberg D: The surgical management of recurrent or persistent pneumothorax: pleuroscopy and talc poudrage. p. 46. In Kittle FC (ed): Current Controversies and Thoracic Surgery. WB Saunders, Philadelphia, 1986

Wied U, Halkier E, Hoeier-Madsen K et al: Tetracycline versus silver nitrate pleurodesis in spontaneous pneumothorax. J Thorac Cardiovasc Surg 86:591, 1983

Wilder RJ, Beacham EG, Ravitch MM: Spontaneous pneumothorax complicating cavitary tuberculosis. J Thorac Cardiovasc Surg 43:561, 1962

Yellin A, Benfield JR: Pneumothorax associated with lymphoma. Am Rev Respir Dis 134:590, 1986

Youmans CR Jr, Williams RD, Monthy RM: Surgical management of spontaneous pneumothorax by bleb ligation and pleural dry sponge abrasion. Am J Surg 120:644, 1970

39

RARE INFECTIONS

Jorge Nin Vivo
Mario Brandolino

PLEURAL HYDATIDOSIS

DEFINITION

Hydatid pleural disease is always secondary to the rupture of hydatid cysts located in adjacent organs such as the lung, the liver, or less commonly, the pericardium, spleen, or chest wall (ribs, spine, or diaphragm). Invasion of the pleural space will result in formation of a new hydatid cyst, which will eventually develop into so-called secondary pleural hydatidosis.

HISTORICAL NOTE

Since the Intercolonial Medical Congress of Australia held in Melbourne in 1889, hydatid cystic disease of the lung has been recognized as a surgical pathologic condition. At that meeting, Thomas (Perez Fontana, 1948) reported a mortality rate of 61.4 percent among 208 patients with hydatic cysts of the lung that had been treated conservatively. He also introduced a surgical technique consisting of pleurotomy, cyst puncture, incision, and marsupialization of the pericyst and evacuation of its content, leaving a chest tube inside the cyst cavity. He later reported a series of 38 patients treated by this technique with 32 good results. Three hydatic cysts of the lung ruptured in the pleura and were treated by pleurotomy.

At about the same time, numerous cases of hydatidosis were also seen in Argentina and Uruguay, where there were two differnt schools of thoughts. Some surgeons performed one-stage procedures (Posadas 1895), with cyst evacuation through the pleural space and pericyst or lung suture to the chest wall with marsupialization, while others carried out surgery in two stages, first inducing pleural adhesions and then evacuating the parasites through these adhesions, thereby avoiding operative pneumothoraces (Fossati, 1943).

In 1937 Dèvé reported 11 cases of secondary pleural hydatidosis, 3 of which being complications of surgery. Armand Ugon (1935) also reported cases of secondary pleural hydatidosis and hydatid pneumothoraces. In 1945 he described pa-tients in whom surgery had been performed with good results, and in 1947 he published his technique for the treatment of hydatid cysts of the lung. The technique consisted of enucleation of the hydatid with partial resection and capitonnage of the emergent pericyst layer. In 1947 Barret described a similar technique.

HISTORICAL READINGS

Armand Ugon V: Equinococosis pleural secundaria. An Dep Cient Salud Publ Montevideo 2:389, 1935

Barret NR: The treatment of pulmonary hydatid disease. Thorax 1:21, 1947

Dèvé F: L'échinococcose secondaire de la plèvre. J Chir (Paris) 49:497, 1937

Fossati A: Quistes hidaticos de pulmon. Metodo de Lamas y Mondino/Tecnica Personal y breve comentario. An Fac Med Montevideo 28:793, 1943

Lamas A: Quelques details a propos du traitement chirurgical au kyste hydatique du poumon. J Chirurgie T.XLI 3, 1933

Perez Fontana V: Nuevo metodo de operar en el quiste hidatico del pulmon. Arch Pediatr Uruguay 19(1):5, 1948

Posadas A: Quistes hidatidicos. An Circulo Med Argent 23:613, 1895

PATHOLOGY

Pleural Complications of Hydatid Cysts of the Lung

Hydatid cysts of the lung are slowly progressive lesions, and their pericyst layer is weak. They can give rise to two varieties of pleural lesions, parahydatid and hydatid pleural complications (Fig. 39-1).

In parahydatid complications the cyst itself is not ruptured, and the clinical manifestations are related either to a pneumothorax (periadventitial complication) or to a serofibrinous pleurisy secondary to mechanical or allergic pleural irritation.

Hydatid pleural complications are produced by the rupture of both the hydatid and the pericyst layer, giving rise to a hydatid hydropneumothorax. When a bronchoadventitial-pleural fistula is also present, secondary infection of the cav-

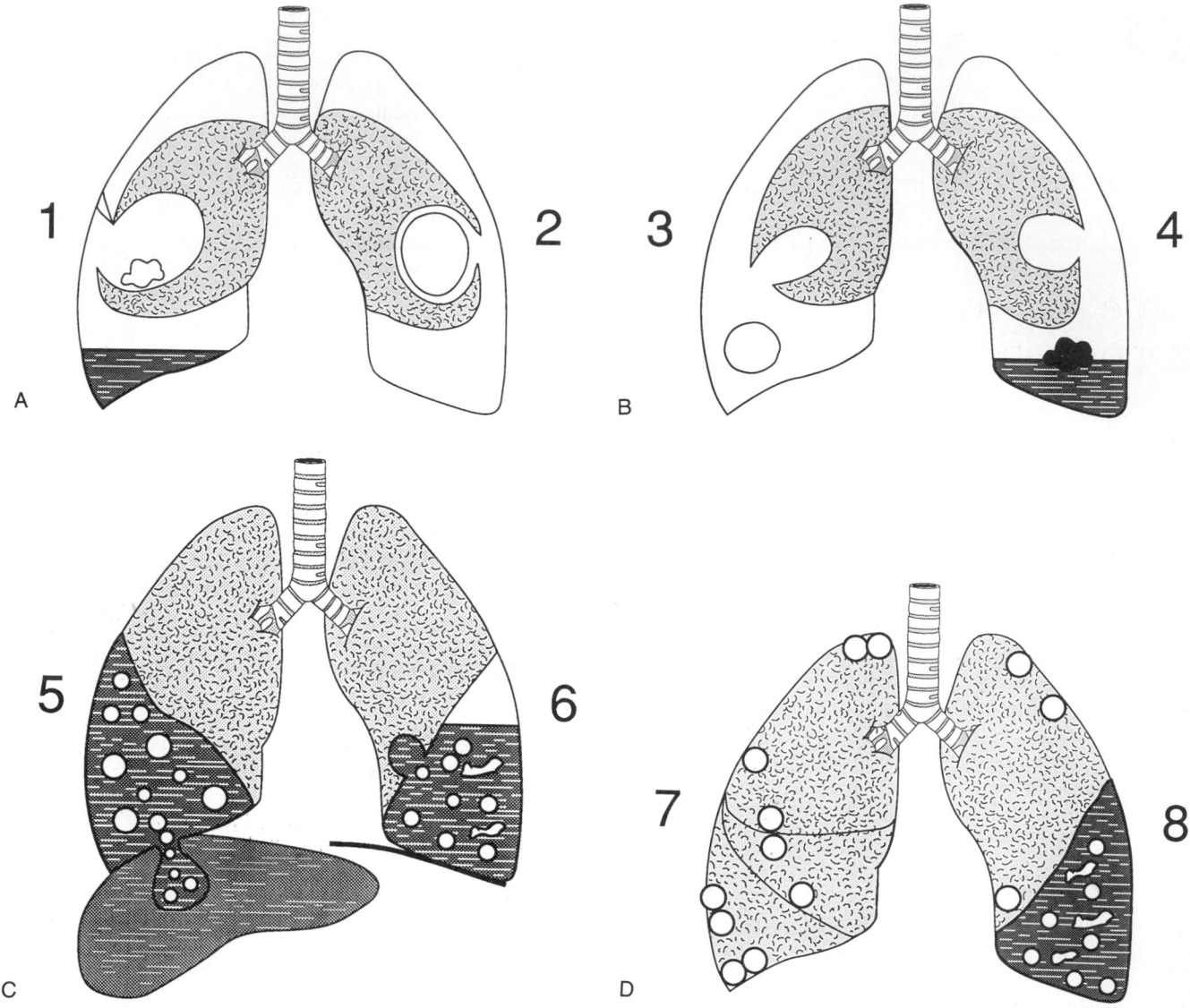

Figure 39-1. Different presentations of hydatid pleural disease. **(A)** 1, Pyopneumothorax (membrane retention); 2, pneumothorax. **(B)** 3, Heterotopic pleural primitive hydatidosis (HPPH); 4, pyopneumothorax (water lily sign). **(C)** 5, Hydatid thorax of hepatic origin; 6, pneumohydatid thorax. **(D)** 7, Hydatid pleural implant; 8, mixed form (hydatid thorax and hydatid pleural implant.)

ity will produce a hydatid pyopneumothorax. Occasionally, the lung will remain collapsed for some time, and its surface will be covered by a fibrinous coat which gives rise to loculated collections of hydatid fluid, air, or pus. With these types of effusions, scolices will grow to become hydatids, this phenomenon being called hydatid thorax. If the bronchopleural fistula closes and the lung reexpands, scolices will remain between the pleural surfaces and eventually grow as independent hydatids. In this form of secondary pleural hydatidosis, which is called hydatid pleural implant and is the form most commonly encountered in clinical practice, cysts are mainly located in dependent areas and at the sites of pleural reflections.

Infrequently, ruptured lung hydatic cysts will simultaneously contaminate both the pleural space and the bronchus,

giving rise to secondary pleural hydatidosis and bronchogenetic secondary pulmonary hydatidosis, also called (Armand Ugon, 1935) massive pleuropulmonary hydatidosis. Accidental surgical rupture of a hydatid cyst of the lung may also produce a secondary pleural hydatidosis. Finally there is a rare variety of secondary pleural hydatidosis called heterotopic pleural primitive hydatidosis, in which isolated pericyst rupture allows passage of the intact hydatid into the pleural cavity.

Pleural Complications of Hepatic Hydatidosis

Pleural complications of hepatic hydatidosis develop in two different stages called the plastic and the perforative stages. During the plastic stage the liver cyst, which is normally located posteriorly and superiorly, will grow upwards, and the diaphragm will progressively contract and become thinner with areas of relative ischemia. During this process infection is common because roughly one-third of hepatic hydatic cysts have already ruptured in the biliary tract. During the perforative stage the pathologic process involves the cyst, the diaphragm, the pleura, and the lung; negative intrapleural pressure elevates the cyst toward the chest, a process helped by the obstructive biliary hypertension. When the diaphragm is perforated (the site of perforation usually does not exceed 2 cm), hydatic collections reach the pleural space, producing a hepatic thoracic transdiaphragmatic pleural hydatidosis.

Pleural Complications Originating in Osseous Echinococcosis

In the spine the parasite can invade the bone, producing necrosis and destruction of trabeculations and generating new spaces in which it will eventually grow in an irregular and asymmetric fashion. If this occurs, the hydatic collection may invade adjacent tissues such as the pleura and become pleural hydatidoses.

DIAGNOSIS

Clinical Features

Initial Pleural Accident

The initial accident is often a dramatic clinical event with sudden and acute thoracic pain, cardiovascular collapse sometimes leading to shock, and hydatid allergy (urticaria, bronchospasm, and fever) (Fig. 39-2). Often the patient will have a tension hydropneumothorax with mediastinal shift. When the lung cyst is accidentally ruptured during a surgical procedure, there are no symptoms, although occasionally the patient will show signs of allergy. Hepatic thoracic transdiaphragmatic hydatidosis may present in an acute fashion, with epigastric pain, cough, fever, shortness of breath, biliphthisis, and anaphylactic reactions.

Secondary Pleural Hydatidosis

With secondary pleural hydatidosis, symptoms often appear years after the initial accident. Hydatid pleural implant is often asymptomatic or produces mild symptoms, while hydatid cysts located in the thoracic vertex can produce symptoms of mediastinal compression. In the hydatid thorax form, the clinical presentation depends on whether secondary infection is present.

Differential Diagnosis

Clinical and radiologic diagnosis of pleural hydatidosis are usually presumptive because only the coughing of hydatid debris or the identification of hydatid elements by thoracentesis is pathognomonic of the disease. The positivity of immunologic testing (hemagglutination, immunofluorescence, and electrosyneresis) varies between 40 and 85 percent. Immuno-electrophoresis testing is useful, but Casoni's reaction and Weinberg's test and the eosinophil count are nonspecific.

Chest radiographs may show a blurred hemidiaphragm or a loculated pleural effusion, and in hydatid pleural implant, the lung may be riddled with multiple rounded opacities projecting into the pleural space. In heterotopic pleural primitive hydatidosis, one can see a hydatid pneumothorax with or without pleural effusion and a ''wanderer'' cyst changing its location with different radiologic positions. Ultrasound and computed tomography (CT) scanning of the thorax and liver may also be of some value to demonstrate the presence of cystic lesions.

MANAGEMENT

Therapy

Treatment of the initial accident is an emergency, and drainage of the pleural contents is mandatory. Definitive therapy, which should be delayed until the anaphylactic reaction is over, consists of removing the parasites, evacuating all pleural contents, and treating the affected lung by meticulous bronchial suturing and capitonnage of the adventitial cavity. The procedure is always completed by profuse pleural swabbing with hydrogen peroxide.

Hydatid pleural implant is a diffuse pleural process (Fig. 39-3), in which cysts can be few or many and can be localized, widespread, or even included in thick and fibrous areas of pachypleuritis. Often this arrangement will tend to make the exploration of the whole pleural cavity very difficult. Since very few of those cysts can be enucleated, most have to be treated by aspiration followed by injection of a parasiticide solution into the cyst.

Thoracotomy alone or with laparotomy is performed electively when the hydatid thorax has originated from a hepatic thoracic transdiphragmatic hydatidosis. The pleural cavity is first totally evacuated and cleaned. An anterolateral radial diaphragmatic incision is then made in such a way as to avoid trauma to the vena cava and suprahepatic veins and at the same time be at a distance from infected tissues. The contents of the hydatid hepatic cyst are suctioned away with a trocar, and the hepatic cavity is opened wide, totally evacuated, cleaned, and drained by two large-bore tubes, which are inserted through a separate abdominal incision. If there is an associated obstruction of the common bile duct, it should be decompressed and drained by simultaneous laparatomy or by endoscopic retrograde cholangiography with papillotomy. Only occasionally will hepatic cysts need to be treated by hepatic resection. Mebendazole and albendazole are useful during the postoperative period to prevent seeded scolices from growing.

Clinical Series

In 1988 we reviewed all 184 patients who had been operated on at Saint Bois Thoracic Department in Montevideo (Nin Vivo, et al., 1990) for thoracic hydatidosis and the 77 who had been seen with pleural complications. The current series includes all previously reported patients plus those seen since

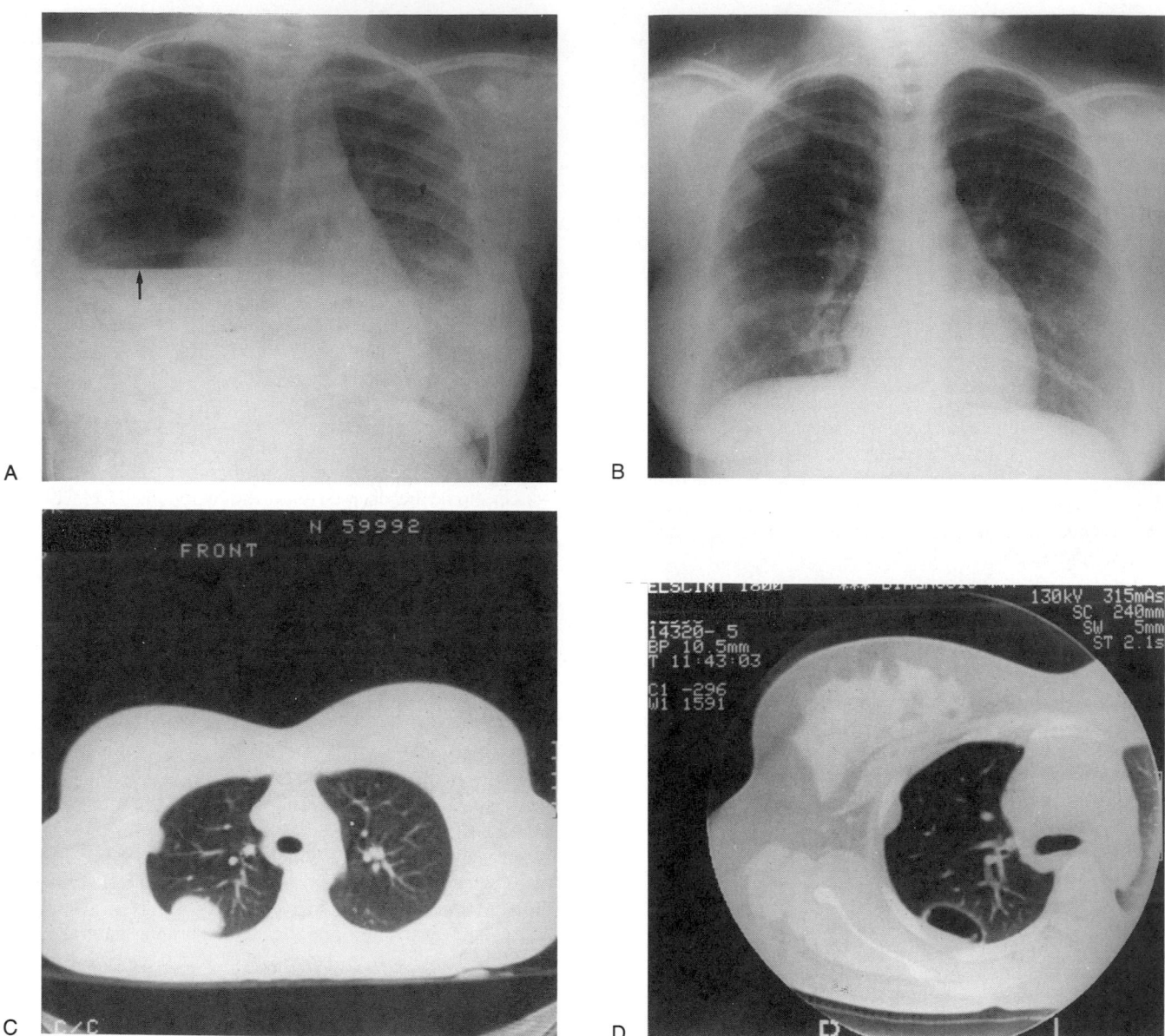

Figure 39-2.   Secondary pleural hydatidosis. **(A)** Standard chest radiograph taken during the initial accident and showing a right pyopneumothorax. The patient underwent thoracotomy, pleural drainage, and cavity treatment. Three years later, **(B)** chest radiograph and **(C)** CT scan show hydatid pleural implants. **(D)** CT scan taken after albendazole treatment. Note that the contents of one cyst were expectorated.

1988. A total of 449 patients were operated on for thoracic hydatidosis, and 46 had pleural complications (Fig. 39-4), which originated from the lung in 23 patients, from an organ located below the diaphragm in 19, from the spine in 2, from the pericardium in 1, and from the diaphgram in 1. Among the 23 patients with previous hydatid cysts of the lung, 2 developed heterotopic pleural primitive hydatidosis, 10 had pleural complications that never progressed to secondary pleural hydatidosis, and 11 developed true secondary pleural hydatidosis. Among the 19 patients with abdominothoracic transdiaphragmatic pleural hydatidosis, this complication

originated from the liver in 16, from a subphrenic hydatic cyst in 2, and from a splenic cyst in 1. All 19 patients reached the stage of secondary pleural hydatidosis, and the two with thoracic vertebral hydatidosis and the one with secondary pericardial hydatidosis also developed secondary pleural hydatidosis. The diaphragmatic cyst secondarily produced a parahydatid pleural effusion. Of the 33 patients who eventually developed secondary pleural hydatidosis, 17 had had previous surgery.

There was no operative mortality during this period, and early complications, which included empyemas, wound in-

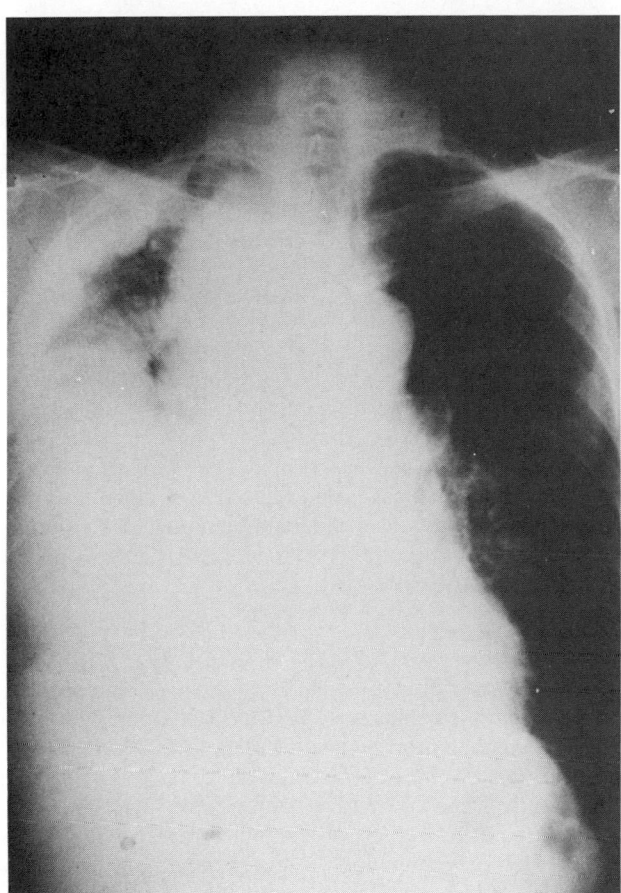

Figure 39-3. Standard chest radiograph showing hydatid pleural implant.

fections, biliary fistulae, and hemorrhage, were all successfully treated. In all of these patients with prior hydatic pleural disease, it is important that follow-up be done at regular intervals because of the possibility of a recurrence of the hydatid disease. In this series, the two patients with secondary pleural hydatidosis of vertebral origin required laminec-

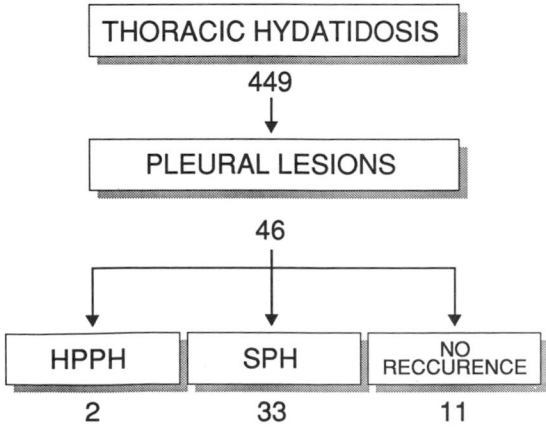

Figure 39-4. Pleural hydatidosis. HPPH, heterotopic pleural primitive hydatidosis; SPH, secondary pleural hydatidosis.

tomy, cord decompression, and vertebral resection, and one of them ended up with permanent paraplegia.

Case Study

This clinical case was chosen to illustrate what Armand Ugon described as massive pleuropulmonary hydatidosis (Fig. 39-5). It is that of a 21-year-old man who presented with dyspnea of acute onset, right-sided chest pain, cough, fever, and a vomica of foul-smelling liquid. Initial chest radiographs showed a pleural effusion with the so-called water lily sign, and thoracentesis confirmed the diagnosis of pleural hydatidosis. A chest tube was inserted, and hydatid membranes with pus were evacuated from the pleural space. The patient made a good recovery, but 18 months later, while in good health, follow-up radiographs showed rounded opacities consistent with the diagnosis of secondary pleural hydatidosis. He then underwent thoracotomy with excision and formolization of 32 hydatid cysts, and 10 days later he had a third space anterolateral thoracotomy with extrapleural excision of 20 additional cysts. After 16 months he presented again with cough, hemoptysis, and abundant expectoration of hydatid membranes, and a mass was noted over the sixth intercostal space. Because of his poor medical status, hydatid debris and pus were evacuated by pleurotomy. However, 2 months later a right pleuropneumonectomy was required, and the postoperative course was uneventful.

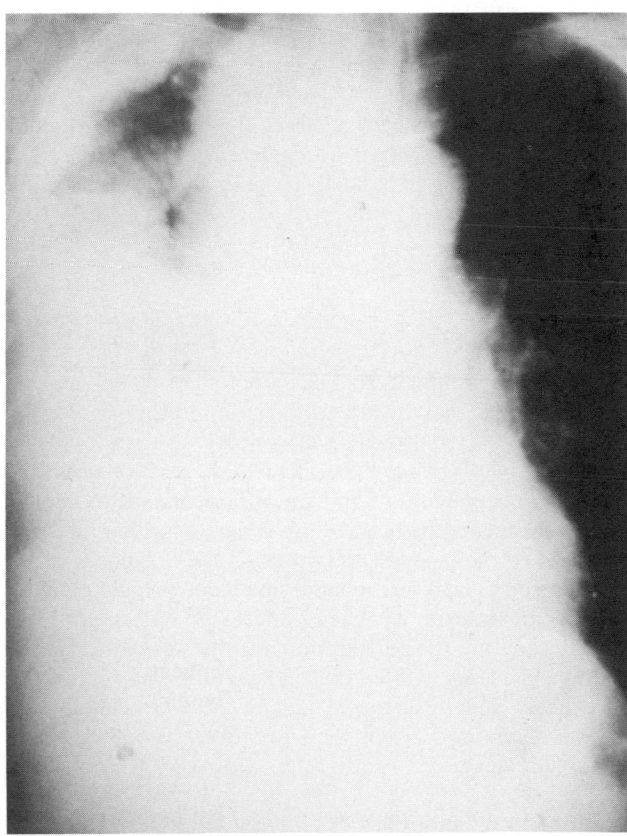

Figure 39-5. Standard chest radiograph showing multiple pulmonary and pleural hydatic cysts. In the vertex and over the mediastinum there are multiple hydatic pleural implants.

PLEURAL AMEBIASIS

DEFINITION AND PATHOLOGY

Amebiasis is a parasitic infection produced by an amoeba called *Entamoeba histolytica*. It is estimated that about 500 million people worldwide are infected and that 10 percent will eventually develop the disease. The expected mortality rate is 0.75 per 100,000 infected persons (Whitton, 1990).

The parasite is mainly transmitted by fecal-oral mechanisms. Once absorbed through the portal system, it migrates to the liver, where it produces abscesses and/or periportal fibrosis. Amebic liver abscesses contain an acellular proteinaceous material, and the trophozoites are located in the periphery of the abscess, where they further invade adjacent tissues. Although periportal fibrosis is common, only 5 percent of patients with symptomatic amebiasis develop true hepatic abscesses. When the abscess ruptures or if it extends to the surrounding tissues, it can produce pleuropulmonary or pericardial complications.

As reported by Ochsner and DeBakey (1943), pleuropulmonary contamination is the most common complication of amebic hepatic abscesses. In their series of over 181 patients with amebiasis-induced hepatic abscesses, 26 had a pleuropulmonary complication (17 pulmonary and 9 pleural) and one a pericardial complication.

The majority of amebic hepatic abscesses develop over the superior and posterior surfaces of the right lobe, and as the abscess enlarges, it includes the diaphragm in its wall. If the abscess develops slowly, it may produce a pleural reaction that will generate adhesions at the base of the right lung and sometimes produce a hepatobronchial fistula. If, on the other hand, the abscess enlarges rapidly, it may rupture in the pleural cavity with consequent empyema. Although less common, amebic hepatic abscesses can also rupture in the pericardial cavity.

DIAGNOSIS

Clinical Features

The most common presenting symptom of pleural amebiasis is right-sided chest pain with radiation to the shoulder. The cough, initially unproductive, is nearly always followed by production of abundant purulent expectorations, which resemble chocolate sauce and are pathognomonic of an amebic hepatobronchial fistula. At this stage, sputum examination can reveal the parasite and establish the diagnosis. Fever is more pronounced with pleural involvement, and there often is general malaise, weakness, anorexia, and weight loss.

Rupture into the pericardium must be suspected when the patient presents with epigastric pain radiating to the base of the neck, severe dyspnea, and fever. Occasionally, acute filling of the pericardial sac will produce symptoms of cardiac tamponade.

Differential Diagnosis

Characteristically, standard chest radiographs show an elevation of the right hemidiaphragm, a pleural effusion, and in the adjacent lung, areas of consolidation with or without cavitation. CT scan, ultrasound, and magnetic resonance imaging (MRI) are mainly used for the detection of hepatic abscesses.

The pleural fluid is generally exudative but it can become secondarily infected by other pathogens. Pleural biopsy or needle biopsy of the wall of the hepatic abscess may reveal the *Entamoeba histolytica*. When there is a pericardial effusion, needle aspiration often yields a fluid which is serofibrinous or "chocolate sauce" pus.

Serologic techniques are very important in the diagnosis of amebiasis because frequently the parasite cannot be isolated. Serology is positive in the majority of thoracic complications and the most commonly used techniques are the indirect hemagglutination test and enzyme-linked immunosorbent assay (ELISA). Double diffusion and counterimmunoelectrophoresis take longer to complete but may also be useful. Agglutination with latex is a simple test but often gives false positive results. In most cases erythrocyte sedimentation rate is elevated and there is a moderate leukocytosis. In pulmonary complications, careful sputum analysis may sometimes reveal the parasite.

MANAGEMENT

The most useful drugs to treat amebiasis are emetine, chloroquine, and metronidazole. Because of its possible cardiotoxicity, emetine must be given with great caution and under electrocardiographic monitoring. Metronidazole is a more effective drug and is less toxic or nontoxic. The usual dosage is 750 mg t.i.d., and when it is combined with drugs of luminal action such as paromomycin, cures are often seen within 10 days of the beginning of treatment. In hepatobronchial fistulae, postural drainage is useful, and all pleural effusions or empyemas must also be drained. Pericardial effusions may require urgent decompression.

INFECTIONS PRODUCED BY HIGHER BACTERIA

Actinomycetes are gram-positive and arborescent bacteria, which reproduce by fission rather than by sporulation as do the fungi. Their growth is inhibited by antibiotics but not by antifungal drugs. In this group human disease is produced by (1) *Actinomyces* and related *Arachnia* spp., which are anaerobic organisms and produce actinomycosis, and by (2) *Nocardia* spp. which are aerobes and produce nocardiosis.

ACTINOMYCOSIS

Pleural actinomycosis is mainly caused by *Actinomyces israelii*, but three other species and related *Arachnia propionica* can also cause actinomycosis with pleural involvement. Thoracic actinomycosis respects no anatomic boundaries and often involves the lung, pleura, mediastinum, and chest wall. It is generally agreed that in at least 50 percent of cases of thoracic actinomycosis there is pleural involvement.

PATHOGENESIS

Actinomycites are normal inhabitants of the oropharynx but they are specially abundant in septic dental processes. The point of entry is usually in the area between skin and mucosal coating, from where the bacteria reach the thorax through aspiration, by local contiguous spreading, or via the bloodstream (hematogenously). Once the disease has reached the lung, it propagates by contiguous spread, tending to externalization through the chest wall or extension to subdiaphragmatic areas.

DIAGNOSIS

Clinical Features

The symptoms of pleural actinomycosis are entirely nonspecific. Chest pain reflects pleural involvement and can be accompanied by dyspnea, fever, cough, hemoptysis, and/or weight loss, all symptoms that can wrongly be interpreted as those of tuberculosis. Poor dentition or skin lesions in the area of the jaw or in the neck may suggest the diagnosis of actinomycosis.

Differential Diagnosis

Standard radiographs often show lung masses that may resemble lung cancer or that may be cavitated, with adjacent pleural thickening and pleural effusion. Chest wall involvement, sometimes with destruction of ribs or even vertebrae, is common. In a majority of cases, however, the definitive diagnosis can only be made by study of the resected specimen (Dambrin, et al., 1957).

Pleural fluid may either be serous or purulent, and typical 1 to 2-mm diameter sulfur granules can be found. These granules are conglomerates of filamentous organisms with characteristically clubbed peripheral radiations. Actinomycosis organisms must be cultured both aerobically and anaerobically. Sulfur granules can also be isolated from sputum, bronchial washings, or pus from dental abscesses or infected cutaneous tracts. In general, erythrocyte sedimentation rate and leukocytosis are elevated. An eosinophil count of 13 percent was found in a patient with a hydatid cavity in which lung actinomycosis had developed with secondary actinomycotic empyema (Cazes, 1965).

MANAGEMENT

The treatment of choice consists of penicillin in doses of up to 30 million units/day given for 5 weeks. In the presence of sepsis and empyema, longer periods of treatment may be required. Erythromycin and tetracyclines have also been successfully used in patients with penicillin allergy. When the pleural effusion is only an exudate, there is usually a good response to antibiotic treatment, but when the pleural fluid is infected, pleural drainage must be instituted. Late sequelae consisting of lung abscesses and chest wall fistulae determine the need for lung and/or chest wall resections.

NOCARDIOSIS

Nocardia spp. are normal inhabitants of the soil, and in tropical countries they constitute the principal cause of foot mycetoma. *N. asteroids* is the organism responsible for pleuropulmonary infections that are clinically and radiologically similar to actinomycosis. It is frequently an opportunistic invader of immunosuppressed patients, and up to 25 percent of patients with lung nocardiosis also have pleural involvement, with effusion, empyema, or bronchopleural fistula. Hematogenous dissemination from the lung frequently affects the central nervous system and the subcutaneous tissues.

DIAGNOSIS

The diagnosis of nocardiosis may be confirmed by identification of the bacteria in the pleural fluid, sputum, or bronchial washings. Because *N. asteroides* is slightly acid-fast, it can be incorrectly identified as *Mycobacterium tuberculosis;* for this reason, acid-alcohol solutions must be used because with these solutions acid-fast characteristics are often lost. Definitive identification of *Nocardia* spp. requires culture under anaerobic conditions (to inhibit actinomycosis) or cultures under aerobic conditions with blood agar in which *Nocardia* spp. will grow.

MANAGEMENT

Sulfonamides are the drugs of choice. Sulfadiazine is usually employed, but trimetoprim-sulfamethoxazole can also be used with similar results. In severe infections and in immunosuppressed patients, use of ampicillin and/or erythromycin along with sulfonamide therapy is also recommended. These drugs should be given for at least 6 weeks and should be continued for 1 year in immunosuppressed patients. The only role of surgery is to drain the pleural space in cases of empyema.

PLEURAL TUBERCULOSIS

Tuberculosis, a disease seldom seen in many areas of the world, occurs with distressing frequency in underdeveloped countries. The amount of tuberculosis bacillus spilling in the pleura and the delayed hypersensitivity of the pleura seem to play a dominant role in determining which disease pattern will occur.

Tuberculous pleurisy generally results from rupture of a subpleural focus of caseous necrosis of the lung. Less commonly, it is secondary to the spillage of a tuberculous node in the pleura; in this process the contamination is light but there is a pleural hypersensitivity reaction with a secondary scarce to moderate aqueous effusion. Most of the time the effusion will regress over 1 to 2 months without treatment. It is the most common form of extrapulmonary tuberculosis and usually occurs within 6 months of the primary infection. Tuberculous pleurisy as a manifestation of primary tuberculosis is more common in adults between 25 and 45 years of age than in older adults and is rarely seen in children.

In tuberculous empyema the pleural contamination is massive, the pleural fluid is purulent, and it is common to find resistant acid-fast bacilli on direct examination or culture of the pleural fluid. Tuberculous empyemas may present as pure empyemas or as pyopneumothoraces. In mixed tuberculous and pyogenic empyemas, bacterial superinfection is produced by a persistent bronchopleural fistula or it occurs secondary to thoracentesis, or chest tube drainage.

DIAGNOSIS

Clinical Features and Differential Diagnosis

Tuberculous Pleurisy

In two-thirds of cases, tuberculous pleurisy presents as an acute infection with low-grade fever, nonproductive cough, pleuritic chest pain, and general malaise. When both cough and pleuritic chest pain are present, the pain usually precedes the cough. In the remaining one-third of patients, the clinical presentation is more insidious and nonspecific, with asthenia, anorexia, weight loss, and nocturnal sweats as the main symptoms. Respiratory symptoms such as cough and chest pain appear only later.

Peripheral white blood cell count is often normal, but the tuberculin skin test is positive in 70 to 80 percent of patients. However, a negative skin reaction does not exclude the diagnosis, because during the acute stage of tuberculous pleuritis, circulating adherent cells suppress the specifically sensitized circulating T lymphocytes. Since those cells are not present in the pleural space (Ellner, 1978), this effect explains why in some cases there is pleural hypersensitivity to the tuberculosis bacillus with cutaneous anergy.

Apart from the moderate and usually unilateral pleural effusion, chest radiographs may be normal. Pulmonary foci are frequently not seen because they are small and peripheral; when present, they are always ipsilateral. In those cases with minimal findings, thoracic CT scan (Hulnick, et al., 1983) and/or thoracoscopy may be more useful in demonstrating the pulmonary lesions. In general, the presence of a massive effusion favors a nontuberculous etiology.

Once a pleural effusion has been diagnosed, fluid must be sampled for analysis. In tuberculous pleurisy the pleural fluid is yellow or sometimes serohemorrhagic with little or no opalescence. The presence of a frankly hemorrhagic effusion eliminates the possibility of tuberculous pleurisy. The fluid is exudative, with a protein content of over 3 and frequently over 5 g/dl.

The remainder of the biochemical workup on the pleural fluid is of little help. Fluid with a pH below 7.3 or with a low glucose level is nonspecific and can be seen in other pathologies, including rheumatoid arthritis and carcinoma. High levels of lactic acid are also nonspecific and not very useful in making the diagnosis of tuberculous pleurisy. Piras, et al. (1978) showed that the more sensitive and useful biochemical markers for tuberculous pleurisy were an increase of the adenosine deaminase level to more than 30 IU/L and an increase in the pleural/serum lysozyme ratio. Lymphocytes are nearly always predominant in the cell count of the pleural fluid (they usually are in the range of 50 to 70 percent) although in the first 2 weeks of tuberculous pleurisy, polymorphonuclear leukocytes may predominate (Berger and Mejia, 1973). When lymphocytes are in excess of 50 to 70 percent, one should suspect the diagnosis of lymphoma. Mesothelial cells are seldom above 5 percent and if eosinophils are found, they are never in excess of 10 percent. Acid-fast bacilli are seldom identified by direct analysis of the pleural fluid or by culture. In order to enhance the chances of isolating acid-fast bacilli, it is advisable to centrifuge all obtained fluid, but even with this technique only 20 to 30 percent of patients will have positive fluid. Percutaneous pleural biopsy with the

Cope or the Abrams needle is one of the better diagnostic methods because it reveals the presence of granulomas in the parietal pleural in 60 to 80 percent of patients. Identification of areas of caseous necrosis or of acid-fast bacilli is helpful but is not absolutely necessary to make the diagnosis.

Pleural biopsies should always be complemented by fluid evacuation, but because chest tubes can promote infection, their use should be discouraged. Thoracoscopic biopsies should be considered when other methods have failed, and this technique has the advantage of providing visualization of all surfaces so that proper areas can be selected for biopsy. In our personal series of 312 thoracoscopies performed for undiagnosed pleural effusions, only 5 turned out to be related to pleural tuberculosis.

A presumptive diagnosis of tuberculous pleural effusion is often enough to initiate treatment, and this diagnosis can be made on the combined basis of a positive tuberculin skin test and a predominantly lymphocytic reaction in the pleural fluid. A biopsy showing caseating or noncaseating epithelioid granulomas is further proof of underlying tuberculosis. However, only direct identification of acid-fast bacilli or culture of these organisms on biopsy specimens provides definitive documentation of tuberculous pleural disease.

Tuberculous Empyema

Tuberculous empyema is much less common than tuberculous pleurisy. In 90 percent of cases it originates from a focus of tuberculous primary infection, and in the remaining 10 percent it is due to reactivation of cavitated or fibrocaseous lesions. Clinically, patients with tuberculous empyemas present with a productive cough, fever, and dyspnea, the severity of symptoms being related to the volume of the empyema. Erythrocyte sedimentation rates are classically above 60 mm/min and are accompanied by leukocytosis and moderate anemia. Resistant acid-fast bacilli are found in the sputum and in the pleural fluid in over 70 percent of patients (Fig. 39-6).

Mixed Empyema

Mixed empyemas are the result of pleural fluid contamination by thoracentesis, chest tube insertion, or bronchopleural fistula. Symptoms are those of the primary tuberculous effusion associated with those of empyema or pyopneumothorax.

MANAGEMENT

Tuberculous Pleurisy

In the therapy of tuberculous pleurisy, the objectives are to prevent tuberculosis from becoming active and to prevent long-term pleural sequelae. In the face of a presumptive diagnosis of pleural tuberculosis with a positive PPD (purified protein derivative) skin test and a predominantly lymphocytic pleural effusion, treatment for 6 to 9 months with a regimen that includes two to four antituberculous drugs is suggested. If the skin test is negative at the start of therapy, the drugs can be stopped after 2 months.

In our clinic we prefer to document the presence of acid-fast bacili either in the sputum or in the gastric contents or to identify tuberculous granulomas by pleural biopsy before

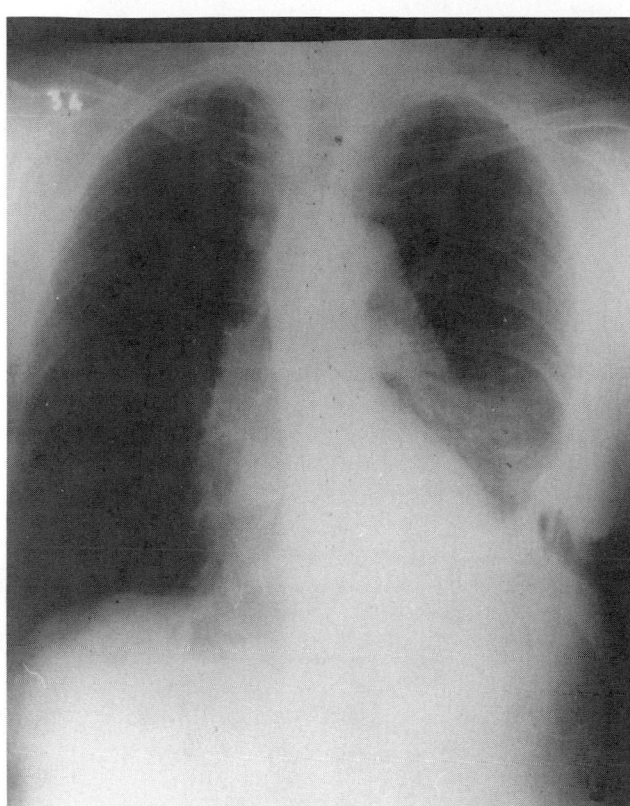

Figure 39-6.   Standard chest radiograph of a patient with tuberculous empyema.

initiating drug therapy. Antituberculous treatment is then given for a total of 7 months starting with the four drugs isoniazid, rifampicin, ethambutol, and pyrazinamide during the first 2 months. During the following 5 months two weekly doses of isoniazid and rifampicin are given. Patients with persistent large effusions and/or intense toxic reactions after adequate antituberculous drug treatment and pleural evacuation may need systemic or intrapleural corticotherapy. Lung decortication is seldom needed, as the pleural process usually resolves with adequate treatment.

Mixed and Tuberculous Empyema

Pleural drainage is indicated in tuberculous empyemas with large effusions and in all mixed empyemas, especially if there is a bronchopleural fistula with its inherent risks of contralateral aspiration. Luizy et al. (1956) described a pleural irrigation technique consisting of continuous aspiration and washing.

When the lung does not expand after drainage or if there is a residual fibrothorax, the condition of the underlying lung should be determined before planning decortication because the presence of fibrotic lesions, cavities, or bronchiectasis can make decortication difficult, impossible, or inadvisable. In those cases pulmonary resection may have to be performed in association with decortication. A review of all available radiographs is important because it will often indicate the topography and evolution of pulmonary lesions. CT scanning

is also useful to determine the nature and extent of pulmonary lesions and to differentiate them from pleural lesions. If pulmonary resection is contemplated, bronchoscopy is imperative in order to document the presence or absence of active endobronchial tuberculosis.

In a classic study, Hood and associates (1986) divided these patients into two groups. The first group included patients with only pleural involvement and the second group those with significant associated parenchymal disease. In the first group, decortication was considered when the constrictive pleuritis extended to 25 to 30 percent of the pleural space or when 25 percent of predicted pulmonary function was lost. Occasionally, smaller collections were also treated surgically because they entailed the risks of tuberculous perforation into the bronchus (bronchopleural fistula) in addition to sometimes interfering significantly with pulmonary function. Decortication was performed when there was no longer evidence of clinical toxicity and tuberculosis was medically controlled. Ideally, the sputum was negative for 4 months preoperatively, and if it had always been negative, antituberculous drug treatment was given for approximately 4 to 6 months prior to surgery. In Hood's second group, patients had severe parenchymal lesions in addition to pleural tuberculosis, and in order to eradicate the disease as well as to prevent reactivation, these patients required pulmonary resection and decortication.

If the empyema is small or loculated, it can be enucleated by the procedure called empyemectomy (Odell, 1990). In most cases, however, pleural decortication is necessary, and it is advisable to decorticate both parietal and visceral surfaces. The diaphragm must also be freed to allow for better mobility, and if the lung does not expand, an individualized thoracoplasty of usually no more than three to five ribs may have to be added to the decortication.

In general, tuberculous lesions predominate in upper lobes, so that this is the most common type of resection performed in association with decortication. Thoracoplasty may also have to be added if there is any doubt about pulmonary reexpansion. Pleuropneumonectomy is rarely indicated and is generally reserved for patients with destroyed lung, empyema, or bronchopleural fistula. In all those cases, special care must be taken to protect the bronchial stump, and pleural drainage with daily irrigations must be maintained for 1 to 3 weeks postoperatively.

Open thoracostomy is indicated when the empyema cannot be managed by closed thoracostomy and when the patient is medically unstable or more importantly, is not considered a candidate for resection. The window thoracostomy should be located in a dependent position, and in patients without important pulmonary lesions, pleural space obliteration can be achieved in 6 to 9 months. For these individuals open thoracostomy is more comfortable than a chest tube, with the added advantage of allowing pleural washing to be performed more easily. If there is a bronchopleural fistula, pleural washings should be done carefully, with the patient always in the upright position and the solution introduced slowly (Fig. 39-7).

Calcified fibrothoraces, which sometimes occur as late sequelae of tuberculous empyemas or of prior therapeutic pneumothoraces, must not be operated on unless absolutely necessary. Decortication is usually neither desirable nor possible,

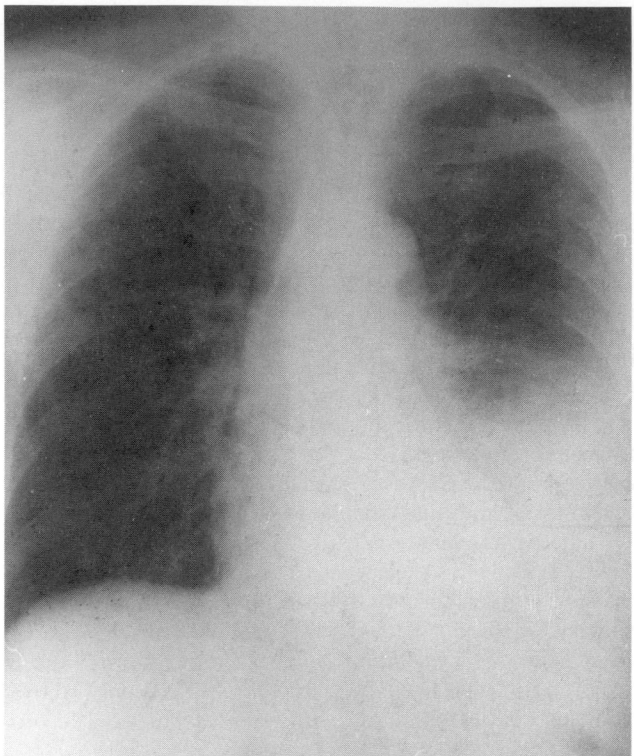

Figure 39-7. Tuberculous empyema treated by open thoracostomy.

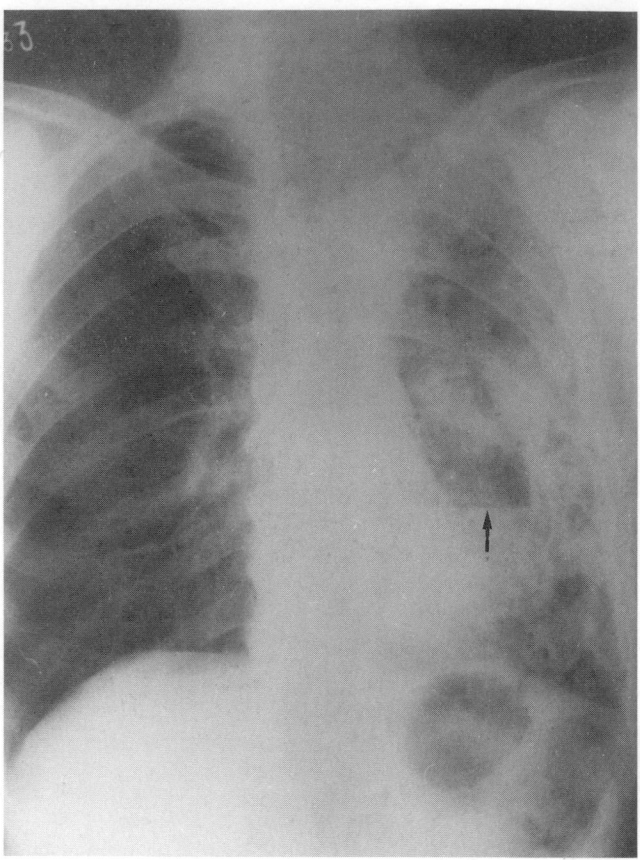

Figure 39-8. Standard chest radiograph showing an empyema with bronchopleural fistula that has developed in an area of calcified pleural sequelae. This patient was treated by open thoracostomy.

and sometimes these patients will present years later with secondary pyogenic empyemas with or without bronchopleural fistula (Fig. 39-8), and they may require pleuropneumonectomy (Fig. 39-9).

NONTUBERCULOUS MYCOBACTERIOSIS

The main causative organisms are *Mycobacterium kansasii,* seen in the urban population, and *Mycobacterium intracellulare* seen more often in rural areas. The symptoms are similar to those seen in association with tuberculosis although they may be somewhat attenuated. The PPD test is negative, but the pleural fluid may have elevated proteins and lymphocytes. Fluid glucose is normal or even decreased, and occasionally, cultures of the biopsy specimen will identify the mycobacterium. Therapy for atypical mycobacterial disease consists of administration of drugs such as rifampicin, ethambutol, and isoniazid until the disappearance of the effusion or until the bacteriology is negative for 6 months.

CRYPTOCOCCOSIS

Cryptococcosis is a disease of universal distribution produced by an opportunistic fungus, *Cryptococcus neoformans.* This organism is widely distributed in nature, its

principal reservoir being dry pigeon excreta. Cryptococcosis is the most common fungal pulmonary infection in the acquired immunodeficiency syndrome (AIDS), and its site of entry is believed to be the respiratory tract. In the early 1950s, 25 percent of patients with cryptococcosis had pulmonary lesions. More recently (1987), Wasser and Talavera reported that in 5 of 11 patients with cryptococcosis and AIDS, pulmonary lesions were the initial manifestation, and that 3 had a pleural effusion (two with pleural fluid positive for cryptococci). Pleural cryptococcosis is usually produced by the extension to the pleura of a subpleurally located lung nodule, and the main symptoms are fever, cough, pleuritic chest pain, dyspnea, and weight loss.

DIAGNOSIS

Although chest radiographs and CT scans may show pulmonary infiltrates or nodules, mediastinal masses, and pleural effusions, the diagnosis of cryptococcosis can only be made by isolating the organism from pulmonary cavities, pleural fluid, or bronchial secretions. By using staining techniques such as hematoxylin-eosin, periodic acid-schiff (PAS), Alcion blue, or Gomori on biopsy specimens, spheroid or ovoid formations of 10 μm average diameter can be seen, sur-

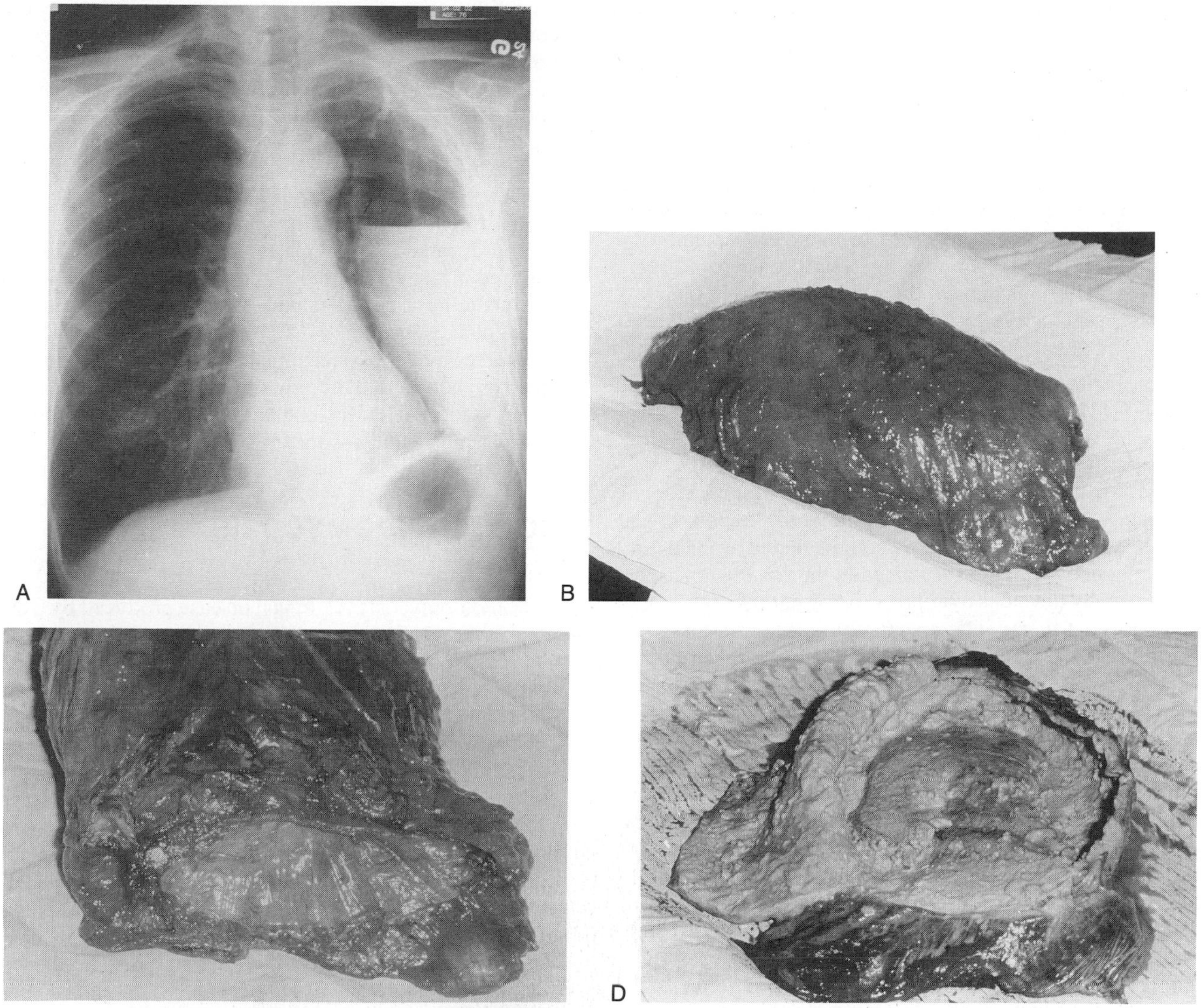

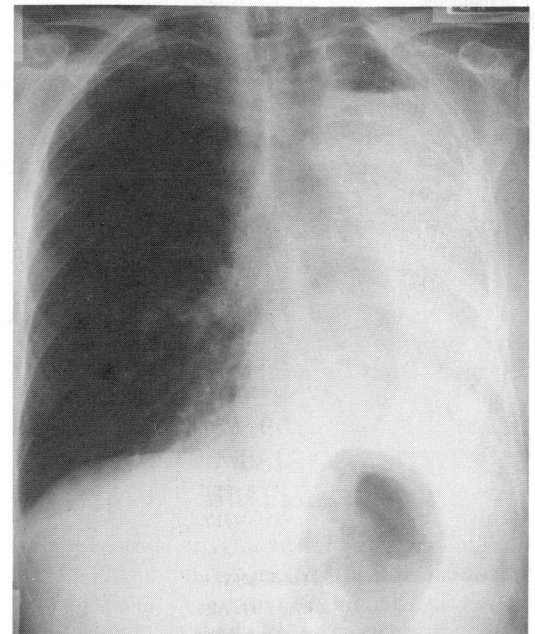

Figure 39-9. **(A)** Standard chest radiograph showing a chronic mixed tuberculous empyema with bronchopleural fistula and an unexpandable lung. The pleuropneumonectomy specimen shows **(B)** the lung, pleura, and peel; **(C)** the portion of the diaphragm that had to be resected to avoid contamination of the space; and **(D)** the inside of the cavity. **(E)** Postoperative chest radiograph showing partial filling of the space.

rounded by a clear halo, which is characteristic of cryptococcosis.

MANAGEMENT

Drug treatment consists of amphotericin b and flucytosine. Fluconazole can also be used, with the same effectiveness but with less side effects on kidneys, liver, and bone marrow. In immunosuppressed patients the treatment must be continued for 6 to 12 months in order to avoid extrapulmonary dissemination. Pleural drainage is generally not necessary. If a previously undiagnosed pulmonary nodule is found at operation to be cryptococcosis, resection must be followed by drug treatment.

ASPERGILLOSIS

Aspergillosis is a disease caused by the opportunistic fungus *Aspergillus fumigatus,* which is adaptive to life both in soil and in organic matter. Humans become infected by inhalation of the conidia, which are suspended in the air. Pleural aspergillosis usually develops over pre-existing pathologies; it may be a sequela of therapeutic pneumothoraces (intra- or extrapleural), residual pleural cavities following pleural or pulmonary surgery, or other pleural diseases (e.g., chronic hemothoraces, pneumothoraces, pleural tuberculosis, or pleural hydatidosis) (Bisson, 1990). In those situations, *Aspergillus* pleural contamination is often secondary to a bronchopleural fistula, which initiates suppuration and aspergillus infection of the pleural residual cavity. Sometimes the fungus may be isolated from the pleural fluid or biopsy specimens of the pulmonary tissues. Serologic studies identifying antibodies against *Aspergillus* are also useful for diagnosis except in immunosuppressed patients, in whom these studies are negative.

In 1992 Massard and colleagues reported a series of 77 patients with pleuropulmonary aspergillomas, of whom 16 had pleural aspergillosis. In 10 of the 16 aspergillosis developed following lobectomy; in one it developed in a residual space after exploratory thoracotomy, in three it followed collapsetherapy, and in two it followed a spontaneous bronchopleural fistula. Chest radiographs showed thickening of the pleura in 10 patients and a pleural effusion that turned out to be an empyema in 6 others. Thirteen patients with pleural aspergillosis were treated by surgery with 2 deaths. The risk is higher in symptomatic patients.

Patients with pleural aspergillosis must be carefully selected for surgery, and whenever possible, radical and agressive operations should be avoided. We prefer to use closed pleural drainage or preferably, open thoracotomy with or without added thoracoplasty. Amphotericin B should be given for several months when necessary.

HISTOPLASMOSIS

Histoplasmosis is the most important fungal disease involving the respiratory system, but pleural involvement is unusual. It is produced by *Histoplasma capsulatum,* a dimorphic fungus living in the soil. Pleural lesions originate from a contiguous pulmonary focus or by hematogenous dissemination (George, 1985).

The most common symptoms associated with pleural histoplasmosis are pleuritic pain, fever, malaise, and signs of a pleural effusion. Diagnosis is based on the identification of the fungus either in the pleural fluid or on biopsy specimens. In 1966, Schub reported four patients with pleural histoplasmosis. In two of them, *Histoplasma* was identified by open pleural or pulmonary biopsies; in a third, *Histoplasma* was cultured in the pleural fluid; and in the fourth, the diagnosis was made by a histoplasmine sensitivity test and elevation of antibody titer.

Small or moderate-size effusions do not need specific therapy. Amphotericin B therapy should be reserved for immunosuppressed patients or for patients with chronic pulmonary histoplasmosis and secondary pleural effusion.

COCCIDIOIDOMYCOSIS

Coccidioidomycosis is a fungal disease produced by a dimorphic fungus called *Coccidioides inmitis*. This fungus, first described in Argentina (Posadas, 1895), grows as a mycelium that eventually develops into arthrospores that are inhaled in the lungs. The incidence of pleural effusion with coccidioidomycosis is about 7 percent (Salkin, 1967).

Pleural effusions may be associated with acute primary coccidioidomycosis. In 1976, Lonky reported that in a series of 28 patients with coccidioidal pleural effusion, in 90 percent it was secondary to direct spread from a contiguous pulmonary infection site. Coccidioidal inmitis was identified in the effusion of only 3 of 15 patients, but in all 8 patients who had pleural biopsies, cultures were positive. In acute disease, the prognosis is excellent, often without specific therapy.

Pleural effusion may also be secondary to chronic pulmonary coccidioidomycosis. In those cases, coccidioidal cavities rupture in the pleural space, where they may produce a pneumothorax, an empyema, or sometimes a bronchopleural fistula. Rapidly, a pleural peel will develop and entrap the lung. The definitive diagnosis can be made by the identification of the fungus in the pleural fluid, by needle biopsy or by culture. A serologic diagnosis can also be obtained by precipitin and complement fixation tests, which are accurate and relatively specific (Hood, et al., 1986).

When a positive diagnosis of pleural coccidioidomycosis is made, specific drug therapy with amphotericin B is indicated. Surgical management also includes tube drainage of pneumothoraces or empyemas and lung decortication or pulmonary resection to manage a bronchopleural fistula.

BLASTOMYCOSIS

Blastomycosis is a fungal infection produced by a dimorphic fungus called *Blastomyces dermatiditis*. This fungus is present in warm and nitrogen-rich soils and has worldwide distribution. Blastomycosis is a less common mycotic infection than either coccidioidomycosis or histoplasmosis. Entry is through inhalation of the conidia into the lungs.

The symptoms are similar to what is seen with other acute fungal infections and include cough, fever, myalgia, erythema nodosum, chest pain, and pleural effusion. In the chronic form of the disease, pleural involvement produces a pleural effusion or an empyema, often without specific symptoms.

Diagnosis can be made by the identification of the fungus in bronchial secretions, pleural fluid, or on pleural biopsies. These are frequently positive either on a smear or by culture. Pleural biopsy may also show granulomas, with stains and cultures of the material defining the etiology. Serologic and skin tests are of limited value. Acute blastomycosis with pleural effusion does not generally require specific therapy. Pleural involvement associated to chronic pulmonary infection must be treated with amphotericin B and tube drainage when necessary.

REFERENCES

Armand Ugon V: Equinococosis pleural secundaria. An Dep Cient Salud Publ Montevideo 2:389, 1935

Barret NR: The treatment of pulmonary hydatid disease. Thorax 1:21, 1947

Berger HW, Mejia E: Tuberculous pleurisy. Chest 63:88, 1973

Bisson A: Pleural aspergillosis. p. 448. In Deslauriers J, Lacquet LK (eds): International Trends in General Thoracic Surgery, Vol. 6. Surgical Management of Pleural Diseases. CV Mosby, St. Louis, 1990

Cazes M: Actinomicosis pleuropulmonar injertada sobre secuela hidatica. ElTorax 14:81, 1965

Dambrin P, Moreau G, Eschapasse H, et al.: Les formes pseudocancéreuses de l'actinomycose pulmonaire. Ann Chir 2:223, 1957

Dèvé F: L'échinococcose secondaire de la plèvre. J Chir (Paris) 49:497, 1937

Ellner JJ: Pleural fluid and peripheral blood lymphocyte function in tuberculosis. Ann Intern Med 89:932, 1978

Fossati A: Quistes hidaticos de pulmon. Met do de Lama y Mondino/ Tecnica Personal y breve comentario. An Fac Med Montevideo 28:793, 1943

George RB, Penn RL, Kinasewitz GT: Mycobacterial, fungal, actinomycotic and nocardial infections of the pleura. Clin Chest Med 6:63, 1985

Hood RM, Antman K, Boyd A, et al.: Surgical Diseases of the Pleura and Chest Wall. WB Saunders, Philadelphia, 1986

Hulnick DH, Naidich DP, McCauley DI: Pleural tuberculosis evaluated by computed tomography. Radiology 149:759, 1983

Lamas A: Auelques details a propos du traitement chirurgical au kyste hydatique du poumon. J Chirurgie T.XLI 3, 1933

Lonky SA, Catanzaro A, Moser KM et al.: Acute coccidioidal pleural effusion. Am Rev Resp Dis 114:681, 1976

Luizy J, Mathey J, Le Brigand H, et al.: Technique d'irrigation pleurale sous dépression continue dans le traitement des pyothorax. Rev Tuberc 30:393, 1966

Massard G. Roeslin N, Wihlm JM, et al.: Pleuropulmonary aspergilloma: clinical spectrum and results of surgical treatment. Ann Thorac Surg 54:1159, 1992

Nin Vivo J, Brandolino MV, Pomi JA, et al.: Hydatid pleural disease. p. 427. In Deslauriers J, Lacquet LK (eds): International Trends in General Thoracic Surgery, Vol 6 Surgical Management of Pleural Diseases. CV Mosby, St. Louis, 1990

Ochsner A, DeBakey M: Amebic hepatitis abscess. Surgery 13:460, 1943

Odell JA: Pleural tuberculosis. p. 459. In Deslauriers J, Lacquet LK (eds): International Trends in General Thoracic Surgery, Vol. 6. Surgical Management of Pleural Diseases. CV Mosby, St. Louis, 1990

Perez Fontana V: Nuevo metodo de operar en el quisto hidatico del pulmon. Arch Pediatr Uruguay 19(1):5, 1948

Piras MA, Gakis C, Budroni M, et al.: Adenosine deaminase activity in pleural effusions: an aid to differential diagnosis. Br Med J 4:1751, 1978

Posadas A: Quistes hidatidicos An Circulo Med Argent 23:613, 1895

Salkin D, Birswer TW, Tarr AD et al.: Roentgen analysis of coccidioidomycosis. In Ajello ED (ed): Coccidioidomycosis. University of Arizona Press, Tucson, 1967

Schub HM, Spivey CG, Baird GD: Pleural involvement in histoplasmosis. Am Rev Resp Dis 94:225, 1966

Wasser L, Talavera W: Pulmonary cryptococcosis in AIDS. Chest 92:692, 1987

Whitton I: Pleural amebiasis. p. 452. In Deslauriers J, Lacquet LK (eds): International Trends in General Thoracic Surgery, Vol. 6. Surgical Management of Pleural Diseases. CV Mosby, St. Louis, 1990

40

ANATOMY OF THE THORACIC DUCT AND CHYLOTHORAX

Richard A. Malthaner
Martin F. McKneally

THORACIC DUCT

HISTORICAL NOTE

Aristotle and the anatomists Herophilos and Erasistratos are said to have described the lymphatic system around 300 B.C. In the sixteenth century, Vesalius, professor of anatomy and surgery at Padua, named the thoracic duct the vena alba thoracis because of the milky white fluid it contained. In Aselli's 1627 illustration of the lymphatic channels in the mesentery of the dog, he traced these vessels into the abdominal receptaculum chyli but mistakenly believed they ended in the liver. In 1651 Pecquet of Paris observed the intestinal lacteal channels emptying into the receptaculum chyli, then into the thoracic duct, and eventually into "the whirlpool of the heart." He confirmed these observations on the body of a criminal autopsied after a large meal. In 1653 Bartholin named these vessels "lymphatics." William Hunter, with his assistants Hewson and Cruikshank at the Hunterian School in 1784, recognized that the lymphatic vessels are the same as the lacteal vessels and "that these altogether with the thoracic duct constitute one great and general system dispersed through the whole body for absorption."

In 1878 Claude Bernard's conception of the mammalian *milieu interieur* and Starling's work (1896) on hydrostatic and colloid osmotic pressure further illuminated the role of the lymphatic channels. Drinker and Field (1931) measured protein flux from the capillaries to the tissues. These workers solidified the concept that the lymphatic channels and the thoracic duct act as vessels that return protein molecules to the central circulation.

Reports on chylothorax were rare before the nineteenth century. Bargebuhr (1894–1895) collected a review of 40 patients with nontraumatic chylothorax from the medical literature dating back to 1691. All had neoplasms of the abdomen and thorax. Although the first traumatic chylothorax was reported by Quinke (1875), Zesas' review (1912) states that Longelot in 1663 probably was the first to describe a traumatic chylothorax. In this collected series of 24 patients, 12 died.

Based on his 1922 review of the literature and personal experimental work on ligation of the thoracic duct, Lee (1922) concluded that injuries should be treated by direct repair when possible and, if not, by ligation. This represented the first challenge to the accepted dogma that the duct was essential to life. In 1936 Blalock, et al. (1936) noted chylothorax following ligation of the superior vena cava. Their attempts at complete lymphatic blockage by duct ligation were successful in only 3 of 72 animals because collateral lymph channels developed rapidly and relieved the obstruction.

Heppner (1934) first pointed out that progressive obliteration of the pleural space around the opening rather than healing of the injured duct was the mechanism of spontaneous resolution of thoracic duct fistulas. Daily thoracenteses were advocated, and many attempts at pleurodesis subsequently failed. Intravenous injection of aspirated chyle was tried in the early 1900s by Oeken but was abandoned following several anaphylactic reactions (Whitcomb and Scoville, 1942). Readministering chyle by mouth or rectum was also found to be unhelpful. Phrenic nerve sectioning also proved to be unsuccessful.

Although Crandall, et al. (1943) successfully treated a thoracic duct fistula in the neck by direct thoracic duct ligation, it was Lampson (1948) who ligated the thoracic duct in the chest and marked the turning point in the therapy of chylothorax. The mortality rate at that time was nearly 100 percent in nontraumatic chylothorax and 50 percent in traumatic chylothorax, with the latter figure indicating that one-half closed spontaneously.

Schumacker and Moore (1951) suggested feeding cream to infants preoperatively to help localize the duct. Klepser and Berry (1954) introduced intraoperative visualization of the duct with lipophilic dyes and early ligation. Their approach through the right chest at the level of the diaphragm regardless of the side of injury, has become one of the most commonly used approaches today for thoracic duct injuries.

HISTORICAL READINGS

Aselli G: De Factibus Sive Lacteis Verris, Quarto Vasorum Mesdarai Corum Genere Novo Invento. JB Bieldellium Mediolani, Milano, 1627

Bernard C: Leçons sur les Phenomènes de la vie Communs aux Animaux et aux Vegetaux. Vol. 1. JB Bailliere et Fils, Paris, 1878

Blalock A, Cunningham RS, Robinson CS: Experimental production of chylothorax by occlusion of the superior vena cava. Ann Surg 104:359, 1936

Lampson RS: Traumatic chylotyhorax—a review of the literature and report of a case treated by mediastinal ligation of the thoracic duct. J Thorac Cardiovasc Surg 17:778, 1948

Lee FC: The establishment of collateral circulation following ligation of the thoracic duct. Bull Johns Hopkins Hosp 33:21, 1922

BASIC SCIENCE

Anatomy

Davis (1915) characterized the anatomy of the thoracic duct as "constant only in its variability." The thoracic duct is the left main collecting vessel of the lymphatic system and is far larger than the right terminal lymphatic duct (Fig. 40-1). The duct originates from the cisterna chyli in the abdomen but may be absent in 1 of 50 people. The cisterna chyli is a globular structure 3 to 4 cm long and 2 to 3 cm in diameter that is found along the vertebral column at the level of L2, but it may be located anywhere between T10 and L3 on the right side of the aorta. From the cisterna chyli, the thoracic duct ascends along the spine to enter the thorax through the aortic hiatus at the level of T10 to T12, just to the right of the aorta. It ascends extrapleurally, along the right anterior surface of the vertebral bodies, posterior to the esophagus, between the aorta and the azygos vein, and anterior to the right intercostal arteries.

At the level of T5 to T7, the duct crosses behind the aorta to the left posterior side of the mediastinum and ascends on the left side of the esophagus beneath the pleural reflection and posterior to the left subclavian artery. In this region the duct is vulnerable during operations involving the aortic arch, left subclavian artery, or esophagus. At a point 4 cm above the clavicle, the duct turns laterally behind the carotid sheath and jugular vein, anterior to the inferior thyroid and vertebral arteries, subclavian artery, and phrenic nerve. At the medial margin of the anterior scalene muscle, it turns inferiorly, entering the venous system at the subclavian–internal jugular vein junction on the left, although it may empty into the left innominate, left internal jugular, left vertebral, or even the right internal jugular vein. The duct contains a variable number of valves throughout its entire course with one consistent valve at the lymphaticovenous junction to protect it against the reflux of blood.

Van Pernis (1949) and Kausel, et al. (1957) noted that variability is common, with 40 to 60 percent of individuals having anomalous collaterals communicating with the azygos, intercostal, and lumbar veins. Meade, et al. (1950) found that 25 to 33 percent of individuals have multiple ducts, at the level of the diaphgram, which has implications if an operation is considered.

The right duct is small, 2 cm in length, and is rarely visualized. It drains lymph from the right side of the head, neck, and chest wall through the jugular trunk and from the right lung, heart, and lower half of the left lung through the bronchomediastinal trunk. Lymph from the dome of the liver, the right diaphragm, and the right upper anterior chest drains through the right internal mammary trunk to the right duct.

These anatomic relationships explain why injury to the duct below the level of T5 to T6 usually results in a right chylothorax and injury above this level results in a left chylothorax. The collateral communications also explain why the duct can be ligated at any point in the chest or neck without impairing the delivery of lymph to the central circulation.

Embryology

The thoracic duct is a bilateral structure, and it may have many varied anatomic patterns. The lymphatic system begins to develop at the end of the fifth week, about 2 weeks later than the cardiovascular system. Sabin (1916) demonstrated that the original lymph sacs arose from the endothelium of the adjacent veins. She described six original lymph spaces (Fig. 40-2). The two jugular sacs arise from the anterior-cardinal vein and the two iliac sacs arise near the junction of the iliac veins and the posterior cardinal veins. The single retroperitoneal sac is situated in the root of the mesentery on the posterior abdominal wall, and the primitive cisterna chyli arises from the mesonephric vein and the veins at the dorsomedial edge of the wolffian bodies. The cisterna chyli is then formed by the union of two lumbar lymphatic trunks and the intestinal trunk within the abdomen. Lymphatic buds appear from the original sacs and follow the tissue planes of least resistance, principally along veins, toward the periphery.

The thoracic duct is formed from a downward growth of the left jugular sac and an upward growth of the right thoracic duct from the cisterna chyli. Initially the duct is represented by a bilateral symmetric plexus of lymph vessels, each side attached to the jugular sac and each having multiple anastomoses between them. The azygos and the intercostal veins also contribute to the formation of a major portion of the duct. This explains the multiple connections between the duct and these vessels that allow chyle to be carried into the blood stream when the duct is ligated. With maturation the upper one-third of the right duct and the lower two-thirds of the left duct are obliterated, but the main communication between them persists to give the adult thoracic duct configuration. If the upper portion on the right side is not obliterated, a right lymphatic duct prevails.

Histology

Lymphatic capillaries consist of single layers of flat endothelial cells, slightly larger and thinner than blood capillary cells. The basement membrane is absent or vestigial, which allows large molecules to permeate the walls easily. The lymphatic capillaries can be distinguished from blood capillaries by the absence of the basement membrane, blind endings, and the lack of arterial and venous connections. Lymphatic capillaries do not have pericytes associated with them, but they do

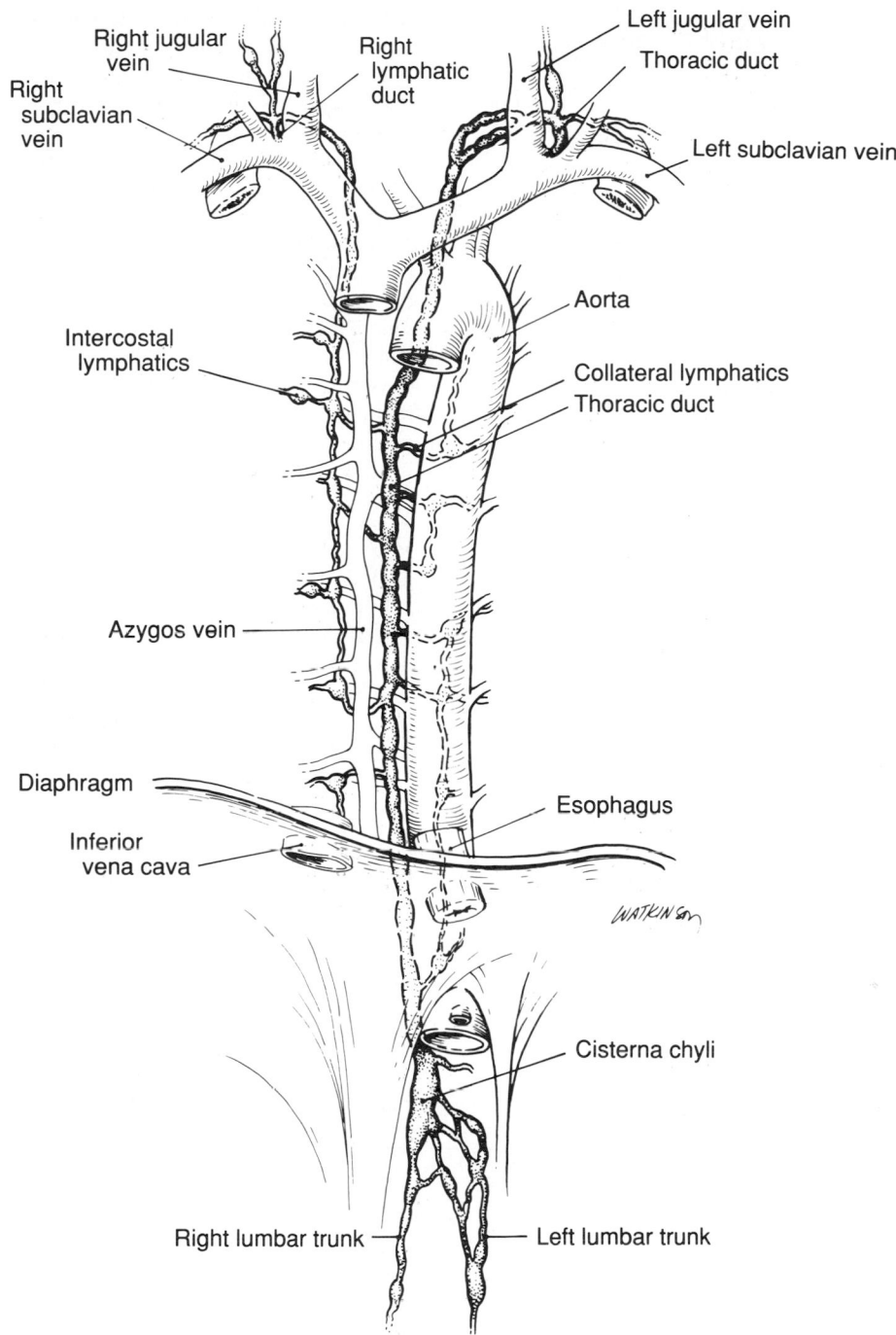

Figure 40-1. Surgical anatomy of the thoracic duct.

have anchoring filaments that attach to the surface of the endothelial cells and extend out into the connective tissue around the capillary. These filaments seem to hold the capillaries open during times when the surrounding edematous pressure might cause them to collapse.

The thoracic duct, however, contains a well-developed basement membrane and has three layers within the wall: intima, media, and adventitia. The intima contains elastic fibers. The media is well developed, consisting of smooth muscle fibers supported by connective tissue containing elastic fibers. It is this well-developed layer that contracts rhythmically to aid in lymph flow. The adventitia is supplied by the vasa vasorum and contains smooth muscle fibers running both longitudinally and obliquely.

The thoracic duct and all lymphatic channels, except the smallest ones, possess valves. The valves have two leaflets, consisting of folds of intima with delicate connective tissue in the middle covered with endothelium. They are more nu-

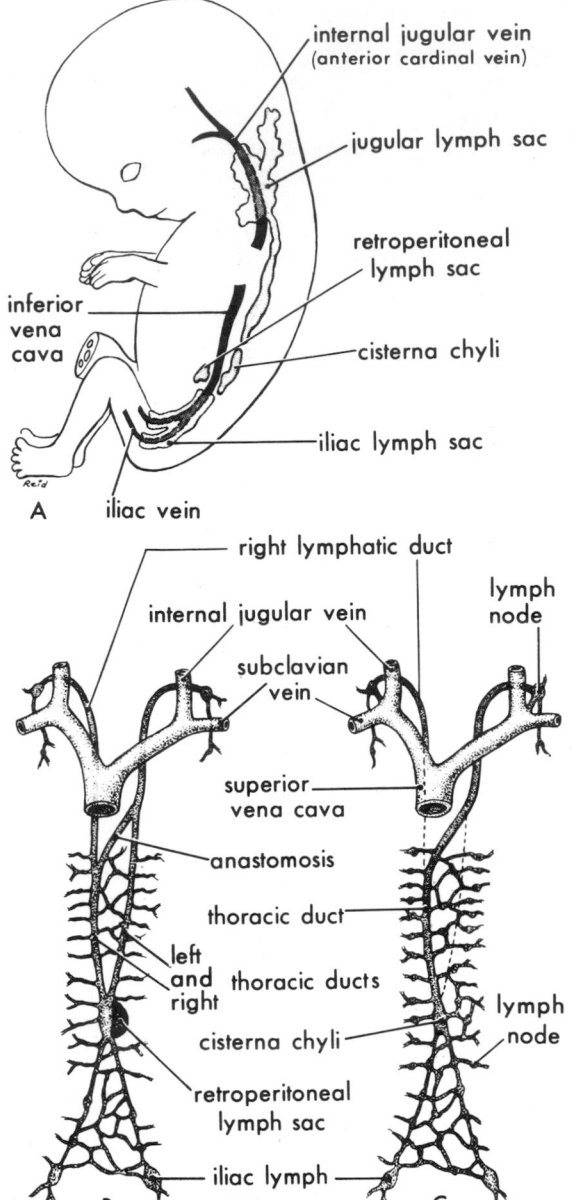

Figure 40-2. Embryologic origin of the lymphatic channels and the thoracic duct in the human embryo. **(A)** Left side of a 7-week-old embryo with the six lymph sacs. **(B)** Ventral view at 9 weeks showing the paired thoracic ducts. **(C)** Later stage showing the formation of the adult thoracic duct and the right lymphatic duct (From Moore KL, Persaud TVN: The Developing Human. 5th Ed. WB Saunders, Philadelphia, 1993, with permission.)

merous and closer together than the valves of veins. The valves are so close together that a distended lymphatic vessel appears beaded because of the dilated sections between the valves.

Physiology

The principal function of the thoracic duct is the transport of digestive fat to the venous system. According to Frazer (1951–1952) small fatty acids with less than 10 carbon atoms are absorbed directly into the portal system, whereas larger lipids are absorbed into the intestinal lymphatic vessels as micelles. The transport time of absorbed fat from the mouth until it appears in the venous blood is less than 1 hour after ingestion, with the peak absorption 6 hours after ingestion.

The volume of lymph flow is estimated to be 1.38 ml/kg of body weight/h. Volumes up to 2,500 ml of chyle in 24 hours have been collected from the cannulated human thoracic duct. Crandall, et al. (1943) found the flow of lymph in the thoracic duct to range from 3.9 ml/min after a meal or during abdominal massage to 0.38 ml/min at rest. It was found that 95 percent of the volume comes from the liver and intestinal lymphatic channels, although the amount from the extremities is negligible. Lymphatic flow in amphibians, reptiles, and some birds is propelled by lymph hearts, whereas mammals have more complex mechanisms. The forward flow of chyle from the abdomen in humans is influenced by four factors:

1. Vis a tergo, from the latin "force exerted from the back," is the transmission of pressure to the cisterna chyli from the intestinal lacteal vessels by the absorption of lymph. This force comes from the inflow of chyle into the lacteal system produced by the intake of food and liquid meals and intestinal movement. It is proportional to the volume of the food and independent of the external pressure or wall pressure.

2. There is a pressure gradient. Negative intrathoracic pressure and positive intra-abdominal pressure create a gradient favoring flow of lymph toward the central circulation.

3. Muscular contractions by the duct itself are probably the most important factor in propelling lymph forward; the valves within the duct prevent retrograde flow. Kinmonth and Taylor (1956) observed that contractions occurred every 10 to 15 seconds, which are independent of respiratory movements. The intraductal pressure ranges from 10 to 25 cmH_2O and may rise to 50 cmH_2O with obstruction, as observed by Shafiroff and Kau (1959). Acetylcholine produced by fibers of the vagus nerve constricts the duct; epinephrine dilates it (Acevedo, 1943).

4. Birt and Connolly (1951–52) believe that there is a Bernoulli suction effect produced by the flow of blood past the lymphaticovenous junction, creating a vacuum.

The lymphatic vessels perform the vital functions of collecting and transporting tissue fluid, extravasated plasma proteins, absorbed lipids, and other large molecules from the interstitial space to the intravascular space. Most of the body's lymphocytes are circulated through the duct.

CHYLOTHORAX

DEFINITION

Chylothorax is the accumulation of excess lymphatic fluid in the pleural space, usually as a result of a leak from the thoracic duct or one of its major branches. The term *chyle* comes from the Latin *chylus,* meaning juice and usually connotes the milky appearance of intestinal lymph caused by the presence of emulsified fats. (Note that chyme is the semifluid mass of partly digested food found in the small intestine.)

BASIC SCIENCE

Etiology

The prevalence of chylothorax ranges from 0.5 to 2.0 percent in selected series, according to Sachs, et al. (1991). Chylothorax is thought to result from either an obstruction or laceration of the thoracic duct. The most common causes are neoplasms, trauma, tuberculosis, and venous thrombosis (Randolph and Gross, 1957; Roy, et al., 1967). A classification adapted from DeMeester (1983) is shown below.

Etiology of Chylothorax

Congenital
   Atresia of thoracic duct
   Thoracic duct-pleural fistula space
   Birth trauma
Traumatic
   Blunt
   Penetrating
   Surgical
      Cervical
         Excision of lymph nodes
         Radical neck dissection
      Thoracic
         Ligation of patent ductus arteriosus
         Excision of coarctation
         Esophagectomy
         Resection of thoracic aortic aneurysm
         Resection of mediastinal tumor
         Left pneumonectomy
         Left subclavian artery operations
         Sympathectomy
      Abdominal
         Sympathectomy
         Radical lymph node dissection
   Diagnostic procedures
      Lumbar arteriography
      Subclavian vein catheterization
      Left-sided heart catheterization
Neoplasms
   Benign
   Malignant
Infections
   Tuberculous lymphadenitis
   Nonspecific mediastinitis
   Ascending lymphangiitis
   Filariasis
Miscellaneous
   Venous thrombosis
      Left subclavian or jugular vein
      Superior vena cava
   Secondary to chylous ascites
   Pancreatitis
   Spontaneous

Congenital Chylothorax

Congenital chylothorax is the leading cause of pleural effusion in the neonate, according to Randolph and Gross (1957). The cause is not always clear, but birth trauma or congenital defects in the duct or both may be precipitating factors. Increased venous pressure during a difficult delivery may cause rupture of the thin walls of the thoracic duct. Malformations of the lymphatic system are rare causes of congenital chylothorax. The anomalous duct may be absent or atretic, or it may have multiple dilated lymphatic channels with abnormal communications between the duct and pleural space. Anomalies of the thoracic duct may be associated with polyhydramnios or lymphedema.

Traumatic Chylothorax

Traumatic injury to the thoracic duct may occur with blunt or penetrating trauma or during surgery (Cevese, et al., 1975). Injury may occur at any point along the course of the duct, making localization difficult. The most common mechanism of nonpenetrating injury is sudden hyperextension of the spine, resulting in the rupture of the duct just above the diaphragm. Birt and Connolly (1951–52) believe this is caused by a shearing of the duct by the right crus of the diaphragm or by sudden stretching over the vertebral bodies. Costal fractures are not necessary to produce this injury.

Penetration by gunshot or stab wounds is rare. These injuries are usually overshadowed by life-threatening damage to other structures. Ductal injury, however, should be considered during the evaluation of a thoracotomy for trauma.

Surgical injury to the thoracic duct has been reported following almost every thoracic surgical procedure, especially those performed in the upper part of the left side of the chest. Surgical injury is possible during procedures on the heart, lungs, aorta, esophagus, sympathetic chain, and subclavian vessels. The duct is the most vulnerable in the upper part of the left chest, during mobilization of the aortic arch, the left subclavian artery, or the esophagus (Higgins and Mulder, 1971).

Injury has also been reported following radical neck dissection and scalene node biopsy. Operations in the abdomen, such as sympathectomy and radical lymph node dissection, also result in damage to the thoracic duct. Diagnostic procedures, such as translumbar aortography and central venous line placement in the jugular or subclavian vein, also cause thoracic duct injuries.

Neoplasms

The thoracic duct can be involved by benign and malignant tumors, lymphatic permeation, direct invasion, or tumor embolus. The most frequent tumors include lymphomas, lymphosarcomas, or primary lung carcinomas. Unilateral or bilateral chylothorax results from the rupture of distended tributaries or erosion into the duct.

Benign lesions of the thoracic duct include lymphangiomas, mediastinal hygromas, and pulmonary lymphangiomyomatosis. The later condition, reported by Cunn, et al. (1973) and Silverstein, et al. (1974), occurs in young women and is associated with pneumothorax and hemoptysis. It is characterized by the proliferation of smooth muscle in the peribronchial, perivascular, and perilymphatic regions of the lung, resulting in the obstruction of the lymphatic channels. Dyspnea is the major symptom, and these women usually die of pulmonary insufficiency within 10 years of presentation (Bradley, et al., 1980).

Tumors cause more than 50 percent of chylothoraces in adults. Roy, et al. (1967) reported that lymphomas were found 75 percent of the time. A chylous effusion should always be evaluated as a possible signal for an unsuspected mediastinal or retroperitoneal malignancy.

Malignant obstruction may occasionally cause leakage of chyle into the pericardium, producing signs and symptoms of cardiac tamponade.

Infections

Infectious causes include tuberculosis, fungal diseases, lymphangiitis, filariasis, and nonspecific mediastinitis, which result in lymph node enlargement and obstruction (Yater, 1935).

Other Causes of Chylothorax

Vomiting or violent coughing can cause a "spontaneous rupture," especially when the duct is full after a fatty meal. However, when rupture does occur after such minor trauma, the possibility of an underlying malignancy must be considered. Thrombosis of the great veins into which the thoracic duct drains can produce a chylous effusion (Ross, 1961).

Chylous effusions in the chest can be the result of chylous ascites, which is usually caused by a malignancy, commonly lymphoma. Primary fistulae and lymphatic disease in children can cause intraperitoneal chylous accumulation. Exudative enteropathy caused by congenital intestinal lymphatic and chylous leaks from the lumen of the bowel are other causes. Amyloidosis can be complicated by chylothorax when the disease process causes ductal obstruction. Chylous ascites also occurs after various abdominal operations and with pancreatitis (Traquair, 1945–46).

Composition of Chyle

Thoracic duct lymph is not pure chyle but a mixture of lymph originating in the lungs, intestine, liver, abdominal wall, and the extremities. The majority is produced in the intestine; the amount of lymph originating from the extremities is negligible under normal circumstances. Chyle is characteristically milky white, odorless, and alkaline. The ductal lymph is clear during fasting and becomes milky following a fatty meal, as observed by Munk and Rosenstein (1891). It is strongly bacteriostatic and contains lipids, proteins, electrolytes, lymphocytes, and various other elements. The normal composition of chyle is shown in Table 40-1.

Lipids

The main component of chyle is fat. Chyle contains from 14 to 210 mM total fat, including neutral fat, free fatty acids, sphingomyelin, phospholipids, cholesterol, and cholesterol esters. Sixty to 70 percent of ingested fat is absorbed by the intestinal lymphatic channels and conveyed to the blood by the thoracic duct. Ross (1961) reported that neutral fat in lymph is transported as chylomicrons, measuring 0.5 mm in diameter. Fatty acids with less than 10 carbon atoms are absorbed directly by the portal venous system. This is the basis of using medium-chain triglycerides as the oral diet in

Table 40-1. Normal Characteristics and Composition of Chyle

Characteristics	Normal Plasma Concentrations
Milky appearance with a creamy layer that clears when fat is extracted by alkali or ether	
pH, 7.4–7.8 (alkaline)	
Odorless	
Specific gravity, 1.012–1.025	
Sterile and bacteriostatic	
Fat globules staining with Sudan III	
Lymphocytes, 400–6800 × 10^6/L	1,500–4,000 × 10^6/L
Erythrocytes, 0.050–0.6 × 10^9/L	4,500–6,500 × 10^9/L
Composition	
Total protein, 21–59 g/L	65–80 g/L
Albumin, 12–41.6 g/L	40–50 g/L
Globulin, 11–30.8 g/L	25–35 g/L
Fibrinogen, 0.16–0.24 g/L	1.5–3.5 g/L
Antithrombin globulin, > 25% plasma concentrate	
Prothrombin, > 25% plasma concentrate	
Fibrinogen, > 25% plasma concentrate	
Total fat, 14–210 mM	
Triglycerides, above plasma value	0.84–2.0 mM
Cholesterol, plasma value or lower	4.4–6.5 mM
Glucose, 2.7–11.1 mM	2.5–4.2 mM
Urea, 1.4–3.0 mM	3.0–7.0 mM
Electrolytes, similar to plasma	
Pancreatic exocrine enzymes present	
Lipoprotein electrophoresis, chylomicron band	
Cholesterol-triglyceride ratio, < 1	

the medical management of chylothorax. The triglyceride content greatly exceeds the cholesterol content.

Protein

The lymphatic vessels are the main pathway for the return of extravascular proteins to the vascular space. Nix, et al. (1957) and Ross (1961) found that the protein content is approximately one-half the plasma concentration, ranging from 22 to 59 g/L. The albumin concentration ranges between 12 and 41.6 g/L and globulin, between 11 and 30.8 g/L.

Electrolytes

The electrolyte composition is similar to that found in plasma; the glucose concentration ranges from 2.7 to 11.1 mM. The predominant ions include sodium, potassium, chloride, calcium, and inorganic phosphorus.

Cellular Elements

Lymphocytes are the main cellular elements in the thoracic duct lymph and arise from the peripheral lymphatic channels and lymphoid organs. Hyde, et al. (1974) found that 90 percent of the lymphocytes are T lymphocytes, and they react differently to antigenic stimulation compared with blood lymphocytes. There is a continuous circulation of cells from blood to lymph and back again. Prolonged drainage can deplete the lymphocytes and impair the immune system. In clear lymph there are 0.05×10^9 erythrocytes per liter, but this may arise to 0.6×10^9 in postabsorptive states, as reported by Shafiroff and Kau (1959).

Miscellaneous Elements

Other components include fat-soluble vitamins, antibodies, urea nitrogen, and enzymes, including pancreatic lipase, alkaline phosphatase, aspartate transaminase, and alanine transaminase.

Pathophysiology

Chylothorax results from a tear or rupture in the thoracic duct. It can cause cardiopulmonary abnormalities and metabolic and immunologic deficiencies. Lymph commonly accumulates in the posterior mediastinum until the mediastinal pleura ruptures, usually on the right side at the base of the pulmonary ligament. The accumulation of chyle in the chest can compress the underlying lung and compromise pulmonary function, resulting in shortness of breath and respiratory distress.

Empyema is a rare complication of chylothorax because of the bacteriostatic actions of lecithin and fatty acids. Sterile chyle is nonirritating and therefore does not cause pleuritic pain or a fibrotic inflammatory reaction.

Although fat is the most conspicuous constituent of chyle, it is the loss of protein and vitamins that is more important in terms of serious metabolic and nutritional defects. Shafiroff and Kau (1959) emphasized the loss of protein, fat-soluble vitamins, lymphocytes, and antibodies from a persistent chyle leak can lead to immunodeficiency, coagulopathy, malnutrition, inanition, and death.

DIAGNOSIS

Clinical Features

The usual presentation of chylothorax is insidious; however, with rapid accumulation, tachypnea, tachycardia, and hypotension can occur. There is often a latent interval of 2 to 10 days before the chylothorax becomes clinically evident because many injured or postsurgical patients receive a restricted diet. Clinical manifestations of chylothorax are initially the result of the mechanical compression of the ipsilateral lung and mediastinum, causing dyspnea, fatigue, and heaviness. The problems of protein, fat-soluble vitamin, and antibody loss can be accentuated by repeated thoracenteses or chronic tube drainage. Fluid losses can reach 2,500 ml of chyle per day and result in cardiovascular instability if they are not replaced. Death is inevitable when supportive treatment fails, unless the fistula closes spontaneously or is ligated surgically.

History

A pleural effusion in a patient with any of the diagnoses associated with chylothorax should always be evaluated for chyle. The history of trauma after a heavy meal or a recent surgical procedure in the distribution of the thoracic duct should raise the suspicion of chylothorax.

Laboratory Studies

Laboratory studies of blood chemistry and hematologic parameters are often normal immediately following traumatic injury to the duct. Chronic effusion or chylothorax in infancy may show hypoproteinemia, decreased triglyceride levels, and lymphocytopenia.

Radiologic Studies

There are no valid radiologic findings to differentiate chylothorax from other pleural effusions. Bipedal lymphangiograms were reported by Sachs, et al. (1991) to be useful in diagnosing thoracic duct laceration. In this procedure 10 ml of ethiodized oil is injected into lymphatic vessels on the dorsum of the foot and followed in 1 to 2 hours later by radiography of the abdomen and chest. This technique, however, may cause pulmonary edema, lymphangiitis, or rarely, cerebral oil embolism. Radionuclide imaging with ^{99}T antimony sulfide colloid, when injected subcutaneously yields images within 3 hours. The radionuclide technique can demonstrate obstruction, but it is limited in localizing the site of leakage (Freundlich, 1975). Computed tomography also has limited use in localizing the site of leakage but may demonstrate a mediastinal mass, enlarged lymph nodes, or a primary lung carcinoma.

Fluid Analysis

Chylothorax is suggested by the presence of nonclotting milky fluid obtained from the pleural space at thoracentesis or chest tube drainage. The characteristics of chyle are listed in Table 40-1. The diagnosis is confirmed by finding free microscopic fat, a fat content that is higher than that of the plasma, and a protein content less than one-half the plasma level. The fat globules clear with alkali or ether and stain with Sudan III. Chyle may be mistaken for pus, but there is no odor, and cultures are negative. Gram staining is helpful because the cells present in chyle are lymphocytes rather than polymorphonuclear leukocytes, and no bacteria are seen.

It is important to recognize that chyle is only milky white when fat is being transported from the gut. Clear or bloody fluid does not rule out a chylous leak. Traumatic injury to the duct in the fasting state may yield chyle, which initially appears blood stained. This may eventually become clear and serous. Lymphocytes are the predominant cells in chyle, and a 90 percent lymphocyte count is virtually diagnostic. In traumatic effusions there is an admixture of erythrocytes and other blood elements.

The diagnosis may be delayed in patients receiving parenteral nutrition and nasogastric suction. Before an effusion is evident, patients may show a widening of the superior mediastinum caused by a chyloma or accumulation of chyle within the mediastinal pleural envelope. The chyloma may drain into the pleural space and develop into a chylothorax, and there often is a decrease in the leukocyte count. This is the result of a selective decrease in the lymphocytes.

Staats, et al. (1980) state chyle has a cholesterol-triglyceride ratio less than 1, whereas nonchylous effusions have a ratio greater than 1. If the fluid has a triglyceride level greater than 1.24 mM, there is a 99 percent chance that the fluid is chyle. If the triglyceride content is less than 0.56 mM, there is only a 5 percent chance that the fluid is chyle (Staats, et al., 1980). An intermediate value requires lipoprotein electrophoresis to verify chylomicrons (Seriff, et al., 1977).

Methylene blue dye may be injected into the lymphatic channel to help visualize the duct and fistula at surgery. Ductal visualization can also be enhanced by the preoperative ingestion of cream or the instillation of methylene blue into the stomach (Murphy and Piper, 1977; Eugevik, 1976). Another useful hint is the rate of fluid accumulation in the chest. A disproportionately high volume of fluid drainage from the chest, averaging 700 to 1,200 ml/day in a patient who has suffered a hyperextension injury or has undergone esophagectomy or thoracic aortic surgery, should be evaluated for a chylous leak.

Differential Diagnosis

In the differential diagnosis of milky effusions, pseudochylothorax and cholesterol pleural effusions need to be considered. Long-standing chronic pleural effusions may have a chylous appearance. These cholesterol effusions are seen in tuberculosis or rheumatoid arthritis and are related to the high cholesterol content of the fluid, as reported by Bower (1968). They do not contain fat globules or chylomicrons.

Boyd (1986) reported that pseudochyle occurs with the thickened or calcified pleura seen with malignant tumors or infections and is milky because of the presence of a lecithin-globulin complex. There is only a trace of fat, and fat globules cannot be seen with Sudan III. It contains less cholesterol and protein than does chyle.

Diagnostic Tests

Gram stain
Complete cell count
pH
Sudan III stain
Triglyceride level
Cholesterol level
Cholesterol-triglyceride ratio < 1
Triglyceride level > 1.24 mM

A complex pleural effusion exists when a thoracic duct leak is present in addition to some other cause of pleural effusion (e.g., congestive heart failure, infections, tumors, or trauma). The analysis may be misleading because of a dilutional effect.

In summary we recommend thoracentesis and fluid analysis for cell count, Gram staining, and lipid levels. This should be diagnostic in the majority of cases.

MANAGEMENT

The management of chylothorax is judgmental, and opinion varies about the aggressiveness and timing of surgery. The modalities used in the management of chylothorax are listed below. Lampson (1948) introduced thoracic duct ligation in 1948. It was shown that the mortality rate decreased from 50 to 15 percent. Nontraumatic chylothorax at that time had a nearly 100 percent mortality rate.

Prevention is important, and injuries need to be recognized or anticipated intraoperatively. Ductal ligation at the aortic hiatus is easily accomplished at the time of esophageal or thoracic aortic dissection. Many surgeons routinely ligate the thoracic duct if an extensive lymphadenectomy or posterior mediastinal node dissection is carried out. Surgical interven-

---

Therapy of Chylothorax

Medical
  Nothing by mouth
  Medium-chain triglycerides
  Central hyperalimentation
  Drainage of pleural space
    Thoracentesis
    Closed chest tube thoracostomy
  Complete expansion of the lung
Surgical
  Direct ligation of thoracic duct
  Mass ligation of thoracic duct tissue
  Pleuroperitoneal shunting
  Pleurectomy
  Fibrin glue
  Thoracoscopy
Radiation therapy
Chemotherapy

tion to ligate the thoracic duct should be performed before the debilitating complications of thoracic duct leakage or its therapy supervene. Although the repair of a ductal fistula has been facilitated by thoracoscopy (Shirai, et al., 1991), the open procedure to ligate the duct through a small right thoracotomy is often easier on the patient than a prolonged course of hyperalimentation. This is particularly true in infants and children, in whom central lines carry significant morbidity rates. Our approach is summarized in Figure 40-3.

Conservative

The diagnosis is established by analysis of the pleural fluid, as described above. Patients with congenital, postoperative, or traumatic chylothorax, in whom immediate thoracotomy for the control of an associated lesion is not required, should be managed initially by conservative treatment (i.e., complete pleural drainage with full reexpansion of the lung to appose the visceral pleura. Multiple thoracocenteses are less adequate than large-bore intercostal tubes and gentle suction.

The most important aspect is nutrition and the correction of fluid and electrolyte imbalance (Bessone, et al., 1971). Enteral formulas with a low fat content supplemented with medium-chain triglycerides are usually recommended but rarely work. Total parental nutrition and nothing by mouth is the most effective (Hashim, et al., 1964). Oral feeding of any kind increases the volume of lymphatic flow, increasing the output through the fistula and perpetuating the leak.

Surgical

There is no consensus on the length of time before surgical therapy. Williams and Burford (1963) and Selle, et al. (1973) recommend 14 days as the maximum limit of conservative management before proceeding with surgical ligation. Twenty-five to 50 percent of leaks will close spontaneously during this interval, and the other 50 to 75 percent require surgical intervention. We favor a shorter course of nonsurgical management, especially in neonates or debilitated patients severely compromised by the lymphocyte, antibody, and protein loss from an active thoracic duct fistula. If spontaneous closure is thought to have occurred, a high-fat challenge meal should be given before removing the chest tube. If the chest tube drainage is consistently greater than 500 ml per day for 2 weeks, surgical intervention is definitely indicated, except for those patients in whom the risk of surgery would be

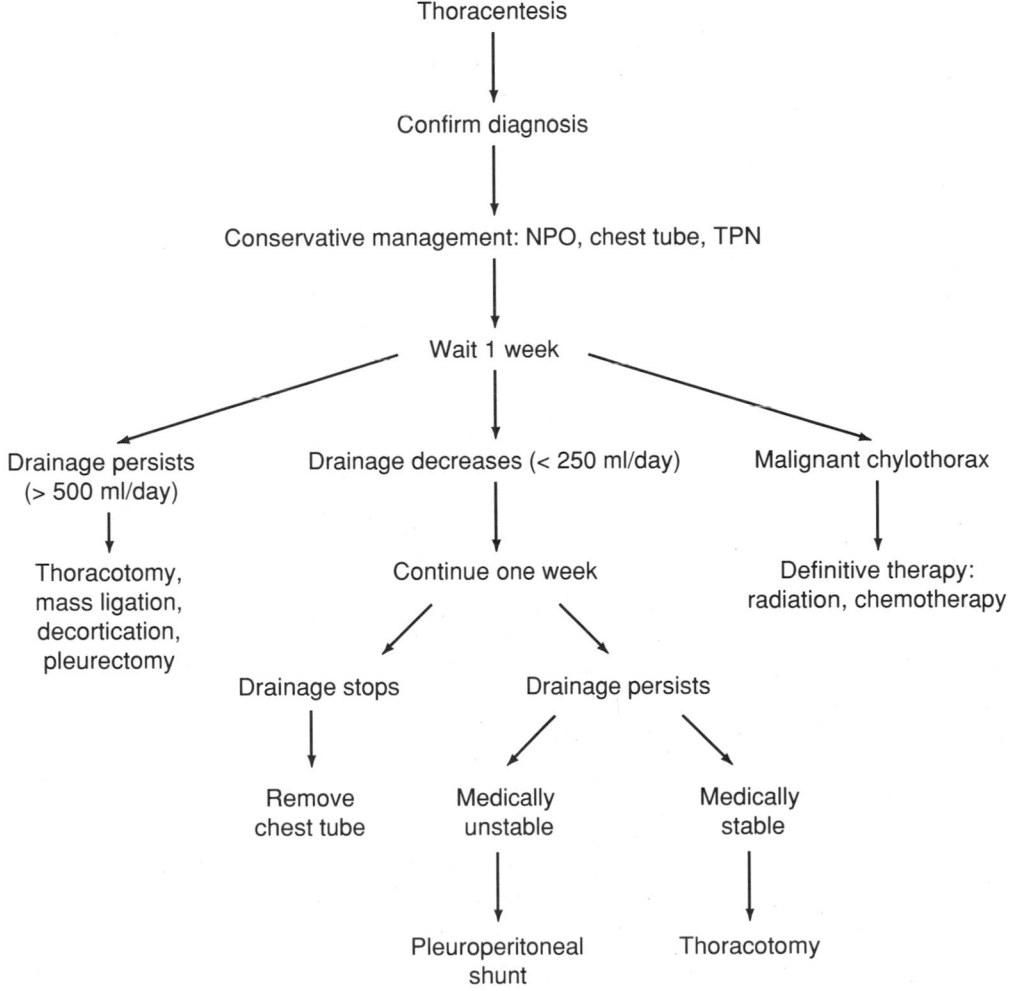

Figure 40-3. Algorithm for the therapy of chylothorax.

outweighed by other considerations, such as vertebral fractures, unresectable tumors, or multiple organ injuries. If a lung is entrapped, malignancy is suspected, or multiple loculations are present, early surgical intervention is appropriate (Brewer, 1955; Goorwitch, 1955).

Operative Techniques

Several techniques have been described: (1) direct ligation of the thoracic duct leak, (2) supradiaphragmatic mass ligation of the thoracic duct, (3) pleuroperitoneal shunting, (4) pleurodesis and pleurectomy, (5) suture ligation of leaking mediastinal pleura, (6) anastomosis of the duct to the azygos vein, (7) decortication, (8) fibrin glue, and (9) thoracoscopy (Cevese, et al., 1975). Many surgeons prefer to perform thoracotomy on the side of the chylothorax, hoping to suture ligate the site of the suspected leak. When extensive nodal dissection has been performed, exposing many potential sites of leakage, as in esophagogastric resection through the left chest, a right-sided supradiaphragmatic approach is more likely to find and ligate the duct. We recommend thoracic duct ligation at the time of the initial thoracotomy whenever an extensive mediastinal dissection is performed or the suspicion of a chyle leak is raised by a continuous accumulation of watery fluid in the thorax. This can be performed supradiaphragmatically through either the right or the left chest by retracting the esophagus to expose the duct as it lies between the aorta and the azygos vein on the vertebral body. Supradiaphragmatic ligation provides a high probability of the elimination of chylothorax on either side (Fig. 40-4).

Ross (1961) suggests instilling 100 to 200 ml of olive oil 2 to 3 hours before the operation through the nasogastric tube. This causes filling of the duct with milky chyle and allows its easy recognition. Any residual oil is aspirated from the stomach prior to the induction of anesthesia. An alternative method is injection of 1 percent aqueous Evans blue dye into the leg. This stains the duct within 5 minutes and lasts about 12 minutes. The disadvantage is that other tissues may also be stained. The preoperative administration of 2 oz of cream 30 minutes prior to thoracotomy has been recommended by Schumacher and Moore (1951). Filling the thorax with saline intraoperatively may facilitate the detection of milky chyle leaking from the duct.

Various surgical approaches to the duct have been well described by Cevese, et al. (1975). We prefer ligation of the thoracic duct just above the diaphragm in the right chest, regardless of the site of the chylous leak. This has been reported by Lampson (1948); Klepser and Berry (1954); Selle, et al. (1973); and Murphy and Piper (1977) and championed by Patterson, et al. (1981) and Milson, et al. (1985). Van Pernis (1949) reported that the duct is a single structure from T12 to T8 in more than 60 percent of patients; therefore, there is an almost 40 percent incidence of duplication of the mediastinal thoracic duct in its caudal portion. We think that mass ligation is important to avoid missing a major channel. A short right anterolateral thoracotomy incision is used. The fibrin deposits on the pleura are removed, and the inferior pulmonary ligament is released. Thickened pleura or enlarged nodes should undergo biopsy to rule out a malignant process causing the chylothorax. We prefer to ligate the duct en

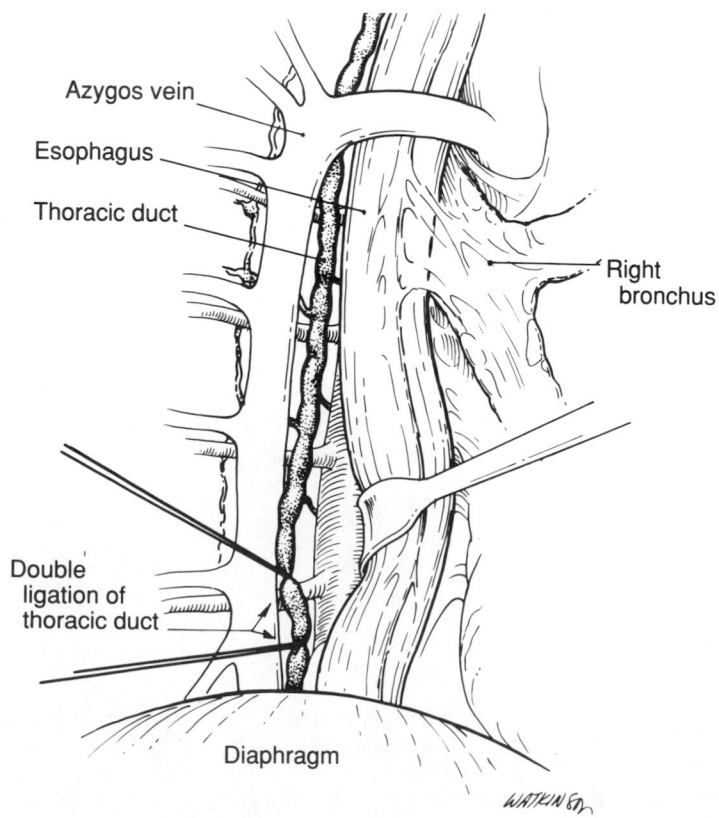

Figure 40-4.   Therapy of chylothorax using mass ligation of the supradiaphragmatic thoracic duct.

masse, along with all the tissue between the azygos vein and aorta, by using nonabsorbable suture material. No attempt is made to close the fistula directly. The minor lymphatic-venous anastomosis between the duct and the azygos, inter-costal, and lumbar veins quickly compensates for this local-ized interruption. In infants, transient edema of the legs and ascites may be seen for several days, which usually then re-solves.

Some believe that the best method is to find the leak and close it with nonabsorbable sutures and Teflon pledgets, allowing the main portion of the duct to remain patent, as discussed by Miller (1989). Reimplantations of the divided duct into a vein or other anastomoses are complicated and un-necessary.

A parietal pleurectomy may be performed to achieve pleu-rodesis but is generally not needed. If the lung is trapped, it may require decortication. The thoracic cavity is drained with chest tubes. Even if the duct cannot be found, mass ligation is successful in 80 percent of patients (Patterson, et al., 1981).

Other Techniques

In nontraumatic chylothorax, the cause must be determined and appropriately treated. Chylous fistulae that result from obstruction by malignancies respond poorly to surgical liga-tion, unless the underlying disease can be treated effectively. For lymphomas or other malignancy, radiation or chemother-apy may be needed. This may not be totally successful. Pleu-roperitoneal shunting with the double-valve Denver shunt has been reported by Milson, et al. (1985); Weese and Schouten (1984); and Miller (1989) in high-risk patients. This may be needed if superior vena caval obstruction is present. This problem is self-limited, and the shunt may be removed in a few months (Azizkhan, et al., 1983; Milsom, et al., 1985). Neoplastic chylothorax usually resounds to irradiation or chemotherapy directed at the primary disease. Pleurodesis with tetracycline, talc, nitrogen mustard, iodine, irradiation, or surgical abrasion may help temporarily. When this fails, thoracic duct ligation can be tried because patients tolerate the operation more readily than the inanition associated with the continuous loss of chyle. The combination of ductal liga-tion with pleurodesis or parietal pleurectomy may be advis-able for chylothorax associated with malignant disease. Sten-zel, et al. (1983) reported the successful use of fibrin glue in one patient. Intrapleural fibrin glue was used by Akaogi, et al. (1989) using thoracoscopy. As our experience increases with this new technique, less invasive methods should be-come the standard in the future.

CONCLUSIONS

Chylothorax is an infrequent but important cause of pleural effusion. The diagnosis is often complicated by the superim-position of other causes of pleural effusion. Early recognition and therapy prevent the nutritional depletion that can result from a continuous chylous leak. Thoracentesis is used for diagnosis, and a chest tube is inserted for drainage and pulmo-nary expansion. This intervention, combined with the elimi-nation of oral feeding and parenteral nutrition, may obliterate the leak if there is no underlying obstruction of lymphatic flow into the central circulation.

Chylothorax in the neonate may respond to drainage, but prompt ligation should be considered if there is continued drainage with high volumes of fluid, cells, and nutrients. When nontraumatic chylothorax is associated with venous or lymphatic obstruction, specific treatment of the underlying process is required for success. If widespread disease is pres-ent, chemical pleurodesis is a reasonable choice before opera-tive intervention is considered. Traumatic leaks may be man-aged with drainage and parenteral support. Thoracoscopic ligation is feasible. Surgical repair is best accomplished by supradiaphragmatic ligation of the thoracic duct through a right thoracotomy, and this should be done early before com-plications set in.

COMMENTS AND CONTROVERSIES

Although chylothorax is more common after surgery of the thoracic aorta, correction of cardiovascular malformations, or resection of the esophagus and lung, injuries to the thoracic duct can complicate any type of intrathoracic operations. With more extensive types of pulmonary resections often involving radical lymph node excisions, the incidence of post-operative chylothoraces is increasing and is currently in the range of 0.3 to 0.5 percent.

Knowledge of the anatomy of the thoracic duct is the key to understanding how this structure can be damaged and how to prevent damage. In most cases of pulmonary resection for lung cancer, intraoperative trauma to the thoracic duct or to collecting trunks occurs during nodal staging or radical node dissection. On the right side, leaks are usually in the posterior mediastinum just below the carina, while on the left, most are secondary to extensive dissections above the aortic arch. As mentioned by Drs. Malthaner and McKneally, many sur-geons, such as Dr. John Wong, Hong Kong, routinely ligate the thoracic duct if an extensive lymphadenectomy is carried out.

Because of reduced lymph flow and pressure, chylous leaks are difficult to recognize intraoperatively if one does not specifically look for them. Postoperatively, the diagnosis is usually made within 48 to 72 hours when the patient resumes a normal diet and the drainage from the chest tube becomes milky. These patients should be started immediately on total parenteral nutrition, since oral prepara-tions containing median-chain triglycerides are generally ineffective. In fact, patients should not be allowed to eat or drink anything, since even the smallest amount of water will increase lymph flow.

When reoperation becomes necessary, I prefer direct liga-tion of the fistula site after the patient has been given 300 ml of 30 percent cream 2 to 3 hours preoperatively. This is done because it is possible that even after ligation of the main duct, lymph will continue flowing through abnormal or secondary ducts.

J.D.

KEY REFERENCES

Bessone LN, Ferguson TB, Burford TH: Chylothorx. Ann Thorac Surg 12:527, 1971

This is a classic in-depth review of the anatomy, pathophysiology, and management of chylothorax. It contains 133 references, and it still remains the most complete review of the subject.

Cevese PG, Vecchioni R, Cordiano C et al.: Surgical techniques for operations on the thoracic duct. Surg Gynecol Obstet 140:958, 1975

This is an excellent compilation of the surgical approaches and techniques related to thoracic duct pathologic conditions. Al-

though more simpler methods are now advised, the background is an essential element in the armamentarium of the thoracic surgeon.

DePalma RG: Disorders of the lymphatic system. p. 1479. In Sabiston DC (ed): Textbook of Surgery. 13th Ed. WB Saunders, Philadelphia, 1987

This chapter summarizes the lymphatic system with respect to the historic and the basic science aspects. It is concise and well written, with 124 references.

REFERENCES

Acevedo D: Motor control of thoracic duct. Am J Physiol 139:600, 1943

Akaogi E, Mitsui K, Sohara Y et al.: Treatment of postoperative chylothorax with intrapleural fibrin glue. Ann Thorac Surg 48:116, 1989

Aselli G: De Factibus Sive Laceteis Verris, Quarto Vasorum Mesarai Corum Genere Novo Invento. JB Bieldellium Mediolani, Milano, 1627

Azizkhan G, Canfield J, Alford BA et al.: Pleuroperitoneal shunts in management of neonatal chylothorax. J Pediatr Surg 18:842, 1983

Bargebuhr A: Chylöse und chyliforme Ergüsse im Pleura un Pericardialraum. Dtsch Arch Klin Med 54:410, 1894–95

Bernard C: Leçons sur les Phenomènes de la vie Communs aux Animaux et aux Vegetaux. Vol. 1. JB Bailliere et Fils, Paris, 1878

Birt AB, Connolly NK: Traumatic chylothorax: a report of a case and a survey of the literature. Br J Surg 39:564, 1951–52

Blalock A, Cunningham RS, Robinson CS: Experimental production of chylothorax by occlusion of the superior vena cava. Ann Surg 104:359, 1936

Bower BC: Chyliform pleural effusion in rheumatoid arthritis. Am Rev Respir Dis 47:4515, 1968

Boyd A: Chylothorax. In Hood RM et al. (eds): Surgical Diseases of the Pleura and Chest Wall. WB Saunders, Philadelphia, 1986

Bradley SL, Dines DE, Soule EH et al.: Pulmonary lymphangiomatosis. Lung 158:69, 1980

Brewer LA: Surgical management of lesions of the thoracic duct. Am J Surg 90:210, 1955

Crandall L Jr, Barker SB, Graham DC: A study of the lymph from a patient with thoracic duct fistula. Gastroenterology 1:1040, 1943

Cunn B, Liebow AA, Friedman PJ: Pulmonary lymphangiomatosis: a review. Am J Pathol 79:398, 1973

Davis MK: A statistical study of the thoracic duct in man. Am J Anat 171:212, 1915

DeMeester TR: The pleura. In Sabiston DC, Spencer FC (eds): Surgery of the Chest. 4th Ed. WB Saunders, Philadelphia, 1983

Drinker CK, Field ME: The protein content of mammalian lymph and the relation of lymph to tissue fluid. Am J Physiol 9:32, 1931

Eugevik L: Traumatic chylothorax. Scand J Thorac Cardiovasc Surg 10:77, 1976

Frazer AC: The mechanism of fat absorption. Biochem Soc Symp 9:5, 1951–52

Freundlich IM: The role of lymphangiography in chylothorax. AJR 125:617, 1975

Goorwitch J: Traumatic chylothorax and thoracic duct ligation. J Thorac Cardiovasc Surg 29:467, 1955

Hashim SA, Roholt RB, Babayan UK et al.: Treatment of chyluria and chylothorax with medium chain triglyceride. N Engl J Med 270:756, 1964

Heppner GJ: Bilateral chylothorax and chyloperiotoneum. JAMA 102:1294, 1934

Hewson W: The Lymphatic System in the Human and Other Animals. J Johnston, London, 1774

Higgins CB, Mulder DG: Chylothorax after surgery for congenital heart diseases. J Thorac Cardiovasc Surg 61:411, 1971

Hunter W: Two Introductory Lectures in His Last Course of Anatomic Lectures at His Theatre in Windmill Street. J Johnston, London, 1784

Hyde PV, Jerky J, Gishen P: Traumatic chylothorax. S Afr J Surg 12:57, 1974

Kausel WH, Reeve TS, Stain AA et al.: Anatomic and pathologic studies of the thoracic duct. J Thorac Cardiovasc 34:631, 1957

Kinmonth JB, Taylor GW: Spontaneous rhythmic contractility in human lymphatics. J Physiol (Lond) 133:3, 1956

Klepser RG, Berry JF: The diagnosis and surgical management of chylothorax with the aid of lipophilic dyes. Dis Chest 25:409, 1954

Lampson RS: Traumatic chylothorax—a review of the literature and report of a case treated by mediastinal ligation of the thoracic duct. J Thorac Cardiovasc Surg 17:778, 1948

Lee FC: The establishment of collateral circulation following ligation of the thoracic duct. Bull Johns Hopkins Hosp 33:21, 1922

Meade RH Jr, Head JR, Moen CW: The management of chylothorax. J Thorac Cardiovasc Surg 19:709, 1950

Miller JI: Chylothorax and anatomy of the thoracic duct. In Shields TW (ed): General Thoracic Surgery. Lea & Febiger, Philadelphia, 1989

Milsom JW, Kron IL, Rheuban KS et al.: Chylothorax: an assessment of current surgical management. J Thorac Cardiovasc Surg 89:221, 1985

Moore KL: The Developing Human. 2nd Ed. WB Saunders, Toronto, 1977

Munk I, Rosenstein A: Zur Lehre von der Resorption ni Darm nach Untersuchungen an einer Lymph (chylus) fistel beim Menschen. Virchows Arch A Pathol Anat Histopathol 123:484, 1891

Murphy TO, Piper CA: Surgical management of chylothorax. Am Surg 43:719, 1977

Nix JT, Albert M, Dugas JE et al.: Chylothorax and chyloascites—a study of 302 selected cases. Am J Gastroenterol 28:40, 1957

Patterson GA, Todd TRJ, Delarue NC et al.: Supradiaphragmatic ligation of the thoracic duct in intractable chylous fistula. Ann Thorac Surg 32:44, 1981

Quinke H: Über fetthaltige Transudate-Hydros chylosus und Hydrops adiposus. Dtsch Arch Klin Med 16:121, 1875

Randolph JG, Gross RE: Congenital chylothorax. Arch Surg 74:405, 1957

Ross JK: A review of the surgery of the thoracic duct. Thorax 16:12, 1961

Roy PH, Carr DT, Payne WS: The problem of chylothorax. Mayo Clin Proc 42:457, 1967

Sabin FR: The origin and development of the lymphatic system. Rep Johns Hopkins Hosp 17:347, 1916

Sachs PB, Zelch MG, Rice TW et al.: Diagnosis and localization of laceration of the thoracic duct: usefulness of lymphaniography and CT. AJR 157:703, 1991

Schumacker HB Jr, Moore TC: Surgical management of traumatic chylothorax. Surg Gynecol Obstet 93:46, 1951

Selle JG, Snyder WH, Schreiber JT: Chylothorax: indications for surgery. Ann Surg 177:245, 1973

Seriff NS, Cohen ML, Samuel P et al.: Chylothorax diagnosis by lipoprotein electrophoresis of serum and pleural fluid. Thorax 32:98, 1977

Shafiroff GP, Kau QY: Cannulation of the human thoracic lymph duct. Surgery 45:814, 1959

Shirai T, Amano J, Takabe K: Thoracoscopic diagnosis and treatment of chylothorax after pneumonectomy. Ann Thorac Surg 52:306, 1991

Silverstein EF et al.: Pulmonary lymphangiomyomatosis. AJR 120: 832, 1974

Staats RA, Ellefson RD, Budahn LL et al.: The lipoprotein profile of chylous and unchylous pleural effusion. May Clin Proc 55:700, 1980

Starling EH: On the absorption of fluid from the connective tissue spaces. J Physiol (Lond) 19:312, 1896

Stenzel W, Rigler B, Tscheliessnig KH et al.: Treatment of post surgical chylothorax with fibrin glue. J Thorac Cardiovasc Surg 31:35, 1983

Traquair K: Chylothorax following traumatic pseudocyst of the pancreas. Br J Surg 33:297, 1945–46

Van Pernis PA: Variation of the thoracic duct. Surgery 26:308, 1949

Weese JL, Schouten JT: Internal drainage of intractable malignant pleural effusions. Wis Med J 83:21, 1984

Whitcomb BB, Scoville WB: Postoperative chylothorax—sudden death following infusion of aspirated chyle. Arch Surg 45:747, 1942

Williams KR, Burford TH: The management of chylothorax related to trauma. J Trauma 3:317, 1963

Yater WM: Non-traumatic chylothorax and chylopericardium; review and report of a case due to carcinomatous thromboangiitis obliterans of the thoracic duct and upper great veins. Ann Intern Med 9:600, 1935

Zesas DG: Die nicht operative entstandenen Verletzungen des Ductus thoracicus. Dtsch Z Chir 115:49, 1912

41

MESOTHELIOMA AND LESS COMMON TUMORS

Valerie W. Rusch

HISTORICAL NOTE

Pleural mesothelioma is an uncommon neoplasm with an estimated annual incidence in the United States of 2,000 to 3,000 cases. The first report of a primary pleural tumor is attributed to Lieutaud in 1767 (Scharifker and Kaneko, 1979), but an accurate pathologic description did not become available until Klemperer and Rabin (1937) classified mesotheliomas as either localized or diffuse. Cell culture experiments by Stout and Murray (1942) in 1942 demonstrated the mesothelial origin of these tumors. The epidemiology of diffuse malignant mesothelioma first became evident in 1960 when Wagner, et al. (1960) and Wagner (1986) reported 33 cases of malignant pleural mesothelioma in asbestos mine workers from the north western Cape Province of South Africa. Subsequent studies, especially work by Selikoff, et al. (1965) in the United States, confirmed that asbestos exposure was the major risk factor for malignant mesothelioma (Whitwell and Rawcliffe, 1971). However, the biology and clinical management of mesothelioma remain a source of confusion and controversy. Pleural mesotheliomas are often classified as benign or malignant. From the standpoint of cause and therapy, however, it is more logical to categorize them as they were originally, that is, as either localized or diffuse.

HISTORICAL READINGS

Klemperer P, Rabin CB: Primary neoplasms of the pleura. A report of five cases. Arch Pathol Lab Med 11:385, 1937
Scharifker D, Kaneko M: Localized fibrous "mesothelioma" of pleura (submesothelial fibroma). Cancer 43:627, 1979
Selikoff IJ, Churg J, Hammond EC: Relation between exposure to asbestos and mesothelioma. N Engl J Med 272:560, 1965
Stout AP, Murray MR: Localized pleural mesothelioma. Arch Pathol Lab Med 34:951, 1942
Wagner JC: Mesothelioma and mineral fibers. Cancer 57:1905, 1986

Illustrations in this chapter were done by the late David H. Dillard, M.D.

Wagner JC, Slaggs CA, Marchand P: Diffuse pleural mesothelioma and asbestos exposure in north western Cape Province. Bre J Ind Med 17:P260, 1960
Whitwell PR, Rawcliffe RM: Diffuse malignant pleural mesothelioma and asbestos exposure. Thorax 26:6, 1971

LOCALIZED MESOTHELIOMA

Localized mesothelimoas are rare tumors, with approximately 600 cases reported to date. They are not associated with asbestos exposure, occur as commonly in women as in men, and are seen predominantly during the sixth and seventh decades of life.

Localized mesotheliomas usually present as discrete encapsulated tumors, but they have a variable histologic appearance. The "patternless pattern," originally described by Stout and Murray (1942), is characterized by a random mixture of fibroblast-like cells and connective tissue and is the most common histologic appearance. A hemangiopericytoma-like pattern is the second most common appearance, but leiomyoma-like or neurofibroma-like patterns are also seen. A mixture of histologic patterns is common and occurs in approximately 40 percent of cases (Wagner, et al., 1960). In contrast to malignant diffuse mesotheliomas, localized mesotheliomas never show any epithelial features histologically, do not stain for keratins on immunohistochemical analysis, and do not have long branching microvilli by electron microscopy (Said, et al., 1984). Localized mesotheliomas are thought to arise from the primitive submesothelial mesenchymal cell rather than from the mesothelial cell itself. Some pathologists believe that localized mesotheliomas are more appropriately termed "localized fibrous tumors of the pleura" (Briselli, et al., 1981) because their pathogenesis is so different from that of diffuse mesotheliomas.

Localized mesotheliomas can be either benign or malignant. The pathologic features that distinguish these two entities are shown in Table 41-1. Benign mesotheliomas are usually pedunculated tumors that arise from the visceral pleura,

Table 41-1. Pathologic Features that Distinguish Benign and Malignant Localized Fibrous Tumor of Pleura

Feature[a]	Benign (n = 141) No.	%	Malignant[a] (n = 82) No.	%
Gross				
Pedunculated	73	52	21	26
Atypical location[b]	67	48	55	67
Size (>10 cm)	34	24	45	55
Necrosis and hemorrhage	21	15	53	65
Microscopic				
Increased cellularity	18	13	62	76
Pleomorphism[c]	14	10	69	84
Mitosis (> 4/10 high-power field)	2	1	63	77

[a] For all features, the differences between benign and malignant tumors are statistically significant by the chi-square test (P < 0.05).

[b] Tumor attached to parietal pleura, fissure, or mediastinum, or inverted into peripheral lung.

[c] Pleomorphism expressed as increased nuclear grades.

(From England DM, Hochholzer L, McCarthy MJ: Localized benign and malignant fibrous tumors of the pleura: a clinico-pathologic review of 223 cases. Am J Surg Pathol 13:647, 1989, with permission.)

measure less than 10 cm in size, are relatively acellular, and have few mitoses (Fig. 41-1). Occasionally, however benign localized mesotheliomas grow to a huge size and fill the entire hemithorax (McNicholas, et al., 1980; Watts, et al., 1989). Localized malignant mesotheliomas are usually larger nonpedunculated tumors that arise from the parietal, mediastinal, or diaphragmatic pleura and have a greater tendency toward increased cellularity, pleomorphism, and frequent mitoses (Fig. 41-2).

Most patients with localized mesotheliomas present with an asymptomatic mass incidentally diagnosed on the chest

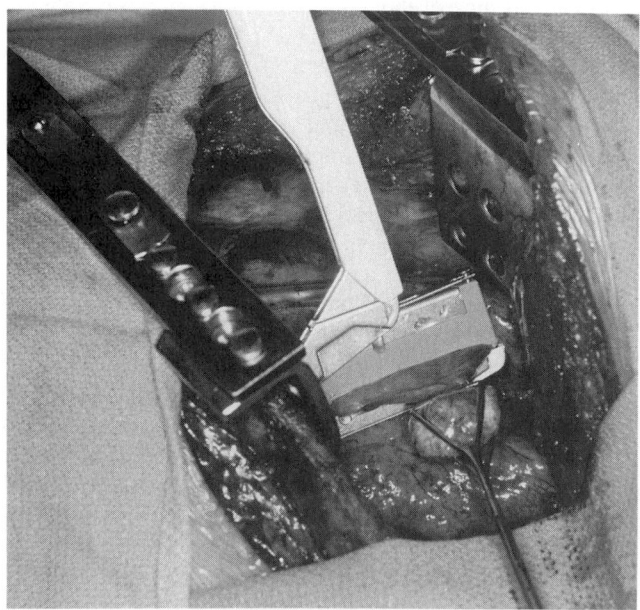

Figure 41-1. Intraoperative photograph of a benign mesothelioma. The stapler is placed across the pulmonary parenchyma just beyond the base of this pedunculated tumor.

radiograph. Among the 30 to 40 percent of patients who have symptoms, cough, chest pain, and dyspnea are the most common complaints, but fever and hypertrophic pulmonary osteoarthropathy and hemoptysis can also occur (Scharifker and Kaneko, 1979; Okike, et al., 1968). The relative incidence rates of these symptoms in 360 cases of localized mesothelioma are shown in Table 41-2. Hypoglycemia is reported in approximately 4 percent of patients and is almost always associated with tumors larger than 10 cm. The mechanism of this hypoglycemia is not fully understood, but it may be related both to the secretion of an insulinlike peptide and to decreased glucagon secretion. The hypoglycemia resolves completely when the tumor is resected (Immerman, et al., 1982). Pleural effusion and clubbing of the fingers are the most common signs associated with localized mesotheliomas but are seen in only 3 to 32 percent of patients. Hemoptysis is thought to occur only with malignant localized mesotheliomas; pulmonary osteoarthropathy has been associated only with benign localized mesotheliomas (Briselli, et al., 1981; England, et al., 1989).

As illustrated in Table 41-3, signs and symptoms occur more often in the malignant than in the benign form of localized mesothelioma. However, neither the pathologic features nor the clinical presentation fully predict the behavior and long-term outcome of localized mesotheliomas. The survival time is directly related to whether or not the tumor can be completely resected. Pedunculated masses, no matter what their size or histologic characteristics, are more easily removed than sessile tumors that invade the diaphragm, chest wall, or mediastinum. With rare exceptions, pedunculated tumors are completely cured by surgical resection. If they recur, they do so locally. Sessile tumors are potentially curable by complete resection. When incompletely resected, they not only recur locally, but also produce widely disseminated metastases, and are invariably fatal within 2 to 5 years of the diagnosis being made. Localized mesotheliomas are so rare that it is impossible to determine whether any adjuvant therapy is beneficial. Complete surgical resection is the mainstay of therapy (Scharifker and Kaneko, 1979; England, et al., 1984; Briselli, et al., 1981; Okike, et al., 1968).

DIFFUSE MESOTHELIOMA

Incidence and Epidemiology

Diffuse mesothelioma is always a malignant tumor. It is a far more common and clinically important entity than localized mesothelioma is, and the term *malignant mesothelioma* is loosely used to refer to the diffuse form. The incidence of this disease has risen steadily since 1970, and there are currently an estimated 2,000 to 3,000 cases annually in the United States. The incidence in women has remained relatively stable at 1 to 2 per million population; the number of cases in men has increased to 15 per million population per year. This trend reflects the impact of occupational asbestos exposure (McDonald and McDonald, 1987). Because the latency period between asbestos exposure and the development of the disease is at least 20 years, the recent surge in the number of cases reflects the widespread unprotected use of asbestos during the 1940s and 1950s, especially in the shipbuilding

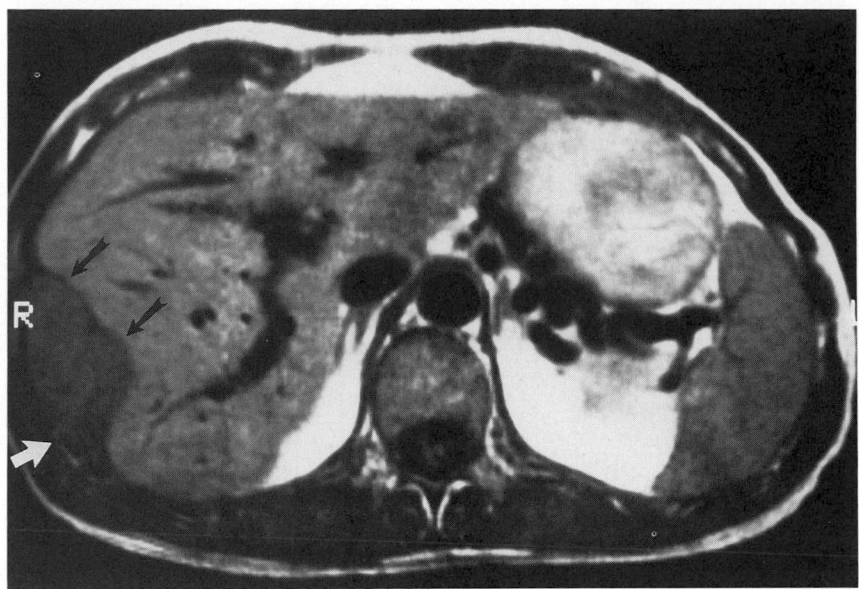

Figure 41-2.   Magnetic resonance scan of a localized malignant fibrosarcomatous mesothelioma (*white arrow*), which originated from the parietal pleura in the right costophrenic angle. The scan shows a distinct plane (*black arrows*) between the mass and the liver. At thoracotomy the tumor did not traverse the diaphragm, and the remainder of the pleura was normal. The patient remains disease-free 2.5 years after wide resection with reconstruction of the chest wall and diaphragm.

industry in World War II. This trend is expected to continue for the next 20 or more years because measures to limit occupational asbestos exposure have been instituted only since the 1970s.

The type of asbestos fiber plays a critical role in this relationship. Asbestos fibers are divided into two major mineralogic groups: amphibole and serpentine. Chrysotile asbestos is the only member of the serpentine group; crocidolite, amosite, tremolite, anthophyllite, and actinolite asbestos belong to the amphibole group. These silicate minerals differ considerably in their structure and composition. Serpentine fibers are large curly fibers that do not travel beyond the major airways; amphibole fibers are narrow and straight fibers that pass into the pulmonary parenchyma and are taken up in the lymphatic vessels (Pooley, 1987). It is the amphibole fibers, especially crocidolite asbestos, that have been most clearly associated with malignant mesothelioma. Crocidolite asbestos is found in South Africa and until recently was also mined in Western Australia (Musk, et al., 1989). Chrysotile accounts for 97 percent of the world's asbestos production, and it is mined principally in the Ural Mountains in Russia, Quebec Province in Canada, Zimbabwe and Swaziland in southern Africa, the Italian Alps, and Cyprus (Wagner, 1986). Chrysotile itself is not thought to cause mesothelioma but is often contaminated with amphibole fibers, such as tremolite or amosite (Churg and De Paoli, 1988). Chrysotile appears to be a far greater risk factor for the development of lung cancer, particularly in patients who are smokers (McDonald, et al., 1989). There are many different situations in which individuals can be exposed to asbestos because it has more than 1,000 uses. However, the areas of the world that have a high incidence of mesothelioma are those with asbestos mines,

asbestos industries, or industries (such as shipyards, insulation, or fireproofing) that use large amounts of asbestos (Andersson and Olsen, 1985). In North America the highest incidence areas include the provinces of Quebec and British Columbia in Canada, which have asbestos mines, and Seattle, Hawaii, San Francisco-Oakland, New York-New Jersey and New Orleans in the United States, which have either large shipyards or asbestos industries (McDonald and McDonald, 1987). It is often difficult to document a relationship between the duration or intensity of asbestos exposure and the development of mesothelioma. Patients with peritoneal mesotheliomas often have a history of heavy exposure, whereas patients with pleural disease may have had brief or indirect exposure (Levine, 1981).

Mesothelioma is also caused by other naturally occurring and human-made fibers that share the physical properties of amphibole asbestos fibers (i.e., have a diameter less than $0.25~\mu m$ and a length greater than $5.0~\mu m$). The most notable example of this is erionite (Wagner, et al., 1975), a zeolite fiber that is found in the volcanic deposits of central Turkey and is the major building material of homes in that area. In Karain, a village with a population of 604, malignant mesothelioma was the single most common cause of death, with 62 cases recorded over the 11-year period from 1970 to 1981 (Baris).

There are other less common causes of malignant mesothelioma. Radiation exposure for periods ranging from 10 to 31 years prior to the development of mesothelioma is the most clearly documented of these causes, but extravasation of radioactive thorium dioxide during radiologic procedures and exposure to isoniazid in utero have also been anecdotally reported (Lerman, et al., 1991; Antman, et al., 1983, 1984;

Table 41-2. Summary of Reported Features in 360 Cases of Solitary Fibrous Tumor of the Pleura

| | No. Patients | Age Range (yr) | Male/Female Ratio | Symptomatic Patients (% of Total) | Prevalence of Various Symptoms (%) | | | | | | Right/Left Ratio | Visceral/ Parietal Pleura Ratio | Benign/Lethal Clinical Behavior Ratio |
					Cough	Chest Pain	Dyspnea	Pulmonary Osteoarthropathy	Fever	Other			
1942–1972	190	12–82 (mean, 50)	84/106	72	39	40	26	47	24	37	61/60	51/28	147/20
1973–1980	170	5–87 (mean, 53)	81/89	54	54	51	49	22	25	25	78/68	90/23	142/18
Total	360	5–87 (mean, 51)	165/195	64	46	44	37	35	24	32	139/128	141/51	289/38

(From Briselli M, Mark EJ, Dickersin GR: Solitary fibrous tumors of the pleura: eight new cases and review of 360 cases in the literature. Cancer 47:2687, 1981, with permission.)

Table 41-3. Initial Clinical Findings in 214 Patients with Localized Fibrous Tumor of the Pleura

Finding	Benign (n = 138)		Malignant (n = 76)	
	No.	% of Total	No.	% of Total
Asymptomatic	92	67	19	25
Symptomatic	46	33	57	75
Chest pain	26	19	31	41
Shortness of breath	15	11	15	20
Cough	16	12	12	16
Hypoglycemia	4	3	8	11
Weight loss	3	2	7	9
Dyspnea on exertion	2	1	4	5
Weakness	1	1	3	4
Hemoptysis	0	0	3	4
Fever	1	1	2	3
Night sweats	1	1	2	3
Signs				
Pleural effusion	11	8	24	32
Clubbing of fingers	4	3	4	5
Others[a]	3	2	2	3

[a] Includes superior vena caval syndrome (three cases: two malignant and one benign); superior sulcus (Pancoast) tumor (benign); and right middle lobe syndrome (benign).

(From England DM, Hochholzer L, McCarthy MJ: Localized benign and malignant fibrous tumors of the pleura: a clinico-pathologic review of 223 cases. Am J Surg Pathol 13:643, 1989, with permission.)

Table 41-4. Nonasbestos Causes of Mesothelioma

Agent	Species Tumor Observed in or Induced in[a]
Naturally occurring mineral fibers	
Zeolites (eronite)	Man, rat
Minerals	
Nickel	Rat
Silica powder	Rat
Beryllium	Rat, ?man
Radiation	Man, rat
Organic chemicals	
Polyurethane, polysilicone	Rat
Sterigmatocystin (aflatoxin B1-related compound)	Rat
Ethylene oxide	Rat
N-Methyl-N-nitrosourea	Guinea pig
N-Methyl-N-nitrosourethane	Mouse
3-Methylcholanthrene	Mouse
Methylnitrosamine	Rat
1-Nitroso-5, 6-dihydrouracil	Rat
Diethylstilbestrol	Monkey
Stilbestrol	Dog
3, 4, 5-Trimethoxycinnamaldehyde	Rat
Mineral oil	Man
Liquid paraffin	Man
Viruses	
MC 29 avian leukosis virus	Chicken
SV 40	Hamster
Chronic inflammation	
Recurrent lung infections	Man
Tuberculous pleuritis	Man
Recurrent diverticulitis	Man
Familial Mediterranean fever	Man
Nonspecific industrial exposure	
Shoe industry workers	Man
Petrochemical-oil industry workers	Man
Stone cutters	Man
Leather factory or textile workers	Man
Occupations involving exposure to copper, nickel, fiberglass, rubber or glass dust	Man
Cocarcinogens	
3-Methylcholanthrene and asbestos	Rat
Radiation and asbestos	Rat
N-Methyl-N-Nitrosourea and asbestos	Rat
Hereditary predisposition	Man

[a] Note: In some instances the tumors induced in animals by various agents may represent sarcomas and not mesotheliomas.

(From Hammar SP, Bolen JW: Pleural neoplasms. p. 979. In Dail DH, Hammar SP (eds): Pulmonary Pathology. Springer Verlag, New York, 1988, with permission.)

Anderson, et al., 1985). A variety of other substances (Malker, et al., 1985; Peterson, et al., 1984), some of which are listed in Table 41-4, have been implicated as possible risk factors for malignant mesothelioma, based on epidemiologic or experimental studies. Of great importance, however, is that smoking does not appear to be a risk factor for malignant mesothelioma. This is in distinct contrast to lung cancer, in which asbestos and smoking act as synergistic carcinogens (McDonald, et al., 1989).

The peak incidence for the majority of individuals who develop mesothelioma is in the sixth decade of life. Malignant mesothelioma is predominantly a disease of adults because of the long latency period between exposure to the causative agents and the development of cancer, but it can occur rarely in childhood (Fraire, et al., 1988). In that setting it seems to be idiopathic. Malignant mesothelioma sometimes develops in young adults because of exposure to risk factors during childhood (Kane, et al., 1990).

Pathology and Molecular Biology

Mesotheliomas arise from multipotential mesothelial or subserosal cells that can develop into either an epithelial or a sarcomatoid neoplasm. In contrast to localized mesotheliomas, diffuse mesotheliomas almost always have an epithelial component. However, they exhibit a wide array of histologic patterns and often have a mixture of epithelial and sarcomatoid features (Hammar and Bolen, 1988). In a review of 819 cases, Hillerdal (1983) reported that 50 percent were of epithelial type, 34 percent were of mixed type, and 16 percent were of the sarcomatoid type. The histologic appearance of mesotheliomas is easily confused with that of other neoplasms, and there is often disagreement among pathologists

when light microscopy is used as the sole method of diagnosis. The reclassification rate of tumors originally diagnosed as mesotheliomas ranges from 30 to 84 percent when these specimens are reviewed by panels of reference pathologists. The challenge for the pathologist is usually to distinguish epithelial mesotheliomas from metastatic adenocarcinomas. However, early mesotheliomas can be difficult to distinguish from benign mesothelial hyperplasia, and the rare desmoplastic form of mesothelioma often resembles benign fibrosis because of its predominantly fibroblastic cell type and sparsely cellular appearance (Hammar and Bolen, 1988; Cantin, et al., 1982). Several standard histochemical stains help to distinguish malignant mesoitheliomas from other tumors.

Histologic Classification of Mesothioma

Epithelial
  Tubulopapillary
  Epithelioid
  Glandular
  Large cell-giant cell
  Small cell
  Adenoid-cystic
  Signet ring
Sarcomatoid (fibrous, sarcomatous, mesenchymal)
Mixed epithelial-sarcomatoid (biphasic)
Transitional
Desmoplastic
Localized fibrous mesothelioma

(From Hammar SP, Bolen JW: Pleural neoplasms. p. 979. In Dial DH, Hammar SP (eds): Pulmonary Pathology. Springer-Verlag, New York, 1988, with permission.)

Pulmonary adenocarcinomas usually stain positively with mucicarmine, whereas mesothelioma does not. About 20 percent of epithelial mesotheliomas produce an acidic mucosubstance, hyaluronic acid, which can be seen either within or between cells with an Alcian blue or colloidal iron stain (Hammar and Bolen, 1988).

However, immunohistochemical analysis and electron microscopy have become the standard approach to diagnosis. Useful immunohistochemical stains include antibodies to high and low molecular weight cytokeratins, vimentin, human milk fat globules, carcinoembryonic antigen (CEA), and Leu-M1 antigen. Mesotheliomas stain positively for low molecular weight cytokeratins, a feature that distinguishes them from sarcomas. They never stain for CEA, a feature that distinguishes them from adenocarcinomas (Battifora and Kopinski, 1985; Mezger, et al., 1990; Wirth, et al., 1991). If immunohistochemical stains yield equivocal results, electron microscopy usually leads to a definitive diagnosis. The most prominent feature of mesotheliomas is that they have numerous long sinuous microvilli; adenocarcinomas have short straight microvilli that are covered by a fuzzy glycocalyx (Burns, et al., 1985; Hammar and Bolen, 1988).

Relatively little is understood about the biology of diffuse malignant mesothelioma. Flow cytometric examination of mesotheliomas surprisingly shows them to be predominantly diploid (approximately 65 percent of cases), with intermediate or low proliferative rates (Burmer, et al., 1989). Molecular biologic information has been derived mostly from mesothelioma cell lines, although chromosomal abnormalities have also been studied in primary tumor specimens. These abnormalities include alterations (usually deletions) on chromosomes 1, 3, 4, 9, 11, 14, and 22 (Hagemeijer, et al., 1990; Popescu, et al., 1988). Additional copies of the short arm of chromosome 7 are also seen and may be an indicator of poor prognosis (Tiainen, et al., 1989). Overexpression of the platelet-derived growth factors and their receptors is a consistent finding in human mesothelioma cell lines compared with normal cell lines (Gerwin, et al., 1987). Abnormalities of the tumor-suppressor gene, p53, were also reported (Cote, et al., 1991). Transfection experiments, using the activated c-Ha-ras oncogene, EJ-ras, in a human mesothelial cell line, suggest that the activation of this oncogene may play a critical role in the malignant transformation of mesothelial cells (Reddel, et al., 1989). How these preliminary pieces of information fit together in the overall sequence of carcinogenesis in mesothelioma remains to be seen.

Clinical Presentation and Diagnosis

The clinical presentation of diffuse malignant mesothelioma is insidious and nonspecific. Because of this the interval between the onset of symptoms and the diagnosis is often 3 to 6 months. Dyspnea and chest pain are the most common symptoms, occurring in 90 percent of patients. Weight loss is seen in about 30 percent of patients. Less common symptoms include cough, weakness, anorexia, and fever. Hemoptysis, hoarseness, dysphagia, Horner's syndrome, and dyspnea (from a spontaneous pneumothorax) occur rarely. The physical examination is usually unrevealing, demonstrating only dullness to percussion and diminished breath sounds over the affected hemithorax. Patients who have locally advanced disease may have a palpable chest wall mass, diffuse infiltration of the chest wall by the tumor, and rarely (palpable supraclavicular lymph nodes (Elmes and Simpson, 1976; Ruffie, et al., 1989; Sheard, et al., 1991).

Paraneoplastic syndromes are uncommon, but autoimmune hemolytic anemia, hypercalcemia, hypoglycemia, inappropriate secretion of antidiuretic hormone (SIADH), and hypercoagulability not related to thrombocytosis have been reported (Gerwin, et al., 1987). Thrombocytosis, defined as a platelet count of 400,000 cells/μl or more, occurs in about 40 percent of patients and can be associated with a leukemoid reaction (Olesen and Thorshauge, 1988).

Patients with mesotheliomas often have abnormal electrocardiographic (ECG) and echocardiographic findings. In a review of 64 patients, Wadler, et al. (1986) found that 55 patients (89 percent) had abnormal ECGs. Sinus tachycardia was seen in 42 percent; nonlife-threatening ventricular or atrial arrhythmias occurred in 17 percent of patients. More than one-third of patients had some form of bundle branch block. Although pericardial invasion or myocardial involvement was a common finding at autopsy in these patients, most ECG abnormalities occurred more than 6 months before death, suggesting that they are not solely related to the presence of advanced disease. Echocardiography was somewhat insensitive but highly specific for involvement of the pericardium or myocardium by tumor. Three patients who had pericardial effusions by echocardiogram had pericardial and myocardial involvement at autopsy, whereas five patients who had pericardial tumors at autopsy had a normal echocardiogram premortem.

There are no tumor markers that are routinely used for malignant mesothelioma. The serum hyaluronan concentration may be elevated in some patients, a not surprising finding given the positive staining for hyaluronic acid seen in many epithelial mesotheliomas. In one study of 37 patients, a rise in the serum hyaluronan level had a sensitivity of 65 percent and a specificity of 85 percent a a predictor of progressive disease. Hyaluronan can be measured using a commercial kit, but this is not readily available in most hospitals (Dahl, et al., 1989). Ca 125 has been anecdotally reported to be a serum marker in malignant mesothelioma, but the utility of this has not been investigated in large numbers of patients (Blackstein M: personal communication, 1989).

Malignant mesothelioma is classically portrayed as a massive tumor involving all pleural surfaces, encasing the lung and chest wall, and producing severe unremitting pain. In fact this appearance is characteristic only of locally advanced mesothelioma. In the early stages of disease, a large pleural effusion is the dominant feature, and this is responsible for

the dyspnea that brings the patient to medical attention. As the tumor grows locally, the pleural effusion becomes loculated, and the pleural tumor becomes confluent. At this stage patients experience vague sensations of chest discomfort along with mild shortness of breath. The massive pleural rind characteristic of locally advanced disease produces dyspnea because of restrictive lung disease and pain because of encasement of the chest wall and infiltration of the intercostal spaces and nerves (Law, et al., 1982b).

The radiographic appearance of malignant mesothelioma is variable and nonspecific. In early-stage mesothelioma a large pleural effusion is often the only sign of disease (Fig. 41-3). Multiple discrete pleural-based masses may be seen

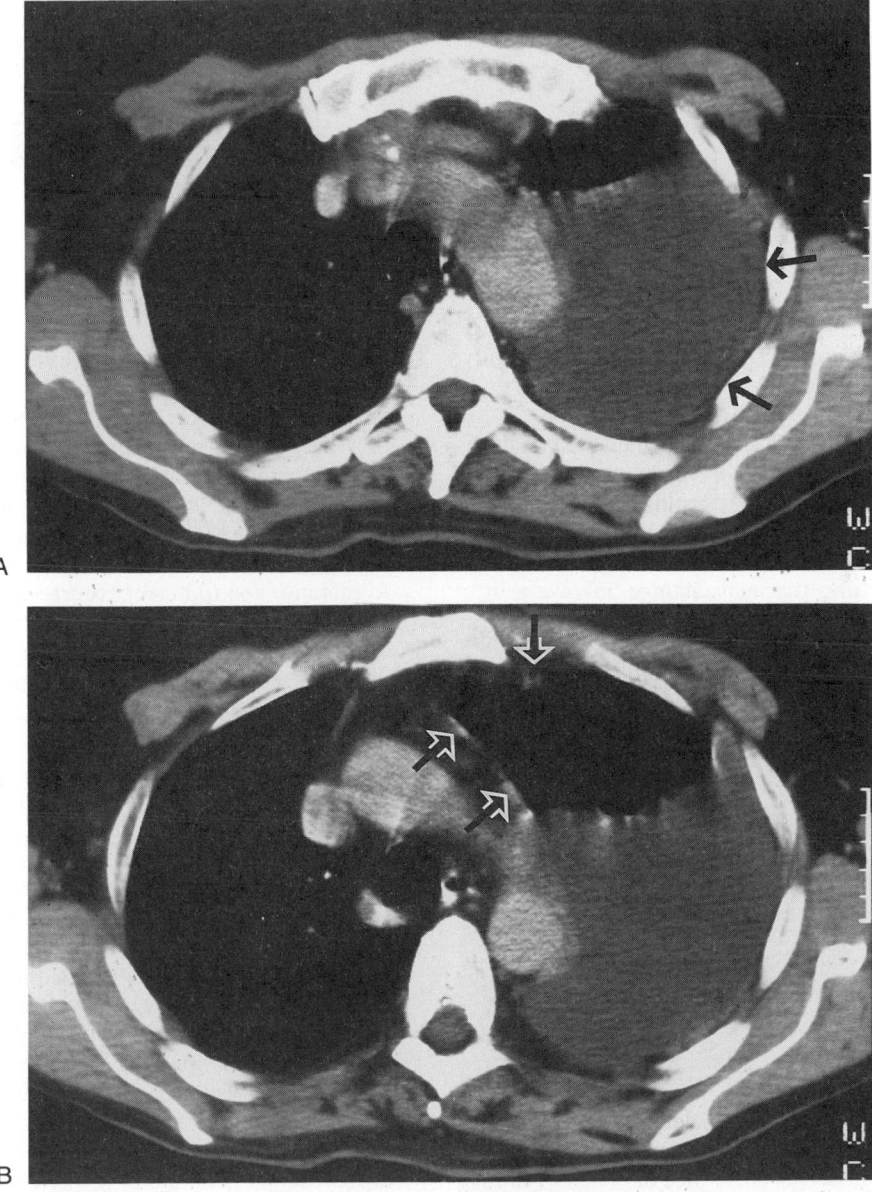

Figure 41-3. CT scan of early-stage diffuse mesothelioma. **(A)** The CT cut at the level of the aortic arch shows a large left pleural effusion (*arrows*) with no evidence of pleural disease. **(B)** The CT cut at the level of the aortopulmonary window shows mild pleural thickening and irregularity (*arrows*) in addition to the effusion. At thoracotomy there was diffuse studding of the pleura with tumor nodules that were 1 to 2 mm in size.

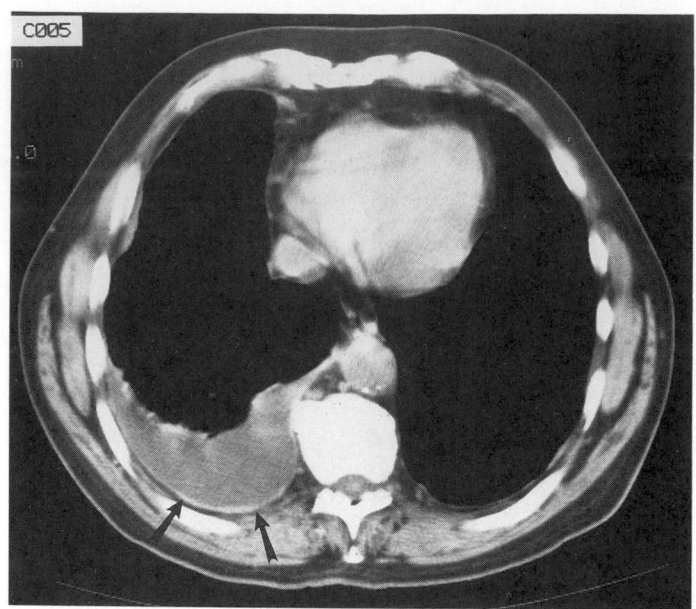 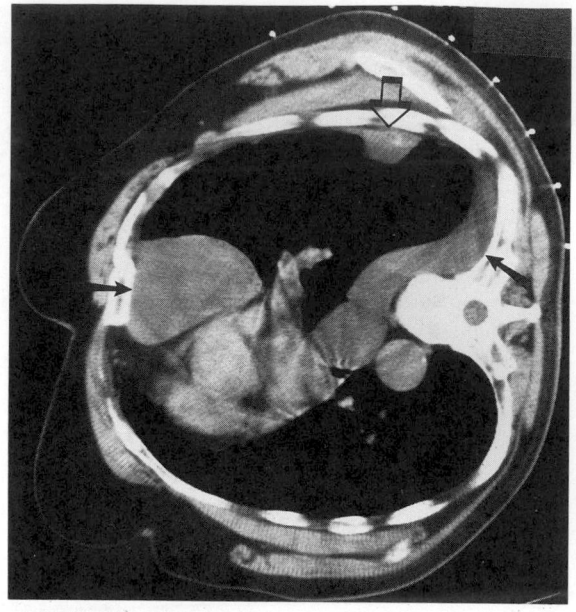

Figure 41-4. CT scan of another early-stage mesothelioma. **(A)** There is a large pleural effusion with diffuse mild pleural thickening and irregularity (*arrows*). **(B)** A CT cut obtained with the patient in the lateral position shows a dominant chest wall mass (*large arrow*) and a freely flowing effusion (*small arrow*).

on by computed tomography (CT) (Figs. 41-4). Subsequently, pleural-based masses become evident, and are often intermixed with multiloculated effusions (Gotfried, et al., 1983). Rarely a dominant pleural-based mass may be the initial presentation, but ultimately the involvement of the pleura is always diffuse. Eventually a thick irregular pleural rind develops, with encasement of the lung and obliteration of the pleural space (Fig. 41-5). Mediastinal adenopathy, direct extension of the tumor into the mediastinum, involvement of

the pericardium with pericardial effusion, and extension into the chest wall or through the diaphragm are seen in locally advanced tumors (Fig. 41-6). CT permits a far better appreciation of the extent of the disease than does plain radiography, which cannot demonstrate many of these abnormalities (Alexander, et al., 1981; Law, et al., 1982a; Mirvis, et al., 1983, Rabinowitz, et al., 1982). CT is currently the most accurate noninvasive way to stage patients, to gauge their responses to therapy, and to detect recurrent disease postoperatively, but it is often inaccurate in diagnosing chest wall involvement or extension through the diaphragm (Rusch, et al., 1988). It is hoped that magnetic resonance imaging will be more accurate in this regard.

A thoracentesis is usually the initial diagnostic procedure because most patients present with a pleural effusion. Pleural fluid cytologic analysis is positive for malignancy in only 30 to 50 percent of patients. Percutaneous pleural biopsy yields a diagnosis of malignancy in up to one-third of cases, but usually it does not provide the pathologist with a large enough specimen on which to perform the immunohistochemical or electron microscopic studies that are so critical to a definitive diagnosis (Lewis, et al., 1981; Ruffie, et al., 1989). Thoracoscopy is the optimal diagnostic procedure because it yields a diagnosis in at least 80 percent of patients but does not commit the patient to a major surgical procedure (Boutin, et al., 1993). The appearance of the pleural space is variable and depends on the extent of disease and the cell type. In the earliest stages of mesothelioma, involvement of the pleura is microscopic, and the only visible finding is a large pleural effusion. As the disease progresses, the thoracoscopic appearance evolves from pleural studding with a free pleural space and a large pleural effusion to larger but still discrete masses with multiloculated pleural effusions to a confluent

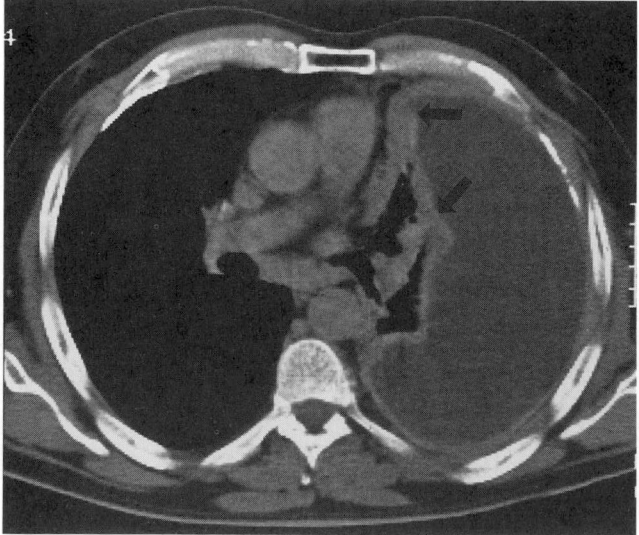

Figure 41-5. CT scan of a more locally advanced mesothelioma. There is a thick confluent pleural peel along the chest wall (*large arrows*), encasing the collapsed lung and extending into the fissure.

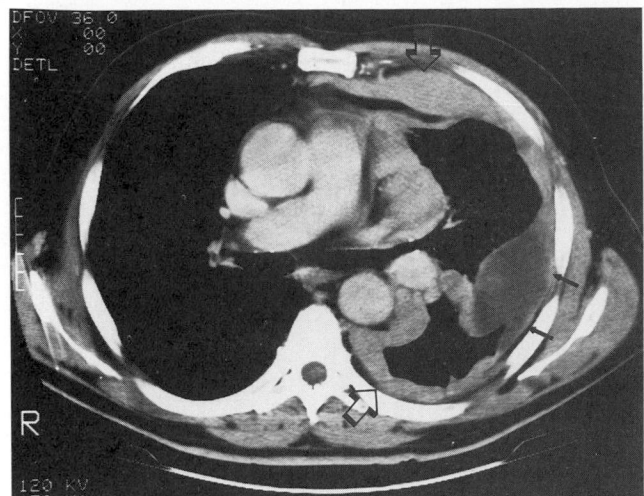 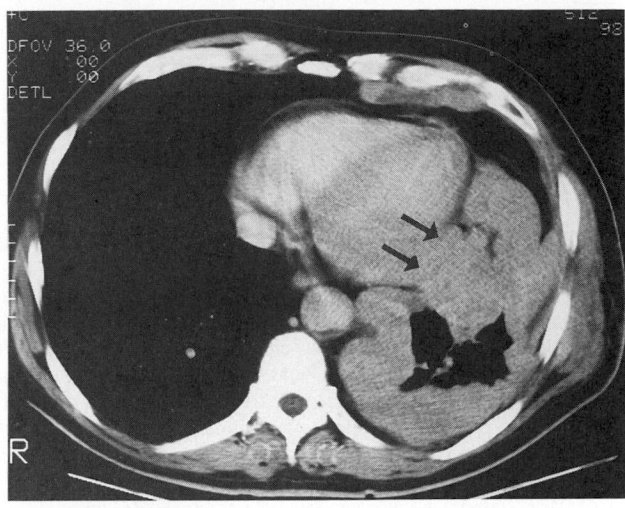

Figure 41-6. CT scan of another locally advanced mesothelioma. **(A)** A cut at the level of the pulmonary artery shows a thick irregular confluent pleural peel (*large arrow*) with a loculated pleural effusion (*small arrow*). **(B)** A cut at the level of the midheart shows massive tumor encasing and collapsing the lung and suggests invasion of the pericardium (*arrows*).

irregular sheet of tumor with obliteration of the pleural space. The tumor ranges in appearance from being soft, friable, and hypervascular to being densely fibrotic, depending on the mixture of cell types (Lewis, et al., 1981). No clinical findings are pathognomonic of malignant mesothelioma.

Thoracoscopy is not technically feasible in the patient whose pleural space is obliterated by a locally advanced tumor. The small incision usually made for thoracoscopy is then simply used for open pleural biopsy. This incision should be placed in line with a possible subsequent thoracotomy incision so that it can be excised at the time of the definitive operation. Mesothelioma has a notorious propensity to implant in the chest wall, and placing the thoracoscopy incision in a random manner complicates the local management of this disease by placing the patient at risk for a site of local chest wall recurrence. Diagnostic thoracotomy is rarely necessary and is ideally avoided because it exposes some patients who have metastatic adenocarcinoma to the unnecessary morbidity of a major operation. Most importantly the surgeon must submit pleural biopsy specimens fresh to the pathologist so that they can be placed in the appropriate fixatives for immunohistochemical analysis and electron microscopy.

Natural History and Staging

An understanding of the natural history is critical to the evaluation and development of therapy for any cancer. Our understanding of the natural history and prognostic factors in malignant mesothelioma is poor because it is an uncommon tumor and there is no accurate universally accepted staging system. The staging system used most often is the one proposed by Butchart, et al. (1976). The descriptors for the primary tumor and the involvement of the lymph nodes are imprecise. A stage I tumor, for instance, could include the disease in patients who have minimal pleural studding, a free pleural space, and a pleural effusion and the disease in patients who have a thick confluent sheet of tumor with

obliteration of the pleural space but without invasion of the mediastinum or opposite pleura. However, clinical experience suggests that the latter represents a much more locally advanced tumor. In addition, the exact incidence of lymph node involvement and its prognostic implications has not been clearly established in malignant mesothelioma. The inclusion of "lymph node involvement within the chest" in stage II and "lymph node involvement outside the chest" is empiric. A recent report of 44 patients, all of whom had Butchart's stage I disease and underwent extrapleural pneumonectomy and adjuvant chemotherapy and radiation, showed a significantly poorer survival rate among the 10 patients who had positive mediastinal nodes (Sugarbaker, et al., 1992). These data need to be confirmed in larger numbers of patients subjected to systematic lymph node dissection.

Staging Proposed by Butchart, et al.

Stage I: Tumor confined within the "capsule" of the parietal pleura (i.e., involving only ipsilateral pleura, lung, pericardium, and diaphragm)

Stage II: Tumor invading chest wall or involving mediastinal structures (e.g., esophagus, heart, opposite pleura); lymph node involvement within the chest

Stage III: Tumor penetrating diaphragm to involve peritoneum; involvement of opposite pleura; lymph node involvement outside the chest

Stage IV: Distant blood-borne metastases

(From Dimitrov NV, McMahon S: Presentation, diagnostic methods, staging and natural history of malignant mesothelioma. p. 233. In Antman K, Aisner J (eds): Asbestos-Related Malignancy. Grune & Stratton, Orlando, FL, 1987, with permission.)

Staging Proposed by Chahinian

Stage I: T1N0M0
Stage II: T1–2N1M0
       T2N0M0
Stage III: T3, any NM0
Stage IV: T4, any NM0, any M1

Abbreviations: T, primary tumor; T1, limited to ipsilateral pleura only (parietal pleura, visceral pleura); T2, superficial local invasion (diaphragm, endothoracic fascia, ipsilateral lung, fissures); T3, deep local invasion (chest wall beyond endothoracic fascia); T4, extensive direct invasion (opposite pleura, peritoneum, retroperitoneum); N, lymph nodes; N0, no positive lymph node; N1, positive ipsilateral hilar nodes; N2, positive mediastinal nodes; N3, positive contralateral hilar nodes; M, metastases; M0, no metastases; M1, metastases, blood-borne or lymphatic.
(From Dimitrov NV, McMahon S: Presentation, diagnostic methods, staging and natural history of malignant mesothelioma. p. 234. In Antman K, Aisner J (eds): Asbestos-Related Malignancy. Grune & Stratton, Orlando, FL, 1987, with permission.)

Staging System Proposed by UICC

T: primary tumor and extent

   Tx: Primary tumor cannot be assessed

   T0: No evidence of primary tumor

   T1: Primary tumor limited to ipsilateral parietal and/or visceral pleura

   T2: Tumor invades any of the following: ipsilateral lung, endothoracic fascia, diaphragm, pericardium

   T3: Tumor invades any of the following: ipsilateral chest wall muscle, ribs, mediastinal organs or tissues

   T4: Tumor extends to any of the following: contralateral pleura or lung by direct extension, peritoneum or intraabdominal organs by direct extension, cervical tissues

N: lymph nodes

   Nx: Regional lymph nodes cannot be assessed

   N0: No regional lymph node metastases

   N1: Metastases in ipsilateral bronchopulmonary or hilar lymph nodes

   N2: Metastases in ipsilateral mediastinal lymph nodes

   N3: Metastases in contralateral mediastinal, internal mammary, supraclavicular or scalene lymph nodes

M: metastases

   Mx: Presence of distant metastases cannot be assessed

(Continues)

M0: No (known) distant metastasis

M1: Distant metastasis present

Mesothelioma staging system[a]

Stage I

   T1N0M0

   T2N0M0

Stage II

   T1N1M0

   T2N1M0

Stage III

   T3N0M0

   T3N1M0

   T1N2M0

   T2N2M0

   T3N2M0

Stage IV

   Any T, N3M0

   T4, any N, M0

   Any T, any N, M1

---

[a] Staging solely on clinical measures is designated cTNM. Staging that can be done on clinical pathologic information is designated as pTNM. Clinical and pathologic groups are identical.
(From Rusch VW, Ginsberg RJ: New concepts in the staging of mesotheliomas. p. 340. In Deslaurier J, Lacquet LK (eds): Thoracic Surgery: Surgical Management of Pleural Diseases. CV Mosby, St. Louis, 1990, with permission.)

Several other staging systems have been proposed, including a tumor-node-metastasis (TNM)-baased system by Chahinian. This system is more precise than the Butchart one but does not fully reflect the usual findings at thoracotomy. For instance, it is uncommon to find patients who have a T1 tumor (as defined by Chahinian), with involvement of the parietal and visceral pleural surfaces but with sparing of the diaphragm, because mesothelioma is a diffuse disease and the area of greatest tumor burden is usually in the lower half of the hemithorax and the diaphragm. In an effort to improve and unify the staging system for malignant mesothelioma, the International Union Against Cancer (UICC) proposed another TNM-based sytem. The T status descriptors are more detailed than in previous systems, and the descriptors for nodal involvement in this system are borrowed directly from the current international staging system for nonsmall cell lung cancer. Even this system is not definitive, however, and needs to be confirmed or modified by careful clinicopathologic correlation.

Another confounding issue is that most published reports do not stage patients by computed tomographic scan. They assess them only by symptoms, physical examination, and chest radiographs. The inaccuracy of such a clinical assessment leads to a heterogeneous patient population. Finally, many series record outcome in small numbers of patients, seen over long periods and treated in a highly individualized manner. Little wonder that reported survival rates vary widely. Law, et al. (1984) reported a median survival of 18 months for 64 patients treated with supportive care, with no differences in survival according to cell types. Twelve of the 64 patients survived longer than 5 years, but the diagnosis of mesothelioma in this study was based on histologic findings alone and less than one-third of all patients were staged by CT scan. Hulks, et al. (1989) reported a median survival of 30 weeks for 68 patients treated with supportive care. They based their pathologic diagnosis on immunohistochemical findings and histologic results. No computed tomographic scanning was performed, and patients were classified principally according to their symptoms. Those who presented with dyspnea lived significantly longer than did patients who presented with pain (median survival, 44 versus 22 weeks), probably reflecting the extent of disease at the diagnosis. The cell type did not appear to influence the survival time.

Other authors have tried to identify prognostic factors in malignant mesothelioma but have done this mainly in the setting of retrospective reviews of patients with different stages of disease, treated with widely varying regimens. Contrary to the data reported by Law, et al. (1984) and by Hulks, et al. (1989), the epithelial histologic type has generally been a favorable prognostic factor. The absence of chest pain and a good performance status are also thought to be favorable prognostic factors, but probably they just reflect an early stage of the disease. Other factors including female gender and age younger than 50 years have incidentally been cited as favorable prognostic factors. In several series a platelet count greater than 400,000 appears to have a negative impact on survival (Adams, et al., 1986; Antman, et al., 1988; Olesen and Thorshouge 1988; Ruffie, et al., 1989).

Malignant mesothelioma was long thought to be a tumor that remained localized to the chest (Nauta, et al., 1982). Several autopsy series have now clearly disproved this. Ruffie, et al. (1989) found that 45 of 92 (49 percent) patients had distant metastases at autopsy. The liver was the most common site, and the contralateral lung was the second most common site of distant disease. However, metastases in sites as widely disseminated as the prostate, brain, and thyroid were also found. Elmes and Simpson (1976) found distant metastases in 48 of 148 (33 percent) patients at autopsy. The metastases were widely disseminated, but the liver and the contralateral lung were once again the most common sites of disease. Similar findings were reported by Roberts (1976) and Whitwell and Rawcliffe (1971). The uncommon but definite occurrence of brain and spinal metastases has been emphasized in several reports (Kaye, et al., 1986; Ruffie, et al., 1989; Walters and Martinez, 1975). Virtually all patients have advanced local or regional disease at death, however. It is the symptoms related to the locoregional tumor that are usually the most difficult to palliate and therefore the most important clinically (Nauta, et al., 1982). Patients with malignant mesothelioma face a dual problem: control of the locoregional tumor throughout the course of their disease and prevention of distant metastases as a late manifestation of their cancer.

Therapy

As in any other cancer, the therapeutic options for malignant mesothelioma include surgery, radiation, chemotherapy, immunotherapy, or some combination of these modalities. However, the choice of therapy is influenced by factors that do not apply to some other malignancies; that is, the location and extent of the tumor and the general medical condition of these patients, who are usually older and often have serious underlying diseases. The assessment of therapeutic regimens for malignant mesothelioma is hampered by a lack of large prospective clinical trials. Most patients have been treated in a highly individualized manner. Reported series are usually small and retrospective.

Radiation

It is difficult to evaluate the success of radiation as the only therapy because it has usually been given in conjunction with surgical resection or chemotherapy. Radiation therapy alone is generally used to palliate an area of symptomatic tumor in the chest wall or mediastinum.

The use of radiation therapy is limited by the volume of the primary tumor, which involves the entire hemithorax, and by proximity of the tumor to many vital structures that are intolerant of high doses of radiation. For the most part, radiation doses to the affected hemithorax have been kept at 4,500 cGy or less to prevent toxicity to the heart, esophagus, lung, and spinal cord (Ball and Cruickshank, 1990; Brady, 1981; Gordon, et al., 1981). Maasilta (1990) documented the severe pulmonary toxicity caused by higher doses of hemithoracic radiation; the radiographic changes, and the deterioration in pulmonary function, in oxygenation that develop over the year following radiation are compatible with a total loss of pulmonary function on the irradiated side. In several studies the toxicity of radiation may also be potentiated by the administration of chemotherapy, including drugs, such as doxorubicin (Sinoff, et al., 1982).

One strategy that has been used to circumvent these problems is to administer radiation after surgical resection of most or all of the gross tumor, using a variety of techniques to minimize the radiation dose to the lung. The largest and most consistent experience with this approach was reported by the Memorial Sloan-Kettering Cancer Center. Gross tumor was resected by pleurectomy and decortication. Unresectable gross tumor present at the completion of the thoracotomy was treated with ^{125}I or ^{192}Ir implants. The patients then received external beam irradiation to the entire hemithorax using a mixed photon-electron beam to a total dose of 4,500 cGy (Hilaris, et al., 1983; Kutcher, et al., 1987). In 105 patients treated from 1976 to 1988, the median surival time was 12.6 months with 1- and 2-year actuarial survival rates of 52 and 23 percent, respectively. However, the 27 patients who had an epithelial histologic type and minimal gross residual disease that required only external beam irradiation without brachytherapy had a median survival time of 15 months, and 1- and 2-year survival rates of 68 and 35 percent, respectively. There were 19 complications, including 12 cases of radiation pneumonitis and 8 patients with pericarditis and tamponade. Local failure occurred in 64 of the 105 patients (63 percent)

(Mychalczak, et al, 1989). Both this clinical experience and some experimental work indicate that a low-dose mixed photon-electron beam may be theoretically attractive but often does not succeed in sparing the underlying pulmonary parenchyma and fails to provide long-term local control for most patients (Soubra, et al., 1989).

Higher doses of external beam radiation can be safely administered when the lung is resected along with the pleural tumor by extrapleural pneumonectomy. At the Dana-Farber Cancer Institute, 31 patients received 5,500 cGy of hemithoracic radiation following extrapleural pneumonectomy without experiencing significant toxicity. These patients had 1- and 2-year survival rates of 70 and 48 percent, respectively, but also received postoperative adjuvant chemotherapy, making it hard to assess the specific contribution of radiation therapy. The sites of relapse were not detailed in this report (Sugarbaker, et al., 1991).

The successful use of fast neutron therapy was described in one report (Blake, et al., 1985). Small series have reported the use of radioactive colloidal compounds, including radioactive gold (^{198}Au) and chromic phosphate (^{32}P), but these appear ineffective in treating any substantial tumor bulk within the pleural cavity (Brady, 1981). Overall the contribution of radiation therapy to the local control of malignant mesothelioma has been disappointing.

Chemotherapy

Numerous phase II studies of chemotherapeutic agents have been performed in malignant mesothelioma. These were well summarized in a recent review (Table 41-5). Response rates as high as 30 to 40 percent were reported in small single institutions studies but were generally in the 20 percent range. The results of these studies are influenced by the inclusion of patients with varying stages of disease and different mesothelioma cell types and by the lack of use of computed tomographic scanning to assess the response. Active agents include doxorubicin, cyclophosphamide, cisplatin, carboplatin, methotrexate, 5-azacytidine, and 5-fluorouracil (Chahinian, et al., 1978; Dabouis, et al., 1981; Dimitrov, et al., 1982; Raghavan, et al., 1990; Umsawasdi, et al., 1991). Combination therapy has not been proved to be superior to single-agent therapy. In a randomized phase II trial comparing the combinations of cisplatin and doxorubicin with cisplatin and mitomycin, the cancer and leukemia Group B initially reported a 13 percent response rate for cisplatin and doxorubicin versus a 28 percent response rate for cisplatin and mitomycin (Chahinian, et al., 1987). The long-term results of this trial have not yet been published. The response rates for currently available chemotherapeutic drugs in malignant mesothelioma remain disappointing.

Immunotherapy

Interferons are known to have a direct antiproliferative effect on mesothelioma cell lines. Studies performed on mesothelioma xenografts in nude mice show the efficacy of recombinant human interferon-α_{2a} combined with mitomycin C (Sklarin, et al., 1988). These experimental data prompted the

Table 41-5. Single-Agent Response Rates (>50% Regression) in Malignant Mesothelioma

Agent	Number Responding/Evaluable
Anthracyclines	
Doxorubicin	29/164
Detorubicine	9/21
Alkylating agents	
Cyclophosphamide	4/14
Mechlorethamine	2/6
Thiotepa	1/7
Melphalan	2/3
Procarbazine	2/6
Mitomycin C	2/12
Dacarbazine	1/4
Cisplatin	5/49
Dibromodulcitol	0/5
Nitrosoureas	
Carmustine	0/2
Semustine	0/3
ACNU	0/2
Streptozocin	0/1
Vincas and related compounds	
Etoposide	0/8
Vindesine	1/37
Antimetabolites	
5-Fluorouracil	4/28
Methotrexate, high dose	4/9
Methotrexate, standard	0/1
Bakers antifol	0/3
Dichloromethotrexate	0/1
5-Azacytadine	0/7
Bleomycin	1/6
Dactinomycin	0/3
Cytarabine, high dose	1/1
Miscellaneous	
Maytansine	0/5
Methyl-G	1/2
Glucosamine	0/2
Hydroxyurea	0/1
DDMP	0/2
Bruceantin	0/1
Amsacrine	1/19
Cycloencine	2/7
Diaziquone	0/20

(Modified from Antman KH, Li FP, Osteen R et al.: Mesothelioma Updates. 3:9, 1989, with permission.)

development of clinical trials using interferon, either alone or in combination with chemotherapy. Two phase II trials designed to evaluate the value of interferon-α in conjunction with chemotherapy in patients with advanced disease are currently in progress. The first trial, being performed at Memorial Sloan-Kettering Cancer Center, combines interferon-α with cisplatin. The second trial, being performed at the National Cancer Institute, combines interferon-α with both cisplatin and tamoxifen. The use of interferon-γ as an intrapleural treatment in patients with early-stage disease was recently reported by Boutin, et al. (1991). Twenty-two patients were treated with a solution of interferon-γ (40 × 106 units) infused into the pleural space twice weekly for 2 months. The response was assessed by serial CT scans and by repeat thoracoscopy. A 56 percent overall response rate was observed. These promising initial results will undoubtedly stimulate additional clinical trials in the next few years.

Surgery

The limitations of radiation and chemotherapy have left surgical resection the mainstay of therapy for malignant mesothelioma. Three operations have been performed: extrapleural pneumonectomy (also termed pleuropneumonectomy), pleurectomy and decortication, and a palliative limited pleurectomy.

Surgical Technique.   Extrapleural pneumonectomy is an en bloc resection of the pleura, the lung, ipsilateral hemidiaphragm, and pericardium. It is performed through an extended posterolateral thoracotomy incision, sometimes with extension into a thoracoabdominal incision, or with a posterior parallel counterincision in the tenth intercostal space to provide access to the diaphragm (Fig. 41-7A). The sixth rib is usually excised to facilitate exposure to the extrapleural

plane (Fig. 41-7B). This approach is slightly lower than for a standard pulmonary resection because the greatest bulk of tumor is usually in the lower half of the hemithorax. Blunt dissection with the fingertips is begun in the extrapleural plane between the parietal pleura and the endothoracic fascia and is continued blindly with a sweeping motion of the hand up to apex of the chest (Fig. 41-7C). A similar dissection is then performed inferiorly from the intercostal incision down to the diaphragm. The dissection is carried anteriorly to the pericardium and posteriorly to the spine. It is important to pack each section of the chest sequentially as this dissection is performed because there can otherwise be substantial blood loss. The argon beam electrocoagulator (Birtcher, Englewood, CO) is helpful in controlling this diffuse chest wall bleeding. When the parietal pleura has been mobilized away from the chest wall, a chest retractor is inserted. The dissection is continued under direct vision, mobilizing the pleura

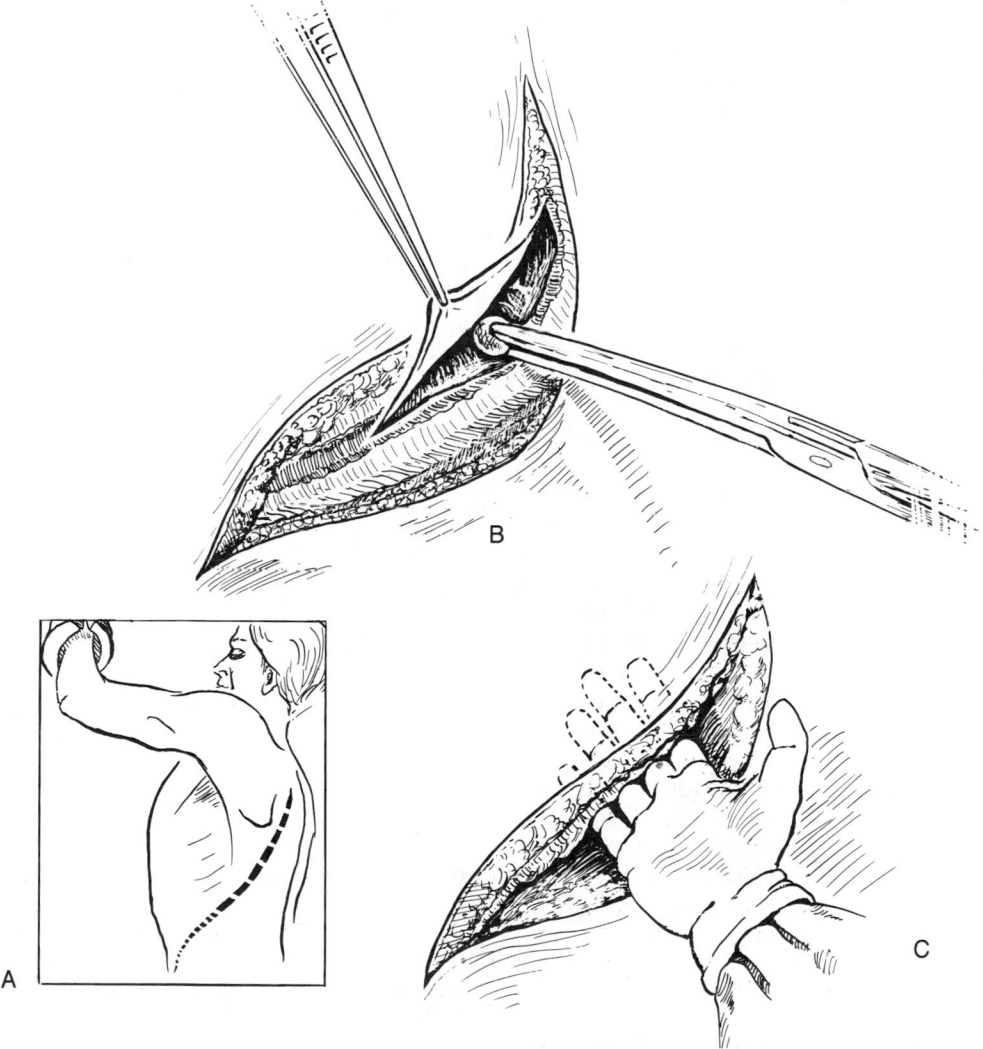

Figure 41-7.   **(A)** Initial approach for a pleurectomy or an extrapleural pneumonectomy. An extended posterolateral thoracotomy or thoracoabdominal incision is performed. A parallel counterincision in the tenth intercostal space, with or without a separate skin incision, can be added to improve exposure to the diaphragm. **(B)** The extrapleural plane is opened after resection of the sixth rib and **(C)** the parietal pleura bluntly dissected away from the endothoracic fascia.

away from the mediastinum superiorly anteriorly and posteriorly (Fig. 41-8). On the left side, care must be taken to identify the esophagus, the plane between the adventitia of the aorta and the tumor, and the origins of the intercostal vessels. It is easy for a surgeon inexperienced in this operation to get into the incorrect plane and cause serious bleeding. On the right side, dissection along the superior vena cava must be performed gently. After this portion of the dissection, the pleura and lung will then have been completely mobilized in the upper half of the chest, exposing the superior and posterior aspects of the hilum. A standard en bloc dissection of the packet of subcarinal lymph nodes is performed for staging purposes and to expose the mainstem bronchus. The lymph nodes are submitted separately, appropriately labeled to the pathologist. In some patients there is a clean plane of dissection between the mediastinal pleura and the pericardium, also allowing exposure of the anterior aspect of the hilum. In other patients this plane is obliterated, and the anterior mediastinal

pleura has to be resected en bloc with the pericardium later in the operation.

Attention is then turned to the resection of the diaphragm. There is always a palpable "edge" between the tumor and normal diaphragmatic muscle or peritoneum. This plane can be entered and the tumor mobilized along the diaphragmatic surface by blunt dissection in much the way that a Kocher maneuver would be performed. With some experience, this portion of the dissection can also be initiated blindly, allowing the use of a slightly more limited thoracotomy incision or omission of the counterincision in the tenth intercostal space. After the tumor has been mobilized from the posterior costophrenic angle, it is rotated up into the thoracotomy incision, rolling it back on itself, and placing strong traction on the diaphragm. The level of dissection varies considerably from one patient to the next. If the involvement of the diaphragm is extensive, the entire thickness of the diaphragm is removed, pealing this away from the peritoneum. If the involvement

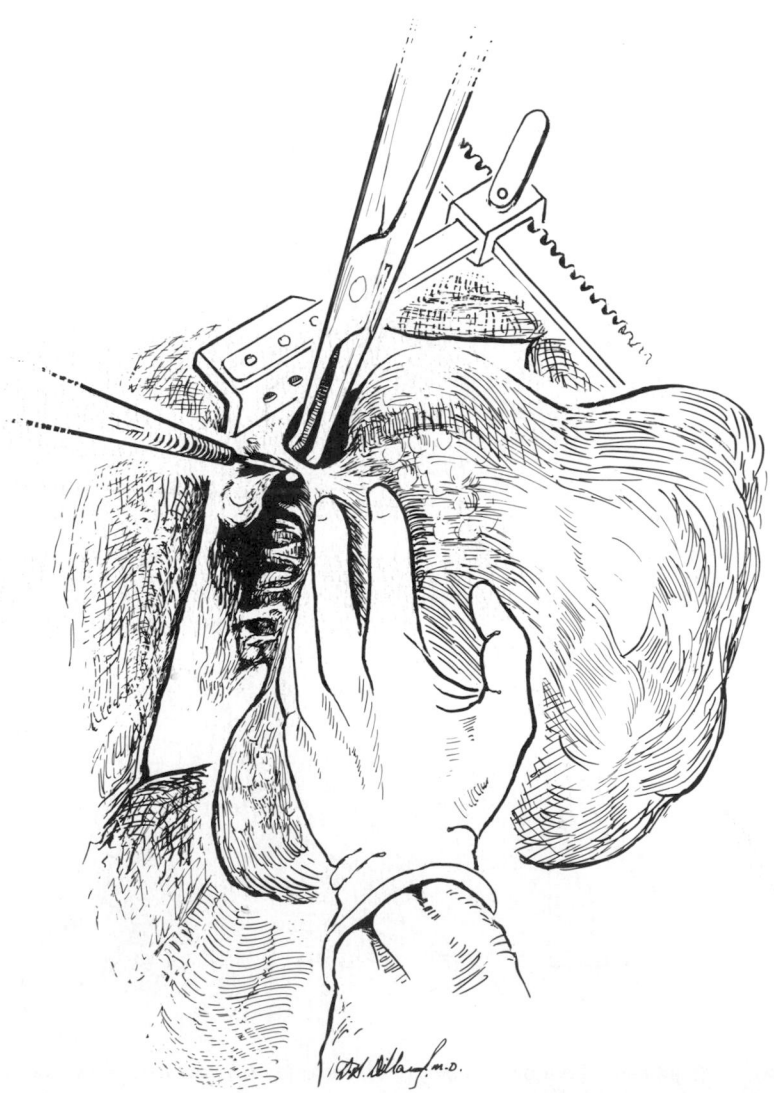

Figure 41-8. After the parietal pleura has been mobilized from the chest wall, a chest retractor is inserted, and the mediastinal pleura is freed from the mediastinal structures under direct vision using a combination of sharp and blunt dissection.

of the diaphragm is superficial, dissection can be carried through the diaphragmatic muscle (Fig. 41-9). Every effort is made not to enter the peritoneum because of the propensity of mesothelioma to produce tumor implants. The most difficult area in which to avoid entering the abdomen is at the level of the central tendon, and often a small opening in the peritoneum is unavoidable but can be immediately repaired primarily. The diaphragmatic portion of the tumor is completely mobilized back to the pericardium medially. The pericardium is entered only when the tumor has been mobilized as fully as possible from all other directions because traction on the pericardium causes arrhythmias and hemodynamic instability (Fig. 41-10). The hilar structures are divided in whatever sequence is technically easiest and requires the least manipulation of the huge tumor mass. Usually this means dividing the inferior pulmonary vein first and then the

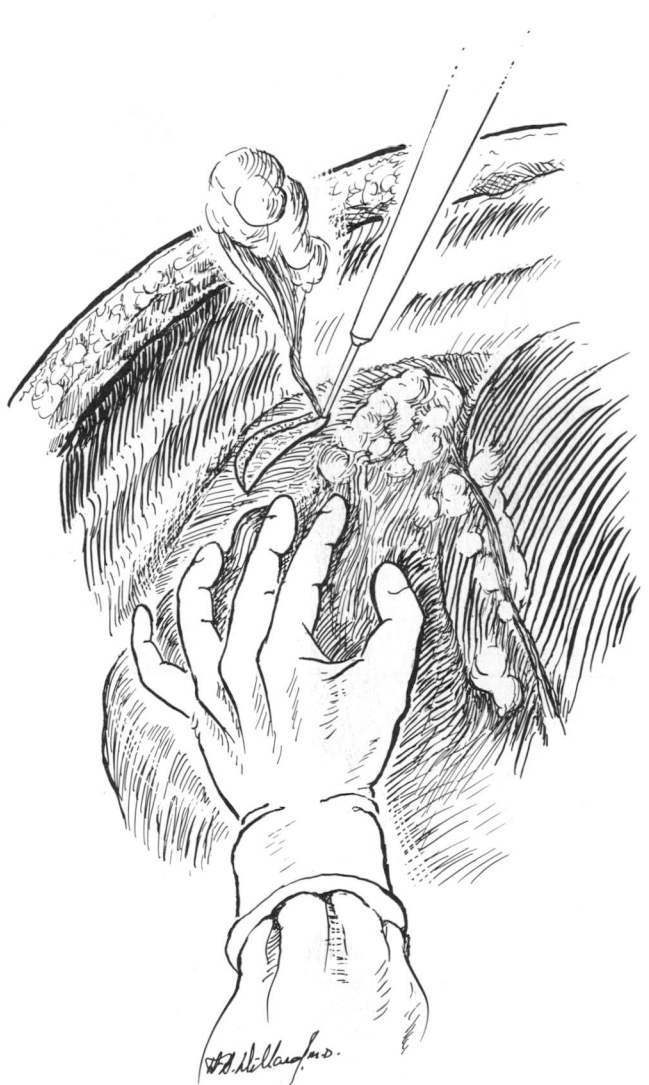

Figure 41-9. The tumor has been bluntly mobilized out of the costophrenic sulcus. Strong traction is placed on the pleural tumor and underlying lung, and cautery is used to dissect the diaphragmatic surface of the tumor away from the diaphragmatic muscle or peritoneum.

superior pulmonary vein. It is sometimes easier to divide the mainstem bronchus, leaving the pulmonary artery until last. The pericardium is gradually opened as this portion of the dissection is carried out. It is important to place traction sutures on the pericardium as it is opened because otherwise the pericardium retracts toward the opposite hemithorax and is difficult to retrieve for reconstruction. Placing these traction sutures under tension also minimizes changes in the position of the heart and reduces hemodynamic instability (Fig. 41-11). The specimen, consisting of pleura, lung, pericardium, and diaphragm, is removed enbloc. Sampling or dissection of the peritracheal lymph nodes if the operation is on the right, or of the aortopulmonary window nodes if the operation is on the left, is performed for staging purposes. Again, these nodes are submitted separately, appropriately labeled to the pathologist.

Reconstruction of the pericardium and diaphragm are then performed (Fig. 41-12). If there is some diaphragmatic muscle remaining, this can usually simply be plicated with interrupted absorbable horizontal mattress sutures without adding prosthetic material. Even if there is only peritoneum remaining, additional reconstruction is unnecessary if the operation has been on the right side. On the left side, prosthetic material is added to prevent herniation of the intra-abdominal contents. Dexon mesh can be used, although many surgeons prefer an impervious material such as Gore-Tex. If the diaphragmatic muscle has been completely resected back to its costal insertion, the prosthesis is secured by placing sutures around the ribs laterally (Fig. 41-13). Posteriorly it is sewn to the crus or gently tacked with fine sutures to the wall of the esophagus. Medially it is sewn to the edge of the pericardium. The pericardium is reconstructed with Dexon mesh. Pericardial reconstruction is particularly important on the right side because the heart can otherwise twist on the axis of the cavae, causing acute and lethal cardiovascular collapse. It is advisable on either side to maintain the heart in as central a position as possible to facilitate postoperative radiation to the hemithorax and minimize the radiation dose to the heart. Meticulous attention is given to obtaining hemostasis throughout the operation and particularly prior to closure of the chest. The thoracotomy incision is closed in the usual manner.

A similar approach is used for the initial portion of the operation for a pleurectomy and decortication. As for an extrapleural pneumonectomy, the intent of a pleurectomy and decortication is to remove all gross tumor, the only difference being that the lung is left in place (Rusch, 1991). The mobilization of the parietal and mediastinal pleura and of the diaphragmatic surface is the same as for an extrapleural pneumonectomy. If the pericardium cannot be easily separated from the pleura, it is also resected and reconstructed as previously described. When all this has been completed, the parietal pleura is opened, and the decortication is begun (Fig. 41-14). The degree to which the parietal and visceral pleura are separable and to which the visceral pleural tumor can be peeled cleanly away from the lung is extremely variable. Sometimes it is necessary to remove large sections of the visceral pleura, leaving the raw pulmonary parenchyma exposed. This is accomplished by a combination of sharp dissection with the electrocautery and gentle dissection with

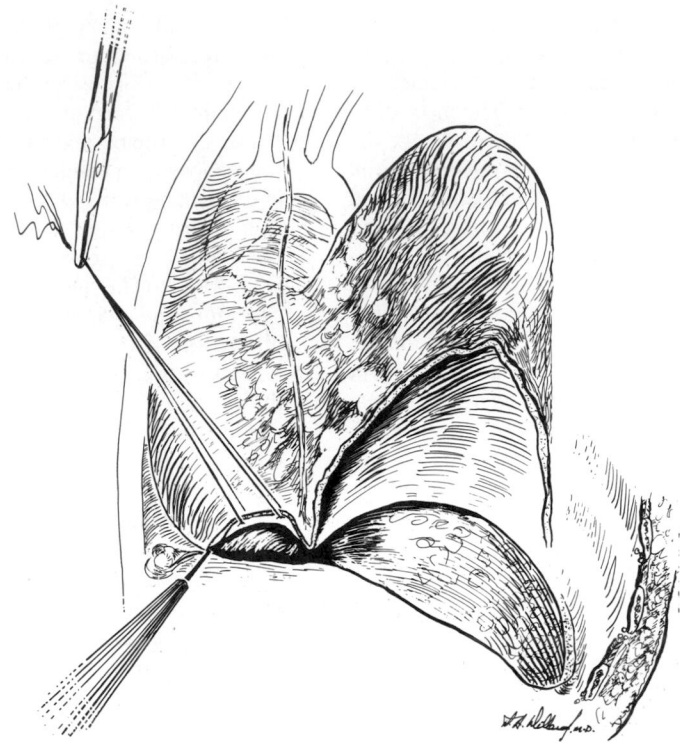

Figure 41-10. The pericardium is opened after the tumor has been completely mobilized from all other directions including the diaphragm.

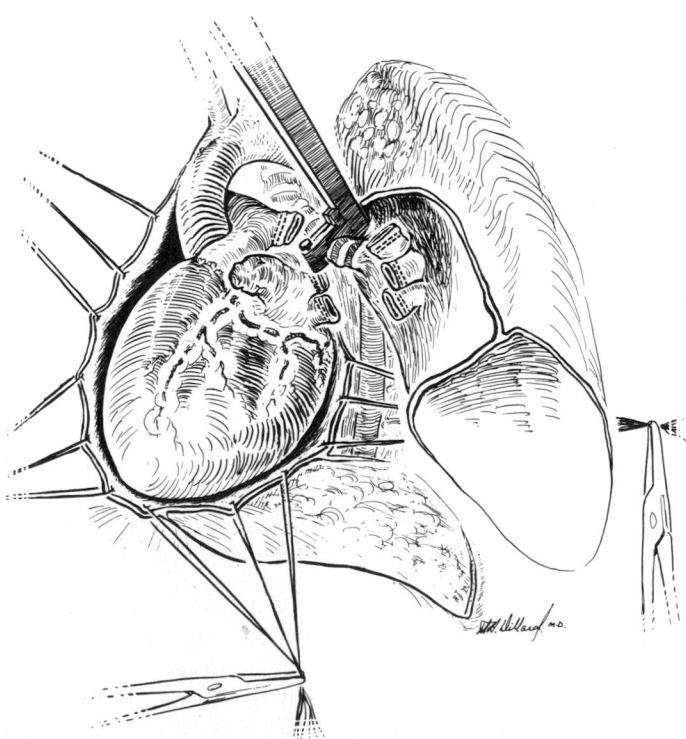

Figure 41-11. The hilar vessels have been divided intrapericardially. Traction sutures have been placed on the edge of the pericardium as it was opened to prevent it from retracting into the contralateral hemithorax.

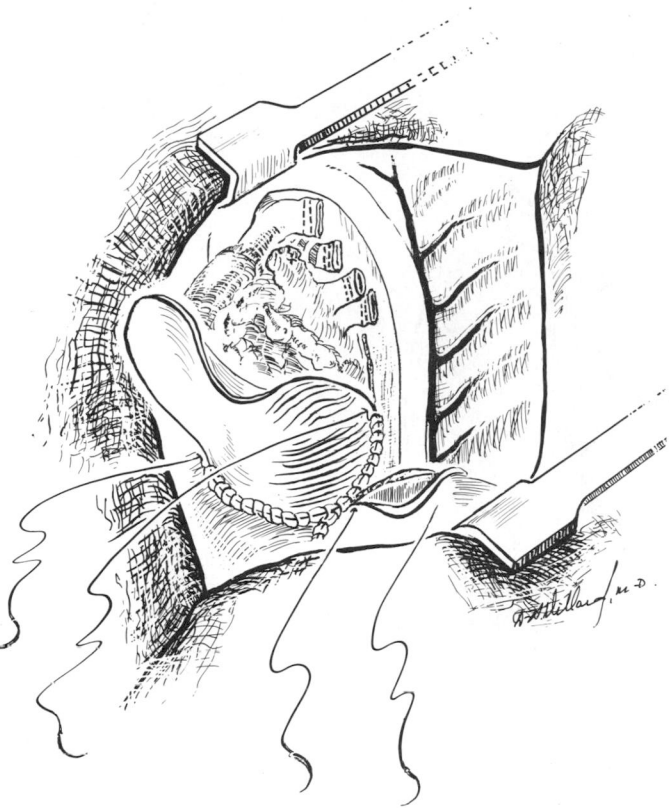

Figure 41-12. The pericardial and diaphragmatic defects are reconstructed with prosthetic material. Reconstruction of the diaphragm is not always necessary, especially on the right side.

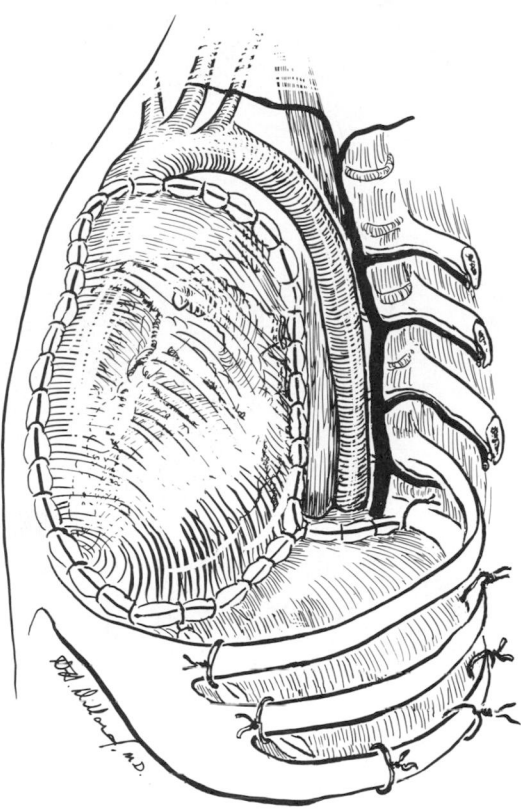

Figure 41-13. The completed pericardial and diaphragmatic reconstruction. If the diaphragm was detached from its costal insertion, the prosthetic material can be secured by sutures placed around the ribs laterally.

a "peanut" sponge. Although the air leaks from the lung surface initially look dramatic, they seal quickly—usually within 72 hours—as long as the lung reexpands fully after the operation. This portion of the operation can be tedious, but if properly performed, it results in the removal of all gross tumor. The parietal pleura is progressively resected in sections as the pleural surfaces are separated and the decortication is performed. Care is taken to remove all tumor from the fissures in which it is often extensive. When all gross tumor has been removed, attention is turned to the diaphragmatic reconstruction. If the diaphragm has been subtotally resected, it can often be closely primarily by plication as described previously (Fig. 41-15). If it has been totally resected, it is reconstructed with Dexon mesh or Gore-Tex, just as is done after an extrapleural pneumonectomy. However, when the lung is left is place, it is important to make this reconstruction taut to prevent the prosthetic diaphragm from rising and causing lower lobe atelectasis. After obtaining careful hemostasis, three chest tubes are inserted, placing one anteriorly up to the apex, another posteriorly, and a right-angle chest tube on the diaphragm. This is to ensure complete reexpansion of the lung and drainage of the pleural space, which is critical in the first few days postoperatively.

The use of a double-lumen endotracheal tube is helpful for both of these operations and is particularly critical for a pleurectomy and decortication. For the decortication, the lung may be alternatively inflated or deflated, depending on what facilitates the dissection technically in each particular case. Deflation minimizes the blood loss; inflation sometimes exposes the plane between the tumor peel and the lung or visceral pleura. Patients are monitored intraoperatively with an arterial line and pulse oximeter as they would be for any other major thoracotomy. A central venous line is often advisable, depending on the patient's age and medical condition. The anesthesiologist should be aware that blood loss for these operations, even when performed carefully, can be as high as 2,000 to 3,000 ml because of diffuse bleeding from the chest wall, and the patient should be transfused accordingly.

The third operation often performed is a palliative pleurectomy. This is really just a parietal pleurectomy performed through a standard thoracotomy incision with the intent of palliating the patient by controlling the pleural effusion. No attempt is made to remove the bulk of the tumor. An alternative approach to palliation of the patient's dyspnea is to control the pleural effusion by performing thoracoscopy and talc poudrage. This approach has not been systematically evaluated but was apparently in 85 percent of 30 patients treated in this manner by Ruffie, et al. (1989). Talc poudrage is not effective or appropriate in patients who have more locally advanced disease with an unexpandable lung because of encasement by tumor.

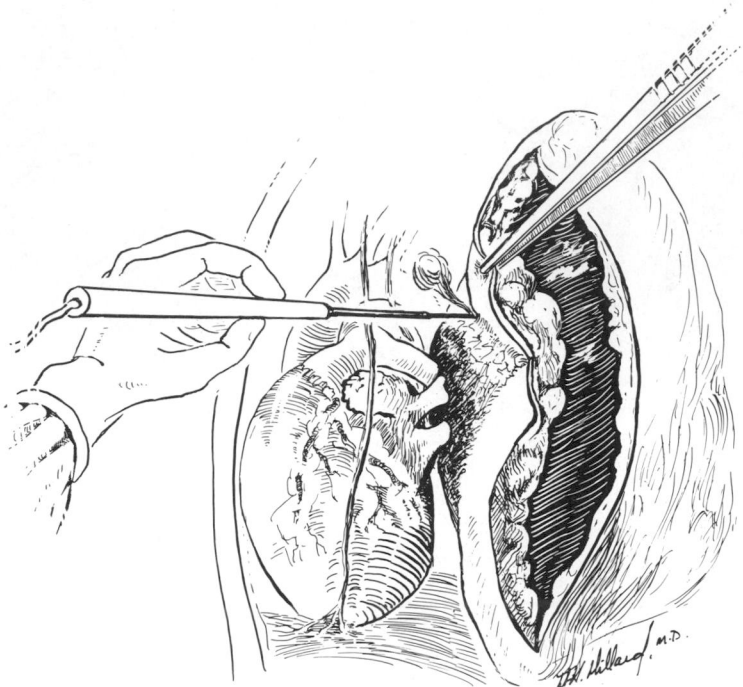

Figure 41-14. Technique of pleurectomy and decortication. The initial dissection shown in Figures 41-7 to 41-9 is identical for a pleurectomy and an extrapleural pneumonectomy. Resection of the pericardium may not be necessary. After the lung and overlying parietal and diaphragmatic pleura have been mobilized, the pleural space is entered and the visceral pleural tumor separated from the underlying lung by a combination of blunt dissection and sharp dissection with cautery.

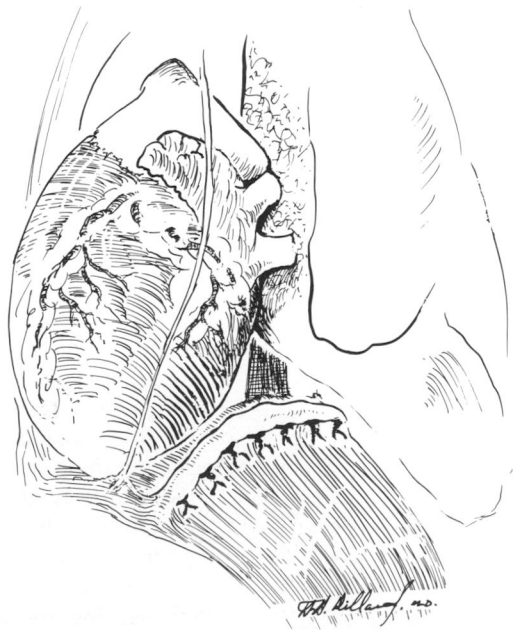

Figure 41-15. If most of the diaphragm has been left intact, it is plicated after the tumor has been removed. This is an important maneuver because, even if the phrenic nerve is anatomically intact, the diaphragm has often been defunctionalized and will rise, causing lower lobe atelectasis postoperatively.

The Role of Surgical Resection. Complete resection of all gross tumor seems to convey a modest but definite improvement in survival in several large series. However, the value of extrapleural pneumonectomy compared with pleurectomy and decortication remains controversial. Extrapleural pneumonectomy has the aesthetic appeal of removing the tumor en bloc, but either operation, if performed well in properly selected patients, allows the removal of all gross tumor. On the other hand, resection of the tumor with microscopically negative margins, as can be achieved with a lung, breast, or colon cancer, is simply not feasible in malignant mesothelioma. The margins of resection are vital structures, such as the aorta, the cavae, and the esophagus.

In an initial report by Butchart, et al. (1976), extrapleural pneumonectomy carried an operative mortality rate of 30 percent. More recent data show a substantial reduction in this mortality rate, probably reflecting better patient selection and improved perioperative care. Preoperative CT scanning, extensive pulmonary function testing, ventilation/perfusion lung scanning, echocardiography, and myocardial thallium scanning now allow us to select patients who have completely resectable tumors and have the cardiopulmonary reserve to tolerate the operation safely. Intraoperative monitoring and anesthetic management are vastly improved compared with that of 20 years ago. In a recent prospective multi-institutional study, the mortality rate was 15 percent (Rusch, et al., 1991). Mortality rates as low as 6 percent have been achieved in single-institution retrospective studies in which patients have been carefully selected and operated on by surgeons specialized in this area (Butchart E: personal communication, 1990; De Laria, et al., 1978; DeValle, et al., 1986; Sugarbaker, et al., 1991). The operative mortality and overall survival rates after extrapleural pneumonectomy as reported in several series are shown in Table 41-6.

In contrast, in the experience reported by Memorial Sloan-Kettering, pleurectomy and decortication was associated with a mortality rate of 1.8 percent (McCormack, et al., 1982). These figures parallel those reported for pulmonary resections for lung cancer, which have shown that the operative mortality rate is directly related to the extent of resection, and is 5 to 10 percent for a standard pneumonectomy. Both operations, and particularly extrapleural pneumonectomy, are complex and are not performed frequently by most surgeons. Therefore, patients benefit by referral to centers dedicated to the treatment of malignant mesothelioma.

Table 41-6. Results of Pleuropneumonectomy

Reference	No. Patients	Mortality Rate	2-Year Survival Rate	Median Survival Time
Worn (1974)	62	Not stated	37%	
Butchart, et al. (1976)	29	31%	10%	4 mo[a]
Davalle (1986)	33	9%	24%	13.5 mo
Vogt Moykopf (1987)	55	5.5%	16% (at 3 yr)	10 mo
Rusch (1991)	20	15%	33%	10 mo
Sugarbaker, et al. (1991)	31	6%	48%	Not stated

[a] For Butchart: overall median, 4 months; median of survivors of surgery, 8 months.

The focus of the controversy with regard to surgical therapy is the relative value of an extrapleural pneumonectomy compared with a pleurectomy and decortication. Is the higher operative mortality rate of extrapleural pneumonectomy justified by a better overall survival rate? One problem is that extrapleural pneumonectomy is applicable to relatively few patients, probably about 20 to 25 percent of all patients with mesotheliomas who have resectable tumors (Butchart E: personal communication, 1991; Rusch, et al., 1991). Underlying cardiopulmonary disease and other medical problems often preclude pneumonectomy in these patients. However, these patients can often tolerate pleurectomy and decortication. On the other hand, pneumonectomy can facilitate some types of adjuvant treatment, especially postoperative radiation, which can be administered to a much higher total dose after pneumonectomy than after pleurectomy and decortication. Some patients do not have a tumor that is technically resectable by pleurectomy and decortication. A confluent sheet of tumor encasing the lung with obliteration of the pleural space is usually resectable only by extrapleural pneumonectomy. This situation can often be recognized by the preoperative CT scan (Figs. 41-8 and 41-9) and by a preoperative ventilation/perfusion lung scan showing minimal function on the affected side. Whether a patient who has early-stage disease that is technically completely resectable by either extrapleural pneumonectomy or by pleurectomy and decortication is better served by one operation versus the other is simply unknown. This question remains unresolved, but ultimately the long-term outcome of such a patient may be determined not by the operation but by the type and effectiveness of the adjuvant therapy.

Combined Modality Therapy

Extrapleural pneumonectomy and pleurectomy and decortication are by definition cytoreductive operations. Patients treated with surgery alone have relapses rapidly. Therefore, most therapeutic regimens have focused on combined modality therapy. Unfortunately it is difficult to evaluate the results of combined modality therapy because most series report small numbers of patients treated in a highly individualized manner over long periods (Achatzy, et al., 1989; Alberts, et al., 1988; Chahinian, et al., 1982). In addition to the Memorial Sloan-Kettering experience with pleurectomy and decortication and radiation described above, another large and relatively uniform experience with combined modality therapy was reported by the Dana-Farber Cancer Center. From 1980 to 1990, 31 patients underwent extrapleural pneumonectomy followed by chemotherapy with cisplatin, doxorubicin, and cyclophosphamide and subsequent hemithoracic radiation. The survival rates were 70 percent at 1 year and 48 percent at 2 years (Butchart, et al., 1976; Sugarbaker, et al., 1991). The Dana-Farber group continue to use this approach and have now seen similar results in a total of 52 patients. In their analysis the epithelial histologic type and a lack of involvement of hilar and mediastinal nodes defined the patient population with the best prognosis.

Finally efforts are ongoing to develop a better staging system and to perform prospective clinical trials in malignant mesothelioma. Several novel therapeutic strategies are currently under investigation. At the National Cancer Institute, a phase I trial evaluating the use of photodynamic therapy after either pleurectomy and decortication or extrapleural pneumonectomy has just been completed (Pass H, 1992). Photodynamic therapy seeks to improve local control by eliminating microscopic residual disease immediately after surgical resection. This approach is based on experimental data with mesothelioma cell lines (Keller, et al., 1990). A previous small clinical trial already suggested the feasibility of this approach (Ris, et al., 1991).

Another novel approach is a phase II trial currently being performed at Memorial Sloan-Kettering Cancer Center. Patients receive a single dose of intrapleural cisplatin (75 mg/m^2) and mitomycin (8 mg/m^2) after complete resection of all gross tumor by pleurectomy and decortication. Additional chemotherapy is then administered systemically starting 1 month postoperatively and using two cycles of cisplatin 50 mg/m^2 per week for 4 weeks and mitomycin 8 mg/m^2 for weeks 1 and 7. This approach of surgical resection and brief but intensive chemotherapy seeks to address the dual problem of local control and eventual distant metastases experienced by most patients with mesotheliomas. It is based on the now well-established use of intraperitoneal chemotherapy in ovarian cancer and on a smaller but successful experience with intracavitary chemotherapy in both pleural and peritoneal mesothelioma (Lederman, et al., 1987; Markman, et al., 1986; Mintzer, et al., 1985). In an early evaluation of the first 23 patients treated on this trial, grade 3 or 4 renal toxicity was seen in 2 patients, and 12 patients were alive and free of disease with a median follow-up of 11.2 months. The sites of relapse were primarily local.

Malignant mesothelioma has long been regarded as an uncommon cancer characterized by a relentless progression of disease. By and large treatment has been haphazard and empiric. Only in the past 10 years has there been an effort to develop a better staging system and to perform carefully designed prospective clinical trials. Innovative strategies to control both local and distant disease are being tested, and a rational approach to the management of malignant mesothelioma is finally beginning to emerge.

OTHER LESS COMMON TUMORS OF THE PLEURA

Primary tumors of the pleura other than mesothelioma are rare and include lipomas, endotheliomas, angiomas, and cysts. Most of these are thought to arise from the subpleural tissues rather than the pleura itself (Le Roux, 1962). Lipomas are the most common among these rare tumors, but a recent review of the 7,751 computed tomographic examinations of the chest found pleural lipomas to be incidentally present in only 0.14 percent of cases (Christ, et al., 1991). Lipomas have a characteristic appearance on the chest radiograph where they are seen as smooth well-defined masses flattened against the chest wall. Pleural cysts usually arise at the pleuropericardial angle and are seen on the chest radiograph as discrete unilocular masses (Le Roux, 1962).

In the past these uncommon pleural-based tumors have been excised mainly for diagnostic purposes because they rarely become symptomatic. The recent advent of video-assisted thoracoscopy may allow the diagnosis and excision of these lesions, thereby obviating the need for exploratory thoracotomy.

COMMENTS AND CONTROVERSIES

This chapter illustrates the numerous difficulties that are routinely encountered in the management of diffuse malignant mesothelioma. The first difficulty is in establishing a positive diagnosis. Optical microscopy is virtually useless; one must rely on electron microscopy and immunohistochemistry performed on large specimens preferably obtained through the thoracoscope. Often, however, the history of asbestos exposure—positive in 50 percent of cases and probable in another 25 percent—the radiologic image of a contracted hemithorax with pleural nodularity, and the thoracoscopic appearance of multiple scattered nodules mostly located at the base will provide good evidence that one is dealing with a mesothelioma. One of the problems associated with thoracoscopy or with other biopsy methods is the high possibility of cutaneous implants of the mesothelioma, a feature which will further complicate management.

As discussed by Dr. Rusch, there is no adequate staging system applicable to mesotheliomas, not only because of the limited number of cases available for study but also because the natural history of this disease is virtually unknown since most of the earlier publications probably included cases of metastatic adenocarcinomas interpreted at the time as mesotheliomas. What staging procedures should be done before therapy is also unknown, although we recommend a full workup, including mediastinoscopy, before proceeding to pleuropneumonectomy.

The exact role of pleuropneumonectomy in the management of malignant mesotheliomas is difficult to determine from the literature. During the early 1980s, there was some enthusiasm for this procedure, but that has decreased considerably in recent years, mostly because there are so few long-term survivors after this operation. It is also worth noting that pleuropneumonectomy is a technically difficult procedure that carries mortality risk of 10 to 15 percent. When making the decision about performing a pleuropneumonectomy, it is worth remembering that 12 to 15 percent of patients have a slow-growing disease and will still be alive without therapy 5 years after diagnosis.

J.D.

REFERENCES

Achatzy R, Beba W, Ritschler R et al.: The diagnosis, therapy and prognosis of diffuse malignant mesothelioma. Eur J Cardiothorac Surg 3:445, 1989

Adams VI, Unni KK, Muhm JR et al.: Diffuse malignant mesothelioma of pleura. Cancer 58:1540, 1986

Alberts AS, Galkson G, Goedhals L et al.: Malignant pleural mesothelioma: a disease unaffected by current therapeutic maneuvers. J Clin Oncol 6:527, 1988

Alexander E, Clark RA, Colley DP, Mitchell SE: CT of malignant pleural mesothelioma. AJR 137:287, 1981

Anderson EA, Hurley WC, Hurley BT, Ohrt DW: Malignant pleural mesothelioma following radiotherapy in a 16-year-old boy. Cancer 56:273, 1985

Andersson M, Olsen JH: Trend and distribution of mesothelioma in Denmark. Br J Cancer 51:699, 1985

Antman K, Shemin R, Ryan L et al.: Malignant mesothelioma: prognostic variables in a registry of 180 patients, the Dana-Farber Cancer Institute and Brigham and Women's Hospital experience over two decades, 1965–1985. J Clin Oncol 6:147, 1988

Antman KH, Blum RH, Greenberger JS et al.: Multimodality therapy for malignant mesothelioma based on a study of natural history. Am J Med 68:356, 1980

Anman KH, Carson JM, Li FP et al.: Malignant mesothelioma following radiation exposure. J Clin Oncol 1:695, 1983

Antman KH, Ruxer RL, Aisner J, Vawter G: Mesothelioma following Wilms' tumor in childhood. Cancer 54:367, 1984

Ball DL, Cruickshank DG: The treatment of malignant mesothelioma of the pleura: review of a 5-year experience, with special reference to radiotherapy. Am J Clin Oncol 13:4, 1990

Baris YI: Asbestos and Erionite Related Chest Diseases. Hacettepe University School of Medicine, Ankara, Turkey,

Battifora H, Kopinski MI: Distinction of mesothelioma from adenocarcinoma. Cancer 55:1679, 1985

Blake PR, Catterall M, Emerson PA: Pleural mesothelioma treated by fast neutron therapy. Thorax 40:72, 1985

Boutin C, Rey F, Gouvernet J et al.: Thoracoscopic diagnosis and staging of pleural malignant mesothelioma: a prospective study of 188 consecutive patients. Cancer 72:389, 1993

Boutin CM, Viallat JR, Van Zandwijk N et al.: Activity of intrapleural recombinant gamma-interferon in malignant mesothelioma. Cancer 67:2033, 1991

Brady LW: Mesothelioma—the role for radiation therapy. Semin Oncol 8:329, 1981

Briselli M, Mark EJ, Dickersin GR: Solitary fibrous tumors of the pleura: eight new cases and review of 360 cases in the literature. Cancer 47:2678, 1981

Burmer GC, Rabionovitch PS, Kulander BG et al.: Fluorcytometric analysis of malignant pleural mesotheliomas. Hum Pathol 20:777, 1989

Burns TR, Greenberg D, Mace ML, Johnson EH: Ultrastructural diagnosis of epithelial malignant mesothelioma. Cancer 56:2036, 1985

Butchart EG, Ashcroft T, Barnsley WC, Holden MP: Pleuropneumonectomy in the management of diffuse malignant mesothelioma of the pleura. Thorax 31:15, 1976

Cantin R, Al-Jabi M, McCaughey WTE: Desmoplastic diffuse mesothelioma. Am J Surg Pathol 6:215, 1982

Chahinian AP, Antman K, Aisner J et al.: Cisplatin with Adriamycin or mitomycin for malignant mesothelioma: a randomized phase II trial. Proc Am Soc Clin Oncol 6:183, 1987

Chahinian AP, Pajak TF, Holland JF et al.: Diffuse malignant mesothelioma: prospective evaluation of 69 patients. Ann Intern Med 96:746, 1982

Chahinian AP, Suzuki Y, Mandel EM, Holland JF: Diffuse pulmonary malignant mesothelioma: response to doxorubicin and 5-azacytidine. Cancer 42:1687, 1978

Christ F, Weinbrenner J, Reiser M: The radiological image of pleural lipomas with special reference to computed tomography. Rofo Fortschr Geb Rontgenstr Neuen Bildgeb Verfahr 155:58, 1991

Churg A, DePaoli L: Environmental pleural plaques in residents of a Quebec chrysotile mining town. Chest 94:58, 1988

Cote RJ, Jhanwar SC, Novick S, Pellicer A: Genetic alterations of the p53 gene are a feature of malignant mesotheliomas. Cancer Res 51:5410, 1991

Dabouis G, LeMevel B, Corroller J: Treatment of diffuse pleural malignant mesothelioma by cis-dichlorodiammine platinum (C.D.D.P.) in nine patients. Cancer Chemother Pharmacol 5:209, 1981

Dahl IMS, Solheim OP, Erikstein B, Muller E: A longitudinal study of the hyaluronan level in the serum of patients with malignant mesothelioma under treatment. Cancer 64:68, 1989

DeLaria GA, Jensik R, Faber LP, Kittle CF: Surgical management of malignant mesothelioma. Ann Thorac Surg 26:375, 1978

DeValle MJ, Faber LP, Kittle CF, Jensik RJ: Extrapleural pneumonectomy for diffuse, malignant mesotheliomas. Ann Thorac Surg 42:612, 1986

Dimitrov NV, Egner J, Balcueva E, Suhrland LG: High-dose methotrexate with citrovorum factor and vincristine in the treatment of malignant mesothelioma. Cancer 50:1245, 1982

Elmes PC, Simpson MJC: The clinical aspects of mesothelioma. Q J Med 45:427, 1976

England DM, Hochholzer L, McCarthy MJ: Localized benign and malignant fibrous tumors of the pleura. Am J Surg Pathol 13:640, 1989

Fraire AE, Cooper S, Greenberg SD et al.: Mesothelioma of childhood. Cancer 62:838, 1988

Gerwin BI, Lechner JF, Reddel RR et al.: Comparison of production of transforming growth factor-β and platelet-derived growth factor by normal human mesothelial cells and mesothelioma cell lines. Cancer Res 47:6180, 1987

Gordon W, Antman KH, Greenberger JS et al.: Radiation therapy in the management of patients with mesothelioma. Int J Radiat Oncol Biol Phys 8:19, 1981

Gotfried MH, Quan SF, Sobonya RE: Diffuse epithelial pleural mesothelioma presenting as a solitary lung mass. Chest 84:99, 1983

Hagemeijer A, Versnel MA, Van Drunen E et al.: Cytogenetic analysis of malignant mesothelioma. Cancer Genet Cytogenet 47:1, 1990

Hammar SP, Bolen JW: Pleural neoplasms. In Dail DH, Hammar SP (eds): Pulmonary Pathology. Springer-Verlag, New York, 1988

Hilaris BS, Nori D, Kwong E et al.: Pleurectomy and intraoperative brachytherapy and postoperative radiation in the treatment of malignant pleural mesothelioma. Int J Radiat Oncol Biol Phys 10:324, 1983

Hillerdal G: Malignant mesothelioma 1982: review of 4710 published cases. Br J Dis Chest 77:321, 1983

Hulks G, Thomas JSJ, Waclawski E: Malignant pleural mesothelioma in western Glasgow 1980–6. Thorax 44:496, 1989

Immerman SC, Sener SF, Khandekar JD: Causes and evaluation of tumor-induced hypoglycemia. Arch Surg 117:901, 1982

Kane MJ, Chahinian AP, Holland JF: Malignant mesothelioma in young adults. Cancer 65:1449, 1990

Kaye JA, Wang A-M, Joachim CL et al.: Malignant mesothelioma with brain metastases. Am J Med 80:95, 1986

Keller SM, Taylor DD, Weese JL: In vitro killing of human malignant mesothelioma by photodynamic therapy. J Surg Res 48:337, 1990

Klemperer P, Rabin CB: Primary neoplasms of the pleura. a report of five cases. Arch Pathol Lab Med 11:385, 1937

Kutcher GJ, Kestler C, Greenblatt D et al.: Technique for external beam treatment for mesothelioma. Int J Radiat Oncol Biol Phys 13:1747, 1987

Law MR, Gregor A, Hodson ME et al.: Malignant mesothelioma of the pleura: a study of 52 treated and 64 untreated patients. Thorax 39:255, 1984

Law MR, Gregor A, Husband JE, Kerr IH: Computed tomography in the assessment of malignant mesothelioma of the pleura. Clin Radiol 33:67, 1982a

Law MR, Hodson ME, Heard BE: Malignant mesothelioma of the pleura: relation between histological type and clinical behavior. Thorax 37:810, 1982b

Lederman GS, Recht A, Herman T et al.: Long-term survival in peritoneal mesothelioma: the role of radiotherapy and combined modality treatment. Cancer 59:1882, 1987

Lerman Y, Learman Y, Schachter P et al.: Radiation assoiated malignant pleural mesothelioma. Thorax 46:463, 1991

Le Roux BT: Pleural tumors. Thorax 17:111, 1962

Levine RL (ed): Asbestos: An Information Resource (NIH publication no. 81–1681). Bethesda, MD: National Institutes of Health, 1981

Lewis RJ, Sisler GE, Mackenzie JW: Diffuse, mixed malignant pleural mesothelioma. Ann Thorac Surg 31:53, 1981

Maasilta P: Deterioration in lung function following hemithorax irradiation for pleural mesothelioma. Int J Radiat Oncol Biol Phys 20:433, 1990

Malker HSR, McLaughlin JK, Erickson JLE, Blot WJ: Occupational risks for pleural mesothelioma in Sweden, 1961–79. J Natl Cancer Inst 75:61, 1985

Markman M, Cleary S, Pfeifle C, Howell SB: Cisplatin administered by the intracavitary route as treatment for malignant mesothelioma. Cancer 58:18, 1986

McCormack PM, Nagasaki F, Hilaris BS, Martini N: Surgical treatment of pleural mesothelioma. J Thorac Cardiovasc Surg 84:834, 1982

McDonald AD, McDonald JC: Epidemiology of malignant mesothelioma. In Antman K, Aisner J (eds): Asbestos-Related Malignancy. Grune & Stratton, Orlando, FL, 1987

McDonald JC, Armstrong B, Case B et al.: Mesothelioma and asbestos fiber type. Cancer 63:1544, 1989

McNicholas KW, Rose EA, Edie RN, Jaretzki A: Resection of giant benign fibrous mesothelioma of pleura. N Y State J Med 80:626, 1980

Mezger J, Lamerz R, Permanetter W: Diagnostic significance of carcinoembryonic antigen in the differential diagnosis of malignant mesothelioma. J Thorac Cardiovasc Surg 100:860, 1990

Mintzer DM, Kelson D, Frimmer D et al.: Phase II trial of high-dose cisplatin in patients with malignant mesothelioma. Cancer Treat Rep 69:711, 1985

Mirvis S, Dutcher JP, Haney PJ et al.: CT of malignant pleural mesothelioma. AJR 140:665, 1983

Musk AW, Dolin PJ, Armstrong BK et al.: The incidence of malignant mesothelioma in Australia, 1947–1987. Med J Aust 150:242, 1989

Mychalczak BR, Nori D, Armstrong JG et al.: Results of treatment of malignant pleural mesothelioma with surgery, brachytherapy, and external beam irradiation. In Proceedings of 12th Midwinter Meeting of the American Endocurietherapy Society, Hilton Head, SC, December 6–9, 1989

Nauta RJ, Osteen RT, Antman KH, Koster JK: Clinical staging and the tendency of malignant pleural mesotheliomas to remain lcoalized. Ann Thorac Surg 34:66, 1982

Okike N, Bernatz PE, Woolner LB: Localized mesothelioma of the pleura. J Thorac Cardiovasc Surg 75:363, 1968

Olesen LL, Thorshauge H: Thrombocytosis in patients with malignant pleural mesothelioma. Cancer 62:1194, 1988

Pass H, Intrapleural photodynamic therapy: results of a phase I trial. Ann Surg Oncol 1:28, 1994

Peterson JT, Greenberg SD, Buffler PA: Non-asbestos related malignant mesothelioma. Cancer 54:951, 1984

Pooley FD: Asbestos mineralogy. In Antman K, Aisner J (eds): Asbestos-Related Malignancy. Grune & Stratton, Orlando, FL, 1987

Popescu NC, Chahinian AP, DiPaolo JA: Nonrandom chromosome alterations in human malignant mesothelioma. Cancer Res 48:142, 198

Rabinowitz JG, Efremidis SC, Cohen B et al.: A comparative study of mesothelioma and asbestosis using computed tomography and conventional chest radiography. Radiology 144:453, 1982

Raghavan K, Gianoutsos P, Bishop J et al.: Phase II trial of carboplatin in the management of malignant mesothelioma. J Clin Oncol 8:151, 1990

Reddel RR, Malan-Shibley L, Gerwin BI et al.: Tumorigenicity of human mesothelial cell line transfected with EJ-*ras* oncogene. J Natl Cancer Inst 81:945, 1989

Ris H-B, Altermatt JH, Inderbitzi R et al.: Photodynamic therapy with chlorins for diffuse malignant mesothelioma: initial clinical results. Br J Cancer 64:1116, 1991

Roberts GH: Distant visceral metastases in pleural mesothelioma. Br J Dis Chest 70:246, 1976

Ruffie P, Feld R, Minkin S et al.: Diffuse malignant mesothelioma of the pleura in Ontario and Quebec: a retrospective study of 332 patients. J Clin Oncol 7:1157, 1989

Rusch V: Pleurectomy/decortication for malignant mesothelioma. Presented at Cine Clinics, Meeting of the American College of Surgeons, Chicago, October 23, 1991

Rusch V, Piantadosi S, Holmes EC: The role of extrapleural pneumonectomy in malignant pleural mesothelioma. J Thorac Cardiovasc Surg 102:1, 1991

Rusch VW, Godwin JD, Shuman WP: The role of computed tomography scanning in the initial assessment and the follow-up of malignant pleural mesothelioma. J Thorac Cardiovasc Surg 96:171, 1988

Said WJ, Nash G, Banks-Schlegel S et al.: Localized fibrous mesothelioma: an immunohistochemical and electron microscopic study. Hum Pathol 15:440, 1984

Scharifker D, Kaneko M: Localized fibrous "mesothelioma" of pleura (submesothelial fibroma). Cancer 43:627, 1979

Selikoff IJ, Churg J, Hammond EC: Relation between exposure to asbestos and mesothelioma. N Engl J Med 272:560, 1965

Sheard JDH, Taylor W, Pearson MG: Pneumothorax and malignant mesothelioma in patients over the age of 40. Thorax 46:584, 1991

Sinoff C, Falkson G, Sandison AG, De Muelenaere G: Combined doxorubicin and radiation therapy in malignant pleural mesothelioma. Cancer Treat Rep 66:1605, 1982

Sklarin NT, Chahinian AP, Feuer EJ et al.: Augmentation of activity of cis-diamminedichloroplatinum(II) and mitomycin C by interferon in human malignant mesothelioma xenografts in nude mice. Cancer Res 48:64, 1988

Soubra M, Dunscombe PB, Hodson DI, Wong G: Physical aspects of external beam radiotherapy for the treatment of malignant pleural mesothelioma. Int J Radiat Oncol Biol Phys 18:1521, 1989

Stout AP, Murray MR: Localized pleural mesothelioma. Arch Pathol Lab Med 34;951, 1942

Sugarbaker D, Strauss G, Lynch T et al.: Trimodality therapy of malignant pleural mesothelioma. J Clin Oncol 11:295, 1992

Sugarbaker DJ, Heher EC, Lee TH et al.: Extrapleural pneumonectomy, chemotherapy, and radiotherapy in the treatment of diffuse malignant pleural mesothelioma. J Thorac Cardiovasc Surg 102;10, 1991

Tiainen M, Tammilehto L, Rautonen J et al.: Chromosomal abnormalities and their correlations with asbestos exposure and survival in patients with mesothelioma. Br J Cancer 60:618, 1989

Umsawasdi T, Dhingra HM, Charnsangavej C, Luna MA: A case report of malignant pleural mesothelioma with long-term disease control after chemotherapy. Cancer 67:48, 1991

Wadler S, Chahnian P, Slater W et al.: Cardiac abnormalities in patients with diffuse malignant pleural mesothelioma. Cancer 58:2744, 1986

Wagner JC: Mesothelioma and mineral fibers. Cancer 57:1905, 1986

Wagner JC, Skidmore JW, Hil RJ, Griffiths DM: Erionite exposure and mesotheliomas in rats. Br J Cancer 51:727, 1975

Wagner JC, Slaggs CA, Marchand P: Diffuse pleural mesothelioma

and asbestos exposure in north western Cape Province. Br J Ind Med 17:260, 1960

Walters KL, Martinez AJ: Malignant fibrous mesothelioma. Acta Neuropathol (Berl) 33:173, 1975

Watts DM, Jones GP, Bowman GA, Olsen JD: Giant benign mesothelioma. Ann Thorac Surg 48:590, 1989

Whitwell F, Rawcliffe RM: Diffuse malignant pleural mesothelioma and asbestos exposure. Thorax 26:6, 1971

Wirth PR, Legier J, Wright GL: Immunohistochemical evaluation of seven monoclonal antibodies for differentiation of pleural mesothelioma from lung adenocarcinoma. Cancer 67:655, 1991

Worn H: Möglickeiten und ergebnisse der chirurgischen behandlung des malignen pleuramesothelioms. Thoraxchir 22:391, 1974

42

FIBROTHORAX AND DECORTICATION

Jean Deslauriers
Louis P. Perrault

Under normal conditions, the pleural space is a virtual cavity interposed between the chest wall and the lung. The visceral and parietal linings of this cavity are 1 to 2 mm thick and serve as permeable membranes for transport of cells and fluid. Under pathologic conditions, these relationships may be altered and lead to the development of chronic infections, trapped lung, and severely impaired respiration. Although infrequently encountered in modern-day thoracic surgery, these pathologies must be well understood, not only because they are of major historical interest but also because they all present challenging management problems.

HISTORICAL NOTE

Between the years 1892 and 1894, Delorme in France and Fowler in America described an operation designed to substitute for the mutilating thoracoplasty of Schede (1890). The purpose of the operation was to promote lung reexpansion instead of letting the chest wall collapse to fill in the space. This procedure came to be called decortication. The exact sequence of these descriptions is still somewhat controversial despite some clarifications offered by Violet (1904).

In a sealed letter deposited at the French Academy of Medicine in June 1892 and at a surgical meeting in April 1893, Delorme, Professeur au Val-de-Grâce, described a personal method for the treatment of chronic empyemas. In a patient with a large chest wall abscess, he performed a scalpel and scissor dissection of the wall of the abscess, which was 1 cm thick and covered the left lung and pericardium. He concluded that he had freed the lung from this "*fausse membrane.*" The apparent success of this procedure and further autopsy work, in which he was able to decorticate encased lung ("*décortiquer une membrane résistante comme du cuir*" and subsequently reexpand healthy lung ("*poumon sain, crépitant et extensible*"), further confirmed his belief that this procedure could be useful for patients with large residual infected intrathoracic spaces.

On January 20th 1894 Delorme performed the first planned decortication, and four days later he reported the case at the Academy. At a French surgical meeting in 1896, he presented 26 cases of pulmonary decortication and concluded that (1) it is possible to free a lung from the membrane that holds it down even long after an operation for an empyema; (2) the method is applicable not only on the right but also on the left side; and (3) it is better than the Estlander operation because it expands and tends to restore the function of an otherwise useless lung (Lund, 1911).

In 1893 Ryerson Fowler also described the operation of decortication, which he had performed for the first time on October 7th 1893 on a woman 35 years of age who had had an empyema with a fistula for 10 years. He dissected out the scar tissue surrounding the fistulous tract and removed the entire mass of fibrous tissue from the diaphragm and lung. He was surprised to discover that the lung began to reexpand as soon as the thick scar tissue was peeled from it (Mayo and Beckman, 1914). His method was applicable to the treatment of chronic empyemas, in which he thought that failure of the lung to reexpand was mostly due to encasement by an inexpandable fibrous peel.

During the early years of the twentieth century and until some years after World War I, the procedure was used sporadically, and finally, because it carried a high fatality rate that results did not appear to justify, it encountered increasing disapproval. Several factors accounted for this lack of enthusiasm, including inadequacy of anesthesia, lack of antimicrobial agents in the face of infection, lack of blood transfusion ability, and lack of technical expertise (Milfeld, et al., 1978). It was often a prolonged and shocking operation. Expansion soon after operation was frequently lost due to wound breakdown from infection. Reexpansion did not always follow successful decortication because of underlying defects such as parenchymal fibrosis, fistulae, or other active diseases (Himmelstein, et al., 1948).

In 1911 Lund reported the experience of Lloyd (1908), who had stated that in the treatment of old empyemas, it was not necessary to remove the pulmonary pleura but simply to break up the adhesions at the borders of the cavity between the parietal and visceral pleurae. Lund also presented seven patients of his own and described the operation performed in the first case: "On splitting this membrane with the scissors and separating carefully from the surface of the lung, the lung began to expand and when the child coughed at the close of the operation, the red velvetly lung blew up like a soap bubble and came up against the chest wall, where it remained."

In 1915 Lilienthal also treated nontuberculous suppurations with decortication. He reported on 23 such patients, among whom there was an operative mortality of 17 percent (4/23) and a good result in all survivors. He insisted on the importance of full lung mobilization and called attention to the dangerous hemorrhage that may follow the tearing away of tough adhesions between the lung and the chest wall.

Other early contributions were those of Mayo and Beckman (1914) and Eggers (1923), who reported shortly after World War I on 146 patients who had undergone decortication for chronic empyemas. He correctly identified the objective of decortication as excision of the peel holding the lung rather than removal of the visceral pleura itself.

The advances in management thoracic trauma that occurred during and after World War II placed further emphasis on decortication of the lung following clotted traumatic hemothorax. Impressive results and new applications of the procedure were reported by Samson and Burford (1947), who formulated the newer concept of early and total decortication of the lung. Samson and associates (1946) showed that complete pulmonary mobilization (decortication) should not be deferred for the length of time usually necessary to transfer the patient to a specialty center (in the "interior" zone in military situations). In those cases early decortication results in immediate pulmonary reexpansion and prevents the development of fibrothoraces. Other investigators such as Patton, et al. (1952) showed that decorticated lungs actually regained function if the underlying parenchyma was free of disease.

HISTORICAL READINGS

Burford TH, Parker EF, Samson PC: Early decortication in the treatment of post-traumatic empyema. Ann Surg 122:163, 1945

Delorme E: Nouveau traitement des empyèmes chroniques. Gaz hop 67:94, 1894

Eggers C: Radical operation for chronic empyema. Ann Surg 77:327, 1923

Estlander JA: Sur la résection des côtes dans l'empyème chronique. Rev Mens 8:885, 1897

Fowler GR: A case of thoracoplasty for removal of a large cicatricial fibrous growth from the interior of the chest, the result of an old empyema. Med Rec 44:838, 1893

Lilienthal H: Empyema. Exploration of the thorax with primary mobilization of the lung. Ann Surg 62:309, 1915

Lloyd S: The treatment of unresolved pneumonia. p. 1977. Sci Med Surg 1908

Lund FB: The advantages of the so-called decortication of the lung in old empyema. JAMA 57:693, 1911

Mayo CH, Beckman EH: Visceral pleurectomy for chronic empyema. Am Surg 59:884, 1914

Patton WE, Watson TR, Gaensler EA: Pulmonary function before and at intervals after surgical decortication of the lung. Surg Gynecol Obstet 95:477, 1952

Samson PC, Burford TH: Total pulmonary decortication. Its evolution and present concepts of indications and operative technique. J Thorac Cardiovasc Surg 16:127, 1947

Samson PC, Burford TH, Brewer LA, Burbank B: The management of war wounds of the chest in a base center. The role of early pulmonary decortication. J Thorac Cardiovasc Surg 15:1, 1946

Schede M: Die Behandlung der Empyeme. Proc 9th Cong Intern Med, Wiesbaden 9:41, 1890

Violet D: De la décortication pulmonaire dans l'empyème chronique. Arch Gen Med 81:657, 1904

BASIC SCIENCE

Definitions

Fibrothorax is the presence of abnormal fibrous tissue within the pleural space, a feature that usually complicates clotted hemothoraces, pleural tuberculosis, or chronic empyemas. As a result of this fibrosis, the lung becomes entrapped and the hemithorax contracts, resulting in reduced mobility. Eventually, there is a marked loss of function in the collapsed lung.

Over the years several terms, listed below, have been used in reference to fibrothoraces. In some cases the visceral peel has been wrongly thought to be thickened pleura (Mayo and Beckman, 1914), and this has contributed to perpetuation of some misunderstandings about this disease. The so-called lung en cuirasse seen in restrictive pleurisy associated with asbestos exposure (Sterling and Herbert, 1980) should also be distinguished from the "peel" seen in fibrothoraces since the latter does not represent thickened pleura.

Decortication, a term derived from Latin, literally means stripping or peeling off of the "bark" from the lung (Lund, 1911). It is a surgical procedure, which consists of removing a restricting fibrotic membrane from the visceral pleural surface of the lung, and its purpose is to free the trapped lung as well as to obliterate the pleural space. It is a different operation than the early thoracotomy done for *deloculation* of the pleural space in cases of fibrinopurulent empyemas (Morin, et al., 1972; Mayo, 1985) or hemothoraces (Beall, et al., 1966). Deloculation consists of cleaning out a cavity littered with fibrous membranes in order to improve on closed drainage. It is not a decortication in the true sense of the word because a mature peel has not yet formed over the lung.

Commonly Used Terminology Referring to Fibrothorax

Trapped lung
Encased lung
Unexpanded lung
Restrictive pleurisy
Constrictive pleurisy/pleuritis/peel
Organizing hemothorax/empyema
Frozen chest
Lung en cuirasse
Pleural constriction

Decortication is also different from empyemectomy, which is the complete excision of the empyema and its contents without entering the cavity itself, the purpose being to avoid soiling the interior of the hemithorax (Leroux, et al., 1986). Finally, decortication is different from the limited decortication described for the management of pediatrc empyema (Kosloke and Cartwright, 1988). This procedure is similar to early deloculation and is used to remove pleural contents that are believed to be in the fibrinopurulent stage and have not yet organized.

Causes of Fibrothorax

The various causes of fibrothorax are listed below. In the earlier parts of the twentieth century, most fibrothoraces were seen in association with tuberculosis, and they resulted from therapeutic pneumothoraces in which the lung became unexpandable or from untreated or unresponsive tuberculous pleurisy or empyema. In recent years classic examples have been those of a trapped lung secondary to chronic empyema, clotted hemothorax, or neglected pleural effusion. In each of these situations the pleural collections of pus, blood, or fluid precipitate into fibrin, which eventually becomes fibrous tissue, and is deposited over the pleural surfaces and the diaphragm.

Rare causes of fibrothoraces include uncommon bacterial and parasitic diseases of the pleural space (see Ch. 39), chylothoraces (Fairfax, et al., 1986), and pleural complications of pancreatitis (Shapiro, et al., 1970). It is also worth noting that in as many as 50 percent of patients with fibrothoraces, no specific cause can be identified either by clinical history or at the time of thoracotomy.

Pathophysiology

While it was originally thought that the fibroblastic reaction in the pleural space was in some way a specific response to the presence of blood, it became rapidly apparent that any insult to the pleura would result in the same reaction (Samson, et al., 1958).

Causes of Fibrothorax

Common causes
    Traumatic or nontraumatic hemothorax
    Chronic empyema
    Chronic pneumothorax
    Sequelae of tuberculosis
        Therapeutic pneumothoraces
        Tuberculous pleurisy or empyema
    Neglected pleural effusion
Uncommon bacterial and parasitic diseases of the pleural space
Rare causes
    Chylothorax
    Pancreatic diseases
    Talc poudrage

Any undrained or untreated pleural collection of fluid, pus, blood, or chyle is always followed by precipitation of fibrin on the exposed surfaces. As the process evolves into the stage of organization, fibroblasts and angioblasts proliferate and the exudate eventually becomes a mature peel, which is composed of adult tissue rich in collagen but relatively poor in blood supply, cells, and elastic fibers. As the peel further thickens, the underlying lung is covered and entrapped and its normal expansion is impeded. Wachsmuth and Schautz (1951) and Rudström and Thoren (1955) have shown that the fully developed parietal peel consists of three poorly defined layers: (1) a layer of comparatively vascular, loosely organized tissue nearest the pleura; (2) a layer of connective tissue containing few vessels and cells, which forms the main bulk of the peel; and (3) an inner layer bounding the central cavity and consisting of necrotic tissues, fibrinoid masses, and detritus with or without bacteria. As the peel ages even more, the fibrotic component increases and the loose layer nearest the pleura becomes thinner and finally disappears. In addition to the peel, there are nearly always dense adhesions between the lung, chest wall, pericardium, diaphragm, and mediastinum.

The parietal peel is always thicker than the visceral peel, and it can reach a thickness of 2 cm or more. Calcifications are common over the inner surface of the peel, and they are usually associated with chronic exudative effusions, hemothoraces, or tuberculous empyemas. Unless the lung has been damaged by tuberculosis or other parenchymal disease, neither the visceral nor parietal pleura becomes thickened, and both remain largely normal membranes.

In patients with small hemothoraces (<200 ml), the continuous movement of the heart and lungs may defibrinate the blood, which will be reabsorbed in a fluid state by the pleural lymphatics. If, however, the hemothorax is larger, if there is continued bleeding, or if air (Drummond and Craig, 1967) or bacteria are also present, a clot with multiple pockets containing air or fluid will form, and eventually this clot will become organized into a peel that will encase the lung.

In empyemas the rapidity of organization varies according to such factors as proper antibiotic treatment, immunologic status of the host, and type of bacteria (Kosloske and Cartwright, 1988). Ultimately, the lung is compressed by the pleural contents, imprisoned by the peel, and restrained by the pleural adhesions (Williams, 1950). Although these factors are not equally important in maintaining the lung in its collapsed state, to be successful the decortication operation must evacuate the pleural contents, remove the peel, and completely mobilize the lung by freeing the adhesions.

Physiologic Consequences

The functional consequences of a fibrothorax are multiple, and several authors have shown that loss of pulmonary function bear no relationship to the degree of pleural thickening as seen on chest radiographs. In other words, a thick pleural peel does not necessarily imply reduced ventilation and perfusion any more than a thin peel (Fraser and Pare, 1979). Other authors have also demonstrated that even a relatively localized pleural restriction may be associated with profound alterations in ventilation and blood flow to the entire lung (Robin, et al., 1966; Autio, 1959; Hughes, et al., 1975).

The physiologic aberrations in pulmonary function seen in patients with fibrothoraces are those of a restriction producing decreased lung volumes, diffusion capacity, and expiratory flows. Patton and colleagues (1952) studied pulmonary function before and at intervals after surgical decortication of the lung. In eight patients, the average maximum breathing capacity was reduced to 68 percent of the predicted normal and the average vital capacity to 65 percent. The almost equal reduction of maximum breathing capacity and vital capacity indicated that the ventilatory defect was of the restrictive type. Bronchospirometric observations showed the ventilatory insufficiency to be almost entirely due to extensive collapse of the involved lung. Similar abnormalities in pulmonary function have been reported by Carroll, et al. (1951) and Siebens, et al. (1956).

Diffusion on the affected side is invariably low, and this is likely due to a reduction in the available alveolocapillary gas exchange surface. As a consequence of mechanical limitation of pulmonary vasculature and hypoxic vasoconstriction, ipsilateral lung perfusion is also decreased. Characteristically, perfusion is decreased out of proportion to ventilation (Grossman, 1979); this reduction is adaptive to the reduced ventilation and is not accompanied by structural arterial changes. Robin and associates (1966) reported four patients in whom severe pulmonary hypertension was associated with chronic constrictive pleuritis, and they speculated about a possible pulmonary vasoconstrictive substance originating in lung tissue, which markedly reduced but still maintained perfusion.

Bolliger and de Kock (1988) have shown that when the movement of the chest wall is impaired by fibrothorax and the lung tissue is not involved, the flow-volume curve has a relatively characteristic pattern, which can be differentiated from that of restrictive lung disease. Another difference between fibrothorax and restrictive parenchymal disease that is revealed in pulmonary function studies is the lack of elevation of maximal static pulmonary recoil pressure observed in patients with fibrothorax (Fraser and Pare, 1979).

DIAGNOSIS

Clinical Features

The clinical presentation of a fibrothorax may vary according to the cause and extent of the process and the presence or absence of underlying parenchymal disease and associated conditions. The most common complaint is that of dyspnea upon exertion, which is typically progressive over a protracted period of time. Occasionally, the patient may experience pain. Right ventricular failure with clinical signs of cor pulmonale may also occur in extreme cases. Physical examination reveals a unilateral fixation of the chest with limited respiratory excursion and atrophy of the overlying musculature. Palpation shows decreased fremitus with dullness to percussion, while auscultation identifies diminished or absent breath sounds.

Fibrothoraces due to tuberculosis may represent a complication of parenchymal disease, and those caused by chronic empyema may be associated with their own complications, such as empyema necessitatis, chondritis, rib osteomyelitis, bronchopleural fistula, pericarditis, or mediastinal abscesses. In those cases signs and symptoms of infections may dominate the clinical picture, and the patient may present with fever, toxicity, and weight loss.

Investigative Techniques

The diagnosis and pathogenesis of a given fibrothorax should always be substantiated by careful review of past medical history and by comparison of old and current chest films and computed tomography (CT) scans. Pulmonary and pleural malignancies must be ruled out, since they often mimic benign fibrothoraces. Diagnostic techniques such as bronchoscopy, ultrasound, nuclear magnetic resonance (NMR) imaging, angiography, percutaneous pleural biopsy, and thoracoscopy will usually serve that purpose.

Standard chest radiographs with posteroanterior (PA) and lateral views often provide clues to the presence of a fibrothorax. The pleura may appear uniformly thickened, initially over the diaphragmatic and lateral surfaces, and this may be visible as a markedly increased water density surrounding the lung in an antigravity distribution (Guenter and Welch, 1982). Later in the process, the entire pleural surface may be obliterated, and other signs of advanced fibrothorax, such as narrowing of the intercostal spaces, diminished size of the involved hemithorax, and ipsilateral displacement of the mediastinum may be present. Mottled calcifications may be seen over the inner aspect of the parietal peel, and these may be used to determine the actual thickness of the parietal peel.

Radiography may contribute to the identification of the causative process in addition to giving clues as to the status of both the involved and the contralateral lung. This evaluation is important, since functional improvement after decortication does not occur if extensive parenchymal disease is present. Morton and co-workers (1970) have demonstrated that absence of underlying parenchymal disease is the best assurance that there will be significant improvement in pulmonary function after operation.

CT scanning is essential to assess the extent and anatomic characteristics of the fibrothorax. Important information concerning the underlying parenchyma may also be obtained by CT scanning, which can identify tuberculous lesions, bronchiectasis, fibrosis, or other conditions that could affect the result of decortication. NMR imaging has not shown any advantage over CT scanning and at present has no precise role in the evaluation of fibrothoraces.

Bronchoscopy, either flexible or rigid, must be performed to ensure the integrity of the bronchus in the entrapped lung (Scannell, 1990). A concomitant carcinoma must be ruled out, and the bronchus of the lung to be decorticated must be free of both active endobronchial tuberculosis and of a cicatricial post-tuberculous bronchial stricture.

Pulmonary function studies, including spirometry, diffusion studies, and exercise tolerance testing are useful to quantify the degree of respiratory impairment, and they also provide for postoperative comparison. Functional and anatomic evaluation may also be useful to predict whether or not decortication will improve dyspnea, whether or not the decorticated lung will reexpand, and whether or not the reexpanded lung will function in a satisfactory manner.

Nutritional assessment may finally be necessary to identify hypovolemia, anemia, and hypoalbuminemia and institute appropriate supportive measures.

MANAGEMENT

Decortication: General Principles

The objectives of decortication are two-fold—first, to reexpand the trapped lung and restore lung, diaphragm, and chest wall function, and second, to obliterate the space and control the infection. In some patients with tuberculosis or chronic empyemas, functional recovery may be a secondary consideration to space obliteration (Ackman and Madore, 1951), since a lung reexpanded after a long period of compression may have impaired ventilation but still be able to fill the space (Okano and Walkup, 1962). In those cases, decortication may obviate the need for more extensive procedures such as thoracoplasty or pleuropneumonectomy. If decortication is performed for an organizing hemothorax, the objectives are to recover function and prevent late suppurative complications.

Mayo, et al., (1982) have described three conditions critical to the optimal success of decortication: it should be the primary surgical procedure; it should be performed at the earliest opportunity; and all elements of the intrathoracic peel should be removed to ensure complete lung reexpansion and both chest wall and diaphragmatic mobility.

Indications for and Timing of Surgery

Indications for Early Deloculation

Early deloculation is indicated in cases of multiloculated empyemas or of hemothoraces when lung expansion cannot be promoted by closed tube thoracostomy alone. Van Way, et al., (1988) reported 40 patients with class III complicated empyemas with multiple loculations. Limited thoracotomy for drainage and placement of tubes was performed in 22 patients, all of whom had resolution of the empyema with no additional procedures. They recommended limited thoracotomy immediately or during the first week of treatment for all multiloculated and complex empyemas (Figs. 42-1 and 42-2). Similarly, Fishman and Ellertson (1977) advocated early decortication for empyemas in immunosuppressed patients. Their approach was based on the following therapeutic principles: (1) early, thorough evacuation of the abscess cavity; (2) obliteration of the cavity by removal of the peel, allowing the restricted lung to inflate; and (3) avoidance of a chest wall sinus tract. Mayo, et al., (1982) reported 21 pediatric patients who had acute or mature empyemas and were treated by open thoracotomy and decortication. There were no deaths or complications, and the authors concluded that early thoracotomy and decortication yielded uniformly good results. It is therefore appropriate to recommend early space deloculation in empyema patients in whom closed thoracostomy does not bring about adequate drainage and lung reexpansion. Personne (1990) also recommends that thora-

cotomy be avoided beyond the third week because at this stage the empyema is not well organized and the peeling of the lung will lead to tearing, bleeding, and prolonged air leaks. He suggests waiting at least 3 months and then proceeding with full decortication.

Culiner, et al., (1959), Beall, et al., (1966) and Milfeld, et al., (1978) have shown that early evacuation of clotted hemothoraces decreases mortality, morbidity, and hospital stay and prevents the development of post-traumatic empyema. In the series of Milfeld et al., 10 patients underwent evacuation of a clotted hemothorax within 5 days of admission, with no mortality and an average hospital stay of 10 days. Among the 41 patients who underwent decortication more than 5 days after injury, there was one death (2.4 percent mortality) and the average period of hospitalization was 25 days. At an early stage simple removal of clots is all that is required, whereas if organization is allowed to occur, formal decortication becomes necessary (Beall, et al., 1966). In an extensive study of 452 patients with traumatic hemothorax, Wilson and associates (1979) concluded that early operative intervention to remove residual blood clot is usually not necessary and that the emphasis of therapy should be on prompt and adequate pleural drainage.

Indications for Decortication

The decision to proceed with decortication in patients with organized fibrothoraces depends on several factors. Since many conditions associated with acute pleural swelling may resolve spontaneously, decortication should only be considered if the pleural thickening has been present for several weeks or months, if the patient's life style is significantly compromised by exertional dyspnea, and if there is evidence of reversible physiologic impairment of the underlying lung. Samson, et al. (1946) summarized the patients with chronic hemothoraces for whom operation is indicated as those in whom there is at least 50 percent compression of the lung, especially if the apex is collapsed, and those in whom aspiration has been unsuccessful and in whom there has been no appreciable pulmonary expansion at the end of 4 to 6 weeks following injury. In those cases one can expect full recovery of function because the lung parenchyma is less likely to have been involved in the disease process. It is important to decorticate early (3 to 5 weeks) in patients with hemothoraces because, with the passage of time, fibrosis may extend into the lung and limit its reexpandability. It is also possible that with time, the plane between visceral pleural and peel will be lost.

In patients with chronic empyemas (Fig. 42-3), the therapeutic aims are (1) to release and expand the collapsed lung if there is marked restriction; (2) to reestablish the intrathoracic spatial relationship so that false reexpansion, characterized by overdistension of the contralateral lung with mediastinal shift, elevation of the diaphragm, and contraction of the chest wall does not occur; and (3) to control infection by evacuation and obliteration of the pleural space. Villalba and colleagues (1979) recommend that once a post-traumatic empyema becomes well established and refractory to standard modalities, decortication with evacuation of the empyema cavity should be performed as soon as possible.

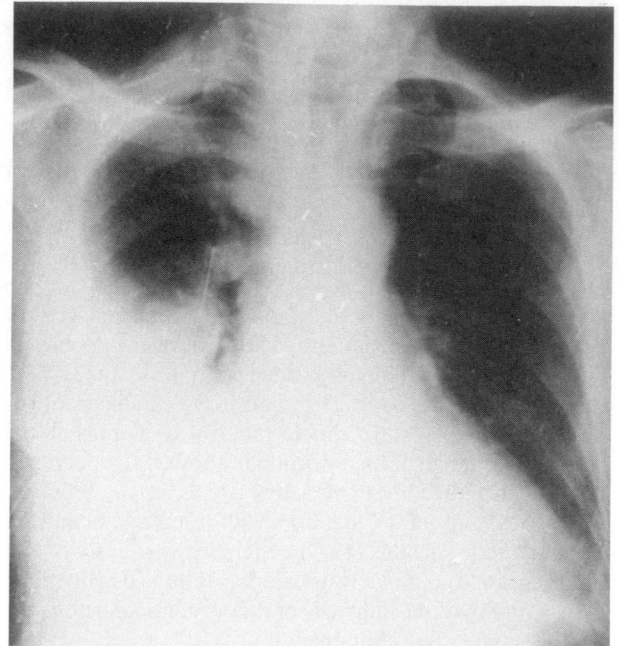
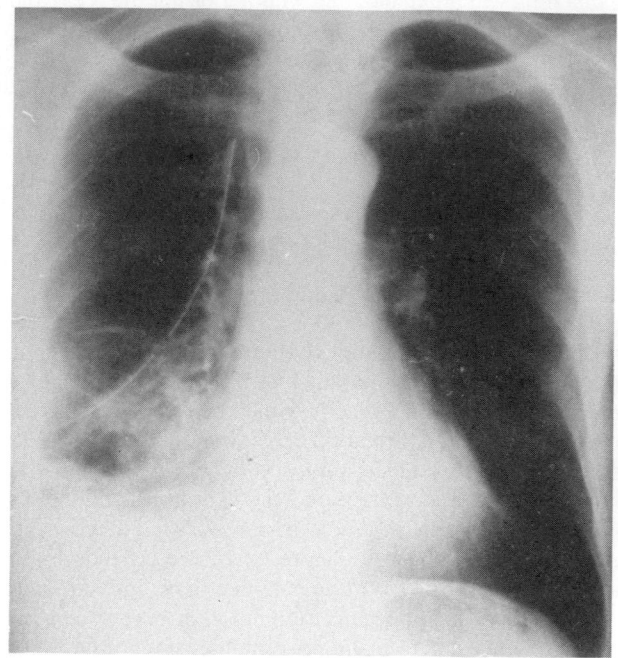
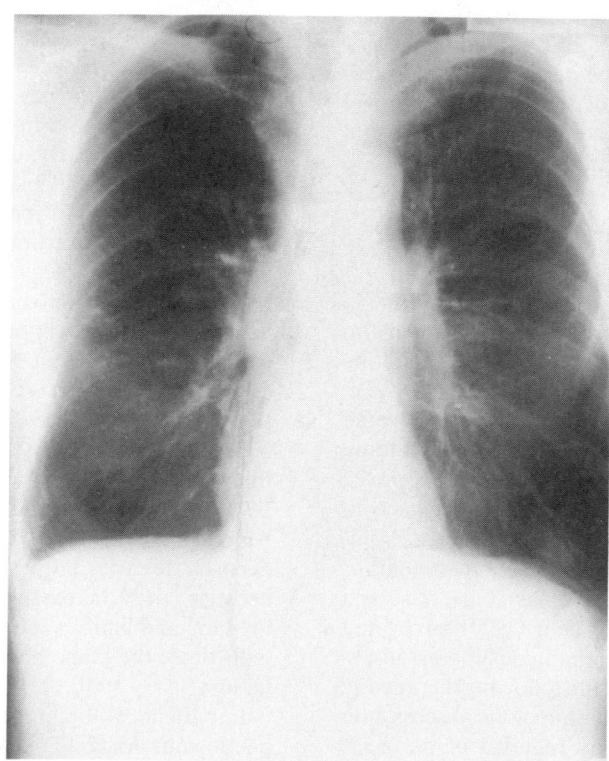

Figure 42-1.   Deloculation for acute empyema. **(A)** Chest radiograph of a 52-year-old man admitted for fever, cough, and right-sided chest pain. **(B)** Chest radiograph following minithoracotomy for deloculation of the empyema. **(C)** Chest radiograph taken 1 year later and showing complete lung reexpansion and obliteration of the space.

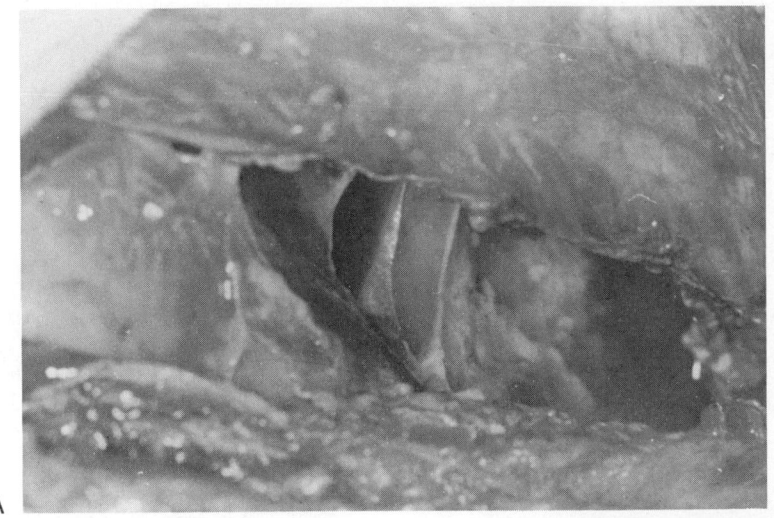

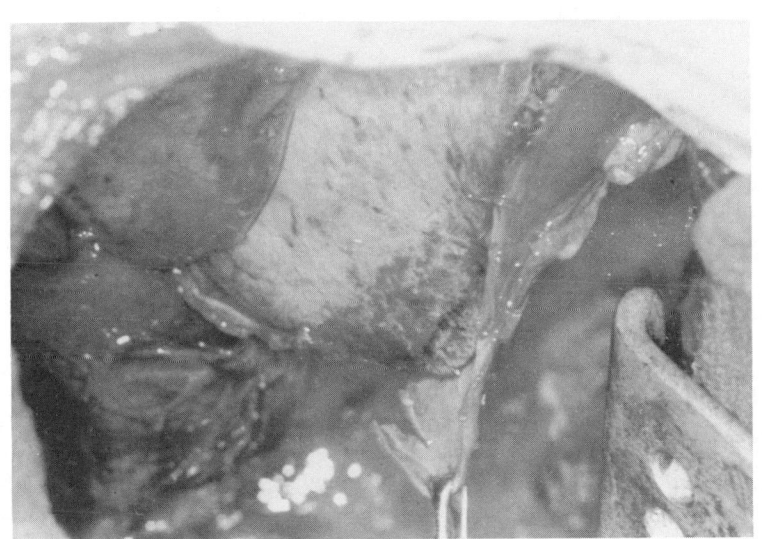

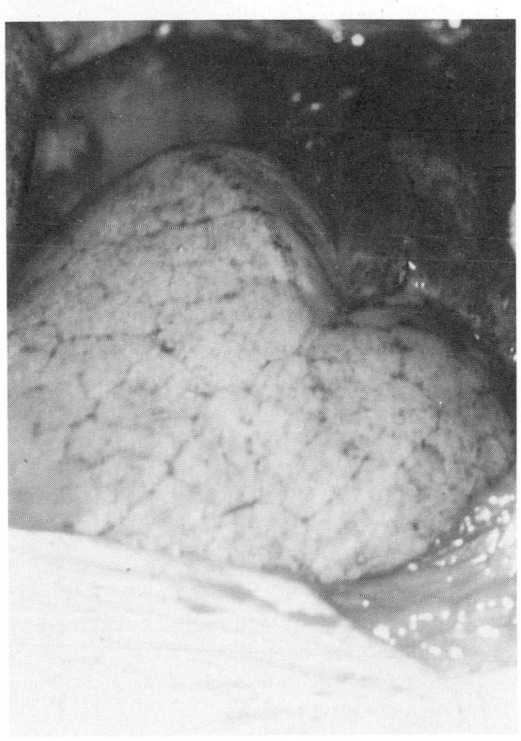

Figure 42-2. Operative photographs showing **(A)** Multiloculated empyema with multiple pockets of fluid and fibrin; **(B)** inflammatory peel being removed from the bisceral pleura; and **(C)** complete reexpansion of the lung. (Courtesy of Dr. Jean Morin.)

It is worth noting that most patients with hemothoraces, pleural effusions, or empyemas will never need decortication if they are properly treated at the onset of disease. In a series of 19 patients, Young and colleagues (1972) reported that in each patient an error in management had been made or a complication had occurred during therapy. They concluded that strict adherence to the principle of complete drainage may require insertion of multiple chest tubes but is necessary if the incidence of trapped lung is to be decreased.

In pleural tuberculosis therapy is primarily medical, and surgical treatment is only used to eliminate or correct those residues of disease that cannot be further altered by chemotherapy (Langston, et al., 1967). In those cases decortication is performed when evidence of toxicity is no longer present, when thoracentesis fails to yield fluid, or when fluid removal fails to alter the radiographic appearance. The extent of pleural involvement should also be taken into consideration and should be equivalent to one-third to one-fourth of the hemithorax and cast a clearly discernible shadow in the lateral projection (Langston, et al., 1967). Decortication may finally be indicated for patients with mixed tuberculous empyemas and for patients with unexpandable lungs secondary to thera-

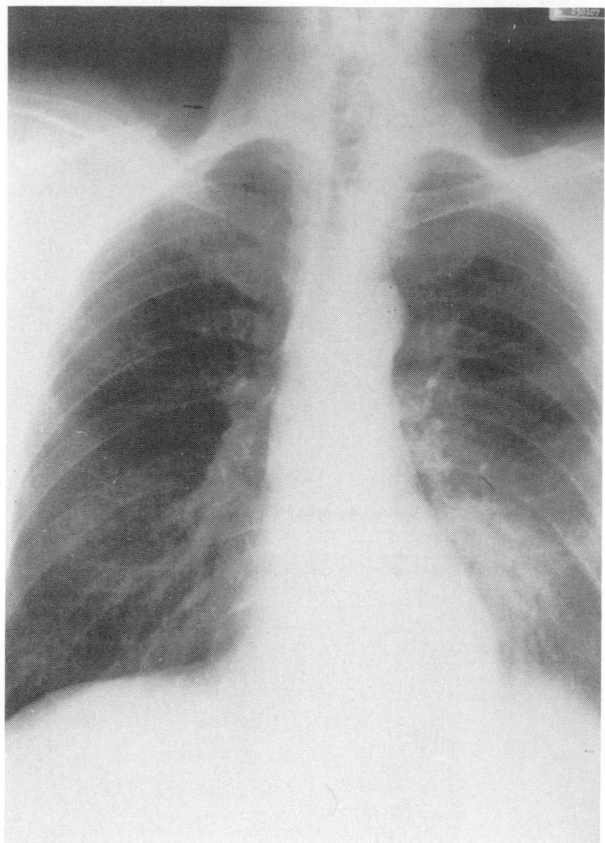
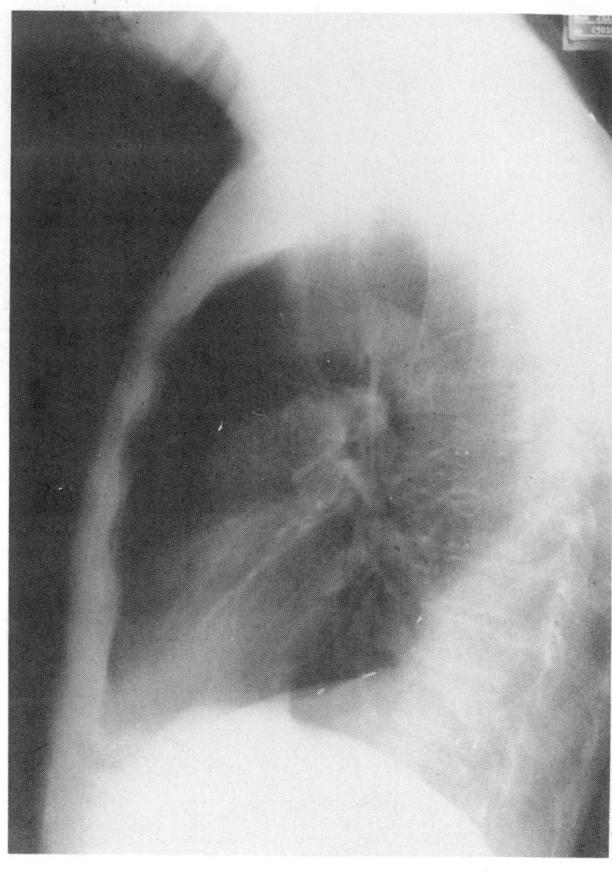

Figure 42-3. Decortication for chronic empyema. Standard **(A)** PA and **(B)** lateral chest radiograph of 49-year-old man admitted for cough, hemoptysis, and purulent sputum of 4 months duration. Note on the lateral radiograph the inverted D-shaped density typical of a chronic empyema. This patient was treated by complete lung decortication.

Indications for Decortication

Early space deloculation (1 to 3 weeks)
    Inadequately drained multiloculated empyema
    Early clotted hemothorax
Decortication (4 to 6 weeks)
    Organizing hemothorax
    Unresolving pleural effusion
    Empyema
Late decortication
    Post-traumatic fibrothorax
    Chronic empyema
    Idiopathic fibrothorax
    Pleural tuberculosis

---

peutic pneumothoraces (Weinberg, et al., 1948; Weinberg and Davis, 1949; Mulvihill and Klopstock, 1948).

Contraindications

Although extensive disease or fibrosis of the lung represents a major obstacle to successful decortication and may even contraindicate its use, the only absolute contraindication to the procedure is a stenosis of a major bronchus feeding the lobe or lung to be decorticated (Savage and Fleming, 1955). O'Rourke, et al., (1949) has shown that major pulmonary lesions, especially those of tuberculous nature, are also contraindications to decortication, owing to their detrimental effect upon reexpansion of the lung and to the risk of a flare-up of the original process. Other relatively absolute contraindications include patients with uncontrolled invasive infection in the lung or pleura, patients with significant operative risks, and debilitated patients. It may also be inappropriate

---

Contraindications for Decortication

Absolute
    Extensive disease in the collapsed lung
    Bronchial stenosis
Relatively absolute
    Uncontrolled invasive infection
    Significant operative risk
    Debilitation
    Contralateral disease
Relative
    Minimal symptoms
    Little evidence of physiologic impairment

Figure 42-4. Limited fibrothorax. CT scan showing a limited fibrothorax at the base of the right lung. There is no significant lung entrapment.

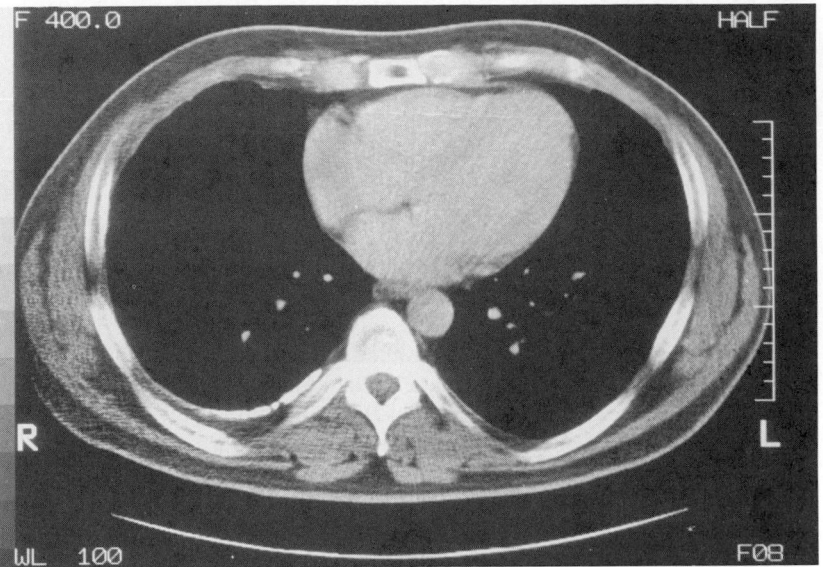

to decorticate a lung when there is significant contralateral disease. Relative contraindications include asymptomatic or minimally symptomatic patients and patients with little evidence of physiologic impairment (Fig. 42-4).

Operative Technique

With few exceptions, the operative technique described by Samson and Burford (1947), Samson (1955), and Williams (1950) is still being followed. The operation requires establishment of a plane between the peel and the visceral pleura, freeing of the lung from all adhesions, and decortication of the diaphragm.

Decortication is performed through a sixth or seventh interspace posterolateral thoracotomy because incision at this lower level offers better exposure of the diaphragm where adhesions are often denser than those encountered elsewhere (Williams, 1950) or worse than preoperatively assessed on chest radiographs. Excision of the sixth rib is not always necessary but may improve exposure, especially when the intercostal spaces have been narrowed by the contractile process of the thickened pleura.

After the intercostal space has been entered, the parietal pleura is separated for a distance of several centimeters on each side of the incision so that a rib spreader can be inserted. If a space is present, it is opened and its contents are thoroughly evacuated. If the contents are purulent, contamination of the operating field will be unavoidable, but this is of little consequence if adequate lung reexpansion is later achieved. When there is no free space, the lung must first be freed from the parietal pleura, starting over the mediastinal surface, where it is usually free from adhesions.

As the next step, the peel is elevated from the visceral pleura. This is done by incising the peel with a scalpel until the visceral pleura, which is thin and pliable, is reached. The edges of the peel are grasped with forceps and are separated from the visceral pleura by gentle blunt dissection with either a "pusher" or a gauzed-covered finger. The initial incision in the peel may be vertical or horizontal or several incisions may be made to start the decortication. Gentle reexpansion of the lung by the anesthesist often facilitates separation of the peel, which must be removed over the entire surface of the lung, including the interlobar fissures. If in some areas thick adhesions to the visceral pleura are encountered, these may be left in situ in order to avoid trauma to the lung or the opening of old tuberculous foci.

The ease of stripping is unpredictable, and a number of tears to the underlying lung will be made. Large tears can be oversewn, while most small tears will heal easily once the lung has achieved complete reexpansion. If the formation of the peel is secondary to an inflammatory process in the lung, separation nearly always presents greater difficulties, because the loose subendothelial layer of the visceral pleura is replaced by fibrous, organized granulation tissue (Rudstrom and Thoren, 1955; Zenker, et al., 1954).

Complete pleurolysis with mobilization of the lung from the diaphragm, pericardium, chest wall, and mediastinum is carried out next. The diaphragm must be decorticated down to the costophrenic angles, which can prove difficult because fibrosis can be very dense at that level and a plane for dissection is seldom found. Although it is important to restore the mobility of the diaphragm, it is sometimes better to leave plaques of thickened pleura than to damage the muscle.

The removal of the parietal peel is subject to controversy. Arguments against performing this step include the possibility that heavy bleeding may occur because the endothoracic fascia may be very vascular and the fact that complete pulmonary reexpansion achieved by visceral decortication may set the stage for resorption of even the thickest of parietal peels. Proponents of removing the parietal peel argue that this is important to restore the full motion of the thoracic cage (Waterman, et al., 1957) and achieve the best functional results. The parietal peel can be excised at the beginning of the operation or after visceral decortication has been completed. When this is done, the plane of dissection is between the parietal pleura and the endothoracic fascia (the parietal pleura cannot be freed from the peel), and in addition to an increased blood loss, technical difficulties can be encountered over the lung apex and mediastinum. At the apex dense adhesions between the upper lobe and the first two ribs may be present, so that pleurolysis or parietal decortication may be difficult. In some cases cavities may have penetrated beyond the pleural layer so that in order to excise them a resection of the costal chest wall, in part at least, may be required (Langston, et al., 1967). Care must be taken not to injure the lower trunk of the brachial plexus, the vagus nerve and subclavian artery on the left side, and the sympathetic chain. Over the mediastinum the dissection is usually considerably easier, but care must be taken to avoid injury to the esophagus, thoracic duct, phrenic nerves, and hilar blood vessels. It is remarkable that not even old and thick peels are bound to large vessels, which usually are surrounded by a layer of loose tissue (Rudstrom and Thoren, 1955). At the end of the procedure, two properly placed chest tubes must be left in the pleural space.

Associated Procedures

If there is a pulmonary lesion, a situation commonly seen with tuberculosis or its sequelae, resection of lung parenchyma may be necessary in addition to decortication. In such cases complete filling of the residual space with the remaining lung must be ensured. If this is not possible, addition of a small tailoring thoracoplasty with preservation of the intercostal muscles, or collapse of the parietal wall without rib resection may obliterate the space (Ilioka, et al., 1985). This has also been used to provide closure of permanent thoracic sinuses (Dowd, 1909). Muscle flaps, such as the latissimus dorsi flap mobilized at the time of decortication, may also be used, thereby avoiding the need for thoracoplasty (Ali and Unruh, 1990).

Thoracoscopy (Video-Assisted Thoracic Surgery) and Decortication

The use of thoracoscopy for early delocation of early-stage empyemas is still a matter of debate. Hutter and colleagues (1985) reported the use of thoracoscopy for delocation and debridement of 12 empyemic cavities. Following lavage of the cavity, the thoracoscope helped in the placement of irrigation drains under direct vision; this resulted in complete cure in 11 of the 12 patients within an average of 20 days after the procedure. One patient required a second thoracoscopy and drainage course but also eventually healed. In 1991 the same group (Ridley and Braimbridge, 1991) reported on a total of 30 patients with a cure rate of 60 percent.

We find video-assisted thoracic surgery (VATS) particularly useful in the management of empyemas seen in early stages (Deslauriers and Mehran, 1993), in which cases the cavity can be delocated under direct vision, the lung reexpanded, and chest drains properly placed at dependent sites. It is also useful for delocation of postpneumonectomy empyemas, since the whole cavity can be explored and debrided and chest tubes can be placed at appropriate sites for lavage and attempted sterilization of the space.

In cases of organized stage 3 empyemas, it may be difficult to obtain a good endothoracic image, and decortication of the lung may be hazardous, traumatic, and of limited value.

Further, the pulmonary decortication that is often required in these situations may not be in the field of expertise of most clinicians performing thoracoscopies. Decortication using the VATS technique has been reported, although no details about the operative techniques have been given (Lewis, et al., 1992; Coltharp, et al., 1992; Mack, et al., 1992).

Results of Decortication

Operative Morbidity and Mortality

In most series the operative mortality varies between 0 and 5 percent. Major postoperative complications include sepsis from a residual empyema or from wound infection, bronchopleural fistula, or peripheral bronchoalveolar air leaks and hemorrhage. The incidence of these complications can be lessened by meticulous surgical technique with intraoperative control of air leaks and hemorrhage, achievement of optimal pulmonary reexpansion, and proper tube drainage. Diaphragmatic avulsion during decortication has been reported by Mayo and associates (1982). In patients with tuberculosis, dissemination of tuberculosis or development of tuberculous sinuses is uncommon if patients are given antituberculous drugs.

Functional Results

Reexpansion of the lung with obliteration of the space is almost always achieved if the underlying parenchyma is normal. This result is usually permanent and is accompanied by subjective improvement, particularly if decortication takes place early in the process of traumatic hemothorax or empyema (Villalba, et al., 1979; Morin, et al., 1972). In 1958 Samson, et al. reported the results of decortication for the pleural complications of pulmonary tuberculosis. Among 104 patients in whom decortication was the main operation, 4 (3.8 percent) died; 79 (77 percent) had a good to excellent result, with prompt pulmonary reexpansion, clear costophrenic sulcus, adequate motion of diaphragm and thoracic cage, and satisfactory improvement in pulmonary function; and 21 (20 percent) had a fair to poor result, due basically in nearly every case to prior disease involving fibrosis of the lung.

Although some authors have reported no or minimal improvement in individual cases (Wright, et al., 1949), decortication is usually followed by improved ventilation and increased lung volumes, measured as improvements in vital capacity, total lung capacity, and maximum breathing capacity. Partial recovery of normal pulmonary blood flow to the diseased side may also be seen (Morton, et al., 1970).

In 1952 Patton and colleagues reported the pulmonary function of 14 patients with unilateral constrictive disease, who were studied before and at intervals up to 3 years after surgical decortication. Restoration of function was closely related to the presence or absence of pre-existing disease, and there was a progressive gain in function during the entire period of observation. The ultimate gain in function was not influenced by the preoperative duration of collapse or by the presence or absence of infection in the pleural fluid, but it bore a close relationship to the amount of reexpansion seen in the chest films. Patients in whom visceral decortication was performed showed improvement comparable with that seen in patients who underwent complete visceral and parietal decortication (Patton, et al., 1952). Other investigators such as Barker and associates (1965) and Carroll, et al. (1951) have shown similar results, rises in vital capacity and maximum breathing capacity and improved oxygen uptake being observed postoperatively. Barker, et al. (1965) even documented apparent improvement in ventilatory function in the uninvolved lung following contralateral simple decortication. However, contrary to the data and opinion of Patton et al. (1952), several investigators have shown that the best results seen after decortication are obtained in patients with pleural disease of short duration (Morton, et al., 1970; Carroll, et al., 1951; Thomas and Jarvis, 1956). Long-term results of decortication in children with empyema showed no limitations of function at intervals of 12 to 18 years after the procedure (Mayo, et al., 1982).

Causes of Failure

Failure of decortication leads to recurrence of the empyema with or without bronchopleural fistula and to possible deterioration of pulmonary function. In all such cases, it is likely that further surgery will be required. The main causes of failure after decortication are listed below. They are numerous, but most are avoidable with adequate preoperative selection and meticulous surgical technique.

The importance of underlying parenchymal disease (Figs. 42-5 and 42-6), especially in cases of decortication performed for tuberculous pleural disease, has been well identified by Gurd (1947), who stated, "When it comes to applying the principles of decortication to typical pulmonary tuberculosis associated with a draining empyema of tuberculous or mixed infection, I would like to sound a note of warning. The prognosis depends chiefly on the extent and severity of the underlying intrapulmonary disease, and is frequently hopeless" (Fig. 42-7). Mulvihill and Klopstock (1948) also described a case of failure to reexpand due to marked fibrosis of the lung. In the 1952 series of Patton et al., patients with advanced

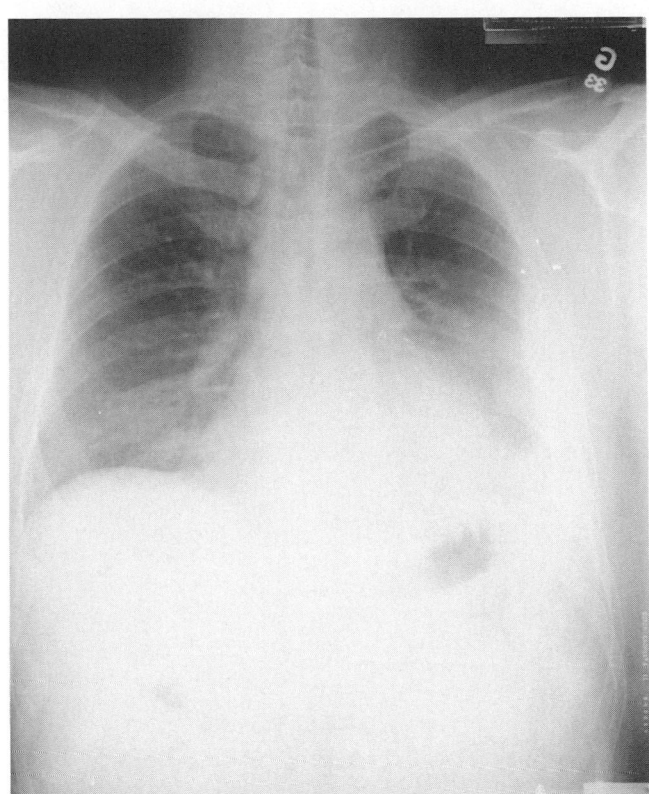

Figure 42-5. Fibrothorax. Standard PA chest radiograph showing an organized left-sided fibrothorax secondary to undrained pleural bleeding following aortocoronary bypass. Note the trapping of the left lung, which appears otherwise normal.

parenchymal disease had a maximum breathing capacity that was 6 percent less and a vital capacity 16 percent less than before decortication. By contrast, patients with little parenchymal disease ultimately showed a mean increase of 47 percent in maximum breathing capacity and a 31 percent increase in vital capacity.

The duration of lung collapse can also play a role in the failure of decortication, and it is generally acknowledged that decortication should be done at the earliest possible time. Several authors have nevertheless reported improvement in pulmonary function studies after decortication performed 10 years or more following lung collapse. In the case presented by Petty et al. (1961), there was improvement in both ventilation and perfusion of a tuberculous lung that had been collapsed for over 20 years.

Technical difficulties are probably the commonest cause of failure after decortication. Sometimes there is inflammatory thickening of the visceral pleura, which makes peel removal very difficult. This condition is likely to be seen in tuberculous lungs or in lungs that have been the site of pneumonic processes. In those cases there will be numerous sites of air leakage and of bleeding on the lung surface, which may compromise lung expansion. If this occurs, the lung must be decorticated very gently, all large tears must be repaired, and the lung must be fully mobilized from all adhesions so

---

Causes of Failure After Decortication

Underlying parenchymal disease
   Tuberculosis (active, fibrosis, bronchiectasis, bronchial stricture)
   Other parenchymal diseases limiting reexpansion
Long duration of lung collapse
Technical difficulties
   Difficulties in removing the peel
   Air leakage
   Poor reexpansion of the lung
   Inadequate postoperative space drainage
   Associated pulmonary resection
   Trauma to the phrenic nerve
Others
   Parietal peel not removed over the diaphragm and/or chest wall
   Postoperative complications

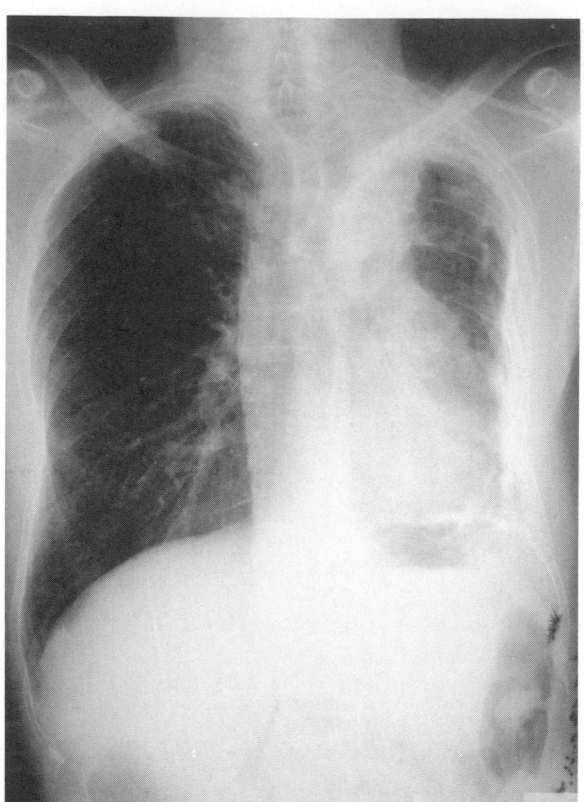

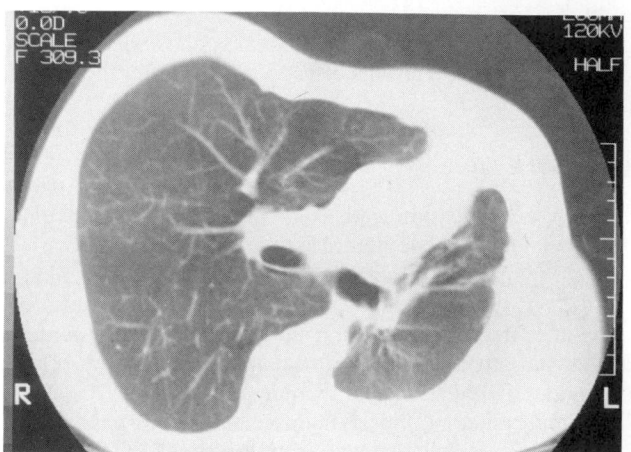

Figure 42-6. Severe fibrothorax with destroyed lung. **(A)** Chest radiograph and **(B)** CT scan of a patient with extensive postuberculous fibrothorax. Note that severe trapping of the left lung and the absence of peripheral blood vessels, indicative of low perfusion.

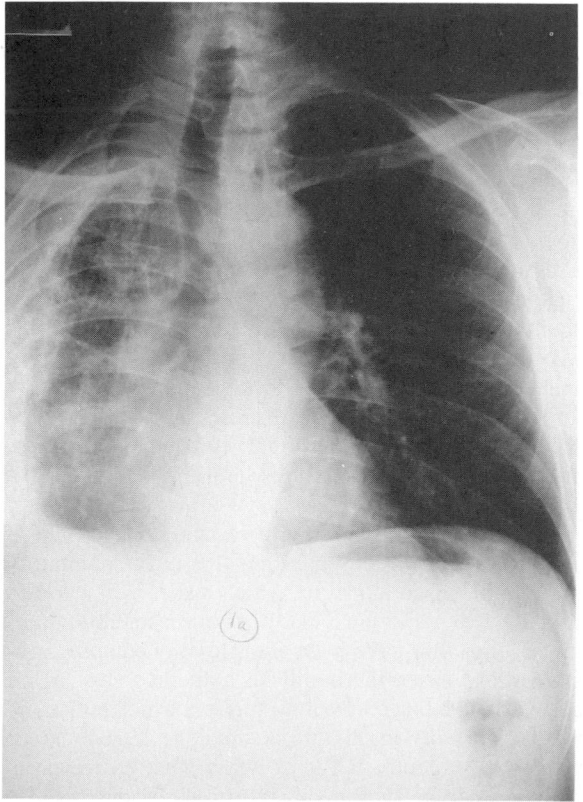

Figure 42-7. Standard PA chest radiograph of a patient with a markedly thickened and calcified pleural peel secondary to tuberculous pleurisy.

that it can reexpand. Bleeding from the surface of the lung is seldom a major problem, but if the lung does not reexpand or if the pleural space is inadequately drained, collections of fluid may occur in the space, with secondary formation of a new fibrothorax.

In all cases the phrenic nerve must be identified so that diaphragmatic function is presented. This is usually fairly easy because the mediastinum is nearly always free of adhesions. Associated pulmonary resections are also a cause of failure, not only because they indicate the presence of lung disease but also because they increase the magnitude of the procedure and reduce the amount of parenchyma available for space filling. In Okano and Walkup's series (1962), major

complications occurred in 35 percent of patients treated by combined decortication and pulmonary resection.

Other factors considered potential factors for failure of decortication are nonremoval of the parietal peel over the diaphragm and thoracic wall, which may impair the mechanics of breathing, and the occurrence of postoperative complications such as empyemas or bronchopleural fistulae. Okano and Walkup (1962) reported significant ventilatory functional improvement and no complications in most of their patients who underwent decortication. On the other hand, patients who had postoperative bronchopleural fistula and empyema requiring thoracoplasty had variable changes, and some had a diminution in function.

REFERENCES

Ackman FD, Madore P: Decortication preceding thoracoplasty for the elimination of long-standing tuberculous empyema. J Thorac Cardiovasc Surg 22:358, 1951

Ali I, Unruh H: Management of empyema thoracis. Ann Thorac Surg 50:355, 1990

Autio V: The reduction of respiratory function by parenchymal and pleural lesions: a broncho spirometric study of patients with unilateral involvement. Acta Tuberc Scand 37:112, 1959

Barker WL, Neuhaus H, Langston HT: Ventilatory improvement following decortication in pulmonary tuberculosis. Ann Thorac Surg 1:532, 1965

Beall AC, Crawford HW, DeBakey ME: Considerations in the management of acute traumatic hemothorax. J Thorac Cardiovasc Surg 52:353, 1966

Bolliger CT, de Kock MA: Influence of a fibrothorax on the flow volume curve. Respiration 54:197, 1988

Burford TH, Parker EF, Samon PC: Early decortication in the treatment of post-traumatic empyema. Ann Surg 122:163, 1945

Carroll D, McClement J, Himmelstein A, Cournand A: Pulmonary function following decortication of the lung. Am Rev Respir Dis 63:231, 1951

Coltharp WH, Arnold JH, Alford WC et al.: Videothoracoscopy: improved technique and expanded indications. Ann Thorac Surg 53:775, 1992

Culinear MM, Roc BB, Grimes OF: The early effective surgical approach to the treatment of traumatic hemothorax. J Thorac Cardiovasc Surg 38:780, 1959

Delorme E: Nouveau traitement des empyèmes chroniques. Gaz hop 67:94, 1894

Deslauriers J, Mehran RJ: Role of thoracoscopy in the diagnosis and management of pleural diseases. Semin Thorac Cardiovasc Surg 5:284, 1993

Dowd CN: Persistent thoracic sinus following empyema: a report of fifteen cases treated by decortication of lung and thoracoplasty. JAMA 53:1281, 1909

Drummond DS, Craig RH: Traumatic hemothorax: complications and management. Am Surg 33:403, 1967

Eggers C: Radical operation for chronic empyema. Ann Surg 77:327, 1923

Estlander JA: Sur la résection des Côtes dans l'empyème chronique. Rev Mens 8:885, 1897

Fairfax AJ, McNabb WR, Spiro SG: Chylothorax: a review of 18 cases. Thorax 41:880, 1986

Fishman VH, Ellertson DG: Early pleural decortication for thoracic empyema in immunosuppressed patients. J Thorac Cardiovasc Surg 74:537, 1977

Fowler GR: A case of thoracoplasty for removal of a large cicatricial fibrous growth from the interior of the chest, the result of an old empyema. Med Rec 44:838, 1893

Fraser RG Pare JA: Diagnosis of diseases of the Chest. Vol. 3. 2nd Ed. WB Saunders Philadelphia, 1979, p. 1780

Grossman GD: Fibrothorax. p. 305. In Cherniak RM (ed): Current Therapy of Respiratory Disease Vol. 3. BC Decker, Philadelphia, 1979

Guenter CA, Welch MH: Pleural Disease in Pulmonary Medicine. 2nd Ed., JB Lippincott, Philadelphia, 1982, p. 597

Gurd FB: Decortication in chronic empyema of tuberculous origin. J Thorac Cardiovasc Surg 16:587, 1947

Himmelstein A, Miscall L, Kirschner PA: Decortication in tuberculosis. Surg Clin North Am 28:1601, 1948

Hughes RL, Jensik RJ, Faber LP, Bliss K: Evaluation of unilateral decortication. Ann Thorac Surg 19:704, 1975

Hutter JA, Harari D, Braimbridge MV: The management of empyema thoracic by thoracoscopy and irrigation. Ann Thorac Surg 39:517, 1985

Ilioka S, Sawanura K, Mori T et al.: Surgical treatment of chronic empyema. A new one stage operation. J Thorac Cardiovasc Surg 90:179, 1985

Kosloke AM, Cartwright KC: The controversial role of decortication in the management of pediatric empyema. J Thorac Cardiovasc Surg 96:166, 1988

Langston AT, Barker WL, Graham AA: Pleural tuberculosis. J Thorac Cardiovasc Surg 54:511, 1967

Leroux BT, Mohlala ML, Odell JA, Whitton ID: Suppurative diseases of the lung and pleural space. I. Empyema, thoracic and lung abscess. Curr Probl Surg 23:27, 1986

Lewis RJ, Caccavale RJ, Sisler GE, Mackenzie JW: One hundred consecutive patients undergoing video-assisted thoracic operations. Ann Thorac Surg 54:421, 1992

Lilienthal H: Empyema. Exploration of the thorax with primary mobilization of the lung. Ann Surg 62:309, 1915

Lloyd S: The treatment of unresolved pneumonia. Sci Med Surg 1908, p. 1977

Lund FB: The advantages of the so called decortication of the lung in old empyema. JAMA 52:693, 1911

Mack MJ, Aronoff RJ, Acuff TE et al.: Present role of thoracoscopy in the diagnosis and treatment of diseases of the chest. Ann Thorac Surg 54:403, 1992

Mayo CH, Beckman EH: Visceral pleurectomy for chronic empyema. Am Surg 59:884, 1914

Mayo P: Early thoracotomy and decortication for nontuberculous empyema in adults with and without underlying disease. Am Surg 51:230, 1985

Mayo WP, Saha SP, McElvein RB: Diaphragmatic avulsion following decortication. Ala J Med Sci 19:81, 1982

Milfeld DJ, Mattox KL, Beall AC: Early evacuation of clotted hemothorax. Am J Surg 136:686, 1978

Morin JE, Munro DD, MacLean LD: Early thoracotomy for empyema. J Thorac Cardiovasc Surg 64:530, 1972

Morton JR, Boushy SF, Guinn GA: Physiological evaluation of results of pulmonary decortication. Ann Thorac Surg 4:321, 1970

Mulvihill DA, Klopstock R: Decortication of the nonexpandable post pneumothorax tuberculous lung. J Thorac Cardiovasc Surg 17:723, 1948

Okano T, Walkup HE: Chronic purulent tuberculous empyema and pulmonary tuberculosis treated by decortication and resections. J Thorac Cardiovasc Surg 43:752, 1962

O'Rourke P, O'Brien E, Tuttle W: Decortication of the lung in patients with pulmonary tuberculosis. Am Rev Respir Dis 59:30, 1949

Patton WE, Watson TR, Gaensler EA: Pulmonary function before and at intervals after surgical decortication of the lung. Surg Gynecol Obstet 95:477, 1952

Personne C: Role of early thoracotomy in the treatment of acute empyema. p. 225. In Deslauriers J, Lacquet LK, (eds): Trends in General Thoracic Surgery Vol. 6. Thoracic Surgery: Surgical Management of Pleural Diseases. CV Mosby, St. Louis, 1990

Petty TL, Filley GF, Mitchell RS: Objective functional improvement by decortication after twenty years of artificial pneumothorax for pulmonary tuberculosis. Report of a case and review of the literature. Am Rev Respir Dis 84:572, 1961

Ridley PD, Braimbridge MV: Thoracoscopic debridement and pleural irrigation in the management of empyema thoracis. Ann Thorac Surg 51:461, 1991

Robin ED, Cross CE, Kroetz F et al.: Pulmonary hypertension and unilateral pleural constriction with speculations on pulmonary vasoconstrictive substance. Arch Intern Med 118:391, 1966

Rudström P, Thoren L: Decortication of the lung. Acta Chir Scand 110:437, 1955

Samson PC: Some surgical considerations in pulmonary decortication. Am J Surg 89:364, 1955

Samson PC, Burford TH: Total pulmonary decortication. Its evolution and present concepts of indications and operative technique. J Thorac Cardiovasc Surg 16:127, 1947

Samson PC, Burford TH, Brewer LA, Burbank B: The management of war wounds of the chest in a base center. The role of early decortication. J Thorac Cardiovasc Surg 15:1, 1946

Samson PC, Merrill DL, Dugan DJ et al: Technical considerations in decortication for the pleural complications of pulmonary tuberculosis. J Thorac Surg Cardiovasc 36:431, 1958

Savage T, Fleming JA: Decortication of the lung in tuberculous disease. Thorax 10:293, 1955

Scannell JG: The captive lung: indication for and techniques of decortication. p. 421. In Deslauriers J, Lacquet LK (eds): Trends in General Thoracic Surgery. Vol. 6. Thoracic Surgery: Surgical Management of Pleural Diseases. CV Mosby, St. Louis, 1990

Schede M: Die Behandlung der Empyeme. Proc 9th Congr Intern Med, Wiesbaden 9:41, 1890

Shapiro DH, Anagnostopoulos CE, Dineen JP: Decortication and pleurectomy for the pleuropulmonary complications of pancreatitis. Ann Thorac Surg 9:76, 1970

Siebens AA, Storey CF, Newman MM et al.: The physiologic effects of fibrothorax and the functional results of surgical treatement. J Thorac Cardiovasc Surg 32:53, 1956

Sterling GM, Herbert A: Lung in cuirasse: restrictive pleurisy associated with asbestos exposure. Thorax 35:715, 1990

Thomas GI, Jarvis FJ: Decortication in primary tuberculous pleuritis and empyema with a study of functional recovery. J Thorac Cardiovasc Surg 32:178, 1956

Van Way C, Narrod J, Hopeman A: The role of early thoracotomy in the treatment of empyema. J Thorac Cardiovasc Surg 96:436, 1988

Villalba M, Lucas CE, Ledgerwood AM, Asfaw I: The etiology of post traumatic empyema and the role of decortication. J Trauma 19:414, 1979

Violet D: De la décortication pulmonaire dans l'empyème chronique. Arch Gen Med 81:657, 1904

Wachsmuth W, Schautz R: Untersuchungen über die Lungen—Pleura-Grenzschicht beider extrapleuralen Dekortikation. Chirurg 22:337, 1951

Waterman DH, Domm SE, Rogers WK: A clinical evaluation of decortication. J of Thorac Cardiovasc Surg 33:1, 1957

Weinberg J, Davis JD: Pleural decortication in pulmonary tuberculosis. Am Rev Respir Dis 60:288, 1949

Weinberg J, Horner JC, Davis JD: Decortication of the unexpanded tuberculous lung following induced pneumothorax. Surg Clin North Am 28:1591, 1948

Williams MH: The technique of pulmonary decortication and pleurolysis. J Thorac Cardiovasc Surg 20:652, 1950

Wilson JM, Boren CH, Peterson SR, Thomas AN: Traumatic hemothorax: is decortication necessary? J Thorac Cardiovasc Surg 77:489, 1979

Wright GW, Yee LB, Filley GF, Stranaham A: Physiologic observations concerning decortication of the lung. J Thorac Cardiovasc Surg 18:372, 1949

Young D, Simon J, Pomerantz M: Current indications for and status of decortication for "trapped lung." Ann Thorac Surg 14:631, 1972

Zenker R, Heberer G, Lohr H: Die Lungenresektionen. Springer-Verlag, Berlin 1954, p.200

43

SURGICAL TECHNIQUES

Closed Drainage and Suction Systems

Jocelyn Grégoire
Jean Deslauriers

The first attempts to drain the pleural space with a tube are credited to Playfair (1875) and Hewett (1876), who both reported, over a century ago, on an underwater seal drainage system for the management of empyemas. Since then the concepts of pleural space drainage have evolved considerably, not only because of a better understanding of pleural space physiology but also because of improved technology and changing needs of physicians.

Despite the claim of many manufacturers, no currently available thoracic drainage system is ideal. Each available system has desirable features, but each also has deficiencies. Two features are, however, particularly important for surgeons: (1) the system must meet the physiologic and therapeutic needs of the patient and (2) its design must be straightforward so that its functioning can be thoroughly understood by the entire surgical team.

HISTORICAL NOTE

Although Hippocrates (Hutchins, 1952) may have been the first to consider drainage of the pleural space when he described incisions, cautery, and metal tubes to drain empyemas (Miller and Sahn, 1987), the concept of closed pleural drainage originated in England in the 1870s. In 1891 Bülau (Fig. 43-1) also described a method of siphon drainage for the management of empyemas. According to his understanding of pleural mechanics and physiology, this method was safer and less complicated than the more radical and then more popular procedure involving resection of the overlying ribs and open drainage of the space. In his original paper, written in German and reported by Meyer (1989), Bülau wrote: "I have always believed that the principal advantage of siphon-drainage is that it lowers the pressure within the pleural space, thereby bringing about re-expansion of the lung."

The importance of closed-tube drainage of empyemas was not recognized until the release of a 1918 survey by the Surgeon General of the U.S. Army, which reported mortality rates for rib resection and open drainage of empyemas to be averaging 30 percent (Graham and Bell, 1918). Because of the creation of an open pneumothorax, death frequently occurred within one-half hour of the operation (Churchill, 1958). The surgeon general appointed the Empyema Commission, headed by Major Evarts A. Graham, which recommended closed drainage in the early stages of empyema. Immediately after adoption of these changes, the mortality of empyema drainage decreased to approximately 3 percent.

The use of chest tubes in postoperative thoracic care was reported by Lilienthal in 1922 and Brunn in 1929. Today, tube thoracostomy is an integral part of treatment for a variety of pleural disorders.

HISTORICAL READINGS

Brunn H: Surgical principles underlying one-stage lobectomy. Arch Surg 18:490, 1929

Bülau G: Für die Heber-Drainage bei Behandlung des Empyems. Z Klin Med 18:31, 1891

Churchill ED: Wound surgery encounters a dilemma. J Thorac Surg 35:279:1958

Graham EA, Bell RD: Open pneumothorax: its relation to the treatment of empyema. Am J Med Sci 156:839, 1918

Hewett CF: Thoracentesis: the plan of continuous aspiration. Br Med J 1:317, 1876

Hippocrates: Writings. p. 142. In Hutchins RA (ed): Great Books

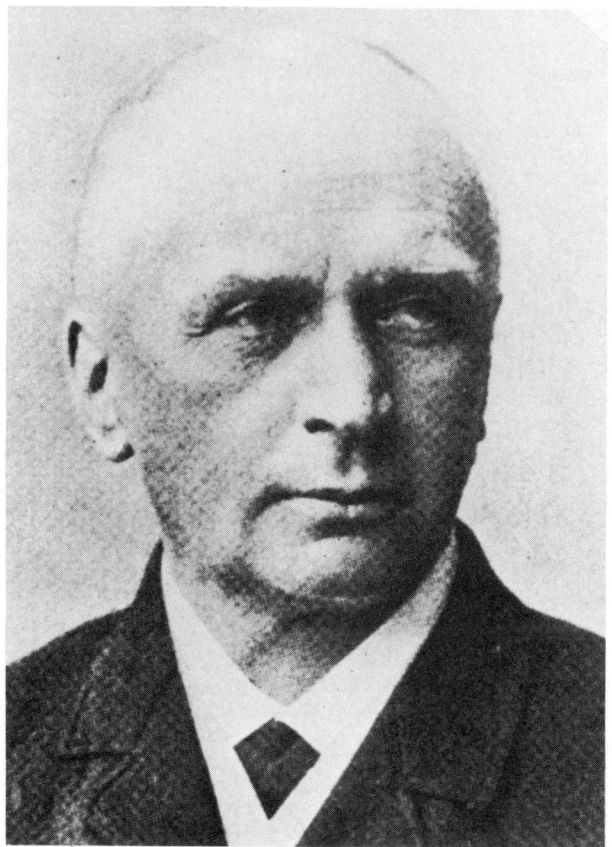

Figure 43-1. Gotthard Bülau (1836–1900) of Hamburg, Germany, originator of the method of closed water-seal drainage of the chest. (From Nissen R, Wilson RHL: Pages in the history of Chest Surgery. Charles C Thomas, Springfield, IL 1960, with permission.)

of the Western World. Vol. 29. Encyclopedia Britannica, Chicago, 1952

Lilienthal H: Resection of the lung for suppurative infections with a report based on 31 consecutive operative cases in which resection was done or intended. Ann Surg 75:257, 1922

Meyer JA: Gotthard Bülau and closed water-seal drainage for empyema, 1875–1891. Ann Thorac Surg 48:597, 1989

Playfair GE: Case of empyema treated by aspiration and subsequently by drainage: recovery. Br Med J 1:45, 1875

INDICATIONS AND CONTRAINDICATIONS FOR CHEST TUBES

Physiology of the Pleural Space

The pleura is a thin and slippery membrane originating from the internal coelom. The parietal segment completely lines the inner surfaces of the ribs, diaphragm, and mediastinum, while the visceral pleura, in continuity with the parietal pleural, begins at the pulmonary hilum and covers all lung surfaces, including the fissures. The two pleural leaflets are separated by a virtual space containing 5 to 15 ml of lubricating fluid. This arrangement provides a smooth and efficient mechanical coupling between the lung, a passive elastic structure, and the chest wall, a dynamic structure activated by respiratory muscles. There are no communications between the left and right pleural spaces.

During quiet breathing, the elastic forces of the lung and chest wall pull in opposite directions, thereby creating a negative intrapleural pressure, which keeps the two pleural surfaces apposed and the lung expanded. In patients with abnormal accumulations of air, blood, or other fluids in the pleural space, the negative pressure is lost and the lung recoils inward, causing hypoxemia and alveolar hypoventilation. Ultimately, this pressure buildup can be large enough to displace the mediastinum to the other side and compromise both the ventilation of the opposite lung and the venous return.

The purpose of thoracic drainage is to promote air or fluid evacuation, lung reexpansion, and restoration of intrapleural negative pressure. Because air has a low density, it tends to accumulate in the upper half of the pleural space, while fluids with a higher density tend to collect in the lower half, inferiorly in the sitting position and posteriorly in the supine position.

Indications for Tube Drainage

In patients with spontaneous pneumothorax, tube drainage is the treatment of choice, not only because it allows for rapid evacuation of air but also because it helps to reexpand the lung. Both tension pneumothorax and open pneumothorax are immediately life-threatening conditions and require emergency pleural drainage. In blunt trauma, pneumothoraces are often the consequence of a fractured rib puncturing the underlying lung, and these pneumothoraces should be drained unless they are small, asymptomatic, and nonprogressive. Most iatrogenic pneumothoraces are secondary to central venous access (Dalbec and Krome, 1986; Herbst, 1978), and they should also be drained. The same policy

---

Indications for Tube Drainage

Pneumothorax
    Spontaneous (primary, secondary)
    Open pneumothorax
    Tension pneumothorax
    Traumatic
    Iatrogenic
        Central venous access procedure
        Thoracentesis, pleural biopsy
        Needle biopsy of lung
        Positive-pressure ventilation

Hemothorax

Empyema
    Parapneumonic effusion
    Frank empyemas

Pleural effusion

Chylothorax

Postoperative drainage
    Thoracic procedures
    Cardiac surgery

applies to patients who develop a pneumothorax while receiving mechanical ventilation. The use of prophylactic tube thoracostomy during administration of positive end-expiratory pressure (PEEP) or continuous positive-pressure breathing is controversial at present (Hayes and Lucas, 1976).

In general, patients with traumatic hemothoraces should have a chest tube to monitor the rate of bleeding, reexpand the lung, and prevent chronic lung entrapment and late empyema. The general issue of how to treat parapneumonic effusions is controversial (Deslauriers, et al., 1987). Light (1985) recommends drainage of parapneumonic effusions when the pleural fluid has a pH below 7.00, a glucose level below 40 mg/dl, or a lactate dehydrogenase (LDH) level above 1,000 units/L, but many surgeons believe that the only absolute indication for tube drainage is the positive identification of bacteria in the effusion. Frank empyemas always require tube drainage whether the tube is inserted under local anesthesia or during thoracoscopy.

Malignant pleural effusions should be drained if they are recurrent and symptomatic or if sclerotherapy is contemplated. Chylothoraces should nearly always be drained. A thoracostomy tube should always be left in the pleural space after any intrathoracic procedure regardless of its magnitude (Watkins, 1961). This is even more important following partial lung resection, which requires air and fluid to be properly evacuated in order to achieve lung reexpansion and sealing of peripheral air leaks. After pulmonary surgery, pleural drainage is also helpful to avoid such complications as bronchopleural fistulae and empyemas (Storey, 1968). After a lobectomy or a lesser pulmonary resection, a single chest tube is usually sufficient to drain the space, but two tubes, one anterior at the apex and one posterior at the base, may be necessary if excessive air leakage or bleeding is anticipated.

Contraindications to Tube Drainage

There are virtually no contraindications to tube drainage although one has to be cautious while inserting a chest tube in a patient with a bleeding disorder or in a patient receiving anticoagulants. The presence of pleural adhesions may sometimes complicate the procedure, and the drainage of multiloculated effusions often requires precise preoperative localization of the collections. Hepatic hydrothorax is a relative contraindication to tube drainage because continuous evacuation of the effusion may lead to massive protein and electrolyte depletion and ultimately to the death of the patient (Runyon, et al., 1986).

TUBE THORACOSTOMY

Chest Tube Sizes

Most chest tubes currently used in North America are made of transparent plastic (Silastic). They have multiple side holes, a radiopaque stripe, and outer diameters ranging from 6 Fr (pediatric) to 40 Fr. As pointed out by Couraud et al., (1990), these tubes are firm but yet pliable. They induce minimal skin or pleural reaction, and they are inexpensive.

Rubber tubes are used only by a handful of surgeons and for the sole purpose of postoperative drainage. There is no clear evidence that the material of a chest tube (rubber or Silastic) has any impact on the recurrence rate of spontaneous pneumothoraces, although Hood and colleagues (1966) have demonstrated a relative lack of tissue reaction associated with polyvinyl as compared with rubber tubes. They suggested that this lack of tissue reaction may reduce pleural surface adhesions and prolong air leaks.

Foley catheters can be used for thoracic drainage, but they have a relatively small lumen and are not radiopaque (Lawrence, 1983). They have, however, the advantage of permitting withdrawal to the inner chest wall, where a partially inflated balloon restrains them from further removal. Tinckler (1976) has also described a self-retaining chest drainage tube that uses an inflatable balloon.

In patients with pneumothoraces, smaller tubes directed toward the lung apex are sufficient to evacuate air from the pleural space. For patients with hemothoraces, malignant effusions, or empyemas, larger tubes (28 to 40 Fr) are preferred because the hemorrhagic fluid or the intense fibrinous reaction tends to occlude smaller-diameter tubes (Deslauriers, 1990). When the tube is occluded, saline irrigation may solve the problem temporarily, but one has to keep in mind that each irrigation increases the risk of contaminating the pleural space.

Chest Tube Insertion

Preoperative Management

A complete history and physical examination should always be done prior to tube thoracostomy. Chest radiographs, computed tomography (CT) scans and ultrasound, if available, should also be reviewed and the exact site of the collection well documented. In cases of pleural effusion, the results of thoracentesis should be available and the exact nature of the effusion known prior to tube drainage. Indeed, some of these effusions may not require drainage at all.

Patients should be informed not only about the indication for tube thoracostomy but also about the technique of tube insertion. Fearful and anxious patients often anticipate this apparently simple operation, a feature that may complicate immensely the procedure.

Insertion Site

For closed thoracostomy, whether for the drainage of a pneumothorax or of pleural fluid, the ideal site of tube insertion is the third or fourth intercostal space in the anterior or midaxillary line immediately behind the pectoralis major fold (Kovarik and Brown, 1969) (Fig. 43-2). In this location the scar is hardly visible, and the technique of tube insertion is easier because there are no muscles other than the intercostals to traverse. If, in addition, the tube has to be left in the pleural space for any length of time, it is more comfortable and less restrictive for such activities as eating, sleeping, or chest physiotherapy. Finally, proper positioning at the apex is easier when the drain is inserted from the axilla because of its natural tendency to slide upward along the curve of the lateral chest wall (Fig. 43-3). The only exception to axillary tube insertion occurs with drainage of loculated pleural

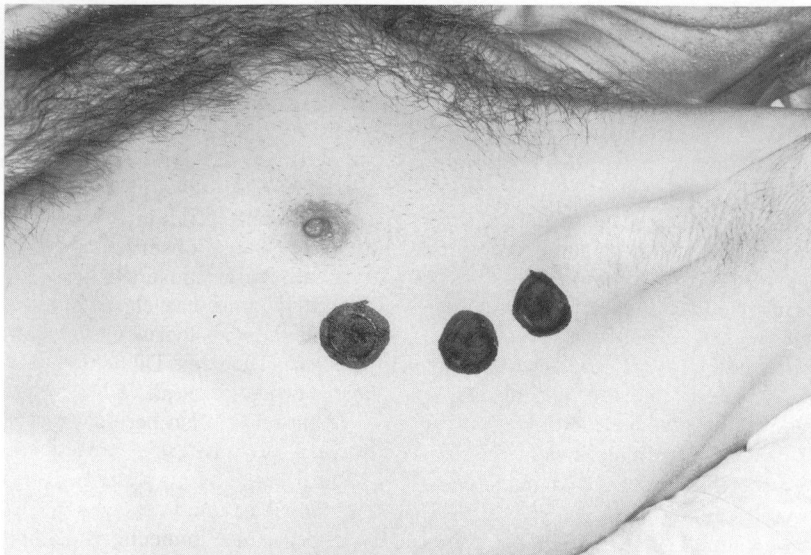

Figure 43-2. The ideal site of tube insertion is the anterior or midaxillary line behind the pectoralis major fold. The dots shown on this picture are acceptable locations for chest tube placement.

fluid, in which situation the chest tube has to be inserted in a specific location as shown by chest films and ultrasound.

The second interspace in the midclavicular line is often mentioned (Miller and Sahn, 1987; Richards, 1978) but seldom used because chest tube placement in this position ne-

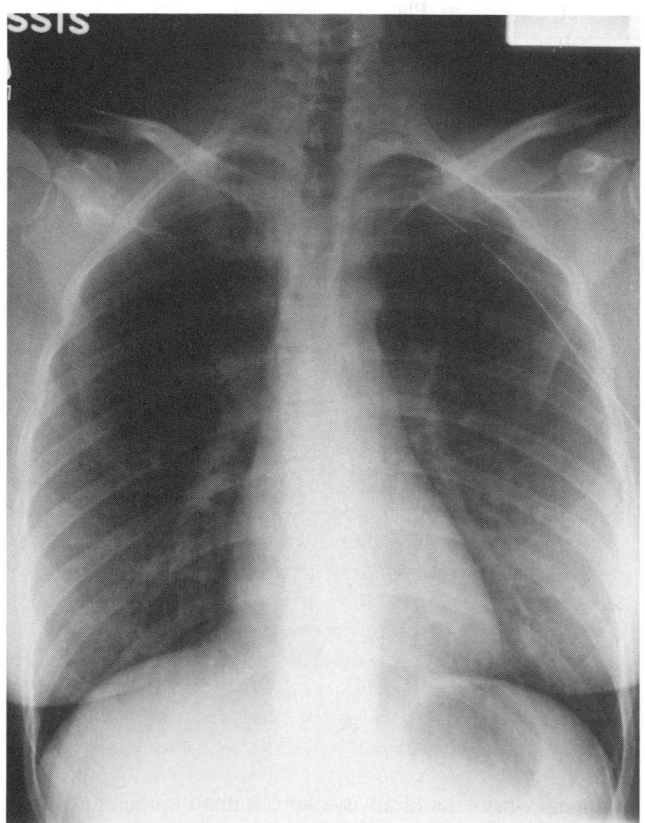

Figure 43-3. Chest radiograph showing a well-positioned tube at the apex.

cessitates dissection through the pectoralis muscle and leaves a highly visible scar. Posterior apical tube placement with an incision in the second or third intercostal space medial to the inner border of the scapula has also been suggested (Aslam, 1970). Again, this is hardly ever indicated because of the difficulties in inserting the tube and unnecessary pain to the patient who must lie on it.

Insertion Technique

Chest tubes are usually inserted under local anesthesia after proper cleansing of the skin with an antiseptic solution. The parietal pleura should be infiltrated generously and aspiration of air or fluid through a needle and syringe is used to confirm the proper location of the drainage site. A 2-cm incision is then made in the interspace, and to avoid injury to the neurovascular bundle, blunt dissection is carried out over the superior border of the rib. It is generally recommended to make the skin incision one space below the interspace to be used, so that an upward diagonal tunnel can be created. This arrangement will provide a better seal when the tube is removed.

Chest tubes can be inserted by the trocar method or by the technique of blunt dissection. The trocar is a sharp-tipped metal rod used to guide the chest tube through the chest wall and parietal pleura. The technique is simple, but since the trocar has to be introduced forcefully into the pleural space, it involves the risk of injuring the underlying lung and/or any other intrathoracic structure. Trocar insertion should be reserved for patients with a large space, although Neptune (1977) and others have found the trocar, when correctly used, to be an efficient, safe, and practical means of inserting a chest tube in the management of spontaneous pneumothorax.

We prefer and recommend blunt dissection of a tunnel through intercostal muscles and parietal pleura with a curved Kelly clamp (Fig. 43-4). With this technique the pleural space can first be inspected with the index finger and the tube then simply advanced in its proper position. The tube is secured and held in place with a skin suture.

In order to facilitate tube insertion with a Kelly hemostat, Ring and Shapiro (1989) and others (Davis, 1987) advocate the use of a tunnel-tip catheter (Fig. 43-5). With this technique there is less dissection of the muscles of the chest wall, and the tip of the tube passes much more easily through the tissues and muscles into the pleural space. Ring and Shapiro (1989) have also observed that there is less air leakage around the catheter because the thoracostomy tract is not as large as with regular catheters. Tunnel-tip thoracic catheters are available (from Sherwood Medical, St. Louis) in straight and right-angled forms. Dilators (Thal and Quick, 1988) and guide wires (Guyton, et al., 1988; Semrad, 1988) to facilitate tube insertion have also been described.

Characteristics of Connecting Tubing

The best tube connectors are made of plastic with serrated ends. It is most important that these connectors have a large internal diameter ($\frac{1}{4}$ inch) and that their ends not be tapered so that the flow of hemorrhagic fluids is not impaired. When more than one chest tube is required, the tubes can be connected to the same unit through a Y connector. Taping the ends of the connector to the connecting tubing does not ensure air tightness but only aids in preventing accidental separation at the site (Miller and Sahn, 1987).

Connecting tubes are made either of clear plastic or of latex. They usually are 5 to 6 feet long with an internal diameter of 12 mm. Plastic tubes have the advantage of water-clear transparency so that the fluctuation of fluid can easily be observed. With Latex tubing, samples of fluid can be directly obtained from the tube through a #18 or 20 needle.

When selecting the size of chest tubes, connectors, and tubing, gas and fluid dynamics must be considered. Batchelder and Morris (1962), in a study of critical factors determining adequate pleural drainage, have shown that gas moving through tubing displays laminar flow and obeys Poiseuille's equation $\dot{V} = \pi r^4 P/8lv$ where $\dot{V}$ is the volume flow rate, l is the length of the tube, v is the viscosity, r is the tube's internal radius, and P is the pressure drop. In this equation the volume of gas in laminar flow through the tube is inversely related to the length of the tube and directly proportional to the fourth power of its radius. Tubes with an internal diameter of $\frac{1}{4}$ inch (6 mm) allow a minimum flow rate of 15 L of air per minute while tubes of $\frac{1}{2}$ inch internal diameter are capable of handling flows of 50 to 60 L/min.

It has also been shown by Swenson and Birath (1957) that moist air has turbulent flow characteristics, which are expressed by the Fanning equation for turbulent flow $v = \pi^2 r^5 P/f\,l$, where f is a friction factor. In this relation the flow rate is proportional to an even higher power of the radius of the lumen.

Tube Management

A chest x-ray should always be obtained immediately after tube insertion so that lung reexpansion and tube position can be assessed. Stark and colleagues (1983) have shown that sometimes both frontal and lateral radiographs are necessary

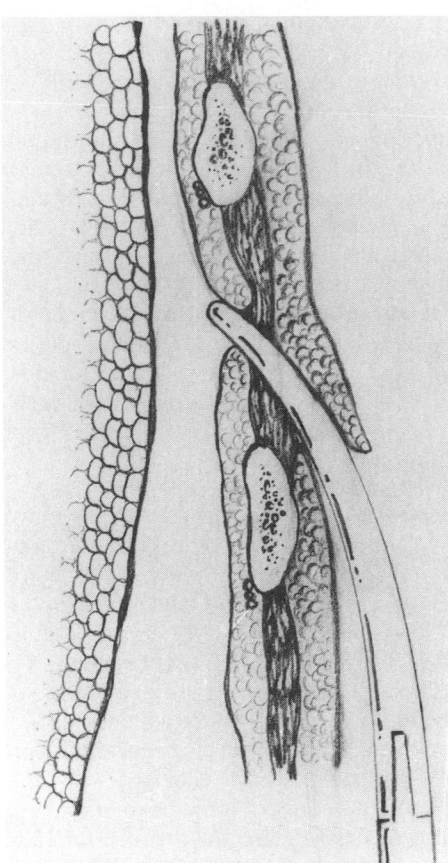

Figure 43-4. Blunt dissection through intercostal muscles with a curved Kelly clamp. Note the upward diagonal tunnel and the dissection, which is carried out over the superior border of the rib.

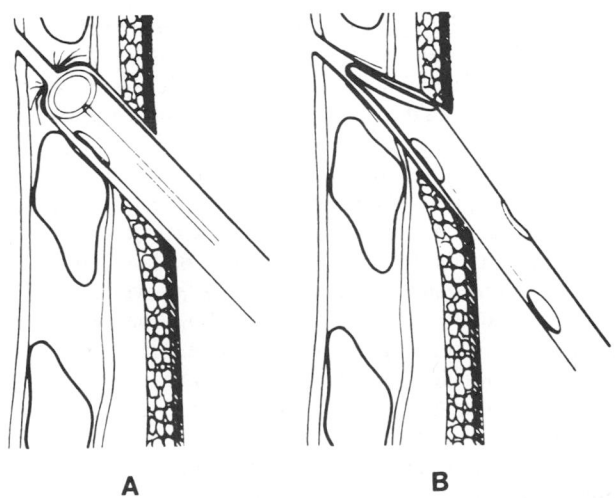

A   B

Figure 43-5. Tube thoracostomy facilitated by using **(B)** a tunnel-tip rather than **(A)** a blunt-tip chest tube. (From Ring EM, Shapiro MJ: The tunnel tip thoracic catheter. Surg Gynecol Obstet 169:553, 1989, with permission.)

Tube Management

Monitoring
  Early and daily chest radiographs
  Nature and volume of air leak and fluid drainage
Clamping of the chest tube
Functional status of the tube
Maintenance of patency
  Milking and stripping
  Irrigation
Airtightness of the system

---

to evaluate thoracostomy tube placement. In their study eight of nine malpositioned chest tubes were only documented on a lateral film. Placement of a chest tube in a lung fissure, for example, can result in inadequate drainage (Maurer, et al., 1982; Webb and Laberge, 1983). Daily chest x-rays and careful monitoring of the nature and volume of fluid drainage are recommended until after the tube has been removed.

Drainage tubes should not be allowed to hang as dependent loops because fluids and clots accumulating in the tubing will increase the resistance of the system. They should almost never be clamped, although Munnell and Thomas (1975), in a survey of 328 thoracic surgeons, have shown that close to 75 percent of experienced thoracic surgeons did in fact clamp tubes at some time during the postoperative period. Chest tubes were clamped for transportation of patients (35 percent), to rule out an air leak (21 percent), to drain a bottle or connecting tube (18 percent), or for patients in whom a tube was used following pneumonectomy (7 percent). Clamping during patient transportation, especially if the patient has an air leak, can be catastrophic because of potential lung collapse, subcutaneous emphysema, or tension pneumothorax. If a chest tube becomes accidentally disconnected from the drainage system, it should simply be reconnected without clamping it before (Morgan and Orcutt, 1972).

When the functional status of a tube is in question, observation of fluid oscillation in the water seal or in the tubing is important. Oscillations that are synchronous with respiratory movements indicate tube patency. If there are no oscillations, the tube may be obstructed, while increased oscillations suggest high negative intrapleural pressures, often associated with atelectasis or incomplete lung reexpansion.

Whether or not a chest tube should be milked or stripped to dislodge clots and debris and maintain patency is a question of controversy (Lim-Levy, et al., 1986). By milking or stripping a chest tube, clots, which may have been attached to the sides of the tube, are mechanically pressed toward the collecting chamber or back into the pleural space (Von Hippel, 1970). In a study done after open heart surgery, Lim-Levy, et al. (1986) showed that chest tubes remained patent with or without milking or stripping. Duncan and Erickson (1982) have also shown that by stripping the entire length of the chest tube, negative intrapleural pressures exceeding 400 cmH_2O can be obtained. Whether these high pressures can cause injury to the lung or to other intrathoracic structures is unknown.

If the system becomes occluded, some authors have suggested use of saline (Miller and Sahn, 1987) or even of fibrinolytic agents (Miller, et al., 1951) to irrigate the tube. Others have suggested the use of a sterile suction catheter introduced into the chest tube through a sterile cap (Halejian, et al., 1988). We do not recommend these procedures because each manipulation increases the risk of contaminating the pleural space.

If air tightness is in question, the unit should be checked by sequentially clamping each of its components while leaving the tube under suction. This will allow for identification of the site of air entry and correction of the problem.

Tube Removal

Chest tubes can be removed when there is no longer a fluctuation in the fluid column of the tube, indicating complete lung reexpansion or tube occlusion, when daily fluid drainage is minimal (<100 ml in 24 hours), and when the air leak has stopped. The proper timing of tube removal is subject to some controversy. Sharma, et al. (1988), for example, showed that in 40 patients subjected to tube thoracostomy for spontaneous pneumothorax, removal of the tube within 6 hours of reexpansion led to recollapse of the lung in 25 percent of cases. None of the patients suffered recollapse when the tube was withdrawn after 48 hours of lung reexpansion.

Most surgeons favor clamping the tube for 12 to 24 hours before removal (Munnell and Thomas, 1975) because clamping allows for identification of a persistent air leak or reaccumulation of fluid. So and Yu (1982) also believe that once the lung has reexpanded and there is no more air leak, the catheter should be clamped for 24 hours before being removed. Clamping before removal may be more important if an air leak has persisted over several days.

Although some authors have suggested that the tube should be removed at end expiration (Miller, 1987) or when performing a Valsava maneuver (Roe, 1965), we believe that it should be at end inspiration. This is based on the observation that patients experiencing an acute pain—like that which may occur on tube removal (Gift, et al., 1991)—tend to inhale rather than exhale, thereby increasing the chances of air entry at the drainage site.

Several techniques can be used to seal the thoracotomy incision at the time of tube removal. Probably the most common method used is the tying down of a U stitch across the wound as the tube is withdrawn. Other methods involve the use of vaseline gauze, skin staples, or adhesive to cover the wound (Lo and Mirza, 1984; Prats, 1990). Whatever method is preferred, the incision should be sealed rapidly in order to prevent any air entry into the pleural space.

A chest radiograph should be obtained 12 to 24 hours after tube removal for observation of possible reaccumulation of air or fluid in the pleural space. Panicek, et al. (1987) and Gilsanz and Cleveland (1978) have shown that chest tube tracks, which are parallel lines corresponding to the prior position of the tube, may persist for some time after the tube is removed. These lines, which represent local pleural

---

Pleural Space Drainage Systems

Passive drainage systems
   Commercially available one-way flutter valves
     (Heimlich valves)
   Homemade emergency one-way valves
   Underwater seal units
     One-bottle units
     Two-bottle units
Active drainage systems
   Three-bottle units
     Homemade systems
     Disposable and commercially available units
   Units with mechanical manometers (dry suction)
   High-pressure systems
Balanced drainage system
   Drainage of the pneumonectomy space
   Drainage following repair of diaphragmatic hernia
Pleuroperitoneal shunt

---

thickening due to the proliferation of mesothelial cells and deposition of fibrin along the course of the tube, have no clinical significance.

DRAINAGE SYSTEMS

Passive Drainage Systems

Passive drainage systems (Couraud, et al., 1990) provide one-way drainage that allows the outflow of gas and/or fluid during expiration but prevents their return into the pleural space during inspiration. These systems are simple and often sufficient to evacuate the pleural space because the slightly positive pressure that prevails during expiration or cough will force out both air and fluid (Von Hippel, 1970, 1975).

The most basic of these drainage systems is the one-way flutter valve (Heimlich, 1968), a device particularly useful in emergency situations or for drainage of uncomplicated pneumothoraces (Fig. 43-6). This flutter valve consists of a piece of rubber tubing, one end of which is compressed and retains its flattened shape. It allows fluid and air to flow out of the chest while preventing their reflux back into the pleural cavity. Mercier, et al. (1976) have shown that outpatient management of individuals with spontaneous pneumothoraces through the use of a flutter valve is safe, efficient, and

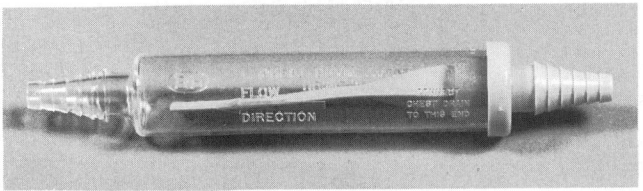

Figure 43-6. Heimlich one-way flutter valve.

economical. If one of these commercially made valves is not available, a homemade system can be fashioned by attaching a surgical glove to the end of the chest tube and puncturing the extremity of one of its fingers. One possible complication of the Heimlich valve is due to improper attachment of the valve to the chest tube. In the two cases reported by Maimimi and Johnson (1990), the valve was inadvertently attached backward, and this resulted in a tension pneumothorax.

With the underwater seal drainage system, water acts as a seal to prevent air from going back up the drain during inspiration. Drainage by means of a single bottle is the simplest of all systems, this single bottle serving as both the collection chamber and the water seal. Drainage is effected by connecting the end of the tubing to a long plastic or glass tube, which reaches the bottom of the bottle containing water to a height of 4 to 5 cm. The extremity of the tube must be at a point below the water level and the bottle itself must be located below the patient's chest in order for the pleural fluid to drain by gravity. Thus, this system employs both the mechanics of respiration (positive expiratory pressure) and gravity to bring about drainage. As air and/or fluids are evacuated, the pleural surfaces are brought together and the intrapleural pressure becomes again negative. A vent is used for the escape of air from the drainage bottle into the atmosphere.

The use of the one-bottle underwater seal drainage unit may be limited, however, by the mounting level of fluid in the bottle, which imposes an increased resistance to drainage. In addition, the foamy drainage that results from the mixing of air and blood in the same bottle may be difficult to measure. To circumvent these problems, a two-bottle system can be fashioned by interposing a collection bottle, which traps fluids and passes air onward, between the patient and the underwater seal bottle. Although this system allows for easier inspection and quantification of drainage, a potential drawback is the additional volume of tubing and dead space, which may sometimes allow reversal of air flow during inspiration (air may flow back into the pleural space).

Active Drainage Systems

Active drainage by the use of continuous suction (Roe, 1958; Pickard and Beall, 1983; Enerson and McIntyre, 1966) is often necessary to achieve and maintain complete reexpansion of the lung and apposition of the visceral and parietal pleural surfaces. This is particularly important when the amount of air leakage exceeds the underwater seal capacity of the system or when the underlying lung is noncompliant and is generating high negative intrapleural pressures exceeding the maximum negative pressure of the unit. Most authors recommend active suction with negative pressures in the neighborhood of -20 cmH$_2$O. Others such as Pecora and Cooper (1981) and Storey (1968), recommend use of higher negative pressures, especially for drainage after thoracotomy.

An ideal active drainage system must be able to evacuate efficiently and thoroughly the contents of the pleural space, whether these are fluids, clots, pus, or air. It must not limit air flow and must be able to reach constant negative suction pressures in the vicinity of -60 cmH$_2$O. It must be compact, unbreakable, easy to set up and use, failsafe in operation, and easy for any member of the management team to understand. It must also have a collection chamber that can be readily emptied. Insofar as possible, active drainage units must also be inexpensive.

Three-Bottle Units

To provide active suction, a third bottle, used for suction control, can be added to the two-bottle water-seal drainage system (Sweet, 1954) (Fig. 43-7). When a built-in wall suction is used for vacuum (unregulated vacuum), this third bottle regulates the amount of suction applied through the entire system. If the vacuum is higher than the desired level of negative pressure (the depth of a central vent below the water level determines the amount of negative pressure), air is drawn from the atmosphere. Bubbling in the suction control bottle indicates that the suction source is applying the right amount of negative pressure, usually -15 to $-20 \text{ cmH}_2\text{O}$. The advantage of the three-bottle units resides in their safety because negative pressures greater than -15 to $-20 \text{ cmH}_2\text{O}$ can never be reached, a feature that may be important if a large bronchopleural fistula develops. The main deficiency of these units is that they may provide inadequate air flow in the event of a large air leak. Additional negative pressure can be added to the three-bottle unit by having a higher column of water in the third bottle, by using mercury instead of water in the suction control bottle (McGrath and Kruger, 1962), or by adding a fourth bottle to the system (Julian and Pennel, 1987). These higher negative pressures are, however, seldom required in a normal thoracic surgical setting.

Disposable units using the same three-bottle suction drainage principles are now used in most institutions. These units are compact, light, and easy to assemble and operate. All are advertised as the ideal system, and each unit is alleged to be superior to the next one. Most have safety devices and/or other components often considered useful by the manufacturer but unnecessary by the surgeon. In fact, some of these devices can make the system so complicated that its functioning is difficult for the surgeon, let alone the staff, to understand. All are relatively expensive.

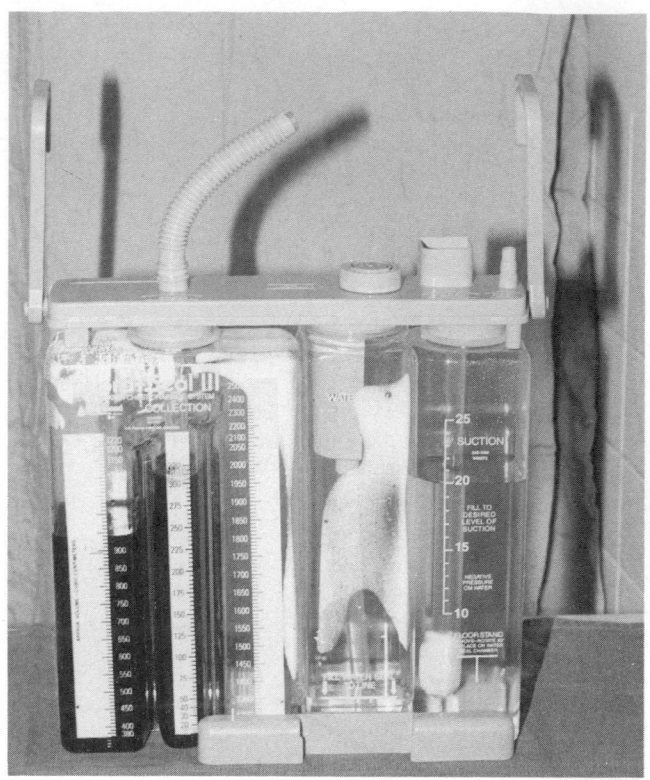

Figure 43-8. Sherwood Medical Thora-Seal III.

Disposable plastic units that duplicate the three-bottle drainage system include the Atrium compact (Atrium Medical Corp., Hollis, NH), the Decknatel Pleur-Evac (Decknatel Inc., Queens Village, NY), the Sherwood Medical Thora-Seal III (Sherwood Medical, St. Louis) (Fig. 43-8), and the Argyle Sentinel Seal (Davol Inc., Cranston, RI). All these disposable plastic units have a collection chamber, a water seal, and a suction control bottle. The Thora-Seal III also has a separate collection bottle (2,500 ml), which can be replaced when required. Most manufacturers include an op-

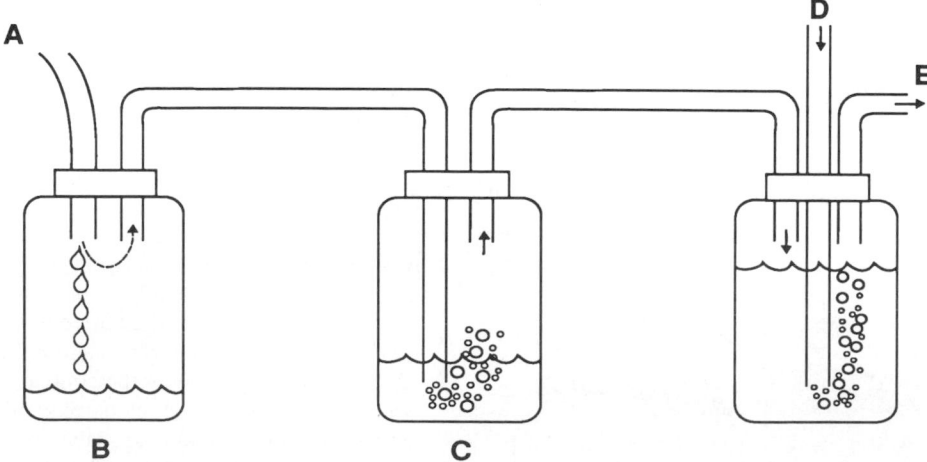

Figure 43-7. Three-bottle water-seal unit, in which the third bottle is used to regulate the amount of suction applied through the entire system (A) from the patient, (B) collecting bottle, (C) water-seal, (D) vent tube, (E) to wall suction.

tional attached container, so that blood drained from the pleural space can be salvaged for autotransfusion.

Dry Mechanical Suction Systems

New drainage units with mechanical manometers are now commercially available. Instead of a third bottle to maintain a constant level of suction, these units have a mechanical suction regulator, which allows for changes in suction level without adding or removing water. In the Decknatel Pleur-Evac unit (Decknatel Inc., Queens Village, NY), the desired level of suction can be reached by adjusting the suction source until the fluorescent indicator appears in the window on the face of the unit (Decknatel advertisement). With this system, higher negative pressures (up to -40 cmH$_2$O) can be safely applied to the system and to the pleural space.

The Thora-Klex chest drainage system (Davol Inc., Cranston, RI) has a rubber diaphragm flutter valve, which is incorporated in the suction port. With this system, fluid drops into the collection chamber and air passes into the air leak indicator and then flows through the one-way valve into the suction source (Davol advertisement). A potential problem of the flutter-valve active drainage unit is that the slit could be held open by clots or debris, thereby allowing to-and-fro air movement.

These dry suction units with mechanical manometers eliminate the noise of bubbling in the third bottle, a feature considered annoying by many. Their problem, however, is the apparent difficulty in maintaining a constant negative pressure when a large air leak is present. In addition, the noise of bubbling in the third bottle may be a desirable feature since it indicates proper functioning of the unit.

High-Volume Systems

When high suction is required to achieve effective evacuation of the pleural space, high-volume systems such as the Emerson pump (JH Emerson Co., Cambridge, MA) can be used (Fig. 43-9). These are capable of reaching negative pressures of the order of -60 cmH$_2$O with air flows of more than 20 L/min. Rusch, et al. (1988) and Capps, et al. (1985) have shown that any pleural drainage unit is effective for the management of small air leaks when it functions with -20 cmH$_2$O of suction. Increasing the suction further to -40 cmH$_2$O does not significantly alter the flow via the chest tube. When a major air leak is present, the high-pressure, high-volume Emerson pump is the only unit capable of absorbing this air flow. Mobile suction units are also available for transportation of patients requiring continuous thoracic suction (Enerson and McIntyre, 1966).

Balanced Drainage

Drainage of the Pneumonectomy Space

Following pneumonectomy, most surgeons do not advocate routine drainage of the pleural space. Air can be removed simply by needle and syringe aspiration at the end of the procedure or by leaving a small thoracic catheter, which is withdrawn in the recovery room. Potential advantages of draining the pneumonectomy space are the possible immedi-

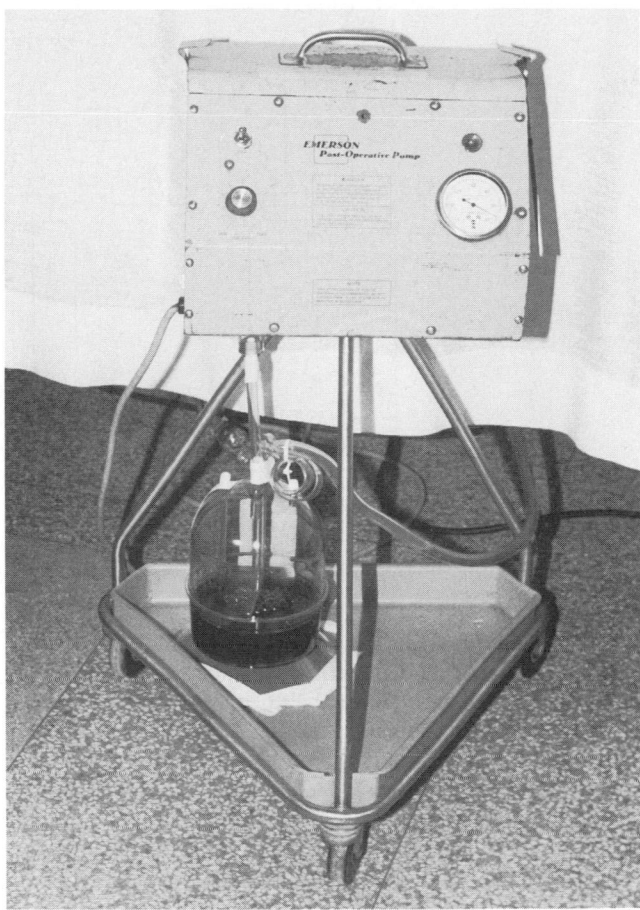

Figure 43-9. Emerson pump.

ate recognition of hemorrhage and the prevention of catastrophic tension pneumothorax should the suture line acutely break down. When a tube is used, it is usually connected to an underwater seal system and kept clamped at all times. It is only unclamped to monitor or evacuate pleural collections or to readjust pleural pressure. Most chest tubes are removed within 48 hours of the pneumonectomy.

Balanced drainage of the pneumonectomy space was described by Storey and Laforet (1953) and Laforet and Boyd (1964) as a method to maintain optimal physiologic position of the mediastinum. The arrangement of the bottles is as shown in Figure 43-10. The first bottle serves as a trap, while the other two bottles serve as pressure regulators. The second bottle or positive-pressure regulator bottle is a simple water-seal, so arranged that any pressure within the system (pleural space) exceeding 1 cmH$_2$O will be vented. The third bottle is a negative-pressure regulator bottle. It is a reverse water seal, so constructed that any pressure more negative than -10 to -15 cmH$_2$O that may develop into the system will automatically be reduced to this level by a compensatory ingress of air. Most balanced drainage units are homemade, although Decknatel Inc. has one such unit commercially available.

One possible disadvantage of the balanced postpneumonectomy drainage system is that extensive subcutaneous emphysema may occur when air is pushed into the soft tissues

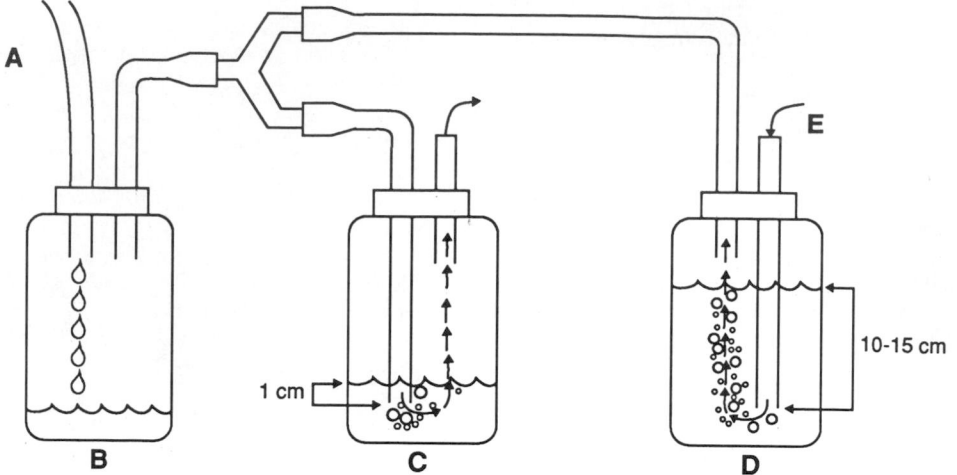

Figure 43-10. Balanced drainage unit for pneumonectomy space drainage: (A) connecting tube from patient, (B) collecting bottle, (C) positive pressure regulator, (D) negative pressure regulator, and (E) air entering system from atmosphere. (Adapted from Laforet EG, Boyd TF: Balanced drainage of the pneumonectomy space. Surg Gynecol Obstet 118:1051, 1964, with permission.)

of the chest wall as a result of coughing. This emphysema tends to increase as additional air is made available from the drainage system. To limit the extent of this problem, Laforet and Boyd (1964) suggest tight and meticulous closure of the pleura, and Pecora and Cooper (1955) also suggest the use of a tight dressing over the excision. Another possible disadvantage of the balanced drainage system is that room air has access to the pleural space, with secondary risk of infection. This may be alleviated by interposing an air filter over the vent of the negative-pressure regulator bottle. Balanced drainage systems can also be useful for draining contaminated pneumonectomy spaces (Miller, et al., 1975).

Drainage Following Repair of Diaphragmatic Hernia

Overdistension of the hypoplastic lung is a major cause of pulmonary injury and death following surgical repair of congenital diaphragmatic hernia in newborns. Tyson and colleagues (1985) have shown that, by maintaining physiologic intrathoracic pressures, balanced thoracic drainage can minimize the risks of further pulmonary injury despite rapidly changing ventilatory or intrathoracic conditions.

Pleuroperitoneal Shunt

The Denver pleuroperitoneal shunt (Denver Biomaterials Inc., Evergreen, CO) is a single-unit medical-grade silicone conduit consisting of a unidirectional-valved pumping chamber located between fenestrated pleural and peritoneal catheters (Fig. 43-11). A barium sulfate stripe in the wall of the proximal and distal catheters permits visualization by chest radiograph or fluoroscopy. Manual compression of the shunt is required 150 to 200 times per day, and each compression transports about 1.5 ml of fluid from the pleural space to the peritoneum. The technique of pumping is neither painful nor difficult to master.

The technique of shunt placement is straightforward and has been well described by Ponn and colleagues (1991). A

short inframammary incision is made over the sixth intercostal space, and a guidewire is passed posteriorly into the pleural space. A contiguous subcutaneous pocket large enough to contain the pump apparatus is then developed inferior to this incision. The pocket needs to be located over the anterolateral costal margin to provide a stable base for external shunt compression. A second upper-quadrant muscle-splitting incision provides access to the peritoneal cavity. The pleural limb of the shunt is then passed into the pleural space through an introducer, and the distal catheter is directed toward the pelvis.

Malignant pleural effusions and chylothoraces are the two indications for use of a Denver pleuroperitoneal shunt. Much has been written about shunting for intractable pleural effusions, the advantages of shunting over the more conventional forms of sclerotherapy being the simplicity of the procedure, the early hospital discharge, and the predictable excellent results. The disadvantages of the technique are the cost of the device, the need for manual pumping, the potential contamination of the peritoneum by malignant cells, and the possible occlusion of the conduit. In a series of 17 patients in whom pleuroperitoneal shunts were implanted for pleural

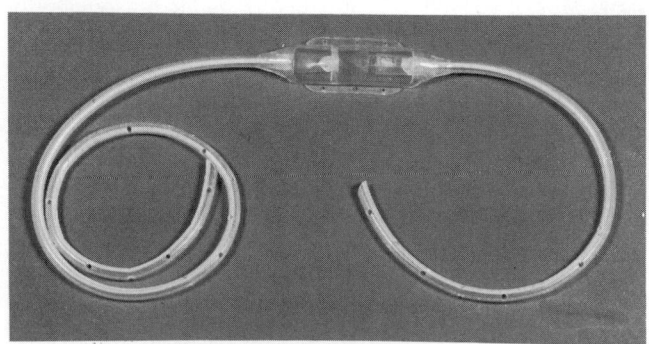

Figure 43-11. Denver pleuroperitoneal shunt.

effusions, Ponn, et al. (1991) reported palliation of dyspnea at rest in all patients. Four shunts became occluded between 1 and 10 months after placement, and two of these had to be replaced. Other series present similar data (Little, et al., 1986; Weese and Schouten, 1984; Tsang, et al., 1990; Cimochowski, et al., 1986). Whether pleuroperitoneal shunting should be the first line of treatment for malignant effusions or whether it should be used only after other methods have failed remains controversial.

Pleuroperitoneal shunting may be useful in the management of persistent chylothorax. In 1989 Murphy and colleagues reported on 16 pediatric patients with refractory chylothoraces due to a variety of causes, in each of whom the chylothorax had been unresponsive to thoracentesis, tube thoracostomy, and dietary manipulations. Of the 16 patients, 12 had excellent results, with complete elimination of the chylothorax and resolution of symptoms following insertion of a pleuroperitoneal shunt.

COMPLICATIONS OF TUBE THORACOSTOMY

A variety of complications have been described in relation to tube thoracostomy. As for most other intrathoracic procedures, the incidence of complications is minimal when the procedure is done with care, when the operator has experience with the technique, and is familiar with the local anatomy of the intercostal space (Moore, 1982).

Misplacement of Thoracostomy Tubes

When inserting a chest tube, the last hole must be well inside the pleural space. When the tube is not advanced far enough, the result may be a false air leak, the development of surgical emphysema, or sometimes physiologic consequences similar

---

Possible Complications of Tube Thoracostomy

Misplacement of the chest tube
  Tube in the soft tissues of the chest wall
  Injury to intrathoracic structures: lung, diaphragm
  Abdominal placement of the tube
Hemorrhage
  Cutaneous
  Intercostal arteries
  Injury to superior vena cava, inferior vena cava, heart
Surgical emphysema
Empyema
Reexpansion pulmonary edema
Intercostal neuralgia and thoracostomy lung herniation
Miscellaneous rare complications
  Horner syndrome
  Diaphragmatic paralysis
  Necrotizing fasciitis
  Chylothorax
  Aortic obstruction

---

to those associated with an open pneumothorax. Tube drainage will obviously be less than optimal if half or the whole of the chest tube is located in the soft tissues of the chest wall. The same kind of problem can result from inadequate suturing of the tube to the thoracostomy incision, accidental pullback by the patient, or loosening of the skin after prolonged drainage. Under those circumstances it is often safer to reinsert another tube through a separate incision rather than risk infection by mobilizing the displaced catheter.

A number of intrathoracic organs may be injured owing to the unchecked passage of chest tubes, usually with the trocar method (Temple, 1975). Lung perforation, for example, has been recognized both in children and adults, and its occurrence is said to be related to pre-existing intrinsic lung disease (Wilson and Krous, 1974; Moessinger, et al., 1978), pleural adhesions, and the use of the trocar catheter. Fraser (1988) reported three cases in adults and suggested that the true incidence of this complication may be greater than appreciated because clear-cut clinical and radiologic evidence of perforation is usually absent. Prophylaxis against lung injury include use of clamp dissection and finger exploration of the pleural space before tube insertion. If lung injury is suspected, one should pull the tube back 1 or 2 inches and then wait until the air leak stops. Occasionally, the tube will be inserted in a large bulla that has been misinterpreted as a pneumothorax. When this is recognized, surgery may be required or it may be decided to leave the tube as it is and wait until the air leak stops. Prophylaxis against this complication includes a high index of suspicion and use of CT scanning before chest drainage.

Diaphragmatic and intra-abdominal injuries are complications bound to happen when the diaphragm is elevated (fourth or fifth interspace), which occurs in obese individuals, in patients with diaphragmatic palsy (Foresti, et al., 1992), or after surgical procedures such as pneumonectomies. Although every organ in the upper abdomen is in jeopardy, the spleen, liver, and stomach are most often injured (Millikan, et al., 1980; Robinson and Brodman, 1981). In such cases the clinical manifestations depend on the organ involved, its vascularity, and the existence of abdominal peritoneal adhesions (Robinson and Brodman, 1981). Some injuries may be apparent immediately while others may not become evident until after removal of tubes. Most of these injuries follow diaphragmatic perforation by the chest tube and can be prevented by high placement of the intercostal tube and finger exploration of the thoracic space prior to tube insertion.

Hemorrhage

Minimal bleeding related to the thoracotomy incision is usually of no consequence. Intercostal artery injury with resulting massive bleeding is also uncommon and is often related to placement of the tube over the inferior border of the rib. It usually occurs in older patients, whose intercostal arteries are more tortuous (Carney and Ravin, 1979).

Massive hemorrhage can be secondary to injury to one of the cavae, right atrium (Meisel, et al., 1990), or right ventricle. These complications are rare and are almost always due to trocar insertion of the chest tube. One known predisposing factor is the extreme mediastinal shift sometimes seen after pneumonectomy or in association with postlobectomy atelectasis. In such circumstances the right ventricle is located underneath the anterolateral chest wall and is susceptible to tube injury, especially if the pericardium has been opened during the prior pulmonary resection. If this type of penetration occurs, the tube should be clamped and the patient brought back to the operating room for immediate repair. At operation, the chest tube track is followed and the laceration repaired with a pledgeted suture. If a cardiac injury is suspected, the tube should never be removed in the patient's room because immediate death is likely to follow.

Surgical Emphysema

Surgical emphysema can occur shortly after chest tube placement or during the days following tube insertion. It is always secondary to inadequate drainage of the pleural space as air reaches the subcutaneous tissues through the perforated pleura at the thoracostomy site. The problem may be due to improper location of the tube in the pleural space, as is seen when pleural adhesions are numerous; to occlusion of the tube or of the connecting tubes; to a large air leak, with inadequate absorption by the drainage unit; or to tube pullback in the soft tissues of the chest wall. When this occurs, the drainage system and thoracostomy site should be first thoroughly checked. If the whole system is airtight and the tube is functioning, the level of suction should be increased. If this does not solve the problem, the tube should be pulled back or another tube inserted.

Empyema

Because the incidence of empyema is low after tube drainage of a sterile collection, prophylactic antibiotic administration is not usually indicated. In a 1971 study Neugebauer, et al. examined the value of routine prophylactic antibiotic therapy following pleural space intubation. Those patients who received prophylactic antibiotic therapy had a higher rate of complications and a longer hospitalization period than those patients who did not receive antibiotics.

The incidence of empyema in acute trauma patients ranges from 1 to 16 percent, with an average of less than 3 percent (Helling, et al., 1989). In those patients tube thoracostomy may contribute to infectious complications by providing a route for contamination, although most empyemas are probably the result of the injury itself or of inadequate drainage with incomplete reexpansion of the lung. In a study by Eddy, et al. (1989), 6 of 12 patients with incomplete evacuation of the pleural space developed empyema while none of the 105 patients with complete evacuation of the pleural space developed this complication. They recommended that if the pleural space cannot be completely evacuated with simple measures such as tube thoracostomy, early limited thoracotomy should be considered. The precise indication for antibiotics in the trauma setting needs further definition (Millikan, et al., 1980), although LoCurto, et al. (1986) have suggested that patients requiring tube thoracostomy for trauma, whether blunt or penetrating, should receive the benefit of systemic prophylactic antibiotic therapy.

Reexpansion Pulmonary Edema

Unilateral pulmonary edema and reexpansion hypotension are rare but potentially lethal complications. They occur when air or fluid is evacuated too rapidly in a patient with lung collapse that has persisted for more than 3 days (Mahfood, et al., 1988). Possible factors implicated in the pathogenesis of this complication include increased pulmonary vascular permeability, airway obstruction, loss of surfactant, and pulmonary artery pressure changes (Pavlin, et al., 1986). The increased pulmonary vascular permeability is a particularly important etiologic factor, with the rapid reexpansion of a collapsed lung causing a rapid increase in pulmonary capillary pressure and blood flow (Ziskind, et al., 1965). This will in turn lead to fluid transportation across the capillary and alveolar membranes and result in an increase in pulmonary extravascular water (Sewell, et al., 1978). Damage to the capillary and alveolar membranes may also be due to oxygen-derived free radicals found when hypoxic areas of the lung are reperfused and reventilated (Mahfood, et al., 1988).

Patients with this problem usually present with uncontrolled and progressive cough and pleuritic pain with unilateral radiologic pulmonary edema. According to Mahfood, et al. (1988), this complication is fatal in about 20 percent of patients. In order to prevent its occurrence, the tube should be clamped and unclamped intermittently until resolution of the pneumothorax or drainage of the effusion is complete.

Intercostal Neuralgia and Thoracostomy Herniation

Placement of a chest tube may result in trauma or even transsection of the intercostal nerve, which can cause persistent postoperative pain. As described in the 1966 edition of *Gray's Anatomy* and by Moore (1982), the main branch of the intercostal nerves (T2 to T11) lies between the ribs rather than in the costal groove, and it may be traumatized during chest tube insertion. When this occurs, the patient will experience intercostal pain radiating anteriorly, and this pain will persist for some time after the tube has been withdrawn. Although these neuralgias can be quite painful on occasion, most are mild and self-limiting. Treatment consists of analgesia and reassurance; intercostal blocks are almost never required.

Intercostal herniation of pleural fluid or lung at the site of drainage is exceedingly rare, and management is generally conservative.

Miscellaneous Rare Complications

Horner syndrome has been reported to occur following tube thoracostomy (Fleishman, et al., 1983; Dutro and Phillips, 1985; Campbell, et al., 1989; Bourque and Paulus 1986; Kahn and Brandt, 1985). It is usually transient and related to direct injury to preganglionic sympathetic fibers coursing near the apex of the lung. Hematoma or pressure ischemia over the sympathetic chain has also been implicated in the pathogenesis of this syndrome. Prophylaxis against this complication involves placement of the tube below the level of the second rib, and if a Horner's syndrome is recognized after tube insertion, the tube should be removed or replaced at another side. Necrotizing fasciitis following tube insertion has been reported by Pingleton and Jeter (1983). In their case the fasciitis followed drainage of an empyema containing anaerobic organisms, and the patient eventually died from multiorgan failure.

In children, reported complications include diaphragmatic paralysis due to injury to the intrathoracic segment of the phrenic nerve (Palomeque, et al., 1990), chylothorax secondary to trauma of the thoracic duct (Kumar and Belik, 1984), and aortic obstruction due to medially deployed thoracostomy tubes (Gooding, et al., 1981).

COMMENTS AND CONTROVERSIES

Insertion of a chest catheter looks beguilingly simple but is fraught with the potential for major troubles. Missing the target of fluid or air is one thing, but spearing a bordering viscus is always serious and may convert what ought to be a small operation into an unexpectedly complicated one. Injury to the spleen or liver usually results from excessive enthusiasm to position the tube "in a dependent position," the operator forgetting that these organs lie underneath the ribs and ignoring the fact that the intubated patient is most likely to be supine anyway.

Less dramatic but important is the bleeding that may result from an undetected or forgotten coagulopathy, the commonest being that induced by aspirin or warfarin. If a bleb is perforated, an air leak may be worsened or a new one created. Additionally, infection of the chest wall, residual numbness, or the memory of a painful insertion are unwelcome concerns.

More egregious errors include the insertion of a chest tube without reviewing the patient's history, physical findings, and chest films. Asking the radiologist to place a radiopaque marker near the target is no substitute for personal verification of the optimal site of the thoracostomy, let alone the need for it in the first place.

To the ordinarily constituted, the prospect of a tube thrust deep into the chest is a matter of gravity. The prescription for allaying apprehension consists of one part sedation, two parts local anesthesia, and a heaping measure of quiet explanation. There is no excuse for allowing the patient to view the tray of surgical instruments.

The first step is to inject 5 to 10 ml of 1 to 2 percent xylocaine around the intercostal nerve and wait several minutes for deep anesthesia to set in before proceeding. It should be remembered that the pleura may still be sensitive; additional infiltration takes only a few seconds. The same needle employed for anesthesia or a slightly larger one may then be used to probe for air or fluid and thus to verify the correctness of the chosen site. A hemostat applied to the needle at the point of penetration serves to steady it and to calibrate the interval from skin to cavity. If the tube is being placed to evacuate a pneumothorax, the patient should be alerted to expect a paroxysm of coughing as the lung reexpands.

Once the tube is in position and draining well, it must be secured so that it does not dislodge when the patient moves or is moved. Nurses need to be reminded that tubes should be fixed to bed linen with rubber bands and safety pins to ensure a straight lie. "Were an imaginary marble placed in the tube it should roll continuously downhill." A sagging, fluid-filled tube works as well as a clamped tube.

Chest tubes should be removed in the morning, lest inadvertent introduction of air or recurrent pneumothorax stress nighttime services. Gloves should be worn! The patient has a right to know what to expect in way of discomfort.

Most of the mentioned problems would be avoided if the invitation to "put in a chest tube" triggered the same sequence of reflection and concerned attention that is part of the routine for major thoracic surgery: Verify the diagnosis. Know the patient. Operate carefully. *And* do no harm.

C.A.H.

KEY REFERENCES

Miller KS, Sahn SA: Chest tubes. Indications, techniques, management and complications. Chest 91:258, 1987

Excellent review article on chest drainage and suction systems.

Munnell ER, Thomas EK: Current concepts in thoracic drainage systems. Ann Thorac Surg 19:261, 1975

Results of a survey done among thoracic surgeons about their views on pleural space drainage. Looks at tubes and drainage systems.

Rusch VW, Capps JS, Tyler ML, Pierson DL: The performance of four pleural drainage systems in an animal model of bronchopleural fistula. Chest 93:859, 1988

Results of a carefully done analysis of the performance of four pleural drainage systems. Discussion on which unit is the best to drain high volume or high pressure leaks.

REFERENCES

Aslam PA, Eastridge CE, Hughes FA: Insertion of apical chest tube. Surg Gynecol Obstet 130:1097, 1970

Batchelder TL, Morris KA: Critical factors in determining adequate pleural drainage in both the operated and non operated chest. Am Surg 28:296, 1962

Bourque PR, Paulus EM: Chest-tube thoracostomy causing Horner's syndrome. Can J Surg 29:202, 1986

Brunn H: Surgical principles underlying one-stage lobectomy. Arch Surg 18:490, 1929

Bulau G: Für die Heber-Drainage bei Behandlung des Empyems. Z Klin Med 18:31, 1891

Campbell P, Neil T, Wake PN: Horner's syndrome caused by an intercostal chest drain. Thorax 44:305, 1989

Capps JS, Tyler ML, Rusch VW, Pierson DJ: Potential of chest drainage units to evacuate broncho-pleural air leaks. Chest 88 (suppl):57, 1985

Carney M, Ravin CE: Intercostal artery laceration during thoracentesis. Chest 75:520, 1979

Cimochowski GE, Joyner LR, Fardin R et al.: Pleuroperitoneal shunting for recalcitrant pleural effusions. J Thorac Cardiovasc Surg 92:866, 1986

Churchill ED: Wound surgery encounters a dilemma. J Thorac Surg 35:279, 1958

Couraud LL, Velly JF, N'Diaye M: Principles and techniques of chest drainage and suction. p. 103. In Delarue NC, Eschapasse H (eds): Thoracic Surgery: Surgical Management of Pleural Diseases. In Deslauriers J, Lacquet LK (eds): International Trends in General Thoracic Surgery. Vol. 6. CV Mosby, St. Louis, 1990

Dalbec DL, Krome RL: Thoracostomy. Emerg Med Clin North Am 1986;4:441–457.

Davis LL: Easier chest tube insertion (letter). Ann Thorac Surg 43:688, 1987

Deslauriers J: More about chest tubes and suction systems. p. 108. In Delarue NC, Eschapasse H (eds): Thoracic Surgery: Surgical Management of Pleural Diseases. In Deslauriers J, Lacquet LK (eds): International Trends in General Thoracic Surgery. Vol. 6. CV Mosby, St. Louis, 1990

Deslauriers J, Liu G, Mousset X et al.: On the use of chest tubes (letter). Chest 92:959, 1987

Duncan C, Erickson R: Pressures associated with chest tube stripping. Heart Lung 11:166, 1982

Dutro JA, Phillips LG: Ipsilateral Horner's syndrome as a rare complication of tube thoracostomy (letter). N Engl J Med 313:121, 1985

Eddy AC, Luna GK, Copass M: Empyema thoracis in patients undergoing emergent closed tube thoracostomy for thoracic trauma. Am J Surg 157:494, 1989

Enerson DM, McIntyre J: A comparative study of the physiology and physics of pleural drainage systems. Thorac Cardiovasc Surg 52:40, 1966

Fleishman JA, Bullock JD, Rosset JS, Beck RW: Iatrogenic Horner's syndrome secondary to chest tube thoracostomy. J Clin Neuro Opthalmol 3:205, 1983

Foresti V, Villa A, Casati O et al.: Abdominal placement of tube thoracostomy due to lack of recognition of paralysis of hemidiaphragm. Chest 102:292, 1992

Fraser RS: Lung perforation complicating tube thoracostomy: pathologic description of three cases. Hum Pathol 19:518, 1988

Gift AG, Bolgiano CS, Cunningham J: Sensation during chest tube removal. Heart Lung 20:131, 1991

Gilsanz V, Cleveland RH: Pleural reaction to thoracotomy tube. Chest 74:167, 1978

Gooding CA, Kerlan RC, Brasch RC, Brito AC: Medially deployed thoracostomy tubes: cause of aortic obstruction in newborns. AJR 136:511, 1981

Goss CM (ed): Gray's Anatomy of the Human Body. 28th Ed. Lea & Febiger, Philadelphia, 1966

Graham EA, Bell RD: Open pneumothorax: its relation to the treatment of empyema. Am J Med Sci 156:839, 1918

Grover FL, Richardson JD, Fewel JG et al.: Prophylactic antibiotics in the treatment of penetrating chest wounds. J Thorac Cardiovasc Surg 74;528, 1977

Guyton SN, Paull DL, Anderson RP: Introducer insertion of minithoracostomy tubes. Am J Surg 155:693, 1988

Halejian BA, Badach MJ, Trilles F: Maintaining chest tube patency. Surgery Gynecol Obstet 167:521, 1988

Hayes DF, Lucas CE: Bilateral tube thoracostomy to preclude fatal tension pneumothorax in patients with acute respiratory insufficiency. Am Surg 42:330, 1976

Heimlich HJ: Valve drainage of the pleural cavity. Chest 53:282, 1968

Helling TS, Gyles NR, Eisenstein CL, Soracco CA: Complications following blunt and penetrating injuries in 216 victims of chest trauma requiring tube thoracostomy. J Trauma 29:1367, 1989

Herbst CA: Indications, management, and complications of percutaneous subclavian catheters. An audit. Arch Surg 113:1421, 1978

Hewett CF: Thoracentesis: the plan of continuous aspiration. Br Med J 1:317, 1876

Hippocrates: Writings. p. 142. In Hutchins RA (ed): Great Books of the Western World. Vol. 29. Encyclopedia Brittanica, Inc., 1952

Hood RH, Dooling JA, Beddingfield GW et al.: Drainage of the pleural space. Drainage tube composition in relation to complications. Ann Thorac Surg 2:94, 1966

Julian JS, Pennell TC: A review of the basics of closed thoracic drainage. NC Med J 48:127, 1987

Kahn SA, Brandt LJ: Iatrogenic Horner's syndrome: a complication of thoracostomy tube replacement (letter). N Engl J Med 312:245, 1985

Kovarik JL, Brown RK: Tube and trocar thoracostomy. Surg Clin North Am 49:1455, 1969

Kumar SP, Belik J: Chylothorax—a complication of chest tube placement in a neonate. Crit Care Med 12:411, 1984

Laforet EG, Boyd TF: Balanced drainage of the pneumonectomy space. Surg Gynecol Obstet 118:1051, 1964

Lawrence GH: Closed chest tube drainage for pleural space problems. The primary therapeutic modality. Major Probl Clin Surg 28:13, 1983

Light RW: Para-pneumonic effusions and empyema. Clin Chest Med 6:55, 1985

Lilienthal H: Resection of the lung for suppurative infections with a report based on 31 consecutive operative cases in which resection was done or intended. Ann Surg 75:257, 1922

Lim-Levy F, Babler SA, De Groot-Kosolcharoen J et al.: Is milking and stripping chest tubes really necessary? Ann Thorac Surg 42:77, 1986

Little AG, Ferguson MK, Golomb HM et al.: Pleuro-peritoneal shunting for malignant pleural effusions. Cancer 58:2740, 1986

Lo LF, Mirza FA: Removal of chest tube using stomadhesive. Surg Gynecol Obstet 158:497, 1984

LoCurto JJ, Tischler CD, Swan KG et al.: Tube thoracostomy and trauma—antibiotics or not? J Trauma 26:1067, 1986

Mahfood S, Hix WR, Aaron BL et al.: Reexpansion pulmonary edema. Ann Thorac Surg 45:340, 1988

Maimimi SE, Johnson FE: Tension pneumothorax complicating small-caliber chest tube insertion. Chest 97:759, 1990

Maurer JR, Friedman PJ, Wing VW: Thoracostomy tube in an interlobar fissure: radiologic recognition of a potential problem. AJR 139:1155, 1982

McGrath D, Kruger BK: Chest suction . . . Using mercury instead of water. Am J Nurs 62:72, 1962

Meisel S, Ram Z, Priel I et al.: Another complication of thoracostomy—perforation of the right atrium. Chest 98:772, 1990

Mercier C, Pagé A, Verdant A et al.: Outpatient management of intercostal tube drainage in spontaneous pneumothorax. Ann Thorac Surg 22:163, 1976

Meyer JA: Gotthard Bülau and closed water-seal drainage for empyema, 1875–1891. Ann Thorac Surg 48:597, 1989

Miller J, Fleming WH, Hatcher CR: Balanced drainage of the contaminated pneumonectomy space. Ann Thorac Surg 19:585, 1975

Miller JM, Ginsberg M, Lipin RJ, Long PH: Clinical experience with streptokinase and streptodornase JAMA 145:620, 1951

Millikan JS, Moore EE, Steiner E: Complications of tube thoracostomy for acute trauma. Am J Surg 140:738, 1980

Moessinger AC, Driscoll JM, Wigger HJ: High incidence of lung perforation by chest tube in neonatal pneumothorax. J Pediatr 92:635, 1978

Moore DC: Anatomy of the intercostal nerve: its importance during thoracic surgery. Am J Surg 144:371, 1982

Morgan CV, Orcutt TW: The care and feeding of chest tubes. Am J Nurs 72:305, 1972

Murphy MC, Newman BM, Rodgers BM: Pleuroperitoneal shunts in the management of persistent chylothorax. Ann Thorac Surg 48:195, 1989

Neptune WB: Trocar for thoracostomy (letter). Ann Thorac Surg 23:195, 1977

Neugebauer MK, Forsburg RG, Trummer MJ: Routine antibiotic therapy following pleural space intubation. J Thorac Cardiovasc Surg 61:882, 1971

Nissen R, Wilson RHL: Pages in the History of Chest Surgery. Charles C. Thomas, Springfield, IL, 1960

Palomeque A, Canadell D, Pastor X: Acute diaphragmatic paralysis after chest tube placement (letter). Intensive Care med 16:138, 1990

Panicek DM, Randall PA, Witanowski LS et al.: Chest tube tracks. Radiographics 7:321, 1987

Pavlin DJ, Raghu G, Rogers TR, Cheney FW: Reexpansion hypotension. A complication of rapid evacuation of prolonged pneumothorax. Chest 89:70, 1986

Pecora DV: Post-thoracotomy suction, (letter). Chest 79:613, 1981

Pecora DV, Cooper P: Pleural drainage following pneumonectomy: description of apparatus. Surgery 37:251, 1955

Pickard LR, Beall AC: Portable suction device for use in patients with postoperative pleural air leaks. Ann Thorac Surg 36:103, 1983

Pingleton SK, Jeter J: Necrotizing fasciitis as a complication of tube thoracostomy. Chest 83:925, 1983

Playfair GE: Case of empyema treated by aspiration and subsequently by drainage: recovery. Br Med J 1:45, 1875

Ponn RB, Blancaflor J, D'Agostino RS et al.: Pleuroperitoneal shunting for intractable pleural effusions. Ann Thorac Surg 51:605, 1991

Prats I: Simplified chest tube removal: a new technique. Curr Surg 47:110, 1990

Richards V: Procedures in family practice. Tube thoracostomy. J Fam Pract 6:629, 1978

Ring EM, Shapiro MJ: The tunnel tip thoracic catheter. Surg Gynecol Obstet 169:553, 1989

Robinson G, Brodman R: Going down the tube (editorial). Ann Thorac Surg 31:400, 1981

Roe BB: Improved technique for closure of thoracostomy incision. Surg Gynecol Obstet 121:845, 1965

Roe BB: Physiologic principles of drainage of the pleural space with special reference to high flow, high vacuum suction. Am J Surg 96:246, 1958

Runyon BA, Greenblatt M, Ming RHC: Hepatic chylothorax is a relative contra indication to chest tube insertion. Am J Gastroenterol 81:566, 1986

Semrad N: A new technique for closed thoracostomy insertion of chest tube. Surg Gynecol Obstet 166:171, 1988

Sewell RW, Fewel JG, Grover FL, Arom KV: Experimental evaluation of reexpansion pulmonary oedema. Ann Thorac Surg 26:126, 1978

Sharma TN, Agnihotri SP, Jain NK et al.: Intercostal tube thoracostomy in pneumothorax—factors influencing re-expansion of lung. Indian J Chest Dis Allied Sci 30:32, 1988

So SY, Yu DYC: Catheter drainage of spontaneous pneumothorax: suction or no suction, early or late removal? Thorax 37:46, 1982

Stark DD, Federle MP, Goodman PC: CT and radiographic assessment of tube thoracostomy. AJR 141:253, 1983

Storey CF: Intrapleural suction. It is being used to best advantage? (editorial). Ann Thorac Surg 6:196, 1968

Storey CF, Laforet EG: The surgical management of bronchiectasis: a review based on the analysis of 100 consecutive resections. US Armed Forces Med J 4:469, 1953

Swenson EW, Birath G: Resistance to air flow in bronchospirometric catheters. J Thorac Surg 33:275, 1957

Sweet RH: Thoracic Surgery. WB Saunders, Philadelphia, 1954, p. 52

Temple LJ: Hazards of Argyll trocar catheter (letter). Br Med J 1:334, 1975

Thal AP, Quick KL: A guided chest tube for safe thoracostomy. Surg Gynecol Obstet 167:517, 1988

Tinckler LF: Self-retaining chest drainage tubes. Br J Surg 63:141, 1976

Tsang V, Fernando IIC, Goldstraw P: Pleuroperitoneal shunt for recurrent malignant pleural effusions. Thorax 45:369, 1990

Tyson KRT, Schwartz MZ, Marr CC: "Balanced" thoracic drainage is the method of choice to control intrathoracic pressure following repair of diaphragmatic hernia. J Pediatr Surg 20:415, 1985

Von Hippel A: Correspondence. Ann Thorac Surg 20:721, 1975

Von Hippel A: Chest Tubes and Chest Bottles. Charles C Thomas, Springfield, IL, 1970

Watkins E: Principles of postoperative management in thoracic surgery. Surg Clin North Am 41:603, 1961

Webb WR, Laberge J: Major fissure tube placement (letter). AJR 140:1039, 1983

Weese JL, Schouten JT: Internal drainage of intractable malignant pleural effusions. Wis Med J 83:21, 1984

Wilson AJ, Krous HF: Lung perforation during chest tube placement in the stiff lung syndrome. J Pediatr Surg 9:213, 1974

Ziskind MM, Weill H, George RA: Acute pulmonary edema following the treatment of spontaneous pneumothorax with excessive negative intra-pleural pressure. Am Rev Respir Dis 62:632, 1965

Open Drainage

Louis F. Jacques
Jean Deslauriers

There are many different options for therapy for empyema thoracis. The management must be individualized according to the underlying disease process, the phase of the empyema (American Thoracic Society, 1962), and the general condition of the patient.

The basic principles of management of empyema are to obtain adequate drainage and sterilization of the empyema cavity, close the bronchopleural fistula if present, and obliterate the pleural space. Drainage can be achieved by thoracentesis, closed-tube thoracostomy, open-tube drainage by rib resection, and in some cases open window thoracostomy.

HISTORICAL NOTE

In 1915 Samuel Robinson (1915, 1916) from the Mayo Clinic, outlined very well the two basic principles of management of chronic empyema: (1) adequate drainage and (2) obliteration of the pleural space. In these classic papers, Robinson described a technique of open drainage and partial obliteration of the cavity with the use of the latissimus dorsi muscle. A U-shaped skin incision was made over the empyema cavity, and portions of the underlying ribs were resected. The latissimus dorsi muscle was then sutured inside the cavity, partially obliterating it. An open window was then fashioned by suturing the edges of the skin and subcutaneous tissue to the walls of the cavity. Unfortunately, this contribution of Robinson is seldom recognized in the literature.

Twenty years later, in an article entitled ''An Operation for Tuberculous Empyema,'' Eloesser (1935) described a technique of open drainage which became known as the Eloesser flap (Fig. 43-12). The procedure consisted of making a U-shaped skin incision, resecting a segment of rib over the most dependent portion of the empyema cavity, suturing the skin flap to the pleura, and suturing the remaining edges of skin together. This flap was designed to act as a tubeless one-way valve. According to Eloesser (1969), successful function of the flap is due to its valve action in that (1) air escapes from the valve opening more readily than it enters, (2) the valve mechanism maintains negative pressure in the pleural cavity in spite of the partially open drainage, and (3) this negative pressure in turn causes the underlying lung to expand until on reaching the chest wall, it seals the inner opening of the flap drainage and obliterates the empyema. As stated by Hurvitz and Tucker (1986, 1990), the illustrations from Eloesser's original paper do not satisfactorily clarify how he accomplished his objective (i.e., the creation of a one-way valve mechanism), and the results of the procedure were never published.

With the availability of antituberculous drugs and antibiotics, the procedure as originally described became obsolete. The only aspect of the original Eloesser operation that still applies today is the concept of providing adequate drainage of an empyema cavity with an epithelialized thoracostomy. From the literature available, it is unclear who is responsible for the modification of the Eloesser flap (Hurvitz and Tucker, 1986). However, the enthusiasm for open drainage was revived in 1963, when Clagett and Geraci described a procedure for the management of postpneumonectomy empyema that is now known as the Clagett procedure.

Since the early 1960s, no major modifications of the technique of open window thoracostomy have been described, and the indications have also remained basically unchanged.

HISTORICAL READINGS

Clagett OT, Geraci JE: A procedure for the management of postpneumonectomy empyema. J Thorac Cardiovasc Surg 45:141, 1963

Eloesser L: An operation for tuberculous empyema. Surg Gynecol Obstet 60:1096, 1935

Eloesser L: Of an operation for tuberculous empyema. Ann Thorac Surg 8:355, 1969

Hurvitz RJ, Tucker BL: The Eloesser flap: past and present. J Thorac Cardiovasc Surg 92:958, 1986

Hurvitz RJ, Tucker BL: The Eloesser flap: past and present. p. 271. In Delarue NC, Eschapasse H (eds): Thoracic Surgery: Surgical Management of Pleural Diseases. In Deslauriers J, Lacquet LK (eds): International Trends in General Thoracic Surgery. Vol. 6. CV Mosby, 1990

Robinson S: The treatment of chronic non-tuberculous empyema. Proc Mayo Clin 7:618, 1915

Robinson S: The treatment of chronic non-tuberculous empyema, Surg Gynecol Obstet 22:557, 1916

OPEN WINDOW THORACOSTOMY

Indications

Although open window thoracostomy is a simple and well tolerated procedure, which allows adequate drainage of a chronic empyema and control of the infection, the indications

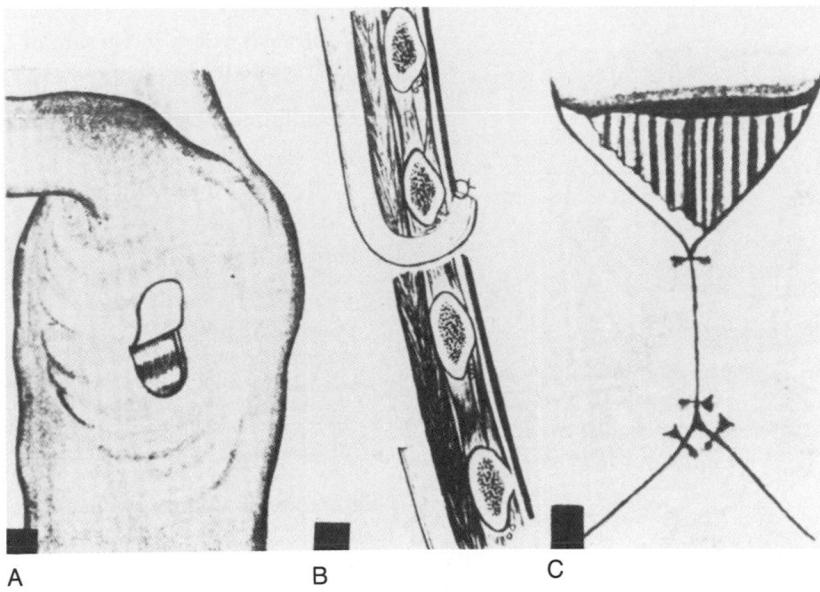

A   B   C

Figure 43-12. Original Eloesser flap. (From Eloesser L: An operation for tuberculous empyema. Surg Gynecol Obstet 60:1096, 1935, with permission.)

for operation are few. It is a valuable option for the treatment of patients with chronic organizing empyemas when long-term or permanent drainage is indicated. It is also indicated for patients with chronic empyemas that do not respond to tube thoracostomy and who are too debilitated to undergo decortication. Open window thoracostomy should be considered to avoid discomfort in patients requiring long-term tube drainage posteriorly or high in the axilla (Le Roux, et al., 1986). Finally, open window thoracostomy is an excellent option for the drainage of postpneumonectomy empyemas with or without bronchopleural fistula.

Technique

Open window thoracostomy is usually performed under general anesthesia, and because a bronchopleural fistula may present, a double-lumen endotracheal tube should always be used.

The site of incision must be carefully planned by review of chest radiographs and thoracic CT scan. Preoperative ultrasound localization and marking of the empyema cavity may also be helpful. Before the incision is made, needle

aspiration of the cavity will confirm adequate localization. Different incisions have been described: U-shaped (Samson, 1971), inverted U-shaped (Symbas, et al., 1971), H-shaped (Hurvitz and Tucker, 1986), and triradiate (Galvin, et al., 1988). Whatever the incision used, the window should be placed at the most dependent portion of the empyema cavity. When the open window thoracostomy is used for postpneumonectomy empyema, the anterior aspect of the thoracotomy incision is usually opened. Because of the elevation of the hemidiaphragm after pneumonectomy, Clagett and Geraci (1963) have shown that this location of the incision will allow satisfactory dependent drainage.

An H-shaped incision 10 to 12 cm long is first made, and musculocutaneous flaps are raised away from the ribs. A 15-cm long segment of two ribs is resected, along with the intercostal muscle, neurovascular bundle, and underlying pleura (Fig. 43-13). The cavity is then drained and debrided avoiding disruption of the visceral pleura or of the pleural adhesions surrounding the cavity. The flaps are then turned into the window and sutured to the parietal pleura, and the cavity is packed with wet gauzes.

Postoperative Care

An open window thoracostomy is easier to care for and generally cleaner than open tube drainage. Attention should be given to the patient's nutritional status and to any associated medical problems that may be present. The dressing is changed at least daily—more often if needed at the beginning—and this can be done at bedside with small doses of analgesics and/or sedatives. Wet-to-dry or lightly moist dressings are preferred as they provide better debridement. Physiological saline solution (Virkkula and Eerola, 1974), povidone-iodine (Betadine) 20 : 1 solution (Pairolero, et al., 1990), and half-strength Dakin's solution (Stafford and Clagett, 1972) have been recommended to irrigate the cavity

---

Indications for Open Window Thoracostomy

Chronic empyema (organizing phase)
    Not responding to conventional therapy
    Patient too debilitated for decortication
    Long-term drainage expected
    Discomfort from tube drainage placed posteriorly
      or in the axillary area
    Postpneumonectomy empyema with or without
      bronchopleural fistula

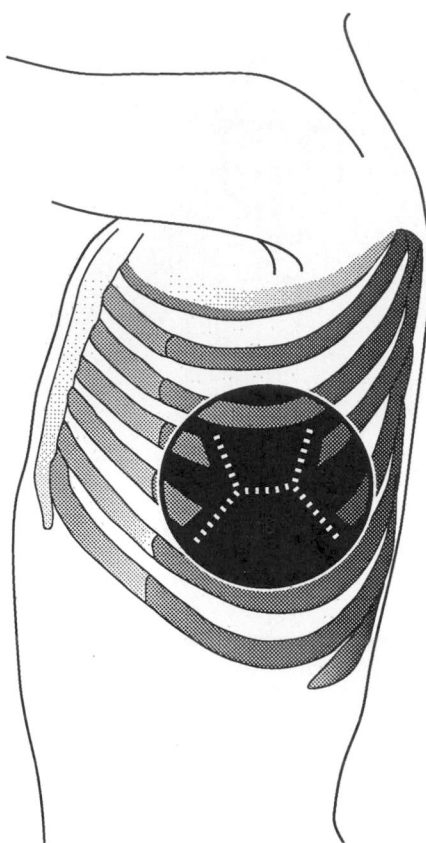

Figure 43-13. Open window thoracostomy. Outline of skin incision, musculocutaneous skin flaps, and rib resection over the empyema cavity.

Contraindications to Closure of Open Window Thoracostomy

Open bronchopleural or esophagopleural fistula
Poor general condition
Evidence of metastatic or locally recurrent cancer
Cavity not clean
Patient's refusal

(Adapted from Virkkula L, Eerola S: Treatment of postpneumonectomy empyema, Scand J Thorac Cardiovasc Surg 8:133, 1974, with permission.)

---

and to moisten the gauzes used to pack the cavity. If the cavity becomes colonized with *Pseudomonas,* gauzes soaked in 1 percent acetic acid should be used. The mechanical debridement by the gauzes themselves is more important than the solution used to moisten the dressing.

Occasionally, the patient is brought to the operating room for a more complete inspection and debridement of the cavity. With time the surface of the cavity will be covered with granulation tissue, and the cavity will become progressively smaller. Given enough time, the cavity can be completely obliterated and reepithlialized, leaving only an indentation on the chest wall (Symbas, et al., 1971). In the majority of patients, mainly those with open window thoracostomy for postpneumonectomy empyema, the cavity is too large and closure should be considered at a later stage. The interval between the making and the closure of the window is variable and depends on the status of the cavity (Virkkula, et al., 1990). However, closure should not be performed if the general condition of the patient is poor, the cavity is not clean, or there is evidence of metastatic or locally recurrent cancer. Before attempting closure, any associated bronchopleural or esophagopleural fistula must also be closed. To achieve successful closure and avoid recurrent empyema, the remaining space must be obliterated. Thoracoplasty, decortication, muscle transposition, and sterilization with antibiotic solution are all options available to obliterate the remaining pleural space.

Results

Adequate drainage of the empyema and local control of the infection are achieved by open window thoracostomy. The systemic signs and symptoms of sepsis will usually subside rapidly. The procedure is well tolerated despite the inconvenience of the daily wound care.

In 1971 Symbas and colleagues reported the results of open window thoracostomy for treatment of empyema in 34 patients. There was only one early death from sepsis. Complete healing of the empyema cavity occurred in all patients within a median time of 3 ½ months after the operation. There were 13 associated bronchopleural fistulae, of which 11 closed spontaneously. All patients had good long-term results, and only two required revision of the stoma because of early closure. In 1982 Weissberg reported the results in 12 empyema patients, 5 of whom had postpneumonectomy empyema, who were treated with open window thoracostomy. In all patients the empyema was controlled and local infection cleared. No complications related to the procedure occurred, and in seven patients an associated bronchopleural fistula closed spontaneously within 4 months. The empyema cavity filled to complete obliteration within 1 to 24 months, depending on the size of the cavity. A permanent open window thoracostomy for postpneumonectomy empyema was provided in six patients by Dorman and colleagues (1973) (Fig. 43-14). They reported five long-term survivors and the permanent open window was well tolerated by all patients. Shamji and colleagues (1983) reported similar results in 11 patients who had permanent open window thoracostomy for postpneumonectomy empyema.

CLAGETT PROCEDURE

As described by Clagett and Geraci in 1963, the Clagett procedure is a two-stage operation designed for the treatment of postpneumonectomy empyema. The first stage is open drainage of the postpneumonectomy empyema cavity, which is then irrigated daily for 6 to 8 weeks. At the second stage the

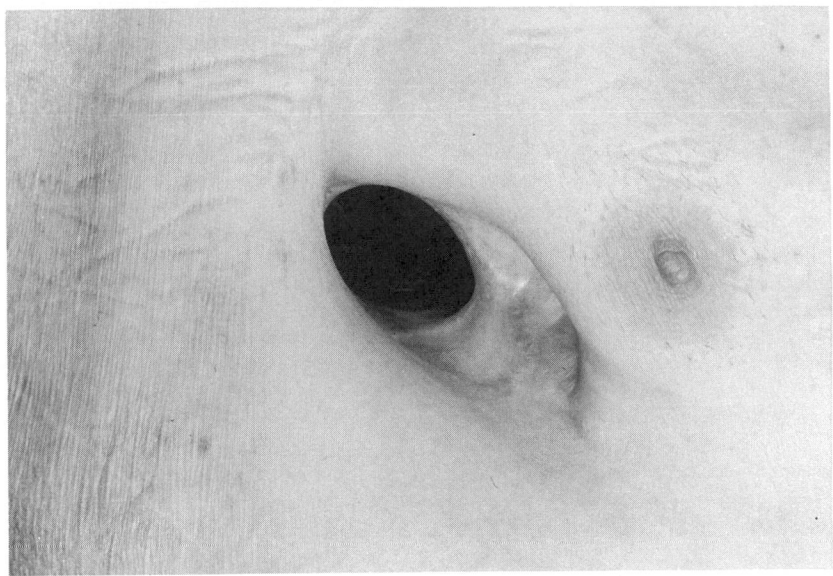

Figure 43-14. Long-term open window thoracostomy in a patient with postpneumonectomy empyema.

edges of the thoracic window are excised and the different layers of the chest wall are mobilized. The cavity is irrigated, cleaned, and filled with saline solution containing 0.25 percent neomycin, and the wound is closed in layers. In their initial report, Clagett and Geraci (1963) described three patients in whom a postpneumonectomy empyema was successfully

Table 43-1. Results of the Clagett Procedure for Therapy for Postpneumonectomy Empyema

Authors (Date)	No. Patients	Overall Success	
		No.	%
Stafford & Clagett (1972)	18	16	88.9
Adler & Plaut (1972)	3	3	100.0
Zumbro, et al. (1973)	3	3	100.0
Barker (1973)	11	9	81.8
Samson (1973)	10	9	90.0
Virkkula & Eerola (1974)	13	10	76.9
Goldstraw (1979)	22	19	86.4
Shamji, et al. (1983)	8	2	25.0
Bayes, et al. (1987)	18	11	61.1
Pairolero, et al. (1990)	31	26	83.9
Virkkula, et al. (1990)	41	32	78.0
Total	178	140	78.6

treated by this procedure. In 1972 Stafford and Clagett reported their experience in 18 patients, in 16 (88.9 percent) of whom successful closure was ultimately obtained. Others have reported similar results with the Clagett procedure (Table 43-1).

Most of the failures are related to a recurrent or persistent bronchopleural fistula. This was recognized by Samson (1973), who advocated direct closure of any associated bronchopleural fistula with intercostal muscle flap reinforcement. This principle is emphasized by Pairolero and colleagues (1990, 1992) in their modification of the Clagett procedure for patients with postpneumonectomy empyemas with bronchopleural fistulae. As an intermediate stage, the bronchopleural fistula is closed directly and the bronchial stump is reinforced by an intrathoracic muscle transposition. Of 28 patients, 21 underwent the three-stage operation, and the procedure was ultimately successful in 20 (95.0 percent) of them (Pairolero, et al., 1990).

CONCLUSIONS

While seldom used, open window thoracostomy is a simple procedure, which is well tolerated by acutely ill patients and which allows adequate drainage of chronic empyemas as well as control of the infection.

KEY REFERENCES

Clagett OT, Geraci JE: A procedure for the management of postpneumonectomy empyema. J Thorac Cardiovasc Surg 45:141, 1963

Original article by Clagett describing the technique of open window thoracostomy to treat post-pneumonectomy empyema.

Hurvitz RJ, Tucker BL: The Eloesser flap: past and present. J Thorac Cardiovasc Surg 92:958, 1986

Describes the modifications in both concept and design that have happened over the years to the Eloesser flap. Excellent description of the history of the flap.

REFERENCES

Adler RH, Plaut ME: Post-pneumonectomy empyema. Surgery 71:210, 1972

American Thoracic Society Subcommittee of Surgery: Management of nontuberculous empyema. Am Rev Respir Dis 85:935, 1962

Barker WL: Discussion of Zumbro GL, Treasure R, Geiger JP, Green DC: Empyema after pneumonectomy. Ann Thorac Surg 15:615, 1973

Bayes AJ, Wilson JAS, Chiu RCJ et al.: Clagett open window thoracostomy in patients with empyema who had and had not undergone pneumonectomy. Can J Surg 30:329, 1987

Dorman JP, Campbell D, Grover FL, Trinkle JK: Open thoracostomy drainage of postpneumonectomy empyema with bronchopleural fistula. J Thorac Cardiovasc Surg 66:979, 1973

Eloesser L: Of an operation for tuberculous empyema. Ann Thorac Surg 8:355, 1969

Eloesser L: An operation for tuberculous empyema. Surg Gynecol Obstet 60:1096, 1935

Galvin IF, Gibbons JRP, Maghout MH: Bronchopleural fistula, a novel type of window thoracostomy. J Thorac Cardiovasc Surg 96:433, 1988

Goldstraw P: Treatment of postpneumonectomy empyema: the case for fenestration. Thorax 34:740, 1979

Hurvitz RJ, Tucker BL: The Eloesser flap: past and present. p. 271. In Delarue NC, Eschapasse H (eds): Thoracic Surgery: Surgical Management of Pleural Diseases. In Deslauriers J, Lacquet LK (eds): International Trends in General Thoracic Surgery. Vol. 6. CV Mosby, St. Louis, 1990

LeRoux BT, Mohlala ML, Odell JA, Whitton ID: Suppurative diseases of the lung and pleural space. Part 1: Empyema thoracis and lung abscess. Curr Probl Surg 23:6, 1986

Pairolero PC, Arnold PG, Trastek VF et al.: Postpneumonectomy empyema: the role of intrathoracic muscle transposition. J Thorac Cardiovasc Surg 99:958, 1990

Pairolero PC, Deschamps C, Allen MS, Trastek VF: Postoperative empyema. Chest Surg Clin North Am 2:813, 1992

Robinson S: The treatment of chronic non-tuberculous empyema. Surg Gynecol Obstet 22:557, 1916

Robinson S: The treatment of chronic non-tuberculous empyema. Mayo Clin Proc 7:618, 1915

Samson PC: Discussion of Zumbro GL, Treasure R, Geiger JP, Green DC: Empyema after pneumonectomy. Ann Thorac Surg 15:615, 1973

Samson PC: Empyema thoracis: essentials of present-day management. Ann Thorac Surg 11:210, 1971

Shamji FM, Ginsberg RJ, Cooper JD et al.: Open window thoracostomy in the management of postpneumonectomy empyema with or without bronchopleural fistula. J Thorac Cardiovasc Surg 86:818, 1983

Stafford EG, Clagett OT: Postpneumonectomy empyema: neomycin instillation and definitive closure. J Thorac Cardiovasc Surg 63:771, 1972

Symbas PN, Nugent JT, Abbot OA et al.: Nontuberculous pleural empyema in adults. Ann Thorac Surg 12:69, 1971

Virkkula L, Eerola S: Treatment of postpneumonectomy empyema. Scand J Thorac Cardiovasc Surg 8:133, 1974

Virkkula L, Eerola S, Varstela E: Surgical approach to the chronic empyema: space sterilization. p. 263. In Delarue NC, Eschapasse H (eds): Thoracic Surgery: Surgical Management of Pleural Diseases. In Deslauriers J, Lacquet LK (eds): International Trends in General Thoracic Surgery. Vol. 6. CV Mosby, St. Louis, 1990

Weissberg D: Empyema and bronchopleural fistula: experience with open window thoracostomy. Chest 82:447, 1982

Zumbro GL, Treasure R, Geiger JP, Green DC: Empyema after pneumonectomy. Ann Thorac Surg 15:615, 1973

Thoracoplasty

Jean Deslauriers
Louis F. Jacques

Thoracoplasty is a surgical measure designed to permanently collapse the lung by removing the ribs from the chest wall. Before the advent of effective chemotherapy for tuberculosis, thoracoplasty was one of several methods used to put the lung to rest with the hope of inactivating the disease. Other, perhaps less aggressive, methods included positioning the patient with the diseased side down, artificial pneumothorax, intrapleural cautery pneumolysis with the thoracoscope, intercostal neurectomy, scalenotomy, phrenic nerve interruption, or bronchial interruption.

Since the early 1960s thoracoplasty has lost much of its popularity, not only because it is considered by many as a mutilating and poorly tolerated procedure but also because of the advent of effective management of tuberculosis and of better techniques of muscle transfer to fill infected spaces. There remain, however, a few patients with chronic infected spaces and with no remaining lung or a lung that cannot be expanded because of intrinsic disease who are potential candidates for thoracoplasty.

HISTORICAL NOTE

Estlander (1879) was the first surgeon to use the term *thoracoplasty* to denote removal of ribs in order to bring the chest wall down to the lung, which would not expand after drainage of an empyema (Young and Moor, 1976). In 1885 de Cerenville of Lausanne also described a technique in which short segments of two or more ribs were resected in order to collapse the chest wall over areas of apical cavitary tuberculosis.

The thoracoplasty described by Schede in 1890 was an operation that included not only multiple rib resections but also the removal of the periosteum, intercostal muscles and nerves, and parietal pleura. According to Kergin (1953), the Schede thoracoplasty was formulated on the basis of accurate knowledge of the pathology of chronic empyemas but it had serious faults: it was shocking and mutilating; it involved the sacrifice of intercostal nerves, with resulting cutaneous anesthesia; and it left a large opened wound, requiring a long period of packing and dressing.

In 1907 Friedrich, following Rudolph Brauer's (an internist) suggestion that thoracoplasty must collapse the diseased lung (Young and Moor, 1976), resected full lengths of the second through the ninth rib with a mortality rate of 43 percent (four of seven patients survived the operation). Subsequently, Wilms (1913) and Sauerbruch (1925) resected the posterior segments of the first 11 ribs by an operation that became the paravertebral thoracoplasty. They pointed out that resection of the posterior ribs would bring about a greater collapse of the underlying lung than resection of the more anterior segments.

All these procedures evolved into the classical three-stage thoracoplasty popularized by Alexander (1937), which involved resecting the posterior segments of the ribs and sometimes portions of the transverse processes but leaving the periosteum to ensure that new bone formation would maintain long-term collapse of the lung.

In 1934 Semb described an important addition to the technique of thoracoplasty, which he called extrafascial apicolysis. His method consisted of extrapleural division of all adhesions between the pleural dome at the apex and the soft tissues around the base of the neck and cervical spine. This dissection, carried out outside the plane of the endothoracic fascia, provided more complete collapse of the lung without having to resect the transverse processes of the vertebrae.

Because conventional thoracoplasty was considered cosmetically unacceptable, other surgeons described plombage thoracoplasty, introduced by Tuffier (1891) as a method of extrapleural pneumolysis in which air was insufflated extrapleurally to maintain lung collapse. Subsequent variations included the use of omentum (Tuffier, 1914) or paraffin extrapleurally or of other products such as plastic balls between the freed periosteum and the ribs.

HISTORICAL READINGS

Alexander J: The collapse therapy of pulmonary tuberculosis. Charles C Thomas, Springfield, IL, 1937

De Cerenville EB: De l'intervention dans les maladies du poumon. Rev Med Suisse Romande 5:441, 1885

Estlander JA: Résection des côtes dans l'empyème chronique. Rev Med Chir (Paris) 3:157, 1879

Friedrich PL: Die operative Beeinflussung einseitiger Lungphthiser durch totale Brustwandmobilisierung Arch Klin Chir 27:588, 1908

Kergin FG: An operation for chronic pleural empyema. J Thorac Surg 26:430, 1953

Sauerbruch F: Die Chirurgie der Brustorgane. Vol. 2. Springer-Verlag, Berlin, 1925, p. 876

Schede M: Die Behandlung der Empyeme. Verh Cong Innere Med Wiesbaden 9:41, 1890

Semb C: Technique of plastic operation of apicolysis. Acta Chir Scand 74:478, 1934

Tuffier T: État Actuel de la Chirurgie Intra-thoracique. Masson, Paris, 1914; pp. 90, 163

Wilms M: Die Pfeilerresektion der Rippen zur Verengerung des Thorax bei Lungentuberculose. Ther Gegehwart 54:17, 1913

Young WG, Moor GF: The surgical treatment of pulmonary tuberculosis. p. 567. In Sabiston DC, Spencer FC (eds): Gibbon's Surgery of the Chest. 3rd Ed. WB Saunders, Philadelphia, 1976

INDICATIONS

Despite the decline in thoracoplasty popularity, four recent studies have shown that it is an excellent therapeutic option for selected patients. In the series of Hopkins et al. (1985), 30 patients were treated with thoracoplasty over a 14-year period. The surgery was performed to close a persistent pleural space in 28 patients and to adapt the thoracic cavity for diminished lung volume concomitantly with pulmonary resection in the other two patients. Among the 28 patients with persistent infected spaces, 24 had an associated bronchopleural fistula and in 19 infection had occurred following an operation. In our own series (Grégoire, et al., 1987), 17 patients underwent thoracoplasty for a postpneumonectomy empyema and 7 had an associated bronchopleural fistula. In 1990 Horrigan and Snow reported a series of 13 patients who underwent thoracoplasty between 1976 and 1989. Five of these patients had chronic apical empyema spaces without prior resection of lung, and all had extensive destruction of upper lobe tissue. Eight patients had undergone prior pulmonary resection and had infected postoperative residual spaces. In the series of Peppas et al. (1993), 19 patients underwent the operation to control complications of resection for lung cancer, and 18 patients had the operation during the course of management of disease not related to lung cancer.

Current indications for thoracoplasty are summarized below. It is worth noting that contrary to what can be achieved with infected apical spaces, thoracoplasty is almost never indicated for the treatment of basal spaces such as those sometimes seen after right and middle lower lobectomies. These lower spaces are better managed by open thoracic window drainage or by filling of the space with muscle flaps, because at the base it is nearly impossible to obtain proper collapse of the chest wall by thoracoplasty. In patients with

Current Indications for Thoracoplasty

Persistent space following pulmonary resection or
    other thoracic procedure
  Apical spaces after upper lobectomy
  Postpneumonectomy empyema space
Unresolving chronic empyemas unrelated to resection
  Apical empyemas with destroyed upper lobe
    (tuberculosis or postpneumonic)
  Empyema in a space following previous therapeutic
    pneumothorax
  Pleural aspergillosis
Patients unfit for pulmonary resection
Tailoring thoracoplasty done concomitantly with
    lung resection

Terminology

Intrapleural thoracoplasty
  Schede (1890): resection of ribs, parietal pleura,
    intercostal muscles, and neurovascular bundles
  Modifications of
    Heller (1934) ⎫ preservation of
    Kergin (1953) ⎭ intercostal muscles
  Horrigan and Snow (1990): limited rib resections
Extrapleural thoracoplasty
  Alexander (1937): resection of ribs but retention of
    periosteum, intercostal muscles, and parietal
    pleura
  Modifications of
    Semb (1935): extrafascial apicolysis
    Björk (1954): osteoplastic thoracoplasty
Plombage thoracoplasty
  Tuffier (1891): extrapleural plombage
  Modern version (1949–1950): extrafascial
    pneumolysis and plombage
  Iioka, et al. technique (1985)
Limited thoracoplasty
  Limited in the number of ribs resected
  Tailoring thoracoplasty: done in association with
    pulmonary resection

postpneumonectomy empyemas, thoracoplasty presents specific advantages over space filling or space sterilization methods (Claggett and Geraci, 1963), and treatment failures are uncommon (Grégoire, et al., 1987). In nonresectional apical empyemas with destroyed upper lobes or in an empyema that has developed in an apical space following previous therapeutic pneumothorax, decortication is inadvisable and will almost inevitably be followed by failure because of the underlying lung disease (see Chap. 42). In these situations thoracoplasty may be indicated to collapse the space. Thoracoplasty may also be indicated in the management of complicated pleuropulmonary aspergillosis (Al-Zeerah and Jeyasingham, 1989). Finally, tailoring thoracoplasty may be indicated after pulmonary resection when it appears that the remaining lobe or lobes will be unable to completely fill the space.

PROCEDURE TYPES

The techniques of thoracoplasty in current use are numerous and varied in their details (Peppas, et al., 1993).

Intrapleural

As described by Schede (1890), intrapleural thoracoplasty involves multiple rib excisions as well as resection of the parietal pleura, periosteum, intercostal muscles, and intercostal neurovascular bundles. Only the skin and thoracic muscles remain to collapse over the residual lung or space, and a large open wound is left, with packing used to fill the space. The Schede thoracoplasty was performed mainly in those patients in whom the walls of the space were so thick that rib resection alone would be insufficient to appropriately collapse the cavity. It was also considered a mutilating operation, and therefore modifications were later proposed by Heller (1934) and Wangensteen (1935). These surgeons described an operation in which, after removal of the ribs overlying the cavity, the rib beds were incised to create a series of ribbons, each consisting of an intercostal muscle with the accompanying vessels, nerve, parietal pleura, and fibrous tissue (Kergin, 1953). These ribbons were dropped into the cavity to act as space fillers.

Kergin himself (1953) described an operation by which he excised the parietal pleura and fibrous tissue from those ribbons so that they became more flexible to adapt to all corners of the empyema cavity (Fig. 43-15). The main advantages of the Kergin thoracoplasty were that the intercostal nerves were preserved and the ribs able to regenerate in order to give stability to the chest wall. In addition, the space was filled with living tissue with excellent vascular supply. Horrigan and Snow (1990) used a similar technique but confined the rib removal below the third rib to the more posterior aspect of the chest. They used adjacent trapezius, latissimus, serratus, or rhomboid muscle to reinforce the fistula closure and fill the space. The results were good and severe deformity was avoided in most patients.

Extrapleural

The extrapleural thoracoplasty was popularized by Alexander (1937) as a procedure that retains the periosteum of the ribs, the intercostal muscles, and the parietal pleura. It provides a lateral collapse of the lung. Because the apex is often held up at the levels of the cervical spine by strong muscular and fibrous bands, Semb (1935) proposed the operation of extrafascial apicolysis, by which vertical relaxation was obtained to complement lateral relaxation. The difficulties inherent in this technique are that the fibrous bands that must be divided to free the apex often surround the subclavian artery and vein and the lower trunks of the brachial plexus. In 1954 Björk described his *osteoplastic* technique of thoracoplasty, whereby a new roof of the thorax was obtained by

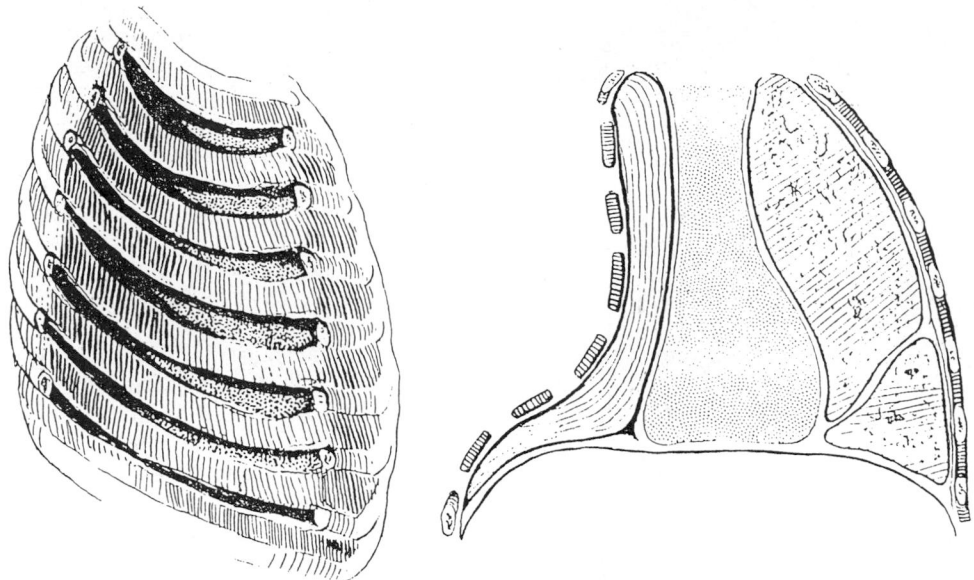

Figure 43-15. After resection of the parietal wall, the muscle bundles are laid in the cavity. (From Kergin FG: An operation for chronic pleural empyema. J Thorac Surg 26:430, 1953, with permission.)

resection of posterior portions of the ribs in increasing lengths from above downward. The ribs were then bent into the costal cartilages and fixed to the posterior end of the uppermost intact rib by stainless steel sutures (Fig. 43-16). By this technique, a stable chest wall was obtained and the lung was prevented from reexpanding above the new roof. A similar technique was described by Barclay and Welch (1957).

Plombage

Plombage thoracoplasty was initiated in 1891 by Tuffier, who described the merits of performing and maintaining an extrapleural pneumothorax to collapse the lung (Tuffier, 1914). The method was simple, and initially Tuffier left the extrapleural space empty. He later inserted air, omentum, or fresh lipomas for this purpose (Horowitz, et al., 1992). In the late 1940s and early 1950s, several articles appeared reporting the same operation but with an extrafascial (outside the endothoracic fascia) rather than an extrapleural pneumothorax. Over the years at least 29 different materials (Horowitz, et al., 1992; Walkup and Murphy 1949) have been used to maintain collapse of affected areas of the lung, including gauze sponge, silk, wax, various oils and gelatin, rubber balloons, drawing crayons, and lead bullets (Horowitz, et al., 1992). These products were inserted between the endothoracic fascia and periosteum on one side and the ribs on the other.

In 1946 Wilson (Horowitz, et al., 1992) reported his experience using balls made of polymethylmethacrylate (Lucite) for plombage (Fig. 43-17). These plombage operations had the advantage of providing good selective collapse without paradoxical respiration but the disadvantage of the patient being prone to infection. In 1985 Iioka, et al., described a technique of collapsing the parietal wall made of parietal pleura, periosteum, and intercostal muscle without rib resection, thereby obliterating the empyema cavity. This collapse

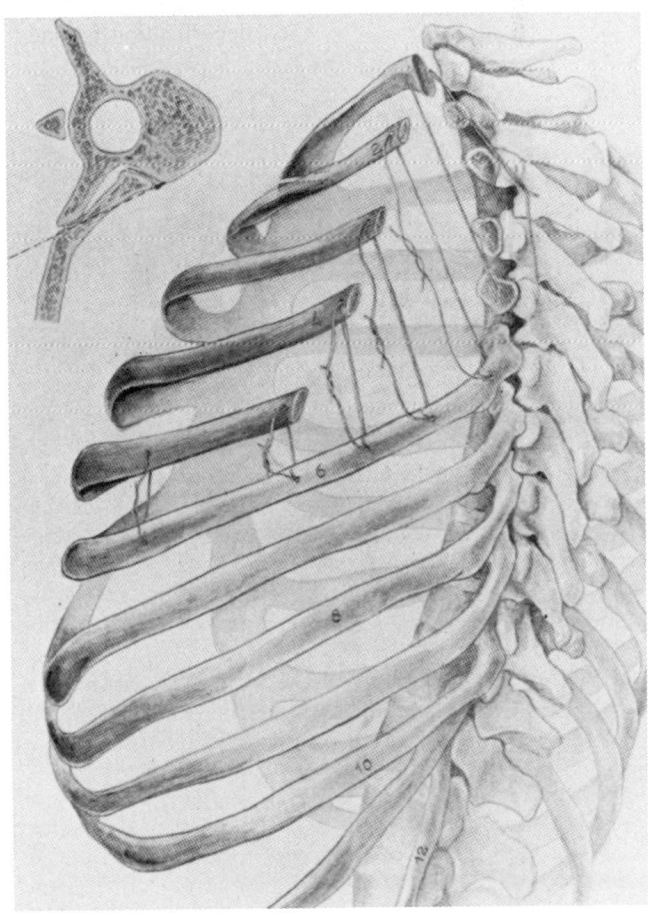

Figure 43-16. The posterior ends of the upper five ribs are resected in increasing lengths. (From Björk VO: Thoracoplasty. A new osteoplastic technique. J Thorac Surg 28:194, 1954, with permission.)

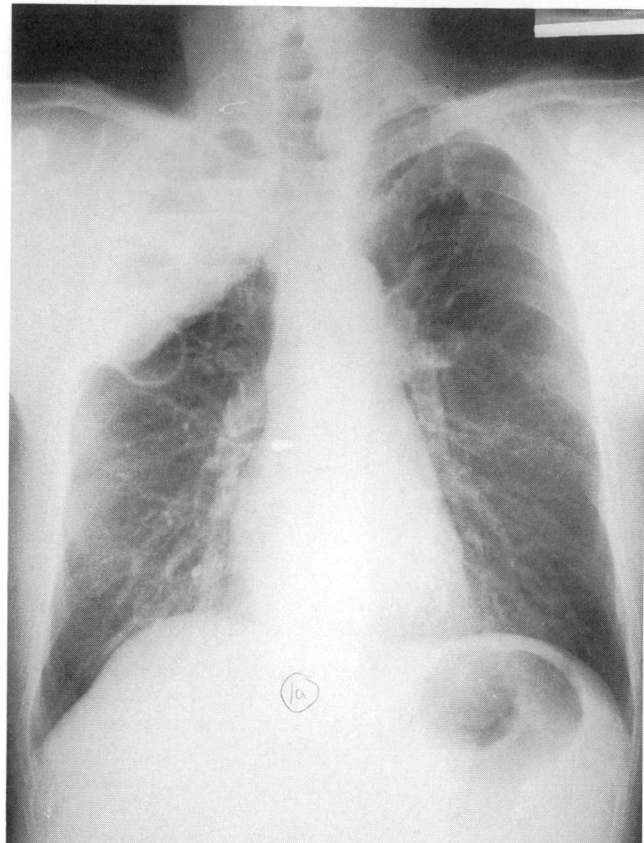

Figure 43-17. Plombage thoracoplasty with Lucite balls. No ribs have been resected.

created an extraperiosteal space, which filled with the patient's own blood and serum.

Limited

A limited thoracoplasty is a procedure that is restricted to the removal of only a few ribs in order to eliminate an infected space. A limited tailored thoracoplasty or tailoring thoracoplasty is done in association with a pulmonary resection in which a space problem is anticipated.

A thoracoplasty is total if the posterior segments of the first eleven ribs are removed and partial if only eight or nine ribs are resected. An extended thoracoplasty removes, in addition to the posterior segments of the ribs, the anterior extremities of the upper ribs (Fey, et al., 1955). Most thoracoplasties are done subperiosteally because the periosteum is left in place so that the rib can regenerate. When both rib and periosteum are removed, the thoracoplasty is called extraperiosteal.

TECHNIQUE

Incisions and Surgical Access

All thoracoplasties are performed under one-lung anesthesia maintained with a double-lumen tube, the use of this tube being important to prevent aspiration of the empyema contents into the contralateral lung.

Thoracoplasty can be done through a posterior or a posterolateral approach or through an axillary incision. The posterior approach was commonly used during the early years of thoracoplasty, but it has now been largely abandoned because it involves division of both the trapezius (superficial layer) and rhomboid (deep layer) muscles, which unite the spine with the lateral border of the scapula. These muscles are important to elevate the scapula and prevent it from free floating. In order to prevent this problem, Brock (1946) and others have shown that the muscles have to be divided close to the spine, thereby avoiding injury to either the spinal nerve or the posterior spinal artery.

In recent years most thoracoplasties are performed through a standard posterolateral thoracotomy, which can be extended vertically upward to provide adequate access to the upper ribs (Peppas, et al., 1993). The posterior division of the latissimus dorsi and the division of the serratus anterior muscles will completely free the scapula, which can then be elevated to expose the ribs. Maintenance of this exposure is achieved by inserting a chest retractor (Finochietto) between a lower rib and the tip of the scapula.

The axillary incision can be used for limited thoracoplasties. It has the advantage of providing good and easy access to the rib cage but the disadvantages of a scapula that cannot be mobilized and of difficult access to the most posterior portion of the ribs.

Conventional Posterolateral Thoracoplasty (Alexander Type)

The procedure consists of extramusculoperiosteal resection of a sufficient number of ribs to completely collapse the space. As originally described by Alexander (1937), it involved the resection of 10 or 11 ribs, and it was done in three stages to prevent paradoxical respiration. Today, most spaces requiring thoracoplasty are the result of postoperative infections, and these can be treated in one stage and with a more limited number of rib resections. If the operation is done in stages, the time between stages varies from 10 to 30 days.

The second to the eighth ribs are usually resected (Fig. 43-18), and it is best to start with the third rib, next resect the second, and then resect the fourth to the seventh or eighth rib. The extent of resection is regulated by the pathologic extent of disease, and as a rule of thumb, one should extend rib resection to one rib below the most inferior area of disease. Sloping resection of the anterior portion of the ribs with progressively less anterior rib being removed will preserve the normal configuration of the anterolateral thoracic wall. This maneuver will also help to decrease the paradox and prevent collapse of the healthy lung, usually located anteriorly. Posteriorly, the ribs should be taken through their neck or head or even be completely disarticulated from the costovertebral joint. To maximize paravertebral collapse and accentuate transverse compression of the lung, part or the whole of the transverse processes may also have to be resected. If the sixth rib is resected, the tip of the scapula may be moving on and off the seventh rib and produce unpleasant sensations. When this is anticipated, the problem can be prevented by resecting either the seventh rib or the lower third of the scapula.

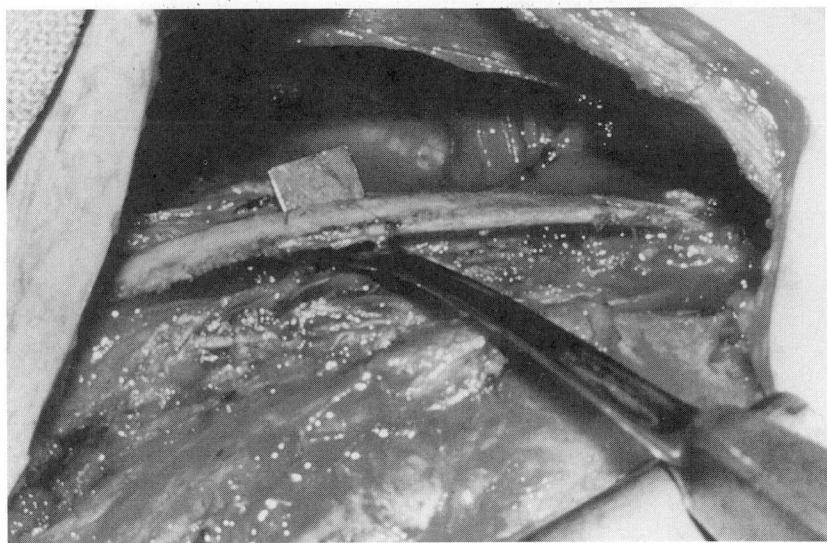

Figure 43-18.   Operative photograph showing rib resection and collapse of the space during thoracoplasty.

There is some controversy as to whether the first rib should be resected. Jaretzki (1991) summarized well the changing attitude toward the resection of the first rib:

> When the classic ten-rib Alexander thoracoplasty was performed in the treatment of tuberculosis, removal of the first rib was necessary to obtain adequate collapse therapy [Fig. 43-19]. However, in performing a limited thoracoplasty to assist in the elimination of an infected space, or a limited tailored thoracoplasty in association with a pulmonary resection where a space problem is anticipated, the first rib should not be removed.

As was shown by Grégoire, et al. (1987), Mansour (1991), and others, preserving the first rib is important in order to

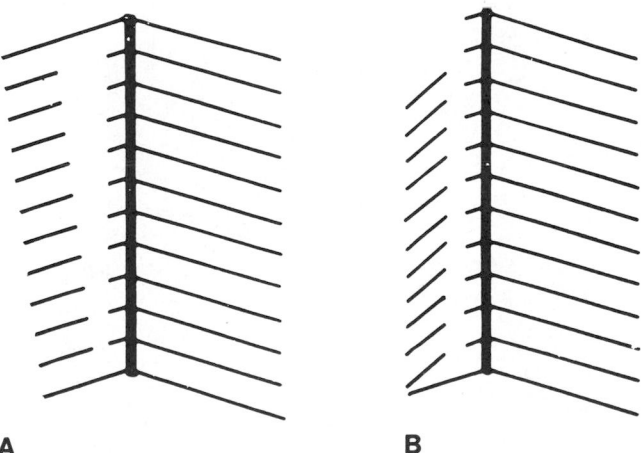

A   **B**

Figure 43-19.   John Alexander's version of the suspensory role of the first rib in thoracoplasty. **(A)** All ribs have been removed except the first, and the collapse is incomplete. **(B)** The first rib has been removed, with more adequate collapse. (From Alexander J: The collapse theory of pulmonary tuberculosis. Charles C. Thomas, Springfield, IL, 1937.)

maintain the integrity of the neck, shoulder girdle, and upper thorax (Fig. 43-20).

Whether or not the first rib is resected, apicolysis is a most important step in the operation of thoracoplasty. It can be done extrapleurally as described by Holst, et al. (1935) or extrafascially (Semb, 1935) (Fig. 43-21). The purpose of apicolysis is to bring the apex of the lung and other soft tissues downward to obliterate the space. It involves division of upper intercostal muscle bundles and fibrous tissue close to the spine and separation of all apical attachments to the chest wall. If the apicolysis is done extrapleurally with the first rib intact, the periosteum over the rib is incised, with use of diathermy, and stripped from its superior surface. Once the rib is freed, the space is collapsed by digital pressure and scissor division of fibrous tissue posteriorly.

There is also some controversy as to whether a bronchopleural fistula, when present, should be closed. It has been our policy (Grégoire, et al., 1987) not to close small bronchopleural fistulae (<2 mm), since collapse of the space will nearly always result in spontaneous closure. If a large fistula is present, a posteriorly pedicled intercostal muscle flap is brought down through the space to cover the bronchial stump. Peppas, et al. (1993) and others have suggested that all fistulae, whether small or large, should be closed by direct suture or by opposition of a myoplastic flap.

Adequate postoperative intra- and extrapleural drainage is mandatory. The intrapleural drain, which is usually in place before the thoracoplasty takes place, is left until complete obliteration of the space is achieved. The extrapleural drain located in the noninfected extrapleural space can be removed within 4 to 5 days of surgery.

MORBIDITY/MORTALITY AND RESULTS

In most recent series, the operative mortality associated with thoracoplasty varies between 0 and 10 percent. Postoperative complications include failure to heal, failure to obliterate the space, failure to control infection, failure to close the

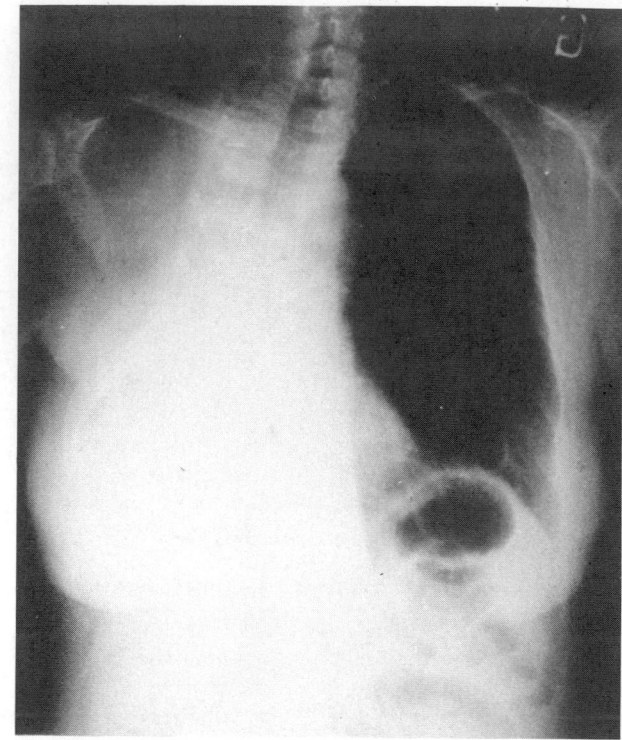

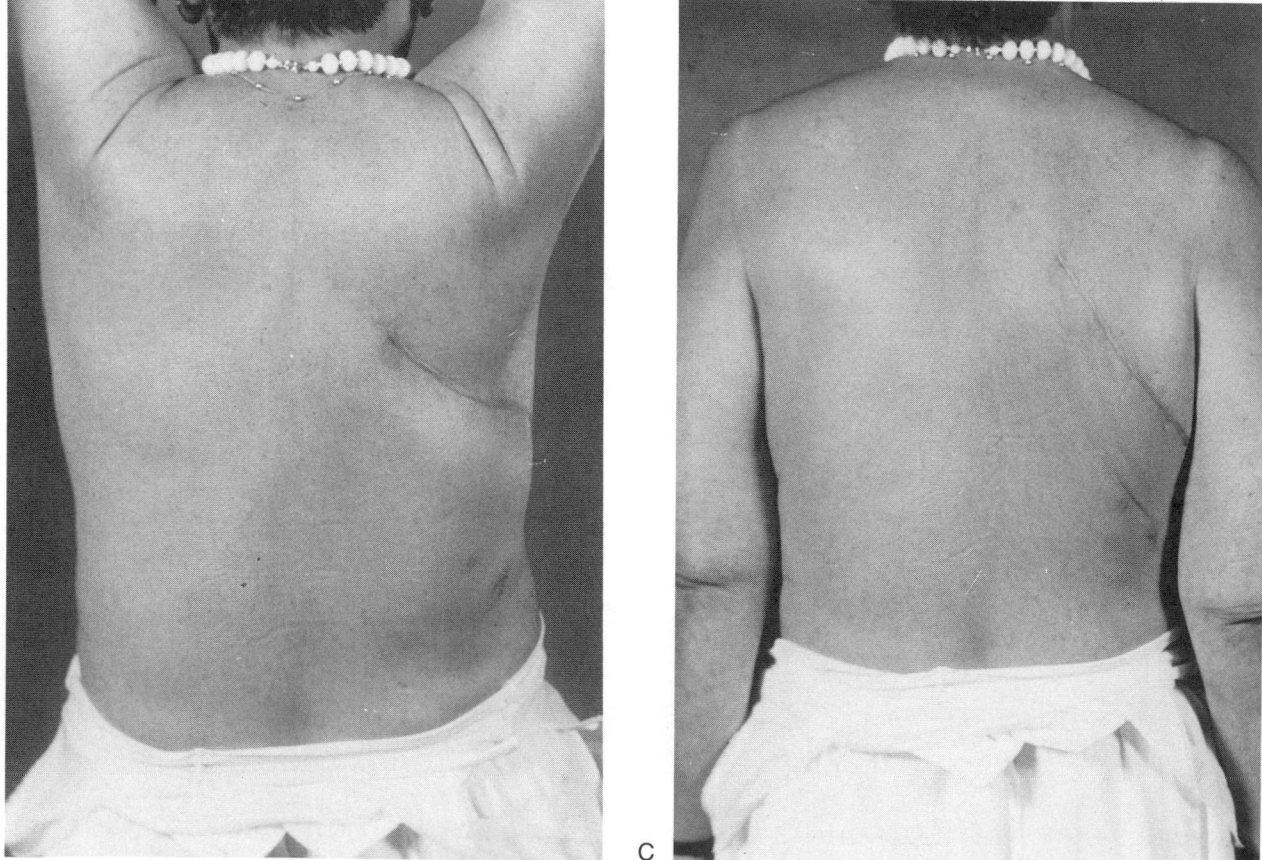

Figure 43-20. **(A)** Chest x-ray film and **(B & C)** photographs of a 53-year-old woman 6 months after right-sided thoracoplasty for a postpneumonectomy empyema. Structural integrity of neck and shoulder girdle is maintained by retaining first rib.

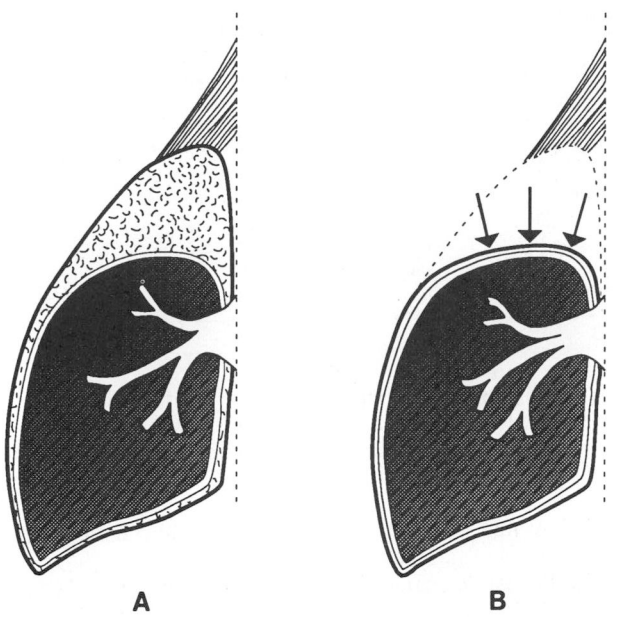

Figure 43-21. (A) Extrapleural apicolysis and (B) extra-fascial apicolysis (Adapted from Fey B, Mocquot P, Oberlin S et al.: Traité de Technique Chirurgicale. Vol. 4. p. 212. Masson, Paris, 1955, with permission.)

bronchopleural fistula, and respiratory failure. Late results show successful collapse and obliteration of the spaces in 80 to 90 percent of patients.

COMPLICATIONS RELATED TO SPECIFIC TYPES OF THORACOPLASTIES

Most thoracoplasties produce some degree of chest wall and shoulder deformities. Progressive scoliosis (Fig. 43-22) may develop if the transverse processes of the spine and the first rib have been resected. Patients may also have chronic postoperative chest pain and hyperanesthesia of the chest wall. With intrapleural types of thoracoplasties such as the Schede, patients have more thoracic deformities, in addition to having cutaneous anesthesia and paresthesias over the lower thoracic and upper abdominal walls. Patients may have restriction of shoulder motion on the involved side because the scapula becomes adherent to the chest wall (Horrigan and Snow, 1990), especially if a portion of that bone has been resected, and the appearance is that of a frozen shoulder. Gaensler and Struder (1951) have finally shown that some patients will develop progressive pulmonary failure. Most of these problems can be avoided by limiting the size of the thoracoplasty, by meticulous surgical technique, and by early postoperative rehabilitation.

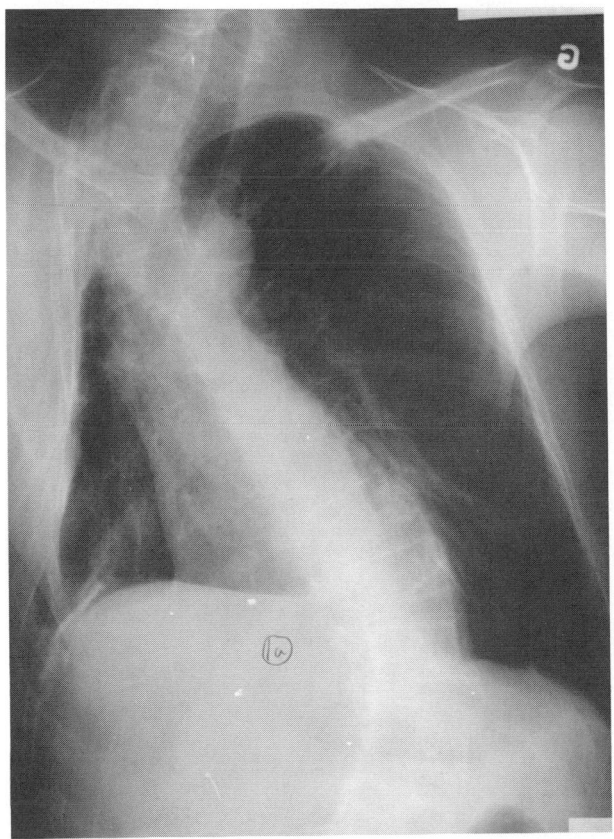

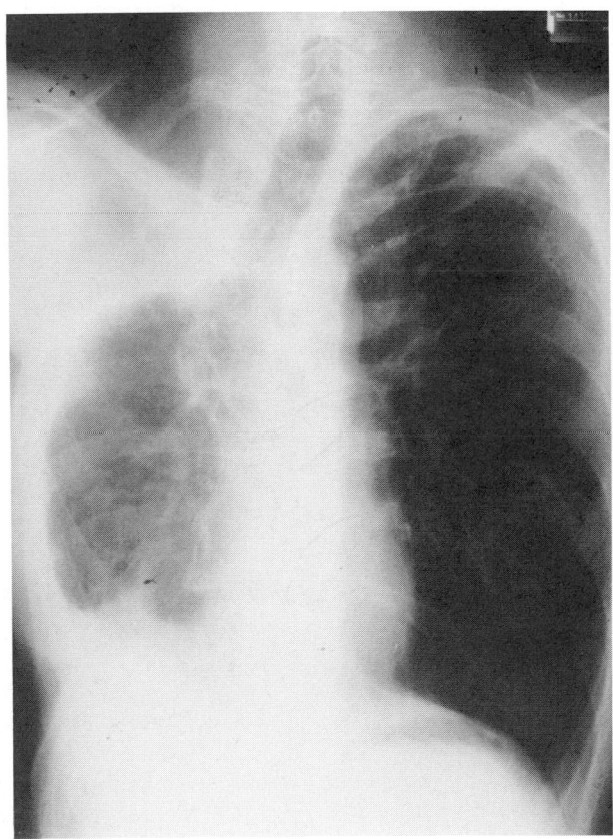

Figure 43-22. (A) Severe scoliosis seen after extensive six-rib thoracoplasty. Note that the first rib has been removed. (B) Less extensive scoliosis, with first rib preservation.

KEY REFERENCES

Hopkins RA, Ungerleider RM, Staub EW, Young WG: The modern use of thoracoplasty. Ann Thorac Surg 40:181, 1985

Excellent review describing modern indications and results of thoracoplasty. Describes the Alexander principles of thoracoplasty.

Peppas G, Molnar TF, Jeyasingham K, Kirk AB: Thoracoplasty in the context of current surgical practice. Ann Thorac Surg 56:903, 1993

This is a review of 37 patients who underwent thoracoplasty between 1975 and 1991. Presents a good discussion of the various types of thoracoplasty and their indications.

REFERENCES

Alexander J: The Collapse Therapy of Pulmonary Tuberculosis. Charles C Thomas, Springfield, IL, 1937

Al-Zeerah M, Jeyasingham K: Limited thoracoplasty in the management of complicated pulmonary aspergillomas. Thorax 44:1027, 1989

Barclay RS, Welch TM: Thoracoplasty with apical fixation. Scott Med J 2:20, 1957

Björk VO: Thoracoplasty. A new osteoplastic technique. J Thorac Surg 28:194, 1954

Brock RC: Musculo-plastic incision for posterior thoracoplasty. J Thorac Surg 15:182, 1946

Claggett OT, Geraci JE: A procedure for the management of postpneumonectomy empyema. J Thorac Cardiovasc Surg 45:141, 1963

De Cerenville EB: De l'intervention dans les maladies du poumon. Rev Med Suisse Romande. 5:441, 1885

Estlander JA: Résection des côtes dans l'empyème chronique. Rev Med Chir (Paris). 3:157, 1879

Fey B, Mocquot P, Oberlin S et al.: Traité de Technique Chirurgicale. Vol. 4. Masson, Paris, 1955 p. 212

Friedrich PL: Die operative Beeinflussung einseitiger Lungphthise durch totale Brustwandmobilisierung. Arch Klin Chir 27:588, 1908

Gaensler EA, Struder JW: Progressive changes in pulmonary function after pneumonectomy: the influence of thoracoplasty, pneumothorax, oleothorax, and plastic sponge plombage on the side of the pneumonectomy. J Thorac Surg 22:1, 1951

Grégoire R, Deslauriers J, Beaulieu M, Piraux M: Thoracoplasty: its forgotten role in the management of non tuberculous postpneumonectomy empyema. Can J Surg 30:343, 1987

Heller H: Ueber Verhutung und Behandlung der Emphysemresthohlen. Chirurg 6:297, 1934

Holst J, Semb C, Frimann-Dahl J: On surgical treatment of pulmonary tuberculosis. Acta Chir Scand 76:1, 1935

Horowitz MD, Otero M, Thurer RJ, Bolooki H: Late complications of plombage. Ann Thorac Surg 53:803, 1992

Horrigan TP, Snow NJ: Thoracoplasty: current application to the infected pleural space. Ann Thorac Surg 50:695, 1990

Iioka S, Sawamura K, Mori T et al.: Surgical treatment of chronic empyema. A new one-stage operation. J Thorac Cardiovasc Surg 90:179, 1985

Jaretzki A: Role of thoracoplasty in the treatment of chronic empyema (letter). Ann Thorac Surg 52:584, 1991

Kergin FG: An operation for chronic pleural empyema. J Thorac Surg 26:430, 1953

Mansour KA: Reply to the editor. Ann Thorac Surg 52:585, 1991

Sauerbruch F: Die Chirurgie der Brustorgane. Vol. 2, Berlin: Springer-Verlag, Berlin, 1925, p. 876

Schede M: Die Behandlung der Empyeme. Verh Cong Innere Med Wiesbaden 9:41, 1890

Semb C: Technique of plastic operation of apicolysis. Acta Chir Scand 74:478, 1934

Semb C: Thoracoplasty with apicolysis. NationaltryKKehut, Oslo, 1935

Tuffier T: État Actuel de la Chirurgie Intrathoracique. Masson, Paris, 1914; pp. 90, 163

Tuffier T: Du décollement pariétal en chirurgie pulmonaire. Arch Med Chir App Respir 1:32, 1926

Walkup HE, Murphy JD: Extrapleural pneumolysis with plombage. Am J Surg 78:245, 1949

Wangensteen OH: The pedicle muscle flap in the closure of persistent bronchopleural fistula. J Thorac Surg 5:27, 1935

Wilms M: Die Pfeilerresektion der Rippen zur Verengerung des Thorax bei Lungentuberculose. Ther Gegenwart 54:17, 1913

Wilson DA: The use of methylmethacrylate plombage in the surgical treatment of pulmonary tuberculosis. Surg Clin North Am 26:1060, 1946

Young WG, Moor GF: The surgical treatment of pulmonary tuberculosis. p. 567. In Sabiston DC, Spencer FC (eds): Gibbon's Surgery of the Chest. 3rd Ed. WB Saunders, Philadelphia, 1976

Therapeutic Thoracoscopy

Jean Deslauriers
Reza John Mehran
Louis F. Jacques

Although pleural diseases are relatively common in the practice of thoracic surgery, their management is often problematic. Spontaneous pneumothoraces, for instance, are easy to diagnose, but therapy often entails open thoracotomy with attendant risks, discomfort, and several days of hospitalization. Empyemas are not only difficult to diagnose but also to drain adequately so that lung reexpansion and space obliteration are achieved. These examples illustrate some of the problems facing the surgeon managing pleural space pathologies, problems that can be included in one of three categories: relative inaccessibility of the pleural space, reliance on diagnostic tools often inaccurate, and the trauma of open thoracotomy.

Videothoracoscopic surgery combines the precision of direct visual inspection with minimal-access surgery. It has expanded the conventional indications for diagnostic thoracoscopy to include therapy of spontaneous pneumothoraces, pleural effusions, and empyemas, as well as of other less common pleural diseases.

HISTORICAL NOTE

In recent years there has been renewed interest in the use of thoracoscopy for management of pleural diseases, a trend that has followed major advances in the field of laparoscopy as well as the development of modern video and endosurgical equipment. There was a time, however, when thoracoscopy independent of laparoscopy was a popular diagnostic and therapeutic tool.

Bozzini in 1807 and Desormeau in 1853 (Bloomberg, 1978) used a hollow tube lighted by a burning light to visualize the bladder. In 1883 Newman incorporated an edisonian light with the cystoscope, and Jacobeus (1910) used a thoracoscope to lyse pleural adhesions in order to improve lung collapse in the treatment of tuberculosis. This procedure was subsequently termed *pneumolysis*. The adhesions were first seen with the thoracoscope and then divided with a diathermic needle inserted through a second orifice. Jacobeus reported 50 consecutive patients, of whom 39 had successful cauterizations and complete collapse of the lung and 35 experienced a favorable clinical response (Oakes, et al., 1984). Between 1936 and 1950 Bloomberg performed or supervised 2,000 thoracoscopies for the lysis of pleural adhesions with good results and minimal complications (Bloomberg, 1978). During the same time, however, the advent of effective antituberculous drugs resulted in the abandonment of induced pneumothorax and of the Jacobeus operation.

In the management of spontaneous pneumothorax, Sattler (1937) was the first to use the thoracoscope, as he recognized that some patients had ruptured emphysematous blebs while others had no such lesions. He also recommended thoracoscopy whenever radiographs demonstrated adhesions, particularly if the lung failed to reexpand promptly (Bloomberg, 1978). In 1974 Swierenga and associates reported thoracoscopic findings in 136 cases of so-called idiopathic spontaneous pneumothorax and on the basis of those findings decided on different methods of therapy.

HISTORICAL READINGS

Bloomberg AE: Thoracoscopy in perspective. Surg Gynecol Obstet 147:433, 1978

Bozzini P: On the Illumination of Internal Cavities. Weimar, 1807

Jacobeus HC: Possibility of the use of cystoscopy in the investigation of serous cavities. Munch Med Wochenschr 40:2090, 1910

Jacobeus HC: The practical importance of thoracoscopy in surgery of the chest. Surg Gynecol Obstet 34:289, 1922

Le Tacon J: La pleuroscopie. Rappel historique. Poumon Coeur 37:5, 1981

Newman D: Lectures on Surgical Diseases of the Kidney. Longmans, Green, London, 1888

Oakes DD, Sherck JP, Brodsky JB, Mark JBD: Therapeutic thoracoscopy. J Thorac Cardiovasc Surg 87:269, 1984

Sattler A: The treatment of spontaneous pneumothorax with special reference to thoracoscopy. Beitr Klin Tuberk 89:395, 1937

Swierenga J, Wagenaar JPM, Bergstein PGM: The value of thoracoscopy in the diagnosis and treatment of diseases affecting the pleura and lung. Pneumologie (Stuttg) 151:11, 1974

INDICATIONS AND TECHNIQUES OF THERAPEUTIC THORACOSCOPY FOR PLEURAL DISEASES

Thoracoscopy for Spontaneous Pneumothorax

Ironically, the earliest indication for therapeutic thoracoscopy was to induce pneumothoraces by the lysis of adhesions in the treatment of tuberculosis (Jacobeus, 1922). Almost the same technique is now being used to manage spontaneous pneumothoraces.

Primary spontaneous pneumothoraces mostly occur in young patients without evidence of coexisting lung disease while secondary pneumothoraces are seen in older individuals with emphysema. Unless there is a complication, most surgeons manage the first episode by conventional tube drainage. Recurrences are usually treated by blebectomy with parietal pleurectomy or pleural abrasion, all of which techniques appear to be safe and are associated with excellent long-term results (Deslauriers, et al., 1980).

Video-Assisted Blebectomy and Apical Pleurectomy for Primary Spontaneous Pneumothorax

Through the videothoracoscopic approach, blebs can be stapled, ligated with the endoloop, or cauterized with electrocautery, the argon beam electrocoagulator, or a laser.

Nathanson and associates (1991) reported two patients with recurrent pneumothorax in whom the lung was collapsed with a carbon dioxide insufflator and the blebs ligated with the endoloop using chronic catgut and a pre-tied Roeder knot. The parietal pleurectomy was done with scissors and grasping forceps. Both patients were cured and benefitted from the decreased trauma of access by reduced pain, rapid recovery, and decreased scarring of the skin. In 1989 Wakabayashi reported his experience with thoracoscopic electrocautery ablation of blebs in the treatment of recurrent or persistent pneumothorax. The procedure involved electrocoagulation of the blebs with a coagulation energy of 30 to 35 W/s. Ablation was successful in 9 of 10 patients. The use of the argon beam coagulator was evaluated by Rusch, et al. (1990), who showed that it is effective both in controlling blood loss and in sealing air leaks. The instrumentation is safe and causes less tissue injury then does standard electrocautery.

Possible Indications for Therapeutic Thoracoscopy in Pleural Diseases

Management of spontaneous pneumothorax and of its complications

Management of early-stage empyemas

Management of recurrent malignant pleural effusions

Other, unusual indications

Tube drainage of a pulmonary bulla

Drainage of hemothoraces and retrieval of foreign bodies

Closure of bronchopleural fistula and leaking thoracic duct

Removal of pleura-based masses

Techniques of VATS Blebectomy

Ligation with endoloop (Nathanson, et al., 1991)

Electrocautery ablation (Wakabayashi, 1989)

Argon beam coagulator (Rusch, et al., 1990)

Laser

Nd : YAG (Torre and Belloni, 1989)

CO$_2$ (Wakabayashi, 1990)

Stapling (Hazelrigg, et al., 1993; Yaita, et al., 1993)

In 1985 Locicero, et al. showed in clinical and experimental studies that both the carbon dioxide and the neodymium : yttrium-aluminum-garnet (Nd : YAG) laser can be used effectively to seal lung blebs. The carbon dioxide laser works better in a bloodless field, while the Nd : YAG laser is more powerful and can be used in the presence of blood. In 1989, Torre and Belloni reported the use of Nd : YAG laser pleurodesis through thoracoscopy in 14 patients. The fiber of the laser was advanced through the operative channel of the thoracoscope, and the blebs were successfully coagulated with low-power laser pulses. The parietal pleura over the first five ribs was then scarified to achieve pleurodesis. There were no side effects, and in 13 patients the therapy was successful without recurrences. Wakabayashi, et al. (1990) reported the use of the carbon dioxide laser in the treatment of patients with apical blebs and diffuse bullous emphysema. The procedure was conducted under general anesthesia with a double-lumen tube, and the entire inner surface of the bullae was exposed to the laser. In their series the air leaks were successfully sealed in all but one patient.

Like Hazelrigg, et al. (1993) and Yaita, et al. (1993), we prefer stapling resection of blebs with the Endo-GIA 30 stapler (Autosuture, U.S. Surgical Corp., Norwalk, CT). General endotracheal double-lumen anesthesia is used in every case, the patient being positioned in the full lateral position with the surgeon operating from the back. We use a Striker camera-lens system of 0 degree angle with an incorporated working channel.

Two to three trocars are necessary to perform the procedure. The first of these, the thoracoscopic trocar, is always inserted in the same location, which is about two fingerbreadth below the tip of the scapula, through the sixth or seventh intercostal space (Fig. 43-23). In that position and once the lung is collapsed, one has access to about 75 percent of the pleural space without any other manipulation, this being a major advantage of video-assisted thoracic surgery (VATS) over the standard axillary approach, by which only the lung apex can be visualized. A second and third trocar are then inserted, one halfway between the posterior border of the scapula and the spine and the other anteriorly to allow for the use of the Endo-GIA stapler (Fig. 43-24) and of grasping forceps. Once the blebs are located, they are grasped with the forceps, excised by multiple (usually two or three) applications of the Endo-GIA stapler, (Fig. 43-25), and removed through the largest incision (Fig. 43-26A).

The best method to predictably achieve optimal pleurodesis is to remove the parietal pleura, a technique originally

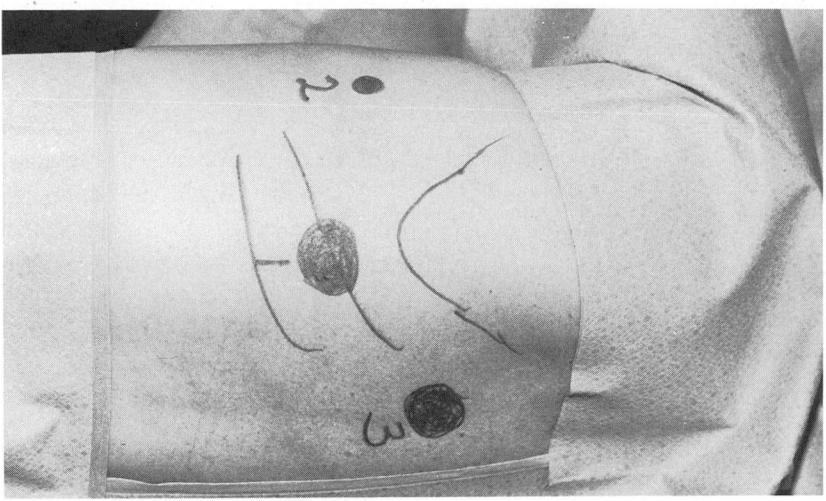

Figure 43-23.   Basic setup for VATS blebectomy and apical pleurectomy. The first port is for the thoracoscope. The Endo-GIA stapler and the grasping forceps can be inserted alternatively from either the second or third working port.

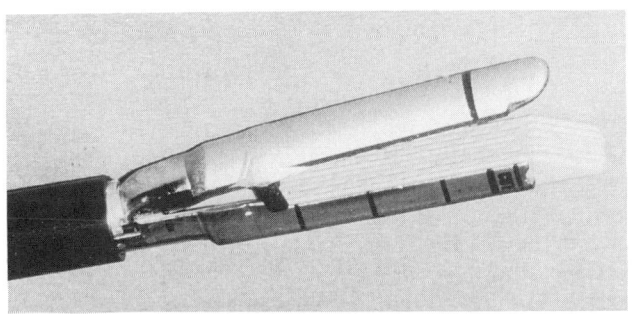

Figure 43-24.   Photograph of the Endo-GIA stapler used for bleb-ectomy.

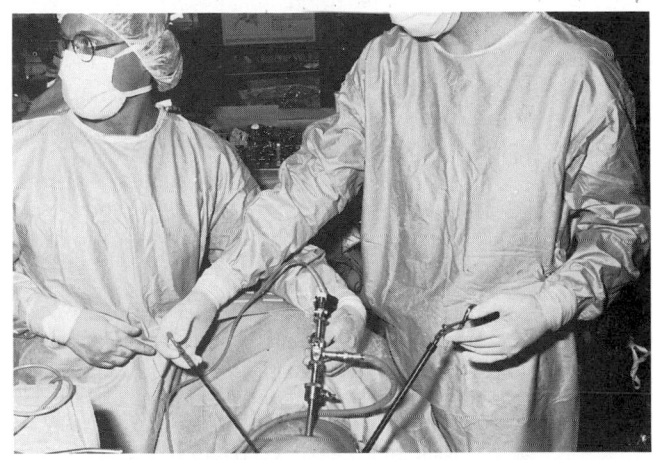

Figure 43-25.   Surgeon and assistant performing VATS bleb-ectomy.

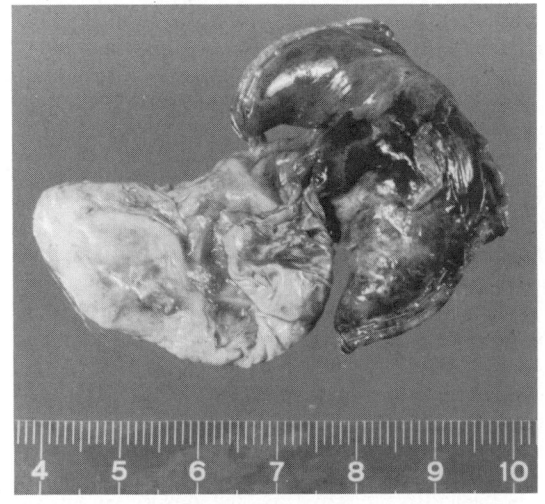

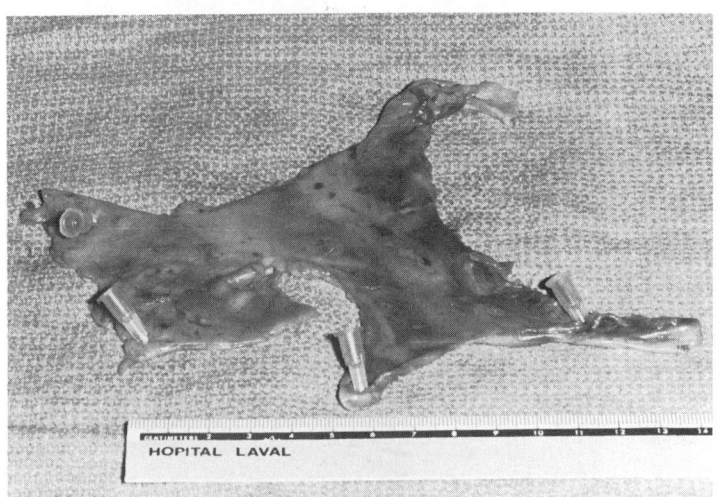

Figure 43-26.   Photographs of **(A)** apical blebs and **(B)** parietal pleura resected by videothoracoscopy.

described by Gaensler (1956), who reported total seal of the pleural space in all seven patients treated by total or subtotal pleurectomy. In patients with recurrent primary spontaneous pneumothorax, the parietal pleura should be removed from the fifth rib up to the apex (Inderbitzi, et al., 1993). It is elevated from the endothoracic fascia starting along the edge of the lower incision and then easily removed by use of endoscissors and dissectors (Fig. 43-26B). During the pleurectomy, constant traction is maintained on the strip of pleura being detached, and care must be taken to preserve the intercostal pedicle as well as to avoid trauma to the sympathetic chain.

As an alternative to pleurectomy, pleural abrasion can be performed with sterile gauze or mesh spread over the entire apical surface of the parietal pleura (Hazelrigg, et al., 1993). Whether pleurectomy or pleural abrasion has been done, the procedure is always completed by the insertion and proper positioning of a 28 Fr chest tube at the apex (Fig. 43-27).

VATS Subtotal Pleurectomy for Secondary Spontaneous Pneumothorax

Although medical conditions of the lung associated with secondary spontaneous pneumothoraces are numerous, most are related to the presence of diffuse emphysema (Fig. 43-28). What makes secondary pneumothoraces different from primary pneumothoraces can be summarized as follow: (1) the site of parenchymal rupture can be anywhere over the lung surface; (2) patients with secondary pneumothoraces are at risk of respiratory failure even with small pneumothoraces; (3) air leaks are often prolonged; (4) secondary pneumo-

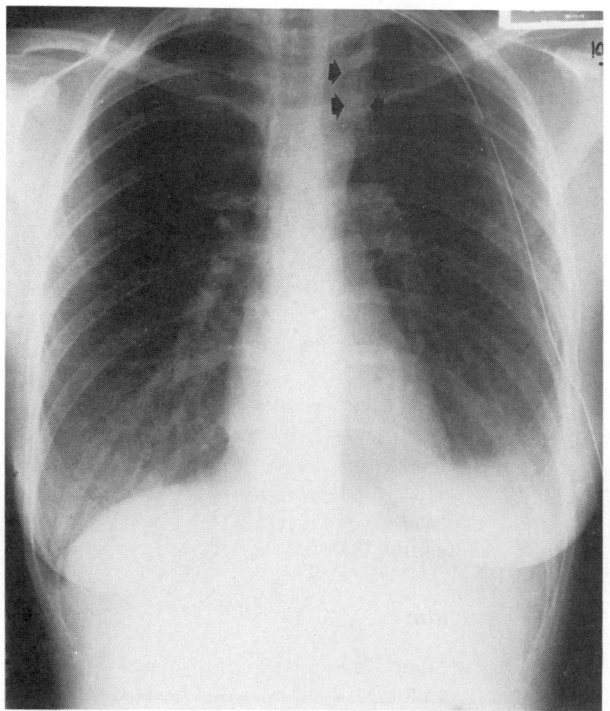

Figure 43-27. Postpleurectomy chest radiograph showing the chest tube placed at the apex and the staple line of the blebectomy (*arrows*).

> **Advantages of Early Thoracoscopic Debridement of Empyema Thoracis**
>
> Disclosure of etiologic factors such as foreign bodies
> Disclosure of causes of treatment failure
> Determination of lung expansibility
> Removal of infected material and fibrin
> Breakdown of pleural adhesions and coagulated pus
> Placement of chest tubes at dependent sites

thoraces have a greater tendency to recur than do primary pneumothoraces; and (5) the operative risk is substantially higher in patients with secondary pneumothoraces than it is in young healthy individuals with apical blebs.

For these reasons, we recommend VATS subtotal pleurectomy and talc insufflation over the diaphragmatic and pericardial pleural surfaces at the time of the first episode. The technique and position of the trocars are the same as has been described for the management of primary spontaneous pneumothoraces. If there are no bullae, a pleurectomy with talc poudrage is performed, great care being taken to avoid trauma to the lung so as to reduce the amount of postoperative air leakage. If bullae are seen, they are excised with the Endo-GIA stapler.

Thoracoscopy for Management of Empyemas

Several papers have reported good results in patients with empyema treated by early thoracoscopic debridement of the space. These techniques emphasize the importance of mechnical removal of infected material together with the breakdown of pleural adhesions and loculated pus to encourage reexpansion of the underlying lung (Ridley and Brainbridge, 1991). In addition, large-diameter drainage tubes can be properly placed at dependent sites (Fig. 43-29). Thoracoscopy may also be useful to drain postthoracotomy empyemas (Fig. 43-30), especially those occurring after pneumonectomy. In this latter situation the whole cavity can be explored an debrided, and chest tubes can be placed at appropriate sites for lavage and attempts at sterilization of the space.

In 1981 Weissberg reported his experience with 19 patients who underwent thoracoscopy for empyema. In 13 of these simple debridement and retrieval of foreign bodies under direct vision followed by drainage resulted in cure. Four patients required open thoracotomy for decortication and one for closure of a bronchopleural fistula. Weissberg suggested that thoracoscopy may be useful for the following reasons: (1) disclosure of etiologic factors such as foreign bodies; (2) facilitation of the search for causes of treatment failures; (3) determination of lung expansibility; (4) drainage; and (5) obliteration of dead space and debridement.

VATS for Early Deloculation

The technique of thoracoscopic debridement of empyema thoracis is basically the same as that described by Ridley and Brainbridge (1991). The empyema space is first delineated

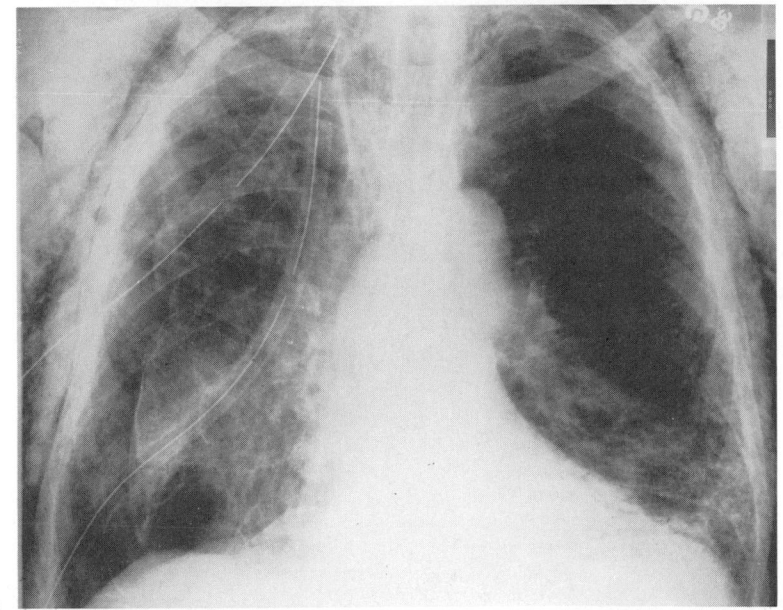

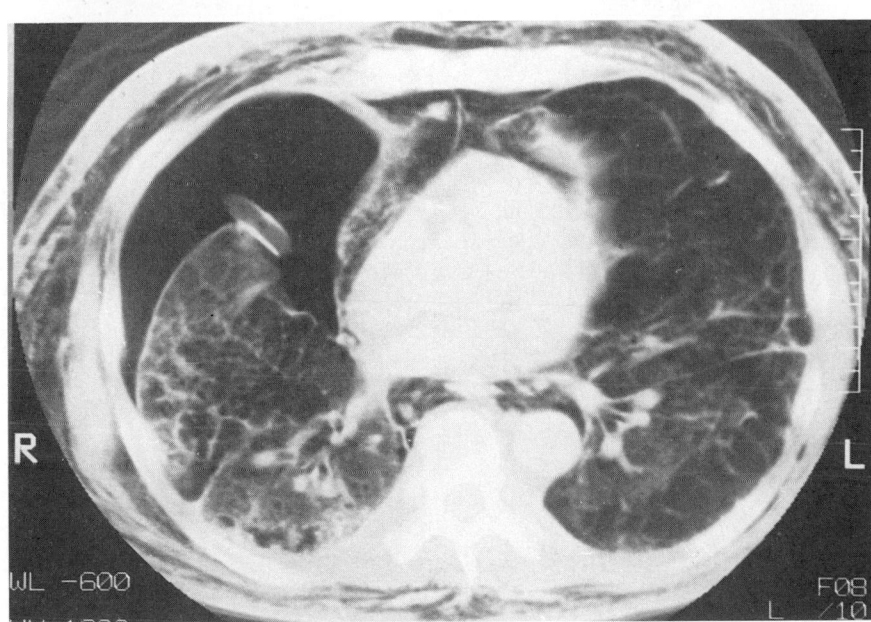

Figure 43-28. **(A)** Standard chest radiograph and **(B)** CT scan of a 60-year-old emphysematous patient with secondary pneumothorax. Note the extensive surgical emphysema, the failure to reexpand despite tube drainage, and the bullae located at the base of the lung.

by ultrasound and/or CT scanning. The patient is then anesthetized via a double-lumen tube and positioned in the lateral position. The use of a double-lumen tube is particularly important in empyema patients because a bronchopleural fistula may be present and with it the risks of contralateral aspiration. The thoracoscopic trocar is inserted below the tip of the scapula and all purulent material aspirated. Under direct vision, the loculations and adhesions are broken down either through the working channel of the thoracoscope or by use of a second port in the posterior axillary line. Once the cavity is dry, it is fully inspected, with special attention to removing fibrin from the lung surface, a procedure made easier by

intermittent inflation of the lung. Finally, the space is thoroughly irrigated and one or two chest tubes are positioned at dependent sites under direct vision.

Late Decortication

In patients with stage III organized empyemas, it is difficult to obtain a good endothoracic image, and furthermore, video-assisted decortication of the lung is hazardous, traumatic, time-consuming, and of limited value. It is far better to perform an open thoracotomy with proper cleaning of the space and decortication of the lung. In addition, decortication is

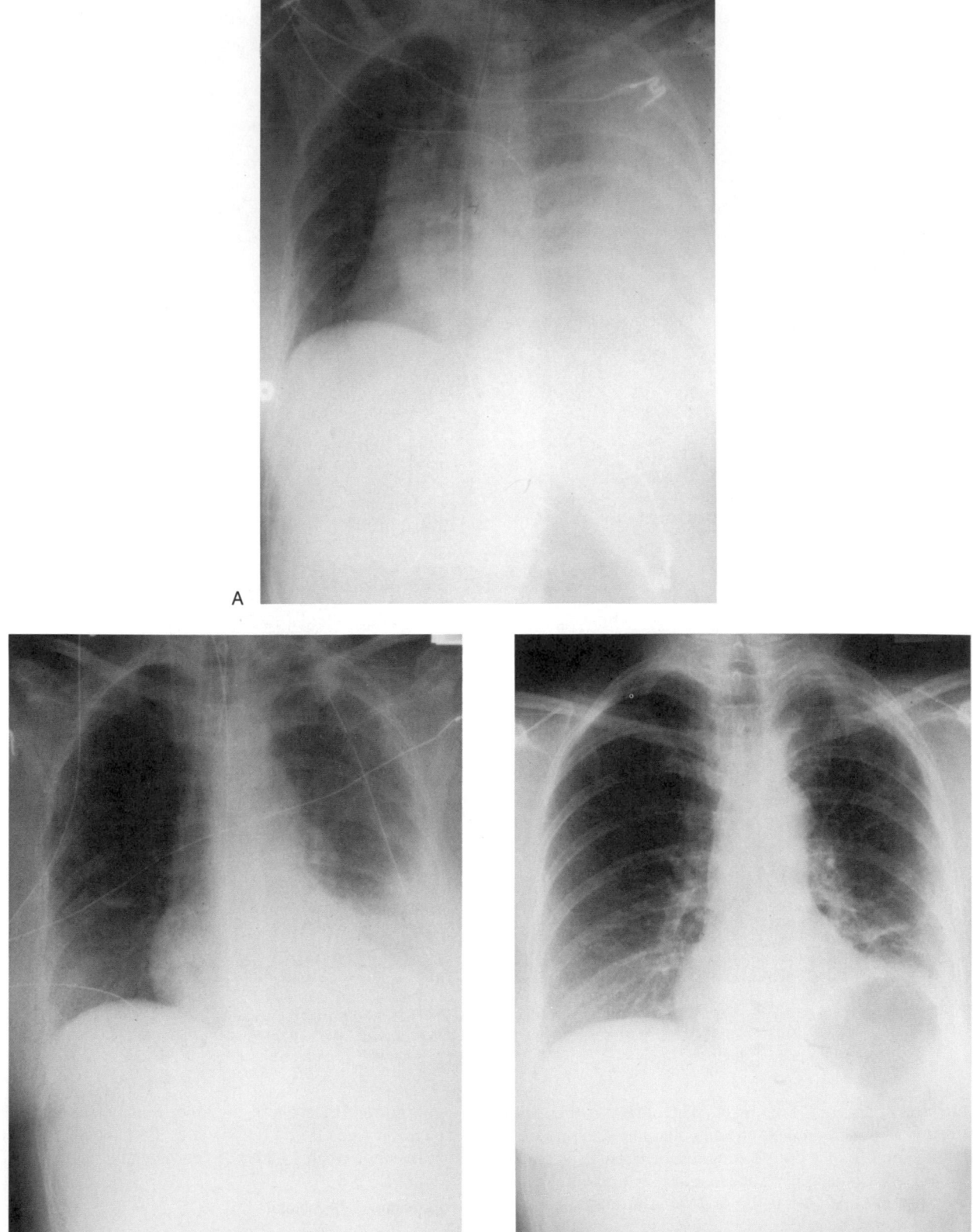

Figure 43-29. **(A)** Standard chest radiograph of a 48-year-old woman with massive parapneumonic empyema; note that the patient is intubated and that the mediastinum is shifted contralaterally. **(B)** Radiograph done early after thoracoscopic drainage of the empyema. **(C)** Radiograph taken 3 weeks later, showing complete space obliteration.

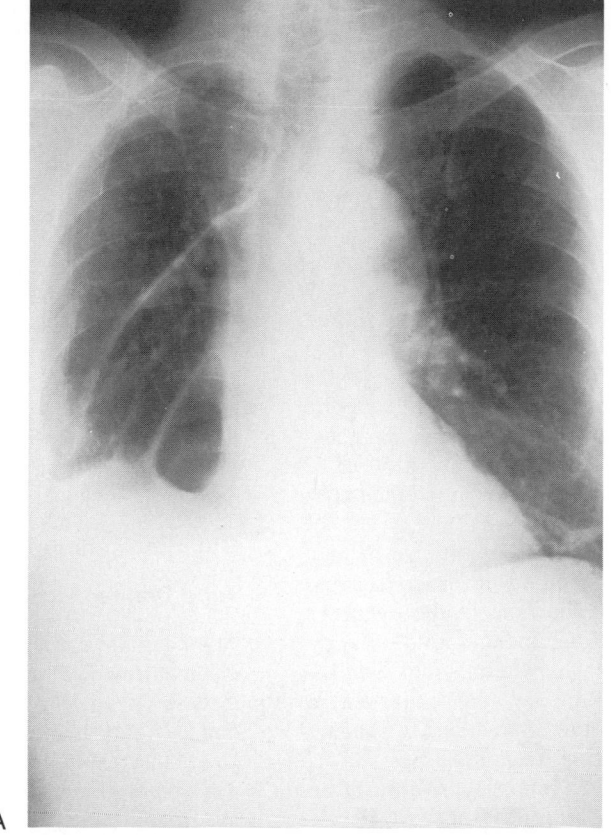

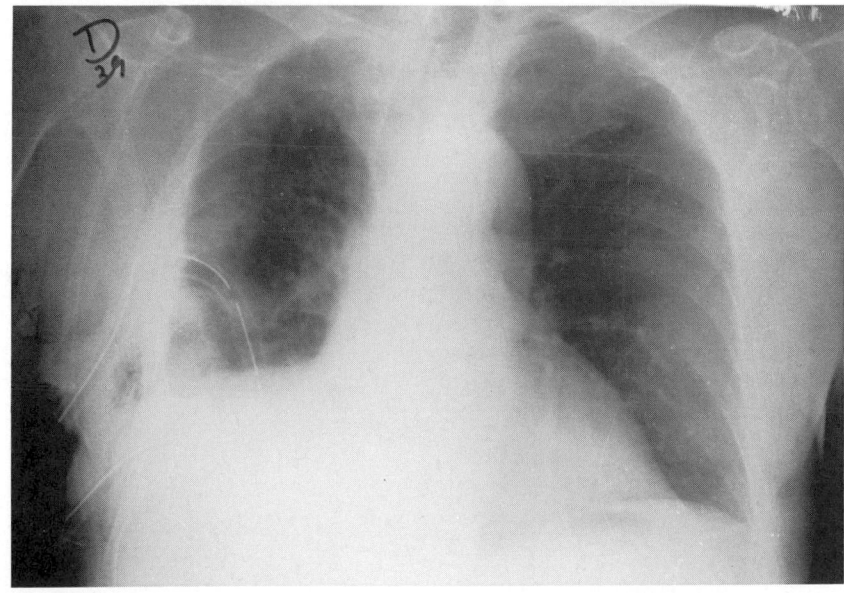

Figure 43-30. **(A)** Standard PA chest radiograph of a 62-year-old man with a basal empyema diagnosed 2 months after lower and middle lobectomy. **(B)** Radiograph taken 5 days after thoracoscopic debridement and drainage. Note that the tubes are placed at dependent sites and that the space is completely obliterated.

not in the field of expertise of most surgeons performing diagnostic thoracoscopies.

Thoracoscopy for Treatment of Malignant Pleural Effusions

In the majority of malignant pleural effusions, the nature of the effusion and the extent of pleural involvement preclude effective and curative therapy. Yet, these effusions are a significant cause of morbidity, with patients suffering from chest pain, dyspnea, or both. They often require repeated thoracentesis, which provides only temporary relief of their symptoms. In this situation palliative therapy should aim at controlling the effusion with the least risk of morbidity to the patient. Many chemicals have been instilled into the pleural space to achieve pleurodesis and control further fluid reaccumulation. Intrapleural tetracycline controls about 50 to 60 percent of pleural effusions, while bleomycin is efficient in approximately 75 to 80 percent of cases.

Bethune in 1935 was the first to report the use of talc, which he insufflated prior to lobectomy in order to avoid collapse of the residual lung at the time of the definitive procedure. Talc induces dense fibrosis of the pleural surfaces, and its efficiency in controlling malignant effusions is in the range of 90 percent (Adler and Rappole, 1967; Sorensen, et al., 1984; Ohri, et al., 1992). In 1990 Daniel and colleagues analyzed the results of thoracoscopic talc poudrage and reported a 90 percent success rate. Similarly, Webb, et al. (1992) showed that iodized talc achieved 100 percent success in controlling recurrent pleural effusions. Boutin, et al., (1985) and Hartman, et al. (1993) finally showed in comparative studies that the efficacy of talc was greater than that of tetracycline.

VATS for Talc Pleurodesis

Thoracoscopy is carried out under general anesthesia with double-lumen endotracheal intubation. The patient is positioned in the lateral decubitus position, and a thoracoscope with an incorporated working channel is inserted in the usual position. Pleural fluid is first aspirated and the cavity completely drained. At this stage further pleural biopsies can be taken and lung reexpansibility checked by having the anesthetist inflate it. Under direct vision, talc powder is insufflated (Fig. 43-31) over the lung and parietal surfaces through the working channel of the thoracoscope or, more often, through a second 10-mm working port. The currently used talc is sterile and free of asbestos fiber, and the amount needed to produce a fine layer of the powder over the surface of the lung seldom exceeds 2 to 5 g. The working trocar is then removed, and a chest tube is inserted under direct guidance of the thoracoscope and left in place until the amount of drainage is less than 100 to 150 ml/day.

Factors that may be associated with failure of talc poudrage to control the effusion are a mesothelioma with entrapped lung (Aelony, et al., 1991), a large tumor mass, a very large or long history of effusion, and age older than 70 years (Ladjimi, et al., 1989).

Other Indications for Therapeutic Thoracoscopy

Tube Drainage of a Bulla

Intracavitary drainage of a bulla can be successful in the elective treatment of symptomatic patients with bullous lung disease (Venn, et al., 1988). In a case reported by Urschel and Dickout (1993), thoracoscopic intravacitary drainage of a large bulla resulted in prompt resolution of the pneumothorax and obliteration of the bulla. The bulla was sutured with an absorbable purse-string suture and a large Foley catheter was inserted. The bulla was then brought up to the chest wall by gentle traction on the inflated Foley catheter.

Therapeutic Thoracoscopy for Hemothorax, Trauma, and Foreign Bodies

Little has been documented about the use of videothorascopy in emergency situations. In 1976 Branco described the use of thoracoscopy in the initial decision making after penetrating injuries to the chest. In 1981 Sattler reported the use of thoracoscopy in a case of hemopneumothorax in which bleed-

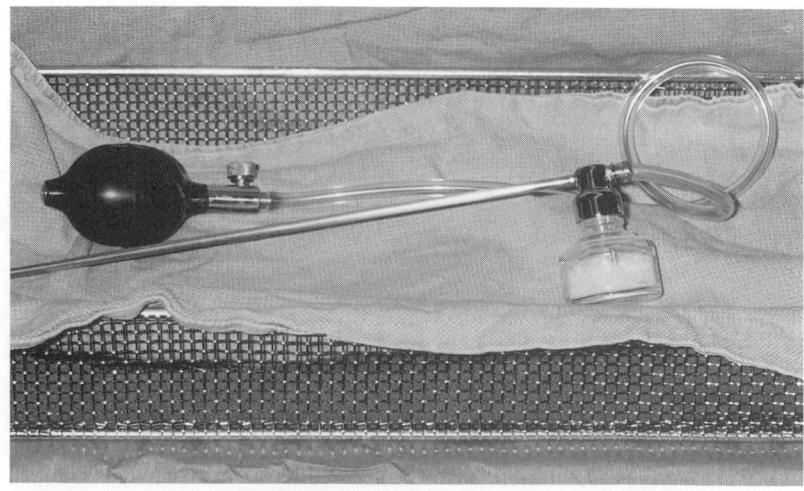

Figure 43-31. A talc insufflator.

ing originating from pleural adhesions was cauterized. In 1991 Duzhyi described thoracoscopy as the method of choice in the investigation of hemopneumothorax, and in 1992 Feliciano suggested the use of thoracoscopy, among other methods, in the diagnosis of thoracic injuries. Thoracoscopy can also be useful in retrieving foreign bodies from the pleural space, as reported by Oakes, et al. (1984) and Get'man (1989). We find VATS particularly useful in the management of post-traumatic clotted hemothoraces, which are susceptible to evolving into the stage of organized fibrothoraces and later requiring lung decortication.

Thoracoscopy for Bronchopleural Fistula and Chylothorax

In 1989 Aasebo reported the application of tissue glue (Histoacryl) via a thoracoscope in three patients with bron-

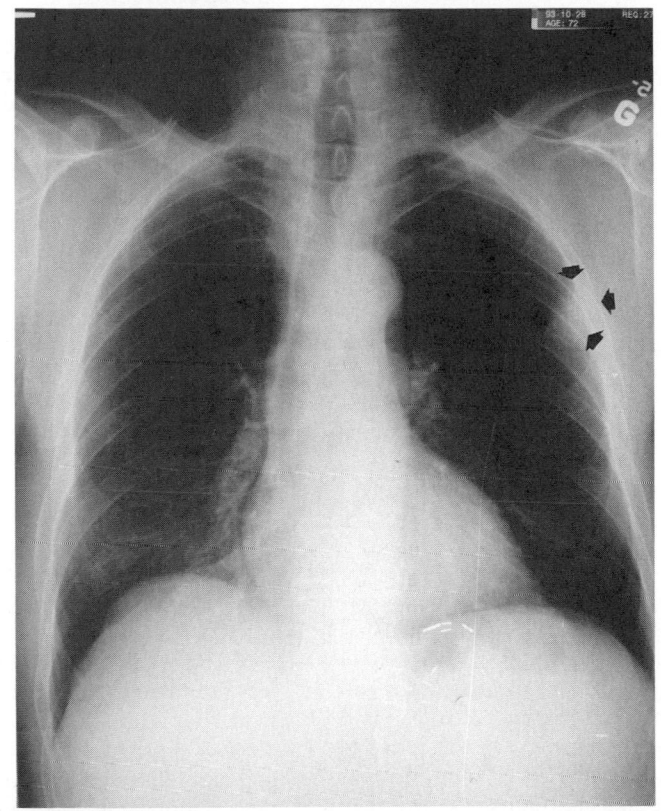

A

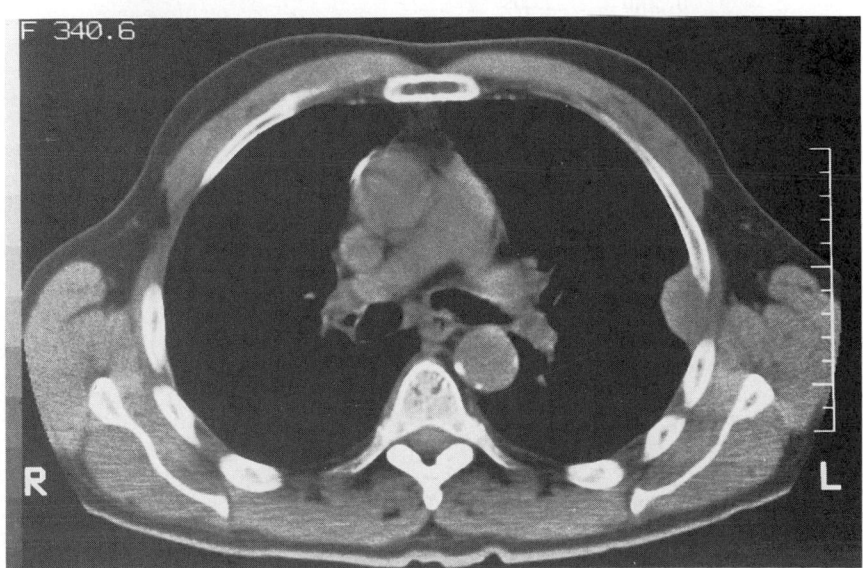

B

Figure 43-32.   **(A)** Standard PA chest radiograph and **(B)** CT scan of a 65-year-old man with an intercostal schwannoma (*arrows*) removed by VATS.

chopleural fistula, with good short-term results. Similarly, Tschopp and colleagues (1990) reported a case of chronic debilitating bronchopleural fistula following right upper lobe resection. The fistula was definitely closed by instillation of talc into the pleura through thoracoscopy. It is conceivable that debridement of a leaking bronchial stump with reclosure by endosuture technique or use of stapling devices may also be possible in the future.

A similar type of application may be used to seal a leaking thoracic duct. Hejgaard and Olsen (1987) controlled a life-threatening chylothorax by thoracoscopic pleurodesis with tetracycline. Morita, et al. (1990), Shirai, et al. (1991), and Inderbitzi, et al. (1992) have also used fibrin glue to successfully seal postoperative chylothoraces. In 1993, Ogawa and colleagues reported the use of a specially designed instrument for spraying aerosolized fibrin glue during thoracoscopy. In order to facilitate identification of the site of leakage, all these procedures should be performed after the patient has been given 200 to 300 ml of 35 percent cream through a nasogastric tube.

Removal of Pleura-based Masses

Videothoracoscopy may be ideal for removing benign pedunculated fibrous mesotheliomas, subpleural lipomas, or intercostal nerve schwannomas (Fig. 43-32).

COMPLICATIONS

Complications of thoracoscopy are uncommon if the technical conditions of the operation are fulfilled (Viskum and Enk, 1981). In a series of 1,820 cases reported by the VATS study group (Hazelrigg, et al., 1993), 24 percent of procedures had to be converted to thoracotomy, and prolonged air leak (>5 days) was the most frequent complication. In the series of 70 patients reported by Mack, et al., (1992), no mortality was associated with the procedure and morbidity was lessened as compared with standard thoracotomy procedures. The postoperative hospital stay after elective procedures performed in well patients averaged 3 days and was often as short as 1 day.

Possible complications of talc insufflation include potentiation of pleural malignancy and long-term deleterious effect on pulmonary function if a fibrothorax is induced by the powder. None of these problems should, however, be encountered if use of talc poudrage is restricted to patients with malignant effusion.

CONCLUSION

Thoracoscopy is a complementary procedure in the evaluation of pleural effusions, in which it helps to clarify the diagnosis in over half the patients still undiagnosed after the usualy methods of investigation. In patients with symptomatic malignant effusions, sclerotherapy can be achieved, and talc pleurodesis appears to be the method of choice. In patients with pneumothoraces secondary to emphysema, video-assisted parietal pleurectomy with or without bullectomy is the therapy of choice.

Thoracoscopy is a procedure of which the mastery and safe application require patience, and one should not despair at the slow rate at which use of a procedure may progress. Although most European descriptions of thoracoscopy have come from pneumologists, without intending disrespect for our colleagues we have to beware of the apparent simplicity of the procedures. Indeed, in order to provide maximum safety for the patient, thoracoscopy should be performed in an equipped operating room by a surgical team that is ready to perform a thoracotomy if a complication occurs or if thoracoscopy is not possible because of adhesions or other technical problem.

VATS is a fine technique, which in selected patients offers less morbidity than the equivalent thoracotomy. This is particularly true in the management of individuals with malignant pleural effusions, secondary spontaneous pneumothoraces, and early-stage empyemas. For patients with recurrent primary spontaneous pneumothorax, the advantages of VATS over axillary pleurectomy have yet to be documented by controlled comparative studies.

REFERENCES

Aasebo U: Thoracoscopic closure of distal bronchopleural fistula, using fibrin glue. Eur Respir J 2:383 1989

Adler RH, Rappole BW: Recurrent malignant pleural effusion and talcum powder aerosol treatment. Surgery 62:1000, 1967

Aelony Y, King R, Boutin C: Thoracoscopic talc poudrage pleurodesis for chronic recurrent pleural effusions. Ann Intern Med 115:778, 1991

Bethune N: Pleural poudrage: new technique for deliberate section of pleural adhesions as preliminary to lobectomy. J Thorac Surg 4:251, 1935

Bloomberg AE: Thoracoscopy in perspective. Surg Gynecol Obstet 147:433, 1978

Boutin C, Rey F, Viallat JR: Étude randomisée de l'efficacité du talcage thoracoscopique et de l'instillation de tétracycline dans le traitement des pleurésies cancéreuses récidivantes. Rev Mal Respir 2:374, 1985

Bozzini P: On the Illumination of Internal Cavities. Weimar, 1807

Branco JMC: Thoracoscopy as a method of exploration in penetrating injuries of the chest. Chest 12:330, 1976

Daniel TM, Tribble CG, Rogers BM: Thoracoscopy and talc poudrage for pneumothoraces and effusions. Ann Thorac Surg 50:186, 1990

Deslauriers J, Beaulieu M, Després JP et al.: Trans-axillary pleurectomy for treatment of spontaneous pneumothorax. Ann Thorac Surg 30:569, 1980

Duzhyi ID: Spontaneous hemopneumothorax. Klin Khir 11:35, 1991

Feliciano DV: The diagnostic and therapeutic approach to chest trauma. Semin Thorac Cardiovasc Surg 4:156, 1992

Gaensler EA: Parietal pleurectomy for recurrent spontaneous pneumothorax. Surg Gynecol Obstet 102:293, 1956

Get'man VG: Diagnosis and removal of foreign bodies in the thoracic cavity using thoracoscopy. Grudn Khir 4:50 1989

Hartman DL, Gaither JM, Kesler KA et al.: Comparison of insufflated talc under thoracoscopic guidance with standard tetracycline and bleomycin pleurodesis for control of malignant pleural effusions. J Thorac Cardiovasc Surg 105:743, 1993

Hazelrigg SR, Landreneau RJ, Mark M et al.: Thoracoscopic stapled resection for spontaneous pneumothorax. J Thorac Cardiovasc Surg 105:389, 1993

Hejgaard N, Olsen PR: Massive Gorham osteolysis of the right hemipelvis complicated by chylothorax: report of a case in a 9 year old boy successfully treated by pleurodesis. J Pediatr Orthop 7:96, 1987

Inderbitzi RGC, Krebs T, Stirnemann T, Althaus V: Treatment of postoperative chylothorax by fibrin glue application under thoracoscopic view with use of local anesthesia (letter). J Thorac Cardiovasc Surg 104:209, 1992

Inderbitzi RGC, Furrer M, Strifyeler H, Althaus V: Thoracoscopic pleurectomy for treatment of complicated spontaneous pneumothorax. J Thorac Cardiovasc Surg 105:84, 1993

Jacobeus HC: The practical importance of thoracoscopy in surgery of the chest. Surg Gynecol Obstet 34:289, 1922

Jacobeus HC: Possibility of the use of cystoscopy in the investigation of serious cavities. Münch Med Wochenschr 40:2090, 1910

Ladjimi S, M'Raihi L, Djemel A et al.: Résultat du talcage pleural sous thoracoscopie au cours des pleurésies néoplasiques. À propos de 218 cas. Rev Mal Respir 6:147, 1989

Le Tacon J: La pleuroscopie. Rappel historique. Poumon Coeur 37:5, 1981

Locicero J, Hartz RS, Frederiksen JA et al.: New applications of the laser in pulmonary surgery: hemostatis and sealing of air leaks. Ann Thorac Surg 40:546, 1985

Mack MJ, Aronoff RJ, Acuff TE et al.: Present role of thoracoscopy in the diagnosis and treatment of diseases of the chest. Ann Thorac Surg 54:403, 1992

Morita R, Akaogi E, Suzuki Y et al.: A case of postoperative chylothorax successfully treated by thoracoscopic fibrin gluing. Nippon Kyobu Gakkai Zasshi 38:3465, 1990

Nathanson LK, Shimi SM, Wood RAB, Cuschieri A: Videothoracoscopic ligation of bulla and pleurectomy for spontaneous pneumothorax. Ann Thorac Surg 52:316, 1991

Newman D: Lectures on Surgical Diseases of the Kidney. Longmans, Green, London, 1888

Oakes DD, Sherck JP, Brodsky JB, Mark JBD: Therapeutic thoracoscopy. J Thorac Cardiovasc Surg 87:269, 1984

Ogawa J, Inoue H, Koide S, Shohtsu A: Newly devised instrument for spraying aerosolized fibrin glue in thoracoscopic operations (letter). Ann Thorac Surg 55:1595, 1993

Ohri SK, Oswal SK, Townsend ER et al.: Early and late outcome after diagnostic thoracoscopy and talc poudrage. Ann Thorac Surg 53:1038, 1992

Ridley PD, Brainbridge MV: Thoracoscopic debridement and pleural irrigation in the management of empyema thoracis. Ann Thorac Surg 51:461, 1991

Rusch VW, Schmidt R, Shoji Y, Fujimara Y: Use of the argon beam electrocoagulator for performing pulmonary wedge resections. Ann Thorac Surg 49:287, 1990

Sattler A: The treatment of spontaneous pneumothorax with special reference to thoracoscopy. Beitr Klin Tuberk 89:395, 1937

Sattler A: La thoracoscopie: intérêt thérapeutique dans les syndromes pleuropulmonaries d'urgence et intérêt diagnostique. Poumon Coeur 37:265, 1981

Shirai T, Amano J, Takabe K: Thoracoscopic diagnosis and treatment of chylothorax after pneumonectomy. Ann Thorac Surg 52:306, 1991

Sorensen PG, Svendsen TL, Enk B: Treatment of malignant pleural effusion with drainage, with and without instillation of talc. Eur J Respir Dis 65:131, 1984

Swierenga J, Wagenaar JPM, Bergstein PGM: The value of thoracoscopy in the diagnosis and treatment of diseases affecting the pleura and lung. Pneumologie (Stuttg) 151:11, 1974

Torre M, Belloni P: Nd: YAG laser pleurodesis through thoracoscopy: new curative therapy in spontaneous pneumothorax. Ann Thorac Surg 47:887, 1989

Tschopp JM, Evéquoz D, Karrer W et al.: Successful closure of chronic BPF by thoracoscopy after failure of endoscopic fibrin glue application and thoracoplasty. Chest 97:745, 1990

Urschel JD, Dickout WJ: Thoracoscopic intracavitary drainage for pneumothorax secondary to bullous emphysema. Can J Surg 36:548, 1993

Venn GE, Williams PR, Goldstraw P: Intracavitary drainage for bullous emphysematous lung disease: experience with the Brompton technique. Thorax 43:998, 1988

Viskum K, Enk B: Complications of thoracoscopy: Poumon Coeur 37:269, 1981

Wakabayashi A, Brenner M, Wilson AF et al.: Thoracoscopic treatment of spontaneous pneumothorax using carbon dioxide laser. Ann Thorac Surg 50:786, 1990

Wakabayashi A: Thoracoscopic ablation of blebs in the treatment of recurrent or persistent spontaneous pneumothorax. Ann Thorac Surg 48:651, 1989

Webb WR, Ozmen V, Moulder PV et al.: Iodized talc pleurodesis for the treatment of pleural effusions. J Thorac Cardiovasc Surg 103:881, 1992

Weissberg D: Pleuroscopy in empyemas: is it ever necessary? Poumon Coeur 37:269, 1981

Yaita H, Ishida T, Sugimachi K: Thoracoscopic surgery of spontaneous pneumothorax with endoscopic GIA stapler. Nippon Kyobu Geka Gakkai Zasshi 7:442, 1993

44

ANATOMY AND PHYSIOLOGY

Geoffrey M. Graeber

INTRODUCTION

The anatomy and physiology of the chest wall are completely intertwined. The musculoskeletal structure of the chest wall has evolved as a mobile but firm encasement of the lungs and thoracic viscera, which provides for functional utility while affording some protection for vital organs. Certain muscles of the upper extremities and the trunk assist the chest wall in performing its physiologic functions under usual circumstances. An appreciation of the embryology of the chest wall helps in understanding its function.

EMBRYOLOGY

The primordial structures that form the chest wall are derived from both the axial and the appendicular skeleton (Graeber, 1986; Arey, 1965; Ravitch, 1977). The sternum arises from the appendicular skeleton, while the ribs and costal cartilages are derived from the axial. Each starts independently, but fusion occurs around the seventh week of gestation, when the primitive ribs and costal cartilages reach the emerging sternum.

The sternum arises from three distinct precursors from the appendicular skeleton. The largest are the two lateral mesenchymal bands, which arise laterally in the body wall in proximity to the emerging pectoralis major muscles at 5 to 6 weeks' gestation. The mesenchymal bands migrate medially and anteriorly to reach the ventral midline, where fusion occurs. The union starts in the cephalad end during the seventh week of gestation and proceeds caudad. The primitive manubrium is formed by fusion of the cephalad medial mesenchymal mass, which most probably corresponds with the presternum of lower animals, with two variable lateral suprasternal elements. Fusion progresses in a craniocaudad fashion until union is complete at 9 weeks.

The ribs, costal cartilages, and associated musculature arise in the posterior common vertebral mass in the axial skeleton at the same time that the lateral sternal bars appear (Graeber, 1986; Arey, 1965; Ravitch, 1977). These primordia grow laterally, anteriorly, and then medially to create the contour of the emerging body wall. By 9 weeks the costal cartilages of ribs one through seven have fused with the sternum. Subsequently the emerging costal cartilages of ribs eight through ten fuse with each other and the sternum to complete skeletal development of the chest wall.

PHYSIOLOGY AND ANATOMY

Chest wall integrity is mandatory for adequate ventilation (Graeber, 1986; Guyton, 1991; West, 1991; Netter, 1979; West, 1979; West, 1977). The best model for conceptual visualization of ventilation is a piston moving up and down in a fixed column. The fixed column is the chest wall; the piston is the diaphragm. When the diaphragm contracts, it draws the central tendon downward in the chest, creating a negative intrathoracic pressure. Since the lung is in contact with the chest wall in the normal physiologic state, contraction of the diaphragm with subsequent migration downward causes the lung to expand. When inspiration is complete, the diaphragm relaxes and the elastic components of the lung allow it to contract to its volume prior to the inspiratory effort. During quiet respiration, the excursion of the diaphragm is all the change in volume necessary to effect adequate ventilation. For the most part the chest wall does not move during quiet respiration. Obviously, the chest wall must maintain its position in order to have the lungs expand properly. The negative pressure created in the chest by the excursion of the diaphragm causes air to come in through the tracheobronchial tree and be distributed to the respective lungs. Deeper inspiration and expiration must be facilitated by movement of the chest wall.

Since the lung follows the chest wall and diaphragm in their movements, the logical way to increase inspiration after the diaphragm has reached maximum contraction is to increase the diameter of the cylinder. By using the same piston model, we can see that if we increase the diameter of the cylinder in which the piston is moving up and down, the volume in the cylinder will increase in proportion to the increase in diameter. The ribs and sternum move in an upward and outward fashion so as to increase the intrathoracic distances and thereby increase expansion of the lung. The sternum has been compared to a handle on a water pump in that it has an upward and downward motion where it is fixed at the top and is most mobile distally. The manubrium articulates with the first rib and the clavicles. Its major motion is upward and anterior with the axis of rotation running through the two heads of the clavicles. The body of the sternum follows the manubrium in an upward and anterior direction. The ribs move much like the handle on a bucket (Fig. 44-1). They are relatively fixed anteriorly and posteriorly in that they articulate with the sternum and the spinal column, respectively. When they are moved upward and outward, they increase the volume within the thorax. The posterior articulation with the spinal column is most fixed, whereas the anterior point of articulation with the sternum does move cephalad and anteriorly with the sternum (Figs. 44-1 and 44-2). Maximum inspiration is achieved when the sternum is elevated anteriorly as far as possible and the ribs are elevated in a similar fashion laterally and cephalad (Figs. 44-3 and 44-4). The accessory muscles of inspiration are responsible for moving the ribs and sternum upward and outward to achieve maximal expansion of the thorax and hence of the lungs (Fig. 44-5).

Maximal expiration is achieved by relaxation of the diaphragm and by downward and inward displacement of the sternum and ribs (Graeber, 1986; Guyton, 1991; West, 1991; Netter, 1979; West, 1979; West, 1977). The downward movement of the sternum causes the posterior and inferior rotation of the manubrium and the posterior and inferior rotation of

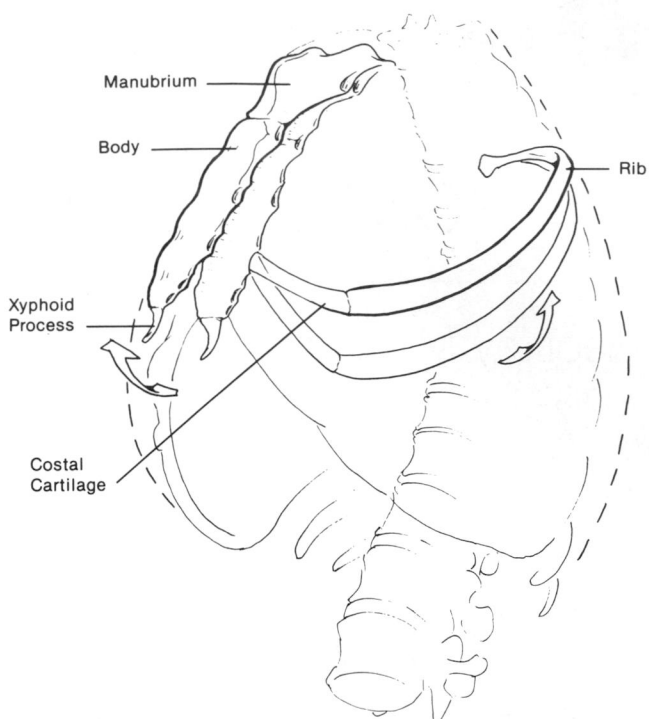

Figure 44-2. The expansion and contraction of the chest wall are governed by the motion of the individual ribs, costal cartilages, and sternum. The sternum works as a handle on a water pump. As it is moved upward, the xyphoid process and body go more anteriorly and cephalad, whereas the manubrium articulates with the first rib and clavicle and rotates anteriorly and cephalad. The bucket handle motion of the ribs and costal cartilages is facilitated by articulations both posteriorly and anteriorly. The posterior articulations of the rib, with the head, the vertebral body, and the articular facet, move against the transverse process of the vertebral body below. The costal cartilage articulates with the sternum and moves upward on forced inspiration and downward on forced expiration.

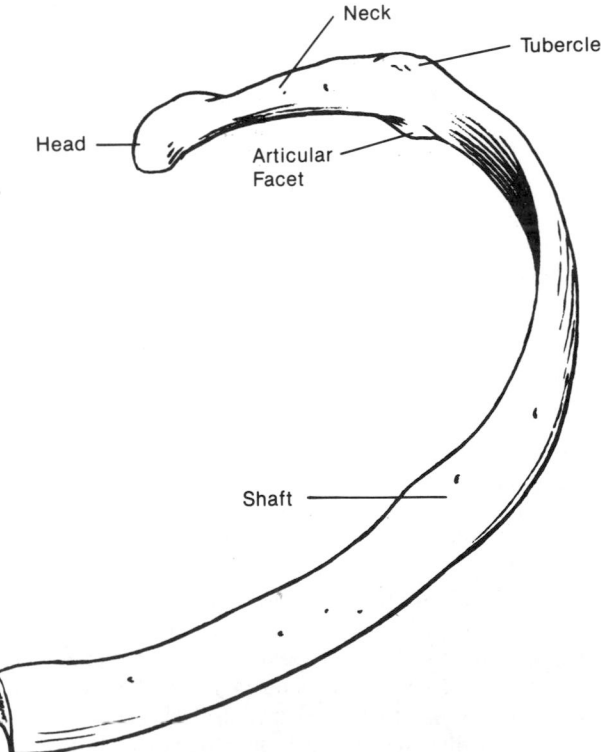

Figure 44-1. The anatomy of a rib. The head abuts on the vertebral body. The articular facet in the region of the tubercle articulates with the transverse process on the vertebral body below. The neck, after it extends to the region of the tubercle and the facet, blends with the elongated shaft. The anterior surface abuts on the corresponding costal cartilage.

the sternal body. The ribs are brought downward and inward so that the internal diameters of the chest are reduced to a minimum. The accessory muscles of expiration are responsible for these movements. The summation of their actions causes a decrease in the volume of the thorax and achieves maximal expiration (Fig. 44-6). These same muscles also press inward on the abdominal viscera and force the relaxed diaphragm upward.

BLOOD SUPPLY AND INNERVATION

The arterial supply to the chest wall arises from the subclavian arteries and the aorta itself. The intercostal arteries, which run under each rib, supply the posterior and lateral aspects of the chest wall (Clemente, 1985b). The internal thoracic artery and the intercostal arteries combine to provide the arterial supply to the anterior portion of the chest wall. The internal thoracic and the highest two intercostals generally arise from the subclavian artery. The lower ten intercostal arteries arise from the descending thoracic aorta and course anteriorly underneath the ribs in the neurovascular

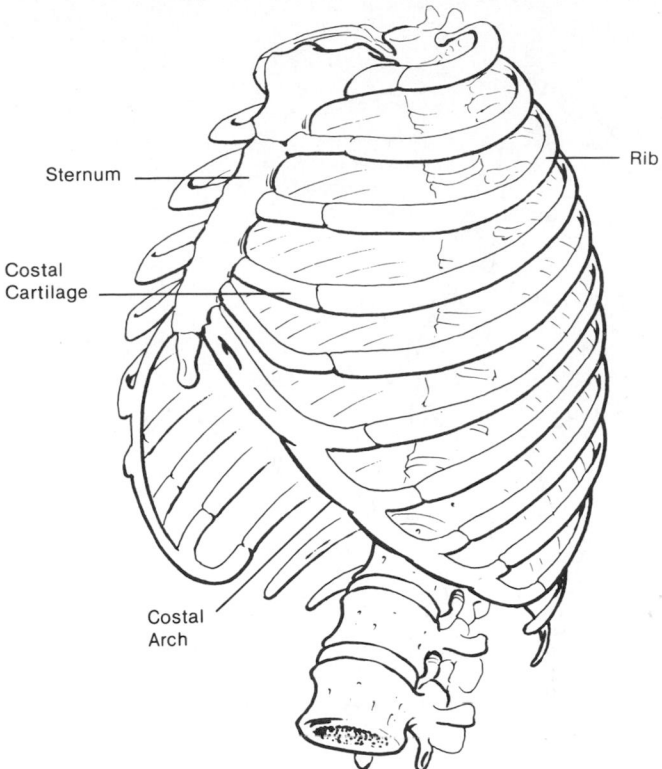

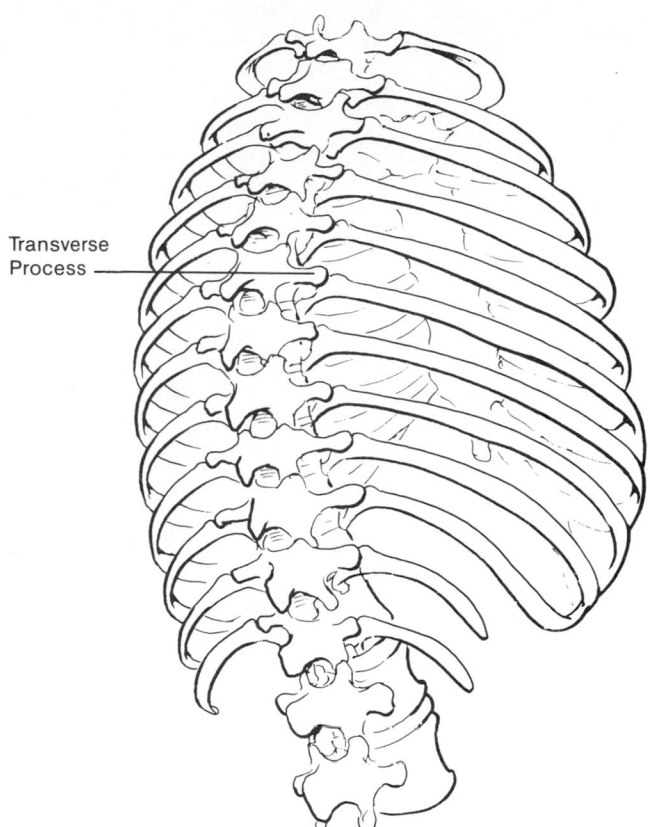

Figure 44-3. The entire bony and cartilaginous thorax is depicted in this left anterior oblique projection. The costal cartilages articulate with the sternum and the individual ribs. In the lower aspects of the costal margin, individual costal cartilages blend. Note that the eleventh and twelfth ribs are completely free of attachment in any way to the sternum. The spine forms the posterior articular aspects for each of the ribs.

Figure 44-4. This right posterior oblique projection shows the relationship of each individual rib to the vertebral bodies and their transverse processes. Note that the head of each rib articulates with the vertebral bodies, whereas the articular processes of each rib articulate with the transverse processes.

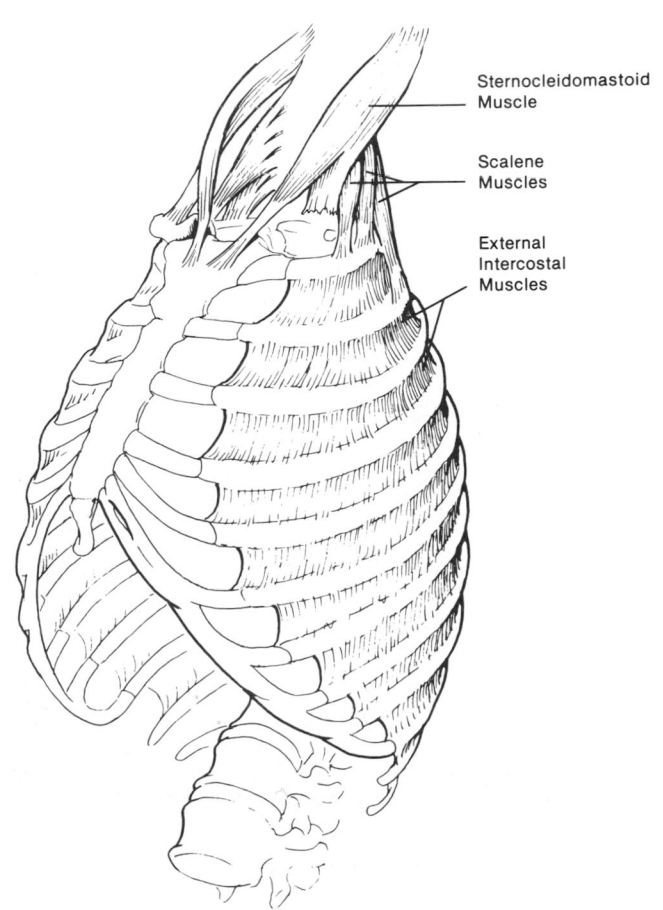

Figure 44-5. Accessory muscles of inspiration. Note that all of this musculature is directed at raising the fibromuscular skeleton and extending it anteriorly. This coordinated motion increases the intrathoracic diameters and allows further expansion of the lungs.

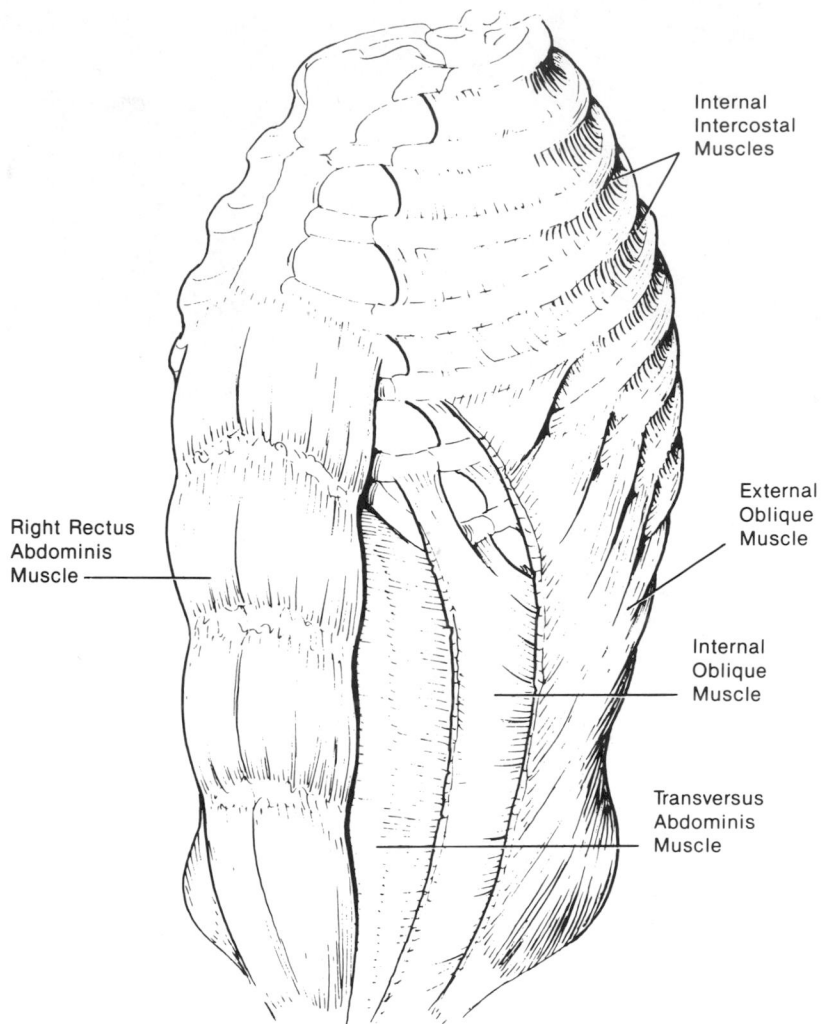

Internal
Intercostal
Muscles

External
Oblique
Muscle

Internal
Oblique
Muscle

Right Rectus
Abdominis
Muscle

Transversus
Abdominis
Muscle

Figure 44-6.   All the accessory muscles of expiration are shown in this left anterior oblique projection. The internal intercostal muscles, the rectus abdominus, and the three flat muscles of the abdomen all draw the ribs, costal cartilages, and the sternum downward and inward to decrease the volume in the entire thoracic cavity.

bundle (Fig. 44-7). The intercostal arteries course anteriorly to anastomose with the internal thoracic at the lateral margin of the sternum. Each of these arteries sends out numerous twigs to the intercostal muscles, the pleura, and the periosteum of the ribs (Fig. 44-7).

Major contributors to the blood supply of the anterior chest wall, and particularly the sternum, are the paired internal thoracic arteries (Fig. 44-8). Each of these vessels arises from the subclavian artery and courses distally along the internal peristernal aspect of the chest (Clemente, 1985b). Distally the internal thoracic artery bifurcates into two major branches: the direct extension, which becomes the superior epigastric artery after it exits the thoracic cavity through the space between the sternal and costal slips of the diaphragm, and the lateral branch, which is the musculophrenic artery. The superior epigastric artery arises from the direct extension of the internal thoracic artery once the internal mammary has gone through the potential foramen of Morgagni and enters the posterior aspect of the rectus sheath. The superior

epigastric further communicates with intercostals coming down from above and with the inferior epigastric artery in the distal end of the rectus sheath. The musculophrenic artery courses laterally toward the costophrenic sinus, where it continues on in the diaphragmatic musculature to anastomose with the distal ends of the intercostal arteries in the lower chest wall. Each internal thoracic artery is the collateral supply for the other. Each one has a major portion of its arterial supply devoted to the sternum. Perforating branches from the anteromedial aspect of each of the internal thoracic arteries supply the respective sides of the sternum. Perforating vessels also go through the intercostal muscles to join with the intercostal arteries underneath each rib and to become the secondary blood supply to the pectoralis major muscle, which lies anteriorly. Another small but important branch of the internal thoracic artery is the pericardiophrenic artery. This artery arises in the proximal portion of the internal thoracic and courses laterally and posteriorly to the phrenic nerve, where it joins the nerve to supply arterial blood to the nerve

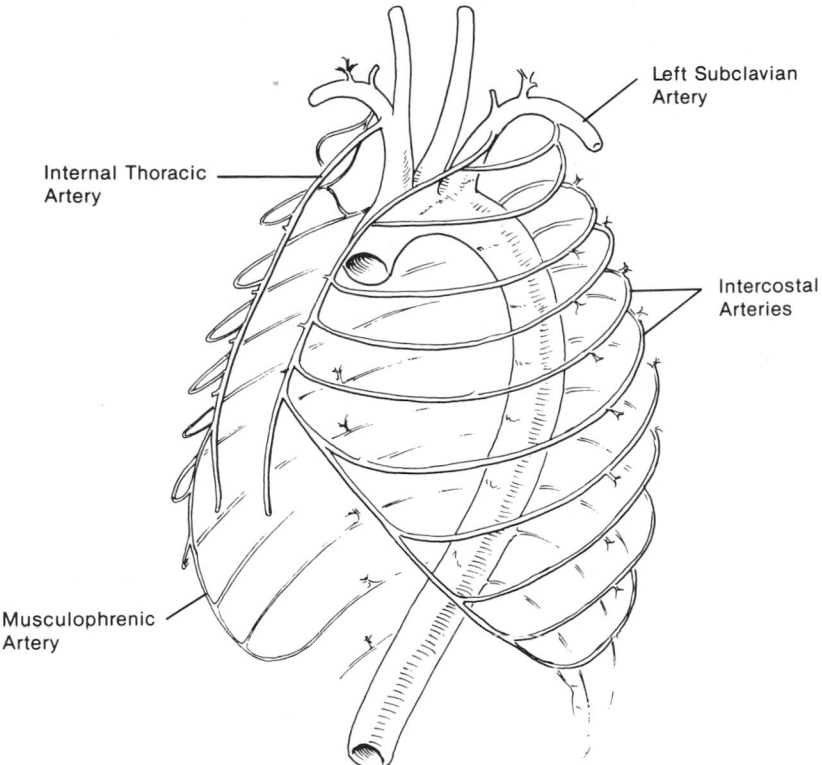

Internal Thoracic Artery

Left Subclavian Artery

Intercostal Arteries

Musculophrenic Artery

Figure 44-7. The arterial supply of the chest wall is shown in this left anterior oblique projection. Note that the intercostal arteries arise from the aorta posteriorly for the lower ten intercostal spaces. The highest intercostal arteries branch off from the subclavian. The paired internal thoracic arteries arise from the subclavian and course down along the posterolateral aspect of the sternum. They give rise to a major branch, the musculophrenic artery, which goes along the costal cartilages to anastomose with the intercostal arteries. The continuation of the internal thoracic artery becomes the superior epigastric artery.

and to a small portion of the diaphragm where the phrenic nerve perforates this structure before innervating its musculature (Fig. 44-8).

The venous drainage of the chest wall consists of numerous intercostal veins, which course with the intercostal arteries underneath the respective ribs (Fig. 44-9). These vessels drain to the hemiazygous and azygous systems, depending on their anatomic position (Clemente, 1985c). The internal thoracic arteries have corresponding paired veins, which drain to the subclavian veins. The veins have anastomotic junctions with the corresponding superior epigastric and musculophrenic veins. Perforating veins from the chest wall also go into the internal mammary veins to drain the anterior portion of the intercostal muscles.

The intercostal nerves provide the primary motor and sensory innervation of the entire chest wall (Clemente, 1985d). They arise within the spinal canal, exit through the intervertebral foramina, and course anteriorly underneath the inferior margin of each of the ribs (Fig. 44-9). There are several important anatomic features of these nerves that need to be mentioned. The sympathetic trunk conveys sympathetic fibers to the nerves just after the nerves exit the spinal canal (Fig. 44-9). The nerves also lie most distad of the three structures of the neurovascular bundle underneath each rib (Fig. 44-9). The intercostal vein is most cephalad, followed pro-

gressively by the intercostal artery and finally the intercostal nerve. The first six to seven intrathoracic nerves supply the sensory innervation and dermatomes ranging from the posterior aspect of the back around to the midline of the sternum. The eighth intercostal nerves supply the anterior wall for sensory fibers around the region of the xiphoid process. The ninth intercostal nerves supply the upper portion of the epigastrium just distal to the xiphoid, and the tenth intercostal is responsible for sensation at the level of the umbilicus. These relationships are important since intrathoracic processes (such as Boerhaave syndrome) may affect the intrathoracic portions of each of these nerves and create symptoms compatible with an intra-abdominal process. Hence, irritation of these nerves posteriorly can create many signs of acute abdomen.

UPPER EXTREMITY MUSCULATURE

A number of upper extremity and abdominal muscles have their origins on the chest wall. Anteriorly the pectoralis major, the pectoralis minor, and the serratus anterior muscles originate and insert onto the upper extremity (Clemente, 1985a). The pectoralis major arises from the lower costal cartilages and ribs, the sternum, and the clavicle to form a unified muscle, which inserts on the humerus. The pectoralis

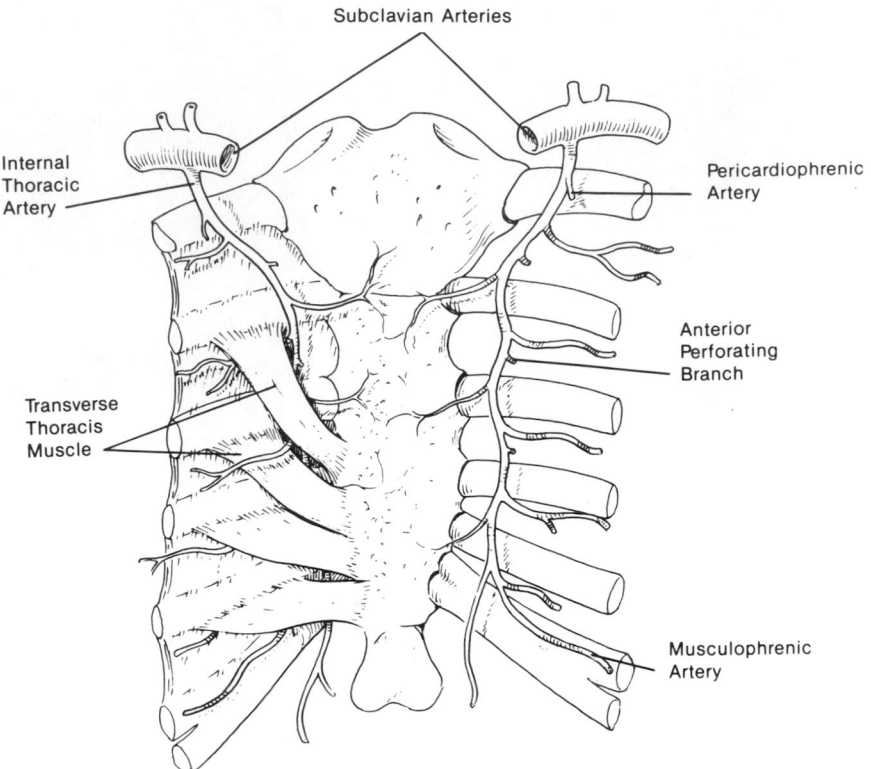

Figure 44-8. This shows the detail of the internal thoracic artery and its major branches. The pericardiophrenic arteries arise from the proximal portion of the internal thoracic arteries. They join with the pericardiophrenic veins, which are usually paired, and progress to the diaphragm with the phrenic nerve. The perforators arising from each internal thoracic are shown, as are the communications with the intercostal vessels. The internal thoracic arteries provide the major blood supply to the sternum. The distal arteries arising from the internal thoracic include the musculophrenic, which goes laterally into the costophrenic sinus at the edge of the diaphragm, and the superior epigastric, which penetrates the diaphragm between the costal and sternal portions of the musculature.

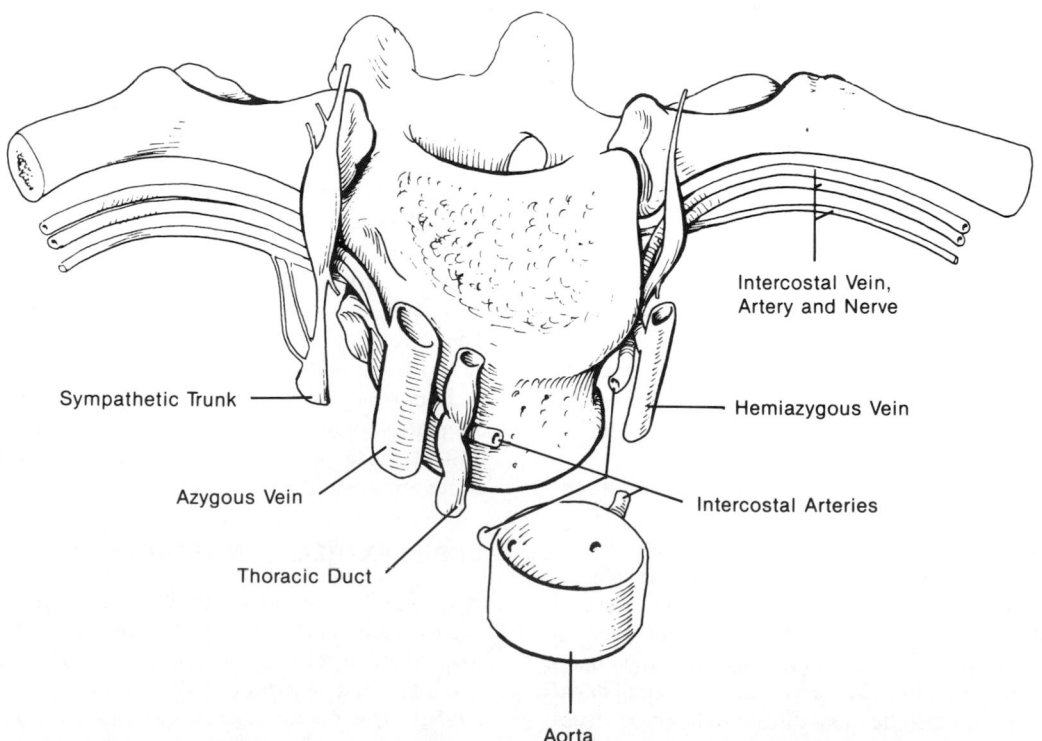

Figure 44-9. The relationship of the intercostal arteries, veins, and nerves is shown. Note that the intercostal arteries are directly caudad to each rib. Sequentially below these are the intercostal artery and nerve. The veins drain into the azygos system on the right and the hemiazygos system on the left. The intercostal nerves arise from the spinal cord, exit the spinal canal, and are joined by communicating branches from the sympathetic trunks.

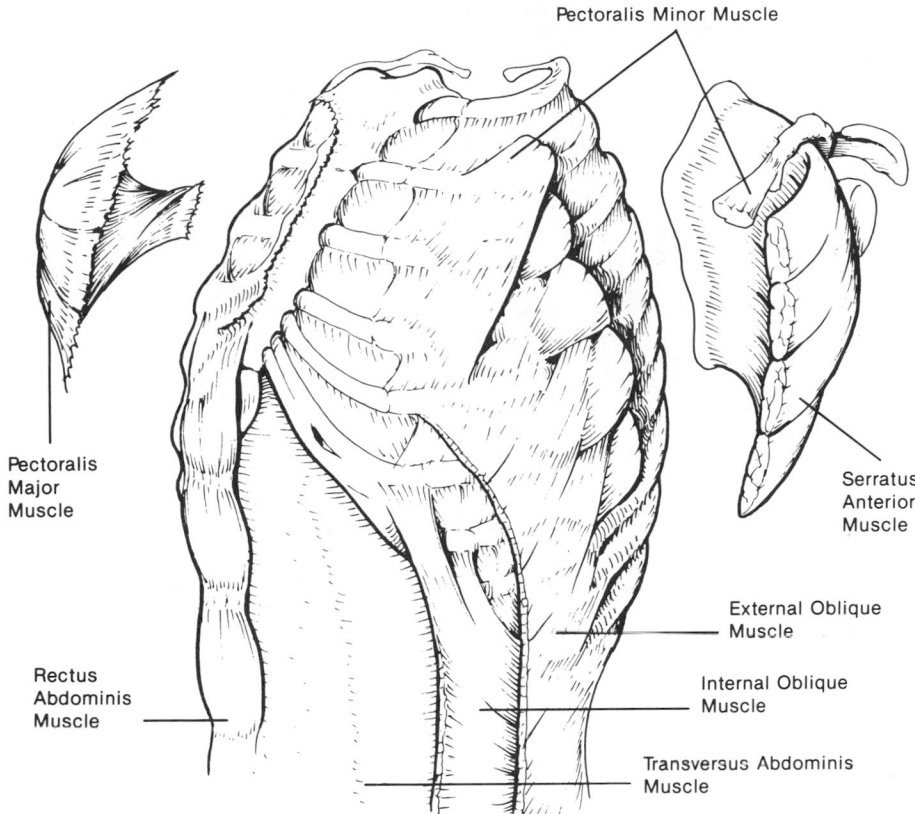

Pectoralis Minor Muscle

Pectoralis Major Muscle

Rectus Abdominis Muscle

Serratus Anterior Muscle

External Oblique Muscle

Internal Oblique Muscle

Transversus Abdominis Muscle

Figure 44-10. The relationship of the major anterior muscles of the pectoral girdle are shown in this left anterior oblique projection. On the right side the pectoralis major muscle is shown elevated away from the chest wall. Its cut origins along the medial aspect of the sternum and costal cartilage on the right side are apparent. The pectoralis major and serratus anterior have been transected on the left side and are placed away from the chest wall for clarity.

minor lies beneath the pectoralis major and has origins on the second through fourth ribs. Its insertion is on the coracoid process of the clavicle. The serratus anterior muscle arises from major muscular slips near the anterior axillary line on the anterior aspect of the ribs and inserts on the scapula (Fig. 44-10). Each of these muscles has obvious importance, not only for governing motion of the upper extremity but also for thoracic surgical incisions. Each of these muscles receives its primary blood supply and innervation from the cephalad aspect of the chest near the axilla.

A number of muscles from the upper extremity have their origins on the posterior aspect of the chest. These are particularly important in creating and reconstructing thoracic surgical incisions (Fig. 44-11). The two most superficial muscles are the trapezius and latissimus dorsi. The latissimus dorsi arises from the lumbodorsal fascia and the fascia of the paraspinous muscles, as well as the aponeurosis going to the iliac crest, and inserts on the humerus. Its blood supply and innervation come from the axilla and proceed downward to the posterolateral aspect of the chest. Thoracotomy incisions that divide this muscle cause a significant alteration in its physiology. When the neuromuscular bundle is divided, the distal portion of the muscle depends on its secondary blood supply for viability. When the distal portion of the muscle has become dependent on the perforating arteries of the lum-

bodorsal fascia, rotation of this muscle as a flap for closure of intrathoracic fistulae or chest wall defects is contraindicated, as this would cause the distal portion of the muscle to die. The proximal portion in these circumstances still maintains the thoracodorsal artery as its primary blood supply. The distal portion of the muscle is no longer dependent on the blood supply arising from above but rather on the secondary supply. Rotation of the entire muscle under these circumstances generally results in necrosis of the distal portion of the muscle. When this is used to close a fistula or to reconstruct a portion of the chest, it causes a severe subsequent complication in that the distal flap generally necroses.

The trapezius muscle, infrequently used in chest wall reconstruction, is more superficial and cephalad; it originates in the paraspinous area and courses laterally to insert on the scapula. The rhomboid muscles lie directly beneath the trapezius and course laterally to insert on the scapula. Directly beneath the rhomboids are the serratus posterior superior muscles, which arise on the spinous processes of the vertebral column and insert on the upper four ribs. The paraspinous muscles, which run the entire length of the spinal column, constitute the deepest layer of the musculature of the back. They run up and down along the spine and connect the vertebral column to the inferior aspects of the ribs. The serratus posterior inferior muscles join the inferior aspects

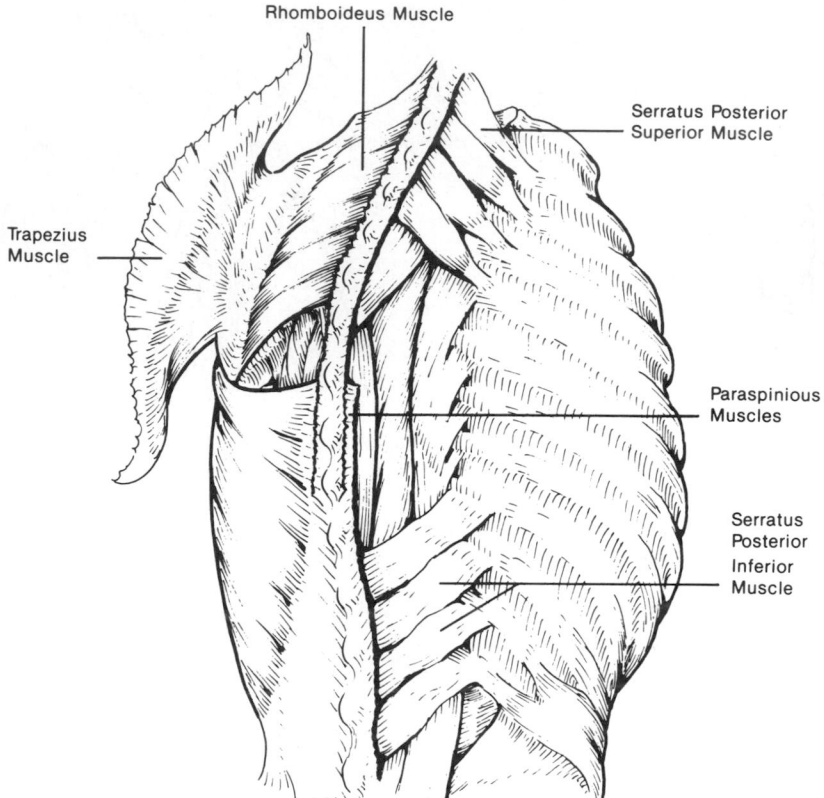

Figure 44-11.   This right posterior oblique view of the torso shows the major musculature on the posterior aspects of the chest wall. Note that the trapezius muscle on the left side has been cut to expose the rhomboid muscles beneath it. The rhomboid major is below and the rhomboid minor is above. These connect the scapula with the spinal column. Beneath the rhomboids are the serratus posterior superior muscles. The latissimus dorsi has been left intact on the right side but has been cut away on the left side to show the serratus posterior inferior muscles. The paraspinus muscles run longitudinally along the spine and connect the spinal column to the individual ribs.

of the lowest four ribs to the lumbar vertebrae. In general, most thoracic incisions do not encounter these muscles, since they are placed so low on the thoracic skeleton. Deep to these muscles lie the lower portions of the paraspinous muscles (Fig. 44-11).

ANATOMY OF SUPERIOR AND INFERIOR APERTURES

The inferior thoracic aperture lies at the boundary between the chest and the abdomen. The anatomy of the diaphragm and the inferior rim of the musculoskeletal thorax is discussed in Chapter 51 on the diaphragm and will not be considered here. The superior thoracic aperture has unique anatomic features, which govern surgical procedures in this region. The main muscles of this region are the sternocleidomastoid and the scalene muscles (Clemente, 1985a). The sternocleidomastoid muscle originates on the temporal bone of the skull and courses inferiorly and anteriorly to insert on the manubrium of the sternum and on the medial third of the clavicle (Fig. 44-12). Its action is to rotate the skull to the opposite side. It also functions as an accessory muscle of respiration in that it elevates the head of the sternum and causes minimal elevation of the clavicle. The three scalene muscles—anter-

ior, middle, and posterior—are also accessory muscles of respiration in that they elevate the first and second ribs and raise them somewhat anteriorly through the bucket handle mechanism. These three muscles originate on the cervical vertebrae and insert on the first two ribs. The anterior and middle scalene muscles insert on the cephalad aspect of the first rib. The posterior scalene muscle inserts on the cephalad aspect of the dorsal third of the second rib.

The major vessels of the head and upper extremities, as well as the trachea and esophagus, exit the thorax through the superior thoracic aperture. In Fig. 44-13 the clavicles and musculature have been removed to show the relationship of the major vessels to the skeletal thorax and to the trachea and esophagus. The subclavian vein is the most anterior vascular structure and lies directly behind the clavicle (Clemente, 1985b). The axillary vein becomes the subclavian vein as soon as it transverses the angle between the first rib and the clavicle. The subclavian vein combines with the internal jugular vein to create the brachiocephalic vein. The subclavian vein also is the point of termination for the thyrocervical trunk, internal thoracic veins, and pericardiophrenic veins. The insertions of these smaller veins onto the larger vessels is somewhat variable. The confluence of the two brachiocephalic veins creates the superior vena cava. As may be noted

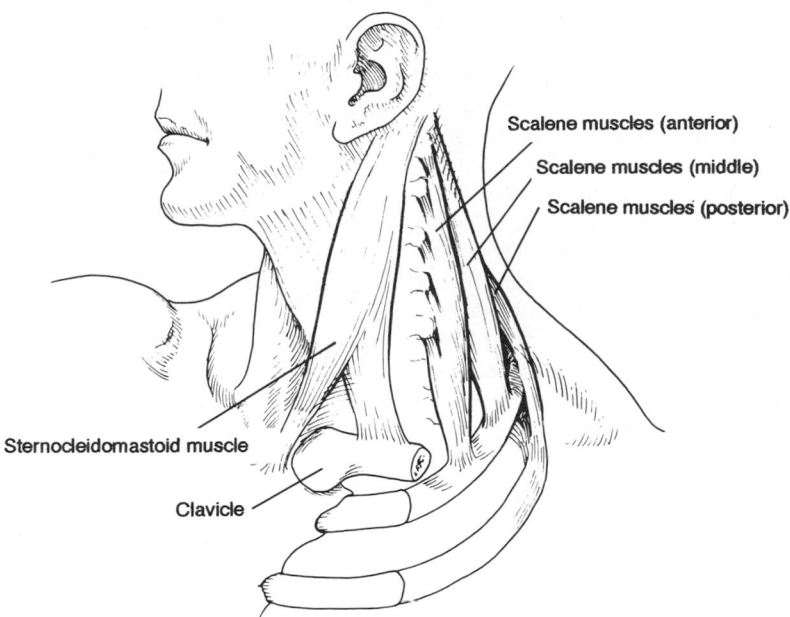

Figure 44-12. The muscles of the superior thoracic inlet are shown here. The sternocleidomastoid muscle has two major heads, one going to the manubrium of the sternum and the second to the clavicle. The scalene muscles—anterior, middle, and posterior—originate from the anterior cervical spine and progress anteriorly and caudad until they insert on the first and second ribs. The anterior and middle scalene muscles join on the first rib; the posterior inserts on the superior aspect of the second rib.

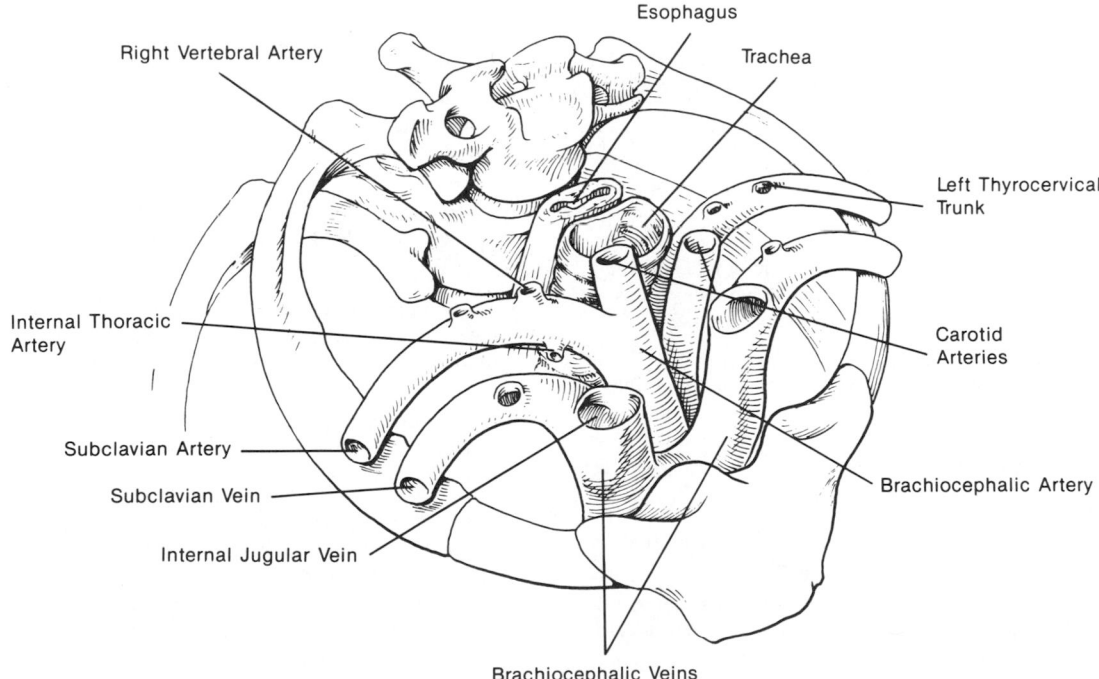

Figure 44-13. The major vascular structures that exit through the superior thoracic aperture are shown in relation to the bony skeleton, the trachea, and the esophagus. Note that the great veins are anterior to the arteries, the arteries are between the great veins and the trachea, and the esophagus lies between the trachea and the spinal column. The clavicles have been removed from this picture for clarity.

in Figure 44-13, the left brachiocephalic vein courses behind the manubrium along its posterior aspect to join the right brachiocephalic vein at the right posterolateral aspect of the manubrium to form the vena cava.

The three great arteries exit the chest through the superior thoracic aperture (West, 1977). The first is the innominate artery (brachiocephalic artery), which gives rise to the right carotid artery and the right subclavian artery. The second branch of the aortic arch exiting through the superior thoracic aperture is the left carotid artery. The left subclavian artery, the third great vessel to arise from the aortic arch, courses medially and caphalad to the apex of the chest and exits over the left first rib just under the clavicle. The paired subclavian arteries each give rise to a vertebral artery, a thyrocervical trunk, and the internal thoracic artery. The first two intercostal arteries generally originate on the inferior aspect of the subclavians. The innominate artery lies directly anterior to the trachea, as is apparent to anyone performing a cervical mediastinoscopy. The proximity of this vessel to the anterolateral wall of the trachea is important, since tracheostomy tubes placed with undue tension on the tube and excessive inflation of the occlusive cuff can result in a trachea–innominate artery fistula. The brachial plexus, although not a true thoracic structure, lies in proximity to the apex of the pleura posteriorly near the first rib. The major trunks of the brachial plexus course posterior to the subclavian artery and travel over the first rib to reach the upper extremity.

ACKNOWLEDGMENT

I would like to express my gratitude to Ms. Joyce A. Elias for her dedication and excellent preparation of this manuscript. Also, I would like to thank Gary G. Wind, M.D., for his creation of the line drawings for this chapter.

KEY REFERENCES

Arey LB: Developmental Anatomy. A Textbook and Laboratory Manual of Embryology. 7th Ed., WB Saunders, Philadelphia 1965

This is a classic work on developmental anatomy. The various aspects of embryologic development are treated in a realistic fashion. A number of specific drawings outline the development of the embryo and are informative regarding the actual relationships of one structure to another.

Clemente CD: Gray's Anatomy. 30th Am. Ed. Lea & Febiger, Philadelphia, 1985

This has for generations been the standard textbook describing the anatomy of the human body. It has thorough descriptions of all structures and appropriate illustrations and correlations of structures with function. It is strongly recommended that this text be consulted concerning the musculature of the chest wall, the bony skeleton of the thorax, or any other anatomic features in the region.

Graeber GM: Embryology, anatomy, and physiology of the chest wall. p. 11. In Seyfer AE, Graeber GM, Wind GG (eds): Atlas of Chest Wall Reconstruction. Aspen Publishers, Rockville, MD, 1986

This chapter outlines the embryology, anatomy, and physiology of the chest wall and the important aspects of chest wall anatomy and physiology used in developing flaps for reconstruction of chest wall defects. Other chapters describe methods for maturing various flaps and their use in repairing chest wall defects.

Guyton AC: Pulmonary ventilation. p. 402. In: Textook of Medical Physiology, 8th Ed. WB Saunders, Philadelphia 1991

A thorough and concise treatment of pulmonary physiology. The roles of the diaphragm, chest wall, and accessory muscles are clearly outlined. An essential preliminary description of respiratory physiology, which serves as an excellent introduction to the topic, is presented.

Netter FM: The Ciba Collection of Medical Illustrations. Vol. 7. Respiratory System. Sect. II, Physiology. Ciba-Geigy Corp. Summit, NJ, 1979

The illustrations of Frank Netter combined with the accompanying text present a dynamic and insightful view of respiratory physiology. The illustrations are particularly exellent, and they demonstrate major principles well. This reference is strongly recommended because the visual images significantly increase understanding of respiratory physiology.

Ravitch MM: Congenital Deformities of the Chest Wall and Their Operative Correction. WB Saunders, Philadelphia, 1977

This is a classic monograph on chest wall abnormalities and their correction, written by one of the true experts in congenital abnormalities of the thorax. The book is richly illustrated with clinical pictures and drawings, which delineate proper reconstruction of the abnormalities.

West JB. Mechanics of breathing. p. 560. In West JB (ed): Best and Taylor's Physiologic Basis of Medical Practice. 12th Ed. Williams & Wilkins, Baltimore, 1991

This reference describes both basic and more advanced pulmonary physiology. It gives dimension and depth to the topic while presenting the material in a straightforward and cogent fashion.

West JB: Respiratory Physiology—The Essentials. 2nd Ed. Williams & Wilkins, Baltimore, 1979

West has a particularly informative and flowing style of writing, which allows him to convey the essentials of respiratory physiology in a particularly lucid fashion. The illustrations clearly illustrate the major points and increase understanding.

West JB: Pulmonary Pathophysiology—The Essentials. 2nd Ed. Williams & Wilkins, Baltimore, 1977

West is particularly adept at describing the pathophysiologic problems of the pulmonary system and how they may present clinically. The illustrations are superlative. His text and illustrations lead to a higher understanding of pulmonary problems and their clinical correlates.

REFERENCES

Clemente CD: Muscles and fasciae. In Clemente CD (ed): Gray's Anatomy. 30th Am. Ed. Lea & Febiger, Philadelphia, 1985a

Clemente CD: The Arteries. In Clemente CD (ed): Gray's Anatomy. 30th Am. Ed. Lea & Febiger, Philadelphia, 1985b

Clemente CD: The Veins. In Clemente CD (ed): Gray's Anatomy. 30th Am. Ed. Lea & Febiger, Philadelphia, 1985c

Clemente CD: The Peripheral Nervous System. Clemente CD (ed): Gray's Anatomy. 30th Am. Ed. Lea & Febiger, Philadelphia, 1985d

45

DIAGNOSTIC MODALITIES

Geoffrey M. Graeber

Pathologic processes that involve the chest wall present numerous perplexing problems to the pulmonologist, radiologist, and thoracic surgeon. The detection, evaluation, and characterization of these processes requires many different diagnostic modalities. The recent expansion of cross-sectional imaging techniques has allowed more precise anatomic definition of chest wall pathologic conditions than was previously available (Schaefer and Burton, 1989). Certain lesions that were difficult, if not impossible, to evaluate two decades ago are now assessed with precision and accuracy (Kuhlman, et al., 1994). The challenge to delineate the full extent of the chest wall pathologic process remains because many vital structures lie in close proximity to the ribs, costal cartilages, and sternum. This chapter discusses most of the methods used to evaluate chest wall disease but focuses on imaging techniques because their importance is paramount. Diagnostic biopsy by both surgical and needle techniques is covered in the chapter on primary chest wall neoplasms (see Ch. 48).

The discussion that follows provides an approach to evaluate the patient with a chest wall pathologic condition in a logical progression. Each patient is subjected to a thorough initial evaluation, which includes standard radiographic techniques. Some traditional imaging modalities still yield valuable information in the assessment of chest wall disease, despite the availability of more sophisticated techniques (Schaefer and Burton, 1989). Axial imaging techniques, such as computed tomography (CT) and magnetic resonance imaging (MRI), have expanded our ability to evaluate chest wall pathologic conditions. The assets and limitations of CT and MRI are compared and contrasted. The potentially confusing presence of healing rib fractures and metastatic neoplasms in the evaluation of chest wall disease is discussed. Chest wall neoplasms may be benign or malignant; they can also result from extension of tumors from adjacent organs and overlying skeletal structures. The pertinent findings associated with chest wall infection are also presented. Finally, the salient features of important congenital chest wall deformities are chronicled. Selected images, mostly taken from the author's recent experience, are used to illustrate major points.

INITIAL EVALUATION AND CONSULTATION

A careful history and physical examination are mandatory in the evaluation of the patient with a suspected chest wall pathologic condition because metastatic neoplasms and healing rib fractures are the most common maladies found in the chest wall (Graeber, et al., 1982). In most instances, a careful history and review of systems reveal signs and symptoms that suggest the presence of neoplastic disease. Similarly, careful questioning evokes any history of trauma, no matter how slight, which could alert the physician to the possibility of healing rib fractures. The physical examination denotes the characteristics of the pathologic type and focuses the physician's thinking toward specific diagnoses. Standard chest radiographs obtained in the posteroanterior and lateral projections often give further information concerning the nature of the pathologic condition (Schaefer and Burton, 1989). When this basic information has been obtained, it is wise to consult with the radiologist concerning which imaging modalities will yield the most information with the least cost.

TRADITIONAL RADIOGRAPHIC TECHNIQUES

Routine chest radiographs taken in the posteroanterior and lateral projections reveal chest wall pathologic findings in many instances. These standard films document the presence of disease and help determine which more sophisticated imaging techniques are required. Most importantly, they provide a set of baseline films to which all subsequent radiographs may be compared. Plain films, moreover, may be able to define whether a tumor is extrapleural (Schaefer and Burton, 1989). The characteristics of subpleural lesions that extend into the pleural cavity include a clearly defined, smooth contour that is convex toward the lung, tapering peripheral margins, and broad-based attachment to the chest wall (Felson, 1973) (Fig. 45-1).

I wish to acknowledge the excellent help of Mrs. Karen DeShong in the preparation of this manuscript and the support of Dr. Debra Granke of the Department of Radiology, West Virginia University Medical Center, in obtaining and interpreting the MRI images that are presented in this chapter.

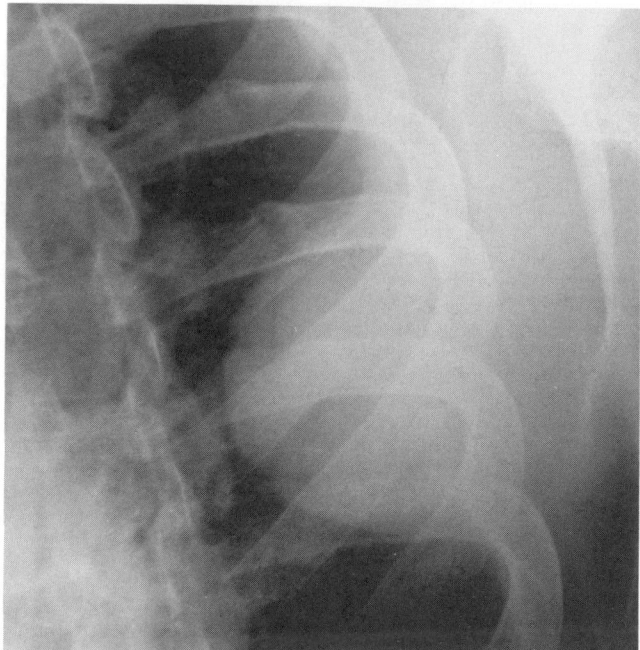

Figure 45-1. This selected radiograph of a neural sheath tumor growing inside the ribs shows the characteristics that define an extrapleural lesion. Note that the mass has a sharp smooth contour, tapering margins along its base on the chest wall, and a broad-based attachment to the chest wall. (From Schaefer PS, Burton BS: Radiographic evaluation of chest wall lesions. Surg Clin North Am 69:911, 1989, with permission.)

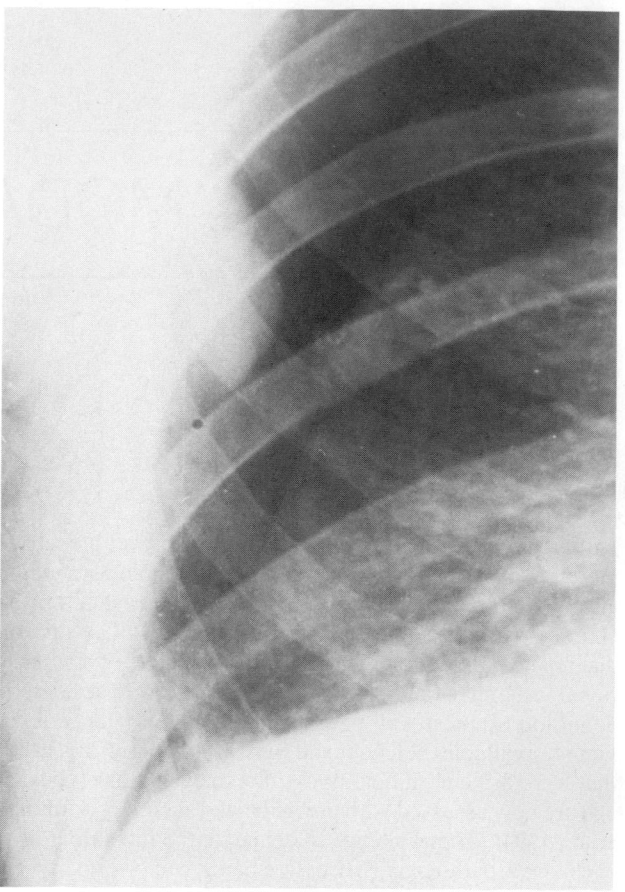

Figure 45-2. This patient underwent induced pneumothorax and chest radiography to determine whether a chest wall mass had its origin in the lung. The lesion (a perineural fibroblastoma) was suspected to be extrapleural, as determined by the characteristics noted in Figure 45-1. The parietal pleura is stretched over the neoplasm. The medial line represents the receding visceral pleura on the lung surface (From Schaefer PS, Burton BS: Radiographic evaluation of chest wall lesions. Surg Clin North Am 69:911, 1989, with permission.)

Routine tomography currently plays a very limited role in the evaluation of chest wall pathologic conditions since CT and MRI have assumed increasing capabilities (Schaefer and Burton, 1989). The newer imaging techniques have surpassed standard tomography in the information they can provide on chest wall disease. Induced pneumothorax, when combined with standard radiographs, may have a limited role in the evaluation of some chest wall pathologic conditions. The induced pneumothorax allows the lung to recede from the chest wall. In many cases, when no adhesions are present, the precise origin of the mass may be defined accurately (Schaefer and Burton, 1989). (Fig. 45-2).

Induced pneumothorax may also be combined with CT to detect the origin of tumors and whether primary pulmonary malignancies invade the chest wall or mediastinum. In one study, the authors used induced pneumothorax combined with CT in 12 patients who had already had initial CT scans that were indeterminate to establish the origin or define the invasion of intrathoracic masses (Watanabe, et al., 1991). In 11 of the 12 patients investigated, correct information, confirmed by surgical exploration, was obtained. In the one patient who had a false-positive reading for mediastinal invasion by lung cancer, adhesions from a previous inflammatory process prevented the lung from receding from the mediastinum. At surgery, the adhesions were transsected, and the malignancy was found to be free of the mediastinum. Yokoi, et al. (1991) have been even stronger advocates of CT in association with induced pneumothorax in the evaluation of invasion of lung cancer into the mediastinum and chest wall.

In their experience with 43 patients, CT in conjunction with pneumothorax was 100 percent accurate for chest wall and 76 percent accurate for mediastinal invasion.

Two other standard techniques that may be used in the evaluation of the extent of thoracic involvement by disease processes that primarily afflict the chest wall are fluoroscopy and decubitus films (Schaefer and Burton, 1989). The integrity of the phrenic nerve and diaphragm to function may be evaluated by fluoroscopy while the patient performs rapid, short inspirations. Decubitus films are also helpful to detect free pleural effusions because the fluid, if not loculated, flows to the most dependent aspect of the chest.

ASSETS AND LIMITATIONS OF COMPUTED TOMOGRAPHY AND MAGNETIC RESONANCE IMAGING

The use of CT and MRI in the evaluation of patients with cancer has yielded more information than plain radiography, but neither modality has provided the diagnostic accuracy anticipated (Kuhlman, et al., 1994). In fact, CT and MRI have fallen short of anticipated goals in the detection of mediastinal or chest wall involvement by pulmonary malignancies (Miller, et al., 1992; Webb, et al., 1991). Indeed, there is no substantial difference between the two modalities in their ability to predict chest wall invasion (Webb, et al., 1991). Both should be considered complementary to one another in the evaluation of chest wall pathologic conditions (Kuhlman, et al., 1994; Schaefer and Burton, 1989). Both continue to undergo evaluation to define their role in the assessment of chest wall disease. Because MRI is newer and has more possible variables to apply, the potential for growth in knowledge is greater with this technique (Templeton, et al., 1990).

At the present time, axial imaging with CT does have some advantages (Kuhlman, et al., 1994). CT has a good capacity to assess cortical bone destruction by neoplastic masses and infection. The changes must be definitive, however, or a firm diagnosis of tumor invasion or osteomyelitis cannot be substantiated (Libshitz, 1990). Pearlberg, et al. (1987) found that definite bony destruction was the only truly reliable finding to substantiate chest wall invasion by a tumor. In some studies, local pain has been as effective as CT in the prediction of chest wall invasion (Gamsu, 1986; Glaser, et al., 1985).

The utility of CT has been extended by specialized techniques to yield somewhat improved results. Mention has already been made of the combination of CT with induced pneumothorax to evaluate tumor invasion of the chest wall and mediastinum (Yokoi, et al., 1991; Wantanabe, et al., 1991). CT has also been used in conjunction with progressive expiration in an attempt to determine chest wall invasion by lung cancer (Murata, et al., 1994). Based on a small number of patients, it appeared that expiratory CT was highly successful in the evaluation of chest wall invasion. Confirmation of these findings awaits a larger series of patients.

CT has also been compared with ultrasound (US) to assess chest wall invasion by lung cancer (Suzuki, et al., 1993). In a series of 120 patients evaluated by both CT and US, 19 had chest wall invasion. The authors found that the sensitivity of US was 100 percent and its specificity was 98 percent. The sensitivity of CT was only 68 percent, and its specificity was 66 percent. The accuracy of US was 98 percent; that of CT was 67 percent. The results of this interesting study await the publication of a larger series and confirmation by other authors.

MRI has some distinct advantages over CT to evaluate primary chest wall neoplasms or the extent of chest wall involvement associated with malignancies of other organs that may extend into the chest wall (Kuhlman, et al., 1994). MRI can image in several planes (coronal, sagittal, and axial) to obtain better definition of neoplastic masses and their relationship to adjacent structures (Kuhlman, et al., 1994; Libshitz, 1990; Templeton, et al., 1990). Because MRI can be adjusted, it is more useful to highlight infiltration of bone marrow and soft tissue invasion (Kuhlman, et al., 1994). Because of these mentioned abilities, MRI is used preferentially to evaluate superior sulcus tumors (Kuhlman, et al., 1994; Templeton, et al., 1990; Libshitz, 1990).

In the final analysis, both imaging techniques should be considered to be complementary modalities, which should be used judiciously and selectively in the evaluation of chest

wall pathologic conditions as part of a thorough and comprehensive workup (Kuhlman, et al., 1994; Templeton, et al., 1990; Libshitz, 1990). Most thoracic surgeons perform standard radiographs and obtain a CT scan, if indicated, as a guide to surgical therapy (Libshitz, 1990; Templeton, et al., 1990). If further delineation of disease is necessary, MRI may be considered to guide definitive therapy (Templeton, et al., 1990). Neither modality by itself or in confirmation with the findings of other diagnostic modalities should be considered absolute or definitive enough to withhold surgical therapy based on images alone (Libshitz, 1990). Indeed, the presence and extent of disease is still determined by tissue biopsy and pathologic examination.

METASTASES TO THE CHEST WALL AND HEALING RIB FRACTURES

As already mentioned, metastases from distant cancers and healing rib fractures are far more common than primary chest wall neoplasms (Graeber, et al., 1982). Because many such lesions may be found on routine chest radiographs, they become an important problem. Differentiation of metastases from healing rib fractures or primary chest wall neoplasms can be impossible with imaging techniques alone (Graeber, et al., 1982; Schaefer and Burton, 1989) (Figs. 45-3 and 45-4). Radiographs and images taken of the chest at some remote prior time may be most helpful to determine the nature of a mass found in the chest wall on a routine radiograph (Schaefer and Burton, 1989). In the absence of previous images, a biopsy may need to be performed to ascertain the exact nature of the pathologic finding. Despite active direct questioning, the patient may deny trauma or minimize its extent such that a biopsy will become necessary.

In the event that the lesion is a metastasis, a biopsy is required to substantiate the disease finding and direct appropriate therapy (Graeber, et al., 1982). The most common offenders that cause metastases in the chest wall are primary malignancies of the breast, lung, kidney, and thyroid, although exceptions occur with reasonable frequency (Fig. 45-5). MRI may be particularly helpful to determine the amount of soft tissue involvement (Fig. 45-6).

Observation of a chest wall lesion is only warranted if its presence has been established on prior radiographic examination and the lesion has been stable for a considerable period (Graeber, et al., 1982). Primary neoplasms and metastases need histologic confirmation and appropriate therapy as soon as possible. Although infectious processes can present as a mass, constitutional symptoms (such as fever and leukocytosis) usually reveal the cause. Because neoplasia, active healing, and infection all arouse active inflammation, masses caused by all three etiologic factors yield a positive bone scan (Fig. 45-3). If there is concern or doubt over the nature of a given lesion or its cause, surgical biopsy is indicated because needle biopsy of chest wall lesions is often imprecise (Graeber, et al., 1982) (Fig. 45-3).

BENIGN PRIMARY CHEST WALL NEOPLASMS

In most series, approximately one-half of all primary chest wall neoplasms are benign (Graeber, et al., 1982; Ryan, et al., 1989). Most of these benign neoplasms are of cartilaginous

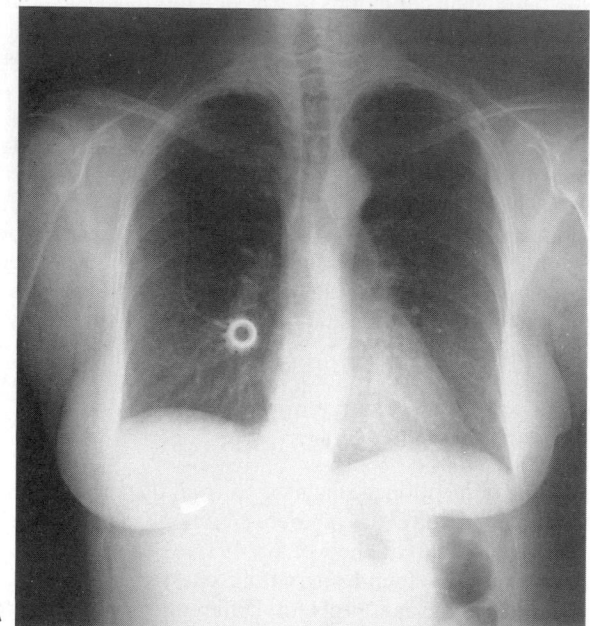
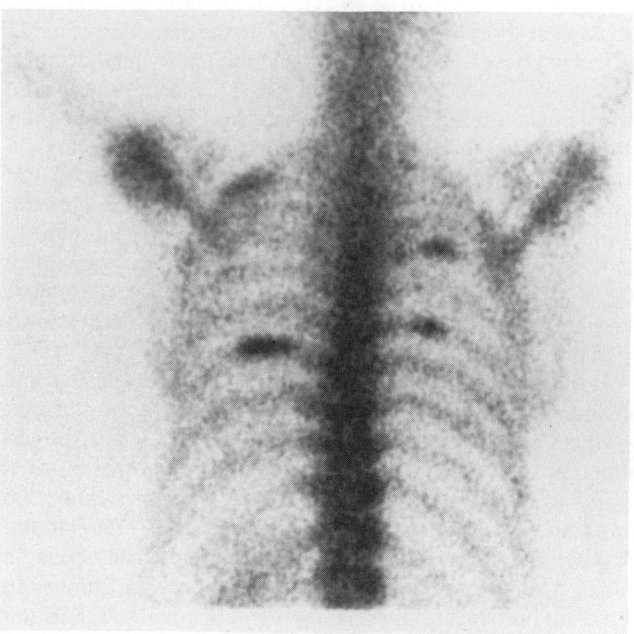

Figure 45-3. **(A)** This posteroanterior radiograph of a 42-year-old woman with known breast cancer shows minimal irregularities in the posterior aspects of the left eight rib. Because the patient had had some posterior tenderness and this irregularity of the eighth rib was detected, the patient was scheduled for a bone scan. It should also be noted that the patient had fallen and landed on her left shoulder approximately 6 months prior to this radiograph. **(B)** This is a posterior projection from the bone scan conducted on the patient whose radiograph is presented in Fig. A. Note that the left eighth rib concentrates the radiopharmaceutical most actively. Three other ribs also concentrate the radiopharmaceutical, as does the head of the left humerus. The patient underwent needle biopsy of the left eighth rib, which showed nonspecific inflammatory changes. An excisional biopsy was performed of the eighth rib, which showed a healing rib fracture.

origin. Enchondromas, juxtacortical chondromas, and osteochondromas are some of the more commonly occurring neoplasms (Fig. 45-7). Many times these lesions present as incidental, asymptomatic findings on routine radiographs or on radiographs conducted to assess other conditions. Several of these neoplasms have radiographic characteristics on plain films that identify them. At times other radiographic techniques, such as CT or MRI, are required to determine the most likely diagnosis. Once the presence of one of these neoplasms has been documented, the treating physician may elect to observe the tumor. If this course is taken, the surveillance must be precise and continuing because malignant degeneration, although rare, does occur (Graeber, et al., 1982). This is particularly true in chondromatous lesions. Observation of such neoplasms must be exceptionally thorough in patients who have certain inherited syndromes, such as multiple hereditary osteochondromatosis or enchondromatosis, because malignant degeneration may occur in 5 to 20 percent of benign neoplasms in these patients (Resnick and Niwayama, 1981). Change in any lesion, particularly expansion accompanied by discomfort, should arouse the physician's serious suspicion of malignant degeneration.

Fibrous dysplasia in some series represented 20 to 30 percent of all benign neoplastic processes found in the chest wall (Teitelbaum, 1972). In reality, the condition probably is not a true neoplasm but rather a developmental abnormality of the bone-forming mesenchyme, which is characterized by filling of the medullary cavity with fibrous tissue and random formation of poor trabeculae (Resnick and Niwayama, 1981). Characteristically, the abnormality often presents as a painless, lytic lesion of the posterior aspect of a rib. Areas of bone expansion may be present. Over time the lesion may progress through increasing density to a ground-glass appearance. Continuation of this process may finally result in a homogeneous sclerosis (Schaefer and Burton, 1989).

Other true, benign neoplasms of the musculoskeletal thorax are less common. These neoplasms, plus other benign conditions that may mimic a neoplasm, are important because in some instances, they may have radiographic characteristics that suggest malignancy. One characteristic that may particularly suggest malignancy is presentation as a lytic area in a rib. Most commonly, however, these lesions present as clearly circumscribed lesions that are discernible on standard chest radiographs. Among these lesions are the eosinophilic granuloma, chondroblastoma, giant cell tumor, hemangioma, aneurysmal bone cyst, and the osteoblastoma (Fig. 45-8). CT may be indicated in any of these conditions to define better the true extent if there is any suggestion of a soft tissue mass or evidence of cortical breakthrough (Schaefer and Burton, 1989).

Probably the most common benign neoplasm of the tissues intimate to the musculoskeletal thorax is the lipoma (Stout and Lattes, 1967). Many arise just outside the parietal pleura. Some have both an intrathoracic and an extrathoracic compo-

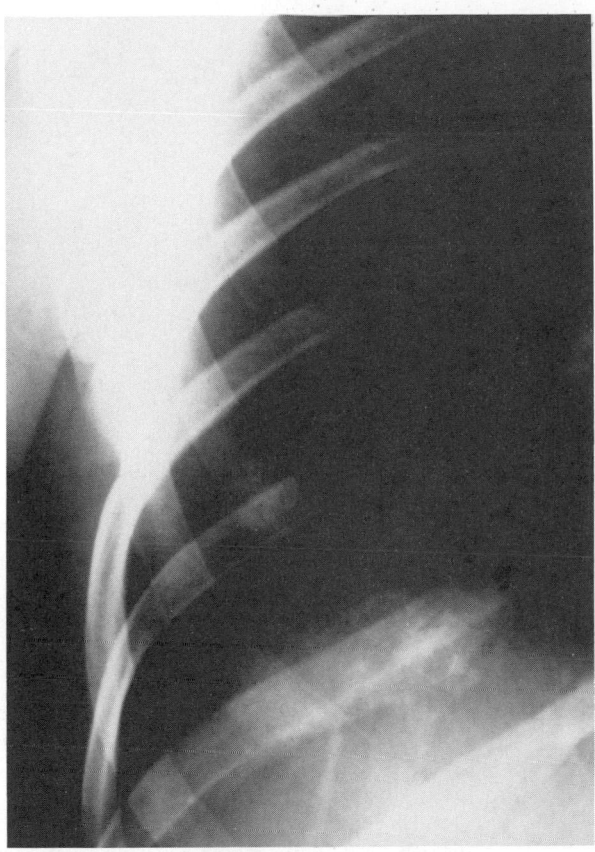

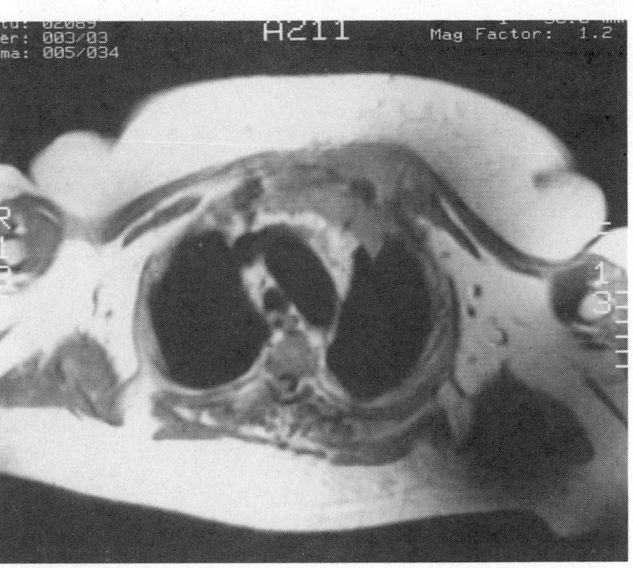

Figure 45-6. MRI may be used to delineate soft tissue involvement by metastatic neoplasms, such as in this patient who has a history of metastatic carcinoma of an unknown primary. This is a thin-density T_1-weighted axial image through the upper thorax that shows a mass involving the chest wall with involvement of the pectoralis major and minor, direct extension into the sternum, and involvement of the anterior mediastinum.

Figure 45-4. This selected radiograph of the ribs demonstrates a mass lesion anteriorly near the costochondral junction. Despite an extensive workup, no other lesions were found. The patient denied any history of significant trauma. The lesion underwent biopsy and was found to be a healing rib fracture.

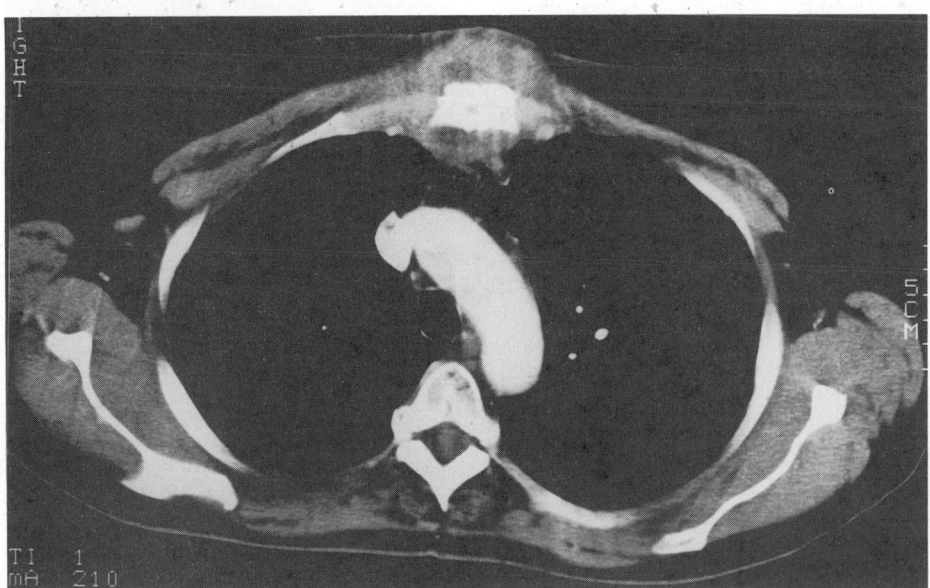

Figure 45-5. This 42-year-old man presented with a recent onset of a painful enlarging mass of his sternum. Radiographically the tumor appeared to be a primary sarcoma of the sternum. An extensive workup did not reveal any other similar lesions or any suggestion of a primary. Biopsy detected a metastatic adenocarcinoma, most likely of colonic origin. Although the primary was never found, multiple other areas of metastasis developed, and the patient died of disseminated disease. This figure shows a representative CT axial image of the chest that demonstrates how the metastatic tumor had enveloped the sternum.

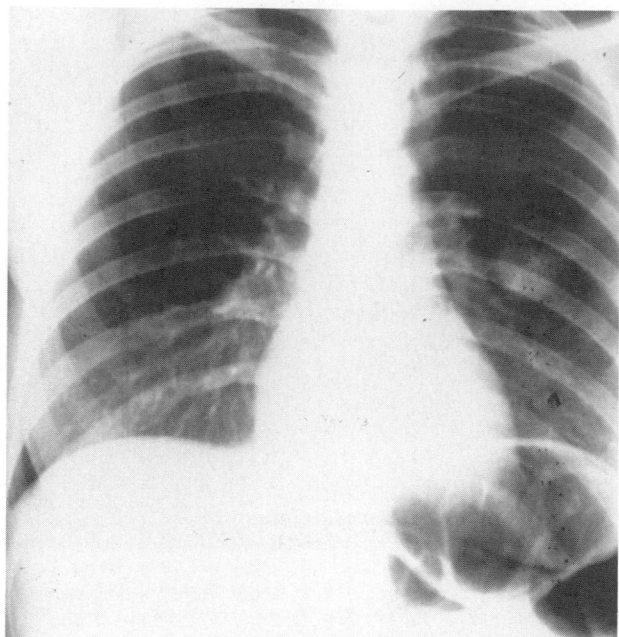

Figure 45-7. This radiograph shows an osteochondroma arising in the region near the posterior aspect of the left sixth rib. Note that the ribs in the area appear to have their cortices intact and that there is no erosion. The lesion is rounded, has a sharp margin, and does not appear to encroach on any other structures.

nent, which are joined by an isthmus that extends between two ribs (Schaefer and Burton, 1989). If the lipoma is of sufficient size, it may be detectable on plain radiographs. They usually appear as a mass of relatively lucent tissue because fat is relatively less dense compared with the other structures of the chest wall. CT can be diagnostic of lipomas in the chest wall because of their low density. CT scanning can generally differentiate between lipomas and liposarcomas because the sarcomas almost always have areas of higher density (Goodwin, 1984).

MALIGNANT PRIMARY CHEST WALL NEOPLASMS

Although certain malignant primary chest wall neoplasms have radiographic characteristics that strongly suggest their type, none has an imaging signature that is unequivocally diagnostic (Graeber, et al., 1982; Schaefer and Burton, 1989). Two malignant primary chest wall neoplasms that have imaging characteristics strongly suggestive of their respective histologic types are osteogenic and Ewing's sarcomas. Both lesions are relatively rare and tend to arise in younger individuals. Ewing's arises principally in the pediatric population and osteogenic sarcoma, usually in young adults. Ewing's sarcoma has a radiographic appearance that suggests multiple layering as a result of its physical characteristics. It may present as a lytic or expansile lesion of a rib or clavicle, which is surrounded by periosteal new bone formation and a soft tissue mass (Franken, et al., 1977). Unfortunately, Ewing's sarcoma is not only the most common malignant primary chest wall neoplasm in children, it is one of the

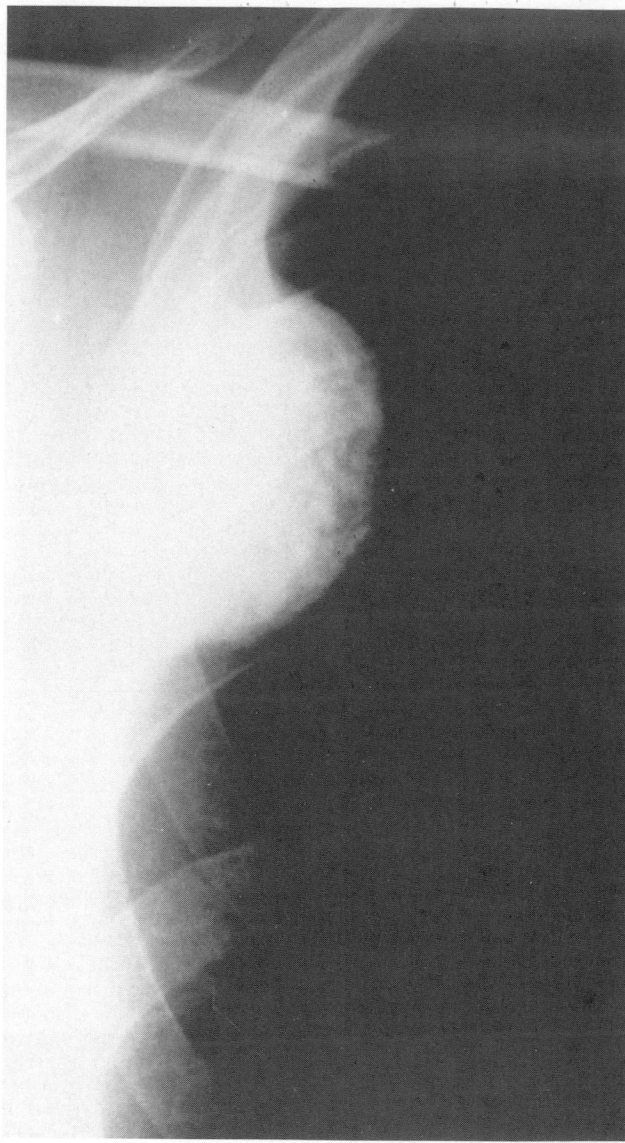

Figure 45-8. This plain chest radiograph of an asymptomatic 44-year-old man revealed this 6-cm mass growing off the right third rib. The flocculent chondroid calcifications are notable. This broad-based lesion with the chondroid calcifications demonstrates all the characteristics of a chondroblastoma. As with all chondromatous lesions, the true nature can only be confirmed after a thorough histologic examination by a pathologist. By the size criteria noted in the text, the lesion should be regarded as a chondrosarcoma until proved otherwise.

more frequent malignancies to metastasize to the bony thorax (Schaefer and Burton, 1989; Larsson and Lorentzon, 1974). Osteogenic sarcomas often have a "sunburst" appearance when they originate from components of the thoracic skeleton. Exceptions to these radiographic characteristics obviously occur.

Among the other malignant primary chest wall neoplasms, general tendencies can be identified, but exceptions are frequent. An obvious example is the chest wall plasmacytoma (Graeber, et al., 1982, Schaefer and Burton, 1989). The solitary chest wall plasmacytoma is often the first sign of systemic myeloma. In the number of instances, the chest wall lesion occurs several years before the systemic disease is apparent (Graeber, et al., 1982). When systemic myeloma has first become apparent in another area, the disease frequently involves several or all ribs and the sternum (Omell, et al., 1973). The CT scan may show subtle lytic lesions in the bone or small soft tissue masses when plain film findings of the chest wall structures are negative (Edelstein, et al., 1985). Solitary plasmacytoma may also present as soft tissue masses or as lytic lesions of the sternum (Fig. 45-9).

Chondrosarcoma, which has frequently been cited as the most common malignant primary chest wall neoplasm, generally presents as a large, lobulated, excrescent mass of the chest wall that shows scattered flocculent calcifications in a characteristic cartilaginous matrix (Schaefer and Burton, 1989). Such a lesion may be particularly indistinguishable from its close relatives, the benign osteochondroma or the enchondroma. Larger lesions, especially those that are greater than 4 cm in greatest extent, are considered malignant until proved otherwise (Marcove, 1971).

Fibrosarcomas are one of the most common chest wall tumors and may be reported as the most frequent primary chest wall malignancy in some series (Graeber, et al., 1982; Threlkel and Adkins, 1971). As has been pointed out, the broad classification of sarcoma in some instances may include other tumors with "spindle cell" histologic types, such as malignant fibrous histiocytoma, malignant schwannoma, and synovial sarcoma (Enzinger and Weiss, 1983). Radiographically, all of these spindle cell tumors appear in virtually identical fashion in that all appear as masses of soft tissue density (Schaefer and Burton, 1989). Necrotic, low-density areas

may be present; these are likely to represent necrosis. If focal areas of calcification are present, they are generally noted on the CT scan.

LUNG CANCER THAT INVOLVES THE CHEST WALL

MRI and CT scans have their assets and liabilities when they are used to assess the amount of chest wall involvement, as has already been described. Two instances that occur infrequently in patients with lung cancer can be more accurately assessed by MRI than by CT because of its multiplanar imaging capacities (Haggar, et al., 1987; Musset, et al., 1986). Tumors of the lung apex can be evaluated to determine involvement of apical thoracic structures and tumors of the lung base, to determine the presence or absence of diaphragmatic invasion. Because superior sulcus neoplasms occur more frequently than tumors that extend into the diaphragm, they have received more attention.

One group investigated 10 patients with superior sulcus tumors with MRI to assess the extent of apical tumor invasion (McCloud, et al., 1989). Five of the 10 patients had chest wall invasion or extension into the base of the neck demonstrated by the contrast between the bright signal intensity of the tumor and the low signal intensity of muscle on T$_2$-weighted images. MRI clearly depicted direct invasion of the mediastinum in three patients because of the inherent contrast between mediastinal fat and neoplastic tissue. In all of the cases studied by these authors, MRI clearly defined the relationship of the tumor to the subclavian artery and the brachial plexus. In two patients, MRI projections confirmed encasement of the artery, and brachial plexus involvement was confirmed in three. One problem noted by these authors

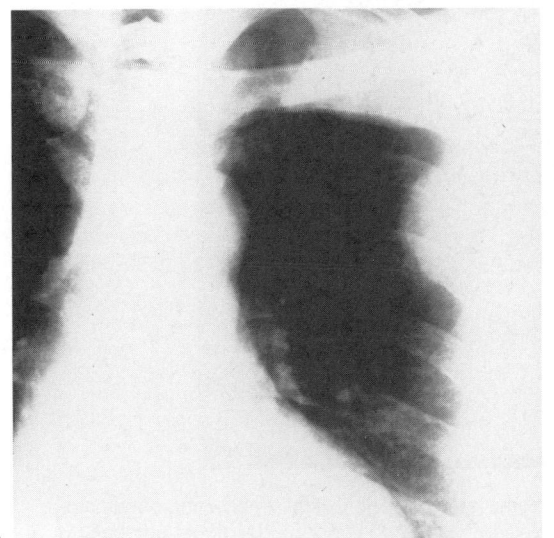

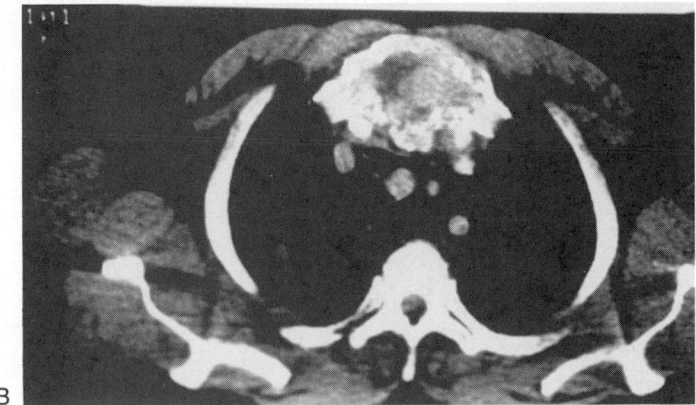

Figure 45-9. **(A)** This section of a posteroanterior chest radiograph shows a mass in the chest wall on the lateral aspect of the left pleura. Note that the mass encroaches on the pleural space. It is contiguous with the chest wall structures. Even though the mass had radiographic characteristics suggestive of a chondrosarcoma, it was found to be a plasmocytoma when it was excised. **(B)** This CT scan shows a large irregular mass that has replaced the entire manubrium of the sternum. Note that it displaces the great vessels posteriorly. This mass, which presented as a rapidly enlarging neoplasm of the sternum, was thought to be a chondrosarcoma. Pathologic examination confirmed that it was a plasmacytoma.

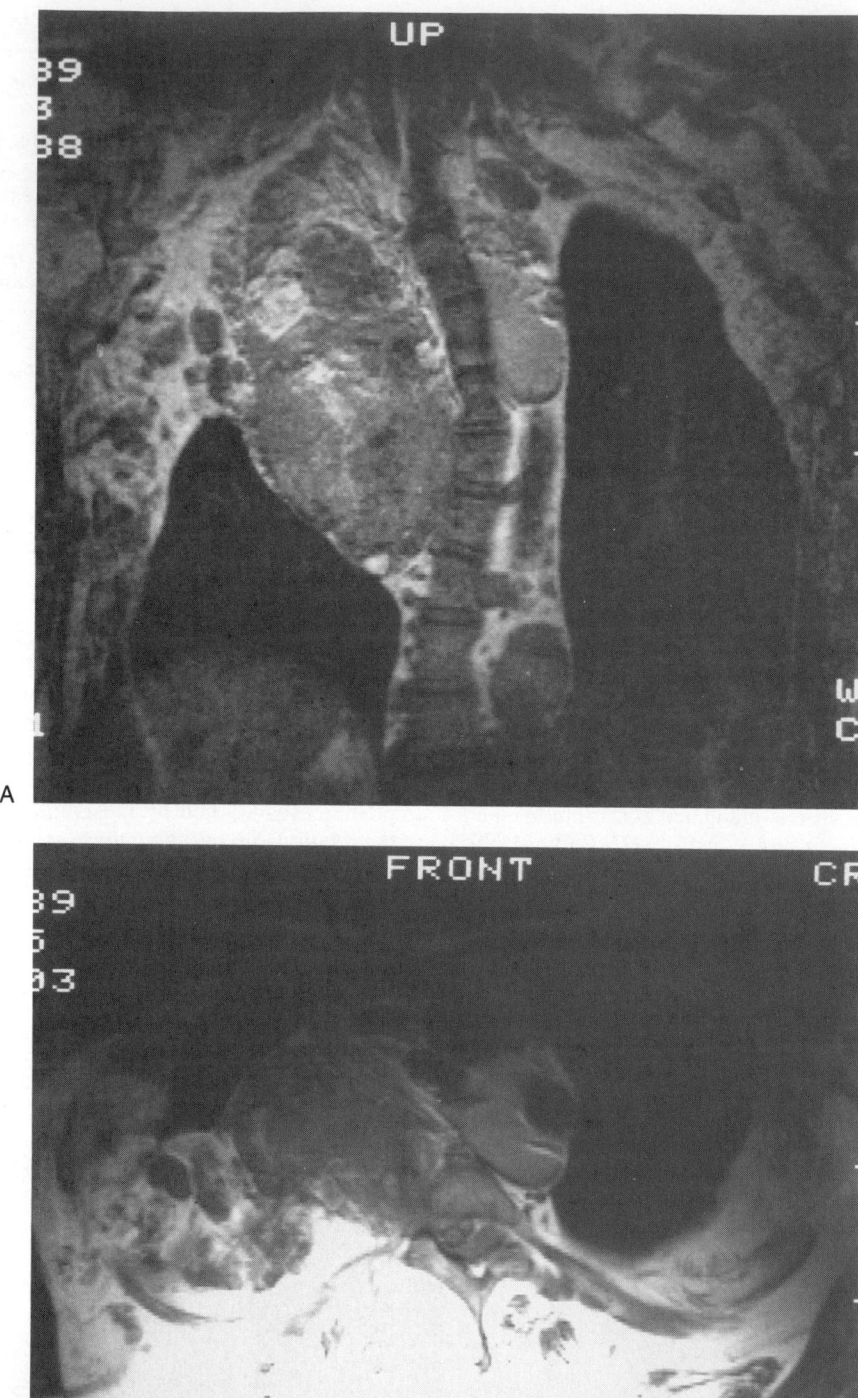

Figure 45-10. **(A)** This coronal T_1-weighted MRI image through the thorax is from a patient with invasive angiolipomatosus. A heterogeneous mass is seen involving the chest wall with extension into the posterior mediastinum adjacent to the spinal column. **(B)** This is an axial T_1-weighted image through the thorax in the same patient as in Fig. A. Note that the image clearly shows a large chest wall mass with mediastinal involvement and evidence for invasion of the spinal canal with spinal cord impingement. The multiple planes available with MRI helped to define the extent of this process.

was that MRI did not detect evidence of rib destruction in five patients who had rib involvement confirmed by other studies. Other authors have confirmed the ability of MRI to assess tumor involvement of apical structures and to detect the presence of spinal canal extension (Kuhlman, et al., 1994). In our own experience, we found MRI to be particularly useful to evaluate the extent of tumor involvement of soft tissues of the mediastinum and base of the neck, the subclavian vessels, and the spinal column (Figs. 45-10 and 45-11). MRI has been particularly helpful to determine the status of a tumor in the spinal canal and its relationship to the spinal cord (Figs. 45-10 and 45-11).

BREAST CANCER THAT INVOLVES THE CHEST WALL

Some studies estimate that 5 to 25 percent of patients treated for breast cancer have local or regional recurrence (Donegan, 1979; Lindfors, et al., 1985). CT scan has been particularly helpful to assess recurrences, document changes in the chest wall anatomy, and follow the progression of breast disease in the chest wall when it is under therapy (Schaefer and Burton, 1989). In several clinical series, it has been shown to be more accurate than physical examination in the assessment of the extent of recurrent disease. Many times CT identifies additional sites of recurrent disease that have not been suspected clinically (Lindfors, et al., 1985; Villari, et al., 1985).

The most common findings of recurrent or residual breast cancer in the chest wall are masses of soft tissue density (Shea, et al., 1987) (Fig. 45-12). Breast cancer may also appear as lytic lesions in the ribs or other bones of the thoracic and axial skeleton. MRI has been particularly helpful to assess recurrent breast disease in the chest wall when CT scan-

ning is not completely able to delineate the extent of recurrent or residual disease. Great care must be taken to confirm the histologic character of the lesions when they have been found. In our experience, the patient who is being treated for breast cancer can have other conditions, which can mimic recurrent disease (Fig. 45-3). Besides healing rib fractures, we must be constantly aware that therapeutic modalities can produce their own problems. One of these problems, which we have seen in several patients, is the destruction of bone by radiotherapy. The lesion presents as a lytic area in bone in the field of previous radiotherapy. The question arises after CT and MRI have been conducted as to whether the lytic area represents recurrent disease (Fig. 45-13). In all instances, the absolute histologic type of the offending lesion should be confirmed before any changes in therapy are instituted.

PYOGENIC INFECTIONS OF THE CHEST WALL

Pyogenic infections of the chest wall can be caused by processes in the chest wall itself or by extensions of intrathoracic problems that arise in the pleura or the underlying lung. In many instances the pyogenic infections may be due to trauma or to a surgical procedure. The diagnosis of early pyogenic infections can be difficult because it is usually 1 to 2 weeks after the onset of symptoms before the characteristic bony changes may be apparent on standard radiographs (Resnick and Niwayama, 1981). The characteristic "moth-eaten" appearance of bones afflicted by osteomyelitis generally occurs after the infection is established and the bone has been thoroughly invaded. Early detection combines careful physical diagnostic procedures to denote the extent of tenderness in the chest wall, the extent of erythema present in the soft

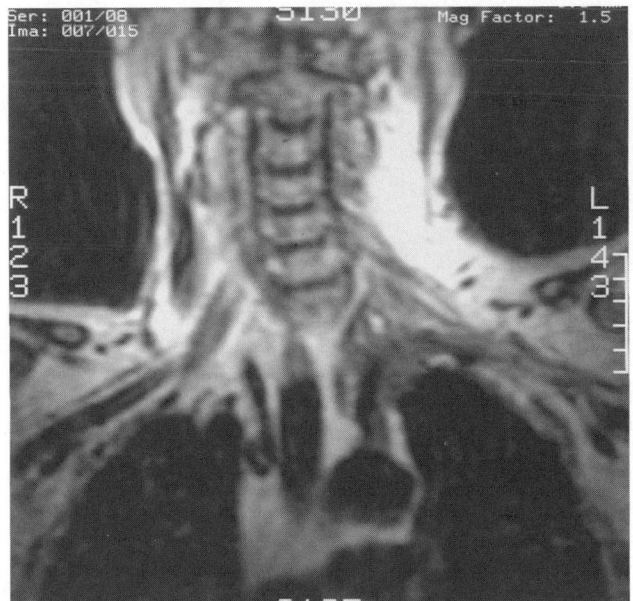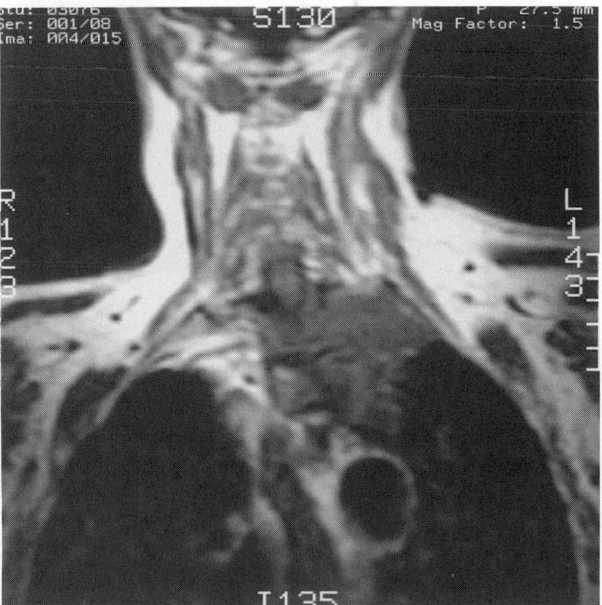

Figure 45-11. **(A)** MRI is most useful to define the structures involved by a superior sulcus tumor. This T_1-weighted coronal image through the lower neck and upper thorax demonstrates a mass at the left lung apex with superior sulcus involvement and encasement of the left subclavian artery. **(B)** This T_1-weighted image demonstrates the mass with involvement of the spinal cord and extension into the region of the brachial plexus.

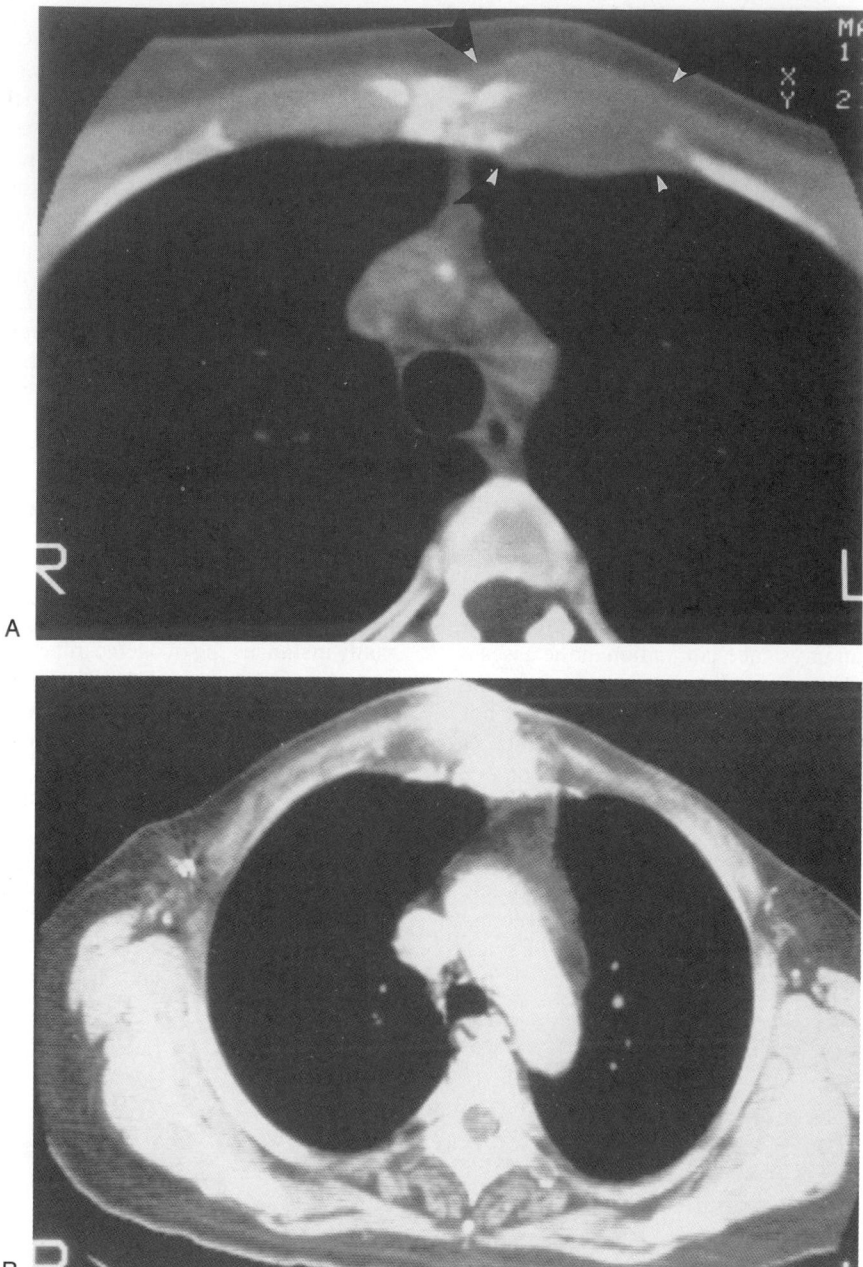

Figure 45-12. **(A)** This axial CT image demonstrates asymmetry of the sternocostochondral junction. There is an apparent soft tissue mass on the left side, which is delineated by arrows. A biopsy conducted subsequently revealed a clinically unsuspected residual carcinoma of the breast. **(B)** This axial CT image taken after bilateral mastectomies demonstrates the presence of a soft tissue mass in the right peristernal region. In this patient, biopsy yielded the diagnosis of recurrent adenocarcinoma of the breast. (From Schaefer PS, Burton BS: Radiographic evaluation of chest wall lesions. Surg Clin North Am 69:911, 1989, with permission.)

tissues, and any evidence of tissue edema. These physical findings, when associated with bone scans, usually allow the clinician to estimate the extent of disease. In fact, radionuclide bone scanning may be particularly helpful when it is combined with a standard ^{99m}T-MPD bone scan with an ^{111}In-labeled leukocyte or ^{67}Ga scan (Schaefer and Burton, 1989). The combination of these modalities may be diagnostic of

osteomyelitis several days or weeks before any conventional or radiographic changes appear on standard radiographs.

CT scan has been particularly helpful to delineate infections of the chest wall because its actual axial projections are extremely sensitive to the changes associated with osteomyelitis. It is particularly effective to localize the infection, identify the limits of the soft tissue process that surrounds

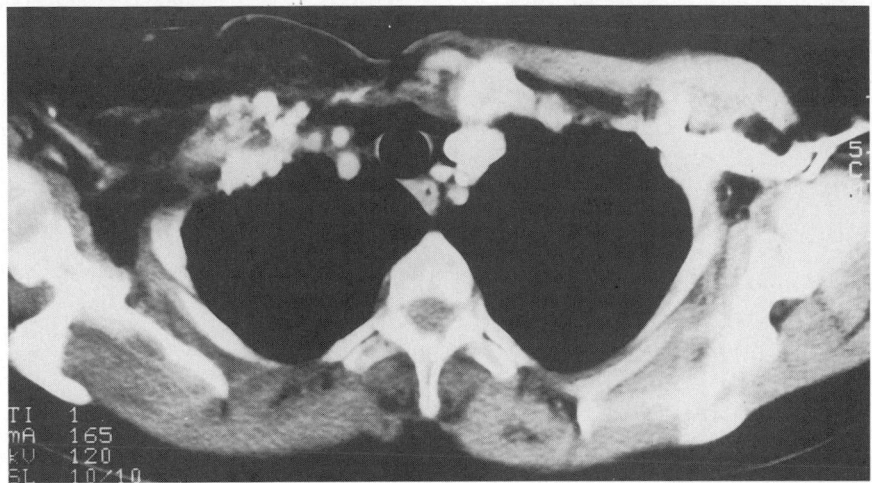

Figure 45-13. This 58-year-old woman had had a mastectomy for carcinoma of the right breast 4 years prior to this examination. She had had a reconstruction of the chest wall with an ipsilateral latissimus dorsi flap and had received substantial radiotherapy to the chest wall. Images taken of the chest wall revealed a lytic lesion in the right clavicle, suggestive of recurrent breast carcinoma. A major operative procedure to resect a portion of the chest wall and perform a secondary reconstruction was contemplated. Fortunately, the excisional biopsy of the lytic area revealed radiation necrosis of the clavicle. There was no evidence of recurrent breast carcinoma. Although radiation-induced chondrosarcomas do occur in heavily radiated bones, there was no evidence of such a sarcoma in this patient.

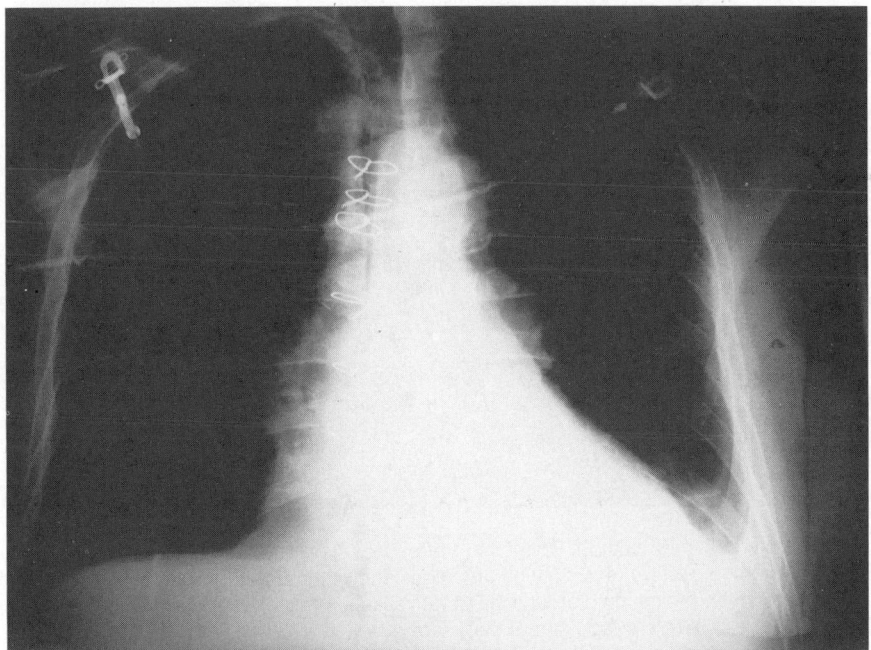

Figure 45-14. This upright portable chest radiograph of a patient 9 days after a myocardial revascularization through a median sternotomy shows an air stripe between the two halves of the sternum. Note also that the sternal wires have either broken or pulled through. The air was introduced in between the two halves of the sternum when fluid drained from the inferior portion of the incision. The patient subsequently underwent rewiring and had aggressive therapy with both topical and systemic antibiotics. The wound healed successfully.

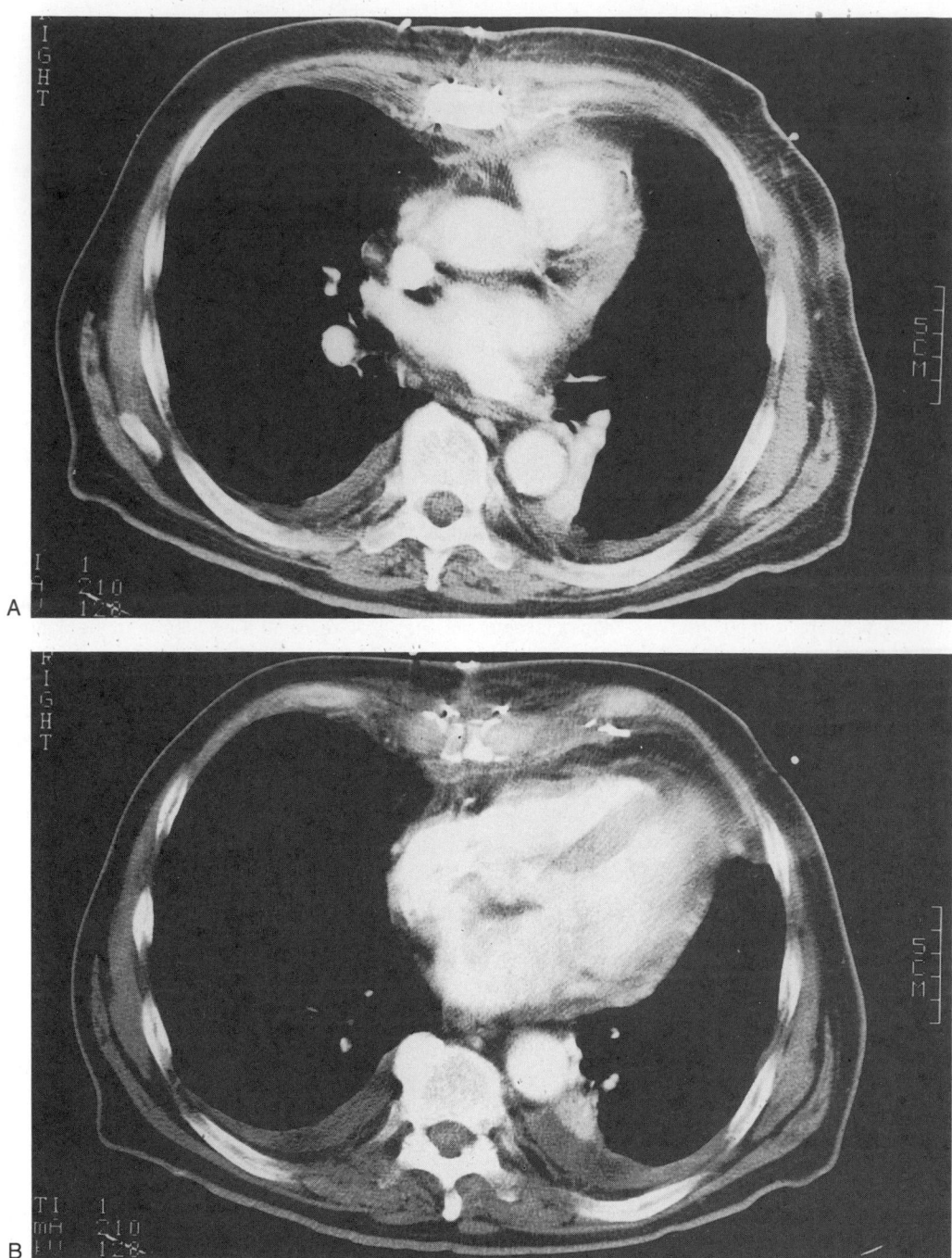

Figure 45-15. These are selected axial CT images of the patient shown in Figure 45-14. These images were taken just prior to the wound draining. Careful examination of images shows air around the healing sternum. **(A)** This image shows air around the sternum and some fluid around the great vessels within the pericardial sack. Note that the sternum has an irregular appearance. **(B)** This image shows that there is air around the sternum and malalignment of the two sternal halves. Fluid is also apparent within the pericardial cavity directly behind the sternum.

the osteomyelitis, and allow a direct guide for drainage (Schaefer and Burton, 1989). The characteristic findings of infection include a bone that has an adjacent soft tissue mass of recent onset, loss of deep soft tissue planes that are normally present, and periosteal elevation on the afflicted bone. These findings are particularly important when they are correlated with the clinical findings.

The most common cause of pyogenic infection of the chest wall at the current time is the dehisced median sternotomy. Plain radiographs may be particularly helpful to suggest this problem because air may be readily apparent between the two halves of the sternum early in a sternal dehiscence. This characteristic dark stripe between the two halves of the sternum suggests not only the nonunion of bone but also reflects

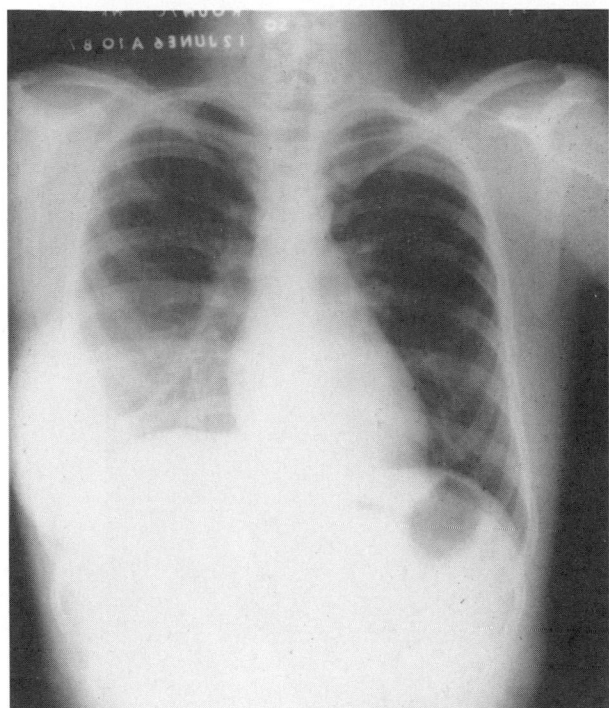

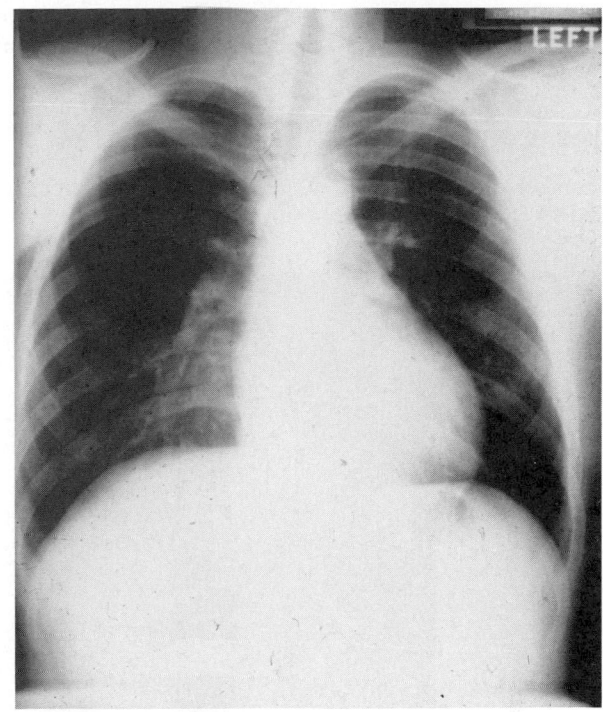

Figure 45-16. **(A)** This shows a posteroanterior radiograph of a young man with Poland syndrome. Note that the ends of ribs 2, 3, and 4 on the right side are either hypoplastic or absent. The corresponding costal cartilages were absent. The pectoralis major and minor and soft tissues in the region were also absent. The absence of these structures caused the hyperlucency seen over the apex of the right lung field. **(B)** Although Poland syndrome occurs more often on the right, this 16-year-old woman presented with a left-sided Poland's syndrome. Note that she has absence of the left breast along with hypoplasia or absence of the anterior segments of ribs 2, 3, and 4. The corresponding pectoralis major and minor were nonexistent. The absence of the normal tissues over the left hemithorax causes the relative hyperlucency of the left lung.

the air that is between the separated sternal halves (Fig. 45-14). In such instances the CT scan may be particularly helpful to show where air is present within the mediastinum, what fluid pockets are present, and where a clot is present. The CT scan is also particularly helpful to follow the progression of therapy because subsequent images will delineate loculated pockets within the pericardium or the mediastinum (Fig. 45-15).

CHEST WALL TUBERCULOSIS

The radiographic picture of chest wall involvement by tuberculosis may vary, just as does the radiographic appearance of this disease when it afflicts soft tissues (Schaefer and Barton, 1989). Tuberculosis may cause lytic lesions of chest wall structures, such as a rib and the sternum. Interestingly, tuberculosis is the most common inflammatory disease to afflict the ribs, and it is second only to metastatic cancer (including myeloma) as a cause of true destruction of ribs (Tatelman and Drouillard, 1953). Tuberculous infection of the sternum and ribs commonly results in sharply demarcated areas of destruction, which may at times have an expansile, cystic appearance (Schaefer and Burton, 1989). Multicystic lesions can occur; sclerotic margins may also be apparent. Although associated soft tissue masses are relatively com-

mon, pathologic fractures are rare (Feigin and Madewell, 1981). The formation of sinus tracts and chest wall abscesses can be demonstrated in approximately 25 percent of patients who present with chest wall involvement (Sinoff and Segal, 1975).

Tuberculosis may afflict the chest wall by extension of infection from an adjacent lung or pleura. More commonly the disease may seed a rib hematogenously without evidence of active pulmonary disease (Schaefer and Burton, 1989). No matter the method of infection, chest wall tuberculosis should be suspected in patients prone to this disease. Today such infection should arouse suspicion of an immunocompromised patient. Appropriate precautions and thorough diagnostic evaluation should be undertaken in such patients.

CT has particular efficacy in the evaluation of the lesions associated with tuberculosis of the chest wall. In one published series based on four patients who were not immunocompromised, the authors concluded that chest wall tuberculosis could result in bone or costal cartilage destruction and soft tissue masses, which have peripheral calcification and rim enhancement with or without evidence of underlying lung or pleural disease (Adler, et al., 1993). In their series, two patients had rib involvement, and one had costal cartilage disease. In the fourth, the sternoclavicular joint was involved. CT demonstrated osseous and cartilaginous destruction in all four, soft tissue masses with calcification in two, and rib enhancement after intravenous contrast administration in two.

FUNGAL INFECTIONS OF THE CHEST WALL

A number of fungal infections may occasionally afflict the chest wall. These include blastomycosis, candidiasis, coccid-

ioidomycosis, cryptococcosis, and nocardiosis (Smilack and Gentry, 1976). Actinomycosis, which usually arises from infected underlying lung and pleura, is more common. It has a well-recognized indolent course, which may result in chest wall fistulae. Imaging techniques are important to define the extent of chest wall disease and direct aspirations and biopsies to document the presence of fungal infection. CT scans and chest radiographs are useful to follow the extent of dis-

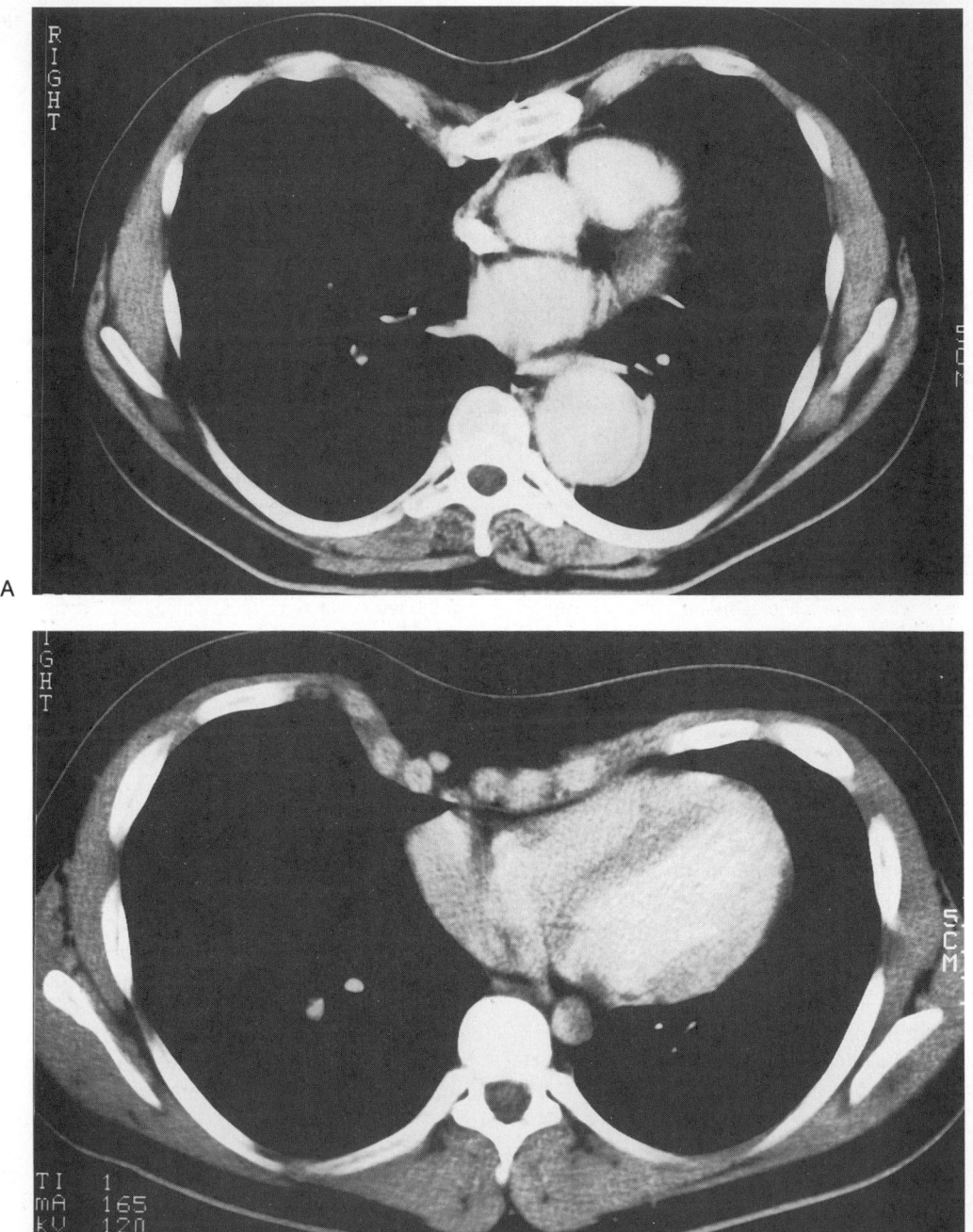

Figure 14-17. **(A)** This axial CT image of an 18-year-old man shows a marked pectus deformity and its relationship to the cardiac silhouette. The patient had no symptoms at the time of the examination but had elected to refrain from vigorous activity because of Marfan syndrome. **(B)** This axial CT image shows a persistent pectus in a 46-year-old man with Marfan syndrome and a repaired ascending aorta. Two years postascending aortic repair, the patient presented with an acute, type I dissection.

ease and its response to treatment (Snape, 1993). A recent study of three patients with Aspergillus chest wall involvement in chronic granulomatous disease suggests that CT and MRI may be complementary and allow progressive assessment of the process as it responds to therapy (Kawashima, et al., 1991).

CONGENITAL ABNORMALITIES OF THE CHEST WALL

In many instances conventional radiographs document the presence of congenital chest wall disease (Schaefer and Burton, 1989). Abnormalities, such as the absence, hypoplasia, or fusion of ribs; cervical ribs; and ankylosed vertebral bodies, are well delineated on standard plain radiographs. The abnormalities generally associated with Poland syndrome are apparent on plain films (Fig. 45-16). In some instances, CT and MRI may be particularly helpful to identify skeletal abnormalities and their relationship to underlying viscera. Compression of the heart may be apparent on axial CT images and may suggest embarrassment of diastolic filling (Fig. 45-17). CT and MRI may also be helpful to assess visceral conditions that may be associated with chest wall abnormalities (Fig. 45-17). An example of this is Marfan syndrome where the major arteries of the body may be followed by axial imaging in conjunction with chest wall abnormalities.

KEY REFERENCES

Kuhlman JE, Bouchardy L, Fishman EK, Zerhouni EA: CT and MR imaging evaluation of chest wall disorders. Radiographics 14:571, 1994

This article discusses the positive and negative aspects of both CT and MR imaging in a number of chest wall disorders. The article is richly illustrated with excellent radiographic material. The authors offer guidelines for detecting different types of suspected chest wall pathologic processes.

Schaefer PS, Burton BS: Radiographic evaluation of chest-wall lesions. Surg Clin North Am 69:911, 1989

This chapter presents a thorough discussion of the different imaging techniques as they are used to evaluate chest wall pathologic conditions. There are a number of illustrations that demonstrate the major points the authors make. The list of references cited is thorough.

Webb WR, Gatsonis C, Zerhouni EA et al: CT and MR imaging in staging non-small cell bronchogenic carcinoma: report of the Radiologic Diagnostic Oncology Group. Radiology 178:705, 1991

This report gives a thorough evaluation of the use of CT and MRI in staging non-small cell bronchogenic carcinoma. It gives good guidelines as to the capabilities and drawbacks of both CT and MRI in the evaluation of non-small cell bronchogenic carcinoma.

REFERENCES

Adler BD, Padley SPG, Miller NL: Tuberculosis of the chest wall: CT findings. J Comput Assist Tomogr 17:271, 1993

Donegan WL: Cancer of the breast: local and regional recurrence. Major Probl Clin Surg 5:484, 1979

Edelstein G, Levitt RG, Slaker DP et al: CT observation of rib abnormalities: spectrum of findings. J Comput Assist Tomogr 9:65, 1989

Enzinger FM, Weiss SW: Soft Tissue Tumors. CV Mosby, St. Louis, 1983

Feigin DS, Madewell JE: Disorders of the chest wall. p. 1323. In Teplick JG, Haskin ME (eds): Surgical Radiology. WB Saunders, Philadelphia, 1981

Felson B: Chest Roentgenology. WB Saunders, Philadelphia, 1973

Franken EA, Smith JA, Smith WL: Tumors of the chest wall in infants and children. Pediatr Radiol 6:13, 1977

Gamsu G: Magnetic resonance imaging in lung cancer. Chest 89:242S, 1986

Glaser HS, Duncan-Meyer J, Aronberg DJ et al: Pleural and chest wall invasion in bronchogenic carcinoma. Radiology 157:191, 1985

Goodwin JD: Computed Tomography of the Chest. JB Lippincott, Philadelphia, 1984

Graeber GM, Snyder RJ, Flemming AW et al: Initial and long-term results in the management of primary chest wall neoplasms. Ann Thorac Surg 34:664, 1982

Haggar AM, Pearlburg JL, Froelich JW et al: Chest wall invasion by carcinoma of the lung: detection by MR imaging. AJR 148:1075, 1987

Kawashima A, Kuhlman JE, Fishman EK et al: Pulmonary Aspergillus chest wall involvement in chronic granulomatous disease: CT and MRI findings. Skeletal Radiol 20:487, 1991

Larsson SE, Lorentzon R: The incidence of malignant primary bone tumors in relation to age, sex, and site. J Bone Joint Surg [Br] 56:534, 1974

Lindfors KK, Meyer JE, Busse PM et al: CT evaluation of local and regional breast cancer recurrence. AJR 145:833, 1985

Libshitz HI: Computed tomography in bronchogenic carcinoma. Semin Roentgenol 25:64, 1990

Marcove RC: Cartilaginous tumors of the ribs. Cancer 27:794, 1971

McCloud TC, Filion RB, Edelman RR, Shepard JA: MR imaging of superior sulcus carcinoma. J Comput Assist Tomogr 13:233, 1989

Miller JD, Gorenstein LA, Patterson GA: Staging: the key to rational management of lung cancer. Ann Thorac Surg 53:170, 1992

Murata K, Takahashi M, Mori M et al: Chest wall and mediastinal invasion by lung cancer: evaluation with multisection expiratory dynamic CT. Radiology 191:251, 1994

Musset D, Grenier P, Carette MF et al: Primary lung cancer staging: prospective comparative study of MR imaging with CT. Radiology 160:607, 1986

Omell GH, Anderson LS, Bramson RT: Chest wall tumors. Radiol Clin North Am 11:197, 1973

Pearlberg JL, Sandler MA, Beute GM et al: Limitations of CT in evaluation of neoplasm involving the chest wall. J Comput Assist Tomogr 11:29, 1987

Resnick DM, Niwayama G (eds): Diagnosis of Bone and Joint Disorders. WB Saunders, Philadelphia, 1981

Ryan MB, McMurtrey MJ, Roth JA: Current management of chest-wall tumors. Surg Clin North Am 69:1061, 1989

Shea WJ, deGneer G, Webb WR: Chest wall after mastectomy. Radiology 162:162, 1987.

Sinoff CL, Segal I: Tuberculous osteomyelitis of the rib. S Afr Med J 49:685, 1975

Smilack JD, Gentry LO: Candida costochondral osteomyelitis. J Bone Joint Surg Am 58:888, 1976

Snape PS: Thoracic Actinomyces: an unusual childhood infection. South Med J 86:222, 1993

Stout AP, Lattes R: Tumors of the soft tissue. p. 17. In Atlas of Tumor Pathology. Series 2. Fascicle 1. Armed Forces Institute of Pathology, Washington, D.C., 1967

Suzuki N, Saitoh T, Kitamura S: Tumor invasion of the chest wall in lung cancer: diagnosis with ultrasound (US). Radiology 187:39, 1993

Tatelman M, Drouillard JP: Tuberculosis of the rib. AJR 70:923, 1953

Teitelbaum S: Twenty years' experience with intrinsic tumors of the bony thorax at a large institution. J Thorac Cardiovasc Surg 63:776, 1972

Templeton PA, Caskey CI, Zerhouni EA: Current uses of CT and MR imaging in staging of lung cancer. Radiol Clin North Am 28:631, 1990

Threlkel JB, Adkins PB: Primary chest wall tumors. Ann Thorac Surg 11:450, 1971

Villari, Fargnoli R, Mungai R: CT evaluation of chest wall recurrence in breast cancer. Eur J Radiol 5:206, 1985

Watanabe A, Shimokata K, Salsa H et al: Chest CT combined with artificial pneumothorax: value in determining origin and extent of tumor. AJR 156:707, 1991

Yokoi K, Mori K, Miyazawa N et al: Tumor invasion of the chest wall and mediastinum in lung cancer: evaluation with pneumothorax CT. Radiology 181:147, 1991

46

CONGENITAL DEFORMITIES

Robert C. Shamberger
W. Hardy Hendren III

PECTUS EXCAVATUM

DEFINITION

Congenital anterior thoracic deformities can be divided into four groups: (1) pectus excavatum, (2) pectus carinatum, (3) Poland syndrome, and (4) sternal clefts and defects, including ectopia cordis. Pectus excavatum (often termed *funnel chest* in English or *Trichterbrust* in German) presents as a depression of the sternum and the lower costal cartilages. The first and second ribs and their costal cartilages as well as the manubrium are usually normal (Fig. 46-1). The extent of sternal and cartilaginous deformity is quite variable. Numerous methods of grading and defining these deformities have been proposed, but none has been universally accepted. Asymmetry is frequently present but may be unappreciated until the time of surgical correction. The right side is often more depressed than the left, with corresponding rotation of the sternum.

HISTORICAL NOTE

Surgical repair of this deformity was first achieved by Meyer and Sauerbruch in 1911 and 1913, respectively. Significant changes in the method of repair have evolved as experience has increased, and the primary components of the deformity have been identified. Ochsner and DeBakey summarized early experience with repair in 1939. Ravitch in 1949 reported a technique that involved excision of all deformed costal cartilages with the perichondrium, division of the xiphoid from the sternum, division of the intercostal bundles from the sternum, and transverse sternal osteotomy, displacing the sternum anteriorly with Kirschner wires in the first two patients and silk sutures in later patients. In 1958 Welch reported a technique for the satisfactory and safe correction of pectus excavatum that emphasized total preservation of the perichondrial sheaths of the costal cartilage, preservation of the upper intercostal bundles, and sternal osteotomy. The technique we use today remains essentially unchanged, more than 700 cases later.

HISTORICAL READINGS

Meyer L: Zur chirurgischen Behandlung der angeborenen Trichterbrust. Verh Berl Med Ges 42:364, 1911

Ochsner A, DeBakey M: Chone-chondrosternon: report of a case and review of the literature. J Thorac Surg 8:469, 1939

Ravitch MM: The operative treatment of pectus excavatum. Ann Surg 129:429, 1949

Sauerbruch F: Die Chirurgie der Brustorgane. J. Springer, Berlin, 1920

Welch KJ: Satisfactory surgical correction of pectus excavatum deformity in childhood: a limited opportunity. J Thorac Surg 36: 697, 1958

BASIC SCIENCE

Etiology

Pectus excavatum may be as common as 1 in 300 to 400 live births (Ravitch, 1977). It is usually noted at birth or within the first year of life in 86 percent of cases and appears in adolescence in less than 5 percent of cases (Shamberger and Welch, 1988a). Transient deformity with vigorous breathing or crying is common in infants. For this reason correction of pectus excavatum should never be performed before 2 years of age. Family history of some form of anterior thoracic deformity is present in 37 percent of patients. Scoliosis has been identified in 26 percent of recent patients with pectus excavatum or carinatum, and in 11 percent of these patients there is a family history of scoliosis.

Patients with Marfan syndrome have a high incidence of severe chest wall deformities, usually accompanied by scoliosis (Fig. 46-2). Patients with abdominal musculature deficiency syndrome (prune belly syndrome) commonly have pectus excavatum; this was the case with 8 of 43 patients in the series of Welch and Kearney (1974).

The etiology of pectus excavatum is unknown. Early investigators (Lester, 1957) attributed its development to an abnormality of the diaphragm, but there has been little evidence to support this theory except for the reported occurrence of

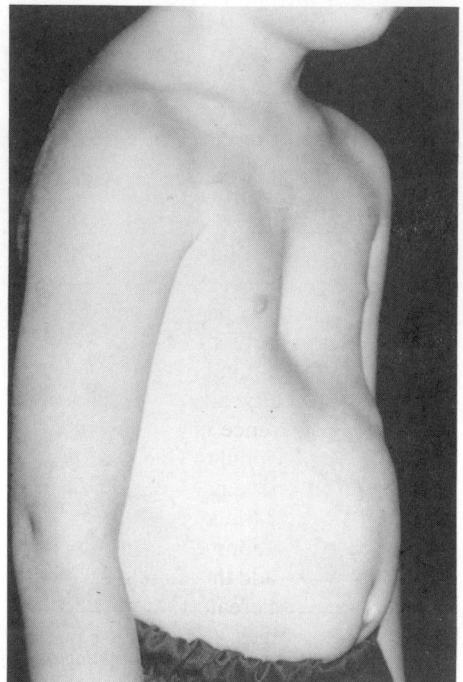 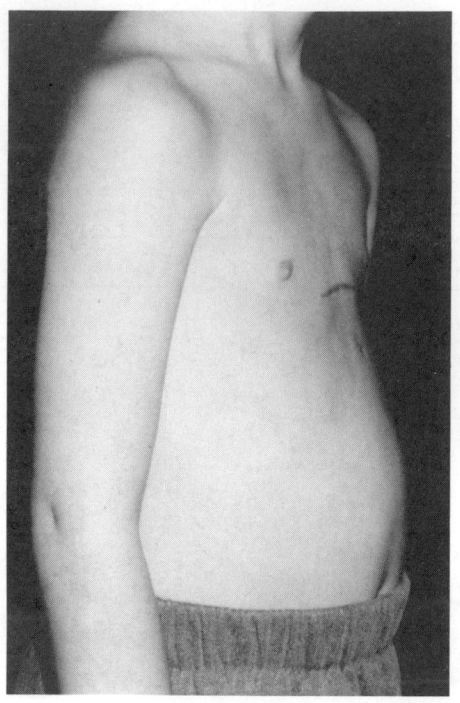

Figure 46-1. **(A)** Preoperative photograph of a 10-year-old boy with a symmetric pectus excavatum deformity. **(B)** The excellent postoperative result is seen.

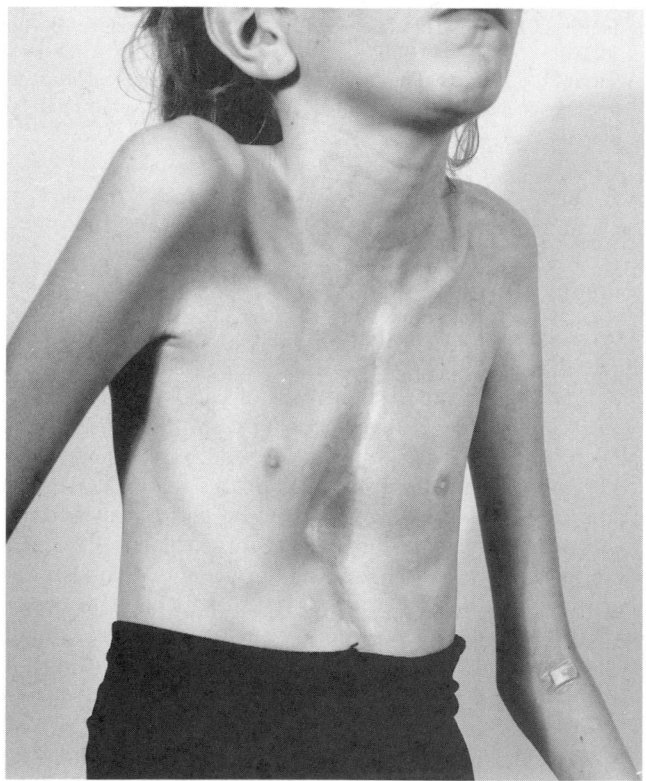

Figure 46-2. An 8-year-old girl with Marfan syndrome. She demonstrated all the characteristic findings of Marfan syndrome, namely extreme laxity of the joints, posterior dislocation of her optic lenses, and cardiac valvular disease. She required mitral valve repair in infancy. Severe excavatum deformity is noted, as well as her prior sternotomy scar.

pectus excavatum in patients with congenital diaphragmatic hernia (Greig and Azmy, 1990).

Pectus excavatum is well tolerated in infancy. Older children may complain of pain in the area of the deformed cartilages or of precordial pain after sustained exercise. A few patients have palpitations or syncope, presumably due to transient atrial arrhythmias. These patients may have mitral valve prolapse, which is associated with atrial arrhythmias and has been identified in patients with pectus excavatum (Shamberger, et al., 1987a).

Pathophysiology

Some authors have stated that no cardiovascular or pulmonary impairment results from pectus excavatum deformity (Haller, et al., 1970). This opinion contrasts, however, with the general clinical impression that many patients have increased stamina following surgical repair. A recent review has summarized clinical studies of these patients (Shamberger and Welch, 1988b).

The symptomatic improvement in patients following surgery for pectus excavatum has been attributed to initial impairment in pulmonary function. Abnormalities in pulmonary function are difficult to demonstrate, however, in view of the wide range of "normal" pulmonary function parameters, which are heavily dependent on physical training and body habitus. Seven patients with pectus excavatum, 4 of whom were symptomatic with exercise, were evaluated in one study by Castile and associates (1982). The mean total lung capacity in the excavatum patients was 79 percent of predicted. The measured oxygen uptake increasingly exceeded predicted values as the work loads approached maximum. This pattern of oxygen uptake differed from that of normal subjects, who had a linear response. The mean oxygen uptake at maximal effort exceeded the predicted values by 25.4 percent in the symptomatic patients. The 3 asymptomatic patients on the other hand demonstrated a normal pattern of linear increase in oxygen uptake during progressive exercise. This increased oxygen uptake in the symptomatic patients suggests that their increased work of breathing was increased, although their vital capacities were only mildly reduced or normal. Cahill, et al. (1984) studied 14 patients with pectus excavatum; maximal voluntary ventilation was significantly improved after repair in all. Exercise tolerance was also improved, as measured by total exercise time and maximal oxygen uptake. Furthermore, there was a consistent decrease in heart rate at a given power output postoperatively, with no change in oxygen consumption. In another report by Blickman and colleagues (1985), xenon 133 perfusion and ventilation scintigraphy were used to study 17 patients. Of 12 patients with regional ventilatory deficits, primarily in the left lower lung, 7 had normal ventilation scans after surgery. Of 10 patients with decreased regional perfusion abnormalities, also primarily in the left lower lung, 6 had normal perfusion scans after surgery. Abnormal ventilation/perfusion ratios became normal in 6 of 10 patients following surgery.

Beiser, et al. (1972) performed cardiac catheterization in 6 patients with moderate degrees of pectus excavatum. Normal pressures were obtained at rest in the supine position. The cardiac index was normal at rest in the supine position, and the response to moderate exercise was within the normal range. The response to upright exercise was below the predicted normal in 2 patients and at the lower limit of normal in 3. Postoperative studies were performed in 3 patients, two of whom achieved a higher level of exercise tolerance following surgery. The cardiac index was increased by 38 percent; the heart rates were unchanged, and the increase resulted from an enhanced stroke volume following surgery.

Peterson, et al. (1985) used first-pass radionuclide angiocardiography to evaluate 13 patients who were upright, both at rest and during bicycle exercise. Although no changes were seen at rest or during exercise in left ventricular ejection fraction or cardiac output, substantial increases were observed in both right and left ventricular volumes postoperatively, which suggests relief of cardiac compression by displacement of the sternum anteriorly. Workload studies were also performed on these patients. Of the 13, 10 were able to reach the target heart rate before surgical repair, 4 without symptoms. After operation all but one patient reached the target heart rate during the exercise protocol, and 9 of 13 reached the target without becoming symptomatic.

SURGICAL REPAIR

In 1958 Welch reported a technique that achieved safe and satisfactory correction of pectus excavatum. He emphasized total preservation of the perichondrial sheaths of the costal cartilage, preservation of the upper intercostal bundles, and anterior fixation of the sternum with silk sutures. This technique has been used at The Children's Hospital in Boston for more than 700 cases in the past three decades. Others (Rehbein and Wernicke, 1957; Adkins and Blades, 1961) have used internal fixation with Kirschner wires or metallic struts,

but no conclusive evidence has been presented to prove that such methods provide better long-term results than those achieved without metal fixation. Willital (1981) reported 92 percent satisfactory results using struts in a large series of 1,112 patients, whereas Hecker, et al. (1981) reported 91 percent satisfactory results in 392 patients using a modification of the Ravitch procedure without struts. Oelsnitz (1981) and Hecker, et al. (1981) reached the same conclusion, namely that internal fixation did not provide a major benefit in their large series, in which satisfactory repairs were achieved in 90 to 95 percent of patients. Nevertheless, one of us (W.H.H.) prefers to use the struts devised by Rehbein to hold the sternum in an anterior position in the belief that it provides stability and greater patient comfort and less chance for recurrence of sternal depression. The struts are removed in the ambulatory operating room 6 to 12 months after repair. We have not seen problems from Rehbein struts placed anterior to the sternum.

Two other variations of repair deserve mention. Haller and associates (1976) add three-point "tripod" fixation by placing an osteotomy and creating oblique chondrotomies of the upper costal cartilages. The medial posterior portion of the costal cartilage will then be anterior to the lateral portion of the cartilages and help support the sternum anteriorly.

Judet and Judet (1956) and Jung, et al. (1964) proposed in the French literature a "sternal turnover" technique. It has been used primarily in Japan by Wada, et al. (1970), who reported a large series. This technique uses a "free graft" of sternum, which is rotated 180 degrees and secured back to the costal cartilages. This method appears radical for children with pectus excavatum in view of the major complications if infection occurs and the generally successful alternatives.

Our operative technique is illustrated in Fig. 46-3. In females particular attention is taken to place the incision within the inframammary fold, thus avoiding the complications of breast deformity and abnormal development. Skin flaps are mobilized primarily in the midline to the angle of Louis superiorly and to the xiphoid inferiorly. Use of Bovie electrocautery minimizes blood loss. Starting medially, the chest wall muscles are detached and retracted to expose the depressed costal cartilages. The lateral extent of muscle elevation is the costochondral junction of the third to fifth ribs and rarely the second. Particular attention is taken to avoid injury to the intercostal bundles, which can result in significant bleeding. Subperichondrial resection of the costal cartilages is performed with removal of the entire third, fourth, and fifth cartilages to the costochondral junctions. Longer (5- to 6-cm) segments of the sixth and seventh cartilages are resected to the point where they flatten to join the costal arch. There are often bridges joining the fifth and sixth costal cartilages lateral to the sternum.

Transverse osteotomy of the anterior table of the sternum is performed with the Hall drill (Zimmer USA, Inc., Warsaw, IN). This allows the lower sternum to be brought forward. The posterior table of the sternum is fractured behind the osteotomy, which must be of adequate size so that the sternum comes forward easily. The rectus muscles are detached from the lower sternum and xiphoid to allow blunt dissection behind the sternum. The xiphoid often projects forward and should be removed. The osteotomy is then closed with heavy silk sutures while holding the sternum forward in a deliberately overcorrected position. Alternatively, struts can be used to hold the sternum forward. Struts are especially helpful when there is extensive sternal rotation or a severe depression. Fixation with struts is also required in patients with Marfan syndrome or other corrective tissue disorders, with which risk of recurrence is higher (Scherer, et al., 1988). In some cases the lowest one or two sets of intercostal bundles (sixth and seventh) are divided from the sternum if required to bring it forward without excessive tension. We limit the

number of perichondrial bundles divided, however, to minimize an unsightly local depression just inferior to the tip of the sternum.

The technique described above provides for precise resection of costal cartilages with preservation of perichondrial sheaths, without injury to mediastinal structures, and usually without pleural or pericardial entry. If the pleura should be entered, the hole should be made large enough to prevent tension pneumothorax intraoperatively and the lungs ventilated with enough positive pressure to maintain inflation. Any

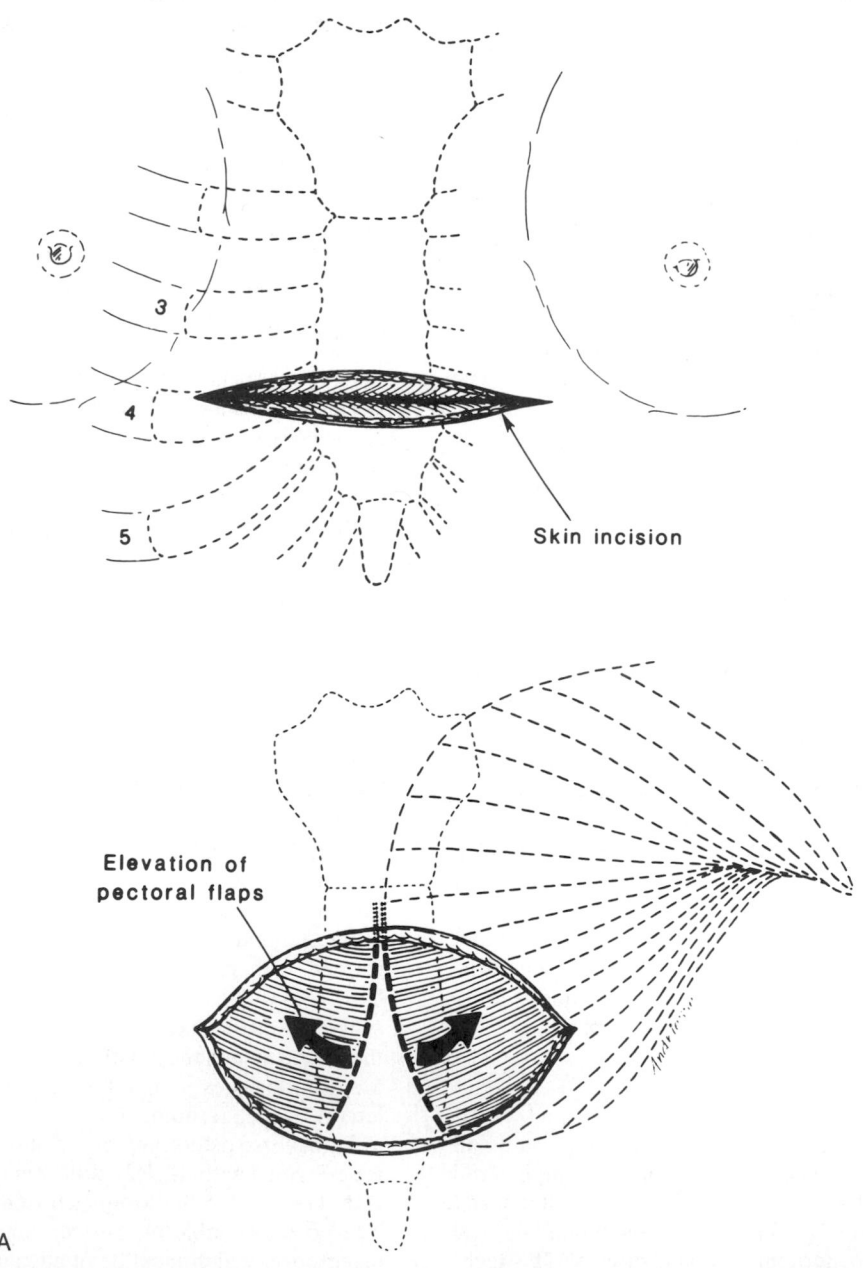

A

Figure 46-3. **(A)** A transverse incision is placed below and well within the nipples at the site of the future inframammary crease. The pectoralis major muscle is detached from the sternum along with portions of the pectoralis minor and serratus anterior muscles and retracted forward and laterally to expose the depressed costal cartilages (usually the third to seventh). (*Figure continues.*)

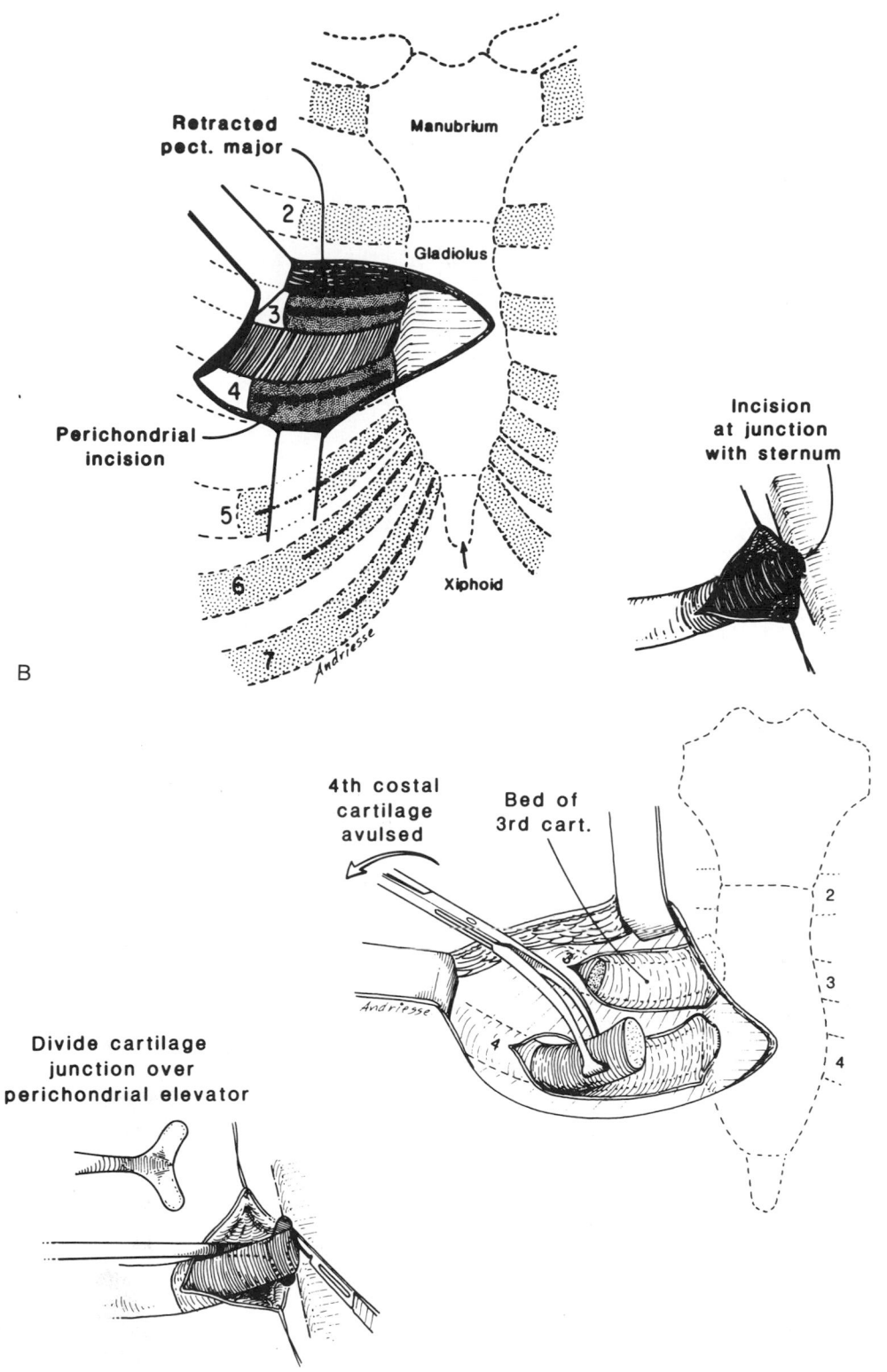

Figure 46-3 (*Continued*).   **(B)** Subperichondrial resection of the costal cartilages is achieved by incising the perichondrium anteriorly. It is then dissected from the costal cartilages in the bloodless plane between perichondrium and costal cartilage. Cutting the perichondrium 90 degrees in each direction at its junction with the sternum (*inset*) facilitates visualization of the back wall of the costal cartilage. **(C)** The cartilages are divided at the junction with the sternum with a Welch perichondrial elevator held posteriorly to elevate the cartilage and protect the mediastinum (*inset*). The divided cartilage can then be held with an Allis clamp, elevated, and avulsed at the costochondral junction. (*Figure continues.*)

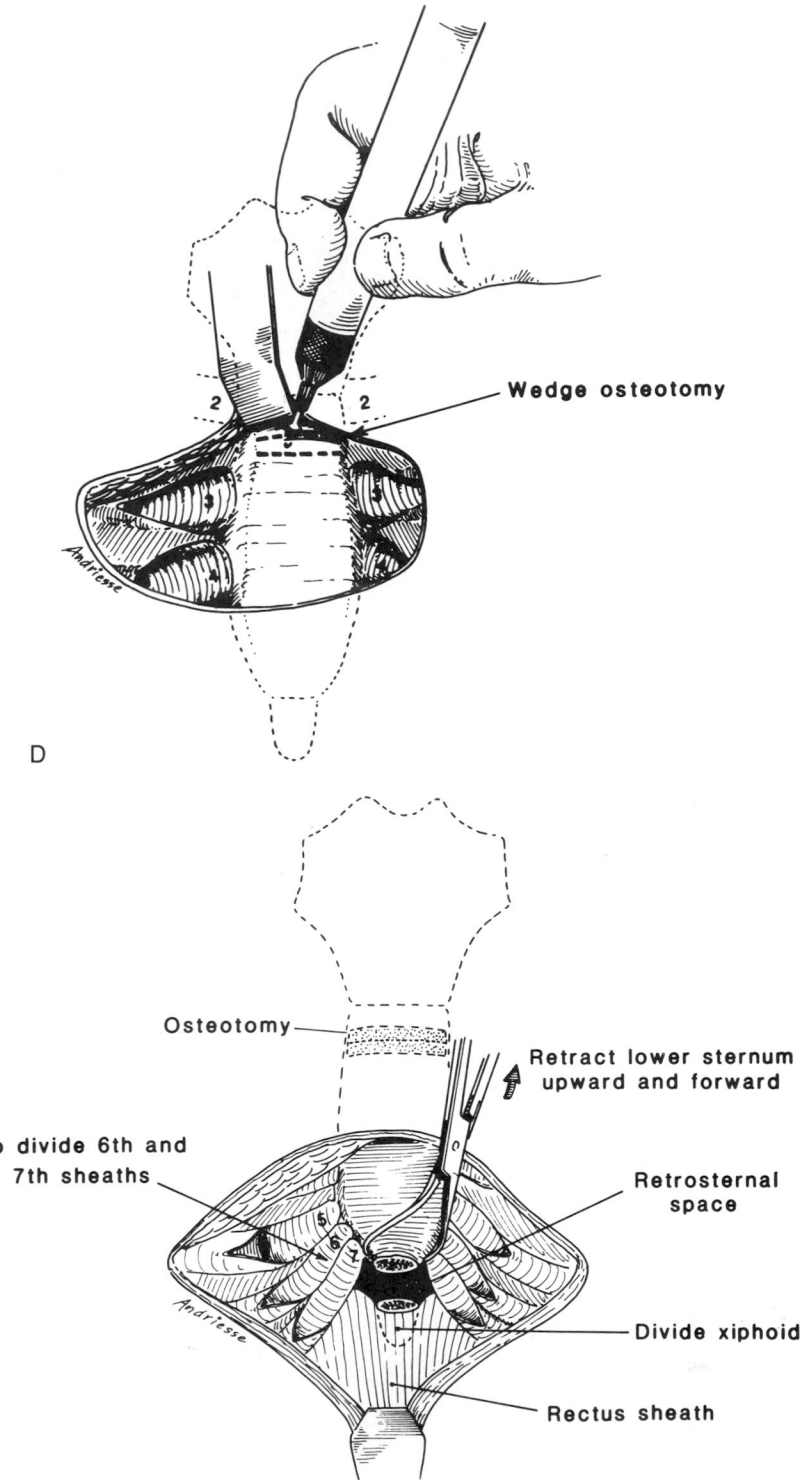

D

E

Figure 46-3 (*Continued*).   **(D)** The sternal osteotomy is created above the level of the last deformed cartilage and the posterior angulation of the sternum, generally the third cartilage but occasionally the second. Two transverse sternal osteotomies are created 2 to 4 mm apart through the anterior cortex with a Hall air drill. **(E)** The base of the sternum and the rectus muscle flap are elevated with two towel clips, and the xiphoid is divided from the sternum with electrocautery. This allows entry into the retrosternal space, and the sixth and seventh perichondrial sheaths can be divided under direct vision, avoiding pleural entry. (*Figure continues.*)

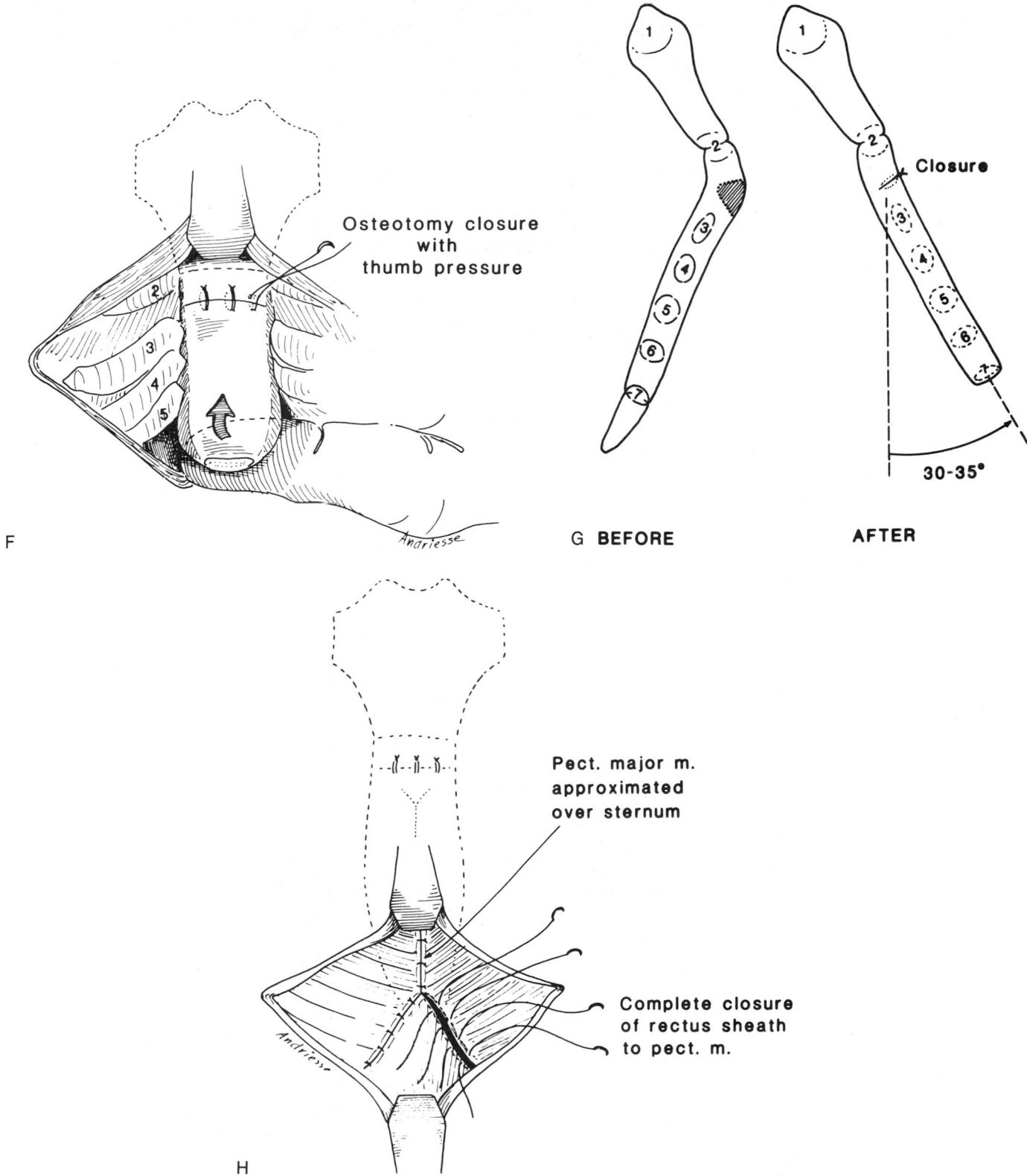

Osteotomy closure
with
thumb pressure

F

G BEFORE

Closure

30-35°

AFTER

Pect. major m.
approximated
over sternum

Complete closure
of rectus sheath
to pect. m.

H

Figure 46-3 (*Continued*).   **(F)** The osteotomy is closed with several heavy silk sutures as the sternum is being elevated with the assistant's thumb. **(G)** Correction of the abnormal position of the sternum is achieved by creation of a wedge-shaped osteotomy, which is then closed, bringing the sternum anteriorly into an overcorrected position. **(H)** The pectoral muscle flaps are secured to the midline of the sternum, while being advanced to provide coverage of the entire sternum. The rectus muscle flap is then joined to the pectoral muscle flaps. (*Figure continues.*)

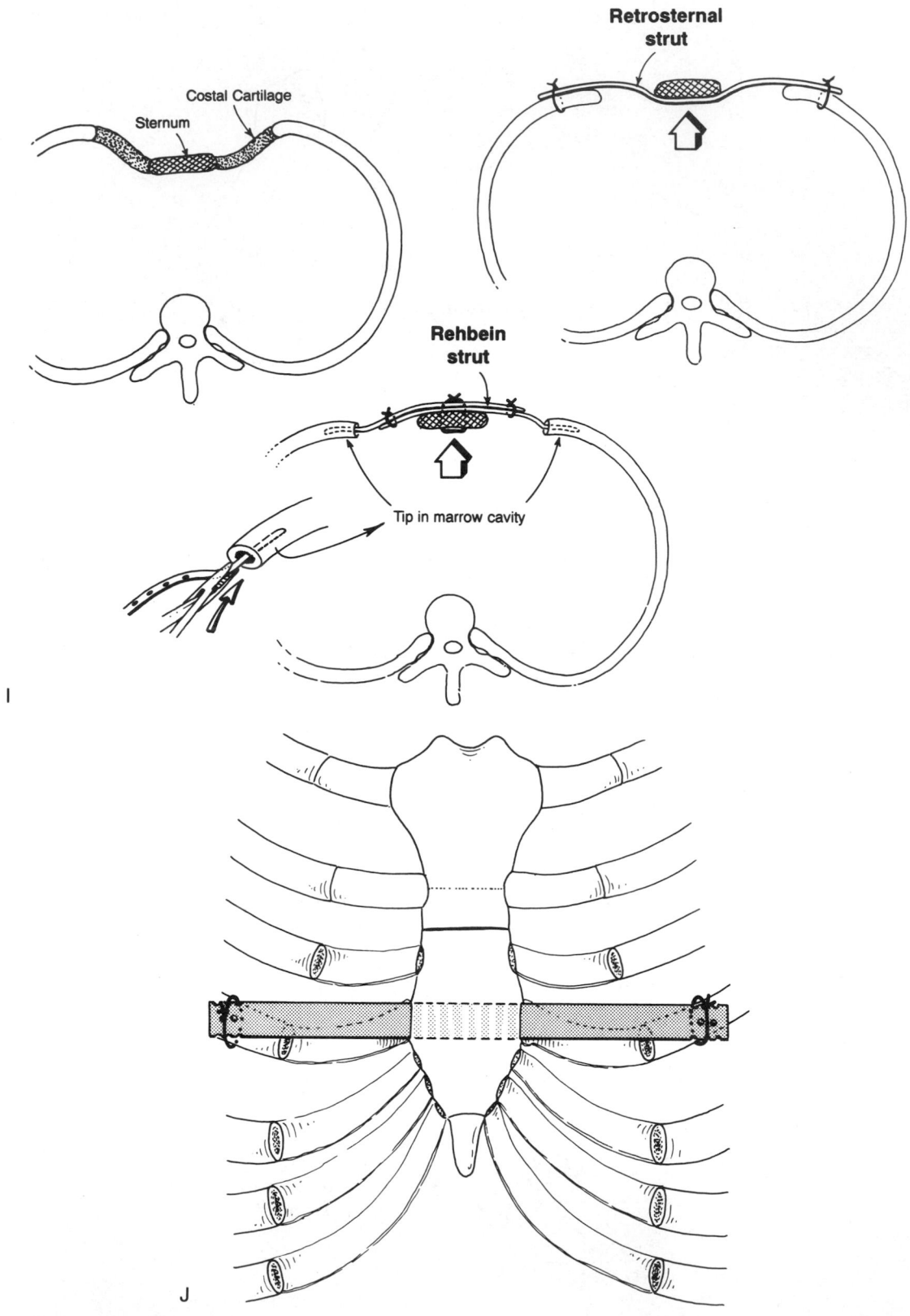

Figure 46-3 (*Continued*). **(I)** Demonstration of the use of both retrosternal struts and Rehbein struts. The Rehbein struts are inserted into the marrow cavity (insert) of the third or fourth ribs and are then joined to each other medially to create a metal arch anterior to the sternum. The sternum is sewn to the arch to secure it in its new forward position. The retrosternal strut is placed behind the sternum and is secured to the rib ends laterally to prevent migration. **(J)** Anterior depiction of the retrosternal struts (V. Mueller). The perichondrial sheath to either the third or fourth rib is divided from its junction with the sternum, and the retrosternal space is bluntly dissected to allow passage of the strut behind the sternum. It is secured with two pericostal sutures laterally to prevent migration. (Fig. H from Shamberger RC, Welch KJ: Surgical repair of pectus excavatum. J Pediatr Surg 23:615, 1988, with permission).

pleural air present is aspirated through a temporary catheter, which is withdrawn when the defect is covered by the pectoralis muscle closure. The wound is flooded with warm saline and cefazolin to remove clots. A single-limb medium Hemovac drain (Snyder Laboratories, Inc., New Philadelphia, OH) is brought through the inferior skin flap with the suction ports in a parasternal position to the level of the highest costal cartilage resection. The pectoralis muscle flaps are sutured to the sternum with advancement of the muscles medially and inferiorly to cover the underlying sternum with muscle. The rectus muscles are then reattached to the lower sternum medially and to the pectoralis muscles laterally. A postoperative chest radiograph is obtained in the recovery room. Perioperative antibiotics are administered, including one dose of cefozolin immediately prior to surgery and three postoperative doses. Blood loss is well below transfusion requirement in patients of all ages. A recent review of this technique in 704 patients at our institution disclosed no deaths and few complications (4.4 percent) (Shamberger and Welch, 1988a). Safe and effective repair is possible at any age.

Complications

Complications of pectus excavatum repair should be few and minor. In 2 percent of patients a limited pneumothorax required aspiration or was simply observed. Tube thoracostomy has not been required in the past decade and was needed by only four patients in our series. Wound infection was rare with the use of perioperative antibiotic coverage.

The most distressing complication following surgical correction of pectus excavatum is major recurrence of the deformity years after the original repair (17 of 704 patients). It is difficult to predict which unfortunate patients will have a major recurrence, but they often seem to have an asthenic or "marfanoid" habitus, with poor muscle development and a narrow anteroposterior chest wall diameter.

PECTUS CARINATUM

DEFINITION

Pectus carinatum is the most accepted term for anterior protrusion deformities of the chest wall. Protrusion deformities are much less frequent in our experience than the depression deformities (constituting 16.7 percent of the total group). The most frequent form of pectus carinatum consists of symmetric anterior displacement of the sternum with concavity of the costal cartilages laterally, a chondrogladiolar defect (Fig. 46-4). Asymmetric deformities with anterior displacement of the costal cartilages on one side, normal cartilages on the contralateral side, and a normally positioned or oblique sternum are much less common. "Mixed" lesions have a carinate deformity on one side and a depression or excavatum deformity on the contralateral side. The upper or chondromanubrial deformities, the so-called pouter pigeon deformities, are the most unusual, with protrusion of the manubrium and second and third costal cartilages and relative depression of the short body of the sternum (Fig. 46-5).

HISTORICAL NOTE

Surgical repair of carinate deformities has had a colorful history, starting with the first reported correction of the upper or chondromanubrial deformity by Ravitch in 1952. He re-

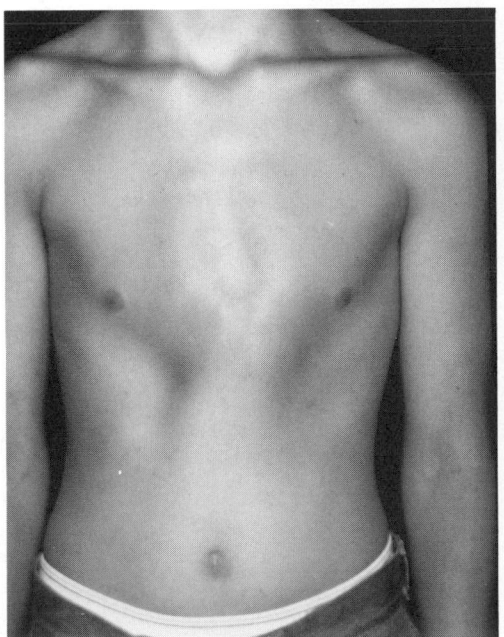 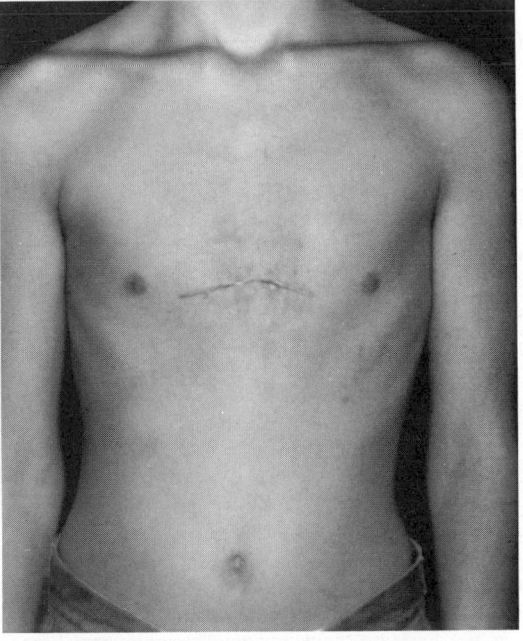

Figure 46-4. **(A)** Preoperative photograph of a patient with a symmetric pectus carinatum deformity, demonstrating symmetric anterior protrusion of the body of the sternum as well as of the costal cartilages. **(B)** The postoperative result shows marked improvement in the chest wall contour.

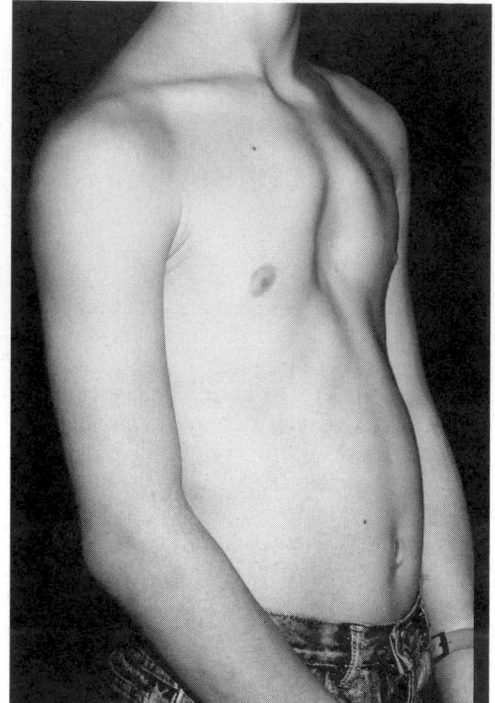 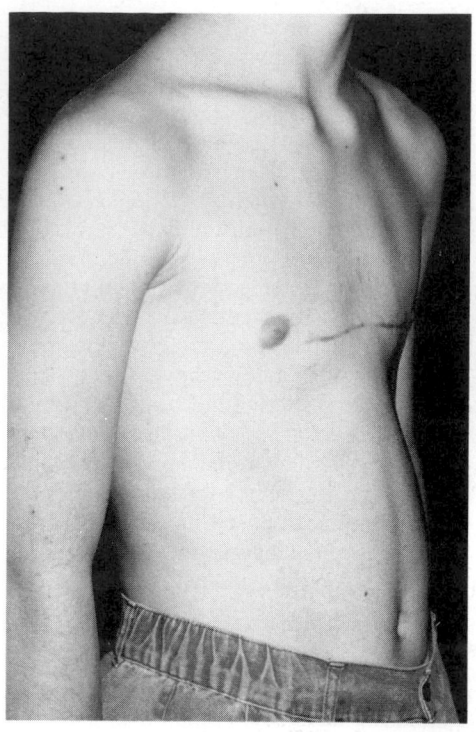

A   B

Figure 46-5. **(A)** Preoperative photograph of a patient with the upper form of pectus carinatum deformity, with marked anterior protrusion of the manubrium and second and third costal cartilages along with depression of the body of the sternum—the "pouter pigeon" deformity. **(B)** The postoperative result shows correction of both the depression and superior protrusion components of the deformity.

sected multiple costal cartilages and performed a double sternal osteotomy. In 1953, Lester reported two methods of repair for chondrogladiolar deformity. The first, involving resection of the anterior portion of the sternum, was abandoned because of excessive blood loss and unsatisfactory results. The second, although a no less radical technique, used subperiosteal resection of the entire sternum. Chin (1957) advanced the transected xiphoid and attached rectus muscles to a higher site on the sternum. This operation, the xiphosternopexy, produced posterior displacement of the sternum in younger patients with a flexible chest wall. Howard (1958) combined this method with subperichondrial costal cartilage resection and a sternal osteotomy. In 1973 Welch and Vos reported an approach to these deformities that we continue to use today.

HISTORICAL READINGS

Chin EF: Surgery of funnel chest and congenital sternal prominence. Br J Surg 44:360, 1957

Howard R: Pigeon chest (protrusion deformity of the sternum). Med J Aust 2:664, 1958

Lester CW: Pigeon breast (pectus carinatum) and other protrusion deformities of the chest of developmental origin. Ann Surg 137:482, 1953

Ravitch MM: Unusual sternal deformity with cardiac symptoms—operative correction. J Thorac Surg 23:138, 1952

Welch KJ, Vos A: Surgical correction of pectus carinatum (pigeon breast). J Pediatr Surg 8:659, 1973

BASIC SCIENCE

Etiology

The etiology of pectus carinatum is no better understood than that of pectus excavatum. It appears as an overgrowth of the costal cartilages with forward buckling and anterior displacement of the sternum. Again, there is a clear-cut family incidence, which suggests a genetic basis. In a review of 152 patients, 26 percent had a family history of chest wall deformity (Shamberger and Welch, 1987b), a family history of scoliosis being obtained in 12 percent of the patients. Pectus carinatum is much more frequent in boys (119 of Shamberger and Welch's patients) than in girls (33 patients). Scoliosis and other deformities of the spine are the most common associated musculoskeletal deformities.

Pectus carinatum usually appears in childhood, and in almost half of the patients the deformity has not been identified until after the eleventh birthday. The deformity may appear in mild form at birth and often progresses, particularly during the period of rapid growth at puberty. The chondromanubrial deformity, linked by Currarino and Silverman (1958) with an increased risk of congenital heart disease, is noted at birth and is associated with a short truncated sternum, with absent sternal segmentation or premature obliteration of sternal sutures. In a prospective review by Lees and Caldicott (1975), 135 patients with sternal fusion anomalies were identified, and 18 percent of these had documented congenital heart disease.

Pathophysiology

Cardiopulmonary impairment has not been demonstrated in patients with pectus carinatum, in contrast with pectus excavatum. Pain from local trauma to the protuberant mass or inability to sleep prone are the most frequent symptoms reported by patients.

SURGICAL REPAIR

A transverse incision is made just below and within the nipples as in repair of pectus excavatum, along with identical mobilization of the pectoral muscle flaps and subperichondrial resection of the deformed costal cartilages. A sternal osteotomy is created with the Hall air drill, allowing the sternum to be fractured and displaced posteriorly into an orthotopic position (Fig. 46-6A). Occasionally, a second osteotomy is required to displace the lower portion of the body of the sternum posteriorly. The upper or chondromanubrial deformity must be managed in a special manner, as described by Shamberger and Welch (1988c). In this situation the costal cartilages must be resected from the second cartilage inferi-

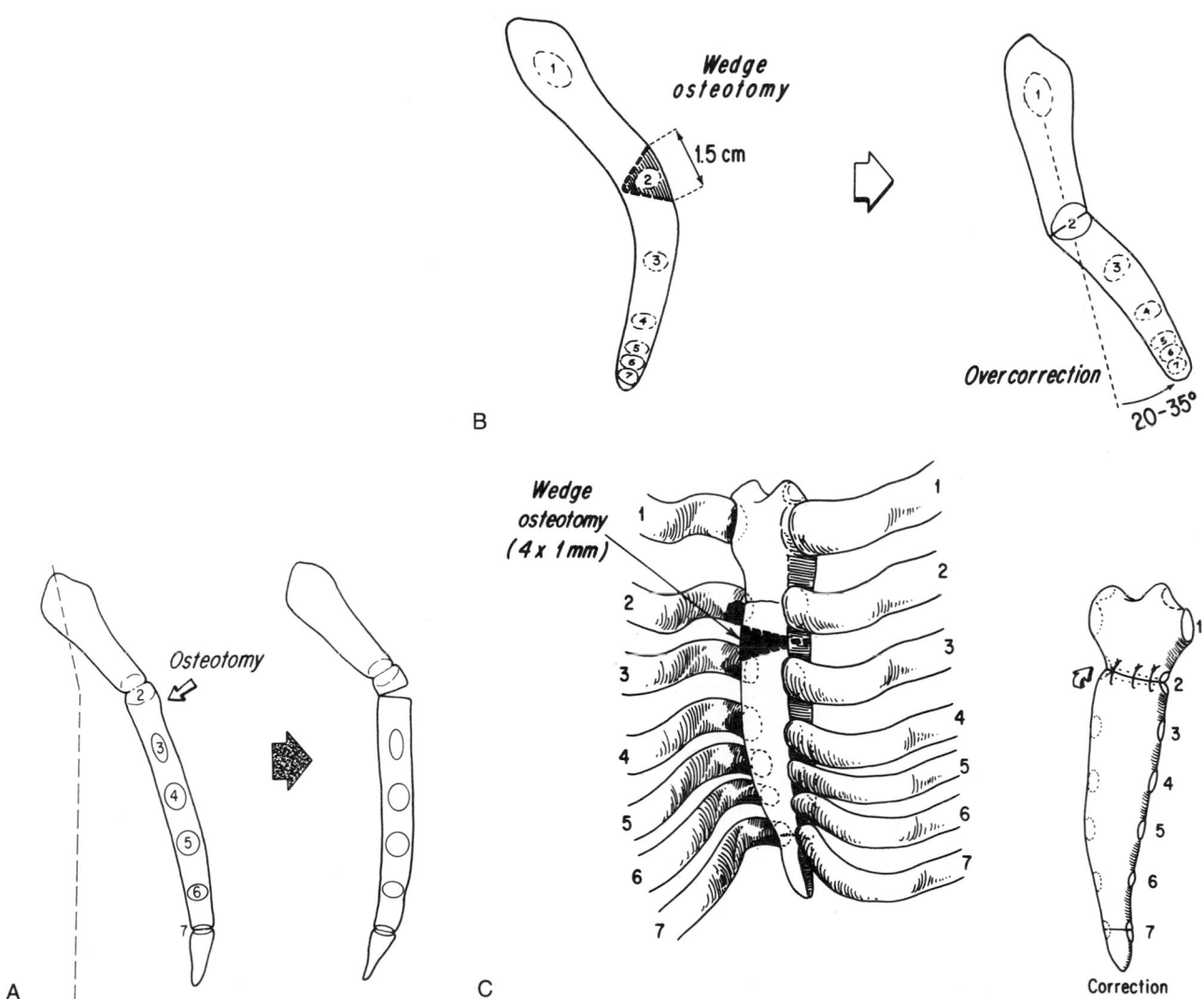

Figure 46-6. **(A)** Chondrogladiolar deformity (90.8 percent of all carinate deformities), symmetric or asymmetric, is managed with a single or double osteotomy after resection of the costal cartilages. This allows posterior displacement of the sternum to an orthotopic position. **(B)** Chondromanubrial deformity is rare. The broad superior osteotomy achieves anterior displacement of the body of the sternum and posterior displacement of the manubrium. **(C)** The mixed pectus deformity is corrected by symmetric resection of the third to seventh costal cartilages followed by transverse offset (0- to 10-degree) wedged-shaped sternal osteotomy. Closure of this defect achieves both anterior displacement and rotation of the sternum. (Fig. B from Shamberger RC, Welch KJ: Surgical correction of chandromanubrial deformity (Currarino Silverman syndrome). J Pediatr Surg 23:319, 1988, with permission. Fig. C from Shamberger RC, Welch KJ: Surgical correction of pectus carinatum. J Pediatr Surg 22:48,1987, with permission.)

orly. A generous wedge osteotomy is then performed at the point of maximal protrusion of the sternum. The superior segment of the sternum can then be displaced posteriorly as the osteotomy is closed, advancing the inferior segment anteriorly (Fig. 46-6B). This method corrects both components of the deformity. Mixed pectus carinatum-excavatum deformities are managed with a transverse wedge-shaped osteotomy, which allows anterior displacement and rotation of the sternum (Fig. 46-6C). Closure and postoperative drainage are performed as in pectus excavatum patients.

Operative Results

Surgical correction of pectus carinatum is very successful. In a recent review by Shamberger and Welch (1987b) of 152 cases, postoperative recovery was generally uneventful. Blood transfusions are rarely required, with none given since the late 1980s. There is a 3.9 percent rate of complications, which have included pneumothorax, wound infection, recurrence, and postoperative pneumonitis. Only three patients have required revision, each having additional lower costal cartilages resected for persistent unilateral malformation of the costal arch.

POLAND SYNDROME

DEFINITION

Alfred Poland in 1841 described congenital absence of the pectoralis major and minor muscles associated with syndactyly. It has become apparent that this entity is a spectrum, often involving chest wall and breast deformities as well. The extent of thoracic involvement may range from hypoplasia

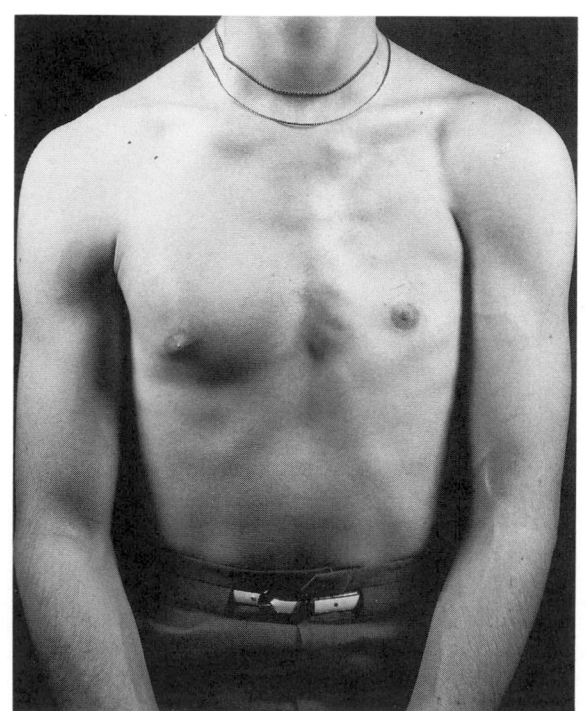

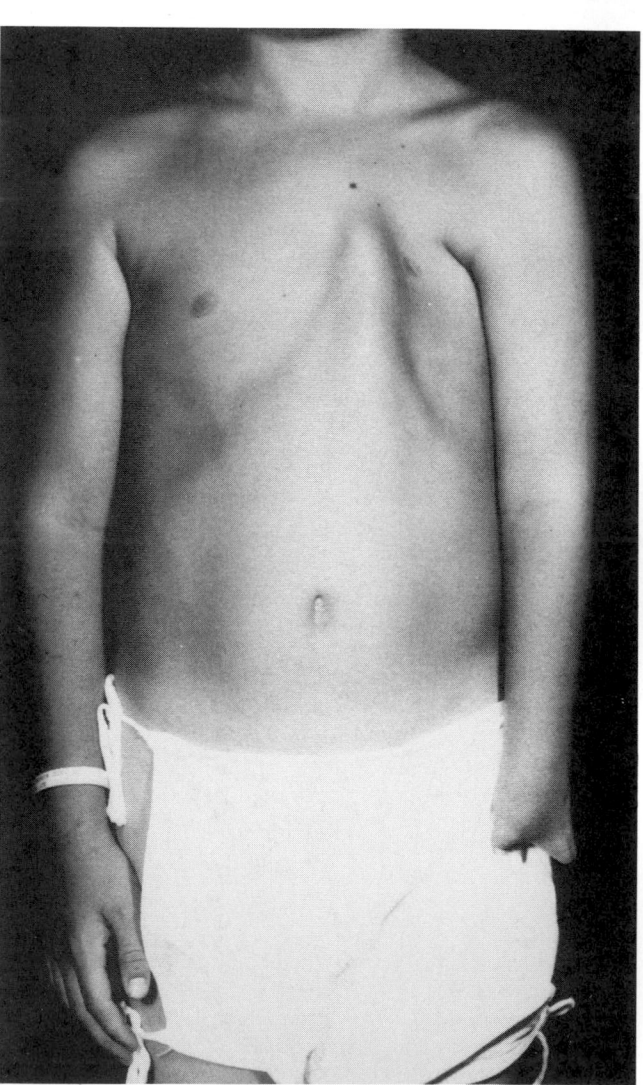

Figure 46-7. **(A)** A 16-year-old boy with Poland syndrome with absent pectoralis major and pectoralis minor muscles. Ribs are intact and in a normal contour. **(B)** A 10-year-old boy with Poland syndrome in whom the anterior third to fifth left ribs are hypoplastic and do not reach the sternum. The left nipple is also hypoplastic and displaced superiorly. This child also had a severe hand deformity with absence of most of the bony elements of the hand and wrist. (From Shamberger RC, Welch KJ, Upton J III: Surgical treatment of thoracic deformity in Poland's syndrome. J Pediatr Surg 24:760, 1989, with permission.)

of the sternal head of the pectoralis major muscle and the pectoralis minor muscle with normal underlying ribs to severe hypoplasia of the ribs with complete absence of the anterior portions of the second to fourth ribs and cartilages (Fig. 46-7). The extent of chest wall involvement is depicted in Figure 46-8, and the findings in our series of 75 patients are shown in Table 46-1 (Shamberger, et al., 1989). Breast involvement is frequent and ranges from mild hypoplasia to complete absence of the breast (amastia) and nipple (athelia). Minimal subcutaneous fat and absence of axillary hair are often found on the involved side. Hand deformities are frequent, as occurred in the patient described by Poland and may include hypoplasia (brachydactyly), fused fingers (syndactyly), and mitten or claw deformity (ectromelia). There is no correlation between the extent of hand, breast, and thoracic deformity.

HISTORICAL NOTE

Poland syndrome is a classic example of the wrong eponym being attached to a syndrome. Alfred Poland in 1841 reported a patient upon whom he performed an anatomic dissection while still a medical student. He found a constellation of anomalies, including absence of the pectoralis major and minor muscles and syndactyly. The syndrome had, however, been previously described by Lallemand (1826) and Froriep (1839) in the French and German literature, respectively. The full spectrum of anomalies was first summarized by Thomp-

Table 46-1. Chest Wall Deformities in 75 Patients with Poland Syndrome

Condition	No. Patients
Normal chest wall	41
Hypoplasia of ribs without depression	10
Depression deformity of ribs	
Major	11
Minor	5
Aplasia of ribs	8
Total	75

son in 1895 prior to Clarkson attributing the syndrome to Poland in 1962.

HISTORICAL READINGS

Clarkson P: Poland's syndactyly. Guy's Hosp Rep 111:335, 1962

Froriep R: Beobachtung eines Falles Von Mangel der Brustdrüse. Notizen Geb Nat Heilk 10:9, 1839

Lallemand LM: Absence de trois côtes simulant un enfoncement accidentel. Ephérmérides Médicales de Monpellier. 1:144, 1826

Poland A: Deficncy of the pectoralis muscles. Guy's Hosp Rep 6:191, 1841

Thomson J: On a form of congenital thoracic deformity. Teratologia 2:1, 1895

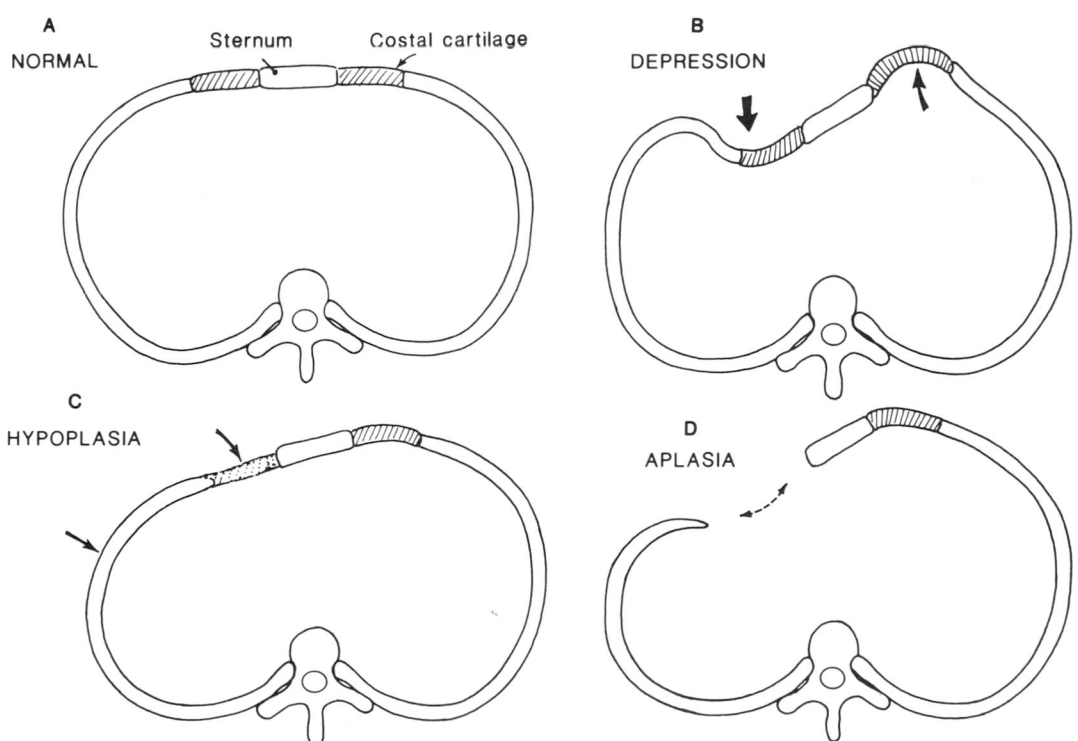

Figure 46-8. The spectrum of rib cage abnormality seen in Poland syndrome. **(A)** Most frequently an entirely normal rib cage is seen with only pectoral muscles absent. **(B)** Depression of the involved side of the chest wall with rotation and often depression of the sternum. A carinate protrusion of the contralateral side is frequently present. **(C)** Hypoplasia of the ribs on the involved side but without significant depression. This usually does not require surgical correction. **(D)** Aplasia of one or more ribs is usually associated with depression of adjacent ribs on the involved side and rotation of the sternum. (From Shamberger RC, Welch KJ, Upton J III: Surgical treatment of thoracic deformity in Poland's syndrome. J Pediatr Surg 24:760, 1989, with permission.)

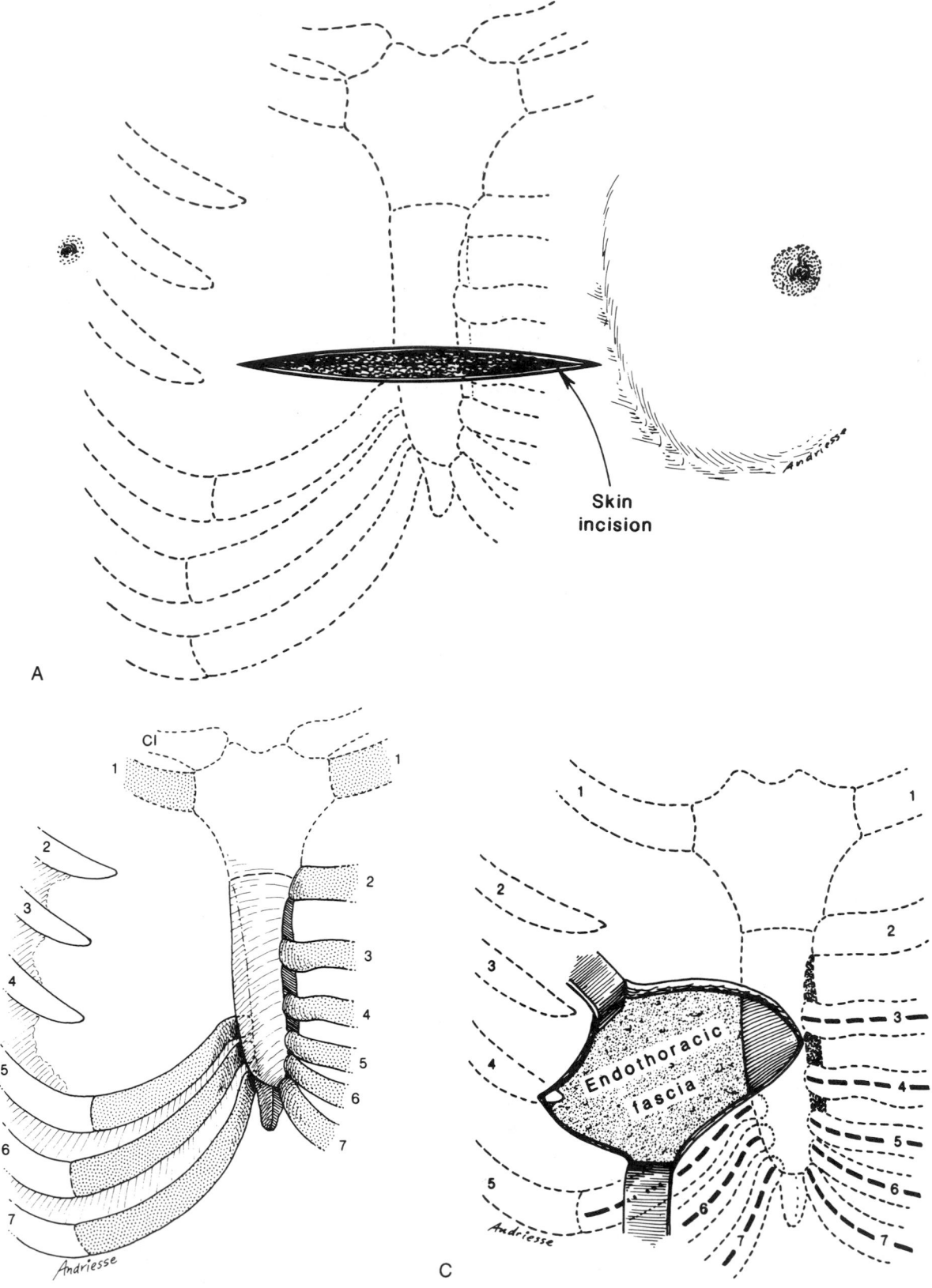

Figure 46-9. **(A)** A transverse incision is placed below the nipple lines and in females in the site of the future inframammary crease. **(B)** Schematic depiction of the deformity with rotation of the sternum, depression of the cartilages of the involved side, and carinate protrusion of the contralateral side. **(C)** In cases with aplasia of the ribs, the endothoracic fascia is encountered directly below the attenuated subcutaneous tissue and pectoral fascia. The pectoral muscle flap is elevated on the contralateral side and the pectoral fasica, if present, on the involved side. Subperichondrial resection of the costal cartilages is then carried out as shown by the dashed lines. Rarely, this must be carried to the level of the second costal cartilage. (*Figure continues.*)

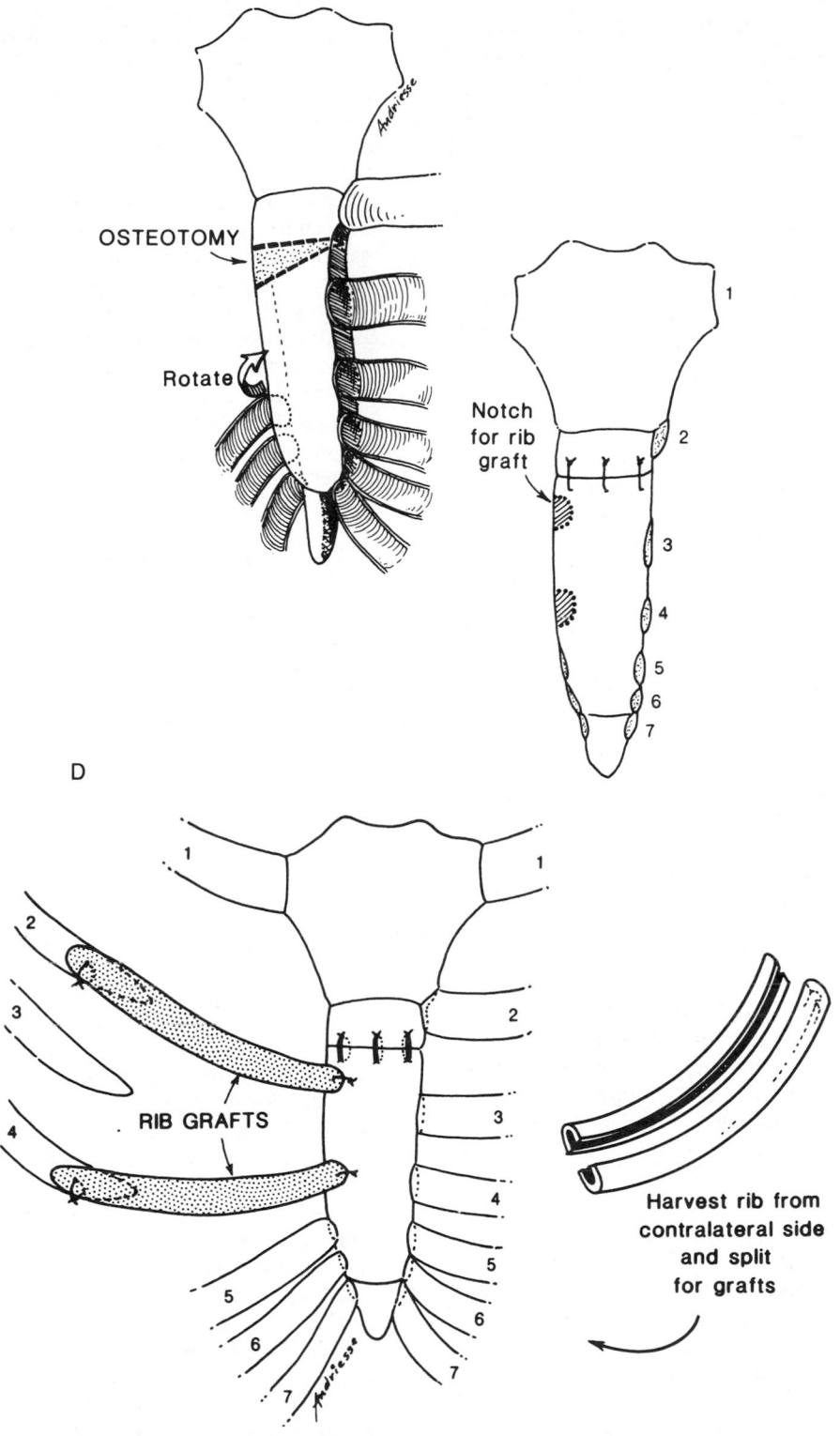

Figure 46-9 (*Continued*).   **(D)** A transverse offset wedge-shaped osteotomy is then created below the second costal cartilage. Closure of this defect with heavy silk sutures corrects both the posterior displacement and the rotation of the sternum. **(E)** In patients with rib aplasia, split rib grafts are harvested from the contralateral fifth or sixth ribs and then secured medially with wire sutures into previously created sternal notches and laterally with wire to the native ribs. Ribs are split as shown along their short axis to maintain maximum mechanical strength. (From Shamberger RC, Welch KJ, Upton J III: Surgical treatment of thoracic deformity in Poland's syndrome. J Pediatr Surg 24:760, 1989, with permission.)

BASIC SCIENCE

This condition is present from birth and has an estimated incidence of 1 in 30,000 to 1 in 32,000 live births (Freire-Maia, et al., 1975; McGillivray and Lowry, 1977). Abnormalities in the breast can be identified at birth by absence of the underlying breast bud and hypoplasia or aplasia of the often superiorly displaced nipple. The etiology is unknown, and cases are sporadic in their occurrence.

SURGICAL REPAIR

Assessment of the extent of involvement of the various musculoskeletal components is critical for optimal thoracic reconstruction. If involvement is limited to the sternal component of the pectoralis major and minor muscles, there is little functional deficit and repair is not necessary except for breast augmentation in girls, which should be performed at full growth. If the underlying costal cartilages are depressed or absent, repair of the chest wall must be considered to minimize the concavity, to eliminate the paradoxic motion of the chest wall, and in girls to provide an optimal base for breast reconstruction. Ravitch (1966) reported correction of posteriorly displaced costal cartilages by unilateral resection of the cartilages, a wedge osteotomy of the sternum allowing rotation of the sternum, and fixation with Rehbein struts and Steinmann pins. We have found that suitable repair can often be achieved with bilateral costal cartilage resection and an oblique osteotomy, as in the patients with the mixed pectus carinatum-excavatum deformity (Shamberger, et al., 1989). This allows correction of the rotational deformity (Fig. 46-9). The sternum is displaced anteriorly, which corrects the posterior displacement of the costal cartilages. An unappreciated carinate deformity is often present on the contralateral side, accentuating the ipsilateral concavity.

Absence of the medial portion of the ribs can be managed with split rib grafts taken from the contralateral side (Fig. 46-9E). These must be secured to the sternum medially and to the hypoplastic rib ends laterally. The grafts can be covered with a prosthetic mesh if needed for further support. In these cases it must be remembered that there is little tissue present between the endothoracic fascia and the fascial remnants of the pectoral muscles. Coverage of this area can be augmented by transfer of a latissimus dorsi muscle flap. This is particularly helpful in girls, who will require breast augmentation (Urschel, et al., 1984). Latissimus transfer is seldom if ever required in boys and has the disadvantage of adding a second thoracic scar as well as removing one of the major functional muscles of the shoulder and arm (Haller, et al., 1984).

STERNAL DEFECTS

CLEFT STERNUM

Deformities involving failure of ventral fusion of the thoracic wall can be divided into three groups: (1) cleft sternum without ectopia cordis, (2) thoracic ectopia cordis, and (3) thoracoabdominal ectopia cordis. Cleft sternum with an orthotopic heart is the simplest of these deformities. The cleft may be complete or incomplete and results from failure of ventral fusion of the sternal bars, which occurs at the eighth week of gestation. In cleft sternum the midline sternal separation is covered, and the pericardium, pleurae, and diaphragm are intact. Omphaloceles do not occur in this entity. Crying or a Valsalva maneuver produces a dramatic increase in the apparent severity of the deformity. Intrinsic congenital heart disease is rare.

Treatment in the newborn period is recommended, when the malformation can be closed primarily without prosthetic materials or cardiac compression. Primary closure in older patients produces excessive cardiac compression. Reconstruction of the anterior chest wall using multiple oblique chondrotomies, as reported by Sabiston (1958), lengthens the costal cartilages and decreases cardiac compression in the older patients with a less flexible chest wall. Autologous grafts, including costal cartilages, split ribs, and resection of the costal arch complex, have been described, but repair in the newborn period is optimal and avoids the need for these methods (Fig. 46-10).

THORACIC ECTOPIA CORDIS

While management of isolated cleft sternum is uniformly successful, only a limited number of patients survive surgical treatment of thoracic and thoracoabdominal ectopia cordis. These patients have a high incidence of associated intrinsic cardiac anomalies in addition to the abnormal cardiac position and surrounding somatic structures. In thoracic ectopia cordis nothing covers the heart, which is external to the thorax, protruding at the upper to mid-thoracic level (Fig. 46-11). The apex of the heart points anteriorly. Attempts to return the heart to the thorax occlude the great vessels and are not tolerated. Only a handful of infants have undergone successful repair, and they generally lack associated cardiac anomalies (Shamberger and Welch, 1990).

THORACOABDOMINAL ECTOPIA CORDIS (CANTRELL'S PENTALOGY)

The features of the Cantrell pentalogy (Cantrell, et al., 1958) are a cleft lower sternum, an anterior diaphragmatic defect due to failure of development of the septum transversum, absence of the parietal pericardium, an adjacent or completely separate omphalocele, and in most patients a cardiac anomaly, frequently the tetralogy of Fallot.

Immediate neonatal intervention to close the abdominal wall is required in patients with an omphalocele and lower sternal cleft (Fig. 46-12). An aggressive approach should be taken with these infants if salvage is to be achieved. After somatic closure, repair of the cardiac defect can be performed.

THORACIC DEFORMITIES IN DIFFUSE SKELETAL DISORDERS

Asphyxiating Thoracic Dystrophy (Jeune Syndrome)

Jeune, et al. in 1954 first described a newborn with a narrow rigid chest and multiple cartilage anomalies, who died early in the perinatal period because of respiratory insufficiency.

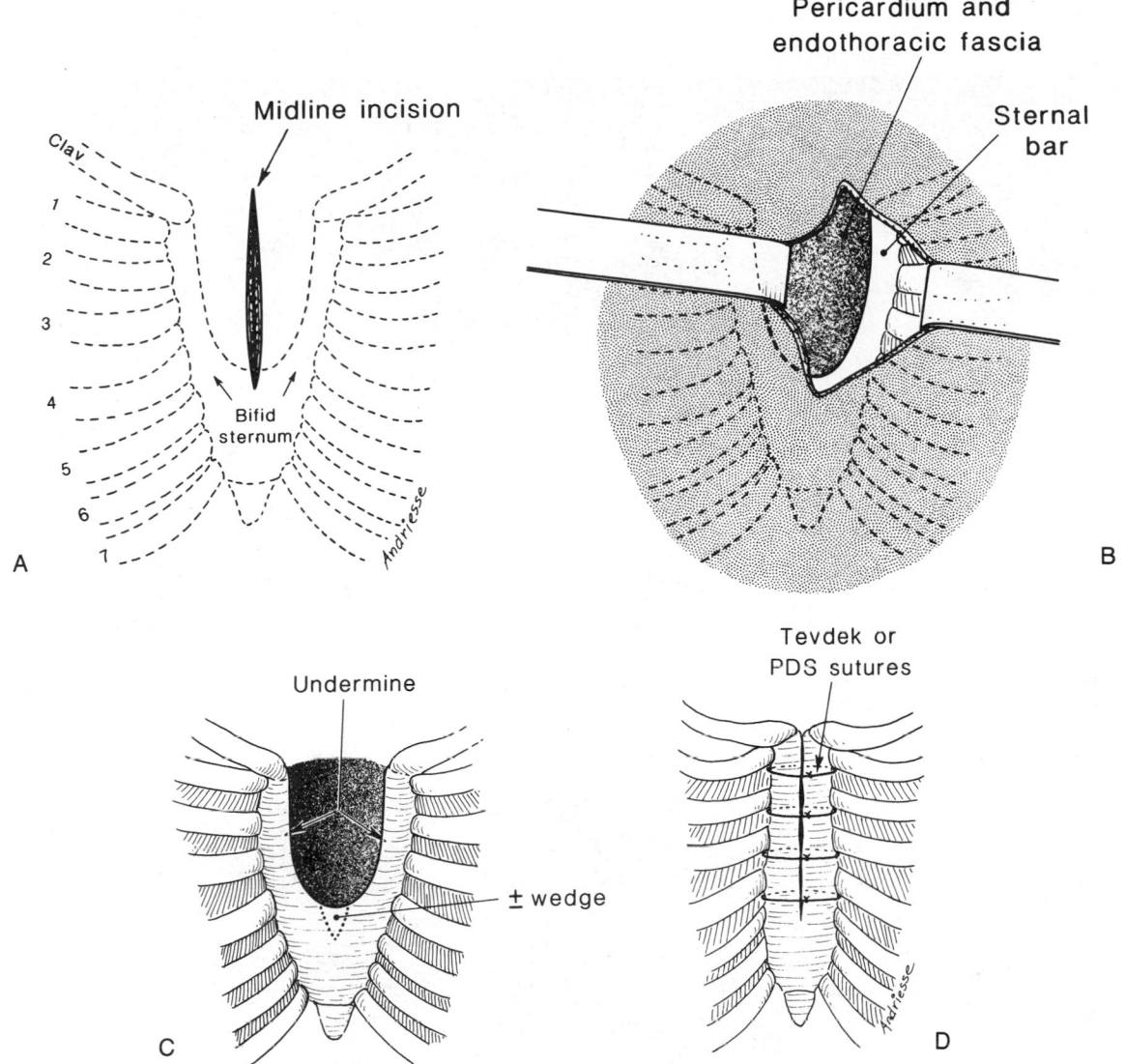

Figure 46-10. **(A)** Repair of bifid sternum is best performed through a longitudinal incision extending the length of the defect. **(B)** Directly beneath the subcutaneous tissues the sternal bars are encountered, with pectoral muscles present lateral to the bars. The endothoracic fascia and pericardium are just below these structures. **(C)** The endothoracic fascia is mobilized off the sternal bars posteriorly with blunt dissection to allow safe placement of the sutures. Approximation of the sternal bars may be facilitated by excising a wedge of cartilage inferiorly. Repair is best accomplished in the neonatal period because of the flexibility of the chest wall. **(D)** The defect is closed with permanent sutures. (From Shamberger RC, Welch KJ: Sternal defects. Pediatr Surg Int 5:156, 1990, with permission.)

Subsequent authors have further characterized this form of osteochondrodystrophy, which has variable skeletal involvement. It is inherited in an autosomal recessive pattern and is not associated with chromosome abnormalities (Tahernia and Stamps, 1977). Its most prominent feature is a narrow "bell-shaped" thorax and protuberant abdomen. The thorax is narrow in both the transverse and sagittal axes and has little respiratory motion owing to the horizontal direction of the ribs (Fig. 46-13). The ribs are short and wide, and the splayed costochondral junctions barely reach the anterior axillary line. The costal cartilage is abundant and irregular like a rachitic rosary. Microscopic examination of the costochondral junction reveals disordered and poorly progressing endochondral ossification, resulting in decreased rib length.

Associated skeletal abnormalities that occur with this syndrome include short and stubby extremities with relatively short and wide bones. The clavicles are in a fixed and elevated position, and the pelvis is small and hypoplastic with square iliac bones.

The syndrome has variable expression and degree of pulmonary impairment. While the initial cases reported resulted in neonatal death, subsequent reports have documented a wide range of survival of patients with this syndrome (Kozlowski and Masel, 1976). The pathologic findings in autopsy cases are variable as well, showing a range of abnormal pulmonary development, although in most cases the bronchial development is normal and there is variable decrease in alveolar divisions (Williams, et al., 1984).

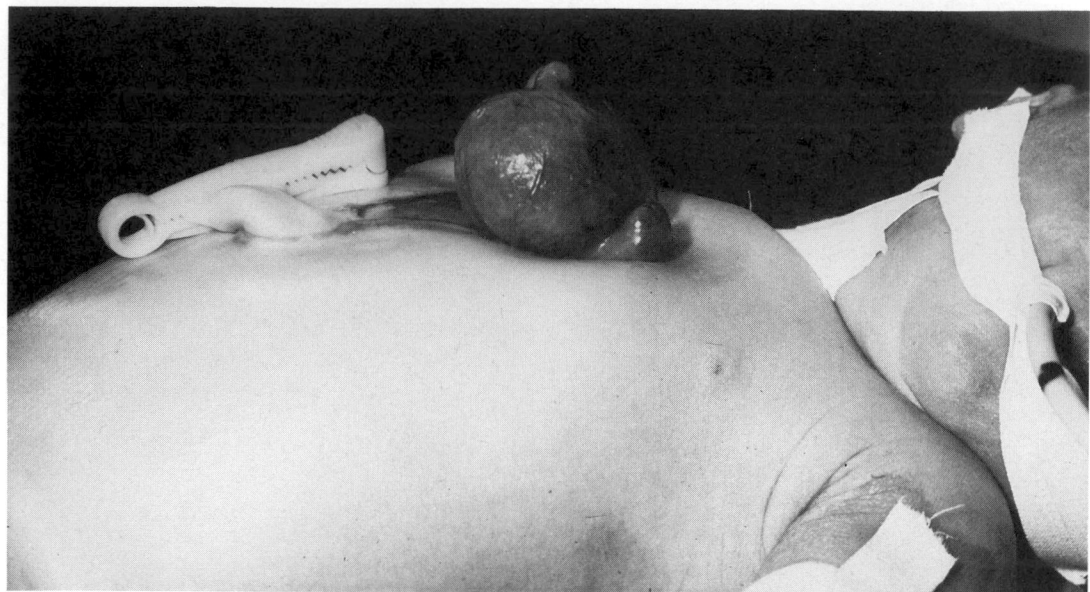

Figure 46-11. Infant with thoracic ectopia cordis with no significant abdominal wall defect present. Characteristic high insertion of the umbilicus.

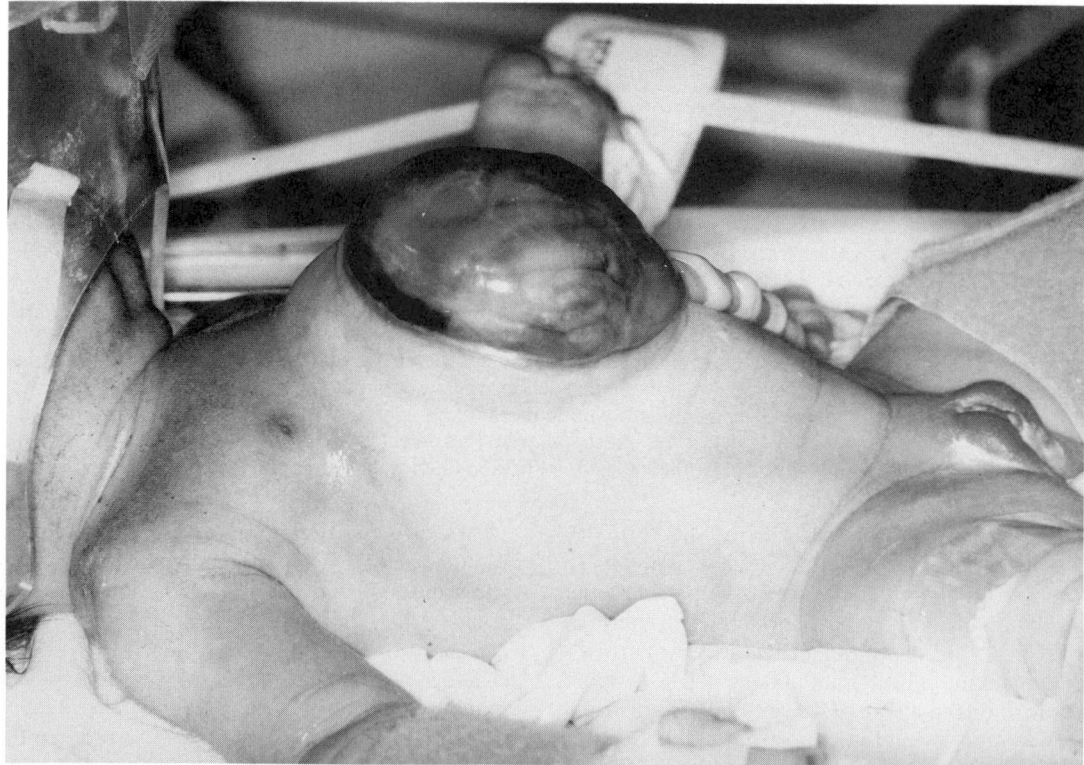

Figure 46-12. Infant with thoracoabdominal ectopia cordis demonstrating high abdominal wall defect and omphalocele below costal arch. Infant's head is to the left, and heart was palpable just below the skin superior to the defect.

Figure 46-13. Infant with asphyxiating thoracic dystrophy (Jeune syndrome). Radiograph shows the short horizontal ribs and narrow thorax with limited lung volumes.

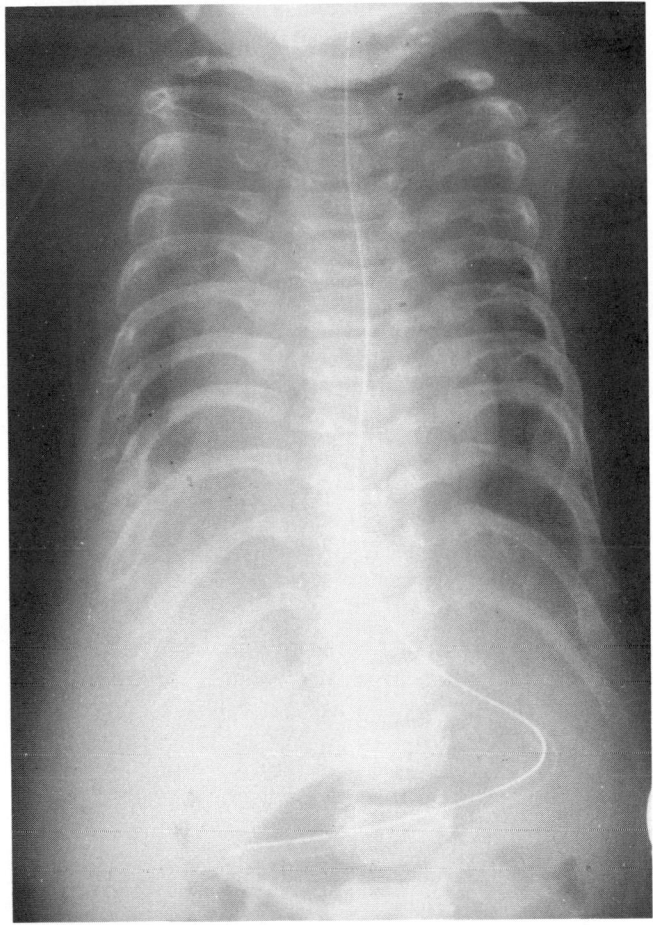

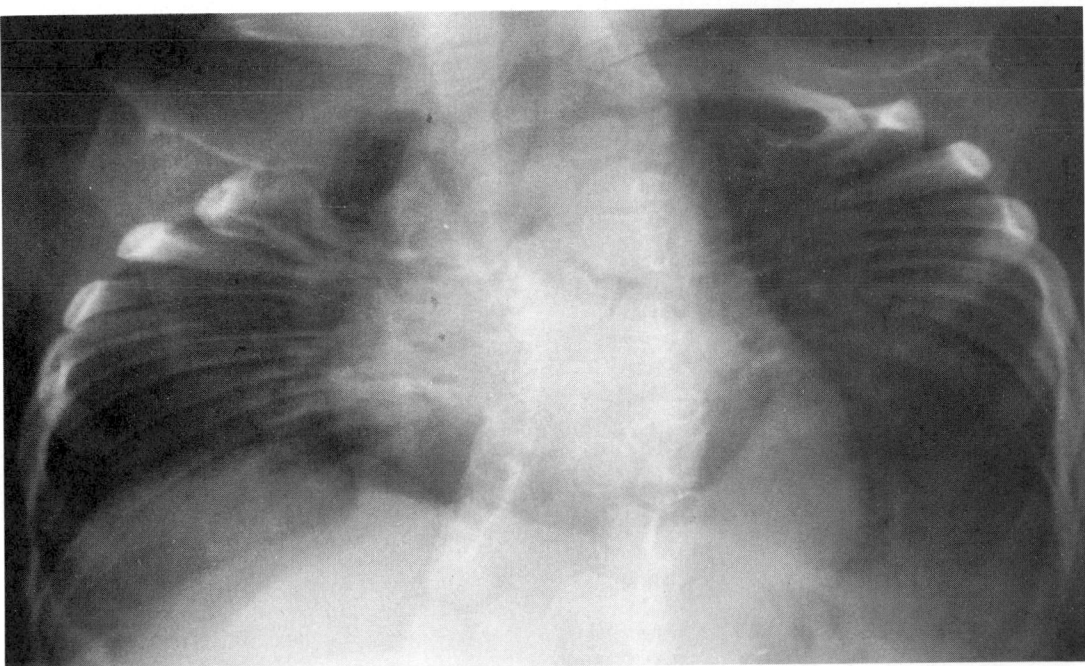

Figure 46-14. Radiograph of infant with spondylothoracic dysplasia (Jarcho-Levin syndrome). Severe abnormality of the spine is apparent, with multiple hemivertebrae and "crablike" ribs, with close approximation posteriorly and splaying out anteriorly.

Surgical interventions for this condition have had very limited success. All have involved splitting the sternum longitudinally and widening the distance between the two sternal halves to increase the intrathoracic volume. Rib grafts, stainless steel struts, iliac bone grafts with metal plate fixation, and polymethylmethacrylate prostheses have all been used to maintain sternal separation. Results of these surgical attempts depend on the degree of underlying pulmonary hypoplasia.

Spondylothoracic Dysplasia (Jarcho-Levin Syndrome)

Spondylothoracic dysplasia is an autosomal recessive deformity in which there are multiple vertebral and rib malformations. Death occurs in early infancy from respiratory failure and pneumonia (Jarcho and Levin, 1983). Patients have multiple alternating hemivertebrae, which affect most if not all of the thoracic and lumbar spine. The vertebral ossification centers rarely cross the midline. Multiple posterior fusions of the ribs as well as remarkable shortening of the thoracic spine results in a "crablike" radiographic appearance of the chest (Fig. 46-14). One-third of patients with this syndrome have associated malformations, including congenital heart disease and renal anomalies. Its occurrence has been reported by Heilbronner and Renshaw (1984), primarily in Puerto Rican families (15 of 18 cases). Bone formation is normal in these patients.

Thoracic deformity is really secondary to the spine anomaly, which results in close posterior approximation of the origin of the ribs. Although most infants with this entity succumb before 15 months of age, no surgical efforts have been proposed or attempted (Roberts, et al., 1988).

COMMENTS AND CONTROVERSIES

The advantages of early repair of pectus excavatum or carinatum minimize pathophysiologic abnormalities, cardiac/pulmonary displacement, and psychological damage secondary to significant deformities as the individual enters puberty and adolescence. Disadvantages of early repair (e.g., at 2 years) revolve around the high recurrence rate because of continuation of growth, particularly of the rib cartilages, which may produce further deformity or recurrence of deformity. From this point of view the best time for repair would be after the main growth has stopped (i.e., after adolescence—in the late teens or early twenties). Although the operation is more traumatic at this time, the results are far better with minimal recurrence.

H.C.U.

KEY REFERENCES

Shamberger RC, Welch KJ: Cardiopulmonary function in pectus excavatum. Surg Gynecol Obstet 166:383, 1988b

This comprehensive summary of all the articles evaluating cardiopulmonary function in patients with pectus excavatum presents a comparison of these studies and attempts to clarify the conflicting reports in the literature.

Shamberger RC, Welch KJ: Sternal defects. Pediatr Surg Int 5:156, 1990

A summary of world literature on sternal defects including bifid sternum, Cantrell's pentology, and thoracic ectopia cordis.

REFERENCES

Adkins PC, Blades B: A stainless steel strut for correction of pectus excavatum. Surg Gynecol Obstet 113:111, 1961

Beiser GD, Epstein SE, Stampfer M et al.: Impairment of cardiac function in patients with pectus excavatum, with improvement after operative correction. N Engl J Med 287:267, 1972

Blickman JG, Rosen PR, Welch KJ et al.: Pectus excavatum in children: pulmonary scintigraphy before and after corrective surgery. Radiology 156:781, 1985

Cahill JL, Lees GM, Robertson HT: A summary of preoperative and postoperative cardiorespiratory performance in patients undergoing pectus excavatum and carinatum repair. J Pediatr Surg 19:430, 1984

Cantrell JR, Haller JA, Ravitch MM: A syndrome of congenital defects involving the abdominal wall, sternum, diaphragm, pericardium and heart. Surg Gynecol Obstet 107:602, 1958

Castile RG, Staats BA, Westbrook PR: Symptomatic pectus deformities of the chest. Am Rev Respir Dis 126:564, 1982

Chin EF: Surgery of funnel chest and congenital sternal prominence. Br J Surg 44:360, 1957

Clarkson P: Poland's syndactyly. Guy's Hosp Rep 111:335, 1962

Currarino G, Silverman FN: Premature obliteration of the sternal sutures and pigeon-breast deformity. Radiology 70:532, 1958

Freire-Maia N, Chautard EA, Opitz JM et al.: The Poland syndrome—clinical and genealogical data, dermatoglyphic analysis, and incidence. Hum Hered 23:97, 1973

Froriep R: Beobachtung eines Falles von Mangel der Brustdruse. Notizen Geb Nat Heilk 10:9, 1839

Greig JD, Azmy AF: Thoracic cage deformity: a late complication following repair of an agenesis of diaphragm. J Pediatr Surg 25:1234, 1990

Haller JA, Peters GN, Mazur D et al.: Pectus excavatum: a 20 year surgical experience. J Thorac Cardiovasc Surg 60:375, 1970

Haller JA Jr, Colombani PM, Miller D et al.: Early reconstruction of Poland's syndrome using autologous rib grafts combined with a latissimus muscle flap. J Pediatr Surg 19:423, 1984

Haller JA Jr, Katlic BA, Shermeta DW et al.: Operative correction of pectus excavatum: an evolving perspective. Ann Surg 184:554, 1976

Hecker WC, Procher G, Dietz HG: Results of operative correction of pigeon and funnel chest following a modified procedure of Ravitch and Haller. Z Kinderchir 34:220, 1981

Heilbronner DM, Renshaw TS: Spondylothoracic dysplasia. J Bone Joint Surg [Am] 66:302, 1984

Howard R: Pigeon chest (protrusion deformity of the sternum). Med J Aust 2:664, 1958

Jarcho S, Levin PM: Hereditary malformation of the vertebral bodies. Johns Hopkins Med J 62:216, 1938

Jeune M, Carron R, Beraud Cl et al.: Polychondrodystrophie avec blocage thoracique d'évolution fatale. Pediatrie 9:390, 1954

Judet J, Judet R: Sternum en entonnoir par résection et retournement. Mem Acad Chir 82:250, 1956

Jung A, Wiest E, Vierling J-P: Traitement par le "retournement pédiculé" de la cuvette sterno-chondrale: résultats éloignés. Rev Chir Orthop 50:446, 1964

Kozlowski K, Masel J: Asphyxiating thoracic dystrophy without respiratory disease: report of two cases of the latent form. Pediatr Radiol 5, 30, 1976

Lallemand LM: Absence detrois côtes simulant un enfoncement accidentel. Ephérmérides Médicales de Montpellier. 1:144, 1826

Lees RF, Caldicott WJH: Sternal anomalies and congenital heart disease. AJR 124:423, 1975

Lester CW: The etiology and pathogenesis of funnel chest, pigeon breast, and related deformities of the anterior chest wall. J Thorac Surg 34:1, 1957

Lester CW: Pigeon breast (pectus carinatum) and other protrusion deformities of the chest of developmental origin. Ann Surg 137:482, 1953

McGillivray BC, Lowry RB: Poland syndrome in British Columbia: incidence and reproductive experience of affected persons. Am J Med Genet 1:65, 1977

Meyer L: Zur chirurgischen Behandlung der angeborenen Trichterbrust. Verh Ber Med Ges 42:364, 1911

Ochsner A, DeBakey M: Chone-chondrosternon: report of a case and review of the literature. J Thorac Surg 8:469, 1939

Oelsnitz G: Fehlbildungen des Brustkorbes. Z Kinderchir 33:229, 1981

Peterson RJ, Young WG Jr, Godwin JD et al.: Noninvasive assessment of exercise cardiac function before and after pectus excavatum repair. J Thorac Cardiovasc Surg 90:251, 1985

Poland A: Deficiency of the pectoralis muscles. Guy's Hosp Rep 6:191, 1841

Ravitch MM: Congenital Deformities of the Chest Wall and Their Operative Correction. p. 78. WB Saunders, Philadelphia, 1977

Ravitch MM: Atypical deformities of the chest wall—absence and deformities of the ribs and costal cartilages. Surgery 59:438, 1966

Ravitch MM: Unusual sternal deformity with cardiac symptoms—operative correction. J Thorac Surg 23:138, 1952

Ravitch MM: The operative treatment of pectus excavatum. Ann Surg 129:429, 1949

Rehbein F, Wernicke HH: The operative treatment of the funnel chest. Arch Dis Child 32:5, 1957

Roberts AP, Conner AN, Tolmie JL et al.: Spondylothoracic and spondylocostal dysostosis: hereditary forms of spinal deformity. J Bone Joint Surg Br 70:123, 1988

Sabiston DC Jr: The surgical management of congenital bifid sternum with partial ectopia cordis. J Thorac Surg 35:118, 1958

Sauerbruch F: Die Chirurgie der Brustorgane. J. Springer, Berlin, 1920, p. 437

Scherer LR, Arn PH, Dressel DA et al.: Surgical management of children and young adults with Marfan syndrome and pectus excavatum. J Pediatr Surg 23:1169, 1988

Shamberger RC, Welch KJ: Surgical correction of pectus excavatum. J Pediatr Surg 23:615, 1988a

Shamberger RC, Welch KJ: Surgical correction of chondromanubrial deformity (Currarino Silverman syndrome). J Pediatr Surg 23:319, 1988c

Shamberger RC, Welch KJ: Surgical correction of pectus carinatum. J Pediatr Surg 22:48, 1987b

Shamberger RC, Welch KJ, Sanders SP: Mitral valve prolapse associated with pectus excavatum. J Pediatr 111:404, 1987a

Shamberger RC, Welch KJ, Upton J III: Surgical treatment of thoracic deformity in Poland's syndrome. J Pediatr Surg 24:760, 1989

Tahernia AC, Stamps P: "Jeune syndrome" (asphyxiating thoracic dystrophy): report of a case, a review of the literature, and an editor's commentary. Clin Pediatr (Phila) 16:903, 1977

Thomson J: On a form of congenital thoracic deformity. Teratologia 2:1, 1895

Urschel HC, Byrd HS, Sethi SM, Razzuk MA: Polanoc's syndrome: improved surgical management. Ann Thorac Surg 37:204, 1984

Wada J, Ikeda K, Ishida T, Hasegawa T: Results of 271 funnel chest operations. Ann Thorac Surg 10:526, 1970

Welch KJ: Satisfactory surgical correction of pectus excavatum deformity in childhood: a limited opportunity. J Thorac Surg 36:697, 1958

Welch KJ, Kearney GP: Abdominal musculature deficiency syndrome: prune belly. J Urol 111:693, 1974

Welch KJ, Vos A: Surgical correction of pectus carinatum (pigeon breast). J Pediatr Surg 8:659, 1973

Williams AJ, Vawter G, Reid LM: Lung structure in asphyxiating thoracic dystrophy. Arch Pathol Lab Med 108:658, 1984

Willital GH: Operationsindikation—Operationstechnik bei Brustkorbdeformierungen. Z Kinderchir 33:244, 1981

47

THORACIC OUTLET SYNDROMES

Susan Mackinnon
G. A. Patterson
Harold C. Urschel, Jr.

DEFINITION

Thoracic outlet syndrome, a term coined by Rob and Standover (1958), refers to compression on the subclavian vessels and brachial plexus at the superior aperture of the chest. It was previously designated according to presumed etiologies as the scalenus anticus, costoclavicular, hyperabduction, cervical rib, or first thoracic rib syndrome. The various syndromes are similar, and the compression mechanism is often difficult to identify. Most compressive factors operate against the first rib (Clagett, 1962; Urschel, et al., 1968) (Fig. 47-1).

HISTORICAL NOTE

Until 1927 the cervical rib was commonly thought to be the cause of symptoms of the thoracic outlet syndrome. Galen and Vesalius first described the presence of a cervical rib (Borchardt, 1901). Hunauld, who published an article in 1742, is credited by Keen (1907) as being the first to describe the importance of the cervical rib in causing symptoms. In 1818 Cooper treated symptoms of cervical rib with some success (Adson and Coffey, 1927), and in 1861 Coote performed the first cervical rib removal. Sir James Paget in 1875 in London and von Schroetter in 1884 in Vienna described this syndrome of thrombosis of the axillary-subclavian vein (which is also known as the Paget-von Schroeter syndrome). Halsted (1916) stimulated interest in dilatation of the subclavian artery distal to cervical ribs, and Law (1920) reported the role of adventitious ligaments in the cervical rib syndrome. Naffziger and Grant (1938) and Ochsner and associates (1935) popularized section of the scalenus anticus muscle. Falconer and Weddell (1943) and Brintnall and associates (1956) incriminated the costoclavicular membrane in the production of neurovascular compression. Wright (1945) described the hyperabduction syndrome with compression in the costoclavicular area by the tendon of the pectoralis minor.

Rosati and Lord (1961) added claviculectomy to anterior exploration, scalentotomy, resection of the cervical rib (when one was present), and section of the pectoralis minor and subclavian muscles, as well as the costoclavicular membrane. The role of the first rib in causing symptoms of neurovascular compression was recognized by Bramwell in 1903. Murphy (1910) is credited with the first resection of the first rib and in 1916 provided a collective review of 112 articles related to compression from the cervical ribs. Brinckner and Milch (1925, 1927), Telford and Stopford (1937), and Telford and Mottershead (1948) suggested that the first rib was the culprit. Clagett (1962) emphasized the first rib and its resection through the posterior thoracoplasty approach to relieve neurovascular compression. Falconer and Li (1962) reported the anterior approach for first rib resection, whereas Roos (1966) introduced the transaxillary route for first rib resection and extirpation. Krusen (1968) and Caldwell, et al. (1971) introduced the measurement of motor conduction velocities across the thoracic outlet in diagnosing thoracic outlet syndrome. Urschel and associates (1976) popularized reoperation for recurrent thoracic outlet syndrome.

HISTORICAL READINGS

Caldwell JW, Crane CR, Drusen EM: Nerve conduction studies in the diagnosis of the thoracic outlet syndrome. South Med J 64:210, 1971

Clagett, OT: Presidential address: Research and prosearch. J Thorac Cardiovasc Surg 44:153, 1962

Paget J: Clinical Lectures and Essays. Longmans-Green, London, 1875

Urschel HC Jr, Razzuk MA, Albers JE, et al.: Reoperation for recurrent thoracic outlet syndrome. Ann Thorac Surg 21:19, 1976

Von Schroetter L: Erkrankungen der Gefässe. In Nathnogel (ed): Handbuch der Pathologie und Therapie. Holder, Vienna, 1884

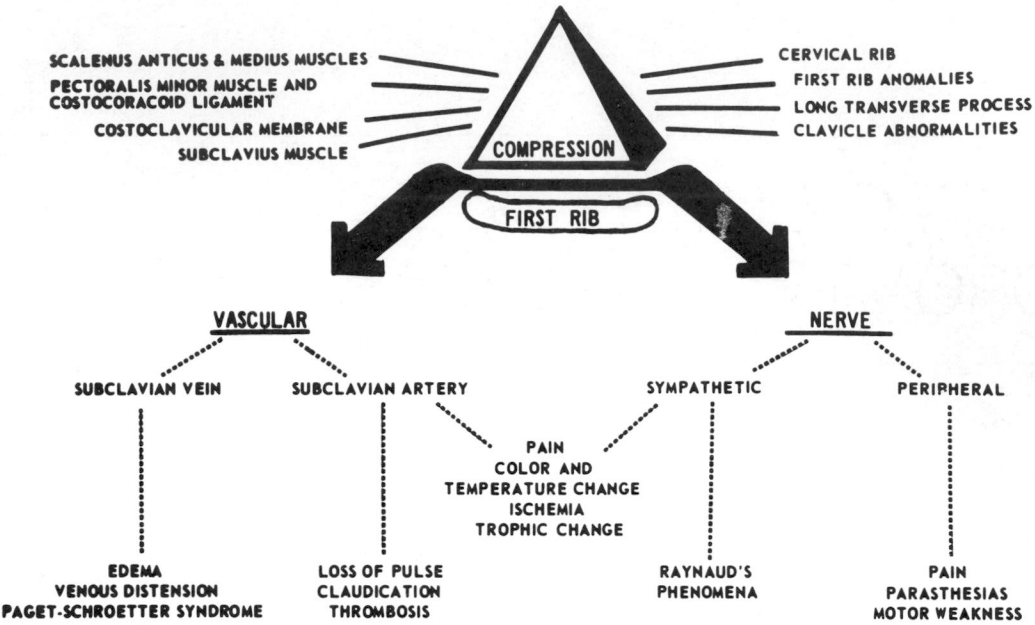

Figure 47-1. The relation of muscle, ligament, and bone abnormalities in the thoracic outlet that may compress neurovascular structures against the first rib.

BASIC SCIENCE

Surgical Anatomy

At the superior aperture of the thorax, the subclavian vessels and the brachial plexus traverse the cervicoaxillary canal to reach the upper extremity. The cervicoaxillary canal is divided by the first rib into two sections: the proximal one, composed of the scalene triangle and the costoclavicular space (the space bounded by the clavicle and the first rib); and the distal one, composed of the axilla (Fig. 47-2). The proximal division is the more critical for neurovascular compression. It is bounded superiorly by the clavicle, inferiorly by the first rib, anteromedially by the costoclavicular ligament, and posterolaterally by the scalenus medius muscle and the long thoracic nerve. The scalenus anticus muscle, which inserts on the scalene tubercle of the first rib, divides the costoclavicular space into two compartments: the anteromedial compartment, which contains the subclavian artery and the brachial plexus; and the scalene triangle, which is bounded by the scalenus anticus anteriorly, the scalenus medius posteriorly, and the first rib inferiorly.

Functional Anatomy

The cervicoaxillary canal, particularly its proximal segment, the costoclavicular area, normally has ample space for passage of the neurovascular bundle with compression. Narrowing of this space occurs during functional maneuvers. It narrows during abduction of the arm because the clavicle rotates backward toward the first rib and the insertion of the scalenus anticus muscle. In hyperabduction, the neurovascular bundle is pulled around the pectoralis minor tendon, the coracoid process, and the head of the humerus. During this maneuver, the caracoid process tilts downward and thus exaggerates the tension on the bundle. The sternoclavicular joint, which ordinarily forms an angle of 15 to 20 degrees, forms a smaller angle when the outer end of the clavicle descends (as in drooping of the shoulders in poor posture), and narrowing of the costoclavicular space may occur (Rosati and Lord, 1961). Normally, during inspiration the scalenus anticus muscle raises the first rib and thus narrows the costoclavicular space. This muscle may cause an abnormal lift of the first rib, as in cases of severe emphysema or excessive muscular development, which is seen in young adults.

The scalene triangle, which is normally located between the scalenus anticus anteriorly, the scalenus medius posteriorly, and the first rib inferiorly, permits the passage of the subclavian artery and the brachial plexus, which are in direct contact with the first rib. The triangle is 1.2 cm at its base and approximately 6.7 cm in height. There is a close-fitting relationship between the neurovascular bundle and this triangular space. Anatomic variations may narrow the superior angle of the triangle, cause impingement on the upper components of the brachial plexus, and produce the upper type of scalenus anticus syndrome, which involves the trunk-containing elements of C5 and C6. If the base of the triangle is raised, compression of the subclavian artery and the trunk-containing components of C7, C8, and T1 results in the lower type of scalenus anticus syndrome. Both types have been described by Swank and Simeone (1944).

Compression Factors

Many factors may cause compression of the neurovascular bundle at the thoracic outlet, but the basic factor is displaced anatomy, to which congenital, traumatic, and occasionally

Figure 47-2. Hyperabduction of the right arm with anatomic structures as noted.

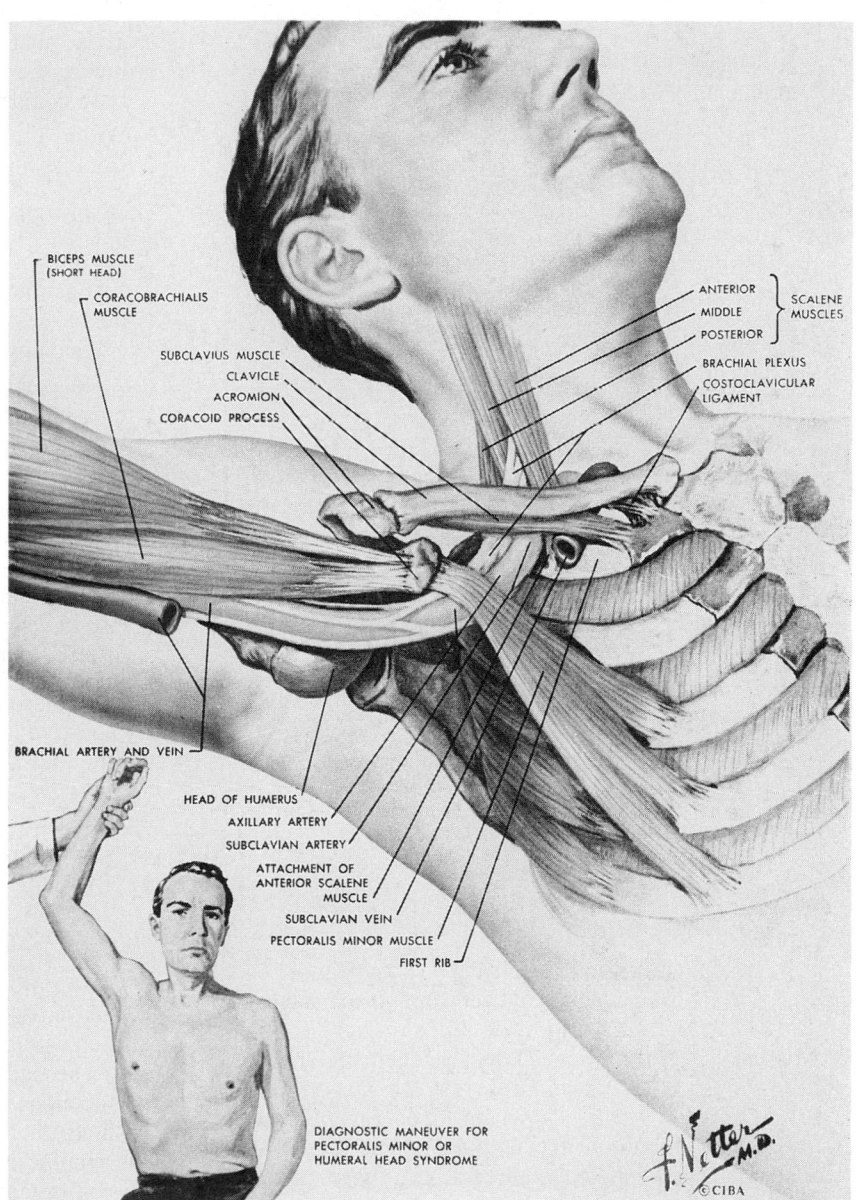

BICEPS MUSCLE (SHORT HEAD)

CORACOBRACHIALIS MUSCLE

SUBCLAVIUS MUSCLE
CLAVICLE
ACROMION
CORACOID PROCESS

ANTERIOR
MIDDLE
POSTERIOR } SCALENE MUSCLES

BRACHIAL PLEXUS
COSTOCLAVICULAR LIGAMENT

BRACHIAL ARTERY AND VEIN

HEAD OF HUMERUS
AXILLARY ARTERY
SUBCLAVIAN ARTERY
ATTACHMENT OF ANTERIOR SCALENE MUSCLE
SUBCLAVIAN VEIN
PECTORALIS MINOR MUSCLE
FIRST RIB

DIAGNOSTIC MANEUVER FOR PECTORALIS MINOR OR HUMERAL HEAD SYNDROME

Neurovascular Compression Factors

Anatomic
    Potential sites of neurovascular compression
        Interscalene triangle
        Costoclavicular space
        Subcoracoid area

Congenital
    Cervical rib and its fascial remnants
    Rudimentary first thoracic rib
    Scalene muscles
        Anterior
        Middle
        Minimus
    Adventitious fibrous bands
    Bifid clavicle
    Exostosis of first thoracic rib
    Enlarged transverse process of C7
    Omohyoid muscle
    Anomalous course of transverse cervical artery
    Brachial plexus postfixed
    Flat clavicle

Traumatic
    Fracture of clavicle
    Dislocation of head of humerus
    Crushing injury to upper thorax
    Sudden, unaccustomed muscular efforts involving
        shoulder girdle muscles
    Cervical spondylosis and injuries to cervical spine

Atherosclerosis

This model has been useful in demonstrating the histopathology of chronic nerve compression and in evaluating current treatment modalities. From these experimental studies, several key points relating to the histopathology have been determined:

1. Histopathology spans a broad spectrum from blood nerve barrier changes to epineural and perineural thickening to segmental demyelination and finally to wallerian degeneration (Fig. 47-3).
2. These changes are slowly progressive and influenced by the degree of compression and the time that the nerve has been compressed.
3. Within the compressed nerve, histologic changes vary from fascicle to fascicle (Figs. 47-4 and 47-5).

These histopathologic findings have significant clinical implications:

1. Just as the histopathology spans a broad spectrum from mild to severe changes, the patient's symptoms and clinical findings vary along a similar continuum (Fig. 47-6).
2. As long as factors that contribute to chronic nerve compression (e.g., provoking job or activity, systemic disease) continue unchanged, the patient will develop progressive problems with nerve compression.
3. The fact that one fascicle within a compressed nerve may be normal while another demonstrates significant histologic changes corresponds with the situation in which the unaffected fascicles are reflected in normal electrical studies, while the patient's symptomatology is related to the fascicles demonstrating nerve damage.

In a fresh cadaver study we biopsied the roots (C5 through T1) and trunks of the brachial plexus. We noted in C8, T1, and the lower trunk the same histomorphologic changes of chronic nerve compression (epineurial thickening, demyelination, a "fallout" of large myelinated fibers and Renaut's bodies) as were noted in other human and experimental studies of chronic nerve compression (Figs. 47-7 and 47-8).

Double and Multiple Crush Syndromes

In their report of the double crush syndrome in 1973, Upton and McComas stated that a proximal source of nerve compression will render the distal nerve segment more susceptible to a second site of compression. They hypothesized that one site alone would not cause clinical disturbance but that the summation of two sites would produce symptomatology. This hypothesis is directly applicable to brachial plexus compression in that several anatomic structures may compress the brachial plexus by amounts that on their own would not be enough to cause symptoms. Similarly, the recognized association between the carpal and cubital tunnel syndromes and the thoracic outlet syndrome is supported by the double crush hypothesis (Fig. 47-9). In our series of workmen's compensation patients with thoracic outlet syndrome, all patients had clinical evidence of either carpal or cubital tunnel syndrome but only 24 percent had electrical evidence of these syndromes.

atherosclerotic factors may contribute (Rosati and Lord, 1961). Bony abnormalities are present in approximately 30 percent of patients, in the form of either cervical rib, bifid first rib, fusion of first and second ribs, clavicular deformities, or the result previous thoracoplasties (Urschel, et al., 1968). These abnormalities can be visualized on the plain posteroanterior chest film, but special radiographic views of the lower cervical spine may be required in some cases of cervical ribs.

Histopathology of Chronic Human Nerve Compression

Nerve compresson is treated with surgical release rather than surgical excision. Thus, there are very few studies providing any documentation of the histopathology of human chronic nerve compression. An experimental rodent and primate model was developed, which reliably produces changes mimicking those seen with chronic human nerve compression.

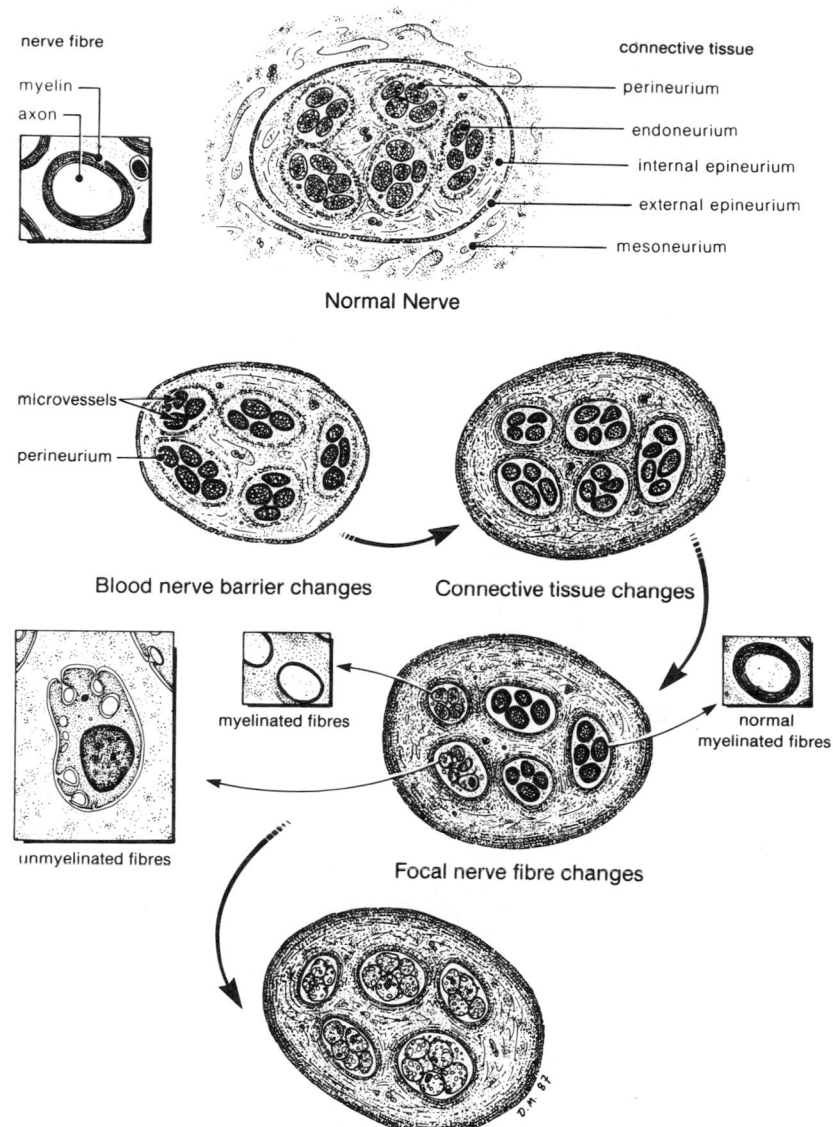

Figure 47-3. The histopathology of chronic nerve compression progresses across a broad spectrum from blood-nerve barrier changes to connective tissue changes to focal nerve fiber changes and finally to wallerian degeneration. (From Mackinnon SE, Dellon AL: Surgery of the Peripheral Nerve. p. 42. Thieme, New York, 1988, with permission.)

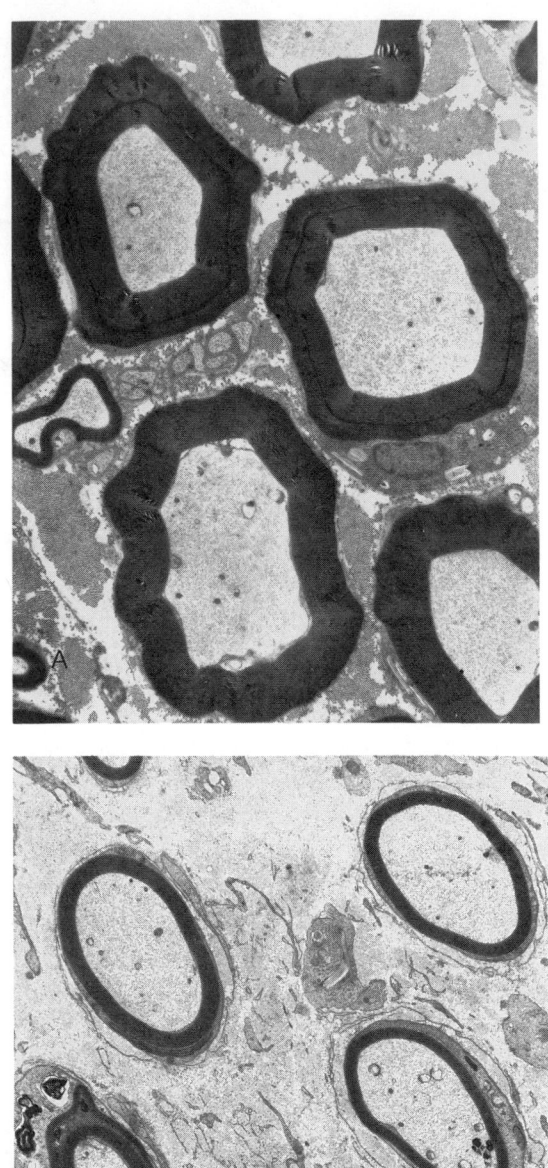

Figure 47-4.   **(A)** A normal myelinated fiber population. **(B)** With chronic nerve decompression, segmental demyelination occurs. The large myelinated fibers are associated with only a thin ring of myelin (From Mackinnon SE, Dellon AL: Chronic human nerve compression: a histological assessment. Neuropathol Appl Neurobiol 12:547, 1986, with permission.)

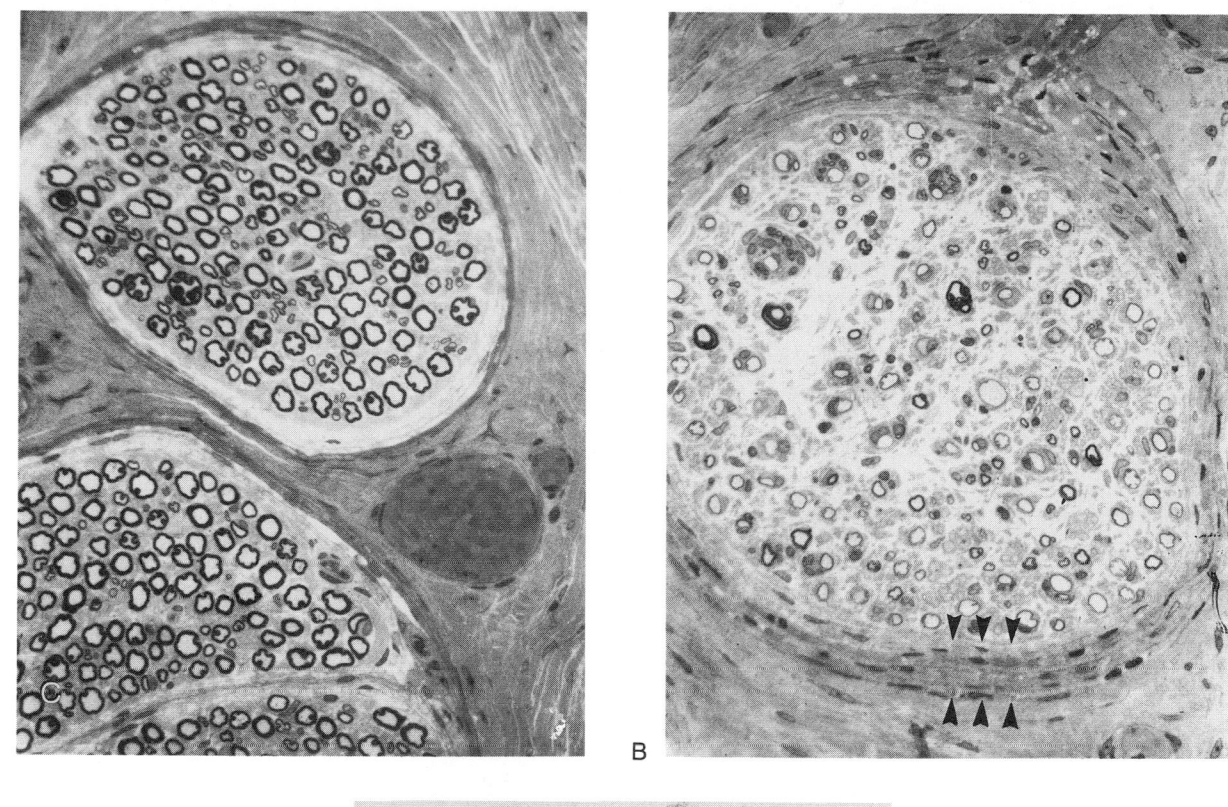

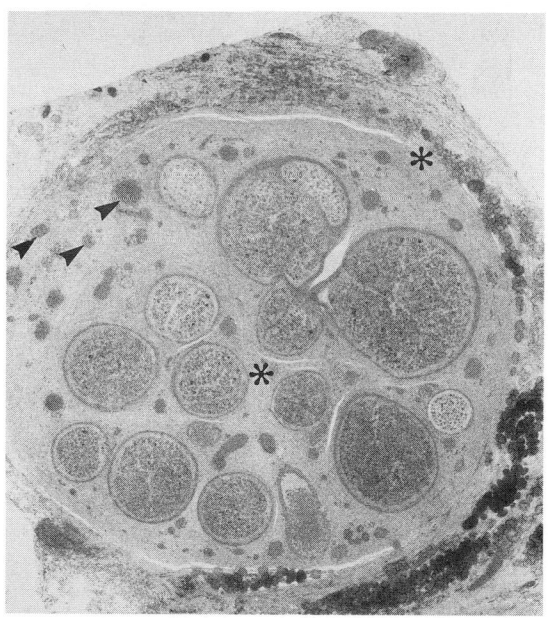

Figure 47-5. **(A)** The cross section of the compressed median nerve in a primate demonstrates increased vascularity and increased epineural connective tissue. **(B)** A fascicle demonstrating wallerian degeneration and severe histologic changes is noted (arrows indicate perineurial thickening). **(C)** Fascicles adjacent to those seen in Fig. 47-4B show a more normal histologic pattern. (From Mackinnon SE, Dellon AL, Hudson AR: A primate model for chronic nerve compression. J Reconstr Microsurg 1:185, 1985, with permission.)

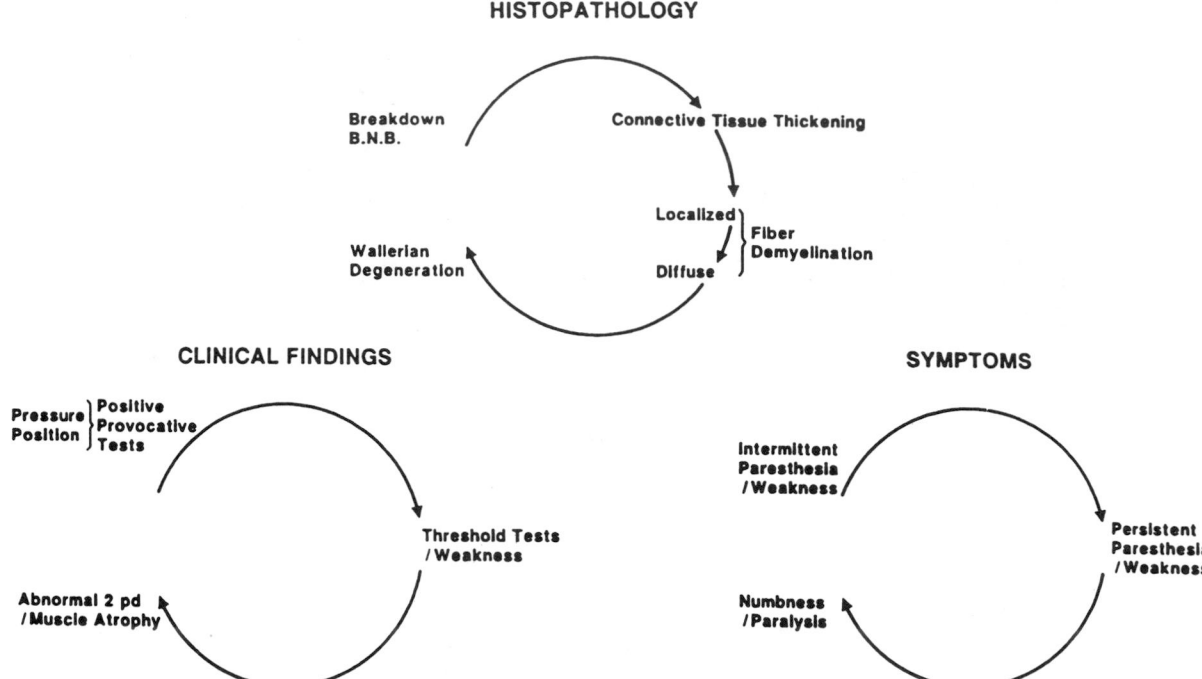

Figure 47-6. The continuum of chronic nerve compression is illustrated. The histopathologic changes begin with breakdown of the blood-nerve barrier and conclude with wallerian degeneration. The patient's presentation, including subjective symptoms and clinical evaluation, will parallel the histopathology of the nerve.

A clinical entity associated with an increase in jobs requiring repetitive activity (assembly lines, keyboarding) and termed *cumulative trauma disorder* or *repetitive stress disorder* is now recognized. A significant component of this disorder relates to multilevel nerve compression. Specific anatomic structures and particular positions of the extremity will increase the pressure around the nerve and ultimately produce symptomatic nerve compression. (If the wrist is in other than a neutral position, pressures increase around the median nerve in the carpal tunnel; elbow flexion produces increased pressure around the ulnar nerve in the cubital tunnel; and elevation of the arms overhead theoretically increases pressure around the lower trunk of the brachial plexus.) Patients with cumulative trauma disorders will frequently have bilateral multilevel nerve compression.

Hand surgeons who are trained to focus on the distal portion of the extremity are encouraged to evaluate their patients for concomitant thoracic outlet syndrome. Similarly, thoracic surgeons treating patients with thoracic outlet syndrome will find a significant association between this syndrome and the carpal and cubital tunnel syndromes. We now recognize that both upper extremities work together as a single functional unit and that problems in one extremity can soon be associated with complaints in the opposite extremity secondary to compensatory overuse. (Similarly, physicians recognize that pathology at an ankle joint can eventually result in pathology at the contralateral hip joint.) The patient should be evaluated for pathology at all points in the "circle" (wrist, elbow,

shoulder, and neck), all components of which are now recognized to be interrelated (Fig. 47-10). Initial conservative management can be directed at several components of this circle. Surgery directed at distal problems in the extremity can result in an improvement in overall function without necessitating proximal surgical intervention. However, if significant pathology exists in the neck or the region of the thoracic outlet, distal procedures may improve but will not completely relieve the patient's symptoms.

DIAGNOSIS

Symptoms and Signs

The symptomatology of thoracic outlet syndrome depends on whether the nerves and/or blood vessels are compressed in the cervicoaxillary canal. Neurogenic manifestations are observed more frequently than vascular ones. Symptoms consist of pain and paresthesias, which are present in approximately 95 percent of cases, as well as motor weakness and occasionally atrophy of hypothenar and interosseous muscles, (the ulnar type of atrophy), which occur in approximately 10 percent. The symptoms occur most commonly in areas supplied by the ulnar nerve, which include the medial aspects of the arm and hand, the fifth finger, and the lateral aspects of the fourth finger. The onset of pain is usually insidiuous and commonly involves the neck, shoulder, arm, and hand. The pain and paresthesias may be precipitated by

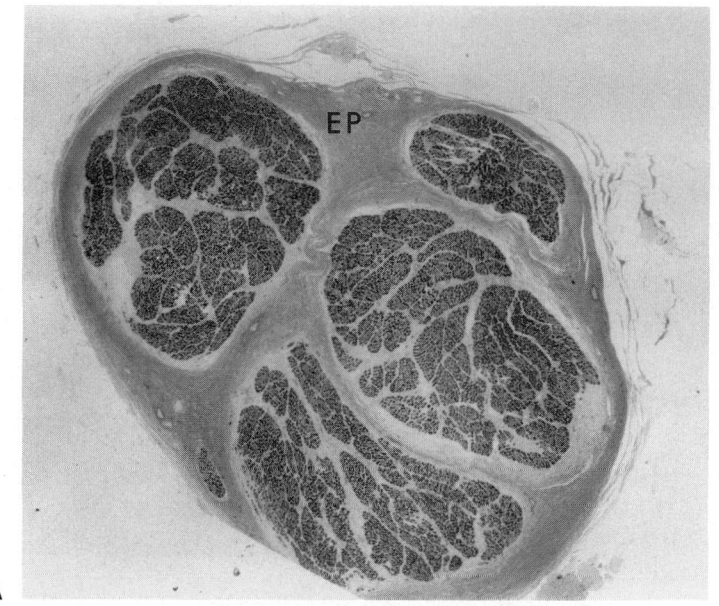

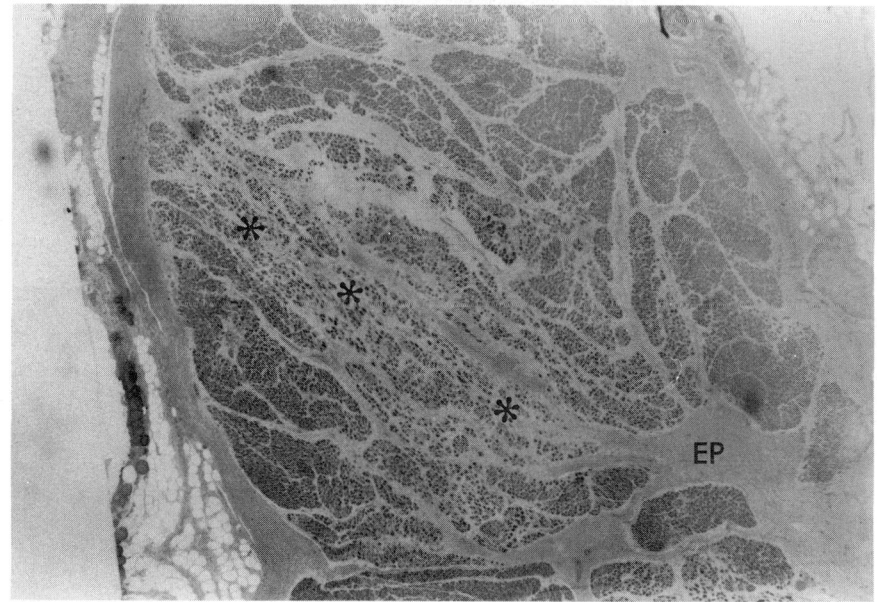

Figure 47-7.   **(A&B)** Photomicrographs of cross section of **(A)** C5 root and **(B)** T1, noting increased epineural (EP) thickening, especially in T1, and fiber fallout in T1 (asterisks). (Toluidine blue, × 88.)

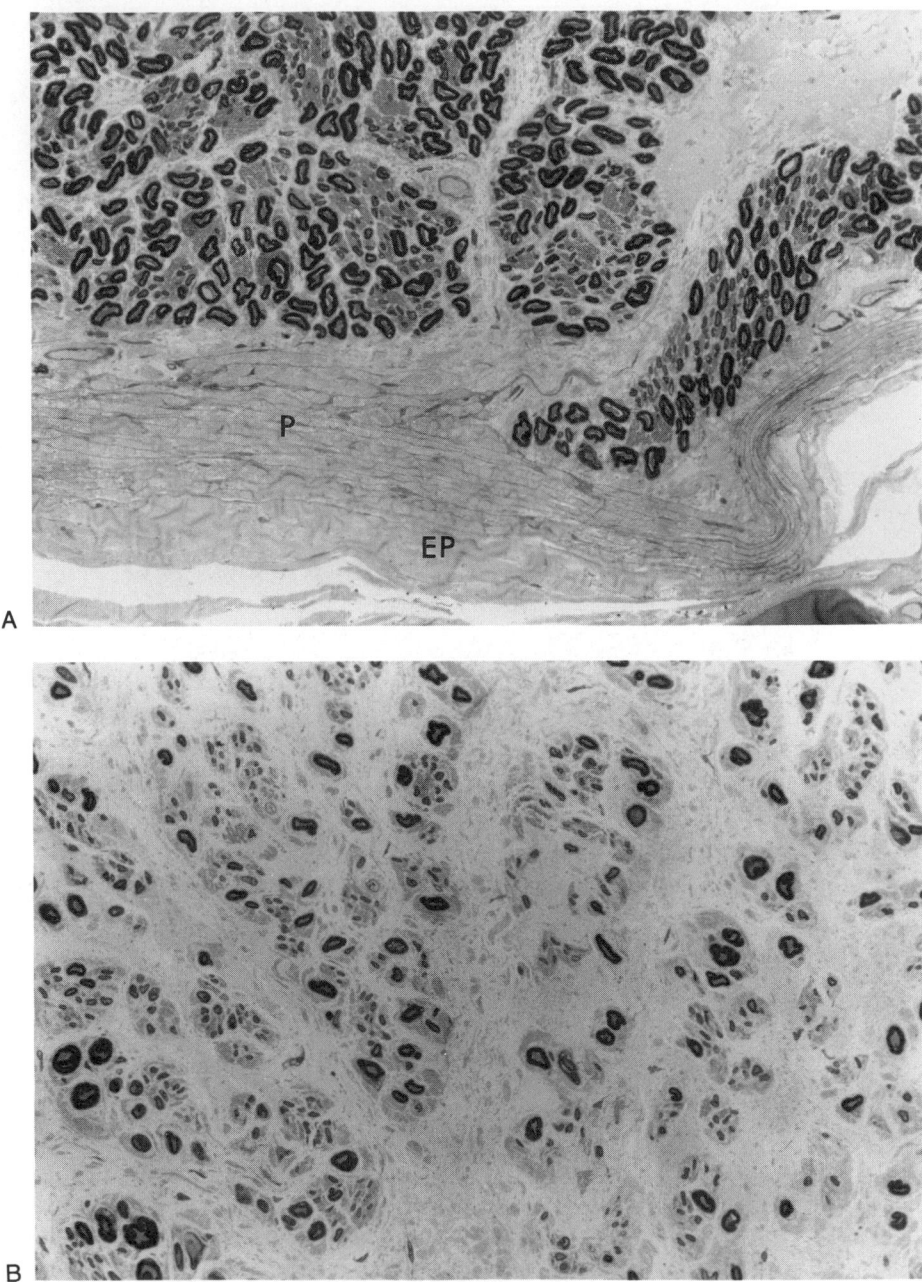

Figure 47-8. Higher-power micrograph of **(A)** C5 and **(B)** T1. Note perineurial (P) thickening in C5 and marked fiber fallout in T1 (Toluidine blue × 140.)

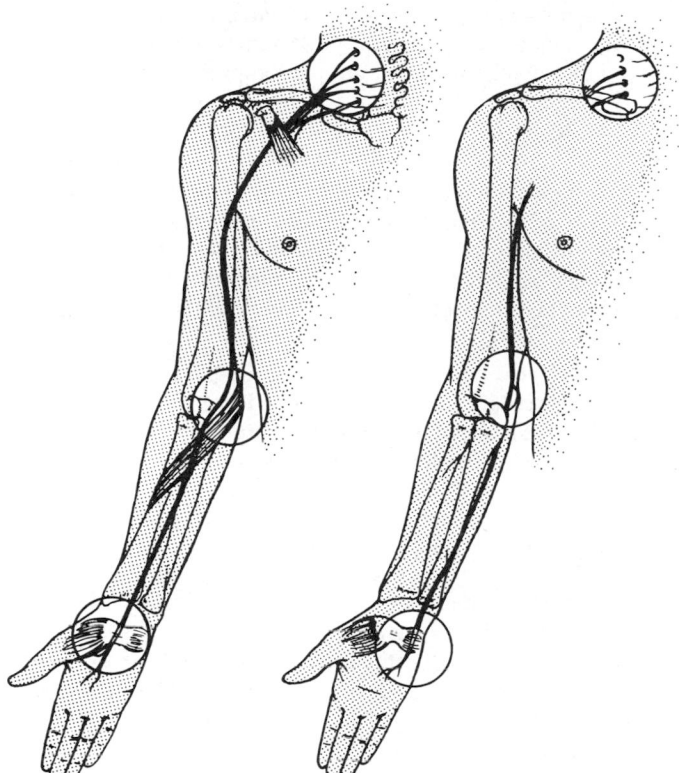

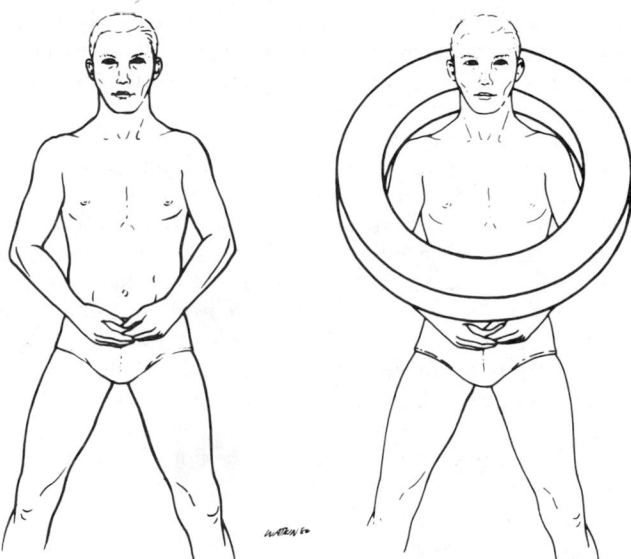

Figure 47-10. The upper extremities and the cervical thoracic region work as a single unit. Pathology anywhere along this "ring" or "circle" will predispose some other area for overuse. The overcompensation can produce symptoms at new sites. Evaluation of patients with upper extremity complaints should include examination for problems at all points on the circle.

Figure 47-9. The double crush hypothesis can be extrapolated to a multiple crush hypothesis. At the left, carpal tunnel is associated with median nerve compression in the forearm and cervical disc disease. At the right, thoracic outlet is associated with cubital tunnel and ulnar nerve compression in Guyon's canal.

strenuous physical exercises or sustained physical efforts with the arm in abduction and the neck in hyperextension. Symptoms may be initiated by sleeping with the arms abducted and the hands clasped behind the neck. In other cases, trauma to the upper extremities or the cervical spine is a precipitating factor. Physical examination may be noncontributory. When present, objective physical findings usually consist of hypesthesia along the medial aspects of the forearm and hand. Atrophy, when evident, is usually described in the hypothenar and interosseous muscles, with clawing of the fourth and fifth fingers. In the upper type of thoracic outlet syndrome, in which components of C5 and C6 nerves are involved in compression, pain is usually in the deltoid area and the lateral aspects of the arm. The presence of this pain should induce action to exclude a herniated cervical disk (Rosati and Lord, 1961). Entrapment of C7 and C8 nerve components that contribute to the median nerve produces symptoms in the index finger and sometimes the middle finger. Components of the C5–T1 nerves can occur at the thoracic outlet because of a cervical rib and can produce symptoms of various degrees in the distribution of these nerves.

In some patients the pain is atypical, involving the anterior chest wall or parascapular area, and is termed *pseudoangina* because it simulates angina pectoris. These patients may have normal coronary arteriograms and ulnar nerve conduction

velocities decreased to 48 m/s or less, which strongly suggests the diagnosis of thoracic outlet syndrome. The shoulder, arm, and hand symptoms that usually provide the clue for the diagnosis of thoracic outlet syndrome initially may be absent or minimal as compared with the severity of the chest pain. The diagnosis of thoracic outlet syndrome is frequently overlooked; many of these patients are committed to becoming "cardiac cripples" without an appropriate diagnosis, or they may develop severe psychological depression when told that their coronary arteries are normal and that they have no significant etiology for their pain (Urschel, et al., 1973).

Symptoms of arterial compression include coldness, weakness, easy fatigability of the arm and hand, and pain that is usually diffuse (Urschel, et al., 1968; Urschel and Razzuk, 1972). Raynaud's phenomenon is noted in approximately 7.5 percent of patients with thoracic outlet syndrome (Urschel, et al., 1968). Unlike Raynaud's disease, which is usually bilateral and symmetric and elicited by cold or emotion, Raynaud's phemonenon in neurovascular compression is usually unilateral and is more likely to be precipitated by hyperabduction of the involved arm, turning of the head, or carrying of heavy objects. Sensitivity to cold may also be present. Symptoms include sudden onset of coldness and blanching of one or more fingers, followed slowly by cyanosis and persistent rubor. Vascular symptoms in neurovascular compression may be precursors of permanent arterial thrombosis (Rosati and Lord, 1961). Arterial occlusion, usually of the subclavian artery when present, is manifested by persistent coldness, cyanosis or pallor of the fingers, and in some cases ulceration or gangrene. Palpation in the parascapular area may reveal prominent pulsation, which indicates poststenotic dilatation or aneyrusm of the subclavian artery.

Less frequently, the symptoms are those of venous obstruction or occlusion, commonly recognized as effort thrombosis or Paget-Schroetter syndrome. The condition characteristically results in edema, dicoloration of the arm, distension of the superficial veins of the limb and shoulder, and some degree of aches and pains. In some patients the condition is observed upon waking; in others it follows sustained efforts with the arm in abduction. Sudden backward and downward bracing of the shoulders, heavy lifting, or strenuous physical activity involving the arm may constrict the vein and initiate venospasm, with or without subsequent thrombosis. In cases of definite venous thrombosis there is usually moderate tenderness over the axillary vein on examination, and a cordlike structure may be felt, which corresponds to the course of the vein. The acute symptoms may subside in a few weeks or days as the collateral circulation develops. Recurrence follows when the collateral circulation is inadequate (Rosati and Lord, 1961).

Objective physical findings are more common in patients with primarily vascular rather than neural compression. Loss or diminution of radial pulse and reproduction of symptoms can be elicited by the three classical clinical maneuvers: the Adson or scalene test (Adson, 1947), the costoclavicular test, and the hyperabduction test (Urschel and Razzuk, 1973a).

Diagnostic Methods

The diagnosis of thoracic outlet syndrome includes history, physical and neurologic examination, films of the chest and cervical spine, electromyogram, and ulnar nerve conduction velocity. In some cases with atypical manifestations, other diagnostic procedures such as cervical myelography, peripheral (Rosenberg, 1966) or coronary arteriography, or phlebography (Adams, et al., 1968) should be considered. A detailed history and physical and neurologic examinations can often result in a tentative diagnosis of neurovascular compression. This diagnosis is strengthened when one or more of the classic clincial maneuvers is positive and is confirmed by the finding of decreased ulnar nerve conduction velocity (Urschel and Razzuk, 1972).

Clinical Maneuvers

The clinical evaluation is best based on the physical findings of loss or decrease of radial pulses and reproduction of symptoms, which can be elicited by the three classic maneuvers and the modified Roos test.

1. The Adson or scalene test (Adson, 1951) (Fig. 47-11A) consists of a maneuver that tightens the anterior and middle scalene muscle and thus decreases the interspace and magnifies any pre-existing compression of the subclavian artery and brachial plexus. The patient is instructed to take and hold a deep breath, extend the neck fully, and turn the head toward the side. Obliteration or decrease of the radial pulse suggests compression (Rosati and Lord, 1961; Urschel and Razzuk, 1973b).

2. In the costoclavicular (Halstead) test, (Fig. 47-11B) the shoulders are drawn downward and backward (military position). This maneuver narrows the costoclavicular space by approximating the clavicle to the first rib and thus tends to compress the neurovascular bundle. Changes in the radial pulse with production of symptoms indicate compression (Rosati and Lord, 1961; Urschel and Razzuk, 1973b).

3. In the hyperabduction test (Wright) (Fig. 47-11C), the arm is hyperabducted to 180 degrees, which pulls the components of the neurovascular bundle around the pectoralis minor tendon, the coracoid process, and the head of the humerus. If the radial pulse is decreased, compression should be suspected (Rosati and Lord, 1961; Urschel and Razzuk, 1973).

4. Roos (1966) has described a test of 90 degrees abduction with external rotation of the shoulder to reproduce symptoms. He has modified this by incorporation of a 3-minute stress test of rapidly closing and opening the hand (Fig. 47-11D).

Radiographic Findings

Films of the chest and cervical spine are helpful in revealing bony abnormalities, particularly cervical ribs and bone degenerative changes. If osteophytic changes and intervertebral space narrowing are present on plain cervical films, a cervical computed tomographic (CT) or magnetic resonance imaging (MRI) scan should be obtained to rule out bony encroachment and narrowing of the spinal canal and the intervertebral foramina.

Electrodiagnostic Testing

Sensory Testing. Just as the histopathology of chronic nerve compression spans a broad spectrum, so will the patient's clinical findings. Initially, patients may be completely asymptomatic at rest and become symptomatic only with positional or pressure provocative maneuvers. With time, patients may have persistent subtle abnormalities in the sensory system, which can only be detected with sensitive tests that determine the threshold of the system by vibratory or pressure threshold measurements. Eventually, there will be nerve injury and loss of nerve fibers, with loss of discriminatory function as measured with two-point discrimination.

Recent efforts have been directed toward developing tests to evaluate sensory function in the hand. The accepted tests and the correlation between these tests and the fiber receptor system are understood.

Provocative tests are used to elicit symptoms from a patient who is asymptomatic at rest. These include percussion of the nerve (Tinel's sign), and pressure and positional provocative tests. In patients with thoracic outlet syndrome, these tests are performed at the common nerve entrapment sites in the upper extremity (carpal tunnel, median nerve in the forearm, cubital tunnel, and brachial plexus). The examiner percusses over the nerve with four to six taps, and the presence or absence of a tingling sensation within the distribution of that nerve is recorded (Tinel's sign). Movement and pressure provocative tests are applied for a total of 60 seconds and are considered positive if parasthesia, numbness, or pain occurs in the appropriate nerve distribution. Movement provocative tests include arm elevation, elbow flexion, and wrist

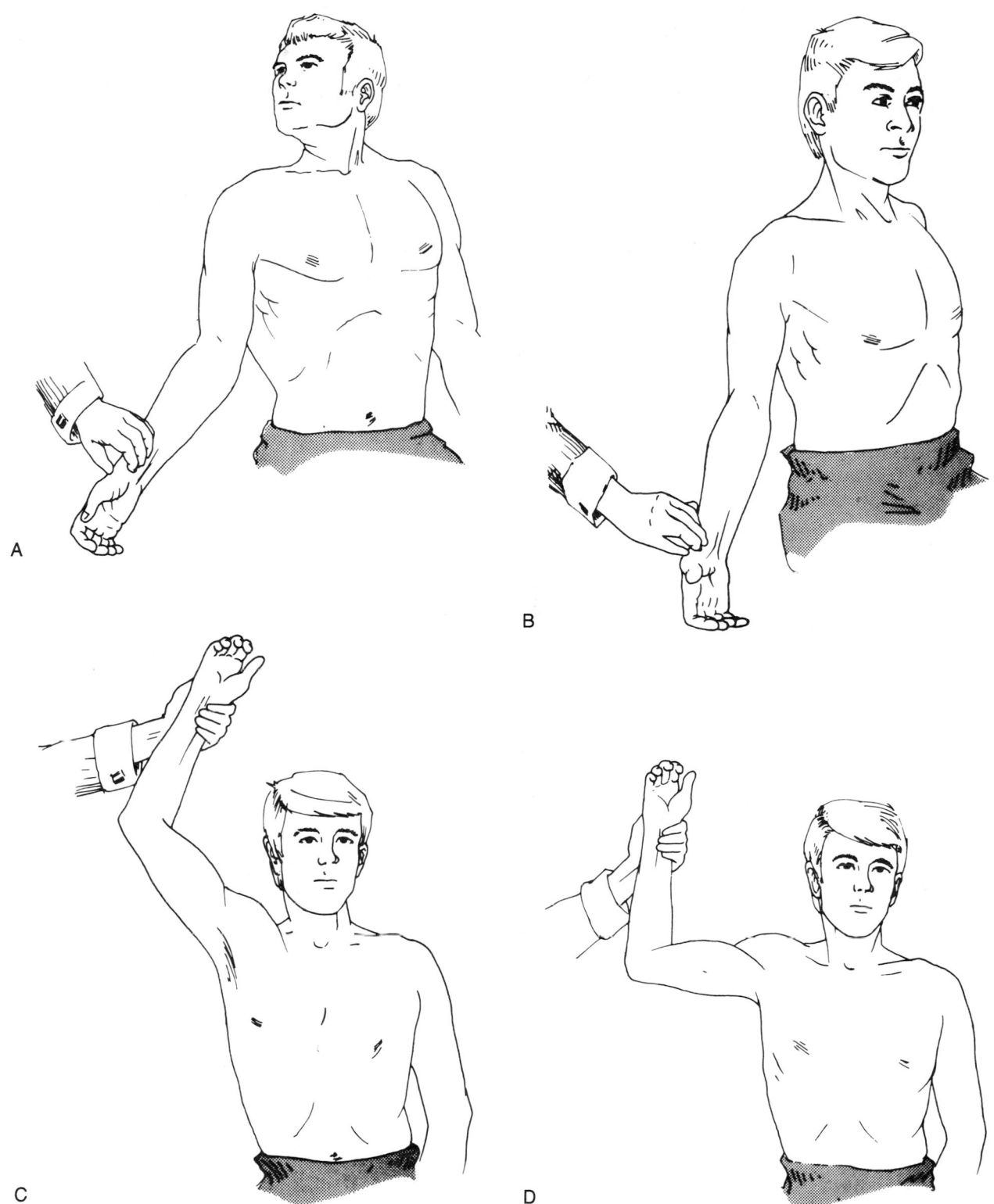

Figure 47-11. **(A)** The Adson maneuver occludes the pulse when the head is turned toward the affected side and the patient inspires deeply. Others have modified this test by turning the head to the unaffected side and requiring reproduction of the patient's symptoms. **(B)** The Halstead maneuver puts the patient in a military position with the shoulders braced down to the side to obliterate the pulse. This test is now considered positive if the symptoms are reproduced. **(C)** Wright described a hyperabduction maneuver to obliterate the pulse, with reproduction of the patient's symptoms being considered a positive test. Wright suggested that the elbows be flexed. We have modified this test to keep the elbows extended, as elbow flexion will reproduce symptomatology with ulnar nerve compression in the cubital tunnel. We consider reproduction of the patient's symptoms after 1 minute of arm elevation to be a positive test. We can decrease the time necessary for a positive test by placing digital pressure over the brachial plexus in the supraclavicular fossa. **(D)** Roos' test has been modified by Roos to add a 3-minute stress test of rapidly opening and closing the hand. The test will be positive if the patient's symptoms are reproduced. (From Luoma A, Nelems B: Thoracic outlet syndrome, thoracic surgery perspective. Neurosurg Clin N Am 2:187, 1991, with permission.)

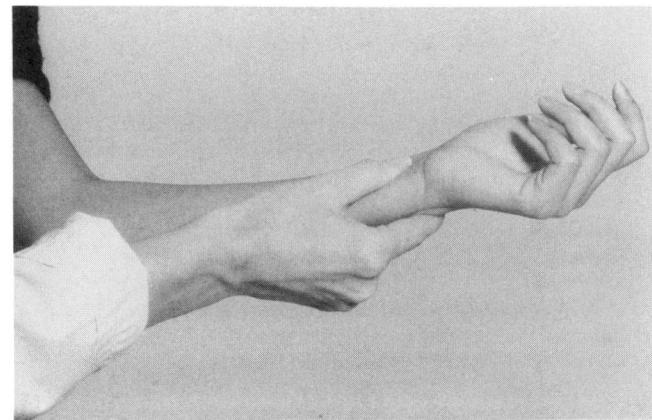

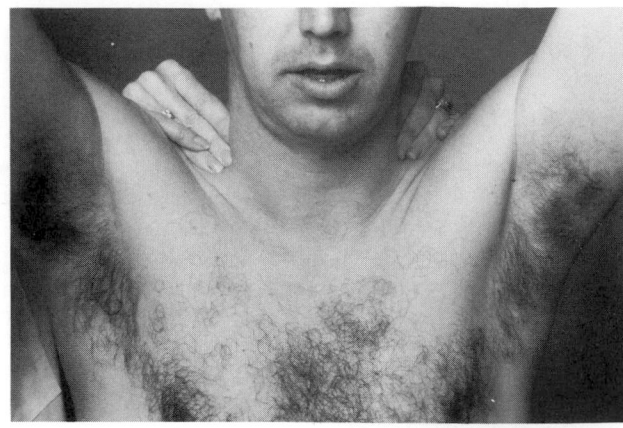

Figure 47-12. **(A)** Pressure provocative tests can be used to reproduce symptomatology; in particular, pressure over the median nerve just proximal to the carpal tunnel will produce paresthesia in the distribution of the median nerve within just a few seconds if the carpal tunnel syndrome is present. This similar test can be used to evaluate cubital tunnel syndrome with pressure over the ulnar nerve in the cubital tunnel. **(B)** Pressure over the brachial plexus and supraclavicular fossa will produce paresthesia in the hand in patients with thoracic outlet syndrome. Symptoms can be accelerated by combining this with elevation of the upper extremities above the head.

flexion (Phalen's sign). The pressure provocative tests include direct pressure with the examiner's thumb or fingertips on the brachial plexus, the ulnar nerve in the cubital tunnel, and the median nerve in the proximal forearm and just proximal to the carpal tunnel (Fig. 47-12). A rest period of approximately 1 minute is permitted between each test to allow return to the asymptomatic state.

Several instruments can be used to measure vibration thresholds (Fig. 47-13A&B). The threshold of the rapidly adapting fiber receptor system can be assessed both qualitatively with a tuning fork and quantitatively with a vibrometer. The "wrong end" of a 256-cps tuning fork is held against the skin. This end of the tuning fork is used in order to provide adequate amplitude for perception of the stimulus. A fixed-frequency (120-cps) variable-amplitude Vibratron II (Sensortek, Clifton, NJ) can be used to quantify the threshold of the quickly adapting fibers. The vibrating portion of the Vibratron II is placed against the skin, and the smallest stimulus perceived is identified as the baseline vibration threshold and recorded in micrometers of motion. (Variable-frequency, variable-amplitude vibrometers are also available that provide a "vibrogram" of the patient's response to a number of frequencies of vibration. As the higher frequencies of vibration are the most sensitive to nerve compression, such an instrument is potentially of great interest in evaluating patients with thoracic outlet syndrome.)

Pressure thresholds can be assessed quantitatively with Semmes-Weinstein monofilaments. These nylon monofilaments are applied perpendicular to the cutaneous surface, and pressure is increased until bending of the monofilament is observed. Probes of increasing weight are used, with the lightest monofilament marked 1.65 and the heaviest marked 6.65. The number of the probe on the filament represents the logarithm of ten times the force in tenths of a milligram that is required to bow the monofilament. The number of the lightest probe that will elicit perception and localization of pressure is recorded (Fig. 47-13C).

An assessment of innervation density provides an indication of the number of innervated receptors. The innervation density of the slowly adapting receptors is measured by a static two-point discrimination test, and that of the rapidly adapting receptors is measured by a moving two-point discrimination test. Moving and static two-point discrimination are assessed with a Disk-Criminator (Neuroregen, Baltimore). The moving discrimination test is carried out by slowly moving the prongs of the Disk-Criminator longitudinally with just enough pressure to elicit a response. The subject is then asked to identify if one or two prongs is felt. The smallest spacing at which the subject is able to correctly identify two of three trials is recorded in millimeters (Fig. 47-14). The simple analogy shown in Fig. 47-15 helps to describe and understand the relationship between innervation density and threshold and the tests used to measure sensibility.

In a prospective study we evaluated 50 patients whom we believed to have thoracic outlet syndrome. The physical examination included provocative tests (positional, percussion [Tinel], and compressive) and sensory evaluation (baseline and postprovocative vibration thresholds and two-point discrimination). In 47 (94 percent) of these patients, provocative position and compression tests were positive (Fig. 47-16), and two-point discrimination was normal in 49 (98 percent). Measurements of sensory thresholds during provocation of symptoms were significantly elevated as compared with thresholds measured at rest.

Somatosensory Potentials. Somatosensory evoked potentials (SSEPs) have been suggested in the diagnosis of thoracic outlet syndrome to deal with the proximal location of the compressive problem. Machleder et al. (1987) demonstrated in a group of 80 patients with thoracic outlet syndrome that 74 percent had abnormal SSEPs. Similarly, Yiannikas and Walsh (1983) found SSEPs to be useful in the diagnosis. By contrast, Borg, et al. (1988) found SSEPs to be abnormal only in patients with positive clinical signs. Both Borg et al.

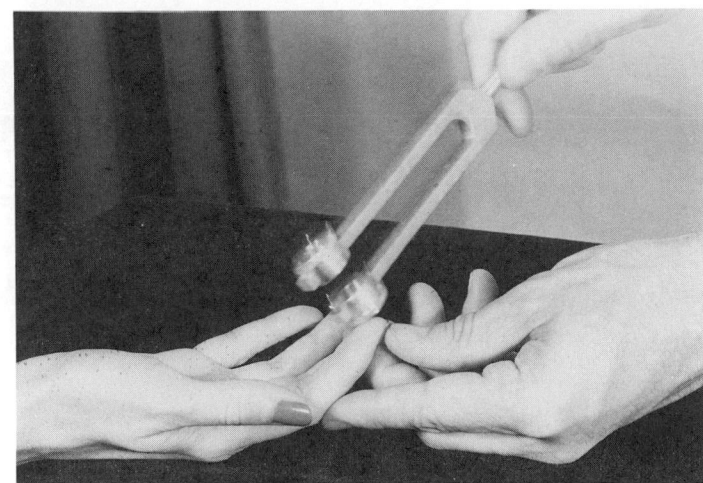

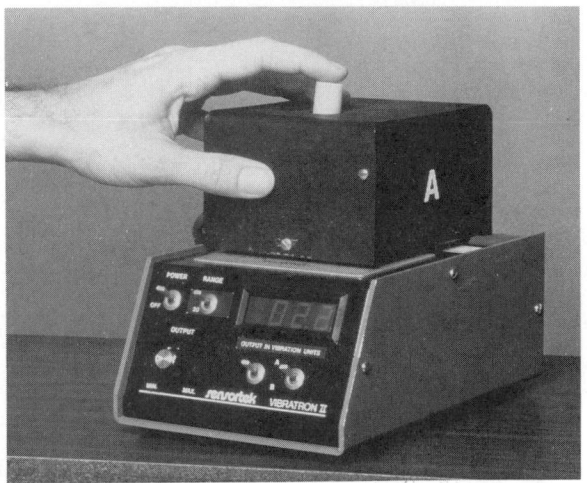

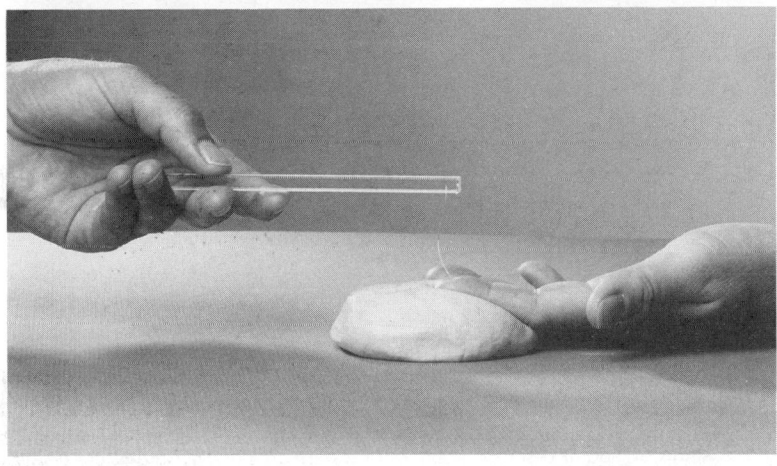

Figure 47-13. **(A)** Threshold testing includes vibration and pressure assessment. Response to vibration can be measured qualitatively with a tuning fork. **(B)** Vibration thresholds can be measured quantitatively with a fixed-frequency variable-amplitude vibrometer. **(C)** Pressure thresholds are measured with Semmes-Weinstein monofilaments (From Mackinnon SE, Dellon AL: Surgery of the Peripheral Nerve. p. 71. Thieme, New York, 1988, with permission.)

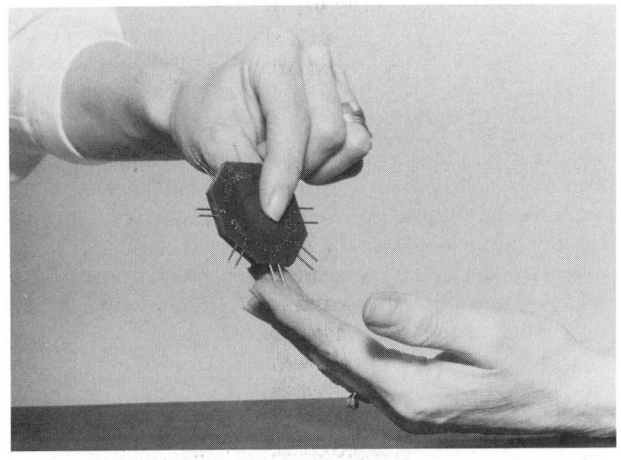

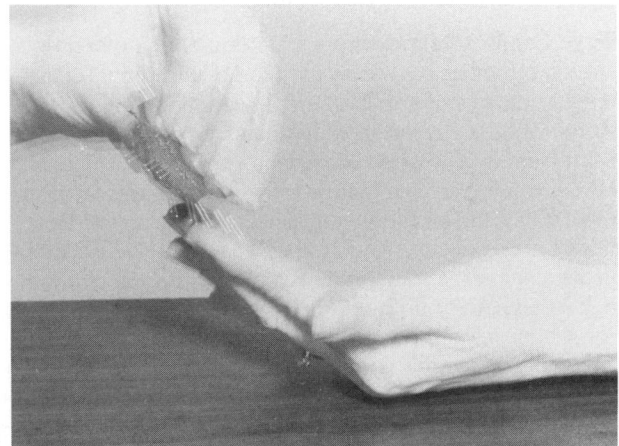

Figure 47-14. **(A)** Two-point discrimination is measured with a Disk-Criminator. **(B)** Moving two-point discrimination is measured by moving the two prongs of the Disk-Criminator across the surface of the skin. (From Mackinnon SE, Dellon AL: Surgery of the Peripheral Nerve. p. 72. Thieme, New York, 1988, with permission.)

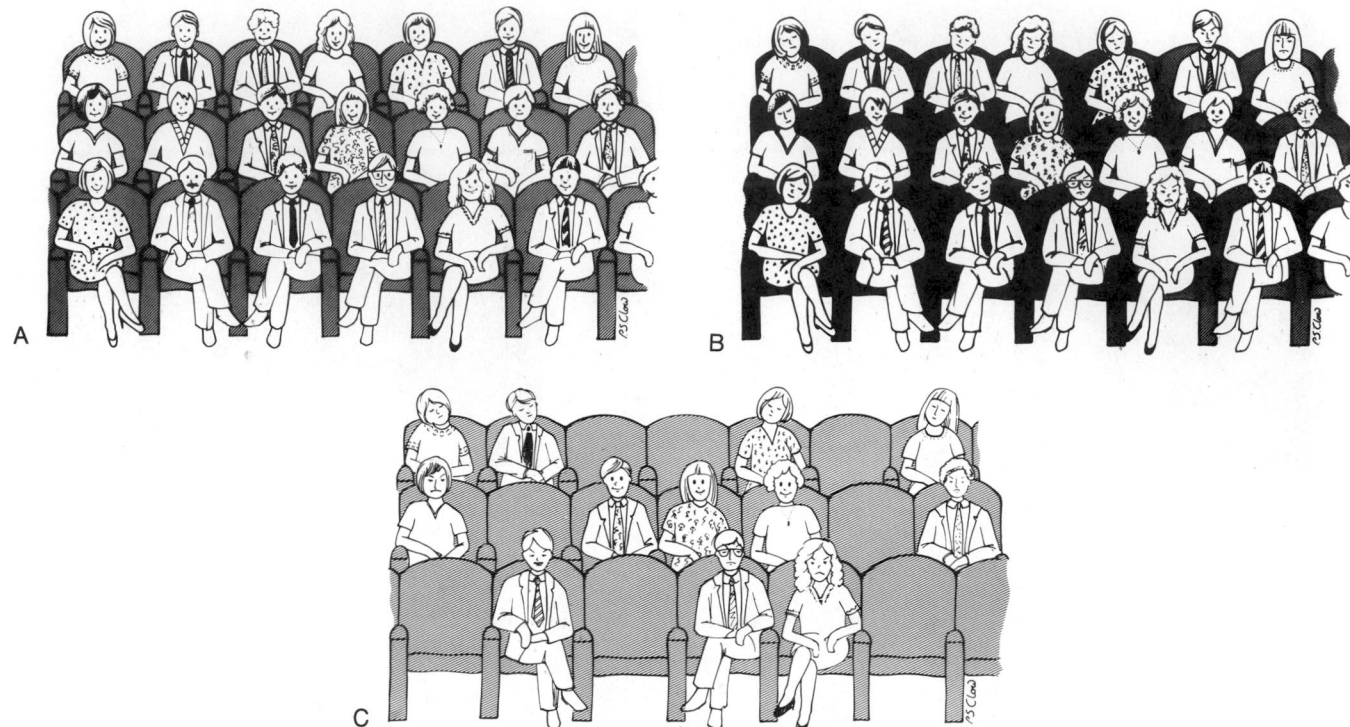

Figure 47-15. **(A)** A simple analogy helps to describe the relationship between innervation density and threshold. If each person in the audience is considered as a single-fiber sensory receptor unit, the number of people present in the audience can be considered the innervation density. A test of threshold will evaluate the "status, health, or well-being" of the individual. If all the seats in the auditorium are full and the individuals in the audience are "awake and content," all testing for fiber receptor function (both innervation density and threshold tests) will be normal. **(B)** Threshold testing will be abnormal (vibration and Semmes-Weinstein monofilaments) if the individuals are not "awake and content" but are "asleep or unhappy." It will take more effort (i.e., greater pressure, larger amplitude) to "wake up" these sleepy receptors. Moving and static two-point discrimination will be normal, since all members of the audience are present and eventually will respond to stimulation. **(C)** If individuals in the audience vacate the auditorium, the innervation density testing (two-point discrimination) will be abnormal. If the remaining individuals are other than happy and content, the threshold tests will be abnormal as well. (From Mackinnon SE: Peripheral nerve injuries in the hand. p. 321. In Vistnes LM (ed): How They Do It: Procedures in Plastic and Reconstructive Surgery. Little, Brown, Boston, 1991, with permission.)

and Machleder, et al. stressed the dynamic nature of this compressive neoropathy by suggesting SSEP assessment in first neutral and then stressed positions.

Nerve Conduction Velocities. Determination of nerve conduction velocities is a widely used test in differential diagnosis of the etiologies of arm pain, tingling, and numbness with or without motor weakness of the hand. Such symptoms may result from compression at various sites: in the spine; at the thoracic outlet; around the elbow, where it causes tardy ulnar nerve palsy; or on the flexor aspects of the wrist, where it produces carpal tunnel syndrome. One author (H.C.U.) relies on the ulnar nerve conduction velocity. The other two authors (S.E.M., G.A.P.) do not. For completeness it is reviewed. For diagnosis and localization of the site of compression, cathodal stimulation is applied at various points along the course of the nerve (Razzuk, et al., in press). Motor conduction velocities of the ulnar, median, radial, and musculocutaneous nerves can be measured reliably (Jebsen, 1967). Caldwell and associates (1971) have improved the technique of measuring ulnar nerve conduction velocity for evaluation of patients with thoracic outlet compression. Conduction veloc-

ities over proximal and distal segments of the ulnar nerve are determined by recording the acting potentials generated in the hypothenar or first dorsal interosseous muscle. The points of stimulation are the supraclavicular fossa, middle upper arm, below the elbow, and at the wirst (Urschel and Razzuk, 1972). Electromyography is usually normal in thoracic outlet syndrome.

Measuring Equipment. Electromyographic examination of each upper extremity and determination of conduction velocities are performed with the Meditron 201 AD or 312 electromyograph; a coaxial cable with three needles or surface electrodes are used to record muscle potentials, which appear on the fluorescent screen.

Technique. The conduction velocity is determined by the Krusen-Caldwell technique (Caldwell, et al., 1971). The patient is placed on the examination table with the arm fully extended at the elbow and in about 20 degrees of abduction at the shoulder to facilitate stimulation over the course of the ulnar nerve.

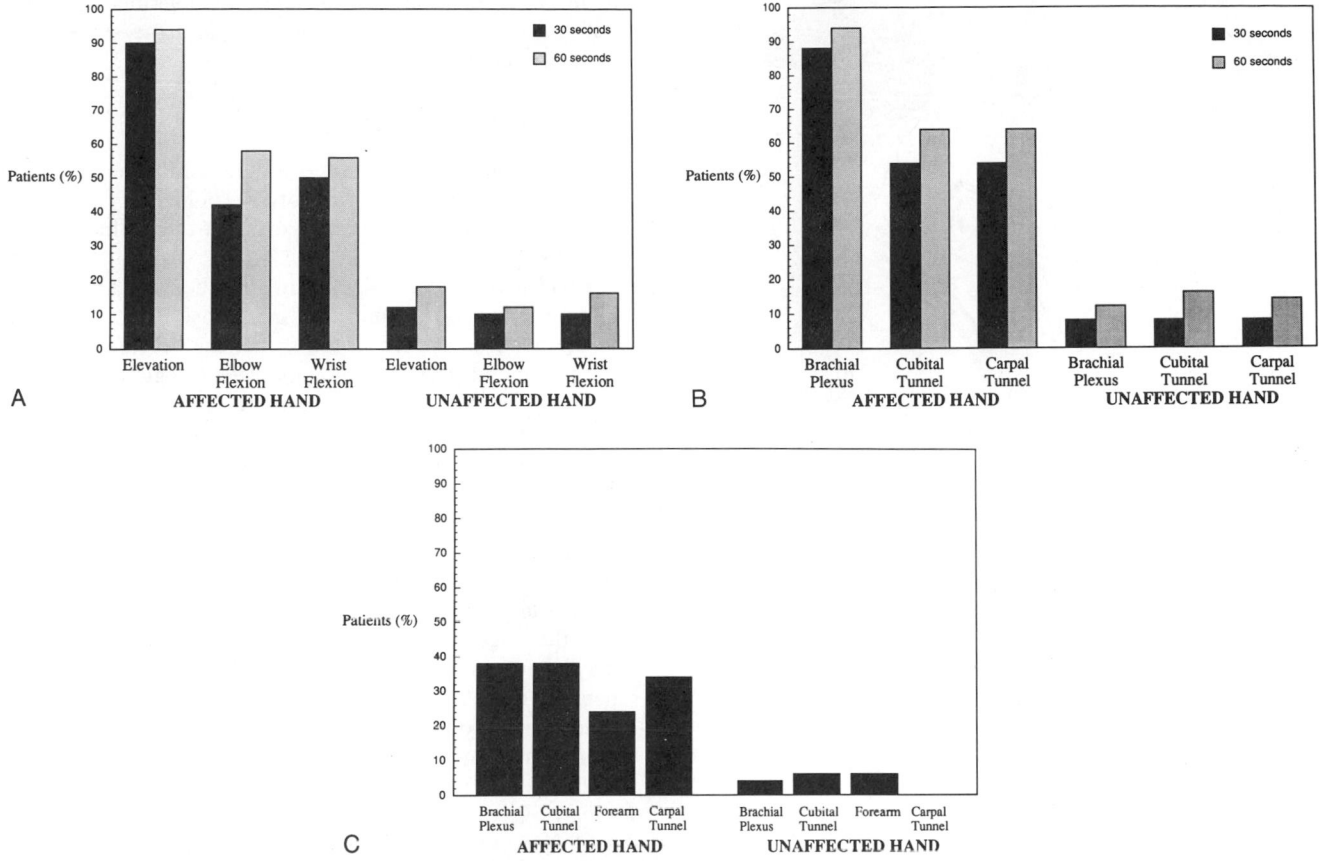

Figure 47-16. **(A)** Distribution of positive provocative movement, showing the percentage of patients represented with positive signs with each provocative movement (arm elevation to reproduce thoracic outlet symptoms, elbow flexion to reproduce cubital tunnel symptoms, and wrist flexion to reproduce carpal tunnel symptoms) within 30 seconds and the total number within 60 seconds. Both affected and unaffected hands are illustrated. **(B)** Distribution of positive pressure provocative movement, showing the percentage of patients with positive signs provoked with pressure of common nerve entrapment sites within 30 seconds and the total number within 60 seconds. **(C)** Distribution of positive Tinel's sign, showing the percentage of patients with a positive Tinel's sign at entrapment sites in the upper extremity (carpal tunnel, forearm, cubital tunnel, and brachial plexus). (From Novak CB, Mackinnon SE, Patterson GA et al: Evaluation of patients for thoracic outlet decompression. J Hand Surg [Am] 18:292, 1992, with permission.)

The ulnar nerve is stimulated at four points by a special stimulation unit, which imparts a 350-V electrical stimulus, which is approximately equivalent to 300 V in view of the patient's skin resistance of 5,000 ohms. Supramaximal stimulation is used at all points to obtain maximal response. The duration of the stimulus is 0.2 ms, except for muscular individuals, for whom it is 0.5 ms. The time of stimulation, conduction delay, and muscle response appear on the electromyograph screen; time markers occur each millisecond on the sweep.

The latency period to stimulation from the four stimulation points to the recording electrode is obtained from the TECA digital recorder or calculated from the tracing on the screen.

Calculation of Velocities. After the latencies, which are expressed in milliseconds, are obtained, the distance in millimeters between two adjacent sites of stimulation is measured with a steel tape. The velocities, which are expressed in meters per second, are calculated by subtracting the distal

latency from the proximal latency and dividing the distance between two points of stimulation by the latency difference (Fig.47-17) according to the formula

Velocity (m/s) =
$$\frac{\text{distance between two adjacent stimulation points (mm)}}{\text{difference in latency (ms)}}$$

Normal Ulnar Nerve Conduction Velocities. The normal values of the ulnar nerve conduction velocities according to the Krusen-Caldwell technique (Caldwell, et al., 1971) are 72 m/s or above across the outlet; 55 m/s or above around the elbow; and 59 m/s or above in the forearm. Wrist delay is 2.5 to 3.5 ms. Decreased velocity in a segment of increased delay at the wrist indicates either compression, injury, neuropathy, or neurologic disorders. Decreased velocity across the outlet is consistent with thoracic outlet syndrome, and decreased velocity around the elbow signifies ulnar nerve entrapment or neuropathy. Increased delay at the wrist is encountered in carpal tunnel syndrome.

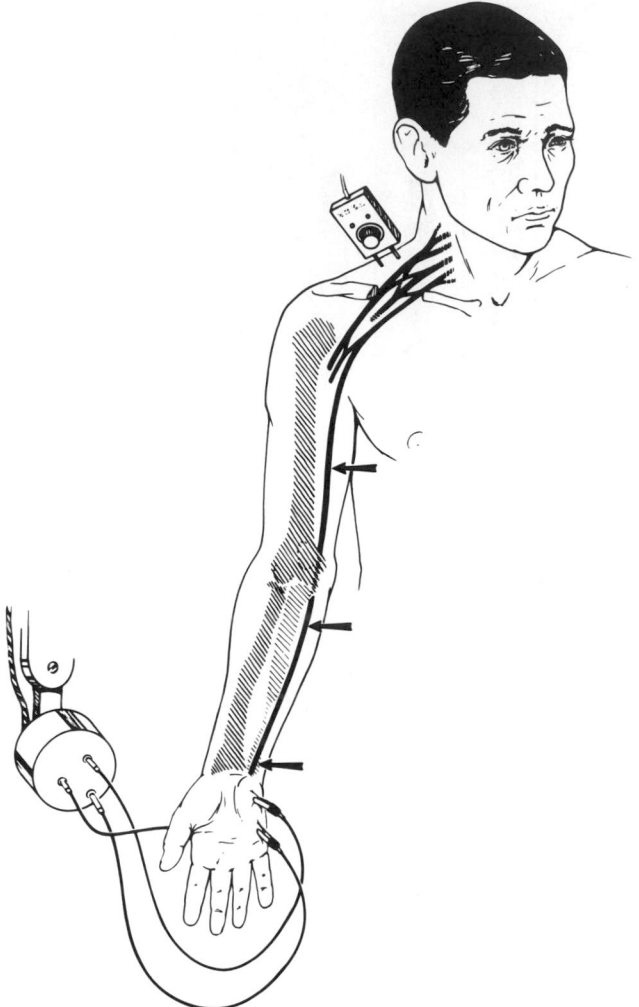

Figure 47-17. Technique for stimulating and recording during the evaluation of nerve conduction velocities.

Grading of Compression. The clinical picture of thoracic outlet syndrome correlates fairly well with the conduction velocity across the outlet. Any value less than 70 m/s indicates neurovascular compression. The severity is graded according to decrease of velocity across the thoracic outlet: compression is called slight when the velocity is 66 to 69 m/s, mild when the velocity is 60 to 65 m/s, moderate when the velocity is 55 to 59 m/s, and severe when the velocity is 54 m/s or less.

Angiography

Simple clinical observations usually suffice to determine the degree of vascular impairment in the upper extremity. Peripheral angiography (Lang, 1962; Rosenberg, 1966) is indicated in some cases, as in the presence of a paraclavicular pulsating mass, the absence of radial pulse, or the presence of supraclavicular or infraclavicular bruits. Retrograde or antegrade arteriograms of the subclavian and brachial arteries should be obtained to demonstrate or localize the pathology (Figs. 47-18 and 47-19). In cases of venous stenosis or obstruction,

as in Paget-Schroetter syndrome, phlebograms are used to determine the extent of thrombosis and the status of the collateral circulation.

Differential Diagnoses

The thoracic outlet syndrome should be differentiated from various neurologic, vascular, cardiac, pulmonary, and esophageal conditions (Rosati and Lord, 1961; Urschel and Razzuk, 1973).

Neurologic causes of pain in the shoulder and arm are more difficult to recognize and may arise from involvement of the nervous system in the spine, the brachial plexus, or the peripheral nerves. A common neurologic cause of pain in the upper extremities is a herniated cervical intervertebral disk. The herniation almost invariably occurs at the interspace between the fifth and sixth or the sixth and seventh cervical vertebrae and produces characteristic symptoms. Onset of pain and stiffness of the neck is manifested with varying frequency. The pain radiates along the medial border of the scapula into the shoulder, occasionally into the anterior chest wall, and down the lateral aspect of the arm, at times into the fingers. Numbness and paresthesias in the fingers may be present. The segmental distribution of pain is a prominent feature. A herniated disk between the C5 and C6 vertebrae, which compresses the C6 nerve root, causes pain or numbness primarily in the thumb and to a lesser extent in the index finger. The biceps muscle and the radial wrist extensor are weak, and the reflex of the biceps muscle is reduced or abolished. A herniated disk between the C6 and C7 vertebrae,

---

Differential Diagnoses

Neurologic phenomena

  Cervical spine: ruptured intervertebral disk, degenerative disease, osteoarthritis, spinal cord tumors

  Brachial plexus: superior sulcus tumors, trauma–postural palsy

  Peripheral nerves: entrapment neuropathy, carpal tunnel–median nerve, ulnar nerve–elbow, radial nerve, suprascapular nerve, medical neuropathies, trauma, tumor

Vascular phenomena

  Arterial: arteriosclerosis–aneurysm (occlusive), thromboangiitis obliterans, embolism, functional (Raynaud's disease), reflex (vasomotor dystrophy), causalgia, vasculitis, collagen disease, panniculitis

  Venous: thrombophlebitis, mediastinal venous obstruction (malignant or benign)

Other diseases

  Angina pectoris

  Esophageal

  Pulmonary

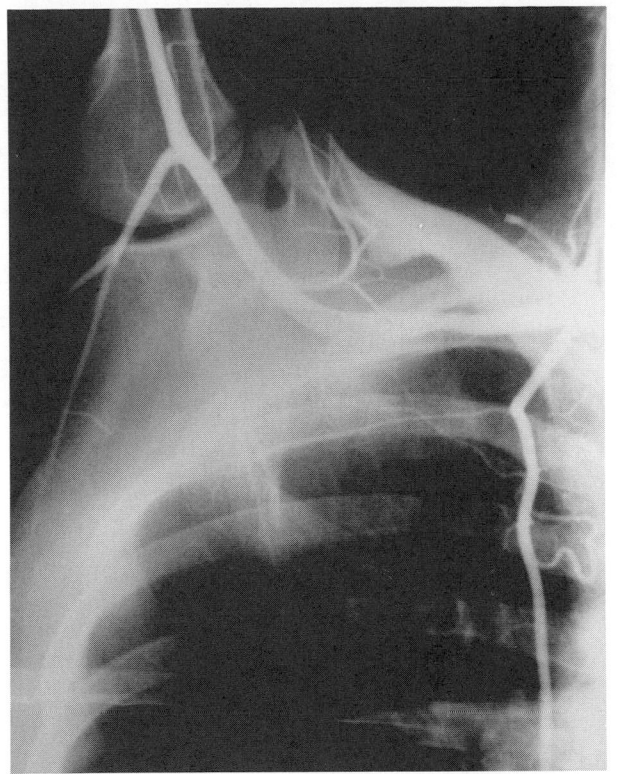

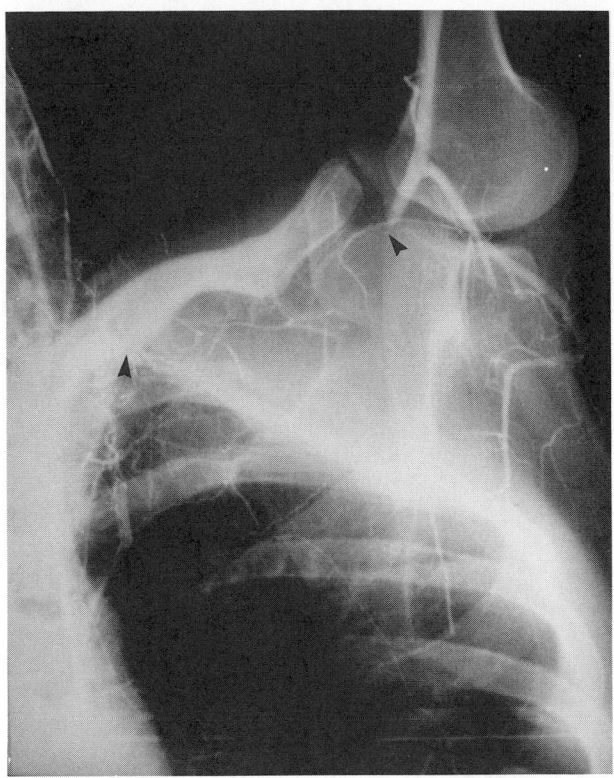

Figure 47-18. In a patient with symptoms of vascular compression in the left upper extremity, an arteriogram with both arms elevated demonstrated **(A)** a patent subclavian artery in the right arm and **(B)** occlusion of the subclavian in the left arm (*arrows*). (Courtesy of P. M. Weeks, M.D., Washington University School of Medicine, St. Louis.)

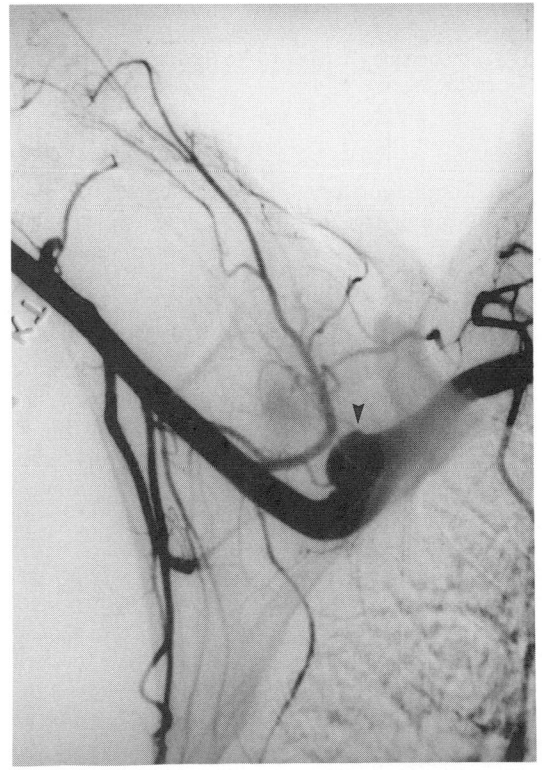

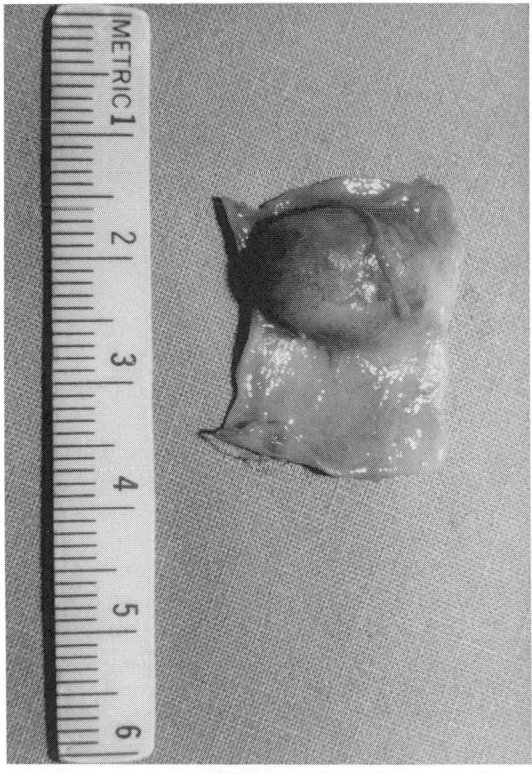

Figure 47-19. Evaluation of vascular thoracic outlet syndrome using an arteriogram may demonstrate unusual findings such as **(A)** this aneurysm (*arrow*), **(B)** which was excised at surgery. (Courtesy of J. J. McDonough, M.D., Cincinnati.)

which compresses the C7 nerve root, produces pain or numbness in the index finger and weakness of index finger flexion and ulnar wrist extension; the triceps muscle is weak, and its reflex is reduced or abolished. Any of these herniated disks may cause numbness along the ulnar border of the arm and hand due to spasm of the scalenus anticus muscle. Rarely, pain and paresthesias in the ulnar distribution may be related to herniation between the C7 and T1 vertebrae, which causes compression of the C8 nerve root. Compression of the latter nerve root produces weakness of intrinsic hand muscles (Krusen, 1968; Rosati and Lord, 1961). Although rupture of the fifth and sixth disks produces hypesthesia in this area, only rupture of the seventh disk produces pain down the medial aspect of the arm. (Rosati and Lord, 1961).

The diagnosis of a ruptured cervical disk is based primarily on the history and physical findings; lateral films of the cervical spine reveal loss or reversal of cervical curvature with the apex of the reversal of curvature at the level of the disk involved. Electromyography can localize the site and extent of the nerve root irritation. When a herniated disk is suspected, cervical myelography should be done to confirm the diagnosis (Krusen, 1968; Rosati and Lord, 1961).

Another condition that causes upper extremity pain is cervical spondylosis, a degenerative disease of the intervertebral disk and the adjacent vertebral margin, which causes spur formation and the production of ridges into the spinal canal or intervertebral foramina. Films and a CT scan of the cervical spine and electromyography help in making the diagnosis of this condition.

Several arterial and venous conditions can be confused with thoracic outlet syndrome; the differentiation can often be made clinically (Rosati and Lord, 1961).

In atypical patients who present with chest pain alone, it is important to suspect the thoracic outlet syndrome in addition to angina pectoris. Exercise stress testing and coronary angiography may exclude coronary artery disease when there is a high index of suspicion of angina pectoris (Urschel and Razzuk, 1973b; Urschel, et al., 1973).

MANAGEMENT

Principles of Management

The initial method of management in the majority of patients with thoracic outlet syndrome is nonoperative. Patients are instructed that overhead activity aggravates their symptomatology. Modifications in their job or even a job change should be attempted. Work that requires overhead activity, heavy lifting, repetitive motions, or use of vibratory tools will aggravate the thoracic outlet syndrome and mitigate against a good long-term surgical result. Rest periods with the arms down are recommended at intervals during the day. Particularly at night, patients tend to sleep with arms above the head, aggravating the thoracic outlet syndrome, with elbows flexed, aggravating the cubital tunnel syndrome, or with wrists off the neutral position, provoking carpal tunnel symptoms. These abnormal sleeping patterns are stressed to the patient and the patient's spouse, and patients are encouraged to develop sleeping patterns with arms by the sides (Fig. 47-20). If patients have concomitant carpal or cubital tunnel

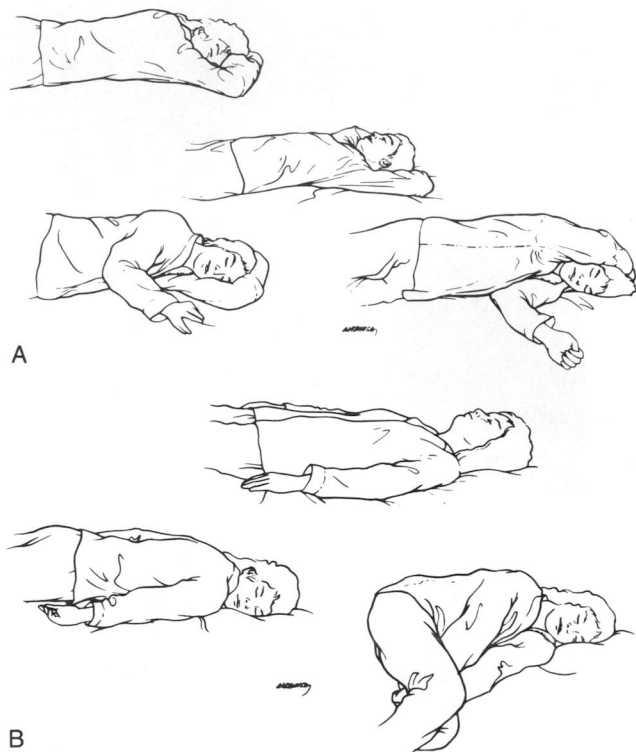

Figure 47-20. **(A)** Certain positions of the extremities put particular nerves at risk for increased pressure. Especially at night, patients assume these postures. Flexion or extension of the wrist aggravates carpal tunnel syndrome, elbow flexion aggravates cubital tunnel syndrome, and elevation of the arms above the head aggravates thoracic outlet symptoms. The sleeping positions illustrated put the nerves at risk for compression. **(B)** Patients should be advised to train themselves to sleep with their arms by their sides and their wrists in neutral.

syndrome, conservative management is directed toward these problems. In particular, night resting wrist splints to maintain the wrist in a neutral position and soft elbow pads to cushion the ulnar nerve and block elbow flexion are recommended. A soft cervical collar made from two rolls of stockinette stuffed with soft gauze pads can be used. An elasticized shoulder harness can be used to condition patients to better posture. Obesity and hypertrophic breasts will aggravate thoracic outlet syndrome, and weight loss plans are recommended. Occasionally breast reduction is indicated and has dramatically improved the patient's symptoms (Fig. 47-21).

Physical Therapy

Many of the symptoms of thoracic outlet syndrome are a consequence of muscle imbalance in the cervicothoracic region. A relaxed forward posture with the head anteriorly displaced in relation to the thorax will result in a shortening of the flexor muscles, weakness of the extensor muscles, and subsequent loss of the cervical lordosis. We follow McKenzie's approach (1983) and recognize three factors that predispose to pain in this region, namely faulty posture, an increased frequency of flexion, and loss of extension. Exercises

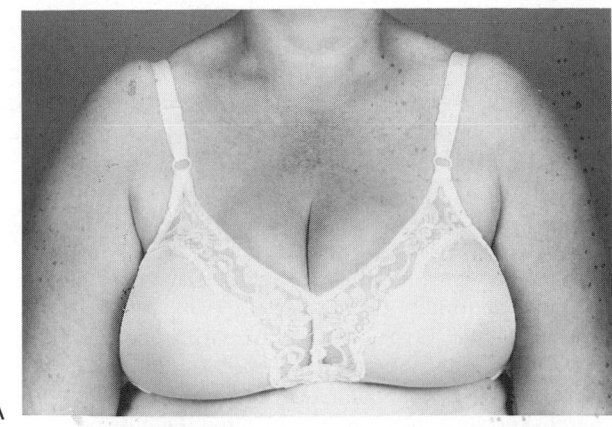

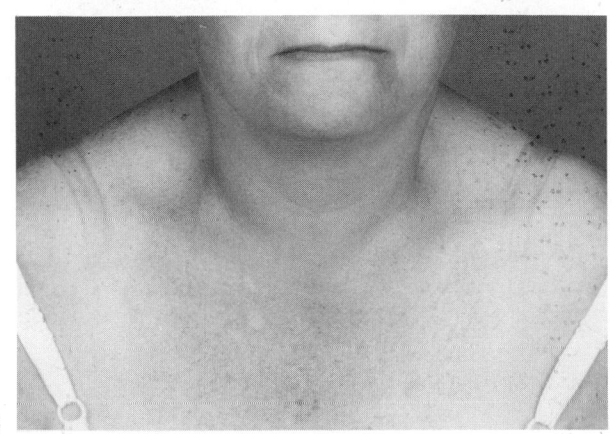

Figure 47-21. **(A)** Occasionally, breast hypertrophy can be a factor in producing thoracic outlet syndrome. In some patients breast reduction can dramatically reduce symptoms. **(B)** Note the strap marks on the patient's shoulders, which although not directly over the brachial plexus, offer evidence for chronic downward pressure on the shoulders.

are recommended to increase neck retraction and correct the cervical lordosis. In addition to posture abnormalities, muscle imbalance is addressed. Muscular assessment will identify muscle imbalance patterns (weakness versus tightness) and also identify referred pain patterns via trigger points. Muscle imbalance occurs when some muscles become tight while others become weak.

Janda (1988) has described a proximal crossed syndrome in the upper extremity in patients with thoracic outlet syndrome in which the pectoralis major and minor, upper trapezius, scalene, and sternaclavamastoid muscles become tight. Weakness occurs in the scapular stabilizers, including the middle and lower trapezius, rhomboid, and serratus anterior muscles. Tightness of these scalene muscles is well recognized as a major contributor to nerve compression of the brachial plexus. Muscles that exhibit decreased range of motion or strength can be evaluated for the presence of hyperirritable fossae (myofascial trigger points).

Patients with very tight and tender scalenes may benefit from local anesthetic block of the scalene muscles at their insertion at the first rib. Travell and Simons (1983) have described a technique for the treatment of trigger points,

including stretching and spraying with fluorimethane. With a decrease in the irritability of the lesion, more aggressive stretching can be implemented, including hold-relaxed techniques (maximal contraction followed by maximal relaxation). Once control of pain and a range of motion are achieved, a progressive strengthening program is instituted, which is directed toward the scapular stabilizers, the upper back, and the posture muscles of the cervical spine (middle and lower trapezius, rhomboids, and serratus anterior). During these strengthening exercises, the stretching and range of motion program is maintained. A successful, conservative physical therapy program for thoracic outlet syndrome requires that patients incorporate these exercises into their daily routine and become responsible for their program.

Abnormal posture patterns are demonstrated to the patients, and efforts are made to correct these. As mentioned above, a soft cervical collar made from two rolls of stockinette stuffed with soft gauze pads can be used, weight loss plans are recommended for obese patients, and occasionally breast reduction is indicated for patients with hypertrophic breasts.

Patients with thoracic outlet syndrome should be given physiotherapy when the diagnosis is made. Proper physiotherapy includes heat massages, active neck exercises, stretching of the scalenus muscles, strengthening of the upper trapezius muscle, and posture instruction. Because sagging of the shoulder girdle, which is common among the middle-aged, is a motor etiologic factor in this syndrome, many patients with less severe cases improve by strenghening the shoulder girdle and by improving posture (Krusen, 1968).

Most patients with thoracic outlet syndrome who have ulnar nerve conduction velocities of more than 60 m/s improve with conservative management. If the conduction velocity is below that level, most patients, may remain symptomatic despite physiotherapy, and surgical resection of the first rib and correction of other bony abnormalities may be needed to provide relief of symptoms (Urschel, et al., 1968, 1971; Urschel and Razzuk, 1972).

If symptoms of neurovascular compression continue after physiotherapy and the conduction velocity shows slight or no improvement or regression, surgical resection of the first rib and the cervical rib, when present, should be considered (Urschel, et al., 1968, 1971; Urschel and Razzuk, 1972). Clagget (1962) popularized the high posterior thoracoplasty approach for first rib resection; Falconer and Li (1962) emphasized the anterior approach; and Roos (1966) introduced the transaxillary route.

Paget-Schroetter Syndrome (Effort Thrombosis)

Effort thrombosis of the axillary subclavian vein (Paget-Schroetter syndrome) is usually secondary to unusual or excessive use of the arm, in addition to the presence of one or more compressive elements in the thoracic outlet (Adams and DeWeese, 1971; Johnston, 1989).

Historically, Sir James Paget in 1875 in London and von Schroetter in 1884 in Vienna described this syndrome of thrombosis of the axillary subclavian vein, which bears their names. The word *effort* (Aziz, et al., 1986) was added to thrombosis because of the frequent association with exertion, producing either direct or indirect compression of the vein. The thrombosis is caused by trauma (Cikrit, et al., 1990) or unusual occupations requiring repetitive muscular activity, as has been observed in professional athletes, linotype operators, painters, and beauticians. Cold and traumatic factors such as carrying skis over the shoulder tend to increase the proclivity for thrombosis (Daskalakis and Bouhoutsos, 1980). Elements of increased thrombogenicity also increase the incidence of the problem and exacerbate its symptoms on a long-term basis.

Adams and DeWeese (1971) and DeWeese, et al. (1970) reported long-term results in patients treated conservatively with elevation and coumadin. There was a 12 percent incidence of pulmonary embolism. Occasional venous distension developed in 18 percent, and late residual arm symptoms of swelling, pain, and superficial thrombophlebitis were noted in 68 percent of the patients (deep venous thrombosis with postphlebitic syndrome). Phlegmasia cerulea dolens was present in one patient.

For many years therapy included elevation of the arm and use of anticoagulants, with subsequent return to work. If symptoms recurred, the patient was considered for a first rib resection, with or without thrombectomy (DeWeese et al., 1970), as well as resection of the scalenus anterior muscle and removal of any other compressive element in the thoracic outlet, such as the cervical rib or abnormal bands [Prescott and Tikoff, 1979; Roos, 1989; Inahara, 1968].

Recent availability of thrombolytic agents (Sundqvist, et al., 1981; Rubenstein and Greger, 1980; Zimmerman, 1981), combined with prompt surgical decompression of the neurovascular compressive elements in the thoracic outlet (Taylor, et al., 1985), have reduced morbidity and the necessity for thrombectomy and have substantially improved clinical results, including the ability to return to work (Urschel and Razzuk, 1991).

One advantage of urokinase over streptokinase is the direct action of urokinase on the thrombosis distal to the catheter, producing a local thrombolytic effect (Becker, et al., 1983; Drury, et al., 1985; Eisenbud, et al., 1990). Streptokinase produces a systemic effect involving potential complications. Heparin decreases the need for thrombectomy after use of the thrombolytic agent followed by aggressive surgical intervention; this is another advantage, as some of the long-term disability is related to morbidity from thrombectomy as well as to recurrent thrombosis (Drapanas and Curran, 1966; Painter and Karpf, 1984, Campbell, et al., 1977).

The natural history of Paget-Schroetter syndrome suggests moderate morbidity (Tilney, et al., 1970) with conservative treatment alone. Bypass with vein or other conduits (Hansen, et al., 1985; Hashmonai, et al., 1976; Jacobson and Haimov, 1977) has limited application. Causes other than thoracic outlet syndrome must be treated individually (Loring, 1952). Intermittent obstruction of the subclavian vein (McLaughlin, 1939) can lead to thrombosis, and decompression should be employed prophylactically (Hashmonai, et al., 1976; Jacobson and Haimov, 1977).

Surgical Management

Several routes have been described to remove the first rib, including posterior, transaxillary, supraclavicular, infraclavicular, transthoracic, and through the bed of the resected clavicle.

Surgical Results

A definitive review of the surgical management of thoracic outlet syndrome has been published by Sanders (1991). Sanders concludes that transaxillary first rib resection, scalenotomy, and supraclavicular first rib resection with scalenotomy give essentially the same results (Fig. 47-22). This is contraindicated by our study and other long-term followup (longer than 10 years) of scalenectomy alone, which demonstrates a 65 percent recurrence rate.

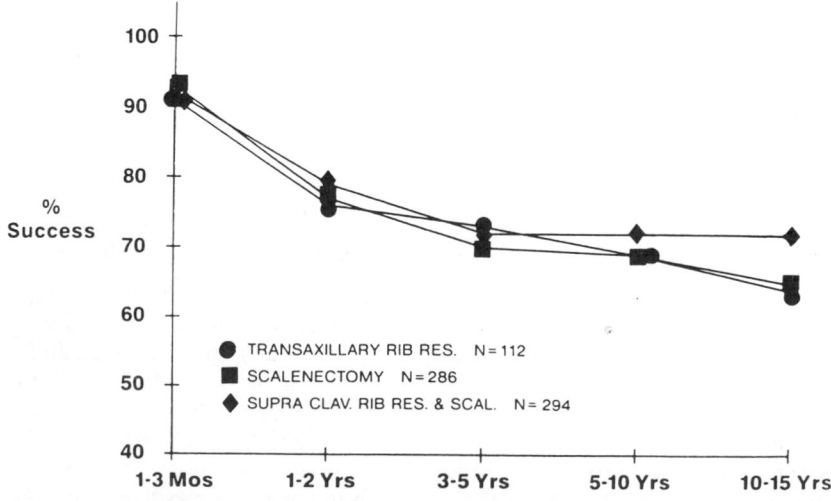

Figure 47-22. Results of the three primary operations for thoracic outlet syndrome. (From Sanders RJ: Thoracic Outlet Syndrome: A Common Sequela of Neck Injuries. p. 182. JB Lippincott, Philadelphia, 1991, with permission.)

Our results after 20 years show 79 percent good results with complete rib resection and only 33 percent good results with scalenectomy. Neither Sanders, Roos, nor most surgeons remove the *complete* first rib in most cases. Sanders states, "Complete removal of the first rib can be a dangerous maneuver." This is the most likely cause for recurrence and best explains why others do *not* have good long-term results.

Reoperation for Recurrent Thoracic Outlet Syndrome

Extirpation of the first rib relieves symptoms in patients with thoracic outlet syndrome not relieved by physiotherapy. Of the surgically treated patients, 10 percent develop various degrees of shoulder, arm, and hand pain and paresthesias, which are usually mild and short-lasting and both respond well to a brief course of physiotherapy and muscle relaxants. In a few patients (1.6 percent), symptoms persist, become progressively more severe, and often involve a wider area of distribution because of entrapment of the immediate trunk in addition to the lower trunk and C8 and T1 nerve roots. Symptoms may recur 1 month to 7 years after rib resection but usually within the first 3 months. Symptoms consist of an aching or burning type of pain, often associated with paresthesias, involving the neck, shoulder, parascapular area, anterior chest wall, arm, and hand. Vascular lesions are uncommon and consist of causalgia minor and an occasional injury of the subclavian artery, with subsequent false aneurysm formation caused by the sharp edge of a remaining posterior stump of an incompletely resected first rib. Recurrence is diagnosed on the basis of history, physical examination, and decreased nerve conduction velocity across the outlet. Diagnostic evaluation should also include thorough neurologic evaluation, chest and cervical spine films, cervical myelography, and subclavian artery angiography when indicated.

Two groups of patients who require reoperation can be identified. Pseudorecurrence has been noted in patients who did not have relief of symptoms after the initial operation. These patients can be identified etiologically as those in whom the second rib was mistakenly resected, leaving a rudimentary first rib. True recurrence has occurred in patients whose symptoms were relieved after the first operation but who retained a significant segment of the first rib and showed excessive scar formation around the brachial plexus.

Physiotherapy should be given to all patients with symptoms of neurovascular compression after first rib resection. If the symptoms persist and the conduction velocity remains below normal, reoperation is indicated.

Reoperation for thoracic outlet syndrome is performed via the posterior thoracoplasty approach to provide better exposure of the nerve roots and brachial plexus, which reduces the danger of injury to these structures and provides adequate exposure of the subclavian artery and vein. This incision also provides a wider field for resection of any bony abnormalities or fibrous bands and allows extensive neurolysis of the nerve roots and brachial plexus, which is not always possible with the limited exposure of the transaxillary approach. The anterior or supraclavicular approach is inadequate for reoperation.

The basic elements of reoperation include resection of persistent or recurrent bony remnants of a cervical or first rib, neurolysis of the brachial plexus and nerve roots, and dorsal sympathectomy. Sympathectomy removes T1, T2, and T3 thoracic ganglia. Care is taken to avoid damage to the C8 ganglion (upper aspect of the stellate ganglion), which produces Horner syndrome. The reoperation provides paresthesias in the supraclavicular and infraclavicular areas. The incidence of so-called postsympathetic syndrome has been negligible in this group of patients. A nerve stimulator is used to differentiate scar from nerve root to avoid damage from reoperation in these patients.

The results of reoperation are good if an accurate diagnosis is made and the proper procedure is used (Urschel and Razzuk, 1986b). More than 800 patients have been followed up for 6 months to 15 years. All patients improved initially after reoperation, and in 79 percent the improvement was maintained for more than 5 years. In 14 percent of the patients, symptoms were managed with physiotherapy, but 7 percent required a second reoperation, in every case because of rescarring. There were no deaths, and only one patient had an infection that required drainage.

SUMMARY

Thoracic outlet syndrome is recognized in approximately 8 percent of the population. Its manifestations may be neurologic, vascular, or both, depending on the component of the neurovascular bundle predominantly compressed. The diagnosis is suspected by determination of the ulnar nerve conduction velocity. Treatment is initially conservative, but persistence of significant symptoms, which occur in approximately 5 percent of patients with diagnosed thoracic outlet syndromes, is an indication for first rib resection. Primary resection is done preferably through the transaxillary approach. Symptoms of various degrees may recur after first rib resection in approximately 10 percent of patients. Most patients improve with physiotherapy, and only 1.6 percent require reoperation. Reoperation for recurrent symptoms is done through a high posterior thoracoplasty incision (Urschel and Razzuk, 1986b; Urschel, et al., 1976).

KEY REFERENCES

Clagett OT: Presidential Address: Research and Prosearch. J Thorac Cardiovasc Surg 44:153, 1962

This is the classic reference explaining the anatomic and pathophysiologic basis for first rib resection to alleviate neurovascular compression in the thoracic outlet. The incision is the high posterior thoracoplasty approach.

Roos DB: Transaxillary approach for first rib resection to relieve thoracic outlet syndrome. Ann Surg 163:354, 1966

The transaxillary approach to first rib resection was initially described by Atkins and popularized by Roose. The technical aspects of this approach and the pathophysiology are described.

Rosati LM, Lord JW: Neurovascular Compression Syndromes of the Shoulder Girdle. Modern Surgical Monographs. Grune & Stratton, Orlando, 1961

Frank Netter's drawings appeared first in this classic monograph demonstrating neurovascular compression. It is the preferred method for diagnosis and management of neurovascular compression syndromes.

Urschel HC Jr, Razzuk MA, Wood RE, Paulson DL: Objective diagnosis (ulnar nerve conduction velocity) and current therapy of the thoracic outlet syndrome. Ann Thorac Surg 12:608, 1971

The first positive objective technique for diagnosing neurologic thoracic outlet syndrome compression is detailed.

Urschel, HC Jr, Razzuk MA: Improved management of the Paget-Schroetter syndrome secondary to thoracic outlet compression. Ann Thorac Surg 52:1217, 1991

This report of the largest series of axillary subclavian vein thromboses describes the current management with urokinase thrombolysis followed by first rib resection.

REFERENCES

Adams JT, DeWeese JA: Effort thrombosis of the axillary and subclavian veins. J Trauma 11:923, 1971

Adams JT, DeWeese JA, Mahoney EB, Rob CG: Intermittent subclavian vein obstruction without thrombosis. Surgery 63:147, 1968

Adson AW: Surgical treatment for symptoms produced by cervical ribs and the scalenus anticus muscle. Surg Gynecol Obstet 85:687, 1947

Adson AW, Coffey IR: Cervical rib: a method of anterior approach for relief of symptoms by division of the scaleneus anticus. Ann Surg 85:839, 1927

Atkins HJB: Peraxillary approach to the stellate and upper thoracic sympathetic ganglia. Lancet 2:1152, 1949

Atkins HJB: Sympathectomy by the axillary approach. Lancet 1:538, 1954

Aziz K, Straenley CJ, Whelan TJ: Effort-related axilla-subclavian vein thrombosis. Am J Surg 152:57, 1986

Becker GJ, Holden RW, Robe FE et al.: Local thrombolytic therapy for subclavian and axillary vein thrombosis. Radiology 149:419, 1983

Borchardt M: Symptomatologie und Therapie der Halsrippen. Berl Klin Wochenschr 38:1265, 1901

Borg K, Persson HE, Lindblom U: Thoracic outlet syndrome: Diagnostic value of sensibility testing, vibratory thresholds and somatosensory evoked potentials at rest and during pertubation with abduction and external rotation of the arm. In Dubner R, Gebhart GF, Bond MR (eds): Proceeding of the Fifth World Congress on Pain. p. 144. 1988

Bramwell E: Lesion of the first dorsal nerve root. Rev Neurol Psychiatr 1:236, 1903

Brinckner WM: Brachial plexus pressure by the normal first rib. Ann Surg 85:858, 1927

Brickner WM, Milch H: First dorsal vertebra simulating cervical rib by maldevelopment or by pressure symptoms. Surg Gynecol Obstet 40:38, 1925

Brintnall ES, Hyndman OR, Van Allen WM: Costoclavicular compression associated with cervical rib. Ann Surg 144:921, 1956

Caldwell JW, Crane CR, Krusen EM: Nerve conduction studies in the diagnosis of the thoracic outlet syndrome. South Med J 64:210, 1971

Campbell BE, Chandler JG, Tegtmeyer CJ: Axillary, subclavian and brachiocephalic vein obstruction. Surgery 82:816, 1977

Cikrit DF, Dalsing MC, Bryand BJ et al.: An experience with upper-extremity vascular trauma. Am J Surg 160:229, 1990

Cooley DA, Wukasch DC: Techniques in Vascular Surgery. WB Saunders, Philadelphia, 1979

Coon WW, Willis PW: Thrombosis of axillary subclavian veins. Arch Surg 94:657, 1966

Coote H: Pressure on the axillary vessels and nerve by an exostosis from a cervical rib; interference with the circulation of the arm; removal of the rib and exostosis, recovery. Med Times Gaz 2:108, 1861

Daskalakis E, Bouhoutsos J: Subclavian and axillary vein compression of musculoskeletal origin. Br J Surg 67:573, 1980

DeWeese JA, Adams JT, Gaiser DI: Subclavian venous thrombectomy. Circulation 16(suppl 2):158, 1970

Drapanas T, Curran W: Thrombectomy in the treatment of "effort" thrombosis of the axillary and subclavian veins. J Trauma 6:107, 1966

Drury EM, Trout HH, Giordono JM et al.: Lytic therapy in the treatment of axillary and subclavian vein thrombosis. J Vasc Surg 2:821, 1984

Eisenbud DE, Brener BJ, Shoenfeld R et al.: Treatment of acute vascular occlusions with intra-arterial urokinase. Am J Surg 160:160, 1990

Falconer MA, Li FWP: Resection of the first rib in costoclavicular compression of the brachial plexus. Lancet 1:59, 1962

Falconer MA, Weddell G: Costoclavicular compression of the subclavian artery and vein: relation to scalenus syndrome. Lancet 2:539, 1943

Galbraith NF, Urschel HC Jr, Wood RE et al: Fracture of first rib associated with laceration of subclavian artery: report of a case and review of literature. J Thorac Cardiovasc Surg 65:4, 1973

Ganong WF: Review of Medical Physiology. 3rd Ed. Appleton & Lange, E. Norwalk, CT, 1967

Halsted, WS: An experimental study of circumscribed dilation of an artery immediately distal to a partially occluding band, and its bearing on the dilation of the subclavian artery observed in certain cases of cervical rib. J Exp Med 24:271, 1916

Hansen B, Feins RS, Detman DE: Simple extra-anatomic jugular vein bypass for subclavian vein thrombosis. J Vasc Surg 2:291, 1985

Hashmonai M, Schramek A, Farbstein J: Cephalic vein cross-over bypass for subclavian vein thrombosis: a case report. Surgery 80:563, 1976

Inahara T: Surgical treatment of "effort" thrombosis of the axillary and subclavian veins. Am Surg 34:479, 1968

Jebsen RH: Motor conduction velocities in the median and ulnar nerves. Arch Phys Med Rehabil 48:185, 1967

Jacobson JH, Haimov M: Venous revascularization of the arm: report of three cases. Surgery 81:599, 1977

Janda V: Muscles and cervicogenic pain syndromes. In Grant R (ed): Physical Therapy of the Cervical and Thoracic Spine. Churchill Livingstone, New York, 1988

Johnston KW: Neurovascular conditions involving the upper extremity. p. 801. In Rutherford RB (ed); Vascular Surgery. 3rd Ed. WB Saunders, Philadelphia, 1989

Keen WW: The symptomatology, diagnosis and surgical treatment of cervical ribs. Am J Sci 133:173, 1907

Krusen EM: Cervical pain syndromes. Arch Phys Med Rehabil 49:376, 1968

Kuntz A: Distribution of the sympathetic rami to the brachial plexus. Arch Surg 15:871, 1927

Lang EK: Roentgenographic diagnosis of the neurovascular compression syndromes. Audiology 79:58, 1962

Law AA: Adventitious ligaments simulating cervical ribs. Ann Surg 72:497, 1920

Litwin MS: Postsympathectomy neuralgia. Arch Surg 84:591, 1962

Lord JW, Urschel HC: Total claviculectomy. Surg Rounds 11:17, 1988

Loring WE: Venous thrombosis in the upper extremity as a complication of myocardial failure. Am J Med 397, 1952

Mackenzie RA: Treat your own neck. Spinal Publications, Waikanes, New Zealand, 1983

Mackinnon SE, Dellon AL: Surgery of the Peripheral Nerve. Thieme, New York, 1988

Machleder HI, Moll F, Nuwer M, Jordan S: Somatosensory evoked potentials in the assessment of thoracic outlet syndrome. J Vasc Surg 6:177, 1987

Martinez NS: Posterior first rib resection for total thoracic outlet syndrome decompression. Contemp Surg 15:13, 1979

McLaughlin CW, Popma AM: Intermittent obstruction of the subclavian vein. JAMA 113:1960, 1939

Murphy T: Brachial neuritis caused by pressure of first rib. Aust Med J 15:582, 1910

Murphy JB. Cervical rib excision: collective review on surgery of cervical rib. Clin John B Murphy 5:227, 1916

Naffziger HC, Grant WT: Neuritics of the brachial plexus—mechanical in origin: the scalenus syndrome. Surg Gynecol Obstet 67:722, 1938

Ochsner A, Gage M, DeBakey M: Scalenous anticus (Naffziger) syndrome. Am J Surg 28:699, 1935

Paget J: Clinical lectures and essays. Longmans Green, London, 1875

Painter TD, Karpf M: Deep venous thrombosis of the upper extremity: 5 years' experience at a university hospital. Angiology 35:743, 1984

Palumbo LT: Anterior transthoracic approach for upper extremity thoracic sympathectomy. Arch Surg 72:659, 1956

Palumbo LT: Upper dorsal sympathectomy without Horner's syndrome. Arch Surg 71:743, 1955

Prescott SM, Tikoff G: Deep venous thrombosis of the upper extremity: a reappraisal. Circulation 59:350, 1979

Rapoport S, Blair DN, McCarthy SM et al.: Brachial plexus: correlation of MR imaging and CT pathologic findings. Radiology 167:161, 1988

Ravitch MM, Steichen FM: Atlas of General Thoracic Surgery. WB Saunders, Philadelphia, 1988

Razzuk MA, Krusen EM, Caldwell JW, Urschel HC Jr: The clinical value and technique of measuring nerve conduction velocities for thoracic outlet syndrome. In Greep JC, Lemmen HAJ, Roos DB, Urschel HC Jr (eds): Pain in Shoulder and Arm. Martinus Nijhoff, The Hague, 1979

Rob CG, Standover A: Arterial occlusion complicating thoracic outlet compression syndrome. Br Med J 2:709, 1958

Roos DB, Owens JC: Thoracic outlet syndrome. Arch Surg 93:71, 1966

Roos D: Thoracic outlet nerve compression. p. 858. In Rutherford RB (ed): Vascular Surgery. 3rd Ed. WB Saunders, Philadelphia, 1989

Rosenberg JC: Arteriography demonstrations of compression syndromes of the thoracic outlet. South Med J 59:400, 1966

Rubenstein M, Greger WP: Successful streptokinase therapy for catheter induced subclavian vein thrombosis. Arch Intern Med 140:1370, 1980

Sanders RJ: Thoracic Outlet Syndrome: A Common Sequela of Neck Injuries. JB Lippincott, Philadelphia, 1991

Smithwick RH: Modified dorsal sympathectomy for vascular spasm

(Raynaud's disease) of the upper extremity. Ann Surg 104:339, 1936

Stoney WS, Addlestone RB, Alford WC Jr et al.: The incidence of venous thrombosis following long-term transvenous pacing. Ann Thorac Surg 22:166, 1976

Sundqvist SB, Hedner U, Kullenberg KHE et al.: Deep venous thrombosis of the arm: a study of coagulation and fibrinolysis. Br Med J 283:265, 1981

Swank WL, Simeone FA: The scalenus anticus syndrome. Arch Neurol Psychiatry 51:432, 1944

Taylor LM, McAllister WR, Dennis DL et al.: Thrombolytic therapy followed by first rib resection for spontaneous subclavian vein thrombosis. Am J Surg 149:644, 1985

Telford ED, Mottershead S: Pressure of the cervicobrachial junction. J Bone Joint Surg [Am] 30:249, 1948

Telford ED, Stopford JSB: The vascular complications of the cervical rib. Br J Surg 18:559, 1937

Tilney NL, Griffiths HFG, Edwards EA: Natural history of major venous thrombosis of the upper extremity. Arch Surg 101:792, 1970

Travell JG, Simons DG: Myofascial Pain and Dysfunction. The Trigger Point Manual. Williams & Wilkins, Baltimore, 1983

Upton ARM, McComas AJ: The double crush in nerve entrapment syndromes. Lancet ii:259, 1973

Urschel HC Jr: Thoracic outlet syndrome. In Gibbons Surgery of the Chest. 5th Ed. WB Saunders, Philadelphia, 1989

Urschel HC Jr: Reoperation for thoracic outlet syndrome. In International Trends in General Thoracic Surgery. Vol. 2. CV Mosby, St. Louis, 1986

Urschel HC Jr, Paulson DL, McNamara JJ: Thoracic outlet syndrome. Ann Thorac Surg 6:1, 1968

Urschel HC Jr, Razzuk MA: Thoracic outlet syndrome. p. 130. In International Trends in General Thoracic Surgery. Vol. 2. CV Mosby, St. Louis, 1986a

Urschel HC Jr, Razzuk MA: The failed operation for thoracic outlet syndrome: the difficulty of diagnosis and management. Ann Thorac Surg 42:523, 1986b

Urschel HC Jr, Razzuk MA: Posterior thoracic sympathectomy. In Malt RA (ed): Surgical Techniques Illustrated: A Comparative Atlas. WB Saunders, Philadelphia, 1985

Urschel HC Jr, Razzuk MA: Thoracic outlet syndrome. In Shields TW (ed): General Thoracic Surgery. 2nd Ed. Lea & Febiger, Philadelphia, 1983

Urschel HC Jr, Razzuk MA: Thoracic outlet syndrome. Surg Annu 5:229, 1973b

Urschel HC Jr, Razzuk MA: Current management of thoracic outlet syndrome. N Engl J Med 286:21, 1972

Urschel HC Jr, Razzuk MA, Albers JE et al.: Reoperation for recurrent thoracic outlet syndrome. Ann Thorac Surg 21:19, 1976

Urschel HC Jr, Razzuk MA, Hyland JW et al.: Thoracic outlet syndrome masquerading as coronary artery disease. Ann Thorac Surg 16:239, 1973

Von Schroetter L: Erkrankungen der Gefässe. In Nathnogel (ed): Handbuch der Pathologie und Therapie. Holder, Vienna, 1884

White JC, Smithwick RH, Simeone FA: The Autonomic Nervous System: Anatomy, Physiology and Surgical Application. 3rd Ed. Macmillan, New York, 1952

Wood RE, Campbell DC, Razzuk MA et al: Surgical advantages of selective unilateral ventilation. Ann Thorac Surg 14:2, 1972

Wright IS: The neurovascular syndrome produced by hyperabduction of the arm. Am Heart J 29:1, 1945

Yiannikas C, Walsh JC: Somatosensory evoked responses in the diagnosis of thoracic outlet syndrome. J Neurol Neurosurg Psychiatry 46:234, 1983

48

PRIMARY NEOPLASMS

Geoffrey M. Graeber
David R. Jones
Peter C. Pairolero

DEFINITION

Chest wall tumors encompass a kaleidoscopic panorama of bone and soft tissue pathologic conditions. Included are primary and metastatic neoplasms of both the bony skeleton and soft tissues and primary neoplasms that invade the thorax from adjacent structures such as the breast, lung, pleura, and mediastinum. Nearly all of these neoplasms have at one time or another been irradiated, and it is fairly common for these patients to present with postradiation necrotic ulceration. The thoracic surgeon is asked to evaluate all of these patients. Most are seen to establish a diagnosis, some to treat for cure, and a few to manage necrotic foul-smelling chest wall malignant ulcers. Primary chest wall neoplasms previously considered unresectable because of their size or extension into adjacent structures are now being resected, and the chest wall is reconstructed with little morbidity. In many patients, surgical extirpation is often the only remaining modality of therapy, and this may be compromised by an incorrect diagnosis or an inability to reconstruct large chest wall defects (Pairolero and Arnold, 1985).

HISTORICAL NOTE

Because primary chest wall neoplasms are uncommon, relatively few series have previously been reported. Moreover, most reports have included only patients with bone tumors (Pascuzzi, et al., 1957; Groff and Adkins, 1967; Stelzer and Gay, 1980). When bone neoplasms are combined with primary soft tissue tumors, however, the soft tissues become a major source of chest wall neoplasms and account for nearly one-half of these tumors treated surgically (Graeber, et al., 1982; Pairolero and Arnold, 1985; King, et al., 1986). The incidence of malignancy in these tumors is variable and has been reported to range from 50 to 80 percent. The higher malignancy rates are found in those series that include soft tissue tumors. When combined, malignant fibrous histiocytoma (fibrosarcoma), chondrosarcoma, and rhabdomyosarcoma are the most frequent primary malignant neoplasms

that the thoracic surgeon is asked to manage. Cartilaginous tumors (osteochondroma and chondroma) and desmoid tumors are the most common primary benign tumors.

HISTORICAL READINGS

Groff DB, Adkins PC: Chest wall tumors. Ann Thorac Surg 4:260, 1967
Pascuzzi CA, Dahlia DC, Clagett OT: Primary tumors of the ribs and sternum. Surg Gynecol Obstet 104:390, 1957
Stelzer P, Gay WA JR: Tumors of the chest wall. Surg Clin North Am 60:779, 1980

CLINICAL FEATURES

The mean age of presentation for a patient with a benign tumor of the chest wall is approximately 15 years younger than for those with primary malignancies. The average patient age for benign tumors is 26 years old; for malignant tumors, the average age is 40 years old (Pass, 1989). The male to female ratio is approximately 2:1 (Graeber, et al., 1982; Gordon, et al., 1991; Sabanathan, et al., 1985) for most tumors, with the exception of the desmoid tumors, which have a 1:2 male to female preponderance (Gordon, et al., 1991; McKinnon, et al., 1989). Chest wall tumors generally present as slowly enlarging masses. Most are initially asymptomatic, but with continued growth, pain invariably occurs. At first, the pain is generalized, and the patient is frequently treated for a neuritis or musculoskeletal complaint. The incidence of a chest wall mass is 70 percent, and pain is seen in 25 to 50 percent of patients (Gordon, et al., 1991; King, et al., 1986). These chest wall masses may be large and have been present for long periods. The size of these tumors may rarely prevent the patient from dressing and thus cause the patient to seek therapy. Pain is more common in malignant tumors but cannot be used to exclude the diagnosis of benignity

---

Primary Chest Wall Neoplasms

Malignant
  Myeloma
  Malignant fibrous histiocytoma
  Chondrosarcoma
  Rhabdomyosarcoma
  Ewing's sarcoma
  Liposarcoma
  Neurofibrosarcoma
  Osteosarcoma
  Hemangiosarcoma
  Leiomyosarcoma
  Lymphoma
Benign
  Osteochondroma
  Chondroma
  Desmoid
  Lipoma
  Fibroma
  Neurilemmoma

---

because one-third of patients with benign chest wall neoplasms have associated pain. Less common symptoms include weight loss, fever, lymphadenopathy, and brachial plexus neuropathy.

DIAGNOSIS

The evaluation of patients with suspected chest wall tumors should include a careful history and physical and laboratory examination followed by conventional plain and tomographic chest radiography. Old chest radiographs are important to determine the growth rate. Computed tomographic scans (CT) should be obtained to delineate soft tissue, pleural, mediastinal, and pulmonary involvement. The role of magnetic resonance imaging (MRI) is not yet fully known, but preliminary evaluation indicates still further enhancement of tissue pathologic findings, which may make it the diagnostic modality of choice in the future. A bone survey should be done if metastases are suspected. Pulmonary function testing should also be obtained.

Most primary chest wall neoplasms should be diagnosed by excisional biopsy. The reasons for excisional biopsy include (1) removal of the entire mass, (2) adequate tissue sampling to establish the tumor's histologic type, and (3) earlier administration of adjuvant therapy if necessary. Cavanaugh, et al. (1986) recommended a limited incisional biopsy to establish the diagnosis and allow appropriate management plans to be made that are based on the histologic type. In this series, 73 percent of the lesions were benign, and no further surgery was performed. In most series, however, the rate of malignancy is 50 to 80 percent, and all require en bloc resection (Graeber, et al., 1982; King, et al., 1986; Pairolero and Arnold, 1985). Incisional biopsies may confuse the histologic diagnosis because certain tumors, particularly chondrosarcomas, have areas that histologically appear be-

nign and other areas in which frank malignancy is present (Graeber, et al., 1982). Clinical decisions based on the wrong pathologic diagnosis may be catastrophic. If an incisional biopsy is performed, it should be made in such a way that the definitive excision will not be compromised. No flaps or extensive dissection should be used to prevent tumor cell seeding. Needle biopsy of a lesion in a patient with a known prior malignancy may be helpful. Ayala and Zornosa (1983) demonstrated a 79 percent accuracy rate in the diagnosis of primary bone tumors with percutaneous needle biopsy. Most thoracic surgeons still prefer excisional biopsy whenever possible.

Laboratory analysis and diagnostic studies should include liver function tests, alkaline phosphatase levels, and a CT or MRI of the chest. Many of these tumors metastasize to the lungs or involve the lung. Involvement of the underlying lung does not preclude resection, but it is associated with a worse prognosis, particularly in a patient with high-grade sarcomas (King, et al., 1986; Perry, et al., 1990). Ultrasound of chest wall tumors helps to localize the tumor's relationship to the pleura and lung parenchyma (Saito, et al. 1988). If the tumor is confined to the chest wall, its movement during respiration is synchronous with the chest wall movement not with the lung parenchyma.

BENIGN TUMORS

Benign chest wall tumors require diagnostic studies similar to those for malignant tumors. Radiographic studies may suggest the diagnosis of benignity, but histologic evidence is necessary. The more common benign chest wall tumors are shown above. Less common benign tumors include lipomas, osteomyelitis, mesenchymomas, fibroxanthomas, hemangioendotheliomas, and some neural tumors.

Chondroma

Chondroma is the most common benign tumor of the chest wall (Graeber, et al., 1982; Sabanathan, et al., 1985; Ryan, et al., 1989). They usually arise in the ribs near the costochondral junction anteriorly. These patients present with a mass that may be painful. Radiographically, the lesion has a lobulated radiodense appearance, which frequently displaces the bony cortex but does not penetrate it (Fig. 48-1). Calcification may be diffuse or focal with a stippled pattern. Histologically, there is mature hyaline cartilage with foci of myxoid degeneration and calcification. These lesions may grow to enormous size if untreated, and the therapy of choice is wide local excision with 2-cm margins.

Fibrous Dysplasia

Fibrous dysplasia occurs in young adults and presents as a painless, asymptomatic mass. It can arise anywhere on the chest wall but occurs frequently in the posterior ribs (Boyd, 1986). There is an association with trauma. Radiographs show a central, fusiform, expanded mass with thinning of the cortex and absence of calcification (Sabanathan, et al., 1985). Cortical bone erosion is not uncommon. Histologically, there is a characteristic fishhook configuration of the trabeculae and

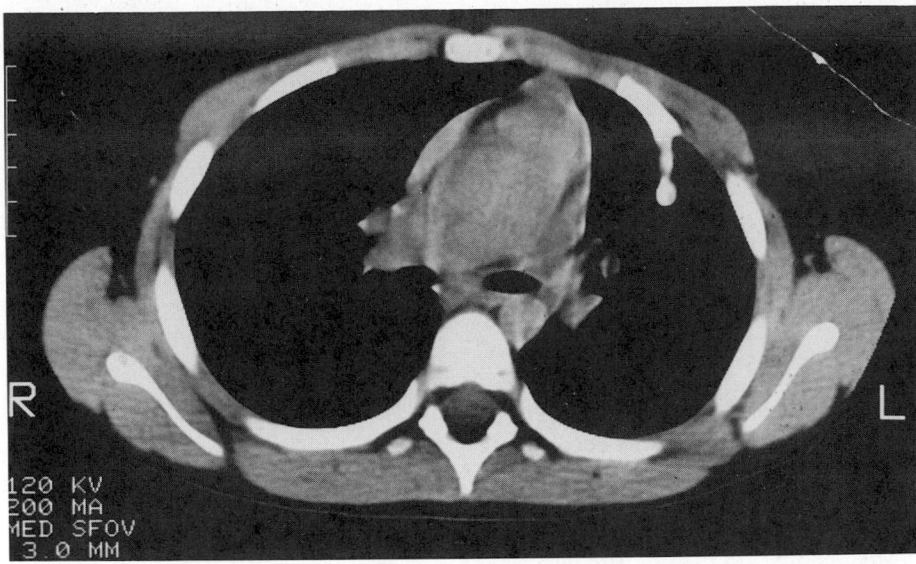

Figure 48-1.   A CT image of a lobulated chondroma in a 42-year-old man arising near the costochondral junction in the left fourth rib. The therapy was resection with adequate margins of excision.

lack of transformation of the coarse bony fibers to lamellar bone. This suggests that fibrous dysplasia represents a maturation defect. Excision of this lesion is curative.

Osteochondromas

Osteochondroma is a rare chest wall tumor that occurs in the first or second decade of life. The radiographic appearance is typical. The lesion, which is usually located in the metaphysis, grows in a direction opposite to that of the adjacent joint (Fig. 48-2). Infrequently, it has a focal radiolucent area surrounded by osteosclerotic tissue (Sabanathan, et al.,

1985). Grossly, the tumor consists of mature bone trabeculae covered by a cartilaginous cap. Most lesions are greater than 4 cm in diameter but may become larger if untreated. Solitary osteochondromas are benign and rarely may degenerate into malignancy. Multiple osteochondromas have a higher incidence of malignancy (Boyd, 1986). The therapy is wide local excision.

Eosinophilic Granuloma

Eosinophilic granuloma is a disease of the lymphoreticular system and not a true bone tumor. It may be solitary or

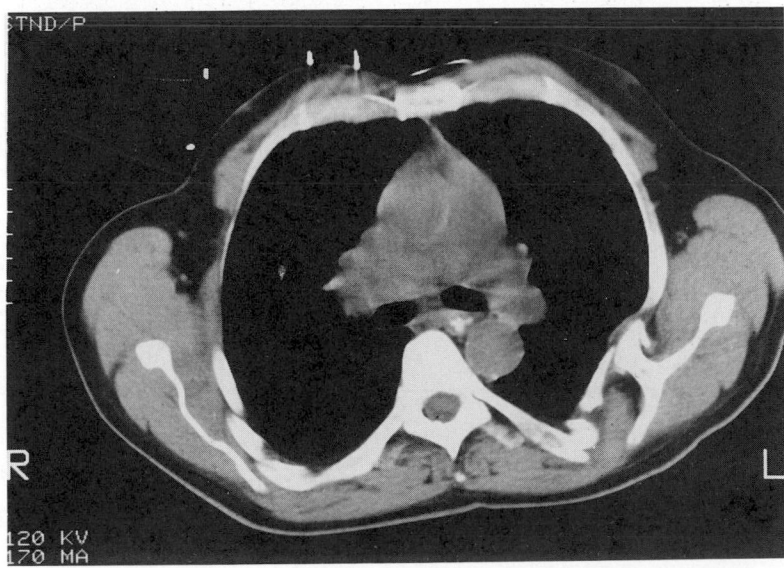

Figure 48-2.   A representative CT scan of a solitary, osteochondroma of the posterior left scapula with displacement of the third rib anteriorly. This produced a dull posterior chest wall pain in the patient.

multifocal and is a unifying feature of the conditions designated as histiocytosis X. Microscopically, there is an abundance of Langerhans cells, giant cells, eosinophils, and neutrophils. The peak incidence is between 5 and 15 years. It occurs in either the metaphysis or diaphysis of the bone and has no malignant potential. These lesions show osteolytic activity with adjacent osteosclerosis by radiography. They are frequently confused with Ewing's sarcoma or osteomyelitis. The therapy consists of either resection or radiotherapy.

Desmoid Tumor

Desmoid tumors occur most commonly in the third to fourth decades of life and have a 2 : 1 female to male predominance. The desmoid tumor is frequently difficult to differentiate from the low-grade fibrosarcoma. Histologically, the desmoid tumor contains sheets of fibroblasts with well-differentiated abundant collagen, which lacks encapsulation. The fibrosarcoma is usually well encapsulated with a herringbone pattern and distinct mitoses (McKinnon, et al., 1989). Although one-third of patients with Gardner syndrome have desmoid tumors, only 2 percent of patients with a desmoid tumor have Gardner syndrome (Hayery and Scheinin, 1988). Desmoids have also been reported to occur after trauma and to be associated with estrogen-induced growth (McKinnon, et al., 1989; Hayery and Scheinin, 1988).

The clinical presentation is usually one of a dull, aching mass, which may be fixed to the underlying tissues but not to the skin (Graeber, et al., 1985). The growth of the mass is slow, and it does not metastasize. There are no characteristic radiographic findings, and the diagnosis should be made by excisional biopsy.

The therapy is wide local excision with margins of at least 4 cm. Because desmoids may spread along fascial planes well beyond the primary, the wider resection margins are recommended. The recurrence rates for desmoid tumors after excision range from 4 percent to as high as 50 percent (McKinnon, et al., 1989; Posner, et al., 1989). The recurrence rates were directly related to resection margin status in McKinnon, et al.'s (1989) study, and 45 percent of patients with positive resection margins had recurrences. Only 4 percent with negative resection margins had relapses. In patients with recurrence or gross residual disease, radiotherapy is effective for local control (Sherman, et al., 1990; Leibel, et al., 1983). The recommended radiation doses of 50 to 60 Gy at 1 : 8 Gy/fraction prevent the dose-related complications of radiotherapy (Sherman, et al., 1990). Chemotherapy plays no role in the therapy of desmoid tumors. Because of the hormonal influence on the desmoid's growth, tamoxifen has been reported to decrease both the size and symptoms of these tumors (Kinzbrunner, et al., 1983).

The actual survival rates after wide local excision are 90 percent at 10 years, with a cause-specific survival rate of 100 percent (Graeber, 1989). Local recurrence remains the most difficult challenge for this locally aggressive, benign tumor.

MALIGNANT TUMORS

Malignant primary chest wall tumors can be cured if certain surgical principles are followed. These tumors may require extensive chest wall resection, but with the aid of muscle flaps, chest wall reconstruction is successful. Adjuvant therapy has become increasingly important in the management of these tumors. The most common primary malignant chest wall tumors were shown previously. Less common malignant tumors include neurofibrosarcomas, malignant hemangioendotheliomas, and leiomyosarcomas. The survival rates after therapy for these tumors vary, but all histologic subtypes have some long-term survivors (Fig. 48-3).

Chondrosarcoma

Chondrosarcoma is the most common primary chest wall malignant tumor. It accounts for 50 percent of the malignant neoplasms and 25 percent of all primary chest wall tumors (Sabanathan, et al., 1985). Eighty percent of these tumors

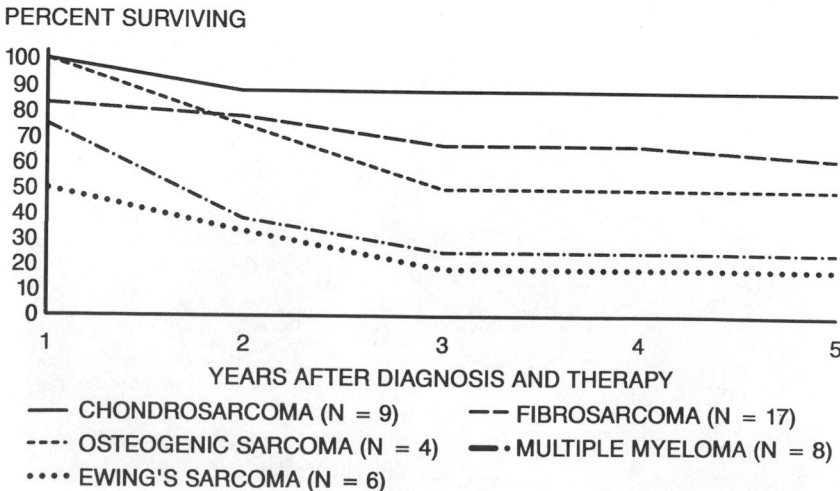

PERCENT SURVIVING

YEARS AFTER DIAGNOSIS AND THERAPY

— CHONDROSARCOMA (N = 9)   – – FIBROSARCOMA (N = 17)

- - - OSTEOGENIC SARCOMA (N = 4)   – • MULTIPLE MYELOMA (N = 8)

•••• EWING'S SARCOMA (N = 6)

Figure 48-3. Survival rates in patients with malignant neoplasms of the chest wall. The total number of patients used to generate this graph was 44 rather than 47 because 2 patients with fibrosarcomas were lost to follow-up and an 84-year-old man with a massive chondrosarcoma of the chest wall was not considered a candidate for resection.

arise in the ribs, and 20 percent arise in the sternum (McAfee, et al., 1985).

Most of these tumors are solitary and have been present an average of 18 months prior to presentation (McAfee, et al., 1985).

The conventional radiographic findings of a chondrosarcoma include a lobulated mass that arises in the medullary portion of the rib or sternum, often with cortical bone destruction. Calcification of the tumor is missed in 45 percent of chest radiographs but detected on chest CT scan. A stippled calcification pattern is most common, but rings and arcs of calcification may be present (Aoki, et al., 1989).

The diagnosis of these tumors should be made by an excisional biopsy. The incisional biopsy has no place in the diagnosis of these lesions because the histologic findings vary from a poorly differentiated cellular appearance to an extremely well-differentiated lesion that is indistinguishable from a benign chondroma (Fig. 48-4) (Sabanathan, et al., 1985; McAfee, et al., 1985). The incidence of chondrosarcomatous change in a solitary osteochondroma is reported to be 1 to 2 percent (Lichtenstin, 1977). The natural history of these tumors is one of slow growth, with frequent local recurrence and late metastasis. Chondrosarcomas have been related to previous chest wall trauma in 12.5 percent of patients (McAfee, et al., 1985).

The therapy of choice is wide local excision, including several partial ribs above and below the lesion, with surgical margins of at least 4 cm. If the lesion originates in the sternum, then a sternotomy with a corresponding resection of the costal arches bilaterally should be performed (Arnold and Pairolero, 1978). Chest wall reconstruction is frequently necessary.

Chondrosarcomas are extremely radio- and chemoresistant. The prognostic factors include the tumor's grade, diameter, and location. Tumors less than 6 cm and sternal tumors have a better patient prognosis. The 10-year survival rates are 96 percent with wide local excision, 65 percent with local

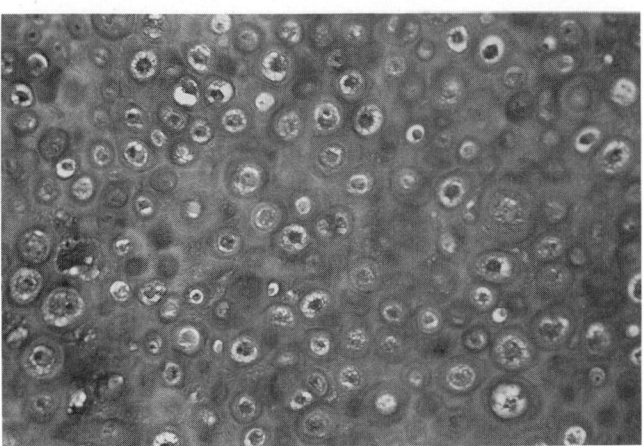

Figure 48-4. This photomicrograph presents a characteristic field from a histologic section of a chondrosarcoma. The histologic characteristics of this tumor include a cartilaginous neoplasm, which has anaplastic cells with one or more bizarre, hyperchromatic nuclei. This malignant neoplasm is also known to have frequent variations in the grade of tumor cells present throughout the presenting mass (H & E, × 200).

excision, and 14 percent with palliative excision (McAfee, et al., 1985). The local recurrence rate is higher with local excision (50 percent) than wide local excision (17 percent). The possibility of late local recurrences of chondrosarcomas necessitates long-term follow-up of these patients (Graeber, et al., 1982).

Ewing Sarcoma and Askin's Tumor

Ewing sarcoma is a small round tumor with characteristics of a primitive neuroectodermal tumor (PNET) and a neural histogenesis, as indicated by experimental studies (Cavazanna, et al., 1987). It is the most common primary chest wall malignancy in children and occurs in 8 to 22 percent of malignant chest wall lesions in adults (Graeber, et al., 1982; Sabanathan, et al., 1985; King, et al., 1986; Shamberger, et al., 1989). The differential diagnosis of small, round cell malignant tumors includes neuroblastomas, embryonal rhabdomyosarcomas, and lymphomas in addition to Ewing sarcomas (Stefanco, et al., 1988). A highly malignant alternative to Ewing sarcoma is the PNET, which was first described by Askin, et al. (1979). PNET is considered similar to Ewing sarcoma because of a common neuroectodermal differentiation and a frequently seen translocation between the long arms of chromosomes 11 and 22 [t(11:22)(q24:q12)] (Turc-Cavel, et al., 1983; Whang-Peng, et al., 1984). PNET and Ewing sarcoma are grouped together because the diagnosis and therapy of each are similar.

Most patients are between 5 and 30 years old and present with progressive chest wall pain with or without the presence of a mass. Some patients have a modest leukocytosis and elevated erythrocyte sedimentation rate. The typical radiographic picture is the characteristic onion-peel appearance, which is produced by multiple layers of periosteal new bone formation (Sabanathan, et al., 1985). Bony destruction, sclerosis of the widened cortex, and a widened medulla are also common radiographic findings. The tumor may involve several ribs but usually is confined to one rib. The diagnosis may be made with percutaneous needle biopsy (Ayala and Zornosa, 1983), but as with other primary chest wall malignancies, an excisional biopsy is best (Fig. 48-5). The preoperative workup should include standard chest imaging and bone marrow aspiration.

These patients are best treated through a multimodality approach. The entire marrow cavity of the rib is considered to be at risk for malignancy; therefore, the entire involved rib is removed along with a partial rib resection above and below the lesion (Shamberger, et al., 1989). Postoperative external beam irradiation to the tumor bed provides excellent local control. If complete surgical resection and irradiation are performed, local control rates of 93 percent have been reported (Thomas, et al., 1983).

Chemotherapy is used to control distant disease and has been shown to decrease the incidence of distant metastases and improve survival rates (Thomas, et al., 1983; Hayes, et al., 1983). Doxorubicin, dactinomycin, cyclophosphamide, and vincristine are the four drugs used in combination most frequently. Failure to include doxorubicin in this combination has detrimental results (Perez, et al., 1981). Preoperative chemotherapy has been reported to facilitate subsequent local therapy, but its use is not well established (Shamberger,

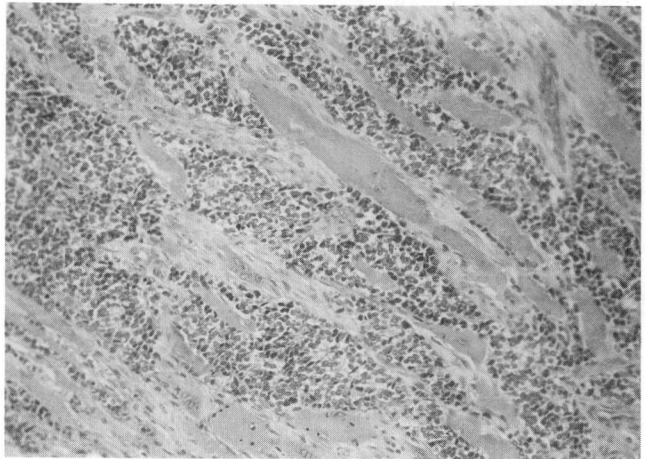

Figure 48-5. This photomicrograph shows a characteristic sample taken from a Ewing sarcoma. The histologic characteristics of this tumor include closely packed small round cells, which are infiltrating muscle fibers (H & E, × 200).

et al., 1989; Brown, et al., 1987). The survival rate was improved with multimodality therapy to 52 percent at 5 years in one study (Hayry and Scheinin, 1988). Patients with distant metastasis rarely survive 5 years.

The complications of extensive chest wall resections in children with Ewing sarcoma include scoliosis and restrictive pulmonary disease (Grosfeld, et al., 1988; Malangoni, et al., 1980). Harrington rod fusion may be necessary for severe scoliosis. The restrictive pulmonary function usually does not result in any long-term respiratory difficulties.

Osteosarcoma

Osteosarcomas occur between the ages of 10 and 25 years and again after age 40 years in association with several other disease processes. They frequently present as a painful mass with a duration of symptoms prior to presentation that lasts from weeks to months. Most osteosarcomas arise de novo and are located in the metaphysial portion of the long bones, such as the femur, tibia, and humerus. They do, however, account for a small but significant number of rib-based malignancies (Fig. 48-6) (Graeber, et al., 1982). There is an associa-

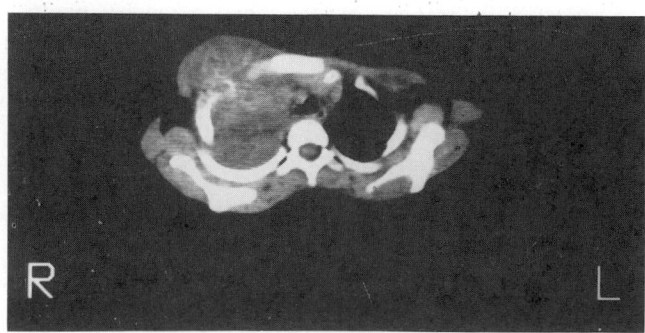

Figure 48-6. Osteosarcoma. A CT scan of a right third rib-based osteosarcoma with destruction of the bone is shown here. The diagnosis was confirmed by an excisional biopsy.

tion between the development of osteosarcomas and previous irradiation, Paget's disease, and chemotherapy (Souba, et al., 1986; Huvos, 1986; Tucker, et al., 1987). The latency period for the development of osteosarcoma after irradiation is approximately 10 years (Huvos, et al., 1985).

The preoperative evaluation of a patient considered to have an osteosarcoma should include an excisional biopsy to confirm the diagnosis. An elevated serum alkaline phosphatase level may be present by laboratory analysis, but this is nonspecific. One study showed that tumors associated with a serum elevation of this enzyme had increased metastatic rates (Raymond, et al., 1987). Radiographically, the classic "sunburst" pattern of new periosteal bone formation is frequently seen (Pass, 1989; Boyd, 1986). Triangular elevation of the periosteum secondary to reactive new bone formation may be seen radiographically and is known as Codman's triangle sign. Histologically, we see eosinophilic staining and a glassy appearance with irregular contours of the osteoid. Interspersed with the osteoblastic cells are foci of fibroblastic and chondroblastic cells, which help divide osteosarcomas into those three subtypes (Fig. 48-7) (Rosai, 1989).

The therapy for osteosarcoma of the chest is preoperative chemotherapy, which usually consists of a combination of doxorubicin, high-dose methotrexate, and cisplatin (Winkler, et al., 1984). This is done to shrink the tumor prior to resection and to evaluate the tumor's response to chemotherapy. Tumors with a significant amount of tumor necrosis postchemotherapy are associated with better patient survival rates (Raymond, et al., 1987). Preoperative intra-arterial chemotherapy with cisplatin has produced significant disease-free survival rates in those patients who have a complete or partial response (Jaffe, et al., 1989). Radiotherapy is usually ineffective for osteosarcomas.

The prognostic factors include the response to preoperative chemotherapy, an association with Paget's disease (worse prognosis), and unifocal osteosarcoma. The addition of multidrug chemotherapy to the therapy of osteosarcoma has in-

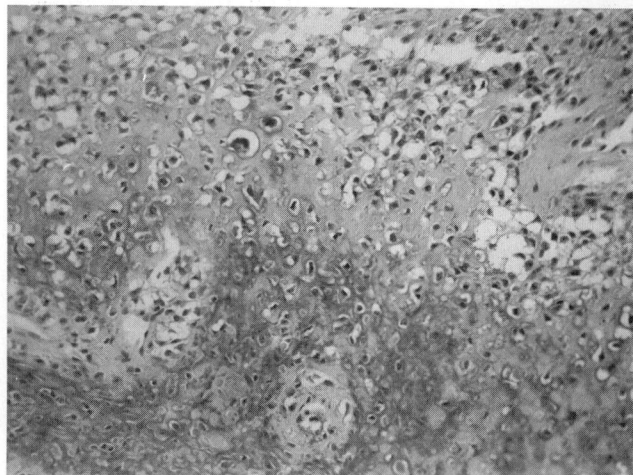

Figure 48-7. This photomicrograph shows a characteristic section taken from an osteosarcoma. The histologic characteristics include anaplastic osteoblasts in an osteoid matrix with atypical calcification (H & E, × 200).

creased 5-year disease-free survival rates to greater than 50 percent (Lane, et al., 1986).

Plasmacytoma

Solitary plasmacytomas that arise in bone account for 10 to 30 percent of primary chest wall malignancies (Pass, 1989; Graeber, et al., 1982). They are more common in male patients and usually present later in life, with a mean age of 60 years (Graeber, et al., 1982). The most common chest wall location is the ribs, followed by the clavicle and sternum. Soft tissue invasion from bone lesions may occur. The radiographic appearance of the plasmacytoma demonstrates an osteolytic process with several paracostal opacities frequently present (Galluccio, et al., 1989).

Confirmation that the plasmacytoma is localized to the chest wall requires several studies. The patient should undergo a bone marrow aspiration, skeletal radiographs, and immunoelectrophoretic examination of the serum and urine. A patient with a solitary plasmacytoma usually has a normal calcium level and is not anemic. Evidence of monoclonality of one of the immunoglobulins with normal levels of the other circulating immunoglobulins strongly suggests that the plasmacytoma is solitary. Serum β_2-microglobulin levels are usually normal in the solitary plasmacytoma. Most bone lesions show a predominance of immunoglobulin reactivity; upper respiratory tract lesions are predominantly immunoglobulin (Rosai, 1989). The diagnosis of a solitary plasmacytoma should be made only if all studies for disseminated disease have negative findings.

Microscopically, plasmacytomas are composed of sheets of plasma cells and are often hypervascular. The nucleoli are prominent and have a characteristic pinwheel appearance. Amyloid may be present in 25 percent of the lesions (Fig. 48-8) (Meis, et al., 1987).

The role of surgery is to establish the diagnosis by excisional biopsy. High-dose radiotherapy (5,000 to 6,000 cGy)

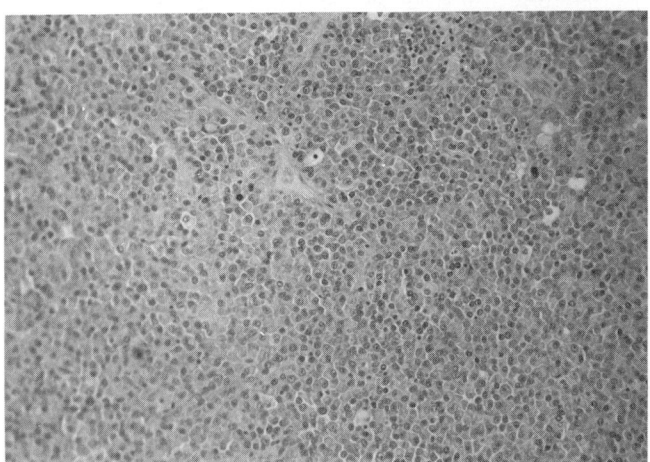

Figure 48-8. This is a representative microphotograph taken from a plasmacytoma. The characteristic features of this neoplasm include a large field of well-differentiated plasma cells that have eccentric nuclei that are surrounded by an adjacent "halo" (H & E, × 200).

has been shown to be successful for the local control of solitary plasmacytomas (Mill and Griffith, 1980). If the lesion is refractory to radiotherapy, then a more extensive surgical excision can be done. Systematic chemotherapy should only be given for evidence of disease progression (Pass, 1989). Local recurrence is uncommon for plasmacytomas. Spontaneous regression of a chest wall plasmacytoma has been reported, but this is rare (Arunabh, et al., 1988). After they are treated for a solitary plasmacytoma, in approximately 35 to 55 percent of patients, multiple myeloma develops, often 10 to 12 years after the initial diagnosis (Meis, et al., 1987). The presence of nuclear immaturity with prominent nucleoli may have a positive predictive value for the development of multiple myeloma. The presence of a monoclonal protein in the serum or urine has no predictive value for the development of multiple myeloma (Rosai, 1989).

The 10-year survival rate for all bony locations of solitary plasmacytoma is 68 percent (Bataille and Sany, 1981). A 25 to 37 percent 5-year survival rate after therapy for primary chest wall plasmacytomas is expected (Graeber, et al., 1982; Gordon, et al., 1991). Close follow-up of these patients with frequent urine and serum electrophoretic studies is necessary because the development of multiple myeloma is fairly common.

Soft Tissue Sarcoma

Primary soft tissue sarcomas of the chest wall are uncommon, and few centers have treated extensive series of these tumors. The more common tumors include fibrosarcomas, liposarcomas, malignant fibrous histiocytomas, rhabdomyosarcomas, dermatofibrosarcomas protuberans, and angiosarcomas (Gordon, et al., 1991; Graeber, et al., 1987). These tumors compromise nearly 50 percent of all primary chest wall sarcomas (Souba, et al., 1986; Ryan, et al., 1989). The factors that may predispose the patient to the development of soft tissue sarcomas include a history of previous irradiation and syndromes such as von Recklinghausen's disease (neurofibromatosis), Gardner's syndrome, and Werner's syndrome (Seyer, 1988; Lynch, et al., 1973).

Fibrosarcomas are large, painful masses that occur in all age groups and often involve adjacent structures (Fig. 48-9) (Boyd, 1986). The radiographic findings show a large irregular mass with frequent destruction of the bone. The therapy includes wide local excision, with tumor-free margins for low-grade sarcomas and the addition of chemotherapy for high-grade lesions (Gordon, et al., 1991). The difficulty in treating this neoplasm is related to the significant incidence of local recurrence and a propensity for the tumor to metastasize to the lungs (Graeber, et al., 1982). The 5-year survival rate is 53 to 86 percent after surgery, with or without adjuvant therapy (Graeber, et al., 1982).

Rhabdomyosarcoma is a rare primary chest wall tumor. It accounts for 4 to 26 percent of primary malignant tumors. These tumors arise from undifferentiated mesoderm and are usually diagnosed after an incisional biopsy. Microscopically, the tumor cells are small and spindle shaped (Fig. 48-10). There are highly cellular regions that surround blood vessels and alternate with abundant parvicellular regions of muscle intercellular material. Immunocytochemical analysis of the

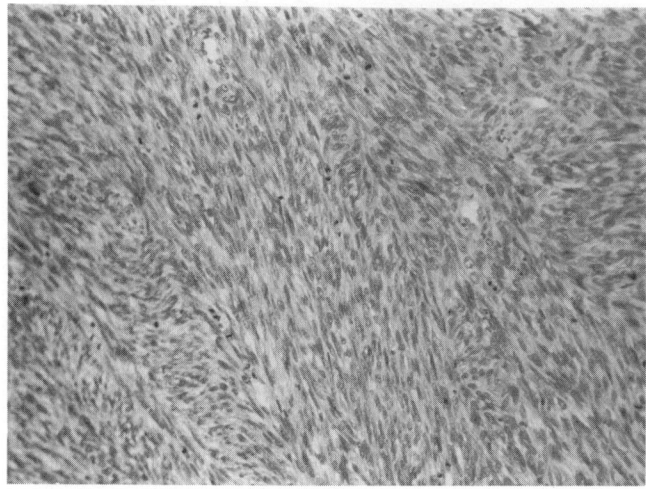

Figure 48-9. This photomicrograph shows a representative sample of a fibrosarcoma. The histologic characteristics of this tumor show malignant spindle cells, which are arranged in a "herringbone" fashion. This alignment is characteristic of the tumor (H & E, × 200).

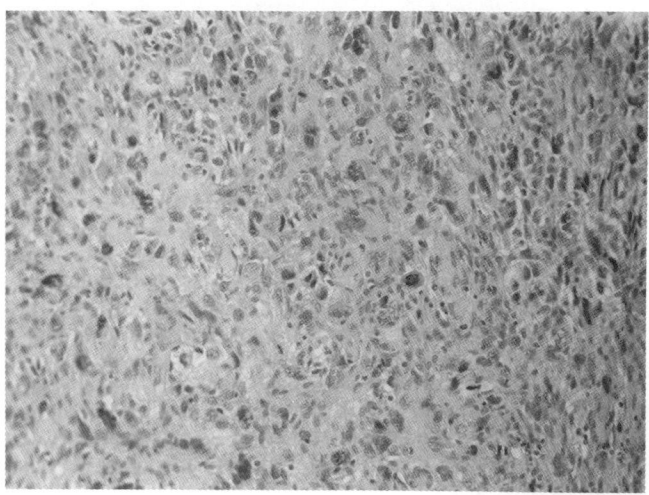

Figure 48-11. This photomicrograph shows a representative field from a MFH. The characteristics of this neoplasm include a pleomorphic tumor, which has many large, bizarre-shaped cells in a fibrous stroma (H & E, × 200).

tissue has been very useful in the diagnosis of rhabdomyosarcoma. The markers used include myoglobin, desmin, myosin, actin, and antiskeletal muscle antibody from myasthenic patients. The therapy is wide surgical excision and multidrug chemotherapy. Radiotherapy is usually not effective in this tumor.

Malignant fibrous histiocytoma (MFH) is an uncommon primary tumor to the chest wall. These tumors arise from tissue histiocytes and have the potential to produce collagen (Fig. 48-11) (Ozzello, et al., 1963). CT scanning aids in the operative planning and in the evaluation of metastatic disease. The therapy is by wide local excision for primary and

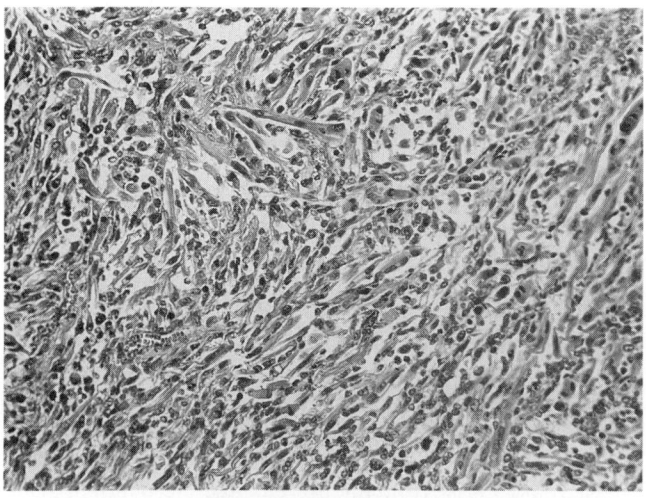

Figure 48-10. This photograph depicts some of the histologic characteristics associated with a rhabdomyosarcoma. Included in the field are large elongated tumor cells that have abundant eosinophilic cytoplasm, raquet cells, and more primitive rhabdomyoblasts (H & E, × 200).

locally recurrent tumors (Venn, et al., 1986). MFH frequently has local recurrence and distant metastasis. However, MFH is generally resistant to chemotherapy. Adjuvant brachytherapy for soft tissue sarcomas has been shown to be beneficial if the patients are undergoing resection for locoregional recurrence in a previously irradiated site (Wallner, et al., 1991). Postoperative external beam radiation may be effective, particularly if the resection margins are inadequate (Venn, et al., 1986; Wallner, et al., 1991).

Liposarcoma accounts for 15 percent of primary chest wall soft tissue sarcomas (Gordon, et al., 1991). Most (70 percent) are low grade, and en bloc resection is the therapy of choice. Local recurrence was found in 33 percent of patients in the study by Greager, et al. (1987), and was treated by wide local excision alone. The presence of local recurrence has no significant effect on the overall survival rate (Gordon, et al., 1991). Radiotherapy may be effective in the control of local recurrence, but its role is unclear. The 5-year survival rate is 83 percent (Graeber, et al., 1982).

The prognostic indicators for primary tissue sarcomas include the tumor grade, presence of distant metastases, and positive surgical resection margins (Gordon, et al., 1991; Graeber, et al., 1982; Perry, et al., 1990). Tumors that are low grade are associated with a 90 percent 5-year survival rate; high-grade sarcomas have a 49 percent 5-year survival rate (Souba, et al., 1986). Positive resection margins negatively affect both the disease-free survival and overall survival rates in high-grade sarcomas, which emphasizes the importance of negative margins (Perry, et al., 1990). Radiotherapy and chemotherapy have no prognostic value for high-grade sarcomas in the adult patient. Because sarcomas tend to metastasize to the lungs, CT scans of the chest should be performed. However, up to 50 percent of lung parenchyma nodules discovered at surgery are not seen on preoperative CT scans (Jablons, et al., 1989). The presence of these synchronous pulmonary metastases is associated with a worse prognosis (Perry, et al., 1990).

SURGERY

Chest Wall Resection

Wide resection of primary malignant chest wall neoplasm is essential to successful management. However, the extent of resection should not be compromised because of an inability to close a large chest wall defect (Pairolero and Arnold, 1985, 1986a, b; Arnold and Pairolero, 1979, 1984a). Opinions differ as to what constitutes wide resection. In a recent report from the Mayo Clinic (King, et al., 1986), which analyzed the effect of the extent of resection on the long-term survival of patients with primary malignant chest wall tumors, 56 percent of patients with a 4-cm or greater margin of resection remained free from recurrent cancer at 5 years compared with only 29 percent for patients with a 2-cm margin (Fig. 48-12). For many surgeons, a resection margin of 2 cm would be considered adequate. Although this margin may be adequate for chest wall metastases, benign tumors and certain low-grade malignant primary neoplasms, such as chondrosarcoma, a 2-cm resection margin is inadequate for more malignant neoplasms, such as osteogenic sarcoma and malignant fibrous histiocytoma, which have the potential to spread within the marrow cavity or along tissue planes, such as the periosteum or parietal pleura. Consequently, all primary malignant neoplasms initially diagnosed by excisional biopsy should undergo further resection to include at least a 4-cm margin of normal tissue on all sides. High-grade malignancies should also have the entire involved bone resected. For neoplasms of the rib cage, this would include removal of the involved ribs, the corresponding anterior costal arches if the tumor is located anteriorly, and several partial ribs above and below the neoplasm. For tumor of the sternum and manubrium, resection of the entire involved bone and corresponding costal arches bilaterally is indicated. Any attached structures, such as the lung, thymus, pericardium, or chest wall muscles, should also be excised.

Consideration for Reconstruction of Chest Wall Defects

Location

Size

Depth
    Partial thickness
    Full thickness

Duration

Condition of local tissue
    Irradiation
    Infection
    Residual tumor
    Scarring

General condition of patient
    Chemotherapy
    Corticosteroid
    Chronic infection

Life-style and type of work

Prognosis

Chest Wall Reconstruction

The ability to close large chest wall defects is of prime importance in the surgical therapy of chest wall neoplasms. The critical questions of whether the reconstructed thorax will support respiration and protect the underlying organs must be answered when we consider that both the extent of resection and dependable reconstruction are the mandatory ingredients for successful therapy. These two important items are accomplished most safely by the joint efforts of a thoracic and a plastic surgeon (Arnold and Pairolero, 1984a).

Reconstruction of chest wall defects involves a consideration of many factors. The location and size of the defect

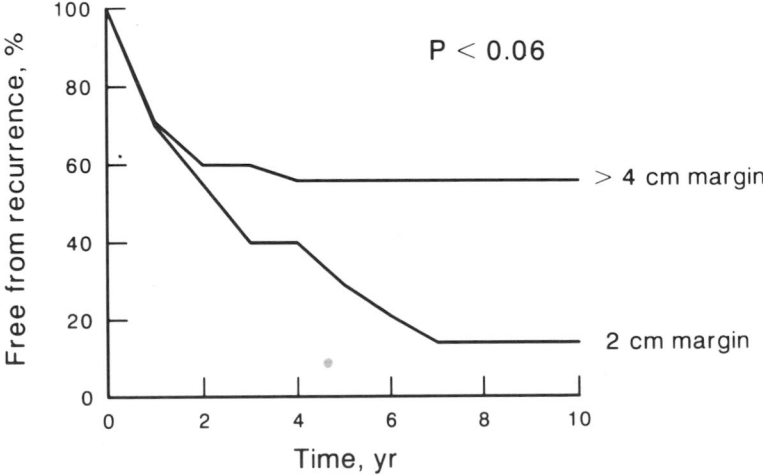

Figure 48-12. Percentage of patients with malignant chest wall tumors free from recurrent tumors by extent of resection margin. Zero time on the abscissa represents the day of the chest wall resection. (From King RM, Pairolero PC, Trastek VH et al: Primary wall tumors: factors affecting survival. Ann Thorac Surg 41:597, 1986, with permission.)

are of the utmost importance, but the medical history and local conditions of the wound may drastically alter a reconstructive choice. Primary closure remains the best option available if possible. If full-thickness reconstruction is required, which is usually the situation in most primary neoplasms that have not been previously treated, consideration must be given to both the structural stability of the thorax and soft tissue coverage.

Skeletal Reconstruction

Reconstruction of the bony thorax is controversial. Differences of opinion exist both as to which patients should undergo reconstruction and what type of reconstruction should be done. The decision not to reconstruct the skeleton depends on the size and location of the defect and whether the wound is infected. In general, infected wounds should not be reconstructed simultaneously. Similarly, defects less than 5 cm in greatest diameter anywhere on the thorax are usually not reconstructed. Likewise, high posterior defects less than 10 cm do not require reconstruction because the overlying scapula provides support. However, if the defect is located near the tip of the scapula, the defect, even if 5 cm or less in size, should be closed to avoid impingement of the tip of the scapula into the chest with movement of the arm. Alternatively, the lower half of the scapula could be resected. Finally, all larger defects located anywhere on the chest should be reconstructed, and either autogenous tissue or prosthetic material may be used.

Stabilization of the bony thorax is best accomplished with prosthetic material, such as Prolene mesh (Ethicon, Somerville, NJ) or 2-mm-thick Gore-Tex (polytetrafluroethylene) soft tissue patch. When either of these materials is placed under tension, the rigidity of the prosthesis is improved in all directions. Currently, the Gore-Tex soft tissue patch is superior because this material has the added advantage of preventing movement of fluid and air across the reconstructed chest wall. Marlex mesh (Daval, Providence, RI) is used less frequently because, when it is placed under tension, this material is rigid in one direction only. Reconstruction with rigid material, such as methylmethacrylate-impregnated meshes is not necessary.

All large full-thickness skeletal defects that result from the resection of a neoplasm in both the sternum and lateral chest wall should be reconstructed if the wound is not contaminated. If the would is contaminated from previous radiation

---

Autogenous Tissue Available for Chest Wall Reconstruction

Muscle
  Latissimus dorsi
  Pectoralis major
  Rectus abdominis
  Serratus anterior
  External oblique
  Trapezius
Omentum

---

necrosis or necrotic neoplasm, reconstruction with prosthetic material is not advised because the prosthesis may subsequently become infected, which would result in obligatory removal. In this situation, reconstruction with a musculocutaneous flap alone is preferred. Similarly, resection of full-thickness bony thorax in a patient who has been previously irradiated may not require skeletal reconstruction because the lung is frequently adherent to the underlying parietal pleura and pneumothorax may not occur with chest wall resection.

Soft Tissue Reconstruction

Both muscle and omentum can be used to reconstruct soft tissue chest wall defects. Muscle can be transposed as muscle alone or as a musculocutaneous flap and is the tissue of choice for closure of most full-thickness soft tissue defects. All major chest wall muscles can be mobilized on a single axis of rotation and transposed to another location of the chest wall (McGraw and Arnold, 1986). If muscle is not available because of previous radiation damage or an operation, free muscle flaps from another location can be reimplanted with the expectation of dependable long-term coverage. The omentum should be reserved for partial-thickness reconstruction or as a back-up procedure when muscle is either not available or has failed in a previous full-thickness repair.

Latissimus Dorsi

The latissimus dorsi is the largest flat muscle in the thorax. Its dominant thoracodorsal neurovascular leash has an arc of rotation that allows coverage of the lateral and central back and the anterolateral and central front of the thorax (Campbell, 1950; Bostwick, et al., 1979). Its dependable musculocutaneous vascular connections permit it to be used also as a reliable musculocutaneous flap. This muscle flap can cover huge chest wall defects because virtually one-half of the back can be elevated on the blood supply of a single latissimus dorsi in the uninjured, nonirradiated patient. The donor site posteriorly may require skin grafting when large musculocutaneous flaps are elevated, but this represents a minior disadvantage when we consider that large, robust flaps can be transposed to either the anterior or the posterior chest for full-thickness reconstruction. If the dominant blood supply has been compromised by previous trauma or surgery, the muscle can still be transposed dependably on the branch of the adjacent serratus anterior (Fisher, et al., 1983).

Pectoralis Major

The pectoralis major is the second largest flat muscle on the chest wall and in many respects is the mirror image of the latissimus dorsi. Its dominant thoracoacromial neurovascular leash, which enters posteriorly about midclavicle, allows both elevation and rotation centrally of the muscle as either a muscle or a musculocutaneous flap (Arnold and Pairolero, 1979). The pectoralis major flap is as reliable as the latissimus dorsi flap. It is of major benefit in the reconstruction of anterior chest wall defects, such as those that result from sternal tumor excisions (Arnold and Pairolero, 1978; Pairolero and Arnold, 1984, 1986). Generally, only the muscle without the overlying soft tissue and skin is transposed, which thereby avoids the distortion created by a centralization of the breast. Reconstruction in this manner is more symmetric and more aesthetically acceptable. If sternal skin must be excised, the symmetry of the breast can still be maintained because the transposed muscle readily accepts and supports a skin graft. If necessary, the muscle may also be transposed on its secondary blood supply through the perforators from the internal mammary vessels.

Rectus Abdominis

Use of the rectus abdominis for chest wall reconstruction is based on the internal mammary neurovascular leash. The inferior epigastric vessels must be divided to allow rotation to the chest wall. This muscle can be mobilized and moved either as a muscle or as a musculocutaneous flap, with the skin component oriented either horizontally, vertically, or both. The vertical skin flap, however, is more reliable because it is oriented along the long axis of the muscle and thus maintains more musculocutaneous perforators. The donor site is usually closed primarily.

The rectus abdominis is most careful in the reconstruction of lower sternal wounds. Either muscle can be used because their arc of rotation is identical. Care must be taken to choose the muscle that has patent and uninjured internal mammary vessels. Angiographic demonstration of vessel patency may be helpful to determine which musculocutaneous unit would be the most reliable, particularly in previously irradiated patients or in patients who had prior coronary artery bypass surgery.

Serratus Anterior

The serratus anterior is a smaller, flat muscle that is located along the midaxillary chest wall. Its blood supply comes from the serratus branch of the thoracodorsal vessels and from the long thoracic artery and vein. Although this muscle can be used alone, it is more commonly utilized in chest wall reconstruction as an adjunctive muscle in tandem with either the pectoralis major or the latissimus dorsi to close larger defects. The muscle also augments the skin-carrying ability of either adjacent muscle (Arnold and Pairolero, 1984b). This muscle is particularly useful as an intrathoracic muscle flap (Pairolero, et al., 1983; Arnold and Pairolero, 1984b).

External Oblique

The external oblique muscle may also be transposed as either a muscle or musculocutaneous flap, and it is most useful in closing defects of the upper abdomen and lower thorax. It reaches the inframammary fold without tension but does not readily extend higher (Hodgkinson and Arnold, 1980). The primary blood supply is from the lower thoracic intercostal vessels. The advantage of this muscle is that lower chest wall defects can be closed without a distortion of the breast.

Trapezius

The trapezius muscle is useful to close defects at the base of the neck or the thoracic outlet, but it is not a consistently useful muscle as far as the remainder of chest wall reconstruc-

tion is concerned. Its primary blood supply is the dorsal scapular vessels.

Omentum

Omental transposition has been useful in the reconstruction of the partial-thickness chest wall defects that may occur with certain soft tissue neoplasms or radiation necrosis (Jurkiewicz and Arnold, 1977; Arnold and Pairolero, 1986). In the latter situation, the skin and soft tissue are debrided down to what remains of the thoracic skeleton, which may be either bone or cartilage but frequently is only irradiated ischemic scar. The transposed omentum, with its excellent blood supply from the gastroepiploic vessels, adheres to the irradiated wound and readily accepts and supports an overlying skin graft. Because the omentum has no structural stability on its own, it is not useful in full-thickness defects because additional support with fascia lata, bone, or prosthetic material would be necessary.

Omental transposition is exceedingly helpful in situations in which planned muscle flaps have been used but have failed because of partial necrosis. Generally, this results in only a soft tissue defect, and a pleural seal with respiratory stability is not required, which thus allows a most threatening situation to be salvaged.

Late Results

During the past 10 years, more than 60 chest wall resections for primary neoplasms were performed at the Mayo Clinic by one team of surgeons (unpublished data). Nearly two-thirds of these neoplasms were malignant. Malignant fibrous histiocytoma and chondrosarcoma were the most common malignant neoplasms, and desmoid tumor was the most common benign tumor. The patients' ages ranged from 12 to 80 years (median, 43.5 years). An average of 3.9 ribs was resected. Total or partial sternectomies were performed in 13 patients. Skeletal defects were closed with prosthetic material in 2 patients and with autogenous ribs in 5. Fifty-four patients underwent 68 muscle transpositions; these included 24 pectoralis major, 23 latissimus dorsi, 6 serratus anterior, 3 external oblique, 2 rectus abdominis, 2 trapezius, and 8 other. The omentum was transposed in eight patients. The median hospitalization was 9 days. There were no 30-day operative deaths. The patients were generally extubated during the evening of the operation or on the following morning. Two patients required tracheostomy. Most other patients had only minor changes in pulmonary function (Meadows, et al., 1985).

The long-term survival of patients with primary chest wall malignant neoplasms is dependent on the cell type and the extent of chest wall resection. In the Mayo Clinic series, the overall 5-year survival rate was 57 percent (King, et al., 1986). Wide resection for chondrosarcoma resulted in a 5-year survival rate of 96 percent (McAfee, et al., 1985) compared with only 70 percent for patients who had local excision (Fig. 48-13). The 5-year overall survival rate for patients with either chondrosarcoma or rhabdomyosarcoma was 70 percent (King, et al., 1986), in contrast to a rate of only 38 percent for patients with malignant fibrous histiocytomas (Fig. 48-14). Recurrent neoplasm, however, was an ominous

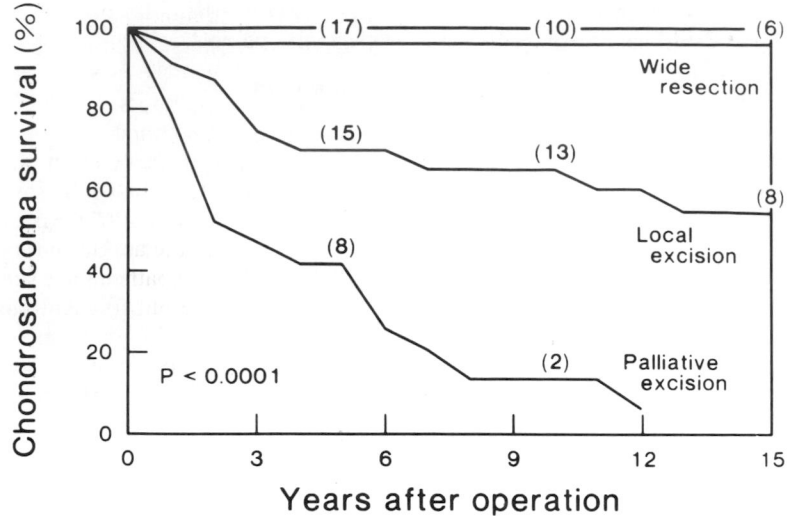

Figure 48-13. Survival of patients with chest wall chondrosarcomas by extent of operation. Zero time on the abscissa represents the day of chest wall resection. (From McAfee MK, Pairolero PC, Bergstrahl EJ et al: Chondrosarcoma of the chest wall: factors affecting survival. Ann Thorac Surg 40:535, 1985, with permission.)

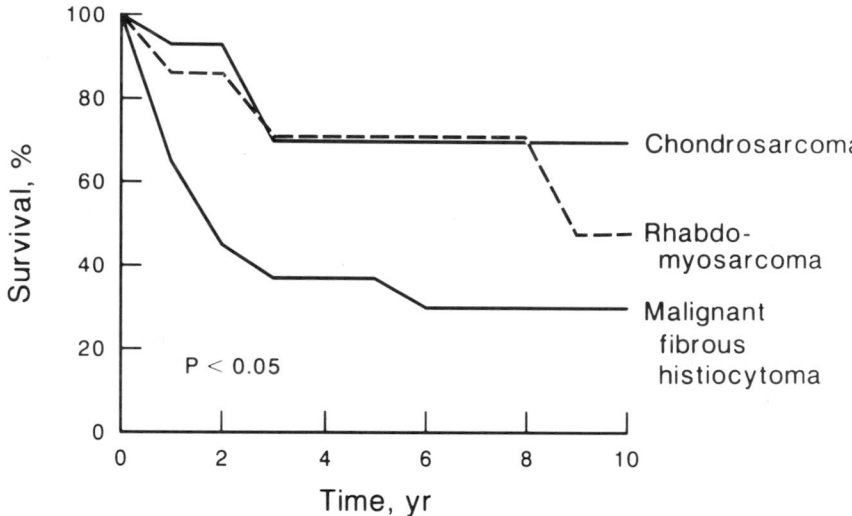

Figure 48-14. Survival for patients with chondrosarcomas and rhabdomyosarcomas compared with malignant fibrous histiocytomas. Zero time on the abscissa represents the day of chest wall resection. (From King RM, Pairolero PC, Trastek VH et al: Primary wall tumors: factors effecting survival. Ann Thorac Surg 41:597, 1986, with permission.)

sign; only 17 percent of patients in whom recurrence developed survived 5 years.

SUMMARY

The key to successful therapy of primary chest wall neoplasms remains early diagnosis and aggressive surgical resection. This procedure can generally be performed in one operation, with minimal respiratory insufficiency and with low operation mortality rates. When combined with current methods of reconstruction, potential cure is likely for most patients with primary chest wall neoplasms.

COMMENTS AND CONTROVERSIES

As documented by Drs. Graeber, Jones, and Pairolero, primary malignant tumors of the chest wall are relatively uncommon. Since almost all primary malignant chest wall neoplasms can be classified as either soft-tissue sarcomas or malignant neoplasms of bone or cartilage, estimates can be made of the number of tumors expected to be diagnosed in

Table 48-1. Estimates of Number of New Cases of Primary Malignant Chest Wall Tumors in the United States in 1993

Tumor	All Sites (No.)	Chest Wall (No.)
Soft-tissue sarcoma	6,000	360
Chondrosarcoma	400	60
Ewing's sarcoma	300	45
Solitary plasmacytoma	125	25
Osteosarcoma	600	18
Total	7,425	508

the United States in 1994 (Boring, et al., 1994; Burt, 1994) (Table 48-1). Approximately 500 new cases of primary malig-

nant chest wall tumors will be diagnosed yearly in the United States. Since it is estimated that there will be 1,170,000 new cases of cancer diagnosed in the United States yearly, primary malignant tumors of the chest wall comprised only 0.04 percent of all new cancers. Since primary malignant tumors of the chest wall are relatively uncommon, data to support therapy options are sparse, but nicely outlined in this chapter.

There is only one area of disagreement, and that is the classification by the authors that chest wall desmoid tumors are benign. Many pathologists currently accept the desmoid tumor as a low-grade fibrosarcoma and not a benign disease (Brodsky, et al., 1992; Posner, et al., 1989).

Michael E. Burt

KEY REFERENCES

Graeber GM, Snyder RJ, Fleming AW et al.: Initial and long-term results in the management of primary chest wall neoplasms. Ann Thorac Surg 34:664, 1982

These authors present the Armed Forces Institute of Pathology's experience with 110 patients with primary chest wall neoplasms. Included are both soft tissue and bone neoplasms. The roles of chemotherapy and radiotherapy for each type of malignant neoplasm are discussed.

King RM, Pairolero PC, Trastek VF et al.: Primary chest wall tumors: factors affecting survival. Ann Thorac Surg 41:597, 1986

This series represents a 20-year experience of chest wall tumors treated at the Mayo Clinic from 1955 to 1975 and includes both soft tissue and bony tumors. Both chondrosarcoma and rhabdomyosarcoma had a better prognosis than did malignant fibrous histiocytoma.

McAfee MK, Pairolero PC, Bergstralh EJ et al.: Chondrosarcoma of the chest wall: factors affecting survival. Ann Thorac Surg 40:535, 1985

These authors present a single institution's experience (96 patients) with chondrosarcoma of the chest wall. This series is the largest series of chest wall chondrosarcoma reported to date and clearly demonstrates that the natural history of chondrosarcoma is one of slow growth and local recurrence.

McGraw JB, Arnold PG: McGraw and Arnold's Atlas of Muscle and Musculocutaneous Flaps. Hampton Press, 1986

The anatomy, indications for, and technique of commonly used muscle flaps in all areas of the body are each summarized, illustrated by color photographs of fresh cadaver dissections, and then supplemented by appropriate intraoperative color photographs of clinical cases. This atlas should be read by every surgeon interested in the reconstruction of the chest wall.

Pairolero PC, Arnold PG: Chest wall tumors: experience with 100 consecutive patients. J Thorac Cardiovasc Surg 90:367, 1985

This series represents a single team of surgeons' experience in the management of 100 consecutive patients with chest wall tumors. This series of patients demonstrates that aggressive resection for a chest wall tumor with reliable reconstruction can be accomplished safely and that early wide resection is potentially curative therapy.

REFERENCES

Aoki J, Moser RP Jr, Kransdorf MJ: Chondrosarcoma of the sternum: CT features. J Comput Assist Tomogr 13:535, 1989

Arnold PG, Pairolero PC: Surgical management of the radiated chest wall. Plast Reconstr Surg 77:605, 1986

Arnold PG, Pairolero PC: The serratus anterior muscle: intrathoracic and extrathoracic utilization. Plast Reconstr Surg 73:240, 1984

Arnold PG, Pairolero PC: Chest wall reconstruction: experience with 100 consecutive patients. Ann Surg 199:725, 1984

Arnold PG, Pairolero PC: Use of pectoralis major muscle flaps to repair defects of anterior chest wall. Plast Reconstr Surg 63:205, 1979

Arnold PG, Pairolero PC: Chondrosarcoma of the manubrium. Resection and reconstruction with pectoralis major muscle. Mayo Clinic Proc 53:54, 1978

Arunabh, Gupta SD, Bal S et al: Spontaneous regression of extramedullary plasmacytoma. A case report. Jpn J Surg 18:455, 1988

Askin FB, Rosai J, Sibley K et al: Malignant small cell tumor of the thoracopulmonary region in childhood. Cancer 43:2438, 1979

Ayala AG, Zornosa J: Primary bone tumors: percutaneous needle biopsy. Radiology 149:675, 1983

Bataille R, Sany J: Solitary myeloma: clinical and prognostic features of a review of 114 cases. Cancer 48:845, 1981

Boring CC, Squires TS, Tong T, Montgomery S: Cancer Statistics, 1994. CA J Clin 44:7, 1994

Bostwick J III, Nahai F, Wallace JG, Vasconez LO: Sixty latissimus dorsi flaps. Plast Reconstr Surg 63:31, 1979

Boyd A: Tumors of the chest wall. p. 239. In Hood RM, Antman K, Boyd A et al. (eds): Surgical Diseases of Pleura and Chest Wall. WB Saunders, Philadelphia, 1986

Brodsky JT, Gordon MS, Hajdu SI, Burt M: Desmoid tumors of the chest wall: a locally recurrent problem. J Thor Cardiovasc Surg 104:900, 1992

Brown AP, Fixen JA, Plowman PN: Local control of Ewing's sarcoma: an analysis of 67 patients. Br J Radiol 60:261, 1987

Burt M: Primary malignant tumors: The Memorial Sloan-Kettering Cancer Center Experience. Chest Surg Clin N Am 4:137, 1994

Campbell DA: Reconstruction of the anterior thoracic wall. J Thorac Surg 19:456, 1950

Cavanaugh DG, Cabellon S Jr, Peake JB: A logical approach to chest wall neoplasms. Ann Thorac Surg 41:436, 1986

Cavazzana AO, Miser JS, Ferreson J, Triche TJ: Experimental evidence for a neural origin of Ewing's sarcoma of bone. Am J Surg Pathol 127:507, 1987

Fisher J, Bostwick J, Powell RW: Latissimus dorsi blood supply after thoracodorsal vessel division: the serratus collateral. Plast Reconstr Surg 72:502, 1983

Galluccio G, Conti L, Fiorucci F, Li Bianchi E: Solitary plasmacytoma of the chest wall. Panminerva Med 31:189, 1989

Gordon MS, Hajdu SE, Bains MS, Burt ME: Soft tissue sarcomas of the chest wall. J Thorac Cardiovasc Surg 101:843, 1991

Graeber GM, Seyfer AE, Shriver CD, Awan M: Desmoid tumor of the paraspinous muscle involving the chest wall. Mil Med 150:458, 1985

Greager JA, Patel MK, Briele HA et al: Soft tissue sarcomas of the adult thoracic wall. Cancer 59:370, 1987

Groff DB, Adkins PC: Chest wall tumors. Ann Thorac Surg 4:260, 1967

Grosfeld JL, Rescoria FJ, West KW et al: Chest wall resection and reconstruction for malignant conditions in childhood. J Pediatr Surg 23:667, 1988

Hayery P, Reitamo JJ, Tofferman S et al: The desmoid tumor II. Am J Clin Pathol 77:674, 1982

Hayes FA, Thompson EI, Hustu HO et al: The response of Ewing's sarcoma to sequential cyclophosphamide and Adriamycin induction therapy. J Clin Oncol 1:45, 1983

Hayery P, Scheinin TM: The desmoid (Reitamo) syndrome: etiology, manifestation, pathogenesis, and treatment. Curr Probl Surg 25:4, 1988

Hodgkinson DJ, Arnold PG: Chest-wall reconstruction using the external oblique muscle. Br J Plast Surg 33:316, 1980

Huvos AG: Osteogenic sarcoma of bones and soft tissues in older person. Cancer 57:1442, 1986

Huvos AG, Woodard HQ, Cahan WG et al: Postradiation osteogenic sarcoma of bone and soft tissues. Cancer 55:1244, 1985

Jablons D, Steinberg SM, Roth J et al: Metastasectomy for soft tissue sarcoma: further evidence for efficacy and prognostic indicators. J Thorac Cardiovasc Surg 97:695, 1989

Jaffe N, Raymond AK, Ayala A et al: Effect of cumulative courses of intraarterial cis-diamminedichloroplatin-II on the primary tumor in osteosarcoma. Cancer 63:63, 1989

Jurkiewicz MJ, Arnold PG: The omentum: an account of its use in the reconstruction of the chest wall. Ann Surg 185:548, 1977

Kinzbrunner B, Ritter S, Domingo J, Rosenthal CJ: Remission of rapidly growing desmoid tumors after tamoxifen therapy. Cancer 52:2201, 1983

Lane JM, Hurson B, Boland PJ, Glasser DB: Osteogenic sarcoma. Clin Orthop 204:93, 1986

Leibel SA, Wara WM, Hill DR et al: Desmoid tumors: local control and patterns of relapse following radiation therapy. Int J Radiat Oncol Biol Phys 9:1167, 1983

Lichtenstein L: Bone Tumors. CV Mosby, St. Louis, 1977

Lynch HT, Krush AJ, Harlan WL, Sharp EA: Association of soft tissue sarcoma, leukemia, and brain tumors in families affected with breast cancer. Am Surg 39:199, 1973

Malangoni MA, Ofstein LC, Grosfeld JL et al: Survival and pulmonary function following chest wall resection and reconstruction in children. J Pediatr Surg 15:906, 1980

McKinnon JG, Neifeld JP, Kay S et al: Management of desmoid tumors. Surg Gynecol Obstet 169:104, 1989

Meadows JA III, Staats BA, Pairolero PC et al: Effect of resection of the sternum and manubrium in conjunction with muscle transposition on pulmonary function. Mayo Clin Proc 60:604, 1985

Meis JM, Butler JJ, Osborne BM, Ordonez NG: Solitary plasmacytomas of the bone and extramedullary plasmacytomas. A clinicopathologic and immunohistochemical study. Cancer 59:1475, 1987

Mill WB, Griffith R: The role of radiation therapy in the management of plasma cell tumors. Cancer 45:647, 1980

Ozzello L, Stout AP, Murray RM: Cultural characteristics of malignant histiocytomas and fibrous xanthomas. Cancer 16:331, 1963

Pairolero PC, Arnold PG: Primary tumors of the anterior chest wall. Surg Rounds 9:19, 1986a

Pairolero PC, Arnold PG: Thoracic wall defects: surgical management of 205 consecutive patients. Mayo Clin Proc 61:557, 1986b

Pairolero PC, Arnold PG: Management of recalcitrant median sternotomy wounds. J Thorac Cardiovasc Surg 88:357, 1984

Pairolero PC, Arnold PG, Piehler JM: Intrathoracic transposition of extrathoracic skeletal muscle. J Thorac Cardiovasc Surg 86:809, 1983

Pascuzzi CA, Dahlin DC, Clagett OT: Primary tumors of the ribs and sternum. Surg Gynecol Obstet 104:390, 1957

Pass HI: Primary and metastatic chest wall tumors. p. 546. In Roth JA, Ruckdeschel JC, Weisenburger TH (eds): Thoracic Oncology. WB Saunders, Philadelphia, 1989

Perez CA, Tefft M, Nesbit M et al: The role of radiation therapy in the management of non-metastatic Ewing's sarcoma of bone. Report of the Intergroup Ewing's Sarcoma Study. Int J Radiat Oncol Biol Phys 7:141, 1981

Perry RR, Venzon D, Roth JA, Pass HI: Survival after surgical resection for high-grade chest wall sarcomas. Ann Thorac Surg 49:363, 1990

Posner MC, Shiu MH, Newsome JL et al: The desmoid tumor: not a benign disease. Arch Surg 124:191, 1989

Raymond AK, Chawla SP, Carrasco CH et al: Osteosarcoma chemotherapy effect. A prognostic factor. Semin Diagn Pathol 4:212, 1987

Rosai J: Ackerman's Surgical Pathology. CV Mosby, St. Louis, 1989

Ryan MB, McMurtrey MJ, Roth JA: Current management of chest-wall tumors. Surg Clin North Am 69:1061, 1989

Sabanathan S, Salama FD, Morgan WE, Harvey JA: Primary chest wall tumors. Ann Thorac Surg 39:4, 1985

Saito T, Kobayashi H, Kitamura S: Ultrasonographic approach to diagnosing chest wall tumors. Chest 94:1271, 1988

Seyer AE: Radiation-associated lesions of the chest wall. Surg Gynecol Obstet 167:129, 1988

Shamberger RC, Grier HE, Weinstein HJ et al: Chest wall tumors in infancy and childhood. Cancer 63:774, 1989

Sherman NE, Romsdahl M, Evans H et al: Desmoid tumors: a 20-year radiotherapy experience. Int J Radiat Oncol Biol Phys 19:37, 1990

Souba WW, McKenna RJ Jr, Meis J et al: Radiation-induced sarcomas of the chest wall. Cancer 57:610, 1986

Stefanko J, Turnbull AD, Helson L et al: Primitive neuroectodermal tumors of the chest wall. J Surg Oncol 37:33, 1988

Stelzer P, Gay WA Jr: Tumors of the chest wall. Surg Clin North Am 60:779, 1980

Thomas PRM, Foulkes MA, Gilula LA et al: Primary Ewing's sarcoma of the ribs. A report from the Intragroup Ewing's Sarcoma Study. Cancer 51:1021, 1983

Tucker MA, D'Angio GJ, Boice JD Jr et al: Bone sarcomas linked to radiotherapy and chemotherapy in children. N Engl J Med 317:588, 1987

Turc-Cavel C, Philip I, Berger M et al: Chromosomal translocations in Ewing's sarcoma. N Engl J Med 309:497, 1983

Venn GE, Gellister J, DaCosta PE, Goldstraw P: Malignant fibrous histiocytoma in thoracic surgical practice. J Thorac Cardiovasc Surg 91:234, 1986

Wallner KE, Nori D, Burt M et al: Adjuvant brachytherapy for treatment of chest wall sarcomas. J Thorac Cardiovasc Surg 101:888, 1991

Whang-Peng J, Triche TJ, Knutsen T et al: Chromosome translocation in peripheral neuroepithelioma. N Engl J Med 311:584, 1984

Winkler K, Beron G, Kotz R et al: Neoadjuvant chemotherapy for osteogenic sarcoma: results of a cooperative German/Austrian study. J Clin Oncol 2:617, 1984

49

RADIONECROSIS AND INFECTION

Robert B. Lee
Joseph I. Miller, Jr.

DEFINITION

Injury to the chest wall is generally a result of neoplasm, trauma, radionecrosis, or infection. Congenital deformity may cause a severe defect with resulting physiologic derangement, but it is not considered damage inflicted to the body by external force. Neoplastic, traumatic, and congenital disease of the chest wall have been dealt with elsewhere in this text. The present discussion focuses on two entities: radionecrosis of the chest wall and infection of soft tissues and supporting structures of the chest wall.

Most of our knowledge and present management techniques for radiation-induced injury comes from the experience gained by resection of chest wall tumors and defects related to radionecrosis (Arnold and Pairolero, 1989; Miller, 1986; Larson, et al., 1982; Seyfer, 1988; Bostwick, et al., 1984). The principles of wide excision of obviously necrotic and questionably viable tissue followed by immediate reconstruction with omentum, muscle, or musculocutaneous flaps are essential to success. The preoperative considerations, techniques of resection and reconstruction, postoperative management, and clinical experience are examined in detail in this chapter.

Chest wall infection involves the skin and soft tissues, the cartilagenous and bony undercarriage, or frequently, a combination of the two. The cause of the infection may be de novo and thus primary in nature or be secondary and result from a previously existing disease or procedure. The management may be simple and require parenteral or intravenous antibiotics or complex and necessitate radical debridement and reconstruction. The causes of chest wall infections are emphasized as are many of the techniques of resection and reconstruction that have been examined in relation to radiation-induced injury.

HISTORICAL NOTE

The historical development of the management of both radionecrosis and infection of the chest wall is based on the two basic techniques: (1) adequate debridement of devitalized defunctionalized necrotic tissue and (2) reconstruction of the structural and physiologic integrity of the chest wall. Halstead established the principles and techniques of debridement. Although new devices, such as the electrocautery and laser scalpels, have come into use, the surgical principles are unchanged. Reconstruction of the chest wall, however, has undergone remarkable evolution during the last 100 years. The management of chest wall radiation injury has paralleled the advancement of reconstruction techniques of the chest wall. Pare remarked that "gangrene and mortification as complications of treatment give more evil to surgeons and patients than the maladies in which they occur" (Woods, et al., 1979). This is certainly the case with radiotherapy, a two-edged sword that not only results in the cessation of primary and recurrent neoplastic growth, but may also induce neoplastic growth in the radiated site (Seyfer, 1988; Bostwick, et al., 1984; Woods, et al., 1979; Larson and McMurtry, 1984). Some changes have occurred in the techniques of radiotherapy that have reduced the severity of the ionizing effects. However, the frequency of injury may actually become increasingly more evident as patients choose breast-conservation procedures and radiotherapy for primary breast malignancies (Lenene, et al., 1977).

Radiation-caused injury was recognized clinically and described histologically in the early 1900s by Wolback (1909). During the late 1960s, it became customary to treat the internal mammary lymph node chain prophylactically when a primary breast carcinoma occurred in the inner quadrant. The axilla was also irradiated (Haagensen, et al., 1969). Some decrease in the severity of injury has been seen with the use of megavoltage compared with the earlier use of orthovoltage. The severity of injury is still less with the newer techniques of cobalt beam therapy and supervoltage (Latham, 1966). Electron linear acceleration may further decrease the toxic effects as the ionizing beam becomes more focused; a report of the long-term follow-up of such therapy is forthcoming. Although these changes have somewhat lessened the severity of the malady of radionecrosis, the most significant advances have come in the reconstruction of the chest wall after resection of the injury. Resection of the chest wall was attempted and described in 1898 by Parham (1898), who echoed the woes of his predecessors when he iatrogenically produced a pneumothorax: "Suddenly was presented to our anxious view one of the most startling clinical pictures that the surgeon can ever be called upon to witness . . . no wonder the old surgeons discountenanced such operations . . . so sudden in my case was the pneumothorax and so striking were the manifestations of profound shock, threatening almost instant dissolution before our eyes, that I resolved to acquaint myself more thoroughly with the dangers of thoracic surgery. . . ." Significant advancement did not occur until the advent of endotracheal intubation, positive pressure ventilation, closed chest drainage, and antibiotic therapy (Arnold and Pairolero, 1984).

Reconstruction of the chest wall began in earnest in 1947 when fascia lata grafts were used for closure of the chest wall by Watson and James (1947). Simultaneously, Maier (1947) was using large cutaneous flaps, which included the opposite breast in patients with defects caused by mastectomies to close the resulting anterior chest wall defects. He also used and reported this technique for the management of chest wall radiation-caused injury. Many autogenous tissues, such as bone, cartilage, and ribs were tried to provide structural support. Prosthetic materials were introduced and tried in the 1940s and 1950s (Sando and Jurkiewicz, 1986). Different cutaneous flaps were proposed. Not a new concept, cutaneous flaps were described in 600 B.C. in the Sushruta Samhita (Kittle, 1986). Campbell (1949) popularized the use of the latissimus dorsi muscular flap, originally described by Tansaii (1906) for chest wall coverage. The use of Marlex was popularized by Usher and Wallace (1959) when they successfully used this more pliable prosthetic material for reconstruction; it became used extensively for the support of the chest wall both as a single layer and with acrylic reinforcement (Kittle, 1986; Usher and Wallace, 1959).

During this period, most reconstructions were multistaged complicated undertakings. Kiricuta (1963) of Rumania performed and described transposition of pedicle omentum for the management of partial-thickness radiation-induced injury in 1963. He previously introduced the techniques in 1956 for the therapy of vesicovaginal fistulas (Arnold and Pairolero, 1989; Kiricuta, 1963). The use of the latissimus dorsi muscle flap, as described by Camel in 1950, was unfortunately essentially unnoticed and ignored for 20 years until the mid-1970s, although many other skin flaps, muscle flaps, and prosthetic materials were tried (Pairolero and Arnold, 1986). Present-day management of the sequelae of chest wall radiotherapy is founded on the aforementioned principles of aggressive resection of necrotic and questionably viable tissue with immediate reconstruction that uses healthy oxygen- and nutrient-carrying muscle. These principles were established by Bostwick and Jurkiewicz at Emory University–affiliated hospitals (Bostwick, et al., 1984), Larson and McMurtry (1984) at M. D. Anderson, and Arnold and Pairolero (Arnold and Pairolero, 1984, 1986, 1989; Pairolero and Arnold, 1986) at the Mayo Clinic. Their philosophies, techniques, and results have been widely accepted and used by plastic and thoracic surgeons and form the basis of the following discussion.

HISTORICAL READINGS

Arnold PG, Pairolero PC: Reconstruction of the radiation-damaged chest wall. Surg Clin 69:1081, 1989

Arnold PG, Pairolero PC: Surgical management of the radiated chest wall. Plast Reconstr Surg 77:605, 1986

Arnold PG, Pairolero PC: Chest wall reconstruction, experience with 100 consecutive patients. Ann Surg 199:725, 1984

Bostwick J, Stevenson TR, Nahai F et al: Radiation to the breast, complications amenable to surgical treatment. Ann Surg 200:543, 1984

Campbell AA: Reconstruction of the anterior thoracic wall. J Thorac Cardiovasc Surg 19:456, 1949

Haagensen CD, Bhonjlay SB, Guttmann RJ et al: Metastasis of carcinoma of the breast to the periphery of the regional lymph node filter. Ann Surg 169:174, 1969

Kiricuta I: C'empoli du grand epiplasm dans la chuurzie du sein cancereux. Presse Med 71:15, 1963

Kittle FC: Muscle flaps and thoracic problems. p. 233. In Current Controversies in Thoracic Surgery. WB Saunders, Philadelphia, 1986

Larson DL, McMurtry MJ: Musculocutaneous flap reconstruction of chest wall defects: an experience with 50 patients. Plast Reconstr Surg 73:734, 1984

Latham WD: Operative treatment for post-radiation defects of the chest wall. Am Surg 32:700, 1966

Lenene MB, Harris JR, Hellman S: Treatment of carcinoma of the breast by radiation therapy. Cancer 39:28840, 1977

Maier HC: Surgical management of large defects of the thoracic wall. Surgery 22:169, 1947

Pairolero PC, Arnold PG: Muscle flaps and thoracic problems: chest wall defects: reconstruction with autogenous tissue. p. 241. In Kittle FC (ed): Current Controversies in Thoracic Surgery. WB Saunders, Philadelphia, 1986

Parham FW: Thoracic resection for tumors growing from the bony wall of the chest. Trans South Surg Gynecol Assoc 11:223, 1898

Sando W, Jurkiewicz MJ: An approach to repairs of radiation necrosis of chest wall and mammary gland. World J Surg 10:206, 1986

Seyfer AE: Radiation-associated lesions of the chest wall. Surg Gynecol Obstet 167:129, 1988

Usher FC, Wallace SA: Tissue reaction to plastics. Arch Surg 76:997, 1959

Watson WC, James AG: Fascia lata grafts for chest wall defects. J Thorac Cardiovasc Surg 16:399, 1947

Wolbach SR: Pathologic history of chronic x-ray dermatitis and early x-ray carcinoma. J Med Res 21:415, 1909

Woods JE, Arnold PG, Masson JK et al: Management of radiation necrosis and advanced cancer of the chest wall in patients with breast malignancy. Plast Reconstr Surg 63:235, 1979

RADIONECROSIS

ETIOLOGY

Radiotherapy has been shown to be effective in controlling certain malignancies of the chest, which include Hodgkin's lymphoma, bronchogenic carcinoma, and mammary carcinoma. The ionizing radiation may control not only a primary malignancy, but it also may eventually induce a secondary malignancy years later (Bostwick, et al., 1984; Latham, 1966; Pizzarello and Witcofoki, 1975). Furthermore, the ionizing radiation is not limited to the neoplastic cells but also affects the undiseased mediastinum and chest wall structures. There are numerous reports of accelerated coronary atherosclerosis (Arsenian, 1991), cardiac valvular disease (Carlson, et al., 1991), and cardiac arrhythmias (Seama, et al., 1991) caused by radiation effects in the literature.

Ionizing rays affect rapidly dividing cells by releasing free radicals and peroxidase and thereby splitting DNA; thus such radiation is lethal to the dividing neoplastic cells. Concurrent transmission of radiation to surrounding vascular structures damages the endothelial cells of small arteries and arterioles, which results in luminal obliteration by myointimal fibrosis and myxoid degeneration of the intima. The resulting occlusion leads to relative tissue anoxemia, which eventually causes ischemic fibrosis. As expected, the less well-vascularized tissues, such as cartilage, tendon, and bone, are particularly vulnerable. The ultimate result is soft tissue ulceration with underlying osteoradionecrosis and chondroradionecrosis (Latham, 1966; Arnold and Pairolero, 1986; MacMillan, et al., 1986; Smith, et al., 1982).

A dose-response relationship appears to exist (Bostwick, et al., 1984). Standard doses of 4,500 to 5,000 cGy that are given over 5 to 6 weeks in 200-cGy increments appear to be associated with less complications (Pantoja, et al., 1978; Meyer, 1978). However, doses as low as 2,200 cGy may cause significant skeletal damage (Smith, et al., 1982; Parker and Berry, 1976). Originally, orthovoltage was used for radiotherapy. As technology advanced, megavoltage was developed. Although the amount of radiation administered was increased, there was believed to be no significant increase in complications (Smith, et al., 1982). Subsequently, it was shown that megavoltage induces damage to deeper tissues, which may lead to lethal changes. Thus, there is no modality that is free of possible ill effects. Even when "safe doses" are given, incorrect dosage calculations, improper machine calibrations, inaccurate field marking, or overlapping of the portals may result in serious radiation-induced injury (Larson, et al., 1982; Pantoja, et al., 1978).

After either low radiation doses or the initial dose, skin erythema may occur; this is called radiodermatitis. The skin may become tender, edematous, and firm from the endothelial injury to arterioles, capillaries, and lymphatic vessels. Higher doses or prolonged administration may result in blistering of the skin, with varying degrees of necrosis. The body's natural repair mechanisms may reverse these superficial changes in a short period of days to weeks. However, because of the vascular injury and induced endarteritis obliterans, the deeper tissue changes persist and progress. The inflammatory response and anoxemia produce fibrosis and scarring. As the subcutaneous tissues undergo fibrosis, the epithelium, now friable, is disrupted, frequently ulcerates, and becomes chronically infected. The underlying structural support of bone and cartilage may become necrotic (Robinson, 1975). Thus, full-thickness injury may occur, which produces devastating tissue loss and a significant challenge for the surgeon.

MANAGEMENT

Preoperative Assessment and Planning

In-depth preoperative assessment and planning is essential for success in this patient population. The typical patient with a chest wall defect from radionecrosis is a 40 to 50-year-old woman who has undergone radical or modified mastectomy followed by postoperative radiotherapy for residual microscopic disease. They generally have large, malodorous, necrotic wounds that do not heal and are surrounded by significant fibrosis. Pain is a prominent component, and these patients require greater than average doses of opioids for relief (Bostwick, et al., 1984; Latham, 1966). Frequently, these patients are chronically depressed as a result of their original disease process, the therapy thereof, and the resulting complications. All too often they have been told that "this is the price to be paid for the cure of the cancer," "recurrent tumor is the cause of the problem," or worse "there is no hope." These patients should be encouraged and given accurate facts and options, thereby allowing them

---

Preoperative Evaluation

History and physical evaluation
  Original primary lesion
  Amount, type, and portals of radiotherapy
  Co-morbid disease processes (i.e., diabetes mellitus)
  Area and depth of destruction
  Involvement of bone, cartilage, or lung
  Limitation of motion of upper extremities
  Exercise tolerance and nutritional status
Radiologic evaluation
  Posteroanterior and lateral chest radiograph with rib detail
  Computed tomographic chest scan
  Bone scan
  Magnetic resonance imaging scan (if spinal column involvement is suspected)
Physiologic evaluation
  Thallium stress test
  Pulmonary function test
  Nutritional status (i.e., concentrations of albumin, prealbumin, and transferrin and skin testing for anergy)
  Biopsy of lesion to determine presence or absence of residual or recurrent tumor

to participate in their care (Seyfer, 1988; Bostwick, et al., 1984; Latham, 1966).

The assessment should include a physical and psychological profile. The history should be ascertained in regard to the amount and type of radiation, recent bleeding from the site, and possible recent changes in cardiac or pulmonary status. Recent sudden or profound bleeding may warn of underlying involvement of the internal mammary vessels, intercostal vessels, or great vessel involvement. Knowledge of coexisting cardiac, pulmonary, renal, and endocrine disease may influence the operative plan. Diabetes, steroid dependency, recent chemotherapy, and obesity may influence the postoperative healing and the choice of flaps (Larson and McMurtry, 1984; Sando and Jurkiewicz, 1986).

The location on the chest wall determines which flaps are available for reconstruction (Larson and McMurtry, 1984; Sando and Jurkiewicz, 1986). The size and depth of the wound determine whether partial- or full-thickness chest wall resection will be required and what amount of tissue will be necessary for the reconstruction. The presence of chronic infection may require preoperative antibiotic therapy and local wound care prior to the surgical intervention. Every effort should be made to determine the presence or absence of malignancy in the wound. The presence of malignancy obviously requires more extensive resection. If malignancy is found, further studies may be necessary to evaluate the extent of invasion (Arnold and Pairolero, 1989; Larson, et al., 1982; Seyfer, 1988; Bostwick, et al., 1984; Larson and McMurtry, 1984).

Plain radiographs may reveal necrosis of bone, which alerts the surgeon to resect deeper tissues. When malignancy is identified or suspected to be in the wound preoperatively, computed tomography or magnetic resonance imaging (MRI) scans may be performed to assess the depth of invasion or involvement of underlying lung or mediastinal structures (Arnold and Pairolero, 1989). It may be necessary to resect underlying lung. Pulmonary function testing provides data to guide the extent of resection. Frequently, the underlying lung is fibrotic from prior radiotherapy and may not contribute to overall pulmonary function. Larsen and McMurtry (1984) showed that chest wall resection for tumor and radionecrosis may be asociated with no change and even an improvement in the forced expiratory volume in 1 second and (vital capacity. The dipyridamole stress thallium test accurately predicts which patients undergoing thoracic procedures are at risk for a cardiac event (Miller, 1992).

Perhaps the most important assessment involves the patient's life-style, ability to work, and prognosis. These patients are generally debilitated and unable to work, either because of the therapy of the primary malignancy or complications of the postoperative radiotherapy. The prognosis for patients with breast cancer that is recurrent in the local chest wall tissues is poor; most die of distant metastasis within 14 months (Larson, et al., 1982; Seyfer, 1988; Larson and McMurtry, 1984). Similarly, postradiation sarcomas are lethal (Larson and McMurtry, 1984). Given this, many surgeons would not undertake extensive resections. However, Woods, et al. (1979) noted that in their series several of the patients undergoing resection and reconstruction died just a few months afterward, but prior to death, they stated that they had great improvement in the quality of their lives after

the removal of the foul-smelling, gangrenous, ulcerating malignant lesions, which indicated that the extensive procedure was indeed worthwhile.

Resection Techniques

Larsen, et al. (1982) succinctly described the purpose of resection as follows: "to rid the patient of the disease process maintaining chest wall and pleural continuity with a single-stage reconstruction, minimizing donor morbidity and thus rehabilitating the patient as quickly as possible" Virtually all authors advocate aggressive resection of the radionecrotic and questionably viable tissue (Arnold and Pairolero, 1989; Seyfer, 1988; Bostwick, et al., 1984; Larson and McMurtry, 1984; Latham, 1966). Simple excision and primary closure are usually not satisfactory (Woods, et al., 1979). To be successful, the resection must encompass all soft tissues, cartilage, and bone of poor quality, turgor, color, and vascularity (Seyfer, 1988). Occasionally, partial-thickness resections can be performed, but more often, full-thickness resection is required to remove all necrotic tissue (Larson, et al., 1982; Seyfer, 1988; Bostwick, et al., 1984; Arnold and Pairolero, 1986). Full-thickness resection of the lesion may require additional resection of normal rib, approximately 2 inches, to allow a comfortable route of entry for the muscle flaps chosen to close the residual space. No residual space should be left, and there must be sufficient transposed tissue to close any intrathoracic space (Miller, 1986).

Full-thickness resection is generally the rule. The surgeon must be prepared to resect underlying vascular structures and pulmonary parenchyma, if necessary, and not to leave nonviable cartilage and bone, which might produce chronic draining fistulae, regardless of the needed coverage. If the pleural space is entered or the pulmonary parenchyma resected, pneumothorax may not occur because the lung is frequently stiff and has undergone fibrosis and the pleural space has been obliterated as a result of the adhesions produced by prior radiotherapy. After all nonviable tissue has been completely resected, reconstruction may proceed.

Reconstruction of Partial-Thickness Defects

Devitalized skin or small ulcerations that are not associated with underlying soft tissue, cartilage, or bony necrosis may be amenable to partial-thickness resection. This usually is not the case, and full-thickness resections are generally required (Arnold and Pairolero, 1984, 1989; Larson, et al., 1982; Pairolero and Arnold, 1986). However, if a partial-thickness resection results in procurement of healthy viable tissue, primary closure of a small superficial wound is preferable (Larson, et al., 1982; Sando and Jurkiewicz, 1986). Primary closure is usually not an option and often compromises resection attempts, thereby eventually failing (Miller, 1986; Larson and McMurtry, 1984). Irradiated tissues appear to respond differently to debridement; therefore, what appears to be adequate at the time of the operation may be necrotic the next day. When the primary wound breaks down, further more aggressive resection is indicated. Topical antibiotics, such as Sefomylon or silver sulfadiazine, may be used to improve wound characteristics in anticipation of a meshed split-thickness skin graft (Sando and Jurkiewicz, 1986).

More often, partial-thickness resection requires reconstruction with transposed tissue. After viable tissues are obtained, omentum may be harvested as a graft on a pedicle and may be brought into the area. Based on the right or left gastric epiploic artery or both, omentum is healthy well-vascularized tissue capable of angiogenesis (Bostwick, et al., 1984; Fix and Vasconez, 1989). The omentum may be used alone or with a split-thickness skin graft (Larson, et al., 1982; Bostwick, et al., 1984; Woods, et al., 1979; Sando and Jurkiewicz, 1986). The techniques for omental usage and harvest have been well documented by Alday (Alday and Goldsmith, 1972).

Bostick, et al. (1984) described the use of the omental free graft for the management of radiation-induced injury. As a free graft, the omentum may be used to cover partial chest wall defects, to wrap the brachial plexus after neurolysis, or to treat radiation-induced hemifacial atrophy (Bostwick, et al., 1984; Arnold and Irons, 1981). Most authors now use omentum for partial-thickness defect reconstruction or as a back-up when flaps fail in the therapy of full-thickness reconstructions (Larson, et al., 1982; Seyfer, 1988; Bostwick, et al., 1984; Woods, et al., 1979).

McMillan, et al. (1986) recently introduced the concept of tissue expanders for the management of the partial-thickness injury. The expander is placed in a nearby area of nonirradiated skin. An advancement flap of sufficient size, which includes skin and subcutaneous tissues, can be "stretched to sufficient size to cover the partial defect" (MacMillan, et al., 1986).

Reconstruction of Full-Thickness Defects

Full-thickness resection of soft tissue, cartilage, and bone destroyed by radionecrosis is required more often than is partial-thickness resection. Radical resection results in defects that can be a reconstructive challenge for the surgeon. Skeletal and supporting elements may need to be supplemented. The surgeon is presented with a wide variety of choices of muscle and myocutaneous flaps (Table 49-1 and Fig. 49-1) (Seyfer, et al., 1986).

Skeletal reconstruction is controversial, and each patient should be assessed individually, based on the site and extent of resection. The preoperative cardiopulmonary status provides data that is important when choosing which patients may need skeletal support. Larger anterior full-thickness re-

sections (more than 5 cm) and complete sternal resections (which have the potential for paradox) may require structural support. A true rib resection laterally or a posterior resection in an area protected by the scapula is usually well tolerated and does not require support (Bostwick, et al., 1984; Pairolero and Arnold, 1986). The chest wall and underlying parenchyma are often fibrotic after radiotherapy, which provides further stability to the chest.

Prolene and Marlex meshes alone or in combination with methyl methacrylate provide excellent stabilization after chest wall resection (McCormack, et al., 1981; Eschapasse, et al., 1981). However, their use should be avoided at all costs in the presence of a contaminated wound, which frequently is associated with osteoradionecrosis. The use of such substances in this setting is associated with high failure rates because of the subsequent infection of the prosthesis. Most authors now believe the use of larger muscle or musculocutaneous flaps results in adequate structural support after full-thickness resection of the chest wall (Seyfer, 1988; Bostwick, et al., 1984; Woods, et al., 1979; Arnold and Pairolero, 1984).

Our current preference for reconstruction of the full-thickness defect is the muscular or musculocutaneous flap, most frequently the latissimus dorsi flap (Bostwick, et al., 1984; Sando and Jurkiewicz, 1986). As described earlier, the size, location, and depth determine which muscle is the most appropriate. Figure 49-2 is a schematic representation of the possible defects and suggested muscle for reconstruction. Each of the possible muscles is briefly described (Table 49-1).

Latissimus Dorsi. The most frequently used flap for lateral and anterior defects is the latissimus dorsi, which is supplied by the thoracodorsal neurovascular bundle. It also receives a blood supply from the branches that supply the serratus anterior and can be based on this vascular pedicle. Excellent musculocutaneous collaterals allow significant skin to be taken with the muscle. It is the largest extrathoracic flap (25 × 35 cm) with a skin area of 30 × 40 cm. It has a large pedicle and a wide arc of rotation. Its origin is T6 to T12, L1 to L4, S1 to S3, and the posterior crest of the ileum. Its insertion is the intertubular groove of the humerus. The donor site rarely causes morbidity but may require a skin graft (Seyfer, 1988; Bostwick, et al., 1984; Larson and McMurtry, 1984; Sando and Jurkiewicz, 1986; Pairolero and Arnold, 1986; Seyfer, et al., 1986; Harashina, et al., 1983).

Table 49-1. Choice of Flaps for Reconstruction of Full-Thickness Defects of the Chest Wall

Muscle	Neurovascular Supply	Origin	Insertion
Latissimus dorsi	Primary: thoracodorsal nerve, artery, and vein Secondary: artery to serratus anterior	T6–S3, posterior crest of ileum	Intratubular groove of the humerus
Pectoralis major	Primary: thoracoabdominal nerve, artery, and vein Secondary: internal mammary and intercostal arteries	Sternum, clavicle, ribs 1–7	Tricipital groove of humerus
Rectus abdominis	Primary: superior and inferior epigastric arteries	Pubic crest	Rib cartilage of ribs 5–7, xiphoid
Serratus anterior	Primary: serratus branch of thoracodorsal artery Secondary: long thoracic artery	Outer surface and superior border of ribs 8–10 intercostal fascia	Scapula tip
External oblique	Primary: lower thoracic intercostal artery, nerve, and vein	External surface and inferior border of ribs 4–12	Iliac crest, lower abdominal process
Trapezius	Primary: transverse cervical artery, nerve, and vein Secondary: occipital branches and intercostal perforators	Occipital bone, C7–T12 spinous processes	Posterior and lateral third of clavicle, acromion, superior lip of scapular spine

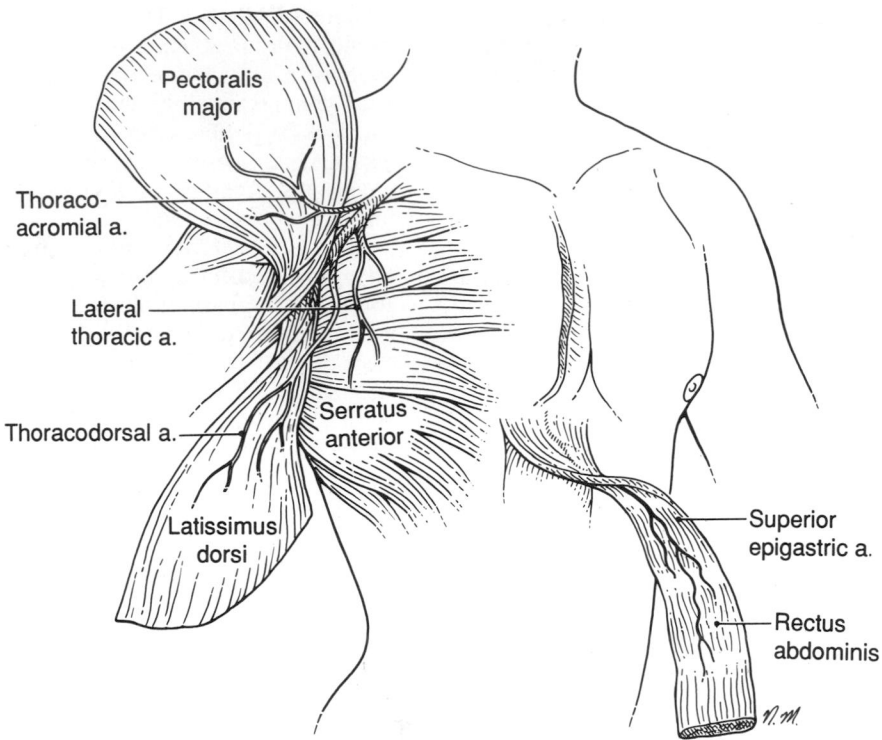

Figure 49-1. Available muscle and musculocutaneous flaps for chest wall reconstruction. Note vascular pedicles.

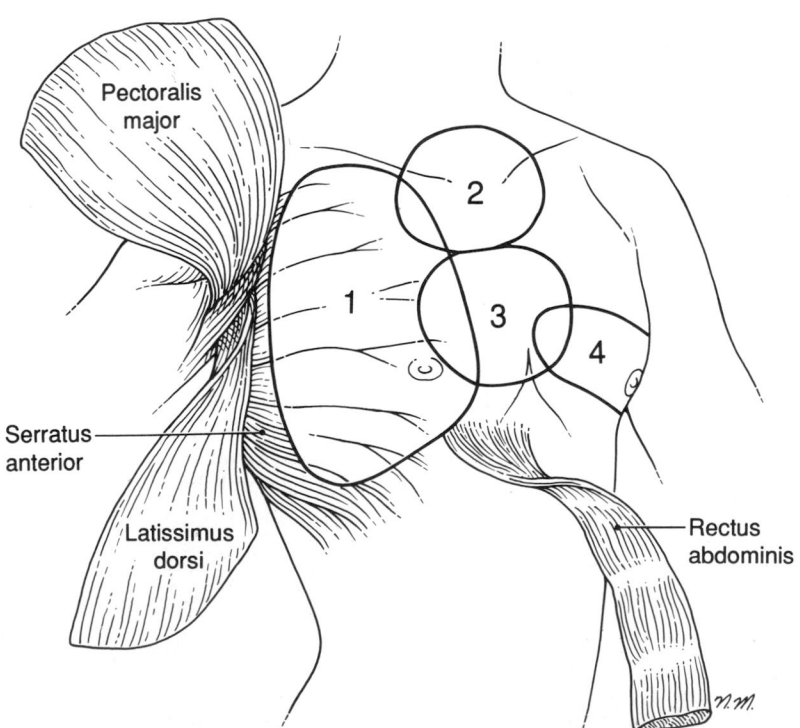

Figure 49-2. Common sites of chest wall defects and available myocutaneous flaps for reconstruction.

Pectoralis Major. The pectoralis major is the second most frequently used flap. It is appropriate for anterior and midline defects. Its primary blood supply is the thoracoacromial neurovascular bundle, which arises at midclavicle. Its secondary blood supply is from the internal mammary artery, lateral intercostal arteries, and lateral thoracic perforators. The pectoralis major is the second largest muscle (15 × 23 cm) with a potential skin area of 20 × 28 cm. Its origin is the sternum, clavicle, and first seven ribs. Its insertion is the bicipital groove of the humerus. It may be used as a graft with a pedicle if the flap is based on the primary blood supply or a "turn-over flap" if the secondary supply is used. The harvest must take into account the possible displacement of the breast and the loss of adduction and medial rotation of the arm. This flap has excellent reliability (Larson, et al., 1982; Bostwick, et al., 1984; Arnold and Pairolero, 1984; Sando and Jurkiewicz, 1986; Seyfer, et al., 1986; Nahai, et al., 1986).

Rectus Abdominis. The third most frequently used flap is the rectus abdominis. It is appropriate for lower anterior chest wall repairs. Two dominant vascular pedicles exist: the superior epigastric artery supply and the deep inferior epigastric. If it is based on the superior epigastric artery, the inferior epigastric artery must be divided. Therefore, adequate flow through the superior epigastric artery through the internal mammary artery must be ensured. Anterior chest wall irradiation may damage the internal mammary artery; therefore, angiography is suggested. The rectus abdominis is a smaller muscle (surface area, 6 × 25 cm), with a potential skin area of 21 × 14 cm. It has a longitudinal pedicle, and the skin flap may be oriented vertically or horizontally. Vertical orientation preserves more musculocutaneous perforators and therefore is safer. Its origin is the pubic crest. Its insertion is rib cartilage of ribs five, six, and seven and the xiphoid. Increased donor site morbidity occurs in obese and diabetic patients as a result of ventral hernia and infection. The relative reliability of the flap is fair, but atrophy occurs because of loss of the innervation that is prerequisite in the harvest (Bostwick, et al., 1984; Larson and McMurtry, 1984; Sando and Jurkiewicz, 1986; Pairolero and Arnold, 1986; Robinson, 1975).

Serratus Anterior. The serratus anterior is less often used for extrathoracic reconstruction. It is located between the latissimus dorsi and pectoralis in the midaxillary line. It is a small muscle that is best suited as an intrathoracic flap. The serratus anterior may be used in combination with the latissimus dorsi or the pectoralis to supplement the blood supply of the cutaneous segments of these larger musculocutaneous flaps. Its primary blood supply is the serratus branch of the thoracodorsal pedicle, and its secondary blood supply is the long thoracic artery. Its origin is the outer surfaces and superior borders of the upper eighth, ninth, and tenth ribs and the intercostal fascia. Its insertion is the tip of the scapula. The blood supply of this flap is reliable, but the bulk of the muscle is small. Therefore, this limits its usefulness as an extrathoracic flap to areas of the axilla (Larson and McMurtry, 1984; Arnold and Pairolero, 1984; Sando and Jurkiewicz, 1986; Seyfer, et al., 1986; Arnold, et al., 1983).

External Oblique. The external oblique is infrequently used. It may be used for upper abdomen and lower thoracic defects as far as the inframammary fold. The primary blood supply is the lower thoracic intercostal vessels. Its origin is the external surface and inferior border of the lower eight ribs. Its insertion is the iliac crest and lower abdominal fascia (Arnold and Pairolero, 1989; Seyfer, et al., 1986).

Trapezius. The trapezius is infrequently used. Occasionally, it is used for upper chest and neck defects. It is most useful for the base of the neck and thoracic outlet defects. Its major pedicle is the transverse cervical artery by the thyrocervical trunk. Its secondary blood supply includes the occipital branches and intercostal perforators. The trapezius is of moderate size and bulk (34 × 18 cm) with potential skin island of 20 × 8 cm. Its origin is the occipital bone, C7, and all thoracic vertebral spinous processes. Its insertion is the posterior and lateral third of the clavicle, the acromian, and the superior lip of the spine of the scapula (Arnold and Pairolero, 1989; Sando and Jurkiewicz, 1986; Seyfer, et al., 1986).

Omentum. Omentum was frequently used early in the history of reconstruction of full-thickness defects. Now it is used for partial-thickness defects and salvage of failed muscle flaps. Its major pedicle is the right and left gastroepiploic arteries. The right pedicle is longer. Its advantages include abundant vascularity, wide arc of rotation, large surface area, and minimal bulk. Its disadvantage is that it requires a laparotomy for harvest (Sando and Jurkiewicz, 1986; Pairolero and Arnold, 1986).

Others. A combination of muscle flaps may be used, for example, latissimus dorsi and pectoralis, or pectoralis and serratus anterior, or pectoralis and rectus abdominis. Three muscle flaps have been used on occasion (generally when primary flaps fail). Latissimus dorsi free flaps and gluteal muscle free flaps have also been used for salvage (Woods, et al., 1979; Sando and Jurkiewicz, 1986).

Postoperative Management

Although these patients generally require major chest wall resection and reconstruction, the postoperative morbidity and mortality rates are low (Larson, et al., 1982; Seyfer, 1988; Woods, et al., 1979; Larson and McMurtry, 1984). Complications are usually due to infection and partial graft failure; total graft failure is uncommon (Larson, et al., 1982; Woods, et al., 1979; Arnold and Pairolero, 1986). After major anterolateral chest wall resection, there may be a brief period of paradoxic chest movement, but large muscle flaps offer good stability for the chest wall. Few patients require prolonged ventilation postoperatively who do not have significant underlying pulmonary disease (Larson and McMurtry, 1984; Arnold and Pairolero, 1986). Tracheostomy was used routinely in early series but is performed uncommonly now (Seyfer, 1988). Chest tubes and suction catheters should be left in place for 7 to 10 days, and antibiotic therapy should be guided by cultures of the wound (Miller, 1986). The hospital stay averages 11 to 21 days; most authors report means of 12 to 14 days (Larson, et al., 1982; Woods, et al., 1979; Arnold and Pairolero, 1984).

Recurrent breast cancer in the chest wall and recurrent malignancy in radionecrotic wounds is associated with a particularly poor outcome and virtually no long-term survivors (Larson, et al., 1982; Seyfer, 1988; Woods, et al., 1979). Therefore, most surgeons believe it is ill advised to put the patient through such a major operative procedure; however, the patients feel great relief and improved well-being when the painful, malodorous lesions have been removed.

CONCLUSION

A number of authors have shown the feasibility and advisability of chest wall resection to remove lesions caused by radionecrosis (Arnold and Pairolero, 1989; Larson, et al., 1982; Bostwick, et al., 1984). Presently, the muscular or musculocutaneous flap is preferred for reconstruction. These procedures can be performed in a well-planned, one-stage operation with minimal morbidity and mortality rates. The quality of life for these patients is significantly improved after surgery.

CHEST WALL INFECTIONS

Chest wall infections secondary to previous procedures, such as median sternotomy and thoracotomy, occur in less than 1.5 to 2.0 percent of the cases. This has been discussed adequately elsewhere. Primary chest wall infections are also uncommon. The true incidence is difficult to establish because of the sporadic nature of the problem and lack of reporting. The management has changed greatly since the antibiotic revolution. Most infections can be treated successfully with the administration of topical or intravenous antibiotics. Some infectious maladies require radical resection. This topic of discussion lends itself to being divided into (1) skin and soft tissue infections and (2) cartilage and bony structure infections.

SKIN AND SOFT TISSUE

Soft tissue infections of superficial abrasions, furuncles, carbuncles, etc. occur in the chest wall with a similar incidence as in other body areas. Herpes zoster ("shingles") occurs in older people who have been previously exposed to herpes simplex type II virus. It occurs along dermatomal paths and is generally self-limited, except in the immunocompromised host. The therapy consists of analgesics, nonsteroidal anti-inflammatory medications, and occasionally acyclovir applied topically. Infrequently when systemic dissemination occurs in the immunocompromised host, systemic acyclovir is indicated.

Soft tissue infections may occur when infectious material is drained by a thoracostomy tube through the chest wall. As reported by Pingleton and Jeter (1983), *Bacteroides mela-*

ninogenicus and *Streptococcus viridans* cause a synergistic gangrene after tube thoracostomy drainage of an empyema, which eventually leads to the patient's death. LoCicero and Vanelko (1985) reported a clostridial myonecrosis at the site of a tube thoracostomy in a patient with Boerhaave syndrome. Infrequently seen but reported cases of anthrax (Navacharoen, et al., 1985), actinomycosis (Golden, et al., 1985), and hydatid cysts (Rami, et al., 1985) can present as pseudotumors or infections of the chest wall.

Mondor's disease is thrombophlebitis of the superficial veins of the breast and anterior chest wall. It is frequently treated as a chest wall infection, but this disease entity results from sclerosing endophlebitis of the affected vein with complete or partial obliteration of the vessel lumen (Farrow, 1955). A spontaneous self-limited condition, it presents as a hard cord in the subcutaneous tissue of the axilla or anterior chest wall, and it is fairly common after mastectomy and breast augmentation (Kikano, et al., 1991; Green and Dowden, 1988). The skin "puckering" produced may be mistaken for inflammatory breast carcinoma, which should be ruled out. Patients may be treated symptomatically with nonsteroidal anti-inflammatory agents. Excision of the affected veins is rarely required.

CARTILAGE AND BONY STRUCTURES

Once frequently seen as a result of the tuberculous bacillus, cartilage and bone infection of the chest wall is now uncommon. The use of prophylactic antibiotics during cardiac and thoracic procedures has virtually eliminated many of the perioperative pathogens. Sternal wound infections following median sternotomy is discussed elsewhere.

Costochondritis, when it occurs apart from surgical procedures, may be due to a wide variety of organisms: staphylococci, streptococci, *Pseudomonas aeruginosa, Escherichia coli, Mycobacterium tuberculosis,* and others. Because the cartilages are fused and continual, a local infection tends to spread that involves all confluent cartilages. These infections are often insidious and indolent and manifest as local pain, swelling, and frequently a draining sinus. The cartilage is avascular and thus is remote from systemic antibiotics. The therapy of choice is radical debridement with reconstruction, as previously discussed.

A particular malady of the chest wall often discussed in the literature is Tietze's syndrome. A benign self-limited entity, it is characterized by nonsupportive, tender, swelling of the costal cartilage (usually the second or third), and the cause is unknown (Jurik and Graudal, 1988). Recent authors have associated the syndrome with seronegative rheumatologic disease (Aeschlimann and Kahn, 1990). The therapy should be conservative with analgesics and nonsteroidal anti-inflammatory agents.

Control of tuberculosis and the sophisticated use of systemic antibiotics has virtually eliminated osteomyelitis of the rib cage that is unassociated with sternal infections. It is occasionally seen associated with open drainage of chronic empyema by the Eloesser technique. When persistent infection occurs, radical debridement is usually required for elimination.

CONCLUSION

Because of the increasing sophistication of antibiotic therapy and refinement in surgical technique, chest wall infections are becoming increasingly uncommon. When they do occur, infections of the cartilage and bone require radical excision and debridement for elimination. Perhaps the most commonly seen chest wall conditions are Mondor's disease and Tietze's syndrome. These two entities are not infections in nature and require only relief of symptoms for resolution.

COMMENTS AND CONTROVERSIES

The most common infection of the chest wall is that of the sternum following median sternotomy for coronary artery bypass or other cardiac surgical procedures. The primary therapy in these cases is resection of necrotic tissue, use of local and systemic antibiotics, and reconstruction with omentum and/or muscle flaps. If no tissue is necrotic, then debridement, antibiotics, and Robicheck weaving of the sternum provide stability and healing.

When there is extensive necrotic infection of the costal cartilages that cannot be treated by simple debridement and reconstruction or other conventional methods because of the poor blood supply, resection of normal cartilage in a perimeter is carried out. This is called "prairie fire containment" by Dr. Robert Shaw and involves cutting out healthy cartilage at the perimeter of the infection to stop the spread of infection, with subsequent reconstruction with omentum and/or muscle flaps.

H.C.U.

KEY REFERENCES

Aesohlimann A, Kahn MF: Tietze's syndrome: a critical review. Clin Exp Rheumatol 8:407, 1990

Drs. Aeschlimann and Kahn have written an excellent review of a frequently underdiagnosed chest wall malady. The article provides guidance for diagnosing and treating Tietze's syndrome.

Arnold PG, Pairolero PC: Reconstruction of the radiation-damaged chest wall. Surg Clin 69:1081, 1989

Drs. Pairolero and Arnold describe the techniques of surgical resection and reconstruction of osteoradionecrosis.

Arnold PG, Pairolero PC: Chest wall reconstruction, experience with 100 consecutive patients. Ann Surg 199:725, 1984

Drs. Pairolero and Arnold describe their vast experience with 100 patients who have required chest wall reconstruction following resection of various chest wall lesions.

Larson DL, McMurtry MJ: Musculocutaneous flap reconstruction of chest wall defects: an experience with 50 patients. Plast Reconstr Surg 73:734, 1984

Drs. McMurtry and Larson describe the resection of lesions secondary to osteoradionecrosis with immediate reconstruction, which was done in one of America's foremost cancer institutes.

Seyfer A, Graeber G, Wind G: Atlas of Chest Wall Reconstruction. Aspen, Rockville, MD, 1986

This is a beautifully illustrated atlas of chest wall reconstructions. It serves as an excellent reference for those who perform reconstructive procedures that require muscle and myocutaneous flaps.

REFERENCES

Alday ES, Goldsmith HS: Surgical technique for omental lengthening based on arterial anatomy. Surg Gynecol Obstet 135:103, 1972

Arnold PG, Irons GB: The greater omentum: extension in transposition and free transfer. Plast Reconstr Surg 67:169, 1981

Arnold PG, Pairolero PC: Surgical management of the radiated chest wall. Plast Reconstr Surg 77:605, 1986

Arnold PG, Pairolero PC, Waldorf JC: The serratus anterior muscle: intrathoracic and extrathoracic utilization. Plast Reconstr Surg 73:240, 1983

Arsenian MA: Cardiovascular sequelae of therapeutic thoracic radiation. Prog Cardiovasc Dis 33:299, 1991

Bostwick J, Stevenson TR, Nahai F et al.: Radiation to the breast, complications amenable to surgical treatment. Ann Surg 200:543, 1984

Campbell AA: Reconstruction of the anterior thoracic wall. J Thorac Cardiovasc Surg 19:456, 1949

Carlson RG, Mayfield WR, Normann S et al.: Radiation-associated vascular disease. Chest 99:538, 1991

Eschapasse H, Gailland J, Henry F et al.: Repair of large chest wall defects: experience with 23 patients. Ann Thorac Surg 32:329, 1981

Farrow JH: Thrombophlebitis of the superficial veins of the breast and anterior chest wall (Mondor's disease). Surg Gynecol Obstet 101:63, 1955

Fix RJ, Vasconez LO: Use of omentum in chest wall reconstruction. Surg Clin 69:1029, 1989

Golden N, Cohen H, Weissbrot J et al.: Thoracic actinomycosis in childhood. Clin Pediatr 24:646, 1985

Green RA, Dowden RV: Mondor's disease in plastic surgery patients. Ann Plast Surg 20:231, 1988

Haagensen CD, Bhonjlay SB, Guttmann RJ et al.: Metastasis of carcinoma of the breast to the periphery of the regional lymph node filter. Ann Surg 169:174, 1969

Harashina T, Takayama S, Yaji I et al.: Reconstruction of chest wall radiation ulcer with free latissimus dorsi muscle flap and meshed skin graft. Plast Reconstr Surg 71:805, 1983

Jurik AG, Graudal H: Sternocostal joint swelling—clinical Tietze's syndrome. Scand J Rheumatol 17:33, 1988

Kikano GE, Caceres VM, Sebas, JA: Superficial thrombophlebitis of the anterior chest wall (Mondor's disease). J Fam Pract 33:643, 1991

Kiricuta I: C'empoli du grand epiplasm dans la chuurzie du sein cancereux. Presse Med 71:15, 1963

Kittle FC: Muscle flaps and thoracic problems. p. 233. In Current Controversies in Thoracic Surgery. WB Saunders, Philadelphia, 1986

Larson DL, McMurtry MJ, Howe HJ et al.: Major chest wall reconstruction after chest wall irradiation. Cancer 49:1286, 1982

Latham WD: Operative treatment for post-radiation defects of the chest wall. Am Surg 32:700, 1966

Lenene MB, Harris JR, Hellman S: Treatment of carcinoma of the breast by radiation therapy. Cancer 39:28840, 1977

LoCicero J, Vanelko RM: Clostridial myonecrosis of the chest wall complicating spontaneous esophageal rupture. Ann Thorac Surg 40:396, 1985

MacMillan RW, Arias JA, Stayman JW: Management of radiation necrosis of the chest wall following mastectomy: a new treatment option. Plast Reconstr Surg 77:832, 1986

Maier HC: Surgical management of large defects of the thoracic wall. Surgery 22:169, 1947

McCormack P, Boins MS, Beattie EJ et al.: New trends in skeletal reconstruction after resection of chest wall tumor. Ann Thorac Surg 31:45, 1981

Meyer JE: Thoracic effects of therapeutic irradiation for breast carcinoma. AJR 130:877, 1978

Miller JI: Thallium imaging in preoperative evaluation of the pulmonary resection candidate. Ann Thorac Surg 54:249, 1992

Miller JI: Muscle flaps and thoracic problems: applicability and utilizations for various conditions. p. 235. In Current Controversies in Thoracic Surgery. WB Saunders, Philadelphia, 1986

Nahai F, Morales L, Bone DK et al.: Pectoralis major muscle turnover flaps for closure of the infected median sternotomy wound with preservation of form and function. Plast Reconstr Surg 70:471, 1986

Navacharoen N, Sirisanthana T, Navacharoen W et al.: Oropharyngeal anthrax. J Laryngol Otol 99:1293, 1985

Pairolero PC, Arnold PG: Muscle flaps and thoracic problems: chest wall defects: reconstruction with autogenous tissue. p. 241. In Kittle FC (ed): Current Controversies in Thoracic Surgery. WB Saunders, Philadelphia, 1986

Pantoja E, Fede T, Kunchaia S: Complications of postoperative radiation in breast cancer. Breast 4:4, 1978

Parham FW: Thoracic resection for tumors growing from the bony wall of the chest. Trans South Surg Gynecol Assoc 11:223, 1898

Parker RG, Berry HC: Late effects of therapeutic irradiation on the skeleton and bone marrow. Cancer 37:1162, 1976

Pingleton SK, Jeter J: Necrotizing fasciitis as a complication of tube thoracostomy. Chest 83:925, 1983

Pizzarello PJ, Witcofoki RL: Basic radiation. In Biology. Lea & Febiger, Philadelphia, 1975

Rami P, Porta R, Bravo-Bravo JL et al.: Tumours and pseudotumours of the chest wall. Scand J Thorac Cardiovasc Surg 19:97, 1985

Robinson DW: Surgical problems in the excision and repair of radiated tissue. Plast Reconstr Surg 55:41, 1975

Sando W, Jurkiewicz MJ: An approach to repairs of radiation necrosis of chest wall and mammary gland. World J Surg 10:206, 1986

Seama MS, LeGulardeo D, Seberg C et al.: Complete arterioventricular block following mediastinal irradiation: a report of six cases. PACE Pacing Clin Electrophysical 14:1112, 1991

Seyfer AE: Radiation-associated lesions of the chest wall. Surg Gynecol Obstet 167:129, 1988

Smith R, Davidson JK, Flatman GE: Skeletal effects of orthovoltage and megavoltage therapy following treatment of nephroblastoma. Clin Radiol 33:601, 1982

Usher FC, Wallace SA: Tissue reaction to plastics. Arch Surg 76:997, 1959

Watson WC, James AG: Fascia lata grafts for chest wall defects. J Thorac Cardiovasc Surg 16:399, 1947

Wolbach SR: Pathologic history of chronic x-ray dermatitis and early x-ray carcinoma. J Med Res 21:415, 1909

Woods JE, Arnold PG, Masson JK et al.: Management of radiation necrosis and advanced cancer of the chest wall in patients with breast malignancy. Plast Reconstr Surg 63:235, 1979

50

SURGICAL TECHNIQUES

Chest Wall Resection

Geoffrey M. Graeber

Chest wall resection is usually performed for one of four reasons: removal of neoplasms, eradication of entrenched infection, excision of radiation injuries, and debridement of traumatic wounds. These indications for chest wall resection are not mutually exclusive, since infection can be a major complication for each of the other three. Recurrent tumor and infection together can complicate radiation injuries. The following discussion delineates the essential surgical principles governing chest wall resection for each of the four major indications. Before any major resection, the surgeon should make a thorough and accurate assessment of the patient in order to avoid major complications (Azarow, et al., 1989; Seyfer, et al., 1986b). In the trauma patient the resection may have to proceed even in victims who are poor operative risks, since allowing devitalized material to remain invites catastrophic infection (Seyfer, et al., 1986c).

RESECTION FOR NEOPLASMS

Before embarking on a biopsy of any chest wall neoplasm, the surgeon must take a complete history and conduct a thorough physical examination with the intent of identifying any history of chest wall trauma and of uncovering any malignancy that could spawn a chest wall metastasis. Metastatic lesions and healing rib fractures are far more prevalent than all primary chest wall neoplasms combined (Graeber, et al., 1982; El-Tamer M, et al., 1989). Either a healing rib fracture or a chest wall metastasis may have many of the same radiographic features as a primary chest wall neoplasm (see Ch. 48). The age of the patient, the presentation of the tumor, its physical location and characteristics on the chest wall, and its radiographic appearance will strongly suggest the true character of the neoplasm (see Ch. 48).

The evaluation of a suspected primary chest wall tumor includes standard chest radiographs plus a computed tomo-

graphic (CT) scan of the thorax that completely images all ribs, the totality of both leaves of the diaphragm, and the entire base of the neck. The treating surgeon should seek several consultations before embarking on a biopsy (Graeber, et al., 1982; Seyfer, et al., 1986d). The first consultation should be with a radiologist who specializes in imaging of the thorax. After the chest radiographs and CT scan have been reviewed by the surgeon and radiologist together, they should determine whether specialized diagnostic imaging techniques could be useful in providing more information about the neoplasm. These specialized studies should be undertaken before any diagnostic biopsy is conducted. The surgeon should also consult with a medical oncologist and a radiation therapist to see if any specialized studies need to be conducted on tissue obtained at the time of biopsy. Finally, a pathologist who regularly reads pathologic specimens containing musculoskeletal neoplasms should be consulted. The pathologist will usually suggest how much tissue will be necessary to perform the tests required to achieve a proper diagnosis. Continuing consultation with the pathologist at the time of surgery is mandatory. Frozen sections are generally of limited value in assessing chest wall neoplasms since so many of them have bony and/or cartilaginous components. The surgeon and the pathologist should work together to obtain enough appropriate material at the time of biopsy to ensure an accurate diagnosis.

The question of how much tumor needs to be biopsied remains controversial (Graeber, et al., 1982; El-Tamer, et al., 1989). The technique of biopsy and how much tumor is removed depends on the suspected type of tumor and the pathologist. At the one extreme is the needle biopsy, a technique that has proved particularly effective for the group at the University of Texas M. D. Anderson Cancer Center in evaluating children with Ewing's sarcoma of the chest wall (Ryan, et al., 1989). In one study of primary bone tumors, needle biopsy accurately diagnosed 83 percent of malignant and 64 percent of benign neoplasms (Ayala and Zornosa, 1983). Incisional biopsy is indicated if the needle biopsy is

I wish to thank Mrs. Karen DeShong for her expert preparation of the manuscript.

1263

not diagnostic or if the pathologist needs more tissue to make a definitive diagnosis. Conduct of the incisional biopsy should be governed by the anticipation of possible radical resection if the tumor proves malignant. The surgeon should bear in mind that 5 cm of clear skin from the margin of the biopsy site should be resected with radical surgical extirpation (Seyfer, et al., 1986d). Meticulous surgical technique is mandatory since hematoma within the wound predisposes to tumor extension. The biopsy site ideally should be closed without a drain because a drain increases the chance of infection, which would complicate definitive resection and reconstruction. Excisional biopsy is indicated for smaller lesions (2 to 3 cm) and also for chondromatous lesions, since these neoplasms may well include benign as well as malignant areas within the same neoplastic mass (Graeber, et al., 1982). Wide excision of osteochondromas and neurofibromas is also indicated, particularly in patients suffering from the familiar syndromes of multiple osteochondromas and neurofibromatosis, as malignant degeneration has been recorded in both entities (Martini, et al., 1969).

Once the true nature of the primary chest wall neoplasm has been established, definitive therapy can be undertaken. Proper resection of benign neoplasms consists of surgical excision with preservation of the overlying skin and surrounding musculature. In the event that the benign neoplasm falls into one of the categories of chondromatous lesions noted above, wider excision should be conducted (Ryan, et al., 1989).

Although there has been some variance in reporting, the generally accepted rate of malignancy for primary chest wall neoplasms is 50 percent (Graeber, et al., 1982; Groff and Adkins, 1967; Stelzer and Gay, 1980). The most common malignancies in most series are the chondrosarcomas, with the incidence of fibrosarcoma not far behind. Adjuvant chemotherapy and radiation therapy have a role in treating some primary chest wall malignancies. For this reason preoperative consultation with a radiation therapist and a medical oncologist is indicated before conducting a radical chest wall resection in any patient suffering from a chest wall neoplasm.

The most common primary chest wall malignancy, chondrosarcoma, is resistant to both chemotherapy and radiotherapy (Ryan, et al., 1989). Appropriate radical resection with tumor-free margins of at least 5 cm has yielded excellent results (Graeber, et al., 1982; Arnold and Pairolero, 1978; Pairolero and Arnold 1985; King, et al., 1986; McAfee, et al., 1985). Survival is related to the tumor's histologic grade and size and the adequacy of resection (Fig. 50-1). In one series, patients with grade I lesions had a 10-year survival rate of 70 percent, and patients with a tumor less than 6.0 cm in greatest dimension had an 87 percent 10-year survival (McAfee, et al., 1985). On the other hand, the same series noted that patients with grade III or dedifferentiated chondrosarcomas had very poor survival.

Primary fibrosarcomas of the chest wall are usually treated with aggressive surgical resection (Graeber, et al., 1982; Martini, et al., 1969). Most chemotherapeutic agents have relatively little effect on these malignancies. Some success has been reported with the use of radiotherapy for lower-grade fibrosarcomas (desmoids) of the chest wall (Ryan, et al., 1989).

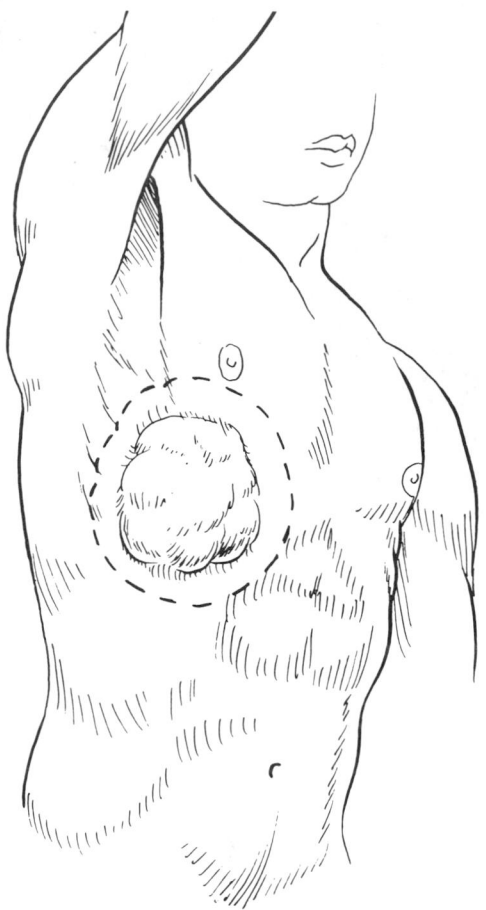

Figure 50-1. Large anterior lateral chest wall neoplastic mass, such as would be seen with a chondrosarcoma. The tumor has obvious physical margins. The dotted line represents the planned area of resection around the tumor, which includes resection of an adequate, approximately 5-cm margin of healthy tissue around the tumor itself. This is the best way to eliminate local recurrence, which is the most common cause of treatment failure in chondrosarcomas. (From Seyfer AE, Graeber GM, Wind GG: Planning the reconstruction. p. 59. In Atlas of Chest Wall Reconstruction. Aspen Publishers, Rockville, MD, 1986e, with permission.)

Preoperative and postoperative chemotherapy appears to be beneficial in treating primary chest wall osteosarcomas (Ryan, et al., 1989). Although most series are small, primary radical surgical resection can yield long-term survivors (Graeber, et al., 1982). Preoperative chemotherapy causes a degree of necrosis in the primary, which may aid in selecting postoperative agents (Martini, et al., 1969). Cisplatin and doxorubicin, either alone or in combination with other agents, appear to be effective (Ryan, et al., 1989).

Ewing's sarcoma generally presents in the second decade of life and is unusual in the ribs (Ryan, et al., 1989). When it presents as a chest wall tumor, it generally has a worse prognosis than when it is a primary in a long bone of an extremity, since metastases to the lungs occur in about half of the cases (Ryan, et al., 1989). When Ewing's sarcoma is localized to the chest wall, the patient is treated with CyVADIC (cyclophosphamide-vincristine-Adriamycin-imidazole carboxamide) induction chemotherapy for two to five cycles before undertaking resection of the primary. In general, the goals of the resection are to excise the primary with minimal soft tissue margins and with the entirety of the affected rib(s) (Ryan, et al., 1989). CyVADIC is then continued for seven to eight cycles postoperatively without administration of radiation therapy (Ryan, et al., 1989). Although some few survivors have been reported with surgery alone, the prudent use of neoadjuvant and adjuvant chemotherapy for treating primary Ewing's sarcoma of the chest wall is strongly indicated (Graeber, et al., 1982; Ryan, et al., 1989). Radiotherapy is reserved only for patients who have residual disease after definitive therapy (Ryan, et al., 1989; Rao, et al., 1988).

Primary solitary plasmacytomas are infrequent chest wall neoplasms, which can be treated by radiotherapy or by resection (Graeber, et al., 1982). In general, the Walter Reed group has favored primary resection with adequate margins for several reasons (Graeber, et al., 1982). Most patients who present with primary chest wall plasmocytomas return with multiple myeloma within 10 years. If the primary has been eradicated by radiotherapy, the amount of subsequent radiotherapy that may be available for the patient may be small or nonexistent. Hence, the patient may present later with severe pain due to myeloma of the thoracic spine and be unable to undergo more radiotherapy because of having already received a maximal dose of radiotherapy to the thorax. Resection is indicated also for larger lesions, since radiotherapy alone often does not eradicate the disease entirely. The patient then presents with a partially treated neoplasm, which has an open necrotic ulcer and infection. Resection and reconstruction in such cases is much more difficult and more likely to have complications.

Wide surgical excision remains the treatment of choice for patients suffering from malignant fibrous histiocytoma (Venn, et al., 1986; Ryan, et al., 1989). Aggressive surgical resection has been successful in selected cases in eliminating locally recurrent disease. These tumors are relatively resistant to radiotherapy and chemotherapy. Consequently, radiotherapy is reserved for residual tumor remaining in margins of resection where total resection was not possible anatomically (Ryan, et al., 1989).

Rhabdomyosarcomas of the chest wall are usually found in the pediatric population. They are responsive to chemotherapy in most cases (Ryan, et al., 1989). Management generally consists of chemotherapy, complete surgical resection, and long-term postoperative chemotherapy. Since radiotherapy is not particularly effective against these tumors, it is employed only in treating lesions for which complete surgical extirpation is not possible or in which the margins of surgical resection are questionable (Ryan, et al., 1989).

Chest wall resection for breast cancer today is most often conducted for recurrent local disease after failure of other forms of therapy (Seyfer, et al., 1986d; Ryan, et al., 1989). Systemic recurrence is common, and chest wall resection is directed at palliating pain, removing friable, ulcerating tumor, and reducing odor. Patients must be selected carefully in the light of survival expectancy. Chemotherapy is beneficial prior to resection and as part of continuing therapy after chest wall resection. The resection should be conducted with the aim of removing all radiation-damaged chest wall since allowing irradiated tissue to remain will often compromise healing. With appropriate chest wall stabilization and rotation of pedicled flap(s) into the resected area, chest wall stability and durability can be achieved. The most gratifying aspect of these resections is the improved quality of life that this resection affords, since pain and tenderness are almost always relieved. The patient's need for analgesics and narcotics is always diminished if not relieved entirely.

Extension of primary lung tumors into the chest wall requires resection in many cases, but chest wall reconstruction is indicated only infrequently (Seyfer, et al., 1986d; El-Tamer, et al., 1989). Patients with primary lung cancers invading the chest wall must be screened carefully before resection to confirm that systemic disease that would preclude meaningful long-term survival is not present. A 5-cm margin of uninvolved chest wall should be resected en bloc with the primary. Entrance into the chest is planned so that neither the tumor itself nor the margin of resection is violated. Tumors that have extended through the chest wall and overlying musculature to invade and/or ulcerate the skin are found infrequently, since the disease is lethal systematically prior to such local extension. Hence, in most cases the overlying muscles of the upper extremity, subcutaneous tissues, and skin will remain intact over the site of chest wall resection, and with so much intact tissue remaining, the need for chest wall stabilization and flap reconstruction is quite rare.

RESECTION FOR INFECTION

Currently the most common indication for chest wall resection is probably infection due to a dehisced median sternotomy incision. With the increase in cardiac surgery and the use of a median sternotomy incision for access to the heart, the absolute number of median sternotomy dehiscences has increased, although the incidence of this occurrence ranges from 1 to 3 percent (Miller and Nahai, 1989). Experimental work in the laboratory on the blood flow to the sternum has shown a marked, precipitous decrease in perfusion of the ipsilateral hemisternum immediately after harvesting of the internal mammary artery (Seyfer, et al., 1988). This is one of many predisposing factors that can increase the incidence of median sternotomy dehiscence. The association of internal mammary artery harvesting with median sternotomy dehiscence remains a clinical problem of continuing concern (Graeber, 1992). The reconstruction of the dehisced median sternotomy incision continues to be an area of interest for numerous investigators (Miller and Nahai, 1989; Seyfer, et al., 1986h; Arnold and Pairolero, 1984; Pairolero and Arnold, 1986).

Initial evaluation of the patient with a dehisced median sternotomy consists of a precise physical examination, which focuses on the median sternotomy wound and its characteristics (Seyfer, et al., 1986h; Miller and Nahai, 1986; Arnold and Pairolero, 1984; Pairolero and Arnold, 1986). Tenderness and erythema generally delineate the margins of the infected tissue. Once these margins have been determined by careful palpation, the anticipated margin of necessary resection to achieve a clean wound and ensure a satisfactory reconstruction is established. The wound is checked for fluctuance, and any fluid that may be expressed from the wound is sent for culture and sensitivities. Crepitus, which may present to varying degrees, usually does not represent clostridial infection but rather reflects air that has entered the wound through the incision itself. When the patient coughs or the ventilator cycles, the sternum is generally unstable. This is heralded by a palpable click, which may be present over varying amounts of the sternum. Determination of exactly how much bone remains unstable within the wound is important, since preservation of as much sternum as possible is beneficial for stabilizing respiratory mechanics.

Several different radiologic techniques have been shown to be of benefit in evaluating these patients (Schaefer and Burton, 1989). Standard posteroanterior and lateral radiographs of the chest will generally show air in the mediastinum and between the two halves of the sternum. Occasionally, air may be seen lateral to the primary incision. When this occurs, the evaluating surgeon can usually suspect either a separation of the bony and cartilaginous elements or the presence of pockets behind the sternum. CT of the chest is helpful in that it delineates any abscess pockets, recesses, and extensions of the infectious process into the mediastinum. Although a CT scan is not always necessary, it may be helpful in determining where fluid collections may be extravasated. Leaving any of these fluid collections, especially if it is infected, will complicate the subsequent reconstruction of the wound.

Fluid and clot sequestrations may also be delineated by echocardiography, which is also beneficial in evaluating ventricular function and whether or not any of the fluid collection present in the mediastinum embarrasses cardiac function in any way. Magnetic resonance imaging (MRI) may in some cases be of assistance in evaluating these wounds. It appears to be most helpful in delineating where fluid collections may be separated from major vascular structures. The risks and benefits of this examination must be considered in the light of the patient's general condition. The presence of wires within the wound also causes a scattering effect on both the CT and MRI procedures. One particularly helpful nuclear medicine test is the bone scan. Because of its ability to delineate active areas of inflammation, it may be very useful in denoting areas of persistent osteomyelitis and chondritis within a chronically infected median sternotomy incision.

Antibiotic therapy in these patients is directed at the specific culture sensitivities and results (Miller and Nahai, 1989). The most commonly offending organisms are *Staphylococcus aureus* and *Staphylococcus epidermidis*. Either Enterobacteriaceae and *Pseudomonas* spp. are the most common gramnegative bacilli that populate these wounds (Miller and Nahai, 1989). Antibiotic therapy should be directed at these species as well as any pathogens that may be specifically delineated on the culture results. The patient should receive systemic antibiotics 6 hours prior to the intended resection, with continuing therapy throughout the time of resection and for 2 days immediately thereafter. The antibiotics are started early so that adequate levels may be maintained in the healthy tissue surrounding the intended area of resection. Postoperative antibiotic coverage is directed at minimizing seeding of other areas within the body associated with bacteremia.

In the operating room several important considerations must be addressed during the positioning and preparation of the patient (Seyfer, et al., 1986h). The patient should be placed in the supine position on the operating table so that the entire anterior thorax is accessible to the operating surgeon for debridement and for possible repair of any cardiovascular injury that may occur during the procedure. Full monitoring is instituted, just as it would be for any patient undergoing a major cardiovascular procedure. This precaution is taken so that if the patient does need to go on cardiopulmonary bypass (a rare occurrence), the surgeon and anesthesiologist are not compromised in their options. One or both groins are prepared for placement of arterial and venous cannulas from a cardiopulmonary bypass machine should bypass be needed. Most surgeons prefer to avoid cannulation through the infected incision, since when tissues are inflamed, they may well be friable, and the repair of the cannulation sites can be extremely difficult. A portion of at least one leg is also prepared in case a segment of saphenous vein should be needed to repair a bypass graft or a major vascular structure.

Once the resection is undertaken, the wound should be actively debrided of all dead tissue (Bellamy and Zajtchuk, 1991b). All nonvital prosthetic tissue and sutures are removed when the wound is opened. Portions of the sternum that show no evidence of bleeding from either the periosteum or the marrow are resected until healthy bleeding is encountered. Any musculature of the chest wall that appears to be compromised is also debrided. In the event that costal cartilages become exposed, the cartilages are resected subperichondrally, since the blood supply to the cartilages is so poor. Once the cartilages are exposed, they should be regarded as infected throughout their entirety. The blood supply to the viable musculature of the chest wall and to any remaining tissues should be preserved scrupulously. Care should be taken to preserve any internal mammary arteries that may be present, since they are the primary blood supply to the rectus abdominis muscles. If one of these muscles is needed as a flap for reconstruction, its arc of rotation is seriously compromised, if not precluded, when the ipsilateral internal mammary artery has been resected or has been used as a cardiac conduit. The ultimate goal of the resection is to remove all tissue that does not have vital capabilities and does not bleed well. Once the resection has been conducted to healthy tissue margins, reconstruction may be contemplated.

In some few cases the margins of resection after debridement of a dehisced median sternotomy may be questionable. In such a case, the wound may be packed with povidone-iodine-soaked gauze and treated as an open wound for 48 hours (Seyfer, et al., 1986h). After the wound has been repacked several times by the surgical team and the patient has been stabilized, the patient may be returned for a secondary debridement and reconstruction. The goal of the secondary debridement is to remove any other tissue that is questionable so that only a healthy margin remains. By use of secondary debridement, persistently infected, recalcitrant median sternotomy infections may be treated successfully. Obviously, retention of any tissue, bone, or cartilage that is devascularized will compromise subsequent reconstruction.

RESECTION FOR RADIATION INJURY

Resection for radiation injuries of the chest wall is usually conducted for palliation. In most such patients there are several concurrent indications for chest wall resection. Many patients will have concurrent infection as well as recurrent tumor in the irradiated field. Complete and thorough evaluation of the patient is necessary, since the benefits and detriments of the resection and reconstruction need to be viewed in the light of the patient's predicted survival. The palliation that will be afforded by the resection in terms of decreased pain, improved cosmesis, and decrease in odor must be weighed against the total survival of the patient. Although a number of chest wall tumors may be irradiated, the malignancy most often associated with chest wall radiation is carcinoma of the breast (Seyfer, 1988). Extensive experiences have been recorded by several institutions in dealing with the irradiated chest wall (Arnold and Pairolero, 1989, 1986; Pairolero and Arnold, 1986; Seyfer, 1988).

Preoperative evaluation of these patients starts with thorough metastatic evaluation. Biopsies are taken from any portions of the irradiated field that are suspected of having recurrent tumor. The chest wall should be evaluated to determine the margins of viable tissue. When doing this, it is very important to consider the contralateral chest as an example of healthy tissue for the region. Once the tissue becomes discolored, the epidermis appears thin, and the vascularity appears abnormal, the tissue should be regarded as tenuous. Evaluation should always be conducted with an eye toward conserving as much healthy tissue as possible, yet not leaving any of the radiation-damaged chest wall behind. Radiation-

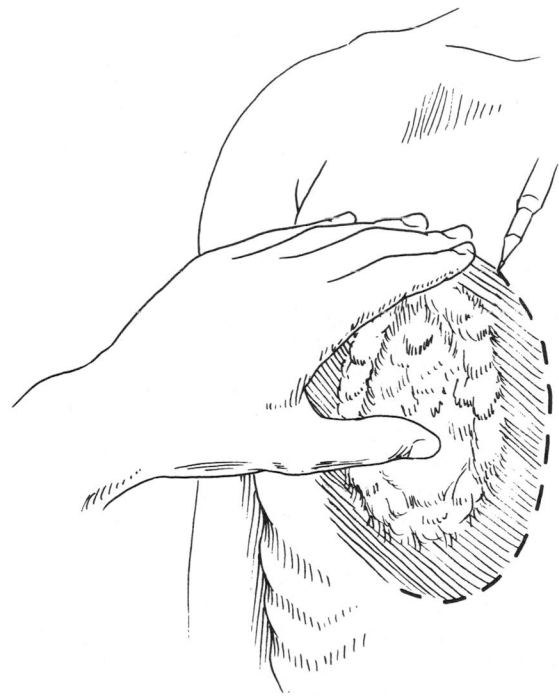

Figure 50-2. Method for determining resection of recurrent cancer in an irradiated field. Note that the line of resection, denoted by the heavy dotted line, is drawn at the margin of skin showing any radiation change. The chest wall excision should include all tissue that is apparently damaged even though the defect may be large. Healing will be better if the flaps are approximated to healthy tissues. (From Seyfer AE, Graeber GM, Wind GG: The rectus abdominis muscle and musculocutaneous flaps. p. 159. In Atlas of Chest Wall Reconstruction. Aspen Publishers, Rockville, MD, 1986e, with permission.)

damaged tissue will provide and unstable margin for reconstruction. In planning the resection, the entire margin of irradiated tissue should be removed (Fig. 50-2).

The same principles that govern surgical resection for infection govern resection for radiation injury, since infection is often present at the time of surgery. Preparation of the patient is similar to that for resection of infection, as described in the previous section. In the case of infection localized to one area of ulceration, we use a double preparation technique. The first step is to prepare the ulcerated, irradiated tissue with a separate instrument set and to isolate this area from the remaining surgical area with a povidone-iodine-impregnated gauze sponge, which is placed in the wound and then covered with a piece of plastic sheeting or rubber glove (Fig. 50-3). A second preparation is then conducted throughout the entire operative field on the patient so that there is no contamination from the infected ulcer. Resection is then carried out to healthy tissue margins (Seyfer, 1988).

Even though the resection may be extensive, it is necessary to achieve healthy margins throughout the wound so that good tissue healing may occur. Radiation-damaged tissue will not heal well, and it offers further chance for breakdown at the margins of the wound. Such tissue will offer poor structural support to the chest wall and will be inadequate to allow firm fixation of any stabilization material. If marginal tissue is retained at the edges of resection, the chances for poor healing between any flaps that may be rotated into the wound and the surgical edges of resection is large.

RESECTION FOR TRAUMA

Traumatic injuries of the chest wall may be broadly categorized as either blunt or penetrating (Pate, 1989). In most cases penetrating wounds are the ones most often responsible for serious chest wall injury requiring surgical repair. Since there has been a tremendous increase in domestic trauma, particularly related to criminal activity, the need for understanding these wounds and treating them appropriately is large (Lo-Cicero and Mattox, 1989). Military weapons, including handguns, shoulder weapons, automatic rifles, and assault weapons, are all being used with greater frequency in domestic violence today. Patients who suffer blast injuries to the chest from detonated ordinance rarely live to reach an emergency center.

Early attempts at treating chest wall injuries were rudimentary at best. In the first part of this century, during World War I, most chest wounds were left open to granulate. If the patient survived, it was purely owing to luck and personal fortitude (Fig. 50-4). Few patients with significant injuries of the chest ever survived during this period. By the time of World War II, there were some organized efforts at treating wounds of the chest effectively. After thorough debridement, local flaps of tissue were advanced to attempt to cover the wound (Fig. 50-5). Currently, effective management consists of thorough debridement and stabilization of the wound followed by flap reconstruction. Since all the wounds are severely infected, chest wall stabilization with synthetic materials is not recommended.

The devastating nature of military and civilian weapons has been well documented (Bellamy and Zajtchuk, 1991a,

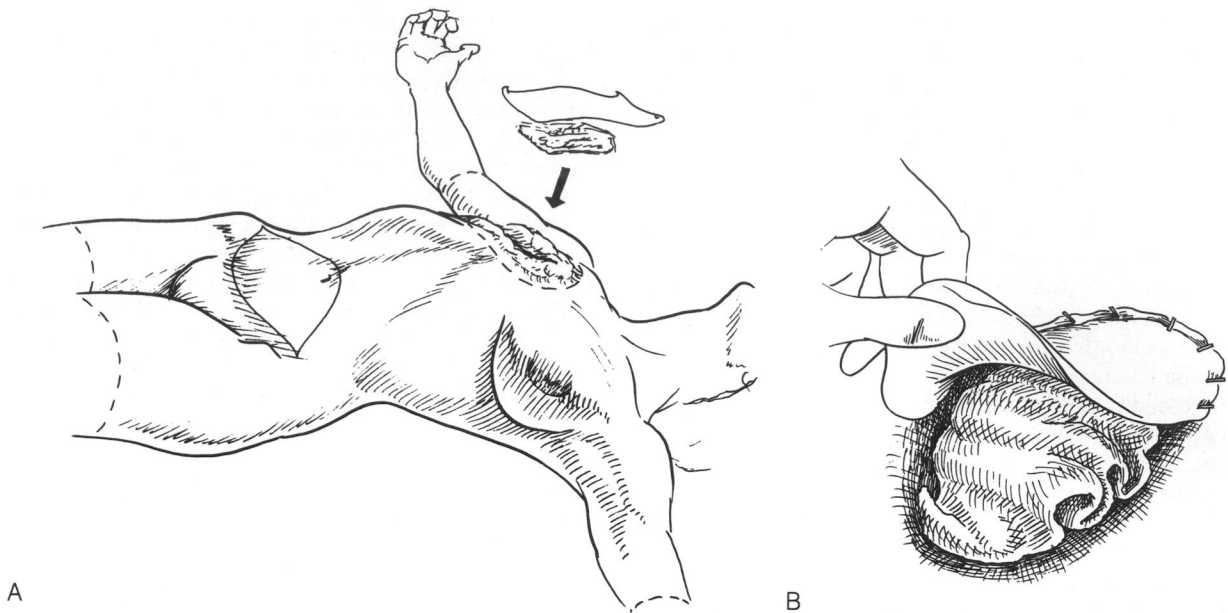

A

B

Figure 50-3. **(A)** The patient has been placed in a supine position on the operating table, and the anticipated margins of resection have been drawn on the chest wall. The dotted lines on the extremities show the preparation of the patient. In this case a transverse musculocutaneous rectus abdominis (TRAM) flap based on the left rectus muscle will be used to reconstruct the defect. The solid line on the lower abdomen depicts the skin island that will be taken with the flap. Preparation of the patient for resection includes a double preparation, the first of which is directed at cleaning the ulcerated wound on the chest. Once this has been closed and covered with a gauze sponge impregnated with povidone-iodine solution, which is covered with a piece of plastic or a section of rubber after being placed in the wound, a second preparation can be conducted over the entire area. **(B)** Close-up of the way the ulcer is filled with the gauze sponge in the defect. Note that the rubber patch, a portion of the glove, or a piece of sterile impermeable drape is stapled in placed so that the entirety of the ulcer is excluded from the field during the second preparation. (Fig. A from Seyfer AE, Graeber GM, Wind GG: The rectus abdominis muscle and musculocutaneous flaps. p. 159. In Atlas of Chest Wall Reconstruction. Aspen Publishers, Rockville, MD, 1986a, with permission. Fig. B from Seyfer AE, Graeber GM, Wind GG: The omentum. p. 141. In Atlas of Chest Wall Reconstruction. Aspen Publishers, Rockville, MD, 1986i, with permission.)

1991b). Detonation of antipersonnel devices such as grenades, mines, and heavy ordinance are rarely encountered in civilian practice; however, in today's world some few patients suffering blast injuries may come to a thoracic surgeon for treatment. The critical effects of blasts have recently been well documented by several authors in military publications (Phillips and Zajtchuk, 1991; Stuhmiller, et al., 1991). Frequently, weapons of civilian origin will also cause significant injuries to the chest wall, which will need resection. The most common weapon of this type is the shotgun, which causes a devastating soft tissue loss of the chest wall while penetrating the lung and underlying viscera.

Preoperative preparation is directed at stabilizing the patient and giving broad-spectrum antibiotics to cover the bacteremia, which is always present with such wounds. The patient is given vigorous fluid resuscitation to restore cardiodynamic integrity and is transported to the operating room as soon as possible. Surgery is directed at stabilizing the life-threatening injuries within the thorax and at debridement of the chest wall. It is necessary to emphasize that the lung should be managed in a conservative fashion since the lung has tremendous regenerative capacity. The need for total

lobectomy and/or pneumonectomy remains infrequent, since the major vessels and bronchi may be closed on the surface of the lung without radical extirpation. Once the lung has been stabilized, it should be ventilated and expanded to its greatest extent. Pleural abrasion is very helpful in securing fixation of the lung to the remaining chest wall. Chest tubes should be placed so that they are not exposed in the open defect but rather drain the inferior as well as the superior portion of the chest of all possible fluid and air that may remain in the pleural cavity (Fig. 50-6).

The resection of the chest wall itself is most important, since removal of all devitalized tissue, foreign material, portions of clothing, dead skin, and hair should be conducted vigorously. The resection should be conducted so that healthy muscle is seen throughout the margin of the wound and there is active bleeding throughout all remaining tissues. The four major qualities consistent with a high degree of viability are color, consistency, contractility, and circulation (Bellamy and Zajtchuk, 1991b). The lung is expanded to the margins of resection and the defect is closed with an impregnated providone-iodine gauze to secure an airtight seal on the chest wall. The chest tubes evacuate any blood or air

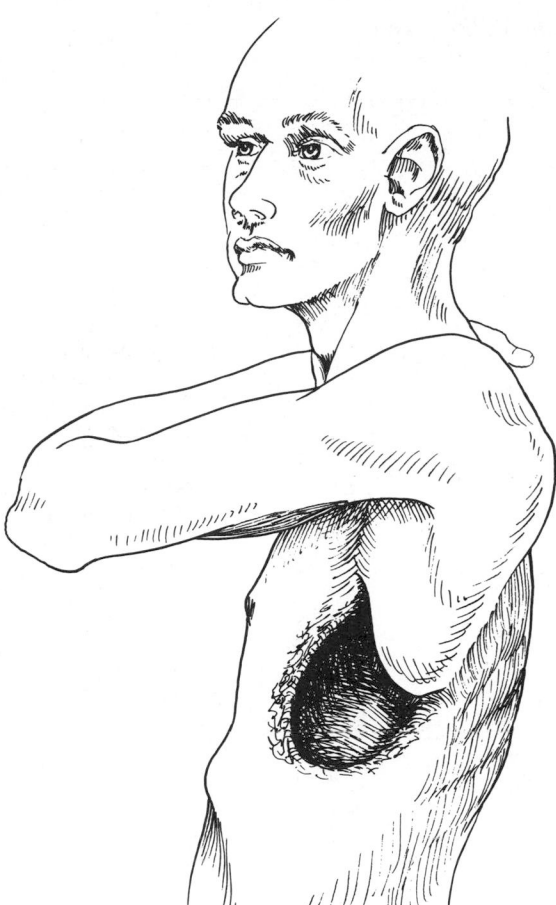

Figure 50-4. Patient with severe chest wall wound, which has been treated in accordance with the principles of military medicine as dictated in the early part of the twentieth century. Note that the wound has been debrided widely and allowed to granulate. Some patients treated in this manner, including soldiers wounded in World War I, survived despite their wounds. The wound continued to granulate and remain superficially infected, causing severe nutritional depletion of the patient. Hence, the patient looked quite cachectic, since this was a long process. Few of these individuals survived the long term. (From Seyfer AE, Graeber GM, Wind GG: Some historical aspects of chest wall reconstruction. p. 3. In Atlas of Chest Wall Reconstruction. Aspen Publishers, Rockville, MD, 1986c, with permission.)

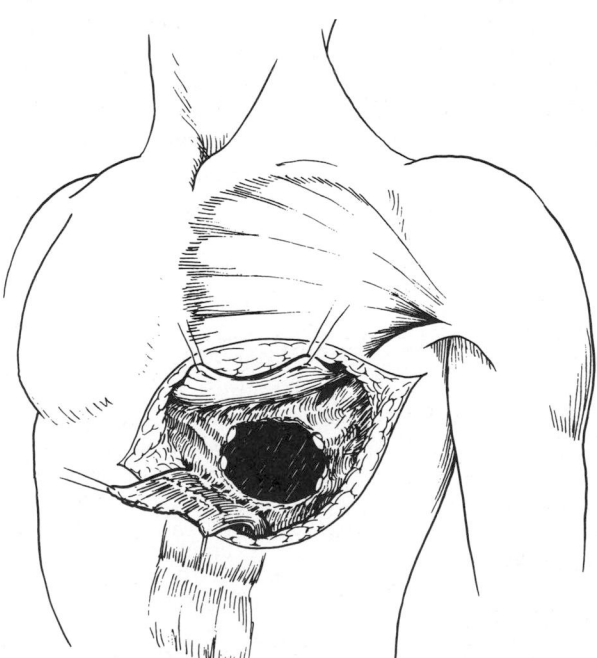

Figure 50-5. Closure of wounds in World War II usually consisted of mobilization of local slips of muscle for closure over the previously debrided defect. This drawing depicts one of the attempts at closure, which was conducted on a patient suffering an anterior thoracic wall wound during World War II. Note that the area had been debrided widely and that closure was attempted only when all evidence of infection had receded. (From Seyfer AE, Graeber GM, Wind GG: Some historical aspects of chest wall reconstruction. p. 3. In Atlas of Chest Wall Reconstruction. Aspen Publishers, Rockville, MD, 1986c, with permission.)

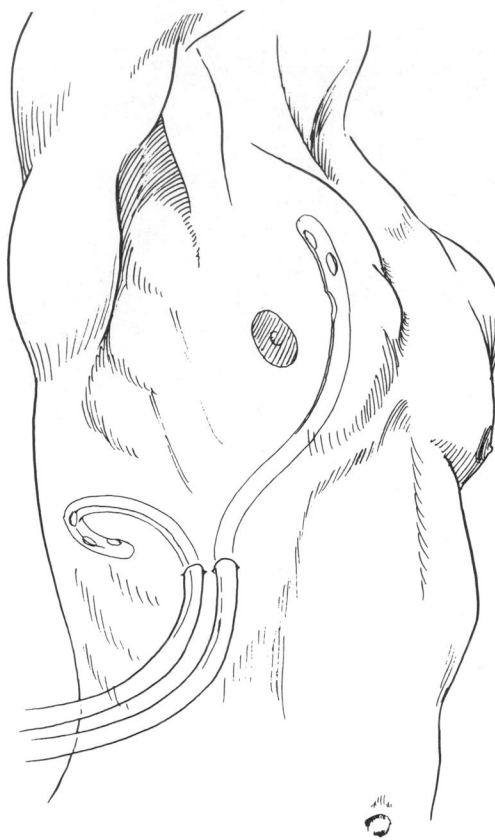

Figure 50-6. Placement of chest tubes as they would be situated for an anterolateral thoracic wound. In placing the tubes, care is taken to remain away from the wound site itself so that the tubes do not traverse the area of the open chest wall. One tube is placed over the apex of the chest to drain any air that may be remaining within the pleural cavity; the other tube is placed low and posterior so that it will evacuate any blood or tissue fluids that may collect in the posterior costophrenic sinus. (From Seyfer AE, Graeber GM, Wind GG: Resection and debridement of the chest wall. p. 75. In Atlas of Chest Wall Reconstruction. Aspen Publishers, Rockville, MD, 1986d, with permission.)

that may accumulate in the pleural cavity and maintain expansion of the lung against the remaining chest wall. A second debridement is often necessary 24 and/or 48 hours after the initial injury since additional tissue may lose viability in this time. The necessity for close observation of the wound and subsequent debridement cannot be underestimated. Retention of foreign material and devitalized tissue within the margins of the wound can lead to clostridial infection and rapid demise of the patient. Fortunately, with adequate initial debridement this is rare.

In the final analysis, the viability of the patient will depend on the individual surgeon's persistence, skill, and creativity. The patient must be observed constantly for any evidence of pending sepsis and evaluated for evidence of crepitus within the margins of the wound. Creativity must be constantly exhibited, since the wound will have to be tailored when it has become stabilized. Constant attention to patients is mandatory since they can deteriorate and die very quickly.

KEY REFERENCES

McCraw JB, Arnold PG: McCraw and Arnold's Atlas of Muscle and Musculocutaneous Flaps, Hampton Press, Norfolk, VA, 1986

This excellent atlas depicts the major muscular and musculocutaneous flaps that may be harvested throughout the human body. Copiously illustrated, this provides an excellent guide for the anatomic dissection of most existing muscular and musculocutaneous flaps. It should be considered an excellent reference for chest wall reconstruction since it depicts both pedicled and free flaps.

Seyfer AE, Graeber GM (eds): Chest wall reconstruction. Surg Clin North Am 69:5, 1989

This monograph specifically addresses chest wall reconstruction in all its major aspects. Major authorities in the field of chest wall reconstructions discuss each of the major flaps that may be used. The specific problems encountered in chest wall reconstruction, such as the dehisced median sternotomy and radiation injuries of the chest wall are covered in depth. The monograph provides an excellent review of the entire field since each of the articles has an extensive list of references.

Seyfer AE, Graeber GM, Wind GG: Atlas of Chest Wall Reconstruction, Aspen Publishers, Rockville, MD, 1986a

This atlas specifically delineates the methods used in chest wall reconstruction. It covers most aspects of chest wall reconstruction, starting from the evaluation of the patient and continuing through postoperative care. Major emphasis is placed on pedicled flap reconstruction and on specific problems afflicting the chest wall. The illustrations depict all the major steps necessary in each of the reconstructions cited.

REFERENCES

Arnold PG, Pairolero PC: Reconstruction of the radiation-damaged chest wall. Surg Clin North Am 69:1081, 1989

Arnold PG, Pairolero PC: Surgical management of the radiated chest wall. Plast Reconstr Surg 77:605, 1986

Arnold PG, Pairolero PC: Chest wall reconstruction: experience with 100 consecutive patients. Ann Surg 199:725, 1984

Arnold PG, Pairolero PC: Chondrosarcoma of the manubrium. Resection and reconstruction with pectoralis major muscle. Mayo Clin Proc 53:54, 1978

Ayala AG, Zornosa J: Primary bone tumors: percutaneous needle biopsy. Radiology 149:675, 1983

Azarow KS, Mallow M, Seyfer AE, Graeber GM: Preoperative evaluation and general preparation for chest wall operations. Surg Clin North Am 69:899, 1989

Bellamy RF, Zajtchuk R: The weapons of conventional land warfare. p. 1. In Bellamy RF, Zajtchuk R (eds): Conventional Warfare: Ballistic, Blast, and Burn Injuries. In Textbook of Military Medicine. Part I: Warfare Weaponry and the Casualty. Vol. 5. Office of the Surgeon General. U.S. Army, Washington, 1991a

Bellamy RF, Zajtchuk R: Assessing the effectiveness of conventional weapons. p. 53. In Bellamy RF, Zajtchuk R (eds): Conventional Warfare: Ballistic, Blast, and Burn Injuries. In Textbook of Military Medicine. Part I: Warfare Weaponry and the Casualty. Vol. 5. Office of the Surgeon General. U.S. Army, Washington, 1991b

Bellamy RF, Zajtchuk R: The physics and biophysics of wound ballistics. p. 107. In Bellamy RF, Zajtchuk R (eds): Conventional Warfare: Ballistic, Blast, and Burn Injuries. In Textbook of Military Medicine. Part I: Warfare Weaponry and the Casualty. Office of the Surgeon General, U.S. Army, Washington, 1991c

Bellamy RF, Zajtchuk R: The management of ballistic wounds of soft tissue. p. 163. In Bellamy RF, Zajtchuk R (eds): Conventional Warfare: Ballistic, Blast, and Burn Injuries. In Textbook of Military Medicine Part I: Warfare Weaponry and the Casualty. Vol. 5. Office of the Surgeon General, U.S. Army, Washington, 1991d

El-Tamer M, Chaglassian T, Martini N: Resection and debridement of chest-wall tumors and general aspects of reconstruction. Surg Clin North Am 69:947, 1989

Graeber GM: Harvesting of the internal mammary artery and the healing median sternotomy, editorial. Ann Thorac Surg 53:7, 1992

Graeber GM, Snyder RJ, Fleming AW et al: Initial and long-term results in the management of primary chest wall neoplasms. Ann Thorac Surg 34:664, 1982

Groff DB, Adkins PC: Chest wall tumors. Ann Thorac Surg 4:260, 1967

King RM, Pairolero PC, Trastek VF et al: Primary chest wall tumors: factors affecting survival. Ann Thorac Surg 41:597, 1986

LoCicero J, Mattox KL: Epidemiology of chest trauma. Surg Clin North Am 69:15, 1989

Martini N, Starzynski TE, Beattie EJ: Problems in chest wall resection. Surg Clin North Am 49:313, 1969

McAfee MK, Pairolero PC, Bergstrahl EJ et al: Chondrosarcoma of the chest wall: factors affecting survival. Ann Thorac Surg 140:535, 1985

Miller JI, Nahai F: Repair of the dehisced median sternotomy incision. Surg Clin North Am 69:1011, 1986

Pairolero PC, Arnold PG: Thoracic wall defects: surgical management of 205 consecutive patients. Mayo Clin Proc 61:557, 1986

Pairolero PC, Arnold PG: Chest wall tumors: experience with 100 consecutive patients. J Thorac Cardiovasc Surg 90:367, 1985

Pairolero PC, Arnold PG: Management of recalcitrant median sternotomy wounds. J Thorac Cardiovasc Surg 88:357, 1984

Pate JW: Chest wall injuries. Surg Clin North Am 69:59, 1989

Phillips YY, Zajtchuk JT: The management of primary blast injury. p. 295. In Bellamy RF, Zajtchuk R (eds): Conventional Warfare: Ballistic, Blast, and Burn Injuries. In Textbook of Military Medicine. Part I: Warfare Weaponry and the Casualty. Vol. 5. Office of the Surgeon General. United States Army, Washington, 1991

Rao BN, Hayes FA, Thompson EI et al: Chest wall resection for Ewing's sarcoma of the rib: an unnecessary procedure. Ann Thorac Surg 46:40, 1988

Ryan MB, McMurtrey MJ, Roth JA: Current management of chest-wall tumors. Surg Clin North Amer, 69:1061, 1989

Schaefer PS, Burton BS: Radiographic evaluation of chest-wall lesions. Surg Clin North Am 69:911, 1989

Seyfer AE, Graeber GM, Wind GG: Preoperative care and considerations. p. 51. In Atlas of Chest Wall Reconstruction. Aspen Publishers. Rockville, MD, 1986b

Seyfer AE, Graeber GM, Wind GG: Some historical aspects of chest wall reconstruction. p. 3. In Atlas of Chest Wall Reconstruction. Aspen Publishers, Rockville, MD, 1986c

Seyfer AE, Graeber GM, Wind GG: Resection and debridement of the chest wall. p. 75. In Atlas of Chest Wall Reconstruction. Aspen Publishers, Rockville, MD, 1986d

Seyfer AE, Graeber GM, Wind GG: Planning the reconstruction. p. 59. In Atlas of Chest Wall Reconstruction. Aspen Publishers, Rockville, MD, 1986e

Seyfer AE, Graeber GM, Wind GG: The rectus abdominis muscle and muscuocutaneous flaps. p. 159. In Atlas of Chest Wall Reconstruction. Aspen Publishers, Rockville, MD, 1986f

Seyfer AE, Graeber GM, Wind GG: The pectoralis major muscle and musculocutaneous flaps. p. 129. In Atlas of the Chest Wall Reconstruction. Aspen Publishers, Rockville, MD, 1986g

Seyfer AE, Graeber GM, Wind GG: The dehisced median sternotomy incision. p. 245. In Atlas of Chest Wall Reconstruction. Aspen Publishers, Rockville, MD, 1986h

Seyfer AE: Radiation-associated lesions of the chest wall. Surg Gynecol Obstet 167:129, 1988

Seyfer AE, Shriver CD, Miller TR, Graeber GM: Sternal blood flow after median sternotomy and mobilization of the internal mammary arteries. Surgery 104:899, 1988

Stelzer D, Gay WA: Tumors of the chest wall. Surg Clin North Am 60:779, 1980

Stuhmiller JH, Phillips YY, Richmond DR: The physics and mechanisms of primary blast injury. p. 244. In Bellamy RF, Zajtchuk R (eds): Conventional Warfare: Ballistic, Blast, and Burn Injuries. In Textbook of Military Medicine Part I: Warfare Weaponry and the Casualty. Office of the Surgeon General. U.S. Army, Washington, 1991

Venn GE, Gellister J, DaCosta PE et al: Malignant fibrous histiocytoma in thoracic surgery practice. J Thorac Cardiovasc Surg 91:234, 1986

Chest Wall Stabilization

Geoffrey M. Graeber

The first step in chest wall reconstruction is preservation of function through stabilization. In some cases the resection itself will not sufficiently compromise chest wall function and thereby also respiratory mechanics to warrant stabilization. If stabilization is necessary, a number of materials have been used successfully to preserve chest wall integrity and respiratory mechanics. Some have remained useful and have earned a secure place in chest wall reconstruction, while others have proved marginally or minimally successful and have been abandoned. The indications for chest wall stabilization as a part of an integrated reconstruction are reviewed below; the materials, both biologic and synthetic, that have been used in this capacity are listed; and the most popular methods as used by surgeons today are summarized.

INDICATIONS FOR STABILIZATION

Chest wall reconstruction is generally viewed as a procedure with two aspects, chest wall stabilization and soft tissue reconstruction. In some cases the consistency of the soft tissue reconstruction will afford satisfactory stabilization to preserve respiratory mechanics (Seyfer, et al., 1986a, 1986b), whereas in others, the flaps used in providing soft tissue coverage have little intrinsic consistency (e.g., omentum flaps) and will usually need stabilization (Seyfer, et al., 1986c; Fix and Vasconez, 1989). In every case the situation must be assessed and handled individually for each patient since respiratory mechanics must be preserved. The final decision as to whether chest wall stabilization will be necessary will involve consideration of multiple factors, the most important of which are the general condition and respiratory capabilities of the patient, the size and location of the resection performed, the integrity and quality of the structures overlying the defect, and the intrinsic qualities of the flaps used for soft tissue coverage. The final goal is to provide a reconstruction that will have minimal if any paradoxic chest wall motion during respiration so that the patient can be weaned from ventilatory support as soon as possible after reconstruction (Seyfer, et al., 1986a and 1986b; McCormack, 1989). Satisfactory cosmesis is an important secondary goal, which merits careful consideration (Seyfer, et al., 1986a and 1986b).

The general condition and respiratory capabilities of the patient are major factors in determining whether chest wall stabilization will be required as a part of chest wall reconstruction (Seyfer, et al., 1986d). The operating surgeon must evaluate the patient who will undergo chest wall resection carefully to determine just how much respiratory embarrassment the patient can tolerate and yet still be able to be weaned from a respirator early in the postoperative period. A reasonable guiding principle is that any patient who would be able to tolerate a pulmonary lobectomy based on pulmonary function studies, arterial blood gas determination, and exercise testing would also be able to tolerate a major chest wall resection (Seyfer, et al., 1986e). Special consideration would have to be given to the unusual patient who needs a pulmonary resection in conjunction with a major chest wall resection and reconstruction. Obviously, a younger, more robust patient with excellent nutrition will tolerate a large resection and reconstruction better than a frail, elderly patient who suffers from cachexia.

The location and size of the chest wall resection are major determinants of whether chest wall stabilization will be required as a part of successful reconstruction. Small defects (5 to 7 cm in greatest diameter) seldom need stabilization, since the amount of paradoxic motion will be small and can be tolerated by most patients (McCormack, 1989; Pairolero and Arnold, 1986). Larger defects almost always need some form of chest wall stabilization to preserve respiratory function (Pairolero and Arnold, 1986; Seyfer, et al., 1986e). Location of the resection is important, since major structures of the ipsilateral upper extremity may provide the necessary overlying support. The scapula is an example of such a structure posteriorly, but its relation to the defect may impinge on the margin requiring partial resection of the inferior scapular pole (Pairolero and Arnold, 1986). Anteriorly the pectoralis major muscle, if it and its overlying skin and subcutaneous tissues are left intact, may provide sufficient support that chest wall stabilization is not necessary. Resections that are lateral and inferoanterior generally require stabilization, since major muscles and bones do not overlie the chest wall in these regions.

The size of the flap employed in soft tissue reconstruction and its intrinsic consistency have direct bearing on whether chest wall stabilization will be required. As noted previously, the omentum usually is very flaccid, with little intrinsic rigidity; hence stabilization will almost always be required when the omentum is used. In contrast, a large musculocutaneous flap (such as a latissimus dorsi) has an intrinsic robust quality, which may allow coverage of a defect without stabilization. All flaps, like any other surgically manipulated tissues, will generate edema within 48 hours of the procedure. Because edema tends to make tissues more rigid, the flap will have less paradoxic motion on the second through fourth postoperative days. The flap will become less robust as the edema fluid is mobilized later in the postoperative period, but usually the patient has been weaned from the ventilator by this time.

MATERIALS USED IN CHEST WALL STABILIZATION

A host of materials have been used to stabilize the chest wall and preserve respiratory mechanics since the inception of chest wall resection and reconstruction. An excellent review by McCormack has summarized most of these and should be consulted (McCormack, 1989). The following discussion is based on experiences recorded in the literature by other authors and on personal observations recorded during major reconstructions performed conducted on patients by myself and colleagues at our respective university institutions. This section presents a classification of materials which have been used to stabilize the chest wall. The last section of this chapter highlights the major methods used in chest wall stabilization which are practiced regularly because of ease in handling, durability, relative radiographic permeability, and superior performance.

The first major category is biologic implants. The assets of the autogenous tissues are availability and biocompatibility. Their liabilities include poor resistance to infection, increased operating time, substantially increased patient discomfort, and relative flaccidity when compared with synthetic materials (Seyfer, et al., 1986a; McCormack, 1989). Their presence in a wound can be disastrous if infection supervenes. Fascia lata is devascularized tissue, which acts as a perfect culture medium for bacteria. Bone chips added to fascia lata provide no stabilization since they are resorbed (McCormack 1989). Their presence on fascia lata compounds the problem of infection, since they act as but another source of devascular-

---

Biologic Materials Used for Chest Wall Stabilization

Human tissues
  Autogenous
    Fascia lata
    Bone grafts
      Ribs, whole and longitudinally split
      Tibia
      Fibula
      Iliac crest
    Composite
  Preserved
    Dura mater
    Fascia
    Pericardium

Preserved animal tissues
  Dura mater
  Pericardium
  Ox fascia

---

ized tissue on which microorganisms can thrive. For all the above reasons, fascia lata alone or in conjunction with bone chips has fallen into disfavor.

Bone grafts can be used judiciously in selected instances for chest wall stabilization. Although portions of tibia, fibula, and iliac crest have been used successfully, their harvesting adds another operative site, with its associated discomfort and potential for complications (Seyfer, et al., 1986a; McCormack, 1989). Rib grafts have the asset of being more likely to follow the natural curvature of the chest wall, but they have significant liabilities. If they are harvested in a subperiosteal fashion, the resultant chest wall instability may be consequential and the rib may regenerate from the remaining periosteum poorly or not at all. Ribs that are partially resected by using a longitudinal line of resection will leave a compromised rib in place at the donor site while providing a graft that is particularly frail. The result will be suboptimal stabilization at both the donor and recipient sites.

The use of rib grafts by my colleagues and me has been limited to carefully selected patients who will need protection for vital intrathoracic structures (such as the heart and great vessels) while maintaining an acceptable cosmetic contour to the reconstruction. The patient must have relatively good pulmonary function, since the discomfort from the donor site, when compounded with that of the reconstruction, can produce a serious decrease in respiratory function. Placement of an epidural catheter to maintain regional anesthesia in the immediate postoperative period has decreased patient discomfort in our experience, so that early weaning from the ventilator is the rule. If the rib grafts are placed properly, marrow from the intact ribs at the margins of the resection will grow into and vascularize the marrow of the graft, ensuring its prolonged viability (Seyfer, et al., 1986a) (Fig. 50-7). Rib grafts in any position are dependent on surrounding tissues, particularly on the rib to which they are attached, for postoperative viability (Graeber, et al., 1985). If a rib graft or any bone graft does not receive a new blood supply, the graft is resorbed by the body, leaving only a fibrous remnant (Graeber, et al., 1985; McCormack, 1989).

Preserved tissues, human or animal, were mostly used before synthetic cloth and sheeting became available and proved so successful (Seyfer, et al., 1986a; McCormack, 1989). There have been some recent proponents of these tissues for chest wall stabilization (Kuakowski and Ruka, 1987). Although these membranes may provide substantial initial stability, they may become flaccid with time owing to peripheral stress on anchoring tissues as well as to intrinsic weakening of structural proteins. The patient's body will react to these materials as it would to any foreign body, with an intense fibrous reaction. The above facts, plus the relatively inferior resistance of these materials to infection, has led to a decrease in their use.

The rise in the use of synthetic materials for chest wall stabilization has been fostered by their variety and availability, their perceived inert nature, and their general ease of handling (Seyfer, et al., 1986a; McCormack, 1989). At the outset, any surgeon should realize that absolutely no material is completely inert when placed in a patient. The patient's natural healing process will at least respond to any foreign material with a fibrous reaction to form a pseudocapsule.

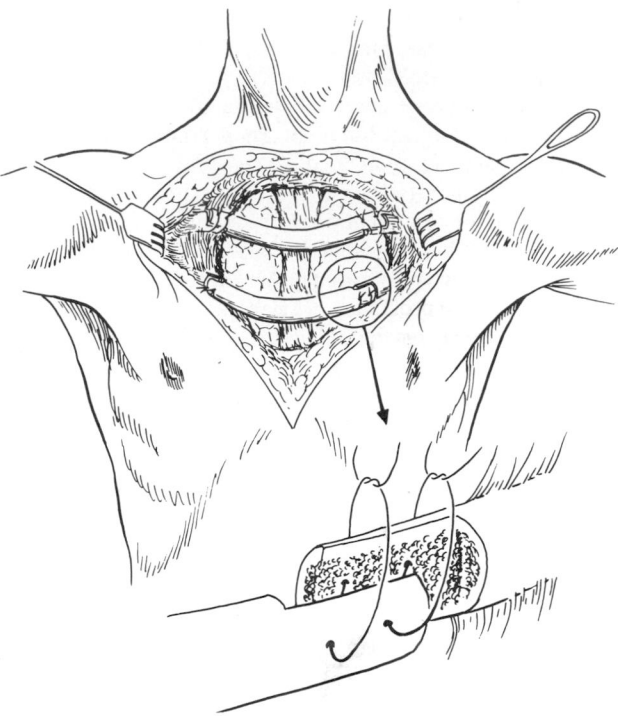

Figure 50-7.   Use of rib grafts in anterior chest wall stabilization. Note that the grafts as well as the ribs are notched so that they can be secured with transfixing permanent sutures. Notching also allows for a greater area of interface between the rib and the graft marrow cavities. The greater interface of the two marrows increases the likelihood that the bone graft will survive, since the marrow of the graft is dependent on ingrowth of cellular material from the end of the rib. (From Seyfer AE, Graeber GM, Wind GG: Planning the reconstruction. p. 59. In Atlas of Chest Wall Reconstruction. Aspen Publishers, Rockville, MD, 1986a, with permission.)

Alloplastic and Synthetic Materials Used in Chest Wall Stabilization

Plates and struts
  Metal
    Tantulum steel
    Stainless steel
  Other materials
    Lucite
    Fiberglass

Synthetic materials
  Sheets and meshes
    Polytetrafluorethylene (Teflon) sheeting and patch
    Nylon
    Polypropylene
    Prolene mesh
    Vicryl mesh
  Solid and firm prosthetics
    Acrylic
    Teflon
    Silastic
    Silicone
  Composite
    Marlex mesh combined } prosthesis
    Methyl methacrylate }

Rigid materials have had some popularity in chest wall reconstruction, but they have some liabilities, which have limited their application (Seyfer, et al., 1986a; McCormack, 1989). Since the chest wall is a dynamic structure, which is constantly active in respiration, rigid materials have a tendency to migrate and fracture. Migration, when it is external, finally causes dermal erosion, which exposes the rigid material. Infection of the entire capsule surrounding the rigid support ensues quickly, requiring removal of the foreign material. If the rigid bar or strut should erode internally, major viscera (such as the lung) and great vessels may be entered and promoting serious if not lethal hemorrhage thereby produced (McCormack, 1989). Metallic struts are for the most part currently limited to stabilization of the sternum after repair of a severe pectus deformity (Garcia, et al., 1989; Seyfer, et al., 1986f). In most cases these struts are not permanent but are removed after the chest wall has become stable (Fig. 50-8).

Most synthetic materials that have been used for human implantation have been produced as sheets or as meshes. Many of these have been employed, with varying degrees of success, as stabilizing membranes in chest wall reconstruction (Boyd, et al., 1981; McCormack, 1989; Pairolero and

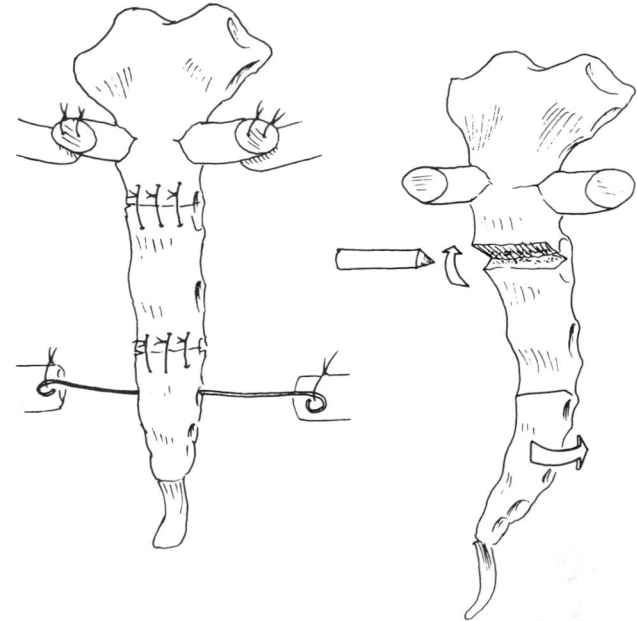

Figure 50-8.   Use of a Steinmann pin in stabilizing a repaired sternum as part of a correction for pectus excavatum. The pin is secured to the ribs lateral to the repair. It will be removed in most cases after the repair has healed. (From Seyfer AE, Graeber GM, Wind GG: Congenital defects: Poland's syndrome, pectus deformities and sternal clefts. p. 229. In Atlas of Chest Wall Reconstruction. Aspen Publishers, Rockville, MD, 1986f, with permission.)

Arnold, 1985 and 1986). Each has its assets and liabilities. For example, Marlex mesh can be stretched along one axis while it is rigid along the perpendicular axis. Prolene mesh is a double-stitch knit, which is rigid along all axes. Gore-Tex, which is very malleable as a soft tissue patch, is impervious to air and water but is most difficult to contour and sew in place tightly. Although each of these materials is relatively inert, they all provoke an intense fibrous reaction when placed in the chest wall. Even polypropylene, which has been touted as quite unreactive, was found to provoke an intense fibrous reaction from the lung and pleura in one experimental model (Graeber, et al., 1985).

A number of synthetic materials can be produced with variable degrees of firmness. Success has been reported with acrylic, silicone, Silastic, and methyl methacrylate prostheses (Eschaposse, et al., 1972; Mendelson and Masson, 1977; Allen and Douglas, 1979; Marcove, et al., 1977). They may be used alone or in composites as prosthetics in chest wall reconstruction (Hochberg, et al., 1994). Although such techniques have been available since well before the early 1980s, recent concerns about silicone, particularly as it has been used in mammary implants, indicate extreme caution in its use (Lavey, et al., 1982; DeComara, et al., 1993). Current Food and Drug Administration guidelines for implanting silicone should be consulted before embarking on such a reconstruction. In current practice, customized prostheses are used for both chest wall stabilization and partial chest wall reconstruction only in selected cases in which standard stabilization and flap reconstruction either has failed or offers exceptionally limited options (Hochberg, et al., 1994). Such individualized prostheses may be created to reconstruct complex defects with rounded contours; however, they are difficult to secure to the chest wall, require sophisticated, computerized techniques to generate the prosthetic, and are subject to all the recognized liabilities of a firm foreign body in the dynamic chest wall. Excellent long-term results have been recorded in carefully selected patients with very special reconstructive needs (Hochberg, et al., 1994).

McCormack and others have had particularly beneficial experience with composite prostheses generated in the operating room from Marlex mesh and methyl methacrylate monomer (McCormack, et al., 1981; McCormack, 1989). A customized prosthesis is made by measuring the size of the defect on the patient, laying a piece of Marlex mesh over a surface of similar contour, applying the methyl methacrylate to the Marlex to match the size and shape of the defect as determined by the previously measured pattern, and then applying another layer of Marlex over the still soft methyl methacrylate so that the Marlex bonds to it. The resulting prosthesis has a firm, contoured center of polymethylmethacrylate, which lies between two layers of Marlex. The 5-cm rim of Marlex that extends beyond the hard central polymethylmethacrylate prosthesis acts as a sewing ring for securing it to the chest wall defect. The prosthesis has several assets: it has an absolutely rigid center, conforms well to the anticipated curve of the chest wall, and has a pliable sewing ring. One of its true liabilities arises with its creation: the reaction leading to the hardening of the methyl methacrylate is extremely exothermic, often reaching temperatures near 140°F. Appropriate curvature may be obtained by shaping the prosthesis over a chest tube collection bottle or over the patient's thigh, which can be protected with towels to prevent the exothermic reaction from causing thermal tissue injury. Once in place, the prosthesis is subject to all the problems, as noted previously, attendant on rigid prostheses in a dynamic environment.

Investigators working at the National Cancer Institute have identified another problem associated with methyl methacrylate prosthesis (Pass, 1989). In their method for creating the prosthesis, the lung is dropped away from the defect in the chest wall and the prosthesis is actually created on the patient from Marlex, steel mesh, and methyl methacrylate. After the prosthesis has been created, the lung is reexpanded against the prosthesis. A metabolic acidosis, which is secondary to anion replacement with methyl methacrylate, ensues. This has to be corrected during the reconstruction.

METHODS OF IMPLANTATION

Chest wall stabilization is necessary to provide a firm surface on which to set the soft tissue flaps that will complete the reconstruction. The key point to remember is that stabilization is directed at reducing paradoxic motion of the chest wall and maintaining its contour. The technical aspects of the three most popular methods of stabilization are discussed below. It should be remembered that creativity is necessary in all aspects of chest wall reconstruction, including achievement of a desired cosmetic result.

There are several important points to consider in implanting the polymethylmethacrylate "sandwich." The prosthesis has a central rigid area, which follows the chest contour and is extremely rigid. The sewing ring, which consists of the 5-cm rim of Marlex around the central hard prosthesis, is used to join the prosthesis to the chest wall. If sutures have to be placed through the central, hard portion of the prosthesis, a tunnel has to be created with a drill to allow passage of the needle since the methyl methacrylate sets to the same consistency as a football helmet.

Stabilization with either mesh or screening requires creative tailoring to suture the material to the chest wall (Fig. 50-9). The margin of resection should be palpated to determine the most stable point, which is usually a rib or a remaining portion of the sternum. A horizontal mattress suture of braided, permanent synthetic material is placed through the edge of the patch or the screening and through the periosteum of the bone and is tied in place. A second suture is placed through the synthetic material so that it can be secured firmly to the most stable point 180 degrees opposite to the original suture. Another set of sutures is placed through the prosthetic material at the edge of the resection so that the material is drawn tight and secured to the periosteum along an axis perpendicular to the line between the first two sutures. Sutures are then placed in a radial fashion so that the material is drawn tightly across the wound. Once the entirety of the prosthesis has been adjusted in place, any excess margins are trimmed.

An alternative method is to start with the firmest point on the margin of resection and secure the prosthesis to the periosteum. Sutures are then placed sequentially in a radial fashion around the defect, drawing the synthetic material

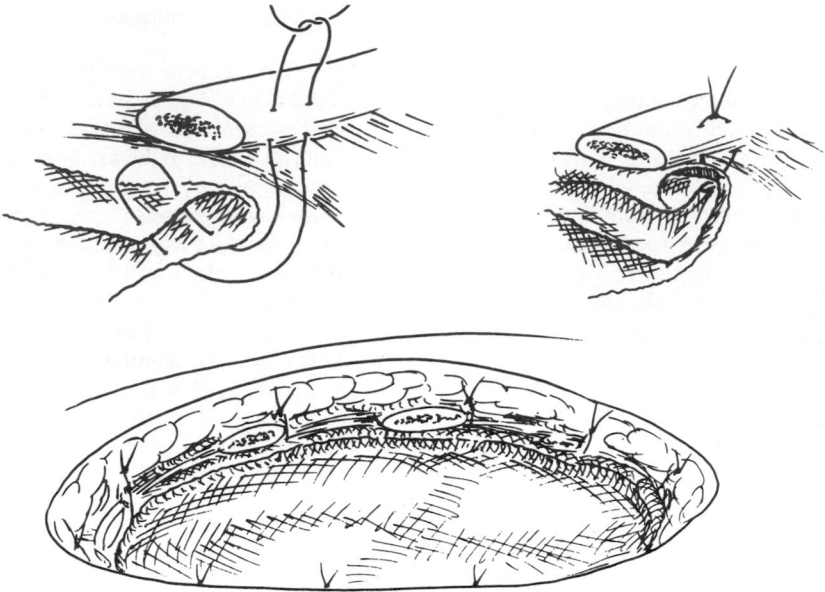

Figure 50-9. A successful method for securing synthetic mesh or sheeting to a chest wall defect to achieve stabilization. Note that the sutures are placed on the cephalad aspect of the ribs to avoid the neurovascular bundles that course along the caudad surfaces of the ribs. Sutures are placed starting at one point in the defect and are placed sequentially and radically to achieve a relatively taut surface on which to place the flap(s) used to reconstruct the soft tissue defect. (From Seyfer AE, Graeber GM, Wind GG: Planning the reconstruction. p. 59. In Atlas of Chest Wall Reconstruction. Aspen Publishers, Rockville, MD, 1986a, with permission.)

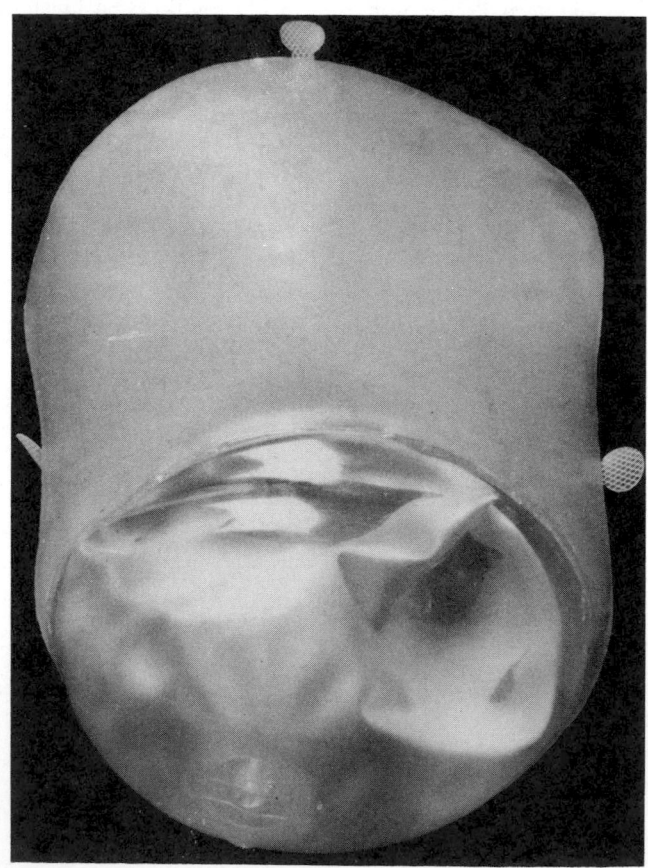

Figure 50-10. Composite prosthesis with two components: a hard Silastic posterior segment, which replaces the upper anterior thoracic wall, and a soft gel prosthesis, which gives contour and shape to the absent breast. Note that there are three integral plastic tabs on the margins of the prosthesis. These plastic tabs are used to secure the prosthesis to bones on the thoracic wall and thereby prevent migration. (From Hochberg J, Ardenghy M, Graeber GM, Murray GF: Complex resconstruction of the chest wall and breast utilizing a customized silicone implant. Ann Plast Surg 32:524, 1994, with permission.)

progressively tighter. Tailoring cuts are made in the prosthetic material after each suture so that the material will tuck underneath the edges of the margin neatly. If the sutures are placed appropriately by either method, a firm, taut surface for accepting the soft tissue flaps is created.

In some patients with very difficult reconstructive problems, a customized prosthesis can be made to achieve chest wall stabilization and replace the soft tissue defect (Fig. 50-10). In such cases there has to be soft tissue coverage of the prosthesis after it is in place. Usually, the soft tissue placed over the prosthesis is the native tissue remaining at the site, but in some cases a musculocutaneous flap is necessary for sufficient coverage. The customized prosthesis is generated via computer modeling: the opposite side of the patient's chest wall is surveyed, measurements are taken, a mirror image of the chest wall is created through a computer model, the dimensions of the model are printed, and a plaster model is created (Hochberg, et al., 1994).

In the case illustrated in Figure 50-10, the patient also needed a breast prosthesis. A silica gel prosthesis was added to the heavy Silastic contoured model of the chest wall. The composite model is custom manufactured, and the prosthesis is sterilized by the manufacturer and delivered to the surgeon for implantation in the patient. Implantation of this model is dependent on integral plastic tabs, which may be seen in Figure 50-10. These tabs are sutured to stable skeletal structures so that the prosthesis does not migrate. In the case cited, the three tabs were secured respectively to the sternum medially, the clavicle superiorly, and the ribs laterally. Heavy, braided synthetic sutures were placed through the plastic tabs and through the periosteum of the bony structures noted. In some situations, as with the clavicle or the sternum, the sutures may actually be placed around the entire structure to provide added security.

One final point cannot be overemphasized. Each reconstruction must be individualized and creative in order to achieve an excellent contour and reduce paradoxic motion in the chest wall to a minimum.

REFERENCES

Allen RG, Douglas M: Cosmetic improvement of thoracic wall defects using a rapid setting silastic mold: a special technique. J Pediatr Surg 14:745, 1979

Boyd AD, Shaw WW, McCarthy JG et al: Immediate reconstruction of full-thickness chest wall defects. Ann Thorac Surg 32:337, 1981

deCamara D, Sheridan JM, Kammer BA: Rupture and aging of silicone gel breast implants. Plast Reconstr Surg 91:828, 1993

Eschaposse M, Gaillard J, Fournial G et al: Use of acrylic prosthesis for the repair of large defects of the chest wall. Acta Chir Belg 76:281, 1977

Fix RJ, Vasconez LO: Use of the omentum in chest-wall reconstruction. Surg Clin North Am 69:1029, 1989

Garcia VF, Seyfer AE, Graeber GM: Reconstruction of congenital chest-wall deformities. Surg Clin North Am 69:1103, 1989

Graeber GM, Cohen DJ, Patrick DR et al: Rib fracture healing in experimental flail chest. J Trauma 25:903, 1985

Hochberg J, Ardenghy M, Graeber GM, Murray GF: Complex reconstruction of the chest wall and breast utilizing a customized silicone implant. Ann Plast Surg 32:524, 1994

Kuakowski A, Ruka W: Dura mater (Lyodural) in reconstruction of the abdominal and chest wall defects after radical excision of soft tissue neoplasms: case reports. Eur J Surg Oncol 23:63, 1987

Lavey E, Apelberg DB, Lash H et al: Customized silicone implants of the breast and chest. Plast Reconstr Surg 69:646, 1982

Marcove RC, Egwele R, Searfoss R et al: Chest wall reconstruction with methyl methacrylate implantation. Compr Ther 3(12):5, 1977

McCormack PM: Use of prosthetic materials in chest-wall reconstruction: assets and liabilities. Surg Clin North Am 69:965, 1989

McCormack PM, Bains MS, Beattie EJ et al: New trends in skeletal reconstruction after resection of chest wall tumors. Ann Thorac Surg 31:45, 1981

Mendelson B, Masson JK: Silicone implants for contour deformities of the trunk. Plast Reconstr Surg, 59:538, 1977

Pairolero PC, Arnold PG: Thoracic wall defects: surgical management of 205 consecutive patients. Mayo Clin Proc 61:557, 1986

Pairolero PC, Arnold PG: Chest wall tumors: experience with 100 consecutive patients. J Thorac Cardiovasc Surg 90:367, 1985

Pass HI: Primary and metastatic chest wall tumors. In Roth JA, Ruchdeschel JC, Weisenferges TH (ed): Thoracic Oncology. WB Saunders, Philadelphia, 1989

Seyfer AE, Graeber GM, Wind GG: Planning the reconstruction. p. 59. In Atlas of Chest Wall Reconstruction, Aspen Publishers, Rockville, MD, 1986a

Seyfer AE, Graeber GM, Wind GG: Postoperative care. p. 87. In Atlas of Chest Wall Reconstruction, Aspen Publishers, Rockville, MD, 1986b

Seyfer AE, Graeber GM, Wind GG: The omentum. p. 141. In Atlas of Chest Wall Reconstruction, Aspen Publishers, Rockville, MD, 1986c

Seyfer AE, Graeber GM, Wind GG: Embryology, anatomy and physiology of the chest wall. p. 13. In Atlas of Chest Wall Reconstruction, Aspen Publishers, Rockville, MD, 1986d

Seyfer AE, Graeber GM, Wind GG: Preoperative care and considerations. p. 51. In Atlas of Chest Wall Reconstruction. Aspen Publishers, Rockville, MD, 1986e

Seyfer AE, Graeber GM, Wind GG: Congenital defects: Poland's syndrome, pectus deformities and sternal clefts. p. 229. In Atlas of Chest Wall Reconstruction. Aspen Publishers, Rockville, MD, 1986f

Soft Tissue Reconstruction

Geoffrey M. Graeber

Soft tissue reconstruction of the chest wall has been revived and expanded since the early 1970s. The concept of pedicled flap reconstruction has been the mainstay of this movement since its inception. Tissue reconstruction has continued to grow, with delineation of new applications of pedicled flaps to repair increasingly complex defects. Free flap transfer has had some limited applications in carefully selected cases. The following discussion presents the major considerations in planning soft tissue coverage of a chest wall defect, the salient characteristics of the pedicled flaps, and the complications associated with specific reconstructions. Several major works have focused on this field, with comprehensive treatments of all aspects of chest wall reconstruction (McCraw and Arnold, 1986; Seyfer, et al., 1986a; Seyfer and Graeber, 1989). Surgeons contemplating chest wall reconstruction should consult these texts for a thorough understanding of the complexities associated with successful thoracic reconstruction.

PLANNING THE RECONSTRUCTION

Pedicled reconstruction of chest wall defects may be conducted on any anatomic region of the chest wall. Certain areas will have more options for reconstruction than others. Selection of appropriate flaps is mandatory since tension on a flap's margin or its pedicle will spell disaster. Designation of secondary flaps in each instance is essential, since one flap may not cover the entire defect without introduction of supplemental tissue and rotation of replacement flaps may become necessary if the primary flap proves unsuitable (Azarow, et al., 1989; Seyfer, et al., 1986b).

Coverage of the anterior and anterolateral chest wall offers the most options because several pedicled flaps may be rotated successfully (Azarow, et al., 1989; Seyfer, et al., 1986b). Major pedicled flaps that may be used in this area include the pectoralis major, rectus abdominis, and latissimus dorsi muscular and musculocutaneous flaps as well as the omentum (Fig. 50-11). The serratus anterior muscular flap may be used in some limited applications.

The lateral chest wall has more limited options for pedicled reconstruction (Azarow, et al., 1989; Seyfer, et al., 1986b).

I wish to thank Ms. Karen DeShong for her assistance in the preparation of this manuscript.

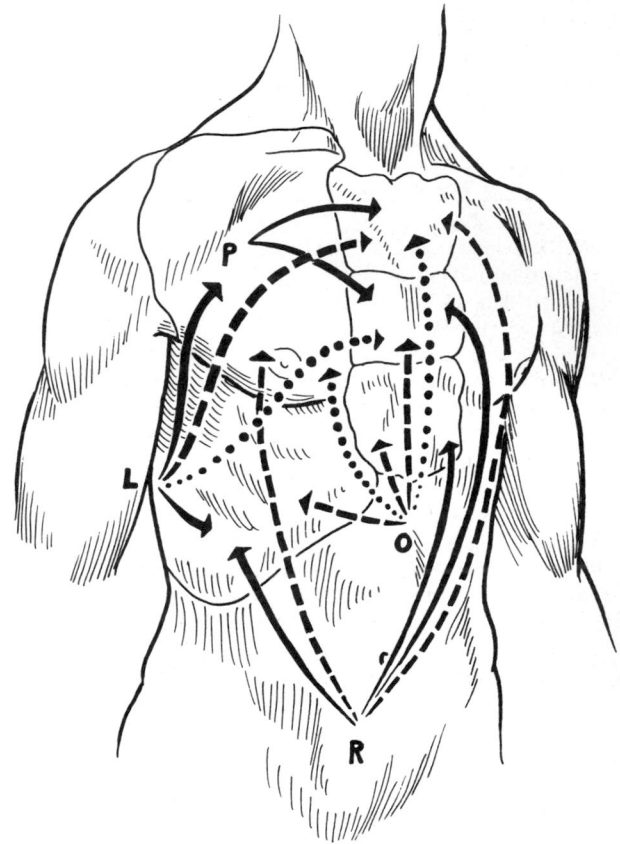

Figure 50-11. Anterior and anterolateral areas of the chest wall and the pedicled flaps that may be used to reconstruct these areas. The sternum has been divided into upper, middle, and lower sections. The area over the pectoralis major muscle has been designated by a solid line extending from the shoulder around the clavicle to the sternum and to just below the breast; this is the upper lateral region. The lower lateral region is directly below this area and covers the rest of the thoracic cage from the anterior axillary line to the sternum. The areas of transfer for each muscle are shown by arrows: the first choice for coverage of a given area is designated by a solid arrow, the second choices by dashed arrows, and the third choices by dotted arrows. Each of the flaps is designated by a letter: L, latissimus dorsi; O, omentum; P, pectoralis major; R, rectus abdominis. (From Seyfer AE, Graeber GM, Wind GG: Planning the reconstruction. p. 59. In Atlas of Chest Wall Reconstruction. Aspen Publishers, Rockville, MD, 1986b, with permission.)

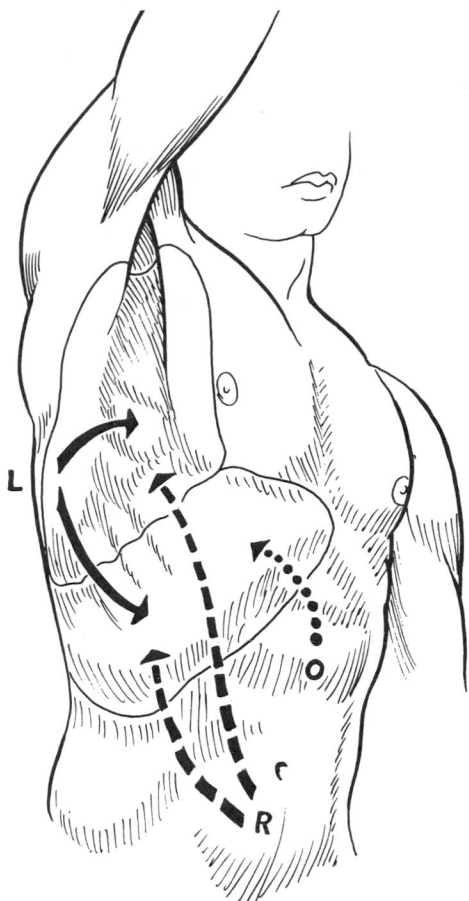

Figure 50-12. The lateral areas of the chest wall may be reconstructed with either latissimus dorsi or rectus abdominis muscular or musculocutaneous flaps or the omentum. The two distinct areas, which are outlined by solid lines, represent an upper and a lower region. Note that the latissimus dorsi (designated by L) is the primary pedicled flap for reconstruction in both areas, the rectus abdominis (designated by R) is the secondary flap, and the omentum (designated by O) is the tertiary flap for reconstructing these areas. The heavy black line designates the latissimus as the primary flap for reconstruction in both areas, the dashed arrows indicate the rectus as the secondary flap, and the dotted line, associated with the omentum, indicates that it is the third choice. (From Seyfer AE, Graeber GM, Wind GG: Planning the reconstruction. p. 59. In Atlas of Chest Wall Reconstruction. Aspen Publishers, Rockville, MD, 1986b, with permission.)

The latissimus dorsi muscular and musculocutaneous flap is the first choice (Fig. 50-12). The rectus abdominis muscular or musculocutaneous flap is the second choice for these areas, and the omentum is the third choice. The serratus anterior flap and abdominal wall flaps have limited roles in this region but may be used if the main options have been exhausted or if their rotation is not possible (McCraw and Arnold, 1986).

Reconstruction of the chest wall posteriorly is more difficult because of limited options (Fig. 50-13). The latissimus dorsi muscular and musculocutaneous flap is clearly the best choice for cephalad rotation. On the upper chest, the trapezius muscle may be rotated to cover spinal and paraspinal defects. In extreme cases, free flap transfer may be used as

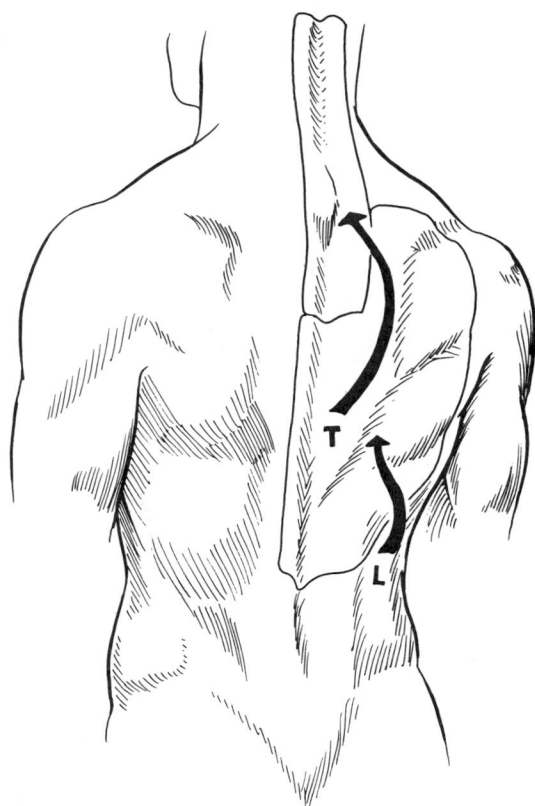

Figure 50-13. The limited options for reconstruction of the posterior aspect of the chest wall are delineated. Note that there are two areas for reconstruction: the upper spinous and paraspinous area and the lower, larger area encompassing most of the back. The primary flap for reconstruction of the upper area is the trapezius muscle (designated by T). The latissimus dorsi (designated by L) is the muscle and musculocutaneous flap that can be used most effectively to cover most of the back. (From Seyfer AE, Graeber GM, Wind GG: Planning the reconstruction. p. 59. In Atlas of Chest Wall Reconstruction. Aspen Publishers, Rockville, MD, 1986b, with permission.)

long as suitable arterial and venous supply is maintained, the pedicle is not placed under tension, and the margins of the flap are not overextended.

Occasionally, a defect may be so large that more than one flap may be necessary to provide for adequate soft tissue coverage (Azarow, et al., 1989; Seyfer, et al., 1986b). In such cases secondary and tertiary flaps may be rotated to achieve satisfactory soft tissue coverage without tension on the pedicle(s) or on the margins of the flaps. In some extreme circumstances, the pedicles of the flaps may be dissected maximally and the size of the flap may extend to its extreme to achieve coverage. Such reconstructions using combined latissimus dorsi and rectus abdominis flaps to close large contralateral defects have been reported (Matsuo, et al., 1991).

FLAPS FOR RECONSTRUCTION

Each of the flaps used in reconstruction of the chest wall has assets and liabilities as well as a defined arc of rotation. Transposition of any of the flaps requires precise understanding of the blood supply. Successful rotation of any flap depends on preservation of the blood supply and prevention of any tension on the pedicle and on the margins of the flap. Previous surgical procedures and pathologic conditions may preclude successful rotation of specific flaps.

Pectoralis Major Muscle

One of the most frequently used muscular and musculocutaneous flaps is the pectoralis major. The utility and durability of this flap has been shown in several series (Arnold and Pairolero 1984; Graeber, et al., 1982; Pairolero and Arnold, 1986). Because of its primary and secondary blood supply, it can be transferred as a pedicled flap based on the thoracoacromial neurovascular bundle or on the perforators arising from the ipsilateral internal mammary artery (Tobin, 1989; Seyfer, et al., 1986b) (Fig. 50-14). It is particularly well suited for use in repairing defects of the upper anterior chest wall and in the upper part of the ipsilateral pleural space (Arnold and Pairolero 1978, 1979) (Fig. 50-15).

Major assets of the pectoralis major muscle and musculocutaneous flap and its ability to be based on two different blood supplies and thus allow successful transfer and its intrinsic ability to be divided into segments so that structure and function may be preserved while maintaining the natural contour of the thoracic wall. It may be moved into the upper portion of the pleural space, into a dehisced median sternotomy incision, or into the head and neck for reconstruction depending on the pathology present (Tobin, 1989; Seyfer, et al., 1986c).

It has relatively few problems, which can be addressed successfully if they are appreciated prior to reconstruction (Tobin, 1989; Seyfer, et al., 1986c). One is elimination of a pedicle due to trauma or removal of the primary blood supply for a pedicle. These complications are quite rare for the primary pedicle, the thoracoacromial neurovascular bundle. They are not uncommon, unfortunately, for the secondary pedicle, the internal thoracic (mammary) artery. If the ipsilateral internal thoracic artery has been harvested for revascularization of the myocardium, rotation of the pectoralis based

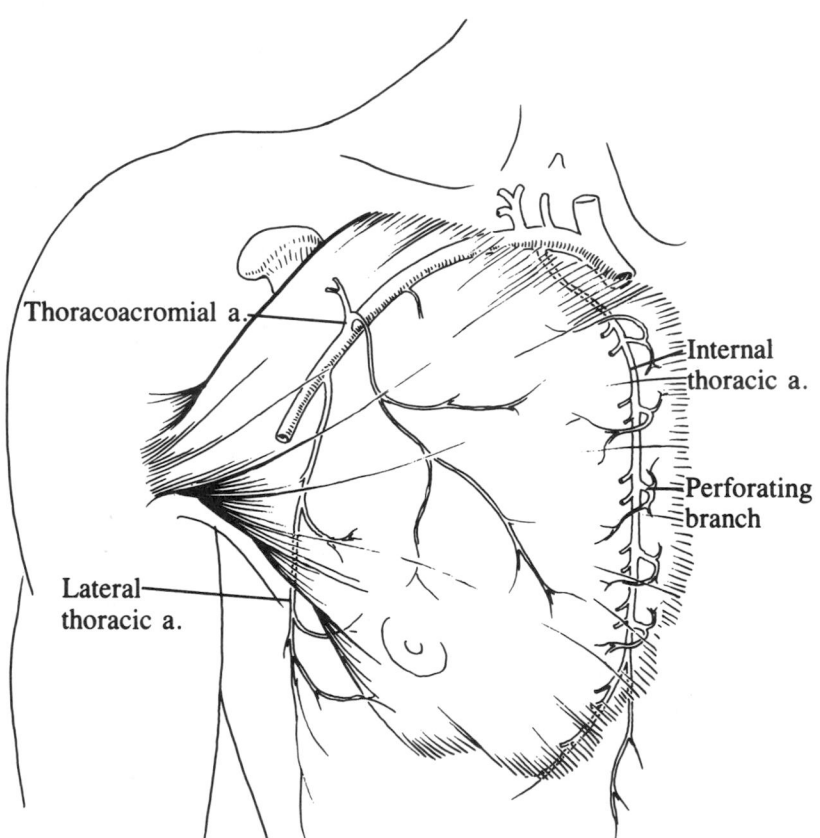

Figure 50-14. The primary and secondary blood supply for the right pectoralis major muscle. Note that the thoracoacromial artery and vein constitute the primary supply, with the major vessel directed from cephalad to caudad. The next most abundant vascular supply to the muscle consists of the internal thoracic artery and vein, which course along the lateral aspect of the sternum to give rise to perforators, which penetrate the intercostal spaces and give blood to the pectoralis major muscle. The tertiary supply consists of some random branches of the lateral thoracic artery and of the intercostal arteries as they give rise to small vessels that perforate the muscle. Pedicled flaps have been described that are based on the thoracoacromial neurovascular bundle and on the internal thoracic artery and its penetrating branches that supply the medial aspect of the pectoralis major muscle. (From Seyfer AE, Graeber GM, Wind GG: The pectoralis major muscle and musculocutaneous flaps. p. 121. In Atlas of Chest Wall Reconstruction. Aspen Publishers, Rockville, MD, 1986c, with permission.)

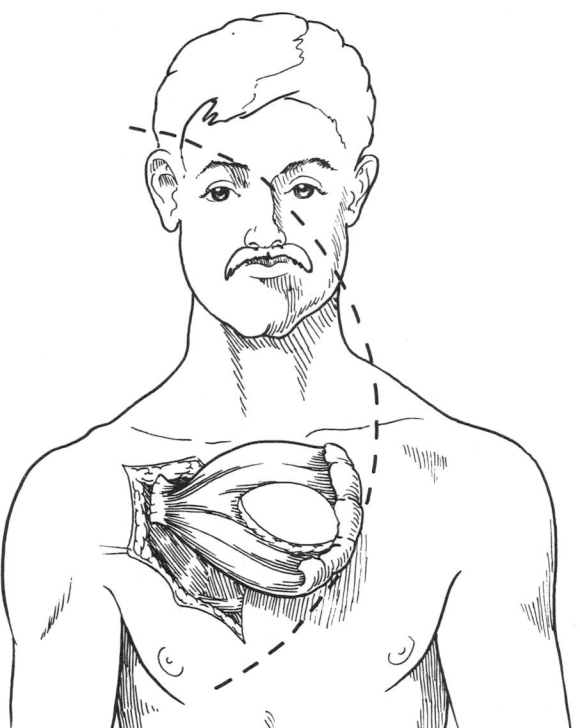

Figure 50-15. The arc of rotation of the pectoralis major muscular and musculocutaneous flap when based on the thoracoacromial neurovascular bundle. Note that the origin and the insertion of the muscle have been cut and have retracted toward the center. The muscle may be rotated over the entire anterolateral chest wall and into the head and neck region. (From Seyfer AE, Graeber GM, Wind GG: The pectoralis major muscle and musculocutaneous flaps. p. 121. In Atlas of Chest Wall Reconstruction. Aspen Publishers, Rockville, MD, 1986c, with permission.)

on the secondary pedicle (ipsilateral internal thoracic artery) is contraindicated, since the muscle pedicle would be based on the tertiary blood supply, the intercostal vessels. Under these conditions, the viability of the flap would be extremely questionable. The blood supply to the flap can also be compromised by a sternal wire that perforates the internal thoracic vessels. Hence, closure of a dehisced median sternotomy incision with pectoralis major muscular flaps based on the ipsilateral internal thoracic artery and vein must be undertaken only after thorough evaluation of the integrity of these vessels.

One of the most common indications for use of the pectoralis major muscular flap is the reconstruction of the dehisced median sternotomy (Miller and Nahai 1989; Pairolero and Arnold 1984, 1986b). One method describes advancement of the pectoralis major muscular flaps into the wound based on their primary pedicles, the thoracoacromial neurovascular bundles. In such cases both muscles in their entirety are dissected free of their origins and insertions and are advanced into the wound together to reconstruct the wound closure (Seyfer, et al., 1986c) (Fig. 50-16). An alternative is to base the flaps on the perforators arising from the respective internal thoracic arteries, divide the thoracromial vessels, and turn the flaps over into the dehisced median sternotomy wound (Morain, et al., 1981; Nahai , et al., 1982) (Fig. 50-17). Variations of these two approaches based on the segmental anatomy of the pectoralis major muscle have been described, in which the first method is used on one side and a variation of the second is used on the contralateral side (Tobin, 1989; Miller and Nahai, 1989).

In addition to reconstruction of the anterior chest wall after tumor resection and reconstruction of the dehisced median sternotomy, the pectoralis major muscular and musculocutaneous flap has been useful in reconstruction of the radiation-

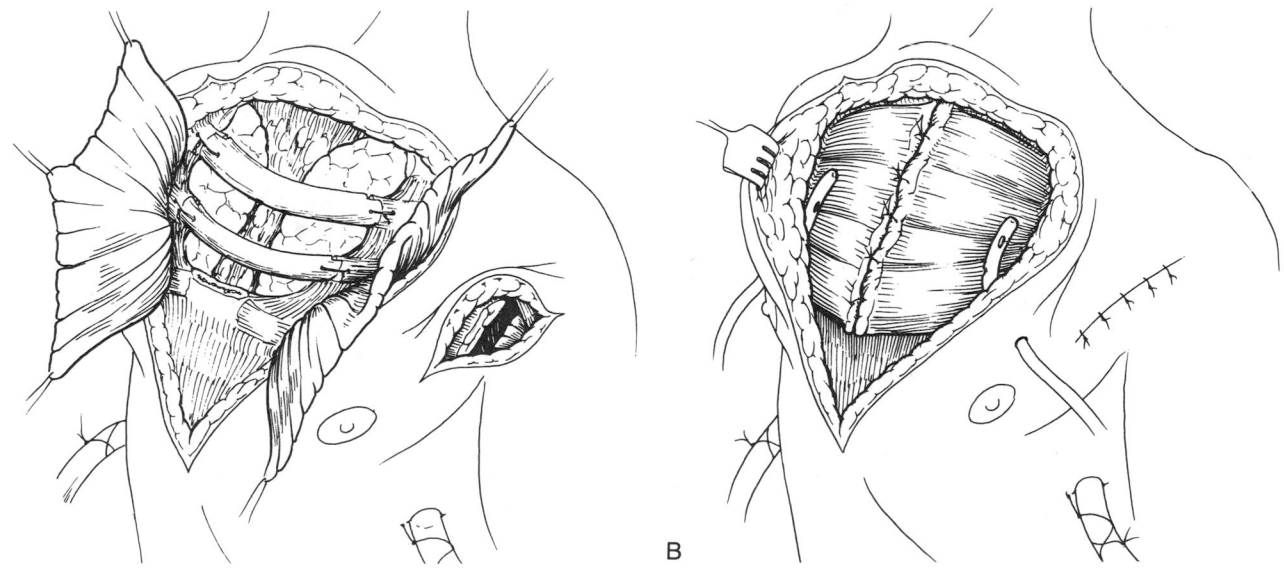

A   B

Figure 50-16. **(A)** Mobilization of the pectoralis major flaps for reconstruction of the upper anterior thorax. Both muscles have been pedicled on their respective thoracoacromial arteries and veins. Note that the origins of both muscles as well as the insertions have been transected. **(B)** Muscles reconstructed over the sternal defect. Note that the pectoralis major muscles join together in the midline to add support to the wound. (From Seyfer AE, Graeber GM, Wind GG: The pectoralis major muscle and musculocutaneous flaps. p. 121. In Atlas of Chest Wall Reconstruction. Aspen Publishers, Rockville, MD, 1986c, with permission.)

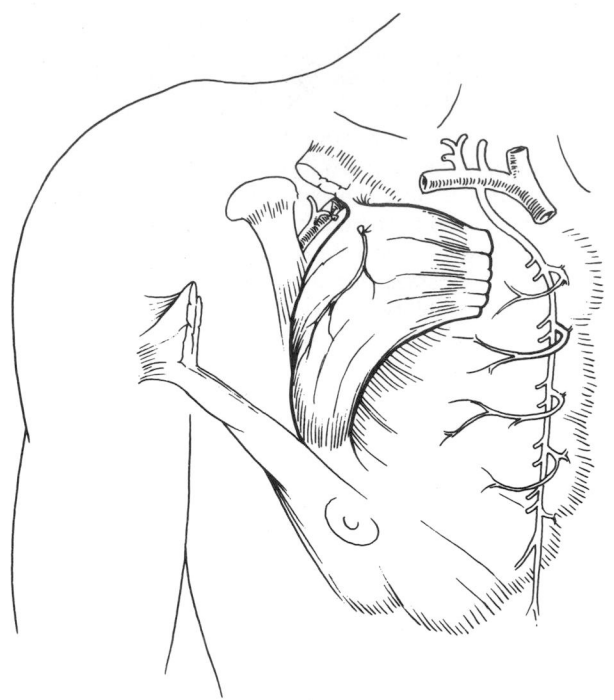

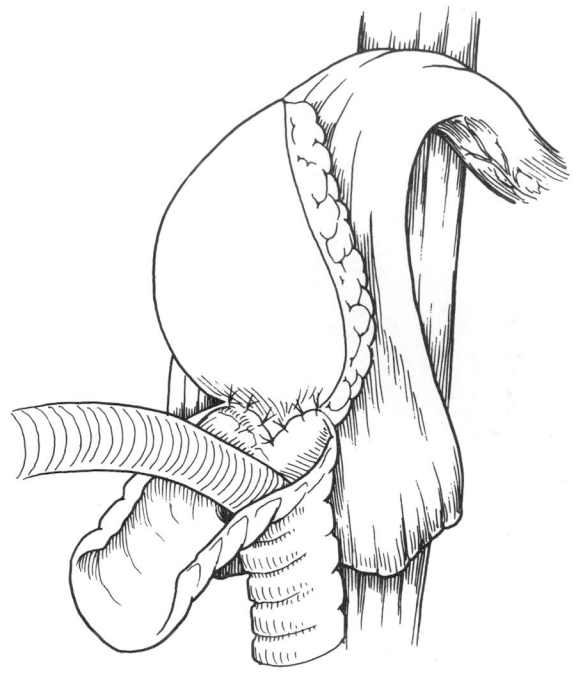

Figure 50-17. The pectoralis major muscular flap may be based on the internal thoracic perforators arising along the origin of the muscle just lateral to the sternum. In this dissection the inferior part of the muscle is saved to preserve function and cosmesis. (From Seyfer AE, Graeber GM, Wind GG: The pectoralis major muscle and musculocutaneous flaps. p. 121. In Atlas of Chest Wall Reconstruction. Aspen Publishers, Rockville, MD, 1986c, with permission.)

Figure 50-18. The pectoralis major musculocutaneous flap has been placed over the repaired esophagus, which is posterior. The skin island is being joined to the open area of the trachea so that the membranous portion is being replaced. Any exposed portion of the muscle that remains after the reconstruction will be covered with meshed, split-thickness skin grafts. (From Seyfer AE, Graeber GM, Wind GG: Tracheoesophageal and bronchopleural/cutaneous fistulas. p. 217. In Atlas of Chest Wall Reconstruction. Aspen Publishers, Rockville, MD, 1986d, with permission.)

damaged chest wall, in treating bronchopleural fistulae and their associated empyemas, and in repairing tracheoesophageal fistulae. In the experience at the Mayo Clinic, the pectoralis major and latissimus dorsi flaps have been the most commonly used in treating patients with radiation damage of the chest wall (Arnold and Pairolero, 1989). The pectoralis major muscular flap has been successful in treating high bronchopleural fistulae and their associated empyemas (Pairolero and Arnold, 1989). For this application the flap has been based on the theracoacromial neurovascular bundle in most cases (Pairolero and Arnold, 1989). Reconstruction of tracheosophageal fistulae has also been successfully performed by using this flap (Seyfer, et al., 1986d). A skin island appended to the flap may be used to reconstruct the membranous trachea, or alternatively, a meshed, split-thickness skin graft may be used for this purpose and for epithelializing any exposed portions of the muscle (Fig. 50-18).

Rectus Abdominis Muscle

The rectus abdominis muscle has been important in chest wall reconstruction both as a muscular and as a musculocutaneous flap. It is a large muscle, with the capacity to carry substantial islands of tissue to repair defects on the chest wall and in the thorax. It can have both a longitudinal and a transverse cutaneous island. Its blood supply is particularly favorable

in that it usually has a balance between the superior and inferior epigastric arteries. The intercostals, which end in the rectus sheaths along the abdominal wall, are the tertiary blood supply. Flaps may be constructed based on the superior or inferior epigastric artery. In some cases involving particularly large defects of the chest wall, flaps have been rotated based on both rectus muscles and both internal thoracic arteries (Glafkides and Toth, 1991). Accurate, comprehensive descriptions of the methodologies for rotating these muscular and musculocutaneous flaps are available (Seyfer, et al., 1986e; Coleman and Bostwick, 1989). This muscle, and particularly its musculocutaneous flap, has been quite useful in reconstruction of the breast, with several authors presenting extensive experiences with this muscle for breast reconstruction (Bunkis, et al., 1983; Dinner, et al., 1982; Hartrampf, et al., 1982; Jacobsen, et al., 1994).

The rectus abdominis muscle has a large arc of rotation, which allows it and/or its musculocutaneous flap to be rotated onto most of the anterior, anterolateral, and lateral thoracic wall (Seyfer, et al., 1986e). The domain of the flap for chest wall reconstruction is extensive and covers virtually all of the anterior and lateral thorax (Fig. 50-19). Besides its significant use in reconstruction of the breast, it has been particularly effective in repair of the dehisced median sternotomy. It must be used carefully in this capacity since its blood supply is dependent on the integrity of the internal thoracic flap must be rotated with great care, since the blood supply must be preserved.

Obviously, previous abdominal incisions can have a deleterious effect on the blood supply to the muscle and hence to the flap. Incisions that may modify or preclude the use of this flap include the paramedian, midline, and upper transverse incisions (Fig. 50-22). The upper transverse incisions, which cross either rectus abdominis muscle, almost always interrupt the superior epigastric vessels so that the muscle distal to the incision becomes dependent on the inferior epigastric vessels for its viability. Cephalad rotation based on the superior epigastric vessels is therefore not indicated, since the distal portion of the muscle will die under these circumstances. A midline incision will limit the amount of subcutaneous tissue and skin that may be transferred on the distal portion of the flap, since the subcutaneous and cutaneous blood supply will be interrupted lateral to the midline incision. Under these circumstances, any soft tissue that is lateral to the midline incision and is transferred with the flap will most

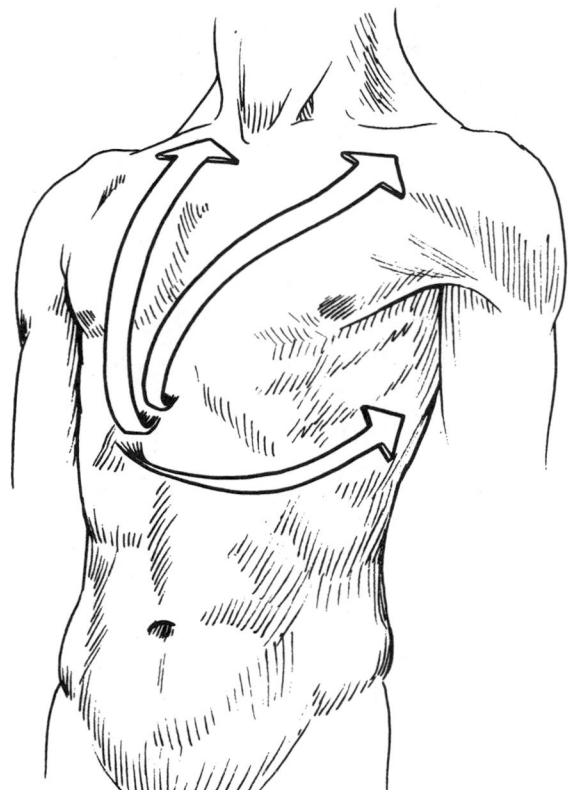

Figure 50-19. The rectus abdominis muscle and musculocutaneous flap are particularly useful in reconstruction of the anterior and lateral chest wall. In all instances of this application, the pedicle is based on the superior epigastric vessels, which are continuations of the internal thoracic (mammary) artery and vein. (From Seyfer AE, Graeber GM, Wind GG: The rectus abdominis muscle and musculocutaneous flaps. p. 159. In Atlas of Chest Wall Reconstruction. Aspen Publishers, Rockville, MD, 1986e, with permission.)

artery (see below). Because of the amount of tissue that can be transferred, the rectus abdominis muscular and musculocutaneous flap has been particularly useful in the reconstruction of anterior and lateral chest wall defects after resection of malignant tumors. These flaps have also been used extensively in reconstruction of the chest wall after radiation injuries, particularly those associated with breast cancer therapy.

The blood supply to the rectus abdominis muscle allows rotation of the entire muscle and an associated subcutaneous and cutaneous island along with the flap onto the greater part of the chest wall (Seyfer, et al., 1986f). The superior epigastric vessels, which are the direct extensions of the internal thoracic artery and vein, are the principal vessels in the pedicle on which this muscular and musculocutaneous flap is based for rotation onto the anterior and lateral thoracic wall (Brown, et al., 1975; Miller, et al., 1988). Because of the rich vascular plexus within the muscle, the entire length of the rectus abdominis may be transferred cephalad with the superior epigastric vessels used as the sole pedicle (Figs. 50-20 and 50-21). In some very rare cases, both rectus abdominis muscles and a large associated subcutaneous and cutaneous island may be rotated onto the anterior thorax based on both pairs of epigastric vessels (Ishii, et al., 1985). This

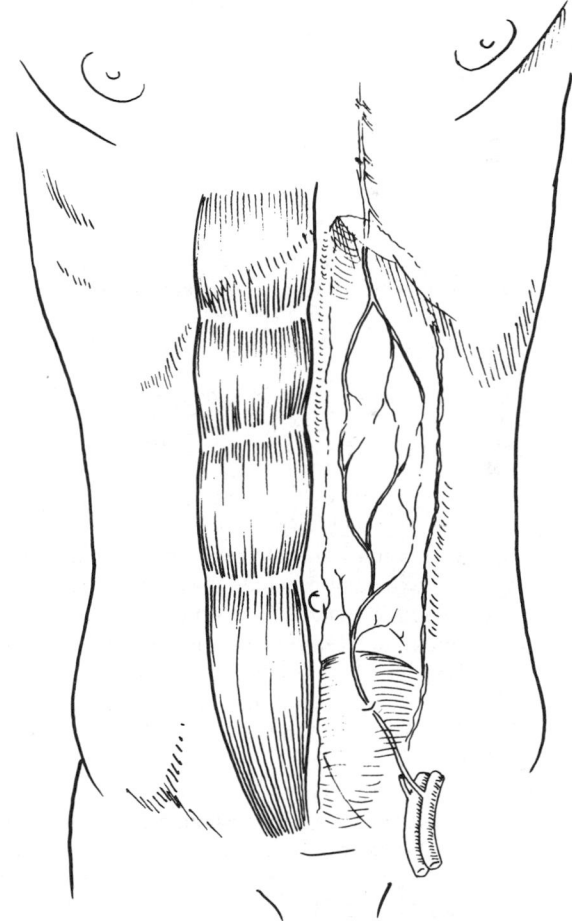

Figure 50-20. The rectus abdominis muscle may be based on either the superior or inferior epigastric vascular pedicles. The rich anastomosis between the vessels, which is in the center portion of the muscle, ensures the viability of the distal portion of the flap when it is based on either pedicle. (From Seyfer AE, Graeber GM, Wind GG: Blood supply to the skin of the chest wall. p. 31. In Atlas of Chest Wall Reconstruction. Aspen Publishers, Rockville, MD, 1986f, with permission.)

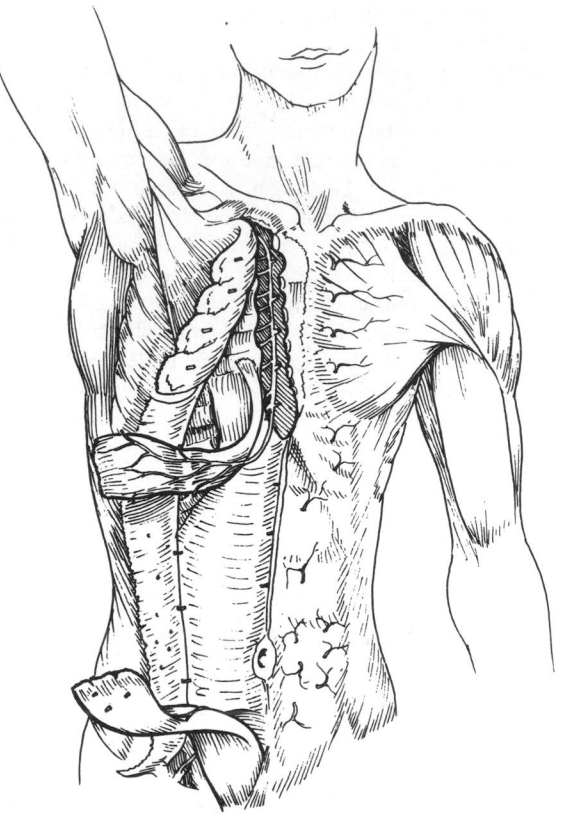

Figure 50-21. This anatomic dissection shows the direct dependence of the superior epigastric vessels on the extension of the internal thoracic artery and vein. The rectus abdominis has been divided in its midportion to show the rich plexus of penetrating vessels, which allow viability of the skin when transferred with the muscular flap. (From Seyfer AE, Graeber GM, Wind GG: Blood supply to the skin of the chest wall. p. 31. In Atlas of Chest Wall Reconstruction. Aspen Publishers, Rockville, MD, 1986f, with permission.)

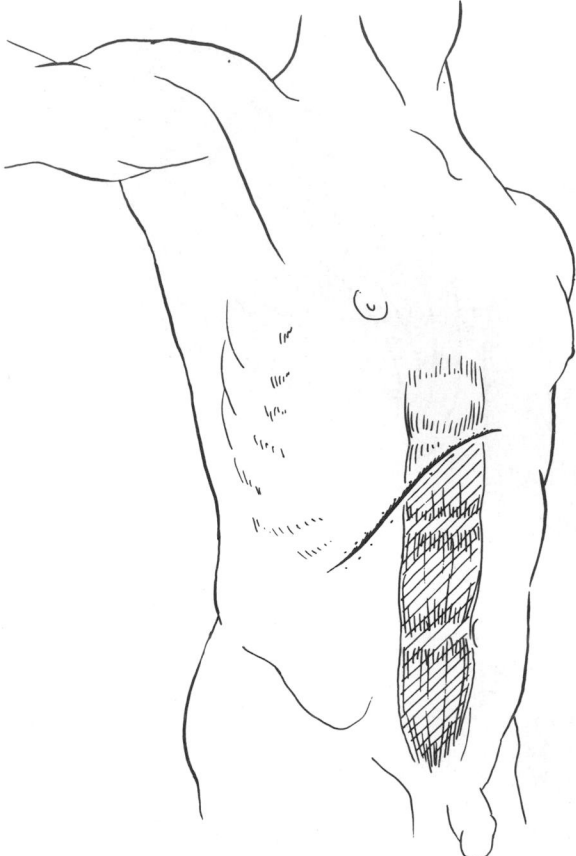

Figure 50-22. Whenever the rectus abdominis muscle is contemplated for reconstruction of the thorax, the surgeon must analyze the previous incisions on the abdomen. In this instance, an upper right subcostal incision precludes the use of the rectus based on the superior epigastric vessels. If a flap based on these vessels were to be rotated, any tissue distal to the line of incision would die, since all this tissue has become dependent on the inferior epigastric vessels after the transverse incision. (From Seyfer AE, Graeber GM, Wind GG: Planning the reconstruction. p. 59. In Atlas of Chest Wall Reconstruction. Aspen Publishers, Rockville, MD, 1986b, with permission.)

likely succumb. Paramedian incisions generally disrupt the entire vascular plexus and preclude successful rotation.

There are several methods for using this muscular and musculocutaneous flap in chest wall reconstruction. The muscle itself may be transposed to fill a dehisced median sternotomy incision. The muscle itself may also be rotated to close a particularly low fistula within the thorax. Most frequently, the rectus is rotated into the chest as a musculocutaneous flap with either a transverse or a longitudinal orientation. The transverse rectus abdominis musculocutaneous (TRAM) flap is very popular for reconstruction of the breast and of radiation injuries of the anterior chest wall (Bunkis, et al., 1983; Dinner, et al., 1982; Hartrampf, et al., 1982; Jacobsen, et al., 1994) (Figs. 50-23 and 50-24). The TRAM flap has been used in many creative ways to reconstruct absent breasts (Figs. 50-25 and 50-26). The longitudinal musculocutaneous flap is particularly beneficial in repairing a severely dehisced median sternotomy incision. The longitudinal island may be rotated with the flap to fill completely a severe defect associated with the severe dehiscence of a median sternotomy wound, such as those more frequently seen in diabetic pa-

tients (Fig. 50-27). If one of the internal mammary arteries has been harvested for myocardial revascularization, the rectus abdominis musculocutaneous flap used for repair of a dehisced median sternotomy should be rotated based on the opposite superior epigastric vessel. If both mammaries have been harvested for myocardial revascularization, the rectus abdominis should not be rotated into the wound, since the muscular or musculocutaneous flap will most likely die in this situation.

The use of the rectus abdominis has been extended by free transfer and by creative vascular anastomoses. Free flap transfers of the rectus abdominis muscle, the omentum, and the latissimus dorsi have been reported in the management of complex intrathoracic problems (Hammond, et al., 1993). These free flaps have been most useful in repairing bronchopleural-cutaneous fistulae. The rectus itself may have its blood supply enhanced and its vertical configuration of tissue transfer enlarged by anastomosing the inferior epigas-

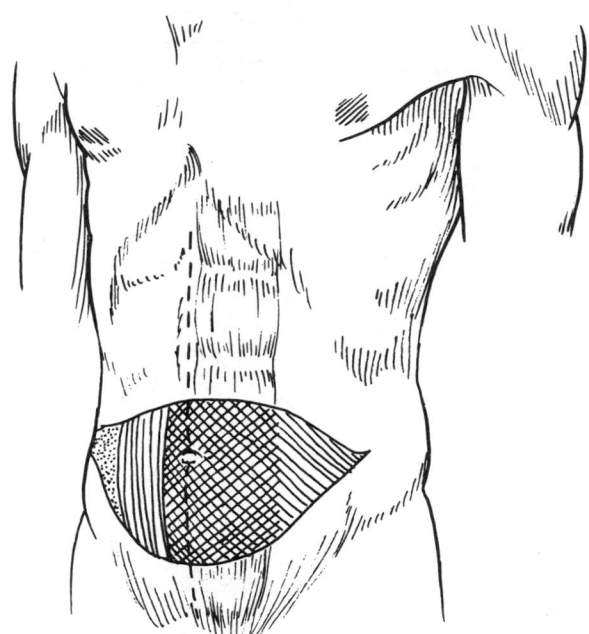

Figure 50-23. The potential viability of skin and subcutaneous tissues when transferred along with the rectus abdominis as a TRAM flap is depicted. The skin and subcutaneous tissues directly overlying the rectus muscle have the highest probability of viability after transfer. These are denoted by the cross-hatched area. Other areas that are directly juxtaposed to this well vascularized tissue may remain viable but can still suffer necrosis under certain conditions. These areas are denoted by the vertical and the oblique lines. The soft tissue that is far distal to the main flap is of questionable viability and should not be used; this area is represented by the stippled area on the right anterior abdominal wall. This drawing depicts a left rectus flap; if a right rectus flap were contemplated, the areas of tissue viability would be the mirror image of that shown here. (From Seyfer AE, Graeber GM, Wind GG: Blood supply to the skin of the chest wall. p. 31. In Atlas of Chest Wall Reconstruction. Aspen Publishers, Rockville, MD, 1986f, with permission.)

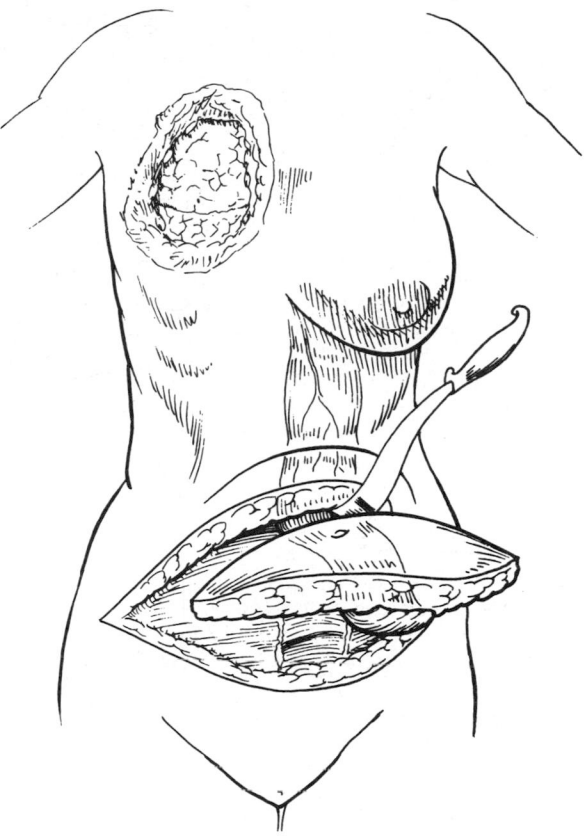

Figure 50-24. TRAM flap being harvested to repair a radiation defect of the right anterior chest wall. Note that the flap is based on the left rectus abdominis muscle and that the distal transverse subcutaneous and cutaneous skin island is being transferred in continuity with the rectus muscle. (From Seyfer AE, Graeber GM, Wind GG: Blood supply to the skin of the chest wall. p. 31. In Atlas of Chest Wall Reconstruction. Aspen Publishers, Rockville, MD, 1986f, with permission.

tric artery and vein to their axillary counterparts (Yamamoto, et al., 1994). Flaps enhanced in this manner have been particularly useful in filling large anterior wall defects.

The Latissimus Dorsi Muscle

Pedicled muscular and musculocutaneous flaps based on the latissimus dorsi muscle have found wide application in chest wall reconstruction, since this muscle has an extensive arc of rotation when the pedicle is based on the thoracodorsal neurovascular bundle (Moelleken, et al., 1989; Seyfer, et al., 1986h) (Fig. 50-28). When a latissimus dorsi muscular or musculocutaneous flap has been based on its primary blood supply, the flap can be used to cover defects on the anterior, lateral, and posterior aspects of the thorax (McCraw, et al., 1978). When the pedicle of a latissimus dorsi flap is based on its secondary blood supply (the ipsilateral ninth through eleventh intercostal arteries and their perforators), the flap's arc of rotation is more limited, and the flap is best suited for posterior intrathoracic applications (Moelleken, et al., 1989).

The primary blood supply to this large, flat muscle located on the posterolateral aspect of the chest wall is the thoracodorsal artery and its associated veins (Rowsell, et al., 1984). In the vast majority of cases, the axillary artery gives rise to the subscapular artery, which divides to create the thoracodorsal artery and the artery or arteries to the serratus anterior muscle (Rowsell, et al., 1984). In 74 percent of cadavers studied by Rowsell et al. (1984), the artery to the serratus anterior was single; in 24 percent it was represented by two or more branches. The thoracodorsal artery, which is a direct extension of the subscapular artery in most cases, descends to the body of the latissimus dorsi, where it most commonly divides into two branches (Fig. 50-29). The more anterior branch descends parallel to the lateral border of the muscle; the medial branch usually traverses more horizontally in the body of the muscle. Both branches form collaterals with the secondary blood supply (the ninth through the eleventh intercostal arteries and their perforators) in the body of the muscle.

The blood supply to the latissimus has allowed some creativity with the primary pedicle. When the subscapular artery

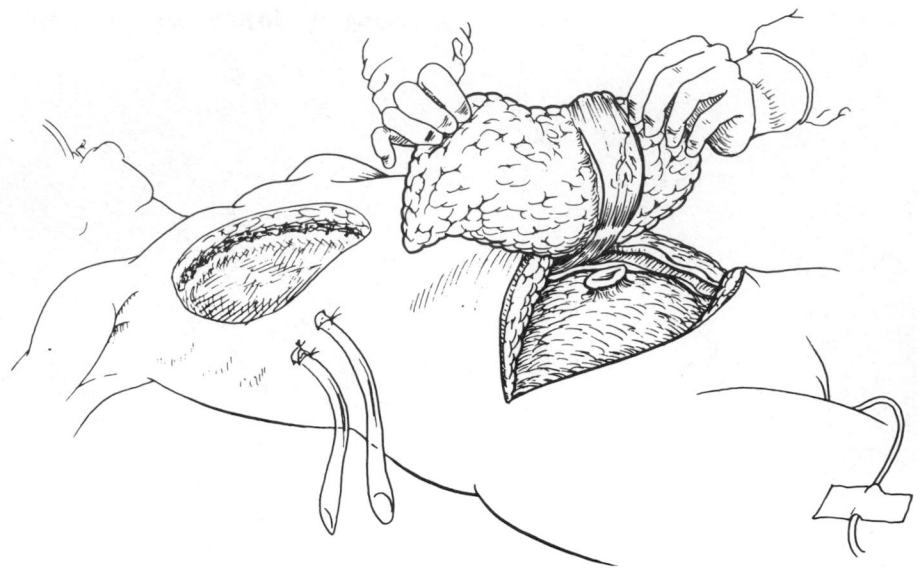

Figure 50-25. A musculocutaneous flap based on the left rectus abdominis muscle has been completed and is ready for transfer into the thoracic defect in the right chest wall. Note that the muscle, the attached subcutaneous tissue, and the skin can all be transposed into the defect by rotation underneath the bridge of intact soft tissue on the upper abdominal wall. (From Seyfer AE, Graeber GM, Wind GG: The rectus abdominis muscle and musculocutaneous flaps. p. 159. In Atlas of Chest Wall Reconstruction. Aspen Publishers, Rockville, MD, 1986e, with permission.)

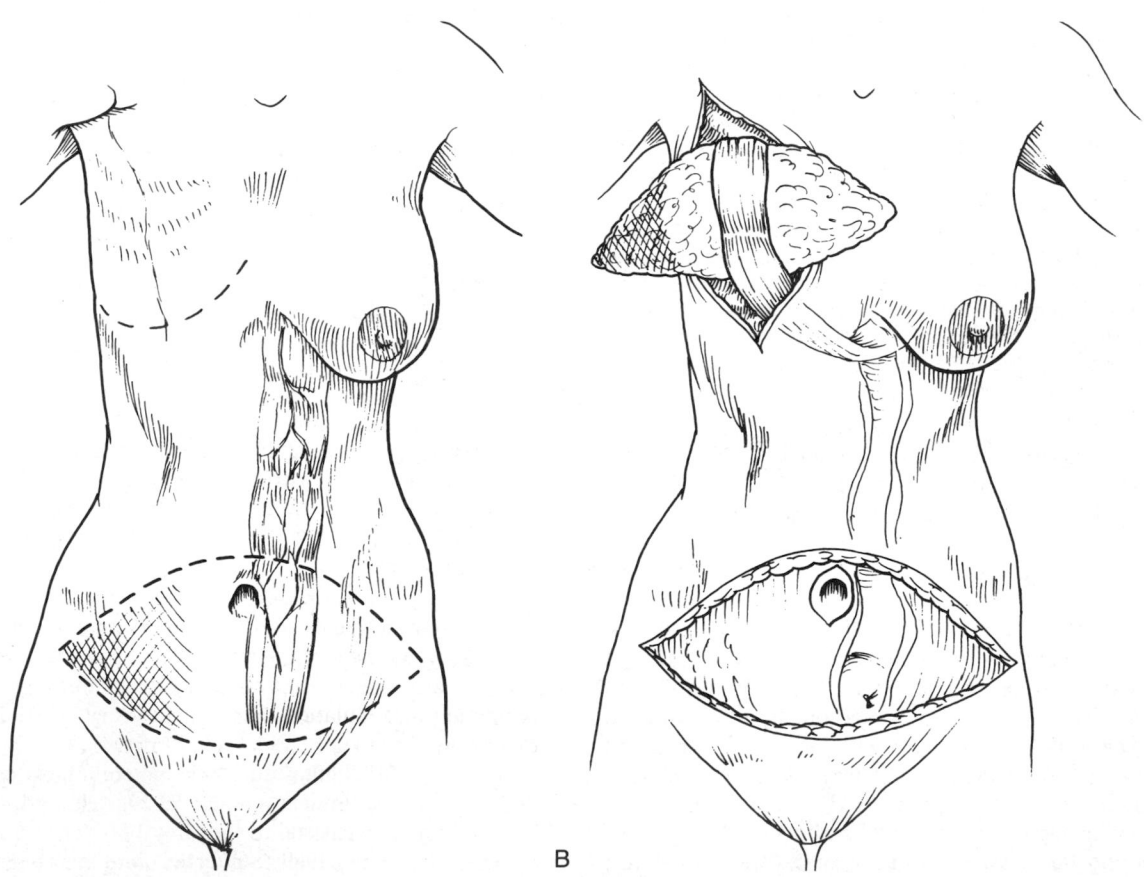

A   B

Figure 50-26. **(A)** Planned reconstruction of the right breast using a left rectus abdominis TRAM flap. There is no associated radiation ulcer of the chest wall. **(B)** The completed left rectus abdominis TRAM flap rotated up into the thoracic defect. The lower abdominal incision can then be closed with preservation of the umbilicus. The flap may be tailored to provide for adequate reconstruction of the breast. (From Seyfer AE, Graeber GM, Wind GG: Reconstruction of the breast following mastectomy. p. 213. In Atlas of Chest Wall Reconstruction. Aspen Publishers, Rockville, MD, 1986g, with permission.)

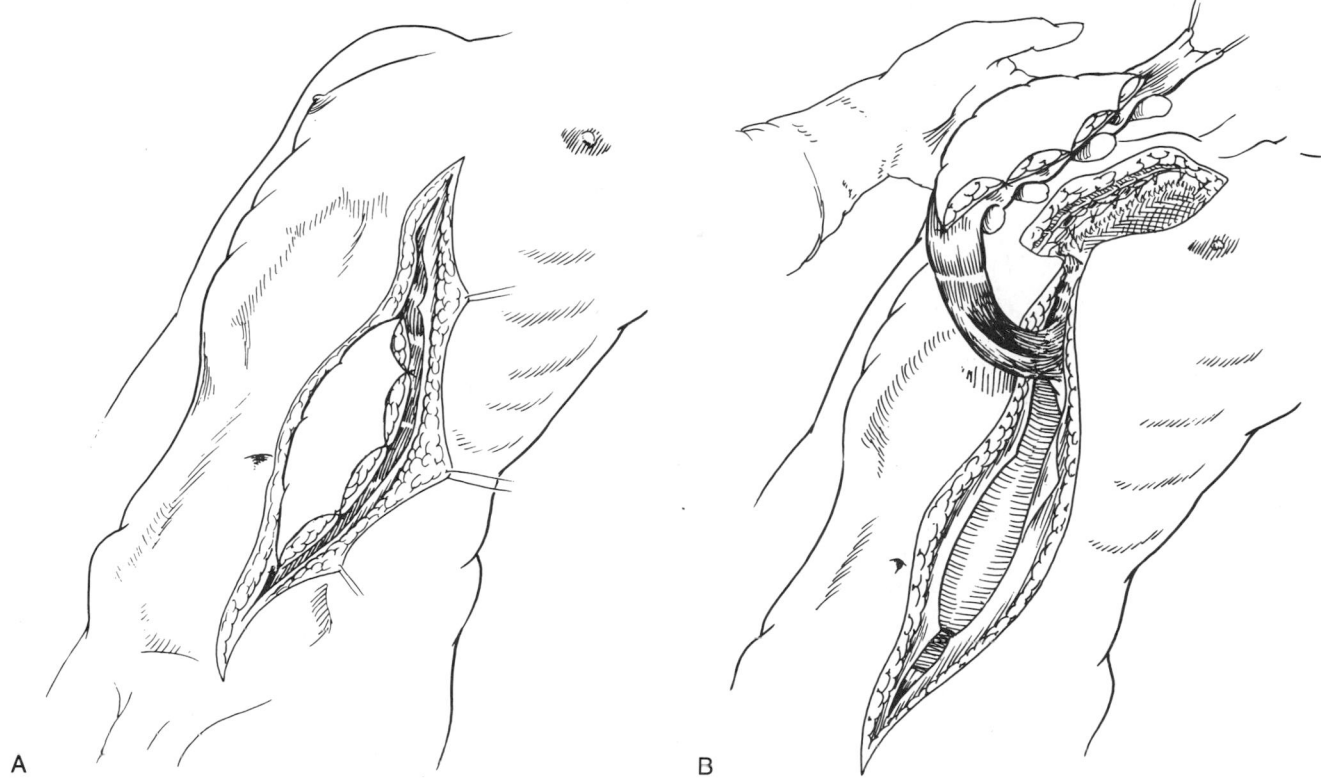

A

B

Figure 50-27. **(A)** The rectus abdominis myocutaneous flap may be used in reconstructing defects of the sternum and the dehisced median sternotomy as long as the ipsilateral internal thoracic vessels are intact. A longitudinal musculocutaneous flap has been fashioned for anterior wall reconstruction in this drawing. **(B)** The completed longitudinal musculocutaneous flap ready to be rotated based on the superior epigastric vessels. The longitudinal flap will be laid into the defect and adjusted to the edges. The blood supply to the musculocutaneous flap must be scrupulously maintained. The viability of the internal thoracic artery for this type of reconstruction is absolutely mandatory. (From Seyfer AE, Graeber GM, Wind GG: The rectus abdominis muscle and musculocutaneous flaps. p. 159. In Atlas of Chest Wall Reconstruction. Aspen Publishers, Rockville, MD, 1986e, with permission.)

has been divided by previous surgery, a latissimus dorsi muscular or musculocutaneous flap may still be rotated by basing it on the continuity of the arteries from the serratus anterior muscle to the thoracodorsal (Moelleken, et al., 1989; Fisher, et al., 1983). When the pedicle for rotation has been created in this fashion, the integrity of the arteries from the serratus anterior must be maintained scrupulously. As might be expected, the arc of rotation in this situation is more limited by the need to preserve the vessels to the serratus anterior.

Some serious limitations to the use of latissimus dorsi muscular and musculocutaneous flaps based on the thoracodorsal pedicle have been found to exist (Moelleken, et al., 1989; Seyfer, et al., 1986h). Previous radiation to the axilla can cause constriction of the thoracodorsal vessels, which limits blood supply and rotation. Probably the most common cause of this problem has been radiation to the chest wall and axilla during therapy for breast carcinoma (Moelleken, et al., 1989). Another serious problem with use of latissimus dorsi arises when a full posterolateral thoracotomy has been performed (Moelleken, et al., 1989; Seyfer, et al., 1986h). Division of the muscle and the thoracodorsal vessels causes the distal part of the muscle to become dependent on the secondary

blood supply. If the entire muscle is raised as flap based on the thoracodorsal vessels, the tissues distal to the scar undergo necrosis. Hence, the entire muscle can no longer be transferred to reconstruct chest wall defects or to repair intrathoracic problems such as bronchopleural-cutaneous fistulae (Fig. 50-30).

A number of authors have favored the use of muscle-sparing thoracotomies so that the blood supply to the latissimus dorsi and the serratus anterior is preserved. The necessity for muscle-sparing incisions is particularly apparent in the pediatric population (Soucy, et al., 1991; Malczyewski, et al., 1994).

Despite these limitations, the latissimus dorsi pedicled muscular and musculocutaneous flaps have found wide appreciation for reconstruction of all types of chest wall defects (Moelleken, et al., 1989; Seyfer, et al., 1986h). The use of these flaps in repairing posterior and spinal defects is well recognized (McCraw, et al., 1978). Even though radiation may have been applied to the axilla in treating mammary or other malignancies, these flaps may still be used quite effectively in breast reconstruction, closure of defects secondary to resection of radiation-induced chest wall necrotic

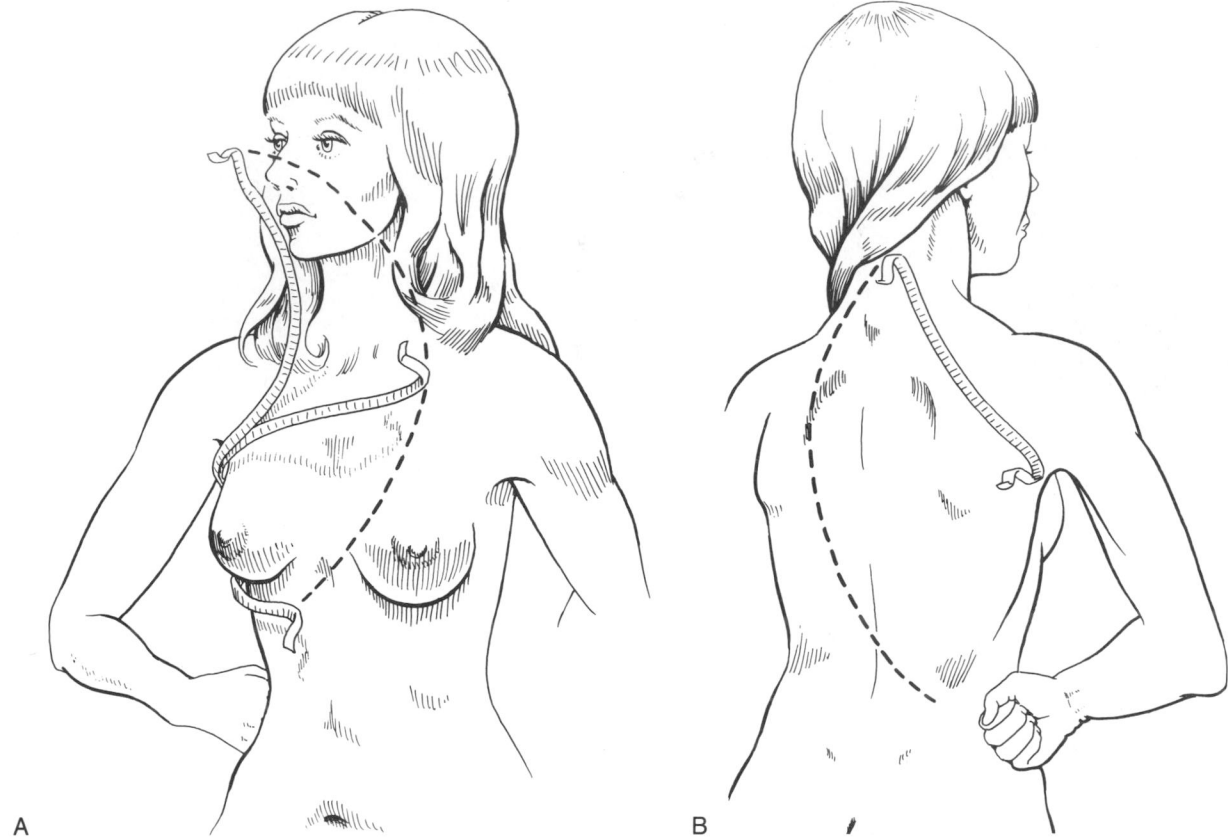

Figure 50-28. **(A)** Arc of rotation over the anterior chest for latissimus dorsi muscular and musculocutaneous flaps based on the thoracodorsal neurovascular pedicle. The tape measure depicts the length of the flap and its rotation when the posterior aspect of the tape is held against the anticipated pedicle. Note that this flap has great ability to reconstruct defects in the lateral, anterior, and superior aspects of the chest wall. This flap is not recommended for covering defects in the region of the distal sternum and xiphoid process. **(B)** The arc of rotation of the latissimus dorsi muscle when it is pedicled on the thoracodorsal neurovascular bundle. This muscular and musculocutaneous pedicle is the most useful one for covering defects of the posterior thoracic wall. (From Seyfer AE, Graeber GM, Wind GG: The latissimus dorsi muscle and musculocutaneous flaps. p. 97. In Atlas of Chest Wall Reconstruction. Aspen Publishers, Rockville, MD, 1986h, with permission.)

tissue, and reconstruction of the axilla (Seyfer, 1988). This musculocutaneous flap may have its capacity for closing defects enhanced by tissue expansion (Slavin, 1994).

Omentum

The omentum may be used in chest wall reconstruction. It has tremendous ability to reach all portions of the anterior and lateral chest wall as well as both pleural spaces (Seyfer, et al., 1986i; Fix and Vasconez, 1989). Indeed, the omentum has been lengthened so that it has been used to repair cervical and cranial defects as well (Fig. 50-31). It has the distinct asset of being able to contain infection well. Since the omentum has no dermal covering, it must be covered to achieve cutaneous continuity; probably the most efficacious method of doing so is application of a meshed, split-thickness skin graft. When the mesh remains small, the continuity of the skin graft follows promptly and provides for a smooth surface.

The blood supply of the omentum is based on the right and left gastroepiploic arteries and veins (Powers, et al., 1976). These vessels create a continuous arcade, which runs along the greater curvature of the stomach. A pedicled flap

may be created that is based on either the right or the left gastroepiploic artery or on both. The caliber of the right and left gastroepiploic arteries may vary from individual to individual. One artery may be larger than the other and therefore may be more suitable as a pedicle on which to base an omental flap. The omentum in any given individual is subject to variation of the blood supply.

The most common anatomic variation has two arcades that are continuous with one another (Fig. 50-32). The omentum may be lengthened by judicious division of the arcades (Alday and Goldsmith, 1972) (Fig. 50-33). Great care should be taken to maintain pulses distally in the omentum when the arcades are divided. Appropriate blood supply may be maintained by testing with a Doppler ultrasound device prior to the division of any of the arcades. The point of division of each of the arcades should be occluded by soft vascular clamps prior to the actual division. If the pulse remains good distal to the anticipated points of division, there is a high probability that the distal portion of the omentum will remain viable.

The blood supply to the omentum also allows free flap transfer to new positions to achieve soft tissue coverage and repair. The omentum has been used as a free flap to cover

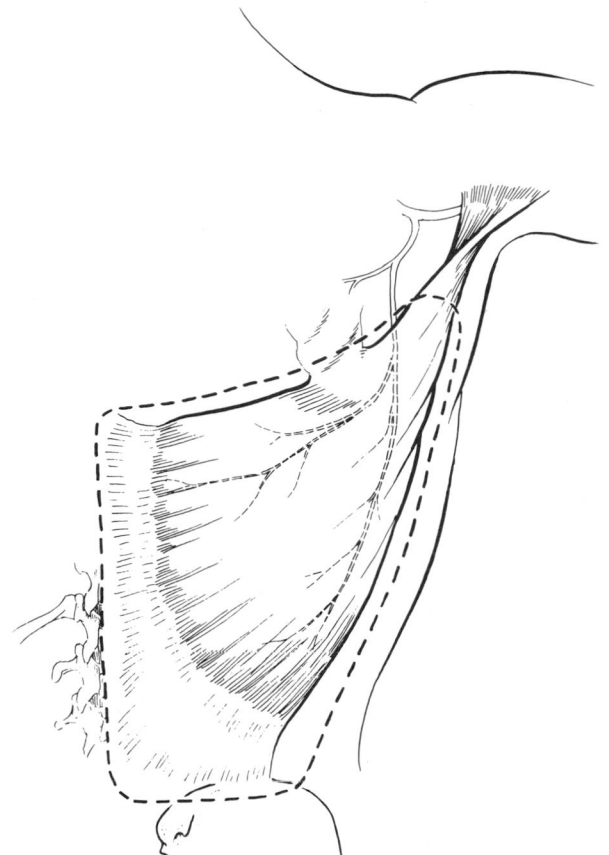

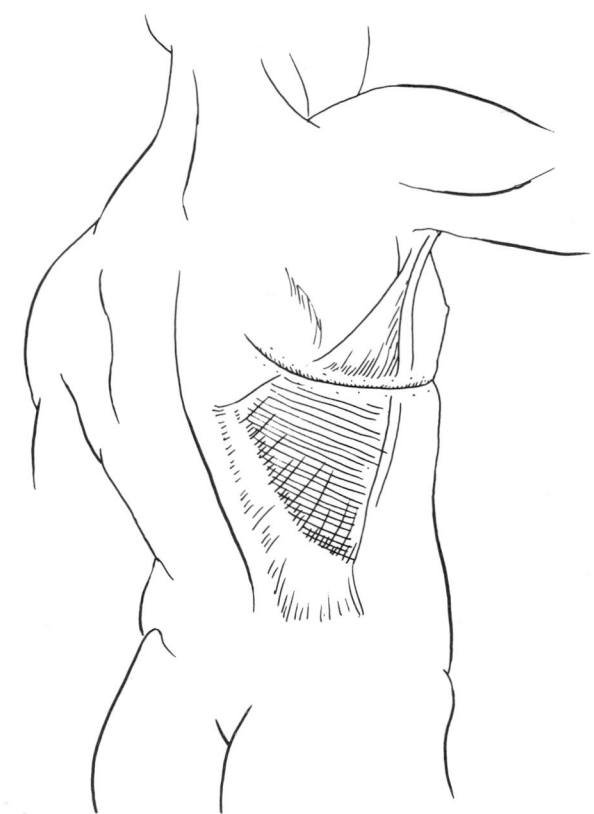

Figure 50-29. Arterial supply to the latissimus dorsi based on the thoracodorsal artery. Note that the subscapular artery originates from the axillary artery. The subscapular artery divides into two branches: a branch that courses medially to the serratus anterior, and the thoracodorsal artery, which is the direct extension of the subscapular artery. Once the subscapular artery enters the latissimus dorsi muscle, it divides into a lateral and a medial branch. The dotted line represents the maximal domain of the cutaneous island that may be carried with this muscle. (From Seyfer AE, Graeber GM, Wind GG: The latissimus dorsi muscle and musculocutaneous flaps. p. 97. In Atlas of Chest Wall Reconstruction. Aspen Publishers, Rockville, MD, 1986h, with permission.)

Figure 50-30. If the patient has had a previous posterolateral thoracotomy incision, the distal portion of the latissimus dorsi muscle and any cutaneous elements that may overlie the muscle receive their blood supply from the secondary vessels that penetrate the lumbodorsal fascia. If the entire muscle were raised on a pedicle based on the thoracodorsal vessels, the distal portion of the muscle beyond the incision would undergo necrosis. Rotation of the entire muscle based on the thoracodorsal pedicle after a posterolateral thoracotomy incision is contraindicated. (From Seyfer AE, Graeber GM, Wind GG: Planning the reconstruction. p. 59. In Atlas of Chest Wall Reconstruction. Aspen Publishers, Rockville, MD, 1986b, with permission.)

defects on the extremities or on the head and neck and to repair intrathoracic problems such as bronchopleural fistulae (Arnold and Irons, 1981; Jurkiewicz and Nahai, 1982). Unique aspects of the omental blood supply, its ability to contain infection, and its malleable nature have allowed creative transfer and sculpting to fill complex defects.

A number of liabilities may be associated with pedicled omental flaps when they are used for chest wall reconstruction (Seyfer, et al., 1986i; Mathiesen, et al., 1988). Previous abdominal surgery or abdominal infection may preclude use of the omentum. Gastric surgery, in particular, may have interrupted the arcades and may eliminate many possibilities for omental transfer. Previous infection may have caused so many adhesions that the omentum cannot be harvested without jeopardizing portions of it. The omentum can also be a channel for spreading infection from the chest to the abdomen; although this complication is rare, it has been docu-

mented. Finally, there is the ever-present complication of chest wall or diaphragmatic hernia associated with thoracic reconstruction using the omentum. The omentum has to be brought to the anterior chest wall through an epigastric hernia. Most often, an iatrogenic anterior defect will have to be created in the diaphragm to allow the omentum to pass into either pleural space. Such defects offer the potential for herniation of abdominal viscera into the thoracic cavity. Obviously, an epigastric hernia may be filled with more than omentum as the healing process progresses.

Despite its liabilities, the greater omentum has been used to cover virtually all possible types of chest wall defects (Mathiesen, et al., 1988). It has been particularly helpful in repairing dehisced median sternotomies and in repairing radiation injuries to the chest wall (Seyfer, 1988; Miller and Nahai, 1989). In such applications its ability to contain infection and to fill irregular defects have proved most useful.

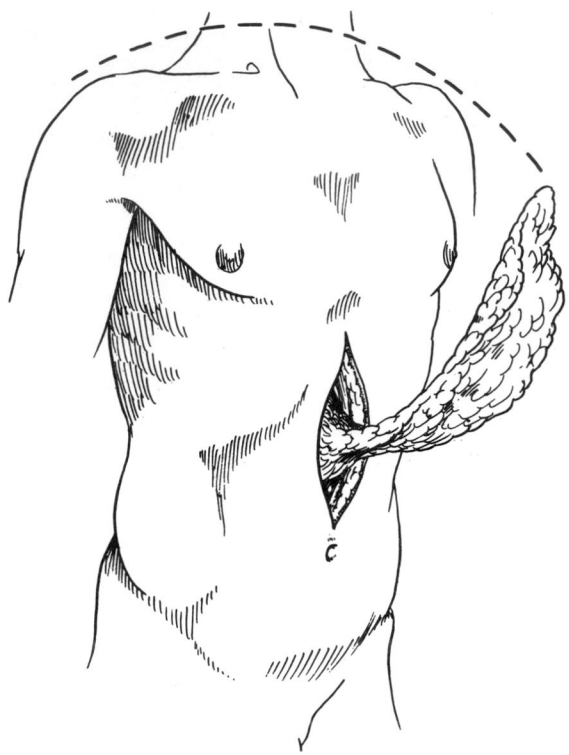

Figure 50-31. The arc of rotation of the omentum is quite large when the pedicle is based on the epiploic vessels. This shows the potential realm of application for the omentum in reconstruction of chest wall defects. The omentum is particularly useful in treating contaminated and infected defects of the anterior and lateral chest wall. (From Seyfer AE, Graeber GM, Wind GG: The omentum. p. 141. In Atlas of Chest Wall Reconstruction. Aspen Publishers, Rockville, MD, 1986i, with permission.)

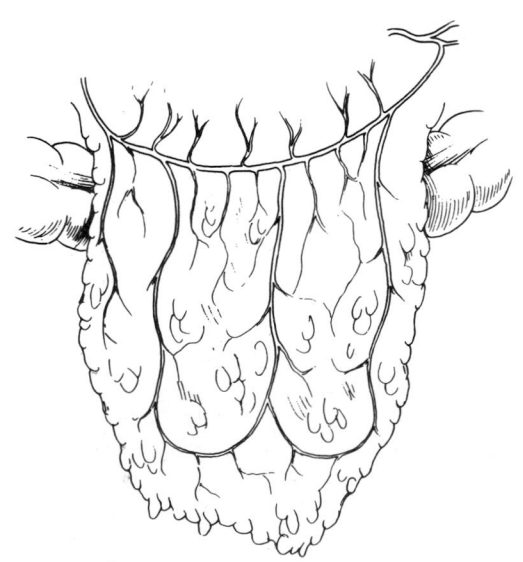

Figure 50-32. The omentum enjoys a dual blood supply, which is based on the right and left gastroepiploic vessels. This drawing represents the arcades that are usually found in the omentum. The main arterial arcade runs along the greater curvature of the stomach and is continuous between the right and left gastroepiploic arteries. There are usually two secondary arterial arcades that descend into the omentum. (From Seyfer AE, Graeber GM, Wind GG: The omentum. p. 141. In Atlas of Chest Wall Reconstruction. Aspen Publishers, Rockville, MD, 1986i, with permission.)

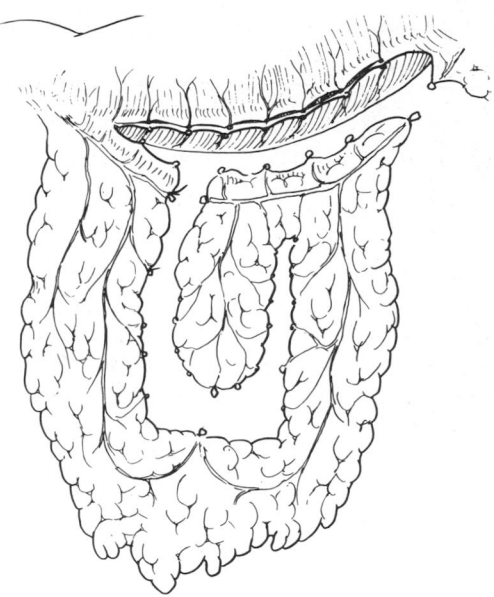

Figure 50-33. One of the most beneficial aspects of the omentum is that it may be tailored to fit irregular defects and lengthened on the basis of the vascular supply. This drawing depicts one of the possible lengthening procedures based on the right gastroepiploic artery. Note that the entire omental arcade has been dissected from the stomach, which is cephalad. The secondary arcades have been divided so that there is continuity of blood flow throughout the omentum. Obviously, because there is variation in the arcades, a continuous pulse must be ascertained before dividing any one of the arcades. Use of fine vascular clamps and Doppler ultrasound allows precise division of these arcades with ensurance of good distal arterial supply. (From Seyfer AE, Graeber GM, Wind GG: The omentum. p. 141. In Atlas of Chest Wall Reconstruction. Aspen Publishers, Rockville, MD, 1986i, with permission.)

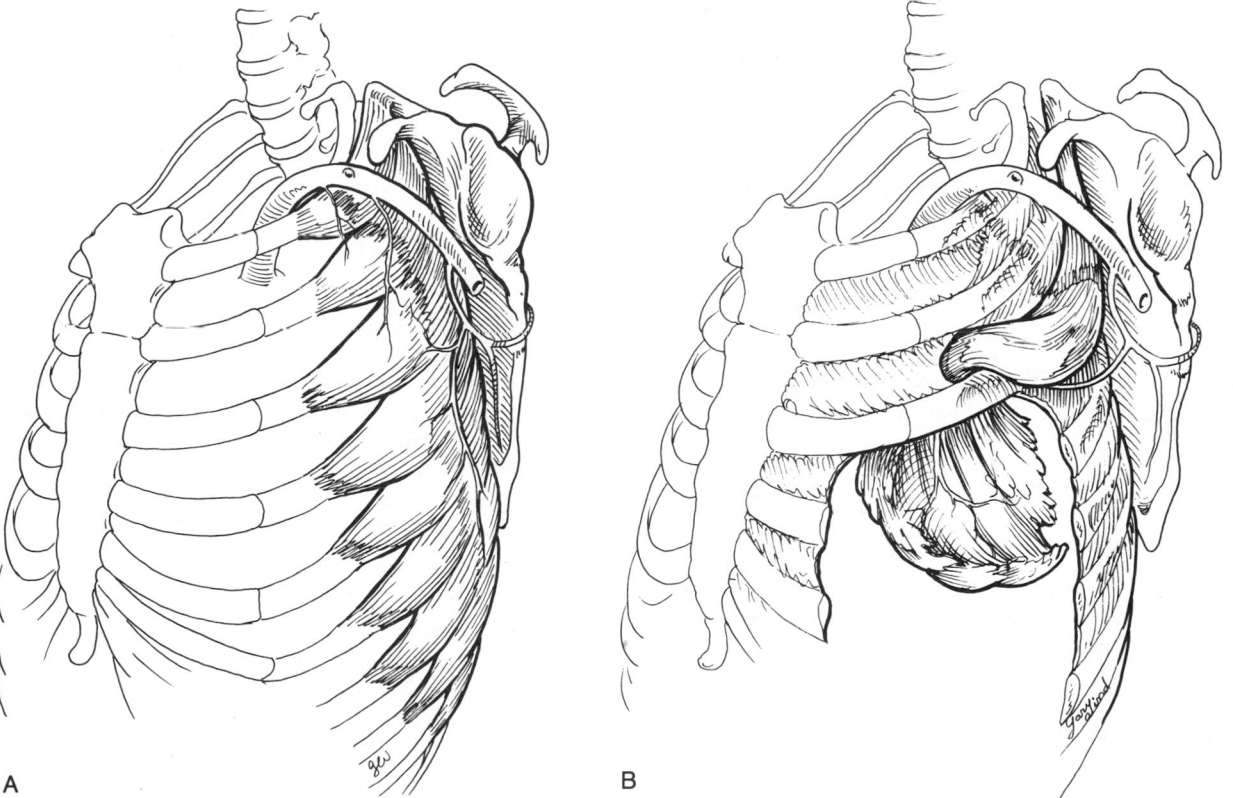

A B

Figure 50-34. **(A)** Arterial supply to the left serratus anterior muscle. The major arterial pedicle comes from the subscapular artery at the origin of the thoracodorsal. Other arteries enter the cephalad aspect of the muscle from the axillary artery. **(B)** Since the serratus anterior is often spared in performing a posterolateral thoracotomy, this muscle may be used effectively in repairing bronchopleural fistulae after pulmonary resection. This line drawing depicts the use of the muscle developed on its primary blood supply arising from the subscapular artery. The muscle has been introduced into the chest through the second intercostal space. Portions of the second and/or third rib may be resected to facilitate transposition of the muscle into the pleural space. As with all muscle transpositions, there should be no tension on the muscle itself or its primary blood supply.

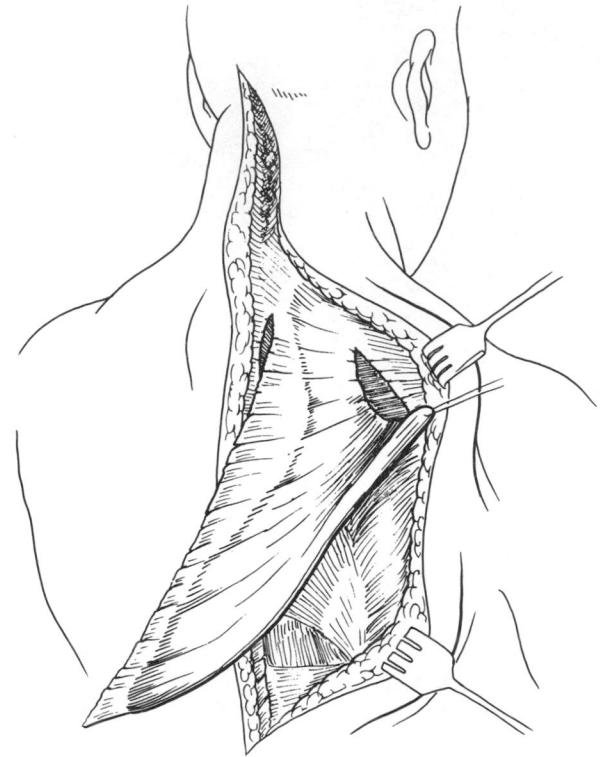

Figure 50-35. The trapezius muscle may be used to reconstruct defects in the region of the shoulder or the spine. Its limited domain of rotation includes the area of the scapula, the apex of the shoulder, and the vertebral region. It is an excellent muscle for closing small defects in these areas. It may be used alone or in addition to a latissimus dorsi flap. (From Seyfer AE, Graeber GM, Wind GG: The trapezius muscle and musculocutaneous flap. p. 183. In Atlas of Chest Wall Reconstruction. Aspen Publishers, Rockville, MD, 1986j, with permission.)

Serratus Anterior

The serratus anterior muscle has found some specific applications in thoracic reconstruction. The most common one is transposition into the thoracic cavity for control of bronchopleural fistulae (Pairolero and Arnold, 1989). Since this muscle is often spared with a lateral or posterolateral thoracotomy, it may be transposed intact with its cephalad blood supply to close chest wall or intrathoracic defects. It has a rather limited arc of rotation since the pedicle must be based on the artery to the serratus anterior, which arises from the subscapular artery (Fig. 50-34). When the serratus anterior is introduced into the chest, the secondary blood supply, which consists of small arteries arising from the axillary artery and some perforators from the intercostals, must be transected. The muscle may be brought through an intercostal space; however, a portion of the second or third rib may be resected to facilitate intrathoracic transposition (Fig. 50-34).

Trapezius

Although posterior defects are generally infrequent, the trapezius muscle offers an option for closure of such defects. The muscle may be used in conjunction with the pedicled latissimus dorsi flap or may be used alone to cover selected defects. This musculocutaneous flap is most useful in covering defects around the shoulder, the suprascapular region, and the perispinous region. It is usually rotated on the descending branch of the transverse scapular artery (Seyfer, et al., 1986i). The muscle also finds some limited use in correcting defects at the extreme apex of the pleural space (Fig. 50-35).

KEY REFERENCES

McCraw JB, Arnold PG: McCraw and Arnold's Atlas of Muscle and Musculocutaneous Flaps. Hampton Press Publishing, Norfolk, VA 1986

This is an excellent atlas that depicts the development and use of all the major pedicled flaps. Excellent dissections are provided to show the major aspects of constructing each flap, and the text is supplemented by clear photographic illustrations of all the flaps. Since most of the flaps were constructed on cadavers, the anatomic landmarks, blood supply, and individual characteristics of each flap are clearly depicted.

Seyfer AE, Graeber GM (eds): Chest Wall Reconstruction. Surg Clin North Am 69(5):1989

This monograph addresses all the major aspects of chest wall reconstruction. A number of authors who have contributed much to the field of thoracic reconstruction have written major chapters. The entire monograph is richly illustrated; the reference lists are extensive; and the text is clear and conveys all major points concerning chest wall reconstruction in a sequential fashion.

Seyfer AE, Graeber GM, Wind GG: Atlas of Chest Wall Reconstruction. Aspen Publishers, Rockville, MD 1986a

This atlas is based on the large experience of the authors at Walter Reed Army Medical Center in Washington, D.C. Each of the flaps is precisely illustrated, and the techniques of developing each one are carefully described. The drawings are particularly helpful, since the artist is also a surgeon.

REFERENCES

Alday ES, Goldsmith HS: Surgical technique for omental lengthening. Surg Gynecol Obstet 135:103, 1972

Arnold PG, Irons GB: The greater omentum: extensions in transposition and free transfer. Plast Reconstr Surg 67:169, 1981

Arnold PG, Pairolero PC: Reconstruction of the radiation-damaged chest wall. Surg Clin North Am 69:1081, 1989

Arnold PG, Pairolero PC: Chest wall reconstruction: experience with 100 consecutive patients. Ann Surg 199:725, 1984

Arnold PG, Pairolero PC: Use of the pectoralis major muscle flaps to repair defects of the anterior chest wall. Plast Reconstr Surg 63:205, 1979

Arnold PG, Pairolero PC: Chondrosarcoma of the manubrium. Resection and reconstruction with pectoralis major muscle. Mayo Clin Proc 53:54, 1978

Azarow KS, Malloy M, Seyfer AE, Graeber GM: Preoperative evaluation and general preparation for chest wall operations. Surg Clin North Am 69:899, 1989

Brown R, Vasconez L, Jurkiewicz M: Transverse abdominal flaps and the deep epigastric arcade. Plast Reconstr Surg 55:416, 1975

Bunkis J, Walton R, Mathes S et al: Experience with the transverse lower rectus abdominis operation for breast reconstruction. Plast Reconstr Surg 72:819, 1983

Coleman JJ, Bostwick J: Rectus abdominis muscle—musculocutaneous flap in chest-wall reconstruction. Surg Clin North Am 69:1007, 1989

Das SK: The size of the human omentum and methods of lengthening it for transplantation. Br J Plast Surg 29:170, 1976

Dinner M, Labandter H, Dowden R: The role of the rectus abdominis myocutaneous flap in breast reconstruction. Plast Reconstr Surg 69:209, 1982

Fisher J, Bostwick J, Powell RW: Latissimus dorsi blood supply after thoracodorsal vessel division: the serratus collateral. Plast Reconstr Surg 72:502, 1983

Fix RJ, Vasconez LO: The use of the omentum in chest-wall reconstruction. Surg Clin North Am 69:1029, 1989

Glafkides MC, Toth BA: Split bipedicle transverse rectus abdominis flaps: expanding their uses in breast reconstruction. Ann Plast Surg 27:9, 1991

Graeber GM, Snyder RJ, Flemming AW et al: Initial and long-term results in the management of primary chest wall neoplasms. Ann Thorac Surg 34:664, 1982

Hammond DC, Fisher J, Meland NB: Intrathoracic free flaps. Plast Reconstr Surg 91:1259, 1993

Hartrampf C, Scheflan M, Black P: Breast reconstruction with a transverse abdominal island flap. Plast Reconstr Surg 69:216, 1982

Ishii C, Bostwick J, Raine T et al: Double-pedicle transverse rectus abdominis myocutaneous flap for unilateral breast and chest wall reconstruction. Plast Reconstr Surg 76:901, 1985

Jacobsen WM, Meland NB, Woods JE: Autologous breast reconstruction with use of transverse rectus abdominis musculocutaneous flap: Mayo Clinic experience with 47 cases. Mayo Clin Proc 69:635, 1994

Jurkiewicz MJ, Nahai F: The omentum: its use as a free vascularized graft for reconstruction of the head and neck. Ann Surg 195:756, 1982

Malczyewski MC, Colony L, Cobb LM: Latissimus-sparing thoracotomy in the pediatric patient: a valuable asset for thoracic reconstruction. J Pediatr Surg 29:396, 1994

Mathiesen DJ, Grillo HC, Vlahakes GJ et al: The omentum in the management of complicated cardiothoracic problems. J Thorac Cardiovasc Surg 95:677, 1988

Matsuo K, Hirose T, Hayashi R, Kiyono M: Reconstruction of large chest wall defects using a combination of a contralateral latissimus dorsi and a rectus abdominis musculocutaneous flap. Br J Plast Surg 44:102, 1991

McCraw JB, Penix JO, Baker JW: Repair of major defects of the chest wall and spine with a latissimus dorsi myocuteneous flap. Plast Reconstr Surg 62:97, 1978

Miller JI, Nahai F: Repair of the dehisced median sternotomy incision. Surg Clin North Am 69:1091, 1989

Miller L, Bostwick J, Hartrampf C et al: The superiorly based rectus abdominis flap: predicting and enhancing its blood supply based on an anatomic and clinical study. Plast Reconstr Surg 81:713, 1988

Moelleken BRW, Mathes SA, Chang N: Latissimus dorsi muscle-musculocutaneous flap in chest-wall reconstruction. Surg Clin North Am 69:977, 1989

Morain WD, Cohen LV, Hutchings JC: The segmental pectoralis major muscle flap: a function-preserving procedure. Plast Reconstr Surg 67:753, 1981

Nahai F, Morales L Jr, Bone DK et al: Pectoralis major muscle turnover flap for closure of the infected sternotomy wound with preservation of form and function. Plast Reconstr Surg 70:471, 1982

Pairolero PC, Arnold PG: Intrathoracic transfer of flaps for fistulas, exposed prosthetic devices and reinforcement of suture lines. Surg Clin North Am 69:1047, 1989

Pairolero PC, Arnold PG: Thoracic wall defects: surgical management of 205 consecutive patients. Mayo Clin Proc 61:557, 1986

Pairolero PC, Arnold PG: Management of infected median sternotomy wounds. Ann Thorac Surg 42:1, 1986

Pairolero PC, Arnold PG: Management of recalcitrant median sternotomy wounds. J Thorac Cardiovasc Surg 88:357, 1984

Pairolero PC, Arnold PG: Bronchopleural fistula: treatment by transposition of pectoralis major muscle. J Thorac Cardiovasc Surg 79:142, 1980

Powers JC, Fitzgerald JF, McAlvanah MJ: The anatomic basis for the surgical detachment of the greater omentum from the transverse colon. Surg Gynecol Obstet 143:105, 1976

Rowsell AR, Davies DM, Eisenberg N et al: The anatomy of the subscapular-thoracodorsal arterial system: study of 100 cadaver dissections. Br J Plast Surg 37:574, 1984

Seyfer AE: Radiation-associated lesions of the chest wall: longitudinal experience with 31 patients. Surg Gynecol Obstet 167:129, 1988

Seyfer AE, Graeber GM, Wind GG: Planning the reconstruction. p. 59. In Atlas of Chest Wall Reconstruction. Aspen Publishers, Rockville, MD, 1986b

Seyfer AE, Graeber GM, Wind GG: The pectoralis major muscle and musculocutaneous flaps. p. 121. In Atlas of Chest Wall Reconstruction. Aspen Publishers, Rockville, MD, 1986c

Seyfer AE, Graeber GM, Wind GG: Tracheoesophageal and bronchopleural/cutaneous fistulas. p. 217. In Atlas of Chest Wall Reconstruction. Aspen Publishers, Rockville, MD, 1986d

Seyfer AE, Graeber GM, Wind GG: The rectus abdominis muscle and musculocutaneous flaps. p. 159. In Atlas of Chest Wall Reconstruction. Aspen Publishers, Rockville, MD, 1986e

Seyfer AE, Graeber GM, Wind GG: Blood supply to the skin of the chest wall. p. 31. In Atlas of Chest Wall Reconstruction. Aspen Publishers, Rockville, MD, 1986f

Seyfer AE, Graeber GM, Wind GG: Reconstruction of the breast following mastectomy. p. 213. In Atlas of Chest Wall Reconstruction. Aspen Publishers, Rockville, MD, 1986g

Seyfer AE, Graeber GM, Wind GG: The latissimus dorsi muscle and musculocutaneous flaps. p. 97. In Atlas of Chest Wall Reconstruction. Aspen Publishers, Rockville, MD, 1986h

Seyfer AE, Graeber GM, Wind GG: The omentum. p. 141. In Atlas of Chest Wall Reconstruction. Aspen Publishers, Rockville, MD, 1986i

Seyfer AE, Graeber GM, Wind GG: The trapezius muscle and musculocutaneous flap. p. 183. In Atlas of Chest Wall Reconstruction. Aspen Publishers, Rockville, MD, 1986j

Slavin SA: Improving the latissimus dorsi myocutaneous flap with tissue expansion. Plast Reconstr Surg 93:811, 1994

Soucy P, Bass J, Evans M: The muscle-sparing thoracotomy in infants and children. J Pediatr Surg 26:1323, 1991

Tobin GR: Pectoralis major muscle-musculocutaneous flap for chest-wall reconstruction. Surg Clin North Am 69:991, 1989

Yamamoto Y, Nohira K, Shintomi Y et al: Turbo-charging the vertical rectus abdominis myocutaneous (turbo-VRAM) flap for reconstruction of extensive chest wall defects. Br J Plast Surg 47:103, 1994

Thoracic Outlet Syndrome: Supraclavicular Approach

Susan Mackinnon
G. A. Patterson

The supraclavicular approach to relieve thoracic outlet syndrome by decompression of the brachial plexus and excision of the first rib releases structures that compress soft tissue in the region of the interscalene portion of the brachial plexus. The lower nerve trunk and C8 and T1 roots can be completely identified and protected as the most posterior aspect of the first rib is resected under direct vision. Any cervical ribs or prolonged transverse processes are easily removed by this supraclavicular approach. This operative procedure is detailed in Figure 50-36.

Loupe magnification ($\times 4.5$) and microbipolar cautery are used and a portable nerve stimulator (Concept 2, Clearwater, FL) is frequently applied throughout the procedure. A sandbag is placed between the scapula and the neck extended to the nonoperative side. Long-acting paralytic agents are avoided. An incision in a neck crease, parallel to and 2 cm above the clavicle, is made in the supraclavicular fossa.

The supraclavicular nerves are identified just beneath the platysma and mobilized in order to allow vessel loop retraction. The omohyoid is divided and the supraclavicular fat pad elevated, after which the scalene muscles and the brachial plexus are easily palpated. The lateral portion of the clavicular head of the sternocleidomastoid is divided and at the end of the procedure is repaired. The phrenic nerve is seen on the anterior surface of the anterior scalene muscle, and similarly, the long thoracic nerve is noted on the posterior aspect of the middle scalene muscle.

The anterior scalene muscle is divided from the first rib. The subclavian artery is noted immediately behind this, and an umbilical tape is placed around the subclavian artery. The phrenic nerve is not mobilized but rather is simply avoided. The upper, middle, and lower trunks of the brachial plexus are easily visualized and gently mobilized. The middle scalene muscle is now divided from the first rib. It has a broad attachment to the first rib, and care must be taken to avoid injury to the long thoracic nerve, which in this position may have multiple branches and may pass through and posterior to the middle scalene muscle. With division of the middle scalene muscle, the brachial plexus is easily visualized and mobilized, and the lower trunk and the C8 and T1 roots are identified above and below the first rib. Congenital bands and thickening in Sibson's fascia are divided.

The first rib is then encircled and divided where easily visible with bone-cutting instruments, and its posterior segment is removed back to its spinal attachments by rongeur technique. By using a fine elevator, the soft tissue attachments to the first rib are separated. Finally, the posterior edge of the first rib is grasped firmly with a rongeur, and then a rocking and twisting motion is used to remove the entire aspect of the rib, so that the cartilaginous components of its articular facets with both the costovertebral and costotransverse joints can be identified on the specimen. The anterior portion of the first rib is removed in a similar fashion in order to decompress the neurovascular elements.

Cervical ribs or long transverse processes are removed by the same technique (Fig. 50-37). We use a technique described by Nelems to open the pleura, facilitating drainage of any postoperative blood collection into the chest cavity rather than allowing the blood to collect in the operative site around the brachial plexus. When the pleura is opened, care is taken to protect the intercostal brachial nerve, which is noted on the dome of the pleura. The wound is closed in a subcuticular fashion, and a simple suction drain is placed and sealed after wound closure and maximal inflation of the lungs by the anesthetist.

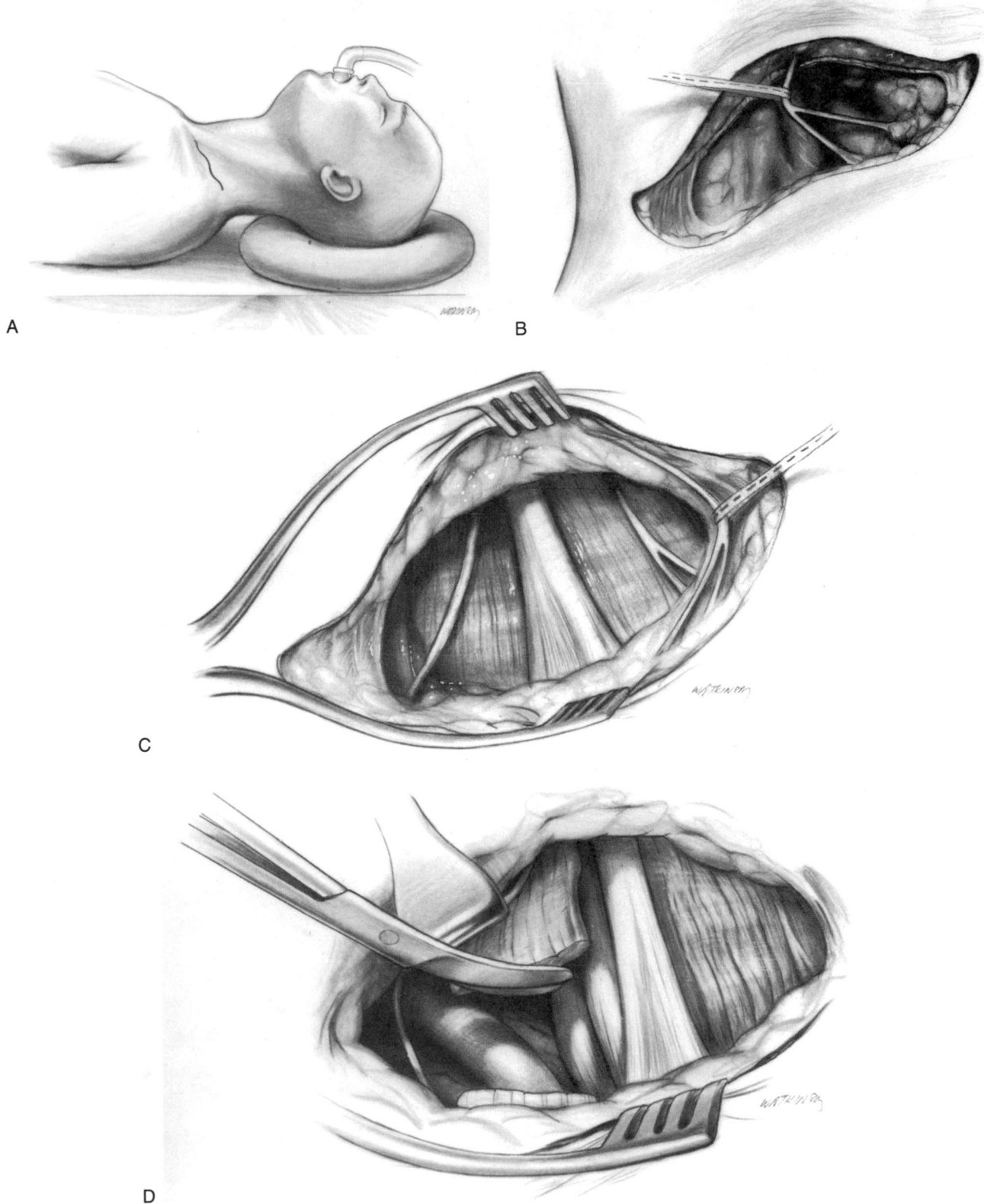

Figure 50-36. **(A)** The surgical incision is parallel to the clavicle. **(B)** The supraclavicular nerves are protected. **(C)** The fat pad has been retracted to identify the phrenic nerve on the scalene anticus muscle and the long thoracic nerve exiting from the posterior border of the scalene medius muscle, with the brachial plexus noted in the interscalene position. **(D)** The phrenic nerve is protected and the scalene anticus divided. The subclavian artery can now be seen in its location behind the scalene anticus muscle. (*Figure continues.*)

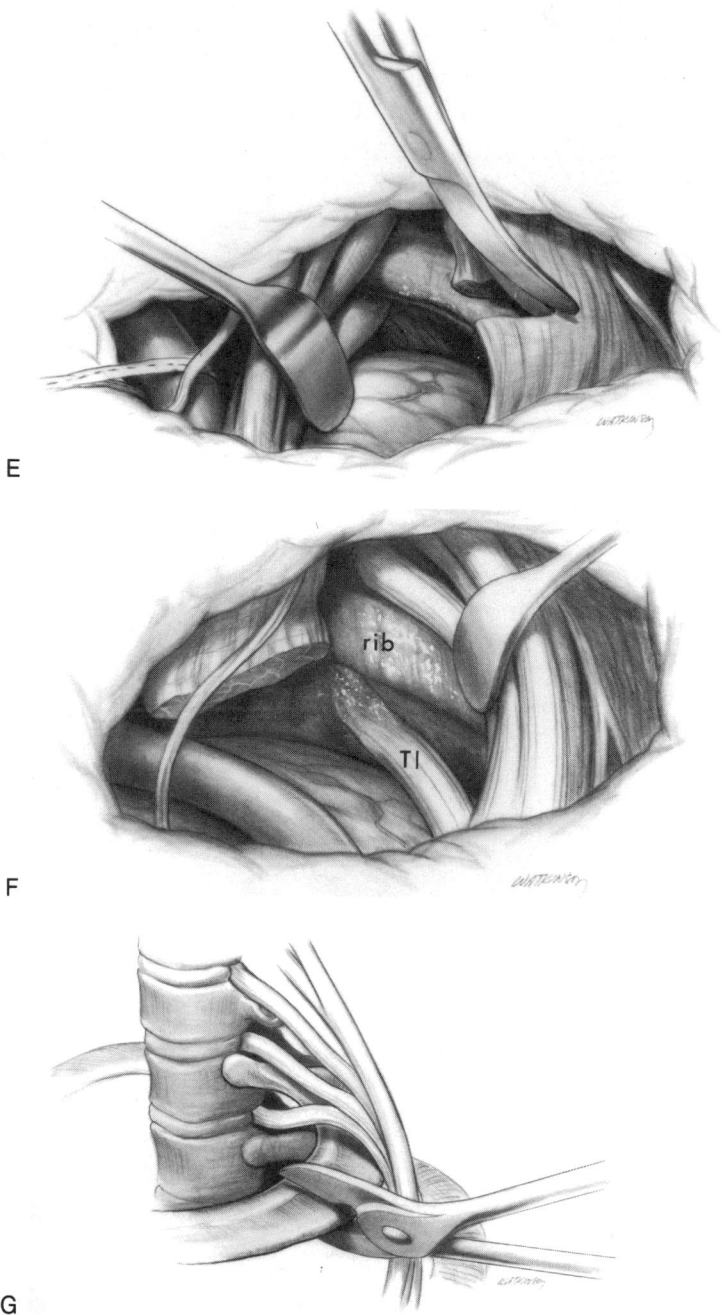

E

F

G

Figure 50-36 (*Continued*).   **(E)** The scalene medius muscle is divided from the first rib with care to protect the long thoracic nerve. **(F)** The upper portion of the brachial plexus is retracted to identify the first rib. T1 can be seen below the first rib. **(G)** The first rib is divided where it is easily visualized, and then the posterior and anterior aspects of the rib are removed. The relationship of T1 and C8 to the head of the first rib can be seen. (*Figure continues.*)

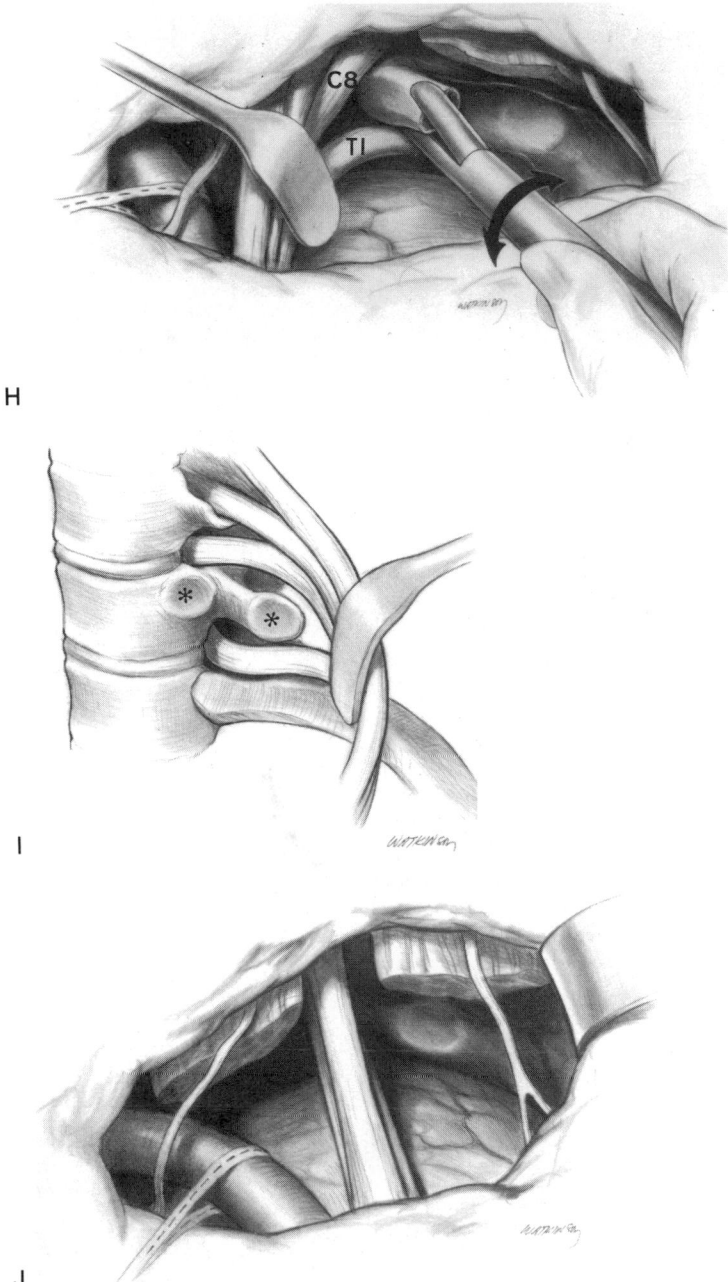

Figure 50-36 (*Continued*).   **(H)** The nerve roots are reflected anteriorly, and with a twisting motion using rongeurs, the posterior aspect of the first rib is removed. **(I)** The entire posterior portion of the first rib is removed so that no residual first rib remains to produce new bone formation and subsequent recurrence of symptoms. The articular facets of the costovertebral and costotransverse joints are noted (*asterisks*). **(J)** The brachial plexus has been completely decompressed. The phrenic and long thoracic nerves have been protected.

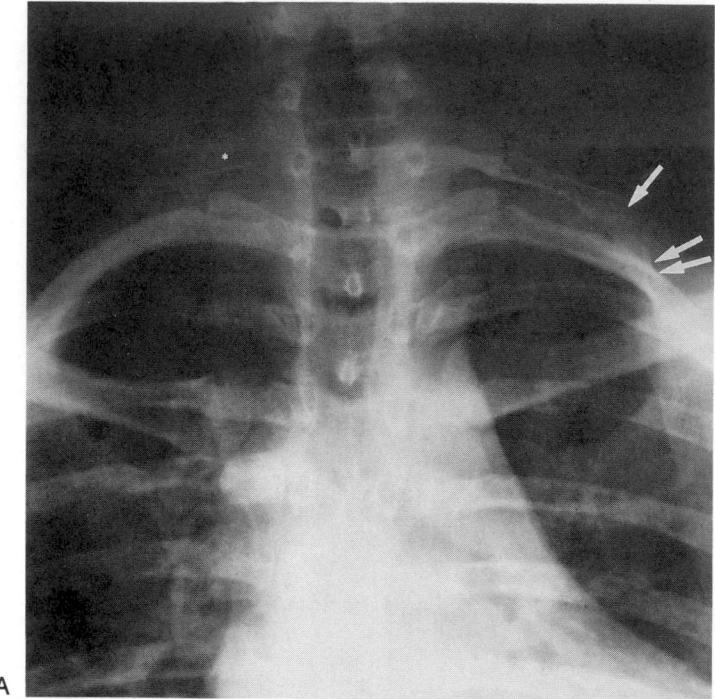

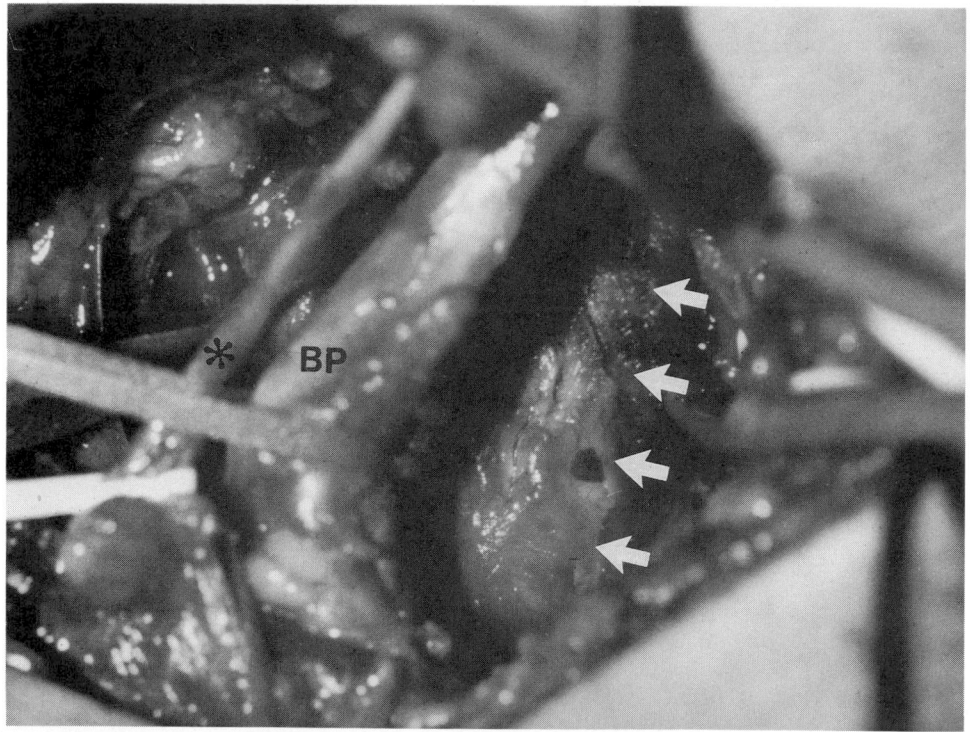

Figure 50-37. **(A)** Radiograph demonstrating a prominent transverse process on the right (*asterisk*) and a large cervical rib on the left. The pseudojoint noted in the cervical rib (*single arrow*) is a frequent finding. The cervical rib can be seen to articulate with the first rib (*double arrow*). **(B)** Operative photograph corresponding to radiograph, demonstrating the relationship between the brachial plexus (BP) and the cervical rib (*arrows*). Note supraclavicular nerve retracted (*asterisk*).

Thoracic Outlet Syndrome: Transaxillary Approach

Harold C. Urschel, Jr.

In surgery to relieve thoracic outlet syndrome, the transaxillary route is an expedient approach for complete removal of the first rib with decompression of the seventh and eighth cervical and first thoracic nerve roots and the lower trunks of the brachial plexus. First rib resection can be done without the need for major muscle division, as in the posterior approach (Clagett, 1962); without the need for retraction of the brachial plexus, as in the anterior supraclavicular approach (Falconer and Li, 1962); and without the difficulty of removing the posterior segment of the rib, as in the infraclavicular approach. In addition, first rib resection shortens postoperative disability and provides better cosmetic results than the anterior and posterior approaches, particularly because 80 percent of patients are female (Urschel, et al., 1968, 1971; Urschel and Razzuk, 1972; Roos, 1966).

The patient is placed in the lateral position with the involved extremity abducted to 90 degrees by traction straps wrapped around the forearm and attached to an overhead pulley. An appropriate weight, usually 3 lb, is used to maintain this position without undue traction. (Urschel and Razzuk, 1973).

A transverse incision is made in the axilla below the hairline between the pectoralis major and the latissimus dorsi muscles and is deepened to the external thoracic fascia (Fig. 50-38). Care should be taken to prevent injury to the intercostobrachial cutaneous nerve, which passes from the chest wall to the subcutaneous tissue in the center of the operative field.

The dissection is extended cephalad along the external thoracic fascia up to the first rib. With gentle dissection, the neurovascular bundle and its relation to the first rib and both scalenus muscles are clearly outlined to avoid injury to its components. The insertion of the scalenus anticus muscle is identified, skeletonized, and divided. The first rib is dissected subperiosteally with a periosteal elevator and separated carefully from the underlying pleura to avoid pneumothorax. A segment of the middle portion of the rib is resected; this is followed by subperiosteal dissection and resection of the anterior portion of the rib at the costochondral junction. After the costoclavicular ligament is cut, the posterior segment of the rib is similarly dissected subperiosteally and resected in fragments, including the articulation with the transverse process, the neck, and the head. The scalenus medius muscle should not be cut from its insertion on the second rib but rather should be stripped with a periosteal elevator to avoid injury to the long thoracic nerve that lies on its posterior margin.

The neck and head of the first rib are removed completely with a long, special double-action pituitary rongeur. The eighth cervical and first thoracic nerve roots may be visualized at this point. If a cervical rib is present, its anterior portion, which usually articulates with the first rib, should be resected at a point at which the middle portion of the first rib is removed. The remaining segment of the cervical rib should be removed after removal of the posterior segments of the first rib.

The wound is drained, and only the subcutaneous tissues and skin require closure because no large muscles have been divided. The patient is encouraged to use the arm for self-care but to avoid heavy lifting until at least 3 months after the operation. Cervical muscle stretching should be started at the end of the first week, and gentle exercising of the arm can be started at the end of the third week after operation.

It is preferable to remove the first rib entirely, including the head and neck, to avoid future irritation of the plexus, because a residual portion, particularly if long, will cause recurrence of symptoms.

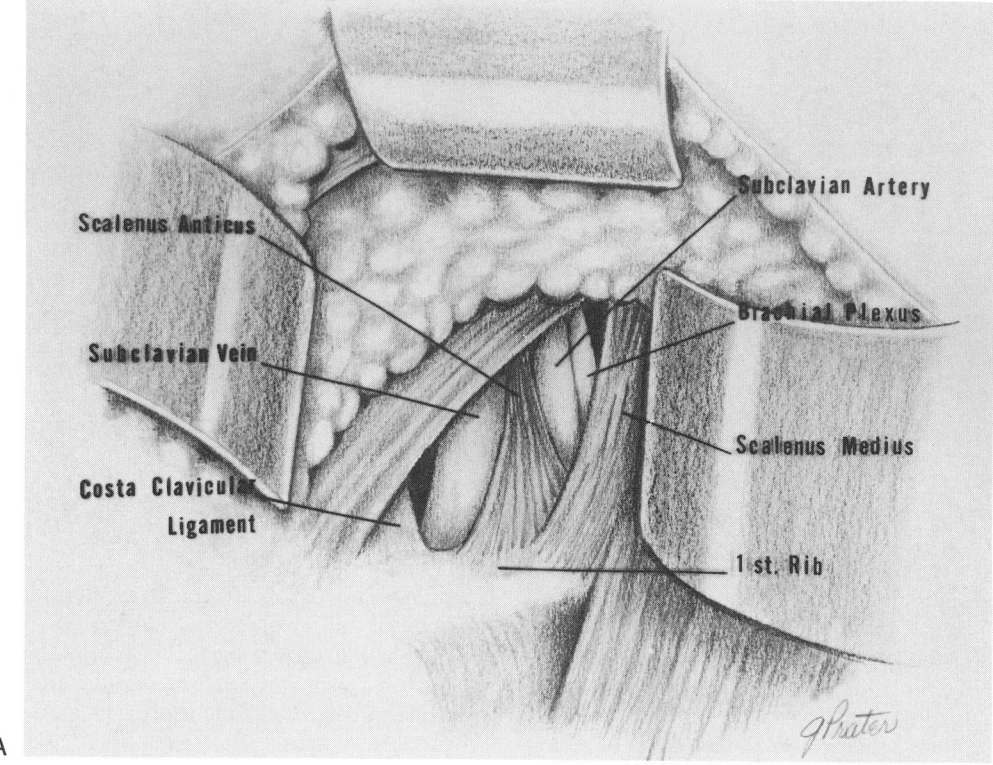

A

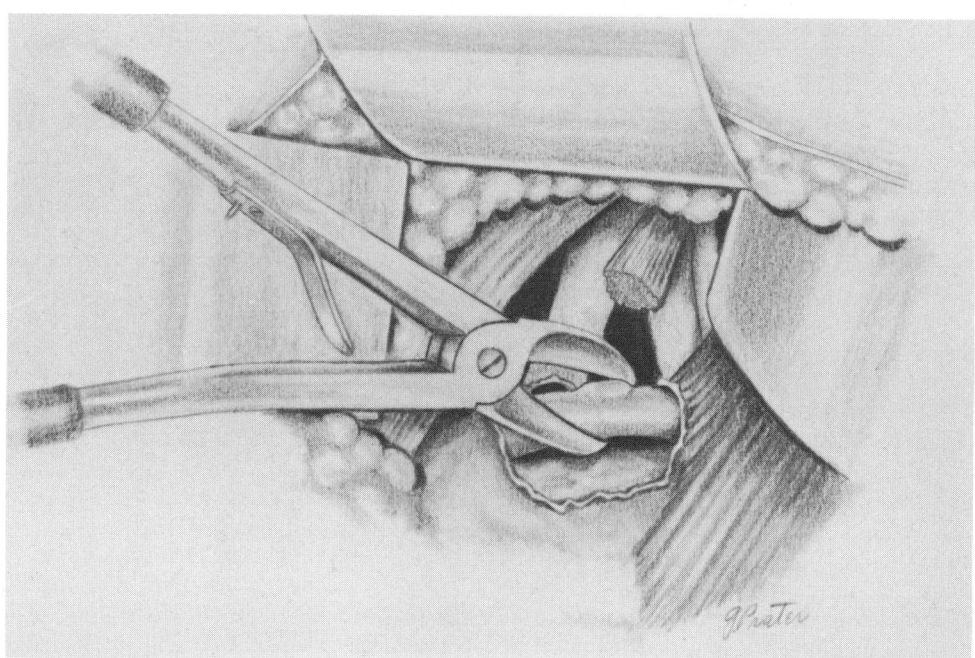

B

Figure 50-38. **(A)** Schematic drawing illustrating the relationship of the neurovascular bundle to scalene muscles, first rib, costoclavicular ligament, and subclavius muscle. **(B)** The scalenus anticus is severed, and the rib is separated from the periosteum and divided at that point. (*Figure continues.*)

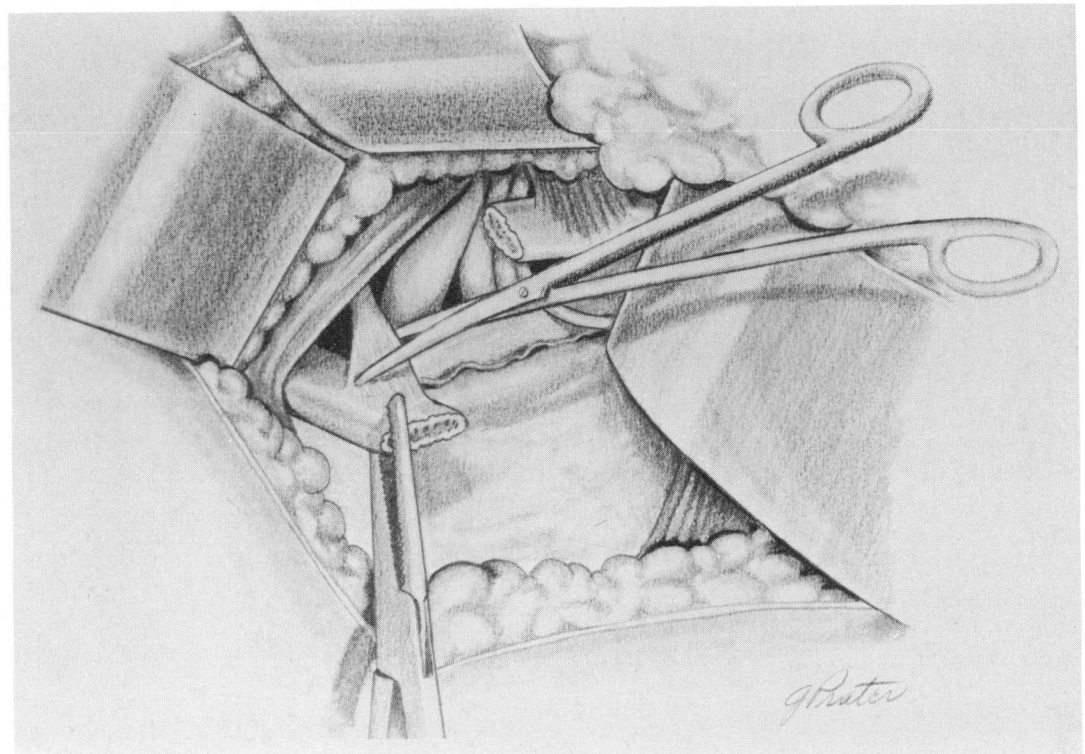

C

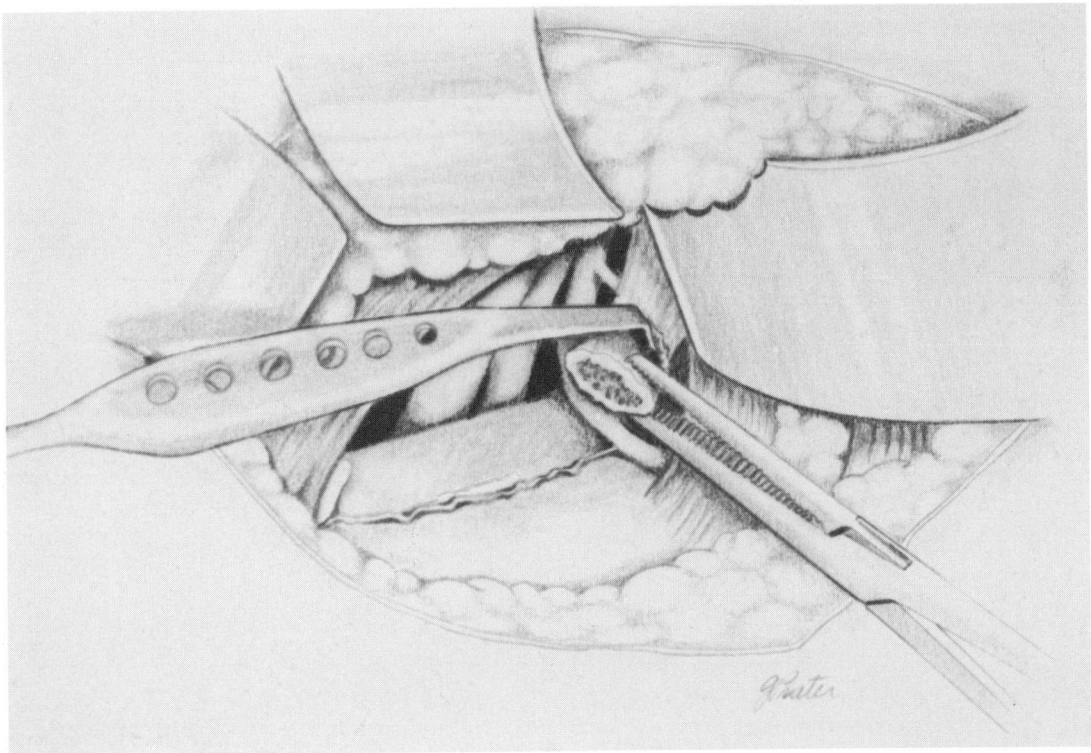

D

Figure 50-38 (*Continued*).   **(C)** The anterior segment of the first rib is pulled away from the subclavian vein, the costoclavicular ligament is cut, and the rib is divided at its medial cartilage attachment. **(D)** The posterior portion of the first rib is carefully dissected in the subperiosteal plane, with avoidance of injury to the subclavian artery and T1 nerve root. (*Figure continues.*)

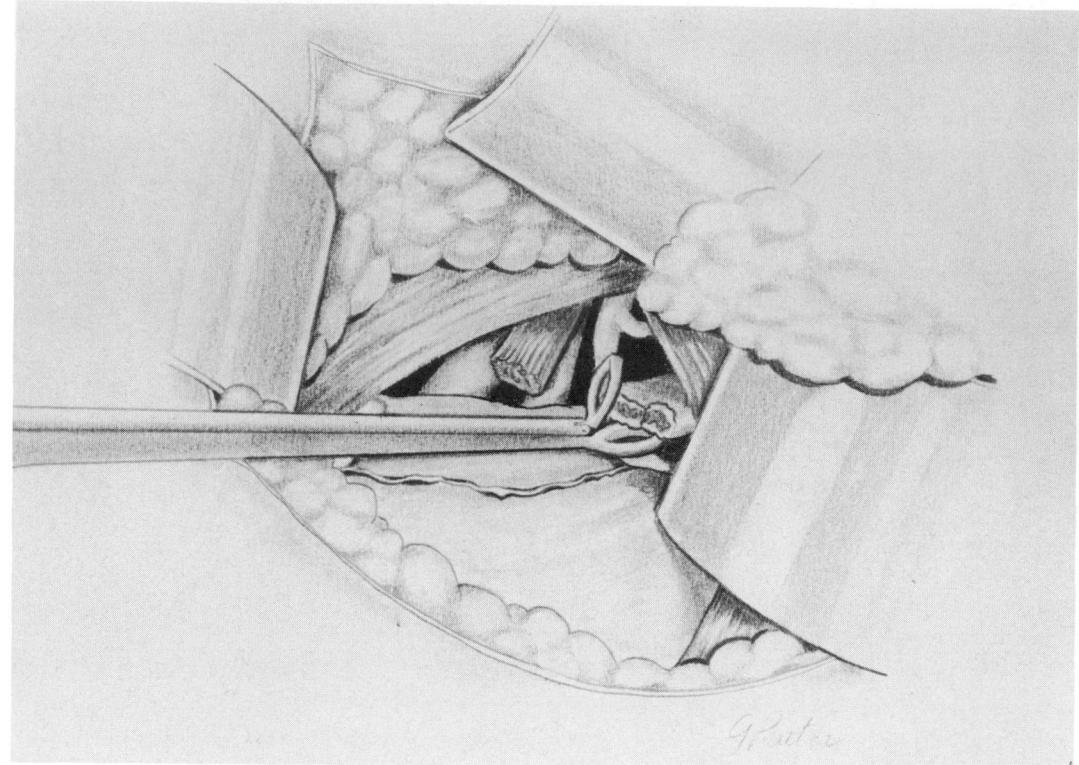

E

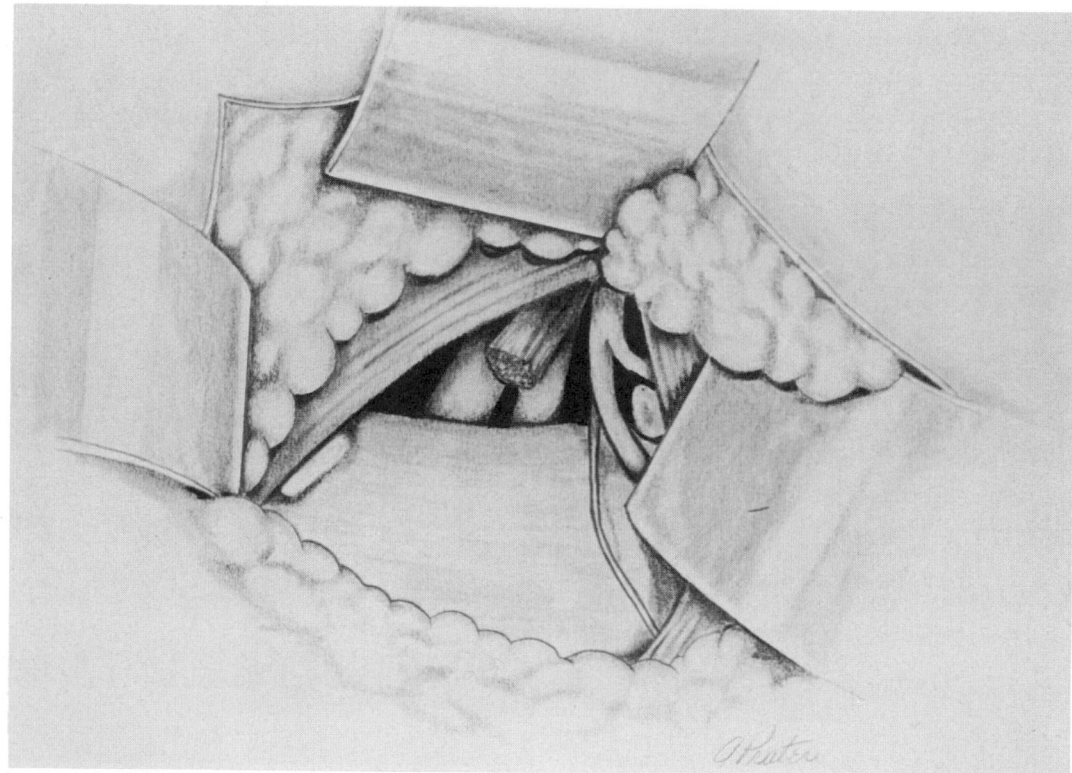

F

Figure 58-38 (*Continued*). **(E)** The posterior portion of the first rib is divided, and its neck and head are removed with a special pituitary rongeur, avoiding injury to the T1 nerve root. **(F)** Completed resection with *complete* first rib removal (including head and neck).

KEY REFERENCES

Clagett OT: Presidential Address: research and prosearch. J Thorac Cardiovasc Surg 44:153, 1962

The classic reference explaining the anatomic and pathophysiologic basis for first rib resection to alleviate neurovascular compression in the thoracic outlet. The incision is the high posterior thoracoplasty approach.

Roos DB: Transaxillary approach for first rib resection to relieve thoracic outlet syndrome. Ann Surg 163:354, 1966

The transaxillary approach to first rib resection was initially described by Atkins and popularized by Roos. The technical aspects of this approach and the pathophysiology are described.

Urschel HC Jr, Paulson DL, McNamara JJ: Thoracic outlet syndrome. Ann Thorac Surg 6:1, 1968

The first positive objective technique for diagnosing neurologic compression in the thoracic outlet syndrome is detailed.

REFERENCES

Falconer MA, Li FWP: Resection of the first rib in costoclavicular compression of the brachial plexus. Lancet 1:59, 1962

Urschel HC Jr, Razzuk MA: Thoracic outlet syndrome. Surg Annu 5:229, 1973

Urschel HC Jr, Razzuk MA: Current Management of thoracic outlet syndrome. N Engl J Med 286:21, 1972

Urschel HC Jr, Razzuk MA, Wood RE, Paulson DL: Objective diagnosis (ulnar nerve conduction velocity) and current therapy of the thoracic outlet syndrome. Ann Thorac Surg 12:608, 1971

51

THE DIAPHRAGM

Embryology, Anatomy, and Incisions

Geoffrey M. Graeber
Joseph I. Miller, Jr.

DEFINITION

The diaphragm is the musculocutaneous structure that separates the peritoneal from the pleural cavities and mediastinum while providing the principal mechanical force of ventilation. Its main anatomic components are a central tendon and radially arranged muscle fibers connecting the central tendon to the thoracic and axial skeleton. Its embryology is key to understanding diaphragmatic anatomy, physiology, and pathology. Successful surgical procedures to correct congenital and acquired abnormalities of this vital structure observe its unique anatomic and physiologic characteristics. Repairs of such defects require preservation of essential anatomic structures that allow continued physiologic performance.

EMBRYOLOGY

The diaphragm is derived from four embryologic precursors: the septum transversum, the paired right and left pleuroperitoneal membranes, and the dorsal mesentery of the esophagus and body wall. The septum transversum appears as a ventral ridge of mesenchymal tissue in the coelomic cavity of the 3-week embryo. By the fourth week it has become a thick, incomplete ventral partition between the emerging peritoneal and pericardial cavities. The septum transversum matures to become the central tendon and fuses with three dorsal structures to form the early diaphragm (Fig. 51-1). One is the dorsal mesentery of the esophagus, which contains the early aorta, inferior vena cava, and esophagus. This early structure matures to become the posterior median portion of the diaphragm (Fig. 51-2). The crura emerge in this structure when developing myoblasts migrate into the dorsal mesentery. Completion of the early fibrous diaphragm occurs during the seventh week, when the right and left pleuroperitoneal folds emerge dorsally and grow medially and anteriorly to fuse with the developing central tendon. The fusion of the four parts completes transection of the maturing coelomic cavity and separates the peritoneum from the pericardium (Fig. 51-2).

The final component necessary to complete the diaphragm is the musculature, which migrates from the third, fourth, and fifth cervical myotomes of the body wall. The developing lung buds, which grow into the body wall after closure of the pericardioperitoneal canal, promote inward migration of the musculature. This final component matures through the developing embryonic stage to provide the majority of the functional muscle tissue in the diaphragm. The emerging phrenic nerves, which will become the major motor and sensory nerves of the diaphragm, arise from the third, fourth, and fifth cervical nerves and migrate distad with the diaphragm. The mature diaphragm as viewed from the peritoneal aspect is presented in Figure 51-3.

Congenital diaphragmatic defects are the result of faulty development and/or fusion of various embryonic components (Moore, 1988; Gray and Skandalakis, 1972) (Fig. 51-4). Such a defect of the pleuroperitoneal membrane results in herniation of the abdominal viscera into the thoracic cavity and is known as congenital posterolateral diaphragmatic hernia of Bochdalek. Diaphragmatic eventration is due to failure of muscularization of the components of the diaphragm, resulting in thin, pliable, sheetlike membrane bulging into the thoracic cavity. The sternocostal hiatus for superior epigastric vessels is formed at the junction of the septum transversum, the anterior thoracic wall, and the lateral components of the diaphragm (Gray and Skandalakis, 1972). Hernia through this congenitally weak area is known as retrosternal hernia of Morgagni. Defects in the septum transversum result in very rare central diaphragmatic hernias.

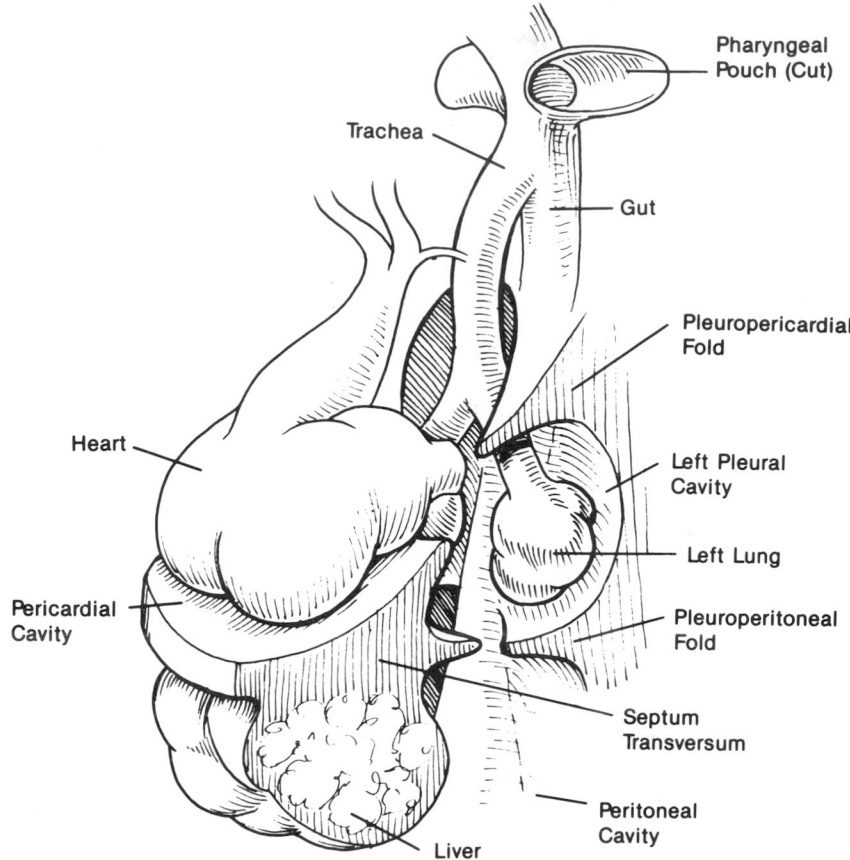

Figure 51-1. This left anterior oblique view of the emerging thoracic organs in the 5- to 6-week-old embryo depicts the early precursors of the diaphragm and their relationship to the heart and lungs. The anterior and lateral portions of the body wall have been removed for clarity. Note that the early septum transversum is migrating dorsad from its anterior origin. The paired left and right pleuroperitoneal folds are emerging from the dorsum and are proceeding in an anteromedial direction to fuse with the septum transversum and the dorsal mesentery, encompassing the esophagus, inferior vena cava, and aorta to complete transverse septation of the coelomic cavity. The pleuropericardial folds migrate anteriorly, mediad, and caudad to form the early pericardial cavity.

ANATOMY

The diaphragm is the major muscle of respiration and separates the peritoneal cavity from the two pleural cavities and the pericardium. When the diaphragm is contracting, the drawing out of its central tendon distally serves to create negative intrathoracic pressure; the lungs then follow the diaphragm in the normal physiologic state. The muscular fibers of the diaphragm are arranged in a radial fashion to cause downward migration of the central tendon of the diaphragm when the muscular fibers contract (Figs. 51-3 to 51-5). The muscles originate along portions of the axial and thoracic skeleton that comprise the lower thoracic inlet. The recognized muscular portions of the diaphragm, from posterior to anterior, are the crura, the segments of muscle arising from the lumbocostal arches, the portions arising from the true ribs, the costal muscles, and the sternal fibers.

The central tendon of the diaphragm is the point of insertion for all the diaphragmatic muscle fibers except for some of the right fibers, which form the esophageal hiatus. The central tendon is a unique fibrous structure, which has three parts.

The two lateral parts are covered on the cephaled aspect by the parietal pleura and on the abdominal aspect by the peritoneum. The middle portion of the central tendon is fused with the pericardium on its cephalad aspect and is covered by the peritoneum and the triangular ligament of the liver inferiorly.

There are three true foramina in the diaphragm (Figs. 51-3 to 51-5). The most cephalad foramen contains only the inferior vena cava. This foramen is situated in the right portion of the central tendon and conveys the inferior vena cava from the peritoneal cavity into the pericardial cavity. The esophageal hiatus is posterior to and slightly to the left of the medial portion of the central tendon. Its boundaries are formed by fibers from the right crus, which forms this foramen exclusively in approximately 85 percent of individuals. Variations obviously occur in the components that form the esophageal hiatus. The esophagus and the two vagus nerves proceed from the mediastinum to the peritoneal cavity through this foramen. The third true foramen is the aortic hiatus, which is bounded by portions of the right and left crus. It conducts the aorta, thoracic duct, and azygos vein and is

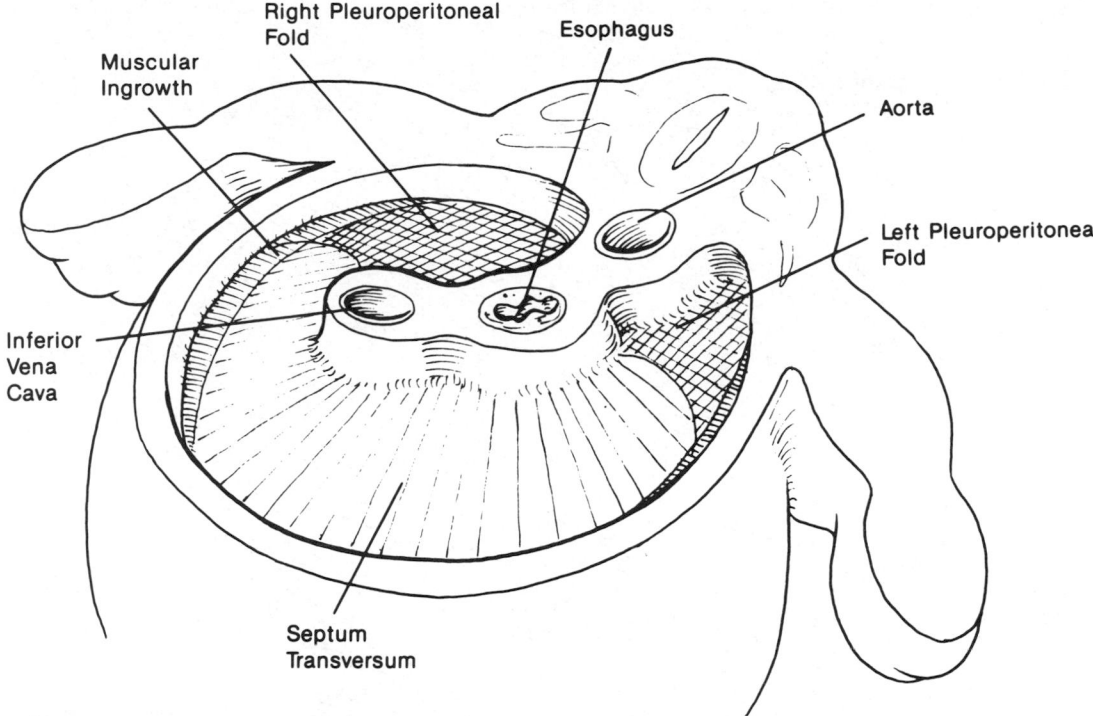

Figure 51-2.   A transverse section of a 10-week embryo reveals the completed diaphragm with its component parts. Muscular ingrowth from the body wall is occurring while continued development of the lungs is forcing them outward into the mesenchymal body walls bilaterally. Final maturation will transform the septum transversum into the majority of the central tendon. The pleuropericardial folds will ultimately be represented by a small portion of the central tendon at the respective posterolateral margins of the lateral leaves. Continued ingrowth of muscle from the body wall will give rise to the radially oriented fibers of the muscular diaphragm. Migration of muscular tissue from the body wall into the dorsal mesentery will give rise to the crura after maturation.

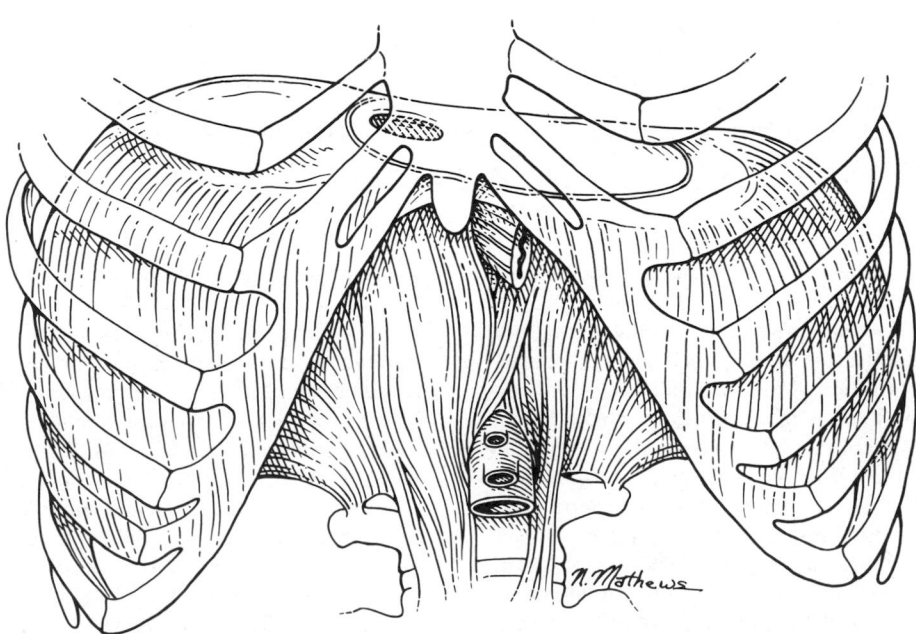

Figure 51-3.   Anatomy of the diaphragm.

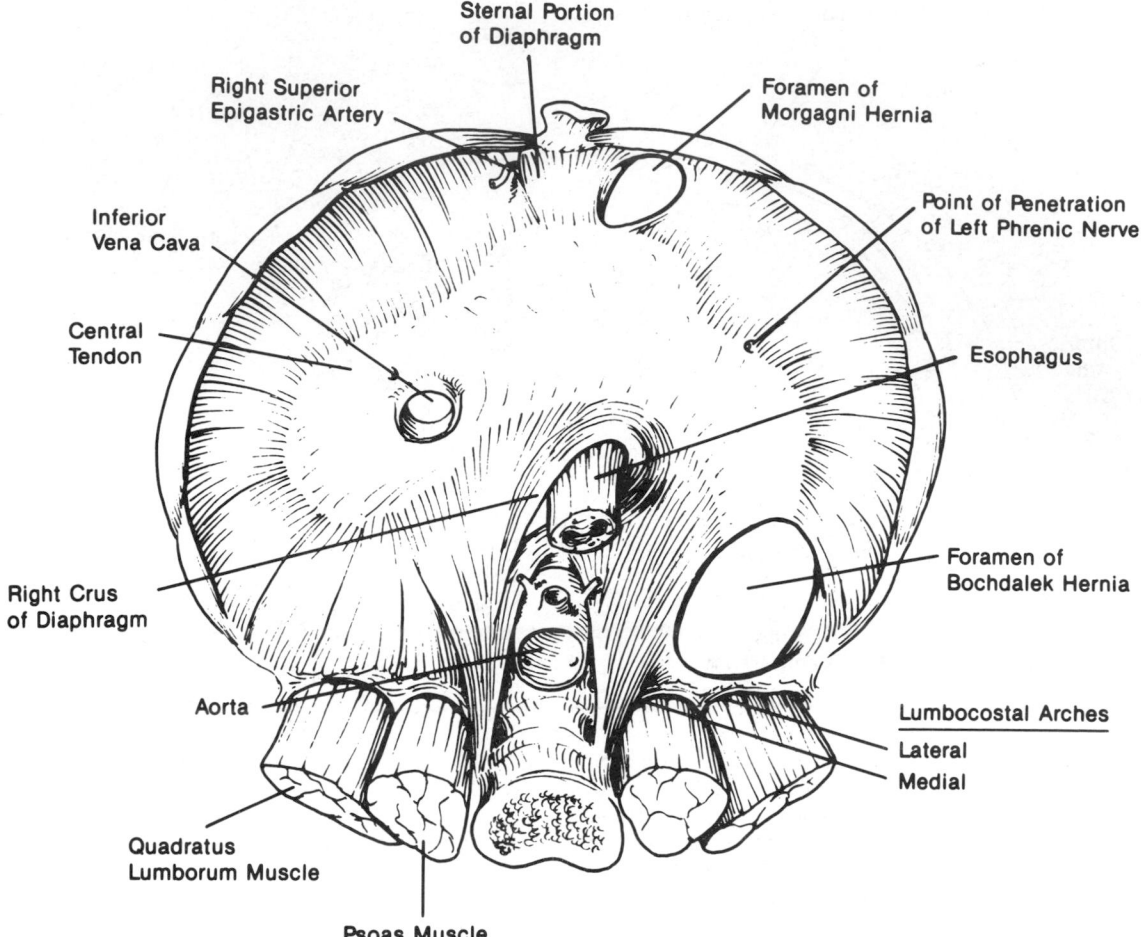

Figure 51-4. This view of the diaphragm from below shows two areas of congenital herniation. The posterior one, the foramen of Bochdalek hernia, is caused by an absence of the pleuroperitoneal membrane or by incomplete migration anteriorly to fuse with the septum transversum. The anterior or foramen of Morgagni hernia arises when there is incomplete fusion of the sternal and costal portions of the diaphragmatic muscle. This occurs at the point where the superior epigastric artery and vein penetrate the diaphragm. The vessels have been left out of the hernia for clarity. Their counterparts on the right side have been included for comparison. The foramen of Morgagni hernia usually has a true peritoneal sac whereas the foramen of Bochdalek does not. The origins of the two inferior phrenic arteries, which arise from the anterior aspect of the aorta, as shown just above the stump of the celiac axis. The leader pointing to the inferior vena cava crosses the point of penetration of the right phrenic nerve anterior and lateral to the cava. The branches of the inferior phrenic arteries, the veins, and the phrenic nerves have been omitted for clarity.

situated just anterior to the vertebral bodies and the anterior longitudinal spinal ligament.

Another potential opening exists between the sternal and costal portions of the muscular diaphragm. This, the foramen of Morgagni, carries the distal internal thoracic artery and vein through the diaphragm to become the superior epigastric artery and vein. The diaphragm is penetrated by two other structures although they do not create a true foramen in any sense. The right and left phrenic nerves penetrate the diaphragm in unique locations. The point of penetration of the right phrenic nerve is just anterior and lateral to the foramen for the inferior vena cava. The left phrenic nerve penetrates the diaphragm at the anterior margin of the left leaf of the central tendon where the central tendon joins the pericardial sac. Both phrenic nerves lie between the pericar-

dium and the parietal pleura above the diaphragm and beneath the peritoneum on the underside.

As we have seen in the embryology of the diaphragm, both phrenic nerves arise from the third, fourth, and fifth cervical levels. Each phrenic nerve innervates the respective muscular portions of the ipsilateral hemidiaphragm (Figs. 51-6 and 51-7). The phrenic nerves branch approximately 2 to 3 cm above their penetration points on their respective sides of the diaphragm to create an anterior and a posterior trunk. The anterior trunk gives rise to a sternal branch, which proceeds anteriorly toward the sternal portion of the diaphragm, and an anterolateral branch, which courses laterally toward the axillary line. The posterior trunk divides into two major branches: the posterolateral branch, which goes across the central tendon and courses toward the posterior axillary line

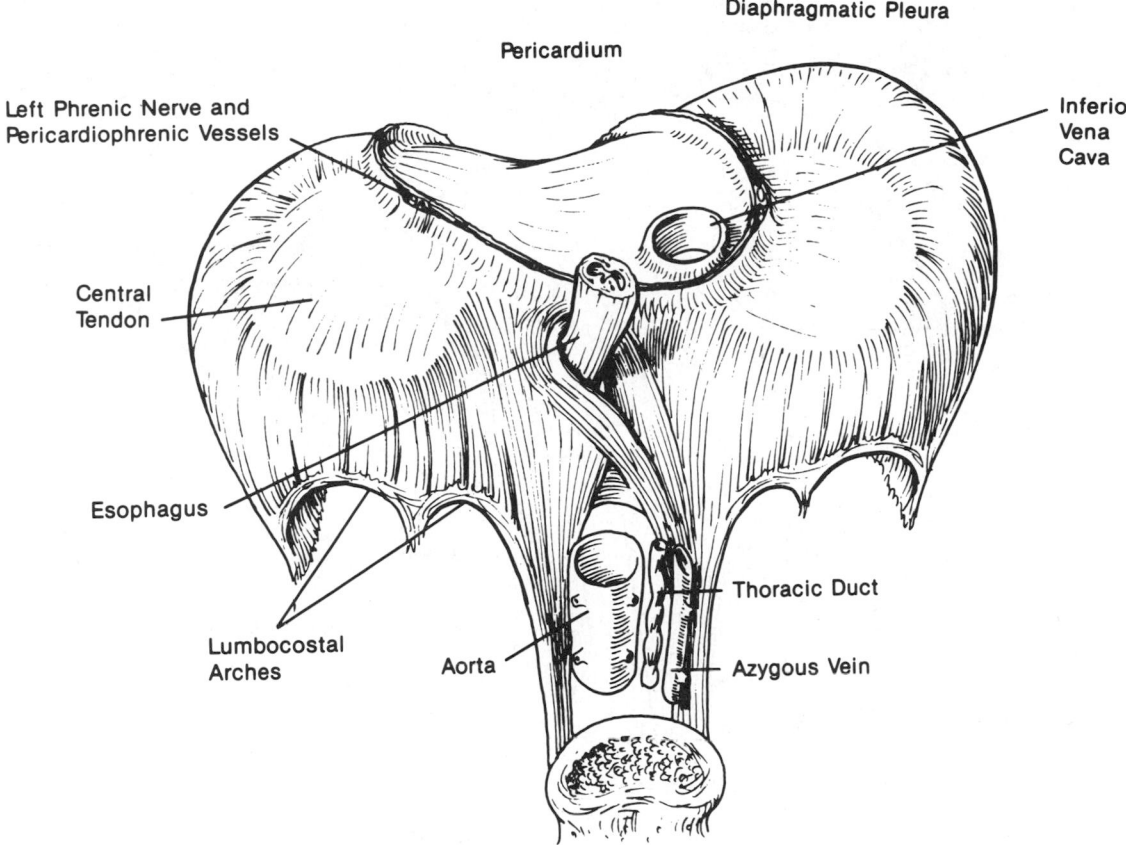

Figure 51-5. This posterior view of the diaphragm shows the placement of the major orifices. Three structures come through the aortic hiatus: the aorta, the thoracic duct, and the azygos vein. The esophageal hiatus, which is slightly higher and anterior to the aortic hiatus, contains the esophagus and the two vagus nerves. Note that the right crus of the diaphragm contributes the vast majority of the muscle fibers forming the esophageal hiatus. The most cephalad and anterior foramen contains the inferior vena cava. Note that the phrenic nerves and the pericardiophrenic vessels pass down along the lateral aspects of the pericardium behind the pleural surfaces. The phrenic nerves begin to branch into rami in most cases about 2 to 3 cm above the point at which they penetrate the diaphragm.

on the body wall, and a crural branch, which descends onto the crus and medial aspects of the musculature arising from the lumbocostal arches. The nerves are similar in their major branches; however, they are unique in their distributions, as may be seen in Figures 51-6 and 51-7.

Incisions in the diaphragm are made with regard to the phrenic nerve anatomy so as to preserve diaphragmatic function. Most of the incisions may be categorized as either circumferential or radial. Circumferential incisions are placed parallel to the rim of the central tendon and the costophrenic sinus to preserve the major branches of the phrenic nerve and the origins of the musculature on the body wall. Radial incisions start centrally and proceed toward the body wall so that the diaphragm is incised without transection of any of the major branches of the phrenic nerve. Combinations of the two types of incisions are used if necessary to achieve the required exposure.

The blood supply of the diaphragm originates from several sources. Probably the largest single source is the paired inferior phrenic arteries, which are below the diaphragm (Figs. 51-6 and 51-7). These arteries course out along the inferior aspect of the diaphragm and supply the diaphragm's medial and posterior portions. The musculophrenic artery originates from the distal portion of the internal thoracic artery, courses down from the internal thoracic artery in the chest along the costophrenic sulcus, and anastomoses with the intercostal arteries of the lower chest. The arch that this forms gives a good collateral blood supply to the sternal, costal, and lateral aspects of the musculature in the diaphragm. The pericardiophrenic arteries originate from the respective internal thoracic arteries high in the chest and course downward with the phrenic nerves to enter the diaphragm at the point of penetration of these nerves. These arteries contribute relatively little to the diaphragmatic blood supply but are essential for preservation of the blood supply to the phrenic nerves. The smaller, paired superior phrenic arteries arise from the aorta above the aortic hiatus and supply a varying portion of the crural fibers.

The venous drainage of the diaphragm is more variable than the arterial supply. Each of the arteries mentioned above has analogous veins; however, their distribution is far more variable than the distribution of the individual arteries. From

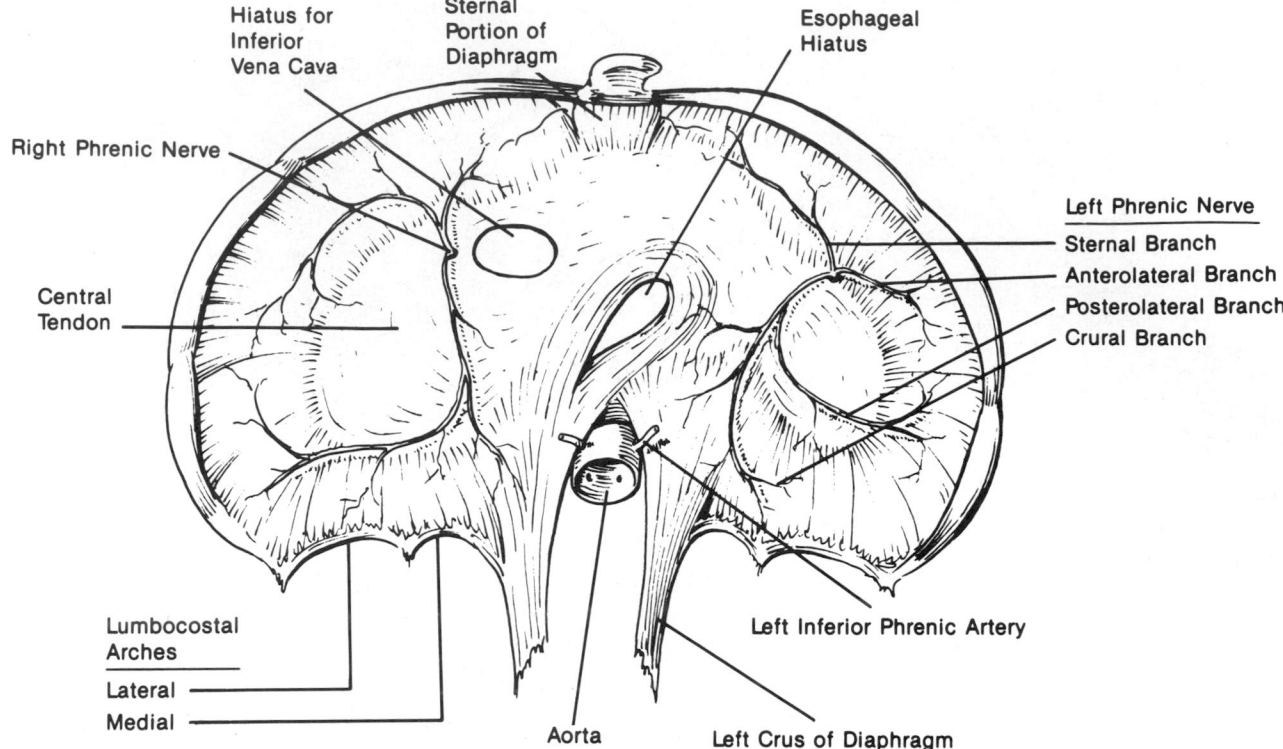

Figure 51-6. This inferior view of the diaphragm shows its innervation. Each phrenic nerve penetrates the diaphragm in a unique position. The right phrenic nerve is directly lateral to the vena cava and bifurcates into an anterior and a posterior branch. The anterior trunk gives off an anterolateral branch and a medial or sternal branch. The posterior trunk gives rise to a posterolateral and a pleural branch. The left phrenic nerve usually separates into two trunks before penetrating the diaphragm just anterior to the central tendon on the anterior aspect of the pericardium. A posterior trunk usually continues for several centimeters to give rise to a posterolateral branch and to a crural branch, which goes into the region of the left crura. The anterior trunk gives rise to a anterolateral branch and a medial or sternal branch going toward the sternum. Some small nerves arising from the chest wall and innervating some of the anterior, costal, and sternal portions of the diaphragm usually penetrate the membrane between the costal and sternal musculature.

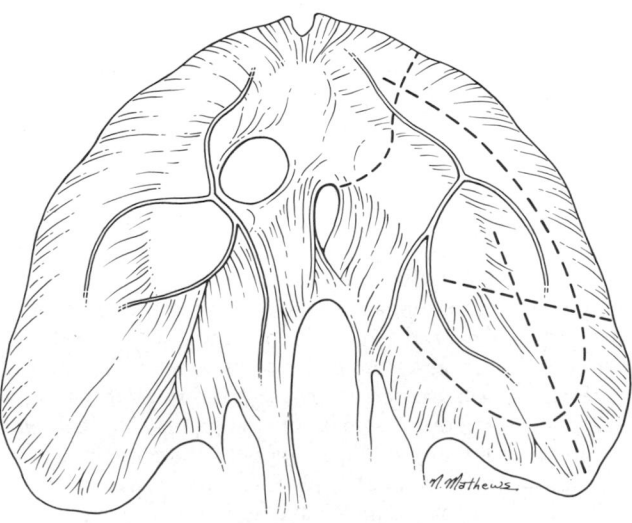

Figure 51-7. Course of phrenic nerves on diaphragm and various types of incisions used for diaphragmatic exposure. (Modified from Merendino KA, Johnson RJ, Skinner HH et al.: The intradiaphragmatic distribution of the phrenic nerve with particular reference to the placement of diaphragmatic incision and controlled segmental paralysis. Surgery 39:189, 1956, with permission.)

the inferior surface of the diaphragm there are paired inferior phrenic veins, which drain into the inferior vena caval system. The veins from the cephalad aspect of the diaphragm drain into the azygous and hemizygous veins. The veins that course with the musculophrenic arcade drain to the intercostal veins in the chest wall.

The diaphragm may be situated at a number of different positions in the chest, depending upon its state of contraction (Fig. 51-8). With maximum inspiration, the central tendon may come down as far as the ninth rib. With maximum expiration using the accessory muscles of expiration, the central tendon may migrate as far cephalad as the fourth rib. The state of contraction of the diaphragm causes motion in the lung by creating a negative intrathoracic pressure. The relation of the lung to the diaphragm is variable, depending on the position of the diaphragm (Fig. 51-9). In extreme expiration the phrenic sulcus of the pleural space may have very little lung tissue in it. When the diaphragm has migrated distally through muscular contraction, the lung obviously fills the sulcus fully.

The diaphragm, because of its unique domed shape and position, lies in an intimate relationship to a number of intrathoracic and intraperitoneal organs (Fig. 51-10). On the thoracic side, the heart and pericardium lie just cephalad to the

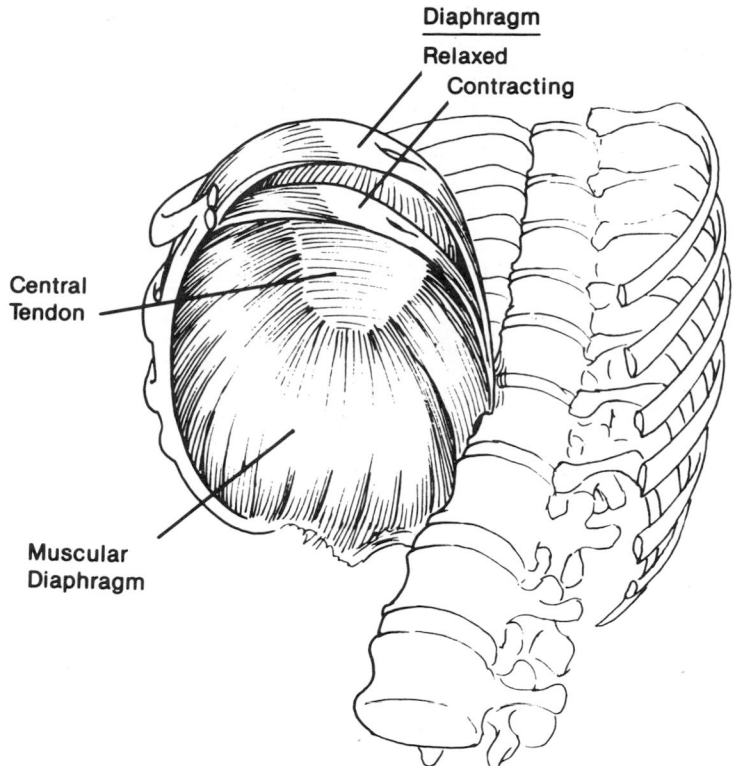

Figure 51-8. The diaphragm is shown in its contracted and relaxed states. In its relaxed state the central tendon of the diaphragm may proceed as high as the fourth or fifth intercostal space. With forced expiration, such as a patient may perform when anticipating a blow, the diaphragm may go as high as the fourth rib.

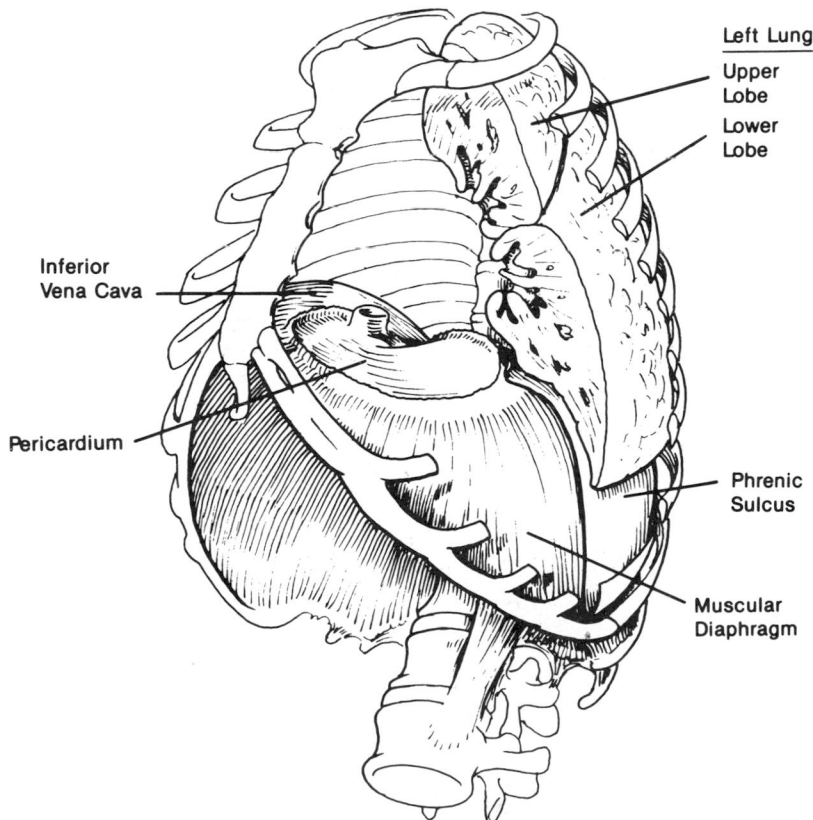

Figure 51-9. The relationship of the chest wall structures to the diaphragm and lung is shown in this left anterior oblique drawing. Note that the left lung protrudes down into the phrenic sulcus for a variable distance depending on the tension exerted by the diaphragm. When the diaphragm is very close to the chest wall, the lung recedes cephalad considerably. Note that the phrenic sulcus goes down to the tenth rib laterally and proceeds posteriorly.

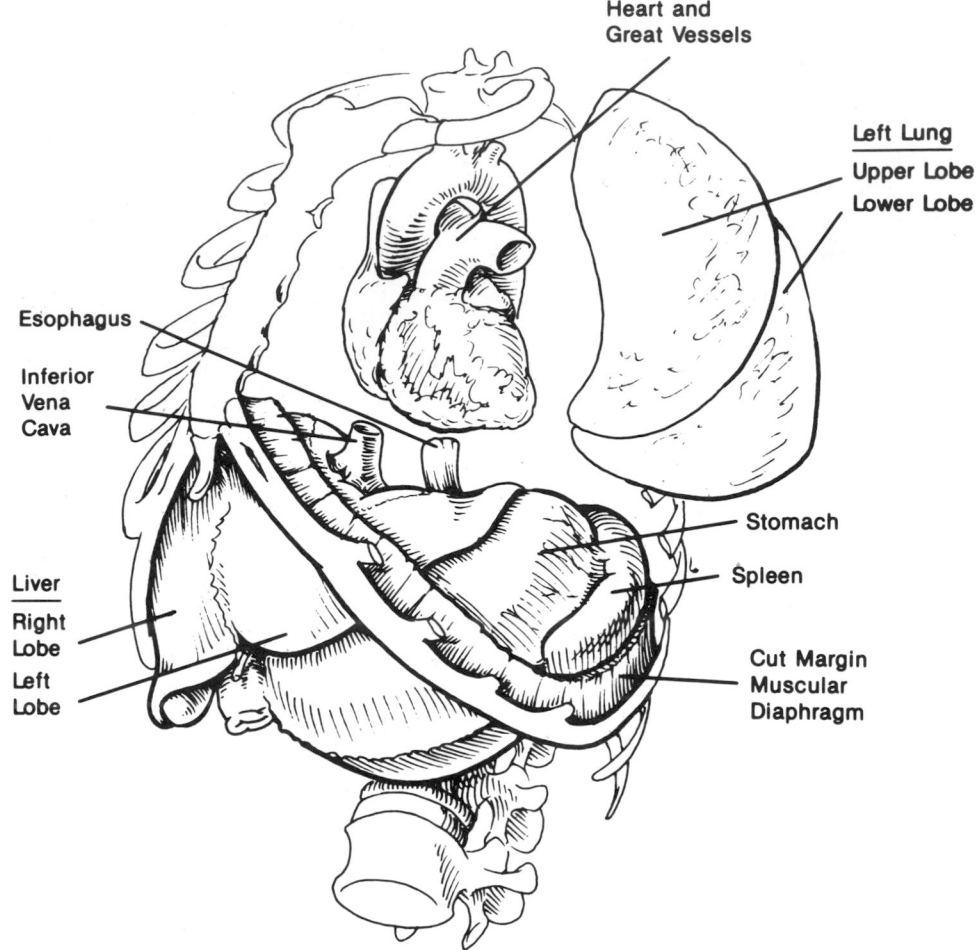

Figure 51-10.   The relationship of the upper abdominal viscera to the diaphragm are shown. The lung and heart have been displaced slightly cephalad and laterally to show their relative position with respect to the abdominal viscera and to promote clarity. Note that the spleen is posterior and lateral and is near the left phrenic sulcus. The stomach abuts on the central portion of the diaphragm and the anterior musculature more medially. The organ that has the largest surface area exposed to the diaphragm is obviously the liver. This structure lies more medial to the stomach and extends laterally toward the right to the costal margin.

medial portion of the central tendon, and the lungs abut on the lateral aspects of the diaphragm. On the peritoneal side, three major organs lie in direct proximity to the diaphragm. The largest of these is the liver, which has segments of both the right and the left lobe directly below the diaphragm (Fig. 51-10). A portion of its cardia and fundus of the stomach abut directly on the diaphragm. The spleen, which is situated laterally and posteriorly, lies directly below the diaphragm on the left side next to the costophrenic sinus. Thoracic surgical procedures on the diaphragm must recognize these important relationships, since injury to the abdominal viscera is a distinct possibility. The organs of the cephalad aspect of the peritoneal cavity may be accessed easily for operative procedures through diaphragmatic incisions.

INCISIONS

The diaphragm can be approached either through the chest or the abdomen. The route of access is dictated by the specific pathology to be corrected and the associated conditions pres-

ent at the time. Knowledge of the anatomy of the diaphragm and topography of the adjacent and traversing organs is a basic requirement. For selected conditions a combined thoracoabdominal approach may be employed.

A transabdominal approach allows easy access to both leaves of the diaphragm and correction of any associated intra-abdominal pathology at the same time. An upper midline or subcostal incision can be used. The lattter incision should be placed about two fingerbreadths below the costal margin to facilitate subsequent closure and avoid a scar over the costal arch. The falciform ligament and the right and left coronary ligaments of the liver may have to be divided for adequate exposure. Access to the diaphragm may be facilitated by use of the "upper hand" retractor.

A transthoracic approach allows excellent exposure of the ipsilateral hemidiaphragm from above. Thoracotomy is performed at or below the sixth intercostal space. By using double-lumen endotracheal intubation and intraoperative collapse of the lung, one can have an unobstructed view of the entire hemidiaphragm and the phrenic nerve. Associated intrathoracic pathology can be corrected at the same time.

Access can be gained to the intra-abdominal organs through carefully placed incisions in the diaphragm itself. The diaphragm can be divided circumferentially about 2 to 3 cm away from the lateral insertions, with complete avoidance of the major branches of the phrenic nerve (Fig. 51-7). Alternatively, the normal or pathologic openings in the diaphragm can be enlarged, or radial incisions may be required. In any case the surgeon must protect the main trunk of the phrenic nerve and have a mental picture of its major truncal branching (Merendino, et al., 1956). The diaphragm should be closed with interrupted nonabsorbable 0 sutures, with consideration of the constant stress on the suture line during respiration. Prosthetic material (Gore-Tex, Marlex) may be required in cases of insufficient tissue for primary closure.

KEY REFERENCE

Merendino KA, Johnson RJ, Skinner HH et al.: The intradiaphragmatic distribution of the phrenic nerve with particular reference to the placement of diaphragmatic incisions and controlled paralysis. Surgery 39:189, 1956

The best description of the phrenic nerve and location of various diaphragmatic incisions.

REFERENCES

Gray SW, Skandalakis JE: The diaphragm. p. 359. In Embryology for Surgeons. The Embryological Basis for the Treatment of Congenital Defects. WB Saunders, Philadelphia, 1972

Moore KL: Development of the diaphragm. p. 164. In The Developing Human. Clinically Oriented Embryology. 4th Ed. WB Saunders, Philadelphia, 1988

Congenital Hernias

Geoffrey M. Graeber   Jacob Davtyan
Joseph I. Miller, Jr.

Congenital diaphragmatic hernias are classified as (1) posterolateral (Bochdalek), (2) retrosternal anterior (Morgagni), (3) septum transversum (central), or (4) esophageal hiatal. The first three are discussed in this chapter. Hiatal hernias are discussed in *Esophageal Surgery*.

POSTEROLATERAL HIATAL HERNIA OF BOCHDALEK

HISTORICAL NOTE

Although Vincent Bochdalek's 1848 description was that of bowel herniation through a dorsal diaphragmatic split into the lumbocostal triangle, the congenital posterolateral diaphragmatic hernia (CPLDH) carries his name. Gross (1946) performed the first successful repair of CPLDH in a newborn in 1946. Bartlett, et al. (1976) reported successful application of extracorporeal membrane oxygenation (ECMO) in infancy. German et al. (1977) reported the first survivor of ECMO in treatment of CPLDH.

CPLDH occurs in 1 in 2,000 to 1 in 5,000 live births (Harrison and de Lorimier, 1981) and is a result of failure of the pleuroperitoneal canal to close at the eighth week of gestation (Gray and Skandalakis, 1972). Of these hernias, 80 percent occur on the left side. Bilateral hernias are extremely rare (Levy, et al., 1969), and very few of these newborns survive (Sokal, et al., 1990). In only 10 percent of cases is there a true hernia sac. The abdominal organs herniate into the chest through the diaphragmatic defect, compressing and retarding the growth and development of the ipsilateral lung. The mediastinum may be shifted to the opposite side, affecting the contralateral lung as well. The morphology of the diaphragmatic muscle is normal (Dietz and Pongratz, 1991). The morphologic and biochemical development of the lungs is retarded in most cases, particularly on the ipsilateral side (Nakamura, et al., 1991). The susceptibility of these babies to bronchopulmonary dysplasia during artificial ventilation is probably related to a defective antioxidant system and defective surfactant production (Molenaar, et al., 1991). Pulmonary hypoplasia is also evident in pulmonary function studies. Nakayama, et al. (1991) showed restrictive lung defects in infants who survived neonatal repair of CPLDH, and Geggel, et al. (1985) reported decrease of the cross-sectional area of the pulmonary arterial bed in infants dying after repair of CPLDH. Associated major anomalies occur in up to 40 percent of live births (Cunniff et al., 1990). Thorp-Beeston, et al. (1989) reported prenatal diagnosis of major abnormalities in 48 percent of fetuses, including chromosomal defects in 31 percent and major malformations in 17 percent. Trisomy 18 and trisomy 13 are the most common chromosomal abnormalities. Cardiac, neural, and genitourinary anomalies are frequent (Adzick, et al., 1989). Malrotation of the bowel is always present.

HISTORICAL READINGS

Bartlett RH, Gazzaniga AB, Jeffries MR et al.: Extracorporeal membrane oxygenation (ECMO): cardiopulmonary support in infancy. Trans Am Soc Artif Intern Organs 22:80, 1976

Cunniff, Jones KL, Jones MC: Patterns of malformation in children with congenital diaphragmatic defects. J Pediatr 116:258, 1990

Dietz HG, Pongratz D: Morphology of the diaphragmatic muscle in CDH. Eur J Pediatr Surg 1:85, 1991

Geggel RL, Murphy JD, Langleben D et al.: Congenital diaphragmatic hernia: arterial structural changes and persistent pulmonary hypertension after surgical repair. J Pediatr 107:457, 1985

German JC, Gazzaniga AB, Amlie R et al.: Management of pulmonary insufficiency in diaphragmatic hernia using extracorporeal circulation with a membrane oxygenator (ECMO). J Pediatr Surg 12:905, 1977

Gray SW, Skandalakis JE: The diaphragm. p. 359. In Embryology for Surgeons. The Embryological Basis for the Treatment of Congenital Defects. WB Saunders, 1972

Gross RE: Congenital hernia of the diaphragm. Am J Dis Child 71:580, 1946

Harrison MR, de Lorimier AA: Congenital diaphragmatic hernia. Surg Clin North Am 61:1023, 1981

Levy JL Jr, Guyner WA, Louis JE et al.: Bilateral congenital diaphragmatic hernias through the foramina of Bochdalek. J Pediatr Surg 4:557, 1969

Molenaar JC, Bos AP, Hazelbrock FWJ, et al.: Congenital diaphragmatic hernia, what defect? J Pediatr Surg 26:248, 1991

Nakamura Y, Yamamoto I, Fukuda S et al.: Pulmonary acinar development in diaphragmatic hernia. Arch Pathol Lab Med 115:372, 1991

Nakayama DK, Motoyama EK, Mutich RL et al.: Pulmonary function in newborns after repair of congenital diaphragmatic hernia. Pediatr Pulmonol 11:49, 1991

Sokal MM, Yellin PB, Mestel AL et al.: Survival after bilateral congenital diaphragmatic hernia. Clin Pediatr (Phila) 29:677, 1990

Thorpe-Beeston JG, Gosden CM, Nicolaides KH: Prenatal diagnosis of congenital diaphragmatic hernia: associated malformations and chromosomal defects. Fetal Ther 4:21, 1989

BASIC SCIENCE

Pathophysiology

The pathophysiology of CPLDH depends on the interplay of pulmonary hypoplasia and pulmonary hypertension. Hypoplastic lungs result in various degrees of hypoxia. In addition, such lungs have increased sensitivity to the stimuli increasing pulmonary vascular resistance, namely hypoxia, acidosis, hypercarbia, hypothermia (Shochat, 1987). The resulting pulmonary hypertension reverses the flow through the patent ductus arteriosus and opens the foramen ovale with right-to-left shunting. Thus, the syndrome of persistent fetal circulation (Gersony, et al., 1969) is established, resulting in the vicious circle of hypoxia, acidosis, even higher pulmonary resistance, and increasing right-to-left shunting, which ultimately culminates in death of these babies.

DIAGNOSIS

The clinical presentation depends on the degree of respiratory compromise, which may vary from severe distress at birth to delayed presentation in infancy or early childhood. The age of the patient at presentation is one of the determining factors of morbidity and mortality (Reynolds, et al., 1984). The newborn with CPLDH is usually dyspneic, tachycardic, and frequently cyanotic with a striking scaphoid abdomen. The trachea and the heart are shifted to the contralateral side. Breath sounds are decreased or absent on the ipsilateral side. Chest x-ray may be diagnostic, with bowel loops in the affected hemithorax and contralateral mediastinal shift. The gastric tube may be seen in the chest, and paucity of gas is noted in the abdomen. On the right the defect may be blocked by the liver, with less extensive herniation and milder respiratory compromise.

The clinical presentation of the infant suffering from foramen of Bochdalek hernia is dependent on the size of the defect and the amount of visceral migration that occurs from the peritoneal cavity to the ipsilateral pleural space. In small hernias the amount of migration of abdominal viscera into the thoracic cavity is minimal. In these cases the patients do not present until later in infancy or even childhood. Symptoms range from discomfort to feeding abnormalities and colicky symptoms with poor progression of growth. Radiographs of the chest generally define these hernias because air is located in one of the viscera that has herniated through the foramen.

Correction of small hernias presenting after the perinatal period is generally conducted through an ipsilateral thoracotomy. The hernia sac, if present, is generally identified, the abdominal viscera are reduced into the peritoneal cavity, the sac is excised, and the defect is closed. Closure is usually affected by horizontal mattress sutures placed over pledgets. Occasionally the repair is reinforced with a running suture line placed superficial to the horizontal mattress sutures. Prosthetic patch reconstruction is seldom necessary. In infants and children presenting in this manner, morbidity and mortality from the condition and its operative correction are minimal. The condition can be severe, however, since severe respiratory distress and even death have been reported with rapid expansion of abdominal viscera into the chest.

Infants who present with large congenital defects of the diaphragm usually have respiratory distress very early in the immediate perinatal period. Auscultation of the chest at that time reveals bowel sounds in the chest on the side of the hernia. In the usual presentation of an infant with this type of hernia, the bowel sounds are in the left chest, and the heart sounds are displaced toward the right side of the chest. The abdomen is scaphoid since the viscera are in the chest. Compression of the ipsilateral lung also causes a severe decrease in or absence of breath sounds on the ipsilateral side. The mediastinum is shifted to the contralateral side, and in severe cases the contralateral lung is also compressed by the shift of the thoracic viscera secondary to the migration of the abdominal viscera into the pleural space. Auscultation of the abdomen demonstrates a relative absence of bowel sounds, which is consistent with the migration of the bowels into the left chest. Confirmation of the diagnosis is usually obtained radiographically. If a nasogastric or orogastric tube has been placed prior to the film, the tip of the tube will be above the diaphragm, particularly with left-sided hernias. This defines the stomach as being in the left pleural space. The radiograph will also demonstrate bowels in the affected pleural space (Fig. 51-11). The infant should not have mask ventilation at this time, since mask ventilation promotes deposition of air in the gastrointestinal tract, which causes further distension of the stomach. The infant should be intubated, an umbilical line should be established, and the patient should be prepared for immediate surgical correction.

MANAGEMENT

Preoperative Management

The clinical suspicion of CPLDH in a newborn with respiratory distress mandates endotracheal intubation, assisted ventilation, and orogastric tube decompression of the gastrointestinal tract to prevent further bowel distension and worsening of respiratory compromise. These babies are maintained with an inspired oxygen fraction (FIO_2) of 1.0, peak

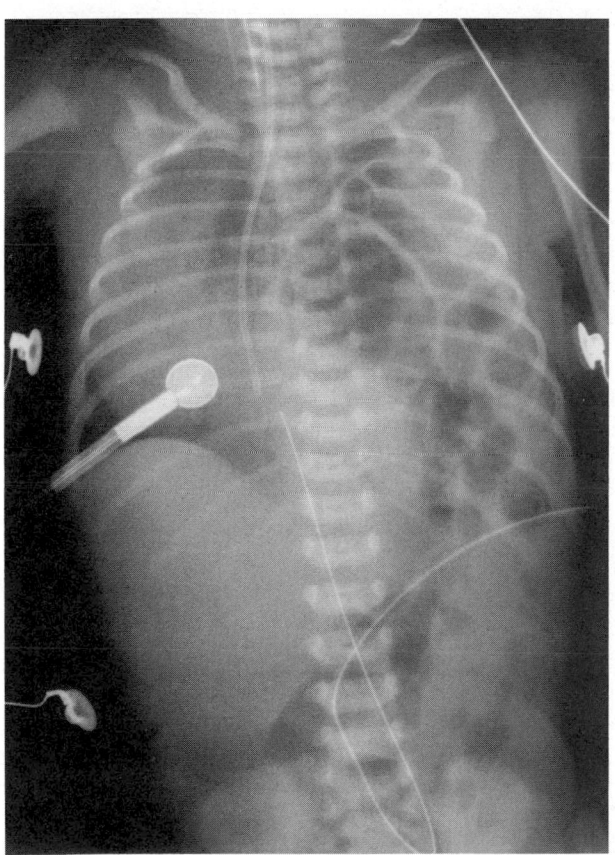 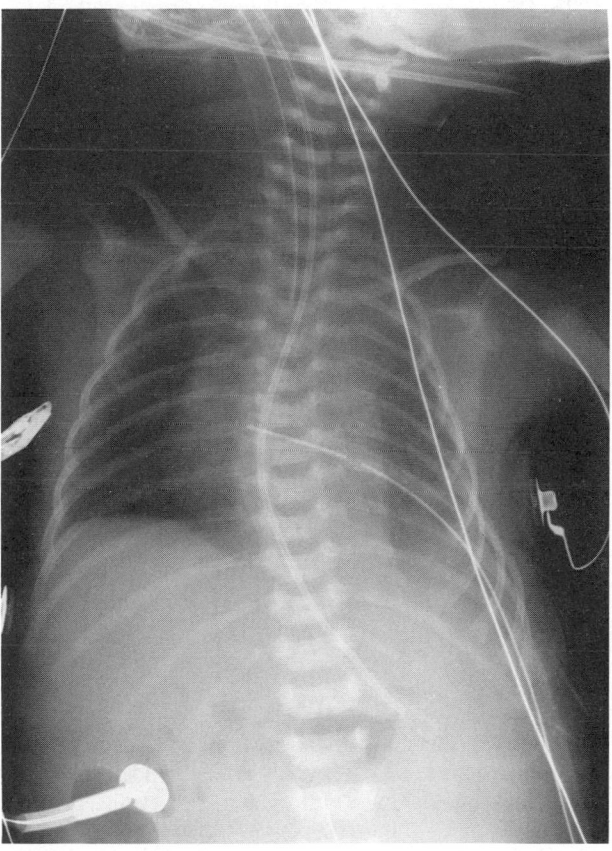

A   B

Figure 51-11. **(A)** This radiograph demonstrates the typical findings of a newborn infant who has a foramen of Bochdalek hernia. Note that the abdominal viscera have migrated through the diaphragm and are occupying the left pleural space. The mediastinal contents, great vessels, and tracheobronchial tree are all shifted to the right. Note that the cardiac silhouette blends with the compressed pulmonary parenchyma on the right side and that the stomach, colon, and small bowel are all in the left chest. The child has been intubated and is being prepared for emergency surgical correction. **(B)** This postoperative chest radiograph shows that the hernia has been corrected and that a chest tube is in place in the left pleural space. Note that the left lung does not totally fill the left pleural space. This is consistent with severe hypoplasia in the lung; the chest tube has been properly placed but does not establish complete expansion of the lung. The tracheal air column, the cardiac silhouette, the great vessels, and the rest of the mediastinal structures have returned to their normal position. Note also that the right lung is fully expanded and is no longer compressed by the displacement of the mediastinal structures.

inspiratory pressure below 30 cmH$_2$O, positive end-expiratory pressure (PEEP) of less than 5 cmH$_2$O, and hyperventilation. High-frequency ventilation may be used. Preductal and postductal arterial blood gases are monitored by right radial and umbilical arterial catheters, respectively. Ideally, postductal arterial oxygen tension (PaO$_2$) is maintained above 100 mmHg, arterial carbon dioxide tension (PaCO$_2$) below 30 mmHg, and pH above 7.50 to prevent and alleviate pulmonary vasospasm. Sodium bicarbonate and tromethamine (THAM) may be used to treat acidosis. Venous access and maintenance of systolic blood pressure higher than 50 mmHg are basic. Fluids are kept to a minimum. Babies should be paralyzed with pancuronium and anesthetized with fentanyl. Fentanyl use is thought to be associated with decreased frequency and severity of episodes of pulmonary hypertension (Vacanti, 1989; Vacanti, et al., 1984) as well as with decreased incidence of pneumothorax, a catastrophic complication (Hansen, et al., 1984).

Multiple attempts have been made to define the predictive factors of mortality of patients with CPLDH (Raphaely and Downes, 1973; Boix-Ochoa, et al., 1974; Boix-Ochoa, et al., 1977; Mishalany, et al., 1979; Ruff, et al., 1980; Manthei, et al., 1983; Wilson, et al., 1991). Admission or preoperative blood gas values, specifically, a pH higher than 7.2, a PaCO$_2$ below 35 mmHg, and a PaO$_2$ above 100 mmHg are associated with an excellent prognosis. Patients with pH below 7.0, PaCO$_2$ above 50 mmHg, and PaO$_2$ below 80 mmHg fare poorly. Vacanti et al. (1984) termed the infants achieving a postductal PaO$_2$ above 100 mmHg with standard therapy *responders* and those who were unable to achieve a postductal PaO$_2$ of 100 mmHg with maximum therapy *nonresponders*. The responders most often survived without ECMO. Nonresponders had more severe pulmonary hyperplasia and pulmonary hypertension not responsive to medical and ventilatory interventions; in the past all these babies died without ECMO (Vacanti, 1989). Bohn (1987) compared preductal PaCO$_2$ levels with ventilatory index (VI). Among those with a PaCO$_2$ of 40 mmHg and a VI over 1,000 there was 100 percent survival. Preoperative alveolar-arterial oxygen difference [P(A-a)O$_2$] calculated from preductal (right radial) arterial blood gas is another predictor of outcome. Survivors have P(A-a)O$_2$ below 200 mmHg; those with P(A-a)O$_2$ above 200 mmHg rarely survive (Bohn, 1987).

Operative Repair

Traditionally the newborns with CPLDH are taken to the operating room as an emergency after expeditious resuscitation. Neck lines should be avoided, preserving the vessels for possible ECMO. A transabdominal subcostal approach is preferred by most for left-sided lesions whereas a transthoracic approach may be more useful for right-sided hernias. Herniated organs are returned to the peritoneal cavity, and the seldom present hernia sac is excised. The lung is inspected, but no attempt should be made to expand the hypoplastic lung. The extralobar pulmonary sequestration, occasionally present, should be excised. The edges of the defect are defined. Frequently, a significant span of the posterior diaphragm can be unrolled after incision of the posterior peritoneum.

Most of the defects can be closed primarily with interrupted nonabsorbable sutures. In rare cases of absent posterior rim, the sutures can be passed around the ribs. Large defects can be closed with a prosthetic patch. The left pleural space is drained with a 12 Fr chest tube, which should be placed to an underwater seal but never to suction. A contralateral chest tube is also placed. If the patient's condition permits, the malrotation should be corrected. The abdomen is closed by using techniques developed for closure of abdominal wall defects and digital stretching of the anterior wall is performed. If primary fascial closure is impossible, only the skin can be closed, leaving ventral hernia to be closed later. Occasionally the "silo" technique has to be used.

Surgical correction of a severe foramen of Bochdalek hernia presenting in the perinatal period is conducted through an upper abdominal approach. After the peritoneal cavity has been opened, the abdominal viscera are reduced from the pleural cavity. If a peritoneal sac is present, it will be resected following the removal of the abdominal viscera from the defect. A 10 Fr chest tube is placed in the pleural cavity to evacuate fluids, to aid in the reexpansion, and to ensure that no pressure occurs in the affected pleural space. Although the chest tube in many cases may not completely reexpand the ipsilateral lung, the equalization of pressure will allow return of the mediastinum to the midline and will remove any pressure on the contralateral lung. Before the defect is repaired, any extralobar pulmonary sequestration that may be present should be surgically removed. If the defect is relatively small, it may be closed by the direct suture technique as outlined previously. If the defect is substantial and can only be closed with tension, synthetic patch reconstruction should be performed. The patch should be sewn to the margin of the defect with permanent horizontal mattress sutures. Some surgeons believe that this suture line should be reinforced with a running, fine Prolene suture superficial to the original layer of horizontal mattress sutures. The peritoneal cavity should then be inspected for obstructing duodenal bands and malrotation of the midgut, which are often present. These conditions should be corrected before closure is started.

Closure of the abdomen can sometimes be difficult, since the abdominal viscera have not matured in the peritoneal cavity. With return of the abdominal viscera into the peritoneal cavity, compression of the diaphragm can occur with a tight abdominal wall closure. Such compression would impede good excursion of the diaphragm and ventilation of the patient. In order to avoid this serious complication, a ventral epigastric hernia may be created. In such cases the fascia and musculature are left open, only the skin being closed. If sufficient relaxing incisions cannot be made by mobilizing only the skin and subcutaneous tissues to close the defect, a surgical gastroschisis is created. In such cases the peritoneal cavity is not large enough to hold the viscera without causing serious encroachment on the diaphragm. The surgical gastroschisis repair is made by using synthetic material to fashion a pouch along the anterior abdominal wall that contains a portion of the viscera. The abdominal viscera are gradually returned to the enlarging peritoneal cavity by gentle, progressive compression of the pouch without causing undue embarrassment of respiratory function.

The management of the chest tube during the operation and in the immediate postoperative period has been a source of some controversy. Some surgeons prefer to leave the chest tube to water seal, whereas others advocate placing a one-way valve in the tube and allowing for manual pressure equalization. Still others advocate gentle negative pressure generated through a water seal system to promote expansion of the lung and relief of pressure in the chest. In general, the majority feel that water seal drainage or gentle suction across a water seal drainage is most beneficial.

Timing of the Operation

As stated earlier, most newborns with CPLDH are operated on emergently. Recently, however, there have been several reports of comparable or even better results with delayed repair after various periods of medical stabilization (Breaux, et al., 1991; Cartlidge, et al., 1986; Langer, et al., 1988; Hazelbrock, et al., 1988; Haugen, et al., 1991; Charlton, et al., 1991). To answer these and many other questions regarding the proper management of newborns with CPLDH, a large, multicenter, prospective randomized study is necessary.

A recent development in the treatment of CPLDH is antenatal surgical therapy (Harrison and deLorimier, 1991; Harrison, et al., 1990a,b). There is an ongoing debate over the feasibility of this experimental therapy (Stolar, 1990). It imposes a risk to the mother as well as to the fetus with potentially fatal results for both. The proper indications for this procedure are yet to be defined (Wenstrom et al., 1991).

Long-term Results

Although some respiratory abnormalities can be found in survivors of CPLDH, they generally have a normal life and carry on normal physical activity (Frenckner and Freyschuss, 1988). Most of these studies were performed in the follow-up of patients operated on in the pre-ECMO era. As more severely affected babies survive the modern therapy, their prognosis may be different (Falconer, et al., 1990).

RETROSTERNAL ANTERIOR DIAPHRAGMATIC HERNIA (MORGAGNI)

BASIC SCIENCE

Retrosternal anterior diaphragmatic hernia was described by Morgagni in 1769. It is much less frequent than posterolateral hernia, accounting for only 1 to 6 percent of all congenital defects of the diaphragm (Cullen, et al., 1985). The herniation occurs between the xiphoid and costochondral attachments of the diaphragm, more frequently on the right side (Gray and Skandalakis, 1972).

In rare cases foramen of Morgagni hernias arise in the potential spaces between the sternum and the costal muscular portions of the diaphragm (Fig. 51-7). These spaces, through which the internal thoracic vessels exit the thorax to become the superior epigastric vessels as they enter the rectus sheath,

exist just lateral to the posterior table of the sternum. On the left side this potential space is partially protected by the pericardium. For this reason herniation through this foramen is more common the right. The visceral peritoneum is usually complete adjacent to both potential spaces. Hence, a foramen of Morgagni hernia usually has a true hernia sac when the abdominal viscera protrude into this space. Any one of the abdominal viscera that has a mesentery may protrude into either one of these potential spaces.

The most frequent organs to protrude into a foramen of Morgagni hernia are the colon, the omentum, the stomach, and the small bowel. Such hernias infrequently present in childhood; more commonly this rare entity presents in the adult with varying symptoms. Obese individuals are more commonly affected than slender patients, and women are more commonly affected than men. Many foramen of Morgagni hernias may be missed because the radiographic indication of a fat pad to the right of the pericardium is mistaken for a pericardial fat pad or a pleuropericardial cyst. Colicky pain is a relatively infrequent finding, as is vascular compromise of the organs herniated into the space. Colonic, gastric, and intestinal volvulus has been reported, although the volvulus is seldom total; rather, the volvulus is relenting in nature, causing the patient to have intermittent symptoms of partial gastric, colonic, or intestinal obstruction. Complete obstruction of any one of these viscera can occur but is extremely rare.

DIAGNOSIS

A strong suspicion of the foramen of Morgagni hernia may be generated by the plain posterior, anterior, and lateral radiographs. An excessively large density in the region of the fat pad on the pericardium should suggest the diagnosis, which can occasionally be confirmed by the plain films alone. Computed tomography (CT), magnetic resonance imaging (MRI), and ultrasound may confirm the diagnosis, depending on what abdominal viscera are in the sac. Occasionally, upper gastrointestinal or colonic contrast radiography will be necessary to confirm the diagnosis by identification of the stomach, small bowel, or colon above the diaphragm in the peristernal position (Fig. 51-12). Often CT scans and/or MRI will make this diagnosis without contrast since loops of bowel will be found in a demonstrable hernia sac. If the patient has only omentum in the hernial sac or the diagnosis is equivocal for any reason, a diagnostic pneumoperitoneum may be conducted to outline the hernia sac. In such cases the hernia sac will be outlined by the air entering the hernia and defining the omentum and/or other structures.

MANAGEMENT

Surgical Repair

An abdominal approach for repair of this hernia is indicated in most instances. An upper abdominal incision based on the patient's body habitus, the size of the hernial contents, and the extent of the hernia sac allows excellent visualization. Foramen of Morgagni hernias have been repaired through subcostal, paramedian, and midline incisions. Once the peritoneal cavity is entered, the abdominal viscera are withdrawn

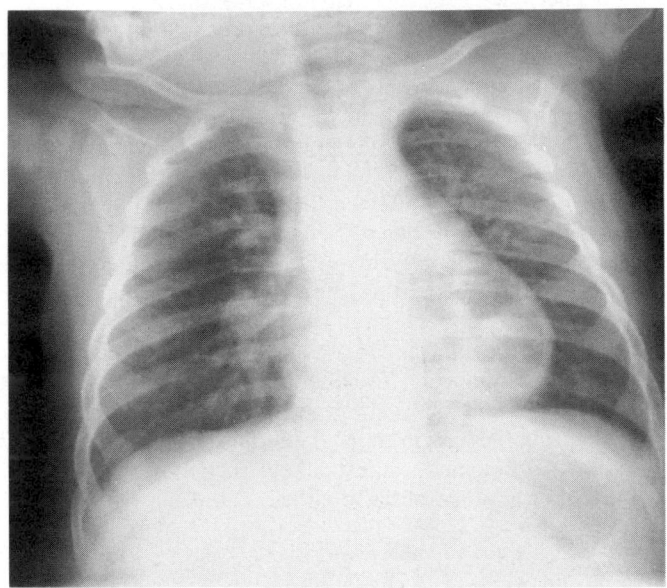

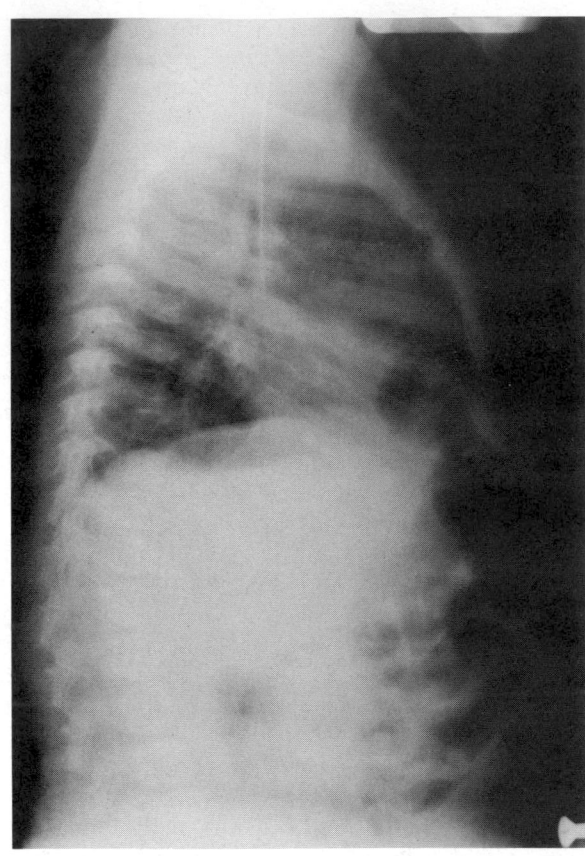

A

B

Figure 51-12. **(A & B)** These radiographs demonstrate a loop of colon filled with air protruding into a foramen of Morgagni hernia. The bowel was not strangulated or obstructed when the examination was performed. The patient suffered from fullness and cramping abdominal pain. An abdominal approach was used in correcting the hernia. The child had an uneventful postoperative course.

from the hernia sac and reduced to their normal anatomic positions. All adhesions are taken down. The hernia sac is then defined, introduced into the peritoneal cavity, and resected. The repair of the defect may be effected by several means.

When the defect is small and the edges are relatively mobile, horizontal mattress sutures of 0-gauge braided permanent material may be placed to close the defect. Some surgeons prefer using polypropylene. In some instances the edges may be oversewn with a running suture superficial to the horizontal mattress suture to further secure closure. Under no circumstances should the edges of the defect be closed under tension since if they are, the hernia has a distinct tendency to recur. Many surgeons prefer to close the defect with synthetic patch material if the defect is too large for the edges to come together without tension. In such cases the prosthetic material is joined to the edges of the diaphragmatic defect and/or the chest wall by permanent synthetic horizontal mattress sutures, which are tied individually. Some surgeons prefer to oversew the suture line with a running polypropylene suture after the horizontal mattress suture layer has been placed. Prosthetic materials that have found favor include polytetrafluoroethylene (PTFE) sheeting, woven Dacron, and various synthetic meshes. Most surgeons now prefer the PTFE sheeting since it has a relatively low

adhesion rate, is pliable, and sutures well to both muscle and the chest wall.

When the foramen of Morgagni hernia is identified through a thoracic incision, the principles of repair are much the same. The hernial sac is entered, the visceral contents are dissected and reduced into the abdomen, the sac is resected, and repair is performed. Under no circumstances should closure be completed under tension. If horizontal mattress sutures will not close the defect appropriately, a soft tissue patch, such as PTFE sheeting, may be used for this purpose. In such instances horizontal mattress sutures of permanent material are placed around the edges. Some practitioners prefer using pledgets on the diaphragmatic surface. Along the chest wall, the sutures may be placed around a rib or costal cartilage to secure the closure. Occasionally sutures have to be placed through the periosteum of the sternum to effect an adequate repair. The primary suture line may then be reinforced, if necessary, with a continuous running suture.

Postoperative Management

Postoperative care is the same as with any other patient who has had major abdominal surgery. The patient is kept NPO until bowel sounds return and flatus is passed per rectum.

Judicious intervenous fluid replacement therapy is maintained. Antibiotics are used appropriately if any one of the abdominal viscera has been opened. If the hernia has been repaired through a thoracic incision, chest tubes are placed to maintain the expansion of the lung. In most cases the patient will enjoy a benign postoperative course and should be discharged within 6 to 10 days after the repair.

SEPTUM TRANSVERSUM (CENTRAL) DIAPHRAGMATIC HERNIA

BASIC SCIENCE

Septum transversum diaphragmatic hernias are extremely rare and are among the midline congenital defects, which may also include omphalocele, sternal defect, and pentalogy of Cantrell (Milne, et al., 1990; Cantrell, et al., 1958). There is a high incidence of gastrointestinal anomalies, absent pericardium, and herniation of the heart through the defect (Wesselhoeft and DeLuca, 1984; Lee, et al., 1991).

Diagnosis

Diagnostic workup may include plain x-rays of the chest and abdomen, ultrasound, contrast studies of the gastrointestinal tract, and nuclear scan. A cardiac workup may be required to delineate the congenital heart defects.

Management

Surgical repair is best done through the abdomen to enable correction of intra-abdominal pathology. The first priority is to reduce the herniated organs into their respective cavities and to close the diaphragmatic defect (Touloukian, 1984)—only then is the omphalocele, if present, dealt with. Congenital heart defects may require repair as well.

KEY REFERENCES

Connors RH, Weber TR, Randolph JG: The diaphragm: developmental, traumatic, and neoplastic disorders. p. 531. In Baue AE, Geha AS, Hammond GL et al. (eds): Glenn's Thoracic and Cardiovascular Surgery, 5th Ed. Appleton & Lange, East Norwalk, CT, 1991

A good reference to general disorders of the diaphragm.

O'Rourke PP, Lillehei CW, Crone RK et al.: The effect of extracorporeal membrane oxygenation on the survival of neonates with high-risk congenital diaphragmatic hernia: 45 cases from a single institution. J Pediatr Surg 26:147, 1991

Excellent review article on the role of ECMO in congenital diaphragmatic hernia.

REFERENCES

Adzick NS, Vacanti JP, Lillehei CW et al.: Fetal diaphragmatic hernia: ultrasound diagnosis and clinical outcome in 38 cases. J Pediatr Surg 24:654, 1989

Bartlett RH, Gazzaniga AB, Jeffries MR et al.: Extracorporeal membrane oxygenation (ECMO): cardiopulmonary support in infancy. Trans Am Soc Artif Intern Organs 22:80, 1976

Bohn D: Blood gas and ventilatory parameters in predicting survival in congenital diaphragmatic hernia. Pediatr Surg Int 2:336, 1978

Boix-Ochoa J, Natal A, Canal J et al.: The important influence of arterial blood gases on the prognosis of congenital diaphragmatic hernia. World J Surg 1:783, 1977

Boix-Ochoa J, Peguero G, Seijo G et al.: Acid-base balance and blood gases in prognosis and therapy of congenital diaphragmatic hernia. J Pediatr Surg 19:49, 1974

Breaux CW Jr, Rouse TM, Cain WS et al.: Improvement in survival of patients with congenital diaphragmatic hernia utilizing a strategy of delayed repair after medical and/or extracorporeal membrane oxygenation stabilization. J Pediatr Surg 26:333, 1991

Cantrell JR, Haller JA, Ravitch MM: A syndrome of congenital defects involving the abdominal wall, sternum, diaphragm, pericardium, and heart. Surg Gynecol Obstet 107:602, 1958

Cartlidge PHT, Mann NP, Kapila L: Preoperative stabilization in congenital diaphragmatic hernia. Arch Dis Child 61:1226, 1986

Charlton AJ, Bruce J, Davenport M: Timing of surgery in congenital diaphragmatic hernia. Low mortality after preoperative stabilization. Anaesthesia 46:820, 1991

Cullen ML, Klein MD, Phillippart AI: Congenital diaphragmatic hernia. Surg Clin North Am 65:1115, 1985

Cunniff, Jones KL, Jones MC: Patterns of malformation in children with congenital diaphragmatic defects. J Pediatr 116:258, 1990

Dietz HG, Pongratz D: Morphology of the diaphragmatic muscle in CDH. Eur J Pediatr Surg 1:85, 1991

Falconer AR, Brown RA, Helms P et al.: Pulmonary sequelae in survivors of congenital diaphragmatic hernia. Thorax 45:126, 1990

Frenckner B, Freyschuss U: Pulmonary function after repair of congenital diaphragmatic hernia—a short review. Pediatr Surg Int 3:11, 1988

Geggel RL, Murphy JD, Langleben D et al.: Congenital diaphragmatic hernia: arterial structural changes and persistent pulmonary hypertension after surgical repair. J Pediatr 107:457, 1985

German JC, Gazzaniga AB, Amlie R et al.: Management of pulmonary insufficiency in diaphragmatic hernia using extracorporeal circulation with a membrane oxygenator (ECMO). J Pediatr Surg 12:905, 1977

Gersony WM, Duc CV, Sinclair JD: "PFC" syndrome (persistence of fetal circulation). Circulation, suppl. III, 39:87, 1969

Gray SW, Skandalakis JE: The diaphragm. p. 359. In Embryology for Surgeons. The Embryological Basis for the Treatment of Congenital Defects. WB Saunders, 1972

Gross RE: Congenital hernia of the diaphragm. Am J Dis Child 71:580, 1946

Hansen J, Jones S, Burrington J et al.: The decreasing incidence of pneumothorax and improving survival in infants with congenital diaphragmatic hernia. J Pediatr Surg 19:385, 1984

Harrison MR, Adzick NS, Longaker MT et al.: Successful repair in utero of a fetal diaphragmatic hernia after removal of herniated viscera from the left thorax. N Engl J Med 322:1582, 1990a

Harrison MR, de Lorimier AA: Congenital diaphragmatic hernia. Surg Clin North Am 61:1023, 1981

Harrison MR, Langer JC, Adzick NS et al.: Correction of congenital diaphragmatic hernia in utero. V. Initial clinical experience. J Pediatr Surg 25:47, 1990b

Haugen SE, Linker D, Eik-Nes S et al.: Congenital diaphragmatic hernia: determination of the optimal time for operation by echocardiographic monitoring of the pulmonary arterial pressure. J Pediatr Surg 26:560, 1991

Hazelbrock FWJ, Tibboel D, Bos AP et al.: Congenital diaphragmatic hernia: impact of preoperative stabilization. A prospective pilot study in 13 patients. J Pediatr Surg 23:1139, 1988

Langer JC, Filler RM, Bohn DJ et al.: Timing of surgery for congenital diaphragmatic hernia: is emergency operation necessary? J Pediatr Surg 23:731, 1988

Lee P, Franks R, Sreeram N: Diaphragmatic hernia with extrathoracic heart. Int J Cardiol 33:176, 1991

Levy JL Jr, Guyer WA, Louis JE et al.: Bilateral congenital diaphragmatic hernias through the foramina of Bochdalek. J Pediatr Surg 4:557, 1969

Manthei U, Vaucher Y, Crowe CP: Congenital diaphragmatic hernia. Immediate preoperative and postoperative oxygen gradients identify patients requiring prolonged respiratory support. Surgery 93:83, 1983

Milne LW, Morosin AM, Campbell JR et al.: Pars sternalis diaphragmatic hernia with omphalocele: a report of two cases. J Pediatr Surg 25:726, 1990

Mishalany HG, Nakkada K, Wooley MM: Congenital diaphragmatic hernias: eleven years experience. Arch Surg 114:1118, 1979

Molenaar JC, Bos AP, Hazelbrock FWJ et al.: Congenital diaphragmatic hernia, what defect? J Pediatr Surg 26:248, 1991

Morgagni GB, Alexander B (transl): Seats and Causes of Disease Investigated by Anatomy. Vol. 3. Miller & Cadell, London 1769, p. 205

Nakamura Y, Yamamoto I, Fukuda S et al.: Pulmonary acinar development in diaphragmatic hernia. Arch Pathol Lab Med 115:372, 1991

Nakayama DK, Motoyama EK, Mutich RL et al.: Pulmonary function in newborns after repair of congenital diaphragmatic hernia. Pediatr Pulmonol 11:49, 1991

Raphaely RC, Downes JJ Jr: Congenital diaphragmatic hernia: prediction of survival. J Pediatr Surg 8:815, 1973

Reynolds M, Luck SR, Lappen R: The "critical" neonate with diaphragmatic hernia: a 21-year perspective. J Pediatr Surg 19:364, 1984

Ruff SJ, Campbell JR, Harrison MW et al.: Pediatric diaphragmatic hernias. Am J Surg 139:641, 1980

Shochat SJ: Pulmonary vascular pathology in congenital diaphragmatic hernia. Pediatr Surg Int 2:331, 1987

Sokal MM, Yellin PB, Meswtel Al et al.: Survival after bilateral congenital diaphragmatic hernia. Clin Pediatr (Phila) 29:677, 1990

Stolar CJH: Repair in utero of a fetal diaphragmatic hernia (letter; comment). N Engl J Med 323:1279, 1990

Thorpe-Beeston JG, Gosden CM, Nicolaides KH: Prenatal diagnosis of congenital diaphragmatic hernia: associated malformations and chromosomal defects. Fetal Ther 4:21, 1989

Touloukian RJ: Discussion of Wesselhoeft CW, DeLuca FG: Am J Surg 147:481,1984

Vacanti JP: Congenital diaphragmatic hernia. In Grillo HC, Austen WG, Wilkins EW et al. (eds): Current Therapy in Cardiothoracic Surgery. DC Decker, Philadelphia, 1989, p. 68

Vacanti JP, Crone RK, Murphy JD et al.: The pulmonary hemodynamic response to perioperative anesthesia in the treatment of high-risk infants with congenital diaphragmatic hernia. J Pediatr Surg 19:672, 1984

Wenstrom KD, Weiner CP, Hanson JW: A five year statewide experience with congenital diaphragmatic hernia. Am J Obstet Gynecol 165:838, 1991

Wesselhoeft CW, DeLuca FG: Neonatal septum transversum diaphragmatic defects. Am J Surg 147:481, 1984

Wilson JM, Lund DP, Lillehei CW et al.: Congenital diaphragmatic hernia: predictors of severity in the ECMO era. J Pediatr Surg 26:1028, 1991

Eventration

Geoffrey M. Graeber   Jacob Davtyan
Joseph I. Miller, Jr.

DEFINITION

Eventration of the diaphragm is broadly defined as an abnormal elevation of the hemidiaphragm. It can be classified into congenital and acquired forms. The acquired form is usually due to injury to the phrenic nerve, and some authors prefer to restrict the term eventration of the diaphragm to the congenital form, which is a result of failure of muscularization of the fetal diaphragm. The peripheral narrow rim has normal musculature which contracts on electrical stimulation (Shah-

Mívany, et al., 1968). As a consequence, the central portion of the affected hemidiaphragm is very thin and pliable. The defect is more common on the left side.

BASIC SCIENCE

Newborns are primarily dependent on diaphragmatic breathing. The intra-abdominal organs can be partially displaced into the chest, which affects to various degrees the growth and development of the lungs. These two factors are the major determinants of the degree of respiratory distress at presentation. The congenital eventration may be associated with prematurity, chromosomal anomalies, or other congenital malformations affecting pulmonary, cardiac, and neural systems and contributing to the mortality and morbidity of these patients (Stokes, 1991; Smith, et al., 1986). Bilateral congenital eventration is rare. When it occurs, the pathophysiology is similar to that of the newborn with CPLDH and is associated with very high mortality (Rodgers and Hawks, 1986).

The acquired form of eventration, which is better termed paralysis of the diaphragm, can be due to trauma to the phrenic nerve during birth or surgical operations for congenital heart disease. As these operations are performed in smaller and smaller newborns, many of whom survive to have reoperations, the danger of phrenic nerve injury due to limited space and extensive scarring is increased. In the acquired form, the embryologic development of the diaphragm is normal. There is, however, neurogenic myopathy with atrophy and degenerative changes, which become more prominent with increasing time following the nerve injury (Obara, et al., 1987).

In adults acute viral inflammation of the phrenic nerve is the most common cause. Open heart surgery and mediastinal fibrosis may be additional etiologic factors. Adults may present with respiratory and gastrointestinal symptoms, including dysphagia, epigastric pain and discomfort, heartburn, and eructation (Sade and Smith, 1989), which are most likely due to the abnormal position of the stomach. Unexplained respiratory insufficiency in a newborn, especially after a difficult delivery, should raise the suspicion of eventration (Symbas et al., 1977).

DIAGNOSIS

The diagnosis of eventration is usually made by the chest x-ray. Fluoroscopy or ultrasound may show abnormal or paradoxic movement of the affected hemidiaphragm. In patients receiving positive pressure-assisted ventilation, the flattened leaf of the diaphragm may be misleading.

MANAGEMENT

Whatever the etiology, the management of eventration is dictated by the severity of respiratory compromise. Indications for surgery are (1) respirator dependence; (2) repeated pulmonary infections; (3) feeding difficulty and failure to thrive secondary to respiratory compromise; and (4) large eventration in an asymptomatic child, which can potentially interfere with lung development (Stokes, 1991).

Thoracotomy through the sixth or seventh interspace is the preferred approach. The diaphragm is plicated with several rows of double-armed nonabsorbable sutures run parallel in the sagittal plane and tied at the end over a pledget. The phrenic nerve and its branches should be preserved. Alternatively, the eventrated diaphragm is grapsed with Babcock clamps and the excess portion is sutured at the base with horizontal nonabsorbable mattress sutures so as to tighten the remainder of the diaphragm almost flat. The edge of the double-layered excess then is folded down on the diaphragm and sutured to the costal margin at the periphery (Symbas, et al., 1977). For the bilateral defects, Rogers and Hawks (1986) recommend a transverse upper abdominal incision allowing access to both hemidiaphragms and permitting exploration and correction of associated gastrointestinal anomalies.

Results

Postoperatively, there is significant improvement of respiratory function in infants and children (Symbas, et al., 1977), but results in adults are less satisfactory (Varpela, et al., 1977).

REFERENCES

Obara H, Hoshina H, Iwai S et al.: Eventration of the diaphragm in infants and children. Acta Paediatr Scand 76:654, 1987

Rodgers BM, Hawks D: Bilateral congenital eventration of the diaphragm: successful surgical management. J Pediatr Surg 21:858, 1986

Sade RM, Smith CD: Diaphragmatic eventration—diaphragmatic plication. p. 71. In Grillo HC, Austen WG, Wilkins EW et al (eds): Current Therapy in Cardiothoracic Surgery. BC Decker, Philadelphia, 1989

Shah-Mivany J, Schmitz GL, Watson RR: Eventration of the diaphram: physiologic and surgical significance. Arch Surg 96:844, 1968

Smith CD, Sade RM, Crawford FA et al.: Diaphragmatic paralysis and eventration in infants. J Thorac Cardiovasc Surg 91:490, 1986

Stokes KB: Unusual varieties of diaphragmatic herniae. Prog Pediatr Surg 27:127, 1991

Symbas PN, Hatcher CR Jr, Waldo W: Diaphragmatic eventration in infancy and childhood. Ann Thorac Surg 24:113, 1977

Varpela E, Laustela EV, Viljeaneu: Acquired eventration of the diaphragm: results of surgery. Ann Chir Gynaecol 66:284, 1977

Diaphragmatic Pacing by Phrenic Nerve Stimulation

Geoffrey M. Graeber
Joseph I. Miller, Jr.

HISTORICAL NOTE

Diaphragmatic pacing by phrenic nerve stimulation has a history dating back hundreds of years. The acute effects of external stimulation were well demonstrated by the turn of the twentieth century. However, clinical applications were not available until the development of modern pacemaker technology. Current concepts and surgical technique and equipment development are largely attributed to Dr. William Glenn and his pioneering efforts at Yale University (Glenn and Phelps, 1985). Historically, Caldeni in 1786 was the first to note movement of the diaphragm with phrenic nerve stimulation (Schecter, 1970). In 1873 Hufeland proposed treatment of asphyxia neonatorium with phrenic nerve stimulation, and in 1878 Puchenne noticed that the phrenic nerve could stimulate normal respiration (Glenn and Phelps, 1985; Hofelance, 1970). In 1968 Judson and Glenn first reported that a phrenic nerve pacemaker had been implanted in a patient for chronic obstructive pulmonary disease, and in 1972 Glenn et al. reported the first pacemaker implant in a quadraplegic patient with ventilatory dependency. Since that time phrenic nerve pacing has been a standard technique for treating ventilatory insufficiency in selected patients.

HISTORICAL READINGS

Caldani LM: Institutiones Physiologine. Penzzana venice, 1786. Cited by Schechter PC: Application of electrotherapy to noncardiac thoracic disorders. Bull N Y Acad Med 46:932, 1970

Glenn WL, Holcomb WG, McLaughlin AJ et al.: Total ventilatory support in a quadraplegic patient with radio frequency electrophrenic respiration. N Engl J Med 286:513, 1972

Glenn WL, Hogan JF, Phelps ML: Ventilatory support of the quadriplegic patient with respiratory paralysis by diaphragmatic pacing. Surg Clin North Am 60:1055, 1980

Glenn WL, Phelps ML: Diaphragm pacing by electrode stimulation of the phrenic nerve. Neurosurgery 17:974, 1985

Hofelance CW: De vsu elec trache in asphyxia experimentis illustrato. Cited by Schechter PC: Application of electrotherapy to non-cardiac thoracic disorders. Bull N Y Acad Med 46:932, 1970

Judson JP, Glenn WL: Radio-frequency electrophrenic respiration. JAMA 203:1033, 1968

BASIC SCIENCE

Interruption of the motor neurons of the phrenic nerve associated with quadraplegia is usually the result of trauma to the spinal cord above the level of C6. Occasionally it may be from tumor invasion, radiation injury, hemorrhage, infarction, syringomyelia, and other demyelinating diseases (Glenn, et al., 1986, 1980). Interruption of the neurotransmission in the spinal cord may be partial or complete. A paralyzed diaphragm can be electronically stimulated if the lower motor neurons and the phrenic nerves are intact and their cell bodies in the C3–C5 segments of the spinal cord are viable.

Indications for Phrenic Nerve Pacing

Indications for phrenic nerve pacing include (1) idiopathic central alveolar hypoventilation; (2) organic lesions of the brain stem; (3) lesions of the cervical cord; (4) certain neuromuscular diseases; and (5) possible chronic obstructive pulmonary disease (Glenn et al., 1986).

Indications for phrenic nerve pacing in quadraplegia are (1) respiratory paralysis requiring artificial ventilation for more than 1 month; (2) a viable phrenic nerve; (3) response of the diaphragm to electrical stimulation on testing; and (4) normal cerebral function of the patient (Glenn, et al., 1980).

Before a patient undergoes implantation of a phrenic nerve pacemaker, a thorough electrophysiologic evaluation is performed to determine eligibility for phrenic nerve pacing. The studies include (1) arterial blood gases at rest; (2) complete pulmonary function testing, consisting of flow volume loops and ventilation/perfusion lung scan; (3) phrenic nerve function to determine viability of the phrenic nerves, which is the most specific test and is done as a diaphragmatic response to percutaneous phrenic nerve stimulation as well as to direct stimulation of the nerve at the time of surgery; and (4) in patients with suspected upper airway obstruction, an upper airway sleep study.

Contraindications to diaphragmatic pacing include nonviable phrenic nerves, generally as a result of injury to the anterior horn cells of the C3–C5 vertebrae or progressive neurologic disease. There may be primary diaphragmatic weakness resulting from myopathies or severe chronic obstructive pulmonary disease, and there may be a major problem with compliant lung secondary to severe parenchymal disease or anatomic thoracic cage deformity.

Transcutaneous phrenic nerve stimulation is achieved by stimulating the phrenic nerve at its motor point in the neck and sensing the diaphragmatic muscle action potential with cutaneous electrodes at the ipsilateral eighth intercostal space. In order to be sure that there are no false negatives, we continuously monitor the patient fluoroscopically at the time of phrenic nerve stimulation. The stimulator delivers impulses of 1-ms duration at a rate of one impulse per second at a current of 1 to 10 mA. If the nerve is viable, brisk contractions will be both observed fluoroscopically and recorded on the oscilloscope. The components of the phrenic nerve pacemaker are an external radio frequency transmitter and an external antenna. There is an implanted radio frequency receiver, an anode plate, and a phrenic nerve electrode, which currently is a unipolar electrode. Factors related to the outcome of the procedure include patient selection, operative technique, pacing regimen, the patient's compliance with the pacing schedule, the family physician's support system for pacing, the functioning of the pacing equipment, and the overall medical status of the patient.

Surgical Technique

The cervical implant technique has been previously reported by Glenn and colleagues (1980). The technique basically consists of a small (2-cm) incision overlying the scalene triangle, with lateral traction of the scalene fat pad and identification of the phrenic nerve as it crosses the anterior scalene muscle. A unipolar phrenic nerve electrode is passed under the phrenic nerve and attached with 3-0 silk sutures to the underlying scalene muscle. The lead is tunneled over the clavicle, and an infraclavicular incision is made approximately 2 cm below the clavicle in the midclavicular line. A pocket is then created that will accommodate the radio receiver unit and the anode ground plate.

The technique for transthoracic implantation of the phrenic nerve pacemaker system has been modified from that originally described by Glenn so that it requires only one incision when a transthoracic approach is used. A 5- to 7-cm transverse incision is made, overlying the second costocartilage and rib. The incision is extended down to the costocartilage and rib surface. The second costocartilage is resected totally and the pleural space entered. A small pediatric retractor is placed into the wound. Ventilation is achieved by the indwelling tracheostomy tube. The lung is packed off superiorly and inferiorly with lap packs. Two traction sutures of 2-0 silk are taken through the pericardium 1 cm above the phrenic bundle. These are elevated and attached with hemostats, therapy lifting the pericardium superiorly. The phrenic nerve can be easily identified running along the anterior surface of the perciardium. On the right side, the ideal site for implantation is just inferior to the junction of the superior vena cava with the right atrium. On the left side, the implantation site is approximately at the level of the left main pulmonary artery as it crosses out from the pericardial reflection.

Once the phrenic nerve is identified, two parallel incisions are made on each side of the phrenic nerve. The entire phrenic bundle, consisting of artery, nerve, and vein, is gently lifted off with a right-angle Gemini clamp. A 0 silk ligature is placed beneath the phrenic nerve. A unipolar electrode is passed with the toe of the electrode coming from below, so that the entire phrenic bundle lies within the U-shaped bend of the phrenic nerve electrode. The electrode is affixed to the pericardium with ligatures of 3–0 silk. At the lateral portion of the thoracic incision, a battery pocket is created to accommodate the ratio receiving unit and anode plate unit.

Once the pacemaker is implanted, the conduct of phrenic nerve pacing and training of the phrenic nerves requires considerable experience and time on the part of the patient, physician, and family. There is a 2-week wait following implantation to allow edema around the phrenic nerve to subside before beginning pacing. The patient is then taken to the fluoroscopic suite in the radiology department to determine the pacing threshold to stimulate the diaphragm as measured. The amount of diaphragmatic excursion is measured, and the pacing threshold is set to achieve 80 to 85 percent of diaphragmatic excursion.

Discussion

Diaphragmatic pacing is only possible if the cell bodies of motor neurons C3 to C5 are still intact following injury or disease process. Phrenic nerve function and diaphragmatic function are assessed by observation of the diaphragm at fluoroscopy and by direct phrenic nerve stimulation studies as previously described. In all patients considered for diaphragmatic pacing, the potential benefits of independence from mechanical ventilation offered by diaphragmatic pacing must outweigh the surgical and anesthetic risk. The following precautions must be taken with diaphragmatic pacing (Glenn et al., 1980): (1) diaphragmatic pacing interference with demand cardiac pacing must be avoided; (2) a permanent tracheostomy is required to obtain adequate ventilation while pacing; (3) the patient's compliance, intelligence, and family support are required; (4) a positive-pressure ventilator must always be available as backup; (5) an apnea alarm system must be available in all cases; (6) a minimum pacing threshold to accomplish diaphragmatic excursion at 80 to 85 percent of measured excursion should be used; (7) unilateral stimulation should not be used for more than 12 hours; and (8) sedation while pacing should be avoided in all patients.

Diaphragmatic pacing may be unsuccessful for the following reasons (Marcy and Oloke, 1987): (1) poor selection of cases; (2) injury to the phrenic nerves at the time of surgical exploration; (3) improper use of the pacemaker, resulting in diaphragmatic fatigue; (4) upper airway obstruction; and/or (5) defective apparatus. Pacing will also fail in conditions marked by progressive disease or injury to the phrenic nerve, lungs, and diaphragm.

KEY REFERENCE

Glenn WL, Phelps ML, Elefteriades JA et al.: Twenty years of experience in phrenic nerve stimulation to pace the diaphragm. Pace 9:789, 1986

The most complete review available of diaphragmatic pacing.

REFERENCES

Caldani LM: Institutiones physiologine. Penzzana Venice, 1786 Cited by Schechter PC: Application of electrotherapy to noncardiac thoracic disorders. Bull N Y Acad Med 46:932, 1970

Glenn WL, Holcomb WG, McLaughlin AJ et al.: Total ventilatory support in a quadriplegic patient with radio frequency electrophrenic respiration. N Engl J Med 286:513, 1972

Glenn WL, Hogan JF, Phelps ML: Ventilatory support of the quadriplegic patient with respiratory paralysis by diaphragmatic pacing. Surg Clin North Am 60:1055, 1980

Glenn WL, Phelps ML: Diaphragm pacing by electrode stimulation of the phrenic nerve. Neurosurgery 17:974, 1985

Hofelance CW: De vsu elec trache in asphyxia experimentis illustrato. Schechter PC: Application of electrotherapy to non-cardiac thoracic disorders. Bull N Y Acad Med 46:932, 1970

Judson JP, Glenn WL: Radio-frequency electrophrenic respiration. JAMA 203:1033, 1968

Marcy TW, Oloke JS: Diaphragm pacing for ventilatory insufficiency. J Intensive Care Med 2:345, 1987

52

ANATOMY AND CLASSIFICATION

Carolyn M. Dresler

DEFINITION

This chapter delineates the surgical anatomy of the mediastinum. The mediastinum is defined as the organs that occupy the space between the thoracic inlet to the diaphragm from the left to the right pleural surfaces. In this chapter the anatomy is described in terms of compartments and includes the thymus, thyroid, parathyroids, lymph nodes, neurogenic and vascular structures, thoracic duct, trachea, and esophagus.

COMPARTMENTS

The anatomy is well defined in the mediastinum, but there is no consensus among thoracic surgeons concerning the actual division of the mediastinum into compartments. This arbitrary division of the mediastinum into compartments is used to assist in the site of origin of abnormalities that are discovered during a diagnostic evaluation.

Probably the oldest division of the mediastinum is the four-compartment model (Fig. 52-1). This consists of superior, middle, anterior, and posterior compartments. The superior compartment extends from a transverse plane through the sternal-manubrial joint and the lower border of T4 to the thoracic inlet. The anterior compartment extends from the superior mediastinum to the diaphragm and between the sternum and pericardium. The posterior compartment of the mediastinum encompasses everything that is posterior to the pericardium. The middle compartment contains all structures between the anterior and posterior compartment.

A more frequently used scheme includes only three compartments, which consist of anterosuperior, medial, and posterior areas of the mediastinum. The anterosuperior compartment extends from the thoracic inlet to the diaphragm inferiorly and from the sternum to the anterior border of the pericardium. The posterior compartment extends from the anterior border of the vertebral bodies posteriorly to the ribs and from the thoracic inlet to the diaphragm. The final compartment, the middle mediastinum, includes all structures between the anterosuperior and posterior mediastinum (Fig. 52-2).

A less commonly used scheme was reported by Heitzman (1977). It describes six separate compartments. They consist of thoracic inlet, anterior mediastinum, superior aortic area, inferior aortic area and supra-aortic area, and supraazygos area, infraazygos area, and hila. This is a detailed division that was developed by a radiologist, but it is too cumbersome for thoracic surgical use.

The final scheme is the one proposed by Shields (1991) in 1972. This is a three-compartment model that consists of the anterior, visceral, and paravertebral sulci compartments. This is probably the simplest system to use and remember (Fig. 52-3). All compartments extend from the thoracic inlet to the diaphragm inferiorly. The anterior compartment encompasses the area from the undersurface of the sternum to a curvilinear border that extends from the pericardium to the anterior surfaces of the great vessels. The visceral compartment includes the thoracic inlet superiorly and extends from the curvilinear border. It defines the posterior aspect of the anterior compartment to the anterior surface of the vertebral bodies. The final compartment, the paravertebral sulci, extends from the visceral compartment posteriorly to the costal vertebral angle.

The division of the mediastinum attempts to simplify the possible origin of mediastinal masses. Table 52-1, utilizing Dr. Shields' (1991) classification, lists the etiology of masses that arise in the different mediastinal compartments.

Thymus

The thymus develops from the third pharyngeal pouch. As the thymus develops, it elongates and migrates inferiorly to rest finally in front of the great vessels in the anterior compartment of the mediastinum. The right and left lobes of the thymus do not fuse and are easily separable with dissection. The two lobes are usually asymmetric; the right is larger than the left.

As the child develops into an adult, the thymus gland gradually regresses in size. The thymus is largest at puberty, with a weight of approximately 30 g. It then gradually evolves to its adult size. Although the thymus grossly appears to consist

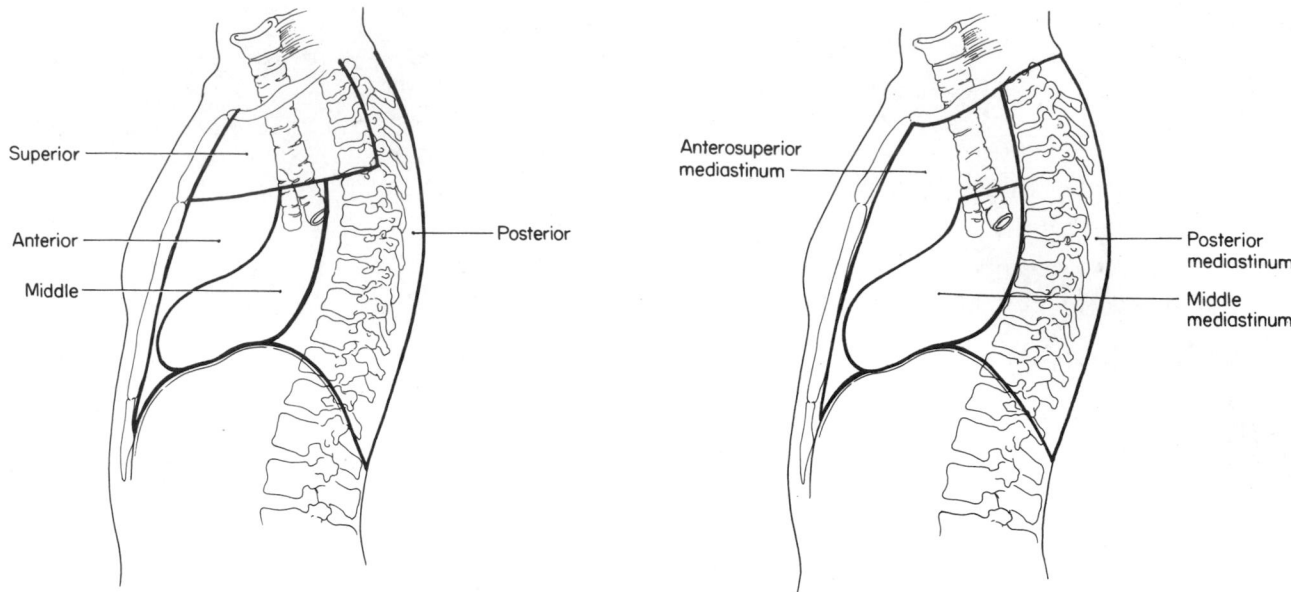

Figure 52-1. Four-compartment model of the mediastinum.

Figure 52-2. Three-compartment model of the mediastinum.

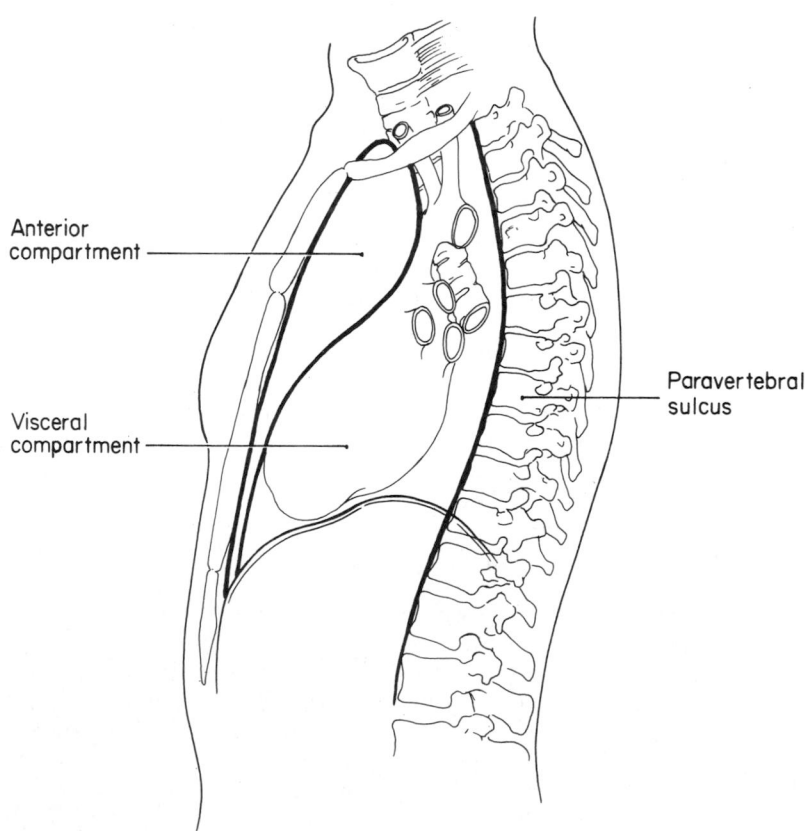

Figure 52-3. Shield's three-compartment model of the mediastinum. (From Shields TW: Mediastinal Surgery. p. 4. Lea & Febiger, Philadelphia, 1991, with permission.)

Table 52-1. Usual Location of the Common Primary Tumors and Cysts of the Mediastinum

Anterior Compartment	Visceral Compartment	Paravertebral Sulci
Thymoma	Enterogenous cyst	Neurilemoma-schwannoma
Germ cell tumor	Lymphoma	Neurofibroma
Lymphoma	Pleuropericardial cyst	Malignant schwannoma
Lymphangioma	Mediastinal granuloma	Ganglioneuroma
Hemangioma	Lymphoid hamartoma	Ganglioneuroblastoma
Lipoma	Mesothelial cyst	Neuroblastoma
Fibroma	Neuroenteric cyst	Paraganglioma
Fibrosarcoma	Paraganglioma	Pheochromocytoma
Thymic cyst	Pheochromocytoma	Fibrosarcoma
Parathyroid adenoma	Thoracic duct cyst	Lymphoma
Aberrant thyroid		

(From Shields TW: The mediastinum and its compartments. p. 5. In Mediastinal Surgery. Lea & Febiger, Philadelphia, 1991, with permission.)

of right and left lobes that extend from the base of the neck down to the pericardium, there may be significant variations in its size, shape, or extent. Of even more importance, however, is the occurrence of isolated thymic tissue. Jaretzki and Wolff (1988) extensively studied the variability of thymic tissue in the cervical and mediastinal areas. They described the frequent occurrence of thymic tissue from the level of the hyoid bone to the diaphragm and beyond either phrenic nerve at the level of the hilum. The importance of these variations is seen during thymectomy for myasthenia gravis. Although the grossly obviously right and left lobes of the thymus are removed, residual thymic tissue in any of the more unusual areas may result in persistent symptoms of myasthenia gravis.

The thymic arterial blood supply arises from the internal mammary arteries. The venous drainage is through the brachiocephalic and internal thoracic veins and may communicate with the internal thyroid veins. The lymphatic drainage flows to the internal mammary, anterior mediastinal, and hilar lymph nodes.

Parathyroids

The parathyroids are usually found in the cervical region; however, they may infrequently be displaced into the mediastinum. The parathyroids arise from the third and fourth pharyngeal pouches. The parathyroids that arise from the fourth pharyngeal pouch usually become cephalad in position and are closely related to the posterior aspect of the thyroid. The lower parathyroids that arise from the third pharyngeal pouch, as does the thymus, usually migrate caudad and are found inferiorly to the upper parathyroids. Usually they are positioned adjacent to the lower pole of the thyroid; however, they may remain related to the thymus and, therefore, be found in the mediastinum. Even more uncommonly, the parathyroids may be found in various other locations, for example, in the visceral compartment (related to either the great vessels, the trachea, or the posterior esophageal space).

The blood supply to the parathyroids usually arises from the inferior thyroid artery and with venous drainage into the inferior thyroid veins.

Thyroid

The thyroid is not generally considered a mediastinal structure. However, aberrant thyroid tissue or a thyroid goiter may extend into the mediastinum significantly. A possible thyroid mass must be part of the differential diagnosis of a mediastinal mass. Generally, the enlarged thyroid that presents as a mediastinal mass appears to be in the anterior compartment. However, because of the fascial planes, it is technically in the visceral compartment, anterior to the trachea, and it splays or displaces the great vessels. The rich blood supply to the thyroid is derived from bilateral superior and inferior thyroid arteries. When the thyroid gland is enlarged and in the mediastinum, the inferior thyroid vessels are dragged down with the mass. Unless there has been a previous thyroid resection, the blood supply should still originate from the neck. Thus, most enlarged thyroids may be resected from a supraclavicular incision.

Lymph Nodes

A knowledge of lymphatic drainage and lymph nodes is important to the thoracic surgeon. It is particularly important because of the involvement of the nodes with metastatic disease, either within the thorax or chest wall, or with changes caused by inflammatory or infectious disease.

To facilitate our discussion, the mediastinal lymph nodes are divided into two groups: the anterior mediastinal and the visceral compartment lymph nodes. The lymph nodes in the anterior compartment drain the anterior chest wall and the medial portions of the breast. They lie firmly adherent to the anterior chest wall extrinsic of the parietal pleura. The drainage from these lymph nodes then proceeds to the cervical nodes on the right or left. In addition, the lymph nodes adjacent to the thymus gland in the anterior aspect of the pericardium drain into adjacent lymph nodes. As noted previously, the anterior compartment lymph nodes are usually important in medial breast carcinoma or chest wall lesions.

The group of lymph nodes that is more critically important to the thoracic surgeon is related to the visceral compartment. These nodes drain the esophagus and lungs. A significant

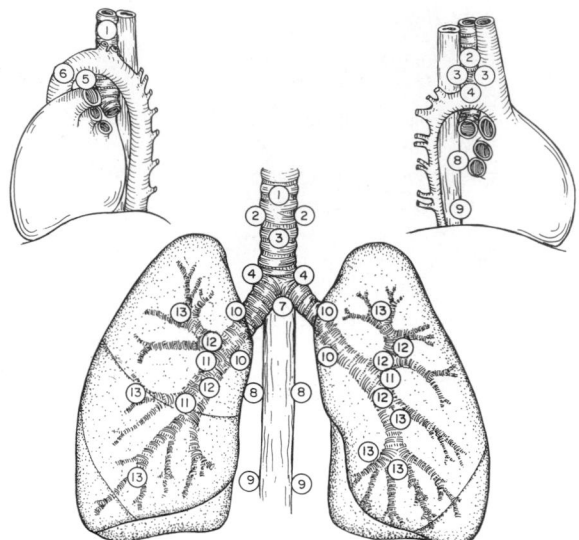

Figure 52-4. Naruke's, et al. mediastinal lymph node map. See Table 52-2 for description.

amount of work has been performed to define the location and drainage of these lymph nodes because of their importance in the staging of both lung and esophageal carcinomas. In particular, Naruke, et al. (1978) defined several stations of mediastinal lymph nodes (Fig. 52-4 and Table 52-2).

For the thoracic surgeons, the lymph nodes that pertain to pulmonary drainage have been labeled N1 and N2 lymph nodes. The N2 lymph nodes are mediastinal nodes; N1 lymph nodes are within the pulmonary parenchyma. Levels 1, 2, 3, and 4 are the paratracheal lymph nodes, as seen in either the Naruke or the American Thoracic Society (ATS) map (Fig. 52-5 and Table 52-3). These four levels describe any lymph node located between the tracheobronchial angle and the thoracic inlet. Levels 5 and 6 occur only on the left side and define the subaortic or aortic (5) window and the para-aortic or ascending (6) aortic lymph node stations. These lymph nodes are particularly important in lesions that drain from the left upper lobe. The inferior mediastinal lymph nodes, levels 7, 8, and 9, define the subcarinal, paraesophageal, and pulmonary ligament lymph nodes, respectively. The subcarinal lymph nodes lie between the left and right mainstem bronchi beneath the carina and above the pulmonary artery;

Table 52-2. Naruke Mediastinal Lymph Node Designation

N2 Nodes	N1 Nodes
1 Highest mediastinal	10 Hilar
2 Upper paratracheal	11 Interlobar
3 Pre- and retrotracheal	12 Lobar
4 Lower paratracheal	13 Segmental
5 Subaortic	
6 Para-aortic	
7 Subcarinal	
8 Paraesophageal	
9 Pulmonary ligament	

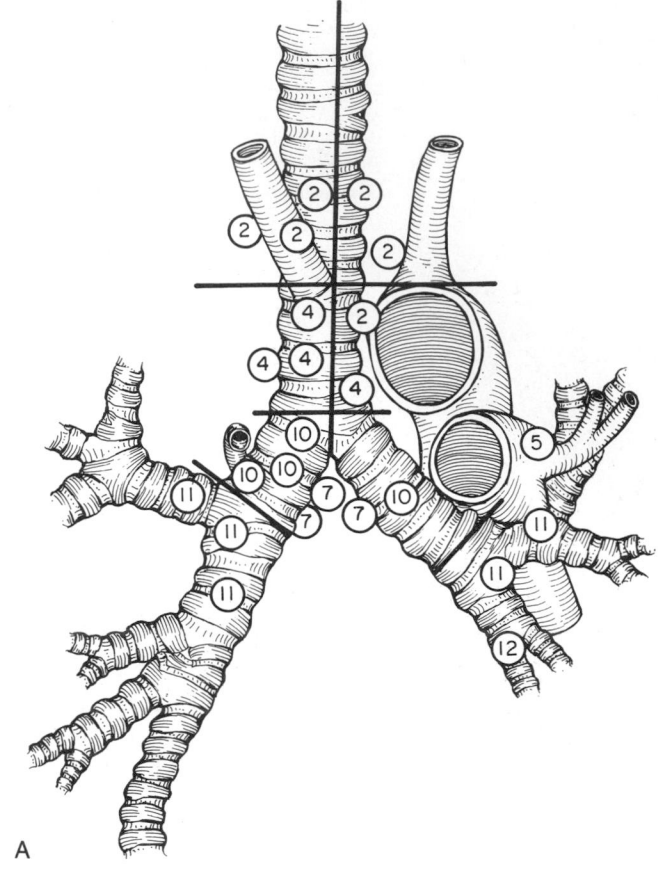

A

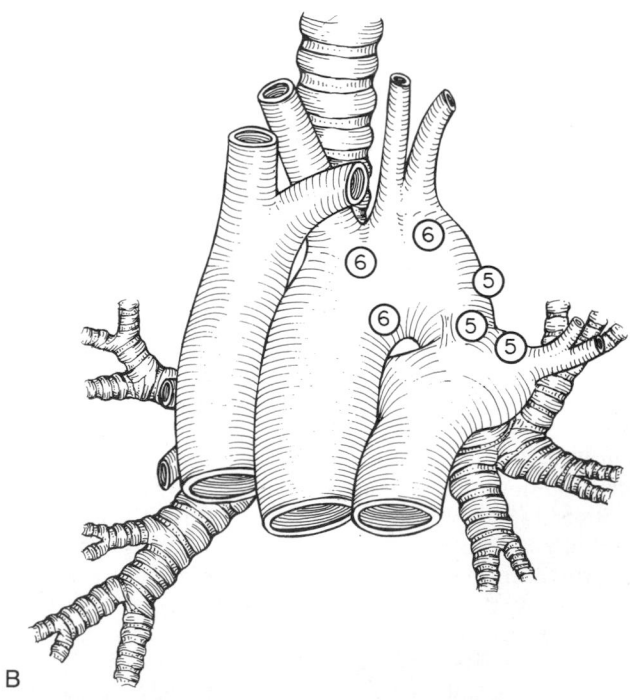

B

Figure 52-5. **(A & B)** ATS mediastinal lymph node map. See Table 52-3 for description.

Table 52-3. American Thoracic Society Lymph Node Designation

N2 Nodes		N1 Nodes	
2R	Right upper paratracheal	11	Interlobar
2L	Left upper paratracheal	12	Lobar
4R	Right lower paratracheal	13	Segmental
4L	Left lower paratracheal	14	Subsegmental
10R	Right tracheobronchial angle		
10L	Left tracheobronchial angle		
5	Aortopulmonary		
6	Anterior mediastinal (anterior to ligamentum arteriosum)		
7	Subcarinal		
8	Paraesophageal		
9	Pulmonary ligament		

they are encased within pretracheal fascia. The subcarinal lymph nodes drain proximally into the right or left tracheobronchial and paratracheal lymph nodes. The paraesophageal lymph nodes occur throughout the length of the esophagus and may drain into either the lymph nodes in the subcarinal space, the paratracheal area, or the base of the neck or distally toward the celiac axis. The pulmonary ligament lymph nodes occur within the pulmonary ligament on either the right or the left side, and they may drain either cephalad to the subcarinal area or distally to the subdiaphragmatic lymph nodes.

The descriptions for level 10, or the tracheobronchial lymph nodes, have been controversial. These lymph nodes lie at the angle between the mainstem bronchi and the trachea. Whether these lymph nodes are mediastinal or hilar in origin is the subject of controversy, particularly on the right side. The right tracheobronchial angle node is described as lying beneath the azygos vein but superior to the right pulmonary artery. This area is difficult to define clearly because of the short distance between levels 4 and 10 on the right during staging by mediastinoscopy. The left tracheal bronchial angle is much easier to define because of the length of the left mainstem bronchus. However, with experience, tracheobronchial angle lymph nodes can be identified and undergo biopsy, and they should be considered to be mediastinal lymph nodes. Therefore, all lymph nodes that are accessible through either a cervical mediastinoscopy, extended mediastinoscopy, or anterior mediastinoscopy (Chamberlain procedure) are definable as N2 or mediastinal lymph nodes. The N1 lymph nodes are defined at thoracotomy. As is described in later chapters, this definition of N1 or N2 lymph nodes stations is critical for accurate staging and therapeutic planning.

The remaining group of lymph nodes are those that occur in the posterior intercostal spaces. These may drain either cephalad to the base of the neck or caudad to the subdiaphragmatic lymph nodes.

Neurogenic Structures

Neurogenic tumors are the most common type of mediastinal tumors. Therefore, it is important to recognize the possible origin of neurogenic structures. The two main nerves of the mediastinum course from the thoracic inlet to the diaphragm in the visceral compartment (Fig. 52-6). The phrenic nerve enters the thoracic inlet on the anterior aspect of the musculus scalenus anterior. As the phrenic nerve enters the thoracic inlet, the pericardiophrenic branch of the internal mammary artery combines with the phrenic nerve to run caudad. On the right side, the phrenic nerve runs along the lateral aspect of the superior vena cava and then continues on, anteriorly to the hilar structures, along the lateral portion of the pericardium. As the phrenic nerves reach the diaphragm, they bifurcate and distribute along the diaphragm. The left phrenic nerve similarly enters the thoracic inlet on the scalenus anterior toward the medial aspect. It then runs under the internal mammary artery, and as the phrenic nerve continues caudad, it crosses anteriorly to the vagus nerve at approximately the level of the origin of the left carotid artery. The nerve goes directly through the middle of the aortic pulmonary window and continues across the anterior hilum of the left lung and then across the lateral aspect of the pericardium. It then reaches the diaphragm and again divides into its terminal branches.

The vagus nerves course through the neck within the carotid sheath. As the right vagus enters the thoracic inlet, which lies anterior to the subclavian and posterior to the innominate artery, the right recurrent nerve is given off. The right recurrent nerve loops around the right subclavian artery to course diagonally toward the tracheoesophageal groove and enter the inner musculature of the larynx.

After it has crossed the anterior aspect of the right subclavian artery and given off the branch to the recurrent nerve, the right vagus passes medially behind the right innominate vein toward the trachea and esophagus. It then continues posteriorly to the trachea and courses down the right lateral aspect of the esophagus. A few branches from the vagus are given off at the level of the trachea and continue caudad to

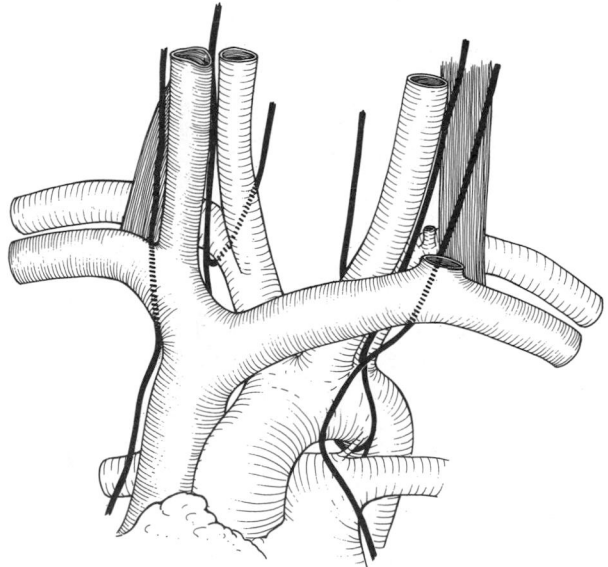

Figure 52-6. Course of intrathoracic nerves. (From Anderson JE: Grant's Atlas of Anatomy. Williams & Wilkins, Baltimore, 1983, with permission.)

the heart to form the cardiac plexuses at the distal aspect of the esophagus (Fig. 52-7). The right vagus curves posteriorly and becomes the posterior vagal trunk to the stomach.

On the left side, the vagus nerve enters the thoracic inlet adjacent to the right carotid artery, exits the carotid sheath, and moves medially to laterally. The vagus nerve then courses across the anterolateral aspect of the aortic arch where the recurrent left laryngeal nerve branches off and continues posteriorly under the aortic arch and ligament arteriosus. It runs cephalad in the tracheoesophageal groove. The remainder of the vagus continues posteriorly to the left pulmonary artery and gives off branches to the anterior and posterior pulmonary plexus. The left vagus continues toward the esophagus and remains on the ventral wall as the anterior esophageal plexus.

The spinal nerves from the vertebral column exit through each intervertebral foramen and form a spinal root. The spinal root then divides, and one ramus runs laterally with the intercostal artery and lies in the intercostal groove. The other division of the spinal root branches and joins the thoracic sympathetic trunk. This thoracic sympathetic trunk is composed of several ganglia that lie on the anterior aspect of the origins of the ribs. The most cephalad ganglia, along with the inferior cervical ganglia, is called the stellate ganglion. The thoracic sympathetic trunk and ganglia give off several branches, which form a rich network of plexus and paraganglia.

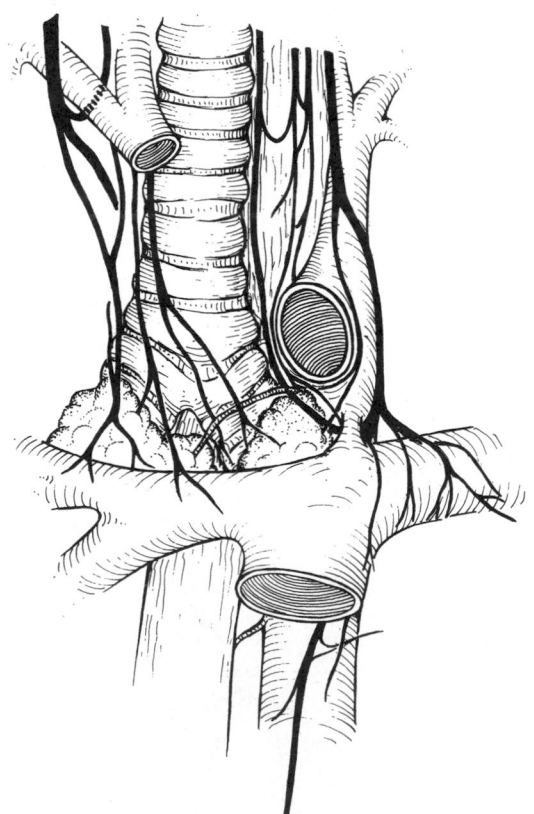

Figure 52-7. Cardiac plexus of vagus. (From Anderson JE: Grant's Atlas of Anatomy. Williams & Wilkins, Baltimore, 1983, with permission.)

Vascular Structures

The largest and most critical blood vessels originate and terminate in the visceral compartment of the mediastinum. The great veins lie anterior to the great arteries. The superior vena cava, which is formed at the junction of the right and left innominate veins at the level of the thoracic inlet, continues caudad along the right lateral aspect of the trachea and enters the right atrium. Just cephalad to the pericardial reflection and entrance of the superior vena cava to the right atrium, at the level of the right tracheobronchial angle, is the confluence of the azygos vein. The aortic arch arises from the left ventricle, courses initially to the right, and then curves posteriorly into the left chest. It runs posteriorly and caudad, lateral to the esophagus. Bronchial arteries arise from the proximal descending aorta and supply the right and left mainstem bronchi.

The pulmonary artery arises from the right ventricle and initially is slightly to the right and anterior to the aorta. As the pulmonary artery arches posteriorly and slightly caudad, it bifurcates into a short left main pulmonary artery and a longer right pulmonary artery. The pulmonary arteries exit the pericardium. On the left immediately outside of the pericardial sac, is the ligament arteriosum, which is draped by the recurrent laryngeal nerve. At this level the left main pulmonary artery is superior to the left mainstem bronchus and superior and slightly posterior to the left superior pulmonary vein.

The right main pulmonary artery courses directly through the subcarinal space and enters the right hilum anteriorly to the right mainstem bronchus but posteriorly and cephalad to the right superior pulmonary vein. The arch of the azygos vein is directly cephalad to the right main pulmonary artery. Directly posterior to the right main pulmonary artery near its origin are the subcarinal lymph nodes.

Bilaterally the pulmonary veins have a superior and inferior division. Both superior veins are the most anterior of the hilar structures. Both inferior pulmonary veins conversely are the most posterior and inferior hilar structures.

On the right, the azygos vein runs along the lateral aspect of the vertebral bodies and receives branches from each intercostal vein. The left hemiazygous system communicates with the left renal vein and continues cephalad along the left ventricular aspect of the vertebral body, which again receives branches from the posterior intercostal veins. Several communications generally occur with the right azygos system with cross-connecting channels.

Thoracic Duct

The thoracic duct (Fig. 52-8) ascends along the vertebral column and arises from the cisterna chyli in the abdomen. It enters the chest through the aortic hiatus; at the level of the diaphragm, it lies on the right lateral aspect of the aorta. As the duct rises cephalad, it begins to curve to the left; at the level of the aortic arch, it becomes a more left-sided structure. The thoracic duct continues to run cephalad between the esophagus and subclavian artery. The thoracic duct curves anteriorly and to the left over the subclavian artery toward the junction of the internal jugular and subcla-

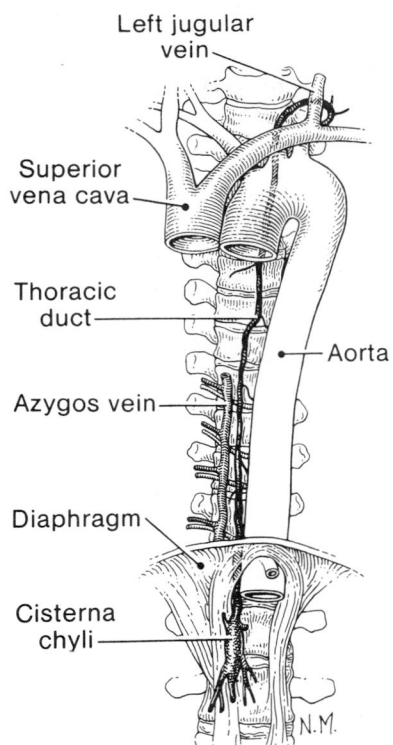

Figure 52-8. Anatomic course of thoracic duct. (From Miller, JI, Jr: Anatomy of the thoracic duct. p. 24. In Shields TW: Mediastinal Surgery. Lea & Febiger, Philadelphia, 1991, with permission.)

Labels on figure: Left jugular vein; Superior vena cava; Thoracic duct; Aorta; Azygos vein; Diaphragm; Cisterna chyli; N.M.

vian veins. The thoracic duct is variable. It may have several branches or a plexus type of formation. The one consistent aspect of the thoracic duct is its inconstant location.

Trachea

The trachea and carina reside in the visceral compartment. The first cartilaginous tracheal ring begins immediately below the cricoid cartilage in the neck. The trachea then descends through the thoracic inlet in the visceral compartment behind the vessels and anterior to the esophagus. The trachea is slightly to the right of midline; the right bronchus bifurcates off in a more vertical direction than the left. For this reason, more aspirations occur on the right than the left. The carina or bifurcation of the trachea occurs at approximately the level of T4. Directly posterior to the carina is the subcarinal space, which contains lymph nodes that drain both the left and right hemithoraces. The pulmonary trunk divides into right and left branches; the right main pulmonary artery traverses the subcarinal space.

The trachea is supplied arterially by bilateral branches of the inferior thyroid, the first intercostal, and the bronchial arteries. The cardiac plexus of nerves intermesh across the anterior aspect of the distal trachea and carina from the right and left vagus and sympathetic nerves.

Esophagus

The esophagus is a muscular conduit that extends from the pharynx in the neck to the gastric cardia. As such, it originates approximately 5 cm above the thoracic inlet as the "cervical" esophagus. It then enters the thoracic inlet in the visceral compartment and is adherent anteriorly to the membranous portion of the trachea. The esophagus descends slightly to the left of the midline when it enters the mediastinum, becomes midline at the level of the carina, and then again begins to deviate slightly to the left and anteriorly to pass through the esophageal hiatus of the diaphragm. Below the trachea and carina, the esophagus is bounded anteriorly by the subcarinal lymph nodes and pericardial sac prior to exiting the mediastinum through the diaphragm. Posteriorly, the esophagus is bounded by the vertebral column.

The left recurrent nerve approaches the tracheal-esophageal groove above the bifurcation of the trachea after it branches off the left vagus and wraps around the ligamentum arteriosum. The right recurrent nerve is found in the cervical tracheoesophageal groove after it divides from the right vagus and loops around the right subclavian artery. The bilateral vagus nerves and branches from the sympathetic chain provide innervation to the smooth muscles of the esophagus. The right and left vagus nerves dive posteriorly distal to the bifurcation of the trachea. The left vagus descends and rotates to lie anteriorly; the right vagus is posterior. However, several branches from each vagus nerve and the sympathetic chain intertwine to innervate the distal esophagus.

The arterial supply of the thoracic esophagus is variable and is derived from two bronchial and two aortic vessels. The arteries form an anastomotic chain that provides a vascular network throughout the esophagus. This form of blood supply allows the thoracic esophagus to be dissected in its entirety without causing significant devascularization.

KEY REFERENCES

Anderson JE: Grant's Atlas of Anatomy. Williams & Wilkins, Baltimore, 1983

This atlas is a well-known general anatomy reference with excellent drawings of the mediastinum.

Marchevsky AM: Surgical Pathology of the Mediastinum. 2nd Ed. Raven Press, New York, 1992

This book begins with a brief section on anatomy but progresses to a thorough and excellent description of pathologic conditions of the mediastinum.

Shields TW: Mediastinal Surgery. Lea & Febiger, Philadelphia, 1991

This publication is current, well researched, and illustrated. It covers the mediastinum in all aspects, from anatomy through pathologic states.

REFERENCES

Heitzman ER: The Mediastinum: Radiologic Correlation with Anatomy and Pathology. CV Mosby, St. Louis, 1977

Jaretzki A III, Wolff M: Maximal thymectomy for myasthenia gravis. Surgical anatomy and operative techniques. J Thorac Cardiovasc Surg 96:711, 1988

Naruke T, Suemasu K, Ishikawa S: Lymph node mapping and curability at various levels of metastasis in resected lung cancer. J Thorac Cardiovasc Surg 76:832, 1978

Tisi GM, et al.: Clinical staging of primary lung cancer. Am Rev Respir Dis 127:659, 1983

53

IMAGING

Gordon L. Weisbrod
Stephen J. Herman

INTRODUCTION

The mediastinum can be divided into anterior, middle, and posterior compartments. The anterior mediastinal compartment is bounded anteriorly by the sternum and posteriorly by the pericardium, aorta, and brachiocephalic vessels. It contains the thymus gland or its remnants, branches of the internal mammary artery and vein, lymph nodes, and variable amounts of fat. The middle mediastinal compartment contains the pericardium and its contents, the ascending and transverse portions of the aorta, the superior and inferior vena cava, the brachiocephalic arteries and veins, the phrenic nerves and upper portion of the vagus nerves, the trachea and main bronchi and their contiguous lymph nodes, and the pulmonary arteries and veins. The posterior mediastinal compartment is bounded anteriorly by the pericardium and extends posteriorly to the chest wall, including the paravertebral gutters. It contains the descending thoracic aorta, esophagus, thoracic duct, azygos and hemiazygos veins, nerves, fat, and lymph nodes (Fraser, et al., 1989).

Once a mediastinal abnormality is identified on conventional radiographs and the cause is not immediately apparent, the most productive procedure to perform next is computed tomography (CT) (Baron, et al., 1981a). CT can differentiate cystic and solid mediastinal masses; localize such masses relative to other mediastinal structures; determine their tissue composition (adipose tissue, calcium, water); assess whether mediastinal widening is pathologic or simply an anatomic variation (i.e., physiologic fat deposition); and differentiate a solid mass from a vascular anomaly or aneurysm.

The impact that magnetic resonance imaging (MRI) will have on the study of the mediastinum has not been firmly established. MRI has the advantages of no ionizing radiation, no intravenous contrast, and multiplanar imaging. Its excellent demonstration of vascular structures is also a decided advantage in showing vascular anomalies or vascular compromise. Its ability to differentiate radiation fibrosis from tumor mass because of differing signal intensities may also prove very useful (Rholl, et al., 1985).

Mediastinal tumors or masses usually show a strong predi-

lection for one of the three mediastinal compartments. Thus, it is logical to classify these masses on the basis of anatomic location. However, overlap from one compartment to another commonly occurs, and therefore the predominant compartment affected should be stated. A 1971 review of the literature documented 34 previous reports of mediastinal tumors in a total of 3,364 patients (Ingels, et al., 1971). Excluding metastatic pulmonary carcinoma and inflammatory conditions, the frequency of tumors was as follows: neurogenic neoplasms, 19.4 percent; lymphoma, 15.8 percent; bronchial and pericardial cysts, 14.2 percent; germ cell tumors, 12.8 percent; thymoma, 11.5 percent; thyroid tumors, 6 percent; and a variety of miscellaneous tumors comprising the remainder. Almost half of all patients with mediastinal masses are asymptomatic, the abnormalities being discovered on a screening chest radiograph (Wychulis, et al., 1971).

ANTERIOR MEDIASTINAL MASSES

Thymic Lesions

Normal Thymus

Before discussing the various diseases that may affect the thymus gland and their radiographic manifestations, it is necessary to review the normal CT appearance of the gland. Baron, et al. (1982b) measured the size and shape of the normal thymus gland in 154 patients in all age groups. The findings were described in terms of the width and thickness of each of the lobes of the gland and were summarized in tabular form for each age group. They found that there was a decrease in the thickness and width of the gland with increasing age, with less variation in the gland thickness within each group. Generally speaking, in those over 20 years of age the upper limit of normal (as defined by the mean thickness plus two standard deviations) was always less than 1.1 cm (1.18 cm for the right lobe in the 20 to 29 age group). In younger patients the gland had the same density as muscle, but with time there was gradual fatty replacement; islands of thymic tissue could be seen within this fat (Fig. 53-1).

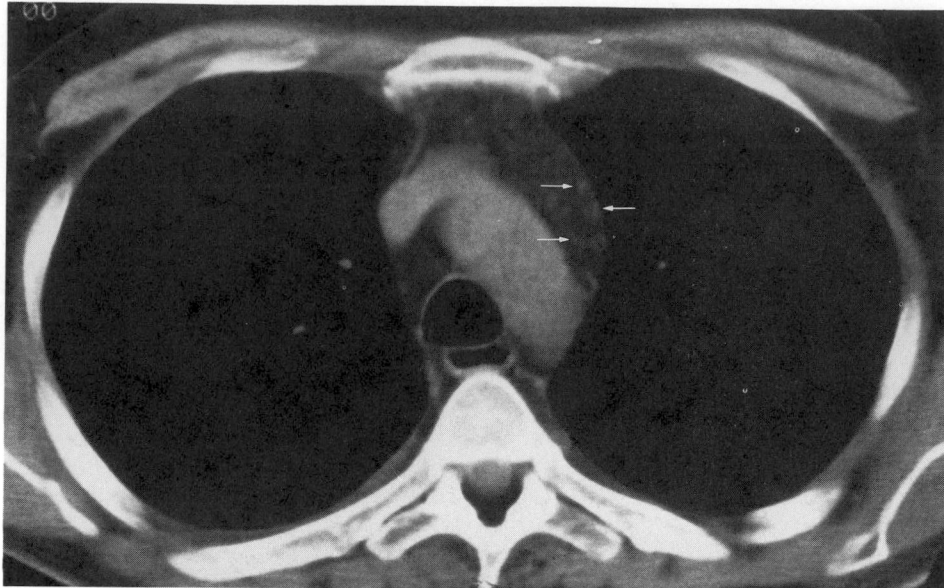

Figure 53-1. CT scan of 43-year-old man with involution of the thymus gland with fatty replacement. The thymus gland has been almost completely replaced by fat. There are only tiny islands of soft tissue density (*arrows*) scattered about the gland.

Heiberg, et al. (1982) described the CT appearance of the thymus gland in 40 patients under age 20, of whom 34 had a normal gland and 6 had a thymoma. The normal gland had smooth lateral margins, which tended to be convex in the very young but became straight or concave with increasing age. The lateral aspect sometimes exhibited a sharp angular contour. This group found higher values for the thickness of the gland than did Baron, et al. (1982b) in the patients aged 10 to 19; both groups claimed that their own values were valid, and no cause for the discrepancy was evident.

A third study described the CT appearance of the thymus in 64 patients in whom the status of the gland was determined by thymectomy or by biopsy at mediastinal exploration (Moore, et al., 1983). The normal gland had a bilobed, arrowhead-shaped appearance. The density was that of soft tissue, and this was gradually replaced by fatty infiltration beginning at age 20. The rate of replacement was most rapid between the ages of 31 and 40, and in most patients over 40 most or all of the gland had been completely replaced by fat. The gland retained its size and shape as fatty involution occurred. A thymoma appeared as a mass, which usually caused a convexity at the mediastinal margin. It was not difficult to recognize it as such in patients over 40 (in whom all of the thymomas in this study occurred), but it could be difficult to distinguish from an island of residual thymic tissue in persons aged 20 to 40 years.

In another study (Francis, et al., 1985), the gland was homogeneous in density in patients under 10 years of age and had a quadrilateral shape with convex (or occasionally straight or concave) margins. The gland enlarged and became more triangular in shape until puberty, after which time it became more inhomogeneous in density as fatty infiltration developed. Over 50 percent of patients over age 40 had total fatty replacement. When thymic tissue did remain, it was in

the form of linear or oval soft tissue densities less than 7 mm in the short axis; occasionally some round tissue was present in this age group but was never larger than 7 mm, and there was never any alteration in contour of mediastinal fat.

In a study examining the thymus by MRI (deGeer, et al., 1986), the gland appeared larger than on CT. This observation was believed to be due to the fact that MRI was able to distinguish between thymic fat and mediastinal fat. The size of the thymus with MRI correlated better with the true anatomic size than did the CT size (the anatomic size was assessed by published values, not by direct correlation with the patients in this study). Thymic fat differed from mediastinal fat in its hydrogen density, and the T_1 relaxation times of the thymus were much longer than those of fat, but this difference decreased with age. The T_2 values of the thymus were about equal to those of fat, and they did not change with age.

Thymoma

Thymomas are neoplasms of the epithelial elements of the thymus and contain variable amounts of infiltration by reactive lymphocytes. They are most common in middle-aged adults, being quite rare in those under 20 years of age. They occur approximately equally in men and women. These tumors are usually well encapsulated and are either spherical or lobulated. The diagnosis of benignancy or malignancy is not made by microscopic examination of the thymus but rather by the operative findings. Cases in which the surgeon notes local invasion through the capsule at the time of sternotomy are considered malignant. However, it should be noted that the tumor can be adherent to adjacent structures without actual tissue invasion being present. Within the thorax, thymoma usually spreads by direct extension into mediastinal fat and to the pleura. Distant metastases are very uncommon.

Patients with thymomas may be asymptomatic, but about one-third will have symptoms due to compression or invasion of adjacent mediastinal structures. These symptoms include dyspnea, chest pain, and cough; however, the most common symptom is weakness due to associated myasthenia gravis, which occurs in about 35 to 50 percent of patients with thymoma. Other associated abnormalities include pure red cell aplasia and hypogammaglobulinemia, along with other rarer conditions.

It has been stated that patients with myasthenia gravis have about a 15 percent chance of having a thymoma. About 60 percent will have thymic lymphoid hyperplasia, and the gland will be atrophic in about 25 percent of patients. These prevalences vary with the age and sex of the patient. Hyperplasia is much more common in females than in males and is rare in patients over 50. Surgical removal of hyperplastic glands results in excellent symptomatic improvement of the myasthenia in most patients. Patients over age 50 have either a thymoma or thymic atrophy, the latter being much more common in men. Surgery is indicated for thymoma but not for atrophy since symptoms are not improved by resecting an atrophic gland.

Radiographically, thymomas appear as a mediastinal mass in the anterior superior mediastinum, near the junction of the heart with the great vessels (Ellis and Gregg, 1964; Good, 1947) (Fig. 53-2). Occasionally they are located adjacent to the heart laterally. They are usually well defined and protrude to one or possibly both sides of the mediastinum. Calcification, either peripheral or scattered throughout the mass, is occasionally seen. Thymomas can be missed on plain film examination, only to be picked up in retrospect when they enlarge or in patients with myasthenia gravis who proceed to CT examination. Reasons for diagnostic error include minimal protrusion of a small convexity into the adjacent lung and confusion as to whether a visible convexity represents a hilar vascular structure or the cardiac margin (Brown, et al., 1980).

Although thymomas may be first detected on the chest radiograph, they are best assessed by CT. This technique can suggest if the tumor is invasive or not and in a patient with myasthenia gravis may reveal a thymoma that is not seen on chest x-ray. When a thymoma is present, it appears as a rounded or lobulated mass of soft tissue density, which bulges the margins of the thymus gland (Fig. 53-3). The mass may be completely separated from adjacent structures by an intact fat plane (Fig. 53-4) or it may be less well defined and in intimate contact with adjacent structures (Fig. 53-5). CT may demonstrate extension of the mass along fascial planes and possibly into the pleural space or lung (Fig. 53-2), features that suggest malignancy. Areas of low density are occasionally noted within the tumor mass, indicating necrosis. Occasionally calcification is present, but this is not of much use either in determining whether the mass represents a thymoma or in suggesting whether it is malignant.

Baron, et al. (1982a) were able to visualize all eight thymomas in their series on CT but only six by chest radiography. Similarly, Moore, et al. (1982) noted that CT detected four of four thymomas, one of which was not seen by chest radiog-

raphy. However, of 19 normal or hyperplastic glands, 2 were called thymoma on CT and 3 on chest x-ray. In a study by Brown et al. (1983) all six thymomas were diagnosed correctly, but there were five false positives (cysts, hyperplasia, hemangioma). In a later study (Ellis, et al., 1988), 17 of 20 thymomas were correctly diagnosed by CT, 12 were seen on chest radiography; there was only one false positive by CT. Three of three malignant thymomas were called malignant on CT, but one benign tumor was also called malignant because of its large size. In a study using MRI, two of two thymomas were diagnosed by chest radiography, CT, and MRI, but MRI was considered to be inferior to CT in studying thymic pathology because of its poorer spatial resolution, longer scan time, and lack of visualization of calcium (Batra, et al., 1987).

In our own group's study of 69 patients with thymic resections, we were able to detect 33 of 34 thymomas (97 percent) by CT (Chen, et al., 1988). In addition, by assessing the presence or absence of the fat plane between the tumor and adjacent mediastinal structure we attempted to determine if the tumor was malignant or not. Of 13 patients with completely preserved fat planes, 12 had no invasion and 1 had focal microscopic capsular invasion. Three patients had complete obliteration of the fat planes, and all of these had malignant tumors. There were 15 tumors with some preserved and some obliterated planes; 7 of these were benign and 8 were malignant.

Thymic Hyperplasia

Thymic lymphoid hyperplasia is the presence of germinal centers in the thymus as seen pathologically. It is the most common thymic disease associated with myasthenia gravis, being seen in about 60 percent of cases. It usually but not always causes enlargement of the gland.

The thymus gland may atrophy in response to stress or following therapy with steroids or chemotherapy; withdrawal of these stimuli may cause so-called rebound thymic hyperplasia (Shin and Ho, 1983b; Carmosino, et al., 1985; Choyke, et al., 1987; Kissin, et al., 1907). This condition is especially frequent in children and young adults. In a study of patients receiving chemotherapy for a variety of neoplasms, a significant volume decrease was observed in almost all patients after administration of chemotherapy (Choyke, et al., 1987). Following this, thymic rebound (defined as a greater than 50 percent increase in thymic size above baseline as assessed by CT) was noted in 5 of 22 patients. In a study of 120 patients receiving chemotherapy for malignant testicular teratomas, thymic enlargement was seen on CT in 14 patients (11.6 percent) (Kissin, et al., 1987).

Thymic lymphoid hyperplasia may be visible as an anterior mediastinal mass on chest x-ray but is best assessed by CT. In pathologically proven cases, the thymus appears abnormally large (best determined by an increase in the thickness of the gland) in about 70 percent of cases (Fig. 53-3B). Rebound thymic hyperplasia may cause thymic enlargement on chest x-ray or CT as well.

In a study by Baron, et al. (1982a), using their own data from normal individuals (Baron, et al., 1982b), six of eight

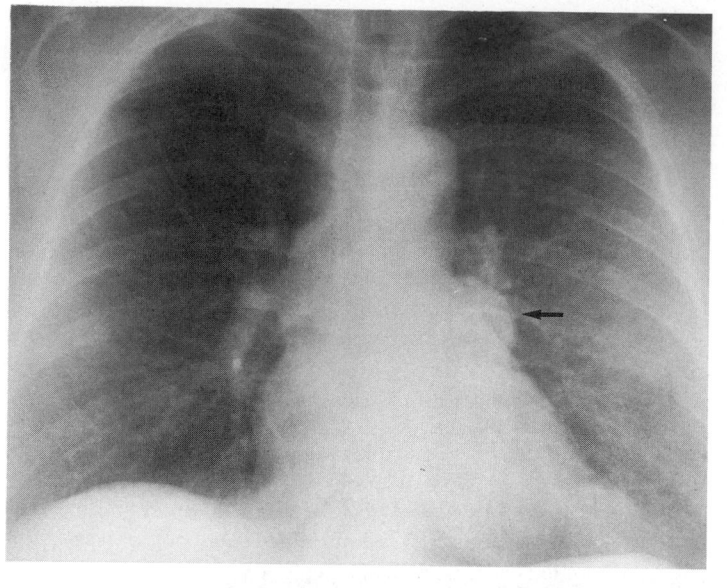
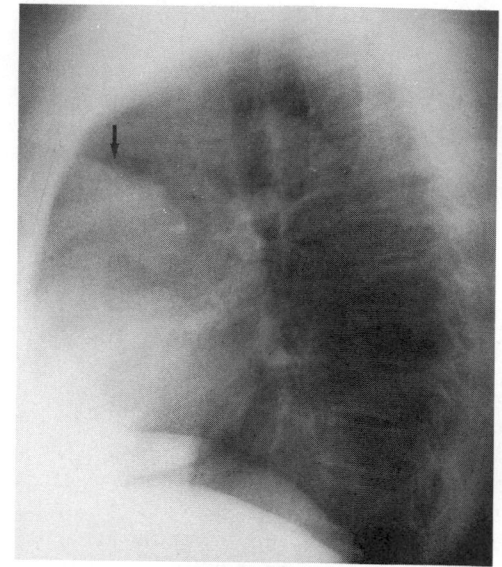
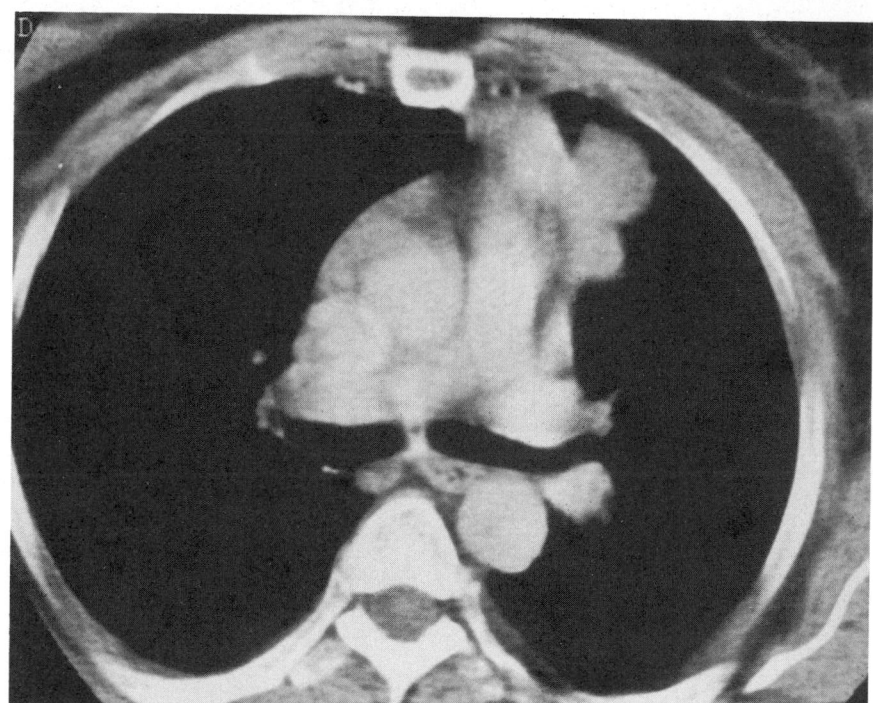

Figure 53-2. Chest x-ray of 55-year-old woman with malignant thymoma, **(A)** PA and **(B)** lateral. Large anterior mediastinal mass (*arrows*) projecting to the left of midline. **(C)** CT scan shows ill-defined anterior mediastinal mass with intact fat plane between the mass and the main pulmonary artery but with extension of tumor into the left anterior lung. At surgery this tumor was noted to be growing through the pleura into the lingula, requiring a wedge resection of lung along with the rest of the mass.

hyperplastic glands were more than 2 standard deviations above normal thickness. Thorvinger, et al. (1987) were able to diagnose six of eight hyperplastic glands by CT. However, Batra, et al. (1987) noted that six of seven hyperplastic glands were normal in size by CT and MRI. In our group's study (Chen, et al., 1988), by using the normal criteria of Baron, et al. (1982b) and designating as abnormal more than 1.5 standard deviations above the mean for each age group, we

correctly detected 20 of 28 cases of hyperplasia (71 percent). One normal was falsely labeled as hyperplastic.

Thymolipomas

Thymolipomas are rare tumors, mentioned here because of their striking radiographic appearance. Because they are soft and pliable, they do not affect adjacent structures and may

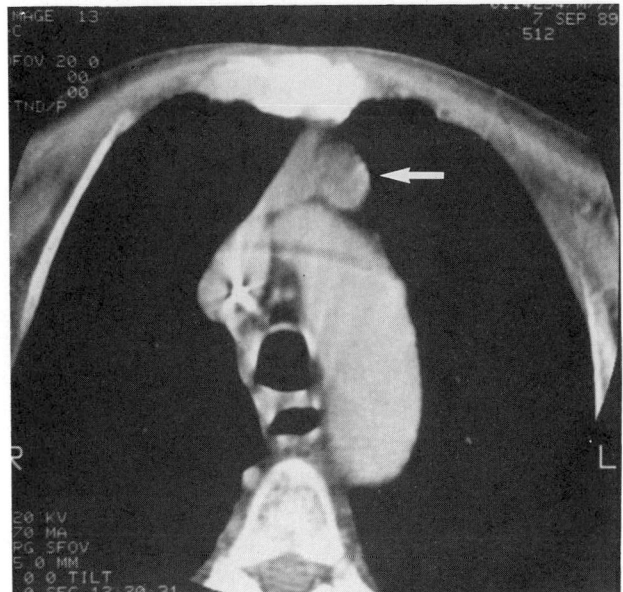

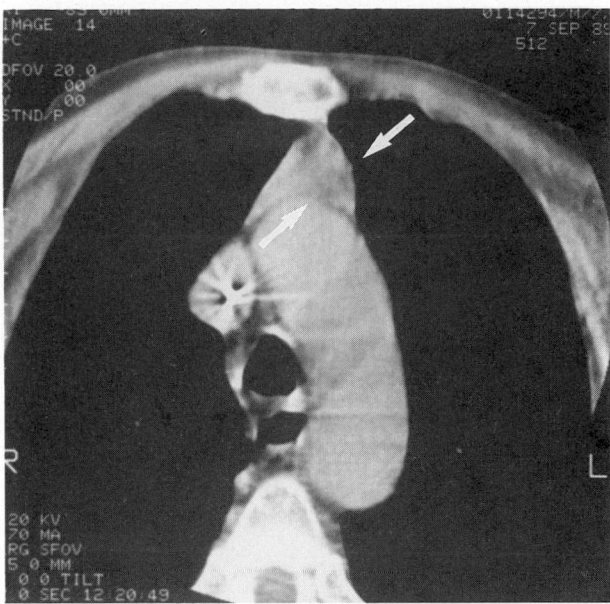

Figure 53-3. This 76-year-old man has myasthenia gravis and a thymoma within a hyperplastic thymus gland. **(A)** CT scan shows a mass (*arrow*) within the left lobe of the thymus gland bulging its margins. **(B)** CT scan 5 mm inferior to Fig. A. Increased thickness (*between arrows*) of left lobe in a person of this age suggests hyperplasia (proven pathologically).

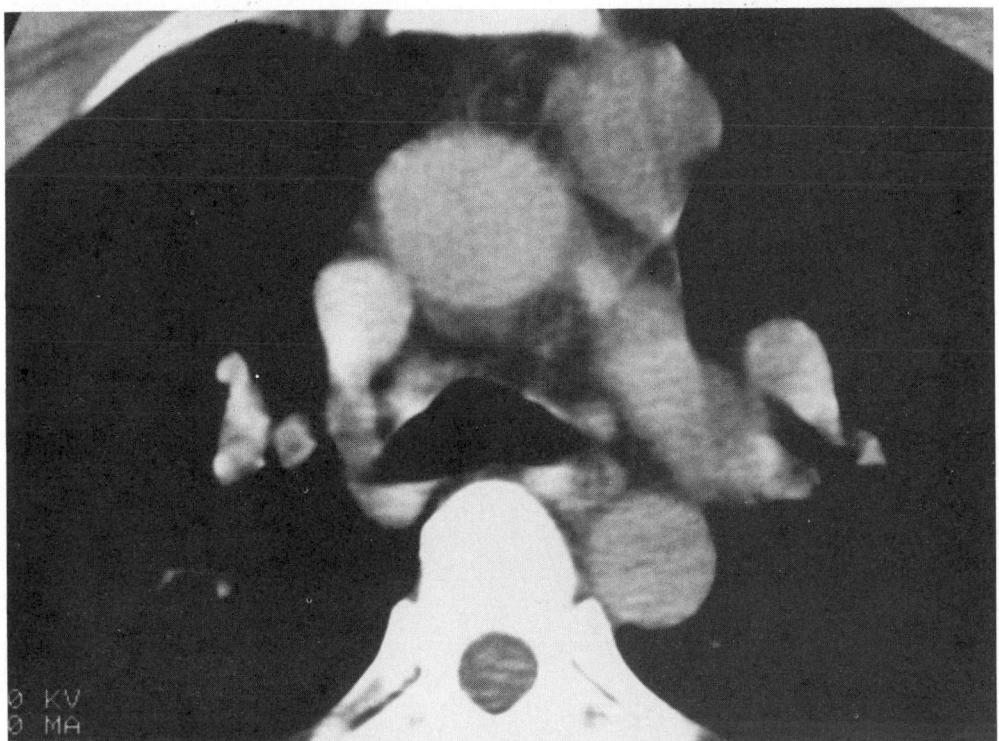

Figure 53-4. In this 44-year-old man with myasthenia gravis and benign thymoma, CT scan shows a slightly lobulated left anterior mediastinal mass. The fat plane between the mass and the adjacent ascending aorta is intact.

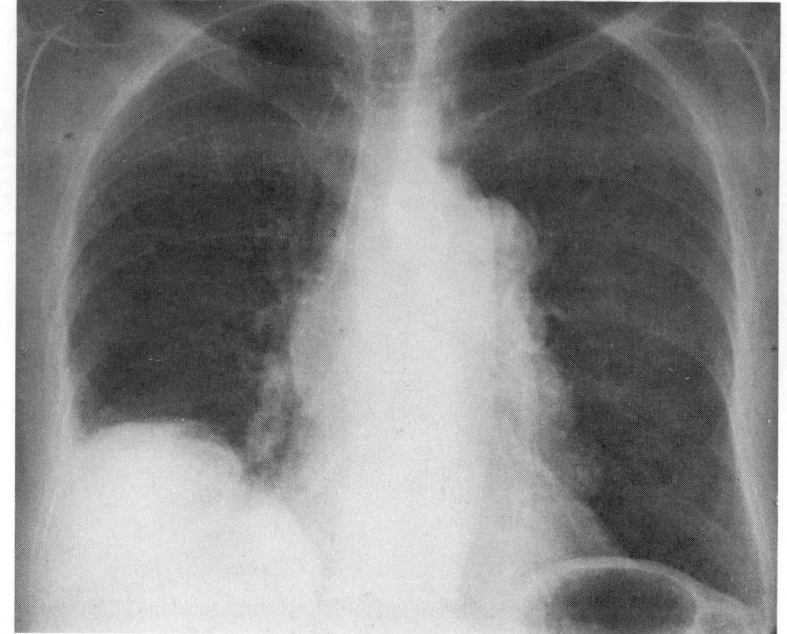

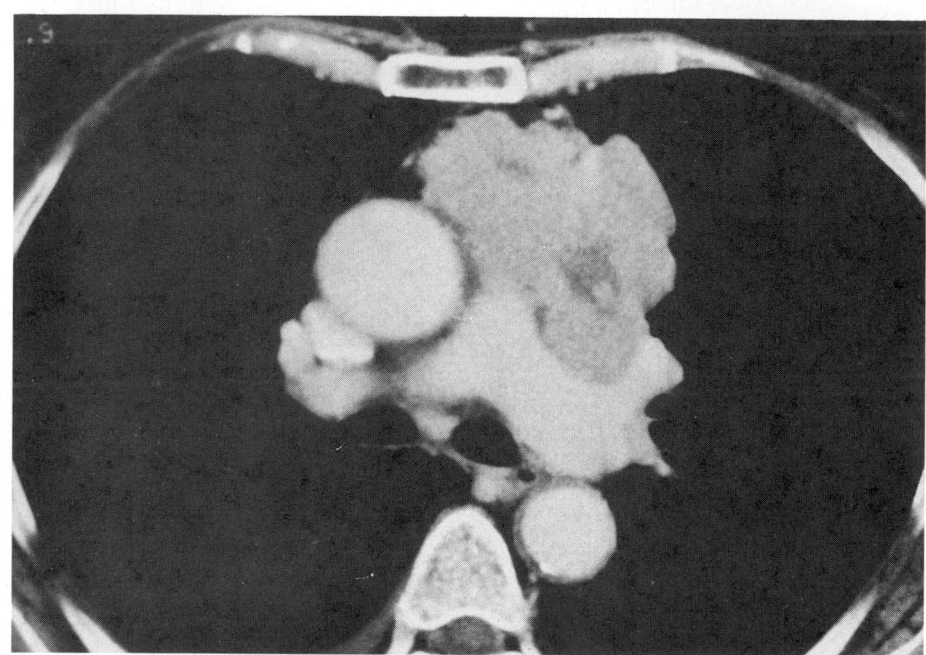

Figure 53-5. In this 70-year-old woman with malignant thymoma, **(A)** PA view of chest shows a long lobulated left-sided mediastinal mass. The large right lower lobe mass is a coincident adenocarcinoma. **(B)** CT scan shows a large lobulated ill-defined mass in the anterior mediastinum located predominantly left of midline. Areas of low density are noted within the mass, which presumably represent necrosis. An intact fat plane is seen between the mass and the ascending aorta, but there is loss of this plane between the mass and the main as well as the left pulmonary artery.

therefore grow to a very large size before being diagnosed. Radiographically they are seen as huge mediastinal masses, which tend to fall away from the superior mediastinum and become most evident in the lower chest, where they drape the heart and may mimic cardiomegaly (Yeh, et al., 1983). CT reveals a huge mass of fat density, with islands of soft tissue density representing thymic tissue.

Thymic Cysts

Thymic cysts are uncommon lesions, which usually are asymptomatic and are discovered by routine radiography. Most often they are simple cysts of no consequence, but they must be distinguished from thymomas, which may contain cystic elements. Occasionally the main portion of the tumor mass is cystic in nature, with only a thin rim of neoplastic tissue (Fig. 53-6). Furthermore, Hodgkin disease involving the thymus may be partially cystic; the cystic component may become especially prominent after therapy (Baron, et al., 1981b; Lindfors, et al., 1985). A thymic cyst appears as a nonspecific anterior mediastinal mass on chest radiography. Although the water density of these cysts is usually evident on CT, occasionally they are soft tissue in density, which suggests solid tumor, if a complication such as hemorrhage into the cyst occurs (Brown, et al., 1983; Dunne and Weksberg, 1983).

Thymic Carcinoid

Carcinoid tumors uncommonly occur in the thymus gland, usually in young men. They may be encapsulated or may invade adjacent structures. Like other mediastinal masses, these may be asymptomatic or may cause symptoms because of compression of adjacent mediastinal structures. Additionally, however, they may be part of a multiple endocrine neoplasia (MEN) syndrome. The most common associated endocrine dysfunction is Cushing syndrome, due to ectopic production of adrenocorticotropic hormone (ACTH). This tumor appears as an anterior mediastinal mass on chest x-ray and CT (Birnberg, et al., 1982) but is frequently missed on chest radiography, and mediastinal CT scanning is suggested early in the course of patients with suspected ectopic ACTH production (Brown, et al., 1982).

Germ Cell Neoplasms

In large series germ cell tumors are almost as common as thymomas, but as opposed to thymomas, most occur in adolescence or young adulthood. For unknown reasons males tend to develop malignant germ cell neoplasms, while in females these tumors tend to be benign. In most series the benign teratoma is the most common of this group, occurring in approximately 70 percent of cases. The most common malignant neoplasm is the seminoma; the other malignant neoplasms include embryonal carcinoma, malignant teratomas, choriocarcinoma, and endodermal sinus tumors. Multiple cell types may be present within the same tumor.

Radiologically, the benign tumors tend to be spherical masses, which grow slowly. They are most commonly seen in the superior mediastinum. Calcification may be present but is usually of no help in diagnosis because it can be seen in other anterior mediastinal masses, including thymoma and thyroid goiter. Occasionally benign teratomas are recognized by the visibility of mature bone or a tooth in the neoplasm. In general, malignant tumors tend to be larger than benign ones, tend to be lobulated, and grow more rapidly (Fig. 53-7). CT may reveal evidence of mediastinal invasion or lymphadenopathy, as well as metastatic disease in lungs, pleurae, or chest wall.

In a report of five benign teratomas of the mediastinum (Brown, et al., 1987), all presented as large (5- to 25-cm diameter) masses on chest x-ray. Four of these were located in the anterior mediastinum, while one was in the right hemithorax. On CT three were predominantly cystic in nature, containing only small soft tissue components (Fig. 53-8), one contained approximately equal amounts cystic and soft tissue components, and the fifth had a whorled, low-density appearance. The density of the cystic regions was higher than that of water. Three of the masses contained a single, dense calcific focus in the periphery of the mass. Similarly, three of six mediastinal teratomas in another report (Suzuki, et al., 1983) had a cystic component, and two of the six contained dense "ossification." In a third study (Mori, et al., 1987), six benign germ cell tumors had a thick wall with homogeneous contents

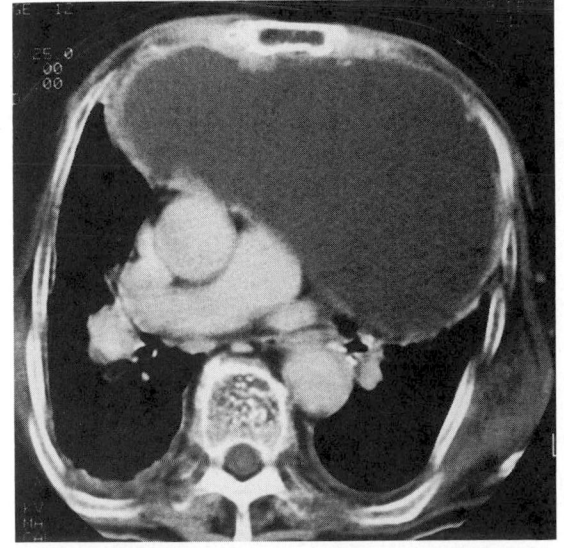
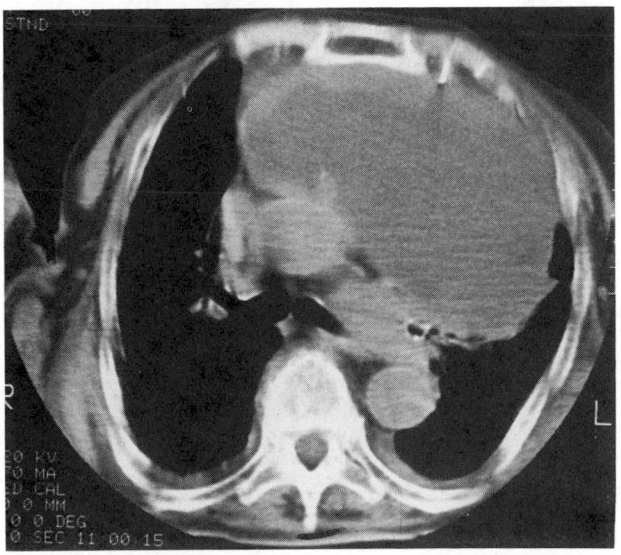

Figure 53-6. **(A)** CT scan of 93-year-old woman with benign thymoma reveals a huge anterior mediastinal mass, which is almost entirely cystic in nature with only a very thin rim of soft tissue. There is significant displacement of the mediastinal vascular structures posteriorly and to the right. **(B)** CT scan showing tip of needle within the soft tissue component of this mass at CT-guided transthoracic needle biopsy (at which time the diagnosis of thymoma was made).

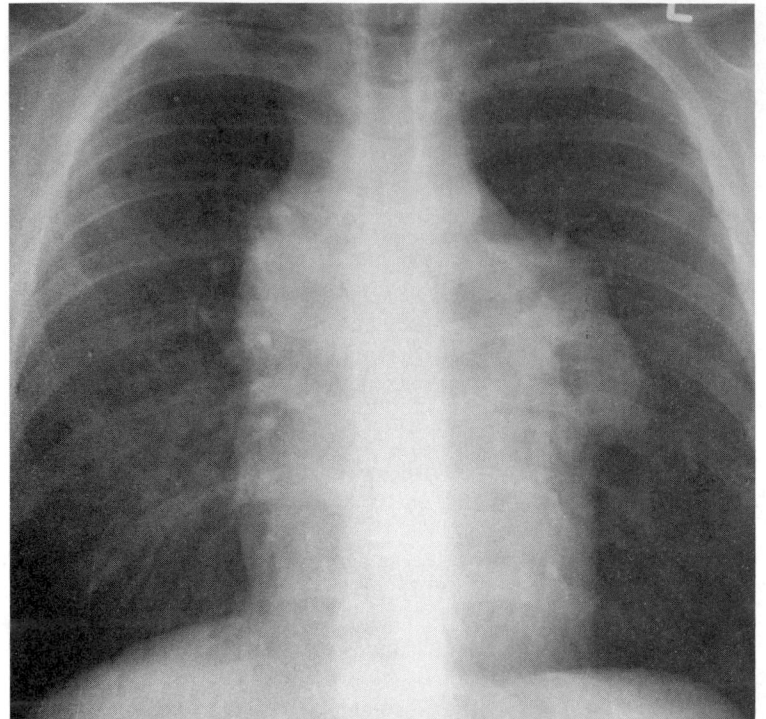
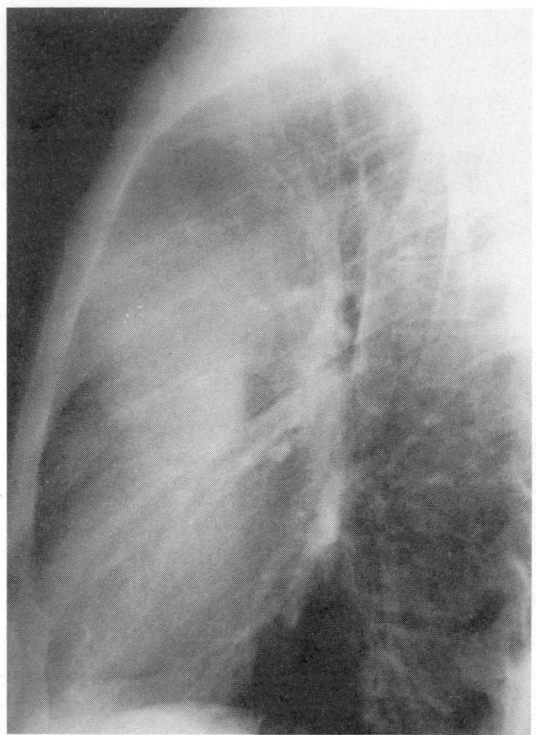
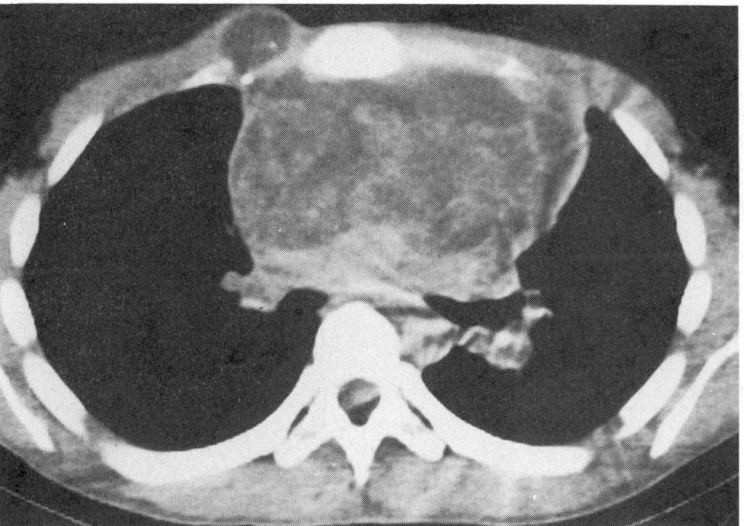

Figure 53-7.   In this 23-year-old man with malignant nonseminomatous germ cell tumor, chest x-rays, **(A)** PA and **(B)** lateral, show a very large lobulated anterior mediastinal mass projecting to both sides of the mediastinum. **(C)** CT scan shows a very large inhomogeneous anterior mediastinal mass containing large areas of necrosis. The fat plane between the mass and the great vessels is obliterated, and the mediastinal structures are displaced posteriorly. Note the extension of the tumor anteriorly into the right chest wall.

slightly higher in density than water. A fat-fluid level has been reported in mediastinal cystic teratomas (Fulcher, et al., 1990). A cystic anterior mediastinal lesion in a patient under 20 years of age, especially if it contains a dense calcific focus peripherally, should be considered to be a cystic teratoma. In this age group thymic cysts and thymomas are very uncommon; bronchogenic cysts rarely occur in the anterior mediastinum.

In one report of four patients with malignant germ-cell tumors, (Levitt, et al., 1984), all neoplasms were very large, obliterated fat planes between the mass and adjacent vessels and tended to extend predominantly along the left side of the mediastinum. All three nonseminomatous tumors contained areas of density near that of water, which were presumed to represent areas of necrosis and hemorrhage. The single seminoma was homogeneous in density. In a report of 13 patients with malignant germ cell tumors of the mediastinum (Lee, et al., 1989) four of five seminomas exhibited obliteration of fat planes and two invaded the chest wall. There were two pleural and one pericardial effusion. Four of the tumors exhibited small areas of low density. Six of eight nonseminomas had spiculated margins, and fat planes were obliterated in seven. More than 50 percent of the mass was of low density in five cases, with these areas containing a septated internal architecture. Five of the eight had pleural and three had

pericardial effusions. In another report of two seminomas (Shin and Ho, 1983a), both were very large with sharply defined margins but with loss of the fat planes between the mass and adjacent structures. Both tumors were homogeneous in density.

In a report of seven endodermal sinus tumors (Fox and Vix, 1980), all presented radiographically as large, lobulated, uncalcified anterior mediastinal masses. Similar radiographic findings were reported in two other patients with this tumor,

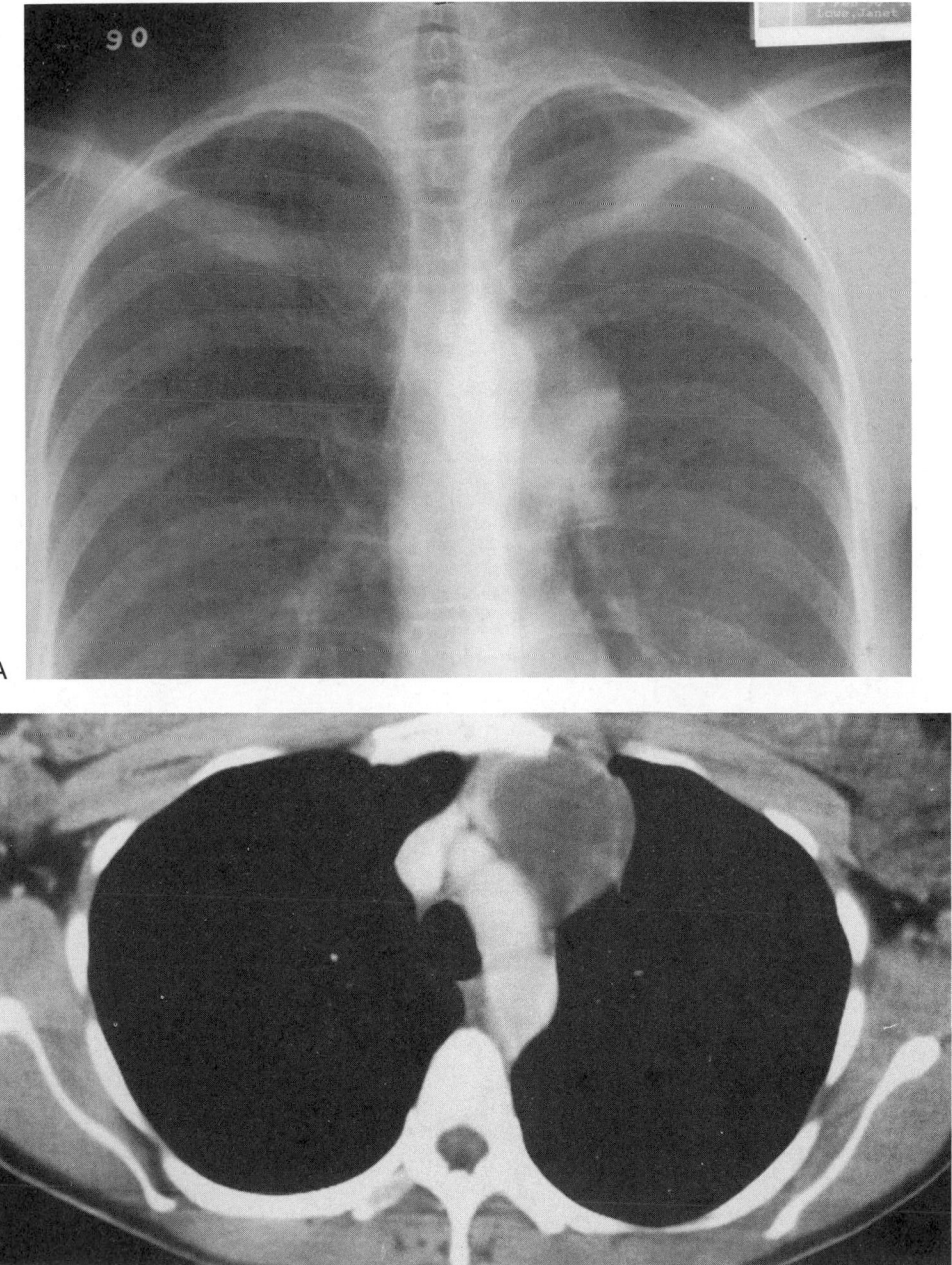

Figure 53-8. **(A)** PA chest radiograph of 29-year-old woman with dermoid cyst shows a well-defined left-sided mediastinal mass, which was noted to be in the anterior mediastinum on the lateral view (not shown). **(B)** CT scan shows left anterior mediastinal mass whose attenuation is slightly greater than water, indicating its cystic nature. A small amount of soft tissue is noted on the right side of the mass.

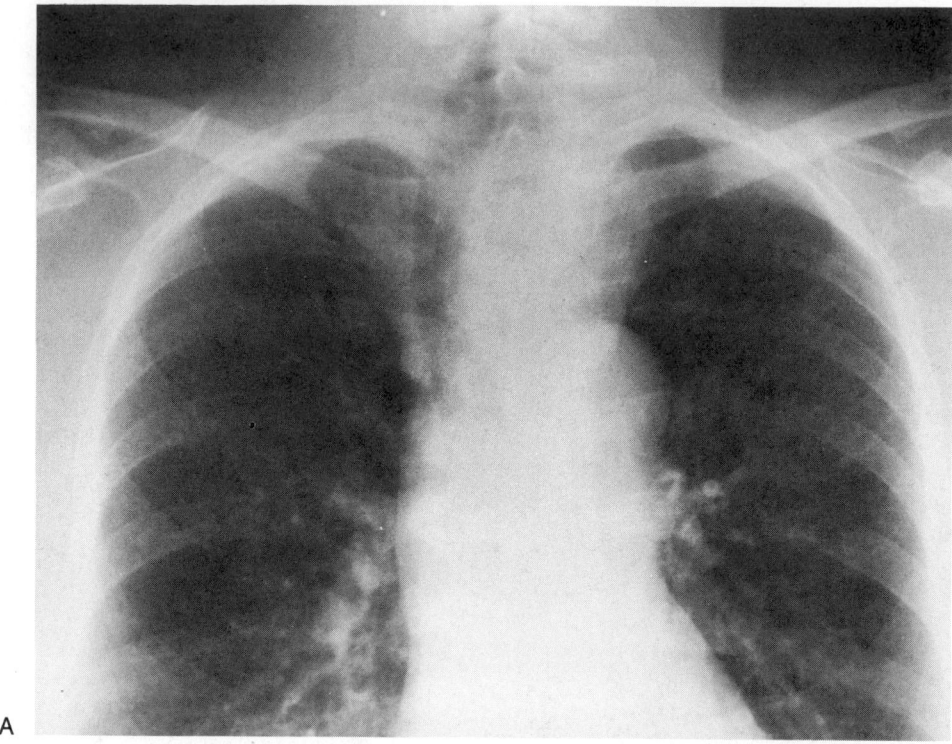

A

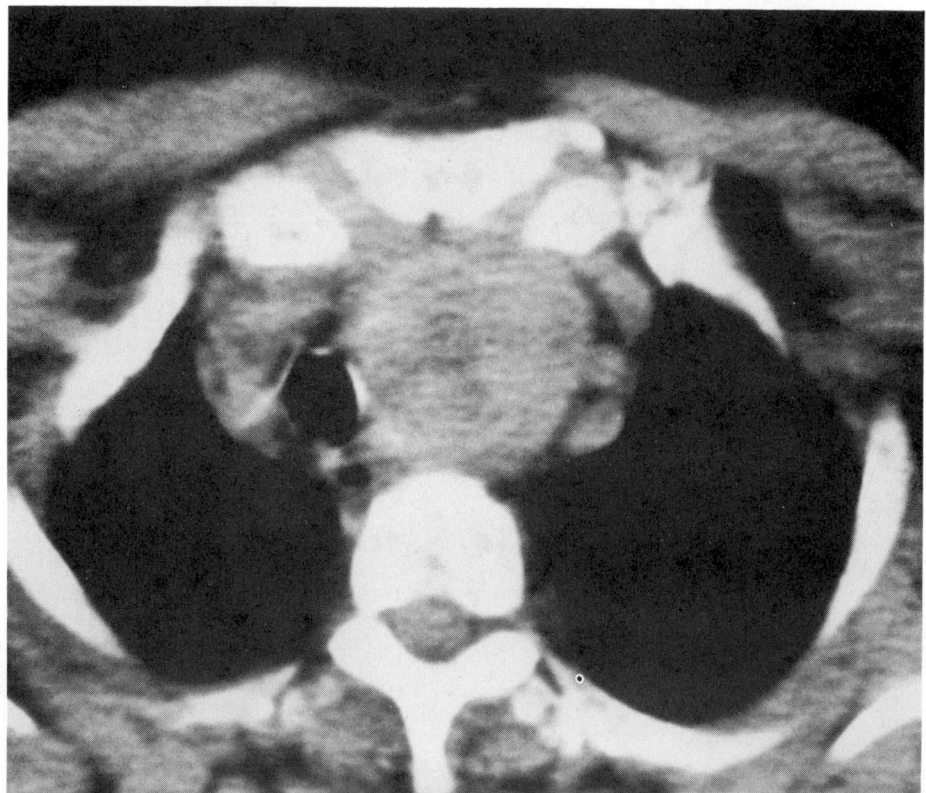

B

Figure 53-9.   Benign goiter in a 70-year-old woman. **(A)** large left paratracheal mass, causing significant displacement of the trachea to the right. **(B)** CT scan shows well-defined left paratracheal mass containing areas of low density centrally. Note the intact fat plane between this mass and the adjacent great vessels, which are displaced laterally.

who also presented with large, lobulated anterior mediastinal masses (Blomlie, et al., 1988). In these patients CT revealed mixed areas of low and high attenuation, and mediastinal fat planes were obliterated. One patient also had pleural and pericardial effusions and invasion of the anterior chest wall.

Thyroid Enlargement

Mediastinal thyroid enlargement is usually due to a nodular goiter; carcinoma is the cause in about 3 percent of cases (Katlic, et al., 1985). The nodular goiters can become quite large and may contain areas of calcification, hemorrhage, and cyst formation. They tend to arise from the inferior aspect of the thyroid gland and extend into the anterior mediastinum anterior to the trachea, but occasionally they occur in a retrotracheal location. Most often they are asymptomatic and discovered on routine radiography, although if large enough they may cause dyspnea, hoarseness, dysphagia, and even the superior vena cava syndrome. On chest x-ray these goiters appear as well-defined, occasionally calcified, lobulated masses in the superior mediastinum. They tend to cause tracheal displacement and occasionally narrowing (Fig. 53-9).

Thyroid scintigraphy has been shown to be very useful in demonstrating that a superior mediastinal mass is due to thyroid tissue and should probably be the next imaging procedure performed once a chest radiograph has revealed a mass that may represent a goiter (Park, et al., 1987). In one study, 93 percent (39/42) of intrathoracic goiters took up radiolabeled agent (^{123}I, ^{131}I, ^{99m}Tc-pertechnetate), while 100 percent (12/12) of nonthyroid masses did not (Park, et al., 1987).

The CT features of mediastinal thyroid have been well-described (Glazer, et al., 1982; Bashist, et al., 1983; Silverman, et al., 1984). These include (1) well-defined borders; (2) definite continuity with the cervical thyroid gland; (3) pretreatment attenuation greater than that of adjacent muscles; (4) an increase in attenuation after injection of intravenous contrast agent; (5) focal, punctate nodular, or curvilinear calcifications; (6) discrete, nonenhancing areas of low attenuation; and (7) insinuation of the mass between the trachea and the great vessels, displacing the latter laterally (rarely, medial vascular displacement can be seen). With significant caudal extension, the mass usually remains posterior to the great vessels and aortic arch; however, it rarely may come to be located anterior to the aortic arch (Glazer, et al., 1982; Bashist, et al., 1983). It is not always possible to distinguish benign from malignant thyroid masses, but CT features suggesting malignancy include (1) ill-defined areas of low attenuation within the gland; (2) adjacent lymphadenopathy; (3) ill-defined margins, with loss of the fat planes between the mass and adjacent mediastinal structures; and (4) destruction of adjacent structures (Silverman, et al., 1984; Pearlberg, et al., 1989) (Fig. 53-10).

More recently, MRI has been shown to provide images of the thyroid that exhibit excellent correlation with pathologic findings (Higgins, et al., 1986; Gefter, et al., 1987; Noma, et al., 1987; Noma, et al., 1988). Tumors generally, but not always, had ill-defined margins and exhibited prolonged T_1 and T_2 values as compared with normal thyroid tissue. Enlarged lymph nodes were clearly visualized, as was the intra-

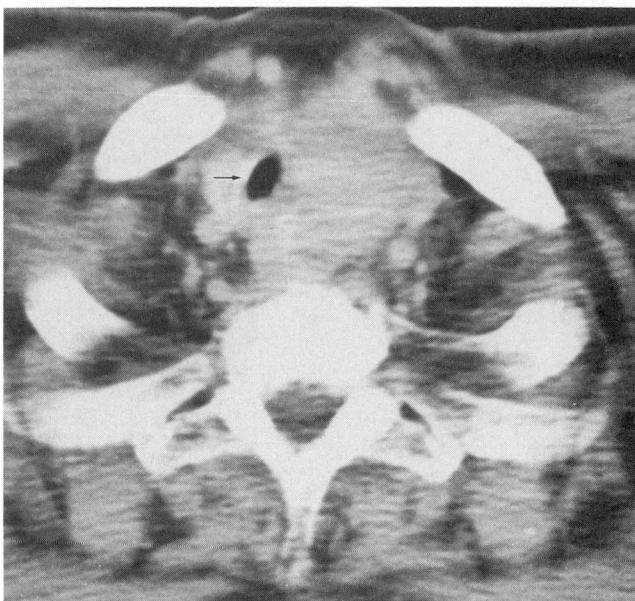

Figure 53-10. CT scan of 85-year-old man with thyroid carcinoma. There is a very ill-defined left paratracheal mass displacing the trachea to the right. There is loss of the fat plane between the mass and the adjacent structures, including the great vessels, and lack of a sharp demarcation between the mass and the adjacent mediastinal fat. The tracheal cartilage has been destroyed by the tumor (note the presence of calcium in the intact tracheal cartilage on the right [*arrow*]).

thoracic extent of the tumor, with coronal and sagittal views being especially helpful in evaluating the latter.

While CT and ultrasound have been shown to be of equal value in most patients with thyroid abnormalities, ultrasound was able to detect some small nodules not imaged by CT, but CT was better at assessing intrathoracic extensions of the gland (Radecki, et al., 1984).

Lymphadenopathy

Lymph node enlargement in the anterior mediastinum is usually caused by lymphoma (Fig. 53-11) or metastatic disease (Fig. 53-12). Other rare causes include Castleman's disease, granulomatous diseases, and angioimmunoblastic lymphadenopathy.

In patients presenting with newly diagnosed Hodgkin's disease, intrathoracic involvement was noted in 67 percent, with 90 percent of these having superior mediastinal adenopathy (Filly, et al. 1976). Similarly, non-Hodgkin's lymphoma patients had thoracic involvement on the initial chest radiograph in 43 percent of cases, with superior mediastinal adenopathy in 46 percent of these. On the chest radiograph, this lymphadenopathy appears as an otherwise typical anterior mediastinal mass. On CT discrete enlarged nodes may be visible or one may note the presence of a large soft tissue mass with ill-defined margins and with loss of the fat plane adjacent to other mediastinal structures (Blank and Castellino, 1987). The mass frequently contains areas of low density representing necrosis; this necrosis does not correlate

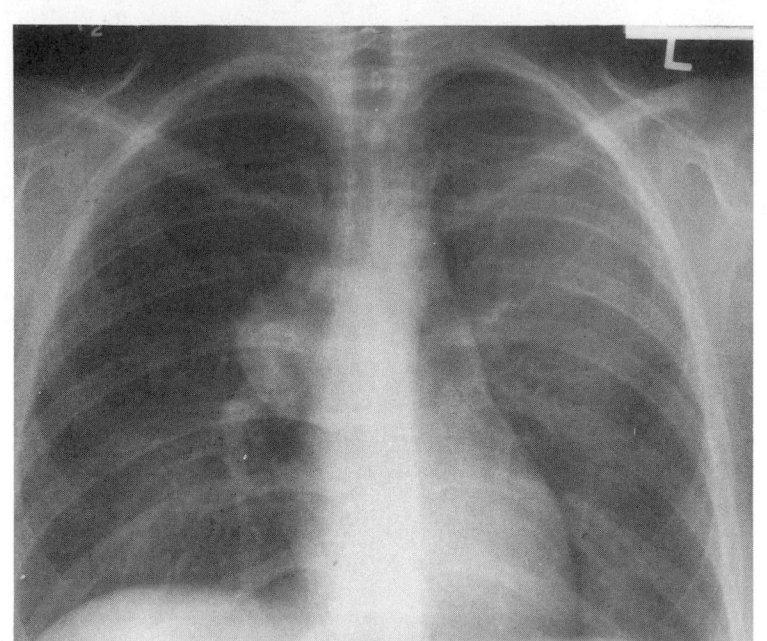
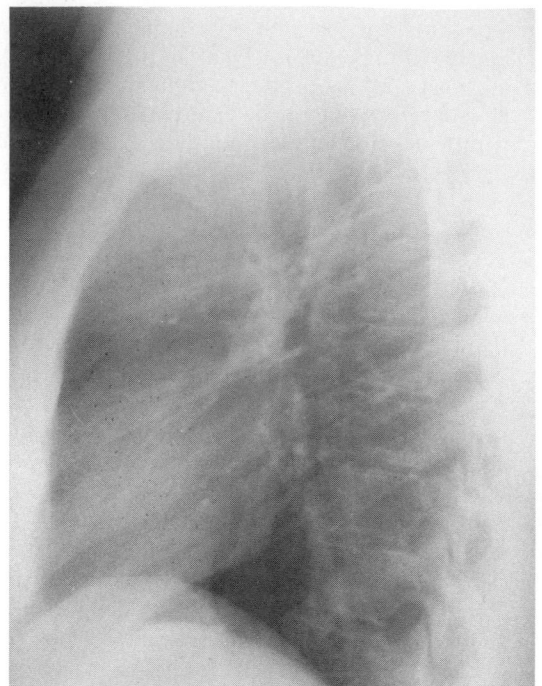
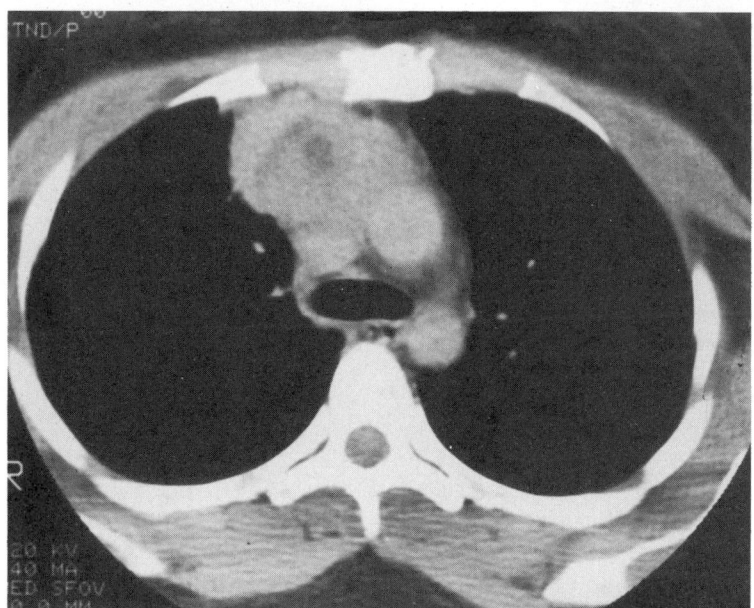

Figure 53-11.   In this 25-year-old asymptomatic woman with Hodgkin's disease, chest x-rays, **(A)** PA and **(B)** lateral, show a right anterior mediastinal mass. **(C)** CT scan shows an ill-defined mass in the anterior mediastinum containing areas of decreased attenuation which presumably representing necrosis. Note loss of fat plane between the posterior aspects of the mass and the superior vena cava and ascending aorta.

with the size of the nodal mass and has no prognostic significance in patients with newly diagnosed Hodgkin's disease (Hopper, et al., 1990). These lymphomatous masses can directly invade the chest wall (Press, et al., 1985; Gouliamos, et al., 1980) and may calcify, even if untreated (Lautin, et al., 1990). A different pattern of involvement is the so-called permeating continuum, which is a large mass lesion with no discernible borders, which blends imperceptibly with the other mediastinal structures.

A cystic form of Hodgkin's disease, which appears as a mass containing large areas with the density of water and which obliterates adjacent fat planes, may mimic germ cell tumors and thymomas (Federle and Callen, 1979). Thymic cysts have been described following successful irradiation of Hodgkin's disease; these appear as smooth, thin-walled structures containing homogeneous water-density material and should not be confused with recurrent tumor (Baron, et al., 1981b).

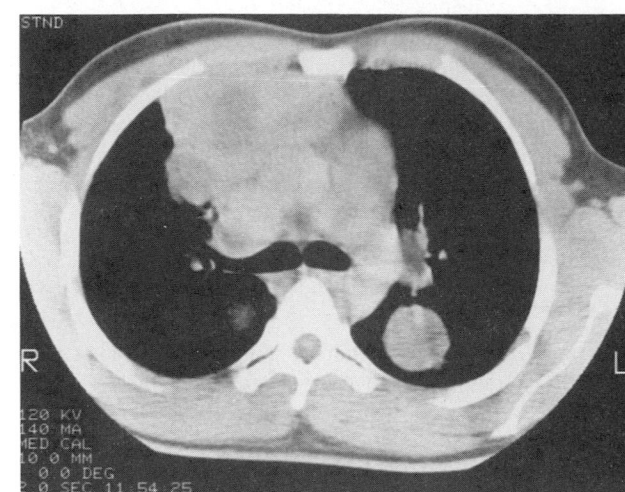
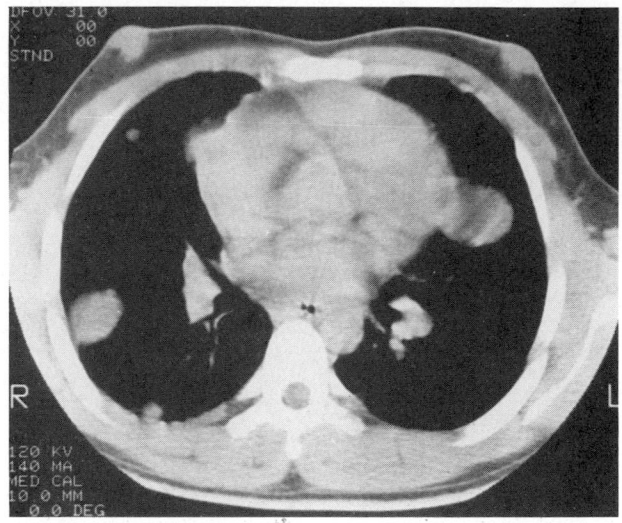

Figure 53-12. **(A)** CT scan in 22-year-old man with testicular choriocarcinoma metastatic to the lungs and anterior mediastinum shows large, right lobulated anterior mediastinal mass. There are areas of low density within this mass, most likely representing necrosis. It is ill-defined where it contacts the adjacent mediastinal structures. **(B)** CT scan 3 cm below Fig. A. There are bilateral pulmonary metastases. Note the bilateral gynecomastia due to the very high levels (greater than 300,000 units) of β-HCG (human chorionic gonadotropin).

Miscellaneous Lesions

Not uncommonly, a chest radiograph can suggest the presence of a mass lesion but no such mass is seen at CT. This may be due to increased amounts of anterior mediastinal fat (Fig. 53-13). A number of other rare causes of anterior mediastinal masses have been described. One of these, which

must always be kept in mind, especially if a biopsy of the mass is contemplated, is an aortic aneurysm. On the chest radiograph an aneurysm of the ascending aorta, which is usually congenital or mycotic in etiology, most often projects to the right of the midline. On CT it can be recognized by the fact that it rapidly takes up intravenous contrast material, although some or most of the aneurysm may be filled with

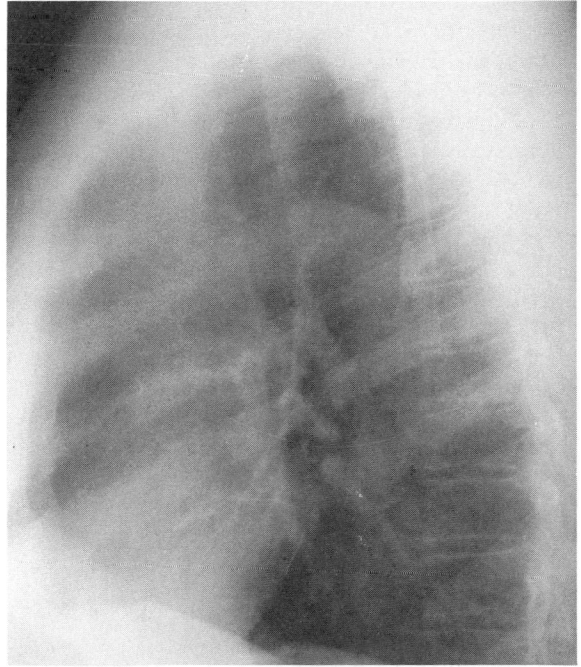
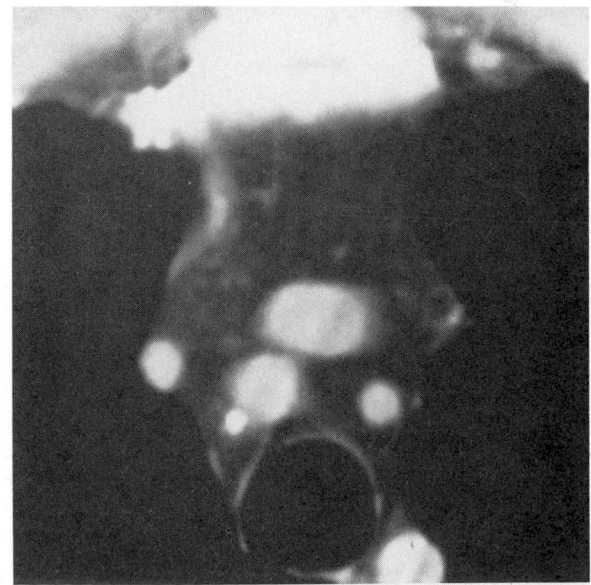

Figure 53-13. This 63-year-old man with mediastinal lipomatosis presented with myasthenia gravis. **(A)** Lateral chest radiograph shows fullness in the anterior mediastinum, suggesting the presence of a mass. **(B)** CT scan indicates that increased amounts of anterior mediastinal fat are causing the plain radiographic findings.

thrombus. Other causes of mass lesions in this location include parathyroid adenoma, cystic hygroma, paraganglioma, hemangioma, lipoma, and liposarcoma.

MIDDLE MEDIASTINAL MASSES

The middle mediastinal compartment contains the heart and pericardium and all the major vessels leaving and entering this organ, plus the trachea and main bronchi, paratracheal and tracheobronchial lymph nodes, phrenic nerves, and the upper portion of the vagus nerves.

Lymph Node Enlargement

Lymph node enlargement is the most common cause of a mediastinal mass and can be caused by lymphoma, metastatic carcinoma, sarcoidosis, and infection (particularly due to *Histoplasma capsulatum* and *Mycobacterium tuberculosis*). Uncommon causes include Castleman's disease (giant lymph node hyperplasia) (Hammond, 1979) (Fig. 53-14), granulomatous mediastinitis (Weinstein, et al., 1983) (Fig. 53-15), and amyloidosis.

Primary Tracheal Neoplasms

Primary tracheal neoplasms are uncommon. Squamous cell carcinoma is the most common, followed by adenoid cystic carcinoma. These may show a subtle alteration in the tracheal air column on routine chest radiography, or if more extensive may cause widening of the upper middle mediastinal soft tissues. In any patient with dyspnea, wheezing, or stridor, the tracheal air column should be carefully scrutinized on conventional radiographs to exclude a subtle mass (Fig. 53-16). CT is superior in showing the extent of tumor involvement (Fig. 53-17). Adenoid cystic carcinomas tend to be very infiltrative tumors, often underestimated in extent even by CT scanning (Spizarny, et al., 1986).

Bronchogenic Cysts

The majority of mediastinal bronchogenic cysts occur around the tracheal carina in relationship to the major airways (Davis and Simonton, 1956). They rarely communicate with the tracheobronchial tree. Radiologically, they occur as a round or oval mass of homogeneous soft tissue density, located just inferior to the carina and often protruding posteriorly and slightly to the right (Reed and Sobonya, 1974) (Fig. 53-18). Calcification of the cyst wall is uncommon (Ziter, et al., 1969). CT scanning may show a cyst of water density. The attenuation is commonly higher than one would associate with a cyst because of the content of thick mucoid material (Mendelson, et al., 1983). Calcium in the cyst contents may also produce high CT numbers (Yernault, et al., 1986). Transthoracic and transbronchial needle aspiration are useful procedures, both diagnostically and therapeutically (Kuhlman, et al., 1988). Mucoid material of varying color and consistency may be aspirated.

MASSES SITUATED IN THE ANTERIOR CARDIOPHRENIC ANGLE

Masses occurring in the anterior cardiophrenic angle can arise from lung parenchyma, pleura, mediastinum, or diaphragm or from beneath the diaphragm. CT is very useful in differential diagnosis of these lesions (Modic and Janicki, 1980). The commonest lesions include a large pleuropericardial fat pad, pericardial cyst, and hernia through the foramen of Bochdalek.

Pericardial Cysts

Pericardial cysts are congenital mesothelial cysts and usually occur as smooth round or oval masses in the right anterior cardiophrenic angle (Feigin, et al., 1977) (Fig. 53-19). The lateral radiograph may show a teardrop configuration as the cyst extends into the interlobar fissure. The cystic nature of these masses can be confirmed by CT (Pugatch, et al., 1978) or ultrasonography. Calcification is rare. Percutaneous fine-needle aspiration shows the contained clear or straw-colored fluid and can be therapeutic as well.

Dilatation of the Major Mediastinal Arteries and Veins

Dilatation of the superior vena cava as a result of raised central venous pressure may cause a smooth widening of the right superior mediastinal soft tissues. Dilatation of the azygos vein may cause a round or oval mass in the right tracheobronchial angle. A dilated vein can be differentiated from a true mass by demonstrating an increase in size of the structure in the supine position as compared with the erect position. The superior vena cava syndrome is characterized by edema of the face, neck, upper extremities, and thorax and dilated chest wall veins. It is caused by obstruction of the superior vena cava, most commonly by bronchogenic carcinoma. Lymphoma, metastatic carcinoma, and chronic sclerosing mediastinitis are uncommon causes. A mass in the right superior mediastinum is usually present. The obstructed vein can be confirmed by CT or venography (Bechtold, et al., 1985).

Aneurysms of the aorta or its major branches may produce a middle (Fig. 53-20) or posterior mediastinal mass. Dynamic CT scanning with bolus injection of contrast agent is very useful in diagnosis of all types of aortic aneurysms. In any patient with a middle or posterior mediastinal mass that could be related to the aorta, CT scanning should be performed prior to invasive procedures such as percutaneous needle biopsy. The aneurysm is frequently occluded by thrombus, so that little if any opacification of the lumen occurs with contrast. MRI is also useful, making aortography unnecessary.

Congenital anomalies of the aorta may present with a middle mediastinal mass (Fig. 53-21). A right aortic arch is the commonest anomaly and presents as a right upper paratracheal mass, displacing the tracheal air column to the left and anteriorly (Shuford, et al., 1970). Usually the diagnosis is evident on plain chest radiographs. CT, aortography, or MRI is diagnostic.

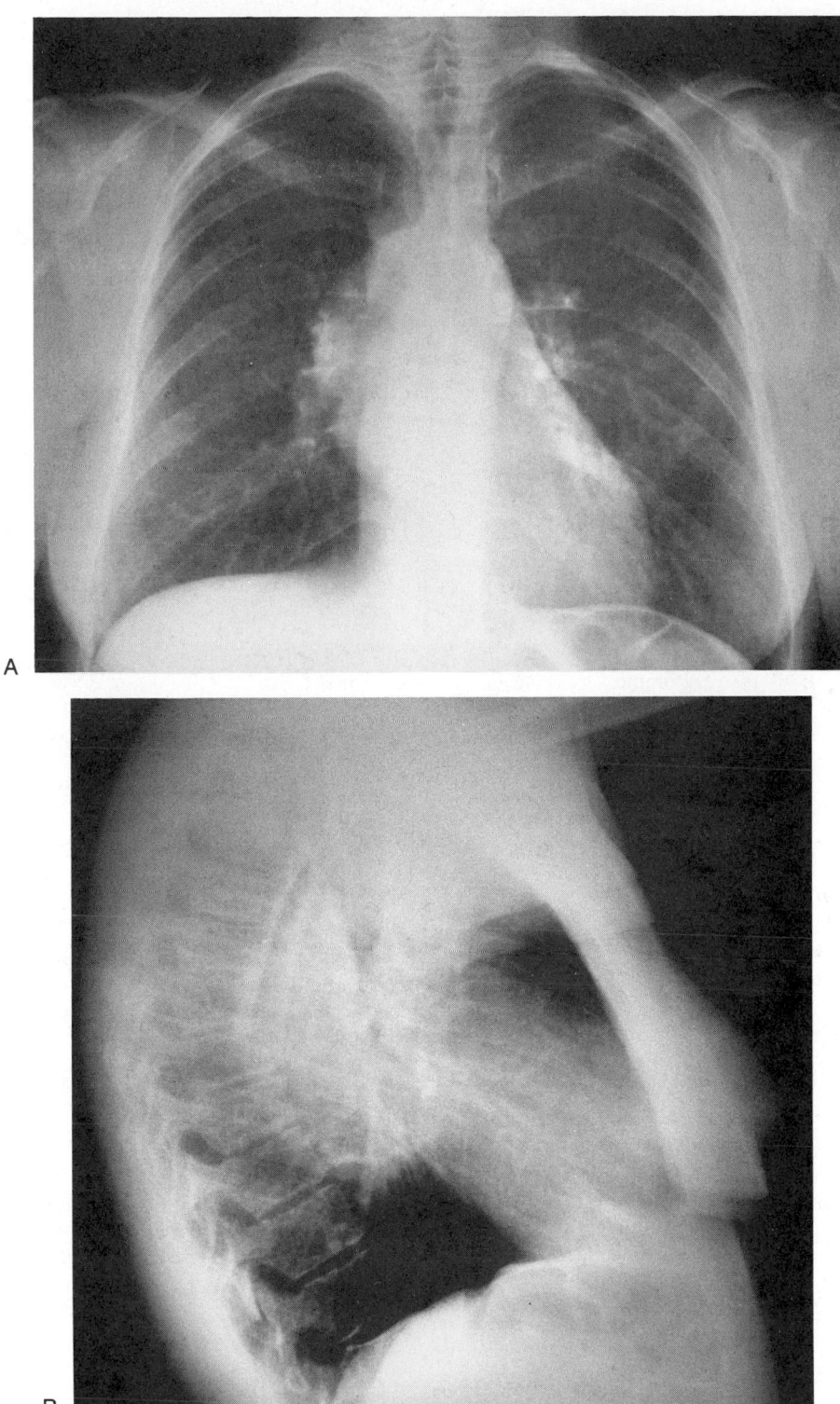

Figure 53-14. A 21-year-old woman was found to have a mediastinal mass on a chest radiograph taken because of an upper respiratory tract infection. **(A)** PA and **(B)** lateral chest radiographs show a large mass arising in the mediastinum just posterior to the distal trachea and upper posterior heart. Thoracotomy revealed a very vascular mass that could not be removed entirely because of bleeding. Biopsy showed giant lymph node hyperplasia (hyaline vascular type).

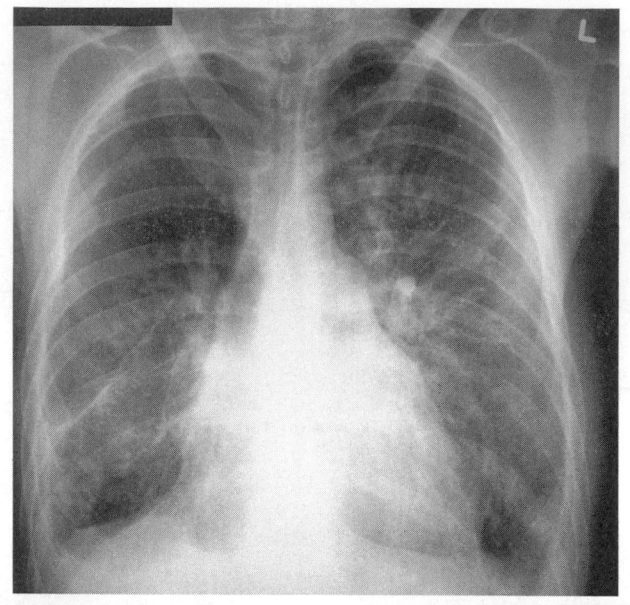

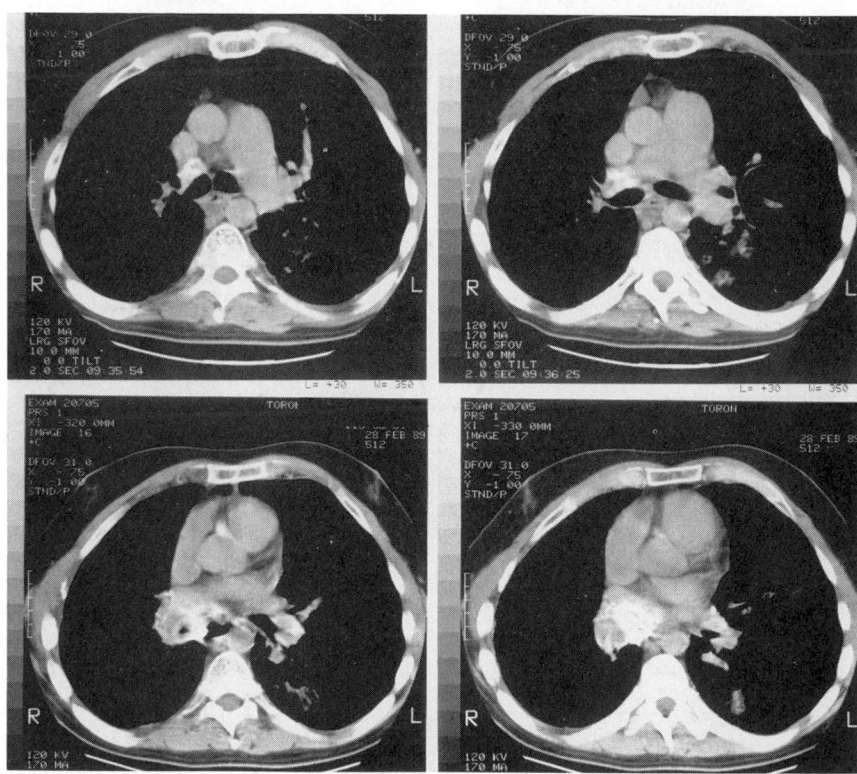

Figure 53-15. A 43-year-old man with a 20-year history of granulomatous mediastinitis. Right thoracotomy and open biopsy of a mediastinal mass in the past showed "burned-out histoplasmosis." At presentation he was severely dyspneic and hypoxemic with pulmonary arterial hypertension. **(A)** PA chest radiograph shows evidence of old right thoracotomy with resection of fifth rib. Increased density is present in the right and left lower lung zones. The right and left lateral costophrenic sulci are blunted by pleural effusions. **(B)** CT scan shows calcified nodal tissue in the right tracheobronchial angle. A large retrocardiac right periesophageal mass is present, containing a large amount of calcification. The main pulmonary artery and central pulmonary arteries are dilated. There is complete obstruction of the bronchus intermedius, and at the origin of the right middle and right lower lobe bronchi. A pulmonary angiogram showed complete obstruction of the right pulmonary artery. The patient died shortly after a left lung transplant. At autopsy, a diagnosis of sclerosing mediastinitis was confirmed. There was encasement of bronchovascular structures at the hila of both lungs, resulting in obstruction of the right pulmonary artery and stenosis of the left pulmonary artery, both pulmonary veins, and main bronchi. Patchy pulmonary congestion, edema, hemosiderosis, and chronic interstitial fibrosis were present.

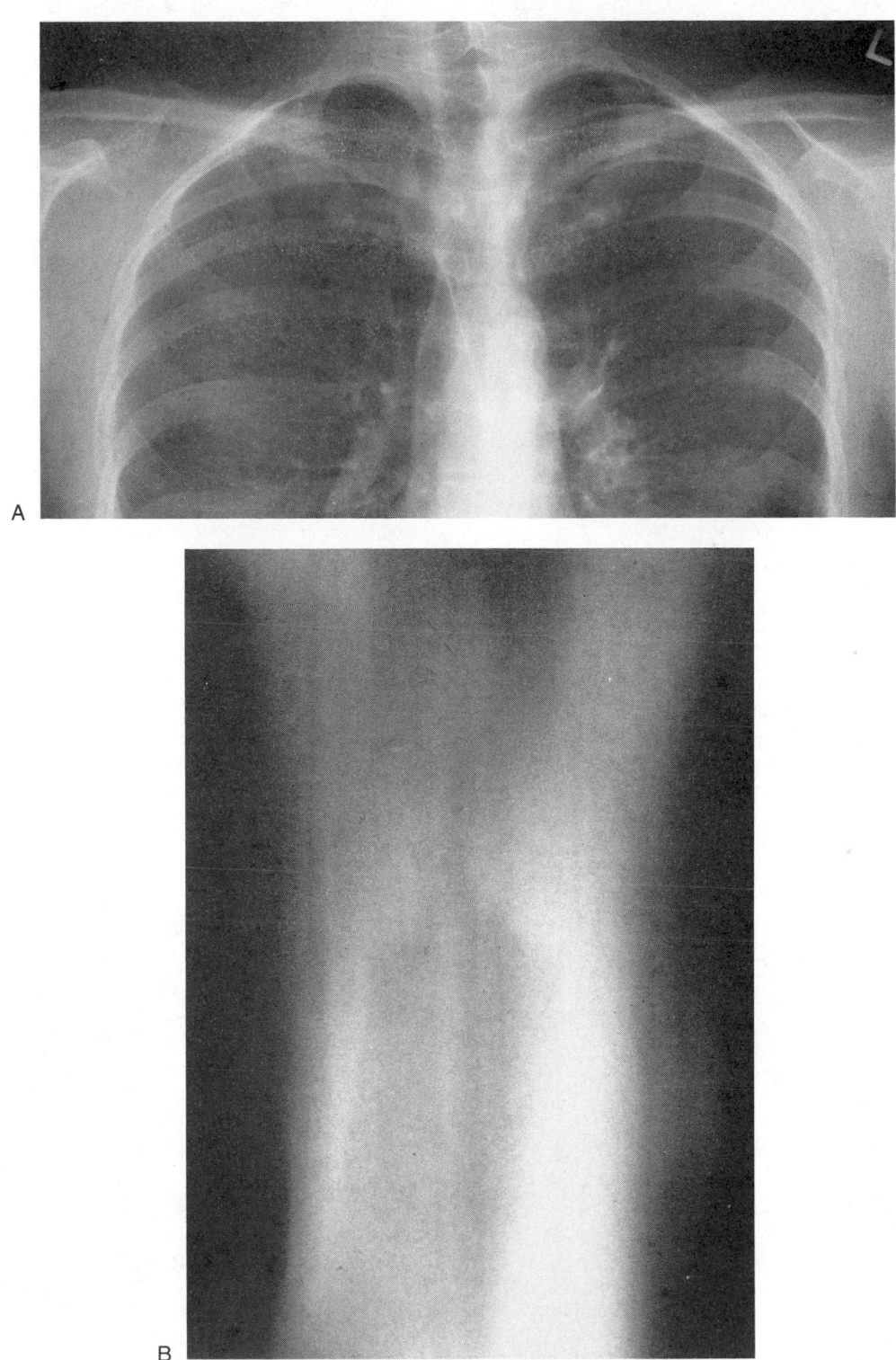

Figure 53-16. A 31-year-old woman with cough and stridor for 1 year. **(A)** PA chest radiograph shows increased density in the midtrachea, with loss of the tracheal outline. **(B)** AP tomogram confirms a mass in the midtrachea. Tracheal resection removed an adenoid cystic carcinoma.

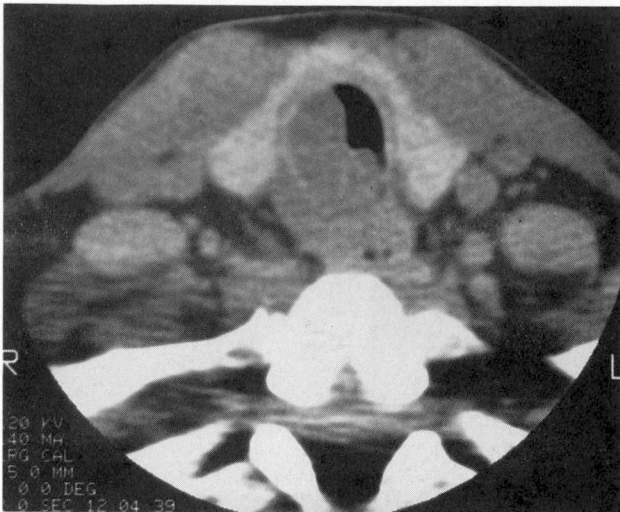

Figure 53-17. This 42-year-old man with stridor shows a large mass occluding much of the upper tracheal lumen. The extratracheal component is well visualized.

POSTERIOR MEDIASTINAL MASSES

Neurogenic Tumors

Neurogenic tumors are a common cause of a posterior mediastinal mass, accounting for almost 20 percent of mediastinal tumors (Ingels et al., 1971). Neurogenic tumors arising from peripheral nerves include neurofibroma, neurilemmoma (schwannoma), and neurogenic sarcoma (malignant schwannoma) (Fig. 53-22). These usually arise from intercos-

tal nerves; vagus and phrenic neurofibromas are rare. Radiologically, these tumors are seen as a well-defined, round or oval mass in the paravertebral region (Fig. 53-23). Calcification is rare. CT may show expansion of the intervertebral foramen. MRI is useful in showing any spinal canal component. Percutaneous fine-needle aspiration biopsy may reveal no diagnostic cells or spindle cells indicative of a spindle cell neoplasm. Cytologically, the differential diagnosis is that of spindle cell tumors, but this, when combined with typical radiology, can be diagnostic of a neurogenic tumor.

Neurogenic tumors originating from sympathetic ganglia include ganglioneuroma, ganglioneuroblastoma, neuroblastoma, and paraganglioma (chemodectoma, pheochromocytoma). Radiologically, these tumors are similar to those of the peripheral nerve group. However, they tend to be more elongated in the cephalocaudal direction, meeting the mediastinum at an obtuse rather than an acute angle (Theros, 1969). Consequently, they are often less easily seen on lateral view (Reed, et al., 1978) (Fig. 53-24). Calcifications are not uncommon; however, bony changes are unusual. Percutaneous fine-needle aspiration biopsy may reveal no diagnostic cells, nondiagnostic spindle cells, or a combination of spindle cells and ganglion cells diagnostic of a ganglioneuroma.

Gastroenteric (Duplication) Cysts

Duplication cysts may cause a middle or posterior mediastinal mass, particularly in the young (Kuhlman, et al., 1985). Histologically, these cysts can be lined by nonkeratinizing squamous, ciliated columnar, gastric, or small intestinal epithelium. They may occur within or adjacent to the wall of the esophagus. Communication with the upper gastrointestinal tract is uncommon (Dresler, et al., 1990) (Fig. 53-25).

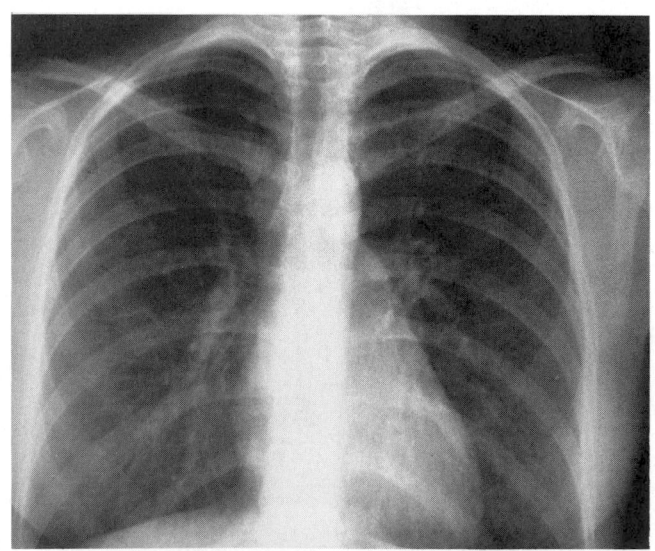

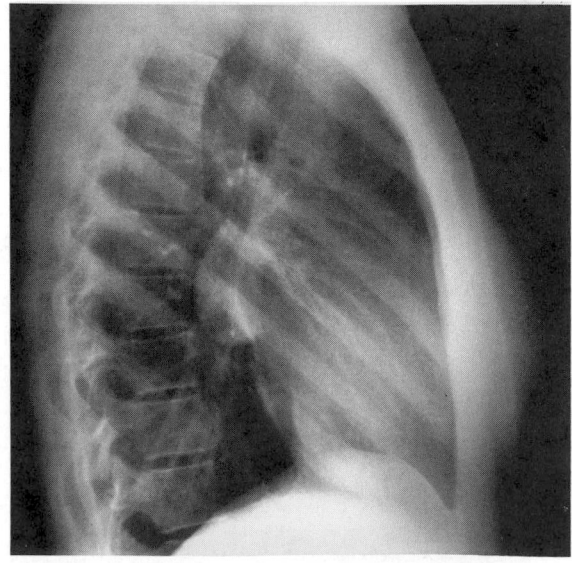

Figure 53-18. This 17-year-old girl with dysphagia was noted to have a middle mediastinal mass. **(A)** PA and **(B)** lateral chest radiographs reveal an oval, well-defined mass occurring in a typical location for bronchogenic cyst, inferior to the carina and projecting posteriorly and to the right. Percutaneous needle aspiration revealed mucus, respiratory epithelial cells, and microcalcifications consistent with a bronchogenic cyst.

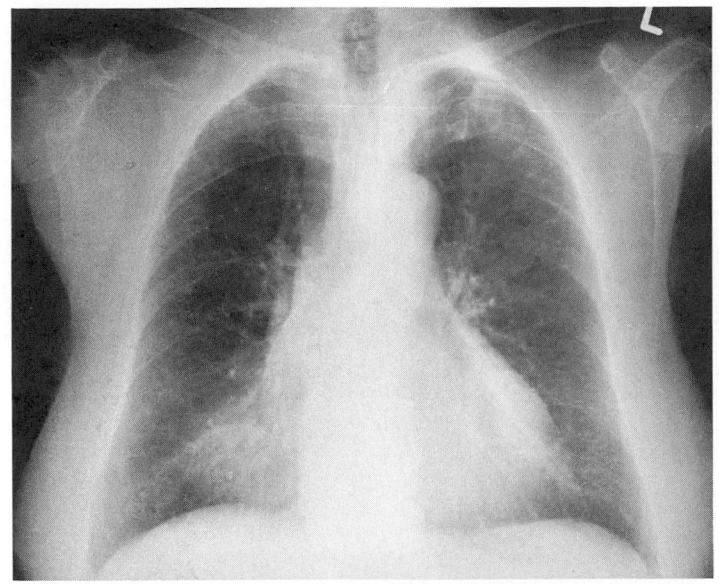
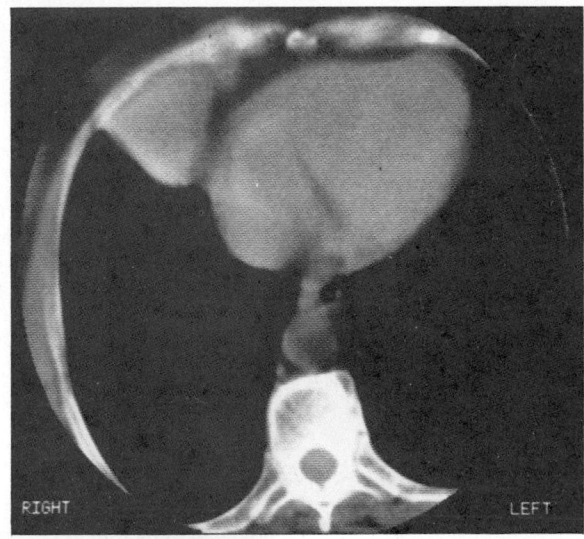
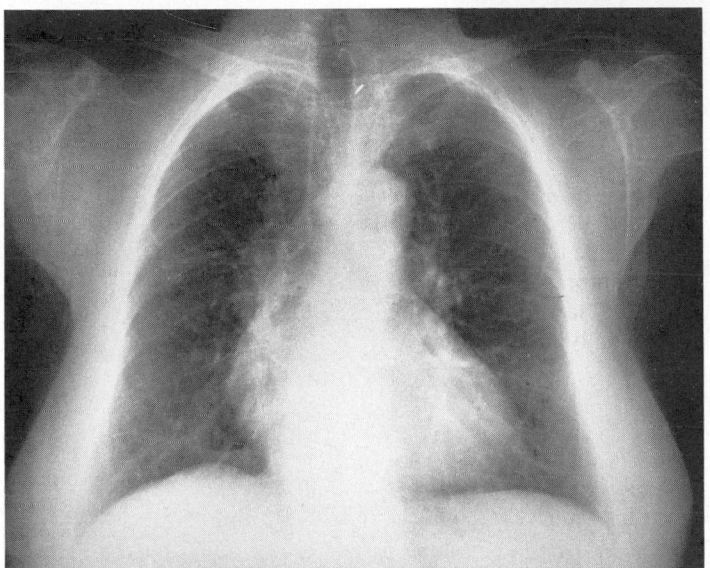

Figure 53-19. **(A)** This 64-year-old asymptomatic woman has a mass in right anterior cardiophrenic angle. **(B)** CT scan shows a mass of water density in this angle. **(C)** PA film taken after aspiration of clear serious fluid shows decrease in size of mass and development of an air-fluid level.

Neurenteric cysts have a connection to the meninges and may be associated with congenital defects of the thoracic spine.

Diseases of the Esophagus

Esophageal neoplasm, diverticulum, hiatus hernia, mega-esophagus, and esophageal varices (Jonsson and Rian, 1970) may cause posterior mediastinal masses in relation to the esophagus. Plain chest radiography is frequently normal in patients with esophageal carcinoma. Abnormalities may be subtle and include a retrocardiac mass (Fig. 53-26A), abnormal azygoesophageal recess interface, widened mediastinum, widened retrotracheal stripe, and esophageal air-fluid level

(Lindell, et al., 1979). CT is very useful in staging of esophageal carcinoma, and it is highly accurate in predicting tumor size and assessing invasion of mediastinum and tracheobronchial tree, as well as spread to the liver, adrenals, and upper abdominal lymph nodes (Picus, et al., 1983) (Fig. 53-26B).

Paravertebral Masses

Primary or metastatic tumors of the thoracic spine may present with a posterior mediastinal paravertebral mass. The bony lesion should be evident radiologically. Lymphomas, particularly Hodgkin's disease, may involve the posterior parietal group of lymph nodes and produce a fusiform para-

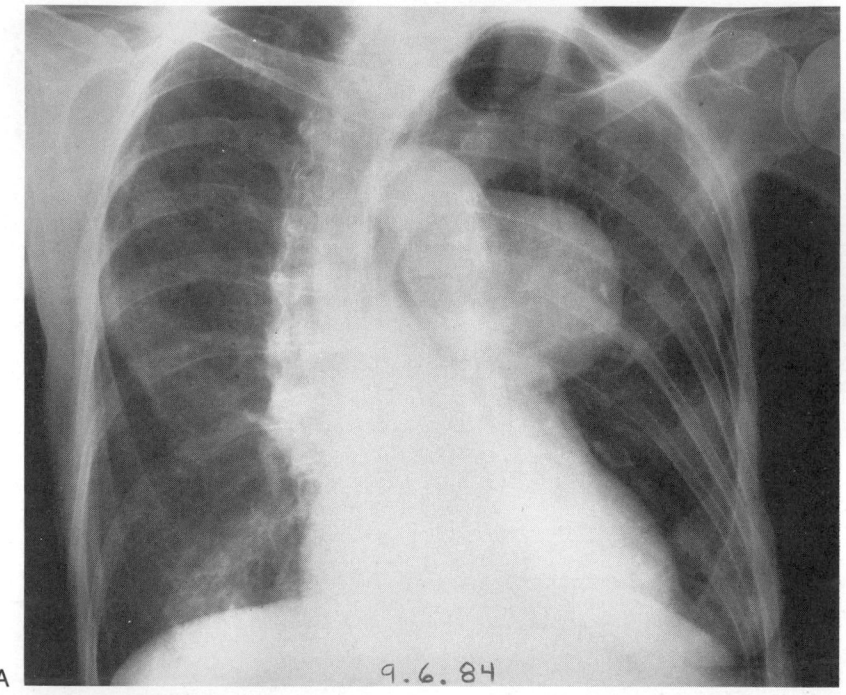

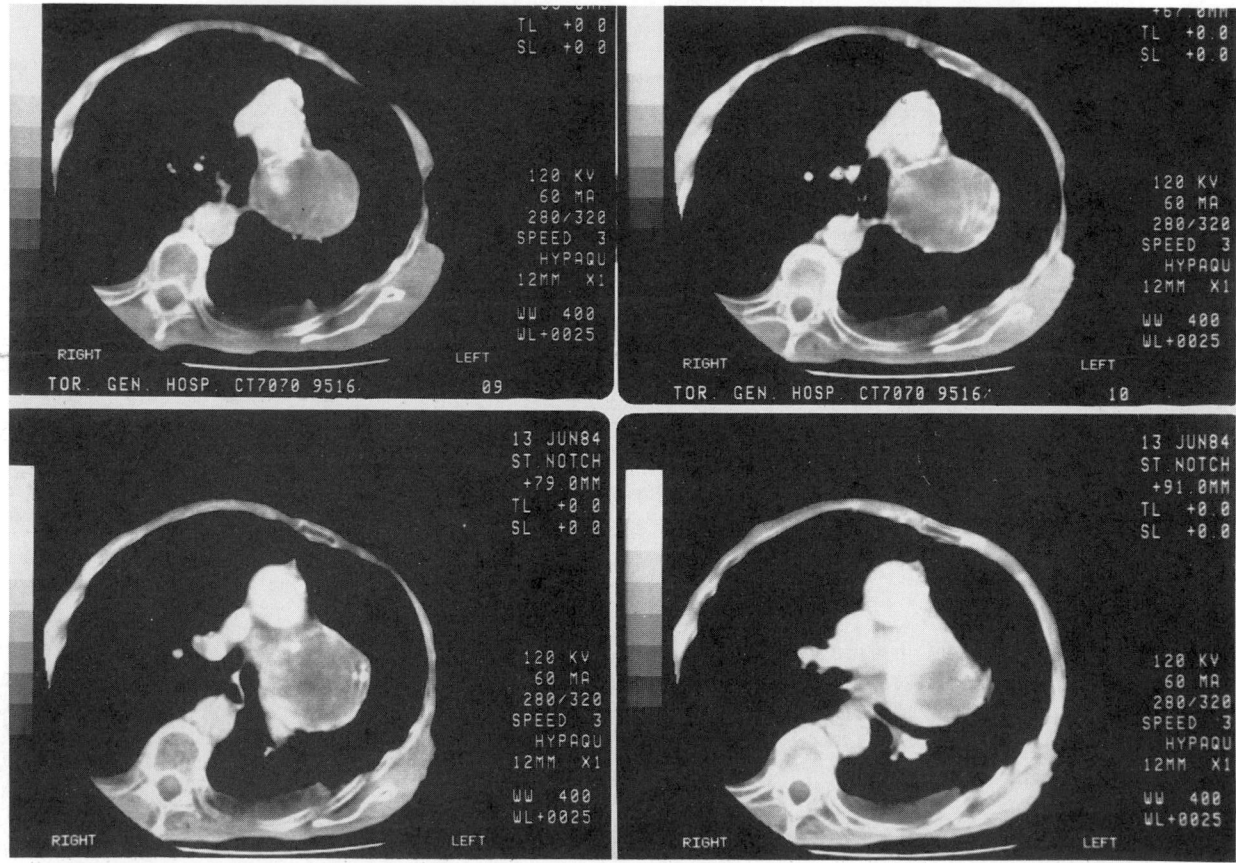

Figure 53-20.   A 73-year-old woman with aortic aneurysm. **(A)** PA chest radiograph shows large round mass occupying the left aorticopulmonary window. Spotty calcification seen within mass laterally. **(B)** CT scan shows very small opacified lumen, with most of the mass occupied by thrombus. The findings were confirmed at autopsy.

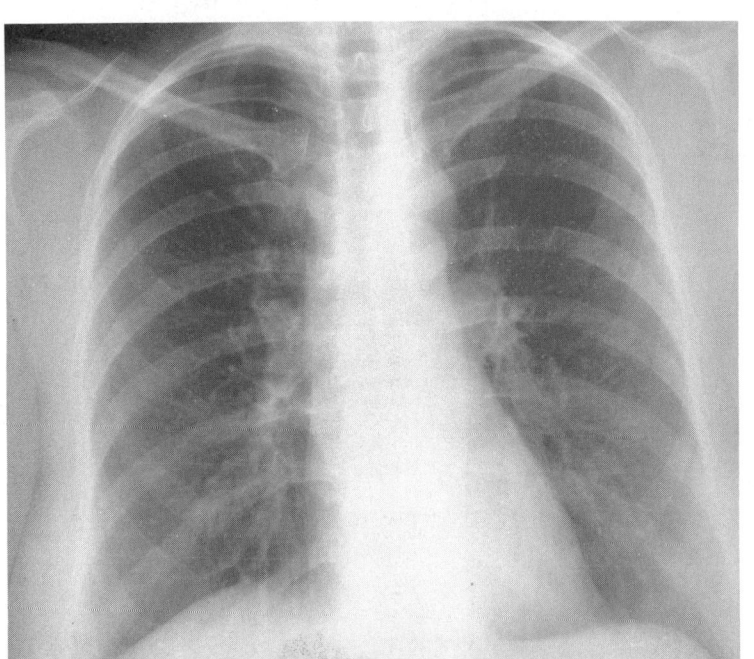
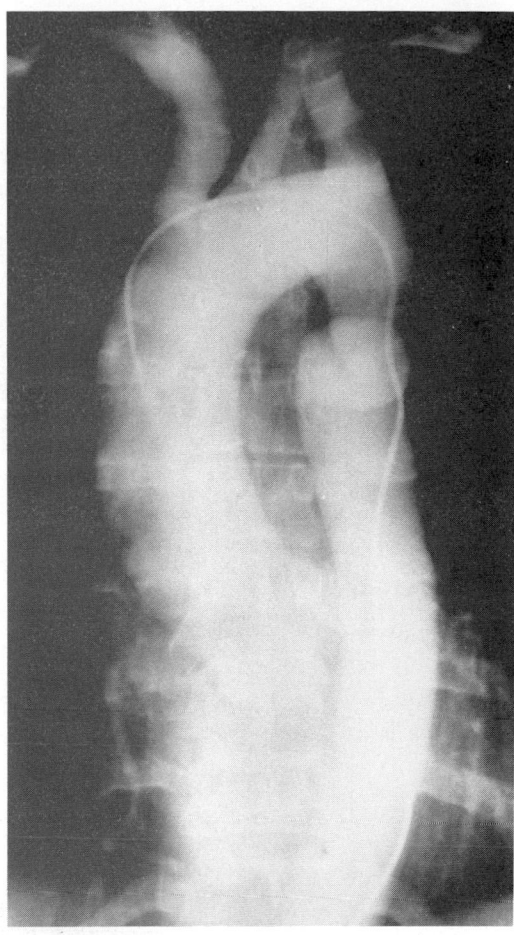

A

B

Figure 53-21. **(A)** PA radiograph of 39-year-old woman shows a left upper middle mediastinal mass. **(B)** Aortogram shows a pseudocoarctation with elongation and buckling distal to the left subclavian artery.

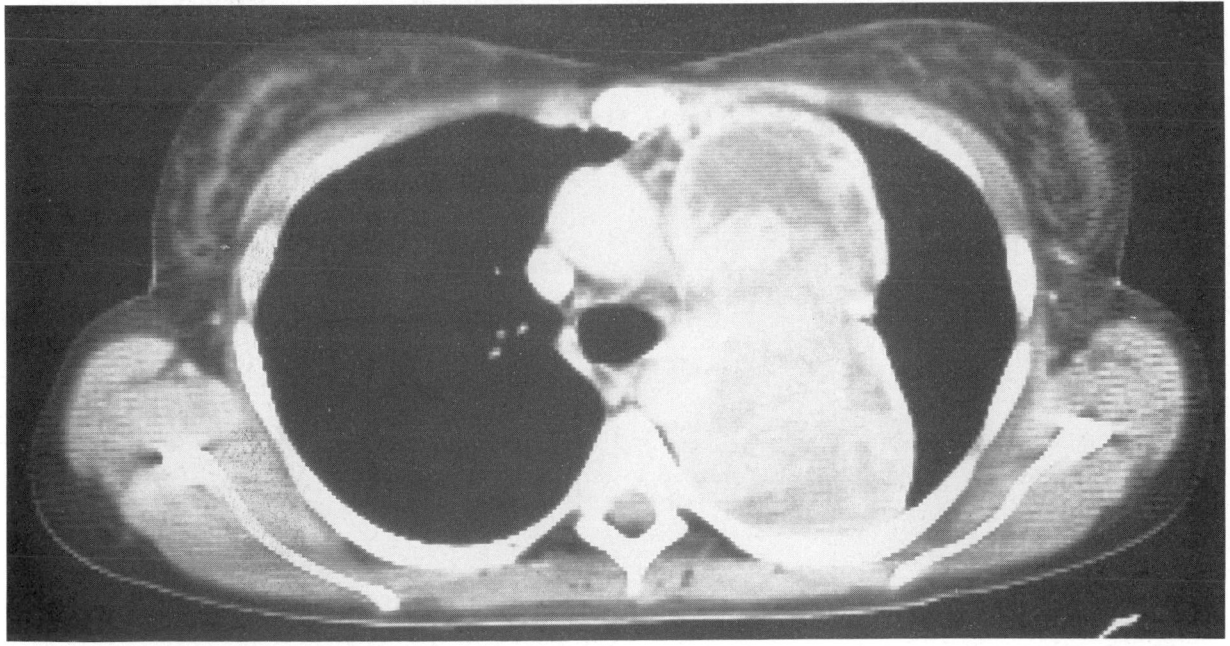

Figure 53-22. CT scan in 47-year-old woman with left chest pain and cough shows large tumor mass of inhomogeneous density (necrosis) occupying the left side of the mediastinum. Other scans showed separate pleural nodules. Left thoracotomy revealed an unresectable neurogenic sarcoma.

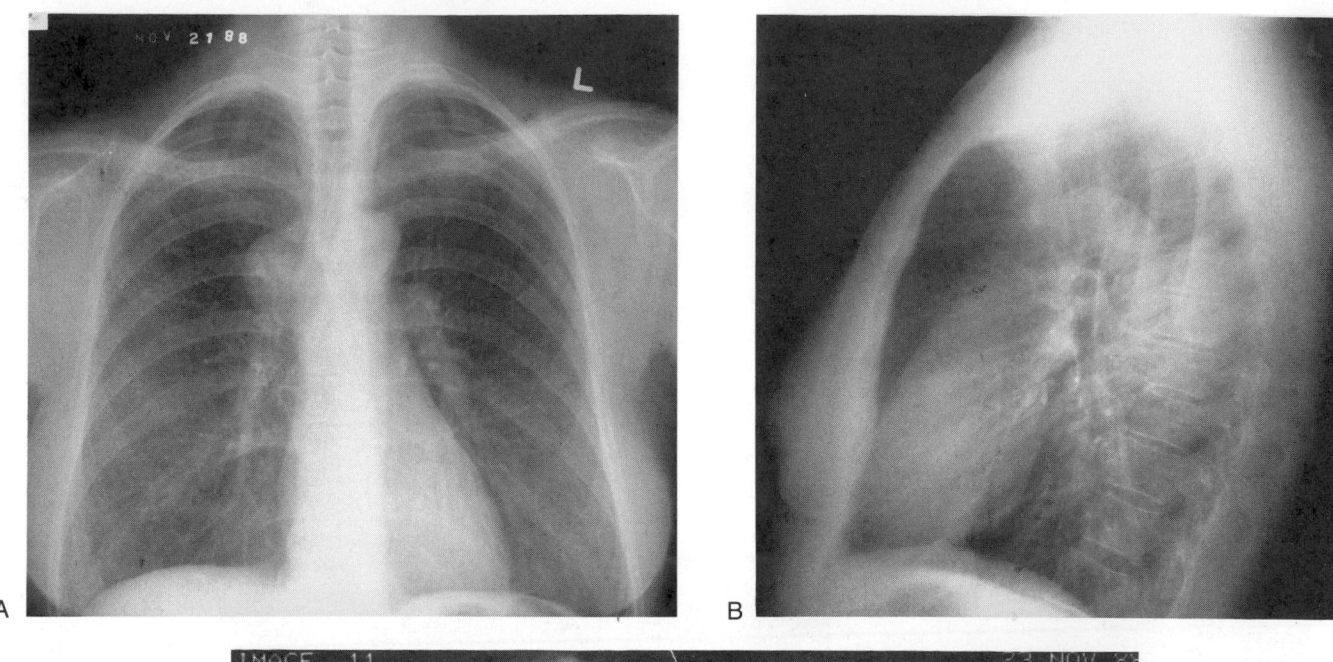

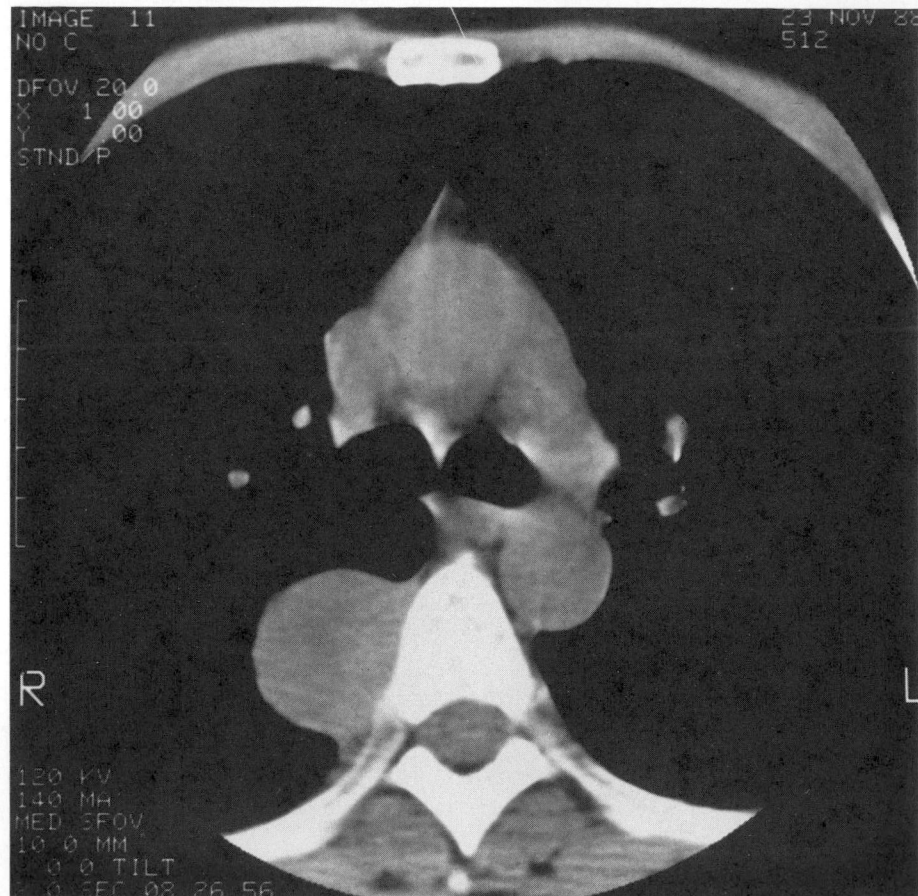

Figure 53-23. A 52-year-old asymptomatic woman with a right posterior paravertebral oval, well-defined mass on **(A)** PA and **(B)** lateral chest radiographs. **(C)** CT shows the typical location of the neurofibroma.

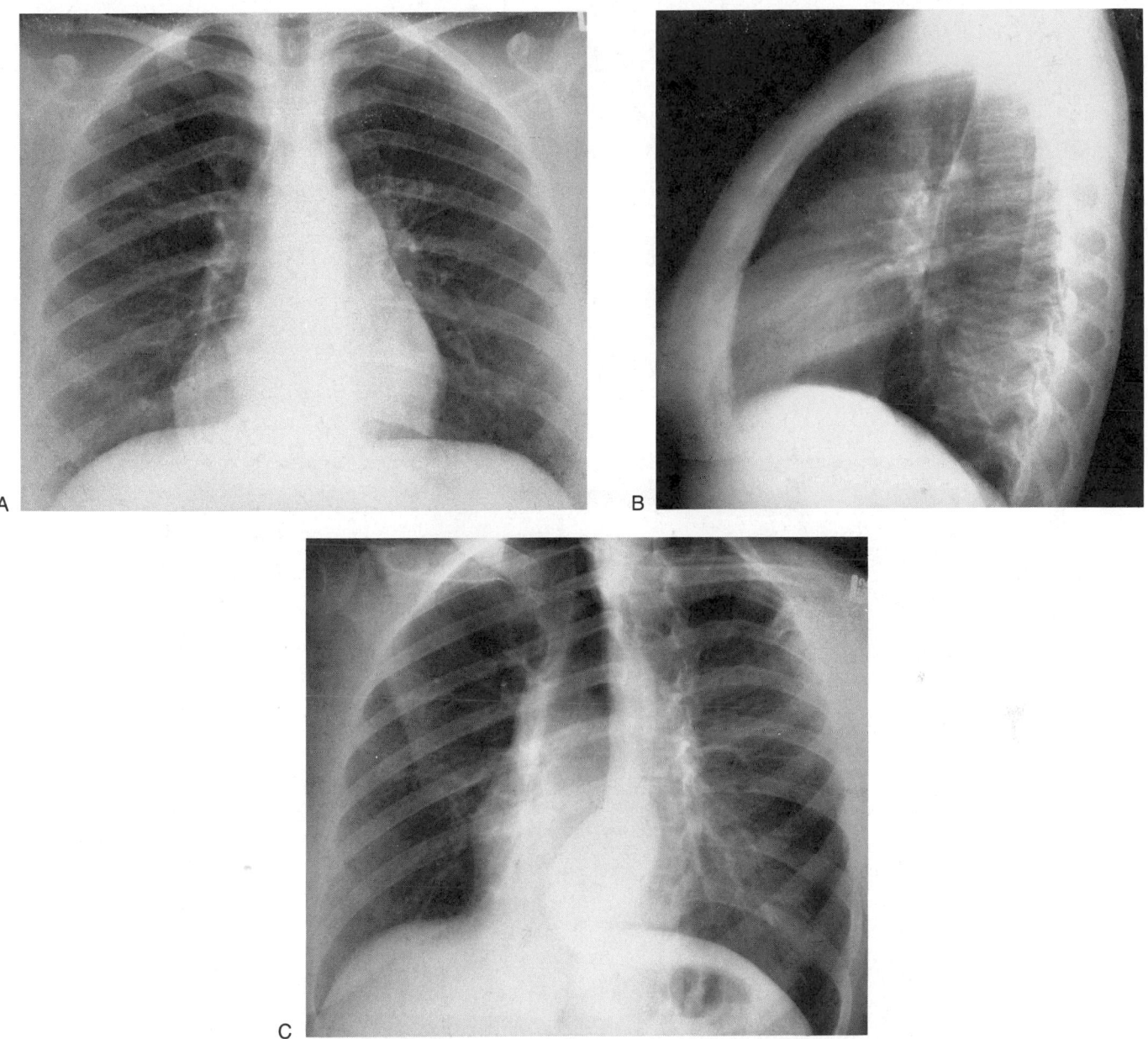

Figure 53-24. **(A)** A 20-year-old asymptomatic woman with a right lower posterior paravertebral mediastinal mass. **(B)** Poorly seen on the lateral radiograph. **(C)** Left anterior oblique radiograph shows the typical well-defined elongated shape of the mass making obtuse angles with the mediastinum.

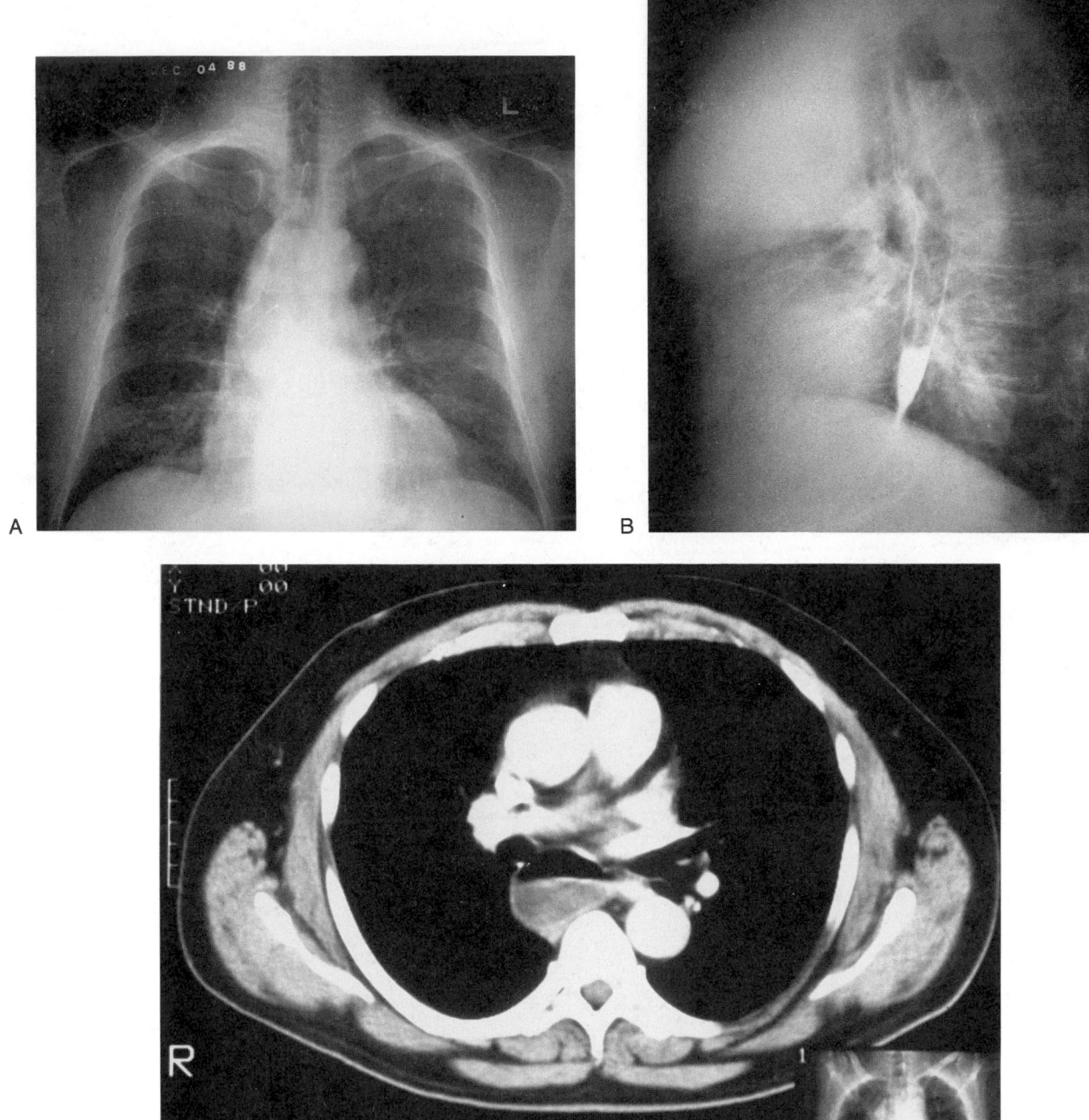

Figure 53-25. A 53-year-old man with iron deficiency anemia. **(A)** PA and **(B)** lateral chest radiographs show a posterior mediastinal mass adjacent to the barium sulfate-filled esophagus. A short air-fluid level is noted in its upper portion. **(C)** CT shows the cystic mass with air-fluid level, which extended the entire length of the posterior mediastinum into the upper abdomen. Barium examination of the upper gastrointestinal tract showed a communication with the second portion of the duodenum, where a diverticulum-like structure was present. Right thoracotomy and laparotomy removed a duplication cyst running from the neck down to the second portion of the duodenum. The cyst was lined by esophageal epithelium in the chest and gastric epithelium in the abdomen. Ulceration was present, likely producing the iron deficiency anemia.

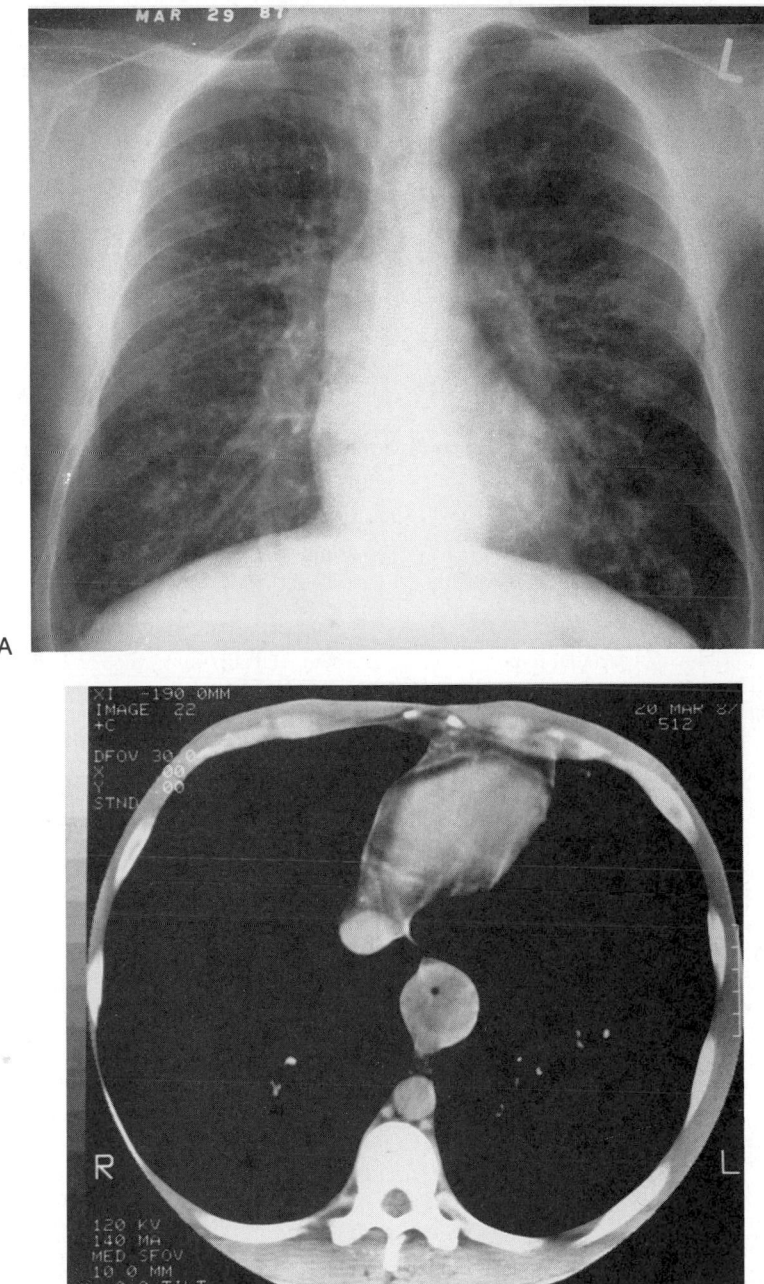

Figure 53-26. **(A)** PA chest radiograph shows a left lower mediastinal retrocardiac mass. **(B)** CT shows a well defined mass in the lower esophagus without invasion of adjacent structures. This proved to be a carcinoma of the lower esophagus.

vertebral soft tissue mass. Infections (e.g., tuberculosis) and post-traumatic hematomas may also cause a paravertebral mass. Rare causes of posterior mediastinal masses include mediastinal extension of a pancreatic pseudocyst (Johnston, et al., 1986), extramedullary hematopoiesis (Ross and Logan, 1969), and meningocele (Edeiken, et al., 1969).

REFERENCES

Baron RL, Lee JKT, Sagel SS, Levitt RG: Computed tomography of the abnormal thymus. Radiology 142:127, 1982a

Baron RL, Lee JKT, Sagel SS, Peterson RR: Computed tomography of the normal thymus. Radiology 142:121, 1982b

Baron RL, Levitt RG, Sagel SS et al.: Computed tomography in the evaluation of mediastinal widening. Radiology 138:107, 1981a

Baron RL, Sagel SS, Baglan RJ: Thymic cysts following radiation therapy for Hodgkin's disease. Radiology 141:593, 1981b

Bashist B, Ellis K, Gold RP: Computed tomography of intrathoracic goiters. AJR 140:455, 1983

Batra P, Herrman C, Mulder D: Mediastinal imaging in myasthenia gravis: correlation of chest radiography, CT, MR, and surgical findings. AJR 148:515, 1987

Bechtold RE, Wolfman NT, Karstaedt N et al: Superior vena caval obstruction: detection using CT. Radiology 157:485, 1985

Birnberg FA, Webb WR, Selch MT et al.: Thymic carcinoid tumors with hyperparathyroidism. AJR 139:1001, 1982

Blank N, Castellino RA: The mediastinum in Hodgkin's and non-Hodgkin's lymphomas. J Thorac Imag 2:66, 1987

Blomlie V, Lien HH, Fossa SD et al.: Computed tomography in primary nonseminomatous germ cell tumors of the mediastinum. Acta Radiol 29:289, 1988

Brown LR, Aughenbaugh GL, Wick MR et al.: Roentgenologic diagnosis of primary corticotropin-producing carcinoid tumors of the mediastinum. Radiology 142:143, 1982

Brown LR, Muhm JR, Aughenbaugh GL et al.: Computed tomography of benign mature teratomas of the mediastinum. J Thorac Imaging 2:66, 1987

Brown LR, Muhm JR, Gray JE: Radiographic detection of thymoma. AJR 134:1181, 1980

Brown LR, Muhm JR, Sheedy PF et al.: The value of computed tomography in myasathenia gravis. AJR 140:31, 1983

Carmosino L, Dibenedetto A, Feffer S: Thymic hyperplasia following successful chemotherapy: a report of two cases and review of the literature. Cancer 56:1526, 1985

Chen J, Weisbrod GL, Herman SJ: Computed tomography and pathologic correlations of thymic lesions. J Thorac Imaging 3:61, 1988

Choyke PL, Zeman RK, Gootenberg JE et al: Thymic atrophy and regrowth in response to chemotherapy: CT evaluation. AJR 149:269, 1987

Davis JG, Simonton JH: Mediastinal carinal bronchogenic cysts. Radiology 67:391, 1956

de Geer G, Webb WR, Gamsu G: Normal thymus: assessment with MR and CT. Radiology 158:313, 1986

Dresler CM, Patterson GA, Taylor BR et al.: Complete foregut duplication. Ann Thorac Surg 50:306, 1990

Dunne MG, Weksberg AP: Thymic cyst: computed tomography and ultrasound correlation. J Comput Assist Tomogr 7:351, 1983

Edeiken J, Lee KF, Libshitz H: Intrathoracic meningocele. AJR 106:381, 1969

Ellis K, Austin JHM, Jaretzki A: Radiologic detection of thymoma in patients with myasthenia gravis. AJR 151:873, 1988

Ellis K, Gregg HG: Thymomas—roentgen considerations. AJR 91:105, 1964

Federle MP, Callen PW: Cystic Hodgkin's lymphoma of the thymus: computed tomography appearance. J Comput Assist Tomogr 3:542, 1979

Feigin DS, Fenoglio JJ, McAllister HA et al.: Pericardial cysts: a radiologic-pathologic correlation and review. Radiology 125:15, 1977

Filly R, Blank N, Castellino RA: Radiographic distribution of intra-thoracic disease in previously untreated patients with Hodgkin's and non-Hodgkin's lymphoma. Radiology 120:277, 1976

Fox MA, Vix VA: Endodermal sinus (yolk sac) tumors of the anterior mediastinum. AJR 135:291, 1980

Francis IR, Glazer GM, Bookstein GL, Gross BH: The thymus: reexamination of age-related changes in size and shape. AJR 145:249, 1985

Fraser RG, Paré JAP, Paré PD et al.: Diagnosis of Diseases of the Chest. 3rd Ed. WB Saunders, Philadelphia, 1989

Fulcher AS, Proto AV, Jolles H: Cystic teratoma of the mediastinum: demonstration of fat/fluid level. AJR 154:259, 1990

Gefter WB, Spritzer CE, Eisenberg B et al: Thyroid imaging with high-field-strength surface-coil MR. Radiology 164:483, 1987

Glazer GM, Axel L, Moss AA: CT diagnosis of mediastinal thyroid. AJR 138:495, 1982

Good CA: Roentgenologic findings in myasthenia gravis associated with thymic tumor. AJR 57:305, 1947

Gouliamos AD, Carter BL, Emami B: Computed tomography of the chest wall. Radiology 134:433, 1980

Hammond DI: Giant lymph node hyperplasia of the posterior mediastinum. J Can Assoc Radiol 30:256, 1979

Heiberg E: Standard for normal thickness of the thymus gland (letter). Radiology 147:887, 1983

Heiberg E, Wolverson MK, Sunaram M, Nouri S: Normal thymus: CT characteristics in subjects under age 20. AJR 138:491, 1982

Higgins CB, McNamara MT, Fisher MR, Clark OH: MR imaging of the thyroid. AJR 147:1255, 1986

Hopper KD, Diehl LF, Cole BA et al.: The significance of necrotic mediastinal lymph nodes on CT in patients with newly diagnosed Hodgkin's disease. AJR 155:267, 1990

Ingels GW, Campbell DC Jr, Giampetro AM et al.: Malignant schwannomas of the mediastinum. Report of 2 cases and review of the literature. Cancer 27:1190, 1971

Johnston RH Jr, Owensby LC, Vargas GM et al.: Pancreatic pseudocyst of the mediastinum. Ann Thorac Surg 41:210, 1986

Jonsson K, Rian RL: Pseudotumoral esophageal varices associated with portal hypertension. Radiology 97:593, 1970

Katlic MR, Wang C, Grillo HC: Substernal goiter. Ann Thorac Surg 39:391, 1985

Kissin CM, Husband JE, Nicholas D et al.: Benign thymic enlargement in adults after chemotherapy: CT demonstration. Radiology 163:67, 1987

Kuhlman JE, Fishman EK, Wang KP et al.: Mediastinal cysts: diagnosis by CT and needle aspiration. AJR 150:75, 1988

Kuhlman JE, Fishman EK, Wang KP et al: Esophageal duplication cyst: CT and transesophageal needle aspiration. AJR 145:531, 1985

Lautin EM, Rosenblatt M, Friedman AC et al.: Calcification in non-Hodgkin's lymphoma occurring before therapy: identification on plain films and CT. AJR 155:739, 1990

Lee KS, Im J, Han CH et al.: Malignant primary germ cell tumors of the mediastinum: CT features. AJR 153:947, 1989

Levitt RG, Husband JE, Glazer HS: CT of primary germ-cell tumors of the mediastinum. AJR 142:73, 1984

Lindell MM Jr, Hill CA, Libshitz HI: Oesophageal cancer: radiographic chest findings and their prognostic significance. AJR 133:461, 1979

Lindfors KK, Meyer JE, Dedrick CG et al.: Thymic cysts in mediastinal Hodgkin disease. Radiology 156:37, 1985

Mendelson DS, Rose JS, Efremidis SC et al.: Bronchogenic cysts with high CT numbers. AJR 140:463, 1983

Modic MT, Janicki PC: Computed tomography of mass lesions of the right cardiophrenic angle. J Comput Assist Tomogr 4:521, 1980

Moore AV, Korobkin M, Olanow W et al.: Age-related changes in the thymus gland: CT-pathologic correlation. AJR 141:241, 1983

Moore AV, Korobkin M, Powers B et al.: Thymoma detection by mediastinal CT: patients with myasthenia gravis. AJR 138:217, 1982

Mori K, Eguchi K, Moriyama H et al.: Computed tomography of anterior mediastinal tumors: differentiation between thymoma and germ cell tumor. Acta Radiol 28:395, 1987

Noma S, Kanaoka M, Minami S et al.: Thyroid masses: MR imaging and pathologic correlation. Radiology 168:759, 1988

Noma S, Nishimura K, Togashi K et al.: Thyroid gland: MR imaging. Radiology 164:495, 1987

Paling MR, Williamson BRJ: Epipericardial fat pad: CT findings. Radiology 165:335, 1987

Park H, Tarver RD, Siddiqui AR et al.: Efficacy of thyroid scintigraphy in the diagnosis of intrathoracic goiter. AJR 148:527–529, 1987

Pearlberg JL, Sandler MA, Talpos GB, Beute GH: Computed tomographic evaluation of intrathoracic thyroid malignancy. Comput Med Imaging Graph 13:411, 1989

Picus D, Balfe DM, Koehler RE et al.: Computed tomography in the staging of esophageal carcinoma. Radiology 146:433, 1983

Press GA, Glazer HS, Wasserman TH et al.: Thoracic wall involvement by Hodgkin's disease and non-Hodgkin lymphoma: CT evaluation. Rdiology 157:195, 1985

Pugatch RD, Braver JH, Robbins AH et al.: CT diagnosis of pericardial cysts. AJR 131:515, 1978

Radecki PD, Arger PH, Arenson RL et al.: Thyroid imaging: comparison of high-resolution real-time ultrasound and computed tomography. Radiology 153:145, 1984

Reed JC, Hallet KK, Feigin DS: Neural tumors of the thorax: subject review from the AFIP. Radiology 126:9, 1978

Reed JC, Sobonya RE: Morphologic analysis of foregut cysts in the thorax. AJR 120:851, 1974

Rholl KS, Levitt RG, Glazer HS: Magnetic resonance imaging of fibrosing mediastinitis. AJR 145:255, 1985

Ross P, Logan W: Roentgen findings in extramedullary hematopoiesis. ARJ 106:604, 1969

Shin MS, Ho K: Computed tomography of primary mediastinal seminomas. J Comput Assist Tomogr 7:990, 1983a

Shin MS, Ho K: Diffuse thymic hyperplasia following chemotherapy for nodular sclerosing Hodgkin's disease: an immunologic rebound phenomenon? Cancer 51:30, 1983b

Shuford WH, Sybers RG, Edwards FK: The three types of right aortic arch. AJR 109:67, 1970

Silverman PM, Newman GE, Korobkin M et al.: Computed tomography in the evaluation of thyroid disease. AJR 141:897, 1984

Spizarny DL, Shepard JO, McLoud TC: CT of adenoid cystic carcinoma of the trachea. AJR 146:1129, 1986

Suzuki M, Takashima T, Itoh H et al.: Computed tomography of mediastinal teratomas. J Comput Assist Tomogr 7:74, 1983

Theros EG: RPC of the month from the AFIP. Radiology 93:677, 1969

Thorvinger B, Lyttkens K, Samuelsson L: Computed tomography of the thymus gland in myasthenia gravis. Acta Radiol 28:399, 1987

Weinstein JB, Aronberg DJ, Sagel SS: CT of fibrosing mediastinitis: findings and their utility. AJR 141:247, 1983

Wychulis AR, Payne WS, Clagett OT et al.: Surgical treatment of mediastinal tumors. A 40 year experience. J Thorac Cardiovasc Surg 62:379, 1971

Yeh H, Gordon A, Kirschner PA et al.: Computed tomography and sonography of thymolipoma. AJR 140:1131, 1983

Yernault J-C, Kuhn G, Dumortier P et al.: "Solid" mediastinal bronchogenic cyst: mineralogic analysis. AJR 146:73, 1986

Ziter FM Jr, Bramwit DN, Holloman KR et al.: Calcified mediastinal bronchogenic cysts. Radiology 93:1025, 1969

54

DIAGNOSTIC TECHNIQUES

Carolyn M. Dresler

INTRODUCTION

Radiologic exploration is by far the most widely used investigational approach for defining diseases of the chest and mediastinum. The routine posteroanterior (PA) and lateral chest x-rays constitute the initial investigative or screening test ordered by either the general physician and/or the specialist. The vast majority of abnormalities are identifiable on the routine chest x-ray. Each of the shadows, lines, densities, and shapes seen on the routine chest x-ray is translatable into identifiable structures. It is the finding on standard chest x-ray that suggests the next appropriate test or investigation in order to further define the abnormality. For example, to examine the abnormalities of the mediastinum, computed tomography (CT) or magnetic resonance imaging (MRI) is usually the next indicated examination. This chapter reviews a multitude of examinations currently available to the physician involved in treatment of the thoracic diseases.

CHEST X-RAYS

The standard examination of the chest consists of a PA projection and a left lateral film. Standardization is extremely important for comparison of films. Therefore, it is critical to ensure that the quality of technique remains constant. The x-ray should be taken with the patient in deep inspiration with a high kilovolt peak between 120 and 145 kvp. The distance of exposure should be 72 in. in order to keep the magnification constant. Even with optimal technique and experience, reading the routine chest x-ray for mediastinal abnormalities may be difficult. As described in Chapter 53, there are several critical and varied organs in the mediastinum, which overlie each other. Neither the PA nor the lateral radiograph is able to well differentiate abnormalities within the mediastinum. Certainly, however, the presence of an abnormality is readily observed on standard PA and lateral films. Further testing is then required to delineate the actual location and etiology of the problem.

LINEAR TOMOGRAPHY

The next technique that was developed to further delineate the structures in the mediastinum was tomography. Linear tomography of the mediastinum is able to describe the site and extension of the lesion more accurately than is standard radiography. It is also quite accurate at decribing calcification or cavitation within the abnormality. Linear tomography eliminates any overlying opacity and thereby exposes the nature of the lesion. Tomography has been particularly useful for examining tracheal tumors and strictures. It is able to accurately define the length and degree of narrowing, perhaps better than CT but similarly to MRI scanning.

TRANSCUTANEOUS ULTRASOUND AND TRANSESOPHAGEAL ECHOCARDIOGRAPHY

Transcutaneous ultrasound is frequently used for diagnostic examination of the heart. It is an inexpensive and accurate test for cardiac evaluation. In addition, it is helpful in identifying loculated fluid collections, either pericardial or pleural, for percutaneous drainage. This technique is useful for marking an appropriate site for percutaneous drainage of a collection by either a chest tube or catheter. It may be used in a mobile examination and therefore is applicable for patients in an intensive care setting. Ultrasound is used less frequently in the United States, however, because of the even better definition of the CT scanner and the lower reliance on technical skill required for adequate examination.

Of even more utility in exploring the mediastinum is transesophageal echocardiography (TEE). TEE has become a standard for evaluation of overall cardiac and specifically valvular function. It not only is used pre- and postoperatively but is increasingly being used intraoperatively. TEE is routinely used to evaluate the adequacy of mitral valve repair, right or left ventricular function, or the presence of shunts. The use of TEE for examination of the aorta and aortic dissection, ascending or descending, is still being evaluated and compared with angiography. In addition, TEE is being evaluated for its ability to delineate mediastinal lymph nodes, both paratracheal and paraesophageal. Paratracheal examination is hampered by both the distance to the pretracheal space from the esophagus and the air density of the trachea. At present, TEE is not better than CT for upper mediastinal lymph node evaluation.

However, paraesophageal demonstration of lymph node size, location, and characteristics and esophageal wall integrity is excellent with TEE. Esophageal masses such as carcionomas or leiomyomas are well defined in their length, circumferential involvement, and degree of invasion. Several studies have addressed the accuracy of T and N status evaluation by TEE, CT scanning, and pathologic stage. The T status is accurately diagnosed in 64 to 89 percent of patients, depending on the degree of wall invasion, as compared with 51 to 59 percent by CT scan. The more invasive the carcinoma, the more accurate the TEE (88 to 100 percent) (Ziegler, et al., 1991; Rice, et al., 1992). Guidelines for determining the actual depth of mediastinal invasion is quite difficult with CT scanning. Picus, et al. (1983) proposed the criterion that a greater than 90-degree angle of contact between the tumor mass and the aorta would predict tumor invasion. Prediction of tumor involvement by CT scanning of the other mediastinal structures is unpredictable and should not preclude exploration.

Similarly, the nodal status is well described by TEE, with accuracies of 51 to 80 percent (Rice, et al., 1992; Ziegler, et al., 1991; Shorvon, 1990). Despite the tendency of esophageal carcinoma to present late with a narrowed lumen, only 8 to 44 percent of patients were unable to undergo passage of the endoscopic ultrasound probe. This technique is growing in importance and is significantly dependent on user expertise. Most users are still at an early part of the learning curve with this modality, and its predictive ability should only improve as expertise increases.

Transesophageal ultrasonography and its usefulness in examining other mediastinal structures such as the ascending or descending aorta and trachea are still in their infancy. As probes of more efficiency are developed to examine these structures, TEE may become a more definitive diagnostic approach to dissection of the aorta and tracheal tumors.

COMPUTED TOMOGRAPHY AND MAGNETIC RESONANCE IMAGING

The two major modalities that are used extensively in more detailed examinations of the mediastinum are the CT scan and MRI. MRI has developed since the introduction of the CT scanner, and the respective roles of the two techniques for various indications are still in the process of being defined. They should be viewed not as competitive but rather as complementary modalities.

CT is excellent for cross-sectional imaging of the chest. Depending on the "generation" of the CT scanner, resolution, particularly in the mediastinum, is excellent. Unfortunately, the cost of this excellent resolution is the use of ionizing radiation and intravenous contrast agents. Mediastinal lymph nodes, which are normally present, may be clearly visualized if they are larger than 0.5 cm. Normal lymph nodes

are usually smaller than 1 to 1.5 cm; therefore, CT scanning should be excellent at demonstrating enlarged adenopathy. Thin-collimation and high-resolution techniques may more clearly demonstrate tracheal or endobronchial tumors. Once an abnormality within the airway has been identified, further fine cuts 0.2 cm apart may be obtained. Cross-sectional definition of the extent of disease is excellent.

Anterior mediastinal masses are clearly delineated on CT scans. Usually their location and the extent of mediastinal involvement give hints of their etiology. Not uncommonly, though, particularly in large lesions, determination of the extent of invasion or identification of margins is difficult. Therefore despite excellent location, biopsy is still required for diagnosis.

Many studies have examined chest x-ray, chest CT, chest MRI, and/or mediastinoscopy in some sort of comparison of efficacy. Batra, et al. (1989), from a comparison of chest x-ray with CT and MRI to evaluate the intrathoracic extent of a lung carcinoma, concluded that all three modalities demonstrated the primary lesion well but that CT scan was more comprehensive. Mediastinal adenopathy was about equally well seen on CT and MRI; however, MRI was better at hilar adenopathy screening. Chest wall invasion was equally well demonstrated on CT and MRI but not by chest x-ray, whereas vertebral involvement was best seen on MRI.

Patterson et al. (1987) compared chest x-ray, CT, MRI, and mediastinoscopy in 84 patients with lung carcinoma. The radiologic comparisons gave results similar to those cited above; however, mediastinoscopy was more accurate (95 percent) than MRI (83 percent) or CT scan (82 percent) for mediastinal lymph node involvement. In a review comparing CT with MRI in patients with lung cancer, Webb (1989) concluded that CT scanning was superior in the peripheral lung lesion but fairly equivalent to MRI for the detection of mediastinal adenopathy. Mediastinal lymph nodes and mediastinal fat have different T_1 values, that of fat being much shorter. Thereore, T_1-weighted images should show mediastinal lymph nodes to be less intense than fat. The spatial resolution of MRI may not be as good as that of CT, which may cause the lymph nodes to blur together. For example, when several small normal lymph nodes are blurred into one apparent larger lymph node on the MRI scan they are identified as abnormal. Also, MRI does not show calcification, which may be critical in defining a benign lymph node. In these situations CT scans are superior to MRI.

MRI, however, is able to demonstrate flow through blood vessels and therefore may be able to delineate lymph nodes in the aortic pulmonary window or subcarinal space better than CT scans. This difference is also quite useful for investigation of superior venal caval syndrome secondary to adenopathy or a primary mass. Flow in a vessel is able to define its margin and thus possible invasion, which is particularly important in proximal tumor involvement of the pulmonary arteries, veins, and superior vena cava. This characteristic of MRI is also helpful in patients with fibrosing mediastinitis. The spin-echo sequence with MRI demonstrates the high flow of the vessels, and thus evidence of obstruction is seen without use of intravenous contrast. However, the lack of visualized calcifications on the MRI makes it in general a less optimal examination than CT scanning for evaluation of fibrosing mediastinitis. The final conclusion has not been reached as to whether CT or MRI is most appropriate to use following standard radiography in the evaluation of the mediastinum. MRI testing is still more expensive and not uncommonly may cause claustrophobic reactions. The CT scan provides excellent answers to many aspects of carcinoma involvement in the majority of situations. When further, more specific information is required, such as possible superior vena caval, brachial plexus, or myocardial invasion, the MRI should then be requested. Also, if other views such as sagittal or coronal sections would be helpful, MRI would be the test of choice.

Abnormalities of the airway, such as benign or malignant tracheal strictures, are most adequately shown on a sagittal or coronal view of an MRI. Mediastinal masses with possible vascular or cardiac involvement are also more clearly seen on an MRI. This reflects the ability of MRI to demonstrate flow in a vessel or cardiac chamber, as described above. MRI is significantly superior to CT in describing possible intervertebral involvement by a posterior mediastinal neurogenic mass.

NEWER IMAGING MODALITIES

Newer modalities of mediastinal imaging are only in their infancy. Single-photon emission computed tomography (SPECT) and positron emission tomography (PET) are able to provide high-contrast but poor-resolution images of lesions based on their functional significance. These investigative techniques are being refined to provide better resolution. A current area of investigation is the differential uptake of glucose among metastatic tumor, mediastinal lymph nodes, and normal background tissue. At present these techniques seem quite promising and exciting but not yet ready for general clinical use.

NUCLEAR MEDICINE

Nuclear medicine investigations in the mediastinum are fairly limited. Blood flow studies may be performed with ^{99m}Tc-labeled red blood cells to examine possible superior vena caval obstruction. This approach may be useful in the patient who is allergic to contrast media, but in others a venogram is probably faster and more definitive. A thyroid scan may be helpful in identifying ectopic thyroid or a substernal goiter. Functioning thyroid tissue may show uptake of ^{99m}Tc or ^{131}I.

Foregut duplications may lead to bronchogenic or enterogenous cysts; the latter cysts may contain mucosa. When they do contain gastric mucosa, ^{99m}Tc will show increased uptake.

Ectopic parathyroids or parathyroid adenomas that occur in the mediastinum may be identified by CT or MRI if they are large enough to be distinguished from surrounding mediastinal fat. Technetium-thallium subtraction scans may also be helpful in identifying the adenomas, and selective venous sampling is useful in aiding localization.

Mediastinal bacterial or fungal infections may be defined with ^{111}In-labeled leukocytes. The patient's blood is drawn (40 ml), and the white blood cells are concentrated, incubated for 20 to 30 minutes with ^{111}In, and then reinjected into the patient. Esophagitis or a nasogastric or endotracheal tube will also result in some small uptake. The true infection or abscess will show more intense uptake, which therefore should be predictive of an actual infection. ^{111}In imaging is probably superior to ^{67}Ga imaging in the mediastinum, as it has a higher target-to-background ratio and requires less time (18 to 24 days versus 2 to 3 days for gallium imaging).

INVASIVE MEDIASTINOSCOPY

In order to examine the mediastinum for diagnosis, the usual radiologic tests are first performed as described in the initial portion of this chapter. Once the abnormality in the mediastinum is identified, an operative procedure for diagnosis may be performed. The two standard explorations of the mediastinum are cervical and anterior mediastinoscopy; a third, less frequently used approach is posterior mediastinoscopy.

Cervical Mediastinoscopy

The cervical mediastinoscopy, as first described by Carlens (1959), is simple to perform; however, it requires significant experience in order to become facile. Cervical mediastinoscopy is indicated for biopsy of a paratracheal mass or more commonly, mediastinal lymph nodes. It is important to explain to the patient preoperatively that the procedure is a standard operation but carries the potential risks inherent in biopsy of a major blood vessel and the risk of injury to the left recurrent nerve. In experienced hands this procedure is extremely safe. However, an appropriate biopsy of a vascular structure, usually venous, may be catastrophic and requires sternotomy for repair. Luke, et al. (1986) reviewed 1,000 patients at the University of Toronto. There were no deaths and a 2.3 percent complication rate. In this series there were only two hemorrhagic complications and no recurrent nerve injuries. The procedure at this university center was performed by thoracic surgeons who were quite experienced with this operation. These results are easily obtainable as one becomes more familiar with the anatomy as seen through the mediastinoscope.

Cervical mediastinoscopy is performed by making a 2-cm incision one fingerbreadth above the sternal notch. The platysma is divided, and the midline fascia between strap muscles is then divided down to the level of the trachea with either sharp or electrocautery dissection. The pretracheal fascia is then bluntly dissected, with the finger progressing caudad underneath the innominate artery. The fasciae on the right and left side of the trachea are bluntly dissected and palpated for adenopathy. The mediastinoscope is inserted, and exploration is conducted with a blunt suction coagulator-dissector. Lymph nodes are then easily dissected along the entire right paratracheal border. Care is taken to identify the azygous vein and pulmonary artery. Dissection can be continued down along the anterior aspect of the right and left mainstem bronchi. The subcarinal lymph nodes are identified once the enveloping pretracheal fascia is opened. Care must be taken along the left paratracheal border, as the left recurrent nerve courses in this location. One must be careful to identify this structure prior to biopsy of adjacent lymph nodes. Little electrocautery, if any, should be used along the left side in order to avoid injury to the left recurrent nerve. Once biopsies are taken of identified lymph nodes, hemostasis is controlled with the electrocautery or by simply packing with a gauze sponge and waiting. Once hemostasis has been achieved, the mediastinoscope can be removed and the platysma and skin reapproximated.

A modification of the cervical mediastinoscopy has been described by Ginsberg (1980). This extended cervical mediastinoscopy is performed through the above-described cervical incision. Following the standard cervical mediastinoscopy dissection, digital dissection of the anterior mediastinum is performed. The small area between the innominate artery and left carotid artery is digitally dissected, and a mediastinoscope is inserted. The area over the aortic arch and into the aortic pulmonary window is examined, and the lymph nodes may then be biopsied in level 5 or 6, as previously described.

Anterior Mediastinoscopy

Left anterior mediastinoscopy, or the Chamberlain approach, is used to biopsy lymph nodes or masses in the left aortic pulmonary window. This area is not reached by standard cervical mediastinoscopy. A 2- to 3-cm incision is made over the second intercostal space and carried down through the pectoralis muscle. The intercostal muscles are divided along the superior aspect of the third rib with care. The pleura need not be entered but may be simply dissected laterally with a peanut dissector. A mediastinoscope is inserted into the second intercostal space and advanced toward the anteroposter-

ior window. Lymph nodes or masses in this area may be readily biopsied. It is not uncommon, however, to open the pleura at the time of intercostal muscle dissection. This actually makes it slightly easier to identify the mediastinal structures through the mediastinoscope. If the pleura is open, closure becomes a simple matter of reapproximating the muscles over a red rubber catheter that has been placed into the chest. Once the muscle and subcutaneous layers are closed, the lung fully re-expanded, and air expelled, the red rubber catheter can be rapidly removed. Anterior mediastinoscopy may also be performed on the right side in exactly the same fashion in order to biopsy any right anterior mediastinal masses.

Posterior Mediastinoscopy

The final approach to the mediastinum is posterior. This is an uncommon technique, which is most likely to be used for drainage of a bacterial mediastinal abscess that has not communicated with the pleura. Such an abscess is fairly uncommon, and standard procedure is to drain it by transthoracic exploration. However, if a posterior mediastinal approach is desired, the ribs over the abscess are identified, and the posterior angles of the ribs are resected. Care is taken to stay out of the pleura by gently dissecting it anteriorly. The posterior mediastinum and the paraesophageal gutter are identified and can be drained to the exterior. This also would be an adequate approach for biopsy of a posteriorly located mass, which, however, is probably more readily performed with a percutaneous needle biopsy.

KEY REFERENCES

Carlens E: Mediastinoscopy. Odense University Press, Denmark, 1971

This short book describes the history, indications, and results of mediastinoscopy from a major enthusiast of the procedure.

Harkens DE, Black H, Claus SR, Farrad RE: A single cervicomediastinal exploration for tissue diagnosis of intrathoracic disease. N Engl J Med 251:1041, 1954

This is a historical article describing cervical mediastinoscopy.

Pearson FG, Nelems JM, Henderson RD, Delarue NC: The role of mediastinoscopy in the selection of treatment for bronchial carcinoma with involvement of superior mediastinal lymph nodes. J Thorac Cardiovasc Surg 64:382, 1972

This article was seminal in making mediastinoscopy a standard part of the evaluation of the mediastinum in patients presenting with lung carcinoma.

REFERENCES

Batra P, Brown K, Collins JD et al.: Evaluation of intrathoracic extent of lung cancer by plain chest radiography, computed tomography, and magnetic resonance imaging. Am Rev Respir Dis 137:1456, 1988

Brown JJ, Barakos JA, Higgins, CB: Magnetic resonance imaging of cardiac and paracardiac masses. J Thorac Imaging 4(2):58, 1989

Carlens E: Mediastinoscopy: a method for inspection and tissue biopsy in the superior mediastinum. Chest 36:343, 1959

Gamsu G, Sostman D: Magnetic resonance imaging of the thorax. Am Rev Respir Dis 139:254, 1989

Luke WP, Pearson FG, Todd TRJ et al.: Prospective evaluation of mediastinoscopy for assessment of carcinoma of the lung. J Thorac Cardiovasc Surg 91:53, 1986

Merine D, Pessar ML, Zerhouni EA et al.: CT and MRI assessment of the mediastinum. p. 67. In Zerhouni EA (ed): CT and MRI of the Thorax. Churchill Livingstone, New York, 1990

Oates E, Ramberg K: Imaging of intrathoracic disease with indium 111-labeled leukocytes. J Thorac Imaging 5(3):78, 1990

Patterson GA, Ginsberg RT, Poon PY et al.: A prospective evaluation of magnetic resonance imaging, computed tomography and mediastinoscopy in the preoperative assessment of mediastinal node status in bronchogenic carcinoma. J Thorac Cardiovasc Surg 94:679, 1987

Picus D, Balfe DM, Koehler RE et al.: Computed tomography in the staging of esophageal carcinoma. Radiology 146:433, 1983

Rankin S: The role of computerized tomography in the staging of oesophageal cancer. Clin Radiol 42:152, 1990

Rice TW, Boyce GA, Sivah MV et al.: Esophageal carcinoma: esophageal ultrasound assessment of preoperative chemotherapy. Ann Thorac Surg 53:972, 1992

Shaffer K, Pugatch RD: Diseases of the mediastinum. p. 171. In Freundlich IM, Bragg DG (eds): A Radiologic Approach to Diseases of the Chest. Williams & Wilkins, Baltimore, 1992

Shorvon PJ: Endoscopic ultrasound in oesophageal cancer: the way forward? Clin Radiol 42:149, 1990

Spritzer C, Gamsu G, Sostman HD: Magnetic resonance imaging of the thorax: techniques, current applications and future directions. J Thorac Imaging 4(2):1, 1989

Swensen SJ, Ehman RL, Brown LR: Magnetic resonance imaging of the thorax. J Thorac Imaging 4(2):19, 1989

Watanabe AT, Teitelbaum GP, Henderson RW, Bradley WG: Magnetic resonance imaging of cardiac sarcomas. J Thorac Imaging 4:90, 1989

Webb WR: Magnetic resonance imaging of the thorax: comparison with CT. p. 525. In Freundlich IM, Bragg DG (eds): A Radiologic Approach to Diseases of the Chest. Williams & Wilkins, Baltimore, 1992

Webb WR: The role of magnetic resonance imaging in the assessment of patients with lung cancer: a comparison with computed tomography. J Thorac Imaging 4(2):65, 1989

Ziegler Z, Sanft C, Zeitz M et al.: Evaluation of endosonography in TN staging of oesophageal cancer. Gut 32:16, 1991

55

INFECTIONS

Bill Nelems

DEFINITION

Mediastinitis can be thought of in three distinctly separate categories: acute bacterial, granulomatous, and sclerosing (Kuhn and Askin, 1990).

Acute bacterial mediastinitis is now most commonly caused by the spread of bacterial infection from the spontaneous or instrumental disruption of the esophagus or from wound contamination following median sternotomy surgery for cardiac or mediastinal disease (Fry and Shields, 1991). Some unusual causes of mediastinal sepsis, such as pneumonia, lung abscess, pleural empyema, and metastatic or dental abscesses, have been virtually eliminated by the present-day availability of antibiotics. These rare possibilities should still be considered, however, when no other more obvious cause is found.

Granulomatous mediastinitis results from the contiguous spread of granulomatous infection of lung to the mediastinal lymph nodes. This most commonly occurs with pulmonary tuberculosis or with histoplasmosis (Goodwin, et al., 1972). This type of inflammatory process has both acute and chronic clinical implications (Kuhn and Askin, 1990).

Sclerosing mediastinitis is a poorly understood clinical entity. Certainly, some patients with this dense relatively acellular fibrosis also have granulomatous inflammation of the mediastinum. Some exhibit calcification; however, many show no association with granulomatous disease at all (Kuhn and Askin, 1990). The clinical manifestations are protean; they vary from mild in severity to fatal (Eggleston, 1980). In about one-half of these cases, histoplasmosis is suspected (Urschel, et al., 1990).

HISTORICAL NOTE

At first glance, a historical perspective on this topic seems elusive because so many different etiologic factors of infection transgress the mediastinal boundaries, but with some introspection, we can view a panorama of many of this century's great medical trends—some hopeful and some ominous. From tuberculosis, which is now partly influenced by the acquired immunodeficiency syndrome (AIDS) epidemic, to tetracycline and from esophageal endoscopes to endocar-

dial exploration, both spectacular and shocking developments have occurred.

As a clinical entity, tuberculosis has a rich and fascinating history (Wilson, 1990). From artificial pneumothorax to plombage and from thoracoplasty to transfusion, the historical development of thoracic surgery as a specialty has no rival. It owes its heritage to the pioneers who toiled against tuberculosis. Today we are experiencing a resurgence of tuberculosis as a modern-day disease, which has occurred in the wake of the worldwide AIDS epidemic (FitzGerald, et al., 1991); Korzeniewsvka-Kosela, et al., 1992; Edlin, et al., 1992). The manifestations of tuberculous mediastinitis have again become fairly common. Today, too, a generation of North American medical students has graduated and entered the practice of medicine with low indices of suspicion for tuberculosis as a diagnostic entity. By the year 2000, it is anticipated that there will be a 10-fold increase in the incidence of tuberculosis in sub-Saharan Africa (FitzGerald, et al., 1991). The emergence of drug-resistant *Mycobacterium tuberculosis* has been reported in patients with AIDS in the United States (Edlin, et al., 1992). As the triple threat of AIDS, drug resistance, and aggressive immunosuppression for transplantation and cancer chemotherapy affects the practice of modern medicine, it would behoove us all to take a refresher course in tuberculosis.

Mycotic diseases of the lung and mediastinum have changed little in their clinical manifestations over time, except that they can be investigated by more precise studies of epidemiology and demography (Kuhn and Askin, 1990).

Modern technology has spawned an era of fiberoptics and membrane oxygenators. The rigid esophagoscope has given way to flexible instruments, with increased patient safety and a decreased incidence of instrumental esophageal perforation (Burnett, et al., 1990; Fleisher, et al., 1994; Urschel, 1974). The development of heart-lung bypass and the proliferation of open heart surgery during the last quarter of a century have been truly amazing. With these developments, however, wound infection has produced a substantial new category of mediastinal infection in a complex subgroup of patients, many of whom have been treated by the insertion of prosthetic valves and delicate grafts (Fry and Shields, 1991). Technology, too, has been important in treating these sources of mediastinitis (Spencer and Grossi, 1990; Gaynes, et al., 1991; Katsal, et al., 1991). What treatise on mediastinal infection would be complete without at least a fleeting reference to the discovery and ongoing refinements of antibiotics and their impact on infection in general?

HISTORICAL READINGS

Eggleston JC: Sclerosing mediastinitis. Prog Surg Pathol 2:1, 1980

FitzGerald JM, Grzybowski S, Allen EA: The impact of human immunodeficiency virus infection on tuberculosis and its control. Chest 1991. 100:191, 1991

Kuhn C, Askin FB: Lung and mediastinum. In Kissane JM (ed): Anderson's Pathology. 9th Ed. CV Mosby, St. Louis, 1990

Light AM: Idiopathic fibrosis of the mediastinum; a discussion of 3 cases and review of the literature. J Clin Pathol 31:78, 1978

Schonengerdt CB, Suyemoto R, Maion FB: Granulomatous and fibrosing mediastinitis. A review and analysis of 180 cases. J Thorac Cardiovasc Surg 57:365, 1979

Wilson LG: The historical decline of tuberculosis in Europe and America; its causes and significance. J History Med Allied Sci 45:366, 1990

BASIC SCIENCE

Acute Mediastinitis

Bacterial contamination of the mediastinum, from whatever source, without prompt recognition, drainage, and therapy, usually leads rapidly to fatal septicemia (Burnett, et al., 1990; Fleisher, et al., 1994).

Granulmatous Mediastinitis

Mediastinitis in acute tuberculosis occurs without major visible parenchymal infection (Korzeniewska-Kasela, et al., 1992). This is particularly so in childhood disease and in patients with AIDS in whom tuberculosis develops. Primary parenchymal infection is often misdiagnosed, and even early adenopathy is often overlooked. However, when extensive mediastinal lymph node inflammation and calcification becomes established, late sequelae may manifest. These may take the form of diffuse sclerosis, or they may cause localized mediastinal problems, such as hemoptysis from calcified nodal erosion of airways or esophageal traction diverticulae (Kuhn and Askin, 1990).

Of the fungal diseases of lung, the organism most likely to cause significant mediastinal complications is *Histoplasma capsulatum* (Urschel, et al., 1990). In its acute phase, histoplasmosis may present with acute adenopathy. In the circumstance in which mediastinoscopy is performed for diagnosis, the fulminating nature of this acute necrotizing inflammation becomes evident. This intense reaction may go on to severe late fibrotic sequelae (Goodwin, et al., 1972; Eggleston, 1980; Dunn, et al., 1990). Some cases may proceed on to a sclerotic phase; in others complications develop from the inflammation or the calcification (Kuhn and Askin, 1990). Late bronchial or tracheal esophageal fistulae may occur. Broncholith forma-

tion may cause hemoptysis with the extrusion of calcified nodes.

With any of the granulomatous cases, masses of large matted lymph nodes may form with caseous necrosis and fibrous encapsulation. Over time, these masses become fibrotic, calcific, or sclerotic (Kuhn and Askin, 1990).

Sclerosing Mediastinitis

This condition is not well understood. Most cases probably follow as late sequelae of granulomatous inflammation (Kuhn and Askin, 1990; Eggleston, 1980). The high incidence of positive Histoplasma complement fixation levels indicates that this particular fungus is responsible for most cases of this condition (Urschel, et al., 1990). The original etiologic factor may have been overlooked, or even if considered, the evidence may be lacking at the time of presentation. Some cases are associated with retroperitoneal fibrosis or Riedel's stroma, which suggests a linkage to a systemic sclerotic process (Light, 1978). Mediastinal and retroperitoneal fibrosis have also been described as complications of methysergide therapy (Kuhn and Askin, 1990).

In this condition, there is a dense white acellular sclerotic inflammation. These patients have two different clinical presentations; these depend on the structures that are involved. The one with upper mediastinal paratracheal involvement tends to present with chronic superior vena caval obstruction, cough, and upper thoracic discomfort. This group has a favorable outcome. The other, which has lower mediastinal fibrosis in the subcarinal region, leads to encasement of the pulmonary arteries and veins, the trachea, and the smaller bronchi. This group tends to fare poorly because they manifest with pulmonary hypertension, pulmonary vein obstruction with thrombi, and fixed smaller airway stenoses. Although the prognosis for the former is fair, for the latter, the outcome may be grim (Kuhn and Askin, 1990; Eggleston, 1980; Dunn, et al., 1990).

MANAGEMENT

Acute Mediastinitis

Esophageal perforation may occur following endoscopic instrumentation, or it may occur spontaneously (Burnett, et al., 1990; Fleisher, et al., 1994). The frequency of instrumental perforation has decreased since the introduction of flexible endoscopes (Fleisher, et al., 1994). The posterior cervical esophagus at the level of C7 and a site some 2 to 3 cm above the gastroesophageal junction represent the areas most vulnerable to perforation by the rigid esophagoscope (Burnett, et al., 1990; Fleisher, et al., 1994). Leakage of contaminated secretions at the level of the cervical esophagus usually results in necrotizing infection and edema in the neck, which may cause respiratory compromise. Cervical drainage with appropriate antibiotic and fluid management is usually sufficient to control the condition (Fry and Shields, 1991; Burnett, et al., 1990; Fleisher, et al., 1994). Thoracic esophageal perforation is usually fatal if it is not recognized and treated promptly. The ensuing mediastinitis is usually also associated with pleural disruption, most commonly on the left side. The therapeutic principles include early recognition, prompt open or closed drainage, closure of early perforations by thoracotomy and exploration, and judicious fluid and antibiotic management.

Instrumental perforation with flexible endoscopy or following pneumatic dilatation in the therapy of achalasia is uncommon (Fleisher, et al., 1994).

Boerhaave's esophageal perforation simulates the clinical findings found with instrumental perforation, but the history of immediate prior emesis facilitates making a diagnosis (Kallis, et al., 1991).

Of the 61 cases of esophageal perforation seen at the Vancouver General Hospital during the past 40 years, 31 were instrumental, and 30 were spontaneous (Fleisher et al., 1994). The instrumentation included rigid esophagoscopy (6), rigid dilatation (5), endoscopy with dilatation (5), foreign body removal (4), pneumatic dilatation for achalasia (4), esophageal biopsy with a rigid endoscope (2), Blakemore tube insertion (1), sclerotherapy for varices (1), endotracheal intubation (1), and flexible endoscopy (1). Thirty-eight patients underwent surgery, and 11 were managed conservatively. In 12 the condition was diagnosed at autopsy. To illustrate the surgical controversy in the management of this disorder, the procedures in this retrospective series included primary closure, closure with buttress, drainage alone, closure with completion myotomy, resection, closure with antireflux procedure, laparotomy and drainage, diversion, and exclusion. The 3 patients with cervical perforation all survived; 4 of 20 surgically treated patients with thoracic instrumental perforation died. Eight of 15 died following surgical therapy after spontaneous perforation. One-half of those patients treated conservatively died. There was a direct correlation between a delay in diagnosis and the mortality rate in all subgroups (Fleisher et al., 1994).

This historical perspective is valuable because it indicates the importance of primary prevention and early diagnosis.

Primary closure with buttress is now viewed as the procedure of choice in the early management of a perforated esophagus.

The clinical features of mediastinal infection following transsternal cardiac and mediastinal surgery have become well recognized during the past three decades. Early recognition, adequate debridement, and appropriate antibiotic management remain the cornerstones of therapy (Fry and Shields, 1991; Spencer and Grossi, 1990; Gaynes, et al., 1991; Katsal, et al., 1991).

Granulomatous Mediastinitis

Mediastinal adenopathy has long been recognized as one of the clinical manifestations of tuberculosis (Korzeniewska-Kosela, et al., 1992). This is also true in children. The chest radiograph in Figure 55-1 demonstrates mediastinal tuberculosis in a 45-year-old woman. Figures 55-2 and 55-3 show the

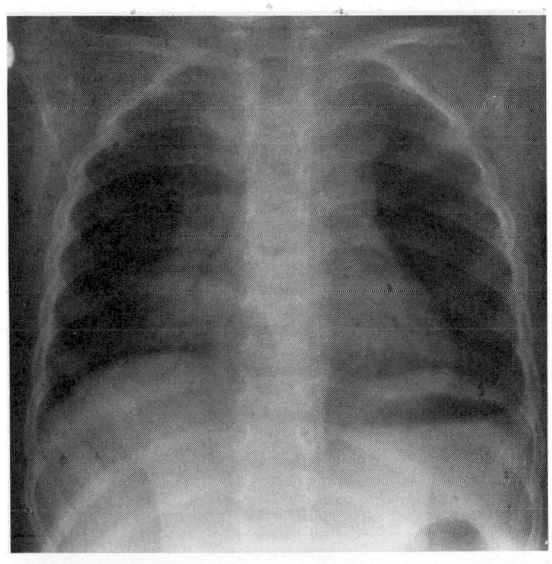
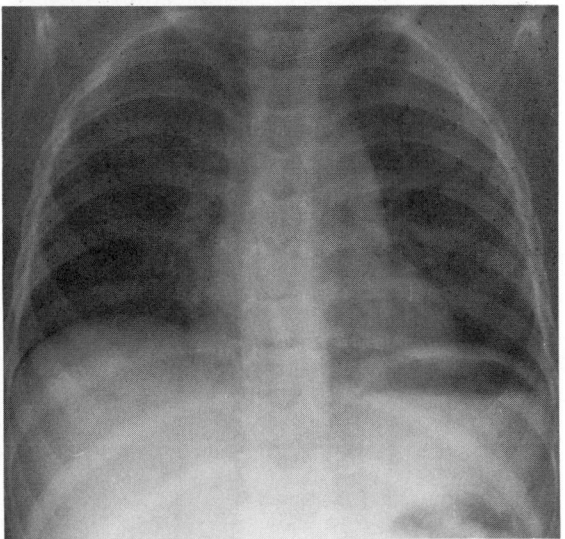

A

B

Figure 55-2. PA chest radiographs of a 4-year-old child with mediastinal tuberculosis: **(A)** before therapy, **(B)** after therapy.

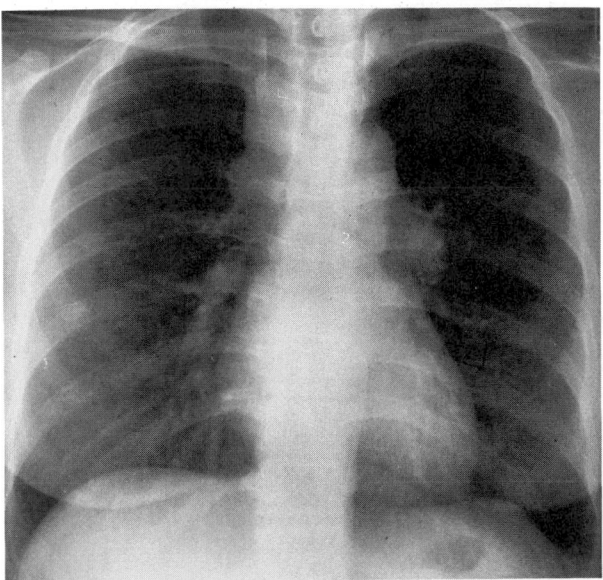

Figure 55-1. PA chest radiograph of a 45-year-old woman with mediastinal tuberculosis.

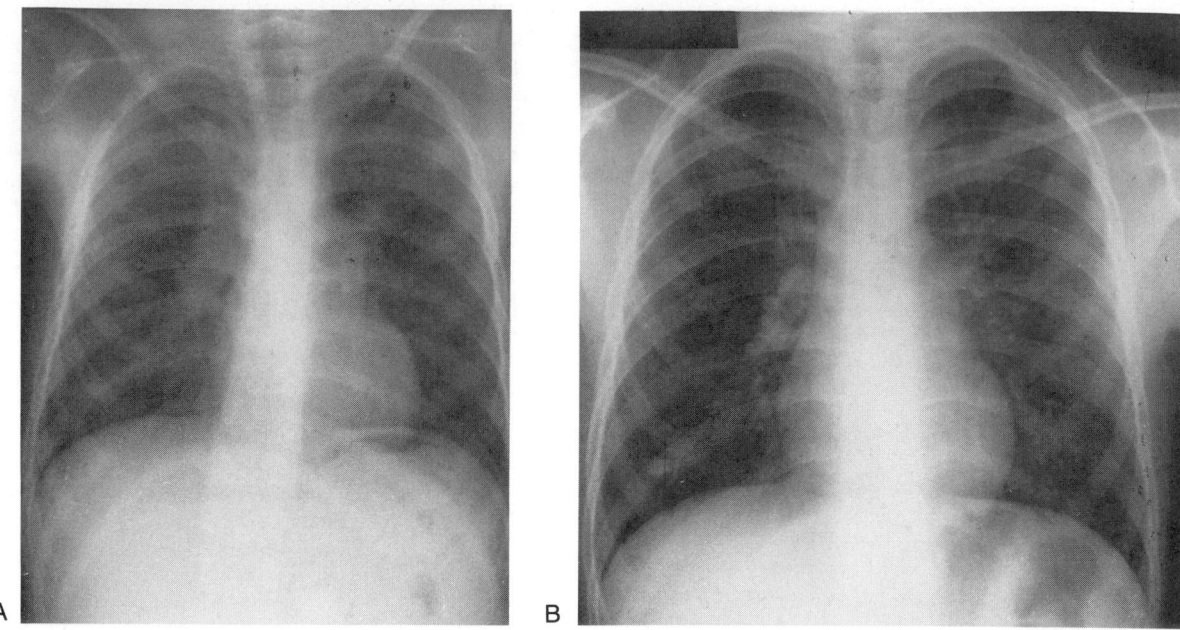

Figure 55-3. PA chest radiographs of a 6-year-old child with mediastinal tuberculosis: **(A)** before therapy, **(B)** after therapy.

before and after therapy radiographs of 4- and 6-year-old children, respectively, with tuberculosis who presented with mediastinal involvement. A mediastinal predilection for tuberculosis is emerging in patients with AIDS. This association is not rare. In a recent review of 40 patients with both AIDS and tuberculosis, 11 presented with striking mediastinal and hilar adenopathy (Korzeniewska-Kasela, et al., 1992).

The therapeutic implications require an increased index of suspicion for the condition, its possible association with AIDS, and an awareness that tuberculosis is making an

alarming reappearance on the world stage (FitzGerald, et al., 1991). Antimicrobial therapy will become more complex with the increased drug resistance that has arisen (Edlin, et al., 1992).

Sclerosing Mediastinitis

Sclerosing or fibrosing mediastinitis results in progressive encasement of vital mediastinal structures (Arnett, et al., 1977; Schonengutt, et al., 1979). Figure 55-4 illustrates supe-

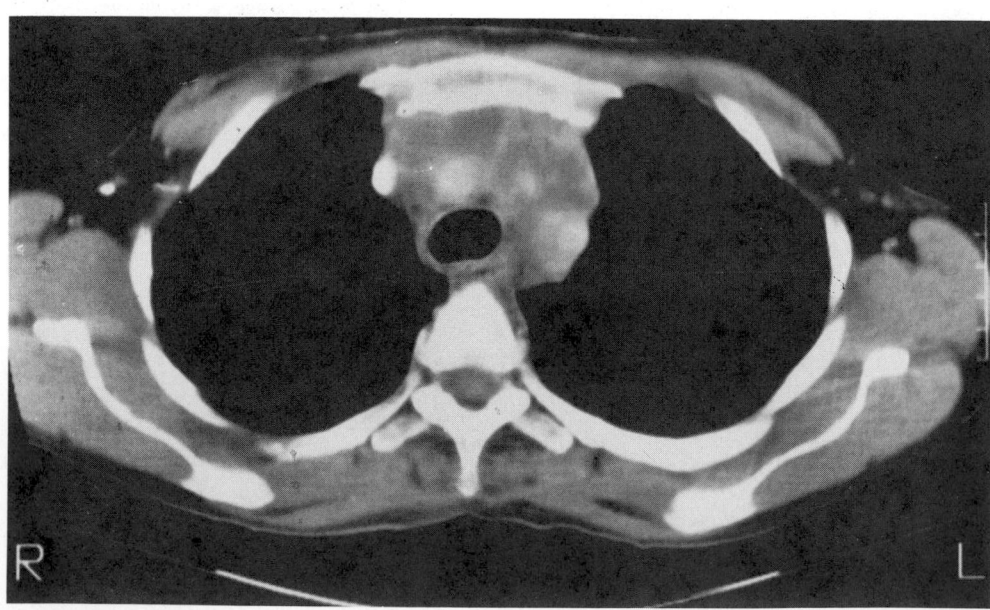

Figure 55-4. Contrast-enhanced 1-cm transverse CT image demonstrates sclerosing mediastinitis that has caused superior vena caval obstruction in a 49-year-old woman.

rior vena caval obstruction in a 49-year-old woman with this condition. One series of 22 patients described compression of the superior vena cava in 13, of the esophagus in 3, of the pulmonary artery and pericardium in 3, and of the trachea in 3. Ketoconazole is reported to decrease the degree of inflammation and subsequent fibrosis (Urschel, et al., 1990).

Surgical therapy may be necessary in cases of tracheal or esophageal obstruction or with superior vena caval or pulmonary arterial obstruction. With persistently elevated Histoplasma complement fixation levels, long-term ketoconazole therapy should be prescribed (Urschel, et al., 1990). Patients with upper mediastinal compression have a better prognosis than do those with lower mediastinal compression (Eggleston, 1980). Over time, collateral circulation develops in caval obstruction. Severe encasement of the pulmonary artery and trachea can be fatal (Eggleston, 1980).

COMMENTS AND CONTROVERSIES

Mediastinal infection will always be a challenge for the thoracic surgeon. Its multiple etiologic sources, the changing clinical patterns, and the high mortality rates of untreated cases will maintain a central place in our specialty.

Primary prevention should characterize our approach to management. Flexible instrumentation has done much to decrease the incidence of esophageal perforation. Prophylactic antibiotic therapy in cardiac and mediastinal surgery, although no substitute for good technique, has been beneficial.

An awareness of modern trends in the management of tuberculosis should enhance the efficient diagnosis and therapy of this mediastinal variant.

The single most useful tool in the medical therapy of sclerosing mediastinitis is the use of ketoconazole when Histoplasma complement levels are elevated. The role of surgical intervention will always be complex and limited.

B.N.

KEY REFERENCES

Burnett CM, Rosemurgy AS, Pfeiffer EA: Life threatening acute posterior mediastinitis due to esophageal perforation. Ann Thorac Surg 49:979, 1990

The authors analyzed the therapy of patients with life-threatening acute postmediastinitis caused by esophageal perforation to elucidate common factors in successful therapy. Thorough mediastinal debridement and wide mediastinal drainage appear to be important in improving the survival times of patients with life-threatening acute posterior mediastinitis.

FitzGerald JM, Grzybowski S, Allen EA: The impact of human immunodeficiency virus infection on tuberculosis and its control. Chest 100:191, 1991

This article describes the impact of human immunodeficiency virus (HIV) infection on tuberculosis and its need for control. Since tuberculosis has long been a source of mediastinitis, it behooves readers to be aware of the negative association between it and HIV infection.

Gaynes R, Marosok R, Moury-Hanly J et al.: Mediastinitis following coronary artery bypass surgery: a 3 year review. J Infect Dis 163:117, 1991

Twenty cases of mediastinitis after coronary bypass graft surgery were reviewed between 1985 and 1987 to determine risk factors.

Two distinct clusters with the methicillin-resistant *Staphylococcus aureus* (MRSA strain) occurred in 1986. This suggests that it is important to follow MSRA strains and to recognize that low preoperative albumin levels are a risk factor for mediastinitis.

Katsal A, Isrisim E, Catav Z et al.: Mediastinitis after open heart surgery. Analysis of risk factors and management. J Cardiovasc Surg 32:38, 1991

Mediastinitis developed following 58 of 8,803 operative procedures that involved median sternotomy, 40 in men and 18 in women. The major risk factors that predisposed patients to mediastinitis in this study were age, sex (men higher), type of procedure, duration of operation, cardiopulmonary bypass, reoperation, and reexploration for postoperative bleeding and cardiac tamponade, diabetes, and low cardiac output states.

Urschel HC, Razzuk MA, Netto GJ et al.: Sclerosing mediastinitis: improved management with histoplasmosis titer and ketoconazole. Ann Thorac Surg 50:215, 1990

In this article, histoplasma complement fixation titers were used to detect unsuspecting subacute disease and to follow the therapeutic adjunctive management with ketoconazole, an oral antifungal agent.

REFERENCES

Arnett EN, Bacos JM, Marsh HB et al.: Fibrosing mediastinitis causing pulmonary artery hypertension without pulmonary venous hypertension. Am J Med 63:634, 1977

Dunn EJ, Ulnicny KS Jr, Wright CB, Gottesman L: Surgical implications of sclerosing mediastinitis. A report of 6 cases and review of literature. Chest 97:338, 1990

Edlin BR, Tohars JI, Grieco MH et al.: An outbreak of multidrug-resistant tuberculosis among hospitalized patients with acquired immunodeficiency syndrome. N Engl J Med 326:1514, 1992

Eggleston JC: Sclerosing mediastinitis. Prog Surg Pathol 2:1, 1980

Fleisher AG, Evans KG, Webber EM et al.: Recommended management of spontaneous and instrumental esophageal perforations. (In preparation).

Fry WA, Shields TW: Acute and chronic mediastinal infections. In Mediastinal Infections.

Goodwin RA, Nichel JA, DesPrez RM: Mediastinal fibrosis complicating healed primary histoplasmosis and tuberculosis. Medicine 51:227, 1972

Kallis P, Bellsham PA, Pepper JR: Spontaneous rupture of the oesophagus (Boerhaave's syndrome): conservative versus surgical management. J R Soc Med 84:690, 1991

Korzeniewska-Kosela M, FitzGerald JM, Vedal S et al.: Spectrum of tuberculosis in patients with HIV infection in British Columbia: report of 40 cases. Can Med Assoc J 146:11, 1992

Kuhn C, Askin FB: Lung and mediastinum. In Kissane JM (ed): Anderson's Pathology. 9th Ed. CV Mosby, St. Louis, 1990

Light AM: Idiopathic fibrosis of the mediastinum; a discussion of 3 cases and review of the literature. J Clin Pathol 31:78, 1978

Schonengerdt CB, Suyemoto R, Maion FB: Granulomatous and fibrosing mediastinitis. A review and analysis of 180 cases. J Thorac Cardiovasc Surg 57:365, 1979

Urschel HC: Improved management of esophageal perforation: exclusion and diversion in continuity. Ann Surg 179:587, 1974

Urschel HC, Razzuk MA, Netto GJ et al.: Sclerosing mediastinitis: improved management with histoplasmosis titer and ketoconazole. Ann Thorac Surg 50:215, 1990

Wilson LG: The historical decline of tuberculosis in Europe and America; its causes and significance. J Hist Med Allied Sci 45:366, 1990

56

PERICARDIAL DISEASE

William G. Jones II

DEFINITION

The pericardium is a serous sac that surrounds, supports, and protects the heart. The smooth pericardial surface adjacent to the heart and the small amount of pericardial fluid normally present within the pericardial sac provide a frictionless chamber for cardiac motion, thus improving the efficiency of myocardial contractions. The pericardium, however, is subject to disease process, including inflammation, infection, trauma, and malignant disease. Impairment of pericardial compliance or intrapericardial fluid accumulation, resulting in reduction of the relative volume of the pericardial space secondary to these disease processes, may lead to pathophysiologic and hemodynamically significant restriction of cardiac function. Prompt recognition and treatment of pericardial disease is often lifesaving.

HISTORICAL NOTE

Hippocrates is credited with the first description of the human pericardium in 460 B.C. Three hundred years later Galen first described inflammatory changes and effusions in animals with pericarditis. Similar studies of pericardial disease in humans, however, did not occur until the seventeenth and eighteenth centuries, when Lower (1669) first described cardiac tamponade secondary to the accumulation of pericardial fluid, and Lancisi and Morgani wrote of the diminution of cardiac function resulting from constrictive pericarditis.

The classic pathologic description of the "bread and butter" appearance of acute pericarditis by Laennec (1819) was later followed by characterization of the pathology of chronic pericarditis associated with hepatic disease by Pick (1886). Knowledge of the pathophysiology of pericardial disease was advanced by the hemodynamic observations of Kussmaul (1873), including the description of pulsus paradoxus in association with tamponade. Modern experimental studies by Beck and others subsequently contributed to our understanding of pericardial disease and led to advances in its treatment.

Early reports of symptomatic relief produced by pericardiocentesis by Karaeneff (1840) introduced the era of treatment of pericardial disease. Rehn and Sauerbrauch (1913) independently described methods for pericardial resection,

followed by modifications by Schmieder and Fischer (1926). Based on the successes of these reports, Churchill (1936) performed the first pericardiectomy in the United States for constrictive disease in 1929.

HISTORICAL READINGS

Beck CS, Griswald RA: Pericardiectomy in the treatment of the Pick syndrome: experimental and clinical observations. Arch Surg 21:1064, 1930

Churchill ED: Pericardial resection in chronic constrictive pericarditis. Ann Surg 104:516, 1936

Karanaeff P: Paracentese des brustkastens und des pericardiums. Med Z 9:251, 1840

Kussmaul A: Ueber schwielige Mediatino-perikarditis und dem Paradoxen Puls. Berl Klin Wochenschr 10:433, 1873

Laennec RTH: Traité d'auscultation médicale et des maladies du poumon et du coeur. Brosson & JS Chaude, Paris, 1819

Lower R: Tractatus de Corde. London, 1669, p 104

Pick F: Ueber chronische, unter dem Bilde der Lebercirrhose Verlaufen der Pericarditis (Pericarditis pseudolebercirrhose) nebst Bemerkungen ueber Zuckergussleber. Z Klin Med 29:385, 1886

Rehn L: Zurexperimentellen pathologie des herzbeutels. Verh Dtsch Ges Chir 42:339, 1913

Sauerbruch F: Die Chirurgie der Brestorgane, Vol II. Berlin, 1925

Schmieder V, Fischer H: Die herzbeutelentzunchung und ihre folgezustande. Ergeb Chir Orthop 19:98, 1926

BASIC SCIENCE

Embryology

The pericardium is derived from membranous partitions, which begin to form between the pleural and peritoneal cavities during the third week of fetal development. By the seventh gestational week, these membranes grow to envelope the fetal heart, ultimately fusing to form the complete pericardial sac. Because of their common origins during development, the pericardium remains intimately associated and in some areas contiguous with the pleurae and diaphragm.

Anatomy

The parietal pericardium consists of a tough fibrous outer layer, with an inner serosal surface composed of cuboidal cells. The serosa of the pericardium is organized into microvilli and cilia, which produce and reabsorb the pericardial fluid. The serosal layer is then reflected into the epicardial surface to form the visceral pericardium and becomes contiguous with the adventitia of the great vessels superiorly. The pericardium is further anchored anteriorly to the sternum by the superior and inferior pericardiosternal ligaments and inferiorly to the diaphagm. The phrenic nerves and associated blood vessels lie within the anterolateral portion of the pericardial fat pad bilaterally.

Physiology

The smooth serosal surface of the pericardial sac provides a frictionless chamber, facilitating cardiac contraction, while the fibrous outer layer provides protection against the spread of infection from the adjacent mediastinum and pleural cavities. The fixed pericardium also supports the heart and prevents cardiac torsion by maintaining the heart in a relatively fixed position despite body motion. The pericardium contributes to the maintenance of a functionally optimal cardiac shape, preventing acute overdilatation, which may damage the myocardium. Negative pressure within the pericardium may also enhance atrial filling to a small degree.

Normally 15 to 20 ml of clear star-colored fluid is present within the pericardial space. Pericardial fluid is produced by the serosal cells and is an ultrafiltrate of plasma (Gibbon and Segal, 1940). Microvilli on the serosal surface both produce and reabsorb pericardial fluid. Although membrane characteristics of these cuboidal serosal cells favor absorption rather than production of fluid (Pegram and Bishop, 1981), the net turnover of pericardial fluid is determined by a number of factors, including intravascular and interstitial oncotic pressure, volume, and composition and the adequacy of the lymphatic drainage of the pericardium.

Histologic section of the fibrous portion of the pericardium reveals that the collagen bundles are arranged in a wavy, "herringbone" pattern (Elias and Boyd, 1960). This configuration gives the pericardium compliance, allowing it to be stretched to where the collagen strands become straightened and aligned. The size of the pericardial sac when the collagen fibers are maximally stretched represents the limiting volume of the pericardial space and the point beyond which further distension is impossible, (Holt, 1970; Ferguson and Willerson, 1991). However, chronic stretching of the pericardium over time results in pericardial hypertrophy and increased pericardial compliance, thus producing a rightward shift in the limiting volume. On the other hand, adherence of the pericardium on the epicardial surface of the heart diminishes the ability of the pericardium to stretch by even small amounts and may ultimately restrict cardiac filling.

The normal pressure within the pericardium is less than atmospheric and is equal to the intrapleural pressure. The normal volume of the pericardial sac exceeds the size of the heart by approximately 20 percent (Shabetai, 1987), allowing physiologic enlargement of the heart to occur without restriction. Additionally, the compliance or distensibility of the normal pericardium allows for relatively large increases to occur in either pericardial fluid volume or cardiac size without an increase in intrapericardial pressure, particularly when such increases occur over time. As pericardial distension approaches the limiting volume, however, intrapericardial pressure begins to rise. Tamponade occurs when the intrapericardial pressure exceeds right ventricular filling pressure. The slope of the pericardial pressure-volume curve and the point at which tamponade occurs thus depends upon the rate of pericardial fluid accumulation, pericardial compliance, and the intravascular volume status, which determines right ventricular filling pressure (Holt, 1970; Shabetai, et al., 1970).

DISEASE CONDITIONS

Acute Pericarditis

Etiology and Pathophysiology

Acute pericarditis may often be the early manifestation of a systemic illness such as connective tissue disease or myocardial infarction. As many as half of all cases of acute pericarditis, however, are due to neoplastic disease, are uremic or infectious in origin, or result from unclear processes and are thus termed idiopathic or nonspecific (Shabetai, 1990). Other less common causes of acute pericarditis are listed below.

Symptoms in acute pericarditis result from inflammation of the pericardium as well as from irritation of adjacent tissues. Pathologic examination of the pericardium during acute pericarditis demonstrates inflammatory cell infiltration and fibrin deposition leading to a characteristic "bread and butter" appearance of the serosal surface.

Diagnosis

Acute pericarditis is often preceded by a prodrome of fever, myalgias, and malaise which may last for 3 to 7 days. As the

---

Less Common Etiologies of Acute Pericarditis

Drug/hypersensitivity reactions
  Procainamide
  Warfarin
  Hydralazine
  Dilantin
  Others
Dissecting aortic aneurysms
Connective tissue diseases
  Arteritis
  Rheumatoid arthritis
  Systemic lupus erythematosus
  Rheumatic fever
Secondary to or post-myocardial infarct or cardiac surgery
Sarcoidosis
Secondary to or postradiation
Secondary to or post-trauma
Myxedema
Amyloidosis

inflammation in the pericardium worsens, chest pain and leukocytosis ensue. The substernal pain associated with acute pericarditis is excruciating and may be confused with angina, although pain associated with pericarditis is usually more pleuritic in nature, increased by supination or deep inspiration. Dyspnea is common and accompanied by a non-productive cough with clear lung fields. The classical friction rub associated with acute pericarditis has been described as resembling the "squeak of leather on a new saddle" (Collin, 1955).

The cardiac silhouette may appear enlarged on chest x-ray, especially when pericarditis is complicated by a large effusion. Electrocardiogram (ECG) changes in pericarditis, consisting of ST segment elevations without Q waves or T-wave inversions, may be helpful in differentiating from an acute myocardial infarction, particularly since pericarditis may rarely result in an elevation of the creatine kinase MB fraction (Shabetai, et al., 1990). An echocardiogram should be obtained in most cases of acute pericarditis to determine the size of the associated effusion and to examine for signs of tamponade when indicated and may be useful in the detection of intrapericardial lymphoma or metastatic disease. If the etiology of acute pericarditis is unclear, minimal workup should include cultures for an infectious etiology, a renal profile, and antibody titers for collagen vascular disease.

Management

In general, acute pericarditis not complicated by tamponade should be treated by bed rest and pain control. Narcotic analgesia is usually required in the early phase and should be supplemented with nonsteroidal anti-inflammatory agents. Severe and persistent pain may require steroids for control. Persistent fevers despite therapy warrant pericardiocentesis to ensure the proper diagnosis and to examine the pericardial fluid for purulence or signs of an infectious etiology. Other indications for pericardiocentesis are to relieve tamponade and to evaluate the etiology in cases in which the effusion persists beyond 2 to 3 weeks.

Infectious pericarditis may result from direct contamination of the pericardial space by penetrating trauma or surgery, from seeding of the pericardium and pericardial fluid during bacteremia, or from rupture of an adjacent infected collection into the pericardial space. Treatment of infectious pericarditis requires control of the primary source of the infection and drainage of the pericardial space. In infectious pericarditis the effusion develops quickly and is often thick and purulent and associated with multiple intrapericardial loculations. Pericardiocentesis, although helpful in establishing the diagnosis, provides inadequate drainage, and pericardiotomy with careful exploration to open all loculated areas is usually needed.

Tuberculous pericarditis requires triple-drug therapy for at least 9 months (Fowler, 1991). Although controversial, addition of steroids to the antituberculin regimen has also been reported to decrease the need for repeated pericardiocentesis procedures in order to control the associated effusion (Strang, et al., 1988). Early operative intervention should also be considered in tuberculous pericarditis, since the dense fibrous pericardial reaction may prevent concentration of antituberculous drugs to eradicate the infection and since

this reaction will ultimately produce a thickened, constrictive pericardium (Larrieu, et al., 1980).

Acute pericarditis has been reported to complicate 5 to 15 percent of all cases of acquired immunodeficiency syndrome (AIDS) at some time during the course of the illness (Acierno, 1989). The etiology of pericarditis in these patients is usually secondary to a viral, fungal, or tuberculous infection or to superimposed neoplasia, and therapy should be directed at the primary cause.

Uremic pericarditis occurs most often in patients with renal failure undergoing hemodialysis. Specific symptoms may be absent until tamponade develops and pericardiocentesis or pericardiotomy is required. Uremic pericarditis without tamponade may respond to more frequent hemodialysis or to a change to peritoneal dialysis (Shabetai, 1990). Intrapericardial instillation of corticosteroids has also been reported to be successful in selected patients (Buselmier, et al., 1976).

Acute pericarditis arises in 10 to 15 percent of patient receiving radiation therapy and may occur months to years after therapy (Applefield, et al., 1981). Radiation-induced pericarditis produces both pericardial effusions and fibrosis and should be treated with systemic steroids. Symptoms of constriction may require pericardiectomy, although great care should be taken to attempt to differentiate constrictive pericarditis from radiation-induced myocardial fibrosis in these patients (Schneider and Edwards, 1979).

Idiopathic acute pericarditis will recur with relapsing episodes in 15 to 30 percent of all cases. Although recurrences are often numerous and may occur over more than 10 to 15 years, the risk of tamponade in recurrent pericarditis is lower than in acute pericarditis (Fowler and Harbin, 1986). Therapy is similar to that for the initial episode, consisting of bed rest and pain control. Steroids are often useful in producing remission, and some patients require long-term steroid courses to prevent recurrence. Colchicine has also been reported to be useful in preventing recurrences (Guindo, et al., 1990). Pericardiectomy will relieve symptoms in 50 to 80 percent of cases (Fowler and Harbin, 1986; Hatcher, et al., 1971) but should be reserved for those patients who develop complications from their steroid therapy or in whom steroids have failed to produce a lasting remission.

Constrictive Pericarditis

Etiology and Pathophysiology

Constrictive pericarditis usually results from acute pericarditis that has progressed to chronic scarring and fibrosis, leading to a thickened and noncompliant pericardium. Presently the most common causes of constrictive pericarditis are neoplastic disease and the effects of mediastinal radiation therapy or chest surgery or trauma (Ferguson and Willerson, 1991). Tuberculous pericarditis, formerly the most common cause of constrictive pericarditis, is now less common in the United States but remains problematic in other areas. Less commonly, constrictive pericarditis may be secondary to uremia and collagen vascular disorders or may follow acute bacterial pericarditis. It is estimated that between 0.02 and 0.3 percent of all cardiac surgical procedures are complicated by pericardial constriction (Miller, et al., 1982; Kutcher, et al., 1982; Marsa, et al., 1979). The development of constrictive pericarditis secondary to cardiac surgery may be related to complete closure of the pericardium following the procedure and to irrigation of the pericardial cavity with irritating solutions (Ribeiro, 1984).

Constriction occurs when a chronically diseased pericardium restricts cardiac function by limitation of diastolic filling. Thickening, fibrosis, and calcification of the pericardium diminish pericardial compliance and result in a fixed, often somewhat contracted intrapericardial volume. As the pericardium becomes more rigid and nondistensible, the limiting volume or ultimate limit of pericardial distension decreases. This leads to an abrupt cessation of the early rapid phase of diastolic filling when the limiting volume of the pericardium is reached. Most commonly the fibrotic process affects most of the pericardial surface and produces a uniform restriction of filling of all heart chambers, resulting in both pulmonary and systemic venous congestion, decreased cardiac output, a fall in systemic blood pressure, and exertional intolerance. Localized constriction and compression may also occur if the disease process in the pericardium is limited.

Diagnosis

Physical examination in constrictive pericarditis reveals evidence of right heart failure, including jugular venous distension, peripheral edema, hepatosplenomegaly, and ascites. Kussmaul's sign, an inspiratory increase in jugular venous pressure, may be present, but pulsus paradoxus does not usually occur. An early diastolic pericardial knock by ascultation and occasionally by palpation is present and corresponds to the cessation of rapid ventricular filling caused by the diminished limiting volume of the constricted pericardium.

Pericardial calcification may be prominent on chest x-ray, especially in the lateral view, (Fig. 56-1). The ECG may display nonspecific ST segment changes but is often only remarkable for low QRS voltages. Other diagnostic studies may be helpful in determining the extent of pericardial disease and the degree of impairment of cardiac function. Echocardiography can document thickening of the pericardium and may demonstrate the abnormal diastolic function in association with normal ventricular systolic function that is characteristic of constriction. Computed tomography (CT) and magnetic resonance imaging (MRI) scans allow measurement of pericardial thickness and assessment of dilatation of the inferior and superior vena cavae and the hepatic veins. Angiography with intrachamber pressure monitoring will demonstrate the abrupt cessation of ventricular diastolic filling and equalization of left and right ventricular diastolic pressure. Angiography may also be helpful in operative planning in older patients if concurrent significant coronary artery disease is suspected.

It may be difficult to differentiate between cardiac dysfunction resulting from constrictive pericarditis and that resulting from a restrictive cardiomyopathy, especially in the patient

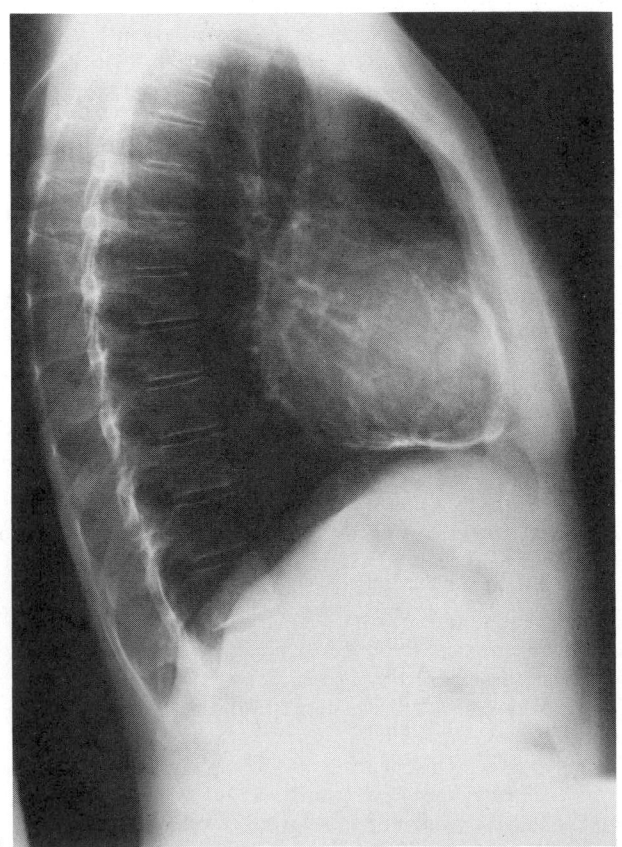
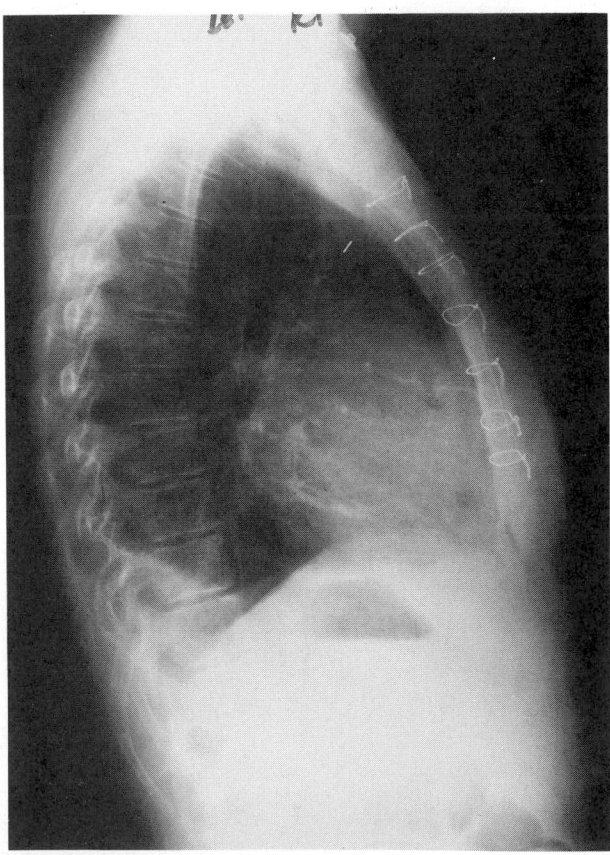

Figure 56-1.   **(A)** Lateral chest radiograph of a patient with constrictive pericarditis, demonstrating extensive calcification of the pericardium. **(B)** The same patient following pericardiectomy.

with disease resulting from prior mediastinal irradiation. Differentiation, however, is crucial, as resection of the constrictive pericardium can be expected to produce a marked resolution of symptoms, while removal of the pericardium in patients in whom the primary problem is restrictive cardiomyopathy will be unsuccessful and poorly tolerated (Hatle, et al., 1989). Restrictive cardiomyopathy results from an infiltrative process in the myocardium, such as amyloidosis or radiation-induced fibrosis, which produces diastolic dysfunction. The resulting hemodynamic pattern may be indistinguishable from constrictive pericarditis. Restrictive cardiomyopathy may, however, affect the left ventricle more than the right and may be associated with signs of other organ involvement in systemic diseases such as amyloidosis. At angiography, restrictive cardiomyopathy may be distinguished from constrictive pericarditis by the presence of right ventricular systolic hypertension. Restrictive cardiomyopathy also result in impaired function throughout diastole, while only the latter portion of the rapid filling phase is affected in constrictive pericarditis.

Management

Thickening, fibrosis, and calcification of the pericardium in constrictive pericarditis are not reversible and therefore require operative intervention if significant. Adequate resection of the pericardium in these cases leads to both immediate relief of symptoms and a later improvement in exercise tolerance (Pugliese, et al., 1984; Seifert, et al., 1985; Copeland, et al., 1975). However, pericardiectomy may be a difficult procedure because the pericardium is often firmly adherent to the epicardial surface, obscuring planes of dissection, and operative mortality of up to 5 percent has been reported (DeValeria, et al., 1991). Failure to improve following pericardiectomy may result from inadequate resection of the visceral portion of the pericardium, leading to continued constriction, or from underlying myocardial disease, atrophy, or fibrosis (Culliford, et al., 1980; Ni, et al., 1990).

Timing of operative intervention remains controversial. Early pericardiectomy, even before the onset of symptoms, has been recommended in pericardial disease processes in which the likelihood that constriction will develop is high as in tuberculous pericarditis (Larrieu, et al., 1980). For most other disease processes operation may be delayed until the patient actually begins to demonstrate signs of early constriction. Serial echocardiograms may be helpful in following these patients and planning intervention. Median sternotomy is the standard surgical approach, although some surgeons perform pericardiectomy through a left anterior thoracotomy if the disease process is limited to the anterior pericardium. However, complete resection of the pericardium from beyond the right phrenic nerve to the left pulmonary vessels with preservation of the phrenic bundles bilaterally is to be recommended to decrease the risk of recurrent constriction, as reoperation for further pericardial resection carries a significantly higher morbidity and mortality (Culliford, et al., 1980). Careful removal of the visceral portion of the pericardium is also crucial in preventing recurrence. Cardiopulmonary bypass should be available at the time of operation in case it is needed to obtain an adequate pericardial resection, but it should probably be avoided if possible to obviate the need for systemic heparinization with its attendant higher risk of bleeding.

Pericardial Effusive Disease and Cardiac Tamponade

Etiology and Pathophysiology

Pericardial effusions result when the net rate of pericardial fluid production exceeds the rate of fluid resorption. The pericardial effusion fluid may be serous, purulent, or hemorrhagic in nature or a combination of the three types. More than 75 percent of pericardial effusions are secondary to malignancy, most commonly of the lung or breast or lymphoma (Press and Livingston, 1987). Benign etiologies of pericardial effusive disease include acute pericarditis, especially if viral and idiopathic in origin or following cardiac surgery; trauma; rupture of an ascending aorta aneurysm or dissection; radiation therapy, and myocardial infarction, particularly in association with anticoagulation.

Irritation and inflammation of the pericardial serosa produce an exudative reaction resulting in increased pericardial fluid. Likewise, implantation of metastatic disease in the serosa leads to exudation of fluid into the pericardial space. When the resorptive capacity of the pericardial serosa is exceeded or inflammatory or neoplastic processes begin to obstruct the venous and lymphatic drainage of the pericardium, a significant effusion develops, which may result in cardiac tamponade when the limiting volume of the pericardium is reached.

The normal function of the heart and circulation is compromised when the presence of fluid under increased pressure within the pericardial space compromises diastolic filling. As the normally compliant pericardium does allow for some distensibility, the rate of pericardial fluid accumulation may be as important as the total amount of fluid present in determining the point at which cardiac function will be compromised. Mild cardiac compression may only produce an elevated central venous pressure with normal systemic blood pressure, as impaired diastolic function may be adequately compensated by a normal heart and circulation. Severe compression leads to further compromise of diastolic filling beyond the compensatory capabilities of the heart and results in tamponade and ultimately in cardiogenic shock.

Diagnosis

Pericardial effusive disease without significant cardiac compromise or tamponade is often asymptomatic. As the development of a pericardial effusion may not diminish the quality of friction rubs or cause ECG changes in acute pericarditis, a high index of suspicion must be maintained for early diagnosis to be made. A pericardial effusion should be suspected when patients with pericarditis, metastatic neoplasms, or uremia and renal failure requiring hemodialysis develop diminished QRS voltages on ECG or an enlarged cardiac silhouette on chest x-ray, especially in association with clear lung fields or an unexplained increase in venous pressure.

Acute cardiac tamponade occurs when a pericardial effusion rapidly develops, as following blunt or penetrating chest trauma, postinfarction ventricular rupture, or intrapericardial rupture of an aortic dissection or from bleeding following cardiac surgery. The central venous pressure markedly increases in association with systemic hypotension. Beck's triad of distended neck veins, muffled heart sounds, and hypotension is characteristic, and pulsus paradoxus may be detectable. Recognition of tamponade in this setting is crucial and should prompt rapid volume infusion to further raise venous pressure to promote diastolic filling, as well as emergent pericardiocentesis for decompression. Definitive identification and correction of the primary abnormality may then be pursued.

Subacute tamponade presents as progressive dyspnea on even minimal activity and should be suspected in hemodynamically compromised patients who have pericarditis, aortic dissections, or known or suspected intrathoracic or metastatic neoplasms or who are during recovering from the chest trauma or cardiac surgery. Hypotension may be present, but the systemic blood pressure may be maintained by elevated peripheral vascular resistance. A narrow pulse pressure accompanied by pulsus paradoxus, distant heart sounds, and an elevated central venous pressure are characteristic. Tachycardia results as a compensatory mechanism to maintain cardiac output, while rales are uncommon. Chest x-rays confirm the presents of an enlarged cardiac silhouette with clear lung fields, while the ECG demonstrates low QRS voltages and ST segment alterations. Electrical alternans, or QRS voltages that vary from beat to beat, may also be present; this reflects swinging of the heart in the pericardial fluid during contractions.

Proper diagnosis of tamponade requires demonstration of a pericardial effusion, demonstration of hemodynamic abnormalities attributable to pericardial fluid under pressure, and improvement of these hemodynamic abnormalities after drainage of the pericardial fluid (Burstow, et al., 1989). Echocardiography (Fig. 56-2), has proved to be the most helpful adjunct in the diagnosis of pericardial effusive disease and tamponade in the subacute setting. M-mode echocardiography allows diagnosis of pericardial effusion by the demonstration of an echo-free space between the heart and pericardium. The heart may be seen to swing freely in the effusion in association with electrical alternans (Vignolo, et al., 1976). The effusion may be characterized as small if present only behind the left ventricle, moderate if also present in front of the right ventricle, and massive if the echo-free area surrounds the heart during all phases of the cardiac cycle (Horowitz, et al., 1977; Martin, et al., 1978). Further, two-dimensional echocardiograms can quantify the amount and location of the effusion, identify loculations and adhesions, and suggest impending tamponade (Martin, et al., 1980).

Hemodynamic compromise and cardiac tamponade may be demonstrated echocardiographically by a decreased right ventricular diameter with compression of the right atrium. Paradoxical septal motion and systolic collapse with inward motion of the right atrial and ventricular walls in early systole suggest severe compromise requiring emergent decompression. Other echocardiographic findings of tamponade may include persistent full distension of the inferior vena cava throughout the entire cardiac cycle and an exaggerated respiratory variation in the velocity of flow through the mitral and tricuspid valves (D'Cruz, et al., 1975).

Management

Treatment for pericardial effusive disease without evidence of hemodynamic compromise may be directed toward the etiology of the effusion alone if the underlying condition is self-limited or responsive to therapy, the effusion does not appear to be enlarging, the patient can be followed for signs of increased effusion or evolving tamponade, and fluid is not necessary to establish a primary diagnosis. The indications for pericardiocentesis in the absence of tamponade are to eliminate the possibility of a purulent effusion requiring operative drainage, to differentiate a neoplastic effusion in patients with malignancy from a reactive effusion following radiation or chemotherapy, and to obtain fluid for proper diagnosis with the etiology of the effusion is unclear or when an exact diagnosis is necessary in choosing therapy (Wenger, 1991).

Signs of impending tamponade on examination or echocardiography are an indication for emergent pericardial decompression by pericardiocentesis or open drainage. While being prepared for drainage, the patient should be treated by volume expansion with saline solutions despite elevated venous pressures. Volume infusion will increase right atrial pressure without affecting intrapericardial pressure, thus promoting diastolic filling. Infusion of dobutamine may also be helpful in the interim management of these patients prior to drainage by decreasing heart size through improved inotropy and systemic vasodilatation. However, it cannot be overemphasized that emergent decompression of the pericardial space is the only maneuver in impending tamponade that is lifesaving.

The choice of pericardiocentesis versus open drainage procedures for tamponade remains controversial and depends upon the etiology of the effusion, the condition of the patient, and the available facilities and physician experience. Pericardiocentesis is less expensive than open drainage and requires

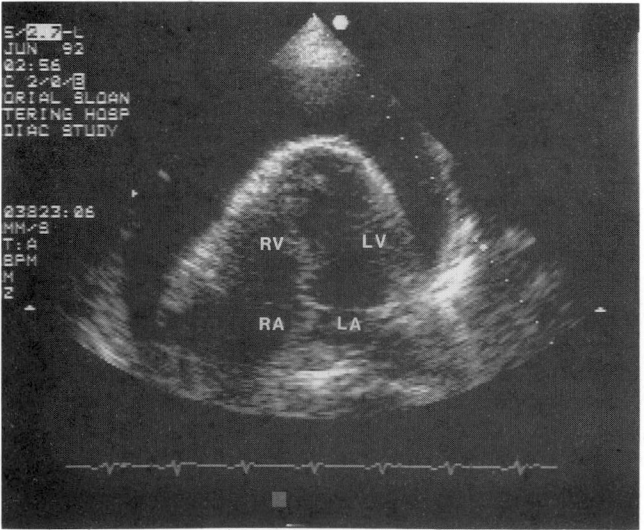

Figure 56-2. Echocardiogram demonstrating a large pericardial effusion in a patient with metastatic breast cancer compressing the right atrium and ventricle at end-diastole.

fewer resources. Placement of a catheter into the pericardial space permits an exact hemodynamic diagnosis to be made and allows for pressure monitoring to evaluate the effects of drainage on hemodynamics. Sclerosis may be subsequently performed for treatment of malignant effusions. Pericardiocentesis is associated with morbidity and occasional mortality from errant catheter placement into the heart or inferior vena cava and from bleeding due to laceration of an epicardial or coronary vessel. Although decompression may be obtained, complete drainage of the effusion, especially if loculated or purulent, may be difficult, necessitating repeated taps or open drainage.

Pericardiotomy may be performed through either a subxiphoid or a left anterior thoracotomy approach. Open drainage through such incisions is performed under direct vision, allows for exploration of the pericardial space, and permits pericardial biopsy if indicated. The incision may be extended if necessary and pericardiectomy performed. Open drainage has the disadvantages that a fully equipped and staffed operating room is required and accurate intraoperative pericardial pressure measurements are difficult to obtain. Furthermore, general anesthesia is necessary, at least for the anterior thoracotomy approach, and anesthetic induction in these hemodynamically compromised patients may be hazardous.

Other Diseases of the Pericardium

Congenital Anomalies

Partial or complete absence of the pericardium is rare and usually asymptomatic. An incomplete defect on the left side is the most common finding and is often associated with other congenital cardiac malformations, including patent ductus arteriosus, atrial septal defect, mitral valve stenosis and prolapse, and tetrology of Fallot (Nasser, 1970). No significant pathophysiology accompanies a pericardial defect unless it is large enough to allow herniation of the left heart or torsion of the great vessels.

Pericardial cysts and diverticula are smooth and rounded structures usually first found on a routine chest x-ray (Klatte and Young, 1972). They most commonly occur in the right cardiophrenic angle anteriorly (Craddock, 1950; Loehr, 1952). The diverticula differ from the cysts by the persistence of a connection to the coelomic cavity (Bates and Lever, 1951). Both uncomplicated cysts and diverticula are asymptomatic but when discovered should be differentiated from neoplasms by CT or occasionally by surgical exploration.

Pericardial Neoplasms

Although metastatic disease of the pericardium is common, primary neoplasms of the pericardium are rare. Mesothelioma is the most common primary pericardial neoplasm, and as with primary pleural mesothelioma, effective therapy producing long-term control is lacking at present. Pericardial resection may be required to control pericardial effusions. Treatment with doxorubicin, cyclophosphamide, and cisplatinum has also met with limited success (Artman, 1980). Other reported primary pericardial neoplasms include lymphagiomas, hemangiomas, teratomas, rhabdomyosarcomas, and lipomas.

As mentioned above, metastatic neoplasms are far more common than primary pericardial tumors. Metastases spread to the pericardium by hematogenous or lymphatic routes or through direct invasion of the pericardium. Common primary tumors that metastasize to or involve the pericardium include lung, breast, colon, esophagus, kidney, ovary, prostate, and stomach neoplasms, leukemia and lymphoma, melanoma, and soft tissue sarcomas (Press and Livingston, 1987). The most common presentation of tumor involving the pericardium is a pericardial effusion, and metastatic disease is the most common etiology of pericardial effusions. The presence of the pericardial effusion almost invariably indicates unresectability for cure. Treatment should be directed toward systemic chemotherapy and effective palliation and control of the effusion by pericardial drainage (Davis, et al., 1978; Hawkins and Vacek, 1989). Sclerosis of the pericardial cavity with tetracycline or bleomycin may be indicated if the effusion is recurrent, enlarging, or hemodynamically significant.

Postpericardiotomy Syndrome

As many as 25 to 30 percent of patients undergoing surgical procedures in which the pericardium is opened will experience symptoms associated with the postpericardiotomy syndrome. Studies have demonstrated elevated antiheart and viral antibody titers in some of these patients (Engle, et al., 1974), but the etiology and pathophysiology of the syndrome remain poorly understood. Symptoms resemble those of acute pericarditis with pleuritic chest pain and dyspnea, a pericardial friction rub, and less frequently fevers and leukocytosis. Most patients are well controlled by administration of nonsteroidal anti-inflammatory agents until symptoms have resolved, although a rare patient may require pulse steroid therapy in order to control symptoms. An occasional patient will relapse with recurrence of symptoms following cessation of therapy and require more prolonged therapy.

PERICARDIOCENTESIS AND PERICARDIAL SURGERY

Preoperative and Anesthetic Considerations

Patients undergoing procedures for decompression of the pericardial space for impending tamponade should be volume-loaded with saline solutions as preparations for the procedure are being made. Volume expansion is crucial, even with already elevated venous pressures, to maintain hemodynamic stability and promote diastolic filling by increasing right atrial pressure above intrapericardial pressure. A careful history for steroid therapy within the past year for pericarditis or underlying disease should be sought, and if it is found, stress steroid therapy should be administered.

Arterial and central venous pressure monitoring is essential for open procedures and highly recommended during pericardiocentesis. Safe anesthetic induction in hemodynamically compromised patients is difficult and requires close cooperation between the surgeon and the anesthesiologist. Sudden loss of vascular tone due to anesthetic administration in patients with impending tamponade will result in hypotension, further hemodynamic compromise, and cardiac arrest if it is not anticipated and proper precautionary actions are not taken. Induction and intubation should not be begun until after the patient is properly positioned on the surgical table with the head elevated. The patient should be prepared and draped awake, and the surgical team should be prepared to commence the operation as the rapid sequence induction is initiated. Pericardiocentesis and partial decompression prior to open drainage may also improve hemodynamic stability and response to anesthesia and surgery.

Pericardiocentesis

Pericardiocentesis is indicated to establish the diagnosis of pericardial disease by examination of effusion fluid, to treat acute or impending tamponade, to differentiate from constriction in the etiology of elevated venous pressures in association with pericardial disease, and as an interim treatment prior to surgical drainage for tamponade to aid anesthetic management (Miller and Hatcher, 1990).

The patient is placed in a semiupright position and the midanterior chest is prepared and draped. A parasternal placement of the catheter through the fourth or fifth intercostal space may be chosen, but the subxiphoid approach is generally easier and safer. An entry point is chosen 2 cm inferior to the xiphoid and to the left of the midline. A 21-gauge spinal needle is directed at a 45-degree angle aimed toward the left shoulder. The direction of the needle may also be guided by ECG monitoring, with deflection looked for as the needle contacts the epicardial surface (Bishop, et al., 1956); by echocardiography (Callahan, et al., 1985); or by fluoroscopy with pressure monitoring in an angiography suite. The needle is continuously aspirated as it is advanced, and once fluid is encountered, the needle may be changed over a guidewire to a flexible Silastic catheter. Returned bloody fluid should be examined carefully for clotting to rule out inadvertent cardiac puncture. A pneumopericardium, produced by insufflation of air into the pericardial space, was often used in the past following completion of drainage of the pericardial fluid to permit determination of pericardial thickness or the presence of masses by plain chest x-ray (Hancock, 1979). This technique has largely been supplanted by the widespread use of echocardiography (Martin, et al., 1980). The catheter may also be left in place for subsequent fluid drainage or sclerosis of the pericardial space.

Bleeding is the most common complication of pericardiocentesis and may result from inadvertent cardiac entry, cardiac or epicardial laceration, or injury to a coronary artery (Scannell, 1989). The risk of cardiac injury and significant hemorrhage is increased in patients with thrombocytopenia, coagulopathies, or small or loculated effusions and when a presumptive effusion is drained without echocardiographic confirmation (Wong, et al., 1979). Vasodilatation secondary to rapid decompression of the pericardial space may also occur and should be treated by volume administration. Failure to adequately drain the effusion or the recurrence of fluid may lead to later tamponade.

The choice of pericardiocentesis over an open surgical drainage procedure depends on the disease process being treated, the availability of facilities, and the experience of the physician performing the procedure. Open drainage should be favored when the accessibility of the effusion by pericardiocentesis is questionable, in the presence of a co-agulopathy or other condition that increases the risk of bleeding, or when constrictive pericarditis, which will require resection, is concomitantly present. Suspicion of the presence of partially clotted blood or purulent fluid within the pericardial space should also prompt an open procedure to ensure adequate drainage.

Pericardiotomy

Open pericardial drainage and pericardiotomy are indicated for pericardial effusions containing clotted blood; for effusions associated with a likely cardiac bleeding site, such as a traumatic injury; for suspected purulent or loculated effusion; for effusions that are recurrent or likely to recur, as in uremic pericarditis; or when pericardial biopsy is required for diagnosis.

Pericardiotomy may be performed by using either a subxiphoid or left anterior thoracotomy incision. The subxiphoid approach may be used with the patient under local anesthesia. A 3- to 4-cm vertical incision is made in the midline just above and inferior to the xiphoid process. Dissection is continued posteriorly and superiorly to the reflection of the pericardium onto the diaphragm. The pericardial space is entered at that point and the effusion drained. The pericardial space is carefully explored to ensure adequate drainage and open loculations. Substernal tubes are then placed for continued drainage and sclerosis if required.

Use of a left anterior thoracotomy approach allows for improved visualization, greater exploration of the pericardial space, and a wider resection of the pericardium, establishing a drainage pathway into the left pleural space. The incision may be extended to perform a pericardiectomy if indicated. General anesthesia is required for the anterior thoracotomy, which is also more painful postoperatively than the subxiphoid procedure. Use of video-assisted thoracic surgery (VATS) instrumentation is now allowing many of the benefits of the thoracotomy approach with reduced postoperative pain and morbidity. Pericardiotomy and partial pericardial resection can easily be performed by the operator skilled in these techniques, although the ability to explore the pericardial space remains limited.

Pericardiectomy

Pericardiectomy is indicated for constrictive pericarditis and in selected cases of recurrent pericarditis or recurrent pericardial effusive disease unresponsive to medical therapy. A median sternotomy approach is preferred, although some surgeons still favor a left anterior thoracotomy incision. Resection of both the parietal and visceral pericardium are necessary for adequate treatment of constrictive pericarditis, while it is less crucial to remove the visceral layer in the treatment of recurrent effusions.

The extent of resection for constrictive disease is usually from the right phrenic nerve to the level of the left pulmonary vasculature anteriorly, to the reflection onto the great vessels superiorly, and to the posterior diaphragm inferiorly. The phrenic nerves and associated blood vessels are preserved bilaterally as 1-cm tissue bridges. The visceral pericardium may then be "teased" from the surface of the epicardium

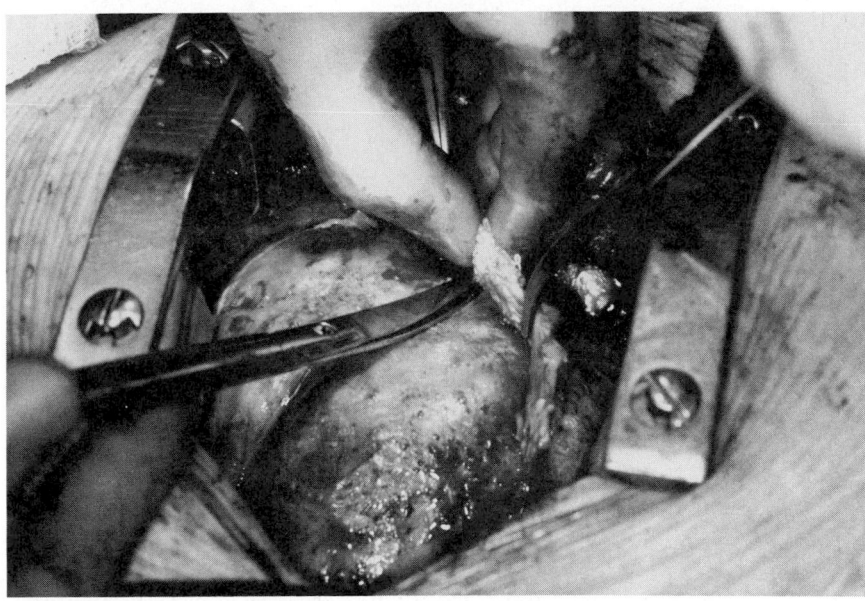

Figure 56-3. Surgical technique of "teasing" the visceral pericardium from the epicardial surface during pericardiectomy for constrictive pericarditis.

with care taken to remain in the proper plane of dissection (Fig. 56-3). The pericardium over the left ventricle is resected when possible before that over the right ventricle to minimize early blood loss, as the latter is the more easily injured of the two chambers. This sequence also theoretically avoids pulmonary congestion, which might occur if right ventricular output were allowed to increase while the left ventricle remained constricted. Following the resection, both pleural cavities should be widely opened to allow for improved postoperative drainage of blood and exudative fluid.

Complications may occur in 10 to 30 percent of cases (Culliford, et al., 1980; DeValeria, et al., 1991). Bleeding may be profuse and may occur from the raw epicardial surface or from laceration of the right atrium, right ventricle, or coronary vessels. Arrhythmias are common and are due to atrial irritability, manipulation of the heart, or injury to branches of the coronary arteries. Some surgeons have recommended the use of cardiopulmonary bypass during pericardiectomy to facilitate control of cardiac lacerations and hemorrhage and to allow safer manipulation of the heart for more complete resection (Copeland, et al., 1975; Culliford, et al., 1980; Pugliese, et al., 1984). However, systemic heparinization may make control of bleeding from the raw epicardial surface more difficult and actually increase operative morbidity. Although the routine use of cardiopulmonary bypass is not indicated, it should be available on a standby basis for all pericardial resections for constrictive disease in case difficulties are encountered.

KEY REFERENCES

Culliford AT, Lipton M, Spencer FC: Operation for chronic constrictive pericarditis: do the surgical approach and degree of pericardial resection influence the outcome significantly? Ann Thorac Surg 29:146, 1980

An excellent study and subsequent discussion of surgical treatment of constrictive pericarditis, weighing the controversies regarding adequate therapy and surgical technique.

Press OW, Livingston R: Management of malignant pericardial effusion and tamponade. JAMA 257:1088, 1987

A well-organized review of etiology and management of malignant pericardial disease, including both medical and surgical treatment options.

Shabetai R, Fowler ND, Gunthenok WG: The hemodynamics of cardiac tamponade and constrictive pericarditis. Am J Cardiol 26:480, 1970

A thorough discussion of pericardial pressure-volume relationships and the hemodynamic consequences of pericardial tamponade and constrictive pericarditis.

REFERENCES

Acierno LJ: Cardiac complications in acquired immunodeficiency syndrome (AIDS): a review. J Am Coll Cardiol 13:1144, 1989

Applefield MM, Slawson RG, Hall-Craigs M et al.: Delayed pericardial disease after radiotherapy. Am J Cardiol 47:210, 1981

Artman K: Current concepts: malignant mesothelioma. N Engl J Med 303:200, 1980

Bates JC, Lever FY: Pericardial coelomic cysts: presentation of 5 new cases and 5 similar cases illustrating difficulty of diagnosis. Radiology 57:300, 1951

Beck CS, Griswald RA: Pericardiectomy in the treatment of the Pick syndrome: experimental and clinical observations. Arch Surg 21:1064, 1930

Bishop LH, Estes EH, McIntosh HD: Electrocardiograms as a safeguard in pericardiocentesis. JAMA 162:264, 1956

Burstow DJ, Oh JK, Bailey KR et al.: Cardiac tamponade: characteristic Doppler observations. Mayo Clin Proc 64:312, 1989

Buselmier TJ, Simmons RL, Najarian JS et al.: Uremic pericardial effusion. Nephron 16:371, 1976

Callahan JA, Seward JB, Nishimura RA et al.: Two-dimensional echocardiographically guided pericardiocentesis: experience with 117 consecutive patients. Am J Cardiol 55:476, 1985

Churchill ED: Pericardial resection in chronic constrictive pericarditis. Am Surg 104:516, 1936.

Collin V, as quoted in Boyd LJ, Elias H: Contributions to disease of the heart and pericardium. Bull N Y Med Coll 18:1, 1955

Copeland JG, Stinson EB, Griepp RB, Shumway NE: Surgical treatment of chronic constrictive pericarditis using cardiopulmonary bypass. J Thorac Cardiovasc Surg 69:236, 1975

Craddock WL: Cysts of the pericardium. Am Heart J 40:619, 1950

D'Cruz IA, Cohen HC, Parbhu R et al.: Diagnosis of cardiac tamponade by echocardiography. Changes in mitral valve motion and ventricular dimensions, with special reference to paradoxical pulse. Circulation 52:460, 1975

Davis S, Sharma SM, Blumberg ED et al.: Intrapericardial tetracycline for the management of cardiac tamponade secondary to malignant pericardial effusion. N Engl J Med 299:1113, 1978

DeValeria PA, Baumgartner WA, Casale AS et al.: Current indications, risks and outcome after pericardiectomy. Ann Thorac Surg 52:219, 1991

Elias H, Boyd LJ: Notes on the anatomy, embryology and histology of the pericardium. J N Y Med Coll 2:50, 1960

Engle MA, McCabe JC, Ebert PA, Zabriskie J: The postpericardiotomy syndrome and antiheart antibodies. Circulation 49:401, 1974

Ferguson JJ, Willerson JT: Constrictive pericarditis. p. 269. In Hurst JW: Current Therapy in Cardiovascular Disease, 3rd Ed. BC Decker, Philadelphia, 1991

Fowler NO, Harbin AD: Recurrent pericarditis: follow-up study of 31 patients. J Am Coll Cardiol 7:300, 1986

Fowler NO: Acute and recurrent pericarditis. p. 260. In Hurst JW: Current Therapy in Cardiovascular Disease. 3rd Ed., BC Decker, Philadelphia, 1991

Gibbon AT, Segal MB: A study of the composition of pericardial fluid with special reference to the probable mechanism of fluid formation. J Physiol 277:635, 1940

Guindo J, Rodriguez de la Seina A, Ramiero J et al.: Recurrent pericarditis: relief with colchicine. Circulation 82:1117, 1990

Hancock EW: Management of pericardial disease. Mod Concepts Cardiovasc Dis 47:1, 1979

Hatcher CR, Logue RB, Logan WD et al.: Pericardiectomy for recurrent pericarditis. J Thorac Cardiovasc Surg 62:371, 1971

Hatle LK, Appleton CP, Popp RL: Differentiation of constrictive pericarditis and restrictive cardiomyopathy by Doppler echocardiography. Circulation 79:357, 1989

Hawkins JW, Vacek JL: What constitutes definitive treatment of malignant pericardial effusion? "Medical" versus surgical treatment. Am Heart J 118:428, 1989

Holt JP: The normal pericardium. Am J Cardiol 26:455, 1970

Horowitz MS, Schultz CS, Stinson EB et al.: Sensitivity and specificity of echocardiographic diagnosis of pericardial effusion. Circulation 72:744, 1977

Karaeneff P: Paracentese des brustkastens und des pericardiums. Med Z 9:251, 1840

Klatte EC, Young HY: Diagnosis and treatment of pericardial cysts. Radiology 104:541, 1972

Kussmaul A: Ueber schwielige Mediatino-perikarditis und dem paradoxen Puls. Berl Klin Wochenschr 10:433, 1873

Kutcher MA, King SB, Alimurung BN et al.: Constrictive pericarditis as a complication of cardiac surgery: recognition of an entity. Am J Cardiol 50:742, 1982

Laennec RTH: Traité d'auscultation medicale et des maladies du poumon et du coeur. Brosson & JS Chaude, Paris, 1819

Larrieu AJ, Tyers FO, Walthams EH, Derrick JC: Recent experience with tuberculous pericarditis. Ann Thorac Surg. 29:464, 1980

Loehr WM: Pericardial cysts. AJR 68:584, 1952

Lower R: Tractatus de corde. London, 1669, p 104

Marsa R, Mehta S, Willis W, Bailey L: Constrictive pericarditis after myocardial revascularization. Report of three cases. Am J Cardiol 44:177, 1979

Martin RP, Bowden R, Filly K et al.: Intrapericardial abnormalities in patients with pericardial effusion. Findings by two-dimensional echocardiography. Circulation 61:568, 1980

Martin RP, Rakowski H, French J et al.: Localization of pericardial effusion with wide angle phased array echocardiography. Am J Cardiol 42:904, 1978

McCaughan BC, Schaff HV, Piehler JM et al.: Early and late results of pericardiectomy for constrictive pericarditis. J Thorac Cardiovasc Surg 89:340, 1985

Miller JI, Hatcher CR: Surgical management of pericardial disease. p. 2185. In Hurst JW: The Heart. Vol. 1. McGraw-Hill, New York, 1990

Miller JI, Mansour KA, Hatcher CR: Pericardiectomy: current indications, concepts and results in a university center. Ann Thorac Surg 34:40, 1982

Nasser WK: Congenital absence of the left pericardium. Am J Cardiol 26:470;1970

Ni Y, von Seegesser LK, Turina M: Futility of pericardiectomy for post-irradiation pericarditis? Ann Thorac Surg 49:445, 1990

Pegram BL, Bishop VS: An evaluation of the pericardial sac as a safety factor during cardiac tamponade. Cardiovasc Res 48:701, 1981

Pick F: Ueber chronische, unter dem Bilde der Lebercirrhose Verlaufen der Pericarditis (Pericarditis pseudolebercirrhose) nebst Bemerkungen ueber Zuckergussleber. Z Klin Med 29:385, 1886

Pugliese P, Bernabei M, Eufrate S: Total pericardiectomy for chronic constrictive pericarditis using femero-femoral bypass. Int Surg 69:39, 1984

Rehn L: Zurexperimentellen pathologie des herzbeutels. Verh Dtsh Ges Chir 42:339, 1913

Ribeiro P: Constrictive pericarditis as a complication of coronary artery bypass surgery. Br Heart J 51:205, 1984

Sauerbruch: Die Chirurgie der Brestorgane. Vol II. Berlin, 1925

Scannell JG: Malignant pericardial effusion. In Grillo HC, Austin WG, Wilkins EW et al. (eds): Current Therapy in Cardiothoracic Surgery. BC Decker, Toronto, 1989, p. 295

Schmieder V, Fischer H: Die herzbeutelentzunchung und irhe folgezustande. Ergeb Chir Orthop 19:98, 1926

Schneider JS, Edwards JE: Irradiation induced pericarditis. Chest 75:560, 1979

Seifert FC, Miller DC, Osterle SN et al.: Surgical treatment of constrictive pericarditis: analysis of outcome and diagnostic error. Circulation 72:264, 1985

Shabetai R: Diseases of the pericardium. In Hurst JW: The Heart. Vol. 1. McGraw-Hill, New York, 1990, p. 1348

Shabetai R: Pericardial and cardiac pressure. Circulation 77:1, 1987

Shepard FA, Morgan C, Evans WK et al.: Medical management of malignant pericardial effusion by tetracycline sclerosis. Am J Cardiol 60:1161, 1987

Strang JIG, Gibson DG, Mitchison DA et al.: Controlled clinical trial of complete open surgical drainage and of prednisolone in the treatment of tuberculous pericardial effusion in Transkei. Lancet 2:759, 1988

Vignolo PA, Pohost GM, Curfrued GD, Myers G: Correlation of echocardiographic and clinical findings in patients with pericardial effusion. Arch Intern Med 136:979, 1976

Wenger NK: Pericardial effusion. In Hurst JW: Current Therapy in Cardiovascular Disease. 3rd Ed. BC Decker, Philadelphia, 1991, p 264

Wong G, Murphy J, Chang CJ: The risk of pericardiocentesis. Am J Cardiol 44:1110, 1979

57

CYSTS

Cysts and Duplications in Infants and Children

Robert C. Shamberger
W. Hardy Hendren III

Cystic masses within the mediastinum are an infrequent problem in infants and children. They are of both neoplastic and congenital origin. Accurate anatomic localization of these cysts often provides a strong indication of both their organ of origin and etiology (Fig. 57-1). Cystic lesions in the anterior mediastinum consist primarily of teratomas or lymphangiomas; less frequently, thymic cysts involve the mediastinum, and rarely, Hodgkin's disease presents as a cystic mass of the thymus. Cystic lesions in the middle mediastinum are primarily bronchogenic cysts, and lesions in the posterior mediastinum are primarily esophageal duplications or neurenteric cysts. These lesions are grouped for presentation by their anatomic location within the mediastinum to facilitate discussion of their symptoms at presentation, differential diagnosis, and therapy (Table 57-1).

ANTERIOR MEDIASTINUM

Teratomas

Mediastinal teratomas are generally benign and may present at any age (Gottschalk, et al., 1980). By definition, teratomas contain derivatives of all three germ cell layers and are frequently cystic. Teratomas are the second most common tumor of the anterior mediastinum, the most common being Hodgkin's disease, which almost invariably occurs as a solid tumor.

Symptoms at presentation are respiratory, the most frequent being cough. Teratomas may become very large and occasionally will produce dyspnea. Because of their cystic nature, tracheal compression and airway compromise rarely occur. Mediastinal teratomas may also become infected or may rupture into the bronchus, pleura, or pericardium, caus-

ing acute inflammatory symptoms (Thompson and Moore, 1969). Computed tomography (CT) best defines the extent of the lesion and excludes any possible tracheal compression. If the calculated tracheal area is less than 50 percent of expected, acute respiratory obstruction may occur on induction of general anesthesia (Shamberger, et al., 1991). Varying the tissue densities and calcification suggest the diagnosis of teratoma (Fig. 57-2).

Surgical resection is usually curative, although malignant elements in the tumor require additional therapy. Teratomas may contain components of either a yolk sac tumor or choriocarcinoma. Because of the possible presence of malignant elements, these lesions should not be followed over a long period. They may be resected through either a midline sternotomy or a thoracotomy. Resection is the definitive therapy except for the infrequent patient with malignant elements, who requires chemotherapy in addition.

Lymphangiomas (Cystic Hygromas)

Lymphangioma is a multilocular, thin-walled cystic mass of lymphatic origin. It develops from lymphatic tissues that become sequestered from the developing lymphatic system during early embryonic life (Childress, et al., 1956). The cyst is filled with serous fluid and lined by a thin, almost transparent membrane. Histologically it consists of a single layer of flattened endothelium with varying amounts of fibrous tissue. It may occur in the anterior mediastinum, and involvement should be considered in all patients with cervical or upper thoracic lymphangiomas (cystic hygromas). Routine chest radiographs should be obtained on any patient who has a lymphangioma in the neck or axilla to define the extent of

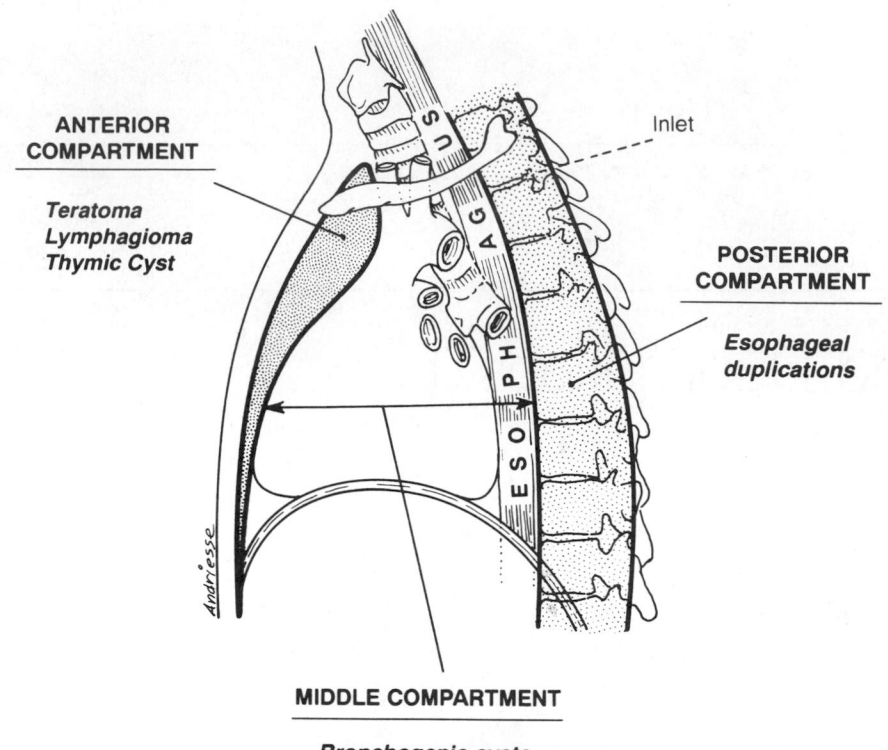

ANTERIOR COMPARTMENT

Teratoma
Lymphagioma
Thymic Cyst

Inlet

POSTERIOR COMPARTMENT

Esophageal duplications

MIDDLE COMPARTMENT

Bronchogenic cysts

Figure 57-1. The three compartments of the mediastinum are shown. The most frequent lesions in the anterior mediastinum are teratomas, lymphangiomas, and thymic cysts. Rarely, Hodgkin's disease involving the thymus presents as a cystic mass. The middle compartment is most frequently involved with bronchogenic cysts or lymphangiomas extending from the anterior mediastinum. The posterior mediastinum most frequently contains esophageal duplications.

any mediastinal involvement, which will occur in up to 10 percent of these patients (Fig. 57-3). Rarely, as described by Perkes and associates (1979), a lymphangioma will be entirely confined to the mediastinum (Fig. 57-4).

Therapy for lymphangioma of the mediastinum is surgical resection. These lesions may extend from the base of the neck to the diaphragm, and while they primarily involve the anterior mediastinum, the middle mediastinum may be involved as well. At resection the lymphangioma is often less discrete than it appears radiographically. Extension of small branches of the lesion in all directions along fascial planes and vital structures may make complete excision impossible. Resection is performed to the greatest extent possible and designed to remove the bulk of the mass that is producing respiratory symptoms or compression of vital structures. Re-

Table 57-1. Summary of Cystic Lesions of the Mediastinum Reported in Six Pediatric Series

Lesion	No. (%)
Teratoma	52 (34)
Lymphangioma	18 (12)
Thymic cyst	9 (6)
Pericardial cyst	2 (1)
Bronchogenic cyst	35 (23)
Esophageal duplication	36 (24)
Total	152

section of these masses may be approached through the neck by excising the external lesion and extending the resection into the anterior mediastinum. Extensive mediastinal involvement requires a posterolateral thoracotomy for resection, as does the entirely mediastinal lymphangioma. Efforts to ligate all the communicating lymphatics will decrease the occurrence or severity of chylothorax following resection.

Thymic Cysts

Thymic cysts are much rarer than teratomas. They can present as lesions at the base of the neck, or they may be entirely intrathoracic. These cysts are lined by epithelium, which is often ciliated. The lining of the wall may contain lymphocytes, as well as cholesterol, crystals, and granulomas. Thymic tissue is always present and is relatively normal in appearance (Lamesch, et al., 1974). These cysts are often asymptomatic and may become fairly large before they produce any symptoms because of their cystic nature.

Thymic cysts may undergo rapid expansion either from hemorrhage or respiratory infections, when they may produce respiratory symptoms (Fig. 57-5). Many are also identified on chest radiographs obtained for other reasons. Their origin is best defined by CT scan and intravenous contrast. The cysts are of homogeneous density in contiguity with the thymus, but often protruding into one hemithorax (Welch, et al., 1979). Resection is curative, as malignant thymomas rarely occur in children or present as cystic lesions. Thymic

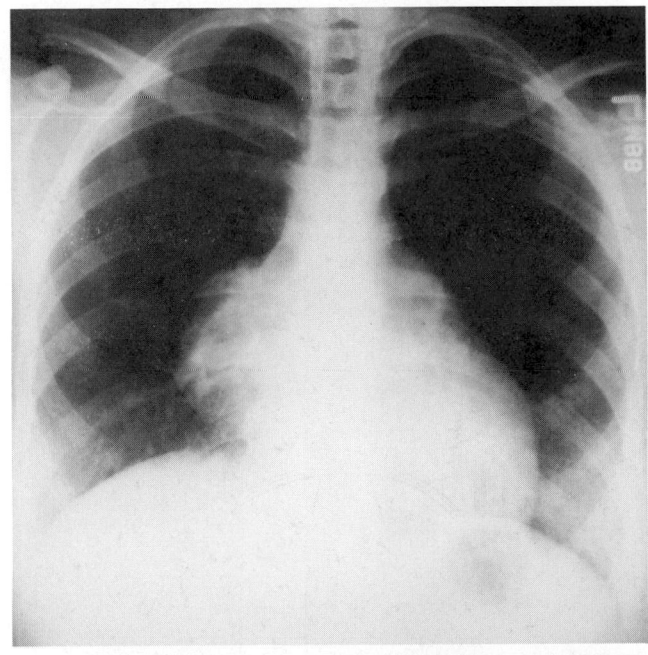

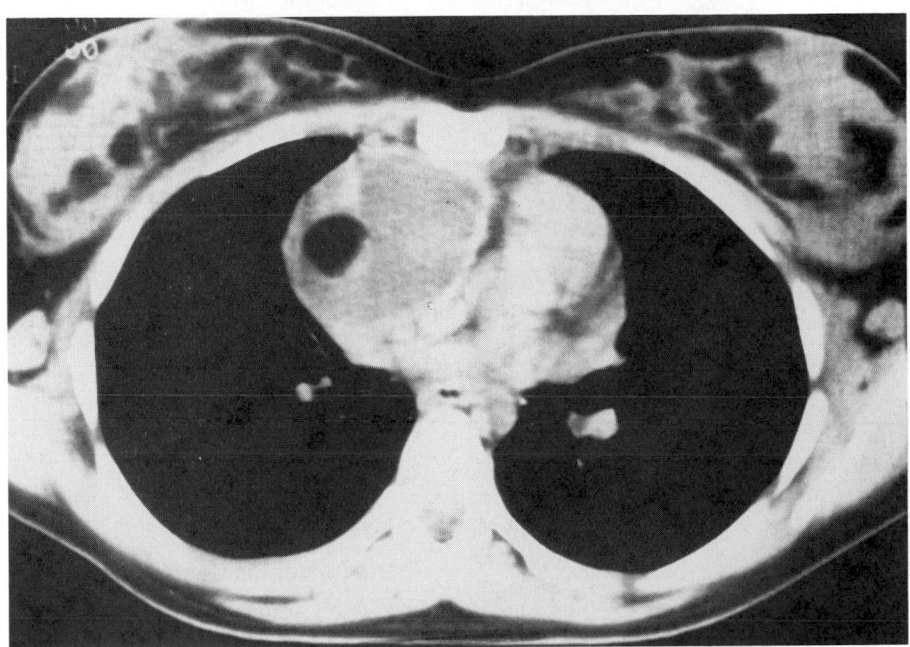

Figure 57-2. **(A)** Chest radiograph of an 18-year-old girl, obtained because of a chronic cough, demonstrates a mass protruding to the right of the heart. **(B)** CT scan demonstrates a partially cystic, partially solid mass of varying densities that is most consistent with a teratoma.

cysts presenting at the base of the neck often can be resected through a transverse cervical incision and do not require thoracotomy (Bower, et al., 1977).

Pericardial Cysts

Pericardial cysts (simple cysts, springwater cysts, coelomic cysts) are benign, unilocular lesions, that are found at the cardiophrenic angle, most frequently the right. These cysts are invariably asymptomatic and are identified on radiographs obtained for other reasons. They are thin-walled, are lined by flattened mesothelium containing clear fluid, and rarely communicate with the pericardium. They may be easily removed, the primary reason for excision being to confirm their innocent nature.

Hodgkin's Disease

Hodgkin's disease generally presents as a solid mass in the anterior mediastinum. Rarely, primary involvement of the

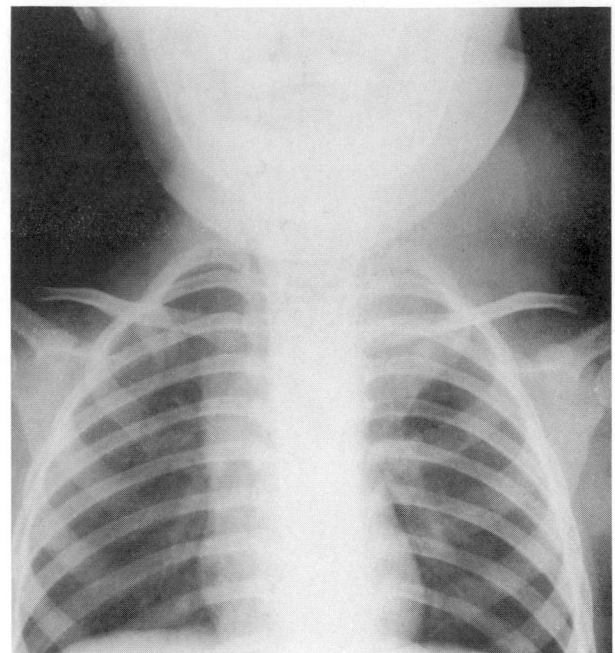

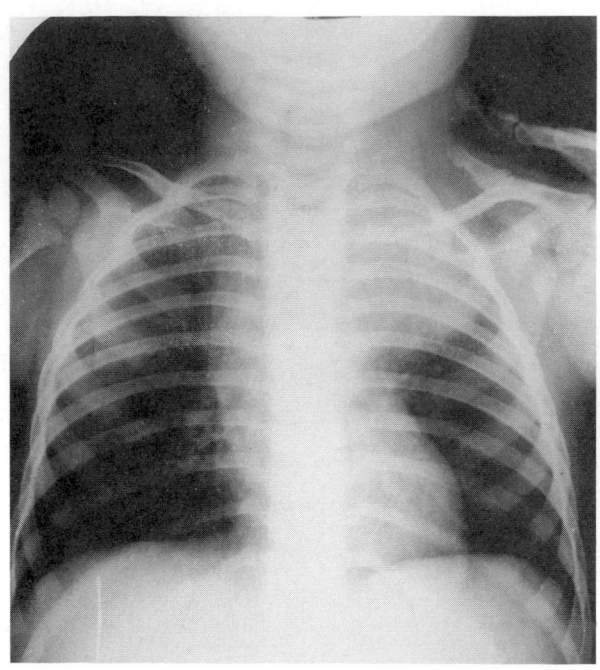

Figure 57-3. **(A)** Chest radiograph of an infant presenting with a lymphangioma of the left neck. It demonstrates extension of the lesion into the left upper anterior mediastinum. **(B)** This radiograph, obtained with manual compression of the cervical mass, is presented to condemn this practice. It can be seen that pressure applied to the cervical mass increases the size of the mediastinal component, which can acutely cause airway obstruction and consequent respiratory distress.

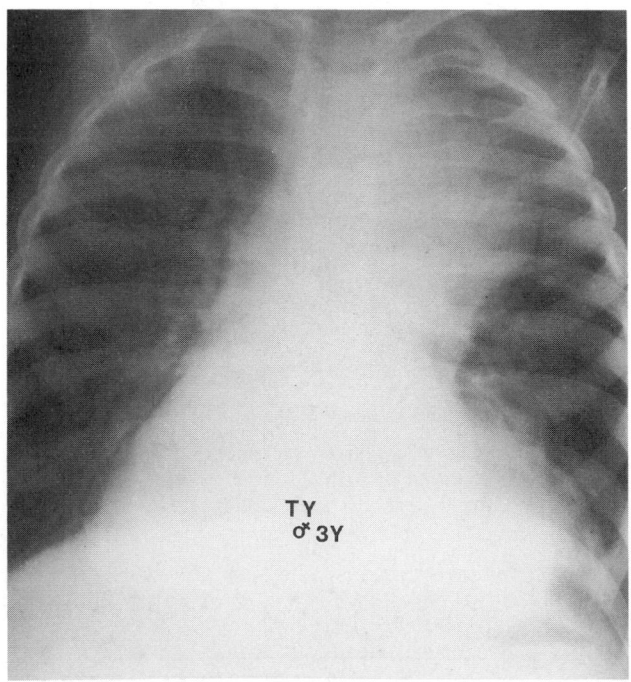

Figure 57-4. Chest radiograph of a 3-year-old boy who presented with mild stridor. The radiograph demonstrated a large anterior mediastinal mass, and no cervical component was present on physical examination. At resection, a large soft, spongy, cystic lesion was resected and found histologically to be a lymphangioma.

thymus may occur (Fig. 57-6), and in these cases it may present as a cystic mass (Nogués, et al., 1987). The diagnosis is often established only after resection of the cystic mass, in contrast with the solid lesions, in which a biopsy establishes the diagnosis. Chemotherapy or radiotherapy, depending on the stage of the disease, is required for definitive treatment.

MIDDLE MEDIASTINUM

Bronchogenic Cysts

Most cystic lesions in the middle mediastinum are of bronchopulmonary origin. They are found in close proximity to the tracheobronchial tree, are often in a perihilar or subcarinal location, and may be found entirely within the lung adjacent to a bronchus. They may produce severe respiratory symptoms in the newborn infant. Bronchogenic cysts are often very difficult to diagnose because subcarinal cysts are hidden by the cardiac silhouette and except for airway compression, which may be difficult to identify, are not demonstrated on standard radiographs. Their presence may be suggested by unilateral emphysema, by air trapping in one lung, or by partial collapse of a lung, depending on the degree of bronchial obstruction (Fig. 57-7).

In a review of 31 infants by Opsahl and Berman (1962), although 25 had respiratory symptoms, the lesion was seen on a standard radiograph in only 14, in 12 of whom it was successfully removed. The 11 symptomatic children for

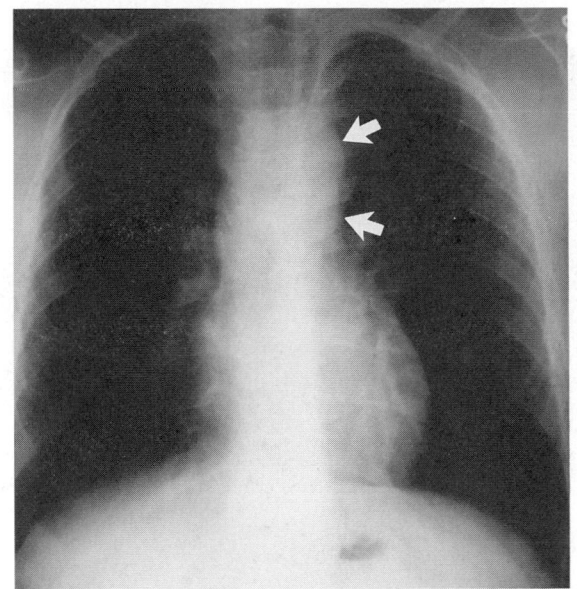
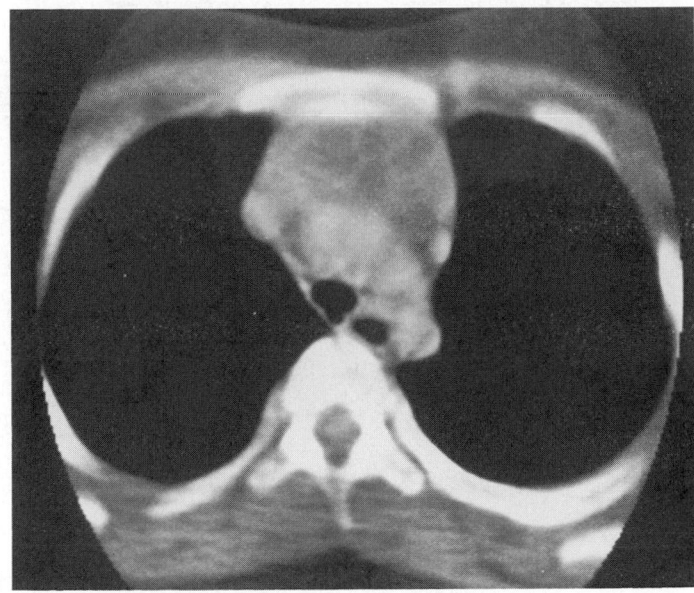

Figure 57-5. **(A)** Chest radiograph of an 11-year-old boy with upper respiratory symptoms and wheezing. It demonstrates a mass in the superior mediastinum (*arrows*). **(B)** A CT scan showed a multilocular, nonenhancing mass, extending from below the thyroid to the region of the great vessels. A multilocular thymic cyst was removed several days later, and the respiratory symptoms entirely resolved.

whom there were not radiographic findings and who did not undergo operation all died. Eraklis, et al. (1969) reported similar findings of 10 infants with bronchogenic cysts, 7 of whom had severe or moderate respiratory distress (Fig. 57-8). The cyst was identified only at autopsy in 4 infants in whom a mediastinal mass was not recognized radiographically or at operation and in 2 additional infants who died without operation.

Bronchogenic cysts and esophageal duplications may arise during embryonic development in the fifth week, when the primitive foregut divides into the laryngotracheal ridge anteriorly and the esophagus posteriorly. Outpouchings of these tissues may become separated and give rise to cystic remnants (Grafe, et al., 1966). The variety of tissues associated with the development of the trachea, bronchus, and esophagus explains why the microscopic appearance of these cysts can be so variable. We believe that bronchogenic cysts and esophageal duplications are best defined by their proximity to the trachea and bronchus or to the esophagus rather than by their histologic appearance as proposed by Reed and Sobonya (1974).

Bronchogenic cysts are usually lined by ciliated, pseudostratified epithelium characteristic of the respiratory tract, although they occasionally may be lined by esophageal or gastric mucosa despite their anatomic location in close proximity to the trachea or bronchus. Cartilage and smooth muscle may also be found within the walls. Communication with the trachea or bronchus is rare. The mucosal lining of these cysts continually produces mucus, thereby increasing the size of the cyst. Rarely, these cysts occur within the pericardial sac (Dabbs, et al., 1957). The ability to obtain CT scans has greatly facilitated identification of occult bronchogenic cysts (Snyder, et al., 1985). Determination of their precise

location to facilitate surgical resection is critical. In older children bronchogenic cysts are often asymptomatic and are identified on radiographs obtained for unrelated symptoms.

Surgical resection is the therapy of choice for bronchogenic cysts. Thoractomy is selected according to the side from which the lesion is most readily accessible. An indication for resection is the concern that progressive fluid collection will produce respiratory symptoms if they are not already present. The development of embryonal rhabdomyosarcoma within a bronchogenic cyst has been reported by Krous and Sexour (1981).

POSTERIOR MEDIASTINUM

Esophageal Duplications

Esophageal duplications, also called enterogenous cysts, gastrogenous cysts, enteric cysts, or neurenteric cysts, account for the bulk of the cystic lesions in the posterior mediastinum. They may produce a variety of symptoms, including respiratory distress or dysphagia if their size is adequate to cause tracheobronchial or esophageal compression. Severe respiratory distress has been reported from tracheal compression of a cervical esophageal duplication (Winslow, et al., 1984). Neurologic symptoms from associated abnormalities of the spine and spinal cord also lead to identification of esophageal duplications. Rarely, bleeding or perforation may produce acute symptoms of pleuritic pain or hemorrhage.

Esophageal duplications are generally in contact with the esophagus but rarely communicate with its lumen. They are identified more frequently on the left than on the right side in the posterior mediastinum. Barium swallow may demon-

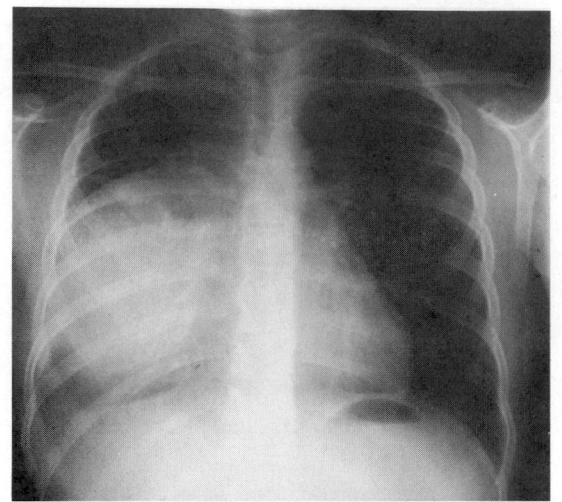

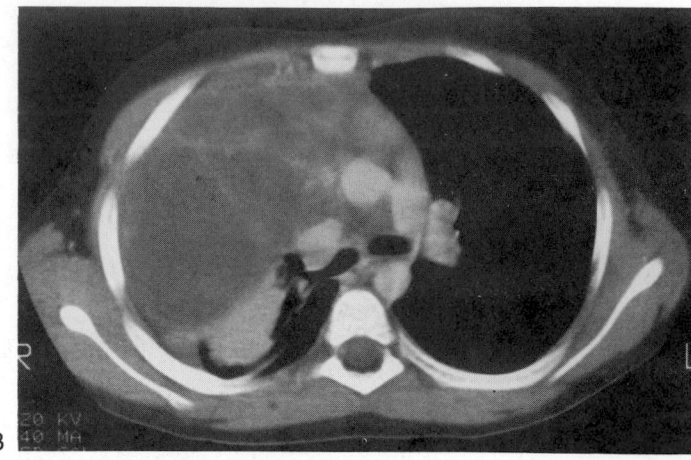

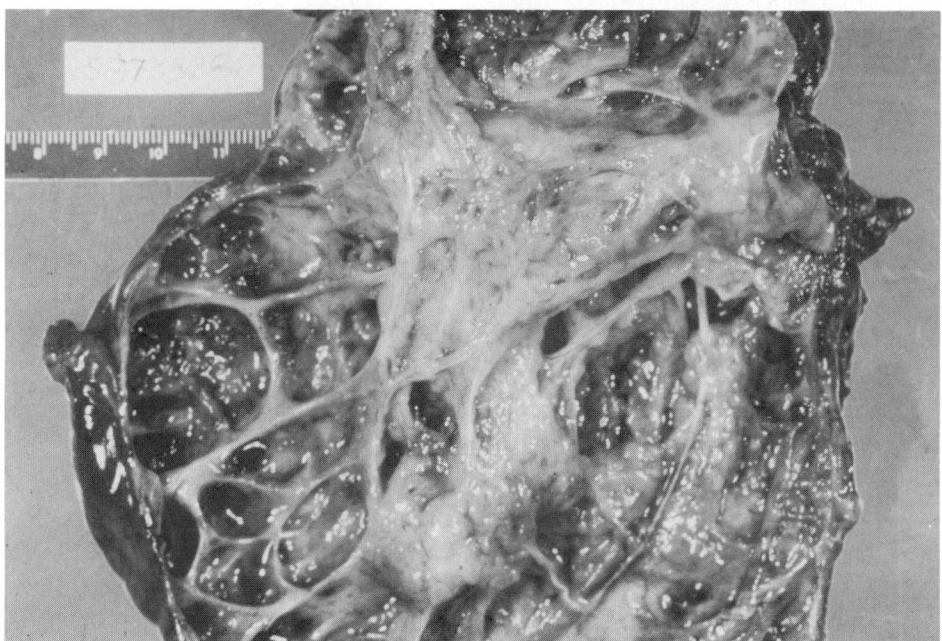

Figure 57-6. **(A)** Chest radiograph of a 10-year-old boy who had a brief episode of right pleural chest pain. On evaluation the absence of breath sounds on the right led to the study, which demonstrated a large right thoracic mass. The patient had had an entirely normal chest radiograph 18 months before this study. **(B)** CT scan shows a cystic mass with multiple septae present. **(C)** Resection of the cystic mass was performed through a right thoracotomy. The mass was found to arise from the thymus and extend into the right pleural space. The walls of the mass were thick and irregular with areas of nodularity, which raised concern about malignancy. Pathologic gross examination of the open specimen shown here revealed a thymic cyst with extensive involvement by Hodgkin's disease.

strate extrinsic compression of the esophagus (Fig. 57-9). CT or magnetic resonance imaging (MRI) scan will readily demonstrate the cystic nature of these lesions and distinguish them from the more frequent neurogenic tumors arising in the posterior sulcus of the chest (Fig. 57-10). The lining of these duplication cysts is usually squamous but may also consist of respiratory epithelium. A surprisingly high frequency of heterotopic gastric mucosa (Fig. 57-11) has been reported, varying from 2 out of 6 lesions in the series by Ildstad, et al. (1988) to 9 out of 15 in that of Superina, et

al., (1984). Two of the lesions in the latter series actually presented with acute perforation. A preoperative technetium pertechnetate scan will demonstrate gastric lining of the cyst (Ferguson, et al., 1973).

Esophageal duplications are generally isolated, but they may occur in association with esophageal atresia (Hemalatha, et al., 1980), and in up to 25 percent a second duplication in the abdominal cavity will be identified (Holcombe, et al., 1989). Vertebral anomalies, including hemivertebrae, spina bifida, and vertebral fusions, occur with a frequency varying

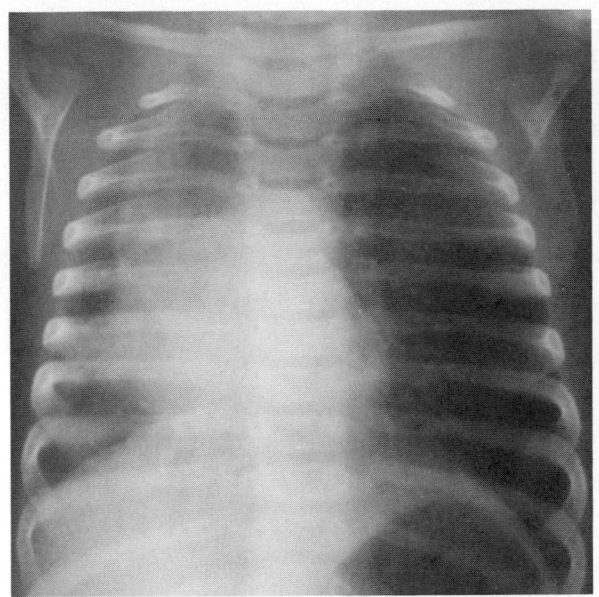
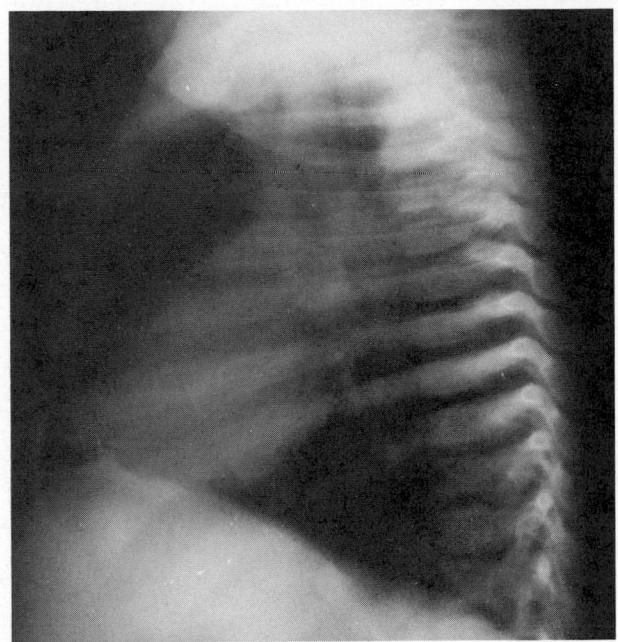

Figure 57-7. **(A)** Chest radiographs of a 3-month-old girl, who presented with cyanotic attacks for 2 months. The infant had always had distinct wheezing. She was extremely dyspneic and had a severe respiratory grunt. Hyperresonance was present on the left side of the chest, and heart sounds were displaced to the right. Radiographs showed gross hyperinflation of the left lung, but no mass lesion was identified on the **(A)** posteroanterior (PA) or **(B)** lateral view. A bronchoscopy was performed to investigate the possibility of a foreign body. Extrinsic compression of the left bronchus was seen. The child died shortly thereafter before a thoracotomy could be performed. Autopsy demonstrated a large subcarinal bronchogenic cyst compressing the left mainstem bronchus. It measured 1.5 cm in diameter and had been completely concealed by the heart on the plain radiographs. A barium swallow, something that was rarely performed in 1927, presumably would have demonstrated compression.

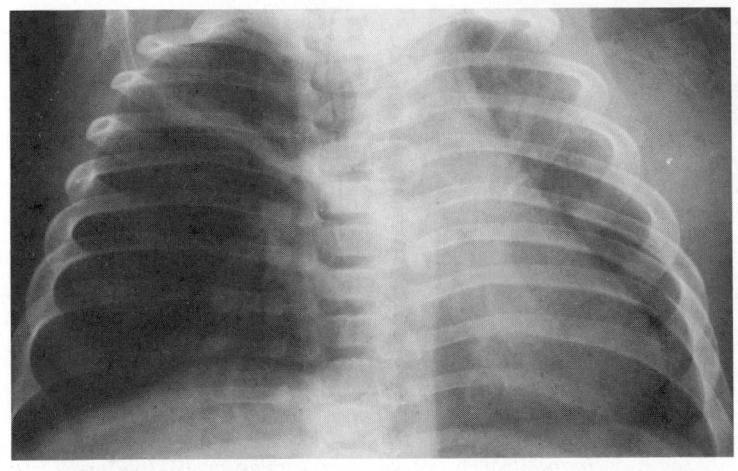
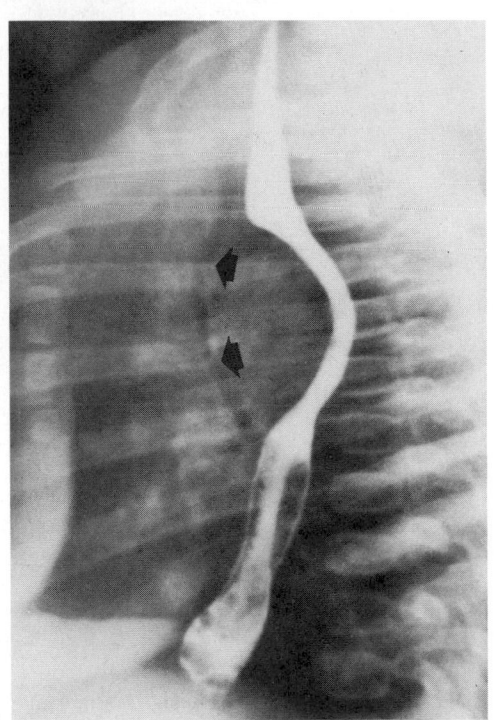

Figure 57-8. **(A)** Chest radiograph of a 6-month-old infant admitted with a history of stridor and labored respiration. Tachypnea and sternal and substernal retractions were first noted at birth. Acute exacerbation of substernal retraction, wheezing, and rhonchi led to evaluation. Chest radiograph revealed hyperinflation of the right lung. **(B)** A barium swallow demonstrated a mass compressing and displacing the trachea anteriorly (*arrows*) and the esophagus posteriorly. A left posterolateral thoracotomy was performed, and a 3.5-cm bronchogenic cyst found densely adherent to the posterior wall of the carina was resected. No communication to the trachea was present. Recovery was uneventful.

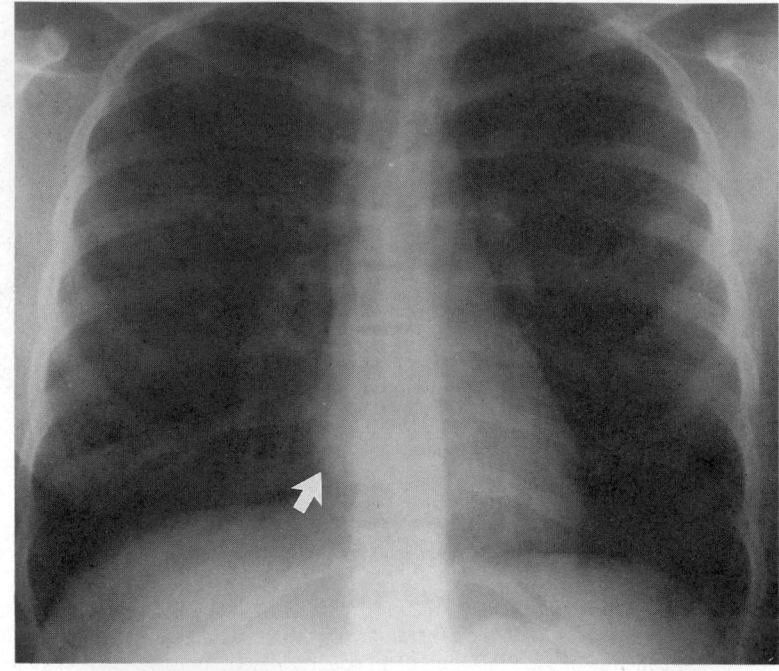

A

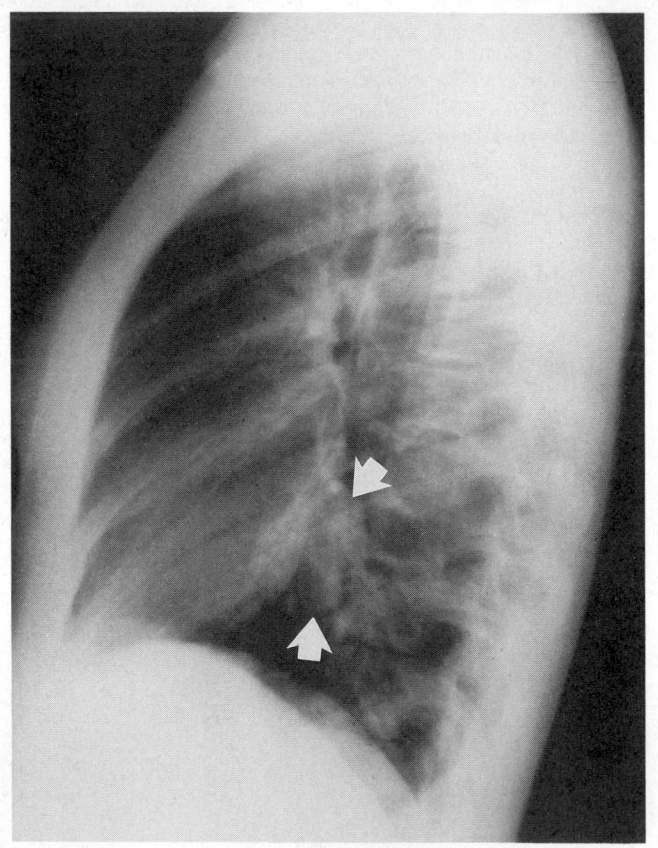

B

Figure 57-9. **(A)** Chest radiograph of a 13-year-old girl, who presented with mild dysphagia, demonstrates a spherical mass protruding at the margin of the right side of the heart (*arrow*), which is best demonstrated on **(B)** the lateral radiograph (*arrows*). (*Figure continues.*)

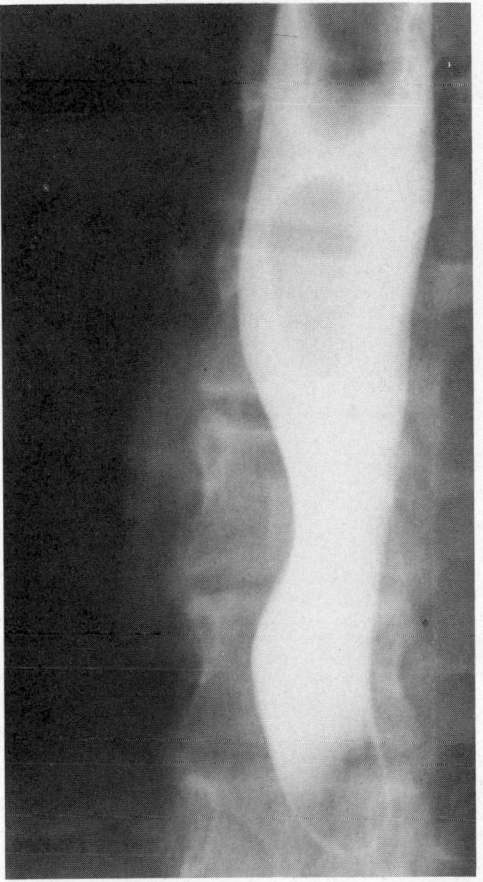

C

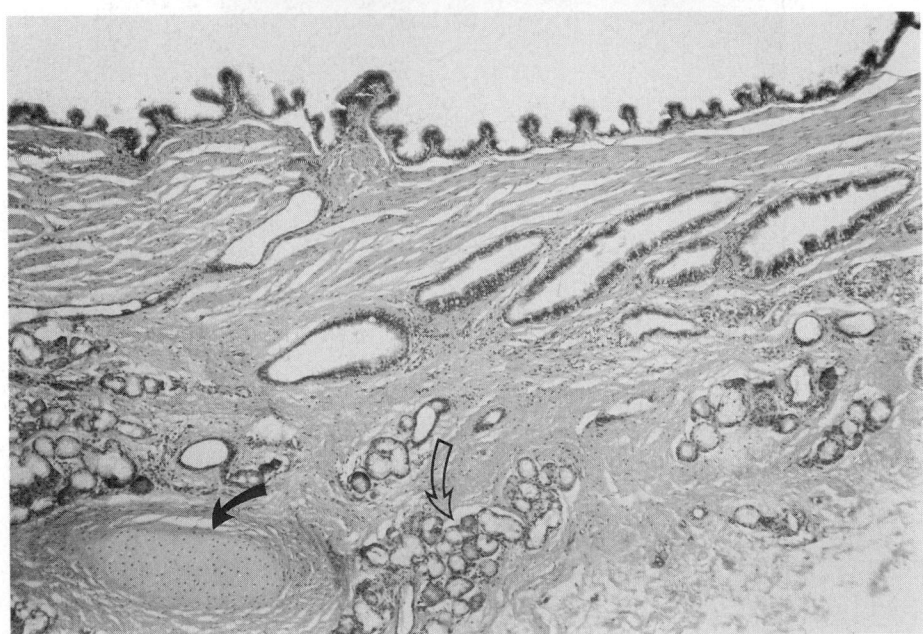

D

Figure 57-9 (*Continued*).   **(C)** Barium swallow demonstrates compression of the esophagus. At resection the cyst was enveloped by esophageal muscles. It was resected in a submucosal fashion, where it was adjacent to the esophagus. The cyst was filled with mucus. **(D)** Pathologic examination demonstrated pseudostratified epithelium and walls with cartilage (*solid arrow*) and mucous glands (*open arrow*) more characteristic of respiratory lining.

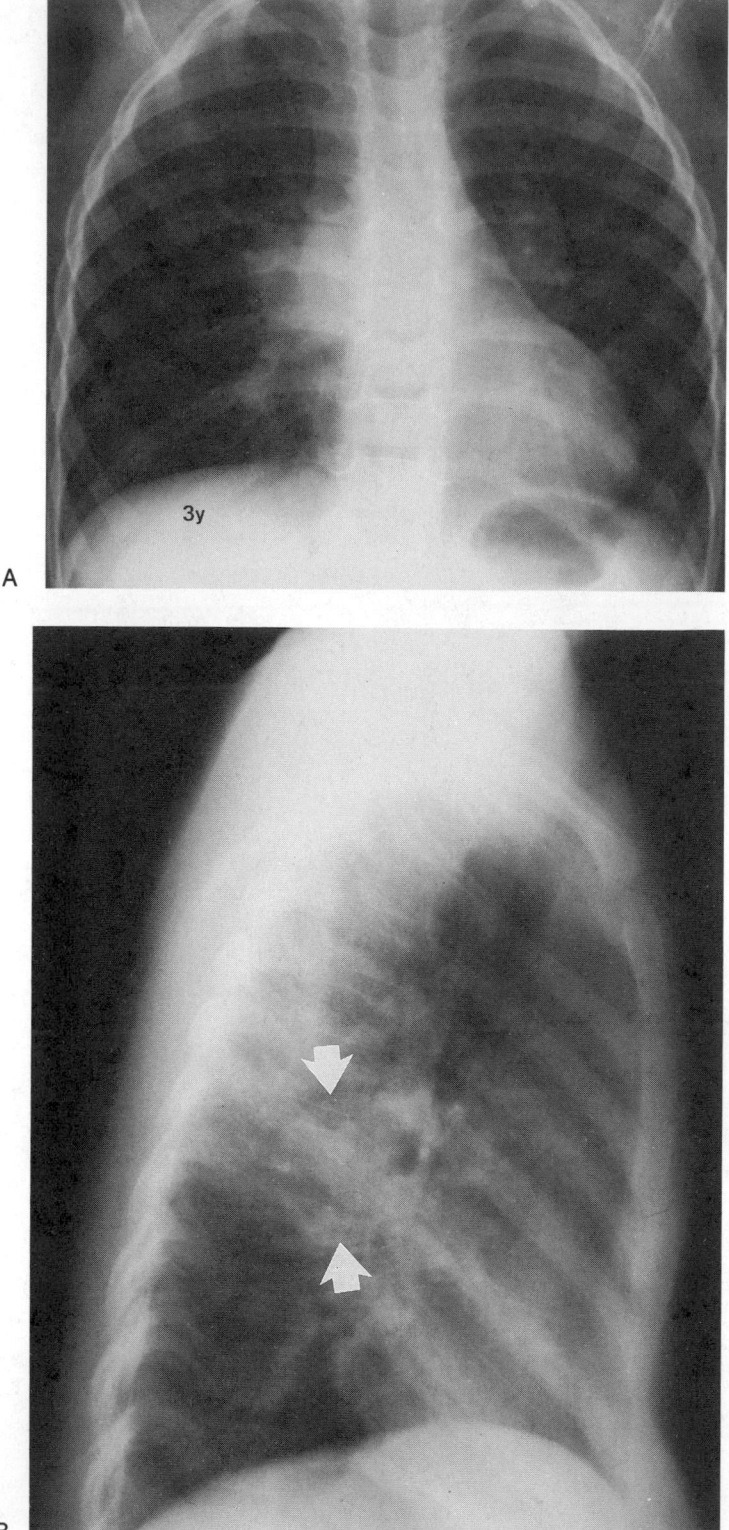

Figure 57-10. **(A)** Chest radiograph of a 3-year-old boy obtained because of mild pectus excavatum. The radiograph demonstrates a right-sided retrohilar mass, also seen on **(B)** the lateral view (*arrows*). Barium swallow showed the mass indenting the esophagus. (*Figure continues*).

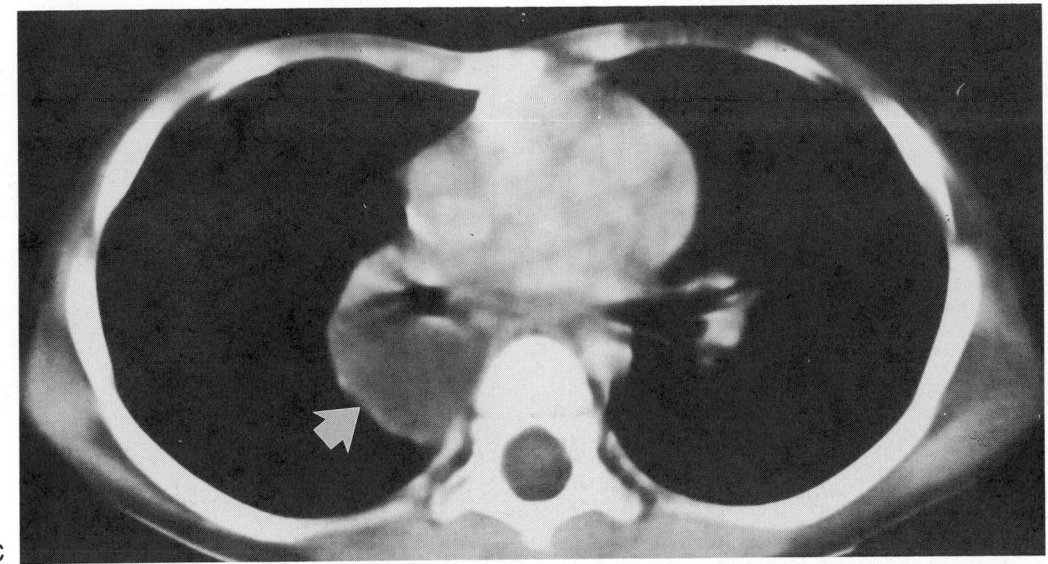

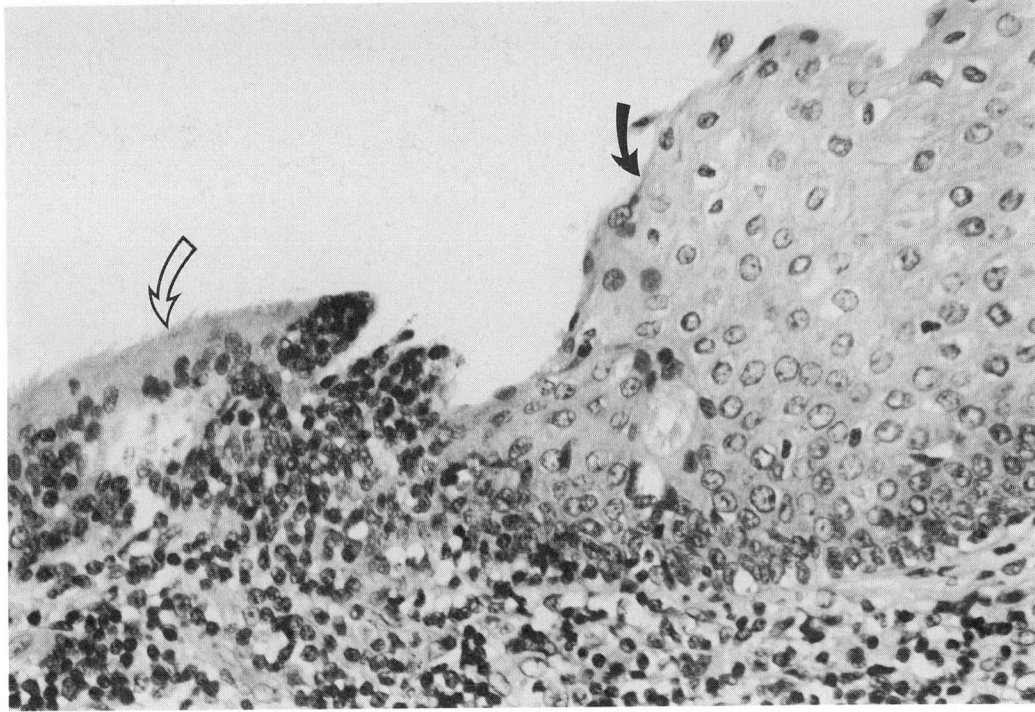

Figure 57-10 (*Continued*).   **(C)** CT scan shows a cystic mass (*arrow*), with no enhancement with intravenous contrast posterior to the right bronchus and adjacent to the esophagus. At resection the mass was closely adherent to the right bronchus, but it was also quite intimately associated with the esophagus, with esophageal muscle coming up onto the posterior aspect of the mass. This case demonstrates the close association and overlap between a bronchogenic cyst and esophageal duplication, since their mechanism of origin is probably identical. **(D)** Histologically the common origin of the cyst is demonstrated as well. The cyst contained both nonkeratinizing stratified squamous epithelium (*solid arrow*) and ciliated pseudostratified columnar epithelium (*open arrow*).

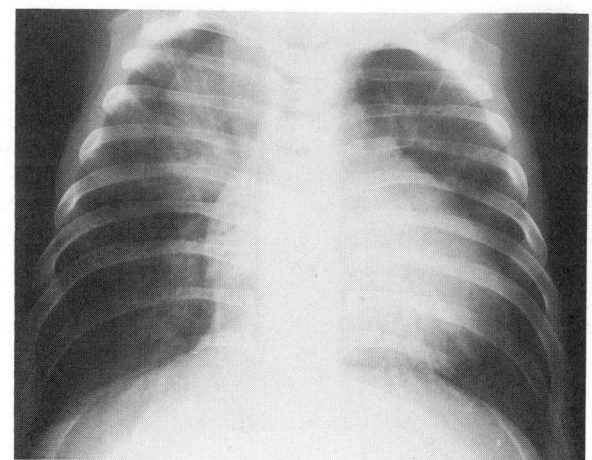

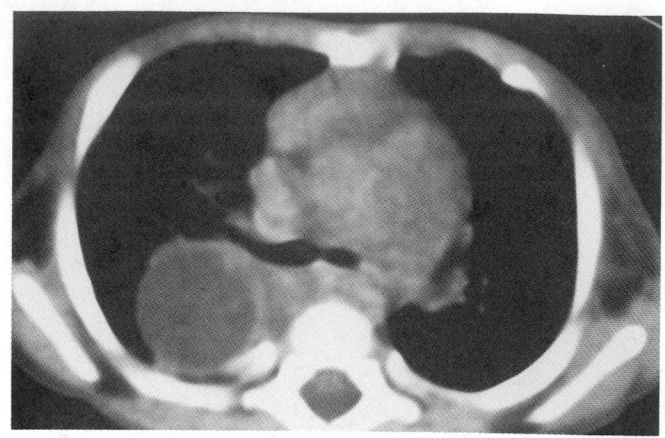

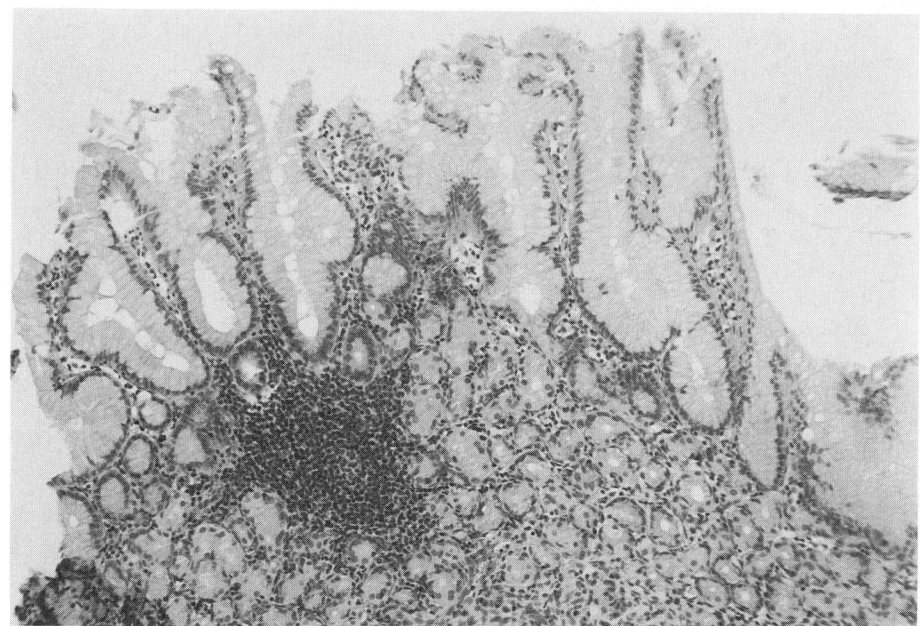

Figure 57-11. **(A)** Chest radiograph of a 7-month-old boy born with trisomy 21, complete atrioventricular canal, and duodenal stenosis shows a right-sided thoracic mass in the right posterior mediastinum. **(B)** CT scan demonstrates a cystic mass in the posterior sulcus, which did not enhance with intravenous contrast. At resection some edema was found around the cyst. The cyst was adjacent to the esophagus but not surrounded by esophageal muscles. Anatomically it lay to the right of the esophagus and posterior to the trachea, and the right mainstem bronchus was draped over its inferior portion. The cyst was not densely adherent, however, to any of these structures. **(C)** Pathologic examination revealed gastric antral-type mucosa surrounded by loose connective tissue and smooth muscles.

from 3 out of 16 (Bower, et al., 1977) to 14 out of 19 patients (Superina, et al., 1984). In the latter series 6 patients presented with neurologic symptoms. Back pain, sensory or motor deficits, or gate disturbances may be the first symptoms of an esophageal duplication.

This association of vertebral anomalies with duplication cysts supports the notochord theory of Veeneklass (1952) for the origin of these mediastinal duplications. The notochord first appears during the third week of embryologic life, wedging itself between cells forming the endoderm and the ectoderm. The theory postulates that if there is an incomplete separation of the notochord from the endoderm, traction may

be exerted upon the primitive gut in such a manner that the outpouching is drawn toward the vertebral bodies. Loss of continuity between the pouch and the primitive gut from which it arose may result in a separate duplication. Rarely, a long tubular esophageal duplication extends through the diaphragm to end in close proximity or even communication with the stomach, pancreas, duodenum, or jejunum. Those duplications not associated with vertebral anomalies presumably arise during separation of the primitive foregut, as discussed above for bronchogenic cysts. This again explains the marked variety of epithelium and components of the cyst wall.

All patients with vertebral anomalies or neurologic symptoms and posterior cystic lesions should have the spinal canal evaluated prior to surgery. In the past myelograms were used, but now MRI scans will easily demonstrate the extent of protrusion of the cyst into the spinal canal, as well as any associated anomalies of the spinal cord.

Surgical resection is the therapy of choice for all esophageal duplications. This is required for four reasons. First, the cyst may progressively increase in size with accumulation of secretions, which may compress the trachea, bronchus, or esophagus. Second, the cyst may become infected by a hematogenous route. Third, malignant lesions may occur in these cysts, including squamous cell carcinoma (Tapia and White, 1985) and adenocarcinoma (Chuang, et al., 1981). Fourth, the cysts, as previously indicated, are frequently lined by gastric mucosa, and hemorrhage or perforation can occur.

Esophageal duplications frequently share a common muscular wall with the esophagus. Resection of only the mucosal portion of the cyst in the area of its contact with the esophagus will avoid entry into the esophageal lumen. Rarely is there a communication between the cyst and the esophagus unless it results from erosion and ulceration from ectopic gastric mucosa, which may cause hemorrhage.

The occasional thoracoabdominal cysts are recognized by their large size and their tubular nature suggesting abdominal extension, in contrast with the more common esophageal duplications limited to the thorax. Successful resection of these lesions was first reported by Gross in 1948. Complete resection to their site of origin at the stomach, duodenum, jejunum, or pancreas is vital. In the collected series reported by Pokorny and Goldstein (1984), the cysts communicated with the gastrointestinal tract in 17 of 25 patients. Patients with these large thoracoabdominal duplications may present with respiratory symptoms secondary to their large size (12 of 25 patients), anemia (10 of 25), melena (8 of 25), emesis (8 of 25), pain (5 of 25), failure to thrive (4 of 25), and/or hemoptysis from peptic ulceration from ectopic gastric mucosa (1 of 25). Younger children and infants present more frequently with respiratory symptoms and older children with anemia, melena, hematemesis, or pain. Either a thoracoabdominal incision or separate thoracic and abdominal incisions may be required for resection, depending on the extent of proximal communication of the lesion (Fig. 57-12).

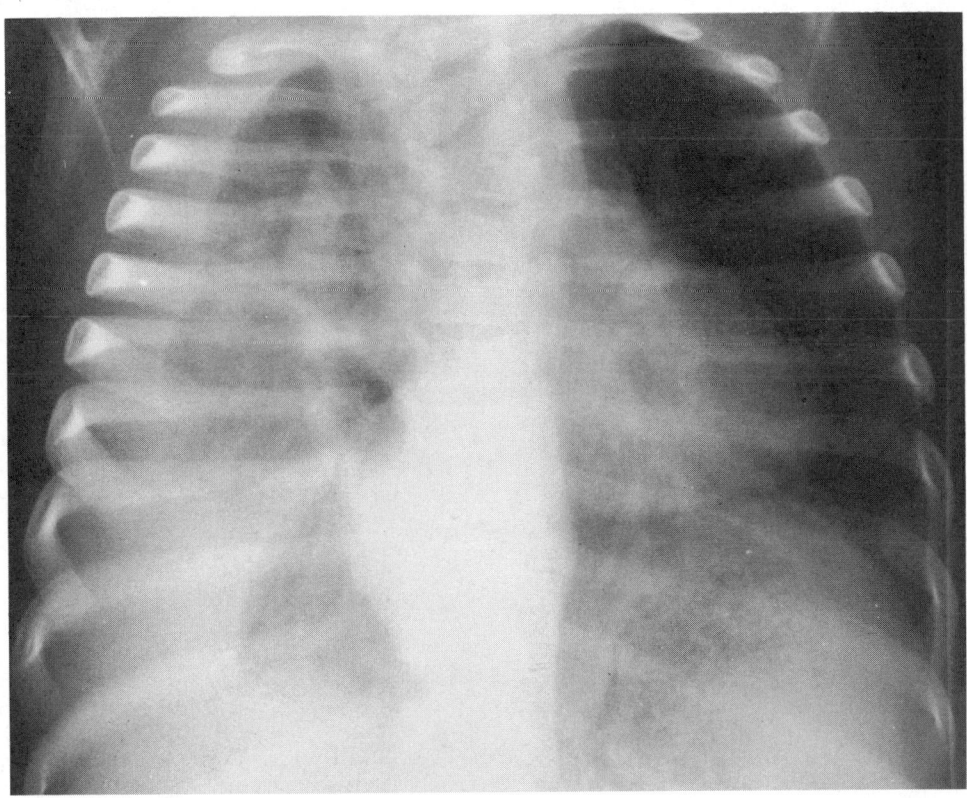

Figure 57-12. Chest radiograph of 1-year-old infant, who developed respiratory difficulty with a large right pleural effusion. Thoracentesis revealed serosanguinous fluid with no bacteria, but a high serum amylase. The chest film also showed vertebral anomalies in the upper thoracic vertebrae. This was a major clue to the presence of a duplication cyst. At thoracotomy the cyst was found to have ruptured into the right cavity. It was resected from its extent up to the inferior cervical vertebral bodies. A soft tissue mass was suggested, with bulging from T6 to T10 along the right parasternal region. A barium swallow and aortogram showed the esophagus and aorta displaced to the left. The cyst was lined by respiratory epithelium, mucous glands, hyaline cartilage, and gastric mucosa.

COMMENTS AND CONTROVERSIES

It is often difficult to differentiate between bronchogenic and esophageal cysts because they are located in the same area of the mediastinum and often have similar histologic features. These cysts, also called foregut cysts, are however all related to developmental anomalies of either the ventral or dorsal foregut. Bronchogenic cysts are derived from the ventral foregut and are thought to be caused by an abnormal budding of the bronchial tree where in cells becomes sequestrated from the main pulmonary branching. If this abnormal budding occurs early during gestation, cysts are located in the mediastinum (75 percent of cases), but if it occurs at a later stage, the cysts are more likely to be located in the lung (25 percent of cases). Most bronchogenic cysts are lined with ciliated columnar epithelium, and their wall contains hyaline cartilage, smooth muscle, and bronchial glands.

Anomalies of the dorsal foregut include esophageal cysts and neurenteric cysts. Esophageal cysts are located within the esophageal wall and are covered by two layers of muscle; their epithelium lining is variable, being squamous, columnar, or gastric. According to most authors, these cysts are due to the persistence in the wall of the foregut of vacuoles, which form when the foregut is in the solid tube stage of development.

Neurenteric cysts are a mixed anomaly of both the dorsal foregut and the primitive notochord. These cysts are adherent to the posterior esophagus but are not included in its wall. They are associated with a high incidence of spinal abnormalities, which may sometimes be very discrete, are covered by well developed muscle walls, and have a gastrointestinal mucosal lining. It is worth noting that the vertebral anomaly may be at an anatomic site different from that of the cyst.

J.D.

REFERENCES

Bower RJ, Sieber WK, Kiesewetter WB: Alimentary tract duplications in children. Ann Surg 188:669, 1977

Childress ME, Baker CP, Samson PC: Lymphangioma of the mediastinum. J Thorac Cardiovasc Surg 31:338, 1956

Chuang MT, Barba FA, Kaneko M, Teirstein AS: Adenocarcinoma arising in an intrathoracic duplication cyst of foregut origin: a case report with review of the literature. Cancer 47:1887, 1981

Dabbs CH, Berg R Jr, Pierce EC II: Intrapericardial bronchogenic cysts: report of two cases and probable embryologic explanation. J Thorac Surg 34:718, 1957

Eraklis AJ, Griscom NT, McGovern JB: Bronchogenic cysts of the mediastinum in infancy. N Engl J Med 281:1150, 1969

Ferguson CC, Young LN, Sutherland JB, Macpherson RI: Intrathoracic gastrogenic cyst—preoperative diagnosis by technetium pertechnetate scan. J Pediatr Surg 8:827, 1973

Gottschalk E, Lichey C, Friedich U: Thorakale Teratome bei Kindern. Z Kinderchir 29:303, 1980

Grafe WR, Goldsmith EI, Redo SF: Bronchogenic cysts of the mediastinum in children. J Pediatr Surg 1:384, 1966

Hemalatha V, Batcup G, Brereton RJ, Spitz L: Intrathoracic foregut cyst (foregut duplication) associated with esophageal atresia. J Pediatr Surg 15:178, 1980

Holcomb GW III, Gheissari A, O'Neill JA et al: Surgical management of alimentary tract duplications. Ann Surg 209:167, 1989

Ildstad ST, Tollerud DJ, Weiss RG et al: Duplications of the alimentary tract: clinical characteristics, preferred treatment, and associated malformations. Ann Surg 208:184, 1988

Krous HF, Sexauer CL: Embryonal rhabdomyosarcoma arising within a congenital bronchogenic cyst in a child. J Pediatr Surg 16:506, 1981

Lamesch A, Capesius C, Theisen-Aspesberro MC: Cervical thymic cysts in infants and children. Z Kinderchir 14:213, 1974

Nogués A, Tovar JA, Suñol M et al: Hodgkin's disease of the thymus: a rare mediastinal cystic mass. J Pediatr Surg 22:996, 1987

Ochsner JL, Ochsner SF: Congenital cysts of the mediastinum: 20-year experience with 42 cases. Ann Surg 136:909, 1966

Opsahl T, Berman EJ: Bronchiogenic mediastinal cysts in infants: case report and review of the literature. Pediatrics 30:372, 1962

Perkes EA, Haller JO, Kassner EG et al: Mediastinal cystic hygroma in infants: two cases with no extension into the neck. Clin Pediatr (Phila) 18:168, 1979

Pokorny WJ, Goldstein IR: Enteric thoracoabdominal duplications in children. J Thorac Cardiovasc Surg 87:821, 1984

Reed JC, Sobonya RE: Morphologic analysis of foregut cysts in the thorax. AJR 120:851, 1974

Shamberger RC, Holzman RS, Griscom NT et al: CT quantitation of tracheal cross-sectional area as a guide to the surgical and anesthetic management of children with anterior mediastinal masses. J Pediatr Surg 26:138, 1991

Snyder ME, Luck SR, Hernandez R et al: Diagnostic dilemmas of mediastinal cysts. J Pediatr Surg 20:810, 1985

Superina RA, Ein SH, Humphreys RP: Cystic duplications of the esophagus and neurenteric cysts. J Pediatr Surg 19:527, 1984

Tapia RH, White VA: Squamous cell carcinoma arising in a duplication cyst of the esophagus. Am J Gastroenterol 80:325, 1985

Thompson DP, Moore TC: Acute thoracic distress in childhood due to spontaneous rupture of a large mediastinal teratoma. J Pediatr Surg 4:416, 1969

Veeneklaas GMH: Pathogenesis of intrathoracic gastrogenic cysts. Am J Dis Child 83:500, 1952

Welch KJ, Tapper D, Vawter GP: Surgical treatment of thymic cysts and neoplasms in children. J Pediatr Surg 14:691, 1979

Winslow RE, Dykstra G, Scholten DJ, Dean RE: Duplication of the cervical esophagus: an unrecognized cause of respiratory distress in infants. Am Surg 50:506, 1984

Cysts and Duplications in Adults

David R. Jones
Geoffrey M. Graeber

INTRODUCTION

Foregut cysts and duplications of the mediastinum are more common in the pediatric population than in adults. Nevertheless, this group of lesions comprises the most common cystic mediastinal masses in adults, accounting for 6 percent of all mediastinal masses. Since these cysts are usually asymptomatic, they may remain undetected until adulthood.

Foregut cysts are divided into bronchogenic or esophageal cysts based on their embryogenesis and histologic features. Other mediastinal cysts rarely encountered in the adult are neuroenteric, hydatid, thoracic duct, thymic, and pericardial cysts. An understanding of the embryogenesis and distinguishing characteristics of each of these mediastinal cysts is important for the thoracic surgeon. Management of these lesions has been increasingly complicated by attempts at percutaneous or endoscopic needle aspiration of the cyst and its contents. A cystic lesion of the mediastinum remains a disease that requires a surgical approach to diagnosis and management.

EMBRYOLOGY AND NOMENCLATURE

At 4 weeks of age the embryo begins to have an outgrowth of the ventral wall of the foregut, which will form the respiratory tree. Initially there is a wide communication between the foregut and this respiratory diverticulum. As the diverticulum extends caudally, it becomes separated from the foregut by two parallel, longitudinal esophagotracheal ridges. Fusion of these ridges forms the esophagotracheal septum, which divides the foregut into a dorsal portion, the esophagus, and a ventral portion, the tracheobronchial tree (Sadler, 1985) (Fig. 57-13).

At 6 weeks the lobar bronchi are present, three on the right and two on the left. Abnormal division or budding of the tracheobronchial tree can result in the formation of bronchogenic cysts. The majority of bronchial cysts occur early in gestation and are located in the mediastinum without any communication to the tracheobronchial tree. If these cysts develop later, they frequently are more peripheral, are lo-

We would like to thank Ms. Karen DeShong for her assistance in the preparation of our contribution to this chapter.

cated in the lung parenchyma, and have a bronchial communication. These intraparenchymal cysts account for approximately 25 percent of all adult bronchogenic cysts (Duranceau and Deslauriers, 1991).

While the trachea and lung buds are developing, the esophagus lengthens with the descent of the heart and lungs. A muscular coat is formed by the surrounding mesenchyme, and innervation is supplied by the vagus nerves and the splachnic plexus (Sadler, 1985).

Esophageal cysts are thought to arise from persistent vacuoles in the wall, which do not coalesce to form the esophageal lumen. They may also arise from abnormal budding of the foregut. Marchevsky and Kaneko (1984) suggest that cysts lined with squamous epithelium result from persistent vacuoles and those lined with ciliated epithelium develop from abnormal foregut budding. For a cyst to be considered an esophageal duplication cyst, it must be contained within the esophageal wall, be covered by two muscle layers, and be lined with an epithelium found in the embryonic foregut. As the esophagus lengthens, the duplication cysts are found inferiorly and more commonly on the right, owing to rightward rotation of the stomach (Murray and Gustafson, 1994).

BRONCHOGENIC CYSTS

Bronchogenic cysts are closed, epithelial-lined sacs that are usually symptomatic in both the pediatric and the adult population. In 1948 Maier classified the location of mediastinal bronchogenic cysts into paratracheal, subcarinal, hilar, paraesophageal, and miscellaneous. The majority of bronchogenic cysts occur in the subcarinal and paratracheal locations followed by paraesophageal and finally hilar locations (St-Georges, et al., 1991; Suen, et al., 1993) (Fig. 57-14). Miscellaneous locations of the cysts include the anterior mediastinum, pericardial cavity, paravertebral sulcus, and abdomen. Rarely, a dumbbell cyst may be present, in which the intrathoracic cyst extends below the diaphragm (Amendola, et al., 1982).

St-Georges, et al. (1991), using the tracheal carina as the dividing point between superior and inferior locations, found

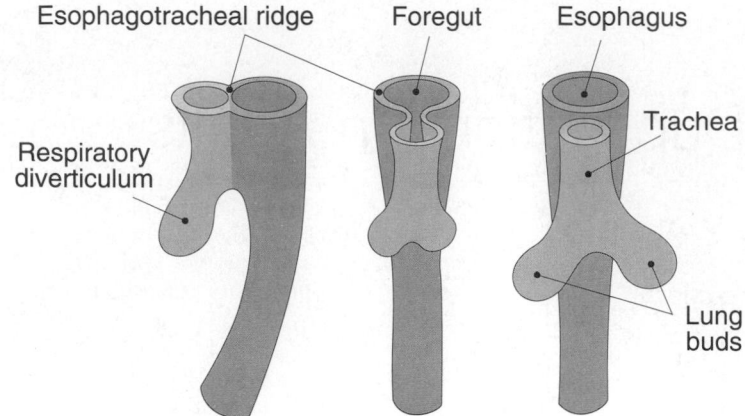

Figure 57-13. (A–C) The successive stages of the development of the respiratory diverticulum. The esophagotracheal ridges eventually fuse to form a septum, which separates the foregut into the esophagus and tracheobronchial tree. (Modified from Sadler TW: Langman's Medical Embryology. 5th Ed. p. 215. Williams & Wilkins, Baltimore, 1985, with permission.)

that 23 percent of cysts were located superiorly and 77 percent inferiorly. In adults 12 to 25 percent of bronchogenic cysts are located within the lung (Duranceau and Deslauriers, 1991; St-Georges, et al., 1991; Suen, et al., 1993). The majority of parenchymal cysts are located in the lower lobes, but they have been found in every lobe (St-Georges, et al., 1991).

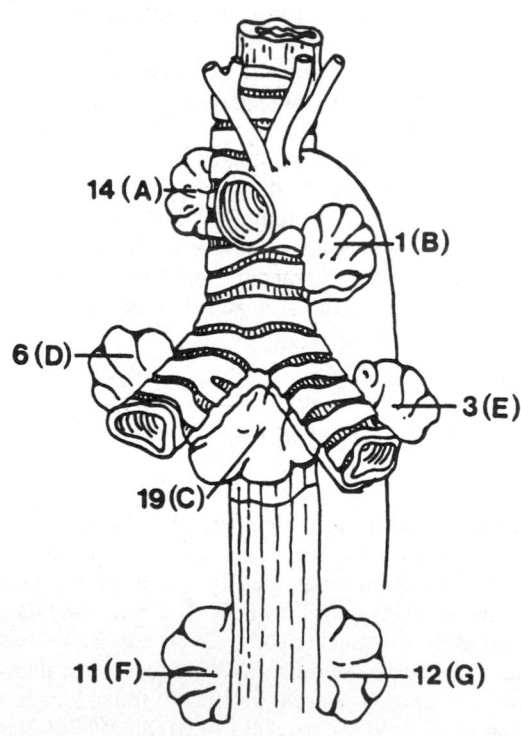

Figure 57-14. Anatomic location of mediastinal bronchogenic cysts according to Maier's classification. A, right paratracheal; B, left paratracheal; C, subcarinal; D, right hilar; E, left hilar; F, right paraesophageal; G, left paraesophageal. (From St-Georges R, Deslauriers J, Duranceau A et al.: Clinical spectrum of bronchogenic cysts of the mediastinum and lung in the adult. Ann Thorac Surg 52:6, 1991, with permission.)

DIAGNOSIS

Clinical Features

Bronchogenic cysts are slightly more common in women than in men (Duranceau and Deslauriers, 1991; St-Georges, et al., 1991; Suen, et al., 1993) and can present from the immediate postnatal period to the seventh decade. Bronchogenic cysts of the mediastinum show progressive symptoms in 50 to 67 percent of patients (St-Georges, et al., 1991; Suen, et al., 1993). The majority of adult patients have more than one symptom. The most common symptom is retrosternal chest pain secondary to inflammation of the mediastinal pleura; other symptoms include dysphagia, dyspnea, cough, fever, and hemoptysis (Table 57-2).

Cysts in the neonate, infant, or young child are almost always symptomatic. These patients frequently present with symptoms of tracheobronchial obstruction, such as respiratory stridor or distress, cyanosis, and severe dyspnea. Hyperinflation, infection, and atelectasis occur in the other lung secondary to obstruction and to the mediastinal shift to the side opposite the lesion.

Parenchymal bronchogenic cysts have a more insidious presentation but are associated with symptoms in over 90 percent of patients (St-Georges, et al., 1991). Fever, recurrent respiratory infections, productive cough, hemoptysis, and dyspnea are frequent complaints of patients with these cysts. This symptom complex is thought to be related to the higher incidence of communication between the cyst and the bronchi in parenchymal bronchogenic cysts.

Pathology

Grossly, bronchogenic cysts are well circumscribed and smooth, with a moderately thick wall. Microscopically, there is an epithelial lining of ciliated columnar cells with associated inflammatory cells (Fig. 57-15). St-Georges, et al. (1991) reported mucosal ulceration in 40 percent of resected bronchogenic cysts. In their series, nests of cartilage were seen in 43 percent of cysts, and other histologic findings included

Table 57-2. Clinical Symptoms in 86 Patients with Bronchogenic Cysts

Characteristic	MBC (n = 66)	LBC (n = 20)	Total[a] (n = 86)
No. of patients with symptoms	44	18	62 (72.1)
No. of patients with more than one symptom	29	17	46 (74.2)
Onset of symptoms			
Acute	7	6	13 (20.9)
Progressive	37	12	49 (79.1)
Severity of symptoms			
Mild	9	4	13 (21)
Moderate	23	12	35 (56.4)
Very severe	12	2	14 (22.6)
Most common symptoms			
Chest pain	27	7	34 (54.8)
Cough	16	15	31 (50)
Dyspnea	16	8	24 (38.7)
Fever	10	10	20 (32.3)
Purulent sputum	5	8	13 (21)
Anorexia and weight loss	9	3	12 (19.4)
Dysphagia	9	0	9 (14.5)
Hemoptysis	3	3	6 (9.7)
Other	7	0	7 (11.3)

Abbreviations: LBC, bronchogenic cyst of the lung; MBC, mediastinal bronchogenic cyst.

[a] Numbers in parenthesis are percentages.

(From St-Georges R, Deslauriers J, Duranceau A et al.. Clinical spectrum of bronchogenic cysts of the mediastinum and lung in the adult. Ann Thorac Surg 52:6, 1991 with permission.)

smooth muscle (59 percent, bronchial glands (41 percent), and nerve tissue (7 percent).

These cysts are almost always benign, but malignant degeneration has been reported (Greenfield and Home, 1965; Chung, et al., 1981). Okubo and associates (1989) reported elevated CA 19-9 levels in an infected bronchogenic cyst that was histologically benign. Elevated serum and cyst fluid levels of this tumor marker appear to be related to its secretion from bronchial glands, with subsequent leakage into the serum after the cyst becomes infected.

Investigative Techniques

Radiographic Studies

Standard chest radiographs identify some abnormality suggestive of a mediastinal mass in the overwhelming majority of patients (Suen, et al., 1993). Bronchogenic cysts are usually present as unilocular, smooth, rounded masses with the fluid density of water (Fig. 57-16). The presence of an air-fluid level suggests a cyst–tracheobronchial tree communication; such a communication is more likely to occur with an intra-

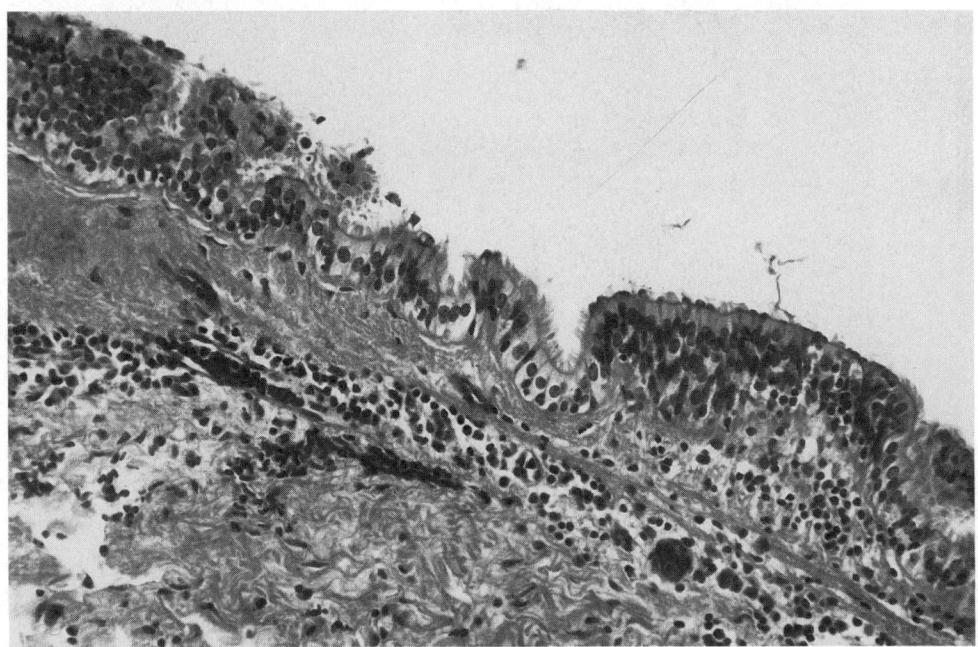

Figure 57-15. Representative photomicrograph of a bronchogenic cyst lining with associated inflammatory cells.

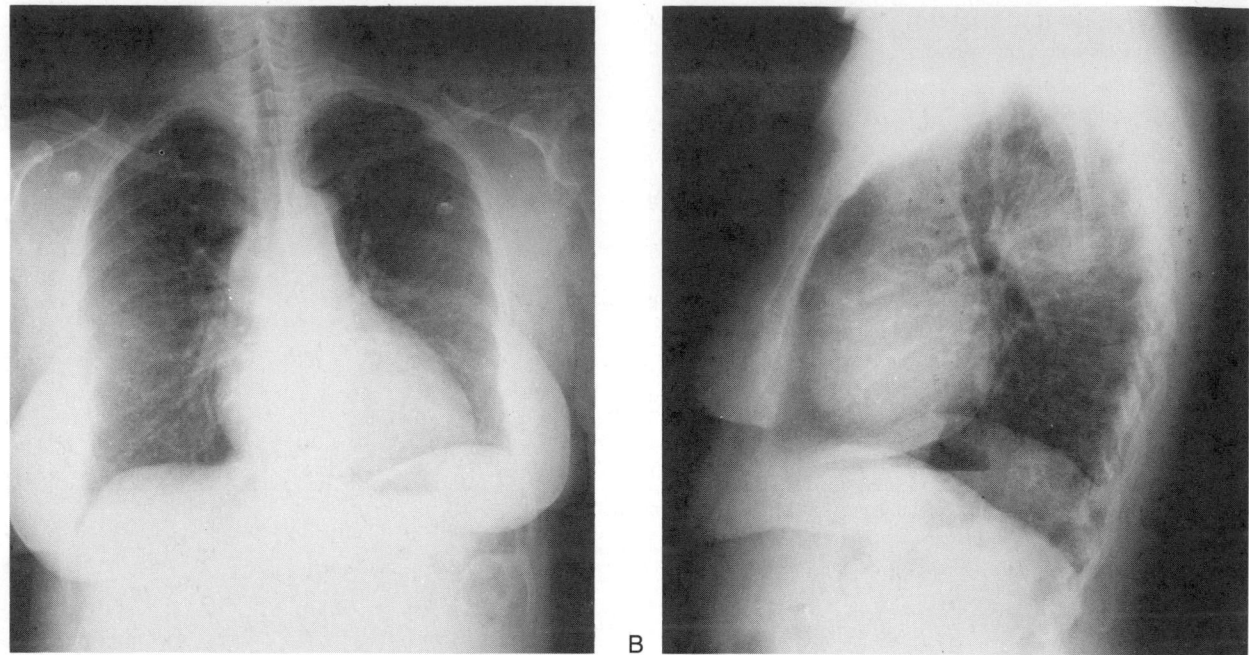

A   B

Figure 57-16. **(A)** PA chest radiograph shows a smooth-contoured mediastinal mass. **(B)** The lateral radiograph shows the mass to be at the level of the carina in the posterior mediastinum. Surgical excision of the mass confirmed the diagnosis of bronchogenic cyst.

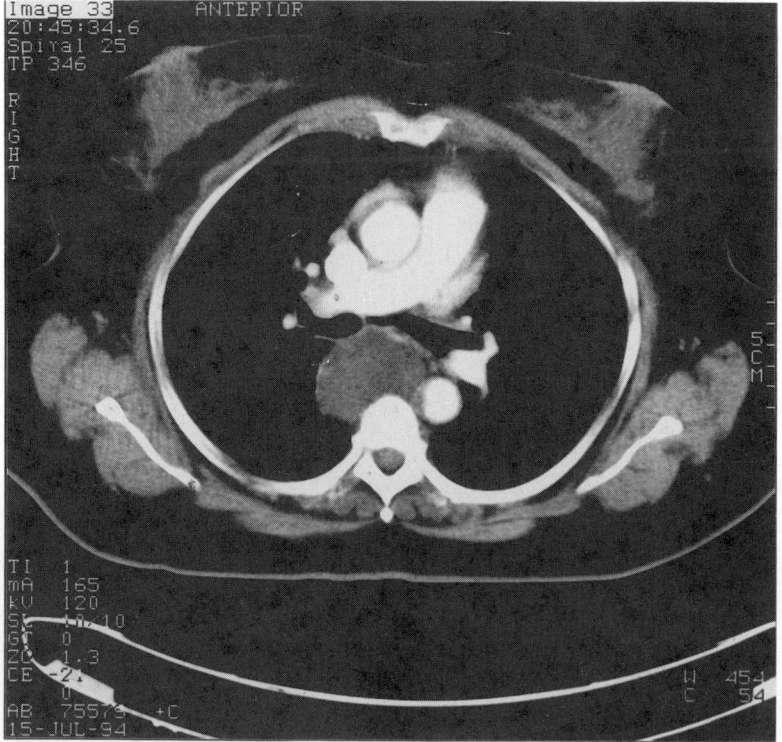

Figure 57-17. CT scan of a mediastinal bronchogenic cyst, showing a well-circumscribed, unilocular, low-Hounsfield-number cyst in the right paraesophageal position.

parenchymal lesion. Lesions not seen on standard radiographs are usually in the subcarinal position.

Barium swallow is abnormal in 54 to 70 percent of patients and shows extrinsic esophageal indentation or displacement (St-Georges, et al., 1991; Suen, et al., 1993). Differentiation between a bronchogenic cyst and a benign esophageal leiomyoma can be difficult on the basis of barium contrast studies only.

Computed Tomography

CT usually shows a round, unilocular, well-circumscribed mass with a density of 0 to 20 Hounsfield units (Suen, et al., 1993). Densities of 130 Hounsfield units have been described, but these are unusual (Mendelson, et al., 1983). Because there is variation in the density of these lesions on CT scan, this diagnostic modality is not absolute. In addition to scanning the chest, the upper abdomen should be evaluated for dumbbell extension of the cyst below the diaphragm (Duranceau and Deslauriers, 1991). In all cysts there is a conspicuous absence of contrast material within the cyst (Fig. 57-17).

Magnetic Resonance Imaging

MRI is rarely used or needed to aid in the diagnosis of bronchogenic cysts. MRI would be indicated in patients who cannot tolerate iodinated contrast agents or who have paravertebral masses (Nakata, et al., 1993). If MRI is performed, there is high signal intensity on both T_1- and T_2-weighted images. The high signal intensity on the T_1 images is thought to be secondary to the large amount of proteinaceous fluid and/or methemoglobin associated with intracystic hemorrhage.

Ultrasound

Ultrasound is an infrequent diagnostic modality for bronchogenic cysts. Perhaps its best use currently is for prenatal diagnosis of such cysts. Large bronchogenic cysts in utero should be suspected when mediastinal shift or obstructive emphysema is seen (Young, et al., 1989). In future, transesophageal ultrasound may be helpful in diagnosing bronchogenic cysts.

Bronchoscopy and Esophagoscopy

Occasionally the cyst may cause symptoms, which warrants esophagoscopy or bronchoscopy. Mediastinoscopy for diagnosis is not needed and should not be performed. Findings on bronchoscopy are related primarily to extrinsic compression of the tracheobronchial tree by the bronchogenic cyst. Blood-tinged or purulent secretions have also been associated with bronchogenic cysts. Rarely, a direct communication between the cyst and the tracheobronchial tree can be visualized bronchoscopically. Findings on esophagoscopy suggestive of a bronchogenic cyst are related to extrinsic compression of the esophagus, a condition that is not unique to bronchogenic cysts and may be secondary to esophageal duplication cysts or esophageal leiomyomas, fibromas, or lipomas.

Aspiration Biopsy

There is no role for needle aspiration biopsy in diagnosis of bronchogenic cysts. The aspirate contains mesothelial cells, lymphocytes, histocytes, and inflammatory cells but no cyst wall tissue. Cytology and further fluid analyses do not help in making the diagnosis. Cohn, et al. (1987) advocated transtracheal aspiration of a bronchogenic cyst, and Zimmer, et al. (1986) recommended percutaneous aspiration of cysts as both diagnostic and therapeutic modalities. These techniques are not recommended because their use has been associated with numerous recurrences due to incomplete resection of the cysts (Duranceau and Deslauriers, 1991). The cyst recurs because the mucosa with its glandular lining is still intact. In addition, attempts to aspirate the cyst can result in secondary infection, which is a serious complication.

MANAGEMENT

Therapy

Bronchogenic cysts should be surgically extirpated, with the entire cyst wall included if possible. The correct preoperative diagnosis of a bronchogenic cyst is made in only 40 to 60 percent of patients (St-Georges, et al., 1991; Suen, et al., 1993), and therefore the diagnosis of a bronchogenic cyst is frequently an intraoperative one. Occasionally, the diagnosis is confirmed only after resection of the mediastinal mass.

The traditional surgical approach to mediastinal bronchogenic cyst is via a posterolateral thoracotomy. The surgeon should be prepared to dissect the cyst from dense attachments to the esophagus, pericardium, lung, or tracheobronchial tree. Aspiration of the cyst fluid may facilitate resection. The fluid should be cultured appropriately if there is any suspicion of infection. Because of dense pericystic adhesions, major operative difficulties or intraoperative complications have been reported in 44 percent of patients undergoing resection of these cysts (St-Georges, et al., 1991). Despite the frequent technical difficulties in removing the cysts, mortality rates are nearly zero and morbidity is 5 to 10 percent. Atelectasis, wound infections, pleural effusions, and, rarely, Horner syndrome are the most common postoperative complications.

Parenchymal bronchogenic cysts are usually symptomatic and often have a fistula with the tracheobronchial tree. These cysts should be surgically removed, segmentectomy or lobectomy being required for adequate cyst removal in these cases. Enucleation may be performed if the patient has inadequate pulmonary reserves to tolerate even a partial lung resection.

The reintroduction of thoracoscopy has led to its diagnostic and therapeutic use for bronchogenic cysts. Several groups have reported small series of patients in whom cysts have been resected with no mortality and minimal morbidity (Hazelrigg, et al., 1993; Lewis, et al., 1992; Kern, et al., 1993). Incomplete resection of the cyst wall has been a potential problem. Cauterization of the mucosa has been proposed to decrease the risk of recurrence in these cases (Lewis, et al., 1992). As more experience with thoracoscopic techniques accumulates and better instrumentation is developed, the majority of bronchogenic cysts will probably be removed by video-assisted thoracoscopic techniques.

Finally, Ginsberg, et al. (1972) have advocated mediastinoscopy as the initial procedure for superior mediastinal bronchogenic cysts. Aspiration followed by attempted resection is the proposed procedure. Failure of this technique is roughly 50 percent in his reported series. Currently we recommend mediastinoscopy as the initial procedure only for the patient too ill to tolerate a thoracotomy. If the patient can tolerate general anesthesia, thoracoscopy would be the preferred approach.

The Asymptomatic Patient

Controversy exists about the correct management of the asymptomatic adult patient with a bronchogenic cyst. Bolton and Shahian (1992) recommend a conservative, nonoperative approach to the asymptomatic patient. Careful surveillance of the patient is maintained, and if the cyst enlarges, develops an air-fluid level, or becomes symptomatic or if a potential malignancy cannot be excluded, surgical removal is indicated.

The majority of authors, including ourselves, recommend surgical excision of all presumed bronchogenic cysts in the asymptomatic adult (St-Georges, et al., 1991; Suen, et al., 1993). Symptoms will develop or the cyst will enlarge in 65 percent of known bronchogenic cysts (St-Georges, et al., 1991) (Table 57-3). It is also known that once symptoms develop, the incidence of pericystic adhesions is higher and operative difficulties are increased (St-Georges, et al., 1991). It is for these reasons that early surgical excision is recommended in the stable asymptomatic patient.

ESOPHAGEAL DUPLICATION CYST

The esophagus is formed after proliferation and later degeneration and vacuolization of epithelial elements of the dorsal foregut. Persistence of one of these vacuoles amid degenerated epithelial masses results in an esophageal duplication cyst (Sirivella, et al., 1985). These cysts account for 0.5 to 2.5 percent of all tumors of the esophagus. The majority present as symptomatic lesions in the neonate or young child but 25 to 30 percent are formed in adults (Whitaker, et al., 1980), in whom they usually are asymptomatic masses and are identified through unrelated diagnostic studies.

The majority (60 percent) of esophageal duplication cysts are located in the lower esophagus, and the remainder are equally divided between the upper and middle thirds. As mentioned previously, they are more common on the right owing to rightward rotation of the stomach (Murray and Gustafson, 1994).

DIAGNOSIS

Clinical Features

If an esophageal duplication produces symptoms in the adult, these symptoms are commonly related to compression of the cyst against structures of the visceral mediastinum. Dysphagia, regurgitation, dyspnea, wheezing, coughing, anorexia, and pain have all been reported. The cyst is thought to enlarge secondary to inflammation, infection, or intracystic hemorrhage. The enlarged cyst then causes these symptoms or produces malfunction of the esophagus at the level of the cyst (Vithespongse and Blank, 1971).

Pathology

Esophageal duplication cysts are well-circumscribed lesions with smooth outer surfaces, which contain brownish, cloudy, serous fluid in most cases. Gross purulence and a necrotic inner lining can be seen if the cyst is infected.

Microscopically the luminal epithelial lining often varies from the single cuboidal to the well-differentiated ciliated respiratory type of epithelium. The presence of ciliated epithelium, even if pseudostratified, does not necessarily indicate a respiratory origin. It is the presence of two layers of muscularis propria in the absence of cartilage formation that confirms that the cyst is esophageal in origin (Whitaker, et al., 1980).

Malignancy has rarely been reported in esophageal duplication cysts. Olsen, et al. (1991) reported a well-differentiated adenocarcinoma in an esophageal duplication cyst in a patient who had been followed clinically for 40 years. Tapia and White (1986) reported a case of squamous cell carcinoma arising in a duplication cyst.

Investigative Techniques

Standard chest radiography may demonstrate the presence of a mediastinal mass, which is seen particularly on the lateral

Table 57-3. Indications for Operation in 86 Patients with Bronchogenic Cysts

Indication	MBC (n = 66)	LBC (n = 20)	Total[a] (n = 86)
Mass previously known	26	11	37 (43)
Stable	11	2	13
Increase in size and/or change in symptomatology	15	9	24
Mass not previously known	39	9	48 (55.8)
Asymptomatic	11	2	13
Symptomatic	28	7	35
Incidental finding during operation for reflux esophagitis	1	0	1 (1.2)

Abbreviations: LBC, bronchogenic cyst of the lung; MBC, mediastinal bronchogenic cyst.

[a] Numbers in parentheses are percentages.

(From St-Georges R, Deslauriers J, Duranceau A et al.: Clinical spectrum of bronchogenic cysts of the mediastinum and lung in the adult. Ann Thorac Surg 52:6, 1991 with permission.)

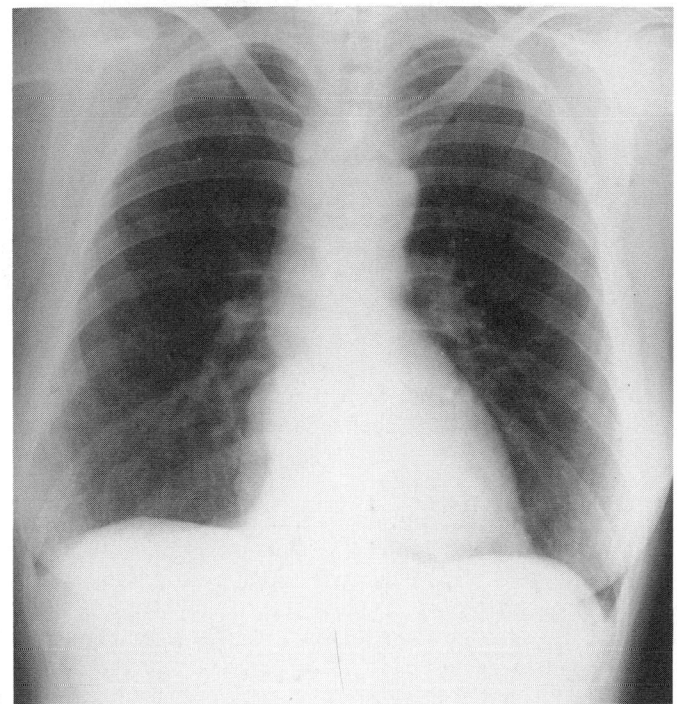
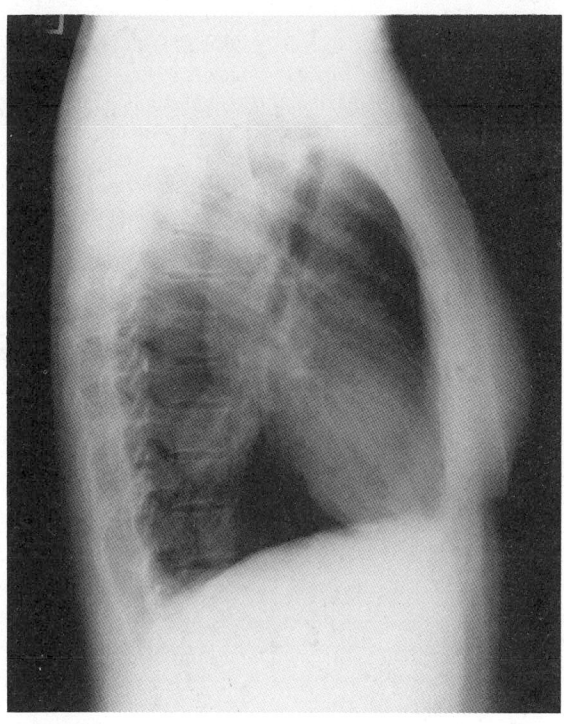

Figure 57-18. **(A&B)** Chest radiographs showing a right-sided tubular esophageal duplication cyst extending from the upper esophagus to the diaphragm. **(B)** Lateral view shows the tubular structure of the cyst better than **(A)** the standard PA exposure.

view (Fig. 57-18). Contrast studies of the esophagus may suggest the diagnosis by revealing focal, smooth compression of the esophagus. Displacement of the esophagus by the duplication cyst can also be seen on contrast esophagography (Fig. 57-19). The esophagogram does not differentiate a cystic lesion of the esophagus from an intramural esophageal leiomyoma.

CT of the chest shows a homogenous, low-attenuation mass with smooth borders (Weiss, et al., 1983). The CT scan cannot definitively distinguish esophageal duplication cysts from benign intramural or paraesophageal lesions such as abscess, old hematoma, neurofibroma, lipoma, or other foregut cysts (Kuhlman, et al., 1985).

MRI of esophageal duplication cysts has been advocated by some to be equal to or better than the CT scan in diagnostic value (Lupetin and Dash, 1987). MRI shows low T_1- and T_2-weighted images of the cyst wall with high-intensity T_1-weighted images of the cyst contents. This high-signal T_1-weighted image is the same as is seen in bronchogenic cysts and mediastinal hematomas (Lupetin and Dash, 1987).

Page, et al. (1989) and Bondestam, et al. (1990) have reported the successful application of transesophageal ultrasound to the diagnosis of these lesions. Ultrasound analysis of intramural cysts usually demonstrates a cystic lesion with occasional echogenic mobile sludge. The cyst does not move with respiratory motions of the pleura nor does it penetrate the esophageal wall (Bondestam, et al., 1990).

Esophagoscopy is a necessary diagnostic study to rule out other esophageal lesions. The smooth, round shape of the

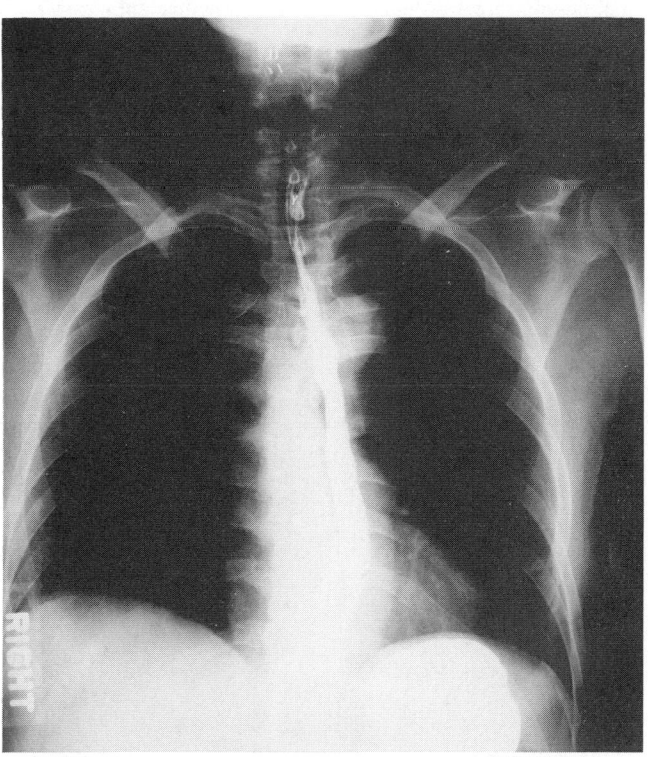

Figure 57-19. A barium swallow shows slight leftward displacement of the esophagus by a large right-sided esophageal duplication cyst.

soft compressible cyst with absent mucosal alterations is the characteristic endoscopic finding. Biopsy of this lesion should be condemned, as the biopsy forceps rarely reaches the lesion and will leave a mucosal laceration, which may lead to subsequent infection of the cyst (Mansour, et al., 1977).

MANAGEMENT

Therapy

Therapy for esophageal duplication cysts is complete surgical excision of the cyst and its contents (Holcomb, et al., 1989; Dresler, et al., 1990). The constant threat of cyst enlargement secondary to intracystic hemorrhage or infection and the possibility of rupture make surgical excision the therapy of choice regardless of the presence or absence of symptoms. The location of the cyst is most commonly intramural or juxtaesophageal but can be retroesophageal or retrocardiac. The surgical principle for removal of these cysts is avoidance of esophageal mucosal injury. The cyst, if small enough, can be enucleated from the wall of the native esophagus without mucosal injury. Long tubular duplications have a common septum separating them from the esophagus. Dissection of this septum can be tedious, but the operator will usually be rewarded for persistence by avoiding mucosal injury or an esophageal resection.

Lewis, et al. (1992) have resected esophageal duplication cysts with video-assisted thoracic surgery. This technique and the necessary instrumentation are still being developed, but it will certainly be used increasingly in the future.

Endoscopic ultrasound with endoscopic needle aspiration has been advocated as an alternative to surgical excision of these lesions (Van Dam, et al., 1992; Page, et al., 1989). This approach may have application in the acutely symptomatic patient who is at high risk for surgery but should not be performed routinely.

After successful removal of the cyst recurrence is extremely rare. The remainder of the gastrointestinal tract should be evaluated radiographically or endoscopically for other duplications. Long-term follow-up for the development of gastroesophageal reflux, is important, as these patients are predisposed to develop reflux after surgery (Salo and Ala-Kulju, 1987).

PERICARDIAL CYSTS

The pericardial sac is formed by the fusion of several different lacunae. Failure of one of these lacunar cavities to merge with others results in the formation of a pericardial (coelomic) cyst, also called pleuropericardial cyst, cardiophrenic angle cyst, and springwater cyst. The majority of these cysts are adjacent to the pericardium and the diaphragm, but occasionally they have been found in a suprapericardial position (Rosai, 1989) (Fig. 57-20). Most of these cysts are found at the right cardiophrenic angle (Lillie, et al., 1950).

The pericardial cyst is usually asymptomatic. Symptoms, if present, are pain, a sensation of heaviness in the chest, and dyspnea. Most cysts are unilocular and are diagnosed with plain chest radiographs and a CT scan of the chest. A teardrop configuration of the cyst on the lateral chest view may be present, as the cyst tends to conform to the medial

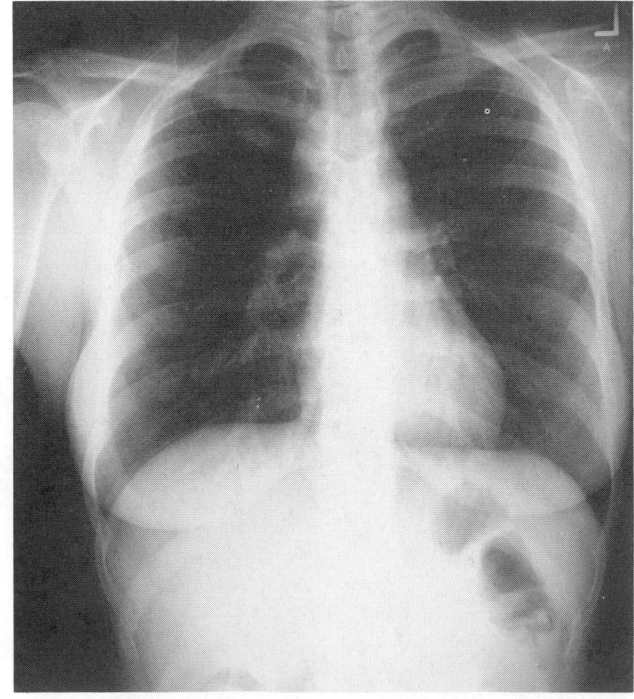
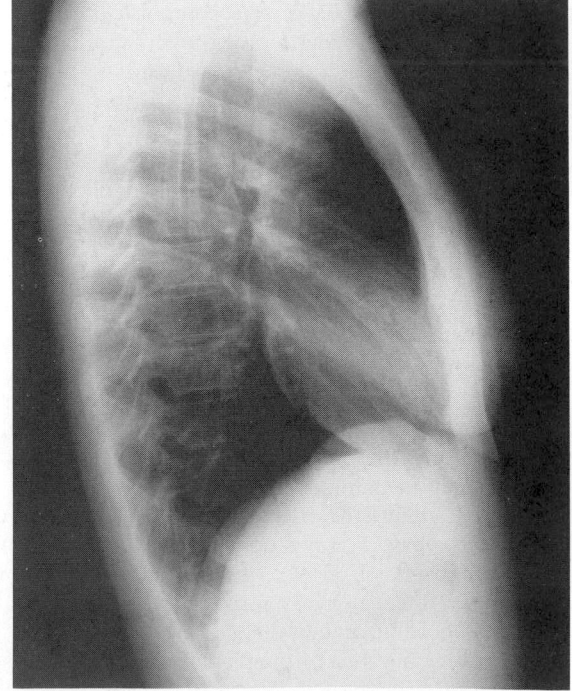

A

B

Figure 57-20. **(A)** PA chest radiograph shows an atypical suprapericardial location of a pericardial cyst. **(B)** The lateral view suggests the presence of a mediastinal mass near the carina.

aspect of the pulmonary fissure (Ochsner and Ochsner, 1966). Most pericardial cysts have a characteristic appearance on CT scan, with a Housfield number very close to zero (Fig. 57-21).

Pathologic examination of the cyst normally demonstrates a unilocular mass with clear intracystic fluid. The blood supply is from the pericardium, and the inner surface of the cyst wall is covered by a thin layer of mesothelium (Rosai, 1989).

Therapy for a pericardial cyst is excision if other mediastinal cystic lesions cannot be excluded. Video-assisted thoracic surgery is rapidly becoming an effective technique for removal of these cysts (Szinicz, et al., 1992; Weder, et al., 1994). Cysts causing altered cardiac function and partial right ventricular erosion have been reported (Shaver, et al., 1965; Chapra, et al., 1991). Removal of these cysts requires formal thoracotomy or median sternotomy, with possible cardiopulmonary bypass.

MISCELLANEOUS CYSTS

NEURENTERIC CYSTS

Neurenteric cysts are formed after a failure of complete separation of the notochord from the foregut. As a result of failure to separate, a split notochord is formed. This embryologic maldevelopment then gives rise to abnormalities of the vertebral column, spinal cord, and alimentary tract (Saunders, 1943). The neurenteric tumors are found in the posterior mediastinum and are most commonly encountered in infants but occasionally, are discovered in adults (Tarnay, et al., 1970).

The neurenteric cyst is usually connected to the vertebral column or spinal canal by a fibrous band or stalk. Vertebral anomalies can occur anywhere along the vertebral column and consist of hemivertebrae, Klippel-Feil syndrome, spina bifida, and scoliosis (Tarnay, et al., 1970).

Diagnostic evaluation includes MRI for possible intraspinal connection of the cyst and for definition of the vertebral body abnormalities. Therapy consists of surgical excision of the cyst and its attachments (Alrabeeah, et al., 1988; Superina, et al., 1984).

THORACIC DUCT CYSTS

A thoracic duct cyst is a rare mediastinal cyst that can occur anywhere along the course of the thoracic duct. CT shows a low attenuated mass, and MRI shows high-intensity signals on T_1- and T_2-weighted images (Lamars and van Belle, 1993). Lymphangiography may be helpful in detecting the communication between the cyst and the thoracic duct (Hori, et al., 1980). Surgical removal of the cyst is curative. Ligation of the thoracic duct may be necessary.

THYMIC CYSTS

Thymic cysts are benign lesions of the thymus and are a result of either a developmental or acquired process (Bieger and McAdams, 1966). They are usually asymptomatic; however, dyspnea, dysphagia, and chest pain have been reported to occur with these cysts (Suster, et al., 1991). The lesions are well circumscribed and lobulated with a thin capsule. Thymic cysts may be unilocular, especially if congenital in etiology, or multilocular if acquired. Radiographically these lesions appear as anterior mediastinal masses on plain x-ray.

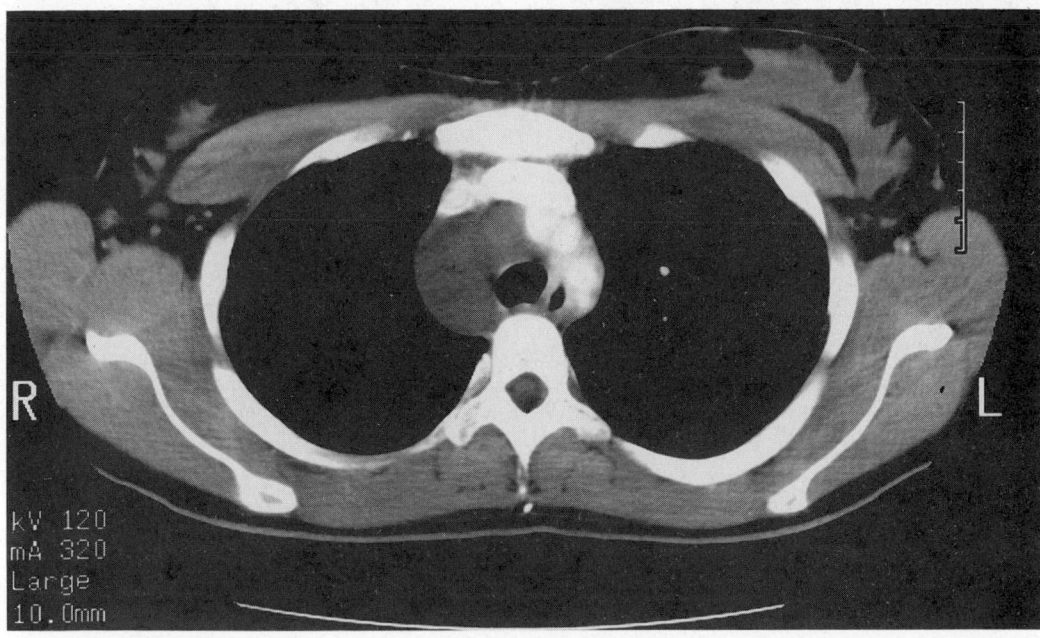

Figure 57-21. CT scan of this pericardial cyst shows its close approximation to the superior portion of the pericardium. It has the radiographic density of water.

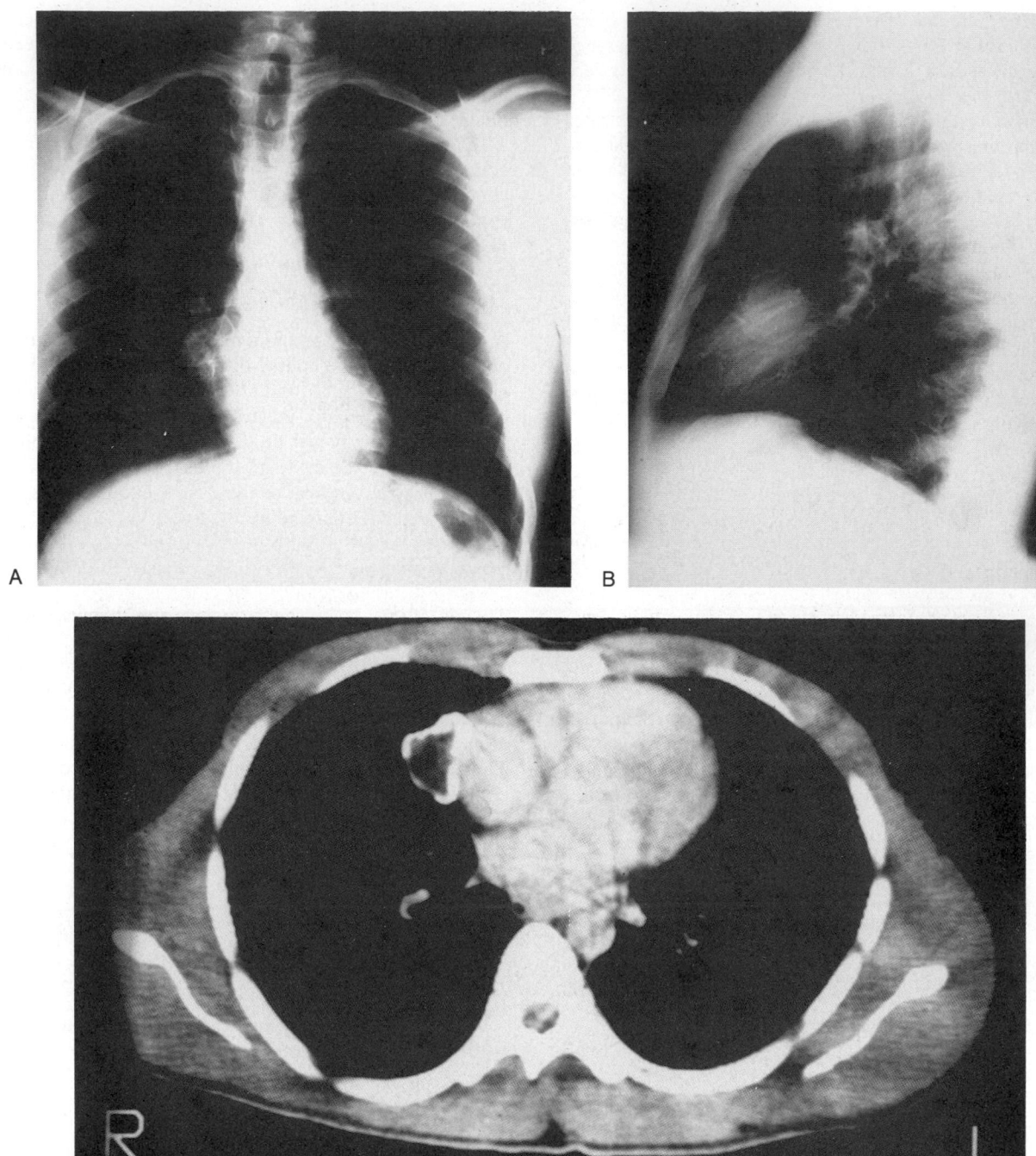

Figure 57-22. **(A)** PA and **(B)** lateral chest films and **(C)** a selected image from a CT scan of a patient with a calcified cyst of the inferior right thymic pole. Note that all the calcification is within the wall of the cyst. The cyst is relatively dense owing to intracystic hemorrhage. (From Graeber GM, Thompson LD, Cohen DJ et al.: Cystic lesions of the thymus. J Thorac Cardiovasc Surg 87:295, 1984, with permission.)

CT scan characteristics of a thymic cyst include a cyst content density near that of water unless intracystic hemorrhage or cell wall degeneration has occurred (Graeber, et al., 1984) (Fig. 57-22). Histologically, the diagnosis of thymic cyst is established by demonstrating continuity of the squamous epithelial lining of the cyst with remnants of normal thymus found within the cyst walls (Suster, et al., 1991). These cysts may be enucleated or excised by open techniques. Video-assisted thoracic surgery may also be employed to perform the thymectomy.

REFERENCES

Alrabeeah A, Gillis DA, Giacomantonio M, Lau H: neuroenteric cysts—a spectrum. J Pediatr Surg 23:752, 1988

Amendola MA, Shirazi KK, Brooks J et al: Transdiaphragmatic bronchopulmonary foregut anomaly: "dumbbell" bronchogenic cyst. AJR 138:1165, 1982

Bieger RC, McAdams AJ: Thymic cysts. Arch Pathol 82:535, 1966

Bolton JWR, Shahian DM: Asymptomatic bronchogenic cysts: what is the best management? Ann Thorac Surg 53:1134, 1992

Bondestam S, Salo JA, Salonen OLM, Lamminen AE: Imaging of congenital esophageal cysts in adults. Gastrointest Radiol 15:279, 1990

Chapra PS, Duke DJ, Pellett JR, Rahko PS: Pericardial cyst with partial erosion of the right ventricular wall. Ann Thorac Surg 51:840, 1991

Chung MT, Barba FA, Kaneko M, Teirstein AS: Adenocarcinoma arising in an intrathoracic duplication cyst of foregut origin. Cancer 47:1887, 1981

Cohn JR, Wechsler R, Zawid J, Brodovsky HS: Resolution of a mediastinal cyst by transtracheal needle aspiration. Pa Med 84:64, 1987

Dresler CM, Patterson GA, Taylor BR, Moote DJ: Complete foregut duplication. Ann Thorac Surg 50:306, 1990

Duranceau ACH, Deslauriers J: Foregut cysts of the mediastinum in the adult. p. 305. In Shields TW (ed): Mediastinal Surgery. Lea & Febiger, Philadelphia, 1991

Ginsberg RJ, Atkins RW, Paulson DL: Case report—a bronchogenic cyst successfully treated by mediastinoscopy. Ann Thorac Surg 13:266, 1972

Ginsberg RJ, Kirby TJ: Bronchogenic cysts. p. 84. In Grillo HC, Austin WG, Wilkens EW Jr et al. (eds): Current Therapy in Cardiothoracic Surgery. BC Decker, Philadelphia, 1989

Graeber GM, Thompson LD, Cohen DJ et al: Cystic lesions of the thymus. J Thorac Cardiovasc Surg 87:295, 1984

Greenfield LJ, Holme HS: Bronchial adenoma within the wall of a bronchogenic cyst. J Thorac Cardiovasc Surg 49:398, 1965

Hazelrigg SR, Landreneau RJ, Mack MJ, Acuff TE: Thoracoscopic resection of mediastinal cysts. Ann Thorac Surg 56:659, 1993

Holcomb GW, Gheissari A, O'Neill JA Jr et al: Surgical management of alimentary tract duplications. Ann Surg 209:167, 1989

Hori S, Harada K, Morimota S et al: Lymphangiographic demonstration of thoracic duct cysts. Chest 78:652, 1980

Kern JA, Daniel TM, Tribble CG et al: Thoracoscopic diagnosis and treatment of mediastinal masses. Ann Thorac Surg 56:92, 1993

Kuhlman JE, Fishman EK, Wang KP, Siegelman SS: Esophageal duplication cyst: CT and transesophageal needle aspiration. AJR 145:531, 1985

Lamars RJS, van Belle AF: Thoracic duct cyst in the middle part of the mediastinum. AJR 161:675, 1993

Lewis RJ, Caccavale RJ, Sisler GE: Imaged thoracic surgery: a new thoracic technique for resection of mediastinal cysts. Ann Thorac Surg 53:318, 1992

Lillie WI, McDonald JR, Clagett OT: Pericardial clonic cysts and pericardial diverticula. A concept of etiology and report of cases. J Thorac Cardiovasc Surg 20:494, 1950

Lupetin AR, Dash N: MRI appearance of esophageal duplication cyst. Gastrointest Radiol 12:7, 1987

Maier HC: Bronchogenic cysts of the mediastinum. Ann Surg 127:476, 1948

Mansour KA, Hatcher CR, Haun CL: Benign tumors of the esophagus: experience with 20 cases. South Med J 70:461, 1977

Marchevsky AM, Kaneko M: Surgical Pathology of the Mediastinum. Raven Press, New York, 1984

Mendelson DS, Rose JS, Efremidis SC et al: Bronchogenic cysts with high CT numbers. AJR 140:463, 1983

Murray GF, Gustafson RA: Benign tumors, cysts, and duplications of the esophagus. p. 1622. In Shields TW (ed): General Thoracic Surgery. 4th Ed. Williams & Wilkins, Baltimore, 1994

Nakata H, Egashira K, Watanabe H et al: MRI of bronchogenic cysts. J Comput Assist Tomogr 17:267, 1993

Ochsner JL, Ochsner SF: Congenital cysts of the mediastinum. Ann Surg 163:909, 1966

Okubo A, Sone S, Ogushi F et al: A case of bronchogenic cyst with high production of antigen CA 19-9. Cancer 63:1994, 1989

Olsen JB, Clemmensen O, Andersen K: Adenocarcinoma arising in a foregut cyst of the mediastinum. Ann Thorac Surg 51:497, 1991

Page JE, Wilson AG, de Belder MA: The value of transesophageal ultrasonography in the management of a mediastinal foregut cyst. Br J Radiol 62:986, 1989

Rosai J: Mediastinum p. 347. In Ackerman's Surgical Pathology 7th Ed. CV Mosby, St. Louis, 1989

Sadler TW: Langman's Medical Embryology. 5th Ed. Williams & Wilkins, 1985, p. 215

Salo JA, Ala-Kulju KV: Congenital esophageal cysts in adults. Ann Thorac Surg 44:135, 1987

Saunders RL: Combined anterior and posterior spina bifida in a living neonatal human female. Anat Rec 87:255, 1943

Shaver VC, Bailey WR, Marrangoni AG: Acquired pulmonic stenosis due to external cardiac compression. Am J Cardiol 16:256, 1965

Sirivella S, Ford WB, Zikria EA et al: Foregut cysts of the mediastinum. Results in 20 consecutive surgically treated cases. J Thorac Cardiovasc Surg 90:776, 1985

St-Georges R, Deslauriers J, Duranceau A et al: Clinical spectrum of bronchogenic cysts of the mediastinum and lung in the adult. Ann Thorac Surg 52:6, 1991

Suen HC, Mathisen DJ, Grillo HC et al: Surgical management and radiological characteristics of bronchogenic cysts. Ann Thorac Surg 55:476, 1993

Superina RA, Ein SH, Humphreys RP: Cystic duplications of the esophagus and neuroenteric cysts. J Pediatr Surg 19:527, 1984

Suster S, Barbuto D, Carlson G, Rosai J: Multilocular thymic cysts with pseudoepitheliomatous hyperplasia. Hum Pathol 22:455, 1991

Szinicz G, Taxer J, Riedlinger J, Erhart K: Thoracoscopic resection of a pericardial cyst. Thorac Cardiovasc Surg 40:190, 1992

Tapia RH, White VA: Squamous cell carcinoma arising in a duplication cyst of the esophagus. Am J Gastroenterol 81:325, 1986

Tarnay TJ, Chang CH, Nugent RG, Warden HE: Esophageal duplication (foregut cyst) with spinal formation. J Thorac Cardiovasc Surg 59:293, 1970

Van Dam J, Rice TW, Sivak MV Jr: Endoscopic ultrasonograpy and endoscopically guided needle aspiration for the diagnosis of upper gastrointestinal tract foregut cysts. Am J Gastroenterol 87:762, 1992

Vithespongse P, Blank S: Ciliated epithelial esophageal cyst. Am J Gastroenterol 56:436, 1971

Weder W, Klatz HP, vanSegesser L, Largiader F: Thoracoscopic resection of a pericardial cyst: a case report. J Thorac Cardiovasc Surg 107:313, 1994

Weiss LM, Fagelman D, Warhit JM: CT demonstration of an esophageal duplication cyst. J Comput Assist Tomogr 7:716, 1983

Whitaker JA, Deffenbaugh LD, Cooke AR: Esophageal duplication cyst. Am J Gastroenterol 73:329, 1980

Young G, L'Heaureux PR, Krueckeberg ST, Swanson DA: Mediastinal bronchogenic cyst: prenatal sonographic diagnosis. AJR 152:125, 1989

Zimmer WD, Kamida CB, McGough PF, Rosenow EC: Mediastinal duplication cyst. Percutaneous aspiration and cystography for diagnosis and treatment. Chest 90:772, 1986

58

TUMORS AND MASSES

Biologic Markers

Leslie J. Kohman
Celeste N. Powers

The mediastinum can host a wide variety of tumors and cysts. These lesions often reside in inaccessible locations and may present considerable problems in identification. New understanding of the basic biology of many of these lesions in recent years has led to techniques that make the mechanism of diagnosis easier for both the patient and the physician. These improvements include targeted radionuclide imaging, discovery of serum and tissue markers specific for tumors, and advances in cytologic techniques. From the following explanation of the development and utility of these procedures, the reader can gain an appreciation of the increasing need for collaboration among radiologist, pathologist, and clinician to provide accurate and specific preoperative diagnosis.

HISTORICAL NOTE

Many mediastinal masses represent ectopic tissue that secretes or takes up various biochemical compounds. Recent advances in radionuclide imaging take advantage of these characteristics to narrow the differential diagnoses. Graham and colleagues (1989) have described the events that led to modern nuclear medicine: the discovery of radioactivity by Becquerel in 1896, the development of the tracer principle, the widespread production of radionuclides during World War II, refinements in scanning from the point counting technique to the rectilinear scanner in 1949, and the development of radiopharmaceuticals during the 1950s. The introduction of the scintillation camera in the 1970s had the greatest impact. More recently we have seen the application of single-photon emission computed tomography (SPECT) and positron emission tomography (PET) to many scans appropriate to the mediastinum, especially monoclonal antibody scanning, which is still in its infancy.

The art of diagnostic histopathology, practiced for well over a century, perhaps truly began with the publication of *Cellularpathologie* by Virchow in 1858. Although methods of tissue fixation, processing, and histochemical stains have advanced, the majority of diagnoses still rely on the pathologist's subjective interpretation, albeit reinforced by over a century of accumulated experience, observations made by using light microscopy. However, since Coons, et al., (1941) first developed and applied the technique of immunofluorescence in the 1940s, the concept of using additional special techniques and/or stains to confirm the diagnosis has become an important aspect of diagnostic histopathology. By the mid-1970s methodologies such as immunohistochemistry, flow cytometry, and image analysis had been developed and refined for diagnostic use.

Immunohistochemistry, like other ancillary diagnostic studies, developed as a technique for use on tissue obtained by surgical biopsy but today is also applied to other cellular preparations, such as fine-needle aspiration (FNA) samples or fluids. The usefulness of these techniques has resulted in the development of a tremendous selection of antibodies directed against a variety of cellular components and products. Several of these apply specifically in the refinement of the diagnosis of mediastinal masses. Beginning in the 1960s (Nordenstrom, 1967), the mediastinum became ever more accessible to needle aspiration to obtain material for such analysis, and now many patients who until recently would have required a surgical biopsy can receive a diagnosis through minimally invasive means.

HISTORICAL READINGS

Coons, AH, Creeh HJ, Jones RN: Immunologic properties of an antibody containing a fluorescent group. Proc Soc Exp Biol Med 47:200, 1941

Graham LS, Keriakes JG, Harris C, Cohen MB: Nuclear medicine from Becquerel to the present. Radiographics 9:1189, 1989

Nordenstrom B: Paraxiphoid approach to the mediastinum for mediastinography and mediastinal needle biopsy: a preliminary report. Invest Radiol 2:141, 1967

Virchow R: Cellular Pathology: as Based Upon Physiological and Pathological Histology. Translated and edited by Frank Chance. Classics in Medicine Library, Division of Gryphon Editions Ltd, Birmingham, AL, 1978

THE BIOLOGIC BASIS FOR IMAGING OF MEDIASTINAL MASSES

Table 58-1 shows several nuclear medicine tests relevant to mediastinal masses. Sorenson and Phelps (1987) provide a thorough background for understanding in their text *Physics in Nuclear Medicine*. The accuracy of all these procedures increases significantly when imaging is by SPECT technology rather than by traditional planar (i.e., two-dimensional) scanning. In SPECT imaging, the patient receives radionuclides that emit single photons, which gamma cameras then detect in a three-dimensional fashion. This methodology can be applied to the various nuclear imaging modalities in common use. PET, on the other hand, determines regional function and biochemistry by imaging of positron-emitting radionuclides of normal components of biologic processes: carbon, nitrogen, oxygen, and fluorine. Most human tumors exhibit accelerated metabolism detectable by PET (Coleman, 1991; Strauss and Conti, 1991). However, this technique is not yet widely available.

A mediastinal mass may represent a substernal goiter or a thyroid tumor. Nuclear thyroid imaging has long been able to delineate the precise location and extent of the patient's functioning thyroid tissue. Most intrathoracic goiters can be diagnosed by this method (Park, et al., 1984). False negatives can occur in the case of a rare hypofunctioning multinodular goiter (rare) or if a large cyst replaces the intrathoracic goiter. The sternum absorbs the low-energy photons of ^{125}I, making it unsuitable for imaging of the substernal and mediastinal thyroid. Likewise, a high blood background from the heart and great vessels interferes with visualization by ^{99m}Tc (Sandler, et al., 1984); SPECT imaging eliminates this problem. Nuclear medicine specialists can largely avoid these errors by use of a parallel-hole collimator (McKitrick, et al., 1985) and an iodine radionuclide, particularly ^{131}I or ^{123}I. SPECT imaging of the scan would provide additional sensitivity and contrast. Thyroid imaging will not work well for 1 to 6 weeks (depending on the agent used) following administration of iodine-containing contrast agents (Spies, 1991), so nuclear scanning should precede any contrast-enhanced computed tomography (CT) scans.

Nuclear imaging can also provide the gallium scan or the indium-labeled white blood cell scan that is useful in detecting

Table 58-1. Nuclear Imaging Relevant to the Mediastinum

Radiopharmaceutical	Isotope	Disease Detected
Iodine	^{123}I, ^{131}I, ^{111}In	Ectopic thyroid; thyroid cancer
Citrate	^{67}Ga	Hodgkins disease, lymphomas
MIBG	^{123}I	Pheochromocytoma
Monoclonal antibodies	^{99m}Tc, ^{123}I, ^{111}In	Specific tumors

Abbreviation: MIBG, metaiodobenzylguanidine.

mediastinal infectious processes as well as certain neoplasms. In the absence of infection, a positive gallium scan probably indicates lymphoma. SPECT imaging of the gallium study significantly enhances the detection of mediastinal and hilar adenopathy (Kostakoglu, et al., 1992).

Other processes in the mediastinum also provide biologic substances capable of detection by radionuclides. A dual radionuclide parathyroid scan may reveal an ectopic parathyroid neoplasm. For this study, ^{201}Tl images both thyroid and parathyroid tissue, a subsequent ^{99m}Tc scan images only thyroid tissue, and a subtraction technique then allows localization of the parathyroid tissue (Broughan, et al., 1987). A scan using MIBG (metaiodobenzylguanidine, a precursor of epinephrine) detects pheochromocytomas and neuroblastomas (Spies, 1991). Scans using ^{99m}Tc pertechnetate can identify gastric mucosa in suspected neuroenteric cysts (Shields, 1991).

Researchers have recently used radionuclide-labeled monoclonal antibodies directed against a wide variety of human tumor antigens (Fischman, et al., 1989). These radiopharmaceuticals may prove useful in the future for imaging such mediastinal neoplasms as lymphoma, invasive lung cancer, and metastases from other sites (Spies, 1991) when imaged by the SPECT technique.

DIAGNOSTIC MODALITIES

Biochemical Markers—Serum

Neoplastic cells have biologic properties that distinguish them from normal cells. These so-called tumor markers may be the expression of new gene products, altered amounts of normal gene products, alterations in chromosomal DNA, or many other structural or functional cellular properties (Robinson and Radosevich, 1991; Fenoglio-Prieser and Willman, 1987). Blood, urine, or tissue may contain these cellular products. Radioimmunoassay (RIA) or enzyme immunoassay (EIA) technologies using monoclonal antibodies help detect products released into the serum. For most of the mediastinal tumors, the serum markers resemble tissue markers (Robinson and Radosevich, 1991). Markers relevant to the mediastinum include α-fetoprotein (AFP), β-human chorionic gonadotropin (β-HCG), catecholamines and their degradation products, parathyroid hormone (PTH), and lactate dehydrogenase (LDH). The pattern of increased serum levels of these proteins can specifically diagnose certain tumors, particularly mediastinal germ cell tumors.

For example, pure seminomas have no AFP and little (< 100 ng/ml) or no β-HCG (Hainsworth and Greco, 1991b). The small amount of β-HCG (present in approximately 10 percent of seminomas) originates in syncytiotrophoblasts scattered throughout the tumor. Higher levels suggest the additional presence of nonseminomatous elements (Hainsworth and Greco, 1991b). More than 90 percent of malignant nonseminomatous germ cell tumors produce either β-HCG or AFP, and 80 to 90 percent of patients with nonseminomatous germ cell tumors also have elevated LDH serum levels, which are directly proportional to tumor volume (Brindley and Francis, 1963; Friedman, et al., 1980). Patients with yolk sac tumor (endodermal sinus tumor), embryonal carcinoma, or teratocarcinoma will have elevated AFP levels, while those with choriocarcinomas have increased β-HCG. Levels of AFP or β-HCG higher than 500 ng/ml are diagnostic of malignant nonseminomatous germ cell tumor, and these patients may receive chemotherapy without biopsy confirmation (Hainsworth and Greco, 1991b). Patients with benign teratoma have no serum tumor markers (Nichols, 1991).

Carcinoembryonic antigen (CEA), an oncofetal antigen useful in the diagnosis of gastrointestinal, breast, and lung malignancies, does not play a part in the diagnosis of malignant mediastinal germ cell tumors (Robinson and Radosevich, 1991). Placental alkaline phosphatase (PLAP), a nonspecific marker, typically contributes little to the diagnosis. Additional serum studies that may help to substantiate various clinical impressions include PTH (for parathyroid tumor), catecholamine levels (for pheochromocytoma), and ferritin (for neuroblastoma or ganglioneuroblastoma).

Analysis of fluid aspirated from cystic lesions may also prove diagnostic. For example a parathyroid cyst, but no other entity, usually contains crystal clear fluid with abundant PTH. In the future we may see even more sophisticated analysis of cyst fluid. Sano, et al. (1991) recently analyzed the fluid from an excised thymic cyst and found high levels of several tumor antigens often found in the serum of cancer patients: sialylated Lewis X-i, carbohydrate antigen 19-9, and tissue polypeptide antigen.

Occasionally, a mediastinal mass will represent metastatic thyroid carcinoma in a patient who has had surgical or radioactive iodine thyroid ablation. Serum thyroglobulin serves as a tumor marker for such cases, particularly of differentiated, nonmedullary thyroid carcinoma (Van Herle and Uller, 1975). Anaplastic thyroid carcinomas and oxyphilic cells present in differentiated thyroid carcinoma may lack the capacity to synthesize thyroglobulin (Müller-Gärtner and Schneider, 1988). In some cases differentiated tumors also fail to produce detectable levels of thyroglobulin. This occurs most commonly in tumors with papillary characteristics, those with metastatic nodes in the neck or mediastinum, and those of small volume. Therefore, evaluation of a mediastinal mass suspected of representing a metastasis from such a tumor should include a determination of the serum thyroglobulin concentrations under endogenous thyrotropic hormone stimulation, as well as a high-resolution ultrasound study of the neck and other imaging studies of the mediastinum (Müller-Gärtner and Schneider, 1988).

If the serum does not contain tumor markers, they may be demonstrated in tissue obtained by FNA or surgical biopsy. Such techniques add greatly to the diagnostic accuracy of histology and cytology.

Tumor Markers/Immunohistochemistry

Although serum studies can prove useful in the diagnostic workup, examination of tissue from the mediastinal mass remains a vital part of definitive diagnosis. Pathologists now routinely supplement standard histologic examination with immunofluorescence and immunohistochemistry, which both rely on the localization of specific antigens by antibodies marked with a visualizable compound. Immunofluorescence uses a fluorochrome responsive to excitation by ultraviolet

Table 58-2. Antibodies Useful in the Diagnosis of Mediastinal Masses

Antibody	Antigen Type	Usefulness
S-100	Ca^{++} binding protein	Melanoma; neural tumors
LCA	Membrane glycoprotein	Lymphomas
Cytokeratin	Intracellular proteins	Epithelial differentiation
Vimentin	Intermediate filament	Especially mesenchymal lesions
Immunoglobulins	Proteins	Subtyping lymphomas
Leu M1	Protein:monocyte/ granulocyte	Hodgkin's disease
α-Thymosin	Thymic hormone	Thymomas (primarily research)
β-HCG	Hormone secreted by syncytiotrophoblasts	Germ cell tumors Especially choriocarcinoma
AFP	Plasma glycoprotein	Especially embryonal carcinoma

Abbreviations: AFP, α-fetoprotein; β-HCG, β-human chorionic gonadotropin; LCA, leukocyte common antigen.

light. Immunohistochemistry uses various chromagens induced through enzymatic reactions, and by virtue of its easier methodology has become a standard diagnostic technique available to most practicing pathologists. It has a high degree of sensitivity and specificity and can be used successfully on formalin-fixed, paraffin-embedded tissue (Taylor, 1978; Hsu, et al., 1981).

The first stage in the diagnosis of any neoplasm involves determination of the broad category to which it belongs (i.e., epithelial, mesenchymal, or hematopoietic). Light microscopy alone can often accomplish this; however, if the tumor is poorly differentiated, an immunohistochemical panel of antibodies directed against various cellular proteins will assist in the classification (Table 58-2). The antibodies selected for these screening panels may vary; four common choices are leukocyte common antigen (LCA) for lymphoma; cytokeratins for carcinoma; vimentin for sarcoma; and S-100, a calcium-binding protein useful in the identification of melanomas and neural lesions (Battifora, et al., 1980; Taylor, 1978).

More specific antibody panels can further subclassify neoplasms. A panel using AFP and β-HCG can often distinguish between the various types of germ cell tumors and indicate the presence of one or more unsuspected components within these tumors (Table 58-3). A lymphocyte-typing panel can likewise subclassify the lymphomas. Such a panel consists

Table 58-3. Tumor Markers in Various Germ Cell Tumors

Germ Cell Tumor	AFP	β-HCG
Embryonal carcinoma	+	−
Embryonal carcinoma with ST	+	+
Choriocarcinoma	−	+
Yolk sac tumor	+	+
Teratoma	−	−
Teratoma with embryonal carcinoma	+	−
Seminoma	−	−
Seminoma with ST	−	+

Abbreviations: AFP, α-fetoprotein; β-HCG, β-human chorionic gonadotropin; ST, syncytiotrophoblasts.

of a variety of surface antigens to distinguish T cells and the various heavy and light chains to further characterize B-cell lymphomas. These immunoglobulin components may include γ and α, IgG, IgA, and the κ and λ light chains.

Although immunohistochemical techniques have improved the field of diagnostic pathology, these techniques also have pitfalls. For example, staining for neuron-specific enolase no longer plays a significant part in tumor identification. Certain isoenzymes of this glycolytic enzyme seem to occur preferentially in neurons and certain endocrine cells, but unfortunately the enzyme has a wide distribution in many types of tissue. This lack of specificity makes this marker of little use in the diagnosis of neuroectodermal and neuroendocrine neoplasms. A thorough knowledge of the various artifacts associated with immunohistochemistry, careful attention to the actual performance of the technique, and use of appropriate controls can avert most of these problems.

Electron Microscopy

Electron microscopy can also provide supplemental information in the workup of neoplasms of the mediastinum (Davis, et al., 1987), although its use has decreased since the advent of immunohistochemistry (Dabbs and Silverman, 1988; Neill and Silverman, 1992; Dardick, et al., 1991; Berkman, et al., 1983; Rosai and Rodriguez, 1968). This technique can classify undifferentiated tumors into one of four major categories: carcinoma, malignant lymphoma, malignant melanoma, and sarcoma. Distinctive cytoplasmic structures observed only at the ultrastructural level may indicate differentiation of the lesion beyond that suspected by light microscopy. For example, light microscopy may reveal a tumor composed of large pleomorphic cells with a high nuclear/cytoplasmic ratio but no other distinctive features that suggest a specific classification. Ultrastructural examination may reveal premelanosomes, which indicate melanoma, or well defined junctional complexes (desmosomes) and scattered tonofibrils, which suggest carcinoma. This technique may also help to further classify small, round cell tumors, neuroendocrine neoplasms, and mesotheliomas (Rosai and Rodriguez, 1968; Taccagni, et al., 1988; Dardick, et al., 1991). Electron microscopy cannot, however, aid in the diagnosis of germ cell tumors, as they do not have any diagnostic ultrastructural features (Hainsworth and Greco, 1991b).

Needle Biopsy—Cytology

Most tumors of the mediastinum require tissue confirmation of the presumed diagnosis prior to specific therapy. Methods of obtaining tissue range from FNA to excisional biopsy. The choice of a particular method depends in large measure on the clinical and radiologic impression, the location of the mass, and the medical condition of the patient.

FNA provides a safe, cost-effective, and rapid means of diagnosis. Clinical indications for this modality have recently expanded rapidly owing to enhanced cytologic characterization of many tumors. The diagnostic accuracy of FNA varies with the experience of those who perform it, as well as those who interpret the material obtained; in general, accuracy rates range between 85 and 95 percent (Ikezoe, et al., 1984;

Ikezoe, et al., 1990; Rosenberger and Adler, 1978; Weisbrod, et al., 1984; Sterrett, et al., 1983; Westcott, 1981). Maximum benefit from the technique requires close communication among pathologist, radiologist, and clinician. In the vast majority of mediastinal lesions, FNA is carried out with radiologic, most commonly CT, guidance (Colquhoun, et al., 1991; Nordenstrom, 1967; Weisbrod, et al., 1984; Moinuddin, et al., 1984; van Sonnenberg, et al., 1988). Ultrasonically guided needle biopsy, either aspiration or cutting, may offer advantages in some cases (Yu, et al., 1991; Sawhney, et al., 1991; Ikezoe, et al., 1984; Pederson, et al., 1986; Ikezoe, et al., 1990; Saito, et al., 1988; Yang, et al., 1992). Ultrasound often gives better definition of some masses than fluoroscopy, avoids the cost of CT, and allows real-time observation of the needle within the mass. However, it cannot be used for lesions in the middle mediastinum or masses that do not abut the chest wall, since aerated lung hinders the signal.

Most mediastinal lesions have well documented diagnostic criteria (Sterrett, et al., 1983; Todd, et al., 1981; Cristallini, et al., 1992; Koss, et al., 1984). FNA can provide an initial classification of the mediastinal mass as a metastatic carcinoma, malignant lymphoma, thymoma, germ cell tumor, or neural lesion when used with rapid staining techniques at the time of biopsy. Certain lesions, such as seminoma, malignant lymphoma, and metastatic small cell carcinoma, have characteristic patterns on aspiration smears that make immediate identification possible. Further study follows the preliminary interpretation, yielding a more definitive diagnosis. This diagnosis, although usually based on light microscopy, may require ancillary studies in difficult cases. Occasionally, errors occur in subclassifications based only on light microscopy. These problems usually arise in cases of insufficient material for supplementary analysis. For example, with no tissue available for marker studies, large malignant cells with no further distinguishing features could represent a poorly differentiated carcinoma or a germ cell tumor, such as embryonal carcinoma (Koss, et al., 1984). A core needle biopsy, processed as a histologic specimen, may provide better diagnostic material than FNA when the lesion is fibrotic or when the FNA yields scant material.

One of the most controversial areas in FNA is the diagnosis of malignant lymphomas. Several studies indicate that malignant lymphomas can be diagnosed as well as subtyped by FNA (Das, et al., 1991; Koo, et al., 1989; Wittich, et al., 1992; Pontifex and Klimo, 1984; Erwin, et al., 1986; Al-Sharabati, et al., 1991; Sneige, et al., 1990). FNA usually yields adequate material for immunohistochemistry and/or flow cytometry. Flow cytometry allows rapid measurements of one or more parameters of individual cells and with appropriate staining (i.e., marking), permits a lymphoma to be typed just as accurately as by immunohistochemistry. This method, however, requires a substantial number of cells, which usually can be obtained by a dedicated pass with the fine needle (Koss, et al., 1989; Diamond, et al., 1982). These methods document monoclonality and also subtype the lymphoma as T-cell or B-cell. Either procedure can further characterize B-cell lymphoma into specific heavy- and light-chain types.

The diagnosis of Hodgkin's disease by FNA also provides a challenge, although specific cytologic criteria, similar to histologic criteria, have been delineated (Friedman, et al., 1980; Kardos, et al., 1986). Reed-Sternberg cells or their variants give the most help, but these cells may occur rarely in aspirates from certain types of Hodgkin's disease. In addition, nodular sclerosing Hodgkin's disease often yields scant material because of the dense sclerotic stroma. Although the FNA analysis may look suspicious for Hodgkin's disease, definitive diagnosis may require open biopsy.

Thymoma presents another type of challenge for the pathologist interpreting mediastinal FNAs. Depending on the tumor type, the aspirate may contain varying numbers of bland epithelial cells and small lymphocytes. Although lymphocytes may predominate in the grade 1 lesion, they are usually small, with regular round nuclei, and easily distinguished from the larger lymphocytes with convoluted nuclei often seen in malignant large cell lymphomas (Millar, et al., 1987; Hoda, et al., 1991; Battifora, et al., 1980).

Aspirates of germ cell tumors usually show large, noncohesive malignant cells, with variable numbers of mature lymphocytes scattered throughout the tumor. While the cytomorphology of these cells may allow correct categorization as a germ cell tumor, immunochemistry will often permit a more specific classification (Battifora, et al., 1984; Miettinem, et al., 1985).

Tumors of peripheral nerve origin, such as those occurring in the posterior mediastinum, may also cause problems in FNA diagnosis. Because these neurogenic tumors often have a firm consistency, the aspirate frequently yields limited material. In addition, cytology alone may not allow distinction between schwannoma and neurofibroma and between ganglioneuroma and ganglioneuroblastoma. Suggestive information may occasionally prove helpful in such cases, but more frequently the patient will proceed to surgical excision without the need for preoperative tissue diagnosis.

Diagnosis by FNA may fail for several reasons. Sometimes the patient cannot achieve or maintain the appropriate position or may not cooperate. Technical problems include air drying of the specimen, dilution of the sample by excessive blood, or difficulty in targeting the lesion. Experience will obviate most of these problems, as well as most interpretive dilemmas.

FNA often provides a reliable diagnosis, with less cost and complications than surgical biopsy of the mediastinum, particularly since many of these lesions require nonsurgical therapy. Rapid staining techniques allow the cytopathologist to render an interpretation of the aspiration specimen within minutes after a radiologically guided FNA. Such rapid assessments can indicate the need for additional material to be mixed as appropriate with glutaraldehyde for electron microscopy, saline for flow cytometry, or tissue culture medium for immunohistochemistry and cytogenetics. Figure 58-1 is an algorithm for processing of tissue obtained by FNA, which will maximize its diagnostic capabilities.

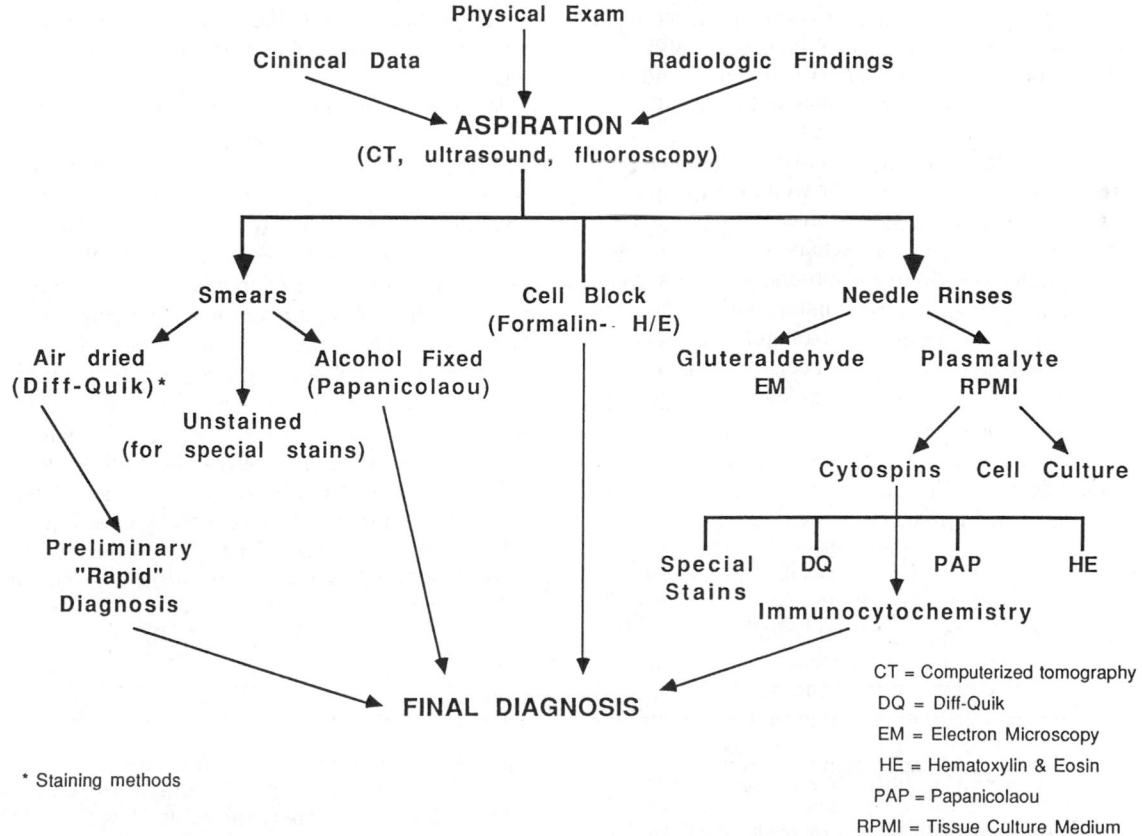

Figure 58-1. Algorithm for the use of fine-needle aspiration biopsy in diagnosis.

Genetic Markers (Cytogenetics)

Hainsworth and Greco (1991a) forecast an increasing role for analysis of specific genetic abnormalities in the diagnosis of poorly differentiated neoplasms. High-resolution chromosomal analysis has detected three specific chromosomal abnormalities, correlated with different histologic subtypes, in tissue from non-Hodgkins lymphoma (Yunis, et al., 1982). Bloomfield and associates (1983) found recurring chromosomal abnormalities in lymphoma samples and concluded that all lymphomas have cytogenetic abnormalities. Detection of gene rearrangements can help to establish a diagnosis of lymphoma in a puzzling neoplasm and to correctly classify T- and B-cell lymphomas (Arnold, et al., 1983).

Germ cell tumors also exhibit cytogenetic abnormalities (Bosl, et al., 1989; Dmitrovsky, et al., 1990). These characteristics may aid in the classification of mediastinal malignancies of uncertain origin, as some patients with such malignancies respond to chemotherapeutic regimens designed for germ cell tumors (Hainsworth and Greco 1991b; Motzer, et al., 1991). As genetic analysis becomes more sophisticated and clinically applicable, some tumors of uncertain origin may be reclassified as germ cell neoplasms. Samaniego and colleagues (1990) reported on a large series of germ cell tumors studied by cytogenetics, including for the first time a series of primary mediastinal tumors. They found distinctive abnormalities of chromosome 12 as well as cytologic evidence of gene amplification. In the future, cytogenetic analysis will certainly contribute to diagnostic accuracy of many mediastinal malignancies.

COMMENTS AND CONTROVERSIES

The utility of fine needle aspiration biopsy has increased in recent years due to two main factors. First, cytologic technique has advanced to the point where explicit cytologic criteria now allow a wide variety of specific diagnoses, both benign and malignant. Second, this minimally invasive and cost-effective procedure has gained the enthusiastic support of patients, physicians, and hospitals. More pathologists now receive specific training in the performance and interpretation of the procedure. Many medical centers have now established FNA biopsy services, headed by someone with special training and interest in this modality, who will also emphasize the collaborative efforts among clinician, radiologist, and pathologist to achieve the best and quickest diagnosis.

The diagnosis and typing of lymphoma by cytology remains a controversial area. According to long-standing dogma, an entire lymph node must be examined to achieve a diagnosis because precise classification depends upon architectural features. Also, pathologists without specific training in cytologic procedures and their interpretation are more comfortable working with tissue than with cells when making a diagnosis. The original classification of lymphoma types did indeed rely upon architecture, but now a pathologist with specific training in these techniques should be able to provide a general classification of lymphomas into large cell, small lymphocytic cell, lymphoblastic, and Hodgkin's categories. Most patients can receive treatment based on such a categorization.

L.J.K.
C.N.P.

The mediastinum is a unique anatomic area! There is probably no other region in the body containing such a diverse group of structures and pluripotential cells that allow for development of such a wide variety of tumors and paraneoplastic syndromes. Because of this, investigation of mediastinal masses requires knowledge of lymphology, endocrinology, embryology, and neoplasia. No other area of the body is so tightly packed with such a variety of organs. Detailed knowledge of anatomy is paramount in developing a differential and specific diagnosis of a presenting lesion, since specific diseases and organs involve specific mediastinal regions.

With the advent of refined imaging (nuclear scans, CT, and magnetic resonance imaging [MRI]), the mysteries of the mediastinum have unfolded. Adding the newer techniques of cytology, immunohistochemistry, and genetic imprinting has only further refined our diagnostic ability.

With all the techniques available today, it is rare that a preoperative diagnosis cannot be made for a presenting mediastinal tumor. A combination of imaging, tumor markers, and FNA biopsy makes it unnecessary in most cases for more invasive diagnostic procedures (e.g., open biopsy). It is important that surgeons have available to them in their hospital these less invasive modalities for diagnosis of these lesions, especially since many tumors presenting as mediastinal masses should not be surgically excised but treated with other modalities as definitive therapy or as induction therapy prior to surgical excision. In the future, the rapidly developing field of cell biology will further open this Pandora's box!

R.J.G.

KEY REFERENCES

Meyers JD: Development and application of immunocytochemical staining techniques. Diagn Cytopathol 5:318, 1989

Concise review of the basic principles in immunochemistry and the various immunostaining techniques currently available. Excellent selection of references.

Sneige N, Dekmezian R, Katz RL et al: Morphologic and immunocytochemical evaluation of 220 fine needle aspirates of malignant lymphoma and lymphoid hyperplasia. Acta Cytol 3403:311, 1990

A comprehensive assessment of the usefulness of FNA in the diagnosis of lymphoma.

Sorenson JA, Phelps ME: Physics in Nuclear Medicine. Grune & Stratton, Orlando, 1987

Key text on the science and technology behind nuclear imaging.

Strauss LG, Conti PS: The applications of PET in clinical oncology. J Nucl Med 32:623, 1991

Thorough summary of current clinical applications of PET in oncology.

Weisbrod GL, Lyons DJ, Tao LC et al: Percutaneous fine-needle aspiration biopsy of mediastinal lesions. AJR 143:525, 1984

Excellent series, with concise discussion of diagnostic accuracy of the various lesions encountered during FNA of mediastinal masses.

REFERENCES

Al-Sharabati M, Chittal S, Duga-Neulat I et al: Primary anterior mediastinal B-cell lymphoma. Cancer 67:2579, 1991

Arnold A, Crossman J, Bakhshi A et al: Immunoglobulin-gene re-arrangements as unique clonal markers in human lymphoid neoplasms. N Engl J Med 309:1593, 1983

Battifora H, Sheibini K, Tubbs RR et al: Antikeratin antibodies in tumor diagnosis: distinction between seminoma and embryonal carcinoma. Cancer 54:843, 1984

Battifora H, Sun TT, Bahu RM, Rao S. The use of antikeratin antiserum as a diagnostic tool: thymoma vs lymphoma. Hum Pathol 11:635, 1980

Berkman WA, Chowdhury L, Brown NL, Padleckas R: Value of electron microscopy in cytologic diagnosis of fine-needle biopsy. AJR 140:1253, 1983

Bloomfield CD, Arthur DC, Frizzera G et al: Nonrandom chromosome abnormalities in lymphoma. Cancer Res 43:2975, 1983

Bosl GJ, Dmitrovsky E, Reuter V et al: i(12p): a specific karyotypic abnormality in germ cell tumors (abstr). Proc Am Soc Clin Oncol 8:131, 1989

Brindley LO, Francis FL: Serum lactate dehydrogenase and glutamine-oxalacetic transaminase correlations with measurements of tumor markers during therapy. Cancer Res 23:112, 1963

Broughan TA, O'Donnell JK, Kropilak MD, Esselstyn CB Jr: Use of thallium-technetium parathyroid scans. Cleve Clin J Med 54:179, 1987.

Coleman RE: Single photon emission computed tomography and positron emission tomography in cancer imaging. Cancer 67:1261, 1991

Colquhoun SD, Rosenthal DL, Morton DL: Role of percutaneous fine-needle aspiration biopsy in suspected intrathoracic malignancy. Ann Thorac Surg 51:390, 1991

Coons AH, Creeh HJ, Jones RN: Immunologic properties of an antibody containing a fluorescent group. Proc Soc Exp Biol Med 47:200, 1941

Cristallini EG, Ascani S, Farabi R et al: Fine needle aspiration biopsy in the diagnosis of intrathoracic masses. Acta Cytol 36:416, 1992

Dabbs DJ, Silverman JF: Selective use of electron microscopy in fine needle aspiration cytology. Acta Cytol 32:880, 1988

Dardick I, Yazdi HM, Brosko RT et al: A quantitative comparison of light and electron microscopic diagnoses in specimens obtained by fine-needle aspiration biopsy. Ultrastruct Pathol 15:105, 1991

Das DK, Gupta SK, Datta BN, Sharma SC: FNA cytodiagnosis of non-Hodgkin's lymphoma and its subtyping under working formulation of 175 cases. Diagn Cytopathol 7:487, 1991

Davis RD Jr, Oldham HN Jr, Sabiston DC Jr: Primary cysts and neoplasms of the mediastinum: recent changes in clinical presentation, methods of diagnosis, management, and results. Ann Thorac Surg 44:229, 1987

Diamond LW, Nathwani BN, Rappaport H: Flow cytometry in the diagnosis and classifications of malignant lymphomas and leukemia. Cancer 50:1122, 1982

Dmitrovsky E, Murty VVVS, Moy D et al: Isochromosome 12p in nonseminoma cell lines: karyologic amplification of c-ki-ras$_2$ without point-mutational activation. Oncogene 5:543, 1990

Erwin BC, Brynes RK, Chan WC et al: Percutaneous needle biopsy in the diagnosis and classification of lymphoma. Cancer 57:1074, 1986

Fenoglio-Preiser CM, Willman CL: Molecular biology and the pathologist. Arch Pathol Lab Med 111:601, 1987

Ferguson MK, Lee E, Skinner DB, Little AG: Selective operative approach for diagnosis and treatment of anterior mediastinal masses. Ann Thorac Surg 44:583, 1987

Fischman AJ, Khaw BA, Strauss HW: Quo vadis radioimmune imaging. J Nucl Med 30:1911, 1989

Friedman A, Vugrin D, Golvey R et al: Prognostic significance of serum tumor biomarkers (TM) alfafetoprotein (AFP), beta subunit chorionic gonadotropin (bHCG) and lactate dehydrogenase (LDH) in non-seminomatous germ cell tumors (abstr.) Proc Am Soc Clin Oncol 21:223, 1980

Friedman M, Kim U, Shimaoka K et al: Appraisal of aspiration cytology in management of Hodgkin's disease. Cancer 45:1653, 1980

Graham LS, Keriakes JG, Harris C, Cohen MB: Nuclear medicine from Becquerel to the present. RadioGraphics 9:1189, 1989

Hainsworth JD, Greco FA: Poorly differentiated carcinoma and germ cell tumors. Hematol Oncol Clin North Am 5:1223, 1991a

Hainsworth JD, Greco FA: General features of malignant germ cell tumors and primary seminomas of the mediastinum. p. 211. In Shields TW (ed): Mediastinal Surgery. Lea & Febiger, Malvern, PA, 1991

Hoda SA, Warren GP, Zaman MB: Extrathoracic metastatic malignant thymoma. Diagnosis by aspiration cytology. Arch Pathol Lab Med 115:399, 1991

Hsu SM, Raine L, Fanger H: Use of avidin-biotin-peroxidase complex (ABC) in immunoperoxidase techniques. J Histochem Cytochem 29:577, 1981

Ikezoe J, Morimoto S, Arisawa J et al: Percutaneous biopsy of thoracic lesions. AJR 154:1181, 1990

Ikezoe J, Sone S, Higashihara T et al: Sonographically guided needle biopsy for diagnosis of thoracic lesions. AJR 143:229, 1984

Kardos TF, Vinson JH, Behm FG et al: Hodgkin's disease: diagnosis by fine-needle aspiration biopsy. Am J Clin Pathol 86:286, 1986

Koo CH, Rappaport H, Sheibani K et al: Imprint cytology of non-Hodgkin's lymphomas. Hum Pathol 20(suppl.):1, 1989

Koss LG, Czerniak B, Herz F, Wersto RP: Flow cytometric measurements of DNA and other cell components in human tumors: a critical appraisal. Hum Pathol 20:528, 1989

Koss LG, Woyke S, Olszewski W: Aspiration Biopsy: Cytologic Interpretation and Histologic Basis. Igaku-Shoin, New York, 1984

Kostakoglu L, Yeh SDJ, Portlock C et al: Validation of gallium-67-citrate single-photon emission computed tomography in biopsy-confirmed residual Hodgkin's disease in the mediastinum. J Nucl Med 33:345, 1992

McKitrick WL, Park HM, Kosegi JE: Parallax error in pinhole thyroid scintigraphy: a critical consideration in the evaluation of substernal goiters. J Nucl Med 26:418, 1985

Miettinem M, Virtanen I, Talerman A: Intermediate filament proteins in human testes and testicular germ cell tumors. Am J Pathol 120:402, 1985

Millar J, Allen R, Wakefield JS et al: Diagnosis of thymoma by fine-needle aspiration cytology: light and electron microscopic study of a case. Diagn Cytopathol 3:166, 1987

Moinuddin SM, Lee LH, Montgomery JH: Mediastinal needle biopsy. AJR 143:531, 1984

Motzer RJ, Rodriguez E, Reuter VE et al: Genetic analysis as an aid in diagnosis for patients with midline carcinomas of uncertain histologies. J Natl Cancer Inst 83:341, 1991

Müller-Gärtner H-W, Schneider C: Clinical evaluation of tumor characteristics predisposing serum thyroglobulin to be undetectable in patients with differentiated thyroid cancer. Cancer 61:976, 1988

Nadji M: The potential value of immunoperoxidase techniques in diagnostic cytology. Acta Cytol 2405:442, 1980

Neill J, Silverman JF: Electron microscopy of fine-needle aspiration biopsies of the mediastinum. Diagn Cytopathol 8:272, 1992

Nichols CR: Mediastinal germ cell tumors: clinical features and biologic correlates. Chest 99:472, 1991

Nordenstrom B: Paraxiphoid approach to the mediastinum for mediastinography and mediastinal needle biopsy: a preliminary report. Invest Radiol 2:141, 1967

Park H-M, Tarver RD, Siddiqui AR et al: Efficacy of thyroid scintigraphy in the diagnosis of intrathoracic goiter. AJR 148:527, 1984

Pedersen OM, Aasen TB, Gulsvic A: Fine-needle aspiration biopsy of mediastinal and peripheral pulmonary masses guided by real-time sonography. Chest 89:504, 1986

Pontifex AH, Klimo P: Application of aspiration biopsy cytology to lymphomas. Cancer 53:553, 1984

Robinson PG, Radosevich JA: Mediastinal tumor markers. p. 62. In Shields TW (ed): Mediastinal Surgery. Lea & Febiger, Malvern PA, 1991

Rosai J, Rodriguez HA: Application of electron microscopy to the differential diagnosis of tumors. Am J Clin Pathol 50:555, 1968

Rosenberger A, Adler O: Fine needle aspiration biopsy in the diagnosis of mediastinal lesions. AJR 131:239, 1978

Saito T, Kobayashi H, Sugama Y et al: Ultrasonically guided needle biopsy in the diagnosis of mediastinal masses. Am Rev Respir Dis 138:679, 1988

Samaniego F, Rodriguez E, Houldsworth J et al: Cytogenetic and molecular analysis of human male germ cell tumors: chromosome 12 abnormalities and gene amplification. Genes Chromosomes Cancer 1:289, 1990

Sandler MP, Patton JA, Sacks GA et al: Evaluation of intrathoracic goiter with I-123 scintigraphy and nuclear magnetic resonance imaging. J Nucl Med 25:874, 1984

Sano T, Kuramochi S, Takahashi M et al: A case of thymic cyst with elevated sialylated Lewis X-i, carbohydrate antigen 19-9 and tissue polypeptide antigen in the cystic fluid with no elevation of serum tumor markers. Jpn J Clin Oncol 21:388, 1991

Sawhney S, Jain R, Berry M: Tru-Cut biopsy of mediastinal masses guided by real-time sonography. Clin Radiol 44:16, 1991

Shields TW: Primary mediastinal tumors and cysts and their diagnostic investigation. p. 111. In Shields TW (ed): Mediastinal Surgery. Lea & Febiger, Malvern PA, 1991

Spies WG: Radionuclide studies of the mediastinum. p. 50. In Shields TW (ed): Mediastinal Surgery. Lea & Febiger, Malvern PA, 1991

Sterrett G, Whitaker D, Shilkin KB, Walters MN: The fine-needle aspiration cytology of mediastinal lesions. Cancer 51:127, 1983

Taccagni G, Cantaboni A, Dell'Antonio G et al: Electron microscopy of fine needle aspiration biopsies of mediastinal and paramediastinal lesions. Acta Cytol 32:868, 1988

Taylor CR: Immunomicroscopy: A Diagnostic Tool for the Surgical Pathologist. WB Saunders, Philadelphia, 1986

Taylor CR: Immunoperoxidase techniques. Arch Pathol Lab Med 102:113, 1978

Todd TRJ, Weisbrod G, Tao LC et al: Aspiration needle biopsy of thoracic lesions. Ann Thorac Surg 32:154, 1981

Van Herle AJ, Uller RP: Elevated serum thyroglobulin: a marker of metastases in differentiated thyroid carcinomas. J Clin Invest 56:272, 1975

van Sonnenberg E, Casola G, Ho M et al: Difficult thoracic lesions: CT-guided biopsy experience in 150 cases. Radiology 167:457, 1988

Virchow R: Cellular Pathology: as Based Upon Physiological and Pathological Histology. Translated and edited by Frank Chance. Classics in Medicine Library, Division of Gryphon Editions Ltd, Birmingham, AL, 1978

Westcott JL: Percutaneous needle aspiration of hilar and mediastinal masses. Radiology 141:323, 1981

Wittich GR, Nowels KW, Korn RL et al: Coaxial transthoracic fine-needle biopsy in patients with a history of malignant lymphoma. Radiology 183:175, 1992

Yang PC, Chang DB, Lee YC et al: Mediastinal malignancy: ultrasound guided biopsy through the supraclavicular approach. Thorax 47:377, 1992

Yu C-J, Yang P-C, Chang D-B et al: Evaluation of ultrasonically guided biopsies of mediastinal masses. Chest 100:399, 1991

Yunis JJ, Oken MM, Kaplan ME et al: Distinctive chromosomal abnormalities in histologic subtypes of non-Hodgkin's lymphoma. N Engl J Med 307:1231, 1982

Thymoma

Earle W. Wilkins, Jr.

DEFINITION

Thymomas have been defined by Levine and Rosai (1978) as thymic epithelial neoplasms with minimal or no cytologic atypia. These authors (Rosai and Levine, 1976) justify interpretation of the thymoma as an epithelial tumor on the basis of "their abnormal arrangement and configuration, their presence in invasive and metastatic areas of the tumor, the occasional occurrence of pure epithelial tumors, and the fact that in the rare cytologically malignant thymomas the anaplastic features are restricted to them."

In this definition, lymphocytes within the tumor are not considered neoplastic; "they do not show biologic properties of neoplastic cells." Malignant lymphomas may be primary within the thymus, particularly Hodgkin's disease. Such a tumor is called precisely that, *Hodgkin's disease of the thymus,* and not, as it once was, "granulomatous thymoma."

Similarly, "a seminomatous thymoma" is a germinoma of the thymus, *not* a thymoma, and "a round cell thymoma" is a neuroendocrine carcinoid of the thymus, *not* a thymoma.

HISTORICAL NOTE

Interest in anterior mediastinal tumors and thymoma paralleled early investigation into the nature of myasthenia gravis. Laquer and Weigert (1901) are credited with first identifying the relationship between the thymus and myasthenia gravis. At the autopsy of a patient who had died of myasthenia gravis, the pathologist Carl Weigert had discovered a 3 cm × 5 cm thymic tumor, typically adherent to pericardium and left lung, and he correctly speculated about the possible correlation of myasthenia gravis and thymoma.

Viets and Schwab (1960), in discussing the history of thymectomy for myasthenia gravis, describe Sauerbruch's early surgery including the first thymectomy (transcervical) in a myasthenia gravis patient on March 6, 1911. The patient's myasthenic symptoms were improved, but the thymus showed only an enlarged, hypertrophic gland and not a tumor.

The landmark operation, however, took place on May 26, 1936, when Blalock successfully removed a thymoma from a 19-year-old myasthenic woman (Blalock, et al., 1939). Safe conduct through the operation was made possible by the recent introduction of the anticholinesterase agent neostigmine bromide. Blalock set a pioneering standard in his use of median sternotomy, now the preferred surgical approach to tumors of the anterior mediastinum.

It was the chain of events relating myasthenia gravis to the thymus and leading to Blalock's historic case that led directly to surgery for anterior mediastinal tumors, whether in the myasthenic or the asymptomatic patient.

HISTORICAL READINGS

Blalock A, Mason MF, Morgan HJ, Riven SS: Myasthenia gravis and tumors of the thymic region. Report of a case in which the tumor was removed. Ann Surg 110:544, 1939

Laquer L, Weigert C: Beiträge zur Lehre von der Erbschen Krankheit. 1. Über die Erbschen Krankheit (Myasthenia gravis). 2. Pathologisch-anatomischer Beitrag zur Erbschen Krankheit (Myasthenia gravis). Neurol Zentralbl 20:594, 1901

Viets HR, Schwab RS: Thymectomy for Myasthenia Gravis. Charles C Thomas, Springfield, IL, 1960

PATHOLOGY

Classification

A basic classification of tumors found in the thymus gland is as follows: (1) Primary only in thymus (thymoma, thymolipoma, carcinoid tumor of the thymus, thymic cyst, thymic carcinoma; (2) primary in thymus or anterior mediastinum (lymphoma, germ cell tumors). In a more detailed classification, Marchevsky and Kaneko (1984) grouped tumors of the thymus into tumors originating from (1) thymic epithelium, (2) neuroendocrine cells, (3) germ cells, (4) lymphoid tissue, (5) adipose tissue, and (6) tumors metastatic to the thymus.

The principal tumor of the thymus gland, however, is the thymoma. It is a tumor arising from thymic epithelium, although its microscopic appearance is one of a mixture of lymphocytes and epithelial cells. Bernatz and colleagues (1961) classified the Mayo Clinic operative series into lymphocytic (30 percent), epithelial (16 percent), mixed (30 percent), and spindle cell (24 percent) tumors. The spindle cell is derived from thymic epithelium.

Assessing Malignancy

Determining the malignancy of a thymoma is difficult, even to the point of controversy. Pathologists have been in general

Classification of Tumors of the Thymus

Tumors of the thymic epithelium
    Benign
        Encapsulated thymoma
            Epithelial
            Lymphocytic
            Mixed lymphocytic and epithelial
    Malignant
        Invasive thymoma
            Epithelial
            Lymphocytic
            Mixed lymphocytic and epithelial
        Thymic carcinoma
            Squamous cell carcinoma
            Lymphoepithelioma-like carcinoma
            Basaloid carcinoma
            Mucoepidermoid carcinoma
            Sarcomatoid carcinoma
            Mixed small-cell–undifferentiated-
              squamous cell carcinoma
            Clear-cell carcinoma
            Undifferentiated carcinoma
Tumors of neuroendocrine cell origin
    Carcinoid
    Oat-cell carcinoma
Tumors of germ cell origin
    Seminoma
    Embryonal carcinoma
    Endodermal sinus tumor
    Teratoma
        Benign cystic teratoma
        Immature teratoma
        Malignant teratoma
    Choriocarcinoma
    Combined germ cell tumors
Tumors of lymphoid origin
    Malignant lymphoma
        Hodgkin's disease
        Non-Hodgkin's lymphomas (lymphoblastic,
            etc.)
Tumors of adipose tissue
    Thymolipoma
Metastatic tumors to the thymus

(From Marchevsky AM, Kaneko M: Surgical Pathology of the Mediastinum. p. 58. Raven Press, New York, 1984, with permission.)

agreement that microscopic examination of the epithelial cell does not provide an easy assessment of malignant potential. Marchevsky and Kaneko (1984) state that "most encapsulated, benign thymomas have identical histologic and cytologic features to invasive malignant thymomas." Rosai and Levine (1976) comment that "the surgeon is usually in a better position to assess the invasive nature of a thymoma from the findings at thoracotomy than the pathologist who examines the specimen after removal."

In a discussion of the role of staging in the prognosis and management of thymoma, Wilkins, et al. (1991) concluded that "pathologic staging of thymomas by the method of Masaoka, et al. (1981) should supplement the gross surgical assessment of encapsulation of tumor versus invasion." The surgeon can determine invasion if there is obvious direct involvement of the innominate vein or the lung, for example. However, only the pathologist can determine microscopic invasion into capsule or mediastinal fat.

Staging

The Masaoka pathologic staging is standard:

Stage I	Macroscopic encapsulation (complete) and *no* microscopic invasion
Stage II	Macroscopic invasion into mediastinal fat or pleura *or* microscopic invasion into capsule
Stage III	Macroscopic invasion into pericardium, great vessels, or lung
Stage IVa	Pleural or pericardial dissemination
Stage IVb	Lymphatic or hematogenous metastases

Malignancy of a thymoma then is manifest by direct invasion, gross or microscopic, or by transpleural seeding (so-called droplet metastasis) to remote pleural surfaces. Lymphogenous metastasis of a thymoma is uncommon.

Recent Microscopic Studies

There has been a recent swing back toward the classification of thymomas on the basis of cell types. Marino and Müller-Hermelink (1986) have proposed a subtyping of cortical thymoma, mixed thymoma, and medullary thymoma. The cortical thymoma is composed of medium to large epithelial cells with round or oval nuclei, prominent central nuclei, finely dispersed chromatin, and poorly defined cytoplasm (Fig. 58-2). These tumors have the potential for malignant spread.

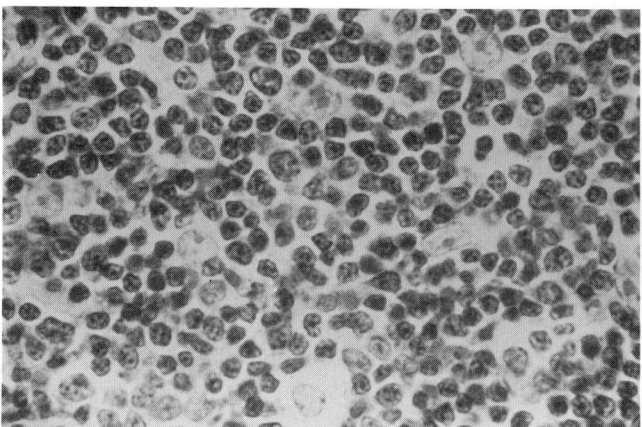

Figure 58-2. Cortical thymoma.

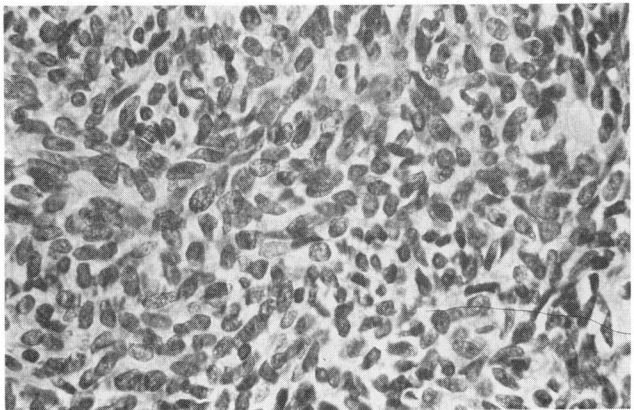

Figure 58-3. Medullary thymoma.

The medullary thymoma is composed of small to medium cells with irregular or spindle-shaped nuclei and no nucleoli (Fig. 58-3). These are benign tumors. The mixed thymoma is obviously a mixture of these two types. A fourth category is the well-differentiated carcinoma, consisting of round-to-oval epithelial cells with mild atypia, sparse mitoses, and very few lymphocytes (Fig. 58-4). It may bear an ominous prognosis, with a likelihood of recurrence.

Pescarmona and associates (1990) have proposed a rather complex prognostic grouping combining the Masaoka pathologic staging and the Marino and Müller-Hermelink cellular classification. Stage I and II medullary thymomas and stage I mixed thymomas have an excellent prognosis; stage III and IV cortical thymomas have a poor prognosis; and stage I and II cortical and plus stage II and III mixed thymomas present an intermediate prognosis.

DIAGNOSIS

The diagnosis of thymoma may be suspected on the basis of its symptoms or of a chest radiograph and suggested by mod-

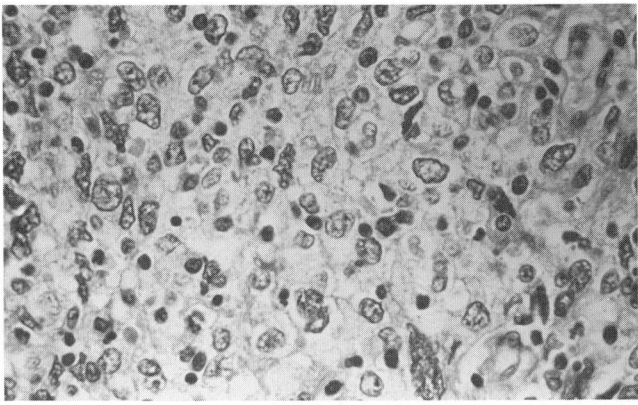

Figure 58-4. Well-differentiated thymic carcinoma.

ern imaging techniques, but it is confirmed only by pathologic evaluation of a specimen.

Clinical Features

A thymoma may be asymptomatic and detected only by routine chest radiography. It may present with symptoms or signs provoked by the local extent of tumor. The more com-

---

Clinical Disorders Associated with Thymomas

Neuromusclular syndromes
    Myasthenia gravis
    Myotonic dystrophy
    Eaton-Lambert syndrome
    Myositis
Hematologic syndromes
    Red cell hypoplasia
    Erythrocytosis
    Pancytopenia
    Megakaryocytopenia
    T-cell lymphocytosis
    Acute leukemia
    Multiple myeloma
Immune deficiency syndromes
    Hypogammaglobulinemia
    T-cell deficiency syndrome
Collagen diseases and autoimmune disorders
    Systemic lupus erythematosus
    Rheumatoid arthritis
    Polymyositis
    Myocarditis
    Sjögren's syndrome
    Scleroderma
Dermatologic diseases
    Pemphigus (vulgaris, erythematosus)
    Chronic mucocutaneous candidiasis
Endocrine disorders
    Hyperparathyroidism
    Hashimoto's thyroiditis
    Addison's disease
    Chemodectoma
Renal diseases
    Nephrotic syndrome
    Minimal-change nephropathy
Bone disorders
    Hypertrophic osteoarthropathy
Malignancy
    Malignant lymphoma (Hodgkin's disease, non-Hodgkin's lymphomas)
    Carcinomas (lung, colon, etc.)
    Kaposi's sarcoma

(From Marchevsky AM, Kaneko M: Surgical Pathology of the Mediastinum. Raven Press, New York, 1984, p. 58 with permission.)

mon of these are chest pain, cough, dyspnea, or in a few cases, venous obstruction. Davis and colleagues (1990) suggest that the absence of symptoms in patients with mediastinal tumors "is reasonably predictive" of a benign neoplasm.

A thymoma may be associated with a systemic or autoimmune disorder. By far the most common of these paraneoplastic syndromes is myasthenia gravis. The presence of this disorder in a patient with an anterior mediastinal tumor is almost always diagnostic of a thymoma. Hematologic syndromes occurring infrequently with thymoma include red blood cell hypoplasia (pure red blood cell agenesis), pancytopenia, and hypogammaglobulinemia. Autoimmune disorders include thyroiditis, systemic lupus erythematosus, polymyositis, myocarditis, and rheumatoid arthritis. A complete listing is provided above.

The 50-year series from 1939 to 1989 from the Massachusetts General Hospital included 164 patients with thymoma, of whom 76 (46 percent) had myasthenia gravis and 88 (54 percent) did not. The presenting chief complaints in this experience are listed in Table 58-4. Fully three-quarters of patients have no local manifestation of thymoma tumor growth.

Natural History

The association of thymoma and myasthenia gravis is still poorly understood. Improvement in the severity of myasthenia, even following total removal of all detectable thymic tissue along with the thymoma, is less likely to occur than following thymectomy in myasthenic patients without tumor. In the Massachusetts General Hospital experience, improvement in myasthenia occurred in 60 percent of patients following thymomectomy, including total thymectomy, compared with 84 percent remission or improvement in nonthymomatous myasthenic patients undergoing thymectomy. Even less understood is the phenomenon of post-thymomectomy development of myasthenia gravis. Five patients in the Massachusetts General Hospital series developed myasthenic symptoms detected only after removal of the thymoma.

No studies have been made of the natural history of the noninvasive thymoma to determine whether an encapsulated stage I tumor may ever progress to an invasive thymoma. Since this is not known, surgical removal of an anterior mediastinal tumor suspected of being a thymoma is recommended for all such patients.

Table 58-4. Presenting Complaints in 164 Patients with Thymoma[a]

Disorder or Symptom	Number	(%)
Myasthenia	76	(46%)
Chest pain	16	
Cough	11	
Dyspnea	10	
Hematologic syndromes[b]	3	
Venous obstruction	2	
Hiccups	1	
Asymptomatic	45	(27%)

[a] Experience at the Massachusetts General Hospital, 1939 to 1989.
[b] One patient each with red cell agenesis, pancytopenia and hypogammaglobulinemia.

Differential Diagnosis

In the differential diagnosis of thymoma (see listing of Murchevsky and Kaneko's classification), the most frequently encountered tumor is the malignant lymphoma, most commonly Hodgkin's disease. It also presents the greatest difficulty in deciding on appropriate management. A useful guideline is that if enlarged regional lymph nodes are identified on CT or physical examination, the tumor is not a thymoma. Other less frequent tumors occurring in the thymus are the carcinoid tumor (Economopoulos, et al., 1990), thymic cyst, and thymolipoma. CT may suggest the diagnosis in the latter two but only excision is confirmatory.

Investigative Techniques

The standard screening study in searching for an anterior mediastinal tumor has always been the biplanar chest x-ray, posteroanterior (PA) and lateral views. The two oblique radiologic views add to the accuracy of detection. CT, however, has become the definitive radiographic study (Fig. 58-5). Spatial resolution and cross-sectional anatomy permit detection of small thymic tumors and the presence of mediastinal adenopathy. It is particularly useful in detecting and differentiating thymic and other mediastinal cysts, such as the pericardial cyst or dermoid. Although disruption of normal fat planes is suggestive of invasion by a thymoma, this must not be considered definitive. The presence of pleural implantation of thymoma is readily identified by CT (Fig. 58-6). Contrast-enhanced CT is useful in assessing vascular invasion, although MRI may provide evidence of vascular involvement without the need for invasive contrast study. In situations of real doubt and concern, such as differentiation of a thoracic aortic aneurysm, angiographic study may be necessary. The angiogram not only provides help in diagnosis but is a reassuring road map for the surgeon.

Radioisotope scanning has limited utility in defining a thymoma from its differential tumors, although where a substernal or ectopic thyroid is a concern, radioactive iodine scanning may be helpful. Pneumomediastinography has never been widely applied, and ultrasound is seldom helpful. Mediastinoscopy leads one into the middle mediastinum; the aortic arch and left innominate vein preclude direct access to the anterior mediastinum. However, mediastinoscopy *is* useful in the search for mediastinal lymph nodes if one suspects Hodgkin's disease.

Direct biopsy, either by percutaneous FNA or by anterior (Chamberlain) mediastinotomy is the only investigative approach providing diagnostic proof. In the former, cytologic differentiation from lymphoma is difficult; in the latter, there is a risk of transpleural implantation of thymoma.

MANAGEMENT

The thymoma is a slowly growing tumor with an overall relatively low malignant potential. Surgical removal is the cornerstone of therapy. In general, biopsy of a thymoma is to be avoided unless the patient is an unsuitable candidate for surgery or unless preoperative radiation therapy is desirable because of the magnitude of tumor involvement. The Toronto

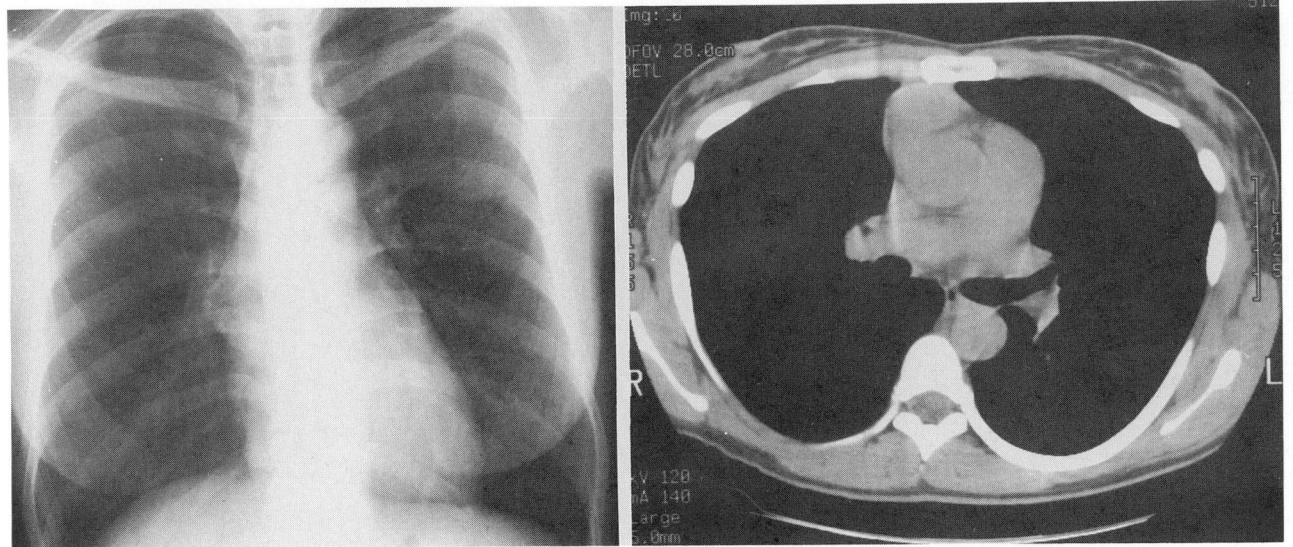

Figure 58-5. **(A)** Posteroanterior chest film and **(B)** CT section demonstrate a moderate-sized asymptomatic thymoma on the right side of the mediastinum.

group (Shamji, et al., 1984) speculated on the use of preoperative radiotherapy for large, apparently invasive thymomas in an effort to reduce the bulk of tumor and "to prevent transpleural metastatic seeding at the time of operation." It is their policy "to use preoperative radiotherapy for large tumors which are believed to be invasive on the basis of roentgenogram, CT scan, or preoperative anterior mediastinotomy for biopsy."

Principles

The basic principles underlying successful surgical therapy are (1) operative access via a complete median sternotomy;

(2) wide opening of both pleural sacs; (3) total thymectomy, including all normal thymic tissue; (4) extended resection of invasive (stage III) tumors, including pericardium, lung, innominate vein, or superior vena cava; and (5) excision of all pleural implants (stage IVa).

Operative Technique

The incisions appropriate for surgery on the thymus are presented in Figure 58-7. The purely cervical approach, which provides acceptable visualization of the nonthymomatous gland in skilled hands, has no role in thymoma surgery. It is seldom necessary as an extension of the median sternotomy

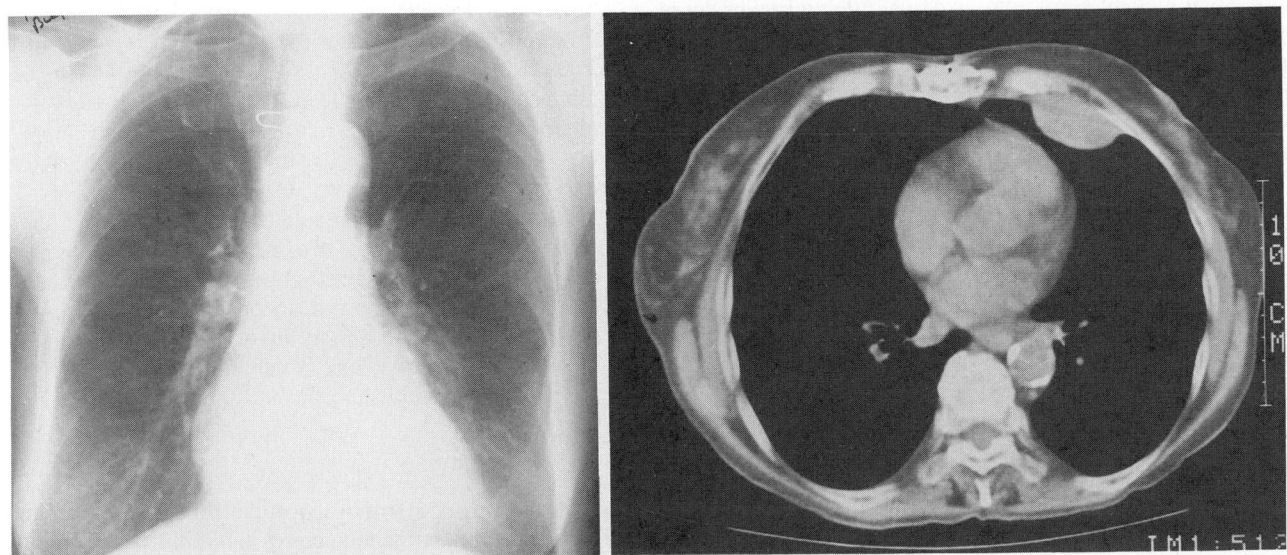

Figure 58-6. **(A)** Recurrent thymoma in a woman with myasthenia gravis; **(B)** CT defines the exact pleural location.

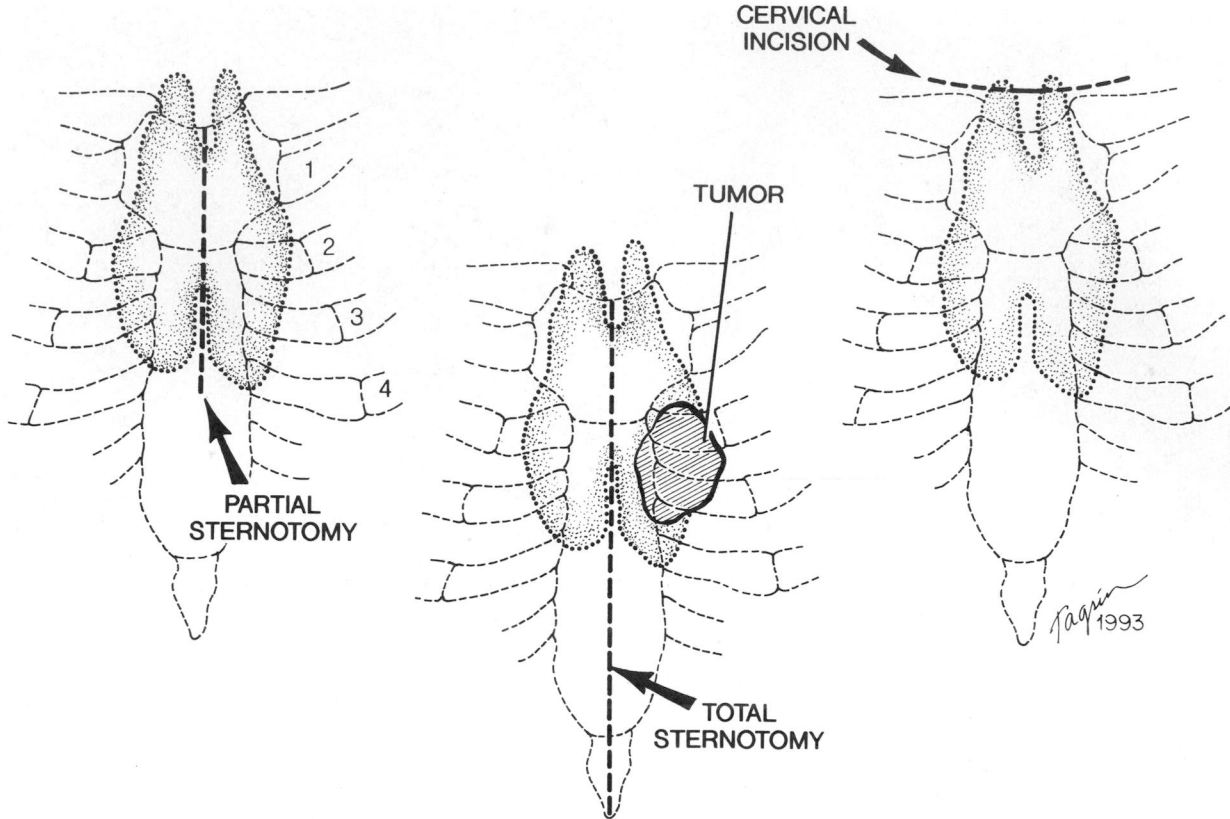

Figure 58-7. The three standard incisional approaches to the thymus gland. In the case of thymoma, only the total median sternotomy permits observation of the essential principles of surgical removal.

incision (the combined cervicosternotomy) unless the tumor extends into the neck itself. The partial sternotomy, which provides excellent exposure for nonthymomatous thymectomy for myasthenia gravis, is not adequate for full assessment of the posterolateral extent of a thymoma, possible involvement of the phrenic nerves, or transpleural implantation. Total median sternotomy carries little additional morbidity as compared with partial upper sternotomy and when combined with bilateral pleurotomy, affords maximal exposure. The surgeon is responsible for gross tumor staging.

Lateral thoracotomy, although it permits easy access to an encapsulated thymoma lying in one lobe, makes total thymectomy more difficult. The occurrence, infrequent as it is, of myasthenia gravis post-thymomectomy, as well as the occasional finding of microscopic tumor in grossly normal thymus, makes total thymectomy desirable. Transverse sternal approaches have no role; the sternum becomes unstable and patient morbidity is high.

Every effort should be made to resect all gross tumor, both that involved by direct invasive extension and that resulting from transpleural seeding. The anterior pericardium can be removed with impunity. Sacrificing a phrenic nerve requires caution, particularly in the myasthenic, emphysematous, or aged patient. In general, it is safe to remove one phrenic nerve, although this may prolong respiratory weaning of the myasthenic patient. Involved lung usually can be resected by wedge stapling, although the surgeon should be prepared

for segmentectomy or lobectomy. Rarely, a pneumonectomy or even extrapleural pneumonectomy may be necessary, but then only in the young or healthy, physiologically uncompromised patient. The left innominate vein can be readily taken, and the superior vena cava too, by lateral excision and patch grafting with pericardium or vein or by total circumferential removal and spiral venous graft replacement. The threat of thrombosis of the graft in the latter maneuver dictates that it should be reserved for those situations in which the thymoma is clearly removable in all its other parameters. Parietal pleural implants can be removed by pleural stripping. Diaphragmatic implants are better removed by full-thickness excision of diaphragm.

A word of caution is necessary. Radiotherapy is a reasonably effective alternative to excision. It may be used preoperatively for large tumors or for those compromising vital structures. I have encountered an operative death in a young patient with marked airway involvement during anesthesia induction; radiation even without biopsy confirmation would have been preferable.

Thoracoscopy

Is there a place for thoracoscopic removal of a thymoma? Not if the surgical tenets expressed in the principles of management above are followed. Nonetheless, thoracoscopic excision of a thymoma is technically possible, as described by

Landreneau and collaborators (1992). Complete removal of a 5-cm encapsulated thymoma was carried out in 245 minutes. Discharge was possible on the third day, with a return to full activity by the fifth. The authors suggest thoracoscopic evaluation followed, if there is no evidence of invasion or tumor implantation, by endoscopic resection. Thus this approach should be limited to stage I lesions. The limitation would seem to depend then on the reliability of endoscopic assessment of stage prior to removal. The pathologic determination of stage II is frequently dependent on microscopic evaluation of not only the tumor but the entire thymus. As Pairolero stated in the invited commentary on the paper by Landreneau, et al., "only time will resolve these issues."

Perioperative Care

Perioperative care is straightforward except in patients with myasthenia gravis, in whom withdrawal of all cholinergic medication is combined with nasotracheal respiratory ventilatory support until extubation is possible. Cholinergic maintenance therapy (Mestinon) is not resumed before 48 to 72 hours postsurgery in the severe myasthenic patient. Preoperative plasmapheresis should be considered; this is usually undertaken as three exchanges in the week prior to surgery.

Early Results

Operative experience at the Massachusetts General Hospital since the establishment of the General Thoracic Surgical Service in 1971 coincides with a period when the care of patients with myasthenia gravis made this condition no longer a threat to survival. This is in contrast to an earlier report (Wilkins, et al., 1966). In a series of 85 consecutive patients from 1972 to 1989 (Wilkins, et al., 1991), 32 with myasthenia gravis and 53 without, there were no operative deaths. The patients ranged in age from 13 to 81 and included 39 males and 46 females. Total removal of gross tumor was possible in 81 patients (95 percent); two patients underwent subtotal removal and two biopsy only. Extended thymomectomy was necessary in 21 patients: lung in 11, phrenic nerve in 5, innominate vein in 3, and pleural implants in 2. Pericardial removal was carried out in 17, although not all for tumor extension. There were four deaths in the first postoperative year, three related to residual thymoma or radiation therapy.

Late Results

In this series there were two thymoma-related deaths within 5 years and four more within 10 years. There is general agreement that the 10-year interval is the proper time standard for measuring success in the surgical therapy of thymoma. Actuarial 10-year survival in relation to the Masaoka pathologic staging is presented in Figure 58-8. There is no statistical difference between the 10-year survival of 45 stage I patients (78 percent) and 23 stage II patients (75 percent). The difference between these stages and 14 stage III patients (21 percent) is significant at a level of $P = .0003$.

Comparable statistics are presented in the report of 52 patients from the University of Toronto group (Shamji, et al., 1984). Cumulative survival at 5 years in stage I patients was 96 percent, in stage II 80 percent, and in stage III 42 percent, as compared with 90, 96, and 58 percent, respectively at Massachusetts General Hospital. They concluded that prognosis "is not significantly influenced by the presence or absence of coexisting myasthenia gravis." This conclusion was also reached in the recent Massachusetts General Hospital series, with the additional finding that this was true regardless of the final pathologic staging of the tumor.

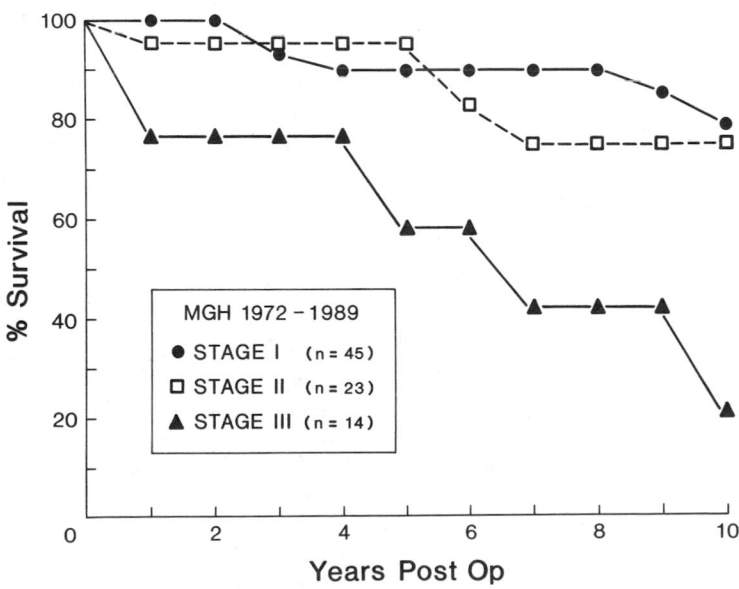

Figure 58-8. The 10-year survival curves for 82 patients with Masaoka stages I to III thymoma reveals no statistical difference between stages I and II but a significant (P = .0003) difference for stage III. (From Wilkins EW Jr, Grillo HC, Scannell JG et al: Role of staging in prognosis and management of thymoma. Am Thorac Surg 51:152, 1991, with permission.)

A recent University of Turin report (Maggi, et al., 1991) of a study of 241 operated cases suggests that thymoma patients with myasthenia gravis actually did better, possibly owing to earlier detection because of the symptoms of myasthenia. Overall survival at 10 years was 87 percent for patients with encapsulated thymoma, 62 percent for those with local inva-sion, and 40 percent for those with pleural seeding. An intriguing finding was the minimal impact of postoperative radiation in the 100 patients with invasive thymoma: tumor relapse occurred in 21 percent of those who received radiotherapy and 25 percent of those who did not.

COMMENTS AND CONTROVERSIES

At this stage in the evaluation of the treatment of thymoma, the Massachusetts General Hospital conclusions (Wilkins, et al., 1991) seem eminently reasonable.

1. Pathologic staging of thymomas by the method of Masaoka should supplement the gross surgical assessment of encapsulation of tumor versus invasion.
2. Stage I thymoma patients do not require adjuvant therapy but all stage II and III patients should receive postoperative radiotherapy.
3. Thymoma patients are at risk for late tumor recurrence and should be carefully followed for at least 10 years. The 10-year actuarial survival is the standard.

It seems clear that surgical extirpation is the treatment of choice for thymoma. A perhaps less clear principle, though certainly not a controversial one, is the possibility of reoperation for recurrence of thymoma, especially if total gross tumor removal was possible at the primary procedure. Among the conclusions drawn by Kirschner (1990) in his review of his personal experience with reoperation in 23 patients with thymoma are (1) "reoperation is a valid accessory to an unsuccessful initial operation"; (2) "reoperation is based on anatomical, pathological, histological, and behavioral features of thymus and thymoma"; (3) the "presence of myasthenia gravis does not have a deleterious effect on reoperation"; and (4) "reoperation is safe." Ohmi and Ohuchi (1990) claim that removing recurrent thymoma from the pleura of three patients was "not only easy to perform but also was extremely effective in improving myasthenic symptoms." This is unusual.

A possibly controversial decision is the need for preoperative tissue confirmation of thymoma. The conclusion that the possibility of risking recurrence is unwarranted is suggested by the combined findings of an anterior mediastinal tumor, the absence of adenopathy on CT study, the propensity for local implantation of tumor, which is increased with biopsy or inadvertent spillage of tumor, and the safety of median sternotomy for thymomectomy. A valid exception, as previously stated, is irradiation for unusually large, bulky, or invasive thymomas.

There is no need for preoperative differentiation of other tumors primary in the mediastinum; the same principles of therapy apply. Occasionally, a pathologist will return a diagnosis of lymphoma, usually Hodgkin's disease. As Keller and Castleman (1974) described in a study of Hodgkin's disease of the thymus gland, it may occur only in the thymus, in both the thymus and regional lymph nodes, or in just the nodes of the anterior mediastinum. CT study should suggest the proper diagnosis in the latter two situations and lead to proper diagnostic biopsy. When Hodgkin's disease is confined to the thymus, however, prognosis is not worsened if mediastinal irradiation and chemotherapy are applied post-thymectomy.

The ability of the pathologist to define malignancy in a thymoma does remain controversial. The conventional wisdom of Rosai and Levine (1976), quoted earlier, is certainly challenged by Müller-Hermelink who, in his lifelong study of the pathology of thymoma, believes his categorization of thymomas into medullary and cortical tumors provides the basis for determining malignant potential (Marino and Müller-Hermelink, 1985). Wick (1990) stated his belief "that staging procedures predicated on the degree of tumor invasion are still the best prognosticators for thymoma."

A final point of controversy is the role of, or need for, radiotherapy postoperatively. The report of Maggi, et al. (1991) suggests a minimal impact of irradiation for patients with invasive thymoma. Yet, Curran and colleagues (1988) reported a relapse rate of 53 percent in patients with invasive thymoma not subjected to postoperative radiotherapy, compared with zero (stage II) and 21 percent (stage III or higher) in patients who did undergo postoperative irradiation. It seems wiser to be generous in the application of radiotherapy—that is, to provide it to all patients in whom any degree of invasion is determined pathologically. A full mediastinal dosage of 4,500 to 5,000 cGy is recommended.

The role of chemotherapy is not controversial; it is just not yet clear. Göldel and colleagues (1989), in a retrospective study of 22 cases, suggested combination chemotherapy as the first-line measure in the management of incompletely removed thymomas. Kirschner (1990) preferred chemotherapy over radiotherapy in patients with initially inoperable thymoma in preparing them for reoperation. In general, combination chemotherapy regimens used for thymoma have been similar to the protocols used in treating malignant lymphoma (e.g., cyclophosphamide, hydroxydoxorubicin, Oncovin, and prednisone [CHOP]). There is need for analysis of results obtained in greater numbers of invasive thymoma patients treated by chemotherapy. This can only be accomplished by a multi-institutional study comparing treated and control groups of patients.

One of the larger reported series is that of Fornasiero and colleagues (1991), who between 1977 and 1990 treated 37 patients with invasive (stage III/IV) thymoma. Their regimen (ADOC) included cisplatin 50 mg/m^2 IV and doxorubicin 40 mg/m^2 on day 1, vincristine 0.6 mg/m^2 on day 3, and cyclophosphamide 700 mg/m^2 on day 4, all given intravenously. This program was recycled at monthly intervals for a median average of five treatments. Complete remission, defined as clinical disappearance of all tumor, was achieved in 43 percent of patients and partial remission in another 49 percent. Two patients in the complete remission group lived in excess of 96 months, and median survival was 12 months. Of the 92 percent of patients responding (complete plus partial remissions), five survived beyond 96 months, and median survival was 15 months. The authors concluded that platinum-containing combinations show "consistent efficacy." They suggest exploratory surgery in these stage III/IV responding patients after four cycles of ADOC.

E.W.W.

KEY REFERENCES

Marino M, Müller-Hermelink HK: Thymoma and thymic carcinoma: relation of thymoma epithelial cells to the cortical and medullary differentiation of thymus. Virchows Arch [A] 407: 119, 1985

An attempt once again to estimate the malignancy of thymoma on its histologic appearance. Müller-Hermelink, the present chief of pathology at University of Würzburg, has spent a lifetime looking at the epithelial cell of the thymus.

Masaoka A, Monden Y, Nakahara K, Tanioka T: Follow-up study of thymoma with special reference to their clinical stages. Cancer 48:2485, 1981

Definition of the factors defining the basic staging of the thymoma. This permits meaningful comparison among reported series.

Pescarmona E, Rendina EA, Venuta F et al: Analysis of prognostic factors and clinicopathologic staging of thymoma. Ann Thorac Surg 50:534, 1990

An integration of the Masaoka staging with the Müller-Hermelink histologic classification for a new, complex prognostic system.

Shamji F, Pearson FG, Todd TRJ et al: Results of surgical treatment for thymoma. J Thorac Cardiovasc Surg 87:43, 1984

A 10-year experience from a leading general thoracic surgical teaching center, with a host of clinical clues and suggestions in management.

Wilkins EW Jr, Grillo HC, Scannell JG et al: Role of staging in prognosis and management of thymoma. Ann Thorac Surg 51:888, 1991

The J. Maxwell Chamberlain Memorial paper at the 1991 meeting of The Society of Thoracic Surgeons. The surgeon's operative assessment combined with microscopic examination of the specimen's margins constitutes the best prognosticator for thymoma.

REFERENCES

Bernatz PE, Harrison EG, Clagett OT: Thymoma: a clinicopathologic study. J Thorac Cardiovasc Surg 42:424, 1961

Blalock A, Mason MF, Morgan HJ, Riven SS: Myasthenia gravis and tumors of the thymic region. Report of a case in which the tumor was removed. Ann Surg 110:544, 1939

Curran WJ, Kornstein MJ, Brooks JJ et al: Invasive thymoma: the role of mediastinal irradiation following complete or incomplete surgical resection. J Clin Oncol 6:1722, 1988

Davis RD Jr, Oldham HN Jr, Sabiston DC Jr: The mediastinum. p. 507. In Sabiston DC Jr, Spencer FC (eds): Surgery of the Chest. WB Saunders, Philadelphia, 1990

Economopoulos GC, Lewis JW Jr, Lee MW, Silverman NA: Carcinoid tumors of the thymus. Ann Thorac Surg 50:58, 1990

Fornasiero A, Daniele O, Ghiotto C et al: Chemotherapy for invasive thymoma. Cancer 68:30, 1991

Göldel N, Böning L, Fredrik A et al: Chemotherapy of invasive thymoma: a retrospective study of 22 cases. Cancer 63:1493, 1989

Keller AR, Castleman B: Hodgkin's disease of thymus gland. Cancer 33:1615, 1974

Kirschner PA: Reoperation for thymoma: report of 23 cases. Ann Thorac Surg 49:550, 1990

Landreneau RJ, Dowling RD, Castillo WM et al: Thoracoscopic resection of an anterior mediastinal tumor. Ann Thorac Surg 54:142 1992

Laquer L, Weigert C: Beiträge zur Lehre von den Erbschen Krankheit. 1. Über die Erbschen Krankheit (Myasthenia gravis). 2. Pathologisch-anatomischer Beitrag zur Erbschen Krankheit (Myasthenia gravis). Neurol Zentralbl 20:594, 1901

Levine GD, Rosai J: Thymic hyperplasia and neoplasia: a review of current concepts. Hum Pathol 9:495, 1978

Maggi G, Casadio C, Cavallo A et al: Thymoma: results of 241 operated cases. Ann Thorac Surg 51:152, 1991

Marchevsky AM, Kaneko M: Surgical Pathology of the Mediastinum. p. 58. Raven Press, New York, 1984

Ohmi M, Ohuchi M: Recurrent thymoma in patients with myasthenia gravis. Ann Thorac Surg 50:243, 1990

Rosai J, Levine GD: Tumors of the thymus. p. 34. In Atlas of Tumor Pathology. 2nd Ser. Fascicle 13. Armed Forces Institute of Pathology, Washington, 1976

Viets HR, Schwab RS: Thymectomy for Myasthenia Gravis, p. 3. Charles C Thomas, Springfield, IL, 1960

Wick MR: Assessing the prognosis of thymomas. Ann Thorac Surg 50:521, 1990

Wilkins EW Jr, Edmunds LH, Castleman B: Cases of thymoma at the Massachusetts General Hospital. J Thorac Cardiovasc Surg 52:322, 1966

Germ Cell Tumors

Paul F. Waters

DEFINITION

Germ cell tumors are a group of neoplasms that usually arise in the gonadal tissues—the ovaries or testicles. Occasionally they arise in extragonadal sites, of which the mediastinum is an example. Indeed, the mediastinum is the most common site of such extragonadal germ cell tumors, which account for approximately 10 percent of primary mediastinal tumors and 20 percent of all anterior and superior mediastinal masses and are the fourth most common tumor of the mediastinum in adults and the third in children. Mediastinal germ cell tumors may be classified as follows:

Teratoma
    Mature, solid
    Cystic (dermoid cysts)
    Immature
    Malignant (teratocarcinoma)
    Mixed
Seminoma (germinoma)
Embryonal carcinoma
Endodermal sinus tumor (yolk sac tumor)
Choriocarcinoma
Mixed germ cell tumor

HISTORICAL NOTE

Kantrowitz (1934), Laipply and Shipley (1945), and Caes and Cragg (1947) described these tumors initially, while the entity of pure mediastinal seminoma was first outlined by Friedman (1951). Fine (1951) suggested that extragonadal malignant germ cell tumors arise from primitive germ cells in the endoderm of the yolk sac or from the urogenital ridge. Normally these cells are expected to migrate into the scrotum during development. When this migration fails and rests remain in the mediastinum, tumors may develop. A different hypothesis was put forth by Schlumberger in 1946. He postulated that totipotential cells that become detached during embryogenesis give rise to primitive rests, which may subsequently develop these germ cell tumors. At the moment neither theory is proven. Most workers accept the postulated extragonadal site of origin of these tumors. However, there remains some question as to whether the tumors represent primaries or metastatic disease from occult gonadal pri-

maries. The latter view is supported by reports of patients with mediastinal germ cell tumors accompanied with small testicular primaries, carcinoma in situ, or fibrous scars, as described by Meares and Briggs (1972), Azzopardi, et al. (1961), and Daugaard, et al. (1987). The former theory, that of an extragonadal origin, is far more attractive as the evidence accumulates. Several autopsy series have examined patients with presumed extragonadal germ cell tumors very extensively and carefully, looking for occult gonadal primaries or even scar tissue to suggest regressed disease. These findings were extraordinarily rare, as described by Oberman and Libcke (1964), Cox (1975), and Luna and Valenzuela-Tamariz (1976). Autopsy reports in patients with testicular germ cell tumors by Lynch and Blewitt (1953) and Luna and Johnson (1975) did not reveal mediastinal metastases in a large number of patients. Additional convincing evidence is provided by patients with mediastinal germ cell tumors treated with radiotherapy who have not developed testicular recurrences. Mediastinal germ cell tumors are therefore regarded and treated as a separate oncologic problem. It is interesting to note that the history of mediastinal germ cell tumors is relatively brief. Advances in the therapy and management of these entities over the last few decades have been dramatic.

HISTORICAL READINGS

Azzopardi JG, Mostofi FK, Theiss EA: Lesions of testes observed in certain patients with widespread choriocarcinoma and related tumors. Am J Pathol 38:207, 1961

Caes JH, Cragg RW: Extragenital choriocarcinoma of the male with bilateral gynecomastia—report of a case. US Navy Med Bull 47:1072, 1947

Cox JD: Primary malignant germinal tumors of the mediastinum. Cancer 36:1162, 1975

Daugard G et al: Carcinoma-in-situ testis in patients with assumed extragonadal germ cell tumors. Lancet 2:528, 1987

Fine F, Smith RW Jr, Pachter MR: Primary extragenital choriocarcinoma in the male subject. Case report and review of the literature. Am J Med 32:776, 1962

Friedman NB: The comparative morphogenesis of extragenital and gonadal teratoid tumors. Cancer 4:265, 1951

Kantrowitz AR: Extragenital chorionepithelioma in a male. Am J Pathol 10:531, 1934

Laipply TC, Shipley RA: Extragenital choriocarcinoma in the male. Am J Pathol 21:921, 1945

Luna MA, Johnson DE: Postmortem findings in testicular tumors. In Johnson DE (ed): Testicular Tumors. Medical Examination Publishing, New York, 1975

Luna MA, Valenzuela-Tamariz J: Germ-cell tumors of the mediastinum, postmortem findings. Am J Clin Pathol 65:450, 1976

Lynch MJG, Blewitt GL: Choriocarcinoma arising in the male mediastinum. Thorax 8:157, 1953

Meares EM, Briggs EM: Occult seminoma of the testis masquerading as primary extragonadal germinal neoplasm. Cancer 30:300, 1972

Schlumberger HG: Teratoma of anterior mediastinum in groups of military age: study of 16 cases and review of theories of genesis. Arch Pathol 41:398, 1946

ETIOLOGY

The cause of malignant germ cell tumors of the mediastinum is unknown. Their incidence is increased, however, in men with Klinefelter syndrome. This syndrome is associated with elevated gonadotropin levels, azoospermia, and hypogonadism. Chromosomal studies reveal an extra X chromosome. Authors describing this increased incidence include Doll, et al. (1976), Sogge, et al. (1979), Curry, et al. (1981), Chaussain, et al. (1980) and Lachman, et al. (1986). The average age of Klinefelter syndrome patients who develop mediastinal germ cell tumors is 10 years younger than that of those who do so without the syndrome. It is postulated that the chromosome abnormality in Klinefelter syndrome may cause an increased incidence of chromosome disjunction and through this mechanism a higher possibility of malignant transformation.

Carrol, et al. (1987) state that many patients who develop extragonadal germ cell tumors will demonstrate other evidence of germ cell defects. They describe patients diagnosed as having extragonadal germ cell tumors, which are associated with infertility and various abnormalities on testicular biopsies. Additionally, these patients often demonstrate ab-

normally low levels of testosterone and increased levels of luteinizing hormone and estradiol. These observations suggest a primary germ cell defect, which may cause defective spermatogenesis and also predispose to extragonadal malignancy.

INCIDENCE

Malignant germ cell tumors of the mediastinum are uncommon. In general, germ cell tumors account for 10 percent of primary mediastinal tumors and 20 percent of all anterior and superior mediastinal masses. From 1 to 5 percent of all germ cell neoplasms occur in the mediastinal location, as reported by Collins and Pugh (1964) and Einhorn and Williams (1980). In earlier studies, inability to distinguish a germ cell tumor by immunohistochemical techniques in cases of poorly differentiated carcinoma in the mediastinum, as well as the lack of other more modern diagnostic tools, probably resulted in underestimation of the incidence of these neoplasms. Malignant germ cell tumors of the mediastinum are very rare in women, usually occurring in men in the 20- to 35-year age range. One-third of all malignant germ cell tumors of the mediastinum are pure seminomatous in histology.

CLINICAL FEATURES

The characteristic presentation of these neoplasms depends on their histology. The benign tumors usually come to attention as asymptomatic mediastinal masses, while those that are malignant may cause symptoms because of compression or invasion of surrounding structures such as the airway, esophagus, and great vessels. With certain of these tumors, serum markers such as AFP, β-HCG, and LDH are markedly elevated. Aside from plain radiographic studies, CT scan and MRI examination have been very useful in determining their precise anatomic relationships and morphologic characteristics (Figs. 58-9 through 58-12). The CT scan is superior. If

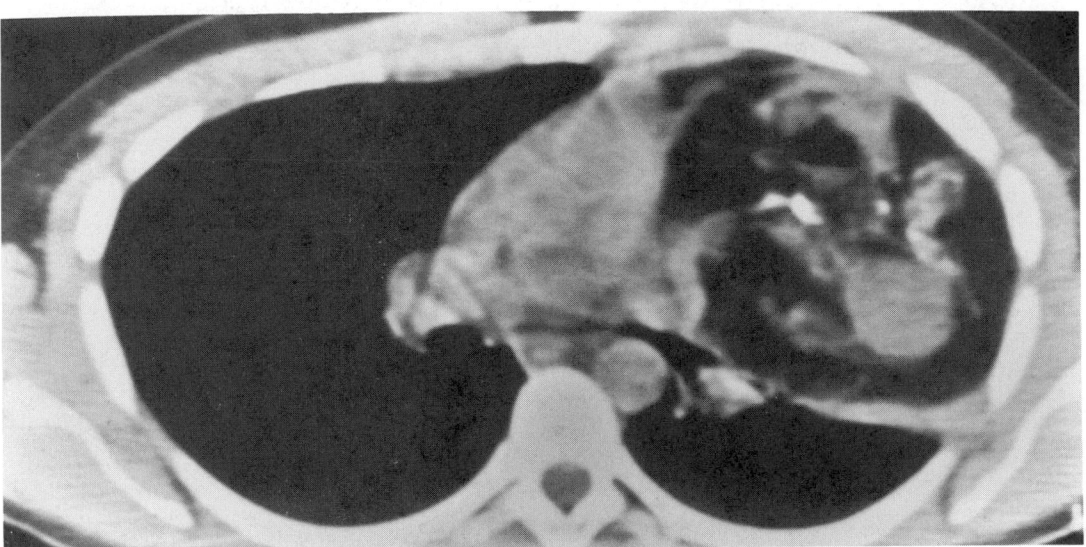

Figure 58-9. CT scan of benign teratoma also shown in Figure 58-13 shows heterogeneous density containing soft tissue elements, fat, and scattered foci of calcification. This is the classic appearance on CT of benign teratoma.

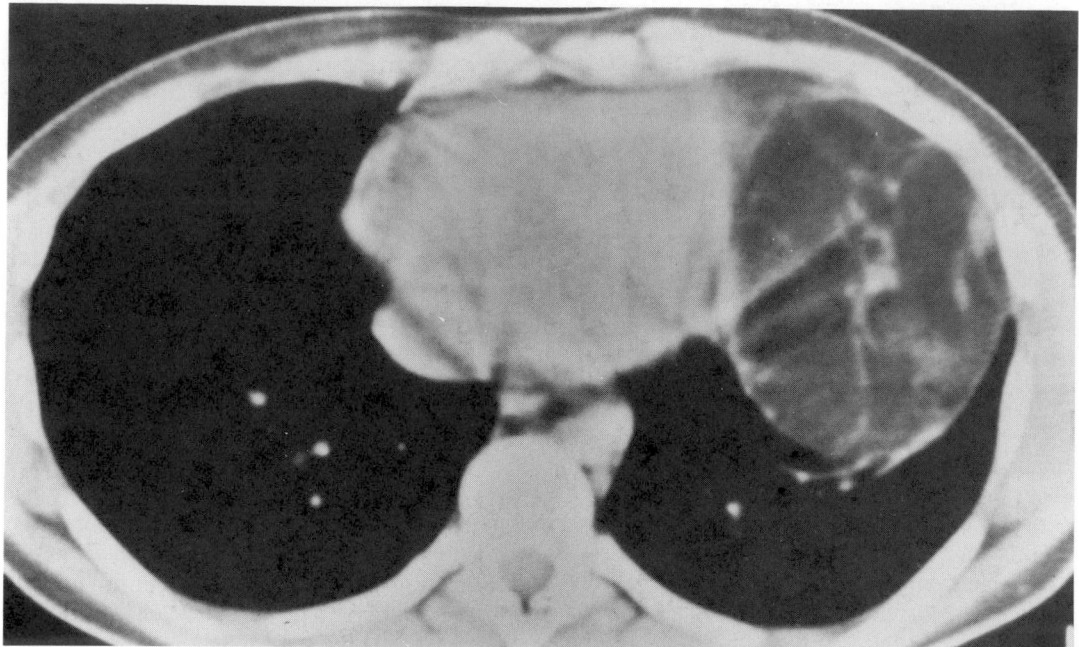

Figure 58-10.   CT scan of the same teratoma at a lower level than in Figure 58-9 shows the tumor to contain predominantly fat in the lower portion.

resection is being considered, angiography, either conventional or MRI, should be considered. Examination of both the pulmonary and left-sided circulations may be necessary.

In general, unless pathognomonic radiologic features are present or serum markers are markedly elevated, tissue will be required for diagnosis. In most institutions the first ap-proach will be a cytologic one. Aspiration needle biopsy may easily be performed percutaneously in most cases. Trans-bronchial needle biopsy is sometimes an option if tumor is seen on the CT scan to be intimately applied to the trachea or carina. The percutaneous route is preferable. Where excel-lent and reliable cytology is available, this will be all that is

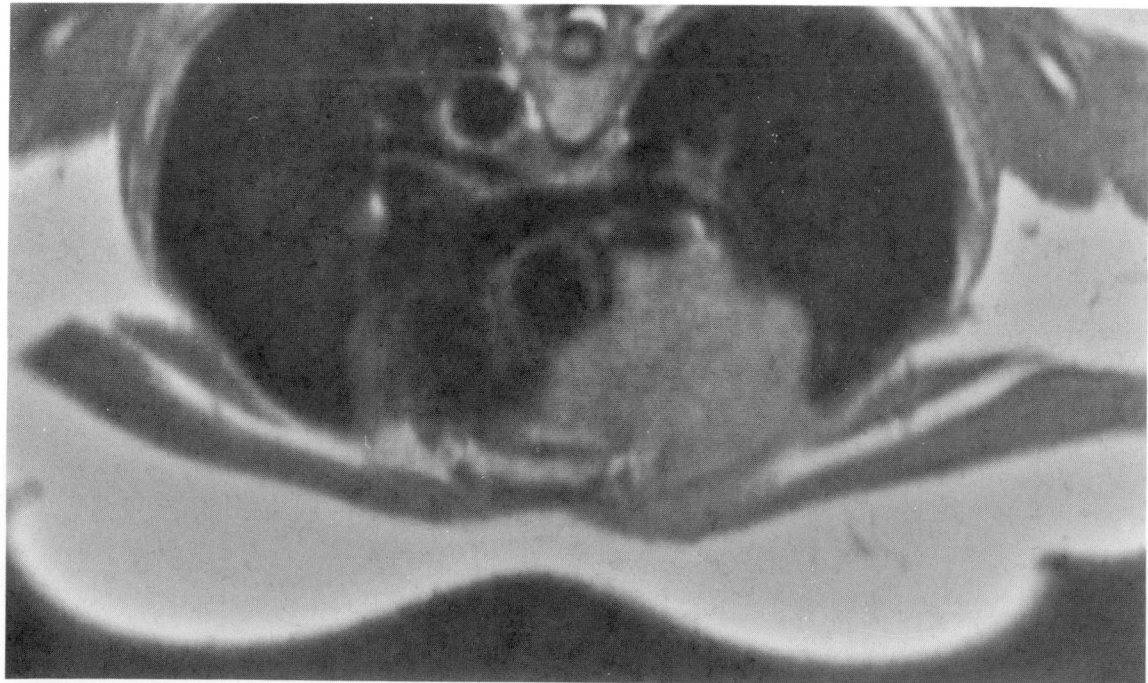

Figure 58-11.   Axial MRI scan (T_1-weighted) of patient in Figure 58-17 demonstrates a large homogeneous mass of intermediate signal density.

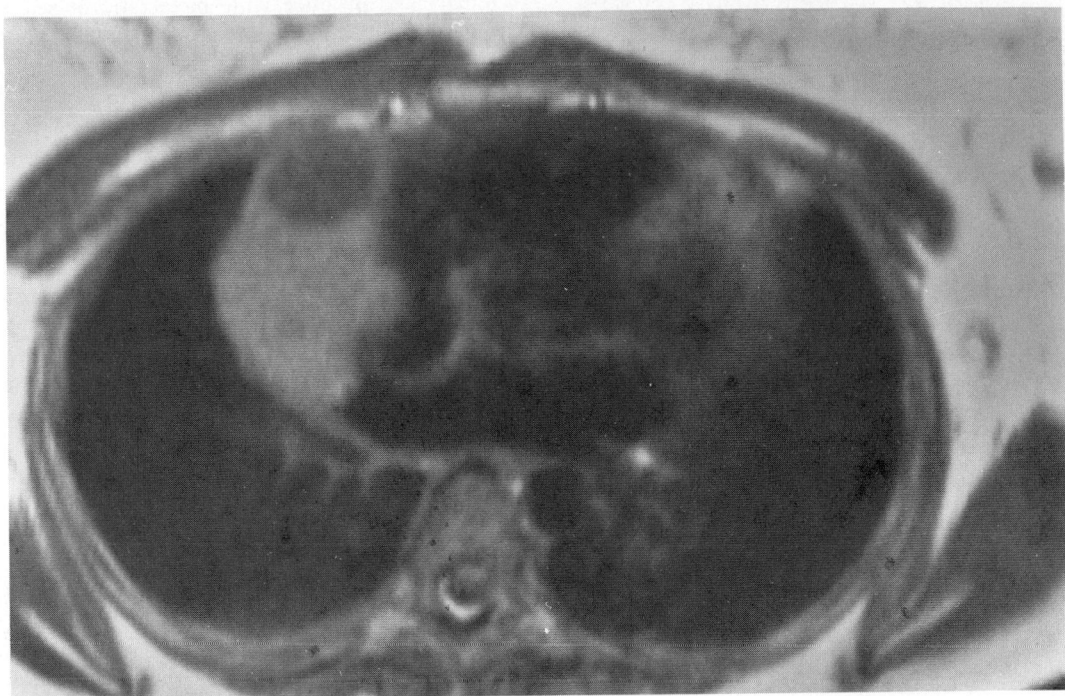

Figure 58-12.   MRI scan of patient in Figure 58-17 at a lower level shows area of low signal intensity, indicating necrosis.

necessary. Cutting needle biopsy is also an acceptable option if more tissue is necessary. Many times these techniques are nondiagnostic or indeterminate, in which case an open biopsy is warranted. Although this is frequently the case, the cytology approach may be all that is required and will thus save an open biopsy and general anesthesia. For this reason, this procedure continues to be part of the diagnostic algorithm. Usually, a small parasternal incision extending between the costal cartilages will lead directly to the tumor as directed by the imaging. It is not necessary to excise costal cartilage. A suitable biopsy can then be taken, frozen section pathology obtained to confirm its adequacy, and suitable special studies ordered. This procedure will require a general anesthetic and may be conducted as an outpatient procedure. Special attention should be paid to airway management, since some large anterior mediastinal masses can exert an important effect on the trachea, the degree of which may not be readily apparent clinically. When the anesthesia and muscle relaxants are given, significant airway compromise may occur. Care should be taken to completely reverse all anesthetic agents before extubation takes place. Rarely, such airway compromise may still present a problem, and techniques such as use of steroids, administration of racemic epinephrine, and even extubation in the prone position will be necessary.

Pathologically, mediastinal germ cell tumors may be indistinguishable from their gonadal counterparts. Part of the workup should include a search, therefore, for occult primary neoplasms in the ovaries or testes. Some authors have suggested a difference in ploidy between mediastinal and gonadal germ cell tumors, which may help to resolve the question (Oosterhuis, et al., 1990).

TERATOMAS

Teratomas represent the most common of the mediastinal germ cell neoplasms (Rusby, 1944; Daniel, et al., 1960; Ovrum and Birkeland, 1979; Parker, et al., 1973). They contain elements of two or three embryonic layers: endoderm, mesoderm and ectoderm. Teratomas may be mature, immature, or malignant.

Almost all benign teratomas are found in the anterior mediastinum (Lewis, ct al., 1983), and in the adult they are asymptomatic about two-thirds of the time. In infants and children the incidence of symptoms, which may include pain, cough, and dyspnea, is higher (Whittaker and Lynn, 1973). Very rarely, rupture may occur into the tracheobronchial tree, with coughing up of the contents into the pericardium to produce tamponade, into the pleural space to cause empyema, and into major vascular structures. Recurrent pericarditis and life-threatening hemoptysis have been described (Aravanis, et al., 1980; Robertson, et al., 1981).

Benign teratoma may be diagnosed by identification of varying tissue densities denoting fat, muscle, bone, and cystic areas on CT scan, which is the imaging technique of choice (Figs. 58-9 and 58-10). The lesion is usually well circumscribed, with smooth margins on both plain chest x-ray and CT. Calcifications may occur within the lesion or as a rim in about one-quarter of the cases (Le Roux, 1960).

The therapy for benign teratoma is surgical removal. The operative approach depends on the precise location and the surgeon's preference, but median sternotomy or posterolateral thoracotomy is most common. Once excised, these tumors do not recur. In adults, immature teratomas may invade

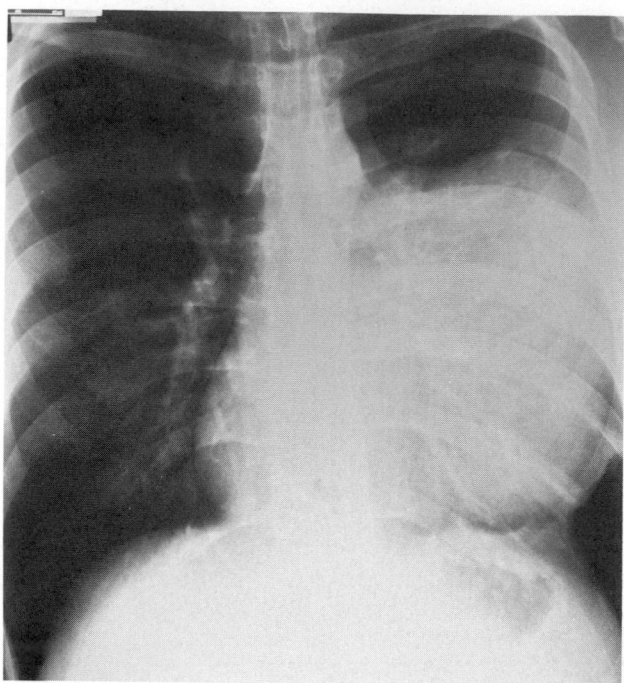

Figure 58-13. Benign teratoma. PA chest radiograph shows large left anterior mediastinal mass, contiguous with the left heart border. There is a suggestion of central calcification.

locally and produce wide metastatic diasease, although in children and adolescents they tend to be encapsulated, local, and amenable to complete excision (Toyofuku, et al., 1987; Saabye, et al., 1987) (Figs. 58-9, 58-10, and 58-13 through 58-16).

Teratocarcinomas of the mediastinum are aggressive, malignant lesions, often widely metastatic at the time of diagnosis. They are rare and carry a very poor prognosis. Various approaches of partial excision and adjuvant or primary chemotherapy and radiotherapy have yielded discouraging results (Bergh, et al., 1978, Irie, et al., 1982). Since teratocarcinomas are usually metastatic at the time of diagnosis, surgical intervention is only warranted to obtain tissue for histology.

Pathologically, mature teratomas may be cystic, hence the term *dermoid cyst*. They are encapsulated, and the capsule may be calcified, a helpful radiologic marker. They contain sebaceous, or oily, gelatinous material of varying colors. The cyst lining is mature stratified squamous epithelium. The cyst contains various elements such as tissue representative of intestinal or bronchial epithelium, bone, cartilage, pancreatic islets, nervous tissue, apocrine glands, thyroid, and others. Certain of these elements may be functional (Suda, et al., 1984; Honicky and DePapp 1973). Immature teratomas have a variegated appearance, exhibiting a wide variety of mature and immature tissues from all three germinal layers. The predominant tissue is usually neural in origin (Carter, et al., 1982). Teratocarcinomas occur when a seminoma, embryonal

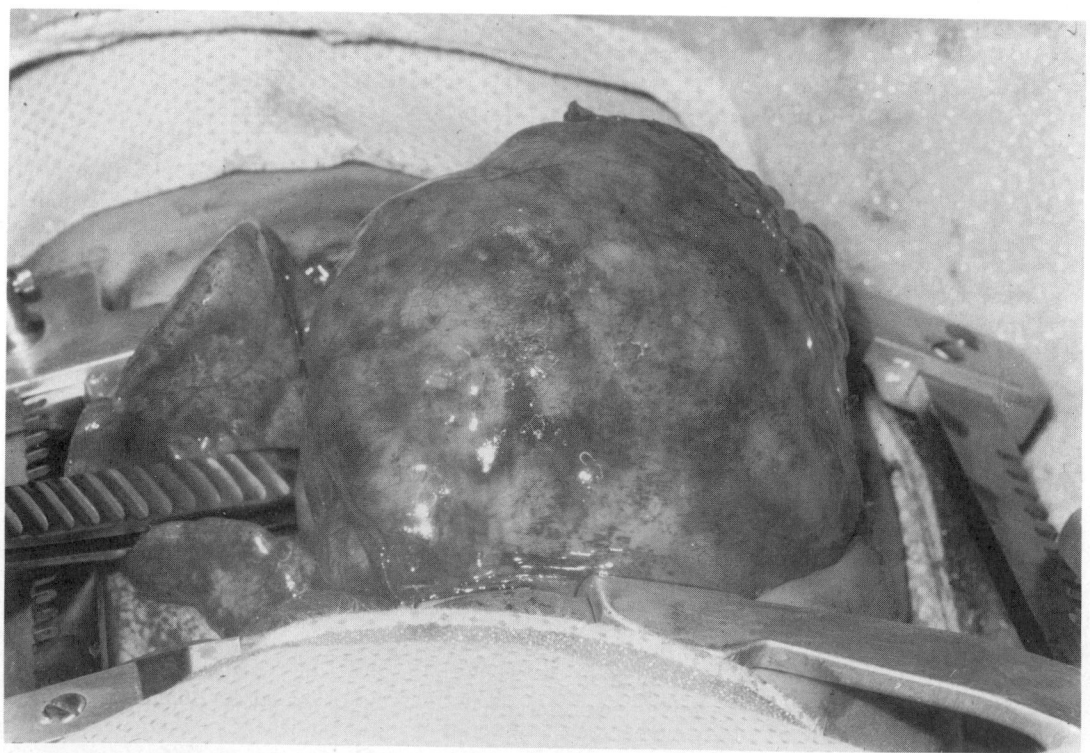

Figure 58-14. Intraoperative photograph of teratoma shown in Figure 58-13. Encapsulated, well-circumscribed tumor is straightforward to remove.

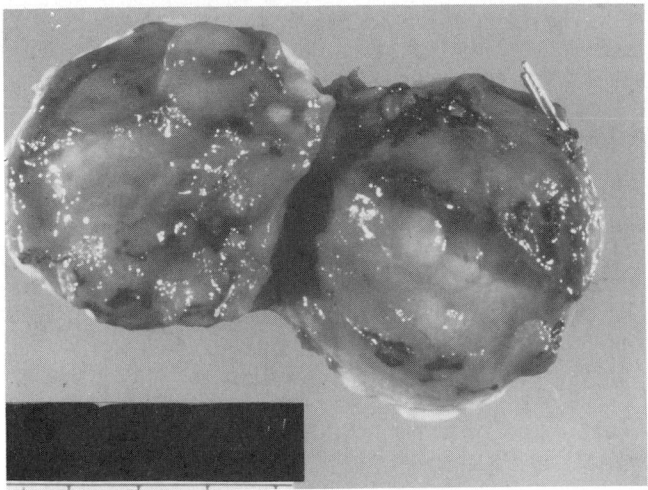

Figure 58-15. Cut surface of tumor in Figure 58-13.

carcinoma, choriocarcinoma, or endodermal sinus tumor develops from a mature or immature teratoma. Their pathologic features depend on the malignant tumor component present.

MEDIASTINAL SEMINOMA

Seminomas, also known as germinomas, make up roughly one-third of malignant mediastinal germ cell tumors (Bush, et al., 1981; Hurt, et al., 1982, Sterchi and Cordell, 1975; Cefaro, et al., 1975). They occur in men in their thirties and forties and are extremely rare in women.

Seminoma may be asymptomatic, presenting as an unexpected radiologic finding in 20 to 30 percent of cases. Tumors can become quite large, (e.g., 20 cm or so in diameter) before they cause symptoms. If symptoms occur, they are due to compression, invasion, or the systemic effect of a malignant illness. Systemic symptoms are very uncommon in mediastinal seminoma. Pain, weight loss, fever, fatigue, and dyspnea have been observed. Adenopathy and superior vena caval obstruction may also be observed in 10 percent of patients. AFP and β-HCG levels are usually not elevated in pure semi-

nomatous tumors, although 10 percent may have modest elevations of β-HCG. If AFP is elevated or β-HCG is markedly elevated, nonseminomatous elements are almost certainly present. Serum LDH is frequently elevated in patients with mediastinal seminoma. There are no pathognomonic radiographic findings. Seminomas present as large, noncalcified anterior mediastinal masses (Figs. 58-11, 58-12, and 58-17). The diagnosis is made by the techniques described previously, usually an anterior mediastinotomy and incisional biopsy.

Current therapy for mediastinal seminoma depends on the features of the presentation at the time of diagnosis. It usually involves some combination of surgery, radiotherapy, and systemic chemotherapy (Nichols, 1991). Surgical therapy as reported by Martini, et al. (1974), Knapp, et al. (1985), Kountz, et al. (1963) and others is associated with unresectable residual tumor in about 50 percent of cases. For this reason surgery is reserved for smaller asymptomatic mediastinal masses that are being excised for diagnosis and therapy. Even in this situation, a high incidence of local recurrence following complete surgical excision alone has been observed, and therefore surgery should be accompanied by adjuvant therapy of some form even if the resection is deemed complete. For some time, primary therapy has involved radical radiotherapy alone, which has yielded a respectable long-term survival of 50 to 60 percent, as reported by Iverson (1956). Effler and McCormack (1956), Polansky, et al. (1979) and Nickels and Franssila (1972). The standard radiotherapy recommendations are 4,500 to 5,000 cGy delivered by external beam megavoltage radiation to the mediastinum, including both supraclavicular areas. It would appear that failure of radiotherapy to cure the disease is due to the development of distant metastases rather than to local recurrence. The combination of radiotherapy and surgery is not logical since both are aimed at achieving local control only. As these

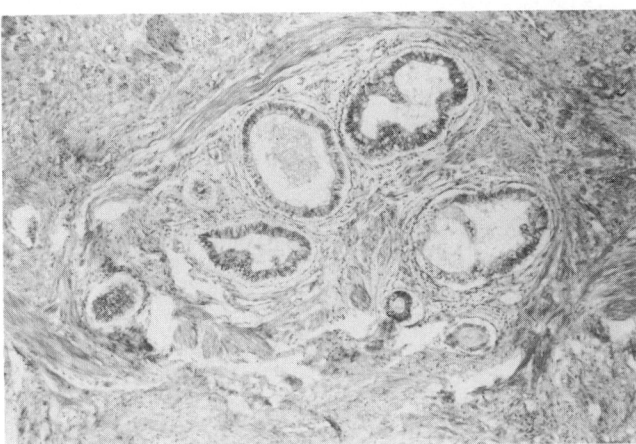

Figure 58-16. Histology of tumor in Figure 58-13, demonstrating various benign tissue elements.

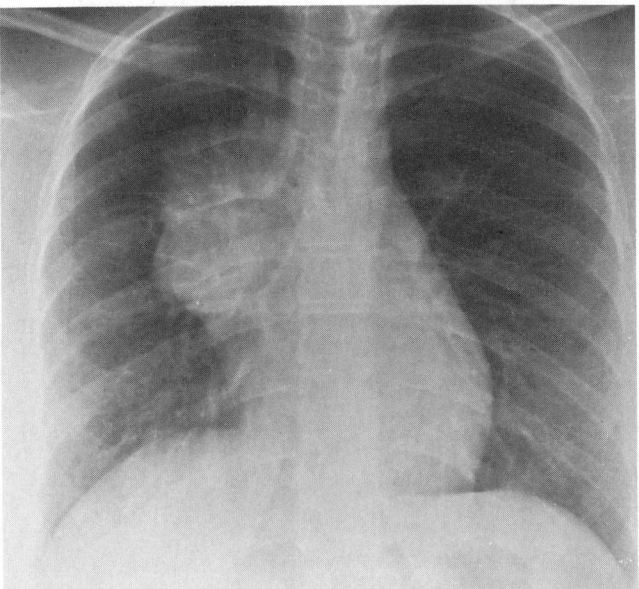

Figure 58-17. Mediastinal seminoma. PA chest radiograph identifies a right anterior mediastinal mass.

tumors are often bulky at presentation, the disease may be difficult to encompass with radiotherapy. There have been several reports of very good results with systemic chemotherapy as the primary treatment (Einhorn and Williams, 1980; Stanton, et al., 1985; Jain, et al., 1984; Loehrer, et al., 1987). These have involved combination regimens based on cisplatin and including bleomycin and either etoposide of vinblastine. Complete response to chemotherapy in the 75 to 100 percent range, has been reported, although these reports describe only a small number of patients. Jain, et al. (1984) compared "up front" chemotherapy with radiotherapy in a nonrandomized fashion, demonstrating better results in the chemotherapy group. The Southeast Cancer Study Group (1987) showed similar results, suggesting the superiority of combination chemotherapy over radiotherapy, but all of these data were obtained on only a small number of patients.

In the light of our current state of knowledge, it is clear that patients with mediastinal seminoma are suitable for aggressive treatment, with high expectations for cure. Careful imaging should be employed to rule out distant metastases and to determine the exact mediastinal extent of the disease. Small, asymptomatic, resectable tumors should be completely resected and treated with postoperative adjuvant radiotherapy. The dose should be in the range of 3,500 to 4,500 cGy. If distant metastases are detected at the time of diagnosis, the patient should be treated with intensive cisplatin-based combination chemotherapy, as described by Einhorn and Donohue (1977), Vugrin, et al. (1981), and Logothetis, et al. (1985).

Residual radiographic findings following completion of therapy present a problem. A small number of patients have been found to have viable seminoma or teratoma in these masses when they are excised. These have usually been larger residual masses of 3 cm or more. Therefore, if a significant mediastinal mass remains after adequate nonsurgical therapy for mediastinal seminoma, it should be excised (Schultz, et al., 1989; Motzer, et al., 1987). Some centers have recommended resection of only larger residual masses, adopting a watchful posture for the small ones, which, however, carries

with it the risk of recurrent disease. It is clear that an excellent survival rate with this disease may be achieved (Kersh, et al., 1990).

Pathologically (Fig. 58-18), mediastinal seminomas are bulky and infiltrate early into adjacent structures. They are composed of large polyhedral or round tumor cells, with distinct cell borders and clear or granular cytoplasm that contains variable amounts of glycogen. The nucleus is central, hyperchromatic, and associated with one or two prominent nucleoli. Sometimes the stroma exhibits a granulomatous reaction. These tumors may also contain large, multinucleated tumor cells, which closely resemble syncytiotrophoblasts.

NONSEMINOMATOUS MALIGNANT GERM CELL TUMORS

As a group, nonseminomatous malignant germ cell tumors are very much less common than pure seminomas and occur rarely in the mediastinum. They predominantly affect young males. Nonseminomatous tumors are divided into embryonal carcinoma (Fig. 58-19), teratocarcinoma (Figs. 58-20 and 58-21), choriocarcinoma (Fig. 58-22, endodermal sinus tumor (Fig. 58-23), and mixed types.

Clinical Presentation

These neoplasms present as space-occupying lesions in the anterior mediastinum and cause symptoms as such. They are more aggressive and grow more rapidly than pure seminomas and more frequently present with established metastatic disease. Metastatic sites include lung, pleura, lymph nodes, and liver. Gynecomastia due to high circulating levels of β-HCG may be present. These patients also present more commonly with constitutional symptoms such as weight loss, fever, and fatigue. Over 90 percent of patients have marked elevations of β-HCG or AFP, as well as LDH.

There appears to be an association of various hematologic malignancies with nonseminomatous tumors of the mediastinum, either synchronously or within 24 months of diagnosis. These include acute nonlymphocyctic leukemia (DeMent, et al., 1985), acute lymphocytic leukemia (Johnson, et al.,

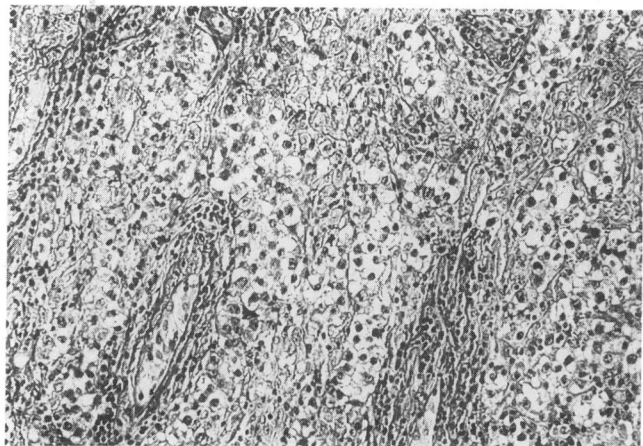

Figure 58-18. Histopathology of tumor in Figure 58-17. Typical appearance for seminoma. Large cells with abundant clear cytoplasm, central hyperchromatic nuclei.

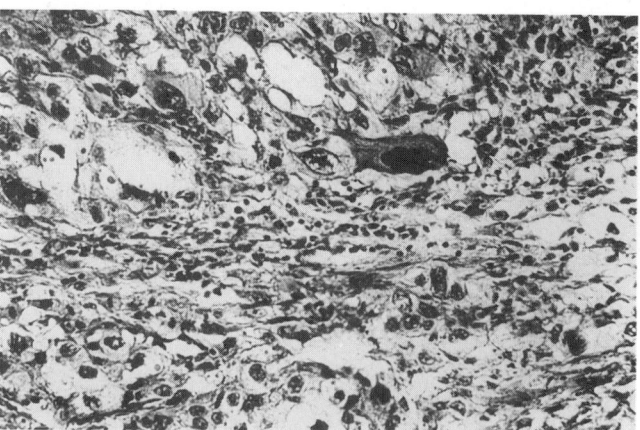

Figure 58-19. Embryonal carcinoma.

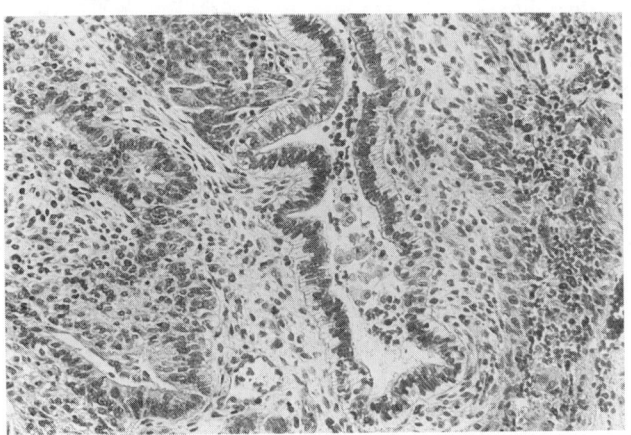

Figure 58-20. Malignant teratoma.

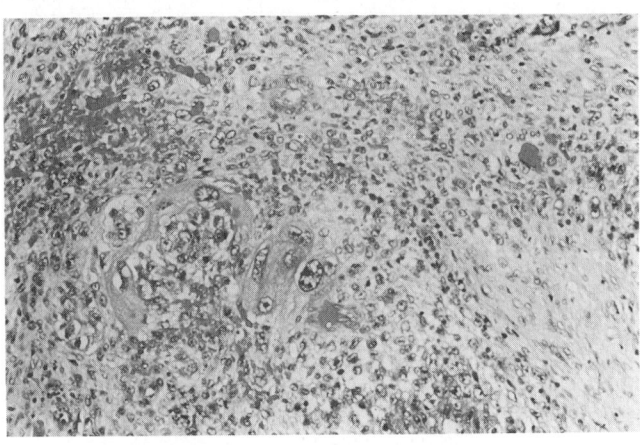

Figure 58-22. Choriocarcinoma.

1980), and malignant histiocytosis (Landanyi and Roy, 1988). Why this association should occur is unknown; it is not thought to be chemotherapy-induced. One theory suggests the presence of malignant hematopoietic cells within the germ cell tumor, as been reported by Larsen, et al. (1984). It is most likely that there is a close relationship between primitive germ cells and hematopoietic cells, which would account for this simultaneous occurrence of malignancy. Garnick and Griffin (1983) and Helman, et al. (1984) describe several examples of idiopathic thrombocytopenia seen in patients with malignant mediastinal germ cell tumors.

Diagnosis

The radiographic examinations should include a CT scan of the abdomen as well as the chest. As compared with seminomatous mediastinal tumors, the nonseminomatous tumors more often appear inhomogeneous, with areas of necrosis and hemorrhage on CT examination. The serum markers are often positive and are usually markedly elevated. Patients with Klinefelter syndrome have an increased incidence of nonseminomatous mediastinal germ cell tumors, as previously noted (Lachman, et al., 1970).

The diagnosis should be made with the least invasive method possible for obtaining material for histologic study. Highly elevated levels of the tumor markers β-HCG and AFP are considered sufficient to make the diagnosis of malignant nonseminomatous germ cell tumor of the mediastinum in the correct clinical setting. Thus, therapy may be initiated on this basis alone.

Management

Local therapeutic modalities, including surgery and radiotherapy, are not indicated in the management of nonseminomatous germ cell tumors of the mediastinum. Single-agent chemotherapy and omission of cisplatin from a combination regimen have both met with failure. There is general agreement that the primary therapy for these lesions is cisplatin-based chemotherapy, followed by complete resection of persistent lesions, which may contain teratoma, persistent tumor, or malignant nongerm elements. A recent review of 31 patients so treated indicated that 58 percent attained disease-free status, the remainder showing partial response (Nichols, et al., 1989). The optimal timing of adjuvant surgical resection is not clear. It is generally accepted

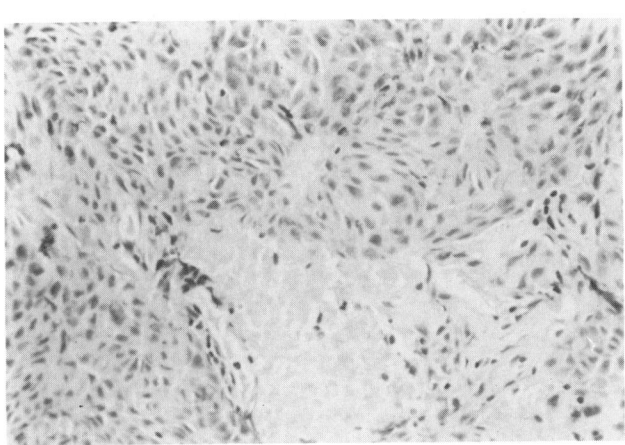

Figure 58-21. Malignant teratoma.

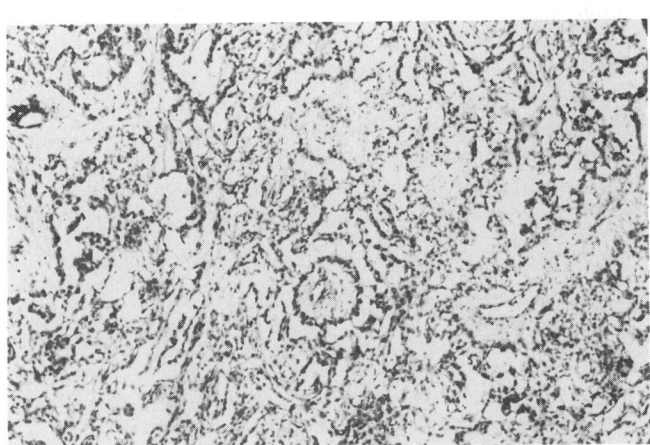

Figure 58-23. Endodermal sinus tumor.

that a 2- to 3-month interval from the completion of therapy, with no further shrinkage observed, is the point at which patients should be considered for removal of residual mediastinal mass. With this type of management, overall survival range can be in the range of 40 to 50 percent. Because these mediastinal tumors are rare and hold a poorer prognosis than their gonadal counterparts, such patients should be entered into clinical trials assessing newer agents. The serum markers are excellent tools for monitoring response to therapy. If they remain elevated, it can be assumed that there is residual active disease and additional chemotherapy can be recommended. Salvage chemotherapy with agents including etoposide, cisplatin, and ifosfamide in combination may produce long-term survival in 20 to 30 percent of patients (Hainsworth, et al., 1985; Loehrer, et al., 1988). If the serum markers revert to normal, along with the radiographs, no further treatment is indicated, and the patient is committed to close follow-up. Surgical resection, as described, is indicated when the markers have resumed normal levels and radiographs identify persistent abnormalities.

Types of Nonseminomatous Malignant Germ Cell Tumors

Embryonal Carcinoma

Embryonal carcinomas are highly malignant tumors. They aggressively infiltrate adjacent structures and metastasize to the lungs, bones, and other solid organs. Pathologically they are composed of solid sheets, acini, anastomosing duct and glands, tubules, or papillary structures composed of very large tumor cells with indistinct cell borders, amphophilic or vacuolated cytoplasm, and irregular round or oval nuclei with prominent nucleoli (Fig. 58-19). As with other nonseminomatous lesions, the primary approach is with chemotherapy followed by excision if possible or necessary. Tumor markers may help confirm the diagnosis and monitor response to therapy.

Endodermal Sinus Tumor

Endodermal sinus tumor was first described in 1959 by Telium. It usually arises in the gonads but may arise in extragonadal sites. Primary mediastinal yolk sac tumor, as this tumor is also known, is an extremely rare malignancy, with only about 70 reported cases in the literature. Management is with chemotherapy followed by surgical resection of residual abnormality; this will yield occasional long-term survival (Saxman, et al., 1991).

Primary Mediastinal Choriocarcinoma

β-HCG will be elevated in primary mediastinal choriocarcinoma, which also is a rare tumor. Males will often exhibit gynecomastia. It is difficult to prove the primary mediastinal nature of this lesion because an occult gonadal primary may be present. Whether primary or secondary, the therapeutic modality is the same, namely, chemotherapy (Kathuria and Jablokow, 1987). The prognosis is poor.

COMMENTS AND CONTROVERSIES

Germ cell tumors of the mediastinum can present as primary lesions or as secondary tumors related to lymphatic metastases from primary testicular sites. In the latter cases, both retroperitoneal and posterior mediastinal lymphatics are involved.

There is increasing evidence that the first-line therapy for seminomas should be chemotherapy. It is the rare case in which small seminomas are surgically resected for diagnosis. In most cases seminomas present as large bulky tumors, requiring chemotherapy as the primary therapeutic modality and possibly radiotherapy for consolidation. Smaller tumors can be cured by radiotherapy alone.

Frequently in nonseminomatous tumors, with complete remission as evidenced by normalization of tumor markers following chemotherapy, resection of residual masses will demonstrate only necrosis or mature teratoma. Whenever possible, surgery is deferred until serum markers are normalized. Persistence of serum markers indicate active disease. On occasion, surgeons are required to remove the residual tumor bulk prior to high-intensity chemotherapy with bone marrow transplantation. Every effort should be made to perform a complete resection in these cases.

Occasionally the primary or secondary mediastinal germ cell tumor is associated with pulmonary metastases, which require concomitant resection after chemotherapy. Despite this intensive therapy, primary mediastinal germ cell tumors do not have as optimistic a prognosis as those arising in the testis or ovary. The overall 5-year disease-free survival following this intensive treatment is reported at 40 to 50 percent. Why these tumors fail to respond to treatment as well as those from other sites is as yet unknown.

R.J.G.

KEY REFERENCES

Knapp RH, Hurt RD, Payne WS et al: Malignant germ cell tumors of the mediastinum J Thorac Cardiovasc Surg 89:82, 1985

This is a comprehensive review of 56 cases from the Mayo Clinic. Although management comments may be a little dated, the accumulated clinical information provides a thorough understanding of the clinical features of the disease.

Nichols CR: Mediastinal germ cell tumors. Clinical features and biologic correlates. Chest 99:472, 1991

A thoughtful, thorough and up-to-date review of the subject from an author who works in the institution where much of the pioneering oncologic work was done.

Nichols CR, Saxman S, Williams SD, et al: Primary mediastinal nonseminomatous germ cell tumors. A modern single institution experience. Cancer 65:1641, 1989

These authors represent Einhorn's group, which has been responsible for much of the current state of the art of the nonsurgical treatment of mediastinal germ cell tumors. This reflects their experience in the nonseminomatous group.

REFERENCES

Aravanis C, Papasteriades E, Steriotis J: Recurrent pericarditis due to cystic teratoma of the mediastinum: a case report. Angiology 31:427, 1980

Azzopardi JG, Mostofi FK, Theiss EA: Lesions of testes observed in certain patients with widespread choriocarcinoma and related tumors. Am J Pathol 38:207, 1961

Bergh NP, Gatzinsky P, Larsson S et al: Tumors of the thymus and thymic region: III. Clinicopathological studies on teratomas and tumors of germ cell type. Ann Thorac Surg 25:107, 1978

Bush SE, Martinez A, Bagshaw MA: Primary mediastinal seminoma. Cancer 48:1877, 1981

Caes JH, Cragg RW: Extragenital choriocarcinoma of the male with bilateral gynecomastia—report of a case. U S Navy Med Bull 47:1072, 1947

Carrol PR, et al: Testicular failure in patients with extragonadal germ cell tumors. Cancer 60:108, 1987

Carter D, Bibro MC, Touloukian RJ: Benign clinical behaviour of immature mediastinal teratoma in infancy and childhood: report of two cases and review of the literature. Cancer 49:398, 1982

Cefaro GA, Luzi S, Turriziani A et al: Primary mediastinal seminoma. Br J Urol 62:461, 1988

Chaussain JL, et al: Klinefelter's syndrome, tumor and sexual precocity. J Pediatr 97:607, 1980

Collins DH, Pugh RCB: Classification and frequency of testicular tumors. Br J Urol 36(suppl.):1, 1964

Cox JD: Primary malignant germinal tumors of the mediastinum. Cancer 36:1162, 1975

Curry WA, et al: Klinefelter's syndrome and mediastinal germ cell neoplasms. J Urol 125:127, 1981

Daniel RA Jr, Diveley WL, Edwards WH et al: Mediastinal tumors. Ann Surg 151:783, 1960

Daugaard G, et al: Carcinoma-in-situ testis in patients with assumed extragonadal germ cell tumors. Lancet 2:528, 1987

DeMent SH, Eggleston JC, Spivak JL: Association between mediastinal germ cell tumors and hematologic malignancies: report of two cases and review of the literature. Am J Surg Pathol 9:23, 1985

Doll DC, Weiss RB, Evans H: Klinefelter's syndrome and extragenital seminoma. J Urol 116:675, 1976

Effler DB, McCormack LJ: Thymic neoplasms. J Thorac Surg 31:60, 1956

Einhorn LH, Donohue JD: Cis-diamminedichloroplatinum, vinblastine, and bleomycin combination chemotherapy in disseminated testicular cancer. Ann Intern Med 87:293, 1977

Einhorn LH, Williams SD: Management of disseminated seminoma. Cancer Clin Trials 3:307, 1980

Einhorn LH, Williams SD: Management of disseminated testicular cancer. p. 117. In Einhorn LH (ed): Testicular Tumors: Management and Treatment. Masson, New York, 1980

Fine F, Smith RW Jr, Pachter MR: Primary extragenital choriocarcinoma in the male subject. Case report and review of the literature. Am J Med 32:776, 1962

Friedman NB: The comparative morphogenesis of extragenital and gonadal teratoid tumors. Cancer 4:265, 1951

Garnick MB, Griffin JD: Idiopathic thrombocytopenia in association with extragonadal germ cell cancer. Ann Intern Med 98:926, 1983

Hainsworth JD, et al: Successful treatment of resistant germinal neoplasms with VP16 and cisplatin; results of a Southeastern Study Group Trial. J Clin Oncol 3:666, 1985

Helman LF, Ozols RF, Longo DL: Thrombocytopenia and extragonadal germ-cell neoplasm. Ann Intern Med 101:280, 1984

Honicky RE, DePapp EW: Mediastinal teratoma with endocrine function. Am J Dis Child 126:650, 1973

Hurt RD, et al: Primary anterior mediastinal seminoma. Cancer 49:1650, 1982

Irie T, Watanabe H, Kawaoi A et al: Alpha-fetoprotein (AFP), human chorionic gonadotropin (HCG), and carcinoembryonic antigen (CEA) demonstrated in the immature glands of mediastinal teratocarcinoma. A case report. Cancer 50:1160, 1982

Iverson L: Thymoma. A review and classification. Am J Pathol 32:695, 1956

Jain KK, Bols GH, Bains MS et al: The treatment of extragonadal seminoma. J Clin Oncol 2:820, 1984

Johnson DC, et al: Acute lymphocytic leukemia developing in a male with germ cell carcinoma: a case report. Med Pediatr Oncol 8:361, 1980

Kantrowitz AR: Extragenital chorionepithelialoma in a male. Am J Pathol 10:531, 1934

Kathuria S, Jablokow VR: Primary choriocarcinoma of mediastinum with immunohistochemical study and review of the literature. J Surg Oncol 34:39, 1987

Kersh CR, Constable WC, Hahn SS et al: Primary malignant extragonadal germ cell tumors. An analysis of the effect of radiotherapy. Cancer 65:2681, 1990

Kountz SL, Connolly JE, Cohn R: Seminoma-like (or seminomatous) tumors of the anterior mediastinum. J Thorac Cardiovasc Surg 45:289, 1963

Lachman MF, Kim K, Koo BC: Mediastinal teratoma associated with Klinefelter's syndrome. Arch Pathol Lab Med 110:1067, 1986

Laipply TC, Shipley RA: Extragenital choriocarcinoma in the male. Am J Pathol 21:921, 1945

Landanyi M, Roy I: Mediastinal germ cell tumor and histiocytosis. Hum Pathol 19:586, 1988

Larsen M, et al: Acute lymphoblastic leukemia: possible origin from a mediastinal germ cell tumor. Cancer 53:441, 1984

Le Roux, BT: Mediastinal teratomata. Thorax 15:333, 1960

Lewis BD, et al: Benign teratomas of the mediastinum. J Thorac Cardiovasc Surg 86:727, 1983

Loehrer PJ, Birch R, Williams SD et al: Chemotherapy of metastatic seminoma: the Southeastern Cancer Study Group experience: J Clin Oncol 5:1212, 1987

Loehrer PJ, et al: Salvage therapy in recurrent germ cell cancer: ifosfamide and cisplatin plus either vinblastine or etoposide. Ann Intern Med 109:540, 1988

Logothetis CJ, et al: Chemotherapy of extragonadal germ cell tumors. J Clin Oncol 3:316, 1985a

Logothetis CJ, et al: Improved survival with cyclic chemotherapy in non-seminomatous germ cell tumors of the testis. J Clin Oncol 3:326, 1985b

Luna MA, Johnson DE: Postmortem findings in testicular tumors.

In Johnson DE (ed): Testicular Tumors. Medical Examination Publishing, New York, 1975

Luna MA, Valenzuela-Tamariz J: Germ-cell tumors of the mediastinum, postmortem findings. Am J Clin Pathol 65:450, 1976

Lynch MJG, Blewitt GL: Choriocarcinoma arising in the male mediastinum. Thorax 8:157, 1953

Marchevsky AM, Kaneko M: Other tumors of the thymus gland. In Surgical Pathology of the Mediastinum. 2nd Ed. Raven Press, New York, 1992

Martini N, et al: Primary mediastinal germ cell tumors. Cancer 33:763, 1974

Meares EM, Briggs EM: Occult seminoma of the testis masquerading as primary extragonadal germinal neoplasm. Cancer 30:300, 1972

Motzer R, Bosl G, Heelan R et al: Residual mass: an indication for further therapy in patients with advanced seminoma following systemic chemotherapy. J Clin Oncol 5:1064, 1987

Nickels J, Franssila K: Primary seminoma of the anterior mediastinum. Acta Pathol Microbiol Scand 80A:260, 1972

Oberman HA, Libcke JH: Malignant germinal neoplasms of the mediastinum. Cancer 117:498, 1964

Oosterhuis JW, Rammeloo RHU, Cornelisse CJ et al: Ploidy of malignant mediastinal germ-cell tumors. Hum Pathol 21:729, 1990

Ovrum E, Birkeland S: Mediastinal tumors and cysts: a review of 191 cases. Scand J Thorac Cardiovasc Surg. 13:161, 1979

Parker D, Holford CP, Bergent FH: Effective treatment for malignant mediastinal teratoma. Thorax 38:897, 1983

Polansky SM, Barwick KW, Ravin CE: Primary mediastinal seminoma AJR 132:17, 1979

Robertson JM, Fee HJ, Mulder DG: Mediastinal teratoma causing life-threatening hemoptysis. Its occurrence in an infant. Am J Dis Child 135:148, 1981

Rusby NL: Dermoid cysts and teratomata of the mediastinum. A review. J Thorac Cardiovasc Surg 13:169, 1944

Saabye J, Elbirk A, Andersen K: Teratomas of the mediastinum. Scand J Thorac Cardiovasc Surg 21:271, 1987

Saxman S, Nichols CR, Williams SD et al: Mediastinal yolk sac tumor. The Indiana University experience, 1976–1988. J Thorac Cardiovasc Surg 102:913, 1991

Schlumberger HG: Teratoma of anterior mediastinum in groups of military age: study of 16 cases and review of theories of genesis. Arch Pathol 41:398, 1946

Schultz SM, Einhorn LH, Conces DH et al: Management of postchemotherapy residual mass in patients with advanced seminoma: Indiana University experience. J Clin Oncol 7:1497, 1989

Sogge MR, McDonald SD, Cofold PB: The malignant potential of dysgenetic germ cell in Klinefelter's syndrome. Am J Med 66:515, 1979

Stanton GF, Bosl GJ, Whitmore WF Jr: VAB-6 as initial treatment of patients with advanced seminoma. J Clin Oncol 3:336, 1985

Sterchi M, Cordell AR: Seminoma of the anterior mediastinum. Ann Thorac Cardiovasc Surg 19:371, 1975

Suda K, Mizuguchi K, Hebisawa A et al: Pancreatic tissue in teratoma. Arch Pathol Lab Med 108:835, 1984

Telium G: Endodermal sinus tumor of the ovary and testis—comparative morphogenesis of the so-called mesonephroma avaii (Schiller) and extraembryonic (yolk-sac, allantoic) structures of the rat's placenta. Cancer 12:1092, 1959

Toyofuku T, Mochizuki I, Kusama S: Mediastinal germ cell tumor in trisomy 8. Eur J Respir Dis 70:245, 1987

Vugrin D, Herr HW, Whitmore WF Jr: VAB-6 combination chemotherapy in disseminated cancer of the testis. Ann Intern Med 95:59, 1981

Whittaker LD, Lynn HB: Mediastinal tumors and cysts in the pediatric patient. Surg Clin North Am 53:893, 1973

Lymphoma

S. B. Sutcliffe

DEFINITION

Lymphomas are malignancies of reticuloendothelial tissues, most commonly lymphocytes. The term *lymphoma* encompasses two major categories of disease. Hodgkin's disease and non-Hodgkin's lymphoma. Hodgkin's disease, an illness with a biphasic age distribution most commonly affecting those in early adult life, commonly presents with supradiaphragmatic adenopathy, has a characteristic histologic presentation involving Reed-Sternberg cells, and has a generally very favorable prognosis with radiation and/or chemother-

apy. Non-Hodgkin's lymphoma is a spectrum of diseases most common in persons over age and in the pediatric age range. It commonly presents as nodal or extranodal disease, demonstrates heterogeneity of lymphoid morphology, and has a variable prognosis, ranging from indolent, incurable conditions to fulminant, rapidly fatal conditions, which, however, may be remarkably responsive to therapy with a curative outcome.

Malignant lymphomas are uncommon diseases with incidence rates of approximately 3 in 100,000 (Hodgkin's disease) and 15 in 100,000 (non-Hodgkin's lymphomas). Although the etiology is unknown, several factors are recognized to be relevant. These include genetically determined or acquired immunodeficiency states (e.g., post-organ transplantation, the acquired immunodeficiency syndrome [AIDS]), viruses (e.g., Epstein-Barr virus, human T-cell lymphoma virus), and chemical exposure (e.g., to hair coloring products, organic solvents, pesticides).

Primary malignant tumors of the mediastinum are uncommon. However, approximately 50 percent of primary mediastinal tumors in children and 20 percent in adults are malignant lymphomas (King et al., 1982; Benjamin, et al., 1972). Despite this apparently high proportion, the presentation of malignant lymphoma as an isolated intrathoracic mediastinal tumor is uncommon, comprising less than 5 percent of supradiaphragmatic presentations of Hodgkin's disease and non-Hodgkin's lymphoma. (Lichtenstein, et al., 1980; Levitt, et al., 1992). Mediastinal adenopathy in association with lymphoma presenting at other extrathoracic sites is well recognized, occurring in 60 to 90 percent of patients with Hodgkin's disease (usually of nodular sclerosing type) (Lukes, et al., 1966; Colby, et al., 1981, Blank and Castellino, 1981) and in 18 to 46 percent of patients with non-Hodgkin's lymphoma (Blank and Castellino, 1987; Jones, et al., 1973). Clearly, the range of incidence data reported reflects technical refinements in imaging and the increased focus since the early 1970s on accurate determination of disease extent as a basis for management.

While primary presentations of lymphoma in the mediastinum, either nodal or thymic, are uncommon, primary extranodal presentations of non-Hodgkin's lymphoma at nonmediastinal sites can account for up to 50 percent of referrals (e.g., gastrointestinal, head and neck, central nervous system, testicular presentations). Primary extranodal presentation of Hodgkin's disease is extremely uncommon.

The term *primary mediastinal lymphoma* designates lymphoma presenting clinically and radiologically as a predominantly intrathroacic neoplasm arising from or with major involvement of the mediastinum, in the absence of peripheral adenopathy or readily detectable or accessible disease beyond the thorax. Within this designation, the principal diagnoses include Hodgkin's disease, mediastinal large cell lymphoma (with or without sclerosis) and lymphoblastic lymphoma. Significant differences in the pattern of presentation, clinical evolution, approach to therapy, and prognosis characterize these malignancies, thereby defining the critical importance of a secure diagnosis as a basis for subsequent management.

HISTORICAL NOTE

Interestingly, the major advances in the management of patients with malignant lymphoma have been achieved without recourse to an understanding of the etiology or biology of the disease.

Histologic Classification and Correlation with Prognosis

The prognostic clinical utility of the Rye classification (Lukes and Butler, 1966) for Hodgkin's disease has been amply demonstrated. Despite its diagnostic and prognostic value, it re-

mains limited by its failure to characterize the origin of the malignant cell, the role of the pleomorphic "normal" cellular infiltrate, and the heterogeneity of outcome within histologic subtypes.

Histologic classification for non-Hodgkin's lymphoma have gone through several iterations (Non-Hodgkins Lymphoma Pathologic Classification Project, 1982). At the morphologic level, key attributes relate to the pattern of architectural effacement of lymphoid tissue (nodular or follicular versus diffuse) and the cytologic features of the malignant cells (small, large, undifferentiated, or mixtures thereof). While such observations underlie the therapeutic approach and prognosis, interobserver variability and subjectivity pose problems that will require more objective measurement (e.g., analytic/flow cytometry, ploidy, DNA measurement) and greater understanding of the biology of the disease (characterization of cell lineage and differentiation).

Staging Classification

The internationally accepted classification for the staging of lymphoma is the Ann Arbor classification (Carbone, et al., 1971). It is based on the anatomic distribution of nodal disease and the distinction of nodal from extranodal disease by either contiguity or dissemination. The usefulness of the classification in management and prognosis has been established for both Hodgkin's and non-Hodgkin's lymphoma. However, it is more appropriate for Hodgkin's disease in view of the high proportion of patients who present with localized nodal disease as compared with the considerably higher proportion of patients presenting with localized extranodal non-Hodgkin's lymphoma, as well as the greater probability of occult hematogenous dissemination by non-Hodgkin's lymphoma, which is unamenable to resolution by conventional imaging techniques.

Radiotherapy

The evolution of radiotherapy practice in relation to the end points of local control, patterns of failure, survival, and toxicity has been clearly characterized, including the appropriate radiation field dispositions, dose-control relationships to achieve high in-field control rates, prognostic factors determining local and distant failure rates with radiation alone, and toxicities relating to therapy. In practice, moderate-dose radiation (about 35 Gy) will achieve a high local control rate with relatively little morbidity, and the principal reason for failure is disease progression to sites distant from the radiation field.

Chemotherapy

The systemic therapy of lymphoma has been characterized by the demonstration that individually active chemotherpeutic agents with differing activities within the cell cycle can be combined into regimens of varying dose intensity (dose, administration schedule) to achieve high levels of disease response (remission, complete or partial) and survival. The issue of dose intensity in patients with relapsed or refractory disease is currently under examination through the approach of high-dose chemotherapy with or without radiotherapy, with autologous bone marrow support.

Biology

Recent developments in immunology, cytogenetics, and molecular genetics have established the clonal origin of malignant lymphoma and provided insight into the genomic events underlying malignant transformation, clonal evolution, phenotypic expression, and disease behavior. Such studies have established that the rearrangement of immunoglobulin genes that occurs under normal circumstances as a regulated event in response to antigenic challenge also occurs in malignant lymphoma, but as an unregulated event, usually in relation to oncogene activity within transposed segments of the immunoglobulin genes. The understanding and characterization of these genomic events presents opportunities for enhanced diagnosis, elaboration of strategies to regulate the dysfunctional genome, and development of immunologic therapies targeted to unique antigenic determinants on the malignant cell surface.

HISTORICAL READINGS

Carbone PP, Kaplan WS, Musshoff et al: Report of the committee on Hodgkin's disease staging classification. Cancer Res. 31:1860, 1971

Chabner BA, Johnson RE, Young RC et al: Sequential non-surgical and surgical staging of non-Hodgkin's lymphoma. Ann Intern Med 85:149, 1976

Lukes RJ, Butler JJ: The pathology and nomenclature of Hodgkin's disease. Cancer Res 26:1063, 1966

Non-Hodgkins Lymphoma Pathologic Classification Project: National Cancer Institute sponsored study of non-Hodgkin's lymphomas: Summary and description of a working formulation for clinical usage. Cancer 49:211, 1982

CLINICAL FEATURES

Symptoms

A minority of patients with primary mediastinal lymphoma—probably not more than 10 percent—present without symptoms on the basis of routine physical examination and chest x-ray. The majority present with symptoms due to local-regional disease, including chest pain (sternal, interscapular, or shoulder, with or without relationship to respiration), cough (usually nonproductive), dyspnea, dysphagia, hoarseness, and facial or arm swelling. Symptoms referable to lymphoma—fever, night sweats, weight loss, and more rarely, pruritus—may also be present.

The pattern of symptomatology differs with the primary diagnosis. Vena caval obstruction and neurologic dysfunction (recurrent laryngeal nerve palsy, Horner syndrome, and cervicothoracic paravertebral gutter symptomatology) are quite uncommon presentations of Hodgkin's disease. Indeed, neurologic symptomatology is quite uncommon in any presentation of lymphoma. Superior vena caval obstruction and symptoms of lymphoma at presentation are more common in non-Hodgkin's lymphoma arising in the mediastinum (Table 58-5).

Cough, chest pain, and dyspnea may arise on the basis of mechanical distortion of the airway, partial or complete lung collapse due to obstruction, or pleural effusion(s) or less commonly, in association with a pericardial effusion.

Physical Signs

The physical findings may include sternal or chest wall deformity with or without venectasia (uncommon) (Fig. 58-24), palpable internal mammary adenopathy (uncommon), tracheal deviation, superior vena caval obstruction, stridor or wheezing, lung collapse or consolidation, pleural effusion(s), or pericardial effusion. Vocal cord dysfunction, Horner syndrome, and brachial plexopathy are unusual findings. A detailed clinical examination for adenopathy beyond the thorax is mandatory but will commonly be negative for most patients with a primary mediastinal presentation.

In many patients with Hodgkin's disease, the presenting features have been present for many months. Primary mediastinal presentation of non-Hodgkin's lymphoma are usually more fulminant, with a median duration of symptoms of 1 to 3 months and more florid findings on examination.

Table 58-5. Principal Characteristics of Primary Mediastinal Lymphoma

Disease	Age	Sex	Symptomatology None	Symptomatology Regional	SVC Obstruction	B Symptoms	Clinical Extranodal Extension	CNS and Bone Marrow	Pattern of Progression	Phenotype
Hodgkin's disease	Early adult	F>M	<20%	>80%	Rare	<30%	<30%	Rare	Commonly localized. Spleen and upper abdominal nodes <30% pretherapy	Nonclonal
Lymphoblastic lymphoma (Nathwani, et al., 1981)	Late teens, early adult	M>F	Rare	Unusual	Not uncommon	30–50%	Common	Common	Rapid systemic progression if untreated. B.M. and sanctuary sites (CNS, testis).	Immature T cell
Mediastinal large cell lymphoma	Adult, median 30–35 yr	F>M	<20%	>80%	30–60%	>50%	>50%	Rare	Progression in retroperitoneal nodes, kidney, pancreas, liver, adrenal	Follicular B cell (variable differentiation)
										Mature T cell

[a] The characteristics noted represent broad generalisations. Statements within individual reports may vary based upon heterogeneity within series and case referral bias. (Data on mediastinal large cell lymphoma from Miller, et al., 1981; Trump and Mann, 1982; Waldron, et al., 1985; Menestrina, et al., 1986; Addis and Isaacson, 1986, Linden, et al., 1986; Perrene, et al., 1986; Scarpa, et al., 1987. Möller, et al., 1987; Jacobson, et al., 1988; Haioun, et al., 1989; Lamarre, et al., 1989; Todeschini, et al., 1990.)

of malignant lymphoma. The discrimination of these features has been enhanced considerably by incorporation of CT and MRI into the evaluation of the thorax (Blank and Castellino, 1987; Nyman, et al., 1989; Salonen, et al., 1987).

Anterior Superior Mediastinal Mass

An anterior superior mediastinal mass may represent an enlarged node or nodal mass or a tumor arising within the thymus. In the absence of other findings, its appearance does not discriminate within the differential diagnosis of malignant mediastinal tumors.

Discrete Mediastinal Adenopathy, with or Without Hilar Adenopathy

Discrete mediastinal adenopathy, particularly in the paratracheal, prevascular, subcarinal, and/or hilar regions, is most consistent with a diagnosis of malignant lymphoma. Enlargement of a single node or nodal group is more common in non-Hodgkin's lymphoma than in Hodgkin's disease.

Contiguous Mediastinal Mass ("Permeating Continuum")

The radiologic presentation termed "permeating continuum" by Blank and Castellino (1987) is that of a contiguous mass involving lymph nodes, possibly arising from the thymus, obscuring the borders of the heart and/or great vessels, and commonly infiltrating into adjacent lung and/or pericardium (Fig. 58-25). Pleural and/or pericardial effusion may be present. Additional features include airway deviation, bronchial narrowing, lung collapse, and anterior extension into the chest wall. This presentation is characteristic of a small proportion of mediastinal lymphoma cases but is not unique to this diagnosis.

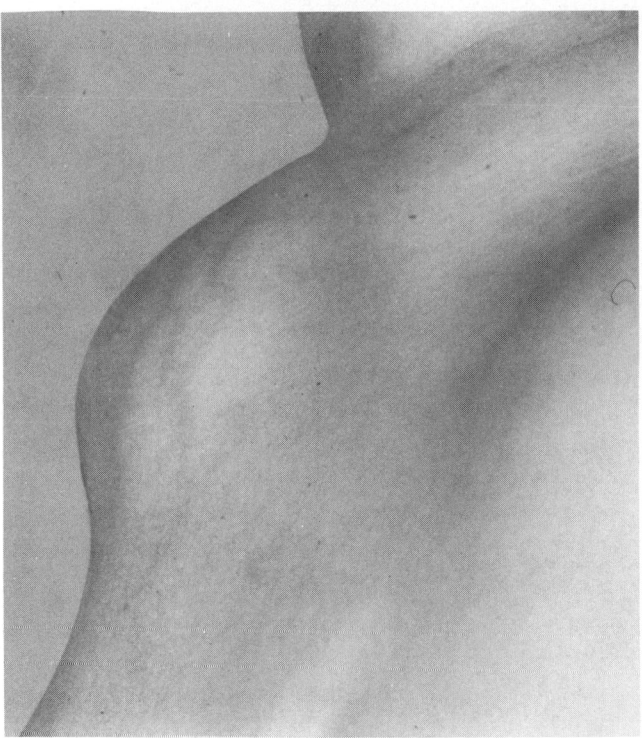

Figure 58-24. Anterior chest wall deformity with venectasia due to sternal and chest wall involvement by an underlying mediastinal mass in a young woman with Hodgkin's disease, diagnosed by biopsy of the mass in the twenty-third week of her first pregnancy.

Radiologic Features

There are probably no unique features that categorically define a diagnosis on the basis of the radiologic features alone. There are, however, certain patterns of radiologic involvement that may be more or less supportive of the diagnosis

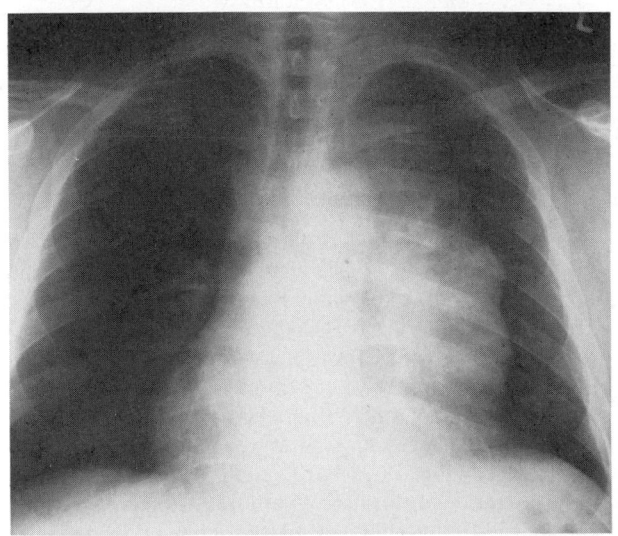

A

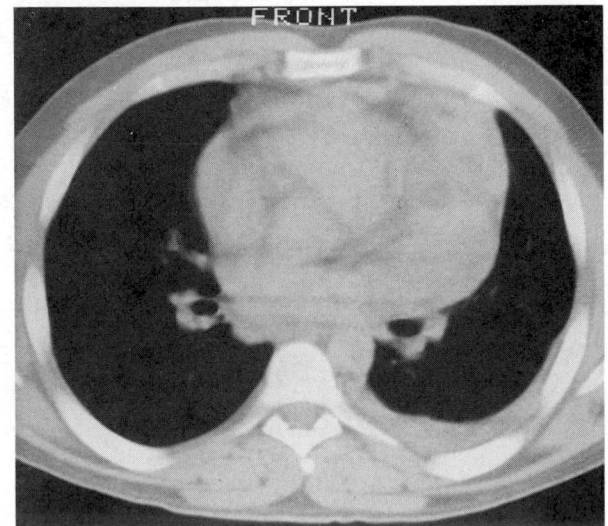

B

Figure 58-25. **(A)** A large irregular mass of lymph nodes occupying the left anterior mediastinum is displayed on the PA chest radiograph. **(B)** On CT scan the lymphadenopathy insinuates among the great vessels, and a right paratracheal and subcarinal adenopathy is identified. The adenopathy extends down over the heart and is associated with a pericardial effusion and a modest left pleural effusion.

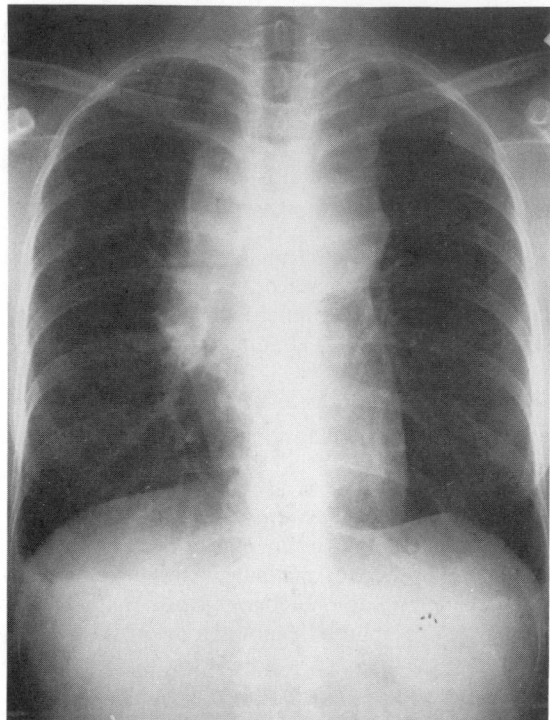

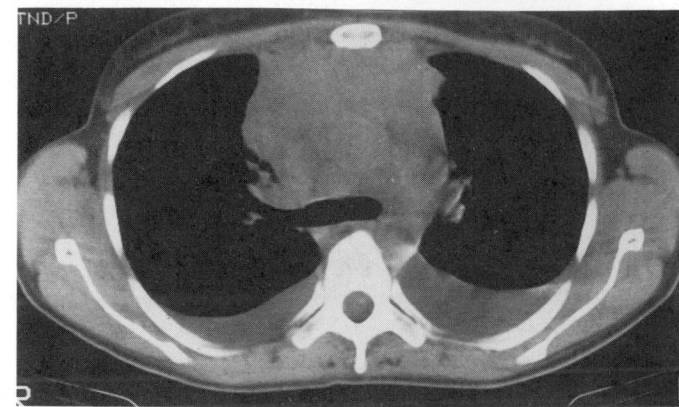

Figure 58-26. **(A)** The PA chest radiograph of a young woman with Hodgkin's disease presenting with cough and anterior chest wall discomfort. A widened mediastinum composed of bilateral paratracheal adenopathy is evident. **(B)** The unenhanced CT scan of the thorax reveals extension of the mass to involve the anterior chest wall. Small bilateral pleural effusions are also present.

Parietal Involvement

Involvement of the sternum and/or sternum chest wall, either by direct anterior extension of a mediastinal mass (Fig. 58-26) or by invasion from involved internal mammary nodes

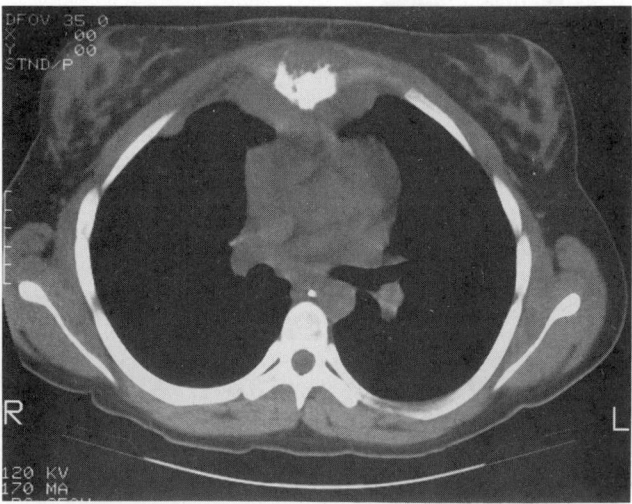

Figure 58-27. A CT scan of the thorax in a patient with Hodgkin's disease, demonstrating a large anterior mediastinal mass associated with internal mammary lymph node enlargement (extending to the diaphragm). In the midportion of the sternum the soft tissue mass extends anteriorly to the sternum, with destruction of the sternal cortex.

(Fig. 58-27), is an important radiologic finding. Breach of the internal mammary chain permits access to intercostal lymphatics and may be a route for spread within the chest wall or to the posterior intercostal nodes, with consequent paravertebral mass formation. Chest wall lymphatic spread or involvement of the pericardium may lead to involvement of the epipericardial nodes, diaphragmatic nodes, and/or diaphragm. While these radiologic features are not unique to lymphoma, they are characteristic of its spread patterns and have particular importance in defining management in that they preclude an effective treatment plan with radiation alone.

Mixed Features of Coincident Pathology

There may be certain radiologic features at presentation that do not appear to be consistent with a single, unifying interpretation (e.g., discrete cystic areas as opposed to the less uniform low-signal areas associated with necrosis, localized, clearly defined mass borders within an otherwise irregular mediastinal lesion) (Fig. 58-28A&B). These features may become more apparent during therapy, when certain components of the mass appear to resolve while others remain unchanged (Fig. 58-28C–E). Such features should stimulate consideration of alternative pathology (e.g., mediastinal cysts (Lindfors, et al., 1985) or paraesophageal cysts. MRI (Fig. 58-29) or transoesophageal ultrasound (Fig. 58-30) may be helpful in distinguishing coexisting lesions that complicate the radiologic interpretation of the mediastinum.

HISTOLOGIC CATEGORIES

Hodgkin's disease, diffuse large cell non-Hodgkin's lymphoma, and lymphoblastic lymphoma comprise over 90 percent of primary mediastinal lymphomas (Benjamin, et al., 1972; Lichtenstein et al., 1980). The principal characteristics of each disease are shown in Table 58-5.

While Hodgkin's disease is recognized to have a bimodal age incidence pattern, primary mediastinal presentations and bulky mediastinal involvement secondary to nodal disease are clearly associated with the early age peak occurring from the late teens to the early thirties. The nodular sclerosing subtype represents by far the most common histologic pattern, and the thymus may be the site of origin of this tumor, previously and erroneously termed "granulomatous thymoma." The characteristic histologic pattern is one of tissue effacement by coarse bands of fibrous tissue, creating a nodular appearance. The cellular content of the nodules comprises a pleomorphic cellular background (lymphocytes, eosinophils, and plasma cells) with mononuclear Hodgkin's cells and the characteristic Reed-Sternberg cells, which in fixed material appear as the so-called lacunar cell variant of the Reed-Sternberg cell. Tissue immunocytochemistry and histochemistry are generally nonspecific inasmuch as no clonal lineage is identified, this parameter serving more to exclude the diagnosis of non-Hodgkin's lymphoma than to confirm the diagnosis of Hodgkin's disease.

Lymphoblastic lymphoma is a highly aggressive tumor arising from the thymus and commonly presenting as a rapidly enlarging mediastinal mass of substantial proportion in ado-lescents and young adults (Nathwani, et al., 1981). The histological appearance is that of a diffuse lymphoma, composed of a polymorphic infiltrate of small to intermediate-size cells with scant cytoplasm and finely divided, often convoluted nuclei containing evenly dispersed chromatin and punctate, inconspicuous nucleoli. The neoplastic cells have an immature T-cell phenotype and characteristically high levels of terminal deoxynucleotidyl transferase (TdT) activity. Lymphoblastic lymphoma has a rapidly fulminant natural history, with early involvement of the central nervous system and bone marrow and progression to a leukemic phase.

Diffuse histiocytic, or large cell, non-Hodgkin's lymphomas of the mediastinum are a more heterogeneous group of lymphomas, whose histolgic diversity is currently being defined through the increasing use of phenotypic and genotypic probes to establish lineage and differentiation. At present, the condition is generally referred to as mediastinal large cell lymphoma, with or without sclerosis, and is subdivided into at least the following three types: follicular center cell tumor with sclerosis, B-cell immunoblastic sarcoma, and T-cell immunoblastic sarcoma.

Follicular Center Cell Tumor with Sclerosis

A tumor of B-cell phenotype, large cell size, and follicular center cell origin occurring with a diffuse pattern (which commonly distinguishes it from secondary mediastinal involvement by systemic follicular center cell lymphoma) is frequently accompanied by organized, "compartmentalizing" sclerosis. This tumor which is more common in women

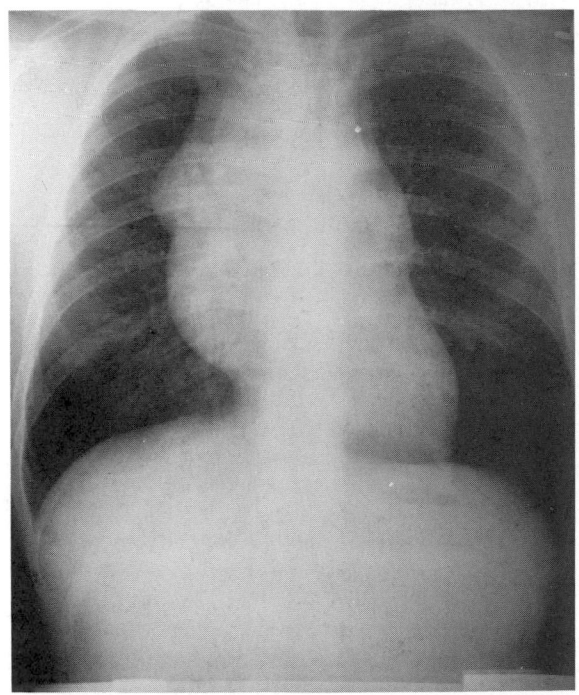
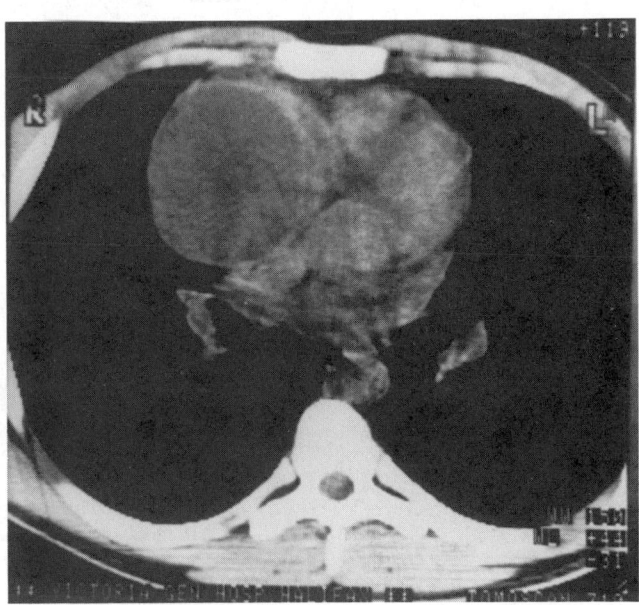

A   B

Figure 58-28. **(A)** A PA chest radiograph of a young man with Hodgkin's disease shows a massively enlarged mediastinum composed of bilateral paratracheal adenopathy and a grossly abnormal right lower paramediastinal-cardiac border. **(B)** The CT scan reveals the right paramediastinal lesion to be circumscribed and of low signal intensity in comparison with the remainder of the mediastinal mass. (*Figure continues.*)

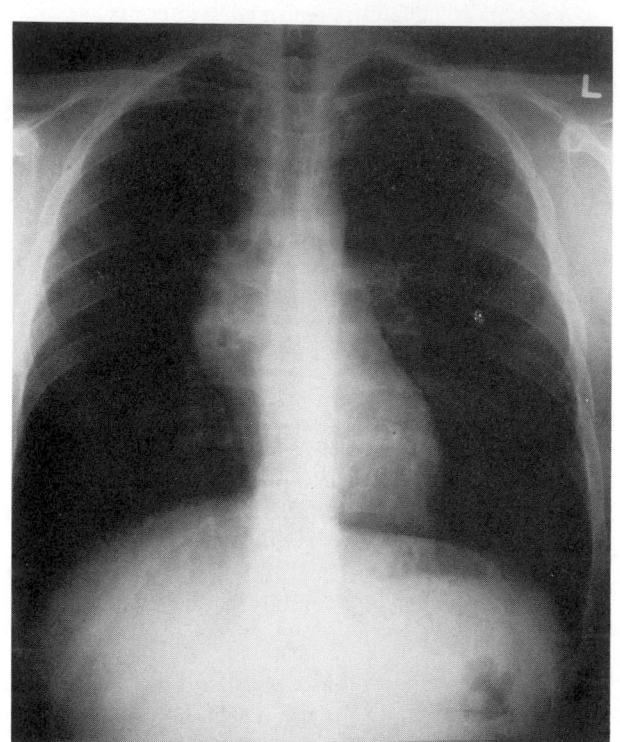

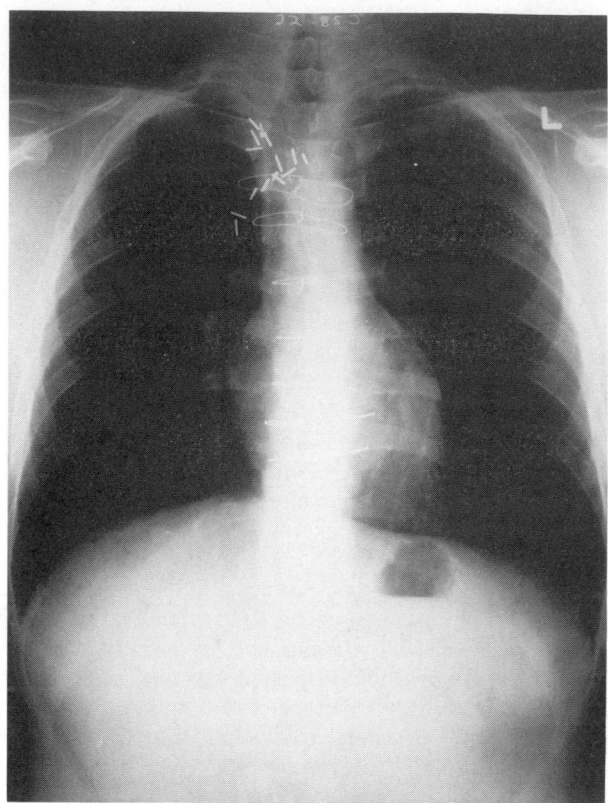

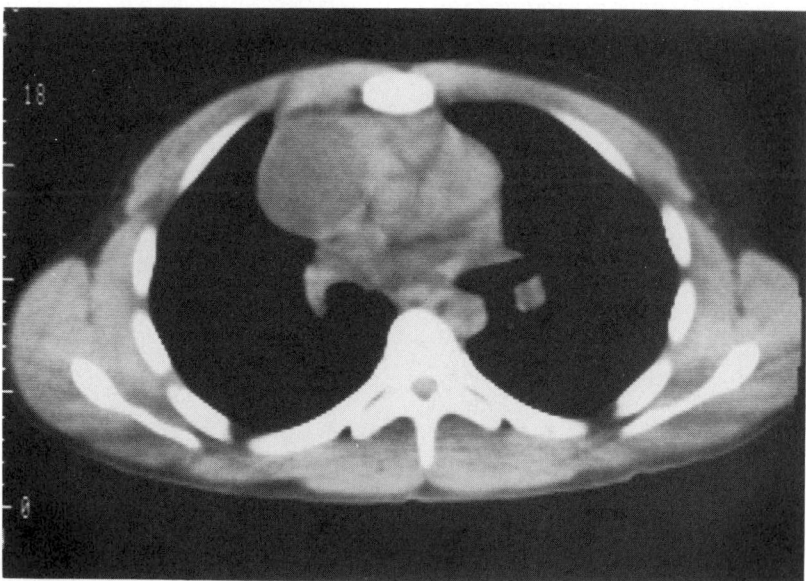

Figure 58-28 (*Continued*). **(C)** PA radiograph and **(D)** CT scan taken 7 months after Figs. A and B, following completion of six cycles of chemotherapy. **(E)** The PA radiograph obtained following midline sternotomy and removal of a thymic cyst. No persisting evidence of Hodgkin's disease was evident in excised tissues.

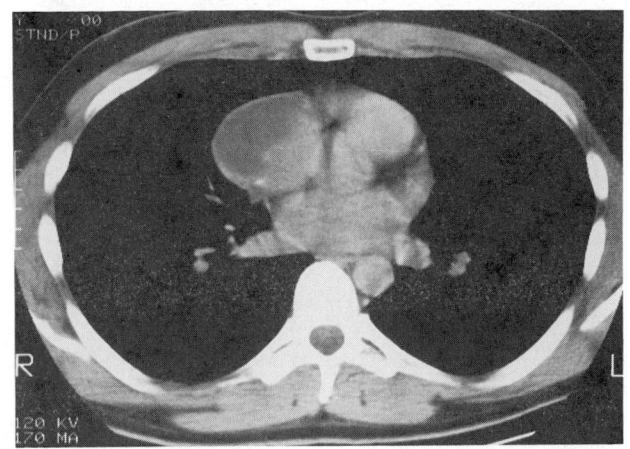

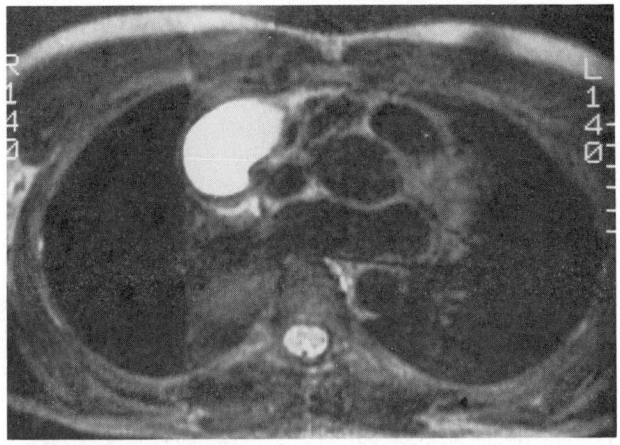

Figure 58-29. **(A)** A mass lesion in the right mediastinum with variable signal intensity is shown on the CT of the thorax of a young man treated with chemotherapy for Hodgkin's disease. **(B)** The lesion, thought to be partially necrotic residual tumor, was demonstrated to be a cyst (probably thymic) on MRI of the thorax (TR 2535; TE 80 2/2).

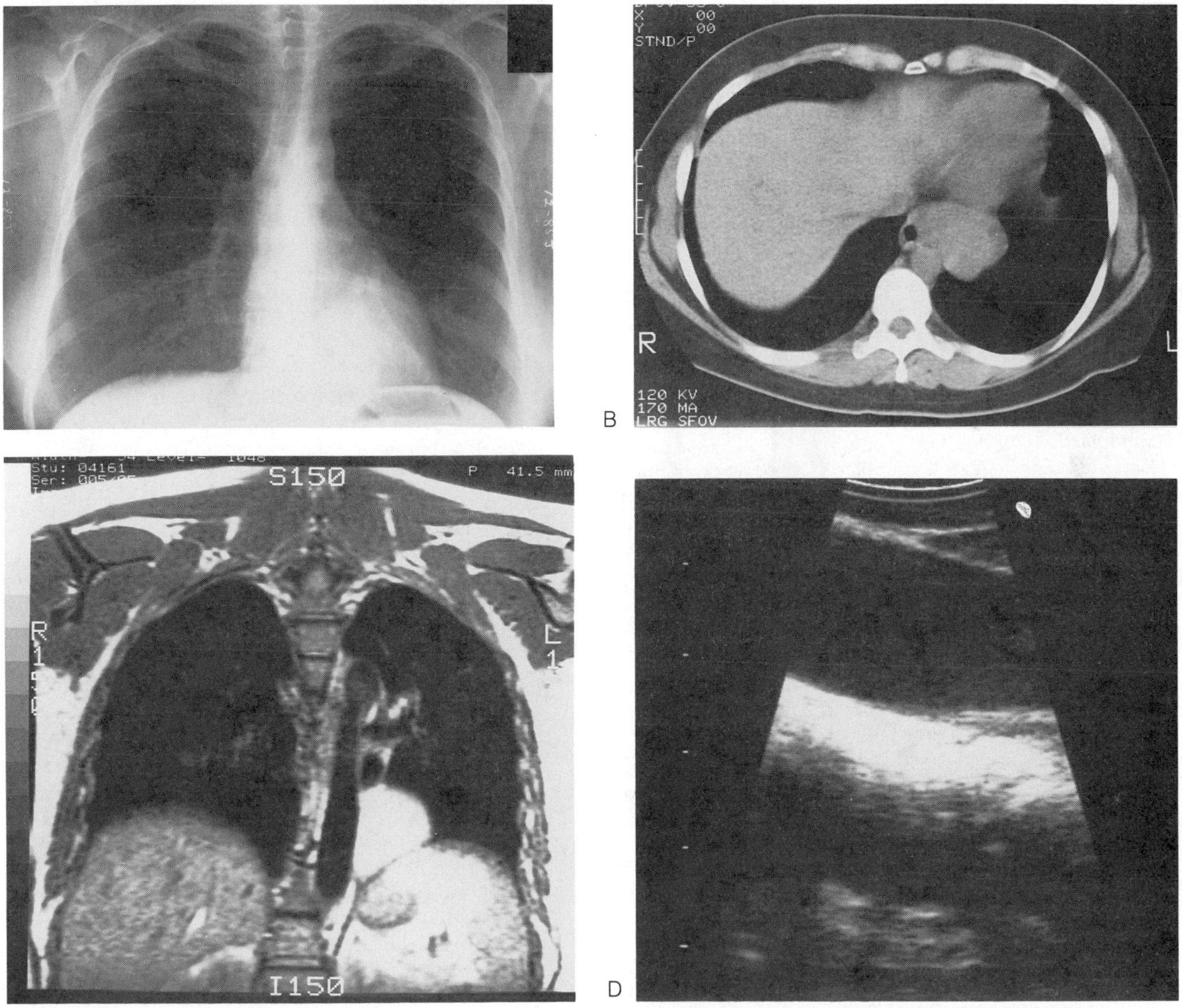

Figure 58-30. **(A)** A PA chest radiograph of a young woman with stage IV B Hodgkin's disease. A retrocardiac mass is evident despite resolution of other mediastinal adenopathy with chemotherapy. **(B)** The location of the mass in relation to the esophagus and aorta is defined on CT. **(C)** The clear delineation of the lesion is shown on coronal MRI [TR 870; TE 30]. **(D)** The lesion was established to be a paraesophageal cyst following transesophageal ultrasound (the transducer is in the esophageal lumen at the superior margin of the figure, and the sonolucent cyst lies adjacent to the esophagus). (Courtesy of Stephanie Wilson, M.D., Toronto Hospital.)

and has a peak incidence in the early thirties (compared with 50 to 60 years for most non-Hodgkin's lymphomas), is frequently accompanied by superior vena caval obstruction, is commonly associated with lymphoma symptoms, and is commonly invasive within the mediastinum. While the lineage is recognized to be of B-cell type, heterogeneity of differentiation is apparent, ranging from a surface immunoglobulin-negative early B-cell to a terminally differentiated, pre-plasma cell phenotype. A proportion of these tumors may, indeed, be primary thymic B-cell lymphomas.

B-Cell Immunoblastic Sarcoma

The B-cell type of immunoblastic sarcoma is a tumor characterized histologically by a diffuse pattern, monomorphous large cells with abundant cytoplasm, round to oval nuclei, predominantly dispersed chromatin, and prominent nucleoli. Sclerosis is less organized in appearance and may be associated with areas of tumor necrosis.

T-Cell Immunoblastic Sarcoma

T-cell immunoblastic sarcomas have the more characteristic appearance of peripheral T-cell lymphoma, with a polymorphic cellular content ranging from small lymphoid cells with "crinkled" nuclear outlines to large cells with abundant cytoplasm and large, lobated nuclei with prominent nucleoli. A stroma rich in postcapillary venules associated with delicate, reticular collagenous fibers is apparent, although the sclerosis appears less organized than the coarse, interanastomosing fibrous bands seen in follicular center cell lymphoma. The phenotype of T-cell immunoblastic sarcoma is characterized by expression of differentiated T-cell antigens, and TdT expression (early phenotype) is absent, in contradistinction to lymphoblastic lymphoma.

There remains a small percentage (<10 percent) of apparently primary mediastinal tumors not encompassed by the above histologic diagnoses. Other diagnoses include small cell lymphocytic lymphoma (the degree to which small cell lymphomas can be considered primarily localized is considered circumspect) and lymphomatoid granulomatosis and angioimmunoblastic lymphadenopathy (both now considered T-cell lymphoma of angiocentric, peripheral T-cell type). The degree to which these diagnoses are distinguishable from the more common categories of non-Hodgkin's lymphoma noted above is dependent on detailed phenotypic-genotypic studies that would underlie a more definitive classification of primary mediastinal non-Hodgkin's lymphoma. Composite tumors comprising Hodgkin's disease and non-Hodgkin's lymphoma have also been recorded (Perrone, et al., 1988).

ROLE OF SURGERY

Presurgery Evaluation

The principal issue facing the surgeon for a patient with a primary mediastinal tumor is the provision of a secure diagnosis upon which to base subsequent management decisions. There is no therapeutic role for total tumor excision or radical node dissection for patients with primary mediastinal lymphoma. Thus, for the patient with mediasinal lymphoma, the questions that the surgeon may address are

Has diagnostic material been obtained?

Has the material been optimally handled to permit a secure diagnosis?

Has sufficient diagnostic tissue been obtained to permit the ancillary histopathologic procedures necessary to achieve a diagnosis within the broad category of mediastinal lymphoma?

These issues are underlined on review of personal experience and the literature on mediastinal lymphoma. Not infrequently, the pathologist's report is tempered by comments relating to "small fragments of tissue" and "extensive crush artifact", "insufficient tissue to undertake special procedures" (e.g., immunohistochemistry and/or cytochemistry, flow cytometric analysis, electron microscopy), and "failure to provide 'fresh' or 'frozen' tissue for further analysis." In addition, the heterogeneity of outcome contained withint reports of therapy for patients with primary mediastinal lymphoma in large part reflects the inability to discriminate among the subtypes of lymphoma with varying untreated and treated natural history (Table 58-5), given either the lack of adequate material or the lack of sufficient material in suitable form to undertake the necessary ancillary procedures for accurate diagnosis. The surgeon should therefore consider these issues in the context of the surgical approach, the type of biopsy, and the acquisition and handling of specimens.

Surgical Approach

The choice of approach—mediastinoscopy, mediastinotomy, upper partial median sternotomy, median sternotomy, or thoracotomy—will be determined by the surgeon on the basis of the distribution of disease as defined by imaging procedures (Yellin, et al., 1987; Ricci, et al., 1990).

Type of Biopsy

In general, material removed by biopsy forceps is limited in its ability to yield high-quality diagnostic information by the small size of the tissue sample, "sampling artifact" (often the tissue fragment contains fibrous, sclerotic tissue representing either capsule or pseudocapsule with little cellular material for diagnostic purposes), "crush artifact," and insufficient material for more discriminating histologic analysis.

Specimen Acquisition and Handling

The surgeon can be assisted by the pathologist in the confirmation that diagnostic materal has been obtained by "quick-section" analysis, that the acquired material is appropriate for further study (i.e., appropriately fixed, fresh and frozen samples), and that adequate material has been taken for further analytic procedures.

Attention to detail on these issues will avoid diagnostic confusion with the attendant risk of inappropriate therapy, the necessity for repeated procedures with additional morbidity, delay in instituting appropriate treatment (Yellin, et al., 1987; Ricci, et al., 1990). The diversity of diagnosis and the implications with respect to treatment and prognosis are identified in Table 58-5.

In addition to the provision of diagnostic material, the surgeon may make an additional valuable contribution through commentary or tissue sampling appropriate to the exposure obtained to the mediastinum. Thus, debulking surgery that does not add appreciably to the morbidity of the diagnostic procedure and commentary and/or tissue biopsies pertaining to spread patterns within the thorax (e.g., lung, pericardium, chest wall, internal mammary nodes, diaphragm) yield valuable information regarding therapeutic approaches and the potential disposition of radiation fields.

Post-Therapy

The surgeon may become involved in the management of patients following therapy for the reasons discussed below.

Assessment of a Persisting Abnormal Mediastinal Contour Post-Therapy

The persistence of a residual radiologic anomaly of the mediastinal contour post-therapy is a well recognized finding in both Hodgkin's disease (Jochelson, et al., 1985; Orlandi, et al., 1990) and non-Hodgkin's lymphoma (Lewis, et al., 1982; Stewart, et al., 1985). These changes may be minor—straightening of the aortopulmonary window, unilateral or bilateral "fullness" of the paratracheal contour—or they may represent obvious and measurable abnormalities and depending upon the imaging procedures employed, may be defined in 30 to 90 percent of those patients presenting with bulky mediastinal disease.

The principal issue raised is whether such abnormalities represent viable, persisting tumor with the attendant therapeutic dilemma of "undertreatment" if a conservative, expectant policy is adopted for persisting disease versus "overtreatment" if a radical treatment is administered for sterilized, nonviable sclerotic tissue. In practice, the majority of such abnormalities represent sclerotic, nonviable tumor, as evidenced by histopathologic evaluation of biopsy material (Lewis, et al., 1982; Stewart, et al., 1985; Surbone, et al., 1988; Durkin and Durant, 1979; Lepage, et al., 1984; Chen, et al., 1987) or by follow-up studies documenting patterns of relapse (Jochelson et al., 1985; Radford, et al., 1988; Orlandi, et al., 1990; Uematsu, et al., 1989). Indeed, all cited evidence would indicate that the thoracic relapse rate does not differ significantly between those patients with normal radiologic examinations post-therapy and those with a persisting stable mediastinal abnormality.

Be that as it may, the intrathoracic relapse rate for patients with presentation of bulky mediastinal disease is 20 percent, and relapse is more likely to occur in those treated with chemotherapy alone. Accordingly, at the individual patient level the issue of a residual mediastinal abnormality and "complete remission status" requires resolution, and this may necessitate histopathologic analysis (Fig. 58-31).

In current practice, this issue cannot be resolved by CT examination. Gallium scanning has been employed to add a functional dimension to the evaluation of radiologic abnormalities. Such studies need to be performed not earlier than 6 weeks following completion of therapy to avoid false negative interpretation and may require delayed and/or serial imaging with SPECT capability. While a negative image may support a diagnosis of completely treated tumor, a positive image is generally considered indicative of residual active tumor. More recently, MRI has been employed to attempt resolution of the issue of viable persistent tumor versus fibrosis, with some indication that change in relative signal intensities may be predictive of treatment response (Nyman, et al., 1989; Webb, 1989). Caution must be exercised, however, in correlating signal parameters with pathologic processes in the absence of histologic verification or detailed, long-term follow-up studies defining patterns of relapse.

In certain circumstances, biopsy(ies) may be required to resolve the issue of persisting tumor post-therapy, where such information cannot be obtained from imaging studies, in order to define appropriate management decisions (Fig. 58-32). The principles defined about pertaining to pretreatment surgicopathologic assessment remain, namely, appropriate exposure to obtain satisfactory samples of tumor tissue and optimal specimen handling. These issues, however, now need to be addressed in the context of additional technical problems due to reduction in tumor bulk, increased fibrosis resulting from therapy, tight adhesions, fragility of vasculature, and loss of tissue cleavage planes (Yellin, et al., 1987; Ricci, et al., 1990).

Management of Disease and Therapy-Related Complications

Constrictive pericarditis is a recognized complication of wide-field supradiaphragmatic radiation. Improvements in the technique of radiotherapy have contributed to a reduction in the incidence of constrictive pericarditis such that it should no longer be a therapy-related complication. These improvements include the use of megavoltage beams at extended source-skin/axis distance, anterior and posterior portals treated daily without differential weighting, fractions size not exceeding 200 cGy tumor dose per day, total tumor does not exceeding 3,500 cGy, and the use of effective chemotherapy to minimize irradiation volumes encompassing the heart. In rare circumstances, however, pericardiectomy may still be required to manage congestive cardiac failure resulting from therapy.

An additional complication related to therapy is the increased relative cardiac death rate for patients with Hodgkin's disease treated by mediastinal irradiation (Boivin and Hutchison, 1982). The development of precocious coronary artery disease in individuals without recognized risk factors other than mediastinal irradiation is being increasingly recognized (Brosius, et al., 1981; Totterman, et al., 1983; Tenet, et al., 1986; Radwaner, et al., 1987). This complication is consistent with the pathology of radiation effect upon vessels within the radiation portals and may become a therapy-related side effect of increasing concern for a patient population spared from dying of their malignant disease.

MANAGEMENT

Although surgical excision has been recorded as a radical therapy for primary mediastinal lymphoma, in an era of effec-

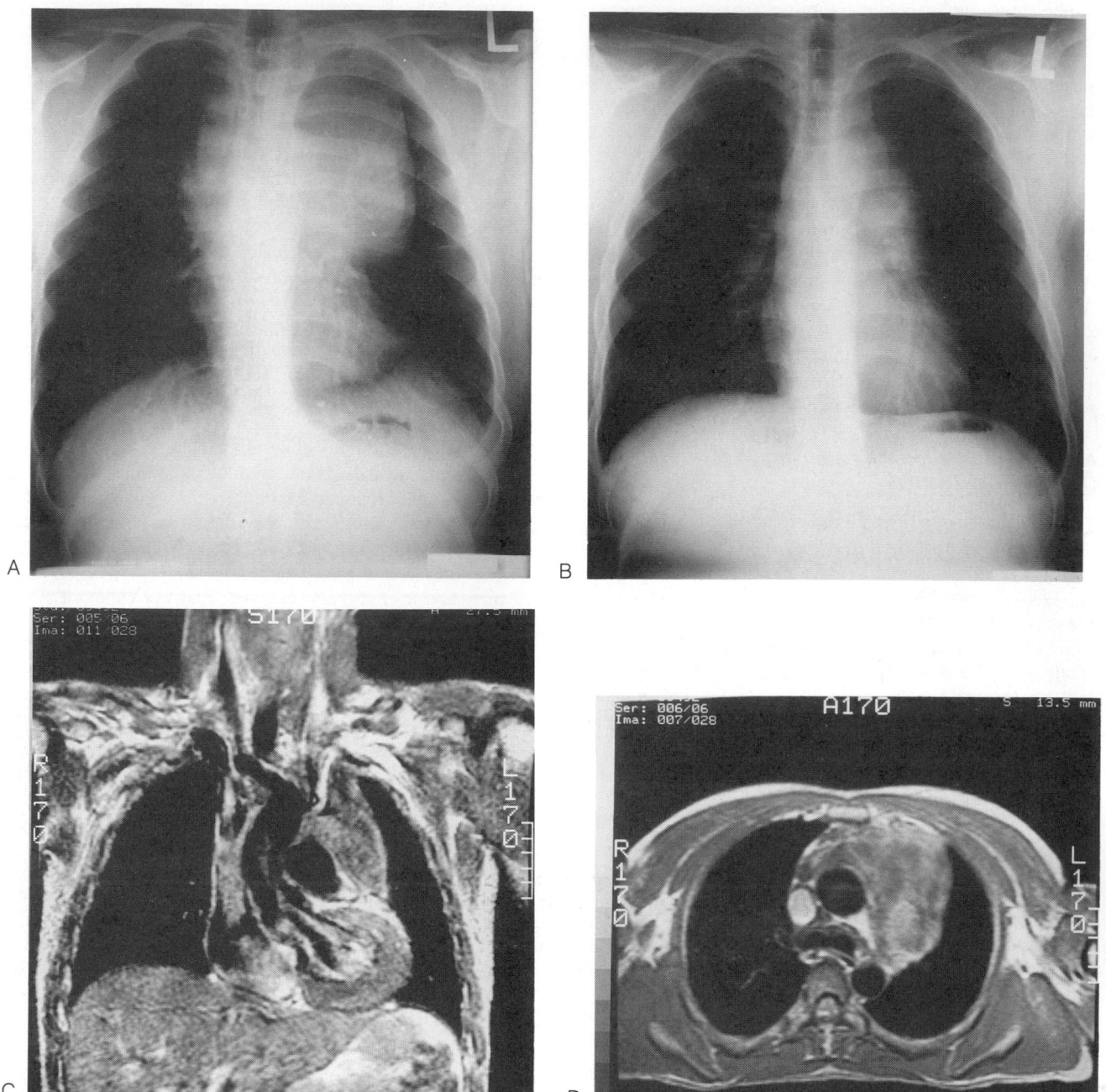

Figure 58-31. **(A)** A PA chest radiograph (taken Nov. 21, 1990) indicating massive mediastinal adenopathy in a young man with clinical stage II B Hodgkin's disease. **(B)** Following six cycles of chemotherapy, the PA chest radiograph (Apr. 4, 1991) revealed substantial, but incomplete resolution of the lesion. **(C)** Coronal and **(D)** sagittal MRI [TR 2105; TE 30½] clearly defined the anatomic dimensions of the lesion and the nonuniform signal characteristics. The lesion was not evident on gallium scanning with SPECT imaging. Generous biopsies through an anterior mediastinotomy revealed fibrous tissue without evidence of active Hodgkin's disease.

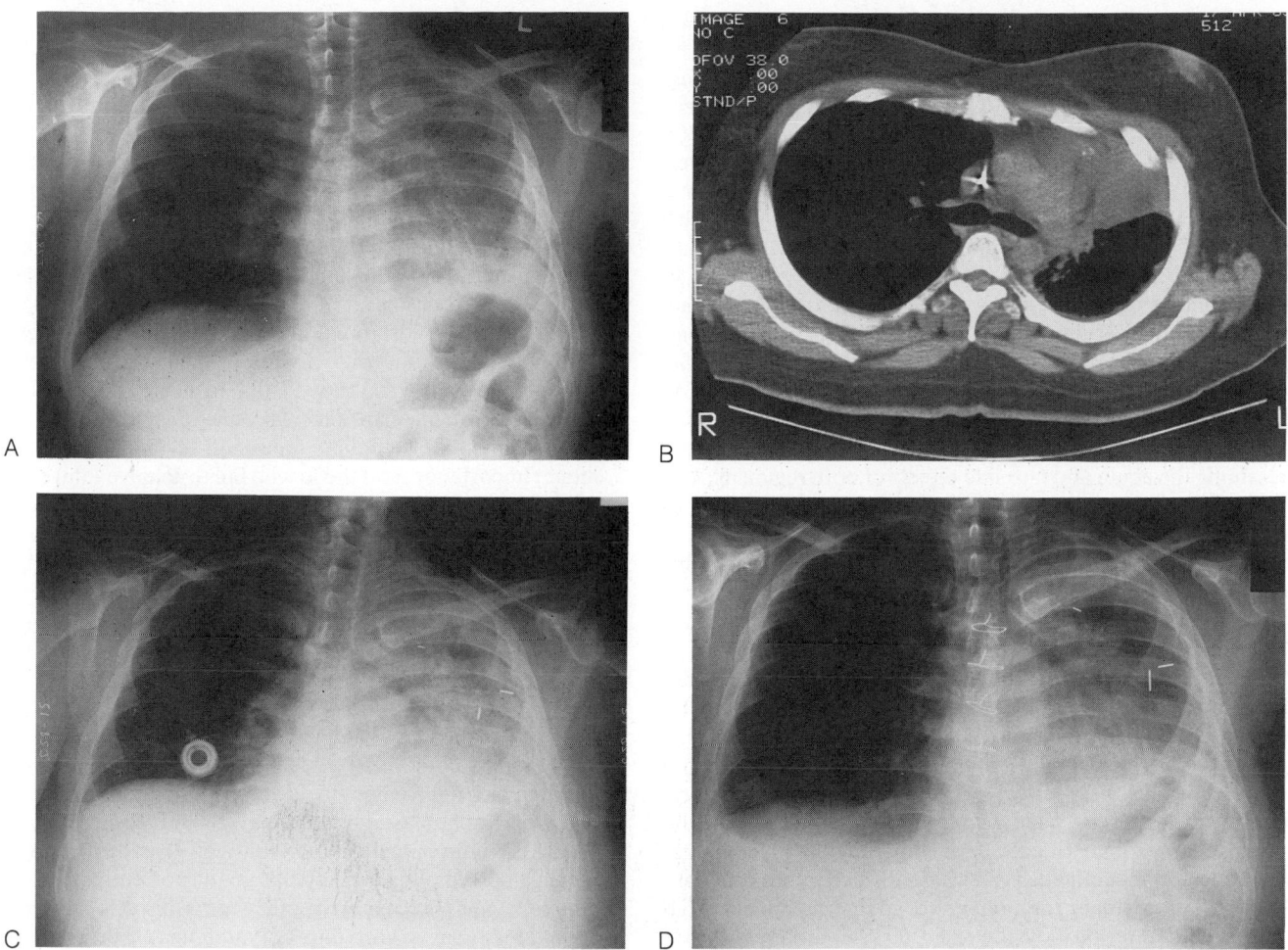

Figure 58-32. PA chest film of a young man referred following previous radiation therapy to a mantle field and a generous portion of the left lung for clinical stage IIA Hodgkin's disease with mediastinal and left hilar adenopathy. Disease recurred in the retronephric, retroperitoneal, and left transdiaphragmatic regions. **(A)** Chest radiograph taken following six cycles of chemotherapy. **(B)** CT scan indicating an abnormality extending from the left cardiac border to the left anterior chest wall. Gross pleural thickening is evident. **(C)** Chest radiograph obtained following a left thoracotomy, which yielded multiple biopsies without evidence of active Hodgkin's disease. **(D)** Chest radiograph taken 3 months later following a midline sternotomy and partial pericardiectomy for rapidly progressive heart failure due to constrictive pericarditis. No evidence of active Hodgkin's disease was obtained from the excised tissues.

tive radiation and chemotherapy it cannot be considered a curative therapy. A radical dissection is rarely ever warranted other than as a debulking procedure without increasing the morbidity beyond a biopsy, and even extensive surgery would not remove the continuing requirement for radiotherapy and/or chemotherapy as the primary curative therapy.

Radiotherapy alone may be employed as a curative therapy for primary mediastinal Hodgkin's disease. Given no evidence of disease beyond the thorax, the principal issues determining curability by radiation are the mass size and the evidence, if any, for extension of disease beyond the confines of the nodal or thymic lesion. The bulk of the mass is important in relation to the physical imposition that it places upon adequate shielding of the lungs (which have a critical limiting tolerance) and also in terms of the predictive power that bulky disease defines for intrathoracic recurrence when conventionally planned supradiaphragmatic radiation fields

are employed. This pattern of failure occurring within the thorax but remote from or marginal to the mass lesion almost certainly indicates the failure to treat occult disease within lymphatic pathways of the chest wall, lung, pericardium, or diaphragm by superimposition of lung shielding blocks. In this circumstance, appropriate management is by modification of radiation technique to provide whole thoracic irradiation within lung tolerance (Lee, et al., 1980) or more commonly, by use of a combined modality approach in which chemotherapy is used to achieve shrinkage or control of the mediastinum prior to radiotherapy.

Chemotherapy has the additional advantage of effectively addressing occult disease beyond the thorax. Given, however, a presentation of primary mediastinal Hodgkin's disease that is technically curable by radiation, supradiaphragmatic disease is managed according to well recognized principles in terms of radiation dose, fractionation, radiation field configuration, and techniques (Hoppe, 1989; Timothy, et al., 1987).

The traditional chemotherapeutic management of Hodgkin's disease has been the MOPP regimen (mustine, vincristine, procarbazine, and prednisone) (DeVita, et al., 1970). Since the mid-1980s, there has been a move toward the alternative ABVD regimen (Adriamycin, bleomycin, vinblastine, and imidazole carboxamide) (Bonadonna, et al., 1975), which has an efficacy superior to that of MOPP (Canellos, et al., 1992) but substantially less long-term morbidity in terms of development of second malignancies and gonadal dysfunction. Another alternative to MOPP alone is use of an alternating sequence of MOPP and ABVD (Bonadonna, et al., 1986) or MOPP and ABV (Klimo and Connors, 1988). These combinations provide greater therapeutic intensity, employing more effective agents in close and alternating sequence but retaining the acute and late side effects of both regimens. The particular significance of the ABVD regimen in the context of irradiation is the potential for enhanced interaction in terms of pulmonary and cardiovascular complications, necessitating consideration of sequence modifications of combined modality therapy, drug dose reductions, and/or radiation dose and volume modifications (Lagrange, et al., 1988).

Given optimal selection of patients with mediastinal Hodgkin's disease for management by radiation alone or by combined-modality therapy, long-term freedom from relapse and survival rates should be approximately 80 percent and 90 percent plus, respectively. Radiation would, almost certainly, no longer be used as the sole curative therapeutic approach for primary mediastinal non-Hodgkin's lymphoma. Several factors mitigate against a satisfactory control rate with radiation alone: the tumors are of intermediate to high grade, with a propensity for rapid dissemination; they are commonly very bulky; extranodal spread beyond the site of origin is common; patients are frequently compromised by local-regional symptomatology and require urgent therapy; and they are frequently symptomatic of lymphoma, an adverse prognostic factor. Prior experience with radiotherapy for apparently localized large cell lymphoma also indicates a very substantial failure rate in the presence of such adverse features, the failure rate involving both local and, more commonly, local-marginal and systemic progression indicative of more extensive disease than clinically apparent at the time of therapy.

Combination chemotherapy has become the therapy of choice, and regimens that are therapy-intensive and based upon Adriamycin have proved most effective (Yi, et al., 1990). The role of adjuvant radiotherapy to the mediastinum has not been established, but such radiation is commonly employed in view the localized nature of the presentation and the likelihood of a significant risk of recurrence at the site of initial bulk disease following chemotherapy. Central nervous system prophylaxis employing intrathecal chemo-

therapy, with or without cranial radiation, is an integral component of the remission induction therapy for lymphoblastic lymphoma but is not required for follicular center cell lymphoma when there is no indication of central nervous system progression as part of the natural history.

Heterogeneity of outcome for patients with primary mediastinal lymphoma is reported in the literature. This may in part reflect heterogeneity of diagnosis. With an intensive combined-modality approach, a cure rate in excess of 50 percent should be achieved (Waldron, et al., 1985; Jacobson, et al., 1988; Todeschini, et al., 1990).

For patients with Hodgkin's disease and non-Hodgkin's lymphoma, total control of disease is mandatory for survival. The prognosis for those who fail to achieve remission is dismal, with a median survival measured in months. The establishment of complete remission is therefore of paramount importance, and those who fail to achieve total control with first-line chemotherapy should proceed to intensive alternate (salvage) therapies, which may include massive chemotherapy with autologous transplantation of tumor-free bone marrow (Canellos, et al., 1988; Crump, et al., 1993).

SUMMARY

Primary malignant mediastinal tumors are uncommon. Lymphomas comprise up to 50 percent of malignancies in children and approximately 20 percent in adults. Hodgkin's disease, lymphoblastic lymphoma, and diffuse large cell non-Hodgkin's lymphomas account for over 90 percent of primary mediastinal lymphomas. Asymptomatic presentations are uncommon, and the majority of patients have local-regional symptomatology. Symptoms of lymphoma (night sweats, fever, and weight loss), superior vena caval obstruction, and extensive extranodal spread beyond the primary mediastinal lesion are more common in non-Hodgkin's lymphoma. Detailed imaging studies employing CT and MRI and gallium scanning are necessary to document extent of disease, define optimal therapy, and document extent of response to therapy. A secure diagnosis is essential for optimal management and is based upon the histopathologic assessment of tissue that is satisfactory in both quality and amount for detailed histologic and immunophenotypic-genotypic studies. Surgical procedures may also be required to establish complete control of mediastinal disease and to correct late complications of therapy.

The principal management strategies are radiation or combined-modality therapy for Hodgkin's disease and combined-modality therapy for non-Hodgkin's lymphoma. Based upon optimal diagnosis and therapy, long-term control rates should exceed 75 percent for Hodgkin's disease and 50 to 60 percent for non-Hodgkin's lymphoma presenting primarily in the mediastinum.

COMMENTS AND CONTROVERSIES

Surgery rarely has more than a diagnostic role in the management of malignant lymphoma. Even for sites at which major resection has traditionally been a component of management

(e.g., gastrointestinal lymphoma, primary bone lymphoma), its role is being challenged in the face of potentially curative chemotherapy and radiation.

Primary mediastinal lymphoma does not differ materially from lymphoma at other nodal or extranodal sites. The role of surgery is largely limited to diagnosis, and while imaging may play an important role in defining disease extent and optimal surgical route, imaging modalities are likely to be most useful in future if they combine a functional analysis of tumor viability with their traditional role in descriptive anatomy (e.g., functional radionuclide imaging, MRI with paramagnetic contrast agents, or PET scanning). Similarly, it is unlikely that there will be major innovations or new understandings in radiotherapy. There has been relatively little advance in conventional chemotherapy since the early to mid-1980s, a plateau in remission and survival rates having been reached. Chemotherapy regimens will continue to be optimized with respect to efficacy and toxicity, and dose intensity will be pursued in the context of autologous marrow/peripheral stem cell or growth factor support. It is likely, however, that such initiatives will optimize therapy for the majority, will benefit a minority who would otherwise fail with conventional therapy, and will fail to materially modify the disease for a further minority who remain refractory to such approaches.

The principal future advances in the management of malignant lymphoma may come from

The early identification and characterization of those patients with disease refractory to standard therapeutic approaches for whom innovative and experimental therapies are required

The identification, following completion of therapy, of those patients with minimal residual occult disease in whom treatment intensification might be effective

An understanding of the molecular basis of transformation, clonal evolution, and genetically determined or acquired drug resistance

Characterization of the regulatory mechanisms of gene function

Regulation of the malignant cell through manipulation of growth at the genomic level or through the use of exogenous growth factors

Alterations to the biology of the cell through immunoregulation or immunocytotoxicity by biologic response modifiers and/or specific immunotherapy employing anti-idiotypic antibodies

Enhancement of therapeutic effects of chemotherapy through regulation of the cell cycle by growth factors, through increasing the bioavailability of effective agents, or through overcoming genetic or acquired drug resistance.

It will be apparent that in the absence of a detailed biologic understanding of malignant lymphoma, the gains of conventional therapy have largely been achieved and have been substantial. Major advance will now require new therapeutic strategies based upon knowledge of malignant cell biology and function and the nature of the tumor-host relationship.

S.B.S.

Dr. Sutcliffe emphasizes the diagnostic role of surgery in the management of malignant lymphomas. He stresses the importance of open biopsy in those lymphomas (especially Hodgkin's disease) for which needle aspiration, cytology, and immunohistochemistry do not yield a positive answer. However, with increasing frequency, especially in pure T- or B-cell lymphomas, cytology and immunohistochemistry can reveal the complete diagnosis without necessitating an open biopsy.

There is nothing more confusing in oncology than the ever-changing classification of lymphomas. With increasing knowledge of cell biology, I hope that in future further changes in this very confusing classification will occur to please us simple surgeons!

Very rarely, the surgeon is asked to debulk nonresponding masses following chemotherapy in order that the radiotherapy fields can encompass the tumor. This, on occasion, is quite justified. In addition, the surgeon is also occasionally required to remove residual masses to identify active disease or recurrent lesions following complete responses or to identify the nature of the new mass before therapy is instituted. In many of these cases, complete resection is impossible and only debulking is appropriate. In managing mediastinal lymphomas when surgery is required, it is very rare that vital structures (e.g., superior vena cava, phrenic or vagus nerves) need to be resected in the therapy. Since these lesions are usually exquisitely sensitive to chemotherapy and radiotherapy, the functional disturbances that occur from this type of aggressive surgical excision militate against its performance.

R.J.G.

KEY REFERENCES

Armitage JO: Chemotherapy for non-Hodgkin's lymphoma. Curr Opinion Oncol 4:840, 1992

A current brief review of chemotherapy for primary treatment and salvage of non-Hodgkin's lymphoma.

Cannellos GP, Anderson, JR, Propert, KJ et al: Chemotherapy of advanced Hodgkin's disease with MOPP, ABVD, or MOPP alternating with ABVD. N Engl J Med 327:1478, 1992

Randomized comparison of the principal chemotherapy regimens for the treatment of advanced Hodgkin's disease.

Carbone PP, Kaplan WS, Musshoff K et al: Report of the committee on Hodgkin's disease staging classification. Cancer Res 31:1860, 1971

A key report defining the evaluation and anatomically based description of disease extent as a basis for of therapy allocation and prognosis for patients with Hodgkin's disease.

Chabner BA, Johnson RE, Young RC et al: Sequential non-surgical and surgical staging of non-Hodgkin's lymphoma. Ann Intern Med 85:149, 1976

An important study emphasizing the higher incidence of occult disease and more advanced stage in non-Hodgkin's lymphoma when subjected to detailed staging evaluation (comparison with Hodgkin's disease).

Jaffe ES: The role of immunophenotypic markers in the classification of non-Hodgkin's lymphoma. Semin Oncol 17:11, 1990

A review of surface antigen expression defined by monoclonal antibodies as a basis for distinction and classification of non-Hodgkin's lymphomas.

Lukes RJ, Butler JJ: The pathology and nomenclature of Hodgkin's disease. Cancer Res 26:1063, 1966

The generally accepted morphologic classification for Hodgkin's disease.

McKeithan TW: Molecular biology of non-Hodgkin's lymphomas. Semin Oncol 17:30, 1990

A current comprehensive review of the molecular events involved in malignant lymphoma of B and T cell types.

Non-Hodgkins Lymphoma Pathologic Classification Project: National Cancer Institute sponsored study of non-Hodgkin's lymphomas: summary and description of a working formulation for clinical usage. Cancer 49:211, 1982

A key study attempting to reconcile existing morphologic concepts

of non-Hodgkin's lymphoma into a clinically and prognostically useful classification.

Sutcliffe SB, Gospodarowicz MK: Clinical features and management of localized extranodal lymphomas. In Keating A, Armitage J, Burnett A, and Newland A (eds): Cambridge Medical Reviews: Haematological Oncology. Vol 2. Cambridge University Press, 1992

A review of localized non-Hodgkin's lymphoma, identifying the diversity of presentations and the variable natural history associated with presentation in various extranodal sites.

Sutcliffe SB, Gospodarowicz MK, Bush RS et al: Role of radiation therapy in localized non-Hodgkin's lymphoma. Radiother Oncol 4:211, 1985

A detailed analysis of local control, relapse-free rate, and survival for patients with non-Hodgkin's lymphoma, with identification of prognostic groups for whom radiation alone is appropriate therapy.

Timothy AR, Van Dyk J, Sutcliffe SB: Radiation therapy for Hodgkin's disease. p. 181. In Selby P, McElwain TJ (eds): Hodgkin's Disease. Blackwell Scientific Publications, Oxford, 1987

A review of radiotherapy management of patients with localized Hodgkin's disease, outlining approaches to evaluation, technique, and results of therapy.

REFERENCES

Addis BJ, Isaacson PG: Large cell lymphoma of the mediastinum: a B-cell tumor of probable thymic origin. Histopathology 10:370, 1986

Benjamin SP, McCormack LJ, Effler DB et al: Primary lymphatic tumors of the mediastinum. Cancer 30:708, 1972

Blank N, Castellino RA: The mediastinum in Hodgkin's and non-Hodgkin's lymphoma. J Thorac Imaging 2:66, 1987

Bonadonna G, Valagussa P, Santoro A: Alternating non-cross-resistant combination chemotherapy or MOPP in stage IV Hodgkin's disease. A report of 8-year results. Ann Intern Med 104:739, 1986

Bonadonna G, Zucali R, Monfardini S et al: Combination chemotherapy of Hodgkin's disease with Adriamycin, bleomycin, vinblastine, and imidazole carboxamide versus MOPP. Cancer 36:252, 1975

Boivin JF, Hutchison GB: Coronary heart disease mortality after irradiation for Hodgkin's disease. Cancer 49:2470, 1982

Brosius FC, Waller BF, Roberts WC: Radiation heart disease. Analysis of 16 young (aged 15 to 33 years) necropsy patients who received over 3,500 rads to the heart. Am J Med 70:519, 1981

Canellos GP, Nadler L, Takvorian T: Autologous bone marrow transplantation in the treatment of malignant lymphoma and Hodgkin's disease. Semin Hematol 25(suppl. 2):58, 1988

Chen JL, Osborne BM, Butler JJ: Residual fibrous masses in treated Hodgkin's disease. Cancer 60:407, 1987

Colby TV, Hoppe RT, Warnke RA: Hodgkin's disease: a clinicopathologic study of 659 cases. Cancer 49:1848, 1981

Crump M, Smith AM, Brandwein J et al: High dose etoposide, melphalan and autologous bone marrow transplantation for patients with advanced Hodgkin's disease: importance of disease status at transplant. J Clin Oncol 11:704, 1993

DeVita VT Jr, Serpick AA, Carbone PP: Combination chemotherapy in the treatment of advanced Hodgkin's disease. Ann Intern Med 73:881, 1970

Durkin W, Durant J: Benign mass lesions after therapy for Hodgkin's disease. Arch Intern Med 139:333, 1979

Haioun C, Gaulard P, Roudot-Thoraval F et al: Mediastinal diffuse large-cell lymphoma with sclerosis: a condition with a poor prognosis. Am J Clin Oncol 12:425, 1989

Hoppe RT: The management of bulky mediastinal Hodgkin's disease. Hematol Oncol Clin North Am 3:265, 1989

Jacobson JO, Aisenberg AC, Lamarre L et al: Mediastinal large cell lymphoma: an uncommon subset of adult lymphoma curable with combined modality therapy, Cancer 62:1893, 1988

Jochelson M, Mauch P, Balikian J et al: The significance of the residual mediastinal mass in treated Hodgkin's disease. J Clin Oncol 3:637, 1985

Jones SE, Fuks Z, Bull M et al: Non-Hodgkin's lymphomas. IV. Clinicopathologic correlation in 405 cases. Cancer 31:806, 1973

King RM, Telander RL, Smithson WA et al: Primary mediastinal tumors in children. J Pediatr Surg 17:512, 1982

Klimo P, Connors JM: An update on the Vancouver experience in the management of advanced Hodgkin's disease treated with the MOPP/ABV hybrid program. Semin Hematol 25(suppl. 2):34, 1988

Lagrange JL, Thyss A, Caldani C et al: Toxicity of a combination of ABVD chemotherapy and mediastinal irradiation for Hodgkin's disease patients with massive initial mediastinal involvement. Bull Cancer (Paris) 75:801, 1988

Lamarre L, Jacobson JO, Aisenberg AC et al: Primary large cell lymphoma of the mediastinum. A histologic and immunophenotypic study of 29 cases. Am J Surg Pathol 13:730, 1989

Lee CK, Bloomfield CD, Goldman AI et al: Prognostic significance of mediastinal involvement in Hodgkin's disease treated with curative radiotherapy. Cancer 46:2403, 1980

Lepage E, Ferme C, Frija J et al: Hodgkin's disease. Residual histologically stable masses after chemotherapy. Presse Med 13:1766, 1984

Levitt LJ, Aisenberg AC, Harris NL et al: Primary non-Hodgkin's lymphoma of the mediastinum. Cancer 50:2486, 1982

Lewis E, Bernardino ME, Salvador PG et al: Post-therapy CT-detected mass in lymphoma patients: is it viable tissue? J Comput Assist Tomogr 6:792, 1982

Lichtenstein A, Levin A, Taylor CR et al: Primary mediastinal lymphoma in adults. Am J Med 68:509, 1980

Linden MD, Tubbs RR, Weick JK: Large-cell lymphoma with diffuse sclerosis. A B-cell neoplasm of late-secretory, preplasma cells. Cleve Clin J Med 53:319, 1986

Lindfors KK, Meyer JE, Dedrick CG et al: Thymic cysts in mediastinal Hodgkin's disease. Radiology 156:37, 1985

Lukes RJ, Butler JJ, Hicks EB: Natural history of Hodgkin's disease as related to its pathological picture. Cancer 19:317, 1966

Menestrina F, Chilosi M, Bonetti F et al: Mediastinal large-cell lymphoma of B-type, with sclerosis: histopathological and immunohistochemical study of eight cases. Histopathology 10:589, 1986

Miller JB, Variakojis D, Bitran JDU et al: Diffuse histiocytic lymphoma with sclerosis: a clinicopathologic entity frequently causing superior venacaval obstruction. Cancer 47:748, 1981

Möller P, Moldenhauer G, Momburg F et al: Mediastinal lymphoma of clear cell type is a tumor corresponding to teminal steps of B cell differentiation. Blood 69:1087, 1987

Nathwani BN, Diamond LW, Winberg CD et al: Lymphoblastic lymphoma: a clinicopathologic study of 95 patients. Cancer 48:2347, 1981

Nyman RS, Rehn SM, Glimelius BL et al: Residual mediastinal masses in Hodgkin's disease: prediction of size with MR imaging. Radiology 170:435, 1989

Orlandi E, Lazzarino M, Brusamolino E et al: Residual mediastinal widening following therapy in Hodgkin's disease. Hematol Oncol 8:125, 1990

Perrone T, Frizzera G, Rosai J: Mediastinal diffuse large-cell lymphoma with sclerosis. A clinicopathologic study of 60 cases. Am J Surg Pathol 10:176, 1986

Radford JA, Cowan RA, Flanagan M: The significance of residual mediastinal abnormality on the chest radiograph following treatment for Hodgkin's disease. J Clin Oncol 6:940, 1988

Radwaner BA, Geringer R, Goldmann AM et al: Left main coronary artery stenosis following mediastinal irradiation. Am J Med 82:1017, 1987

Ricci C, Rendina EA, Venuta F et al: Surgical approach to isolated mediastinal lymphoma. J Thorac Cardiovasc Surg 99:691, 1990

Salonen O, Kivisaari L, Standertskjöld-Nordenstam CG et al: Chest radiography and computed tomography in the evaluation of mediastinal adenopathy in lymphoma. Acta Radiol 28:747, 1987

Scarpa A, Bonetti F, Menestrina F et al: Mediastinal large-cell lymphoma with sclerosis. Genotypic analysis establishes its B nature. Virchows Arch [A] 412:17, 1987

Stewart FM, Williamson BR, Innes DJ et al: Residual tumor masses following treatment for advanced histiocytic lymphoma. Diagnostic and therapeutic implications. Cancer 55:620, 1985

Surbone A, Longo DL, DeVita VT Jr et al: Residual abdominal masses in aggressive non-Hodgkin's lymphoma after combination chemotherapy: significance and management. J Clin Oncol 6:1832, 1988

Tenet W, Missri J, Hager D: Radiation-induced stenosis of the left main coronary artery. Cathet Cardiovasc Diagn 12:169, 1986

Timothy AR, VanDyk J, Sutcliffe SB: Radiation therapy for Hodgkin's disease. p. 181. In Selby P, McElwain TJ (eds): Hodgkin's Disease. Blackwell Scientific Publications, Oxford, 1987

Todeschini G, Ambrosetti A, Meneghini V: Mediastinal large-B-cell lymphoma with sclerosis: a clinical study of 21 patients. J Clin Oncol 8:804, 1990

Tötterman KJ, Pesonen E, Siltanen P: Radiation-related chronic heart disease. Chest 83:875, 1983

Trump DL, Mann RB: Diffuse large cell and undifferentiated lymphomas with prominent mediastinal involvement. Cancer 50:277, 1982

Uematsu M, Kondo M, Tsutsui T et al: Residual masses on follow-up computed tomography in patients with mediastinal non-Hodgkin's lymphoma. Clin Radiol 40:244, 1989

Waldron JA, Dohring EJ, Farber LR: Primary large cell lymphomas of the mediastinum: an analysis of 20 cases. Semin Diagn Pathol 2:281, 1985

Webb WR: M.R. imaging of treated mediastinal Hodgkin's disease (editorial). Radiology 170:315, 1989

Yellin A, Pak HY, Burke JS, et al: Surgical management of lymphomas involving the chest. Ann Thorac Surg 44:363, 1987

Yi PI, Coleman M, Saltz L et al: Chemotherapy for large cell lymphoma: a status update. Semin Oncol 17:60, 1990

Thyroid

Thomas W. Shields

A thyroid mass, most often a nontoxic colloid goiter or occasionally an adenoma, is not an unusual finding below the level of the thoracic inlet. As a result of partial or complete location of the mass within the mediastinum, the substernal thyroid mass is readily mistaken for a primary mediastinal tumor. It has been estimated by Creswell and Wells (1992) that these thyroid masses comprise 5.8 percent of all mediastinal lesions. In fact, however, almost all such masses descend from the original cervical location of the gland and as such are not truly primary tumors of the mediastinum.

HISTORICAL NOTE

The various definitions of substernal thyroid masses were in question during the early part of the twentieth century, and many confusing and conflicting classifications were suggested. However, the seminal report of Wakeley and Mulvany (1940), which divided intrathoracic thyroid masses into three types, can be accepted as a reasonable and logical classification. Their three types are (1) "small substernal extension" of a mainly cervical thyroid mass; (2) "partial" intrathoracic, where the major portion of the mass is situated within the thorax; and (3) "complete," in which all of the mass lies within the thoracic cavity. Although in these authors' report, all the thyroid masses were colloid goiters, whereas at the present intrathoracic thyroid masses comprise a variety of thyroid pathologic conditions, this changing pathologic pattern does not invalidate their classification.

Approximately 80 percent of the substernal thyroid masses in most all series are of the small substernal extension type, 15 percent are partial and only 2 to 4 percent are completely within the thorax. Most of these are in the anterior compartment, with only a small percentage retrotracheal or in the posterior mediastinum (Sweet, 1949). In Wakeley and Mulvany's (1940) series, the overall incidence of all substernal goiters was 8.7 percent, the incidences of the three aforementioned types being 81.9, 15.3, and 2.7 percent, respectively. The latter two categories, the ones the thoracic surgeon is concerned with, comprised only 1.6 percent of all goiters. A similar incidence, 1.4 percent in 9,100 patients with goiter, was reported by DeAndrade (1977). McCort (1949) reported an incidence for the partial and complete lesions of over 3 percent, but still this represents only a small percentage of patients with thyroid disease.

HISTORICAL READINGS

Kocher T: Bericht uber ein zweites Tausend Kropfexcisionen. Arch Exp Klin Chir 64:454, 1901

Lahey FH: Intrathoracic goiters. Surg Clin North Am 25:609, 1945

McCort JL: Intrathoracic goiter: its incidence, symptomatology, and roentgen diagnosis. Radiology 53:227, 1949

Sweet RH: Intrathoracic goiter located in the posterior mediastinum. Surg Gynecol Obstet 89:57, 1949

Wakeley CPG, Mulvany JH: Intrathoracic goiter. Surg Gynecol Obstet 70:702, 1940

EMBRYOLOGY

Embryologically the thyroid anlage arises from a midline diverticulum of the floor of the pharynx at a level between the first and second pharyngeal pouches. This site is identified subsequently as the foramen cecum of the tongue. The tissue develops into a bilobed structure, which ends its descent at the level of the laryngeal primordium. In the adult, the lower poles of the gland usually reach the level of the first tracheal ring, although abnormal descent to the sixth ring has been recorded. The major ectopic locations of thyroid tissue are from the upper poles of the gland to the base of the tongue. It is possible that tissue from the lower poles may be carried into the anterior compartment along with the thymus and the developing heart. However, in contrast to the presence of ectopic parathyroid tissue in or adjacent to the thymus, there are only rare reports of isolated normal thyroid tissue in such a location. An illustration of an ectopic thyroid follicle located in the parathymic mediastinal fat was published by Meissner and Warren (1969). How common this occurrence is remains unknown. A report of extensive dissection of the anterior mediastinal area by Jaretzki and Wolff (1988) fails to note the identification of thyroid tissue located in the mediastinal fat removed during the operation. Gilmour (1937), in an extensive study of the parathyroid glands in a large series of autopsy specimens, mentioned the occasional difficulty of gross distinction of parathyroid tissue from accessory thyroid nodules but failed to describe the anatomic location of these accessory nodules. However, as noted by Meissner and Warren (1969), such nodules are most commonly located adjacent to the normal thyroid gland in the neck; it may be assumed that few if any were found in the mediastinum.

ECTOPIC THYROID TISSUE IN THE MEDIASTINUM

From the data available, even though ectopic thyroid tissue can occur in the mediastinum, it is exceedingly rare for a true ectopic thyroid mass arising in the anterior compartment of the mediastinum. Cove (1988) states that thyroid tissue can be displaced inferiorly during the embryogenesis of the heart, and ectopic thyroid tissue has infrequently been found at the aortic root, in the pericardium, or even within the cardiac muscle or in the esophageal wall. However, such ectopic tissue is rare indeed, although Rogers and Kesten (1962), as well as Willis (1962), have described several examples of ectopic thyroid tissue in these locations. Ectopic thyroid tissue has not been identified paratracheally within the thorax. It is possible that ectopic tissue from the bilateral postbronchial bodies from the rudimentary fifth pharyngeal pouches, which are believed normally to become incorporated and differentiated into normal thyroid, could be carried down into either the anterior or visceral compartments. According to Rogers (1978), if these postbronchial bodies fail to be incorporated into the thyroid, differentiation into thyroid tissue does not occur. However, such tissue may give rise to a small cystic structure adjacent to the trachea in the neck or in the visceral compartment of the mediastinum.

The presence of a true ectopic thyroid lesion in the mediastinum has been debated for years. Whereas Lahey (1945) reported that he had never encountered one in over 24,000 goiter operations, other authors have noted its occurrence, albeit very rarely. Unfortunately, the documentation of a true ectopic origin of a thyroid mass in the mediastinum is lacking in most all cases so reported. The only criteria frequently employed are that the thyroid tissue be completely separated from the gland in the neck and that its blood supply be from vessels arising with the thorax rather than from the inferior thyroid vessels. These criteria are insufficient, and to them must be added the following: (1) the thyroid gland in the neck should be normal or completely absent; (2) no prior surgical removal of the "whole" or portion of the cervical gland should have been done in the past; (3) no invasive malignancy of the thyroid gland should be present or have been present in the past; and (4) no similar pathologic process should be present in both the cervical gland and the "ectopic" tissue. With these strict criteria, very few of the case reports of a so-called ectopic thyroid mass can be substantiated. For example, only one case of the several reported by LeRoux (1961) and of those reported by Salvatore and Gallo (1975) and by Sussman and associates (1986) meets these criteria. Likewise, I have had one such case initially recorded in 1972. Most cases, including the more recent cases reported by Mishriki, et al. (1983) and Hall, et al. (1988), do not meet the aforementioned criteria and should not be classified as ectopic lesions. However, the ectopic nature of a mediastinal thyroid mass is really the least of the many controversies associated with substernal thyroid masses.

ANATOMIC LOCATION

A major controversy associated with substernal thyroid masses is: What is the true location of the mass? This controversy has been the result of a number of factors, two of which are the presence of numerous different classifications of the mediastinal compartments and the failure to appreciate that the thoracic inlet consists almost entirely of the superior aspect of the visceral compartment of the mediastinum. The anterior, or prevascular, compartment begins well below the sternal notch, and no posterior compartment exists. The term *superior mediastinum,* unless used specifically to modify the anterior or visceral compartment, only adds to the confusion.

In many series of substernal goiters, such as that of Dahan and colleagues (1989), the majority of substernal goiters have been reported to be located in the anterior (prevascular) compartment. Most of the thoracic goiters that are classified as being in the anterior compartment are of the small substernal type. These are actually, in most cases, situated anteriorly in the visceral compartment and lie in contact with the undersurface of the manubrium on the cephalad aspect of the great vessels. These vessels may be displaced caudad and even somewhat dorsad. The impression is then gained that the goiter has descended into the prevascular (anterior) mediastinal compartment. However, as a rule the anterior substernal extension remains in the visceral compartment, being confined anteriorly by the pretracheal fascia. The goiter is thus prevented from entering the prevascular space that lies between this fascial layer and the more superficial investing layer of the deep cervical fascia.

The descent of a partial or complete intrathoracic goiter into the prevascular space is uncommon. Most examples of extension into the prevascular space have been recorded in patients with prior thyroid surgery, in whom the fascial planes sealing this compartment undoubtedly had been violated by the previous procedure. Ellis and associates (1952) reported that all nine patients in their series with goiters in this location had had previous thyroid operations. Examples of a complete substernal thyroid mass in the prevascular compartment by CT scan were published by both Glazer, et al. (1982) and Bashist, et al. (1983). In the former report no history was given for the patient, but in the latter report the patient had a definite history of previous goiter removal. An invasive malignant tumor of the thyroid, either a primary or a recurrent lesion, may also invade into the anterior compartment. Finally, although this is an infrequent occurrence, a partial or complete intrathoracic goiter on the right that is anterior or partially anterolateral to the trachea may originally enter the mediastinum via the visceral compartment, but once within the thorax, the lower aspect of the mass may pass in front of the ascending arch of the aorta. Thus, its lowermost portion may come to lie in the anterior compartment below the innominate vessels at the inlet.

In contrast to the exceptional location of a partial or complete substernal thyroid mass within the anterior compartment, the vast majority of such masses are within the visceral compartment. As such, they are located behind and medial to the great vessels as the goiter descends into the thorax in close relationship to the trachea. McCort (1949) initially made this observation and rightly stated that the vessels in the superior portion of the mediastinum were the border-forming structures of the substernal thyroid goiters. His observation has been amply documented by the CT characteristics of these lesions in the studies of Glazer, et al. (1982) and Bashist, et al. (1983), as well as by others, including my own similar

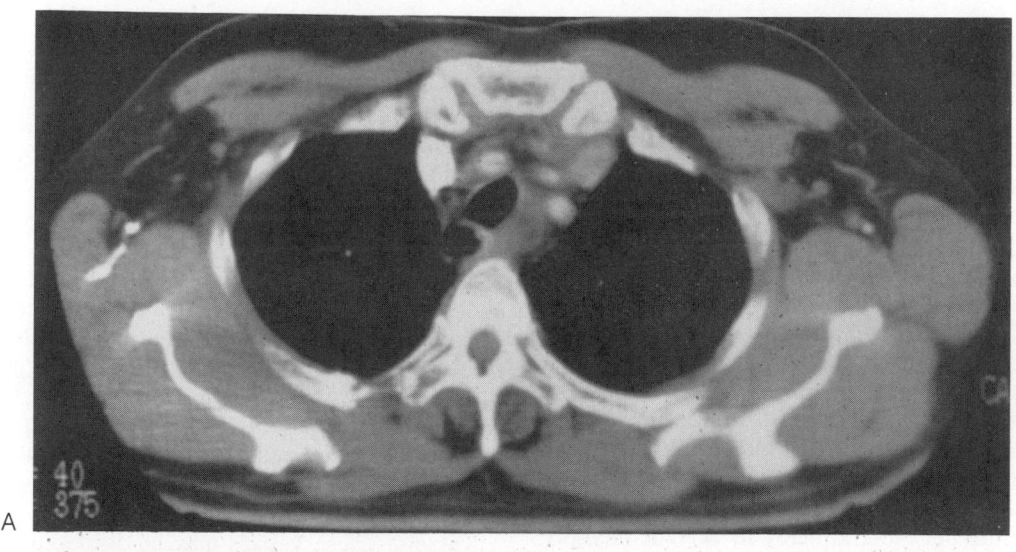

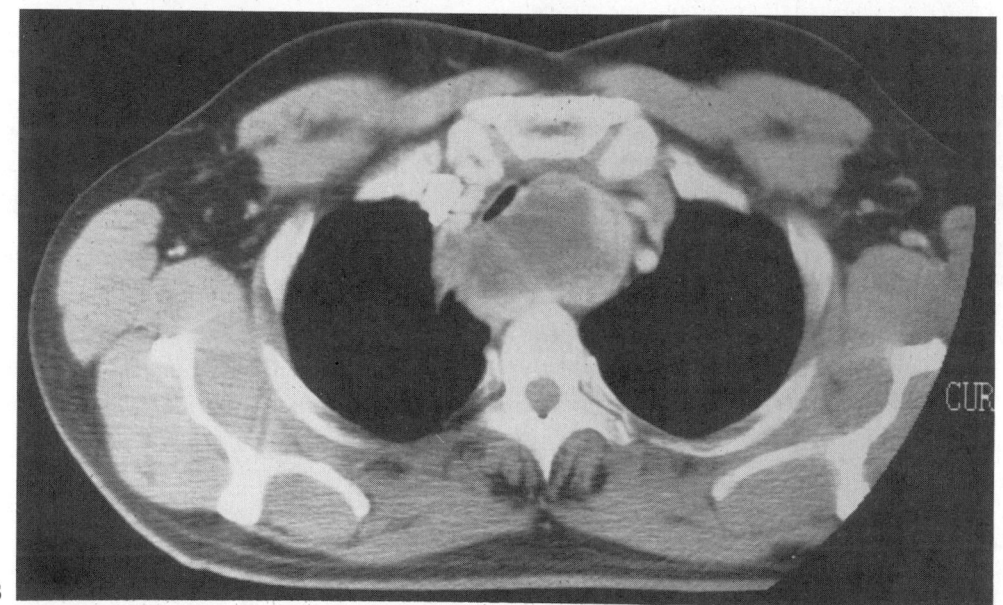

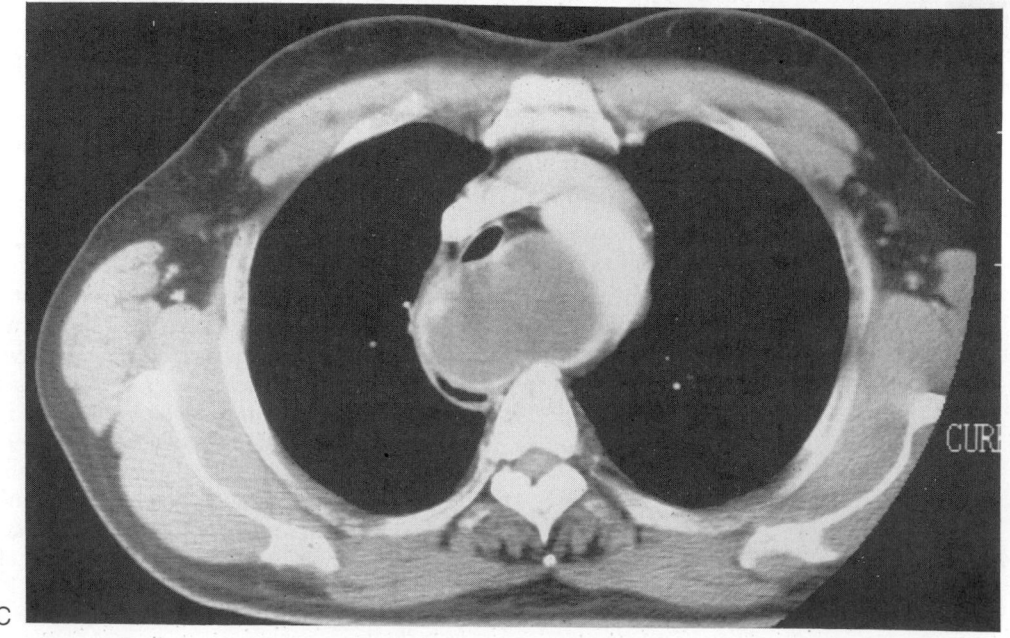

observations (Shields, 1991) (Fig. 58-33). The vessels, especially the veins, are displaced laterally and may become compressed against the bony structures of the thoracic inlet. In this latter situation the findings of a superior vena cava syndrome may be mimicked.

The vast majority of true partial and completely intrathoracic goiters or other thyroid lesions remain in continuity with the trachea. Very infrequently the substernal thyroid mass may become retroesophageal in location. In McCort's (1949) series of 28 partial or complete intrathoracic goiters, 4 were located anterior, 12 anterolateral, 3 bilateral, and 6 posterior to the trachea, with the remaining 3 located posterior to the esophagus. Thus, 9 (32 percent) of the 28 patients had retrotracheal lesions, often referred to as "posterior" goiters in the literature. Dahan and associates (1989) reported that of their 75 posterior substernal goiters, approximately 86 percent were retrotracheal, almost always on the right side, 4 percent were retroesophageal, 4 percent were anterior and to the right of the trachea although arising from the left lobe, and 6 percent were circumferential ("ring shaped") about the trachea.

With goiters in this posterior location, the carotid vessels and recurrent laryngeal nerves are located anterior to the mass rather than in their normal position dorsal to the gland. Consequently, the nerves are difficult to identify, and frequent injury to these nerves during removal of posterior goiters has been reported by Ellis and colleagues (1952), as well as by others.

The greater number of partial and complete goiters, even some of those arising from the left lobe, are located on the right. This is believed to result from the position of the arch of the aorta on the left. Regardless of the lobe of origin, the partial or complete substernal extension is confined, in most cases, within the basket formed by the great vessels anterior to the trachea. Most of the lesions are located above the level of the arch of the aorta, but some may descend to the level of the arch, and a few have even descended to the level of the diaphragm.

The arterial blood supply of almost all the partial and complete intrathoracic goiters arises from the inferior thyroid vessels in the neck. In a few patients with the complete variety, particularly those that descend beyond the level of the midthorax, and in some patients who have had previous thyroid surgery, the vascular supply from these inferior thyroid vessels may be absent. In these cases, neovascular supply and drainage may be from or to one or more of the great vessels within the thorax. However, this variance in blood supply in itself does not indicate that the site of origin of the goiter was not the original thyroid tissue in the neck.

PATHOLOGY

In most of the early series of substernal thyroid masses, the pathology of the lesion was that of a nontoxic multinodular colloid goiter. Toxic hyperplasia was uncommon, as it still is. However, Higgins (1927) reported 3 percent of the lesions to be toxic, and in addition he noted a 16 percent incidence of fetal adenomas in his series. More recently, Katlick and associates (1985) in a series of 80 patients at the Massachusetts General Hospital, reported an incidence of multinodular goiter of 51 percent, follicular adenoma 44 percent, and Hashimoto's thyroiditis 5 percent. Of the follicular adenomas 23 were classified as simple, 4 as fetal, 2 as colloid, 2 as embryonal, and 3 as Hurthle cell lesions. In two patients an occult papillary carcinoma was identified, for an incidence of 2.5 percent, which was not dissimilar to the incidence reported by Wakeley and Mulvany (1940) but somewhat less than the 5 percent incidence reported by Dahan and colleagues (1989). Allo and Thompson (1983) reported an incidence of malignancy of 16 percent, and Sanders and associates reported one of 21 percent. However, in the latter series, nine of the malignant lesions, including three cases of lymphoma involving the thyroid, were clinically significant, and in only two patients (4.6 percent) was an occult tumor discovered at the time of the removal of the substernal thyroid goiter.

CLINICAL FEATURES

Most patients with substernal thyroid masses are in the sixth or a later decade of life. Women are affected two to four times as often as men. A greater or lesser degree of kyphosis is often observed, as is the finding of a short, thick neck. Obesity is common. A variable number of patients report a history of one or more previous thyroid operations. In the series of Katlick, et al. (1985) and Sanders et al. (1992), the incidence was 20 percent exclusive of those patients with clinically suspicious malignant lesions.

In patients with small substernal extension of a cervical goiter, there are few if any clinical features related to the substernal extension. The clinical features are those of the cervical mass. The majority of patients with partial or complete substernal masses are symptomatic as the result of the substernal mass, although according to Rietz and Werner (1960), Rieve, et al. (1962), Lamke, et al. (1979), and Katlick, et al. (1985), 15 to 30 percent of the patients may be asymptomatic. Sanders and colleagues (1992) reported half of their patients to be asymptomatic.

In the symptomatic patients, a mass of variable size can be palpated in the midline or adjacent to it above the sternal notch. A cervical mass may be lacking in patients with previ-

Figure 58-33.   Typical location of a partial substernal thyroid mass in the visceral compartment. **(A)** CT scan reveals that the gland at the level of the inlet is enlarged posterolaterally to the trachea and is confined by the superior branches of the aortic arch. **(B)** At a slightly lower level within the thorax, the thyroid gland has assumed a primarily retrotracheal position, with displacement of the trachea to the right and anteriorly and marked narrowing of the tracheal lumen. The esophagus has been displaced posteriorly and to the right. The gland remains confined in the visceral compartment as the great vessels have been laterally and anteriorly displaced by the thyroid mass. **(C)** The retrotracheal goiter is confined anteriorly by the aortic arch, the left innominate vein, and the superior vena cava; no obstruction of these vessels is present.

ous thyroid surgery, in those with a so-called plunging goiter (goiter plongeant), which ascends into the lower neck only when the patient strains or coughs, and in those with a "complete substernal thyroid lesion.

The majority of patients, however, present with one or more complaints of a cervial mass, a choking sensation, dyspnea, cough, and voice change or hoarseness. Dysphagia is not uncommon when the patient eats solid foods. Wheezing and stridor may be present, and upper airway obstruction can occur acutely. This may result as a sequel of an acute respiratory infection or a spontaneous hemorrhage within the mass. LeRoux and colleagues (1984) reported that acute airway obstruction can occur after administration of ^{131}I owing to temporary enlargement of the goiter. Acute airway obstruction can lead to sudden death, as reported by Warren (1979) as well as other authors. Warren recorded one death in four patients who developed acute airway obstruction. The management of this emergent event has been discussed in detail by Shaha and colleagues (1989b). The airway must be promptly established by intubation and urgent thyroidectomy carried out.

On physical examination, in addition to a cervical mass that often moves on swallowing, deviation of the trachea away from the mass is common. A cervical scar from previous thyroid surgery is not uncommonly present, in which case a cervical mass may be absent. Facial flushing and distended neck and anterior chest wall veins can be occasionally observed. This superior vena cava-like venous obstruction is seen in 1 to 5 percent of patients.

Most patients are euthyroid, and rarely are signs or symptoms of frank hyperthyroidism present. Shaha and associates (1989a) reported hyperthyrodism in only 1.6 percent of their patients. However, Allo and Thompson (1983) reported that hyperactivity of the gland was present in 10 (20 percent) of the 50 patients in their series. They suggested that this hyperactivity probably was the result of autonomously functioning "hot" nodules or of the total bulk of functioning thyroid tissue within the mass. In most patients the thyrotoxicosis was manifested by heart failure, cardiac arrhythmia, or a wasting syndrome, the so-called apathetic thyrotoxicosis.

In most series, except those of Allo and Thompson (1983) and Sanders and associates (1992) at the Lahey Clinic, evidence of malignant disease has been absent and the few tumors discovered have been occult in nature. However, in the series of Sanders and associates (1992), four of the nine patients with malignancy had suspicious lesions clinically, and in the other five, the malignant nature of the thyroid mass was readily apparent at the time of operation. Hoarseness due to vocal cord paralysis is a strong indicator of the possibility of a malignant tumor, but it can occur with a benign lesion as well, so that even though it is suggestive of malignancy it is not diagnostic.

DIAGNOSTIC PROCEDURES

Standard Radiographs

Chest and neck radiographs are usually diagnostic for the partial substernal thyroid lesions. The mass occupies the superior portion of the chest and extends upward into the neck. Calcifications may be recognized in the mass in a vari-

able number of patients. Lateral deviation of the trachea is almost always present (in 80 to 95 percent of patients), and in contrast to primary mediastinal masses confined to mediastinum, the tracheal deviation begins in the neck above the thoracic inlet (Fig. 58-34). In patients with complete substernal thyroid lesions, tracheal deviation may be absent, but when present it is often seen only on the lateral radiographs of the chest, the trachea being displaced in an anterior or a posterior rather than in a lateral direction. In this situation the radiographs are not diagnostic, as they are for a partial substernal thyroid mass.

Contrast Studies

A barium swallow readily demonstrates esophageal displacement and extrinsic compression, particularly in the patient with retrotracheal or retroesophageal (posterior) thyroid masses (Fig. 58-35). A venacavogram, although not often indicated, may reveal displacement or even obstruction of the innominate and internal jugular veins as they are compressed against the thoracic inlet. The superior vena cava, however, remains intact (Fig. 58-36).

Computed Tomography

CT scans are obtained routinely although not always required. However, this study confirms the position of the lesion within the visceral compartment of the mediastinum in most cases and its relationship to the great vessels in the thorax, as previously noted (Fig. 58-37). Glazer, et al. (1982) and Bashist, et al. (1983) have described the usual CT findings. These consist of (1) a clear continuity of the mediastinal mass with the cervical gland; (2) well-defined borders, (3) the frequent presence of punctate, coarse, or ringlike calcifications; (4) the nonhomogeneity of the mass; (5) the presence of nonenhancing low-density areas; (6) precontrast attenuation greater than for the adjacent muscles and even greater enhancement after the injection of iodinated contrast

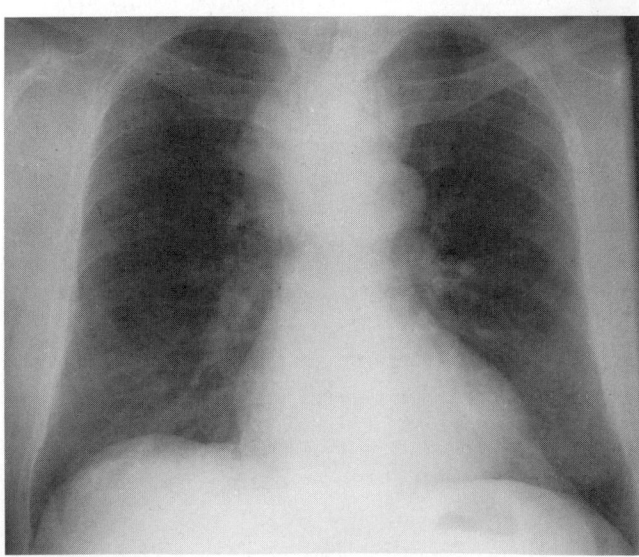

Figure 58-34. Large partial substernal mass with deviation of the trachea to the right. The deviation is noted as being above the thoracic inlet.

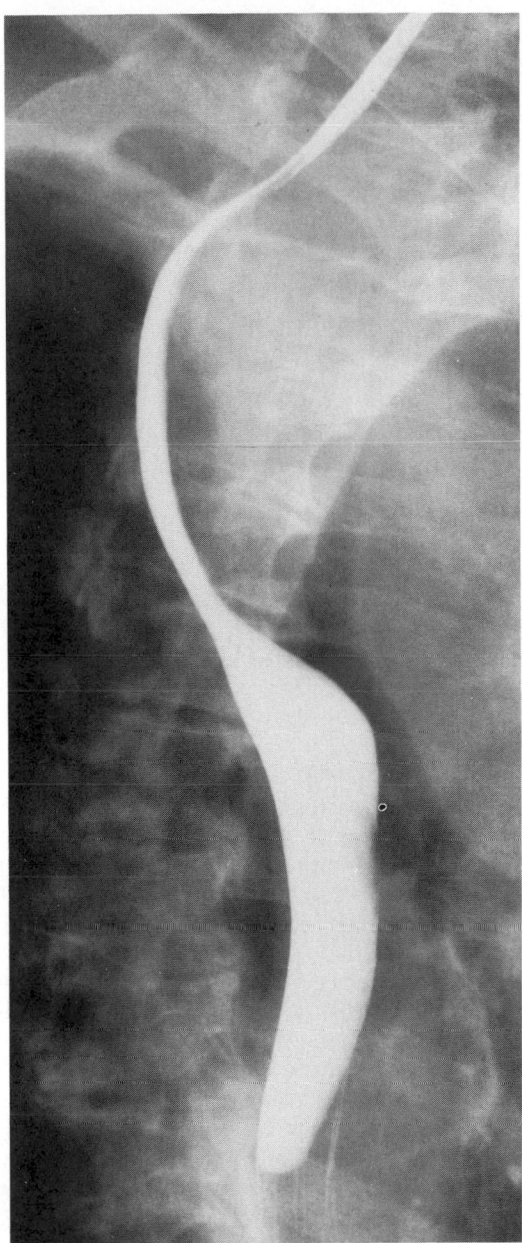

Figure 58-35. Barium swallow reveals marked displacement by the substernal mass seen in Figure 58-34.

medium; and (7) most importantly, the characteristic pattern of lateral and anterior displacement of the vessels in the superior portion of the visceral compartment of the mediastinum with cradling of the mass by the right and left brachiocephalic vessels. The CT scan may be less diagnostic when the mass is complete in nature and is retrotracheal or retroesophageal in location or infrequently, is present in the anterior compartment.

Magnetic Resonance Imaging

MRI is usually unnecessary, although as reported by von Schulthess, et al. (1986), it permits excellent delineation of the great vessels and their relationship to the mass. The other findings are similar to those obtained by CT scanning except for one important feature, the demonstration of "flow voids" within the mass due to the marked vascularity of the substernal thyroid tissue. This feature should be especially helpful in patients with either the rare complete anterior compartment or posterior retrotracheal or retroesophageal masses (Fig. 58-38).

Thyroid Scintigraphy

Thyroid scintigraphy may be accomplished with ^{99m}Tc pertechnetate or either ^{131}I or ^{123}I but must be done before a CT scan with contrast enhancement has been carried out. As a rule, the procedure is unnecessary except in some complete goiters the diagnosis of which remains in doubt despite the aforementioned examinations. Unfortunately, the results of the examination are generally less than ideal—less than 50 percent identification of thyroid tissue in most reports in the literature—although Park and colleagues (1987) report a much higher percentage of positive results if strict attention is paid to the details of the technique used.

Fine-Needle Aspiration Biopsy

Although Lamke and associates (1979) recommended FNA biopsy to confirm the nature of the mass, this procedure is unnecessary and is not recommended except under very unusual circumstances. Despite the presence of occult tumor in 1 to 2 percent of patients, random biopsy is unrewarding in identifying such an occult lesion. Only if a dominant cold nodule is present or if preoperative findings are unequivocally suggestive of a malignancy, should a needle biopsy be considered.

MANAGEMENT

The therapy for a partial or complete intrathoracic thyroid mass is surgical resection. The use of radioactive iodine is contraindicated: not only may it initially aggravate any preexisting tracheal compression, but as noted by Beierwalters (1978), radioactive iodine rarely, if ever, alleviates tracheal deviation or compression caused by a large multinodular goiter. L-Thyroxine likewise is of no avail to suppress a thyroid goiter.

Anesthetic management is best accomplished with an endotracheal tube and general anesthesia. The initial surgical incision is a low transverse collar (thyroid) incision, since over 95 percent of substernal goiters may be removed through this approach. DeAndrade (1977), Katlick, et al. (1985), and Sanders, et al. (1992) reported the necessity of only a cervical incision in 95.3, 97.5, and 94.4 percent of their cases, respectively. Reasons for the cervical approach that are just as or even more compelling are the facts that in almost all patients the blood supply of the intrathoracic mass is from the inferior thyroid arteries and injury to the recurrent laryngeal nerve is less likely to occur with this approach.

In those few cases in which additional exposure becomes necessary, a partial sternal splint, initially advocated by Lilienthal (1915), is the procedure used by most thoracic surgeons. However, it is to be noted that in most cases in which this is necessary, the great vessels are in front of the

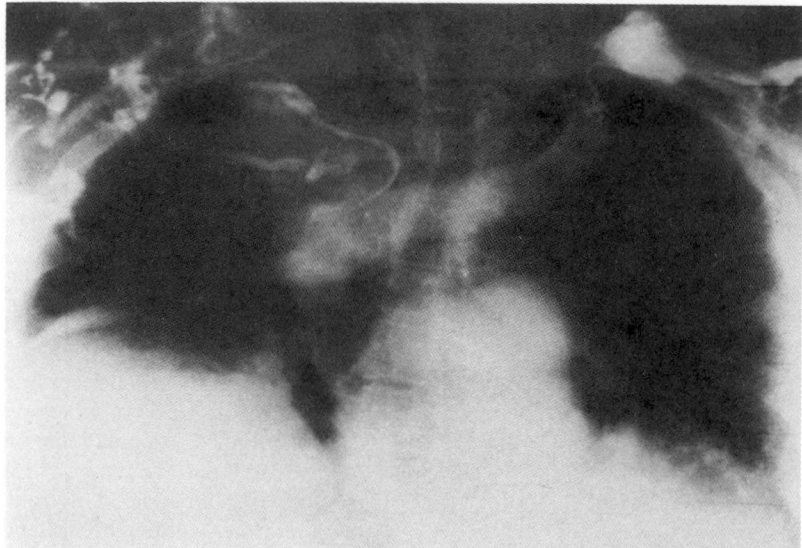

Figure 58-36. Intravenous contrast study in a patient with a large partial substernal thyroid mass. Complete obstruction of right innominate vein with collateral vessels is evident. Distal portion of left innominate vein is almost completely obstructed at the thoracic inlet, but the major portion of this vein and the superior vena cava, although displaced, are widely patent. (From Silverstein GE, et al: Superior vena caval system obstruction caused by benign endothoracic goiter. Chest 56:519, 1969, with permission.)

intrathoracic mass (Fig. 58-39) and not behind it, as described by Creswell and Wells (1992). Gourin and associates (1971) suggested a combined cervicomediastinal approach for all partial and complete intrathoracic goiters. This would seem to be totally unnecessary in view of the aforementioned data. In addition, Le Roux and colleagues (1984) stated that they found the use of a sternal split to be of little help in mobilizing a gland that could not be extracted through the standard cervical approach. Landreneau and associates (1991) have stated that it is important to break the negative intrathoracic

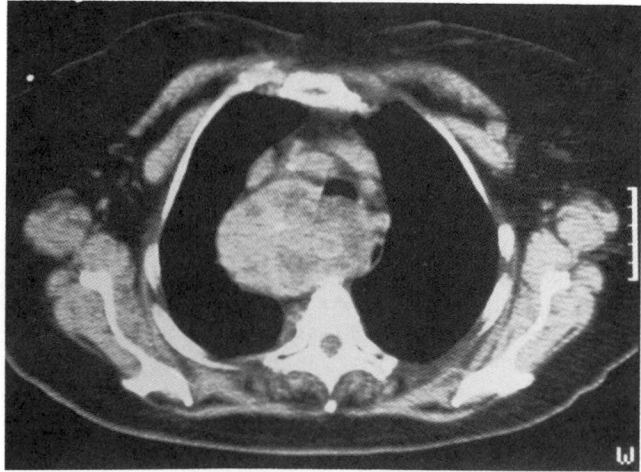

Figure 58-37. CT scan of large retrotracheal goiter, showing its position in the visceral compartment and relationship to the adjacent vessels. The mass has well-defined borders, contains a ringlike area of calcification, and is nonhomogeneous in density.

negative pressure to facilitate removal of the substernal portion of the gland. They accomplished this decompression by use of a sterile spoon, but I am sure that any blunt instrument would do as well. Actually, the use of a special "goiter spoon" was reported by Kocher in 1901.

Rather than a sternal split, Johnston and Twente (1956) advocated a combined cervicoanterior thoracic approach because they believed that a better exposure of the enlarged gland could be obtained by this method (Fig. 58-40). This approach has also been advocated by DeAndrade (1977). In addition to the better exposure, gentle upward pressure on the goiter to deliver it into the cervical incision is readily accomplished. A posterior lateral thoracotomy approach, as suggested by Sweet (1949) and subsequently reported by Ellis and co-workers (1952), for posterior intrathoracic goiters is to be avoided if at all possible. Appropriate control of the vascular supply from the neck is difficult at best, and a high incidence of recurrent nerve injury, approximately 27 percent, has been recorded by Ellis and associates (1952) and others with the use of this approach. To avoid these problems, Shahian and Rossi (1988) agree with Hilton and Griffin (1968) and Maurer (1955) as to the efficiency of a simultaneous cervical and thoracic approach for contralateral retrotracheal or retroesophageal posterior thyroid masses, since this permits control of any mediastinal as well as the cervical vessels and adequately protects the recurrent nerve.

In the standard cervical approach, the superior cervical blood supply to the involved lobe is identified and controlled, at least one superior parathyroid gland is identified, and if possible at this time, the vascular supply via the inferior thyroid vessels to the substernal portion of the gland is also controlled and the recurrent nerve identified. These latter steps may not be possible until the substernal portion of

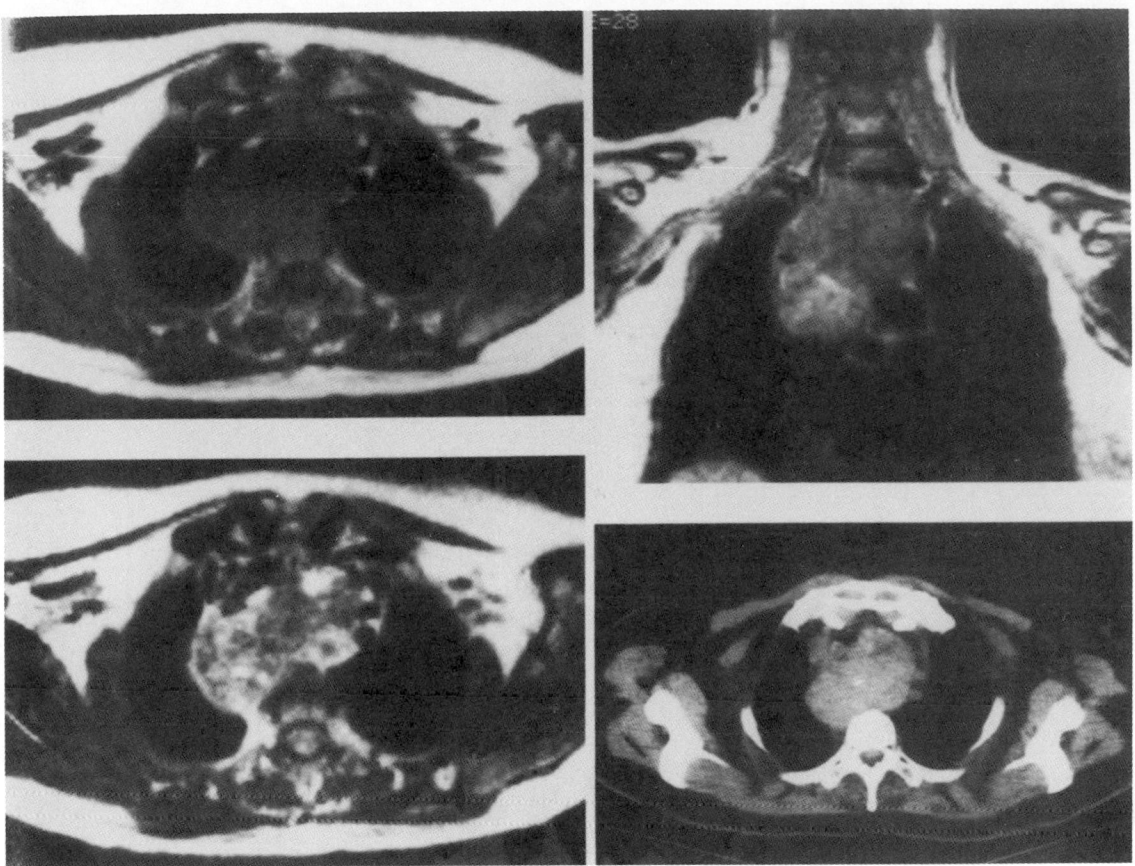

Figure 58-38. MRI of substernal thyroid mass, compared with CT of the mass (lower right-hand corner), reveals relationship of the mass to the adjacent vessels and the multiple flow void present within the mass on the MRI scan.

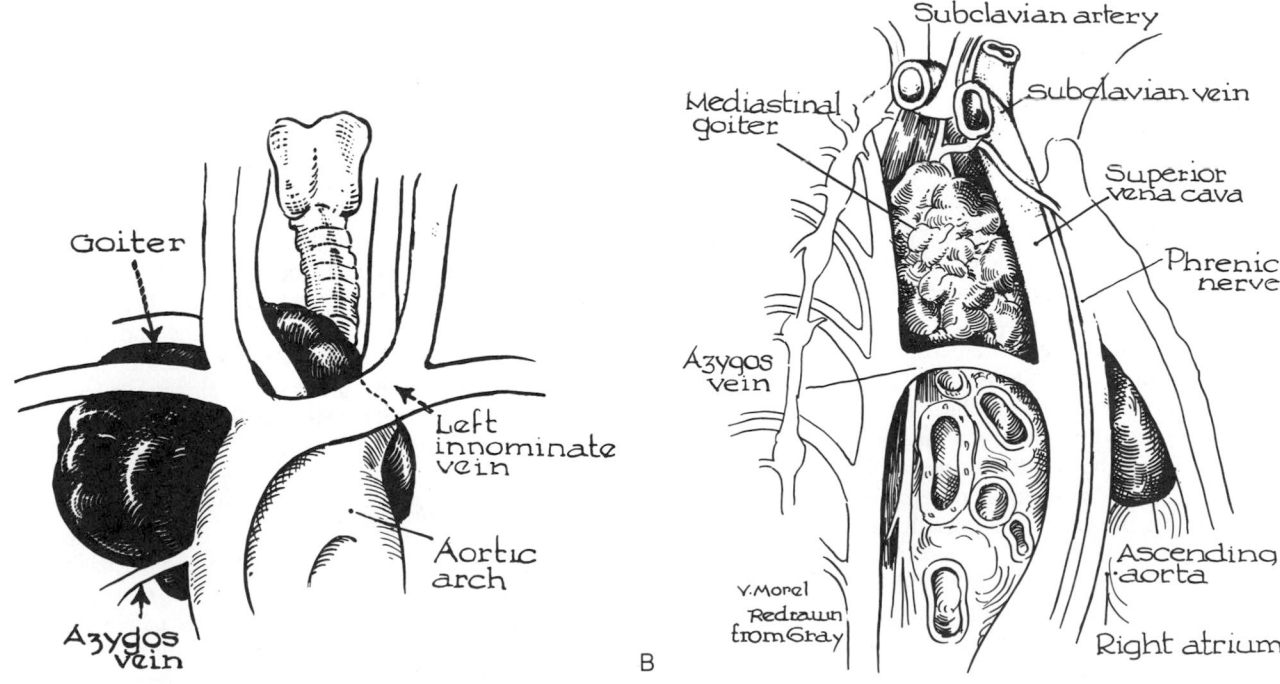

Figure 58-39. **(A & B)** Schematic illustrations from the frontal and lateral aspects of a partial intrathoracic goiter lying in the visceral compartment of the mediastinum, resting on the border of the vertebrae behind the superior vena cava and the innominate vessels above the azygos vein. (From Johnston JH Jr, Twente GE: Surgical approach to intrathoracic (mediastinal) goiter. Ann Surg 143:572, 1956, with permission.)

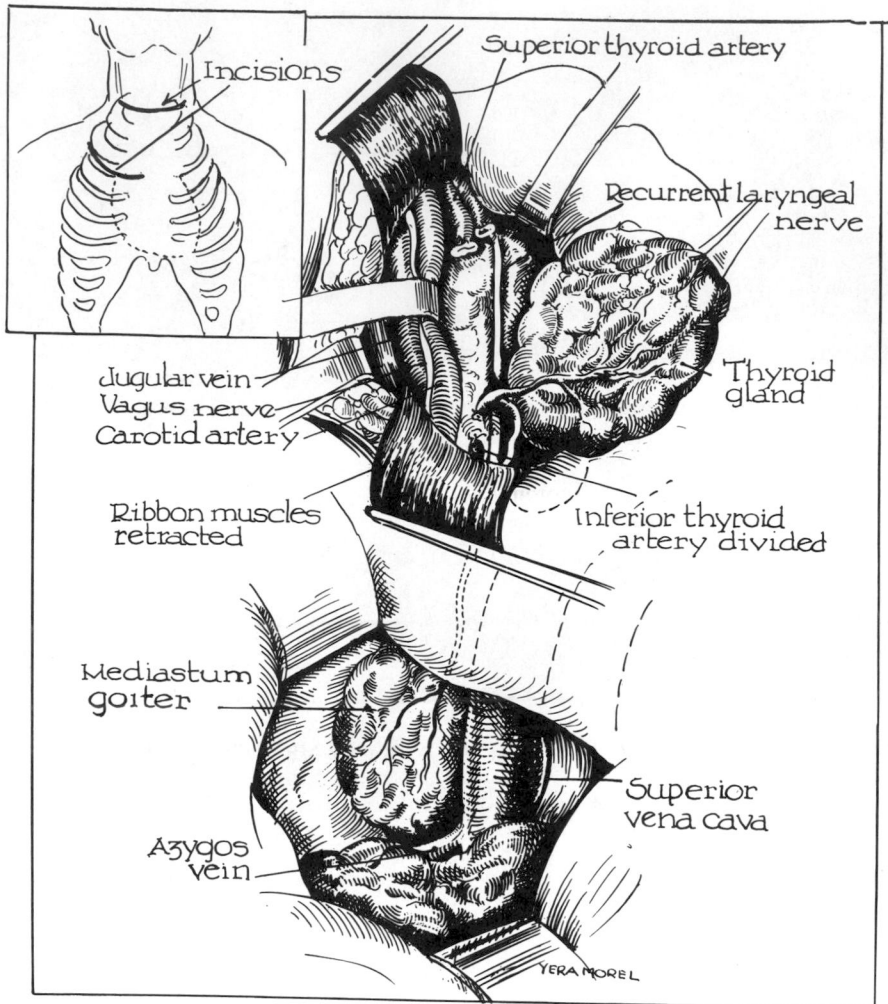

Figure 58-40. Schematic illustration of combined cervicoanterior approach to substernal goiters that cannot be removed through a cervical approach alone. (From Johnston JH Jr, Twente GE: Surgical approach to intrathoracic (mediastinal) goiter. Ann Surg 143:572, 1956, with permission.)

the gland is removed from the mediastinum. This step is accomplished by finger or pledget dissection within the capsule of the goiter to prevent injury to either the nerve or vessels. Infrequently, as noted, it is necessary to provide additional exposure by either a partial upper median sternotomy or a small anterior thoracotomy incision on the appropriate side in the second or third interspace to complete the mobilization. Morcellation of the goiter, as suggested by Lahey (1945), is to be avoided in order to lessen the possibility of bleeding, which may be difficult to control, and because of the possible presence of an occult carcinoma within the gland. After mobilization of the intrathoracic thyroid mass, the inferior thyroid vessels, if not already controlled, are ligated and divided, and the mass is removed.

Collapse of the tracheal wall due to tracheomalacia is frequently feared but rarely observed. When tracheal obstruction does occur, Allo and Thompson (1983) believe this is more likely the result of kinking of the elongated, distorted trachea. To prevent the occurrence of kinking, they suggest tacking the trachea anteriorly to one of the strap muscles in

the neck before closure of the incision. It is a prudent precaution to inspect the tracheal lumen by flexible fiberoptic endoscopy prior to removal of the endotracheal tube; if any narrowing or compromise is suspected, the endotracheal tube should be left in place for 24 to 48 hours postoperatively. Tracheostomy may be indicated if airway obstruction persists. The mediastinal space is drained in all cases to prevent accumulation of fluid within the mediastinal space.

Morbidity and Mortality

Watt-Boolsen and associates (1981) noted permanent unilateral vocal cord paralysis in 10 percent of their patients, but it was not stated if these were patients who had undergone a lateral thoracotomy. This latter approach, as noted, has a high incidence of recurrent nerve injury. Dahan and associates (1989) reported a 6 percent incidence of recurrent nerve paralysis. Katlick and associates (1985), on the other hand, reported no instances of vocal cord paralysis.

Postoperative mortality is rare. DeAndrade (1977) reported only one death in 128 patients (an 0.7 percent incidence) with a partial or complete intrathoracic goiter. Dahan and associates (1989) reported a mortality rate of 2.8 percent. Most authors have reported mortality rates within the range of these two reports.

Results

Recurrent substernal goiter is uncommon. Unfortunately a frankly malignant lesion may recur. Thyroid function is usually normal, as is parathyroid function, as was noted by Watt-Boolsen and colleagues (1981) in their long-term follow-up study.

COMMENTS AND CONTROVERSIES

In 35 years of clinical experience with substernal thyroidectomy, it has never been necessary to split the sternum. This includes the rare retrotracheal tumor as well. If a sternotomy should be necessary, a complete sternotomy provides much better access and is easier to close expeditiously than a partial sternotomy. The recommendation for partial sternotomy is left over from previous years, when the fear of infection or dehiscence was significant. A posterolateral thoracotomy for a retrotracheal goiter has not been necessary in our experi-ence, although Dr. Richard A. Sweet, who made the recommendation, certainly was a giant in the field of substernal thyroid surgery. Although tracheomalacia can produce clinical stridor, it is extremely rare, as pointed out by Dr. Shields. Use of a membranous tracheal stent from either rib or Marlex has been successful, in addition to the use of muscle, which he described to prevent complete collapse of the trachea on expiration.

H.C.U.

REFERENCES

Allo MD, Thompson NW: Rationale for operative management of substernal goiters. Surgery 94:969, 1983

Bashist B, Ellis K, Gold RP: Computed tomography of intrathoracic goiters. AJR 140:455, 1983

Beierwalters WH: The treatment of hyperthyroidism with iodine 131. Semin Nucl Med 8:95, 1978

Cove H: The mediastinum. In Coulson WF (ed): Surgical Pathology. 2nd Ed. JB Lippincott, Philadelphia, 1988

Creswell LL, Wells SA Jr: Mediastinal masses originating in the neck. Chest Surg Clin North Am 2:23, 1992

Dahan M, Gaillard J, Eschapasse H: Surgical treatment of goiters with intrathoracic development. In Thoracic Surgery: Frontiers and Uncommon Neoplasms. In Delarue NC, Eschapasse H (eds): International Trends in General Thoracic Surgery. Vol 5. CV Mosby, St. Louis, 1989

DeAndrade MA: A review of 128 cases of posterior mediastinal goiter. World J Surg 1:789, 1977

Dundas P: Intrathoracic aberrant goiter. Acta Chir Scand 128:729, 1964

Ellis FH Jr, Good CA, Seybold WD: Intrathoracic goiter. Ann Surg 135:79, 1952

Gilmour JR: The embryology of the parathyroid glands, the thymus and certain associated rudiments. J Pathol 45:507, 1937

Glazer GM, Axel L, Moss AA: CT diagnosis of mediastinal thyroid. AJR 138:495, 1982

Gourin A, Garzon A, Karlson KE: The cervicomediastinal approach to intrathoracic goiter. Surgery 69:651, 1971

Hall TS, Caslowitz P, Popper C et al: Substernal goiter versus intrathoracic aberrant thyroid: a critical difference. Ann Thorac Surg 46:684, 1988

Higgins CC: Intrathoracic goiter. Arch Surg 15:895, 1927

Hilton HD, Griffin WT: Posterior mediastinal goiter. Am J Surg 116:891, 1968

Jaretzki A III, Wolff M: "Maximal" thymectomy for myasthenia gravis. Surgical anatomy and operative technique. J Thorac Cardiovasc Surg 96:711, 1988

Johnston JH Jr, Twente GE: Surgical approach to intrathoracic (mediastinal) goiter. Ann Surg 143:572, 1956

Katlick MR, Grillo HC, Wang C: Substernal goiter: analysis of 80 patients from Massachusetts General Hospital. Am J Surg 149:283, 1985

Kocher T: Bericht uber ein zweites Tausend Kropfexcisionen. Arch Exp Klin Chir 64:454, 1901

Lahey FH: Intrathoracic goiters. Surg Clin North Am 25:609, 1945

Lamke LO, Bergdahl L, Lamke B: Intrathoracic goiter: a review of 29 cases. Acta Chir Scand 145:83, 1979

Landreneau RJ, Nawarwong W, Boley TM et al: Intrathoracic goiter: approaching the posterior mediastinal mass. Ann Thorac Surg 52:134, 1991

LeRoux BT: Heterotopic mediastinal thyroid. Thorax 16:192, 1961

LeRoux BT, Kallichurum S, Shama DM: Mediastinal cysts and tumor. Curr Probl Surg 21:11, 1984

Lilienthal H: A case of mediastinal thyroid removed by transternal mediastinotomy. Surg Gynecol Obstet 20:589, 1915

Maurer ER: The surgical treatment of retrotracheal intrathoracic goiter. Arch Surg 71:357, 1955

McCort JL: Intrathoracic goiter: its incidence, symptomatology, and roentgen diagnosis. Radiology 53:227, 1949

Meissner WA, Warren S: Tumors of the thyroid gland. In Atlas of Tumor Pathology, 2nd Ser., Fascicle 4. Armed Forces Institute of Pathology, Washington, 1969

Mishriki YY, Lane BP, Lozowski MS, Epstein H: Hurthle-cell tumor arising in the mediastinal ectopic thyroid and diagnosis by fine needle aspiration: light microscopic and ultrastructural features. Acta Cytol 27:188, 1983

Morris UL, Colletti PM, Ralls PW et al: CT demonstration of intrathoracic thyroid tissue. J Comput Assist Tomogr 6:821, 1982

Nwafo DC: Heterotopic mediastinal goitre. Br J Surg 65:505, 1978

Park HM, Tarver RD, Siddiqui AR et al: Efficacy of thyroid scintigraphy in the diagnosis of intrathoracic goiter. AJR 148:527, 1987

Rietz KA, Werner B: Intrathoracic goitre. Acta Chir Scand 119:379, 1960

Rieve TS, et al: The investigation and management of intrathoracic goitre. Surg Gynecol Obstet 115:223, 1962

Rogers W: Anomalous development of the thyroid. In Werner SC,

Ingbar SH (eds): The Thyroid. 5th Ed. Harper & Row, New York, 1978

Rogers WM, Kesten HD: Embryologic bases for thyroid tissue in the heart. Anat Rec 142:323, 1962

Salvatore M, Gallo A: Accessory thyroid tissue in the anterior mediastinum. J Nucl Med 16:1135, 1975

Sanders LE, Rossi RL, Shahian DM, Williamson WA: Mediastinal goiters. The need for an aggressive approach. Arch Surg 127:609, 1992

Shaha AR, Alfonso AE, Jaffe BM: Operative treatment of substernal goiters. Head and Neck 11:325, 1989a

Shaha AR, Burnett C, Alfonso A, Jaffe BM: Goiter and airway problems. Am J Surg 158:378, 1989b

Shahian DM, Rossi RL: Posterior mediastinal goiter. Chest 94:599, 1988

Shields TW: Lesions masquerading as primary mediastinal tumors or cysts. p. 118. In Shields TW (ed): Mediastinal Surgery, Lea & Febiger, Philadelphia, 1991

Shields TW: Primary tumors and cysts of the mediastinum. p. 931. In Shields TW (ed): General Thoracic Surgery. 1st Ed. Lea & Febiger, Philadelphia, 1972

Silverstein GE, et al: Superior vena caval system obstruction caused by benign endothoracic goiter. Chest 56:519, 1969

Sussman SK, Silverman PM, Donnal JF: CT demonstration of isolated mediastinal goiter. J Comput Assist Tomogr 10:863, 1986

Sweet RH: Intrathoracic goiter located in the posterior mediastinum. Surg Gynecol Obstet 89:57, 1949

von Schulthess GK, et al: Mediastinal masses: MR imaging. Radiology 158:289, 1986

Torres A, Arroyo J, Kastanos N et al: Acute respiratory failure and tracheal obstruction in patients with intrathoracic goiter. Crit Care Med 11:265, 1983

Wakeley CPG, Mulvany JH: Intrathoracic goiter. Surg Gynecol Obstet 70:702, 1940

Warren CPW: Acute respiratory failure and tracheal obstruction in the elderly with benign goiters. Can J Med 121:191, 1979

Watt-Boolsen SW et al: Surgical treatment of benign nontoxic intrathoracic goiter: a long-term observation. Am J Surg 141:721, 1981

Willis RA: The Borderland of Embryology and Pathology. Butterworths, London, 1962

Parathyroids

Carl E. Bredenberg
Clement A. Hiebert

INTRODUCTION

The thoracic surgeon should possess detailed knowledge of parathyroid anatomy, physiology, and pathology to be prepared for five contingencies:

1. A mediastinal hunt for the elusive quarry may be suggested by an endocrinologist or surgeon following an unsuccessful search for a hyperfunctioning gland or glands in the neck. Before embarking on what may be a difficult and lengthy procedure, the thoracic surgeon must confirm the diagnosis and, if possible, ascertain the location of what often is a small and exasperatingly well-camouflaged tumor.

2. A mediastinal mass found on routine chest x-ray may unexpectedly prove at operation to be a parathyroid cyst or tumor. Concomitant biopsy of cervical glands may be indicated to obviate the possibility of leaving hyperplastic tissue behind.

3. Failure to identify and reimplant parathyroid tissue during extensive resections of malignant growths of the cervical esophagus may result in life-threatening hypocalcemia afterward. The surgeon needs to be familiar with the appearance and normal location of these lilliputian glands.

4. Hyperparathyroidism may be mimicked by other diseases, including squamous cancers of the lung and esophagus.

5. The thoracic surgeon must be aware that mediastinal parathyroid tumors usually are more accessible through a cervical incision than via a sternotomy or lateral thoracotomy and that the recurrent laryngeal nerve is especially vulnerable when the approach is via a right thoracotomy.

DEFINITION

Primary hyperparathyroidism is a disease caused by a tumor or hyperplasia of the parathyroid glands. PTH increases serum ionized calcium, and it is the hypercalcemia that causes most of the symptoms and complications of the disease. Other diseases such as sarcoid, hypernephroma, and metastatic cancer may cause hypercalcemia, and some, particularly squamous cell carcinomas of the lung or esophagus, produce a peptide that binds to PTH receptor and mimics some of the actions of PTH.

Secondary hyperparathyroidism is hyperplasia of the parathyroid glands with increased PTH secretion in response to chronic hypocalcemia usually caused by calcium loss. This is most often seen in patients with chronic renal failure. In most of these patients successful renal transplantation removes the stimulus for parathyroid hypersecretion, and PTH levels return to normal within 6 months (Friesen and Thompson, 1990). In tertiary hyperparathyroidism, however, hypercalcemia persists following successful renal transplantation.

There are normally four parathyroid glands, and as the name suggests, their proper residence is close by the thyroid. In 2 to 6 percent of unselected subjects, there is an extra gland, and in less than 3 percent of otherwise normal individuals, a fourth gland is impossible to find (Akerstrom, et al., 1984; Wang 1976). The hyperfunctioning gland or glands are found in the mediastinum in 11 to 22 percent of patients, but fewer than 4 percent of all patients require a thoracotomy for excision (Russell, et al., 1981; Wang 1986; Clark 1988; Conn, et al., 1991; Hiebert, unpublished data on 191 consecutive parathyroid operations).

HISTORICAL NOTE

The first detailed gross and microscopic description of the parathyroid glands in humans was made in 1877 by a Swedish medical student, Ivar Sandstrom (Thompson 1990).

It took a number of years to establish the physiologic and pathologic role of the parathyroid glands. Halsted at Johns Hopkins in 1906 relieved clinical tetany after thyroidectomy by giving a patient dietary supplements of parathyroid glands harvested from cattle and later confirmed these observations in experimental animals (Halsted, 1961). Also at Johns Hopkins and contemporary with Halsted's work, MacCallum, then a young pathologist, demonstrated experimentally that the parathyroid's major role was control of calcium metabolism and that tetany occurring after total parathyroid excision was caused by hypocalcemia (Halsted, 1961).

The first excision of a parathyroid tumor was for relief of demineralizing bone disease and was performed in 1924 by Felix Mandel in Vienna. Ironically, Mandel's patient had been treated for more than a year with parathyroid extracts and implantation of parathyroid glands following the mistaken diagnosis of the bone disease as a result of parathyroid insufficiency (Cady and Rossi, 1991).

Collip at the University of Alberta, isolated PTH in 1924, and Aub, an endocrinologist at the Massachusetts General Hospital, began using PTH to hasten the elimination of lead from the bones of patients with lead poisoning (Cope, 1966). In so doing Aub demonstrated the increase in serum calcium, fall in serum phosphate, and increase in urinary elimination of calcium that came to be recognized as characteristic of hyperparathyroidism. This experience allowed Aub in 1926 to diagnose the source of the bone disease in Charles Martel, a sea captain, as a hyperfunctioning parathyroid gland, which led to the first operation in North America for hyperparathyroidism. A total of six neck explorations looking for an en-

larged parathyroid gland were made in Captain Martel, beginning in 1926, each without success. In 1928 Bulger and colleagues at Washington University in St. Louis, stimulated in part by discussions with Aub, diagnosed hyperparathyroidism in a 57-year-old woman with bone disease, and I. Y. Olch successfully removed the first parathyroid adenoma in North America (Barr, et al., 1929). In 1930, despite several unsuccessful neck explorations in Captain Martel, neck explorations were carried out in two additional patients at the Massachusetts General Hospital, and a parathyroid adenoma was found in one of them.

Persisting and building on the solid endocrinology base of Aub and his medical colleagues Bauer and Albright, Edward Churchill at the Massachusetts General Hospital in 1931 directed Oliver Cope, then his resident, to study the anatomic distribution of parathyroid glands in the autopsy suite. On the basis of the experience obtained in the postmortem dissections, Cope and Churchill in 1932 began a systematic development of surgery for parathyroid disease, and it was these two surgeons who performed the last three of the six unsuccessful cervical explorations in Captain Martel. The relationship of the bone disease and a hyperactive parathyroid gland was so soundly based on the physiologic understanding of their endocrinology colleagues that Cope and Churchill, on the basis of embryologic studies, finally explored the mediastinum of Martel and found the parathyroid tumor "just lateral to the superior vena cava." Its successful removal was the first excision of mediastinal parathyroid adenoma, and the patient's calcium promptly fell to tetanic levels (Cope, 1966).

HISTORICAL READINGS

Cope O: The Story of Hyperparathyroidism at the Massachusetts General Hospital. N Engl J Med 274:1171, 1966

Halsted WE: Surgical papers. p. 150. Vol. 2. 3rd Printing. Johns Hopkins Press, Baltimore, 1961

Thompson NW: The history of hyperparathyroidism. Acta Chir Scand 156:5, 1990

BASIC SCIENCE

Most of the clinical manifestations of primary hyperparathyroidism are caused by hypercalcemia. PTH increases serum calcium by three mechanisms (Cady and Rossi 1991; Clark 1985; Friesen and Thompson, 1990):

1. By stimulating the activity of osteoblasts and osteoclasts, PTH causes calcium release from bone during remodeling, and this process leads to the demineralizing bone disease of hyperparathyroidism first described by von Recklinghausen.

2. In addition, PTH increases reabsorption of calcium from the renal tubules.

3. Finally, PTH increases the renal conversion of vitamin D to a metabolically more active form, which in turn increases intestinal absorption of calcium.

PTH also decreases renal tubular reabsorption of phosphorus and bicarbonate. Low serum phosphate may be present in up to half of patients with primary hyperparathyroidism, and in advanced cases bicarbonate loss may lead to metabolic acidosis.

Pathology

Of patients with primary hyperparathyroidism, 80 to 85 percent have a solitary adenoma, 12 percent have hyperplasia of all four glands, and about 1 percent have parathyroid cancer (Thompson, et al., 1982). Multiple adenomas have been described in 3 percent, which may represent true multiple adenomas or hyperplasia of more than one gland (Friesen and Thompson, 1990). The pathology of abnormal mediastinal glands in primary hyperparathyroidism is similar, with 80 to 90 percent adenomas and the balance hyperplasia (Clark, 1988; Wang, et al., 1986; Hiebert, 1993).[*] If patients with secondary hyperparathyroidism are included, the proportion of hyperplasia in the mediastinal glands may rise to 40 percent (Clark, 1988). Although histologic criteria have been offered to distinguish between adenoma and hyperplasia—such as cellular density, amount of interstitial fat, and a rim of ''normal'' parathyroid around an abnormally dense nodule of parathyroid tissue—none of these histologic findings absolutely distinguishes between the two processes (Bonjer, et al., 1992; Wells, et al., 1985).

Traditionally, the diagnosis of adenoma required identification by the surgeon of one enlarged parathyroid gland and at least one other normal-sized gland. Recent work, however, has pointed out that classification of hyperfunctioning parathyroids as either adenoma(s) or four-gland hyperplasia may be an oversimplification. Wells, et al. (1985) described a series of patients with primary hyperparathyroidism in which 65 percent of patients had single-gland ''adenomas,'' 10 percent had four-gland ''hyperplasia,'' and 25 percent had either two- or three-gland hyperplasia. This variation has led some investigators of primary hyperparathyroidism to favor the terms *single-gland* or *multiple-gland disease* over the traditional distinction between adenoma and hyperplasia (Bonjer, et al., 1992; Wells, et al., 1985). The distinction between single-gland and multiple-gland disease can be difficult, leading many surgeons to advocate routine identification of all four parathyroids (Wells, et al., 1985).

Carcinoma occurs in 1 percent or less of patients with primary hyperparathyroidism. Histologically the diagnosis is difficult to make on cellular morphology alone and usually requires the identification of invasion of adjacent soft tissue or the finding of metastatic disease.

Embryology

The surgical anatomy of the parathyroid glands is best understood on the basis of embryology. The parathyroid glands arise from the third and fourth branchial pouches during the fifth week of embryogenesis (Moore, 1988). The parathyroids

---

* The 1993 reference to Hiebert consists of his collection of unpublished data on 191 consecutive parathyroid operations.

of the fourth branchial pouches (parathyroid IV) arise contiguous with the lateral components of the thyroid, and they normally come to lie on the posterolateral surface of the thyroid gland above the crossing of the recurrent laryngeal nerve by the inferior parathyroid artery, where they normally become the superior parathyroid (Fig. 58-41).

Parathyroid III arises with the thymus from common primordia in the third pharyngeal pouch and migrates with the future thymus into the lower neck and superior mediastinum (Fig. 58-41). Parathyroid III thus becomes the lower parathyroid and most often settles at the cephalad end of the thymus immediately below the thyroid's lower pole. Not always, however, for during the descent of the thymus, anlage scraps of the future lower parathyroids drop off and tumble like pebbles from an advancing glacier. The surgeon must know both the route of the thymus glacier and where the randomly displaced parathyroids are likely to come to rest. It is equally important that the thoracic surgeon know if the search is for

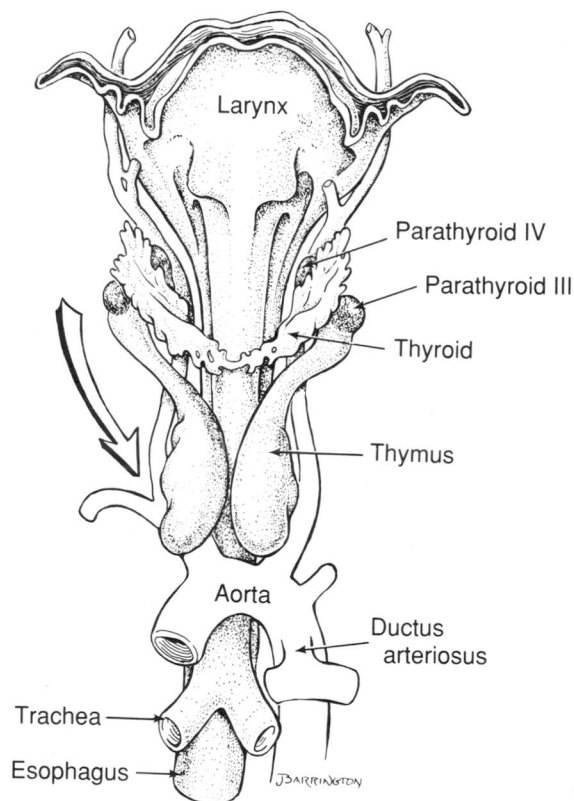

Figure 58-41. Drawing of 23-mm embryo, illustrating embryologic relationships of parathyroids, thyroid, and thymus. Parathyroid IV has come to rest on the posterolateral aspect of the thyroid, which was formed by the union of two lateral components with a midline component. Parathyroid III is still contiguous with the cephalad end of the thymus, and both are in the process of descent into the lower neck and superior mediastinum. Parathyroid III anlage may come to rest anywhere in the thymus itself, on the anterior superior pericardium, or adjacent to the aorta and great arteries and veins of the superior mediastinum. See Figure 58-43 for the same projection in the adult. (Adapted from Weller GL: Development of the thyroid, parathyroid and thymus glands in man. Contrib Embryol 141:95, 1933, with permission.)

parathyroid III or parathyroid IV, so that the most productive moraine is searched first.

Surgical Anatomy

Most mediastinal parathyroid glands are found in one of the following four anatomic territories (Figs. 58-42 and 58-43):

1. Anterior mediastinum within or adjacent to the thymus
2. Superior mediastinum associated with the ascending aorta, aortic arch, and proximal brachial cephalic arteries
3. Posterior mediastinum related to the esophagus
4. Midmediastinal glands

Ectopic lower parathyroids (embryologically parathyroid III) are shown in Figures 58-42 and 58-43. If outside the thymus, they are most frequently at the level of the innominate vein, either anterior or posterior to the thymus. About one-third of normal lower parathyroid glands are found below the lower pole of the thyroid in the cervical tongue of the thymus or in the thyroid-thymic tract of fat, fascia, and vein that extends from the lower pole of the thyroid to the tip of

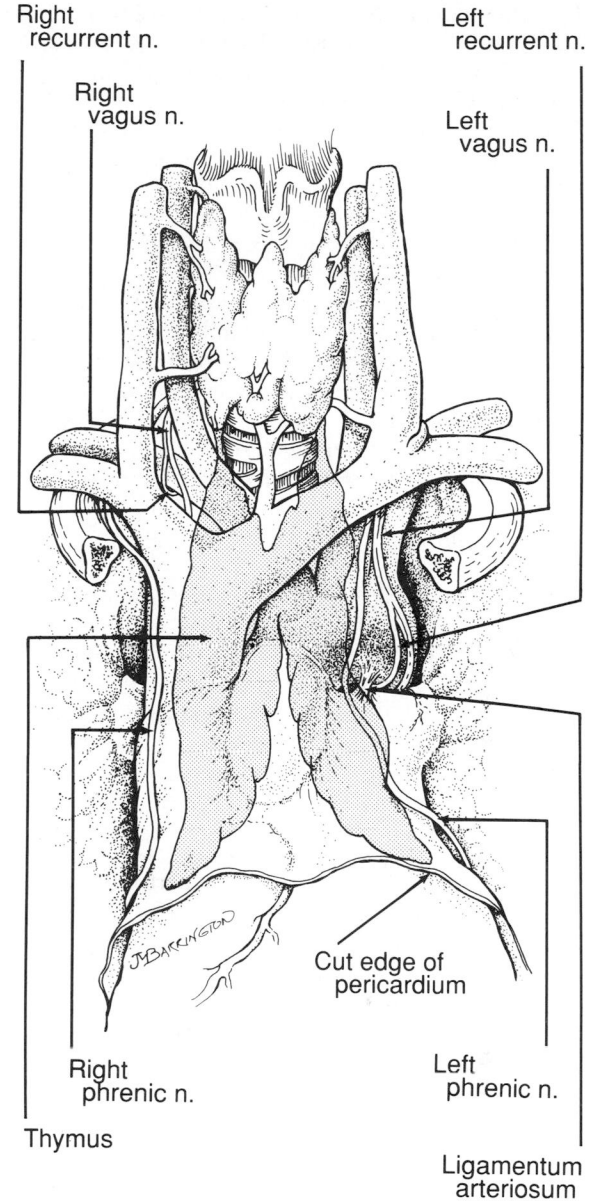

Figure 58-43. The moraine of the embryologic descent of the thymic glacier, which includes the sites of the mediastinal ectopic lower parathyroid (III). The pericardium and major vascular structures provide the key landmarks. Note the phrenic, vagus, and recurrent laryngeal nerves, which must be protected on each side. The search may extend onto the anterior surface of the left pulmonary artery or may require division of the ligamentum arteriosum to gain full exposure of the aortopulmonary window. Beneath the aortic arch is the left-sided extension of the "midmediastinal" location of ectopic parathyroids.

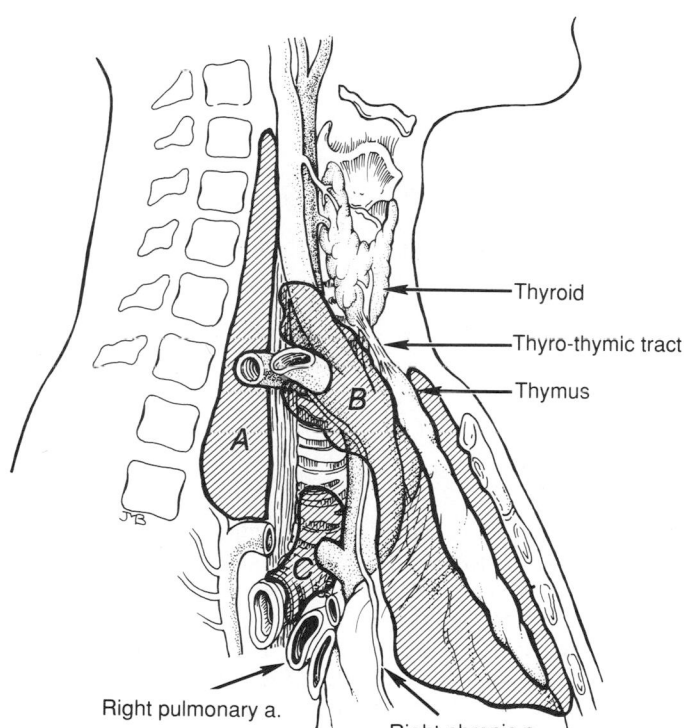

Figure 58-42. The three regions in which mediastinal ectopic parathyroid glands are found: **(A)** retro- and paraesophageal region, which spans both the neck and the upper mediastinum down to the level of the carina (ectopic upper parathyroid IV); **(B)** anterior mediastinum, including thymus and posteriorly the pericardium, the aortic arch, and the great vessels of the upper mediastinum (ectopic lower parathyroid III); **(C)** midmediastinal compartment in front of carina and mainstem bronchi. Note close proximity anteriorly of the right pulmonary artery. This area extends out of view along the left main bronchus underneath the aortic arch into the aortopulmonary window (see Fig. 58-43).

the mediastinal thymus (Akerstrom, et al., 1984; Wang, 1976; Gilmour, 1937).

In a series of 112 reoperations (mainly cervical) for missing parathyroid glands (Wang, 1977) one-third of the pathologic glands were found within the thymus, of which 40 percent were in the cervical thymus and 60 percent were in the mediastinal thymus. In less frequent surgical explorations of the mediastinum through a sternotomy, half to over three-fourths of hyperfunctioning mediastinal parathyroids have been found within the thymus (Russell, et al., 1981; Norton, et al., 1985; Conn, et al., 1991; Wang, et al., 1986).

Ectopic lower parathyroids may also lie between the thymus and the great vessels or pericardium (Figs. 58-42 and 58-43). Caudad to the thymus they may lodge on the pericardium; they may also land lateral to the superior vena cava (as in Captain Martel's case) or adjacent to the left or right innominate vein. Distribution points along the aorta include the origin and proximal innominate and right and left common carotid arteries, as well as the anterolateral aspect of the arch extending back to the ligamentum arteriosum within the mediastinal pleural reflection. Parathyroid glands have been found in the concavity of the aortic arch in the aortopulmonary window, and slightly caudad on the anterior surface of the left pulmonary artery within the mediastinal pleural reflection. Although the possibility of intrapericardial parathyroids has been mentioned, embryologically this should be impossible (Gilmour, 1937; Weller, 1933; Norton, et al., 1985).

Posterior mediastinal glands are generally superior parathyroids (embryologically parathyroid IV). It is thought that the size and weight of the enlarged gland, combined with negative intrathoracic pressure, cause the enlarged gland to fall posteriorly and inferiorly toward the esophagus and posterior mediastinum (Wang, et al., 1986). These posterior mediastinal glands are found in the retroesophageal space, laterally along the esophagus, or in the tracheoesophageal groove. Some surgeons (Thompson, et al., 1982) categorize all these glands as posterior mediastinal in location, although strictly speaking many are located in the neck (Fig. 58-44). Others (Wang, 1977) do not consider these as mediastinal since they can be almost uniformly extracted via a cervical incision. At reoperation for persistent hyperparathyroidism one-third of missing glands have been found in the retro- or paraesophageal area, either in the neck or further down in the posterior mediastinum (Wang, 1977).

On rare occasions the middle mediastinum hides the missing parathyroid, usually in one of two areas (Curley, et al., 1988). One area is located posteriorly along either side of the transverse aortic arch near the ligamentum arteriosum in the aortopulmonary window. In this position they are outside the pericardium and within the mediastinal reflections of the pleura. Embryologically this may be simply an extension of the superior mediastinal location of parathyroid III, as described above. The other location is in front of the carina or right or left mainstem bronchi posterior to the pericardium and pulmonary artery (Fig. 58-42) (Clark, 1988; Wang, et al., 1986; Russell, et al., 1981; Norton, et al., 1985; Conn, et al., 1991; Hiebert, 1993). The embryologic origin of these parathyroids is uncertain.

Finally, a word about supernumerary glands. When four biopsy-proven glands have been uncovered without correcting the hyperparathyroidism, the presence of a fifth gland may be assumed. Two-thirds of such unwelcome tumors will be found below the thyroid, associated with the thymus or the thyroid-thymic tract. Most remaining supernumary glands are found in the neck between the normal locations of the upper and lower parathyroids (Akerstrom, et al., 1984, Russell, et al., 1982).

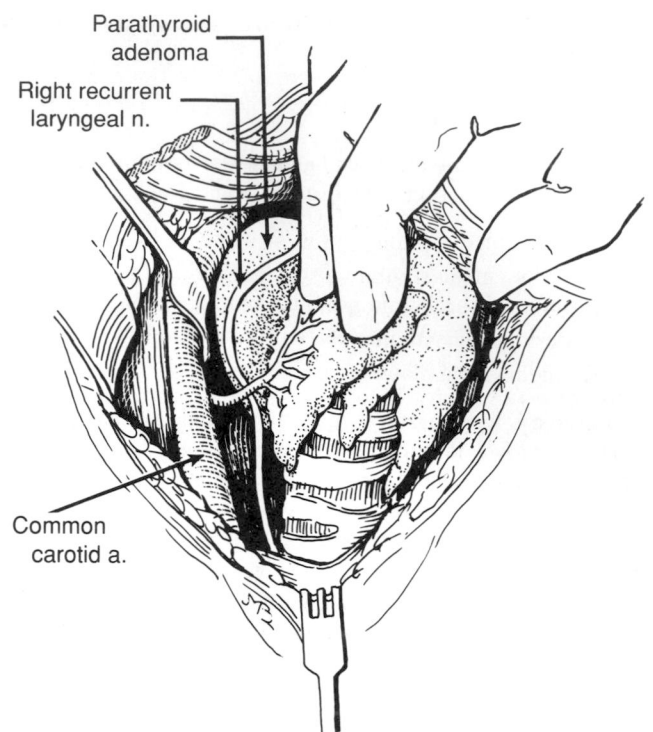

Figure 58-44. Drawing of a large superior parathyroid adenoma lying behind the right recurrent laryngeal nerve above the crossing of the inferior thyroid artery and extending back into the retroesophageal space. This space extends caudally into the posterior mediastinum and is a frequent ectopic site of superior parathyroid glands (parathyroid IV). Posterior glands such as these, whether in the neck or lower in the posterior mediastinum, can be removed via a cervical incision. (From Thompson NW, Eckhauser FE, Harnes JK: The anatomy of primary hypoparathyroidism. Surgery 92:814, 1982, with permission, and Hiebert CA: unpublished data on 191 consecutive parathyroid operations, 1993.)

DIAGNOSIS

Hyperparathyroidism is a condition with a wide variety of symptoms and associated diseases. In general, patients with more severe symptoms have both higher serum calcium levels and larger glands. The classic clinical problems of hyperparathyroidism include bone disease and renal complications. The demineralizing bone disease caused by a direct effect of PTH on bone osteoblasts and osteoclasts gives symptoms of bone pain, tenderness, and susceptibility to fractures (Cady and Rossi, 1991). Renal and ureteral calculi were once frequent presenting signs of hyperparathyroidism. Functional abnormalities of the kidney are more frequently found today, arising from renal tubular abnormalities, including decreased reabsorption of bicarbonate and decreased ability to concentrate urine. Thus, dehydration and metabolic acidosis can be part of the clinical presentation of severe hyperparathyroidism.

A number of other diseases are associated with hyperparathyroidism, although the exact mechanisms of these links are unclear (Clark, 1985; Cady and Rossi, 1991). Peptic ulcer disease, hypertension, and pancreatitis all occur with increased frequency. Subtle psychiatric symptoms are common, including difficulty in concentration or mild depression. Mild proximal muscle weakness may also be present. Joint complications, with pain and effusions from calcification of articular cartilage, as well as true gout and pseudogout, may occur.

Patients with serum calcium levels below 11 mg/dl may be asymptomatic. Patients with calcium between 11 and 14.5 mg/dl may have lethargy, anorexia, weight loss, weakness, and fatigue, in addition to any of the forgoing symptoms. Hypercalcemic crisis occurs at serum levels above 14.5 mg/ dl and may be associated with anorexia leading to nausea and vomiting, fatigue, confusion, and ultimately stupor and coma (Clark, 1985; Cady and Rossi, 1991). Hypercalcemic crisis is a life-threatening emergency, therapy of which includes hydration with isotonic saline solution, with vigorous diuresis to increase urinary excretion of calcium.

Urgent diagnostic workup looking for the etiology of the hypercalcemia must be carried out. This is illustrated by a case managed by one of us (C.A.H., in which a 62-year-old woman presented with nausea, vomiting, lethargy, weakness, and orthostatic hypotension secondary to dehydration. There was a history of fractures with minimal trauma. Bone pain was present in the left femur, and routine electrolyte determinations disclosed a serum calcium of 22 mg/dl. Saline hydration and vigorous diuresis with furosemide brought the serum calcium down to 16 mg/dl. A CT scan showed a prominent retrotracheal mass extending from the lower neck down the posterior mediastinum to the level of the carina (Fig. 58-45). With no other evidence of malignancy, diagnosis of primary hyperparathyroidism was made, and a pathologically benign parathyroid adenoma was removed through a neck incision in an emergency operation. The tumor was 7 cm in length and weighed 31 g. Following its removal, the patient's serum calcium quickly returned to normal levels.

Differential Diagnosis

The causes of hypercalcemia, of which malignancy and hyperparathyroidism are the most common, are summarized in Table 58-6. Malignancy is more common in hospitalized patients, while hyperparathyroidism is more frequently seen in outpatients newly presenting with hypercalcemia. The hypercalcemia of malignancy may be due to bony metastasis or to tumors such as some squamous carcinomas, which secrete a PTH-like substance. In either case, hypercalcemia from malignancy rarely occurs with a tumor volume less than 250 cm^3 (Clark, 1985). These tumors are usually evident on careful physical examination and routine laboratory tests and radiography. The most common occult tumors that cause hypercalcemia are squamous cell carcinomas of the lung, hypernephromas, multiple myeloma, and lymphoma. Chest x-ray, urinalysis, intravenous pyelography or kidney ultrasound, complete blood count, and serum electrophoresis are helpful in excluding these malignancies (Clark, 1985). After exclusion of other causes of hypercalcemia, the diagnosis of primary hyperparathyroidism is confirmed by the findings of sustained elevations in serum calcium and elevated serum PTH levels (Cady and Rossi, 1991; Clark, 1985; Friesen and Thompson, 1990).

Usually the thoracic surgeon is consulted when hypercalce-

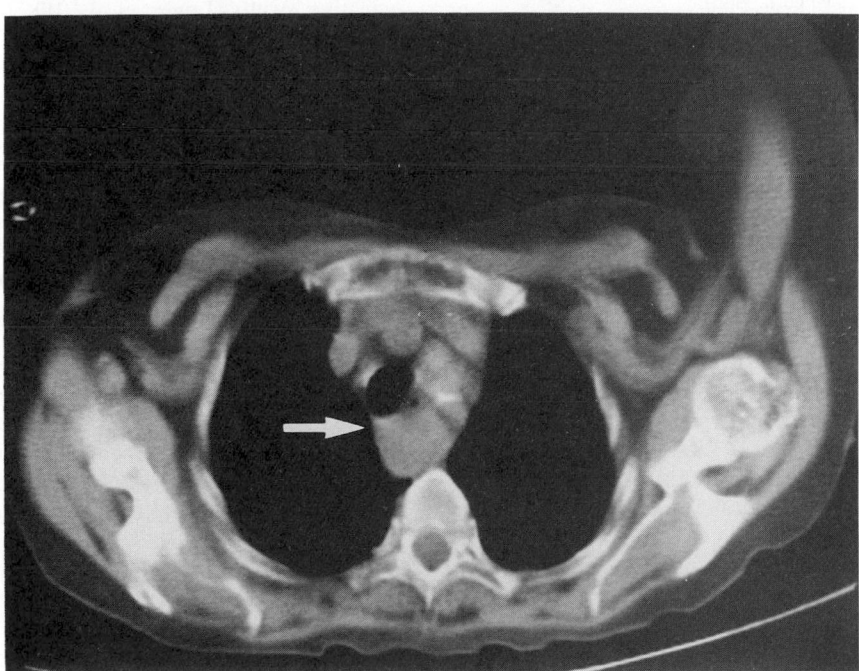

Figure 58-45. CT scan of a patient with large retrotracheal, retroesophageal mediastinal adenoma (*arrow*). Just anterior to the tumor mass and adjacent to the posterolateral angle of the trachea is a smaller air shadow in the lumen of the esophagus. This tumor, like nearly all posterior mediastinal parathyroids, was removed via a cervical incision. (From Hiebert, CA: unpublished data on 191 consecutive parathyroid operations, 1993.)

Table 58-6. Causes of Hypercalcemia

Condition	Approximate Frequency (%)
Malignancy	35
Breast cancer	
Metastatic tumor	
PTH-secreting tumor	
Multiple myeloma	
Acute and chronic leukemia	
Hyperparathyroidism	30
MEA syndrome[a]	
Artifact (e.g., laboratory error, dirty glassware, cork stopper, tight tourniquet)	10
Increased intake	10
Milk-alkali syndrome	
Vitamin D and A overdose	
Thiazide diuretics	
Lithium	
Aluminum	
Granulomatous diseases	5
Sarcoidosis	
Tuberculosis	
Berylliosis	
Other endocrine disorders	5
Hyperthyroidism	
Hypothyroidism	
Addison's disease	
VIP-secreting tumor	
Miscellaneous	5
Immobilization	
Paget's disease	
Idiopathic hypercalcemia of infancy	
Benign familial hypocalciuric hypercalcemia	

Abbreviations: PTH, parathyroid hormone; MEA, multiple endocrine adenomatosis; VIP, vasoactive intestinal polypeptide.
[a] Hyperparathyroidism as a manifestation of MEA syndrome is beyond the scope of this chapter.
(From Clark OH, Siperstein AE: The hypercalcemic syndrome: hyperparathyroidism. In Friesen SR, Thompson NW (eds): Surgical Endocrinology. 2nd Ed. JB Lippincott, Philadelphia, 1990, with permission.)

mia persists or recurs following one or more unsuccessful surgical explorations of the neck. Since a small percentage of failed operations for abnormal parathyroid glands are the result of diseases other than hyperparathyroidism, the original diagnosis should be reconfirmed if there is any doubt. With the diagnosis of primary hyperparathyroidism secure, the principal diagnostic problem is anatomic localization of the hyperfunctioning parathyroid gland(s).

Localizing studies are not routinely advocated prior to initial cervical exploration. However, reexploration of the neck is far more tedious than initial exploration and exposes the patient to a greater likelihood of complications such as recurrent nerve injury. Mediastinal exploration is an even larger operation, requiring an extensive and often lengthy search. Hence, use of multiple modalities to attempt to localize the parathyroids is generally advised: localization studies include thallium-technetium scans, ultrasound, CT scan, MRI, arteriography, and selective venous sampling for PTH levels.

The thyroid gland concentrates both thallium and technetium, and the parathyroid gland accumulates only thallium. After injection of thallium both the thyroid and parathyroid are imaged; technetium, which displays only the thyroid, is then injected, and this image is "subtracted" from the composite image, permitting visualization of the parathyroid and its relationship to the thyroid.

Although thallium-technetium scanning has been reported to localize parathyroid tumors in 75 to 90 percent of cases (Clark, 1985; Cady and Rossi, 1991; Levin, et al., 1987), its ability to localize parathyroid adenoma in the previously operated neck is reduced to the range of 27 to 64 percent (Cady and Rossi, 1991). When the parathyroid target is small, the sensitivity of the test is low. The same is true for specificity when the thyroid is nodular or carcinomatous (Clark, 1985; Cady and Rossi, 1991).

Ultrasound with use of a 10 MHz probe may be useful in the neck but is not useful in the mediastinum, and moreover, the acoustic shadow of the air-filled trachea reduces its sensitivity in searching the retroesophageal area (Clark, 1985; Friesen and Thompson, 1990). Lymph nodes, tortuous vessels, and thyroid nodules all may be mistaken for parathyroid disease. Because of these deficiencies in ultrasound, CT scan and MRI are more useful in localizing abnormal parathyroid glands in the mediastinum.

CT scan or MRI can occasionally detect parathyroid tumors as small as 0.6 to 0.8 cm (Levin, et al., 1987; Friesen and Thompson, 1990). In a group of patients undergoing mediastinal exploration by sternotomy, CT scan, MRI, and thallium-technetium scan each accurately identified the location of the gland in only 46 to 65 percent of the cases with 13 to 18 percent false positive and 18 to 39 percent false negative results (Levin, et al., 1987).

Selective arteriography has been reported to have a 60 to 77 percent sensitivity in detecting abnormal parathyroid glands (Cady and Rossi, 1991). Selective injection is made of internal mammary arteries, both thyrocervical trunks, both inferior thyroid arteries, and if necessary, both superior thyroid arteries. Serious complications can occur from selective angiography, particularly spinal cord damage from inadvertent injection of spinal branches from the costocervical or thyrocervical trunks. The superior thyroid artery arises from the origin of the internal carotid artery, and catheter manipulation there can induce embolization and stroke.

Digital angiography in which the injection is made in the aortic arch or common carotid artery is safer, but digital subtraction angiography will correctly identify parathyroid tumors only about 30 percent of the time (Clark, 1985; Cady and Rossi, 1991). The main use for digital angiography is to map out the venous pattern for subsequent selective venous sampling of PTH levels.

Venous samples are obtained from all available thyroid, vertebral, thymic, and internal mammary veins. Because of collateral drainage, localization is not precise, but at least it may lateralize the abnormal gland to one side or another. However, differentiating between mediastinal and cervical locations may not be possible because mediastinal glands may drain into either cervical or mediastinal veins. Interpretation is further obfuscated by altered flow patterns around previously ligated veins.

However, the test remains valuable. Experienced arteriographers using selective venous PTH measurements can localize abnormal parathyroid glands in 70 to 80 percent of cases (Friesen and Thompson 1990). In one series 57 percent of those tumors not identified by other noninvasive techniques were localized by selective venous catheterization (Levin, et al., 1987). Selective venous sampling, however, is technically difficult and time-consuming and requires experienced personnel (Cady and Rossi, 1991).

In summary, all localization studies have substantial shortcomings, making it desirable to have at least two tests provide confirmatory information preoperatively. This may be possible in only one-third of patients (Levin, et al., 1987).

MANAGEMENT

At reexploration most "missing" parathyroid glands are found in the neck or can be extracted from the upper mediastinum via the cervical incision. Clark (1988) found that 38 percent of patients requiring reexploration had glands in the mediastinum, the remaining glands being discovered in the neck. Half of the mediastinal glands discovered at reoperation were removed through a cervical incision. In 112 reoperations, Wang (1977) found 81 percent of the previously hidden glands via a cervical reexploration and 19 percent via median sternotomy. In 38 percent of the neck reoperations, the missing gland was found in the superior or posterior mediastinum just below the thoracic inlet. Conversely, at median sternotomy two-thirds of the glands were found in the upper anterior mediastinum or mediastinal thymus, potentially within reach of cervical exploration (Wang 1977). In the series of Norton et al. (1985) which comprised 33 patients undergoing median sternotomy, two-thirds also underwent concomitant cervical incision, and 18 percent of the glands were found in the neck.

In the initial neck exploration for primary hyperparathyroidism, an even greater percentage of mediastinal glands can be extracted via the neck incision. Although 10 to 20 percent of patients with primary hyperparathyroidism have abnormal glands located in the mediastinum, only 3.5 percent or less of patients require a thoracotomy or sternotomy (Wang, et al., 1986; Russell, et al., 1981; Norton, et al., 1985; Hiebert, 1993). Hence, before transternal mediastinal exploration is undertaken, one must establish the adequacy of the previous neck exploration(s).

Adequate neck exploration includes transcervical thymectomy, retropharyngeal-esophageal exploration, and transcervical exploration of the superior mediastinum down to the aortic arch. Other unusual cervical locations should also be searched, including those near or within the carotid sheath. Other uncommon cervical hiding places range from as high as the angle of the jaw to as low as the supraclavicular fat pad. Use two power optical loupes! Be on the lookout for vascular tethers stretching from the thyroid arteries! Be methodical, and above all, don't hurry! (Thompson, et al., 1982; Friesen and Thompson, 1990; Wang, 1977; Hiebert, 1993). The superior parathyroid gland may be found beneath the capsule of the thyroid, which makes it difficult to see until that capsule is incised; 2 to 5 percent of lower parathyroid glands have been found within thyroid parenchyma (Wang, 1976; Thompson, et al., 1982) and have either been removed by thyroid lobectomy or enucleated after incision of the thyroid parenchyma. At least three or more normal parathyroid glands should have been identified before the neck is ruled out as the source of the missing gland. Following this protocol, Thompson et al., (1982) had a failure rate of initial cervical exploration of only 4 percent.

Using a collar incision to remove certain mediastinal parathyroid tumors is analogous to withdrawing a substernal goiter from the neck. Not only is it less traumatic overall to do so, but the recurrent laryngeal nerves may stand a better chance of surviving. This is especially so on the right.

If the prior neck exploration(s) are inadequate, the initial reexploration should be through a neck incision unless preoperative studies convincingly locate the missing gland in the mediastinum. This cervical reexploration should include visual and digital exploration of the prevertebral space, search of ectopic areas in the neck, and a digital exploration of the anterior mediastinum down to the aortic arch and along the brachiocephalic arteries. If it has not already been performed at a prior operation, transcervical thymectomy may be done now. The technique of transcervical thymectomy is described in Chapter 59.

If thorough neck reexploration and transcervical exploration of the upper mediastinum are negative, opinion is divided as to whether to proceed at the same operation to sternotomy and definitive mediastinal exploration or alternatively to close and bring the patient back at a later date. Most surgeons prefer to close the reoperated neck and return at a later date for mediastinal exploration. The unsuccessful cervical exploration has usually already been tedious and frustrating, which may hamper immediate detailed mediastinal exploration. Other surgeons (Norton, et al., 1985) note the improved exposure of the anatomic interface between neck and mediastinum afforded by a combined incision, but a higher wound complication has also accompanied this approach. Because mediastinal exploration is a bigger operation and has a higher failure rate, nonoperative management and simple observation may be elected in the asymptomatic patient with minimally elevated serum calcium (<11 mg/dl) (Wang, 1977; Wang, et al., 1986). The rationale is that this mild degree of hyperparathyroidism is rarely life-threatening. Furthermore, with this mild disease the missing gland is generally small and thus more difficult to find at mediastinal exploration or cervical reexploration.

Unless confident preoperative localization warrants a different approach, median sternotomy offers the most versatile incision for mediastinal exploration for missing parathyroid glands. A right lateral thoracotomy, in particular, endangers the recurrent laryngeal nerve (Fig. 58-46). If the posterior mediastinal retroesophageal space has been thoroughly explored at a previous neck exploration, the most likely site of the missing gland will be in the anterior mediastinum in the embryologic distribution of the thymus. If complete thymectomy has not been performed previously, it should be done now. The search should include the anterior superior surface of the pericardium and superior mediastinum, including all sides of the left and right innominate vein; the pericardium covering the superior vena cava and down over the anterior surface of the right hilum; the pericardium overlying the ascending aorta, the aortic arch, and proximal brachio-

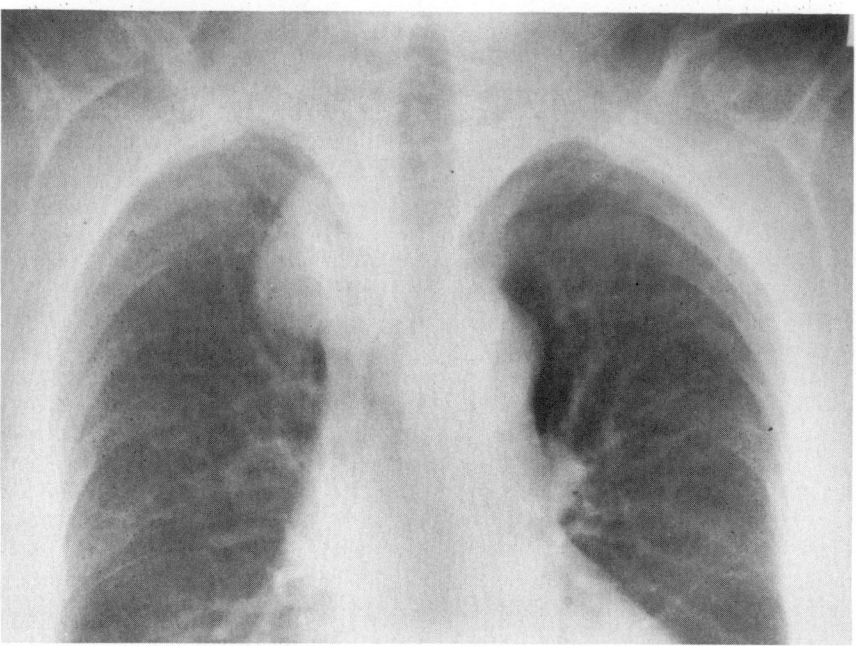

Figure 58-46. Chest x-ray of a 57-year-old woman with a 20-year history of nephrolithiasis and a parathyroid tumor in the upper mediastinum. Awkward exposure through a right lateral thoracotomy resulted in inadvertent division of the recurrent laryngeal nerve as it looped around the lower margin of the growth.

cephalic arteries and back along both sides of the arch to the aortopulmonary window and down onto the anterior surface of the left pulmonary artery (Fig. 58-43). Protect the phrenic nerves!

The remaining area to be searched lies deep in the aortopulmonary window behind the ligamentum arteriosum and in front of the distal trachea and proximal mainstem bronchi (Fig. 58-42). Division of the ligamentum arteriosum may disclose the gland in front of the left mainstem bronchus underneath the aortic arch on the superior surface of the bifurcation of the main pulmonary artery or the surface of the proximal left main pulmonary artery (Figs. 58-42 and 58-43). The left recurrent laryngeal nerve passes under the aortic arch just posterolateral to the ligamentum arteriosum and must be carefully protected (Fig. 58-43). The distal trachea, carina, and origins of the right and left mainstem bronchi can be exposed behind the pericardium by first opening the anterior pericardium and retracting the aortic arch to the left and the superior vena cava to the right to open the posterior pericardium above the right main pulmonary artery (Perleman technique). An alternative approach is to stay completely outside the pericardium, identifying the trachea by retracting the innominate artery to the patient's left and retracting the superior vena cava and right innominate vein to the right after division of the left innominate vein. The anterior surface of the carina is then carefully approached from above and behind the ascending aorta. The fragile right main pulmonary artery lies anterior to the midmediastinal parathyroid territory (Fig. 58-42) (Curley, et al., 1988). In either approach, paratracheal and subcarinal lymphadenopathy may obscure immediate identification of the abnormal parathyroid.

One cannot emphasize too much either the value of thorough neck exploration at the first operation or the ability to retrieve most mediastinal glands from this initial neck operation if appropriately carried out. In one of the authors' (C.A.H.) personal (unpublished) series of 191 patients with primary hyperparathyroidism (Hiebert, 1993), 21 abnormal glands (11 percent) were found in the mediastinum at the primary operation. Almost two-thirds were found in the anterior mediastinum, either within the thymus or in tissue adjacent to the thymus, and slightly less than one-third were found in the retroesophageal or paraesophageal posterior mediastinum (10 additional abnormal glands were found in the retroparaesophageal region high enough to be considered within the neck). One gland was found on the superior aspect of the aortic arch, another was found at the origin of the left internal carotid from the aortic arch, and one large adenoma was located behind the tracheal bifurcation. All these abnormal mediastinal glands were successfully removed at the primary operation from the neck incision, with restoration of normal calcium levels. In these 191 patients only a single gland, located on the anterior pericardium just caudad to the mediastinal thymus, required subsequent sternotomy for excision. This gland was a fifth, supernumerary gland, found in the mediastinum after four normal parathyroids had been identified in the neck (Hiebert, 1993).

Outcome

Even in the most experienced hands mediastinal exploration for missing parathyroids fails to find an abnormal gland in one-third of cases (Conn, et al., 1991; Russell, et al., 1981; Wang, et al., 1986). In one series of mediastinal explorations,

85 percent of patients had an abnormal parathyroid gland removed, but only 70 percent had the gland removed from the mediastinum, the remainder having been found in the neck through a concomitant cervical incision (Norton, et al., 1985). In another series of transternal mediastinal explorations one-third of the failures subsequently had the missing gland found in a later neck exploration (Wang, et al., 1986). A small number of patients end up by having another etiology of their hypercalcemia established (Thompson, et al., 1982; Wang, et al., 1986).

Postoperative Concerns

Serum calcium levels fall following parathyroidectomy, usually reaching a nadir about 48 to 72 hours following operation. Transient hypocalcemia may occur postoperatively as a consequence of prior suppression of normal parathyroid tissue by hyperfunctioning glands. Also, patients with severe bone disease from hyperparathyroidism can develop ''bone hunger'' postoperatively, and with the bones taking up calcium and phosphorus, the fall of serum calcium and phosphorus is apt to be rapid (Cady and Rossi, 1991; Clark, 1985). Permanent hypoparathyroidism can result from excising or devascularizing too much parathyroid tissue. This is more apt to be a problem in surgically treating hyperplasia, since the usual goal is to remove three and one-half parathyroids. Take biopsies away from the vascular pedicle, and avoid grasping the gland with forceps!

The clinical manifestations of acute hypocalcemia include numbness around the mouth, paresthesia of fingers and toes, muscle cramps, and carpopedal spasms. Laryngospasm with airway obstruction may also complicate hypocalcemia. Profound hypocalcemia may lead to tetany (i.e., seizures) and opisthotonos (a form of tetanic spasm of the entire body, in which the head and heels are bent backward and the body bowed forward (Cady and Rossi, 1991; Clark, 1985). Hyper-

ventilation with alkalosis further reduces the ionized calcium and can aggravate symptoms, whereas renal failure with acidosis may mask hypocalcemia temporarily. Chvostek's sign can be elicited by tapping the patient in the preauricular area over the facial nerve and observing a twitching of the ipsilateral corner of the mouth. This test is positive in 10 percent of normal persons (Cady and Rossi, 1991). Trousseau's sign is the observation of carpal spasms with flexion of the metacarpopharyngeal joints and extension of the interpharyngeal joints after inflation of an arm tourniquet above systolic pressure for 3 minutes. This test may be painful to the patient.

Low serum magnesium levels may also cause tetany, and thus both serum magnesium and calcium levels should be checked. Treatment of mild hypocalcemia (serum calcium approximately 7.5 mg/dl) can be treated with oral calcium (calcium carbonate 2.5 g q4h). More severe hypocalcemia and/or tetany is treated with intravenous calcium, usually 10 to 20 ml of 10 percent calcium chloride or 20 to 30 ml of 10 percent calcium gluconate, given slowly by intravenous push over 5 minutes. An intravenous calcium drip is then started. Chronic hypoparathyroidism will require the administration of both oral calcium and vitamin D or its active component, calcitriol (Rocaltrol), 0.25 μg bid (Cady and Rossi, 1991; Clark, 1985).

A strategy for prevention of permanent hypoparathyroidism when one is uncertain of the adequacy of residual functioning tissue is to transplant parathyroid tissue to an easily accessible site such as the forearm or antecubital fossa, where 1-mm slices can be deposited in small muscle pockets and marked for future excision should recurrent hyperparathyroidism develop (Wells, et al., 1979). Parathyroid tissue can also be frozen and cryopreserved for later surgical autotransplantation if necessary (Norton, et al., 1985; Wells, et al., 1979). These techniques are modern updates of Halsted's experimental work at the beginning of the century.

COMMENTS AND CONTROVERSIES

Probably the greatest need for future development is for improved techniques of preoperative localization of parathyroids, particularly smaller glands and particularly in the reoperative neck or the mediastinum.

Recently angiographic techniques have been used to obliterate enlarged and hyperfunctioning mediastinal parathyroids. Large doses of ionic contrast material are deliberately injected into the appropriate artery, perfusing the enlarged gland. This technique requires a gland large enough and well enough vascularized to be identified by contrast staining. It also requires radiologists who are skilled and experienced in highly selective arteriography. The technique was successful in obliterating the function of 63 percent of the patients in whom it could be accomplished and did not appear to interfere

with subsequent surgical excision in those in whom it failed. Failure in superselective catheterization can lead to contrast injection of arteries feeding the spine and to spinal complications, but none occurred in the hands of this experienced group (Doherty, et al., 1992).

The parathyroids are routinely ignored in major extirpative operations in the neck in which the thyroid is excised along with various combinations of larynx, trachea, and esophagus. The consequences of this neglect and strategies for prevention have only recently begun to be addressed (Baumann and Wells, 1993).

C.A.B.
C.A.H.

KEY REFERENCES

Thompson NW, Eckhauser FE, Harnes JK: The anatomy of primary hyperparathyroidism. Surgery 92:814, 1982

From one of the world's leading endocrine surgery services, a review of the pathology and anatomic location of abnormal parathyroids in 273 patients with primary hyperparathyroidism. Their 96 percent success rate of surgical exploration for primary hyperparathyroidism sets a standard.

Wang CA: Parathyroid re-exploration: a clinical and pathological study of 112 cases. Ann Surg 186:140, 1977

A review of 45 years of experience at the Massachusetts General Hospital in reoperation following one or more failed cervical explorations for abnormal hyperfunctioning parathyroids. This study documents the cervical and mediastinal location of abnormal glands found at reexploration and outlines management principles for reoperative parathyroid surgery.

Wang CA: The anatomic basis of parathyroid surgery. Ann Surg 183:271, 1976

A well written and clearly illustrated summary of the location of normal adult parathyroid glands found in the dissection of 160 cadavers. The adult anatomy is clearly related to embryology.

Wang CA, Gaz RD, Moncure AC: Mediastinal parathyroid exploration: a clinical and pathologic study of 47 cases. World J Surg 10:687, 1986

A review of nearly 60 years of experience at the Massachusetts General Hospital, going back to the very first mediastinal exploration on Captain Martel in 1926. A clear description of the pathology and most importantly, the anatomic locations of abnormal parathyroids that were found at median sternotomy. Of a total of 1,200 patients with hyperparathyroidism surgically treated during that interval, 47 underwent mediastinal exploration.

Weller GL: Development of the thyroid, parathyroid and thymus glands in man. Contrib Embryol 141:95, 1933

The fundamental study documenting the embryologic development of the parathyroid glands. It also includes the embryology of the thyroid and thymus glands and is invaluable for understanding the anatomy of these structures.

REFERENCES

Akerstrom G, Malmaeus J, Bergstrom R: Surgical anatomy of human parathyroid glands. Surgery 95:14, 1984

Barr DP, Bulger HA, Dixon HH: Hyperparathyroidism. JAMA 29:951, 1929

Baumann DS, Wells SA: Parathyroid autotransplantation. Surgery 113:130, 1993

Bonjer HJ, Bruining HA, Birkenhager JC: Single and multigland disease in primary hyperparathyroidism: clinical follow-up, histopathology, and flow cytometric DNA analysis. World J Surg 16:737, 1992

Cady B, Rossi RL: Surgery of the Thyroid and Parathyroid Glands. 3rd Ed. WB Saunders, Philadelphia, 1991

Clark OH: Mediastinal parathyroid tumors. Arch Surg 123:1096, 1988

Clark OH: Endocrine Surgery of the Thyroid and Parathyroid Glands. CV Mosby, St. Louis, 1985

Clark OH, Siperstein AE: The hypercalcemic syndrome: hyperparathyroidism. In Friesen SR, Thompson NW (eds): Surgical Endocrinology. 2nd Ed. JB Lippincott, Philadelphia, 1990

Conn JM, Goncalves MA, Mansour KA, McGrity WC: The mediastinal parathyroid. Am Surg 57:62, 1991

Cope O: The story of hyperparathyroidism at the Massachusetts General Hospital. J Med N Engl 274:1171, 1966

Curley IR, Wheeler MH, Thompson NW et al: The challenge of the middle mediastinal parathyroid. World J Surg 12:818, 1988

Doherty GM, Doppman JL, Miller DL et al: Results of a multidisciplinary strategy for management of mediastinal parathyroid adenoma as a cause of persistent primary hyperparathyroidism. Ann Surg 215:101, 1992

Doppman JL, Marx SJ, Brennan MF et al: The blood supply of mediastinal parathyroid adenomas. Ann Surg 488, 1977

Friesen SR, Thompson NW: Surgical Endocrinology: Clinical Syndromes. 2nd Ed. JB Lippincott, Philadelphia, 1990

Gilmour JR: The gross anatomy of the parathyroid glands. J Pathol 46:133, 1938

Gilmour JR: The embryology of the parathyroid glands, the thymus and certain associated rudiments. J Pathol 45:507, 1937

Halsted WS: Surgical Papers. Vol. 2. 3rd Printing. Johns Hopkins Press, Baltimore, 1961

Levin KE, Gooding GAW, Okerlund M et al: Localizing studies in patients with persistent or recurrent hyperparathyroidism. Surgery 102:917, 1987

Moore KL: The Developing Human: Clinically Oriented Embryology. 4th Ed. JB Lippincott, Philadelphia, 1988

Nathaniels EK, Nathaniels AM, Wang CA: Mediastinal parathyroid tumors: a clinical and pathological study of 84 cases. Ann Surg 171:165, 1970

Norton JA, Schneider PD, Brennan MF: Median sternotomy in reoperations for primary hyperparathyroidism. World J Surg 9:807, 1985

Rothmund M, Diethelm L, Brunner H, Kummerle F: Diagnosis and surgical treatment of mediastinal parathyroid tumors. Ann Surg 183:139, 1976

Russell CF, Edis AJ, Scholz DA et al: Mediastinal parathyroid tumors: experience with 38 tumors requiring mediastinotomy for removal. Ann Surg 193:805, 1981

Russell CF, Grant CS, Van Heerden JA: Hyperfunctioning supernumerary parathyroid glands. Mayo Clin Proc 57:121, 1982

Thompson NW: The history of hyperparathyroidism. Acta Chir Scand 156:5, 1990

Wells SA, Leight GS, Hensley M, Dilley, WG: Hyperparathyroidism associated with the enlargement of two or three parathyroid glands. Ann Surg 202:533, 1985

Wells SA Jr, Ross AJ III, Dale JK, Gray RS: Transplantation of the parathyroid glands: current status. Surg Clin North Am 59:167, 1979

Neurogenic Tumors

Bill Nelems

DEFINITION

Neurogenic tumors of the thorax arise from peripheral nerves, sympathetic ganglia, or the mediastinal chemoreceptive paraganglion system (Kissane, 1990). The peripheral nerve lesions occur most commonly in adults in the paravertebral sulci of the mediastinum (Ringertz and Lindholm, 1956) and less commonly in the brachial plexus and the intercostal nerves. In children the highly aggressive neuroblastoma and ganglioneuroblastoma are of sympathetic origin, as is the less hostile ganglioneuroma, which can be seen in both teenagers and young adults (Cohen and Israel). This group of lesions occur almost exclusively in the paravertebral sulci. Paragangliomas are rare and tend to occur in the visceral and anterior compartments of the thorax. Most are hormonally inactive, but catecholamine-secreting thoracic pheochromocytomas can cause hypertension (Kissane, 1990).

The following discussion is intended to summarize the salient features of neurogenic tumors for practicing thoracic surgeons, to review the diagnostic criteria, and to assist in the preoperative planning so essential to the successful outcome for this interesting group of patients.

BASIC SCIENCE AND CLINICAL FEATURES

Table 58-7 classifies the origin of these tumors, revealing their individual identities and their benign or malignant natures (Kissane, 1990; Cohen and Israel; Shields, 1989; Weller, 1990).

Table 58-7. Tumors of the Thoracic Peripheral Nervous System[a]

Origin	Benign	Malignant
Nerve sheath	Neurilemoma (schwannoma)	Malignant schwannoma
	Neurofibroma[b]	Malignant schwannoma[b]
Sympathetic ganglia	Ganglioneuroma	Ganglioneuroblastoma[c]
		Neuroblastoma[c]
Paraganglion system		
Chromaffin secreting	Pheochromocytoma	Malignant pheochromocytoma
Non-chromaffin-secreting	Paraganglioma	Malignant paraganglioma

[a] Askin tumor not included.
[b] Also seen with von Recklinghausen's disease.
[c] Most frequent in childhood.

Nerve sheath tumors may arise from Schwann cells of neuroectodermal origin or from the mesodermally derived perineural cells (Kissane, 1990). Both cell types are thought to be pluripotential in nature and capable of forming collagen, bone, cartilage, muscle, and adipose tissue. Some of the malignant neurogenic tumors exhibit this heterogeneity. The two most common nerve sheath tumors are neurilemmomas (also known as schwannomas) and neurofibromas.

Neurilemmomas are almost always benign. Malignant schwannoma transformation, while described, remains very infrequent (Kissane, 1990). These tumors are usually single and are most commonly found on routine radiography. When large, they may evoke pressure symptoms, eroding bone and displacing soft tissues. They may generate pain and paraesthesias. Patients of all ages have been reported with this neoplasm, but most are older than 40 years. There is no sex predominance (Kissane, 1990). They can occur anywhere in soft tissues or viscera; the most common thoracic site is the posterior sulcus, brachial plexus and intercostal nerves being less frequent locations. Figures 58-47 and 58-48 demonstrate a PA chest radiograph and a coronal MRI of a brachial plexus neurilemmoma in a patient presenting with symptoms of tho-

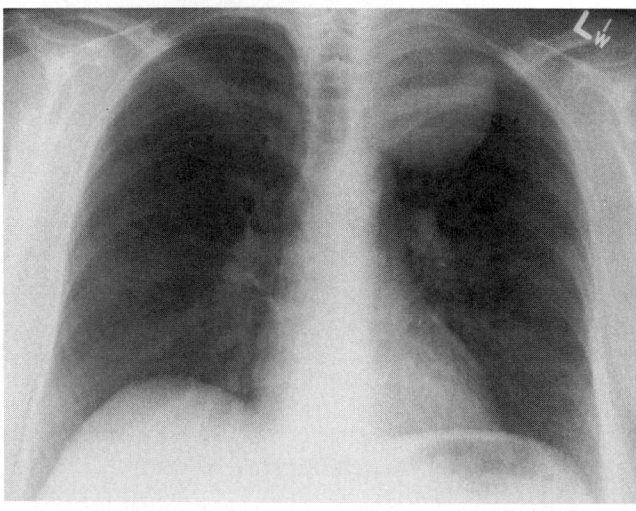

Figure 58-47. A PA chest radiograph showing a brachial plexus neurilemmoma in a patient presenting with lower root thoracic outlet syndrome.

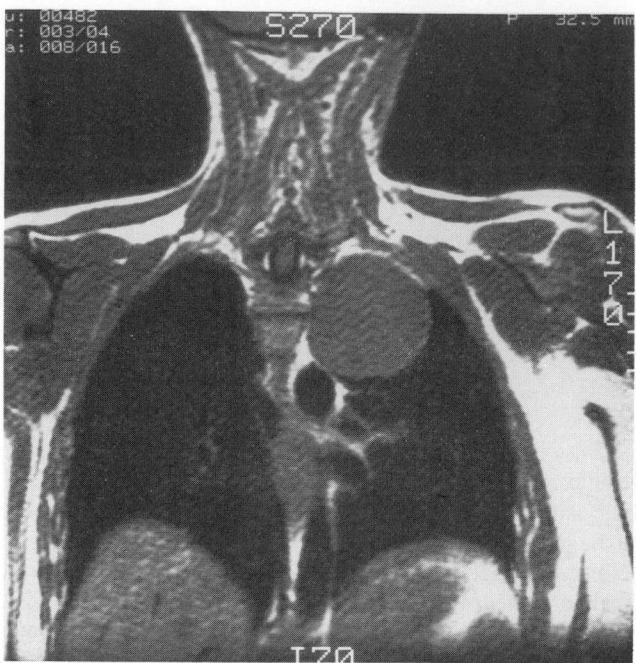

Figure 58-48. Coronal T$_1$-weighted (TR 800/TE 20) MRI demonstrates a heterogenous mass in the left thoracic apex in the same patient illustrated in Figure 58-47.

racic outlet symdrome. Figure 58-49 demonstrates the wasting of hand intrinsic muscles 1 year after resection of this T1 nerve root tumor. Adequate local excision is almost always curative. Sometimes the peripheral nerve can be spared.

The relationship between Schwann cells and perineural cells is still debated by pathologists, but electron microscopy has established that neurilemmomas are almost entirely made up of Schwann cells. Immunofluorescent staining techniques are also helpful in establishing cell types (Kissane, 1990).

Neurofibromas are distinctly different from neurilemmomas, not only in their histopathology but also in their clinical significance. While sharing common sites of origin, neurofibromas tend to occur in younger patients, tend to be multiple in many cases, and may be associated with the autosomally dominant von Recklinghausen's disease, in which brain and spinal cord tumors predominate over those at thoracic sites (von Recklinghausen, 1882). This condition must be considered when café au lait skin lesions are seen (Brasfield and DasGupta, 1972).

Neurofibromas have a more varied cell population than neurilemmomas. Electron microscopy reveals both Schwann and perineural cells in equal proportion (Kissane, 1990). Single lesions again tend to be asymptomatic, and recurrence after excision is rare. Patients with multiple lesions or with von Recklinghausen's disease, however, are at significant risk of developing malignant degeneration (Kissane, 1990).

The designation of malignant tumors of the peripheral nerves causes some semantic confusion. In the benign end of the spectrum the word schwannoma is used interchangeably with neurilemmoma, a tumor that very rarely indeed undergoes malignant degeneration. In the unusual event that it does so, it would be called a malignant schwannoma. However, since the neurofibroma also contains an abundance of Schwann cells, its malignant form is also called schwannoma.

Having resolved this confusion of words, we now discover that the pathology of these tumors is most complex. Some lesions show sarcomatous features, while others exhibit undifferentiated pleomorphism, with a variety of mesenchymal and epithelioid components (Kissane, 1990). Suffice it to say that patients with multiple neurofibromatosis have been re-

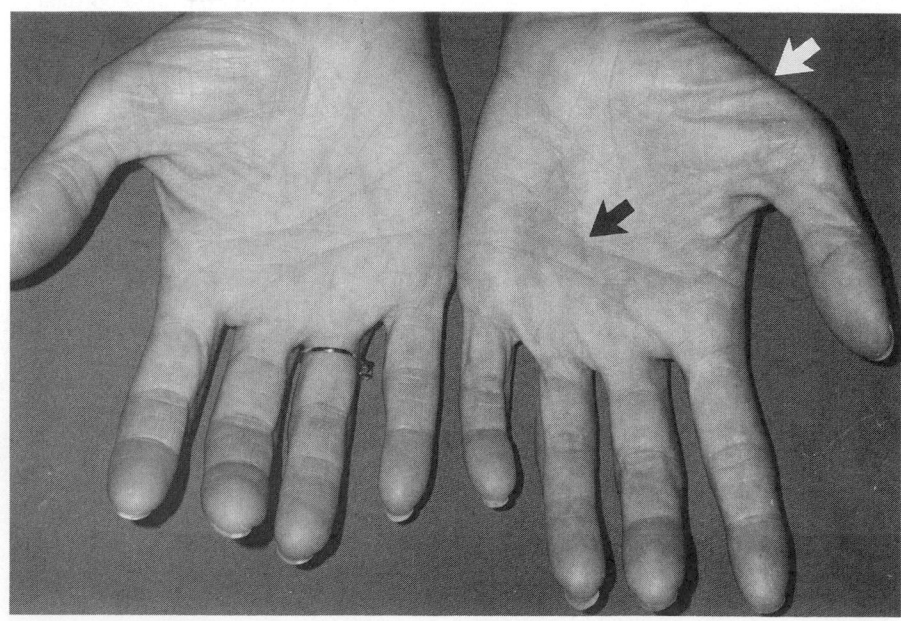

Figure 58-49. Clinical photograph of the hand of the patient illustrated in Figures 58-47 and 58-48, taken 1 year after resection of the T1 nerve root neurilemmoma. Note the wasting in the abductor pollicis brevis muscle and the intrinsic muscles of the hand.

ported to develop malignancy in 4 to 29 percent of cases (Brasfield and DasGupta, 1972). Five-year survival rates, even with appropriate therapy, are quoted at 35 to 65 percent of cases (White, 1971; Sordillo, et al., 1981; Bojsen-Mollor and Myhre-Jensen, 1984). It is not uncommon for local recurrence or distant metastases to manifest 5 to 10 years after therapy (Kissane, 1990).

Sympathetic nerve and ganglia tumors are frequently highly aggressive, and for the most part, they afflict children more often than adults (Cohen and Israel).

Neuroblastomas, while usually of adrenal gland origin, may also be found in areas where embryonic neuroblasts migrate from neural crests. Specifically, they can be seen in relation to the sympathetic trunks and plexuses in the neck, thorax, abdomen, and pelvis. They are infrequent in the mediastinum, where they occur almost exclusively in the paravertebral sulci adjacent to the sympathetic chain (Cohen and Israel). These neoplasms are most frequent in infancy and early childhood, with 86 percent occurring in the first 2 years of life and adult cases being very exceptional (Kissane, 1990). Furthermore, they comprise 7 to 10 percent of all childhood malignancies. Clinically, they present with local tumor masses or with evidence of metastatic disease. The 2-year survival rates following chemotherapy and surgery is 10 to 15 percent (Grosfield and Baehner, 1980).

Ganglioneuromas and their malignant counterparts, the ganglioneuroblastomas, may arise in the adrenal glands, but they are found more frequently elsewhere along the sympathetic chains. The former are slow-growing, may become quite large and encapsulated, and are seen in young adults. They are asymptomatic or present with localized pressure symptoms. Adequate excision is curative. Ganglioneuroblastomas are rare but also more aggressive, presenting generally in early childhood with direct invasion or with metastases (Kissane, 1990).

The extra-adrenal paraganglion system is distributed widely in the peripheral portions of the autonomic nervous system. It consists of macroscopic bodies and microscopic cell clusters of nervous tissue. The major sites for paraganglion tumors are the glomus jugulare, the carotid bodies, the aortic arch, and the abdominal aorta. Glenner and Grimley (1974) divide the intrathoracic paraganglion system into four groups based on anatomic distribution, innervation, and microscopic structure; these they term the branchiometric (derived from branchial arch structures), intravagal, aorticosympathetic, and visceral autonomic paraganglia (Glenner and Grimley, 1974).

These paraganglia act as chemoreceptors, storing catecholamine granules, which are most easily seen on electron microscopy. They may or may not secrete these catecholamines. The catecholamine-secreting pheochromocytoma with its hypertension-producing tendency can arise from this system (Kissane, 1990). The association of thoracic tumor and hypertension, together with measurement of the catecholamine metabolites vanillylmandelic acid and metanephrines in the urine, should establish the rare diagnosis (Cohen and Israel). The nonfunctioning paraganglioma grows slowly and can be difficult to resect in cases in which it becomes intricately enmeshed with the vital structures of the mediastinum and heart. In the world's published experience

of 70 cases, Lamy, et al. quote survival at 78 percent following complete resection, but only 42 percent following partial excision or biopsy. Therefore total excision should be attempted wherever possible. Lamy, et al. have described the excision in a case that required cardiopulmonary bypass to resect such a tumor. Figure 58-50 demonstrates the lesion excised by Lamy, et al.

Ten percent of pheochromocytomas, regardless of their location, are familial. These syndromes include simple familial pheochromocytoma, multiple endocrine neoplasia types II and III, neurofibromatosis, and von Hippel-Lindau disease (Levine and McDonald, 1984). Both pheochromocytomas and paragangliomas have been reported to undergo malignant change (Kissane, 1990).

One remaining and rare tumor needs to be included here. The peripheral neuroepithelioma of the thoracopulmonary window, also known as Askin's tumor, has not been included in Table 58-7 because its histopathology remains controversial (Cohen and Israel). Histologically, undifferentiated small blue cells intermingle with cells with varying degrees of neuronal differentiation. Electron microscopy reveals a unique chromosomal translocation (Whang-Peng, et al., 1984). These features suggest that this lesion arises from a different peripheral nerve cell from that in which the neuroblastoma originates (Thiele, et al., 1987). The clinical course of this tumor tends to be aggressive, and the prognosis is poor. The tumor occurs in childhood and young adult life, presenting with pleura-based masses, with rib erosion, or with paravertebral encroachment. Urine catecholamine excretion is absent. Treatment tends to be multimodal, including surgical resection where possible and chemotherapy.

INVESTIGATIVE TECHNIQUES

Radiologic techniques are used almost exclusively to establish the location and extent of this group of tumors. For

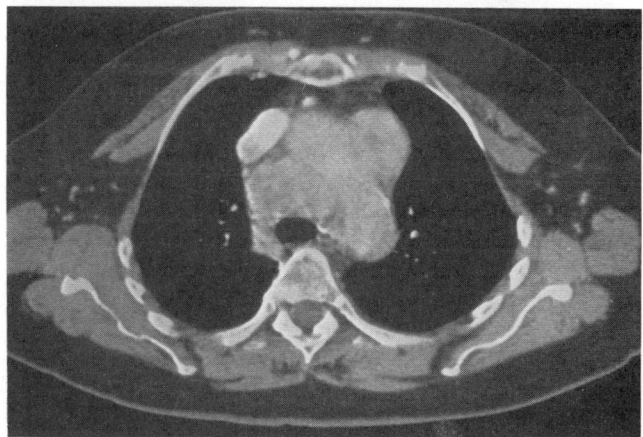

Figure 58-50. Contrast-enhanced 1-cm transverse CT image demonstrates a mediastinal paraganglioma tumor encasing the aorta and pericardium. This patient required cardiopulmonary bypass for complete resection. (From Lamy A, Fradet G, Luoma A, Nelems B: Aortic body tumor (paraganglioma): complete surgical resection is the treatment of choice. Ann Thorac Surgery (accepted for publication), with permission.)

all paravertebral sulcus lesions, standard chest radiographs locate the primary tumor site. Oblique views of the spinal nerve foramina may be helpful in determining central extent. However, with the advent of CT and MRI, the uncertainties of tumor extent have largely been eliminated (Ricci, et al., 1990). The same can be said of lesions that arise in the anterior or visceral mediastinal compartments and for brachial plexus and chest wall neurogenic tumors. Figures 58-51 through 58-53 demonstrate the precision of such imaging techniques.

MANAGEMENT

Pediatric management mainly involves the care of malignant disease. Combined tumor group participation by radiation oncologist, chemotherapist, and surgeon is often helpful in these cases. In adults the management is mostly surgical in nature. Meticulous preoperative planning is essential for good outcome. In cases of locally invasive or distant malignant disease, radiotherapy and/or chemotherapy will be necessary.

Anterior and visceral compartment tumors are best approached anteriorly through the neck or by sternotomy. Invasive mediastinal and intracardiac lesions may be difficult to resect and may require cardiopulmonary bypass (Lamy, et al.).

Vertebral sulcus tumors are now easily divided into two groups, on the basis of CT and MRI findings, namely, purely intrathoracic tumors and tumors with spinal canal extension through the intervertebral foramina. The latter group includes 10 percent of vertebral sulcus tumors, and 60 percent of this group present with neurologic symptoms or signs (Grillo and Ojemann, 1989).

For those tumors that are confined exclusively to the thorax, I prefer to use serratus anterior-splitting or latissimus dorsi-retracting muscle-sparing lateral incisions, depending

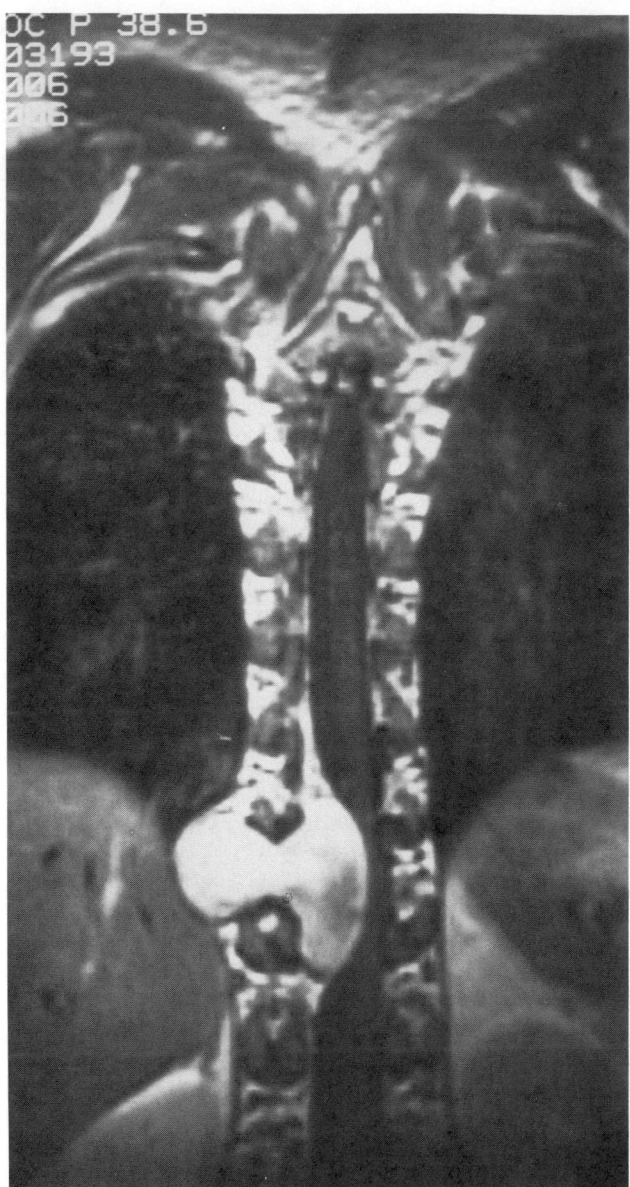

Figure 58-52. Coronal T_1-weighted (TR 600, TE 20) MRI shows a dumbbell-shaped neurofibroma of predominantly high signal intensity, extending through the neural foramen into the spinal canal and causing weakness in the legs.

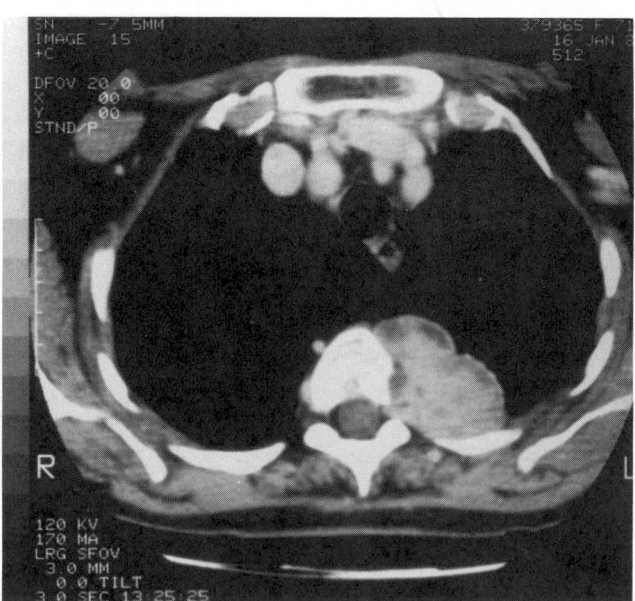

Figure 58-51. Contrast-enhanced 3-mm transverse CT image demonstrates a neurogenic tumor extending into the neural foramen. This lesion was resected by thoracotomy and without laminectomy.

on the tumor site. For tumors with intraspinal extension, we are helped by the recommendations of Akwari, et al. (1978), Grillo and Ojemann, (1989), and Grillo, et al. (1983). Akwari, et al. suggested that the spinal component should be exposed first through a paravertebral incision. The laminectomy should be performed and the intraspinal dissection completed prior to a lateral thoracotomy for removal of remaining tumor. Grillo and associates (1983) recommend a combined approach, with a posterior exposure that allows for both posterior thoracotomy and spinal laminectomy. Ricci, et al. (1990) suggest that each case should be individualized. In most cases the Grillo technique seems to be optimal. However, Ricci, et al. suggest that when more than one foramen is involved or when three or more laminectomies are required, a vertical

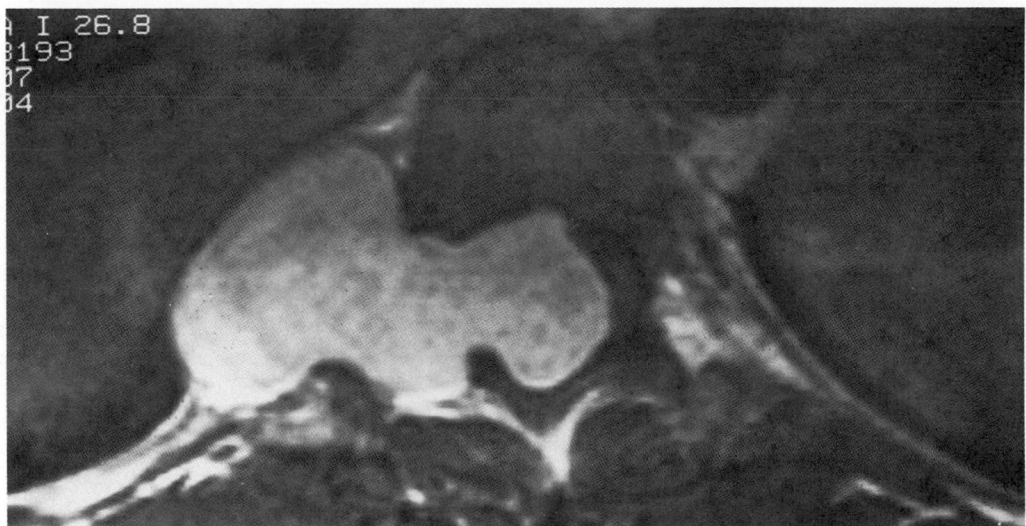

Figure 58-53. Transverse T₁-weighted (TR 800, TE 20) MRI of the patient illustrated in Figure 58-52, also showing the intraspinal extent of tumor.

posterior incision is needed for muscle mobilization. They used the technique of Grillo, et al. in three of five cases and the approach of Akwari, et al., in the other two.

I personally prefer Grillo's one-incision style. His illustration shows that with vertical extension of the skin incision, sufficient space becomes available for laminectomy. In my own experience I have found transsection of the paraverte-

bral musculature to be more valuable than retraction, as it allows for linkage of the posterior thoracotomy and the laminectomy aspects of the surgical field, thereby providing better visualization of the tumor under resection. For lesions above the scapular tip, the upward-curving incision of Grillo, et al. is ideal. For lower lesions, a horizontal incision may suffice (Fig. 58-54).

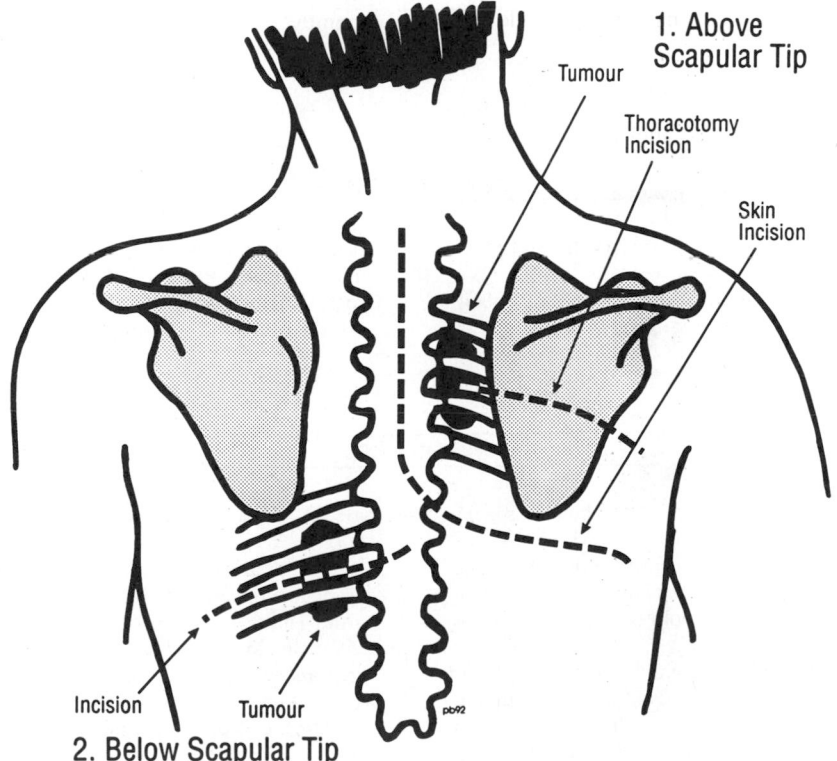

Figure 58-54. The right side illustrates the one-incision approach of Grillo, et al. for lesions above the scapular tip. The left side illustrates a horizontal incision for lesions below the scapula. Division of the paravertebral muscles facilitates the procedure. (Adapted from Grillo HC, Ojemann RG, Scannell JG, Zervais NT: Combined approach to "dumbbell" intrathoracic and intraspinal neurogenic tumors. Ann Thorac Surg 36:402, 1983, with permission.)

COMMENTS AND CONTROVERSIES

This uncommon group of neoplasms will continue to challenge all who encounter them. Those aspects that pertain to the management of malignancy, particularly in children, will require the most attention. The understanding of basic pathology is quite advanced. This is not a disease for which life-style couseling is needed. Genetic counseling may be important in von Recklinghausen's disease, the autosomal dominant nature of which must be considered.

Radiologic techniques, particularly the development of CT and MRI, have revolutionized the diagnostic and surgical planning aspects of all neurogenic tumors. For localized lesions, even with spinal extension, surgical resection remains the preferred treatment, offering high cure rates. The combine neurosurgery-thoracic approach of Grillo and associates deals effectively with these lesions.

B.N.

Neurogenic tumors are among the commonest primary neoplasms of the mediastinum. The majority are benign, but in 8 to 10 percent of cases, there is extension of the intrathoracic component through the intervertebral foramen, resulting in the so-called dumbbell tumor. In modern thoracic surgery, failure to fully investigate the local extension of any posterior mediastinal mass before thoracotomy should be considered negligent. This investigation is important, not only because 40 to 50 percent of dumbbell tumors are asymptomatic, but also because the unexpected finding of spinal extension during removal may contribute to permanent spinal canal drainage.

Most neurogenic tumors are detected on routine chest radiographs, where the tumor is seen as a smoothly rounded mass located in the posterior mediastinum. All patients with these findings must undergo CT because this technique is more sensitive than plain radiography in detecting enlargement of the foramen and possible extension of the tumor into the spinal canal. If CT clearly shows that the tumor is extradural and extraspinal, no further investigation is required. If CT is inconclusive, MRI should be done, because it accurately defines the existence and extension of the intraspinal component of the tumor. With the use of MRI, myelography is seldom necessary. The role of thoracic aortography to document the site of origin of the artery of Adamkiewicz, which supplies the anterior spinal artery, is controversial. Some surgeons, particularly those in Europe, always perform thoracic aortography before surgery, and if the artery of Adamkiewicz is found to arise in the area of the tumor, excision is not recommended unless absolutely necessary. If the artery is found to arise at a distance from the tumor, surgery can proceed without concern for possible damage to the blood supply of the spinal cord.

Although observation alone is a reasonable course of action for tumors that have been stable for years, the majority of neurogenic tumors should be resected because of uncertain diagnosis, location near or in the spinal canal, or possible malignancy.

J.D.

KEY REFERENCES

Brasfield RD, Das Gupta TK: Von Recklinghausen's disease, a clinical pathological study. Ann Surg 175:86, 1972

Grillo HO, Ojemann RG: Mediastinal and intraspinal "dumbbell" neurogenic tumors. p. 205. In Thoracic Surgery: Frontiers and Uncommon Neoplasms. In International Trends in General Thoracic Surgery. Vol 5. CV Mosby, St. Louis, 1989.

Grosfeld JL, Baehner RL: Neuroblastoma; an analysis of 160 cases. World J Surg 4:29, 1980

REFERENCES

Akwari OE, Payne WS, Onofrio BM et al: Dumbbell neurogenic tumors of the mediastinum. Mayo Clin Proc 53:353, 1978

Bojsen-Moller M, Myhre-Jensen O: A consecutive series of 30 malignant schwannomas. Survival in relation to clinico-pathological parameters and treatment. Acta Pathol Microbiol Scand[A] 92:147, 1984

Cohen PS, Israel MA: Biology and treatment of thoracic tumors of neural crest origin. p. 520. In Malignancies of the Mediastinum.

Glenner GG, Grimley PM: Tumors of the extra-adrenal paraganglion system (including chemoreceptors). In Atlas of Tumor Pathology 2nd Ser., Fascicle 9. Armed Forces Institute of Pathology, Washington, 1974

Grillo HC, Ojemann RG, Scannell JG, Zervas NT: Combined approach to "dumbbell" intrathoracic and intraspinal neurogenic tumors. Ann Thorac Cardiovasc Surg 36:402, 1983

Kissane JM (ed): Anderson's Pathology. CV Mosby, St. Louis, 1990

Lamy A, Fradet G, Luoma A, Nelems B: Aortic body tumour (paraganglioma): complete surgical resection is the treatment of choice Ann Thorac Surg (accepted for publication)

Levine SN, McDonald JC: The evaluation and management of pheochromocytomas. Adv Surg 17:281, 1984

Ricci C, Rendina EA, Venuta F et al: Diagnostic imaging and surgical treatment of dumbbell tumors of the mediastinum. Ann Thorac Surg 50:586, 1990

Ringertz N, Lindholm SO: Mediastinal tumors and cysts. J Thorac Cardiovasc Surg 31:45, 1956

Shields TW: Primary tumors and cysts of the mediastinum. p. 1096. In Shields TW (ed): General Thoracic Surgery. 3rd Ed. Lea & Febiger, Philadelphia, 1989

Sordillo PP, Helson L, Hadju SI et al: Malignant schwannoma—clinical characteristics, survival, and response to therapy. Cancer 47:2503, 1981

Thiele CJ, McKeon C, Triche TJ et al: Differentiation of protooncogene expression characterizes histopathologically indistinguishable tumors of the peripheral nervous system. J Clin Invest 80:804, 1987

Von Recklinghausen, FD: Ueber die multiplen Fibrome der Haut und ihre Beziehung zu den multiplen Neuromen. Berlin, 1882

Weller RO: Tumors of the nervous system. p. 466, 494. In Weller RO (ed): Nervous System, Muscle, and Eyes. In Systemic Pathology. 3rd Ed. Vol. 4. Churchill Livingstone, New York 1990

Whang-Peng J, Triche YJ, Knutsen T et al: Chromosomal translocation in peripheral neuroepithelioma. N Engl J Med 311:584, 1984

White HR: Survival in malignant schwannoma. An 18 year study. Cancer 27:720, 1971

59

SURGICAL TECHNIQUES

Thymectomy

Earle W. Wilkins, Jr.

HISTORICAL NOTE

Interest in anterior mediastinal tumors and thymoma paralleled early investigation into the nature of myasthenia gravis. Laquer and Weigert (1901) are credited with first identifying the relationship between the thymus and myasthenia gravis. On autopsy of a patient who died of myasthenia gravis, Carl Weigert, a pathologist, discovered a 3 × 5 cm thymic tumor, typically adherent to pericardium and left lung; he correctly speculated about the possible correlation of myasthenia gravis and thymoma.

Viets and Schwab (1960), in discussing the history of thymectomy for myasthenia gravis, described Sauerbruch's early surgery, including the first thymectomy (transcervical) on March 6, 1911, in a patient with myasthenia gravis. The patient's myasthenic symptoms were improved, but the thymus showed only an enlarged, hypertrophic gland and not a tumor.

However, the landmark operation took place on May 26, 1936, when Blalock (1939) successfully removed a thymoma from a 19-year-old myasthenic woman. Safe conduct through the operation was made possible by the recent introduction of the anticholinesterase agent neostigmine bromide. Blalock set a pioneering standard in his use of median sternotomy, now the preferred surgical approach to tumors of the anterior mediastinum.

The application of thymectomy to myasthenic patients without thymoma was Blalock's (1941) creatively innovative next step. In 1941 he described the use of thymectomy in 6 patients without tumor. His assumption that the thymus gland was in some way responsible for the block at the myoneural junction remains a hypothesis and the basis for thymectomy in myasthenia gravis today.

HISTORICAL READINGS

Blalock A, Harvey AM, Ford FR, Lilienthal JL Jr: The treatment of myasthenia gravis by removal of the thymus gland. JAMA 117:1529, 1941

Blalock A, Mason MF, Morgan HJ, Riven SS: Myasthenia gravis and tumors of the thymic region. Report of a case in which the tumor was removed. Ann Surg 110:544, 1939

Laquer L, Weigert C: Beiträge zur Lehre von der Erbschen Krankheit. 1. Über die Erbschen Krankheit (Myasthenia gravis). 2. Pathologisch-anatomischer Beitrag zur Erbschen Krankheit (Myasthenia gravis). Neurol Zentralbl 20:594, 1901

Viets HR, Schwab RS: Thymectomy for Myasthenia Gravis. CC Thomas, Springfield, IL, 1960

THYMECTOMY

In patients with myasthenia gravis, thymectomy may be carried out by the transcervical approach or by midline sternotomy. (Transverse sternotomy should never be used for simple thymectomy.) In general, sternotomy is chosen by those thoracic surgeons who prefer a more open, direct operative field or who are uncomfortable with the visual limitations of the purely cervical incision. The thymus gland is a cervicomediastinal structure that can be totally exposed by a limited partial upper sternotomy. Jaretzki, et al. (1977) proposed total median sternotomy as "a rational approach to total thymectomy in the treatment of myasthenia gravis" because of the frequency of ectopic foci of thymic tissue. His approach is based on the eminently reasonable tenet that thymectomy in the management of myasthenia gravis should be total, including removal of all such ectopic foci.

ANESTHESIA

Endotracheal intubation is essential because either one or both pleural spaces may be inadvertently entered during the dissection. The intubation may be carried out transnasally if the myasthenia is severe and it is anticipated that the patient may require postoperative ventilator support. With the advent of preoperative plasmapheresis, usually employed as three exchanges on alternate days in the week before operation, prompt extubation is now usually possible, however.

The usual anesthetics are a rapidly acting barbiturate, such as thiopental sodium, for induction and a general anesthetic, such as fluothane. Muscle-relaxing drugs are not necessary and indeed are contraindicated. Standard monitoring includes cardiac evaluation by continuous electrocardiography and blood pressure and oxygenation by a radial artery line.

Anticholinesterase drugs are never administered during thymectomy for myasthenia gravis.

PARTIAL STERNOTOMY

The patient is placed supine and the proposed incision marked to avoid a skewed scar when one arm is extended on an arm board. Details of the approach were described very early by Sweet (1950) and more recently by Wilkins (1981).

The midline skin incision may be as short as 8 cm. When it is carried down to the sternum itself, the skin and subcutaneous tissue can then be retracted upward or downward to provide necessary exposure of the bone. Alternatively, a standard supraclavicular cervical incision may be used with elevation of the lower skin flap for exposure of the upper sternum (Fig. 59-1). Finally, a transverse submammary incision is possible, with elevation of an extensive upper soft tissue dissection. All these approaches are directed at better cosmetic results than the lengthy, full median sternotomy incision. I much prefer the direct limited midline incision.

The sternotomy is accomplished easily by dividing the cortical bone of the manubrium with the Lebsche shears and then splitting the sternum distally with the Lebsche knife to the level of the fourth anterior rib. The Striker power-driven saw may be preferred. The application of a Gelfoam strip on either side against the cut sternal edges under wound-protecting gauzes minimizes vascular ooze. A small Finochietto or Tuffier spreader provides the desired exposure of the anterosuperior mediastinum and base of the neck.

The thymus gland is identified by its characteristic grayish pink color, which distinguishes it from the yellow fat of the mediastinum. It is grasped with a Babcock- or Duval-type forceps, which permits the appropriate elevating tension for easy extracapsular separation of the gland from the mediastinal pleura laterally and from the pericardium posteriorly. The actual dissection is begun from below upward. An effort is made to push away the mediastinal pleura without entering it; if inadvertent entry should result, no attempt is made to suture and close the defect.

The principal arterial supply from each internal mammary artery is identified and divided (Fig. 59-2). In further lateral dissection toward each lung root, extreme care is taken to avoid damage to the phrenic nerves. Diaphragmatic palsy can present a major post-thymectomy management problem in the myasthenic patient. The venous drainage via one or two sizable veins into the inferior aspect of the left innominate vein is divided (Fig. 59-3). This permits ready exposure and dissection of the two upper poles extending into the base of the neck. One or both poles may occasionally pass posterior to the innominate vein. Care is taken to avoid removal of an inferior parathyroid gland.

The mediastinal thymic bed is carefully inspected in search of ectopic thymic tissue or residual bleeding. Sternal bleeding is controlled with cautery. The sternum is reapproximated with two or three stainless steel wires placed either through or around the sternum, with use of appropriate care to avoid laceration of the internal mammary vessels. Particular attention is paid to inverting the twisted wire ends in order to minimize the postoperative annoyance of sensitively palpable wire ends. Running subcuticular Dexon skin closure is helpful in providing a cosmetically acceptable scar.

Mediastinal drainage is usually unnecessary; a suprasternal suction catheter of the Jackson-Pratt or Hemovac type may be used. Pleural drainage is also unnecessary even when pleural entry has occurred. In these cases positive pressure ventilation by the anesthesiologist at the time of sternal closure permits full lung expansion.

TOTAL STERNOTOMY

The approach for the Jaretzki "maximal" thymectomy is also illustrated in Figure 59-1. The cervical collar extension facilitates the search for ectopic thymic foci in the neck. In a later report Jaretzki and Wolff (1988) describe separate cervical and thoracic incisions; the T incision "is used for large or malignant thymomas, reoperations, and for obese patients with a short neck."

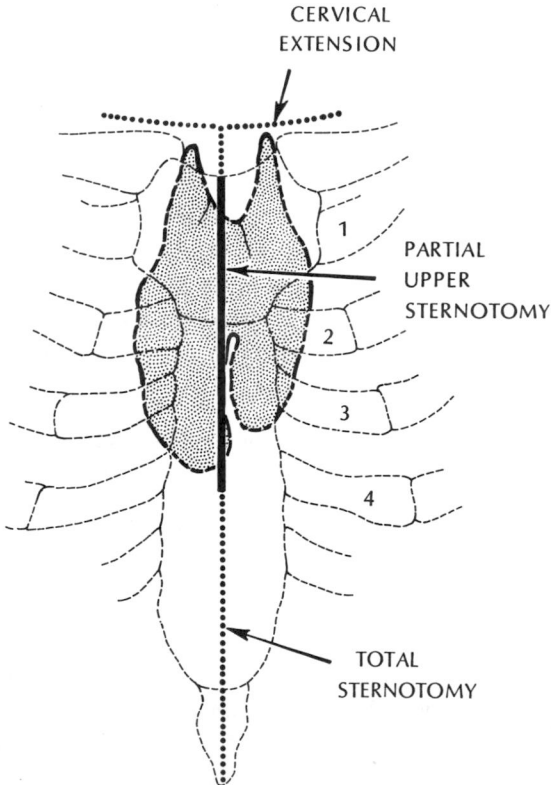

Figure 59-1. The limited partial upper sternotomy is illustrated with the straight black line. The median total sternotomy includes this black line plus the dotted line extending inferiorly. When a cervical extension is necessary, this is made as illustrated at the top. In the Jaretzki procedure the cervical incision is made separate from the median sternotomy without the short dotted line connecting the two incisions. (From Wilkins EW Jr: Thymectomy. Modern technics in surgery. p. 38-1. In Cohn LH (ed): Cardiac/Thoracic Surgery. Futura Publishing, Mt. Kisco, NY, 1981, with permission.)

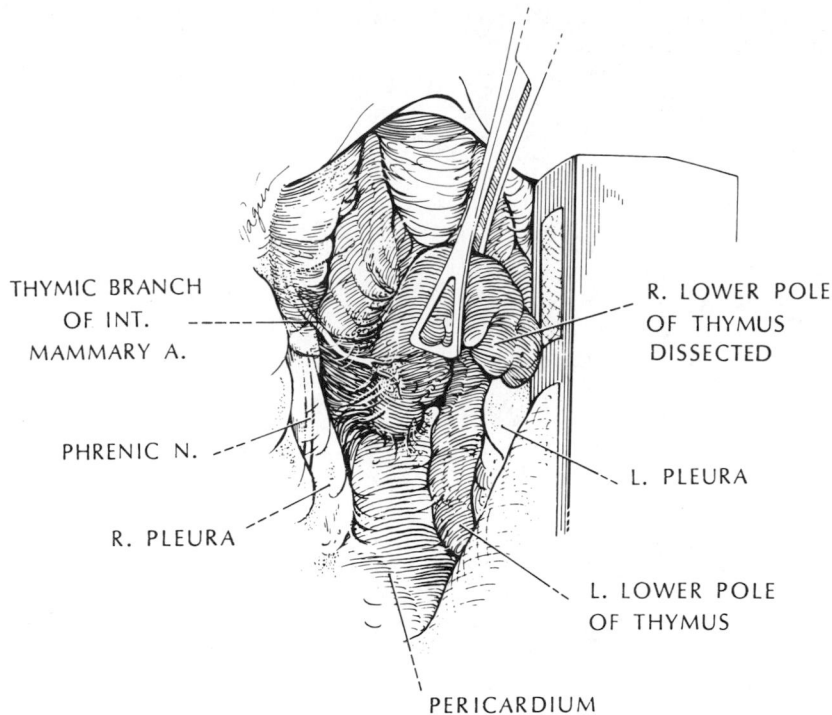

THYMIC BRANCH
OF INT.
MAMMARY A.

PHRENIC N.

R. PLEURA

R. LOWER POLE
OF THYMUS
DISSECTED

L. PLEURA

L. LOWER POLE
OF THYMUS

PERICARDIUM

Figure 59-2. The dissection of the thymus is begun from below upward; the thymic branch of the internal mammary artery is illustrated (From Wilkins EW Jr: Thymectomy. Modern technics in surgery. p. 38-1. In Cohn LH (ed): Cardiac/Thoracic Surgery. Futura Publishing, Mt. Kisco, NY, 1981, with permission.)

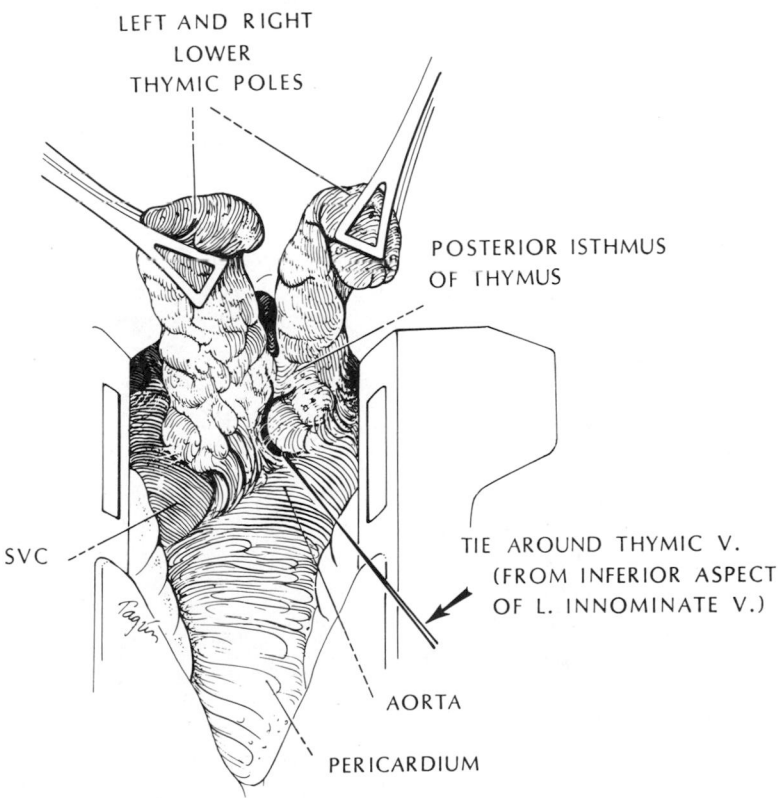

LEFT AND RIGHT
LOWER
THYMIC POLES

POSTERIOR ISTHMUS
OF THYMUS

SVC

TIE AROUND THYMIC V.
(FROM INFERIOR ASPECT
OF L. INNOMINATE V.)

AORTA

PERICARDIUM

Figure 59-3. The lower poles have been dissected free and the internal mammary artery branches divided. The principal venous drainage is illustrated as a single tributary into the left innominate vein. (From Wilkins EW Jr: Thymectomy. Modern technics in surgery p. 38-1. In Cohn LH (ed): Cardiac/Thoracic Surgery. Futura Publishing, Mt. Kisco, NY, 1981, with permission.)

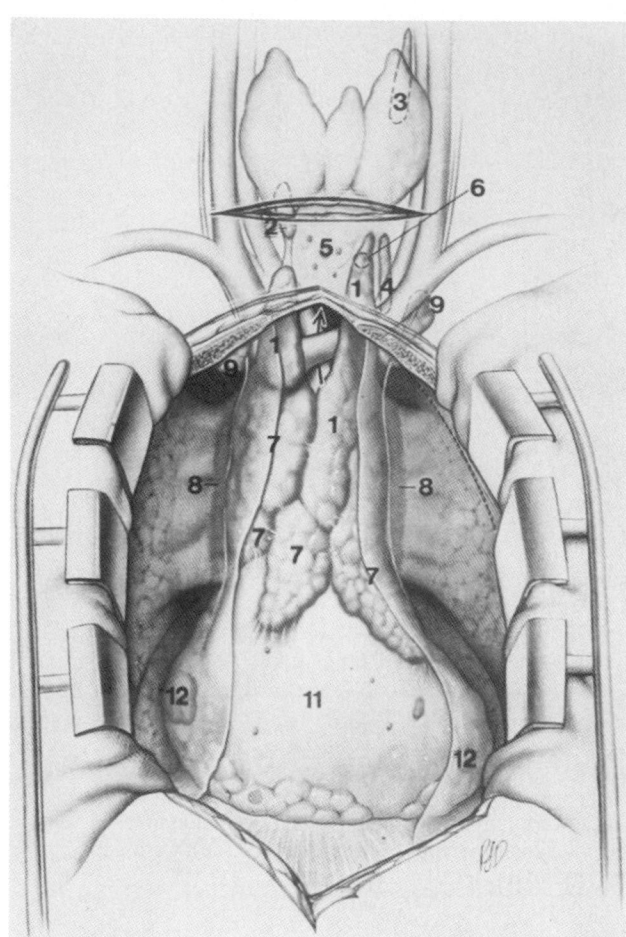

Figure 59-4. In a composite anatomy based on 50 consecutive Jaretzki resections, the locations of thymic tissue are numbered: 1, cervical mediastinal lobes; 2, cervical extension; 3, retrothyroid location; 4, unilateral cervical lobe; 5, pretracheal fat containing thymus; 6, parathyroid tissue in specimen removed; 7, additional mediastinal lobes (other than 1, 8, and 9); 8, under the phrenic nerves; 9, behind the innominate vein and the aortopulmonary window region; 11, anterior mediastinal fat; 12, lobule in cardiophrenic fat. (From Jaretzki A III, Bethea M, Wolff M et al.: A rational approach to total thymectomy in the treatment of myasthenia gravis. Ann Thorac Surg 24:120, 1977, with permission.)

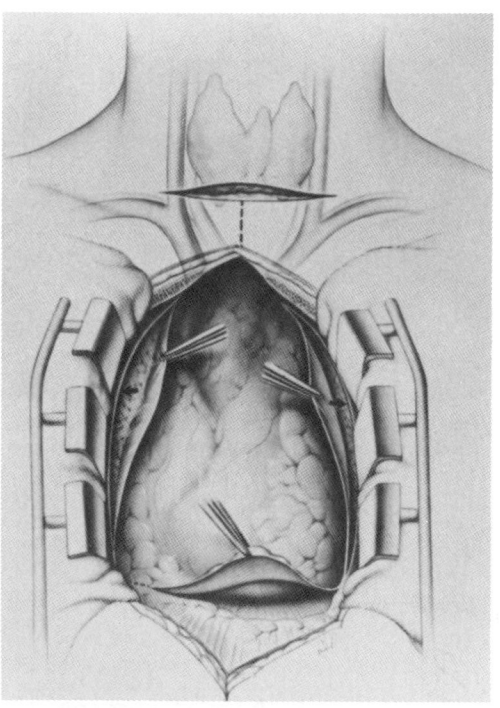

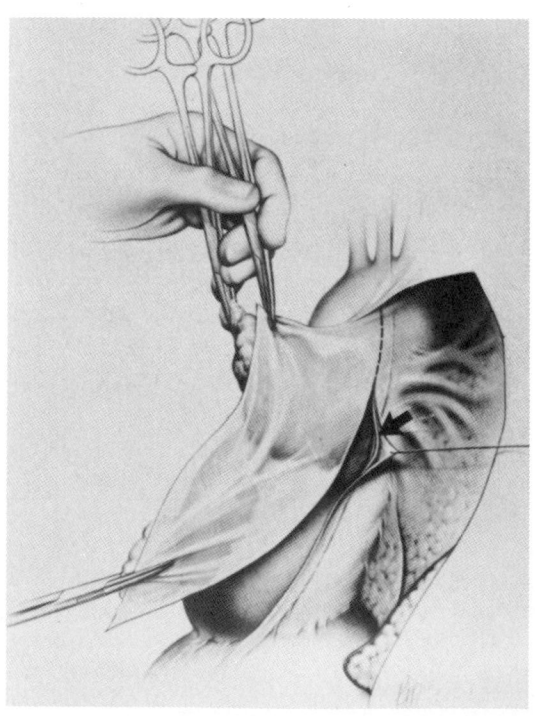

A

B

Figure 59-5. The mediastinal pleural incisions. **(A)** Cervical and thoracic incisions. The arrows indicate the initial pleural incisions. **(B)** The second mediastinal pleural incision anterior to the phrenic nerve. The phrenic nerves are elevated and dissected off underlying fatty thymic tissue. (From Jaretzki A III, Bethea M, Wolff M et al.: A rational approach to total thymectomy in the treatment of myasthenia gravis. Ann Thorac Surg 24:120, 1977, with permission.)

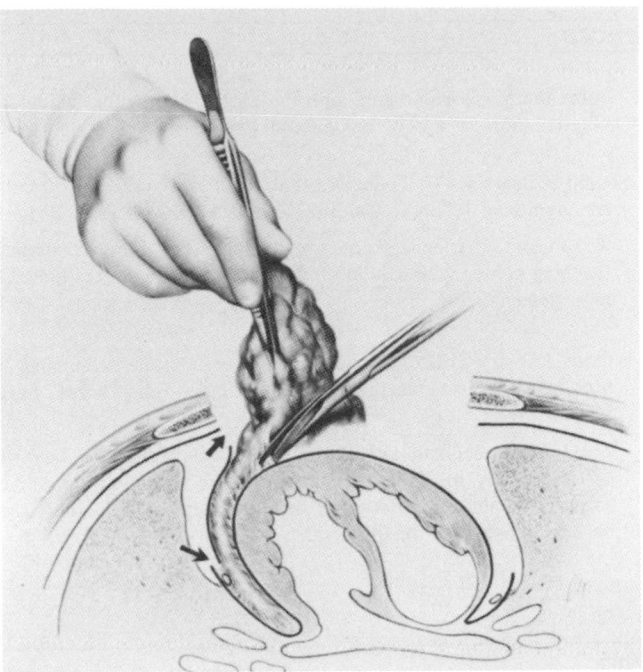

Figure 59-6. En bloc resection from hilum to hilum laterally and from diaphragm to innominate vein superiorly. The arrows indicate the two pleural incisions on the right. Fatty thymic tissue is removed from the aortopulmonary window on the left and the aortocaval groove on the right. (From Jaretzki A III, Bethea M, Wolff M et al.: A rational approach to total thymectomy in the treatment of myasthenia gravis. Ann Thorac Surg 24:120, 1977, with permission.)

The mediastinal pleura is incised bilaterally retrosternally from the level of the thoracic inlet to the diaphragm and again approximately 1 cm anterior to the phrenic nerve (Fig. 59-5). The posterior mediastinal pleura with adherent phrenic nerve is elevated bilaterally from the underlying fatty thymic tissue. An en bloc dissection from diaphragm to innominate vein and from hilum to hilum is then undertaken by means of sharp dissection on the pericardium (Fig. 59-6). All thymus, suspected thymus, and mediastinal fat (including both mediastinal pleural sheets) are removed. Included in the specimen are the anterior pericardiophrenic fat, the fatty thymic tissue lying in the sulcus between the superior vena cava and the aorta, the fatty thymic tissue in the region of the aortopulmonary window deep under the innominate vein extending to the aorta and pulmonary artery (*the left phrenic and vagus nerves are especially at risk here*), and the lappets of pericardium extending into the thymus. The innominate vein is identified and the thymus separated from it by dividing thymic veins. Chest tubes are placed bilaterally. Cephalad to the innominate vein, the en bloc dissection is continued posterior to the strap muscles, medial to the recurrent nerves, and anterior to the trachea and is terminated at the level of the thyroid isthmus.

The maximal thymectomy is predicated on the postulates that (1) complete removal of thymic tissues is the goal of surgery for myasthenia gravis and (2) better results are possible than those involving incomplete removal (Jaretzki and Wolff, 1988). Variation in the anatomic location of thymic tissue is widespread. In the neck it has been found above or behind the thyroid, behind the left innominate vein, or in pretracheal fat; in the mediastinum, it has been found under the phrenic nerves, in the aortopulmonary window or aortocaval groove, and in anterior mediastinal or cardiophrenic fat (Fig. 59-4).

Jaretzki and Wolff (1988) describe their technique as follows:

POSTOPERATIVE CARE

In patients with moderately severe or severe myasthenia gravis, cholinergic medication is withdrawn for a minimum of 3 days after operation. This may result in the need for ventilatory support, which is preferable to the difficulties encountered in managing cholinergic crises. In milder cases or in patients in whom plasmapheresis has induced a temporary "remission," extubation may be possible upon completion of surgery. In either event, Mestinon therapy should be resumed cautiously, beginning with small oral doses.

Other than cholinergic crisis, the complications following thymectomy for myasthenia gravis via sternotomy include atelectasis, pneumonia, pneumothorax, hydrothorax, and phrenic palsy. Sepsis and pulmonary embolism are uncommon. Prophylactic antibiotics are used intravenously beginning prior to anesthetic induction and continuing 48 hours postoperatively. Vigorous respiratory therapy is essential.

COMMENTS AND CONTROVERSIES

Bias has much to do with the decision of which approach to use in performing thymectomy. The cervical approach requires special training, which obviously will be achieved more easily with video-assisted thoracoscopic methodology. Many surgeons will still prefer a direct transsternal operative field. In terms of possible risks, particularly those of damage to the vagus, recurrent, or phrenic nerves, the maximum thymectomy may not have significant additional benefits over partial sternotomy to warrant its routine use. My current vote is for the limited partial sternotomy, performed through either a small midline or low supraclavicular collar incision.

E.W.W.

KEY REFERENCES

Marino M, Müller-Hermelink HK: Thymoma and thymic carcinoma: relation of thymoma epithelial cells to the cortical and medullary differentiation of thymus. Virchows Arch [A] 407:119, 1985

An attempt to once again estimate the malignancy of thymoma on its histologic appearance. Müller-Hermelink, the present chief of pathology at Wurzburg, has spent a lifetime looking at the epithelial cells of the thymus.

Masaoka A, Monden Y, Nakahara K, Tanioka T: Follow-up study of thymoma with special reference to their clinical stages. Cancer 48:2485, 1981

Definition of the factors determining the basic staging of the thymoma. This permits meaningful comparison among reported series.

Pescarmona E, Rendina EA, Venuta F et al: Analysis of prognostic factors and clinicopathologic staging of thymoma. Ann Thorac Surg 50:534, 1990

Joins the Masaoka staging with the Müller-Hermelink histologic classification for a new, complex prognostic system.

Shamji F, Pearson FG, Todd TRJ et al: Results of surgical treatment for thymoma. J Thorac Cardiovasc Surg 87:43, 1984

A 10-year experience from a leading general thoracic surgical teaching center with a host of clinical clues and suggestions for management.

Wilkins EW Jr, Grillo HC, Scannell JG et al: Role of staging in prognosis and management of thymoma. Ann Thorac Surg 51:888, 1991

The J. Maxwell Chamberlain Memorial paper at the 1991 meeting of the Society of Thoracic Surgeons. The surgeon's operative assessment plus microscopy of the specimen margins offers the best prognosticator for thymoma.

REFERENCES

Jaretzki A III, Bethea M, Wolff M et al: A rational approach to total thymectomy in the treatment of myasthenia gravis. Ann Thorac Surg 24:120, 1977

Jaretzki A III, Wolff M: "Maximal" thymectomy for myasthenia gravis. Surgical anatomy and operative technique. J Thorac Cardiovasc Surg 96:711, 1988

Sweet RH: Thoracic Surgery. pp. 75–78, 192–195. WB Saunders, Philadelphia, 1950

Wilkins EW Jr: Thymectomy. Modern technics in surgery. p. 38-1. In Cohn LH (ed): Cardiac/Thoracic Surgery, Futura Publishing, Mt. Kisco, NY, 1981

Thoracoscopy

Michael Mack

DEFINITION

Thoracoscopy or video-assisted thoracic surgery (VATS) encompasses intrathoracic procedures that are performed with a thoracoscope attached to a camera and video monitor for visualization. With recent advances in video technology and multichip minicameras as well as improvements in endoscopic instrumentation, many disease processes in the mediastinum are now approachable by video-assisted techniques. Pericardial disease and pericardial effusions of diverse etiologies, anterior and posterior mediastinal masses, and mediastinal lymphadenopathy and cysts, as well as conditions for which thoracic dorsal sympathectomy has been demonstrated to be beneficial, can now all be approached by thoracoscopic techniques. This chapter part discusses pericardial disease, mediastinal masses, and upper extremity pain syndromes relative to the thoracoscopic approaches that have proved useful for their management. A more complete discussion of anatomy, pathophysiology, and surgical management by other than thoracoscopic techniques is contained in fuller detail in Chapters 57, 59, and 61, which deal specifically with these conditions.

PERICARDIAL DISEASE

DEFINITION

For the purpose of discussing thoracoscopic approaches to the pericardium, pericardial disease will be considered to be either effusive pericarditis or postcardiotomy tamponade. Effusive pericarditis is an inflammatory, nonconstrictive process involving the pericardium, which can be due to either benign or malignant conditions. It is usually manifested by a pericardial effusion that causes cardiac tamponade at the time surgical management is required. Postcardiotomy tamponade is a low cardiac output state due to blood and/or clot in the pericardial space after a recent cardiac surgical procedure.

HISTORICAL NOTE

Surgical drainage of the pericardium was first described by Larrey (1829), a French physician during the Napoleonic wars. Allengham (1900) further popularized the subxiphoid approach for pericardial drainage as originally described by Larrey. For most of the twentieth century, however, *transthoracic* drainage of the pericardial space, by either a pericardiectomy or creation of a pericardial window, became the preferred method for treating effusive pericarditis. In the early 1960s Fontenelle and colleagues (1970) introduced the subxiphoid approach for the management of effusive pericardial disease, and this technique has continued to remain quite useful, especially in debilitated patients with malignant pericardial effusions. Pericardiectomy has also been performed by a median sternotomy; however, this approach has been reserved mostly for constrictive pericarditis. Although thoracoscopy was initially described in 1910 by Jacobaeus (1922), it remained primarily a diagnostic procedure until recently. The first thoracoscopic approaches were described by Azorin, et al. (1986) and Vogel and Mall (1990) as the latest surgical methods of draining the pericardial space for effusive pericardial disease.

HISTORICAL READINGS

Allengham H: Drainage of the pericardium. Lancet 1:639, 1900

Azorin J, Lamour A, Destable MD, de Saint-Florent G: Pericardioscopy: definition, value and limitation. Rev Pneumol Clin 42:138, 1986

Fontenelle LJ, Cuello L, Dooley BN: Subxiphoid pericardial window. Am J Surg 120:679, 1970

Jacobaeus HC: The practical importance of thoracoscopy in surgery of the chest. Surg Gynecol Obstet 34:289, 1922

Larrey DJ: New surgical procedure to open the pericardium and determine the cause of fluid in its cavity. Clin Chir 36:303, 1829

BASIC SCIENCE

Anatomically, the pericardial sac is located in the lower anterior portion of the mediastinum, behind and to the left of the sternum. However, drainage by video-assisted thoracoscopic techniques can be accomplished through either the right or the left hemithorax. Most frequently, thoracoscopic pericardial drainage is accomplished through the left chest, but when the pericardial sac is distended from effusive pericarditis, the procedure can be difficult to perform because of lack of room to maneuver instruments within the left hemithorax. For this reason some surgeons prefer to approach the pericardium from the right chest cavity. This is easily accomplished despite the fact that the pericardial sac is primarily located to the left of midline. The right approach allows ease of trocar placement without injury to the distended pericardium and allows ample room for manipulation of instruments in the chest.

Extensive resection of the pericardium can be accomplished through either approach. Relevant anatomy for the thoracoscopic approach through either hemithorax includes the location of the phrenic nerve on the pericardial surface. The phrenic nerve is identified initially upon entry of the pericardial cavity, and an appropriate bridge of pericardium is left so that injury to the phrenic nerve does not occur.

Often, when patients present for surgical drainage of the pericardial space, it is after an unsuccessful pericardiocentesis. This is frequently due to the fact that the effusion is loculated, mainly in the posterior pericardium. Confirmation of this posterior loculation can be demonstrated by either transthoracic or transesophageal echocardiography. When this situation occurs, thoracoscopy offers the optimal surgical approach, as access to the posterior pericardial space is easier by thoracoscopy than by other surgical techniques.

The character of the pericardial fluid varies with the disease process and can affect the ease or difficulty of the video-assisted procedure. When the pericardium is thin and relatively noninflamed and there is a large effusion present, the pericardiectomy is relatively simple to perform. However, in some of the more chronic conditions such as uremic pericarditis, in which "bread and butter" pericarditis occurs and there is a very thick pericardium with extensive adhesions to the epicardium and little fluid, the procedure can still be performed, albeit with more difficulty. My colleagues and I have discussed this in detail (Mack, et al., 1993).

DIAGNOSIS

For the purposes of discussing the thoracoscopic approach, pericardial disease will be divided into (1) benign, effusive pericarditis, (2) malignant pericardial effusions, and (3) postcardiotomy delayed tamponade. Diagnosis and management of constrictive pericardial disease will not be addressed in this chapter part. The standard clinical presentation of effusive pericarditis requiring surgical drainage as elucidated by Kirklin and Barratt-Boyes (1993), whether benign or malignant, includes signs of low cardiac output, relative systemic hypertension, pulsus paradoxus, jugular venous distension, ascites, and hepatomegaly. The initial diagnostic investigation includes a chest x-ray, which will usually show a large cardiac silhouette with a globular appearance. Confirmation of effusive pericardial disease can be obtained with a computed tomography (CT) scan, which will demonstrate a thickened pericardium, fluid in the pericardial space, and usually a normal size heart. Electrocardiography may show diffuse ST segment elevation or electrical alternans. Transthoracic or transesophageal echocardiography is often helpful to demonstrate fluid accumulation in the pericardial space and is often valuable in quantifying the amount and character of the fluid present and the location in the pericardial space (i.e., primarily anterior or posterior). This is helpful information in determining the correct approach for management (i.e., pericardiocentesis or surgical drainage). Diagnostic cardiac catheterization can be helpful if the diagnosis is in doubt by demonstrating equalization of pressures between the different chambers of the heart.

The differential diagnosis of effusive pericardial disease is between a constrictive pericardial process or occasionally a cardiomyopathy. A careful clinical history regarding the acute nature or the chronicity of the process and any prior history of malignancy or radiation therapy, together with use of the diagnostic methods outlined, usually results in a successful differential diagnosis. The natural history of pericardial effusive disease depends on the etiology of the pericardial effusion. It is usually insidious in onset and early in its course can be manifested only by malaise and pericardial discomfort, as discussed by DeValeria, et al. (1991). Benign, effusive pericarditis is frequently self-limited and can be managed by conservative medical therapy. Malignant pericardial effusions most commonly occur in patients with a prior history of malignancy. The most common malignancies causing effusive pericardial disease, according to Chan, et al. (1991), are breast cancer, lung cancer, and lymphoma. On occasion, the pericardial effusion in a patient with malignancy may be due not to the malignant process itself but to pericarditis induced by the radiation therapy used to treat the patient (Mack, et al., 1993).

When delayed tamponade exists following open heart surgery, its manifestation can be somewhat obscured by the other facets of the patient's recovery. When the usual recovery is not as rapid as anticipated, especially in a patient requiring postoperative systemic anticoagulation for prosthetic valve placement, delayed tamponade can be suspected. The diagnostic procedures are the same as those outlined for benign and malignant pericardial effusive disease. However, quite frequently the pericardial blood or clot is loculated in a posterior location. Transesophageal echocardiography is quite helpful in this determination.

Other pericardial disease processes that occasionally can be managed by the thoracoscopic techniques include uremic pericarditis, which is more frequently manifested by the "bread and butter" type pericardial thickening and inflammation than by a purely effusive process, and purulent pericarditis, which also is not a purely effusive process and usually manifests before a significant degree of cardiac tamponade occurs. Presenting signs in children in whom this occurs include fever, tachypnea, tachycardia, and hepatomegaly (Majid and Omar, 1991).

MANAGEMENT

Benign effusive pericarditis is frequently self-limited and can be managed by conservative medical therapy with systemic nonsteroidal anti-inflammatory agents. If this conservative

management fails after 7 to 10 days, Kirklin and Barratt-Boyes (1993) recommend a surgical approach. Subxiphoid pericardiocentesis with instillation of steroids into the pericardial space has been demonstrated to be occasionally effective in managing benign processes but is seldom used. Although malignant pericardial effusions can be managed temporarily with pericardiocentesis and systemic chemotherapy or instillation of sclerosing agents into the pericardial space, as described by Chan, et al., (1991), more complete surgical drainage has commonly been necessary in the experience of Landreneau, et al. (1993).

Once surgical drainage of the pericardial space has been deemed necessary, several operative approaches are available. The subxiphoid approach is appropriate for debilitated patients with malignant disease in whom general endotracheal anesthesia and single-lung ventilation is deemed risky. Naunheim, et al. (1991) have demonstrated that the subxiphoid technique offers the ability to perform the procedure under local anesthesia with minimal postoperative morbidity. However, the exposure is limited, minimal pericardium can be resected, and recurrence rates as high as 20 percent have been reported (Piehler, et al., 1985). Transthoracic pericardiectomy is the most commonly performed option and is usually performed by a limited anterior thoracotomy, as discussed by Miller, et al. (1982) and Austudillo and Ivert (1989). The advantages of this approach are good visualization and the ability to perform wide pericardial resection, but there is significant morbidity associated with even a limited incision. General endotracheal anesthesia is required.

A median sternotomy is used in constrictive processes, as reported by McCaughan, et al. (1984), and is the standard approach for the patient with delayed tamponade after open heart operations. There is, however, an increased risk of wound infection and sternal dehiscence associated with reentry through the previous incision.

Thoracoscopy allows excellent visualization of the pericardium both anterior and posterior to the phrenic nerve with less postoperative morbidity than a thoracotomy, even if limited. Video-assisted thoracoscopic pericardiectomy may be performed from either the right or the left thorax and has the additional advantage of being able to drain any associated pleural effusions, which often occur with malignant disease. The disadvantage of thoracoscopy for drainage of pericardial space is the requirement for general anesthesia and single-lung ventilation. This can present significant management problems for the unstable or debilitated patient.

Operative Technique

Operative management of the patient for thoracoscopic pericardiectomy can be aided by preoperative pericardiocentesis. This allows the patient to remain hemodynamically stable during the peripheral vasodilatation that occurs with induction of general anesthesia. The patient is intubated with a double-lumen endotracheal tube to allow ipsilateral lung collapse. Hemodynamic monitoring of arterial blood pressure is performed, and if the patient is unstable, central venous pressure or pulmonary capillary wedge pressure measurement is also used. The patient is placed in the right lateral position, the chest is widely prepared for conversion to an open thoracotomy if necessary, and ventilation to the ipsilateral lung is stopped.

A 1-cm incision is made in the seventh intercostal space posterior to the midaxillary line, as described by Landreneau, et al. (1992). The intercostal muscle is spread with a hemostat and the pleural cavity is entered and initial pneumothorax induced. Digital exploration with a finger is undertaken to ensure that lung collapse has occurred and pleural symphysis is not present. Digital exploration can also determine whether this initial trocar site has been positioned too close to a distended pericardium before instrumentation is placed. A 10-mm trocar is then placed through the incision to create access for a thoracoscope and video camera. A 10-mm, zero-degree rigid thoracoscope is introduced through this entry site, and exploratory thoracoscopy is undertaken to identify any associated pleural, pulmonary, or mediastinal pathology. Appropriate sites are then selected for further trocar placement; most commonly, these sites are in the fifth and ninth intercostal spaces in the posterior axillary line (Fig. 59-7). If visualization of the pericardium is a problem because of the lower lobe of the lung, an additional trocar can be placed in the seventh intercostal space in the posterior axillary line for placement of an endoscopic retractor. Insufflation with carbon dioxide is *not* usually necessary; however, if the lung is not adequately collapsed, insufflation up to a pressure of 8 to 10 cm H_2O can help enhance the atelectasis of the left lung and aid visualization.

Once satisfactory visualization of the pericardium has been obtained (Fig. 59-8), the distended sac is approached. Unless a preoperative pericardiocentesis has been performed, it may be difficult to grasp a tense pericardium. A laparoscopic needle can be introduced through one of the trocar sites and, under direct visualization, aspiration of the pericardial space can be performed (Fig. 59-9). A grasping instrument can now be placed through the lower trocar site to hold the pericardium. Endoscopic scissors are then directed through the most

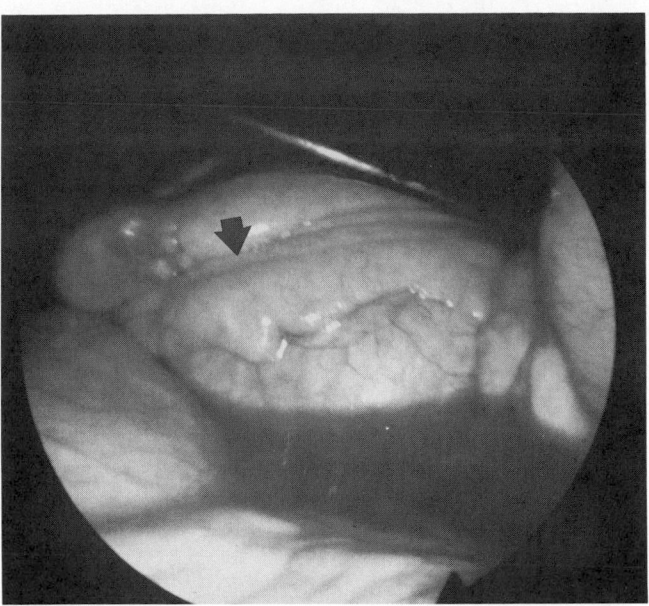

Figure 59-8. View of the pericardial sac through a thoracoscope in the left chest. Arrow indicates left phrenic nerve.

cephalad port, and an initial incision of the pericardium is made (Fig. 59-10). If extensive inflammation of the pericardium is present and a cut edge bleeds easily, electrocautery through the endoscopic scissors can be used to obtain hemostasis once the pericardium has been tented away from the heart. Wide swatches of pericardium, 10 to 12 cm² in area, can be excised both anterior and posterior to the phrenic nerve (Fig. 59-11) and removed through one of the trocar sites. Care is taken to avoid injury to the left atrial appendage as the pericardial resection is carried superiorly. Cardiac defibrillator and paddles are available in case an inadvertent

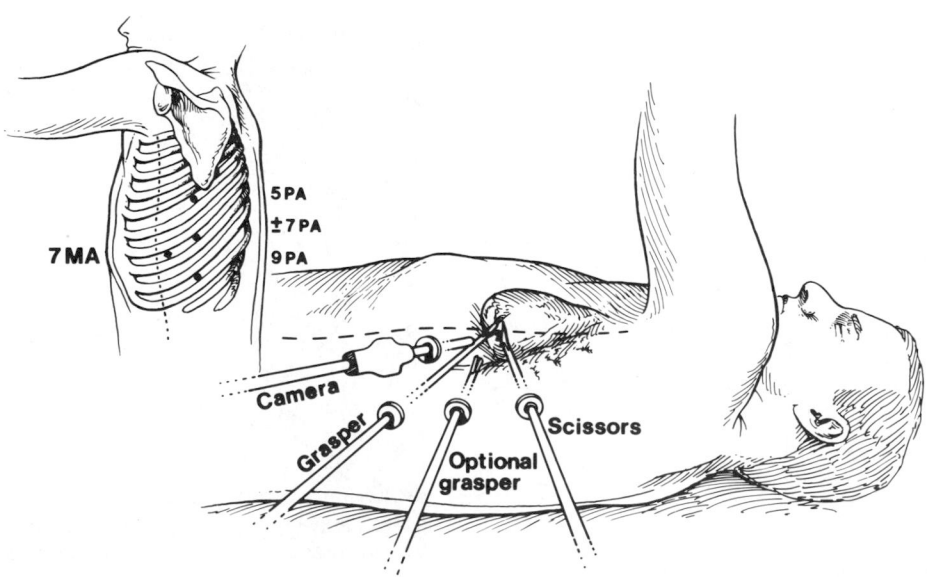

Figure 59-7.   Typical trocar placement for performance of a left thoracoscopic pericardiectomy.

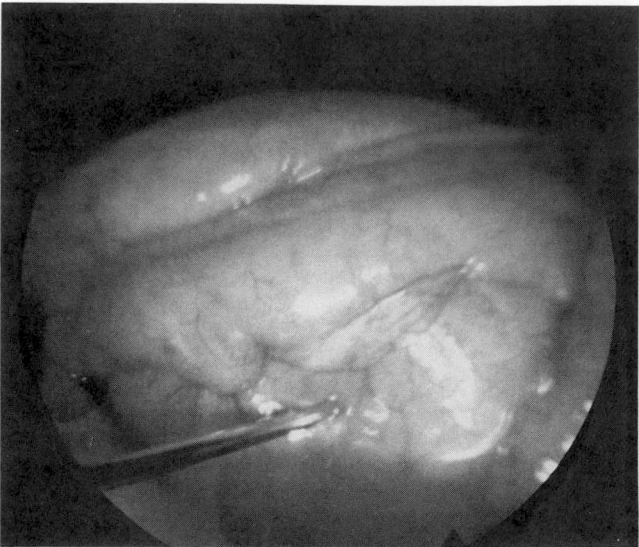

Figure 59-9. Needle aspiration under direct visualization of the pericardial sac.

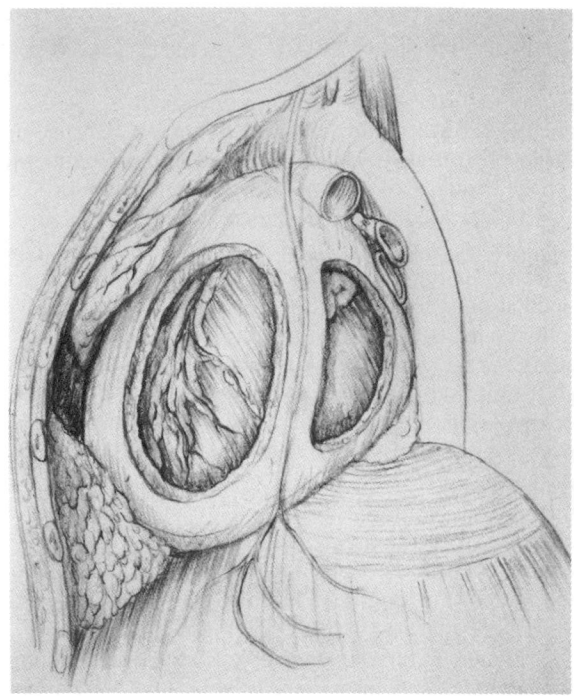

Figure 59-11. Representation of the amount of pericardium typically excised by left thoracoscopy.

cardiac arrhythmia is induced. Upon completion of the procedure, a chest tube is inserted through one of the lower trocar sites and placed under direct vision in the proximity of the pericardium. If an associated pleural effusion is present, it is completely drained, and a chemical or mechanical pleurodesis can be performed at this time. The remaining trocar sites are then closed with an absorbable, subcuticular suture.

Some authors prefer approaching the pericardium through the right pleural cavity. The benefit of this approach is ease of maneuverability of endoscopic instruments and camera in the less confined right pleural space. A wide incision of the pericardium both anterior and posterior to the phrenic nerve can be performed by this approach, with adequate drainage of the pericardial space.

In patients who have developed delayed tamponade after open heart procedures, the pericardial space can be drained by VATS techniques. This is most easily accomplished by excising the pericardium posterior to the phrenic nerve (Fig. 59-12). Usually, there is organized thrombus adherent to the epicardial surface, which can be carefully teased off by endo-

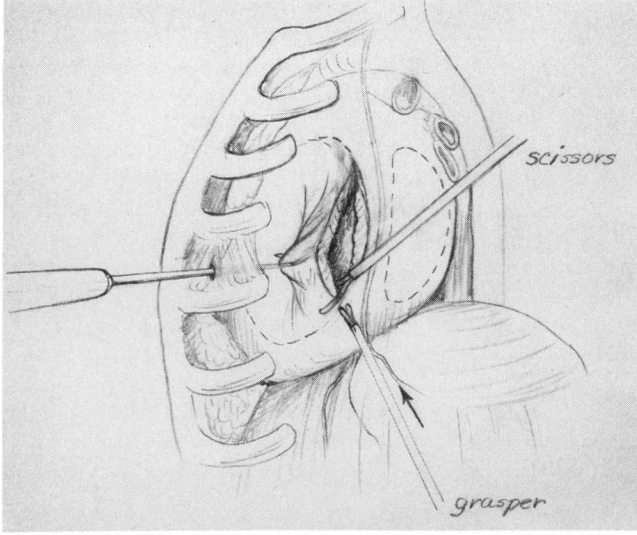

Figure 59-10. Diagrammatic representation of the initiation of a pericardiectomy.

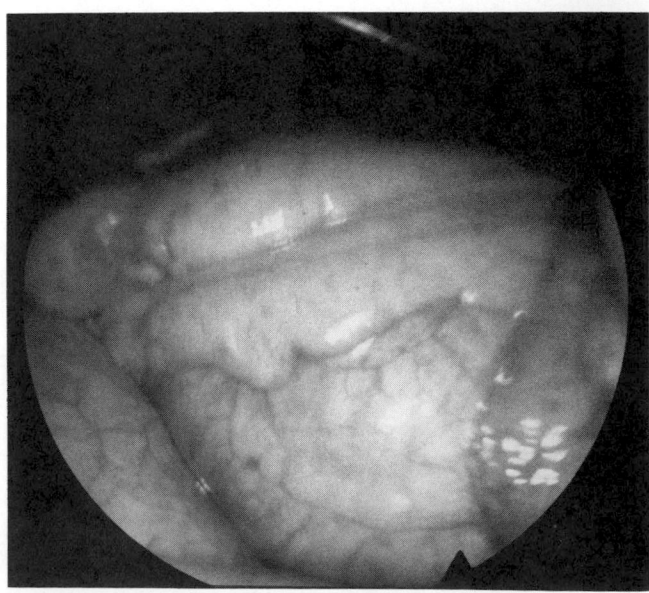

Figure 59-12. Typical view of the pericardium through the left chest. Note how the pericardium posterior to the phrenic nerve is easily exposed and therefore approached and drained.

scopic grasping instruments and frequent irrigation. Occasionally, placement of a standard Yankeur suction tip or standard ring forceps through one of the trocar sites can aid in removing this clot.

Postoperatively, the chest tube is left in place until drainage is less than 150 ml in a 24-hour period. Addition of ketorolac or other nonsteroidal anti-inflammatory agent is helpful in the management of postoperative pain. Parenteral narcotics are helpful in the immediate postoperative period but seldom necessary beyond the first 24 to 48 hours.

In my experience with a series of 22 video-assisted thoracoscopic pericardial resections performed for effusive, nonconstrictive pericarditis, the average duration of chest tube use was 2 days, and the average hospital stay for patients with benign pericardial disease was 4 days (Mack, et al., 1993). Patients with malignant pleural effusions remained hospitalized for longer periods, either because of their debili-

tating illness or to receive further antitumor therapy. There have been no recurrences of the effusion in an average follow-up of 7.5 months after thoracoscopic drainage in my experience.

We have also had experience with relief of tamponade several weeks after open heart surgery in five patients, including two who had undergone coronary artery bypass, two who had undergone valve replacement with a mechanical prosthesis and received postoperative anticoagulant therapy, and one cardiac transplant patient who had received a small donor heart that was placed in a large recipient pericardial space. This mismatch helped contribute to a large pericardial fluid collection, which required surgical drainage. All pericardiectomies were successfully performed by VATS techniques, and repeat sternotomy was avoided. The average hospital stay was 3 days after the thoracoscopy, and there was no recurrence at an average follow-up of 4.5 months.

COMMENTS AND CONTROVERSIES

Improvement in video endoscopic equipment and instrumentation as well as surgical expertise gained in thoracoscopic techniques has expanded thoracoscopy from a limited role for the diagnosis of intrathoracic disease processes to a therapeutic approach for many intrathoracic problems, as our initial experience has shown (Mack, et al., 1992). Pericardiectomy is now routinely and safely performed by thoracoscopic techniques. Until the advent of the thoracoscopic approach, a limited anterior thoracotomy was our standard approach for pericardiectomy. We reserved the subxiphoid approach for patients who are significantly debilitated or ill from end-stage malignancy with a poor prognosis. We still use the subxiphoid approach for these patients, who are too ill to withstand a general anesthetic or who have a life expectancy of less than 3 to 6 months. However, for patients with benign effusive pericarditis, radiation-induced pericardial disease, or purulent pericarditis, as well as in patients with delayed (not immediate) tamponade after open heart surgery, the thoracoscopic approach has become the preferred method of drainage of the pericardial space in our surgical armamentarium. It has the benefit of being safe, effective, and expeditious and allows management of simultaneous pleural disease. There appears to be less postoperative morbidity, as manifested by less pain and shortened hospital stay, than with standard open approaches when experience (Mack, et al., 1993) with other published series (Miller, et al., 1982).

There remains, however, a strong argument for the subxiphoid approach. Although Piehler, et al. (1985) and others (Santos and Frater, 1977) have demonstrated a recurrence rate as high as 20 percent, Naunheim, et al. (1991) have reported a recurrence rate of 7 percent for subxiphoid drainage and 4 percent for transthoracic procedures. Hankins, et al. (1980), Ghosh, et al. (1985), Gregory, et al. (1985), Mills, et al. (1989), and Palatianos, et al. (1989) have also reported good results with the subxiphoid approach. Despite the small window of pericardium excised, extensive lymphatic absorption of pericardial fluid appears to occur, as elucidated by Sugimoto, et al. (1990). In our experience, however, the ability to excise large portions of the pericardium with mini-

mal morbidity tends to favor the video-assisted thoracoscopic approach in all but the gravely ill patients with malignancy and a poor prognosis.

We also caution against the use of thoracoscopic pericardiectomy on thick-walled pericardial processes with minimal effusion or in the presence of significant epicardial adhesions. If concern exists regarding the ability to safely remove the pericardium, then conversion to an open thoracotomy should be performed.

In our short experience, the thoracoscopic approach for drainage of the postoperative cardiac surgery patient has proved to be helpful. The ability to completely drain the pericardial space without reentry through the median sternotomy site has the potential benefit of avoiding added morbidity. This would appear to be especially helpful in the immunosuppressed transplant population.

The video-assisted technique appears to offer a minimally invasive approach, which can completely drain the pericardial space in many patients with benign and malignant effusive pericardial disease. There may also be a role for this technique in the postoperative cardiac patient with delayed tamponade.

M.M.

The ideal approach for pericardial biopsy or decompression is from the right rather than the left side. The left approach has been classical because it is closer to the skin for direct surgical procedures. However, following the principle that it is better to have the camera as far away as possible from the lesion in the chest, the right side gives a better perspective for thoracoscopic evaluation and treatment of pericardial disease.

Additionally, the use of argon beam cautery provides a distinct advantage, since it tends not to fibrillate the heart when it cauterizes blood vessels near the myocardium.

The subxiphoid approach with a xiphoid resection offers an equally advantageous situation to a pericardial window within the chest. It does have the problem of contamination because of external drainage.

H.C.U.

KEY REFERENCES

Landreneau RJ, Mack MJ, Hazelrigg SR et al: Video assisted thoracic surgery: basic technical concepts and intercostal approach strategies. Ann Thorac Surg 54:800, 1992

Review article, which addresses the basic concepts integral to initiating most video-assisted thoracic procedures. The principles outlined here serve as a strong foundation for performing thoracoscopic surgery.

Landreneau RJ, Mack MJ, Hazelrigg SR et al: The role of thoracoscopy in the management of intrathoracic neoplastic processes. Semin Cardiothorac Surg 5:219, 1993

Defines in depth the place for thoracoscopy in the management of malignant pericardial effusions as well as in other neoplastic situations. Explains well the advantages of VATS techniques versus conventional approaches.

Mack M, Landreneau RJ, Hazelrigg SR, Acuff TE: Video thoracoscopic management of benign and malignant pericardial effusions. Chest 103:3905, 1993

Describes technique of video-assisted pericardiectomy and an early multi-institutional experience with the technique. The first 22 patients undergoing this approach are discussed.

Miller JI, Mansour KA, Katcher CR: Pericardiectomy: current indications, concepts, and results in a university center. Ann Thorac Surg 34:40, 1982

Classic review series, which serves as the current standard for pericardiectomy results.

Naunheim KS, Kesler KA, Fiore AC et al: Pericardial drainage: subxiphoid vs. transthoracic approach. Eur J Cardiothorac Surg 5:99, 1991

The extensive experience reported makes a strong case for the subxiphoid approach for pericardiectomy. Broad review of the literature regarding results of different techniques.

REFERENCES

Allengham H: Drainage of the pericardium. Lancet 1:639, 1900

Astudillo R, Ivert T: Late results after pericardiectomy for constrictive pericarditis via left thoracotomy. Scand J Thorac Cardiovasc Surg 23:115, 1989

Azorin J, Lamour A, Destable MD, de Saint-Florent G: Pericardioscopy: definition, value and limitation. Rev Pneumol Clin 42:138, 1986

Chan A, Rischin D, Clarke CP, Woodruff RK: Subxiphoid partial pericardiectomy with or without sclerosant instillation in the treatment of symptomatic pericardial effusions in patients with malignancy. Cancer 68:1021, 1991

DeValeria PA, Baumgartner WA, Casale AS et al: Current indications, risks, and outcome after pericardiectomy. Ann Thorac Surg 52:219, 1991

Fontanelle LJ, Cuello L, Dooley BN: Subxiphoid pericardial window. Am J Surg 120:679, 1970

Ghosh SC, Larrieu AJ, Ablaza SGG, Grana VP: Clinical experience with subxiphoid pericardial decompression. Int Surg 70:5, 1985

Gregory JR, McMurtrey MJ, Mountain CJ: A surgical approach to the treatment of pericardial effusion in cancer patients. Am J Clin Oncol 8:319, 1985

Hankins JR, Satterfield JR, Aisner J et al: Pericardial window for malignant pericardial effusion. Ann Thorac Surg 30:465, 1980

Jacobaeus HC: The practical importance of thoracoscopy in surgery of the chest. Surg Gynecol Obstet 34:289, 1922

Kirklin JW, Barratt-Boyes BG: Cardiac Surgery, 2nd Ed. Vol. 1. Churchill Livingstone, New York, 1993, p. 1684

Larrey DJ: New surgical procedure to open the pericardium and determine the cause of fluid in its cavity. Clin Chir 36:303, 1829

Mack MJ, Aronoff RJ, Acuff TE et al: Present role of thoracoscopy in the diagnosis and treatment of diseases of the chest. Ann Thorac Surg 54:403, 1992

Majid AA, Omar A: Diagnosis and management of purulent pericarditis. J Thorac Cardiovasc Surg 102:413, 1991

McCaughan BC, Schaff HV, Piehler JM et al: Early and late results of pericardiectomy for constrictive pericarditis. J Thorac Cardiovasc Surg 89:340, 1984

Mills SA, Julian S, Holliday RH et al: Subxiphoid pericardial window for pericardial effusive disease. J Cardiovasc Surg 30:768, 1989

Palatianos GM, Thurer RJ, Pompeo MQ, Kaiser GA: Clinical experience with subxiphoid drainage of pericardial effusions. Ann Thorac Surg 48:381, 1989

Piehler JM, Pluth JR, Schaff HV et al: Surgical management of effusive pericardial disease. J Thorac Cardiovasc Surg 90:506, 1985

Sugimoto JT, Little AG, Ferguson MK et al: Pericardial window: mechanisms of efficacy. Ann Thorac Surg 50:442, 1990

Santos GH, Frater RWM: The subxiphoid approach in the treatment of pericardial effusion. Ann Thorac Surg 23:467, 1977

Vogel B, Mall W: Thoracoscopic pericardial fenestration—diagnostic and therapeutic aspects. Pneumologie (Stuttg) 44 (suppl 1): 184, 1990

MEDIASTINAL DISEASE

DEFINITION

While VATS has been useful for the diagnosis and management of many pleural conditions, it recently has been expanded to have a role in the diagnosis and management of many intrathoracic conditions including mediastinal pathology. For purposes of diagnosis and surgical intervention, the mediastinum has traditionally been divided into three compartments: anterior, middle, and posterior. Since the disease processes are different in each, the thoracoscopic techniques used for approaching these compartments varies. Each is discussed separately in this section. Although thoracoscopy is still primarily a diagnostic procedure for mediastinal disease, its possible role as a therapeutic procedure for the management of some conditions is also discussed.

HISTORICAL NOTE

Surgical approaches to the mediastinum historically have been used either for performance of thymectomy for myasthenia gravis or for the biopsy of mediastinal nodes or masses. Blalock first performed a successful thymectomy in Baltimore in 1936 on a 19-year-old woman with thymoma associated with myasthenia gravis (Blalock, et al., 1936). He subsequently (Blalock, 1944) described his experience with 20 cases of myasthenia gravis that had been managed by thymectomy. Surgical approaches to the mediastinum for myasthenia gravis were subsequently changed to median sternotomy by most surgeons and were then further by Jaretzki et al., who in 1977 described a combined transcervical and transsternal approach for total thymectomy. Numerous other surgical series exist attesting to the role of surgery for the management of myasthenia gravis with and without thymoma, including that of Papatestas, et al. (1987).

Mediastinoscopy was described in 1949 by Carlens as a method for examining and biopsying tissue in the superior mediastinum from the neck. Another surgical approach, the anterior mediastinotomy for the diagnosis of mediastinal masses and lymphadenopathy, was described by McNeill and Chamberlain in 1966 as a relatively noninvasive method of diagnosing mediastinal disease and evaluating and staging lymph nodes in primary lung cancer.

More recently, thoracoscopic techniques have begun to be applied to mediastinal disease, as described by Deslaurier, et al. (1976) and Landreneau, et al. (1992b, 1993b).

HISTORICAL READINGS

Blalock A, Mason MF, Morgan HJ, Riven SS: Myasthenia gravis and tumors of the thymic region. Report of a case in which the tumor was removed. Ann Surg 110:544, 1939

Blalock A: Thymectomy in the treatment of myasthenia gravis. Report of twenty cases. J Thorac Surg 13:316, 1944

Carlens E: Mediastinoscopy. A method for inspection and tissue biopsy in the superior mediastinum. Chest 35:343, 1949

Jaretski A III, Bethea M, Wolff M, et al.: A rational approach to total thymectomy in the treatment of myasthenia gravis. Ann Thorac Surg 2:120, 1977

McNeill T, Chamberlain J: Diagnostic anterior mediastinotomy. Ann Thorac Surg 2:532, 1966

BASIC SCIENCE

For diagnostic and surgical purposes, specific anatomic compartments of the mediastinum have been defined (Pearson, 1992). The anterior mediastinum is bounded by the sternum anteriorly, by the anterior surfaces of the great vessels and pericardium posteriorly, and by the mediastinal pleura on each side. The anterior mediastinal compartment can be further subdivided into superior and inferior components. The middle mediastinum is demarcated by the esophagus posteriorly and by the mediastinal pleura laterally. The posterior aspect of the heart and great vessels form the anterior boundary of the middle mediastinum. The posterior mediastinum includes the esophagus and is limited posteriorly by the spine and paravertebral gutters.

In adults anterior mediastinal masses account for 50 to 60 percent of all mediastinal masses. Approximately 60 percent of all masses in this compartment are malignant, and lymphoma, thymoma, and germ cell neoplasms predominate (Rice, 1992). The majority of these tumors occur in the superior anterior mediastinum, thymoma being the only type that may present in the inferior compartment. The middle mediastinum accounts for 20 to 25 percent of mediastinal masses, the majority of which are benign and cystic, as described by Rice (1992). Bronchogenic and pericardial cysts are the most common of these cysts. The middle mediastinum also contains the greatest concentration of lymphatics and lymph nodes and is the most common site for primary lymphomas of the mediastinum as well as for metastatic lymphadenopathy from lung cancer and other tumors, according to Pearson (1992). Posterior mediastinal masses account for 25 to 30 percent of mediastinal lesions and are usually benign (Rubish, et al., 1973). Almost all neurogenic tumors of the mediastinum occur in the posterior compartment, although mediastinal cysts have been described in all three compartments (Rice, 1992).

DIAGNOSIS

Most mediastinal disease is asymptomatic. When symptoms do occur, they usually result from compression or invasion of adjacent mediastinal structures or from the systemic symptoms of myasthenia gravis associated with thymoma or thymic hyperplasia. Compression symptoms can include those of superior vena cava syndrome from vascular compression as well as persistent cough, dyspnea, or stridor from airway compression. If significant impingement upon the esophagus occurs, dysphagia can be a presenting symptom. If a malignant mediastinal tumor invades the adjacent sternum, spine, chest wall, or diaphragm, pain can be produced. On occasion, if significant pleural or pericardial invasion occurs or if significant lymph node obstruction occurs from tumor, pleural and/or pericardial effusions with associated clinical signs of dyspnea or tamponade may result. Occasionally, hoarseness may be the presenting symptom of lung cancer metastatic to the mediastinal lymph nodes.

Initial evaluation of mediastinal disease is usually radiologic. If the disease is asymptomatic, often the initial diagnosis is made as an incidental finding on chest x-ray. Because of the radiopacity of normal mediastinal structures, including heart, pericardium, and great vessels, definitive information regarding the mass is seldom evident on plain chest x-rays. A CT scan is almost always necessary for further evaluation of suspected mediastinal disease and gives significantly helpful information regarding the character of the mass—that is, whether it is solid or cystic and its size, density, and other anatomic relations, according to Weisbrod and Herman (1992). A magnetic resonance imaging (MRI) scan can, on occasion, provide some additional helpful information. Most commonly, the MRI is helpful in differentiating hilar and mediastinal lymphadenopathy from adjacent vascular structures. MRI has also been helpful for evaluating dumbbell lesions of posterior mediastinal tumors due to extension through the intervertebral foramina to the spinal canal.

The use of radionuclide scans for the evaluation of mediastinal masses is occasionally helpful. The ^{131}I scan may be helpful for identifying substernal or ectopic thyroid tissue. Technetium/thallium scans are occasionally helpful in locating ectopic parathyroid glands. Less often, technetium scans to identify gastric mucosal and neuroenteric cysts, gallium scans to differentiate inflammatory masses of the anterior mediastinum, and the ^{131}I metaiodobenzylguanidine (MIGB) scan for pheochromocytoma evaluation can be used, according to Weisbrod and Herman (1992).

Immunoassays for evaluation of germ cell neoplasms, including α-fetoprotein and β-human chorionic gonadotropic (β-HCG) are used if these tumors are high on the differential diagnosis list, as described by Ginsberg (1992).

Fluoroscopic or CT-guided fine-needle aspiration biopsy can be performed either percutaneously or by the transesophageal or transbronchial route. Skill in performing this technique is necessary, but an experienced cytopathologist is even more crucial, according to Weisbrod and Herman (1992). The main difficulty is in differentiating lymphoma from thymoma, which is crucial in the evaluation of anterior mediastinal masses.

Despite this myriad of diagnostic procedures, surgical intervention is usually necessary to establish a definitive diagnosis of a mediastinal mass. For masses that are clearly cysts and are asymptomatic, simple observation and serial follow-up is a reasonable option. However, for the evaluation of solid masses in the mediastinum, a definitive surgical diagnosis is necessary.

The usual surgical approach to mediastinal masses is either cervical mediastinal exploration or anterior mediastinotomy. The cervical approach provides access to the middle mediastinum and to the upper portion of the anterior mediastinum, as originally described by Carlens (1949). For masses that are in the more inferior portion of the anterior mediastinum, a second, left intercostal space anterior mediastinotomy provides adequate access to obtain tissue for biopsy, as first described by McNeill and Chamberlain (1966). One of the problems of this approach, however, is the placement of the surgical incision in the area where postoperative radiation portals are placed, which causes an occasional problem with wound healing (Landreneau, et al., 1993a).

MANAGEMENT

Most mediastinal disease processes are approachable by thoracoscopy. Certain generalizations are common to all thoracoscopic procedures. Like most thoracoscopic operations, all procedures on the mediastinum are performed under general endotracheal anesthesia with a double-lumen tube to maintain single-lung ventilation and obtain ipsilateral lung collapse. The patient is placed in the lateral position. For procedures on the posterior mediastinum, the patient is canted slightly posteriorly so that a more anterior approach can be used. In a similar manner, the patient is rotated slightly

forward for posterior access to anterior mediastinal masses. For procedures in the upper mediastinum, the patient is placed in the reverse Trendelenburg position, so that the lung becomes more dependent. For procedures on the posterior mediastinum near the diaphragm, the gravitational benefit of the Trendelenburg position is utilized. The patient is then fully prepared as for a standard thoracotomy, according to Landreneau, et al. (1992a).

Intercostal approach strategies and trocar placement are determined the compartment in which the target pathology is located and will be discussed in detail for the individual compartments. However, certain principles apply to strategic placement of trocars. Careful preoperative planning is necessary so that trocars are placed widely apart. Placement too close together causes "sword fighting" of instrumentation or obstruction of the visual field. Care should also be taken to place access at a fair distance from the target pathology since too close placement does not allow for maneuverability of instruments. In addition, the thoracoscope and instruments should all face and work in the same direction to prevent the "mirror imaging" that occurs if the instruments are working toward the thoracoscope. Once the incision is made for the initial trocar placement, the intercostal muscle is spread with a hemostat and the pleural cavity is entered. A finger is placed through the incision, and digital exploration is performed to ensure pleural symphysis is not present. When a free pleural space has been ascertained, an open 10-mm trocar (Thoracoport, AutoSuture, United States Surgical Corp., Norwalk, CT) is placed, since carbon dioxide insufflation is usually not necessary. A 10-mm rigid zero-degree telescope is satisfactory for most procedures and is placed through this trocar. An exploratory thoracoscopy is then performed, target pathology is identified, and unexpected disease is ruled out. Subsequent trocars for access for endoscopic surgical instrumentation are then placed under direct vision at appropriate sites (see below). After completion of the planned procedure, a tube for pleural drainage is placed only if significant air or fluid accumulation is anticipated and is therefore unnecessary for most mediastinal procedures. The lung is then inflated under direct vision and the incisions are closed with a subcuticular suture.

Posterior Mediastinum

Most posterior mediastinal masses in adults are benign, neurogenic tumors and are amenable to thoracoscopic excision. Removal is indicated for confirmation of diagnosis, symptoms referable to the lesion, or evidence of growth. Preoperative assessment with CT or MRI is essential to rule out direct intraspinal extension of tumor. The technique was first reported by Landreneau, et al. (1993b).

Once general anesthesia has been induced and the patient properly positioned (lateral decubitus with slight posterior cant), the first trocar is placed in the fifth intercostal space in the midaxillary line. Subsequent trocars are placed in the second intercostal space in the anterior axillary line and in the fourth intercostal space in the anterior axillary line (Fig. 59-13). An additional access site can be provided in the sixth intercostal space if retraction of the lung is necessary. By using a grasping forceps placed through one trocar and an

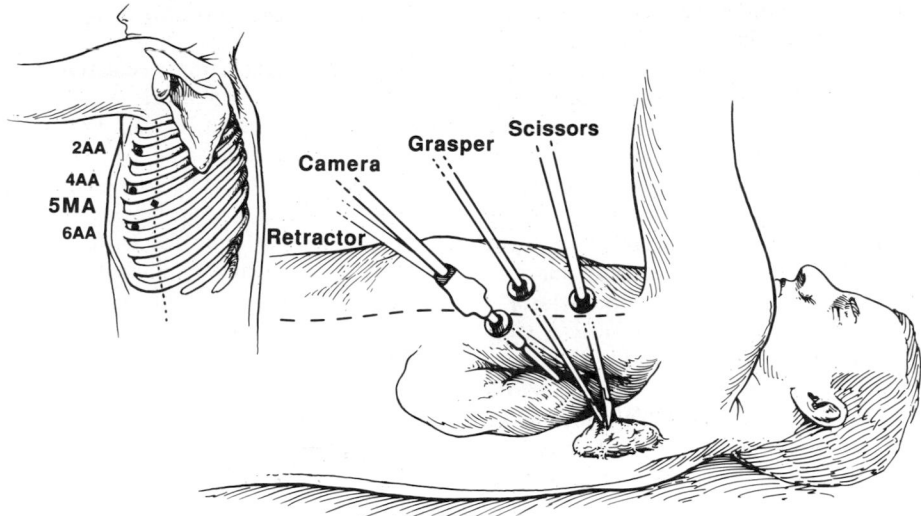

Figure 59-13. Trocar placement for optimal approach to a posterior mediastinal mass.

endoscopic scissors with electrocautery attachment in the other, the parietal pleura adjacent to the tumor is incised. Care is taken to identify and ligate with endoscopic clips any adjacent vertebral veins, since bothersome bleeding may occur unless such veins are ligated early. Dissection under direct vision is continued underneath the tumor until it has been completely excised. The tumor is placed in a specimen bag for removal through the chest wall. The surgical site is inspected for hemostasis and the procedure is concluded. Pleural drainage is not usually necessary. Postoperative care in an intensive care unit is not necessary, and parenteral narcotics are seldom needed after 24 hours. Postoperative hospital stay is usually 1 to 2 days.

Middle Mediastinum

The majority of masses in the middle mediastinum are cystic in nature and can easily be removed by thoracoscopic tech-

niques, as described by Lewis, et al. (1992). The most common cysts in this location are bronchogenic, esophageal, neuroenteric, and pericardial. Rarely is intraluminal communication present, and surgical excision is recommended only for symptoms or complications. When removal is indicated, thoracoscopy provides an excellent method of excision.

Preoperative examination indicating no luminal communication for bronchogenic or esophageal duplication cysts is necessary. The patient is then placed in the lateral position, and the same anesthetic management and preoperative preparation are used as with posterior mediastinal masses. Usually, three trocars are placed, as indicated in Figure 59-14. The first trocar for the thoracoscope is usually placed in the fifth intercostal space in the midaxillary line, and access ports for a grasping instrument and endoscopic scissors are placed in the third and fifth intercostal spaces in the anterior line. If optimal collapse of the lung has not been obtained by the endotracheal intubation procedure alone, the addition of a

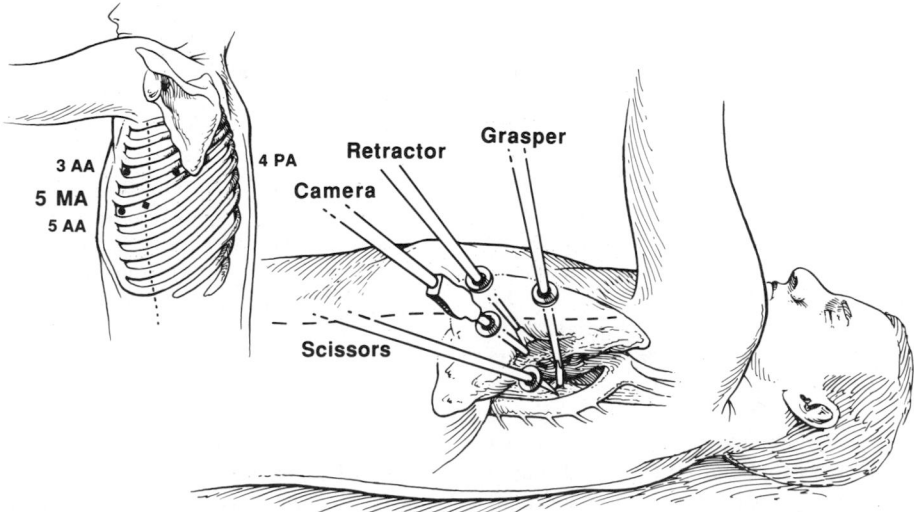

Figure 59-14. Trocar placement for approaching both mediastinal cysts and the aortopulmonary window.

brief period of carbon dioxide insufflation or placement of a fourth trocar, more posteriorly, for insertion of an endoscopic fanlike retractor can be helpful. Exploratory thoracoscopy is then performed and the location of the cyst is ascertained. It is helpful to aspirate the cyst under direct visualization to avoid spillage and to make grasping of the cyst easier, as well as to allow eventual removal from the chest cavity through a trocar access site. Occasionally, complete aspiration is not possible because of the thick, viscous nature of the cyst contents. Complete excision of the cyst is usually possible by sharp and blunt dissection with an endoscopic scissors. If a portion of the cyst wall is densely adherent to a vital structure, that part can be left and the mucosal wall obliterated with an electrocautery, laser, or argon beam coagulator. Pleural drainage is only necessary if blood or fluid accumulation is anticipated or if inadvertent lung injury has occurred. Postoperative care is the same as for other thoracoscopic procedures, with prompt removal of the chest tube and hospital discharge on the first or second postoperative day.

Aortopulmonary Window and Hilum

Accurate evaluation of the mediastinum for the staging of lung cancer carries prognostic and therapeutic significance (Naruke, et al., 1978; American Thoracic Society, 1983; Mountain, 1986; Shields, 1990). Although all lymph node-bearing areas of the mediastinum can be evaluated by thoracoscopy, the thoracoscopic approach is especially helpful to evaluate lymph nodes in the aortopulmonary window (level 5), subcarinal area (level 7), and paraesophageal region (level 8). Even though all nodal regions of the mediastinum can be evaluated by thoracoscopy, cervical mediastinal exploration remains the most appropriate, least invasive surgical means of evaluating paratracheal nodes. Thoracoscopy should not replace this approach for mediastinal evaluation, according to Landreneau, et al. (1993a). In cases in which we previously would have performed an anterior mediastinotomy (Chamberlain procedure), we now approach thoracoscopically. We have found that thoracoscopy provides better visualization of these areas and permits staging can be performed more safely, as well as making it possible to place the incisions out of the field of potential radiation therapy. Thoracoscopy also offers an excellent method of evaluating aortopulmonary window or hilar masses, as originally described by Paris, et al. (1985), and of providing adequate tissue for pathologic examination, especially when lymphoma or sarcoidosis is under consideration.

Trocar placement is similar to that for mediastinal cysts, with a viewing port placed in the fifth or sixth intercostal space in the midaxillary line and working ports placed in the fourth intercostal space in the posterior axillary line or even more posteriorly in the auscultatory triangle and in the intercostal space in the anterior axillary line (Fig. 59-14). Lung retraction is almost always necessary to adequately visualize the aortopulmonary window, and a fourth trocar is therefore placed anteriorly and inferiorly in the fifth intercostal space. In addition to the usual grasping instrument and endoscopic scissors, an endoscopic clip applier is usually necessary for control of the nodal blood supply.

Anterior Mediastinal Masses

Masses in the anterior mediastinum can be biopsied and in some instances completely excised by thoracoscopic techniques (Landreneau, et al., 1992b). The usual differential diagnosis of anterior mediastinal masses includes thymoma, teratoma, substernal thyroid goiter, and lymphoma. In addition, thoracoscopy can be employed for exploration of the anterior mediastinum for ectopic parathyroid tissue (Landreneau, personal communication). Mandatory preoperative evaluation includes CT or MRI. Other preoperative diagnostic tests that may be helpful, as discussed earlier, include ^{131}I scans for substernal goiter, technetium/thallium scans for ectopic parathyroid, and tumor markers (α-fetoprotein, β-HCG) for suspected germ cell neoplasms.

In addition, thoracoscopic thymectomy has been performed for the removal of stage I thymomas and in the management of myasthenia gravis (Mack, et al., 1992). Although total removal of the thymus gland can technically be achieved by thoracoscopy (Fig. 59-15) and complete remission of the disease accomplished, experience is brief and follow-up short (1 year). The appropriate role of thoracoscopy for thymectomy in the management of myasthenia gravis remains to be determined.

When anterior mediastinal masses are approached by thoracoscopy, the general thoracoscopic principles are applied for anesthetic management, positioning, and trocar placement. The mediastinum can be approached from either the right or left pleural cavity. The side on which the mass to be biopsied is most prominent is usually chosen. If a thymectomy is to be performed, the left side is usually chosen. Optimal trocar placement is achieved by placing the first trocar in the fifth intercostal space in the midaxillary to posterior axillary line (Fig. 59-16). Second and third ports are placed in the fourth intercostal space in the anterior axillary line and in the third intercostal space in the midaxillary line. If the patient is placed in the reverse Trendelenburg position and canted slightly posteriorly, the lung retracts inferiorly and posteriorly, allowing better visualization of the anterior mediastinum. A grasping instrument is placed through one working port and an endoscopic scissors through the other. The usual initial exploratory thoracoscopy is performed, and mediastinal structures, including pericardium, aortic arch, subclavian artery, and phrenic nerves, are identified. If a biopsy of a mass or lymphadenopathy is to be performed, the incision is made with judicious use of electrocautery to achieve hemostasis yet not disrupt the pathologic examination. If a thymectomy is to be performed for thymoma, a judgment is made regarding the invasive nature of the tumor. If the tumor is judged to be an invasive thymoma, the patient is best managed by conversion to an open procedure via median sternotomy so that complete excision can be performed. If thymectomy is performed for an encapsulated stage 1 thymoma or in the setting of myasthenia gravis, dissection is begun inferiorly along the anterior border of the phrenic nerve. By using both sharp and blunt dissection, all mediastinal tissue, including fat, is swept away from the phrenic nerve (Figs. 59-17A and 59-18).

Dissection is next continued posteriorly and laterally across the midline to the right side, elevating the tissue off

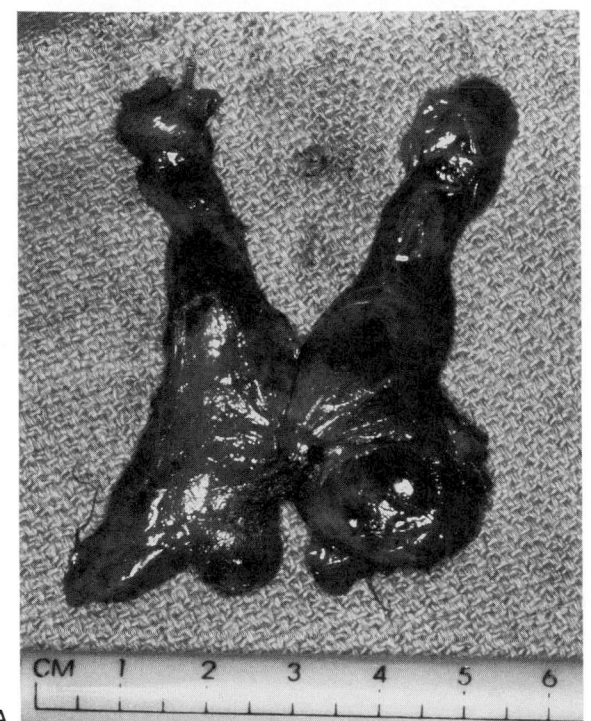 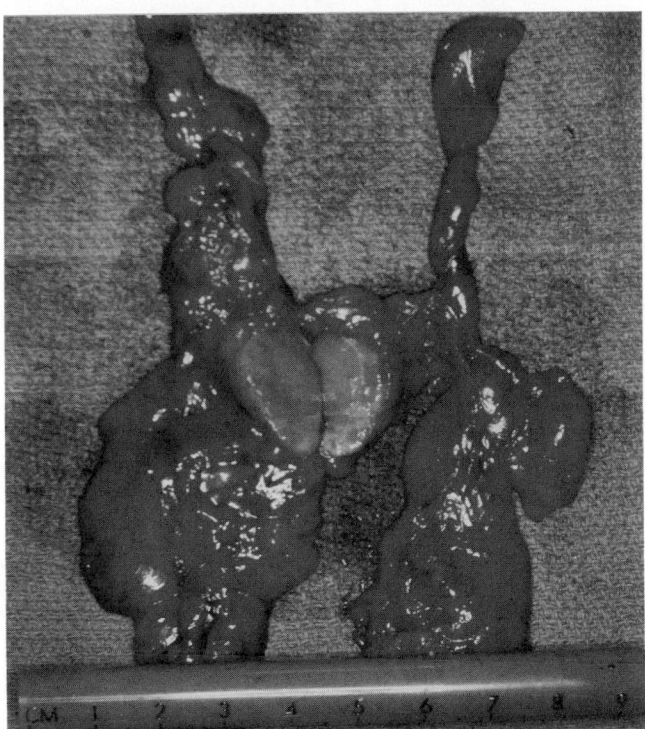

Figure 59-15. Specimens obtained from thoracoscopic thymectomy for myasthenia gravis. Specimen revealed **(A)** hyperplasia and **(B)** an encapsulated stage 1 thymoma.

the pericardium and away from the sternum (Figs. 59-19 and 59-20). As the resection of anterior mediastinal tissue continues, blunt dissection of the tissue from the retrosternal area is rather expeditiously accomplished. Dissection is continued along the right mediastinal pleura with care not to enter the pleura or to damage the right phrenic nerve. Once the inferior portion of the gland has been mobilized, the innominate vein with thymic vein branches is identified. The thymic veins

are ligated with endoscopic clips (Fig. 59-17B) and divided. Dissection is then continued cephalad superior to the innominate vein into the lower cervical area. The most difficult area to visualize and dissect is the recess at the angle of the innominate vein and superior vena cava. The arterial blood supply to the thymus gland, which arises from the left and right internal mammary arteries, is next identified and divided with endoscopic clips (Fig. 59-17C). The remainder of the

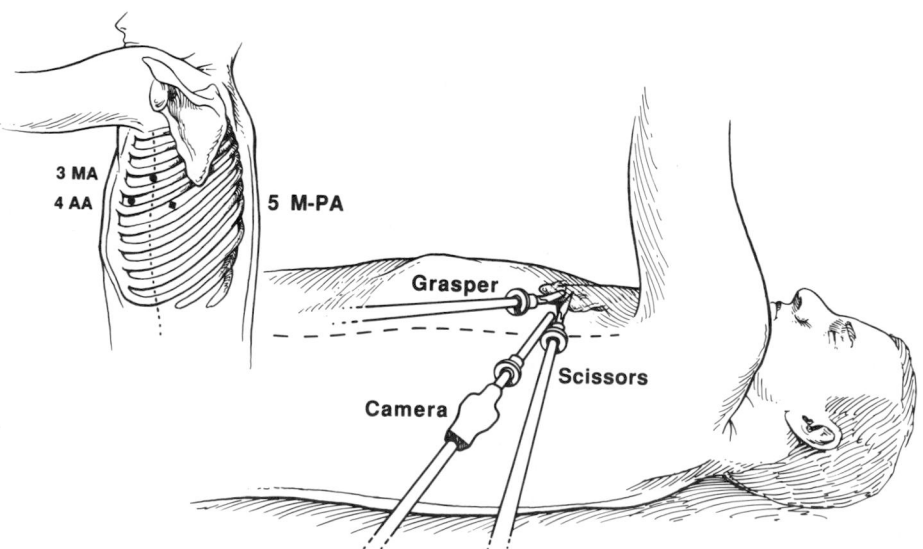

Figure 59-16. Trocar placement for approaching the anterior mediastinum.

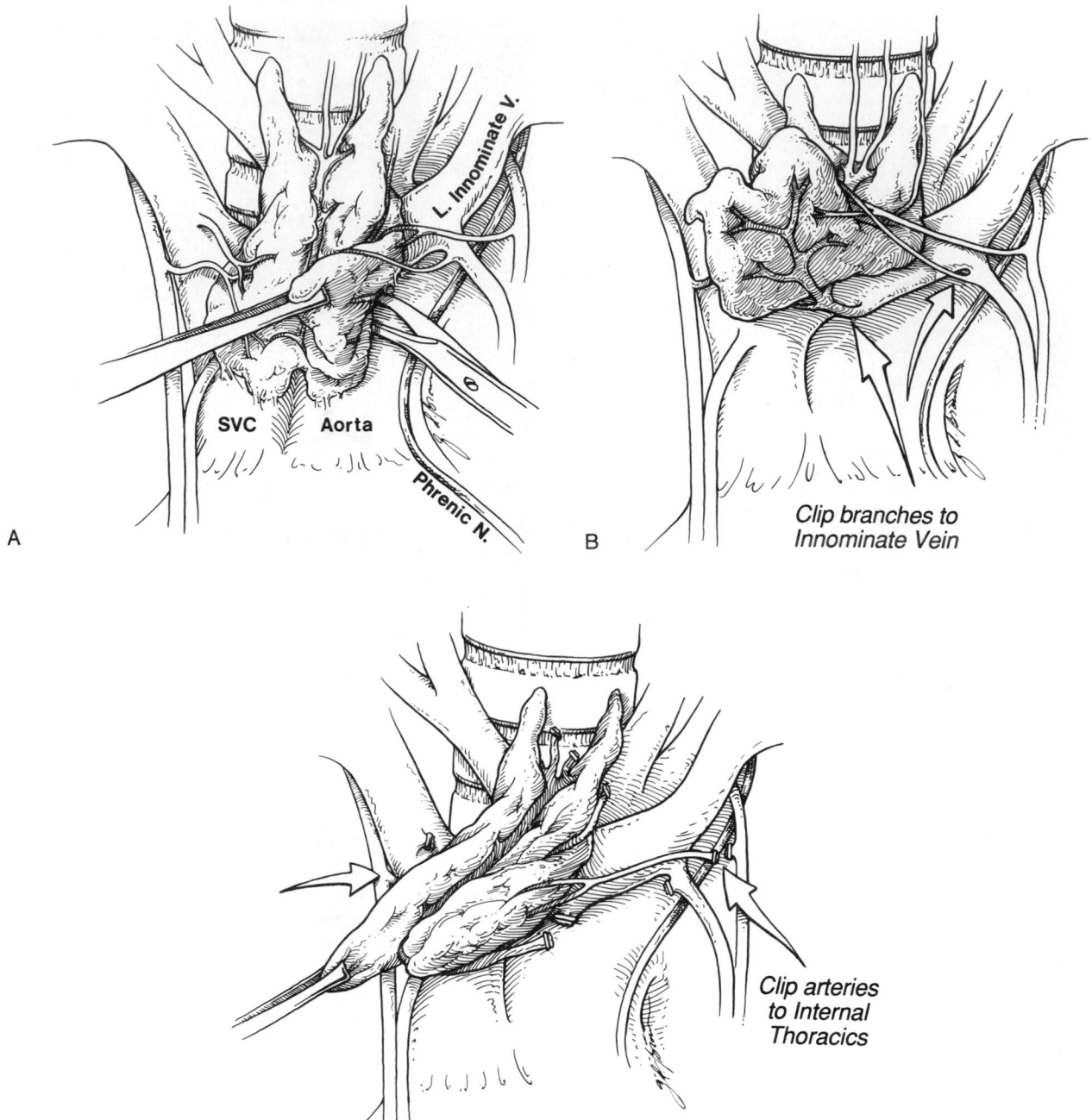

Figure 59-17. **(A)** Initial dissection during thymectomy performed by left thoracoscopic approach. **(B)** After the initial mobilization of the gland, the venous drainage into the innominate vein is identified, ligated, and divided. **(C)** The arterial supply from the internal thoracic arteries is identified and controlled.

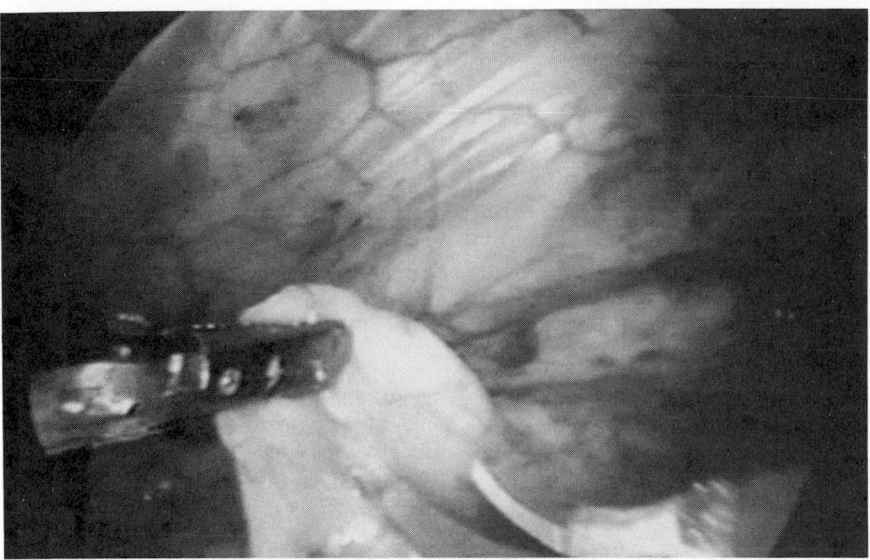

Figure 59-18. View of the left inferior pole of the thymus gland as dissection is initiated (Fig. 59-17A).

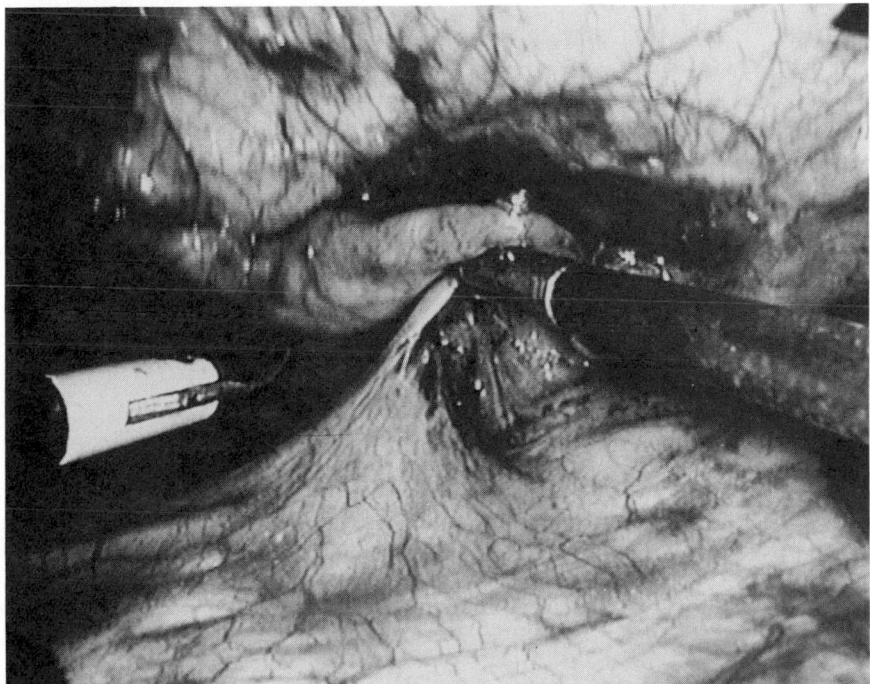

Figure 59-19. Thymic dissection is continued by sweeping the gland away from the sternum.

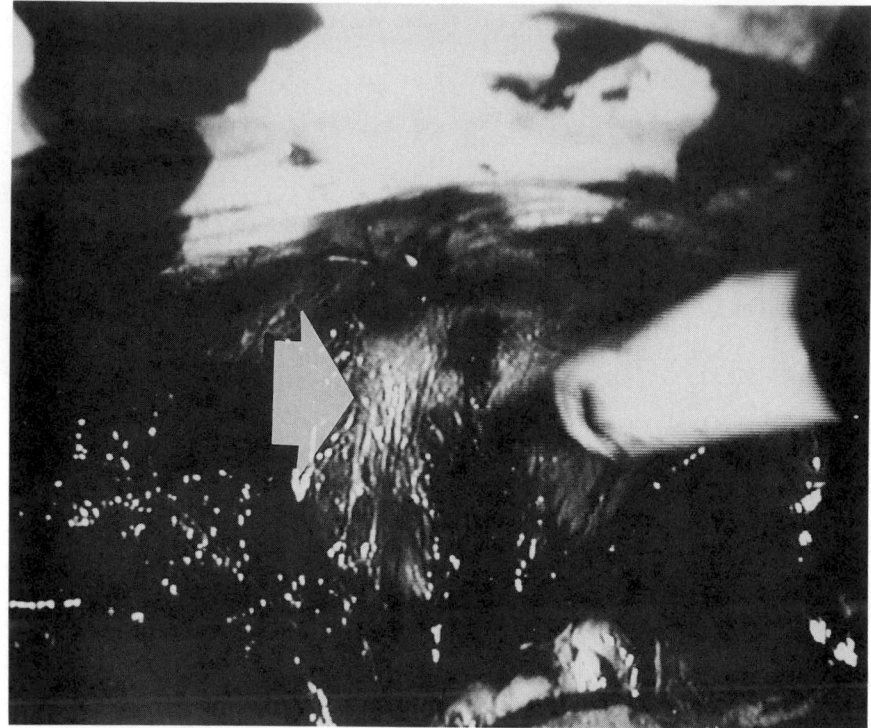

Figure 59-20.   View of the right pleural (*arrow*) as the thymus is dissected away.

dissection is concluded by identifying the superior poles of the gland and dividing the fascial attachments. The skin of the cervical area can be transilluminated with the thoracoscope at this point to confirm the superior extent of dissection. The intact specimen is then removed through the anterior trocar site, where the intercostal space is wider. If the specimen is too large, a finger can be used to slightly enlarge the access site. The specimen is examined to ensure that the whole gland has been removed, and the anterior mediastinal bed is inspected to ensure hemostasis and complete exenteration of all mediastinal tissue. A pleural drainage tube may be placed but is not necessary. The lung is reinflated under direct visualization, and trocar sites are closed with an absorbable suture. Postoperative care in an intensive care unit is necessary only if the patient has myasthenia gravis, so that the respiratory status can be closely monitored postanesthesia. Hospitalization is usually required for 24 to 48 hours.

COMMENTS AND CONTROVERSIES

The role of thoracoscopy for the management of the posterior and middle mediastinal compartments is relatively straightforward, and controversial issues are virtually nonexistent. Since most tumors of the posterior mediastinum are benign and if intraspinal extension of the tumor has been ruled out preoperatively, surgical excision is technically straightforward and the patient is spared the morbidity of an open thoracotomy. For masses of the middle mediastinum, which are almost always cystic, if surgical intervention is elected, the thoracoscopic approach is again minimally invasive and techniques are fairly standard.

However, in the surgical diagnostic evaluation and therapeutic excision of masses of the anterior mediastinal compartment, the approaches are much less resolved, the issues much more controversial, and the recommendations far from complete. Minimally invasive surgical approaches to the anterior mediastinum for diagnostic biopsy are already available either through the cervical mediastinal approach or by means of an anterior mediastinotomy. Both procedures require only small incisions, do not require intubation with a double-lumen tube or arterial line placement for hemodynamic monitoring, and require relatively short postoperative hospitalization. However, visualization of anatomic and pathologic structures in the mediastinum is relatively limited, and the placement of incisions may not be cosmetically acceptable and may also be in postoperative radiation portals.

The thoracoscopic approach to the anterior mediastinum has the disadvantages of requiring intubation with a double-lumen tube, arterial line monitoring, and a transpleural approach. It has advantages, however, of offering superior visualization of all mediastinal structures and lymph node-bearing areas with a high degree of confidence that diagnostic tissue has been safely obtained. In addition, the surgical incisions are usually in cosmetically more acceptable areas and not in portals of postoperative radiation.

The issue of the use of VATS techniques for performance

of thymectomy is certainly one that will generate interest, controversy, and commentary for years to come. Although it has been amply demonstrated by a number of investigators that a total thymectomy can be technically performed by thoracoscopic techniques, the long-term benefit of such techniques, especially in the management of myasthenia gravis, can only be demonstrated by longitudinal studies. Only when a large surgical series has been compiled and 5-year follow-up results are available will it be possible adequately to compare thoracoscopy with either the transcervical or transsternal approach for thymectomy. The long-term results of both these approaches are well documented accurately in multiple series (Andersen, et al., 1986; Hebra, et al., 1990; Kark and Kirschner, 1971; Maggi, et al., 1989; Molnar and Szobor, 1990; Wechsler and Olanow, 1981; Whyte, et al., 1989). The thoracoscopic approach is less invasive than the transsternal approach and offers superior visualization, at least of the lower portion of the thymus gland, as compared with the transcervical approach. However, much more experience and significantly longer follow-up are necessary before it can be recommended as a standard therapeutic alternative for thymectomy, especially in patients with myasthenia gravis.

M.M.

Thymectomy should be complete whether it be done for tumor or for myasthenia gravis. Leaving part of the thymus often creates problems at a later time. The problem with removing the thymoma by thoracoscopy is the possibility of seeding the pleural space with the tumor.

A second interspace incision can sometimes best be managed by thoracoscopy if general anesthesia is used.

Thoracoscopic sympathectomy can be performed through the transthoracic approach as described. Many foreign authors simply cauterize the sympathetic chain; however, in the United States because of the medical/legal aspects, ganglion cells must be documented on frozen section, and therefore a resection, rather than a simple cauterization, is necessary.

The combination of first rib resection with extrapleural sympathectomy is advantageous and less painful than the transpleural approach (Urschel, 1993).

H.C.U.

KEY REFERENCES

Landreneau RJ, Hazelrigg SR, Mack MJ, et al.: Thoracoscopic mediastinal lymph node sampling: a useful approach to mediastinal lymph node stations inaccessible to cervical mediastinoscopy. J Thorac Cardiovasc Surg 105:554, 1993a

Extensive presentation of the argument for use of thoracoscopy as an adjunct in mediastinal staging.

Landreneau RJ, Mack MJ, Hazelrigg SR, et al.: Video assisted thoracic surgery: basic technical concepts and intercostal approach strategies. Ann Thorac Surg 54:800, 1992a

Review article that addresses the basic concepts integral to initiating most video-assisted thoracic procedures. The principles outlined here serve as a strong foundation for performing thoracoscopic surgery.

Naruke T, Suemasu K, Ishikawa S: Lymph node mapping and curability at various levels of metastasis in resected lung cancer. J Thorac Cardiovasc Surg 76:832, 1978

Classic paper defining the importance of lymph node staging of lung cancer.

Pearson FG: Mediastinal tumors. Semin Thorac Cardiovasc Surg V 4: 1, 1992

Comprehensive issue devoted totally to the diagnosis and management of mediastinal masses. Experience antedates the role of thoracoscopy but serves as a valuable compendium for management of mediastinal disease.

Shields T: The significance of ipsilateral mediastinal lymph node metastasis (N2 disease) in non–small cell carcinoma of the lung. J Thorac Cardiovasc Surg 99:48, 1990

Further support for the importance of lymph node staging.

REFERENCES

American Thoracic Society: Clinical staging of primary lung cancer. Am Rev Respir Dis 127:659, 1983

Andersen M, Jorgensen J, Clausen PP: Transcervical thymectomy in patients with nonthymomatous myasthenia gravis. Scand J Thorac Cardiovasc Surg 20:233, 1986

Bell ET: Tumour of the thymus in myasthenia gravis. J Nerv Ment Dis 45:130, 1917

Blalock A: Thymectomy in the treatment of myasthenia gravis. Report of twenty cases. J Thorac Surg 13:316, 1944

Blalock A, Mason MF, Morgan HJ, Riven SS: Myasthenia gravis and tumours of the thymic region. Report of a case in which the tumour was removed. Ann Surg 110:544, 1939

Carlens E: Thymectomy for myasthenia gravis with the aid of mediastinoscopy. Opuscule Med 13:175, 1968

Carlens E: Mediastinoscopy. A method for inspection and tissue biopsy in the superior mediastinum. Chest 35:343, 1949

Crile G: Thymectomy through the neck. Surgery 59:213, 1966

Deslaurier J, Beaulieu M, Dufour C, et al.: Mediastinopleuroscopy: a new approach to the diagnosis of intrathoracic diseases. Ann Thorac Surg 22:265, 1976

Ginsberg RJ: Mediastinal germ cell tumors: the role of surgery. Semin Thorac Cardiovasc Surg 4:51, 1992

Ginsberg RJ: Evaluation of the mediastinum by invasive techniques. Surg Clin North Am 67:1025, 1987

Hebra AH, Reed CE, Heldmann M, Black MJ: Myasthenia gravis: a review with emphasis on the potential role of thymectomy. J S C Med Assoc 86:392, 1990

Jaretzki A III, Bethea M, Wolff M, et al.: A rational approach to total thymectomy in the treatment of myasthenia gravis. Ann Thorac Surg 2:120, 1977

Kark AE, Kirschner PA: Total thymectomy through the transcervical approach. Br J Surg 58:321, 1971

Landreneau RJ, Dowling RD, Castillo W, Ferson PF: Thoracoscopic resection of an anterior mediastinal mass. Ann Thorac Surg 54:142, 1992b

Landreneau RJ, Dowling RD, Ferson PF: Thoracoscopic resection of a posterior mediastinal mass. Chest 1993b (in press)

Lewis RJ, Caccavale RJ, Sisler GE: Imaged thoracoscopic surgery: a new thoracic technique for resection of mediastinal cysts. Ann Thorac Surg 53:318, 1992

Mack MJ, Aronoff RJ, Acuff TE, et al.: Present role of thoracoscopy in the diagnosis and treatment of diseases of the chest. Ann Thorac Surg 54:403, 1992

Maggi G, Casadio C, Cavallo A, et al.: Thymectomy in myasthenia gravis: results of 662 cases operated upon in 15 years. Eur J Cardiothorac Surg 3:504, 1989

McNeill T, Chamberlain J: Diagnostic anterior mediastinotomy. Ann Thorac Surg 2:532, 1966

Molnar J, Szobor A: Myasthenia gravis: effect of thymectomy in 425 patients—a 15-year experience. Eur J Cardiothorac Surg 4:8, 1990

Mountain CF: A new international staging system for lung cancer. Chest 89:225 (suppl), 1986

Papatestas AE, Genkins G, Korafeld P, et al.: Effects of thymectomy in myasthenia gravis. Ann Surg 206:79, 1987

Paris F, Garcia-Zarza A, Canto A, et al.: Hilioscopy as a staging procedure. p. 54. In Delarue NC, Eschapasse H (eds): International Trends in General Thoracic Surgery. Vol. 1. Lung Cancer, WB Saunders, Philadelphia, 1985

Patterson GA: Significance of metastatic disease in subaortic lymph nodes. Ann Thorac Surg 43:155, 1987

Pearson FG: Surgical therapy of mediastinal (N2) disease. p. 201. In Bitran JD, Golomb HM, Little AG, Weichselbaum RR (eds): Lung Cancer: a Comprehensive Treatise. WB Saunders, Philadelphia, 1988

Rice TW: Benign neoplasms and cysts of the mediastinum. Semin Thorac Cardiovasc Surg 4:25, 1992

Rubish JL, Gardner IR, Boyd WC, Ehrenhaft JL: Mediastinal tumors. J Thorac Cardiovasc Surg 65:216, 1973

Urschel HC Jr: Dorsal sympathectomy and management of thoracic outlet syndrome with VATS. Ann Thorac Surg 50:717, 1993

Wechsler AS, Olanow CW: The surgical management of myasthenia gravis. In Sabiston DC, Jr (ed): Davis-Christopher Textbook of Surgery. 12th Ed. Vol. 2. WB Saunders, Philadelphia, 1981

Weisbrod GL, Herman SJ: Mediastinal masses: diagnosis with noninvasive techniques. Semin Thorac Cardiovasc Surg 4:3, 1992

Whyte RI, Kaplan DK, Deegan SP, Donnelly RJ: Cervical thymectomy in the treatment of myasthenia gravis. J R Coll Surg Edinb 34:74, 1989

THORACOSCOPIC SYMPATHECTOMY

DEFINITION

This section discusses the use of VATS techniques for performance of sympathectomy in the thoracic cavity. Equivalent terms for the procedure have included dorsal sympathectomy or cervical thoracic sympathectomy for denervation of the upper extremity. Surgical sympathectomies have been performed to treat a variety of conditions of the upper extremities, including pain management syndromes such as reflex sympathetic dystrophy, vasculopathies including Raynaud's disease and Buerger's disease, and hyperhidrosis of the arm and hand. This section describes the thoracoscopic technique for performance of sympathectomy and addresses some of the relevant issues of this procedure.

HISTORICAL NOTE

The sympathetic trunk was originally described by Galen, who recognized the superior cervical, the middle cervical, and the inferior cervical ganglia. Galen apparently did not appreciate that the vagus nerve was not part of the sympathetic system, and it was left to Stephanes to distinguish between the vagus nerve and the sympathetic trunk. The term *sympathetic trunk* was first used in 1732 by J. B. Winslow, and the functional significance of the sympathetic trunk was first recognized by Claude Bernard in 1852. Post-traumatic pain syndromes were first described by Mitchell, et al. (1864) in their account of Civil War injuries.

The first surgical intervention on the sympathetic trunk was performed by Alexander in 1889. This procedure, as well as subsequent operations by Jonnesco in 1916, were attempts to treat epilepsy. Jaboulay (1899) was the first to suggest that sympathectomy might improve circulation in the upper extremity. The anterior approach for sympathectomy was pioneered by Jonnesco, who in 1916 performed a sympathectomy in an attempt to relieve angina pectoris. The use of sympathectomy for upper extremity vascular disorders was first applied by Leriche and Fontaine in 1932.

Many surgical approaches have been described for performance of a sympathectomy. The initial approaches were anterior and were used by Jonnesco, Leriche, Royle, Gask, and Fontaine in the early 1930s. In the anterior approach as originally described, a transverse supraclavicular incision is made. The clavicular head of the sternocleidomastoid muscle is divided, the carotid sheath and phrenic nerve are retracted medially, and the anterior scalene muscle is divided. The subclavian artery is retracted, and the stellate ganglion is located behind the vertebral artery adjacent to the seventh cervical and first thoracic vertebral bodies.

The next approach to be described was the posterior approach, initially described by Adson and Brown (1929). By this approach the second rib posteriorly is resected and the posterior mediastinum entered. Occasionally this approach was varied to include resection of the first rib and transverse process of the vertebral body. Numerous variations of this operation were subsequently described, including a preganglionic sympathectomy by Telford in 1935 and by Smithwick in 1936. Goetz and Marr (1944) performed a second thoracic ganglionectomy. This was extended by Goetz in 1948 to include the third and fourth thoracic ganglia. Subsequent alternative surgical approaches include the posterolateral approach, which is performed by a paravertebral incision, division of the trapezius muscle, retraction of the scapula, and resection of the third or fourth rib. An easier approach consists of bilateral paravertebral incisions in prone position performed by resection of the second rib, and sympathectomy of the T1, T2, and T3 ganglia (Urschel and Razzuk, 1985).

Another alternative approach is the transaxillary transpleural approach, which until this time has been the most common approach used because of the superior visualization of the sympathetic chain and the ability to perform a more extensive sympathectomy. Removal is also possible following transaxillary first rib resection and extrapleural sympathectomy (Urschel, 1993a).

The first endoscopic approach to the thoracic sympathetic trunk was described by Hughes (1942). Subsequent descriptions include those of Kux in 1954, 1955, and again in 1978 (Kux, 1978). As originally described by Hughes, the sympathetic trunk is approached through an endoscope placed in the third intercostal space in the anterior axillary line with the patient in the supine position. The sympathetic chain is then visualized after a pneumothorax is induced. The technique was not routinely used because of concern about proximity to the stellate ganglion and to the vertebral artery.

Resurgence in this endoscopic technique has occurred because of the addition of better illumination, improved optics, and video magnification. This combines the benefit of a minimally invasive approach with superior visualization. The first reports of video endoscopic techniques were by Lin (1990), Kao (1992), and Edmondson, et al. (1992).

HISTORICAL READINGS

Adson AW, Brown GE: The treatment of Raynaud's disease by resection of the upper thoracic and lumbar sympathetic ganglia and trunks. Surg Gynecol Obstet 48:577, 1929

Jaboulay M: Le traitment de quelques troubles trophiques de le pied et de la jambe par la dénudation de l'artère et la distension des nerfs vasculaires. J Med Lyon 91:467, 1899

Kux M: Thoracic endoscopic sympathectomy in palmar and axillary hyperhidrosis. Arch Surg 113:264, 1978

Mitchell SW, Morehouse GR, Keen WW: Gunshot wounds and other injuries of nerves. JB Lippincott, Philadelphia, 1864

Urschel HC Jr, Razzuk MA: Posterior thoracic sympathectomy. In Malt RA (ed): Surgical Techniques Illustrated: A Comparative Atlas. WB Saunders, Philadelphia, 1985

Urschel HC Jr: Dorsal sympathectomy and management of thoracic outlet syndrome with VATS. Ann Thorac Surg 56:717, 1993

BASIC SCIENCE

The sympathetic chain runs the total length of the cervical and thoracic spinal cord as far as the second lumbar nerves inferiorly. The sympathetic chain, with its associated ganglia, are located over the head of the ribs at their articulation with the transverse process of the vertebral bodies (Fig. 59-21). The inferior cervical ganglia and the first thoracic ganglion fuse to form the stellate ganglion over the head of the first rib. The first thoracic ganglion supplies sympathetic innervation to the head and neck, including the pupil of the eye. Most of the innervation to the hand originates in the second and third ganglia, with the innervation of the axilla provided

by the fourth and fifth thoracic ganglia of the sympathetic chain. It is estimated that in approximately 10 percent of patients T1 ganglionic fibers also supply sympathetic impulses to the arm. In addition, postganglionic fibers from the second and third thoracic ganglia may combine to form an intrathoracic nerve, the nerve of Kunt, which passes to the T1 root, bypassing the stellate ganglion and carrying sympathetic fibers to the inferior portion of the brachial plexus. This variation in normal anatomy is what makes it unclear whether any of the stellate ganglion needs to be divided in order to obtain complete sympathetic denervation of the upper extremity.

In upper extremity syndromes, sympathectomy is usually only effective when end arterioles are capable of vasodilatation. In conditions such as Raynaud's disease, because maximal vasodilatation has already occurred, the benefits of sympathectomy are usually short-lived. However, in other ischemic syndromes of the upper extremity, including thromboangiitis obliterans, or other upper extremity occlusive syndromes of the hand or digits in which reconstructive surgery is not feasible, sympathectomy has been demonstrated to show good and lasting results.

Thoracic sympathectomy has also been performed for the relief of visceral abdominal pain, especially that due to advanced pancreatic disease (Stone and Chauvin, 1990; Mannell, et al., 1988; Lebovits and Lefkowitz, 1989). The celiac plexus is innervated by the greater splanchnic nerve (T5–T10), the lesser splanchnic nerve (T10–T11), and the least splanchnic (T12). The sympathetic system has been demonstrated to be the primary pathway for pain sensation in these patients. Therefore, a number of centers have begun to use thoracoscopy for performing a splanchnicectomy for pain control in these patients (Landreneau, personal communication, 1993). The greater splanchnic nerves can be readily identified at thoracoscopy on the left side.

DIAGNOSIS

The most common indications for surgical sympathectomy have been post-traumatic pain syndromes. Reflex sympathetic dystrophy (RSD) is the name most commonly used to describe this condition, although the terms *causalgia, shoulder-hand syndrome,* and *Sudeck's atrophy* have also been applied to it. Three stages of RSD have been described by Drucker, et al. (1959). Stage 1 is the acute stage and usually persists for 1 to 3 months. Symptoms include burning, pain, hyperthermia, edema, erythema, muscle spasms, hyperhidrosis, and hyperalgesia. Spontaneous resolution frequently occurs during this stage and surgical intervention is seldom necessary. Stage 2, the dystrophic phase, follows the acute phase and also usually lasts 3 months. During this phase, spontaneous resolution seldom occurs. Symptoms include continuous pain, coolness of the extremity, and often edema and cyanosis. Stage 3, the atrophic phase, usually results in pain that occurs well beyond the site of original injury. Extensive muscular atrophy occurs, and this stage is irreversible. Initial treatment of RSD includes percutaneous stellate ganglion blocks, usually with local anesthetics. Permanent ablation with percutaneous stellate ganglion blocks can also be obtained with injection of alcohol. Physical therapy is also an important component of conservative treat-

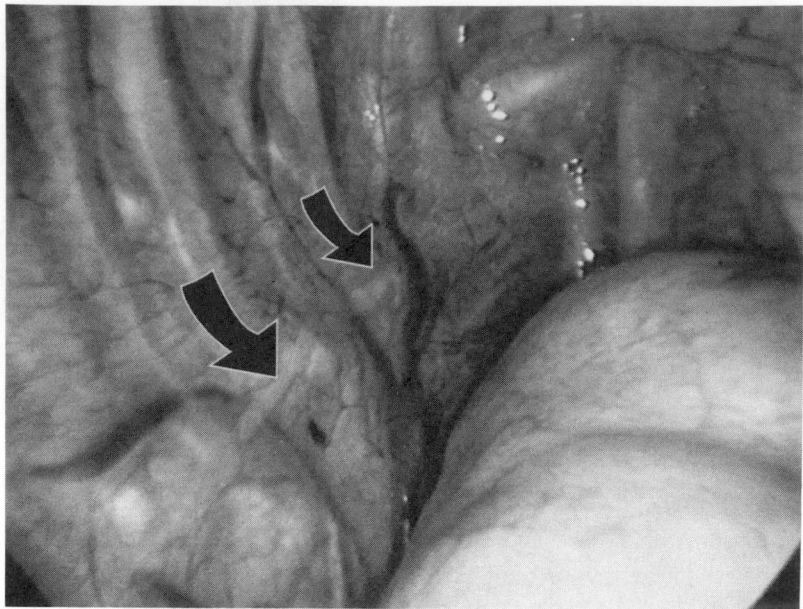

Figure 59-21. Thoracoscopic view of the sympathetic chain (*arrows*) in the right chest.

ment, and it is generally believed that 50 to 70 percent of patients respond to conservative, nonsurgical therapy, according to Patman, et al. (1973).

For those in whom conservative therapy fails, surgical sympathectomy is usually recommended. Results in most series consistently demonstrate a good or excellent result in over 90 percent of patients who have been properly selected (Olcott, et al., 1991; Patman, et al., 1973; Urschel, 1993b). It is crucial that preoperative relief of symptoms by a percutaneous stellate ganglion block be demonstrated. The shorter the duration of the RSD, the better the surgical result.

Hyperhidrosis

Hyperhidrosis occurs from excessive sweating from the eccrine glands of the upper extremity. The excessive sweating of the hand often results in occupational and social problems. There is an increased incidence of the disorder among some Middle Eastern Jews as well as in the Japanese, as described by Salob, et al. (1991); however, most cases are idiopathic. Systemic disorders such as hyperthyroidism, menopause, pheochromocytoma, and anxiety need to be ruled out, however. Conservative management is usually with a topical application of aluminum chloride compounds as drying agents. Systemic anticholinergics have been used in an attempt to block postganglionic acetylcholine receptors. However, systemic side effects of blurred vision, dry mouth, and urinary retention usually limit their benefit. Coagulation of eccrine glands by iontophoresis has had some limited success. For axillary hyperhidrosis, local excision of the glands has also been used.

Surgical sympathectomy has been the best method for long-term relief of palmar hyperhidrosis. The amount of sympathetic chain excised or ablated varies but usually includes the T2 through the T5 level of sympathetic ganglia. The suc-

cess rate has ranged from 85 to 95 percent in different series (Kao, 1992; Lin, 1990). Potential complications include Horner syndrome if the first thoracic ganglion is excised, as well as gustatory sweating, recurrent palmar hidrosis, and compensatory sweating in other areas of the body, the mechanism of which is not clear.

Ischemic Syndromes

Application of sympathectomy for treatment of upper extremity vascular disorders is generally indicated in those ischemic syndromes for which revascularization techniques are not possible. Vasospastic disorders, including collagen vascular diseases, Raynaud's phenomenon, and Buerger's disease are all occasional indications for sympathectomy; however, the results are not uniformly as good as in reflex sympathetic dystrophy or hyperhidrosis.

Preoperative noninvasive tests predictive of a good result from sympathectomy most commonly include percutaneous medical stellate ganglion block. Since sympathectomy is generally only beneficial when vasodilatation of end arterioles or capillaries is possible, tests such as plethysmographic pulse monitoring before and after sympathetic block may occasionally be helpful if the benefit is not clearly demonstrable clinically.

MANAGEMENT

Conservative Management

Conservative management of RSD consists of physical therapy of the upper extremity and administration of nonsteroidal anti-inflammatory agents, as well as temporary percutaneous stellate ganglion blocks with local anesthetics. Upon failure of standard conservative measures, some pain management anesthesiologists perform alcohol denervation of a stellate ganglion; however, most authorities prefer surgical sympathetic ablation.

For hyperhidrosis of the upper extremity, additional conservative measures include antiperspirants and other topical agents (e.g., aluminum chloride), as well as anticholinergic medication and on occasion psychotherapy). Once these conservative measures have failed, operative intervention is appropriate.

Operative Technique

Although multiple surgical approaches have been used, including anterior, lateral, axillary, and posterior approaches, the thoracoscopic approach offers the significant comparative advantages of diminished postoperative pain and improved cosmesis. The procedure is most commonly performed under general endotracheal anesthesia with a double-lumen tube to effect collapse of the ipsilateral lung, and hemodynamic monitoring with an arterial line is routinely performed. There is, however, extensive European experience with performance of the procedure under local anesthesia in the spontaneously breathing patient. In this technique, the patient receives intravenous sedation, and a partial pneumothorax is induced on the operative side.

The patient is placed in the lateral position, and the chest is widely prepared in case conversion to a thoracotomy is necessary. If a bilateral sympathectomy is to be performed, the patient is instead positioned in the supine position and both sides are prepared. In the most common method of placing trocars for access to the thoracic cavity, one 10-mm trocar for access of the telescope and video camera is placed in the fourth intercostal space in the mid- to anterior axillary line (Fig. 59-22), after which two additional trocars are placed in the third intercostal space, one at the anterior border of the trapezius and the other in the anterior axillary line just

at the posterior border of the pectoralis muscle. Care is taken to avoid crowding of the trocars so that visualization is not obscured by the instruments in the visual field of the telescope and so that the instruments do not crowd one another inside the thoracic cavity. This slightly anterior placement of the trocars allows direct visualization of the sympathetic trunk, which overlies the heads of the ribs at the junction with the transverse processes of the vertebral bodies. The sympathetic trunk is readily apparent through the parietal pleural. Occasionally, retraction of the apex of the lung is necessary, especially if the resorptive atelectasis is not complete. However, visualization can sometimes be improved by placing the patient in the Trendelenburg position and allowing the lung to drop out of the way by gravity.

Once the sympathetic trunk has been clearly identified, the parietal pleura overlying the chain is excised along the full length of anticipated resection. Endoscopic scissors with electrocautery capability and a grasping instrument are most effective for opening up the parietal pleura. The sympathetic trunk is further visualized by blunt dissection of the surrounding soft tissue until the inferior portion of the stellate ganglion overlying the head of the first rib is clearly identified. There is usually a vein overlying the sympathetic chain between the second and third ganglia (Figure 59-23). To prevent bothersome bleeding, this vein is next ligated with endoscopic clips and divided before further dissection is performed. Next, the trunk is transected at the desired inferior level, which most commonly is below the T4 sympathetic ganglion. For hyperhidrosis syndromes in which denervation of the axilla is important, this inferior extent of resection is carried to the T5 level. The chain is usually simply divided without placing clips on it because of concern of causing postsympathectomy neuralgia. With judicious use of cautery as well as blunt and sharp dissection, the trunk is mobilized cephalad. Once the chain has been fully mobilized, it is our preference to divide the trunk at the inferior border of the stellate ganglion to prevent Horner syndrome. Because of the 10 percent

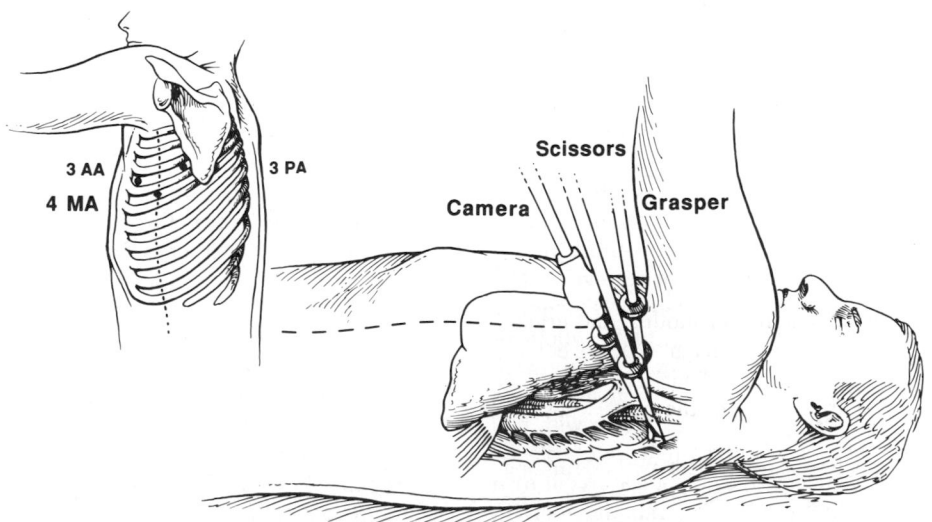

Figure 59-22.   Optimal trocar placement for performing thoracic sympathectomy.

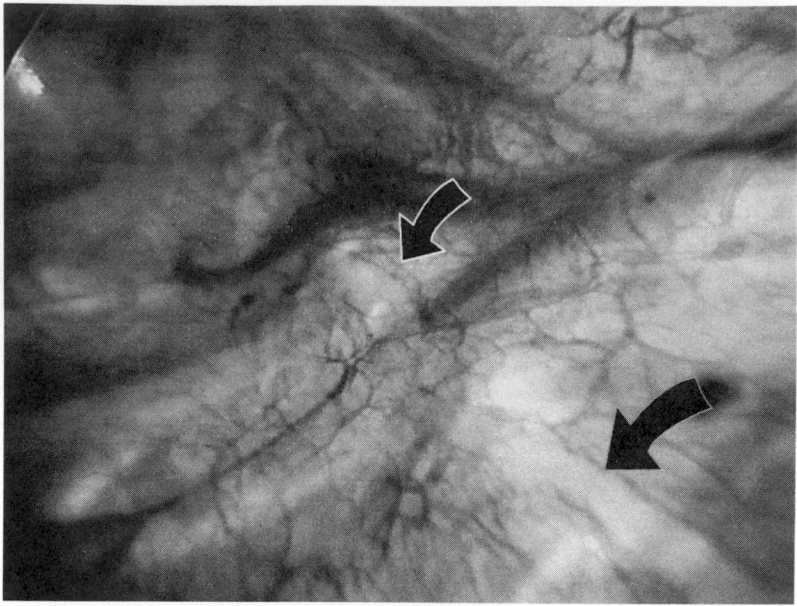

Figure 59-23. Close-up view of the sympathetic chain (*arrows*) through the parietal pleura. Note the vein overlying the chain above the upper arrow.

of patients in whom sympathetic innervation to the upper extremity does occur through the stellate ganglion, some investigators have believed that excision of at least a portion of the stellate ganglion is crucial. Because occurrence of Horner syndrome with surgical excision of the stellate ganglion is almost universal, we have not included this as a part of our standard sympathectomy. After the trunk has been divided superiorly, the chain is removed through one of the trocar sites. Hemostasis is obtained with judicious use of monopolar electrocautery. A chest tube is not necessary unless inadvertent injury to the lung has occurred during retraction. Reexpansion of the lung is directly ob-

served, and the trocar sites are closed with a subcuticular suture. Postoperative management usually includes intravenous morphine for 24 hours and a hospital stay of 1 to 2 days.

Splanchnicectomy for relief of intractable abdominal pain is performed by a left thoracoscopic approach. The ports are placed more caudal in the seventh or eighth intercostal space. The greater splanchnic nerve originating from T5 to T10 and the lesser splanchnic nerve (T10–T11) are identified and cut. Often the lesser nerve is difficult to identify. Vagotomy, which has been advocated by some, is not recommended since it may cause gastric stasis.

COMMENTS AND CONTROVERSIES

Although surgical sympathectomy has been well defined for most of this century, the operation has not gained wide use, especially in the management of patients with pain syndromes of the upper extremity. The morbidity associated with standard open surgical approaches has usually negated the beneficial effect of the sympathectomy. The post-thoracotomy pain associated with open approaches has not been viewed by patients or their pain management physicians as acceptable morbidity in these conditions. The benefit of the thoracoscopic approach is the lessened postoperative morbidity associated with it in these patients with difficult to manage pain syndromes. The minimal postoperative morbidity with this approach has led, in our brief experience, to a wider role for sympathectomy in pain management syndromes. In our own experience of 30 cases of thoracoscopic sympathectomy in less than 2 years, we have achieved a good or excellent result in 94 percent of patients with RSD or hyperhidrosis.

Postoperative morbidity or prolonged postoperative pain has been virtually nonexistent.

The extent of the sympathetic chain to be excised remains controversial. Because some sympathetic innervation of the upper extremity occurs through the first thoracic ganglion in approximately 10 percent of patients, some authors believe that excision of the inferior portion of the stellate ganglion is mandatory for good clinical results. It is also considered that the Horner syndrome associated with this extent of excision is acceptable morbidity. It is our own personal experience that good clinical results can be obtained without excising any portion of the stellate ganglion so that the significant morbidity of a postoperative Horner syndrome is avoided. It is our belief that Horner syndrome is not acceptable morbidity in a significant number of patients.

Another issue to be addressed is the technique of performing sympathectomy. The techniques include simple excision of the trunk, ablation of the trunk with either electrocautery or laser as used by Kao (1992), or simple division of the preganglionic fibers to the sympathetic trunk. We believe that simple surgical excision of the sympathetic trunk is technically easy and accurately documents the extent of the sympathectomy that has been performed. Because of concern about the use of monopolar cautery adjacent to the spinal column, we only use electrocautery judiciously for hemostasis and do not use it for ablation of the trunk.

In conclusion, thoracoscopic sympathectomy is an effective therapeutic modality in RSD, hyperhidrosis, and ischemic syndromes of the upper extremity when more conservative modalities have failed. The endoscopic approach appears to have less morbidity than any of the more standard approaches for surgical sympathectomy and therefore has led to wider use of surgery for the management of these syndromes in a very short time. In addition, use of thoracoscopy for performance of splanchnicectomy for chronic visceral abdominal pain syndromes also appears to offer palliative benefit.

M.M.

Thoracoscopic sympathectomy can be performed through the transthoracic approach as described. Many foreign authors simply cauterize the sympathetic chain. In the United States, however, because of the medico/legal aspects, ganglion cells must be documented on frozen section, and therefore resection, rather than simple cauterization, is necessary.

The combination of first rib resection with extrapleural sympathectomy is advantageous and less painful than the transpleural approach (Urschel, 1993a).

H.C.U.

KEY REFERENCES

Drucker WR, Hubay CA, Holden WD, Bukovnic JA: Pathogenesis of post-traumatic sympathetic dystrophy. Am J Surg 97:454, 1959
  Original and most comprehensive description of the etiology of post-traumatic pain syndromes. The classification into three stages forms the current algorithm for management.

Kux M: Thoracic endoscopic sympathectomy in palmar and axillary hyperhidrosis. Arch Surg 113:264, 1978
  First description of the endoscopic technique for performance of sympathectomy.

Lin CC: Extended thoracoscopic T$_2$-sympathectomy in treatment of hyperhidrosis: experience with 130 consecutive cases. J Laparoendosc Surg 2:1, 1992
  Broad experience of using the thoracoscopic approach to perform sympathectomy for hyperhidrosis. Among the first descriptions of the use of video assistance for the endoscopic approach.

Urschel HC Jr: Dorsal sympathectomy and management of thoracic outlet syndrome with VATS. Ann Thorac Surg 56:717, 1993b

---

REFERENCES

Adson AW, Brown GE: The treatment of Raynaud's disease by resection of the upper thoracic and lumbar sympathetic ganglia and trunks. Surg Gynecol Obstet 48:577, 1929

Edmondson RA, Banerjee AK, Rennie JA: Endoscopic transthoracic sympathectomy in the treatment of hyperhidrosis. Ann Surg 215:289, 1992

Fairbairn JF, Juergens JL, Spittell JA: Surgical procedures of the sympathetic nervous system for peripheral vascular disease. p. 687. In Allen C, Barker S, Hines M (eds): Peripheral Vascular Diseases. 4th Ed. WB Saunders, Philadelphia, 1972

Goetz RH, Marr JA: The importance of the second thoracic ganglion for the sympathetic supply of the upper extremities with a description of two new approaches for its removal in cases of vascular disease: a preliminary report. Clin Proc 3:102, 1944

Hughes J: Endothoracic sympathectomy. J R Soc Med 35:585, 1942

Jaboulay M: Le traitement de quelques troubles trophiques du pied et de la jambe par la denudation de l'artère et la distension des nerfs vasculaires. J med Lyon 91:467, 1899

Kao MC: Video endoscopic sympathectomy using a fiberoptic CO_2 laser to treat palmar hyperhidrosis. Neurosurgery 30:131, 1992

Lebovits AH, Lefkowitz M: Pain management of pancreatic carcinoma: a review. Pain 36:1, 1989

Lin CC: A new method of thoracoscopic sympathectomy in hyperhidrosis palmaris. Surg Endosc 4:224, 1990

Malone PS, Duignan JP, Hederman WP: Transthoracic electrocoagulation (TTEC)—a new and simple approach to upper limb sympathectomy. Ir Med J 75:20, 1982

Mannell A, Adson MA, McIlrath DC et al: Surgical management of chronic pancreatitis: long term results in 141 patients. Br J Surg 75:467, 1988

Mitchell SW, Morehouse GR, Keen WW: Gunshot Wounds and Other Injuries of Nerves. JB Lippincott, Philadelphia, 1864

Olcott C. Eltherington LG, Wilcosky BR et al. Reflex sympathetic dystrophy—the surgeon's role in management. J Vasc Surg 14:488, 1991

Patman RD, Thompson JE, Persson AV: Management of post-traumatic pain syndromes: report of 113 cases. Ann Surg 177:780, 1973

Salob SP, Atherton DJ, Kiely EM: Thoracic endoscopic sympathectomy for palmar hyperhidrosis in an adolescent female. J R Soc Med 84:114, 1991

Stone HH, Chauvin EJ: Pancreatic denervation for pain relief in chronic alcohol associated pancreatitis. Br J Surg 77:303, 1990

Urschel HC Jr: Video-assisted sympathectomy and thoracic outlet syndrome. Chest Surg Clin North Am 3(2):299, 1993a

Urschel HC Jr: Dorsal sympathectomy and management of thoracic outlet syndrome with VATS. Ann Thorac Surg 56:717, 1993b

Urschel HC Jr, Razzuk MA: Posterior thoracic sympathectomy. In Malt RA (ed): Surgical Techniques Illustrated: a Comparative Atlas. WB Saunders, Philadelphia, 1985

60

SURGERY OF MYASTHENIA GRAVIS

Jeffrey A. Hagen
G. A. Patterson

DEFINITION

Myasthenia gravis is a neurologic disorder that is defined clinically on the basis of weakness or fatigability following repetitive exercise, which resolves with rest. It is an autoimmune disorder of neuromuscular transmission in which antibodies reduce the number of functional acetylcholine receptors at the neuromuscular junction. The clinical course in patients with myasthenia gravis is unpredictable, with frequent spontaneous remissions followed by relapses. The response to therapy is also unpredictable, and specifically with regard to thymectomy, it may be delayed.

The initiating events and the factors that sustain this autoimmune attack on the neuromuscular junction are unknown. The thymus gland is believed to play an important role for several reasons. First, it has been observed, especially in young patients, that the thymus gland is either hyperplastic or contains a thymoma in up to 80 percent of cases (Buckberg, et al., 1967). Second, antibodies to acetylcholine receptors (Almon, et al., 1974) and antibodies to other striated muscle antigens (Williams and Lennon, 1986) have been demonstrated in the thymus of patients with myasthenia. It is believed that the myoid cells present in the thymus may serve as the antigenic source of these autoantibodies. Finally, the importance of the thymus gland in the pathogenesis of myasthenia is supported by the beneficial effect observed following thymectomy.

Myasthenia gravis is a relatively uncommon disorder occurring in 0.5 to 5 per 100,000 population. It can occur at virtually any age; the peak age of onset is of 20 to 30 years in women and older than 50 in men. Overall it is more common in women; there is a female predominance of 3:2. The disease is nonfamilial in most cases. A genetic predisposition has been suggested, however, by the associations observed between histocompability antigen (HLA)-B8 and myasthenia gravis in young patients and by the association between HLA-A2 and -A3 and myasthenia associated with thymoma in older patients (Seybold and Lindstrom, 1982). The disease is more common in patients with other autoimmune disorders, such as Graves disease, Hashimoto's thyroiditis, rheumatoid arthritis, systemic lupus erythematosus, and pernicious anemia (Seybold, 1983). There are no known racial or geographic predilections.

Although the incidence in the general population is low, myasthenia gravis is one of the more common disorders of neuromuscular transmission and one of the most clearly understood physiologically. There remains a great deal of controversy, however, in regard to the diagnosis and therapy of this disorder. Much of this controversy is related specifically to the role of thymectomy in these patients.

HISTORICAL NOTE

Clinical recognition of the disorder now known as myasthenia gravis dates back to 1877 when Wilks (1877) reported on a patient with progressive weakness who ultimately died of respiratory paralysis. Autopsy revealed no evidence of a central nervous system cause. Over the next several years, similar case reports appeared in the literature of patients who died of respiratory paralysis without central nervous system causes. Goldflam (1893) summarized these case reports, along with his own collected series of patients. He described the clinical findings in common in these patients; these findings became known as the Erb-Goldflam symptom complex. Two years later, in his classic description of the decremental response to repetitive tetanic stimulation in these patients, Jolly (1895) coined the term *myasthenia gravis pseudoparalytica.*

The therapy of these patients dates back to 1934 when Walker (1934) first used anticholinesterase drug therapy. Following her subsequent report in 1935, prostigmine remained the drug of choice until Osserman, et al. (1954) reported on the use of pyridostigmine bromide, which remains the standard therapy to this day. The idea of surgical therapy of patients with myasthenia gravis began with the recognition by Weigert (1901) of a thymoma in a patient who died of myasthenia gravis. Subsequently Bell (1917) reported on a series of cases collected at autopsy, which revealed thymic abnormalities in 27 of 57 patients who died of myasthenia gravis. During this same period, the first thymectomy operations were being developed. Originally performed by the transcervical route, thymectomy was most often performed in patients with thyrotoxicosis. Von Haberer (1917) reported on 40 such operations, these included one performed in a patient with myasthenia gravis. Following thymectomy, the patient's myasthenic symptoms improved. It was Blalock, et al. (1939) who first intentionally removed the thymus in a young woman who had a thymoma and myasthenia gravis. The thymus was removed because of the tumor, not as specific therapy for her myasthenia. She experienced improvement in her myasthenic symptoms, which encouraged the performance of six more thymectomies in patients without thymomas that Blalock, et al. (1941) reported on in 1941. By 1944, Blalock (1944) had accumulated a total of 20 patients who had undergone thymectomy. He emphasized that the results were best in patients with a short duration of myasthenia, and he cited the importance of complete thymectomy, two observations that remain important to this day.

Although the initial surgical approach was transcervical, the work of Blalock and the series by Keynes (1955) that reported on 260 cases led to adoption of the median sternotomy approach. The transcervical method of thymectomy was reintroduced by Akakura (1965), Crile (1966), and Carlens, et al. (1967). This technique became attractive because it minimized surgical morbidity and increased patient acceptance. The major limitation to this approach was recognized by Henze, et al. (1984), who noted that removal of persistent thymic tissue in patients with persistent myasthenic symptoms following transcervical thymectomy led to substantial improvement in their symptoms. Recently modifications in technique, such as those reported by Cooper, et al. (1988), have resulted in improved exposure and more complete thymectomy by the transcervical route.

HISTORICAL READINGS

Blalock A: Thymectomy in the treatment of myasthenia gravis: report of twenty cases. J Thorac Cardiovasc Surg 13:316, 1944

Goldflam S: Ueber einen scheinbar heilbaren bulbar paralytischen symptomen Complex mit Beteiligung der Extremitaten. Dtsch Z Nervenheilkd 4:312, 1893

Keynes G: Investigations into thymic disease and tumor formation. Br J Surg 62:449, 1955

Walker MB: Treatment of myasthenia gravis with physostigmine. Lancet 1:1200, 1934

BASIC SCIENCE

To appreciate the important aspects of the diagnosis and therapy of patients with myasthenia gravis, it is important to have an understanding of a few fundamentals of the normal physiology of neuromuscular transmission. In contrast to the complex integration of impulses at other synapses, neuromuscular transmission involves a relatively simple process of relays between motor neuron terminals and the postsynaptic receptors on the muscle cell. In response to nerve stimulation and calcium entry into the motor neuron, acetylcholine is released. This diffuses across the synaptic cleft where it binds to receptors on the muscle cell (Fig. 60-1). Binding to the receptor creates an ion channel that allows the influx of positively charged ions, principally sodium, down the normal electrochemical gradient. This influx of positively charged ions results in localized depolarization of the muscle cell membrane, which is referred to as a miniature endplate potential. If the sum of several of these miniature endplate potentials is of sufficient amplitude, which is dependent on the amount of acetylcholine bound to receptors, the threshold for activation of the muscle cell is reached. This results in the generation of an action potential and calcium influx by activation of membrane calcium channels, which causes muscle contraction (Keesey, 1989).

Under normal circumstances, more acetylcholine is released from the motor neuron than is necessary to create an action potential in the muscle cell. In addition, many times the number of acetylcholine receptors are present on the motor endplate than are needed. These two factors provide a safety factor (Waud and Waud, 1975), which ensures neuromuscular transmission under normal circumstances. Alterations in this safety factor cause disorders of neuromuscular transmission, such as myasthenia gravis.

The autoimmune nature of myasthenia gravis was suggested by Seybold (1983), who identified antibodies to acetylcholine in up to 80 percent of patients with myasthenia gravis. Pestronk, et al. (1985) localized these antibodies to the neuromuscular junction in patients with myasthenia gravis, which further supports the autoimmune hypothesis. The number of acetylcholine receptors in these patients has also been shown to be reduced. The result is that, although normal amounts of acetylcholine are released from the motor neuron, the number of resultant miniature endplate potentials is decreased because of the reduced number of functional acetylcholine receptors. As a result, the endplate potentials generated may not reach the threshold for action potential generation. This results in failed neuromuscular transmission. Drachman, et al. (1980) proposed three mechanisms for this antibody-mediated interference in neuromuscular transmission. First, cross-linking of receptors may result in accelerated degradation of acetylcholine receptors. Second, antibodies may bind to receptor sites, which would render them unavailable for acetylcholine binding. Third, binding of antibodies may produce complement activation. This would result in degradation of the acetylcholine binding site.

This process of binding to or destruction of acetylcholine receptors is not uniform. As a result, two or more muscle fibers that are innervated by a single motor neuron may show variation in the number of miniature endplate potentials that occur in response to acetylcholine binding and hence in the timing of action-potential generation. This variability in action-potential formation is manifested on single-fiber electromyography (EMG) as "jitter," which is characteristic of myasthenia gravis. When this variability in response between muscle cells reaches 80 to 100 ms, one of the pair of muscle cells innervated by the motor neuron may not generate an action potential. This phenomenon, known as blocking, is

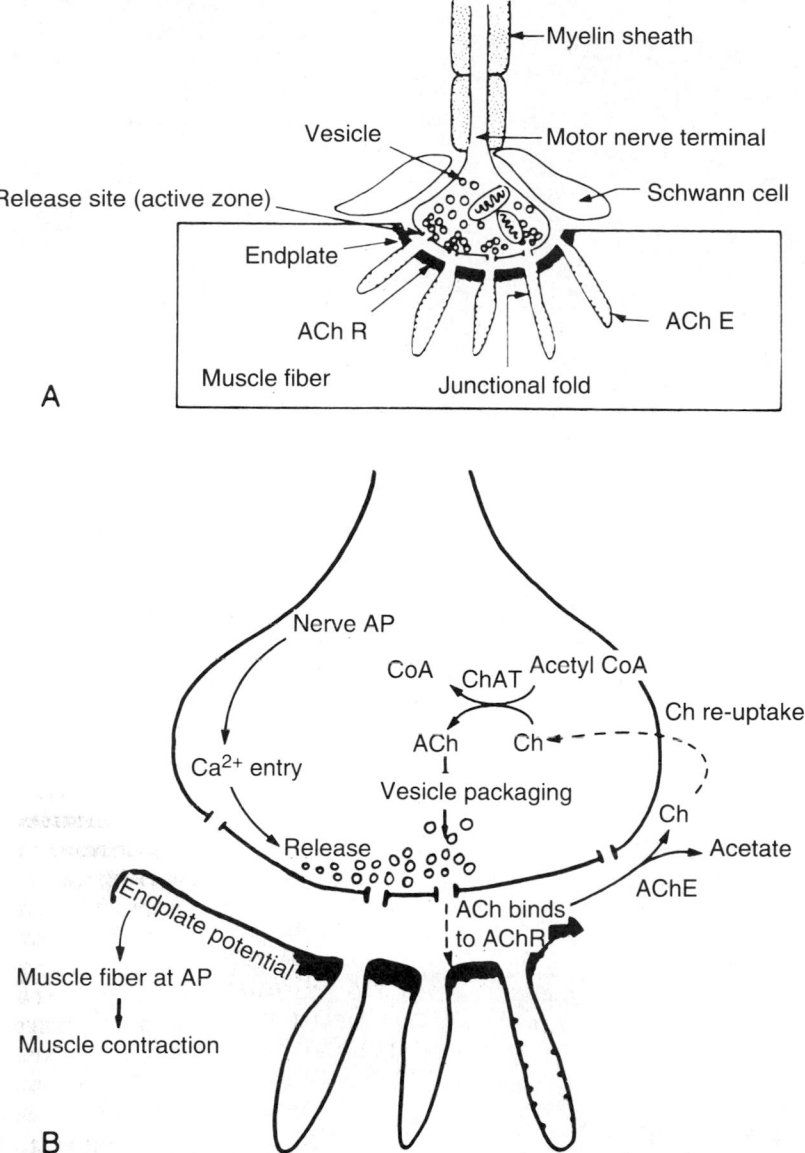

Figure 60-1. **(A)** Schematic representation of the neuromuscular junction. **(B)** Magnification showing details of the mechanisms of acetylcholine release, degradation, and binding to receptors, leading to muscle contraction. (From Pascuzzi RM: Introduction to the neuromuscular junction and neuromuscular transmission. Semin Neurol 10:1, 1990, with permission.)

the cellular cause for the decremental response to repetitive stimulation seen on standard electromyography, and it results in the fatigue seen following repetitive exercise in patients with myasthenia.

Pathologically, abnormalities of the thymus gland are well recognized in patients with myasthenia gravis. The most common abnormality seen is follicular lymphoid hyperplasia (Fig. 60-2), which is present in up to 60 percent of patients. These lymphoid follicles have been shown by Pahwa, et al. (1979) to contain B lymphocytes, which produce antibodies to acetylcholine receptors. An additional 10 to 25 percent of patients with myasthenia gravis have thymomas (Rivner and Swift, 1990), and 30 to 60 percent of patients with thymomas have myasthenia gravis. Given the high prevalence of thy-

moma, all patients whose conditions are diagnosed as myasthenia gravis should have a computed tomographic (CT) scan performed at the time of diagnosis. The thymus gland in a typical patient is depicted in Figure 60-3; this shows the uniform enlargement of the thymus without focal enlargement, which suggests a thymoma. The pathologic features of thymoma and the anatomic considerations of the thymus gland are considered in Chapters 58 and 59.

DIAGNOSIS

The diagnosis of myasthenia gravis is suspected on the basis of clinical findings of fluctuating weakness and early fatigue following repetitive exercise, which improves with rest. In

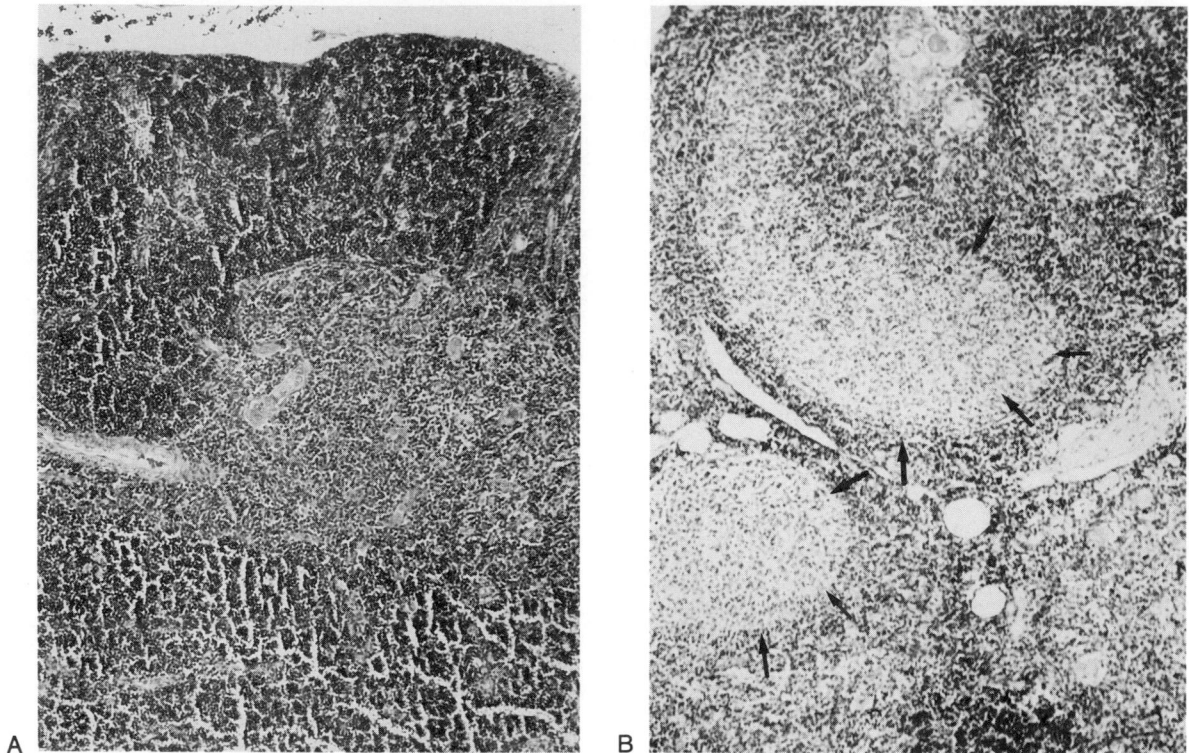

Figure 60-2. **(A)** Photomicrograph of normal thymus. Note the absence of lymphoid follicles (H&E, × 80). **(B)** Photomicrograph from a patient with myasthenia gravis. Note the prominent pale staining germinal centers *(arrows)* that represent follicular lymphoid hyperplasia (H&E, × 80).

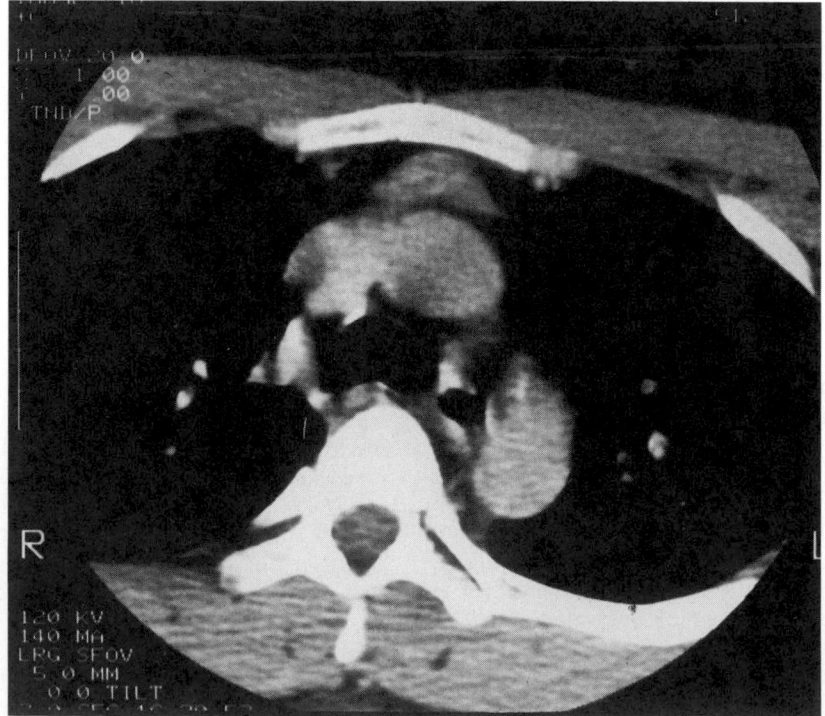

Figure 60-3. T scan with contrast revealing uniform enlargement of the thymus in a patient with myasthenia gravis.

individual patients the variability of the muscle groups involved and their extent of involvement over time is considerable. Typically symptoms begin with transient episodes of weakness, which become progressively more severe over time. Muscles innervated by cranial nerves are most commonly involved initially. This may result in ptosis and diplopia in the case of extraocular muscle involvement; weakness with prolonged mastication with involvement of jaw muscles; or dysphagia, choking, or nasal regurgitation. In 85 percent of patients, the disease progresses to generalized muscle involvement (Osserman and Genkins, 1971), which tends to involve proximal muscle groups predominantly, often in an asymmetric fashion. The weakness is often subtle and requires repetitive activity to allow detection. A convenient system to classify the pattern of clinical involvement was described by Osserman and Genkins (1971) and is depicted below.

The natural history of myasthenia gravis is not well documented; early studies suggest a mortality rate of 30 to 60 percent (Kennedy and Moersch, 1937). However, these studies were performed prior to the existence of intensive care units and the use of mechanical ventilation. More recent data in regard to the natural history are lacking because medical therapy with cholinesterase inhibitors became commonplace in 1934 and thymectomy has been used with increasing frequency since 1939.

A large retrospective series by Grob, et al. (1987) highlights some features of the natural history of this disease. They found that ocular complaints were the most common initial symptoms; they occurred in 53 perent of patients. Bulbar dysfunction occurred as the presenting symptom in 11 percent, leg weakness in 10 percent, and generalized muscle weakness in 9 percent. Within 1 month, only 40 percent of patients had purely ocular symptoms; generalized muscle weakness was present in 40 percent of patients. Long term, only 14 percent continued to have only ocular symptoms. The rate of progression to generalized weakness varied; 87 percent of patients had progression within the first year. They reported a spontaneous remission rate of 10 percent.

Similar findings in regard to the natural history were found by Bever, et al. (1983). Ocular symptoms were present in 84 percent; roughly one-half of patients had only ocular symptoms. Forty-nine percent of those who presented with ocular symptoms progressed to generalized weakness, with 85 percent doing so in the first 2 years. They also noted that 17 of 20 patients in whom myasthenic crisis developed did so within 2 years of the onset of disease. The rate of spontaneous remission was 17 percent; 30 percent of these occurred in the first year. However, spontaneous remission occurred as late as 13 years following the onset of illness.

The differential diagnosis of myasthenia gravis includes such disorders of neuromuscular transmission as botulism and the Lambert-Eaton syndrome. Botulism is a disease of neuromuscular transmission caused by the toxin of the bacterium *Clostridium botulinum*. The bacteria can either be ingested in contaminated food or can be produced in anaerobically infected wounds. The result is typically a descending paralysis that involves the eye muscles first and then the other muscles of the head and neck, followed by generalized skeletal muscle weakness. The defect in neuromuscular

---

Summary of Osserman and Genkins Classification System

I. Pediatric MG
  A. Neonatal MG (1%)
    1. Occurs in offspring of myasthenic mothers
    2. Self-limited (< 6 weeks)
    3. Due to placental transfer of antibodies
    4. Progression to juvenile or adult forms is rare
  B. Juvenile MG (9%)
    1. Onset from birth to puberty
    2. Tends to be permanent
    3. Differentiated from neonatal form by permanency and lack of maternal disease
    4. Subclassified by nature and degree of defect as in adult forms

II. Adult MG
  A. Ocular MG (20%)
    1. Disease limited to ocular involvement
    2. Carries excellent prognosis
    3. Rarely progresses after 2 years of isolated ocular symptoms
  B. Mild generalized MG (30%)
    1. Initial ocular symptoms progress gradually to generalized symptoms
    2. Respiratory muscles are spared
    3. Good response to medical therapy
  C. Moderate generalized MG (20%)
    1. More severe generalized involvement
    2. Bulbar symptoms are common
    3. Relative sparing of respiratory muscles
    4. Less responsive to medical therapy
  D. Acute fulminating MG (11%)
    1. Rapid onset of severe generalized weakness
    2. Prominent respiratory symptoms
    3. Highest association with thymoma
    4. Mortality high rate
    5. Poor response to therapy
  E. Late severe MG (9%)
    1. Patients with severe symptoms developing more than 2 years after onset of ocular or mild myasthenia gravis
    2. Thymoma common
    3. Poor response to therapy

MG, myasthenia gravis.

(From Osserman KE, Genkins G: Studies in myasthenia gravis: review of twenty year experience in over 1200 patients. Mt Sinai J Med 38:497, 1971, with permission.)

---

transmission involves impairment of acetylcholine release from the motor neurons (Simpson, 1986) in contrast to the impaired binding to receptors seen in myasthenia gravis. EMG in these patients reveals an incremental response to repetitive testing.

The Lambert-Eaton syndrome is a myasthenic syndrome that involves fluctuating weakness of the proximal muscle groups. The weakness may involve the facial muscles, but to a lesser extent than seen in myasthenia gravis. This syndrome, presumed to be autoimmune in origin, is associated with an underlying malignancy in most cases. Small cell cancer is the most common; it occurs in 70 percent of patients (Lambert, 1986). In contrast to patients with myasthenia gravis, patients with Lambert-Eaton syndrome have diminished deep tendon reflexes, and autonomic symptoms are fairly common. EMG shows an incremental response in the compound muscle action potential compared with the decremental response seen in myasthenia gravis.

Although suggested as the basis of symptoms, the diagnosis of myasthenia gravis is confirmed electrophysiologically on the basis of testing, pharmacologically by the response to acetylcholinesterase drugs, or immunologically based on antibody levels. None of these tests give uniformly positive results in all patients with myasthenia gravis.

Since the first description of the classic decremental response on EMG by Harvey and Masland (1941), the techniques of EMG have been refined, which has improved the accuracy of this test in myasthenia gravis. Phillips and Melnick (1990) recently reviewed the diagnostic tests applicable in patients with myasthenia gravis. For all patients with myasthenia, they found a sensitivity rate of 34 percent for standard EMG; there was a sensitivity rate of 76 percent in patients with generalized disease. A technique of single-fiber EMG has been developed, which by the detection of jitter or blocking, may allow the identification of subclinical cases of myasthenia gravis. Single-fiber EMG may also improve the sensitivity and specificity of EMG testing. It has been shown to have abnormal findings in approximately 90 percent of patients with mild generalized myasthenia and in virtually 100 percent of those with moderate to severe disease (Massey, 1990). In patients with isolated ocular myasthenia, single-fiber EMG gives positive results in 60 to 75 percent (Stalberg and Sanders, 1981).

Shortly after EMG was introduced as a diagnostic test, the use of short-acting edrophonium (Tensilon) was introduced by Osserman and Kaplan (1952) as a diagnostic test for myasthenia gravis. When administered intravenously, Tensilon results in significant improvement in muscle strength, usually within 30 to 60 seconds. Although the exact sensitivity and specificity are unknown, Phillips and Melnick (1990) estimate a sensitivity of 85 percent for ocular myasthenia gravis and 95 percent for generalized myasthenia.

Finally, the diagnosis of myasthenia gravis can be confirmed on the basis of elevated acetylcholine antibody titers. First detected by Almon, et al. (1974), the presence of elevated titers of acetylcholine antibodies is highly specific for myasthenia gravis. The sensitivity ranges from 64 percent in patients with ocular disease to as high as 89 percent in patients with generalized disease (Phillips and Melnick, 1990).

MANAGEMENT

The therapeutic options for patients with myasthenia gravis include medical therapy with anticholinesterase medication, immunosuppression, plasma exchange, and surgical therapy by thymectomy (Finley and Pascuzzi, 1990). There is considerable controversy with regard to the various combinations of these therapies and their sequence of use. Much of this controversy centers around difficulties in classifying the extent of disease to allow a comparison of various modes of therapy. In addition, the variable natural history of this disease, with its remissions and relapses, makes the benefits of any therapeutic modality difficult to discern.

Drug Therapy

Although it has no direct effect on the underlying disease, anticholinesterase therapy can lead to substantial improvement in symptoms in patients with myasthenia gravis. These drugs work by decreasing the hydrolysis of acetylcholine at the motor endplate. Pyridostigmine (Mestinon) is the most commonly used agent; it has a relatively long duration of action. Neostigmine, with its more rapid onset and shorter duration of action, may be more useful in the perioperative period. Edrophonium (Tensilon), with its rapid onset and short duration of action, is used mostly as a diagnostic test. The optimum doses of these preparations vary widely from patient to patient and require careful adjustment to achieve the maximal response while the muscarinic side effects of abdominal cramping, diarrhea, excessive salivation, diaphoresis, and bradycardia are minimized.

A particularly feared complication of cholinesterase inhibition therapy is the development of a so-called cholinergic crisis. The mechanism for this profound weakness is unknown, but it may be due to excessive accumulation of acetylcholine at the neuromuscular junction, which results in a depolarizing blockade. Differentiation of this drug-induced cholinergic crisis from myasthenia crisis on clinical grounds can be difficult. The administration of the short-acting drug edrophonium results in an improvement in strength in patients who have a myasthenic crisis; there is no improvement in those with a cholinergic crisis. This method allows these two conditions to be differentiated in most cases.

Corticosteroid therapy has been reported to result in improvement in up to 80 percent of patients with myasthenia gravis (Pascuzzi, et al. 1984), although no controlled trials exist to document this benefit. Usually reserved for patients who do not respond to anticholinesterase therapy or those in whom intolerable side effects develop, steroids have also been used in the preparation of patients for thymectomy. The side effects of long-term corticosteroid therapy limit their usefulness, and relapses are common following discontinuation.

Immunosuppression with azathioprine has also been advocated as an alternative in patients who do not respond to, or are intolerant of, anticholinesterase therapy. Again, there are relatively few controlled studies to document the usefulness of azathioprine, although response rates in retrospective studies range from 71 percent (Matell, 1987) to 83 percent (Witte, et al., 1984). Side effects are common and lead to a dosage reduction or discontinuation of therapy in many patients.

The role of plasma pheresis to treat myasthenia remains uncertain. Although Pinching, et al. (1976) and several others have reported successful clinical results with this technique, no controlled trials have been performed to document this benefit. Typically four or five exchanges are required over 10 days to 2 weeks to obtain a clinical response, which typically lasts 2 to 3 weeks. The most common indications for plasma pheresis are in myasthenia crisis to assist in weaning the patient from mechanical ventilation and in the preparation for thymectomy in patients with severe generalized weakness. Cost, and the prevalence of complications, prohibit the use of this technique for long-term management of myasthenia gravis.

Thymectomy

Following the report by Blalock et al., in 1941, a number of series have been reported that demonstrate a favorable response to thymectomy in patients with myasthenia gravis. Although it is generally agreed that thymectomy is beneficial to many patients, its precise role in the therapy of patients with myasthenia gravis remains uncertain because of the lack of controlled studies to identify those patients who are likely to respond. In addition, the mechanism by which thymectomy exerts its beneficial effect is unknown. Most authors consider patients for thymectomy when medical therapy is unsuccessful or when side effects limit the usefulness of medication. In addition, many authors (Jaretzki, et al., 1988; Cooper, et al. 1988) consider patients for operation early in the presence of generalized symptoms. This is based on the observation, made initially by Blalock (1944), and repeatedly observed by others, that the patient with a short duration of illness is most likely to benefit from an operation.

Prior to the operation, the patient's symptoms should be controlled medically, usually by anticholinesterase therapy. In some cases, steroids are administered, although if possible these are to be avoided by using preoperative plasma pheresis instead. Particular attention should be paid to pulmonary mechanics, especially if a sternotomy is contemplated. A CT scan is performed in all cases to rule out the presence of thymoma. The choice of operation varies from transcervical thymectomy, as advocated by Kirshner, et al. (1969) and Cooper, et al. (1988), to a more radical thymectomy performed through a median sternotomy, as advocated by Jaretzki, et al. (1988). Advocates of the transcervical approach emphasize the decreased morbidity associated with the less invasive procedure, although satisfactory remission and response rates are still achieved, which are comparable to those seen following transsternal resection (Table 60-1). Jaretzki,

Table 60-1. Results of Recent Series of Thymectomy for Myasthenia Gravis

Author	Remission (%)	Benefit (%)	Mortality Rate (%)	Morbidity Rate (%)
Jaretzki, et al. 1977–85 (1988)	40	94	0	7
Mulder, et al. 1954–81 (1983)	51	87	1	N/A
Mulder, et al. 1981–87 (1989)	36	80	0	N/A
Huang, et al. 1977–84 (1988)	46	95	0	12
Halton, et al. 1972–87 (1989)	28	72	2	15
Cooper, et al. 1977–86 (1988)	52	95	0	2

[a] Refers to total number of patients with improved symptoms or complete remission.

et al. (1977), citing the common anomalies of thymic anatomy, emphasized the importance of removing all adjacent mediastinal fat that might contain aberrant thymic tissue. Because there are no direct comparative studies, the optimal surgical technique remains to be identified. There is no doubt, however, that the single most important principle of surgical therapy, regardless of the approach taken, is the complete removal of the thymus.

Transsternal Thymectomy

The technique of transsternal thymectomy involves the performance of a standard median sternotomy. The mediastinal extension of the deep cervical fascia is identified on the undersurface of the sternothyroid muscle. This fascia layer is incised at the midline to expose the thymus gland. Each lower pole is then dissected bluntly from the undersurface of this fascia, from the pericardium posteriorly, and from the extrapleural fascia laterally. As the dissection proceeds superiorly, one or two arterial branches to the thymus that arise from the internal mammary arteries are identified and divided. When the dissection is continued superiorly, with downward traction on the gland, the superior poles can be brought into the wound. At the apex of each superior pole, there is usually an arterial branch, which arises from the inferior thyroid artery. Finally, blunt dissection posterior to the gland separates the thymus from the innominate vein. It is here that the venous drainage, that is, one or two branches that drain directly into the innominate vein, can be ligated. The anterior mediastinum is drained (as are the pleural spaces if they are entered), and the wound is closed with sternal wires and appropriate subcutaneous and skin sutures.

Maximal Thymectomy

The "maximal thymectomy" approach described by Jaretzki, et al. (1988) combines a horizontal cervical incision with a median sternotomy to allow "removal of all thymic tissue predictably." This approach was based on their observations in regard to the variability of the anatomy of the thymus that were published in 1977 (Jaretzki, et al., 1977). In this operation, all mediastinal tissue anterior to the pericardium and great vessels is removed. The dissection extends laterally to a point located posterior to the phrenic nerves. The resection includes removal of the mediastinal pleura. In the neck, the upper poles are removed en bloc with the adjacent fatty tissue. They reported complete remission rates of 46 percent and an overall response rate of 96 percent in first-time operations when this technique was used.

Transcervical Thymectomy

The transcervical approach, because of its less invasive nature, has continued to receive interest. As mentioned, this was the initial approach historically; it was replaced by the transsternal approach by Blalock (1944) and others. Interest in the transcervical approach was rekindled by articles by Carlens, et al. (1967), Crile (1966), and Akakura (1965). Kirshner, et al. (1969) reported on 40 patients treated by transcervical thymectomy, and this was soon followed by a report by Papatestas, et al. (1987) that involved more than

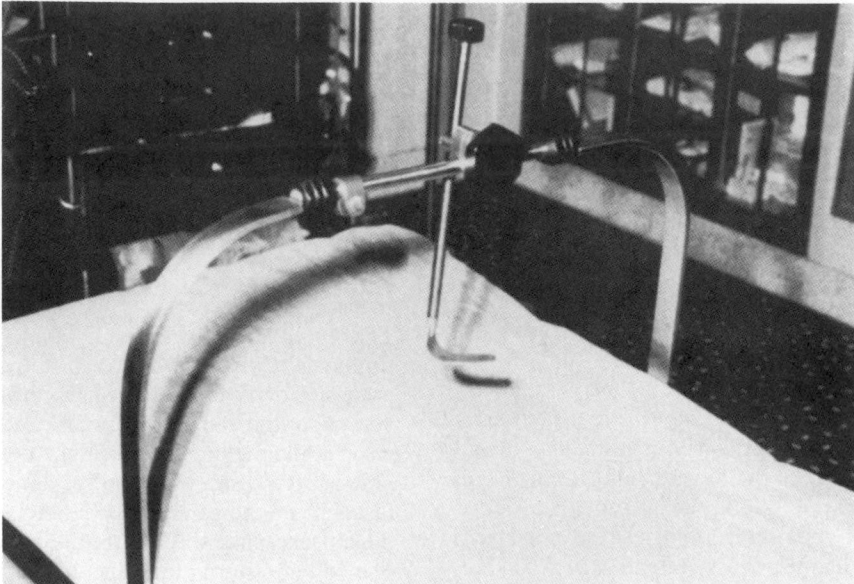

Figure 60-4. Specially designed right-angle retractor attached to an overhead bar. The retractor is placed behind the manubrium to provide upward lift on the sternum. (From Cooper JD, Al-Silaihana AN, Pearson FG et al: An improved technique to facilitate transcervical thymectomy for myasthenia gravis. Ann Thorac Surg 45:242, 1988, with permission.)

700 cases of myasthenia treated by transcervical thymectomy. The technique was further enhanced by a report by Cooper, et al. (1988) of the use of a specially designed retractor, which facilitates exposure to ensure a more complete transcervical thymectomy.

The operative technique is as follows. The patient is placed supine with the shoulders elevated on an inflatable bag and the head resting at the top of the operating table in a "donut." An intravenous line is placed in the right arm, and the blood pressure is measured on the patient's left arm. The patient should be prepared as if a sternotomy is to be performed should it become necessary. The skin incision is made along a skin crease approximately 2 cm above the sternal notch; this is extended laterally to each sternocleidomastoid muscle. Flaps are raised superiorly to the level of the thyroid gland and inferiorly to the level of the sternum, in a plane beneath the platysma. The strap muscles are split vertically at the midline, and the thymus gland is identified immediately beneath the sternothyroid muscle. The uppermost aspect of the left upper pole is identified near the inferior thyroid vein where it is ligated. The ligature is left attached for purposes of traction. The right upper pole is similarly dissected and ligated prior to division. The upper poles are then bluntly dissected free to the level of the sternal notch where they typically fuse anterior to the innominate vein. A finger is inserted into the mediastinum anterior to the gland to dissect it from the undersurface of the sternum. When the superior pole is retracted anteriorly at this point, the veins that drain to the innominate vein are easily identified, ligated, and divided.

At this point a specially designed narrow right-angle retractor is placed beneath the sternum (Cooper Thymectomy Retractor, Pilling Company, Ft. Washington, PA) and attached to a Poly-Tract (Pilling Company) overhead bar (Fig. 60-4). After the sternum is lifted with this apparatus, the inflatable pillow beneath the shoulders is deflated; this allows the shoulders to fall backward and improves the exposure. When this technique is used, the entire mediastinal portion of the thymus can be dissected under direct vision. The dissection begins on the right lateral aspect of the gland and extends inferiorly to the limits of the right lower pole. The gland is then swept off the anterior surface of the aorta and pericardium, which mobilizes finally the left lower pole and includes the tail of tissue, which often extends downward toward the aortopulmonary window. After the gland has been removed entirely (Fig. 60-5), the remaining mediastinal fat is removed

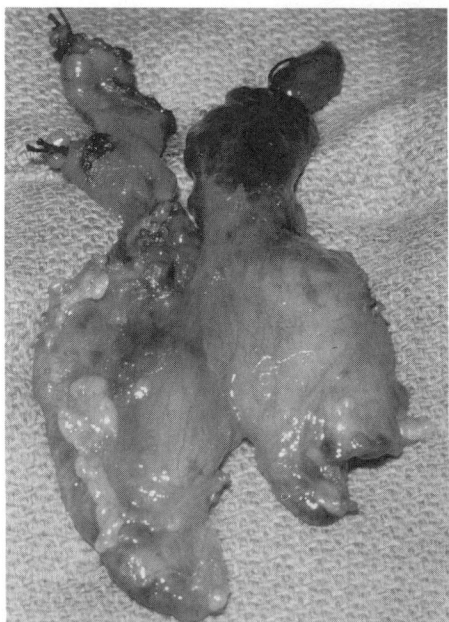

Figure 60-5. Photograph of thymectomy specimen from patient in Figure 60-3, removed by transcervical thymectomy.

on both sides extending to the mediastinal pleura. The wound is then closed in layers over a red rubber catheter. This catheter is removed as the platysma is closed, with the lungs held in static inflation. With this technique, a chest tube is rarely required, even if one or both pleural spaces were entered.

Postoperative Care

The essentials of postoperative care center around early extubation, aggressive attention to the patient's pulmonary status, and early ambulation, whether a transmediastinal or transcervical approach has been used. Anticholinesterase medication is resumed when the patient is extubated; attempts to wean patients from medical therapy are delayed for several weeks following the procedure. Early postoperative results from this approach have been satisfying, with mortality rates in the range of 0 to 2 percent and morbidity rates between 2 and 15 percent of patients in the recently reported series (Table 60-1).

Results of Surgery

The long-term results of thymectomy in patients with myasthenia gravis are more difficult to identify with precision. This is due in part to the uncertainty in regard to the natural history of untreated myasthenia gravis, the unpredictable rate of progression of disease, and the unpredictable occurrence of spontaneous remission. In addition, a comparison between series is complicated by difficulties encountered in classifying the extent of disease in a given patient population. In a large retrospective series published by Buckingham, et al. (1976) that compared medical versus surgical therapy, the authors found complete remission in 33 percent of patients following thymectomy compared with an 8 percent complete remission rate with medical therapy. There was also a significant survival advantage associated with the performance of thymectomy.

With regard to patients with isolated ocular symptoms, the results of surgical therapy are less clear. One study, published by Schumm, et al. (1985), reported on 18 patients, with clinical improvement noted in 80 percent and a complete remission rate of 17 percent. These results are slightly less than the rate of clinical improvement and complete remission observed following thymectomy for generalized disease but compare favorably with the results of medical therapy.

Specific predictors of improvement following thymectomy were addressed in a recent publication by Frist, et al. (1994), which reported a series of 46 patients. Age younger than 45 years was found to be an independent predictor of improved outcome following thymectomy. However, other series, such as those of Olanow, et al. (1987) and Papatestas, et al. (1987) have found no association between age and outcome. Female gender was also identified in this series as an independent predictor of a favorable response to surgery. This finding was also observed by Hatton, et al. (1989), but not in the series by Jaretzki, et al. (1988) or Papatestas, et al. (1987). The preoperative stage of disease was found to predict a favorable outcome in Frist, et al.,'s (1994) series. In most recent series, the duration of symptoms alone does not appear to be an independent predictor of outcome (Frist, et al., 1994; Huang, et al., 1988; Jaretzki, et al., 1988. The presence of a thymoma is in general believed to be associated with lesser degrees of improvement following resection compared with that in nonthymomatous myasthenia gravis.

COMMENTS AND CONTROVERSIES

Although it has been nearly 100 years since the condition was first recognized and more than 50 years since the medical and surgical therapies were defined, there remains a great deal of uncertainty in regard to the diagnosis, natural history, and therapy of myasthenia gravis. At present, the diagnosis depends not on the results of any single test, but rather on a battery of test findings combined with careful clinical evaluation. Because there are no controlled trials, the optimal combination of therapeutic strategies remains undefined.

Recent advances in the understanding of the immunology of this disorder may resolve some of the uncertainty in regard to the therapy of these patients as specific immunotherapy becomes available. On the surgical side, thoracoscopic removal of the thymus has been described (Sugarbaker, 1993); however, proof of its usefulness awaits large-scale application, which would include follow-up data. Complete thymectomy by a lesser procedure, such as transcervical or video-assisted thoracoscopic thymectomy, has the obvious attraction of being more acceptable to patients at an earlier stage of disease. It appears that the earlier resection is undertaken, the better the result will be.

J.A.H.
G.A.P.

Despite the fact that the three approaches that are now accepted for thymectomy for myasthenia gravis (transsternal, maximal, and transcervical) have been in use for up to 50 years, there is no unanimity of opinion as to which is the best approach. All three techniques seem to have similar long-term results. Whether or not every last thymocyte has to be removed to obtain these results is really unknown.

The recent introduction of video-assisted thoracoscopic techniques to remove the thymus gland does not take into account the cervical extension of the gland. Proponents of this approach are now adding a cervical incision to remove the upper poles. It would seem to be wiser to use video-assisted techniques when a transcervical approach has difficulty reaching the lowest regions of the inferior poles and when difficulty arises in removing them. It is fair to say, however, that most surgeons still practice transsternal total thymectomy but not the maximal approach of Jaretzki, et al. (1988).

An interesting phenomenon is the occasional occurrence of myasthenia gravis following the removal of thymomas. This seems to be most prevalent when a thymoma is removed without the addition of a complete thymectomy.

H.C.U.

KEY REFERENCES

Finley JC, Pascuzzi RM: Rational therapy of myasthenia gravis. Semin Neurol 10:70, 1990

This is a thorough discussion of the natural history of, and therapeutic options available for, myasthenia gravis. It includes an extensive list of references that cover all available therapeutic modalities.

Keesey JC: Electrodiagnostic approach to defects in neuromuscular transmission. Muscle Nerve 12:613, 1989

This is a comprehensive reference that summarizes the rationale behind the use of single-fiber EMG and repetitive nerve stimulation in diseases of neuromuscular transmission.

Osserman KE, Genkins G: Studies in myasthenia gravis: review of a twenty year experience in over 1200 patients. Mt Sinai J Med 38:497, 1971

This classic reference includes observations in regard to the important aspects of diagnosis and therapy of patients with myasthe-

nia gravis from the myasthenia gravis clinic at Mount Sinai Hospital. A classification system is described, and the results of therapy are outlined based on the largest reported series of myasthenic patients.

Pascuzzi RM: Introduction to the neuromuscular junction and neuromuscular transmission. Semin Neurol 10:1, 1990

This is a concise informative overview of the mechanisms of neuromuscular transmission. It includes a discussion of the principles of EMG.

Phillips LH, Melnick PA: Diagnosis of myasthenia gravis in the 1990's. Semin Neurol 10:62, 1990

A concise summary of the diagnostic tests available for myasthenia gravis, this article includes the rationale behind their application, an interesting analysis of the clinical decision-making process, and a proposed decision-making strategy.

REFERENCES

Akakura I: Mediastinoscopy. Presented at the XI International Congress of Bronchoesophagology, Hakone, Japan, 6, 1965.

Almon RR, Andrew AG, Appel SH: Serum globulin in myasthenia gravis: inhibition of l-bungarotoxin to acetylcholine receptors. Science 186:55, 1974

Bell ET: Tumors of the thymus in myasthenia gravis. J Nerv Ment Dis 45:130, 1917

Bever CT Jr, Aquino AV, Penn AS et al.: Prognosis of ocular myasthenia. Ann Neurol 14:516, 1983

Blalock A: Thymectomy in the treatment of myasthenia gravis: report of twenty cases. J Thorac Cardiovasc Surg 13:316, 1944

Blalock A, Harvey AM, Ford RF, Lilienthal JL Jr: The treatment of myasthenia gravis by removal of the thymus gland. JAMA 117:1529, 1941

Blalock A, Mason MF, Morgan HJ, Riven SS: Myasthenia gravis and tumors of the thymic region. Report of a case in which the tumor was removed. Ann Surg 110:544, 1939

Buckberg GD, Herrmann C, Dillon JR, Mulder DG: A further evaluation of thymectomy for myasthenia gravis. J Thorac Cardiovasc Surg 53:401, 1967

Buckingham JM, Howard FM Jr, Bernatz PE et al.: The value of thymectomy in myasthenia gravis: a computer assisted matched study. Ann Surg 184:453, 1976

Carlens E, Johansson L, Olsson P: Mediastinoscopy auxiliary to thymectomy by the cervical route. Bronches 17:408, 1967

Crile G Jr: Thymectomy through the neck. Surgery 59:213, 1966

Cooper JD, Al-Jilaihawa AN, Pearson FG et al.: An improved technique to facilitate transcervical thymectomy for myasthenia gravis. Ann Thorac Surg 45:242, 1988

Drachman DB, Adams RN, Stanley EF, Pestronk A: Mechanisms of acetylcholine receptor loss in myasthenia gravis. J Neurol Neurosurg Psychiatry 43:601, 1980

Frist WH, Thirumalai S, Doehring CB et al.: Thymectomy for the myasthenia gravis patient: factors influencing outcome. Ann Thorac Surg 57:334, 1994

Goldflam S: Ueber einen scheinbar heilbaren bulbar paralytischen symptomen Complex mit Beteiligung der Extremitaten. Dtsch Z Nervenheilkd 4:312, 1893

Grob D, Arsura EL, Brunner NG, Namba T: The course of myasthenia gravis and therapies affecting outcome. Ann N Y Acad Sci 505:472, 1987

Hatton PD, Diehl JP, Daly BDP et al.: Transsternal radical thymectomy for myasthenia gravis: a 15 year review. Ann Thorac Surg 47:838, 1989

Harvey AM, Masland RL: The electromyogram in myasthenia gravis. Bull Johns Hopkins Hosp 69:1, 1941

Henze A, Biberfeld P, Christensson B et al.: Failing transcervical thymectomy in myasthenia gravis: an evaluation of transternal re-exploration. Scand J Thorac Cardiovasc Surg 18:235, 1984

Huang M, King K, Ksu W et al.: The outcome of thymectomy in nonthymomatous myasthenia gravis. Surg Gynecol Obstet 166:436, 1988

Jaretzki A, Bethea M, Wolff M et al.: A rational approach to total thymectomy in the treatment of myasthenia gravis. Ann Thorac Surg 24:120, 1977

Jaretzki A, Penn AS, Younger DS et al.: "Maximal" thymectomy for myasthenia gravis. J Thorac Cardiovasc Surg 95:747, 1988

Jolly F: Ueber Myasthenia gravis pseudoparalytica. Klin Wochenschr 32:1, 1895

Kennedy FS, Moersch FP: Myasthenia gravis: a clinical review of 87 cases observed between 1915 and the early part of 1932. Can Med Assoc J 37:217, 1937.

Keynes G: Investigations into thymic disease and tumor formation. Br J Surg 62:449, 1955

Kirschner PA, Osserman KE, Kark AE: Studies in myasthenia gravis: transcervical total thymectomy. JAMA 209:906, 1969

Lambert EH: The Lambert-Eaton myasthenic syndrome: clinical features and pathophysiology. Presented at the Seventh International Conference on Myasthenia Gravis, New York Academy of Sciences, New York, March 6, 1986

Massey JM: Electromyography in disorders of neuromuscular transmission. Semin Neurol 10:6, 1990

Matell G: Immunosuppressive drugs: azathioprine in the treatment of myasthenia gravis. Ann N Y Acad Sci 505:588, 1987

Mulder DG, Graves M, Herrmann C: Thymectomy for myasthenia gravis: recent observations and comparisons with past experience. Ann Thorac Surg 48:551, 1989

Mulder DG, Herrmann C Jr, Keesey J, Edwards H: Thymectomy for myasthenia gravis. Am J Surg 146:61, 1983

Olanow CW, Wechsler AS, Siratkin-Roses M et al.: Thymectomy as primary therapy in myasthenia gravis. Ann N Y Acad Sci 505:595, 1987

Osserman KE, Kaplan LI: Rapid diagnostic test for myasthenia gravis: increased muscle strength without fasciculations after intravenous administration of edrophonium (Tensilon) chloride. JAMA 150:265, 1952

Osserman KE, Teng P, Kaplan LI: Studies in myasthenia gravis: preliminary report on therapy with mestinon bromide. JAMA 155:961, 1954

Pahwa R, Ikehara S, Pahwa SG, Good RA: Thymic function in man. Thymus 1:27, 1979

Papatestas AE, Genkins G, Kornfeld P et al.: Effects of thymectomy in myasthenia gravis. Ann Surg 206:79, 1987

Pascuzzi RM, Coslett HB, Johns TR: Long-term corticosteroid treatment of myasthenia gravis: report of 116 patients. Ann Neurol 15:291, 1984

Pestronk A, Drachman DB, Self SG: Measurement of junctional acetylcholine receptors in myasthenia gravis: clinical correlates. Muscle Nerve 8:245, 1985

Pinching AJ, Peters DK, Newsom-Davis J: Remission of myasthenia gravis following plasma exchange. Lancet 2:1373, 1976

Rivner MH, Swift TR: Thymoma: diagnosis and management. Semin Neurol 10:83, 1990

Schumm JF, Wietholter H, Fateh-Moghadam A, Dichgans J: Thymectomy in myasthenia with pure ocular symptoms. J Neurol Neurosurg Psychiatry 48:332, 1985

Seybold ME: Myasthenia gravis: a clinical and basic science review. JAMA 250:2516, 1983

Seybold ME, Lindstrom JM: Immunopathology of acetylcholine receptors in myasthenia gravis. Springer Semin Immunopathol 5:389, 1982

Simpson LL: Molecular pharmacology of botulinum toxin and tetanus toxin. Annu Rev Pharmacol Toxicol 26:427, 1986

Stalberg E, Sanders DB: Electrophysiologic tests of neuromuscular transmission. In Stalberg E, Young RR (eds): Clinical Neurophysiology. Butterworth, London, 1981

Sugarbaker DJ: Thoracoscopy in the management of anterior mediastinal masses. Ann Thorac Surg 56:653, 1993

Von Haberer A: Zur klinischen Bedeutung der Thymus Drüse. Arch Klin Chir 109:193, 1917

Walker MB: Treatment of myasthenia gravis with physostigmine. Lancet 1:1200, 1934

Waud DR, Waud BE: In vitro measurement of margin of safety of neuromuscular transmission. Am J Physiol 229:1632, 1975

Weigert C: Pathologisch-anatomischer Beitrag zur Erb-schen Krankheit (myasthenia gravis). Neurol Zentralbl 20:597, 1901

Wilks S: On cerebritis, hysteria and bulbar paralysis. Guy's Hosp Rep 22:7, 1877

Williams CL, Lennon VA: Thymic B lymphocyte clones from patients with myasthenia gravis secrete monoclonal striational antibodies reacting with myosin, alpha actin, or actin. J Exp Med 164:1043, 1986

Witte AS, Cornblath DR, Parry GJ et al.: Azathioprine in the treatment of myasthenia gravis. Ann Neurol 15:602, 1984

61

PATHOPHYSIOLOGY AND INITIAL MANAGEMENT

David A. Fullerton
Frederick L. Grover
Martin F. McKneally

The spectrum of traumatic chest injuries is broad, ranging from simple rib fractures to exsanguinating major vascular injuries. Approximately 25 percent of traumatic deaths result from chest injury, yet more than 85 percent of chest injuries undergoing hospital evaluation are appropriately managed with no more than a closed-tube thoracostomy (Lewis, 1982). It is important to emphasize that two-thirds of all traumatic deaths secondary to chest injuries occur after the patient reaches the hospital and may therefore be preventable. Herein lies the challenge to the thoracic trauma surgeon, that is, maintaining a high index of suspicion in the evaluation of thoracic trauma to avoid missing the uncommon lethal injury.

HISTORICAL NOTE

Thoracic trauma has been an integral component of medicine, providing the foundation for understanding of the physiology of the chest for more than 5,000 years. The Smith Papyrus, written prior to 3000 B.C., contains reports of three chest injuries: two large penetrating wounds treated with a wound covering of fresh meat, grease, honey, and lint and rib fractures for which no treatment was advised (Breasted, 1930). Homer described a variety of chest wounds sustained during the siege of Troy in 950 B.C., including death from a penetrating cardiac injury. Theodoric espoused the advantages of primary closure of chest wall wounds in 1267 (Campbell and Colton, 1955). In 1346 firearms were first used in the battle of Crecy (Meade, 1961). Since that time gunshot wounds to the chest have continued to grow in medical importance, both during war and in civilian life. In the Crimean War, it was estimated that 6 to 8 percent of all wounds were blunt and penetrating chest wounds, with a 79 percent mortality rate. In the American Civil War, the incidence was 8 percent of all wounds, with a 63 percent mortality rate. In World War I, chest wounds accounted for approximately 2 to 5 percent of wounds, with a 25 percent mortality rate. In World War II, rapid evacuation of the wounded, recommended originally by Napoleon's surgeon Larrey (1700s) and by Letterman during the American Civil War, was instituted. In World War II, the incidence of chest wounds was about 8 percent, with only a 12 percent mortality rate. This drop in mortality rate during World War II was attributed to the physiologic principle of immediate closure of chest wounds and major advances in the immediate therapy of the wounded. The placement of thoracic surgeons in military field hospitals also contributed to this improvement in survival (Meade, 1961). These principles were furthered in subsequent wars. The mortality rate from penetrating thoracic wounds in the Viet Nam War was estimated to be as low as 2 percent.

HISTORICAL READINGS

Breasted JH: The Edwin Smith Surgical Papyrus. University of Chicago Press, Chicago, 1930
Campbell E, Colton J: The Surgery of Theodoric. Appleton-Century-Crofts, Norwalk, CT, 1955
Meade RH: A History of Thoracic Surgery. Charles C Thomas, Springfield, IL, 1961

PATHOPHYSIOLOGY

The immediate objective of all trauma care is resuscitation of cardiac and pulmonary physiology to restore and maintain oxygen delivery to vital organs. Trauma to the chest may have immediate and uniquely life-threatening physiologic consequences because of the close relationship between the structure of the thoracic cavity and the physiologic function of the heart and lungs.

Because the physiology of the chest is central to the survival to the patient, appropriate therapy of thoracic injuries should be physiologically based. An understanding of the cardiovascular and pulmonary pathophysiology produced by chest trauma provides a rationale for therapy. The pulmonary insufficiency and cardiovascular compromise produced by a relatively large variety of chest injuries are ultimately mediated through common pathophysiologic mechanisms.

Pulmonary insufficiency and respiratory distress produced by chest injuries ultimately result from disturbance of the mechanics of ventilation or from ventilation/perfusion mismatching. The mechanics of ventilation are dependent on the structural integrity and ridigity of the thorax and airway. A problem with the mechanics of ventilation is easily recognized when the flow of air into the lung is precluded by injury to the larynx or trachea, resulting in airway collapse.

The loss of integrity of the rigid thorax and mechanical interference with pleural dynamics by blood or air in the pleural space are more subtle mechanical problems that must be considered, diagnosed, and treated. For inspiration to occur, a pressure gradient from the mouth to the alveoli must be generated. Alveolar pressure is atmospheric, and the intrapleural pressure is subatmospheric in the uninjured chest. This subatmospheric pressure is generated at rest by the balance of the opposing forces of the elastic recoil of the lung and the resistance of the rigid chest wall. The elastic recoil of the lung provides an inward force that is countered by the outward force of the chest wall. With inspiration the diaphragm contracts and descends as the intercostal muscles contract and elevate the ribs laterally. Increasing the outward forces of the expanding thorax lowers the pressure within the pleural space and generates the pressure gradient from mouth to alveoli necessary for inhalation (Comroe, 1974).

With chest injury subatmospheric pressure may not be generated within the pleural space, and alveolar ventilation is compromised by several mechanisms. If air is introduced into the pleural space (closed or open pneumothorax), the subatmospheric pressure of the intrapleural space is lost, and the intrapleural pressure may rise to an atmospheric level, eliminating the pressure gradient from the mouth to the alveolus. With a tension pneumothorax, the air pressure within the chest cavity rises above atmospheric pressure, impeding alveolar and venous filling. As the intrapleural pressure continues to rise, the mediastinum, a mobile complex, is displaced toward the contralateral hemithorax. This mediastinal shift may ultimately kink the venae cavae, further decreasing venous return to the heart.

A second pathophysiologic mechanism of pulmonary insufficiency results from ventilation/perfusion mismatching, resulting in hypoxemia. Significant ventilation/perfusion mismatching may be produced by injuries that prevent alveolar ventilation because of lung collapse (atelectasis or pneumothorax) or because the lung is unable to expand because of extrinsic compression by tension pneumothorax, hemothorax, or intra-abdominal contents herniated through a diaphragmatic rupture. Diffuse intraparenchymal hemorrhage associated with pulmonary contusion may result in significant ventilation/perfusion mismatching and hypoxemia.

The cardiovascular system may be injured in a variety of ways, but the hemodynamic compromise is ultimately mediated by either inadequate circulating blood volume (hemorrhagic shock) or primary or secondary cardiac dysfunction (cardiogenic shock). Major thoracic vascular injury, whether to the aorta, the great vessels, or the major pulmonary vessels, may produce rapid exsanguination into the chest and hemorrhagic shock. The pathophysiology of such injuries is the same as hemorrhage produced elsewhere. Primary cardiogenic shock may result from ventricular dysfunction produced by myocardial contusion, direct penetrating injury to the heart, coronary arterial injury, or valvular injury. Tension pneumothorax may produce secondary cardiogenic shock by impairment of venous return to the heart, which is caused by compression or distortion of the venae cavae.

Secondary cardiogenic shock from pericardial tamponade results from excessive blood in the pericardial sac. The compliance of the pericardium allows filling to its elastic limit with little change in hemodynamics. Beyond this point the addition of only a small amount of blood causes a rapid rise in intrapericardial pressure. When this occurs the myocardium is compressed during diastole, and filling of the heart is impaired, resulting in a lethal reduction in forward flow (Bashore, 1989). The compensatory mechanisms to maintain cardiac output are an increase in sympathetic nervous output and increased circulating catecholamine levels. These mechanisms maintain blood pressure by increasing peripheral vasoconstriction, heart rate, and myocardial contractility. Compensation may be lost abruptly if anesthesia is induced in a trauma patient who has unrecognized pericardial tamponade.

A relatively broad spectrum of chest injuries ultimately produce harm through a small number of final common pathways of pathophysiology. Knowledge of this pathophysiology enables the thoracic surgeon to approach injuries to the chest in a systematic fashion, regardless of the specific injury. This approach should begin in the prehospital phase of trauma care (Fig. 61-1).

PREHOSPITAL CARE

The delivery of trauma care varies between communities, depending largely on the regional population and the proximity of a level I trauma center. In optimal systems trauma care is initiated at the injury scene by fire fighters and police officers who provide basic trauma life support (BTLS) by controlling external hemorrhage, stabilizing long bone fractures, providing oxygen, and extricating the patient from the site of injury while protecting the spine. Paramedics are summoned to the scene to initiate advanced trauma life support (ATLS) and to transport the patient to a hospital. Paramedics use radio communication with their hospital base to provide the trauma surgeon with an assessment of the patient and to act on the medical directives of the trauma surgeon. Opinions differ among adherents of various trauma systems about the role the paramedics should play in the resuscitation of trauma patients. In virtually all systems, the paramedics advise the trauma surgeon of the extent and potential severity of injuries to the patient prior to arrival at the hospital. In some systems the paramedics provide the ABCs of resuscitation (airway, breathing, and circulation), begin fluid resuscitation, and apply military antishock (MAST) trousers. In other systems the paramedics simply "load and run" the trauma victim to the hospital.

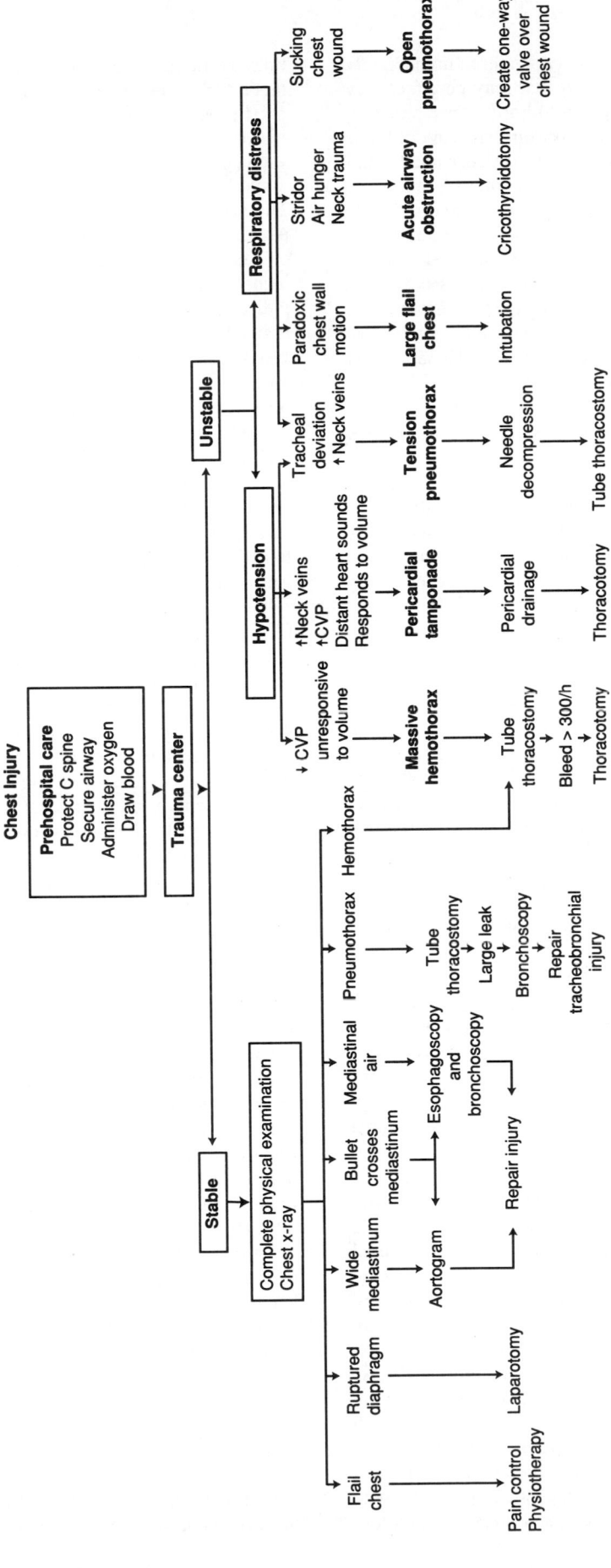

Figure 61-1. A general algorithm for initial management in the field and the trauma room.

During the prehospital phase, there are three immediately life-threatening injuries to the chest that may be effectively treated by paramedics: tension pneumothorax, open pneumothorax, and a large flail chest. The patient with any of these injuries may be in significant respiratory distress and should have the airway secured. A pneumothorax may be temporarily but effectively treated in the field by placement of a needle flutter valve in the second intercostal space in the midclavicular line. An open pneumothorax may be controlled by rapid placement of a one-way valve on the wound, as described below. Endotracheal intubation and oxygen administration is first-line therapy for a large flail chest and respiratory distress. Definitive therapy of these injuries can be performed after arrival at the trauma center (Fig. 61-1).

EMERGENCY DEPARTMENT MANAGEMENT AND THE ROLE OF THE THORACIC SURGEON

On arrival at the trauma center, evaluation and resuscitation of all traumatized victims is optimal when conducted in a consistently systematic manner, as outlined by the ATLS protocols (Thal, et al., 1988). The trauma team must first secure the airway, breathing, and circulation (ABCs) before attention is directed toward individual organ system injuries. Throughout the evaluation and resuscitation, a cervical spine injury must always be assumed to be present until proved otherwise by radiography. The neck must be immobilized with a cervical collar. The ABCs are followed by a rapid primary survey of the patient, as outlined by the ATLS protocol, to identify life- and limb-threatening injuries. Following this survey the initial resuscitation phase is begun. Intravenous access with two large-bore intravenous lines is obtained, fluid resuscitation is started, and blood is drawn for typing and cross matching. A central venous catheter is placed to monitor central venous pressure. Simultaneously therapy of life- and limb-threatening injuries is initiated.

As the resuscitation proceeds, the secondary survey of the patient is conducted. This is a thorough evaluation during which more information is obtained including an in-depth physical examination from head to toe, a review of the patient's medical history with family or friends, and an analysis of radiographs, electrocardiograms, and other laboratory data.

Thoracic surgeons are invaluable members of the trauma team because of their unique expertise in the anatomy, physiology, and therapy of injuries to the chest. As the evaluation of the traumatized patient proceeds from the primary survey into the resuscitation phase and the secondary survey, the thoracic surgeon must constantly review the patient's global condition and the impact of the thoracic injuries. The specific focus of the thoracic surgeon is recognition and treatment of immediately life-threatening chest injuries, such as airway obstruction, tension pneumothorax, open pneumothorax, massive hemothorax, flail chest, and cardiac tamponade. As the patient's evaluation progresses, the thoracic surgeon must then focus on potentially life-threatening injuries, such as pulmonary contusion, aortic disruption, tracheobronchial disruption, diaphragmatic rupture, and myocardial contusion (Thal, et al., 1988). This is best accomplished by a systematic approach beginning with the history and physical examina-

tion, recognizing that in certain emergent circumstances, more than one aspect of the evaluation and resuscitation must proceed simultaneously.

Airway

The first priority of the ABCs is to secure the airway. If the patient is struggling for air, apneic, tachypneic, stridorous, or has evidence of laryngeal trauma or an expanding neck hematoma, prompt tracheal intubation is indicated. Other indications for tracheal intubation include hypoxemia, significant head injury, shock, and loss of the thoracic bellows mechanism (Phillips, 1991). In the patient with a depressed level of consciousness, the upper airway may be acutely obstructed by the tongue, teeth, vomitus, or debris. In the patient with trauma to the upper chest and neck, delayed upper airway obstruction secondary to injury to the larynx must be suspected. Laryngeal injury may produce submucosal hemorrhage and swelling, which may later produce upper airway obstruction. A high index of suspicion must be maintained for this development in the patient with possible laryngeal injury.

The initial maneuver to secure the airway is the "jaw lift" (ATLS). This maneuver brings the mandible anteriorly, lifting the tongue, and thereby augments the upper airway. Teeth, vomitus, and foreign material may then be cleared.

Endotracheal intubation should be performed immediately if the jaw lift does not secure the airway. The nasotracheal or orotracheal route of intubation is chosen, depending on the personal experience of the surgeon, the presence of significant facial trauma, and the level of suspicion of cervical spine injury. In the patient breathing spontaneously, especially if a cervical spine injury is suspected, nasotracheal intubation is the method of choice. This technique is blind and requires the patient to ventilate spontaneously. In experienced hands, successful nasotracheal intubation may be accomplished in greater than 90 percent of cases (Iverson, 1981) without neck displacement, thereby avoiding potential exacerbation of cervical spinal cord injury. In patients without spontaneous ventilation or in whom nasotracheal intubation cannot be performed, orotracheal intubation should be conducted with a 7.5- or 8.0-mm tube. If muscle relaxation is required, succinylcholine (1 mg/kg IV) may be given. An assistant must apply cricothyroid pressure to minimize the risk of aspiration if succinylcholine is used. Prior to paralyzing patients pharmacologically, surgeons must be certain that they will be able to secure the airway, either by endotracheal intubation or surgically.

The traditional recommendation for orotracheal intubation of the trauma patient when a cervical spine injury has not been ruled out is for an assistant to provide axial traction on the cervical spine (Thal, et al., 1988). Recently evidence generated in victims of trauma with unstable cervical spine fractures has suggested that axial traction may not completely immobilize an unstable cervical spine fracture during orotracheal intubation (Bivins, et al., 1988). The surgeon should be aware of this but must not be dissuaded from securing the airway to sustain life.

If endotracheal intubation cannot be achieved, the airway must be secured surgically. In such emergent circumstances,

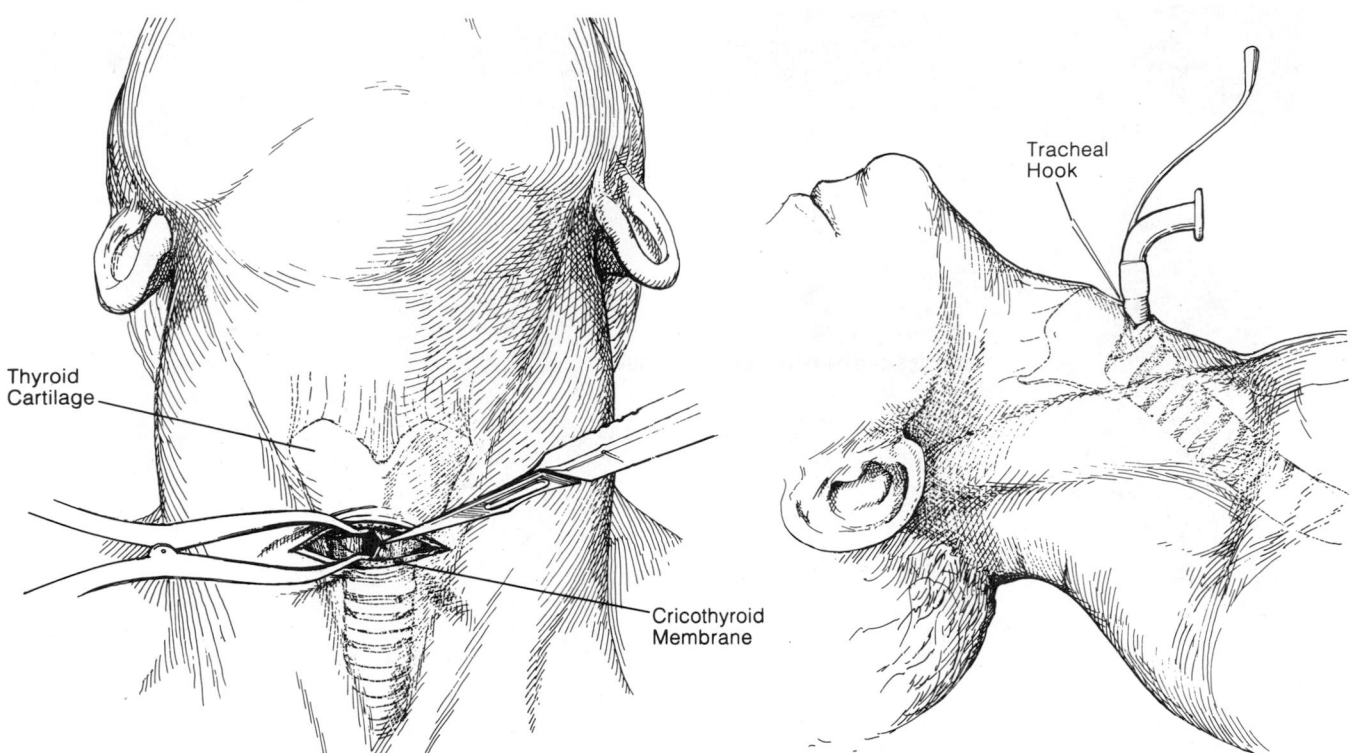

Figure 61-2. Technique for cricothyroidotomy. A transverse skin incision is made over the cricothyroid membrane, which is then incised with the knife. If traction devices are not available, the blunt end of the knife handle may be placed through the defect in the membrane and rotated 90 degrees to open the membrane, and then the tracheostomy tube is inserted. (From Moore FA, Moore EE: Trauma resuscitation. p. 5. In Wilmore DN, Brennan MF, Harken AH et al. (eds): Care of the Surgical Patient. Scientific American, New York, 1989, with permission.)

cricothyroidotomy can be performed quickly and easily and is recognized as the procedure of choice. Cricothyroidotomy is indicated in patients with significant maxillofacial injury combined with suspected cervical spine injury (Moore and Moore, 1989) (Fig. 61-2).

Immediate Life-Threatening Injuries

During the primary survey, the thoracic surgeon must identify chest injuries that may be immediately life threatening. These injuries should be treated with the fastest and simplest techniques.

Tension Pneumothorax

Tension pneumothorax is one such injury. Normally the pressure within the pleural space is subatmospheric. If atmospheric pressure enters the pleural space, this subatmospheric pressure is lost, and the elastic recoil of the lung results in pulmonary collapse. If a one-way valve exists through the lung, airway, or chest wall, atmospheric air entering the pleural space cannot escape. Not only does the lung collapse, but the pressure within the pleural space continues to rise as air accumulates. With increased pressure within the hemithorax, venous return to the heart fails. The mediastinum shifts contralaterally, distorting the trachea and venae cavae. This distortion of the venae cavae further decreases

venous return to the heart, compromising cardiac output. Tension pneumothorax should be suspected in the patient with respiratory distress, hypotension, distended neck veins, and tracheal deviation away from the hemithorax with no breath sounds and hyper-resonance on percussion. The immediate life-saving therapy is to decompress the hemithorax by placement of a needle into the involved chest in the second intercostal space in the midclavicular line. This converts the tension pneumothorax into an open pneumothorax, usually providing immediate improvement. Definitive therapy may then be performed by thoracostomy tube placement (Fig. 61-3).

Open Pneumothorax

An open pneumothorax or "sucking chest wound" must be immediately recognized and treated. An open pneumothorax results from a large penetrating defect in the chest wall that allows an equilization of the intrapleural pressure and atmospheric pressure. As the patient inhales, the inspired air travels down the path of least resistance. Therefore, if the diameter of the chest wall defect is greater than two-thirds the diameter of the trachea, most of the patient's tidal volume traverses the chest wall, resulting in severe respiratory distress (Eddy, et al., 1991). An open pneumothorax can result in a to-and-fro shifting of the mediastinum with the patient's exaggerated respiratory effort, distorting the venae cavae

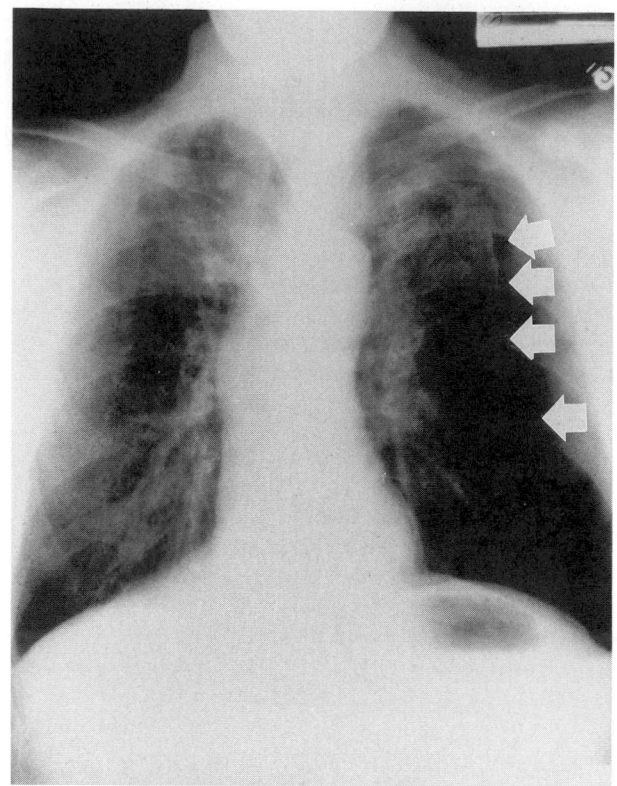

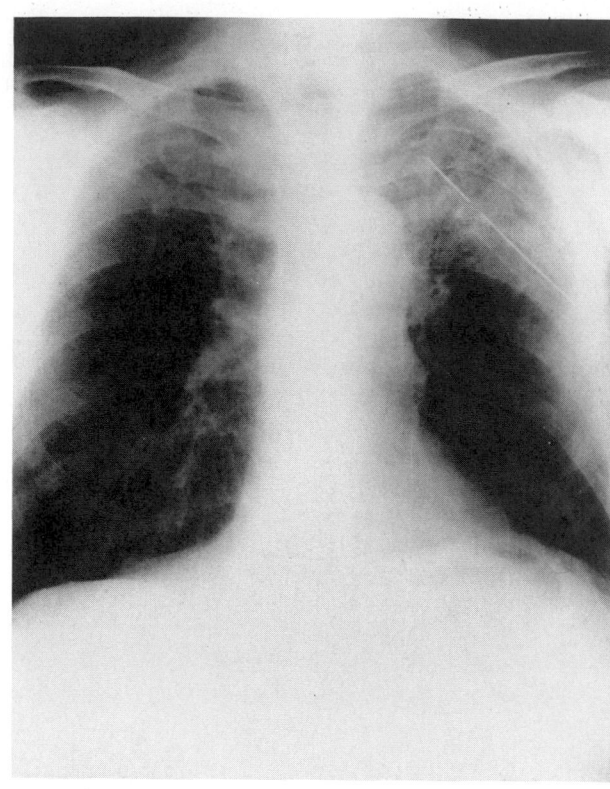

Figure 61-3.   Tension pneumothorax. **(A)** Chest radiograph of a 60-year-old man involved in a car accident showing a left side tension pneumothorax. **(B)** Complete lung reexpansion following tube drainage.

and compromising venous return to the heart. This injury is easily recognized on visual inspection of the chest in the patient in respiratory distress and is easily treated immediately by taping a rubber glove over the defect with the tip of one finger cut off. Alternatively a plastic drape may be taped on three sides over the defect. In either case, a one-way valve is created that allows air to exit the chest cavity but not enter. If performed quickly, these maneuvers allow the patient to recover from severe respiratory distress. A thoracostomy tube may then be placed under more controlled conditions and the chest wall repaired.

Flail Chest

During the initial evaluation, the surgeon specifically examines the chest wall for a flail segment. A flail chest is created when multiple rib fractures separate a segment of the chest wall from continuity with the remainder of the chest. The flail segment moves paradoxically with respiration and dissipates the subatmospheric pressure normally generated with inspiration. In an effort to compensate, the patient must exert tremendous effort to generate enough negative intrapleural pressure to inhale. The force required to create the flail segment usually causes significant pulmonary contusion of the underlying lung, which further compromises oxygenation. Combined with the pain produced by trying to breathe effectively, this injury may produce severe respiratory distress,

frequently associated with both hypoxemia and hypercarbia. This injury is recognized on the initial physical examination of the patient in respiratory distress as a chest wall deformity, which moves paradoxically with respiration. On palpation it is associated with chest wall crepitance, pain, and deformity. The immediate therapy of this injury is determined by the degree of respiratory distress. The patient should be intubated and mechanically ventilated if hypoxemic or hypercarbic, but prolonged ventilatory support is not required if the chest wall can be stabilized and pain controlled (Fig. 61-4).

Massive Hemothorax

The chest trauma patient in shock should be suspected of having a massive hemothorax. This may be suspected on physical examination by diminished or absent breath sounds and dullness to percussion, but it is confirmed by chest radiography. This injury usually results from exsanguinating hemorrhage into the chest cavity from either penetrating or blunt injury of the aorta, its branches, or a major pulmonary vessel. In massive hemothorax, the pressure developed within the chest cavity may partially tamponade the bleeding vessel. If this tamponade is released by tube thoracostomy placement, the bleeding may actually increase significantly. The surgeon should wait to place a chest tube until ready to transfuse the patient rapidly. If the hemodynamic condition worsens as blood exits through the chest tube, the tube should be

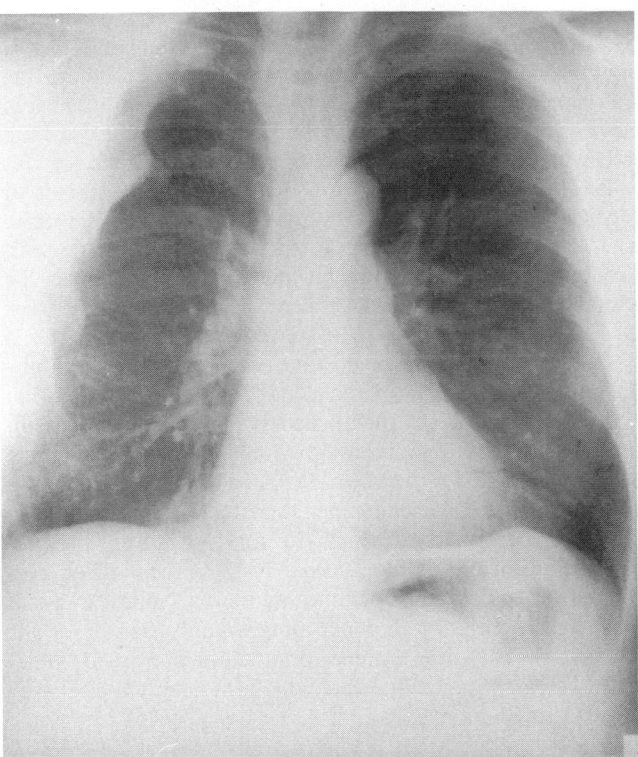

Figure 61-4. Flail chest. Chest radiograph of a 48-year-old man who fell from a height of 80 feet. Note the caved-in right chest due to fractures of ribs one through seven.

Initial Management Pitfalls for the Unwary

Intubation may convert a cervical fracture to paraplegia. Assume the cervical spine is unstable. For urgent intubation before spine radiographs, use the nasotracheal route, intubate over a flexible bronchoscope, or perform cricothyroidotomy.

Intubation may disrupt a tracheal transsection. Intubate over a flexible bronchoscope if airway injury is suspected.

Hemothorax and ruptured diaphragm both produce dullness to percussion. Obtain chest radiograph prior to tube thoracostomy.

Many critical components of the chest injury can be missed if the patient is not prepared for the chest radiograph. *Mark entry and exit wounds* with radiopaque markers prior to the chest radiograph. *Place a radiopaque nasograstric tube* prior to the chest radiograph to outline the aorta and aid in the diagnosis of diaphragmatic rupture.

clamped in an effort to try to tamponade the bleeding. This situation is associated with a very high mortality rate and may require immediate emergency room thoracotomy in an effort to control hemorrhage. However, the likelihood of survival is extremely low (Fig. 61-5).

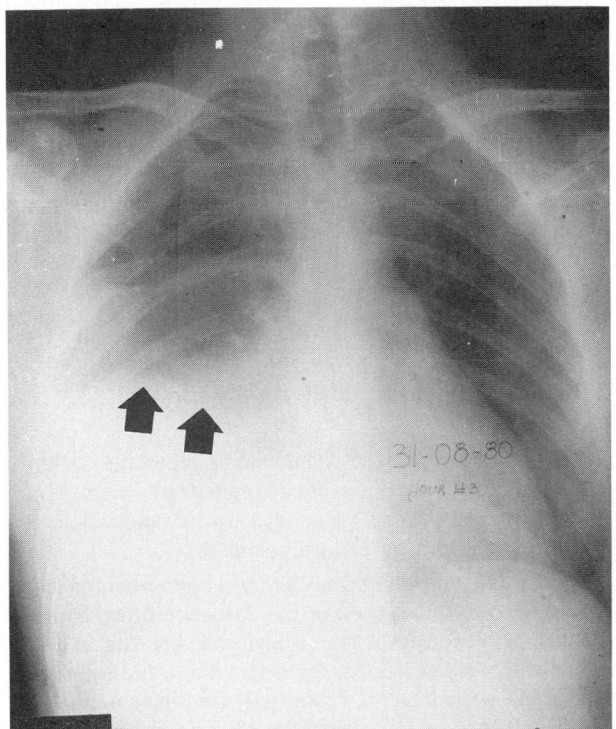

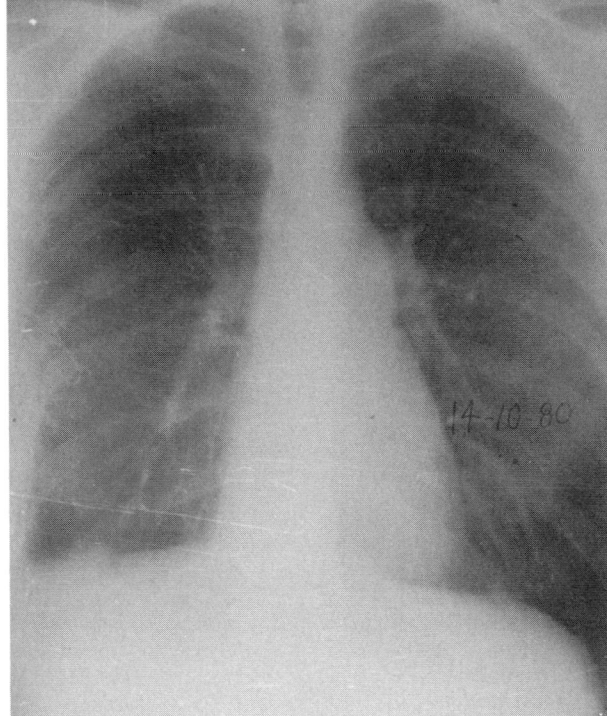

Figure 61-5. Hemothorax. **(A)** Chest radiograph of a 35-year-old man involved in a motorcycle accident. He has rib fractures on the right side and a 2,000 ml hemothorax. **(B)** Chest radiograph showing complete resolution after tube drainage.

Cardiogenic Shock

Cardiogenic shock must be immediately recognized. The distinction from hemorrhagic shock may be difficult. The patient in cardiogenic shock has a high central venous pressure, despite hypotension. This may be evidenced by distended neck veins on physical examination. Direct measurement of central venous pressure is extremely valuable in distinguishing cardiogenic shock (central venous pressure [CVP] >15 mmHg) from hypovolemic shock (CVP <5 mmHg). If cardio-

genic shock is present, pericardial tamponade is suggested by distant heart sounds on auscultation. Pulsus paradoxus is another valuable physical finding in tamponade, defined as a 10-mmHg drop in systolic pressure during inspiration. It is caused by shifting of the intraventricular septum toward the left, with a resultant decrease in left ventricular stroke volume. In a noisy trauma room, it is extremely difficult to recognize pulsus paradoxus without an intra-arterial catheter. The diagnosis of pericardial tamponade may be made with accuracy if echocardiography is immediately available in the trauma room. If not, pericardiocentesis may be both diagnostic and therapeutic (Figs. 61-6 and 61-7).

The patient in shock should have both chests vented empirically to release any component of pneumothorax. If still in shock that is refractory to volume administration, an immediate left anterolateral thoracotomy should be performed. Open cardiac massage is more effective than closed-chest compression, and aortic cross-clamping may effectively increase coronary and cerebral perfusion. The survival rate for trauma-room thoracotomy is approximately 50 percent when performed for shock from penetrating cardiac injuries, but it falls to 20 percent for all penetrating wounds (Baxter, et al., 1988). Survival after trauma-room thoracotomy for blunt trauma is rare (Fig. 61-8). Emergent thoracotomy is discussed in detail in Chapter 65.

History

While the airway is being secured and life-threatening injuries treated, information about the patient should be obtained directly from the patient or from the family by another member of the trauma team. In seriously injured patients, this information is commonly relayed by paramedics transporting the patient to the trauma center or from a bracelet that may be worn by the patient informing of a significant medical condition. Early in the patient's initial evaluation, valuable time should not be lost in extensive discussion, but the surgeon should make an attempt to learn the patient's significant medical history, including any allergies and current medications. Medications, such as β-blockers, diuretics, insulin, and antihypertensives, may have significant impact on the

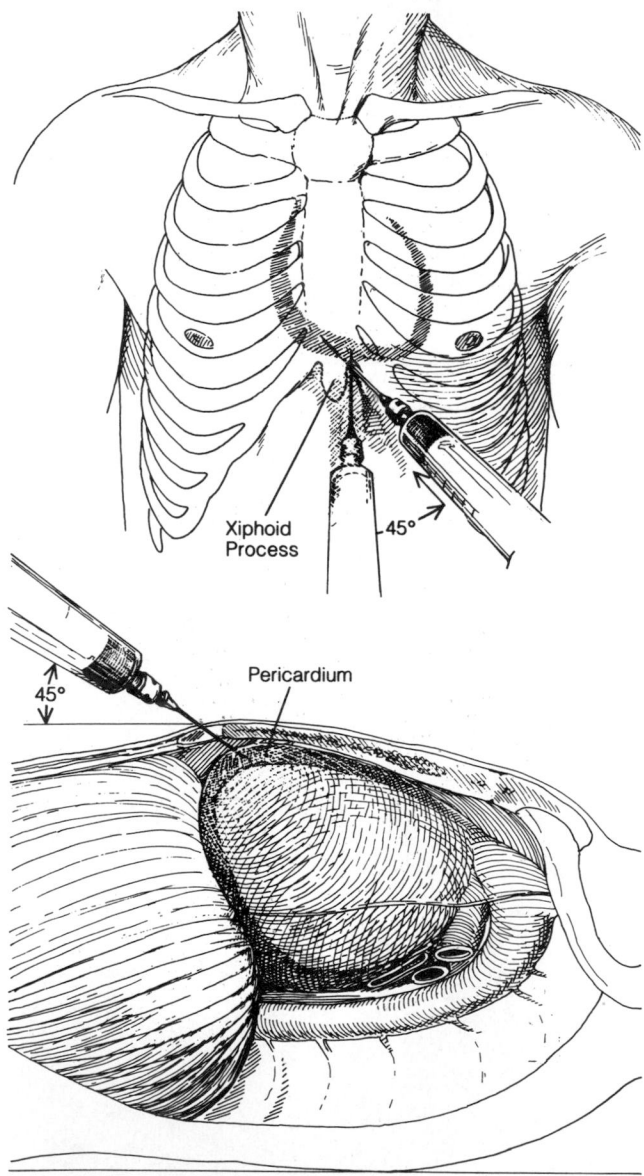

Xiphoid Process — 45°

Pericardium — 45°

Figure 61-6. Technique for pericardiocentesis. An 18-gauge spinal needle is used to enter the pericardium through the subxiphoid approach. The angle of approach is at 45 degrees to both the patient and the xiphoid process. A "pop" is usually felt on penetrating the pericardium. (From Moore FA, Moore EE: Trauma resuscitation, p. 5. In Wilmore DN, Brennan MF, Harken AH et al. (eds): Care of the Surgical Patient. Scientific American, New York, 1989, with permission.)

Cardiogenic Shock: Pitfalls for the Unwary

Pericardial tamponade and tension pneumothorax both produce hypotension and distended neck veins. Rule out pneumothorax by needle aspiration or chest radiograph before pericardiocentesis.

Pericardial tamponade may be misdiagnosed if the CVP reading is falsely elevated. Measure after zeroing when the patient is not struggling to breathe. A diagnostic pericardiocentesis may yield a false-positive result if the heart is punctured, creating a new problem because of the misdiagnosis. Obtain an echocardiogram when possible to avoid empiric pericardiocentesis.

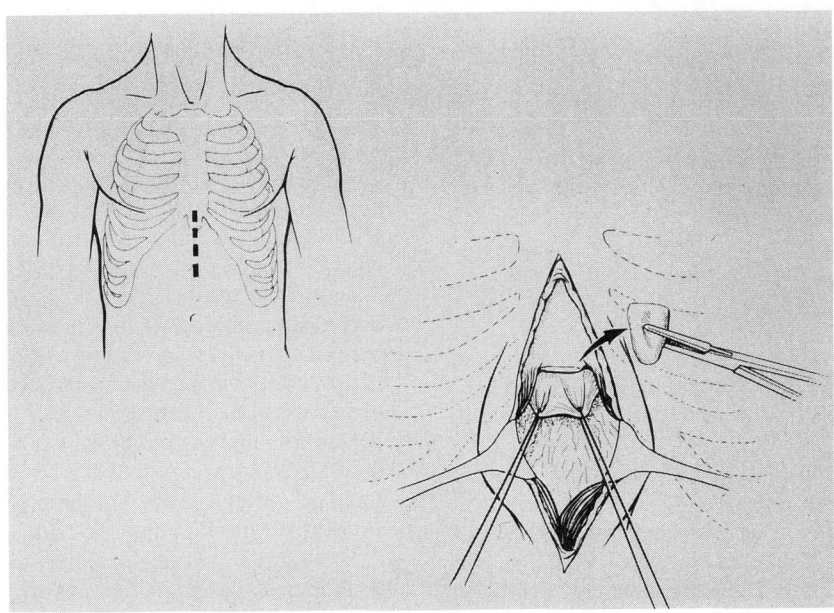

Figure 61-7. Subxiphoid pericardiotomy. This technique may be preferable if pericardiocentesis produces insufficient relief of tamponade. An incision is made over the xiphoid process, which is excised exposing the pericardium.

patient's response to both injury and resuscitation. It is especially important for the surgeon to know about significant illnesses, particularly ischemic heart disease, hypertension, congestive heart failure, chronic pulmonary disease, and diabetes mellitus.

The history of the events surrounding the traumatic injury is crucial and may usually be obtained from police or para-

medics involved in prehospital transportation to the trauma facility. Knowledge of the mechanism of injury allows the surgeon to infer the likelihood of specific injuries. In motor vehicle accidents, vehicular speed, the direction of impact, whether the patient was restrained, and the condition of the vehicle, especially the steering wheel, are important. Deceleration injuries suggest the possibility of thoracic aortic trans-

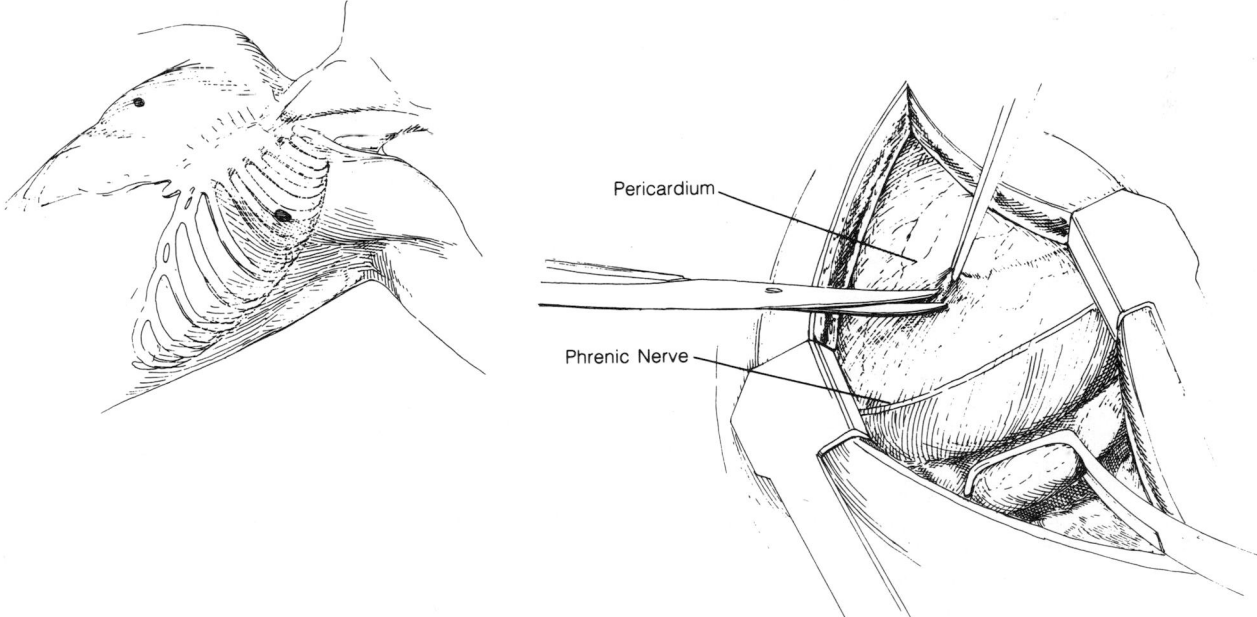

Figure 61-8. Trauma department thoracotomy. A left anterior thoracotomy incision is made with the patient in the supine position. The fourth intercostal space is entered, and the descending thoracic aorta is cross-clamped. Care is taken to avoid injury to the esophagus. The pericardium is opened to initiate internal cardiac massage. From Moore FA, Moore EE: Trauma resuscitation, p. 5. In Wilmore DN, Brennan MF, Harken AH et al. (eds): Care of the Surgical Patient. Scientific American, New York, 1989, with permission.)

section. A bent steering wheel suggests cardiac contusion or rupture. Crushing chest injuries suggest possible traumatic asphyxiation or cardiac or pulmonary contusion. In cases of penetrating thoracic trauma, specific knowledge of the weapon is valuable. The size of a knife or other penetrating object allows an estimation of the extent of internal injury. The caliber of the gun and the proximity of the assailant allow a better estimate of the injury produced by a thoracic gunshot wound.

Physical Examination

After the airway has been secured, attention is directed to the patient's breathing. The patient should be ventilated or supplemented with 100 percent oxygen during the resuscitation phase and secondary survey. The physical examination should proceed expeditiously, beginning with inspection of the head, neck, and chest.

The head and neck should be inspected for evidence of maxillofacial trauma, including subtle evidence of injury to the larynx or cervical trachea. The patient may have bruising of anterior neck or an expanding cervical hematoma. The trachea should be in the midline on inspection; tracheal deviation from the midline may indicate tension pneumothorax. The neck should be inspected for distended veins, indicating impaired venous return to the heart from pericardial tamponade or tension pneumothorax. Plethora of the head and neck, combined with subconjunctival hemorrhage, may result in "traumatic asphyxia," a syndrome of capillary and venous bleeding in the distribution of the superior vena caval watershed from a sudden crushing injury to the chest. After inspection the neck should be palpated for swelling and subcutaneous emphysema, with laryngeal or airway injury.

The chest should be specifically inspected to ensure symmetric expansion of the hemithoraces with ventilation. If asymmetric motion of the hemithoraces is noted, it may indicate improper endotracheal tube position or failure of lung expansion secondary to pneumothorax, hemothorax, or intra-abdominal contents herniated through a diaphragmatic rupture. A segment of chest wall moving paradoxically represents a flail chest. The chest is inspected both anteriorly and posteriorly for penetrating thoracic wounds. Their size and location must be noted with specific reference to possible intrathoracic visceral injury. An open pneumothorax found on inspection must be treated immediately.

The soft tissues of the chest should be palpated for crepitance and subcutaneous emphysema. Likewise the ribs, sternum, and clavicles should be palpated for localized pain, tenderness, and deformity, which are consistent with fracture.

The chest should be percussed again to ensure symmetry. Hyper-resonance of a hemithorax may indicate a pneumothorax. This finding may help distinguish tension pneumothorax from pericardial tamponade in a patient with neck vein distension. Dullness may indicate hemothorax or herniated intra-abdominal contents through a ruptured diaphragm.

Auscultation of the chest may be difficult amid the noisy activity of a busy trauma room resuscitation, but it is a valuable part of the physical examination. Absent or diminished breath sounds may represent a malpositioned endotracheal tube, hemo- or pneumothorax, or diaphragmatic rupture. Dis-

tant heart sounds suggest pericardial tamponade when combined with hypotension and distended neck veins.

Chest Radiographic Evaluation

The chest radiograph is the diagnostic modality by which potentially life-treatening injuries are usually discovered. It is an essential component of the evaluation and therapy of all chest injuries. A portable chest radiograph should be obtained in the trauma room as soon as the airway has been secured and immediate life-threatening injuries have been at least temporarily treated. It is preferably taken after nasogastric or orogastric tube placement because the radiodense tube serves as an excellent marker of mediastinal position. For penetrating injuries a radiopaque marker should be taped to the skin over entrance and exit wounds. In our institution the standard portable chest radiograph is taken from a distance of 36 inches from the patient's chest and during inspiration.

The surgeon should examine the chest radiograph in a systematic fashion to avoid missing an injury. The following points must be determined.

1. *Correct position of the endotracheal tube:* The surgeon must be certain that the tube is neither up too high in the trachea, near the larynx, risking inadvertent extubation, or down too far, usually in the right mainstem bronchus.

2. *Pneumothorax:* This finding may be easily missed by a hurried examination of a portable radiograph. Lung markings should be traced to the periphery of the lung bilaterally. An often subtle finding is hyperlucency of the costophrenic angle.

3. *Tension pneumothorax:* Although this injury is usually identified during the primary survey, the radiographic findings are striking. The ipsilateral hemothorax is lucent, the diaphragm is depressed, and the trachea and mediastinum (easily marked by the radiodense nasogastric tube) are shifted contralaterally.

4. *Hemothorax:* This is visualized radiographically by opacification of the hemithorax. With massive hemothorax the entire hemithorax may be radiodense from blood. However, with lesser degrees of bleeding, the finding may be subtle. One trick is to compare the density of each hemithorax against the other. If the chest radiograph is taken in the supine position, the blood may layer out posteriorly, creating a slightly more dense appearance, despite demonstrating aeration of the lung.

5. *Pulmonary contusion:* This injury may not be evident on the initial radiographic evaluation. However, a diffuse density in the lung parenchyma suggests the diagnosis.

6. *Mediastinal emphysema:* The tissues of the mediastinum and cervical facia should be scrutinized for air. When combined with a pneumothorax, which is refractory to chest tube suction, this radiographic finding should raise the question of tracheobronchial disruption.

7. *Intra-abdominal contents displaced into the chest:* Diaphragmatic injury may result in herniation of virtually any of the intra-abdominal viscera into the chest. On the left a gas-filled loop of bowel may easily be confused

with a pneumothorax. This is another reason to place the nasogastric tube prior to chest radiography; if the stomach is displaced into the chest, the radiodensity of the tube helps to identify this injury. Chest radiographic diagnosis of a right diaphragmatic rupture may be subtle. Because the liver is usually the organ that herniates, the radiographic appearance may simply be that of an elevated right hemidiaphragm.

8. *Fractures:* Costal fractures are notoriously difficult to visualize on a chest radiograph; the diagnosis is primarily made on physical examination. However, a large flail segment is frequently identifiable on a chest radiograph. The thoracic spine should be studied on the chest radiograph for fracture or dislocation, as should the clavicles and humeral heads.

9. *Bullets:* The intrathoracic course of a bullet must be ascertained. Particularly if no exit wound has been identified, the location of the bullet is important. If the bullet has crossed the mediastinum, the aorta, esophagus, and trachea, all must be evaluated by further studies to exclude injury. If the bullet resides or passed below the diaphragm, laparotomy is indicated.

10. *Widened mediastinum:* A widened mediastinum is the hallmark of aortic disruption. If the portable chest radiograph suggests mediastinal widening, an upright posterolateral chest radiograph should be obtained. A mediastinum wider than 8 cm is highly suggestive of aortic transsection and merits aortography. Other radiographic findings consistent with this diagnosis include a loss of sharp contrast of the aortic-pulmonary window, depression of the left mainstem bronchus, deviation of the nasogastric tube to the right, left rib fractures, and left hemothorax.

Triage and Transfer

After the diagnosis of thoracic injuries has been made and immediate life-threatening injuries have been treated by temporizing measures, definitive therapy of these injuries must be accomplished. The thoracic surgeon coordinates the operative strategy for the repair of thoracic injuries with the other surgical specialties of the trauma team. The severity of all injuries must be prioritized. Hemorrhage in the chest or elsewhere must be controlled as the first priority. Likewise, pericardial tamponade must be definitively treated immediately. To guarantee the security of the airway, tracheobronchial injuries should be repaired prior to repair of intra-abdominal viscera but under the same anesthesia.

The natural history of traumatic aortic transsection is well defined; it progresses to rupture in the majority of patients. Therefore this injury must be repaired promptly after the diagnosis has been confirmed by aortography. A challenging dilemma exist when a patient has both intra-abdominal hemorrhage and aortic transsection. If the aorta is not actively bleeding, the intra-abdominal hemorrhage should be stopped quickly, and then attention should be directed to the aortic repair. If the aorta is frankly ruptured, it should be repaired first.

As noted the majority of all chest injuries may be managed with tube thoracostomy alone. Injuries, such as simple pneumothorax, simple hemothorax, mild cardiac contusion, and mild pulmonary contusion, may be appropriately managed in most hospitals, and the expertise of a thoracic surgeon may not be required. On the other hand, virtually all complex thoracic injuries, particularly those requiring thoracotomy, should be handled in the facilities available in a trauma center by a thoracic surgeon. If the admitting hospital is not so equipped, the patient should be transferred after stabilization to a capable facility. Prior to transfer chest tubes should be placed to treat documented or suspected pneumothorax. If air transportation is required, the patient should be provided 100 percent oxygen to breathe. The cabin should be pressurized to avoid exacerbation of pressure effects on loculated pneumothorax and ensure optimal availability of oxygen. Most fixed-wing aircraft are pressurized to only 8,000 feet above sea level, a significant reduction for some patients.

Key Elements in the Trauma Room Chest Radiograph

Endotracheal tube: Ensure that it is neither too high nor too low.

Pneumothorax: Lung markings should reach the periphery, without costophrenic hyperlucency.

Hemothorax: Subtle increase in opacification of one lung on a supine film signifies blood in the pleural space.

Lung contusion: A pattern of pneumonia or atelectasis at this stage usually indicates contusion.

Tension pneumothorax: This shifts the diaphragm and mediastinum, however slight.

Ruptured diaphragm: Look for abdominal gas in the chest or elevation of the right diaphragm.

Mediastinal emphysema: This should be carefully sought as a sign of esophageal or airway injury.

Fractures: Ribs, clavicles, humeri, and sternum are better seen when the film is rotated 90 or 180 degrees to allow undistracted attention to bony structure.

Bullets: Their intrathoracic course as well as their location should be assessed.

Aorta: A superior mediastinum wider than 8 cm, depressed left bronchus, blurred aortic knob, and deviation of the nasogastric tube suggest rupture.

CONCLUSION

Initial management that is based on careful, systematic assessment and an understanding of the common pathophysiologic mechanisms in chest injury leads to a high salvage rate in this challenging group of patients. Subsequent chapters will discuss the details of definitive therapy of specific injuries to the airway and thorax. The final three chapters of this section review the current management of complications of chest injury and their sequelae.

COMMENTS AND CONTROVERSIES

Thoracic injury is common in traumatized patients, but thoracic trauma without injury to the heart and great vessels rarely requires operative surgical intervention. When there is no vascular or cardiac injury, the majority of traumatic injuries to the chest are managed by chest tube drainage and supportive care. For this reason, general thoracic surgeons in many centers have abdicated trauma management to a "trauma team," which is composed of general surgeons and intensivists, excusing themselves from active participation in an interesting and sometimes dramatically challenging category of thoracic surgical practice.

Many intensive care units were started by thoracic surgeons, and their contributions to the care of the traumatized patient with thoracic injuries have been substantial and lasting. This chapter illustrates the valuable contributions of thoracic surgeons to the management of trauma and its sequelae. Sharing in responsibility for surgical intensive care on a rotating basis offers thoracic surgeons a broad exposure to the problems of traumatized patients, including some of the most demanding problems of respiratory and multiple organ system failure.

Because trauma is a descriptor of cause, its discussion crosses structural organization in the way that a section devoted to infection or cancer might. For this reason the topic is widely dispersed throughout this textbook as an important consideration in the differential diagnosis or pathogenesis of many of the disorders discussed.

This section offers a general approach to thoracic trauma and reviews some unique aspects of management and complications that are not discussed systematically in other chapters. Some material developed more fully elsewhere is repeated here to provide continuity. The chapters on penetrating and blunt trauma are derived from the experience of surgeons at leading trauma centers and necessarily include some overlapping material. The sequelae of trauma to the chest, including adult respiratory distress syndrome, sepsis, multiple organ failure, and rehabilitation, are mentioned in the trauma section for completeness, although the discussion of these subjects is pertinent to a variety of other clinical settings.

M.F.M.

KEY REFERENCES

Baxter BT, Moore EE, Cleveland HC et al: Emergency department thoracotomy following injury: critical determinants for survival. World J Surg 12:671, 1988

The authors reviewed their experience with 632 emergency department thoracotomies—50 percent for blunt trauma, 35 percent for gunshot wounds and 15 percent for stab wounds. If vital signs were present on arrival, survival was 32 percent for stab wounds, 15 percent gunshot wounds, and only 5 percent for blunt trauma. Without signs of life on arrival, survival was 10 percent for stab wounds, 1 percent for gunshot wounds, and 1 percent for blunt trauma. The authors advocate a selective approach to emergency-department thoracotomy: survival is nil when thoracotomy is performed for blunt trauma in patients without signs of life, but one-third of patients presenting in extremis from stab wounds survived.

Survival is greatest when the procedure is performed for penetrating rather than blunt trauma.

Moore FA, Moore EE: Trauma resuscitation. In Wilmore DW, Brennan MF, Harken AH et al. (eds): Care of the Surgical Patient. Scientific American, New York, 1989

The authors provide excellent instruction for the initial management of the trauma patient.

Thal ER: Advanced Trauma Life Support Course for Physicians, Subcommittee Trauma, 1987–1988, American College of Surgeons, Chicago, 1988

This manual provides the classic algorithms for initial trauma management.

REFERENCES

Bashore T: Invasive Cardiology Principles and Technique. BC Decker, New York, 1989

Bivins HG, Ford S, Bezmalinovic Z et al.: The effect of axial traction during orotracheal intubation of the trauma victim with an unstable cervical spine. Ann Emerg Med 17:25, 1988

Breasted JH: the Edwin Smith Surgical Papyrus. University of Chicago Press, Chicago, 1930

Campbell E, Colton J: The Surgery of Theodoric. Appleton-Century-Crofts, Norwalk, CT, 1955

Comroe JH: Mechanical factors in breathing. p. 94. In Comroe JH (ed): Physiology of Respiration. 2nd Ed. Year Book Medical Publishers, Chicago, 1974

Eddy CA, Carrico CJ, Rusch VW: Injury to the lung and pleura. p. 358. In Moore EE, Mattox KL, Feliciano DV (eds): Trauma. Appleton and Lange, Norwalk, CT, 1991

Iverson KV: Blind nasotracheal intubation. Ann Emerg Med 10:468, 1981

Lewis RF: Thoracic trauma. Surg Clin North Am 69:97, 1982

Meade RH: A History of Thoracic Surgery. Charles C Thomas, Springfield, IL, 1961

Phillips TF: Airway management. p. 142. In Moore EE, Mattox, KL, Feliciano DV (eds): Trauma. Appleton and Lange, Norwalk, CT, 1991

62

TRAUMA TO THE LARYNX

Ian J. Witterick
Patrick J. Gullane
Jonathan C. Irish

Management of the acutely injured larynx remains a diagnostic and therapeutic challenge. Frequently a laryngeal injury is only one of several injuries sustained in the multiply traumatized patient, and it is only when the patient cannot be extubated or decannulated that thought is given to the possibility of laryngeal injury. Failure of early recognition can turn a relatively simple definitive repair into a more complicated procedure with a less successful outcome. It is essential therefore to consider laryngotracheal trauma in patients with a history of neck trauma, especially if they require intubation or tracheotomy because of upper airway obstruction.

BASIC SCIENCE

Etiology

Blunt trauma most commonly results from motor vehicle accidents; however, sports injuries, strangulation, recreational vehicle accidents, and child abuse all can result in significant laryngeal injury. Laryngotracheal separation may occur from collision with a clothes line or fence wire, which are often difficult to see and usually struck at high speeds. Most blunt injuries occur when the larynx is compressed against the rigid vertebral column, fracturing the cartilages and contusing or lacerating the mucosal lining. The appearance of the neck can be misleading because a severe blunt laryngotracheal injury may be concealed beneath what appears to be normal overlying tissue (Nahum, 1969). In blunt trauma the surrounding neurovascular and digestive structures are usually flexible enough to avoid significant injury, except for the cervical spine.

Seat belts have a major influence on the type of injury sustained in motor vehicle accidents (Fig. 62-1). The use of lap belts and shoulder straps has significantly reduced the incidence of maxillofacial trauma and blunt laryngeal injury.

Penetrating trauma may be secondary to firearms, knives, and other sharp objects available in an altercation. The extent of damage may not be apparent from the entrance or exit wounds (Stanley, et al., 1988). Esophageal injuries are frequently associated with penetrating laryngotracheal trauma and early recognition is essential to prevent postoperative complications (Minard, et al., 1992).

Demographics

Laryngotracheal trauma is a more frequent occurrence in male patients because they are more commonly involved in motor vehicle accidents and violence. Overall it is a rare injury, accounting for less than 1 percent of the trauma cases seen in most major centers (Gussack and Jurkovich, 1988). In recent years the incidence of laryngeal trauma seems to be decreasing, possibly as a result of speed-limit reductions and mandatory seat belt laws (Schaefer and Close, 1989; Miller, 1990). A lack of recognition of minor laryngotracheal trauma in the patient with multiple injuries may lead to underreporting of this entity. In addition, the incidence of clinically presenting laryngeal fractures may be further reduced because of death at the scene from asphyxiation. The experience of any one surgeon is therefore limited, resulting in management controversies.

Pathophysiology

Blunt and penetrating trauma interrupt the normal functions of the larynx in respiration, phonation, prevention of aspiration, and the ability to perform the Valsalva maneuver. The mandible affords some protection superiorly and the sternum inferiorly, but this protection is often bypassed in motor vehicle accidents because the neck is extended during sudden deceleration, resulting in an exposed neck striking the steering wheel or dashboard. The submucosal tissues of the larynx are distensible, particularly in the supraglottic portions, permitting the rapid accumulation of fluid and blood. The mucosal lining of the larynx and pharynx is easily torn by traumatic forces, leading to subcutaneous emphysema and contamination of the deep tissues of the neck. An environment is set up for the development of cellulitis, abscess formation, and perhaps fistulous tracts.

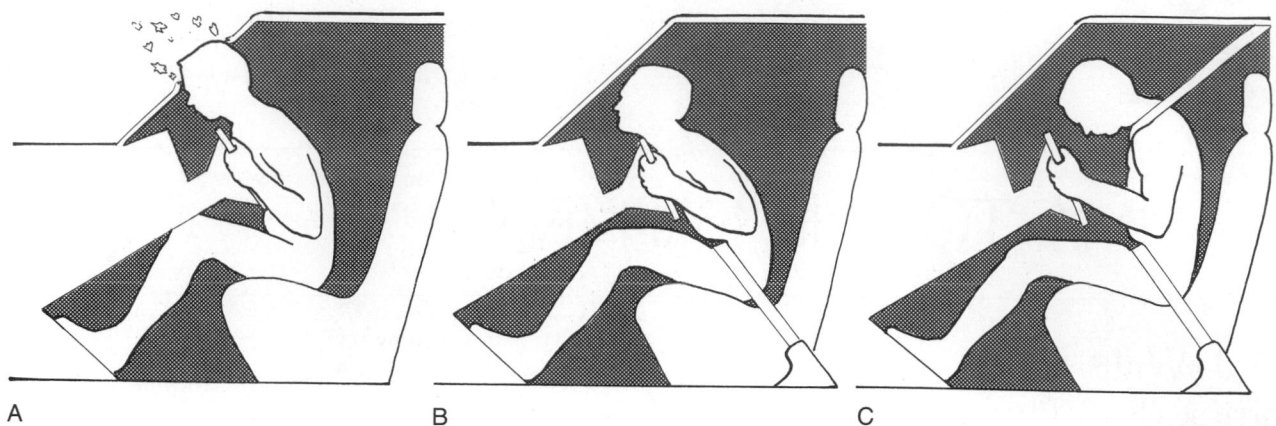

A   B   C

Figure 62-1. Injury patterns associated with seat belt use in automobile accidents. **(A)** When no seat belt is worn, injuries to the chest, head, and face are more common. **(B)** Lap belts can cause neck and upper aerodigestive tract trauma. **(C)** Lap and shoulder belts can cause injury to the upper aerodigestive tract from the shoulder belt, but usually the injury is much less severe.

Laryngeal fractures and joint dislocations occur in a wide variety of patterns but tend to be more severe in the less resilient, calcified cartilages of the elderly patient. The patterns of injury were described under actual and experimental situations (Lee, 1992). Injury may lead to subperichondrial hematoma and ischemic necrosis of cartilage followed by perichondritis and chondritis. Laryngeal injuries heal by granulation tissue and eventual fibrosis because the wounds are usually secondarily infected. Epithelialization may be delayed, resulting in excessive fibrous tissue, deformity, and considerable permanent alteration in laryngeal function. The larynx can usually be restored to relatively normal function if primary healing is allowed to take place by repairing the torn mucosa and reducing and stabilizing cartilaginous fractures in a timely fashion.

Classification

There is no universally accepted classification scheme for laryngotracheal trauma. Laryngotracheal injury has been classified by location (Bryce, 1979), severity (Olson, 1982), and combinations of these parameters and others (Ogura, et al., 1973; Richardson, 1981; Biller and Lawson, 1985; Schaefer, 1992). It would seem logical to classify these injuries as to the type of wound (blunt or penetrating) and the anatomic sites affected.

DIAGNOSIS

Clinical Presentation and Examination

Symptoms indicating possible laryngeal injury include increasing airway obstruction with dyspnea and stridor, dysphonia or aphonia, cough, hemoptysis, neck pain, dysphagia, and odynophagia. Clinical signs can include deformities of the neck, with swelling and alterations in its contour (Fig. 62-2), subcutaneous emphysema, laryngeal tenderness, and bony crepitus. The presence of airway obstruction and subcutaneous emphysema is diagnostic of a severe disruption of laryngeal or tracheal structures.

Laryngeal injuries with an open wound are rarely misdiagnosed, and airway obstruction if present can often be relieved by intubation through the laceration. The presence of an open wound usually dictates exploration of the wound, whereas closed injuries present the clinician with the problem of whether or not to perform a surgical exploration (Biller and Lawson, 1985). Indirect mirror or flexible laryngoscopy can be helpful in deciding the necessity for exploration. It is important to assess vocal cord mobility, the presence of edema, hematoma, mucosal tears, exposed cartilage, or evidence of dislocation of the arytenoid cartilages. Direct laryngoscopy under general anesthesia may be required to evaluate the larynx properly in addition to the pharynx and esophagus. A tracheotomy should be performed if required for safe adequate direct laryngoscopy. It is particularly important to evaluate the patient for symptoms or signs of vascular, digestive tract, or neurologic injuries. The patient should be assumed to have a cervical spine injury until it is proved otherwise.

Imaging

Computed tomography (CT) is an excellent noninvasive technique for examining the laryngeal skeleton and has largely replaced laryngograms, tomograms, and xerograms

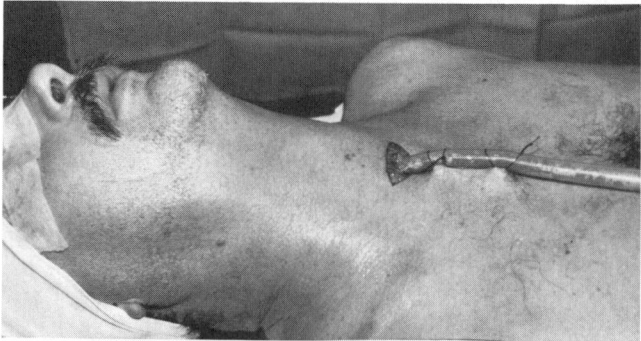

Figure 62-2. Blunt laryngeal injury with marked neck edema and loss of thyroid prominence from subcutaneous emphysema. Tracheotomy is performed prior to surgical exploration.

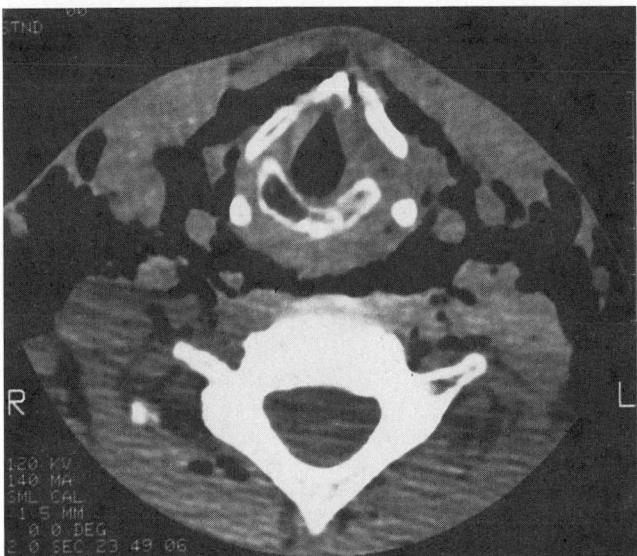

Figure 62-3. Axial CT scan demonstrating marked subcutaneous emphysema following blunt laryngotracheal trauma.

(Mancuso and Hanafee, 1979) (Fig. 62-3). Many authors do not recommend CT scanning in severe soft tissue damage or obvious cartilaginous fracture-dislocation because such patients require exploration and repair anyway (Miller, 1990; Stanley, 1984; Schaefer, 1991). Others find valuable information for preoperative counseling if the surgical management is likely to involve extensive tissue resection, such as partial laryngectomy (Marceri, et al., 1992). The therapy for laryngotracheal trauma is less clearly defined for mild to moderate damage in which the clinical findings are equivocal for cartilaginous damage. In these instances CT is recommended to assess for cartilaginous fractures or dislocations, which may influence the need for surgical exploration (Fig. 62-4). Three-dimensional CT may be superior to conventional two-dimensional CT in assessing laryngeal fractures and differentiating them from anatomic variants (Meglin, et al., 1991).

Cervical spine and chest radiographs are required to exclude associated injuries to the cervical spine and chest. Contrast studies during swallowing are helpful in demonstrating an associated perforation of the pharynx or esophagus.

MANAGEMENT

General Principles

Any acute laryngeal injury requires the establishment of an adequate airway, which may necessitate tracheotomy, intubation, or in an urgent situation, cricothyroidotomy. Following stabilization of the patient, the injuries are assessed, and a plan is formulated for definitive therapy. This may be immediate or delayed, as dictated by the clinical picture. Early therapy is best to avoid the loss of laryngeal function, leading to problems of stenosis, aspiration, and altered voice (Pearson, et al; 1986).

Penetrating trauma is usually obvious, and surgical exploration is normally performed without delay. In blunt laryngotracheal trauma, it is generally agreed that more serious injur-

---

Indications for Surgical Exploration in Laryngotracheal Trauma

Airway obstruction sufficient to warrant tracheotomy (if not the result of edema alone)

Progressive subcutaneous emphysema

Extensive mucosal lacerations and/or exposure of cartilage

Palpable fracture of the laryngeal skeleton or displaced fracture seen by CT

Doubt as to the extent of injury

---

ies should be treated surgically, whereas minor injuries can be treated medically. There is a gray area between these two extremes in which management controversy exists. Indirect mirror or flexible laryngoscopy, CT and direct endoscopy are helpful in determining the need for surgical exploration in these cases.

The indications for surgical exploration are outlined below. The presence of airway obstruction, bare cartilage in the laryngeal lumen, or cricoid collapse require early and aggressive treatment (Olson, 1978). The less severely injured larynx with mild edema, minor endolaryngeal hematoma formation, small lacerations with no anterior commissure involvement, mobile vocal cords, and no airway compromise can be managed medically (Stanley, 1984; Snow, 1984). This includes observation in the hospital, elevation of the head of the bed, voice and bed rest, humidity, and possibly antibiotics and steroids.

Surgical therapy is usually performed through a horizontal skin incision with midline division and retraction of the strap muscles. The larynx is exposed and entered, mucosal

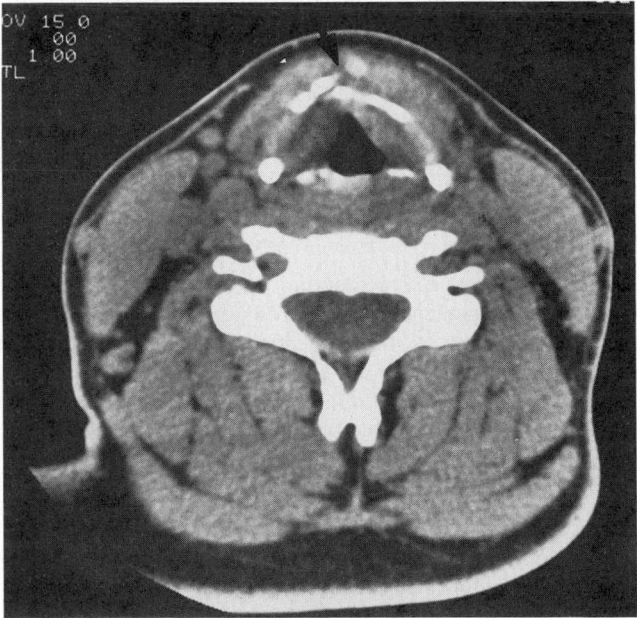

Figure 62-4. Axial CT scan demonstrating minimally displaced thyroid cartilage fracture (*arrow*) following blunt laryngeal trauma.

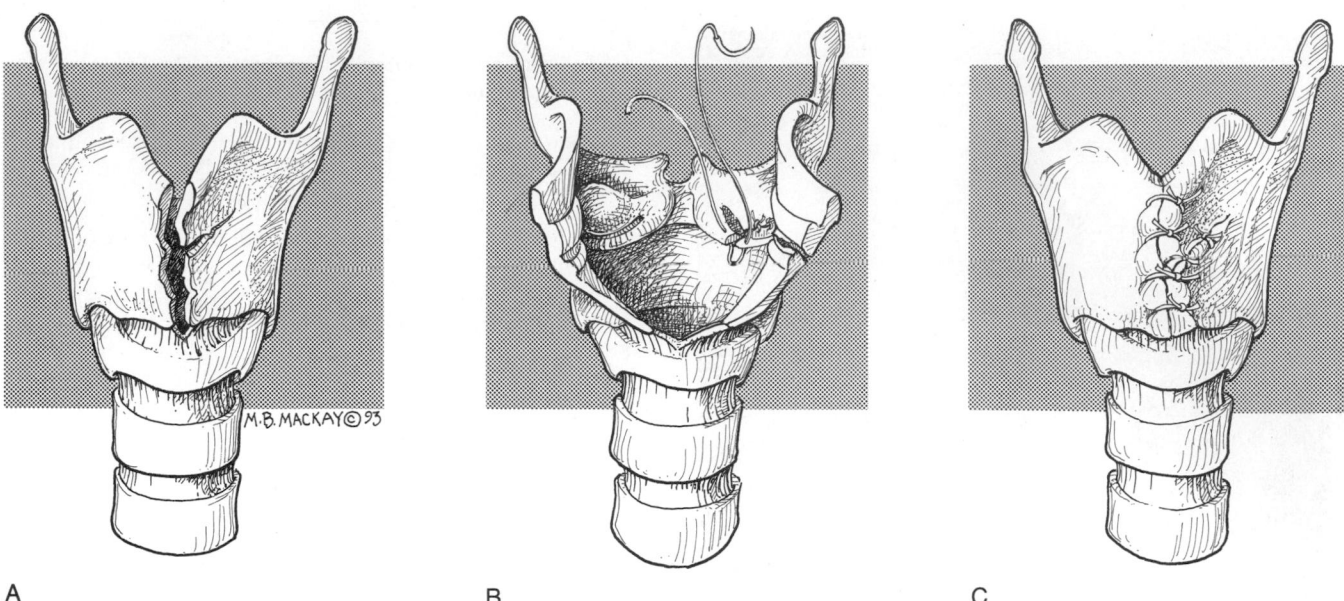

Figure 62-5. Repair of laryngeal fractures. **(A)** Laryngeal framework is exposed. **(B)** The larynx is entered through a midline thyrotomy (or suitable fracture if present). Mucosal tears are repaired with absorbable suture. **(C)** Cartilaginous fractures are reduced and secured with wire or nonabsorbable suture.

tears are repaired with absorbable suture, exposed cartilage is provided with an epithelial cover, and the cartilaginous fractures are reduced and secured with wire or nonabsorbable suture (Fig. 62-5). Dislocated arytenoid cartilages are reduced or removed if avulsed. An internal laryngeal stent may be required to stabilize the repair (Fig. 62-6).

The larynx is commonly entered by making an incision in the cricothyroid membrane and performing a midline thyrotomy (laryngofissure) using an oscillating saw in ossified cartilage or a scalpel in children and young adults. The anterior commissure is divided sharply under direct vision. At the commissure the incision is carried laterally to the epiglottis to avoid dividing it. This approach may have to be modified, based on the location and direction of any cartilaginous fractures. It may even be necessary to explore the larynx through one of the fractures. An attempt is made to preserve all pieces of cartilage, particularly if they are attached to perichondrium.

Controversies

There is no prospective randomized controlled trial dealing with the management of the injured larynx. There continues to be controversy as to the best management strategies in dealing with these injuries. These dilemmas include how to control the airway; the timing of repair; the need for grafts; and the use of stents, corticosteroids, and antibiotics.

Control of Airway

Controversy exists as to whether to perform endotracheal intubation or tracheotomy to manage the compromised airway. Many authors advocate tracheotomy under local anesthesia because intubation may create false passages and further disrupt already damaged mucosa (Schaefer and Close, 1989; Casiano and Goodwin, 1991; Gill, 1969; Harris and

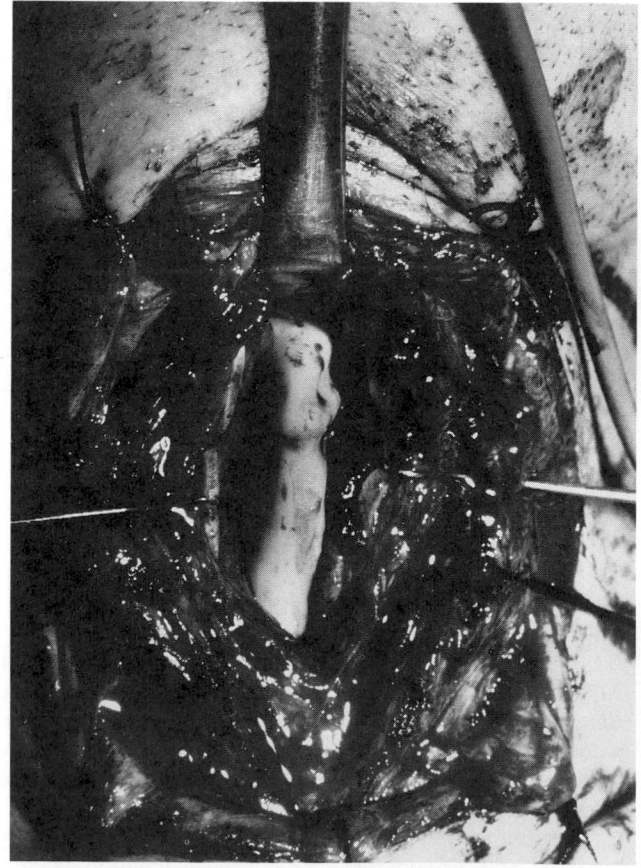

Figure 62-6. Silastic stent that conforms to the shape of the internal larynx. The stent is secured in position by nonabsorbable sutures placed through the stent and thyroid cartilage and brought out on each side of the neck. The ends of the sutures are secured over Silastic buttons on the skin surface.

Aimworth, 1965). This can convert a partially obstructed airway into a completely obstructed airway. Other authors point out that orotracheal intubation under direct visualization by the most experienced physician is usually safe and minimizes the risk of further damage (Schaefer and Close, 1989; Gussack, et al., 1986; Sheely, et al., 1974). Blind intubation should be avoided (Yarington, 1979).

Our bias is for tracheotomy under local anesthesia, especially if indirect laryngoscopy cannot visualize the larynx. If the laryngeal injury is minor, as judged by indirect laryngoscopy with or without CT scanning, and the patient requires general anesthesia for the therapy of other injuries, then careful intubation by an experienced physician is acceptable.

Timing of Repair

It is generally agreed that early repairs yield the best results. There is some controversy as to what constitutes "early" repair. Some authors emphasize repair within the 1st week following the injury (Biller and Lawson, 1985; Potter, et al., 1978; Pennington, 1972). Others emphasize repair within 24 hours (Schaefer, 1982; Leopold, 1983). Other authors recommend waiting 3 to 5 days to permit the edema to resolve (Nahum, 1968; Olson, 1978; Olson and Miles, 1971).

Need for Mucosal or Skin Grafts

It is generally recognized that exposed cartilage should be covered by soft tissue. Preferably a laceration is repaired primarily with absorbable suture or a local flap of mucosa. Alternatively a free mucosal graft is harvested from the pyriform sinus, epiglottis, or buccal mucosa and used to cover the defect (Casiano and Goodwin, 1991). Split-thickness skin grafts may be required to cover exposed cartilage. Olson (1991) and Olson and Miles (1971) recommend placing a finger cot stent surrounded by a split-thickness skin graft with the dermis side facing outward. It is thought that this provides an epithelial lining to areas where closure of normal mucosa is tenuous, impossible, or might fall apart. Grafts may not be necessary, as evidenced by the work of Schaefer and Close (1989), who accumulated experience with 120 cases of laryngotracheal trauma over 23 years and never required skin or mucous membrane grafts.

Stenting

Controversy exists as to the type of stent used, the length of time the stent should remain in the larynx, and whether a stent is required at all. The purpose of a stent is to stabilize the laryngeal skeleton, maintain the internal configuration of the larynx, and prevent scarring between endolaryngeal lacerations. There are no specific guidelines as to whether a stent is required, and its use usually rests with the experience and bias of the surgeon. In general stents are used for more severe trauma with multiple cartilaginous fractures and when the anteroposterior dimension of the larynx must be maintained because of cartilage loss and foreshortening.

No particular type of stent is universally accepted, and all seem to produce satisfactory results. The more popular varieties consist of a finger cot filled with a soft material, such as Ivalon sponge or foam rubber (Miller, 1990), a Portex endotracheal tube cut and shaped to the interior of the larynx

(Schaefer and Close, 1989), or a commercially available solid molded silicone stent (Gluckman, 1981). The length of time recommended to leave the stent in the larynx before removing it transorally includes 1 week (Miller, 1990), 2 weeks (Schaefer and Close, 1989), 2 to 4 weeks (Casiano and Goodwin, 1989), 6 weeks (Snow, 1984), and 3 months (Gluckman, 1981). Clinical experience has usually shown no significant problems with short-term stenting, but experimental laryngeal injuries in dogs have demonstrated an increased incidence of infection and granulation tissue with a variety of "soft stents" (Thomas and Stevens, 1975).

Corticosteroids and Antibiotic Prophylaxis

Corticosteroids are used in an inconsistent manner in most series. Many surgeons view the primary role of steroids as the reduction of edema and inflammation, others use them if there is a delay in surgical exploration in the hope of slowing granulation tissue and collagen deposition (Olson, 1978).

Most authors recommend prophylactic antibiotics for laryngotracheal trauma, but there are no specific clinical trials to substantiate their effectiveness in preventing infection. Experience has been gained from other studies in which prophylactic antiobiotics show a reduction in the infection rate with surgical incisions into contaminated areas or across mucosal edges (Johnson, 1989). Recommendations in cases of laryngotracheal trauma include administering a cephalosporin for 2 to 10 days postoperatively and even longer for some patients with stents or those in whom cartilage remains exposed internally (Schaefer and Close, 1989; Casiano and Goodwin, 1991).

Specific Injuries

Acute Supraglottic Injury

Acute supraglottic injury is usually associated with a fracture of the hyoid bone and horizontal fracture of the thyroid cartilage, producing a loss of the thyroid prominence and displacement of the epiglottis posteriorly and superiorly (Bryce, 1972). During indirect laryngoscopy the displaced epiglottis may obscure the anterior cords, and only the posterior aspect of the vocal cords is visualized. Direct laryngoscopy may miss the injury because the anterior lip of the laryngoscope can correct the posterior displacement of the epiglottis during the examination.

In a pure supraglottic injury, the larynx can be approached through an anterior pharyngotomy. If the tissues are not amenable to primary repair because of a severe injury, a supraglottic laryngectomy can be performed. Supraglottic laryngectomy is contraindicated if the vocal cords are immobile or there is an associated glottic injury (Harris, 1972).

Acute Glottic Injury

Acute glottic injury typically accompanies fractures of the thyroid cartilage that are horizontal, vertical, or cruciate (Fig. 62-7). The airway may become obstructed by vocal cord edema, and the voice is poor. Mucosal tears of the true cords are common, and there may be disruption of the anterior commissure with foreshortening of the anteroposterior diameter of the larynx. One or both vocal cords may be immobile

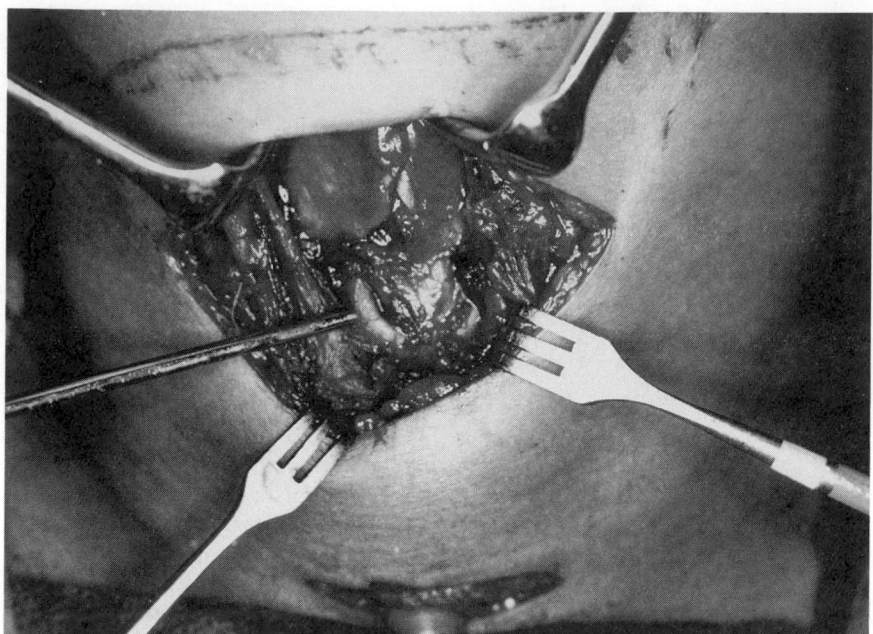

Figure 62-7. Fractured thyroid cartilage following blunt trauma. The sucker points to a segment of right inferior thyroid ala, which has been displaced inferiorly.

because of recurrent laryngeal nerve damage or disruption of the cricoarytenoid joint. The injuries are approached through a midline thyrotomy. It is important to reapproximate the true cords to the thyroid cartilages or perichondrium in the midline and insert a keel or stent to prevent anterior commissure webbing.

Acute Subglottic Injury

Acute subglottic injury involves injury to the cricoid cartilage and often the cervical trachea. The cricoid prominence is lost to palpation, and as subglottic edema increases, the airway becomes severely compromised. Hoarseness is usually not marked unless the recurrent laryngeal nerves have been injured. If the anterior arch is depressed, it can usually be elevated and a stent inserted. If there is comminution and loss of the anterior arch, it is preferable to perform a thyrotracheal anastomosis.

Laryngotracheal Separation

Laryngotracheal separation is a specialized form of subglottic injury in which the cricoid cartilage may be avulsed from the trachea (Fig. 62-8). The strap muscles, recurrent laryngeal nerves, and esophagus may be divided in the process (Lejeune, 1978). The usual mechanism of injury is from the shearing force of a restraining cable against the upper trachea. Airway obstruction develops rapidly, and if suspected an emergency tracheotomy or intubation of the distal trachea through a laceration is required. It is important to determine if vocal cord mobility is intact because of the high incidence of avulsion of the recurrent laryngeal nerves in this injury.

During exploration the trachea is mobilized superiorly, and a cricotracheal anastomosis is performed. It is important to

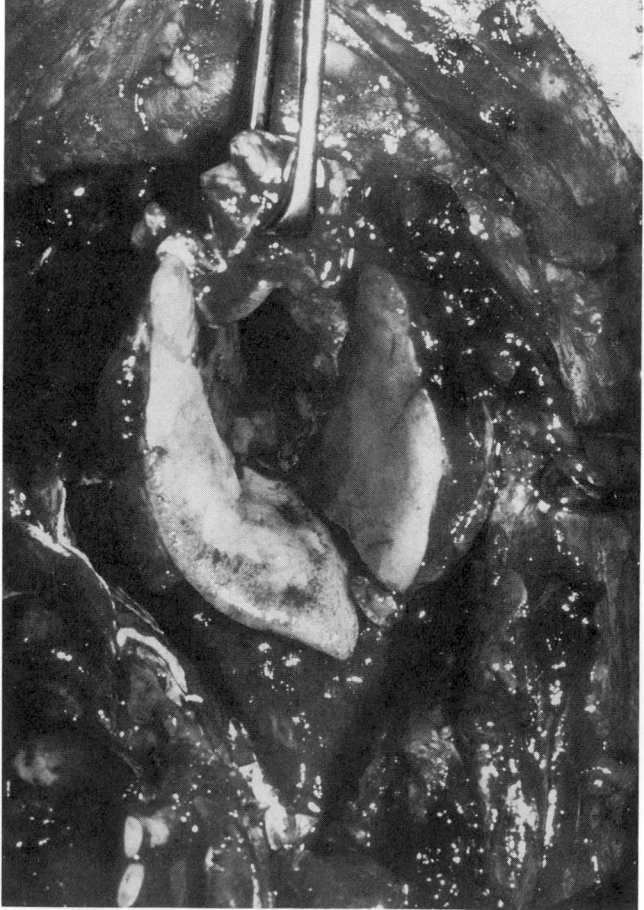

Figure 62-8. Laryngotracheal separation. The cricoid ring is viewed from inferiorly looking into the larynx. Note the denuded mucosa and exposed fractured cricoid cartilage.

place a stent or T tube to reduce the incidence of subglottic stenosis (Alonso, et al., 1974). If the esophagus requires repair, the strap muscles can be interposed between the trachea and esophagus to prevent fistula formation.

The ideal solution for the problem of recurrent laryngeal nerve transsection remains elusive (Miehlke, 1974; Sato, et al., 1974). It is controversial whether to repair the transsected ends of this nerve if they can be found. Some success with the repair of transsected recurrent laryngeal nerves has been achieved (Doyle, et al., 1967) but many believe the procedure is not effective in achieving abduction of the vocal cord (Tucker, 1980). Animal studies show that adductor function returns fairly reliably but abductor function does not (Murakami and Kirchner, 1971). This is thought to occur because there is an approximately 3:1 predominance of adductor nerve fibers in recurrent laryngeal nerves compared with abductor fibers. During regeneration, the adductor fibers are more likely to reach their motor end plates. It may be better to implant the avulsed end of the nerve into the posterior cricoarytenoid muscle, which is the primary abductor of the larynx (Snow, 1984; Miglets, 1974). The superior laryngeal nerves are usually intact; therefore, adduction can still be achieved by tension of the cricothyroid muscles. Casiano and Goodwin (1991) believe it is reasonable to repair the nerve, even though the possibility of the return of function is poor. If any of these measures fail, a permanent tracheotomy or vocal cord lateralizing procedure is required.

Dislocation of Cricoarytenoid Joint

Arytenoid function may be difficult to evaluate immediately after an injury because poor function can be caused by nerve or joint injury. When the arytenoid is avulsed completely, it is best to remove it. When only partially disrupted, the arytenoid may be relocated. A secondary arytenoidectomy can always be performed at a later date if an inadequate airway results.

Fractured Hyoid Bone

A fracture of the hyoid bone may occur alone or in association with other fractures. The most common area to be fractured is the central body. This results in pain and swelling over the upper anterior neck, and bony crepitus is noted on palpation and swallowing. It is important to look for an associated avulsion of the epiglottis. The hyoid bone is intimately related to the muscles of deglutition, causing movement at the fracture sites and delayed or nonunion. It is possible to reduce and stabilize some fractures, but more commonly the area of fractured hyoid bone is resected with little sequelae.

Minimally Displaced Thyroid Cartilage

In the past it has generally been thought that nondisplaced or minimally displaced thyroid cartilage fractures did well with medical therapy alone. The voice may sound normal by subjective criteria, but in one case of a paramedian thyroid fracture reported by Hirano, et al. (1985), there was a significant improvement in fundamental frequency, range, and phonation intensity after open reduction. Schaefer and Close (1989) recommend that any single displaced thyroid cartilage fracture should be managed surgically.

Prognosis

The patient's ultimate vocal quality and airway function following laryngotracheal trauma are influenced by the management of this laryngeal and related injuries, especially the central nervous system and the pulmonary system. The resulting vocal and respiratory functions of the larynx depend on the severity of the initial injury. Poor prognostic signs include early airway obstruction (implying more severe injury), denuded cartilage in the laryngeal lumen, and fracture or collapse of the cricoid cartilage (Olson, 1978). Decannulation and good voice are expected in more than 80 percent of all patients managed with early surgical intervention (Schaefer, 1992; Casiano and Goodwin, 1991).

KEY REFERENCES

Casiano RR, Goodwin WJ: Restoring function to the injured larynx. Otolaryngol Clin North Am 24:1215, 1991

This article is a good reference to accompany this chapter, which addresses the principles of managing laryngeal injuries.

Pearson FG, Brito-Filomeno L, Cooper JD: Experience with partial cricoid resection and thyrotracheal anastomosis. Ann Otol Rhinol Laryngol 95:582, 1986

This article details the management techniques of tracheal and subglottic resection by primary thyrotracheal anastomosis for various pathologic conditions, including cricotracheal disruption caused by blunt trauma. The authors outline how consistently good results can be achieved for this rare but challenging problem.

Schaefer SD: The acute management of laryngeal trauma: a 27 year experience. Arch Otolaryngol Head Neck Surg 118:598, 1992

This article outlines a 27-year experience in the management of 139 consecutive patients with external laryngeal trauma principally by one physician. The rationales for changes in the therapeutic protocol over this period based on patient outcome are discussed. This is an excellent reference for any clinician interested in the diagnostic and therapeutic principles of laryngotracheal trauma.

REFERENCES

Alonso WA, Pratt LL, Zollinger WK, Ogura JH: Complications of laryngotracheal disruption. Laryngoscope 84:1276, 1974

Biller HF, Lawson W: Management of acute laryngeal trauma. p. 149. In Bailey BJ, Biller HF (eds): Surgery of the Larynx. WB Saunders, Toronto, 1985

Bryce DP: Laryngeal trauma and stenosis. In Maran AGD, Stell PM (eds): Clinical Otolaryngology. Blackwell Scientific Publications, Oxford, 1979

Bryce DP: The surgical management of laryngotracheal injury. J Laryngol Otol 86:547, 1972

Doyle PJ, Brummett RE, Everts EC: Results of surgical section and repair of the recurrent laryngeal nerve. Laryngoscope 77:1245, 1967

Gill AJ: Rupture of the cervical trachea and esophagus. Arch Otolaryngol Head Neck Surg 90:95, 1969

Gluckman JL: Laryngeal trauma: surgical therapy in the adult. Ear Nose Throat J 60:366, 1981

Gussack GS, Jurkovich GJ: Treatment dilemmas in laryngotracheal trauma. J Trauma 28:1439, 1988

Gussack GS, Jurkovich GJ, Luterman A: Laryngotracheal trauma: a protocol approach to a rare injury. Laryngoscope 96:660, 1986

Harris HH: Management of injuries to the larynx and trachea. Laryngoscope 82:1924, 1972

Harris HH, Aimworth JZ: Immediate management of laryngeal and tracheal injuries. Laryngoscope 75:1103, 1965

Hirano M, Kurita S, Terasawa R: Difficulty in high-pitched phonation by laryngeal trauma. Arch Otolaryngol Head Neck Surg 111:59, 1985

Johnson JT: Perioperative antibiotics in head and neck surgery. p. 109. In Cummings CW, Fredrickson JM, Harker LA et al (eds): Otolaryngology—Head and Neck Surgery Update I. CV Mosby, Toronto, 1989

Lee SY: Experimental blunt injury to the larynx. Ann Otol Rhinol Laryngol 101:270, 1992

Lejeune FE: Laryngotracheal separation. Laryngoscope 88:1956, 1978

Leopold DA: Laryngeal trauma. A historical comparison of treatment methods. Arch Otolaryngol Head Neck Surg 109:106, 1983

Maceri DR, Mancuso AA, Canalis RF: Value of computed axial tomography in severe laryngeal injury. Arch Otolaryngol Head Neck Surg 108:449, 1982

Mancuso AA, Hanafee WN: Computed tomography of the injured larynx. Radiology 133:139, 1979

Meglin AJ, Biedlingmaier JF, Mirvis SE: Three-dimensional computerized tomography in the evaluation of laryngeal injury. Laryngoscope 101:202, 1991

Miehlke A: Rehabilitation of vocal cord paralysis. Studies using the vagus recurrent bypass anastomosis type ramus posterior shunt. Arch Otolaryngol Head Neck Surg 100:431, 1974

Miglets AW: Functional laryngeal abduction following reimplantation of the recurrent laryngeal nerves. Laryngoscope 84:1996, 1974

Miller RH: Acute laryngeal trauma. p. 362. In Gates GA (ed): Current Therapy in Otolaryngology—Head and Neck Surgery. Vol. 4. BC Decker, Toronto, 1990

Minard G, Kudsk KA, Croce MA et al: Laryngotracheal trauma. Am Surg 58:181, 1992

Murakami Y, Kirchner JA: Vocal cord abduction by regenerated recurrent laryngeal nerve. An experimental study in the dog. Arch Otolaryngol Head Neck Surg 94:64, 1971

Nahum AM: Immediate care of acute blunt laryngeal trauma. J Trauma 9:112, 1969

Ogura JH, Heeneman H, Spector GV: Laryngotracheal trauma: diagnosis and treatment. Can J Otolaryngol 2:112, 1973

Olson NR: Skin grafting of the larynx. Otolaryngol Head Neck Surg 104:503, 1991

Olson NR: Acute laryngeal trauma. p. 1982. In Gates GA (ed): Current Therapy in Otolaryngology—Head and Neck Surgery. CV Mosby, St. Louis, 1982

Olson NR: Surgical treatment of acute blunt laryngeal injuries. Ann Otol Rhinol Laryngol 87:716, 1978

Olson NR, Miles WK: Treatment of acute blunt laryngeal injuries. Ann Otol Rhinol Laryngol 80:704, 1971

Pennington CL: External trauma of the larynx and trachea. Immediate treatment and management. Ann Otol Rhinol Laryngol 81:546, 1972

Potter CR, Sessions DG, Ogura JH: Blunt laryngotracheal trauma. Otolaryngology 86:909, 1978

Richardson MA: Laryngeal anatomy and mechanisms of trauma. Ear Nose Throat J 60:346, 1981

Sato I, Harvey JE, Ogura JH: Impairment of function of the intrinsic laryngeal muscles after regeneration of the recurrent laryngeal nerve. Laryngoscope 84:53, 1974

Schaefer SD: Use of CT scanning in the management of the acutely injured larynx. Otolaryngol Clin North Am 24:31, 1991

Schaefer SD: Primary management of laryngeal trauma. Ann Otol Rhinol Laryngol 91:399, 1982

Schaefer SD, Close LG: Acute management of laryngeal trauma. Ann Otol Rhinol Laryngol 98:98, 1989

Sheely CH II, Mattox KL, Beall AC Jr: Management of acute cervical tracheal trauma. Am J Surg 128:805, 1974

Snow JB: Diagnosis and therapy for acute laryngeal and tracheal trauma. Otolaryngol Clin North Am 17:101, 1984

Stanley RB: Value of computed tomography in management of acute laryngeal injury. J Trauma 24:359, 1984

Stanley RB, Crockett DM, Persky M: Knife wounds into the airspaces of the laryngeal trapezium. J Trauma 28:101, 1988

Thomas GK, Stevens MH: Stenting in experimental laryngeal injuries. Arch Otolaryngol Head Neck Surg 101:217, 1975

Tucker HM: Nerve-muscle pedicle reinnervation for paralysis of the vocal cord. p. 43. In Snow JB Jr (ed): Controversy in Otolaryngology. WB Saunders, Philadelphia, 1980

Yarington CT: Trauma involving the air and food passages. Otolaryngol Clin North Am 12:321, 1979

63

TRACHEOBRONCHIAL TRAUMA

David S. Mulder
Salim Ratnani

DEFINITION

As discussed in this chapter, tracheobronchial injury is defined as any traumatic injury to the trachea or bronchi from the level of the cricoid cartilage to the division of the lobar bronchi into segmental branches. It includes all etiologic agents that cause direct injury. Trauma to the larynx is discussed separately in Chapter 62, and trauma to the lung is considered in Chapter 64.

HISTORICAL NOTE

One of the earliest recorded patients with a traumatic rupture of the bronchus was an Indian man who suffered a crushing injury to the chest and abdomen when he was run over by a cart. Autopsy revealed a ruptured liver and a ruptured left mainstem bronchus (Webb, 1848).

Winslow (1871) recorded the survival of a canvasback duck following a left bronchial injury, which he noted had healed spontaneously with preserved distal pulmonary function. The first human survivor was reported by Krinitzki (1927), who described a traumatic rupture of the right mainstem bronchus in a 30-year-old woman who was crushed by a wine keg when she was 10 years old. His report suggested that not all of these injuries are fatal initially and that humans may have the same ability as the canvasback duck to heal a major injury to the bronchial tree. Nissen (1931) observed a delayed stricture at the site of a complete rupture of a mainstem bronchus, which was subsequently treated successfully by pneumonectomy.

Sanger (1945) reported the successful suture of a major bronchial laceration. Kinsella and Johnsrud (1947) described the successful repair of a complete bronchial rupture caused by blunt trauma. Griffith (1949) successfully resected a post-traumatic bronchial stricture with preservation of pulmonary function, and Beskin (1959) sutured a total rupture of the trachea with a successful outcome.

These brief historical observations reinforce modern-day management of airway injuries and emphasize that early recognition and surgical therapy lead to a favorable outcome in a high percentage of patients.

HISTORICAL READINGS

Griffith JL: Fracture of the bronchus. Thorax 4:105, 1949
Krinitzki SI: Zur Kasuistik einer vollstandingen Zerreibung der rechten Luftrohrenastes. Virchows Arch A Pathol Anat Histopathol 266:815, 1927
Sanger PW: Evacuation hospital experience with war wounds and injuries of the chest. Ann Surg 122:147, 1945
Webb A: Pathologica Indica of the Anatomy of Indian Diseases. 2nd Ed. Thacker, Calcutta, 1848
Winslow WH: Rupture of bronchus from wild duck. Philadelphia Medical Times 1:225, April 15, 1871

BASIC SCIENCE

Etiologic Classification

The etiologic classification of tracheobronchial injury can be listed as follows.

1. Blunt trauma caused by crushing, acceleration or deceleration, or a fall from height
2. Inhalation injuries caused by smoke, noxious gas, or chemical inhalation
3. Penetrating stab or gunshot wounds
4. Iatrogenic injuries caused by endotracheal intubation with regular or double-lumen tubes, bronchoscopy, long-term ventilatory support or barotrauma, laser injuries, or injury

during adjacent or related surgery (such as mediastinoscopy, esophagectomy, and thyroidectomy)

Blunt Trauma

There are three traditional mechanisms postulated to explain tracheobronchial injury after blunt trauma:

1. A sudden anteroposterior compression of the chest increases the transverse diameter of the thoracic cavity. Because the lungs remain in contact with the chest wall as a result of the negative intrapleural pressure, they become forcefully pulled laterally, placing traction on the relatively fixed carina. If the injuring force exceeds the elasticity of the tracheobronchial tree, rupture occurs, usually in a transverse or circumferential manner (Deslauriers, 1987).
2. Schonberg (1912) hypothesized that a blunt impact to the chest occurring with a closed glottis produces a sudden rise in airway pressure, which is greatest in the large-diameter airways (Laplace's law) and results in a disruption near the carina. This type of injury may be longitudinal and contained by mediastinal structures.
3. A rapid deceleration type of injury results in shearing forces on the airway and at the areas of fixation, namely, the carina and the cricoid cartilage. This may contribute to the high incidence of airway injuries centered on the carina in the thoracic cavity and just below the cricoid area in the neck.

Inhalation Injury

Moylan and Chan (1978) described a greatly increased incidence of inhalation injuries following thermal trauma. The airway may also be injured following the inhalation or aspiration of noxious gases or chemicals, such as acids or alkalis. The availability of the fiberoptic bronchoscope has revealed a threefold increase in inhalation injury, and the authors describe three distinct patterns: (1) upper airway, (2) major intrathoracic airways, and (3) a distal parenchymal injury.

Penetrating Injury

Penetrating injuries may involve the airway in the neck or thoracic cavity, depending on the muzzle velocity and trajectory of the wounding missile (Symbas, et al., 1976). More than 80 percent of the penetrating airway injuries involve the trachea in the neck, and the majority of the intrathoracic penetrating injuries involve the trachea or major bronchi concentrated in the carinal area.

Associated Injuries

The magnitude of trauma required to produce an injury to the airway is great, and thus associated injuries are common and frequently determine the ultimate outcome in terms of the patient's survival and morbidity (Symbas, et al., 1992). Head, facial, and cervical spine injuries are frequently described as associated injuries and important predictors of mortality and morbidity rates. Traumatic rupture of intra-abdominal solid organs, such as the liver and spleen, are commonly associated with major blunt chest trauma. Associated injuries of structures adjacent to the major airway include the esophagus and great vessels (Feliciano, et al., 1985; Glatterer, et al., 1985). A tracheoesophageal fistula has occurred in slightly more than 50 patients with blunt chest trauma (Mulder and Barkun, 1986). Injuries to the great vessels and the aorta distal to the subclavian artery are the common major vascular injuries associated with both blunt and penetrating airway injury. Pericardial and cardiac injuries have also been described.

Pathophysiology

Autopsy studies following blunt trauma that emphasize airway injury suggest that hypoxemia is still the most common cause of death (Bertelsen and Howitz, 1972; Kemmerer, et al., 1961). Hypoxemia results from mechanical disruption of the airway, with a resultant inability to ventilate the lung tissue distal to the injury. A secondary and common consequence of injury is bleeding into the airway from injured bronchial arteries or adjacent structures. Blood in the airway may clot and obstruct large segments of the airway distal to the injury itself. Trauma of the magnitude required to rupture an airway almost always causes pulmonary contusion, which further contributes to the hypoxemia.

Many of the clinical manifestations depend on the location and severity of the airway injury. Airway injuries in the cervical trachea or larynx produce small amounts of subcutaneous emphysema initially, and the major threat is to the integrity of the airway itself. Injury to the airway in the thorax with a large pleural communication demonstrates a massive pneumothorax on the involved side along with a pneumomediastinum and massive subcutaneous emphysema. An intrathoracic airway injury that is contained by the mediastinum is characterized by an extensive pneumomediastinum with subcutaneous emphysema, depending on the size of the airway injury (Fig. 63-1). A small contained airway injury may present little in the way of physiologic consequences unless the injury produces granulation tissue and subsequent stenosis of the airway.

Thus, the common final pathway in airway injury is hypoxemia from multiple contributing factors. The resulting dyspnea may produce hypocapnia such as that seen with hyperventilation. Hypercapnia has also been described ($PaCO_2 > 40$ mmHg), which is associated with a high mortality rate, and severe hypoxia, which usually requires an FIO_2 of 50 percent or higher to maintain a PaO_2 of 65 mmHg. This group of patients also shows secondary alterations in the relationships between $PaCO_2$ and the base excess, suggesting that the hypercapnia is a consequence of impaired gas exchange. These changes were noted to be almost immediately reversible following endobronchial intubation.

DIAGNOSIS

Clinical Presentation

Davies and Hopkins (1973) categorized bronchial injuries into two types. In type I the injury to the airway opens directly into the pleural cavity, producing a massive pneumothorax,

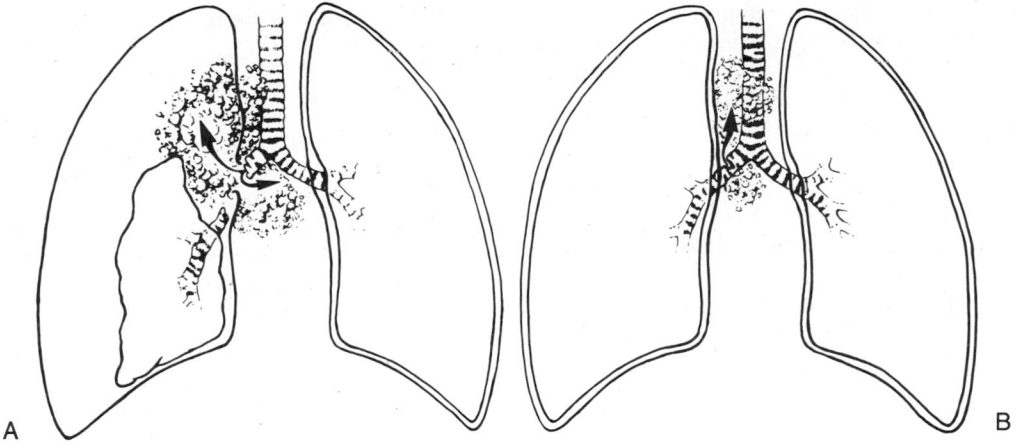

Figure 63-1. **(A)** Intrapleural bronchial disruption with a drop of the right hilum and a massive pneumothorax. **(B)** Rupture of a bronchus contained by mediastinal structures with mediastinal emphysema.

which may be refractory to chest tube drainage. In type II the airway injury produces little communication with the pleural cavity and is sealed off by the mediastinum. They describe instances in which this type of lesion did not require surgical closure. The distal airway and the lung parenchyma may be injured at any level, and this type of injury is usually associated with the formation of a parenchymal hematoma.

The airway is thus subject to a wide variety of mechanisms of injury. Most intrathoracic airway injuries caused by blunt trauma involve the trachea or mainstem bronchi within 2.5 cm of the carina. The proximal right mainstem bronchus appears to be involved more frequently than the left. The left mainstem bronchus has a longer mediastinal course, and a partial injury may result in a contained pneumomediastinum. Incomplete injuries to a major airway may result in subsequent formation of a granuloma and secondary stenosis of the bronchus, producing a pattern of recurrent pneumonia in the involved pulmonary segment.

Incidence

The true incidence of tracheobronchial injury is difficult to establish because many patients with blunt trauma caused by motor vehicle accidents die before reaching the hospital. There is, however, general agreement that the incidence of both blunt and penetrating tracheobronchial injury is increasing as the result of several factors. First, there has been a dramatic improvement in prehospital care through North America. This has resulted in an increased number of more seriously injured patients reaching hospital emergency rooms alive. Second, the development of trauma centers has resulted in a relative concentration of the most seriously injured patients within an organized trauma system. Third, there has been an absolute increase in the amount of penetrating trauma as a result of knife and gunshot wounds.

One of the better studies on the incidence of airway injury reviewed the postmortem reports of 1,178 patients who died of blunt trauma in Denmark (Bertelsen and Howitz, 1972). They noted an incidence of tracheobronchial injury to be 2.8 percent (33 patients); 27 of the 33 patients died instantly prior

to any hospital care. Six patients arrived at the hospital and died within 2 hours following admission but prior to definitive surgical therapy. Bertelsen and Horwitz emphasized the importance of aspirated blood in otherwise normal lungs as a contributing factor to the hypoxemia and high mortality rate. They inferred that a surgical solution was feasible.

Kemmerer et al. (1961) studied 585 deaths following traffic accidents in metropolitan New Orleans. They noted five patients (1 percent) with tracheobronchial rupture, four of whom died at the scene of the accident. One patient reached the hospital alive and died during an attempted surgical repair of a bronchial injury.

Many recent case reports, series, and collective reviews confirm an increased incidence in injury to the trachea and major bronchi. They all emphasize that, although this lesion continues to be rare, it demands early recognition and prompt surgical therapy for a successful outcome (Burke, 1962; De la Rocha and Kayler, 1985; Symbas, et al., 1982).

History and Examination

The early diagnosis begins with a careful history as to the nature of the injury, such as a sudden deceleration injury related to motor vehicle trauma, ejection from a vehicle, or a fall from a height. The trajectory and muzzle velocity of any missile are important factors in raising the possibility of an airway injury. There may be an inhalation component to many thermal injuries and also with the ingestion of acids or alkalis.

Dyspnea and various degrees of respiratory distress are the most common symptoms associated with an airway injury. Stridor may be present if the larynx or upper trachea are involved. Hemoptysis is commonly associated with airway injuries at any level (Wilson, et al., 1987).

Subcutaneous emphysema and evidence of respiratory distress are the most common findings on the physical examination. The degree of subcutaneous emphysema varies with the location and magnitude of the airway injury. There is frequently a pneumothorax present, particularly if the injury communicates freely with the pleural space. The development of a pneumothorax following endotracheal intubation or positive pressure ventilation is another common finding with airway injuries. A persistent massive air leak and the failure of a pulmonary expansion after tube thoracostomy are further evidence for a major airway injury. Several authors have described an increase in dyspnea following chest tube insertion, particularly if suction is applied (Baumgartner, et al., 1990; Shimazu, et al., 1988; Wilson, et al., 1985).

The characteristic findings of dyspnea, cyanosis, subcutaneous and mediastinal emphysema, hemoptysis, pneumothorax, and fractured ribs are seen in approximately one-third of patients. Dyspnea and hemoptysis are indications for an early diagnostic bronchoscopy.

Major thermal injuries are associated with inhalation or airway sequelae in 11 to 33 percent in the majority of cases of significant airway injury (Lund, et al., 1985; Haponik, et al., 1988). There is external evidence of thermal trauma involving the external nares orthe oropharyngeal mucosa. There may also be associated carbonaceous material in the nasal cavity or in the airway itself. These observations are important because they are frequently associated with upper airway obstruction, which requires intubation.

In the case of the ingestion of acids and alkali, there may be an inhalation component or an involvement of the true and false vocal cords, resulting in an immediate threat to the airway (Postlethwait, 1979).

Laboratory Studies

The most consistent finding associated with tracheobronchial injuries is a significantly lower arterial PaO_2 on admission compared with that of other patients with chest trauma. The level of arterial $PaCO_2$ is related to the degree of hyperventilation and also the extent of impaired ventilation.

Hemoglobin and hematocrit levels are frequently reduced as a result of the associated injuries that produce intra-abdominal or intrathoracic hemorrhage.

Radiologic Examination

Chest Radiographs

The upright posteroanterior chest film remains one of the most valuable diagnostic studies in blunt chest trauma. The most common findings are subcutaneous emphysema, pneumothorax, pneumomediastinum, and a pleural effusion (Figs. 63-2 and 63-3) (Reynolds and Christiensen, 1986).

The lateral cervical spine film may reveal air along the prevertebral fascia and is good indirect evidence of the possibility of an airway or an esophageal injury (Fig. 63-4). A penetrating missile may directly enter the trachea or bronchus (Fig. 63-5).

Several early radiologic signs, indicating the possibility of a traumatic transsection of an airway, have been described. Although most of these signs provide only indirect evidence of bronchial rupture, they may add to the common clinical picture of an uncontrolled pneumothorax.

Kumpe, et al. (1970), Oh, et al. (1969), and Endress, et al. (1991) described typical radiologic evidence for unilateral complete bronchial avulsion. The affected lung on the involved side is not only collapsed but falls inferior to its normal point of hilar attachment. This is in contrast to a simple pneumothorax in which the apex of the lung remains above the level of the main bronchus. In the supine position, the lung is noted to fall laterally and posteriorly away from the mediastinum. In a simple pneumothorax, the lung collapses medially onto the hilum. The hilar structures in a completely detached lung are also less visible as a result of the bronchial laceration and the inferior position of the remaining lung. Disruption of the tracheal air column is the most specific radiographic sign of a tracheal transsection.

Computed Tomography

The precise role of a CT scan and the diagnosis of a bronchial rupture is not clear at this time in spite of recent reports

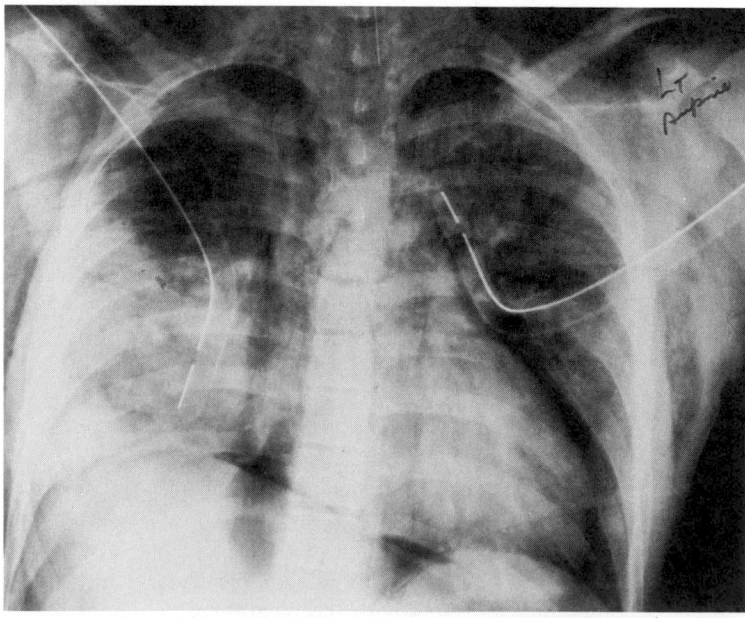

Figure 63-2. Massive mediastinal and subcutaneous emphysema and bilateral pneumothoraces poorly controlled with bilateral chest tubes.

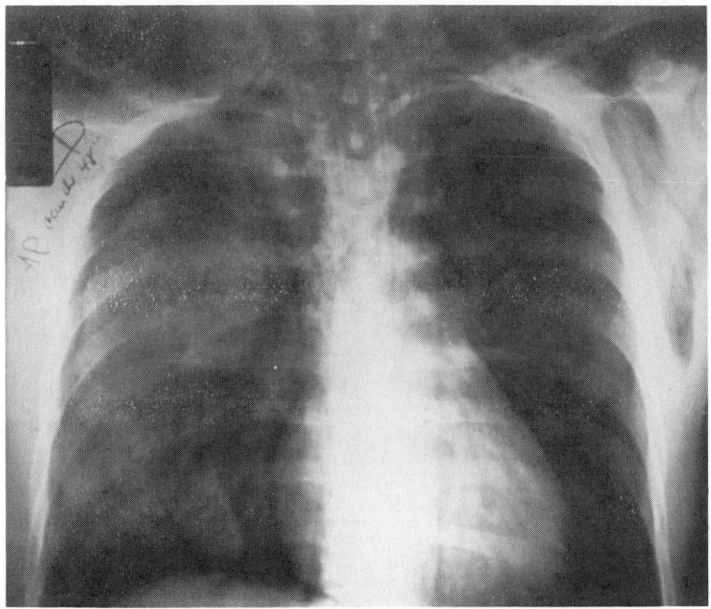

Figure 63-3. Pneumothorax on right with lung parenchymal and mediastinal hematoma.

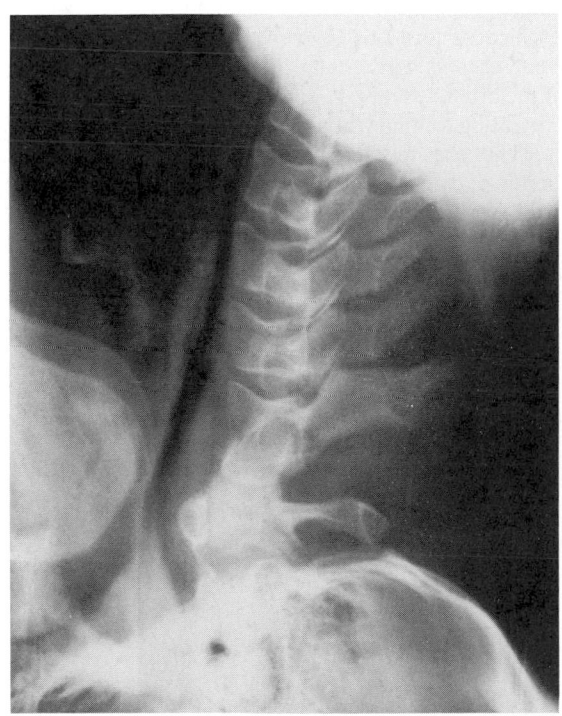

Figure 63-4. Demonstrates air in the prevertebral space associated with an injury to the membranous trachea.

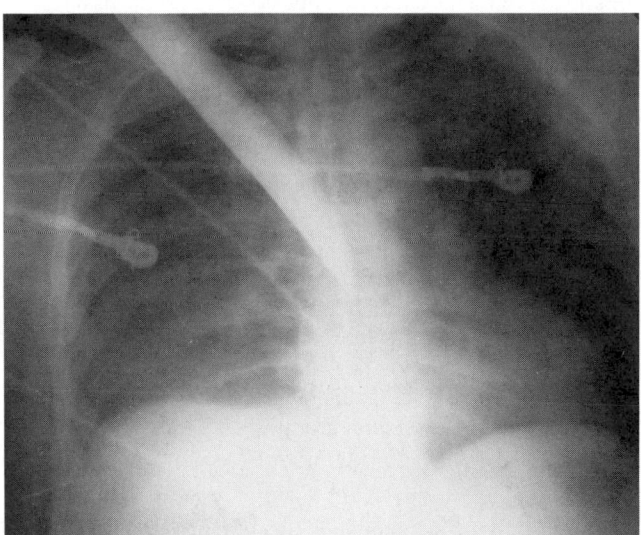

Figure 63-5. A stab wound of posterior thorax partially transsected the right upper lobe bronchus.

Early Radiologic Signs of Bronchial Rupture

Indirect signs
    Tension pneumothorax, uni- or bilateral
    Fracture of upper ribs (one to three)
    Mediastinal emphysema
    Deep cervical emphysema
More direct signs
    Obstruction of an air-filled bronchus
    Sleeve of air surrounding the ruptured bronchus
Direct signs
    Affected lung drops inferiorly

(Weir, et al., 1988). Its greatest value lies in detecting the presence of a mediastinal hematoma and the possibility of associated injuries of great vessels. A CT scan may also define the anatomic relationships of the trachea and the mainstem bronchi.

The signs of a ruptured left mainstem bronchus, as seen on a CT scan, include the deviation of the trachea and the right mainstem bronchus to the right, with the remainder of the mediastinum and the consolidated left lung being shifted to the left, along with an abrupt tapering of the left mainstem bronchus. CT has also been useful in the long-term follow-up of bronchial repairs, particularly to document the presence of a bronchial granuloma or a stricture.

A negative CT finding does not obviate the need for bronchoscopy or further diagnostic studies.

Contrast Studies

Bronchography

A bronchogram is rarely valuable in the acute setting, and in fact it may be contraindicated. Some authors have described using it for more distal airway injuries when flexible and rigid bronchoscopic results have been negative. They suggest the use of the contrast agent Dionosil because the water-soluble contrast media may be more irritating to the lung parenchyma. Bronchography has also been useful in the later phases of follow-up of a distal bronchial repair or in the documentation of bronchial granulomas or strictures.

Esophagogram

An esophagogram is valuable in the case of a suspected associated esophageal injury. It is particularly valuable in the face of a penetrating injury to the trachea. We prefer the initial use of dilute barium as the contrast medium of choice. It is useful to carry out both anteroposterior and lateral projections to rule out smaller esophageal injuries or the presence of a tracheoesophageal fistula.

Angiography

Angiography remains the procedure of choice in terms of the investigative studies for a widened mediastinum, suspicious mediastinal hematoma, or the absence of upper limb pulses.

An angiogram may also be valuable in ruling out other arterial injuries in the neck, abdomen, or even intracranial lesions.

Endoscopy

The increased incidence of blunt chest trauma and penetrating injuries that may involve the airway have greatly liberalized the role of bronchoscopy and esophagoscopy, both pre- and postoperatively.

Early bronchoscopy is the single most effective diagnostic study in a patient with suspected airway injury. Many such patients have concomitant head and cervical spine injuries, and thus fiberoptic bronchoscopy can be accomplished with on-line traction in place to minimize the risk of compounding a spinal cord injury. Bronchoscopy can also be therapeutic when the fiberoptic bronchoscope is armed with an endotracheal tube. The flexible bronchoscope can be used as a stent or guide to cross a transsection of the thoracic cervical or thoracic trachea or to intubate a mainstem bronchus selectively (Fig. 63-6). This avoids a blind intubation with its associated complications. Ideally the bronchoscopy is best performed in an operating room environment in which surgical control of the airway by tracheostomy or thoracotomy can be accomplished. An important part of the diagnostic bronchoscopy is the evaluation of the hypopharynx and particularly vocal cord function.

In our critical care trauma unit, we have made flexible fiberoptic bronchoscopy almost routine in major blunt trauma or penetrating trauma when the trajectory suggests an airway injury. The classic indications for bronchoscopy include pneumomediastinum, a refractory pneumothorax, unexplained persistent atelectasis, hemoptysis, and marked subcutaneous emphysema in a patient with a history of chest trauma. Careful attention is always directed to the cervical and intrathoracic trachea and the proximal mainstem bronchi in which the majority of airway injuries occur. These injuries may be masked by the presence of an endotracheal tube, making the entire larynx and proximal trachea difficult to evaluate. We recently observed a complete transsection of

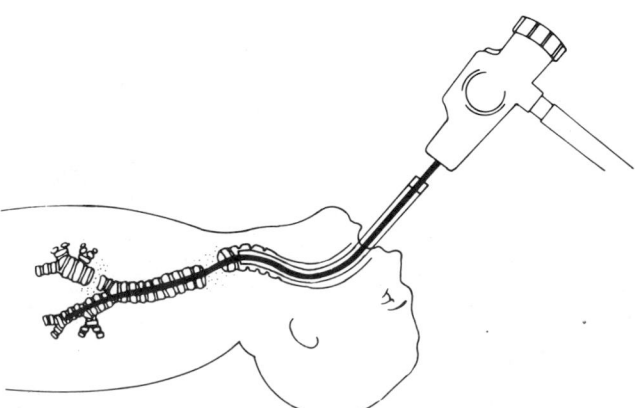

Figure 63-6. Fiberoptic bronchoscope armed with an endotracheal tube used to cross a tracheal rupture or intubate the left mainstem bronchus selectively in the presence of a right mainstem bronchial disruption.

the trachea, which was detected 24 hours following laparotomy for major hepatic trauma. The endotracheal tube had bridged the gap and allowed effective ventilation for the operation to proceed. A pre-extubation bronchoscopy quickly made the appropriate diagnosis. Some authors combine bronchoscopy with the injection of methylene blue or a contrast agent, particularly in the diagnosis of more peripheral airway injuries or if there is a possibility of a small tracheoesophageal fistula.

It is our policy to carry out early tracheobronchoscopy in any serious inhalational burn injury or following the ingestion of acid or alkali in which a laryngeal injury may be present. This examination is always carried out following vigorous oxygenation with a mask and bag if endotracheal intubation has not been required.

Although it is our preference to use flexible fiberoptic bronchoscopy in the trauma patient to minimize the risk of compounding a spinal cord injury, there are situations in which rigid bronchoscopy is indicated. The presence of massive bleeding or copious secretions are best handled with a rigid bronchoscope under general anesthesia.

The liberal use of flexible fiberoptic bronchoscopy has increased our diagnostic yield of airway injuries and has also controlled many airway emergencies, particularly in the face of laryngeal or cervicotracheal injuries. It is also an invaluable technique during the postoperative period in which it facilitates tracheobronchial toilet and allows repeated examination of the airway repair.

MANAGEMENT

The initial evaluation of the severely traumatized patient is accomplished best by using the ABCs of resuscitation, as outlined in the Advanced Trauma Life Support Guidelines of the American College of Surgeons (Committee on Trauma, 1989). The highest priority in this system is placed on the establishment and maintenance of an adequate airway, which is a particular challenge with a tracheobronchial injury.

A high index of suspicion should be maintained in the patient with severe blunt chest trauma and the symptoms of dyspnea, hemoptysis, and subcutaneous emphysema. A pneumothorax refractory to drainage with one or two chest tubes is also highly suggestive of a major airway injury. These patients require immediate fiberoptic bronchoscopy, both for diagnostic and therapeutic purposes. The fiberoptic bronchoscope allows the diagnosis of the level and extent of injury and at the same time facilitates stenting of the lacerated or transsected trachea or mainstem bronchus. This allows controlled ventilation prior to a definitive surgical procedure.

There are certain associated injuries, such as laceration of the great vessels, major intrathoracic hemorrhage, or the presence of a massive tracheoesophageal fistula, in which immediate thoracotomy becomes an integral part of the resuscitation. Major intratracheal or intrabronchial bleeding may be controlled by selective intubation and ventilation of the right or left mainstem bronchus. Bronchial blockers may also be an important adjunct in this situation.

After the diagnosis of a major airway injury is made, definitive surgical therapy should be planned. A patient with multiple systemic injuries frequently presents a dilemma in terms of prioritization and sequencing of the operative procedures. Thus the effective ventilation made possible with selective intubation of a bronchus allows decompression of an epidural hematoma or control of major intra-abdominal bleeding from solid organs or major vascular injuries. It is our preference then to proceed to the definitive repair of the airway as rapidly as possible following the management of life- or organ-threatening injuries.

Other types of tracheobronchial injuries, such as a laser-induced endobronchial burn, require specific immediate intervention (Sosis, 1990). This requires immediate removal of any combustible endobronchial material, including endotracheal tube, fiberoptic bronchoscope, laser fibers, and suction catheters. Any flames should be extinguished with injections of saline. Ventilation may be accomplished temporarily by a mask. The airway should then be carefully examined for the presence of foreign material, clearance of blood and mucus plugs, and a complete assessment of the extended injury. A chest radiograph is extremely useful in this instance. Aggressive tracheobronchial toilet should be instituted in the postoperative period, including humidification, hydration, aerosols with mucolytic and B_2-adrenergic agonists agents, and vigorous chest physiotherapy.

Injury to the trachea or bronchi during other surgical procedures, such as thyroidectomy, esophagectomy, or mediastinoscopy, is usually quickly recognized and can be dealt with directly at the time of the operation (Puhakka, 1989). An occasional injury manifests later and requires specific investigation and therapy, depending on the extent and level of the injury.

In the case of a thermal inhalation burn, any question of upper airway edema or injury should lead to endotracheal intubation until the exact extent of the injury can be determined.

Anesthesia Considerations

In every instance of major airway injury, whether in the neck or intrathoracic area, there must be extremely close cooperation between the anesthesiologist and surgeon in regard to the ultimate management. The anesthesiologist may be invaluable in assisting with airway control and selective intubation of the airway. The choice and timing of muscle relaxants, the type of endotracheal tubes used, and the possibility for using a double ventilation system with intrathoracic placement of an endotracheal tube in either mainstem bronchus must be considered.

High-frequency jet ventilation is another option in the management of tracheobronchial trauma, both intra- and postoperatively, because it provides effective ventilation with relatively lower airway pressures without the necessity for inflation of an endotracheal cuff against a tracheal suture line or airway laceration (Brimioulle, et al., 1990). High-frequency jet ventilation also lowers the tidal volume and intra-airway pressures, minimizing the risk of barotrauma or the disruption of airway suture lines.

There are extremely rare instances in which the proposed surgical procedure must be carried out with cardiopulmonary bypass. Symbas, et al. (1992) discussed the role of cardiopulmonary bypass in complex injuries involving the carina or associated with great vessel or aortic injuries. They used femorofemoral bypass prior to instituting any anesthetic procedure, again requiring close cooperation with the anesthesiologist. A major drawback to cardiopulmonary bypass following major blunt trauma is the potential for exacerbating intracerebral or intra-abdominal hemorrhage, which is related to systemic heparinization.

Operative Management

The principles of operative repair of airway injuries include adequate debridement, mucosa-to-mucosa repair, and some type of protective wrap for the airway anastomosis. The debridement varies depending on the location and mechanism of the injury. A knife laceration of the trachea requires minimal debridement, whereas a gunshot wound may require extensive debridement, depending on the muzzle velocity. In blunt trauma there is frequently an area of the injured bronchus that is devascularized, and it is important to carry out adequate debridement in this instance. Precise debridement minimizes the incidence of postoperative granuloma and stricture formation.

Our recent approach to a mucosa-to-mucosa repair of the trachea uses interrupted absorbable sutures. Some authors have used continuous suture on the membranous portion of the trachea or mainstem bronchus. Other authors suggest a telescoping technique, such as that used during lung transplantation (Calhoon, et al., 1991). The repair can be covered with appropriate adjacent tissue, such as intercostal muscle, pleura, pericardium, mediastinal fat, strap muscles, or a portion of the sternocleidomastoid muscle (Grillo and Mathieson, 1988). This is particularly important when concurrent injuries of the esophagus and major vessels are repaired.

Injuries to the trachea in the neck are usually best dealt with by a transverse collar incision 2 to 3 cm above the level of the jugular notch (Angood, et al., 1985). The neck incision may be altered in the presence of a gunshot wound, as related to the trajectory of the bullet and the suspected injuries. A collar incision allows excellent exposure of the cervical trachea and larynx and permits a laryngeal or hyoid release in which significant segments of trachea are removed. Wherever possible, we attempt to avoid a tracheostomy, except in the case of a laryngeal injury or an anterior gunshot wound of the trachea in which the area of injury can be used as a tracheostomy site.

Injuries to the distal trachea and mainstem bronchus are best dealt with through a standard posterolateral thoracotomy through the fourth or fifth intercostal space. A right thoracotomy is preferred for the mediastinal trachea and the right mainstem bronchus and partial injuries of the proximal left mainstem bronchus. We prefer a left posterolateral thoracotomy for a complete or major injury of the left mainstem bronchus. A median sternotomy may be used with a tracheal or proximal mainstem bronchial injury, which is associated with injury to the innominate artery or vein.

The key component of any airway repair involves close cooperation with the anesthesiologist in maintaining effective ventilation (Glatterer, et al., 1985; Brimioulle, et al., 1990; Pate, 1989). A complete tracheal transsection in the neck or in the mediastinum can be dealt with by directing the endotracheal tube across the injury and carrying out the repair with the endotracheal tube in place. A complete transsection of the right mainstem bronchus is best treated using by selective intubation of the left mainstem bronchus and single-lung anesthesia. A major injury or transsection at the level of the carina requires separate intraoperative intubation of the left and right mainstem bronchi and the use of two anesthesia machines on rare occasions.

On completion of the debridement, repair, and wrap of the injured airway (Grillo and Mathieson, 1988), the pleural space is always drained with at least two chest tubes. We advocate early removal of the endotracheal tube whenever possible. This depends on the associated injuries, the degree of parenchymal lung injury, and the extent of postoperative bronchorrhea. It has been our practice to perform a completion bronchoscopy at the conclusion of all airway repairs, using the fiberoptic bronchoscope.

There are complex injuries of the carina or mainstem bronchi and adjacent great vessels in which cardiopulmonary bypass is essential for the operative repair. This has been rarely required in our experience, although Symbas, et al. (1992) reported its use in complex airway injuries on several occasions. This group advocates delaying the induction of general anesthesia until after the establishment of femorofemoral bypass through the groin, which is done under local anesthesia. The conduct of the operative procedure must be carefully individualized and depends on the hemodynamic and ventilatory stability of the patient.

Postoperative Management

Basic postoperative management following repair of an airway injury includes vigorous tracheobronchial toilet, prevention of infection, careful control of pain, and effective ventilation and oxygenation (Mathieson, et al., 1987; Ramzy, et al., 1988). Most of our patients are managed with an epidural catheter in place through which local anesthesia or an opioid could be used to obtain excellent pain relief. This facilitates coughing and the clearance of tracheobronchial secretions. During the first 24 hours, careful suctioning and aspiration of blood and other secretions are carried out through the endotracheal tube. Fiberoptic bronchoscopy is used liberally. All patients receive a prophylactic broad-spectrum antibiotic.

The high association of costal fractures, pulmonary contusions, and flail chest with major tracheobronchial injuries makes effective pain control a high priority. If an epidural anesthetic is not possible, then multiple intercostal blocks may be used.

It is our preference to remove the endotracheal tube as early as possible when the tracheal secretions are under control and chest wall stability allows effective ventilation. Selected patients require prolonged ventilation, and at some point, a decision is required that is related to the indication for tracheostomy.

Role of Conservative Management

Selected patients with small tracheobronchial lacerations may be managed nonoperatively. Conservative therapy is reserved for patients who are hemodynamically stable, have no major associated intrathoracic injuries, and in whom the laceration of the tracheobronchial tree is small, as demonstrated by bronchoscopy. It is contraindicated when a prolonged period of positive pressure ventilation is attempted.

Some authors also advocate conservative therapy if a major bronchial tear involves less than one-third of the circumference of the bronchus or is limited to a small defect in the membranous portion of the bronchus (De la Rocha and Kayler, 1985; Symbas, et al., 1976; Flynn, et al., 1989). A key indicator is the ability to reexpand the involved lung and maintain expansion with a single chest tube.

Patients treated conservatively should receive prophylactic antibiotics and be observed carefully for airway obstruction and pulmonary and mediastinal sepsis.

Results

The ultimate prognosis following airway injury is usually dependent on the associated injuries, particularly closed head injuries. Four of 30 patients in our series were left in a vegetative state with excellent functional airways (Angood, et al., 1985).

A most important factor in determining the outcome of a tracheal injury in the neck is related to the integrity of the recurrent laryngeal nerves. Our experience with 20 laryngeal and upper tracheal injuries was associated with a 40 percent incidence of dysphonia, primarily related to anatomic involvement of the larynx or an injury to recurrent laryngeal nerves (Angood, et al., 1985). The most important direct airway complication is related to the development of a granuloma or stenosis. We observed complete stenosis of the right mainstem bronchus 6 weeks following resection and repair of a complete blunt transection. This required reresection, and it was believed at the time of reoperation that a contributing factor was an inadequate debridement of the devascularized mainstem bronchus on the right side. Tracheal stenosis has also been observed following tracheal repairs, and its incidence is higher in the patients who require long-term ventilation or tracheostomy. An established tracheal stenosis may be treated conservatively or surgically. Conservative measures include bronchoscopic dilatation or laser resections. Some strictures may require a long-term stent or T tube, as advocated by Dumon, et al. (1991–1992). Definitive surgical therapy of a tracheal or bronchial stricture depends on the location of the stricture and the failure of conservative measures. The techniques for the repair of stenosis of the cervical and mediastinal trachea are described in the tracheal surgery chapters in this text.

Case Studies

Blunt Airway Injury

Two illustrative clinical problems are presented: one representing blunt trauma to the right mainstem bronchus and one representing penetrating trauma to the trachea.

The first patient was a 20-year-old university student who was a passenger in a vehicle involved in a head-on collision. The driver was killed instantly. The right front seat passenger was ejected. He was taken to a local hospital where he was noted to have massive subcutaneous emphysema (Fig. 63-2), a closed head injury, and a fractured left femur. Two chest tubes inserted on the right side did not reexpand the lung. He was transferred 75 miles to our critical care trauma unit, where he went into cardiorespiratory arrest immediately on arrival. Obstruction of the endotracheal tube with dried blood was recognized and treated. Reintubation and effective ventilation allowed his resuscitation. Bronchoscopy through the endotracheal tube revealed a free passage of the bronchoscope into the right pleural space. The endotracheal tube was advanced into the left mainstem bronchus. His femur was stabilized with a K wire in the distal tibia with traction, and he was promptly taken to the operating room.

A right posterolateral thoracotomy through the fifth intercostal space revealed a complete transection of the right mainstem bronchus. There was significant parenchymal hematoma. The great vessels and esophagus were normal. The trachea was debrided flush with the carina. The right mainstem bronchus was debrided, and an anastomosis was carried out using interrupted Prolene sutures. His immediate postoperative course was satisfactory, and he was discharged from hospital on the tenth postoperative day.

He returned to hospital 5 weeks later with a high spiking temperature, and radiography revealed the collapse of the right lower lobe (Fig. 63-7). Bronchoscopy revealed a high-grade stricture at the anastomotic site. He required a reoperation, resection of the stricture, and a new end-to-end anastomosis. This anastomosis was carried out with absorbable sutures. His postoperative course was benign. He was discharged on the tenth postoperative day and has remained well (Fig. 63-8). This patient illustrates the valuable role of controlling the airway initially by selective intubation of the left mainstem bronchus. It was our belief that the initial debridement was probably inadequate and contributed to the early stricture. The use of nonabsorbable Prolene sutures may also have been a factor. The patient also illustrates the need for long-term bronchoscopic follow-up after bronchial repair.

Penetrating Airway Injury

A 39-year-old professional musician at the peak of a psychotic depression plunged a 12-inch scissors into her chest through the jugular notch. The trajectory of the scissors was downward and toward the right. She immediately coughed up blood and collapsed. She was seen in the emergency room within 15 minutes, at which time she was short of breath and had a rapid heart rate and blood pressure of 90/70 mmHg. She underwent the usual advanced trauma life support protocol of resuscitation, including blood volume replacement and a chest radiograph (Fig. 63-3), which revealed a small pneumothorax on the right side and the suggestion of a parenchymal hemorrhage in the right upper lobe and mediastinum. She continued to have mild hemoptysis, and an angiogram was contemplated. She then developed significant hemoptysis and

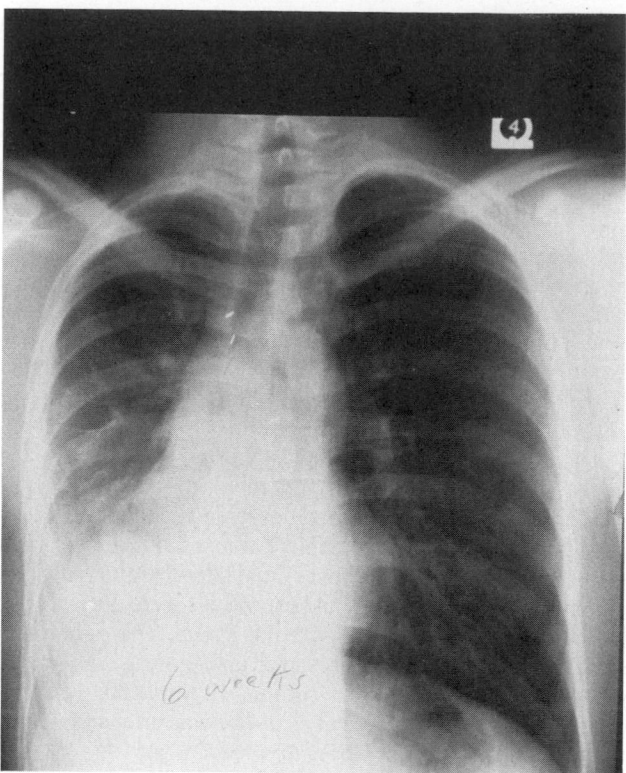

Figure 63-7. Six weeks after the postoperative repair of right mainstem bronchus. The patient was febrile with stricture of the intermediate bronchus seen by bronchoscopy.

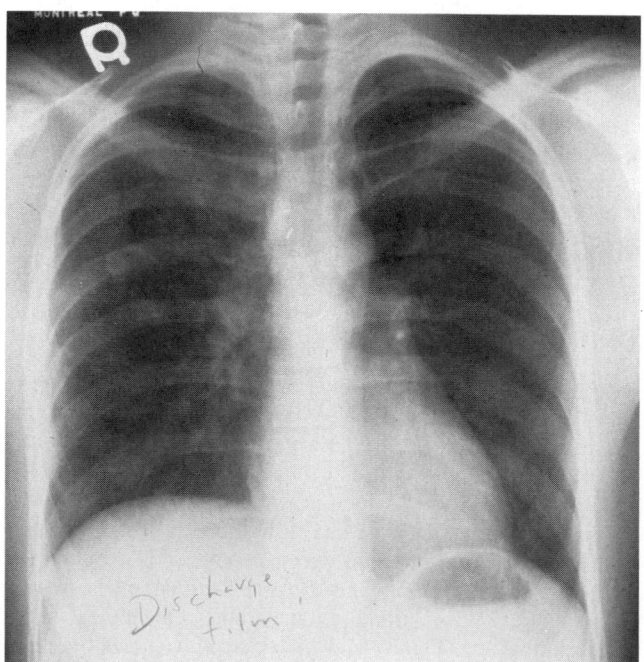

Figure 63-8. Discharge radiograph following excision of stricture and reanastomsis of the right intermediate bronchus.

was rushed to the operating room. She was intubated, and by hyperinflating the cuff and slowly withdrawing the endotracheal tube, the hemorrhage from the airway could be controlled. A rapid median sternotomy revealed a complete transsection of the innominate vein and a partial laceration of the innominate artery. The cuff of the endotracheal tube could be seen protruding through a tangential laceration of the trachea. Digital control allowed dissection for proximal and distal clamping of the innominate artery. This was repaired using 4–0 Prolene vascular sutures. The tracheal wound was explored by advancing the endotracheal tube so that the full extent of the injury could be visualized. The laceration involved approximately 40 percent of the tracheal circumference and was repaired with interrupted absorbable sutures. The innominate vein was then repaired using a continuous 5–0 Prolene suture. The remaining thymic tissue was dissected inferiorly to superiorly as a flap and placed over the tracheal repair between the trachea and the innominate artery repair to prevent late erosion and fistula formation.

Her postoperative course was complicated by copious tracheobronchial secretions requiring frequent bronchoscopy in the first 24 to 48 hours. Subsequently, she could be extubated and was discharged on the ninth postoperative day. Her follow-up bronchoscopy revealed a cleanly healed tracheal repair.

This patient illustrates the importance of associated injuries, particularly those involving adjacent great vessels. This case also emphasizes the valuable role of hyperinflation of the endotracheal tube with positioning to control major airway hemorrhage.

SUMMARY

Major injuries to the airway in the neck and the thorax are seen with increasing frequency as the result of improved prehospital care, allowing more seriously injured patients to reach the emergency room alive. Regionalization of trauma care results in a concentration of such seriously injured patients in level I or II trauma centers. The key to a successful outcome is a high level of suspicion and the early use of fiberoptic bronchoscopy, both for diagnosis and selective intubation to establish effective ventilation. There is a high incidence of serious associated injuries, which frequently predict the final outcome.

The management of the airway is based on well-established principles of adequate debridement, mucosa-to-mucosa repair, and a protective wrap of the surgically repaired airway. Vigorous tracheobronchial toilet, including frequent fiberoptic bronchoscopy, is an important part of postoperative care. Granuloma formation and stricture of the airway are significant sequelae that require a well-planned postoperative follow-up to ensure a good outcome.

The final functional result is usually related to associated injuries, such as severe craniofacial trauma, major pelvic or orthopaedic injuries, or injuries to the great vessels. A most important factor related to the airway in terms of long-term results is the presence of a major laryngeal or cricoid component to the injury and injury to the recurrent laryngeal nerves. Dysphonia is a common late sequela. Most injuries that are limited to the major airways are associated with an excellent functional outcome provided they are recognized immediately and effective surgical therapy is provided.

KEY REFERENCES

Beskin CA: Rupture-separation of the cervical trachea following a closed chest injury. J Thorac Cardiovasc Surg 34:392, 1959

Griffith JL: Fracture of the bronchus. Thorax 4:105, 1949

Sanger PW: Evacuation hospital experience with war wounds and injuries of the chest. Ann Surg 122:147, 1945

These references document the rationale for and the initial attempt at surgical repair of the injured trachea or bronchus, and they provide the basis for modern surgical management.

REFERENCES

Angood PB, Attia EL, Brown RA, Mulder DS: Civilian trauma to the larynx and the cervical trachea. J Trauma 26:869, 1985

Baumgartner F, Sheppard B, de Virgilio C et al: Tracheal and main bronchial disruption after blunt chest trauma: presentation and management. Ann Thorac Surg 50:569, 1990

Bertelsen S, Howitz P: Injuries to the trachea and bronchi. Thorax 27:188, 1972

Brimioulle S, Rocmans P, de Rood M et al: High frequency jet ventilation in the management of tracheal laceration. Crit Care Med 18:338, 1990

Burke JF: Early diagnosis of traumatic rupture of the bronchus. JAMA 181:682, 1962

Calhoon JH, Grover FL, Gibbons WJ et al: Single lung transplantation: alternative indications and technique. J Thorac Cardiovasc Surg 101:816, 1991

Committee on Trauma, American College of Surgeons: Advanced Trauma Life Support Program Instructor's Manual. American College of Surgeons, Chicago, IL, 1989

Davies D, Hopkins JS: Patterns in traumatic rupture of the bronchus. Injury 4:261, 1973

De la Rocha AG, Kayler D: Traumatic rupture of the tracheobronchial tree. Can J Surg 28:68, 1985

Deslauriers J, Beaulieu M, Archambault G et al.: Diagnosis and long-term follow-up of major bronchial disruptions due to nonpenetrating trauma. Ann Thorac Surg 33:32, 1982

Dumon C, Viallat JR, Aelony Y: Practical Thoracoscopy. Springer-Verlag, New York, 1991–92

Endress C, Guyot DR, Engels JA: The "fallen lung with absent hilum" signs of complete bronchial transection. Ann Emerg Med 20:317, 1991

Feliciano DV Jr, Bitondo CG, Mattox KL et al: Combined tracheoesophageal injuries. Am J Surg 150:710, 1985

Flynn AE, Thomas AN, Schecter WP: Acute tracheobronchial injury. J Trauma 29:1326, 1989

Glatterer MS Jr, Toon RS, Ellestad C et al: Management of blunt and penetrating external esophageal trauma. J Trauma 25:784, 1985

Grillo HC, Mathieson DJ: Surgical management of tracheal strictures. Surg Clin North Am 68:3, 1988

Haponik EF, Crapo RO, Herndon DN et al: Smoke inhalation. Am Rev Respir Dis 138:1060, 1988

Kemmerer WT, Eckert WG, Gathright JB et al: Patterns of thoracic injuries in fatal traffic accidents. J Trauma 1:595, 1961

Kinsella TJ, Johnsrud LW: Traumatic rupture of the bronchus. J Thorac Cardiovasc Surg 16:571, 1947

Krinitzki SI: Zur Kasuistik einer vollstandingen Zerreibung der rechten Luftrohrenastes. Virchows Arch A Pathol Anat Histopathol 266:815, 1927

Kumpe DA, Oh KS, Wyman SM: A characteristic pulmonary finding inunilateral complete bronchial transection. AJR 110:704, 1970

Lund T, Goodwin CW, McManus WF et al: Upper airway sequelae in burn patients requiring endotracheal intubation or tracheostomy. Ann Surg 201:374, 1985

Mathieson DJ, Grillo H et al: Laryngotracheal trauma. Ann Thorac Surg 43:254, 1987

Moylan JA, Chan CK: Inhalation injury—an increasing problem. Ann Surg 188:34, 1978

Mulder DS, Barkun JS: Injury to the trachea, bronchus and esophagus. In Mattox KL, Moore EE, Feliciano DV (eds): Definitive Trauma Care. Appleton-Century-Crofts, New York, 1986

Nissen R: Total pneumonectomy. Ann Thorac Surg 29:390, 1980

Oh KS, Fleischner FG, Wyman SM: Characteristic pulmonary finding in traumatic complete transection of main stem bronchus. Radiology 92:321, 1969

Pate JW: Tracheobronchial and esophageal injuries. Surg Clin North Am 69:1, 1989

Postlethwait RW: Chemical burns of the esophagus. p. 286. In Surgery of the Esophagus. Appleton-Century-Crofts, New York, 1979

Puhakka HJ: Complication of mediastinoscopy. J Laryngol Otol 103:312, 1989

Ramzy AI, Rodriguez A, Turney SZ: Management of major tracheobronchial ruptures in patients with multiple system trauma. J Trauma 28:1353, 1988

Reynolds J, Christiensen EE: Early radiological signs of bronchial rupture. Tex Med 64:50, 1986

Schonberg S: Bronchial rupturen bei thorax kompression. Klin Wochenschr 49:2218, 1912

Shimazu et al: Tracheobronchial rupture caused by blunt chest trauma: acute respiratory management. Am J Emerg Med 6:427, 1988

Sosis MB: Airway fire during CO_2 laser surgery using Xomed laser endotracheal tube. Anesthesiology 72:747, 1990

Symbas PN, Hatcher CR Jr, Bochm GAW: Acute penetrating tracheal trauma. Ann Thorac Surg 22:473, 1976

Symbas PN, Hatcher CR Jr, Vlasis SE: Bullet wounds of the trachea. J Thorac Cardiovasc Surg 83:235, 1982

Symbas PN, Justicz AG, Ricketts RR: Rupture of the airways from blunt trauma: treatment of complex injuries. Ann Thorac Surg 54:177, 1992

Vierheilig J: Die Subkutane Bronchuszerreibung. Beitr Klin Chir 93:201, 1914

Webb A: Pathologica Indica of the Anatomy of Indian Diseases. 2nd Ed. Thacker, Calcutta, 1848

Weir IH, Muller NL, Connell DG: CT diagnosis of bronchial rupture. J Comput Assist Tomogr 12:1035, 1988

Wilson RF, Soullier GW, Wiencek RG: Hemoptysis in trauma. J Trauma 27:1123, 1987

Wilson RF, Steiger Z: Thoracic Injuries: Emergency Medicine: A Comprehensive Study Guide. 2nd Ed. McGraw-Hill, New York, 1985

Winslow WH: Rupture of bronchus from wild duck. Philadelphia Medical Times 1:225, April 15, 1871

64

BLUNT TRAUMA

Trauma to the Chest Wall

David A. Fullerton
Frederick L. Grover

Injury to the chest wall is extremely common in blunt and penetrating thoracic injuries. Knife and gunshot wounds account for the majority of penetrating injuries, motor vehicle accidents produce approximately 75 percent of blunt chest wall injuries (Shorr, et al., 1987). Despite their relative frequency, these injuries are rarely immediately life threatening.

The musculature and skeleton of the chest wall provide excellent protection for its contents. Even more importantly, the integrity of the chest wall is critical for the physiologic function of the organs contained within it. With inhalation the rigid chest wall expands laterally as the diaphragm descends, increasing the intrathoracic volume and generating the negative intrapleural pressure required to bring atmospheric air into the alveoli and return venous blood to the heart. Loss of the rigidity of the chest wall may preclude the generation of negative intrapleural pressure. Because the chest wall must expand laterally with respiration, significant pain with this motion from chest wall fractures may limit the mechanics of respiration.

Chest wall injuries are virtually always accompanied by associated injuries; isolated injuries occur in only 16 percent of cases (Shorr, et al., 1987). For this reason and because chest wall injuries are rarely life threatening, they should be noted, but the focus of the primary survey of the patient evaluation should be on potential intrathoracic injuries. Two chest wall injuries may be immediately life threatening: an open pneumothorax and a large flail chest. These injuries can produce acute respiratory distress and require immediate therapy (see Ch. 62).

HISTORICAL NOTE

The earliest medical literature contains reference to the therapy of chest wall injuries. In the Smith papyrus (3,000 B.C.), Imhotep recommended that rib fractures required no therapy

(Breasted, 1930). In the first century A.D., Galen described sternal and pericardial excision for abscess formation following sternal injury (Meade, 1961). Theodoric described a technique for splinting a fractured sternum and open reduction and extraction of fragments of rib fractures in 1267 (Campbell and Colton, 1955). Bromfield described subcutaneous emphysema following rib fractures in 1773 and recommended skin incision to allow the air to escape (Meade, 1961). In 1792 Munro described an operative technique to control bleeding from intercostal vessels by encircling the involved rib (Meade, 1961). The famous British military surgeon Guthrie advised neglect for blunt chest injuries in 1815 (Hochberg, 1960). During the Civil War, Billings described rupture of the thoracic viscera without rib fractures (Meade, 1961). Tracheotomy for the therapy of flail chest was introduced by Carter and Giuseffi (1951).

HISTORICAL READINGS

Breasted JH: The Edwin Smith Surgical Papyrus. University of Chicago Press, Chicago, 1930

Campbell E, Colton J: The Surgery of Theodoric. Appleton-Century-Crofts, Norwalk, CT, 1955

Carter BN, Giuseffi J: Tracheotomy: useful procedure in thoracic surgery with particular reference to employment in crushing injuries of the thorax. J Thorac Cardiovasc Surg 21:495, 1951

Hochberg LA: Thoracic Surgery Before the 20th Century. Vantage Press, New York, 1960

Meade RH: A History of Thoracic Surgery. Charles C. Thomas, Springfield, IL, 1961

CLAVICULAR FRACTURES

Clavicular fractures are among the most common injuries to the chest wall, either as isolated injuries or in association with other chest injuries. These fractures are generally produced in falls or by blows to the lateral shoulder. The fracture most commonly occurs in the midshaft region, with only 15 to 20 percent of clavicular fractures occurring in either the medial or lateral thirds of the bone. Uncommonly the underlying subclavian vessels or brachial plexus may be injured (Costa, 1988). A careful neurologic and vascular examination of the ipsilateral upper extremity must be carried out.

Clavicular fracture should be suspected by the presence of localized deformity, pain, and tenderness. The fracture is usually readily visible on chest radiography, and the initial portable chest radiograph taken in the trauma department should be scrutinized for this fracture. Although this injury may be uncomfortable for the patient, it is almost always successfully treated by fracture immobilization with a figure-eight strap around the shoulders. The prognosis of these fractures is generally excellent. One possible long-term disability is the late development of thoracic outlet syndrome. The formation of excessive callus surrounding the fracture site, possibly from fracture malunion, may lead to compression of the underlying trunks of the brachial plexus and subclavian vessels (Barger, 1984). Patients with clavicular fractures should be made aware of this potential complication.

STERNAL FRACTURE

Although occasionally produced by a direct sternal blow, sternal fractures are usually produced in the course of deceleration injury, most frequently as the driver of a motor vehicle strikes the steering column (Buckman, et al., 1987; Wojcik and Morgan, 1988). Fractures generally occur in the upper midsternal body and are only rarely comminuted (Wojcik and Morgan, 1988). Sternal fractures are frequently associated with rib (40 percent) or long bone (25 percent) fractures (Buckman, et al., 1987; Wojcik and Morgan, 1988). At least 20 percent are associated with significant head injury (Wojcik and Morgan, 1988). Unless the sternal fracture is open or badly displaced and causing significant pain, there is no need for open reduction and internal fixation, and the long-term outcome without operative intervention is excellent (Harley and Mena, 1986).

The presence of a sternal fracture should raise concern about a potential underlying blunt cardiac injury; 61 percent of patients with sternal fracture had electrocardiographic changes (Buckman, et al., 1987), and 91 percent of patients with sternal fracture were found to have abnormal left and right ventricular radionuclide ejection fraction scan results (Harley and Mena, 1986). Although the diagnosis is difficult to make with certainty, at least 18 pecent of patients with sternal fracture may have myocardial contusion (Wojcik and Morgan, 1988). The management of this problem is discussed later in this chapter.

STERNOCLAVICULAR DISLOCATION

Separation of the sternoclavicular joint is rare. On physical examination anterior dislocation is recognized by pain, tenderness, and a protrusion over the joint. Posterior dislocation is recognized by a depressed deformity over the joint. The mechanism of injury producing anterior dislocation is an ante-

rior blow to the shoulder. A posterior dislocation is produced by an anterior blow to the medial clavicle or a posterior blow to the shoulder.

Therapy for this injury is closed reduction, under either general or sometimes local anesthesia. After sterile preparation a penetrating towel clamp is used to grasp the clavicular head and to reduce the fracture while the shoulder joint is distracted laterally. After the dislocation is reduced, the ipsilateral shoulder should be immobilized.

The thoracic surgeon must be particularly sensitive to potential underlying injury with a posterior dislocation. The patient must be carefully examined for evidence of injury to the subclavian artery or vein or the brachial plexus. Tracheal compression has also been reported (Buckerfield, 1984) (Fig. 64-1).

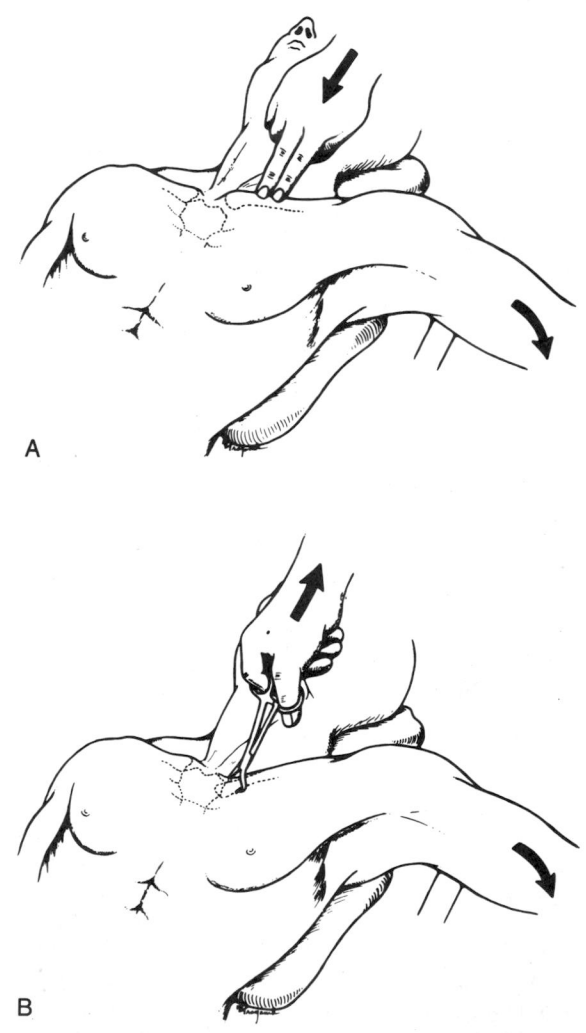

Figure 64-1. **(A)** Reduction of a posterior sternoclavicular dislocation. **(B)** Under anesthesia and after sterile preparation, the clavicular head is grasped with a penetrating towel clamp as the arm is extracted laterally. (From Cogbill TH, Landercasper J: Injury to the chest wall. p. 334. In Moore EE, Mattox KL, Feliciano DV (eds): Trauma. 2nd Ed. Appleton & Lange, Norwalk, CT, 1991, with permission.)

COSTAL FRACTURES

The most common blunt chest injury is costal fracture, usually incurred by direct impact. Most commonly ribs four through nine are broken. Fractures typically occur over the lateral chest wall and may not be visualized well on the chest radiograph. The diagnosis is made clinically by an appropriate history accompanied by localized pleuritic pain, tenderness, and often crepitance in the fracture region. Aside from underlying injuries, significant pain with respiration is the principal morbidity of costal fractures. Pain may lead to chest wall splinting, reduced respiratory excursion, atelectasis, and pneumonia. In patients with compromised pulmonary function, these pulmonary complications may be life threatening. For this reason the mortality rate of costal fractures in patients older than 80 years of age is 20 percent (Trinkle, et al., 1988). Successful management of such fractures requires adequate pain control. This may be effectively accomplished with a combination of systemically administered analgesics and intercostal nerve blocks. For severe injuries epidural analgesia appears to offer superior pain relief and may be particularly valuable if pulmonary status is greatly compromised by pain (Mackersie, et al., 1987; Dittmann, et al., 1982) (Fig. 64-2).

As with other chest wall injuries, the surgeon must be vigilant to detect and treat underlying visceral injuries. Costal fractures accompanied by a hemothorax, a pneumothorax, or both should be treated with tube thoracostomy. The underlying lung may be contused, requiring careful management, as described below. Fractures of ribs nine through twelve may be associated with occult injury to the kidney, liver, or especially the spleen. These fractures warrant hospitalization of serial examinations of the abdomen and monitoring of hematocrit levels.

Because of their protected location, fractures of the first and second ribs require significant force, and they are frequently the hallmark of severe injury (Richardson, et al., 1975; Wilson, et al., 1978). Fractures of the first rib occur in up to 9 percent of blunt chest injuries (Wilson, et al., 1978). Earlier data suggested a mortality rate of 36 percent associ-

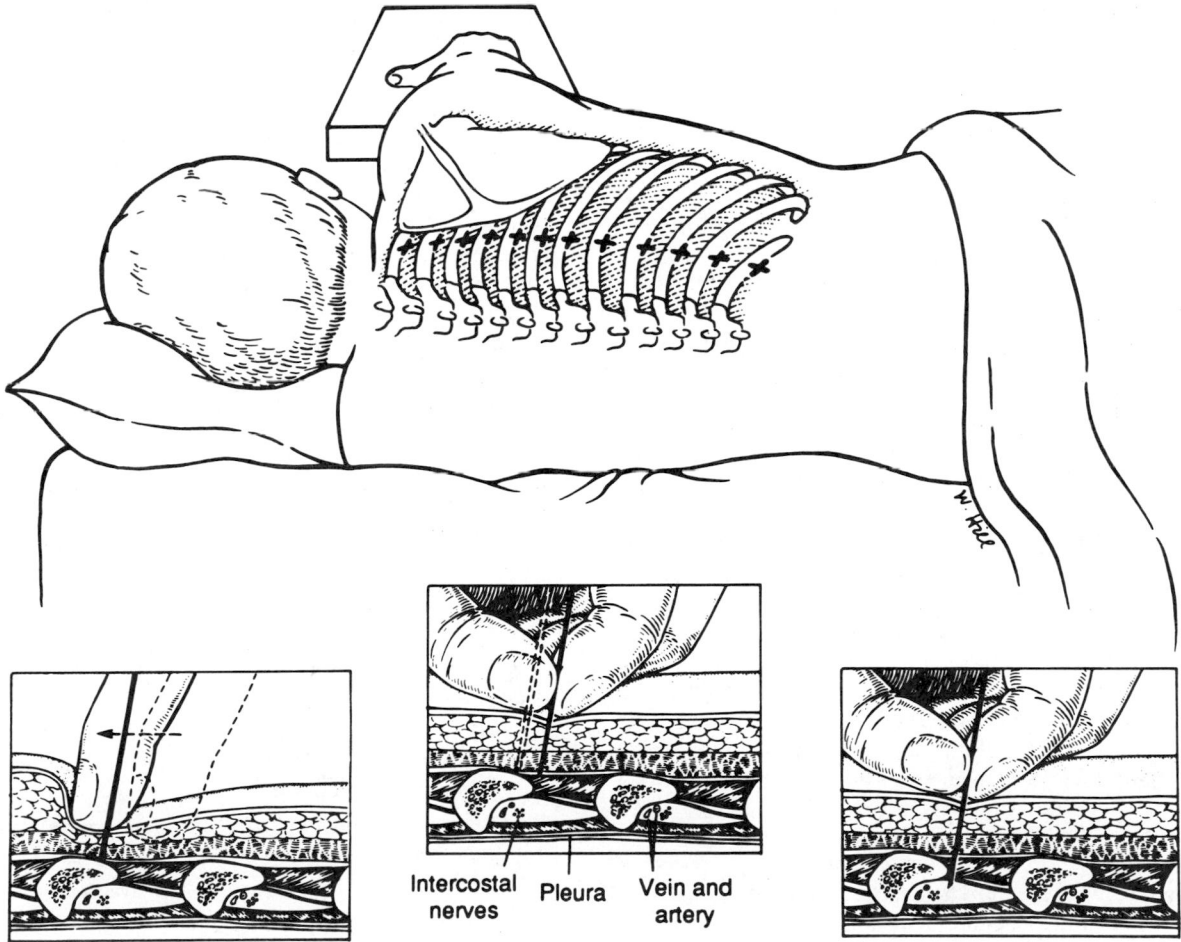

Intercostal nerves   Pleura   Vein and artery

Figure 64-2. Technique for performing intercostal nerve blocks. The patient is placed in the lateral position with arm extended to pull the scapula anteriorly. Local anesthetic is injected just below the inferior edge of the rib. (From Chung KS: Intercostal nerve block. p. 360. In Sinatra RS, Hord AH, Ginsberg B, Preble LM (eds): Acute Pain—Mechanisms and Management. Mosby-Year Book, St. Louis, 1992, with permission.)

ated with fractures of the first or second ribs, primarily from severe head, chest, or abdominal injuries (Richardson, et al., 1975; Wilson, et al., 1978). A 6 percent incidence of major thoracic vascular injury associated with fractures of the first rib led to earlier recommendations for routine aortography (Albers, et al., 1982; Fisher, et al., 1982; Logrove, et al., 1982; Phillips, et al., 1981; Woodring, et al., 1982). However, more recent data suggest that these fractures alone are not independent predictors of major vascular injury, and more recent reports estimate mortality rates associated with fractures of the first or second ribs to be approximately 5 percent (Albers, et al., 1982; Logrove, et al., 1982; Phillips, et al., 1981).

FLAIL CHEST

Flail chest is defined as a segment of chest wall that moves paradoxically with respiration. It is usually caused by costal fractures, resulting from direct impact and occurs in up to 13 percent of blunt chest injuries (LoCicero and Mattox, 1989). As in most fractures, the force required to produce a flail segment is inversely related to age. The diagnosis may be subtle and requires careful physical examination and observation of respiration. The diagnosis is delayed in up to 14 percent of cases (Shackford, et al., 1981).

The morbidity and potential mortality rates of flail chest stem from pulmonary compromise. This compromise was thought for many years to be secondary to rebreathing air tidally exchanged between the normal lung and the air space beneath the flail segment, the so-called pendelluft phenomenon (Trinkle, et al., 1988). This hypothesis has been experimentally disproved (Maloney, et al., 1961). It is now recognized that the pulmonary compromise results from the underlying pulmonary contusion. Pulmonary contusion is a significant risk factor for the development of adult respiratory distress syndrome (Pepe, et al., 1984) with a potential mortality rate of 50 percent (Montgomery, et al., 1985). This complication is discussed in detail in Chapter 68.

For many years the standard therapy of flail chest in some trauma centers was internal stenting of the flail segment by endotracheal intubation and mechanical ventilation (Avery, et al., 1956). More recent studies show that more selective and restrictive use of intubation and mechanical ventilation reduces the incidence of both pneumonia and the mortality rate of flail chest (Landercasper, et al., 1984; Richardson, et al., 1982; Shackford, et al., 1976, 1981; Trinkle, et al., 1975). Currently the therapy of flail chest is based on the selective use of mechanical ventilation, and the indication for endotracheal intubation and mechanical ventilation is an inability to oxygenate or ventilate the patient (Shackford, et al., 1981; Trinkle, et al., 1988) rather than the mere presence of a flail segment.

A large flail chest may produce rapid respiratory deterioration and require prompt endotracheal intubation and positive pressure ventilation. Fewer than one-half of all patients with flail chest require endotracheal intubation (Richardson, et al., 1982). Those who are not in immediate respiratory distress, requiring endotracheal intubation, should be admitted to an intensive care unit for observation for evidence of respiratory

deterioration and aggressive pulmonary toilet. Humidified supplemental oxygen should be administered to maintain an arterial oxyhemoglobin saturation of at least 90 percent. Adequate pain control is essential; intercostal nerve blocks and epidural analgesia are particularly valuable (Dittman, et al., 1982; Mackersie, et al., 1987). These patients frequently require assistance in clearing pulmonary secretions, and vigorous chest physiotherapy and postural drainage is an invaluable component of their care. Flexible bronchoscopy may be valuable to help clear secretions.

If the patient develops respiratory distress despite optimal pulmonary toilet, endotracheal intubation and mechanical ventilation should be instituted. Specific indications for endotracheal intubation include a tidal volume of less than 5 ml/kg, respiratory rate more than 35 breaths/min, partial carbon dioxide pressure more than 55 mmHg, and/or an arterial oxyhemoglobin saturation less than 90 percent. *Even those patients requiring intubation may generally be extubated within 72 hours* (Richardson, et al., 1982) and returned to the regimen described above. It is inappropriate to persist with mechanical support until the flail segment stabilizes.

Operative fixation of the flail segment is rarely indicated. Prospective trials have shown no advantage over nonoperative therapy (Menard, et al., 1983; Moore, 1975; Paris et al., 1975; Thomas, et al., 1978), except in unusual situations, such as large unstable segments of the chest wall in patients with borderline pulmonary function. This subgroup of patients may benefit from optimizing their mechanics of ventilation and accelerating weaning from the ventilator. A second indication for internal fixation of the flail segment is in the patient undergoing ipsilateral thoracotomy for another reason. In such patients the flail segment may be internally stabilized with little addition to the planned operation using Kirschner wires, Rush medullary nails, or Jergesen orthopaedic plates (Grover, 1989).

The outcome of therapy of flail chest is largely dependent on the severity of associated injuries (Clark, et al., 1988; Pinilla, 1982; Reliham and Litwin, 1973; Sankaran and Wilson, 1970). At least 75 percent of patients sustain major ortho-

---

Chest Wall Trauma: Pitfalls and Points to Remember

Clavicular fracture seems relative innocuous; injury to the subclavian artery or brachial plexus may be overlooked, and thoracic outlet syndrome may develop as a late complication.

Cardiac contusion is extremely common with sternal fracture.

Look for underlying injury to the trachea or major vessels with medial sternoclavicular dislocation.

Splenic and hepatic lacerations should be ruled out when the lower ribs are fractured.

Flail chest is commonly overtreated by intubation and mechanical ventilation.

paedic injury; 35 percent sustain major neurologic injury (Clark, et al., 1988; Shackford, et al., 1981). Approximately 15 to 50 percent contract pneumonia (Clark, et al., 1988; Reliham, and Litwin, 1973). The average mortality rate is 16 percent. Increased risk is associated with advanced age, the number of ribs fractured, and the severity of the pulmonary contusion (Clark, et al., 1988; Johnson, et al., 1986; Landercasper, et al., 1984; Pinilla, 1982; Reliham and Litwin, 1973; Richardson, et al., 1982; Sankaran and Wilson, 1970). Late sequelae of this injury are discussed in Chapter 70.

TRAUMATIC ASPHYXIA

Traumatic asphyxia may result from a crush injury to the chest. The sharp rise in intrathoracic pressure, especially when the glottis is closed, results in a markedly increased intrathoracic venous pressure, which stops or even reverses venous drainage of the head and neck (Cogbill and Landercasper, 1991). This profound increase in venous pressure results in capillary rupture, producing the classic physical findings of edema and cyanosis of the head and neck, petechiae, and subconjunctival hemorrhage (Williams, 1968). Impairment of cerebral venous outflow may increase intracranial pressure enough to cause a depressed level of consciousness, seizures, and temporary or permanent blindness (Landercasper, et al., 1984).

Despite the dramatic initial appearance of the patient, the prognosis is usually excellent (Landercasper, et al., 1984). The patient's neurologic status should be monitored closely, and the head of the patient's bed should be elevated to promote venous drainage. The surgeon should look closely for intrathoracic injuries, particularly cardiac and pulmonary contusion. Therapy should be directed toward these injuries.

COMMENTS AND CONTROVERSIES

Tracheal intubation and prolonged ventilation was introduced for management of flail chest, and belief in the pendelluft phenomenon fostered its overutilization for a substantial period in the United States. Canadian surgeons and intensivists did not adopt this strategy but remained selective in their use of ventilatory support. More recently moderation has arrived in the United States through the influential work of Trinkle and Grover. Through the skillful application of the same techniques used to manage post-thoracotomy pain, they were able to treat patients without using a ventilator or to wean them from respiratory support rapidly.

Thoracic surgeons need to be proficient and well informed about the management of chest wall pain. This area of knowledge, so critical in the management of chest wall injury, is best developed by hands-on management of thoracotomy pain in the immediate postoperative period. Delegation of this experience to a pain service in the anesthesiology department should not be allowed to deprive residents in training from becoming expert in the management of chest wall pain. Pain management is an important consideration when making an emergency room decision about the management of an elderly patient with one or two costal fractures. If the pain management required to promote deep breathing and coughing cannot be conducted reliably at home, admission for a few days of instruction and care will prevent retention of secretions leading to atelectasis, pneumonia, and possibly to death.

M.F.M.

KEY REFERENCES

Albers JE, Rath RK, Glaser RS, Poddar PK: Severity of intrathoracic injuries associated with first rib fractures. Ann Thorac Surg 33:614, 1982

This study demonstrated that fracture of the first rib was not an independent risk factor for major vascular injury or death.

Cogbill TH, Landercasper J: Injury to the chest wall. p. 327. In Moore EE, Mattox KL, Feliciano DV (eds): Trauma, 2nd Ed. Appleton and Lange, Norwalk, CT, 1991

This chapter is an excellent review of chest wall trauma and its management and associated extrathoracic injuries.

Trinkle JK, Richardson JD, Franz JL et al.: Management of flail chest wthout mechanical ventilation. Ann Thorac Surg 19:355, 1975

This study demonstrated that, in patients with flail chest, the incidence of pneumonia and the mortality rate was less if selective use of mechanical ventilation was used.

REFERENCES

Avery EE, Morch ET, Benson DW: Critically crushed chests: a new method of treatment with continuous mechanical hyperventilation to produce alkalotic apnea and internal pneumatic stabilization. J Thorac Cardiovasc Surg 32:291, 1956

Bargar NL, Marcus RE, Ittleman FP: Late thoracic outlet syndrome secondary to pseudoarthosis of the clavicle. J Trauma 24:857, 1984

Breasted JH: The Edwin Smith Surgical Papyrus. University of Chicago Press, Chicago, 1930

Buckman R, Trooskin SZ, Flancbaum L, Chandler J: The significance of stable patients with sternal fractures. Surg Gynecol Obstet 164:261, 1987

Campbell E, Colton J: The Surgery of Theodoric. Appleton-Century-Crofts, Norwalk, CT, 1955

Carter BN, Giuseffi J: Tracheotomy: useful procedure in thoracic surgery with particular reference to employment in crushing injuries of the thorax. J Thorac Cardiovasc Surg 21:495, 1951

Clark GC, Schecter WL, Trunkey DD: Variables affecting outcome in blunt chest trauma: flail chest vs. pulmonary contusion. J Trauma 28:298, 1988

Costa MC, Robbs JV: Nonpenetrating subclavian artery trauma. J Vasc Surg 8:71, 1988

Dittmann M, Steenblock U, Kranzlin M et al.: Epidural analgesia or mechanical ventilation for multiple rib fractures. Intensive Care Med 8:89, 1982

Fisher RG, Ward RE, Ben-Manachem Y et al.: Arteriography and the fractured first rib: too much for too little? AJR 138:1059, 1982

Grover FL: Flail chest. p 152. In Pickard LR (ed): Decision Making in Surgery of the Chest. WB Saunders, Philadelphia, 1989

Harley DP, Mena I: Cardiac and vascular sequelae of sternal fractures. J Trauma 26:553, 1986

Hochberg LA: Thoracic Surgery Before the 20th Centery. Vantage Press, New York, 1960

Johnson JA, Cogbill TH, Winga ER: Determinants of outcome after pulmonary contusion. J Trauma 26:695, 1986

Landercasper J, Cogbill TH, Lindermoth LA: Long-term disability after flail chest. J Trauma 24:410, 1984

LoCicero J III, Mattox KL: Epidemiology of chest trauma. Surg Clin North Am 69:15, 1989

Logrove S, Harley DP, Grinnell VS et al.: Should all patients with first rib fractures undergo arteriography? J Thorac Cardiovasc Surg 83:532, 1982

Mackersie RC, Shackford SR, Hoyt DB, Karagianes TG: Continuous epidural fentanyl analgesia: ventilatory function improvement with routine use in treatment of blunt chest injury. J Trauma 27:1207, 1987

Maloney JV, Schmutzer KJ, Raschke E: Paradoxical respiration and "pendelluft." J Thorac Cardiovasc Surg 41:291, 1961

Meade RH: A History of Thoracic Surgery. Charles C Thomas, Springfield, IL, 1961

Menard A, Tentart J, Phillipe JM, Grist P: Treatment of flail chest with Judet's struts. J Thorac Cardiovasc Surg 86:300, 1983

Montgomery AB, Stager MA, Carrico CJ, Hudson LD: Causes of mortality in patients with the adult respiratory distress syndrome. Am Rev Respir Dis 132:485, 1985

Moore BP: Operative stabilization of nonpenetrating chest injuries. J Thorac Cardiovasc Surg 70:619, 1975

Paris F, Tarazona V, Blasco E et al.: Surgical stabilization of traumatic flail chest. Thorax 30:521, 19745

Pepe PE, Hudson LD, Carrico CJ: Early application of positive end-expiratory pressure in patients at risk for the adult respiratory distress syndrome. N Engl J Med 311:281, 1984

Phillips EH, Rogers WF, Gasper MR: First rib fractures: incidence of vascular injury and indications for angiography. Surgery 89:42, 1981

Pinilla JC; Acute respiratory failure in severe blunt chest trauma. J Trauma 22:221, 1982

Reliham M, Litwin MS: Morbidity and mortality associated with flail chest injury: a review of 85 cases. J Trauma 13:663,1973

Richardson JD, Adams L, Flint LM: Selective management of flail chest and pulmonary contusion. Ann Surg 196:481, 1982

Richardson JD, McElvein RB, Trinkle JK: First rib fracture: a hallmark of severe trauma. Ann Surg 181:251, 1975

Sankaran S, Wilson RF: Factors affecting prognosis in patients with flail chest. J Thorac Cardiovasc Surg 60:420, 1970

Shackford SR, Smith DE, Zarins CK et al.: The management of flail chest: a comparison of ventilatory and nonventilatory treatment. Am J Surg 132:759, 1976

Shackford SR, Virgilio RW, Peters RM: Selective use of ventilatory therapy in flail chest injury. J Thorac Cardiovasc Surg 81:194, 1981

Shorr RM, Crittenden M, Indects et al.: Blunt thoracic trauma: analysis of 515 patients. Ann Surg 206:200, 1987

Thomas AN, Blaisdell FN, Lewis FR, Schlobolm RM: Operative stabilization for flail chest after blunt trauma. J Thorac Cardiovasc Surg 75:793, 1978

Trinkle JK, Harman PK, Grover FL: Chest trauma, p. 2448. In Fishman AP (ed): Pulmonary Diseases and Disorders. McGraw-Hill, New York, 1988

Wilson JM, Thomas AN, Boodman PC, Lewis FR: Severe chest trauma: morbidity implications of first and second rib fracture in 120 patients. Arch Surg 113:846, 1978

Wojcik JB, Morgan AS: Sternal fractures—the natural history. Ann Emerg Med 17:912, 1988

Woodring JH, Fried AM, Hatfield DR et al.: Fractures of first and second ribs: predictive value for arterial and bronchial injury. AJR 138:211, 1982

Trauma to the Lung and Pleura

David A. Fullerton
Frederick L. Grover

The majority of injuries to the lung and pleural are appropriately treated with tube thoracostomy alone. However, their importance should not be minimized. These injuries may produce significant immediate morbidity and may be the precursors of potentially life-threatening complications, such as adult respiratory distress syndrome or empyema. Prompt recognition and therapy of lung and pleural injuries is essential because they account for one-half of all fatal thoracic injuries (Kemmerer, et al., 1961).

HISTORICAL NOTE

Morgagni, Pare, and Hewson each described pulmonary disruption secondary to blunt chest trauma and open pneumothorax in the eighteenth century (Meade, 1961). In 1767 Hewson described a soldier who could not breathe with an open chest wound but did so readily if the wound was closed. Although known from the time of Hippocrates and popularized during the mid-eighteenth century, thoracentesis was rarely applied during the American Civil War. Thoracentesis came into wide use as a therapy for hemothorax during World War I. Later in that war, thoracotomy was performed to evacuate clotted hemothorax. During World War II, decortication for clotted hemothorax and trapped lung was standard therapy. Pulmonary blast injuries were described among British bombing victims of World War II, and surgical intervention was applied with increasing confidence and success to a variety of pulmonary and pleural problems.

HISTORICAL READING

Meade RH: A History of Thoracic Surgery. Charles C Thomas, Springfield, IL, 1961.

PNEUMOTHORAX

In blunt thoracic trauma, pneumothorax results from direct lung puncture (usually by broken ribs), a shearing lung laceration caused by rapid deceleration, or an abrupt rise in intrathoracic pressure against a closed glottis (Thal, et al., 1988). In the latter mechanism, the acute rise in airway pressure causes rupture of distal alveolar air spaces. Air tracks proximally along the bronchial tree into the mediastinum. If sufficient air collects within the mediastinum, the mediastinal pleural may rupture, producing pneumothorax.

Pneumothorax is extremely common in blunt and penetrating trauma. It should be suspected in the initial evaluation of all traumatized patients. Signs on physical examination include dyspnea, hyper-resonance of the chest to percussion, and diminished or absent breath sounds. Tension pneumothorax is life-threatening and should be suspected in any patient with hemodynamic compromise, tracheal shift, and absent breath sounds (Thal, et al., 1988). This same constellation of physical signs may also be produced by massive hemothorax or diaphragmatic rupture. If the patient's condition permits and chest radiography is immediately available, the diagnosis should be confirmed radiographically prior to tube thoracostomy. Otherwise, a needle should be placed into the chest in the second intercostal space in the midclavicular line. This maneuver is diagnostic if there is a large rush of air, and it may also be therapeutic. After the diagnosis is confirmed, either radiographically or by needle, a careful tube thoracostomy should be performed. To evacuate air, the tube is best placed in the fourth or fifth intercostal space in the anterior or midaxillary line and directed anteriorly (Hughes, 1965). If the lung does not completely reexpand or a large or continuous air leak is present, a major airway injury should be suspected (Figs. 64-3 and 64-4).

Thoracotomy is rarely if ever indicated for the control of a parenchymal air leak. If a parenchymal air leak is identifiable at the time of thoracotomy for another reason, it is advisable to close the leak surgically during that operation. The region of the parenchymal laceration should be grasped with Duvall lung clamps and fine absorbable suture passed through the pulmonary parenchyma just beneath the clamps. Alternatively, control of a parenchymal laceration may be achieved by application of surgical staples just beneath the clamps, but lung resection is virtually never indicated (Graham, et al., 1979; Sherman, 1966).

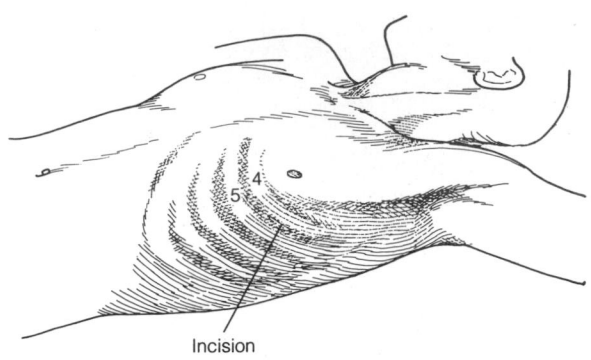

Incision

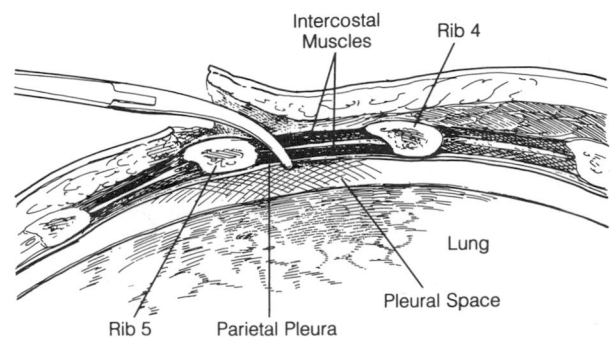

Intercostal Muscles   Rib 4

Lung

Pleural Space

Rib 5   Parietal Pleura

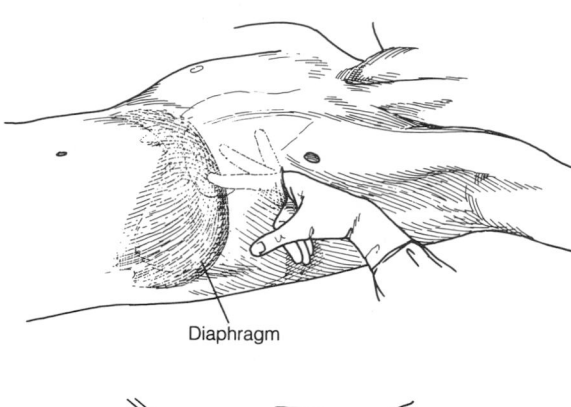

Diaphragm

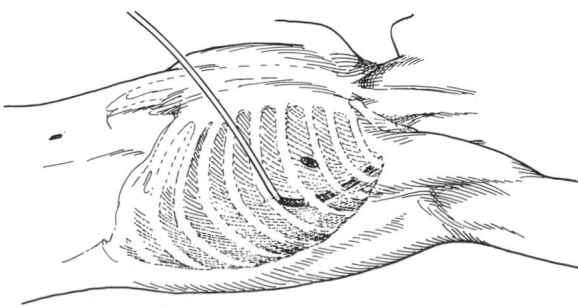

Figure 64-3. Technique for tube thoracostomy. When placed acutely for trauma, an incision is made in the anterior axillary line. The fourth intercostal space is entered. A clamp and finger exploration is performed to be certain that the pleural space is entered. The tube is directed to the apex of the chest. (From Moore FA, Moore EE: Trauma resuscitation. p. 5. In Wilmore DN, Brennan MF, Harken AH et al (eds): Care of the Surgical Patient. Scientific American, New York, 1989, with permission.)

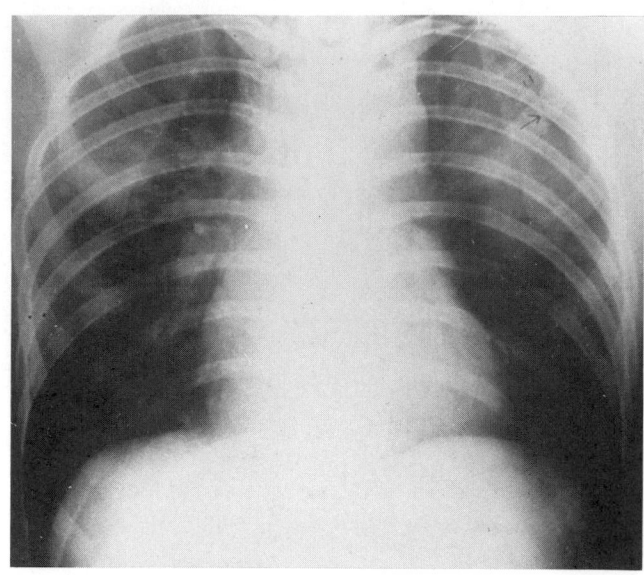

Figure 64-4. Subtle pneumothorax. The chest radiograph must be carefully studied for pneumothorax. This patient had bilateral pneumothoraces, evident only by the hyperlucency of both costophrenic angles.

HEMOTHORAX

Hemothorax usually results from parenchymal laceration, intercostal vessel injury, chest wall injury, bronchial arterial injury, or major thoracic vascular injury (Hughes, 1965). When identified on the chest radiograph, a tube thoracostomy should be performed. To evacuate blood the tube is best placed in the fifth or sixth intercostal space and directed posteriorly. A large-bore (36 Fr) tube should be used (Fig. 64-5).

If greater than 1,000 ml of blood is immediately evacuated and bleeding continues at a rate of greater than 100 to 200 ml/h, emergent thoracotomy should be performed (Richardson, 1985). Likewise, even if significantly less than 1,000 ml is immediately evacuated but bleeding continues at a rate of 100 to 200 ml/h for several hours, the patient should undergo thoracotomy for the control of hemorrhage.

It is essential that all blood be evacuated. If the first chest tube does not completely evacuate the pleural space, a second and if necessary a third large-bore tube should be placed. Experimental data demonstrate that some pleural blood may be lysed and reabsorbed across the mesothelial pleural layer (Condon, 1968; Culiner, et al., 1959). However, failure to evacuate hemothorax runs the risk of producing a clotted hemothorax (Gray, et al., 1960; Jones, et al., 1967). Several studies show that incomplete evacuation of traumatic hemothorax is a major risk factor for the development of post-traumatic empyema (Eddy, et al., 1989). At least 10 to 15 percent of patients with a clotted hemothorax develop empyemas or significant fibrothoraces with resultant trapped lung (Kish, et al., 1976).

Some controversy surrounds the management of clotted hemothorax. Some advocate limited thoracotomy and surgical evacuation of the hemothorax (Collins, et al., 1978; Coselli,

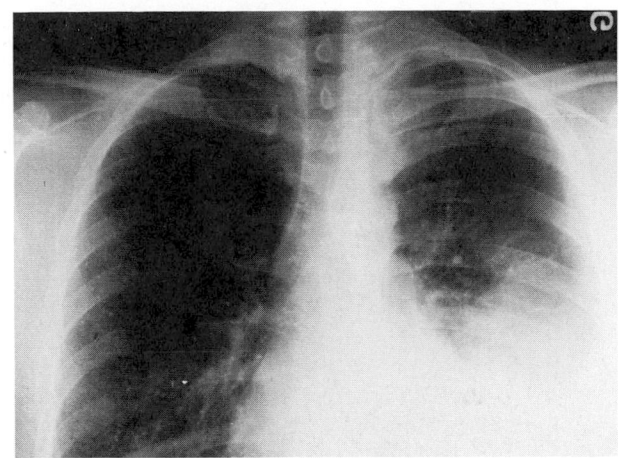
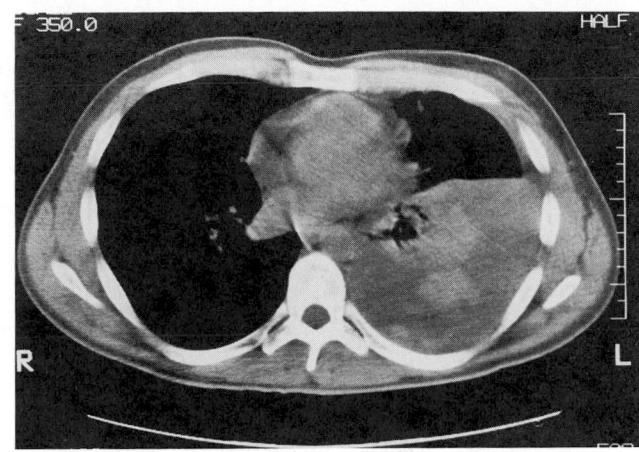

Figure 64-5. Hemothorax. **(A)** Chest radiograph and **(B)** CT scan showing massive left-sided post-traumatic hemothorax.

et al., 1984; Culiner, et al., 1959). These authors cite limited morbidity to the procedure, elimination of the risk for empyema, shorter hospital stay, and potentially improved patient outcome. Other authors acknowledge the potential risk of empyema but prefer to reserve thoracotomy for specific indications, such as the presence of empyema (evidenced by fever and leukocytosis) or lung entrapment (evidenced by at least a 25 percent reduction in ipsilateral lung volume) (Arom, et al., 1977; Wilson, et al., 1979). The posterior lower lobe is the region most commonly collapsed (Arom, et al., 1977).

It seems reasonable to individualize the management of clotted hemothorax. In those patients with a significant volume of clotted hemothorax or suspected pleural sepsis, surgical evacuation is advisable when an anesthetic and a limited thoracotomy are believed to pose minimal morbidity. In the multiple injury patient with significant pulmonary dysfunction requiring high levels of support from mechanical ventilation, the risks of transport to the operating room, anesthesia, and potential intraoperative lung injury may outweigh the potential benefits of thoracotomy. In the latter situation, reserving thoracotomy for a specific indication is appropriate.

If surgical evacuation of the clotted hemothorax is to be performed, it should be performed early. Within the first 7 days, the clot is relatively easy to scoop out through a limited thoracotomy (Coselli, et al., 1984). Thereafter, the clot begins to organize and becomes adherent to both the lung and chest wall, making extraction more difficult and traumatic. Beyond 4 to 6 weeks following injury, a fibrous peel develops creating a fibrothorax, which may require a more difficult decortication (Collins, et al., 1978).

Empyema following chest trauma is usually caused by gram-positive cocci (Levitsky, et al., 1970). If the abdominal viscera are injured, the incidence of enteric gram-negative empyema is markedly increased (Caplan, et al., 1984). If pneumonia develops, the bacteria causing the pneumonia may be expected to infect the hemothorax. Although some authors recommend the routine use of prophylactic antibiotics surrounding the use of chest tubes, there is no convincing evidence that this reduces the risk of empyema (Eddy, et al., 1989), and we recommend that their use be reserved for specific indications.

PULMONARY HEMATOMA, CONTUSION, AND LACERATION

Pulmonary hematoma is usually identified on the chest radiograph as a rather indistinct alveolar infiltrate (Hankins, et al., 1973). Despite a somewhat unimpressive initial radiographic appearance, the injury represents a significant collection of intraparenchymal blood. It may not become visible radiographically for 24 to 72 hours following trauma resuscitation, during which time it increases insidiously. Interestingly pulmonary hematomas generally do not interfere with gas exchange, nor do they produce significant intrapulmonary shunting (Eddy, et al., 1991). However, a pulmonary hematoma is a major risk factor for infection and lung abscess formation (Hankins, et al., 1973).

In contrast, pulmonary contusion is a more serious lung injury because it is not a distinct collection of blood in a cleft or tear in the parenchyma but a diffuse infiltration of blood and proteinaceous fluid within the preserved alveolar architecture. Contusions cause significant intrapulmonary shunting with resultant hypoxemia (Carrico and Hudson 1984; Pepe, et al., 1984; Roscher, et al., 1974). Like hematomas, pulmonary contusions may not be visualized on initial chest radiographs, but 24 to 48 hours may be required for their appearance. Because of the detrimental impact on oxygenation, patients with pulmonary contusion more frequently require endotracheal intubation and mechanical ventilation, thereby incurring the augmented risks of barotrauma and nosocomial pneumonia (Carrico, et al., 1984). Patients with pulmonary contusion should not be intubated prophylactically. The indications for endotracheal intubation with this injury include inability to oxygenate or ventilate the patient. Pulmonary contusion has been identified as a major risk factor for the development of adult respiratory distress syndrome (Pepe, et al., 1984).

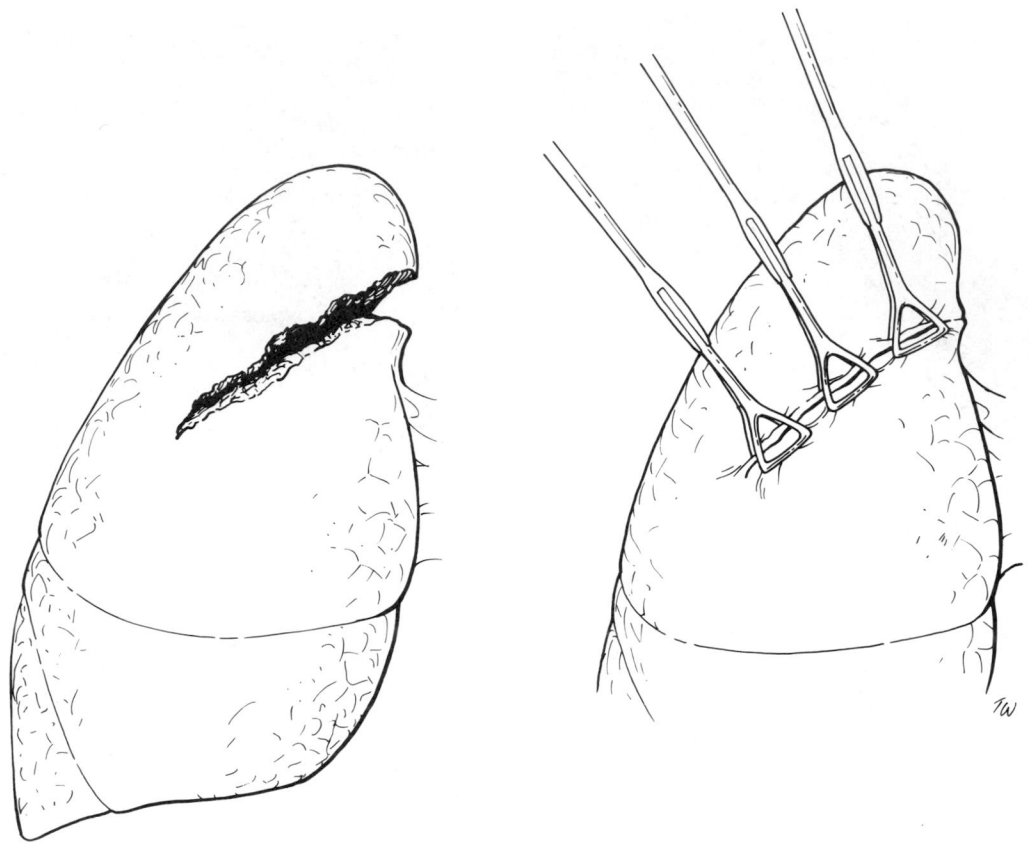

Figure 64-6. Duvall lobe forceps used for hemostasis closure of a large lung laceration.

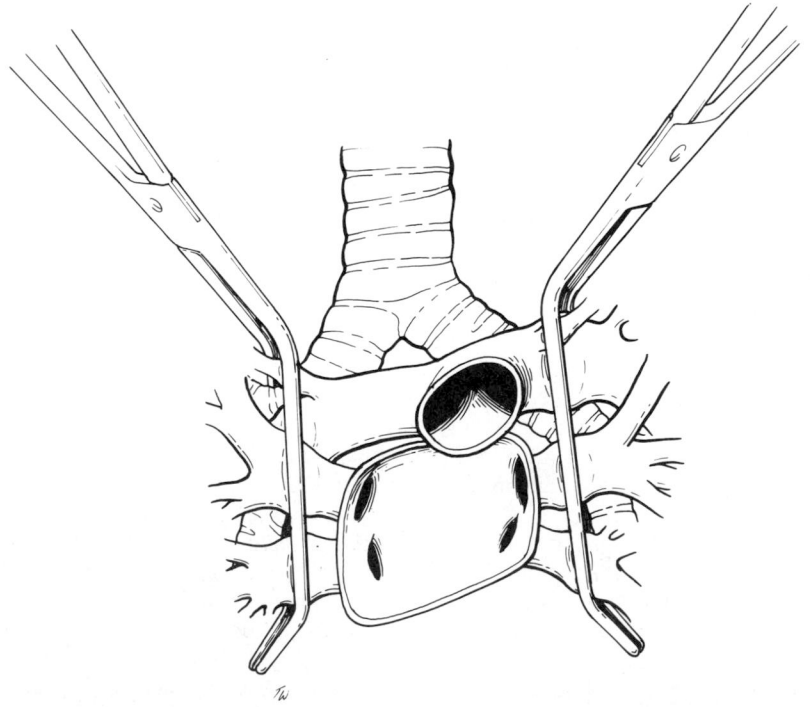

Figure 64-7. Technique to stop major pulmonary vascular hemorrhage. The entire pulmonary hilum is grasped with one hand as a large vascular clamp is applied across the hilum with the other hand.

If either pulmonary hematoma or pulmonary contusion is identified at the time of thoracotomy, the surgeon should resist the temptation to resect the involved lung. Despite the gross appearance, there is rarely an indication for the resection of an injury lung (Fisher, et al., 1974; Sherman, 1966; Graham, et al., 1979), unless there are associated significant injuries to the airway or pulmonary vessels.

Large lacerations of the lung may bleed briskly. Closure with a line of Duvall lobe forceps can give immediate control of hemorrhage and air leak. The laceration should then be oversewn with a running Prolene suture, reinforced with mattress sutures as needed (Fig. 64-6).

PULMONARY VASCULAR INJURY

Vascular injury within the pulmonary parenchyma occurs within a low-pressure system compressed by the surrounding parenchyma. Such hemorrhage generally stops with complete expansion of the lung (Beall, et al., 1966; Graham, et al., 1979; Sherman, 1966). However, uncorrected injury to the main pulmonary arteries or veins or their principal lobar branches is usually lethal from rapid exsanguination because these structures bleed freely into the pleural space and extrapleural spaces. These injuries rarely produce massive hemoptysis. Major pulmonary vascular injuries usually result from sudden deceleration. Mortality rates for pulmonary arterial or venous injuries exceed 75 percent. Therefore patients rarely live to reach a trauma center (Mattox, et al., 1989).

If major pulmonary vascular injury is diagnosed or suspected, immediate thoracotomy should be performed. Temporary vascular control may be obtained at the pulmonary hilum by clamping the entire hilum. Through a thoracotomy incision, the hilum of the lung is grasped firmly with one hand as the surgeon uses the other hand to apply a long vascular clamp across the entire pulmonary hilum. (Fig. 64-7). This maneuver excludes the main pulmonary artery and veins from the circulation. This may prevent exsanguination and provide time to resuscitate the patient. If there is a

---

Pulmonary Vascular Injury: Pitfalls and Points to Remember

Pneumothorax may not be present on the initial chest radiograph. Obtain serial radiographs.

Pneumothorax may be subtle on the initial portable chest radiograph. Study the costophrenic angles.

A hollow viscus in the chest may resemble a pneumothorax.

Use finger exploration to be certain the pleural space, not the peritoneal space, is entered when placing a chest tube.

Place at least two large chest tubes (36 Fr) for a large hemothorax in an unstable patient. The first tube may clog.

Pulmonary contusion may not be visible on the initial chest radiograph. Obtain serial radiographs.

Badly damaged lung tissue invites resection. Resist the temptation; the lung will remodel and control or prevent pleural complications.

If venous drainage is sacrificed, resect the involved lung to avoid infarction.

---

significant amount of blood in the airway, a double-lumen endotracheal tube or a bronchial blocker may be used to protect the opposite lung from the blood. Next the vascular injury should be isolated and repaired using standard vascular techniques (Carr, 1980). If a lobar pulmonary artery is irreparable, it may be ligated without fear of pulmonary necrosis. The bronchial blood supply is usually sufficient to maintain parenchymal viability (Wolf and Sabiston, 1980). If the venous drainage to a parenchymal region must be sacrificed, the involved parenchyma should be resected to prevent the complications of infarction (Carr, 1980).

KEY REFERENCES

Coselli JS, Mattox KL, Beall AC: Re-evaluation of early evacuation of clotted hemothorax. Am J Surg 148:785, 1984

The authors demonstrate the advantages of early evacuation of clotted hemothorax.

Richardson JD: Indications for thoracotomy in thoracic trauma. Curr Surg 42:361, 1985

The author offers standardized guidelines for thoracotomy for hemothorax.

REFERENCES

Arom KV, Grover FL, Richardson JD, Trinkle JK: Post-traumatic empyema. Ann Thorac Surg 23:254, 1977

Beall AC, Crawford HW, DeBakey ME: Considerations in the management of acute traumatic hemothorax. J Thorac Cardiovasc Surg 52:351, 1966

Caplan ES, Hoyt NJ, Rodriquez A et al.: Empyema occurring in the multiply traumatized patient. J Trauma 24:785, 1984

Carr RE: Injuries to the pulmonary parenchyma and vasculature. In Daughtry DC (ed): Thoracic Trauma. Little, Brown, Boston, 1980

Carrico CJ, Hudson LD: Post-injury acute pulmonary failure. In Shires GT (ed): Principles of Trauma Surgery. 3rd Ed. McGraw-Hill, New York, 1984

Collins MP, Shuck JM, Wachtel TL et al.: Early decortication after thoracic trauma. Arch Surg 113:44, 1978

Condon RE: Spontaneous resolution of experimental clotted hemothorax. Surg Gynecol Obstet 126:505, 1968

Culiner MM, Roe BB, Grimes OF: The early elective surgical approach to the treatment of traumatic hemothorax. J Thorac Cardiovasc Surg 38:780, 1959

Eddy AC, Luna GK, Copass MK: Factors affecting the incidence of empyema thoracic in patients undergoing emergent closed tube thoracostomy for thoracic trauma. Am J Surg 157:494, 1989

Eddy CA, Carrico CJ, Rusch VW: Injury to the lung and pleura. p. 358. In Moore EE, Mattox KL, Feliciano DV (eds): Trauma. Appleton and Lange, Norwalk, CT, 1991

Fischer RP, Geiger JP, Guernsey JM: Pulmonary resections for severe pulmonary contusions secondary to high velocity missel wounds. J Trauma 14:293, 1974

Graham JM, Mattox KL, Beall AC: Penetrating trauma of the lung. J Trauma 19:655, 1979

Gray AR, Harrison WH, Couves CM et al.: Penetrating injuries to the chest: clinical results in the management of 769 patients. Am J Surg 100:709, 1960

Hankins J, Attar S, Turndy S et al.: Differential diagnosis of pulmonary parenchymal changes in thoracic trauma. Am Surg 39:309, 1973

Hughes RK: Thoracic trauma. Ann Thorac Surg 1:778, 1965

Jones RJ, Samson PC, Dugan DJ: Current management of civilian thoracic trauma. Am J Surg 114:289, 1967

Kemmerer WT, Eckert WG, Garthright JB et al.: Patterns of thoracic injuries in fatal traffic accidents. J Trauma 1:595, 1961

Kish G, Kozloff L, Joseph WL, et al.: Indications for early thoracotomy in the management of chest trauma. Ann Thorac Surg 22:23, 1976

Levitsky S, Annable CA, Thomas PA: The management of empyema after thoracic wounding. J Thorac Cardiovasc Surg 59:630, 1970

Mattox KL, Feliciano DV, Beall AC, et al.: Five thousand seven hundred sixty cardiovascular injuries in 4459 patients: epidemiologic evolution 1958-1988. Ann Surg 209:698, 1989

Meade RH: A History of Thoracic Surgery. Charles C Thomas, Springfield, IL, 1961

Pepe PE, Hudson LD, Carrico CJ: Early application of positive end-expiratory pressure in patients at risk for the adult respiratory distress syndrome. N Engl J Med 311:281, 1984

Roscher R, Bittner R, Stockmann U: Pulmonary contusion: clinical experience. Arch Surg 109:508, 1974

Sherman RT: Experience with 472 civilian penetrating wounds of the chest. Mil Med 131:63, 1966

Thal ER, Ramenofsky MI et al.: Advanced Trauma Life Support Course for Physicians, Subcommittee Trauma, 1987-1988. American College of Surgeons, Chicago, 1988

Wilson JW, Boren CH Jr, Peterson SR, Thomas AN: Traumatic hemothorax: is decortication necessary? J Thorac Cardiovasc Surg 77:489, 1979

Wolf W, Sabiston DC Jr (eds): Chronic pulmonary embolism and cor pulmonale. In: Pulmonary Embolism. Little, Brown, Boston, 1980

Trauma to the Diaphragm, Esophagus, and Thoracic Duct

David A. Fullerton   Geoffrey M. Graeber
Frederick L. Grover   Joseph I. Miller, Jr.

DIAPHRAGMATIC INJURY

The diaphragm separates the abdominal and thoracic cavities, inserting along its perimeter into the lower ribs laterally, the lower sternum anteriorly, and the periosteum of the first three lumbar vertebral bodies posteriorly. Physiologically the diaphragm functions as the primary muscle of respiration, descending with inhalation to generate more subatmospheric pressure in the pleural space and ascending with expiration. At end expiration the dome of the diaphragm rises anteriorly as high as the fifth intercostal space on the right and the fourth intercostal space on the left, making it susceptible to penetrating injuries through the lower chest and the upper abdomen.

HISTORICAL NOTE

Traumatic diaphragmatic injuries have been recognized in the medical literature for more than 450 years. Postmortem findings of diaphragmatic hernia following penetrating injury were described in 1541 by Sennertus and in 1579 by Ambrose Pare (Orringer, et al., 1975). In 1785 Duncan described a diaphragmatic hernia in a soldier injured in the Battle of Quebec (Meade, 1961). The famous military surgeon Guthrie (1853) described multiple cases of penetrating diaphragmatic injuries in the ninteenth century British campaigns in Europe. In that year, Bowditch suggested that operative repair of diaphragmatic hernias should be performed. In 1889 Walker performed a successful repair of a diaphragmatic hernia in a patient crushed by a falling tree. Billings described more than

100 cases of diaphragmatic penetration and diaphragmatic rupture during the American Civil War (Meade, 1961). With the development of radiology in the late 1800s, successful antemortem diagnosis became more feasible and remains the mainstay of diagnosis today. The series compiled by Bernatz, et al. (1958) and Hood (1971) describe twentieth century surgical experience with these injuries.

HISTORICAL READINGS

Bernatz PE, Burnside AF Jr, Clagett OT: Problem of the ruptured diaphragm. JAMA 168:877, 1958

Guthrie GJ: Commentaries on the Surgery of the War in Portugal, Spain, France and The Netherlands. 5th Ed. Renshaw, London, 1853

Hood RM: Traumatic diaphragmatic hernia (collective review). Ann Thorac Surg 12:311, 1971

Meade RH: A History of Thoracic Surgery. Charles C Thomas, Springfield, IL, 1961

Orringer MB, Kirsch MM, Sloan H: Congenital and traumatic diaphragmatic hernias exclusive of the hiatus. Curr Probl Surg 3:3, 1975

BLUNT DIAPHRAGM RUPTURE

The mechanism of blunt diaphragmatic rupture is a rapid increase in intra-abdominal pressure, creating a large pressure gradient between the abdominal and thoracic cavities. The stress of this pressure results in rupture, usually through the central portion of the diaphragm. This injury is commonly produced by rapid deceleration in a motor vehicle accident, but any injury that produces a sudden force to the torso, such as a fall from a significant height or a crush injury to the abdomen, may cause diaphragmatic rupture.

Estera, et al. (1979) reported an equal incidence of left and right blunt diaphragmatic injuries in an autopsy series. In most clinical series, the left hemidiaphragm is reported to be injured far more commonly than the right, probably because of the greater difficulty in making the radiographic diagnosis of right-sided injuries. The liver is believed to dissipate the force and protect the right diaphragm from injury (Brooks, 1978; Orringer, et al., 1975).

Rupture of the diaphragm results in the herniation of intra-abdominal contents into the chest. On the left the most common organs to herniate are the stomach, spleen, colon, omentum, and small bowel. On the right, the liver and colon herniate most frequently (Orringer, et al., 1975). Rarely, intrapericardial rupture may occur (Van Loenhout, et al., 1978).

The diagnosis may be difficult, requiring a high index of suspicion. The initial chest radiograph must be studied carefully. It may be normal in as many as 38 percent of patients with diaphragmatic rupture (Wise, et al., 1973). During the initial evaluation, it is extremely helpful to place a nasogastric tube prior to taking the chest radiograph; the tube within the stomach may be radiographically visible in the chest. Subtle radiographic signs on the chest radiograph that suggest the diagnosis include an elevated hemidiaphragm, pleural effu-

sion, platelike atelectasis above an indistinct diaphragm, and mediastinal shift away from the injured side (Payne and Yellin, 1982). The diagnosis may be obvious if the chest radiograph demonstrates abdominal viscera within the left chest cavity. On the right making a diagnosis from the chest radiograph is especially difficult; only 17 percent of chest radiographs in patients with right-sided rupture are strongly suspicious of diaphragmatic rupture. Protrusion of the liver through the hemidiaphragm may give the radiographic appearance of an elevated right hemidiaphragm (Fig. 64-8).

Acute diaphragmatic rupture and herniation of intra-abdominal contents into the chest may result in dramatic cardiopulmonary compromise. The diagnosis must be considered in any victim of blunt trauma in respiratory distress. Because of the pressure gradient between the peritoneal and pleural cavities, the intra-abdominal contents may be pulled through the diaphragmatic defect and into the chest. A large volume of abdominal contents that herniates acutely may not only compress the ipsilateral lung, but it may also cause mediastinal shift away from the injured side, also compressing the contralateral lung. Together these may produce significant respiratory distress. As in tension pneumothorax, the shift of the mediastinum may compromise venous return to the heart and reduce cardiac output.

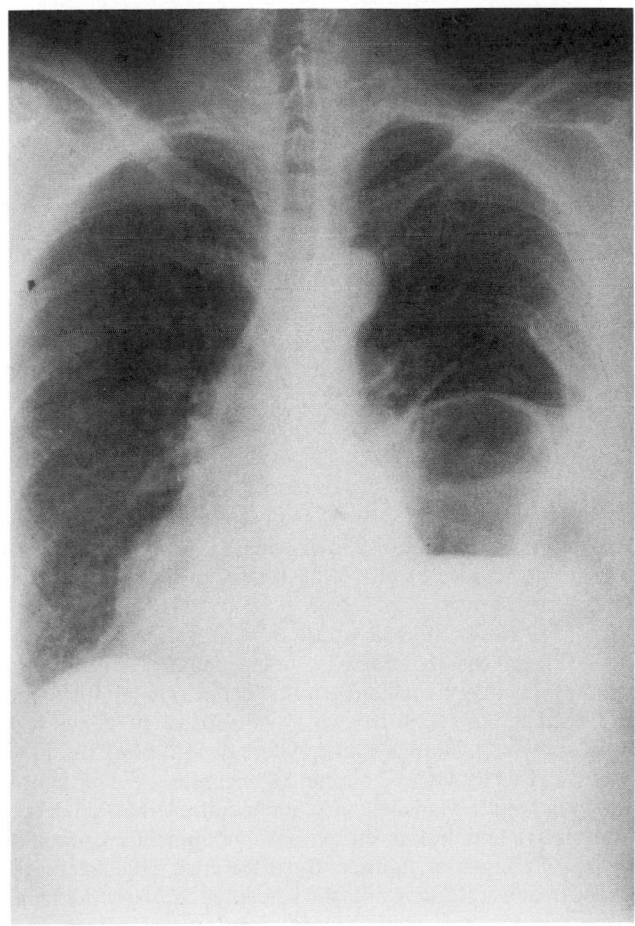

Figure 64-8. Chest radiograph of a 62-year-old woman with a ruptured left hemidiaphragm.

Acute management includes nasogastric suction to decompress the proximal gut and endotracheal intubation to provide positive pressure ventilation (Miller, et al., 1984). Positive pressure ventilation minimizes the pressure gradient from the abdomen to the thorac, diminishing the herniation of abdominal contents. The surgical approach for the repair of the ruptured diaphragm is dictated by whether the injury is acute or chronic. The repair of acute injuries should be performed by laparotomy because acute diaphragmatic injury is associated with intra-abdominal injury in approximately 90 percent of cases (Orringer, et al., 1975). On the other hand, adhesions between the herniated viscera and lung or mediastinum may be most effectively controlled through the chest. Chronic injuries (those more than a few weeks old) should be repaired through a thoracotomy incision. The diaphragmatic tear should be repaired with interrupted figure-eight 0 non-absorbable suture. In rare instances of significant tissue loss, a prosthetic material may be required. If there is contamination, autologous tissue should be used.

Patients requiring immediate laparotomy for blunt trauma should have both diaphragmatic leaves examined for injury. The tear should be repaired at that time if found. Patients not requiring immediate laparotomy but in whom the diagnosis is suspected should undergo additional studies. Thoracoscopy, fluoroscopy, radionuclide liver and spleen scan (Harman, et al., 1981) and upper or lower gastrointestinal tract contrast studies (Madden, et al., 1989) may be helpful. Computed tomography (CT) and magnetic resonance imaging (MRI) have been reported to diagnose large diaphragmatic tears (Aronoff, et al., 1982; Mirvis, et al., 1988), although the sensitivity of these techniques is uncertain.

Patients with blunt diaphragmatic trauma have a high mortality rate, which is related to the severity of associated injuries rather than to the diaphragmatic tear itself. Mortality rates range from 19 to 40.5 percent; in Beal, et al.'s (1988) series, 87 percent of those who died were in profound shock on arrival.

ACUTE PENETRATING DIAPHRAGMATIC TRAUMA

Penetrating trauma is the most common cause of diaphragmatic injury in most series (Chen and Wilson, 1991; Miller, et al., 1984; Symbas, et al., 1986; Wise, et al., 1973). The proportion of patients with penetrating versus blunt injury depends on demographics. Penetrating injuries are more frequent in areas of violent urban crime (Symbas, et al., 1986). Penetrating trauma to the lower chest carries an especially high risk. Moore, et al. (1980) reported injury to the diaphragm in 15 percent of lower thoracic stab wounds and 46 percent of lower thoracic gunshot wounds.

The size of the diaphragmatic tear secondary to a penetrating injury is much smaller than that caused by blunt trauma. In Wise, et al.'s (1973) report, 84 percent of penetrating injuries were less than 2 cm in length. None of the blunt ruptures was less than 2 cm, and 60 percent were more than 10 cm in length. Consequently, immediate herniation occurs rarely after penetrating injury, and the clinical presentation is that of coexisting injuries. Symbas, et al. (1986) reported injury to one additional organ in 43 percent, two to four major organs in 45 percent, and more than four major organs in 1.6 percent of patients with acute penetrating diaphragmatic injury. Patients may present with abdominal pain, dyspnea, or shock. The initial chest radiograph may not be diagnostic. It was normal in at least 28 percent of patients reported by Symbas, et al. (1986), although 61 percent of patients had hemopneumothoraces. Miller, et al. (1984) repoted 43 percent normal chest radiographs in their series on penetrating diaphragmatic trauma. An abnormal diaphragmatic contour may be a helpful finding (Minagi, et al., 1977).

The majority of these patients are operated on for suspected or known injuries of other organs. Both leaves of the diaphragm should be carefully examined and appropriately repaired, as described for blunt injuries. In patients suspected of having diaphragmatic injury but not requiring emergency surgery, additional tests may be performed to rule out injury, as described earlier. Thoracoscopy and laparoscopy may be particularly useful.

The mortality rate of patients with penetrating diaphragmatic trauma is much less than that of those with blunt injuries and is related to the severity of associated injuries. Symbas, et al. (1986) reported a 2.2 percent mortality rate in 185 patients, all from complications of associated injuries.

CHRONIC TRAUMATIC DIAPHRAGMATIC HERNIA

Miller, et al. (1984) estimated that, without immediate exploration, about 13 percent of injuries to the diaphragm are missed. Because blunt defects are larger than penetrating ones, most of the missed hernias presenting late are secondary to penetrating trauma (Hegarty, et al., 1978). It is doubtful whether a defect in a constantly moving diaphragm will ever heal unless it is obliterated by an adherent adjacent viscus (Symbas, 1989). An important factor in the development of diaphragmatic hernia is the negative pleuroperitoneal gradient, which ranges from 7 to 20 cm H_2O during quiet respiration but may increase to more than 100 cm H_2O during maximal inspiratory effort (Marchand, 1957). The larger the defect and the longer the time since injury are, the higher the chance is of herniation with resulting complications of incarceration, strangulation, gastrointestinal obstruction, or respiratory compromise. These complications dictate the clinical presentation. An asymptomatic hernia may be found on a routine chest radiograph. Graivier and Freeark (1963) suggested that the diagnosis of chronic diaphragmatic hernia should be considered in any of the following four circumstances: (1) bowel obstruction with a history of thoracic trauma, particularly stab wounds; (2) bowel obstruction and changes at the left base on the chest radiograph: (3) small bowel obstruction without hernias or abdominal scars; and (4) large bowel obstruction in young patients.

In a patient with a history of thoracoabdominal trauma and a clinical suspicion of diaphragmatic hernia, a chest radiograph should be the first test; it is usually abnormal. Barium studies of the gastrointestinal tract, a liver and spleen scan, or ultrasound further define the extent of herniation.

Patients are taken to the operating room after appropriate preparation and resuscitation, if necessary. The approach should be through a posterolateral thoracotomy in the sixth or seventh interspace for the safe lysis of adhesions. After the organs are freed and the edges of the defect are defined, the herniated organs are returned to the peritoneal cavity, and the defect is repaired with figure-eight 0 nonabsorbable sutures. In rare instances of inability to close the defect primarily, an autologous or prosthetic patch can be used (Symbas, 1989).

The mortality rate may be high in the presence of gangrenous visicera in the chest. Hegarty, et al. (1978) reported 20 percent overall mortality rate, which increased to 80 percent when gangrene was present. Further discussion on the diaphragm is found in Chapter 51.

ESOPHAGEAL INJURY

HISTORICAL NOTE

The Smith papyrus describes an esophagocutaneous fistula from an esophageal perforation (Witte, and Pratshehke, 1991). The earliest surgical procedures on the esophagus were performed to retrieve foreign bodies. In 1676 Wiseman advised suture closure of an esophageal injury and a "thin diet." In 1695 Purmann acknowledged the difficulties that may be encountered in an effort to expose an injured esophagus and recommend that "it be left to the patient's good constitution to contribute to the cure" (Hochberg 1960). In 1792 Munro, A Scottish surgeon, advocated that longitudinal esophageal wounds best healed without assistance. Late in the nineteenth century, the first attempts were made to operate in the posterior mediastinum, and Bryant and Potarca described posterior approaches to the thoracic esophagus (Hochberg, 1960). Brewer and Burford (1965) reported the successful repair of a traumatic esophageal perforation in 1947.

HISTORICAL READINGS

Brewer LA, Burford TH: Special types of thoracic wounds. p. 269. In Medical Department: U.S. Army Surgery in World War II, Thoracic Surgery. 38th Ed. Washington, D.C, U.S. Government Printing Office, 1965

Hochberg LA: Thoracic Surgery Before the 20th Century. Vantage Press, New York, 1960

Witte J, Pratshehke E: Esophageal perforations. p. 669. In Baue AE, Geha AS, Hammond et al (eds): Glenn's Thoracic and Cardiovascular Surgery. 5th Ed. Appleton and Lange, Norwalk, CT, 1991

TRAUMATIC ESOPHAGEAL INJURIES

Esophageal injuries are uncommon. Overall, fewer than 20 percent of all esophageal perforations are secondary to trauma (Jones and Ginsberg, 1992). The low incidence of traumatic esophageal injuries is attributed to the well-protected location of the esophagus in the posterior mediastinum and the frequency of injuries to adjacent structures resulting in the early death of these patients (Bombeck, et al., 1972; Jones and Samson, 1975). The cervical esophagus is the most commonly injured site in virtually all series. Of all cervical esophageal perforations, 40 percent result from trauma, in

contrast in 16 percent of all thoracic esophageal perforations. Because of its protected position, only 4 to 5 percent of penetrating cervical injuries involve the esophagus (Weaver, et al., 1971; Blass, et al., 1978; Bladergroen, et al., 1986) (Fig. 64-9).

Penetrating injuries typically result from gunshot wounds, and at least 60 percent of these injuries occur in the cervical esophagus (Glatterer, et al., 1985; Symbas, et al., 1980). Blunt injuries to the esophagus are rare, with an incidence among traumatized patients that is below 0.1% (Kemmerer, et al., 1961). Although these injuries are infrequent, a high index of suspicion of their presence must be maintained. A delay in the diagnosis of thoracic esophageal perforation beyond 24 hours carries a high mortality rate. A chemical mediastinitis is incited with progression to multiple organ failure. When traumatic esophageal injuries occur, more than 50 percent are associated with tracheal injury (Beal, et al., 1988; Nissen, 1980). Patients found to have thoracic tracheobronchial injury should be considered to be at risk for an associated esophageal injury and should undergo esophagoscopy.

Patients with penetrating thoracic trauma to the posterior mediastinum, particularly from gunshot wounds that traverse the mediastinum, must be evaluated for esophageal injury. Physical findings include fever, pain and crepitance in the neck, or pain in the upper abdomen. The diagnosis may be suggested on the initial chest radiograph by the presence of pneumomediastinum or pleural effusion. However, in both

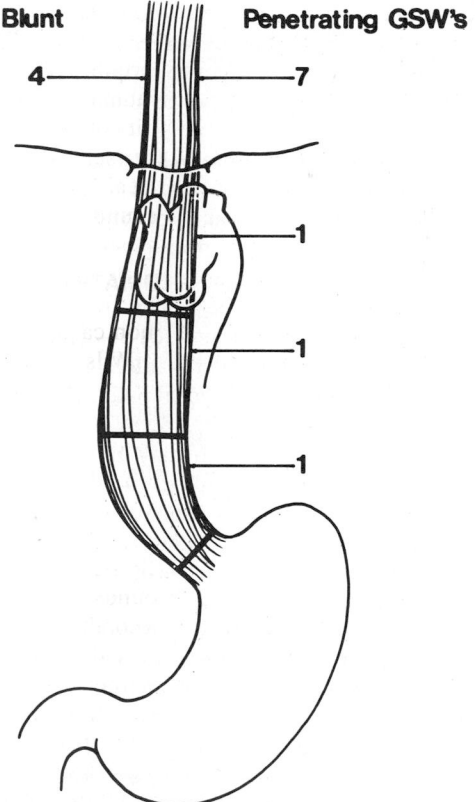

Figure 64-9.   The cervical esophagus is most commonly injuried. (Data from Glatterer MS Jr, Toon RS, Ellestad C, et al: Management of blunt and penetrating external esophageal trauma. J Trauma 25:784, 1985.)

blunt and penetrating injuries, up to one-third of patients have a normal initial chest radiograph (Glatterer, et al., 1985). Adjunctive studies are needed.

Contrast esophagography, particularly when Gastrografin is used, is notoriously insensitive in making the diagnosis, with false-negative rates ranging from 0 to 50 percent (Attar, et al., 1991; Cheadle and Richardson, 1982; Glatterer, et al., 1985; Popovsky, 1984; Symbas, et al., 1980). Esophagoscopy should be performed; visualization of a tear or of localized blood is diagnostic. Unfortunately the false-negative rate for esophagoscopy has ranged from 0 to 40 percent (Cheadle and Richardson, 1982; Defore, et al., 1977; Glatterer et al., 1985; Sawyers, et al., 1975; Sheely, et al., 1975). If the diagnosis is entertained, it is best evaluated by a combination of esophageal endoscopy and barium esophagography when feasible (Kemmerer, et al., 1961). A pleural effusion containing high levels of amylase should be considered diagnostic in this setting.

Although successful nonoperative management of small iatrogenic esophageal perforations has been reported, these data should not be considered applicable to the trauma patient. The extent of both penetrating and blunt esophageal injuries is much less predictable than in simple iatrogenic perforations. We think that all traumatic esophageal injuries should be explored early. Cervical esophageal injuries may be debrided and closed primarily with drainage of the paraesophageal space. A fifth or sixth intercostal space incision is performed for suspected injuries to the mid- to distal esophagus. An incision in the right third or fourth intercostal space may be advantageous for injuries to the upper thoracic esophagus. Primary one- or two-layered esophageal closure and wide mediastinal drainage should be accomplished (Nesbitt and Sawyer, 1987).

If primary esophageal closure cannot be satisfactorily attained, it may be possible to approximate the wound edges over a T tube placed into the lumen of the esophagus through the perforation, which is then brought out the chest wall to divert saliva from the mediastinum (Mulder and Barkun, 1991). This procedure should be combined with gastrostomy drainage and feeding jejunostomy tube placement. Wide mediastinal drainage is essential. Perforation of the distal esophagus may best be handled by serosal patch closure provided by the gastric fundus.

Cervical esophageal diversion may be necessary in the patient with the diagnosis of esophageal perforation who has extensive mediastinitis. This is usually seen in cases with a significant diagnostic delay of greater than 12 to 24 hours. The procedure requires (1) a cervical esophagostomy to divert salivary flow, (2) a thoracotomy to accomplish wide mediastinal debridement of devitalized tissue and wide mediastinal drainage, and (3) placement of a gastrostomy drainage tube and a feeding jejunostomy tube. Prevention of gastroesophageal reflux by occlusion of the esophagus distal to the perforation was recommended by Urschel, et al. (1974). The latter may be accomplished by ligation of the esophagus with umbilical tape. This requires a second procedure at a later date to remove the tape. Alternatively, the esophageal hiatus may be occluded by wrapping it with absorbable suture material (Popovsky, 1984). This avoids a second operative procedure and therefore seems preferable. Although esophageal diversion may be life-saving in some circumstances, the mortality rate is very high, and a subsequent reconstructive procedure is frequently required. Successful exclusion with late restoration of function has been achieved by Lewis (1985) using Rummell tourniquets and catheter drainage.

Because of the association with tracheal injuries, tracheoesophageal fistula formation may result from esophageal trauma. These fistulae are found in the distal trachea. Their initial presentation is usually one of subcutaneous emphysema, followed by aspiration when the patient beings to drink. Their repair should include debridement and primary closure of both the trachea and esophagus with interposition of an intercostal muscle flap or pericardial flap between the two repairs. For an additional discussion of esophageal injuries, the reader may consult Chapter 35 in *Esophageal Surgery*.

THORACIC DUCT INJURY

Traumatic injury to the thoracic duct may occur with blunt or penetrating trauma (Cevese, et al., 1978) at any point along the course of the duct, making localization difficult. Hyperextension of the spine may cause rupture of the duct just above the diaphragm. Penetration by gunshot or stab wounds is usually overshadowed by life-threatening damage to other structures, but it is a good habit to look for thoracic duct injury after definitive therapy of these injuries, just before placement of drains and closure of the thoracotomy. The anatomy and management of thoracic duct injury is discussed in more detail in Chapter 40.

Trauma to Diaphragm, Esophagus, and Thoracic Duct: Points to Remember

Herniation of a hollow viscus may resemble pneumothorax.

Place a radiopaque nasogastric tube prior to the initial chest radiograph.

Any penetrating injury below the fourth intercostal space can lacerate the diaphragm and abdominal organs.

Consider diaphragmatic hernia in the patient with bowel obstruction and a history of trauma.

Rule out esophageal laceration in any patient with a penetrating thoracic wound and pneumomediastinum

Perform both esophagoscopy and barium esophagraphy to assess injuries to the esophagus.

KEY REFERENCES

Jones WG, Ginsberg RJ: Esophageal perforation: a continuing challenge. Ann Thorac Surg 53:534, 1992

This is a thorough review of surgical options for the therapy of traumatic and iatrogenic esophageal perforations.

Orringer MB, Kirsch MM, Sloan H: Congenital and traumatic diaphragmatic hernias exclusive of the hiatus. Curr Probl Surg 3:3, 1975

This is an excellent, comprehensive review.

REFERENCES

Aronoff RJ, Reynolds J, Thal E: Evaluation of diaphragmatic injuries. Am J Surg 144:671, 1982

Attar S, Hankins JR, Suter CM et al: Esophageal perforation: a therapeutic challenge. Ann Thorac Surg 50:45, 1991

Beal SL, Pottmeyer EW, Pisso S: Esophageal perforation following external blunt trauma. J Trauma 28:1425, 1988

Bernatz PE, Burnside AF Jr, Clagett OT: Problem of the ruptured diaphragm. JAMA 168:877, 1958

Bladergroen MR, Lowe JE, Postlethwait RW: Diagnosis and recommended management of esophageal perforation and rupture. Ann Thorac Surg 42:235, 1986

Blass DC, James EC, Reed RJ III et al: Penetrating wounds of the neck and upper thorax. J Trauma 18:2, 1978

Bombeck CT, Boyd DR, Nyhus LM: Esophageal trauma. Surg Clin North Am 52:219, 1972

Brewer LA, Burford TH: Special types of thoracic wounds. p. 269. In Medical Department: US Army Surgery in World War II, Thoracic Surgery. 38th Ed. Washington, DC, Government Printing Office, 1965.

Brooks JN: Blunt traumatic rupture of the diaphragm. Ann Thorac Surg 26:199, 1978

Cevese PG, Vecchioni R, Cordiano C et al: Surgical techniques for operations on the thoracic duct. Surg Gynecol Obstet 140:958, 1978

Cheadle W, Richardson JD: Options in management of trauma to the esophagus. Surg Gynecol Obstet 155:380, 1982

Chen JC, Wilson SE: Diaphragmatic injuries: recognition and management in 62 patients. Am Surg 57:810, 1991

Defore WW Jr, Mattox KL, Hansen HA et al: Surgical management of penetrating injuries of the esophagus. Am J Surg 134:72, 1977

Estera AS, Platt MR, Mills LJ: Traumatic injuries of the diaphragm. Chest 75:306, 1979

Glatterer MS Jr, Toon RS, Ellestad C et al: Management of blunt and penetrating external esophageal trauma. J Trauma 25:784, 1985

Graivier L, Freeark RJ: Traumatic diaphagmatic hernia. Arch Surg 86:363, 1963

Guthrie GJ: Commentaries on the Surgery of the War in Portugal, Spain, France and The Netherlands. 5th Ed. Renshaw, London, 1853

Harman PK, Mentzer RMJ, Weinberg AD et al: Early diagnosis by liver scan of a right-sided traumatic diaphragmatic hernia. J Trauma 21:489, 1981

Hegerty MM, Bryer JM, Angorn IB et al: Delayed presentation of traumatic diaphragmatic hernia. Ann Surg 188:229, 1978

Hochberg LA: Thoracic Surgery Before the 20th Century. Vantage Press, New York, 1960

Hood RM: Traumatic diaphragmatic hernia (collective review). Ann Thorac Surg 12:311, 1971

Jones RJ, Samson PC: Esophageal injury. Ann Thorac Surg 19:216, 1975

Kemmerer NT, Eckert WG, Gathright JB et al: Patterns of thoracic injuries in fatal accidents. J Trauma 1:595, 1961

Lewis RJ, Sisler GE: Reversible total esophageal exclusion. Ann Thorac Surg 39:476, 1985

Madden M, Paull D, Shires GT et al: Occult diaphragmatic injury from stab wounds to the lower chest and abdomen. J Trauma 29:292, 1989

Marchand P: A study of the forces productive of gastroesophageal regurgitation and herniation through the diaphragmatic hiatus. Thorax 12:189, 1957

Meade RH: A History of Thoracic Surgery. Charles C Thomas, Springfield, IL, 1961

Miller L, Bennett EV, Root HD et al: Management of penetrating and blunt diaphragmatic injury. J Trauma 24, 1984

Minagi H, Brody WR, Laing FC: The variable roentgen appearance of traumatic diaphragmatic hernia. Can Assoc Radiol 28:124, 1977

Mirris SE, Keramati J, Buckman R et al: MR imaging of traumatic diaphragmatic rupture. J Comput Assist Tomogr 12:147, 1988

Moore JB, Moore EE, Thompson JS: Abdominal injuries associated with penetrating trauma in the lower chest. Am J Surg 140;724, 1980

Mulder DS, Barkun JS: Injury to the trachea, bronchus and esophagus. p. 348. In Moore EE, Mattox KL, Feliciano DV (eds): Trauma. Appleton and Lange, Norwalk, CT, 1991

Nesbitt JC, Sawyers JL: Surgical management of esophageal perforation. Am Surg 53:183, 1987

Nissen R: Total pneumonectomy. Ann Thorac Surg 29:390, 1980

Payne JH, Yellin AE: Traumatic diaphragmatic hernia. Arch Surg 117:18, 1982

Popovsky J: Perforations of the esophagus from gunshot wounds. Trauma 24:337, 1984

Sawyers JL, Lane CE, Foster JH et al: Esophageal perforation—an increasing challenge. Ann Thorac Surg 19:233, 1975

Sheely CH II, Mattox KL, Beall AC et al: Penetrating wounds of the cervical esophagus. Am J Surg 130:707, 1975

Symbas PN: Diaphragmatic injuries. p. 344. In Symbas PN (ed): Cardiothoracic Trauma. WB Saunders, 1989

Symbas PN, Hatcher CR Jr, Vlasis SE, Esophageal Gunshot injuries. Ann Surg 191, 703, 1980

Symbas PN, Vlasis SE, Hatcher CR Jr: Blunt and penetrating diaphragmatic injuries with or without herniation of organs into the chest. Ann Thorac Surg 42:158, 1986

Urschel HC Jr, Razzuk MA, Wood RE et al: Esophageal perforation: exclusion and diversion in continuity. Ann Surg 179:587, 1974

Van Loenhout RMM, Shiphors TJMJ, Wittens CHA et al: Traumatic intrapericardial diaphragmatic hernia. J Trauma 26:271, 1978

Weaver AW, Sankaran S, Fromm SH et al: The management of penetrating wounds of the neck. Surg Gynecol Obstet 133:49, 1971

Wise L, Connors J, Hwang YH et al: Traumatic injuries to the diaphragm. J Trauma 13:946, 1973

Witte J, Pratshchke E: Esophageal perforations. p. 669. In Baue AE, Geha AS, Hammond GL et al: (eds)]: Glenn's Thoracic and Cardiovascular Surgery. 5th Ed. Appleton and Lange, Norwalk, CT, 1991

Trauma to the Heart and Great Vessels

David A. Fullerton
Frederick L. Grover

This chapter discusses blunt cardiac and major vessel trauma. Penetrating injuries are discussed in Chapter 66.

HISTORICAL NOTE

Death from cardiovascular trauma has been described throughout the history of warfare. In the second century, Galen believed that all cardiac wounds were fatal and noted in gladiators that penetrating wounds of the left ventricle produced rapid death but that death from wounds of the right ventricle was delayed (Meade, 1961). In the sixteenth century, Hollerius noted that cardiac wounds were not necessarily fatal. In 1624 Cabriolanus described two hearts at autopsy with healed wounds, confirming that cardiac wounds were not always fatal. Nonetheless, cardiac injuries were commonly believed fatal until the early 1800s. Larrey in 1810 and Romero in 1814 were the first to perform surgical pericardiotomy for cardiac injury. The term *tamponade of the heart* was coined in 1894 by the German surgeon Rose. In 1896 Paget expressed exasperation that cardiac wounds were untreatable and wrote that "no new discovery can overcome the natural difficulties that attend a wound of the heart." At approximately the same time, however, Rehn (Frankfurt), Cappelen (Norway), and Farina (Rome) all successfully suture repaired a cardiac stab wound (Shumaker, 1992). During World War II, Harken performed the incredible surgical accomplishment of removing foreign bodies from the hearts of wounded soldiers. The first successful repair of a traumatic aortic aneurysm was by Bahnson in 1952.

HISTORICAL READINGS

Meade RH: A History of Thoracic Surgery. Charles C Thomas, Springfield, IL, 1961
Shumaker HB Jr: The Evolution of Cardiac Surgery. Indiana University Press, Bloomington, IN, 1992

BLUNT CARDIAC INJURIES

The incidence of blunt cardiac injuries is generally considered to be low (Hood, 1983; Liedtke and DeMuth, 1973), but cardiac injuries account for at least 5 percent of all blunt trauma deaths (Osborn and Meld 1943; Slatis, 1962). Most blunt cardiac injuries are caused by rapid decleration in motor vehicle accidents (Kirsh and Sloan, 1977). The heart may be injured in falls or by direct blows to the chest.

The spectrum of blunt cardiac injuries is broad. The most common injury is myocardial contusion (Kumar, et al., 1983; Saunders and Doty, 1977; Tenzer, 1985), but trauma may result in chamber rupture (Calhoon, et al., 1986; Madoff and Desforges, 1972; Smith, et al., 1976), acute coronary artery occlusion (Stern, et al., 1974), or injury to any valve or valve apparatus (Caudros, et al., 1984; Havada, et al., 1977; Munim and Chodoff,1983; Selmonsoky and Ellison, 1972). Atrial or ventricular septal injury may occur with resultant left-to-right shunt. Because of the central hemodynamic importance of the heart, even what might otherwise be relatively minor cardiac injuries may have a significant impact on the overall hemodynamic status of trauma victims, most of whom require a relatively high cardiac output to survive (Shoemaker, et al., 1988).

Myocardial Contusion

Because most patients with rupture of a cardiac chamber die almost immediately, myocardial contusion is the most common cardiac injury among patients who survive long enough to reach a trauma center (Kumar, et al., 1983; Saunders and Doty, 1977; Tenzer, 1985). The right ventricular free wall is the most commonly contused region of the heart because of its anterior location. The spectrum of contusion ranges from minor epicardial ecchymosis to full-thickness contusion and necrosis (Jones, 1970). The diagnosis should be suspected in all patients with an appropriate mechanism of injury and in those with evidence of significant chest trauma. The diagnosis must be sought especially in patients with sternal fracture, fracture of the first rib, aortic tear, and bronchial rupture (Hamilton, et al., 1984; Robbs and Baker, 1984).

The pathophysiology of myocardial contusion differs from that of myocardial infarction. Myocardial infarction by definition entails myocytic death, almost invariably consequent to acute coronary arterial occlusion (DeWood, et al., 1980). On the other hand, myocardial contusion is a concussion-like injury of the heart that produces some degree of bleeding into the myocardium without coronary occlusion (Saunders and Doty, 1977). The amount may range from scant epicardial staining to hemorrhage throughout the full thickness of the wall. Because of the inherent difference in the underlying pathophysiology, the diagnosis of myocardial contusion is more difficult to make than the diagnosis of myocardial infarction.

Myocardial infarction is suggested by typical electrocardiogram (ECG) changes and confirmed by the release of the myocardial isozyme of creatine phosphokinase (CPK-MB fraction), indicative of myocytic death (Pasternack, et al., 1988). Because myocardial contusion does not necessarily result in myocytic death, these tests are much less sensitive in the diagnosis of myocardial contusion (Blair, et al., 1971; Sutherland, et al., 1981). Because of their specificity for myocardial necrosis, these tests should be performed in patients undergoing evaluation for myocardial contusion. Myocardial contusion may cause cardiac dysrhythmias within the first 48 to 72 hours following injury; therefore, electrocardiographic monitoring is appropriate.

Myocardial contusion results in varying degrees of mural motion abnormality. The most sensitive tests in the diagnosis are those that assess mural motion, namely echocardiography and gated blood pool scanning (King, et al., 1983; Mattox, et al., 1985b; Robbs and Baker, 1984; Sutherland, et al., 1983). Because EKG can be performed at the bedside, this is the preferred diagnostic modality (King, et al., 1983). Transesophageal EKG provides superior cardiac imaging and should be used if available. In summary ECG monitoring, cardiac enzyme levels, and echocardiography are indicated in patients suspected of having this diagnosis. There is virtually no role for cardiac catheterization in the diagnostic evaluation of myocardial contusion.

The clinical course of patients with myocardial contusion is usually stable from a cardiac standpoint, and the majority of such injuries are otherwise subclinical, despite recognizable mural motion abnormalities on echocardiography (Shoemaker, et al., 1988). These patients should be monitored for cardiac dysrhythmias for at least 48 to 72 hours. In the absence of other significant injuries, monitoring may be done on a telemetry unit. Severe contusions may produce significant cardiac compromise (Harman and Trinkle, 1991), requiring aggressive hemodynamic support, including a flow-directed pulmonary arterial catheter and an indwelling arterial line. The information derived can be applied to optimize cardiac output by control of ventricular preload and afterload. Inotropic support may be necessary. When aggressive inotropic support does not restore satisfactory cardiac function, intra-aortic balloon counterpulsation has been used successfully in the therapy of severe myocardial contusion (Saunders and Doty, 1978).

It is particularly unfortunate that the right ventricle is the most frequently injured in the trauma setting. The rise in pulmonary vascular resistance that typically develops following severe trauma (Sturm, et al., 1979) may exacerbate the right ventricular dysfunction caused by myocardial contusion, resulting in right ventricular failure. In patients with significant right ventricular contusion, all efforts should be made to minimize pulmonary vascular resistance to optimize right ventricular function. Mean airway pressure should be minimized (Fishman, 1985), and high-frequency jet ventilation should be considered in severe cases of right ventricular dysfunction if mechanical ventilation is required.

If emergency surgery is performed in patients with myocardial contusion, the perioperative hemodynamic and anesthetic management should be based on the principles applied in patients with recent myocardial infarction (Flancbaum, et al., 1986). A pulmonary arterial catheter and an indwelling arterial line should be used to allow for tight pharmacologic control of hemodynamic variables (Fullerton and Harken, 1991; Rao, et al., 1983).

Other Cardiac Injuries

Although the overwhelming majority of patients with blunt cardiac rupture die before they reach a trauma center, patients may survive if the pericardium remains intact, and pericardial tamponade develops (Moreno, et al., 1986). The left atrium is particularly susceptible to rupture because it is compressed against the spine. The mechanism is acute elevation of intrathoracic pressure because the glottis is closed by the patient just prior to impact, and then anteroposterior force is applied to the chest (Kumar, et al., 1983; Madoff and Desforges, 1972; Tenzer, 1985). This typically occurs with deceleration in a motor vehicle accident.

For repair or cardiac rupture, patients should be taken immediately to the operating room, and a median sternotomy should be performed. Although it is optimal to have cardiopulmonary bypass available, there is frequently not enough time, and most blunt cardiac injuries can be repaired without the need for cardiopulmonary bypass (Calhoon, et al., 1986; Smith, et al., 1976). A useful technique is temporary inflow occlusion provided by transient occlusion of the superior and inferior venae cavae (Fig. 64-10). Most injuries can be repaired by primary closure, controlling hemorrhage with vascular clamps for atrial injuries and digital pressure in ventricular injuries. Autotransfusion should be available.

Simple right atrial perforations and perforations of either atrial appendage may usually be closed with simple suture repair without cardioplegic arrest of the heart. Most extensive left atrial perforations and virtually all ventricular injuries requiring cardiopulmonary bypass should be repaired on the nonbeating heart, and the use of cardioplegic arrest is indicated (Calhoon, et al., 1986). If a ventricular perforation is not amenable to simple closure, the repair may be reinforced by sewing through felt strips placed along either side of the defect for additional support.

Blunt injuries to cardiac valves or valvular apparatus are rare (Caudros, et al., 1984; Havada, et al., 1977; Munim and Chodoff, 1983; Selmonsoky and Ellison, 1972). These injuries should be suspected in the presence of cardiac failure and a murmur following trauma. Minor injuries, especially to the tricuspid valve, may present late following trauma (Sheikhzadeh, et al., 1984). Most valvular, atrial, or ventricular septal injuries may be diagnosed by echocardiography. It is preferable to avoid a surgical approach to such injuries in the acute setting, and they should be managed medically if at all possible. If medical management fails, the valve injury should be addressed surgically with the use of cardiopulmonary bypass. To minimize the operative time and the complications of

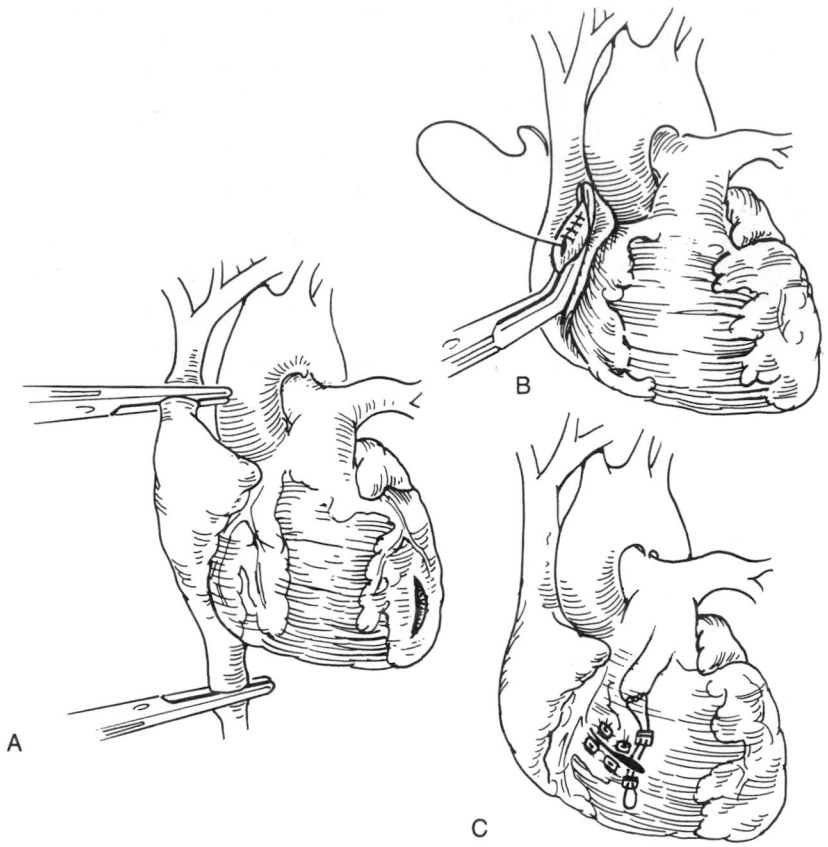

Figure 64-10. Techniques to repair simple blunt cardiac injuries without cardiopulmonary bypass. (From Mattox KL: Injury to the thoracic great vessels. p. 394. In Moore EE, Mattox KL, Felicino DV (eds): Trauma. Appleton & Lange, Norwalk, CT, 1991, with permission.)

cardiopulmonary bypass in these patients, valve replacement rather than valve repair should be performed in all but the most straightforward injuries.

INJURIES TO THE GREAT VESSELS

The incidence of blunt injuries to the thoracic great vessels has progressively risen over the past three decades with the rise in motor vehicular trauma. At least one-third of all patients undergoing thoracotomy for trauma do so for major vascular injury (Rapport, et al., 1982). The aorta and the subclavian artery are the most frequently injured great vessels, and combined they account for more than one-half of all major vascular injuries (Mattox, 1989a,b). Injury to the thoracic aorta accounts for at least 16 percent of deaths from motor vehicle accidents (Greendyke, 1966).

Aortic Injury

Although the aorta may be injured as a result of compression against the spine (Klotz and Simpson, 1932; May, 1975; Symbas, 1978), the most common mechanism of injury involves rapid deceleration, usually from a motor vehicle accident. An aortic tear must be considered in any patient with a deceleration injury. A high index of suspicion must be maintained

because up to 50 percent of patients with a traumatic aortic tear have no external signs of intrathoracic injury (Kirsch, et al., 1976; Mattox, 1991; Pickard, et al., 1977; Paton, et al., 1971; Plume and DeWeese, 1979; Rittenhouse, et al., 1969). Frequently associated injuries include costal fractures, long bone fractures, closed head injury, myocardial contusion, and intra-abdominal injuries.

The mainstay of the diagnosis is the chest radiograph (Fig. 64-11). The radiographic findings that suggest an aortic tear include a superior mediastinum wider than 8 cm, depression of the left mainstem bronchus, fractures of the first or second ribs, left apical capping, left hemothorax, tracheal or esophageal deviation to the right, and obliteration of the contour of the aortic knob. The most sensitive of these signs appears to be an obliteration of the contour of the aortic knob; there are many other signs that may be associated with aortic injury (Mattox, 1991). Radiographically, however, the injury may be subtle because approximately 25 percent of patients with these injuries have a normal initial chest radiograph (Kirsch, et al., 1976). If the initial chest radiograph is normal, it should be repeated several times over the next 12 to 24 hours.

Preoperative localization of the site of injury is important to guide the choice of incision. A left thoracotomy is used to repair an injury at the aortic isthmus; a median sternotomy is used to repair an injury to the aortic root. If a patient is

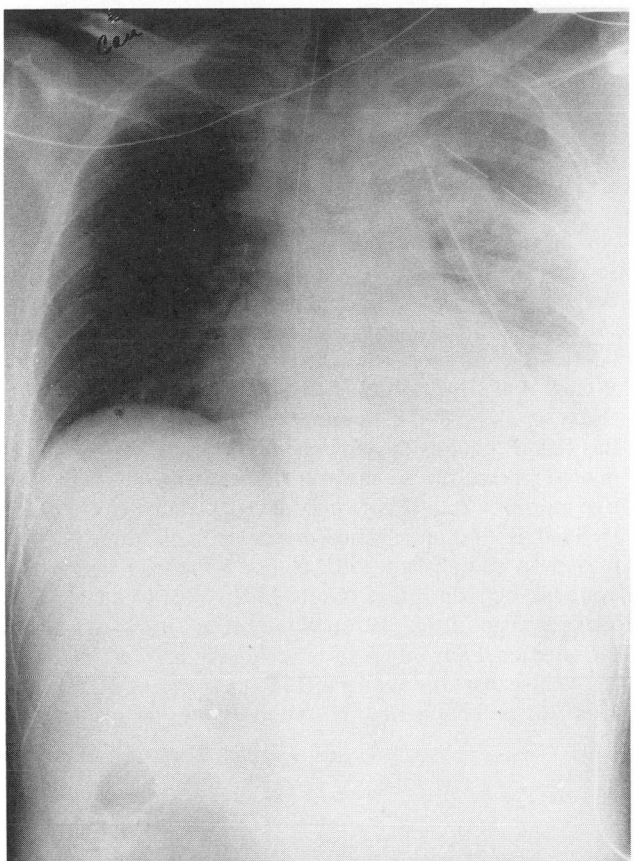

Figure 64-11. Chest radiograph showing a widened mediastinum in a 30-year-old patient previously involved in a car accident.

Radiographic Findings Consistent with Great Vessel Injury and Mediastinal Hematoma

1. Widening of superior mediastinum >8 cm
2. Depression of left mainstem bronchus >140 degrees
3. Obliteration of the aortic knob
4. Deviation of the nasogastric tube, endotrachial tube, or trachea to the right
5. Fracture of the first or second rib, scapula, or sternum
6. Left apical hematoma
7. Obliteration of the aortopulmonary window on lateral chest radiograph
8. Anterior displacement of the trachea on lateral chest radiograph
9. Fracture-dislocation of the thoracic spine
10. Calcium layering in the aortic knob area
11. Double contour of the aorta
12. Multiple rib fractures
13. Massive hemothorax

(From Mattox KL: Injury to the thoracic great vessels. p. 394. In Moore EE, Mattox KL, Feliciano DV (eds): Trauma. Appleton & Lange, Norwalk, CT, 1991, with permission.)

actively bleeding in the left chest, an emergent left thoracotomy should be performed without the delay required to obtain an imaging study. Aortography remains the procedure of choice among diagnostic modalities and should be performed if either the chest radiograph suggests the presence of an aortic injury or the mechanism of injury suggests the possibility of such an injury (Fig. 64-12). Both CT and MRI scanning are insensitive in making the diagnosis, and valuable time should not be lost on these studies (Miller, et al., 1989). CT may be useful as a screening test in a patient in whom there is a low level of suspicion or in whom an aortogram is equivocal or contraindicated on medical grounds.

Approximately 85 percent of patients with blunt thoracic aortic injuries die before they reach the hospital (Parmley, et al., 1958). The natural history of the 10 to 15 percent of patients who survive long enough to reach a trauma center is one of steadily increasing mortality rates from aortic rupture with at least 50 percent of patients dying within the next 48 hours. The injury must be successfully diagnosed and treated within a short period following arrival at a trauma center. From the time that the diagnosis is suspected, the blood pressure must be controlled to prevent hypertension (Kirsch, et al., 1976).

Autopsy data suggest that traumatic aortic tears usually occur in three locations: the aortic root at its juncture with the heart, at the aortic isthmus, and at the diaphragm (Kirsch,

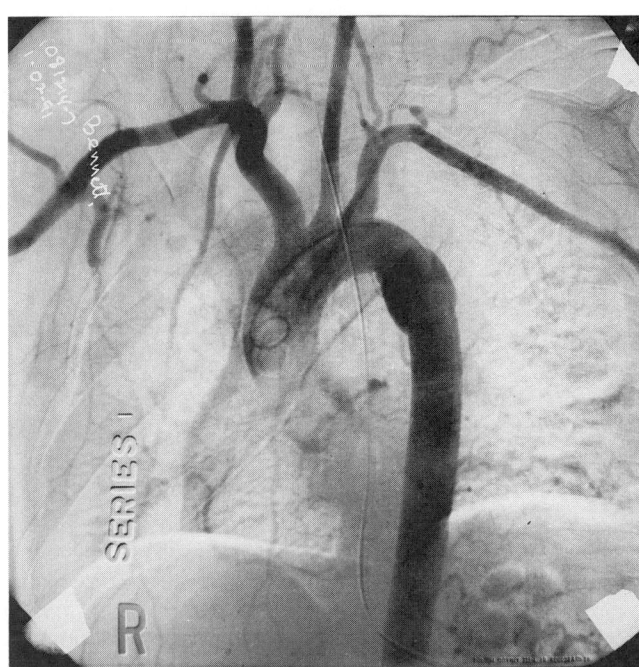

Figure 64-12. Aortogram of patient in Figure 64-11. Aorta is torn just distal to the left subclavian artery.

et al., 1976; Parmley, et al., 1958). Although only 50 percent of all blunt aortic injuries occur at the aortic isthmus, 97 percent of patients with blunt aortic tears who are alive on arrival at a trauma center have the tears located at the aortic isthmus (Fischer, et al., 1990). Most tears at the diaphragm and in the ascending aorta cause immediate exsanguination.

After the diagnosis has been confirmed by aortography, repair should be accomplished expeditiously. Considerable judgment must be used to treat the patient with multiple injuries requiring operative therapy of associated injuries. If the aortic injury is not actively bleeding, intra-abdominal bleeding or intracranial bleeding should be stopped prior to addressing the aortic injury.

The repair usually requires replacement of the torn segment of aorta with a tube graft, although some simple noncircumferential injuries may be repaired primarily. The mortality rate associated with operative repair ranges from 5 to 25 percent (Mattox, et al., 1985a), largely determined by the severity of associated injuries. The most feared complication of operative repair is paraplegia. The incidence of postoperative paraplegia ranges from 8 to 30 percent (Mattox, et al., 1985a; Mattox, et al., 1989; Verdant, 1990; Williams, et al., 1980).

Many recommend repair by simply clamping the aorta during repair (Mattox, et al., 1985a). Advocates of this technique cite its speed and simplicity as distinct advantages. Furthermore data suggest that the spinal cord is able to tolerate up to 30 minutes of ischemia with a small risk of paraplegia (Laschiger, et al., 1983). Therefore, those who believe the repair may be accomplished within this time frame prefer this technique (Mattox, et al., 1985a,b, 1989; Graham, 1980; Graham, 1982).

However, in an effort to minimize the risk of postoperative paraplegia, some authors advocate bypassing the occluded segment of aorta during the repair. Techniques that have been used include cardiopulmonary bypass (Beall, et al., 1969), heparinized shunts from ascending to descending aorta (Gott, 1972; Murray, et al., 1971; Wakabayashi, et al., 1976; Wolfe, et al., 1977), and left atrial to femoral artery bypass (Hess, et al., 1989). The use of cardiopulmonary bypass for this repair requires systemic heparinization. In the multiply injured patient, its use has been associated with a high operative mortality rate (Mattox, et al., 1985a) and is not recommended. Both shunting and left atrial to femoral artery bypass may be accomplished with relative simplicity and without systemic heparinization (Gott, 1972; Murray, et al., 1971; Wakabayashi, et al., 1976; Wolfe, et al., 1977). They offer the additional advantage of relieving the marked increase in left ventricular afterload inherent in aortic occlusion. This afterload reduction may be advantageous in patients with

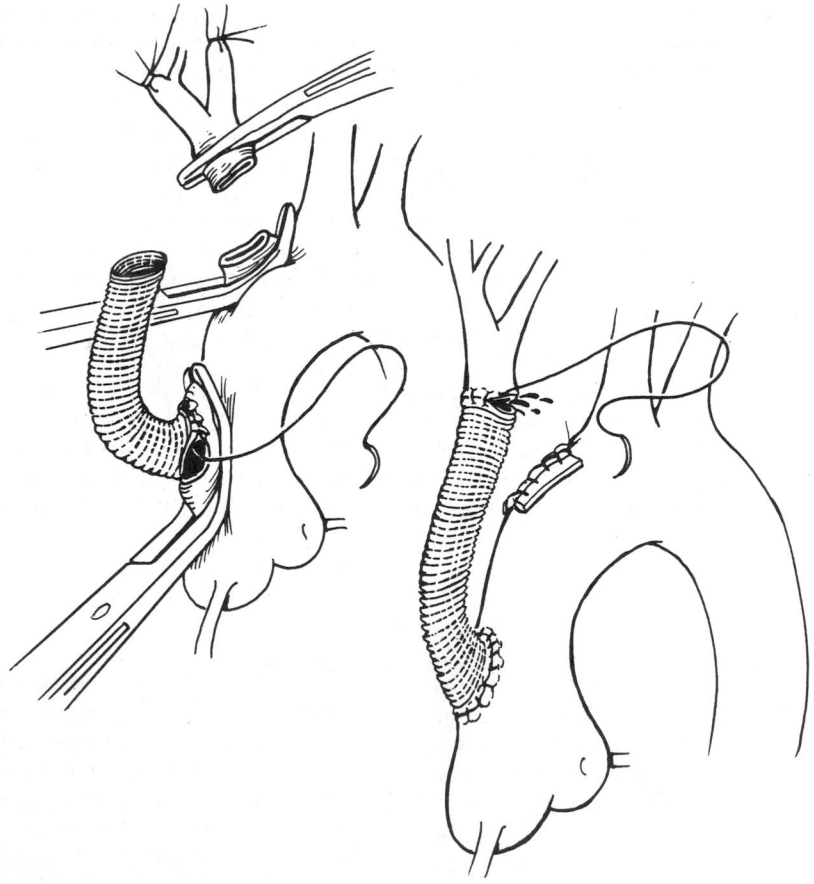

Figure 64-13. Technique to repair injury to innominate artery without cardiopulmonary bypass. (From Mattox KL: Injury to the thoracic great vessels. p. 394. In Moore EE, Mattox KL, Feliciano DV (eds): Trauma. Appleton & Lange, Norwalk, CT, 1991, with permission.)

myocardial dysfunction secondary to contusion or in the patient with coronary artery disease at risk for myocardial ischemia during clamping of the aorta.

Despite the theoretical attractiveness of these techniques, it has not been possible to demonstrate a statistically significant reduction in the incidence of postoperative paraplegia with their use compared with simple clamping and repair (Mattox, et al., 1989). In fact the incidence of paraplegia is generally reported to be higher with the use of shunts (Mattox, et al., 1985a). Perhaps some of this statistical difficulty reflects the many variables that may play a role in the development of postoperative paraplegia. Such factors as unpredictable spinal cord blood supply, perioperative hypotension or shock, operative spinal cord ischemic time, preoperative neurologic status, the length of aorta isolated between vascular clamps, and permanent interruption of spinal cord blood supply by the operative procedure all contribute variability, which cannot be controlled from one study to the next (Crawford and Rubio, 1983; Colliford, et al., 1983; Kirsch, et al., 1976; Mattox, et al., 1985a; Williams, et al., 1980).

Other Major Vascular Injuries

Injuries to either the subclavian or innominate arteries are usually suspected on the basis of upper extremity ischemia, pulse deficit, bruit, adjacent hematoma, extrapleural apical hematoma, and a wide superior mediastinum. These are confirmed by aortography. The repair of subclavian arterial injuries may be performed by obtaining proximal control by an

---

> **Major Vascular Injuries: Points to Remember**
>
> Use echocardiography to diagnose myocardial contusion.
>
> If emergent surgery is required in the setting of myocardial contusion, manage the patient as if a recent myocardial infarction were present.
>
> Suspect traumatic aortic tear in any deceleration injury.
>
> The initial chest radiograph may be normal. Look closely for blurring of the aortopulmonary window.

---

anterior lateral thoracotomy in conjunction with a clavicular incision. If necessary a segment of the clavicle may be removed to facilitate exposure. Repair may be accomplished by either graft interposition or primary repair.

Innominate arterial injury usually occurs at its origin from the ascending aorta. Exposure is best obtained by a median sternotomy. The innominate vein may be divided if necessary for optimal exposure. A straightforward approach without the use of cardiopulmonary bypass entails partial occlusion of the aorta at the origin of the innominate artery, dividing the innominate artery after distal control is obtained, oversewing its origin at the aorta, and placing a tube graft from the proximal ascending aorta to the distal innominate artery (Reyes, et al., 1975) (Fig. 64-13).

COMMENTS AND CONTROVERSIES

Significant controversy surrounds the optimal surgical technique to be used in the repair of traumatic aortic tear. Although Mattox reported excellent results by using the clamp and repair technique, we favor the use of left heart bypass during the repair. Left heart bypass may be used safely and without systemic heparinization. If offers the hemodynamic advantage of left ventricular afterload reduction during the repair and maintains blood flow to the mesentery, kidneys, and spinal cord during the period of aortic clamping. If problems occur during the aortic repair, the period of aortic clamping may exceed 30 minutes, which is commonly believed to be the upper limit of ischemic time tolerated by the spinal cord. In this situation left heart bypass is valuable because it maintains distal perfusion during this extended period.

If the surgeon must operate for frank rupture of the aorta, then time should not be lost by instituting left heart bypass. Under these circumstances the clamp and repair technique should be used. However, if the aortic injury is contained and the patient is otherwise stable enough for the institution of left heart bypass, we recommend its use.

D.A.F.
F.L.G.

Paraplegia is an unsolved problem that develops in a small minority of patients rescued by surgical intervention from the otherwise lethal injury of aortic transsection. Multifactorial causation is illustrated by the variety of current research approaches to solve this problem. These include studies of spinal fluid oxygenation and pressure and a variety of pharmacologic agents.

Because of the permanence and severity of the injury, which frequently occurs in young patients, litigation against the surgeon who performed the operation to save the patient's life is common. The experience is emotionally traumatic for all involved, including the surgeon. It is inherent in the litigation process that adversarial distortion of the sum of knowledge on the subject is used to convince jurors that the surgeon, by choosing the wrong method, is culpable for the injury. It is not accurate to conclude that there is a unique correct method that must be applied in every case or that deviation from a practice recommended here or elsewhere constitutes malpractice or failure to provide diligent and prudent care.

M.F.M.

KEY REFERENCES

Mattox KL: Fact and fiction about management of aortic transection. Ann Thorac Surg 48:1, 1989b

This is a critical review of the controversy surrounding the operative approach to aortic transsection.

Parmley LF, Mattingly TW, Marian WC et al.: Nonpenetrating traumatic injury of the aorta. Circulation 17:1026, 1958

This classic article outlines the natural history of this injury and documents the importance of diagnosis and therapy.

REFERENCES

Beall AC Jr, Argegast NR, Ripepi AL et al.: Aortic laceration due to rapid deceleration. Arch Surg 98:595, 1969

Blair E, Topuzlu C, David JH: Delayed or missed diagnosis in blunt chest trauma. J Trauma 11:129, 1971

Calhoon JH, Hoffman TH, Trinkle JK et al.: Management of blunt rupture of the heart. J Trauma 26:495, 1986

Caudros CL, Hutchinson JE, Mostader AH: Laceration of a mitral papillary muscle and the aortic root as a result of blunt trauma to the chest. J Thorac Cardiovasc Surg 88:134, 1984

Colliford AT, Ayvaliotic TS, Shemin R et al.: Aneurysm of the descending aorta. J Thorac Cardiovasc Surg 85:98, 1983

Crawford ES, Rubio PA: Reappraisal of adjuncts to avoid ischemia in the treatment of aneurysm of descending thoracic aorta. J Thorac Cardiovasc Surg 66:693, 1983

DeWood MA, Spores J, Notske R et al.: Prevalence of total occlusion during the early hours of transmural myocardial infraction. N Engl J Med 303:897, 1980

Fischer RP, Pepe PE, Porks DH et al.: Academic consequences of a trauma system failure. J Trauma 30:784, 1990

Fishman AP: Pulmonary circulation. p. 93. In Fishman AP (ed): Handbook of Physiology: The Respiratory System. Vol. 1. Am Physiological Society, Bethesda, MD, 1985

Flancbaum L, Wright J, Siegel HH: Emergency surgery in patients with post-traumatic myocardial contusion. J Trauma 26:795, 1986

Fullerton DA, Harken AH: Cardiac insufficiency. In Wilmore DW, Brennan MF, Harken AH et al (eds): Care of the Surgical Patient. Scientific American, New York, 1991

Gott VL: Heparinized shunts for thoracic vascular operations. Ann Thorac Surg 14:219, 1972

Greendyke RM: Traumatic rupture of aorta: special reference to automobile accidents. JAMA 195:119, 1966

Hamilton JR, Dearden C, Rutherford WH: Myocardial contusion associated with fractures of the sternum: important features of the seat belt syndrome. Injury 16:155, 1984.

Harman PK, Trinkle JK: Injury to the heart. p. 382. In Moore EE, Mattox KL, Feliciano DV (eds): Trauma. Appleton and Lange, Norwalk, CT, 1991

Havada M, Osawa M, Kosukegawa K: Isolated mitral valve injury from non-penetrating cardiac trauma. J Cardiovasc Surg 18:459, 1977

Hess PJ, Howe HR, Robicsek F et al.: Traumatic tears of the thoracic aorta: improved results using the Bimedicus pump. Ann Thorac Surg 48:6, 1989

Hood RM: Trauma to the chest. p. 299. In Sabiston DC, Spencer FG (eds): Surgery of the chest. WB Saunders, Philadelphia, 1983

Jones FL Jr: Transmural myocardial necrosis after non-penetrating cardiac trauma. Am J Cardiol 26:419, 1970

King RM, Macha P Jr, Seward JB et al.: Cardiac contusion: a new diagnostic approach utilizing two-dimensional echocardiography. J Trauma 23:510, 1983

Kirsch MM, Behrendt DM, Orringer MB et al.: The treatment of acute traumatic rupture of the aorta. Ann Surg 184:308, 1976

Kirsch MM, Sloan H: Blunt Chest Trauma. General Principles of Management. Little, Brown, Boston, 1977

Klotz O, Simpson W: Spontaneous rupture of the aorta. Am J Med Sci 184:455, 1932

Kumar S, Puri V, Mittal V, Cortez J: Myocardial contusion following nonfatal blunt chest trauma. J Trauma 23:327, 1983

Laschinger JC, Cunningham JN Jr, Nathan IM et al.: Experimental and clinical assessment of the adequacy of partial bypass in maintenance of spinal cord flow during operations on the thoracic aorta. Ann Thorac Surg 36:417, 1983

Liedtke AJ, DeMuth WE: Nonpenetrating cardiac injuries: a collective review. Am Heart J 86:687, 1973

Madoff IM, Desforges G: Cardiac injuries due to nonpenetrating thoracic trauma. Ann Thorac Surg 14:504, 1972

Mattox KL: Injury to the thoracic great vessels. p. 394. In Moore EE, Mattox KL, Feliciano DV (eds): Trauma. Appleton and Lange, Norwalk, CT, 1991

Mattox KL: Approaches to trauma involving the major vessels of the thorax. Surg Clin North Am 69:77, 1989a

Mattox KL, Feliciano DV, Beall AC et al.: Five thousand seven hundred sixty cardiovascular injuries in 4459 patients: epidemiologic evolution, 1958-1988. Ann Surg 209:698, 1989

Mattox KL, Holtzman M, Pickard LR et al.: Clamp/repair: a safe technique for treatment of blunt injury to the descending thoracic aorta. Ann Thorac Surg 40:456, 1985a

Mattox LK, Limacher MC, Feliciano DV et al.: Cardiac evaluation following heart injury. J Trauma 25:758, 1985b

May ET: Clinical Evaluation of the Critically Injured. Charles C Thomas, Springfield, IL, 1975

Meade RH: A History of Thoracic Surgery. Charles C Thomas, Springfield, IL, 1961

Miller FB, Richardson JD, Thomas HA: Role of CT in the diagnosis of major arterial injury after blunt thoracic trauma. Surgery 106:596, 1989

Moreno C, Moore EE, Majure JA, Hopeman AR: Pericardial tamponade: a critical determinant of survival following penetrating cardiac wounds. J Trauma 26:821, 1986

Munim A, Chodoff P: Traumatic acute mitral regurgitation secondary to blunt chest trauma. Crit Care Med 11:311, 1983

Murray GF, Brawley RK, Gott VL: Reconstruction of the innominate artery by means of a temporary heparin-coated shunt bypass. J Thorac Cardiovasc Surg 62:34, 1971

Osborn GR, Meld MB: Findings in 262 fatal accidents. Lancet 2:277, 1943

Pasternack RC, Braunwald E, Sobel BE: Acute myocardial infarction. P. 1238. In Braunwald E (ed): Heart Disease. WB Saunders, Philadelphia, 1988

Paton BC, Elliot DP, Tauman JO, Owens JC: Acute treatment of traumatic aortic rupture. J Trauma 11:1, 1971

Pickard LR, Mattox KL, Espada R: Transection of the descending thoracic aorta secondary to blunt trauma. J Trauma 17:749, 1977

Plume S, DeWeese JA: Traumatic rupture of the thoracic aorta. Arch Surg 114:240, 1979

Rao TLK, Jacobs KIT, El-Etr AA: Reinfarction following anesthesia in patients with myocardial infarction. Anesthesiology 59:499, 1983

Rapport A, Feliciano DV, Mattox KL: An epidemiologic profile of urban trauma in American. Tex Med 78:44, 1982

Reyes LH, Rubio PA, Korampai FL et al.: Successful treatment of transection of aortic arch and innominate artery. Ann Thorac Surg 19:468, 1975

Rittenhouse EA, Dillard DH, Winterscheid LC, Merendino KA: Traumatic rupture of the thoracic aorta: a review of the literature and a report of five cases with attention to special problems in early surgical management. Ann Surg 170:87, 1969

Robbs JV, Baker LW: Cardiovascular trauma. Curr Probl Surg 21:1, 1984

Saunders CR, Doty DB: Myocardial contusion: effect of intra-aortic balloon counter pulsation on cardiac output. J Trauma 18:706, 1978

Saunders CR, Doty DB: Myocardial contusion. Surg Gynecol Obstet 144:595, 1977

Selmonsoky CA, Ellison RG: Traumatic mitral valve incompetence: case report: J Trauma 12:632, 1972

Sheikhzadeh A, Langbehn F, Ghabusi P et al.: Chronic traumatic tricuspid insufficiency. Clin Cardiol 7:299, 1984

Shoemaker WC, Appel PL, Kram HBB et al.: Prospective trial of super normal values of survivors as the therapeutic goals in high risk surgical patients. Chest 94:1176, 1988

Shumaker HB Jr: The Evolution of Cardiac Surgery. Indiana University Press, Bloomington, IN, 1992

Slatis P: Injuries in fatal traffic accidents. Acta Chir Scand 297:9, 1962

Smith JM III, Grover FL, Marcos et al.: Blunt traumatic rupture of the atria. J Thorac Cardiovasc Surg 71:617, 1976

Stern T, Wolf RY, Reichart B et al.: Coronary artery occlusion resulting from blunt trauma. JAMA 230:1308, 1974

Sturm JA, Lewis FR, Trentz O et al.: Cardiopulmonary parameters and prognosis after severe multiple trauma. J Trauma 19:305, 1979

Sutherland GR, Calvin JD, Driedger AA et al.: Anatomic and cardiopulmonary responses to trauma with associated blunt chest injuries. J Trauma 21:1, 1981

Sutherland GR, Driedger AA, Holliday RL et al.: Frequency of myocardial injury after blunt trauma as evaluated by radionuclide angiography. Am J Cardiol 52:1099, 1983

Symbas PN: Trauma to the Heart and Great Vessels. Grune & Stratton, New York, 1978

Tenzer ML: The spectrum of myocardial contusion: A review. J Trauma 25:620, 1985

Verdant A: Traumatic rupture of the thoracic aorta. Ann Thorac Surg 49:686, 1990

Wakabayashi A, Connoly JE, Stemmer EA et al.: Prevention of paraplegia associated with resection of extensive thoracic aneurysms. Arch Surg 111:1186, 1976

Williams TE, Vasko JS, Kakos GS et al.: Treatment of acute and chronic traumatic rupture of the descending thoracic aorta. World J Surg 4:545, 1980

Wolfe WG, Klainman LA, Sabiston DC Jr: Heparin coated shunts for lesions of the descending aorta. Arch Surg 112:1481, 1977

65

PENETRATING TRAUMA

Kenneth L. Mattox
Robert H. Johnston, Jr.
Matthew J. Wall, Jr.

Penetrating thoracic injury may be the result of stab wounds from a sharp object or weapon, low- or high-velocity missile, shotgun wounds, or iatrogenic injury. The incidence of low- and high-velocity gunshot wounds and iatrogenic injury is increasing. Most penetrating injury is secondary to social violence and is potentially preventable (LoCicero, et al., 1989).

Iatrogenic penetrating thoracic injury occurs during various diagnostic and therapeutic procedures. Percutaneous aspiration of lung masses can produce pneumothorax and pulmonary hemorrhage and occasionally systemic air embolism. Penetration of subclavian, cervical, and mediastinal vascular structures by percutaneously inserted trocars, catheters, pacemaker lead wires, introducers, and other instruments can result in significant hemorrhage and death. Percutaneously introduced balloon-directed catheters may cause injury to the superior vena cava, right atrium, right ventricle, or pulmonary arteries. These iatrogenic injuries may occur in environments in which no surgical personnel are available, and surgeons are frequently summoned too late to reverse an iatrogenic vascular catastrophe. In spite of the trend away from this procedure, pericardiocentesis is included in the American College of Surgeons' Advanced Life Support course. Iatrogenic injury to the heart and coronary vessels is occurring with increasing frequency from this maneuver. Careless placement of a tube thoracostomy may produce injury. Because partial pleural symphysis is present in 25 percent of the population, puncture of the lung with resultant pulmonary hematoma, arteriovenous fistula, and air embolism can occur.

HISTORICAL NOTE

The insulting victor with disdain bestrode
The prostrate prince, and on his bosom trod.
Then withdrew the weapon from his panting heart,
The reeking fibers clinging to the dart;
From the wide wound gush'd out a stream of blood,
And the soul issued in the purple flood.

—*The Iliad,* Homer

Penetrating wounds of the thorax have been the subject of medical writings, ancient literature, and works of art since antiquity. The Edwin Smith and Evers papyri of Egypt described the consequences of penetrating thoracic wounds.

During each period artists in Europe have depicted thoracic penetration by knives, spears, and musket balls. The first recorded operation for penetrating chest trauma in North America occurred in Texas. Cabeza de Vaca wrote in his diary in 1535 of the extraction of an arrowhead from the sternum of an Indian (Sparkman, et al., 1965). One of the early and incapacitating injuries reported with survival was William Beaumont's (1833) famous patient, Alexis Saint Martin, who sustained a traumatic lung herniation at the entrance site of a musket ball.

The mortality rate from thoracic wounds decreased with each ensuing major war. Although many patients with penetrating thoracic injury died shortly after injury, Harken (1946) was able to tabulate 134 operations for the removal of foreign bodies in and around the heart and great vessels without a single death among this group arriving at his thoracic surgery referral center in World War II. Through the 1960s, pericardiocentesis, rather than thoracotomy and cardiorrhaphy, was the preferred method of treating pericardial tamponade from penetrating injury. In the 1970s and 1980s, large series, primarily from inner-city trauma centers, reported significant numbers of patients with penetrating thoracic injury. At that time thoracotomy and cardiorrhaphy replaced pericardiocentesis. A high-velocity gunshot wound to the chest nearly took the life of Governor Connally at the time of the assassination of President John F. Kennedy in 1963. An injury to the chest from a handgun seriously injured President Ronald Reagan. Both required thoracotomy.

HISTORICAL READINGS

Beaumont W: Experiments and Observations on the Gastric Juice and Physiology of Digestion. FP Allen, Pittsburgh, 1833

Harken DE: Foreign bodies in, and in relation to, thoracic blood vessels and heart. I. Techniques for approaching and removing foreign bodies from chambers of the heart. Surg Gynecol Obstet 83:117, 1946

Sparkman RS, Nixon PI, Crosthwait RW et al.: The Texas Surgical Society, The First Fifty Years. Texas Surgical Society, Dallas, 1965

INVESTIGATIVE TECHNIQUES

Penetrating injuries require a precise definition of the anatomy. Arteriography is useful in the evaluation of the hemodynamically stable trauma patient with suspected vascular injuries, whether it be a transsected aorta or innominate artery, or a cervical injury. Arteriography for these conditions is usually performed in the arteriography suite. The option of the retrograde brachial-axillary arteriogram for selected subclavian and axillary artery injuries should be considered. These arteriograms can be performed in the emergency center by surgical personnel (Itani, et al., 1992). In general the usefulness of arteriography for penetrating trauma is limited to suspected innominate, carotid, or subclavian artery injury to guide the proper choice of incision. Arteriography for penetrating thoracic aortic injury may yield false-negative results related to prior sealing of the penetration or inadequate projections. Neither computed tomography (CT) nor magnetic resonance imaging (MRI) has been shown to be as effective as arteriography for diagnosing aortic injuries (Miller, et al., 1989). Transesophageal endocardiography has been reported to be useful in demonstrating internal flaps and mediastinal hematomas. However, this technique appears to be overly sensitive and often requires angiography for clarification, a duplication of effort.

INDICATIONS FOR THORACOTOMY

Following penetrating chest trauma, 85 percent of patients can be treated with either observation or tube thoracostomy and surgery for concomitant cervical or abdominal injury. Only 15 percent require thoracotomy.

Urgent thoracotomy is usually performed in the emergency center on patients who arrive in extremis or who have an arrest shortly after arrival. Emergency-center thoracotomy should be performed by surgical personnel familiar with this procedure. It should not be performed on unintubated patients who have undergone prehospital cardiopulmonary resuscitation (CPR) for longer than 5 minutes or intubated patients with prehospital CPR in progress longer than 10 minutes (Durham, et al., 1992). Anterolateral thoracotomy is performed through a fourth interspace incision (below the inframammary crease in female patients), with transsternal

extension if necessary. The descending thoracic aorta may be cross-clamped to increase cerebral and coronary flow, effective open cardiac massage may be instituted, the pericardium may be entered, and cardiorrhaphy may be performed. For such urgent procedures, the survival rate may be as high as 30 percent following stab wounds and 8 percent following gunshot wounds to the heart.

Acute indications for thoracotomy include post-traumatic cardiovascular collapse, pericardial tamponade, vascular injury to the thoracic outlet, traumatic thoracotomy, massive air leak, proven tracheobronchial injury, proven esophageal injury, suspected great vessel injury, continuing hemothorax, a bullet path traversing the mediastinum, bullet embolism, and systemic air embolism. Chronic conditions requiring thoracotomy include unevacuated clotted hemothorax, chronic traumatic diaphragmatic hernia, chronic cardiac septal or valvular injuries, chronic false aneurysm of the thoracic aorta, chronic nonclosure of thoracic duct fistula, chronic empyema, infected intrapulmonary hematomas, missed tracheal bronchial lesions, and traumatic arteriovenous fistula. A small-volume hemothorax, thoracoabdominal wounding alone, a bullet in proximity to a major vessel, tension pneumothorax, and pneumomediastinum are not appropriate indications for thoracotomy following trauma (Mattox, 1989).

CHEST WALL PENETRATION

Penetrating injury to the chest wall from knives and low-caliber missiles rarely produces loss of chest wall substance but may require thoracotomy to control injuries to the intercostal vascular bundle or the internal mammary artery. High-velocity missiles and shotgun blasts can cause extensive loss of chest wall tissue, leaving a traumatic open thoracotomy. In such injuries the underlying lung and other adjacent structures are likely to be severely injured. Plastic sheets, such as Saran Wrap or sterile plastic drapes, can be used to close these defects temporarily until the definitive procedure can be done. At times such surgical procedures as acute thoracoplasty or immediate reconstruction of the chest wall with plastic surgery techniques may be required.

Injuries to the internal mammary artery or intercostal bundle are frequently found at the time of thoracotomy for continued hemothorax. The internal mammary artery can simply be suture ligated, with control of the bleeding. The intercostal bundle may require a secondary intercostal incision approached through the same skin incision or a ligature encircling the rib proximal and distal to the area of the bleeding because suture ligature and clips may not control the hemorrhage.

Cardiac and Pericardial Penetration

Penetrating cardiac injury is being seen more frequently. At the Ben Taub General Hospital in Houston, four to five patients per month are treated for penetrating injury to the heart or pericardium. Of this group, the largest number of injuries are stab wounds, with gunshot wounds accounting for most of the remainder. The diagnosis of cardiac injury must be considered any time the chest is penetrating by a missile or knife. This is especially true when the entry is medial to the nipple anteriorly or medial to the scapula posteriorly. If this type of injury is accompanied by restlessness and hypotension, the diagnosis of pericardial tamponade must be strongly considered. The patient with these injuries most commonly presents with cardiac tamponade, in extremis, with vital signs still present, or with CPR in progress.

Patients with penetrating chest trauma have the best results from emergency-department thoracotomy. This is especially true in patients with cardiac wounds. Most patients with this injury present with cardiac tamponade, and a significant number are in extremis. Emergency-department thoracotomy allows the release of the pericardial tamponade, assessment of cardiac function, and control of the cardiac injury. If needed, open cardiac massage and cross-clamping of the descending thoracic aorta can be accomplished.

To perform the urgent thoracotomy, the patient is positioned supine on the operating table, with the left side tilted slightly up. The incision of choice is a left anterolateral thoracotomy. If the injury requires access to the right heart, this incision can be extended to the right, across the sternum, and into the right chest. Should access to the descending aorta be required, the incision can be taken posteriorly to expose the descending thoracic aorta. Rapid access to the heart can be gained through this incision. After the chest is opened, the pericardium is easily visualized. If blood is present, the pericardium will be distended and have a blue appearance. The pericardium is opened anterior to the phrenic nerve with a large incision. After this is done, the cardiac action is assessed, and the site of preparation is identified and controlled. Subxiphoid pericardiotomy is not recommended because it may convert a contained hemorrhage into an exsanguinating hemorrhage with no means of rapid control.

The most common site of penetrating injury is the right ventricle because it has greatest anterior exposure, followed by the left ventricle and then the right atrium. Digital pressure is used to control the injury until adequate suture control can be accomplished. Metal skin staples have been used in some cases to protect the surgeon from needle sticks. The myocardium can be either penetrated or lacerated without complete cavitary penetration. These injuries may penetrate the septum, producing a traumatic ventricular septal defect, and may result in a shunt between chambers. Patients surviving penetrating cardiac injury should undergo daily evaluations of heart sounds. Special attention should be given to "new" murmurs because septal perforation may manifest

itself late. Most septal injuries from penetrating trauma close spontaneously. No patient should be considered for operation acutely. Only after several months of observation should surgery be considered, and then only if a significant intracardiac shunt greater than 2 : 1 is confirmed by cardiac catheterization. If a coronary artery injury is found, it must be repaired because ligation of a proximal coronary artery leads to myocardial infarction and death in a high percentage of patients. Valve penetration can occur but is very rare in our experience.

A significant number of patients have only pericardial injuries. Should the wound be a stab wound with the knife still in place, the weapon is left in place until the patient reaches the operating room, where operative control of the penetrating injury can be accomplished.

Some cardiac injury results in marked swelling of the heart, often secondary to excessive fluid administration. On occasion the thoracotomy cannot be closed without adverse cardiac compression. These patients are managed by leaving the sternum and chest open and sewing sterile plastic material into the incision, allowing transfer to the intensive care unit (ICU) until swelling abates. They can be returned to the operating room later for definitive closure of the thoracotomy.

GREAT VESSEL PENETRATION

Penetrating injury to thoracic vessels is usually obvious on presentation. The prehospital phase of assessment and management includes the initial level of hypotension and fluid volume required for resuscitation and stability during transfer. Examination of all entrance and exit wounds may give some indication of the missile's trajectory, although a missile, after it enters the body, can deviate markedly from a straight line between entry and exit sites. Should the entry be medial to the nipples anteriorly or medial to the scapula posteriorly, major mediastinal vascular injury is highly probable. If the mediastinum has been traversed by a missile, exploration is required. Auscultation of the chest and an assessment of distal pulses are helpful if the blood pressure is sufficient to produce extremity pulses. The chest radiograph demonstrates an enlarging mediastinal hematoma or hemothorax if present.

If the patient is stable enough, arteriography gives significant information about the extent of injury. It demonstrates a false aneurysm, arteriovenous fistula, intimal disruption, and arterial occlusion. Arteriography is reserved for the more stable patient; the majority of these patients are too unstable to permit this examination. Arteriography has a low diagnostic yield for penetrating aortic injury.

After the patient reaches the emergency center, injuries are rapidly assessed as are airway patency, systemic blood pressure, blood volume loss, and the presence of external hematomas, hemothorax, cardiac tamponade, or pneumothorax. Intravenous access and frequently endotracheal intubation are required. Resuscitation of the patient includes restoration of circulating blood volume with aggressive fluid and colloid management. A chest radiograph is obtained and an arterial blood gas evaluation. Chest-tube insertion may be required. At this point patients can be stratified into three categories. Patients in extremis, but with signs of life, are in the first category and require an emergency-center thoracotomy. The objective of this maneuver is to release pericardial tamponade, control intrathoracic hemorrhage, provide access for temporary clamping of the descending aorta to raise the central blood pressure, and give access for open cardiac massage. Patients in the second category are those who are unstable following volume replacement or may have an expanding hematoma. This group requires immediate thoracotomy in the operating room. The stable patient falls into the third category. In this group the physician has time to perform aortography, endoscopy, and esophography.

After a patient reaches the operating room, the surgeon must have an idea of the pattern of injury. If the surgeon is faced with uncontrolled bleeding from an unknown site, the recommended incision is a left anterolateral thoracotomy. The chest is prepared so an incision can cross the midline and be converted into a bilateral anterior thoracotomy by crossing the sternum. In the case of an anterior injury to the ascending aorta or great vessels, the incision should be a median sternotomy, which easily can be extended into the neck for access to the innominate or the right subclavian arteries. Should the injured vessel be the descending aorta, a posterolateral thoracotomy incision is required. One of the more difficult surgical exposures is that required to repair the proximal left subclavian artery. For proximal control a high (third intercostal space) left anterolateral thoracotomy is used. The injury is then approached by a supraclavicular incision. On rare occasions these incisions may need to be joined to create a ''book'' or ''trap door'' type of incision. The medial end of the clavicle can be resected for better exposure of this area.

In patients with ascending aortic injury, good exposure can be obtained through a median sternotomy. The injury is initially controlled by digital pressure, and 4–0 monofilament sutures are used to oversew the injury as the finger is withdrawn. The evaluation of other vessels for injury after the control of the initial bleeding point is imperative. Should the injury be in the aortic arch, the sternotomy incision is extended into the neck for better exposure. The bracheocephalic vein is divided, and occasionally if digital control cannot be obtained, a balloon catheter or Hegar dilator can be inserted into the defect to facilitate tamponade control of the bleeding point.

Descending thoracic aortic injury is associated with a high prehospital mortality rate of 85 percent (Parmely, et al., 1958). If this injury is not discovered during the initial assessment of the trauma patient, the hospital mortality rate is 50 percent in the first 48 hours. This injury can be associated with a large hemothorax on the left. The approach to the descending aorta is through a left posterolateral thoracotomy incision. For penetrating trauma proximal and distal control is gained, the aorta is clamped, and lateral repair is accomplished.

Penetrating injury to the innominate artery usually occurs in its distal portion; however, the injury can be located in any portion. The innominate artery can be visualized in its entirety through a median sternotomy with neck extension. If the injury is small, a primary repair can be accomplished.

However, if a segment is missing or a large defect is present, then the bypass principle is used. A polytetrafluoroethylene (PTFE) graft is attached on the ascending aorta wih a side-biting clamp and then anastomosed to the distal innominate artery. Complex techniques, using hypothermia, temporary shunting, or heparinization, are not required for this operation. The bracheocephalic vein can be ligated and divided with impunity for better visualization.

The subclavian arteries are the more difficult to expose, and gaining proximal control is of the utmost importance. Control of the proximal right subclavian artery is accomplished through a median sternotomy with a right neck extension. The bracheocephalic vein or the jugular vein may be divided, and then the first part of the right subclavian artery can be seen. The artery is then isolated with a tape for clamp control when needed. The proximal left subclavian artery is exposed through a left anterolateral thoracotomy incision placed in the third or fourth interspace. The left subclavian artery is easily visualized as it arises from the aorta. The middle and distal subclavian artery is exposed through a supraclavicular incision, whether injury is on the right or left side, and exposure for repair may require removal of a segment of the clavicle. The incision can be made over the course of the subclavian artery, dissecting down until both the proximal and distal ends of the artery are exposed. Injuries to the subclavian artery frequently require graft replacement. Both autogenous saphenous vein and 6-mm Gore-Tex grafts have been used for this purpose. A notable potential pitfall to this repair is injury to the brachial plexus, vagus, phrenic, or recurrent laryngeal nerves. On the left side, the thoracic duct should be identified and avoided, as should the jugular duct on the right.

An intrapericardial injury to the pulmonary artery or vein is usually best managed by bilateral anterior thoracotomy incision because these patients are usually in extremis on admission to the emergency center. Bleeding may be profuse, and control of the injury may be difficult. Usually digital control can be gained and suture repair accomplished. A significant problem seen with this injury and injury to the pulmonary hilum is air embolization. The use of cardiopulmonary bypass has not improved the outcome for the patient with an air embolus (Graham, et al., 1977).

Injury to the superior vena cava is often associated with injury to the innominate artery and jugular or bracheocephalic veins. Although the jugular or bracheocephalic vein can be ligated, the superior vena cava must be reconstructed. Previous experience with the use of prosthetic material in the superior vena cava has not yielded long-term patency (Doty, 1976). Construction of a conduit using the spiral saphenous vein technique (Doty, 1976) or substituting another vein, such as the common femoral vein, has been recommended for the repair of the superior vena cava. Shunting of the blood may be required while this repair is being accomplished in the acute setting.

Injuries of the intrapericardial inferior vena cava have a very high mortality rate, especially when the injury occurs at the junction of the inferior vena cava and right atrium. Management is likely to require cardiopulmonary bypass with repair accomplished transatrially. Injury to the azygos vein is potentially fatal and is usually associated with another injury, especially to the innominate artery, trachea, bronchus, or superior vena cava. Injury to the azygos vein can be difficult to control through a median sternotomy incision, and a right anterolateral or a right posterolateral thoracotomy incision is preferred. The azygos vein is then suture ligated for control.

Penetrating injury to the great vessels in the chest must be approached with a high index of suspicion by a surgical team ready and able to perform a definitive life-saving thoracotomy in the emergency center or the operating room. An aggressive approach to these injuries is advised. For patients presenting with signs of life and arrest secondary to pericardial tamponade, emergency-center thoracotomy has yielded a survival rate of 8 percent (Durham, et al., 1992).

PENETRATING TRACHEOBRONCHIAL INJURIES

Penetrating injury of the vascular structures of the pulmonary hilum is usually manifested by massive hemothorax, incomplete evacuation of hemothorax, or hemothorax with continued active bleeding. Patients with these injuries can be surprisingly stable initially, but thoracotomy should not be delayed when indicated. Penetrating injury to tracheobronchial structures of the pulmonary hilum usually presents as respiratory distress and inability to ventilate the patient adequately (Ecker, et al., 1971; Pate, 1989). If the injury is intrapleural, it may present as pneumothorax or a large air leak after tube thoracostomy with incomplete expansion of the lung. If the injury is extrapleural, it may present as pneumomediastinum with subcutaneous and cervical emphysema. The procedure of choice for the diagnosis of this injury is bronchoscopy. The bronchoscope may be used therapeutically to pass an endotracheal tube through the disrupted trachea. The bronchoscope can also be used to pass an uncut endotracheal tube selectively into the uninjured bronchus. A large amount of bleeding into the pulmonary parenchyma is always associated with this injury, and aggressive tracheobronchial suction is required. If the patient is stable enough to permit it, selective bronchial intubation with a double-lumen endotracheal tube is a helpful adjunct. Many of the details of the operative technique and ventilation are discussed in Chapter 63.

Positioning

For proximal tracheal injuries, the patient is positioned supine with the neck extended and the head elevated to decrease the central venous pressure. The neck and entire chest should be prepared and draped. The groin should be prepared for cannulation for cardiopulmonary bypass, although it is not commonly needed. For distal tracheal and bronchial injuries, the patient is positioned in the standard posterolateral thoracotomy position. The patient in extremis is placed in the supine position and prepared and draped from the neck to the groin so that a rapid anterolateral thoracotomy can be performed.

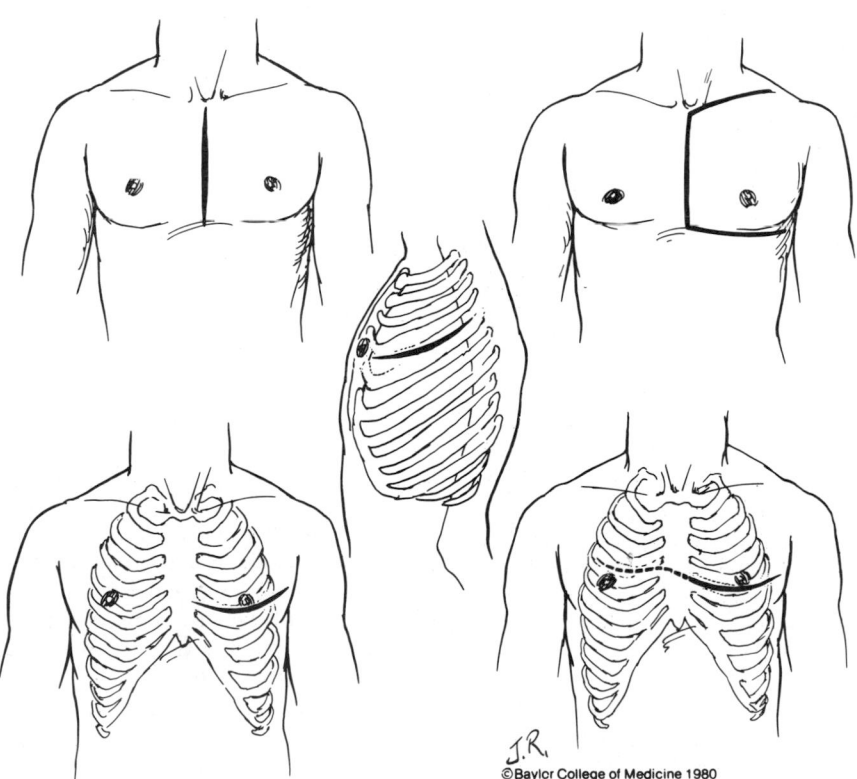

J.R.
©Baylor College of Medicine 1980

Figure 65-1.   Incision option that might be used in penetrating thoracic trauma.

Incisions

The patient in extremis from hemorrhage is approached by an anterolateral thoracotomy on the appropriate side. In the stable patient with isolated proximal tracheal injuries, the repair is accomplished through a cervical collar incision at the level of the injury. Superior and inferior flaps are raised for exposure, and knowledge of the anatomy of the neck is essential. The chest is prepared so that a median sternotomy can be performed if needed. For distal tracheal or bronchial injuries, a right standard posterolateral thoracotomy is the incision of choice, allowing access to the distal trachea, carina, and the right mainstem bronchus. For the left mainstem bronchus beyond the carina, a left posterolateral thoracotomy incision is performed (Fig. 65-1).

Technique

The principle for tracheobronchial repair is mucosa-to-mucosa apposition. The repair of tracheal or bronchial transsection requires adequate debridement without interruption of the blood supply, with anastomosis performed in one layer using interrupted absorbable sutures. This can be reinforced with a pleural or intercostal muscle patch. Standard bronchoplasty techniques can be used as needed. Cardiopulmonary bypass can be used selectively in these patients; however, this adjunct has its own set of complications. Alternatives to cardiopulmonary bypass may be the intubation of each bronchus with selective ventilation during repair. Penetrating and blunt injuries to the pulmonary hilum require rapid control by digital compression followed by hilar cross-clamping. The patient's condition commonly necessitates pneumonectomy, and time should not be wasted attempting a lesser resection in a critically ill trauma patient.

Injuries to the tracheobronchial tree result in mortality rates ranging from 0 to 30 percent. The risk of death depends on the anatomy, initial condition of the patient, and whether the injury is secondary to blunt or penetrating injury (Burke, 1962; De La Rocha and Kayler, 1982; Deslauriers, et al., 1982; Grover, et al., 1979; Jones, et al., 1984; Mills, et al., 1982; Pate, 1989).

ESOPHAGEAL INJURY

The management of esophageal injury is discussed in Chapter 64 and in *Esophageal Surgery* in Chapter 35. The essential step in management is alertness in looking for the injury at the time of presentation. Closure of penetrating injuries is usually readily done by using a two-layered interrupted suture technique.

BULLET EMBOLISM

Intravascular migratory missiles produce confusing clinical findings because the entrance site is often misleading. Symptoms and physical findings do not match anticipated and projected injuries. In the chest missile emboli may lodge either in the right ventricle or the pulmonary arteries. Missiles entering the heart and aorta may embolize to distant sites,

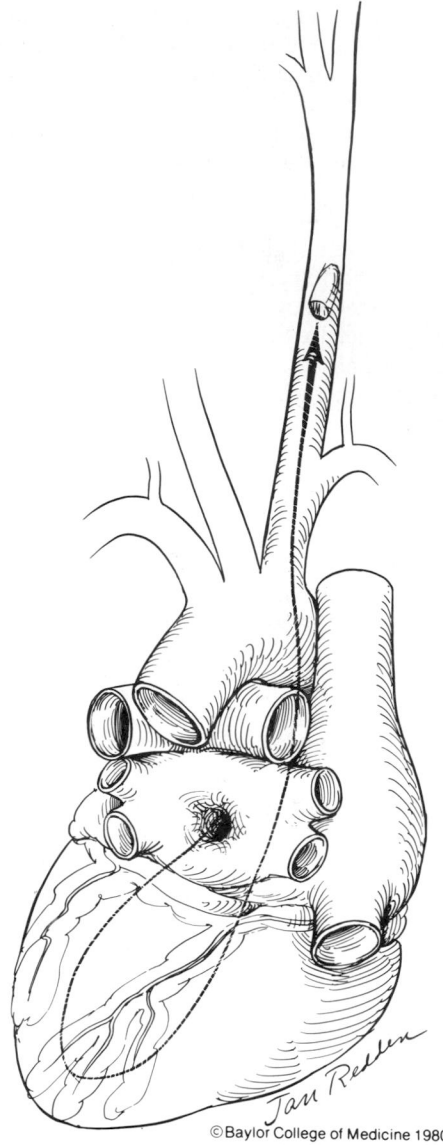

© Baylor College of Medicine 1980

Figure 65-2. A bullet embolizing from the heart to the carotid artery.

such as the carotid and iliac artery (Fig. 65-2). In all instances, control of the entrance site is achieved first, and then the embolized missile is removed. In general, missile emboli are removed from the heart using cardiopulmonary bypass, although nonbypass and angiographic means have been used. A missile embolus in the heart should be removed to prevent complications of endocarditis, tricuspid valve dysfunction, cardiac arrhythmias, and secondary embolization to pulmonary and systemic arteries. A radiologic clue that suggests a bullet embolus to the heart is a bullet appearing out of focus (secondary to the beating heart) while the rest of the radiograph is in focus (Fig. 65-3). Bullet emboli to the pulmonary arteries should be removed with the patient in a supine position to prevent the bullet from falling into the dependent lung during lateral thoracotomy. Very small emboli, such as small pellets from a shotgun wound, can be left undisturbed.

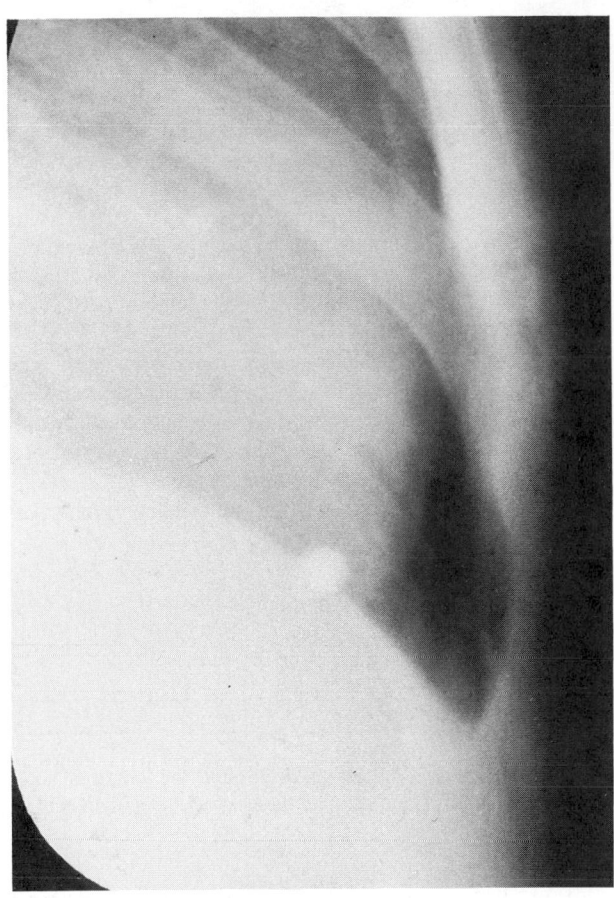

Figure 65-3. Radiograph of the chest showing a bullet embolism to the right ventricle; note that the bullet appears to be out of focus.

AIR EMBOLISM

The physiology of the pulmonary vasculature and current techniques for positive pressure-assisted ventilation are conducive to the formation of a systemic air embolism. The normal pressures within the pulmonary artery are 25/5 to 15/0. The pressures within the pulmonary veins are frequently 5 cmH$_2$O. During positive pressure breathing, pressure at the site of the endotracheal tube normally peaks at 30 cmH$_2$O. During resuscitation in ambulances and emergency centers, the current ventilatory bags are capable of delivering pressures in excess of 120 cmH$_2$O (Fig. 65-4). During the last 10 years, many manufacturers of ventilatory bags have removed the pop-off valve that prevented positive pressure ventilation in excess of 50 mmHg. Numerous clinical and experimental studies have documented that systemic air embolism can occur when pressure in the positive pressure ventilatory circuit exceeds 60 cmH$_2$O. In this situation, a fistula is created between the bronchioles and adjacent pulmonary veins, with air then going to the aorta, coronary arteries, cerebral circulation, and other areas in the body (Graham, et al., 1977).

UNRESOLVED ISSUES

Unresolved areas for focused future research and dialogue include (1) the appropriate volume of fluid to administer to patients with penetrating chest trauma (Martin, et al., 1992), (2) the development and application of techniques to prevent systemic air emboli, (3) appropriate approaches for the management of penetrating wounds of the thoracic inferior vena cava, and (4) reconstructive techniques for injuries to the superior vena cava and the innominate vein.

Figure 65-4. Mechanism of systemic air embolism from a penetrating lung injury.

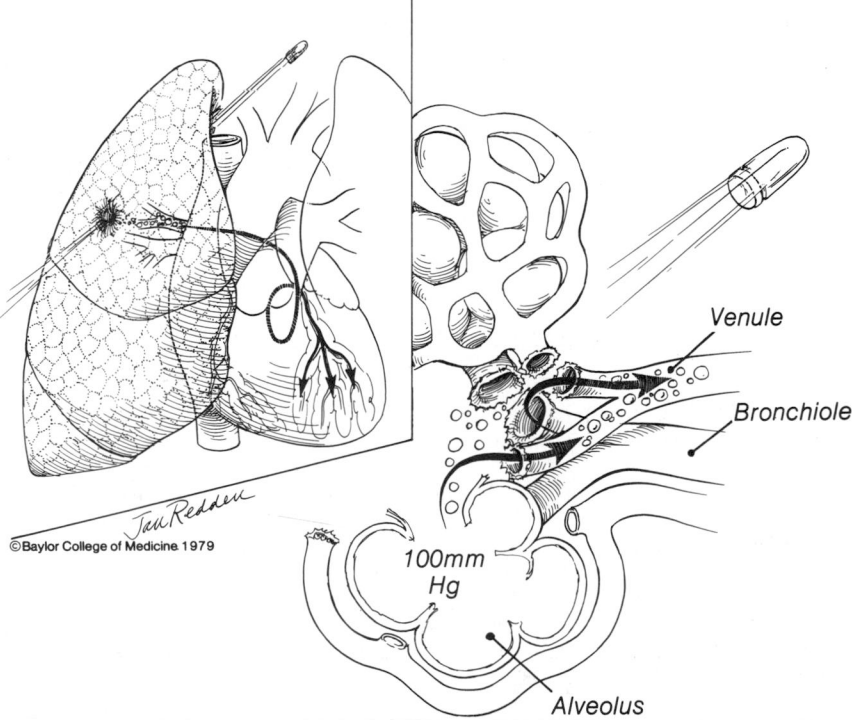

COMMENTS AND CONTROVERSIES

This chapter reviews the practical management of an epidemic problem of injury to the chest by knives and guns, derived from the extensive experience and thoughtful analysis of Dr. Mattox and his colleagues in Houston. There is a difference in the opinions expressed regarding the approach to hemopericardium. Dr. Mattox recommends against subxiphoid drainage, favoring anterior thoracotomy to allow immediate placement of a pledgetted suture, which is commonly needed with penetrating wounds. Transverse sternotomy is added for the less common penetrating injury requiring cardiopulmonary bypass.

In contrast Grover, et al. endorse subxiphoid pericardial drainage in the chapters on initial management of trauma and the management of blunt cardiac injury, with median sternotomy as the next step if the pericardium continues to fill (see Ch. 65). The probability of needing cardiopulmonary bypass rather than digital pressure and a pledgetted suture is probably higher with a blunt injury, which causes persistent pericardial bleeding. The ease and familiarity of the median sternotomy for this purpose is certainly advantageous. Thus, both approaches have merit and a rational basis for application.

Recently the use of externally stented Gore-Tex grafts has been associated with improvement in the patency rate when superior vena caval replacement is required (Dartevelle, et al., 1991). This is an encouraging development because the spiral vein graft technique of Doty, which works well, is time consuming and demanding.

Hyperbaric oxygen treatment should be considered in patients with air embolism following penetrating trauma. Good results have been reported in patients with systemic air embolism from other causes, and hyperbaric oxygen was responsible for recovery in a patient treated 23 hours after massive air embolism unresponsive to cardiopulmonary bypass (Lar, et al., 1990).

M.F.M.

KEY REFERENCES

Durham LA, Richardson RJ, Wall MJ et al.: Emergency center thoracotomy: impact of prehospital resuscitation. J Trauma 32:775, 1992

Patients with penetrating thoracic trauma requiring prehospital CPR (who are not intubated) for more than 5 minutes or more than 10 minutes (intubated) do not survive. Extensive resuscitative efforts must be carefully chosen.

LoCicero J, Mattox K: Epidemiology of chest trauma. Surg Clin North Am 69:15, 1989

In civilian practice, penetrating thoracic trauma is on the increase. Twenty-five percent of the 150,000 annual U.S. deaths caused by trauma have thoracic injury as a cause.

Martin RR, Bickell WH, Pepe PE et al.: Prospective evaluation of preoperative fluid resuscitation in hypotensive patients with penetrating trauma injury: a preliminary report. J Trauma 33:1, 1992

Preoperative crystalloid fluid restriction (during the ambulance ride and in the emergency center) decreases the incidence of adult respiratory distress syndrome (ARDS) and the length of stay in the ICU. It increases the survival time in patients with penetrating thoracic trauma.

Mattox KL: Indications for thoracotomy: decision to operate. Surg Clin North Amer 69:53, 1989

Only 15 percent of patients with penetrating thoracic trauma require a formal thoracotomy. A decision to operate follows precise and reproducible indications.

Mattox KL, Feliciano DV, Beall AC et al.: Five thousand seven hundred sixty cardiovascular injuries in 4459 patients: epidemiologic evolution 1958–1988. Ann Surg 209:698, 1989

Although military vascular injuries occur in the extremities more than 90 percent of the time, in civilian vascular trauma cases, penetrating injury is seen in the trunk in more than 60 percent of the cases. Penetrating thoracic vascular injury produces especially complex lesions.

REFERENCES

Beaumont W: Experiments and Observations on the Gastric Juice and Physiology of Digestion. FP Allen, Pittsburgh, NY, 1833

Burke JK: Early diagnosis of traumatic rupture of the bronchus. JAMA 181:682, 1962

Dartevelle P, Chapelier A, Pastorino U et al.: Long-term follow-up after prosthetic replacement of the superior vena cava combined with resection of mediastinal-pulmonary malignant tumors. J Thorac Cardiovasc Surg 102:159, 1991

DeLa Rocha AG, Kayler D: Traumatic rupture of the tracheobronchial tree. Can J Surg 28:68, 1982

Deslauriers J, Beaulieu M, Archambault G et al.: Diagnosis and long-term follow-up of major bronchial disruptions due to nonpenetrating trauma. Ann Thorac Surg 33:32, 1982

Doty DB: Bypass of superior vena cava: six years experience with spiral vein graft for obstruction of superior vena cava due to benign and malignant disease. Ann Thorac Surg 22:490, 1976

Ecker RR, Libertine RV, Rea WJ et al.: Injuries of the trachea and bronchi. Ann Thorac Surg 11:289, 1971

Graham JM, Beal AC Jr, Mattox KL, Vaughn GD: Systemic air embolism following penetrating trauma to the lung. Chest 72:449, 1977

Grover FL, Ellestad C, Arom KV et al.: Diagnosis and management of major tracheobronchial injuries. Ann Thorac Surg 28:384, 1979

Harken DE: Foreign bodies in, and in relation to, thoracic blood vessels and heart. I. Techniques for approaching and removing foreign bodies from chambers of the heart. Surg Gynecol Obstet 83:117, 1946

Itani KMF, Burch JM, Richardson R et al.: Emergency center arteriography. J Trauma 32:302, 1992

Jones WS, Mavroudis C, Richardson JD et al.: Management of tracheobronchial disruption resulting from blunt trauma. Surgery 95:319, 1984

Lar LW, Lai LC, Ren LW: Massive arterial air embolism during cardiac operation: successful treatment in a hyperbaric chamber under 3 ATA. J Thorac Cardiovasc Surg 100:928, 1990

Miller FB, Richardson JD, Thomas HA: Role of CT in the diagnosis of major arterial injury after blunt thoracic trauma. Surgery 106:596, 1989

Mills SA, Johnston FR, Hudspeth AS et al.: Clinical spectrum of blunt tracheobronchial disruption illustrated by seven cases. J Thorac Cardiovasc Surg 84:4, 2982, 1982

Parmely LF, Mattingly TW et al.: Non-penetrating traumatic injury of the aorta. Circulation 17:1086, 1958

Pate JW: Tracheobronchial and esophageal injuries. Surg Clin North Am 69:111, 1989

Sparkman RS, Nixon PI, Crosthwait RW et al.: The Texas Surgical Society, the First Fifty Years. Texas Surgical Society, Dallas, 1965

66

FOREIGN BODIES IN THE RESPIRATORY TRACT

Alma Smitheringale

Foreign bodies are often aspirated into the aerodigestive tract, and 20 (Webb, 1988) to 30 percent (Helinger, 1962) become impacted in the larynx or tracheobronchial tree, of which 20 percent lie in the glottis and supraglottis; 7 percent, in the trachea; 48 percent, in the right mainstem bronchus; and 25 percent in the left mainstem bronchus (Helinger, 1962). The symptoms and morbidity and mortality rates depend on the size, type, and location of the foreign body, with large objects in the glottis presenting the greatest emergency.

HISTORICAL NOTE

Prior to the advent of illuminated rigid bronchoscopy, death from aspiration of large or sharp objects was almost certain, and the morbidity rate associated with the aspiration of small objects increased with the duration of their presence. In 1936 Chevalier Jackson (1936) reported that the mortality rates had dropped from 24 percent to 2 percent among his patients, and the use of his new bronchoscope was successful in 98 percent of cases. In a recent study of 400 aspirated foreign bodies, the mortality rate associated with removal by means of rigid bronchoscopy was 0.25 percent (Mu, 1991). Results have improved further since this era, caused in part by the improved fiberoptic distal illumination of bronchoscopes and telescopic magnifications but also by the increased awareness on the part of practitioners and improved radiographic diagnostic techniques.

HISTORICAL READINGS

Jackson C: Diseases of the Air and Food Passages of Foreign Body Origin. WB Saunders, Philadelphia, 1936

Mu L: Inhalation of foreign bodies in Chinese children: a review of 400 cases. Laryngoscopy 101:657, 1991

INCIDENCE

Seventy percent of all foreign bodies are aspirated by children (Jackson and Jackson, 1951), of whom three-quarters are younger than age 4 years (Holinger, 1990). The other popula-

tion at risk are elderly patients, especially those who wear dentures or who have a neurologic deficit. For infants younger than 1 year of age, suffocation from inhalation of foreign objects is the leading cause of accidental death (National Safety Council, 1981).

The typical materials aspirated by infants into the trachea or bronchi are peanuts and hard vegetables (carrots, celery, watermelon seeds, and apple cores) and small plastic toy pieces. Safety pins used to be a common culprit but are rarer since the advent of disposable diapers. Adults more commonly choke on meat, dentures, or bottle tops at the level of the larynx.

SYMPTOMS AND SIGNS

The acute symptoms of aspirating material into the larynx are coughing, gagging, choking, hoarseness, and cyanosis. If the object is large and totally occludes the airway, then there may be no sound at all, just wild gesticulations and progressive cyanosis. If this is witnessed, the Heimlich maneuver (Heimlich, 1975) is the safest therapy to expel the object. Alternatively, if the foreign body is aspirated below the cords into the subglottis or trachea, there is a harsh inspiratory biphasic stridor with continued paroxysms of coughing. If it passes into the bronchi (the right side being more common because it is larger and more vertically continuous with the trachea (Fig. 66-1), then there may ensue a silent phase of minimal symptoms, other than a unilateral expiratory wheeze. Coughing bouts may only occur with exercise, which loosens and dislodges the object.

COMPLICATIONS

The chronic symptoms of a distal foreign object, which may remain for weeks or months, may present eventually as atypical asthma. The clinician should always suspect a foreign body in a child with unilateral or asymmetric "asthma." Recurrent lobar pneumonia occurs when only one bronchial orifice is blocked. However, irritant chemicals, such as small alkaline disc batteries or acidic arachnadoic oil from peanuts,

1591

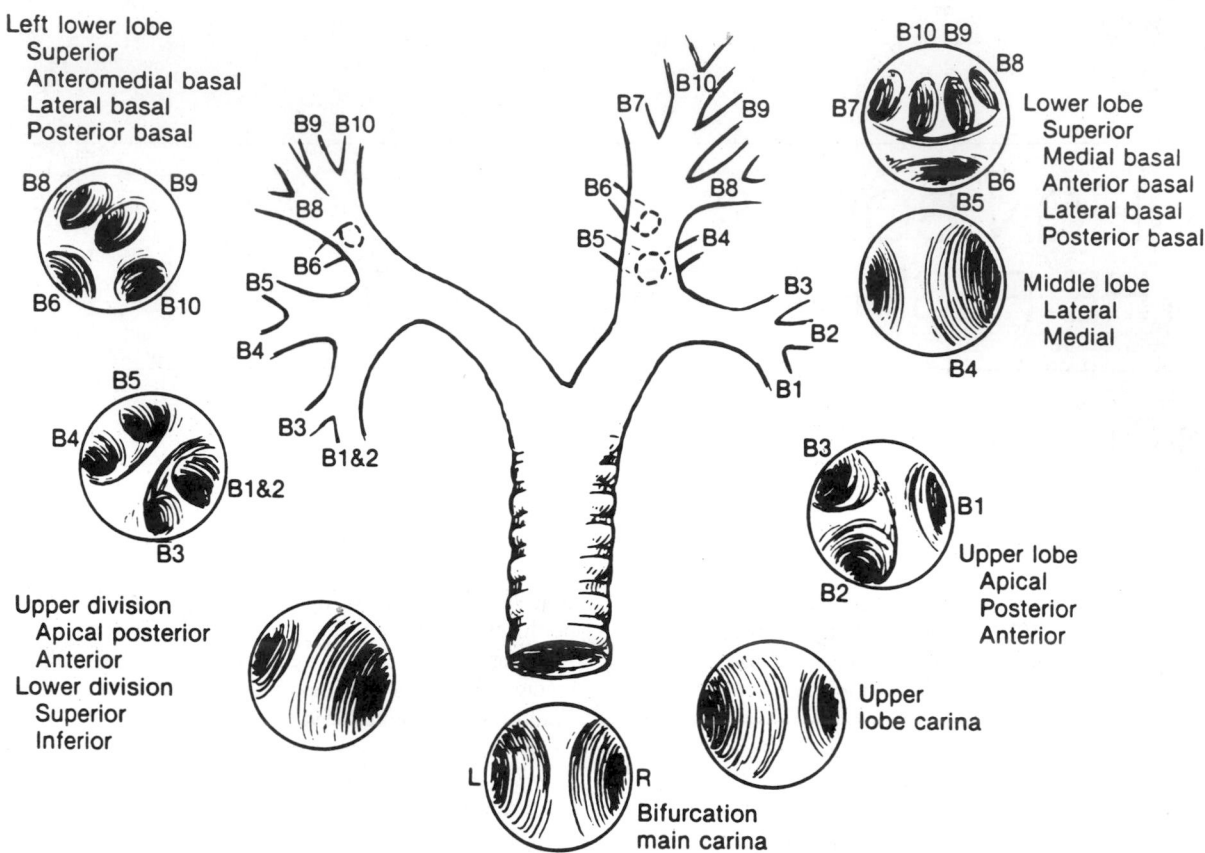

Figure 66-1. Anatomy of the tracheobronchial tree.

cause local inflammation, granulation tissue formation with total occlusion and an atelectatic lobe, pneumonitis, or even vessel erosion and hemoptysis. Spiked or pointed material, typically tips of Christmas trees or timothy grass (Fig. 66-2), may gradually work their way more distal with movement and enter the small distal bronchi or parenchyma, causing atelectasis (Fig. 66-2A) or hemoptysis. These are almost impossible to remove endoscopically and may necessitate a lobectomy for removal (Jewett and Butsch, 1965; Dudgeon, et al., 1980). Another complication to be aware of is tension pneumothorax, which can occur when a smooth object (peanut or ball bearing) blocks a bronchus on expiration, but not totally on inspiration, causing a ball-valve phenomenon, which leads to increasing air trapping in that lung, while pushing the mediastinum over and compressing the other lung until respiratory distress and cyanosis occur (Fig. 66-3). Sharp objects may erode through the trachea or bronchi and cause pneumomediastinum (Burton and Riggs, 1989), mediastinitis, or surgical emphysema with subcutaneous crepitation (Fig. 66-4).

RADIOGRAPHIC EVALUATION

Plain soft tissue radiographs of the neck (anteroposterior and lateral) and plain chest radiographs (inspiration and expiration) are most helpful. They may show the object if it is radiopaque (Fig. 66-5), or they may demonstrate a lowered nonmobile ipsilateral hemidiaphragm with tracheal shift to the contralateral side (Fig. 66-6) if there is any degree of air trapping and hyperinflation distal to the object (Jackson, 1936). This obstructive emphysema is evident in 40 percent of patients with tracheobronchial foreign bodies (Kim, et al., 1973). If it is bilateral it may be difficult to recognize, as in a patient with peanuts in both mainstem bronchi (Fig. 66-7). Baraka (1974) noted normal chest radiographs in the first 24 hours for 86 percent of children who had aspirated foreign objects, but after 48 hours 90 percent were abnormal, many with developing lobar atelectasis.

Bronchograms are rarely necessary today but are occasionally helpful for delineating a radiolucent foreign body that is too peripheral for endoscopic visualization. Video-assisted fluoroscopy, as a dynamic examination, is advantageous to observe the diaphragmatic movements and any obstruction to air flow at a bronchial orifice (McGill, 1986) or to aid retrieval intraoperatively. The use of computed tomographic (CT) scans and magnetic resonance imaging (MRI) is increasing for the purpose of exposing a radiolucent foreign body, together with any surrounding granulation tissue reaction, fibrosis, or adjacent vessels. Pulmonary function studies may also help to identify the asthma or emphysema caused by the chronic foreign body. A barium swallow may be helpful in the case of a bulky esophageal foreign body that compresses the overlying trachea and gives rise to airway compromise symptoms (Fig. 66-8).

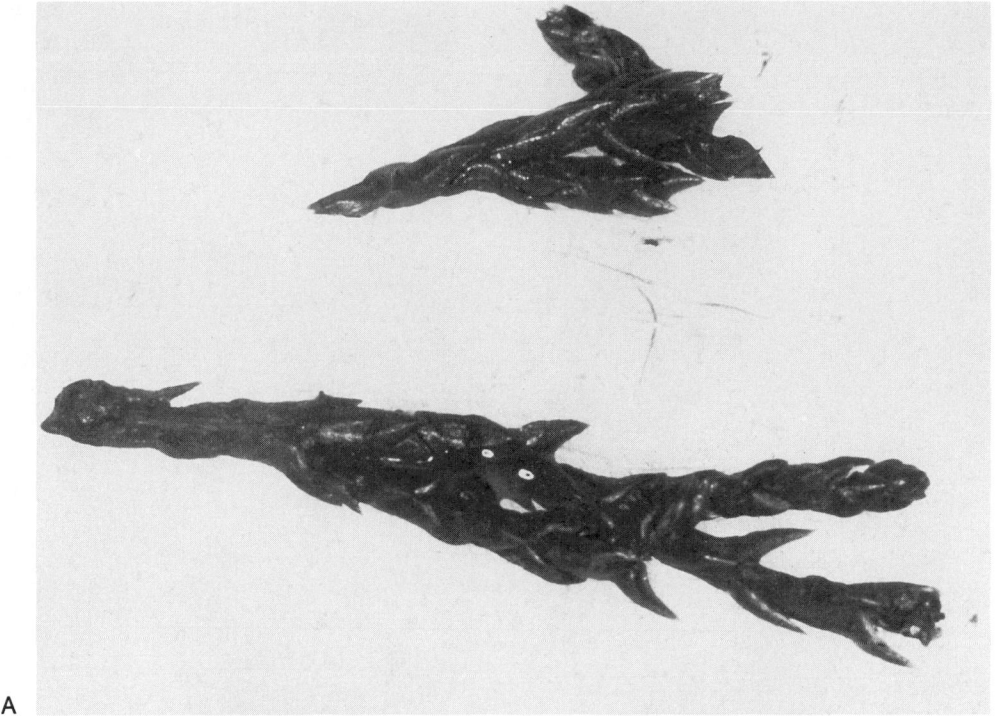

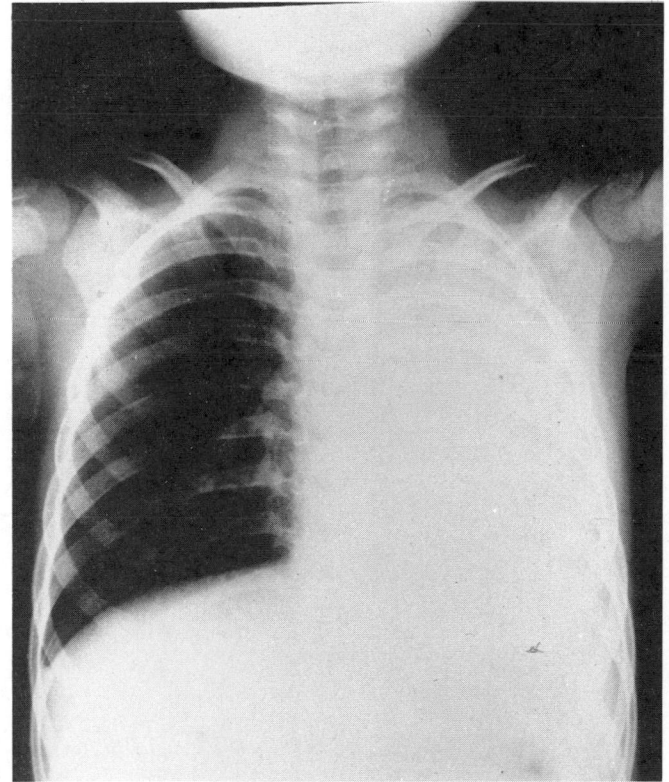

Figure 66-2. **(A)** Aspirated fir tree twigs. **(B)** Left lung atelectasis from aspirated fir tree twigs.

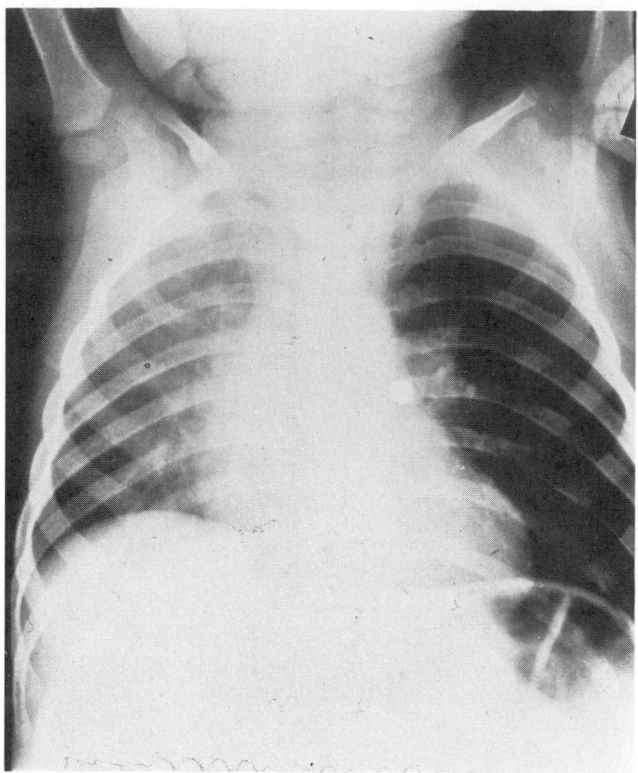

Figure 66-3. Left tension pneumothorax, with tracheal shifting to the right, from a piece of carrot "ball-valving" the left mainstem bronchus.

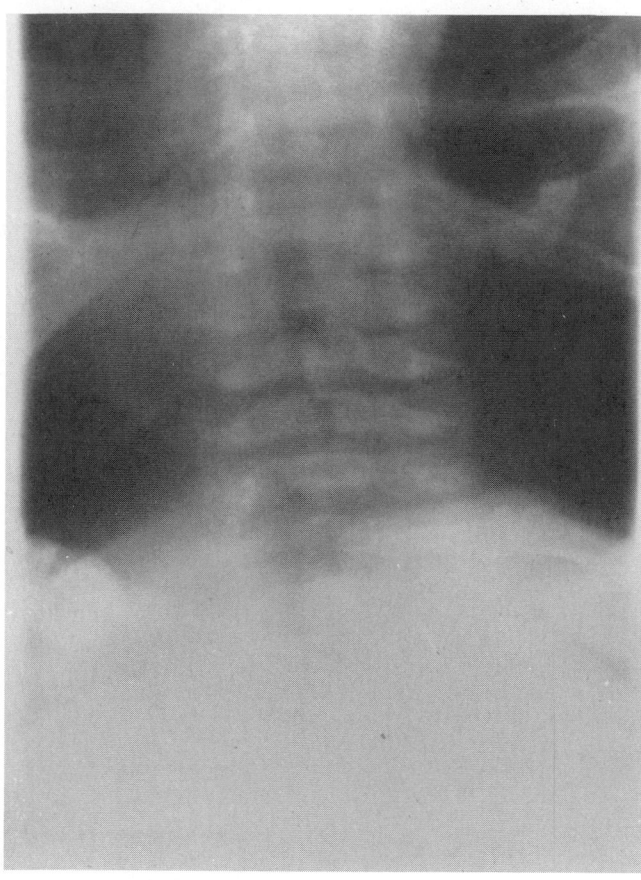

Figure 66-5. Radiopaque foreign body in midtrachea, causing an audible and palpable slapping sound on expiration.

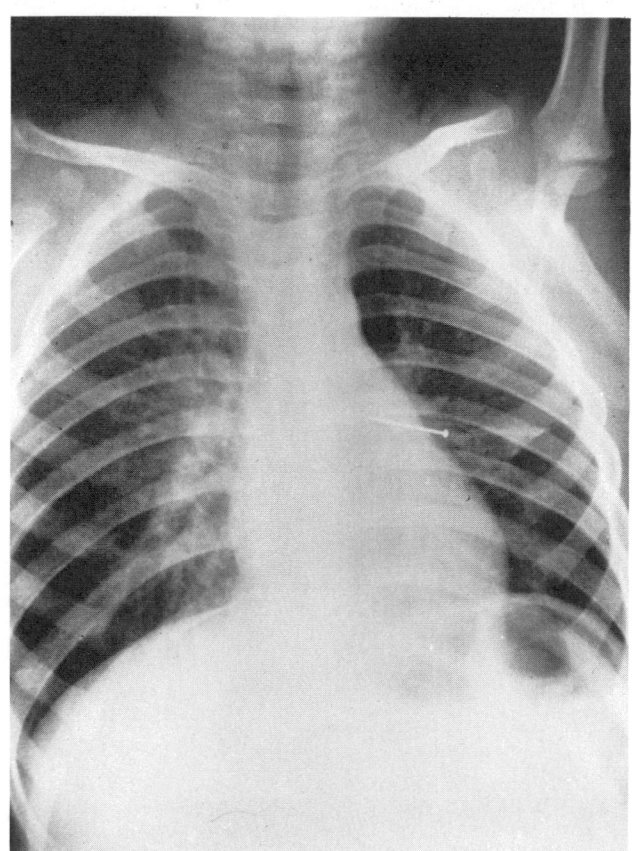

Figure 66-4. Pin in left upper lobe bronchus.

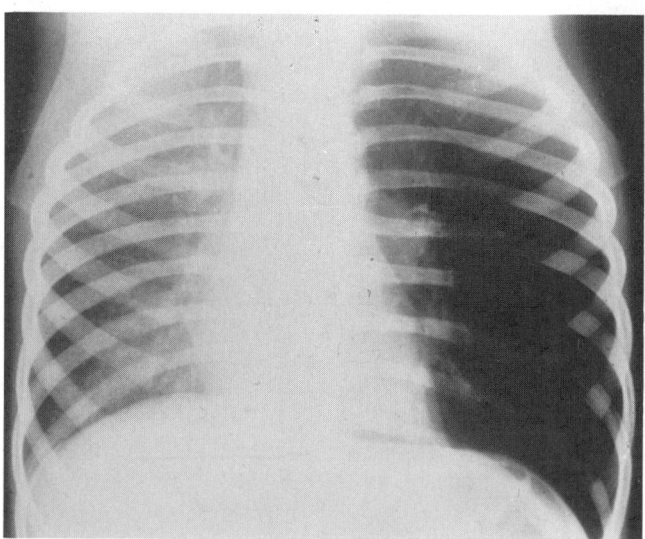

Figure 66-6. Immobile left hemidiaphragm, with tracheal shift to the right.

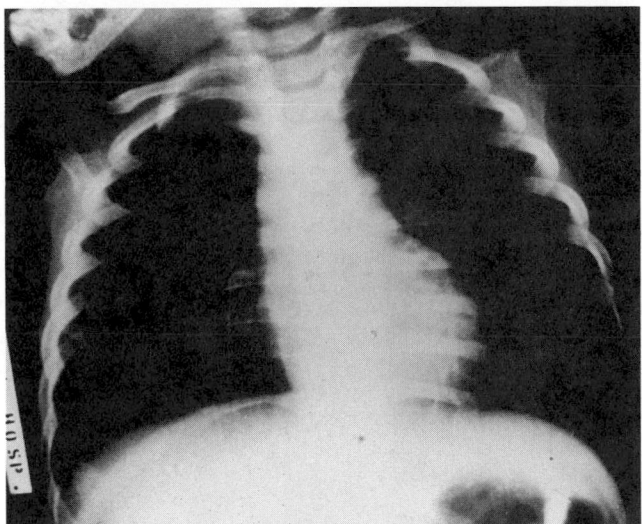

Figure 66-7. Bilateral hyperinflation from peanuts in both mainstem bronchi.

DIFFERENTIAL DIAGNOSIS

A foreign body in different locations may mimic many other pathologic conditions. If a large piece of plastic, cellophane wrap, or balloon is swallowed by a child and is caught in the supraglottis, the oropharyngeal gurgling stridor may mimic epiglottitis, together with the drooling and muffled voice. Typically, however, the onset is too sudden, and there is no associated fever nor leukocytosis (Fig. 66-9). If a foreign body is lodged at the glottis or in the ventricles (e.g., wire or a fishbone), it may produce hoarseness, mimicking laryngitis or nodules (Fig. 66-10). When an object is caught in the subglottis or trachea, it may give rise to a harsh inspiratory stridor and dyspnea, similar to croup. However, on auscultation, an audible slap is often heard, and a thud can be palpated over the trachea where the stridor is maximal (Fig. 66-5).

A bronchial foreign body may be present for many weeks or months, especially in children, if the initial choking episode is not witnessed, and approximately 25 percent may present with the chronic symptoms, mimicking asthma, chronic cough, or current pneumonia (Steen and Zimmermann, 1991). Penetrating foreign bodies in the distal bronchi or lung parenchyma can lead to abscess formation and bronchiectasis (Denny, et al., 1968). The resulting cough, fever, hemoptysis, and radiographic findings may mimic tuberculosis or chornic cystic fibrosis. All these late manifestations may be obscured by prior therapy with antibiotics, steroids, and bronchodilators before the true diagnosis is suspected.

MANAGEMENT

Glottic and Supraglottic Foreign Bodies

Glottic and supraglottic foreign bodies represent the greatest emergency, and if large enough to obliterate the airway, the Heimlich maneuver should be performed. It is unwise to put

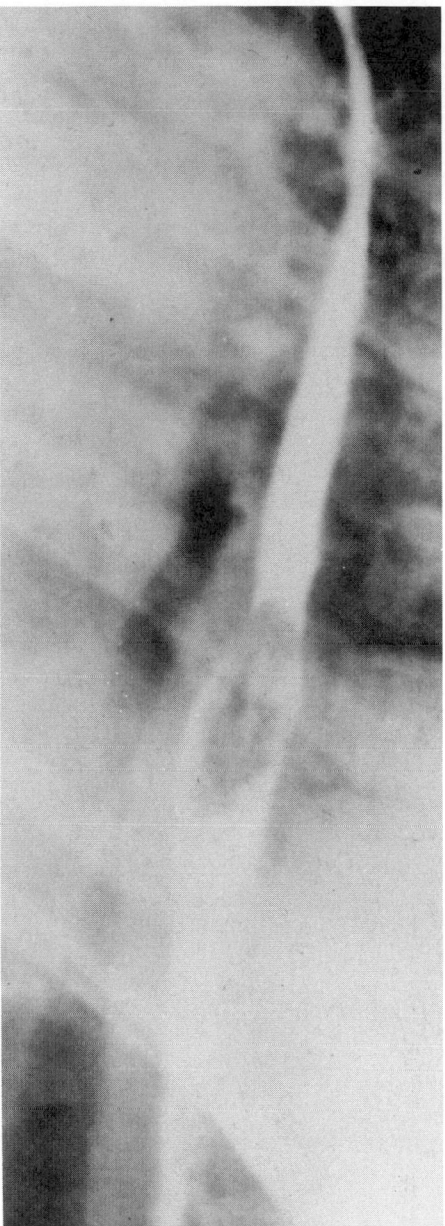

Figure 66-8. Barium swallow demonstrating a bulky radiolucent foreign body in the esophagus, compressing the overlying trachea.

a finger into the oropharynx, unless under direct visualization with a lit laryngoscope and Macgill forceps to avoid pushing the object deeper into the larynx.

Tracheobronchial Foreign Bodies

If the patient is still breathing, however stridorous, it is advisable to avoid any maneuvers other than application of oxygen by mask until the patient reaches the operating room. In particular inverting the patient and slapping the back should be avoided because this may dislodge an object from the trachea or bronchi, causing it to lie in the glottis or subglottis and totally obstruct the airway.

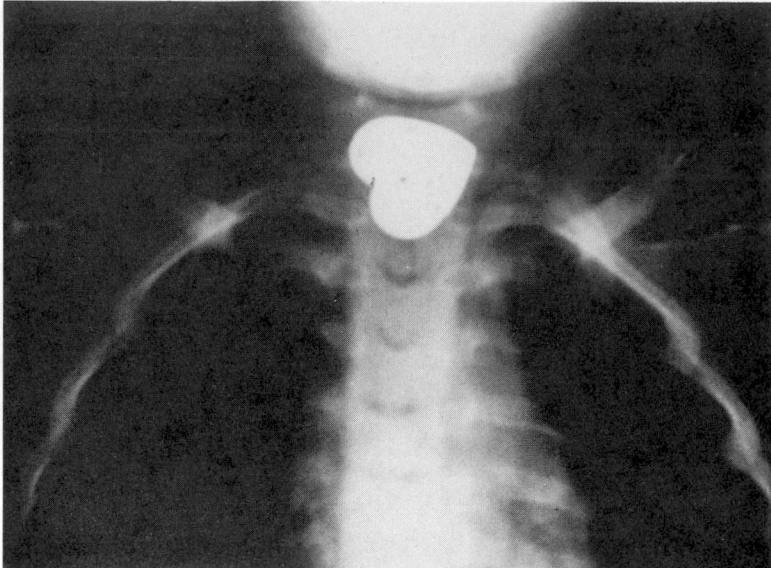

Figure 66-9.   Foreign body (silver locket) in the laryngeal inlet. Drooling and stridor can mimic epiglottitis.

The safest method of removal is under general anesthesia, using a laryngoscope, a rigid bronchoscope, and forceps. If the object is known or an exact replica can be produced, then the most suitable grasping forceps can be chosen, ensuring that they can also fit down the correct-diameter bronchoscope and are long enough to extend beyond it to the lower bronchi (Fig. 66-11). When the object has migrated distally to peripheral bronchi beyond visualization, it can be visualized by positioning the patient on the opposite side and using chest physioslapping. If it is metal, a strong external magnet can be used to stroke it into the lumen. If available, a 70- or 30-degree Hopkins rod telescope or a 2.5-mm flexible bron-

choscope can be passed through the rigid bronchoscope to visualize an upper or middle lobe bronchial orifice. When the foreign body has been in site for a long period, it may have become soft, and removal with a wide-bore open-end suction is easiest.

In cases in which an object has become embedded in the mucosa, a foreign-body granulation tissue reaction may totally obscure it. This granulation tissue is often friable and bleeds easily. It should be removed with cup forceps, and a 1 : 1,000 epinephrine-soaked cottonoid micropledget (on a long string) can be applied with pressure through the bronchoscope. The foreign object can then be visualized and

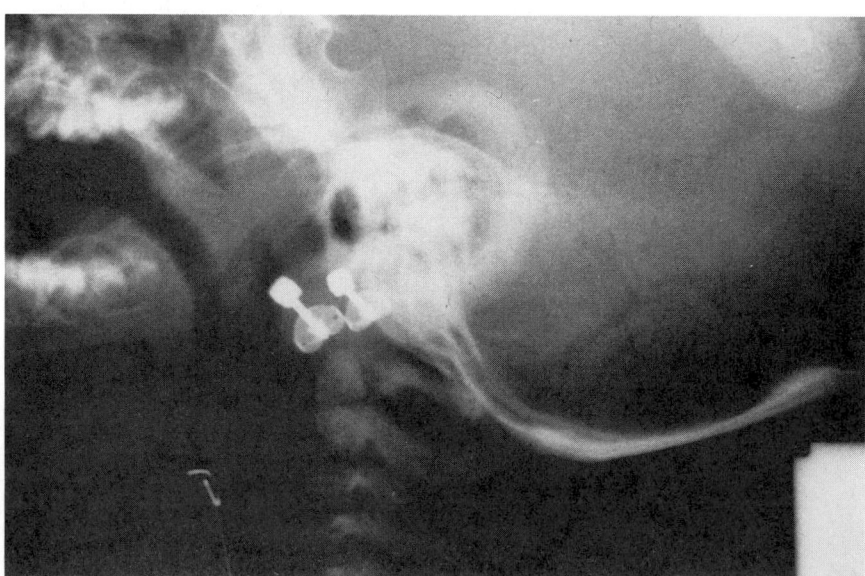

Figure 66-10.   Foreign body (wire) caught across the laryngeal ventricles and protruding through the glottis. Presenting symptoms were cough and hoarseness.

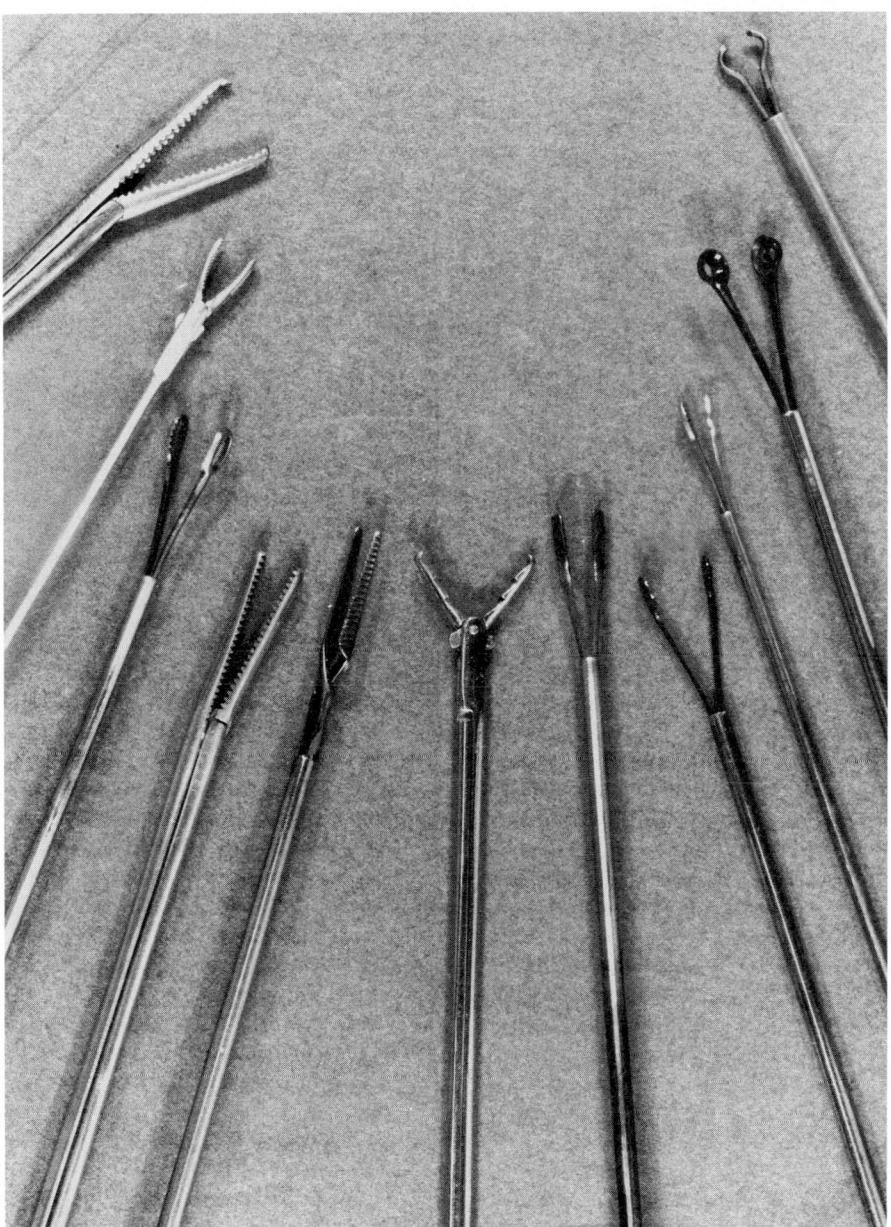

Figure 66-11. A selection of bronchoscopic foreign body forceps.

removed. A foreign body that is firmly impacted can be dislodged by passing a fine Fogarty catheter beyond it and inflating and withdrawing it gradually (Vane and Pritchard, 1988).

If the foreign object has a sharp point, this should be gently disengaged from the mucosa, covered by the forceps, and withdrawn into the lumen of the bronchoscope. (Figs. 66-4 and 66-12). After removal with the foreign body, the bronchoscope should always be reinserted to check for mucosal damage or perforation or the possible presence of a second foreign object. Any mucosal breach should prompt a postoperative chest radiograph to check for a pneumothorax.

ANESTHESIA CONSIDERATIONS

The ideal and safest situation occurs when the patient is breathing spontaneously with a deep inhalation anesthetic, using a bronchodilator agent (e.g., halothane) with a topical spray of lidocaine on the vocal cords and carina to minimize laryngospasm and coughing. The anesthetic can be continued through the side vent of the rigid bronchoscope, and when the 2.5 to 3.5-mm pediatric scopes are used, additional positive end-expiratory pressure ventilation (PEEP) may be required when the telescope is reducing the lumen. It should

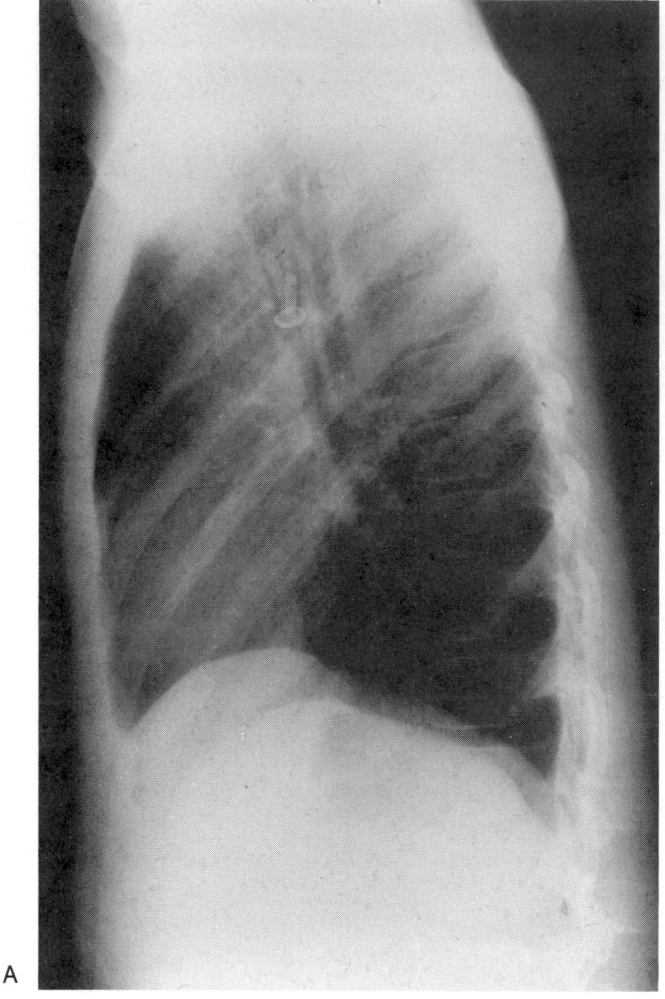
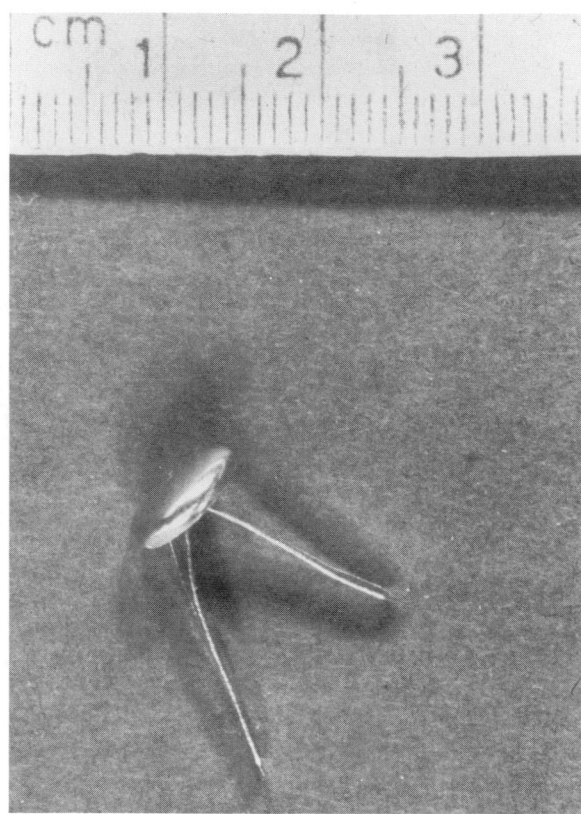

Figure 66-12. **(A)** Sharp foreign body (paper tack) embedded in the tracheal mucosa at the carina. **(B)** Paper tack removed from trachea.

always be remembered that when the scope is in the bronchus containing the foreign object, gas exchange is minimal. Therefore, when the oxygen saturation falls below 90 percent, the scope should be withdrawn above the carina to oxygenate the other lung. If airway mucosal edema is anticipated, then racemic epinephrine in a nebulizer can be administered preoperatively; this reduces the stridor and may disimpact the foreign body (Bready, et al., 1986). I would not recommend Venturi jet ventilation anesthesia because the jet can push the foreign body more distally, and tension pneumothorax is a potential risk in infants (Ostfeld and Ovadia, 1984).

COMMENTS AND CONTROVERSIES

Controversy exists regarding the suitability of the flexible bronchoscope for foreign body removal. I do not think there is ever any justification for its use because the airway cannot be protected in the vent of a large obstructing foreign body or a significant hemorrhage. The only indication for flexible

POSTOPERATIVE CARE

Humidification of the inspired air is always recommended postoperatively and where there is any stridor. Racemic epinephrine inhalations are most helpful. If mucosal swelling is anticipated, prophylactic parenteral steroids are advisable. Prophylactic antibiotics (e.g., cephalosporins) are usually administered if the foreign body has been indwelling for a long time or if there is a mucosal tear. In the latter instance, mediastinitis is a possible sequela. Therefore, regular vital signs and chest radiographs should be performed.

bronchoscopy is the case in which the foreign object is tiny particular matter (e.g., sand) that cannot be removed by bronchial lavage.

Fluoroscopic imaging is required where a radiopaque object has become embedded under granulation tissue or mucosa or has passed into distal bronchi beyond visualization. It is also helpful in identifying asymmetric diaphragmatic movement from air trapping and mediastinal shift (Black and Choi, 1984; Laks and Barzilay, 1988; Mu, 1991). Foreign body forceps combined with telescopic rods give the best visualization, but there is little variety of jaw shapes and sizes available. Therefore, the traditional nonfiberoptic forceps are still preferable in some cases or for very small infants (2.5 or 3.0-mm bronchoscope).

In the hands of well-trained bronchoscopists, the retrieval of foreign bodies from the trachea or bronchi by means of rigid bronchoscopy, under general anesthesia, is a reliable and safe method (Mu, 1991). Increased morbidity is associated with missed diagnoses in which the indwelling object produces mucosal swelling, infection, and erosion.

A.S.

KEY REFERENCES

Holinger LD: Foreign bodies of the larynx, trachea and bronchi. In Bluestone and Stool (eds): Pediatric Otolaryngology, Bluestone and Stool. 2nd Ed. WB Saunders, Philadelphia, 1990

This chapter gives a comprehensive overview of all types of foreign body aspirations, including the clinical presentation, complications, and general philosophy of endoscopic management.

Kim IG, Brunsitt WM, Humphrey A et al: Foreign bodies in the airway: a review of 202 cases. Laryngoscope 83:347, 1973

This paper discusses the presentation of respiratory foreign bodies and the radiologic findings, stating that hyperinflation and mediastinal shift, or diaphragm stenting should be looked for 40 percent of patients had obstructive emphysema.

Steen KH, Zimmerman T: Tracheobronchial aspiration of foreign bodies in children: a study of 94 cases. Laryngoscope 100:525, 1991

This paper alerts us to the fact that many aspirated foreign bodies may be missed and may present with chronic symptoms of cough, atypical asthma, or recurrent pneumonia and bronchiectasis.

REFERENCES

Baraka A: Bronchoscopic removal of inhaled foreign bodies in children. Br J Anaesth 46:124, 1974

Black RE, Choi KJ: Bronchoscopic removal of aspirated foreign bodies in children. Am J Surg 148:778, 1984

Bready LL, Orr MD, Petty C: Bronchoscopic administration of nebulized racemic epinephrine to facilitate removal of aspirated peanut fragments in pediatric patients. Anesthesiology 65:523, 1986

Burton EM, Riggs W Jr: Pneumomediastinum caused by foreign body aspiration in children. Pediatr Radiol 20:45, 1989

Denny MK, Berkas EM, Snider TH et al.: Foreign body bronchiectasis. Dis Chest 53:613, 1968

Dudgeon DL, Parker FB, Frittelli G: Bronchiectasis in pediatric patients resulting from grass inflorescences. Arch Surg 115:979, 1980

Heimlich HJ: A life-saving maneuver to prevent food choking. JAMA 234:398, 1975

Helinger PH: Foreign bodies in the air and food passages. Trans Am Acad Ophthalmol Otolaryngol 66:193, 1962

Jackson C: Diseases of the Air and Food Passages of Foreign Body Origin. WB Saunders, Philadelphia, 1936

Jackson C, Jackson CL: Bronchoesophagology (Experiences of over 4000 Cases). WB Saunders, Philadelphia, 1951

Jewett TC Jr, Butsch WL: Trials with treacherous timothy grass. J Thorac Cardiovasc Surg 50:124, 1965

Laks Y, Barzilay Z: Foreign body aspiration in childhood. Pediatr Emerg Care 4:102, 1988

McGill TJ: Foreign bodies in the aerodigestive tract. In Cummings (ed): Otolaryngology—Head and Neck Surgery, CV Mosby, St. Louis, 1986

Mu L: Inhalation of foreign bodies in Chinese children: a review of 400 cases. Laryngoscopy 101:657, 1991

Ostfeld E, Ovadia L: Bilateral tension pneumothorax during pediatric bronchoscopy (high-frequency jet injection ventilation). Int J Pediatr Otorhinolaryngol 7:301, 1984

Vane DW, Pritchard J: Bronchoscopy for aspirated foreign bodies in children. Experience in 131 cases. Arch Surg 123:885, 1988

Webb WA: Management of foreign bodies of the gastrointestinal tract. Gastroenterology 94:204, 1988

67

ADULT RESPIRATORY DISTRESS SYNDROME

Thomas R. J. Todd
A. C. Ralph-Edwards

In Chapter 6 we discussed the perioperative prophylactic measures that might be used to avoid postoperative respiratory failure. This complication can be particularly devastating after major pulmonary resection because the respiratory reserve has been already permanently altered by the resection itself. When it occurs following esophageal surgery, it is usually the result of sepsis from anastomotic separation or nosocomial pneumonia. Frequently multiple system organ failure ensues. The mortality rate is thus high, as are the number of days in intensive care long for those who survive. This chapter deals with the management of the patient in incipient and established respiratory failure and provides special emphasis on adult respiratory distress syndrome (ARDS).

HISTORICAL NOTE

The definition and management of respiratory failure has undergone many changes since the inception of volume-cycled ventilatory support during the polio epidemic. We have come to realize that there are several mechanisms involved in the development of respiratory failure and that they require specific and often different means of support. In particular the role of endothelial lung injury after trauma and sepsis was defined in the classic article of Asbaugh, et al. (1967) and later summarized with great clarity by Francis Moore (1969) in his monograph. It was left to Pepe, et al. (1982) to note the major association between what would become known as ARDS and sepsis.

Alternatives to volume-cycled mechanical ventilation have occupied intensive care physicians since the 1970s in an effort to support patients for longer periods and to reduce the barotrauma that has been recorded by several authors after the inspiratory pressures increase (Tzuno, et al., 1991). Particularly noteworthy are the efforts of Bartlett, et al. (1977) in the establishment of extracorporeal membrane oxygenation (ECMO), and the reader is referred to the landmark study

of Zapol, et al. (1979), which concluded that ECMO provided no survival benefit over conventional forms of ventilation. The latter study, although often quoted, was undertaken without a sample size calculation and has an inherently large beta error; that is, the chance that there was a positive result not recorded by the study because of insufficient numbers is quite high. Carlon, et al. (1981) is credited with bringing high-frequency ventilation (HFV) to our attention, and it plays a significant role in the management of patients with bronchopleural fistulae. These means of ventilatory support are discussed in the section on ventilatory support that follows.

HISTORICAL READINGS

Asbaugh DG, Bigelow DB, Petty TL et al: Acute respiratory distress in adults. Lancet 2:319, 1967

Bartlett RH et al: Extracorporeal membrane oxygenation support for cardiopulmonary failure. J Thorac Cardiovasc Surg 73:375, 1977

Carlon GC et al: Clinical experience with high frequency jet ventilation. Crit Care Med 9:1, 1981

Moore F: Clinical pathologic ARDS. In Moore, Lyons, Pierce, et al (eds): Post-Traumatic Pulmonary Insufficiency. WB Saunders, Philadelphia, 1969

Pepe PE, Potkin RT, Reus DH et al: Clinical predictors of the adult respiratory distress syndrome. Am J Surg 144:124, 1982

Tzuno K, Miura K, Takeya M et al: Histopathological pulmonary changes from mechanical ventilation at high peak airway pressures. Am Rev Respir Dis 1543:1115, 1991

Zapol WM et al: Extracorporeal membrane oxygenation in severe acute respiratory failure. JAMA 193:2193, 1979

RESPIRATORY FAILURE

Despite adequate perioperative evaluation and preparation, respiratory failure may still develop in the postoperative period. It is useful to classify respiratory failure as in Table

Table 67-1. Respiratory Failure Classification

Type	Measurement	Condition
Ventilatory failure	$\uparrow PaCO_2$	Proximal airway obstruction Narcotic overdosage Anesthesia excess Fatigue Bronchospasm Pneumothorax Bronchopulmonary fistula
Ventilation perfusion abnormality	$\downarrow PaO_2$	Pneumonia Atelectasis Pneumothorax Bronchospasm Pulmonary embolism Pulmonary edema Adult respiratory distress syndrome
Mixed	$\uparrow PaCO_2$ $\downarrow PaO_2$	Respiratory fatigue Large pulmonary embolus Acute upon chronic failure Combinations of above

67-1 because the diagnosis may be facilitated by an appreciation of the pathophysiology.

Pure ventilatory failure usually occurs in the immediate postoperative period secondary to inadequate reversal of anesthesia, opiate overdosage, unrecognized pneumothorax, or airway obstruction. As a result, early assessment of arterial blood gasses in the recovery room is important. If the initial arterial carbon dioxide tension ($PaCO_2$) is normal, then further assessments of a gas exchange can probably be achieved with noninvasive oxygen saturation monitoring. However, if the $PaCO_2$ is elevated, careful evaluation of the patient, further blood gas assessment, and possibly the administration of narcotic antagonists or the further reversal of muscle relaxation are indicated. The latter is particularly indicated when there is significant respiratory acidosis (pH < 7.20). Under such circumstances pharmacologic intervention or reintubation is required. Pneumothorax is usually readily apparent on physical examination or on the first postoperative chest radiograph. Airway obstruction that results in pure ventilatory failure is usually proximal in location. In the early postoperative period, it is usually secondary to laryngeal trauma and glottic edema. Tracheal obstruction is uncommon unless the surgical procedure was for a primary tracheal pathologic condition. Glottic or subglottic obstruction may be present following intubation and ventilation in the operating room or in the postextubation period in the intensive care unit, and this should lead us to administer racemic epinephrine by mask nebulizer and oxygen in combination with helium (Heliox). The latter is commercially available in a mixture of 30 percent oxygen and 70 percent helium, although with adjustments to gas flow, 40 percent oxygen can be achieved. As helium is less dense than nitrogen, turbulence is minimized, and the gas flow through a restricted orifice is maximized. Such interventions are usually successful, and reintubation can be avoided in most cases. The role of prophylaxis should, however, be emphasized. Following tracheal intubation edema of the upper airway can occur in a matter of hours, even though it is more commonly seen in a patient ventilated for several days. As a result, it is a worthwhile precaution always to assess the adequacy of the airway before extuba-

tion. This can be achieved by deflating the cuff of the endotracheal tube and determining whether there is a leak present during either inspiration or expiration. Failure to demonstrate a leak should alert the physician to the possibility of laryngeal edema because it would appear that the endotracheal tube is completely occluding the airway in the absence of cuff inflation. Under such circumstances laryngoscopy, preferably through a flexible bronchoscope, should be performed, and extubation should be delayed. The role of corticosteroids in this condition has not been firmly established. The most important consideration is time.

Ventilatory failure later in the postoperative period most commonly occurs in a mixed fashion with associated hypoxemia. The most common causes are respiratory muscle fatigue, bronchial spasm, pneumonia, and bronchopleural fistula. Often the clinician is under the impression that pure ventilatory failure is present because supplemental oxygenation has achieved a satisfactory arterial oxygen tension (PaO_2) and/or oxygen saturation as the $PaCO_2$ is rising. In the patient with marginal preoperative pulmonary function, the one with postoperative atelectasis, pneumonia, pulmonary edema, etc.; or the one with poor relief of pain, respiratory muscle fatigue may eventually develop. Fatigue may be clinically manifest by the development of tachypnea, confusion, somnolence, or the use of the accessory muscles of respiration. A more specific indicator of fatigue and the need for ventilatory support is the presence of abdominal-chest wall respiratory paradox. The latter can often be assessed visually in obvious cases, or in its more subtle form, by placing a hand on the chest and another hand on the abdomen during spontaneous breathing. During normal spontaneous inspiration, both the chest wall and the abdomen expand—the latter is secondary to diaphragmatic descent. With the development of respiratory muscle fatigue, the diaphragm no longer functions properly. As a result, as the chest expands from the contraction of the chest wall muscles, the diaphragm is drawn upward as pleural pressure falls. Thus, during clinical assessment, the hand on the abdomen follows the abdomen inward as the hand on the chest expands. Although new $PaCO_2$ elevations that occur in association with ventilation/perfusion abnormalities may alert the clinician to the onset of a mixed respiratory failure pattern, the presence of chest wall-abdominal paradox indicates established respiratory fatigue and the need for reintubation and ventilatory support.

Hypoxemic respiratory failure is fairly common. Supplemental oxygenation is often required in the first 24 hours because of atelectasis and excessive extravascular water in the lung. The latter is often secondary to excessive fluid administration, cardiac failure, or alterations in pulmonary capillary permeability. Chest physiotherapy, adequate pain relief, and diuretic therapy usually result in an improvement in alveolar arterial oxygen gradients. In the first few days following surgery, however, sputum retention and resultant microatelectases or the aspiration of gastric contents may lead to further impairments of oxygenation or the establishment of pneumonia. The therapy is both supportive and specific. The specific therapy of the particular clinical condition is covered in subsequent chapters. The supportive therapy involves supplemental oxygen administration, chest physiotherapy, adequate analgesia, inhalation therapy, bronchoscopy, and diuretic therapy when applicable. The latter three deserve further comment. Inhalation therapy is important. These patients frequently have small airways disease, and bronchospasm is exacerbated in the postoperative period from sputum retention, bronchial infection, and fluid overload. As a result albuterol therapy through an ultrasonic nebulizer is an important adjunct. The ultrasonic nebulizer ensures adequate deposition of the bronchodilator compared with the standard hand-held inhalers that depend on the patient's performance. Acetylcysteine (Mucomyst) is a further aid when secretions are thick and tenacious. Although it can cause bronchial irritation and bronchospasm, this complication is unusual if it is given with albuterol. Bronchoscopy through the fiberscope can be undertaken in a step-down area or intensive care unit to aid in the elimination of secretions or to obtain specimens in the diagnosis of pulmonary sepsis. It is important to remember that, in the face of significant hypoxemia, bronchoscopy is not without risk. As a result, it should be performed under controlled circumstances with adequate local analgesia, oxygen supplementation, and oxygen saturation monitoring. If hypoxemia requires high-flow oxygen (>60 percent), endotracheal intubation should be considered to permit safe bronchoscopy. Diuresis is often necessary because most postoperative pulmonary bronchial disease is complicated by extravascular fluid accumulation. As noted above, the permeability characteristics of the pulmonary capillary are altered by mechanical trauma during surgery, infection, aspiration, and sepsis. The filtration of fluid across the pulmonary capillary is described by the Starling equation as follows

$$FM = K[(P_c - P_{is}) - \sigma(P_c - P_{is})]$$

where FM = the fluid movement across the capillary, K = the permeability coefficient of the membrane, P_c = capillary hydrostatic pressure, and P_{is} = interstitial hydrostatic pressure. Gamma (σ) = the osmotic reflection coefficient of the membrane, P_{is} = the capillary osmatic pressure, and P_{is} = interstitial osmotic pressure.

When the permeability coefficient is altered, the major determinants of transcapillary fluid movement are hydrostatic capillary pressure and capillary osmotic pressure. There is really no recognized therapeutic maneuver to alter osmotic pressure, except temporarily. Hydrostatic pressure can, however, be modified by fluid restriction and diuretic therapy. Thus diuresis is a useful therapeutic adjunct whenever the extravascular fluid accumulation is secondary to fluid overload or altered permeability.

Adult Respiratory Distress Syndrome

The term *ARDS* was coined by Ashbaugh, et al. (1967) to describe a clinicopathologic entity of acute lung injury. Frances Moore (1969) provided a comprehensive review of the knowledge at that time. He identified several clinical stages in the disorder from an initial stage of respiratory distress, which is indistinguishable from acute pulmonary edema, to a late stage characterized by stiff poorly compliant lungs and both hypercarbia and hypoxia. The pathologic descriptions of the latter stages perfectly paralleled those described in subsequent reports. The clinical situations associated with

ARDS are legion and have led to considerable confusion in regard to the pathophysiologic conditions. Shock, pancreatitis, and perfusion-reperfusion injuries (such as in transplantation, multiple blood transfusions, trauma, and, most importantly, sepsis) have all been associated with the development of ARDS. Sepsis is perhaps the most frequent predisposing situation (Pepe, et al., 1982). The common clinical picture involves the rapid development of hypoxemia and diffuse pulmonary infiltrates 24 to 48 hours after the inciting event. Frequently, the clinical picture is confused with either pulmonary edema secondary to cardiac failure or with pulmonary sepsis. There are initially few systemic signs of sepsis unless it is also the inciting event, and the left ventricular preload is normal. As a result, accurate assessment of preload (often with a pulmonary artery catheter) is essential in the diagnostic workup. Pulmonary sepsis can usually be eliminated as the cause of the respiratory failure by an appreciation of the radiographic features and the use of invasive diagnostic methods for the diagnosis of pneumonia. The radiographic features peculiar to ARDS, as opposed to pneumonia, are the diffuse nature of the alveolar infiltrate, presence of interstitial edema, and the occasional appearance of peribronchial cuffing (although the latter is more commonly seen with cardiac edema). It is important to remember that pneumonia may complicate established ARDS, particularly in the ventilated patient, and is the most important prognostic index of survival.

The numerous predisposing factors suggest either that the lung has one pathophysiologic response or that there is a common pathway of biochemical injury to the alveolar-capillary membrane. Common to all the predisposing entities is the clinical and radiologic picture of pulmonary edema. The lungs are poorly compliant and filled with copious frothy pink secretions. It was initially suggested that the pulmonary edema was secondary to an increase in microvascular pressure (Kusajima, et al., 1974; Webb, 1982). However, capillary pressures in both humans and experimental models of ARDS were subsequently shown to be normal or low (Todd, et al., 1968; Brigham, et al., 1974). Staub, et al. (Brigham, et al., 1974; Ureim and Staub, 1976) demonstrated that, in awake sheep, pulmonary capillary permeability was altered. A summary of the available literature suggests that neutrophils and macrophages are required to produce the permeability defect. It would appear that this occurs by virtue of the inflammatory mediators that these cells produce. The complement system has also received a great deal of attention, but its involvement is likely to be related to the stimulation of leukocytes. In addition, arachidonic acid metabolites (Fig. 67-1) appear to be responsible for many of the physiologic alterations noted in the clinical and the experimental disorder. The degradation of arachidonic acid results in the production of several compounds that have profound effects on vascular reactivity, inflammation, and capillary permeability. In particular experimental observation has focused on the generation of thromboxane A_2 and prostacyclin. The latter has been shown to initiate platelet aggregation (White, et al., 1978) and dilatation of both the systemic and the pulmonary vascular trees (Watkins, et al., 1980). On the other hand, thromboxane A_2 is a potent vasoconstrictor and a stimulus to platelet aggregation (Oats, et al., 1988). Both of these metabolites are released

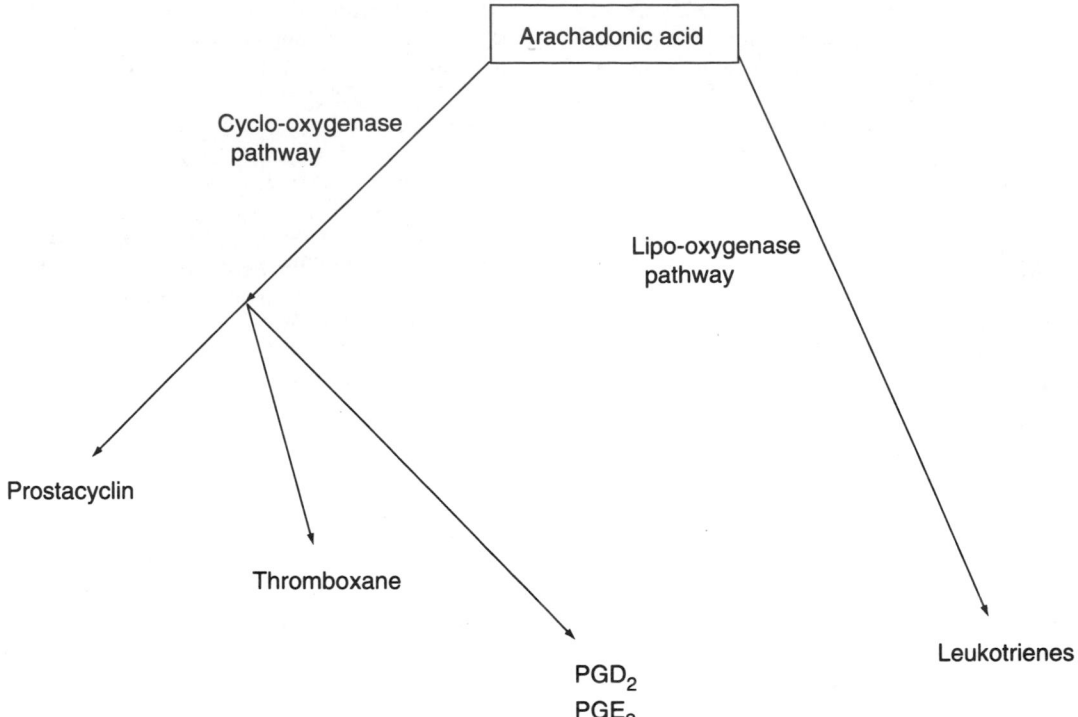

Figure 67-1. Arachidonic acid metabolism.

from the lung, probably from the vascular endothelium during the injection of endotoxin or bacteria into the circulation (Demling, et al., 1981). In experimental models the appearance of prostanoids is temporarily correlated with pulmonary changes that mimic ARDS in humans. In addition, the inhibition of cyclo-oxygenase by nonsteroidal anti-inflammatory drugs (NSAIDs) has been shown to blunt the pulmonary hypertensive response and resultant arterial hypoxemia that were noted in the early stages of all animal models of ARDS. This observation is consistently noted both pretreatment and post-treatment with these mediators (Metz and Sibbald, 1991). The degree of protection afforded by NSAIDs is variable. It is greatest with ibuprofen, which suggests that such drugs individually possess properties beyond their observed effects on cyclo-oxygenase. This latter point is emphasized by the relatively poor effects of corticosteroids in the early phase I stage of experimental ARDS. NSAIDs also have been shown to ameliorate the phase II arterial oxygen desaturation phase of ARDS.

An important role for leukocytes has been suggested by the observation that they are sequestered in the lung after endotoxemia, bacteremia, or the administration of compounds that activate the complement system (Smith, et al., 1981). This particular feature appears to be consistent in most animal models of ARDS. Leukocytes adhere to the pulmonary endothelium, and the oxidative burst that follows their activation can certainly produce the permeability changes noted in the full-blown syndrome. Several studies in human subjects support a prominent role for leukocytes in the pathogenesis of ARDS (Nahum, et al., 1991; Rivkind, et al., 1981; Simms and Damico, 1991; Tagan, et al., 1981). These reports have compared the expression of leukocyte

antigen and the incidence of white cell activation in patients with ARDS or at risk for ARDS with similar parameters in nonseptic control subjects. In some animal models of ARDS, depletion of white cells prior to the induction of injury has prevented or attenuated the defect (Egan, et al., 1985).

Recognition of an important role for tumor necrosis factor (TNF) or cachectin has focused attention on the macrophage. TNF is a 15-amino acid polypeptide that is released by macrophages in response to various stimuli. Responsible for several biologic interactions, it can mediate the adhesion of leukocytes to endothelial cells (Gamble, et al., 1985), and its levels have been shown to increase dramatically during experimental sepsis (Leeper-Woolford, et al., 1991). After the white blood cells adhere to the pulmonary endothelium, a superoxide release occurs that appears to be augmented by TNF and can lead to significant pulmonary destruction (Tracey, et al., 1987). Of considerable interest is the fact that anti-TNF monoclonal antibodies have been shown to prevent the pulmonary complications and ventilatory failure associated with a 50 percent lethal dose intravenous injection of live bacteria in baboons. Elevation of the TNF level has been observed in the bronchoalveolar lavage fluid and serum of patients with established ARDS and also in those at risk of this syndrome (Hers, et al., 1991). In summary it would appear that there are a series of interrelated events and pathways. As noted by Metz and Sibbald (1991), the two main components are the inflammatory process (as represented by the stimulation of the complement system and leukocytes) and the generation of the products of arachidonic acid metabolism.

Supportive measures are the mainstay of therapy, as outlined in the following ventilation section. Although there is no definitive evidence that more specific intervention is valuable, there is nonetheless a voluminous body of literature on the subject. Intervention is directed at the interruption of the pathophysiologic changes. For the most part, it has been concerned with the blockade of the proposed mediators discussed above. Experimentation with corticosteroids in animal models, either therapeutically or prophylactically, has not produced consistent results (Begley, et al., 1984; Demling, et al., 1980; Modig and Bord, 1985; Treber, et al., 1984). Clinical trials of methylprednisolone in patients with ARDS or at risk of acquiring it have not demonstrated a beneficial effect (Bernard, et al., 1987; Bone, et al., 1987; Luce, et al., 1988), and thus it is not possible to support its use at the present time. There is a wealth of experimental literature on the use of NSAIDs as preventive therapy or postinjury therapy in ARDS. The most impressive evidence for their therapeutic role has been found with the use of ibuprofen. In experimental models, pretreatment with ibuprofen in bacteriologically induced ARDS has uniformly resulted in significant amelioration of the pulmonary vascular responses and resultant hypoxemia (Balk, et al., 1984; Barke et al., 1983; Kaplovic, et al., 1984). There have been two clinical reports of ibuprofen therapy in human lung injury. One showed no benefit, but the other—an anecdotal report—suggested that there was considerable improvement in both pulmonary vascular pressures and hypoxemia (Hallemans, et al., 1984; Hasselstrom, et al., 1985).

There have been no clinical trials of the other half of the arachidonic acid metabolic pathway, that is, the lipo-oxygenase pathway. Experimentation in animal models has been limited compared with that is cyclo-oxygenase blockade. Pretreatment has been the rule, and attenuation of the pathophysiologic changes, but no complete protection, has been observed (Cohn, et al., 1991; Turner, et al., 1991). Other prostanoids have been used in the therapy of ARDS, particularly prostaglandin E_1 (PGE_1). Holcroft, ct al. (1986) conducted a randomized trial of PGE_1 in ARDS and reported a significant improvement in the mortality rate. The trial involved a small group of patients in whom remarkable improvement occurred. A large randomized trial was not able to duplicate these results, although the trial did conclude that PGE_1 had a beneficial effect on oxygen transport (Silverman, et al., 1990). If PGE_1 is beneficial in this disorder, its effect is likely to be secondary to pulmonary and systemic vasodilatation, with a resultant reduction in right ventricular afterload and improvement in oxygen delivery. Prostacyclin has also been reported to have beneficial effects in experimentally induced ARDS (Slotman, et al., 1982), but to date there are no clinical studies to support its use.

Recently interest has been generated in the use of nitric oxide. Roissant, et al. (1993) demonstrated an improvement in gas exchange without an influence on the overall mortality rate.

The search continues for a therapy that is specific and can interrupt the sequence of events that leads to ARDS. The most exciting recent prospect is the development of a monoclonal antibody against TNF. In a rabbit model of endotoxic shock, administration of anti-TNF antibodies prevented the deposition of fibrin in the lung and the appearance of pulmonary edema (Mathison, et al., 1988). Similar results were observed in baboons that were given a lethal injection of bacteria; pulmonary edema and subsequent ventilatory failure did not occur (Tracey, et al., 1987).

VENTILATION

Tracheal Intubation

Despite prophylactic measures, respiratory failure may ensue, which would require the institution of mechanical ventilation. Clinical judgment rather than plain numbers would determine when conservative methods of support are inadequate. The increased work of breathing is signaled by accessory muscle recruitment. Progression to discoordinated breathing patterns in which abdominal-diaphragmatic excursion is paradoxic to chest wall movement is a certain sign of impending respiratory failure. Tachypnea and a rising $PaCO_2$ should prompt action. Hypoxemia refractory to conservative therapy indicates a continued loss of alveolar volume and functional residual capacity (FRC), which would require positive-pressure ventilation for correction. The combination of hypoxemia and hypercarbia should signal the need for immediate reintubation. The fatigued patient often presents the most difficult problem. When does the clinician decide that it is time for mechanical support? Often the patients are the best guide. The finding of lucid patients who can speak in sentences and report that they are the same or better provides a reliable index for continued conservative therapy. The onset of confusion, agitation, and inability to speak in sentences in the previously lucid patient indicates that reintubation is now essential. A combination of impending respiratory failure and hemodynamic instability can be lethal and warrants tracheal intubation and ventilatory support at an earlier stage. In general ongoing and frequent reevaluation of the patient and arterial blood gases provides the best guide. The rapidity of change is of prognostic importance. Under such circumstances early reintubation and ventilation before overt signs are present is preferable to a respiratory or cardiopulmonary arrest.

At the time of intubation, it is imperative that the clinician have readily available all the equipment that might be required should difficulties arise. Most hospitals have accumulated this equipment into a specific intubation tray. Reintubation for ventilatory or respiratory failure is best done with the patient awake but sedated. During awake intubation patients must be subjected to minimal trauma and stress. The act of intubation itself can activate ventricular arrhythmias, cause aspiration, and exacerbate hypoxemia. The procedure should be explained to the patient in a reassuring manner. Intravenous diazepam, at a dose of 5 to 10 mg, induces light sedation and relieves anxiety. A short-acting intravenous analgesic, such as fentanyl (50 to 100 mg), may further reduce the patient's awareness. The mouth is suctioned to remove secretions, and the back of the throat is sprayed with a 1 percent lidocaine aerosol. The laryngoscope blade is inserted, and the vocal cords are visualized and sprayed with the local anesthetic. This takes time. The lidocaine should be applied to the pharynx and larynx intermittently, with 100 percent oxygen supplied by a tandem setup between applications. A pulse oximeter can ensure that oxygen saturation is appropriate throughout the procedure. During the application of the local anesthetic, the patient's own respiration should be assisted by an Ambu bag. It is important to ensure synchrony with the patient's own efforts. Under such circumstances oxygenation can usually be maintained and reassurance of the same obtained with continuous noninvasive saturation monitoring. In addition, the patient should not be positioned supine because the diaphragm is then placed in a disadvantageous position, which further increases the work of breathing. Rather, position the patient in a high Fowler's position. Not only will it be easier to assist the patient's respiratory effort, but in addition, the intubation itself will be facilitated, particularly if a pillow remains behind the head to ensure that the oropharynx and glottis are in alignment.

Most patients can accommodate at least a 7.5-mm diameter endotracheal tube, but an 8- to 9-mm tube is preferable. Smaller tubes either do not accept the fiberoptic bronchoscope or do so only at the expense of severe limitation in air flow. Paralyzing agents are seldom required, but if used, they should be of the ultrashort-acting nondepolarizing type, such as atracurium.

An alternate approach is nasotracheal intubation. The nares and the throat must be anesthetized with lidocaine spray. A 7.5- to 8-mm tube is usually well tolerated. Successful blind intubation requires practice, although with Magill forceps and a laryngoscope, the tube can often be guided into the proper position. Again with the patient in a Fowler's position, the endotracheal tube is positioned through the nares into the oropharynx. By listening over the end of the tube, the clinician can appreciate the point at which the tube lies over the vocal cords. It is imperative that the clinician ensure that the endotracheal tube has not already been cut, in which case it may be too short to reach from the anterior nares to the upper trachea.

Because flexible bronchoscopes are available to the thoracic surgeon, intubation should be neither blind nor difficult. Flexible bronchoscopy can be used for either oral or nasal routes. Pharmacologic management is the same as described. The bronchoscope is passed through the endotracheal tube and then placed into the mouth or nostril. Once the vocal cords have been visualized, 5 ml of 1 percent lodicaine is flushed through the suction port to anesthetize the cords. The scope is then passed between the cords into the upper trachea and into either mainstem bronchus with or without supplemental lidocaine. In this position the bronchoscope acts as a stent, and the endotracheal tube is advanced into the airway. Should difficulty be encountered on advancing the endotracheal tube, a rotation of the tube usually ensures that the tip does not "hang up" on the arytenoid cartilages or the vocal cords. The proper position is confirmed by withdrawal of the bronchoscope into the endotracheal tube, and the distance of the latter above the tracheal carina is noted. If flexible bronchoscopy is unavailable or is unsuccessful because of the patient's anatomy, rigid bronchoscopy may be attempted, particularly as the surgeon is both familiar and adept at its passage in the face of airway obstruction. The adaptor cap for attachment to the ventilator tubing should be removed from the endotracheal tube because this piece limits the internal diameter. A 7-mm rigid bronchoscope will pass through a 7.5-mm endotracheal tube. The principles of intubation are the same as for flexible bronchoscopy. Obvi-

ously the nasal approach cannot be used. The rigid scope, however, can be used as a laryngoscope to lever the tongue and epiglottis out of the way to view the vocal cords better. After the scope has been passed through the cords, ventilation can be initiated with the Venturi technique to relieve hypoxemia caused by the intubation attempts. Again, an oximeter, if available, should be used to monitor saturation during the reintubation attempt.

Should all attempts at reintubation fail and a surgical airway seem necessary, apneic oxygenation may provide support until proper ventilation can be established. This can be achieved with the insertion of an Intracath through the cricothyroid membrane. The catheter is then connected to wall oxygen at 6 to 10 L/min. Such endotracheal gas flow usually provides satisfactory oxygenation, which is similar to that provided during an apnea test for brain death. Although the $PaCO_2$ level continues to rise, oxygen saturation can be restored and/or maintained.

Ventilator Settings

The following is designed as a pragmatic approach to ventilatory management. This information reflects our personal bias, and it is recognized that there are several means to achieve the same end. The objectives of ventilatory management are improvement in oxygenation, as assessed by PaO_2, and the maintenance of appropriate ventilation, as assessed by both the $PaCO_2$ and maintenance of arterial pH in an acceptable range. Before discussing the different modes of ventilatory support, we should note those settings that are intrinsic to all modern ventilators and with which the surgeon should have some familiarity. The important settings to remember on any ventilator are the fraction of respired oxygen (FIO_2), the peak airway pressure (PAW), positive end-expiratory pressure (PEEP), and flow. To determine the ventilatory settings and the hemodynamic management of the patient, it is useful to remember the rule of lowest therapeutic intervention. This involves the achievement of the lowest FIO_2, the lowest PAW, and the lowest left ventricular preload to maximize therapy and avoid the complications of therapy itself.

Achieving the Lowest Therapeutic Intervention

Means of lowering fraction of inspired oxygen
    Positive end-expiratory pressure
    Diuresis
    Postural changes
    Ventilatory changes (e.g., high-frequency jet ventilation or inverse ratio)
Means of lowering airway pressure
    ↑ Rate and ↓ tidal volume
    Permissive hypercarbia
    Bronchoscopy
    Pleural drainage
    High-frequency jet ventilation
Means of lowering preload
    Diuresis and fluid restriction
    β-adrenergic agents (e.g., dopamine)

Oxygen has a variety of deleterious effects, particularly when the FIO_2 exceeds 50 percent (Fox, et al., 1981; Sackner, et al., 1976). The surgeon should thus attempt to achieve the lowest possible FIO_2 that produces an oxygen saturation of 90 percent. There are several avenues available. First and foremost is PEEP. There is no question that under most circumstances PEEP improves (A-a) DO_2 and hence permits a decrease in FIO_2. PEEP, however, can produce deleterious effects; the two principal features are a fall in cardiac output and an increase in barotrauma. The former is unusual if PEEP is less than 10 cmH_2O. Above this level it is advisable to measure cardiac output by the thermodilution technique that uses the Swan-Ganz catheter. Barotrauma is an important complication, and PEEP can certainly adversely affect peak airway pressure and thus contribute to the development of pneumothorax, subcutaneous emphysema, or more subtle parenchymal damage. Other measures to lower the FIO_2 are noted below. In situations in which excessive lung water has accumulated (e.g., pulmonary edema and ARDS), diuresis improves lung compliance and ventilation perfusion equally. Parenchymal lung disease is rarely homogeneous. Some areas of the lung are more severely affected than are others. If the ventilation/perfusion relationship in one lung is superior to that on the contralateral side, then nursing the patient on that side may improve oxygenation by ensuring that pulmonary arterial blood flow is favored to the side that receives the most efficient alveolar ventilation. In addition, if the patient's position is alternated between supine and prone on a circle electric or Stryker frame, this can also improve ventilation/perfusion mismatching. With time the dependent area of the lung becomes more atelectatic because of the accumulation of secretions and the effect of the pleural hydrostatic pressure gradient, but the dependent area of the lung receives most of the pulmonary arterial blood flow. A quick change from supine to prone brings the previously nondependent but well-ventilated area into a dependent position where the blood supply is optimal for gas exchange. The improvement is short lived, but the maneuver can be repeated every 3 to 4 hours. Respiratory failure that requires excessive levels of FIO_2 may suggest that alternative means of ventilation, such as inverse ratio or high-frequency jet ventilation (HFJV), should be used. Although each can at times lower the FIO_2, there is no convincing evidence that the outcome is altered. Nitric oxide has recently been shown in selective patients to have beneficial effects on gas exchange (Roissant, et al., 1934). This would appear to be secondary to its vasodilatory properties on the pulmonary circulation. The role of nitric oxide in the therapy of respiratory failure requires delineation.

High peak airway pressures may result in pneumothoraces, or worse still, the separation of bronchial anastomosis or the disruption of bronchial stumps. Tzuno, et al. (1992) reported on the deleterious effects on the pulmonary parenchyma of modest increases in peak airway pressure. The peak pressure can be lowered by decreasing the tidal volume. To maintain the same $PaCO_2$, the minute ventilation must be preserved by increasing the ventilatory rate. The required change is quickly calculated from the following:

$$\text{Minute ventilation} = \text{tidal volume} \times \text{rate}$$

More recently, several authors have argued that $PaCO_2$ is unimportant and can be allowed to increase as long as the pH is maintained at 7.2 (Hickling, 1990; Darioli and Perret, 1984). Such permissive hypercarbia has been successfully used in ARDS and asthma. Simple measures, such as bronchoscopy and drainage of pneumothoraces, are obvious interventions. Bronchoscopy is warranted whenever the peak airway pressure exceeds 40 cmH_2O for a sustained period. HFJV delivers tidal volumes that are less than dead space at high rates (80 to 250 breaths/min). The peak airway pressure is low, but the mean airway pressure increases. Intuitively we would expect barotrauma to be lessened, but there are no good data to suggest this. In our series of more than 70 cases of HFJV for hypoxemic respiratory failure, the incidence of pneumothorax was identical to that seen in patients with peak area pressures in excess of 45 cmH_2O.

The preload can be obtained either through central venous pressure (CVP) or pulmonary arterial wedge pressure, measured by a Swan-Ganz catheter. As noted above, even if excessive water in the lung is the result of altered permeability, a reduction in preload can reduce the amount of extravascular water. Fluid restriction and diuresis are the simplest means to achieve this end. The addition of β-adrenergic doses of dopamine helps to preserve renal cortical flow and urine output. In essence we should strive to obtain the lowest wedge pressure that is compatible with normal renal function.

Modes of Ventilation

In initiating ventilator therapy, respiratory rate, tidal volume, inspiratory time, PEEP and FIO_2 are adjusted, based on the surgeon's clinical knowledge of the patient. Subsequent adjustments are made by following serial arterial blood gases. Changes in oxygenation are made by adjusting FIO_2 or PEEP; the $PaCO_2$ is altered by varying the respiratory rate or tidal volume. In making subsequent adjustments, the surgeon strives to achieve the lowest FIO_2 and the lowest possible peak airway pressure. In general only one variable should be changed at a time to avoid unpredictable interactions.

Volume Cycle Ventilation

Volume cycle ventilators are the mainstay of modern ventilatory therapy. These machines deliver a preset tidal volume at a specified respiratory rate. Generally the inspiratory time is short—0.5 to 1.0 second—and the gas is delivered in a sine wave pattern. Because the ventilator is designed to deliver constant volumes, high peak airway pressures may be generated during the inspiratory cycle if the compliance of the lung-chest wall interface is poor. All machines have built-in pressure limits to prevent excessive barotrauma. Precise adjustments of FIO_2, PEEP, inspiration-expiration ratio, tidal volume, and respiratory rate can be made on all standard ventilators. An important hidden factor must be remembered when the tidal volume is adjusted. Although the machine delivers a constant preset volume to the system, the patient does not receive the entire amount. Changes in the volume of the ventilator tubing—compression volume—account for the rest of the breath. Bartel, et al. (1985) showed that up to 20 percent of the delivered tidal volume can be sequestered within the tubing in patients with low lung compliance. Most volume cycle ventilators offer several modes of ventilator support.

Control Ventilation

Control ventilators initiated by the patient are not sensed by the machine. A preset tidal volume is delivered at a constant respiratory rate. This style of ventilation is generally reserved for patients who are apneic because of anesthesia, muscle relaxant therapy, or head injury.

Assist Control Ventilation

Preset respiratory rates and volumes are again delivered, as in the control method. The machine also senses the patient's respiratory effort and delivers the same preset volume for all patient-driven breaths. Minute ventilation, therefore, depends on the effort of the patient, but a lower limit is ensured by the preset rate. The sensitivity of the machine to a patient-initiated breath can be altered. This most common mode of ventilation is used routinely in the postoperative period and for patients with prolonged respiratory failure.

Intermittent Mandatory Ventilation

For intermittent mandatory ventilation (IMV), the ventilator is set to deliver a specific tidal volume at a predetermined rate. In this mode, the ventilator also senses the patient-initiated breath, as it does in the assist control mode. Unlike the latter, however, the tidal volume delivered to the patient during these breaths depends entirely on the magnitude of the patient's respiratory effort. When the machine senses an inspiration, a fresh gas flow valve opens, which allows the patient to take a breath. No preset tidal volume is delivered during the patient-initiated breath. In the IMV setting, minute ventilation is determined not only by the number of patient-initiated breaths but also by their force. Again a minimum volume is ensured by the preset IMV rate. IMV is frequently used postoperatively when extubation is expected within 24 hours, and it is also used as a weaning strategy in prolonged respiratory failure.

Inverse Ratio Ventilation

Inverse ratio ventilation is used infrequently and is reversed for those situations in which oxygenation is severely impaired, usually as a result of poor lung compliance and a loss of pulmonary volume. Under normal circumstances the ventilator is cycled to allow expiration to be longer than inspiration. When the inspiratory-expiratory ratio is reversed, more of the total time is spent on inspiration on the assumption that the inspired volume is more evenly distributed and that the pulmonary volume will be maintained by the shortening of expiration. Intrathoracic volume and pressure are increased by this maneuver, and thus it should only be undertaken by an experienced critical care physician.

Pressure-Limited Ventilation

There are several forms of ventilation (e.g., permissive hypercarbia, pressure preset ventilation, and pressure-limited ventilation) that differ from each other in relatively minor ways.

Common to each is the goal of limiting the peak inflation pressure or the mean airway pressure. On the basis of the work of several authors, as noted above, the advocates of these modes of ventilatory support suppose that barotrauma is perhaps responsible for additive pulmonary parenchymal damage after the initiation of ventilatory support for other reasons. As a result, an effort is made to limit the airway pressure.

Marini, et al. (1989) introduced a concept of pressure preset ventilation, a square wave form of ventilatory drive that focuses on three parameters: a preset pressure, an inspiratory time fraction, and frequency. PEEP is usually set a 10 to 12 cmH_2O, and hence ventilatory pressure becomes the difference between the preset pressure and PEEP. This is a reliable means of ventilatory support that should limit or reduce barotrauma.

The inspiratory time fraction is a particularly intriguing parameter the benefits of which were largely unappreciated until they were better defined by Marini, et al. (1992). Basically the authors demonstrated that an extension of the inspiratory time fraction results in an improvement in arterial oxygenation unless the minute ventilation was already high. It is postulated that a slowing in inspiratory time may permit a better distribution of ventilation. This is particularly appealing in ARDS in which there may be lung units with vastly different time constants. It was previously demonstrated (Pesanti, et al., 1985) that increases in inspiratory time would improve alveolar ventilation. However, if the minute ventilation is already high, such a maneuver may result in an increase in auto-PEEP (auto-PEEP is defined as the increase in end-expiratory pressure that is generated unintentionally by the ventilator when the expiratory time is insufficient to allow for full expiration of the expired gas). This circumstance, rather than improving alveolar ventilation, should result in an increase in dead space.

At high frequencies, therefore, pressure preset ventilation may result in hypercarbia. Such, however, should not be considered a failure of ventilatory support as long as the metabolic compensation is sufficient to prevent respiratory acidosis below a pH of 7.20. Indeed, a ventilatory mode termed "permissive hypercarbia or pressure-limited ventilation" has become increasingly popular. This involves limiting the inflation pressure irrespective of tidal volume. Initial requirements for increased ventilation can be achieved by increases in rate. However, if the $PaCO_2$ is allowed to rise gradually, renal compensation should prevent a major deterioration in the acid-base balance. It would appear that a pH of 7.2 is well tolerated without undue hematologic or hemodynamic sequelae. If it is done gradually, the $PaCO_2$ may rise to substantial levels. Favorable results with this form of ventilatory support have been reported in asthmatic patients (Darioli and Perret, 1984) and in ARDS (Hickling, 1990).

High-Frequency Ventilation

HFV offers an alternative when conventional ventilation fails and gas exchange is insufficient. The delivery of small tidal volumes at high frequencies may improve alveolar mixing and alleviate the gas exchange problem. Such is achieved with the maintenance of the mean airway pressure but a reduction of peak airway pressure. There are several forms

Table 67-2. Comparison of Arterial Blood Gases Under Two Forms of Ventilation

Arterial Blood Gases	Volume Cycle Ventilation	High-Frequency Jet Ventilation
Rate	20	120
Tidal volume	1.0 L	—
Positive end-expiratory pressure	10 cmH$_2$O	10 cmH$_2$O
Fraction of inspired oxygen	0.60	0.60
Pounds per square inch	—	10
pH	7.23	7.37
Arterial carbon dioxide tension	102 mmHg	63 mmHg
Arterial oxygen tension	57 mmHg	85 mmHg

of HFV. High-frequency positive-pressure ventilation (HFPPV) refers to conventional ventilators set to deliver small tidal volumes at rates that exceed 40 breaths/min. This technique is useful for bronchoscopy and some open chest operations, as Malina, et al. (1981) showed. To avoid overextension of the lungs, sufficient time for exhalation must be allowed.

High-frequency oscillation (HFO) delivers some volumes of fresh gas at rates of 900 to 3,000 breaths/min. The gas flow is rapidly interrupted by a piston or ball to produce oscillations. The mechanism for gas exchange is unclear. Molecular diffusion of gas in the airways may be enhanced by the turbulence generated by the oscillations.

During HFJV, jets of gas at rates of 80 to 400 breaths/min are delivered through a small cannula into the distal trachea. By the Venturi principle, additional gas is drawn into the airway—the biased gas flow. Traditionally, these systems have been open; the biased gas is drawn from the atmosphere or from an oxygen source. Because the degree of mixing of jet-stream gas and biased gas remained unknown, the true

F$_{IO_2}$ was also uncertain. These systems have been particularly useful in the ventilatory management of patients with large bronchopleural fistulae. Table 67-2 displays the arterial blood gases associated with ventilation by a standard volume cycle ventilator and then by HFJV in a patient with an iatrogenically created defect in the trachea and left mainstem bronchus after complicated esophageal surgery, as reported by Panos, et al. (1986). These systems have, however, been hampered by several difficulties. As noted, the mixing of based gas and jet gas leads to an unknown F$_{IO_2}$. In addition, humidification of the biased gas is often difficult, which results in drying of the airways. An important factor is that many of these systems lack disconnect and high-pressure alarms. It is, however, possible to use a standard volume cycle ventilator set in an IMV mode (at 2 to 6 breaths/min and a tidal volume of 200 ml) as the source of the biased gas flow. Thus a constant F$_{IO_2}$, adequate humidification, and the alarm systems of a conventional ventilator are supplied. This method also allows the surgeon to use PEEP to a greater extent should that be desired.

Although general agreement exists about the efficacy of HFJV in the management of bronchopleural fistulae, controversy concerning its role in hypoxemic respiratory failure continues. McIntyre, et al. (1986) did not demonstrate any advantage of HFJV over conventional ventilators in their patients with respiratory failure. Carlon, et al. (1981) documented their experience in 17 patients with various abnormalities that caused hypoxemia that was refractory to conventional ventilation. Of these 17, 8 patients improved and survived as a result of HFJV, and none of the 17 patients experienced a deterioration when switched to HFJV. Experimental work by Lucking, et al. (1986) demonstrated an improvement in cardiac output and systemic hemodynamic parameters with maintenance in gas exchange in dogs with induced right ventricular dysfunction. In our experience the closed system alluded to above has provided improved gas exchange even in hypoxemic respiratory failure. Figures 67-2 and 67-3 demonstrate the rapid improvement in PaO$_2$

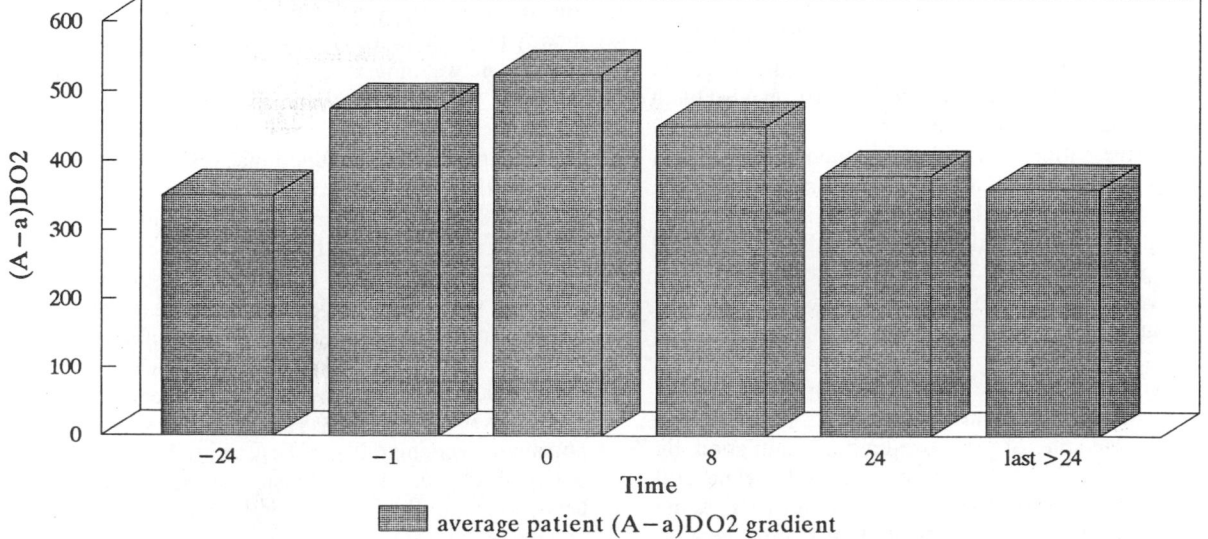

average patient (A−a)DO2 gradient

Figure 67-2. (A-a) DO$_2$ average gradient in 67 patients with hypoxemic respiratory failure subjected to high-frequency jet ventilation. At time 0 ventilation was instituted. Note the rapid improvement of (A-a) DO$_2$ following such ventilation.

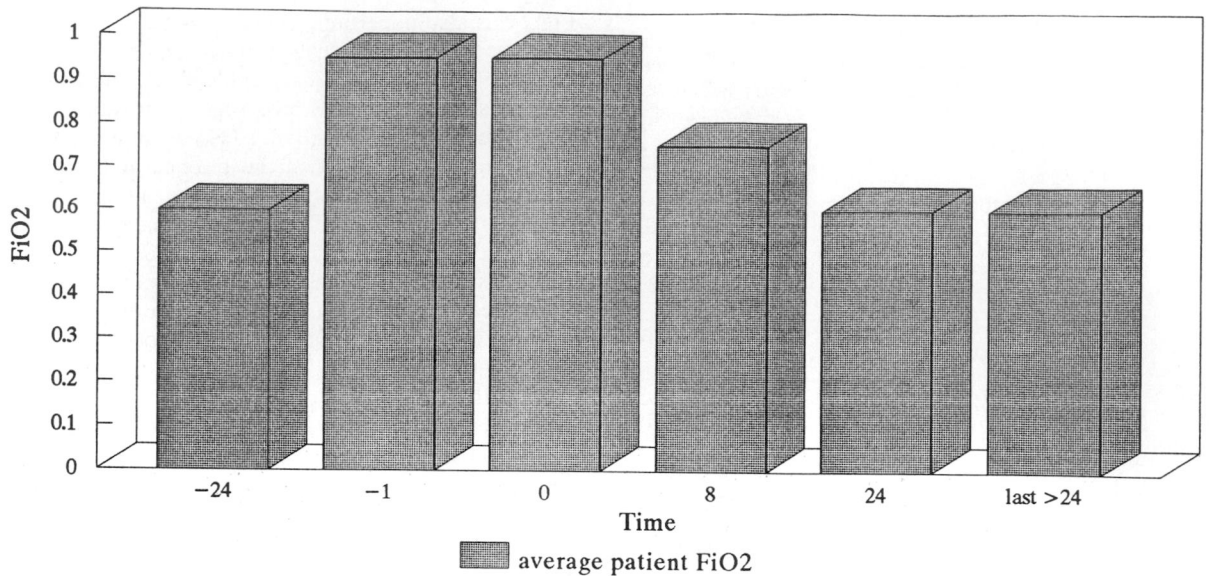

Figure 67-3. Average change in FiO_2 after institution of high-frequency jet ventilation in a group of patients with hypoxemic respiratory failure. At time 0 ventilation was begun. Within 24 hours the FiO_2 was lowered to less than 0.6.

and the ability to decrease FiO_2 to acceptable limits. Such improvement is not, however, universal.

Extracorporeal Membrane Oxygenation

Occasionally, maximum ventilatory support, which includes the use of HFJV, is insufficient to reverse hypoxemia, hypercarbia, or both. ECMO may salvage a few of these patients in terminal respiratory failure. A multicenter National Institutes of Health trial reported by Zapol, et al. (1979) concluded that ECMO provided no survival advantage over continued conventional ventilatory support. The study had a large beta error; that is, the risk of not demonstrating a true benefit from the therapy was high, given the sample size. Several authors, including Solca, et al. (1985); Egan, et al. (1988); and Bartlett, et al. (1977), reported their success with varying forms of ECMO.

A technique for the rapid institution of ECMO with percutaneous catheters and a Bio-Medicus pump, the so-called mini-membrane, has been developed. Girotti, et al. (1986) described the techniques, and Rice, et al. (1986) presented the results in five patients. Rapid percutaneous cannulation of the femoral veins provided venous drainage. Blood was returned through a canula placed in the internal jugular vein. Oxygenation improved from 37 mmHg pre-ECMO to 186 mmHg post-ECMO. The carbon dioxide level was normalized in all cases. Three of the five patients survived their pulmonary insult and were discharged from the hospital.

A further refinement of the use of extracorporeal circuits has been formalized by Gattanoni, et al. (1986). They extended the principle of pressure-limited ventilation by removing CO_2 through extracorporeal circuits while still providing the support of oxygenation (at least to some degree) with a low-frequency positive pressure ventilation system.

WEANING

Most patients who require mechanical assistance for respiratory failure present different challenges because varying degrees of continued parenchymal disease, increased bronchial reactivity, respiratory muscle debility, and cardiovascular compromise demand a more cautious approach to weaning. The initial problem is to identify that weaning has become possible. This is usually signaled by a FiO_2 less than 50 percent. PEEP less than or equal to 7 cmH_2O, and clearing of infiltrates on chest radiography. Further support for the initiation of the weaning effort can be obtained in the conscious patient who has the ability to generate a forced vital capacity of at least 7 ml/kg of body weight and a minimal negative inspiratory force of -15 cmH_2O. There are several methods of weaning. We focus on the classic method, IMV, and pressure support. Although weaning through an open airway (T-piece method) has often been quoted as a variant of a classic weaning method, it possesses no distinct advantage. On the contrary there are potential disadvantages in that the removal of end-expiratory pressure results over time in a progressive fall in functional residual capacity and the pretentiation of ventilation/perfusion mismatching. Annest, et al. (1980) and Quan, et al. (1981) showed that this leads to an increased work of breathing. The continuous positive airway pressure (CPAP) method (or classic method) places the entire ventilatory responsibility on the patient. It provides for intermittent stresses with periods of complete rest at levels of assisted ventilation. Theoretically this maximal stress followed by rest should provide beneficial respiratory muscle exercise. When using the classic technique, it is important to recognize that patients initially tolerate CPAP for only a short time. The extension of the interval should proceed slowly; patients should not be stressed to the point of impending failure. Cohen, et al. (1982) described the clinical signs of respiratory muscle fatigue. An increased respiratory rate is followed by an alteration between rib cage and abdominal breathing, which they termed "respiratory alternans," the paradoxic abdominal-chest wall motion we described earlier, and finally decreased PaO_2 accompanied by a fall in minute ventilation and hypercarbia. Electromyographic recordings from their patients revealed high- and low-frequency discharges from the intercostal muscles. A fall in the ratio of high- to low-frequency power indicated fatiguing muscle and preceded the clinical signs of failure. Clinically, a simple guide to a patient's tolerance of the weaning process can be obtained by a measurement of vital capacity and negative inspiratory force at the beginning and at the end of the CPAP weaning. The weaning period should not be extended unless the beginning and end values are comparable.

During the use of the IMV technique, a patient must work constantly and may not be able to sustain the effort. As noted, failure occurs when fatigue results in diminishing tidal volumes, which in turn reduces functional residual capacity. Gas exchange becomes increasingly impaired. In addition, the ventilator may itself impose an increased burden on the work of breathing. Marini, et al. (1986) demonstrated higher workloads during patient-triggered ventilatory breaths than during spontaneous breathing. Part of the explanation for this phenomenon lies in the resistance threshold in the ventilator itself. The resistance within the internal circuitry of respirators varies greatly. For this reason, when CPAP is used, it is wise to use external circuits.

Pressure support ventilation and the use of pressure support during weaning has become popular. We have previously discussed the theory behind pressure support ventilation. During weaning the amount of pressure support is gradually decreased until it is eliminated or at least until 10 cmH$_2$O

has been achieved. This is a well-tolerated form of weaning. However, as with the classic method, adequate rest with maximal pressure support is a prerequisite between weaning intervals.

Failure to wean should prompt further investigations to reveal possible causes. A finding of a dead space to tidal volume ratio (VD/VT) of greater than 0.7 suggests an inability to wean. However, this is a dynamic measurement, and patients often improve over time. It is an accurate measurement of subtle improvement in long-term patients who have severe inspiratory insults. In our experience it may require up to 3 months of stable respiratory maintenance before VD/VT improves and the criteria for weaning are reached. Open lung biopsy sometimes reveals unsuspected and treatable disease, but this is less useful than it was in the past given the advent of protected specimen brushing and bronchoalveolar lavage. Ventilation/perfusion scanning may show areas of gross mismatch that contribute to the intrapulmonary shunt. Several patients are unable to be weaned because of hemodynamic instability, which is evident only during the weaning period. Insertion of a pulmonary artery catheter may uncover significant pulmonary arterial hypertension, which can be corrected with appropriate vasodilator therapy. Figure 67-4 documents the results seen in a patient with left ventricular dysfunction and mitral valve replacement. Several weaning attempts had failed in this patient over several weeks. After pulmonary artery pressures were controlled, weaning proceeded rapidly and successfully.

Aubier, et al. (1987) showed that digoxin improved diaphragmatic strength by 19.5 percent in ventilated patients with chronic obstructive pulmonary disease. The mechanism of action is unclear.

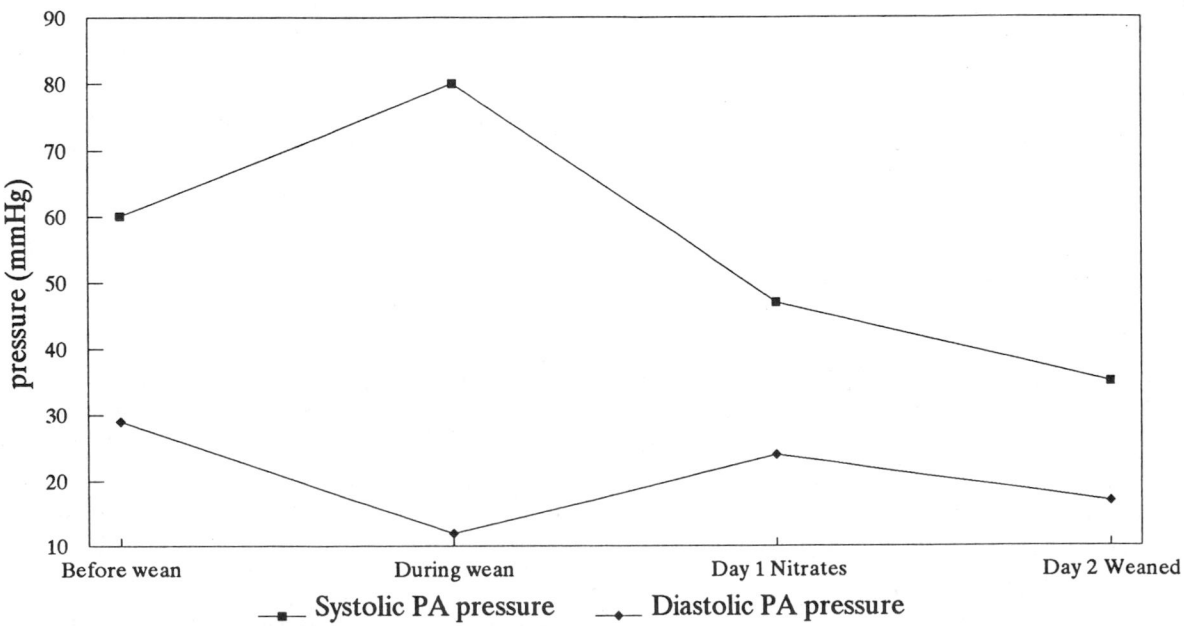

Figure 67-4. Systolic and diastolic pulmonary artery pressures after prolonged mechanical ventilatory support. Note the increase in systolic pressure observed with weaning; this was accompanied by pulmonary edema. Weaning proceeded smoothly with the use of nitrates.

REFERENCES

Annest SJ et al: Detrimental effects of removing end-expiratory pressure prior to extubation. Ann Surg 191:539, 1980

Ashbaugh DG, Bigelow DB, Petty TL: Acute respiratory distress in adults. Lancet 2:319, 1967

Aubier M et al: Effects of digoxin on diaphragmatic strength generation in patients with chronic obstructive pulmonary disease during acute respiratory failure. Am Rev Respir Dis 135:544, 1987

Balk RA, Tryka AF, Bone RC: The effect of ibuprofen on endotoxin induced sheep. Am Rev Respir Dis 129 (suppl):A144, 1984

Barke RA, Dunn RL, Dalmasso P: Effects of ibuprofen treatment versus ibuprofen pretreatment of pulmonary micro-vascular permeability and pulmonary function following escherichia coli peritoneal contamination. Surg Forum 34:144, 1983

Bartel LP, Bazik JR, Powner DJ: Compression volume during mechanical ventilation: comparison of ventilators and tubing circuits. Crit Care Med 13:851, 1985

Bartlett RH et al: Extracorporeal membrane oxygenation support for cardiopulmonary failure. J Cardiovasc Thorac Surg 73:375, 1977

Begley CJ, Ogletree ML, Meyrick BO: Modification of pulmonary response to endotoxemia in awake sheep by steroidal and nonsteroidal anti-inflammatory agents. Am Rev Respir Dis 130:1140, 1984

Bernard JR, Luce JM, Sprung CL: High dose corticosteroids in patients with the adult respiratory distress syndrome. N Engl J Med 317:1365, 1987

Bone RC, Hisha JR, Clemer TP: Early methylprednisolone treatment for septic syndrome in the adult respiratory distress syndrome. Chest 92:1032, 1987

Brigham KR, Wolverton WC, Blake JH: Increased sheep lung vascular permeability caused by Pseudomonas. J Clin Invest 54:792, 1974

Carlon GC et al: Clinical experience with high frequency jet ventilation. Crit Care Med 9:1, 1981

Cohen CA et al: Clinical manifestations of inspiratory muscle fatigue. Am J Med 73:308, 1982

Cohn SM, Cruithoff KL, Rothchild HR: Beneficial effects of LY203647, a novel leukotriene C4/D4 antagonist, on pulmonary function and mesenteric perfusion in a porcine model of endotoxin shock in ARDS. Circ Shock 33:7, 1991

Darioli R, Perret C: Mechanical controlled hypertension in status asthmaticus. Am Rev Respir Dis 129:385, 1984

Demling RH, Smith M, Gunther R: Pulmonary injury and prostaglandin production during endotoxemia in conscious sheep. Am J Physiol 240:H238, 1981

Demling RJ, Proctor R, Grossman J: Comparison of systemic and pulmonary vascular response to plasma and lung lymph lysosomal enzyme release—the effects of steroid treatment. Circ Shock 7:317, 1980

Egan T et al: Experience with ECMO for hypoxemic respiratory failure. Chest 94:681, 1988

Egan TM, Saunders NR, Dubois P: Contribution of circulating formed elements to prostanoid production in complement mediated lung injury in sheep. Surgery 98:350, 1985

Fox RB, Shasti DM, Harada N: A novel mechanism for pulmonary oxygen toxicity—phagocyte mediated lung injury. Chest 80(suppl):35, 1981

Gamble JR, Harlan JM, Klebanoff SI: The stimulation of the adherence of neutrophils to umbilical vein endothelium by human recombinant tumor necrosis factor. Proc Natl Acad Sci USA 82:8667, 1985

Gattinoni L et al: Low frequency positive pressure ventilation with extracorporeal CO_2 removal in severe acute respiratory failure. JAMA 256:881, 1986

Girotti MJ et al: Simultaneous use of membrane oxygenation and high-frequency jet ventilation in acute pulmonary failure. Crit Care Med 14:511, 1986

Hallemans R, Naelje R, Malot C: Do cyclo-oxygenase products mediate hypoxic pulmonary vasoconstriction in man? Am Rev Respir Dis 129 (suppl):A341, 1984

Hasselstrom LJ, Ekkasen K, Mogensen T: Lowering pulmonary arterial pressure in a patient with severe acute respiratory failure. Intensive Care Med 11:48, 1985

Hers TM, Tricomi SM, Dettenmeir PA: Tumor necrosis factor levels in serum and broncho-alveolar lavage fluid of patients with the adult respiratory distress syndrome. Am Rev Respir Dis 144:268, 1991

Hickling KG: Permissive hypercarbia. Intensive Care Med 16:219, 1990

Holcroft JW, Vassar MJ, Weber CJ: Prostaglandin E_1 and survival in patients with the adult respiratory distress syndrome—a prospective study. Ann Surg 203:371, 1986

Kapolovic R, Thrallkill KM, Martin DT: Effects of ibuprofen on a porcine model of acute respiratory failure. J Surg Res 36:300, 1984

Kusajima K, Waks SP, Webb WR: Effect of methylprednisolone on the pulmonary microcirculation. Surg Gynecol Obstet 139:1, 1974

Leeper-Woolford SK, Carey PE, Byrne K: Tumor necrosis factor, alpha and beta subtypes appear in circulation during the onset of sepsis induced lung injury. Am Rev Respir Dis 143:1076, 1991

Luce JM, Montgomery AB, Marks JD: Ineffectiveness of high dose methylprednisolone in preventing parenchymal lung injury and in improving mortality in patients with septic shock. Am Rev Respir Dis 138:62, 1988

Lucking SE et al: High-frequency ventilation versus conventional ventilation in dogs with right ventricular dysfunction. Crit Care Med 14:798, 1986

MacIntyre NR et al: Jet ventilation at 100 breaths per minute in adult respiratory failure. Am Rev Respir Dis 134:897, 1986

Malina JR et al: Clinical evaluation of high-frequency positive pressure ventilation (HFPPV) in patients scheduled for open chest surgery. Anesth Analg 60:324, 1981

Marini JJ, Crooke PS, Truwitt JD: Determinants and limits of pressure preset ventilation: a mathematical model of pressure control. J Appl Physiol 67:1081, 1989

Marini JJ et al: New approaches to the ventilatory management of the adult respiratory distress syndrome. J Crit Care 7:256, 1992

Marini JJ, Rodriguez M, Lamb V: The inspiratory workload of patient-initiated mechanical ventilation. Am Rev Respir Dis 134:902, 1986

Mathison JC, Wolfson E, Ulevitch RJ: Participation of tumor necrosis factor in the mediation of gram negative bacterial lipopolysaccharide induced injury in rabbits. J Clin Invest 81:1925, 1988

Metz C, Sibbald WJ: Anti-inflammatory therapy of acute lung injury. Chest 100:1110, 1991

Modig J, Bord T: High dose methylprednisolone in a porcine model of ARDS induced by endotoxemia. Acta Chir Scand 526:94, 1985

Moore F: Clinical pathologic review ARDS. In Moore, Lyons, Perce et al. (eds): Post-Traumatic Pulmonary Insufficiency. WB Saunders, Philadelphia, 1969

Nahum A, Chamberlain W, Sznajder J: Differential activation of mixed venous and arterial neutrophils in patients with sepsis syndrome and acute lung injury. Am Rev Respir Dis 143:1083, 1991

Oats JA, Fitzgerald GA, Branch RA: Clinical implications of prostaglandin and thromboxane A_2 formation. N Engl J Med 319:689, 1988

Panos A, Demajo W, Todd TR: High frequency jet ventilation in the management of bronchopleural fistula (BPF). Chest 89(suppl):521S, 1986

Pepe PE, Potkin RT, Reus DH: Clinical predictors of the adult respiratory distress syndrome. Am J Surg 144:124, 1982

Pesanti A et al: Mean airway pressure vs positive end expiratory pressure during mechanical ventilation: a review of 39 cases. Crit Care Med 13:34, 1985

Quan SF, Falltrick RT, Schlobolm RM: Extubation from ambient or expiratory positive airway pressure in adults. Anesthesiology 55:53, 1981

Rice TW et al: The mini-membrane—a new method of extracorporeal membrane oxygenation (ECMO) for profound acute respiratory failure. Clin Invest Med 9:A8, 1986

Rivkind AE, Seigel GH, Littleton M: Neutrophil oxidative burst activation and the pattern of respiratory physiological abnormalities in the fulminant post traumatic adult respiratory distress syndrome. Circ Shock 33:48, 1981

Roissant R, Falke KJ, Lopez F: Inhaled nitric oxide for the adult respiratory distress syndrome. N Engl J Med 328:399, 1934

Sackner MA, Landa J, Hirsh J: Pulmonary effects of oxygen breathing—a 6 hour study in normal men. Ann Intern Med 82:40, 1976

Silverman HJ, Slotman G, Maunder R: Effects of prostaglandin E_1 on oxygen delivery and consumption in patients with adult respiratory distress syndrome. Chest 98:405, 1990

Simms HH, Damico R: Increased polymorphonuclear CD11B/CD18 expression following post traumatic ARDS. J Surg Res 50:362, 1991

Slotman G, Machiedo JW, Casey KF: Histological and hemodynamic effects of prostacyclin and prostaglandin E_1 following oleic acid infusion. Surgery 92:93, 1982

Smith ME, Gunther R, Gee M: Leukocytes, platelets and thromboxane A_2 in endotoxin induced lung injury. Surgery 90:102, 1981

Solca M et al: Multidisciplinary approach to extracorporeal respiratory assist for acute pulmonary failure. Int Surg 70:9, 1985

Tagan MC, Maibert M, Smaller MD: Oxidative metabolism of circulating granulocytes in adult respiratory distress syndrome. Am J Med 91:72S, 1981

Todd TRJ, Baile EM, Hogg JC: Pulmonary arterial wedge pressure in hemorrhagic shock. Am Rev Respir Dis 118:613, 1968

Traber DL, Adam J, Sziieber TL: Failure of a protease inhibitor to effect a cardiopulmonary response to endotoxin when combined with a cyclo-oxygenase inhibitor. Circ Shock 13:319, 1984

Tracey KJ, Fong Y, Hesse DG: Anti-cachetin/TNF monoclonal antibodies prevent septic shock during lethal bacteremia. Nature 330:662, 1987

Turner CR, Lackey MN, Quinlan MF: Therapeutic intervention in a rat model of adult respiratory distress syndrome. II. Lipo-oxygenase pathway inhibition. Circ Shock 34:263, 1991

Tzuno K, Miura K, Takeya M: Histopathological pulmonary changes from mechanical ventilation at high peak airway pressures. Am Rev Respir Dis 1543:1115, 1992

Vreim CE, Staub NC: Protein composition of lung fluid in acute alloxan edema in dogs. Am J Physiol 230:376, 1976

Watkins WD, Peterson MD, Crane RK: Prostacyclin and prostaglandin E_1 for severe idiopathic pulmonary hypertension. Lancet 1:1083, 1980

Webb WR: Adult respiratory distress syndrome. p. 58. In Delarue N (ed): Clinical Facets in International Trends in Thoracic Surgery. CV Mosby, St. Louis, 1982

Whittle E, Moneada S, Vane JR: Comparison of the effects of prostacyclin (PGI_2), prostaglandins E_1 and D_2 on platelet aggregation in different species. Prostaglandins 16:1373, 1978

Zapal WW et al: Extracorporeal membrane oxygenation in severe acute respiratory failure: a randomized prospective study. JAMA 242:2193, 1979

68

MULTIPLE ORGAN DYSFUNCTION SYNDROME

Avery B. Nathens
John C. Marshall

Thoracic surgical patients admitted to an intensive care unit rarely die as a direct consequence of the disease responsible for their hospitalization. When it occurs death is more commonly a result of respiratory insufficiency, cardiac infarction, or a poorly characterized syndrome involving progressive impairment of vital organ function that is variously known as multiple organ failure (Eiseman, et al., 1977), multiple systems organ failure (Fry, et al., 1980), or the multiple organ dysfunction syndrome (MODS) (American College of Chest Physicians/Society of Critical Care Medicine Consensus Conference, 1992). MODS develops as a consequence of physiologic instability and the interventions required to manage the unstable patient. In this sense, it is an iatrogenic disorder. The syndrome has emerged as a clinically important problem only because the intensive care unit (ICU) provides the technologic capacity to support organ system function during a period of otherwise lethal physiologic insufficiency. As the processes responsible for organ injury become better understood, it is becoming clear that the evolution of MODS reflects a pesistent and excessive response to an inflammatory stimulus.

Earlier chapters addressed some of the specific complications of thoracic surgical interventions (Ch. 6) and the management of ventilatory failure and the adult respiratory distress syndrome (ARDS) (Ch. 67). This chapter reviews the clinical features and epidemiology of MODS, briefly considers the complex interactions between the endogenous mediators (which are believed responsible for the propagation of the syndrome), and highlights the therapeutic principles of relevance to the management of the critically ill thoracic surgical patient with evolving MODS.

DEFINITION

There has been considerable controversy regarding the definition of multiple organ failure and the clinical phemomenon of sepsis with which it is so intimately related (Bone, 1991;

Sibbald, et al., 1991). This controversy is not merely semantic; it reflects a fundamental shift in understanding of the host response to infection and has important implications for the clinical management of this complex group of patients. A consensus on definitions is evolving but is incomplete (American College of Chest Physicians/Society of Critical Care Medicine Consensus Conference, 1992). The definitions used in this chapter are outlined below; Figure 68-1 summarizes schematically the relationship of MODS to the response to a major homeostatic insult.

Infection

Infection is the invasion of normally sterile host tissues by microorganisms or their toxins. Under normal circumstances, tissue invasion evokes a coordinated series of cellular and biochemical responses in the host; these responses produce the clinical manifestations of sepsis. Sepsis, therefore, is a host-based phenomenon, the clinical response to an infectious stimulus. Infection can occur without a characteristic septic response, a situation commonly encountered in the patient receiving steroids or in the neutropenic patient. Similarly, a clinical syndrome identical to sepsis can arise in response to noninfectious stimuli, such as ischemia, tissue injury, hemorrhage, or sterile inflammation (Marshall, et al., 1990). The clinical response, independent of its trigger, has been termed the systemic inflammatory response syndrome (SIRS); sepsis denotes this syndrome arises as a consequence of infection (American College of Chest Physicians/Society of Critical Care Medicine Consensus Conference, 1992).

Multiple Organ Dysfunction Syndrome

MODS is a clinical syndrome characterized by the development of progressive but potentially reversible physiologic dysfunction in two or more organs or organ systems, arising in the wake of an acute threat to homeostasis. MODS may

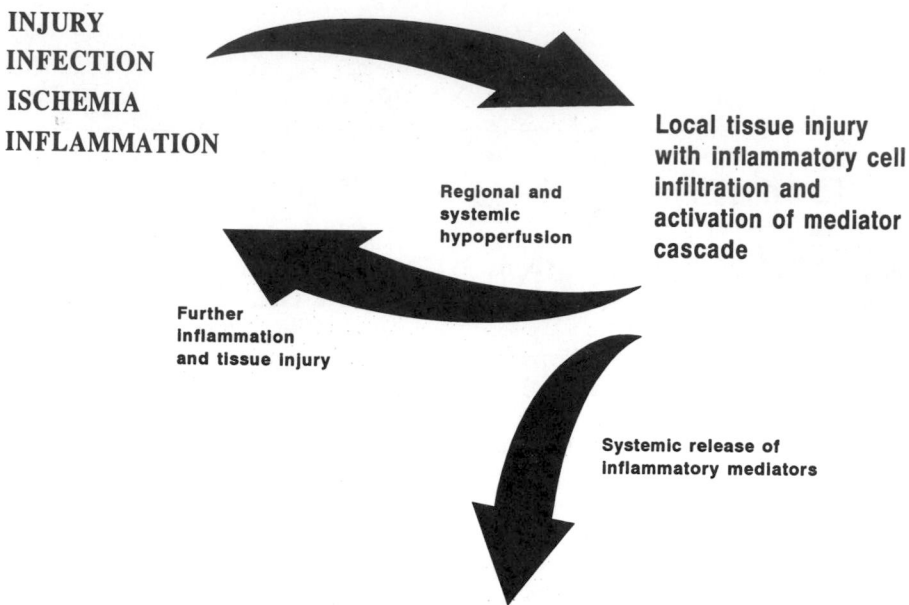

INJURY
INFECTION
ISCHEMIA
INFLAMMATION

Local tissue injury
with inflammatory cell
infiltration and
activation of mediator
cascade

Regional and
systemic
hypoperfusion

Further
inflammation
and tissue injury

Systemic release of
inflammatory mediators

SYSTEMIC INFLAMMATORY RESPONSE SYNDROME

Figure 68-1.   Local tissue injury resulting from infection, ischemia, or immunologic stimulation triggers an inflammatory response that is characterized by the release of endogenous mediator molecules from host cells. These mediators alter the local milieu, favoring the recruitment of additional immunologically activated cells to the site and setting the stage for the eradication of the injury and subsequent tissue repair. The release of these mediators into the systemic circulation results in changes in systemic homeostasis and the clinical syndrome of sepsis, characterized by alterations in hemodynamic, metabolic, and immunologic function. This systemic syndrome, however, can result in further tissue injury by amplifying local or remote processes of ischemia, inflammation, or immune system activation. This process of systemic or remote organ injury, resulting in the wake of the activation of an appropriate inflammatory response, is the clinical syndrome of multiple organ failure (MODS).

be primary or secondary. Primary MODS is organ system dysfunction that develops as a direct consequence of the physiologic insult, for example, coagulopathy resulting from the depletion of platelets and coagulation factors in the patient who is bleeding or pulmonary dysfunction resulting from contusion or hemorrhage. The most common initiating mechanisms confronting the thoracic surgeon are probably trauma and mediastinal contamination following perforation or anastamotic leak from the esophagus. Secondary MODS arises as a consequence of the systemic inflammatory response syndrome, for example, coagulopathy in association with intravascular consumption or pulmonary dysfunction as part of the adult respiratory distress syndrome. The distinction between primary and secondary MODS is neither absolute nor always clinically obvious.

There is little consistency from one report to the next regarding the systems whose dysfunction comprises MODS or the criteria for establishing failure in any given system. Moreover the severity of organ dysfunction in any given patient can be expressed as the number of failing systems (Fry, et al., 1980; Faist, et al., 1993) or as the global degree of dysfunction using a numeric score (Goris, et al., 1985, Marshall, et al., 1988).

HISTORICAL NOTE

Until recently, critically ill patients died from the uncontrolled progression of their underlying disease process rather than as a result of the delayed sequelae of resuscitation and

support. Although potentially life-threatening complications following resuscitation from trauma have been recognized since Curling's (1842) report of fatal duodenal ulceration and bleeding in burn victims, organ system insufficiency became a significant clinical problem only after the development of the intensive care unit.

During World War I, refractory shock was the leading cause of post-trauma death. Research into the cause of wound shock as the result of blood loss led to the emergence of rational fluid replacement strategies and to the use of whole blood for resuscitation (Blalock, 1934). By the time of World War II and the Korean conflict, early deaths from irreversible shock had given way to late deaths from renal failure. Research into the pathophysiology of post-traumatic renal insufficiency by Howard (1955) and others refined the strategies of volume replacement using crystalloid to replace third-spce losses and achieve adequate urine output; the development of techniques of hemodialysis permitted the prolonged survival of the patient with established renal failure. By the time of the Vietnam War, deaths from shock and renal failure had been reduced, only to be replaced by a new challenge: ARDS or Da Nang lung. Coincident with the development of improved techniques of mechanical ventilatory support came the first reports suggesting that the unsolved challenge was the simultaneous failure of two or more organ systems (Skillman, et al., 1969; Tilney, et al., 1973) and the articulation of the concept of multiple organ failure by Baue (1975). The emergence of this new syndrome was an inevitable result of successive triumphs in overcoming the immediate threats to the survival of the multiply injured and critically ill patient.

Studies by Eiseman, et al. (1977) and Fry, et al. (1980) demonstrated that death in the patient with organ failure depended on the number of failing systems. These authors, along with Polk and Shields (1977), showed that the development of unexplained organ dysfunction in the critically ill patient may be a harbinger of occult infection. This observation prompted a brief period of enthusiasm for empiric or "blind" laparotomy in patients with organ system dysfunction and no defined focus of infection (Ferraris, 1983). Later studies by Faist, et al. (1983); Goris, et al. (1985); and Marshall, et al. (1988) showed that uncontrolled infection was present in a minority of patients dying with organ failure. Norton (1985) noted that the control of infection does not necessarily result in the reversal of the syndrome. It is now believed that MODS does not arise because of uncontrolled infection but rather because of the persistent and uncontrolled septic response of the host, and that this response can be triggered by both infectious and noninfectious stimuli (Goris, et al., 1985; Marshall, 1991; Deitch, 1992).

HISTORICAL READINGS

American College of Chest Physicians/Society of Critical Care Medicine Consensus Conference: Definitions for sepsis and organ failure and guidelines for the use of innovative therapies in sepsis. Crit Care Med 20:864, 1992

Baue AE: Multiple, progressive, or sequential system failure: a syndrome for the 1970's. Arch Surg 110:779, 1975

Fry DE, Pearlstein L, Fulton RL, Polk HC: Multiple system organ failure: the role of uncontrolled infection. Arch Surg 115:136, 1980

Tilney NL, Bailey GL, Morgan AP: Sequential system failure after rupture of abdominal aortic aneurysms: an unsolved problem in postoperative care. Ann Surg 178:117, 1973

BASIC SCIENCE

Pathophysiology

Secondary MODS arises as a result of the host's response to infection, injury, inflammation, or ischemia (Carrico, et al., 1986). The cascade of endogenous mediators, which has been linked to organ injury, is intimidatingly complex. In the absence of effective specific mediator-directed therapy, however, the details of this cascade are less important than the underlying concepts. Our focus here is on the principles that have evolved from the study of the host's response to infection but that are generalizable to the biologic response to injury, ischemia, and sterile inflammation.

Infection, the invasion of microorganisms into normally sterile tissues, evokes a predictable response in the host that results in the recruitment of polymorphonuclear neutrophils and monocytes to the site, in phagocytosis, and in the killing of the organism. During this process a specific immune response involving B and T lymphocytes is activated, that augments the clearance of bacteria while minimizing bystander injury to the host's tissues. Coordination of the processes responsible for immune cell localization and activation at the site of an infection is accomplished through the release

of an extraordinary array of biochemical mediators, more than 100 of which have been identified to date. These substances act as chemoattractants and produce the local changes in blood flow and vascular permeability that favor the influx of immune cells to the site of infection. They alter the adhesive properties of immune cells and vascular endothelium to facilitate immune cell entry to the site of the infection and play a critical role in activating recruited cells to enhanced bacterial killing. Finally they alter the systemic milieu of the host in a manner that tips the balance in favor of the host and away from the bacterium, for example, by inducing the release of neutrophils from the bone marrow, elevating the core temperature, changing the patterns of intermediary metabolism, evoking changes in stress hormone release, reducing peripheral vascular resistance, and downregulating the expression of the immune responses at sites remote from the challenge. It is now apparent that the entire spectrum of the clinical process of sepsis is mediated by products of the host rather than by toxins derived from bacteria.

This response is not specific for infection. The clinical manifestations of gram-positive bacterial (Wiles, et al., 1980) or viral infection (Deutschman, et al., 1987) are indistinguishable from those of gram-negative bacterial infection. Moreover an identical clinical response can be induced by noninfectious stimuli, such as salicylates (Leatherman and Schmitz, 1991), etiocholanolone (Watters, et al., 1986), infusion of the mediators themselves (Michie, et al., 1988), and even exercise (Camus, et al., 1992). Although the biology of this mediator cascade is incompletely understood, several components merit special mention because they point to new avenues of therapy, which are currently undergoing clinical trials.

Proteins known collectively as cytokines are particularly important mediators of the host's response. Endotoxins from gram-negative bacteria induce macrophages to release a protein, variously known as tumor necrosis factor (TNF) for its tumoricidal activities in vitro and cachectin for its effects on metabolism and its role in cancer cachexia. TNF is an early mediator of the host's response to infection and in turn triggers the release of a cascade of other cytokines. The administration of TNF to animals results in a clinical process remarkably similar to human MODS; blockade of TNF activity by anti-TNF antibodies prevents the development of such changes in response to endotoxin (Beutler and Cerami, 1987). TNF thus appears to an important early mediator of MODS, although whether its effects are mediated directly or indirectly through the release of secondary mediators is unknown. Experience with TNF blockade in humans is limited. Anti-TNF antibody has been shown to lessen myocardial dysfunction in sepsis (Vincent, et al., 1992a), and a phase 2 study suggests that it may improve the outcome for some patients with sepsis syndrome (Fisher, et al., 1993). In animal models divergent results occur, depending on the nature of the experimental insult. TNF blockade improves survival during endotoxemia (Tracey, et al., 1987), but actually increases mortality rates in intra-abdominal infection produced by cecal ligation and puncture (Eskandari, et al., 1992).

Interleukin-1 (IL-1) is a macrophage product released in response to bacteria and TNF. IL-1 was previously known as endogenous pyrogen in recognition of its role as the endogenous mediator of fever and as lymphocyte activating factor because of its role in lymphocyte activation (Dinarello, 1984). The infusion of IL-2 can induce a shocklike state in experimental animals; blockade of IL-1 with a naturally occurring antagonist known as the IL-1 receptor antagonist improves the survival rate in a variety of animal models of infection and has shown preliminary promise in a phase II study in human sepsis syndrome (Fisher, et al., 1991). Like TNF the effects of IL-1 augmentation or blockade are strongly influenced by the experimental model. Although IL-1 blockade with IL-1 receptor antagonist improves the outcome in animal models of experimental infection (Arend, 1991), Alexander, et al. (1991) reported improved survival rates in both endotoxemia and intra-abdominal infection by pretreatment of mice with IL-1.

The definition of the clinical role of mediator manipulation awaits a better clinical characterization of the complex processes for which these strategies might be used. Table 68-1 summarizes some of the more important endogenous mediators of the host's septic response. These substances, in the setting of an exaggerated or prolonged resposne, can produce the clinical manifestations of MODS.

Clinical Features

There are no published series describing the prevalence or clinical features of MODS in a thoracic surgical population, although there is no reason to believe that the syndrome would differ substantially from that described in the heterogeneous groups of patients in medical or surgical intensive care units who have formed the basis of previous published reports.

We studied the epidemiology of MODS in a population of 692 patients admitted to a surgical intensive care unit (Marshall, 1994). Of these patients, 118 were admitted under the care of a thoracic surgeon, either following a thoracic

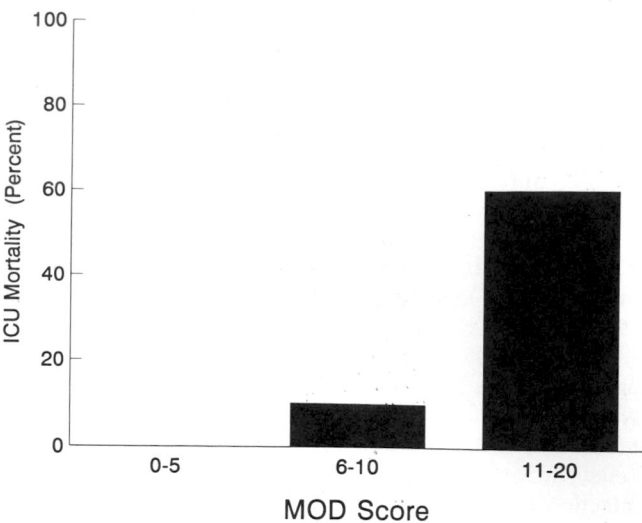

Figure 68-2. Organ dysfunction and ICU mortality rates for 118 patients admitted to the unit under the care of a thoracic surgeon. Organ dysfunction scores were calculated as described in Table 69-2; the mortality rate increases progressively as global organ system dysfunction worsens.

surgical procedure or as a consequence of multiple trauma necessitating ICU support. The mean age of this subgroup was 57.2 ± 17.4 years; eight patients died (7.3 percent). The severity of MODS was measured using a numeric score that grades dysfunction into six separate organ systems—respiratory, renal, hepatic, cardiovascular, central nervous system, and hematologic—on a scale of increasing severity from 0 to 4. As seen in Figure 68-2, ICU mortality increased with the increasing severity of MODS. The admission diagnoses for the nine patients with MODS scores of greater than 10 are summarized in Table 68-2. It is apparent that tissue injury,

Table 68-1.   Some Endogenous Mediators of the Host's Septic Response

Mediator	Biologic Effects
Cytokines:	
Interleukin-1	Induction of fever, release of neutrophils from bone marrow, hypoferremia, hypozincemia; hypotension follows bolus administration
Interleukin-2	T-cell activation; systemic infusion results in generalized increase in vascular permeability, immune suppression, and multiple organ dysfunction
Interleukin-6	Stimulates production and release of acute phase reactants by the liver in association with a reduction in serum albumin levels; levels are high in septic shock, although the pathologic significance of these elevations is uncertain
Interleukin-8	Induces chemotaxis and migration of neutrophils to the site of inflammation
Interleukin-10	Downregulates the release of a number of other proinflammatory mediators
Tumor necrosis factor	Induces a shocklike state and triggers the release of later inflammatory mediators; primes neutrophils for enhanced antimicrobial activity, and induces necrosis of tumors and cachexia
Transforming growth factor-β	Suppresses immune responses, induces fibrosis, and initiates tissue repair
Eicosanoids	
Thromboxane A_2	Constricts bronchial and vascular smooth muscle, increases vascular permeability, and augments platelet and neutrophil aggregation
Prostaglandin E_2	Increases body temperature and capillary permeability; suppresses a number of immunologic responses; and inhibits macrophage release of the proinflammatory cytokines interleukin-1 and -6 and tumor necrosis factor
Leukotrienes	Alters vascular reactivity and microvascular permeability and regulates the aggregation and activation of inflammatory cells
Platelet-activating factor	Triggers neutrophil chemotaxis and degranulation, increases microvascular permeability, and primes monocytes for augmented release of tumor necrosis factor and interleukin-1
Nitric oxide	Induces the relaxation of vascular smooth muscle, producing a generalized reduction in systemic vascular resistance; depresses myocardial function; and downregulates immune responses

Table 68-2. Admission Diagnoses for Patients with Multiple Organ Dysfunction Syndrome Score More Than 10[a]

Diagnosis	No. Patients
Multiple trauma	3
Pneumonia	2
Endocarditis	1
Sepsis with no focus	1
Esophageal varices	1
Postoperative esophagectomy or malnutrition	1

[a] Nine of 110 thoracic surgical intensive care unit patients.

Table 68-3. Prognosis in the Multiple Organ Dysfunction Syndrome

No. of Failing Systems	Mortality Rate (%)
0	3
1	30
2	50–60
3	85–100
4	72–100
5 or more	100

(Adapted from Nathens AB, Marshall JC: Multiple Organ Dysfunction Syndrome. In Wilmore DW, Brennan MF, Harken AH et al. (eds): Scientific American Medicine: Care of the Surgical Patient. Scientific American, New York, 1989, with permission.)

infection, and chronic disease were important preludes to the development of MODS in thoracic surgical patients.

The temporal evolution of MODS has not been well characterized, and the clinical presentation of the syndrome is highly variable. In the young trauma patient with normal physiologic reserve, there may be a predictable pattern to organ system failure. Fry, et al. (1980) evaluated the temporal relationships of organ failure from the onset of the septic state and determined that pulmonary failure occurred early, within the first 2 or 3 days, followed by hepatic failure, gastrointestinal bleeding, and finally renal failure during the second week. The degree of physiologic reserve influences the timing of the appearance of organ dysfunction. Cirrhosis, pre-existing chronic pulmonary disease, or renal insufficiency lead to earlier decompensation of these organ systems.

Risk factors for the development of MODS have been studied by several authors. Knaus, et al. (1985) showed the risk of organ system failure to be higher in those patients with nonoperative diagnoses, advanced age (older than 65 years of age), pre-existing chronic disease, and an admission diagnosis of sepsis or cardiac arrest. Fry, et al. (1980); Eiseman, et al. (1977); and Bell, et al. (1983) reported that the development of MODS correlated strongly with the presence of uncontrolled infection. Henao, et al. (1991) studied risk factors for MODS and found hypovolemic shock, infection, and delay in therapy to be independent risk factors for the development of the syndrome.

The Temporal Sequence of Organ Dysfunction in Multiple Organ Dysfunction Syndrome (Median Interval to Onset)

Respiratory: 2–3 days

Hematologic: 3–5 days

Renal: 4–5 days

Hepatic: 6–7 days

Central nervous system: 7–9 days

(Adapted from Nathens AB, Marshall JC: Multiple Organ Dysfunction Syndrome. In Wilmore DW, Brennan MF, Harken AH et al. (eds): Scientific American Medicine: Care of the Surgical Patient. Scientific American, New York, 1989, with permission.)

Despite the absence of consensus on the criteria used to define MODS, a universal finding of studies of the syndrome is that death is a function of the severity of the process, whether quantified as the number of failing systems (Table 68-3) or as the global severity of dysfunction using a numeric score (Fig. 68-2).

MANAGEMENT

Prevention

MODS can be prevented or minimized by careful attention to well-established principles of surgical and ICU supportive care. Because MODS arises as a consequence of injury, infection, ischemia, and inflammation, measures taken to prevent or reverse these insults rapidly can be expected to reduce the severity of the syndrome.

The restoration and maintenance of optimal homeostasis is the cornerstone of the prevention of MODS. In the setting of the elective operation, gentle but decisive techniques to minimize injury to normal tissues, combined with expert cardiorespiratory support under anesthesia, are the best form of prophylaxis against MODS. For the management of the emergency case, the rapid restoration of physiologic stability and early definitive control of deranged anatomy and physiology are the critical factors in minimizing MODS. Goris (1987); Johnson, et al. (1985); and Seibel, et al. (1985) all showed that organ system dysfunction following multiple trauma can be minimized by early definitive therapy of long bone injuries. Similarly, early burn wound excision in thermal injury, debridement of necrotic tissue in pancreatitis, or wide debridement and drainage of the mediastinum after esophageal injury or leakage may obviate the development of organ dysfunction.

Timely recognition of the operative complications or missed injuries and rapid and adequate correction of the problem can also abort the development of MODS. Clinical evidence of deteriorating organ function should raise the possibility of an occult complication and trigger an appropriate clinical and radiographic investigation. With the widespread availability of high-resolution computed tomography (CT) scanners, there is little justification for the practice of empiric or blind laparotomy (Bunt, 1985); however, early directed surgical intervention is an important component of the prevention of MODS in the complex postoperative patient.

Anastomotic leaks, iatrogenic hollow viscus injuries, and missed injuries following trauma are the most common correctable causes of evolving organ dysfunction. Monomicrobial bacteremia with enteric organisms, such as *Escherichia coli* or anerobes, should raise the possibility of a significant breach of the gastrointestinal tract. Ing, et al. (1981) suggested that polymicrobial bacteremia frequently indicates the presence of uncontrolled intra-abdominal infection. It must be recognized, however, that in many patients, a satisfactory explanation for evolving MODS is never found.

The maintenance of optimal tissue perfusion to minimize ischemia and subsequent reperfusion injury is an important component of the prevention of MODS. Shoemaker, et al. (1988) championed the practice of maximizing oxygen delivery to end organs through a combination of fluids, inotropes, and vasopressors and showed that such an approach may improve ICU survival rates. Optimization of oxygen delivery necessitates invasive hemodynamic monitoring with a Swan-Ganz catheter; such physiologic parameters as blood pressure and urine output do not adequately reflect oxygen delivery when hemodynamic homeostasis is altered, as it is in critical illness. Fiddian-Green (1991) and Gutierrez, et al. (1992) suggested that the use of a tonometer to monitor gastric intramucosal pH as a reflection of the adequacy of splanchnic oxygen delivery may facilitate the hemodynamic management of the complex critically ill patient and improve the outcome.

Metabolic support to meet the demands of the hypercatabolic state is central to the prevention of MODS. Injury and its sequelae result in the depletion of protein stores and in the impairment of the host's defenses, retardation of wound healing, and subclinical organ dysfunction (Cerra, 1988). Both Alexander, et al. (1980) and Moore and Moore (1991) showed that nutritional support in this setting can reduce infectious complications and maintain immunocompetence. Until recently parenteral and enteral nutrition were believed to be equally effective; the parenteral route was often chosen because of its ease of use and a concern about the reliability of absorption in the presence of altered gut function. Recent reports suggest that initiating enteral nutrition early following injury results in a reduction in septic morbidity rates, and that the enteral route is readily tolerated (Border, et al., 1987; Moore, et al., 1992). Kudsk, et al. (1992) recommends that enteral access be established at the time of the initial celiotomy for trauma and demonstrates the greatest benefit in the most severely injured patients. Parenteral nutrition may actually augment the catabolic response to trauma and infection. Lowry (1990) observed that parenterally fed patients exhibit an exaggerated response to an endotoxin challenge, and Hoshino, et al. (1991) demonstrated an exaggerated response to TNF in rats following the administration of total parenteral nutrition (TPN). Conversely enteral feeding has a beneficial impact on local gut immunity. Secretory immunoglobulin A plays a vital role in mucosal defense by preventing binding of endotoxin and microorganisms to the intestinal mucosa. Enteral feeding in the rat maintains normal biliary levels of secretory immunoglobulin A (Alverdy, et al., 1985) and prevents the translocation of viable bacteria from the gut into regional mesenteric lymph nodes (Alverdy, et al., 1988).

Thus, the maintenance of gut barrier function appears to play a pivotal role in the metabolic and immunologic support of the critically ill patient (Wilmore, et al., 1988).

Specific Organ Dysfunction

Adult Respiratory Distress Syndrome

ARDS is a common manifestation of MODS. It is characterized by the development of hypoxemia, noncardiogenic pulmonary edema, and reduced pulmonary compliance and usually arises within 72 hours of a definable risk factor (Montgomery, et al., 1985). Its manifestation of primary MODS may occur as a direct result of aspiration or pulmonary contusion. Alternatively, the lung may be injured indirectly through the activation of a systemic inflammatory response, a phenomenon frequently seen in secondary MODS. Histologically, ARDS is characterized by endothelial cell injury and destruction, deposition of platelet and leukocyte aggregates in clots of fibrin and cellular debris, and patchy destruction of type I pneumocytes. Ventilation/perfusion mismatch, an elevated shunt fraction, and pulmonary hypertension are characteristic of the syndrome, although they correlate poorly with the radiologic appearance.

The therapy for ARDS is supportive. The objective of pulmonary support is to permit adequate oxygen uptake in the pulmonary capillary while minimizing iatrogenic injury from mechanical ventilation. Its ventilatory management is discussed in greater detail elsewhere (Ch. 67). In general terms, however, these objectives can be accomplished by limiting inspired oxygen concentrations to avoid hyperoxic lung injury and by using ventilatory modes, such as pressure control ventilation, to minimize barotrauma. Although useful in the management of isolated lung injury, extracorporeal membrane oxygenation (ECMO) appears to play a limited role in adult respiratory distress syndrome associated with MODS (Zapol, et al., 1979). The role of new modalities, such as intravascular oxygenation (High, et al., 1992) or the use of inhaled nitric oxide (Rossaint, et al., 1993), remains to be defined.

Hepatic Dysfunction

Biochemical evidence of hepatic dysfunction occurs in up to 54 percent of patients admitted to a general intensive care unit (Howarth, et al., 1990). Two clinical syndromes of hepatic dysfunction have been described. Ischemic hepatitis or "shock liver," the hepatic injury of primary MODS, characteristically follows an episode of hypotension and is related to a discrete episode of hepatic ischemia. Marked elevations of serum transaminase levels occur within 24 hours and may be associated with mild elevations in prothrombin time and hypoglycemia. Centrilobular necrosis is seen histologically. Successful resuscitation of the shock state results in the normalization of the transaminase concentrations over the ensuing several days (Hawker, 1991).

ICU jaundice is the more common of the two syndromes and usually occurs 1 to 2 weeks after the inciting physiologic insult. This type of jaundice is characterized by conjugated hyperbilirubinemia with bilirubin levels commonly increasing to 150 to 300 μM. Elevations of serum transaminase levels and prothrombin time are less marked (Zimmerman, et al., 1979). The histologic features include intrahepatic cholestasis, steatosis, and Kupffer cell hyperplasia (Neale, et al., 1966). The pathogenesis is multifactorial; ongoing hepatic ischemia, TPN-induced cholestasis, and drug effects have all been implicated as contributory factors, although the molecular basis of injury is unknown (Hawker, 1991). In contrast to the management of ARDS or acute renal failure, there is no effective therapy for hepatic dysfunction in MODS. It may be possible to increase splanchnic blood flow and oxygen delivery with low-dose dopamine; the discontinuation of hepatotoxic drugs and the reduction of cholestasis by the early institution of enteral feeding in preference to parenteral nutrition are intuitively attractive approaches to minimize organ injury. Techniques of extracorporeal support of the failing liver have been described (Nyberg, et al., 1992). However, these are not available clinically, and their potential role in the ICU setting has never been studied.

It has been suggested that the liver plays a significant role in the propagation of MODS through the activation of hepatic Kupffer cells and hepatocyte-Kupffer cell interactions (Keller, et al., 1985). Impaired Kupffer cell function, which is related to hypoxemia and ischemia (Jones, et al., 1988), results in the loss of the normal clearing of endotoxin from portal blood, giving rise to systemic endotoxemia (Miyata, et al., 1989). Portal endotoxemia in vivo reproduces both the immunologic (Marshall, et al., 1987) and metabolic (Arita, et al., 1988) manifestations characteristic of critical illness; stimulation of Kupffer cell-hepatocyte cocultures with endotoxin in vitro produces changes in protein synthesis and mediator release similar to those seen in the critically ill patient (West, et al., 1988).

Renal Dysfunction

Clinical or subclinical renal dysfunction is a common occurrence in the ICU. Two temporally different patterns of dysfunction have been described. Early-onset renal dysfunction results from renal hypoperfusion secondary to a hypotensive event preceding or coinciding with ICU admission. The cause of late-onset renal failure is multifactorial and includes prerenal factors (decreased cardiac output, hypovolemia, and altered renal blood flow) and the cumulative effect of nephrotoxic agents, such as aminoglycosides and amphotericin B. Histologic studies show evidence of acute tubular necrosis with a disruption of the basement membrane, patchy necrosis of tubules, interstitial edema, and tubular casts (Tilney and Lazarus, 1983).

The prevention of renal dysfunction depends on careful fluid resuscitation and careful use of nephrotoxic drugs. Uncontrolled clinical trials of low-dose dopamine (3 to 5 μg/kg/min) either alone or in conjunction with the loop diuretic, furosemide, have been effective in inducing diuresis; however, they have not established that this strategy preserves renal function or alters the clinical outcome (Corwin and Bonventre, 1988). The indications for dialytic therapy in the critically ill patient are similar to conventional indications for dialysis, although the particular objectives of therapy differ. Massive fluid overload secondary to resuscitation and altered vascular permeability is a common problem that must be treated to facilitate the administration of nutrition, blood products, and medication. Efficient clearance mechanisms are required to remove the products of accelerated protein breakdown and tissue catabolism in MODS, and dialysis may be necessary. Conventional pump-driven intermittent hemodialysis can aggravate hypotension in the critically ill patient in whom fluid shifts, reduced systemic vascular resistance, and autonomic dysfunction all contribute to hemodynamic instability (Schetz, et al., 1989). Ischemic lesions have been documented in the kidney during the course of acute renal failure treated with hemodialysis and are related to the inability of the failed kidney to autoregulate blood flow (Dickson and Hillman, 1990).

These problems can be partially overcome by the use of continuous modalities of renal replacement therapy, including slow continuous ultrafiltration (SCUF) and continuous arteriovenous hemodiafiltration (CAVHD) (Fig. 68-3). Both techniques use an extracorporeal circuit through which blood passes across a low-resistance hemofilter, driven by the arteriovenous pressure gradient. Hydrostatic pressure across the membrane results in the ultrafiltration of plasma. With fluid removal the hydrostatic pressure falls, resulting in a reduction in the amount of fluid removed. This capacity for autoregulation permits the maintenance of hemodynamic stability and allows for continuous hemofiltration in patients with a systolic blood pressure as low as 50 to 70 mmHg (Golper, 1985). SCUF is used exclusively for fluid removal. The addition of a dialysate to the system (CAVHD) permits the clearance of solutes, regulation of acid-base balance, and removal of uremic "toxins." The access for both SCUF and CAVHD is readily accomplished by the placement of femoral arterial and venous catheters in the ICU. The complications of SCUF and CAVHD are primarily those of vascular access and include limb ischemia, hemorrhage, and arteriovenous fistula formation (Nahman and Middendorf, 1990). The need for anticoagulation to prevent filter occlusion and clotting of the circuit may pose problems in the early postoperative period.

Cardiovascular Dysfunction

Both myocardial and peripheral vascular function are altered in MODS (Siegal, et al., 1976). An increase in cardiac output with a modest reduction in systemic vascular resistance is the earliest measurable abnormality. If the inciting physiologic insult is corrected, hemodynamic function normalizes, usually within 72 hours. If not and provided that adequate hemodynamic support is provided, the cardiac output increases to supranormal levels in association with a marked reduction in systemic vascular resistance. Although cardiac output is increased, myocardial contractility is generally believed to be impaired, with right ventricular function showing the most marked degrees of abnormality (Sturm, 1979; Vincent, et al., 1992b). In the preterminal state, the cardiac index may drop precipitously; the maintenance of adequate blood pressure is impossible despite the use of large doses of inotropes and vasoconstrictors. Myocardial dysfunction associated

CAVHD

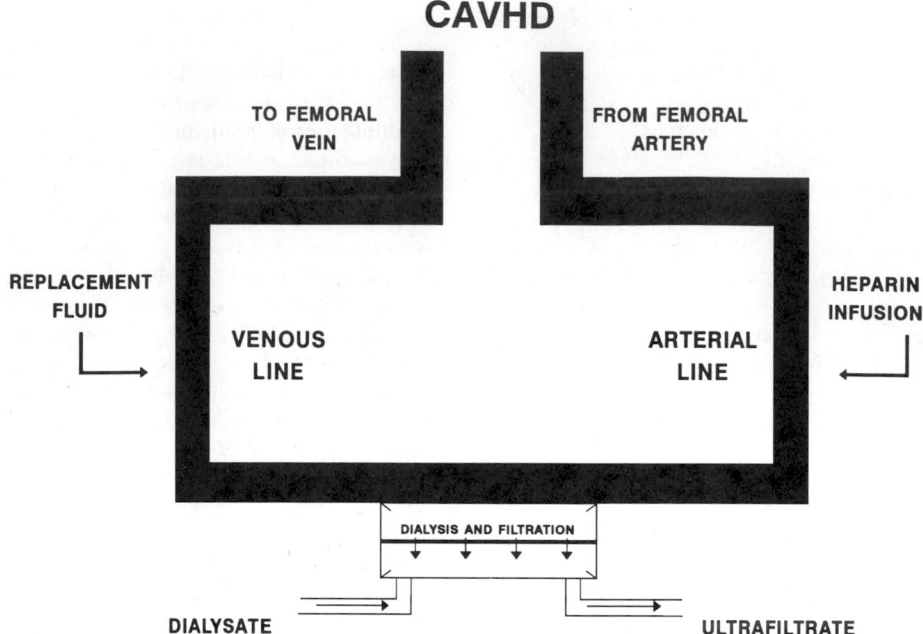

Figure 68-3. Schematic of a circuit used in continuous renal replacement in the critical care setting. Vascular access is achieved, usually through the femoral route, and the arterial blood is heparinized and passed through an extracorporeal circuit where both ultrafiltration and dialysis occur. Flow through the circuit is maintained by the arteriovenous pressure gradient and is thus autoregulatory.

with sepsis may be a consequence of circulating TNF (Hollenberg, et al., 1988) or endotoxin (Carmona, et al., 1985). The negative inotropic effects of circulating cytokines appear to be mediated in turn through nitric oxide (Finkel, et al., 1992).

This characteristic hemodynamic pattern reflects derangements in oxygen delivery and consumption at the tissue level, and these derangements are the target of therapeutic intervention. In the normal subject, oxygen uptake is maintained at a constant value, despite variability in oxygen delivery through concomitant increases in oxygen extraction by the tissues, a phenomenon termed supply independent oxygen consumption. The level of oxygen delivery below which oxygen uptake begins to fall is referred to as the critical threshold, and at this point, oxygen consumption becomes supply dependent (Fig. 68-4). In patients with MODS, supply dependence occurs over a wide range of oxygen delivery, including levels that normally are more than sufficient to meet tissue metabolic demands. This pathologic supply dependency implies the existence of an oxygen debt that may contribute to the development of MODS. Whether pathologic supply dependency is a fundamental abnormality of MODS or an artifact resulting from mathematical coupling of shared variables in the equations used to calculate oxygen delivery and consumption (Ronco, et al., 1993) is controversial. Shoemaker, et al. (1988) demonstrated improved survival when therapy was titrated to maximize oxygen delivery and proposes that oxygen delivery should be increased to supranormal values with the objective of raising the cardiac index to greater than 4.5 L/min/m², oxygen delivery to more than 600 ml/min/m², and oxygen consumption to more than 170 ml/min/m². This

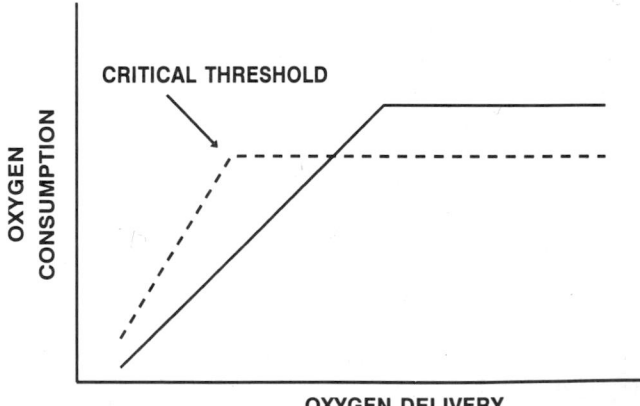

Figure 68-4. The relationship between oxygen consumption and delivery in the normal state *(solid line)* and in the critically ill patient with MODS *(dashed line)*. Supply dependence is demonstrated by the ascending portions of the curve. Note that supply dependence occurs over a much wider range of oxygen delivery than it does in normal individuals. In normal subjects such supply dependence is demonstrated in classic situations of tissue ischemia, such as a cardiogenic or hypovolemic shock. The critical threshold is that point at which oxygen uptake becomes supply dependent.

objective can usually be accomplished by a combination of volume resuscitation and inotropic support, maintenance of oxygen saturation in excess of 90 percent by mechanical ventilation, and transfusion to greater than 10 g/dl (Heard and Fink, 1992). Although patients attaining this level of supranormal hemodynamic hemostasis are more likely to survive their ICU stay (Shoemaker, et al., 1988), it is unclear that this is a consequence of the intervention. A hyperdynamic response to resuscitation may identify a group of patients with better intrinsic myocardial reserve, and the phenomenon may thus be a marker for, rather than a mechanism of, improved survival.

Gastrointestinal Dysfunction

Stress-related upper gastrointestinal bleeding has been the classic manifestation of gastrointestinal failure in MODS; however, ileus and intolerance of enteral feedings are more sensitive indicators of mild dysfunction (Chang, et al., 1987). Prior to the widespread use of stress ulcer prophylaxis in the 1970s, gastrointestinal bleeding was a common problem in the ICU setting, occurring during up to 25 percent of all ICU admissions. Prophylaxis with antacids and H_2-blockers caused a significant reduction in this risk (Cook, et al., 1991). More recently the incidence of clinically significant bleeding has declined, independent of the effects of prophylaxis. A recent Canadian study showed the rate of clinically significant bleeding to be less than 4 percent overall and even lower in low-risk patients not receiving prophylaxis; the risk factors for bleeding were a requirement for ventilatory support for more than 48 hours or the presence of coagulopathy (Cook, et al., 1994). It would appear that routine prophylaxis can be withheld from the majority of patients admitted to a contemporary ICU.

Mucosal ischemia associated with splanchnic hypoperfusion has been implicated as the principal factor in the development of erosive gastritis (Fiddian-Green, et al., 1983), and it is likely that improved hemodynamic management and the earlier diagnosis of infection have been the most important reasons for the reduction in rates of gastrointestinal bleeding in the ICU. An increased awareness that gastric acid is a vital component of a normal host's defenses against bacterial colonization has shifted attention to the possible risks of prophylactic alkalinization (du Moulin, et al., 1982; Driks, et al., 1987; Garvey, et al., 1989). Subclinical aspiration is common in the critically ill patient (Kingston, et al., 1991) and is generally believed to be the most important etiologic factor in the development of ICU-acquired pneumonia (Craven and Driks, 1987). Whether the use of the cytoprotective agent, sucralfate, for stress ulcer prophylaxis can cause a significant reduction in the rates of nosocomial pneumonia is not known (Driks, et al., 1987; Cook, et al., 1991). Avoidance of stress ulcer prophylaxis entirely or the early institution of acidified enteral feeds (Heyland, et al., 1992) may emerge as the standard of care in the future. At present prophylaxis should be reserved for individuals at high risk, that is, those with extensive burns, central nervous system injury, prolonged hypotension, sepsis, uncorrectable coagulopathy, or acute respiratory or hepatic failure (Schuster, et al., 1984).

Neurologic Dysfunction

MODS is associated with a decreased level of consciousness in 7 to 30 percent of patients (Dorinsky and Gadik, 1990). Multiple factors contribute to the evolution of altered neurologic function in the critically ill patient, including sedative drugs, global or regional ischemia, hypoxia, and encephalopathy related to hepatic and/or renal failure. An autopsy study by Jackson, et al. (1985) documented disseminated cerebral microabscesses in 75 percent of patients dying with a diagnosis of MODS associated with sepsis. Additional findings included cerebral infarcts, purpura, multiple small white matter hemorrhages, and central pontine myelinosis, despite normal CT head scans. Electroencephalograms revealed diffuse or multifocal abnormalities; cerebrospinal fluid examinations were unremarkable. Peripheral neuropathy has also been documented in the critically ill patient and may complicate weaning from prolonged mechanical ventilation (Bolton, et al., 1984).

Hematologic Dysfunction

The most common hematologic abnormality of MODS is thrombocytopenia. The cause is multifactorial and includes consumption and intravascular sequestration secondary to an activated septic response, bone marrow depression, and the effects of pharmacologic therapy. Abnormalities of the prothrombin and partial thromboplastin times occur less frequently; in conjunction with increases in fibrin degradation products, they comprise disseminated intravascular coagulation (DIC), the most fulminant expression of hematologic dysfunction in MODS. Anemia is common in critical illness and arises, not only as a consequence of chronic diagnostic blood letting, but also as a manifestation of the acute phase response, mediated in part by IL-1, which is known to induce hypoferremia (Dinarello, 1984). Folate deficiency secondary to nutritional deprivation and hemolysis resulting from medications or blood transfusions may also contribute to anemia in the critically ill patient. Transient leukopenia is a classic manifestation of early endotoxemia (Suffredini, 1992) and occurs in response to the release of TNF (Michie, et al., 1988); more commonly the white blood cell count is elevated as part of a systemic septic response. Lymphopenia is another common finding, variously attributed to sepsis and nutritional deprivation.

Immune Dysfunction and Nosocomial Infection

ICU-acquired infection complicates one-third of all admissions (Nathens, et al., 1992) and may play a role in the initiation and propagation of MODS. The nonspecific immunologic barrier provided by intact skin and mucous membranes is commonly disrupted in the critically ill patient. Violation of the skin and mucous membranes with intravascular devices, urinary catheters, and endotracheal tubes provides a portal of entry for organisms. Gut barrier function is compromised by the lack of enteral nutrition and hypoperfusion, resulting in alterations in the indigenous flora and bacterial translocation.

MODS is associated with a complex spectrum of systemic immune abnormalities, the most prominent of which are abnormalities of cell-mediated immunity. MacLean, et al. (1975) demonstrated that the delayed-type hypersensitivity (DTH) response to common recall antigens is depressed following trauma and sepsis and showed that anergy to DTH cutaneous testing identifies a group at increased risk of morbidity and death. Christou (1985) correlated the degree of suppression of DTH responsiveness with the risk of infectious complications and death. Suppression of in vitro lymphocyte proliferation has been well documented in burn patients (Munster, et al., 1980) and in patients with hemorrhagic shock (Chaudry, et al., 1990). Alterations in humoral immunity are more variable and include impairment of specific immunity to T-cell-dependent antigens (Nohr, et al., 1984; Wood, et al., 1986) but not to B-cell-dependent antigens (Nohr, et al., 1986).

The development of ICU-acquired infection can be considered another manifestation of MODS. In the preantibiotic era, gram-positive cocci and the tubercle bacillus were the predominant organisms implicated in infections in hospitalized patients (Rogers, 1959). With the widespread introduction of antimicrobial therapy, endogenous gram-negative organisms and fungi assumed greater importance (Altemeier, et al., 1967). Although classic surgical pathogens, such as enteric gram-negative bacteria, anaerobes, and enterococcis are the most common organisms isolated in infections leading to ICU admission, Marshall, et al. (1988) demonstrated that the predominant flora of ICU-acquired infection is strikingly different. ICU-acquired infections are most commonly caused by organisms of low intrinsic pathogenicity, in particular, coagulase-negative staphylococci, Candida, Pseudomonas, and the enterococci. These organisms are also the predominant isolates from the proximal gastrointestinal tract, suggesting that the gut is an important occult reservoir of such pathogens in the critically ill patient (Marshall, et al., 1993). Indiscriminate antibiotic use is probably a factor in the emergence of this spectrum of organisms, which are typically resistant to first-line antimicrobial therapy.

The support of the immune system is best accomplished by the prevention of nosocomial infection through such measures as the sparing use of invasive devices, the prevention of pathologic gut colonization by early enteral nutrition and restricted use of systemic antibiotics, and the institution of handwashing policies to minimize patient-to-patient spread of pathogens. Selective decontamination of the digestive tract is a novel regimen using oral nonabsorbable antibiotics to eliminate gram-negative aerobes and fungi while maintaining the normal anaerobic flora of the gut. It has been shown to reduce the incidence of nosocomial infections but has not yet been demonstrated to reduce mortality rates or length of stay in the ICU (Reidy and Ramsay, 1990). Its benefits are greatest for patients admitted to the ICU following trauma or transplantation.

Systemic Therapy

At present the therapy of MODS is limited to measures to support the function of failing organ systems. Although significant progress has been made in elucidating the molecular mediators of the syndrome, therapeutic strategies aimed at modulating the systemic mediator cascade remain experimental.

The neutralization of circulating bacterial products, particularly endotoxin, showed promise in clinical trials using both polyclonal immunoglobulins (Schedel, et al.,1991) and monoclonal antibody directed against endotoxin (Ziegler, et al., 1991). These therapies are expensive, and later trials of anti-endotoxin therapy have not duplicated the results of earlier studies (Greenman, et al., 1991). Their role remains undefined. Polymyxin B, an antibiotic that can chelate endotoxin in doses low enough to avoid systemic toxicity, has shown some benefit in the management of burn victims (Munster, et al., 1989), but it has not been studied in other settings. A naturally occurring endotoxin chelator, the neutrophil-derived protein, bactericidal-permeability increasing protein, has shown efficacy in animal studies but has yet to be studied in humans (Marra, et al., 1992).

Therapy directed against the host-derived mediators of MODS remains experimental. Corticosteroids result in suppression of TNF release by macrophages but have not been shown to improve outcome in randomized clinical trials (Bone, et al., 1987; Hinshaw, 1987). A phase 2 trial of a naturally occurring antagonist of IL-1, known as the IL-1 receptor antagonist, showed a striking reduction in the mortality rate of treated patients (Fisher, et al., 1991). A large multicenter trial of this agent has just been completed, and although therapeutic benefit is documented, the effects are much less impressive than those originally reported. Antibody to TNF has been shown to improve the altered hemodynamics of sepsis (Vincent, et al., 1992a); a large multicenter study is in progress. It is to be anticipated that the next decade will see the emergence of a number of new therapeutic approaches, based on the manipulation of the host's response. For the present, however, many fundamental questions regarding the techniques of, and even the indications for, mediator manipulation remain unanswered. Suppression of the host's response may be beneficial in some circumstances, or its augmentation may be desirable in others. TNF and other cytokines are some of the most strongly conserved genes in mammalian evolution and play an important role in the host's response to infection (Michie and Wilmore, 1990). Clarification of the nature of this role awaits the results of more carefully designed clinical trials.

Therapeutic measures to support the gut mucosal barrier and to prevent gut microbial overgrowth, although theoretically attractive, have not yet been shown to prevent the development of organ dysfunction or to modulate the course of established multiple organ failure. Although early enteral feeding can reduce rates of nosocomial ICU-acquired infection (Kudsk, et al., 1992), Cerra, et al., (1988) did not show any significant impact of enteral nutrition on the development of MODS. Similarly, although selective digestive tract decontamination can reduce the rates of nosocomial pneumonia, its impact on minimizing organ dysfunction is uncertain.

Careful surgical technique and adherence to time-honored principles of surgical care are an important and often unappreciated component of the therapy of MODS. Timely operative intervention with the control of shock, drainage of infection, debridement of necrotic tissue, and basic nutritional support all have a positive influence on the host's immune response (Meakins, 1991).

KEY REFERENCES

Baue AE: Multiple Organ Failure. Patient Care and Prevention. Mosby Year Book, St. Louis, 1990

This is an excellent compendium detailing the clinical setting, prevention, therapy, and pathophysiology of both MODS and the individual organ system abnormalities that comprise the syndrome, written by the surgeon who first proposed the concept of multiple organ failure. This book provides a wealth of information: historical, theoretic, and clinical.

Carrico CJ, Meakins JL, Marshall JC et al.: Multiple-organ-failure syndrome. Arch Surg 121:196, 1986

This is a review of the clinical features of multiple organ failure and of three different hypotheses regarding its pathogenesis: the roles of the gastrointestinal tract, circulating mediators, and altered immune cell function.

Deitch EA: Multiple organ failure. Ann Surg 216:117, 1992

This is an exhaustive and up-to-date overview of current hypotheses regarding the pathogenesis of multiple organ failure and their potential implications for future therapy.

Marshall JC: Multiorgan failure. In Wilmore DW, Brennan MF, Harken AH et al. (eds): American College of Surgeons. Care of the Surgical Patient. Vol. 1. Scientific American Medicine, New York, 1991

Updated every few years, this chapter provides a clinical approach to the patient with MODS, discussing principles of patient care, controversies in clinical management, and competing hypotheses of pathogenesis. Other chapters in this highly recommended text detail the clinical approach to the failure of specific organ systems.

REFERENCES

Alexander HR, Doherty GM, Fraker DL et al: Human recombinant interleukin-1α protection against the lethality of endotoxin and experimental sepsis in mice. J Surg Res 50:421, 1991

Alexander JW, Macmillan BG, Stinnett JD et al.: Beneficial effects of aggressive protein feeding in severely burned children. Ann Surg 192:505, 1980

Altemeier WA, Todd JC, Inge WW: Gram-negative septicemia: a growing threat. Ann Surg 166:530, 1967

Alverdy J, Chi HS, Sheldon GF: The effect of parenteral nutrition of gastrointestinal immunity. Ann Surg 202:681, 1985

Alverdy JC, Aoys E, Moss GS: Total parenteral nutrition promotes bacterial translocation from the gut. Surgery 104:185, 1988

American College of Chest Physicians/Society of Critical Care Medicine Consensus Conference: Definitions for sepsis and organ failure and guidelines for the use of innovative therapies in sepsis. Crit Care Med 20:864, 1992

Arend WP: Interleukin 1 receptor antagonist. A new member of the interleukin 1 family. J Clin Invest 88:1445, 1991

Arita H, Ogle CK, Alexander JW, Warden GD: Induction of hypermetabolism in guinea pigs by endotoxin infused through the portal vein. Arch Surg 123:1420, 1988

Baue AE: Multiple, progressive, or sequential system failure: a syndrome for the 1970's. Arch Surg 110:779, 1975

Bell RC, Coalson JJ, Smith JD, Johanson WG: Multiple organ system failure and infection in adult respiratory distress syndrome. Ann Intern Med 99:293, 1983

Beutler B, Cerami A: Cachectin: more than a tumor necrosis factor. N Engl J Med 316:379, 1987

Blalock A: Acute circulatory failure as exemplified by shock and hemorrhage. Surg Gynecol Obstet 58:551, 1934

Bolton CF, Gilbert JJ, Hahn AF, Sibbald WJ: Polyneuropathy in critically ill patients. J Neurol Neurosurg Psychiatry 4:1223, 1984

Bone RC, Fisher CJ, Clemmer TP et al: The Methylprednisolone Severe Sepsis Study Group: A controlled clinical trial of high-dose methylprednisolone in the treatment of severe sepsis and septic shock. N Engl J Med 317:653, 1987

Bone RC: Let's agree on terminology: definitions of sepsis. Crit Care Med 19:973, 1991

Border R, Hassett J, LaDuca J et al: The gut origin septic states in blunt multiple trauma (ISS = 40) in the ICU. Ann Surg 206:427, 1987

Bunt TS: Urgent relaparotomy: the high risk, no choice operation. Surgery 98:555, 1985

Camus G, Pincemail J, Lamy M: Sepsis and strenuous exercise: common inflammatory factors. In Lamy M, Thijs LJ (eds): Mediators of Sepsis. Update in Intensive Care and Emergency Medicine. Springer-Verlag, New York, 1992

Carmona R, Tsao T, Dae M et al: Myocardial dysfunction in septic shock. Arch Surg 120:30, 1985

Cerra FB: Hypermetabolism, organ failure, and metabolic support. Surgery 104:917, 1988

Cerra FB, McPherson JP, Konstantinides FN et al: Enteral nutrition does not prevent multiple organ failure syndrome (MOFS) after sepsis. Surgery 104:727, 1988

Chang RWS, Jacobs S, Lee B: Gastrointestinal dysfunction among intensive care unit patients. Crit Care Med 15:909, 1987

Chaudry IH, Ayala A, Ertel W et al: Hemorrhage and resuscitation: immunological aspects. Am J Physiol 28:R663, 1990

Christou NV: Host defense mechanisms in surgical patients: a correlative study of the delayed hypersensitivy skin-test response, granulocyte function and sepsis. Can J Surg 28:39, 1985

Cook DJ, Fuller H, Guyatt GH: The Canadian Critical Care Trials Group: Risk factors for gastrointestinal bleeding in critically ill patients. N Engl J Med 330:377, 1994

Cook DJ, Witt LG, Cook RJ, Guyatt GH: Stress ulcer prophylaxis in the critically ill: a meta-analysis. Am J Med 91:519, 1991

Corwin HL, Bonventre JV: Acute renal failure in the intensive care unit. Part 2. Intensive Care Med 14:86, 1988

Craven DE, Driks MR: Nosocomial pneumonia in the intubated patient. Semin Respir Infect 2:20, 1987

Curling TB: On acute ulceration of the duodenum in cases of burns. Med.-Chir. Tr. London 25:260, 1842

Deutschmann CS, Konstantinides FN, Tsai M et al: Physiology and metabolism in isolated viral septicemia. Further evidence of an organism-independent, host-dependent response. Arch Surg 122:21, 1987

Dickson DM, Hillman KM: Continuous renal replacement in the critically ill. Anaesth Intensive Care 18:76, 1990

Dinarello CA: Interleukin-1 and the pathogenesis of the acute phase response. N Engl J Med 311:1413, 1984

Dorinsky PM, Gadek JE: Multiple organ failure. Clin Chest Med 11:581, 1990

Driks MR, Craven DE, Celli BR et al.: Nosocomial pneumonia in intubated patients given sucralfate as compared with antacids or histamine type 2 blockers. N Engl J Med 317:1376, 1987

du Moulin GC, Hedley-White J, Paterson DG, Lisbon A: Aspiration of gastric bacteria in antacid-treated patients: a frequent cause of postoperative colonisation of the airway. Lancet 1:242, 1982

Eiseman B, Beart R, Norton L: Multiple organ failure. Surg Gynecol Obstet 144:323, 1977

Eskandari MK, Bolgos G, Miller C et al: Anti-tumor necrosis factor antibody fails to prevent lethality after cecal ligation and puncture or endotoxemia. J Immunol 148:2724, 1992

Faist E, Bauer AE, Dittmer H, Heberer G: Multiple organ failure in polytrauma patients. J Trauma 23:775, 1983

Ferraris VA: Exploratory laparotomy for potential abdominal sepsis in patients with multiple organ failure. Arch Surg 118:1130, 1983

Fiddian-Green RG: Should measurements of tissue pH and PO$_2$ be included in the routine monitoring of intensive care unit patients? Crit Care Med 19:141, 1991

Fiddian-Green RG, McGough E, Pittenger G, Rothman E: Predictive value of intramural pH and other risk factors for massive bleeding from stress ulceration. Gastroenterology 85:613, 1983

Finkel MS, Oddis CV, Jacob TD et al.: Negative inotropic effect of cytokines on the heart mediated by nitric oxide. Science 257:387, 1992

Fisher CJ, Opal SM, Dhainaut J-F et al.: Influence of an anti-tumor necrosis factor monoclonal antibody on cytokine levels in patients with sepsis. Crit Care Med 21:318, 1993

Fisher CJ, Slotman GJ, Opal S et al.: Interleukin 1 receptor antagonists (IL-1ra) reduces mortality in patients with sepsis syndrome. Presented at the 1991 meeting of the American College of Chest Physicians, San Francisco, November 1991

Fry DE, Pearlstein L, Fulton RL, Polk HC: Multiple system organ failure: the role of uncontrolled infection. Arch Surg 115:136, 1980

Garvey B, McCambley JA, Tuxen DV: Effects of gastric alkalinization on bacterial colonization in critically ill patients. Crit Care Med 17:211, 1989

Golper TA: Continuous arteriovenous hemofiltration in acute renal failure. Am J Kidney Dis 6:373, 1985

Goris RJ: Prevention of ARDS and MOF by prophylactic mechanical ventilation and early fracture stabilization. Prog Clin Biol Res 163:236B, 1987

Goris RJ, Beokhorst PA, Nuytinck KS: Multiple organ failure: generalized autodestructive inflammation. Arch Surg 120:1109, 1985

Greenman RL, Schein RMH, Martin MA et al.: A controlled clinical trial of E5 murine monoclonal IgM antibody to endotoxin in the treatment of gram-negative sepsis. JAMA 266:1097, 1991

Gutierrez G, Palizas F, Doglio G et al.: Gastric intramucosal pH as a therapeutic index of tissue oxygenation in critically ill patients. Lancet 339:195, 1992

Hawker F: Liver dysfunction in critical illness. Anaesth Intensive Care 19:165, 1991

Heard SO, Fink MP: Multiple organ failure syndrome—part II: prevention and treatment. J Intensive Care Med 7:4, 1992

Henao FJ, Daes JE, Dennis RJ: Risk factors for multiorgan failure: a case-control study. J Trauma 31:74, 1991

Heyland D, Bradley C, Mandell LA: Effect of acidified enteral feedings on gastric colonization in the critically ill patient. Crit Care Med 20:1388, 1992

High KM, Snider MT, Richard R et al.: Clinical trial of an intravenous oxygenator in patients with adult respiratory distress syndrome. Anesthesiology 77:856, 1992

Hinshaw L, Peduzzi P, Young E et al: The Veterans Administration Systemic Sepsis Coopertive Study Group: Effect of high-dose glucocorticoid therapy on mortality in patients with clinical signs of systemic sepsis. N Engl J Med 317:659, 1987

Hollenberg SM, Cunnion RE, Lawrence M et al.: Tumor necrosis factor depresses myocardial contractility: results using an in vitro assay of myocyte performance. Clin Res 37:528A, 1989

Hoshino E, Pichard C, Greenwood CE et al.: Body composition and metabolic rate in rats during a continuous infusion of cachectin. Am J Physiol 260:E27, 1991

Howard JM (ed): Battle Casualties in Korea: Studies of the Surgical Research Team: IV. Post-Traumatic Renal Insufficiency. US Government Printing Office, Washington, D.C., 1955

Howarth DM, Sampson DC, Hawker FH et al: Digoxin-like immunoreactive substances in the plasma of ICU patients: relationship to organ dysfunction. Anaesth Intensive Care 18:45, 1990

Ing AFM, McLean APH, Meakins JL: Multiple-organism bacteremia in the surgical intensive care unit: a sign of intraperitoneal sepsis. Surgery 90:779, 1981

Jackson AC, Gilbert JJ, Young B et al: The encephalopathy of sepsis. Can J Neurol Sci 12:303, 1985

Johnson KD, Cadambi A, Seibert GB: Incidence of adult respiratory distress syndrome in patients with multiple musculoskeletal injuries: effect of early operative stabilization of fractures. J Trauma 25:375, 1985

Jones EA, Summerfield JA: Kupffer cells. In Arias IM, Jakoby WB, Popper H (eds): The Liver: Biology and Pathobiology. Raven Press, New York, 1988

Keller GA, West MA, Cerra FB, Simmons RL: Multiple systems organ failure. Modulation of hepatocyte protein synthesis by endotoxin activated Kupffer cells. Ann Surg 201:87, 1985

Kingston GW, Phang PT, Leathley MJ: Increased incidence of nosocomial pneumonia in mechanically ventilated patients with subclinical aspiration. Am J Surg 161:589, 1991

Knaus WA, Draper EA, Wagner DP, Zimmerman JE: Prognosis in acute organ-system failure. Ann Surg 202:685, 1985

Kudsk KA, Croce MA, Fabian TC et al: Enteral versus parenteral feeding. Ann Surg 215:503, 1992

Leatherman JW, Schmitz PG: Fever, hyperdynamic shock, and multiple-system organ failure. A pseudo-sepsis syndrome associated with chronic salicylate intoxication. Chest 100:1391, 1991

Lowry SF: The route of feeding influences injury responses. J Trauma 30:S10, 1990

MacLean LD, Meakins JL, Taguchi K et al: Host resistance in sepsis and trauma. Ann Surg 182:207, 1975

Marra MN, Wilde CG, Collins MS et al.: The role of bactericidal/permeability-increasing protein as a natural inhibitor of bacterial endotoxin. J Immunol 148:532, 1992

Marshall JC: A scoring system for the multiple organ dysfunction syndrome (MODS). p. 38. In Reinhart K, Eyrich K, Sprung C (eds): Sepsis: Current Perspectives in Pathophysiology and Therapy. Springer-Verlag, New York, 1994

Marshall JC, Lee C, Meakins JL et al: Kupffer cell modulation of the systemic immune response. Arch Surg 122:191, 1987

Marshall JC, Meakins JL: Multiorgan failure. Chapter 2. In Wilmore DW, Brennan MF, Harken AH, Holcroft JW, Meakins JL (eds): American College of Surgeons. Care of the Surgical Patient. Vol. 1: Critical Care. Scientific American Medicine, New York, 1989

Marshall JC, Sweeney D: Microbial infection and the septic response in critical surgical illness: sepsis, not infection determines outcome. Arch Surg 125:17, 1990

Meakins JL: Surgeons, surgery and immunomodulation. Arch Surg 126:494, 1991

Michie H, Wilmore D: Sepsis, signals, and surgical sequelae. Arch Surg 125:531, 1990

Michie HR, Spriggs DRG, Manogue KR et al: Tumor necrosis factor and endotoxin induce similar metabolic responses in human beings. Surgery 104:280, 1988

Miyata T, Yokoyama I, Todo S et al: Endotoxemia, pulmonary complications and thrombocytopenia in liver transplantation. Lancet 2:189, 1989

Montgomery AB, Stager MA, Carrico CJ et al: Causes of mortality in patients with the adult respiratory distress syndrome. Am Rev Respir Dis 132:485, 1985

Moore EE, Moore FA: Immediate enteral nutrition following multisystem trauma. J Am Coll Nutr 10:633, 1991

Moore FA, Feliciano DV, Andrassy RJ et al: Early enteral feeding, compared with parenteral, reduces postoperative septic complications. Ann Surg 216:172, 1992

Munster AM, Winchurch RA, Birmingham WJ, Keeling P: Longitudinal assay of lymphocyte responsiveness in patients with major burns. Ann Surg 192:772, 1980

Munster AM, Xiao GX, Guo Y et al: Control of endotoxemia in burn patients by the use of polymyxin B. J Burn Care Rehabil 10:327, 1989

Nahman NS, Middendorf DF: Continuous arteriovenous hemofiltration. Med Clin North Am 4:975, 1990

Nathens AB, Chu PTY, Marshall JC: Nosocomial infection in the surgical intensive care unit. Infect Dis Clin North Am 6:657, 1992

Neale G, Caughey DE, Mollin DL et al: Effects of intrahepatic and extrahepatic infection on liver function. BMJ 1:382, 1966

Nohr CW, Christou NV, Rode H et al: In vivo and in vitro humoral immunity in surgical patients. Ann Surg 200:373, 1984

Nohr CW, Latter DA, Meakins JL, Christou NV: In vivo and in vitro humoral immunity in surgical patients: antibody response to pneumococcal polysaccharide. Surgery 100:229, 1986

Norton LW: Does drainage of intraabdominal pus reverse multiorgan failure? Am J Surg 149:347, 1985

Nyberg SL, Shatford RA, Hu W-S et al: Hepatocyte culture systems for artificial liver support: implications for critical care medicine (bioartificial liver support). Crit Care Med 20:1157, 1992

Polk HC, Shields CL: Remote organ failure: a valid sign of occult intraabdominal infection. Surgery 81:310, 1977

Reidy J, Ramsay G: Clinical trials of selective decontamination of the digestive tract: review. Crit Care Med 18:1449, 1990

Rogers DE: The changing pattern of life threatening microbial disease. N Engl J Med 261:677, 1959

Ronco JJ, Fenwick JC, Wiggs BR et al: Oxygen consumption is independent of increases in oxygen delivery by dobutamine in septic patients who have normal or increased plasma lactate. Am Rev Respir Dis 147:25, 1993

Rossaint R, Falke KJ, Lopez F et al.: Inhaled nitric oxide for the adult respiratory distress syndrome. N Engl J Med 328:399, 1993

Schedel I, Dreikhausen U, Nentwig B et al: Treatment of gram-negative septic shock with an immunoglobulin preparation: a prospective, randomized clinical trial. Crit Care Med 19:1104, 1991

Schetz M, Lauwers PM, Ferdinande P: Extracorporeal treatment of acute renal failure in the intensive care unit: a critical view. Intensive Care Med 15:349, 1989

Schuster DP, Robley H, Feinstein S et al: Prospective evaluation of the risk of upper gastrointestinal bleeding on admission to a medical intensive care unit. Am J Med 76:623, 1984

Seibel R, LaDuca J, Hassett JM et al: Blunt multiple trauma (ISS 36), femur traction, and the pulmonary failure-septic state. Ann Surg 202:283, 1985

Shoemaker WC, Appel PL, Kram HB et al: Prospective trial of supranormal values of survivors as therapeutic goals in high-risk surgical patients. Chest 94:1176, 1988

Sibbald WJ, Marshall J, Christou N et al: "Sepsis"—clarity of existing terminology . . . or more confusion? Crit Care Med 19:996, 1991

Siegal JH, Cerra FB, Coleman B et al: Physiologic and metabolic correlations in human sepsis. Surgery 86:163, 1976

Skillman JJ, Bushnell LS, Goldman H, Silen W: Respiratory failure, hypotension, sepsis, and jaundice. A clinical syndrome associated with lethal hemorrhage from acute stress ulceration of the stomach. Am J Surg 117:523, 1969

Sturm JA, Lewis FR, Trentz O et al: Cardiopulmonary parameters and prognosis after severe multiple trauma. J Trauma 19:305, 1979

Suffredini AF: Endotoxin administration to humans: a model of inflammatory responses relevant to sepsis. p. 13. In Lamy M, Thijs LG (eds): Mediators of Sepsis. Springer-Verlag, New York, 1992

Tilney NL, Bailey GL, Morgan AP: Sequential system failure after rupture of abdominal aortic aneurysms: an unsolved problem in postoperative care. Ann Surg 178:117, 1973

Tilney NL, Lazarus JM: Acute renal failure in surgical patients: causes, clinical patterns and care. Surg Clin North Am 63:357, 1983

Tracey KJ, Fong Y, Hesse DG et al: Anti-cachectin/TNF monoclonal antibodies prevent septic shock during lethal bacteremia. Nature 330:662, 1987

Veterans Administrative Systemic Sepsis Cooperative Study Group: Effect of high-dose glucocorticoid therapy on mortality in patients with clinical signs of systemic sepsis. N Engl J Med 317:659, 1987

Vincent JL, Bakker J, Marecaux G: Administration of anti-TNF antibody improves left ventricular function in septic shock patients. Chest 101:810, 1992a

Vincent JL, Gris P, Coffernils M et al: Myocardial depression characterizes the fatal course of septic shock. Surgery 111:660, 1992b

Watters JM, Bessey PQ, Dinarello CA et al: Both inflammatory and endocrine mediators stimulate host responses to sepsis. Arch Surg 121:179, 1986

West MA, Billiar TR, Mazuski JE et al: Endotoxin modulation of hepatocyte secretory and cellular protein synthesis is mediated by Kupffer cells. Arch Surg 123:1400, 1988

Wiles JB, Cerra FB, Siegel JH, Border JR: The systemic septic response: does the organism matter? Crit Care Med 8:55, 1980

Wilmore DW, Smith RJ, O'Dwyer ST et al: The gut: a central organ after surgical stress. Surgery 104:917, 1988

Wood JJ, O'Mahoney JB, Rodrick ML et al: Abnormalities of antibody production after thermal injury. Arch Surg 121:108, 1986

Zapol WM, Snider MT, Hill JD et al: Extracorporeal membrane oxygenation in severe respiratory failure. A randomized prospective study. JAMA 42:2193, 1979

Ziegler E, Fisher C, Sprung C et al: Treatment of gram-negative bacteremia and septic shock with HA-1A human monoclonal antibodies against endotoxin. N Engl J Med 324:429, 1991

Zimmerman HJ, Fang M, Utili R et al: Jaundice due to bacterial infection. Gastroenterology 77:362, 1979

69

LATE SEQUELAE
AND REHABILITATION

Louis F. Jacques
Denis Desaulniers
Jean Deslauriers

The incidence of late sequelae associated with thoracic trauma is relatively low, and most are unavoidable. Often they are the result of undue delay in diagnosing the initial injury or of inadequate early management. A classic example is the incompletely drained hemothorax, which may eventually lead to a trapped lung, post-traumatic empyema, or both. This chapter reviews the pathophysiology, diagnosis, and management of some of the most common sequelae of thoracic trauma. Emphasis will be given to their prophylaxis.

TRAUMA TO THE CHEST WALL

Complications of Bony Fractures

Malunion or nonunion at the site of fracture of a costal cartilage, costochondral junction, or rib may result in chronic costochondral separation or pseudoarthrosis of the rib. The symptoms associated with these problems are local tenderness, often increased by movement or cough, and sometimes the feeling of motion over the involved cartilage or rib. Therapy consisting of subperichondrial resection of the involved cartilage or resection of the involved segment of rib is curative in most cases. Late sequelae associated with first rib fracture include brachial plexus injuries with neurologic deficits in the upper limbs, Horner syndrome, unrecognized arterial injuries, and thoracic outlet syndrome (Richardson, et al., 1975). Delayed nerve symptoms may also be due to nerve compression from a callus at the site of a first rib fracture.

Most sternal fractures heal primarily without sequelae. Late complications include nonunion or overriding of the fragments with thoracic deformity (Fig. 69-1). Surgical correction by open reduction and sternal wiring is indicated when the symptoms of tenderness, deformity, or abnormal motion are present and incapacitating. In the series reported by Gibson, et al. (1962) of 80 sternal fracture patients, normal union of "undisplaced" fracture occurred in 6 weeks or less

in nearly all surviving patients. There was only one patient in whom pain related to the fracture persisted for a period of 5 months. All other patients were considered to have no disability for heavy work 3 months after injury. Of the 25 patients with "displaced" fractures, 8 had pain and disability for longer than 6 weeks but only 1 for more than 3 months (Gibson, et al., 1962). In contrast to the series of Gibson, et al., Richardson, et al. (1975) recommend early operation for patients with sternal fractures that have overriding defects, are unstable at the fracture site, are causing severe pain, or result in a major deformity of the sternum. In our opinion, most sternal fractures can be managed conservatively and very few will develop complications or require surgery.

Chest Wall Infection

Most post-traumatic infections of the chest wall are the result of penetrating injuries with or without retained foreign bodies. Occasionally they can also be due to blunt trauma with destruction of the perichondrium and necrosis of the cartilage (Brown and Trenton, 1952; Pontius, et al., 1959; Payne, et al., 1973; Miller, et al., 1978). Costal cartilages are particularly prone to infection because they are poorly vascularized, and once they have undergone necrosis, they act as foreign bodies and contribute to the chronicity of the problem. Symptoms of infection include fever, chills, local tenderness, swelling, and draining sinuses of the chest wall. Payne, et al. (1973) noted that in several cases of post-traumatic chest wall infection, the draining sinus first appeared months or years after apparent complete healing and recovery from the initial trauma.

Management is by surgical debridement and specific antibiotic therapy. When carrying out debridement, it is most important to remove all infected and devitalized bone, cartilage, soft tissue, and foreign bodies, as well as the full length of the involved cartilage(s). If the cartilages of the sixth to tenth

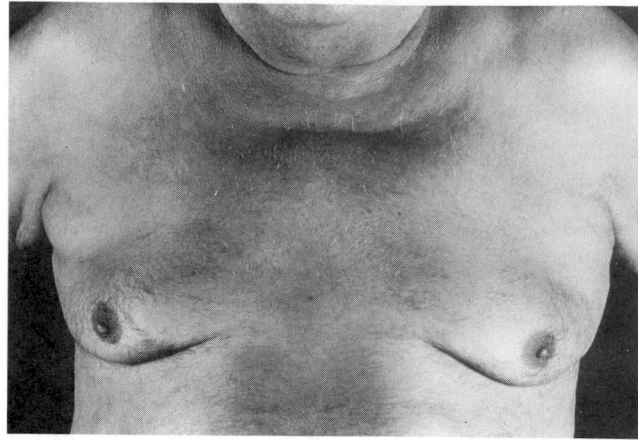

Figure 69-1. Photograph of a patient with an anterior chest wall deformity secondary to a sternal fracture with overriding of the fragments.

ribs are involved, resection of the entire costal arch may be necessary. The wound can then be kept open until it is clean and covered with granulation tissue, at which time reconstruction is completed by transposition of well vascularized adjacent soft tissues or distant myocutaneous flaps. With modern techniques of chest wall reconstruction, infected wounds can now be closed primarily with the use of transposed muscle flaps (Fig. 69-2) with or without cutaneous islands. Prosthetic materials such as Gore-Tex or Marlex mesh should be avoided, and indeed these prostheses are usually unnecessary because chronically infected wounds are already fibrotic and contracted.

Intercostal Hernias

Intercostal pulmonary hernias are rare (Table 69-1), and most result from complications related to chest trauma. They are located parasternally or paravertebrally (Munnel, 1968; Salter and Hapton, 1969), are small, and usually are relatively asymptomatic. Surgery, consisting of plication of the hernial sac and repair of the intercostal defect with autogenous tissue or synthetic materials, is only recommended for large and symptomatic hernias.

Rarely, a combination of diaphragmatic and intercostal defects will occur, causing abdominal contents to herniate through the intercostal space (Fig. 69-3). Like simple lung hernias, these occur anteriorly (costochondral junction to sternum) because of the absence of external intercostal muscle or posteriorly (costal angle to vertebra) because of the absence of internal intercostal muscles (Cole, et al., 1986; Saw, et al., 1976). Transdiaphragmatic intercostal hernias are repaired by closure of both the diaphragmatic and intercostal defects (Cole, et al. 1986).

Other Complications of Trauma to the Chest Wall

Arteriovenous fistulae of the internal mammary or intercostal vessels are uncommon (Ketharanathan and Westlake, 1969; Rubino and Milnes, 1971; Holland, 1960) and have been reported following both blunt and penetrating trauma. A continuous murmur and thrill over the fistula are the characteristic findings on physical examination. The diagnosis can usually be confirmed by arteriography, and therapy consists of ligation of the feeding vessels with excision of the fistula.

Chronic Chest Wall Pain

Chronic thoracic pain is a common and most challenging problem to investigate and treat. It occurs in approximately 30 percent of victims of thoracic trauma and can last for months or even years. It can be accompanied by numbness or paresthesias in the cutaneous dermatomes of the involved intercostal nerve.

Therapy can be frustrating because in the majority of cases the exact cause of pain is unknown (see Ch. 28). Initially, it should be conservative and one must take time to reassure the patient about the absence of any serious underlying problem. Mild non-narcotic analgesics can be given, but the use of narcotics should be restricted. Other options include physical therapy, heat massages, and ultrasound. Non steroidal antiflammatory drugs (NSAIDs) may be added to the physical therapy. The use of transcutaneous electrical nerve stimulation (TENS) is also recommended, especially in the presence of a myofascial pain syndrome.

If the pain still persists, management benefits from a multidisciplinary approach, in which the anesthesiologist usually plays a key role in the developing a plan of therapy. Intercostal neurectomy can be considered if the pain is neurogenic or musculoskeletal in origin but should only be performed in patients in whom intercostal nerve blocks have produced temporary but significant relief. Not only may neurectomy not relieve the symptoms, but it commonly results in dysesthesias that are often worse than the original pain.

TRAUMA TO MAJOR AIRWAYS

Larynx and Upper Trachea

Unrecognized injuries to the larynx and cervical trachea may result in late subglottic or tracheal stenosis with progressive airway obstruction. In most cases an emergency tracheotomy has been performed at the time of the initial trauma and the underlying laryngotracheal injury has been overlooked.

The management of these chronic injuries is difficult, and the expertise of both the thoracic surgeon and the otorhinolaryngologist is required. The repair should be attempted only when the patient no longer requires mechanical ventilation and when all associated injuries have resolved. Preoperatively the extent of injury and involvement of associated structures must be carefully evaluated radiographically and endoscopically, and the functional status of the larynx must also be assessed. A barium swallow to rule out a tracheoesophageal fistula will complete the investigation.

There are two major series reporting the results of subglottic tracheal resection for sequelae of blunt trauma. In the series of Maddaus, et al. (1992) eight patients underwent subglottic resection for lesions resulting from blunt trauma, and in all there was complete transection of the airways at the cricotracheal junction, fracture of the cricoid, and permanent disruption of both recurrent laryngeal nerves. In

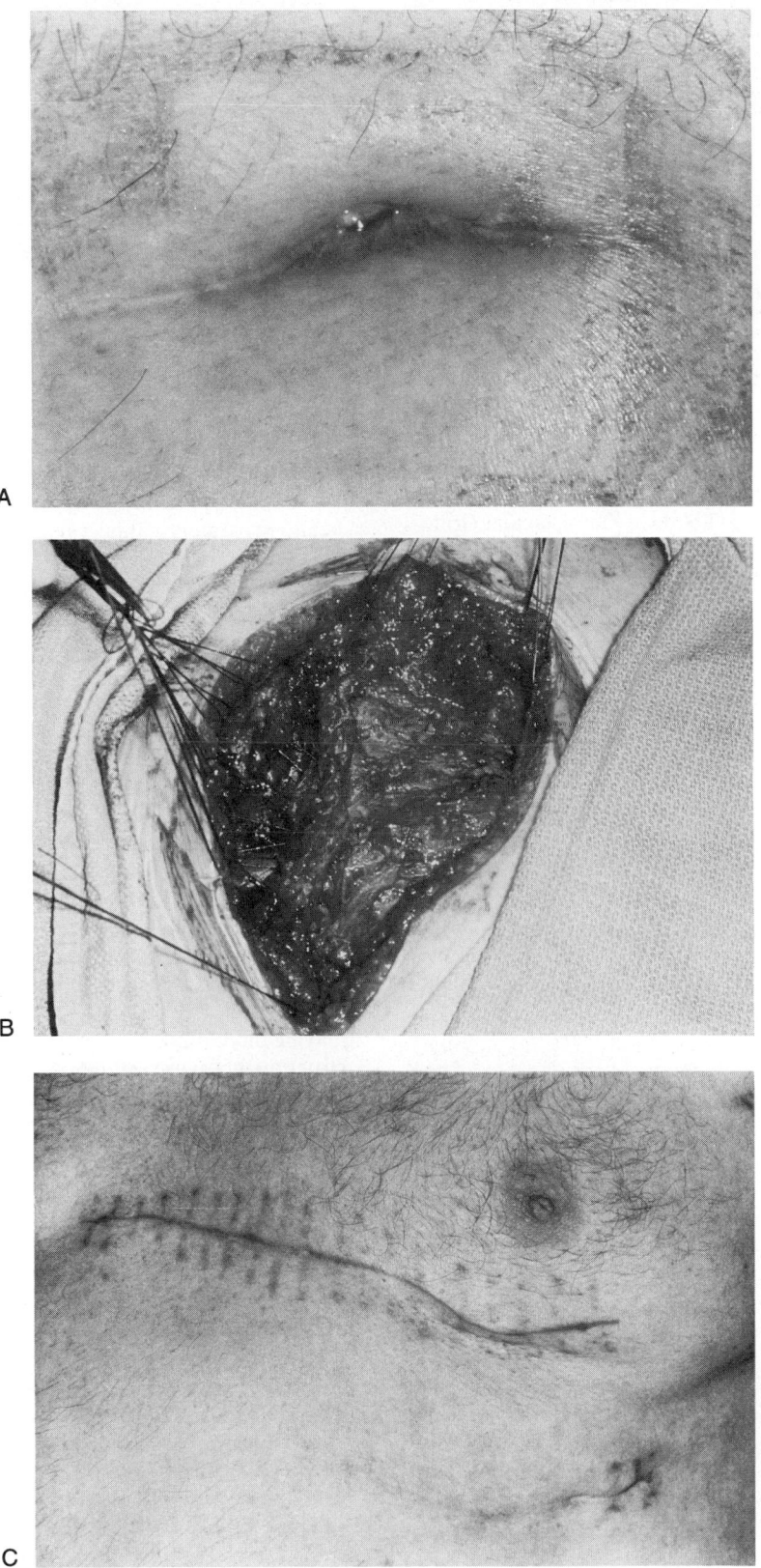

Figure 69-2. Chest wall infection: (**A**) Photograph of a chronic sinus of the anterior chest wall still draining despite previous attempts at resection. (**B**) Pectoralis major muscle flap used to reconstruct the defect after wide excision of all necrotic cartilages. (**C**) Complete healing of the wound.

Table 69-1. Etiologic Classification[a] of Lung Hernias with Relative Frequencies

Type	Frequency
Congenital: Rib or intercostal hypoplasia or agenesis	18%
Acquired:	
Traumatic	52%
Pathologic or spontaneous	30%

[a] Classification based on that of Morel-Lavelle A: iternies du poumon. Bull Soc Chir Paris 1:75, 1847

(Data from Hiscoe Band Digman J: Types and incidence of lung hernias. J Thorac Cardiovasc Surg 30:335, 1955; and from Forty J, Wells FC: Traumatic intercostal pulmonary hernia. Ann Thorac Surg 49:670, 1990.)

addition, four of the eight patients had a vertical fracture of the posterior cricoid plate with a tracheoesophageal fistula. All these patients were successfully managed by tracheal and subglottic resection (Fig. 69-4), with reconstruction by primary laryngeal anastomosis (Maddaus et al., 1992; Pearson et al, 1986; Pearson et al, 1975). In Mathisen and Grillo's series (1987), 17 patients were treated for delayed traumatic laryngotracheal stenosis, and the laryngotracheal junction or

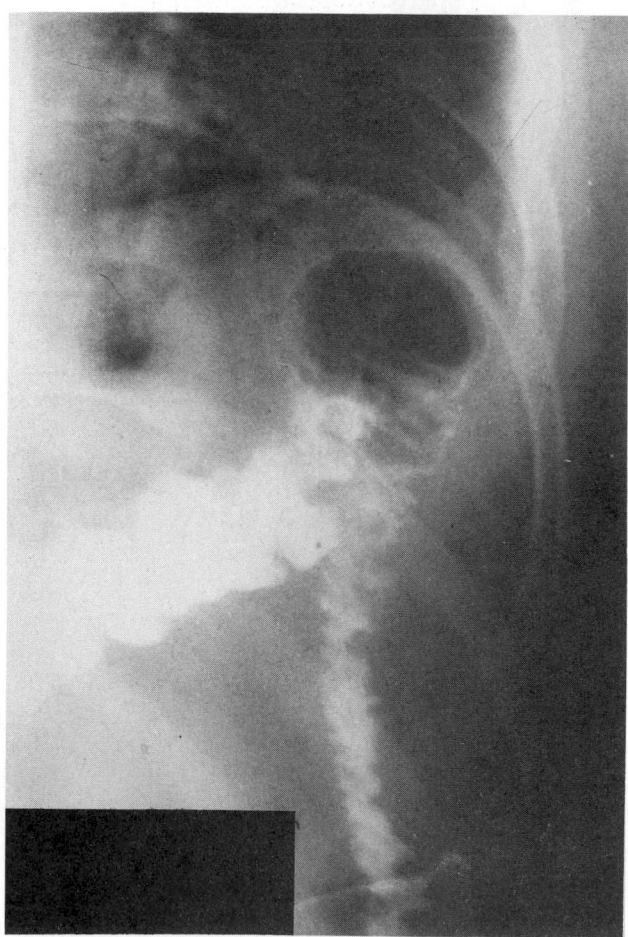

Figure 69-3. Transdiaphragmatic intercostal hernia: barium enema showing a left-sided diaphragmatic hernia and a defect in the anterolateral chest wall in a 33-year-old man previously involved in a car accident.

upper trachea was involved in 11 patients. Results of surgery were good in 16 of the 17 patients, with the airway not limiting them in their activities.

Intrathoracic Trachea and Main Bronchi

Most intrathoracic tracheobronchial injuries occur within 2.5 cm of the carina. In the acute phase, the clinical presentation depends on the size and location of the rupture and most importantly, on the presence or absence of free communication with the pleural space.

If the rupture does not communicate with the pleural space and bronchial continuity is preserved by surrounding peribronchial tissues, the clinical presentation may be subtle and the diagnosis can be missed (Deslauriers, 1987). A stricture will develop at the site of rupture. Within 4 to 6 weeks saccular bronchiectasis and irreversible parenchymal damage may develop (Fig. 69-5).

When complete rupture is missed, each of the two stumps heals separately, this eventually causes obstruction of the airway, with distal atelectasis. These patients either may be asymptomatic or they may present with signs of arterial desaturation secondary to intrapulmonary shunting (Deslauriers, et al, 1981; Deslauriers, 1987).

Management depends on the presence or absence of distal suppuration. If there is no infection, lung preservation is usually possible no matter how long the interval between the initial injury and the repair (Fig. 69-6). Pulmonary resection is usually required when there is distal suppuration. When a pulmonary resection is carried out, reinforcement of the bronchial stump with well vascularized autologous local tissues such as the intercostal muscle should be considered.

The surgical principles involved in the repair of posttraumatic bronchial strictures are the same as in any other tracheobronchial reconstruction. Proper exposure of the site of injury is essential, but extensive dissection with bronchial devascularization should be avoided. Suturing may be more difficult than in other cases of bronchial reconstruction becsause of dense peribronchial scarred tissues (Deslauriers and Bussières, 1989). Occasionally, fibrosis and loss of elasticity of the lung will prevent re-expansion despite adequate reconstruction. In these cases resection may be necessary.

Lynn and Iyengar (1972) reported excellent functional results in most patients who underwent reconstruction within 6 months of injury. They found, from a literature review (Lynn and Iyengar 1972), that early repair is best, not only to ensure more complete recovery of function but also to prevent irreversible fibrosis or pulmonary infection. In 1953 Webb and Burford reported the results of their experimental studies of the re-expanded lung after prolonged atelectasis. Dog lungs that had been atelectatic for 3, 3½, and 7½ months re-expanded readily and completely, had a normal pattern of blood flow by angiocardiogram, and oxygenated the blood flowing through the lung.

Mahaffey, et al. (1956), Logeais, et al. (1970), and Nonoyama, et al. (1976) reported successful reconstruction of the airway 4, 8, and 9 years, respectively, after the initial injury. The patient reported by Nonoyama, et al. (1976) showed progressive improvement in pulmonary function following

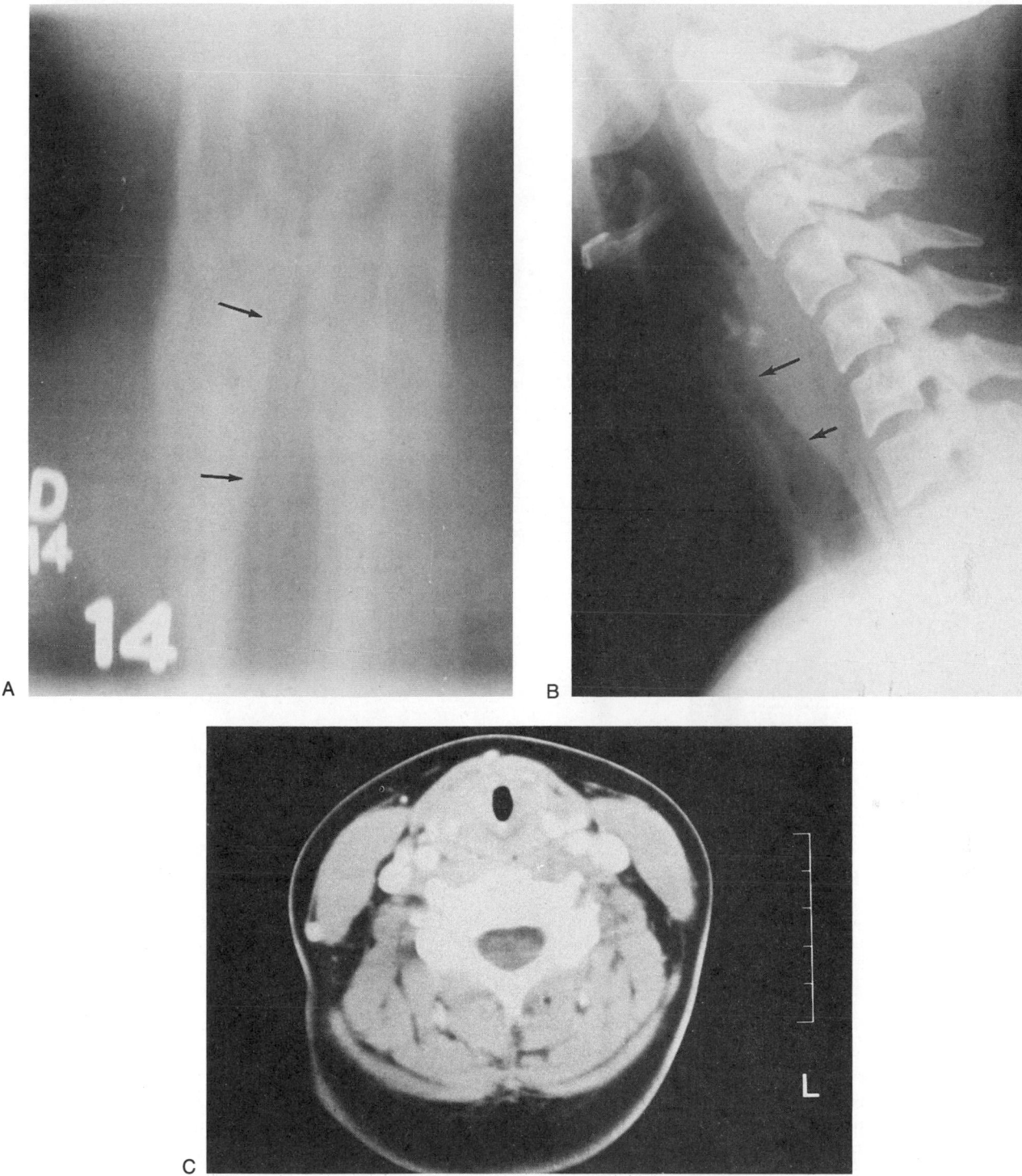

Figure 69-4. Post-traumatic subglottic stricture: (**A**) Posteroanterior and (**B**) lateral tomograms and (**C**) computed tomography (CT) scan of an 18-year-old woman with a post-traumatic subglottic stricture (*arrows* in Fig. A and Fig. B). The trauma had occurred at age 7 and the patient had been relatively asymptomatic for over 10 years. (*Figure continues.*)

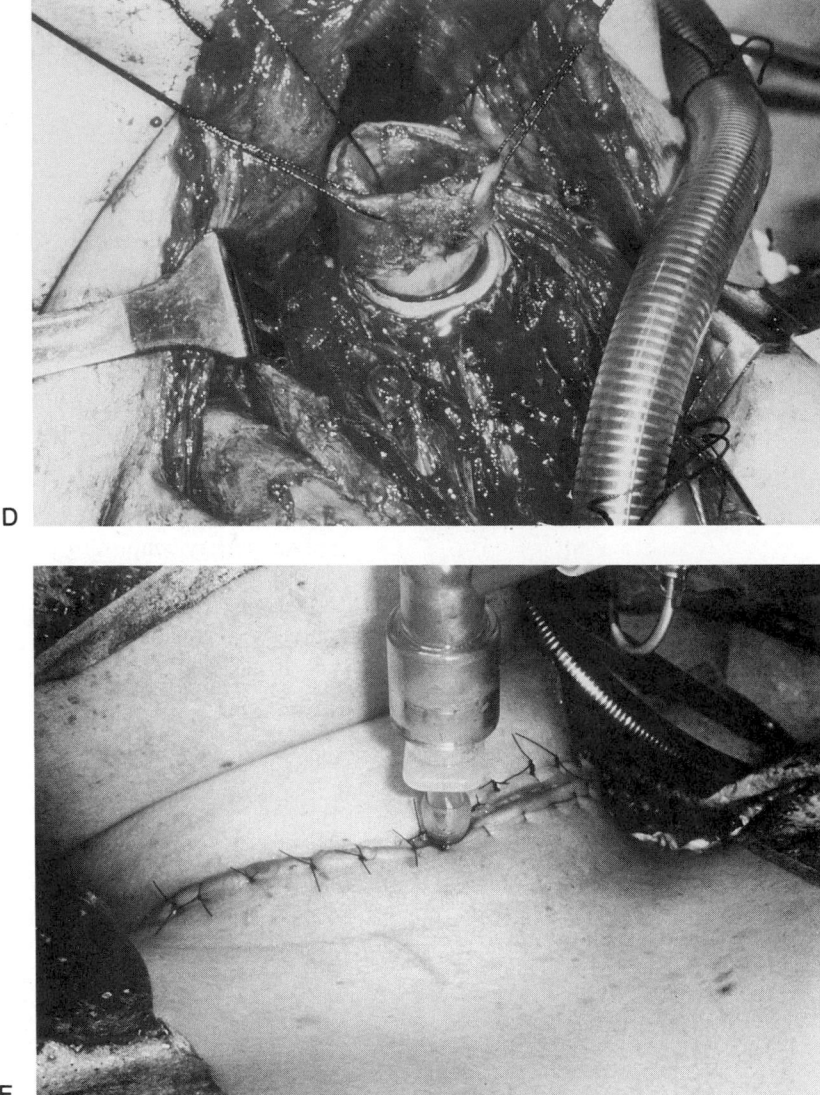

Figure 69-4 (*Continued*). (**D**) Operative photograph showing the distal trachea, which had been transected and intubated, and the proximal segment mobilized to the inferior border of the cricoid cartilage. The lower border of the cricoid plate has been exposed subperichondrially, and a rim of white posterior cartilage is clearly seen. (Courtesy of M. A. Maddaus, M.D., and F. G. Pearson, M.D.). (**E**) Completed operation with a Montgomery T tube.

delayed repair 9 years after injury. Although they were slightly reduced from predicted, oxygen uptake and vital capacity in the reimplanted lung returned to almost normal 2 months after direct anastomosis. Partial return of pulmonary function should therefore be expected following resection of a post-traumatic bronchial stricture even after prolonged intervals between injury and repair (Deslauriers, et al., 1981).

Tracheoesophageal and Bronchoesophageal Fistulae

Most combined injuries to the trachea and esophagus associated with penetrating cervical trauma are recognized and repaired early (Kelly, et al., 1987). Following blunt trauma, injuries to the trachea and esophagus may not be immediately

recognized, either because of lack of symptoms or because of the extent of associated injuries.

Tracheoesophageal fistulae may develop in the upper cervical region in association with fracture of the cricoid cartilage and cricotracheal separation or as a complication of prolonged intubation. They may also occur at or near the carina, where they are secondary to a tear of the membranous trachea, with partial disruption of the esophageal wall, necrosis, and eventually fistula formation. Layton, et al. (1980) have shown that at the moment of impact, there is an immediate laceration of the membranous trachea, which seals rapidly, and a contusion of the anterior wall of the esophagus, which progresses to necrosis, probably accelerated by infection. In 3 to 5 days a fistula between the trachea and esophagus is

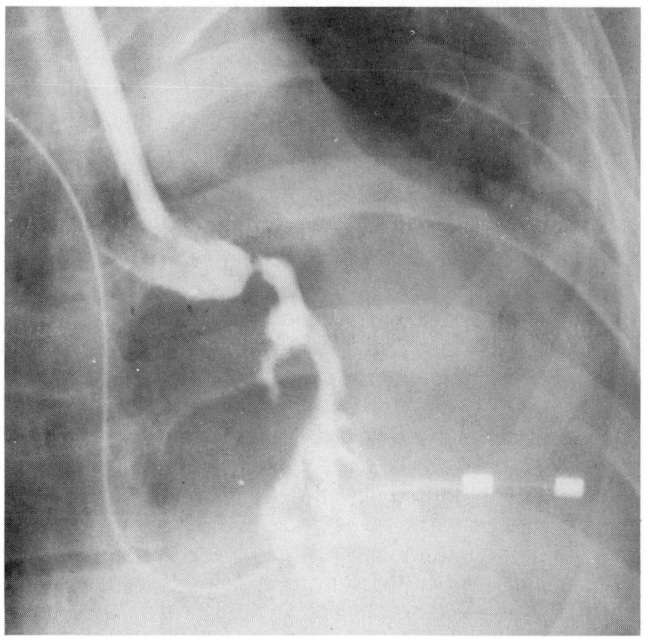

Figure 69-5. Post-traumatic bronchial stricture: Post-traumatic left main bronchial stricture with distal bronchiectasis. This patient required a left pneumonectomy.

established. In a review of the literature (Layton, et al., 1980), 71 percent of fistulae (24 of 35) were at or just above the carina, and in five cases the fistula was located in the cervical esophagus.

A collar incision is used for a cervical fistula, and a right posterolateral thoracotomy is the best approach for a thoracic fistula. The fistula is first identified and divided, and the esophageal wall is then closed in two layers of interrupted silk sutures. The trachea often needs to be locally resected and reconstructed. Interposition of well vascularized tissues such as pleura, pericardium, or intercostal muscle between the suture lines is highly recommended in the repair of intrathoracic fistulae.

TRAUMA TO THE LUNG

Pulmonary Contusion

Although blunt thoracic trauma and missile injury often cause acute pulmonary contusion, significant late sequelae are rare even if the contused lung becomes infected. Hanning, et al. (1981) noted, however, that over half of the survivors of pulmonary contusion may have increased respiratory symptoms, presenting as worsening of productive cough and wheezing. In their series prevalence of respiratory symptoms after injury was greater than expected, with 23 survivors (27 percent) claiming a persistent productive cough, 18 (21 percent) a persistent wheezing, and 22 (26 percent) grade 2

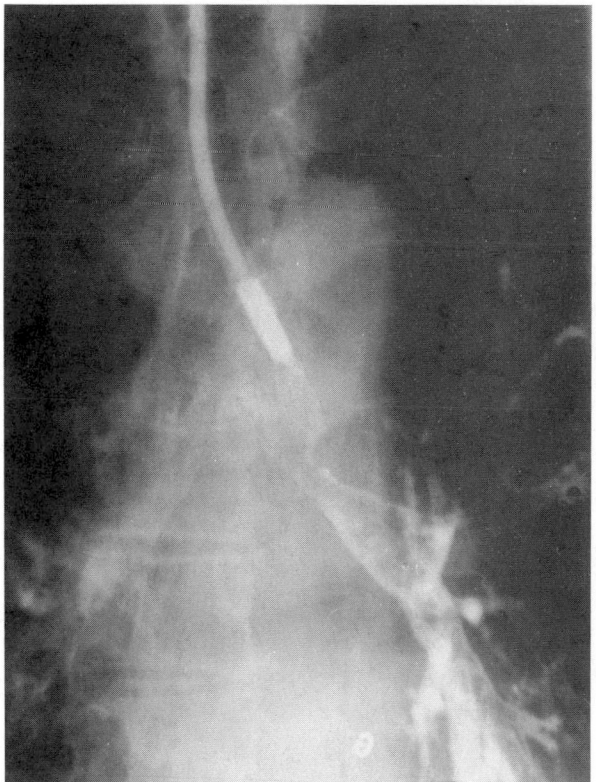

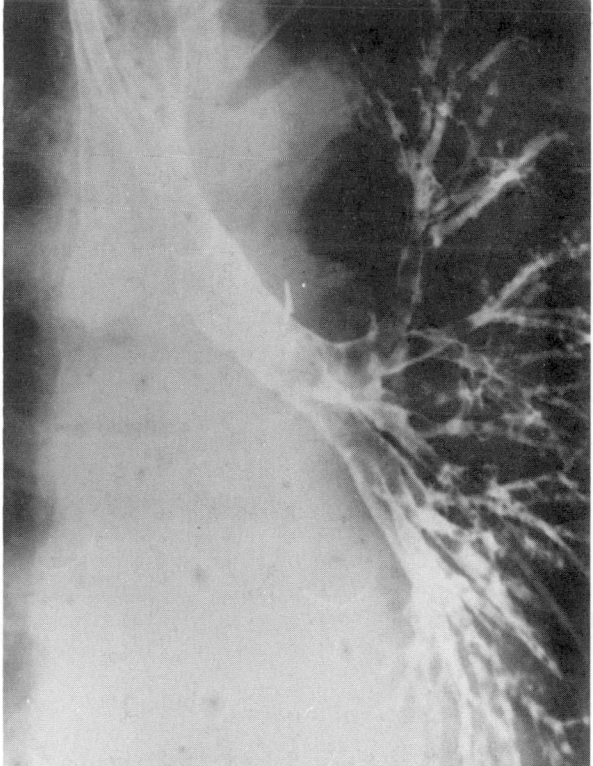

A

B

Figure 69-6. Post-traumatic bronchial stricture: (**A**) Bronchogram showing a post-traumatic stricture of the left main bronchus. (**B**) Repeat bronchogram 4 years after resection and reanastomosis.

dyspnea. Persistent productive cough (P <0.05) and occasional wheezing (P <0.01) were more common among smokers and exsmokers than among nonsmokers (Haning, et al., 1981).

Pseudocyst and Hematoma

Traumatic pulmonary pseudocyst and lung hematoma are closely related sequelae of shearing injury to the pulmonary tissue. If the lesion has no communication with an airway, a pulmonary hematoma will develop; if it communicates with the airway, a traumatic pulmonary pseudocyst will be formed (Kato, et al., 1989). If there is hemorrhage or exudation into the pseudocyst, an air-fluid level will be visible until blood or exudate is reabsorbed or drained. Other possible mechanisms of post-traumatic pulmonary pseudocyst formation include disruption of the wall of the small bronchus in conjunction with increased intrabronchial pressure (Fagan, 1966) or increased pressure with rupture in areas distal to a traumatically occluded bronchus (Fagan and Swischuk, 1976). In a review of the literature, Santos and Mahendra (1979) noted that most reported traumatic lung pseudocysts occurred in children or young adults, suggesting that the lung is more fragile in young individuals than in older patients.

The clinical picture depends on the size of the cavity and the importance of the associated pulmonary contusion. About 40 percent of patients present with cough or hemoptysis. Unless they become infected, most pseudocysts resolve spontaneously over a period of a few months. In the series of Kato et al. (1989), all 12 traumatic pulmonary pseudocysts resolved without any specific treatment, and late sequelae were only those of radiologic scarring in an area of previous lung injury. In 1990 Ulstad, et al. reported a patient whose bilateral post-traumatic paramediastinal lung cysts were presumed to be bilateral hemidiaphragmatic hernias, which led to unnecessary surgery.

Pulmonary Arteriovenous Fistula and Pulmonary Artery Aneurysm

Rarely, penetrating or blunt trauma to the thorax will cause a pulmonary arteriovenous fistula or a pulmonary artery aneurysm. These lesions should be suspected in patients with a history of trauma, signs and symptoms of pulmonary arteriovenous fistula with shunting (Arom and Lyons, 1975), and chronic residual, well circumscribed density on chest x-ray. The diagnosis can be confirmed by pulmonary arteriography. Excision of the lesion with preservation of the lung whenever possible or resection of the involved lobe is the therapy (Symbas, et al., 1980) of choice. Embolization by coils or other foreign material has seldom been reported in the management of past-traumatic pulmonary arteriovenous fistulae.

TRAUMA TO THE PLEURAL SPACE

Chronic empyemas and fibrothoraces with entrapped lung are often the result of undrained or inadequately drained traumatic hemothoraces. Incomplete drainage leads to clot formation, loculation of the pleural space, and organization of the collection (see Chs. 37 and 42).

Hemothorax

Culiner, et al. (1959), Milfeld, et al. (1978) and Coselli, et al. (1984) have recommended early thoracotomy for residual hemothoraces because of their significant potential for empyema and/or fibrothorax development. In the series of Milfeld et al. (1978), 85 (3.3 percent) of 3,000 patients with hemothorax or pneumohemothorax developed a clotted hemothorax or post-traumatic empyema. Among 10 patients undergoing evacuation of a clotted hemothorax within 5 days of admission, there was zero mortality and an average hospital stay of 10 days. Among 41 patients undergoing decortication more than 5 days after injury, there was one death (for a 2.4 percent mortality), while among 34 patients requiring decortication and drainage of empyema, 4 died (12 percent mortality), and the average hospital stay was 41 days. By contrast, Wilson, et al. (1979) concluded that early thoracotomy was often unneccessary. They reviewed the management and results in 452 patients with hemothorax caused by penetrating ($n = 338$) or blunt trauma ($n = 114$). The overall incidence of empyema was 4.9 percent, and this incidence was not changed by thoracotomy or by the presence of residual hemothorax. Shock, pleural contamination, pneumonia, and duration of pleural catheter drainage were found to be significant variables. We currently use videothoracoscopic techniques to remove residual clots that may still remain in the pleural space after trauma. This technique is far less invasive than thoracotomy, and probably achieves the same overall result.

Empyema

Post-traumatic empyema is defined as an empyema that develops secondary to infection of a traumatic hemothorax (Symbas, 1989). It is usually related to incomplete drainage of intrapleural blood, with contamination either from an open thoracic wound, from the chest tube, or from an infection in the adjacent lung. Predisposing factors (box 1) include delay in initial chest tube insertion, improper positioning or unnecessary manipulations of the tube, tube occlusion, prolonged drainage (Eddy, et al., 1989) or the presence of an intrapleural foreign body. Larger hemothoraces (more than 500 ml) are more likely to become infected (Young, et al., 1972; Ogilvie, 1950) (Table 69-2) than smaller ones. Residual pneumothorax

---

Predisposing Factors for the Development of Post-traumatic Empyemas

Delay in initial chest tube insertion
Improper positioning of the tube
Manipulations of the tube
Tube occlusion
Large hemothoraces (>500 ml)
Pneumohemothoraces
Foreign body driven into pleural space
Open thoracic wounds
Bronchopneumonia
Diaphragmatic perforation
Extrapleural hematomas

Table 69-2. Size of Hemothorax in Relation to Pleural Infection

| | Number of Hemothoraces | | | Percentage |
Size	Sterile	Infected	Total	Infected
Large	123	43	166	26%
Small	57	7	64	11%
Total	180	50	230	22%

(From Ogilvie AG: Final results in traumatic haemothorax: a report of 230 cases. Thorax 5:116, 1950, with permission.)

(incomplete reexpansion of the lung or loculated spaces), missed diaphragm perforation, lung contusion, and extrapleural hematomas are other factors considered important in the development of post-traumatic empyemas (Hix, 1984; Villalba, et al., 1979).

Post-traumatic empyemas should be treated in the same way as empyemas of other etiologies. The principles of management include adequate drainage of the collection, lung re-expansion, and obliteration of the pleural space. Arom, et al. (1977) recommend early decortication as soon as pleural infection is evident and cannot be controlled by closed tube drainage. With early decortication and immediate removal of infected peel, chronic empyema with additional weeks of disability is prevented, and the patient is spared considerable discomfort (Arom, et al., 1977). Neef (1991) also recommends early debridement if suction drainage does not achieve complete expansion of the lung.

Fibrothorax

Post-traumatic fibrothorax is the presence of abnormal fibrous tissue within the pleural space. As an end-stage manifestation of an undrained or incompletely drained hemothorax, it causes entrapment and loss of function of the lung (see Ch. 42).

Decortication is indicated to remove the fibrous tissue and allow the lung to re-expand. Successful surgery will generally improve pulmonary function and lower the incidence of infection in the underlying lung (Petty, et al., 1961; Siebens, et al., 1956).

Chylothorax

Traumatic chylothorax is an accumulation of chyle in the pleural space secondary to an injury to the thoracic duct. Although most of these injuries are iatrogenic, chylothoraces can occur with vertebral fractures, with hyperextension injuries of the spine, or even after violent coughing or vomiting. Penetrating trauma of the thoracic duct is highly unusual. Chylothoraces will often only become apparent and/or symptomatic 4 to 6 weeks after the injury.

TRAUMA TO THE ESOPHAGUS

Because of its protected position, small size, and resiliency, the esophagus is rarely the site of trauma. In 1973 Andréassiam, et al. reported 63 cases (collective review), and most were secondary to blunt thoracic trauma incurred in high-speed motor vehicle accidents. Isolated ruptures of the cervical esophagus (Niezgoda, et al., 1990) or of the abdominal esophagus (Barrié, et al., 1961) are extremely unusual.

Late sequelae of esophageal injuries include stricture or fistula formation. Strictures are secondary to ischemia or initial loss of tissue, and most can be treated by dilatation alone, although resection and reconstruction of the esophagus may occasionally be necessary. Fistulae between the esophagus and the pleural space, airway, aorta, and pericardium have all been described as results of undetected perforations of the esophagus due to external trauma.

Most esophagopleural fistulae present as empyemas, and their diagnosis can readily be confirmed by a barium swallow. As with any other type of esophageal perforation, management of an established esophagopleural fistula depends on the location and extent of injury, the local inflammatory reaction, the degree of pleural contamination, the significance of associated injuries, and the overall condition of the patient.

TRAUMA TO THE DIAPHRAGM

Like many other injuries previously considered rare, diaphragmatic rupture is being reported with increasing frequency (see Ch. 51). This relates not only to a net increase in the number of high-speed motor vehicle accidents but also to a higher index of suspicion of this type of injury. When the diagnosis of blunt diaphragmatic injury is missed, the most likely sequela is either a chronic herniation of abdominal contents in the pleural space or an eventration.

Diaphragmatic Hernia

Chronic post-traumatic diaphragmatic hernias are usually seen in patients previously involved in deceleration injuries. Because of the extent of associated injuries, the diagnosis is overlooked at the time of injury, and often the typical radiologic signs are obscured by the presence of atelectasis, hemopneumothorax, pulmonary contusion, or subcutaneous emphysema. Patients with chronic post-traumatic diaphragmatic hernia may be asymptomatic or may present with minor symptoms such as postprandial chest pain and dyspnea (Childress and Grimes, 1961). The time between injury and diagnosis ranges from months to years before, but an average figure in the literature is about 10 years after the initial trauma (Mansour, et al., 1975). At this stage the diagnosis can again be missed because the radiologic signs are falsely attributed to late pleural sequelae. However, the diagnosis should be suspected when standard chest radiographs show elevation of the diaphragmatic shadow, an abdominal viscus within the pleural space, or a contralateral mediastinal shift. Additional studies that may be helpful are computed tomography (CT) scanning, gastroesophageal contrast studies, and pneumoperitoneum. This last study, in which 500 ml of air is introduced into the peritoneal cavity, is diagnostic in virtually all cases. When the diagnosis is still not made or the hernia is unrepaired, the patient will eventually go on to incarcerate or strangulate the contents of the hernia, an event more likely to occur with left-sided hernias (Estrera, et al., 1985).

Because of the high likelihood of incarceration (Fig. 69-7) or strangulation, surgical repair of a traumatic diaphragmatic

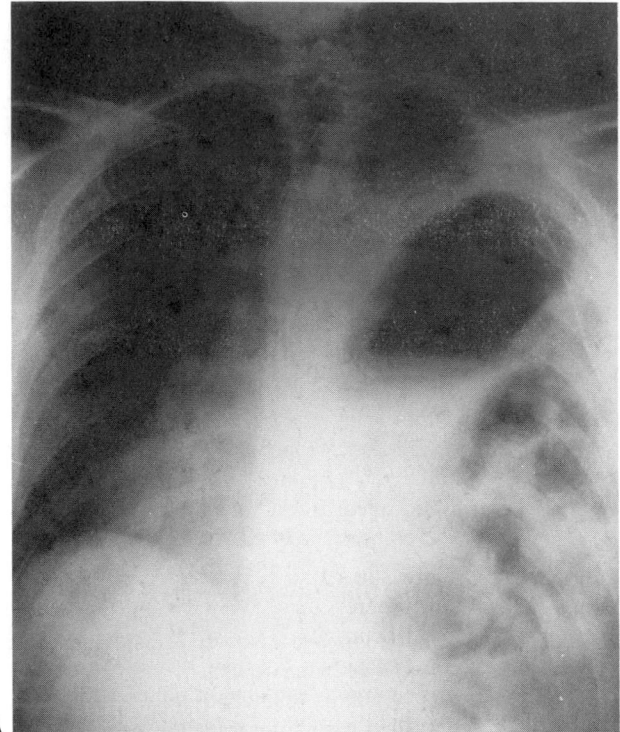
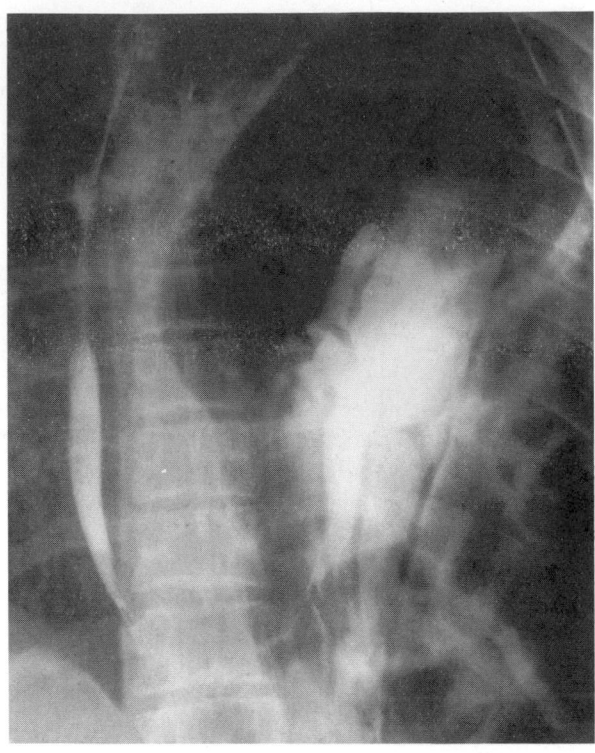

Figure 69-7. Chronic diaphragmatic hernia. (**A**) Posteroanterior chest radiograph and (**B**) barium swallow of a 25-year-old man with incarcerated stomach in a left-sided traumatic diaphragmatic hernia. (*Figure continues.*)

hernia is always indicated when the diagnosis is made. On the right side, the repair is best accomplished through a right posterolateral seventh interspace thoracotomy, whereas on the left side, controversy exists as to whether it should be done by the transthoracic or transabdominal route. Because of often dense adhesions between the contents of the hernia and the lung, we prefer the transthoracic approach. Unless infected or necrotic tissues exist within the hernia, the morbidity and mortality rates associated with the repair of a diaphragmatic hernia are low and the long-term results excellent.

Diaphragmatic Eventration

Post-traumatic eventration of the diaphragm can be caused either by an injury to the phrenic nerve or by partial disruption of the diaphragmatic muscle itself (Waldschmidt and Laws, 1980). The chest x-ray shows an elevated hemidiaphragm, and paralysis of the diaphragm can be confirmed by fluoroscopy. Surgical correction is never indicated before 6 to 8 months have elapsed after the injury, because the diaphragm will often resume its normal position and function during this interval. Plication of the diaphragm may be indicated in patients in whom there is evidence of respiratory restriction due to lung compression.

TRAUMA TO THE HEART AND GREAT VESSELS

Late sequelae of thoracic injuries to the heart and the great vessels are rare and have generated very few reports (Sturaitis, et al., 1986; Antunes, et al., 1988; Hix and Aaron, 1987;

Deslauriers, et al., 1991). Less than 5 percent of survivors from penetrating wounds of the heart and great vessels will have symptomatic sequelae up to 10 years after the injury. Complete recovery from myocardial contusion associated with blunt chest trauma is also the rule if complications are promptly recognized and properly managed (Sturaitis, et al., 1986).

Penetrating Cardiac Trauma

Because of the initial cardiac tamponade, intra- or extracardiac shunts may be unrecognized at the time of trauma, only to become symptomatic and functionally significant when the perforation becomes larger as a result of fibrous contraction of its edges. Although the prevalence of extracardiac shunts is unknown, Antunes, et al. (1988) reported an incidence, as late sequelae, of 42 percent in a series of 31 patients.

Symptoms are usually those of congestive heart failure, and the shunt can easily be documented by noninvasive techniques such as Doppler echocardiography (Sturaitis, et al., 1986; Antunes, et al., 1988; Kirklin and Barratt-Boyes, 1993). Intracardiac shunts include ventricular septal defects and fistulae between the aorta and either the right atrium or the right ventricle or between the left ventricle and the right atrium. The most common post-traumatic extracardiac shunts are between the aorta and the innominate vein or between the aorta and the main pulmonary artery. Surgical repair is always indicated and should be carried out by standard techniques.

Lacerations of cardiac valves, particularly of the tricuspid or pulmonary valves, can also occur and be diagnosed late

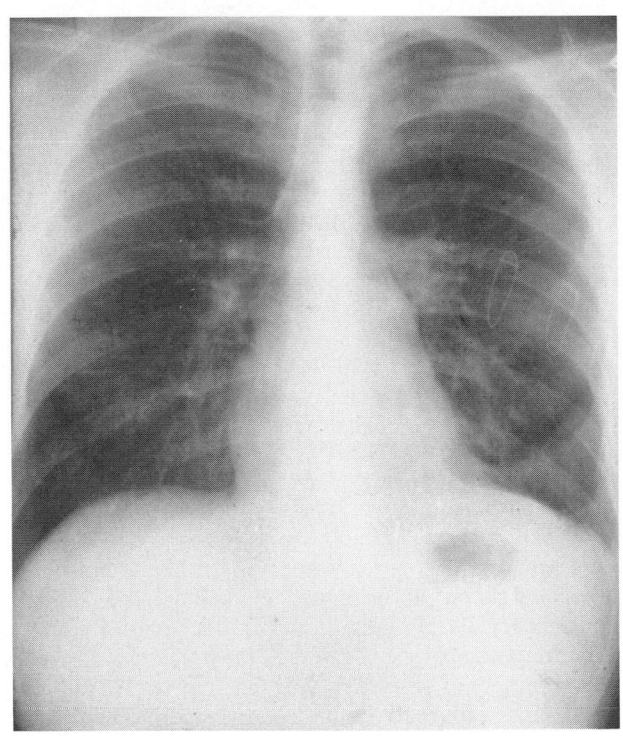

C

Figure 69-7 (*Continued*). (**C**) Postoperative chest radiograph showing the repaired hemidiaphragm in normal position.

after the trauma. These lacerations can be safely repaired (Antunes, et al., 1988; Symbas, 1989), although recovery may be impaired by traumatic neurosis, a syndrome similar to that seen in patients who have sustained violent and major abdominal trauma (Abbott, et al., 1978).

Blunt Cardiac Trauma

Post-traumatic left ventricular aneurysms were described in 1892, but since then very few cases have been reported. In a recent literature review only 35 documented cases could be found (Grieco, et al., 1989). In this review, the interval between injury and diagnosis ranged from 5 days to 18 years (with a median of 3 months), and in most cases associated coronary artery disease rather than myocardial contusion was implicated as the possible cause of aneurysm. The thin walls of post-traumatic ventricular aneurysms and their liability to rupture indicate surgical resection in most patients with this problem (Kirklin and Barratt-Boyes, 1993). Grieco, et al. (1989) noted that 10 of 12 patients treated conservatively died from complications directly attributed to the aneurysm.

Tricuspid incompetence from chordal or papillary muscle rupture is rare, and progression from injury to severe disability may take as long as 5 or even 10 years (Kirklin and Barratt-Boyes, 1993). Because of the severe disability of these patients by the time they are referred for surgery and because of the technical difficulties associated with the repair of tricuspid chordal or papillary muscles, tricuspid valve replacement by a bioprosthetis is the procedure of choice.

Coronary artery injuries may cause angina or heart failure as late sequelae of blunt trauma, usually in patients with previous arteriosclerotic coronary artery disease. In such patients both the intimal tear with secondary thrombosis and platelet aggregation and the myocardial contusion contribute to occlude the coronary artery. Blunt chest trauma may also occlude aortocoronary bypass grafts.

Coronary artery fistulae have been reported as sequelae of penetrating trauma (Lowe, et al., 1983). In the series of Lowe, et al., the cause of fistula was a penetrating trauma in 80 percent of patients and a blunt injury in 20 percent. The right and left coronary arteries were equally involved, and the fistula was between the coronary artery and right ventricle in 50 percent of patients and between the coronary and right atrium in 35 percent.

Atrial septal rupture is a rare sequela, which has been diagnosed from months up to 5 years after trauma. The delay in diagnosis is often related to the severity of associated injuries, as trauma of major proportion is required to rupture the atrial septum (Jenson, et al., 1993).

Great Vessels

Traumatic rupture of the thoracic aorta is responsible for approximately 10 percent of all deaths due to blunt trauma (Desaulniers and Bruneau, 1972), but because of associated injuries or lack of suspicion, the diagnosis is often overlooked or missed completely at the time of injury. Indeed, Utley (1987) reported that the interval between trauma and diagnosis of aneurysm is longer than 10 years in about half of the patients. Symptoms are usually those of compression of adjacent organs, such as the lung, esophagus, or recurrent nerve.

Post-traumatic aneurysms of the descending aorta should always be resected, even in asymptomatic patients, because in contrast with arteriosclerotic aortic aneurysms, the aortic wall is held in place only by the adventitia, these aneurysms being in fact false aneurysms. We recommend that while repairing a chronic post-traumatic aneurysm, a temporary shunt (Verdant, et al., 1988) or partial heart-lung bypass be used in association with an autotransfusion system. Since this is an elective procedure, every precaution to prevent spinal cord ischemia and blood loss should be taken. Because of significant operative morbidity and mortality, resection of arch aneurysms is only indicated in patients in whom the lesion is symptomatic or enlarging.

Pericardium

Post-traumatic constrictive pericarditis was first described by Goldstein and Yu (1965). It is rare, probably secondary to a local post-traumatic immune reaction (Blake, et al., 1983). Indications for pericardectomy are based on clinical and hemodynamic symptoms. Results of surgery are similar to those obtained after pericardectomy for pericarditis due to other causes.

MISCELLANEOUS COMPLICATIONS OF TRAUMA TO THE CHEST

Traumatic Asphyxia

In 1837 Ollivier d'Angers described the syndrome of traumatic asphyxia on the basis of autopsy results in 23 patients who had suffered thoracic compression as victims of a panic in Paris (Glinz, 1991). The term *traumatic asphyxia* was introduced by Burrell and Crandon (1899) to designate the clinical picture of bluish-red discoloration of the head and neck caused by petechiae secondary to acute, severe compression by the chest, which produces a massive increase of intrathoracic pressure, resulting in increased central venous pressure (Glinz, 1991). Most patients will survive the acute episode and the syndrome will gradually disappear. Late sequelae are rare, but lasting neurologic impairment (Sandiford and Sickler, 1974) or chronic vena cava thrombosis (Daughtry, 1980) have been reported. Because of this last potential problem, patients may benefit from long-term anticoagulation.

Thoracic Outlet Syndrome

In 1973 Mulder, et al. reported seven patients who developed varying forms of the thoracic outlet syndrome following trauma to the clavicle, shoulder, first rib, or cervical spine. The signs and symptoms were different for each patient and depended on the location and degree of neurovascular compression. Traumatic disruption of the first rib potentially narrows the interscalene triangle and may result in mechanical compression of the brachial plexus and subclavian artery, while injuries to the clavicle compromise the costoclavicular space (Mulder, et al., 1973). Management of these patients is the same as that of patients with thoracic outlet syndrome due to other causes. Untreated effort thrombosis of the axillary vein can lead to chronic venous insufficiency of the involved limb.

Thoracic Splenosis

Thoracic splenosis is a rare entity in which autotransplantation of splenic tissue occurs in the pleural cavity after combined splenic and diaphragmatic injury (Roucos, et al., 1990). It was first reported by Shaw and Shafi (1937). Preoperative diagnosis of thoracic splenosis depends on a high index of suspicion in patients who have a mass or masses in the left hemithorax that on CT scan appear to be subpleural and scattered in the chest who also have a history of thoracoabdominal trauma with splenectomy (Roucos, et al., 1990). If the diagnosis of thoracic splenosis is well documented, surgery is usually unnecessary.

CONCLUSION

Late sequelae of thoracic trauma are rare and most can be prevented by proper understanding and management of the initial injury. When they do occur, successful therapy depends on a complete evaluation of the problem before undertaking surgery or other measures that may lead to more damage. This is especially true in complicated problems related to sequelae of airway trauma, where hurried surgery may lead to irreversible disabilities.

KEY REFERENCES

Hix WR: Residua of thoracic trauma. Surg Gynecol Obstet 158:295, 1984

Collective review summarizing all late sequelae of thoracic injuries. Good description of pathogenesis and principles of management.

Hix WR, Aaron BL: Residua of Thoracic Trauma. Futura Publishing, Mount Kisco, NY 1987

Excellent volume detailing all sequelae of thoracic injuries.

Maddaus MA, Toth JLR, Gullane PJ, Pearson FG: Subglottic tracheal resection and synchronous laryngeal reconstruction. J Thorac Cardiovasc Surg 104:1443, 1992

Excellent review of indications for surgery, operative techniques, and results for patients with postintubation or post-traumatic laryngotracheal strictures.

REFERENCES

Abbott JA, Cousineau BS, Cheitlin M et al: Late sequelae of penetrating cardiac wounds. J Thorac Cardiovasc Surg 75:510, 1978

Andréassiam B, Lacombe M, Nussaume O et al: Ruptures de l'oesophage par traumatisme fermé. Ann Chir 12:409, 1973

Antunes MJ, Fernandes LE, Oliveira JM: Ventricular septal defects and arteriovenous fistulas, with and without valvular lesions, resulting from penetrating injury to the heart and aorta. J Thorac Cardiovasc Surg 95:902, 1988

Arom KV, Grover FL, Richardson JD, Trinkle JK: Post-traumatic empyema. Ann Thorac Surg 23:254, 1977

Arom KV, Lyons GW: Traumatic pulmonary arteriovenous fistula. J Thorac Cardiovasc Surg 70:918, 1975

Barrié J, Sarrazin R, Bonnett-Eymard J: Rupture traumatique de l'oesophage abdominal. Mem Acad 87:662, 1961

Blake S, Bonar S, O'Neill H et al: Aetiology of chronic constrictive pericarditis. Br Heart J 50:273, 1983

Brown RB, Trenton J: Chronic abscesses and sinuses of the chest wall. Ann Surg 135:44, 1952

Burrell HL, Crandon LRG: Traumatic apnea or asphyxia. Boston Med Surg J 51:599, 1899

Campbell DC, Swindell HV, Dominy DE: Delayed repair of rupture of the bronchus. J Thorac Cardiovasc Surg 43:320, 1962

Childress ME, Grimes OF: Immediate and remote sequelae in traumatic diaphragmatic hernia. Surg Gynecol Obstet 113:573, 1961

Cole FH, Miller MP, Jones CV: Transdiaphragmatic intercostal hernia. Ann Thorac Surg 41:565, 1986

Coselli JS, Mattox KL, Beall AC Jr: Reevaluation of early evacuation of clotted hemothorax. Am J Surg 148:786, 1984

Culiner MM, Roe BR, Grimes OF: The early elective surgical approach to the treatment of traumatic hemothorax. J Thorac Cardiovasc Surg 38:780, 1959 d'Angers O: Relation médicale des événements survenus au Champ-de-Mars 14 juin 1837. Ann Hyg Publique Med Legale 18:485, 1837

Daughtry DC: Thoracic Trauma. Little, Brown, Boston, 1980, p. 198

Desaulniers D, Bruneau L: Rupture traumatique de l'aorte thoracique. Union Med Can 101:1055, 1972

Deslauriers J: Bronchial rupture. p. 246. In Grillo HG, Eschapasse H (eds): Major Challenges. In International Trends in General Thoracic Surgery. Vol. 2. CV Mosby. St. Louis, 1987

Deslauriers J, Beaulieu M, Archambault G et al: Diagnosis and long-term follow-up of major bronchial disruptions due to nonpenetrating trauma. Ann Thorac Surg 33:32, 1981

Deslauriers J, Bussières J: Bronchial rupture. p. 42. In Grillo HC, et al. (eds): Current Therapy in Cardiothoracic Surgery. BC Decker, Philadelphia, 1989

Deslauriers J, Desaulniers D, Pomerleau S, Sasseville N: Late sequelae of thoracic injuries. p. 513. In Webb WR, Besson A (eds): Thoracic Surgery: Surgical Management of Chest Injuries. Vol. 7. In International Trends in General Thoracic Surgery. CV Mosby, St. Louis, 1991

Eddy AC, Luna GK, Copass M: Empyema thoracis in patients undergoing emergent closed tube thoracostomy for thoracic trauma. Am J Surg 157:494, 1989

Estrera AS, Landay MJ, McClelland RN: Blunt traumatic rupture of the right hemidiaphragm: experience in 12 patients. Ann Thorac Surg 39:525, 1985

Fagan CT: Traumatic lung cyst. AJR 97:186, 1966

Fagan CT, Swischuk LE: Traumatic lung and para mediastinal pneumatoceles. Radiology 120:11, 1976

Fallahnejad M, Kutty ACK, Wallace HW: Seconary lesions of penetrating cardiac injuries. Ann Surg 191:228, 1980

Forty J, Wells FC: Traumatic intercostal pulmonary hernia. Ann Thorac Surg 49:670, 1990

Gibson LD, Carter R, Hinshaw DB: Surgical significance of sternal fracture. Surg Gynecol Obstet 144:443, 1962

Glinz W: Acute thoracic compression syndrome—"traumatic asphyxia". p. 344. In Webb WR, Besson A (eds): Thoracic Surgery: Surgical Management of Chest Injuries. In International Trends in General Thoracic Surgery. Vol. 7. CV Mosby, St. Louis, 1991

Goldstein S, Yu PN: Constrictive pericarditis after blunt chest trauma. Am Heart J 69:544, 1965

Grieco JG, Montoya A, Sullivan HJ et al: Ventricular aneurysm due to blunt chest injury, Ann Thorac Surg 47:322, 1989

Grillo HC, Moncure AC, McEnany MT: Repair of inflammatory tracheoesophageal fistula. Ann Thorac Surg 22:112, 1976

Hanning CD, Ledingham E, Ledingham IM: Late respiratory sequelae of blunt chest injury: a preliminary report. Thorax 36:204, 1981

Hiscoe B, Digman J: Types and incidence of lung hernias. J Thorac Cardiovasc Surg 30:335, 1955

Holland RH: Arteriovenous fistula of the left internal mammary vessels stimulating a patent ductus arteriosus. J Thorac Cardiovasc Surg 39:767, 1960

Jenson BP, Hoffman I, Follis FM: Surgical repair of atrial septal rupture due to blunt trauma. Ann Thorac Surg 56:1172, 1993

Kato R, Horinouchi H, Maenaka Y: Traumatic pulmonary pseudocyst. J Thorac Cardiovasc Surg 97:309, 1989

Kelly P, Webb WR, Moulder PV: Management of airway trauma. II: Combined injuries of the trachea and esophagus. Ann Thorac Surg 43:160, 1987

Ketharanathan V, Westlake GW: Traumatic arteriovenous fistula between the internal thoracic artery and vein. Aust N Z J Surg 38:278, 1969

Kirklin JW, Barratt-Boyes BG: Cardiac Surgery. Churchill Livingstone, New York, 1993

Layton TR, Dimarco RF, Pellegrini RV: Tracheoesophageal fistula from nonpenetrating trauma. J Trauma 20:802, 1980

Logeais Y, DeSaint Florent G, Danrigal A et al: Traumatic rupture of the right main bronchus in an 8 year old child successfully repaired 8 years after injury. Ann Surg 172:1039, 1970

Lowe JE, Adams DH, Cummings RG et al: The natural history and recommended management of patients with traumatic coronary artery fistulas. Ann Thorac Surg 36:295, 1983

Lynn RB, Iyengar R: Traumatic rupture of the bronchus. Chest 61:81, 1972

Mahaffey DE, Creech O, Boren HG, Debakey ME: Traumatic rupture of the left main bronchus successfully repaired eleven years after injury. J Thorac Surg 32:312, 1956

Mansour KA, Clements JL, Hatcher CR et al: Diaphragmatic hernia caused by trauma: experience with 35 cases. Am Surg 13:97, 1975

Mathisen DJ, Grillo H: Laryngotracheal trauma. Ann Thorac Surg 43:254, 1987

Milfeld DJ, Mattox KL, Beall AC Jr: Early evacuation of clotted hemothorax. Am J Surg 136:686, 1978

Miller DR, Murphy K, Cesario T: Pseudomonas infection of the sternum and costal cartilages. J Thorac Cardiovasc Surg 76:723, 1978

Morel-Lavelle A: Hernies du poumon. Bull Soc Chir Paris 1:75, 1847

Mulder DS, Greenwood AH, Brooks CE: Post-traumatic thoracic outlet syndrome. J Trauma 13:706, 1973

Munnell ER: Herniation of the lung. Ann Thorac Surg 5:204, 1968

Neef H: Post-traumatic and post-operative empyema. p. 253. In Webb WR, Besson A (eds): Thoracic Surgery: Surgical Management of Chest Injuries. In International Trends in General Thoracic Surgery. CV Mosby, St. Louis, 1991

Niezgoda JA, McMenamin P, Graeber GM: Pharyngoesophageal perforation after blunt neck trauma. Ann Thorac Surg 50:615, 1990

Nonoyama A, Masuda A, Kasahara K et al: Total rupture of the left main bronchus successfully repaired 9 years after injury. Ann Thorac Surg 21:445, 1976

Ogilvie AG: Final results in traumatic haemothorax: a report of 230 cases. Thorax 5:116, 1950

Payne WS, Cardoza F, Weed LA: Chronic draining sinuses of the chest wall. Surg Clin North Am 53:927, 1973

Pearson FG, Brito-Filomeno L, Cooper JD: Experience with partial cricoid resection and thyrotracheal anastomosis. Ann Otol Rhinol Laryngol 95:582, 1986

Pearson FG, Cooper JD, Nelems JM, Van Nostrand AWP: Primary tracheal anastomosis after resection of the cricoid cartilage with preservation of the recurrent laryngeal nerves. J Thorac Cardiovasc Surg 70:806, 1975

Petty TL, Filley GF, Mitchell RS: Objective functional improvement by decortication after twenty years of artificial pneumothorax for pulmonary tuberculosis. Report of a case and review of the literature. Am Rev Respir Dis 84:572, 1961

Pontius JG, Clagett OT, McDonald JR: Costal chondritis and perichondritis. Surgery 45:852, 1959

Ribet M: Traumatic pulmonary pseudocyst (letter). J Thorac Cardiovasc Surg 99:171, 1990

Richardson JD, Grover FL, Trinkle JK: Early operative management of isolated sternal fractures. J Trauma 15:156, 1975

Richardson JD, McElvein RB, Trinkle JK: First rib fracture: a hallmark of severe trauma. Ann of Surg 181:251, 1975

Roucos S, Tabet G, Jebara VA et al: Thoracic splenosis. Case report and literature review. J Thorac Cardiovasc Surg 99:361, 1990

Rubino PJ, Milnes RF: Internal artery arteriovenous fistula. Int Surg 55:404, 1971

Salter DG, Hapton DS: Traumatic intercostal hernia without penetrating injury in a child. Br J Surg 56:550, 1969

Sandiford JA, Sickler D: Traumatic asphyxia with severe neurological sequelae. J Trauma 14:805, 1974

Santos GH, Mahendra T: Traumatic pulmonary pseudocysts. Ann Thorac Surg 27:359, 1979

Saw EC, Yokoyama T, Lee BC et al: Intercostal pulmonary hernia. Arch Surg 111:548, 1976

Shaw AFB, Shafi A: Traumatic autoplastic transplantation of splenic tissue in man with observations on the late results of splenectomy in six cases. J Pathol 45:215, 1937

Siebens AA, Storey CF, Newman MM et al: The physiologic effects of fibrothorax and the functional results of surgical treatment. J Thorac Cardiovasc Surg 32:53, 1956

Sturaitis M, McCallum D, Cheung H et al: Lack of significant long-term sequelae following traumatic myocardial contusion. Arch Intern Med 146:1765, 1986

Symbas PN: Cardiothoracic Trauma. WB Saunders, Philadelphia, 1989

Symbas PN: Residual or delayed lesions from penetrating cardiac wounds. Chest 66:408, 1974

Symbas PN, Goldman M, Erbesfeld MH, Vlasis SE: Pulmonary arteriovenous fistula, pulmonary artery aneurysm and other vascular changes of the lung from penetrating trauma. Ann Surg 191:336, 1980

Ulstad DR, Bjelland JC, Quan SF: Bilateral para-mediastinal post-traumatic lung cysts. Chest 97:242, 1990

Utley JR: Residua of trauma to the heart and great vessels. p. 171. In Residua of Thoracic Trauma. Futura Publishing, Mount Kisco, NY, 1987

Verdant A, Pagé A, Cossette R et al: Surgery of the descending thoracic aorta: spinal cord protection with the Gott shunt. Ann Thorac Surg 46:147, 1988

Villalba M, Lucas CE, Ledgerwood AM, Asfaw I: The etiology of post-traumatic empyema and the role of decortication. J Trauma 19:414, 1979

Waldschmidt ML, Laws HL: Injuries of the diaphragm. J Trauma 20:587, 1980

Webb WR, Burford TH: Studies of the reexpanded lung after prolonged atelectasis. Arch Surg 66:801, 1953

Wiesel W, Jake RJ: Anastomosis of right bronchus to trachea forty-six days following complete bronchial rupture from external injury. Ann Surg 137:270, 1953

Wilson JM, Boren CH, Peterson SR, Thomas AN: Traumatic hemothorax: is decortication necessary? Journal Thorac Cardiovasc Surg 77:489, 1979

Young D, Simon J, Pomerantz M: Current indications for and status of decortication for "trapped lung." Ann Thorac Surg 14:631, 1972

70

REQUIREMENTS FOR PRACTICE AND TRAINING IN THORACIC SURGERY

Joel D. Cooper

For the past 25 years, as a resident, fellow, and faculty member, my primary professional interest has been in the field of general thoracic surgery. During this time, I have had the privilege of learning, practicing, and teaching in various institutions, each of which had a specialized interest in this field. These included a tuberculosis sanitorium, a regional thoracic surgical referral center in England, and three outstanding university hospitals, the Massachusetts General Hospital, the Toronto General Hospital, and Barnes Hospital. From my experience, I have become convinced that a well-organized, properly equipped thoracic surgical unit provides the optimal environment for patient care. When located in a teaching hospital, such a unit provides training for medical students, residents, nursing staff, and paramedical personnel and further stimulates rsidents and fellows to consider a career in general thoracic surgery.

FACILITIES, ORGANIZATIONS, AND EQUIPMENT FOR A THORACIC SURGICAL UNIT

With the exception of trauma patients and other emergency admissions, the practice of general thoracic surgery generally involves elective or semielective surgery for both benign and malignant conditions of the chest. More so than with many other surgical specialties, the effect of such procedures is to make the patient physiologically much worse. Patients—often older ones and those with a smoking history—are subjected to prolonged anesthesia, painful thoracotomy, and in the case of pulmonary resection, the removal of a significant portion of the lung. Such patients usually have chronic pulmonary disease preoperatively. The prompt complication-free recovery of such patients requires highly specialized care. This is best provided in a dedicated nursing unit in which the staff are thoroughly familiar with the care of such patients, including the proper positioning, pain relief, chest physiotherapy, early ambulation, and the prompt recognition of impending respiratory failure. The balance between effective pain control and excessive sedation is crucial and is more likely to be accomplished on a unit where the senior staff have considerable experience with the management of such patients. In the first few days following thoracotomy, most patients now receive analgesia either by means of an epidural catheter or by a patient-controlled analgesia system. The safe administration of these systems is likewise best managed on an experienced nursing unit.

In my opinion, no single aspect of postoperative care is more important for complication-free recovery than is properly applied chest physiotherapy. This includes the proper positioning for postural drainage, vibration, and/or percussion and assistance with coughing by means of chest stabilization. Optimum chest physiotherapy requires a dedicated team of physiotherapists working in concert with the nursing staff. Proper timing and the frequency of chest physiotherapy requires individuals who are skilled in auscultation, familiar with radiographic interpretation, knowledgeable in pulmonary anatomy, and experienced regarding postoperative care and the complications that may arise following major esophageal and pulmonary procedures. A dedicated pain service can also play a supportive role in the mangement of thoracic surgical patients.

A step-down or intermediate care unit as part of the thoracic nursing unit further improves patient care and reduces the cost of hospitalization. Such a unit cares for patients for the initial 1 to 3 postoperative days and, for patients not requiring ventilatory assistance following their operations, often eliminates the need for a stay in a surgical intensive care unit. Needed is monitoring equipment for electrocardiography and pulse oximetry and for the maintenance of arterial lines. The optimum nurse-to-patient ratio is 1:2. With such a unit, few patients require a stay in the intensive care unit. Without such a unit, most patients who have undergone thoracotomies are cared for overnight in an intensive care

---

Equipment for Clinical Nursing and Intermediate Care Units

Clinical nursing unit

    Rigid bronchoscope

    Flexible bronchoscope

    Right-angle telescope for laryngoscopy

    Equipment for early ambulation of patients with chest tubes, including suction apparatus, supportive walking frame on wheels with attachments for oxygen supply, drainage bags, chest bottles, etc.

    Portable pulse oximeter for ambulation

    Crash cart with equipment prepared for emergency intubation

    Intermediate care or step-down unit

    Each bed equipped with monitoring equipment, including electrocardiography and pulse oximetry

    Immediate access to equipment listed above on nursing unit

    Central monitoring station

---

unit. Furthermore, effective pain relief and early mobilization of the patient are more likely to be accomplished in this setting. A partial list of the equipment needed in a clinical nursing unit and an intermediate care unit is presented above.

A surgical intensive care unit is an essential component of a thoracic surgical service and should be used for patients who are hemodynamically unstable and for those requiring ventilatory assistance, either for mechanical support or for pulmonary dysfunction. Patients requiring inotropic support and those requiring careful hemodynamic monitoring, including the use of a Swan-Ganz catheter, should also be managed in such a unit. The traditional interest of thoracic surgeons in respiratory care has been manifested by their active participation as directors or codirectors of intensive care units. The organization of the surgical intensive care unit should permit an active role for a member of the thoracic surgical team who has an active interest in respiratory intensive care.

Operating Facilities

The practice of thoracic surgery involves both major and minor procedures, the latter including endoscopic procedures on both an ambulatory and inpatient basis, and the use of either topical or general anesthesia. For procedures under general anesthesia, it is most efficient for the surgeon if both a major and a minor operating room are available, preferably near each other. The overall case load, the distribution between major and minor procedures, and the availability of operating room space are the primary determining factors. Either way, dedicated space and time are essential for the efficient practice of this specialty, which generally involves cases that can be scheduled days or even weeks in advance.

One of the most interesting and important aspects of the practice of thoracic surgery is the diagnostic evaluation of the patient. This requires the surgeon to be expert in all aspects of both flexible and rigid bronchoscopy and upper gastrointestinal endoscopy. Flexible endoscopy is often performed on an outpatient basis and is also practiced by pulmonary physicians and gastroenterologists. To retain their traditional and important expertise in this field, thoracic surgeons require facilities for the efficient provision of endoscopy services on a timely basis. This is best provided by means of a dedicated endoscopy suite, often shared with pulmonary and gastrointestinal medicine. Alternatively a separate endoscopy suite located in the operating room area has certain advantages, including the efficient interposition of major and minor procedures in the operating schedule and the avoidance of a costly duplication of endoscopic and video equipment, which is required in the operating room for procedures done under general anesthesia.

Below is a partial list of necessary endoscopic equipment.

Thoracoscopy Equipment

The development of thoracoscopic procedures, based on improved imaging techniques, is currently in its infancy. Cameras, monitoring equipment, and recording devices are similar to those used for laparoscopic procedures. Specially designed equipment for thoracic surgery is currently being developed. Unlike laparoscopic surgery, however, video-assisted thoracic surgical procedures do not require the maintenance of a gas-tight entrance porthole, and thus in many instances, ordinary thoracic surgical instruments can be introduced through small incisions, with procedures carried out by using standard instruments and techniques.

Esophageal Investigational Laboratory

The practice of esophageal surgery has been firmly rooted in thoracic surgery in North America and England, whereas in many other countries, it is practiced by gastrointestinal surgeons exclusively. With the resurgence of general thoracic surgery, the involvement of the surgeon in all diagnostic aspects of esophageal disease is essential. Just as the indications and use of upper gastrointestinal endoscopy may differ between the surgeon and gastroenterologist, so too does the use of esophageal function studies. For this reason thoracic surgical involvement in an esophageal diagnostic laboratory should be encouraged. The equipment for such a laboratory is listed below.

Pulmonary Rehabilitation Unit

Many patients requiring thoracic surgical procedures have chronic obstructive pulmonary disease and may be active cigarette smokers at the time of the initial consultation. Pulmonary complications are especially prone to occur in such high-risk patients following thoracotomy. Smoking cessation coupled with an outpatient pulmonary rehabilitation program can reduce postoperative morbidity and mortality rates and shorten the hospital stay. Such a program, which is administered by a trained nurse or physiotherapist, with input from

Necessary Endoscopic Equipment

Endoscopy facility—for procedures under topical anesthesia

- Flexible bronchoscope (4.8 mm and 5.8-mm dual-channel)
- Flexible esophagoscope (adult and pediatric sizes)
- Set of mercury-weighted tapered (Maloney) esophageal dilators
- Video equipment, including camera for video projection, video tape recording, and still photography

Equipment for procedures under general anesthesia or sedation

- Rigid bronchoscopes (sizes 5 to 9)
- Ventilatory adaptor for ventilation through the open bronchoscope
- Rigid bronchoscopic telescopes (0- and 90-degree angle)
- Rigid esophagoscopes including 35- and 50-cm lengths and oversized (Jessburg or other type) for foreign body retrieval and direct dilatation with larger sized bougies
- Complete set of gum elastic-tipped dilators
- Complete set of tapered mercury-weighted (Maloney) dilators
- For esophageal dilatation, balloons ranging in diameter from 1 to 3.5 cm
- For airway dilatation, balloons ranging in size from 1 to 2 cm

Equipment for placement of endoesophageal prostheses

- Video equipment for projecting an image on a monitor and obtaining video tape recordings and still recording
- Laser apparatus (yttrium aluminum garnet laser generally preferred)

Equipment Necessary for a Diagnostic Esophageal Laboratory

- Equipment for simultaneously obtaining and recording esophageal pressures from at least three sites and esophageal pH at one site
- Portable equipment for inpatient or outpatient continuous monitoring of esophageal pH with subsequent playback and analysis functions

the thoracic surgeon and pulmonary medicine practitioner, provides optimal preparation. It is my practice to delay major surgery, even in the case of malignant pulmonary or esophageal disease, until high-risk patients are optimized in terms of exercise tolerance. The equipment for such an outpatient unit includes a treadmill (with variable speed and inclination), a bicycle ergometer, an arm ergometer, and a pulse oximeter. A graded exercise program under close supervision can usually increase the patient's performance significantly within 2 to 3 weeks.

Support Services

Support services are required for a thoracic surgical unit. Among these are members of the departments of anesthesia, radiology, pathology, medical oncology, radiation oncology, pulmonary medicine, and gastroenterology.

Thoracic anesthesia requires particular expertise in the management of double-lumen tubes; the use of bronchial blockers, Venturi tube for rigid bronchoscopy, and high-frequency jet ventilation for complicated airway surgery; a general knowledge of thoracic anesthesia techniques; and in the insertion of thoracic and lumbar epidural catheters. A special interest in thoracic anesthesia should be encouraged in one or more members of the anesthesia staff.

A radiologist with a special interest in pulmonary and esophageal disease who is skilled in diagnostic procedures, such as aspiration needle biopsy, is essential. On occasion the placement of a catheter into a confined pleural space is best achieved under fluoroscopic guidance by a skilled radiologist. The prompt viewing of daily chest radiographs is an essential clinical need, and efficient organized retrieval and display of radiographs is mandatory.

A pathologist who is skilled and interested in thoracic surgical diseases is one of the most important support services required by a general thoracic unit. A cytologic evaluation for intraoperative and outpatient specimens is essential. An accurate rapid histologic interpretation of frozen sections is essential. Ideally the pathology laboratory is close to the operating suite, facilitating communication between the pathologist and surgeon and processing of the frozen-section specimens.

Malignant disease of thoracic organs constitutes the most common indication for diagnostic and therapeutic thoracic surgical procedures. Appropriate patient care requires the combined input of specialists in thoracic surgery, medical oncology, and radiation oncology. A medical oncologist and a radiation oncologist with a particular interest and expertise in thoracic malignancies greatly contribute to patient care.

The fields of general thoracic surgery and pulmonary medicine closely complement each other, and a close working relationship between these specialties is generally the rule. A pulmonary physician can be especially supportive to the thoracic surgical service in the areas of preoperative pulmonary rehabilitation, assessment of pulmonary and general medical status, consultation for patients with respiratory failure in the intensive care unit, management of infectious complications, and the evaluation and long-term therapy of patients with diffuse pulmonary disease.

Although there is considerable overlap in the diagnostic studies provided by specialists in gastroenterology and general thoracic surgery, a mutually supportive role is a great advantage to both services. For the thoracic surgeon, the gastroenterologist may provide important input regarding the medical management of gastroesophageal reflux, gastric motility disorders, and various functional gastrointestinal disorders that may be associated with reflux disease or result in postoperative complications of upper gastrointestinal surgery.

Lung Transplantation

When a lung transplant program exists, few additional requirements are necessary if the above facilities and personnel are available. However, the additional workload imposed on the pulmonary physician is significant and, depending on the size of the program, may require the full-time involvement of such an individual.

TRAINING REQUIREMENTS FOR GENERAL THORACIC SURGERY

There has been significant discussion over the past decade as to the training of general thoracic surgeons and the relationship of general thoracic surgery to the overall specialty of cardiothoracic surgery (Grillo, et al., 1984; Orringer, 1991; Orringer, et al., 1989; Paulson, 1981). Although cardiac and general thoracic surgery have common origins, both components of cardiothoracic surgery have significantly expanded, making it unlikely that one individual can master all aspects. Cardiac surgery now involves heart and heart-lung transplantation, the use of internal and external ventricular-assist devices, and complex surgery for arrhythmias, valvular disease, disease of the great vessels, and coronary artery bypass. The field of congenital cardiac surgery has become, at most centers, a subspecialty. In contrast to cardiac surgery, general thoracic surgery involves a knowledge of thoracic oncology, including the staging of tumors, and combined modality therapy. The maintenance of a referral practice for esophageal disease requires particular commitment, one that is difficult to fit into the demands of a busy cardiac surgical practice. The introduction of thoracoscopic techniques further distinguishes between general thoracic and cardiovascular practice. On the other hand, lung transplantation bridges the two arms of our specialty. In my opinion, the optimum training of a general thoracic surgeon requires a familarity with all aspects of cardiothoracic surgery.

Not every training program in cardiothoracic surgery will wish or be able to provide the facilities and adequate case load volume to train individuals who wish to specialize in general thoracic surgery. It is essential, however, that an adequate number of institutions maintain the interest, facilities, and staff to ensure the continued production of those who will become the teachers, researchers, and clinical authorities of the future. Furthermore, this environment will stimulate advances in research and clinical care. Such institutions will maintain active research laboratories focused on problems relevant to general thoracic surgery, such as cell biology, oncology, lung transplantation, respiratory and esophageal physiology, and others. The ideal environment for training or general thoracic surgeons involves a teaching unit staffed by two or more faculty members whose predominant or sole practice is in the field of general thoracic surgery. The trainee should receive a minimum of 12 months of experience in general thoracic surgery and a minimum of 6 months of adult cardiac experience. Additional training in cardiac surgery, including congenital cardiac surgery, is required, as determined by the standards set by the certifying body for the specialty. While on the general thoracic surgery rotation, the clinical activities of the trainee should be exclusively devoted to general thoracic surgery. A dedicated nursing unit and operating room time and space for general thoracic surgery should be provided. A series of teaching rounds should be held on a weekly basis. In my experience, the following rounds are particularly appropriate.

Case presentation rounds for the discussion of the management of problem cases or recent cases of interest to the resident

Combined thoracic surgery, pathology, and radiology rounds for the presentation and discussion of radiologic, operative, and pathologic findings in selected cases of interest

Combined medical oncology, radiation oncology, and thoracic surgical rounds for the presentation and decision making in regard to the optimum management of patients currently under consideration

Combined pulmonary medicine, thoracic surgery, and radiology rounds for the presentation of interesting radiologic findings and diagnostic challenges

Thoracic morbidity and mortality conference (every 1 to 3 months)

Trauma

The thoracic surgical service should be consulted on all (noncardiac) trauma cases and should play the primary role in emergency thoracotomies. This is in the best interest of our patients and further provides an essential ingredient in the training of thoracic surgeons.

Outpatient and Follow-Up Clinic

"The follow-up clinic is the shoals upon which founder many attractive theories in surgery."

—Ronald Belsey

The training of general thoracic surgeons is incomplete without first-hand involvement in the evaluation of new patients and in the postoperative and long-term follow-up of patients undergoing operative procedures. This is best provided in a joint follow-up clinic at which all faculty members and resident staff participate. All previous radiographs should be available in addition to the patient's file, including the pathologic report and summary of the radiotherapy or chemotherapy used. Long-term follow-up is particularly important for patients undergoing surgery for functional diseases of the esophagus.

COMMENTS AND CONTROVERSIES

Dr. Cooper's summary emphasizes essential ingredients: facilities, equipment, a dedicated nursing unit, and teaching rounds. In addition, the prescription for an academic thoracic program should include a pervasive spirit of dedication to thoracic surgery as the primary mission of the service. Such a spirit has an important formative influence on trainees and students as they develop their career goals and self-concept.

I believe that the outstanding contribution of the Belsey and Pearson schools of thoracic surgery has been the exposure of trainees to role models who held general thoracic surgery above and apart from all of surgery, allowing its full development as a specialty. The urgent call for help from the cardiac patient or staff surgeon has kept many residents in combined cardiothoracic programs from concentrating on the solution of thoracic surgical problems. When the services and faculty are sufficiently separated, outstanding advances in general thoracic surgery can be expected, as illustrated by the contributions throughout this text.

Training in critical care can add another important dimension to strengthen the specialist in general thoracic surgery. Training and knowledge of intensive care played a pivotal role in the initial and continuing success of the Toronto group in lung transplantation and in the development of solutions to other complex thoracic surgical problems.

M.F.M.

REFERENCES

Grillo HC, Benfield JR, Faber LP et al.: General thoracic surgery in cardiothoracic surgery: the search for balance (editorial). J Thorac Cardiovasc Surg 88:321, 1984

Orringer MB: General thoracic surgery—issues and direction. Ann Thorac Surg 51:814, 1991

Orringer MB, Cooper JD, Magovern G et al.: The continuing dilemma of general thoracic surgery—where to now? J Thorac Cardiovasc Surg 97:649, 1989

Paulson DL: A time for assessment. J Thorac Cardiovasc Surg 82:163, 1981

71

STATISTICS

Statistical Terminology
and Definitions

Steven Piantadosi
John Kirklin
Eugene Blackstone

The purpose of this chapter section is twofold: (1) to provide definitions of statistical terms that are commonly encountered and (2) to provide additional details about statistical concepts that are helpful for understanding the literature related to clinical trials methods. There are numerous references that describe specific mathematic and statistical applications in medicine but few that explicitly define their terminology. The definitions offered here are not authoritative in the sense of representing a consensus of experts. However, they are internally consistent and are defined in ways consistent with common usage.

In the following list, the defined terms are in **boldface.** Comments, clarifications, and examples are in *italics.*

TERMINOLOGY AND CONCEPTS

Adjustment: Use of any of several statistical methods to account for the effect of **prognostic factors** when estimating differences attributable to therapies or other prognostic factors. Adjustments may be non–risk-adjusted (**stratification**) or risk-adjusted (**multiple regression** equations or nomograms of multiple regression equations).

Bias: Systematic (nonrandom) error in the **estimate** of a **therapeutic effect** of clinical interest.

Clinical trial: A planned study in humans.

Confidence interval (informal definition): A region in which the investigator believes a true parameter value will lie with some specified probability.

Confidence interval (formal definition according to frequentist statisticians): A region that will contain the true parameter with a specified probability if the experiment were repeated a large number of times. Thus, informally a confidence interval is a probability statement about the true parameter's value. However, in reality it is a probability statement about the region. *It is customary to report confidence intervals whose coverage probability is 95 percent (i.e., such an interval would enclose the true parameter value 95 percent of the time if the experiment were repeated a large number of times). Approximate 95 percent confidence intervals can be constructed by taking the mean ±2 standard deviations. However, there are circumstances in which intervals other than 95 percent are useful.*

Confounder: A **prognostic factor** that is associated with both therapy and outcome and can affect both.

Dichotomous: Having only two possible values.

End point: A clinical or laboratory outcome that yields the definitive information about the result of therapy for an individual study subject. *For example, death or survival time is a frequently used end point. In theory the investigator need not follow the subject past the end point (if this were even possible); however, intermediate end points are sometimes used because of their strong association with more definitive outcomes. Examples of intermediate end points are CD4 + lymphocyte counts in acquired immunodeficiency syndrome (AIDS), prostate-specific antigen levels in prostate cancer, and blood pressure in cardiovascular disease.*

Estimate (verb): The process of determining the value for an unknown **parameter** that satisfies prespecified criteria.
Estimate (noun): The numeric value for an unknown parameter that satisfies prespecified criteria.

Eligibility: A list of criteria to be satisfied for each patient before the person is treated during a clinical study.

Evaluability: A list of criteria to be satisfied before considering that the patient has had a legitimate trial on the therapy. *Unfortunately evaluability is partially an outcome of therapy and is therefore not a proper basis for excluding patients from analysis.*

Fully sequential: Clinical trial designs that permit the evaluation of study results after *every* patient has been accrued. Such designs can provide convincing evidence of efficacy at the earliest possible time, provided the type I error is properly controlled. *To use such a design, end points must be ascertained quickly before the next patient is accrued.*

Group sequential: Clinical trial designs similar to **fully sequential** ones, except that therapeutic comparisons are made after groups of patients have been accrued. These designs also terminate early when therapeutic differences are large.

Hazard: The risk of failure when the time to failure (e.g., survival) is the **end point.** For a cohort being followed, the overall hazard can be estimated by

$$\lambda = \frac{d}{\Sigma t_i}$$

where d is the number of events during the observation period and Σt_i is the sum of all the observation times of the patients. *This estimate of the overall hazard is sometimes termed the "linearized rate."*

Hazard function regression: A method for analysis of a time-related event and its correlates that accounts simultaneously for the distribution of times until the event in terms of a biomathematic **model** and for **prognostic factors** in terms of one or more regression models that modulate parameters of the biomathematic model.

Hazard ratio: The **hazard** in one group divided by the hazard in another group. A hazard ratio of 1 implies no difference in risk. *A hazard ratio of 1.8, for example, implies that the numerator group is at persistently higher risk of failure than the denominator group. The clinical significance of an elevated hazard ratio depends on other evidence, including the absolute risk, the significance level, and the clinical context.*

Inference: Conclusion drawn while accounting for **random variability.**

Intent to treat: The idea that patients assigned to therapies in randomized clinical trials should be analyzed according to the assigned therapeutic group rather than according to the therapy actually received. *Clinicians sometimes disagree with this perspective, which views clinical trials as tests of therapeutic policy rather than tests of the therapy received. However, the clinical trials literature supports the validity of the intention to treat (ITT) principle because it yields valid tests of the null hypothesis of no therapeutic difference. In studies in which a large fraction of patients do not receive the assigned therapy, neither the ITT nor the therapy received analyses necessarily yield the most clinically relevant conclusions. The ITT analysis does not correspond closely to efficacy because many patients did not receive the intended therapy, and the therapy received*

analysis is potentially biased because patients may switch therapies for reasons associated with outcome.

Interim analysis: An analysis of an ongoing clinical trial, particularly one that might stop the trial if convincing evidence of efficacy is seen.

Logistic regression: A statistical **model** in which the log **odds** of the response probability is predicted from a set of **prognostic factors:**

$$\log\left\{\frac{P}{1-P}\right\} = \beta_0 + \beta_1 X_1 + \beta_2 X_2 + \ldots$$

where P is the probability of response; X_1, X_2, . . . are the predictor (explanatory) variables; and β_1, β_2, . . . are **parameters** to be estimated from the data. Thus, the effect of each prognostic factor is to multiply the baseline log odds.

Model: A logical mathematic construct, generally containing **parameters** (β_1 above) and **variables** (X_1 above) (place marks for data values). *When data have been entered and the values for parameters have been estimated by statistical techniques, the model, which is generic, becomes a specific equation.*

Monitoring: Observing the conduct of an ongoing clinical trial according to a set of predefined guidelines.

Multiple comparisons: The problem that arises when attempting to interpret the results of numerous hypothesis tests in the same study. By chance, 5 percent of tests will reject the **null hypothesis** if all tests are performed at the 5 percent significance level. To preserve the overall **type I error** rate at 5 percent, each test might be performed at a significance level less than 5 percent.

Multiple regression: Use of statistical **models** to account for the effects of several **prognostic factors** simultaneously. *Linear* regression relates the response variable to the predictor variables through a linear function of **parameters:**

$$Y = \beta_0 + \beta_1 X_1 + \beta_2 X_2 + \ldots + \varepsilon$$

where Y is the response variable; X_1, X_2, . . . are the predictor variables; β_0, β_1, β_2, . . . are the parameters to be estimated from the data, and ε is a random error term.

Multivariable: Analyzing several *predictor* (explanatory) variables simultaneously. *Suppose that a univariable analysis suggests that therapy A is better than therapy B. The hazard ratio is 2.2 (95 percent confidence interval, 1.5 to 2.9) and P = 0.02. However, when we simultaneously account for the effects of sex and therapy using multivariable analysis, we estimate the adjusted hazard ratio to be 1.35 (95 percent confidence interval, 0.75 to 1.95) and P = 0.45. We might conclude from these results that the apparent univariable effect of therapy is due to sex and that therapy A is not likely to be of real benefit.*

Multivariate: Analyzing several *outcome* variables simultaneously, all as a function of one or more predictor variables. *Note that multivariate does not mean "several predictor variables," as it is often informally used, but refers to several outcome variables. When there are several predictors, the term "multiple" and "multivariable" are probably better descriptors.*

Null hypothesis: In statistical hypothesis tests, the hypothesis of no difference between the comparison groups. It is usually established as a "straw man" to be disproved.

Observational study: A study design in which the investigator does not control the assignment of therapy to individual study subjects.

Odds: The probability of an outcome divided by the probability of not having that outcome. If P is the probability of the outcome, the odds equals $P/(1 - P)$. *This is the ordinary betting odds.*

Odds ratio: **Odds** in one group divided by the odds in another group. The odds ratio is commonly used for categorical data, which might be summarized as

		Outcome	
		Yes	No
Condition	Yes	a	b
	No	c	d

where a, b, c, and d are the counts in the various categories. The odds of outcome when the condition is present is

$$\frac{\dfrac{a}{a + b}}{\dfrac{b}{a + b}} = \frac{a}{b}$$

When the condition is absent, the odds of outcome are:

$$\frac{\dfrac{c}{c + d}}{\dfrac{d}{c + d}} = \frac{c}{d}$$

Thus the odds ratio is:

$$\frac{ad}{bc}$$

The odds ratio is related to the risk ratio or relative risk in that when the probability of the outcome is small (i.e., a much less than b and c much less than d), the odds ratio approximately equals the risk ratio:

$$\frac{\dfrac{a}{a + b}}{\dfrac{c}{c + d}}$$

However, the odds ratio is a useful measure of difference between groups even when it does not approximate the relative risk and arises naturally in important statistical models, such as logistic regression. An odds ratio of 1 implies no difference in risk between the groups. An odds ratio of 2.3, for example, implies that the numerator group is at higher risk than the denominator group. The clinical significance of an elevated odds ratio depends on other evidence, including the absolute risk, the significance level, and the clinical setting.

Parameter: A constant in a **model.**

Phase I study: A **clinical trial** designed to measure the distribution, metabolism, excretion, and toxicity of a new drug.

Phase II study: A **clinical trial** designed to test the feasibility of, and level of activity of, a new agent or procedure.

Phase III study: A **clinical trial** designed to estimate the relative efficacy of a therapy against a standard or alternative therapy or a placebo.

Power: The chance of detecting a difference of a specified size as being statistically signifcant. If the **type II error** probability is β, the power $= 1 - \beta$.

Precision: The certainty with which a measurement or **estimate** is made. *A precise measurement may not be accurate (unbiased).*

Prognostic factor: A variable that carries information about future clnical outcomes. Baseline prognostic factors have values fixed at study onset and never change. Time-dependent prognostic factors have values that change over time and are considerably more difficult to model statistically.

Proportional hazards: A mathematic assumption used in survival models in which the **hazard ratio** between two groups is assumed to be constant over time, although the baseline hazard can fluctuate. For example, the usual assumption is

$$\log\left\{\frac{\lambda(t)}{\lambda_0(t)}\right\} = \beta_1 X_1 + \beta_2 X_2 + \ldots$$

where $\lambda_0(t)$ is the baseline hazard function, which can vary over time; $\lambda(t)$ is the hazard function in the test group; $X_1, X_2, \ldots$ are the predictor variables; and $\beta_1, \beta_2, \ldots$ are **parameters** to be estimated from the data. Thus, the effect of each prognostic factor is to multiply the baseline hazard function.

Protocol: The detailed written plans for conducting an **experiment,** clinical study, or **clinical trial.**

Publication bias: The tendency for studies with positive results (i.e., those finding significant differences) to be published in journals in preference to those with negative findings. Whcn journals arc rcvicwed for summarizing study results (metanalysis), a biased impression of therapeutic efficacy might then result.

***P* value:** The probability that the observed effect (or one larger) is due to chance if the **null hypothesis** is true.

Random: The result of chance alone.

Randomization: Assignment of patients or experimental subjects to two or more therapies by chance alone. *In comparative studies, the important consequence of randomized assignments is that confounding factors are not permitted to influence the choice of therapy. This means that therapeutic differences are attributable either to chance or to true therapeutic differences. In a designed clinical trial, the effects of chance are quantifiable, which leads to reliable inferences about therapeutic differences. This is true even if the confounding factors are unobserved. Control over unknown confounders is the principal advantage of randomized clinical trials. Although haphazard therapeutic assignment can be random or unbiased, it is not convincingly so. Thus, the use of randomization enhances the reliability and credibility of inferences.*

Risk ratio: The probability of a specified outcome in one group divided by the probability of the outcome in another group. A risk ratio of 1 implies no difference in risk.

Sample size: The number of patients or experimental subjects on a study. *Ideally the sample size is determined as a consequence of the need for precision in the estimate of therapeutic difference. However, in many cases the sample size is determined by cost, time, or other mundane constraints.*

Statistical significance: The quantitative degree, as measured by the *P* value, to which a difference is likely to be the result of chance, assuming the **null hypothesis** is true. *Conventionally* P *values less than 0.05 are judged to be "significant." However,* P *values are influenced by several factors, making universal criteria impossible.*

Trial: A study in which the investigator controls three elements of design: (1) the therapy assigned to the subject(s), (2) ascertainment of outcomes, and (3) analysis of results. *We have carefully chosen the word* assigned *rather than*

using applied *because, at least in humans, if not in all trials and experiments, the investigator cannot guarantee the application of an intended therapy.*

Type I error: Concluding that a **therapeutic effect** or difference exists when, in reality, it does not (false positive).

Type II error: Concluding that a **therapeutic effect** or difference does not exist when, in reality, it does (false negative).

Univariable: Analyzing one *explanatory* variable at a time.

Univariate: Analyzing one *outcome* variable at a time.

Variability: Unaccounted for fluctuation (random error) in the estimate of a **therapeutic effect** or measurement of a variable.

Variable: A measurement that can take on different values for each experimental subject or observation.

Statistical Issues Arising in Thoracic Surgery Clinical Trials

Steven Piantadosi
Mitchell H. Gail

INTRODUCTION

The purpose of this chapter section is to review biostatistical concepts that are helpful to clinicians in planning, conducting, and assessing clinical trials and to outline the role of the statistician as a member of a team of investigators studying thoracic disease. We describe questions and issues that require statistical thinking and areas in which a statistical perspective can improve the design, execution, analysis, and interpretation of clinical studies. Our emphasis is on major concepts. We refer the reader to several excellent texts and expository articles to provide additional discussion of these concepts and details of statistical calculations. These include history and policy (Bull, 1959; Office of Technology Assessment, 1983; Packard, 1921; Haygarth, 1800; Fisher and MacKenzie, 1923; Amberson, et al., 1931; Food and Drug Admin-

istration, 1963; Louis, 1936; Miké, 1982; Fisher, 1966; Doll, 1992; Medical Research Council, 1951; Streptomycin in Tuberculosis Trials Committee, 1948), general discussions (Meinert, 1986; Silverman, 1985; Shapiro and Louis, 1983; Pocock, 1983; Freidman, et al., 1981; Armitage, 1979; Olak and Chiu, 1993; Louis, et al., 1982; Lewis, 1983; Peto, et al., 1976, 1977; Armitage and Berry, 1987), cancer trials (Buyse, et al., 1984; Leventhal and Wittes, 1988; Leventhal and Piantadosi, 1988; Piantadosi, 1988; Piantadosi, et al., 1992; Simon, 1989; Green, 1981), randomization and therapeutic allocation (Byar, et al., 1976; Taves, 1974), ethics (Schafer, 1977; Burkhardt and Kienle, 1983; Vere, 1983; National Commission for the Protection of Human Subjects of Biomedical and Behavioral Research, 1978; Levine, 1986; Simberkoff, et al., 1993), prognostic factor analyses (Byar, 1984; George, 1988), and reporting and summarizing results

(International Committee of Medical Journal Editors, 1988; Bailar and Mosteller, 1988; Altman, et al., 1983; Mosteller, et al., 1980; Berry 1986, 1987; Der Simonin, et al., 1982; Simon, 1986; Gardner and Altman, 1986; Braitman, 1988; Berger, 1986; Berger and Sellke, 1987; Rothman, 1986). For the clinician, particularly accessible reading includes the book by Silverman (1985) and that edited by Shapiro and Louis (1983).

Much of this chapter section pertains to study design, implementation, and quality control. We emphasize these features because a well-designed and well-executed trial that addresses an important therapeutic or management question usually provides cogent evidence without an elaborate analysis. In fact statistical analysis can do little to make the results of a poorly designed or executed trial compelling. This is not to say that analysis and interpretation are unimportant. An improper analysis can distort the findings of a well-designed and executed trial.

After a brief historical perspective on clinical trials, we discuss several types of studies used to identify promising therapies and associated problems and uncertainties in inferring therapeutic efficacy from such studies. Then we discuss four areas of statistical activity that are important to the success of a program of studies in the management of thoracic disease.

One activity is helping to identify and refine an important therapeutic question through the use of pilot studies and "phase II" trials to determine if a proposed therapy has sufficient promise to warrant further study.

Helping to design a comparative ("phase III") trial to compare a new therapy with conventional ones is a major responsibility of the statistician. The statistician must make sure that the objectives of the trial are clearly stated and that the quantities measured will provide the evidence needed to meet those objectives. This process typically involves detailed discussions with other investigators to define such issues as (1) what population should be studied, (2) are the therapies unambiguously defined, (3) how will therapy be assigned, (4) how will patient responses be measured and what can be done to ensure that measurements will be obtained uniformly on all patients regardless of therapeutic assignment, (5) are sufficient numbers of patients available to meet the scientific objectives of the study, and (6) what can be done to minimize loss to follow-up and to promote compliance to the therapeutic protocol.

Once the trial has been planned, the statistician plays an important role in implementing the trial and ensuring quality control. The statistical office can check that only eligible patients are randomized or registered and can ensure the reliability of this process. Monitoring accrual and incoming data can identify protocol violations and other data management problems and can resolve problems before they threaten the validity of the trial. The monitoring of toxicity and therapeutic effects is an important safeguard for participants.

Statisticians can contribute importantly to the analysis of the trial results and preparation of publications. They are well equpped to describe the quantitative methods used, to assess the strength of the evidence and sources of uncertainty, and to make sure that the analysis and data descriptions clearly address the trial objectives.

HISTORICAL NOTE

Many medical advances have been made without the need for concurrently controlled clinical experiments. When the effects of therapies or interventions are large and the natural history of the disease is well known, informal methods of assessment and analysis, or observation alone, may provide convincing evidence of efficacy. One of the earliest examples of such a circumstance was the observations of Ambrose Paré (1510–1590), a French surgeon at the Battle of Villaine (1537), who was accustomed to treating wounds with boiling oil. When the supply of oil was exhausted, he used an alternative, which consisted of egg yolks, oil of roses, and turpentine (Packard, 1921):

> I raised myself very early to visit them, when beyond my hope I found those to whom I had applied the digestive medicament feeling but little pain, their wounds neither swollen nor inflamed, and having slept through the night. The others to whom I had applied boiling oil were feverish with much pain and swelling about their wounds. Then I determined never again to burn . . . the poor wounded . . . .

As uncertainty in medical thinking slowly replaced authoritarian influences, structured experiments became more common. An example was provided by Haygarth (1740–1827) who studied Perkin's tractors, metallic rods that were used to treat inflamed joints and other disorders (Haygarth, 1800). Haygarth stated

> Let their merit be impartially investigated, in order to support their fame, if it be well founded, or to correct the public opinion, if merely formed upon delusion. Such a trial may be accomplished in a most satisfactory manner, and ought to be performed without any prejudice. Prepare a pair of false, exactly to resemble the true Tractors. Let the secret be kept inviolable, not only from the patient, but from every other person. Let the efficacy of both be impartially tried; beginning always with the false Tractors. The cases should be accurately stated, and the reports of the effects produced by the true and false Tractors be fully given, in the words of the patients.

The results of placebo therapy were

> On the 7th of January 1799, the wooden Tractors were employed. All the five patients, except one, assured us that their pain was relieved . . .

The results of "active" therapy were

> All the patients were in some measure, but not more relieved by the second application, except one, who received no benefit from the former operation, and who was not a proper subject for the experiment, having no existing pain, but only stiffness of her ankle.

Louis (1836) introduced the "numerical method" for estimating the effects of therapy by carefully comparing results for large numbers of patients treated one way with those of patients treated another way. This method led him to the surprising conclusion that bloodletting was not nearly as effective in the therapy of inflammatory disorders as he had anticipated and contributed to a growing skepticism in regard to the available medical therapies (Miké, 1982). Louis (1836) was cognizant of the criticism that patients treated with bloodletting did not resemble those not given bloodletting perfectly, but he hoped to overcome this bias through the use of large therapeutic groups. He wrote

> . . . and it is precisely on this account that enumeration becomes necessary; by doing so, the errors (which are inevitable) being the same in the two groups of patients subjected to different treatment, mutually compensate each other, and they may be disregarded without sensibly affecting the exactness of the results.

In the 1920s Fisher and MacKenzie (1923) used randomization as a means to achieve therapeutic comparability in agricultural field trials and showed how the randomization procedure itself induced a valid basis for testing the hypothesis of no therapeutic effect (Fisher, 1966). Fisher and MacKenzie (1923) also suggested that randomization should be used in human studies.

In 1931, Amberson, et al. (1931) used randomization to assign one group of study subjects to therapy as follows:

> The 24 patients were then divided into two approximately comparable groups of 12 each. The cases were individually matched, one with another, in making the division. . . . Then, by a flip of the coin, one group became identified as group I (sanocrysin-treated) and the other as group II (control). The members of the separate groups were known only to the nurse in charge of the ward and to two of us. The patients themselves were not aware of any distinctions in the treatment administered.

This example illustrates the concepts of matching patients, masking therapy, and using randomization to achieve good therapeutic balance on prognostic factors not controlled by matching.

However, it was not until 1946 that the method of randomization became a widely accepted tool in investigational therapeutics. In that year, Sir A. B. Hill persuaded committees of the Medical Research Council (1951) in Great Britain to test the value of pertussis vaccine and, later, to test the efficacy of streptomycin treatment for tuberculosis (Streptomycin in Tuberculosis Trials Committee, 1948) in randomized trials. An interesting article by Doll (1992) describes Sir A. B. Hill's contributions to clinical trial methodology and other aspects of medical statistics.

Another landmark in the development of modern clinical trials occurred in 1962 with the Kefauver-Harris amendment to the 1938 U.S. Food, Drug, and Cosmetic Act (Food and Drug Administration, 1963). This amendment defines a standard of evidence for drug approval based on clinical trials as follows:

> The term "substantial evidence" means evidence consisting of adequate and well controlled investigations, including clinical investigations, by experts qualified by scientific training and experience to evaluate the effectiveness of the drug involved, on the basis of which it could fairly and responsibly be concluded by such experts that the drug will have the effect it purports or is represented to have under the conditions of its use prescribed, recommended, or suggested in the labeling or proposed labeling thereof.

Clinical trial methodology continues to evolve today. The journal *Controlled Clinical Trials* was founded in 1980 and the Society for Clinical Trials began annual meetings in 1982. Multicenter clinical trials, many of which use unbiased methods of therapeutic allocation and ethically oriented monitoring procedures, are common in the development and testing of new therapies in cancer, cardiovascular disease, AIDS, neurologic disease, and vaccines in both North America and Europe.

HISTORICAL READINGS

Amberson JB Jr, McMahon BT, Pinner M: A clinical trial of sancrysin in pulmonary tuberculosis. Am Rev Respir Dis 24:401, 1931

Doll R: Sir Austin Bradford Hill and the progress of medical science. BMJ 305:1521, 1992

Fisher RA: The Design of Experiments. Hafner Publishing Co., New York, 1966

Fisher RA, MacKenzie WA: Studies in crop variation: II. The manurial response of different potato varieties. J Agricultural Sci 13:311, 1923

Food and Drug Administration: Procedural and interpretive regulations: investigational use. Fed Reg 28:179, Jan. 8, 1963

Haygarth J: Of the Imagination as a Cause and as a Cure of Disorders of the Body: Exemplified by Ficticious Tractors and Epidemical Convulsions. R. Cruttwell, Bath, UK, 1800

Louis PCA: Researches on the Effects of Bloodletting in Some Inflammatory Diseases and on the Influence of Tartarized Antimony and Vessication in Pneumonitis. Hilliard Gray and Co., Boston, 1836

Medical Research Council Whooping-Cough Immunization Committee: The prevention of whooping-cough by vaccination. BMJ 1:1463, 1950

Miké V: Clinical studies in cancer: a historical perspective. p. 111. In Miké V, Stanley, KE (eds): Statistical Issues in Medical Research. Methods and Issues, with Applications in Cancer Research. New York, Wiley, 1982

Packard FR: Life and Times of Ambroise Paré, 1510–1590. Paul B. Hoeber, New York, 1921

Streptomycin in Tuberculosis Trials Committee: Streptomycin treatment of pulmonary tuberculosis. BMJ 2:769, 1948

SOURCES OF UNCERTAINTY IN TREATMENT STUDIES

In the following discussion, we emphasize sources of uncertainty that arise in comparisons of the effectiveness of one therapy with another. Such comparative studies are subject to two main sources of uncertainty: *bias* and *random uncertainty*. Random uncertainty can be reduced by enlarging the study population, whereas fundamental changes in the experimental design or analysis are usually requried to control bias. The concepts of bias and random uncertainty also apply to noncomparative studies, such as phase II cancer trials (to estimate the proportion of patients who respond to a new therapy) or case series (to estimate the rate of therapeutic response in the absence of a control group).

Biases Associated with Various Types of Studies

Nonrandomized Studies of Therapy

Many sources of information can be useful to advance a program of therapeutic research (Table 71-1). A single case report may indicate a possible new therapeutic strategy, and case series may provide some evidence as to the rate of success of a given therapeutic approach. However, such studies cannot be relied on to yield reliable estimates of the therapeutic effect because the patients selected may be unusual in some respects and because results from concurrent control patients treated with standard methods are not usually available. Reliance on the experience of previously treated patients ("historical controls") can be misleading for several reasons. Improvements in ancillary care tend to favor the more recently treated patients. Refinements in diagnostic techniques and staging procedures have the paradoxic effect of improving the prognosis in each stage of disease. For example, the use of modern imaging techniques detects evidence of regional spread of disease that was formerly undetectable. Thus a patient who may have previously been classified as having stage I disease would be reclassified as having stage II or III disease. The impact of this technology is that patients classified as having stage I disease recently would have less advanced disease than patients classified as having stage I disease previously. Likewise, today's patients with stage II disease would have less advanced stage II disease than previously, and so forth (Byar, 1979). Such factors tend to make results from recently treated patients appear better than those from historical controls, even in the absence of a true improvement in therapeutic efficacy. These effects of patient selection, improvements in ancillary care, and refinements in staging produce bias, namely a systematic artifact that tends to make current therapies appear better (or worse) than standard ones. Such bias is not ameliorated by increasing the size of the study. Larger samples only yield more precise estimates of the biased result.

Sometimes investigators attempt to make therapeutic comparisons using data from databases constructed for general purposes (Table 71-1). Often the data quality in such studies is poor because the type of data needed and the type of follow-up required were not specified in advance. Sometimes observational data are gathered prospectively as part of a carefully planned study. In this case the quality of information on measured covariates, such as the stage of disease, and on outcomes, such as the time to recurrence, may be good. Such data may provide useful leads for further study. However, even in well-conducted prospective observational studies, the possibility for *selection bias* remains. Patients given the new therapy may have been selected specifically because they were thought to be likely to benefit from it.

Even in well-conducted observational studies in which high-quality data have been collected on clinical outcomes and on baseline covariates, attempts to adjust the therapeutic comparisons for imbalances on measured patient characteristics are not usually convincing. For example, Byar, et al. (1979) compared the survival of patients treated for thyroid cancer by surgery with that of patients treated by radiotherapy. The survival rate in the surgery group exceeded that in the radiation group, and the difference was highly "statistically significant," even after adjustment for imbalances on the known prognostic factors of age, sex, cell type, nodal status, and whether or not there were distant metastases. Nonetheless, these investigators did not conclude that surgery was the superior therapy because they were concerned that the results reflected *residual selection bias*. For example, patients with subtle extensions of disease that were not operable may have been treated with radiation. Such selection biases have also been described as "confounding by indication" (Miettinen, 1983) because in observational studies therapy is tailored to the particular prognostic indications and preferences of the patient.

Thus case reports, case series, reviews of data base experience, and prospective observational studies may generate useful therapeutic hypotheses for further study, but they are rarely convincing in themselves. An exception would be an observational study in which the observed therapeutic effects were so large that they could not be explained by selection bias or other biases. However, human populations are so heterogeneous in their response to disease that most therapeutic effects of interest are comparable to or smaller than the potential selection biases.

Randomized Therapeutic Comparisons

There is one way to avoid selection bias, and that is to allocate therapy randomly to study subjects. This technique was introduced into clinical therapeutics in the late 1940s by Bradford

Table 71-1. Types of Studies of Therapeutic Effects

Type of Study	Evaluation
Case report	Demonstrates that some clinical event is possible. No estimate of the frequency of the event. No concurrent comparison group.
Case series	Gives an estimate of the rate of occurrence of some clinical event. Contains potential serious selection bias. No concurrent controls. Historical controls may be used.
Unplanned data base study	Data quality often poor and subject to ascertainment biases. Required data on covariates often missing.
Prospective observational study	Concurrent therapeutic comparisons possible but subject to important selection biases. Data quality may be good, but covariate information still may be inadequate to overcome selection bias.
Randomized clinical trial	Randomization precludes selection bias. Well-executed studies minimize loss to follow-up and bias in response ascertainment, and the main analysis is defined in advance.

Hill (Doll, 1992) and has revolutionized clinical trial practice. However, even a clinical trial with random patient allocation to a new or standard therapy is subject to potential biases.

One important bias to be avoided in randomized trials is the *response measurement bias*. Such a bias can arise if the timing and measurement of outcome responses differs in the two therapeutic groups. For example, a trial comparing adjuvant chemotherapy with no further therapy may yield biased estimates of the effects on time to recurrence if the patients in the cancer chemotherapy group are examined more frequently than patients in the control group. Strategies to avoid response measurement bias are discussed in the section on Measuring End Points.

A well-executed randomized trial will only yield unbiased estimates of therapeutic effects if an appropriate analysis is performed that takes into account all patients randomized (May, et al., 1981; Gail, 1985). Improper exclusion of subsets of randomized patients from the analysis can lead to important biases, particularly if the causes for exclusion are related both to the therapy assigned and to the clinical outcome. An extreme version of this type of bias is represented by the following quote, attributed to Galen, "All who drink of this remedy recover in a short time, except those whom it does not help, who all die. Therefore, it is obvious that it fails only in incurable cases." By this reasoning an analyst wishing to prove that a new therapy is preferable to a standard one need only exclude from the analysis all patients who did not respond to the new therapy.

Excluding patients who did not comply with the assigned therapy can also produce biases because the patients who do not comply may have been just those patients who were doing poorly.

A related difficulty of interpretation associated with randomized clinical trials should be mentioned. Randomization only ensures an unbiased comparison of all those originally assigned to each therapeutic arm, and the analysis of all randomized patients (ITT analysis) provides an unbiased comparison of the new therapeutic policy compared with the standard one. If the investigator is interested in the biologic effects of a given therapy rather than the clinical effectiveness of a given therapeutic policy, the ITT analysis, which is based on all randomized patients, may yield misleading results, particularly if large numbers of patients do not comply with the therapeutic protocol. Thus a randomized trial may yield an unbiased estimate of the effectiveness of a therapeutic policy but produce a biased estimate of the hypothetic effect that would have been observed in perfectly compliant patients. This is not a defect of randomization but rather a limitation of the experiment itself. It is usually unethical to design a study specifically to evaluate biologic effects by enforcing compliance to the protocol. Schwartz and Lellouch (1967) point out that most clinical trials are better suited to the study of "pragmatic" clinical questions about therapeutic policies rather than of "explanatory" questions about how a therapy works or would have worked under ideal conditions.

Another limitation of a clinical trial is that estimates of therapeutic effect from the trial may not be applicable to a broader population. Typically clinical trial participants are selected for their ability and willingness to adhere to the protocol and remain in follow-up. Other restrictions based on age and concomitant diseases may be imposed. The *internal validity* of the therapeutic comparison among trial participants is protected by randomization and other aspects of the design to ensure an unbiased estimate of the therapeutic effect in the study population. However, this result may overestimate the effectiveness of therapy as administered in the general population. One approach to this issue is to relax the eligibility requirements to include large numbers of patients from the general population in the trial (Yusuf, et al., 1984), but this use of "large simple trials" may not be feasible for technical, logistic, or other reasons. Another approach is to replicate the trial in several different types of populations. In the rest of this article, we emphasize measures to protect internal validity, even though the issue of *generalizability* of the result is important.

Random Errors

Even if a study is well designed and executed so as to yield unbiased estimates of therapeutic effect, the results may be subject to large random error. This reflects the great variability of human responses to disease. For example, some women treated for breast cancer will have rapid recurrences, whereas other women, with the same initial stage of disease, may be cured. It is difficult to detect modest therapeutic effects, such as a 10 percent improvement in 5-year survival rates, against this background of heterogeneous response.

There are three basic strategies to control the effects of heterogeneity and limit random error. One approach is to limit the study population to a homogeneous subgroup. However, this approach may not be feasible if the subgroup constitutes a small proportion of all patients. A more important criticism is that the results in a homogeneous subgroup may not be generalizable. Furthermore, there remains substantial heterogeneity of clinical response within most subgroups, which are defined by prognostic variables.

A second approach is to assume good therapeutic balance within strata, as defined by prognostic subgroups ("blocked" or "balanced" randomization), and to adjust for any residual therapeutic imbalances in prognostic factors in the analysis. However, efforts to improve the efficiency by balancing and/or covariate adjustment tend to produce relatively minor improvements in efficiency for some types of responses, such as survival times with rare outcomes (Beach and Meier, 1989).

The principal tool used to control random variation is to increase the size of the study population. The standard deviation of an average response in a noncomparative study is inversely proportional to the square root of the population's size. In a study that compares two groups of equal size, the standard deviation of the estimated therapeutic effect is likewise inversely proportional to the square root of the size of the common sample. Thus increasing the sample size from 100 to 400 will double the precision of the estimated therapeutic effect.

Often studies are designed to test a specific "null hypothesis." For example, a preliminary phase II study of a promising cancer therapy may be designed to test the null hypothesis that the probability of a complete or partial response to therapy is 0.20 or less. Rejection of this null hypothesis might encourage the investigators to proceed to a larger (phase III) trial to compare survival rates using this new therapy with those of the standard one. The null hypothesis for this comparative study might be that the two therapies have the same distributions of survival times (i.e., the same "survival curves"). If one therapy had a more favorable survival experience than the other, this null hypothesis would be rejected, and the therapy with the better survival rate would usually be adopted, provided its toxicity and the patient's quality of life were acceptable.

We can make mistakes by applying hypothesis tests (Table 71-2). Even in bias-free randomized studies, random variation can lead to a false rejection of the null hypothesis, H_0, (a type I error) or false acceptance of H_0 (a type II error). In simplest terms, type I errors find an effect or benefit when one is not truly present. Type II errors do not find a benefit when one is truly present. We might call a type I error a false-positive trial result because a therapeutic effect will be claimed when none exists. Similarly we may call a type II error a false-negative result.

The chance of making a type I error is under the control of the investigator. By selecting an appropriately stringent significance level, such as 0.05, the investigator can ensure that the chance of a type I error is no greater than 0.05, for example. This control of type I error is lost, however, if the analyst performs many comparisons. For example, if the analyst did not reject the null hypothesis for the main trial comparison but then looked for a therapeutic effect in many subgroups, it is likely that the null hypothesis would be rejected for some subgroup, even if the therapy has no effect. For this reason, it is important to specify a few main hypotheses and analyses in advance.

A second type of *multiple comparison* that can threaten control of the type I error arises in sequential monitoring of accumulating clinical trial data. Depending on how frequently the data are monitored and the rules used to stop the trial, the type I error can exceed nominal levels, unless appropriate adjustments are made.

The type II error is a false-negative result that arises when investigators do not detect a therapeutic effect that is present. The *power* of a clinical trial is the chance that the null hypothesis will be rejected when there is a therapeutic effect, namely the chance of not making a type II error. The power depends on the size of the therapeutic effect, on the background variability of clinical responses, and on the sample size. The power can be large even when the sample size is small if the therapeutic effect is large compared with the background variability in the clinical response. However, except in unusual cases, clinically worthwhile therapeutic effects are much smaller than background variability in responses. To have good power to detect such therapeutic effects, there-fore, large samples are required. Many trials are much too small to detect clinically worthwhile improvements in therapy. When such trials do not reject the null hypothesis, it may be the result of type II error. Such small negative trials are often interpreted as indicating "no therapeutic effect." However, the confidence intervals on the estimated therapeutic effect are often very wide in such trials and include a range of potentially worthwhile therapeutic effects. Thus a small study has little power to detect worthwhile therapeutic effects and yields imprecise estimates of them. We indicate how to calculate appropriate sample sizes in greater detail in the sections on phase II trials and randomized comparative trials.

The type I and II errors have interesting consequences for the seemingly inconsistent results of some clinical trials. For example, we consider a trial of bacillus Calmette-Guerin vaccine immunotherapy (McKneally, et al., 1976) that concluded that there was a significant benefit and a second trial of the same therapy that demonstrated no benefit (Oldham, et al., 1982). Although several explanations for this occurrence are possible, we consider the possibility that the first result was a false positive. Suppose we make the following assumptions: (1) the chance of discovering a beneficial therapy is only 5 percent; (2) all trials are performed with a two-sided type I error rate of 5 percent, but we declare a therapeutic effect only when the trial favors immunotherapy; (3) the power of the studies is 30 percent (i.e., the trials performed are small); and (4) 1,000 trials are performed. Of the 1,000 trials, 950 are of ineffective immunotherapies. These yield $950 \times 0.05 \times 0.5 = 24$ false-positive trials. Fifty studies are of effective immunotherapies, yielding $50 \times 0.3 = 15$ true-positive trials. Thus of the 39 positive trials, 24 or 61 percent are false positives. Even if the power of the studies was 90 percent, the false-positive rate would be 35 percent. This example demonstrates the likelihood that the original report of immunotherapy benefit was a false positive and the difficulty in detecting true therapeutic advances when the chance of developing an effective therapy is small.

PRELIMINARY STUDIES

Preliminary studies are necessary to identify and refine promising therapies before a more definitive comparison is attempted with other available therapies in a comparative phase III trial. Many of the ideas used in the preliminary assessment of medical interventions are applicable to surgical interventions. However, certain differences should be kept in mind. Surgical procedures are often harder to standardize than are medical interventions. There may be considerable flexibility in modifying surgical procedures during the pilot phase of development. Patients who are well enough to participate in pilot studies of surgical interventions are usually healthier than are those who might qualify for pilot studies of a medical therapy for cancer. There may be a greater immediate perioperative risk in surgical pilot studies than in pilot studies of medical interventions.

Statistical thinking plays a role in several aspects of the preliminary development of surgical inventions, including (1) the assessment and summary of available medical knowledge,

Table 71-2. Errors in Hypothesis Testing

Result of hypothesis test	True state of nature	
	H_0 true	H_0 false
Reject H_0	Type I error	No error
Do not reject H_0	No error	Type II error

(2) the design and analysis of pilot studies to refine a new therapy, and (3) the design and interpretation of noncomparative (phase II) trials to determine whether the new therapy is promising enough to warrant further study.

Assessment of Scientific Knowledge

Two essential elements in a successful program of therapeutic research are the identifications of (1) important clinical problems that require improvements in therapy and (2) promising new therapies. An experienced thoracic surgeon will be all too aware of clinical problems for which improved therapies are needed. However, an organized review of the epidemiologic and clinical literature will be needed to define how common a particular problem is and the distribution of clinical outcomes for patients with this problem who are treated using conventional methods. Statistical methods may be useful in describing and synthesizing such evidence.

Literature review and other channels of scientific communication may suggest ideas for promising experimental approaches (E). In some cases there may have been a number of previous studies with the proposed therapy E, but the evidence in favor of E compared with conventional therapy (C) may not yet be regarded as convincing. Before initiating another trial of therapy E versus C, an effort should be made to review the evidence from all previous randomized comparisons, including some that may never have been published. Formal statistical methods for combining data from such trials have been called metanalysis (Dickersin and Berlin, 1992). In some situations the combined evidence from a number of studies that were previously unconvincing in isolation may provide strong evidence in favor of E, obviating the need for further study.

Often, however, there has been little previous experience with the proposed new therapy E, or features of previous studies differ in important respects from the planned study. In this setting it is important to conduct preliminary studies to determine whether the therapy E is feasible and promising enough to warrant study in a comparative clinical trial.

Pilot Studies

Pilot studies are needed to determine whether a proposed therapy is even feasible. For example, suppose a new therapy E involves preoperative radiotherapy and chemotherapy before attempted resection of stage III non-small cell lung cancer. If such a preoperative therapy leads to numerous catastrophic surgical complications in pilot studies, it would need to be modified or abandoned. Pilot studies are needed to modify the therapy to make it tolerable and feasible. By changing the dose of radiotherapy or chemotherapy in the previous example, it may be possible to find conditions that avoid serious surgical complications. It is probably a good idea to conduct pilot studies of a proposed regimen in more than one clinical center if the therapy is intended for further study in a cooperative clinical trial.

Medical oncologists often use the term *phase I trial* to describe pilot studies designed to assess the toxicities and maximum tolerated doses associated with a new drug or drug combination. Usually such studies are carried out on patients with advanced, intractable disease. Formal statistical methods have been proposed to escalate and titrate the dose until intolerable toxicity is reached (Simon, 1989). Similar approaches might be useful in pilot studies of postsurgical adjuvant chemotherapy. However, regimens that involve surgery and other therapeutic modalities are complicated and diverse. Thus stylized methods of drug escalation may not be applicable. Despite these difficulties a formal protocol is useful for planning pilot studies involving surgical components and for specifying the approach to therapeutic modification, if it is needed.

Noncomparative (Phase II) Trials to Demonstrate that the New Therapy Has Promise

After pilot studies have defined a tolerable regimen that embodies a new therapeutic approach, E, further preliminary testing is needed to establish that therapy E has at least a minimal promise of biologic activity or effectiveness. In medical oncology such phase II trials are often designed to determine whether a new drug or drug combination shrinks the size of a tumor or completely eliminates evidence of tumors in some proportion of subjects. Unless it can be shown that the proportion of such "complete or partial tumor responses" exceeds some minimal percentage, such as 20 percent, the investigators will abandon therapy E and avoid the substantial effort and use of medical and patient resources needed to carry out a randomized comparative study.

Phase II trials usually rely on measures of biologic activity that can be determined in a short period, such as tumor shrinkage. These measures may not reflect the therapy's ultimate effectiveness on a more meaningful measure of clinical response, such as long-term survival rates. Nonetheless such short-term surrogate end points are thought to be useful to weed out unpromising therapies.

We imagine that a tolerable preoperative regimen with chemotherapy and radiotherapy has been devised in pilot studies applied to patients with non-small cell lung cancer that would usually be regarded as inoperable. A possible end point for a phase II study would be whether or not the lesion was apparently resectable after such preoperative therapy, as in the study by Eagan, et al. (1987). It is harder to define appropriate phase II end points for adjuvant chemotherapies for patients whose tumors have been resected because we cannot measure tumor response in such patients. In this setting we would usually adopt chemotherapies that had been proved to be clinically effective or biologically active in other types of patients.

One approach to the determination of the sample size required for a phase II study is to specify the required precision of the estimated response rate. Consider a trial in which patients with esophageal cancer are treated with chemotherapy prior to surgical resection. A *complete response* is defined as the absence of macroscopic and microscopic tumor at the time of surgery. We suspect that this might occur 35 percent of the time and would like the 95 percent confidence interval of our estimate to be $\hat{p} \pm w = \hat{p} \pm 0.15$, where $\hat{p}$ is the observed proportion of responses and $w = 0.15$ is the half-width of the confidence interval. Approximate 95 percent confidence intervals for a proportion, $\hat{p}$, are:

$$\hat{p} \pm 1.96 \times \sqrt{\frac{\hat{p}(1-\hat{p})}{n}}$$

where n is the number of patients tested. Substituting $\hat{p} = 0.35$ and $w = 0.15$ into this formula yields $0.15 = 1.96 \times \sqrt{0.35(1-0.35)/n}$. It follows that $n = 39$ patients are required to meet the requirements for precision. Because 0.35 is just an estimate of the proportion and some patients may not complete the study, the actual sample size used might be increased slightly. For example, if $\hat{p} = 0.5$ instead of 0.35, $n = 43$ patients would be required to attain precision ± 0.15. Instead if we desired a precision of ± 0.10 on the estimated proportion with a complete response, $n = 88$ patients would be needed. This degree of precision may not be required to determine whether a new therapy is worth studying further, particularly because we are relying on surrogate information (complete response) rather than on definitive clinical outcomes, such as survival time.

Medical oncologists often use multistage designs that offer a chance to reduce the number of patients studied in phase II trials. For example, Gehan (1961) proposed that 14 patients be studied initially. If there are no successes, the trial is stopped because such an event would be very unlikely if the true success rate were 20 percent or more. If there are one or more successes among the first 14 subjects, an additional 11 patients are studied to achieve a 95 percent confidence interval precision of ± 19.6 percent. Other multistage approaches that are based on hypothesis testing are reviewed by Simon (1987). These procedures are designed to guarantee that if the new agent has a success rate of p_0 or less, the new agent will be rejected for further study with high probability $1 - \alpha$, and if the new agent has a success rate of p_1 or more, the new agent will be accepted for further study with high probability $1 - \beta$. For example, Fleming (1982) considered this approach with $p_0 = 0.2$ and $p_1 = 0.4$. First, 25 patients are studied. If five or fewer successes are observed, we reject the drug. If 10 or more successes are observed, we accept the drug. Otherwise we study an additional 20 patients. If the total successes in the 45 patients are 13 or fewer, we reject the drug. Otherwise we accept the drug as effective and worthy of further evaluation in a comparative clinical trial. This procedure ensures that the chance of accepting a bad drug with success rate $p_0 = 0.2$ or less is smaller than $\alpha = 0.055$, and the chance of rejecting a good drug with success probability $p_1 = 0.4$ or greater is no more than $\beta = 0.091$.

Although required sample sizes can sometimes be reduced by using multistage designs, larger samples are often useful because they provide (1) greater precision of the estimated therapeutic success rate and (2) an additional opportunity to learn about toxicities or unforeseen complications. These opportunities may be especially important for complicated therapeutic strategies involving surgery and other modes of therapy. This experience can be incorporated in the refining of the therapeutic procedure to be tested in a comparative clinical trial.

DESIGNING A COMPARATIVE (PHASE III) TRIAL

After preliminary studies have defined the need for and promise of a new therapy, a comparative (phase III) trial is needed to compare the new therapy, E, with the standard one, C. The purpose of the trial is frequently to determine if E produces a better response than C on a major outcome variable such as survival. Sometimes phase III trials are conducted to determine whether E produces an equivalent response to C ("equivalency trial"). Equivalency trials are useful because, even though E may confer no survival advantage compared with C, for example, E may be preferable because it is less toxic or more easily tolerated.

Intense collaborative effort is often required to design a phase III trial because investigators must agree on the purpose of the trial, details of therapy, and many other elements. The product of this collaborative planning effort is a written protocol that will guide the activities of all participants, including medical and nursing staff, laboratory staff, statisticians, and study subjects. Thus it is important that the investigative team consider and debate key elements of the protocol and finally agree to abide by it.

A phase III protocol should contain the elements listed below. We shall discuss many of these elements, with emphasis on statistical and design considerations. The following items are not necessarily listed in chronologic order for purposes of designing a trial. In fact a number of these issues will need to be considered jointly to achieve a good design.

Some Elements of a Protocol for a Phase III Trial

Background, rationale, and ethical considerations

Specific objectives

Eligibility and exclusion criteria to define the study population

Detailed therapeutic protocol

Therapeutic modifications

Schedule for following patients and procedures for measuring clinical response

Study design, including diagram to indicate therapeutic comparisons and randomization

Required baseline and follow-up clinical and laboratory data

Statistical considerations
    Main analyses planned to meet the specific objectives
    Sample size requirements and feasibility assessment
    Description of the randomization procedure
    Plans for monitoring intercurrent trial results

Plans for quality control and data management, including forms

References

Informed consent

Names and means of contacting key personnel

Background, Rationale, and Ethical Considerations

The proposed trial must be justified on scientific and ethical grounds. Based on preliminary studies, we should be convinced that (1) the proposed trial addresses an important therapeutic issue; (2) the proposed experimental therapy, E, has a reasonable prospect of benefitting or at least not harming trial participants compared with standard therapies treatments, C; (3) there is sufficient scientific uncertainty regarding the relative merits of therapies E and C to justify the need for a formal study; and (4) the proposed study will add substantial, interpretable scientific data to help determine the relative merits of E and C.

These features are important to ensure the scientific merit of the proposed trial, but they also address important ethical requirements of *beneficence* and *nonmaleficence* (National Commission for the Protection of Human Subjects of Biomedical and Behavioral Research, 1978; Levine, 1986). Beneficence requires that investigators attempt to achieve a favorable balance between risks and benefits for study participants and that the trial be well grounded scientifically so as to provide information that will advance medical science or patient care. Nonmaleficence requires that investigators take every measure to avoid harming study participants, although it is understood that some risks are unavoidable or cannot be anticipated. A third ethical requirement is *justice,* namely that study participants be selected for study in an unbiased manner, that study participants be treated fairly, and that study participants have equal chances of exposure to the risks and benefits of the study. A final ethical criterion is *autonomy,* which requires that study subjects understand the nature of the trial and its potential risks and benefits. Autonomy also requires that no coercion is used to recruit study subjects and, in particular, that potential study subjects will be offered good medical care regardless of whether they elect to participate in the study or decide for some reason to drop out of the study. *Informed consent* documents are designed to protect patient autonomy, but a continuing process of communication is required to maintain patient autonomy. If new information becomes available, based on intercurrent trial results or results from other trials, special efforts may be needed to inform trial participants and to solicit their continued participation (Simberkoff, et al., 1993).

It is sometimes argued that randomization is unnecessary. However, randomization controls selection bias and leads to relatively assumption-free methods of statistical inference (Leventhal and Pientadosi, 1988), thus providing strong evidence regarding therapeutic comparisons that is not provided by other types of study. If the major purpose of the trial is to determine the merits or defects of a new therapy and to convince others of the validity of the findings, then randomization usually plays an essential role.

The argument is sometimes made that physicians cannot ethically recommend that their patients participate in a randomized clinical trial. An informed physician probably has an opinion as to which therapy is preferable, and a physician must seek the optimal therapy for each patient. Therefore, it is argued, physicians must recommend the therapy they believe to be superior rather than allow the therapy to be determined at random. However, such physicians are doing their patients no favor if they persistently recommend an inferior therapy out of ignorance. Provided the physician and patient have substantial uncertainty as to which therapy is preferable and provided the study is properly designed to gather information that may benefit trial participants and other patients, a randomized experiment is practicable and consistent with the ethical desiderata above.

Although the introduction and background portions of a protocol usually emphasize scientific rather than ethical considerations, attention to ethical principles should be implicit, if not explicit. Indeed, if the needs of study participants are not kept in mind when the study is designed, the trial may not achieve its scientific objectives because patients will not agree to participate or to comply with the assigned therapy.

Quantifying Study Objectives

One of the most difficult tasks in the design of a clinical trial is to define clinical objectives precisely and to choose quantitative outcome measurements that reflect these clinical objectives. For example, we might be interested to know whether a certain surgical procedure "results in lower perioperative and postoperative morbidity." However, the measurement of morbidity requires definition, particularly if the study involves more than one surgeon. At least three aspects of morbidity must be defined. The first is the window of time during which adverse events can plausibly be attributed to the operative procedure. The second is a list of specific diagnoses or complications to be included. The third is a list of procedures required to establish each diagnosis definitively. As another example, "improved survival" might mean prolonged median survival, a higher 5-year survival rate, or a lower death rate in the first year. It is important for the statistician to consult with medical investigators to determine which criterion best meets clinical objectives and to explain to the medical investigators how the choice of a particular response measurement will affect the design and analysis of the trial, including the required sample size and trial duration.

The choice of response measurement has important implications for the monitoring of the trial. For example, if it is decided to compare recurrence-free survival rates in therapy E versus therapy C using standard methods for comparing survival curves, such as the log-rank test, the trial may need to be stopped early on the basis of earlier recurrences in one or the other therapeutic group in the first year or two of the trial. Such early stopping would be a serious mistake if the medical investigators really needed to learn about the impact of E on long-term survival rates. If the clinical objectives center on long-term survival, the protocol should emphasize this end point rather than disease-free survival in the first year or two.

Another consideration in the choice of a response measurement (end point) for the study is how reliable the measurement is and how complete the response data are likely to be. For example, the date of death will be obtained accurately on nearly every study participant, but an end point such as the time to recurrence depends on how closely the patients are followed and how carefully diagnostic procedures are performed and interpreted. Sometimes, however, a subjective or variable end point measurement, such as "quality of life," may be the only type of measurement that adequately addresses the clinical objectives.

These examples are meant to emphasize that the proper choice of the primary response measurement is crucial in making sure that the trial meets its clinical objectives. The choice of the most informative and efficient end point to meet the clinical objectives requires close collaboration between the medical investigators and the statistician.

Defining the Study Population

The protocol should carefully describe all eligibility criteria and exclusionary criteria so that someone reading about the study would have a good idea of the types of patients who participated. The types of patients admitted to a trial can have an important impact on the results, particularly in non-comparative phase II trials.

Ethical considerations can dictate eligibility requirements. In the first place, only patients who give informed consent should be eligible to participate. Furthermore, patients who are likely to be harmed by trial participation should be excluded. Whenever possible such exclusions should be made on the basis of direct observations. For example, it is preferable to exclude patients with a creatinine level above 2 mg/100 ml or with a Karnofsky performance status of 7 or less (Karnofsky, et al., 1948), rather than to exclude patients with a vaguely defined "life expectancy of 6 months or less."

Patients are also excluded to improve the reliability of the assessment of the main end point. For example, patients with nonpulmonary malignancies within the previous 5 years may be excluded to minimize the possibility of lung metastases from nonpulmonary tumors and to permit a more reliable assessment of recurrence-free survival after the resection of lung cancer.

Eligible patients are often defined by the stage of disease. This restriction has the advantage of reducing heterogeneity of responses, thus making it easier to detect an effect of therapy. However, a good argument can be made that such restrictions needlessly reduce accrual to the trial and limit the generalizability of the trial results. It is argued that studying larger number of patients will overcome the disadvantages of heterogeneity of responses by studying a more diverse patient population, especially if adjustment procedures are used to account for the stage of disease in the analysis of trial results. Perhaps the best rationale for restricting patients to a given stage of disease is that the therapeutic approach might be expected to benefit only patients with that stage of disease. For example, we might not wish to subject patients with resected stage $T_1N_0M_0$ squamous cell lung cancer to a debilitating adjuvant chemotherapeutic regimen designed for patients with stage III disease.

Defining Therapies

The protocol should carefully describe the therapies that are being compared and the measures that will be taken to modify therapies in the event of anticipated toxicities. In describing the compared therapies, there will usually need to be some flexibility to allow for medical discretion and judgment while the essential features of the therapies are preserved. For example, in a study of pleurodesis with lung expansion as the primary outcome measurement, the protocol might compare specific sclerosing agents. However, it would not be wise or necessary to specify the antibiotic to be used if complicating pneumonia occurred.

Physicians who participate in trials are always obligated to replace protocol therapies with others when they believe that it is in the best interest of the patient. However, sufficient flexibility in the therapeutic specification, especially in regard to complications, toxicity, or side effects, may permit most patients to continue to comply with the therapy assigned by the protocol. Thus some flexibility in defining the therapeutic regimen can improve compliance and increase the credibility of the study report.

Measuring End Points

In the section called Quantifying Study Objectives, we stressed the paramount importance of the selection of an outcome measurement (end point) that meets the scientific objectives of the study. It is also important that the protocol specify precisely how the measurement is to be made and that measurement bias be avoided by attempting to carry out the measurements in the same way on all patients, regardless of therapy. Before we discuss these issues, we mention three generic types of response measurements.

Continuous response measurements, such as forced expiratory volume or weight, may be used to compare therapies. For example, forced expiratory volume might be used in a study to determine whether a limited wedge resection preserves more lung function than does a lobectomy. The therapeutic effects will often be gauged by a comparison of the mean responses at the end of the study or the mean changes in the measurements at the end of the study. Regression methods, including analysis of covariance, are often used to adjust such therapeutic differences in the means for baseline imbalances on prognostic factors.

Sometimes responses are categorical. For example, "normal, mild dyspnea, moderate dyspnea, and severe dyspnea" define an ordered ("ordinal") categorical response measure. Unordered categorical response measurements, such as the toxicities, "cardiac, pulmonary and other," may also be used. The most widely used type of categorical response is dichotomous, such as whether or not the patient survived 30 days. The therapeutic comparisons for dichotomous outcomes are often based on differences in proportions with a given outcome or on the odds ratios. For example, if $P_E = 0.9$ is the proportion of patients surviving after receiving therapy E and $P_C = 0.7$ is the proportion surviving after C, the therapeutic effect might be measured as the difference $0.9 - 0.7 = 0.2$ or as the odds ratio $(0.9/0.1)(0.7/0.3) = 3.86$. Note that $0.9/0.1 = 9$ is the odds of a patient surviving after therapy E and $0.7/0.3 = 2.33$ is the odds of surviving after C. Odds ratios are useful because logistic-regression models can be used to adjust odds ratios for therapeutic imbalances on baseline covariates (Cox, 1970). Similar models are available to analyze categorical data with more than two categories.

Measurements of the time to a clinical event, such as the time to death or the time to the earlier of death or recurrence, are widely used end points. The distinguishing feature of time to event data is that the event may not be observed before the end of the study. When this happens the data are said to be "censored" because all that is known is that the event did not occur before the point at which observation ceased. Standard methods of analysis can be misleading when they are applied to censored data. In particular usual comparisons of means are inappropriate. Specialized methods are needed to estimate the distribution of survival times (the survival curves) properly in the separate therapeutic groups. From such survival curves, we can estimate quantities such as the proportion of patients who survive 5 years or the median survival time, even though some study participants were censored before 5 years or before the median survival time. Two therapies can then be compared in terms of the difference or ratio of median survival times or in terms of the difference in 5-year survival rates, for example. Another measure of therapeutic effect is the "hazard ratio," also known as the "relative risk." The hazard at time t multiplied by a small time increment dt is the probability of having the event in a small time interval [t, t + dt) given that the subject has not had the event up until time t. The ratio of two such hazards can be used as a summary measure of therapeutic effect, provided this hazard ratio remains reasonably constant over time. Covariate adjustment methods based on Cox's (1972) proportional-hazards model are based on this assumption. A simple procedure to test whether the hazard ratio is 1.0 (the null hypothesis), is called the log-rank test (Kalbfleisch and Prentice, 1980).

Three important factors affect the quality of the response measurement data: completeness, freedom from bias, and repeatability. If response data are missing on a substantial portion of subjects, no statistical analysis can rule out the possibility that those who were not measured were nonrepresentative. In this case a therapeutic comparison of only those who were measured can be misleading. For example, suppose that 100 patients are assigned to therapies E and C but that outcomes are only observed on 80 patients in each group (Table 71-3). In the observed data, it appears that E and C have equal effectiveness because 70 successful results are observed with each therapy. However, although the proportion missing was the same with each therapy (20 percent), the types of people missing were different. In therapy E, 50 percent of those missing had a good outcome, whereas in therapy C only 25 percent of those missing had a good outcome. In fact the true success rate with E was 80/100 = 80 percent compared with 75/100 = 75 percent with C. Thus the analysis of only the observed data was misleading, even

though the amount of missing data was the same in both therapeutic groups. The implication is that every effort should be made to measure the response on every study participant.

To avoid response measurement bias, the protocol should specify that measurements be performed in the same way on every subject, regardless of therapy. Thus the measurements should be scheduled identically for both therapeutic groups, and the same devices and procedures should be used to make measurements on all patients whenever possible. If different measurement instruments need to be used in various institutions, they should be carefully and repeatedly calibrated. Blocking the randomization to ensure equal therapeutic balance within an institution can minimize measurement bias because, if an instrument is not properly calibrated in a given institution, the bias will apply equally to both therapies and measures of therapeutic effect, such as differences in mean responses, may be unbiased.

Equal scheduling of procedures to determine the time tó recurrence are required to avoid bias. For example, in comparing surgery alone with surgery plus adjuvant chemotherapy, it is important that the schedule of radiographs, blood tests that could detect metastases, and other tests for recurrence be equal in both therapeutic groups. Otherwise the more frequently tested group will tend to have shorter apparent times to recurrence, even if there is no therapeutic effect.

Subjective end points, such as the degree of dyspnea or severity of pain or disability, may yield biased results if the patient or the observer who is making the assessment is aware of the therapy the patient received. Sometimes it is feasible to mask the therapy given so that the patient and/or observer is unaware ("blind") of the therapeutic assignment. Although blinding may be feasible in the comparison of drugs with similar toxicities and effects, it may not be possible to blind patients or observers to the type of surgical procedure performed or the type of multimodality therapy used. In such circumstances we may place heavier reliance on less subjective end points, such as laboratory measurements or survival time.

Even if measurement response biases have been avoided, the trial may be weakened if the measurements are not repeatable. Such measurement variability can be reduced by the investigator perfecting measuring devices to reduce the variability and by the monitoring of the performance of measuring devices to detect quickly when they go out of calibration. Training and quality control workshops can also be helpful in improving observer agreement. For example, pathologists in a collaborative group may find it useful to define and refine diagnostic criteria and to compare opinions in regard to difficult cases. Such activities may improve the consistency of diagnoses by individual pathologists and may improve agreement among different observers. Similar quality control activities may be useful to train medical personnel who are trying to assess quality of life or other subjective end points.

Study Design and Random Therapeutic Allocation

Every protocol should include a description of the study design. A simple diagram can indicate which patients are eligible, what therapies are being compared, the point at which random therapeutic assignment occurs, procedures

Table 71-3. Effect of Missing Information on Interpretation of Dichotomous Data

	Observed		Missing		Total	
	E	C	E	C	E	C
Success	70	70	10	5	80	75
Failure	10	10	10	15	20	25
Total	80	80	20	20	100	100

Abbreviations: E, new therapy; C, standard therapy.

(such as stratification or balancing) that may be used to improve therapeutic balance on important prognostic factors, and the type of response measurement.

Several aspects in regard to randomization should be stressed. The eligibility of the patient should be confirmed before randomization to avoid controversies that arise when ineligible randomized patients are excluded. An excellent way to accomplish this task is to have investigators call a central statistical office to obtain a random therapeutic assignment. The statistical office personnel will ask for information regarding eligibility before assigning the therapy. This procedure reduces the chance that ineligible patients will be entered on study, and it protects the randomization process. Alternative randomization procedures, in which physicians are given packets of envelopes with therapeutic assignments, for example, are subject to conscious or unconscious abuses.

The randomization should take place just before experimental therapies are initiated if possible. For example, suppose it is desired to determine whether adjuvant chemotherapy prolongs life after the resection of stage II squamous cell lung cancer and that chemotherapy is to begin 2 weeks after surgery. It is preferable to randomize the patient to receive chemotherapy or placebo therapy 2 weeks after surgery rather than before surgery. The implied therapeutic question of interest is, "among patients who have survived surgery and are well enough to undergo chemotherapy, is adjuvant chemotherapy preferable to placebo therapy?"

Some effort to achieve good therapeutic balance within an institution and possibly within a stratum that is defined by one or two important prognostic factors may be worthwhile in smaller trials. Blocked stratified randomization or other balancing schemes can be used for this purpose. In trials that involve several hundred patients, simple randomization without blocking achieves adequate therapeutic balance (Peto, et al., 1976; Lachin, 1988).

Sample Size Requirements and Study Feasibility

We first consider trials designed to determine if E is superior to C. Suppose D measures the effect of therapy. For example, $D = \overline{X}_E - \overline{X}_C$ measures the mean difference in responses to the two therapies, $D = \hat{P}_E - \hat{P}_C$ measures the difference in proportions with successful therapeutic outcomes, or $D =$ logarithm of the estimated hazard ratio that compares C with E in the proportional-hazards model measures the effect of therapy on survival. In each case D has an expected value δ and a variance σ^2. The null hypothesis of no therapeutic effect is $\delta = 0$, and it is judged to be worthwhile to be able to detect a value δ_a greater than 0 (the "alternative" hypothesis). Sample sizes are often chosen to guarantee that a two-sided α level test will have a power $1 - \beta$ to detect the therapeutic effect δ_a. The requirement is that the sample size, n, in each group be sufficient to guarantee that

$$\delta_a^2/\mathrm{Var}(D) = (Z_\alpha + Z_\beta)^2 \qquad (1)$$

where Z_α and Z_β are the $1 - \alpha$ and $1 - \beta$ quantiles from the standard normal distribution. For $\alpha = 0.05$ and power = $0.9 = 1 - \beta$, $Z_\alpha = 1.96$ and $Z_\beta = 1.282$. This equation determines the required sample size n because Var(D) decreases as n increases. For example, suppose the variance of forced

expiratory volume in the population is 500 ml and suppose we desire to be able to detect an improvement $\delta_a = 250$ ml. Then $\mathrm{Var}(D) = \mathrm{Var}(\overline{X}_E - \overline{X}_C) = 500/n + 500/n$. From the previous equation, $n = (1{,}000/250)^2(1.96 + 1.282)^2 = 169$ subjects are required in each therapeutic group. Similar calculations apply to the difference in proportions, except then $\mathrm{Var}(D) = \{P_E(1 - P_E) + P_C(1 - P_C)\}/n$.

An alternative sample size criterion is that the estimate of the therapeutic effect, D, be sufficiently precise to put tight confidence limits about the true therapeutic effect δ. Suppose the half-width of the 95 percent confidence interval is required to be w or less. Then we would need n to be large enough so that $1.96\sqrt{\mathrm{Var}(D)}$ is less than or equal to w. This was the type of criterion described for phase II trials, except that in phase II trials we want a precise estimate of the response rate, whereas in phase III trials we want a precise estimate of the effect of therapy on the response rates.

Time-to-event (survival) data pose special problems in sample size calculation because some event times are censored. However, to detect a hazard ratio r_a that is different from unity, we can calculate the total number of *required events*, e, from $e = 4(Z_\alpha + Z_\beta)^2/\log^2(r_a)$ (George and Desu, 1974; Schoenfeld, 1981). This result can be derived from Equation 1 by setting $D = \log$ (estimated hazard ratio) and noting that Var(D) is approximately (4/e) and $\delta_a = \log(r_a)$. For example, suppose it is desired to test the null hypothesis $\delta = \log(1) = 0$ against the alternative $\delta_a = \log(r_a) = \log(1.75)$ using a two-sided $\alpha = 0.05$ level test with power 0.9. Then $e = 4(1.96 + 1.282)^2/\log^2(1.75) = 135$ events are required.

How many patients need to be entered into the trial to obtain 135 events depends on the planned trial duration and on the chance that an event will develop during the trial. For example, a rapidly fatal disease with a 20 percent mortality rate in 2 years would require roughly $135/0.2 = 675$ patients (338 in each therapeutic group) to yield the required number of deaths, whereas a rarely fatal disease with a 2 percent mortality rate in 2 years would require 6,750 patients. Prolonging the observation period can reduce the required number of patients. For example, a 4-year trial would require roughly $6{,}750/2 = 3{,}375$ patients. These calculations are very rough because it was assumed that all patients were entered into the study at the same time. Actually patients accrue to the study over time, and some patients are lost to follow-up or die from causes not under study. More careful analysis is required to calculate sample sizes accurately (Rubenstein, et al., 1981).

Required sample sizes can be affected by other factors. Some adjustment should be made for patients who will drop out of the study before an end point measurement is provided. Noncompliance to the assigned therapy can *seriously dilute* the power of the study and require larger sample sizes. For example, if we anticipate that a substantial number of patients assigned to receive adjuvant chemotherapy will refuse to come for therapy, the expected therapeutic benefit from adjuvant chemotherapy would be reduced. In this setting we would want to increase the study size to be able to detect a therapeutic benefit, even in the presence of noncompliance.

Sample size considerations are different for equivalency trials. The null hypothesis is no longer that there is no therapeutic effect, $\delta = 0$. Instead we test the null hypothesis that the new therapy E is worse than the standard one C, namely δ is less than or equal to $-\delta_a$. For example, if the proportion of patients surviving after receiving C is 0.50, we might accept E to be "equivalent" if the proportion surviving after E was proved to be at least 0.45. Then $\delta_a = 0.45 - 0.50 = -0.05$. If we reject the null hypothesis δ is less than or equal to $-\delta_a$, we can accept the new therapy as almost as good or better (δ greater than $-\delta_a$) than C, namely equivalent. Equation 1 can be used with $\delta = -\delta_a$ to determine the required sample size (Blackwelder and Chang, 1984).

Estimating Accrual and Study Feasibility

After the sample sizes needed to meet the study objectives have been calculated, we must assess whether the anticipated accrual rate is sufficient to make the trial feasible. One unfortunate and preventable mistake is to plan and initiate a study, only to have it terminate early because of low accrual. This situation can be avoided with some advance planning.

First, investigators should be aware of the accrual rate required to complete a study in a desirable fixed period. Most researchers would like to see comparative therapeutic trials completed within 5 years and pilot or feasibility studies finished within 1 to 2 years. Disease prevention trials may take longer. In any case the accrual rate required to complete a study within the time targeted can be estimated from the total sample size required.

Second, investigators must obtain *realistic* estimates of accrual rates. The raw number of patients with a specific diagnosis can often be determined easily from hospital or clinic records, but such numbers grossly overestimate the potential study accrual. Only a fraction of these patients will meet the eligibility criteria, and only a fraction of those eligible will be willing to participate in the trial and consent to randomization. This latter proportion is usually less than one-half. Thus the accrual rate is usually only one-half to one-quarter of the raw rate at which patients come for therapy.

Third, investigators should project the trial's duration based on a worst-case accrual. The study may still be feasible under such plans. If not, plans for terminating the trial because of low accrual are needed to avoid a waste of resources.

A formal survey of patients in potential participating clinics may be helpful to gauge potential accrual. As patients are seen, a record can be kept to see if they match the eligibility criteria. To estimate the proportion willing to give consent, we could briefly explain the proposed study to sampled patients and ask if they would hypothetically be willing to participate.

On the basis of such analysis, it may be decided that the original trial design is not feasible. One solution may be to expand participation in the trial by forming a cooperative study that involves several research institutions. Alternatively it may be decided that the trial can be stretched out over a longer period than originally desired. A third alternative is to relax the sample size requirements to produce a less precise estimate of therapeutic effect or to have the power to detect only large therapeutic effects. Such decisions have major implications for trial design, management, and scientific impact and should not be taken lightly. The best course may

be to decide that the trial should not be attempted with the available resources.

Plans for Data Management and Quality Control

The most critical data elements required to meet scientific objectives should be identified, and the protocol should indicate when these data should be gathered. Simple self-coding data forms or methods for direct computer entry should be devised and tested to make sure they are easily understood. Nurses and data managers should be trained in the use of these forms and other data management activities. The quality control and data management activities described in the next section require careful planning and testing when the trial is designed.

TRIAL IMPLEMENTATION

Quality Control and Data Management

Quality control activities should be designed to prevent problems or errors, to detect errors when they arise, and to change procedures to avoid such errors in the future. The scope of these activities depends on the complexity and size of the trial.

Making sure that only eligible patients are entered in the study and that the validity of the randomization is protected is an essential quality control function that can be performed by the staff in a statistical and data management office.

A collaborative effort by medical, statistical, and data management staff is needed to develop and implement checks on data quality. Audits of primary medical data sources can be used to verify that the data are being properly interpreted and entered onto the data forms. The medical staff may provide special training to make sure that those who are abstracting the data from the clinical record have an adequate understanding of the medical terms and the purpose of the protocol. The medical staff may suggest special checks of relationships between data items, based on medical knowledge. These checks can be incorporated in automated data editing systems. For example, a TNM classification may be inconsistent with a given definition of the disease stage. The medical staff may also be useful for validating crucial end point data, such as the date of recurrence, and for resolving data inconsistencies detected by a data management system.

The data management system should be able to identify errors or compliance problems quickly and track their resolution. Simple checks for the completeness of data and the validity of individual items (e.g., age must be less than 110 years) can be performed by the data entry personnel and computer and quickly resolved by direct communication with those charged with filling out the forms. A system is required to track the resolution of more subtle problems that can be detected by automated checks for data consistency (e.g., therapy occurs before randomization) or from bizarre results in interim analyses.

The data management system should identify patients who are late for follow-up, and special efforts should be made to contact such patients.

An important benefit of interim reporting is that it offers investigators a chance to review the data on potential problems, such as low accrual rates, noncompliance with therapy, unusual toxicities, and incomplete follow-up. It is crucial that such problems be recognized and dealt with as soon as possible.

These examples illustrate that quality control activities are dynamic and require extensive communication among all members of the investigative team for adequate resolution. Periodic meetings among data managers, medical and nursing staff, and statisticians can help improve data quality. Personnel with special training and experience in data management will usually be needed.

Monitoring the Progress of the Trial

Many studies of chronic diseases take several years to complete. It is necessary to review the progress of such trials periodically to detect problems that might threaten the scientific value of the study and to protect patients from unexpected toxicities or from allocation to a therapy that has been convincingly shown to be inferior during the course of the trial.

It is a good idea to establish a data monitoring board (DMB) whose primary responsibilities are to protect patient interests and to stop the trial as soon as the study objectives have been met or as soon as it is clear that the trial has serious deficiencies that will prevent its ever meeting the scientific objectives. The DMB should include experienced investigators from several disciplines, including statistics and the relevant medical subspecialties. Information on end point response data should only be made available to the DMB and not to the investigators with the responsibility for patient management. Some members of the DMB should have no direct involvement with the trial to help ensure objectivity.

The DMB reviews the general progress of the trial, including accrual rates, protocol violations, noncompliance with therapy, loss to follow-up, and the rate of acquisition of the end point data. As mentioned in the section on Quality Control and Data Management, this review is essential to proper quality control and should lead to prompt corrective action. The DMB may decide to terminate the trial if such problems cannot be rectified. Such information may be distributed to trial investigators to promote a discussion of the ways to improve the problems.

The DMB monitors toxicity and end point data to determine whether convincing differences are emerging in favor of one therapy. Interim end point data must be viewed cautiously for two reasons. First the data may be incomplete or may contain more errors than would be expected of a final planned analysis. Second it is known that if data is looked at repeatedly over time, some dramatic differences will appear by chance alone. Therefore, more stringent criteria for rejecting the null hypothesis are required at interim data inspections than would be required if the data were inspected only at the planned termination of the study. For example, Armitage, et al. (1969) found that if the accumulating data were examined five times and a conventional two-sided $\alpha = 0.05$ level test was used each time, the null hypothesis would be rejected 14 percent of the time, instead of the desired 5 percent, in the absence of therapeutic effects. Some of the statistical methods used to avoid this problem and protect the type I error level are described in DeMets (1987) and Gail (1982). These statistical prescriptions should be used as guidelines to prevent an overzealous interpretation of accumulating information, rather than as rigid stopping rules. The actual decision to stop the trial is complex and involves an assessment of how well the trial has met its scientific objectives, other information that may arise outside the trial, and the welfare of trial participants.

ANALYSIS AND PUBLICATION

The published article should be written so that a reader can easily understand the motivation and essential elements of the study, the results, and the major uncertainties and unresolved issues. In the following sections, we comment on contributions that a statistician can make to the Introduction, Methods, Results, and Discussion portions of a scientific report. We emphasize phase III trials, although many of the same elements are needed to describe other studies.

Introduction

The statistician may provide statistical information or summaries that are useful in defining the importance of the scientific problem, preliminary quantitative information concerning the promise of the proposed therapy, and some discussion of the need for a randomized phase III study. Most importantly the statistician should ensure that the objectives of the trial are clearly stated and correspond directly to the subsequent analyses and descriptions of results.

Methods

The statistician should check that the sources of the study population and eligibility criteria are clearly described, together with randomization procedures, including stratification or other balancing methods. The end point measurements should be clearly defined, including schedules for follow-up. Special measures to reduce the possibility of response measurement bias, such as blinding, should be described. Statistical guidelines used to monitor the trial should be mentioned, and methods used for statistical analyses should be cited.

Results

Before we describe the analyses and results, we reiterate the importance of carefully checking the raw data. This step is especially useful for small or single-investigator studies that are not supported by professional data management staff and quality control procedures. Many errors can be detected by examining lists, simple tabulations, and plots. These techniques can identify available data that are inadvertently coded as missing, incorrect decimal points, incorrect use of missing data codes, and other miscodings. We assume that these approaches and more extensive data edits have been performed in what follows.

Describing the Study Population

The study population should be described in terms of its distributions of baseline characteristics, such as age, sex, stage of disease, and other prognostic factors. These distributions of baseline covariates should be compared between therapies. Serious imbalances may indicate a violation of randomization procedures that threatens the validity of the entire study.

A table or description should be presented that accounts for all randomized patients and indicates protocol violations and losses to follow-up. In Table 71-4 note that 3 patients were inadvertently randomized to a trial for which they were ineligible, 12 others did not complete their assigned therapies, and 11 patients were lost before their end point could be measured. Data of this type are essential to assess whether the study is seriously weakened by noncompliance with therapy or by missing data. More elaborate descriptions of the degree of therapeutic compliance and the completeness of follow-up are also often useful.

Analyses Directed at the Principal Study Objectives

The protocol should specify a few central questions that the study is designed to investigate, and these central issues should be addressed by corresponding analyses. For example, the most important question may be, "Does the policy of administering therapy E lead to prolonged survival compared with the policy of administering therapy C?" In Table 71-4, we suppose that the 11 patients who were lost were never seen after randomization and so provided no useful survival data. The analysis is therefore restricted to the remaining $93 + 107 = 200$ patients who provided survival information. However, as mentioned in sections on bias and quantification of study objectives, if those who were lost during therapy with E tended to be healthy, whereas those who were lost during therapy with C tended to be sick, a bias could be introduced in favor of therapy E.

We must still decide which of the 200 patients with survival data to include in the analysis. The ITT analysis requires that we include all randomized patients, as discussed in the section on bias. It is possible that the nine patients receiving therapy E who did not receive complete therapy were patients with poor prognoses. In this case to exclude them could induce a bias in favor of therapy E. In general any exclusions based on data that arise after randomization can lead to subgroup comparisons that are not fully protected by the randomization (Braitman, 1988; Berger, 1986).

Suppose that the three ineligible patients were thought to have had non-small cell lung cancer initially, but a subsequent pathologic review detected the presence of small cell cancer. The trial was intended for non-small cell lung cancer. An argument can be made that these patients should still be included in the trial because these patients looked as if they were eligible, and the results are meant to apply to patients who seem to have non-small lung cancer at the time of the initial therapy before a definitive pathologic review with special laboratory procedures can take place. However, if the pathologic review was based on pathologic material obtained before randomization and carried out by pathologists who did not know the patients' clinical outcomes or therapeutic assignments, it is unlikely that the exclusion of the patients would cause bias. To cause bias the exclusion must be both related to the therapy and to the clinical outcome.

To answer the main pragmatic therapeutic question, we recommend the ITT analysis based on all randomized patients (Schwartz and Lellouch, 1967). This analysis can be supplemented by an analysis that excludes only those ineligible patients who were inadvertently enrolled in the trial by a gross error and who should have been excluded based on information known before randomization. Aside from the bias that analyses not based on the ITT can introduce, the ITT principle yields estimates of therapeutic benefit that are likely to generalize to new patients in the clinic. For example, when the surgeon encounters a new patient, the knowledge of compliance with the intended therapy is not available. The ITT analysis would yield the probability that this patient benefits from the therapy.

Continuing this example, we find that 77 of the 93 patients with follow-up data after therapy E died during the trial compared with 87 of 107 patients who received C (Table 71-5). For now we focus on the rows labeled "Total" in Table 71-5. The corresponding hazard rates were estimated by dividing the total number of deaths by the total person-years of exposure time. For example, someone who dies after 1.5 years contributes 1.5 years of exposure, and someone who is alive at the end of the study 3 years after the date of randomization contributes 3 years. Hazard ratios are obtained by division.

Table 71-4. Protocol Violations Among Randomized Patients

	E		C	
	Complete End Point Assessment	Lost Before End Point Assessment[a]	Complete End Point Assessment	Lost Before End Point Assessment
Full therapy not received	9	1	2	0
Full therapy received but ineligible at entry	1	0	2	0
Treated, eligible	83	4	103	6
Total randomized	93	5	107	6

Abbreviations: E, new therapy; C, standard therapy.

[a] For time-to-event end points, a complete end point assessment only requires that the patient complied with the follow-up schedule not that the event occurred before the study ended.

Table 71-5. Hypothetical Comparison of Survival Data

	Therapy	Total	Exposure Time (Person-Years)	Deaths	Hazard Rates (Person-Years)	Hazard Ratio (Relative Risk)	95% CI
Age <60 yrs	E	43	393	35	0.089	0.61	(0.40, 0.95)
	C	54	325	47	0.145		
Age ≥60 yrs	E	50	251	42	0.167	0.79	(0.51, 1.22)
	C	53	189	40	0.211		
Total	E	93	645	77	0.119	0.70	(0.52, 0.96)
	C	107	514	87	0.169		
"Adjusted" for therapeutic imbalances on age						0.70	(0.51, 0.95)

Abbreviations: E, new; C, standard; CI, confidence interval.

For example, the hazard ratio 0.119/0.169 = 0.70 indicates that therapy E appears to have a somewhat protective effect overall. Using standard methods appropriate for exponentially distributed survival data, we obtain the 95 percent confidence interval (0.52, 0.96) (Kalbfleisch and Prentice, 1980). Because this confidence interval excludes 1.00, we can reject the null hypothesis of no therapeutic effect (relative risk = 1.00 or log relative risk = 0).

Note that the hazard rates tend to be smaller for patients under age 60 (Table 71-5) and that proportionately more younger patients were assigned to receive therapy C (54/ (54 + 53) = 50 percent) than E (43/(43 + 50) = 46 percent). This mild disproportion may be due to chance. If we perform analyses separately within strata defined by age, we obtain similar hazard ratios, taking random error into account, in each stratum. Formal stratification procedures to "adjust" the estimate of therapeutic effect for imbalances on covariates such as age usually produce only modest changes in randomized trials. In this case the estimated hazard ratio was not changed, and the confidence interval was changed only slightly by an adjustment for the imbalance on age compared with the unadjusted value.

Similar analyses and adjustments for imbalances on baseline covariates can be performed by using the proportional-hazards model of Cox (1972) for survival data, logistic regression for dichotomous outcomes (Cox, 1970), and classic regression ("analysis of covariance") for continuous outcome data. Two caveats should be stressed in regard to covariate adjustment. First, adjustments should only be performed on baseline covariates when the effects of therapy are estimated. If we adjust for factors, such as pulmonary function, that are measured after randomization, we can seriously distort the estimate of therapeutic effects and obtain highly misleading results. Second, we should not select baseline covariates for adjustment by searching for covariates that change the apparent therapeutic effect. It is preferable to perform an unadjusted analysis and one adjusted analysis that includes factors, such as stratification factors, that are known a priori to be highly prognostic. Randomization allows us to reduce our reliance on adjustment procedures by inducing a good balance of covariates across therapies. Indeed valid hypothesis tests are possible with no adjustment (Byar, et al., 1976).

Table 71-5 illustrates the descriptive value of parameter estimates with confidence intervals rather than simple P values. If the 95 percent confidence interval excludes the null parameter value, we have "statistically significant" evidence against the null hypothesis. A P value only indicates whether the null hypothesis has been rejected; it gives no information on the size of the therapeutic effect. Thus confidence intervals provide useful information about the largest and smallest therapeutic effects that could be reasonably supported by the data. If the confidence interval excludes clinically meaningful therapeutic effects, we can be reasonably sure that they do not exist. Conversely if the confidence interval includes clinically important effects, we might consider obtaining additional data before drawing final conclusions.

Graphs are also useful for presenting the distributions of responses, rather than simple summary statistics such as the means or hazard rates. Plots of survival curves would usually be needed to provide a description of the distribution of survival times related to each therapy. Differences between survival curves are often tested for statistical significance using "nonparametric" tests (i.e., those that make no assumptions about the mathematic form of the distributions). Two such tests are frequently used, the log rank (Mantel and Haenszel, 1959) and the Wilcoxon (Gehan, 1965). Because of slight differences in the way the statistics are calculated, the Wilcoxon test tends to emphasize differences that occur relatively early in follow-up; log-rank analysis tends to give equal weighting to differences over the entire survival curves.

When we interpret graphs of survival curves, it is often helpful to keep in mind the difference between "actual survival" and "actuarial survival." Actual survival is the number of study subjects alive divided by the number studied. Actuarial survival is determined by the survival curve. Both depend on the follow-up experience of the population. Physicians are often concerned that the actuarial estimates become less precise with increasing follow-up time (i.e., in the "tail" of the survival curve). Although this is true, the actual survival estimates are also variable and have the added disadvantage that they ignore differences in follow-up time.

To summarize, the main analyses should be clearly identified and easy to understand. They should include the ITT analysis of the main end points without any adjustment and with adjustments for a few baseline covariates known from other studies to be highly prognostic. The investigator's emphasis should be on describing therapeutic effects and presenting confidence intervals. The presentation of P values alone is inadequate. Graphic presentation of data, such as survival curves, is helpful; actuarial survival estimates are the most useful.

Toxicity Data

It is important to describe information on the toxicity and the effects of therapy on performance status or other measures of quality of life, if these are available. Such analyses are needed to arrive at a balanced view of therapeutic costs and benefits.

Exploratory Analyses

A clinical trial data set offers many opportunities to test ideas for further study. For example, we can look for subgroups of patients who seem to have benefitted from therapy E, even though no benefit was demonstrated overall. If we examine many subsets, we are likely to find a provocative result. However, such findings are likely to be the result of chance and require confirmation by independent data.

We may decide to compare those patients who complied fully with therapy E against those who complied fully with therapy C, in an effort to reach explanatory conclusions rather than pragmatic conclusions (Schwartz and Lellouch, 1967). However, such analyses are subject to the biases mentioned in that section.

A fruitful use of clinical trial data is to identify prognostic factors that can be used in subsequent studies. Biologic materials can also be stored for future testing of new potentially prognostic assays. However, these analyses and activities would usually not be described in the main article.

Discussion

The statistician can contribute to the interpretation of trial results by assessing random and systematic sources of uncertainty in the estimates of therapeutic effect. Variance estimates and the widths of confidence intervals provide a useful indication of the extent of random uncertainty. The evaluation of possible systematic biases, including biases induced by missing data, is more difficult. Sometimes special analyses can yield insight into the sensitivity of the conclusions to possible biases.

The statistician may provide additional perspective on the trial results by comparing and possibly combining them with data from other similar clinical trials (Dickerson and Berlin, 1992).

SUMMARY

We have tried to indicate the usefulness of statistical methods and perspectives in carrying out a program of research involving thoracic surgery clinical trials. It seems that statisticians can be most effective when they work closely with other members of the study team on many activities, including preliminary studies, trial design, implementation, quality control, analyses, and publication.

COMMENTS AND CONTROVERSIES

In this chapter statistical theory and its practical applications in thoracic surgical studies were presented by two close friends of thoracic surgery. Dr. Piantadosi served as a surgical intern under Dr. John Kirklin and subsequently joined Dr. Mitchell Gail as a biostatistical coinvestigator in the Lung Cancer Study Group. Their discussion of trials methodology is balanced, clear, and sensitive to the nuances of surgical trials.

A recent development in trials methodology is the requirement for the inclusion of women and minorities in clinical research mandated by the 1993 National Institutes of Health guidelines in the United States. It is required that any clinical research project be "carried out in a manner sufficient to provide for a valid analysis of whether the variables . . . affect women or members of minority groups . . . differently than other subjects in the research" (U.S. Congress, Public Law 103-43, June 10, 1993). This requirement for designed therapy-covariate interaction analysis is a political objective and is not necessarily scientifically worthwhile (Piantadosi and Wittes, 1993). Nevertheless, as law, it could be influential on the way in which clinical trial resources are used in the near future.

Metanalysis, briefly discussed in this chapter, is a relatively new technique for the synthesis of the literature with strict weighting criteria and rules for inclusion, an important advance over the haphazard or biased selection and evaluation process commonly used in the scientific literature. Opponents of metanalysis argue against its overemphasis on statistical methodology and "significance" and underemphasis on the magnitude and direction of observed therapeutic effects.

A middle ground between traditional reviews and metanalysis is *best evidence synthesis* (Slavin, 1986), a technique that emphasizes the discussion of criteria for inclusion that minimize reviewer bias, the presentation of enough original evidence to allow the reader to evaluate the study, the germaneness and substance of a study, and the avoidance of pooling and of undue emphasis on statistical significance.

It is interesting that no metanalyses or best evidence syntheses appear in this textbook. We asked our authors to follow the traditional review format and to defend their own bias about the choice of therapy. This approach is most familiar and comfortable and has much to recommend it. It is "the way of our people."

As costs rise, new technology evolves, and an aging population seeks more care, challenges to our more traditional thinking are being posed by analytic statistical reviews produced by representatives of payers and government. We will learn to use the methods of analytic literature synthesis to respond effective, just as we have learned from our colleagues Piantadosi and Gail to use sound statistical methods to design and analyze individual studies.

M.F.M.

KEY REFERENCES

Olak, Chiu: Surgeon's guide to biostatistical inferences. Bull Amer Coll Surg 78:1, 1993

This is a readable survey of biostatistical methods oriented toward a surgical audience.

Silverman WA: Human Experimentation: A Guided Step into the Unknown. Oxford University Press, Oxford, 1985

This book is inexpensive and covers many of the important concepts in clinical trials without using statistics. Many examples are drawn from the author's experience with pediatric studies.

Buyse ME, Staquet MJ, Sylvester RJ (eds): Cancer Clinical Trials. Methods and Practice. Oxford University Press, Oxford, 1984

This is an excellent introduction to clinical trials. The chapters are written by knowledgeable experts, and it contains numerous excellent examples. Although oriented toward cancer, it contains useful information for all types of clinical trials.

International Committee of Medical Journal Editors: Uniform requirements for manuscripts submitted to biomedical journals. Ann Intern Med 108:258, 1988

Surgeons would benefit from the reasonable advice and guidelines provided in this reference. It emphasizes the need to report estimates of therapeutic effect rather than relying only on *P* values. Broader issues of reporting are considered.

The National Commission for the Protection of Human Subjects of Biomedical and Behavioral Research: The Belmont Report: Ethical Principles and Guidelines for the Protection of Human Subjects of Research. DHEW publication no. (OS) 78-0012. Appendix I, DHEW publication no. (OS) 78-0013; Appendix II, DHEW publication no. (OS) 78-0014. U.S. Government Printing Office, Washington, D.C., 1978.

This is virtually required reading for anyone participating in clinical trials.

Byar DP: The necessity and justification of randomized clinical trials. p. 75. In Tagnon HJ, Staquet J (eds): Controversies in Cancer. Mason, New York, 1979

This is a lively and eloquent defense of clinical trials in a time when some objections are being raised.

REFERENCES

Altman D, Gore S, Gardner M, Pocock S: Statistical guidelines for contributors to medical journals. BMJ 286:1489, 1983

Amberson JB Jr, McMahon BT, Pinner M: A clinical trial of sancrysin in pulmonary tuberculosis. Am Rev Respir Dis 24:401, 1931

Armitage P: The design of clinical trials. Aust J Stat 21:266, 1979

Armitage P, Berry G: The design of experiments. p. 172. In Statistical Methods in Medical Research, Blackwell Scientific, Oxford, 1987

Armitage P, McPherson CK, Rowe BC: Repeated significance tests on accumulating data. J R Stat Soc Series A 132:235, 1969

Bailar J, Mosteller F: Guidelines for statistical reporting for medical journals: amplifications and explanations. Ann Intern Med 108:266, 1988

Beach ML, Meier P: Choosing covariates in the analysis of clinical trials. Controlled Clin Trials 10:161S, 1989

Berger J: Are p-values reasonable measures of accuracy? In Francis BI, Manly Lam FC (eds): Pacific Statistical Congress. Elsevier, North Holland, 1986

Berger J, Sellke T: Testing a point null hypothesis: the irreconcilability of p-values and evidence. J Am Stat Assoc 82:112, 1987

Berry G: Statistical guide-lines and statistical guidance. Med J Aust 146:408, 1987

Berry G: Statistical significance and confidence intervals. Med J Aust 144:618, 1986

Blackwelder WC, Chang MA: Sample size graphs for "proving the null hypothesis." Controlled Clin Trials 5:97, 1984

Braitman L: Confidence intervals extract clinically useful information from data. Ann Intern Med 108:296, 1988

Bull JP: The historical development of clinical therapeutic trials. J Chronic Dis 10:218, 1959

Burkhardt R, Kienle G: Basic problems in controlled trials. J Med Ethics 9:80, 1983

Byar DP: Identification of prognostic factors. p. 210. In Buyse ME, Staquet MJ, Sylvester RJ (eds): Cancer Clinical Trials: Methods and Practice. Oxford University Press, Oxford, 1984

Byar DP, Green SB, Dor P et al: A prognostic index for thyroid cancer. A study of the E.O.R.T.C. Thyroid Cancer Cooperative Group. Eur J Cancer 15:1033, 1979

Byar DP, Simon RM, Friedewald WT et al: Randomized clinical trials: perspectives on some recent ideas. N Engl J Med 295:74, 1976

Cox DR: Regression models and life tables (with discussion). J R Stat Soc Series B 34:187, 1972

Cox DR: The Analysis of Binary Data. Chapman and Hall, London, 1970

DeMets DL: Practical aspects in data monitoring: a brief review. Stat Med 6:753, 1987

DerSimonian R, Charette LJ, McPeek B, Mosteller F: Reporting on methods in clinical trials. N Engl J Med 306:1332, 1982

Dickersin K, Berlin J: Meta-analysis: state of the science. Epidemiol Rev 14:154, 1992

Doll R: Sir Austin Bradford Hill and the progress of medical science. BMJ 305:1521, 1992

Eagan RT, Rudd C, Lee RE et al: Pilot study of induction therapy with cyclophosphamide, doxorubicin, and cisplatin (CAP) and chest irradiation prior to thoracotomy in initially inoperable stage III M0 non-small cell lung cancer. Cancer Treat Rep 71:895, 1987

Fisher RA: The Design of Experiments. Hafner Publishing Co., New York, 1966

Fisher RA, MacKenzie WA: Studies in crop variation: II. The manurial response of different potato varieties. J Agric Sci 13:311, 1923

Fleming TR: One-sample multiple testing procedure for phase II clinical trials. Biometrics 38:143, 1982

Food and Drug Administration: Procedural and interpretive regulations: investigational use. Fed Reg 28:179, Jan. 8, 1963

Freidman LM, Furberg CD, DeMets DL: Fundamentals of Clinical Trials. John Wright, Boston, 1981

Gail MH: Eligibility exclusions, losses to follow-up, removal of randomized patients, and uncounted events in cancer clinical trials. Cancer Treat Rep 69:1107, 1985

Gail M: Monitoring and stopping clinical trials. p. 455. In Mike V, Stanley KE (eds): Statistics in Medical Research. Wiley, New York, 1982

Gardner MJ, Altman DG: Confidence intervals rather than P values: estimation rather than hypothesis testing. BMJ 292:746, 1986

Gehan EA: A generalized Wilcoxon test for comparing arbitrarily singly-censored samples. Biometrika 52:203, 1965

Gehan EA: The determination of the number of patients required in a preliminary and follow-up trial of a new chemotherapeutic agent. J Chronic Dis 13:346, 1961

George SL: Identification and assessment of prognostic factors. Semin Oncol 15:462, 1988

George SL, Desu MM: Planning the size and duration of a clinical trial studying the time to some critical event. J Chronic Dis 27:15, 1974

Green SB: Randomized clinical trials: design and analysis. Semin Oncol 8:417, 1981

Haygarth J: Of the Imagination as a Cause and as a Cure of Disorders of the Body: Exemplified by Ficticious Tractors and Epidemical Convulsions. R. Cruttwell, Bath, 1800

Kalbfleisch JD, Prentice RL: The Statistical Analysis of Failure Time Data. Wiley, New York, 1980

Karnovsky DA, Abelmann WH, Craver LF et al: The use of nitrogen mustards in the palliative treatment of cancer. Cancer 1:634, 1948

Lachin JM: Properties of simple randomization in clinical trials. Controlled Clin Trials 9:312, 1988

Leventhal BG, Wittes RE: Research Methods in Clinical Oncology. Raven Press, New York, 1988

Leventhal BL, Piantadosi S (eds): Issues in clinical research. Semin Oncol 15:1, 1988

Levine RJ: Ethics and the Regulation of Clinical Research. 2nd Ed. Urban and Schwarzenberg, Baltimore, 1986

Lewis JA: Clinical trials: statistical developments of practical benefit to the pharmaceutical industry (with discussion). J R Stat Soc Series A 146:362, 1983

Louis PCA: Researches on the Effects of Bloodletting in some Inflammatory Diseases and on the Influence of Tartarized Antimony and Vessication in Pneumonitis. Hilliard Gray and Co., Boston, 1836

Louis, TA, Mosteller F, McPeek B: Timely topics in statistical methods for clinical trials. Annu Rev Biophys Biphys Chem 11:81, 1982

Mantel N, Naenszel W: Statistical aspects of the analysis of data from retrospective studies of disease. J Natl Cancer Inst 22:719, 1959

May GS, Chir B, DeMets DL et al: The randomized trial: bias in analysis. Circulation 64:669, 1981

McKneally MF, Maver C, Kausel HW, Alley RD: Regional immunotherapy with intrapleural BCG for lung cancer. Surgical considerations. J Thorac Cardiovasc Surg 72:333, 1976

Medical Research Council: Whooping-Cough Immunization Committee: The prevention of whooping-cough by vaccination. BMJ 1:1463, 1951

Meinert CL: Clinical Trials. Oxford University Press, Oxford, 1986

Miettinen OS: The need for randomization in the study of intended effects. Stat Med 2:267, 1983

Miké V: Clinical studies in cancer: a historical perspective. p. 111. In Miké V, Stanley KE (eds): Statistical Issues in Medical Research. Methods and Issues, with Applications in Cancer Research. Wiley, New York, 1982

Mosteller F, Gilbert J, McPeek B: Reporting standards and research strategies for controlled clinical trails; agenda for the editor. Controlled Clin Trials 1:37, 1980

Office of Technology Assessment, U.S. Congress: The Impact of Randomized Clinical Trials of Health Policy and Medical Practice: Background Paper. Publication no. OTA-BP-H-22. U.S. Government Printing Office, Washington, D.C., 1983

Oldham RK, Gail MH, Baker MA et al.: Immunological studies in a double-blind controlled trial comparing intrapleural BCG against placebo in patients with resected stage I non-small cell lung cancer. Cancer Immunol Immunother 13:164, 1982

Packard FR: Life and Times of Ambroise Paré, 1510-1590. Paul B. Hoeber, New York, 1921

Peto R, Pike MC, Armitage P et al.: Design and analysis of randomized clinical trials requiring prolonged observations of each patient: II. Analysis and examples. Br J Cancer 35:1, 1977

Peto R, Pike MC, Armitage P et al.: Design and analysis of randomized clinical trials requiring prolonged observation of each patient: I. Introduction and design. Br J Cancer 34:585, 1976

Piantadosi S: Principles of clinical trial design. Semin Oncol 15:423, 1988

Piantadosi S, Saijo N, Tamura T: Basic design considerations for clinical trials in oncology. Jpn J Cancer Res 83:547, 1992

Piantadosi S, Wittes J: Politically correct clinical trials (letter). Controlled Clin Trials 14:562, 1993

Pocock SJ: Clinical Trials: A Practical Approach. John Wiley, New York, 1983

Rothman K: Significance questing. Ann Intern Med 105:445, 1986

Rubinstein LV, Gail MH, Santner TJ: Planning the duration of a comparative clinical trial with loss to follow-up and a period of continued observation. J Chronic Dis 34:469, 1981

Schafer A: The ethics of the randomized clinical trial. N Engl J Med 307:719, 1977

Schoenfeld D: The asymptotic properties of nonparametric tests for comparing survival distributions. Biometrika 68:316, 1981

Schwartz D, Lellouch J: Explanatory and pragmatic attitudes in therapeutic trials. J Chronic Dis 20:637, 1967

Shapiro SH, Louis TA (eds): Clinical Trials: Issues and Approaches. Marcel Dekker, New York, 1983

Simberkoff MS, Hartigan PM, Hamilton JD et al.: Ethical dilemmas in continuing a zidovudine trial after early termination of similar trials. Controlled Clin Trials 14:6, 1993

Simon R: Design and conduct of clinical trials. p. 396. In Devita, VT, Jr, Hellman S, Rosenberg SA (eds): Cancer: Principles and Practice of Oncology. Vol. 1. JB Lippincott, Philadelphia, 1989

Simon R: How large should a phase II trial of a new drug be? Cancer Treat Rep 71:1079, 1987

Simon R: Confidence intervals for reporting results of clinical trials. Ann Intern Med 105:429, 1986

Slavin RE: Best evidence synthesis: an alternative to meta-analytic and traditional reviews. Educ Res 15:5, 1986

Streptomycin in Tuberculosis Trials Committee: Streptomycin treatment of pulmonary tuberculosis. BMJ 2:769, 1948

Taves DR: A new method of assigning patients to treatment and control groups. Clin Pharmacol Ther 15:443, 1974

Vere DW: Problems in controlled trials—a critical response. J Med Ethics 9:85, 1983

Yusuf S, Collins R, Peto R: Why do we need some large, simple randomized trials? Stat Med 3:409, 1984

72

RESEARCH

Martin F. McKneally

INTRODUCTION

The thrill that comes from advancing medical practice through research is one of the most exhilarating experiences of the human mind and spirit. Consider the moment of John Hunter's realization that his research demonstration of collateral circulation in the antler of the deer could provide a scientific basis for his heroic decision to ligate a popliteal aneurysm rather than amputate the leg (Kobler, 1960). Imagine the feelings that came to Alfred Blalock (Blalock and Taussig, 1945) when he realized that his laboratory model of subclavian to pulmonary artery anastomosis, developed for research on pulmonary hypertension, could find an application in bringing blood flow to the lungs in the tetralogy of Fallot.

Innovation and imaginative problem solving is an important part of the daily practice of clinical thoracic surgery and a source of great satisfaction for surgeons as they exercise their creative intuition. Systematic scientific problem solving in a research environment as a continuous process of consecutive thinking is a privilege limited to a minority of surgeons, usually only experienced during a brief sabbatical period during residency training.

The role of research training in the education of a surgeon is to provide guidance for taking responsible initiatives to change established rules and practices, reinterpret the information from which surgical principles are derived, or develop new information. Research methods teach the surgeon to collect credible and representative data, perform reliable analyses, and draw reasonable inferences. Research provides the foundation for future developments in surgery because of its emphasis on the validation of new interpretations of reality. Using measurement as its cardinal procedure, research "seeks to ascertain the actual relationship between phenomena. Uncritical reliance on initial observations potentially distorted by bias can lead to a systematic divergence from the truth" (Sackett, 1979). Rigorous research methods are devised precisely to counter the tendency to mistake a mere semblance of correlation for a fact.

Exposure to research teaches surgeons how to test new hypotheses and to reexamine old ones, using principles derived from the scientific method. Well-studied and generally accepted techniques for validating measurements, outcomes, and beneficial or harmful effects provide the basis for a broader education that equips surgeons to expand their knowledge, eliminate error based on previous misinterpretations, and deal effectively with new problems for which previous experience provided no specific guidelines.

Research is valued in many training programs for its critical role in developing inquisitive attitudes in trainees (Wechsler, 1991) but is not a standard component of a thoracic surgical education. In thoracic surgery divisions with research programs, emphasis is placed on cardiac surgical problems studied in the past several decades. A renaissance of enthusiasm and support for research in general thoracic surgery dawned during the era of lung transplantation.

DEFINITION

Research is defined in *Webster's Ninth New Collegiate Dictionary* (1990) as "1. careful or diligent search; 2. studious inquiry or examination, especially investigation or experimentation aimed at the discovery and interpretation of facts, revision of accepted theories or laws in the light of new facts, or practical application of such new or revised theories or laws; 3. the collecting of information about a particular subject."

Diligent systematic investigation may be carried out as bench research in a thoracic surgical laboratory where a particular procedure or intervention commonly used in thoracic surgery can be assessed more systematically than it might be in human patients by controlling variables that are potentially confounding. Standardization and replication increase the reliability of inferences derived from data points measured in these experiments.

Basic science research related to thoracic surgical problems is performed in laboratories with a strong emphasis on physiologic, cellular, or molecular mechanisms that are investigated for reasons that transcend their relationship to thoracic surgery.

Clinical research generally consists of archival reviews of experience or prospective reviews of interventions that compare one technique with another. The extent to which scientific laboratory research principles are incorporated into clinical studies strengthens the inferences derived from their analysis and increases their influence on clinical practice.

Kirklin (1993) provides clear and useful definitions of many of the components of research:

> Information is a collection of material and observations. Data consist of organized discrete values or observations, usually expressed numerically. Data include derivations (expressions) from information that summarize parts or all of the data and express its variability. Analysis is a process, often prolonged and repeated, by which the component parts of the whole are identified, their relations clarified and quantified, and the degree of uncertainty expressed. Inferences are simple summarizing statements derived from information, data, and analysis, drawn with varying and preferably stated confidences that they are true. Knowledge is the totality of the data and inferences. Secure inferences and knowledge can be applied to a number of processes in health care, including: (1) generating new concepts and paradigms; (2) improving outcomes obtained by individuals and institutions; (3) making individual patient care decisions; (4) obtaining informed consent from patients; (5) determining the quality and appropriateness of care; and (6) making regulatory decisions.

> Speculations are statements suggested by the data, or by abstract reasoning, without rigorously defined supportive data or knowledge. Hypotheses are statements to be tested, made on the basis of abstract reasoning or of previously derived data, knowledge, and inferences.

HISTORICAL NOTE

Pioneering thoracic surgical laboratory research by Sauerbruch and O'Shaughnessy (1937) and others led circuitously to the development of safe anesthesia for thoracic surgery.

The anatomic and physiologic studies of Heuer and Reinhoff (Reinhoff, et al., 1935) on the anatomy of the lung provided the basis for the introduction of safe techniques of pulmonary resection. The development of more refined techniques of lobar and segmental resections by Churchill and Belsey (1939) and Blades and Kent (1940) were based on carefully researched anatomic studies.

The development of cardiac surgery led to an enormous expansion of research related to interventions on the heart and great vessels, which is outside the scope of this chapter. During this period and subsequently, some surgeons dedicated to the solution of difficult problems in general thoracic surgery continued to perform productive research, particularly in the area of tracheal injury, tracheal reconstruction, lung transplantation, and gastroesophageal reflux disease.

HISTORICAL READINGS

Blades B, Kent EM: Individual ligation technique for lower lobe lobectomy. J Thorac Cardiovasc Surg 10:84, 1940

Churchill E, Belsey HR: Segmental pneumonectomy in bronchiectasis. Ann Surg 109:481, 1939

Rienhoff WF, Reichert FL, Heuer GJ: Compensatory changes in the remaining lung following total pneumonectomy. Bull Johns Hopkins Hosp 67:373, 1935

Sauerbruch F, O'Shaughnessy L: Thoracic Surgery. Edward Arnold, London, 1937

CURRENT RESEARCH TOPICS

There have been many workers in the vineyard of thoracic surgical research. A chapter of this size cannot provide an encyclopedic review or do justice to their contributions. This is a descriptive discussion of some of the contributions of only a few of the thoracic surgeons who have influenced the specialty through their scholarly studies. It was not possible to trace "thoracic surgical research" through any index retained by funding agencies or prepared by any journal or textbook. Much of the work that thoracic surgeons do in the area of research is collaborative, particularly in the modern era. Funding for such research comes from programs devoted to an analysis of the problems of cancer, transplantation, sepsis, and other broad categories. Even tracking "surgical research" (McKneally, 1991; McKneally, et al., 1991) within the National Institutes of Health proved to be a daunting problem. Many illuminating observations of a fundamental nature have been contributed by surgeons in pursuit of practical goals of tumor control, eradication of infection, improvement of circulation, or the safe conduct of surgery.

Lung Transplantation

Applied thoracic surgical research led to the development of safe techniques for lung transplantation (Lima, et al., 1981, 1982; Morgan, et al., 1983; Goldberg, et al., 1983; Dubois, et al., 1984; Dark, et al., 1986; Patterson, et al., 1988). Studies on lung preservation and the immunology of rejection have been performed using the best techniques of the basic science and surgical laboratories. Lung transplantation has provided a productive field of laboratory and clinical research, which has reinvigorated thoracic surgery. Benfield (1976) prepared a complete and thoughtful review of the early clinical and laboratory studies in this field. Subequent work on lung preservation, technical problems of implantation, and management of rejection are discussed by Cooper and Patterson in Chapter 33. Like cardiac transplantation, the clincial introduction of lung transplantation came before the solutions to critical problems were sufficiently advanced in the research laboratory and before rigorous stable teams of clinical scientists were assembled to deal with the new problems generated by the application of this new technology in humans. The success of the Toronto group, led by Cooper and firmly based in systematic laboratory study and a well-developed team effort, paralleled the success of the Stanford heart transplantation group led by Shumway and his colleagues in the preceding decade.

Infection

Infection, particularly pleural infection, has been studied by thoracic surgeons for many years. Important contributions were made by the Empyema Commission in World War I, based on clinical research that defined optimal care and set the standard for management of empyema (Berry, 1963). More recent studies of early decortication (Fishman and Ellertson, 1977) and muscle flap closure (Miller, et al., 1984) brought the management of even the most complex cases of empyema to a satisfactory level.

Esophageal Disorders

Esophageal research studies, which focused on the analysis of disorders of motility and reflux disease and their response to surgical interventions, have been a sustained and important area of surgical research for the past several decades (DeMeester, et al., 1979; O'Sullivan and DeMeester, 1982; Duranceau, et al., 1983). More recent studies of oncogene expression (Casson, 1992) and the epidemiology and biochemical analysis of the causative mechanism of esophageal cancer (Chang-Claude, et al., 1990) are exciting developments in esophageal research. Clinical studies of Barrett's epithelium have stimulated potentially important changes in our thinking about screening and early resection (Streitz, et al., 1993).

Gastroesophageal Reflux

Some experimental work has of necessity been conducted exclusively in humans, such as the solution to the problem of a congenital tracheoesophageal fistula (Haight, 1957). Research on the clinical problem of gastroesophageal reflux and its surgical therapy was performed primarily by observational studies of outcome in patients. The studies of Nissen (1956, 1961); Hill (1967); and Hill, et al., (1970); DeMeester, et al. (1974, 1976); and Pearson and Henderson (1973, 1976) are notable examples.

Pulmonary Function

Pulmonary function laboratories originated in response to the thoracic surgeons' need to measure preoperative function and estimate residual postoperative function through the application of objective measuring techniques. An analysis of the data from these studies provided guidelines for a safe resection, based on the relationship between pulmonary function and mortality rates contributed by Gaensler, et al., (1955); Wernley, et al. (1980); and others. More recent refinements have expanded the safe limits of pulmonary resection through the application of the differential analysis of the contribution of each lung and lobe to overall function (Miller, 1992).

Intensive Care Unit Issues

Thoracic surgeons in the intensive care unit (ICU) made important contributions to the understanding and practical management of flail chest (Trinkle, et al., 1975) and adult respiratory distress syndrome (ARDS) (Ch. 67). Clinical research by thoracic surgeons can be credited for the many advances leading to the current effectiveness of intensive care units, particularly in the management of acute respiratory failure. Important contributions to the development of ventilation and extracorporeal oxygenation techniques have been driven by the thoracic surgeon when caring for desperately ill patients. Diaphragmatic pacing, pioneered by Glenn, et al. (1972), is a fascinating example of the thoracic surgeon at work on the frontier of surgical knowledge. The pacing techniques for the diaphragm were adapted from those developed for heart block induced by surgical interventions to close ventricular septal defects (Lillehei, et al., 1964).

Tracheal Injury

Tracheal injury from prolonged intubation was analyzed in research studies by Cooper and Grillo (1969a,b), Pearson and Andrews (1971), and Andrews and Pearson (1971). These studies led to changes in clinical practice, which have dramatically reduced the incidence of these complications. Reconstruction of the trachea developed from laboratory and clinical research in Boston (Maeda and Grillo, 1972; Grillo, 1982a,b) and Toronto (Pearson, et al., 1975).

Thoracic Oncology

Thoracic oncology has been an important focus of research in thoracic surgery. The analytic studies of Abbey-Smith (1978) on the appropriate limits of surgical intervention, and the studies of Pearson, et al. (1982) on the significance of a positive mediastinoscopy saved a large number of patients from the disabling consequences of nonresecting thoracotomies. Studies by Naruke and Suemasu (1976), Naruke, et al. (1988), and Martini, et al. (1980, 1983) on radical node dissection focused attention on the role of surgical resection for the control of lung cancer after nodal spread. This important research question remains unsettled (McKneally, 1988).

Analytic epidemiologic studies by Mountain, et al. (1974), Mountain (1986), and Shields, et al. (1980) led to the development of a staging system for lung cancer that provides a sound basis for a comparison of results between institutions and between treatment strategies (Miller, et al., 1989).

A small randomized trial of intrapleural bacillus Calmette-Guérin (BCG) (McKneally, et al., 1976) led to the development of the collaborative Lung Cancer Study Group sponsored by the National Institutes of Health. This outstanding surgical study group effectively refuted the apparent advantages of such treatment. More importantly it standardized therapies and assessed a variety of interventions in a systematic series of studies over a 10-year period. These investigations provide reliable information on the patterns of recurrence (Feld, et al., 1984), postoperative radiation therapy (Weisenburger, et al., 1986), postoperative chemotherapy (Holmes, et al., 1986), induction chemotherapy (Egan, et al., 1987; Weiden, et al., 1987), immunotherapy (Mountain, et al., 1981), limited resection (Ginsberg, et al., 1991), blood transfusion (Moores, et al., 1989), and other important questions about lung cancer management. A valuable handbook was developed to strengthen the reliability of thoracic oncology trials (Rusch, et al., 1993).

Recent studies by the Radiation Therapy Oncology Group, the Eastern Cooperative Oncology Group, the Southwestern Oncology Group, and others represent more fragmented attempts at the systematic study of the management of lung cancer and other thoracic malignancies. They are flawed by variations of small consequence between protocols. Efforts by Rusch, Ginsberg, and Feins to bring these disparate programs under common intergroup protocols and thus reproduce the advantages of the Lung Cancer Study Group effort represent an important leadership step by thoracic surgeons that should be endorsed and supported (Wechsler, 1991; Feins, 1992).

The Video Assisted Thoracic Surgery Study Group (Joseph LoCicero III, MD, New England Deaconess Hospital, Suite 2C, 110 Francis St., Boston, MA 02215), through its registry and therapeutic protocols, provides a research venue for analyzing the effect of the recent introduction of video-assisted technology on the practice of thoracic surgery under the aegis of the American Association for Thoracic Surgery/Society of Thoracic Surgeons Joint Committee on Video Assisted Thoracic Surgery.

THE FUTURE OF THORACIC SURGICAL RESEARCH

The success of thoracic surgery requires the education of our practitioners in research, using a contemporary and effective process. In the past we have taught research through the preceptorship approach, which has been abandoned as a standard method of education for the practice of surgery. It is time for us to broaden the education of our residents to include a structured and well-planned exposure to research. At a minimum every resident should have the opportunity to prepare and publish a peer-reviewed article. The European approach of requiring a thesis based on three peer-reviewed articles is a worthwhile consideration for residents bound for an academic position. Courses in research are just starting to appear at some of our meetings and in some of our institutions. The textbook *Principles and Practice of Research: Strategies for Surgical Investigators* (Troidl, et al., 1991) includes three thoracic surgeons among its editors; this is the first such text to appear for many years. A designated forum for presenting research articles was recently introduced at our national meetings. We must create more accessible sites for the presentation of research and reinforce its significance. It is remarkable that the American College of Surgeons has had a research forum on fundamental problems in surgery for more than 50 years. The Society of Thoracic Surgeons introduced a research forum at its national meetings only in the past decade, and the American Association for Thoracic Surgery has had a research forum for only 6 years. Some productive laboratories believe that the available sites for the presentation and discussion of research techniques and results are too narrow in thoracic surgery. They prefer to submit their research abstracts to the American College of Surgeons forum on fundamental problems in surgery or to the American Thoracic Society to allow young surgeons in the laboratory an opportunity to present and discuss their work as part of their training at an early stage in their development.

An Environment for Research

Creating the environment for research requires positive reinforcement of the curiosity and inventiveness of thoracic surgeons who seek to expand knowledge of the specialty. Role models in thoracic surgery need to be provided and supported through well-planned programs to develop and sustain surgeon scientists.

The emergence of biology clubs for cardiothoracic surgeons, at the suggestion of John Waldhausen during his presidency of the American Association for Thoracic Surgery, will strengthen and promote the research environment. A General Thoracic Surgical Biology Club has been initiated for the presentation and discussion of research topics in a forum of limited size (G. A. Patterson, MD, Division of Cardiothoracic Surgery, Suite 3108 Queeny Tower, One Barnes Hospital Plaza, St. Louis, MO 63110-1013).

Education and Training

Education and training in research should be available to all thoracic residents as a component of their surgical program. Some should have more extensive exposure if they show a proficiency and enthusiasm for scientific research. A few should have the opportunity to study in a basic sciences laboratory and learn the technology and thinking of their colleagues in related disciplines. During such periods they should not lose touch with clinical activities, although they should be protected from the urgent call of the patient in distress. It is good for them to have some continuing clinical exposure, for example, to the esophageal function laboratory, to organ harvesting or to controlled opportunities to assist in the operating room to maintain a sense of continuity with surgery. A durable relationship with basic scientists can grow out of this period of scientific training, facilitating optimal collaboration and the transfer of leading-edge technology to clinical investigations.

The Marburg experiment is a formalized model of a durable interaction between the surgeon/scientist and the basic scientist (Lorenz, et al., 1991). The immunologist Adriana Zieve, collaborating with Bartley Griffith and his colleagues on the transplantation service in Pittsburgh, and John Hammond, working on lung carcinogenesis with John Benfield in Sacramento, are examples of this kind of productive interaction. We need to foster more of these durable relationships with fundamental science collaborators and incorporate them into the structure of thoracic surgical divisions.

Funding

More funding for surgeon/scientists in the thoracic field is required. The American Association of Thoracic Surgery has provided 2-year research scholarships for one surgeon studying a general thoracic subject and for four surgeons studying cardiac surgical subjects over the past 8 years and sponsored 37 Graham Fellows to come to North American centers to study a variety of clinical and research subjects over the past 38 years. Although admirable, this represents a very small investment of the overall budget of thoracic surgery in research and development.

For success in business it is axiomatic that at least 7 percent of revenues should be invested in research. The specialty of thoracic surgery must look to its own members and to external sources for funding of research. Funding from the National Institutes of Health and other peer-reviewed extramural sources is less available at the present time in the United States and throughout the world because of the worldwide recession. Voluntary agencies, such as the American Cancer Society and the American and Canadian Lung Associations, award grants in smaller amounts. A continuing disadvantage for thoracic surgical applicants is that both the federal and voluntary agencies tend to emphasize basic science rather than clinically oriented research, which is often viewed as less worthy than "fundamental" research. Collaboration with investigators in basic science disciplines strengthens a thoracic surgical research application. The number of grant applications to voluntary agencies from surgeons is relatively low, and surgical investigators should be encouraged to apply to these sources for smaller grants of start-up funds.

Endowed foundations, such as the Rockefeller, Kaiser, and the Robert Wood Johnson Foundations, provide relatively larger grants with uncomplicated application forms, but they are presently funding research into health-care delivery systems, rather than clinical or basic medical research. Innovative thoracic surgeons should consider adapting their clinical research questions to the societal goals favored by these foundations.

Industry has a long record of support for surgical research and the resources to provide substantial amounts of funding. The contribution of industry is important, especially in the area of technology-intensive fields, such as artificial organs and new device development. The problems associated with industry as a source of funding include potential conflicts of interest, the "strings" attached to the funding (which might limit the reporting of data in a timely and objective manner), and the negative image generated by these potential conflicts. A frank discussion with enlightened managers, clearly defined contracts, and the provision of funds through third-party organizations can minimize these problems.

The recent emphasis on cost cutting and the need for faculty surgeons to support their medical schools through clinical revenue has undercut research efforts by reducing available time and discretionary money for research. The contributions of patients to support research are important,

particularly in the United States, where a tradition of philanthropy and tax incentives facilitate this revenue stream.

Hospitals can contribute to the infrastructure for controlled research trials through an interesting organizational innovation described by Neuhauser (1990). Changes in therapeutic policies are randomly allocated to hospital teams or "firms" at the Cleveland Metropolitan Hospital, facilitating the performance of health policy research with a minimum of dislocation or extramural support. This type of research structure is well suited to comparing strategies of prophylaxis for phlebitis, infection, dysrhythmia, and other common perioperative problems (McPeek, et al., 1989).

Recently the Thoracic Surgery Foundation for Research and Education was formed (401 North Michigan Avenue, Chicago, IL 60611-4267), based on the highly successful model of the Orthopedic Research and Education Foundation. This foundation relies on surgeons, patients, and industry to provide support that can be directed to thoracic surgeons performing research in their field. The management of industrial funds through the Foundation will alleviate the potential problems discussed earlier. The Foundation provides funding to thoracic surgeons from a source sympathetic to their needs. Applications are peer reviewed by an outstanding panel of thoracic surgical researchers. This new initiative deserves the support of all thoracic surgeons.

CONCLUSIONS

The remarkable accomplishments of surgery in the past three decades (Austen, 1992) and those recounted and illustrated in this book of thoracic surgery emphasize the importance of reviewing and expanding the knowledge base for thoracic surgery. A proactive and systematic approach to research by surgeons, their patients, and their societies ensures the continued success of our specialty. Research is the foundation and source of inspiration for the specialty, and thoracic surgeons can plan on growth and expansion in the future in proportion to their commitment to research.

KEY REFERENCES

Abbey-Smith R: The importance of mediastinal lymph node invasion by pulmonary carcinoma in selection of patients for resection. Ann Thorac Surg 25:5, 1978

This classic observational study is a model of clinical research by an individual practitioner, who learned and taught based on careful study of his patients.

Benfield JF: Transplantation of the lung. In Lenfant C, Kirkpatrick CH, Reynold HY (eds): Immunologic and Infectious Reactions in the Lung. Marcel Dekker, New York, 1976

This careful and thoughtful review illuminates the state of the art of lung transplantation before the era of cyclosporine.

Cooper JD, Grillo HC: Experimental production and prevention of injury due to cuffed tracheal tubes. Surg Gynecol Obstet 129:1235, 1969a

This experimental study illustrates the process of taking a clinical problem to the laboratory for analysis and solution. Subsequent clinical application of the principles derived from these experiments has virtually eliminated the problem of cuff-induced tracheal strictures.

Troidl, H, Spitzer WO, McKneally MF et al. (eds): Principles and Practice of Research; Strategies for Surgical Investigators. 2nd Ed. Springer-Verlag, New York, 1991

This is a textbook written for the surgeon-scientist that presents a practical approach to a broad range of issues, including training, funding, planning, conducting, presenting, and publishing clinical and laboratory research.

REFERENCES

Andrews MJ, Pearson FG: The incidence and pathogenesis of tracheal injury following cuffed tube tracheostomy with assisted ventilation: analysis of a two-year prospective study. Ann Surg 173:249, 1971

Austen WG: Presidential address: surgery is a great career. Bull Am Coll Surg 77:7, 1992

Berry FB: Historical note. In Medical Department, United States Army: Surgery in World War II. Vol. 1. Office of the Surgeon General, Dept. of the Army, Washington, D.C., 1963

Blades B, Kent EM: Individual ligation technique for lower lobe lobectomy. J Thorac Surg 10:84, 1940

Blalock A, Taussig HB: The surgical treatment of malformations of the heart in which there is pulmonary stenosis or pulmonary atresia. JAMA 128:189, 1945

Casson A: Oncogene Activation in Esophageal Cancer. RG Landes, Austin, 1992

Chang-Claude JC, Wahrendorf J, Liang QS et al.: An epidemiological study of precursor lesions of esophageal cancer among young persons in a high-risk population in Huixian, China. Cancer Res 50:2268, 1990

Churchill E, Belsey HR: Segmental pneumonectomy in bronchiectasis. Ann Surg 109:481, 1939

Cooper JD, Grillo HC: The evolution of tracheal injury due to ventilatory assistance through cuffed tubes. A pathologic study. Ann Surg 196:334, 1969b

Dark JH, Patterson GA, Al-Jilaihawi AN et al.: Experimental en bloc double-long transplantation. Ann Thorac Surg 42:394, 1986

DeMeester TR, Johnson LF, Joseph GJ et al.: Patterns of gastroesophageal reflux in health and disease. Ann Surg 184:459, 1976

DeMeester TR, Johnson LF, Kent AH: Evaluation of current operations for the prevention of gastroesophageal reflux. Ann Surg 180:511, 1974

DeMeester TR, Wernly JA, Bryant GH et al.: Clinical and in vitro determinants of gastroesophageal competence: a study of the principles of antireflux surgery. Am J Surg 137:39, 1979

Dubois P, Choiniere L, Cooper JD: Bronchial omentopexy in canine lung allotransplantation. Ann Thorac Surg 38:211, 1984

Duranceau A, Rheault MJ, Jamieson GG: Physiologic response to cricopharyngeal myotomy and diverticulum suspension. Surgery 96:655, 1983

Eagan RT, Ruud C, Lee R et al.: The Lung Cancer Study Group. A pilot study of induction therapy with CAP chemotherapy and chest irradiation prior to thoracotomy in initially inoperable stage III M0 non-small cell lung cancer. Cancer Treat Rep 71:895, 1987

Feld R, Rubinstein LV, Weisenburger TH, The Lung Cancer Study Group: Sites of recurrence in resected stage I non-small lung cancer: a guide for future studies. J Clin Oncol 2:1352, 1984

Feins RH: Thoracic surgery participation in cooperative group studies of cancer therapy. Ann Thorac Surg 53:9, 1992

Fishman NG, Ellertson DG: Early pleural decortication for thoracic empyema in immunosuppressed patients. J Thorac Cardiovasc Surg 74:537, 1977

Gaensler EA, Cugell DW, Lingren I et al.: The role of pulmonary insufficiency in mortality and invalidism following surgery for pulmonary tuberculosis. J Thorac Cardiovasc Surg 29:163, 1955

Ginsberg R, Rubenstein L, The Lung Cancer Study Group: A randomized trial of lobectomy versus limited resection in patients with T1 N0 non-small cell lung cancer (abstr). Lung Cancer 7:83, 1991

Glenn WWL, Holcomb WG, McLaughlin AJ et al.: Total ventilatory support in a quadriplegic patient with radiofrequency electrophrenic respiration. N Engl J Med 286:513, 1972

Goldberg M, Lima O, Morgan E et al.: A comparison between cyclosporin A and methylprednisolone plus azathioprine on bronchial healing following canine lung allotransplantation. J Thorac Cardiovasc Surg 85:821, 1983

Grillo HC: Primary reconstruction of airway after resection and subglottic laryngeal and upper tracheal stenosis. Ann Thorac Surg 33:3, 1982a

Grillo HC: Carinal reconstruction. Ann Thorac Surg 34:356, 1982b

Haight C: Some observations on esophageal atresias and tracheoesophageal fistulas of congenital origin. J Thorac Cardiovasc Surg 34:141, 1957

Hill LD: An effective operation for hiatal hernia: an eight year appraisal. Ann Surg 166:681, 1967

Hill LD, Gelfand M, Bauermeister D: Simplified management of reflux esophagitis with stricture. Ann Surg 172:638, 1970

Holmes EC, Gail M, The Lung Cancer Study Group: Surgical adjuvant therapy for stage II and stage III adenocarcinoma and large-cell undifferentiated carcinoma. J Clin Oncol 4:710, 1986

Kirklin JW: The generation of knowledge from information, data, and analyses. In Kirklin JW, Barratt-Boyes BG (eds): Cardiac Surgery. 2nd Ed. Churchill Livingstone, New York, 1993

Kobler J: The Reluctant Surgeon; A Biography of John Hunter. Doubleday, New York, 1960

Lillehei CS, Levy MJ, Bonnabeau MD Jr et al.: The use of a myocardial electrode and pacemaker in the management of acute postoperative and postinfarction complete heart block. Surgery 56:463, 1964

Lima O, Cooper JD, Peters WJ et al.: Effects of methyl-prednisolone and azathioprine on bronchial healing following lung autotransplantation. J Thorac Cardiovasc Surg 82:211, 1981

Lima O, Goldberg M, Peters WJ et al.: Bronchial omentopexy in canine lung transplantation. J Thorac Cardiovasc Surg 83:418, 1982

Lorenz W, Troidl H, Rothmund M: The Marburg experiment: developing the new specialty of theoretical surgery. In Troidl H, Spitzer WO, McKneally MF et al. (eds): Principles and Practice of Research; Strategies for Surgical Investigators. Springer-Verlag, New York, 1991

Maeda M, Grillo HC: Tracheal growth following anastomosis in puppies. J Thorac Cardiovasc Surg 64:304, 1972

Martini N, Flehinger BJ, Zaman MB, Beattie EJ Jr: Results of resection in non-oat cell carcinoma of the lung with mediastinal lymph node metastases. Ann Surg 198:386, 1983

Martini N, Flehinger BJ, Zaman MB, Beattie EJ Jr: Prospective study of 445 lung carcinoma with mediastinal lymph node metastases. J Thorac Cardiovasc Surg 80:390, 1980

McKneally MF: Research challenges and solutions in the United States. In Troidl H, Spitzer WO, McKneally MF et al. (eds): Principles and Practice of Research; Strategies for Surgical Investigators. Springer-Verlag, New York, 1991

McKneally MF: Invited comments to Naruke T et al.: The importance of surgery to non-small cell carcinoma of lung with mediastinal lymph node metastasis. Ann Thorac Surg 46:603, 610, 1988

McKneally MF, Maver C, Kausel HW: Regional immunotherapy of lung cancer with intrapleural BCG. Lancet 1:377, 1976

McKneally MF, Troidl H, Mulder DS et al.: Common characteristics and distinctive diversity in surgical research: some international comparisons. In Troidl H, Spitzer WO, McKneally MF et al. (eds): Principles and Practice of Research; Strategies for Surgical Investigators. Springer-Verlag, New York, 1991

McPeek B, Mosteller F, McKneally M: Randomized clinical trials in surgery. Int J Technol Assess Health Care 5:317, 1989

Miller JI: Physiologic evaluation of pulmonary function in the lung resection candidate (abstr). Presented at the American Association for Thoracic Surgery, Los Angeles, CA, April 26–29, 1992

Miller JI, Mansour KA, Nahai F et al.: Single-stage complete muscle flap closure of the post pneumonectomy empyema space: a new method and possible solution to a disturbing complication. Ann Thorac Surg 38:227, 1984

Miller SJ, Moores DWO, McKneally MF: Staging of lung cancer. In Roth JA, Ruckdeschel JC, Weisenburger TH (eds): Thoracic Oncology. WB Saunders, Philadelphia, 1989

Moores DWO, Piantadosi S, McKneally MF, The Lung Cancer Study Group: Effect of perioperative blood transfusion on outcomes in surgically resected lung cancer patients. Ann Thorac Surg 47:346, 1989

Morgan WE, Lima O, Goldberg M et al.: Improved bronchial healing in canine left lung reimplantation using omental pedical wrap. J Thorac Cardiovasc Surg 85:139, 1983

Mountain CF: A new international staging system for lung cancer. Chest 89(suppl):225S, 1986

Mountain CF, Carr DT, Anderson WAD: A system for the clinical staging of lung cancer. AJR 120:130, 1974

Mountain CM, Gail MH, The Lung Cancer Study Group: Surgical adjuvant intrapleural BCG treatment for stage I non-small cell lung cancer. J Thorac Cardiovasc Surg 82:649, 1981

Naruke T, Goya T, Tsuchiya R, Suemasu K: The importance of surgery to non-small cell carcinoma of lung with mediastinal lymph node metastasis. Ann Thorac Surg 46:603, 1988

Naruke T, Suemasu K: Surgical treatment for lung cancer with metastasis to mediastinal lymph nodes. J Thorac Cardiovasc Surg 71:279, 1976

Neuhauser D: The Metro Firm trials and ongoing patient randomization. In Tanur JM, Mosteller F, Kruskal WH, et al (eds): Statistics, a Guide to the Unknown. 3rd Ed. Brooks/Cole, Pacific Grove, CA, 1990

Nissen R: Gastropexy and "fundoplication" in surgical treatment of hiatal hernia. Am J Dig Dis 6:954, 1961

Nissen R: Eine einfache Operation zur Beeinflussung der Reflux-oesophagitis. Schweiz Med Wochenschr 86:590, 1956

O'Sullivan GC, DeMeester TR: The interaction between distal esophageal sphincter pressure and length of the abdominal esophagus as determinants of gastroesophageal competence: a clinical study. Am J Surg 143:40, 1982

Patterson GA, Cooper JD, Goldman B et al.: Technique of successful clinical double lung transplantation. Ann Thorac Surg 45:626, 1988

Pearson FG, Andrews MJ: Detection and management of tracheal stenosis following cuffed tube tracheostomy. Ann Thorac Surg 12:359, 1971

Pearson FG, Cooper JD, Nelems JM, van Nostrand AWP: Primary tracheal anastomosis after resection of cricoid cartilage with preservation of recurrent laryngeal nerves. J Thorac Cardiovasc Surg 70:806, 1975

Pearson FG, Delarue NC, Ilves R et al.: Significance of positive superior mediastinal nodes identified at mediastinoscopy in patients with resectable cancer of the lung. J Thorac Cardiovasc Surg 83:1, 1982

Pearson FG, Henderson RD: Long-term follow-up of peptic strictures managed by dilatation, modified Collis gastroplasty, and Belsey hiatus hernia repair. Surgery 80:396, 1976

Pearson FG, Henderson RD: Experimental and clinical studies of gastroplasty in the management of acquired short esophagus. Surg Gynecol Obstet 136:737, 1973

Rienhoff WF, Reichert FL, Heuer GJ: Compensatory changes in the remaining lung following total pneumonectomy. Bull Johns Hopkins Hosp 67:373, 1935

Rusch VW, Ginsberg RJ, Holmes EC (eds): A Thoracic Surgical Handbook for Clinical Trials. Memorial Sloan-Kettering Cancer Center, New York, 1993

Sackett DL: Bias in analytic research. J Chronic Dis 32:60, 1979

Sauerbruch F, O'Shaughnessy L: Thoracic Surgery. Edward Arnold, London, 1937

Shields TW, Humphrey EW, Matthews M et al.: Pathological stage grouping of patients with resected carcinoma of the lung. J Thorac Cardiovasc Surg 80:400, 1980

Streitz JM Jr, Andrews CW Jr, Ellis FH Jr: Endoscopic surveillance of Barrett's esophagus: does it help? J Thorac Cardiovasc Surg 105:383, 1993

Trinkle JK, Richardson JD, Franz JL et al.: Management of flail chest without mechanical ventilation. Ann Thorac Surg 19:355, 1975

Wechsler AS: Cardiothoracic research. Presented at the Planning Session of the American Association of Thoracic Surgery, Snowbird, UT, September 20–22, 1991

Weiden P, The Lung Cancer Study Group: Preoperative chemoradiotherapy in stage III non-small cell lung cancer: a phage II study of the Lung Cancer Study Group. Proc Am Soc Clin Oncol 6:185, 1987

Weisenburger TH, Gail M, The Lung Cancer Study Group: Effects of postoperative mediastinal radiation on completely resected stage II and stage III epidermoid carcinoma of the lung. N Engl J Med 315:1377, 1986

Wernly JA, DeMeester TR, Kirchner P et al.: Clinical value of quantitative ventilation-perfusion lung scans in the surgical management of bronchogenic carcinoma. J Thorac Cardiovasc Surg 80:535, 1980

INDEX

Page numbers followed by *f* indicate figures; page numbers followed by *t* indicate tables.